Brief Contents

MEDICAL-SURGICAL NURSING

Focus on Clinical Judgment

THIRD EDITION

MEDICAL-SURGICAL NURSING

Focus on Clinical Judgment

THIRD EDITION

LINDA HONAN, RN, PhD, CNS-BC, ANEF, FAAN
Professor Emerita
Yale University School of Nursing
New Haven, Connecticut

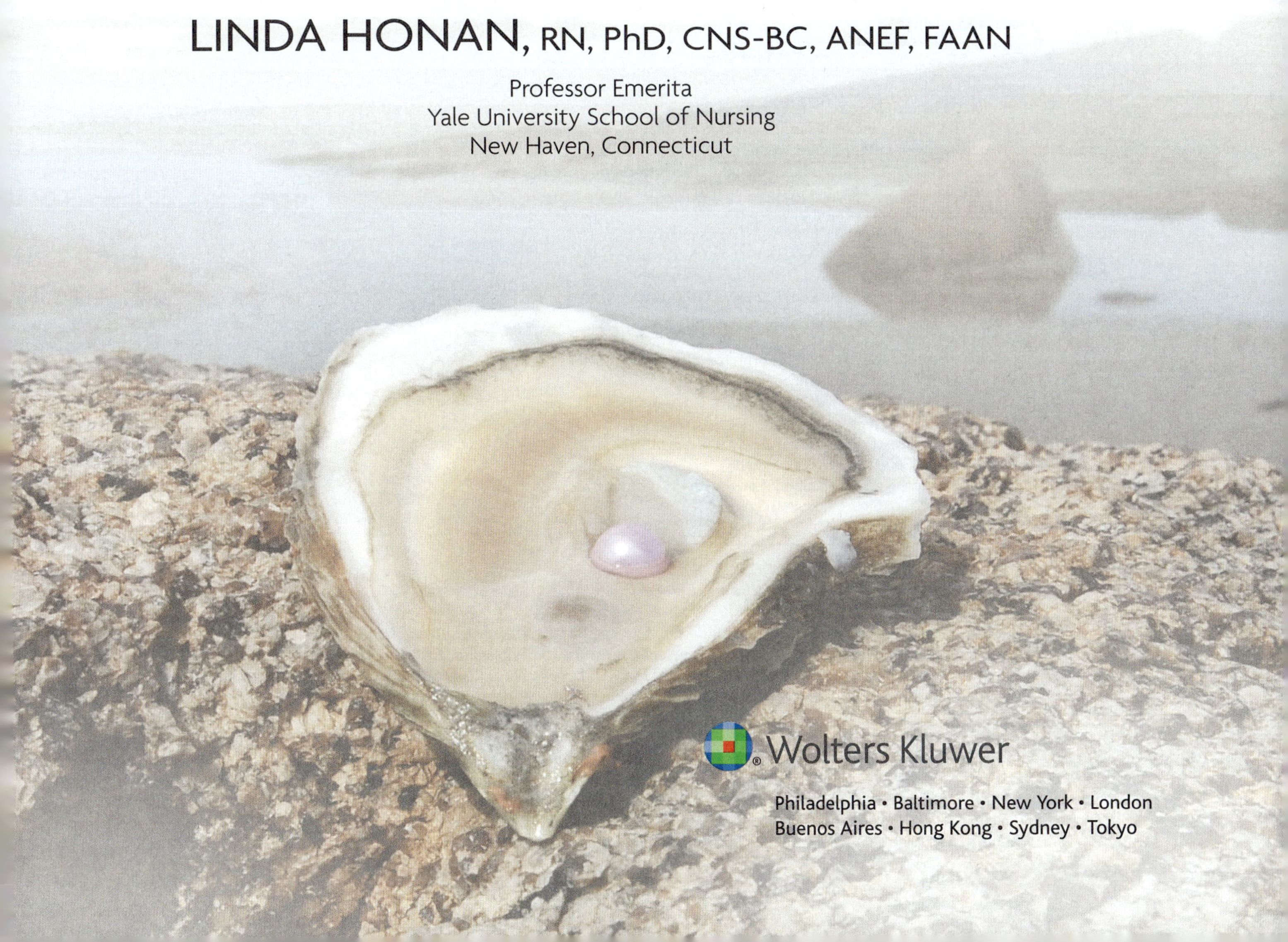

Wolters Kluwer
Philadelphia • Baltimore • New York • London
Buenos Aires • Hong Kong • Sydney • Tokyo

Vice President, Nursing Segment: Julie K. Stegman
Manager, Nursing Education and Practice Content: Jamie Blum
Senior Acquisitions Editor: Susan Hartman
Senior Development Editor: Julie Vitale
Editorial Coordinator: Caroline Define
Marketing Manager: Greta Swanson
Editorial Assistant: Devika Kishore
Production Project Manager: Frances M. Gunning
Manager, Graphic Arts and Design: Stephen Druding
Art Director: Jennifer Clements
Manufacturing Coordinator: Margie Orzech-Zeranko
Prepress Vendor: Aptara, Inc.

3rd Edition

9 8 7 6 5 4 3 2 1

Printed in the United States of America

Library of Congress Cataloging-in-Publication Data

Names: Honan, Linda, 1955- editor.
Title: Medical-surgical nursing : focus on clinical judgment / [edited by] Linda Honan.
Other titles: Focus on adult health.
Description: Third edition. | Philadelphia : Wolters Kluwer, [2024] | Preceded by: Focus on adult health : medical-surgical nursing / [edited by] Linda Honan. Second edition. 2019. | Includes bibliographical references and index. | Summary: "The third edition includes The Nurse's Role and Health Education and Health Promotion combined to provide more concise coverage of this material. This edition includes bias-free, gender-neutral language used throughout the text. All NEW content on social and structural determinants of health, COVID-19, continued focus and enhancement of clinical judgment, updated Determinants of health align with new standards outlined in Healthy People 2030, LGBTQIA updated content is reflected in applicable chapters. Each chapter contains all NEW end-of-chapters questions in NexGen (NGN) formatting in those question types that we could translate well for print for every chapter, along with Brand NEW Clinical Judgment Case Studies, incorporating NCSBN's Clinical Judgment Measurement Model, written by Dr. Honan"– Provided by publisher.
Identifiers: LCCN 2023020349 (print) | LCCN 2023020350 (ebook) | ISBN 9781975190941 (hardback) | ISBN 9781975190965 (epub)
Subjects: MESH: Medical-Surgical Nursing | Nursing Care–methods | Nursing Process | BISAC: MEDICAL / Nursing / Medical & Surgical
Classification: LCC RD99.24 (print) | LCC RD99.24 (ebook) | NLM WY 150 | DDC 617/.0231–dc23/eng/20230620
LC record available at https://lccn.loc.gov/2023020349
LC ebook record available at https://lccn.loc.gov/2023020350

shop.lww.com

MPP0823

For Ryan and Katie

About the Author

Linda Honan is a Professor Emerita at Yale University School of Nursing. She taught in the Graduate Entry Prespecialty in Nursing (GEPN) program since 1989, served as Curriculum Coordinator and Director and consults nationally to nursing programs in other universities. She taught anatomy, medical-surgical nursing and was Associate Director of the Interprofessional Longitudinal Clinical Experience (ILCE) where she was responsible for the clinical curriculum for all first-year medical, nursing, and Physician Associate students at Yale.

Dr. Honan obtained her nursing diploma from the Meriden-Wallingford Hospital School of Nursing, a BS in nursing from Southern Connecticut State University, and her MSN from Yale University School of Nursing as a general surgery Clinical Nurse Specialist. She received her PhD from the University of Connecticut where she studied the experiences of students enrolled in Graduate entry programs. Her research interests are on the education of adult learners, creative teaching strategies, and narrative inquiry. She is a nurse scholar and a clinical educator dedicated to understanding and developing effective and innovative techniques for clinical education in a multidisciplinary environment.

Known for her creativity and the development of novel and effective teaching strategies for adult learners, Dr. Honan has received numerous awards including *The Josephine S. Dolan Award* for Outstanding Contributions to Nursing Education, the *Donna Diers Mentorship Award*, the *Annie W. Goodrich Award* for Excellence in Teaching, Yale University *Leadership Award*, *Connecticut Teachers Association Salutes Award*, *Inspiring Yale*, State of Connecticut, *"Nightingale Award"* for Excellence in Nursing, Yale University *Daisy Award*, University of Connecticut School of Nursing *"Beverly Koerner Outstanding Alumni Award"* for Education in Nursing, Robert Wood Johnson, New Careers in Nursing*: Innovation Award* and the *Seton Ivy Award* from Yale University. She is a Fellow of the NLN Academy of Nursing Education and a Fellow in the American Academy of Nursing.

Dr. Honan spearheaded the development of a creative writing award and created the books; *Do you see what I see?* which are compilations of years of student journaling chapbooks. She developed the *looking is not seeing and listening is not hearing program* at YSN which uses art and music to support the development of nursing students' physical assessment skills. Her research reveals that diagnostic observations can be significantly improved by training in the visual examination of works of art, that the narratives of student experiences can give insight into the process of learning nursing, and that aural training with music improves auscultative abilities.

Contributors

Deborah S. Adelman, PhD, RN, NE-BC
Professor
Graduate Nursing Program
Purdue University Global
Springfield, Illinois
Chapter 55, Nursing Management: Emergencies and Disasters

Patricia Aguinaldo, DNP, FNP-C, CCRN
Critical Care Nurse Practitioner
Cedars-Sinai Medical Center
Los Angeles, California
Chapter 17, Nursing Management: Patients With Vascular Disorders and Problems of Peripheral Circulation

Laura Kierol Andrews, PhD, APRN, ACNP-BC
Associate Professor and Adult/Gerontology Specialty Director
Yale School of Nursing
Orange, Connecticut
Chapter 9, Nursing Management: Patients With Chest and Lower Respiratory Tract Disorders
Chapter 54, Nursing Management: Critical Care

Kassandra August-Marcucio, DNP, APRN, RN, ACNP-BC, CUNP
Nurse Practitioner
Department of Urology
Department of Veterans Affairs, VACT
Yale University School of Nursing
West Haven, Connecticut
Chapter 27, Nursing Management: Patients With Urinary Disorders
Chapter 33, Nursing Management: Care of the Assigned Male at Birth (AMAB) Patients With Reproductive Disorders

Donna M. Avanecean, DNP, FNP-BC, FNAP
APRN Neuro-oncology
Hartford Healthcare Medical Group
Hartford, Connecticut
Chapter 42, Nursing Assessment: Neurologic Function

Stephanie A. Barrett, MSN, BSN, ONC
Nursing Professional Development Specialist
Orthopedics & Spine Yale New Haven Hospital
New Haven, Connecticut
Chapter 40, Nursing Management: Patients With Musculoskeletal Disorders

Mary E. Bartlett, DNP, FNP-BC, CNE
Assistant Professor
Department of Family Medicine
Oregon Health and Sciences University
Portland, Oregon
Chapter 35, Nursing Assessment: Immune Function
Chapter 36, Nursing Management: Patients With Immunodeficiency, HIV Infection, and AIDS

Cynthia Bautista, PhD, APRN, FNCS, FCNS
Associate Professor
Egan School of Nursing and Health Studies
Fairfield University
Fairfield, Connecticut
Chapter 40, Nursing Management: Patients With Musculoskeletal Disorders
Chapter 44, Nursing Management: Patients With Neurologic Trauma
Chapter 45, Nursing Management: Patients With Neurologic Disorders

Yolanda Bone, DNP, MSN, BSN, ADN, APRN, FNP-BC, AOCNP
Oncology Nurse Practitioner
W. Temple Webber Cancer Treatment Center, Medical Oncology
Christus St. Michael Health System
Texarkana, Texas
Chapter 32, Nursing Management: Patients With Breast and Female Reproductive Disorders

Leonie L. Rose Bovino, PhD, APRN, AGACNP-BC, FAHA
Nurse Practitioner
Department of Cardiology
Hartford Healthcare, St. Vincent's Medical Center
Bridgeport, Connecticut
Chapter 15, Nursing Management: Patients With Structural, Inflammatory and Infectious Cardiac Disorders

Margaret T. Bowers, DNP, FAANP, FAAN, FNP-BC
Associate Professor
Division of Cardiology
Duke University School of Nursing
Durham, North Carolina
Chapter 14, Nursing Management: Patients With Complications From Heart Disease

Carolynn Spera Bruno, PhD, APRN, CNS, FNP-C
Clinical Associate Professor of Nursing
New York University Rory Meyers College of Nursing
New York, New York
Chapter 48, Nursing Management: Patients With Eye and Vision Disorders
Chapter 49, Nursing Management: Patients With Hearing and Balance Disorders

Gwen M. Cassidy, APN, MSN, MFA
Nurse Practitioner
Digestive Health Center
Northwestern Medicine
Chicago, Illinois
Chapter 22, Nursing Management: Patients With Gastric and Duodenal Disorders

Naomi Cazeau, RN, MSN
Adult Nurse Practitioner
Memorial Sloan Kettering Cancer Center
New York, New York
Chapter 19, Nursing Management: Patients With Hematologic Disorders

Jose Chavez, DNP, RN, ACCNS-AG, CCRN, AACC
Critical Care Clinical Nurse Specialist
Cardiac Intensive Care Unit and Cardiac Surgery Intensive Care Unit
Cedars-Sinai Medical Center
Los Angeles, California
Chapter 13, Nursing Management: Patients With Coronary Vascular Disorders

Lauren Collin, MS, PA-C
Physician Assistant
Pulmonary Department
Hartford Healthcare
Hartford, Connecticut
Chapter 10, Nursing Management of Patients Diagnosed With Chronic Obstructive Pulmonary Disease and Asthma

Nicole C. Colline, DNP, APRN, FNP-C, MSN
Family Nurse Practitioner
Yale University, School of Nursing
Orange, Connecticut
Chapter 37, Nursing Management: Patients With Allergic Disorders

Audrey Coolman, BS, MPH
Health Equity and Community Engagement Lead
Office of Medical Student Engagement
Washington University in St. Louis
St. Louis, Missouri
Chapter 1, The Nurse's Role in Adult Health Nursing

Sharon Druce, MSN, RN
Associate Faculty
Department of Health Sciences and Human Services
Saddleback College
Mission Viejo, California
Chapter 55, Nursing Management: Emergencies and Disasters

Mary Dudley, MSN, APRN, ANP-BC, ACNP-BC, RN-BC
Retired APRN Pain Medicine Service
Department of Anesthesiology
Yale University
New Haven, Connecticut
Chapter 6, Pain Management

Linda S. Dune, PhD, RN, CNL, BSN, MS(n)
Associate Professor, Director
Department of Natural Sciences
Department of Nursing
University of Houston Downtown
Houston, Texas
Chapter 47, Nursing Assessment: Sensorineural Function

Gregory Eichelzer, MSN, RN, CEN
Associate Director, Clinical Operations
Gastrointestinal Endoscopy
Cedars-Sinai Medical Center
Los Angeles, California
Chapter 24, Nursing Management: Patients With Hepatic and Biliary Disorders

Christa Palancia Esposito, DNP, MSN, CNM
Assistant Professor
Egan School of Nursing and Health Studies
Fairfield University
Fairfield, Connecticut
Chapter 34, Nursing Management: Patients With Sexually Transmitted Infections

Deborah Bain Fahs, DNP, MSN, FNP-BC
Associate Professor (retired)
Yale University School of Nursing
Orange, Connecticut
Chapter 20, Nursing Assessment: Digestive, Gastrointestinal, and Metabolic Function
Chapter 25, Nursing Assessment: Renal and Urinary Tract Function

Jessica Goldberg, PhD, RN, AGPCNP-BC, ACHPN
Nurse Practitioner
Supportive Care
Memorial Sloan Kettering Cancer Center
New York, New York
Chapter 2, Chronic Illness and End-of-Life Care

Lindsay R. Grasso, DNP, FNP-BC, RN
Nurse Practitioner
Department of Colorectal Surgery
Yale-New Haven Health
New Haven, Connecticut
Chapter 23, Nursing Management: Patients With Intestinal and Rectal Disorders

Linda Honan, RN, PhD, CNS-BC, ANEF, FAAN
Professor Emerita
Yale University School of Nursing
New Haven, Connecticut
Chapter 1, The Nurse's Role in Adult Health Nursing
Chapter 3, Fluid and Electrolyte and Acid–Base Imbalances
Chapter 7, Nursing Assessment: Respiratory Function
Chapter 10, Nursing Management of Patients Diagnosed With Chronic Obstructive Pulmonary Disease and Asthma
Chapter 11, Nursing Assessment: Cardiovascular and Circulatory Function
Chapter 26, Nursing Management: Patients With Renal Disorders
Chapter 39, Nursing Assessment: Musculoskeletal Function
Chapter 41, Nursing Management: Patients With Musculoskeletal Trauma
Chapter 53, Nursing Management: Shock and Multisystem Failure

Jill Keller, RN, MSN, FNP-BC, AONCP-BC, AOCNP
Nurse Practitioner—Oncology
Yale New Haven Health, Smilow Cancer Hospital
Bridgeport, Connecticut
Chapter 43, Nursing Management: Patients With Oncologic Disorders of the Brain and Spinal Cord

Honore Garrin Kotler, ACNP, CCTC, BSN, MSN, PhD(c)
Associate Director
Department of Transplant Surgery
Cedars-Sinai Medical Center
Los Angeles, California
Chapter 24, Nursing Management: Patients With Hepatic and Biliary Disorders

Zachary R. Krom, PhD, RN, CCRN, CHSE, NPD-BC
Nurse Scientist
Department of Critical Care Nursing
Cedars-Sinai Medical Center
Los Angeles, California
Chapter 21, Nursing Management: Patients With Oral and Esophageal Disorders and Patients Receiving Gastrointestinal Intubation, Enteral, and Parenteral Nutrition

Jacqueline Laird, BSN, CNML
Nurse Manager
Connecticut Burn Center
Bridgeport Hospital, Yale New Haven Health
Bridgeport, Connecticut
Chapter 52, Nursing Management: Patients With Burn Injuries

Gayge J. Maggio, MSN, FNP-BC, AAHIVS
Medical Provider
Callen-Lorde Community Health Center
New York, New York
Chapter 28, Nursing Assessment: Endocrine Function

Andrea Rothman Mann, MSN, RN
Professor of Practice
Gwynedd Mercy University
Frances M. Maguire School of Nursing and Health Professions
Gwynedd Valley, Pennsylvania
Chapter 26, Nursing Management: Patients With Renal Disorders

Kelly Martinez, EdD, MSN, APRN, FNP
Assistant Professor
School of Nursing, College of Health and Human Services
Southern Connecticut State University
New Haven, Connecticut
Chapter 8, Nursing Management: Patients With Upper Respiratory Tract Disorders

Philip R. Martinez, Jr., EdD, MSN, APRN-BC
Nurse Practitioner
Department of Pulmonary and Critical Care Medicine
Middlesex Hospital
Middletown, Connecticut
Chapter 3, Fluid and Electrolyte and Acid–Base Imbalances
Chapter 53, Nursing Management: Shock and Multisystem Failure

Elissa Mastrangelo, MS, BSN, RN, BC
Clinical Coordinator Regional Anesthesia
Anesthesia Department
Yale University/Yale New Haven Health
New Haven, Connecticut
Chapter 6, Pain Management

Jeanine L. May, APRN, MSN, MPH
Nurse Practitioner
Yale University School of Medicine
New Haven, Connecticut
Chapter 15, Nursing Management: Patients With Structural, Inflammatory and Infectious Cardiac Disorders

Kara H. McGee, MA, AGNP, ACHPN
Nurse Practitioner Specialist
Supportive Care Service
Memorial Sloan Kettering Cancer Center
New York, New York
Chapter 2, Chronic Illness and End-of-Life Care

Erin M. Morelli, PhD(c)
Associate Dean of Student Life
Yale University School of Nursing
Orange, Connecticut
Chapter 31, Nursing Assessment: Assigned Female at Birth (AFAB) and Assigned Male at Birth (AMAB) Reproductive Function

Maura Murphy Abbott, PhD, AOCNP, CPNP
Assistant Dean, Associate Professor, Oncology Nurse Practitioner
Columba University School of Nursing
New York, New York
Chapter 32, Nursing Management: Patients With Breast and Female Reproductive Disorders

Karin V. Nyström, MSN, APRN, FAHA
Stroke Program Manager
Yale New Haven Hospital
New Haven, Connecticut
Chapter 46, Nursing Management: Patients With Cerebrovascular Disorders

Daphny Grace M. Peneza, MSN, RN, CNOR, CSSM, FAORN
Perioperative Services Manager
Neurosurgery and Otolaryngology
Vanderbilt University Medical Center
Nashville, Tennessee
Chapter 4, Perioperative Nursing

Jennifer Picagli, MA, MSN, AGACNP-BC
Advanced Practice Registered Nurse
Department of Neurology, Stroke Center
Yale University, Yale New Haven Hospital
New Haven, Connecticut
Chapter 46, Nursing Management: Patients With Cerebrovascular Disorders

Linda Alessie Podolak, DNP, MSN, BSN
Nursing Director
Yale New Haven Health Bridgeport Hospital
Bridgeport, Connecticut
Chapter 38, Nursing Management: Patients With Rheumatic Disorders

Vanessa Pomarico-Denino, EdD, FNP-BC, FAANP
APRN/Lead Clinician, Diversity, Equity and Inclusion, Northeast Medical Group; Faculty, Fitzgerald Health Education Associates
Northeast Medical Group/Fitzgerald Health Education Associates
Hamden, Connecticut/North Andover, Massachusetts
Chapter 32, Nursing Management: Patients With Breast and Female Reproductive Disorders

Susanne A. Quallich, PhD, ANP-BC, NP-C, CUNP, FAANP
Editor, Urologic Nursing
Assistant Professor of Urology
Andrology Nurse Practitioner
Division of Andrology, General and Community Health
Department of Urology, Michigan Medicine
University of Michigan Health
Ann Arbor, Michigan
Chapter 31, Nursing Assessment: Assigned Female at Birth (AFAB) and Assigned Male at Birth (AMAB) Reproductive Function

Kaytlin Reedy-Rogier, MSW
Pipeline to Compassionate Care Project Coordinator
The St. Louis Integrated Health Network
St. Louis, Missouri
Chapter 1, The Nurse's Role in Adult Health Nursing

Kristen V. Roche, MSN
Assistant Clinical Professor
Yale University School of Nursing
Orange, Connecticut
Chapter 5, Cancer Care
Chapter 18, Nursing Assessment: Hematologic Function

Elaine Siow, PhD
Associate Professor
Department of Health and Social Sciences
Singapore Institute of Technology
Singapore
Chapter 30, Nursing Management: Patients With Endocrine Disorders

Michelle L. Telfer, DNP, MPH, CNM, FACNM
Assistant Professor, Co-Director of the Midwifery Program
Midwifery and Women's Health Nurse Practitioner
Yale School of Nursing
West Haven, Connecticut
Chapter 31, Nursing Assessment: Assigned Female at Birth (AFAB) and Assigned Male at Birth (AMAB) Reproductive Function

Kathryn Shugrue Tierney, MSN, APRN, FNP-BC, FAANP
Nurse Practitioner
Department of Endocrinology
Middlesex Health
Middletown, Connecticut
Chapter 29, Nursing Management: Diabetes Mellitus

Captain Patina S. Walton-Battle, DNP, APRN, FNP-C, PMHNP, GERO-BC, CWCN-AP, CFCN, CCHP-MH
Advanced Practice Nurse IV
Department of Health Services
United States Public Health Services/Federal Bureau of Prisons-Edgefield
Edgefield, South Carolina
Chapter 50, Nursing Assessment: Integumentary Function
Chapter 51, Nursing Management: Patients With Dermatologic Problems

Carol Ann Wetmore, MSN, RN
Assistant Professor
University of Connecticut
Storrs, Connecticut
Chapter 1, The Nurse's Role in Adult Health Nursing
Chapter 12, Nursing Management: Patients With Hypertension

Dawn Wicker, BS
Level 3 Neuroscience Physical Therapist
Department of Rehabilitation Services
Yale New Haven Hospital
New Haven, Connecticut
Chapter 46, Nursing Management: Patients With Cerebrovascular Disorders

Catherine G. Winkler, PhD, MPH, BSN, NP-BC
Nurse Practitioner
Medical Staff
Nuvance Health
Danbury, Connecticut
Chapter 16, Nursing Management: Patients With Arrhythmias and Conduction Problems

Reviewers

REVIEWERS FOR THIRD EDITION

Sherry Barnard, EdD, MSN, APRN
Vermont Technical College
Randolph, Vermont

Joan Boyd, MSN, MBA/HCA, RN
Florida State College at Jacksonville
Jacksonville, Florida

Kimberly Day, DNP, MSN-Ed, BSN, ADN
Clinical Assistant Professor
Edison College-Nursing Prelicensure
Phoenix, Arizona

Heraldine Flores, MSN, RN, CHSE, CNE, CPN
Baker College
Hills, Michigan

Tabitha Legambi, DNP, RN, CEN, CNE
University of Maryland School of Nursing
Baltimore, Maryland

Elizabeth Swinny, DNP, APRN, FNP-C, CCRN, CDCES
Baptist Health System, School of Health Professions
San Antonio, Texas

Laura Vasel, PhD, RN, CPNP, CNE
Randolph-Macon College
Ashland, Virginia

REVIEWERS FOR SECOND EDITION

Joyce Brasfield Adams, EdS
Instructor
Hinds Community College
Jackson, Mississippi

Hannah M. Anderson, MSN, RN-BC
Associate Professor and Nursing Program Coordinator
Thomas Nelson Community College
Hampton, Virginia

Sheri L. Banovic, MSN, RN, FNP-BC
Associate Professor and Nursing Program Coordinator
Lewis and Clark Community College
Godfrey, Illinois

Wanda G. Barlow, MSN, RN, FNP
Nursing Instructor
Winston-Salem State University
Winston-Salem, North Carolina

Joyce Basham, MN, CNS
Nursing Instructor
Midlands Technical College
Columbia, South Carolina

Mary Bergmann, MSN, RN
Professor
San Antonio College
San Antonio, Texas

Roberta Bernardini, MSN, BSN
Professor
Tidewater Community College
Portsmouth, Virginia

Sabrina T. Beroz, MSN, RN
Professor
Montgomery College
Takoma Park, Maryland

Jason Berry, MSN, BSN
Nursing Instructor
Winston-Salem State University
Winston-Salem, North Carolina

Sophia Beydoun, MSN, RN
Nursing Faculty
Henry Ford Community College
Dearborn, Michigan

Deborah A. Beyer, MSN, RN
Assistant Professor
Miami University
Hamilton, Ohio

Carol Blakeman, MSN, ARNP
Professor
College of Central Florida
Ocala, Florida

Jill E. Bobb, RN, BSN
Program Administrator of Nursing
Edison State Community College
Piqua, Ohio

Joy Borrero, MSN, RN, APRN
Instructor
Suffolk County Community College in Brentwood
Brentwood, New York

Cynthia A. Bowman, MSN, RNC, CNE
Nursing Instructor
Penn State
Altoona, Pennsylvania

Rebecca Bowman, MSN, BSN
Professor of Nursing
Florida State College at Jacksonville
Jacksonville, Florida

Angie Brindowski, MSN, BSN, RN
Clinical Assistant Professor
Carroll University
Waukesha, Wisconsin

Victoria Brioso-Ang, MSN, RN, CNE
Associate Professor
Sentara College of Health Sciences
Chespeake, Virginia

Michele Bunning, MSN, RN
Associate Professor
Good Samaritan College of Nursing & Health Science
Cincinnati, Ohio

Schvon Bussey, MSN, FNP
Instructor
Albany Technical College
Albany, Georgia

Darlene M. Cantu, MSN, RNC
Assistant Professor
San Antonio College
San Antonio, Texas

Theresa Capriotti, DO, MSN, RN, CRNP
Clinical Associate Professor
Villanova University
Villanova, Pennsylvania

Cecelia Carew, MA, RN-BC, CNE, CCRN, CPAN, CEN, LNC
Associate Professor
Department of Nursing
Bronx Community College
Bronx, New York

Kristine Carey, MSN, RN
Nursing Faculty
Normandale Community College
Bloomington, Minnesota

Arica Carter
Instructor
Atlanta Technical College
Atlanta, Georgia

Mary Rose Chasler, MSN, RN
Associate Professor of Nursing
Jamestown Community College
Jamestown, New York

Fran Cherkis, DHSc, RN, CNE
Instructor
Farmingdale State College
Farmingdale, New York

Maria J. Colón, MSN, RN
Faculty Professor
Inter American University of Puerto Rico—Metropolitan Campus
San Juan, Puerto Rico

Ruth S. Conner, PhD(c), RN, FNP-BC
Instructor
Medical University of South Carolina
Charleston, South Carolina

Patricia Dale Cork, MS, BSN, RN
Assistant Director
Riverside School of Professional Nursing and Riverside School of Practical Nursing
Newport News, Virginia

Theresa Delahoyde, EdD, RN
Dean of Nursing and Associate Professor of Nursing
BryanLGH College of Health Sciences
Lincoln, Nebraska

Fernande E. Deno, MSN, RN
Instructor
Anoka Ramsey Community College
Coon Rapids, Minnesota

Larinda Dixon, EdD, MS, RN
Professor of Nursing
College of DuPage
Matteson, Illinois

Sarah J. Doty, MSN, BSN, BSW
Instructor and Student Health
Southeast Missouri Hospital College of Nursing and Health Sciences
Cape Girardeau, Missouri

Linda K. Dunaway, MSN, RN, SANE
Professor
Maysville Community and Technical College
Maysville, Kentucky

David Dunham, DHEd, MSN, RN
Instructor
Hawaii Pacific University
Honolulu, Hawaii

Shelba Durston, MSN, RN, CCRN, SAFE
Instructor
San Joaquin Delta College
Stockton, California

Carrin Dvorak, MSN, RN, CNE
Assistant Professor of Nursing
Cuyahoga Community College
Cleveland, Ohio

Ellen Elder, MSN, RN
Instructor
Georgia Southwestern State University
Americus, Georgia

Jennifer Ellis, DNP, MSN, RN
Instructor
University of Cincinnati Blue Ash College
Blue Ash, Ohio

Susan Estes, MSN, BSN
Clinical Associate Professor
Georgia Baptist College of Nursing of Mercer University
Atlanta, Georgia

Stacey Estridge, MN, RN
Nursing Faculty
Midlands Technical College
Columbia, South Carolina

Patricia Ferrell, BSN, RN
Nursing Instructor
San Jacinto College North
Houston, Texas

Julie A. Fisher, PhD, MSN, BSN, RNC
Professor of Nursing
Wesley College
Dover, Delaware

Rebecca Flynn, MSN, ARNP, CPNP
Assistant Professor of Nursing
Mercy College of Health Sciences
Des Moines, Iowa

Kristi France, MS, BSN, RN
National Director of Product Development–Nursing & Allied Health
Lincoln Educational Services
West Orange, New Jersey

Margie Francisco, EdD, MSN, RN
Instructor
Illinois Valley Community College
Oglesby, Illinois

Connie P. Gazmen, MS, RN, OCN
Instructor and Program Director of Adult Health Clinical Nurse Specialist Program
School of Nursing and Dental Hygiene
University of Hawaii at Manoa
Honolulu, Hawaii

Christy Gee, MSN, RN, FNP-BC
Doctoral Student
South College
Asheville, North Carolina

Gwendolyn Greene, MSN/ED, BSN, RN
Nursing Instructor
Midlands Technical College
Columbia, South Carolina

Karla Hall, MSN, RN
Assistant Professor
Mercy College of Health Sciences
Des Moines, Iowa

Janet R. Hamilton, MSN, RN
Allied Health Department Chair
And
Assistant Professor
Lamar State College
Port Arthur, Texas

Janice Hancock, MS, BS, RN
Faculty
North Hennepin Community College
Brooklyn Park, Minnesota

Carol Ann Hanna, PhD, BC, RN
Faculty
Delaware County Community College
Media, Pennsylvania

Elaine C. Hannigan, MSN, RN
Continuing Lecturer
Purdue University
West Lafayette, Indiana

Karla Hanson, MSN, RN
Instructor
College of Nursing at South Dakota State University
Brookings, South Dakota

Lisa Harding, MSN, RN, CEN
Associate Professor
Bakersfield College
Bakersfield, California

Janice Hausauer, MSN, FNP, APRN-BC
Instructor
Montana State University in Bozeman
Bozeman, Montana

Celia G. Hay, PhD, RN
Chair of Nursing Department
LaGrange College
LaGrange, Georgia

Lori Hendrickx, EdD, RN, CCRN
Associate Professor
College of Nursing at South Dakota State University
Brookings, South Dakota

Janet Hertlzer, MSN, FNP-BC
Instructor
Marian University
Indianapolis, Indiana

Barbara A. Hoglund, EdD, MSN, RN, FNP-BC
Associate Professor of Nursing
Bethel University
St. Paul, Minnesota

Nina J. Hollifield, MS, RN
Assistant Professor
College of Southern Idaho
Twin Falls, Ohio

Barbie Hoover, MSN, RN
Instructor
School of Health Sciences
School of Nursing
Pennsylvania College of Technology
Williamsport, Pennsylvania

Laura J. Hope, MSN, RN, CDE
Nursing Faculty
Florence-Darlington Technical College
Florence, South Carolina

Catherine Howell, MSN, RN
Professor of Nursing Education
San Diego City College
San Diego, California

Claudette Jacobs, DNP, MS, BSN, RN-BC
Instructor of Nursing
Howard Community College
Columbia, Maryland

Uletha M. Jones, MSN, CCRN
Nursing Faculty
Pensacola State College
Pensacola, Florida

Melanie M. Jorgenson, BSN, RN
Nursing Instructor
North Seattle Community College
Seattle, Washington

Denise Pruskowski Kavanagh, MSN, RN
Professor
La Salle University
Philadelphia, Pennsylvania

Katie Kay, MSN
Faculty Manager
Chamberlain College of Nursing
Chicago, Illinois

Penny Kessler, DNP, RN
Clinical Assistant Professor
School of Nursing
University of Minnesota
Minneapolis, Minnesota

Jonni K. Pielin Kircher, MSN, RN, CSN
Assistant Professor of Nursing
Westmoreland County Community College
Youngwood, Pennsylvania

Andrea Knesek, DNP, MSN, RN, BC
Nursing Faculty
Macomb Community College
Clinton Township, Michigan

Stephen D. Krau, PhD, RN, CNE
Associate Professor
School of Nursing
Vanderbilt University Medical Center
Nashville, Tennessee

Donna Kubesh, PhD, MS, RN
Associate Professor
Luther College
Decorah, Iowa

Karen Kulhanek, MEd, BSN, RN
Nursing Professor
Kellogg Community College
Battle Creek, Michigan

Marjorie J. Kurt, MSN, RN
Clinical Professor
Indiana University School of Nursing
Indianapolis, Indiana

Jill J. Lambert, MSN, RN, GNP/CNS
Associate Professor
Charity School of Nursing
Delgado Community College
New Orleans, Louisiana

Marci L. Langenkamp, MS, BSN, RN (AD)
Assistant Professor of Nursing
Edison Community College
Piqua, Ohio

Ronnette C. Langhorne, MS, RN
Assistant Professor
Thomas Nelson Community College
Hampton, Virginia

Kelly T. Lawson, MSN, RN
Instructor of Nursing
Francis Marion University
Florence, South Carolina

Kathy Leach, PhD, RN
Adjunct Assistant Professor
St. Louis University
St. Louis, Missouri

Heidi Loucks, MS, RN, CNE
Nurse Educator
Casper College
Casper, Wyoming

Lynn Lowery, MSN, RN, FCN, CCHC, CDE
Associate Professor
Charity School of Nursing
Delgado Community College
New Orleans, Louisiana

Jennifer Lunny, MSN, RN
Assistant Professor of Nursing
Broward College
Coconut Creek, Florida

Elisa Mangosing-Lemmon, MSN, BSN, RN, CMSRN
Nursing Instructor
Riverside School of Health Careers
School of Professional Nursing
Newport News, Virginia

Patricia Ann Martin, MSN, RN, FNP-BC, CNE
Associate Professor
West Kentucky Community and Technical College
Paducah, Kentucky

Ellen McAcoy, MA, RN, CNE
Associate Professor
Hillsborough Community College
Tampa, Florida

Connie McFadden, MSN, RN, CNE
Assistant Professor
The Christ College of Nursing and Health Sciences
Cincinnati, Ohio

Barbara McGraw, MSN, RN, CNE
Nursing Instructor and Curriculum Coordinator
Central Community College
Grand Island, Nebraska

Anthony McGuire, PhD, RN, CCRN, ACNP-BC
Nursing School Lecturer
California State—Long Beach
Long Beach, California

Mary McKay, DNP, ARNP, CNE
Associate Clinical Professor
University of Miami
Coral Gables, Florida

Mary Elizabeth McKenna-Dailey, APRN-BC
Professor and Nurse Education/Family Nurse Practitioner
North Shore Community College
Danvers, Massachusetts

Heather M. McKnight, MSN, RN
Assistant Professor
Texarkana College
Texarkana, Texas

Kathleen McNeese, MN, RN, CNS
Tenured Faculty
Glendale Community College
Glendale, California

Susan McReynolds, MS, RN, CNE
Instructor
Blessing-Rieman College of Nursing
Quincy, Illinois

Dona Molyneaux, PhD, MSN, BSN, RN, ONC
Associate Professor
Gwynedd Mercy University
Gwynedd Valley, Pennsylvania

Cynthia Moore, MSN, RN, PLNC
Nursing Faculty
Minnesota State Community and Technical College
Detroit Lakes, Minnesota

Mary Moseley, EdD, MN, BSN
Professor
Northern Virginia Community College
Springfield, Virginia

Ann Motycka, MSN, RN, CNE
Instructor
Ivy Tech State College, Southwest
Evansville, Indiana

Cindy Neely, MSN, RN
Campus Clinical Lab Coordinator and Professor of Nursing
Oklahoma City Community College
Oklahoma City, Oklahoma

Susan E. Nelson, MSN, RN, WCC, CLNC
Regional Nursing Department Chair
Ivy Tech Community College
Anderson, Indiana

Kathy Newton, MSN, BSN, RN
Nurse Educator
Kellogg Community College
Battle Creek, Michigan

Lynn Noell, MSN, RN
Associate Professor
Department of Nursing Education
Joliet Junior College
Joliet, Illinois

Karen Noss, MSN, RN, OCN
Associate Professor
Luzerne County Community College
Nanticoke, Pennsylvania

Annette Oberhaus, MSN, RN
Clinical Teaching Assistant
Northwest State Community College
Archbold, Ohio

Crystal O'Connell-Schauerte, MSCN, BSCN
Coordinator and Professor
Algonquin College
Ottawa, Ontario

Patricia Brown O'Hara, PhD, RN
Associate Professor of Nursing
Gwynedd Mercy University
Gwynedd Valley, Pennsylvania

Catherine J. Pagel, MSN, RN
Assistant Professor of Nursing
Mercy College of Health Sciences
Des Moines, Iowa

Karen Parker
Professor and Clinical Coordinator
Lorain County Community College
Elyria, Ohio

LaVinda Pearson, PhD, RN, CRRN, CNE
Instructor
St. Catherine University
St. Paul, Minnesota

Michelle M. Pelter, PhD, RN
Assistant Professor
Orvis School of Nursing
University of Nevada
Reno, Nevada

Catherine Pence, MSN, RN
Associate Professor
Northern Kentucky University
Highland Heights, Kentucky

Sherily Pereia, PhD, MSN, RNA
Instructor
Medical Sciences Campus and School of Nursing
University of Puerto Rico
San Juan, Puerto Rico

Norma Jean Peters, MSN
Nursing Instructor
Madison College—Reedsburg
Reedsburg, Wisconsin

Vicki Plagenz, MSN, RN
Assistant Professor
Montana State University Northern
Lewistown, Montana

Julia R. Popp, MSN, RN
Professor of Nursing
Owens Community College
Toldeo, Ohio

Dale Powis, MSN, RN
Professor
Community College of Rhode Island
Warwick, Rhode Island

Kathleen Puri, MSN, RN
Associate Professor
Chattanooga State Community College
Chattanooga, Tennessee

Loretta G. Quigley, MS, RN
Associate Dean
St. Joseph's College of Nursing
Syracuse, New York

Sharon Rappold, MSN, RN, BC
Instructor
Wharton County Junior College
Wharton, Texas

Lucille Rayford, MSN
Adjunct Faculty
California State University—Dominguez Hill
Carson, California

Emily Reece, PhD, MSN, RN
Nursing Professor
El Centro College
Dallas, Texas

Gwendolyn E. Richardson, RN, ACNS-BC
Instructor of Nursing
Midlands Technical College
Columbia, South Carolina

Jennifer Robinson, MSN
Instructor of Nursing
Washington Health System
Atlanta, Georgia

Noelle Rohatinsky, PhD, MN, BSN, RN
Assistant Professor
University of Saskatchewan
Saskatoon, Saskatchewan

Tami Rogers, DVM, MSN, CNE
Lead Nursing Professor, Adult Health
Keiser University
Orlando, Florida

Martha Kathryn Findley Roper, MSN, RN
Nursing Instructor
Wallace State Community College
Hanceville, Alabama

Kathleen S. Rose, MSN, BSN, RN
Associate Professor of Nursing
Coordinator for LPN and Paramedic to RN Transition Programs
Chattanooga State Community College
Chattanooga, Tennessee

Kristin E. Sandau, PhD, RN
Associate Professor of Nursing and Staff RN at United Hospital
Department of Nursing
Bethel University
St. Paul, Minnesota

Joanne Serembus, EdD, RN, CNE, CCRN
Associate Clinical Professor
College of Nursing and Health Professions
Drexel University
Philadelphia, Pennsylvania

Kathy Sheats, MSN, RN
Associate Professor
University of the Virgin Islands
Kingshill, United States Virgin Islands

Leslee H. Shepard, EdD, MSN, RN, CMSRN
Assistant Professor of Nursing
Winston-Salem State University
Winston-Salem, North Carolina

Margaret Sherer, MS, RN, CEN, CNE
Nursing Faculty
Portland Community College
Portland, Oregon

Mandy M. Sheriff, MSN, RN
Instructor
Western Illinois University
School of Nursing
Macomb, Illinois

Karin Sherill, MSN, RN, CNE
Faculty Nursing Educator and Simulation Coordinator
Maricopa Nursing at Mesa Community College
Mesa, Arizona

Louise A. Shirk, MSN
Instructor, Medical-Surgical Nursing
Midlands Technical College
Columbia, South Carolina

Michelle Sink, MSN, RN
Professor of Nursing
Florida State College at Jacksonville
Jacksonville, Florida

Julie Skrabel, MSN, RN
Assistant Professor
Bryan LGH College of Health Sciences
Lincoln, Nebraska

June R. Soto, MEd, RN, APRN
Assistant Professor of Nursing
Borough of Manhattan Community College
New York, New York

Lisa Sparacino, PhD, MS, RN, CCRN
Instructor
New York Institute of Technology
New York, New York

Denise Spohler, MSN, RN
Professor of Nursing
Owens Community College
Toledo, Ohio

Jodie Steblay, MSN
Instructor
Hibbing Community College
Hibbing, Minnesota

Mary Stedman, EdD, RN
Instructor
Farmingdale State College
Farmingdale, New York

Nancy Steffen, MSN, RN
Nursing Instructor
Century College
White Bear, Minnesota

Elizabeth Zion Stratton, MS, RN
Assistant Professor of Nursing
Monroe Community College
Rochester, New York

Megan Talbot, DNP, MSN, BSN, RN, CNE
Instructor
Merritt College-Oakland
Oakland, California

Stephanie B. Turner, EdD, MSN, RN
Nursing Instructor
Wallace State Community College
Hanceville, Alabama

Patricia Voelpel, EdD
Clinical Assistant Professor
Stony Brook University
Stony Brook, New York

Timothy J. Voytilla, MSN, ARNP
Nursing Program Director
Keiser University–Tampa Campus
Tampa, Florida

Gerry Walker, DHEd, MSN, RN
Nursing Program Chair and Assistant Professor of Nursing
Park University
Parkville, Missouri

Terri L. Walker, MSN, RN
Assistant Nursing Program Director and Team Leader NPIV
Oklahoma City Community College
Oklahoma City, Oklahoma

Kathleen Warner, MSN, RN
Assistant Professor of Nursing
Viterbo University
La Crosse, Wisconsin

Cynthia L. Williams, MS, RN, CMSRN
Professor of Nursing
Oklahoma City Community College
Oklahoma City, Oklahoma

Cheryl Winter, MSN, RN, FNP-BC
Associate Professor of Nursing
Erma Byrd Higher Education Center
Bluefield State College
Beaver, West Virginia

Christine Wood, MSN, RN
Nursing Professor
Des Moines Area Community College
Ankeny, Iowa

Mary E. Wright, MSN, RN, BSN, PHN
Professor of Nursing Medical Surgical
Mount San Jacinto College
Menifee, California
MiraCosta College
Oceanside, California

Regina L. Wright, MSN, RN
Assistant Professor of Nursing
Neumann University
Aston, Pennsylvania

Jamie Zwicky, MSN-Ed, RN
Faculty
Bryant and Stratton College
Waukesha, Wisconsin

Preface

Welcome to the third edition of *Medical-Surgical Nursing: Focus on Clinical Judgment.*

A NOTE FROM THE AUTHOR

As the long and rightly held "canaries in the coal mine," it is no wonder nurses are leading the charge in rethinking how clinical practice can be better, and spotlighting the importance of developing "clinical judgment." This may be the term *du jour*, and for good reason, but it describes something primordial about our profession: It is the fundamental faculty of observation, allowing us to respond even more dynamically and adaptively to the ever-changing clinical setting. At our core, nurses are the noticers, the ones who are always present.

In the third edition of this textbook, the primary aim was still the same—to distill the essential, need-to-know content—but I wanted to tweak things, and to encourage you, the reader, to help in lifting up the lens; in seeing the broader context where complex structures produce inequalities and barriers to health. I created *Pearls for Practice: Lifting the Lens* that are interspersed throughout the chapters.

While other *Pearls for Practice* highlight pathophysiology, technical skills, clinical presentation, nutrition, etc., all were created from nearly five decades in clinical practice, and in seeing where the glitches in learning occur with my students over three decades of teaching. Thus, *Pearls for Practice* are bountiful in this edition.

Importantly, I had to move beyond the notion that I know clinical judgment when I see it and instead detail via cases the process or reasoning one works through in deciphering actual clinical examples. More than 20 cases were created to walk the students through the complexities of clinical reasoning. Additionally, I wanted expert clinicians to write this book. Nurses who continue to live in the real world of clinical practice and have strong opinions about essential nursing knowing. You, the reader, will be the judge of our success.

The third edition includes The Nurse's Role and Health Education and Health Promotion combined to provide more concise coverage of this material. This edition includes bias-free, gender-neutral language used throughout the text. All NEW content on social and structural determinants of health, COVID-19, continued focus and enhancement of clinical judgment, updated Determinants of health align with new standards outlined in Healthy People 2030, LGBTQIA+ updated content is reflected in applicable chapters. Each chapter contains all NEW end-of-chapter questions in NexGen (NGN) formatting in those question types that we could translate well for print for every chapter, along with brand NEW Clinical Judgment Case Studies, incorporating National NCSBN's Clinical Judgment Measurement Model.

INCLUSIVE LANGUAGE

A note about the language used in this book. Wolters Kluwer recognizes that people have a diverse range of identities, and we are committed to using inclusive and nonbiased language in our content. In line with the principles of nursing, we strive not to define people by their diagnoses, but to recognize their personhood first and foremost, using as much as possible the language diverse groups use to define themselves, and including only information that is relevant to nursing care.

We strive to better address the unique perspectives, complex challenges, and lived experiences of diverse populations traditionally underrepresented in health literature. When describing or referencing populations discussed in research studies, we will adhere to the identities presented in those studies to maintain fidelity to the evidence presented by the study investigators. We follow best practices of language set forth by the *Publication Manual of the American Psychological Association, 7th edition* but acknowledge that language evolves rapidly, and we will update the language used in future editions of this book as necessary.

FEATURES

We have designed some special features to help engage you, the reader, and assist you in your understanding of the content and the nurse's role in caring for patients.

Guidelines for Nursing Care provide steps and rationales for important procedures.

Focused Assessment boxes summarize important assessment criteria and significant findings related to a particular disorder.

Risk Factors provide a bulleted list of risk factors for a particular disorder, drawing attention to factors that can impair health.

Patient Education summarizes patient teaching, home care, and discharge planning.

Health Promotion reviews important points the nurse should discuss with the patient to prevent common health problems from developing.

NEW! Lifting the Lens highlights the impact of upstream factors on our patients, their diseases, and communities.

Gerontologic Considerations highlight information that pertains specifically to the care of older adults who comprise the fastest-growing segment of our population.

Laboratory and Diagnostic Tests tables list common lab tests for particular disorders along with normal values, critical values, and nursing implications.

Nursing Research: Bridging the Gap to Evidence-Based Practice demonstrates the nursing implications of important research.

Pearls for Practice: Pathophysiology highlights and describes important pathophysiologic processes.

Pearls for Practice: Nutrition highlights nutritional considerations for particular disorders.

Nursing Pearls for Practice offer brief tips or highlight red-flag warnings for clinical practice.

DRUG ALERTS highlight key nursing considerations and drug safety information.

Unfolding Patient Stories feature patients from Wolters Kluwer's *vSim for Nursing.*

A COMPREHENSIVE PACKAGE FOR TEACHING AND LEARNING

Ancillary Package

To further facilitate teaching and learning, a carefully designed ancillary package has been developed to assist faculty and students.

Instructor Resources

Tools to assist you with teaching your course are available upon adoption of this book on thePoint® at http://thepoint.lww.com/Honan3e.

A **Test Generator** features National Council Licensure Exam (NCLEX)-style questions mapped to chapter learning objectives.

- **PowerPoint Presentations** provide an easy way to integrate the textbook with your students' classroom experience; multiple-choice and true/false questions are included to promote class participation.
- **Guided Lecture Notes** are organized by outcome and provide corresponding PowerPoint slide numbers to simplify preparation for lecture.
- **Discussion Topics** (and suggested answers) can be used in the classroom or in online discussion boards to facilitate interaction with your students.
- **Assignments** (and suggested answers) include group, written, clinical, and web assignments to engage students in varied activities and assess their learning.
- **Case Studies** with related questions (and suggested answers) give students an opportunity to apply their knowledge to a client case similar to one they might encounter in practice.
- **Care Plans** created for instructors to guide their students through real-life nursing plans of care in preparation for clinical nursing.
- **Answers to the Think Critically questions in the book** reinforce key concepts.
- Sample **Syllabi** are provided for 7-week and 15-week courses.
- An **American Association of Colleges of Nursing (AACN) Essentials Competency Map** identifies book content related to the AACN Essentials.
- An **Image Bank** provides access to the photographs and illustrations from this textbook to use in your course materials.
- **Learning Objectives** from the book are provided for your convenience.
- An **ebook** serves as a handy resource.
- Access to all **Student Resources** is provided so that you can understand the student experience and use these resources in your course as well.

Student Resources

An exciting set of free learning resources is available on thePoint® to help students review and apply vital concepts in adult health: medical-surgical nursing. Multimedia engines have been optimized so that students can access many of these resources on mobile devices. Students can access all these resources at http://thepoint.lww.com/Honan3e using the codes printed in the front of their textbooks.

- **Journal Articles** offer access to current research relevant to each chapter and available in Wolters Kluwer journals to familiarize students with nursing literature.
- **Interactive Learning Resources** appeal to a variety of learning styles.
- **Heart and Breath Sounds** are provided for your convenience.

Student Ancillaries

- **Concepts in Action Animations** bring physiologic and pathophysiologic concepts to life.
- **Practice & Learn Case Studies** present case scenarios and offer interactive exercises and questions to help students apply what they have learned.
- **Watch & Learn Video Clips** reinforce skills from the textbook and appeal to visual and auditory learners.
- Nursing Care Plans for selected chapters
- Suggested Readings for students.

vSim for Nursing

Available for separate purchase, vSim for Nursing, jointly developed by Laerdal Medical and Wolters Kluwer Health, offers innovative scenario-based learning modules consisting of web-based virtual simulations, course learning materials, and curriculum tools designed to develop critical thinking skills and promote clinical confidence and competence. vSim for Nursing | Medical-Surgical includes 10 cases from the *Simulation in Nursing Education—Medical-Surgical scenarios*, authored by the National League for Nursing. Students can progress through suggested readings, pre- and postsimulation assessments, documentation assignments, and guided reflection questions and will receive an individualized feedback log immediately upon completion of the simulation. Throughout the student learning experience, the product offers remediation back to trusted Lippincott resources, including Lippincott Nursing Advisor and Lippincott Nursing Procedures—two online, evidence-based clinical information solutions used in health care facilities throughout the United States. This innovative product provides a comprehensive patient-focused solution for learning and integrating simulation into the classroom.

Contact your Wolters Kluwer sales representative or visit http://thepoint.lww.com/vsim for options to enhance your medical-surgical nursing course with vSim for Nursing.

Lippincott DocuCare

Available for separate purchase, Lippincott DocuCare combines web-based academic electronic health record (EHR) simulation software with clinical case scenarios, allowing students to learn how to use an EHR in a safe, true-to-life setting while enabling instructors to measure their progress. Lippincott DocuCare's nonlinear solution works well in the classroom, simulation lab, and clinical practice.

Contact your Wolters Kluwer sales representative or visit http://thepoint.lww.com/DocuCare for options to enhance your pediatric nursing course with DocuCare.

A COMPREHENSIVE, DIGITAL, INTEGRATED COURSE SOLUTION: LIPPINCOTT® CoursePoint+

Lippincott® CoursePoint+ is an integrated, digital curriculum solution for nursing education that provides a completely interactive experience geared to help students understand, retain, and apply their course knowledge and be prepared for practice. The time-tested, easy-to-use and trusted solution includes engaging learning tools, evidence-based practice, case studies, and in-depth reporting to meet students where they are in their learning, combined with the most trusted nursing education content on the market to help prepare students for practice. This easy-to-use digital learning solution of *Lippincott® CoursePoint+*, combined with unmatched support, gives instructors and students everything they need for course and curriculum success!

Lippincott® CoursePoint+ includes:

- Leading content provides a variety of learning tools to engage students of all learning styles.
- A personalized learning approach gives students the content and tools they need at the moment they need it, giving them data for more focused remediation and helping to boost their confidence and competence.
- Powerful tools, including varying levels of case studies, interactive learning activities, and adaptive learning powered by PrepU, help students learn the critical thinking and clinical judgment skills to help them become practice-ready nurses.
- Preparation for Practice tools improve student competence, confidence, and success in transitioning to practice.
  - vSim® for Nursing: Co-developed by Laerdal Medical and Wolters Kluwer, vSim® for Nursing simulates real nursing scenarios and allows students to interact with virtual patients in a safe, online environment.
  - Lippincott® Advisor for Education: With over 8,500 entries covering the latest evidence-based content and drug information, Lippincott® Advisor for Education provides students with the most up-to-date information possible, while giving them valuable experience with the same point-of-care content they will encounter in practice.
- Unparalleled reporting provides in-depth dashboards with several data points to track student progress and help identify strengths and weaknesses.
- Unmatched support includes training coaches, product trainers, and nursing education consultants to help educators and students implement CoursePoint+ with ease.

Linda Honan, RN, PhD, CNS-BC, ANEF, FAAN

Acknowledgments

I must acknowledge and thank the following people who helped clear cobwebs in my understanding. They include Walter Zawalich and Sharen McKay who always came through with answers to my pathophysiology questions; Lisa B. Meland, my pharmacology guru who answered questions from standard dosages to interactions, and everything in between; my anatomy sages William Stewart and Charles Duncan, MD for all their assistance and friendship, and my orthopedic expert, Dr. Gary Friedlaender, who edited and refined Clinical Judgment cases. Finally, to Audrey Coolman and Kaytlin Reedy-Rogier who edited and improved each lifting the lens feature in this edition. To all the patients I cared for over 45 years, the nursing staff on 6-4 at Yale New Haven Hospital and all the GEPNs who honed my skills as a nurse and educator for over 30 years. I am in your debt. To Julie Vitale and Caroline Define who edited this edition with care. Finally, my thanks to all the clinician colleagues who wrote chapters about their day-to-day practice so that this book is grounded in the real world of clinical.

New Features Guide

Medical-Surgical Nursing: Focus on Clinical Judgment, 3rd edition contains many accessible features to help students grasp the important content.

Greater breadth and depth of content emerge as the reader continues; although still striving for compelling context, which provides a greater wealth of information.

NEW FEATURES

NEW! CLINICAL JUDGMENT CASES can be found in numerous chapters, which encompass the National Council State Board of Nursing (NCSBN) Clinical Judgment Measurement Model within each and every case. Each case incorporates each step of the measurement model and writes out what it means to a student (written in second person to engage students).

Clinical Judgment Case

Your patient is 66 years old and is 5 days postlaryngeal surgery for cancer, where a partial laryngectomy was performed (a portion of the larynx is removed, along with one vocal cord and the tumor; all other structures remain). Medical history includes hypertension, chronic obstructive pulmonary disorder (COPD) with a 30-pack year smoking history (1 pack per day [PPD] ×'s 30 years), and type 2 diabetes; home medications include hydrochlorothiazide, metformin, and albuterol. The patient rang the call bell stating, "I think I choked on my tea, I can't breathe." Upon walking in the room, you find the patient leaning forward on the edge of the bed and note respiratory distress, characterized by dyspnea, use of accessory muscles, intercostal retractions, nasal flaring, mouth breathing, coughing of tea colored fluid followed by frothy secretions. You hear crackles in the right lower lobe (RLL) and scattered rhonchi and wheezing throughout. The patient's skin is warm and dry with delayed skin turgor and vital signs are as follows: 100.7°F, HR 112 and regular, 28 RR with an oxygen saturation of 90% on room air and the blood pressure is 132/78. Heart Sounds are S1 S2 without murmur, gallop or rub; neck veins are flat. There is no peripheral edema, capillary refill is 2 seconds and dorsalis pedis and posterior tibial pulses are 2+ to 3+ bil. The patient is anxious and restless.

Step One: Recognize cues where relevant and important information is identified from different sources, such as medical history or vital signs.

NEW! LIFTING THE LENS provides a view into social and structural determinants of health written to deliver information to the students on patients, their diseases, and communities.

Pearls for Practice: Lifting the Lens

Note in the image above the impact of climate change on health. Rising temperatures worsen air quality (increases respiratory difficulty), increase pollen count (increases allergic reactions and asthma attacks in some), and increase ground-level ozone pollution (particularly in heavily populated urban areas) that reduces lung function, and increase the risk of asthma attacks and exacerbation of other chronic lung diseases (Anderko & Pennea, 2022; CDC, 2022c). An additional threat is wildfires that reduce air quality, both locally and in areas downwind of fires (CDC, 2022c). Nurses will need to educate patients about preventive measures in extreme heat; such measures include increasing hydration, use of electric fans and/or air conditioning, staying indoors and avoiding outdoor activities where possible, and wearing cool and sun-protective clothing (Liu et al., 2021). The nurse offers resources to patients and families related to air pollution and health.

Here are resources for patients and families:

Air Quality

Check air quality (www.airnow.gov/sites/default/files/2018-06/aqi-forecasts.pdf)

Clinical **PEARLS FOR PRACTICE** offer brief tips or highlight red-flag warnings for clinical practice.

Pearls for Practice

Obesity (BMI of 35% or higher) in and of itself is associated with all-cause mortality regardless of level of physical activity. Questions exist regarding whether obesity itself is a risk factor for CAD or cardiovascular events, or if it is the relationship of obesity to glucose intolerance, insulin resistance, HTN, physical inactivity, and dyslipidemia that increases risk. Given the significant risk that DM, HTN, and hyperlipidemia impose on coronary disease, nurses need to make efforts toward increasing awareness of the crucial role that these disorders have on cardiovascular mortality and morbidity.

DRUG ALERTS highlight key nursing considerations and drug safety information.

> ***Drug Alert***
> ***Epinephrine results in α- and β-adrenergic effects, resulting in vasoconstriction and bronchial smooth-muscle relaxation. Epinephrine works rapidly to reduce throat swelling, open up the airways, and maintain blood pressure in patients. Age is not a barrier to IM epinephrine injections in patients with anaphylaxis (Rowe & Gaeta, 2020).***

BOX 44-9 **Pearls for Practice: Nutrition**

Nutritional Support Following Traumatic Brain Injury

- Patients with traumatic brain injury (TBI) have increased metabolic expenditure so they have high caloric needs.
- Full nutritional support should be begun no later than 72 hours after the injury to achieve full caloric replacement by postinjury day 7.
- Protein should comprise 15% of total calories.
- When feedings are initiated, glucose levels should be closely monitored as hyperglycemia is associated with worse outcomes.
- Consultation with a dietician is recommended to provide optimal nutritional support.

Contents

UNIT ONE

Basics of Adult Health Nursing

A 70-year-old patient diagnosed with hypertension is being seen in the health clinic. When gathering information on the patient, the nurse notes a definite problem with medication adherence. The patient states, "I just forget to take the medication. It's no big deal!" The patient's current BP is 170/90, and the medical record notes a history of previous transient ischemic attacks (TIAs) and a cerebral vascular accident (CVA) or stroke with resulting visual and hearing deficits.

- **What areas of health education would be important to emphasize for this patient?**
- **Discuss variables that could affect this patient's medication adherence.**
- **What teaching strategies could be incorporated into the plan of care for this 70-year-old patient?**

CHAPTER 1

The Nurse's Role in Adult Health Nursing

Linda Honan • Kaytlin Reedy-Rogier • Audrey Coolman • Carol Ann Wetmore

Learning Objectives

After reading this chapter, you will be able to:

1. Define nursing.
2. Define the nursing process and clinical judgment.
3. Differentiate health, wellness, and health promotion.
4. Describe factors causing significant changes in the health care delivery system and their impact on the health care field and the nursing profession.
5. Describe structural and social determinants of health and their impact on patients' health.
6. Describe the purposes and significance of health education.
7. Describe strategies that facilitate adults' learning abilities.
8. Describe the relationship of health education to the nursing process.
9. Develop a teaching plan for a patient.
10. Define health promotion and discuss the role of the nurse related to it.

NURSING DEFINED

Since Florence Nightingale wrote (1859) that the goal of nursing was "to put the patient in the best condition for nature to act upon him," nursing leaders have described nursing as both an art and a science. In the 20th century, Virginia Henderson (1966) defined nursing as the profession that "[assists] the individual, sick or well, in the performance of those activities contributing to health or its recovery (or to peaceful death) that he would perform unaided if he had the necessary strength, will, or knowledge. This is done in such a way as to help him gain independence as rapidly as possible." The American Nurses Association (ANA), which is the professional organization representing the interests of the nation's 3.8 million registered nurses (RNs) defines our profession as "Nursing integrates the art and science of caring and focuses on the protection, promotion, and optimization of health and human functioning; prevention of illness and injury; facilitation of healing; and alleviation of suffering through compassionate presence. Nursing is the diagnosis and treatment of human responses and advocacy in the care of individuals, families, groups, communities, and populations in recognition of the connection of all humanity" (ANA, 2019, 2021). The definition of nursing, while always evolving, maintains some vestiges from the time of Florence Nightingale, and the ANA delineates essential features of professional nursing.

Nursing:

- Integrates the art and science of caring
- Protects, promotes, and optimizes health and human functioning
- Prevents illness and injury
- Facilitates healing
- Alleviates suffering through compassionate presence

Nursing is:

- the diagnosis and treatment of human responses and
- advocacy in the care of individuals, families, groups, communities, and populations in recognition of the connection of all humanity (ANA, 2021).

General Professional Nursing

Each individual nurse has the responsibility to carry out their role as described in the Scope and Standards of Nursing Practice (ANA, 2021) and to comply with the Code for Nurses (ANA, 2015) and the Nurse Practice Act of the state in which they practice. These documents support the definition of nursing and the claim that nurses must be actively

BOX 1-1

American Nurses Association Code of Ethics for Nurses

1. The nurse practices with compassion and respect for the inherent dignity, worth, and unique attributes of every person.
2. The nurse's primary commitment is to the patient, whether an individual, family, group, community, or population.
3. The nurse promotes, advocates for, and protects the rights, health, and safety of the patient.
4. The nurse has authority, accountability, and responsibility for nursing practice; makes decisions; and takes action consistent with the obligation to promote health and provide optimal care.
5. The nurse owes the same duties to self as to others, including the responsibility to promote health and safety, preserve wholeness of character and integrity, maintain competence, and continue personal and professional growth.
6. The nurse, through individual and collective effort, establishes, maintains, and improves the ethical environment of the work setting and conditions of employment that are conducive to safe, quality health care.
7. The nurse, in all roles and settings, advances the profession through research and scholarly inquiry, professional standards development, and the generation of both nursing and health policy.
8. The nurse collaborates with other health professionals and the public to protect human rights, promote health diplomacy, and reduce health disparities.
9. The profession of nursing, collectively through its professional organizations, must articulate nursing values, maintain the integrity of the profession, and integrate principles of social justice into nursing and health policy (ANA, 2015).

involved in the decision-making process regarding ethical concerns surrounding health care and human responses.

The Code of Ethics (Box 1-1), established by the ANA, consists of ethical standards, each with its own interpretive statements. The interpretive statements provide guidance in addressing nursing responsibilities and ethical decision making.

The role of nurses is specified by individual state boards of nursing and is termed *scope of practice*. Only licensed providers (RNs, LPNs) have a scope of practice. Scope of practice is used to delineate actions that are legally permitted for a particular profession, based on specific educational qualifications. Nurses need to know and understand their scope of practice, as well as those of other professions with which they interact during patient care. Some actions are described as *dependent*, meaning that a specific action depends upon an order from a medical doctor (MD) or licensed independent practitioner (LIP), such as a nurse practitioner (NP). An example of a dependent action is a task, such as administering medications that have been ordered. Other actions are *interdependent* and are done in a collaborative manner with others. Interdependent actions might include medication titration or participation in interdisciplinary rounds. *Independent* actions can be performed by the RN without input from others. Independent actions include performing nursing assessments and patient education.

Delegation is a tool that nurses use and is defined as the process by which a nurse assigns or directs another member of the health care staff to perform nursing activities (ANA & National Council of State Boards of Nursing [NCSBN], 2019). Delegation is a complex skill that must be taught and practiced to develop proficiency in the delivery of nursing care. Delegation is not as simple as assigning the "task" of obtaining vital signs to an assistant. For example, *IF* the patient is stable AND *IF* circumstances have not changed AND *IF* the RN has already assessed the patient, then the vital signs can be delegated. Clearly, there are *Ifs* that the nurse must consider before delegating! It is crucial that the nurse understands that when delegating "a task" to another, the delegating nurse remains ultimately responsible for both the action and its outcome (Box 1-2). The RN uses critical thinking and professional judgment when following the Five Rights of Delegation (right task; under the right circumstances; to the right person; with the right directions and communication; and under the right supervision and evaluation) (ANA & NCSBN, 2019).

The Nursing Process and Clinical Judgment

The nursing process consists of five steps:

1. Assess the patient, family, caregivers, group, or community;
2. Consider all the data you have collected and arrive at a diagnosis (can be an actual problem or a problem you have determined the patient is at risk for);
3. Plan your care, which includes prioritization of the problems with goal setting for each one;
4. Perform the interventions that based on your clinical judgment will achieve the goals of care; and
5. Evaluate the patient, family, group, or community's response to your interventions.

It is an iterative process and begins anew with each step.

You are beginning to build your knowledge base related to medical-surgical nursing, which is a vast amount of information, and soon you will possess what feels like an extraordinary fund of knowledge. But your ability to make thoughtful decisions that promote positive patient outcomes will depend on your clinical judgment. And that judgment is dependent on what you know and how you reason.

The first step is for you to build your understanding about a variety of disorders, their risk factors, clinical presentations,

BOX 1-2
Nursing Delegation

Who?

The RN
To the LPN or nursing assistant or other (e.g., transport aide)

What?

Gives authority to a competent individual to perform a selected nursing task
Each task falls within the Nursing Scope of Practice, but can be done by another

Where?

On the nursing unit

When?

When the nurse requires
When the person performing the task has been trained and is deemed competent
When the patient is stable, without unexpected changes in condition

Why?

To achieve a desired patient outcome
To efficiently and effectively make use of personal, financial, and material resources
To efficiently and effectively deliver patient care

How?

Assess the patient need(s), the task(s) required, and the ability of another to perform the task(s)
Delegate the task with clear directions as to priority, timing, and communicating the outcome
Monitor the process of task performance and its completion
Evaluate the patient outcome

Examples of Tasks that Can Be Delegated

Vital signs
Assisting patient out of bed to a chair or to the bathroom
Assisting patient with activities of daily living
Feeding a patient
Measuring and recording fluid intake and output

diagnostic findings, treatments, and potential complications associated not only with the condition but with your treatment. For without that knowledge, there is no ability to make appropriate, safe clinical judgments.

In nursing education, we do not simply teach you cognitive information; we bring you into the clinical arena, where we will begin to see your content knowledge in vivo, build your expertise, technical skills, and affective skills—your competencies. With each patient, you are generating insight into the wide variety of clinical presentations for specific disorders, and patient responses to your actions. You are creating your database that will inform your decisions or judgments about the data that you have collected and what actions you will enact to avoid a potential problem, treat a problem, or resolve a patient problem (Jessee, 2021). Thus, clinical judgment "is your interpretation or conclusion about a patient's needs, concerns or health problems, and/or decisions to take action (or not), use or modify standard approaches, or improvise new ones as deemed appropriate by the patient's response" (Tanner, 2006, p. 204). In Tanner's Model of Clinical Judgment, there are four processes: noticing, interpreting, responding, and reflecting. The act of noticing is observing, "seeing." As Florence Nightingale noted, "the most important practical lesson that can be given to nurses is to teach them what to observe—how to observe—what symptoms indicate improvement—what the reverse—which are of importance" (Nightingale, 1859, p. 59). From noticing, you interpret meaning from the data, and respond (or not) based upon your interpretation of that data. In the final process you evaluate the patient's response to your intervention(s). Consider a few years back when COVID-19 emerged. Answers were unknowable, yet it was the ability of nurses, advanced practice registered nurses (APRNs), physicians, respiratory therapists, dieticians, social workers, pharmacists, and researchers to use their clinical judgment that resulted in us all navigating the new unknown virus. It is your clinical judgment that will determine whether you act or not, based on the outcomes of using your thinking and reasoning. It is indeed a complex, multilayered process that includes the cognitive knowledge this book aims to provide. It also includes your individual reflection about a clinical situation, determining what the priorities are and creating solutions. Rather than a simple decision, it is an iterative process, and your clinical judgment will improve with knowledge, time, and experience. Next Generation NCLEX (which is the exam you will take upon completion of your program) outlines six steps in the clinical reasoning model (Ignatavicius, 2021; NGN, 2019).

Scenario: You have made plans for a road trip to see your nursing school colleague who lives 2 hours away. You have the entire day planned, so you get up early, excited about the day ahead. You jump in your car and start on your journey. A few miles after you merge onto the highway, you notice that the steering wheel is shaking a bit and you feel slight vibrations.

Step One: Recognize cues where relevant and important information is identified from different sources, such as medical history or vital signs.

In our example, you notice the slight tremor of the steering wheel and the vibrations. You "noticed" these cues; that is step one.

Step Two: Analyze cues. In the clinical setting, this means organizing and linking the recognized cues to the patient's clinical presentation. In this example you recognize that the symptoms of a shaking steering wheel and vibrations may mean something is wrong with the car's engine, suspension, or tires, or that the highway needs to be repaved. You are trying to link what you are experiencing with the actual or potential causes.

Step Three: Prioritize hypotheses, where hypotheses are evaluated and ranked according to priority. This can include urgency, likelihood, risk, difficulty, and/or time. In this phase, you cluster your findings to arrive at a list of problems (actual and/or potential problems) you believe the patient is experiencing and determine the importance or urgency. What do you think is of greatest concern?

In our situation, you have clustered the data and considered you have two options. Option one is that you continue on your trip and hope that the pavement will smooth out and the road will be better soon. Option two is to pull off the highway and get to a garage. Maybe there is a problem with the car, or maybe the highway is just full of potholes. You are deciding which of your options you should do first.

Step Four: Generate solutions. Identify expected outcomes. Hypotheses help to define a set of interventions for the expected outcomes.

For example, you reason that for option one, you keep going so you will arrive on time to see your friend and then you can figure out what is happening, or in option two, you need to get off the highway now because you don't want the car to blow up on the highway! Those are your two solutions, and your expected outcome is to get to your friend, sooner or later.

Step Five: Take action, where the solutions that address the highest priorities are implemented.

In this situation, you have decided your priority action is to pull off the highway and check your car. Because just like in nursing, your priority is preventing harm to others and you.

Step Six: Evaluate outcomes. Compare observed outcomes against expected outcomes.

As you pull off the exit a little alert lights up on your dashboard and as you exit the car you notice your left front tire is deflated. You have now learned that when the tire is deflated, vibrations are felt in the steering wheel because of misalignment. And you are thankful you made the decision to pull off and be two hours late to see your friend, rather than have a flat tire on the highway.

We recognize learning nursing can seem overwhelming as you are just beginning to build your knowledge base, including an array of kinesthetic, communication and sensory (observation, auscultative, palpation, percussion) skills, but you begin to build your knowledge, skills and aptitudes starting now. And over the course of your education, the scaffolding of each course will lead you to the ultimate goal of becoming an RN, ready to deliver safe and effective nursing care! In Table 1-1, the nursing process is compared to Tanner's model and the National Clinical Judgment Measurement Model (NCJMM) which will be used on your RN licensing exam (Ignatavicius, 2019).

THE PATIENT

The central figure in health care services is the patient. The term *patient* is derived from a Latin verb meaning "to suffer." It has traditionally been used to describe those who are recipients of care. Patients' needs vary, depending on their roles (as a member of a family, as a member of a particular community), associated circumstances, and past experiences, as well as the problem or problems for which they sought health care. Among the nurse's important functions in health care delivery is obtaining an understanding of the patient's situation and identifying their immediate needs, in order to address them.

Certain needs are basic to all people. Noted psychologist Abraham H. Maslow (1954) developed a theory describing basic human needs and how these needs build upon one another to achieve physical, social, and spiritual health and well-being. This model is now known as Maslow's *hierarchy of needs* (Fig. 1-1). Maslow ranked human needs as

TABLE 1-1 Comparing the Nursing Process Against Tanner's Model and the National Clinical Judgment Measurement Model (NCJMM)

Nursing Process	Tanner's Clinical Judgment Model	National Clinical Judgment Measurement Model
Assessment	Noticing	Recognize cues
Analysis	Interpreting	Analyze cues
Analysis	Interpreting	Prioritize hypothesis
Planning	Responding	Generate solutions
Implementation	Responding	Take action
Evaluation	Reflecting	Evaluate outcomes

Reprinted from Ignatavicius, D. D. (2021). Preparing for the new nursing licensure exam: The next-generation NCLEX. *Nursing*, *51*(5), 34–41. https://doi.org/10.1097/01.NURSE.0000743100.95536.9b

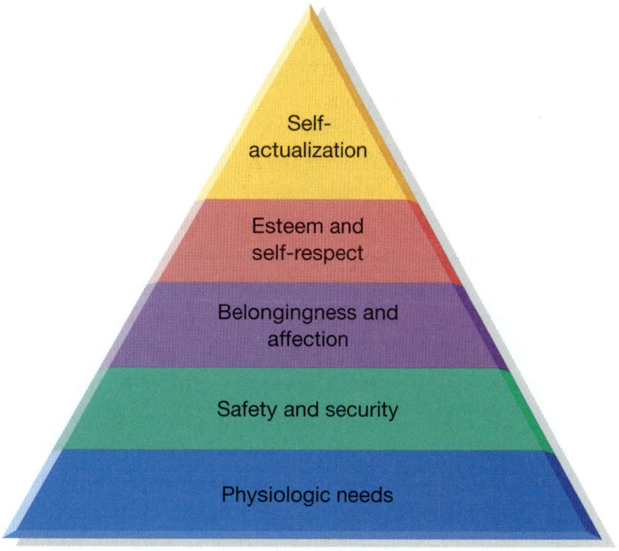

FIGURE 1-1 **Maslow's hierarchy of needs.**

physiologic needs, safety and security, sense of belonging and affection, esteem and self-respect, and self-actualization. This last level—self-actualization—refers to fulfilling one's individual potential and includes the desire to know and understand, as well as aesthetics. Once a basic or essential need is met, people usually experience a need on the next level. Depending on an individual's certain situation (e.g., minor vs. major illness or injury), they may move among levels. Lower-level needs always remain, but a person's ability to pursue higher-level needs generally indicates movement toward improved health and well-being. This hierarchy provides a useful framework that can be applied to the patient when assessing strengths, limitations, and needs as a consumer of nursing and health care.

The patient who seeks care for a health issue is also an individual person, a member of a family, and a citizen of the community. The ultimate goal of care is to return the patient to the various roles they hold in life. Many patients, as consumers of health care, have become more knowledgeable about health care options and are assuming a collaborative approach with the nurse and the health care system.

Consumers of nursing and health care are as varied as their numbers. There are countless differences in demographics, personalities, and abilities that must be understood so that the patient can participate in their own health care decisions. A basic tenet of nursing is to determine the consumers' needs and wants, in order to guide them through their health care experience.

HEALTH, WELLNESS, AND HEALTH PROMOTION

The health care system of the United States, which traditionally has been disease oriented, is placing increasing emphasis on health and health promotion. Many nurses who would formerly have been involved in the care of acutely ill patients are engaged in health promotion and illness prevention. Further, there is a movement toward outpatient care for both acute and chronic conditions.

Health

How health is perceived depends on how health is defined. The WHO, in the preamble to its constitution, defines health as a "state of complete physical, mental, and social well-being and not merely the absence of disease and infirmity" (WHO, 1948). Although this definition of health does not allow for any variation in degrees of wellness or illness, the concept of a health–illness continuum allows for a greater range in describing a person's health status. By viewing health and illness on a continuum, it is possible to consider a person as being neither completely healthy nor completely ill (see Chapter 2). Instead, a person's state of health is ever-changing and has the potential to range from high-level wellness to extremely poor health and imminent death. Use of the health–illness continuum makes it possible to view a person as simultaneously possessing degrees of both health and illness.

Wellness

Wellness has been thought of as being equivalent to health but is more comprehensive and interrelational and includes various aspects of life that lead to health: emotional, environmental, financial, intellectual, occupational, physical, social, and spiritual. In addition, wellness is sought not just on an individual micro level but on the macro, societal level, whereas health is limited to an individual's overall state of illness or lack thereof (IsHak et al., 2020). It is the goal of wellness that we are constantly moving toward. As health care providers, our goal is to promote positive changes that are directed toward health and well-being of the individual and society.

Health Promotion

Today, increasing emphasis is placed on health, health promotion, wellness, and self-care. Health is seen as resulting from a lifestyle oriented toward wellness. The result has been the evolution of a wide range of health-promotion strategies, including screening, genetic testing, lifetime health monitoring, environmental and mental health programs, risk reduction, and nutrition and health education.

A growing interest in self-care skills is evidenced by the large number of health-related publications, internet sites, conferences, and workshops designed for the lay public. These programs are designed to promote self-care education, often emphasizing health promotion and disease prevention. As people become increasingly knowledgeable about their health, they often take more interest in and responsibility for their health and well-being.

Special efforts need to be made by health care professionals to determine which organizations, websites, and other venues are providing peer-reviewed and up-to-date information, to ensure people's ability to obtain accurate information concerning health-promoting behaviors. Health-related information and sources of health promotion, whether received from health care professionals, through self-help groups, or from publications, are intended to reach and motivate members of various cultural and socioeconomic groups about lifestyle and health practices.

INFLUENCES ON HEALTH CARE DELIVERY

Scientific and technologic advances throughout the 21st century have led to social, political, and economic changes. These profound changes have forced the health care industry in general, and nursing practice in particular, to adapt.

Population Demographics

There have been many significant shifts in the demographics of the United States. First of these includes the U.S. Census Bureau (2021) estimation of population increase from 331 million in 2021 to nearly 400 million by the year 2060. That said, it should be noted that the U.S. population grew at the lowest rate in a century because there were fewer births, more deaths, and less immigration (Johnson, 2020).

Immigration and Diversity

The United States has been home to an increasingly culturally diverse population, as growing numbers of people from different national backgrounds enter the country. In fact, the U.S. Census Bureau revealed that the U.S. population is much more multiracial and diverse than past measurements indicated due to improved census question design (Jones et al., 2021).

As the cultural composition of the population changes, it is increasingly important to address cultural considerations in the delivery of health care. Patients from diverse sociocultural groups not only bring various health care beliefs, values, and practices to the health care setting, but they may also have a variety of social and structural determinants for some disease conditions and unique reactions to treatment. These determinants significantly affect an individual's responses to health care problems or illnesses, to caregivers, and to the care itself. Unless these factors are understood, respected, and considered by health care providers, the care delivered may be ineffective, and health care outcomes may be negatively affected. In addition, the profession of nursing has set a goal of parity between the nursing workforce and the population of the United States. Thus, a priority is encouraging and fostering the education of a culturally diverse workforce that mirrors the nation's change in demographics. If achieved, the health care professional staff will reflect the actual population it serves.

Acknowledging and adapting to the cultural needs of patients and significant others are important components of nursing care. In addition, facilitating access to culturally appropriate health care is critical if nursing care is to be holistic. Nursing care that utilizes cultural humility is a dynamic process that requires an openness to the ongoing learning of culture-specific information and an awareness of and sensitivity to the effect that culture has on the care situation. Exploring one's own cultural beliefs and how they might differ from the beliefs of the patient being cared for is a first step toward practicing cultural humility. Specific areas to be considered when providing care include the amount of space and distance needed to feel comfortable, the amount of eye contact, attitudes related to time, the use of touch, body language, observance of civil and religious holidays, and the cultural meanings associated with food. Because the nurse–patient interaction is the focal point of nursing, nurses should consider their own cultural orientation and continually monitor for bias when conducting assessments of patients and patients' families and friends. The guidelines in Box 1-3 may prove useful to nurses providing culturally appropriate care. Box 1-4 provides suggestions on overcoming language barriers.

BOX 1-3 Culturally Appropriate Care

- Know your own cultural attitudes, values, beliefs, and practices.
- Maintain a broad, open attitude. Expect the unexpected. Enjoy surprises.
- Avoid seeing all people as alike; that is, avoid cultural stereotypes.
- Try to understand the reasons for any behavior by discussing commonalities and differences.
- If a patient has said or done something that you do not understand, ask for clarification. Be a good listener. Most patients will respond positively to questions that arise from a genuine concern for and interest in them.
- If at all possible, speak the patient's language (even simple greetings and social courtesies are appreciated). Avoid feigning an accent or using words that are ordinarily not part of your vocabulary.
- Do not make assumptions about a person's sexual orientation or gender identity based on appearance. Recognize that self-identification and behaviors do not always align.
- Be yourself. There is no right or wrong way to learn about cultural diversity.
- Use resources available, consider the site by U.S. Health and Human Services (http://www.thinkculturalhealth.hhs.gov) which offers the latest resources and tools to promote cultural competence in health care and includes free online courses accredited for continuing education credit to help promote respectful, culturally congruent, high-quality care to an increasingly diverse patient population (Williams, 2020).

The more recent move in education is from developing cultural humility in health care providers to "structural competency," which consists of training in: (1) recognizing the structures that shape clinical interactions (e.g., the price of medications impacts patient adherence; it is about recognizing how decisions about resources, and the political economy of health care in the United States, impact you as well as your patients); (2) developing an extraclinical language of structure (e.g., begin to see how the patients, diseases, and attitudes that you see can be better understood as the product of social structures interacting with biologies such as the effect of racism on your patients and communities); (3) rearticulating "cultural" formulations in structural terms (e.g., recognition of the deeper ways in which complex cultural structures produce inequalities and create barriers to health); (4) observing and imagining structural interventions (e.g., this relates to you recognizing that structures that shape health and illness can be changed since they reflect specific financial, legislative, or cultural decisions made at particular moments in time); and (5) developing structural humility (e.g., recognize that the skills you are developing "are the beginning points of conversations rather than endpoints") (Metzl & Hansen, 2014, p. 131).

BOX 1-4

Overcoming Language Barriers

- Greet the patient using the last or complete name. Avoid being too casual or familiar. Point to yourself and say your name. Smile.
- Proceed in an unhurried manner. Pay attention to any effort by the patient or family to communicate.
- Speak in a low, moderate voice. Avoid talking loudly. Remember that there is a tendency to raise the volume and pitch of your voice when the listener appears not to understand. The listener may perceive that you are shouting and/or angry.
- Organize your thoughts. Repeat and summarize frequently. Repeat the message in different ways if necessary. Use audio-visual aids when feasible.
- Use short, simple sentence structure and speak in the active voice.
- Use simple words, such as "pain" rather than "discomfort." Avoid medical jargon, idioms, and slang. Avoid using contractions, such as *don't, can't, won't.*
- Use nouns repeatedly instead of pronouns. *Example*: Do not say: "He has been taking his medicine, hasn't he?" Do say: "Does Juan take medicine?"
- Pantomime words (use gestures) and simple actions while verbalizing them.
- Give instructions in the proper sequence. *Example*: Do not say: "Before you rinse the bottle, sterilize it." Do say: "First, wash the bottle. Second, rinse the bottle."
- Discuss one topic at a time, and avoid giving too much information in a single conversation. Avoid using conjunctions. *Example*: Do not say: "Are you cold and in pain?" Do say (while pantomiming/gesturing): "Are you cold?" "Are you in pain?"
- Talk directly to the patient, rather than to the person who accompanied them.
- Validate whether the person understands by having them repeat instructions, demonstrate the procedure, or act out the meaning.
- Use any words you know in the person's language. This indicates that you are aware of and respect the patient's primary means of communicating.
- Be aware that 65% of the message received in communication is nonverbal (Hall, 1966). Seek congruence between your body language or motions (kinetic behavior), facial expression, and words.
- Try a third language. Many world populations are multilingual.
- Be aware of culturally based gender and age differences and diverse socioeconomic, educational, and tribal/regional differences when choosing an interpreter.
- Use interpreters to improve communication. Using plain language with the interpreter assists in providing a clear and accurate conversion.
- Obtain phrase books from a library or bookstore, make or purchase flash cards. Although they are costly, some telecommunication companies provide translation services.

Lifting the Lens: Upstream versus Downstream Means What?

The metaphor of a stream is used to discuss public health with upstream factors bringing downstream effects (Kuehnert et al., 2022; McKinlay, 1979). The story begins with a baby found floating down a river. Villagers swim into the river to save the baby, but soon there are two babies in the river, and again villagers rush out to save them. Each day more and more babies are seen in the river, and the villagers now decide to station teams of people at an outlook post to rush into the water to save the babies. And this continues day after day; the villagers are exhausted, and then one person screams out, "Who the hell is upstream pushing them all in?" (McKinlay 1986, p. 48). It is then that they realize their focus needs to shift upstream. Who is tossing the babies in the river in the first place? For until you focus on that, you will not be able to save all the babies. So too, until we focus on the conditions that make people sick, we cannot improve the health of society. What you will soon see when you enter clinical practice is the downstream manifestations of the impact of all structural and social determinants of health, and while you are busy building your knowledge about nursing, learning how to swim and how to care for patients "in the stream," we encourage you to

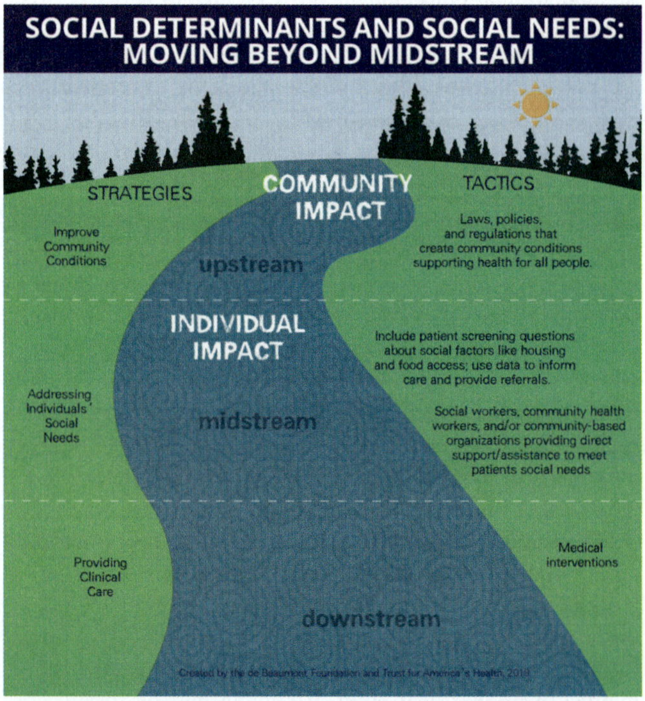

Reproduced with permission from Castrucci, B., & Auerbach, J. (2019). Meeting individual social needs falls short of addressing social determinants of health. *Health Affairs Forefront*. https://www.healthaffairs.org/do/10.1377/forefront.20190115.234942/

consider that the river is long, and as nurses we need to advocate to upstream efforts which will reach as high as our planet's health.

The Older Population

An unprecedented increase in the number of older adults in the United States has one in seven people over the age of 65 years, representing 16% of the population (2022). This trend is expected to continue, and it is projected that by 2060, older adults will make up nearly 25% of the U.S. population. The health care needs of older adults are often chronic in nature, with intermittent exacerbations or acute episodes. This makes their care more complex and demands significant human, material, and financial investment by the health care industry.

Social and Structural Determinants of Health

"The social determinants of health are the circumstances in which people are born, grow up, live, work and age, and the systems put in place to deal with illness. These circumstances are in turn shaped by a wider set of forces: economics, social policies, and politics" (WHO, n.d.). It is understood that social, economic and environmental factors impact your patient's health and well-being. A consensus paper was recently released by nursing experts to establish conceptual clarity and consensus for what social determinants of health mean for nursing (Kuehnert et al., 2022). They defined six key dimensions for nursing: (1) economic stability, (2) education access and quality (including health literacy), (3) health care access and quality, (4) neighborhood and the built environment, (5) social and community context, and (6) planetary conditions (e.g., the health of our planet). You will notice the focus is on upstream factors in the six key areas to improve population health. And you will soon learn in other nursing courses about the national goals for improving the health of all Americans via a national agenda every decade in the form of Healthy People 2030 (ODPHP, 2022b). In the most recent initiative, social determinants of health are broken into six key areas: (1) Safe housing, transportation, and neighborhoods, (2) Racism, discrimination, and violence, (3) Education, job opportunities, and income, (4) Access to nutritious foods and physical activity opportunities, (5) Polluted air and water, (6) Language and literacy skills.

Structural determinants of health are the systemic inequities in health or the "political determinants of health which involve the systematic processes of structuring relationships, distributing resources, and administering power, operating simultaneously in ways that mutually reinforce one another to shape opportunities that advance health equity or create, perpetuate, and exacerbate health inequities" (Dawes, 2020, p. 146). As noted earlier, structural competency means we will over the course of your education and clinical training aim to lift your lens up to intervene at the level of social structures, institutions, and policies that must be altered to improve population health and promote health equity (Hansen & Metzi, 2016).

Changing Patterns of Disease

The past century has seen a dramatic shift in disease patterns. Perusal of literature and popular media leads us to ask about the impact of major issues on our health: population growth, aging, urbanization, immigration, new novel viruses, environmental challenges, and increasing costs of mitigating their effects. The good news is that innovation continues and science and technology are giving us ever-new ways of preventing, treating, and/or living with illness and injury.

Advances in Technology

As Florence Nightingale noted "There are two classes of people in this world—those who take the best and enjoy it and those who wish for something better and try to create it. The world needs the appreciation of the first and the discontent of the second (Nightingale, 1969, p. 29)." That discontent has led to advances in technology with greater frequency during the past several decades than in all other periods of civilization. Sophisticated devices have revolutionized how disease is prevented, how patients are diagnosed and treated, and even how communication to and about patients is conducted. Advanced technology has provided access to faster, less invasive, and less painful testing and procedures. In fact, many tests and procedures that once required a hospital stay are performed routinely on an outpatient basis. A disorder that once may have required an operation for diagnosis many times can be diagnosed via computed tomography (CT) or magnetic resonance imaging (MRI). Computers are also significantly changing workflow, as medical records become completely electronic, in order to improve communication among caregivers, make documentation more efficient, and ease medical investigation and research. However, the electronic medical record (EMR) has led to a burden on health professionals. As an example, in a recent publication from the National Academy of Medicine it was found that, on average, nurses and doctors spend 50% of their workday treating the screen, not the patient, and the increased work burden associated with EMRs is one of the factors for burnout (NAM, 2019). Clearly, we have miles to go before we can be satisfied with electronic records. In addition, artificial intelligence (AI) and machine learning (ML) technology are being developed at a rapid pace to help predict and identify health emergencies, disease populations, and disease state and immune response, among other applications resulting in the need to educate nurses on how to work safely and effectively with ML and AI (Gray et al., 2021).

Public Safety

The U.S. health care system is based on public trust. This translates to people's confidence that the care they will receive in a hospital or other health care setting will meet legal and social

BOX 1-5
QSEN Competencies

Patient-Centered Care

Recognize the patient or designee as the source of control and full partner in providing compassionate and coordinated care based on respect for patient's preferences, values, and needs.

Teamwork and Collaboration

Function effectively within nursing and interprofessional teams, fostering open communication, mutual respect, and shared decision making to achieve quality patient care.

Evidence-Based Practice

Integrate best current evidence with clinical expertise and patient/family preferences and values for delivery of optimal health care.

Quality Improvement

Use data to monitor the outcomes of care processes and use improvement methods to design and test changes to continuously improve the quality and safety of health care systems.

Safety

Minimizes risk of harm to patients and providers through both system effectiveness and individual performance.

Informatics

Use information and technology to communicate, manage knowledge, mitigate error, and support decision making.

Reproduced, with permission, from Cronenwett, L., Sherwood, G., Barnsteiner, J., Disch, J., Johnson, J., Mitchell, P., Sullivan, D. T., & Warren, J. (2007). Quality and safety education for nurses. *Nursing Outlook*, *55*(3), 122.

standards. Thus, this large and diverse system is charged with the protection and maintenance of these standards when providing a safe work environment for employees and a healing environment for clients and patients.

The QSEN project has established standards for educating RNs at the baccalaureate and master's levels. In this model, clearly delineated knowledge, skills, and attitudes were developed so that you can continuously improve the quality and safety of the health care systems where you will work. The six major categories delineate the knowledge, skills, and attitudes for each section (Box 1-5).

Regulatory Bodies

To ensure that minimum standards are maintained, governing and oversight bodies regulate the health care system. Agencies involved in oversight include those in the following discussion.

Occupational Safety and Health Administration

Under the Occupational Safety and Health Act of 1970, employers are responsible for providing a safe and healthy workplace for their employees. The role of the Occupational Safety and Health Administration (OSHA) is to promote the safety and health of working people by setting and enforcing standards; providing training, outreach, and education; establishing partnerships; and encouraging continual process improvement in workplace safety and health.

The Joint Commission

The Joint Commission (TJC) is an independent, nonprofit organization whose mission is to "continuously improve health care for the public, in collaboration with other stakeholders, by evaluating health care organizations and inspiring them to excel in providing safe and effective care of the highest quality and value (TJC, n.d.a)." At present, TJC accredits approximately 80% of the nation's hospitals (TJC, n.d.c).

Patient Protection and Affordable Care Act of 2010

The Patient Protection and Affordable Care Act (PPACA), also known as "health care reform," "Obamacare," "Affordable Care Act," or the "ACA," is a law enacted on March 23, 2010, which issued rules and guidelines on the offering, administration, and acceptance of health care coverage in the United States (Healthcare.gov, n.d.). It was designed to improve the health of the population at reduced per capita cost. This is to be accomplished by increasing the number of people with health insurance, improving the insurance policies and reimbursing facilities (hospitals, etc.) based on the quality of care. While the ACA was largely successful in reducing the number of uninsured adults in the United States (3% or approximately 10 million people receive their care and insurance through the ACA [Watson, 2017]), barriers remain. Issues of insurance companies pulling out of the exchanges have only heightened the pressure to either repeal the law or improve the act. The act has been the target of numerous legal and political challenges since its inception and likely will continue to face challenges for the foreseeable future.

Centers for Medicare and Medicaid Services

The Centers for Medicare and Medicaid Services (CMS) is the federal agency that manages Medicare, which is the health insurance program for people over 65 years of age, people under age 65 with certain disabilities, and those with end-stage kidney disease (ESKD). The CMS also manages Medicaid, which is a state-administered program for low-income individuals and families who fit into an eligibility group recognized by federal and state law. In addition, the CMS manages the children's health insurance program (CHIP), which provides coverage for millions of uninsured children. The CMS exists to ensure effective up-to-date health care coverage and to promote quality care for beneficiaries.

Department of Public Health

Each state has its own Department of Public Health (DPH) with its own mission. They all are generally charged with the protection of the health and well-being of the state's population and environment. The State Board of Nursing falls within this department and serves to regulate the practice of nursing and the licensing of individual nurses.

HEALTH EDUCATION

Teaching, as a function of nursing, is included in all state nurse practice acts and in the *Scope and Standards of Clinical Nursing Practice* of the American Nurses Association (ANA, 2021). **Health education** is an independent function of nursing practice and is a primary nursing responsibility. All nursing care is directed toward promoting, maintaining, and restoring health; preventing illness; and helping people adapt to the residual effects of illness. Many of these nursing activities are accomplished through health education or patient teaching. Nurses who serve as teachers are challenged to focus on the educational needs of communities, as well as on specific patient and family educational needs. Health education is important to nursing care because it affects the abilities of people and families to perform important self-care activities.

Every contact an individual nurse has with a health care consumer, whether or not that person is ill, should be considered an opportunity for health teaching. Although people have a right to decide whether or not to learn, nurses have the responsibility to present information that motivates people to recognize the need to learn. Therefore, nurses must use opportunities in all health care settings to promote **wellness**. Educational environments may include homes, hospitals, community health centers, community fairs, schools, places of business, service agencies, shelters, and consumer action or support groups.

Trends in Health Education, Communication, and Patient Safety

Much of the core of health education today is focused on increasing patient involvement and accountability for individual care and treatment plans. Health education programs are often designed as patient safety initiatives and are geared toward encouraging increased communication between patients and care providers. The effect of improved communication between patients and providers is multifaceted and includes improved patient outcomes, patient safety, and patient perception of quality. TJC has found consistently that adverse events are caused by breakdowns in communication among caregivers and between caregivers and patients (2017). Therefore, there has been much collaboration to develop processes that encourage improved communication.

Pearls for Practice

A common communication issue occurs during hand-offs, or hand-overs, when expectations can be out of balance between the message sender and the receiver. Understanding that effective communication is brief and concise, you may learn of a structured communication tool using the mnemonic ISBAR to alleviate communication errors where I stands for Identification, S refers to the Situation, B relates to the background, A is your Assessment, and R is your Recommendation or Request. To detail, you will Identify yourself and your role, and you will detail the Situation requiring your call (e.g., a sudden change in the patient condition, a transfer to a different unit, a reaction to a medication or intervention). Background will include the patient's significant past history (medical, surgical, social), medications, recent procedure, diagnostic and laboratory results, and/or recent situation (e.g., fall). Your Assessment of the current patient condition that necessitated your call will likely include vital sign changes, physical examination findings, laboratory data, and your Recommendation or request for next steps for patient treatment.

The mission of the Agency for Healthcare Research and Quality (AHRQ) is to produce evidence to make health care safer, higher quality, more accessible, equitable, and affordable, and to work within the U.S. Department of Health and Human Services and with other partners to make sure that the evidence is understood and used (2021b). They lead in helping both providers and patients to not only understand how important communication is but also develop tools and programs to improve those skills and have a variety of resources according to settings (hospitals, emergency rooms, long-term care, ambulatory care, end-stage renal disease clinics, pharmacies and multiple settings).

Purpose of Health Education

The goal of patient and family education is to improve patient outcomes. For purposes of this discussion, family shall be considered to be the person(s) who plays a significant role in the patient's life. This may include person(s) not legally related to the patient. Effective health education lays a solid foundation for individual and community wellness. Teaching is an integral tool that all nurses use to assist patients and families in developing effective health behaviors and in altering lifestyle patterns that predispose people to health risks.

People with chronic illnesses and disabilities are among those most in need of health education. As the lifespan of the population increases, the number of people with such illnesses also increases. People with chronic illness need health care information to participate actively in and assume responsibility for much of their own care (refer to Chapter 2). Health education can help change a patient's behavior favorably, increase the ability to cope with and manage health, and improve understanding of the options, risks, and benefits of care, treatment, and services. It can also prevent crisis situations and reduce the potential for rehospitalization resulting from inadequate information about self-care. The goal of health education is to teach people to live life to its healthiest—that is, to strive toward achieving their maximum health potential.

In addition to the public's right to and desire for health education, patient education is also a strategy for promoting self-care at home and in the community, reducing health care costs by preventing illness, avoiding expensive medical treatments, decreasing lengths of hospital stays, and facilitating earlier discharge.

Adherence to the Therapeutic Regimen

As noted by Yale School of Nursing's first dean, Annie Warburton Goodrich, "in order to effectively interpret the truly great role [of nursing] ...you must be master of two tongues, the tongue of science and that of the people" (Goodrich, 1933, p. 14). To fulfill our role of patient educator, we must be able to interpret the science, avoid medical jargon, and meet the patient where they are. That is, understand the patient perspective, what is influencing them, and the impact of the diagnosis personally. If patients don't understand their diagnosis or treatment plan, how do you expect to impact their health outcomes?

One of the goals of patient education is to encourage people to adhere to their **therapeutic regimen**. **Adherence** to treatment usually requires that a person make one or more lifestyle changes to carry out specific activities that promote and maintain health. In addition, the term *adherence* implies a collaborative relationship with the patient, together determining the treatment regimen rather than acquiescing to the health care provider's suggestions. Adherence denotes awareness of and agreement to adopt a behavior or plan of action. Common examples of behaviors facilitating health include taking prescribed medications, maintaining a healthy diet, increasing daily activities and exercise, self-monitoring for signs and symptoms of illness, practicing specific hygiene measures, seeking recommended health evaluations and screenings, and performing other therapeutic and preventive measures.

Many people do not adhere to their prescribed regimens; rates of adherence vary depending on the setting, treatment plan, and population, but are generally low, especially when the regimens are complex or of long duration. Nonadherence to prescribed therapy has been the subject of many studies; a wide range of variables (patient, disease, condition, social/economic, and health system–related) appears to influence the degree of adherence (Cea-Calvo et al., 2020), including the following:

- Inadequate cognitive, psychomotor, or language skills
- Personal values, beliefs, misconceptions, and attitudes coupled with their associated anxiety, depression, and/or fear
- Distrust if loss of control occurs in the decision-making process
- Lack of involvement in shared decision-making
- Difficulty in adopting recommended changes
- Insufficient social support or outright sabotage by that support
- Economic factors such as high co-payment amount

Nurses' success with promoting adherence can be improved by creating a collaborative relationship that addresses patient's priorities, circumstances, and goals. Motivational interviewing (MI) is a collaborative cost-effective conversational technique intended to strengthen a patient's motivation to change. It has been shown to be effective in addressing many different lifestyle problems as well as in chronic disease management, and many disease prevention guidelines promote use of motivational interviewing. There are four key interrelated elements: partnership (you and the patient are seen as equal), acceptance (there is mutual trust, understanding, autonomy of self, and accurate empathy [not sympathy]) between the patient and the nurse, compassion (priority is given to the patient's needs), and evocation (this is what allows the patient to articulate positive reasons for change) (Porterfield & Heyne, 2020). The communication skills often employed include: (1) listening to the patient, (2) asking open-ended questions rather than instructing the patient on what they should do, (2) affirming the patient's responses, (3) applying accurate reflections, and (4) providing summaries when necessary (Porterfield & Heyne, 2020).

It is also important to note that adherence does not just relate singularly to patients and may be used when we consider why nurses and providers do or do not adhere to guidelines and checklist "bundles" that are intended to provide evidence-based recommendations for the prevention of disease. A bundle is a set of interventions that, when used together, significantly improve patient outcomes and have been developed for ventilator care, central line management, and management of sepsis, among others.

Health Literacy and Willingness to Learn

Before initiating a teaching–learning program, it is important to assess the person's physical and emotional readiness to learn, as well as their ability to learn what is being taught. This information then becomes the basis for establishing goals that can motivate the person. Involving learners in establishing mutually acceptable goals serves the purpose of encouraging active involvement in the learning process and shared responsibility for learning.

Health literacy is the degree to which an individual has the capacity to obtain, communicate, process, and understand basic health information and services to make appropriate health decisions. Low literacy affects individuals' ability to participate in health decisions and influences health outcomes (Mannoh et al., 2021). It is linked to poor health outcomes such as higher rates of hospitalization, increased emergency department use, inappropriate use of medications, misunderstanding of follow-up instructions, higher health care costs and less frequent use of preventive services

(Ling, 2021). Considering the complexity of medication regimens (dosing, timing, calculations), informed consent, and technology (peak flow meters, glucose monitoring devices, etc.), it is important for the nurse to have insight into how health literacy impacts the patient's well-being. TJC requires all health providers assess patient's learning needs and health literacy when providing culturally competent care (Price, 2021; TJC, n.d.b), and Healthy People 2030 has established health literacy as a national priority for health improvement (ODPHP, 2022).

Current evidence shows that health care providers overestimate patients' health literacy consistently and, therefore, may be unaware of creating difficulties for their patients by not providing adequate information or assuming the patient knows more than they do (Voigt-Barbarowicz & Brütt, 2020). There are four methods that can be used to quickly assess a patient's health literacy, including the Rapid Estimate of Adult Literacy in Medicine—Short Form (REALM-SF), the Short Assessment of Health Literacy–Spanish and English (SAHL–S&E), Ask Me 3, and the Newest Vital Sign or "ice cream label assessment". THE REALM-SF is a seven-item word recognition test to provide health providers with a valid quick assessment of patient health literacy. Words include "exercise," "antibiotics," and "jaundice" for example. It can be accessed at https://www.ahrq.gov/health-literacy/research/tools/index.html#rapid. The SAHL–S&E is available from AHRQ at https://www.ahrq.gov/health-literacy/research/tools/index.html. It is available in English and Spanish and consists of 18 key words such as "kidney" or "constipation," and the patient is presented with two words, one with a related meaning and a distractor unrelated in meaning to the test term. For example, for kidney, the patient selects between the words urine and fever. This test takes only 2 to 3 minutes to administer. Me 3 asks three primary questions: (1) What is my main problem? (2) What do I need to do? and (3) Why is it important for me to do this? While this tool is a great starting point for patient education, it does not gauge patient's understanding of the providers responses. The Newest Vital Sign, also known as the "ice cream label assessment" is distributed by Pfizer and available at https://www.pfizer.com/health/literacy/public-policy-researchers/nvs-toolkit. With this tool, a patient and/or significant other look at the nutrition label from a container of ice cream and answer six questions. These questions include numeracy skills (calculating the number of calories in the container) and general knowledge (should a patient who is allergic to peanuts eat this ice cream?). It is available in Spanish and English and can be completed within 3 minutes. In addition, health literacy resources for developing patient education material (written and audiovisual) can be accessed at the AHRQ website or the Office of Disease Prevention and Health Promotion website: http://health.gov/healthliteracyonline.

Box 1-6 provides guidance for patient education in the older adult population.

BOX 1-6

Gerontologic Considerations

Older people frequently have one or more chronic illnesses that are managed with numerous medications and complicated by periodic acute episodes. Older people also may have other problems that affect adherence to therapeutic regimens, such as increased sensitivity to medications and their side effects, difficulty in adjusting to change and stress, financial constraints, inadequate support systems, lifetime habits of self-treatment with over-the-counter medications, visual and hearing impairments, and mobility limitations. An important predictor of patient adherence to a therapeutic regimen is concordance of the patient's and providers' perception of their health.

Changes in cognition with age may include slowed mental functioning; decreased short-term memory, abstract thinking, and concentration; and slowed reaction time. Often these changes are accentuated by the health problems that cause the older person to seek health care in the first place. Effective teaching strategies include finding out what the patient wants to learn, presenting small amounts of material at a slow-pace, frequent repeating information (at least three times) (Steinhauser, 2019), and using reinforcement techniques, such as audio-visual and written materials and repeated practice sessions. Present information in several forms, for example written material, discussion, video and audiotape, and photos and pictures (Steinhauser, 2019). Distracting stimuli should be minimized as much as possible in the teaching environment; for example, turn off the TV/radio.

Sensory changes associated with aging also affect teaching and learning. Teaching strategies to accommodate decreased visual acuity include large-print and easy-to-read materials printed on nonglare paper. To maximize hearing, speak distinctly with a normal or lowered pitch, facing the person so that speech reading can occur as needed. Visual cues often help to reinforce verbal teaching. Check for patient understanding by asking them to explain in their own words what was taught.

Family members should be involved in teaching sessions when possible. They provide another source for reinforcement of material and can help the older person recall instructions later. Also family members can provide valuable assessment information about the person's living situation and related learning needs.

When nurses, families, and other involved health care professionals work collaboratively to facilitate the older person's learning, chances of success are maximized. Successful learning for older adults should result in improved self-care management skills, enhanced self-esteem, confidence, and a willingness to learn in the future. Above all, health care professionals must work together to provide continuous, coordinated care; otherwise, the efforts of one health care professional may be negated by those of another.

NURSING PROCESS
Patient Teaching

The steps of the nursing process—assessment, diagnosis, planning, implementation, and evaluation—are used when constructing a teaching plan to meet people's teaching and learning needs (Box 1-7).

ASSESSMENT

Assessment in the teaching–learning process is directed toward the systematic collection of data about the person's learning needs and style and readiness to learn, as well as the family's learning needs. Box 1-8 discusses the Stages of Change model in relation to teaching and behavior change.

LEARNING READINESS

Due to nurses' extensive patient contact, we are able to assess patients' needs and readiness to learn, which is one of the most significant factors influencing learning. Learning readiness is a crucial step in the assessment process. If patients are not ready to learn, change, or alter their behavior, education can be fruitless. For adults, readiness is based on culture, attitude, personal values, physical and emotional status, and past experiences in learning. Experiential readiness to learn refers to past experiences that may influence a person's ability to learn. Previous educational experiences and life experiences in general are significant determinants of a person's approach to learning. People with little or no formal education may not be able to understand the instructional materials presented. People who have had difficulty learning in the past may be hesitant to try again. Many behaviors required for reaching maximum health potential require knowledge, physical skills, and positive attitudes. In their absence, learning may be very difficult and very slow. For example, a person who does not understand the basics of normal nutrition may not be able to understand the restrictions of a specific diet. A person who does not view the desired learning as personally meaningful may reject teaching efforts. A person who is not future-oriented may be unable to appreciate

BOX 1-7 **Patient Education**

A Nursing Process Guide to Patient Education

Assessment

1. Assess the person's readiness for health education.
   A. What are the person's health beliefs and behaviors?
   B. What physical and psychosocial adaptations does the person need to make?
   C. Is the learner ready to learn?
   D. Is the person able to learn these behaviors?
   E. What additional information about the person is needed (such as availability of resources and tools)?
   F. Are there any variables (e.g., hearing or visual impairment, cognitive issues, and literacy issues) that will affect the choice of teaching strategy or approach?
   G. What are the person's expectations?
   H. What does the person want to learn?
2. Organize, analyze, synthesize, and summarize the collected data.

Planning and Goals

1. Specify the learning goals established by teacher and learner together.
2. Identify teaching strategies appropriate for goal attainment.
3. Establish expected outcomes.
4. Develop the written teaching plan.
   A. Include diagnoses, goals, teaching strategies, and expected outcomes.
   B. Put the information to be taught in logical sequence.
   C. Write down the key points.
   D. Select appropriate teaching aids.
   E. Keep the plan current and flexible to meet the person's changing learning needs.
5. Involve the learner, family or significant others, nursing team members, and other health care team members in all aspects of planning.

Implementation

1. Put the teaching plan into action.
2. Use language the person can understand.
3. Use appropriate teaching aids and provide Internet resources if appropriate.
4. Use the same equipment that the person will use after discharge.
5. Encourage the person to participate actively in learning.
6. Record the learner's responses to the teaching actions.
7. Provide feedback.

Evaluation

1. Collect objective data.
   A. Observe the person.
   B. Ask questions to determine whether the person understands.
   C. Use rating scales, checklists, anecdotal notes, and written tests when appropriate.
2. Compare the person's behavioral responses with the expected outcomes. Determine the extent to which the goals were achieved.
3. Include the person, family or significant others, nursing team members, and other health care team members in the evaluation.
4. Identify alterations that need to be made in the teaching plan.
5. Make referrals to appropriate sources or agencies for reinforcement of learning after discharge.
6. Continue all steps of the teaching process: assessment, diagnosis, planning, implementation, and evaluation.

BOX 1-8

Stages of Change

An approach to health teaching is the use of the transtheoretical model developed to conceptualize the process of intentional behavior change. This model considers decisional balance (weighing the pros and cons of the proposed behavioral change), self-efficacy (confidence in one's ability to change), and the relationship between stage of change and behavior (Prochaska & Prochaska, 2014). The model considers educational interventions that are not "one size fits all" but rather individualized interventions based upon a patient's current stage of readiness to learn or motivational readiness. Transtheoretical model-based measures have been developed for smoking, alcohol use, sun exposure, and exercise, to name a few. The model is not linear but expects that patients will move between stages until successful behavioral changes are established. The nurse considers the patient's current stage when planning educational needs.

- Precontemplation (the patient is not considering any change in behavior [defined as within the next 6 months]). Patients often do not perceive their behavior as problematic or do not factor negative consequences.
- Contemplation (the patient has serious consideration of change in the next 6 months).
- Preparation (the patient has taken initial behavioral steps toward change and intends to make changes in the next 30 days). Small steps may be taken toward the behavior change which patients believe can lead to a healthier life.
- Action (concrete activities that lead to the desired change have been made for less than 6 months).
- Maintenance (active efforts to sustain the changes made for more than 6 months).

The expectation would be for the patient in the precontemplation stage to disagree with suggestions that a change in behavior is needed. The patient would not be expected to exert effort toward making changes in the "risk" behavior. At this stage, the nurse would offer suggestions and material for the patient to consider the need for behavior change and encourage the patient to consider changes in the future. At the preparation phase the nurses would assist in developing a plan regarding the lifestyle change (e.g., smoking cessation, diet changes). On the other hand, the nurse may expect an individual in the action stage to endorse the need for change and engage in specific behaviors that would lead to behavioral change. Engagement in educational activities would be expected at this stage. Of note, unmotivated smokers were proactively recruited and engaged to quit smoking, and the most influential factor to patient engagement was person-centered communication by the health care provider (e.g., good listener, nonjudgmental, pleasant, and respectful) (Mena et al., 2017).

many aspects of preventive health teaching. Experiential readiness is closely related to emotional readiness, because motivation tends to be stimulated by an appreciation for the need to learn and by those learning tasks that are familiar, interesting, and meaningful.

A practical way of assessing the patient's learning readiness is to ask how they view their health-related problem and what actions they see that can be taken. Other open-ended questions that might be asked include, "What changes would you like to make now?" and "Are there any problems that prevent you from learning right now?" Research continues to find that these questions are best asked early in a meeting with a patient. In addition, asking "Do you have any other concerns?" as opposed to "Do you have any other questions?" will illicit more information. In summary, a wide variety of factors are considered when assessing the patient readiness to learn including their emotions, perception of need, importance, and attitudes to and previous experiences of learning, when setting achievable, learner-directed goals (Thompson et al., 2020).

DETECTING COMMUNICATION ISSUES

Lack of communication skills is one of the most significant barriers to patient education. This can include both a patient's reading and computer skills. Patients who struggle with written material may appear disinterested in learning rather than admitting that they may not understand. Watch a patient's eyes while they are "reading"; the eyes should move left to right as the document is read. Using computerized resources to support learning with inexperienced users requires careful assessment and planning. Computer-based education will work best and make the most efficient use of time when it is matched to the skill level of the patient.

Improved health outcomes are achieved when culturally competent nurses acknowledge the patient's culture care values and preferred care practices, and incorporate them into their patient's plan of care. Completing a cultural assessment will allow the nurse to adapt information and delivery to a patient's cultural beliefs and preferences (Box 1-9). An individual's culture can affect their viewpoint in many ways, such as the meaning of a diagnosis, the expectation of reporting symptoms, how much information is desired, how death and dying will be managed, gender roles, family participation, and decision making. Culturally competent communication skills play an important role in your success in influencing your patients' health.

There are a number of cultural mores and rules that a nurse can learn and follow:

- Understand nonverbal behavior (e.g., the cultural meaning of touch, eye contact)
- Allow time to build a relationship and establish a rapport:
  - exchange information
  - greet and respond in culturally appropriate ways
  - be genuine
  - pay attention to children
  - listen carefully, don't interrupt or put words in one's mouth
  - value stories
- Notice eye contact and body language
- Reach out to the appropriate family member

(*continued on page 16*)

BOX 1-9

Cultural Assessment Components to Consider When Formulating a Teaching Plan

When formulating a teaching plan, consider the patient's beliefs about:

- Body size, shape, boundaries, and functions
- Beauty and strength
- Value of the mind or brain
- Nature and function of blood
- Diet and nutrition
- Communication
- Gender
- Family and social support
- Physical health and illness
- Mental health and illness
- Age-related changes
- Pain
- Medicine, herbs, and talismans
- Spirituality or religion

- Check for understanding and ask questions
- Avoid jargon and stereotyping
- Do not impose your personal values, morals, or beliefs on to your patients

A balance is necessary; it is important to avoid overemphasizing culture-specific beliefs so as not to reinforce stereotypes.

Language barriers, once identified, must be addressed. In 2010, The Joint Commission (TJC) developed patient-centered communication standards that detail hospital staff's obligation to respect patients' right to and need for effective communication, including the provision of interpreter and translation services when needed (TJC, 2021). Hospitals are required to provide professional language services to every patient with limited English proficiency (LEP) and tailor written materials to the patient's age, language, and ability to understand. Interpreters must be competent and trained as medical interpreters. If you are bilingual or multilingual, you are not prohibited from communicating directly with a patient in another language while providing care. However, TJC does recommend that your organization has a process to make sure that communication with the patient in the non-English language is effective and meets the patient's needs (TJC, 2021). Using family members or even untrained support staff as interpreters raises quality, ethical, and possible legal issues. Family members, including children, may incorporate bias into their interpretations, and patient confidentiality is compromised. Issues about sharing sensitive, private matters with family or friends or their withholding of bad news or information should also be considered. Often interpreter services are delivered via the telephone or remote video-phone; however, this method of communication does not have applicability for all patients (e.g., for patients who are deaf, where eye contact and nonverbal gestures are essential). Box 1-10 discusses using interpreter services effectively. The recent pandemic magnified inequities in health care where patients with English as a Second Language (ESL) received "lower-quality health care and experience[d] poorer outcomes" (Velasquez et al., 2021, p. 93). The authors suggest that efforts such as interpreter services and linguistically tailored health information do not address the upstream factors. Rather, health care providers should also consider upstream efforts such as teaching ESL by partnering with hospitals, community-based institutions and leveraging Medicare and insurers to improve health care delivery for populations with limited English proficiency. Table 1-2 details strategies for patients with disabilities.

DIAGNOSIS

Diagnoses related to health education may include:

- Altered health-seeking behaviors
- Altered health maintenance
- Readiness for enhanced health management
- Knowledge, deficiency (specify)
- Readiness for enhanced knowledge
- Readiness for enhanced health literacy

PLANNING

Once assessment data are collected, the planning component of the teaching–learning process is established in accordance with the steps of the nursing process:

1. Specify the immediate, intermediate, and long-term goals of learning.
2. Identify specific teaching strategies appropriate for attaining goals.
3. Specify the expected outcomes.
4. Document the goals, teaching strategies, and expected outcomes of the teaching plan.

Developing the plan and goals of teaching should be a joint effort by the nurse and the patient and family members. Consideration must be given to the urgency of the patient's learning needs; the most critical needs should receive the highest priority. The nurse should also differentiate between factual (declarative) knowledge and practical (procedural) knowledge (Thompson et al., 2020). For example, disease-specific information on diabetes mellitus versus the procedural skill of blood glucose testing. For declarative or factual knowledge the patient must construct meaning themselves, organize their knowledge, and store it so that information is easily retrievable, whereas procedural knowledge is what is necessary to complete practical tasks, and extends to shaping the skill, recognizing how to vary the procedure if needed, and learning how to avoid common errors. It involves practicing the skill until it becomes automatic (Thompson & Thompson, 2014; Thompson et al., 2020). After the learning priorities have been established, it is important to identify the immediate and long-term goals and the teaching strategies appropriate for attaining those goals. Learning begins with the establishment of goals that are appropriate to the situation and realistic in terms of the patient's ability and desire to achieve them. Involving the patient and family in establishing goals and in planning teaching strategies promotes their cooperation in implementing the

BOX 1-10

Working Effectively Through an Interpreter

Knowing the patient:
- Determine ethnicity and nationality of the patient.
- Determine what language(s) the patient speaks, and preferred language.
- Offer an interpreter to all patients where English is not their first language.
- Determine patient preference for face-to-face or telephone interpreter service.

Preparing for the meeting:
- Ensure a private, quiet environment, with space for all meeting participants.
- Gather any needed decision aids. Make sure they match the communication needs of your patient (and their companions).
- Maintain a warm, nonrushed environment where patient and interpreter can raise concerns.
- Meet with the interpreter before the meeting to discuss the goals of the meeting and the process (such as pausing for interpretation); if repeat meetings are required, try to use the same interpreter.
- Explain that interpreters are bound by their code of ethics to treat everything that is said as confidential.

Seating arrangements:
- Ensure that the seating is arranged to facilitate communication. When the meeting involves only a client, interpreter, and a clinician, arrange seating in a triangle formation.
- When interpreting with family, caregivers, or more than two people, it is advisable to arrange the seating in a horseshoe or circle formation, with the interpreter seated next to the clinician.
- In a large or group meeting situation, arrange the seating in a circular formation; seat the interpreter next to the clinician and close to the client so they are able to understand the proceedings with minimum disruption to others.
- For telephone interpreting, use a dual handset or hands-free phone, and sit facing your client.

Verbal and nonverbal communication (telephone and face-to-face interpreter):
- Ensure your patient knows the interpreter's name and what the interpreter will do.
- Explain to your patient that the interpreter is required to maintain patient privacy and will not share any of the information.
- Speak directly to the patient, not to the interpreter.
- Maintain eye contact and face your patient.
- Speak more slowly rather than more loudly.
- Keep your sentences or questions brief.
- Pause at the end of each statement to allow the interpreter time to interpret, explaining the need to pause to the client.
- Be aware that the interpreter may sometimes have to clarify a statement or answer with the client, family member, or caregiver.

During the medical interview:
- Assume, and insist, that everything you say, everything the patient says, and everything that family members say is interpreted.
- Do not hold the interpreter responsible for what the patient says or doesn't say. The interpreter is the medium, not the source, of the message.
- If you feel that you are not getting the type of response you were expecting, restate the question or consult with the interpreter to better understand if there is a cultural barrier that is interfering with communication.
- Be aware that many concepts you express have no linguistic or conceptual equivalent in other languages. The interpreter may have to paint word pictures of many terms you use. This may take longer than your original speech.
- Respond to nonverbal cues (e.g., quizzical or frightened look, stiffening of body posture)
- If you need to ask questions that may be extremely personal or sensitive, explain to the patient that doing so is part of your evaluation and reiterate that the information will remain private.
- Avoid: highly idiomatic speech, complicated sentence structure, sentence fragments, changing your idea in the middle of a sentence, and asking multiple questions at one time. Also avoid making assumptions or generalizations about your patients or their experiences. Common practices or beliefs in a community may not apply to everyone in that community.
- Encourage the interpreter to ask questions and to alert you about potential cultural misunderstandings that may come up. Respect an interpreter's judgment that a particular question is culturally inappropriate and either rephrase the question or ask the interpreter's help in eliciting the information in a more appropriate way.
- Ask the patients what they believe the problem is, what causes it, and how it would be treated in their country of origin.
- Ask the patient to repeat back important information that you want to make sure is understood. Use teach-back to assess patient understanding. Have your patient explain to you, in their own words, what was said. Ask the interpreter to tell you exactly what your patient said so you can check for comprehension.
- Be patient. Providing care across a language barrier takes time. However, the time spent up front will be paid back by good rapport and clear communication that will avoid wasted time and dangerous misunderstandings later in the process.

Data from AHRQ (2020a), Kaur (2014), Miletic et al. (2006), pp. 18–26.

teaching plan. A partnership between patients and providers, based on both shared decision making and two-way communication, will develop your patient's skills and confidence needed to self-manage their health.

Expected outcomes of teaching strategies can be stated in terms of behaviors of patients, families, or both. Outcomes should be realistic and measurable, and the critical time periods for attaining them should be identified. The desired outcomes

(continued on page 19)

TABLE **1-2 Teaching People with Disabilities**

Type of Disability	Teaching Strategy
Physical, Emotional, or Cognitive Disability	Adapt information to accommodate the person's cognitive, perceptual, and behavioral disabilities. Give clear written and oral information. Highlight significant information for easy reference. Avoid medical terminology.
Hearing Impairment	Use slow, directed, deliberate speech. Use sign language or interpreter services if appropriate. For lip reading and/or hearing augmented by hearing aids: Position yourself so that the person can see your mouth; do not chew gum or food. Speak slowly and distinctly; do not exaggerate your pronunciation. Use smallest number of words to convey the message. Maintain eye contact. Use telecommunication devices (TTY[a] or TDD[b]) for the hearing impaired. Consider a battery-powered microphone with earpiece if applicable. Use written materials and visual aids, such as models and diagrams. Use captioned videos, films, and computer-generated materials. Teach on the side of the "good ear" if unilateral deafness is present.
Visual Impairment	Use optical devices such as a magnifying lens. Use proper lighting and proper contrast of colors on materials and equipment. Use large-print materials. Use Braille materials if appropriate. Convert information to auditory and tactile formats. Obtain audiotapes and talking books. Explain noises and sensations associated with procedures, equipment, and treatments. Arrange materials in clockwise pattern.
Learning Disabilities	
Input disability—process of recording information in the brain, perceptual disability	If visual perceptual disorder: • Explain information verbally, repeat, and reinforce frequently. • Use audiotapes. • Encourage learner to verbalize information received. If auditory perceptual disorder: • Speak slowly with as few words as possible, repeat, and reinforce frequently. • Use direct eye contact to focus person on task. • Use demonstration and return demonstration such as modeling, role playing, and hands-on experiences. • Use visual tools, written materials, and computers.
Output disability—communication of information from the brain to other people or translation of the information into action, by means of words—language output—or through muscle activity, such as writing, drawing, gesturing, and so forth—motor output	Use all senses as appropriate. Use written, audiotape, and computer information. Review information and give time to interact and ask questions. Use hand gestures and motions.
Developmental disability	Base information and teaching on developmental stage, not chronologic age. Use nonverbal cues, gestures, signing, and symbols as needed. Use simple explanations and concrete examples with repetition. Encourage active participation. Demonstrate information and have the person perform return demonstrations.

[a]TTY, a special device that lets people who are deaf, hard of hearing, or speech-impaired use the telephone for communication needs (messages are typed back and forth).

[b]TDD, operates similarly to a TTY but is a much smaller desktop machine.

and the critical time periods serve as a basis for evaluating the effectiveness of the teaching strategies.

During the planning phase, the nurse must consider the sequence in which the subject matter is presented in each of the teaching strategies. Critical information (e.g., procedural knowledge of blood glucose monitoring for a patient with diabetes) and material that the person or family identifies to be of particular importance will be high priority and, thus, should be presented earlier than other information. An outline is often helpful for arranging the subject matter and for ensuring that all necessary information is included. In addition, appropriate teaching aids to be used in implementing teaching strategies are prepared or selected at this time.

THE LEARNING ENVIRONMENT

Although learning can take place without teachers, most people who are attempting to learn new or altered health behaviors benefit from the services of nurses. The interpersonal interaction between the person and the nurse who is attempting to meet the person's learning needs may be formal or informal, depending on the method and techniques of teaching.

Learning may be optimized by minimizing factors that interfere with the learning process. For example, the room temperature, lighting, noise levels, and other environmental conditions should be appropriate to the learning situation.

TIMING

The time selected for teaching should be suited to the needs of the individual person. Scheduling a teaching session at a time of day when a patient is fatigued, uncomfortable, or anxious about a pending diagnostic or therapeutic procedure, or when visitors are present, is not conducive to learning. However, if the family is to participate in providing care, the sessions should be scheduled when family members are present, so that they can learn any necessary skills or techniques.

TEACHING TECHNIQUES

Teaching techniques and methods enhance learning if they are appropriate to the patient's needs. It is important that we note here that it is not a "one size fits all" approach. Rather, the nurse considers the uniqueness of the individual patient, and teaching techniques will be selected "from where each person is" and adapted to the patient's specific health needs aligned to their experiences and abilities (Pueyo-Garrigues et al., 2019). Numerous techniques are available, including lectures, group teaching, and demonstrations with teach back method, all of which can be enhanced with specially prepared teaching materials.

Learning is exceedingly complex, and we have yet to elucidate its intricacies. As James Watson (one of the proposers of the double helix structure of the DNA molecule) noted, "The brain is the last and grandest biologic frontier, the most complex thing we have yet discovered in our universe. It contains hundreds of billions of cells interlinked through trillions of connections. The brain boggles the mind" (Watson, 1992). The following axiom regarding what types of information we retain is not grounded in any scientific sense. We place it here, fully aware that there is no research or evidence on the percentages. However, it serves as a useful classification scheme for the various types of learning experiences based on the work of Edgar Dale (1946). Retained information of learning activities:

- 10% of what is read
- 25% of what is heard
- 45% of what is seen
- 65% of what is heard and seen
- 70% of what is said and written
- 90% of what is said as a task is performed

The lecture or explanation method of teaching is commonly used but should always be accompanied by discussion. Discussion is important because it affords learners opportunities to express their feelings and concerns, to ask questions, and to receive clarification. Group teaching is appropriate for some people because it allows them not only to receive needed information but also to feel secure as members of a group. People with similar issues or learning needs have the opportunity to identify with each other and gain moral support and encouragement. Recently, the use of online health communities (OHCs) offers opportunities for people with chronic diseases such as diabetes to share information and experiences for self-improvement (Aghdam et al., 2021). The use of a health literacy, chronic disease self-management, and social support intervention for older people delivered by group videoconferencing into the home demonstrated improved health literacy behaviors and self-management skills, and participants reported improved perception of companionship, emotional, and informational support (Banbury et al., 2020). This study also demonstrated that older people with little or no experience with technology can be supported to use technology. Group visits (whether in person or online) allow interactions in a more natural setting, and conversations between patients help them feel less isolated and, possibly, less threatened. If group teaching is used, assessment and follow-up are imperative to ensure that each person has gained sufficient knowledge and skills. Demonstration and practice are essential ingredients of a teaching program, especially when the nurse is teaching skills to the patient. It is best to demonstrate the skill and then give the learner ample opportunity for practice.

When teaching a patient and special equipment is involved, such as syringes, colostomy bags, dialysis equipment, dressings, or suction apparatus, it is important to teach with the same equipment that will be used in the home setting. Learning to perform a skill with one kind of equipment and then having to change to a different kind may lead to confusion, frustration, and mistakes.

A tool such as the plan-do-study-act (PDSA) model is a framework for quality improvement activities. The PDSA model, or others like it, is used often by health care organizations to approach performance improvement work in a consistent way. Before implementing PDSA, three questions are asked: What is the goal of the project (in this case teaching)? How will one

(*continued on page 20*)

know whether the goal was reached? and What will be done to reach the goal? The PDSA model is a way to engage patients with their own care and have a role in developing their own plan. Patients should help prioritize items for best time management. A communication/demonstration technique known as *ask–tell–ask–close the loop (or teach back, discussed shortly)* can help improve communication and patient understanding:

- *Ask* permission to give information about a topic of importance to the patient.
- *Tell:* Explanations and written materials are most effective when given in response to the patient's expressed agenda and tailored to their ability to understand.
- *Ask* for understanding, and provide additional information or clarification as necessary.
- *Close the loop:* Ask the patient to restate the information as the patient understands it

Teaching aids used to enhance learning include books, pamphlets, pictures, models, programmed instruction, or multimedia formats (videos, web-based, or smartphones). These are made available as needed for home, clinic, or hospital use, and they allow review and reinforcement of content and enhanced visual and auditory learning. Such teaching aids are invaluable when used appropriately and can save a significant amount of personnel time and related cost. However, all such aids should be reviewed before use to ensure that they meet the patient's learning needs. Developing tools as part of a multidisciplinary group also has been shown to yield benefits not only for patients who will use the tools but for the staff involved in creating them. Table 1-3 offers guidelines for developing patient education materials. In addition, there is a growing approach to educating patients using digitally connected coaches or virtual communities available from employers and insurance companies such as Diabetes Prevention Program (Marcotte & Dugdale, 2019).

Reinforcement and follow-up are important because learning takes time. Allowing ample time to learn, and then reinforcing what is learned, are important teaching strategies; rarely is a single teaching session adequate. Follow-up sessions are imperative to promote the learner's confidence in their abilities and to plan for additional teaching sessions. For hospitalized patients who may not be able to transfer what they have learned in the hospital to the home setting, follow-up after discharge is essential to ensure that they have realized the full benefits of a teaching program.

The entire planning phase of the teaching–learning process concludes with the documentation of the teaching plan. This teaching plan communicates information to all members of the nursing and health care team. Documentation enhances the continuity of care for the patient and communication among caregivers. Documentation should include:

- The learner, instructor, and interpreter (if used)
- The patient's need assessment
- Learning objectives and goals
- Information and skills taught
- Teaching methods used
- Teaching materials provided or used
- Patient and family response to teaching
- Evaluation of what the patient learned
- Further learning needs
- Revised goals (if necessary)

TABLE **1-3 Guidelines for Developing Patient Education Materials**

- Use visuals as much as possible (DVDs or printed illustrations) of anatomical features of the specific system that relates to the patient's problem or need
- Choose books, pamphlets, and/or brochures that are written at a third to fifth grade level
- Use short sentences (10 words or less) when developing printed materials
- Write paragraphs with no more than two or three sentences with one key point per paragraph
- Focus efforts on key bullet points of "must know" information
- Use visual terms such as "runny nose" and "redness"
- Explain measurements, e.g., "pain that lasts more than 30 minutes"
- Clearly list when the patient needs to call the health care provider and what phone number to call
- Focus on actions patients should do using familiar words
- Use plain language: Define any terms that are difficult to understand
- Have patient and family members "teach back" the information to you to ensure understanding
- Be aware of language, customs, and values to create a culturally sensitive and effective tool
- Use wide margins and leave white space between sections
- Find an advocate for the person with low literacy who will ensure that the individual understands and follows through with instructions

The American Academy of Ambulatory Care Nursing Patient Education Special Interest Group (AAACN). (n.d.). Guidelines for developing patient education materials. https://www.aaacn.org/guidelinesdeveloping-patient-education-materials

IMPLEMENTATION

In the implementation phase of the teaching–learning process, the patient, the family, and other members of the nursing and health care team carry out the activities outlined in the teaching plan. The nurse coordinates these activities.

During the implementation phase of the teaching–learning process and throughout the ongoing assessment of patient responses to the teaching strategies, flexibility is indispensable to support modification of the teaching plan as necessary. Creativity is essential in promoting and sustaining the patient's motivation to learn. Be sure to consider new learning needs that may arise after discharge from the hospital or after home care visits have ended.

Feedback about progress also motivates learning. Such feedback should be presented in the form of positive reinforcement when the learner is successful and in the form of constructive suggestions for improvement when they are unsuccessful.

The implementation phase ends when the teaching strategies have been completed and when the patient's responses

BOX 1-11

Teach-Back Method

- Keep in mind this is not a test of the patient's knowledge. It is a test of how well you explained the concept.
- Plan your approach. Think about how you will ask your patients to teach back the information. For example:
  - "We covered a lot today and I want to make sure that I explained things clearly. So let's review what we discussed. Can you please describe the 3 things you agreed to do to help you control your diabetes?"
- "Chunk and Check." Don't wait until the end of the visit to initiate teach-back. Chunk out information into small segments and have your patient teach it back. Repeat several times during a visit.
- Clarify and check again. If teach-back uncovers a misunderstanding, explain things again using a different approach. Ask patients to teach-back again until they are able to correctly describe the information in their own words. If they parrot your words back to you, they may not have understood.
- Start slowly and use consistently. At first, you may want to try teach-back with the last patient of the day. Once you are comfortable with the technique, use teach-back with everyone, every time!
- Practice. It will take a little time, but once it is part of your routine, teach-back can be done without awkwardness and does not lengthen a visit.
- Use the show-me method. When prescribing new medicines or changing a dose, research shows that even when patients correctly say when and how much medicine they'll take, many will make mistakes when asked to demonstrate the dose. You could say, for example:
  - "I've noticed that many people have trouble remembering how to take their blood thinner. Can you show me how you are going to take it?"
- Use handouts along with teach-back. Write down key information to help patients remember instructions at home. Point out important information by reviewing written materials to reinforce your patients' understanding. You can allow patients to refer to handouts when using teach-back, but make sure they use their own words and are not reading the material back verbatim.

From AHRQ. (2020b). Health Literacy Universal Precautions Toolkit, 2nd Edition, Use the Teach-Back Method: Tool #5. https://www.ahrq.gov/health-literacy/improve/precautions/tool5.html

to the actions have been recorded. This record serves as the basis for evaluating how well the defined goals and expected outcomes have been achieved.

EVALUATION

Evaluation of the teaching–learning process determines how effectively the patient has responded to teaching and to what extent the goals have been achieved. An evaluation must be made to determine what was effective and what needs to be changed or reinforced. It cannot be assumed that patients have learned just because teaching has occurred; learning does not automatically follow teaching. An important part of the evaluation phase addresses the question, "What can be done to improve teaching and enhance learning?" Answers to this question direct the changes to be made in the teaching plan.

A variety of measurement techniques can be used to identify changes in patient behavior and evaluation of learning. These techniques include directly observing the behavior; using rating scales, checklists, or anecdotal notes to document the behavior; and indirectly measuring results using oral questioning and written tests. The teach back method is a way for you to assess whether your patient understands your teaching. It is not a test or quiz! It is an evidence-based technique for educating patients by verifying their understanding of your teaching by asking the patient, family member, or caregiver to repeat the information provided in the recipient's own words. It has demonstrated increased patient understanding, trust, and patient satisfaction (see Box 1-11) (AHRQ, 2020a; Nickles et al., 2020). Using more than one measuring technique enhances the reliability of the resulting data and decreases the potential for error from a measurement strategy.

In many situations, measurement of actual behavior is the most accurate and appropriate technique. In other cases, indirect measurement may be used such as patient satisfaction surveys, attitude surveys, and instruments that evaluate specific health status variables.

However, measurement is only the beginning of evaluation, which must be followed by data interpretation and value judgments about learning and teaching. These aspects of evaluation should be conducted periodically throughout the teaching–learning program, at its conclusion, and at varying periods after the teaching has ended.

Evaluation of learning after hospitalization is highly desirable because the analysis of teaching outcomes must extend into home care. With shortened lengths of hospital stay and with short-stay and same-day surgical procedures, follow-up evaluation in the home is especially important. Coordination of efforts and sharing of information between hospital- and community-based nursing personnel facilitate postdischarge teaching and home care evaluation.

Evaluation is not the final step in the teaching–learning process, but the beginning of the iterative process of a new patient assessment. The information gathered during evaluation should be used to redirect teaching actions, with the goal of improving the patient's responses and outcomes.

HEALTH PROMOTION

Health teaching and **health promotion** are linked by a common goal—to encourage people to achieve as high a level of wellness as possible so that they can live maximally healthy lives and avoid preventable illnesses. Patients are the primary managers of their health conditions. Nurses are in an ideal position to provide the kind of support that patients need to manage their conditions. Health promotion has become a cornerstone in health policy because of the need to control costs and reduce unnecessary sickness and death.

The U.S. Department of Health and Human Services' Healthy People initiative was designed to establish a program of nationwide health-promotion and disease-prevention goals. The goals established in the publication *Healthy People 2000* focused on disease prevention. *Healthy People 2030* builds on past achievements, reaffirming the overarching goals from the past decades (Fig. 1-2). Given the health inequities that worsened during the COVID-19 pandemic and the greater attention to racial and social justice, there is an increased focus on social determinants of health and health equity. The number of objectives in Health People 2030 (2020) was decreased to improve prioritization of the most pressing public health issues. Healthy People 2030 (2020) also includes well-being as a defined measure.

Definition

Health promotion is defined as the process of enabling people to increase control over their health and its determinants, thereby improving their health (World Health Organization [WHO], 2016). The WHO (2016) identified three elements of health promotion: good governance for health, health literacy, and healthy cities. The purpose of health promotion is to focus on the person's potential for wellness and to encourage

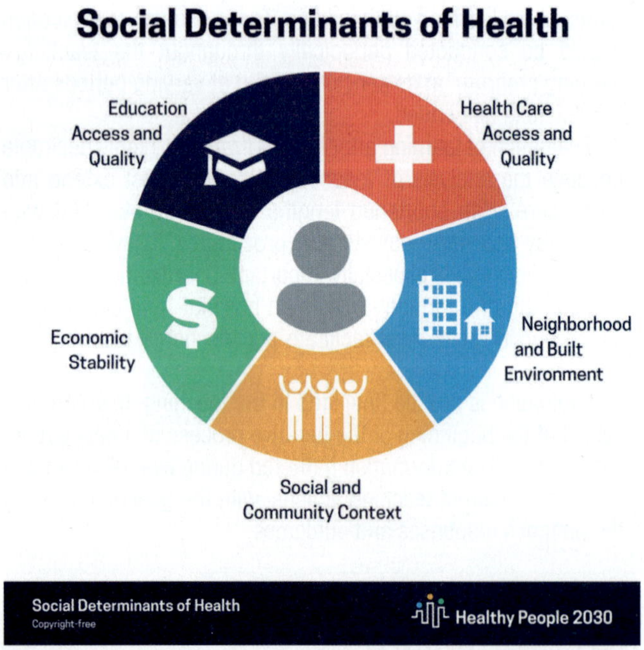

FIGURE 1-2 Social determinants of health from Healthy People 2030. (From Healthy People 2030, U.S. Department of Health and Human Services, Office of Disease Prevention and Health Promotion. Retrieved April 14, 2022, from https://health.gov/healthypeople/objectives-and-data/social-determinants-health)

appropriate alterations in personal habits, lifestyle, and environment in ways that reduce risks and enhance health and well-being. Health promotion is an active process; that is, it is not something that can be prescribed or dictated. It is up to each person to decide whether to make changes to promote a higher level of wellness. Only the individual can make these choices.

The concepts of health, wellness, health promotion, and disease prevention have been a topic of extensive discussion in the lay literature and news media, as well as in professional journals. As a result, public demand for health information has increased, and health care professionals and agencies have responded by providing this information. As employers strive to reduce costs associated with absenteeism, health insurance, hospitalization, disability, excessive turnover of personnel, and premature death, the workplace has become an important site for health-promotion programs (Schaap et al., 2020). The concept of health promotion has evolved because of a changing definition of health and an awareness that wellness exists at many levels of functioning. Health is viewed as a dynamic, ever-changing condition that enables people to function at an optimal potential at any given time. The ideal health status is one in which people are successful in achieving their full potential, regardless of any limitations they might have.

Wellness, as a reflection of health, involves a conscious and deliberate attempt to maximize one's health. Wellness does not just happen; it requires planning and conscious commitment and is the result of adopting lifestyle behaviors for the purpose of attaining one's highest potential for well-being. Wellness is not the same for every person. The person with a chronic illness or disability may still be able to achieve a desirable level of wellness (refer to Chapter 2). The key to wellness is to function at the highest potential within the limitations over which there is no control. The interaction between mental health, well-being, and physical health appears to be interconnected. Park and Lee (2019) found that higher levels of spiritual peace and social support each uniquely predicted increased positive states of mind, and that social support predicted improved physical health-related quality of life.

Unfolding Patient Stories: VB • Part 1

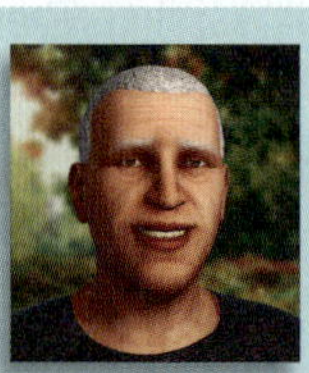

VB, a 67-year-old with chronic obstructive pulmonary disease (COPD), is experiencing increased fatigue. The patient spends most of the day in a recliner chair watching television, smoking 1–2 packs per day with a limited nutritional intake due to shortness of breath. What patient education can the nurse provide to promote self-care behaviors for symptom improvement and a healthier lifestyle? (VB's story continues in Chapter 50.)

Care for VB and other patients in a realistic virtual environment: ***vSim** for Nursing* (thepoint.lww.com/vSimMedicalSurgical). Practice documenting these patients' care in DocuCare (www.lww.com/DocuCareEHR).

Health Promotion

Health promotion is a concept and a process that extends throughout the lifespan. Any number of clinical organizations and, in particular, the U.S. Preventive Services Task Force (USPSTF) review research and literature and work to improve the health of people by making evidence-based recommendations about clinical preventive services. At any stage of the lifespan, health promotion includes health screening. Screenings are tests that look for diseases before symptoms are present. In general, screening tests can find diseases early, when they are easier to treat. Some conditions that health care providers commonly screen for include breast cancer and cervical cancer in females, prostate cancer in males, as well as colorectal cancer, diabetes, high blood pressure, high cholesterol, osteoporosis, and obesity. Tests needed depend on age, sex, family history, and whether there are risk factors for certain diseases. The USPSTF offers a website where the public can obtain specific recommendations based upon age, sex, and risk factors for clinical counseling, preventive medications, and screening services.

People of all ages are challenged to find the best way to make health behavior changes. Downes and Foote (2019) found any number of barriers in the way of healthy behaviors and practices such as lack of trust in health professionals; denial; sense of invincibility; poor mental health; social isolation with no incentive for good health and well-being, past or present trauma; erratic lifestyle; unstable living conditions; negative influence of partner, family, friends and social media; poor literacy skills; and English as a second language.

Even when highly motivated, people can find it difficult to achieve and/or sustain success. According to Ross et al. (2020), people of all ages are more likely to participate in spiritual growth and interpersonal relationships than in physical activity, health responsibility, and stress reduction programs. The physical health of people is an important determinant of participation in health-promoting behaviors. People starting a health journey in poor health are less likely during high stress times to make improvements in healthy living. Nurses can serve as health coaches, assisting patients to meet small, attainable health goals, which can help increase client self-efficacy (Ross et al., 2020).

It is also critical to be aware of cultural aspects that are important to our patients. Blacks are the second largest minority group in the United States and are disproportionately burdened with chronic diseases such as obesity, heart disease, cancer, and type 2 diabetes (HHS, 2021b). It is important that our educational interventions are provided where our patients "work, live and play" (Palmer et al., 2020, p. 2). Faith-based organizations are an integral part of communities for females and older adults and are often tasked with community outreach initiatives. Barbershops for males and hair salons for females are sociologically important places in Black communities that have been shown to have significant impact on health-promotion activities over the last decade (Palmer et al., 2020). When considering health promotional interventions, it is important to meet the patient where they are.

Young and Middle-Age Adults

Frequently, adults are motivated to change their lifestyles in ways that they believe will enhance their health and wellness. Middle to older adults' beliefs can have a moderating effect because beliefs about susceptibility to health issues become more real with age. Many adults who wish to improve their health turn to health-promotion programs to help them make the desired changes in their lifestyles. Many have responded to programs that focus on topics such as general wellness, smoking avoidance or cessation, exercise, physical conditioning, weight control, conflict resolution, and stress management. Because of the nationwide emphasis on health during the reproductive years, young adults actively seek programs that address prenatal health, parenting, family planning, and female health issues.

Health-promotion efforts and information can often be found in workplaces. Estrella et al. (2018) studied the association between employment status and ideal cardiovascular health (CVH) scores. In the study, males employed either part time or full time had higher ideal CVH scores. Females employed outside the home full time had higher CVH scores than other females. Although availability of health insurance may also play a role in these results, there is also an opportunity to target CVH factors and behaviors according to sex, employment status, and age to maximize health education impact.

The use of health coaches is another intervention that can improve health behaviors. These programs have become increasingly accessible through insurance plans. McQueen et al. (2020) identified preferred health coach characteristics includes expertise in the subject matter, experience in helping clients, excellent communication and interpersonal skills, empathy, and not being bossy or too aggressive. In addition, the ideal health coaching program characteristics include some in-person interaction between a coach and client, client input in determining the frequency and modality of coach–client interactions, and multiple options for learning about, entering into, and engaging with a health coaching program. Those who access their coaching program through a Medicaid plan also emphasized that coaches should take their life context into account by understanding their job demands, childcare responsibilities, financial hardship, or need for social support. Coaches should also personalize recommendations by understanding the resources available to clients.

Older Adults

Health promotion is as important for older adults as it is for other adults and children. Although their chronic illnesses and disabilities cannot be eliminated, these adults can benefit from activities that help them maintain independence and achieve an optimal level of health. Older adults have different health and social circumstances compared to younger people. Because of these differences, there are other strategies that can be used to help promote healthy behaviors. The WHO has identified reducing ageism as a way to improve health because ageism, in the form of negative stereotypes, prejudice, and discrimination, increases the risks to older people's physical and mental health. Interventions that combine elements of both education and intergenerational contact have the largest effect on people's attitudes toward older adults.

Physical activity contributes to better mental and physical well-being in older adults. There are both barriers and facilitators to participation in exercise. Palmer (2020) identified that minimizing the barriers and accentuating the opportunities can be key to increasing older adult participation, leading to the positive outcomes. The opportunities that lead to greater participation include the individual's motivation to maintain physical and mental health, access to appropriate affordable services, the physical ability to access services, and trained staff to guide exercise and support motivation, encourage the social aspect, help set realistic goals, track progress, assist in working through barriers to exercise, and offer regular verbal encouragement (Palmer, 2020).

Pettigrew et al. (2021) reported that older people can be receptive to promotional advertisements that depict their peers engaging in the desired health behaviors like moderate to vigorous forms of activity. An innovative teaching–earning strategy was described by Elliott (2020) that incorporated group work, public service announcements (PSAs), and developing teaching tools for older adults as an active learning project for baccalaureate nursing students. The project was impactful and provided a positive experience for older adults and nursing students. The adults felt empowered by providing input on teaching tools designed for their population. They also were exposed to the critical information carried by the PSAs. Students felt empowered with new knowledge and gained a greater respect for older adults (Elliott, 2020).

Nursing Implications

Nurses have a unique relationship with the American public, topping Gallup's Honesty and Ethics ranking of professions every year but one since they were added to the list in 1999. The exception is 2001, when firefighters were included on the list on a one-time basis, shortly after the September 11 terrorist attacks. "The fact that this is the 20th year in a row that the American public has voted nurses #1 is a testament to nurses' consistent professionalism, despite the challenges of the persistent pandemic" (ANA, 2022). By virtue of nurses' expertise in health and health care and our long-established credibility with consumers, nurses play a vital role in health promotion. In many instances, nurses have initiated health-promotion and health-screening programs or have participated with other health care personnel in developing and providing wellness services in a variety of settings. As health care professionals, nurses have a responsibility to promote activities that foster well-being, self-actualization, and personal fulfillment. Every interaction with consumers of health care must be viewed as an opportunity to promote positive health attitudes and behaviors. And our continued privileged place in the eyes of patients depends on each nurse encountered. It is up to you to maintain the trust our patients have placed in us.

CHAPTER REVIEW

NCLEX-Style Review Questions

1. Which of the following influences are impacting health care today and in the foreseeable future? Select all that apply.
   a. Fewer individuals with chronic disease
   b. Increased aging population
   c. An awareness that social, economic, and environmental factors impact patient health
   d. Lengthened hospital stays
   e. Increasingly culturally diverse population

2. Nurses should consider their own cultural orientation when interacting with patients. Which of the following is a technique that can be used to overcome a language barrier when interacting with a patient? Select all that apply.
   a. Talk loudly so that the patient will understand.
   b. Give the patient a substantial amount of information.
   c. Give instructions in proper sequence.
   d. Talk directly to the person that accompanied the patient.
   e. Proceed in an unhurried manner

3. A nurse is providing discharge teaching for an older patient who is fully dressed, watching television, and waiting for family. The nurse sits in a chair facing the patient and shows the patient a handout. The patient squints while reading and periodically looks at the television. The nurse is about to review the information and determine the patient's understanding of the material when the family enters the room. The nurse determines the need for further education due to learning barriers. Which barriers affected the patient's ability to comprehend the information? Select all that apply.
   a. Patient is watching television.
   b. The patient is older.
   c. The patient squints while reading.
   d. The family entered the room while teaching.
   e. The patient is fully dressed.

4. The nurse is to provide discharge teaching to a patient with newly diagnosed coronary artery disease. In what order should the following steps be prioritized and completed?
   a. Implement teaching plan.
   b. Collect and analyze data regarding the patient's knowledge of coronary artery disease.
   c. Form nursing diagnoses related to patient teaching.
   d. Reassess patient's knowledge as needed.
   e. Develop teaching plan.
   f. Identify learning needs.
   g. Update and change plan.

5. In the situations below, select which examples of tasks could be delegated to the nurses' assistant. Select all that apply.
   a. Feeding to a newly admitted patient with a diagnosis of left CVA with right hemiparesis
   b. Ambulating a stable patient post left hip replacement who is post-op day 2
   c. Measuring output from a Foley bag of a postoperative patient admitted to your unit
   d. Bathing to a patient admitted for chronic obstructive pulmonary disease (COPD)
   e. Performing a physical examination of a newly admitted patient

REFERENCES AND SELECTED READINGS

References and selected readings associated with this chapter can be found on the website that accompanies the book. Visit **http://thepoint.lww.com/Honan3e** to access the references and other additional resources associated with this chapter.

CHAPTER 2

Chronic Illness and End-of-Life Care

Kara H. McGee • Jessica Goldberg

Learning Objectives

After reading this chapter, you will be able to:

1. Define "chronic illness."
2. Identify factors related to the increasing incidence of chronic diseases.
3. Describe the characteristics of chronic illness and its impact on patients.
4. Describe implications of caring for patients with chronic illnesses for nursing practice.
5. Define and compare palliative and hospice care.
6. Describe the principles and components of hospice care.
7. Identify barriers to improving care at the end of life.
8. Identify and describe eight tasks that are essential for nurses to manage at the end of a patient's life.
9. Apply skills for communicating with terminally ill patients and their families or other caregivers.

Chronic diseases account for seven of the ten leading causes of death in the United States, including the four most frequently occurring diseases (heart disease, stroke, cancer, and diabetes) that may result from preventable causes (tobacco use, unhealthy diet and physical inactivity, and alcohol use). Chronic illnesses affect people of all ages, and of all ethnic, cultural, and racial groups, although some illnesses occur more frequently in some groups than in others (Boersma et al., 2020). The nonclinical characteristics of a person's life, including poverty, food insecurity, and education level, create disparities in the development of chronic illnesses (Butkus et al., 2020).

Many people with chronic illnesses function independently with only minor inconvenience to their everyday lives; others require frequent and close monitoring or placement in long-term care facilities. Certain illnesses require advanced technology for survival, as in the late stages of amyotrophic lateral sclerosis (ALS) or end-stage kidney disease (ESKD), or intensive care for periods of weeks or months. People with diseases such as these have been described as chronically critically and progressively ill. Some chronic illnesses have little effect on quality of life, but others have a significant impact because they can result in a progressive decline. The nurse recognizes that many patients admitted to acute care institutions have pre-existing chronic diseases that must continue to be managed along with their acute illnesses.

OVERVIEW OF CHRONICITY

Although each chronic disease has its own specific physiologic characteristics, chronic diseases do share common features. For example, many chronic diseases have pain and fatigue as associated symptoms. Usually, some degree of physical decline is present in severe or advanced chronic illness, limiting the patient's participation in many activities. Many chronic diseases require therapeutic regimens to keep them under control. Unlike the term "acute," which implies a reversible and relatively short course of disease, the term "chronic" describes a long course of disease and illnesses that may be incurable. This often makes managing chronic illnesses challenging for those who must live with them.

People who develop chronic illnesses may react with shock, disbelief, depression, anger, resentment, or any number of emotions. How people react to and cope with chronic illness is usually similar to how they react to other difficult events in their lives. Each person's individual coping style depends, in part, on their understanding of the illness and their perceptions of its potential impact on their own and their family's lives. Adjustment to chronic illness is affected by various factors:

- Suddenness, extent, and duration of lifestyle changes caused by the illness

- Family and individual resources for coping with stress
- Stage of individual/family life cycle
- Previous experience with illness and crises
- Underlying personality characteristics
- Unresolved anger or grief from the past

Psychological, emotional, and cognitive reactions to chronic illnesses are likely to occur at the onset of the illness and recur if symptoms worsen or reappear after a period of remission. Often symptoms associated with chronic illnesses are unpredictable and may be perceived as crisis events by patients and their families, who must contend with both the uncertainty of the chronic illness and the unexpected changes it brings to their lives. These possible effects can guide nursing assessment and interventions for the patient who has a chronic illness.

Definition of Chronic Illnesses

The literature does not support a single uniform definition for chronic disease. Recurrent themes include the non–self-limited nature, the association with persistent and recurring health problems, the need to be constant with treatment, and a duration measured in months and years, not days and weeks (Schmidt, 2016; Stutzin, 2021). Traditionally, chronic diseases have focused on individual chronic pathologies. Now, however, health initiatives have expanded to include not only chronic disease but also chronic conditions such as functional limitations; anatomic problems that are not manifestations of physical disease but are permanent or long-standing; and a broad spectrum of behavioral health problems, some of which have traditionally not been classified as diseases. The specific condition may be a result of illness, genetic factors, or injury; it may be a consequence of illnesses or unhealthy behaviors that began during childhood and young adulthood. Management of chronic illness includes adjusting to symptoms and identity changes resulting from life as a chronically ill person. It also consists of carrying out the lifestyle changes and regimens designed to control symptoms and to prevent complications (Schulman-Green et al., 2016; Stutzin, 2021). Although some people assume what might be called a "sick role" identity, most people with chronic illness wish to be involved in health care decision-making, and perform as active participants in their health care with preferences for their treatment and management of disease.

Prevalence and Causes of Chronic Illnesses

Chronic illnesses occur in people of every age group, socioeconomic level, and culture. In the United States, as of 2018, about half of all adults—129 million people—had one or more chronic health conditions. One of four adults had two or more chronic health conditions (Table 2-1) (Boersma et al., 2020). As the incidence of chronic illnesses increases, the costs associated with these illnesses (e.g., hospital costs, equipment, medications, supportive services) also increase; expenditures for health care for people with chronic illnesses exceed billions of dollars every year (CDC, 2022; Figueroa et al., 2021).

TABLE 2-1 Percentage of Adults with Chronic Diseases in the United States (2019)

Chronic Diseases	Adults with the Disease (%)[a]
Arthritis	23.5
Asthma	9.9
Chronic obstructive pulmonary disease among adults >= 45 years	9.0
Chronic kidney disease	2.6
Cardiovascular Disease	
Hypercholesterolemia	30.6
Hypertension	29.8
Diabetes	9.6

[a]Age-adjusted prevalence%.
Adapted from CDC (2022a).

Although some chronic health illnesses cause little or no inconvenience, others are severe enough to cause major activity limitations. When people with activity limitations are unable to meet their needs for health care and personal services, they may be unable to carry out their therapeutic regimens or have their prescriptions filled on time, may miss appointments and office visits with their health care providers, and may be unable to carry out their activities of daily living (ADLs).

Chronic disease is a global issue that affects both rich and poor nations. With the advent and distribution of highly active antiretroviral therapies and other treatments for communicable diseases, and thus longer lifespans, the incidence of chronic illness is increasing in developing countries of the Global South, even while they try to cope with new and emerging infectious diseases. In developed Western countries of the Global North, chronic illnesses have become the major cause of health-related problems. The Global North represents the world's more economically developed societies, including Europe, North America, Australia, Israel, and South Africa, while the Global South represents the economically developing or less-developed countries of Africa, India, China, Brazil, and Mexico, among others.

Causes of the increase in the number of people with chronic illnesses include the following:

- A decrease in mortality from infectious diseases, such as smallpox, diphtheria, and other serious illnesses
- Longer lifespans because of advances in technology and pharmacology, improved nutrition, safer working conditions, and greater access (for some people) to health care
- Improved screening and diagnostic procedures, enabling early detection and treatment of diseases

- Prompt and aggressive management of acute illnesses, such as myocardial infarction and AIDS-related infections
- The tendency to develop chronic illnesses with advancing age
- Lifestyle factors, such as smoking, chronic stress, and a sedentary lifestyle, which increase the risk for chronic health problems such as respiratory disease, hypertension, cardiovascular disease, and obesity

Consequences of unhealthy lifestyles include an increase in the incidence of diabetes, hypertension, obesity, and cardiac and chronic respiratory disorders. Physiologic changes in the body often occur before the appearance of symptoms of chronic disease. Therefore, the goal of emphasizing healthy lifestyles early in life is to improve overall health status and slow or prevent the development of such disorders.

Characteristics of Chronic Illnesses

Sometimes it is difficult for people who are disease-free to understand the often-profound effect of chronic illness on the lives of patients and their families. Health professionals may inadvertently focus on the illness itself while overlooking the personhood of the individual who has the disorder. In all illnesses, but even more so with chronic illnesses, the illness cannot be separated from the person. People with chronic illness must contend with it daily. To relate to what people must cope with or to plan effective interventions, nurses must understand what it means to have a chronic illness. Characteristics of chronic illness include the following:

- Managing chronic illness involves more than managing medical problems. Associated psychological and social problems must be addressed because living for long periods with illness symptoms and disability can threaten identity, bring about role changes, alter body image, and disrupt lifestyles. These changes require continuous adaptation and accommodation, depending on age and situation in life. Each decline in functional ability requires physical, emotional, and social adaptation for patients and their families.
- Over the course of a person's lifetime, chronic illnesses usually involve many different phases, including acute periods, stable and unstable periods, flare-ups, and remissions. Each phase brings its own set of physical, psychological, and social problems, and each requires its own regimens and types of management. Table 2-2 describes the phases in the trajectory model of chronic illness.
- Managing chronic illness requires persistent adherence to therapeutic regimens. Inconsistent or nonadherence to a treatment plan increases the risks of developing complications and accelerating the disease process. However, the realities of daily life, including the impact of culture, values, and socioeconomic factors, affect the degree to which people adhere to a treatment regimen. Managing a chronic illness takes time, requires knowledge and planning, and can be uncomfortable and inconvenient. It is not unusual for patients to stop taking medications or alter dosages because of side effects that are more disturbing or disruptive than symptoms of the illness, or to cut back on regimens they consider overly time-consuming, fatiguing, or costly. In fact, up to 50% of those with chronic illness will be nonadherent to long-term treatment plans; this contributes to high rates of premature death and poor health outcomes (Stutzin, 2021).
- One chronic disease can lead to the development of other chronic illnesses. Diabetes, for example, can affect many parts of the body and is associated with serious complications, such as heart disease and stroke, blindness, kidney failure, and lower-limb amputation. The presence of a chronic illness also contributes to a higher risk of morbidity and mortality in patients admitted to the intensive care unit with acute health illnesses.
- Chronic illness affects the entire family. Family life may be dramatically altered as a result of role reversals, unfilled roles, loss of income, time required to manage the illness, decreases in family socialization activities, and the costs of treatment. Stress and caregiver fatigue are common with severe chronic illnesses, and the entire family rather than just the patient may need care. However, some families dealing with chronic illness are able to master the treatment regimen and successfully incorporate the changes that accompany chronic illness into the routine of daily life. Furthermore, they are able to prevent the chronic illness from becoming the focal point of family life (Schulman-Green et al., 2021).
- The daily management of illness is largely the responsibility of people with chronic disorders and their families. As a result, the home, rather than the hospital, is the center of care in chronic illnesses. Hospitals, clinics, providers' offices, nursing homes, nursing centers, and community agencies (home care services, social services, and disease-specific associations and societies) are considered adjuncts or backup services to daily home management.
- The management of chronic illnesses is a process of discovery. People can be taught how to self-manage their illnesses. However, each person must discover how their own body reacts under varying circumstances—for example, what it is like to be hypoglycemic, what activities are likely to bring on chest pain, and how these or other illnesses can best be prevented and managed.
- Managing chronic illnesses must be a collaborative process in which many different health care professionals, patients, and their families work together to provide the full range of services that are typically needed for home management. Often the medical, social, and psychological aspects of chronic health problems are complex, especially in severe illnesses. The ultimate goal is to help patients to self-manage and take full responsibility for their own health.

TABLE **2-2 Phases in the Trajectory Model of Chronic Illness**

Phase	Description	Focus of Nursing Care
Pre-trajectory	Genetic factors or lifestyle behaviors that place a person or community at risk for a chronic condition	Refer for genetic testing and counseling if indicated; provide education about prevention of modifiable risk factors and behaviors
Trajectory onset	Appearance or onset of noticeable symptoms associated with a chronic disorder; includes period of diagnostic workup and announcement of diagnosis; may be accompanied by uncertainty as patient awaits a diagnosis and begins to discover and cope with implications of diagnosis	Provide clear explanations of diagnostic tests and procedures and reinforce information and explanations given by health care providers; provide emotional support to patient and family
Stable	Illness course and symptoms are under control as symptoms, resulting disability, and everyday life activities are being managed within limitations of illness; illness management is centered in the home	Reinforce positive behaviors and offer ongoing monitoring; provide education about health promotion and encourage participation in self-management, health-promoting activities, and health screening
Unstable	Characterized by an exacerbation of illness symptoms, development of complications, or reactivation of an illness in remission Period of inability to keep symptoms under control or reactivation of illness; difficulty in carrying out everyday life activities May require more diagnostic testing and trial of new treatment regimens or adjustment of current regimen, with care usually taking place at home	Provide guidance and support; reinforce previous teaching
Acute	Severe and unrelieved symptoms or the development of illness complications necessitating hospitalization, bed rest, or interruption of the person's usual activities to bring illness course under control	Provide direct care and emotional support to the patient and family members
Crisis	Critical or life-threatening situation requiring emergency treatment or care and suspension of everyday life activities until the crisis has passed	Provide direct care, collaborate with other health care team members to stabilize patient's condition
Comeback	Gradual recovery after an acute period and learning to live with or to overcome disabilities and return to an acceptable way of life within the limitations imposed by the chronic condition or disability; involves physical healing, limitations stretching through rehabilitative procedures, psychosocial coming-to-terms, and biographical reengagement with adjustments in everyday life activities	Assist in coordination of care; rehabilitative focus may require care from other health care providers; provide positive reinforcement for goals identified and accomplished
Downward	Illness course characterized by rapid or gradual worsening of a condition; physical decline accompanied by increasing disability or difficulty in controlling symptoms; requires biographical adjustment and alterations in everyday life activities with each major downward step	Provide home care and other community-based care to help patient and family adjust to changes and come to terms with these changes; assist patient and family to integrate new treatment and management strategies; encourage identification of end-of-life preferences and planning
Dying	Final days or weeks before death; characterized by gradual or rapid shutting down of body processes, biographical disengagement and closure, and relinquishment of everyday life interests and activities	Provide direct and supportive care to patients and their families through hospice programs

Adapted from Corbin, J. M. (1998). The Corbin and Strauss chronic illness trajectory model: an update. *Scholarly Inquiry for Nursing Practice*, *12*(1), 33–41.

- The management of chronic illnesses is expensive. Many of the expenses incurred by an individual patient (e.g., costs for hospital stays, diagnostic tests, equipment, medications, and supportive services) may be covered by health insurance and by federal and state agencies. However, the cost increases affect society as a whole as insurance premiums increase to cover these costs. Cost increases at the government level decrease resources that might benefit society. In addition, many out-of-pocket expenses are not reimbursed. Many people with chronic disorders, including older individuals and people who are working, are uninsured or underinsured and may be unable to afford the high costs of care often associated with chronic illnesses. Absence from work because of chronic disorders may jeopardize job security and income, and consequently health coverage. The financial toxicities associated with chronic illness are a significant concern for many, particularly in light of rising health care costs (CDC, 2022).
- Chronic illnesses raise difficult ethical issues for patients, health care professionals, and society. Problematic questions include how to establish cost controls, how to allocate scarce resources (e.g., organs for transplantation), what constitutes quality of life, and when life-sustaining therapies should be withdrawn.
- Living with chronic illness means living with uncertainty. Although health care providers may be aware of the usual progression of a chronic disease such as Parkinson disease, no one can predict with certainty a person's illness course because of individual variation. Even when a patient is in remission or symptom-free, they often fear that the illness will reappear.

Implications of Managing Chronic Illnesses

Chronic illnesses have implications for everyday living and management for people and their families, as well as for society at large. Most importantly, individual efforts should be directed at chronic illness prevention because many chronic illnesses or disorders are linked to unhealthy lifestyles or behaviors such as smoking, inactivity, and overeating. Therefore, changes in lifestyle can prevent some chronic disorders, or at least delay onset until a later age. Because most people resist change, bringing about alterations in people's lifestyles is a major challenge for nurses today.

Once a chronic condition has emerged, the focus shifts to managing symptoms, avoiding complications (e.g., eye complications in a person with diabetes), and avoiding the development of other acute illnesses (e.g., pneumonia in a person with chronic obstructive pulmonary disease). Health-promoting behaviors, such as exercise, are essential to quality of life in people who have chronic illnesses because regular exercise helps to maintain functional status. Encouraging discussions about quality of life, often overlooked by health professionals in their approach to people with chronic illnesses, is also important, especially in the later stages of a chronic illness.

Although coworkers, extended family, and health care professionals are affected by chronic illnesses, the problems of living with chronic illnesses are most acutely experienced by patients and their immediate families. Chronic illness forces patients and families to make lifestyle modifications that directly impact quality of life. Nurses provide direct care, especially during acute episodes, but they also provide teaching, help secure resources, and provide other supports that enable people to integrate their illness into their lives and to have an acceptable quality of life despite the illness. To understand what nursing care is needed, it is important to recognize and appreciate the issues that people with chronic illness and their families contend with and manage, often on a daily basis. The challenges of living with chronic illnesses include the need to accomplish the following:

- Alleviate and manage symptoms
- Psychologically adjust to and physically accommodate disabilities
- Prevent and manage crises and complications
- Adhere to regimens as prescribed
- Validate individual self-worth and family functioning
- Manage threats to identity
- Normalize personal and family life as much as possible
- Live with altered time, social isolation, and loneliness
- Establish networks and resources to support and enhance quality of life
- Return to an acceptable way of life after an acute debilitating episode (e.g., another myocardial infarction or stroke) or reactivation of a chronic condition
- Die with dignity and comfort

Many people with chronic illness must face the additional challenge of living with more than one chronic illness at a time. Multiple illnesses are termed *comorbidities*. The symptoms or treatment of a second chronic condition may aggravate the first chronic condition. Patients need to be able to deal with their various chronic illnesses separately as well as in combination. Furthermore, the effects of increasing longevity among Americans are likely to increase health care costs in the future.

Even more challenging for many people with chronic illness is the need to hire and oversee caregivers who come into their homes to assist with ADLs and instrumental activities of daily living (IADLs). ADLs and IADLs are the activities that let an individual live independently in a community, such as preparing meals, shopping, telephone use, and taking medications correctly. It is difficult for many people to be in a position of hiring, supervising, and sometimes firing people who may provide them with intimate physical care. The need to balance the dual role of care recipient and care manager may lead to blurring of role boundaries.

The challenges of living with and managing a chronic illness are well known, and people with chronic illnesses often report receiving inadequate care, information, services, and counseling. This provides an opportunity for nurses to address many of the issues experienced, to coordinate care, and to serve as an advocate for patients and their families who need additional assistance to manage the patient's illness while maintaining a quality of life that is acceptable to all of them.

Phases of Chronic Illnesses

Chronic illnesses can pass through different phases, as described in Table 2-2. However, this course may be too uncertain to predict with any degree of accuracy. The course of an illness can be thought of as a trajectory that can be managed or shaped over time, to some extent, through proper illness management strategies. It is important to keep in mind that not all phases occur in all patients; some phases do not occur at all, and some phases may recur. Each phase is characterized by different medical and psychosocial issues. For example, the needs of a patient with a stroke who is a good candidate for rehabilitation are very different from those of a patient with terminal cancer. By thinking in terms of phases and individual patients within a phase, nurses can target their care more specifically to each person. Not every chronic condition is necessarily life-threatening, and not every patient passes through each possible phase of a chronic condition in the same order.

Using the trajectory model enables the nurse to put the current situation into the context of what might have happened to the patient in the past—that is, the life factors and understandings that might have contributed to the current state of the illness. In this way, the nurse can more readily address the underlying issues and problems.

NURSING CARE OF PATIENTS WITH CHRONIC ILLNESSES

Nursing care of patients with chronic illnesses is varied and occurs in a variety of settings. Care may be direct or supportive. *Direct care* may be provided in the clinic or health provider's office, the hospital, or the patient's home, depending on the status of the illness. Examples of direct care include assessing the patient's physical status, providing wound care, managing and overseeing medication regimens, and performing other technical tasks. The availability of this type of nursing care may allow the patient to remain at home and return to a more normal life after an acute episode of illness. *Supportive care* may include ongoing monitoring, teaching, counseling, serving as an advocate for the patient, navigating the system to coordinate care, making referrals, and case-managing. Providing supportive care is just as important as giving technical care. For example, through ongoing home or clinic monitoring, a nurse might detect early signs of impending complications and make a referral (i.e., contact the provider or consult the medical protocol in a clinic) for medical evaluation, thereby preventing a lengthy and costly hospitalization.

Working with people with chronic illness requires not only dealing with the medical aspects of their disorders but also working with the whole person—physically, emotionally, and socially. This holistic approach to care requires nurses to draw on their knowledge and skills, including knowledge from the social sciences and psychology. Although quality of life usually is affected by chronic illness, especially if the illness is severe, patients' perceptions of what constitutes quality of life often drive their management behaviors or affect how they view advice about health care. Nurses and other health care professionals should recognize this, even though it may be difficult to see patients make unwise choices and decisions about lifestyles and disease management. People have the right to receive care without fearing ridicule or refusal of treatment, even if their behaviors (e.g., smoking, substance abuse, overeating, and failure to follow health care providers' recommendations) may have contributed to their chronic disorder.

Unfolding Patient Stories: S.H. • Part 1

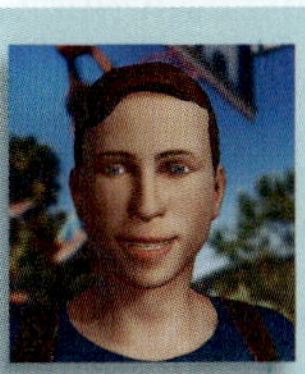

S.H. is an 18-year-old patient recently diagnosed with type 1 diabetes, who lives with two younger siblings and their parents and is active in high school sports. The patient now requires insulin injections, glucose monitoring, and a diabetic diet. Examine how the psychological, physical, and teaching needs for managing a new diagnosis can be a great source of stress to the patient and family. How can the nurse enhance their ability to cope with and adapt to diabetes management? (S.H.'s story continues in Chapter 29.)

Care for S.H. and other patients in a realistic virtual environment: ***vSim** for Nursing* (thepoint.lww.com/vSimMedicalSurgical). Practice documenting these patients' care in DocuCare (thepoint.lww.com/DocuCareEHR).

Skills for Communicating With the Chronically Ill

Nurses need to develop skill and comfort in assessing patients' and families' responses to chronic illness and planning interventions that will support their values and choices throughout the continuum of care. Patients and families need ongoing assistance: telling a patient something once is not teaching, and hearing the patient's words is not the same as active listening. Throughout the course of illness, patients and their families encounter complicated treatment decisions, bad news about disease progression, and recurring emotional responses. In addition to the time of initial diagnosis, lack of response to the treatment course, decisions to continue or withdraw particular interventions, and decisions about hospice care are examples of critical points on the treatment continuum that require patience, empathy, and honesty from nurses. Discussing sensitive issues such as progressive illness, hopes for survival, and fears associated with death is never easy. However, the art of therapeutic communication can be learned and, like other skills, must be practiced to gain expertise. Similar to other skills, communication should be practiced in a "safe" setting, such as a classroom or clinical skills laboratory with other students or clinicians.

Although communication with each patient and family should be tailored to their particular level of understanding and values concerning disclosure, general guidelines for nurses include the following:

- Deliver and interpret the technical information necessary for making decisions without hiding behind medical terminology.
- Realize that the best time for the patient to talk may be when it is least convenient for you.
- The importance of being fully present and using active listening techniques cannot be overstated.
- Allow the patient and family to set the agenda regarding the depth of the conversation.
- Realize that beginning the conversation requires a willingness to continue it, despite any personal inconvenience or discomfort on the part of the nurse.

When Patients and Families Receive Bad News

Communicating about a life-threatening diagnosis or about disease progression is best accomplished by the interdisciplinary team in any setting: a physician, advanced practice nurse, nurse, and social worker should be present whenever possible to provide information, facilitate discussion, and address concerns. Most importantly, the presence of the entire team conveys caring and respect for the patient and family. If the patient wishes to have family present for the discussion, arrangements should be made to have the discussion at a time that is best for everyone. A quiet area with a minimum of disturbances should be used. All team members present should turn off beepers, cell phones, and other electronic devices for the duration of the meeting and should allow sufficient time for the patient and family to absorb and respond to the news. Finally, the space in which the meeting takes place should ideally be conducive to seating all participants at eye level.

After the initial discussion of a life-threatening illness or progression of a disease, the patient and family often have many questions and may need to be reminded of factual information. Coping with news about a serious diagnosis or poor prognosis is an ongoing process. The nurse should be sensitive to these ongoing needs and may need to repeat previously provided information or simply be present and allow for pauses or silence while the patient and family react emotionally. Seriously ill patients and their families need time and support to cope with the changes brought about by changes in the patient's condition and the prospect of impending death. The nurse who is able to sit comfortably with another's suffering, time and time again, without judgment and without the need to solve the patient's and family's problems, provides an intervention that is a gift beyond measure.

THE CHANGING TRAJECTORY OF CHRONIC ILLNESS TO END-OF-LIFE CARE

As individuals become chronically ill, their health shifts between stable and unstable and acute and crisis events. During these periods of health status changes, patients will use increased health care services to regain their balance and recover. There are peaks and valleys to these patterns, and eventually patients reach a point from which they do not rebound, and they become progressively ill, decline, and die. It is during these periods of time when chronically ill patients come in contact with members of the health care team who should evaluate them for unmet palliative care needs to enhance their care and improve and sustain their quality of life.

Providing end-of-life care for someone chronically ill is very different from providing it to someone who dies suddenly from an accident, trauma, disaster, or homicide. When a death is sudden, there is tremendous shock and disbelief by the person's survivors that the person has died. The shock is compounded if the death was thought to be preventable, or if it resulted from a reckless act of irresponsibility, such as from a drunk driving crash. When a person has a chronic disease that progresses with a predictable trajectory, it gives the patient and family members opportunities to plan and participate in decisions about their goals and values, treatment choices, and resources for enhancing their quality of life individually and as a family.

Sociocultural Context

Although each person experiences terminal illness uniquely, that illness is also shaped substantially by the social and cultural contexts in which it occurs. In the United States, life-threatening illness, life-sustaining treatment decisions, dying, and death occur in a social environment in which illness is largely considered a foe and battles are either lost or won (Hui et al., 2018; Swiss Academy of Medical Sciences, 2021). A care–cure dichotomy emerged early on in modern medicine, in which health care providers may view cure as the ultimate goal and care as second best and only acceptable when cure is no longer possible. In this model of health care, alleviating suffering is not as valued as curing disease, and patients who cannot be cured feel distanced from the health care team, concluding that when treatment has failed, they too have failed. Patients and families who have internalized the socially constructed meaning of care as second-best to cure may fear that any shift from curative goals in the direction of comfort-focused care will result in no care or lower-quality care, and that the providers on whom they have come to rely will abandon them if they withdraw from the battle for cure. The fear of provider abandonment can be alleviated in part by a compassionate, reassuring nursing presence during difficult transitional periods (Back et al., 2009; Shalev et al., 2022).

The reduction of patients to their diseases is exemplified in the frequently relayed message in late-stage illness that "nothing more can be done." This all-too-frequently used statement communicates the belief of many providers that there is nothing of value to offer patients who are beyond cure. In a care-focused perspective, mind, body, and spirit are inextricable, and treating the body without attending to the mind and spirit is considered inadequate to evoke true healing. The idea of healing as care, along with and beyond cure, implies that healing can take place throughout life and outside the boundaries of contemporary medicine. In this expanded definition, there continue to be opportunities for physical, spiritual, emotional, and social healing, even as body systems begin to fail at the end of life.

Providers' attitudes toward the terminally ill and dying remain the greatest barrier to improving care at the end of life. Kübler-Ross illuminated the concerns of the seriously ill and dying in her seminal work, *On Death and Dying,* published in 1969. At that time, it was common for patients to be kept uninformed about life-threatening diagnoses, particularly cancer, and for physicians and nurses to avoid open discussion of death and dying with their patients. Kübler-Ross taught the health care community that having open discussion about life-and-death issues did not harm patients and that the patients, in fact, welcomed such openness. She was openly critical of what she called "a new but depersonalized science in the service of prolonging life rather than diminishing human suffering" (Kübler-Ross, 1969). She taught the health care community that healing could not take place in a conspiracy of silence, and that as providers break the silence and enter the patient's world, they too can be enriched by being partners with their patients. Her work revealed that, given adequate time and some help in working through the process, patients could reach a stage of acceptance in which they were neither angry nor depressed about their fate.

Providers' reluctance to discuss disease and death openly with patients may stem from their own anxieties about death, as well as misconceptions about what and how much patients want to know about their illnesses. In a seminal study of care of the dying in hospital settings, sociologists Glaser and Strauss (1965) identified that health care professionals in hospital settings avoided direct communication about dying in hopes that the patient would discover it on their own. They identified four "awareness contexts" that described awareness of the patient's status by providers, patients, and family members.

- *Closed awareness,* in which the patient is unaware of their terminal state
- *Suspected awareness,* in which the patient suspects what others know and attempts to find out details about their condition
- *Mutual pretense,* in which the patient, family, and providers are aware that the patient is dying but all pretend otherwise
- *Open awareness,* in which the patient, family, and providers are aware that the patient is dying and openly acknowledge that reality (Glaser & Strauss, 1965).

The two major reasons they identified for which providers avoided direct communication with patients about the seriousness of their illness were (1) patients already knew the truth or would ask if they wanted to know; or (2) patients would subsequently lose all hope, give up, or be psychologically harmed by disclosure. Glaser and Strauss' findings were published decades ago, yet their observations remain valid today. Although a growing number of health care providers are becoming comfortable with assessing patients' and families' information needs and disclosing honest information about the seriousness of illness, many still avoid the topic of death in hope that the patient will ask or find out on their own. Despite progress on many health care fronts, those who work with dying patients have identified the persistence of a "conspiracy of silence" about dying.

The Importance of Palliative Care in Chronic Illness

As patients decline and treatments become complex, there has been an international recognition of the need to help patients transition from a cure orientation to one of care. Palliative care and hospice care have been recognized as important bridges between a medical bias in the direction of cure-oriented treatment and the needs of terminally ill patients and their families for comprehensive care in the final years, months, or weeks of life. This bridge has been built by experts in the field who advocate that palliative care needs to be extended throughout the course of life-threatening illness from the time when the patient is first diagnosed and not limited to end-of-life care (Bickel et al., 2016; Kmetec et al., 2022). It is a common misconception among patients, families, and even some health care professionals that palliative care is only for those at end-of-life. In fact, palliative care should be offered at diagnosis to anyone living with any serious illness—at any age, any stage, any diagnosis.

Palliative care encompasses a wide range of therapeutic interventions that aim to prevent and relieve suffering caused by multiple issues that patients and family caregivers face at any stage during an acute or chronic illness. In providing palliative care to the whole person (Ferrell et al., 2018b), health care providers attend to all domains of the human experience of illness that may be involved: physical, psychological, social, and spiritual. A number of models of care have described the difference in these approaches to treatment. An exclusively "cure-oriented" approach to chronic illness care

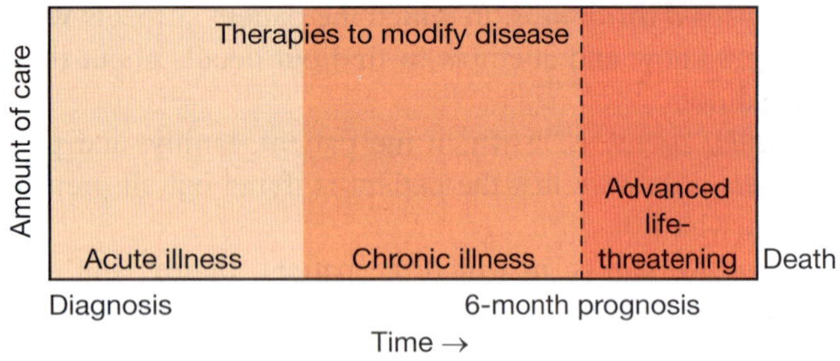

FIGURE 2-1 **Model of cancer care in which only therapies directed at the disease are considered as part of standard care. (From Irwin, S. A., & von Guntun, C. F. [2010]. The role of palliative care in cancer care transitions. In J. C. Holland, W. S. Bretibart, P. B. Jacobsen, M. S. Lederberg, M. J. Loscalzo, & R. McCorkle [Eds.], *Psycho-oncology* [2nd ed., pp. 277–283]. Oxford University Press.)**

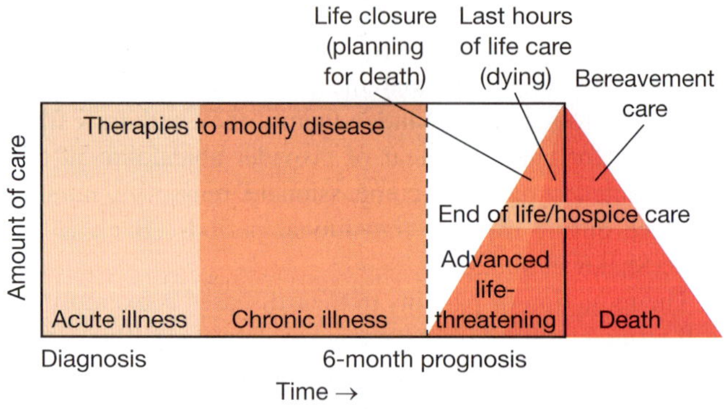

FIGURE 2-3 **Model of cancer care in which palliative care begins after efforts directed at the disease end. (From Irwin, S. A., & von Guntun, C. F. [2010]. The role of palliative care in cancer care transitions. In J. C. Holland, W. S. Bretibart, P. B. Jacobsen, M. S. Lederberg, M. J. Loscalzo, & R. McCorkle [Eds.], *Psycho-oncology* [2nd ed., pp. 277–283]. Oxford University Press.)**

can be conceptualized in Figure 2-1; here, the treatment is compartmentalized by the type of illness and disease events. In Figure 2-2, the treatment of a disease diminishes over time as treatment becomes less effective. In Figure 2-3, "comfort care" is instituted when the patient with a chronic illness is not responding to the previous treatments, and additional symptom management efforts are needed. Figure 2-4 illustrates how palliative care can begin at diagnosis and become integrated throughout the entire course of the chronic illness trajectory for the patient and family caregiver. Ideally, palliative care should precede the time when the provider recognizes that hospice care is needed. When palliative care coexists with disease-oriented treatment, patients and their families benefit from the more comprehensive management of the illness experience.

Goal Setting in Palliative Care

As treatment goals begin to shift in the direction of comfort-focused care over aggressive disease-directed treatment, symptom relief and patient- and family-defined quality of life assume greater prominence in treatment decision-making. Patients, families, and health care providers all may be accustomed to an almost automatic tendency to pursue exhaustive diagnostic testing to locate and treat the source of patients' illnesses or symptoms. Each decision to withdraw treatment or discontinue diagnostic testing may be an extremely emotional one for the patient and family. They may fear that the support from health care providers on whom they have come to rely will be withdrawn along with the treatment.

Throughout the course of the illness, and especially as the patient's functional status and symptoms indicate approaching death, the provider should help the patient and family weigh the benefits of continued diagnostic testing and disease-focused medical treatment against the burdens of those activities. The patient and family may be extremely reluctant to forego monitoring that has become routine throughout the illness (e.g., blood testing, x-rays) but that may contribute little to comfort. Likewise, health care providers from other disciplines may have difficulty discontinuing such diagnostic testing or medical treatment.

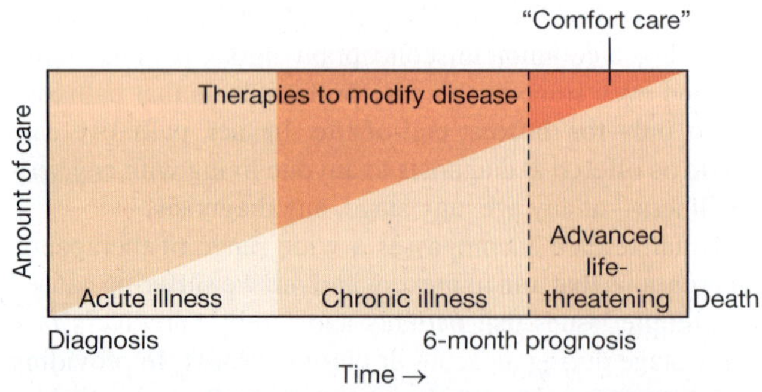

FIGURE 2-2 **Model of cancer care in which antidisease treatment diminishes over time as it becomes less and less effective. (From Irwin, S. A., & von Guntun, C. F. [2010]. The role of palliative care in cancer care transitions. In J. C. Holland, W. S. Bretibart, P. B. Jacobsen, M. S. Lederberg, M. J. Loscalzo, & R. McCorkle [Eds.], *Psycho-oncology* [2nd ed., pp. 277–283]. Oxford University Press.)**

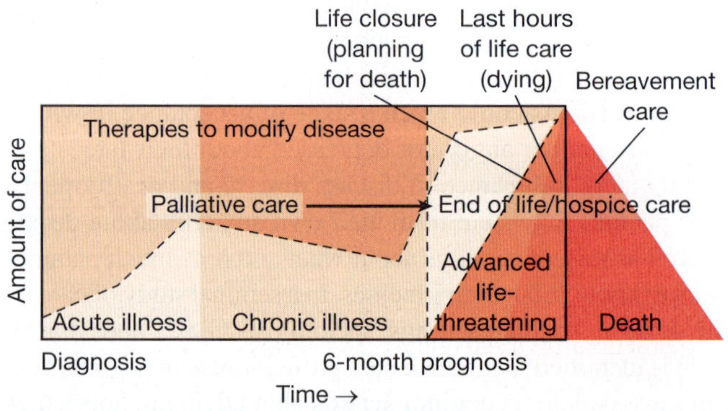

FIGURE 2-4 **Model of cancer care in which palliative care begins at diagnosis and is integrated throughout the course of treatment. (From Irwin, S. A., & von Guntun, C. F. [2010]. The role of palliative care in cancer care transitions. In J. C. Holland, W. S. Bretibart, P. B. Jacobsen, M. S. Lederberg, M. J. Loscalzo, & R. McCorkle [Eds.]. *Psycho-oncology* [2nd ed., pp. 277–283]. Oxford University Press.)**

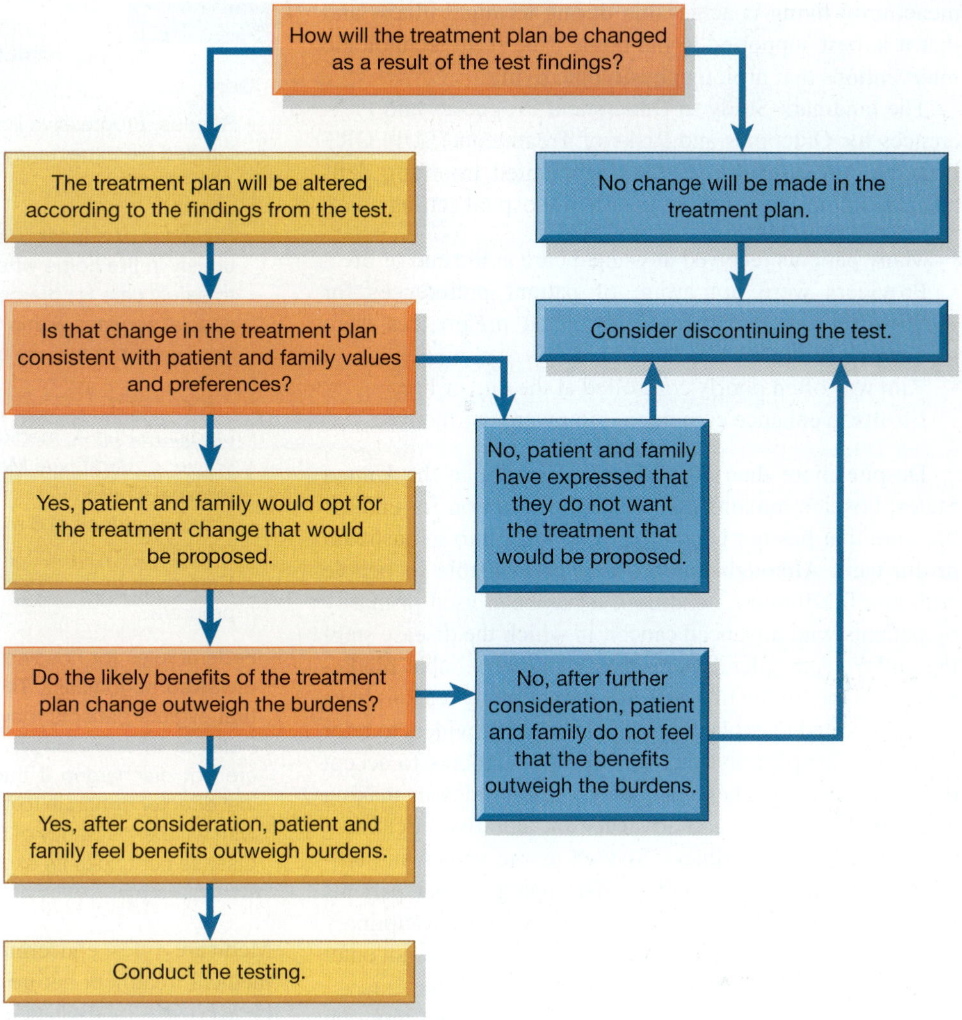

FIGURE 2-5 An algorithm for decision-making about diagnostic testing at the end of life.

Specifically, the nurse should collaborate with other members of the interdisciplinary team to share assessment findings and develop a coordinated plan of care (Fig. 2-5). In addition, the nurse should help the patient and family clarify their goals, expected outcomes, and values as they consider treatment options (Box 2-1). The nurse should work with interdisciplinary colleagues to ensure that the patient and family are referred for continuing psychosocial support, symptom management, and assistance with other care-related challenges (e.g., arrangements for home care or hospice support, referrals for financial assistance).

Hospice Care in the United States

The broadening of the concept of palliative care followed the development of the hospice movement in the United States. Hospice care is, in fact, palliative care. The difference is that hospice care is associated solely with the end of the patient's life, and although it focuses on quality of life, hospice care by necessity usually includes realistic emotional, social, spiritual, and financial preparation for death. The hospice movement in the United States is based on the belief that

BOX 2-1

Assessing the Patient and Family Perspective: Goal Setting in Palliative Care

Patient and Family

- **Awareness of diagnosis, illness stage, and prognosis:** "Tell me your understanding of your illness right now."
- **Values:** "Tell me what is most important to you as you are thinking about the treatment options available to you/your loved one."
- **Preferences:** "You've said that being comfortable and pain-free is most important to you right now. Where would you like to receive care (home, hospital, long-term care facility, doctor's office), and how can I help?"
- **Expected/desired outcomes:** "What are your hopes and expectations for this (diagnostic test [e.g., CT scan] or treatment)?"
- **Benefits and burdens:** "Is there a point at which you would say that the testing or treatment is outweighed by the burdens it is causing you (e.g., getting from home to the hospital, pain, nausea, fatigue, interference with other important activities)?"

meaningful living is achievable during terminal illness and that it is best supported in the home, free from technologic interventions that prolong physiologic dying.

The landmark Study to Understand Prognoses and Preferences for Outcomes and Risks of Treatments (SUPPORT Principal Investigators, 1995) documented troubling deficiencies in the care of dying people in hospital settings:

- Many patients received unwanted care at the end of life.
- Providers were not aware of patient preferences for life-sustaining treatment, even when preferences were documented in the clinical record.
- Pain was often poorly controlled at the end of life.
- Efforts to enhance communication were ineffective.

Despite more than 40 years of existence in the United States, hospice remains an underutilized option for end-of-life care that has not been integrated fully into mainstream health care. Although hospice care is available to people with any life-limiting condition, it has been used primarily by patients with advanced cancer, in which the disease staging and trajectory lend themselves to more reliable prediction about the timing of a person's dying. Many reasons have been suggested to explain the reluctance of providers to refer patients to hospice and the reluctance of patients to accept this form of care. These include the difficulties in making a terminal prognosis and advances in "curative" treatment options in late-stage illness, as well as the values and attitudes of health care providers. The result is that patients who could benefit from the comprehensive, interdisciplinary support offered by hospice programs frequently do not enter hospice care until their final days (or hours) of life.

After hospice care was recognized as a distinct program of services under Medicare in the early 1980s, organizations providing hospice care were able to receive Medicare reimbursement if they could demonstrate that the hospice program met the Medicare "conditions of participation." State Medical Assistance (Medicaid) also provides coverage for hospice care, as do most commercial insurers. Federal reimbursement for hospice care ushered in a new era in hospice, in which program standards developed and published by the federal government codified what had formerly been a grassroots, loosely organized, and somewhat undefined ideal for care at the end of life. In many aspects, Medicare standards have come to largely define hospice philosophy and services.

In most programs, the Medicare definitions for patient eligibility are used to guide all enrollment decisions. According to Medicare, the patient who wishes to use their Medicare Hospice Benefit must be certified by a physician as terminally ill, with a life expectancy of 6 months or less if the disease follows its natural course (Box 2-2). Thus, hospice has come to be defined as care provided to terminally ill persons and their families in the last 6 months of the patient's life. Most hospice care is provided at the "routine home care" level and includes the services depicted in Box 2-3. Because of additional Medicare rules concerning completion of all cure-focused medical treatment before the Medicare Hospice Benefit may be accessed, many patients delay enrollment in hospice programs until very close to the end of life. This enrollment delay is common in terminal cancer patients wishing to pursue cancer-directed treatment with the hope of slowing disease progression or those enrolled in clinical trials. Patients are reassessed for extension of eligibility at regular intervals, and

BOX 2-2

Eligibility Criteria for Hospice Care

General

- Serious, progressive illness
- Limited life expectancy

Hospice-Specific

- Presence of a family member or other caregiver continuously in the home when the patient is no longer able to safely care for themself (some hospices have created special services within their programs for patients who live alone, but this varies widely)

Medicare and Medicaid Hospice Benefits

- Medicare Part A; medical assistance eligibility
- Waiver of traditional Medicare/Medicaid benefits for the terminal illness
- Life expectancy of 6 months or less
- Provider certification of terminal illness
- Care must be provided by a Medicare-certified hospice program

Federal rules for hospices require that patients' eligibility be reviewed periodically. There is no limit to the length of time that eligible patients may continue to receive hospice care. Patients who live longer than 6 months under hospice care are not discharged if their provider and the hospice medical director continue to certify that the patient is terminally ill with a life expectancy of 6 months or less, assuming that the disease continues its expected course.

BOX 2-3

Home Hospice Services Covered Under the Medicare/Medicaid Hospice Benefit Routine Home Care Level

- Nursing care provided by or under the supervision of a registered nurse, available 24 hours a day
- Medical social services
- Physician's services
- Counseling services, including dietary counseling
- Home health aide/homemaker
- Physical/occupational/speech therapists
- Volunteers
- Bereavement follow-up (for up to 13 months after the death of the patient)
- Medical supplies for the palliation of the terminal illness
- Medical equipment for the palliation of the terminal illness
- Medications for the palliation of the terminal illness

then there is no limit on the amount of time a patient can spend under hospice care (Greenstein et al., 2019).

NURSING CARE OF TERMINALLY ILL PATIENTS

Nurses can have a significant and lasting effect on the way in which patients live until they die, the manner in which the death occurs, and the enduring memories of that death for the patient's survivors. Knowledge about end-of-life principles of care and patients' and families' unique responses to death is essential to supporting their unique values and goals (Box 2-4). There is an opportunity to bring research, education, and practice together to change the culture of dying, bringing much needed improvement to care that is relevant across practice settings, age groups, cultural backgrounds, and illnesses. A skillful, compassionate nursing presence at end-of-life can make the difference between a "good death" and a bad one.

Factors that Influence Dying

Many factors can directly or indirectly affect how a person dies and what happens to one's body and one's survivors after death. It is useful for nurses to think of these factors as those that cannot be changed by one's actions and those that can be influenced in some fashion.

Unalterable Factors

Unalterable factors are those that are constant, including the age, gender, and personality of the dying person. Cultural attitudes toward death and dying also cannot be changed and must be taken into account in providing care. Other factors that need to be assessed, and that may affect a person's dying or bereavement, are previous experiences with illness and death, the type of disease of the dying person and its expected course, and the actual cause of death. Death by suicide or from neglected care will affect the family's recovery and grief process negatively compared to a death that is expected. The survivors of people who die suddenly or take their own lives may have more emotional and physical problems than do survivors of people with long-term illnesses. In contrast, an expected death provides opportunities for the family to bring closure to their relationships and participate in maintaining the dying person's comfort. Certain diseases are associated with a likely trajectory or expected course of dying. Some patients will die very suddenly, and others will have ample time to participate in decisions surrounding their care. The nurse needs to understand the natural course of diseases and the changes that can be expected from treatment regimens in tandem with the responses of those family members left behind.

Changeable Factors

Changeable factors are those that can be influenced by nurses. These factors need ongoing reassessment because they *are* subject to change. These factors include the dying person's previous and current relationship with health care providers; the medical management of the illness; treatment effects; the projected prognosis; the meaning the dying person invests in the experience; and the resources

BOX 2-4 **Nursing Research**

Bridging the Gap to Evidence-Based Practice

Stokman, A., Brown, S., & Seacrist, M. (2021). Baccalaureate nursing students' engagement with end-of-life curriculum: A grounded theory study. *Nurse Education Today*, *102*, Article 104914.

Purpose

The art of being prepared to support patients and their families during end-of-life experiences is not always emphasized in nurse education. Despite the efforts from the American Association of Colleges of Nursing and End of Life Nursing Education Consortium (ELNEC), only 25% of nursing schools across the United States are using their modules. The purpose of this study was to explore how student nurses engage with end-of-life education.

Design

Qualitative study using a grounded theory approach. Baccalaureate nursing program located in the rural agricultural western United States. Using a grounded theory approach, student experiences and engagement with the curriculum were explored. Using the constant comparative method, three researchers coded the data independently and then came together to reach consensus on themes and for the development of the conceptual model.

Findings

Three categories emerged from the data to describe student engagement with the curriculum: Novice, Evolving, and Prepared. The central theme for the Novice students was *Being Afraid*. Students expressed fear over the unknown and not knowing what to say or do. *Becoming Aware* was the central theme for the Evolving students; this included a blend of being aware of their deficiencies as well as the important aspects of end-of-life care. The final category was Prepared. The theme for this category was *Becoming Accomplished*, which included recognition of respectful care, disrespectful care, team work, and advocacy.

Nursing Implications

There is an overall lack of consistent education across the nation on end-of-life and/or palliative care for nursing students. Yet, this education is essential for nursing students to provide appropriate care at end of life, as well as for providing improved knowledge, attitudes, and confidence of students. The End of Life Nursing Education Consortium modules, placed strategically within the curriculum, allow nursing students to move through the process of *Being Afraid*, to *Becoming Aware*, and finally *Becoming Accomplished* upon graduation.

available for support, including the primary caregiver's health and willingness to provide care. The overwhelming majority of patients repeatedly report they prefer to die at home, and if these factors are assessed and the patient's wishes are considered, dying at home may likely be possible for those patients who work together with their families and the nurse and medical staff to accomplish the patient's goals of care.

Critical Time Periods of Terminal Care

There are three critical time periods during terminal care: before death, the death event, and bereavement. In each period, guiding principles can direct nursing care for people who are dying and for their survivors (Berry & Griffie, 2019). Although a dying person and the survivors progress sequentially through the three time periods of terminal care, unfortunately the same nurse does not care for the patient and family throughout all three phases; therefore, it is essential that there is consensus about the critical aspects of care so that continuity can be provided to the patient and family regardless of who the health care provider is.

Predeath Period

Quint-Benoliel (1967), in her landmark study of the nurse and the dying patient, determined that progressively ill patients need the opportunity for three kinds of experiences that may be difficult to achieve in today's society. They need to (1) know what is happening to them and be able to talk about its reality with someone who will listen, (2) be allowed to experience the pain of "feeling bad" instead of having to hide their feelings to protect other people from the pain of their own feelings, and (3) participate in the decisions affecting how they will live their final days and how they will die (Quint, 1967). The primary responsibility of the nurse during the predeath period is to establish a relationship with the dying person. Through this relationship, the nurse should share information with the dying person about what is happening to them, as well as the available choices for care. It is important to establish this relationship while the dying person feels well enough to converse with the nurse about their goals and values as death approaches. It is primarily a time of assessment, not action, in which the nurse gathers data on how the person and family are coping with what is happening and how the options available fit within the person's lifestyle and goals for the future. Documentation regarding the person's disease state, responses to treatment, personal goals, and changes in family interactions is essential so that consistent care can be provided over time. As symptoms occur or change, the nurse elicits the meaning of the experience and helps the patient be informed about alternatives in treatment. Specific interventions are planned and evaluated after discussing with the patient the alternatives available, their effects, and long-term consequences.

The Death Event

Many people have misconceptions about how people die and whether dying patients are aware of what is happening to them. Most health care providers have seen people die only in institutional settings and when advanced medical technology had been used to sustain life. Most health care providers have not had an opportunity to witness a person dying without medical intervention and in the natural setting of home or another place of preference. Gradually, as the patient becomes more socially and physically dependent on others for assistance, the dying person and the family need increased supervision by providers. The primary purpose in being present as death becomes imminent is to anticipate problems, such as distressing symptoms or family disruptions, before they interfere with the dying person's wishes. The best of plans, well made over a period of months or weeks of preparation, can easily and unintentionally be undermined by any member of the health care team or family. Distressing symptoms that warrant hospitalization generally can be prevented if the nurse and provider are working closely together and the family has the resources for maintaining the person in the home. Some patients may prefer to die in an inpatient setting because they do not want to be a burden on their family or because their symptoms cannot be managed safely at home.

If possible, the nurse is present when the patient dies, or arranges to be called shortly thereafter, to assist with the preparation of the body and to support the family. If the patient dies in the hospital, the family may request ample time in private to be with the body. The nurse assists the family with answering questions, making telephone calls, and expressing grief. Depending on the patient's and family's cultural or religious beliefs, the nurse may be asked to provide help providing post-mortem care, or such care may only be permitted by certain family members. Nothing should be done without the family's permission, including helping to clean the patient's room after the death. Some families may want these tasks done for them, and others have a need to do them themselves. Once the death event is over, most nurses need an opportunity to debrief with someone they trust about the experience. It is important for nurses to develop a support network of their own to share their feelings and validate their care with others. Social workers, chaplains, and the palliative care or hospice team can be helpful in arranging a formal debrief for particularly challenging cases.

Bereavement

The third critical time period is the time after the death. Most members of the family may need several opportunities to relive the events surrounding the death, and the nurse is in a unique position to listen, having been a part of the experience. Often family and friends do not want to relive the events over and over and frequently send both overt and passive messages that the grieving person should get on with living. Part of the support given in reliving the death experience involves reinforcing the family's sense that they supported the dead person's wishes and communicating to the family that everything was done that could be done. The nurse should praise the family's efforts to be present and care for their loved one at the end of life. The length of time a nurse sees a family for bereavement varies. Usually, at least 3 months are needed to assist with making decisions and disposing of the dead person's belongings as well as to assess the family's coping with the loss; the COVID-19 pandemic has impacted the length and complexity of both the grieving process for victims' families and the general post-mortem logistics of death in the United States (Wallace et al., 2020). Family members need encouragement not to act impulsively and to think through the consequences of their decisions. The nurse helps the family to discuss options available and to talk not only about the major loss associated with the death but also the consequential losses (e.g., financial, emotional, and social). If a family member needs additional help, the nurse can make a referral to a mental health provider, support group, or primary care provider.

Communicating with the Terminally Ill

To develop a level of comfort and expertise in communicating with seriously and terminally ill patients and their families, nurses and other providers should first consider their own experiences with and values concerning illness and death. Reflection, reading, and talking with family members, friends, and colleagues can help nurses examine beliefs about death and dying. Talking with people from different cultural backgrounds can help nurses view personally held beliefs through a different lens and can help nurses become sensitive to death-related beliefs and practices in other cultures. Discussion with nursing and non-nursing colleagues also can be useful; it may reveal the values shared by many health care professionals and identify diversity in the values of patients in their care. Values clarification and personal death awareness exercises can provide a starting point for self-discovery and discussion. Asking a person to share a personal experience of someone who has died and what that experience was like for the person is a place to start.

Ethical Decision-Making in End-of-Life Care

Nurses are responsible for educating patients about the possibilities and probabilities inherent in their illness and their life with the illness, and for supporting them as they conduct life review, values clarification, treatment decision-making, and end-of-life closure. The only way to do this effectively is to try to appreciate and understand the illness from the patient's perspective. It is also important that patients have had an opportunity to identify their preferences for how decisions are made at the end of life through legal documents recognized on a federal and state level (Box 2-5).

BOX 2-5

Methods of Stating End-of-Life Preferences

Advance directives: Written documents that allow the individual of sound mind to document preferences regarding end-of-life care that should be followed when the signer is terminally ill and unable to communicate their wishes verbally. In general, the documents are completed in advance of serious illness but may be completed after a diagnosis of serious illness if the signer is still of sound mind. The most common types are the durable power of attorney for health care and the living will.

Durable power of attorney for health care: A legal document through which the signer appoints and authorizes another individual to make medical decisions on their behalf when they are no longer able to speak for themselves. This is also known as a *health care power of attorney* or a *proxy directive.*

Living will: A type of advance directive in which the individual documents treatment preferences. It provides instructions for care in the event that the signer is terminally ill and not able to communicate their wishes directly and often is accompanied by a durable power of attorney for health care. This is also known as a *medical directive* or *treatment directive.*

Information about the advance care planning and state-specific advance directive documents and instructions are available from the website of Caring Connections (http://caringinfo.org). The legality of these documents may vary across states and within institutions, and it is important that people have someone they have spoken to and trust who can advocate for individual preferences if needed.

At the same time, nurses should be both culturally aware and sensitive in their approaches to communication with patients and families about death. Attitudes toward open disclosure about terminal illness vary widely among different cultures, and direct communication with patients about such matters may be viewed as harmful. To provide effective patient- and family-centered care at the end of life, nurses must be willing to set aside their own assumptions and attitudes so that they can discover what type and amount of disclosure is most meaningful to each patient and family within their unique belief systems.

Providing Culturally Sensitive Care at the End of Life

Although death, grief, and mourning are universal aspects of living, one's values, expectations, and practices during serious illness, as death approaches, and after death are culturally bound and expressed. Health care providers may share very similar values concerning end-of-life care or may find that they are inadequately prepared to assess for and implement care plans that support culturally diverse perspectives. Historical mistrust of the health care system and unequal access to even basic medical care may underlie the beliefs and attitudes among ethnically diverse populations. In addition, limited health care literacy or knowledge about end-of-life care treatment options and language barriers influence decisions among many socioeconomically disadvantaged groups.

Much of the formal structure concerning health care decisions in the United States is rooted in the Western notions of autonomy, truth telling, and the acceptability of withdrawing or withholding life-prolonging medical treatment at the end of life. In many cultures, however, interdependence is valued over autonomy, leading to communication styles that favor relinquishment of decision-making to family members or to perceived authority figures, such as physicians or religious leaders. In addition, there is variation in preference regarding the use of life-prolonging medical treatments such as cardiopulmonary resuscitation and artificially provided nutrition and hydration at the end of life; some groups are less likely to agree with withholding or withdrawing such life supports from the patient with a terminal illness.

The nurse's role is to assess the values, preferences, and practices of every patient, regardless of ethnicity, socioeconomic status, or background. The nurse can share knowledge about a patient's and family's cultural beliefs and practices with the health care team and facilitate the adaptation of the care plan to accommodate these practices. For example, a nurse may find that a male patient prefers to have his eldest son make all of his care decisions. Institutional practices and laws governing informed consent are also rooted in the Western notion of autonomous decision-making and informed consent. If this patient wishes to defer decisions to his son, the nurse can work with the team to negotiate informed consent, respecting the patient's right not to participate in decision-making and honoring his family's cultural practices.

The nurse should assess and document the patient's and family's specific beliefs, preferences, and practices regarding end-of-life care, preparation for death, and after-death rituals. The nurse must use judgment and discretion about the timing and setting for eliciting this information. Some patients may wish to have a family member speak for them or may be unable to provide information because of advanced illness. The nurse should give the patient and family a context for the discussion, such as, "It is very important to us to provide care that addresses your needs and the needs of your family. We want to honor and support your wishes and want you to feel free to tell us how we are doing and what we could do to better meet your needs. I'd like to ask you some questions; what you tell me will help me to understand and support what is most important to you at this time. You don't need to answer anything that makes you uncomfortable. Is it all right to ask some questions?" The assessment of end-of-life beliefs, preferences, and practices probably should be carried out in short segments over a period of time (e.g., across multiple days of an inpatient hospital stay or in conjunction with multiple patient visits to an outpatient setting). The discomfort of novice nurses with asking questions and discussing this type of sensitive content can be reduced by prior practice in a classroom or clinical skills laboratory, observation of interviews conducted by experienced nurses, and partnering with experienced nurses during the first few assessments.

Symptom Management

Many patients suffer unnecessarily when they do not receive adequate attention for the symptoms accompanying serious illness. Careful evaluation of the patient should include not only the physical problems but also the psychological, social, and spiritual dimensions of the patient's and family's experience of serious illness. This approach contributes to a more comprehensive understanding of how the patient's and family's lives have been affected by illness and leads to nursing care that addresses the needs in every dimension.

Clinical depression should not be accepted as an inevitable consequence of dying, nor should it be confused with sadness and anticipatory grieving, which are normal reactions to the losses associated with impending death. Emotional and spiritual support and control of distressing physical symptoms are appropriate interventions for situational depression associated with terminal illness. Cancer patients in advanced stages of the disease are especially vulnerable to delirium, depression, suicidal ideation, and severe anxiety. Higher levels of debilitation predict higher levels of pain and depressive symptoms, and the presence of pain increases the likelihood of developing major psychiatric complications of illness. Patients and their families must be given space and time to experience sadness and to grieve, but patients should not have to endure untreated depression at the end of their life. An effective combined approach to clinical depression includes relief of physical symptoms, attention to emotional and spiritual distress, and pharmacologic interventions.

Patients approaching the end-of-life experience many of the same symptoms, regardless of their underlying disease processes. Symptoms in terminal illness may be caused by the disease, either directly (e.g., dyspnea due to chronic obstructive pulmonary disease) or indirectly (e.g., nausea and vomiting related to pressure in the gastric area); by the treatment for the disease; or by a coexisting disorder that is unrelated to the disease. Some of the most frequently encountered symptoms as death approaches include pain, dyspnea, anorexia and cachexia, delirium, and depression (Berry & Griffie, 2019). Chapter 6 presents assessment principles for pain that include identifying the effect of the pain on the patient's life, the importance of believing the patient's report of the pain and its effect, and the importance of systematic assessment of pain. Similarly, symptoms such as dyspnea, nausea, weakness, and anxiety should be carefully and systematically assessed and managed. Questions that guide the assessment of symptoms are listed in Box 2-6.

The patient's goals should guide symptom management. Medical interventions may be aimed at treating the underlying

BOX 2-6

Assessing Symptoms Associated with Serious Illness

Questions to consider:

- When did the symptom start?
- How long has the symptom been present?
- Has the symptom changed in any way?
- Is the symptom intermittent or constant/continuous?
- Are there any other symptoms?

(if symptom is pain specific)

- Does the pain radiate or move anywhere?
- What makes the pain worse or better?
- What has been tried to treat the pain? Has it helped? Are there side effects? What are the scheduled doses?
- What are the patient's goals and expectations regarding pain management for comfort and function? What about those of the family/caregivers?
- How much distress is the pain causing?
- What does the patient think that the pain means (e.g., tumor spread)?
- Who does the patient have for support? Are family members or others available?
- What are cultural, spiritual, or religious concerns about pain?

Adapted from Fink, R. M., Gates, R. A., & Jeffers, K. D. (2019). Pain assessment. In B. R. Ferrell & J. A. Paice (Eds.), *Oxford textbook of palliative nursing* (5th ed., pp. 98–115). Oxford University Press. https://doi.org/10.1093/med/9780190862374.003.0033.

causes of the symptoms or reducing the impact of symptoms. For example, a medical intervention such as thoracentesis (an invasive procedure in which fluid is drained from the pleural space) may be performed to relieve dyspnea temporarily in a patient with pleural effusion secondary to lung cancer. Pharmacologic and nonpharmacologic methods for symptom management may be used in combination with medical interventions to modify the physiologic causes of symptoms. For example, in addition to having a thoracentesis, many patients find symptoms are reduced using a handheld fan, which has been associated with a reduction in breathlessness (Gupta et al., 2021). In addition, pharmacologic management with a low-dose oral opioid is very effective in relieving dyspnea, and guided relaxation may reduce the anxiety associated with the sensation of breathlessness. As is true with pain, the principles of pharmacologic symptom management call for the use of the smallest dose of the medication to achieve the desired effect, avoidance of polypharmacy, anticipation and management of medical side effects, and creation of a therapeutic regimen that is acceptable to the patient based on their goals for maximizing quality of life.

The patient's goals take precedence over the providers goals to relieve all symptoms at all costs. Although providers may believe that symptoms must be relieved completely whenever possible, the patient might choose to decrease symptoms to a tolerable level rather than to relieve them completely if the side effects of medications are unacceptable to them. This often allows the patient to have greater independence, mobility, and alertness and to devote attention to issues that they consider of higher priority and greater importance.

Anticipating and planning interventions for symptoms that have not yet occurred is a cornerstone of end-of-life care. Both patients and family members and other caregivers cope more effectively with new symptoms and exacerbations of existing symptoms when they know what to expect and how to manage the symptoms. Hospice programs typically provide "emergency kits" containing ready-to-administer doses of a variety of medications that are useful to treat symptoms in advanced illness. For example, a kit might contain small doses of oral morphine liquid for pain or shortness of breath, a benzodiazepine for restlessness, and an acetaminophen suppository for fever. Family members and other caregivers can be instructed to administer a prescribed dose from the emergency kit, often avoiding prolonged suffering for the patient as well as rehospitalization for symptom management.

Pain Management

Numerous studies have shown that patients with advanced illness, particularly cancer, experience considerable pain. Pain is a significant symptom for many cancer patients throughout their treatment and disease course; it results from both the disease and the modalities used to treat it. Pain and suffering are among the most feared consequences of cancer. Poorly managed pain affects the psychological, emotional, social, and financial well-being of patients and families.

Patients who are taking an established regimen of analgesics should continue to receive those medications as they approach the end of life. Inability to communicate pain should not be equated with the absence of pain. Although most pain can be managed effectively using the oral route, as the end of life nears, patients may be less able to swallow oral medications due to somnolence or nausea. Patients who have been receiving oral opioids should continue to receive equianalgesic doses via rectal, sublingual, or intravenous routes. Concentrated opioid solutions (i.e., morphine, oxycodone) can be delivered very effectively by the sublingual route because the small liquid volume is well tolerated even if swallowing is not possible. As long as the patient continues to receive opioids, a regimen to combat constipation must be implemented. If the patient cannot swallow laxatives or stool softeners, rectal suppositories or enemas may be necessary.

The nurse should teach the family about continuation of comfort measures as the patient approaches the end of life, how to administer analgesics via alternative routes, and how to assess for nonverbal signs of pain when the patient cannot verbally report pain intensity. Because the analgesics administered orally or rectally are short-acting and typically scheduled as frequently as every 3 to 4 hours around the clock, there is always a strong possibility that a patient approaching the end of life will die in close proximity to the time of analgesic administration. If the patient is at home, family members administering analgesics should be prepared for this possibility. They need reassurance that they did not "cause" the death of the patient by administering a dose of analgesic medication.

Nutrition and Hydration at the End of Life

Anorexia and cachexia are common problems in seriously ill people. The profound changes in the patient's appearance and the concomitant lack of interest in the socially important rituals of mealtime are particularly upsetting to families. The approach to this problem varies depending on the patient's stage of illness, level of disability associated with the illness, and desires. The anorexia–cachexia syndrome is characterized by disturbances in carbohydrate, protein, and fat metabolism; endocrine dysfunction; and anemia. The syndrome results in severe asthenia (loss of energy).

Although causes of anorexia may be controlled for a period of time, progressive anorexia is an expected and natural part of the dying process. Anorexia may be related to or exacerbated by situational variables (e.g., the ability to have meals with family vs. eating alone in the "sick room"), progression of the disease, treatment for the disease, or psychological distress. The patient and family should be instructed in strategies to manage the variables associated with anorexia (Table 2-3).

A number of pharmacologic agents are commonly used to stimulate appetite in anorexic patients. Commonly used medications for appetite stimulation include dexamethasone, megestrol acetate, and dronabinol. Although several of these agents may result in temporary weight gain, their use is not associated with an increase in lean body mass in the terminally ill patient and therefore will be unlikely to reverse anorexia-cachexia.

Dexamethasone initially increases appetite and may provide short-term weight gain in some patients. However, therapy may need to be discontinued in patients with a longer life expectancy because after 3 to 4 weeks, corticosteroids interfere with the synthesis of muscle protein.

Megestrol acetate produces temporary weight gain of primarily fatty tissue with little effect on protein balance. Because of the time required to see any effect from this agent, therapy should not be initiated if life expectancy is less than 30 days.

Dronabinol is a psychoactive compound found in cannabis that may be helpful in reducing nausea and vomiting, appetite loss, pain, and anxiety, thereby improving food and fluid intake in some patients. However, dronabinol is not as effective as other agents for appetite stimulation in most patients.

Cachexia

Cachexia refers to severe muscle wasting and weight loss associated with illness. Although anorexia may exacerbate cachexia, it is not the primary cause. Cachexia is associated with changes in metabolism that include hypertriglyceridemia, lipolysis, and accelerated protein turnover, leading to depletion of fat and protein stores. However, the pathophysiology of cachexia in terminal illness is not well understood. In terminal illness, the severity of tissue wasting is greater than would be expected from reduced food intake alone; typically increasing appetite or food intake does not reverse cachexia in the terminally ill.

Anorexia and cachexia differ from starvation (simple food deprivation) in several important ways. In the case of anorexia and cachexia, appetite is lost early in the process, the body becomes catabolic in a dysfunctional way, and supplementation by gastric feeding (tube feeding) or parenteral nutrition in advanced disease does not replenish lean body mass that has been lost. At one time, it was believed that cancer patients with rapidly growing tumors developed cachexia because the tumor created an excessive nutritional demand and diverted nutrients from the rest of the body. Research links cytokines produced by the body in response to a tumor to a complex inflammatory-immune response present in patients whose tumors have metastasized, leading to anorexia, weight loss, and altered metabolism. It can be important for the nurse to educate the patient and family about the difference between anorexia-cachexia and starvation at end of life.

Artificial Nutrition and Hydration

Along with breathing, eating and drinking are essential to survival throughout life. Near the end of life, the body's nutritional needs change, and the desire for food and fluids may diminish. People may no longer be able to use, eliminate, or store nutrients and fluids adequately. For patients with progressive illness, food preparation and mealtimes often become battlegrounds in which well-meaning family members argue, plead, and cajole to encourage ill people to eat. It is not unusual for seriously ill patients to lose their appetites entirely, to develop strong aversions for foods they have enjoyed in the past, or to crave a particular food to the exclusion of all other foods.

Although nutritional supplementation may be an important part of the treatment plan in early or chronic illness, unintended weight loss and dehydration are expected sequelae of progressive illness. As illness progresses, patients, families, and providers may believe that, without artificial nutrition and hydration, terminally ill patients will "starve," causing profound suffering and hastened death. However, starvation should not be viewed as the failure to implant tubes for nutritional supplementation or hydration of terminally ill patients with irreversible progression of disease. Studies have demonstrated that terminally ill patients who were hydrated had neither improved biochemical parameters nor improved states of consciousness. Similarly, survival was not increased when terminally ill patients with advanced dementia received enteral feeding. Furthermore, in patients who are close to death, there are beneficial effects to withholding or withdrawing artificial nutrition and hydration, such as

TABLE **2-3 Measures for Managing Anorexia**

Nursing Interventions	Patient and Family Teaching Tips
Initiate measures to ensure adequate dietary intake without adding stress to the patient at mealtimes.	Reduce the focus on "balanced" meals; offer the same food as often as the patient desires it.
Assess the impact of medications (e.g., chemotherapy, antiretrovirals) or other therapies (e.g., radiation therapy, dialysis) that are being used to treat the underlying illness. Administer and monitor effects of prescribed treatment for nausea, vomiting, and delayed gastric emptying.	Increase the nutritional value of meals. For example, add dry milk powder to milk, and use this fortified milk to prepare cream soups, milkshakes, and gravies.
Encourage the patient to eat when effects of medications have subsided.	Allow and encourage the patient to eat when hungry, regardless of usual mealtimes.
Assess and modify the environment to eliminate unpleasant odors and other factors that cause nausea, vomiting, and anorexia.	Eliminate or reduce noxious cooking odors, pet odors, or other odors that may precipitate nausea, vomiting, or anorexia.
Remove items that may reduce appetite (soiled tissues, bedpans, emesis basins, clutter).	Keep the patient's environment clean, uncluttered, and comfortable.
Assess and manage anxiety and depression to the extent possible.	Make mealtime a shared experience away from the "sick" room whenever possible. Reduce stress at mealtimes. Avoid confrontations about the amount of food consumed. Reduce or eliminate routine weighing of the patient.
Position the patient to enhance gastric emptying.	Encourage the patient to eat in a sitting position; elevate the head of the patient's bed. Plan meals (food selection and portion size) that the patient desires.
Assess for constipation and/or intestinal obstruction.	Provide small, frequent meals if they are easier for the patient to eat. Ensure that the patient and family understand that prevention of constipation is essential, even when the patient's intake is minimal.
Prevent and manage constipation on an ongoing basis, even when the patient's intake is minimal.	Encourage adequate fluid intake, dietary fiber, and use of a bowel program to prevent constipation.
Provide frequent mouth care, particularly following nourishment.	Assist the patient to rinse after every meal. Avoid mouthwashes that contain alcohol or glycerine, which dry mucous membranes.
Ensure that dentures fit properly.	Weight loss may cause dentures to loosen and cause irritation. Remove them to inspect the gums and to provide oral care.
Administer and monitor the effects of topical and systemic treatment for oropharyngeal pain.	The patient's comfort may be enhanced if medications for pain relief given on an as-needed basis for breakthrough pain are administered before mealtimes.

decreased complications associated with tube feeding or total parenteral nutrition, which include dislodgement, infection, discomfort, and aspiration (Berry & Griffie, 2019).

As the patient approaches the end of life, the family and health care providers should offer the patient what the patient prefers and can tolerate most easily. The nurse should instruct the family how to separate feeding from caring and to demonstrate love and sharing by being with the loved one in other ways. Preoccupation with appetite, feeding, and weight loss diverts energy and time that the patient and family could use in other meaningful activities. Here are tips to promote nutrition for terminally ill patients:

- Offer small portions of favorite foods.
- Do not be overly concerned about a "balanced" diet.
- Cool foods may be better tolerated than hot foods.
- Offer cheese, eggs, peanut butter, mild fish, chicken, or turkey. Meat (especially beef) may taste bitter and unpleasant.
- Add milkshakes, powdered instant drinks, or other liquid supplements.

- Add dry milk powder to milkshakes and cream soups to increase protein and calorie content.
- Place nutritious foods at the bedside (fruit juices, milkshakes in insulated drink containers with straws).
- Schedule meals when family members can be present to provide company and stimulation.
- Avoid arguments at mealtime.
- Help the patient to maintain a schedule of oral care. Rinse the mouth after each meal or snack. Avoid mouthwashes that contain alcohol. Use a soft toothbrush. Treat oral ulcers or lesions. Make sure dentures fit well.
- Treat pain and other symptoms.
- Offer ice chips made from frozen fruit juices.
- Allow the patient to decline foods and fluids.

Changes in Consciousness and Delirium

Many patients remain alert, arousable, and able to communicate until very close to death. Others sleep for long intervals and awaken only intermittently, with eventual somnolence until death. Delirium refers to concurrent disturbances in level of consciousness, psychomotor behavior, memory, thinking, attention, and sleep–wake cycle. In some patients, a period of agitated delirium precedes death, sometimes causing families to be hopeful that patients who are suddenly active may be getting better. Confusion may be related to underlying treatable conditions such as medication side effects or interactions, pain or discomfort, hypoxia or dyspnea, or a full bladder or impacted stool. In patients with cancer, confusion may be secondary to brain metastases. Delirium also may be related to metabolic changes, infection, and organ failure.

Patients with delirium may become hypoactive or hyperactive, restless, irritable, and fearful. Sleep deprivation and hallucinations may occur. If treatment of the underlying factors contributing to these symptoms brings no relief, a combination of pharmacologic intervention with neuroleptics or benzodiazepines may be effective in decreasing distressing symptoms. Haloperidol may reduce hallucinations and agitation. Benzodiazepines (e.g., lorazepam) can reduce anxiety but do not clear the sensorium and may contribute to worsening cognitive impairment if used alone. In patients with advanced cancer and agitated delirium at end of life, the concomitant administration of haloperidol and lorazepam may be useful in controlling the symptoms of agitation or delirium; however, further high-quality evidence is needed to support or refute the use of pharmacologic therapies for delirium in terminally ill adults (Bramati & Bruera, 2021).

Nursing interventions are aimed at identifying the underlying causes of delirium, acknowledging the family's distress over its occurrence, reassuring family members about what is normal, teaching family members how to interact with and ensure safety for the patient with delirium, and monitoring the effects of medications used to treat severe agitation, paranoia, and fear. Confusion may mask the patient's unmet needs and fears about dying. Spiritual intervention, music therapy, gentle massage, and therapeutic touch may provide some relief. Reduction of environmental stimuli, avoidance of harsh lighting or very dim lighting (which may produce disturbing shadows), presence of familiar faces, and gentle reorientation and reassurance are also helpful.

Dyspnea

Dyspnea is an uncomfortable awareness of breathing or breathlessness that is common in patients approaching the end of life. Dyspnea is a highly subjective symptom that often is not associated with visible signs of distress, such as tachypnea, diaphoresis, or cyanosis. Patients with primary lung tumors, lung metastases, pleural effusion, or obstructive lung disease may experience significant dyspnea. Although the underlying cause of the dyspnea can be identified and treated in some cases, the burdens of additional diagnostic evaluation and treatment aimed at the physiologic problem may outweigh the benefits. The treatment of dyspnea varies depending on the patient's general physical condition and imminence of death. For example, a blood transfusion may provide temporary symptom relief for a patient with anemia earlier in the disease process; however, as the patient approaches the end of life, the benefits are typically short-lived or absent. As with assessment and management of pain, reports of dyspnea by patients must be believed. As is true for physical pain, what dyspnea means to an individual patient may increase their suffering. For example, the patient may interpret increasing dyspnea as a sign that death is approaching. For some patients, sensations of breathlessness may invoke frightening images of drowning or suffocation, and the resulting cycle of fear and anxiety may increase the sensation of breathlessness, or "air hunger." Therefore, the nurse should conduct a careful assessment of the psychosocial and spiritual components of the dyspnea. Physical assessment parameters include:

- Symptom intensity, distress, and interference with activities (scale of 0 to 10)
- Auscultation of lung sounds
- Assessment of fluid balance
- Measurement of dependent edema (circumference of lower extremities)
- Measurement of abdominal girth
- Temperature
- Skin color
- Sputum quantity and character
- Cough

To determine the intensity of dyspnea and its interference with daily activities, the nurse can ask the patient to report the severity of the dyspnea using a scale of 0 to 10, where 0 is no dyspnea and 10 is the worst imaginable dyspnea. Ongoing objective evidence for the efficacy of the treatment plan is provided by the patient's baseline measurement before treatment and then subsequent measurements taken during exacerbation of the symptom, periodically during treatment, and whenever the treatment plan changes. In addition, physical assessment findings may assist in locating the source of the dyspnea and selecting appropriate nursing interventions to relieve the symptom. The components of the assessment change as the patient's condition changes. Like other symptoms at the end of life, dyspnea can be managed effectively in the absence of assessment and diagnostic data that are standard when a patient's illness or symptom is reversible (e.g., arterial blood gases).

Nursing management of dyspnea at the end of life is directed toward administering medical treatment for the underlying pathology, monitoring the patient's response to treatment, helping the patient and family manage anxiety (which exacerbates dyspnea), altering the perception of the symptom, and conserving energy (Box 2-7). Pharmacologic intervention is aimed at modifying lung physiology and improving performance, as well as altering the perception of the symptom. Bronchodilators and corticosteroids are examples of medications used to treat underlying obstructive pathology, thereby improving overall lung function. Low doses of opioids are very effective in relieving dyspnea, although the mechanism of relief is not entirely clear. Although dyspnea in terminal illness is typically not associated with diminished blood oxygen saturation, low-flow oxygen often provides psychological comfort to both patients and families, particularly in the home setting.

As previously mentioned, dyspnea may be exacerbated by anxiety, and anxiety may trigger episodes of dyspnea, setting off a respiratory crisis in which the patient and family may panic. For patients receiving care at home, patient and family instruction should include anticipation and management of crisis situations and a clearly communicated emergency plan. The patient and family should be instructed about medication administration, condition changes that should be reported to the provider and nurse, and strategies for coping with diminished reserves and increasing symptomatology as the disease progresses. The patient and family need reassurance that the symptom can be managed effectively at home without the need for activation of the emergency medical services or hospitalization, and that a nurse will be available at all times via telephone or to make a visit.

BOX 2-7

Palliative Nursing Interventions for Dyspnea

Decrease Anxiety

- Administer prescribed anxiolytic medications as indicated for anxiety or panic associated with dyspnea.
- Assist with relaxation techniques, guided imagery.
- Provide the patient with a means to call for assistance (call bell/light within reach in a hospital or long-term care facility; handheld bell or other device for home).

Treat Underlying Pathology

- Administer prescribed bronchodilators and corticosteroids (obstructive pathology).
- Administer blood products, erythropoietin as prescribed (typically not beneficial in advanced stages of disease).
- Administer prescribed diuretics and monitor fluid balance.

Alter Perception of Breathlessness

- Administer prescribed oxygen therapy via nasal cannula if tolerated; masks may not be well tolerated.
- Administer prescribed low-dose opioids
- Provide air movement in the patient's environment with a portable fan or a cool draft of air as from a handheld fan.

Reduce Respiratory Demand

- Teach the patient and family to implement energy conservation measures.
- Place needed equipment, supplies, and nourishment within reach.
- For home or hospice care, offer a bedside commode and/or electric bed (with head that elevates).

Secretions

If family members have been prepared for the time of death, they are less likely to panic and are better able to be with their loved ones in a meaningful way. Noisy, gurgling breathing or moaning is generally most distressing to family members. In most cases, the sounds of breathing at the end of life are related to oropharyngeal relaxation and diminished awareness. Family members may have difficulty believing that the patient is not suffering or drowning or that the patient's breathing could not be improved by suctioning secretions. Patient positioning and family reassurance are the most helpful responses to these symptoms.

When death is imminent, patients may become increasingly somnolent and unable to clear sputum or oral secretions, which may lead to further impairment of breathing from pooled or dried and crusted secretions. Often the sound ("terminal bubbling") and appearance of the secretions are more distressing to family members than is the presence of the secretions to the patient. Family distress over the changes in the patient's condition may be eased by supportive nursing care. Continuation of comfort-focused interventions and reassurance that the patient is not in any distress can do much to ease family concerns. Gentle mouth care with a moistened swab or very soft toothbrush helps maintain the integrity of the patient's mucous membranes. In addition, gentle oral suctioning, positioning to enhance drainage of secretions, and sublingual or transdermal administration of anticholinergic drugs reduce the production of secretions and provide comfort to the patient and support to the family. Deeper suctioning may cause significant discomfort to the dying patient and is rarely of any benefit because secretions reaccumulate rapidly. When anticholinergic drugs are used prophylactically prior to secretions occurring, there is an increased chance of being effective (van Esch et al., 2021). Refer to Table 2-4 for pharmacologic management of excess oral/respiratory secretions with dying patients.

TABLE 2-4 **Pharmacologic Management of Excess Oral/Respiratory Secretions When Death Is Imminent**

Medication	Dose
Atropine sulfate drops 1%	1 or 2 drops 1% PO/sublingual q4–6h p.r.n. or around the clock (ATC) up to 12 drops/d
Atropine injection	0.4–0.6 mg IV/SC/IM q4–6h p.r.n. or ATC (if PO therapy is ineffective)
Glycopyrrolate	1–2 mg PO/rectal/sublingual TID p.r.n. or ATC (maximum dose 6 mg/d)
Hyoscyamine	0.125–0.25 mg PO/sublingual q4–6h p.r.n. or ATC (maximum dose 1.5 mg/d)
Scopolamine	1–3 patches q3d (maximum dose 3 patches every 72 hours)

Reprinted with permission from ExcelleRx, Inc. (2008). *Hospice Pharmacia pharmaceutical care tool kit* (9th ed.). Author.

Palliative Sedation at the End of Life

Effective control of symptoms can be achieved under most conditions, but some patients may experience distressing, intractable symptoms. Although **palliative sedation** remains controversial, it is offered in some settings to patients who are close to death or who have symptoms that do not respond to conventional pharmacologic and nonpharmacologic approaches, resulting in unrelieved suffering. Palliative sedation is distinguished from **euthanasia** or physician-assisted suicide in that the intent of palliative sedation is to relieve uncontrolled, refractory symptoms, not to hasten death. Palliative sedation is most commonly used when the patient exhibits intractable pain, dyspnea, seizures, or delirium, and it is generally considered appropriate in only the most difficult situations. Before implementing palliative sedation, the health care team should assess for the presence of underlying and treatable causes of suffering, such as depression or spiritual pain. Finally, the patient and family should be informed fully about the use of this treatment and alternatives.

Palliative sedation is accomplished through infusion of sedative drugs such as benzodiazepines to achieve the desired level of sedation to provide relief from the refractory symptoms in the last hours and days of life (Beler et al., 2022; Garetto et al., 2018). Nurses are important members of the interdisciplinary health care team, providing emotional support to patients and families, facilitating clarification of values and preferences, and providing comfort-focused physical care. Once sedation has been induced, the nurse should continue to comfort the patient, monitor the physiologic effects of the sedation, support the family during the final hours or days of their loved one's life, and maintain communication within the health care team and between the team and family. When caring for patients with refractory symptoms at end of life, nurses may be asked to administer escalating doses of potentially sedating medications, such as opioids and benzodiazepines, in an effort to alleviate and prevent suffering. Such medications are given only in an effort to alleviate and prevent suffering, never to hasten death. The risk of hastening death by increasing sedating medications is morally permissible as the intent is not to harm, but to help. The nurse caring for patients at end of life should understand the rule of double effect, a philosophical principle applied to medical ethics to justify certain actions that may have a foreseeable negative outcome (Chessa & Moreno, 2019).

NURSING CARE OF PATIENTS AND FAMILIES IN THE FINAL HOURS OF LIFE

Providing care to patients who are close to death, being present when patients die, and helping to ensure a good death can be one of the most rewarding experiences a nurse can have. Patients and their families are understandably fearful of the unknown, and the approach of death may prompt new concerns or cause previous fears or issues to resurface. Family members who have a history of poor communication or who are part of families in which there are old resentments may experience heightened difficulty as their loved one nears death. In contrast, the time at the end of life can also afford opportunities to resolve old conflicts and learn new ways of being a family. Regardless of the setting, skilled practitioners can make the dying patient comfortable, make space for their loved ones to remain present when they wish, and give family members the opportunity to experience growth and healing. Likewise, regardless of setting, the patient and family may be less apprehensive near the time of death if they know what to expect and how to respond.

Expected Physiologic Changes

As death approaches and organ systems begin to fail, observable, expected changes in the body take place. Nursing care measures aimed at patient comfort should be continued: pain medications (administered rectally, intravenously, or sublingually), turning, mouth care, eye care, positioning to facilitate draining of secretions, and measures to protect the skin from urine or feces (if the patient is incontinent) should be continued. The nurse should consult with the provider about discontinuing measures that no longer contribute to patient comfort, such as drawing blood, administering tube feedings, suctioning (in most cases), and invasive monitoring. The nurse should prepare the family for the normal, expected changes that accompany the period immediately preceding death. Although the exact time of death cannot be predicted, it is often possible to identify when the patient is very close to death. Hospice programs frequently provide written information for families so they know what to expect and what to do as death nears (Box 2-8).

BOX 2-8

Patient Education

Signs of Approaching Death

The person will show less interest in eating and drinking. For many patients, refusal of food is an indication that they are close to death. Fluid intake may be limited to that which will keep the mouth from feeling too dry.

- What you can do: Offer, but do not force, fluids and medication. Sometimes, pain or other symptoms that have required medication in the past may no longer be present. For most patients, pain medications still will be needed and can be provided by concentrated oral solutions placed under the tongue, by rectal suppository, or intravenously.

Urinary output may decrease in amount and frequency.

- What you can do: No response is needed unless the patient expresses a desire to urinate and cannot. Call the hospice nurse for advice if you are not sure.

As the body weakens, the patient will sleep more and begin to detach from the environment. They may refuse your attempts to provide comfort.

- What you can do: Allow your loved one to sleep. You may wish to sit with them, play soft music, or hold hands. Your loved one's withdrawal is normal and is not a rejection of your love.

Mental confusion may become apparent as less oxygen is available to supply the brain. The patient may report strange dreams or visions.

- What you can do: As they awaken from sleep, remind them of the day and time, where they are, and who is present. This is best done in a casual, conversational way.

Vision and hearing may become somewhat impaired, and speech may be difficult to understand.

- What you can do: Speak clearly but no more loudly than necessary. Keep the room as light as the patient wishes, even at night. Carry on all conversations as if they can be heard, because hearing may be the last of the senses to cease functioning.
- Many patients are able to talk until minutes before death and are reassured by the exchange of a few words with a loved one.

Secretions may collect in the back of the throat and rattle or gurgle as the patient breathes through the mouth. They may try to cough, and their mouth may become dry and encrusted with secretions.

- What you can do: If the patient is trying to cough up secretions and is experiencing choking or vomiting, call the hospice nurse for assistance.
- Secretions may drain from the mouth if you place the patient on their side and provide support with pillows.
- Cleansing the mouth with moistened mouth swabs will help to relieve the dryness that occurs with mouth breathing.
- Offer water in small amounts to keep the mouth moist. A straw with one finger placed over the end can be used to transfer sips of water to the patient's mouth.

Breathing may become irregular with periods of no breathing (apnea). The patient may be working very hard to breathe and may make a moaning sound with each breath. As the time of death nears, the breathing remains irregular and may become more shallow.

- What you can do: Raising the head of the bed may help the patient to breathe more easily. The moaning sound does not mean that the patient is in pain or other distress; it is the sound of air passing over very relaxed vocal cords.

As the oxygen supply to the brain decreases, the patient may become restless. It is not unusual for the patient to pull at the bed linens, to have visual hallucinations, or even to try to get out of bed at this point.

- What you can do: Reassure the patient in a calm voice that you are there. Prevent them from falling out of bed. Soft music or a back rub may be soothing.

The patient may feel hot one moment and cold the next as the body loses its ability to control its temperature. As circulation slows, the arms and legs may become cool and bluish. The underside of the body may darken. It may be difficult to feel a pulse at the wrist.

- What you can do: Provide and remove blankets as needed. Avoid using electric blankets, which may cause burns because the patient cannot tell you if they are too warm.
- Sponge the patient's head with a cool cloth if this provides comfort.

Loss of bladder and bowel control may occur around the time of death.

- What you can do: Protect the mattress with waterproof padding and change the padding as needed to keep the patient comfortable.

As people approach death, many times they report seeing gardens, libraries, or family or friends who have died. They may ask you to pack their bags and find tickets or a passport. Sometimes they may become insistent and attempt to do these chores themselves. They may try getting out of bed (even if they have been confined to bed for a long time) so that they can "leave."

- What you can do: Reassure the patient that it is all right; they can "go" without getting out of bed. Stay close, share stories, and be present.

Used with permission from the Family Home Hospice of the Visiting Nurse Association of Greater Philadelphia.

Although every death is unique, it is often possible for experienced providers to assess that the patient is "actively" or imminently dying and to prepare the family in the final days or hours leading to death. As death nears, the patient may withdraw, sleep for longer intervals, or become somnolent. Family members should be encouraged to be with the patient, to speak and reassure the patient of their presence, to stroke or touch the patient, or to lie alongside the patient (even in the hospital or long-term care facility) if the family members are comfortable with this degree of closeness and can do so without causing discomfort to the patient.

The family may have gone to great lengths to ensure that their loved one will not die alone. However, despite the best intentions and efforts of the family and providers, the patient may die at a time when no one is present. In any setting, it is unrealistic for family members to be at the patient's bedside 24 hours a day, and it is not unusual for a patient to die when family members have stepped away from the bedside just briefly. Experienced hospice providers have observed and reported that some patients appear to "wait" until family members are away from the bedside to die, perhaps to spare their loved ones the pain of being present at the time of death. Nurses can reassure family members throughout the death vigil by being present intermittently or continuously, modeling behaviors (such as touching and speaking to the patient), providing encouragement in relation to family caregiving, providing reassurance about normal physiologic changes, and encouraging family rest breaks. If a patient dies while family members are away from the bedside, the family may express feelings of guilt and profound grief and may need emotional support. If this occurs, it is important both to normalize the events surrounding the death and the family's feelings and to partner with the family in their experience to avoid perceived abandonment.

After-Death Care

The time of death is generally preceded by a period of gradual diminishment of bodily functions in which increasing intervals between respirations, a weakened and irregular pulse, diminishing blood pressure, and skin color changes or mottling may occur. For patients who have received adequate management of symptoms and for families who have received adequate preparation and support, the actual time of death is commonly peaceful and occurs without struggle. Nurses may or may not be present at the time of a patient's death. In many states, nurses may be authorized to make the pronouncement of death and sign the death certificate. The determination of death is made through a physical examination that includes auscultation for the absence of breathing and heart sounds. Home care or hospice programs in which nurses make the time-of-death visit and pronouncement of death have policies and procedures to guide the nurse's actions during this visit. Immediately on cessation of vital functions, the body begins to change. It becomes dusky or bluish, waxen-appearing, and cool; blood darkens and pools in dependent areas of the body (e.g., the back and sacrum if the body is in a supine position); and urine and stool may be evacuated.

Immediately after death, family members should be allowed and encouraged to spend time with the deceased person. Normal responses of family members at the time of death vary widely and range from quiet expressions of grief to overt expressions that include wailing and prostration. The family's desire for privacy during their time with the deceased should be honored. Family members may wish to independently manage or assist with care of the body after death. If the death occurs in a long-term care facility, nurses follow the facility's procedure for preparation of the body and transportation to the facility's morgue. However, the needs of families to remain with the deceased, to wait until other family members arrive before the body is moved, and to perform after-death rituals should be honored. When an expected death occurs in the home setting, the funeral director often transports the body directly to the funeral home or mortuary.

Loss, Grief, and Bereavement

A wide range of feelings and behaviors are normal, adaptive, and healthy reactions to the loss of a loved one. **Grief** refers to the personal feelings that accompany an anticipated or actual loss. **Mourning** refers to individual, family, caregiver, group, and cultural expressions of grief and associated behaviors. **Bereavement** refers to the period of time during which mourning takes place. Both grief reactions and mourning behaviors change over time as people learn to live with the loss. Although the pain of the loss may be tempered by the passage of time, loss is an ongoing developmental process, and time may never heal the bereaved individual completely. That is, the bereaved do not get over a loss entirely, nor do they return to who they were before the loss. Rather, they develop a new sense of who they are and where they fit in a world that has changed dramatically and permanently without their loved one and that relationship.

Anticipatory Grief and Mourning

Denial, sadness, anger, fear, and anxiety are typical grief reactions in people with life-threatening illness and those close to them. Kübler-Ross (1969) described five common emotional reactions to dying that are applicable to the experience of any loss: denial, anger, bargaining, depression, and acceptance. Kübler-Ross cautioned that not every patient or family member experiences every stage; many patients never reach a stage of acceptance, and patients and families fluctuate sometimes on a daily basis in their emotional responses. Individual and family coping with the anticipation of death is complicated by the varied and conflicting trajectories that grief and mourning may assume in families. For example, although the patient may be experiencing sadness while contemplating role changes that have been brought about by the illness, the patient's spouse or partner may be expressing or suppressing feelings of anger about the current changes in role and impending loss of the relationship. Others in the family may be engaged in denial (e.g., "Dad will get better; he just needs to eat more"), fear ("Who will take care of us?" or "Will I get sick too?"), or profound sadness and withdrawal. Although each of these behaviors is normal, tension may arise when one or more family members perceive that others are less caring, too emotional, or too detached.

The nurse should assess the characteristics of the family system and intervene in a manner that supports and enhances the cohesion of the family unit. The nurse can encourage family members to talk about their feelings and help them understand what is happening to them in the broader context of anticipatory grief and mourning. Acknowledging and expressing feelings, continuing to interact with the patient in meaningful ways, and planning for the time of death and bereavement are adaptive family behaviors. Professional support provided by grief counselors, chaplains, and social workers, whether in the community, at a local hospital, in the long-term care facility, or associated with a hospice program, can help both the patient and the family sort out and acknowledge feelings and make the end of life as meaningful as possible.

Grief and Mourning After Death

When a loved one dies, the family members enter a new phase of grief and mourning as they begin to accept the loss, feel the pain of permanent separation, and prepare to live a life without the deceased. Even if the loved one died after a long illness, preparatory grief experienced during the terminal illness does not preclude the grief and mourning that follow the death. With a death after a long or difficult illness, family members may experience conflicting feelings of relief that the loved one's suffering has ended, compounded by guilt and grief related to unresolved issues or the circumstances of death. Grief work may be especially difficult if a patient's death was painful, prolonged, accompanied by unwanted interventions, or unattended. Families who had no preparation or support during the period of imminence and death may have a more difficult time finding a place for the painful memories.

Although some family members may experience prolonged or complicated mourning, most grief reactions fall within a "normal" range or uncomplicated grief. The feelings are often profound, but bereaved people eventually reconcile the loss and find a way to reengage with their lives. Grief and mourning are affected by several factors, including individual characteristics, coping skills, and experiences with illness and death; the nature of the relationship to the deceased; factors surrounding the illness and the death; family dynamics; social support; and cultural expectations and norms. Uncomplicated grief and mourning are characterized by emotional feelings of sadness, anger, guilt, and numbness; physical sensations such as hollowness in the stomach and tightness in the chest, weakness, and lack of energy; cognitions that include preoccupation with the loss and a sense of the deceased as still present; and behaviors such as crying, visiting places that are reminders of the deceased, social withdrawal, and restless overactivity.

After-death rituals, including preparation of the body, funeral practices, and burial rituals, are socially and culturally significant ways in which family members begin to accept the reality and finality of death. Preplanning of funerals is becoming increasingly common, and hospice professionals in particular help the family make plans for death, often involving the patient, who may wish to play an active role. Preplanning of the funeral relieves the family of the burden of making decisions in the intensely emotional period after a death.

In general, the period of mourning is an adaptive response to loss during which mourners come to accept the loss as real and permanent, acknowledge and experience the painful emotions that accompany the loss, experience life without the deceased, overcome obstacles to adjustment, and find a new way of living in a world without the loved one. Particularly, immediately after the death, mourners begin to recognize the reality and permanence of the loss by talking about the deceased and telling and retelling the story of the illness and death. Societal norms in the United States are frequently at odds with the normal grieving processes of people; time excused from work obligations is typically measured in days, if granted at all, and often mourners are expected to get over the loss quickly and get on with life.

The work of grief and mourning takes time, and avoiding grief work after death often leads to long-term adjustment difficulties. Mourning for a loss involves the "undoing" of psychosocial ties that bind mourners to the deceased, personal adaptation to the loss, and learning to live in the world without the deceased. In his classic work, Worden (1991) described four tasks of mourning:

- Acceptance of the reality of the loss
- Working through the pain of grief
- Adjusting to the environment from which the deceased has gone
- Emotional "relocation" of the deceased to move on with life

Although many people complete the work of mourning with the informal support of families and friends, many find that talking with others who have had a similar experience, such as in formal support groups, normalizes the feelings and experiences and provides a framework for learning new skills to cope with the loss and create a new life. Hospitals, hospices, religious organizations, and other community organizations often sponsor bereavement support groups. Groups for parents who have lost a child, children who have lost a parent, widows, widowers, and members of the LGBTQIA$^+$ community who have lost a loved one are some examples of specialized support groups available in many communities.

Complicated Grief and Mourning

Complicated grief and mourning are characterized by prolonged feelings of sadness and feelings of general worthlessness or hopelessness that persist long after the death, prolonged symptoms that interfere with ADLs (anorexia, insomnia, fatigue, panic), or self-destructive behaviors such as alcohol or substance abuse and suicidal ideation or attempts. Complicated grief and mourning require a referral for a psychiatric assessment and evaluation to determine if pharmacologic and additional psychological interventions are needed. It is important that family members at risk for complicated grief be recognized early so that resources can be identified and mobilized.

COPING WITH DEATH AND DYING: PROFESSIONAL CAREGIVER ISSUES

Whether practicing in the trauma center, intensive care unit or another acute care setting, home care, hospice, long-term care, or the many locations where patients and their families receive ambulatory services, the nurse is closely involved with complex and emotionally laden issues surrounding loss of life. To be most effective and satisfied with the care provided, the nurse should attend to their own emotional responses to the losses witnessed every day. Like family members, nurses need opportunities to grieve and express sorrow at the losses experienced and the sadness associated with a person dying before fulfilling one's dreams, leaving children prematurely, or completing one's commitments. Well before the nurse exhibits symptoms of stress or burnout, they should acknowledge the difficulty of coping with others' pain on a daily basis and put healthy practices in place that guard against emotional exhaustion. In hospice settings, where death, grief, and loss are expected outcomes of patient care, interdisciplinary colleagues rely on each other for support, using meeting time to express frustration, sadness, anger, and other emotions; to learn coping skills from each other; and to speak about how they were affected by the lives of those patients who have died since the last meeting. In many settings, staff members organize or attend memorial services to support families and other caregivers, who find comfort in joining each other to remember and celebrate the lives of patients. Finally, healthy personal habits, including diet, exercise, stress reduction activities (e.g., dance, yoga, tai chi, meditation), and sleep, help guard against the detrimental effects of stress. Health care professionals, in particular nurses, are bearing the emotional brunt of caring for the victims of COVID-19 at end of life. Due to the immense psychological toll of working under challenging conditions, there is a new focus on supporting health care workers with resources for emotional support and burnout prevention (Rosa et al., 2020).

SUMMARY

Chronic illnesses, those that last longer than 3 months, may be caused by injury or disease. Some of these diseases may be the result of genetic factors, while others may be the result of unhealthy lifestyles and behaviors earlier in life. Chronic illness is not merely a disease that has an irreversible pathology; it is also the slow, progressive decline in normal function that brings with it disability and the need for long-term surveillance. Given its prevalence, chronic illness touches many lives, meaning nurses encounter many people who have been living with the symptoms or disabilities that accompany chronic illness. When they do, nurses will encounter people who are living with uncertainty. Chronic illness waxes and wanes, and with these modulations come a different set of health care regimens and types of management, often placing variable demands on family caregivers. Nurses need to be aware of the phases of the trajectory model of chronic illness, and they need to tailor the care they give to the care demanded, depending on the phase.

As people with chronic illness move in and out of the different phases of the trajectory model of care, and treatments become more complex, focus shifts from cure to care. There has been an international movement to recognize the need to help patients and families transition from cure to care. The goal of this movement is a seamless integration of palliative care into treatment from the beginning—at the time of diagnosis. Palliative care, encompassing a wide range of therapeutic interventions, seeks to prevent and relieve suffering. Because suffering has many and varied sources, nurses who provide palliative care should attend to the whole patient—that is, to the physical, psychological, social, and spiritual domains of human experience. As patients move into the downward phase of chronic illness, they need hospice or hospice-like care. Hospice care includes palliative care, but unlike palliative care, hospice care is associated with the patient's end of life: it helps patients and families prepare for death—emotionally, socially, spiritually, and financially. Nurses who provide end-of-life care have eight tasks: (1) They provide pain and symptom management. (2) With an ease that comes from expertise, they communicate effectively with dying patients and their families. (3) They educate patients and families about end-of-life decision-making and (4) help other professional caregivers to develop a coordinated plan of care that aligns with the wishes of patients and families. (5) They provide care to patients who are close to death, and (6) often, are present at death. (7) After death, they attend to families' loss, grief, and bereavement. (8) Finally, they achieve quality of care at the end of life by providing culturally sensitive care throughout the entire hospice-care experience.

Providing nursing care for patients and families who live with chronic illness is nursing at its fullest and deepest, for from the onset of disease to the end of life, care of the chronically ill centers on the whole person.

CHAPTER REVIEW

NCLEX-Style Review Questions

1. When educating patients about chronic diseases, such as diabetes, which of the following should the nurse include in the rationale for effective management of the disease? Select all that apply.

a. An unmanaged chronic disease may lead to the development of other chronic illnesses.
b. When a patient is admitted to the ICU with a comorbid chronic disease, that patient faces a greater risk of morbidity and mortality.
c. Although chronic disease affects the entire family system, management of the disease is solely the patient's responsibility.
d. By managing a chronic disorder early in the disease process, the patient may be able to save themself the high costs associated with the sequelae of unmanaged disease.
e. Chronic illness management is not influenced by lifestyle changes.

2. A patient is nearing death from metastatic cancer and is receiving hospice care in the home. The home care nurse visits. The patient's family caregiver states that the patient has not eaten well for the last several days and rarely wishes to drink, only sucking on ice now and then. The caregiver thinks that it is cruel to let the dying patient starve to death or die from dehydration. Which would the nurse's best response be? Select all that apply.

a. "I think it is cruel, too. If this were my mother, I would not let her die like that."
b. "Tell me why you feel that way?"
c. "It's okay, because this may hasten death and relieve suffering."
d. "This is what happens when people die."
e. "Can you tell me about your concerns?"

3. The sounds of breathing, including terminal secretions, at the time of death may be distressing for families to hear. When the nurse hears these sounds, which of the following actions should be performed? Select all that apply.

a. Reposition the patient in an attempt to move secretions out of the oropharynx.
b. Educate the family about what they are hearing and that the sound does not mean that the patient is in any distress.
c. Suction the patient deeply and often to rid the oropharynx of the build-up of secretions.
d. Suggest to the provider that now is the time for an anticholinergic drug (such as glycopyrrolate).

4. Chronic illnesses are characterized by which of the following? Select all that apply.

a. An irreversible pathology
b. A slow, progressive decline in normal physiologic function
c. A decreasing prevalence nationally and internationally
d. Necessity of long-term surveillance

5. A dying patient has sudden onset of confusion, waxing and waning consciousness, and loss of orientation, thinking they are at home when they are in the hospital. The nurse recognizes this as ______________ and knows that the most appropriate pharmacologic treatment for it may include ______________.

a. Dementia, acetylcholinesterase inhibitor
b. Delirium, benzodiazepine
c. Delirium, haloperidol
d. Dementia, haloperidol

REFERENCES AND SELECTED READINGS

References and selected readings associated with this chapter can be found on the website that accompanies the book. Visit **http://thepoint.lww.com/Honan3e** to access the references and other additional resources associated with this chapter.

UNIT TWO

Concepts and Challenges in Patient Management

A 45-year-old patient who has recently been diagnosed with brain cancer will be undergoing surgery, followed by chemotherapy. The patient is very anxious and has fears about the overall prognosis.

- **What psychosocial aspects may be affected by this diagnosis?**
- **Explain postoperative risks that may occur following surgery.**
- **Discuss the special needs of a patient undergoing chemotherapy.**

CHAPTER 3

Fluid and Electrolyte and Acid–Base Imbalances

Philip R. Martinez, Jr. • Linda Honan

Learning Objectives

After reading this chapter, you will be able to:

1. Differentiate between osmosis, diffusion, filtration, and active transport.
2. Describe the role of kidneys, lungs, and endocrine glands in regulating the body's fluid composition and volume.
3. Identify the effects of aging on fluid and electrolyte regulation.
4. Plan effective care of patients with the following imbalances: hypovolemia, hypervolemia, hyponatremia, hypernatremia, hypokalemia, and hyperkalemia.
5. Describe the cause, clinical manifestations, management, and nursing interventions for the following imbalances: hypocalcemia, hypercalcemia, hypomagnesemia, hypermagnesemia, hypophosphatemia, hyperphosphatemia, hypochloremia, and hyperchloremia.
6. Explain the roles of lungs, kidneys, and chemical buffers in maintaining acid–base balance.
7. Compare metabolic acidosis and alkalosis with regard to causes, clinical manifestations, diagnosis, and management.
8. Compare respiratory acidosis and alkalosis with regard to causes, clinical manifestations, diagnosis, and management.
9. Interpret arterial blood gas measurements.
10. Describe measures used for preventing complications of IV therapy.

Fluid and electrolyte balance is a dynamic process that is crucial for life and **homeostasis**. Potential and actual disorders of fluid and electrolyte balance occur in every setting, with nearly every disorder, and with a variety of changes that affect healthy people as well as those who are ill. The blood's acid–base balance is precisely controlled, and because deviations from the normal pH range of 7.35 to 7.45 can cause severe effects in body function, the nurse needs to competently interpret arterial blood gases (ABGs).

FUNDAMENTAL CONCEPTS

AMOUNT AND COMPOSITION OF BODY FLUIDS

Approximately 60% of the weight of a typical adult consists of fluid (water and electrolytes). Factors that influence the amount of body fluid are age, gender, and body fat. In general, younger people have a higher percentage of body fluid than older people due to progressive loss of muscle mass, and males have proportionately more body fluid than females (e.g., 60% vs. 50%). People who are obese have less fluid than those who are thin because fat cells contain little water.

Body fluid is located in two fluid compartments: the intracellular space (ICS, fluid inside the cells) and the extracellular space (ECS, fluid outside the cells). Approximately two thirds of body fluid is intracellular fluid (ICF) and is located primarily in the skeletal muscle mass; approximately one third is in the extracellular fluid (ECF).

The ECF compartment is further divided into the intravascular, interstitial, and transcellular fluid spaces. The intravascular space (IVS, the fluid within the blood vessels) contains plasma. Plasma is water, along with molecules, electrolytes, and proteins, minus blood cells and platelets. Approximately 3.5 L of the total blood volume (~5 to 6 L) is made up of plasma, which has a straw-colored appearance. The remainder consists of erythrocytes (red blood cells [RBCs]), leukocytes (white blood cells [WBCs]), and

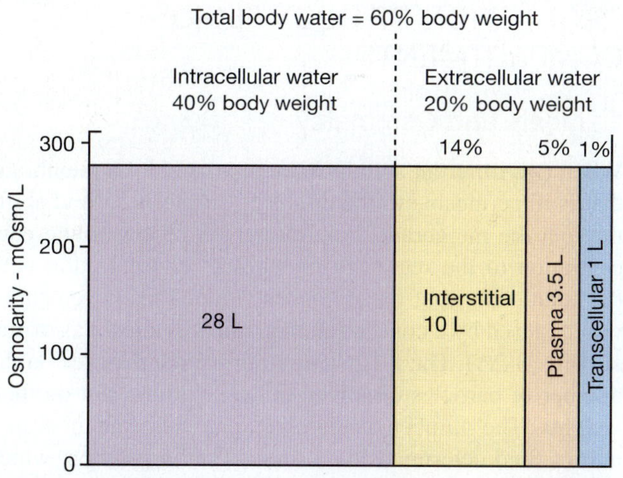

FIGURE 3-1 Approximate size of body compartments in a 70-kg male. (From Porth, C. M., & Matfin, G. (2009). *Pathophysiology: Concepts of altered health status* (8th ed.). Lippincott Williams & Wilkins.)

thrombocytes (platelets). The interstitial space contains the fluid between the cells, tissues, organs, and blood vessels and totals about 10 L in an adult. Lymph fluid is an interstitial fluid. The transcellular space is the smallest division of the ECF compartment and contains approximately 1 L. However, transcellular fluid can increase significantly in disease states (e.g., bowel obstruction or cirrhosis with ascites), and is formed at the expense of the remaining interstitial and plasma volumes (Delaney & Finfer, 2019). Examples of transcellular fluids are cerebrospinal, pericardial, synovial, intraocular, pleural, and the peritoneal cavity. Figure 3-1 demonstrates the composition of body compartments.

Body fluid normally shifts between the two major compartments or spaces (ICS and ECS) in an effort to transport gases, nutrients, and wastes while maintaining overall bodily function. Loss of fluid from the body can disrupt this equilibrium. Sometimes, fluid is not lost from the body but is unavailable for use by either the ICF or ECF. Loss of ECF into a space that does not contribute to equilibrium between the ICF and the ECF is referred to as an *interstitial and transcellular fluid shift,* or *third-spacing.*

Pearls for Practice

Early evidence of third-space fluid shifting is a decrease in urine output despite adequate fluid intake. Urine output decreases because fluid shifts out of the IVS; the kidneys then receive less blood and attempt to compensate by decreasing urine output. Other signs and symptoms of third-spacing that indicate an intravascular fluid volume deficit (FVD) include increased heart rate, decreased blood pressure, decreased central venous pressure (CVP), edema, and imbalances in fluid intake and output (I&O). Third-space shifts into the transcellular spaces occur in ascites, burns, peritonitis, bowel obstruction, and massive bleeding into a joint or body cavity.

Electrolytes in body fluids are active chemicals (cations that carry positive charges and anions that carry negative charges). The major cations in body fluid are sodium (Na^+), potassium (K^+), calcium (Ca^{+2}), magnesium (Mg^{+2}), and hydrogen (H^+) ions. The major anions are chloride (Cl^-), bicarbonate (HCO_3^-), phosphate (PO_4^{3-}), sulfate (SO_4^{2-}), and proteinate ions.

These chemicals unite in varying combinations. Therefore, electrolyte concentration in the body is expressed in terms of milliequivalents (mEq) per liter, a measure of chemical activity, rather than in terms of milligrams (mg), a unit of weight. More specifically, a milliequivalent is defined as being equivalent to the electrochemical activity of 1 mg of hydrogen. In a solution, cations and anions are equal in milliequivalents per liter.

Although all body fluid contains equal amounts of cations and anions, the electrolyte concentrations in the ICF are markedly different from those in the ECF, as reflected in Table 3-1. Sodium ions, which are positively charged, far outnumber the other cations in the ECF. Because sodium concentration affects the overall concentration of the ECF, sodium is important in regulating the volume of body fluid. Approximately 90% of the serum osmolality (discussed later) is determined by the serum sodium level. Retention

TABLE 3-1 Approximate Major Electrolyte Content in Body Fluid

Electrolytes	mEq/L[a]
Extracellular Fluid (Plasma)	
Cations	
Sodium (Na^+)	142
Potassium (K^+)	5
Calcium (Ca^{+2})	5
Magnesium (Mg^{+2})	2
Total cations	154
Anions	
Chloride (Cl^-)	103
Bicarbonate (HCO_3^-)	26
Phosphate (PO_4^{3-})	2
Sulfate (SO_4^{2-})	1
Organic acids	5
Proteinate	17
Total anions	154
Intracellular Fluid	
Cations	
Potassium (K^+)	150
Magnesium (Mg^{+2})	40
Sodium (Na^+)	10
Total cations	200
Anions	
Phosphates and sulfates	150
Bicarbonate (HCO_3^-)	10
Proteinate	40
Total anions	200

[a]Values may vary depending on the method of analysis used.

of sodium is associated with fluid retention, and conversely, excessive loss of sodium is usually associated with decreased volume of body fluid.

As shown in Table 3-1, the major electrolytes in the ICF are potassium and phosphate. The ECF has a low concentration of potassium and can tolerate only small changes in potassium concentrations. Therefore, any condition that causes the release of large stores of intracellular potassium (e.g., trauma to the cells and tissues) can be extremely dangerous.

Pearls for Practice

*The nurse understands that the **intracellular** concentration of K^+ is approximately 140 to 150 mEq/L and that the kidneys are primarily responsible for K^+ excretion. The nurse recognizes that hyperkalemia (generally defined as a plasma K^+ of greater than 5.0 mEq/L) is associated with cardiac arrhythmias (discussed in Chapter 16), muscle weakness, and acute muscle damage from rhabdomyolysis (discussed in Chapter 41), kidney failure (discussed in Chapter 26), and acidosis (discussed later in this chapter). One of the most common metabolic causes of cardiac arrest is hyperkalemia, which is associated most frequently in patients with kidney failure.*

The body expends a great deal of energy maintaining the high extracellular concentration of sodium and the high intracellular concentration of potassium. It does so by means of cell membrane pumps that exchange sodium and potassium ions.

Normal movement of fluid through the capillary wall into the tissues is dependent on two primary forces (called Starling forces): (1) the capillary hydrostatic pressure generated by cardiac contraction and exerted by plasma fluids on the walls of the blood vessel, and (2) the plasma oncotic (colloid osmotic) pressure, exerted by plasma proteins (primarily by capillary-impermeable albumin). At the arterial end of the capillary bed, fluids are filtered because the hydrostatic pressure exceeds the oncotic pressure; thus, water and electrolytes leave the capillary and enter the interstitial space and/or ICS. Because hydrostatic pressure decreases as blood moves along the capillary bed, the relatively constant plasma oncotic pressure exceeds the hydrostatic pressure at the venous end of the capillary; therefore, fluids now re-enter the capillary. In many capillary beds, the forces favoring filtration slightly exceed those that favor reabsorption. However, excessive interstitial fluid accumulation is prevented since the lymphatic drainage returns this excess fluid to the systemic circulation.

In addition to electrolytes, the ECF transports other substances, such as enzymes and hormones. It also carries blood components, such as RBCs, WBCs, and platelets, throughout the body.

REGULATION OF BODY FLUID COMPARTMENTS

Osmosis and Osmolality

When two different solutions are separated by a membrane that is impermeable to the dissolved substances, fluid shifts through the membrane from the region of low solute concentration to the region of high solute concentration until the solutions are of equal concentration. The movement of water caused by a concentration gradient is known as **osmosis** (Fig. 3-2A). The magnitude of this force depends on the number of particles dissolved in the solutions, not on their weights. The number of dissolved particles contained in a unit of fluid determines the osmolality of a solution, which influences the movement of fluid between the fluid compartments. **Tonicity** is the ability of all the solutes to cause an osmotic driving force that promotes water movement from one compartment to another (Norris, 2019). Intravenous (IV) solutions are termed isotonic, hypotonic, or hypertonic. If a solution is isotonic (e.g., 0.9% sodium chloride [NaCl]), it has a close approximation to normal serum osmolarity (308 milliosmoles per liter [mOsm/L] in 0.9% NaCl vs. 275 to 295 mOsm/L in plasma). Sodium, mannitol, glucose, and sorbitol are all effective osmoles (capable of affecting water movement; see later discussion of IV solutions). Osmolarity (mOsm/L) and osmolality (mOsm/kg) are used interchangeably in clinical practice; however, most calculations of body fluids are based on osmolality (Noble, 2021).

Pearls for Practice

It is important to understand osmotic diuresis, which is an increase in urine output caused by the excretion of substances such as glucose, mannitol, or contrast agents in the urine, which exert an osmotic pull on water. For example, because glucose is an osmotic agent (capable of affecting water movement), when glucose is excreted in the urine, it will bring water with it, causing polyuria with resulting FVD.

Diffusion

Diffusion is the natural tendency of a substance to move from an area of higher concentration to one of lower concentration (see Fig. 3-2B). Examples of diffusion are the exchange of oxygen and carbon dioxide between the pulmonary capillaries and alveoli.

Pearls for Practice

Let us consider that your patient has a nasogastric (NG) or nasal jejunal (NJ) tube in place that is connected to suction or gravity drainage. You may need to irrigate the tube to ensure its patency. What solution will you use? Tap water from the sink or normal saline irrigation? In this situation, you will use normal saline because it is isotonic and therefore will prevent

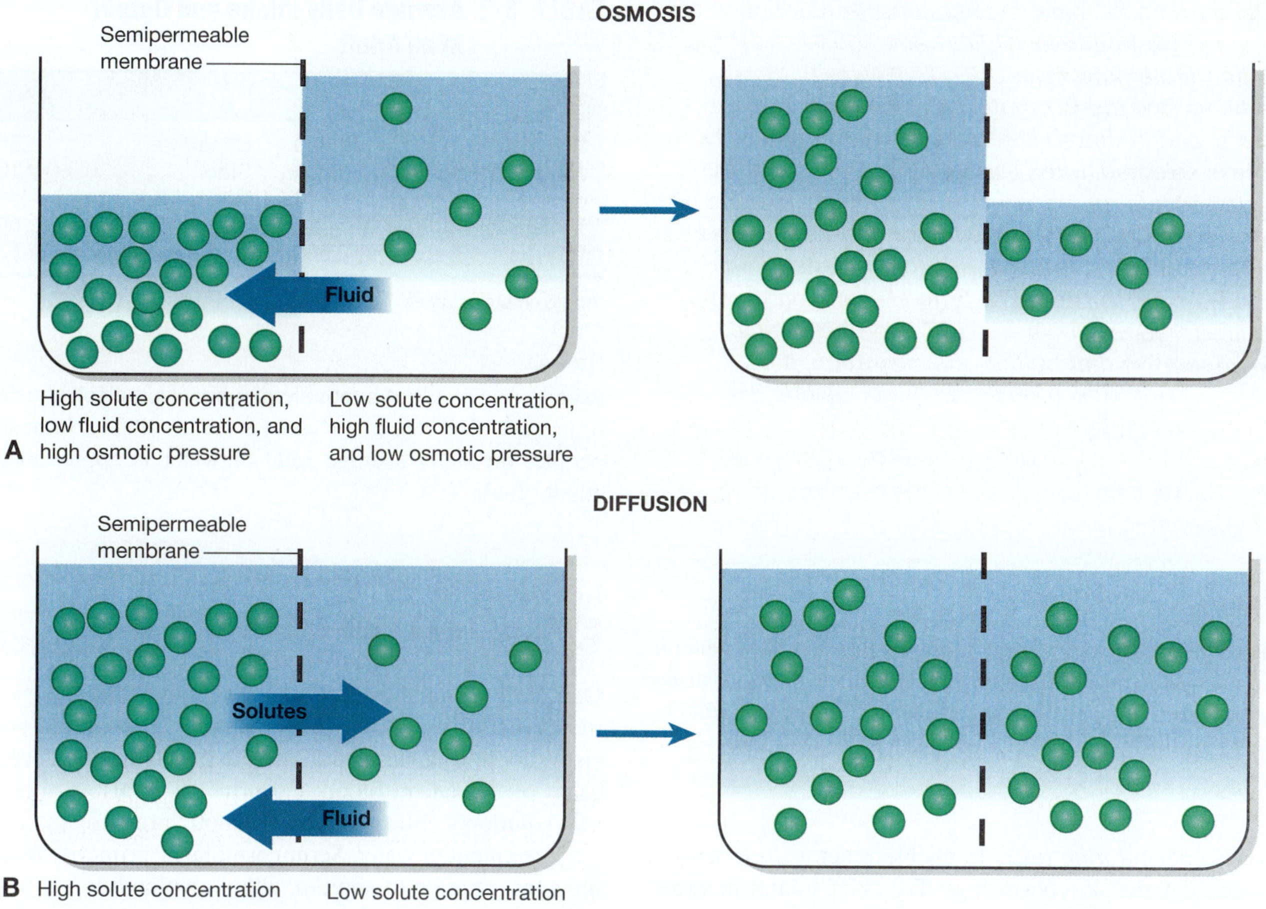

FIGURE 3-2 **A. Osmosis: Movement of fluid from an area of lower solute concentration to an area of higher solute concentration with eventual equalization of the solute concentrations. B. Diffusion: Movement of solutes from an area of greater concentration to an area of lesser concentration, leading ultimately to equalization of the solute concentrations.**

electrolyte wash out which would occur if you used tap water (Haugen & Galura, 2020). Does that make sense to you? Consider what you just learned about diffusion. Visualize all the electrolytes in the stomach or jejunum and irrigating with an equal number of electrolytes versus irrigation with only water. More electrolytes would be lost with irrigation of water; thus, all tubes are irrigated with normal saline when the NG or NJ tube is connected to suction. When the tube is used for feeding, water is used.

Filtration

Hydrostatic pressure in the capillaries tends to filter fluid out of the intravascular compartment into the interstitial fluid. Movement of water and solutes occurs from an area of high hydrostatic pressure to an area of low hydrostatic pressure. Filtration allows the kidneys to filter 180 L of plasma per day.

Sodium–Potassium Pump

As previously stated, the sodium concentration is greater in the ECF than in the ICF, and, because of this, sodium tends to enter the cell by diffusion. This tendency is offset by the sodium–potassium pump, which is located in the cell membrane and actively moves sodium from the cell into the ECF. Conversely, the high intracellular potassium concentration is maintained by pumping potassium into the cell. By definition, **active transport** implies that energy must be expended for the movement to occur against a concentration gradient.

ROUTES OF GAINS AND LOSSES

Water and electrolytes are gained in various ways. A healthy person gains fluids by drinking and eating. Fluids may also be provided by the parenteral route (IV or subcutaneously) or by means of an enteral feeding tube in the stomach or intestine.

Pearls for Practice

What is the difference between parenteral and enteral nutrition? Parenteral refers to fluids or medications or nutrition in the form of total parenteral nutrition (TPN) or peripheral parenteral nutrition (PPN) that is administered via an IV catheter into the bloodstream.

Enteral refers to fluids, medications, or nutrition using the gastrointestinal (GI) tract. You will hear the adage, "if the gut works-USE IT." However, there are times that the PO route, NG tube, or NJ tube is unsafe, and in those situations, the parenteral or IV route is selected. Each carries risks. Parenteral will be discussed later in this chapter, and enteral feeding is reviewed in Chapter 21. It is important to recognize that enteral fluids, medications (oral), or nutrition can NEVER be administered IV. Enteral— and parenteral—administered products are NOT interchangeable. It is imperative that before administration, the nurse validates the specific products labeling for administration. The nurse understands the Rights of Medication Administration include the right patient, drug, ***route****, time, dosage, and form, as well as the right documentation and responses.*

Kidneys

The usual daily urine volume in the adult is 1.5 L. A general rule is that the output is approximately 0.5 to 1 mL of urine per kilogram of body weight per hour (0.5 to 1 mL/kg/hr) in all age groups, with boundaries of 0.5 to 2 mL/kg/hr.

Skin

Sensible perspiration refers to visible water and electrolyte loss through the skin (sweating). The chief solutes in sweat are sodium, chloride, and potassium. Actual sweat loss can vary from 0 to 1 to 3 L/hr, depending on the environmental temperature (Norris, 2019). Continuous water loss by evaporation (approximately 600 mL/day) occurs through the skin as insensible perspiration, a nonvisible form of water loss. Fever greatly increases insensible water loss through the lungs and the skin by 75 mL per 1°F increase in temperature (Lough, 2022), as does loss of the natural skin barrier (e.g., through major burns). Although sodium content in sweat is low (ranging from approximately 20 to 50 mmol/L), with increased sweat loss, sodium deficit and FVD can occur (Surapongchai et al., 2021).

Lungs

The lungs normally eliminate water vapor (insensible loss) at a rate of approximately 400 mL every day. The loss is much greater with increased respiratory rate or depth, or in a dry climate.

Gastrointestinal Tract

The usual loss through the GI tract is only 100 mL daily, even though approximately 8 L of fluid circulates through the GI system every 24 hours. Because the bulk of fluid is normally reabsorbed in the small intestine, diarrhea and fistulas cause large losses. To illustrate, worldwide, infectious diarrhea is associated with 1.5 to 2.5 million deaths per year

TABLE **3-2 Average Daily Intake and Output in an Adult**

Intake (mL)			
Oral liquids	1,300	Urine	1,500
Water in food	1,000	Stool	100
Water produced by metabolism	300	Insensible Lungs	400
		Skin	600
Total gain[a]	2,600	Total loss[a]	2,600

[a]Approximate volumes.

usually as a result of hypovolemia; however, electrolyte disorders are also common (Sattar & Singh, 2021). In healthy people, the daily average I&O of water is approximately equal (Table 3-2).

LABORATORY TESTS FOR EVALUATING FLUID STATUS

Osmolality is the concentration of fluid that affects the movement of water between fluid compartments by osmosis. Osmolality measures the solute concentration per kilogram of solvent in blood and urine. It is also a measure of a solution's ability to create osmotic pressure and affect the movement of water. Serum osmolality primarily reflects the concentration of sodium, although blood urea nitrogen (BUN) and glucose also play a major role in determining serum osmolality (Norris, 2019). Urine osmolality is determined by urea, creatinine, and uric acid. When measured with serum osmolality, urine osmolality is the most reliable indicator of the concentrating ability of kidneys. Osmolality is reported as milliosmoles per kilogram of water (mOsm/kg).

Osmolarity, another term that describes the concentration of solutions, is measured in milliosmoles per liter (mOsm/L). The term *osmolality* is used more often in clinical practice. Normal serum osmolality is 275 to 295 mOsm/kg, and normal urine osmolality is 50 to 1,400 mOsm/kg in a random urine test and 300 to 900 mOsm/kg in a 24-hour urine collection (Fischbach et al., 2022); there are variations in ranges based on the clinical laboratory standard values.

Pearls for Practice

When concerned about renal concentrating ability, a serum and urine osmolality test is obtained at the same time. In general, the normal ratio of urine and serum is 3:1. Higher ratios are seen in concentrated urine, whereas lower ratios are seen with poor concentrating ability.

Factors that increase and decrease serum and urine osmolality are identified in Table 3-3. Serum osmolality may be

TABLE **3-3 Factors Affecting Serum and Urine Osmolality**

Fluid	Factors Increasing Osmolality	Factors Decreasing Osmolality
Serum (275–295 mOsm/kg water)	• Severe dehydration • Free water loss • Diabetes insipidus • Hypernatremia • Hyperglycemia • Stroke or head injury	• Fluid volume excess • Syndrome of inappropriate antidiuretic hormone (SIADH) • Kidney failure • Adrenal insufficiency • Hyponatremia • Overhydration
Random Urine (50–1,200 mOsm/kg water)	• Fluid volume deficit (FVD) • SIADH • Acidosis	• Diabetes insipidus • Hyponatremia • Fluid volume excess

measured directly through laboratory tests or estimated at the bedside by doubling the serum sodium level or by using the following formula:

$$\text{Plasma osmolality (mOsm/kg)} = 2\,[\text{serum sodium}] + \text{Glucose}/18 + \text{BUN}/2.8$$

The calculated value usually is within 10 mOsm of the measured osmolality.

The specific gravity of urine measures the kidneys' ability to excrete or conserve water. The specific gravity of urine is compared to the weight of distilled water, which has a specific gravity of 1.000. The normal range of urine specific gravity is 1.010 to 1.025. Specific gravity of urine can be measured by placing a calibrated hydrometer or urinometer in a cylinder of approximately 20 mL of urine, or with a refractometer or dipstick with a reagent for this purpose. Specific gravity varies inversely with urine volume; normally, the larger the volume of urine, the lower the specific gravity, whereas a high specific gravity indicates concentrated urine.

Pearls for Practice

Specific gravity is a less reliable indicator of concentration than urine osmolality because it is influenced by both the number and size of particles in urine; increased glucose or protein in urine can cause a falsely elevated specific gravity. Factors that increase or decrease urine osmolality are the same as those for urine specific gravity. In addition, a fixed specific gravity that does not vary with fluid intake implies early kidney dysfunction, suggesting the kidneys are unable to excrete or resorb water and solutes.

The laboratory value BUN, part of the basic metabolic panel, is made up of urea, which is an end product of the metabolism of protein (from both muscle and dietary intake) by the liver. The normal BUN is 6 to 20 mg/dL (2.1 to 7.2 mmol/L). The BUN level varies with urine output. Factors that increase BUN include decreased kidney function, GI bleeding, dehydration, increased protein intake, fever, and sepsis. Any condition that increases tissue necrosis and protein catabolism will cause the BUN to rise; a critical value for BUN is when it is over 100 mg/dL (Fischbach et al., 2022). Those factors that decrease BUN include end-stage liver disease, a low-protein diet, starvation, syndrome of inappropriate antidiuretic hormone (SIADH), and any condition that results in expanded fluid volume (e.g., pregnancy).

Creatinine is the end product of muscle metabolism. Creatinine is a better indicator of kidney function than BUN because it does not vary with protein intake and metabolic state. The normal serum creatinine is approximately 0.6 to 1.3 mg/dL (53 to 115 mmol/L); however, its concentration depends on lean body mass and varies from person to person (Fischbach et al., 2022). Serum creatinine levels increase when kidney function decreases.

Hematocrit (Hct) measures the volume percentage of RBC (erythrocytes) in whole blood and normally ranges from 42% to 52% for males and 36% to 48% for females (Fischbach et al., 2022). Conditions that increase the Hct value are dehydration and polycythemia, and conditions that decrease Hct are overhydration and anemia. A Hct below 20% can lead to cardiac failure and death, whereas a Hct >60% can cause spontaneous clotting of blood (Fischbach et al., 2022).

Urine sodium values change with sodium intake and the status of fluid volume: as sodium intake increases, excretion increases; as the circulating fluid volume decreases, sodium is conserved. Normal urine sodium levels range from 40 to 220 mEq every 24 hours (40 to 220 mmol/day). A random specimen usually contains more than 40 mEq/L of sodium. Urine sodium levels may be used to assess volume status and are useful in the diagnosis of hyponatremia, SIADH, and acute kidney failure (AKF).

HOMEOSTATIC MECHANISMS

The body is equipped with remarkable homeostatic mechanisms to keep the composition and volume of body fluid within narrow limits of normal. Organs involved in homeostasis include the kidneys, lungs, heart, adrenal glands, parathyroid glands, and pituitary gland.

Kidney Functions

Vital to the regulation of fluid and electrolyte balance, the kidneys normally filter 180 L of plasma every day in the adult, while excreting only 1.5 L of urine. They act both autonomously and in response to blood-borne messengers, such as aldosterone and antidiuretic hormone (ADH) (Norris, 2019). Major functions of the kidneys in maintaining normal fluid balance include the following:

- Regulation of ECF volume and osmolality by selective retention and excretion of body fluids;
- Regulation of electrolyte levels in the ECF by selective retention of needed substances and excretion of unneeded substances;
- Regulation of pH of the ECF by excretion or retention of hydrogen ions and/or bicarbonate ions (HCO_3^-);
- Excretion of metabolic wastes and toxic substances.

Given these functions, it is readily apparent that kidney failure results in multiple fluid and electrolyte abnormalities. Kidney function declines with advanced age, as does muscle mass and daily exogenous creatinine production. Therefore, high-normal and minimally elevated serum creatinine values actually may indicate substantially reduced kidney function in older individuals.

Heart and Blood Vessel Functions

The pumping action of the heart circulates blood through the kidneys under sufficient pressure to allow for urine formation. Failure of this pumping action interferes with renal perfusion and thus with water and electrolyte regulation.

Lung Functions

The lungs are also vital in maintaining homeostasis. Through exhalation, the lungs remove approximately 400 mL of water daily in a normal adult. Abnormal conditions, such as hyperpnea (abnormally deep respiration) or continuous coughing, increase this loss; mechanical ventilation with excessive moisture decreases it. The lungs also play a major role in maintaining acid–base balance. Normal aging results in decreased respiratory function, causing increased difficulty in pH regulation in older adults, especially those with major illness or trauma.

Pituitary Functions

The hypothalamus manufactures ADH, which is stored in the posterior pituitary gland and released as needed. ADH is sometimes called the *water-conserving hormone* because it causes the body to retain water. Functions of ADH include maintaining the osmotic pressure of the cells by controlling the retention or excretion of water by the kidneys and by regulating blood volume (Fig. 3-3).

Adrenal Functions

Aldosterone, a mineralocorticoid secreted by the zona glomerulosa (outer zone) of the adrenal cortex, has a profound effect on fluid balance. Increased secretion of aldosterone causes sodium retention (and, thus, water retention) and potassium loss. Conversely, decreased secretion of aldosterone causes sodium and water loss and potassium retention.

Cortisol, another adrenocortical hormone, has only a fraction of the mineralocorticoid potency of aldosterone. However, when secreted in large quantities (or administered as corticosteroid therapy), it can also produce sodium and fluid retention.

Parathyroid Functions

The parathyroid glands, embedded in the thyroid gland, regulate calcium and phosphate balance by means of parathyroid hormone (PTH). PTH influences bone resorption (movement of calcium out of bone to the blood), calcium absorption from the intestines, and calcium reabsorption from the renal tubules. A decrease in serum calcium is the primary stimulus for PTH secretions, whereas a rise in serum calcium inhibits secretion.

Other Mechanisms

Changes in the volume of the interstitial compartment within the ECF can occur without affecting body function. However, the vascular compartment cannot tolerate change as readily and must be carefully maintained to ensure that tissues receive adequate nutrients.

Baroreceptors

The baroreceptors or pressoreceptors are small nerve receptors in the walls of the blood vessels and heart that detect changes in pressure within blood vessels and transmit this information to the central nervous system (CNS), specifically the medulla oblongata (brainstem). They are responsible for monitoring the circulating volume, and they regulate sympathetic and parasympathetic neural activity. They are categorized as either low-pressure or high-pressure baroreceptors. Low-pressure baroreceptors are in the cardiac atria, ventricles, and pulmonary vasculature (Armstrong et al., 2021). High-pressure baroreceptors are nerve endings in the aortic arch and the carotid sinus, as well as in the afferent arteriole of the juxtaglomerular apparatus of the nephron.

As arterial pressure decreases, baroreceptors transmit fewer impulses from the carotid sinuses and the aortic arch to the vasomotor center. A decrease in impulses stimulates the sympathetic nervous system and inhibits the parasympathetic nervous system. The outcome is an increase in cardiac rate, conduction, and contractility as well as an increase in circulating blood volume. Sympathetic stimulation constricts renal arterioles; this increases the release of aldosterone, decreases glomerular filtration, and increases sodium and

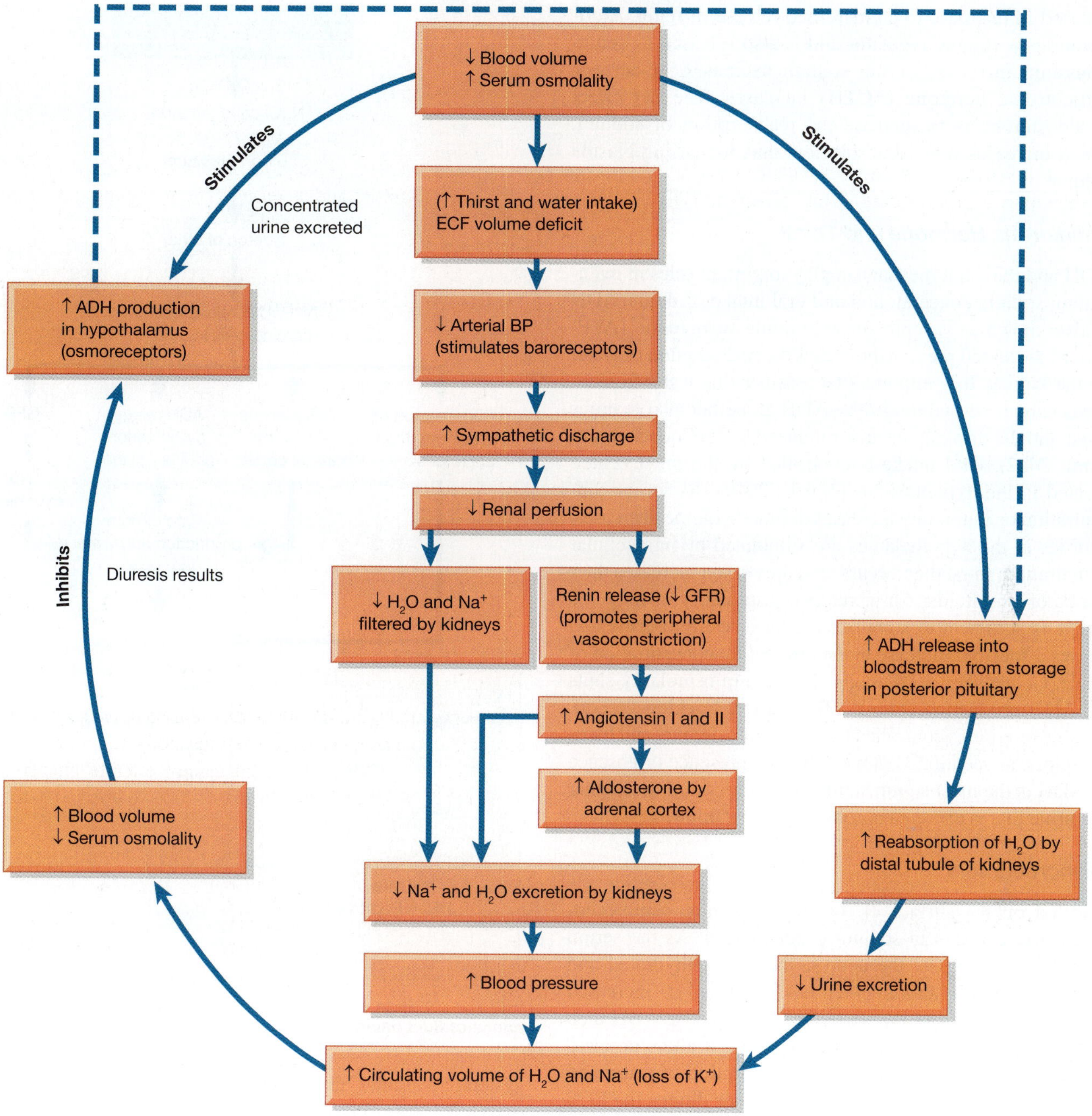

FIGURE 3-3 **Fluid regulation cycle.**

water reabsorption and potassium loss (discussed below). Conversely, if high-pressure baroreceptors are stimulated, such as in fluid volume excess, the baroreceptor response results in parasympathetic activity of a lowered heart rate and lowered blood vessel resistance. These baroreceptor responses occur very rapidly, most often within seconds to minutes (Carbino, 2020).

Renin–Angiotensin–Aldosterone System

Renin is an enzyme that converts angiotensinogen, an inactive substance formed by the liver that continuously circulates in the plasma, into angiotensin I (AI) (Fountain & Lappin, 2022). Renin is released by the juxtaglomerular cells of the kidneys in response to decreased renal perfusion. Angiotensin-converting enzyme (ACE), which is found primarily in the vascular endothelium of the lungs and kidneys, converts AI to angiotensin II (AII). AII, with its vasoconstrictor properties, increases arterial perfusion pressure and also stimulates thirst and increased water intake. It also stimulates the release of ADH by the posterior pituitary, which increases water reabsorption in the kidneys, specifically in the distal tubule and collecting duct (Fountain & Lappin, 2022). When the sympathetic nervous system is stimulated, aldosterone is released in response to an increased release of renin. Aldosterone is a volume regulator and is also released as serum potassium increases, serum sodium decreases, or adrenocorticotropic hormone (ACTH) increases. The net effect of aldosterone is to increase the reabsorption of sodium, which increases water reabsorption, thus increasing plasma volume.

Antidiuretic Hormone and Thirst

ADH and the thirst mechanism play important roles in maintaining sodium concentration and oral intake of fluids. ADH is also known as vasopressin or arginine vasopressin (AVP) and, as discussed previously, causes the reabsorption of water by the kidney. It is important to consider that water homeostasis cannot be maintained by ADH alone but also requires thirst and the drinking behavior induced by it (Cooper & Van Uum, 2022). Oral intake is controlled by the thirst center, located in the hypothalamus (Norris, 2019). As serum concentration or osmolality increases or blood volume decreases, neurons in the hypothalamus are stimulated by intracellular dehydration; thirst then occurs, and the person increases their intake of oral fluids. An increase in osmolality of only 1% to 2% is sufficient to stimulate a strong desire to drink and causes a fourfold increase in the circulating concentration of ADH. Conversely, a 1% to 2% decrease in osmolality shuts off ADH production entirely (Toffaletti & Rackley, 2022a). Water excretion is controlled by ADH, aldosterone, and baroreceptors, as mentioned previously. The presence or absence of ADH is the most significant factor in determining whether the urine that is excreted is concentrated or dilute.

Osmoreceptors

Located on the surface of the hypothalamus, osmoreceptors sense changes in sodium concentration. As the serum osmolality increases, the neurons become dehydrated and quickly generate action potentials resulting in increased release of ADH from the posterior pituitary. The ADH then travels in the blood to the kidneys, where it alters permeability to water, causing increased reabsorption of water and decreased urine output. The retained water dilutes the ECF and returns its concentration to normal. Restoration of normal serum osmolality provides feedback to the osmoreceptors to inhibit further ADH release (see Fig. 3-3).

Release of Atrial Natriuretic Peptide

Atrial natriuretic peptide (ANP), also called *atrial natriuretic factor,* is a hormone synthesized, stored, and released by muscle cells of the atria of the heart in response to several factors. ANP secretion is enhanced by increases in atrial pressure, hypernatremia (discussed shortly), any condition that results in volume expansion or hypervolemia (e.g., pregnancy), increased cardiac filling pressures (e.g., high sodium intake, heart failure [HF], chronic kidney failure [CKF], decreased cardiac output, vasoconstriction, and increased

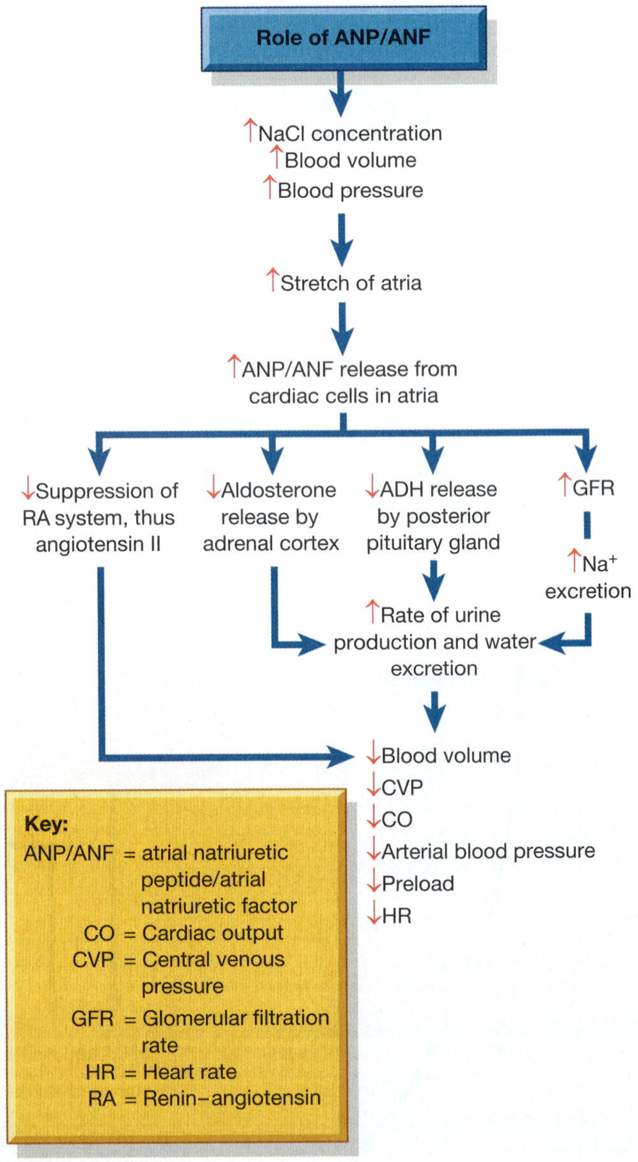

FIGURE 3-4 Role of atrial natriuretic peptide (ANP) in maintenance of fluid balance.

systemic vascular resistance) (Lough, 2022). The action of ANP is the direct opposite of the renin–angiotensin–aldosterone system (RAAS); ANP decreases blood pressure and volume by initiating vasodilation and stimulating increased sodium and water excretion by the collecting ducts of the kidney (Fig. 3-4) (Lough, 2022). The ANP measured in plasma is normally 20 to 77 pg/mL (20 to 77 ng/L) (Pagana et al., 2023). This level increases in paroxysmal atrial tachycardia, hyperthyroidism, subarachnoid hemorrhage, and small-cell lung cancer. In HF and cirrhosis with ascites, ANP is elevated but not sufficiently to prevent fluid volume excess (FVE). Brain natriuretic peptide (BNP) that is stored primarily in ventricular myocardium and released when ventricular diastolic pressure rises has actions similar to **ANP**. Normal BNP levels are less than 100 pg/mL (Pagana et al., 2023). For reasons that are not understood, the renal effects of the natriuretic peptides appear to become dampened with advancing HF, leaving the effects of RAAS unopposed.

Pearls for Practice

BNP correlates well with left ventricular pressures and is a good marker for HF. The higher the levels of BNP, the more severe the HF. In emergency room settings, when a patient complains of shortness of breath (SOB), a BNP will be drawn. If the BNP is elevated, the SOB is secondary to HF. If the BNP is normal, the cause of SOB is not cardiac, and other etiologies are considered (e.g., pulmonary causes). Thus, this test is useful in evaluating SOB in patients with cardiac and chronic lung disease as well as evaluation of treatment and therapeutic response of patients with HF (Pagana et al., 2023).

GERONTOLOGIC CONSIDERATIONS

Normal physiologic changes of aging, including reduced cardiac, kidney, and respiratory function and reserve, as well as alterations in the ratio of body fluids to muscle mass, may alter the responses of older people to fluid and electrolyte changes and acid–base disturbances. For example, with age, the GFR declines by approximately 0.75 mL/min/yr (Lough, 2022). In addition, the frequent use of medications in the older adult can affect kidney and cardiac function and fluid balance, thereby increasing the likelihood of fluid and electrolyte disturbances. Routine procedures, such as the vigorous administration of laxatives before GI studies, may produce a serious FVD, necessitating the use of IV fluids to prevent hypotension and other effects of hypovolemia.

Alterations in fluid and electrolyte balance that may produce minor changes in young and middle-aged adults have the potential to produce profound changes in older adults, accompanied by a rapid onset of signs and symptoms. In older patients, the clinical manifestations of fluid and electrolyte disturbances may be subtle or atypical. For example, fluid deficit may cause confusion or cognitive impairment in the older person, whereas in the young or middle-aged person, the first sign commonly is increased thirst. Rapid infusion of an excessive volume of IV fluids may produce fluid overload and cardiac failure in the older patient. These reactions are likely to occur more quickly and with the administration of smaller volumes of fluid than in healthy young and middle-aged adults because of the decreased cardiac reserve and reduced kidney function that accompany aging. Dehydration in older people is common as a result of decreased reserve capacity of the kidney from the aging process, disease, and use of medications.

Increased sensitivity to fluid and electrolyte changes in older patients requires careful assessment, with attention to I&O of fluids from all sources and to changes in daily weight, careful monitoring of side effects and interactions of medications, and prompt reporting and management of disturbances.

FLUID VOLUME DISTURBANCES

Appendix A summarizes the major fluid and electrolyte imbalances that are described in this chapter.

HYPOVOLEMIA

FVD, or hypovolemia, occurs when loss of ECF volume exceeds the intake of fluid. It occurs when water and electrolytes are lost in the same proportion as they exist in normal body fluids, so that the ratio of serum electrolytes to water remains the same. FVD should not be confused with the term *dehydration,* which refers to loss of water alone, resulting in increased serum sodium levels and hemoconcentration. FVD may occur alone or in combination with other imbalances. Unless other imbalances are present concurrently, serum electrolyte concentrations remain essentially unchanged.

Pearls for Practice

The nurse is aware that the Hct is the proportion of RBCs present in the bloodstream or intravascular space (IVS) and is expressed as a percentage (e.g., Hct of 45% indicates that 45% of the whole blood is comprised of RBCs). In patients with normal fluid balance, the Hct is approximately three times the hemoglobin level (Lough, 2022). When the Hct increases, the nurse associates the finding with a fluid volume deficit (less water in the bloodstream so the percentage of RBCs in blood increases). This is termed hemoconcentration. The nurse expects that since water is lacking in the bloodstream, other lab findings will also be elevated (e.g., sodium, BUN). However, you are aware that there is a disorder of RBC production called polycythemia that can also increase Hct level (Fischbach et al., 2022). Conversely, a decreased Hct can indicate fluid volume excess because of the dilutional effect of the extra fluid load. There is now more water in the bloodstream, so the percentage of RBCs in blood decreases. Again, the nurse expects that with hemodilution, other lab findings will also be decreased (e.g., sodium, BUN). Other causes of a decreased Hct include blood loss, anemia, chronic disease, or hemolytic reactions (Fischbach et al., 2022). When the Hct is decreasing but the hemoglobin concentration remains constant, the cause is fluid volume overload, whereas a decreased Hgb and Hct indicates a true RBC loss (Lough, 2022).

Pathophysiology

FVD results from loss of body fluids and occurs more rapidly when coupled with decreased fluid intake. FVD can develop from inadequate intake alone if the decreased intake is prolonged. The nurse considers NPO status of patients for diagnostic tests, those with difficulty swallowing, nausea, decreased level of consciousness (LOC), or depression when IV fluids are not administered. Older individuals are at risk for FVD because of poor oral intake and potential difficulty gaining access to water. Causes of FVD also include abnormal fluid losses, such as those resulting from vomiting, diarrhea, GI suctioning (nasogastric or intestinal tubes, drains [biliary, pancreatic]), fever, and diaphoresis (sweating). Additional risk factors include burns, surgery, diabetes insipidus (DI), adrenal insufficiency, osmotic diuresis, hemorrhage, and coma. Third-space fluid shifts, or the movement of fluid from the vascular system to other body spaces (e.g., with edema formation in burns, ascites with liver dysfunction), also cause FVD because although the fluid has not left the body, it is not available in the IVS.

Clinical Manifestations and Assessment

FVD can develop rapidly and can be mild, moderate, or severe, depending on the degree of fluid loss. Important signs include acute weight loss; decreased skin turgor; oliguria (urinary output below 400 mL/day); concentrated urine with a high specific gravity; postural hypotension (a 20 mm Hg decrease in systolic pressure or a 10 mm Hg decrease in diastolic pressure with position change); a weak, rapid heart rate; flattened neck veins; decreased CVP; cool, clammy skin related to peripheral vasoconstriction; a smaller tongue with additional longitudinal furrows; dry oral mucous membranes; delayed capillary refill (greater than 2 seconds); altered sensorium; and thirst. The eyeballs may appear sunken into the orbital cavities (Castera & Borhade, 2021). Diagnostic testing includes BUN and its relation to serum creatinine concentration. A volume-depleted patient has a BUN elevated out of proportion to the serum creatinine (ratio greater than 20:1). The BUN can also be elevated because of decreased renal perfusion and function. The cause of abnormal laboratory findings may be determined through the health history and physical findings.

Pearls for Practice

The nurse compresses the nail bed to produce blanching; the release of this pressure should result in the return of blood flow and baseline nail color in less than 2 seconds. A capillary refill >5 seconds is associated with severe organ failure and increased mortality (Lough, 2022).

The Hct level is greater than normal in dehydration because the RBC becomes suspended in a decreased plasma volume, which is also known as *hemoconcentration.*

Serum electrolyte changes may also exist. Potassium and sodium levels can be reduced (hypokalemia, hyponatremia) or elevated (hyperkalemia, hypernatremia):

- Hypokalemia occurs with GI and kidney losses;
- Hyperkalemia occurs with adrenal insufficiency;
- Hyponatremia occurs with increased thirst and ADH release;
- Hypernatremia results from increased insensible losses and DI.

Specific gravity of urine is increased in relation to the kidneys' attempt to conserve water and decreased with DI (more details on DI are found in Chapter 30). The range of urine specific gravity will vary with

- the hydration status of the patient (increased with FVD, decreased with FVE),
- the volume of urine (increased specific gravity with decreased urine output, decreased specific gravity with increased urine output), and
- the number of the particles in the urine (increased with increased particles, decreased with fewer particles).

A urine specific gravity of 1.005 or less indicates the diluting ability of the kidney, whereas 1.020 or greater indicates concentrating ability of the kidney. For example, a patient with preserved kidney function who is volume depleted will have a specific gravity greater than 1.020 because the patient is able to concentrate their urine. However, there are times that the specific gravity is falsely elevated, such as during kidney excretion of radiopaque x-ray contrast (high-molecular-weight substance). Thus, a urine osmolality test is a more exact measurement than specific gravity and may be required when assessment of the concentrating or diluting function of the kidney is needed.

Medical Management

When planning the correction of fluid loss for the patient with FVD, the health care provider considers the usual maintenance requirements of the patient and other factors (e.g., fever) that can influence fluid needs. If the deficit is not severe, the oral route is preferred, provided the patient can drink. However, if fluid losses are acute or severe, the IV route is required. Isotonic electrolyte solutions (e.g., lactated Ringer solution, 0.9% sodium chloride) are frequently used to treat the hypotensive patient with FVD because those solutions expand plasma volume. The ICS is essentially sodium free; thus, for every liter of 0.9% sodium chloride administered, 1,000 mL will remain in the ECS, of which approximately 250 mL will remain in the IVS, re-expanding the plasma volume. Because this solution can expand the IVS, patients must be assessed for signs and symptoms of FVE (discussed shortly). As soon as the patient becomes normotensive (normalization of their blood pressure), a hypotonic electrolyte solution (e.g., 0.45% sodium chloride) is often used to provide both electrolytes and water for renal excretion of metabolic wastes. These and additional fluids are discussed later in the chapter.

Pearls for Practice

The nurse understands that when the patient is hypotensive, restoration of the IVS is imperative. If an isotonic solution such as Dextrose 5% Water (D5W) (primarily water as the sugar is metabolized quickly) was administered, two thirds of the fluid would move to the ICS (~666 mL); recall the discussion earlier when we noted two thirds of the water in the body is intracellular, which will not increase the blood pressure! The remaining 333 mL will be in the ECS, but approximately 75% will move to the interstitial space, leaving only 83 mL in the IVS, which is unlikely to increase the blood pressure significantly. Thus, in emergency situations, a solution such as normal saline (0.9% NaCl) is selected because 75% of the solution will move to the interstitial space, leaving 25% in the circulating blood volume or ~250 mL in the IVS.

Accurate and frequent assessments of I&O, weight, vital signs, CVP, LOC, breath sounds, and skin color should be performed to determine when therapy should be slowed to avoid volume overload. The rate of fluid administration is based on the severity of loss and the patient's hemodynamic response to volume replacement.

If the patient with severe FVD is not excreting enough urine and is, therefore, oliguric (less than 400 mL/24 hrs), the health care provider needs to determine whether the depressed function is caused by reduced renal blood flow secondary to FVD (prerenal azotemia or increased nitrogen levels in the blood) or, more seriously, by acute kidney injury (AKI) from prolonged FVD (further details on AKI can be found in Chapter 26). The test used in this situation is referred to as a *fluid challenge test.* During a fluid challenge test, volumes of fluid are administered at specific rates and intervals while the patient's hemodynamic response to this treatment is monitored (i.e., vital signs, breath sounds, sensorium, CVP, pulmonary capillary wedge pressure values, and urine output).

An example of a typical fluid challenge involves administering 100 to 250 mL (4 to 6 mL/kg) of normal saline solution over a maximum of 20 minutes (Wilkinson et al., 2020). The goal is to provide fluids rapidly enough to attain adequate tissue perfusion without compromising the cardiovascular system. The response by a patient with FVD but normal kidney function is increased urine output and an increase in blood pressure, mean arterial pressure (MAP), and CVP (Trinooson & Patel, 2023). For calculation and meaning of MAP, refer to Chapter 11. It is understood that in patients whose baseline CVP is between 0 and 5 mm Hg (normal CVP is 2 to 8 mm Hg), up to 25% do not elevate with a fluid challenge (Lough, 2022). In this situation, the nurse will look at other indices of poor tissue perfusion such as an elevated lactate level (Chapter 53), low base deficit (discussed later in this chapter), or decreased urine output. In addition, rather than administering IV fluid, a passive leg raise can be used to assess fluid responsiveness. Venous compression stockings should be removed before the nurse raises the lower extremities and the patient's elevated legs should be supported to allow the venous blood from the lower extremities and abdominal compartment to flow rapidly into the vena cava and return to the right heart (Lough, 2022). A passive leg raise has the effect of essentially giving an IV fluid bolus without the fluid administration and is equivalent to administering 200 mL to 250 mL of blood to the central circulation (Johnson et al., 2019). If CVP increases with this maneuver, it suggests a positive response to an IV fluid bolus would occur. The passive leg raise is useful in those with known cardiac disease, frail or older individuals, and those whose volume status is uncertain, to prevent iatrogenic HF by administering fluid bolus (Schriger, 2020). Contraindications to the passive leg raise include head trauma or intracranial pressure issues, lower extremity deep vein thrombosis, severe hypovolemia and/or hemorrhage, and lower extremity amputations (Lough, 2022).

Shock can occur when the volume of fluid lost exceeds 25% of the intravascular volume, or when fluid loss is rapid. Shock and its causes and treatment are discussed in detail in Chapters 19 and 53.

Nursing Management

Assessing Fluid Status

To assess for FVD, the nurse monitors and measures fluid I&O at least every 4 to 8 hours; depending on the patient's status, the assessment may be done hourly. As FVD develops, body fluid losses exceed fluid intake. This loss may be in the form of excessive urination (polyuria), diarrhea, vomiting, and so on. Later, after FVD progresses, the kidneys attempt to conserve needed body fluids, leading to a urine output of less than 30 mL/hr in an adult or less than 0.5 mL/kg/hr. Urine in this instance is concentrated; the specific gravity generally is greater than 1.020, indicating healthy renal conservation of fluid.

Daily body weights are monitored; an acute loss of 1 lb represents a fluid loss of approximately 500 mL, whereas 1 L is approximately 1 kg or 2.2 lb.

Pearls for Practice

Patients should be weighed on admission to provide a baseline assessment. One of the most sensitive indicators of fluid status is the daily weight, which should be obtained at the same time, in the same clothes, and with the same scale. Weight gains or losses of more than 1 kg/day usually indicate fluid rather than nutritional factors (Lough, 2022).

Pearls for Practice

The nurse recognizes that the FVD is associated with weight loss; however, if the patient is edematous or third-spacing (e.g., developing ascites), weight gain may be seen despite FVD.

Vital signs are closely monitored. The nurse observes for a weak, rapid pulse and postural hypotension (i.e., a decrease in systolic pressure exceeding 20 mm Hg or decrease of 10 mm Hg of diastolic pressure when the patient moves from a lying to a sitting position). Skin and tongue turgor is monitored on a regular basis. In a healthy person, pinched skin immediately returns to its normal position when released. This elastic property, referred to as *turgor,* is partially dependent on interstitial fluid volume. In a person with FVD, the skin flattens more slowly after the pinch is released. In a person with severe FVD, the skin may remain elevated or tented for many seconds. Skin turgor is best measured by pinching the skin over the sternum, inner aspects of the thighs, or forehead.

Pearls for Practice

Skin turgor is a less valid assessment in the older patient because the skin has lost some of its elasticity due to the decreased number of papillae and collagen fibers; therefore, other assessment measures become more useful in detecting FVD (e.g., slowness in filling of veins of the hands and feet: veins in hands generally fill within 3 to 5 seconds; if filling takes longer than 5 seconds, consider FVD or hypovolemia). In older patients, skin turgor is best tested over the forehead or the sternum because alterations in skin elasticity are less marked in these areas. In addition, if the hand is elevated and the veins in the hands do not disappear within 5 seconds, FVE is suspected (Lough, 2022).

Tongue turgor is not affected by age. In a normal person, the tongue has one longitudinal furrow. In the person with FVD, there are additional longitudinal furrows, and the tongue is smaller because of fluid loss. The degree of oral mucous membrane moisture is also assessed; a dry mouth may indicate either FVD or mouth breathing.

Mental function is eventually affected in severe FVD as a result of decreasing cerebral perfusion. Decreased peripheral perfusion can result in cold extremities. In patients with relatively normal cardiopulmonary function, a low CVP is indicative of hypovolemia. Patients with acute cardiopulmonary decompensation require more extensive hemodynamic monitoring of pressures in both sides of the heart to determine if hypovolemia exists.

Preventing Fluid Volume Deficit

To prevent FVD, the nurse identifies patients at risk and takes measures to minimize fluid losses. The nurse recognizes that patients who are semidependent on another for care (related to sensorium or mobility) are at a higher risk for limited fluid intake. For example, if the patient has diarrhea, diarrhea-control measures should be implemented and replacement fluids administered. These measures may include administering antidiarrheal medications and small volumes of oral fluids at frequent intervals or, if necessary, IV therapy. Given the typical sensible and insensible loss of approximately 2,600 mL/day, if a patient is NPO, the nurse expects that the total daily water requirement for a 70-kg male is about 2 to 3 L/day, which translates to approximately 25 to 35 mL/kg/day (Trinooson & Patel, 2023). However, fluid and electrolyte therapy should be individualized based on physical examination findings, daily weight, and serum electrolytes.

Pearls for Practice

The nurse is aware that when a patient has an increased insensible loss, it is associated with FVD. As an example, when the patient has an elevated temperature between 101°F and 103°F, an increase of 1,000 mL of fluid may be needed; fluid needs also increase in clinical scenarios such as diarrhea, vomiting, and an increased respiratory rate (greater than 35 breaths per minute).

Pearls for Practice

A positive fluid balance exists when intake (PO, tube feedings, IV fluid) exceeds output (urine, diarrhea, vomiting, NG/NJ tube drainage, ostomy, drains). In AKI, the positive fluid volume results in FVE. Conversely, if output (via fever, increased insensible loss, increased respiratory rate, diuretic therapy, urine, vomiting, diarrhea, gastric suction) exceeds intake, a negative fluid balance, or FVD, exists.

Correcting Fluid Volume Deficit

When administering oral fluids, consideration is given to the patient's likes and dislikes. The type of fluid the patient has lost is also considered, and attempts are made to select fluids most likely to replace the lost electrolytes. If the patient is reluctant to drink because of oral discomfort, the nurse assists with frequent mouth care and provides nonirritating fluids. If nausea is present, antiemetics may be ordered and administered before oral fluid replacement is initiated.

If the patient cannot eat and drink, fluid may need to be administered by an alternative route (enteral or parenteral) until adequate circulating blood volume and renal perfusion are achieved. Isotonic fluids are prescribed to increase ECF volume.

Pearls for Practice

When fluid balance is critical, all routes of gain and all routes of loss must be recorded and all volumes compared. Organs of fluid loss include the kidneys, skin, lungs, and GI tract.

HYPERVOLEMIA

FVE, or hypervolemia, refers to an isotonic expansion of the ECF caused by the abnormal retention of water and sodium in approximately the same proportions in which they normally exist in the ECF. It is always secondary to an increase in the total body sodium content, which, in turn, leads to an increase in total body water. Because there is isotonic retention of body substances, the serum sodium concentration remains essentially normal.

Pearls for Practice

There are conditions that cause retention of water relative to sodium, such as SIADH. In these situations, hemodilution of the ECF will be reflected by decreased sodium, as well as BUN, and Hct. The term used for this situation is hypervolemic (increased volume) hyponatremia (decreased sodium related to dilution). Refer to Chapter 30 for more details on SIADH.

Pathophysiology

The maintenance of an effective circulating volume—that part of the "extracellular fluid that is in the arterial system and, therefore, effectively perfusing tissues" (Rennke & Denker, 2020)—is essential to sustain blood pressure to ensure organ vitality is monitored and tightly regulated. It may be increased in a number of situations, including fluid overload, excessive water ingestion, iatrogenic overadministration of IV fluids, or the ectopic secretion of ADH. Since the kidneys are responsible for regulating fluid excretion, kidney failure, either acute or chronic, is also associated with FVE. Excessive salt intake or the administration of sodium-containing fluids in a patient with impaired renal regulatory mechanisms may predispose the patient to serious FVE. On the other hand, a decrease in the effective circulating volume results in activation of the RAAS. Consider that since circulation is critical for survival, if the heart pump does not work effectively to generate enough volume for perfusion and function of vital organs, this "underfilling" results in activation of RAAS. This activation of RAAS results in increased circulating ADH or AVP and aldosterone, which increases sodium reabsorption and renal water reabsorption. This occurs in situations where cardiac output is decreased (HF) or when the patient suffers from hypovolemia (blood loss), increased capillary permeability (anaphylaxis), or extreme vasodilation (neurogenic shock).

Pearls for Practice

The nurse understands that a normal serum sodium is 135 to 145 mEq/L (135 to 145 mmol/L) and that normal saline or 0.9% NaCl has 154 mEq/L of sodium; thus, overadministration of normal saline leads to hypernatremia and potential for FVE.

Clinical Manifestations and Assessment

Clinical manifestations of FVE stem from expansion of the ECF and include edema, distended neck veins or jugular vein distention (JVD), and crackles (abnormal lung sounds) in lung fields. Other manifestations include tachycardia; increased blood pressure, pulse pressure, and CVP; increased weight; increased urine output (with normal kidney function); and shortness of breath and/or wheezing (Fig. 3-5).

Laboratory data useful in diagnosing FVE include BUN and Hct levels. In FVE, both of these values may be decreased because of plasma dilution, termed *hemodilution.* Other causes of abnormalities in these values include low protein intake and anemia. Azotemia (increased nitrogen levels in the blood) can also occur with FVE when urea and creatinine are not excreted due to decreased perfusion by the kidneys and decreased excretion of wastes. In CKF, both serum osmolality and the sodium level are decreased due to excessive retention of water (inability of the kidneys to excrete the normal 1.5 L/day). The urine sodium level is increased if the kidneys are attempting to excrete excess volume. Chest x-rays may reveal pulmonary congestion. Hypervolemia occurs when aldosterone is chronically stimulated (i.e., cirrhosis, HF, and nephrotic syndrome). Therefore, the urine sodium level does not increase in these conditions.

Medical Management

Management of FVE is directed at the causes. If the fluid excess is related to excessive administration of sodium-containing fluids, discontinuing the infusion may be all that is needed. Symptomatic treatment consists of administering diuretics and restricting fluids and sodium.

Pharmacologic Therapy

Diuretics are prescribed when dietary restriction of sodium alone is insufficient to reduce fluid excess, which inhibits the reabsorption of sodium and water by the kidneys. The choice of diuretic is based on the severity of the hypervolemic state, the degree of impairment of kidney function, and the potency of the diuretic. Thiazide diuretics block sodium reabsorption in the distal tubule, where only 5% to 10% of filtered sodium is reabsorbed. Loop diuretics, such as furosemide, or bumetanide, can cause a greater loss of both sodium and water because they block sodium reabsorption in the ascending limb of the loop of Henle, where 20% to 30% of filtered sodium is normally reabsorbed. In general, thiazide diuretics, such as hydrochlorothiazide or metolazone, are prescribed for mild to moderate hypervolemia and loop diuretics for severe hypervolemia.

Electrolyte imbalances may result from the effect of the diuretic. Hypokalemia can occur with all diuretics except those that work in the last distal tubule of the nephrons (e.g., spironolactone). Potassium supplements can be prescribed to avoid this complication. Hyperkalemia can occur with diuretics that work in the last distal tubule, especially in patients with decreased kidney function.

Hemodialysis

If kidney function is so severely impaired that pharmacologic agents cannot act efficiently, other modalities are considered

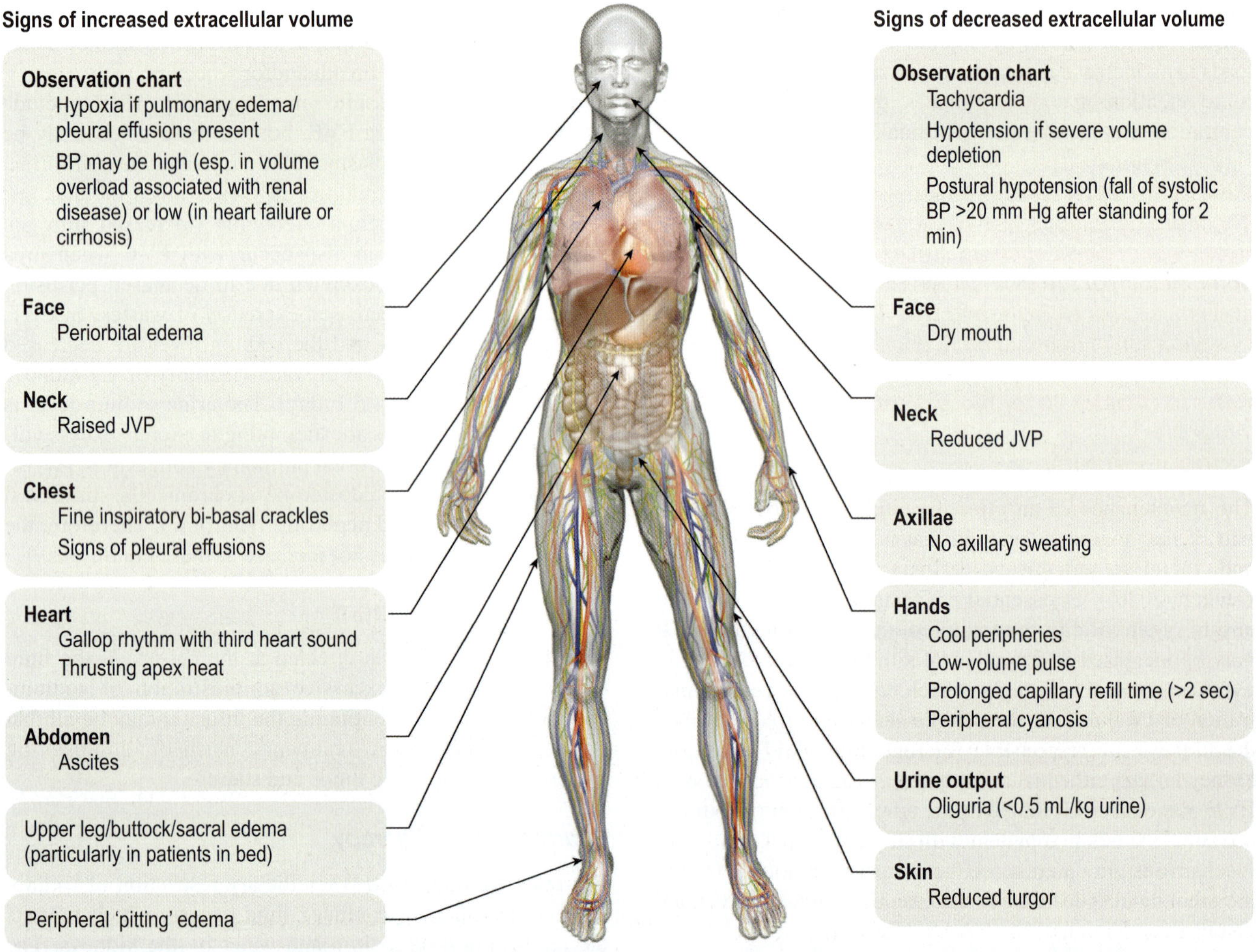

FIGURE 3-5 Signs of fluid volume excess (FVE) versus fluid volume deficit (FVD). (Adapted from Yaqoob, M., & McCafferty, K. [2021]. Water balance, fluids and electrolytes, In *Kumar and Clark's clinical medicine* [10th ed., ch. 9, pp. 169–202]. Elsevier Inc.)

to remove sodium and fluid from the body. Hemodialysis or peritoneal dialysis may be used to remove nitrogenous wastes and control potassium and acid–base balance, and to remove sodium and fluid. Continuous renal replacement therapy may also be required. See Chapter 26 for discussion of these treatment modalities.

Nutritional Therapy

Treatment of FVE usually involves dietary restriction of sodium. Research reveals that Americans consume sodium at or above the recommendation level of <2,300 mg/day according to the Chronic Disease Risk Reduction advice (FDA, nd; Oria et al., 2019; Rozga et al., 2022), whereas the maximum level for low-sodium diets varies based upon the patient's disease process and can range from a mild restriction (<2,300 mg/day) to as little as 250 mg/day, depending on the patient's needs. Of note, in a recent study on fast-food offerings in the United States, sodium content and portion size increased in entrées, sides, and desserts, adding to the problem of increased dietary sodium (McCrory et al., 2019). A mild sodium-restricted diet allows only light salting of food (about half the usual amount) in cooking and at the table as well as no addition of salt to commercially prepared foods that are already seasoned. Of course, foods high in sodium must be avoided. Most of the dietary sodium (over 70%) comes from eating packaged and prepared foods, and patients are instructed to read food labels carefully to determine salt content (FDA, nd).

Reducing ingested sodium in the form of table salt and other seasonings can play a major role in decreasing sodium intake. Patients are educated to use alternative seasoning such as lemon juice, onions, and garlic to enhance the flavors of food. Some patients prefer salt substitutes; however, most salt substitutes contain potassium and, therefore, must be used cautiously by patients taking potassium-sparing diuretics (e.g., spironolactone, triamterene, amiloride). They should not be used at all in conditions associated with potassium retention, such as advanced kidney disease. Salt substitutes containing ammonium chloride can be harmful to patients with liver damage.

Although the EPA has recommended that sodium levels in water not exceed 20 mg/L for those on a "no salt diet," in some communities, the drinking water may contain too much sodium for a sodium-restricted diet. Bottled water can have a sodium content from 0 to 680 mg/L; therefore, if sodium is restricted, the label must be examined carefully for sodium content before purchasing and drinking bottled water. Many brands are available that are below the EPA recommendation. Also, patients on sodium-restricted diets should be cautioned to avoid water softeners that add sodium to water in exchange for other ions, such as calcium.

Nursing Management

Assessing the Patient

To assess for FVE, the nurse measures I&O at regular intervals to identify excessive fluid retention. The patient is weighed daily, and acute weight gain is noted. An acute weight gain of 2.2 lb (1 kg) is equivalent to a gain of approximately 1 L of fluid. The nurse also needs to assess breath and heart sounds at regular intervals in at-risk patients (those with limited cardiac and renal reserves), particularly if parenteral fluids are being administered. Fine inspiratory bibasilar (both bases) crackles and an S3 gallop is suggestive of HF (refer to Fig. 3-5). The nurse monitors the degree of edema in the most dependent parts of the body, such as the feet and ankles in ambulatory patients and the sacral region in patients confined to bed. The degree of pitting edema is assessed, and the extent of peripheral edema is monitored by measuring the circumference of the extremity or the abdomen (in ascites) with a tape marked in millimeters. It is important to mark the abdomen so that future nurses are using the same area so that comparing measurements of diameter over time can be made. In general, edema that is apparent is associated with a minimum of 2.5 L of fluid in the interstitial space, and pitting edema is associated with a gain of 4.5 L (~10 lb) (Suneja et al., 2020). Often, a history of weight gain will correlate with the edema.

Pearls for Practice

The etiology of edema—visible or palpable (pitting) tissue swelling produced by the expansion of interstitial fluid volume—is not as simple as it may appear. Edema occurs in response to many factors, including increased venous pressure, as with a deep vein thrombosis (DVT) or venous clot; lymphatic drainage obstruction (often an unwanted side effect of removal of the breast [mastectomy] and underarm lymph tissue or lymph node infection, tumor, inflammation); decreased plasma albumin oncotic pressure (seen in malnutrition, nephrotic syndrome, or liver damage); increased capillary leakage (caused by burns, sepsis); local injury (a result of sprains, fractures, surgery); infection (cellulitis); FVE (HF, AKI, CKF, hypervolemia); or inadequate valves in the venous system (chronic venous insufficiency) (Kibble, 2020). The nurse must consider a variety of etiologies when assessing edema.

Preventing Fluid Volume Excess

Specific interventions vary somewhat with the underlying condition and the degree of FVE. However, most patients require sodium-restricted diets in some form, and adherence to the prescribed diet is strongly recommended. Patients are instructed to avoid over-the-counter medications without first checking with a health care provider because these substances may contain sodium. If fluid retention persists despite adherence to a prescribed diet, hidden sources of sodium, such as the water supply or use of water softeners, should be considered.

Correcting Fluid Volume Excess

It is important to detect FVE before the condition becomes critical. Interventions include restricting sodium intake, monitoring parenteral fluid therapy, and administering appropriate medications.

Sodium and fluid restriction should be instituted as indicated. Because most patients with FVE require diuretics, the patient's response to these agents is monitored. The rate of parenteral fluids and the patient's response to these fluids are also closely monitored. If dyspnea or orthopnea is present, the patient is placed in a semi-Fowler position to promote lung expansion. The patient is turned and positioned at regular intervals, and skin is assessed at regular intervals because edematous tissue is fragile and more prone to skin breakdown than normal tissue. Because conditions predisposing to FVE are likely to be chronic, patients are taught to monitor their response to therapy by monitoring their fluid I&O and documenting daily body weight changes.

Teaching Patients About Edema

Because edema is a common manifestation of FVE, patients need to recognize its symptoms and understand its importance. As noted earlier, edema can occur as a result of increased capillary fluid pressure, decreased capillary oncotic pressure, or increased interstitial oncotic pressure, causing expansion of the interstitial fluid compartment (Kibble, 2020). Edema can be localized (e.g., in an extremity, as in a fracture) or generalized (as in cardiac and kidney failure). Thus, edema can be dependent, unilateral, bilateral, generalized, localized, and pitting or nonpitting (Lough, 2020). Severe generalized edema is called *anasarca*.

Edema occurs when there is a change in the capillary membrane, increasing the formation of interstitial fluid or decreasing the removal of interstitial fluid. Sodium retention is a frequent cause of the increased ECF volume.

Burns and infection are examples of conditions associated with increased interstitial fluid volume. Obstruction to lymphatic outflow, decreased plasma albumin levels, or a decrease in plasma oncotic pressure contributes to increased interstitial fluid volume. The kidneys retain sodium and water when decreased ECF volume occurs as a result of decreased cardiac output from HF. A thorough medication history is necessary to identify any medications that could cause edema, such as nonsteroidal anti-inflammatory drugs (NSAIDs), estrogens, corticosteroids, and antihypertensive agents.

Ascites is a form of edema in which fluid accumulates in the peritoneal cavity; it results from nephrotic syndrome, cirrhosis, and some malignant tumors. The patient commonly reports shortness of breath and a sense of pressure because of pressure on the diaphragm.

Edema usually affects dependent areas. It can be seen in the ankles, sacrum, scrotum, or the periorbital region of the face. Recall that if the patient is confined to bed, edema of the flank area or sacrum can be seen. Pitting edema is so named because a pit forms after a finger is pressed into edematous tissue. In pulmonary edema, the amount of fluid in the pulmonary interstitium and the alveoli increases. Manifestations include shortness of breath, increased respiratory rate, diaphoresis, and crackles and wheezing on auscultation of the lungs. Decreased Hct resulting from hemodilution as well as decreased serum sodium and osmolality from retention of fluid may occur with edema. The goal of treatment is to preserve or restore the circulating intravascular fluid volume. In addition to treating the cause, other treatments may include diuretic therapy, restriction of fluids and sodium, elevation of the extremities, application of elastic compression stockings, paracentesis, dialysis, and continuous renal replacement therapy in cases of kidney failure or life-threatening fluid volume overload.

Pearls for Practice

Edema does not always mean FVE. Consider the patient that has an overwhelming infection that is causing increased capillary permeability, allowing the albumin to escape the capillary and enter the interstitial space. Without the albumin to "pull" the water back into the capillary, generalized edema will occur, and the intravascular volume is depleted, causing a reduction in preload or volume of blood in the heart and cardiac output! Thus, the patient is edematous but actually has a significant fluid volume deficit. Remember, edema is a symptom that requires further analysis to determine the etiology.

ELECTROLYTE IMBALANCES

Disturbances in electrolyte balances are common in clinical practice and must be corrected for the patient's health and safety.

SODIUM IMBALANCES

Sodium is the most abundant electrolyte in the ECF; its concentration ranges from 135 to 145 mEq/L (135 to 145 mmol/L). Consequently, sodium is the primary determinant of ECF osmolality. Sodium plays a major role in controlling water distribution throughout the body because it does not easily cross the intracellular membrane and because of its abundance and high concentration in the body. Sodium also functions in establishing the electrochemical state necessary for muscle contraction and the transmission of nerve impulses. Sodium is regulated by the kidneys, the adrenal glands (aldosterone secretion), the posterior pituitary (ADH), thirst, and the RAAS. A loss or gain of sodium is usually accompanied by a loss or gain of water.

The sodium imbalances commonly seen are: sodium deficit (hyponatremia) and sodium excess (hypernatremia).

HYPONATREMIA (SODIUM DEFICIT)

Hyponatremia refers to a serum sodium level that is below normal (less than 135 mEq/L [135 mmol/L]). It is one of the most common electrolyte abnormalities, seen in almost 14% of hospitalized patients, and nearly 50% can be attributed to SIADH (Farber & Yee, 2022).

Pathophysiology

Plasma sodium concentration represents the ratio of total body sodium to total body water. A decrease in this ratio can occur because of salt loss that is greater than water loss (e.g., diarrhea, diuretics, NG tube suctioning), or there is an excess of water relative to total body sodium (e.g., HF, cirrhosis of the liver, excessive water intake without salt, SIADH). Therefore, a hyponatremic state can be superimposed on an existing FVD or FVE.

Sodium may be lost by way of vomiting, diarrhea, fistulas, or prolonged or excessive sweating, or it may be lost as the result of the use of diuretics, particularly in combination with a low-salt diet. A deficiency of aldosterone, as occurs in adrenal insufficiency, also predisposes a patient to sodium deficiency. Potomania, otherwise known as beer potomania, due to the chronic consumption of large amounts of beer (a hypotonic solution) and protein malnutrition, may also cause hyponatremia due to an inability of the kidneys to excrete free water.

In dilutional hyponatremia (water intoxication), the patient's serum sodium level is diluted by an increase in the ratio of water to sodium. Dilutional hyponatremia, therefore, results from an increased ECF volume and a normal or increased total body sodium. Predisposing conditions for this type of hyponatremia include cirrhotic ascites; SIADH; hyperglycemia, which causes increased water to be drawn into the IVS; and increased water intake through the administration of electrolyte-poor parenteral fluids, the use of tap-water enemas, or the irrigation of nasogastric tubes with water instead of normal saline solution. Water may be gained abnormally by the excessive parenteral administration of hypotonic solutions such as dextrose and water solutions, particularly during periods of stress. It may also be gained by compulsive water drinking (psychogenic polydipsia).

Pearls for Practice

Psychogenic polydipsia has been linked to a number of psychiatric conditions; however, it can also occur in a variety of individuals, including high-endurance athletes, and users of 3,4-Methylenedioxymethamphetamine (MDMA, commonly known as ecstasy) (Clinical Overview, 2022a).

The basic physiologic disturbances in SIADH are excessive ADH activity, with water retention and dilutional hyponatremia, and inappropriate urinary excretion of sodium in the presence of hyponatremia. SIADH can be the result of either sustained secretion of ADH by the hypothalamus or production of an ADH-like substance from a tumor (aberrant ADH production). Conditions associated with SIADH include oat-cell lung tumors (AKA small-cell carcinoma), head injuries, endocrine and pulmonary disorders, physical or psychologic stress, and a variety of medications (e.g., vincristine, phenothiazines, tricyclic antidepressants, thiazide diuretics, anticonvulsants, nicotine). SIADH is discussed in more detail in Chapter 30.

Clinical Manifestations and Assessment

Clinical manifestations of hyponatremia depend on the cause, magnitude, and speed with which the deficit occurs. Patients can present with FVD, as euvolemic which refers to normal fluid balance (SIADH), or with FVE. With true salt loss, a number of conditions occur, including poor skin turgor, dry mucosa, headache, decreased saliva production, orthostatic blood pressure (decreased with position changes), nausea, and abdominal cramping. With water gain in excess of sodium, clinical manifestations are associated with FVE, such as edema, crackles, ascites, and JVD. Symptoms of hyponatremia are primarily neurologic due to brain cell swelling. This is related to osmotic water shift as water from the relatively dilute ECF is pulled into the cell, leading to increased ICF volume, specifically brain cell swelling or cerebral edema (Fig. 3-6). The skull limits the brain's ability to expand, which results in increased intracranial pressure (ICP), the precursor to brain damage. Neurologic changes include altered mental status, headache, lethargy, seizures, and a progressively decreased LOC eventuating in coma. When the serum sodium level decreases to less than 115 mEq/L (115 mmol/L), signs of increasing intracranial pressure may occur, such as lethargy, confusion, muscle twitching, focal weakness, hemiparesis, papilledema, and seizures. In general, patients with an acute decrease in serum sodium levels have more cerebral edema and higher mortality rates than those with more slowly developing hyponatremia. Acute decreases in sodium, developing in less than 48 hours, may

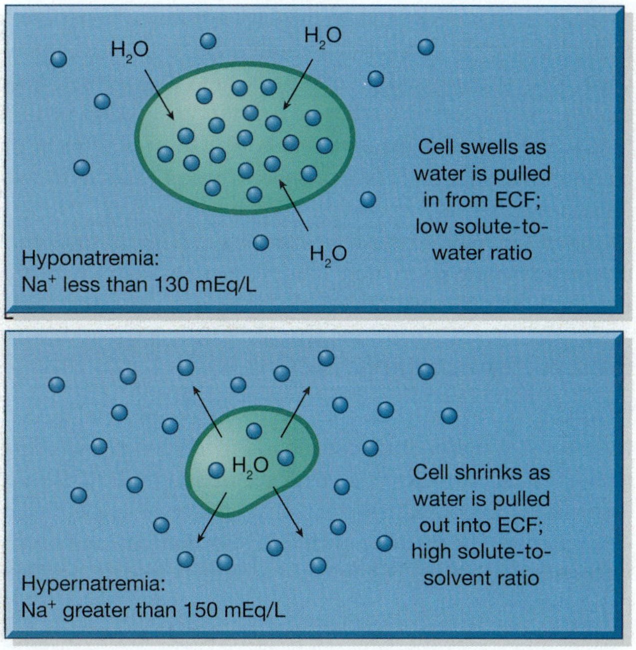

FIGURE 3-6 **Effect of extracellular sodium level on cell size.**

be associated with brain herniation and compression of midbrain structures.

Regardless of the cause of hyponatremia, the serum sodium level is less than 135 mEq/L. When the sodium level is between 130 and 134 mEq/L, it is termed mild hyponatremia, a sodium level of 120 to 129 mEq/L is moderate hyponatremia, and a sodium <120 mEq/L is severe hyponatremia (Sterns, 2022). When hyponatremia is due primarily to sodium loss, the urinary sodium content is less than 20 mEq/L (20 mmol/L), suggesting increased renal reabsorption of sodium secondary to ECF volume depletion, and the specific gravity is low (1.002 to 1.004). However, when hyponatremia is due to SIADH, the urinary sodium content is greater than 20 mEq/L, and the urine specific gravity is usually greater than 1.012. Refer to Chapter 30 for details on urine sodium in SIADH. Although the patient with SIADH retains water abnormally and, therefore, gains body weight, there is no peripheral edema; instead, fluid accumulates equally within the three compartments (intracellular, interstitial, and intravascular).

Medical Management

Treatment depends on the cause of the hyponatremia, the amount of time the individual has had hyponatremia, and the presence of signs and symptoms. Hyponatremia is considered acute if it developed within the last 48 hours and chronic if the duration of time since the initiation of hyponatremia is more than 48 hours or unknown. It is important to recognize that complications caused by either undertreatment of hyponatremia or from overcorrection of hyponatremia are most common in those with sodium levels <120 mEq/L (severe hyponatremia) (Sterns, 2022a).

Treatment will depend on the cause of the hyponatremia. If the etiology is related to sodium and (to a lesser extent) water loss, sodium and water replacement is expected; if the etiology is related to water intoxication, restriction of fluid intake and diuretics are anticipated. For example, when the cause of hyponatremia is an excess of water relative to total body sodium or hypervolemic hyponatremia (e.g., HF, cirrhosis of the liver, excessive water intake without salt), then treatment is fluid restriction, diuretic therapy, sodium restriction, and management of underlying cause.

Sodium Replacement

In mild hyponatremia, the intention is to identify and discontinue (or substitute) drugs contributing to hyponatremia, limit further intake of water (e.g., fluid restriction [<800 mL/day], discontinue hypotonic IV infusions), and/or increase dietary salt (Sterns, 2022a). For patients who can eat and drink, sodium is easily replaced because sodium is consumed abundantly in a normal diet.

For those patients who are hypovolemic and hyponatremic (e.g., vomiting, diarrhea, NG tube suctioning), isotonic saline (0.9% sodium chloride) solution may be prescribed until the blood pressure and perfusion are restored (Clinical Overview, 2022a).

If acute hyponatremia is present, a bolus (50 to 100 mL) of 3% saline (i.e., hypertonic saline) may be administered to prevent the serum sodium from falling further (Sterns, 2022a; Clinical Overview, 2022a). It is important not to correct the sodium level too rapidly; serum sodium must not be increased by more than 6 to 8 mEq/L in the first 24 hours to avoid neurologic damage due to osmotic demyelination. This condition, termed osmotic demyelination syndrome (ODS), formerly referred to as *central pontine myelinolysis (CPM),* may occur when the serum sodium concentration is overcorrected too rapidly, causing a relatively hypotonic ICS compared to the ECS. This causes water to flow from the ICS to the ECS, causing cell volume collapse. Symptoms typically appear 2 to 6 days after the overcorrection and include flaccid paralysis, dysarthria (speech that is slurred, slow, and difficult to produce), dysphagia (difficulty in swallowing), seizures, lethargy, confusion, paraparesis, quadriparesis, and coma which are frequently irreversible (Sterns, 2022b). To minimize the risk of ODS, the rate of correction of hyponatremia should not exceed 6 to 8 mEq/L in any 24-hour period (Sterns, 2022b).

In patients with severe symptoms of hyponatremia, such as seizures or obtundation, or in patients with acute hyponatremia, administration of hypertonic saline solution may be ordered to stabilize the patient and prevent brain herniation. In this setting, the goal increase of sodium may be lowered to 4 to 6 mEq/L and a maximum of 8 mEq/L in a 24-hour period; however, these values are often debated and subject to change; the nurse follows institutional guideline. The adage of "go slow" has particular utility in symptomatic hyponatremia. Refer to Chapter 30 for treatment of SIADH.

Water Restriction

In a patient with normal or excess fluid volume, hyponatremia is treated by restricting fluid to a total of 800 mL in 24 hours. This is far safer than sodium administration and is usually effective. However, if neurologic symptoms are present, it may be necessary to administer small volumes of a hypertonic sodium solution, such as 3% sodium chloride. Incorrect use of these fluids is extremely dangerous because 1 L of 3% sodium chloride solution contains 513 mEq of sodium with an osmolality of 1,026! Recall normal serum osmolality is 275 to 295 mOsm/kg. A 3% saline solution is three times higher; thus, if administered rapidly, the blood osmolality would increase dramatically. However, because of the blood–brain barrier, the osmolality in the brain would be the same; thus, intracellular water would attempt to try to dilute the bloodstream causing ODS (see alert below).

Pearls for Practice

A 3% saline solution has an osmolality of 1,026 mOsm/kg. A normal serum osmolality varies from approximately 275 to 295 mOsm/kg. Thus, a 3% saline solution is >3 times more concentrated than normal blood osmolality. Rapid administration would have an adverse impact on the brain. The blood osmolality would increase dramatically. However, because the blood–brain barrier limits capillary sodium but not water permeability, the movement of interstitial and neuronal intracellular water into the capillary may potentially culminate in cerebral shrinkage, osmotic demyelination, and the constellation of clinical symptoms (including paraparesis, dysphagia, and coma) known as ODS. In addition, a solution this concentrated must be administered via a central IV line because it is too concentrated for peripheral veins; it is tolerated when administered in central lines because it is diluted by vena cava blood.

Nursing Management

The nurse needs to identify patients at risk for hyponatremia so that they can be monitored. Early detection and treatment of this disorder are necessary to prevent serious consequences. For patients at risk, the nurse monitors fluid I&O as well as daily body weight. It is also necessary to note abnormal losses of sodium or gains of water as well as GI manifestations such as anorexia, nausea, vomiting, and abdominal cramping. The nurse must be particularly alert for CNS changes, such as lethargy, confusion, muscle twitching, and seizures. In general, more severe neurologic signs are associated with very low sodium levels that have fallen rapidly because of fluid overloading. Serum sodium is monitored very closely in patients who are at risk for hyponatremia; when indicated, urine sodium and specific gravity are also monitored.

Hyponatremia is a frequently overlooked cause of confusion in older patients, who have an increased risk for hyponatremia because of changes in kidney function and subsequent decreased ability to excrete excessive water loads. Administration of medications causing sodium loss or water retention is a predisposing factor.

Correcting Hyponatremia

For a patient who is experiencing abnormal losses of sodium and can consume a general diet, the nurse encourages foods and fluids with a high sodium content. For example, broth made with one beef cube contains approximately 900 mg of sodium; 8 oz of tomato juice contains approximately 700 mg of sodium. The nurse also needs to be familiar with the sodium content of parenteral fluids (see later discussion and Table 3-6 on page 98).

For the patient taking lithium, the nurse understands that this medication decreases sodium reabsorption in the renal tubules, resulting in sodium depletion (Standard, 2022a). Therefore, it is vital for patients to maintain a normal diet, including sodium. Because diuretics also promote sodium loss, the patient taking lithium is instructed not to use diuretics without close medical supervision.

Excess water supplements are avoided in patients receiving isotonic or hypotonic enteral feedings, particularly if abnormal sodium loss occurs or water is being retained abnormally (as in SIADH). Actual fluid needs are determined by evaluating fluid I&O, urine specific gravity, and serum sodium levels.

HYPERNATREMIA (SODIUM EXCESS)

Hypernatremia is a higher-than-normal serum sodium level (exceeding 145 mEq/L [145 mmol/L]).

Pathophysiology

Hypernatremia can be caused by a gain of sodium in excess of water or by a loss of water in excess of sodium. It can occur in the euvolemic patient or in those with FVD or FVE. With a water loss, the patient loses more water than sodium; as a result, the serum sodium concentration increases and the increased concentration pulls fluid out of the cell. This is both an extracellular and an intracellular FVD. In sodium excess, the patient ingests or retains more sodium than water.

A common cause of hypernatremia is fluid deprivation in unconscious patients who cannot perceive, respond to, or communicate their thirst (Kumbar et al., 2022). Most often affected are patients who are very old, are very young, or have cognitive impairment. Administration of hypertonic enteral feedings without adequate water supplements leads to hypernatremia, as does watery diarrhea and greatly increased insensible water loss (e.g., hyperventilation, denuding effects of burns).

DI, a deficiency of ADH or AVP from the posterior pituitary gland, leads to hypernatremia if the patient does not experience, or cannot respond to, thirst or if fluids are excessively restricted. Neurogenic or nephrogenic causes of DI should be considered in the assessment (refer to Chapter 30).

IV administration of hypertonic saline, hypertonic feeding preparations, or excessive use of sodium bicarbonate can also cause hypernatremia. Hypokalemia and hypercalcemia cause polyuria and therefore can be a risk factor for hypernatremia (Boling, 2023). It is also seen in hyperglycemia with osmotic diuresis.

Clinical Manifestations and Assessment

The clinical manifestations of hypernatremia are primarily neurologic and are the consequence of increased plasma osmolality caused by an increase in plasma sodium concentration. Water moves out of the ICS into the ECS, resulting in cellular dehydration (see Fig. 3-6). Clinically, these changes may be manifested by restlessness and weakness in moderate hypernatremia and by disorientation, delusions, and hallucinations in severe hypernatremia. Dehydration (resulting in hypernatremia) is often overlooked as the primary reason for behavioral changes in older patients. If hypernatremia develops rapidly, the brain shrinks, which puts traction on intracranial veins and venous sinuses, leading to intracranial hemorrhage (Trinooson & Patel, 2023).

A primary characteristic of hypernatremia is thirst. Thirst is such a strong defender of serum sodium levels in healthy people that hypernatremia never occurs unless the person is unconscious or does not have access to water. However, ill people may have an impaired thirst mechanism. Other signs include a dry, swollen tongue and sticky mucous membranes. Flushed skin, peripheral and pulmonary edema, postural hypotension, and increased muscle tone and deep tendon reflexes are additional signs and symptoms of hypernatremia. Body temperature may increase mildly, but it returns to normal after the hypernatremia is corrected. In hypernatremia, the serum sodium level exceeds 145 mEq/L (145 mmol/L), and the serum osmolality exceeds 300 mOsm/kg (300 mmol/L). The specific gravity and osmolality of urine are increased as the kidneys attempt to conserve water (provided the water loss is from a route other than the kidneys). In addition, polydipsia and polyuria will be seen in DI (discussed in Chapter 30).

Medical Management

Treatment of hypernatremia consists of a gradual lowering of the serum sodium level by the infusion of a hypotonic electrolyte solution or an isotonic nonsaline solution (e.g., dextrose 5% in water [D5W]). D5W is indicated when water needs to be replaced without sodium. Many clinicians consider a hypotonic sodium solution (e.g., 0.45% NaCl or ½ normal saline) to be safer than D5W because it allows a gradual reduction in the serum sodium level, thereby decreasing the risk of cerebral edema. It is the solution of choice in severe hyperglycemia with hypernatremia. If possible, fluids should be administered orally or via a feeding tube whenever possible. When a hypotonic IV solution is used, the nurse is aware that a rapid reduction in the serum sodium level temporarily decreases the plasma osmolality below that of the fluid in the brain tissue, causing dangerous cerebral edema. Rapid correction causes cerebral edema as the water moves from the serum into the brain cells, seizures may occur, and permanent brain damage (Sonani et al., 2022). Diuretics also may be prescribed to treat the sodium gain. Rarely, hemodialysis may be used to lower serum sodium concentration (Goshima et al., 2022). Repeated serum sodium measurements are necessary every 1 to 3 hours to ensure that serum sodium concentration is falling at the desired rate (Sterns & Hoorn, 2022).

There is no consensus about the exact rate at which serum sodium levels should be reduced. As a general rule, in acute hypernatremia, the serum sodium level is reduced by 1 to 2 mEq/L/hr and to restore a normal serum sodium in less than 24 hours, whereas in chronic hypernatremia the goal of this regimen is to lower the serum sodium by approximately 10 mEq/L in a 24-hour period (Sterns & Hoorn, 2022). This is suggested to allow sufficient time for readjustment through diffusion across fluid compartments. Treatment of DI is reviewed in Chapter 30.

Pearls for Practice

One of the most common causes of hypernatremia is the inadequate intake of free water. Consider that if you or I had an increased salt load, our sense of thirst would be stimulated, and we would drink water, which would lower our serum sodium into the normal range. We would not develop hypernatremia. It occurs (primarily) in those who are unable to sense thirst or respond to thirst normally. This occurs in the extremes in age from the infant to the older adult and in those with impaired mental status, impaired physical limitations, and on mechanical ventilation. Although the etiology is not known, older adult patients have a diminished thirst response to osmotic stimulation via an unknown mechanism. The nurse is also alert to iatrogenic causes of hypernatremia such as excessive sodium bicarbonate administration or hypertonic fluid infusions (recall that normal saline is hypertonic with a sodium content of 154 mEq/l compared to a normal serum sodium of 135 to 145 mEq/l), especially when combined with the patient's inability for adequate water intake (Sonani et al., 2022).

Nursing Management

As in hyponatremia, fluid losses and gains are carefully monitored in patients who are at risk for hypernatremia. The nurse should assess for abnormal losses of water or low water intake and for large gains of sodium as might occur with ingestion of over-the-counter medications that have high sodium content (e.g., Alka-Seltzer). In addition, the nurse obtains a medication history because some prescription medications have high sodium content. The nurse also notes the patient's thirst or elevated body temperature and evaluates it in relation to other clinical signs. The nurse monitors for changes in behavior, such as restlessness, disorientation, and lethargy.

Preventing Hypernatremia

The nurse attempts to prevent hypernatremia by offering fluids at regular intervals, particularly in debilitated patients who may be unable to perceive or respond to thirst. If fluid intake remains inadequate, the nurse consults with the provider to plan an alternative route for intake, either by enteral feedings or by the parenteral route. If enteral feedings are used, sufficient water should be administered to keep the serum sodium and BUN within normal limits. As a rule, the higher the osmolality of the enteral feeding, the greater the need for water supplementation.

For patients with DI, adequate water intake must be ensured. If the patient is alert and has an intact thirst mechanism, merely providing access to water may be sufficient. If the patient has a decreased LOC or other disability interfering with adequate fluid intake, parenteral fluid replacement may be prescribed. This therapy can be anticipated in patients with neurologic disorders, particularly in the early postoperative period.

POTASSIUM IMBALANCES

Potassium is the major intracellular electrolyte; in fact, 98% of the body's potassium is inside the cells. The remaining 2% is in the ECF, and it is this 2% that is important in neuromuscular function. The normal serum potassium concentration ranges from 3.5 to 5.2 mEq/L (3.5 to 5.2 mmol/L), and even minor variations are significant; there are variations in ranges based on the clinical laboratory standard values (Fischbach et al., 2021).

To maintain potassium balance, the renal system must function because ~90% of the potassium excreted daily leaves the body by way of the kidneys; the other 10% is lost through the bowel. Intestinal fluid may contain 40 to 60 mEq/L of potassium (Norris & Tuan, 2020). However, the kidneys are the primary regulators of potassium balance; they accomplish this by adjusting the amount of potassium that is excreted in the urine. Aldosterone also increases the excretion of potassium by the kidney. Because the kidneys do not conserve potassium as well as they conserve sodium, potassium may still be lost in urine in the presence of a potassium deficit. Potassium imbalances are commonly associated with a variety of diseases, injuries, medications (diuretics, laxatives, antibiotics, insulin, theophylline), pH, and special treatments such as parenteral nutrition and chemotherapy.

HYPOKALEMIA (POTASSIUM DEFICIT)

Hypokalemia (below-normal serum potassium concentration) usually indicates an actual deficit in total potassium stores. However, it may occur in patients with normal potassium stores, such as when alkalosis is present, since it causes a temporary shift of serum potassium into the cells (see later discussion). It is classified as mild when the serum potassium level is 3 to 3.4 mmol/L, moderate when the serum potassium level is 2.5 to 3 mmol/L, and severe when the serum potassium level is less than 2.5 mmol/L (Castro & Sharma, 2022).

Pathophysiology

Hypokalemia (less than 3.5 mEq/L) is a common imbalance. It is associated with conditions that cause an increased output of K^+ (diuretic use, diarrhea, laxative use, vomiting, gastric suction, recent ileostomy, intestinal drains, villous adenoma [a tumor of the intestinal tract characterized by excretion of potassium-rich mucus]); decreased intake (NPO, anorexia, vomiting, alcoholism, fasting diets); or redistribution of K^+ (metabolic alkalosis).

The nurse considers clinical conditions that cause increased loss. Approximately 5 to 10 mEq/L K^+ are found in upper GI fluid, whereas 30 to 50 mEq/L are lost with diarrhea (Mount, 2022). Thus, relatively large amounts of potassium are lost in intestinal fluids.

Potassium-losing diuretics, such as the thiazides, can induce hypokalemia, particularly when administered in large doses to patients with inadequate potassium intake. Other medications that can lead to hypokalemia include corticosteroids and amphotericin B.

Increased loss is also seen with hyperaldosteronism, which causes reabsorption of sodium and renal excretion of K^+. Primary hyperaldosteronism is seen in patients with adrenal adenomas. Secondary hyperaldosteronism occurs in disorders that activate RAAS to maintain serum sodium concentrations such as cirrhosis, nephrotic syndrome, or HF.

Decreased intake occurs in patients who are unable or unwilling to eat a normal diet. This may occur in debilitated older adults, patients with alcohol use disorder, and patients with anorexia nervosa. It can also occur in those receiving IV fluids without K^+ replacement. In addition to poor intake, people with bulimia frequently suffer increased potassium loss through self-induced vomiting and abuse of laxatives and diuretics.

Redistribution is associated with alterations in acid–base balance or certain medications, such as insulin. In general, a hypokalemia is associated with an alkalosis and, in turn, an alkalosis can cause hypokalemia. The mechanism involves shifts of hydrogen and potassium ions between the ICS and the ECF. For example, hydrogen ions move out of the cells in alkalotic states to help correct the high pH, and potassium ions move in to maintain an electrically neutral state (see later discussion of acid–base balance).

Pearls for Practice

*To help you remember, think of alkalosis as Al K^+ (potassium) **LOW** sis; thus, when the K^+ is low, alkalosis exists, and when alkalosis is present, look for hypokalemia.*

Because insulin promotes the entry of potassium into skeletal muscle and hepatic cells (primarily by increasing the activity of the Na-K-ATPase pump), patients with persistent insulin hypersecretion may experience hypokalemia, which is often the case in patients receiving high-carbohydrate parenteral fluids (as in parenteral nutrition) and IV insulin administration in diabetic ketoacidosis (DKA) and hyperosmolar, hyperglycemia nonketotic syndrome (HHNS). The nurse anticipates that patients requiring IV insulin are at risk for hypokalemia.

Finally, a magnesium depletion can cause a renal potassium loss and must be corrected or loss of potassium in the urine will continue. If hypomagnesemia exists along with hypokalemia, potassium replacement can only be corrected after the magnesium deficit is corrected (Clinical Overview, 2021).

Clinical Manifestations and Assessment

Potassium deficiency can result in widespread derangements in physiologic function. Severe hypokalemia can cause death through cardiac or respiratory arrest. Clinical signs rarely develop before the serum potassium level has decreased to less than 3 mEq/L (3 mmol/L) unless the rate of decline has been rapid. Manifestations of hypokalemia include fatigue, anorexia, nausea, vomiting, muscle weakness, leg cramps, decreased bowel motility, paresthesias (numbness and tingling), arrhythmias, and increased sensitivity to digitalis. Rare complications associated with hypokalemia include rhabdomyolysis (see Box 41–9), ascending paralysis, and progression to respiratory arrest due to diaphragmatic paralysis and cardiac arrest (Kerner, 2021).

If prolonged, hypokalemia can lead to an inability of the kidneys to concentrate urine, causing dilute urine (resulting in polyuria, nocturia) and excessive thirst. Potassium depletion depresses the release of insulin and results in glucose intolerance. Decreased muscle strength and tendon reflexes can be found on physical assessment.

Electrocardiographic (ECG) changes can include flat T waves or inverted T waves or both, suggesting ischemia, and depressed ST segments (Fig. 3-7). An elevated U wave (a positive deflection after the T wave on the ECG) should alert the clinician to check the serum potassium level for hypokalemia; this pattern is often seen in the lateral precordial leads of V4 to V6 (Lough et al., 2022). Hypokalemia increases sensitivity to digitalis, predisposing the patient to digitalis toxicity at lower digitalis levels. It does this by increasing binding of digoxin to cardiac cells, potentiating its action and decreasing its clearance (Yaqoob & McCafferty, 2022).

Medical Management

If hypokalemia cannot be prevented by conventional measures, such as increased intake in the daily diet, it is treated

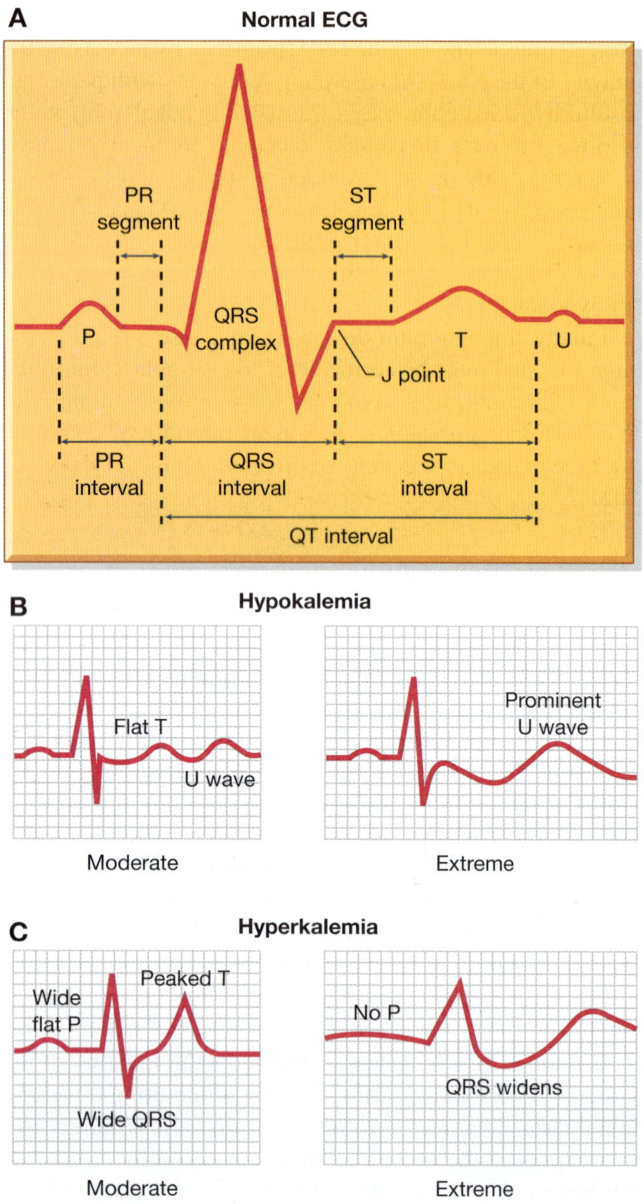

FIGURE 3-7 **Effect of potassium on the electrocardiogram (ECG). A. Normal tracing. B. Hypokalemia: Serum potassium level below normal. Left: Flattening of the T wave and the appearance of a U wave. Right: further flattening with prominent U wave. C. Hyperkalemia: Serum potassium level above normal. Left: moderate elevation with wide, flat P wave, wide QRS complex, and peaked T wave. Right: ECG changes seen with extreme potassium elevation: widening of QRS complex and absence of P wave.**

with oral or IV replacement therapy. Potassium loss must be corrected daily; administration of 40 to 100 mEq/day of potassium by mouth in divided doses (with or after a meal due to gastric mucosa irritation) is adequate in the adult if there are no abnormal losses of potassium. The maximum single oral dose is 40 mEq and should not exceed 200 mEq/day (Standard, 2022b).

For patients who are at risk for hypokalemia, a diet containing sufficient potassium should be provided (e.g., dried fruits [prunes, raisins, and dates], nuts, spinach, potatoes, cantaloupe, bananas). See Box 3-1.

Many salt substitutes contain potassium. The amounts vary and can range from 5 to 40 mEq of per teaspoon, which may be sufficient to prevent hypokalemia.

If oral administration of potassium is not feasible, the IV route is indicated. The IV route is mandatory for patients with severe hypokalemia (e.g., serum level of less than 2.5 mEq/L).

Pearls for Practice

Potassium should be administered in normal (0.9%) saline because using a glucose solution would stimulate insulin release that will cause intracellular shifting of potassium, making the loss of K^+ worse.

Pearls for Practice

Serum potassium levels on average will rise by .1 mEq/L for each 10 mEq of potassium given to a patient.

Nursing Management

Because hypokalemia can be life-threatening, the nurse needs to monitor for its early presence in patients who are at risk. Fatigue, anorexia, muscle weakness, decreased bowel motility, paresthesias, and arrhythmias are signals that warrant assessing the serum potassium concentration. When available, the ECG may provide useful information. For example, patients receiving digitalis who are at risk for potassium deficiency should be monitored closely for signs of digitalis toxicity, because hypokalemia potentiates the action of digitalis.

Preventing Hypokalemia

Measures are taken to prevent hypokalemia when possible. Prevention may involve encouraging the patient at risk to eat foods rich in potassium (when the diet allows). If the hypokalemia is caused by abuse of laxatives or diuretics, patient education may help alleviate the problem.

Pearls for Practice

Sources of potassium include fruit and fruit juices (bananas, melon, citrus fruit, avocado, coconut water), fresh and frozen vegetables, fresh meats, milk, and processed foods.

Correcting Hypokalemia

Great care should be exercised when administering potassium, particularly in older adults who have lower lean body mass and total body potassium levels and, therefore, lower potassium requirements. In addition, because of the physiologic loss of kidney function with advancing years, potassium may be retained more readily in older than in younger people.

BOX 3-1
Potassium Content of Selected Food

Food	Milligrams (mg) per Serving	Percent DV*
Apricots, dried, ½ cup	755	16
Lentils, cooked, 1 cup	731	16
Squash, acorn, mashed, 1 cup	644	14
Prunes, dried, ½ cup	635	14
Raisins, ½ cup	618	13
Potato, baked, flesh only, 1 medium	610	13
Kidney beans, canned, 1 cup	607	13
Orange juice, 1 cup	496	11
Soybeans, mature seeds, boiled, ½ cup	443	9
Banana, 1 medium	422	9
Milk, 1%, 1 cup	366	8
Spinach, raw, 2 cups	334	7
Chicken breast, boneless, grilled, 3 ounces	332	7
Yogurt, fruit variety, nonfat, 6 ounces	330	7
Salmon, Atlantic, farmed, cooked, 3 ounces	326	7
Beef, top sirloin, grilled, 3 ounces	315	7
Molasses, 1 tablespoon	308	7
Tomato, raw, 1 medium	292	6
Soymilk, 1 cup	287	6
Yogurt, Greek, plain, nonfat, 6 ounces	240	5
Broccoli, cooked, chopped, ½ cup	229	5
Cantaloupe, cubed, ½ cup	214	5
Turkey breast, roasted, 3 ounces	212	5
Asparagus, cooked, ½ cup	202	4
Apple, with skin, 1 medium	195	4
Cashew nuts, 1 ounce	187	4
Rice, brown, medium-grain, cooked, 1 cup	154	3
Tuna, light, canned in water, drained, 3 ounces	153	3
Coffee, brewed, 1 cup	116	2
Lettuce, iceberg, shredded, 1 cup	102	2
Peanut butter, 1 tablespoon	90	2
Tea, black, brewed, 1 cup	88	2
Flaxseed, whole, 1 tablespoon	84	2
Bread, whole-wheat, 1 slice	81	2
Egg, 1 large	69	1
Rice, white, medium-grain, cooked, 1 cup	54	1
Bread, white, 1 slice	37	1
Cheese, mozzarella, part skim, 1½ ounces	36	1
Oil (olive, corn, canola, or soybean), 1 tablespoon	0	0

Source: National Institutes of Health (NIH): Office of Dietary Supplements. (2022). Potassium: Fact Sheet for Health Professionals; https://ods.od.nih.gov/factsheets/Potassium-HealthProfessional/

Pearls for Practice

Oral potassium supplements can produce small-bowel lesions; therefore, the patient must be assessed for and cautioned about abdominal distention, pain, or GI bleeding. In addition, the nurse observes for potassium chloride–induced esophagitis. Symptoms include sudden onset of pain when swallowing (odynophagia), retrosternal pain, and dysphagia (difficulty swallowing). Risk factors for esophagitis include taking the medication without water and taking the medication at night (Standard, 2022b). Symptoms usually resolve within days to weeks after discontinuing the medication.

Potassium should be administered only after adequate urine flow has been established. A decrease in urine volume to less than 0.5 mL/kg/hr for 2 consecutive hours is an indication to reassess renal function and potassium level. Recall that potassium is primarily excreted by the kidneys; therefore, when oliguria occurs, potassium administration can cause the serum potassium concentration to rise dangerously. Each health care facility has its own standard of care for the administration of potassium, which should be consulted; however, the maximum concentration of potassium that should be administered on a medical-surgical unit through a peripheral IV line is 10 mEq/100 mL at a rate no faster than 10 mEq/hr. Pain and phlebitis usually occur with peripheral IV infusions when infusion rates exceed 10 mmol per hour (Castro & Sharma, 2022). Concentrations of potassium greater than 20 mEq/100 mL should be administered through a central IV catheter using an infusion pump with the patient monitored by ECG. Caution must be used when selecting the correct premixed solution of IV fluid containing potassium chloride as the concentrations range from 10 to 40 mEq/100 mL. IV bags of 1,000 mL of fluid containing potassium are also available with 20 to 40 mEq/L. IV pumps should always be used with potassium administration. Rapid infusion can cause sudden hyperkalemia and cardiac arrest. Repeat evaluation of potassium levels are recommended to prevent inadvertent iatrogenic hyperkalemia secondary to potassium replacement (Kuiper, 2020). Kidney function should be monitored through BUN and creatinine levels and urine output if the patient is receiving potassium replacements, and the provider should be notified of changes in kidney function to prevent complications.

Pearls for Practice

*Potassium is **never** administered by IV push or intramuscularly. Injection of concentrated potassium solution has been instantaneously fatal (Standard, 2022b). IV potassium is available as a premixed solution; the nurse is aware that it must be administered using an infusion pump.*

Pearls for Practice

Potassium supplements are extremely dangerous for patients who have impaired kidney function and thus decreased ability to excrete potassium. Even more dangerous is the IV administration of potassium to such patients because serum levels can rise very quickly. Aged (stored) blood should not be administered to patients with impaired kidney function because the serum potassium concentration of stored blood increases as the cold storage time increases, a result of deterioration of RBCs. It is possible to exceed the renal tolerance of any patient with rapid IV potassium administration, as well as when large amounts of oral potassium supplements are ingested.

HYPERKALEMIA (POTASSIUM EXCESS)

Hyperkalemia (greater-than-normal serum potassium concentration) seldom occurs in patients with normal kidney function.

Pathophysiology

Like hypokalemia, hyperkalemia is often caused by iatrogenic (treatment-induced) causes. Although hyperkalemia is less common than hypokalemia, it is usually more dangerous because cardiac arrest is more frequently associated with high serum potassium levels.

Pseudohyperkalemia, also known as spurious hyperkalemia (a variation of hyperkalemia), has a number of causes. The most common causes are the use of a tight tourniquet around an exercising extremity while drawing a blood sample or prolonged tourniquet time, fist clenching during phlebotomy, and hemolysis of the sample before analysis (delay in processing the sample). Other causes include marked leukocytosis as in leukemia (leukemic lymphocytes are fragile and release potassium during centrifugation, tube transport in the hospital, and when shaken) or thrombocytosis (platelet count exceeding 500,000) (Clinical Overview, 2022b); drawing blood above a site where potassium is infusing; and familial pseudohyperkalemia, in which potassium leaks out of the RBC while the blood is awaiting analysis. Failure to be aware of these causes of pseudohyperkalemia can lead to aggressive treatment of a nonexistent hyperkalemia, resulting in serious lowering of serum potassium levels. Therefore, measurements of grossly elevated levels should be verified by retesting.

Pearls for Practice

When the laboratory reports hyperkalemia but the patient has no underlying kidney disease, the ECG is normal and patient is asymptomatic, the nurse considers pseudohyperkalemia as the cause of hyperkalemia and alerts the provider to repeat the electrolytes.

Hyperkalemia (K^+ greater than 5.2 mEq/L or in some institutions >5.5 mEq/L) is associated with increased K^+ intake, reduced renal excretion of K^+ or redistribution (shifting of K^+ out of the cells into the extracellular fluid). Increased intake may be related to use of salt substitutes or potassium supplements; administration of medications that increase K^+ load such as penicillin-K^+; K^+-sparing diuretics such as spironolactone and ACE inhibitors; or cell injuries such as crushing injuries, burns, trauma, intravascular hemolysis, rhabdomyolysis (see Chapter 41), or chemotherapy with cell lysis. Decreased K^+ output is associated with kidney disease (AKI/CKF) and hypoaldosteronism; while redistribution is associated with acute acidosis.

The major cause of hyperkalemia is decreased renal excretion of potassium, commonly seen in patients with untreated kidney failure, particularly those in whom potassium levels increase as a result of infection or excessive intake of potassium in food or medications. In addition, patients with hypoaldosteronism or Addison disease are at risk for hyperkalemia because of deficient aldosterone.

Although a high intake of potassium can cause severe hyperkalemia in patients with impaired kidney function, hyperkalemia rarely occurs in people with normal kidney function. However, improper use of potassium supplements predisposes all patients to hyperkalemia, especially if salt substitutes are used. Not all patients receiving potassium-losing diuretics require potassium supplements, and patients receiving potassium-conserving diuretics should not receive supplements.

In **acidosis**, potassium moves out of the cells and into the ECF. This occurs as hydrogen ions enter the cells, a process that buffers the pH of the ECF (see later discussion). An elevated ECF potassium level should be anticipated when extensive tissue trauma has occurred, as in burns, crushing injuries, or severe infections. Similarly, it can occur with lysis of malignant cells after chemotherapy.

Clinical Manifestations and Assessment

The most important consequence of hyperkalemia is its effect on the myocardium. The effect of hyperkalemia in the heart may be seen with potassium levels >5.2 mEq/L; at levels >7 mEq/L, hyperkalemia is considered life-threatening due to cardiac arrhythmias, particularly ventricular fibrillation (Clinical Overview, 2022b). As the plasma potassium level rises, disturbances in cardiac conduction occur. The earliest changes, often occurring when the serum potassium reaches 5.5 to 6.5 mEq/L, are peaked, narrow T waves. If the serum potassium level continues to increase, the PR interval becomes prolonged and is followed by disappearance of the P waves and widened QRS complexes (when the level reaches 6.5 to 8.0 mEq/L) (Kuiper, 2020) (see Fig. 3-7). Ventricular arrhythmias and cardiac arrest may occur at any point in this progression. Severe hyperkalemia causes skeletal muscle weakness (usually affecting lower limbs first) and even paralysis, related to a depolarization block in muscle. Similarly, ventricular conduction is slowed. Although hyperkalemia has marked effects on the peripheral nervous system, it has little effect on the CNS. Rapidly ascending muscular weakness leading to flaccid quadriplegia has been reported in patients with very high serum potassium levels. Paralysis of respiratory and speech muscles can also occur. In addition, GI manifestations, such as nausea, intermittent intestinal colic, and diarrhea, may occur in hyperkalemic patients. Serum potassium levels and ECG changes are crucial to the diagnosis of hyperkalemia, as discussed previously. ABG analysis may reveal metabolic acidosis; in many cases, hyperkalemia occurs with acidosis, owing to shifts of hydrogen and potassium ions between the ICS and the ECF. For example, hydrogen ions move into the cells in acidotic states to help correct the low serum pH, and potassium ions move out of the cells in exchange, causing hyperkalemia.

Medical Management

In nonacute situations, that is, the absence of symptoms or ECG abnormalities, hyperkalemia is treated conservatively with restriction of dietary potassium and potassium-containing medications. For example, eliminating the use of potassium-containing salt substitutes in a patient who is taking a potassium-conserving diuretic may be all that is needed to deal with mild hyperkalemia.

Prevention of serious hyperkalemia by the administration, either orally or by retention enema, of cation exchange resins may be necessary in patients with renal impairment. For example, the cation exchange resin sodium polystyrene acts by binding potassium within the bowel and excreting it within the stool. Once in the GI lumen, the insoluble resin in sodium polystyrene swells, allowing for the sodium contained within the polymer to be exchanged for potassium, and the K^+ now bound to the polymer is excreted in feces (Tang, 2022). Its onset of action is delayed and is approximately 1 to 2 hours after administration; it is contraindicated in patients with GI obstruction or obstructive bowel disease since complications include intestinal necrosis and other serious GI adverse events such as bleeding, ischemic colitis, and perforation (Standard, 2022c). Due to concerns about colonic necrosis associated with sodium polystyrene, the mixture with 70% sorbitol has been banned, but versions with 33% sorbitol are still commonly used (Kerner, 2021). Patiromer is another ion exchange resin that exchanges calcium for potassium in the GI tract, which reduces potassium levels by binding to potassium in the GI tract. However, the onset of action for patiromer is 7 hours (Kovesdy, 2023). Sodium zirconium cyclosilicate (SZC), a novel nonabsorbed, nonpolymer zirconium silicate compound, exchanges hydrogen and sodium for potassium and ammonium that has the advantage of an onset of action within 1 hour (Tang, 2022). Because of the delay in onset of action in cation exchange resins, other emergency treatment is required for life-threatening hyperkalemia.

Emergency Pharmacologic Therapy

If serum potassium levels are dangerously elevated, it may be necessary to administer IV calcium gluconate. Within minutes after administration, calcium antagonizes the action of hyperkalemia on the heart. Infusion of calcium does not reduce the serum potassium concentration, but it immediately antagonizes the adverse cardiac conduction abnormalities. Calcium chloride and calcium gluconate are not interchangeable: calcium gluconate contains 4.6 mEq of calcium, and calcium chloride contains 13.6 mEq of calcium; therefore, caution must be used (Standard, 2022d, e).

Monitoring the blood pressure is essential to detect hypotension, which may result from the rapid IV administration of calcium gluconate. The ECG should be monitored continuously during administration; the appearance of bradycardia is an indication to stop the infusion. The myocardial-protective effects of calcium are transient, lasting about 30 to 60 minutes. The dose of either formulation can be repeated after 5 minutes if the ECG changes persist or recur (Tang, 2022). Extra caution is required if the patient has been "digitalized" (i.e., has received accelerated dosages of a digitalis-based cardiac glycoside to reach a desired serum digitalis level rapidly) because parenteral administration of calcium sensitizes the heart to digitalis and may precipitate digitalis toxicity.

IV administration of sodium bicarbonate may be necessary to alkalinize the plasma and cause a temporary shift of potassium into the cells. Also, sodium bicarbonate furnishes sodium to antagonize the cardiac effects of potassium. Effects of this therapy begin within 30 to 60 minutes and may persist for hours; however, they are temporary. In addition, sodium bicarbonate should not be used in FVE patients, since the high sodium content may precipitate pulmonary edema and HF.

IV administration of regular insulin and a hypertonic dextrose solution causes a temporary shift of potassium into the cells. Glucose and insulin therapy has an onset of action within 30 minutes and lasts for several hours. Loop diuretics, such as furosemide, increase excretion of water by inhibiting sodium, potassium, and chloride reabsorption in the ascending loop of Henle and distal renal tubule. This treatment can be used in patients without severe kidney function impairment.

Beta-2 agonists, such as albuterol, can be effective in decreasing potassium; however, large doses are needed to elicit potassium shifting into the cells. They work by increasing the activity of the Na-K-ATPase pump in skeletal muscle, thereby driving potassium into the cells (Mount, 2022). The nurse is aware that beta-2 agonists may cause tachycardia and the possibility of angina; therefore, it is important to observe the cardiac response to treatment. Additionally, the provider may consider other options in the patient with ischemic cardiac disease. Administration of these medications is a stopgap measure that only temporarily protects the patient from hyperkalemia. If the hyperkalemic condition is not transient, actual removal of potassium from the body is required; this may be accomplished by using hemodialysis or other forms of renal replacement therapy.

Nursing Management

Patients at risk for potassium excess (e.g., those with kidney failure) should be identified so that they can be monitored closely for signs of hyperkalemia. The nurse observes for signs of muscle weakness and arrhythmias. The presence of paresthesias and GI symptoms, such as nausea and intestinal colic, should be monitored for and reported if identified.

Because measurements of elevated serum potassium levels may be erroneous, highly abnormal levels should always be verified by repeating the test. To avoid false reports of hyperkalemia, prolonged use of a tourniquet while drawing the blood sample is avoided, and the patient is cautioned not to exercise the extremity immediately before the blood sample is obtained. The blood sample is delivered to the laboratory as soon as possible because hemolysis of the sample results in a falsely elevated serum potassium level.

Preventing Hyperkalemia

Measures are taken to prevent hyperkalemia in patients at risk, when possible, by encouraging the patient to adhere to the prescribed potassium restriction. Potassium-rich foods to be avoided include many fruits and vegetables, legumes, whole-grain breads, meat, milk, eggs, coffee, tea, and cocoa (see Box 3-1). Conversely, foods with minimal potassium content include butter, margarine, cranberry juice or sauce, ginger ale, gumdrops or jellybeans, hard candy, root beer, sugar, and honey.

Correcting Hyperkalemia

As previously stated, it is possible to exceed the tolerance for potassium in any person if it is administered rapidly by the IV route. Therefore, great care should be taken to administer and monitor potassium solutions closely, paying attention to the solution's concentration and rate of administration. Today, premixed solution of IV potassium chloride is available; however, if your institution does not have premixed solution, check with a pharmacist before mixing a medication in an IV container. If a pharmacist confirms that you need to prepare the medication (emergency situation), ask another nurse to verify your medication calculations and have that nurse watch you during the entire procedure to ensure that you prepare the medication safely (Perry et al., 2022a). To ensure the potassium is mixed with the fluid, invert the bottle several times. Potassium chloride should never be added to a hanging bottle because the potassium might be administered as a bolus (potassium chloride is heavy and settles to the bottom of the container).

It is important to caution patients to use salt substitutes sparingly if they are taking other supplementary forms of potassium or potassium-conserving diuretics. Also, potassium-conserving diuretics, potassium supplements, and salt substitutes should not be administered to patients with kidney dysfunction.

CALCIUM IMBALANCES

More than 99% of the body's calcium is located in the skeletal system, where it provides strength and stability to the skeletal system and serves as a source for extracellular calcium (Norris & Tuan, 2020). Approximately 0.1% to 0.2% of calcium (8.5 to 10.5 mg/dL) circulates in the serum, 40% is bound to plasma proteins (mostly albumin), 10% is complexed or chelated with substances such as phosphate and sulfate, and approximately 50% is ionized or free to leave the bloodstream and participate in cellular function (Norris & Tuan, 2020). Calcium plays a major role in the transmission of nerve impulses, regulation of muscle contraction and relaxation including cardiac muscle, and coagulation pathways; thus, it is important for cardiac conduction, neuromuscular activity, and blood clotting. Calcium is also instrumental in activating enzymes that stimulate many essential chemical reactions in the body. Because many factors affect calcium regulation, both hypocalcemia and hypercalcemia are relatively common disturbances.

Calcium is absorbed from foods (milk and milk products) in the presence of normal gastric acidity and vitamin D. Calcium is excreted in feces and urine. The serum calcium level is controlled by PTH and calcitonin. As ionized or free serum calcium decreases, the parathyroid glands secrete PTH. This, in turn, increases calcium absorption from the GI tract (mediated by an increase in renal vitamin D synthesis), increases calcium reabsorption from the renal tubule, and releases calcium from the bone. The subsequent increase in calcium ion concentration suppresses PTH secretion. When calcium increases excessively, the thyroid gland secretes calcitonin, the antagonist of PTH. It briefly inhibits calcium reabsorption from bone, encourages calcium salt deposits in the bone matrix, and decreases the serum calcium concentration. In addition, blood phosphate (most phosphorus is present as phosphate) levels have a reciprocal relationship with calcium levels. Increases in blood phosphate result in a fall in free calcium concentrations. PTH secretion is stimulated, and this reduces renal excretion of calcium and increases renal phosphate excretion. These adaptations prevent the potentially damaging effects of calcium phosphate crystal deposition that can form in soft tissues when the normal calcium–phosphorus ratio is disturbed.

Pearls for Practice

In conditions such as kidney failure, excess phosphate is not excreted, nor is vitamin D activated, which decreases absorption of calcium. This excess phosphate binds with free calcium, forming an insoluble compound that can be deposited in the heart, lungs, eyes, kidneys, skin, and soft tissues.

The subsequent fall in serum calcium increases PTH secretion, which dissolves more calcium from the bone to attempt to maintain a normal serum calcium level. The net effect is the development of hyperparathyroidism and a variety of symptoms (renal osteodystrophy, bone pain, fractures, and bleeding) (see Chapters 26 and 30).

HYPOCALCEMIA (CALCIUM DEFICIT)

Hypocalcemia (lower-than-normal serum concentration of calcium), or less than 8.5 mg/dL and an ionized calcium of less than 4.6 mg/dL, occurs in a variety of clinical situations (Fischbach et al., 2021). Normal values vary greatly, so check with your laboratory.

Pathophysiology

Factors associated with hypocalcemia include inadequate calcium intake, increased calcium loss, malabsorption of calcium, and increased binding of calcium. Inadequate intake is associated with alcohol use disorder and malnutrition. Increased calcium loss is associated with pancreatic insufficiency and acute pancreatitis. It is thought that calcium ions combine with the fatty acids released by lipolysis, forming soaps. As a result of this process, hypocalcemia occurs and is common in pancreatitis. However, the exact mechanism is not known but may include parathyroid dysfunction, calcitonin release, and endotoxin release (Toffaletti & Rackley, 2022b). Recently, research suggested that pancreatitis may cause calcium deposition in the abdominal cavity as a result of ongoing inflammation with subsequent serum hypocalcemia (Muhammed et al., 2022). Inadequate secretion of PTH by the parathyroid gland results in hypocalcemia and can be related to hypoparathyroidism or other parathyroid gland disorders, use of certain drugs, surgery of the thyroid gland with inadvertent removal of the parathyroids, radiation injury to the thyroid, and radical neck dissection. This is likely to occur in the first 24 to 48 hours postoperatively. In addition, hypomagnesemia inhibits PTH release and impairs its action on bone resorption. Until the magnesium is replaced, it is difficult to treat the hypocalcemia (Norris & Tuan, 2020).

Malabsorption of calcium may be seen in severe diarrhea, laxative abuse, decreased exposure to sunlight or conditions that impair vitamin D, high phosphorus level in the intestines, reduced gastric acidity, and kidney failure. In kidney failure, hypocalcemia is seen related to the impaired phosphate elimination which (because of the inverse relation) causes the calcium level to decrease, as well as an inability to activate vitamin D. In addition, hypoalbuminemia, alkalosis, and massive blood transfusion are associated with hypocalcemia. Recall that approximately 40% of calcium is bound to albumin; thus, a decrease in serum albumin will result in a decrease in total serum calcium, but it does not affect the concentration of the ionized form of calcium that is essential for body function (Fischbach et al., 2021). When the arterial pH increases (alkalosis), more calcium binds to protein. As a result, the ionized portion decreases; thus, symptoms of hypocalcemia may occur with alkalosis. Transient hypocalcemia can occur with massive administration of citrated blood, because citrate can combine with ionized calcium and temporarily remove it from the circulation. This may occur in adults who experience massive hemorrhage and shock, as citrate is used in blood transfusions to prevent blood clotting. Finally, medications predisposing the patient to hypocalcemia include aminoglycosides, anticonvulsants (phenytoin and phenobarbital due to impairment of vitamin D), chemotherapy (cisplatin), and bisphosphonates and denosumab (inhibit osteoclastic bone resorption) (Goyal et al., 2022).

Clinical Manifestations and Assessment

If ionized calcium level is normal despite low total calcium levels, patients are generally asymptomatic, whereas large changes in ionized calcium levels lead to a variety of symptoms associated with neuromuscular hyperactivity and cardiovascular effects detailed below. Tetany (the most characteristic manifestation of hypocalcemia) and convulsions are seen when the total calcium level is less than 4.4 mg/dL and/or the ionized calcium is less than 2.0 mg/dL (Fischbach et al., 2021). *Tetany* refers to the entire symptom complex induced by increased neural excitability. These symptoms are caused by spontaneous discharges of both sensory and motor fibers in peripheral nerves. Sensations of tingling may occur in the tips of the fingers, around the mouth, and, less commonly, in the feet. Spasms of the muscles of the extremities and face may occur. Pain may develop as a result of these spasms.

Trousseau sign (Fig. 3-8) can be elicited by inflating a blood pressure cuff on the upper arm 10 to 20 mm Hg above the systolic pressure for 3 minutes; carpal spasm (adducted thumb, flexed wrist and metacarpophalangeal joints, extended interphalangeal joints with fingers together) occurs as ischemia of the ulnar nerve develops. *Chvostek*

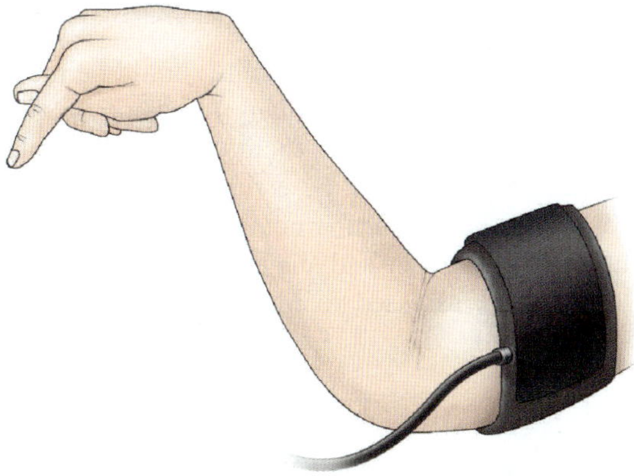

FIGURE 3-8 **Trousseau sign. Ischemia-induced carpal spasm can occur with hypocalcemia or hypomagnesemia. Occluding the brachial artery with a blood pressure cuff for 3 minutes can produce carpal spasm that mimics the spasm that occurs with hypocalcemia or hypomagnesemia.**

sign consists of twitching of muscles supplied by the facial nerve when the nerve is tapped about 2 cm anterior to the earlobe, just below the zygomatic arch.

Seizures occur because hypocalcemia causes irritability of the CNS as well as of the peripheral nerves. Other changes associated with hypocalcemia include mental changes, such as depression, impaired memory, confusion, delirium, and even hallucinations. A prolonged QT interval is seen on the ECG due to prolongation of the ST segment, which predisposes patients to a form of ventricular tachycardia called *torsades de pointes* (see Chapter 16). Respiratory effects with decreasing calcium include dyspnea and laryngospasm (stridor). Signs and symptoms of chronic hypocalcemia include hyperactive bowel sounds, dry and brittle hair and nails, and abnormal clotting. When evaluating serum calcium levels, variables such as the serum albumin level and the arterial pH must be considered. Because abnormalities in serum albumin levels may affect interpretation of the serum calcium level, it may be necessary to calculate the corrected serum calcium if the serum albumin level is abnormal. For every decrease in serum albumin of 1 g/dL below 4 g/dL, the total serum calcium level is underestimated by approximately 0.8 mg/dL. The following is a quick method to calculate the corrected serum calcium level:

$$\text{Corrected calcium} = \text{measured calcium} + 0.8\,(4.0 - \text{measured serum albumin})$$

An example of the calculations needed to obtain the corrected total serum calcium level is as follows: A patient's reported serum albumin level is 2.5 g/dL; the reported serum calcium level is 10.5 mg/dL. First, the decrease in serum albumin level from normal (i.e., the difference from the normal albumin concentration of 4 g/dL) is calculated: 4 g/dL − 2.5 g/dL = 1.5 g/dL. Next, multiply 0.8 (1.5) = 1.2.

Finally, 1.2 mg/dL is added to 10.5 mg/dL (the reported serum calcium level) to obtain the corrected total serum calcium level: 1.2 mg/dL + 10.5 mg/dL = 11.7 mg/dL.

The ionized calcium level is usually normal in patients with reduced total serum calcium levels and concomitant hypoalbuminemia.

Ideally, the ionized level of calcium should be measured in the laboratory. However, in many laboratories, only the total calcium level is reported; therefore, the concentration of the ionized fraction must be estimated by simultaneous measurement of the serum albumin level as described above. In addition, PTH levels and magnesium and phosphorus levels need to be assessed to identify possible causes of decreased calcium.

Medical Management

Acute symptomatic hypocalcemia is life-threatening and requires prompt treatment with IV administration of calcium. Although calcium chloride produces a significantly higher ionized calcium level than calcium gluconate, it is not used as often because it is more irritating to the vasculature and can cause sloughing of tissue if it infiltrates. Administering IV calcium too rapidly can cause cardiac arrest, which may be preceded by bradycardia in patients. IV administration of calcium is particularly dangerous in patients receiving digitalis-derived medications because calcium ions exert an effect similar to that of digitalis and can cause digitalis toxicity, with adverse cardiac effects. Therefore, calcium should be diluted in D5W or normal saline and administered via a slow IV infusion using a volumetric infusion pump (Goltzman, 2022). The IV site must be observed often for any evidence of infiltration because of the risk of extravasation and resultant cellulitis or necrosis. Solutions containing phosphates or bicarbonate should not be used with calcium because they cause precipitation when calcium is added. The nurse must clarify with the provider which calcium salt to administer because calcium gluconate yields 4.6 mEq of calcium, and calcium chloride provides 13.6 mEq of calcium. Because calcium can cause postural hypotension, the patient is kept in bed during IV replacement, and blood pressure is monitored.

Vitamin D therapy may be instituted to increase calcium absorption from the GI tract. Phosphate binders may be prescribed to decrease elevated phosphorus levels before treating hypocalcemia in the patient with CKF (see Chapter 26). Increasing the dietary intake of calcium to at least 1,000 to 1,200 mg/day in the adult is recommended. Calcium-containing foods include milk products; green, leafy vegetables; canned salmon; sardines; and fresh oysters. Hypomagnesemia can also cause tetany; if the tetany does not respond to IV calcium, then a low magnesium level is considered as a possible cause.

Nursing Management

It is important to observe for hypocalcemia in patients at risk. Seizure precautions are initiated if hypocalcemia is severe. The status of the airway is closely monitored because laryngeal stridor can occur. A tracheotomy tray should be kept at the bedside and a manual resuscitation bag nearby in case of laryngospasm in patients with audible stridor. Safety precautions are taken, as indicated, if confusion is present. Because of the cardiac complications, ECG monitoring should be instituted to detect changes in heart rate and rhythm, especially if the patient is receiving digoxin.

People who have a high risk for osteoporosis are instructed about the need for adequate dietary calcium intake; it is important to teach the patient which foods are rich in calcium. The nurse must also advise the patient to consider calcium supplements if sufficient calcium is not consumed in the diet. Such supplements should be taken in divided doses with meals. In addition, the value of regular weight-bearing exercise in decreasing bone loss should be emphasized, as well as the effect of medications on calcium balance. For example, alcohol and caffeine in high doses inhibit calcium absorption, and moderate cigarette smoking increases urinary calcium excretion. Teaching also includes strategies to reduce the risk of falls. The patient is also cautioned to avoid the overuse of laxatives and antacids that contain phosphorus because their use decreases calcium absorption.

HYPERCALCEMIA (CALCIUM EXCESS)

Hypercalcemia (excess of calcium in the plasma) is a dangerous imbalance. Mild hypercalcemia is a calcium level of 10.5 to 11.9 mg/dL, moderate is 12.0 to 13.9 mg/dL, and hypercalcemic crisis is 14.0 to 16.0 mg/dL or greater (Sadiq et al., 2021). Hypercalcemic crisis (an acute increase in calcium level) has an extremely high mortality rate if not corrected promptly, often related to life-threatening cardiac tachyarrhythmia, coma, AKF, and ileus with abdominal distention (Smith & Schreiber, 2022).

Pathophysiology

Ninety percent of hypercalcemia cases are related to either malignancy or hyperparathyroidism (Smith & Schreiber, 2022; Sadiq et al., 2021). Considered an oncologic emergency, hypercalcemia occurs in 10% to 20% of patients with advanced cancer (Norris & Tuan, 2020). It is associated with increased osteoclast activity resulting in bone demineralization, direct bone destruction by tumor cells and subsequent release of calcium, and/or tumor-produced factors that affect bone resorption and/or tubular calcium reabsorption. Tumor cells can secrete PTH-related protein, resulting in increased serum calcium. The excessive PTH secretion associated with hyperparathyroidism causes increased release of calcium from the bones and increased intestinal and renal absorption of calcium.

Bone mineral is lost during immobilization, and, sometimes, this causes elevation of total (and especially ionized) calcium in the bloodstream. Symptomatic hypercalcemia from immobilization is rare; when it does occur, it is virtually limited to people with high calcium turnover rates (e.g., adolescents during a growth spurt). Most cases of hypercalcemia secondary to acute immobility occur after severe or multiple fractures, spinal cord injury, head injuries, and burns (Goltzman, 2021). This hypercalcemia of immobilization resolves with return to normal weight-bearing activity (Smith & Schreiber, 2022).

Thiazide diuretics can cause a slight elevation in serum calcium levels because they potentiate the action of PTH on the kidneys, reducing urinary calcium excretion. A rare condition, called *milk–alkali syndrome,* has occurred in patients with peptic ulcer treated previously for a prolonged period with large amounts of calcium together with sodium bicarbonate, particularly calcium carbonate. While the exact mechanism is unknown, hypercalcemia, kidney failure, and metabolic alkalosis are seen in this syndrome (Smith & Schreiber, 2022). Vitamin A and D intoxication, as well as the use of lithium, can cause calcium excess.

Clinical Manifestations and Assessment

As a rule, the symptoms of hypercalcemia are proportional to the degree and rate of elevation of the serum calcium level. Hypercalcemia reduces neuromuscular excitability because it suppresses activity at the myoneural junction. Symptoms such as muscle weakness, incoordination, anorexia, and constipation may be caused by decreased tone in smooth and striated muscle. Cardiovascular effects include hypertension and a shortened QT interval, which can cause increased sensitivity to digitalis and vascular calcification (Chonchol et al., 2020).

Anorexia, nausea, vomiting, and constipation are common symptoms of hypercalcemia. Abdominal and bone pain may also be present. Abdominal distention and paralytic ileus may complicate severe hypercalcemic crisis. Excessive urination due to disturbed renal tubular function produced by hypercalcemia may occur. In fact, nephrogenic DI can be seen in patients with this disorder (Clinical Overview, 2022c). Severe thirst secondary to the polyuria caused by the high solute (calcium) load is expected. Although uncommon, patients with chronic hypercalcemia may develop symptoms similar to those of peptic ulcer because hypercalcemia increases the secretion of acid and pepsin by the stomach.

Confusion, impaired memory, slurred speech, lethargy, acute psychotic behavior, or coma may occur. In patients with calcium >14 mg/dL, there is often progression of symptoms (Shane, 2022). However, some patients become profoundly disturbed with serum calcium levels of only 12 mg/dL. These symptoms resolve as serum calcium levels return to normal after treatment.

Hypercalcemic crisis refers to an acute rise in the serum calcium level. Severe thirst and polyuria are often present. Other findings may include muscle weakness, intractable nausea, abdominal cramps, obstipation (very severe constipation) or diarrhea, peptic ulcer symptoms, and bone pain. Lethargy, confusion, and coma may also occur. This condition is very dangerous and may result in cardiac arrest. Persistent hypercalcemia or persistently elevated calcium–phosphorus can cause calcium deposits in tissues throughout the body. This may take the form of calcified blood vessel walls associated with necrotic skin lesions in calciphylaxis (see Chapter 26) (Klemm et al., 2022).

Serum PTH levels, calcium, phosphorus, magnesium levels are obtained. PTH levels are increased in primary or secondary hyperparathyroidism and suppressed in malignancy. X-rays may reveal the presence of osteoporosis if the patient has hypercalcemia secondary to a malignancy or bone cavitation. A 24-hour urine calcium collection may be ordered; hypercalciuria is defined as calcium excretion of greater than 350 mg/day (Fischbach et al., 2021).

Pearls for Practice

The mnemonic "bones (bone pain), stones (kidney), groans (pain), and psychic moans (anxiety, psychiatric symptoms)" may be helpful to recall the cascade of symptoms associated with hypercalcemia.

Medical Management

Therapeutic aims in hypercalcemia include decreasing the serum calcium level and reversing the process causing hypercalcemia. Treating the underlying cause (e.g., chemotherapy for a malignancy, partial parathyroidectomy for hyperparathyroidism) is essential. For example, drugs such as thiazides and vitamin D compounds, as associated with hypercalcemia, may be discontinued, dietary calcium restricted, and hydration of at least six to eight glasses of water per day to decrease the risk of nephrolithiasis (kidney stones) (Shane & Berenson, 2022).

General measures include the simultaneous administration of IV fluids, a bisphosphonate, and subcutaneous calcitonin. Isotonic saline (0.9% sodium chloride) temporarily dilutes the serum calcium level and increases urinary calcium excretion by inhibiting tubular reabsorption of calcium. While furosemide enhances renal excretion of calcium, it is associated with a paradoxical hypercalcemia due to bone resorption, thus should only be used in those with renal insufficiency or HF to avoid FVE associated with saline administration (Sadig et al., 2021).

Calcitonin works by increasing renal calcium excretion and decreasing bone resorption via interference with osteoclast function. When administered (SQ or IM) with IV saline, a substantial reduction in serum calcium concentrations should be seen within 12 to 48 hours and a bisphosphonate which inhibits osteoclast activity has efficacy by the second to fourth day and provides a more sustained effect (Shane & Berenson, 2022). Dialysis using a low or zero calcium dialysate should be considered if these treatments are not effective or if the patient has kidney disease or HF. Additional measures include mobilizing the patient and restricting intake of fluids and medications that contain calcium. When the acute management of hypercalcemia has been completed, appropriate treatment for the underlying cause needs to be undertaken.

For patients with cancer, treatment is directed at controlling the condition by surgery, chemotherapy, or radiation therapy. Refer to Chapter 5 for more details.

Nursing Management

It is important to monitor for hypercalcemia in patients who are at risk. Interventions such as increasing patient mobility and encouraging fluids can help prevent hypercalcemia, or at least minimize its severity. Fluids containing sodium should be administered unless contraindicated because sodium favors calcium excretion. Patients are encouraged to drink three to four quarts of fluid daily. Adequate fiber should be provided in the diet to offset the tendency for constipation. Safety precautions are implemented, as necessary, when mental symptoms of hypercalcemia are present. The patient and family are informed that these mental changes are reversible with treatment. Increased calcium potentiates the effects of digitalis; therefore, the patient is assessed for signs and symptoms of digitalis toxicity. Because ECG changes (premature ventricular contractions, paroxysmal atrial tachycardia, and heart block) can occur, the cardiac rate and rhythm are monitored for any abnormalities.

MAGNESIUM IMBALANCES

Magnesium is the most abundant intracellular cation after potassium. It acts as an activator for many intracellular enzyme systems and plays a role in both carbohydrate and protein metabolism. The normal serum magnesium level is 1.3 to 2.3 mEq/L (1.8 to 3.0 mg/dL; 0.8 to 1.2 mmol/L). Approximately one third of serum magnesium is bound to protein; the remaining two thirds exists as free cations—the active component (Mg^{+2}). Magnesium balance is important in neuromuscular function. Because magnesium acts directly on the myoneural junction, variations in the serum concentration of magnesium affect neuromuscular irritability and contractility. Magnesium produces its sedative effect at the neuromuscular junction, probably by inhibiting the release of the neurotransmitter acetylcholine.

Magnesium exerts effects on the cardiovascular system, acting peripherally to produce vasodilation. Magnesium is thought to have a direct effect on peripheral arteries and arterioles, which results in a decreased total peripheral resistance. IV magnesium may also be helpful in patients with acute asthma by potentially improving both bronchodilation and airflow. Magnesium is predominantly found in bone and soft tissues. It is primarily eliminated by the kidneys.

HYPOMAGNESEMIA (MAGNESIUM DEFICIT)

Hypomagnesemia refers to a below-normal serum magnesium concentration (<1.3 mEq/L; <1.8 mg/dL; <0.8 mmol/L). Magnesium is similar to calcium in two aspects: (1) it is the ionized fraction of magnesium that is primarily involved in neuromuscular activity and other physiologic processes, and (2) magnesium levels should be evaluated in combination with albumin levels. Low serum albumin levels decrease total magnesium.

Pathophysiology

Hypomagnesemia is a common yet often overlooked imbalance in people with acute and critical illness. It may occur with decreased intake (alcohol use disorder, chronic disease, and administration of tube feedings or parenteral nutrition) or increased GI or renal loss. Loss of magnesium from the GI tract may occur with gastric suctioning, diarrhea, or fistulas. Because fluid from the lower GI tract has a higher concentration of magnesium (up to 15 mEq/L of magnesium) than fluid from the upper tract (1 to 2 mEq/L), losses from diarrhea and intestinal fistulas are more likely than gastric suction to induce magnesium deficit. Although magnesium losses are relatively small in gastric suctioning, hypomagnesemia will occur if losses are prolonged and magnesium is not replaced through IV infusion. Because the distal small bowel is the major site of magnesium absorption, any disruption in small-bowel function, as in intestinal resection or inflammatory bowel disease, can lead to hypomagnesemia.

Alcoholism is currently the most common cause of symptomatic hypomagnesemia in the United States. Hypomagnesemia is particularly troublesome during treatment of alcohol withdrawal. Therefore, the serum magnesium level should be measured routinely in patients undergoing withdrawal from alcohol. The serum magnesium level may be normal on admission but may decrease as a result of metabolic changes, such as the intracellular shift of magnesium associated with IV glucose administration.

During nutritional replacement, the major cellular electrolytes move from the serum to newly synthesized cells. Patients on enteral (feeding that uses the GI tract) or parenteral (delivery of calories and nutrients into a vein, i.e., TPN, PPN) feedings should have magnesium levels measured routinely, as serious hypomagnesemia can occur with magnesium-deficient formulas, especially in those who have undergone a period of starvation. Other causes of hypomagnesemia include the administration of loop and thiazide diuretics, proton pump inhibitors, aminoglycosides, cyclosporine, cisplatin, diuretics, digitalis, and amphotericin, as well as the rapid administration of citrated blood, especially to patients with kidney or hepatic disease (Gragossian et al., 2022). Magnesium deficiency often occurs in DKA, secondary to increased renal excretion during osmotic diuresis and shifting of magnesium into the cells with insulin therapy. Other contributing causes are sepsis, burns, and hypothermia.

Clinical Manifestations and Assessment

Clinical manifestations of hypomagnesemia are largely confined to the neuromuscular system. Some of the effects are due directly to the low serum magnesium level; others are due to secondary changes in potassium and calcium metabolism. Symptoms do not usually occur until the serum magnesium level has dropped to less than 1 mEq/L (0.5 mmol/L).

Among the neuromuscular changes are hyperexcitability with muscle weakness, tremors, and *athetoid movements* (slow, involuntary twisting and writhing). Others include tetany, generalized tonic–clonic or focal seizures, laryngeal stridor, and positive Chvostek and Trousseau signs (see earlier discussion on calcium), which occur, in part, because of accompanying hypocalcemia.

Hypomagnesemia may be accompanied by marked alterations in mood. Apathy, depression, apprehension, and extreme agitation have been noted, as well as ataxia, dizziness, insomnia, and confusion. At times, delirium, auditory or visual hallucinations, and frank psychoses may occur.

On laboratory analysis, the serum magnesium level is less than 1.3 mEq/L or 1.8 mg/dL (0.75 mmol/L). Hypomagnesemia is frequently associated with hypokalemia and hypocalcemia. About 25% of magnesium is protein bound, principally to albumin. A decreased serum albumin level can, therefore, reduce the measured total magnesium concentration. ECG evaluations reflect magnesium, calcium, and potassium deficiencies, tachyarrhythmias, prolonged PR and QT intervals, widening QRS, depression of the ST segment, flattened T waves, and a prominent U wave. Torsades de pointes is associated with a low magnesium level. Premature ventricular contractions, paroxysmal atrial tachycardia, and heart block may also occur. Digitalis toxicity is associated with low serum magnesium levels. This is important because patients receiving digoxin are also likely to be receiving diuretic therapy, predisposing them to renal loss of magnesium. Urine magnesium levels may be helpful in identifying causes of magnesium depletion and are measured after a loading dose of magnesium sulfate is administered.

Medical Management

Mild magnesium deficiency can be corrected by diet alone. Principal dietary sources of magnesium, which is a component of chlorophyll, are green leafy vegetables, nuts, seeds, legumes, whole grains, and seafood. Magnesium is also plentiful in peanut butter and cocoa.

If necessary, magnesium salts can be administered orally in an oxide or gluconate form to replace continuous excessive losses. Diarrhea is a common complication of excessive ingestion of magnesium. Patients receiving parenteral nutrition require magnesium in the IV solution to prevent hypomagnesemia. Magnesium sulfate must be administered intravenously by an infusion pump typically at a rate of 1 to 2 g over an hour. If the patient is hemodynamically unstable, or in cardiac arrest with pulseless VT with torsade de pointes, the IV magnesium (1 to 2 g diluted in 10 mL solution [5% dextrose or normal saline]) can be administered over 15 minutes (Yu, 2022). A bolus dose of magnesium sulfate given too rapidly can produce alterations in cardiac conduction, leading to heart block or asystole. Vital signs must be assessed frequently during magnesium administration to detect changes in cardiac rate or rhythm, hypotension, and respiratory distress. Monitoring urine output is essential before, during, and after magnesium administration; the provider is notified if urine volume decreases to less than 0.5 mL/kg/hr. Calcium gluconate must be readily available to treat hypocalcemia-induced tetany or hypermagnesemia. Serial measurements of serum magnesium levels can be used to regulate the dosage.

Nursing Management

The nurse should be aware of patients who are at risk for hypomagnesemia and observe them for its signs and symptoms. Patients receiving digitalis are monitored closely because a deficit of magnesium can predispose them to digitalis toxicity. If hypomagnesemia is severe, seizure precautions are implemented. Other safety precautions are instituted, as indicated, if confusion is observed.

Because difficulty in swallowing (dysphagia) may occur in magnesium-depleted patients, a swallowing evaluation should be performed before oral medications or foods are offered. Dysphagia is probably related to the athetoid or *choreiform* (rapid, involuntary, and irregular jerking) movements associated with magnesium deficit. To determine neuromuscular irritability, the nurse needs to assess and grade deep tendon reflexes (refer to Chapter 42).

Teaching plays a major role in treating magnesium deficit, particularly that resulting from abuse of diuretic or laxative medications. In such cases, the nurse instructs the patient about the need to consume magnesium-rich foods. For patients experiencing hypomagnesemia from alcohol use disorder, the nurse provides teaching, counseling, support, and possible referral to alcohol abstinence programs or other professional help.

HYPERMAGNESEMIA (MAGNESIUM EXCESS)

Hypermagnesemia is a rare electrolyte abnormality because usually, the kidneys are efficient in excreting magnesium. A serum magnesium level can appear falsely elevated if blood specimens are allowed to hemolyze or are drawn from an extremity with a tourniquet that was applied too tightly or for too long a period of time prior to blood draw.

Pathophysiology

By far, the most common cause of hypermagnesemia is kidney failure. In fact, most patients with advanced kidney failure have at least a slight elevation in serum magnesium levels. This condition is aggravated when such patients receive magnesium to control seizures or inadvertently take one of the many commercial antacids that contain magnesium salts.

Hypermagnesemia can occur in a patient with untreated DKA when catabolism causes the release of cellular magnesium that cannot be excreted because of profound fluid volume depletion and resulting oliguria (less than 400 mL/24 hrs). An excess of magnesium can also result from excessive magnesium administered to treat hypertension of pregnancy or to treat low hypomagnesemia. Increased serum magnesium levels can also occur in adrenocortical insufficiency, Addison disease, or hypothermia. Excessive use of antacids, laxatives, and medications that decrease GI motility, including opioids and anticholinergics, can also increase serum magnesium levels. Decreased elimination of magnesium or its increased absorption due to intestinal hypomotility from any cause can contribute to hypermagnesemia. Lithium intoxication can also cause an increase in serum magnesium levels.

Clinical Manifestations and Assessment

Acute elevation of the serum magnesium level depresses the CNS as well as the peripheral neuromuscular junction. At mildly increased levels, there is a tendency for lowered blood pressure because of peripheral vasodilation. Nausea, vomiting, weakness, soft tissue calcifications, facial flushing, and sensations of warmth may also occur. At higher magnesium concentrations, lethargy, difficulty speaking (dysarthria), and drowsiness can occur. Deep tendon reflexes are lost, and muscle weakness and paralysis may develop. The respiratory center is depressed when serum magnesium levels exceed 10 mEq/L (5 mmol/L). Coma, atrioventricular heart block, and cardiac arrest can occur when the serum magnesium level is greatly elevated and not treated. High levels of magnesium also result in platelet clumping and delayed thrombin formation. On laboratory analysis, the serum magnesium level is greater than 2.5 mEq/L or 3.0 mg/dL (1.25 mmol/L). Increased potassium and calcium are present concurrently. ECG findings may include a prolonged PR interval, tall T waves, a widened QRS, and a prolonged QT interval, as well as an atrioventricular block.

Medical Management

Hypermagnesemia can be prevented by avoiding the administration of magnesium to patients with kidney failure and by carefully monitoring patients with a serious illness who are receiving magnesium salts. In patients with severe hypermagnesemia, all parenteral and oral magnesium salts are discontinued. In emergencies, such as respiratory depression or defective cardiac conduction, ventilatory support and IV calcium gluconate (to reverse the neuromuscular and cardiac effects of hypermagnesemia) are indicated. In addition, hemodialysis with a magnesium-free dialysate can reduce the serum magnesium to a safe level within hours. Administration of loop diuretics (furosemide) and IV isotonic fluids (e.g., normal saline) enhances magnesium excretion in patients with adequate kidney function.

Nursing Management

Patients at risk for hypermagnesemia are identified and assessed. The nurse monitors the vital signs, noting hypotension and shallow respirations, or ECG abnormalities. The nurse also observes for decreased deep tendon reflexes and changes in the LOC. Medications that contain magnesium are not administered to patients with kidney failure or compromised kidney function, and patients with kidney failure are cautioned to check with their health care providers before taking over-the-counter medications. Caution is essential when preparing and administering magnesium-containing fluids parenterally because available parenteral magnesium solutions (e.g., 2 mL ampules, 50 mL vials) differ in concentration.

PHOSPHORUS IMBALANCES

Phosphorus is a critical constituent of all the body's tissues. It is essential to the function of muscle and RBC; the formation of adenosine triphosphate (ATP) and of

2,3-diphosphoglycerate, which facilitates release of oxygen from hemoglobin; and the maintenance of acid–base balance, as well as to the nervous system and the intermediary metabolism of carbohydrate, protein, and fat. It provides structural support to bones and teeth in the form of phosphate. Phosphorus is the primary anion of the ICF. About 85% of phosphorus is located in bones and teeth, 14% in soft tissue, and less than 1% in the ECF. The normal serum phosphorus level is 2.5 to 4.5 mg/dL (0.8 to 1.45 mmol/L).

HYPOPHOSPHATEMIA (PHOSPHORUS DEFICIT)

Pathophysiology

Hypophosphatemia (<2.5 mg/dL) can be caused by decreased phosphate intake, decreased intestinal absorption, increased phosphate excretion (primarily via the kidneys), or acute movement of extracellular phosphate into the cells.

Hypophosphatemia may occur during the administration of calories to patients with severe protein–calorie malnutrition. It is most likely to occur with overzealous intake or administration of simple carbohydrates. This syndrome can be induced in anyone with severe protein–calorie malnutrition, such as patients with anorexia nervosa or alcohol use disorder, or in older debilitated patients with decreased oral intake. Approximately 50% of patients hospitalized due to chronic alcoholism have hypophosphatemia.

Marked hypophosphatemia may develop in malnourished patients who receive parenteral nutrition if the phosphorus loss is not adequately corrected. Other causes of hypophosphatemia include pain, heat stroke, prolonged intense hyperventilation, alcohol withdrawal, poor dietary intake, DKA (insulin is a strong stimulus for shifting phosphate into cells), hepatic encephalopathy, and major thermal burns. Low magnesium levels, low potassium levels, and hyperparathyroidism related to increased urinary losses of phosphorus contribute to hypophosphatemia. Loss of phosphorus through the kidneys also occurs with acute volume expansion, osmotic diuresis, use of carbonic anhydrase inhibitors (acetazolamide), and some malignancies. Respiratory alkalosis can cause a decrease in phosphorus because of an intracellular shift of phosphorus, which often stimulates intracellular glycolysis.

Excess phosphorus binding by antacids containing magnesium, calcium, or albumin may decrease the phosphorus available from the diet to an amount lower than required to maintain serum phosphorus balance. The degree of hypophosphatemia depends on the amount of phosphorus in the diet compared to the dose of antacid. Phosphate loss can occur with chronic diarrhea or through severe potassium restriction. Vitamin D regulates intestinal ion absorption; therefore, a deficiency of vitamin D may cause decreased GI absorption of calcium and phosphate (phosphorus), which may lead to osteomalacia (softened, brittle bones).

Clinical Manifestations and Assessment

A wide range of neurologic symptoms may occur, including irritability, fatigue, apprehension, weakness, numbness, paresthesias, dysarthria, dysphagia, diplopia, confusion, seizures, and coma. Low levels of diphosphoglycerate may reduce the delivery of oxygen to peripheral tissues, resulting in tissue anoxia. Hypoxia then leads to an increase in respiratory rate and respiratory alkalosis, causing phosphorus to move into the cells and potentiating hypophosphatemia. Hemolytic anemia may lead to pale skin and conjunctivae. It is thought that hypophosphatemia may predispose a person to infection due to a decrease in granulocyte function.

Muscle damage may develop as the ATP level in the muscle tissue declines. Clinical manifestations are muscle weakness, which may be subtle or profound and may affect any muscle group; muscle pain; and at times acute rhabdomyolysis (disintegration of striated muscle). Weakness of respiratory muscles may greatly impair ventilation. Hypophosphatemia also may predispose a person to insulin resistance and thus hyperglycemia. Chronic loss of phosphorus can cause bruising and bleeding from platelet dysfunction.

On laboratory analysis, the serum phosphorus level is less than 2.5 mg/dL (0.80 mmol/L) in adults. When reviewing laboratory results, the nurse should keep in mind that glucose or insulin administration causes a slight decrease in the serum phosphorus level. If hypophosphatemia is associated with hyperparathyroidism, the serum PTH levels are increased. Likewise, if etiology of hypophosphatemia is related to increased osteoblastic activity the serum alkaline phosphatase is increased. X-rays may show skeletal changes of osteomalacia or rickets.

Medical Management

Prevention of hypophosphatemia is the goal. In patients at risk for hypophosphatemia, serum phosphate levels should be monitored closely and correction initiated before deficits become severe. Adequate amounts of phosphorus should be added to parenteral solutions, and attention should be paid to the phosphorus levels in enteral feeding solutions.

Severe hypophosphatemia is dangerous and requires prompt attention. Aggressive IV phosphorus correction is usually limited to the patient whose serum phosphorus levels decrease to less than 1 mg/dL (0.3 mmol/L) and whose GI tract is not functioning. IV preparations of phosphorus are available as sodium or potassium phosphate, although sodium phosphate is preferred; it must be diluted before administered and infused slowly; it is contraindicated in patients with renal insufficiency or hypercalcemia (Yu & Stubbs, 2022; Lexicomp, 2022; Yu, 2020). IV phosphate is potentially dangerous since it can precipitate with calcium and produce a variety of adverse effects including hypocalcemia due to binding of calcium (resulting in tetany), kidney failure due to calcium phosphate precipitation in the kidneys, calcifications in tissues (blood vessels, heart, lung, eyes), and possibly fatal arrhythmias (Yu & Stubbs, 2022). The IV site should be monitored carefully because tissue sloughing and necrosis can occur with infiltration, and continuous cardiac monitoring is required with IV administration (Lexicomp, 2022). In less acute situations, oral phosphorus replacement is usually adequate.

Nursing Management

The nurse identifies patients who are at risk for hypophosphatemia and monitors them. Because malnourished patients receiving parenteral nutrition are at risk when calories are introduced too aggressively, preventive measures involve gradually introducing the solution to avoid rapid shifts of phosphorus into the cells.

For patients with documented hypophosphatemia, careful attention is given to preventing infection because hypophosphatemia may alter the granulocytes. In patients requiring correction of phosphorus losses, the nurse frequently monitors serum phosphorus levels and documents and reports early signs of hypophosphatemia (apprehension, confusion, change in LOC). If the patient experiences mild hypophosphatemia, foods such as milk and milk products, organ meats, nuts, fish, poultry, and whole grains should be encouraged. With moderate hypophosphatemia, supplements such as Neutra-Phos capsules (250 mg phosphorus/capsule) or Fleet's Phospho-Soda (815 mg phosphorus/5 mL) may be prescribed.

HYPERPHOSPHATEMIA (PHOSPHORUS EXCESS)

Hyperphosphatemia is a serum phosphorus level that exceeds normal. Various conditions can lead to this imbalance, but the most common cause is kidney failure. Other causes include increased intake, decreased output, or a shift from the ICS to ECS, as well as chemotherapy for neoplastic disease, hypoparathyroidism, metabolic or respiratory acidosis, high phosphate intake, and increased phosphorus absorption. High intake of phosphate can result with excessive use of phosphate-containing laxatives or enemas and vitamin D intoxication since the vitamin increases intestinal phosphate absorption (Goyal & Jiala, 2022). Excessive phosphate load can occur when there is massive tissue breakdown due to a variety of causes (e.g., rhabdomyolysis, [refer to Chapter 41], tumor lysis syndrome [see Chapter 5], acute hemolysis), leading to the release of intracellular phosphate into the extracellular fluid (Goyal & Jiala, 2022). Shift of phosphorus from the ICS to ECS can rarely be caused by lactic acidosis and DKA. The primary complication of increased phosphorus is metastatic calcification (soft tissue, joints, and arteries), which occurs when the calcium—magnesium product (calcium × magnesium) exceeds 70 mg/dL.

Clinical Manifestations and Assessment

An increased serum phosphorus level causes few symptoms. Symptoms that do occur usually result from decreased calcium levels and soft tissue calcifications. The most important short-term consequence is tetany. Because of the reciprocal relationship between phosphorus and calcium, a high serum phosphate level tends to cause a low serum calcium concentration. Tetany can result, causing tingling sensations in the fingertips and around the mouth. Anorexia, nausea, vomiting, bone and joint pain, muscle weakness, hyperreflexia, and tachycardia may occur.

The major long-term consequence is soft tissue calcification, which occurs mainly in patients with a reduced glomerular filtration rate. High serum levels of inorganic phosphorus promote precipitation of calcium phosphate in nonosseous sites, decreasing urine output, impairing vision, and producing palpitations.

On laboratory analysis, the serum phosphorus level exceeds 4.5 mg/dL (1.5 mmol/L) in adults. Serum phosphorus levels are normally higher in children presumably because of the high rate of skeletal growth. The serum calcium level is useful also for diagnosing the primary disorder and assessing the effects of treatments. X-ray studies may show skeletal changes with abnormal bone development. PTH levels are decreased in hypoparathyroidism. BUN and creatinine levels are used to assess kidney function. Renal ultrasonography may be indicated as part of the diagnostic assessment for kidney failure; bone studies and coronary calcification studies also provide information about the chronicity and prognosis of kidney failure.

Medical Management

When possible, treatment is directed at the underlying disorder. For example, hyperphosphatemia may be related to volume depletion or respiratory or metabolic acidosis. If renal function is adequate, a phosphate restrictive diet along with the use of saline infusion and diuretics can increase renal phosphate excretion (Goyal & Jiala, 2022). In kidney failure, elevated PTH production contributes to a high phosphorus level and bone disease. Measures to decrease the serum phosphate level in these patients include phosphate restriction, phosphate binders, and vitamin D preparations, such as calcitriol or synthetic vitamin D analogs, which is available in both oral and parenteral forms. IV administration of calcitriol does not increase the serum calcium unless its dose is excessive. However, these measures should not be administered unless the serum phosphate concentration is <5.5 mg/dL and the serum calcium is less than 9.5 mg/dL, because they can increase the serum calcium and phosphate, leading to vascular calcification (Goyal & Jiala, 2022). Surgery may be indicated for removal of large calcium–phosphorus deposits.

Nursing Management

The nurse monitors patients at risk for hyperphosphatemia. If a low-phosphorus diet is prescribed, the patient is instructed to avoid phosphorus-rich foods such as hard cheese, cream, nuts, meats, whole-grain cereals, dried fruits, dried vegetables, kidneys, sardines, sweetbreads, and foods made with milk. When appropriate, the nurse instructs the patient to avoid phosphate-containing substances such as laxatives and enemas. The nurse also teaches the patient to recognize the signs of impending hypocalcemia and to monitor for changes in urine output.

CHLORIDE IMBALANCES

Chloride, the major anion of the ECF, is found more in interstitial and lymph fluid compartments than in blood. Chloride is also contained in gastric and pancreatic juices, sweat, bile, and saliva. The choroid plexus, where cerebrospinal fluid forms in the brain, depends on sodium and chloride to attract water to form the fluid portion of the cerebrospinal fluid. Sodium and chloride in water make up the composition of the ECF and assist in determining osmotic pressure. The serum level of chloride reflects a change in dilution or concentration of the ECF and does so in direct proportion to the sodium concentration. Serum osmolality parallels chloride levels as well. The normal serum chloride level is 96 to 106 mEq/L (96 to 106 mmol/L) (Fischbach et al., 2021). Inside the cell, the chloride level is 4 mEq/L.

Plasma bicarbonate has an inverse relationship with chloride, that is, as the bicarbonate rises, the chloride decreases and vice versa. For example, the carbonic anhydrase reaction in RBCs generates both hydrogen and bicarbonate from metabolically produced CO_2. Hydrogen facilitates the dissociation of oxygen from hemoglobin. The intracellular accumulation of bicarbonate is prevented by its movement out of the cell into the plasma. To maintain electrical neutrality, chloride enters the RBC, a response referred to as the *chloride shift*. It is important to note that when the level of one of these three electrolytes (sodium, bicarbonate, or chloride) is disturbed, the other two are also affected. Chloride is important not only in maintaining acid–base balance, but it also mediates the hyperpolarizing effect of many neurotransmitters on the membrane potential. Chloride is primarily obtained from the diet as table salt.

HYPOCHLOREMIA (CHLORIDE DEFICIT)

Chloride control depends on the intake of chloride and the excretion and reabsorption of its ions in the kidneys. Chloride is produced in the stomach, where it combines with hydrogen to form hydrochloric acid. A small amount of chloride is lost in the feces. GI tube drainage and severe vomiting and diarrhea, laxatives, ileostomy, and fistulas are risk factors for hypochloremia. Administration of chloride-deficient formulas, low sodium intake, decreased serum sodium levels, metabolic alkalosis, prolonged therapy with IV dextrose (water intoxication), diuretic therapy, burns, and fever may also cause hypochloremia. As chloride decreases (usually because of volume depletion), sodium and bicarbonate ions are retained by the kidney to balance the loss. Bicarbonate accumulates in the ECF, which raises the pH and leads to hypochloremic metabolic alkalosis. In addition, in chronic respiratory acidosis, since metabolic compensation increases renal HCO_3^- reabsorption, the urinary loss of chloride is increased (Toffaletti & Rackley, 2022).

Clinical Manifestations and Assessment

Because hypochloremia rarely occurs in the absence of other abnormalities, signs and symptoms of hypochloremia are associated with hyponatremia, hypokalemia, and metabolic alkalosis. Metabolic alkalosis is a disorder that results in a high pH and a high serum bicarbonate level as a result of excess alkali intake or loss of hydrogen ions. With compensation, the partial pressure of carbon dioxide in arterial blood ($PaCO_2$) increases to >45 mm Hg. Hyperexcitability of muscles, tetany, hyperactive deep tendon reflexes, weakness, twitching, and muscle cramps may result. Hypokalemia can cause hypochloremia, resulting in cardiac arrhythmias. In addition, because low chloride levels parallel low sodium levels, a water excess may occur. Hyponatremia can cause seizures and coma.

In addition to the chloride level, sodium and potassium levels are also evaluated because these electrolytes are lost along with chloride. ABG analysis identifies the acid–base imbalance, which is usually metabolic alkalosis.

Medical Management

Treatment involves correcting the cause of hypochloremia and the contributing electrolyte and acid–base imbalances. If the hypochloremia is mild, it may be corrected by consuming more NaCl salt (Toffaletti & Rackley, 2022). For more severe hypochloremia, normal saline (0.9% sodium chloride) or half-strength saline (0.45% sodium chloride) solution may be administered by IV to replace the chloride. The provider may re-evaluate whether the patient receiving a diuretic (loop, osmotic, or thiazide) should discontinue the medications or change to another diuretic.

Foods high in chloride are provided; these include tomato juice, bananas, dates, eggs, cheese, milk, salty broth, canned vegetables, and processed meats. A patient who drinks free water (water without electrolytes) or bottled water excretes large amounts of chloride; therefore, the patient is instructed to avoid this kind of water. Ammonium chloride, an acidifying agent, may be prescribed to treat metabolic alkalosis; the dosage depends on the patient's weight and serum chloride level. This agent is metabolized by the liver, and its effects last for about 3 days. Its use should be avoided in patients with impaired liver or kidney function.

Nursing Management

The nurse monitors the patient's I&O, ABG values, and serum electrolyte levels as well as LOC and muscle strength and movement. Changes are reported to the provider promptly. Vital signs are monitored, and respiratory assessment is carried out frequently. The nurse teaches the patient about foods with high chloride content.

HYPERCHLOREMIA (CHLORIDE EXCESS)

Hyperchloremia exists when the serum level of chloride exceeds 106 mEq/L (106 mmol/L).

Pathophysiology

Because chloride has an affinity for sodium and an inverse relationship with bicarbonate, hyperchloremia is related to hypernatremia, bicarbonate loss, and metabolic acidosis. Hyperchloremic metabolic acidosis is also known as *normal anion gap acidosis* (see later discussion). It is usually caused by the loss of bicarbonate ions via the kidney or the GI tract via diarrhea with a corresponding increase in chloride ions. Chloride ions in the form of acidifying salts accumulate, and acidosis occurs with a decrease in bicarbonate ions. Hyperchloremia results from increased intake either by mouth or by isotonic or hypertonic IV fluid administration (e.g., 9% NaCl has a chloride content of 154 mEq/L). Since normal chloride is 96 to 106 mEq/L, the nurse recognizes that prolonged administration of normal saline can result in hyperchloremic metabolic acidosis (electroneutrality is maintained by a decrease in the serum HCO_3^- [bicarbonate or base] concentration in the presence of a high chloride level, so a hyperchloremic acidosis ensues). It can also result from decreased chloride excretion as in hyperparathyroidism, hyperaldosteronism, and kidney failure.

Clinical Manifestations and Assessment

The signs and symptoms of hyperchloremia are the same as those of metabolic acidosis, hypervolemia, and hypernatremia and can include tachypnea; weakness; lethargy; deep, rapid respirations; diminished cognitive ability; and hypertension. If untreated, hyperchloremia can lead to a decrease in cardiac output, arrhythmias, and coma. A high chloride level is often accompanied by a high sodium level and fluid retention. Laboratory analysis reveals the serum chloride level of >106 mEq/L (108 mmol/L), the serum sodium level >145 mEq/L (145 mmol/L), the serum pH <7.35, and the serum bicarbonate level <22 mEq/L (22 mmol/L).

Medical Management

Correcting the underlying cause of hyperchloremia and restoring electrolyte, fluid, and acid–base balance are essential. Hypotonic IV solutions may be given to restore balance. Lactated Ringer solution may be prescribed to convert lactate to bicarbonate in the liver, which increases the base bicarbonate level and corrects the acidosis. IV sodium bicarbonate may be administered to increase bicarbonate levels, which leads to the renal excretion of chloride ions as bicarbonate and chloride compete to combine with sodium. Diuretics may be administered to eliminate chloride as well. Sodium, chloride, and fluids are restricted.

Nursing Management

Monitoring vital signs, ABG values, and the patient's I&O status is important to assess the patient's status and the effectiveness of treatment. Assessment findings related to respiratory, neurologic, and cardiac systems are documented, and changes are discussed with the provider. The nurse teaches the patient about the diet that should be followed to manage hyperchloremia and maintain adequate hydration.

ACID–BASE DISTURBANCES

Acid–base disturbances are commonly encountered in clinical practice. Identification of the specific acid–base imbalance is important in identifying the underlying cause of the disorder and determining appropriate treatment.

Plasma pH is an indicator of hydrogen ion (H^+) concentration. Homeostatic mechanisms keep pH within a normal range (7.35 to 7.45). These mechanisms consist of buffer systems, the kidneys, and the lungs. The H^+ concentration is extremely important: the greater the concentration, the more acidic the solution and the lower the pH; the lower the H^+ concentration, the more alkaline the solution and the higher the pH. The process causing an acidemia (condition when the blood is acidic) is termed either *metabolic* or *respiratory acidosis,* whereas the process causing an alkalemia (condition when the blood is alkaline) is either *metabolic* or *respiratory alkalosis.* Blood pH must be kept within narrow limits because a pH outside the range of 6.8 to 7.8 is incompatible with life.

Buffer systems prevent major changes in the pH of body fluids by removing or releasing H^+; they can act quickly to prevent excessive changes in H^+ concentration. Hydrogen ions are buffered by both intracellular and extracellular buffers. The body's major extracellular buffer system is the bicarbonate–carbonic acid buffer system, which is assessed when ABGs are measured. The sources for bicarbonate (HCO_3^-) are the intestinal lumen, pancreas, kidney, and, to a lesser extent, diet. The role of the kidneys is to reabsorb filtered bicarbonate and make new bicarbonate. The bicarbonate ion acts as a H^+ ion acceptor and is responsible for buffering the majority of the hydrogen ions in blood. Normally, there are 20 parts of bicarbonate (HCO_3^-) to one part of carbonic acid (H_2CO_3). If this ratio is altered, the pH will change. It is the ratio of HCO_3^- to H_2CO_3 that is important in maintaining pH, not absolute values. Carbon dioxide (CO_2) is regulated by the lungs and, when dissolved in water, becomes carbonic acid ($CO_2 + H_2O = H_2CO_3$). Therefore, when CO_2 is increased, the carbonic acid content is also increased, and vice versa. If either bicarbonate or carbonic acid is increased or decreased so that the 20:1 ratio is no longer maintained, an acid–base imbalance will result. Less important buffer systems in the ECF include the inorganic phosphates and the plasma proteins. Intracellular buffers include proteins, organic and inorganic phosphates, and, in RBC, hemoglobin.

The kidneys regulate the bicarbonate level in the ECF; they can regenerate bicarbonate ions as well as reabsorb them from the renal tubular cells. In respiratory acidosis, the kidneys respond to the increased CO_2 (carbon dioxide) and decreased pH by excreting hydrogen ions and conserving bicarbonate ions to help restore balance. Conversely, in respiratory alkalosis, the kidneys' response to the decreased CO_2 and increased pH is to retain hydrogen ions and excrete bicarbonate ions to help restore balance. However, the renal compensation for imbalances described above is relatively slow (a matter of hours or days).

The lungs, under the control of the pons and the medulla, regulate the CO_2 and, thus, the carbonic acid content of the ECF. They do so by adjusting ventilation in response to the amount of CO_2 in the blood. A rise in the partial pressure of CO_2 in arterial blood ($PaCO_2$) is a powerful stimulant to respiration. Of course, the partial pressure of oxygen in arterial blood (PaO_2) also influences respiration. However, its effect is not as marked as that produced by the $PaCO_2$.

In metabolic acidosis, the respiratory rate increases, causing greater elimination of CO_2 (to reduce the acid load). In contrast, in metabolic alkalosis, the respiratory rate decreases, causing CO_2 to be retained (to increase the acid load). Both mechanisms are an attempt to return the pH to normal, and the respiratory response is instantaneous.

To review, a normal pH is 7.35 to 7.45 and is associated with three conditions: (1) a normal level of acid and base; (2) an abnormal process in which too many bases are produced (alkalosis), and the body counteracts this base load by allowing more acids to accumulate (20 base to 1 acid ratio maintained); (3) an abnormal process in which too many acids are produced, and the body counteracts by allowing more base to accumulate (20 base to 1 acid ratio maintained). The second and third conditions are considered compensation and will be discussed later in the chapter. If the pH is greater than 7.45, an alkalemia (blood is excessively alkaline) exists. If the pH is less than 7.35, an acidemia (blood is excessively acid) exists.

BASE BICARBONATE IMBALANCES

Metabolic Acidosis (Base Bicarbonate Deficit)

Metabolic acidosis is a clinical disturbance characterized by a low pH (increased H^+ concentration) and a low plasma bicarbonate concentration (less than 22 mEq/L). It can be produced by a gain of hydrogen ions or a loss of bicarbonate, and it is divided clinically into two forms according to the values of the serum anion gap: high anion gap acidosis and normal anion gap acidosis. The anion gap reflects unmeasured anions (phosphates, sulfates, and proteins) in plasma. Recall cations are positively charged ions (Na^+, K^+, H^+), and anions are negatively charged ions (HCO_3^-, Cl^-). Under normal conditions, the ratio of cation to anion is not equal; that is, the Na^+ and K^+ levels are greater than the number of HCO_3^- and Cl^-. In actuality, the ECF is, under normal circumstances, electroneutral, and the sum of cations does equal the sum of anions. However, since not all anions are measured, there is a gap. The anion gap can be calculated by either one of the following equations:

$$(Na^+ + K^+) - (HCO_3^- + Cl^-)$$

or

$$Na^+ - (HCO_3^- + Cl^-)$$

Potassium is often omitted from the equation because of its low level in the plasma; therefore, the second equation is used more often than the first.

The normal value for an anion gap is about 8 to 12 mEq/L (8 to 12 mmol/L) without potassium in the equation. If potassium is included in the equation, the normal value for the anion gap is 12 to 16 mEq/L (12 to 16 mmol/L). An anion gap greater than 16 mEq/L (16 mmol/L) is termed a *high anion gap metabolic acidosis* and results from excessive accumulation of fixed acid. High anion gap occurs in the ketoacidosis of uncontrolled diabetes or starvation, lactic acidosis, the late phase of salicylate poisoning, uremia, and methanol or ethylene glycol toxicity. In each of these situations, the excess hydrogen is buffered by HCO_3^-, causing the bicarbonate concentration to fall. This is the reason for the high anion gap. See Box 3-2 for major causes of high anion gap acidosis.

Normal anion gap acidosis results from the direct loss of bicarbonate, and can occur in diarrhea, lower intestinal fistulas, ureterostomies, diuretic therapy, early renal insufficiency, excessive administration of chloride (recall 0.9% NaCl contains 154 mEq of Cl^- per liter), and the administration of parenteral nutrition without bicarbonate or bicarbonate-producing solutes (e.g., lactate). Pancreatic drains are also associated with the direct loss of bicarbonate. In these situations, the direct loss of HCO_3^- is associated with an increase in plasma chloride, and the anion gap remains normal. This condition is also referred to as *hyperchloremic acidosis.* Refer to Box 3-2 for major causes of normal anion gap acidosis

Pearls for Practice

Metabolic acidosis (high anion gap) is frequently due to lactic acid (lactic acidosis), due to anaerobic (without oxygen) metabolism that occurs during shock states or following cardiac arrest. Thus, lactic acid is a marker for anaerobic glycolysis (to try to give the body

BOX 3-2

Mnemonics for Anion Gap Metabolic Acidosis: CAT MUDPILES and Normal Anion Gap Metabolic Acidosis: HARDUP

Mnemonic for Anion Gap Metabolic Acidosis: CAT MUDPILES

- **C:** **C**yanide and **C**arbon monoxide poisoning
- **A:** **A**rsenic, **A**lcohol ketoacidosis, **A**cetaminophen in fulminant hepatic failure
- **T:** **T**oluene (used as a solvent, and antiknock agent for gasoline, also in herbicides, pesticides, organic solvents, painting materials)
- **M:** **M**ethanol (wood alcohol), **M**etformin
- **U:** **U**remia (kidney failure)
- **D:** **D**iabetic ketoacidosis (DKA)
- **P:** **P**araldehyde
- **I:** **I**ron, INH
- **L:** **L**actic acidosis
- **E:** **E**thylene glycol (antifreeze)
- **S:** **S**alicylates (late)

Mnemonic for Normal Anion Gap Metabolic Acidosis (Hyperchloremic Metabolic Acidosis): HARDUP

- **H**yperalimentation/**H**ospital-acquired administration of saline (hyperchloremia)
- **A**cid infusion/**A**ddison disease/carbonic **A**nhydrase inhibitors
- **R**enal tubular acidosis (RTA) (failure of the kidneys to excrete acid)
- **D**iarrhea (loss of bicarbonate via GI system)
- **U**reterosigmoidostomy (and ileal diversion)
- **P**ancreatic drainage/fistula

Adapted from McCoin & Self, (2023). Acid base disorders, In Ron Walls (Ed), *Rosen's emergency medicine: Concepts and clinical practice*, 10th ed., Elsevier Inc.

energy during this crisis). The higher the lactic acid level and the longer it takes to correct, the higher the mortality rate (Burger & Shaller, 2022). For example, lactate levels greater than 4 mmol/L (normal value is 0.5 to 1.0 mmol/L are associated with a fivefold increase in mortality (Kupchik, 2021).

Clinical Manifestations and Assessment

Signs and symptoms of metabolic acidosis vary with the severity of the acidosis and the etiology. They may include headache, lethargy, confusion, sluggishness, increased respiratory rate and depth, nausea, and vomiting. As the acidosis worsens, significant neurologic, cardiac, and metabolic effects are seen such as obtundation and coma, decreased myocardial contractility, arrhythmias, decreased cardiac output, and hyperkalemia.

ABG measurements reveal a low bicarbonate level (less than 22 mEq/L) and a low pH (less than 7.35). Hyperkalemia may accompany metabolic acidosis as a result of the shift of potassium out of the cells. Later, as the acidosis is corrected, potassium moves back into the cells and hypokalemia may occur. Hyperventilation decreases the CO_2 level as a compensatory action. As stated previously, calculation of the anion gap is helpful in determining the cause of metabolic acidosis. An ECG detects arrhythmias caused by the associated increased serum potassium.

Medical and Nursing Management

Treatment is directed at correcting the underlying cause. When the problem results from excessive intake of chloride, treatment is aimed at eliminating the source of the chloride (discontinuation of offending medication). When necessary, in general, bicarbonate is administered if the pH is less than 7.1 and the serum bicarbonate level is less than 6 mEq/L (Wiederkehr & Emmett, 2022). Although hyperkalemia occurs with acidosis, hypokalemia may occur with reversal of the acidosis and subsequent movement of potassium back into the cells. Therefore, the serum potassium level is monitored closely, and hypokalemia is corrected as acidosis is reversed.

METABOLIC ALKALOSIS (BASE BICARBONATE EXCESS)

Metabolic alkalosis is a clinical disturbance characterized by a high pH (decreased H^+ concentration) and a high plasma bicarbonate concentration. It can be produced by a gain of bicarbonate or a loss of H^+.

Pathophysiology

A common cause of metabolic alkalosis is related to volume depletion from vomiting or gastric suction, with loss of stomach acid (hydrogen and chloride ions). The disorder also occurs in pyloric stenosis, in which only gastric fluid is lost. Gastric fluid has an acid pH (usually 1 to 3), and loss of this highly acidic fluid increases the risk of alkalosis. Other situations predisposing the patient to metabolic alkalosis include those associated with loss of potassium, such as diuretic therapy that promotes excretion of potassium (e.g., thiazides, furosemide), and excessive adrenocorticoid hormones (as in hyperaldosteronism and Cushing syndrome).

Hypokalemia produces alkalosis in two ways: (1) the kidneys conserve potassium, and, therefore, H^+ excretion increases; and (2) cellular potassium moves out of the cells into the ECF in an attempt to maintain near-normal serum levels (as potassium ions leave the cells, hydrogen ions must enter to maintain electroneutrality). As discussed earlier, a helpful cue to recall the association of a decreased K^+ to alkalosis is "al-K^+-low-sis."

Excessive alkali ingestion from antacids containing bicarbonate or from use of sodium bicarbonate during cardiopulmonary resuscitation can also cause metabolic alkalosis.

Pearls for Practice

You will notice that the patient's chemistry panel includes Na (sodium), K (potassium), Cl (chloride), and CO_2, which is measured as total CO_2. The total CO_2 has three components: HCO_3^-, dissolved CO_2, and carbonic acid, but because more than 80% of the total CO_2 is base bicarbonate, we refer to it as the bicarbonate level. When you obtain ABGs, you will notice the bicarbonate (HCO_3^-) (which is a calculated value) is lower by 1 to 2 mEq/L than the venous HCO_3^- or venous CO_2 from the chemistry panel. That is because the venous CO_2 also includes dissolved CO_2 and carbonic acid; thus, the venous total CO_2 concentration is higher than the calculated HCO_3^-.

Clinical Manifestations and Assessment

In mild metabolic alkalosis (pH <7.50), patients are usually asymptomatic (Seifter, 2020). However, symptoms are primarily related to decreased calcium ionization, such as tingling of the fingers and toes, dizziness, and hypertonic muscles. The ionized fraction of serum calcium decreases in alkalosis as more calcium combines with serum proteins. Because it is the ionized fraction of calcium that influences neuromuscular activity, symptoms of hypocalcemia are often the predominant symptoms of alkalosis. Respirations are depressed as a compensatory action by the lungs. As the alkalosis worsens, atrial tachycardia, hypokalemia, and ventricular disturbances may occur. Decreased motility and paralytic ileus may also occur. As the serum potassium decreases, frequent premature ventricular contractions or U waves are seen on the ECG.

Evaluation of ABG reveals a pH greater than 7.45 and an elevated serum bicarbonate concentration. The $PaCO_2$ increases as the lungs attempt to compensate for the excess bicarbonate by retaining CO_2. This hypoventilation is more pronounced in semiconscious, unconscious, or debilitated patients than in alert patients. The former may develop hypoxemia as a result of hypoventilation. Hypokalemia and hypocalcemia are expected.

Pearls for Practice

Consider that chloride and bicarbonate tend to be inversely related; therefore, when the chloride level is low (hypochloremia), the HCO_3^- rises, causing metabolic alkalosis. Conversely, when the HCO_3^- falls, the chloride level rises, causing hyperchloremic metabolic acidosis (or normal anion gap acidosis). Last, gastric suction and vomiting causes the loss of stomach acid (HCl), resulting in alkalosis.

Medical and Nursing Management

Treatment of metabolic alkalosis is aimed at correcting the underlying cause (e.g., treat the cause of vomiting, stop or reduce the removal of gastric secretions, and, if possible, discontinue the loop or thiazide diuretics) (Mehta & Emmett, 2022). Because of volume depletion from GI loss, the patient's fluid I&O must be monitored carefully.

Sufficient chloride must be supplied for the kidney to absorb sodium with chloride (allowing the excretion of excess bicarbonate). Treatment also includes restoring normal fluid volume by administering sodium chloride fluids (because continued volume depletion serves to maintain the alkalosis). In patients with hypokalemia, potassium is administered as KCl to replace both K^+ and Cl^- losses. Carbonic anhydrase inhibitors are useful in treating metabolic alkalosis since inhibiting the carbonic anhydrase enzyme allows more bicarbonate (HCO_3^-) to be released into the filtrate resulting in an alkaline diuresis; they are useful in those who cannot tolerate rapid volume expansion (e.g., patients with HF).

CARBONIC ACID IMBALANCES

RESPIRATORY ACIDOSIS (CARBONIC ACID EXCESS)

Respiratory acidosis is a clinical disorder in which the pH is less than 7.35 and the $PaCO_2$ is greater than 45 mm Hg. It may be either acute or chronic.

Pathophysiology

Respiratory acidosis is always due to inadequate excretion of CO_2 with inadequate ventilation, resulting in elevated plasma CO_2 concentrations and, consequently, increased levels of carbonic acid. Any condition that causes hypoventilation is associated with an elevated $PaCO_2$, and usually a decrease in PaO_2. Acute respiratory acidosis occurs in emergency situations, such as aspiration of a foreign object, atelectasis, diaphragmatic paralysis, overdose of sedatives, sleep apnea syndrome, administration of high-flow oxygen to a patient with chronic hypercapnia (excessive CO_2 in the blood), severe pneumonia, and acute respiratory distress syndrome. Respiratory acidosis can also occur in diseases that impair respiratory muscles, such as muscular dystrophy, myasthenia gravis, and Guillain–Barré syndrome.

Mechanical ventilation may be associated with hypercapnia if the rate of effective alveolar ventilation is inadequate (respiratory rate or tidal volume too low).

In addition, some disorders, such as pulmonary edema and pneumothorax, may initially cause hyperventilation, but as respiratory fatigue develops, the CO_2 level will rise and acidosis will develop. Therefore, the nurse cannot assume that a clinical condition will cause a predicted disturbance. Rather, the nurse considers whether the respiratory center is capable of continuing to exhale the respiratory acid.

Clinical Manifestations and Assessment

Clinical signs in acute and chronic respiratory acidosis vary. Sudden hypercapnia (elevated $PaCO_2$) can cause increased pulse and respiratory rate, mental cloudiness, dull headache, or weakness. An elevated $PaCO_2$ causes cerebrovascular vasodilation and increased cerebral blood flow, particularly when it is greater than 60 mm Hg. Ventricular fibrillation may be the first sign of respiratory acidosis in anesthetized patients.

If respiratory acidosis is severe, intracranial pressure may increase, resulting in papilledema and dilated conjunctival blood vessels. Hyperkalemia may result as the hydrogen concentration overwhelms the compensatory mechanisms and H^+ moves into cells, causing a shift of potassium out of the cell.

Chronic respiratory acidosis occurs with pulmonary diseases such as chronic emphysema and bronchitis, obstructive sleep apnea, and obesity. As long as the $PaCO_2$ does not exceed the body's ability to compensate, the patient will be asymptomatic. However, if the $PaCO_2$ increases rapidly, cerebral vasodilation will increase the intracranial pressure, and cyanosis and tachypnea will develop. Patients with chronic obstructive pulmonary disease (COPD) who gradually accumulate CO_2 over a prolonged period (days to months) may not develop symptoms of hypercapnia because compensatory renal changes have had time to occur.

ABG analysis reveals a pH lower than 7.35, a $PaCO_2$ greater than 45 mm Hg, and a variation in the bicarbonate level, depending on the duration of the acute respiratory acidosis. When compensation (renal retention of bicarbonate) has fully occurred, the arterial pH may be within the lower limits of normal. Depending on the cause of respiratory acidosis, other diagnostic measures would include monitoring of serum electrolyte levels, chest x-ray for determining any respiratory disease, and a drug screen if an overdose is suspected. An ECG to identify any cardiac arrhythmias may be indicated.

Medical and Nursing Management

Treatment is directed at treating the cause of the hypoventilation; exact measures vary with the cause of inadequate ventilation. Pharmacologic agents are used as indicated. For example, bronchodilators help reduce bronchial spasm, antibiotics are used for respiratory infections, and thrombolytics or anticoagulants are used for pulmonary emboli.

Pulmonary hygiene measures are initiated, when necessary, to clear the respiratory tract of mucus and purulent drainage. Adequate hydration (2 to 3 L/day) is indicated to keep the mucous membranes moist and thereby facilitate the removal of secretions as long as not contraindicated by cardiac, liver, or kidney disease. Supplemental oxygen is administered as necessary.

Pearls for Practice

If the $PaCO_2$ is chronically higher than 50 mm Hg, the respiratory center becomes relatively insensitive to CO_2 as a respiratory stimulant, leaving hypoxemia as the major drive for respiration. Oxygen administration may remove the stimulus of hypoxemia, and the patient develops "carbon dioxide narcosis" unless the situation is quickly reversed. Additional theories for the increased CO_2 seen with oxygen administration are that oxygen administration increases the release of CO_2 from hemoglobin (which would cause the CO_2 to rise) or that oxygen administration abolishes the compensatory response of pulmonary vasoconstriction. With O_2 administration, pulmonary arteriolar vasodilation increases perfusion to poorly ventilated alveoli causing a rise in the CO_2 (Stacy, 2022). While the exact etiology has not been elucidated for carbon dioxide narcosis, it is prudent to administer the amount of oxygen necessary to improve the patient's oxygen saturation to approximately 90%. Typically low-flow oxygen (24% or 28% or 1 to 2 L/min) is administered; however, oxygen administration may need to be above this level. Therefore, the nurse recognizes that failure to achieve appropriate oxygenation is an indication for assisted ventilation.

Mechanical ventilation may be required to improve pulmonary ventilation. Inappropriate mechanical ventilation (e.g., increased dead space, insufficient rate or volume settings, high fraction of inspired oxygen [FiO_2] with excessive CO_2 production) must be corrected with appropriate changes to the ventilator setting. Proper patient positioning in a semi-Fowler position facilitates expansion of the chest wall.

RESPIRATORY ALKALOSIS (CARBONIC ACID DEFICIT)

Respiratory alkalosis is a clinical condition in which the arterial pH is greater than 7.45 and the $PaCO_2$ is less than 35 mm Hg. As with respiratory acidosis, acute and chronic conditions can occur.

Pathophysiology

Respiratory alkalosis is always caused by hyperventilation, which causes excessive "blowing off" of CO_2 and, hence, a decrease in the plasma carbonic acid concentration. Causes of respiratory alkalosis can include extreme anxiety, hypoxemia, the early phase of salicylate intoxication (since the medulla is directly stimulated by the drug and the respiratory rate increases), high fever, gram-negative bacteremia, or inappropriate ventilator settings that do not match the patient's requirements. Acute exposure to a high altitude also can result in a hypoxia-induced hyperventilation, which can take several days before the patient is fully adapted.

Clinical Manifestations and Assessment

Clinical signs consist of lightheadedness due to vasoconstriction and decreased cerebral blood flow, inability to concentrate, numbness and tingling from decreased calcium ionization, tinnitus, and, sometimes, loss of consciousness. Recall that cerebral blood flow is significantly decreased by hypocapnia, which is a potent vasoconstrictor; thus, many of the clinical manifestations of respiratory alkalosis are related to the CNS and reduced free calcium. Cardiac effects of respiratory alkalosis include tachycardia and ventricular and atrial arrhythmias.

Analysis of ABG reveals an elevated pH (greater than 7.45) as a result of a low $PaCO_2$ (less than 35 mm Hg) and a normal bicarbonate level. (The kidneys cannot alter the bicarbonate level quickly; it may take up to 3 days for compensation to occur.) The response of the kidneys will be to reduce hydrogen ion excretion (holding on to acids to maintain the 20:1 relationship) and increase bicarbonate excretion. In the compensated state, the kidneys have had sufficient time to lower the bicarbonate level to a near-normal level. Evaluation of serum electrolytes is indicated to identify a decrease in potassium as hydrogen is pulled out of the cells in exchange for potassium. As the blood pH rises and blood becomes more alkaline, proteins such as albumin become more negatively charged, causing a higher affinity for binding with free calcium in the bloodstream. As a result, the ionized portion of calcium decreases, and symptoms of carpopedal spasms and tetany occur. A toxicology screen should be performed to rule out salicylate intoxication.

Medical and Nursing Management

Treatment depends on the underlying cause of respiratory alkalosis. If the cause is anxiety, the patient is instructed to breathe more slowly to allow CO_2 to accumulate. A sedative may be required to relieve hyperventilation in very anxious patients. Treatment of other causes of respiratory alkalosis is directed at correcting the underlying problem such as reducing the respiratory rate and/or tidal volume when on mechanical ventilation.

MIXED ACID–BASE DISORDERS

Patients can simultaneously experience two or more independent acid–base disorders. A normal pH in the presence of changes in the $PaCO_2$ and plasma HCO_3^- concentration immediately suggests a mixed disorder. The only mixed disorder that cannot occur is a mixed respiratory acidosis and alkalosis because it is impossible to have alveolar hypoventilation and hyperventilation at the same time. An example of a mixed disorder is the simultaneous occurrence of metabolic acidosis and respiratory acidosis during respiratory and cardiac arrest.

Compensation

In general, the pulmonary and renal systems compensate for each other to return the pH to normal. In a single acid–base disorder, the system not causing the problem will try to compensate by returning the ratio of bicarbonate to carbonic acid to the normal 20:1. The lungs compensate for metabolic disturbances by changing CO_2 excretion. The kidneys compensate for respiratory disturbances by altering bicarbonate retention and H^+ secretion.

TABLE 3-4 **Acid–Base Disturbances and Compensation**

Disorder	Initial Event	Compensation
Respiratory acidosis	↓ pH, ↑ or normal HCO_3^-, ↑ $PaCO_2$	↑ Renal acid excretion and ↑ serum HCO_3^-
Respiratory alkalosis	↑ pH, ↓ or normal HCO_3^-, ↓ $PaCO_2$	↓ Renal acid excretion and ↓ serum HCO_3^-
Metabolic acidosis	↓ pH, ↓ HCO_3^-, ↓ $PaCO_2$	Hyperventilation with resulting ↓ $PaCO_2$
Metabolic alkalosis	↑ pH, ↑ HCO_3^-, ↑ $PaCO_2$	Hypoventilation with resulting ↑ $PaCO_2$

In respiratory acidosis, excess hydrogen is excreted in the urine, and bicarbonate is retained. In respiratory alkalosis, the renal excretion of bicarbonate increases, and hydrogen ions are retained. In metabolic acidosis, the compensatory mechanisms increase the ventilation rate; in metabolic alkalosis, the respiratory system compensates by decreasing ventilation to conserve CO_2 and increase the $PaCO_2$. Because the lungs respond to acid–base disorders within minutes, compensation for metabolic imbalances occurs faster than does compensation for respiratory imbalances. Table 3-4 summarizes compensation effects.

Blood Gas Analysis

Blood gas analysis is often used to identify the specific acid–base disturbance and the degree of compensation that has occurred (see Boxes 3-3 and 3-4). The analysis is usually based on an arterial blood sample, but if an arterial sample cannot be obtained, a mixed venous sample may be used. Results of ABG analysis provide information about alveolar ventilation, oxygenation, and acid–base balance. The health history, physical examination, previous blood gas results, and serum electrolytes should always be part of the assessment used to determine the cause of the acid–base disorder. Before obtaining an ABG from the radial artery, the nurse assesses patency of the ulnar artery by performing the Allen test (refer to Chapter 11). Treatment of the underlying condition usually corrects most acid–base disorders. Table 3-5 compares normal ranges of venous and ABG values.

PARENTERAL FLUID THERAPY

When no other route of administration is available, fluids are administered intravenously in hospitals, outpatient diagnostic and surgical settings, clinics, and homes to replace fluids, administer medications, and provide nutrients. An algorithm

BOX 3-3
Assessing Arterial Blood Gases

The following steps are recommended to evaluate arterial blood gas (ABG) values. They are based on the assumption that the average values are:

pH = 7.4
$PaCO_2$ = 40 mm Hg (normal 35 to 45 mm Hg)
HCO_3^- = 24 mEq/L (normal 22 to 26 mEq/L)

First, note the pH. It can be high, low, or normal as follows:

pH greater than 7.4 (alkaline side of normal or if >7.45 alkalosis)
pH less than 7.4 (acid side of normal or if <7.35 acidosis)
pH equal to 7.4 (normal)

A normal pH may indicate perfectly normal blood gases, or it may be an indication of a compensated imbalance. A compensated imbalance is one in which the body has been able to correct the pH by either respiratory or metabolic changes (depending on the primary problem). For example, a patient with primary metabolic acidosis starts out with a low bicarbonate level but a normal CO_2 level. Soon afterward, the lungs try to compensate for the imbalance by exhaling large amounts of CO_2 (hyperventilation). As another example, a patient with primary respiratory acidosis starts out with a high CO_2 level; soon afterward, the kidneys attempt to compensate by retaining bicarbonate. If the compensatory mechanism is able to restore the bicarbonate to carbonic acid ratio back to 20:1, full compensation (and thus normal pH) will be achieved.

The next step is to determine the primary cause of the disturbance. This is done by evaluating the $PaCO_2$ and HCO_3^- in relation to the pH.

Example: pH greater than 7.4 (alkalosis)

a. If the $PaCO_2$ is less than 35 mm Hg, the primary disturbance is respiratory alkalosis. (This situation occurs when a patient hyperventilates and "blows off" too much CO_2. Recall that CO_2 dissolved in water becomes carbonic acid, the acid side of the "carbonic acid–bicarbonate buffer system.")
b. If the HCO_3^- is greater than 26 mEq/L, the primary disturbance is metabolic alkalosis. (This situation occurs when the body gains too much bicarbonate, an alkaline substance. Bicarbonate is the basic or alkaline side of the "carbonic acid–bicarbonate buffer system.")

Example: pH less than 7.4 (acidosis)

a. If the $PaCO_2$ is greater than 45 mm Hg, the primary disturbance is respiratory acidosis. (This situation occurs when a patient hypoventilates and thus retains too much CO_2, an acidic substance.)
b. If the HCO_3^- is less than 22 mEq/L, the primary disturbance is metabolic acidosis. (This situation occurs when the body's bicarbonate level drops, either because of direct bicarbonate loss or because of gains of acids such as lactic acid or ketones.)

The next step involves determining if compensation has begun. This is done by looking at the value other than the primary disorder. If it is moving in the same direction as the primary value, compensation is under way. Consider the following gases:

pH	$PaCO_2$	HCO_3^-
(1) 7.2	60 mm Hg	24 mEq/L
(2) 7.4	60 mm Hg	37 mEq/L

The first set (1) indicates acute respiratory acidosis without compensation (the $PaCO_2$ is high, the HCO_3^- is normal). The second set (2) indicates chronic respiratory acidosis. Note that compensation has taken place; that is, the HCO_3^- has elevated to an appropriate level to balance the high $PaCO_2$ and produce a normal pH.

Two distinct acid–base disturbances may occur simultaneously. These can be identified when the pH does not explain one of the changes.

Example: Metabolic and respiratory acidosis

a. pH	7.2 decreased acid
b. $PaCO_2$	52 increased acid
c. HCO_3	13 decreased acid

This is an example of metabolic and respiratory acidosis.

known as the 5 Rs has been created to guide safe and effective use of IV fluids; the 5 Rs include resuscitation, routine maintenance, replacement, redistribution, and reassessment (see Fig. 3-9). Typical indications for giving a fluid bolus include hypotension, low urine output, inadequate cardiac output for tissue needs, and restoration of intravascular

BOX 3-4
Factors in Selecting a Venipuncture Site

The following factors should be considered when selecting a site for venipuncture:

- Condition of the vein
- Type of fluid or medication to be infused
- Duration of therapy
- Patient's age and size
- Whether the patient is right- or left-handed
- Patient's medical history and current health status
- Skill of the person performing the venipuncture

TABLE 3-5 **Normal Values for Arterial and Mixed Venous Blood**

Parameter	Arterial Blood	Mixed Venous Blood
pH	7.35–7.45	0.03–0.05 pH units lower than the arterial pH
$PaCO_2$	35–45 mm Hg	4–5 mm Hg higher than the arterial pH
PaO_2[a]	80–100 mm Hg	35–40 mm Hg
HCO_3^-	22–26 mEq/L	22–26 mEq/L
Base excess/deficit	±2 mEq/L	±2 mEq/L
Oxygen saturation	over 95%	75%

[a]At altitudes of 3,000 feet and higher, the values for oxygen are decreased.

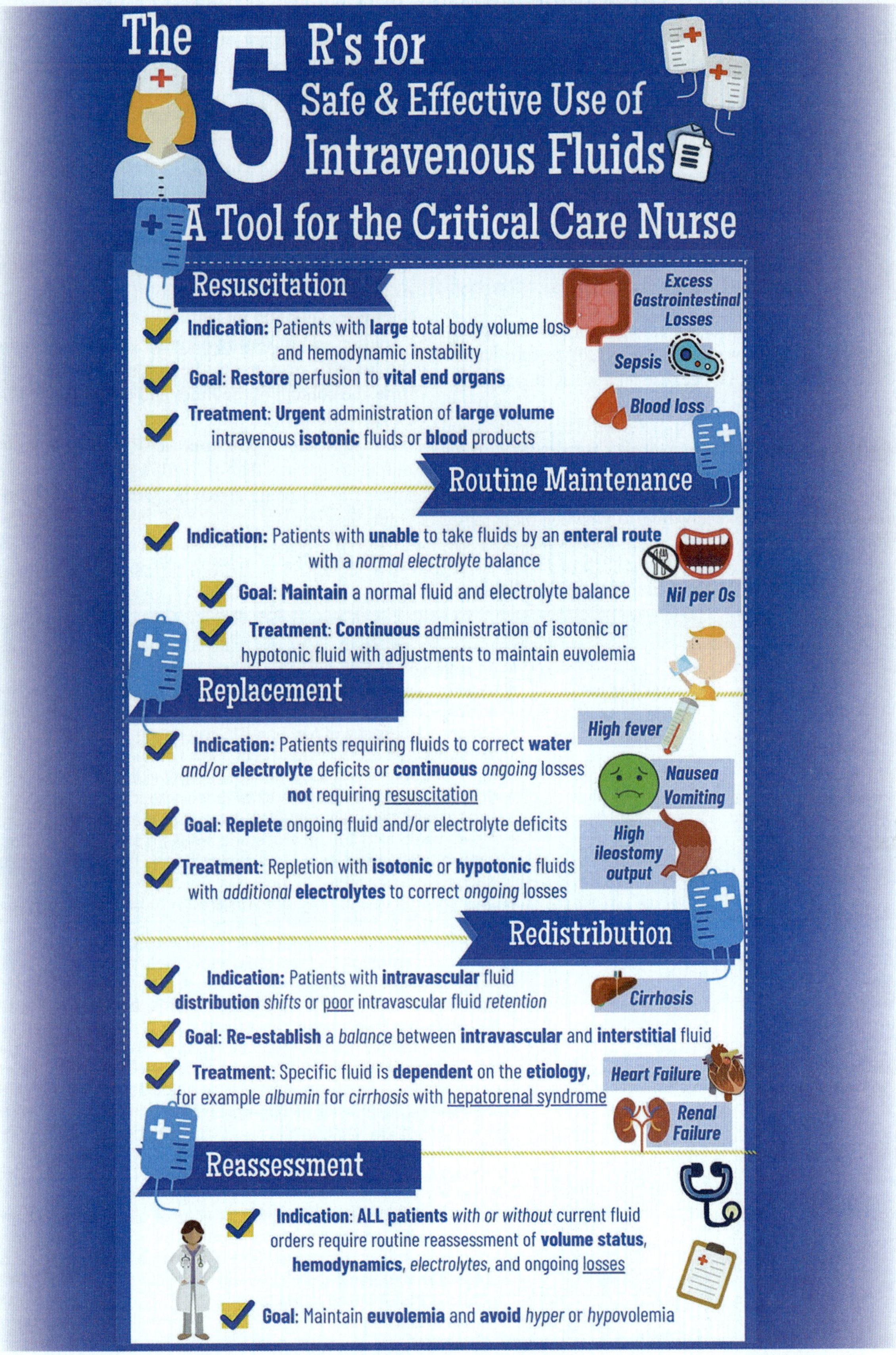

FIGURE 3-9 Algorithm known as the 5 Rs to guide safe and effective use of IV fluids. (From Barlow, A., Barlow, B., Tang, N., Shah, B. M., & King, A. E. [2020]. Intravenous fluid management in critically ill adults: A review. *Critical Care Nurse*, *40*[6], e17–e27. doi: 10.4037/ccn2020337 © 2020 by the American Association of Critical-Care Nurses. All rights reserved. Used with permission.)

volume in patients with life-threatening hypovolemia and compromised end-organ perfusion (Barlow et al., 2020).

Purpose

The choice of an IV solution depends on the purpose of its administration. In general, IV fluids are administered to achieve one or more of the following goals:

- To provide water, electrolytes, and/or nutrients to meet daily requirements;
- To replace water and correct electrolyte deficits;
- To administer medications and blood products.

IV solutions contain dextrose or electrolytes mixed in various proportions with water. Pure, electrolyte-free water can never be administered IV because it enters RBCs rapidly and causes them to rupture.

Types of IV Solutions

Crystalloid solutions are often categorized as **isotonic**, **hypotonic**, or **hypertonic**, according to whether their total osmolality is the same as, less than, or greater than that of plasma (see earlier discussion of osmolality). Crystalloid fluids generally contain three basic components: water, electrolytes, and sugar (dextrose).

Electrolyte solutions are considered isotonic if the total electrolyte content (anions + cations) ranges from 240 to 340 mEq/L, hypotonic if the total electrolyte content is less than 240 mEq/L, and hypertonic if the total electrolyte content is greater than 340 mEq/L (Noble, 2022). The nurse must also consider a solution's osmolality, keeping in mind that the osmolality of plasma is 275 to 295 mOsm/kg. For example, a 10% dextrose solution has an osmolality of approximately 505 mOsm/L.

When administering parenteral fluids, the nurse monitors the patient's response to the fluids, considering the fluid volume, the content of the fluid, and the patient's clinical status. Effectiveness of IV fluid therapy is frequently defined as an increase in blood pressure, MAP, cardiac output, and urine output to greater than 0.5 mL/kg/hr, or decrease in lactate level (Barlow et al., 2020). Refer to Table 3-6 for various IV solutions.

TABLE 3-6 **Selected Water and Electrolyte Solutions**

Solution	Comments
Isotonic Solutions 0.9% NaCl (isotonic, also called normal saline [NS]) Na^+ 154 mEq/L Cl^- 154 mEq/L (308 mOsm/L) Also available with varying concentrations of dextrose (the most frequently used is a 5% dextrose concentration)	• An isotonic solution that expands the ECF volume • Used in hypovolemic states, resuscitative efforts, shock, diabetic ketoacidosis, metabolic alkalosis, hypercalcemia, mild Na^+ deficit • Supplies an excess of Na^+ and Cl^-; can cause FVE and hyperchloremic metabolic acidosis if used in excessive volumes, particularly in patients with compromised kidney function, heart failure, or edema • Not desirable as a routine maintenance solution as it provides only Na^+ and Cl^- (and these are provided in excessive amounts) • When mixed with 5% dextrose, the resulting solution becomes hypertonic in relation to plasma and, in addition to the above described electrolytes, provides 170 cal/L • Only solution that may be administered with blood products
Lactated Ringer solution Na^+ 130 mEq/L K^+ 4 mEq/L Ca^{+2} 3 mEq/L Cl^- 109 mEq/L Lactate (metabolized to bicarbonate) 28 mEq/L (274 mOsm/L) Also available with varying concentrations of dextrose (the most common is 5% dextrose)	• An isotonic solution that contains multiple electrolytes in roughly the same concentration as found in plasma (note that solution is lacking in Mg^{+2}), provides 9 cal/L • Used in the treatment of hypovolemia, burns, fluid lost as bile or diarrhea, and for acute blood loss replacement • Lactate is rapidly metabolized into HCO_3^- in the body. Previously, it was felt lactated Ringer solution should be avoided in septic patients secondary to the fear of worsening lactic acidosis; new research reveals this solution limits acidosis during sepsis (Singh, Kerndt, & Davis, 2022). However, lactate metabolism is impaired in chronic liver disease patients; thus, the acidosis prevention effect of lactated Ringers in chronic liver disease patients is questionable (Tseng, Chen, Chan, Chen, Wu et al., 2021). • Not to be given with a pH over 7.5 because bicarbonate is formed as lactate breaks down, causing alkalosis • Should not be used in kidney failure (because it contains 4mEq/L of potassium and can cause hyperkalemia) or in liver disease (because lactate is metabolized in the liver) • Similar to plasma

Solution	Comments
5% dextrose in water (D5W) No electrolytes 50 g of dextrose	• Initially an isotonic solution, once the dextrose is metabolized it becomes a hypotonic solution that supplies 170 cal/L and free water to aid in renal excretion of solutes • Used in treatment of hypernatremia, fluid loss, and dehydration • Should not be used in excessive volumes in the early postoperative period (when antidiuretic hormone secretion is increased due to stress reaction) • Should not be used solely in treatment of FVD because it dilutes plasma electrolyte concentrations • Contraindicated in head injury because it may cause increased intracranial pressure • Should not be used for fluid resuscitation because it can cause hyperglycemia and will not expand the IVS • Should be used with caution in patients with kidney or cardiac disease because of risk of fluid overload • Electrolyte-free solutions may cause peripheral circulatory collapse, anuria in patients with sodium deficiency, and increased body fluid loss • Over time, D5W without NaCl can cause water intoxication (ICF volume excess [FVE]) because the solution is hypotonic
Hypotonic Solutions 0.45% NaCl (half-strength saline) Na^+ 77 mEq/L Cl^- 77 mEq/L (154 mOsm/L) Also available with varying concentrations of dextrose (the most common is a 5% concentration)	• Provides Na^+, Cl^-, and free water • Free water is desirable to aid the kidneys in elimination of solute • Lacking in electrolytes other than Na^+ and Cl^- • When mixed with 5% dextrose, the solution becomes slightly hypertonic to plasma and, in addition to the above-described electrolytes, provides 170 cal/L • Used to treat hypertonic dehydration, Na^+ and Cl^- depletion, and gastric fluid loss • Not indicated for third-space fluid shifts or increased intracranial pressure • Administer cautiously because it can cause fluid shifts from vascular system into cells, resulting in cardiovascular collapse and increased intracranial pressure.
Hypertonic Solutions 3% NaCl (hypertonic saline) Na^+ 513 mEq/L Cl^- 513 mEq/L (1,026 mOsm/L)	• Used to increase ECF volume, decrease cellular swelling • Highly hypertonic solution used only in critical situations to treat hyponatremia • Must be administered slowly and cautiously because it can cause intravascular volume overload and pulmonary edema • Supplies no calories • Assists in removing ICF excess
5% NaCl (hypertonic solution) Na^+ 855 mEq/L Cl^- 855 mEq/L (1710 mOsm/L)	• Highly hypertonic solution used to treat symptomatic hyponatremia in extremely critical situations • Administered slowly and cautiously because it can cause intravascular volume overload and pulmonary edema • Supplies no calories
Colloid Solutions Dextran in NS or 5% D5W Available in low-molecular-weight (Dextran 40) and high-molecular-weight (Dextran 70) forms	• Colloid solution used as volume/plasma expander for intravascular part of ECF • Affects clotting by coating platelets and decreasing ability to clot • May cause anaphylaxis in patients • Remains in circulatory system up to 24 hours • Used to treat hypovolemia in early shock to increase pulse pressure, cardiac output, and arterial blood pressure • Improves microcirculation by decreasing RBC aggregation • Contraindicated in hemorrhage, thrombocytopenia, kidney disease, and severe dehydration • Not a substitute for blood or blood products

Pearls for Practice

When administering fluids to patients with cardiovascular disease, the nurse assesses for signs of circulatory overload (e.g., cough, dyspnea, puffy eyelids, dependent edema, weight gain in 24 hours). The lungs are auscultated for crackles. Extreme care is taken when administering highly hypertonic sodium fluids (e.g., 3% or 5% sodium chloride) because these fluids can be lethal if infused carelessly.

Isotonic Fluids

Isotonic fluids have a total osmolality close to that of the ECF and do not cause RBCs to shrink or swell. The composition of these fluids may or may not approximate that of the ECF. Isotonic fluids expand the ECF volume. One liter of isotonic fluid expands the ECF by 1 L; however, it expands the plasma by only 0.25 L because it is a crystalloid fluid and diffuses quickly into the ECF compartment.

D5W

A solution of D5W has a serum osmolality of 252 mOsm/L. Once administered, the glucose is metabolized rapidly, and this initially isotonic solution then disperses as a hypotonic fluid, one third extracellular and two thirds intracellular. It is essential to consider this action of D5W, especially if the patient is at risk for ICP. During fluid resuscitation, this solution should not be used because of its limited ability to expand the intravascular volume. Therefore, D5W is used mainly to supply water and to correct an increased serum osmolality. About 1 L of D5W provides fewer than 200 kcal and is a minor source of the body's daily caloric requirements.

Normal Saline Solution

Normal saline (0.9% sodium chloride) solution has a total osmolality of 308 mOsm/L. Because the osmolality is contributed entirely by electrolytes, the solution remains within the ECF. For this reason, normal saline solution is often used to correct an extracellular volume deficit. Normal saline contains only sodium and chloride and does not actually simulate the ECF. It is used with administration of blood transfusions and to replace large sodium losses, as in burn injuries. It is not used for HF, pulmonary edema, kidney impairment, or sodium retention. Normal saline does not supply calories. Historically, in patients with trauma or penetrating injury, initial treatment consisted of large amounts of isotonic saline administration to maintain a systolic blood pressure greater than 90 mm Hg, MAP >65 mm Hg and hourly urine output >0.5 mL/kg/hr.

Other Isotonic Solutions

Several other solutions contain ions in addition to sodium and chloride and are somewhat similar to the ECF in composition. Lactated Ringer solution contains potassium and calcium in addition to sodium and chloride and can be used to correct dehydration and sodium depletion or to replace GI losses. Lactated Ringer solution contains bicarbonate precursors as well. Lactated Ringer is typically not used in patients with severe acidosis or in advanced liver disease, which can affect lactate metabolism.

Pearls for Practice

The rate of IV fluid administration should be individualized depending upon the underlying problem, the rate of fluid loss, estimated total body deficit, underlying electrolyte abnormalities, and predicted future losses, which is challenging to predict if fluid loss continues from persistent bleeding or third space sequestration (Mandel & Palevsky, 2022). There is no one ideal initial rate, so nurses must monitor for signs of persistent FVD versus the development of FVE (particularly in those with cardiac and kidney disease).

Hypotonic Fluids

One purpose of hypotonic solutions is to replace cellular fluid. Another is to provide free water for excretion of body wastes. At times, hypotonic sodium solutions are used to treat hypernatremia and other hyperosmolar conditions. Half-strength saline (0.45% sodium chloride) solution, with an osmolality of 154 mOsm/L, is frequently used. Multiple-electrolyte solutions are also available. Excessive infusions of hypotonic solutions can lead to intravascular fluid depletion by causing a fluid shift from blood vessels to cells, resulting in decreased blood pressure, cellular edema, and cell damage. These solutions exert less osmotic pressure than the ECF.

Hypertonic Fluids

When normal saline solution or lactated Ringer solution contains 5% dextrose, the total osmolality exceeds that of the ECF. However, the dextrose is quickly metabolized, and only the isotonic solution remains. Therefore, any effect on the intracellular compartment is temporary.

Higher concentrations of dextrose, such as 50% dextrose in water, are administered to help meet caloric requirements or to treat hypoglycemia in the NPO patient. These solutions are strongly hypertonic and must be administered into central veins so that they can be diluted by rapid blood flow.

Saline solutions are also available in osmolar concentrations greater than that of the ECF. These solutions draw water from the ICF to the ECF and cause cells to shrink. If administered rapidly or in large quantity, they may cause an extracellular volume excess and precipitate circulatory overload. As a result, these solutions must be administered cautiously and usually only when the serum osmolality has decreased to dangerously low levels. Hypertonic solutions exert an osmotic pressure greater than that of the ECF.

Pearls for Practice

Highly hypertonic sodium solutions (3% and 5% sodium chloride) should be administered only in intensive care settings under close observation because only small volumes are needed to elevate the serum sodium concentration. These fluids are administered slowly and in small volumes, and the patient is monitored closely for fluid overload. Frequent checks of the patient's electrolyte panel are warranted. The purpose is to relieve acute manifestations of cerebral edema and to prevent neurologic complications rather than to specifically correct the sodium concentration. Along with the sodium solution, the patient may receive a loop diuretic to prevent ECF volume overload and to increase water excretion.

Other IV Substances

When the patient's GI tract is unable to tolerate food, nutritional requirements are often met using the IV route. Parenteral solutions may include high concentrations of glucose, protein, or fat to meet nutritional requirements (see Chapter 21). The parenteral route may also be used to administer colloids, plasma expanders, and blood products including packed RBCs, fresh frozen plasma, and platelets.

Many medications are also delivered by the IV route, either by infusion or directly into the vein. Because IV medications enter the circulation rapidly, administration by this route is potentially very hazardous. While all medications may produce reactions, IV medications are especially dangerous due to the rapid introduction and absorption within the bloodstream. Astute nursing includes knowledge of the administration rates and recommended dilutions for any medication given.

Nursing Management of the Patient Receiving IV Therapy

The ability to perform venipuncture to gain access to the venous system for administering fluids and medication is an expected nursing skill in many settings. This responsibility includes selecting the appropriate venipuncture site and type of cannula and being proficient in the technique of vein entry. This skill should be mastered by all bedside nurses, and it is up to each individual nurse to seek out the opportunity to learn and practice venipuncture.

Preparing to Administer IV Therapy

Before performing venipuncture, the nurse performs hand hygiene, applies gloves, and informs the patient about the procedure. Next, the nurse selects the most appropriate insertion site and type of cannula for a particular patient. See Box 3-3 for the factors that influence these choices. Some institutions have organized specialized "IV therapy" teams who assist in IV placement and management.

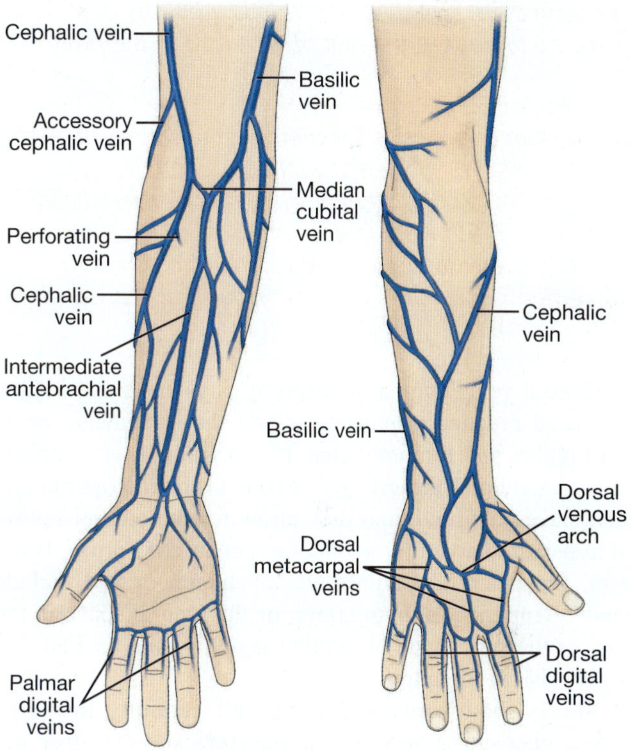

FIGURE 3-10 Site selection for peripheral cannulation of veins: anterior (palmar) veins at left, posterior (dorsal) veins at right. (Adapted from Agur, A. M. R., Lee, M. J., & Boileau Grant, M. J. [1999]. *Grant's atlas of anatomy* [10th ed.]. Lippincott Williams & Wilkins.)

Choosing an IV Site

Veins of the extremities are designated as peripheral locations and are ordinarily the only sites used by nurses. Because they are relatively safe and easy to enter, upper extremity veins are most commonly used (Fig. 3-10). The metacarpal, cephalic, basilic, and median veins and their branches are recommended sites because of their size and ease of access. More distal sites should be used first whenever possible, with more proximal sites used subsequently as new IVs are needed. Leg veins should rarely, if ever, be used because of the high risk of thromboembolism. Additional sites to avoid include veins distal to a previous IV infiltration or phlebitic area, sclerosed or thrombosed veins, an arm with an arteriovenous shunt or fistula, an arm on the same side where lymph nodes were previously removed (e.g., during a mastectomy), and an arm affected by edema, infection, blood clot, or skin breakdown.

Pearls for Practice

Due to the interruption in the lymphatic system in patients who have had a mastectomy or lymph node removal, blood pressure measurements (both manual and automatic) or IV therapy placement should not occur on the same side. Performing either of these procedures on the affected arm can cause fluid to back up in the arm, and lymphedema (accumulation of lymph fluid) can develop. This is a painful condition that also increases the risk of infection to the patient.

Pearls for Practice

When selecting an IV site, veins that are straight, distal (farthest away), and nonbranched (venous valves are commonly near branching points) are preferred (Beecham & Tackling, 2021). Joints or areas of flexion should be avoided, since these sites are prone to movement, occlusion, and dislodgement (Panepinto et al., 2021).

Central veins commonly used by physicians and trained advanced practice providers include the subclavian, internal jugular, and femoral veins. It is possible to gain access to (or cannulate) these larger vessels even when peripheral sites have collapsed, and they allow for the administration of hyperosmolar solutions and vasoconstrictive drugs. However, the potential hazards are much greater and include inadvertent entry into an artery, or the pleural space in the case of the subclavian or internal jugular veins, as well as a higher risk of infection.

Ideally, both arms and hands are carefully inspected before choosing a specific venipuncture site that does not interfere with mobility. For this reason, the antecubital fossa is avoided, except as a last resort. The most distal site of the arm or hand is generally used first so that subsequent IV access sites can be moved progressively upward. Refer back to Box 3-3 for factors to consider in selecting an IV site.

The tourniquet is applied so it is tight enough to engorge the veins but not interfere with arterial blood flow into the extremity. After applying a tourniquet, the nurse palpates and inspects the vein. The vein should feel firm, elastic, engorged, and round—not hard, flat, or bumpy. Because arteries lie close to veins in the antecubital fossa, the vessel should be palpated for arterial pulsation (even with a tourniquet on), and cannulation of pulsating vessels should be avoided. Once the vein is cannulated, the tourniquet is released.

Pearls for Practice

It is suggested that no more than two attempts at peripheral IV insertion should be made by a single nurse and no more than four attempts in total access since it can be painful to the patient, delay treatment, and increase costs (Panepinto et al., 2021).

Using Venipuncture Devices

Cannulas. Most peripheral access devices are cannulas. "Catheter" and "cannula" are terms that are used interchangeably. General guidelines for selecting a cannula include the following:

- Length: 0.75 to 1.25 in long
- Diameter: Narrow diameter of the cannula to occupy minimal space within the vein
- Gauge: 20 to 22 gauge for most IV fluids, a larger gauge for caustic or viscous solutions, 14 to 18 gauge preferred for trauma patients and those undergoing surgery, and blood administration can now safely use as small as a 24-gauge needle. While a smaller gauge IV can be used, consider diluting the blood with compatible IV fluids (normal saline) to ease the flow of the blood component, as long as the patient can tolerate the additional volume and the provider agrees (Kyles, 2021). It is preferable to use a larger gauge IV catheter for blood transfusion.

Cannulas have an obturator inside a tube that is later removed. The main types of cannula devices available are those referred to as indwelling plastic cannulas that are inserted over a steel needle, indwelling plastic cannulas that are inserted through a steel needle, or winged infusion sets (butterfly) with a steel needle or as over-the-needle catheters with wings. Scalp vein or butterfly needles are short steel needles with plastic wing handles. These are easy to insert, but because they are small and nonpliable, infiltration occurs easily. The use of these needles should be limited to obtaining blood specimens and not for IV medications because they increase the risk of vein injury and infiltration.

Plastic cannulas inserted through a hollow needle are usually called *intracatheters*. They are available in long lengths and are well suited for placement in central locations. Because insertion requires threading the cannula through the vein for a relatively long distance, these can be difficult to insert. The most commonly used infusion device is the over-the-needle catheter. A hollow metal stylet is preinserted into the catheter and extends through the distal tip of the catheter to allow puncture of the vessel in an effort to guide the catheter as the venipuncture is performed. The vein is punctured and a flashback of blood appears in the closed chamber behind the catheter hub. Once the flashback has occurred, the catheter is threaded through the stylet into the vein, and then the stylet is removed. All institutions should carry safety over-the-needle catheter designs with retracting stylets to protect health care workers from needlestick injuries.

Many types of cannulas are available for IV therapy. Some of the variations in these cannulas include the thickness of the cannula wall (affects rate of flow), the sharpness of the insertion needles (determines needle insertion technique), the softening properties of the cannula (influences the length of time the cannula can remain in place), safety features (minimizes risk of needlestick injuries and bloodborne exposure), and the number of lumens (determines the number of solutions that can be infused simultaneously).

Needleless IV Delivery Systems. The federal Needlestick Safety and Prevention Act, which was signed into law in November 2000, requires needleless systems in an effort to decrease needlestick injuries and exposure to human immunodeficiency virus (HIV), hepatitis, and other bloodborne pathogens. These systems have built-in protection against needlestick injuries and provide a safe means of using and disposing of an IV administration set (which consists of tubing, an area for inserting the tubing into the container of IV fluid, and an adapter for connecting the tubing to the needle). Numerous companies produce needleless components. IV-line connectors allow the simultaneous infusion of IV medications and other intermittent medications (known as a *piggyback delivery*) without the use of needles. Many examples of these devices are on the market. Each institution must evaluate products to determine its own needs based on Occupational Safety and Health Administration (OSHA) guidelines and the institution's policies and procedures.

Peripherally Inserted Central Catheter or Peripheral-Midline Catheter Access Lines. Patients who need moderate- to long-term parenteral therapy often receive a peripherally inserted central catheter (PICC line) or a peripheral-midline catheter. These catheters are also used for patients with limited peripheral access who require IV antibiotics, blood, vasopressors, or parenteral nutrition. For these devices to be used, the median cephalic, basilic, and cephalic veins must be patent and undamaged. Typically, insertion of these catheters is performed by specialized nurses who are trained in their insertion and the use of ultrasonography (which is used to visualize the vein to be cannulized).

If these veins are damaged, then central venous access via the subclavian, internal jugular, or femoral vein, or surgical placement of an implanted port or a vascular access device must be considered as an alternative. Table 3-7 compares peripherally inserted central and peripheral-midline catheters.

The provider prescribes the line and the solution to be infused. Insertion of these types of catheters requires sterile technique. The size of the catheter lumen chosen is based on the type of solution, the patient's body size, and the vein to be used. The patient's consent is obtained before use of these catheters. The right arm is preferred as it provides a straighter venous path to the superior vena cava (Montanarella et al., 2022). Contraindications to arm choice include prior mastectomy, pacemaker placement, hemiparesis, dialysis shunt, coagulopathy, infection at the insertion site, history of surgical manipulation, or trauma at the insertion site (Leib et al., 2021). Review each institution's policy regarding PICC lines for further contraindications.

Teaching the Patient

Except in emergency situations, a patient should be prepared in advance for an IV infusion. The venipuncture, the expected length of infusion, and activity restrictions are explained. Then, the patient should have an opportunity to ask questions and express concerns.

Preparing the IV Site

Before preparing the skin, the nurse should ask the patient whether they are allergic to latex, commonly used in products in preparation for IV therapy. Excessive hair at the selected

TABLE 3-7 Comparison of Peripherally Inserted Central and Peripheral-Midline Catheters

	Peripherally Inserted Central Catheter (PICC)	Peripheral-Midline Catheter
Indications	Parenteral nutrition; IV fluid replacement; administration of chemotherapy agents, analgesics, and antibiotics; removal of blood specimens	Parenteral nutrition; IV fluid replacement; administration of analgesics and antibiotics (no solution or medications with a pH less than 5 or greater than 9 or osmolarity greater than 500 mOsm/L); removal of blood specimens
Features	Single- and double-lumen catheters available 40–60 cm long; gauge variable (16–24 gauge)	Single- and double-lumen catheters available 7.5–20 cm long; gauge variable (16–24 gauge). Can increase two gauges in size as it softens
Material	Radiopaque, polymer (polyurethane), Silastic materials. Flexible.	Silicone, polyurethane, and their derivatives; available impregnated with heparin to ↓ thrombogenicity (radiopaque or clear, with radiopaque strip)
Insertion sites	Venipuncture performed in the antecubital fossa, above or below it into the basilic, cephalic, or axillary veins of the dominant arm. The median basilic is the ideal insertion site.	Venipuncture performed 1½ in above or below the antecubital fossa through the cephalic, basilic, or median cubital vein.
Catheter placement	The tip of the catheter lies in the superior vena cava. The catheter is placed via the basilic or cephalic vein at the antecubital fossa.	Between the antecubital area and the head of the clavicle (tip in axilla region). The tip terminates in the proximal portion of the extremity below the axilla and proximal to central veins and is advanced 3–10 in

(*continued*)

TABLE **3-7 Comparison of Peripherally Inserted Central and Peripheral-Midline Catheters (*continued*)**

	Peripherally Inserted Central Catheter (PICC)	Peripheral-Midline Catheter
Insertion method	Through-the-needle technique, with or without a guide wire, breakaway needle with introducer or cannula with introducer (peel-away sheath). (A peripherally inserted central catheter can also be used as a midline catheter.)	No separate guide wire or introducer is needed. Stiff catheter is passed using the catheter advancement tab.
	Insertion can be accomplished at the bedside using sterile technique. Arm to be used should be positioned in abduction to 90-degree angle. Consent is required	Insertion can be accomplished at the bedside using sterile technique. Arm to be used should be positioned in abduction to 45-degree angle. Consent is required
	Catheter may stay in place for up to 12 months or as long as required without complications	Catheter may stay in place for 2–4 weeks
Potential complications	Malposition, pneumothorax, hemothorax, hydrothorax, arrhythmias, nerve or tendon damage, respiratory distress, catheter embolism, thrombophlebitis, or catheter occlusion. Compared with centrally placed catheters, venipuncture in the antecubital space reduces risk of insertion complications	Thrombosis, phlebitis, air embolism, infection, vascular perforation, bleeding, catheter transection, occlusion
Contraindications	Dermatitis, cellulitis, burns, high fluid volume infusions, rapid bolus injections, hemodialysis, and venous thrombosis. No clamping of this catheter or splinting of the arm permitted. No blood pressure or tourniquets to be used on extremity where PICC is inserted.	Dermatitis, cellulitis, burns, high fluid volume infusions, rapid bolus injection, hemodialysis, and venous thrombosis. No blood pressure or tourniquet to be used on extremity where midline catheter is placed
Catheter maintenance	Sterile dressing changes according to agency policy and procedures. In general, dressing is changed every 2–3 days or when wet, soiled, or nonocclusive. Line is flushed every shift with 3 mL normal saline. The nurse follows institutional policy for flushing catheter	Sterile dressing changes according to agency policy and procedures. In general, dressing is changed every 2–3 days or when wet, soiled, or nonocclusive. Line is flushed after each infusion or every shift with 5–10 mL normal saline. Catheter must be anchored securely to prevent its dislodgment. The nurse follows institutional policy for flushing catheter
Postplacement	Ultrasound or chest x-ray needed to confirm placement of catheter tip	Chest x-ray to assess placement may be obtained if unable to flush catheter, if no free flow blood return, if difficulty with catheter advancement, or if guide wire is difficult to remove or bent on removal
Assessment	Daily measurement of arm circumference (4 in above insertion site) and length of exposed catheter	Daily measurement of arm circumference (4 in above insertion site) and length of exposed catheter
Removal	Catheter should be removed when no longer indicated for use, if contaminated, or if complications occur	Catheter should be removed when no longer indicated for use, if contaminated, or if complications occur
	Arm is abducted during removal. Patient should be in a dorsal recumbent position with head of bed flat and should perform the Valsalva maneuver while catheter is withdrawn	Arm is abducted during removal
	Pressure is applied on removal with a sterile dressing and antiseptic ointment to site. Dressing is changed every 24 hours until epithelialization occurs	Pressure is applied on removal with a sterile dressing and antiseptic ointment to site. Dressing is changed every 24 hours until epithelialization occurs
Advantages	Reduces cost and avoids repeated venipunctures compared with centrally placed catheters. Decreases incidence of catheter-related infections	Reduces cost and avoids repeated venipunctures compared with centrally placed catheters. Decreases incidence of catheter-related infections

site may be removed by clipping to increase the visibility of the veins and to facilitate insertion of the cannula and adherence of dressings to the IV insertion site. Shaving should not be performed due to increased risk of infection.

Because infection can be a major complication of IV therapy, the IV device, the fluid, the container, and the tubing must be sterile. The insertion site is scrubbed with a sterile pad soaked in chlorhexidine gluconate solution for 30 seconds, and allowed to air dry for approximately 2 minutes. The site should not be wiped with 70% alcohol because the alcohol negates the effect of the disinfecting solution. (However, if the patient is allergic to chlorhexidine or povidone-iodine [betadine, which although no longer routinely used may still be present on the clinical unit], the nurse can cleanse the skin with alcohol pledgets for 30 seconds instead.) After cleaning, the site should not be palpated again before insertion to prevent infection (Panepinto et al., 2021). The nurse must perform hand hygiene and put on gloves. Gloves (nonsterile, disposable) must be worn during the venipuncture procedure because of the likelihood of coming into contact with the patient's blood.

Pearls for Practice

When cleaning the skin for peripheral IV insertion, the circular motion (begin at the center of the circle, moving in an outward direction cleaning approximately 2 to 3 inches around the center of the circle) has long been believed to be effective in removing bacteria from the top layer of skin (Stonecypher, 2009). While the CDC guidelines do not specify how to clean the insertion site, the Infusion Nurses Society recommends a back-and-forth scrubbing technique because this technique was more effective at removing bacteria than the circular motion. However, the original research by Stonecypher is dated (2009) and additional research comparing these two cleaning techniques using chlorhexidine and alcohol would help strengthen evidence-based standards for PIV insertion (Panepinto et al., 2021).

Performing Venipuncture

IV therapy initiation is a specialized nursing skill. Institutional policies and procedures determine whether all nurses must be certified to perform venipuncture. A nurse certified in IV therapy or an IV team can be consulted to assist with initiating IV therapy when available. Refer to each institution's guidelines on venipuncture for specific policies regarding this skill.

Understanding Factors Affecting Gravity Flow

Gravity flow of an IV infusion is governed by the same principles that govern fluid movement in general. Flow is directly proportional to the height of the infusion. Raising the infusion bag may improve sluggish flow. The clamp on IV tubing regulates the flow by changing the tubing diameter. In addition, the flow is faster through large-gauge rather than small-gauge cannulas. Issues such as length of IV tubing and viscosity of the fluid being infused may also affect the flow rate.

Monitoring Flow

Because so many factors influence gravity flow, a solution does not necessarily continue to run at the speed originally set. Therefore, the nurse monitors IV infusions frequently to make sure that the fluid is flowing at the intended rate. The IV container should be marked with tape to indicate at a glance whether the correct amount has infused. The flow rate is calculated when the solution is originally started and then monitored at least hourly. To calculate the flow rate, the nurse determines the number of drops delivered per milliliter; this varies with equipment and is usually printed on the administration set packaging. In an effort to decrease the amount of medication errors, it has become standard for all intermittent IV infusions to be given with an electronic infusion device.

A variety of electronic infusion devices are available to assist in IV fluid delivery. These devices allow more accurate administration of fluids and medications than is possible with routine gravity-flow setups. A pump is a positive-pressure device that uses pressure to infuse fluid at a pressure of 10 psi; newer models use a pressure of 5 psi. The pressure exerted by the pump overrides vascular resistance (increased tubing length, low height of the IV container).

Volumetric pumps calculate the volume delivered by measuring the volume in a reservoir that is part of the set and is calibrated in milliliters per hour (mL/hr). A controller is an infusion assist device that relies on gravity for infusion; the volume is calibrated in drops (gtt) per minute. A controller uses a drop sensor to monitor the flow. Factors essential for the safe use of pumps include alarms to signify the presence of air in the IV line or an occlusion. The standard for the accurate delivery of fluid or medication via an electronic IV infusion pump is plus or minus 5%. The manufacturer's directions must be read carefully before use of any infusion pump or controller because there are many variations in available models. Use of these devices does not eliminate the need for the nurse to monitor the infusion and the patient frequently; however, it does limit the amount of bedside drug calculations and medication administration errors.

Flushing of a vascular device is performed to ensure patency and to prevent the mixing of incompatible medications or solutions. This procedure should be carried out at established intervals, according to hospital policy and procedure, especially for intermittently used catheters. Most manufacturers and researchers suggest the use of saline for flushing. The volume of the flush solution should be at least twice the volume capacity of the catheter. The catheter should be clamped before the syringe is completely empty and withdrawn to prevent reflux of blood into the lumen, which could cause catheter clotting and infiltration.

Discontinuing an Infusion

The removal of an IV catheter is associated with two possible complications: bleeding and catheter embolism. To prevent excessive bleeding, a dry, sterile pressure dressing should be held over the site as the catheter is removed. Firm pressure is applied until hemostasis occurs.

If a plastic IV catheter is severed, the patient is at risk for catheter embolism. To detect this complication when the catheter is removed, the nurse compares the expected length of the catheter with its actual length. Plastic catheters should be withdrawn carefully and their length measured to make certain that no fragment has broken off in the vein.

Great care must be exercised when using scissors around the dressing site. If the catheter clearly has been severed, the nurse can attempt to occlude the vein above the site by applying a tourniquet to prevent the catheter from entering the central circulation (until surgical removal is possible). However, as always, it is better to prevent a potentially fatal problem than to deal with it after it has occurred. Fortunately, catheter embolism can be prevented easily by following simple rules:

- Avoid using scissors near the catheter.
- Avoid withdrawing the catheter through the insertion needle.
- Follow the manufacturer's guidelines carefully (e.g., cover the needle point with the bevel shield to prevent severance of the catheter).

Managing Systemic Complications

IV therapy predisposes the patient to numerous hazards, including both local and systemic complications. Systemic complications occur less frequently but are usually more serious than are local complications. They include circulatory overload, air embolism, febrile reaction, and infection.

Overloading the circulatory system with excessive IV fluids can cause an increase in preload and blood pressure. Signs and symptoms of fluid overload include moist crackles on auscultation of the lungs (suggestive of pulmonary edema), peripheral edema, weight gain, jugular vein distention, dyspnea, and respirations that are shallow and have an increased rate. Possible causes include rapid infusion of an IV solution or hepatic, cardiac, or kidney disease. The risk of fluid overload and subsequent pulmonary edema is especially increased in older patients with cardiac disease; this is referred to as *circulatory overload.*

The treatment for circulatory overload is decreasing the IV rate or discontinuing the IV infusion, monitoring vital signs frequently, assessing breath sounds, and placing the patient in a high Fowler position. The provider is contacted immediately. This complication can be avoided by using an infusion pump for infusions and by carefully monitoring all infusions.

The risk of air embolism is rare but ever-present. It is most often associated with cannulation of central veins. During insertion of a catheter, air can enter through a disconnected or broken catheter by means of an open stopcock, or once the catheter is removed, air could enter along the path of a removed central venous catheter (CVC) (Lough et al., 2022). Manifestations of air embolism include dyspnea and cyanosis; hypotension; weak, rapid pulse; loss of consciousness; and chest, shoulder, and low back pain. A large heart murmur that sounds machinery-like or churning over the middle chest may be heard, it is termed a mill wheel murmur and reflects the large obstruction to right ventricular outflow (Lough et al., 2022; Kerrigan & Cooper, 2022). Treatment calls for immediately clamping the cannula and replacing a leaking or open infusion system, placing the patient on the left lateral decubitus position, assessing vital signs and breath sounds, and administering 100% oxygen. The oxygen administration is to correct the hypoxia/hypoxemia as well as decrease the size of the bubble due to a diffusion gradient allowing nitrogen to leave the gas embolus (recall that room air is 21% oxygen and 78% nitrogen) (Kerrigan & Cooper, 2022). Air embolism can be prevented by using a Luer Lock adapter on all lines, filling all tubing completely with solution, and using an air detection alarm on an IV pump. Complications of air embolism include shock and death. The amount of air necessary to induce death in humans is not known (in animal studies, it is projected to 4 mL/kg); however, the rate of entry is probably as important as the actual volume of air (Lough et al., 2022).

Pyrogenic substances in either the infusion solution or the IV administration set can induce a febrile reaction and septicemia. Signs and symptoms include an abrupt temperature elevation shortly after the infusion is started, backache, headache, increased pulse and respiratory rate, nausea and vomiting, diarrhea, chills and shaking, and general malaise. In severe septicemia, vascular collapse and septic shock may occur. Causes of septicemia may include contamination of the IV product or a break in aseptic technique, especially in immunocompromised patients. Treatment is symptomatic and includes culturing of the IV cannula, tubing, or solution if it is suspect, as well as establishing a new IV site for medication or fluid administration. See Chapter 53 for a discussion of septic shock. Long-term complications of central vein catheters include catheter-related upper extremity deep venous thrombosis, which can result in pulmonary embolism. Figure 3-11 details immediate and long-term complications of CVCs.

Infection ranges in severity from local involvement of the insertion site to systemic dissemination of organisms through the bloodstream, as in septicemia. Measures to prevent infection are essential at the time the IV line is inserted and throughout the entire infusion. Prevention includes the following:

- Careful hand hygiene before every contact with any part of the infusion system or the patient
- Examining the IV containers for cracks, leaks, or cloudiness; these findings may indicate a contaminated solution

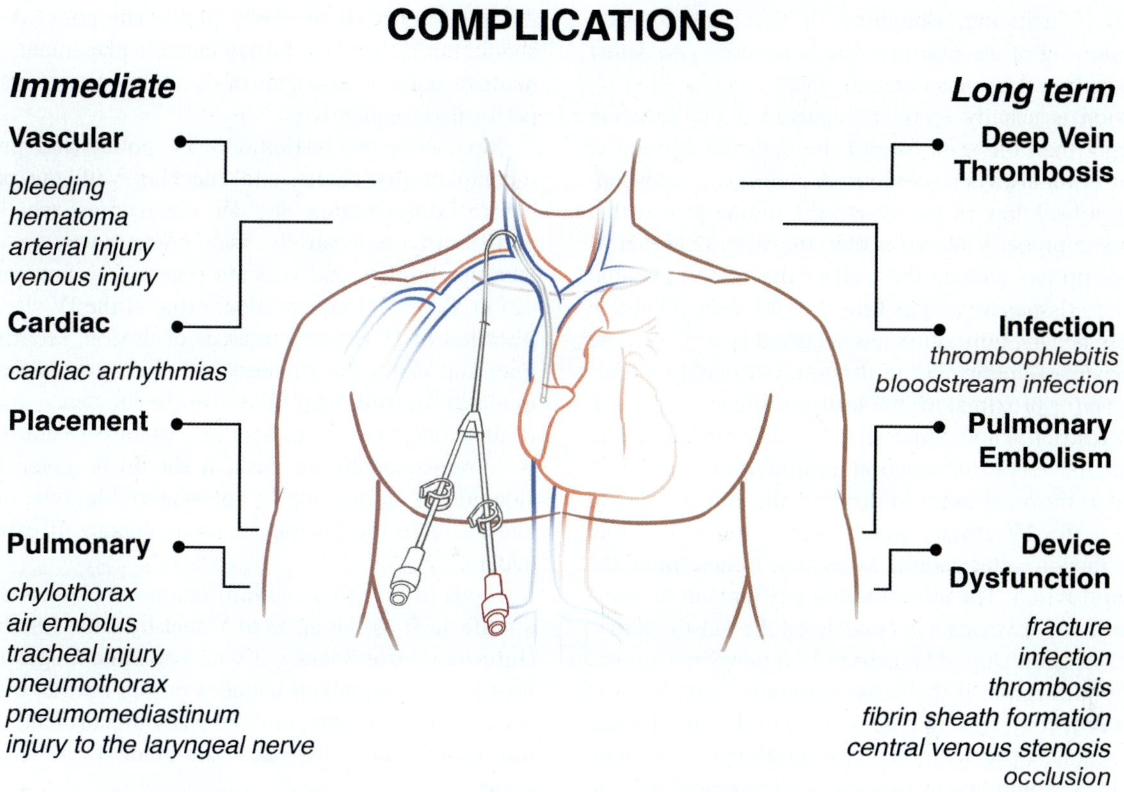

FIGURE 3-11 **The immediate and long-term complications of central venous catheters. (From Conoscenti, E., & Blot, S. [2020]. A necessary evil: Central venous catheters. *Intensive & Critical Care Nursing*, *57*, 102810. doi: 10.1016/j.iccn.2020.102810)**

- Using strict aseptic technique
- Firmly anchoring the IV cannula to prevent to-and-fro motion
- Inspecting the IV site daily and replacing a soiled or wet dressing with a dry, sterile dressing (antimicrobial agents that should be used for site care may include alcohol, chlorhexidine gluconate, or, less likely, 2% tincture of iodine or 10% povidone iodine, used alone or in combination per the institution's policy)
- Disinfecting injection/access ports with antimicrobial solution before use
- Removing the IV cannula at the first sign of local inflammation, contamination, or complication
- Replacing the peripheral IV cannula no less than every 72 to 96 hours, or as indicated (Webster et al., 2019)
- Replacing the IV cannula inserted during emergency conditions (with questionable asepsis) as soon as possible
- Using a 0.2-μm air-eliminating and bacteria/particulate-retentive filter with non–lipid-containing solutions that require filtration. The filter can be added to the proximal or distal end of the administration set. If added to the proximal end between the fluid container and the tubing spike, the filter ensures sterility and particulate removal from the infusate container and prevents inadvertent infusion of air. If added to the distal end of the administration set, it filters air particles and contaminants introduced from add-on devices, secondary administration sets, or interruptions to the primary system. The nurse would choose where to place the filter depending on whether the administration set is on a dedicated line.
- Replacing the solution bag and administration set in accordance with agency policy and procedure
- Infusing or discarding medication or solution within 24 hours of its addition to an administration set
- Changing primary and secondary continuous administration sets every 96 hours, or immediately if contamination is suspected (Duncan et al., 2018; Perry et al., 2022b)
- Changing primary administration sets containing lipid-based solutions every 24 hours, or immediately if contamination is suspected (Duncan et al., 2018; Perry et al., 2022c)

Managing Local Complications

Local complications of IV therapy include infiltration and extravasation, phlebitis, thrombophlebitis, hematoma, and clotting of the needle.

Infiltration is the unintentional administration of a nonvesicant solution or medication into surrounding tissue. This can occur when the IV cannula dislodges or perforates the wall of the vein. Infiltration is characterized by edema around the insertion site, leakage of IV fluid from the insertion site, discomfort and coolness in the area of infiltration, and a significant decrease in the flow rate. When the solution is particularly irritating, sloughing of tissue may result. Close monitoring of the insertion site is necessary to detect infiltration before it becomes severe.

Infiltration is usually easily recognized if the insertion area is larger than the same site of the opposite extremity; however, it is not always so obvious. A common misconception is that a backflow of blood into the tubing proves that the catheter is properly placed within the vein. However, if the catheter tip has pierced the wall of the vessel, IV fluid will seep into tissues as well as flow into the vein. Although blood return occurs, infiltration has occurred as well. A more reliable means of confirming infiltration is to apply a tourniquet above (or proximal to) the infusion site and tighten it enough to restrict venous flow. If the infusion continues to drip despite the venous obstruction, infiltration is present.

As soon as the nurse notes infiltration, the infusion should be stopped, the IV discontinued, and a sterile dressing applied to the site after careful inspection to determine the extent of infiltration. The infiltration of any amount of blood product, irritant, or vesicant is considered the most severe.

The IV infusion should be started in a new site or proximal to the infiltration if the same extremity must be used again. A warm compress may be applied to the site if small volumes of noncaustic solutions have infiltrated over a long period or if the solution was isotonic with a normal pH; the affected extremity should be elevated to promote the absorption of fluid. If the infiltration is recent and the solution was hypertonic or had an increased pH, a cold compress may be applied to the area. Infiltration can be detected and treated early by inspecting the site every hour for redness, pain, edema, coolness at the site, and IV fluid leaking from the IV site. Using the appropriate size and type of cannula for the vein prevents this complication.

Extravasation is similar to infiltration with an inadvertent administration of vesicant or irritant solution or medication into the surrounding tissue. Medications such as dopamine, calcium preparations, and chemotherapeutic agents can cause pain, burning, and redness at the site. Blistering, inflammation, and necrosis of tissues can occur. The extent of tissue damage is determined by the concentration of the medication, the quantity that extravasated, the location of the infusion site, the tissue response, and the duration of the process of extravasation. The nurse's first action is to stop the infusion and notify the provider promptly. The agency's protocol to treat extravasation is initiated; the protocol may indicate specific treatments, including antidotes specific to the medication that extravasated, and may indicate whether the IV line should remain in place or be removed before treatment. The protocol often specifies infiltration of the infusion site with an antidote prescribed after assessment by the provider, removal of the cannula, and application of warm compresses to sites of extravasation from vinca alkaloids or cold compresses to sites of extravasation from alkylating and antibiotic vesicants (Kim et al., 2020). The warm or cold compress is applied for 15 to 20 minutes, every 4 hours, for 24 to 48 hours (Kim et al., 2020). The affected extremity should not be used for further cannula placement. Thorough neurovascular assessments of the affected extremity must be performed frequently.

Reviewing the institution's IV policy and procedures, incompatibility charts, and checking with the pharmacist before administering any IV medication, whether given peripherally or centrally, is a prudent way to determine incompatibilities and vesicant potential to prevent extravasation. Careful, frequent monitoring of the IV site, avoiding insertion of IV devices in areas of flexion, securing the IV line, and using the smallest catheter possible that accommodates the vein help minimize the incidence and severity of this complication. In addition, when vesicant medication is administered by IV push, it should be given through a side port of an infusing IV solution to dilute the medication and decrease the severity of tissue damage if extravasation occurs.

Signs of phlebitis and infiltration may be assessed using a scale such as the updated Visual Infusion Phlebitis Scale (Infusion Nurse Society, 2021). The scale ranges from 0, or no edema, to 4, which includes pitting edema, moderate to severe pain at the site, or circulatory impairment. Extravasation should always be rated as a grade 4 on the infiltration scale.

Phlebitis is defined as inflammation of a vein, which can be categorized as chemical, mechanical, or bacterial; however, two or more of these types of irritation often occur simultaneously. Chemical phlebitis can be caused by an irritating medication or solution (increased pH or high osmolality of a solution), rapid infusion rates, and medication incompatibilities. Mechanical phlebitis results from long periods of cannulation, catheters in flexed areas, catheter gauges larger than the vein lumen, and poorly secured catheters. Bacterial phlebitis can develop from poor hand hygiene, lack of aseptic technique, failure to check all equipment before use, and failure to recognize early signs and symptoms of phlebitis. Other factors include poor venipuncture technique, catheter in place for a prolonged period, and failure to adequately secure the catheter. Phlebitis is characterized by a reddened, warm area around the insertion site or along the path of the vein, pain or tenderness at the site or along the vein, and swelling. The likelihood of phlebitis increases with the length of time the IV line is in place, the composition of the fluid or medication infused (especially its pH and tonicity), the size and site of the cannula inserted, ineffective filtration, inadequate anchoring of the line, and the introduction of microorganisms at the time of insertion. Treatment consists of discontinuing the IV and restarting it in another site as well as applying a warm, moist compress to the affected site. Phlebitis can be prevented by using aseptic technique during insertion, using the appropriate-size cannula or needle for the vein, considering the composition of fluids and medications when selecting a site, observing the site hourly for any complications, anchoring the cannula or needle well, and changing the IV site according to agency policy and procedures.

Thrombophlebitis refers to the presence of a clot plus inflammation in the vein. It is evidenced by localized pain, redness, warmth, and swelling around the insertion site or along the path of the vein, immobility of the extremity because of discomfort and swelling, sluggish flow rate, fever, malaise, and leukocytosis.

Treatment includes discontinuing the IV infusion; applying a cold compress first, to decrease the flow of blood and increase platelet aggregation, followed by a warm compress; elevating the extremity; and restarting the line in the opposite extremity. If the patient has signs and symptoms of thrombophlebitis, the IV line should not be flushed (although flushing may be indicated in the absence of phlebitis to ensure cannula patency and to prevent mixing of incompatible medications and solutions). The catheter must be removed promptly. In some circumstances, the catheter tip may be sent to the laboratory for culture, and it should be removed and placed in a sterile container prior to sending to the lab. Thrombophlebitis can be prevented by avoiding trauma to the vein at the time the IV is inserted, observing the site every hour, and checking medication additives for compatibility.

A hematoma results when blood leaks into tissues surrounding the IV insertion site. Leakage can result if the opposite vein wall is perforated during venipuncture, the needle slips out of the vein, or insufficient pressure is applied to the site after removal of the needle or cannula. The signs of a hematoma include ecchymosis, immediate swelling at the site, and leakage of blood at the insertion site.

Treatment includes removing the needle or cannula and applying light pressure with a sterile, dry dressing; applying ice for 24 hours to the site to avoid extension of the hematoma; elevating the extremity; assessing the extremity for any circulatory, neurologic, or motor dysfunction; and restarting the line in the other extremity if indicated. A hematoma can be prevented by carefully inserting the needle and by using diligent care with patients who have a bleeding disorder, are taking anticoagulant medication, or have advanced liver disease.

Blood clots may form in the IV line as a result of kinked IV tubing, a very slow infusion rate, an empty IV bag, or failure to flush the IV line after intermittent medication or solution administrations. The signs are decreased flow rate and blood backflow into the IV tubing. If blood clots in the IV line, the infusion must be discontinued and restarted in another site with a new cannula and administration set. The tubing should not be irrigated or milked. Neither the infusion rate nor the solution container should be raised, and the clot should not be aspirated from the tubing. Clotting of the needle or cannula may be prevented by not allowing the IV solution bag to run dry, taping the tubing to prevent kinking and maintain patency, maintaining an adequate flow rate, and flushing the line after intermittent medication or other solution administration. In some cases, a specially trained nurse or provider may inject a thrombolytic agent.

CHAPTER REVIEW

NCLEX-Style Review Questions

1. A patient is admitted with severe dehydration. Which of the following laboratory findings should the nurse anticipate related to hemoconcentration? Select all that apply.

a. Decreased BUN
b. Decreased creatinine
c. Elevated serum osmolality
d. Elevated BUN
e. Elevated sodium

2. As part of a large hospital's IV team, two nurses are responsible for inserting peripherally inserted central catheters (PICCs) at the bedside for patients who require this form of venous access. Which of the following patients would most likely require a PICC? Select all that apply.

a. A patient requiring long-term IV antibiotic administration
b. A patient who has been admitted from the community with a fluid volume deficit
c. A patient with hypocalcemia requiring a stat infusion of calcium gluconate
d. A patient who has just been ordered total parenteral nutrition (TPN)
e. A patient who recently suffered a pelvic fracture in a motor vehicle accident

3. A patient arrives in the emergency department complaining of weakness, nausea, vomiting, and abdominal distention for 3 days. The 12-lead ECG shows sinus bradycardia with prominent U waves.

Na+ 145 mEq/L
K+ 2.7 mEq/L
Glucose 110 mg/dL
BUN 38 mg/dL
Creatinine 1.0 mg/dL
Hematocrit (Hct) 55%

What laboratory findings and ECG findings are priorities for your intervention? Select all that apply.
a. Hypokalemia
b. Increased serum osmolality
c. Hyperglycemia
d. Azotemia
e. Hypernatremia

4. Patients with which of the following conditions are at risk for hyperkalemia? Select all that apply.
a. Rhabdomyolysis
b. Diarrhea
c. Alkalosis
d. Kidney failure
e. Hypoaldosteronism

5. Which of the following intravenous fluids should be considered in the patient diagnosed with hypovolemia (fluid volume deficit)? Select all that apply.
a. Lactated Ringer
b. D5W
c. Half-normal saline (0.45% sodium chloride)
d. 3% saline
e. Normal saline (0.9% sodium chloride)

REFERENCES AND SELECTED READINGS

References and selected readings associated with this chapter can be found on the website that accompanies the book. Visit **http://thepoint.lww.com/Honan3e** to access the references and other additional resources associated with this chapter.

CHAPTER 4

Perioperative Nursing

Daphny Grace M. Peneza

Learning Objectives

After reading this chapter, you will be able to:

1. Define the three phases of perioperative nursing.
2. Discuss key strategies in the management of the surgical patient in the preoperative, intraoperative, and postoperative phases.
3. Identify the nurse's role in ensuring patient safety and quality care in the perioperative setting.
4. Describe a comprehensive preoperative assessment to identify surgical risk factors.
5. Recognize legal and ethical considerations related to informed consent.
6. Illustrate the principles of surgical asepsis.
7. Enumerate the types of anesthetic approaches and the implications for nursing care in the perioperative setting.
8. Discuss potential adverse effects of anesthesia and surgical procedures.
9. Describe perioperative nursing measures that decrease the risk for complications.
10. Identify strategies that will facilitate the perioperative team's preparedness and efficiency in a surgical trauma emergency.

Surgery, whether elective or emergent, is a stressful, complex event. Perioperative care continues to evolve as the demand for health care services increases every. Nurses must adapt to advocate for patients and their families and caregivers in every perioperative phase.

INTRODUCTION

Phases

Perioperative and perianesthesia nursing addresses the nursing roles relevant to the three phases of the surgical experience: preoperative, intraoperative, and postoperative. Each phase begins and ends at a particular point in the sequence of events that constitutes the surgical experience, and each includes a wide range of activities that the nurse performs using the nursing process and based on the standards of practice (American Society of Perianesthesia Nurses [ASPAN], 2018). Box 4-1 represents nursing activities characteristic of the three perioperative phases of care.

Surgical Settings

Today, as a result of advances in surgical techniques and instrumentation, as well as in **anesthesia**, the number of surgeries, imaging studies, and diagnostic tests performed outside of hospitals is growing rapidly. These procedures are primarily moving to **ambulatory surgery centers** (ASCs), which provide outpatient surgical services not requiring an overnight stay, independent diagnostic and testing facilities, and health providers' offices. Innovation in medical technology and surgical techniques, along with the preferences of multiple players in the health care system, has driven the migration of care to nonhospital settings. Less invasive surgical techniques and advances in anesthesia have made it possible for more procedures to be performed in outpatient settings, where recovery time is limited. As a result, today many patients arrive at the hospital on the morning of surgery and go home after recovering from the anesthesia in the postanesthesia care unit (PACU). Often, surgical patients who require hospital stays are trauma patients, acutely ill patients, and/or patients undergoing major surgery.

BOX 4-1

Examples of Nursing Activities in the Perioperative Phases of Care

Preoperative Phase

Preadmission Testing

1. Initiates initial preoperative health history and physical assessment
2. Initiates teaching appropriate to patient's needs
3. Involves family in interview
4. Verifies completion of preoperative testing
5. Verifies understanding of surgeon-specific preoperative orders (e.g., bowel preparation, preoperative shower)
6. Discharge planning—assesses patient's need for postoperative transportation and care

Admission to Surgical Center or Unit

1. Verifies patient identification and expected procedure
2. Completes preoperative assessment
3. Assesses patient's status, including nutritional status and baseline level of pain
4. Assesses for risks for postoperative complications
5. Assesses for and manages perioperative nomothermia
6. Reports unexpected findings or any deviations from normal
7. Verifies that operative consent and all appropriate documents have been signed
8. Coordinates patient teaching with other nursing staff and reinforces previous teaching
9. Explains phases in perioperative period and expectations; answers patient's and family's questions
10. Develops a plan of care
11. Removes and secures prostheses, dentures, glasses, jewelry
12. Ensures interpreter is present if patient requires
13. Encourages patient to void immediately pre-op
14. Establishes IV line
15. Obtains pre-op blood glucose or pregnancy testing as ordered
16. Administers medications if prescribed, reminds patient not to get OOB after premedicated
17. Takes measures to ensure patient's comfort
18. Provides psychological support
19. Communicates patient's emotional status to other appropriate members of the health care team

Intraoperative Phase

Maintenance of Safety

1. Maintains aseptic, controlled environment
2. Effectively manages human resources, equipment, and supplies for individualized patient care
3. Transfers patient safely and securely to operating room bed or table
4. Safely positions the patient:
   a. Confirms functional alignment and secures patient to operating room table
   b. Initiates pressure ulcer reduction and skin injury processes
   c. Ensures appropriate exposure of surgical site
5. Applies grounding device to patient
6. Ensures that the sponge, needle, and instrument counts are correct
7. Ensures that the collaborative surgical team final verification (time out) is conducted and documented
8. Completes intraoperative documentation
9. Maintains an environment to support patient's body temperature per procedural protocol
10. Ensures that a postprocedure debriefing is conducted to verify blood loss, fluid status, specimen (if applicable), surgical procedure performed, patient disposition, and any change of patient status

Psychological Support (Before Induction and When Patient Is Conscious)

1. Provides emotional support to patient
2. Stands near or touches patient during procedures and induction
3. Continues to assess patient's emotional status

Postoperative Phase

Transfer of Patient to Postanesthesia Care Unit

1. Communicates intraoperative information via hand off circulating to recovery room nurse
   a. Identifies patient with at least two patient identifiers
   b. States type of surgery performed
   c. Identifies type of anesthetic used
   d. Reports patient's response to surgical procedure and anesthesia
   e. Describes intraoperative factors (e.g., insertion of drains or catheters; administration of blood, analgesic agents, or other medications during surgery; occurrence of unexpected events)
   f. Describes physical limitations
   g. Reports patient's preoperative level of consciousness
   h. Communicates necessary equipment needs
   i. Communicates presence of family and/or significant others

Postoperative Assessment Recovery Area

1. Determines patient's immediate response to surgical intervention
2. Integrates data received at transfer of care
3. Monitors patient's physiologic status
4. Assesses patient's pain level and administers appropriate pain relief measures
5. Maintains patient's safety (airway, circulation, prevention of injury)
6. Administers medications, fluid, and blood component therapy, if prescribed
7. Provides oral fluids if prescribed for ambulatory surgery patient
8. Assesses patient's readiness for transfer to in-hospital unit or for discharge home based on institutional policy

Surgical Unit

1. Continues close monitoring of patient's physical and psychological response to surgical intervention
2. Assesses patient's pain level and administers appropriate pain relief measures
3. Provides teaching to patient during immediate recovery period
4. Assists patient in recovery and preparation for discharge home
5. Determines patient's psychological status
6. Assists with discharge planning

Home or Clinic

1. Provides follow-up care during office or clinic visit or by telephone contact
2. Reinforces previous teaching and answers patient's and family's questions about surgery and follow-up care
3. Assesses patient's response to surgery and anesthesia and their effects on body image and function
4. Determines family's perception of surgery and its outcome

TABLE **4-1 Categories of Surgery Based on Urgency**

Classification	Indications for Surgery	Examples
I. Emergent—Patient requires immediate attention; disorder may be life-threatening	Without delay	Severe bleeding Bladder or intestinal obstruction Fractured skull Gunshot or stab wounds Extensive burns
II. Urgent—Patient requires prompt attention	Within 24–30 hours	Acute gallbladder infection Kidney or ureteral stones
III. Required—Patient needs to have surgery	Plan within a few weeks or months	Prostatic hyperplasia without bladder obstruction Thyroid disorders Cataracts
IV. Elective—Patient should have surgery	Failure to have surgery not catastrophic	Repair of scars Simple hernia
V. Optional—Decision rests with patient	Personal preference	Cosmetic surgery

Although each setting (ambulatory, outpatient, or inpatient) offers its own unique advantages for the delivery of patient care, they all require comprehensive preoperative nursing assessment and nursing interventions, and a sound knowledge of all aspects of perioperative and perianesthesia nursing.

Surgical Classifications

A surgical procedure may be diagnostic (e.g., biopsy, exploratory laparotomy), curative (e.g., excision of a tumor or an inflamed appendix), or reparative (e.g., multiple wound repair). It may be reconstructive or cosmetic (e.g., mammoplasty or a facelift) or palliative (e.g., to relieve pain or correct a problem—for instance, a gastrostomy tube may be inserted to compensate for the inability to swallow food). Surgery may also be classified according to the degree of urgency involved (Table 4-1).

Emergency Surgery

Emergency surgeries are unplanned and occur with little time for preparation of the patient or the perioperative team. The unpredictable nature of trauma and emergency surgery poses unique challenges to the nurse throughout the perioperative period. All of the factors that affect patients preparing to undergo surgery apply to these patients, usually in a very condensed time frame. There may be only one preoperative assessment, and it may take place at the same time as resuscitation in the emergency department. For the unconscious patient, informed consent and essential information, such as pertinent past medical history and allergies, need to be obtained from a family member, if one is available. A quick visual survey of the patient is essential to identify all sites of injury if the emergency surgery is due to trauma. The patient, who may have undergone a very frightening experience, may need extra support, including an explanation of the surgery.

Special Populations

Patients Who Are Older

Advances in nutrition, public health, education, and social services have produced a major change in human longevity in industrialized societies, and the number of Americans aged 65 and older is expected to nearly double from 52 million in 2018 to 95 million by 2060, which will increase the number of 65-and-older age group's share of the total population from 16% to 23% (U.S. Census Bureau, 2022). Demographers have termed this the *greying of America.* Nurses need to consider that the vast majority of this population have at least one chronic condition, and many have multiple conditions that contribute to frailty and disability, which leads to the finding that older adults experience disproportionate levels of postoperative mortality and morbidity (Allen, 2023; Kumar et al., 2018). Although the decision to operate lies within the purview of the surgeon, perioperative nurses should be aware of the surgery's implications. Surgical intervention should be tailored to the patient's symptoms, overall functional and health status, and predicted benefit of the intervention. Important factors that need to be evaluated are (1) disease course versus life expectancy, (2) state of independence, (3) personal motivation, and (4) surgical risk factors versus nonoperative management (Rothrock, 2019).

Preoperative pain assessment and teaching are important in older patients. The older person undergoing surgery may have a combination of chronic illnesses and health issues in addition to the specific one for which surgery is indicated. Older people frequently do not report symptoms, perhaps because they fear a serious illness may be diagnosed or because they accept such symptoms as part of the aging process. Subtle clues alert the nurse to underlying problems. A complete assessment and review of the patient's medical history will assist with identifying the risk for postoperative complications. Delirium is a common but often undiagnosed complication in an older person following a major operation.

Health care staff must remember that the hazards of surgery for older people are proportional to the number and severity of coexisting health problems and the nature and duration of the operative procedure. The underlying principle that guides the preoperative assessment, surgical care, and postoperative care is that the older patient has less physiologic reserve (the ability of an organ to return to normal after a disturbance in its equilibrium) than does a younger patient. Refer to Table 4-2 for the implications of aging on operative course. The nurse plans interventions based on the patient's medical history, clinical presentation, and knowledge of the physiologic impact of aging. For example, arthritis is common in older people and may affect mobility, making it difficult for the patient to turn from one side to the other or ambulate without discomfort. The older patient has less subcutaneous fat, poor skin turgor, and tissue fragility. Aging-related changes in the musculoskeletal system accentuate bony prominences and decrease range of motion. These changes, along with limitations imposed by chronic pain, make positioning one of the most important considerations for this population of surgical patients. Protective measures include adequate padding for tender areas, moving the patient slowly, and protecting bony prominences from prolonged pressure. Precautions are taken when moving an older person because of the fragility of skin, and a lightweight cotton blanket is an appropriate cover when the patient is moved to and from the operating room because of temperature sensitivity.

In addition, many older people have experienced personal illnesses and possibly life-threatening illnesses of friends and family. Such experiences may result in fears about the surgery and about the future. By providing an opportunity for the patient to express these fears, the nurse enables the patient to gain some peace of mind.

TABLE **4-2 GERONTOLOGIC CONSIDERATIONS / Age-Related Changes and Impact on Operative Course**

Structural or Functional Change	Impact
Increased incidence of coexisting disease	Higher risks from anesthesia and surgery than younger adult patients
Aging heart and blood vessels	Decreased ability to respond to stress
Reduced cardiac output and limited cardiac reserve	Increased vulnerability to changes in circulating volume and blood oxygen levels. In addition, excessive or rapid administration of IV solutions can cause pulmonary edema.
Decreased ability to compensate for hypoxia	Increased risk of cerebral ischemia, thrombosis, embolism, infarction, and anoxia
Decrease in the percentage of lean body tissue and a steady increase in fatty tissue (from 20 to 90 years of age).	Anesthetic agents that have an affinity for fatty tissue concentrate in body fat and the brain. The older patient needs fewer and smaller amounts of anesthetic agents to produce anesthesia and eliminates the anesthetic agent over a longer period of time, compared with a younger patient.
If malnourished or has low plasma protein levels (hypoalbuminemia)	With decreased plasma proteins, more of the anesthetic agent remains free or unbound, resulting in more potent action.
Reduced liver size and potential for reduced kidney function	Decreases the rate at which the liver can inactivate many anesthetic agents, and decreased kidney function slows the elimination of waste products and anesthetics
Impaired ability to increase metabolic rate and impaired thermoregulatory mechanisms	Increased susceptibility to hypothermia
Bones become susceptible to fracture; this susceptibility doubles every 5 years after 50 years of age (Allen, 2023)	Increased risk of musculoskeletal problems postoperatively
Loss of collagen and muscle; thinning, sagging skin	Increased risk of skin complications
Impaired vision or hearing and reduced tactile sensitivity	Increased potential for communication issues, increased risk of skin complications
Increased tooth loss and periodontal disease, increased incidence of dental devices (dentures, partial plates, crowns)	Increased risk of airway occlusion due to dental device dislodgement

Because the older patient may face greater risks during the perioperative period, the following factors are critical: (1) skillful preoperative assessment and treatment, (2) adept anesthesia and surgery, and (3) meticulous and competent postoperative management. In addition, the nurse should incorporate pain management information and pain communication skills when teaching the older patient how to obtain greater postoperative pain relief.

Patients Who Are Obese

Like age, obesity increases the risk and severity of complications associated with surgery. During surgery, fatty tissues are especially susceptible to infection. In addition, obesity increases technical and mechanical problems related to surgery. Therefore, dehiscence (wound separation) and wound infections are more common. Moreover, the obese patient may be more difficult to care for because of the added weight. The patient tends to have shallow respirations when supine, which increases the risk of hypoventilation and postoperative pulmonary complications. It has been estimated that for each 30 lb of excess weight, about 25 additional miles of blood vessels are needed, and this places increased demands on the heart. Thus, nursing management includes careful assessment of the cardiopulmonary status of obese patients and thorough wound assessments.

Patients with Disabilities

Special considerations for patients with mental or physical disabilities include the need for appropriate assistive devices, modifications in preoperative teaching, and additional assistance with and attention to positioning or transferring. Assistive devices include hearing aids, eyeglasses, braces, prostheses, and other devices. People who are hearing-impaired may need a sign interpreter or some alternative communication system perioperatively. If the patient relies on signing or speech (lip) reading, and their eyeglasses or contact lenses are removed or the health care staff members wear surgical masks, an alternative method of communication will be needed. These needs must be identified during the preoperative evaluation and clearly communicated to the appropriate personnel. Specific strategies for accommodating the patient's needs must be identified in advance. Ensuring the security of assistive devices is important because these devices are expensive and can be misplaced easily.

Most patients are directed to move from the stretcher to the OR table and back again. In addition to being unable to see or hear instructions, the patient with a disability may be unable to move without special devices or a great deal of assistance. The patient with a disability that affects body position (e.g., cerebral palsy, post-polio syndrome, and other neuromuscular disorders) may need special positioning during surgery to prevent pain and injury. Moreover, these patients may be unable to sense whether their extremities are positioned incorrectly.

Patients with respiratory problems related to a disability (e.g., multiple sclerosis, muscular dystrophy) may experience pulmonary difficulties unless the problems are made known to the anesthesia provider, who can make adjustments. These factors need to be identified clearly in the preoperative period and communicated to the appropriate personnel.

PREOPERATIVE NURSING

The **preoperative phase** begins when the decision to proceed with surgical intervention is made and ends with the transfer of the patient onto the OR table. The nursing roles during this phase focus on assessing the patient and developing a plan of care. This process is performed utilizing diverse modalities. Telephone interviews, face-to-face assessments, computer-aided tools, and video teleconferences with language interpreters are used to review the physical, psychological, sociocultural, and spiritual needs of the patient. Preadmission units or anesthesia clinics work collaboratively with anesthesia providers to interview and assess the patient to identify potential or actual problems that may occur. The goals of preoperative assessment are to reduce the patient's surgical and anesthetic perioperative morbidity or mortality. Medical history, laboratory values, and diagnostic tests help clinicians evaluate the patient. Preadmission nurses actively participate in pre-op education to prepare the patient and family to take an active role in their experience.

The Enhanced Recovery After Surgery (ERAS) programs includes procedure-specific bundled elements (i.e., pathways), designed to standardize patient care within a specific cohort, thereby improving targeted patient metrics/outcomes. Examples may include protocols such as perioperative counseling, decreased preoperative fasting, anti-emetic prophylaxis, and multimodal anesthesia (Wicklin, 2023). ERAS program-associated patient benefits may vary depending on the procedure as well as institution-specific care elements included within each pathway.

Preoperative patient and caregiver/significant other (SO) preparation, including education, may decrease preoperative delays, enhance understanding of the surgery, increase feelings of control, decrease postoperative anxiety, anti-emetic and analgesic use, and decrease hospital length of stay. In addition, preoperative teaching that includes postoperative expectations may improve overall patient satisfaction and decrease complications in the postoperative period.

Informed Consent

The surgical experience, except in extreme emergencies, begins after a patient has consented to a recommended surgical procedure. Voluntary and written **informed consent** from the patient is necessary before nonemergent surgery can be performed. The Department of Health and Human Services, Centers for Medicare and Medicaid Services (CMS), believes that a patient or their representative (as allowed under state law) has the right to make informed decisions regarding the patient's care. The guidelines further indicate that, for the surgical patient, a properly executed informed consent form for the operation must be in the patient's chart prior to surgery, except in emergencies. The primary purpose of the informed consent process is to ensure that the patient, or the patient's representative, is provided information necessary to enable them to evaluate the proposed surgery before agreeing to it; all procedures, regardless of associated risk, require patient consent (Center for Medicare and Medicaid Services, 2017; Hillanbrand, 2023). Informed consent also outlines the risks, benefits, and alternative treatment options that are available (Hillanbrand, 2023). A written consent protects the patient from unsanctioned surgery and protects the surgeon from claims of an unauthorized operation (The Joint Commission [TJC], 2022a). It is normally the responsibility of the performing surgeon to obtain the informed surgical consent, which should consist of the following four basic elements:

1. The surgeon documents that the patient or surrogate has decision-making capacity, which is distinct from the legal concept of competency as determined by courts. Adults are presumed to be legally competent unless declared otherwise by a court (Emanuel, 2020).
2. The surgeon discloses to the patient details regarding the diagnosis and treatment options sufficiently for the patient to make an informed choice.
3. The patient demonstrates understanding of the disclosed information.
4. The patient freely authorizes a specific treatment plan voluntarily without undue influence, coercion, or manipulation by the physician (Emanuel, 2020).

Informed consent is necessary in a variety of circumstances which include:

- Invasive procedures, such as a surgical incision, a biopsy, a cystoscopy, or paracentesis
- Procedures requiring sedation and/or anesthesia
- A nonsurgical procedure, such as an arteriography, that carries more than slight risk to the patient
- Procedures involving radiation
- Research protocols, clinical trials (Barlow, 2020)

If the patient has doubts and has not had the opportunity to investigate alternative treatments, a second opinion may be requested. Refusing to undergo a surgical procedure is a person's legal right and privilege.

The consent process can be improved by providing audiovisual materials to supplement discussion, by ensuring that the wording of the consent form is understandable, and by using other strategies and resources as needed to help the patient understand its content. It is required to have the consent available in multiple languages or have a trained medical interpreter available for non–English-speaking patients. In many cases, it is required to have alternative forms of communication (e.g., Braille, large print, sign interpreter) for the older or disabled patient.

Pearls for Practice

Consent materials should be written at a fifth-grade or lower reading level in order to meet health literacy requirements. Materials should be designed with bullet points to divide complex material and translated into the patient's preferred language whenever possible (Hillanbrand, 2023). A certified medical interpreter should be used for non–English-speaking patients (Munroe, 2021).

Preoperative Health Assessment

Before any surgical treatment is initiated, a health history is obtained, a physical examination is performed during which vital signs are noted, and a database is established for future comparisons. Preoperative blood tests, x-rays, and other diagnostic tests are obtained as needed.

The goal in the preoperative period is for the patient to have as many positive health factors as possible. Many risk factors may lead to complications (Box 4-2). Every attempt

BOX 4-2 Risk Factors for Surgical Complications

- Hypovolemia
- Dehydration or electrolyte imbalance
- Nutritional deficits
- Extremes of age (very young, very old)
- Extremes of weight (emaciation, obesity)
- Infection and sepsis
- Toxic conditions
- Immunologic abnormalities
- Pregnancy (because of diminished maternal physiologic reserve)
- Cerebrovascular disease
- Pulmonary disease:
  - Obstructive disease
  - Restrictive disorder
  - Respiratory infection
- Renal or urinary tract disease:
  - Decreased renal function
  - Urinary tract infection
  - Obstruction
- Cardiovascular disease:
  - Coronary artery disease or previous myocardial infarction
  - Cardiac failure
  - Arrhythmias
  - Hypertension
  - Prosthetic heart valve
  - Thromboembolism
  - Hemorrhagic disorders
- Endocrine dysfunction:
  - Diabetes mellitus
  - Adrenal disorders
  - Thyroid malfunction
- Hepatic disease:
  - Cirrhosis
  - Hepatitis
  - Pre-existing mental or physical disability

is made to stabilize those conditions that otherwise hinder recovery.

Nutritional and Fluid Status

Optimal nutrition is an essential factor in promoting healing and resisting infection and other surgical complications. Assessment of a patient's nutritional status identifies factors that can affect the patient's surgical course, such as obesity, under nutrition, weight loss, malnutrition, deficiencies in specific nutrients, metabolic abnormalities, and the effects of medications on nutrition. Nutritional needs may be determined by measurement of body mass index (BMI) and waist circumference (U.S. Department of Health and Human Services, 2022). A BMI of 18.5 to 24.9 is normal; less than 18.5 is underweight, greater than 25 is overweight, greater than 30 is obese, and 40 and greater is extreme obesity. A waist circumference measurement of greater than 40 inches in males and 35 inches in females is associated with increased cardiac risk.

If possible, any nutritional deficiency, such as malnutrition, should be corrected before surgery to provide adequate protein for tissue repair. The nutrients needed for wound healing are summarized in Table 4-3. Dehydration, hypovolemia, and electrolyte imbalances can also lead to significant problems in patients with comorbid medical conditions or in patients who are older. Common electrolyte abnormalities associated with malnutrition include hypokalemia (low potassium), hypocalcemia (low calcium) and hypomagnesemia (low magnesium; refer to Chapter 3; Phillips &

TABLE **4-3 Nutrients Important for Wound Healing**

Nutrient	Rationale for Increased Need
Protein	To allow collagen deposition and wound healing to occur; clotting factor production; white blood cell (WBC) production and migration; cell-mediated phagocytosis; fibroblast proliferation; granulation tissue formation; neovascularization. Traditionally, dietary distribution of macronutrients is 40–60% carbohydrates, 25–30% fat, and 15–20% protein, but protein needs are increased during all phases of wound healing by up to 250% (Ghaly et al., 2021).
Arginine (amino acid)	To provide necessary substrate for collagen synthesis and nitric oxide (crucial for wound healing) at wound site To increase wound strength and collagen deposition To stimulate T-cell response To support a variety of essential reactions of intermediary metabolism
Carbohydrates and fats	To be a primary source of energy in the body and, consequently, in the wound-healing process To meet the demand for increased essential fatty acids needed for cellular function after an injury To spare protein Fibroblast proliferation is sensitive to glucose deficiencies.
Water	To maintain homeostasis
Vitamin C	To support capillary formation, tissue synthesis, and wound healing through collagen formation affecting the proliferative and remodeling phases To allow for antibody formation, WBC production. Deficiency is associated with abnormal scar tissue formation.
Vitamin B complex	To influence host resistance, indirectly supporting wound healing
Vitamin E	An antioxidant responsible for normal fat metabolism and collagen synthesis
Vitamin A	Increases inflammatory response in wounds, reduces anti-inflammatory effects of corticosteroids on wound healing; is essential for epidermal proliferation, reepithelialization, and epithelium maintenance
Vitamin K	Important for normal blood clotting To help avoid impaired intestinal synthesis associated with the use of antibiotics
Magnesium	Essential cofactor for many enzymes that are involved in the process of protein synthesis and wound repair
Copper	Responsible for collagen cross-linking and erythropoiesis
Zinc	A cofactor for collagen formation, also metabolizes protein, liberates vitamin A from storage in the liver, interacts with platelets in blood clotting, and assists in immune function; plays a role throughout all phases of wound healing, affecting immunity and aiding fibroblast proliferation, collagen synthesis, and epithelization (Ghaly et al., 2021)

Hornacky, 2021a). The severity of fluid and electrolyte imbalances is often difficult to determine. Mild volume deficits may be treated during surgery; however, additional time may be needed to correct pronounced fluid and electrolyte deficits to promote the best possible preoperative condition.

Drug or Alcohol Use

People who use illicit drugs or alcohol frequently deny or attempt to hide it. In such situations, the nurse who is obtaining the patient's health history needs to ask frank questions with patience, care, and a nonjudgmental attitude. Because acutely intoxicated people are at higher risk for potential injury, surgery is postponed if possible. If emergency surgery is required, local, spinal, or regional block anesthesia is used for minor surgery. Otherwise, to prevent vomiting and potential aspiration, a nasogastric tube is inserted before general anesthesia is administered.

The person with a history of chronic alcohol use disorder often suffers from malnutrition and other systemic problems that increase surgical risk. In addition, postoperative morbidity and mortality rates are increased in alcohol use disorder due to the association with impaired wound healing, infection, bleeding, pneumonia, and further hepatic decline (Odom-Forren & O'Brien, 2023). Alcohol withdrawal syndrome or delirium tremens (DTs) may be anticipated, although the onset time interval is variable. DTs usually occurs within 1 week after reduction or cessation of heavy alcohol intake and persists for 1 to 3 days (Ferri, 2023a). DTs is associated with a significant mortality rate when it occurs postoperatively.

Pearls for Practice

The nurse is aware that withdrawal symptoms usually appear within 8 hours after blood alcohol levels decrease; peak at about 72 hours of withdrawal; and are often preceded by tremulousness, anxiety, and insomnia, progressing to tachycardia, diaphoresis, anorexia, agitation, headache, and gastrointestinal distress. Late symptoms include visual hallucinations, delirium, or seizures (Ferri, 2023a). Many institutions use the Clinical Institute Withdrawal Assessment-Alcohol (CIWA-A) scale to measure the severity of alcohol withdrawal. The CIWA-A scale consists of 10 symptoms, and treatment is either a fixed-dose regimen or individualized benzodiazepine administration dose.

Respiratory Status

The goal for surgical patients is optimal respiratory function. Because adequate ventilation is potentially compromised during all phases of surgical treatment, surgery is usually postponed if the patient has a respiratory infection. Patients with underlying respiratory disease (e.g., asthma, chronic obstructive pulmonary disease [COPD], pulmonary fibrosis) are assessed carefully for current threats to their pulmonary status. Patients should be evaluated for conditions such as respiratory infection and neuromuscular diseases, such as Parkinson disease, which may affect respiratory function.

The use of tobacco is an important risk factor but one that usually cannot be influenced. Even among smokers who have not developed chronic lung disease, smoking is associated with significant changes in lung function. While cessation for 2 days prior to surgery is recommended, a seminal study by Warner et al. (1984) revealed that smoking cessation for up to 8 weeks was necessary to reduce the rate of postoperative pulmonary complications. While the ideal duration of cessation of smoking before surgery remains unclear, longer periods of smoking cessation (≥8 weeks) outcomes include marked improvement in pulmonary mechanics such as boosted ciliary function, decreased mucous secretion and small airway obstruction, and boosted immune function (Sheets, 2023). What it known is that patients who smoke have almost six times the number of pulmonary complications, such as pneumonia and atelectasis (Odom-Forren & O'Brien, 2023). Patients should be encouraged to stop smoking at least 12 to 48 hours before surgery to reduce the effects of nicotine, decrease carbon monoxide levels, improve oxygen delivery which improves vasodilatation, and decrease toxic substances that impair wound healing (Sheets, 2023).

Pearls for Practice

Smoking impacts the patient's postoperative progress via a variety of effects. Namely, the vasoconstriction associated with smoking decreases blood supply and wound oxygenation. In addition, the carbon monoxide (CO) in smoke binds with hemoglobin (forming carboxyhemoglobin), which reduces oxygenation to the tissues (Sheets, 2023). The nurse also considers that increased mucus in the airways associated with smoking can cause forceful coughing, raising intra-abdominal pressure, which increases the strain on a wound and impair healing (Phillips & Hornacky, 2021b). The nurse, while acknowledging how difficult smoking cessation is, informs patients that stopping for even one night before surgery decreases their heart rate, blood pressure (BP), and circulating catecholamine levels and lets the carboxyhemoglobin values return to normal levels (Sheets, 2023).

Cardiovascular Status

The goal in preparing any patient for surgery is to ensure a well-functioning cardiovascular system to meet the oxygen, fluid, and nutritional needs of the perioperative period. If the patient has uncontrolled hypertension, surgery may be postponed until the blood pressure is stabilized. At times, surgical treatment can be modified to meet the cardiac tolerance of the patient. For example, in a patient with obstruction of the descending colon and coronary artery disease, a temporary simple colostomy may be performed rather than a more extensive colon resection that would require a prolonged period of anesthesia.

Hepatic and Kidney Function

The presurgical goal is optimal function of liver and kidney function so that medications, anesthetic agents, body wastes, and toxins are adequately processed and removed from the body.

The liver is important in the biotransformation of anesthetic compounds. Therefore, any disorder of the liver has an effect on how anesthetic agents are metabolized. The limited ability of a failing liver increases the perioperative risks and presents significant challenges. In addition, increased surgical and anesthesia-related morbidity and mortality is associated with varying degrees of liver insufficiency; thus, it is important to quantify and grade preoperative liver dysfunction using various serum liver function tests (Collins et al., 2023). Because the kidneys are involved in excreting anesthetic medications and their metabolites, and because acid–base status and metabolism are also important considerations in anesthesia administration, an evaluation of recent laboratory measurements (i.e., electrolytes, coagulation, BUN and creatinine), coexisting diseases, and current medications is essential. If patients have end-stage kidney disease, specific information gathered should include the serum potassium, the type of and schedule for dialysis, and volume status (dry weight) (Morse, 2023). Surgery may be contraindicated if a patient has acute nephritis, acute kidney injury with oliguria or anuria, or other acute kidney problems. The exception is surgery that is performed as a life-saving measure or that is necessary to improve urinary function, as in the case of an obstructive uropathy.

Endocrine Function

Diabetes is the most common endocrinopathy and has both acute and chronic disease manifestations. Because of this and other factors, patients with diabetes are more likely to require surgery. Most patients with diabetes develop disease in more than one body system; thus, a thorough assessment of major organ disease (cardiac, renal, peripheral vascular) must be identified and managed carefully during the perioperative period. The patient with diabetes who is undergoing surgery is at risk for hypoglycemia and hyperglycemia. Hypoglycemia may develop during anesthesia or postoperatively from inadequate carbohydrates or excessive administration of insulin. Hyperglycemia, which can increase the risk for surgical wound infection, and fluid and electrolyte loss may result from the stress of surgery because it triggers increased release of catecholamines. An increase in catecholamines contributes to an elevation in the blood glucose level. Previously, blood sugar was tightly controlled with intensive insulin therapy—this practice is no longer recommended routinely. Surgical patients with type 1 diabetes are also at risk for developing ketoacidosis. Refer to Chapter 29 for details on management of patients with diabetes.

Patients who have received corticosteroids are at risk of adrenal insufficiency. Therefore, the use of corticosteroids for any purpose during the preceding year must be reported to the anesthesia provider and surgeon. The patient is monitored for signs of adrenal insufficiency, which frequently presents with hyponatremia, hypoglycemia, hyperkalemia, and complaints of weakness and fatigue (see Chapter 30).

Patients with uncontrolled thyroid disorders are at risk for thyrotoxicosis (with hyperthyroid disorders) or respiratory failure (with hypothyroid disorders). Therefore, the patient is assessed for a history of these disorders. Refer to Chapter 30 for further discussion of endocrine disorders.

Immune Function

The nurse determines the presence of allergies. It is especially important to identify and document any sensitivity to medications and past adverse reactions to these agents. The nurse asks the patient to identify any substances that precipitated previous allergic reactions, including medications, herbal supplements, blood transfusions, contrast agents, latex, and food products, and to describe the signs and symptoms produced by these substances. A sample latex allergy screening questionnaire is shown in Figure 4-1.

Immunosuppression is common with corticosteroid therapy, kidney transplantation, radiation therapy, chemotherapy, and disorders affecting the immune system, such as AIDS and leukemia. The mildest symptoms or slightest temperature elevation must be investigated. Because patients who are immunosuppressed are highly susceptible to infection, the health care team should take great care to ensure strict asepsis.

Medication Use

A medication history is obtained from each patient because of the possible effects of medications on the patient's perioperative course, including the possibility of drug interactions. Any medication the patient is using or has used in the past is documented, including the frequency with which the medication is used. Potent medications have an effect on physiologic functions; interactions of such medications with anesthetic agents can cause serious problems, such as arterial hypotension and circulatory collapse.

The potential effects of prior medication therapy are evaluated by the anesthesia provider, who considers the length of time the patient has used the medication, the physical condition of the patient, and the nature of the proposed surgery. Medications that cause particular concern are listed in Table 4-4.

In addition, many patients take self-prescribed or over-the-counter (OTC) medications. Aspirin is a common OTC medication that inhibits platelet aggregation; therefore, it is prudent to stop aspirin at least 7 to 10 days before surgery if possible, especially for surgeries in which excess bleeding would cause significant complications, such as brain or spinal cord surgeries. Because of the effects of aspirin or other OTC

Ask the patient the following questions. Check "Yes" or "No" in the box.	YES	NO
1. Has a doctor ever told you that you are allergic to latex?		
2. Do you have on-the-job exposure to latex?		
3. Were you born with problems involving your spinal cord?		
4. Have you ever had allergies, asthma, hay fever, eczema, or problems with rashes?		
5. Have you ever had respiratory distress, rapid heart rate, or swelling?		
6. Have you ever had swelling, itching, hives, or other symptoms after contact with a balloon?		
7. Have you ever had swelling, itching, hives, or other symptoms after a dental examination or procedure?		
8. Have you ever had swelling, itching, hives, or other symptoms following a vaginal or rectal examination or after contact with a diaphragm or condom?		
9. Have you ever had swelling, itching, hives, or other symptoms during or within 1 hour after wearing rubber gloves?		
10. Have you ever had a rash on your hands that lasted longer than 1 week?		
11. Have you ever had swelling, itching, hives, runny nose, eye irritation, wheezing, or asthma after contact with any latex or rubber product?		
12. Have you ever had swelling, itching, hives, or other symptoms after being examined by someone wearing rubber or latex gloves?		
13. Are you allergic to bananas, avocados, kiwi, or chestnuts?		
14. Have you ever had an unexplained anaphylactic episode?		

Preop RN Signature: ______________________

Patient Name: ______________________

Procedure: ______________________

Scheduled Date / Time: ______________________

Surgeon: ______________________

FIGURE 4-1 **Example of a latex allergy assessment form. (Courtesy of Inova Fairfax Hospital, Falls Church, Virginia.)**

medications and possible interactions with prescribed medications and anesthetic agents, it is important to ask a patient about their use. The information is noted in the patient's chart and conveyed to the anesthesia provider and surgeon.

The use of herbal medications is widespread among patients; because of their potential effects on coagulation and potentially lethal interactions with other medications, the nurse must ask surgical patients specifically about the use of these agents, document their use, and inform the surgical team and anesthesia provider. Those who use herbal remedies may be at an "increased risk of intraoperative complications such as increased blood loss, cardiac instability, prolongation of anesthesia, and adverse drug interactions" (Donoghue, 2018, p. 243). Decisions should be made by the surgical team about the discontinuation of herbal medications prior to surgery. In general, while it is prudent for patients to stop taking herbal medications 1 to 2 weeks before surgery to avoid potential cardiovascular, central nervous system (CNS), and bleeding effects, it is unlikely that the patient will be seen by an anesthesia provider 2 weeks before the operative event, which complicates management for anesthesia providers (Donoghue, 2018).

Psychosocial Factors

All patients have some type of emotional reaction before any surgical procedure, be it obvious or hidden, normal or abnormal. For example, preoperative anxiety may be an anticipatory response to an experience the patient views as a threat to their customary role in life, body integrity, or life itself. Psychological distress directly influences body functioning. In addition to providing anticipatory guidance about what the patient will experience during the operative procedure, the nurse provides opportunities for the patient to ask questions, so that concerns can be addressed.

Most patients who are about to undergo surgery have fears, including fear of the unknown, of death, of anesthesia, of pain, or of cancer. Concerns about loss of work time, loss of job, increased responsibilities or burden on family members, and the threat of permanent incapacity further contribute to the emotional strain created by the prospect of surgery. Less obvious concerns may occur because of previous experiences with the health care system and people the patient has known with the same condition.

People express fear in different ways. For example, some patients may repeatedly ask many questions, even though answers were given previously. Others may withdraw, deliberately avoiding communication, perhaps by reading, watching television, or talking about trivialities. Assessing the patient's readiness to learn and determining the best approach to maximize comprehension provides the basis for preoperative patient education. Consequently, the nurse must be empathetic, listen well, and provide information that helps alleviate concerns.

An important outcome of the psychosocial assessment is the determination of the extent and role of the patient's support network. The value and reliability of all available support systems are assessed. Other information, such as usual level of functioning and typical daily activities, may assist in the patient's care and rehabilitation plans.

Spiritual and Cultural Beliefs

Spiritual beliefs play an important role in how people cope with fear and anxiety. Regardless of the patient's religious affiliation, spiritual beliefs can be as therapeutic as medication. Every attempt must be made to help the patient obtain

TABLE **4-4 Examples of Medications with the Potential to Affect the Surgical Experience**

Agent	Effect of Interaction with Anesthetics
Corticosteroids Prednisone	Cardiovascular collapse can occur if discontinued suddenly. Therefore, a bolus of corticosteroid may be administered intravenously immediately before and after surgery.
Diuretics Hydrochlorothiazide	During anesthesia, may cause excessive respiratory depression resulting from an associated electrolyte imbalance
Phenothiazines Chlorpromazine	May increase the hypotensive action of anesthetics
Tranquilizers Diazepam	May cause anxiety, tension, and even seizures if withdrawn suddenly
Insulin	Interaction between anesthetics and insulin must be considered when a patient with diabetes is undergoing surgery. IV insulin may need to be administered to keep the blood glucose within the normal range.
Antibiotics Erythromycin	When combined with a curariform muscle relaxant, nerve transmission is interrupted and apnea from respiratory paralysis may result.
Anticoagulants Warfarin	Can increase the risk of bleeding during the intraoperative and postoperative periods; should be discontinued in anticipation of elective surgery. The surgeon will determine how long before the elective surgery the patient should stop taking an anticoagulant, depending on the type of planned procedure and the medical condition of the patient.
Antiseizure Medications	IV administration of medication may be needed to keep the patient seizure-free in the intraoperative and postoperative periods.
Monoamine Oxidase (MAO) Inhibitors Phenelzine sulfate	May increase the hypotensive action of anesthetics
Thyroid Hormone Levothyroxine sodium	IV administration may be needed during the postoperative period to maintain thyroid levels.

the spiritual support that they request. Faith has great sustaining power. Therefore, the beliefs of each patient should be respected and supported. In addition, the nurse needs to communicate and document if the patient declines blood transfusions for religious reasons (Jehovah's Witnesses), as this information needs to be clearly identified in the preoperative period. Some nurses avoid the subject of a clergy visit lest the suggestion alarm the patient. Asking whether the patient's spiritual advisor knows about the impending surgery is a caring, nonthreatening approach.

Showing respect for a patient's cultural values and beliefs facilitates rapport and trust. Some areas of assessment include identifying the ethnic group to which the patient relates and the customs and beliefs the patient holds about illness and health care providers. For example, patients from some cultural groups are unaccustomed to expressing feelings openly. Nurses need to consider this pattern of communication when assessing pain. Nurses should familiarize themselves with culturally competent guidelines (see Box 1-3 in Chapter 1).

Perhaps the most valuable skill at the nurse's disposal is listening carefully to the patient, especially when obtaining the history. Invaluable information and insights may be gained through effective communication and interviewing skills. An unhurried, understanding, and caring nurse promotes confidence on the part of the patient.

Presence of Genetic Disorders

In the preoperative period, attention needs to be paid to patients with various genetic disorders (listed below) since surgical outcomes may be altered related to complications with anesthesia.

- Malignant hyperthermia (MH) (discussed on page 139)
- Central core disease (CCD), is a genetic disorder that presents in the neonatal period or infancy with muscle

weakness and hypotonia and mild facial weakness. This condition increases the risk of developing MH.

- Duchenne muscular dystrophy and Becker dystrophy are two types of muscular dystrophies associated with risk of developing MH. Congenital myopathies have also been implicated as a risk factor for MH (Gregory & Weant, 2021).
- Hyperkalemic periodic paralysis is a genetic disorder that causes episodes of extreme muscle weakness and occasionally hyperkalemia. It is also associated with MH. Other risk factors include a history of unexplained fevers with thorough workup and no diagnosis, previous episode of rhabdomyolysis with thorough workup and no diagnosis, history of dark-colored urine, and history of heat stroke (Gregory & Weant, 2021).
- King–Denborough syndrome, a rare genetic disorder associated with musculoskeletal abnormalities, is associated with MH.

Preoperative Nursing Management

Providing Preoperative Teaching

Preoperative education is important for improved patient outcomes. Each patient is taught as an individual, with consideration for any unique concerns or learning needs. Preoperative teaching is initiated as soon as possible, includes different modalities (verbal, written, electronic, smartphone app, web-based videos, return demonstration), and should be tailored to the needs of the patient (Fraile et al., 2022). It should start in the surgeon's office or at the time of Pre-Admission Testing (PAT), continue until the patient arrives in the OR, and extend to and through discharge.

Timing and Technique

It is best to begin teaching early, when the patient and family may be less anxious and can make adjustments or prepare for the postoperative period more effectively. The ideal timing for preoperative teaching is not on the day of surgery but during the preadmission visit, when diagnostic tests are performed. At this time, the nurse or resource person answers questions and provides important patient teaching. During this visit, the patient can meet and ask questions of the perioperative nurse and health care team members, view audiovisual resources, receive written materials, and be given the telephone number to call as questions arise closer to the date of surgery. Many institutions provide access to websites where patients can view and review written instructions, communicate electronically, and ask questions with caregivers.

Teaching should go beyond descriptions of the procedure and should include explanations of the sensations the patient will experience. For example, telling the patient only that preoperative medication will cause relaxation before the operation is not as effective as also noting that the medication may result in lightheadedness and drowsiness. Knowing what to expect will help the patient anticipate these reactions and, thus, attain a higher degree of relaxation than might otherwise be expected. Knowing ahead of time about the possible need for a ventilator, drainage tubes, or other types of equipment helps decrease anxiety in the postoperative period. In addition, preoperative teaching includes instruction in the breathing and leg exercises used to prevent postoperative complications such as pneumonia and deep vein thrombosis (DVT). These exercises may be performed in the hospital or at home. The nurse should guide the patient through the experience and allow ample time for questions. For some patients, overly detailed descriptions increase anxiety; the nurse should be sensitive to this and provide as much detail as necessary to ensure patient preparation.

Deep Breathing, Coughing, and Incentive Spirometry

One goal of preoperative nursing care is to teach the patient how to promote optimal lung expansion and consequent blood oxygenation after anesthesia. The patient assumes a sitting position to enhance lung expansion. The nurse then demonstrates how to take a deep, slow breath and how to exhale slowly (see Box 10-8 in Chapter 10). After practicing deep breathing several times, the patient is instructed to breathe deeply, exhale through the mouth, take a short breath, and cough deeply (see Box 4-3). In addition to enhancing respiration, these exercises may help the patient relax. The nurse also demonstrates how to use an incentive spirometer, a device that provides measurement and feedback related to breathing effectiveness.

If a thoracic or abdominal incision is anticipated, the nurse demonstrates how to splint the incision to minimize pressure and control pain. The patient should put the palms of both hands together, interlacing the fingers snugly. Placing the hands across the incisional site acts as an effective splint when coughing. In addition, the patient is informed that medications are available to relieve pain and should be taken regularly for pain relief, so that effective deep breathing and coughing exercises can be performed. The goal in promoting coughing is to mobilize secretions so that they can be removed. Deep breathing before coughing stimulates the cough reflex. If the patient does not cough effectively, atelectasis (collapse of the alveoli), pneumonia, or other lung complications may occur.

Promoting Mobility

The goals of promoting mobility postoperatively are to improve circulation, prevent venous stasis, and promote optimal respiratory function. The nurse explains the rationale for frequent position changes after surgery and then shows the patient how to turn from side to side and how to assume the lateral position without causing pain or disrupting IV lines, drainage tubes, or other equipment. The nurse uses proper body mechanics when turning the patient and instructs the patient to do the same. Whenever the patient is positioned, their body needs to be properly aligned.

BOX 4-3 **Patient Education**

Preoperative Instructions to Prevent Postoperative Complications

Coughing

1. Lean forward slightly from a sitting position in bed, interlace your fingers together, and place your hands across the incisional site to act as a splint-like support when coughing.

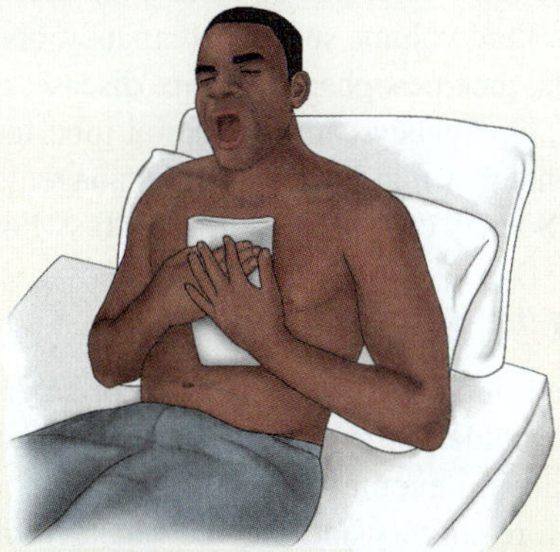

Splinting of chest when coughing

Leg Exercises

1. Lie in a semi-Fowler position and perform the following simple exercises to improve circulation.
2. Bend your knee and raise your foot—hold it a few seconds, then extend the leg and lower it to the bed.

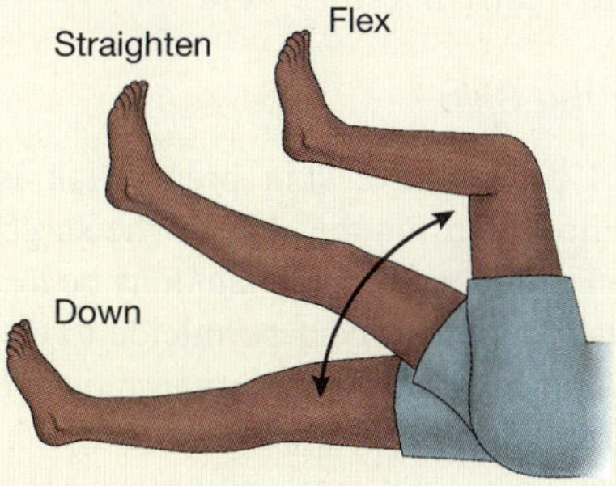

Leg exercises

3. Do this five times with one leg, and then repeat with the other leg.
4. Then trace circles with the feet by bending them down, in toward each other, up, and then out.
5. Repeat these movements five times.

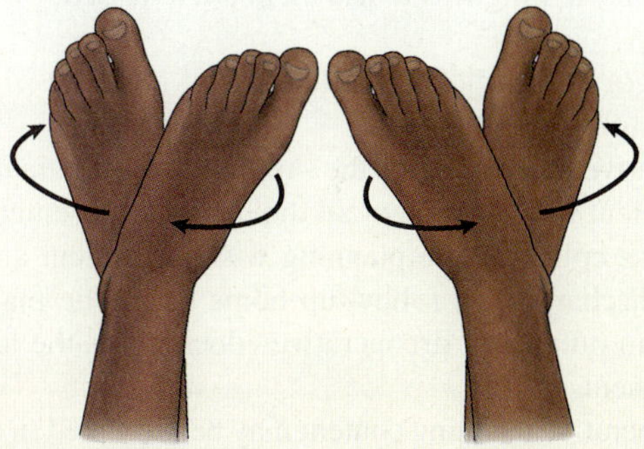

Foot exercises

Turning to the Side

1. Turn on your side with the uppermost leg flexed most and supported on a pillow.
2. Grasp the side rail as an aid to maneuver to the side.
3. Practice coughing while on your side.

Getting Out of Bed

1. Turn on your side.
2. Push yourself up with one hand as you swing your legs out of bed.

In addition, some patients require instruction about special positions that are required after surgery (e.g., abduction or elevation of an extremity). The importance of maintaining as much mobility as possible despite restrictions is discussed. Reviewing the process before surgery is helpful because the patient may be too uncomfortable or drowsy after surgery to absorb new information.

Exercise of the extremities includes extension and flexion of the knee and hip joints (similar to bicycle riding while lying on the side). The foot is rotated as though tracing the largest possible circle with the great toe (see Box 4-3). The elbow and shoulder are also put through their range of motion. At first, the patient is assisted and reminded to perform these exercises. Later, the patient is encouraged to do them independently. Muscle tone is maintained so that ambulation will be easier.

Pain Management

The nurse is guided by the recommendations of TJC that "Pain assessment tools are generally evidence-based and often include, at a minimum, an evaluation of pain intensity, location, quality, and associated symptoms. An accurate pain screening and assessment is the foundation on which an individualized, effective pain management plan is developed" (TJC, 2022b). A pain assessment should include differentiation between acute and chronic pain. A pain intensity scale should be introduced and explained to the patient to promote more effective postoperative pain management.

Once a patient answers yes to whether they have pain, the nurse should perform a comprehensive pain assessment and select an appropriate pain assessment scale (see Chapter 6).

Patients are informed that medications will be administered to relieve pain and maintain comfort without compromising the cardiopulmonary and neurologic status. Anticipated methods of administration of analgesic agents for inpatients include patient-controlled analgesia (PCA), epidural catheter bolus or infusion, peripheral nerve blockades, or patient-controlled epidural analgesia (PCEA). A patient who is expected to go home likely will receive local anesthetic and oral analgesic agents. These methods are discussed with the patient before surgery, and the patient's interest and willingness to use them are assessed.

Instruction for Patients Undergoing Ambulatory Surgery

Preoperative education for the same-day or ambulatory surgical patient is composed of all the material presented above as well as collaborative planning with the patient and family for discharge and follow-up home care. The major difference in outpatient preoperative education is the teaching environment.

Preoperative teaching content may be presented in a group class, on a videotape, over the web or via an app, at preadmission testing, or by telephone in conjunction with the preoperative interview. In addition to answering questions and describing what to expect, the nurse tells the patient when and where to report, what to bring (insurance card, copayment, and list of medications [prescribed and over the counter], COVID immunization status, and allergies), what to leave at home (jewelry, watch, medications, contact lenses), and what to wear (loose-fitting, comfortable clothes; flat shoes). During the final preoperative telephone call, teaching is completed or reinforced as needed, and last-minute instructions are given. The patient is reminded not to eat or drink as directed.

Unfolding Patient Stories: V.W. • Part 1

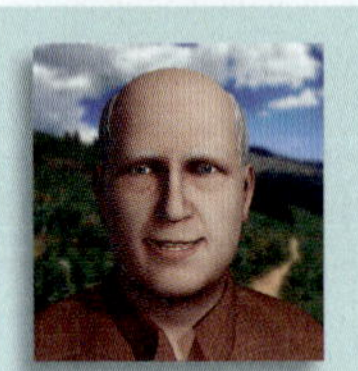

V.W., a 69-year-old patient, came to the emergency department with severe abdominal pain, and a bowel perforation was diagnosed. The patient is being prepared for surgery. Significant medical history includes controlled hypertension and smoking for 50 years. What preoperative education should the nurse discuss with V.W. prior to their emergent surgery? (V.W.'s story continues in Chapter 48.)

Care for V.W. and other patients in a realistic virtual environment: ***vSim*** *for Nursing* (thepoint.lww.com/vSimMedicalSurgical). Practice documenting these patients' care in (thepoint.lww.com/DocuCareEHR).

Managing Nutrition and Fluids

The major purpose of withholding food and fluid before surgery is to prevent aspiration. Until recently, fluid and food were restricted preoperatively overnight and often longer. However, the American Society of Anesthesiologists (ASA) reviewed this practice and has made new recommendations for people undergoing elective surgery who are otherwise healthy.

The ASA (2017) published practice guidelines pertaining to preoperative fasting in nonlaboring individuals undergoing elective procedures. The recommended fasting period after consuming clear fluids for all patients is 2 hours. In general, the volume of liquid ingested is less important than the type of liquid ingested (e.g., clear liquids vs. milk products). However, they acknowledge that modifications may be necessary for patients who have disorders or conditions that impact gastric emptying or fluid volume such as pregnancy, obesity, diabetes, hiatal hernia, gastroesophageal reflux disease, ileus or bowel obstruction, emergency care, or enteral tube feeding, as well as for patients that may have airway management difficulties (American Society of Anesthesiologists Task Force, 2017).

Preparing the Bowel

Enemas are not commonly prescribed preoperatively unless the patient is undergoing abdominal or pelvic surgery. In this case, a cleansing enema or laxative may be prescribed the evening before surgery and may be repeated the morning of surgery. The goals of this preparation are to allow satisfactory visualization of the surgical site and to prevent trauma to the intestine or contamination of the peritoneum by feces. Unless the condition of the patient presents some contraindication, the toilet or bedside commode, rather than the bedpan, is used for evacuating the enema if the patient is hospitalized during this time. In addition, antibiotics may be prescribed to reduce intestinal flora.

Preparing the Skin

The goal of preoperative skin preparation is to decrease bacteria without injuring the skin. If the surgery is not performed as an emergency, the patient may be instructed to use a soap containing a detergent-germicide to cleanse the skin area for several days before surgery to reduce the number of skin organisms; this preparation may be carried out at home.

In general, hair is not removed preoperatively unless the hair at or around the incision site is likely to interfere with the operation. If hair must be removed, electric clippers are used for safe hair removal immediately before the operation in the preoperative area or in the OR using a clipper and vacuum device to suction clipped hair.

Providing Immediate Preoperative Care

The patient changes into a hospital gown that is tied loosely and opens in the back. The patient with long hair may braid it, remove hairpins, and cover the head completely with a disposable bouffant cap.

The mouth is inspected, and dentures or plates are removed. If left in the mouth, these items could easily fall to the back of the throat during induction of anesthesia and cause respiratory obstruction.

Jewelry is not worn to the OR; wedding rings and jewelry of body piercings should be removed to prevent injury (The Association of PeriOperative Registered Nurses [AORN],

2022a). If a patient objects to removing a ring, some institutions allow the ring to be securely fastened to the finger with tape. All articles of value, including assistive devices, dentures, glasses, cell phones, and prosthetic devices, are given to family members or are labeled clearly with the patient's name and stored in a safe and secure place according to the institution's policy.

All patients (except those with urologic disorders) should void immediately before going to the OR to promote continence during low abdominal surgery and to make abdominal organs more accessible. Urinary catheterization is performed in the OR as necessary.

Maintaining the Preoperative Record

Since the release of the World Health Organization's Surgical Safety Checklist in 2009, surgical safety checklists have been used to foster an environment of teamwork and communication while ensuring that staff members consistently adhere to safety standards (Fig. 4-2). The nurse completes the preoperative assessment and plan of care, as well as the portion of the universal protocol/safety checklist that focuses on patient identification, correct documents, and patient understanding of the surgical procedure. The surgical site should be marked by the surgeon during this phase if the surgery involves laterality, and the marking is documented by the admitting nurse. The completed chart (with the preoperative checklist and verification form) accompanies the patient to the OR with the most recent history and physical (within the past 30 days), anesthetic assessment, and surgical consent form attached, along with all laboratory reports and nurses' records per hospital policy. Any unusual last-minute observations that may have a bearing on anesthesia or surgery are

Before induction of anaesthesia → **Before skin incision** → **Before patient leaves operating room**

Before induction of anaesthesia
(with at least nurse and anaesthetist)

Has the patient confirmed their identity, site, procedure, and consent?
☐ Yes

Is the site marked?
☐ Yes
☐ Not applicable

Is the anaesthesia machine and medication check complete?
☐ Yes

Is the pulse oximeter on the patient and functioning?
☐ Yes

Does the patient have a:

Known allergy?
☐ No
☐ Yes

Difficult airway or aspiration risk?
☐ No
☐ Yes, and equipment/assistance available

Risk of >500ml blood loss (7ml/kg in children)?
☐ No
☐ Yes, and two IVs/central access and fluids planned

Before skin incision
(with nurse, anaesthetist, and surgeon)

☐ **Confirm all team members have introduced themselves by name and role.**

☐ **Confirm the patient's name, procedure, and where the incision will be made.**

Has antibiotic prophylaxis been given within the last 60 minutes?
☐ Yes
☐ Not applicable

Anticipated Critical Events

To Surgeon:
☐ What are the critical or non-routine steps?
☐ How long will the case take?
☐ What is the anticipated blood loss?

To Anaesthetist:
☐ Are there any patient-specific concerns?

To Nursing Team:
☐ Has sterility (including indicator results) been confirmed?
☐ Are there equipment issues or any concerns?

Is essential imaging displayed?
☐ Yes
☐ Not applicable

Before patient leaves operating room
(with nurse, anaesthetist, and surgeon)

Nurse Verbally Confirms:

☐ The name of the procedure

☐ Completion of instrument, sponge and needle counts

☐ Specimen labeling (read specimen labels aloud, including patient name)

☐ Whether there are any equipment problems to be addressed

To Surgeon, Anaesthetist and Nurse:

☐ What are the key concerns for recovery and management of this patient?

This checklist is not intended to be comprehensive. Additions and modifications to fit local practice are encouraged.

FIGURE 4-2 **Surgical safety checklist. Based on the WHO Surgical Safety Checklist, http://whqlibdoc.who.int/publications/2009/9789241598590_eng_Checklist.pdf. (© World Health Organization [WHO], 2008. All rights reserved.)**

noted prominently at the front of the chart. Many institutions document these preoperative requirements electronically. To support this process, institutions are required to ensure that a standard hand-off process is in place to communicate critical and pertinent information to the next caregiver.

Administering Preanesthetic Medication

The rare use of preanesthetic medication is a minimal dose with ambulatory or outpatient surgery. If prescribed, it is usually administered in the preoperative holding area. If a preanesthetic medication is administered, the patient is kept in bed with the side rails raised because the medication can cause lightheadedness or drowsiness. During this time, the nurse observes the patient for any untoward reaction to the medications. The immediate surroundings are kept quiet to promote relaxation.

Pearls for Practice

Protecting patients from injury is one of the major roles of the perioperative nurse. Specific nursing interventions to decrease the risk of falling after the premedication is administered are to raise the side rails of the bed, provide the call light if available, and remind the patient that out of bed (OOB) activity is not permitted due to potential medication side effects such as dizziness.

Transporting the Patient to the Presurgical Area

Patient safety in the preoperative area is a priority. Use of a process to verify patient identification, the surgical procedure, and the surgical site is imperative to maximize patient safety. This process should be performed at the time of admission in the presurgical unit and during all hand-offs from caregiver to caregiver. This allows for prompt intervention if any discrepancies are identified.

Attending to Family Needs

Most hospitals and ASCs have a waiting room where family members and significant others can wait while the patient is undergoing surgery. This room may be equipped with comfortable chairs, television, telephones, and facilities for light refreshment. Volunteers may remain with the family, offer them coffee, and keep them informed of the patient's progress. After surgery, the surgeon should meet the family in the waiting room or call the family and discuss the outcome.

The family and significant others should never judge the seriousness of an operation by the length of time the patient is in the OR. A patient may be in surgery much longer than the actual operating time for several reasons:

- Patients are routinely transported well in advance of the actual operating time.
- The anesthesia provider often makes additional preparations that may take 30 to 60 minutes.
- Patient positioning may take up to 45 minutes prior to procedure start time.
- The surgeon may take longer than expected with the preceding case, which delays the start of the next surgical procedure.

After surgery, the patient is taken to the PACU to ensure safe emergence from anesthesia. Family members and significant others waiting to see the patient after surgery should be informed that the patient may have certain equipment or devices (e.g., IV lines, indwelling urinary catheter, nasogastric tube, oxygen lines, monitoring equipment, blood transfusion lines) in place when they return from surgery. Many hospitals now adopt the model of patient- and family-centered care and allow visitations in the PACU for short periods after the patient is stabilized and made comfortable. In ambulatory surgery and pediatric settings, family members are brought in early in the recovery process and are integral to the preparation for discharge. When the patient returns to the room, the nurse provides explanations regarding the frequent postoperative observations that will be made. However, it is the responsibility of the surgeon, not the nurse, to relay the surgical findings and the prognosis, even when the findings are favorable.

INTRAOPERATIVE NURSING

The **intraoperative phase** begins when the patient is transferred onto the OR table and ends with admission to the PACU. In this phase, the scope of nursing activities includes:

- providing for the patient's safety
- maintaining an aseptic environment
- ensuring proper function of equipment
- providing the surgeon with specific instruments and supplies for the surgical field
- completing appropriate documentation
- providing emotional support during induction of general anesthesia
- assisting in positioning the patient on the OR table using appropriate principles of body alignment
- acting as scrub nurse, circulating nurse, or registered nurse first assistant (RNFA)

The intraoperative experience has undergone many changes that make it safer and less disturbing to patients. However, even with these advances, anesthesia and surgery place the patient at risk for several complications or adverse events. Consciousness or full awareness, mobility, protective biologic functions, and personal control are totally or partially relinquished by the patient when entering the OR. Staff from the departments of anesthesia, nursing, and surgery work collaboratively to implement professional standards of care, to control iatrogenic (adverse condition in a patient resulting from treatment) and individual risks, to prevent complications, and to promote high-quality patient outcomes.

TABLE **4-5 The Surgical Team**

Team Member	Responsibilities
Circulating nurse (Circulator)	Using the nursing process to develop individualized plans of care Checking and managing the OR conditions (ensuring cleanliness, proper temperature, humidity, lighting, safe function of equipment, and the availability of supplies and materials) Continually assessing the patient for signs of injury and implementing appropriate interventions Verifying consent and ensuring documentation is correct Coordinating the team Monitoring aseptic practices to avoid breaks in technique while coordinating the movement of related personnel (medical, x-ray, and laboratory) Implementing fire safety precautions and accounting for all surgical counts in collaboration with scrub person Ensuring that the second verification of the surgical procedure and site takes place and is documented Managing specimens
Scrub person	Performing a surgical hand scrub Setting up the sterile tables Preparing sutures, ligatures, and special equipment (e.g., laparoscope) Anticipating the instruments and supplies that will be required, such as sponges, drains, and other equipment As the surgical incision is closed, counting all needles, sponges, and instruments with the nurse to be sure they are accounted for and not retained as a foreign body within the patient's body
Registered nurse first assistant (RNFA)	Handling tissue Providing exposure at the operative field Suturing Maintaining hemostasis
Surgeon (a licensed physician, osteopath, oral surgeon, or podiatrist who is specially trained and qualified)	Performing the surgical procedure Heading the surgical team
Anesthesia provider—Anesthesiologist (a physician specifically trained in the art and science of anesthesiology) and anesthetist (a qualified health care professional who administers anesthetics; most are certified registered nurse anesthetists [CRNAs])	Assessing the patient before surgery Selecting the anesthesia and administering it Intubating the patient if necessary Managing any technical problems related to the administration of the anesthetic agent Supervising the patient's condition throughout the surgical procedure

The Surgical Team

The surgical team includes the **circulating nurse** (also known as the **circulator**), the **scrub person** (may be a nurse or a scrub technologists), first assistant (RN first assistant or physician assistant), surgeon, and anesthesia providers. Table 4-5 summarizes the roles of each member. Every member of the surgical team verifies the patient's name, procedure, and surgical site using objective documentation and data before beginning the surgery, as mandated by TJC. This is referred to as the "time out" or final pause and must be performed prior to incision, preferably with the patient involved; if patient's surgical site was marked, the mark should be visible.

The Surgical Environment

The surgical environment is known for its stark appearance and cool temperature. The surgical suite is behind double doors, and access is limited to authorized personnel. To provide the best possible conditions for surgery, the OR is situated in a location that is central to all supporting services (e.g., pathology, x-ray, laboratory). The OR has special air filtration devices to screen out contaminating particles, dust, and pollutants.

Maintaining the Environment

Most of TJC's 2023 National Patient Safety Goals pertain to the perioperative areas (see Box 4-4). External precautions include adhering to principles of surgical asepsis, and strict control of the OR environment is required, including traffic pattern restrictions. Policies governing this environment address such issues as the health of the staff; the cleanliness of the rooms; the sterility of equipment and surfaces; processes for scrubbing, gowning, and gloving; and OR attire.

BOX 4-4

Hospital National Patient Safety Goals for 2023

- Identify patients correctly
- Improve staff communication
- Use medicines safely
- Use alarms safely
- Prevent infection
- Identify patient safety risks
- Prevent mistakes in surgery

From https://www.jointcommission.org/-/media/tjc/documents/standards/national-patient-safety-goals/2023/2023-hap-npsg-goals-102122_simple.pdf

Preventing Surgical Fire

Fire is a risk to both patients and personnel in the operating room due to the three elements of the fire triangle that are necessary for a fire: a fuel source (alcohol-based skin preparation agents, surgical gowns, drapes, towels), oxidizer (gaseous oxygen, nitrous oxide), and ignition source (electrosurgery, laser, electrocautery) (Culp & Muse, 2021). Although rare, surgical fires can result in devastating disfigurement, serious injury, and death. Fires can occur at any time in the OR; for example, surgical drapes provide an opportunity for oxygen to concentrate; a stray spark could easily ignite a fire. To evaluate safety in the facility, electrical hazards, emergency exit clearances, and storage of equipment and anesthetic gases are monitored periodically by official agencies, such as the state department of health and TJC. All operating room personnel must be familiar with and educated about fire prevention and how to respond in the event that a fire should occur in the operating room. A fire risk assessment should be completed and communicated to the surgical team prior to the start of a procedure (AORN, 2022a).

Donning Proper Attire

To help decrease microbes, the surgical area is divided into three zones: the **unrestricted zone**, where street clothes are allowed; the **semi restricted zone**, where attire consists of scrub clothes and caps; and the **restricted zone**, where scrub clothes, shoe covers, caps, and masks are worn. The surgeons and other surgical team members wear additional sterile clothing and protective devices during the operation.

The Association of Perioperative Registered Nurses, formerly known as the Association of Operating Room Nurses (still abbreviated as AORN), recommends specific practices for personnel wearing surgical attire to promote a high level of cleanliness in a particular practice setting (AORN, 2022a, 2022b). Shirts and waist drawstrings should be tucked inside the pants to prevent accidental contact with sterile areas and to contain skin shedding. Wet or soiled garments should be changed.

Masks are worn at all times in the restricted zone of the OR. High-filtration masks decrease the risk of postoperative wound infection by containing and filtering microorganisms from the oropharynx and nasopharynx. Masks should fit tightly; should cover the nose and mouth completely; and should not interfere with breathing, speech, or vision. Masks must be adjusted to prevent venting from the sides. Disposable masks have a filtration efficiency exceeding 95%. Masks are changed between patients and should not be worn outside the surgical department. The mask must be either on or off; it must not be allowed to hang around the neck.

Headgear should cover the hair completely (head and neckline, including beard), so that single strands of hair, bobby pins, clips, and particles of dandruff or dust do not fall on the sterile field.

Shoes should be comfortable and supportive. Shoe covers are worn when it is reasonably anticipated that spills or splashes will occur or if shoes are worn outside of the OR suite. Shoe covers should be changed when they become wet, torn, or soiled (AORN, 2022a).

Barriers such as scrub attire and masks do not entirely protect the patient from microorganisms. Upper respiratory tract infections, sore throats, and skin infections in staff and patients are sources of pathogens and must be reported.

Because artificial fingernails harbor microorganisms and can cause nosocomial infections, a ban on artificial nails by OR personnel is supported by the Centers for Disease Control and Prevention (CDC), AORN, and the Association of Professionals in Infection Control. Short, natural fingernails are encouraged.

Using Environmental Controls

In addition to the protocols described previously, surgical asepsis requires meticulous cleaning and maintenance of the OR environment. Floors and horizontal surfaces are cleaned frequently with detergent, soap, and water or with a detergent germicide. Sterilizing equipment is inspected regularly to ensure optimal operation and performance.

All equipment that comes into direct contact with the patient must be sterile. Sterilized linens, drapes, and solutions are used. Instruments are cleaned and sterilized in Central Sterile Services (CSS). Individually wrapped sterile items are used when additional individual items are needed.

Air quality is a major factor that can contribute to surgical site infections (SSIs). To decrease the amount of bacteria in the air, numerous controls have been designed and are being improved upon to maintain clean air in the operating room. Standard OR ventilation provides 15 air exchanges per hour, at least 3 of which are fresh air (CDC, 2019). A temperature of 20° to 24° C (68° to 73° F), humidity between 30% and 60%, and positive pressure relative to adjacent areas are maintained (CDC, 2019). Additional measures may include laminar air flow, UV germicidal lamps, portable negative pressure units containing HEPA and carbon filters, and monitoring systems (Carroll & Kirschman, 2022). Some ORs have laminar airflow units. These units provide more than 300 air exchanges per hour (Jain & Reed, 2019). The goal for a laminar airflow–equipped OR is an infection rate of less than 1%. An OR equipped with this unit is frequently used for total joint replacement or organ transplant surgery.

Staff members shed skin scales that carry bacteria-carrying particles (or colony-forming units [CFUs]), and measures such as the use of long sleeves and gloves while applying the skin preparation solution have demonstrated decreased particulate and microbial shedding (Markel et al., 2018). The use of a head cover when entering the semi-restricted and restricted areas is recommended (Elmously et al., 2019). Unnecessary personnel and physical movement may be restricted to minimize bacteria in the air and achieve an OR infection rate no greater than 3% to 5% in clean, infection-prone surgery. Constant surveillance and conscientious technique in carrying out aseptic practices are necessary to reduce the risk of contamination and infection.

Health Hazards Associated with the Surgical Environment

Safety issues in the OR include exposure to blood and body fluids, latex and adhesive substances, radiation, toxic agents, and laser plumes. Internal monitoring of the OR includes the analysis of surface swipe samples and air samples for infectious and toxic agents. In addition, policies and procedures have been established for minimizing exposure to body fluids and reducing the dangers associated with lasers and radiation.

An additional hazard is the unintentional leaving of an object in a person during a surgical procedure. The risk that foreign objects may be left in a person increases in the following situations: when the procedure is performed on an emergency basis, when there is an unplanned change in the procedure, and when the patient has a high BMI. Surgical sponges are the most frequently retained foreign object (Grant et al., 2020). Many complications can occur from the retention of an object, and the patient is subjected to the risk of an additional surgical procedure.

Exposure to Blood and Body Fluids

OR attire has changed dramatically since the advent of HIV/AIDS. Double-gloving is routine in trauma and other types of surgery where sharp bone fragments are present. Goggles, or a wrap-around face shield, are worn to protect against splashing when the surgical wound is irrigated or when bone drilling is performed. In hospitals where numerous total joint procedures are performed, a complete face shield may be used. This shield provides full-barrier protection from bone fragments and splashes. Ventilation is accomplished through an accompanying hood with a separate air-filtration system.

Latex Allergy

The AORN has recommended standards of care for the patient with latex allergy (AORN, 2022a). These recommendations include early identification of patients with latex allergies, preparation of a latex allergy supply cart, and maintenance of latex allergy precautions throughout the perioperative period. Because of the increased number of patients with latex allergies, most products are latex free. For safety, manufacturers and hospital material managers need to take responsibility for identifying the latex content in items used by patients and health care personnel. Additional discussion of latex allergy can be found in Chapter 37.

Laser Risks

The AORN has recommended practices for laser safety. While lasers are in use, warning signs must be posted clearly to alert personnel. Safety precautions are implemented to reduce the possibility of exposing the eyes and skin to laser beams, to prevent inhalation of the laser plume (smoke and particulate matter), and to protect the patient and personnel from fire and electrical hazards. Several types of lasers are available for clinical use; perioperative personnel should be familiar with the unique features, specific operation, and safety measures for each type of laser used in the practice setting.

All personnel wear special protective goggles specific to the type of laser used in the procedure (Anicoche & Mamaril, 2021).

Whether protection is needed to avoid the laser plume and the effects of its inhalation is controversial. Smoke evacuators are used in some procedures to remove the laser plume from the operative field. In recent years, this technology has been used to protect the surgical team from the potential hazards associated with the generalized smoke plume generated by standard electrocautery units.

The Surgical Experience

During the surgical procedure, the patient will need sedation, anesthesia, or some combination of these. In addition, strict surgical asepsis is maintained.

Anesthesia and Sedation

Anesthesia today is very safe. Anesthesia-related morbidity and mortality is difficult to quantify; however, in a recent study representing the full range of anesthesia practices and locations in the Southeastern United States, the rate of preanesthetic death was 0.509 in 100,000 (Pollard et al., 2018). When the patient arrives in the OR, the anesthesia provider reassesses the patient's physical condition immediately prior to initiating anesthesia. For the patient, the anesthesia experience consists of having an IV line inserted, if it was not inserted earlier; receiving a sedating agent prior to induction with an anesthetic agent; losing consciousness; being intubated, if indicated; and then receiving a combination of anesthetic agents. Typically, the experience is a smooth one, and the patient has no recall of the events. The main types of anesthesia are general anesthesia, regional anesthesia, moderate sedation, monitored anesthesia care, and local anesthesia.

During surgery, the anesthesia provider monitors the patient's blood pressure, pulse, and respirations as well as

BOX 4-5

Stages of General Anesthesia

- *Stage I: Beginning anesthesia.* As the patient breathes in the anesthetic mixture, warmth, dizziness, and a feeling of detachment may be experienced. The patient may have a ringing, roaring, or buzzing in the ears and, although still conscious, may sense an inability to move the extremities easily. During this stage, noises are exaggerated; even low voices or minor sounds seem loud and unreal. For this reason, unnecessary noises and motions are avoided when anesthesia begins.
- *Stage II: Excitement.* The excitement stage, characterized variously by struggling, shouting, talking, singing, laughing, or crying, is often avoided if the anesthetic is administered smoothly and quickly. Because of the possibility of uncontrolled movements of the patient during this stage, the anesthesia provider must always be assisted by someone ready to help restrain the patient. The patient should not be touched except for purposes of restraint, but restraints should not be applied over the operative site.
- *Stage III: Surgical anesthesia.* Surgical anesthesia is reached by continued administration of the anesthetic vapor or gas. The patient is unconscious and lies quietly on the table. With proper administration of the anesthetic, this stage may be maintained for hours in one of several planes, ranging from light (1) to deep (4), depending on the depth of anesthesia needed.
- *Stage IV: Medullary depression.* This stage is reached when too much anesthesia has been administered. Cyanosis develops and, without prompt intervention, death follows rapidly. If this stage develops, the anesthetic is discontinued immediately and respiratory and circulatory support is initiated to prevent death. Stimulants, although rarely used, may be administered; narcotic antagonists can be used if the overdosage is due to opioids.

When opioid agents (narcotics) and neuromuscular blockers (relaxants) are administered, several of the stages are absent. During smooth administration of an anesthetic, there is no sharp division between stages I, II, and III, and there is no stage IV. The patient passes gradually from one stage to another, and it is through close observation of the signs exhibited by the patient that an anesthesia provider controls the situation. The responses of the pupils, the blood pressure, and the respiratory and cardiac rates are among the most reliable guides to the patient's condition.

the electrocardiogram (ECG), blood oxygen saturation level, tidal volume (the amount of air that moves in or out of the lungs with each respiratory cycle; approximately around 500 mL), blood gas levels, blood pH, alveolar gas concentrations, and body temperature. Monitoring by electroencephalography (measure of brain waves) is sometimes required. Levels of anesthetics in the body also can be determined; a mass spectrometer can provide instant readouts of critical concentration levels on display terminals. This information helps personnel assess the patient's ability to breathe unassisted or the need for mechanical assistance if ventilation is poor and the patient is not breathing well independently. Even with the availability of automatic monitoring equipment, the anesthesia provider and/or nurse must remain in close contact with the patient to observe any significant physiologic changes immediately.

General Anesthesia

Anesthesia is a state of narcosis (severe CNS depression produced by pharmacologic agents), analgesia, relaxation, and reflex loss. Patients under general anesthesia are not arousable, not even to painful stimuli. They lose the ability to maintain ventilatory function and require assistance in maintaining a patent airway. Cardiovascular function may be impaired as well.

General anesthesia consists of four stages, each associated with specific clinical manifestations (Box 4-5; Rothrock, 2019).

Anesthetic agents used in general anesthesia are inhaled or administered by IV (Fig. 4-3). Anesthetics produce anesthesia because they are delivered to the brain at a high partial pressure that enables them to cross the blood–brain barrier. Relatively large amounts of anesthetic must be administered

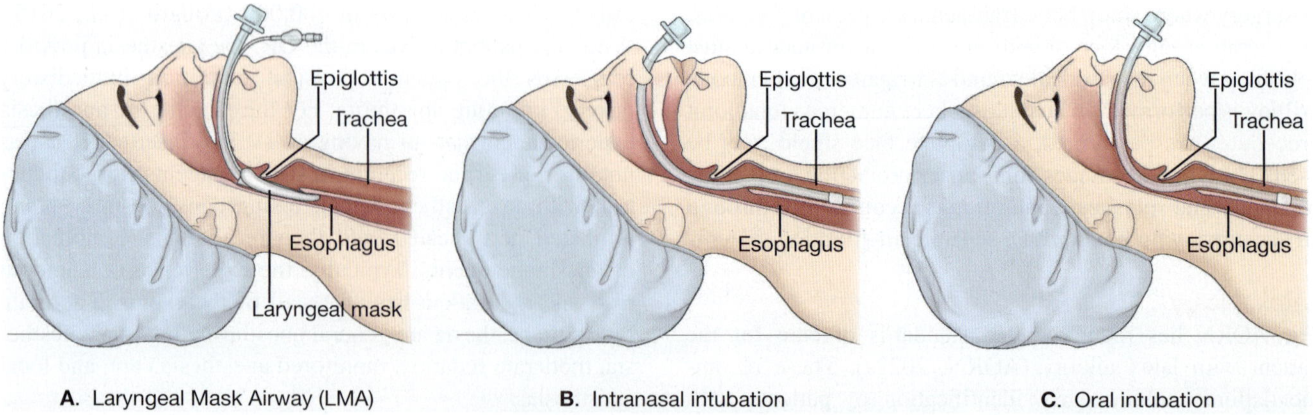

FIGURE 4-3 **Anesthetic delivery methods: (A) laryngeal mask airway (LMA), (B) nasal endotracheal catheter (in position with cuff inflated), and (C) oral endotracheal intubation (tube is in position with cuff inflated).**

during induction and the early maintenance phases because the anesthetic is recirculated and deposited in body tissues. As these sites become saturated, smaller amounts of the anesthetic agent are required to maintain anesthesia because equilibrium or near equilibrium has been achieved among brain, blood, and other tissues.

Any condition that diminishes peripheral blood flow, such as vasoconstriction or shock, may reduce the amount of anesthetic required. Conversely, when peripheral blood flow is unusually high, as in a muscularly active or apprehensive patient, induction is slower, and greater quantities of anesthetic are required because the brain receives a smaller quantity of anesthetic.

Inhaled Administration. Inhalation anesthetics are commonly used for the provision of general **anesthesia**. With the addition of a volatile (readily vaporized) anesthetic to inspired oxygen, a state of unconsciousness and amnesia can be established. When combined with additional medications (e.g., opioids and benzodiazepines), further sedation/hypnosis and amnesia are established. They are considered easy to administer across a diverse surgical population, inexpensive, and reliable in terms of ability to monitor their effects (Nagelhout, 2023). In addition, they are important in situations where there is a lack of venous access and anticipated airway difficulty.

Lifting the Lens

Nurses are aware of the global impact of climate change; a key contributor is the emission of greenhouse gases (GHGs). The release of waste anesthetic gases (WAGs) from surgical procedures into the environment contributes, albeit a small portion, to GHGs emission. Operating room nurses recognize that there is strong evidence supporting the importance of minimizing WAG release into the environment, which will also reduce occupational exposure and the risk of adverse effects (Varughese & Ahmed, 2021).

Intravenous Administration. General anesthesia can be produced by the IV administration of various substances, such as barbiturates, benzodiazepines, nonbarbiturate hypnotics, dissociative agents, and opioid agents. Table 4-6 lists commonly used IV anesthetic and analgesic agents, including IV medications used as muscle relaxants in the intraoperative period. These medications may be administered to induce (initiate) or maintain anesthesia. Although they are often used in combination with inhalation anesthetics, they may be used alone. They may also be used to produce moderate sedation.

An advantage of IV anesthesia is that the onset of anesthesia is pleasant; there is none of the buzzing, roaring, or dizziness known to follow administration of an inhaled

TABLE **4-6 Commonly Used Intravenous Medications**

Medication	Common Usage	Advantages	Disadvantages	Comments
Opioid Analgesics				
Morphine sulfate (MS)	Perioperative pain; premedication	Inexpensive; duration of action 4–5 hours; euphoria; good cardiovascular stability	Nausea and vomiting; histamine release; respiratory depression; postural ↓ BP and ↓ SVR	Used intrathecally and epidurally for postoperative pain; elimination half-life 90 minutes
Alfentanil	Surgical analgesia in ambulatory patients	Duration of action 0.5 hour; used as bolus or infusion		Potency: 750 µg = 10-mg morphine sulfate; elimination half-life 1.6 hours
Fentanyl	Surgical analgesia: epidural infusion for postoperative analgesia; add to SAB	Good cardiovascular stability; duration of action 0.5 hour		Most commonly used opioid; potency: 100 µg = 10-mg morphine sulfate; elimination half-life 3.6 hours
Remifentanil	IV infusion for surgical analgesia; small boluses for brief, intense pain	Easily titratable; metabolized by blood and tissue esterases; very short duration; good cardiovascular stability	New; expensive; requires mixing; may cause muscle rigidity	Potency: 25 µg = 10-mg morphine sulfate; 20–30 times the potency of alfentanil; elimination half-life 3–10 minutes
Sufentanil	Surgical analgesia	Good cardiovascular stability; duration of action 0.5 hour; prolonged analgesia	Prolonged respiratory depression	Potency: 15 µg = 10-mg morphine sulfate; elimination half-life 2.7 hours

(continued)

TABLE **4-6 Commonly Used Intravenous Medications (*continued*)**

Medication	Common Usage	Advantages	Disadvantages	Comments
Nondepolarizing Muscle Relaxants—Intermediate Onset and Duration				
Rocuronium	Intubation; maintenance of relaxation	Rapid onset (dose dependent); elimination via kidney and liver	Vagolytic; may ↑ HR	Duration similar to atracurium and vecuronium
Vecuronium	Intubation; maintenance of relaxation	No significant cardiovascular or cumulative effects; no histamine release	Requires mixing	Mostly eliminated in bile, some in urine
Intravenous Anesthetics				
Etomidate	Induction	Good cardiovascular stability; fast, smooth induction and recovery	May cause pain with injection and myotonic movements	May cause adrenal suppression
Diazepam	Amnesia; hypnotic; preoperative medication	Good sedation	Prolonged duration	Residual effects for 20–90 hours; increased effect with alcohol
Ketamine	Induction, occasional maintenance (IV or IM)	Short acting; patient maintains airway; good in small children and burn patients	Large doses may cause hallucinations and respiratory depression	Need darkened, quiet room for recovery; often used in trauma cases
Midazolam	Hypnotic; anxiolytic; sedation; often used as adjunct to induction	Excellent amnesia; water-soluble (no pain with IV injection); short acting	Slower induction than thiopental	Often used for amnesia with insertion of invasive monitors or regional anesthesia
Propofol	Induction and maintenance; sedation with regional anesthesia or MAC	Rapid onset; awakening in 4–8 minutes	May cause pain when injected	Short elimination half-life (34–64 minutes)
Sodium methohexital	Induction	Ultrashort-acting barbiturate	May cause hiccups	Can be given rectally
Thiopental sodium	Induction	Induction	May cause laryngospasm; large doses may cause apnea and cardiovascular depression	Can be given rectally

BP, blood pressure; HR, heart rate; IM, intramuscular; IV, intravenous; MAC, monitored anesthesia care; SAB, subarachnoid block; SVR, stroke volume ratio.

anesthetic. For this reason, induction of anesthesia usually begins with an IV agent; this often is preferred by patients who have experienced various methods. The duration of action is brief, and the patient awakens with little nausea or vomiting.

The IV anesthetic agents are nonexplosive, require little equipment, and are easy to administer. The low incidence of postoperative nausea and vomiting (PONV) makes the method useful in eye surgery because in this setting vomiting would increase intraocular pressure and endanger vision in the operated eye. IV anesthesia is useful for short procedures but is used less often for the longer procedures of abdominal surgery. It is not indicated for children, who have small veins, or for those who require intubation because of their susceptibility to respiratory obstruction.

A disadvantage of an IV anesthetic such as thiopental (Pentothal) is its powerful respiratory depressant effect. It must be administered by a skilled anesthesia provider and only when some method of oxygen administration is available immediately in case of difficulty. Sneezing, coughing, and laryngospasm are sometimes noted with its use.

IV neuromuscular blockers (muscle relaxants) block the transmission of nerve impulses at the neuromuscular junction of skeletal muscles. Muscle relaxants are used to relax muscles in abdominal and thoracic surgery, relax eye muscles in certain types of eye surgery, facilitate endotracheal

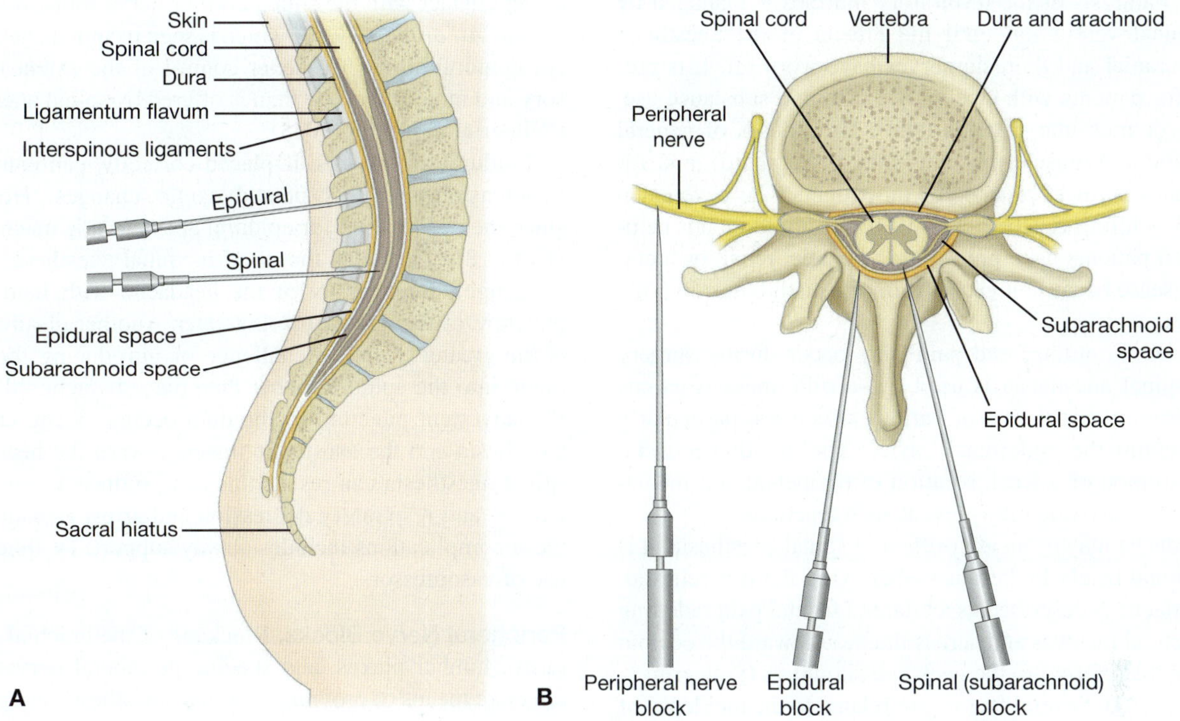

FIGURE 4-4 (A) Injection sites for spinal and epidural anesthesia. (B) Cross-section of injection sites for peripheral nerve, epidural, and spinal blocks.

intubation, treat laryngospasm, and assist in mechanical ventilation.

Local Anesthesia

Local anesthesia is used to block nerves in the peripheral nervous system and CNS. Local anesthesia provides anesthesia and analgesia by blocking the transmission of pain sensation along nerve fibers. The degree of blockage depends on both drug concentration and volume.

Local anesthesia can be used alone or in conjunction with other types of anesthesia. Usually it is administered by the surgeon to a specific area of the body by topical application or local infiltration. In most cases, the patient will be monitored by a nurse. To ensure safety and quality of care, the AORN has developed recommended practices for nurses who monitor patients receiving local anesthesia (AORN, 2022c). The nurse should also monitor the quantity of medication administered since toxic reactions are dose related (AORN, 2022c).

Regional Anesthesia. Regional anesthesia is a form of local anesthesia in which an anesthetic agent is injected around nerves so that the area supplied by these nerves is anesthetized. The most common techniques are spinal, epidural, and peripheral nerve blocks (PNBs). Regional anesthesia is an attractive anesthetic option for many types of operative procedures and has been shown to decrease opiate use, lower the incidence of PONV, shortes the recovery period, and reduce PACU stay in selected patients (Ward, 2023). The effect will depend on the type of nerve involved. A local anesthetic blocks motor nerves least readily and sympathetic nerves most readily. An anesthetic cannot be regarded as having worn off until all three systems (motor, sensory, and autonomic) are no longer affected.

The patient receiving regional anesthesia is awake and aware of their surroundings unless medications are given to produce mild sedation or to relieve anxiety. The nurse must avoid careless conversation, unnecessary noise, and unpleasant odors; these may be noticed by the patient in the OR and may contribute to a negative response to the surgical experience. A quiet environment is therapeutic. The diagnosis must not be stated aloud if the patient is not to know it at this time.

Spinal Anesthesia. Spinal anesthesia is an extensive conduction nerve block that is produced when a local anesthetic is introduced into the subarachnoid space at the lumbar level, usually between L4 and L5 (Fig. 4-4). It produces anesthesia of the lower extremities, perineum, and lower abdomen. For the lumbar puncture procedure, the patient usually lies on their side in a knee-to-chest position. Sterile technique is used as a spinal puncture is made and the medication is injected through the needle. As soon as the injection has been made, the patient is positioned on their back. If a relatively high level of block is sought, the head and shoulders are lowered.

A few minutes after induction of a spinal anesthetic, anesthesia and paralysis affect the toes and perineum and then gradually the legs and abdomen. If the anesthetic reaches the upper thoracic and cervical spinal cord in high concentrations, a temporary partial or complete respiratory paralysis results. Paralysis of the respiratory muscles is managed by mechanical ventilation until the effects of the anesthetic on the cranial and thoracic nerves have worn off. It is preferred for patients with alcohol use disorder, substance use, obesity or muscular patients (since large doses of general anesthetic and muscle relaxants may be required), and for emergency surgical procedures on patients who have eaten recently (Phillips & Hornacky, 2021c). In addition, it is helpful when patients have pre-existing hepatic, renal, or metabolic disease because it causes minimal disturbance in body chemistry.

Nausea, vomiting, and pain may occur during surgery when spinal anesthesia is used. As a rule, these reactions result from manipulation of various structures, particularly those within the abdominal cavity. The simultaneous IV administration of a weak solution of thiopental and inhalation of nitrous oxide may prevent such reactions.

Headache may be an after-effect of spinal anesthesia. It is a positional headache because when lying flat it is relieved; the headache is described as a bilateral frontal pain radiating from behind the eyes and across the head toward the occiput and may be referred to the neck and shoulders (Pellegrini & Conley, 2023). Several factors are related to the incidence of headache: the size of the spinal needle used, the leakage of fluid from the subarachnoid space through the puncture site, and the patient's hydration status. Measures that increase cerebrospinal pressure are helpful in relieving headache. These include maintaining a quiet environment, keeping the patient lying flat, keeping the patient well hydrated, oral analgesics, and the administration of caffeine (Pellegrini & Conley, 2023). Caffeine has demonstrated the ability to eliminate headache in up to 70% of patients, but this effect may be temporary (Pellegrini & Conley, 2023). Refractory postspinal headache may be treated by an epidural blood patch in which 5 to 10 mL of the patient's own blood is administered at the puncture site (resulting in clot formation that seals the dural puncture), resulting in headache relief in 90% of patient (Phillips & Hornacky, 2021c; Pellegrini & Conley, 2023).

In continuous spinal anesthesia, the tip of a plastic catheter remains in the subarachnoid space during the surgical procedure so that more anesthetic may be injected as needed. This technique allows greater control of the dosage, but there is greater potential for postanesthetic headache because of the large-gauge needle used.

Epidural Anesthesia. Epidural anesthesia, a commonly used conduction block, is achieved by injecting a local anesthetic into the epidural space that surrounds the dura mater of the spinal cord (refer to Fig. 4-4). In contrast, spinal anesthesia involves injection through the dura mater into the subarachnoid space surrounding the spinal cord. Epidural anesthesia blocks sensory, motor, and autonomic functions; it differs from spinal anesthesia by the site of the injection and the amount of anesthetic agent used. Epidural doses are much higher because the epidural anesthetic does not make direct contact with the spinal cord or nerve roots; thus, it is not an "*All or none block*" which is seen in spinal anesthesia. An epidural allows for better control of the extent of sensory and motor blockade than is offered by spinal anesthesia (Pellegrini & Conley, 2023).

Epidural anesthetics, if placed correctly, can cause less hypotension and less hemodynamic changes. However, since the needle used for epidural anesthesia is much larger (17 to 18 gauge) than that used in spinal anesthesia (22 to 24 gauge), the severity of the headache with inadvertent puncture of the dura is much greater. Another disadvantage is the greater technical challenge of introducing the anesthetic into the epidural rather than the subarachnoid space. If inadvertent puncture of the dura occurs during epidural anesthesia and the anesthetic travels toward the head, high spinal anesthesia can result; this can produce severe hypotension and respiratory depression and arrest. Treatment of these complications includes airway support, IV fluids, and use of vasopressors.

Peripheral Nerve Blocks. Blockade of the brachial plexus (arm), lumbar plexus, and specific peripheral nerves is an effective means of providing surgical anesthesia and postoperative analgesia for many surgical procedures involving the upper and lower extremities. The advantages of PNB include reduced physiologic stress in comparison to spinal or epidural anesthesia, avoidance of airway manipulation and the potential complications associated with endotracheal intubation, and avoidance of potential side effects associated with general anesthesia. The use of ultrasound-guided regional anesthesia (UGRA) has become routine and may become the gold standard for performing nerve blocks; however, to date it has not resulted in a decreased incidence of nerve injury (Pellegrini & Conley, 2023). All patients undergoing PNB should receive a full perioperative evaluation under the assumption that general anesthesia could be used if the block is inadequate. Examples of common local conduction blocks are:

- Brachial plexus block, which produces anesthesia of the arm
- Paravertebral anesthesia, which produces anesthesia of the nerves supplying the chest, abdominal wall, and extremities
- Transsacral (caudal) block, which produces anesthesia of the perineum and, occasionally, the lower abdomen
- Femoral nerve block, which produces anesthesia of the nerves supplying the leg

Moderate Sedation and Analgesia and Monitored Anesthesia Care

It is important to distinguish between moderate sedation and analgesia (MSA) and **monitored anesthesia care**. *MSA* is a term used by the ASA in their practice guidelines for sedation and analgesia by nonanesthesiologists. *Monitored anesthesia care* implies the potential for a level of sedation

BOX 4-6

Basic Guidelines for Maintaining Surgical Asepsis

All practitioners involved in the intraoperative phase have a responsibility to provide and maintain a safe environment. Adherence to aseptic practice is part of this responsibility. Here are the basic principles of aseptic technique:

- All materials in contact with the surgical wound or used within the sterile field must be sterile. Sterile surfaces or articles may touch other sterile surfaces or articles and remain sterile; contact with unsterile objects at any point renders a sterile area contaminated.
- Gowns of the surgical team are considered sterile in front from the chest to the level of the sterile field. The sleeves are also considered sterile from 2 in above the elbow to the stockinette cuff.
- Sterile drapes are used to create a sterile field. Only the top surface of a draped table is considered sterile. During draping of a table or patient, the sterile drape is held well above the surface to be covered and is positioned from front to back.
- Items are dispensed to a sterile field by methods that preserve the sterility of the items and the integrity of the sterile field. After a sterile package is opened, the edges are considered unsterile. Sterile supplies, including solutions, are delivered to a sterile field or handed to a scrubbed person in such a way that the sterility of the object or fluid remains intact.
- The movements of the surgical team are from sterile to sterile areas and from unsterile to unsterile areas. Scrubbed persons and sterile items contact only sterile areas; circulating nurses and unsterile items contact only unsterile areas.
- Movement around a sterile field must not cause contamination of the field. Sterile areas must be kept in view during movement around the area. At least a 1-foot distance from the sterile field must be maintained to prevent inadvertent contamination.
- Whenever a sterile barrier is breached, the area must be considered contaminated. A tear or puncture of the drape permitting access to an unsterile surface underneath renders the area unsterile. Such a drape must be replaced.
- Every sterile field is constantly monitored and maintained. Items of doubtful sterility are considered unsterile. Sterile fields are prepared as close as possible to the time of use.

deeper than that provided by sedation/analgesia and is always administered by an anesthesiologist (AORN, 2022c). **Moderate sedation and analgesia (MSA)**, previously referred to as *conscious sedation or procedural sedation*, and monitored anesthesia are forms of anesthesia that involve the IV administration of sedatives and/or analgesic medications to reduce patient anxiety and control pain during diagnostic or therapeutic procedures. They are being used increasingly for specific short-term surgical procedures in hospitals and ambulatory care centers (Williams, 2022). The goal is to depress a patient's level of consciousness (LOC) to a moderate level to enable surgical, diagnostic, or therapeutic procedures to be performed while ensuring the patient's comfort during and cooperation with the procedures. MSA allows the patient to maintain a patent airway, retain protective airway reflexes, respond to verbal and physical stimuli, and recover more rapidly postprocedure.

MSA can be administered by an anesthesiologist, anesthetist, or other specially trained and credentialed physician or nurse. The patient receiving moderate sedation is never left alone and is closely monitored by a physician or nurse who is knowledgeable and skilled in detecting arrhythmias, administering oxygen, and performing resuscitation. The continual assessment of the patient's vital signs, LOC, and cardiac and respiratory function is an essential component of care. Pulse oximetry, an ECG monitor, and frequent measurement of vital signs are used to monitor the patient. The regulations for use and administration of moderate sedation differ from state to state, and its administration is addressed in standards issued by TJC and by institutional policies and nursing specialty organizations, including the AORN (Williams, 2022).

Surgical Asepsis

Surgical asepsis prevents the contamination of surgical wounds. The patient's natural skin flora or a previously existing infection may cause postoperative wound infection. Rigorous adherence to the principles of surgical asepsis by OR personnel is basic to preventing SSIs.

Traditionally, the surgeon, surgical assistants, and nurses prepared themselves by scrubbing their hands and arms with antiseptic soap and water, but this traditional practice is being challenged by research investigating the optimal length of time to scrub and the best preparation to use. Also, consider that despite the hand- and arm-cleansing process, skin is never rendered sterile, and tap water is not sterile; thus, surgical scrubbing is not a sterile procedure (Phillips & Hornacky, 2021d). Many institutions have now introduced a scrubless process for cleaning the hands prior to surgery. Box 4-6 provides guidelines for maintaining surgical asepsis.

Intraoperative Nursing Management

The major goals for care of the patient during surgery are to reduce the patient's anxiety, keep the patient free of perioperative injury related to positioning, avoid threats to safety, maintain patient dignity, and avoid complications associated with operative events.

Reducing Anxiety

The OR environment can seem cold, stark, and frightening to the patient, who may be feeling isolated and apprehensive. Introductions, addressing the patient by name warmly and frequently, verifying details, providing explanations,

A. Patient in position on the operating table for a laparotomy. Note the strap above the knees.

B. Patient in Trendelenburg position on operating table. Note padded shoulder braces in place. Be sure that brace does not press on brachial plexus.

C. Patient in lithotomy position. Note that the hips extend over the edge of the table.

D. Patient lies on unaffected side for kidney surgery. Table is spread apart to provide space between the lower ribs and the pelvis. The upper leg is extended; the lower leg is flexed at the knee and hip joints; a pillow is placed between the legs.

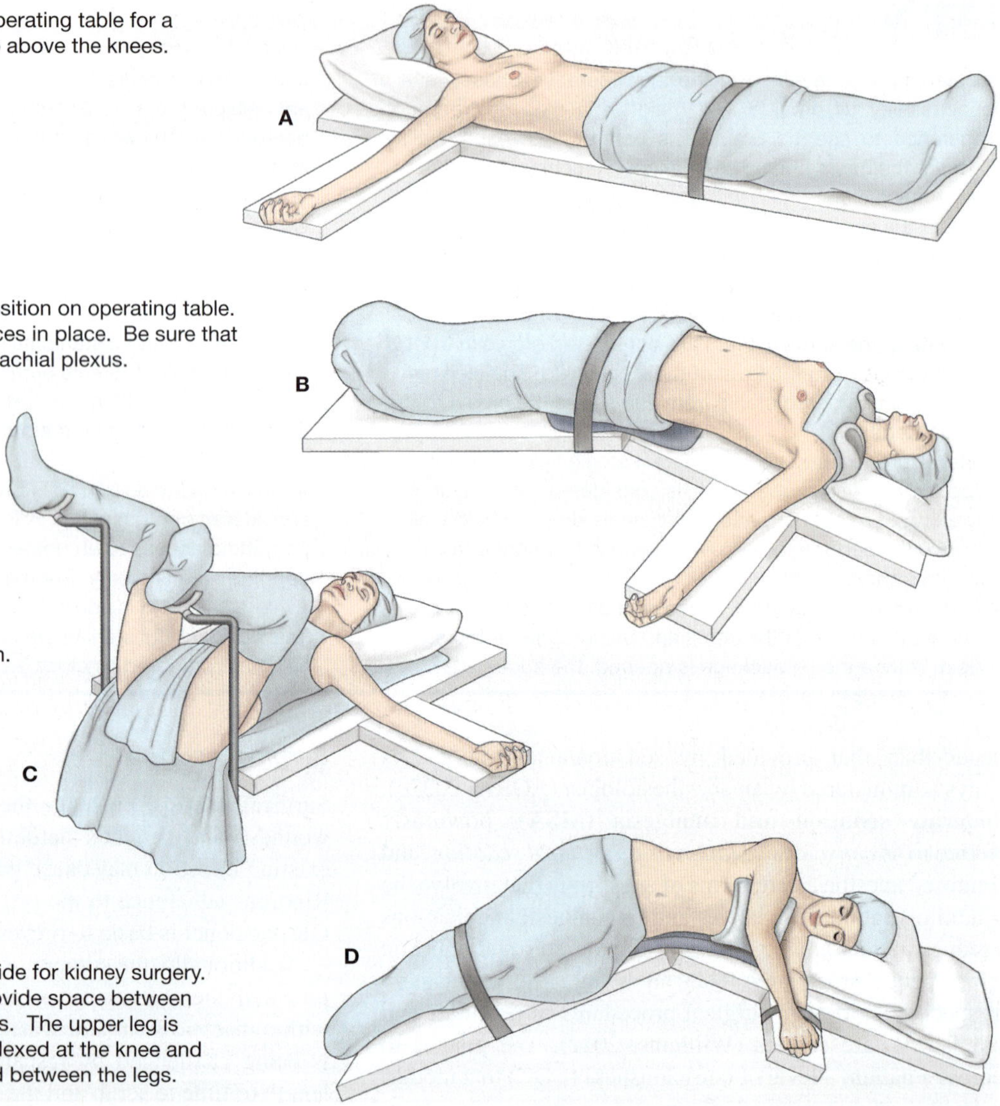

FIGURE 4-5 **Positions on the operating table. Captions call attention to safety and comfort features. All surgical patients wear caps to cover the hair completely.**

and encouraging and answering questions convey a sense of professionalism and friendliness that can help the patient feel secure. When discussing what the patient can expect in surgery, the nurse uses basic communication skills, such as touch and eye contact, to reduce anxiety. Attention to physical comfort (warm blankets, position changes) helps the patient feel more comfortable. Telling the patient who else will be present in the OR, how long the procedure is expected to take, and other details helps the patient prepare for the experience and gain a sense of control.

Preventing Intraoperative Positioning Injury

The patient's position on the operating table depends on the surgical procedure to be performed as well as on the patient's physical condition (Fig. 4-5). The potential for transient discomfort or permanent injury is present because many positions are awkward. Hyperextending joints, compressing arteries, or pressing on nerves and bony prominences usually results in discomfort simply because the position must be sustained for a long period of time (Rothrock, 2019). Factors to consider include the following:

- The patient should be in as comfortable a position as possible, whether conscious or unconscious.
- The operative field must be exposed adequately.
- An awkward position, undue pressure on a body part, or use of stirrups or traction should not obstruct the vascular supply.
- Respiration should not be impeded by pressure of arms on the chest or by a gown that constricts the neck or chest.
- Nerves must be protected from undue pressure. Improper positioning of the arms, hands, legs, or feet can cause serious injury or paralysis. Shoulder braces must be well padded to prevent irreparable nerve injury, especially when the Trendelenburg position (head down) is necessary. The

postoperative complication of compartment syndrome is associated with intraoperative positioning (AORN, 2022d). Refer to Chapter 41 for information related to clinical manifestations of compartment syndrome.
- Precautions for patient safety must be observed, particularly with thin, older, or obese patients as well as those with a physical deformity.
- The patient may need light restraint before induction in case of excitement.

The usual position for surgery, called the dorsal recumbent position, is flat on the back. One arm is positioned at the side of the table, with the hand placed palm down; the other is carefully positioned on an arm board to facilitate IV infusion of fluids, blood, or medications. This position is used for most abdominal surgeries except for surgery of the gallbladder or pelvis (see Fig. 4-5A).

The Trendelenburg position usually is used for surgery on the lower abdomen and pelvis to obtain good exposure by displacing the intestines into the upper abdomen. In this position, the head and upper body are lowered. The patient is held in position by padded shoulder braces (see Fig. 4-5B).

The lithotomy position is used for nearly all perineal, rectal, and vaginal surgical procedures (see Fig. 4-5C). The patient is positioned on the back with the legs and thighs flexed. The position is maintained by placing the feet in stirrups.

The Sims or lateral position is used for renal surgery. The patient is placed on the nonoperative side with an air pillow or beanbag 12.5 to 15 cm (5 to 6 in) thick under the loin, or on a table with a kidney or back lift (see Fig. 4-5D).

Other procedures, such as neurosurgery or abdominothoracic surgery, may require unique positioning and supplemental apparatus, depending on the operative approach.

Protecting the Patient from Injury

A variety of activities are used to address the diverse patient safety issues that arise in the OR. The nurse protects the patient from injury by providing a safe environment. Verifying information, checking the chart for completeness, and maintaining surgical asepsis and an optimal environment are critical nursing responsibilities. Verifying that all required documentation is completed is one of the first functions of the intraoperative nurse. The patient is identified, and the planned surgical procedure, correct surgical site, and type of anesthesia are verified. It is important to review the patient's record for the following:

- Correct informed surgical consent, with patient's and surgeon's signatures
- Completed records for health history and physical examination
- Results of diagnostic studies
- Allergies (including latex)

In addition to checking that all necessary patient data are complete, the perioperative nurse obtains the necessary equipment specific to the procedure. The need for nonroutine medications, blood components, instruments, and other equipment and supplies is assessed, and the readiness of the room; completeness of physical setup; and completeness of instrument, suture, and dressing setups are determined. Any aspects of the OR environment that may negatively affect the patient are identified. These include physical features, such as room temperature and humidity; electrical hazards; potential contaminants (dust, blood, and discharge on floor or surfaces, uncovered hair, faulty attire of personnel, jewelry worn by personnel); and unnecessary traffic. The circulating nurse also sets up and maintains suction equipment in working order, sets up invasive monitoring equipment, assists with insertion of vascular access and monitoring devices (arterial, Swan-Ganz, central venous pressure, IV lines), and initiates appropriate physical comfort measures for the patient.

Preventing physical injury includes using safety straps and side rails and not leaving the sedated patient unattended. Transferring the patient from the stretcher to the OR table requires safe transferring practices. Other safety measures include properly positioning the grounding pad under the patient to prevent electrical burns and shock, removing excess antiseptic solution from the patient's skin, and promptly and completely draping exposed areas after the sterile field has been created to decrease the risk for hypothermia.

The importance of nursing measures to prevent "never events" in surgery such as prevention of retained foreign objects, wrong site surgery, and pressure ulcers cannot be overemphasized. TJC and the AORN have developed guidelines that should be implemented in each facility to prevent these from occurring. There are also technologic devices that can support the safe counting of surgical instruments and supplies to prevent retention of foreign objects. The unintended retention of foreign objects (URFOs)—also called retained surgical items (RSIs)—after invasive procedures can cause death, and surviving patients may sustain both physical and emotional harm, depending on the type of object retained and the length of time it is retained (TJC, 2022c). The risk of URFOs increases during certain surgical conditions (Box 4-7).

Nursing measures to prevent injury from excessive blood loss include blood conservation using equipment such as a cell-saver (a device for recirculating the patient's own blood

BOX 4-7

Risk Factors for Unintended Retention of Foreign Objects (URFOs)

- The absence of policies and procedures
- Failure to comply with existing policies and procedures
- Problems with hierarchy and intimidation
- Failure in communication with physicians
- Failure of staff to communicate relevant patient information
- Inadequate or incomplete education of staff

From The Joint Commission (2016).

cells) and administration of blood products. Few patients undergoing an elective procedure require blood transfusion, but those undergoing higher-risk procedures (such as orthopedic or cardiac surgeries) may require an intraoperative transfusion. The circulating nurse anticipates this need, checks that blood has been cross-matched and held in reserve, and is prepared to support the anesthesia provider with administration when needed.

Serving as Patient Advocate

Because the patient undergoing general anesthesia or moderate sedation experiences temporary sensory/perceptual alteration or loss, there is an increased need for protection and advocacy. Patient advocacy in the OR entails maintaining the patient's physical and emotional comfort, privacy, rights, and dignity. Patients, whether conscious or unconscious, should not be subjected to excess noise, inappropriate conversation, or, most of all, derogatory comments. It has been found that banter in the OR occasionally includes jokes about the patient's physical appearance, job, personal history, and so forth. Cases have been reported in which seemingly deeply anesthetized patients recalled the entire surgical experience, including disparaging personal remarks made by OR personnel. As an advocate, the nurse never engages in this conversation and discourages others from doing so. Other advocacy activities include minimizing the clinical, dehumanizing aspects of being a surgical patient by making sure the patient is treated as a person, respecting cultural and spiritual values, providing physical privacy, and maintaining confidentiality.

Monitoring and Managing Potential Complications

It is the responsibility of the surgeon, anesthesia provider, and the circulating nurse to monitor and manage complications. Important nursing functions include being alert to and reporting changes in vital signs and symptoms of nausea and vomiting, anaphylaxis, hypoxia, hypothermia, MH, or disseminated intravascular coagulation (DIC) and assisting with the management of those complications. Each of these complications will be discussed shortly. It is the responsibility of all members of the health care team to maintain asepsis.

Nausea and Vomiting

Nausea and vomiting, or regurgitation, may affect patients during the intraoperative period. If gagging occurs, the patient is turned to the side, the head of the table is lowered, and a basin is provided to collect the vomitus. Suction is used to remove saliva and vomited gastric contents. The advent of new anesthetics has reduced the incidence; however, there is no single way to prevent nausea and vomiting. An interdisciplinary approach involving the surgeon, anesthesia provider, and nurse is best.

In some cases, the anesthesia provider administers antiemetics preoperatively or intraoperatively to counteract possible aspiration. If the patient aspirates vomitus, it will trigger an asthma-like attack with severe bronchial spasms and wheezing. Pneumonitis and pulmonary edema can subsequently develop, leading to extreme hypoxia. Increasing medical attention is being paid to silent regurgitation of gastric contents (not related to preoperative fasting times), which occurs more frequently than previously realized. The volume and acidity of the aspirate determine the extent of damage to the lungs.

Anaphylaxis

Anaphylaxis is an acute life-threatening allergic reaction to a specific antigen or hapten (a small molecule that can cause an immune response when bound to a protein) resulting in urticaria (hives), pruritus (itching), or angioedema (swelling beneath the skin rather than on the surface), quickly deteriorating to vascular collapse, shock, and respiratory distress. Any time the patient comes into contact with a foreign substance, there is the potential for an anaphylactic reaction. Because medications are the most common cause of anaphylaxis, intraoperative nurses must be aware of the type and method of anesthesia used as well as the specific agents. An anaphylactic reaction can occur in response to many medications, latex, or other substances. Chapter 37 provides additional detail on anaphylaxis.

Hypoxia and Other Respiratory Complications

Inadequate ventilation, occlusion of the airway, inadvertent intubation of the esophagus, and hypoxia are significant potential complications associated with general anesthesia. Many factors can contribute to inadequate ventilation. Respiratory depression caused by anesthetic agents, aspiration of respiratory tract secretions or vomitus, and the patient's position on the operating table can compromise the exchange of gases. Anatomic variation can make the trachea difficult to visualize, resulting in the artificial airway being inserted into the esophagus rather than into the trachea. In addition to these dangers, asphyxia can occur from foreign bodies in the mouth; spasm of the vocal cords; relaxation of the tongue; or aspiration of vomitus, saliva, or blood. Brain damage from hypoxia occurs within minutes; therefore, vigilant monitoring of the patient's oxygenation status is a primary function of the anesthesia provider and the circulating nurse. Peripheral perfusion is checked frequently, and pulse oximetry values are monitored continuously.

Hypothermia

During anesthesia, the patient's temperature may fall. This condition is called *hypothermia* and is indicated by a core body temperature that is lower than normal (36.6° C [98.0° F] or less). Inadvertent hypothermia may occur as a result of a low temperature in the OR, infusion of cold fluids, inhalation of cold gases, open body wounds or cavities, decreased muscle activity, advanced age, or the pharmaceutical agents used (e.g., vasodilators, phenothiazines, general anesthetics). Also, hypothermia may be induced intentionally in selected surgical procedures (e.g., cardiac surgeries requiring cardiopulmonary bypass) to reduce the patient's metabolic rate and energy demands.

Preventing unintentional hypothermia is a major objective. If hypothermia occurs, the goal of intervention is to minimize or reverse the physiologic process. If hypothermia is intentional, the goal is safe return to normal body temperature. Environmental temperature in the OR can be set temporarily at 25° to 26.6° C (78° to 80° F). IV and irrigating fluids are warmed to 37° C (98.6° F). Wet gowns and drapes are removed promptly and replaced with dry materials because wet linens promote heat loss. Whatever methods are used to rewarm the patient, warming must be accomplished gradually, not rapidly. Conscientious monitoring is required for core temperature, urinary output, ECG, blood pressure, arterial blood gas (ABG) levels, and serum electrolyte levels.

Pearls for Practice

Shivering is associated with hypothermia. The nurse is aware that shivering can increase oxygen demand by 300% to 400%; thus, supplemental oxygen should be administered, and oxygen saturation monitoring should be continuous.

Malignant Hyperthermia

MH is a rare inherited muscle disorder that is chemically induced by the administration of a volatile anesthetic agent with or without succinylcholine, but in a small percentage of cases, MH appears to be triggered by succinylcholine alone in the absence of a volatile agent (Litman et al., 2019). In the 1970s, mortality rates exceeded 80% whereas in recent years it has decreased to approximately 1.4% to 10% even with proper treatment (Bin et al., 2022). This decrease is largely due to the introduction of dantrolene sodium in 1979, the development of genetics testing, early detection, education, and treatment with specific institutional protocols. Identification of patients at risk for MH is imperative. Susceptible people include those with strong and bulky muscles, familial genetic mutations as described earlier, first-degree relatives who have been diagnosed or suspected of MH, and an unexplained death of a family member during surgery that was accompanied by a febrile response. It is important to note that previous history of exposure to triggering agents without developing MH does not exclude the possibility of a future MH crisis since half of afflicted patients may have had a prior uneventful exposure (Hajmohamed & Suh, 2023).

During anesthesia, potent agents such as inhalation anesthetics (halothane, enflurane) and muscle relaxants (succinylcholine) may trigger the symptoms of MH (refer to Table 4-6 for list of anesthetic agents). Stress and some medications, such as sympathomimetics (epinephrine), theophylline, aminophylline, anticholinergics (atropine), and cardiac glycosides (digitalis), can induce or intensify such a reaction. The pathophysiology is related to a hypermetabolic condition in skeletal muscle cells that involves altered mechanisms of calcium function at the cellular level. This disruption of calcium causes clinical symptoms of hypermetabolism, which, in turn, increases muscle contraction (rigidity). The sustained muscle contraction causes hyperthermia (fever may exceed 110° F) and subsequent damage to the CNS.

The skeletal muscle cells, when depleted of their source of cellular energy (adenosine triphosphate [ATP]), break down and release the muscle cell contents, including myoglobin (a protein released from muscle when injury occurs), creatine phosphokinase (CPK), and potassium into the systemic circulation. The resulting hyperkalemia has a dramatic effect on the heart, causing ventricular arrhythmias. The muscle pigment myoglobin has an affinity for the kidneys, resulting in potential for kidney failure (refer to Chapter 41, Box 41-9 for details). If untreated, cardiac arrest, kidney failure, blood coagulation problems, internal hemorrhage, brain injury, liver failure, and death can result.

The initial symptoms of MH are related to cardiovascular and musculoskeletal activity. Tachycardia (heart rate >150 bpm) is often the earliest sign. In addition to the tachycardia, sympathetic nervous stimulation leads to ventricular arrhythmia, hypotension, decreased cardiac output, oliguria (less than 400 mL), and, later, cardiac arrest. With the abnormal transport of calcium, rigidity or tetanus-like movements occur, often in the jaw. The rise in temperature is actually a late sign that develops rapidly, and higher core body temperature correlates with increased morbidity; body temperature can increase 1.8° F (1° C) every 5 minutes if untreated (Hajmohamed & Suh, 2023; Phillips & Hornacky, 2021e). The core body temperature can reach or exceed 42° C (104° F) in a very short time and must be properly monitored and recorded during surgery. Clinical signs of patients with MH include: hypercarbia (elevated carbon dioxide in the blood); sinus tachycardia; rapidly increasing temperature; elevated temperature; masseter muscle spasm, also known as masseter muscle spasm after succinylcholine administration (the muscle covering the side of the jaw nearest the ear, responsible for mastication [chewing]); generalized muscular rigidity; tachypnea (increased respiratory rate); profuse diaphoresis; cola-colored urine; cyanosis; skin mottling; cardiac arrhythmias; excessive bleeding; and unstable blood pressure (Phillips & Hornacky, 2021e; Watt & McAllister, 2022). The entire health team is alert for the presence of any of the aforementioned signs.

Recognizing symptoms early and discontinuing anesthesia promptly are imperative. The immediate response is the discontinuation of the triggering agent and hyperventilation of the patient with 100% oxygen to treat the effects of hypercapnia, metabolic acidosis, and increased oxygen consumption and immediate administration of at least 2.5 mg/kg of dantrolene sodium intravenously (Watt & McAllister, 2022). Additional incremental doses may be required until the signs of MH are controlled. Because dantrolene is available in 20-mg multidose vials that must be reconstituted with 50 mL of sterile water only, it is expected that at least two nurses will be reconstituting the drug during the crisis. Because large volumes of medications and IV fluids are required, a central line is initiated (Phillips & Hornacky, 2021e). Cold normal saline is adminstered IV at a rate of 15 mL/kg every 15 minutes for at least 45 minutes; Ringer solution is not recommended because each liter contains 4 mEq/L of potassium, and there is concern over increasing the level of metabolic acidosis (Phillips & Hornacky, 2021e). If the patient is hyperthermic, active cooling is initiated with iced saline lavage of the stomach, bladder, rectum, and open body cavities if appropriate with iced saline, use of a hypothermia blanket, and use of ice packs. It is essential to monitor the patient's temperature to assess treatment efficacy and avoidance of hypothermia. The cooling measures are continued until the patient's core temperature reaches 38° C (100.4° F) (Spruce, 2020). Antiarrhythmic medications, such as amiodarone, are expected for management of ventricular arrhythmias; infusion by IV glucose and insulin, as well as calcium chloride, is anticipated for the hyperkalemia. Sodium bicarbonate may be administered to treat the metabolic acidosis based upon ABG analysis. In addition, mannitol and diuretics may be administered to assist with the clearance of filtered myoglobin into the urine; hourly urine output and color of urine are observed closely (Watt & McAllister, 2022).

Goals of treatment are to decrease metabolism, reverse metabolic and respiratory acidosis, correct arrhythmias, decrease body temperature, provide oxygen and nutrition to tissues, and correct electrolyte imbalance. The Malignant Hyperthermia Association of the United States (MHAUS) publishes a treatment protocol that should be posted in the OR and be readily available on an MH cart. Although MH is uncommon, all providers must identify patients at risk, recognize the signs and symptoms, have the appropriate medication and equipment available, and be knowledgeable about the protocol to follow. This preparation may be life-saving for the patient.

Disseminated Intravascular Coagulation

DIC is a dynamic systemic disorder that results in widespread hemorrhage and microthrombosis with ischemia. It can be a side effect of MH or a precursor to the development of MH. The mortality rate exceeds 75%, and clinical manifestations may be bleeding from mucous membranes, venipuncture sites, and the GI and urinary tracts (Cohn & Gultawatvichai, 2022). Bleeding can range from minimal occult internal bleeding to profuse hemorrhage from all orifices. It is important that all providers are alert for the subtle cues of developing DIC. Refer to Chapter 19 for complete details of DIC.

POSTOPERATIVE NURSING

The **postoperative phase** begins when the patient is transferred to the PACU and report is given by the anesthesia provider and circulating nurse to the perianesthesia nurse. The postoperative phase ends when the patient is discharged from all phases of postoperative care. The scope of nursing care in this phase covers a wide range of activities, including maintaining the patient's airway, monitoring vital signs, assessing the effects of the anesthetic agents, assessing the patient for complications, and providing comfort and pain relief. Nursing activities also focus on promoting the patient's recovery and initiating the teaching, follow-up care, and referrals essential for recovery and rehabilitation after discharge.

Nursing Management During Postanesthesia Care

Postanesthesia care in some hospitals and ambulatory surgical centers is divided into two phases. In **phase I PACU**, which is the immediate recovery phase, intensive nursing care is provided. In **phase II PACU**, the patient is prepared for self-care or care in the hospital, an extended-care setting, or discharge. Recliners rather than stretchers or beds are standard in many phase II units. In facilities without separate phases, the patient remains in the PACU and may be discharged home directly from this unit.

The nursing management objectives for the nurse in the PACU are to provide care until the patient has recovered from the effects of anesthesia (e.g., until resumption of motor and sensory functions), is oriented or returns to baseline cognition, has stable vital signs and adequate pain control, and shows no evidence of hemorrhage or other complications. All PACU nurses have special skills, including strong assessment skills. The PACU nurse provides frequent monitoring (every 15 minutes) of the patient's pulse, ECG, respiratory rate, blood pressure, and pulse oximeter value (blood oxygen level). In some cases, the end-tidal carbon dioxide ($ETCO_2$) level is monitored as well. The patient's airway may become obstructed because of the latent effects of recent anesthesia, and the PACU nurse must be prepared to assist in reintubation and in handling other emergencies that may occur. Nurses in PACUs must also possess excellent patient teaching skills.

Admitting the Patient to the PACU

Transferring the postoperative patient from the OR to the PACU is the responsibility of the anesthesia provider. During transport from the OR to the PACU, the anesthesia provider remains at the head of the stretcher (to maintain the airway), and a surgical team member remains at the opposite end. Transporting the patient involves special consideration of the incision site, potential vascular changes, and exposure. The surgical incision is considered every time the postoperative patient is moved; many wounds are closed under considerable tension, and every effort is made to prevent further strain on the incision. The patient is positioned so that they are not lying on or obstructing drains or drainage tubes. Serious orthostatic hypotension may occur when a patient is moved too quickly from one position to another (e.g., from a lithotomy position to a horizontal position or from a lateral to a supine position), so the patient must be moved slowly and carefully. As soon as the patient is placed on the stretcher or bed, the soiled gown is removed and replaced with a dry gown. The patient is covered with lightweight blankets and warmed. Three side rails may be raised to prevent falls.

Assessing the Patient

The cornerstones of nursing care in the PACU are frequent, skilled assessments of the blood oxygen saturation level, pulse rate and regularity, depth and nature of respirations, skin color, LOC, and ability to respond to commands. The nurse performs a baseline assessment and then checks the surgical site for drainage or hemorrhage and makes sure that all drainage tubes and monitoring lines are connected and functioning. The nurse checks any IV fluids or medications currently infusing and verifies dosage and rate.

After the initial assessment, the patient's vital signs and general physical status are assessed at least every 15 minutes. Patency of the airway and respiratory function are always evaluated first, followed by assessment of cardiovascular function, the condition of the surgical site, and function of the CNS. Any surgical procedure has the potential for injury due to disrupted neurovascular integrity resulting from prolonged awkward positioning in the OR, manipulation of tissues, inadvertent severing of nerves, or tight bandages. Any orthopedic surgery or surgery involving the extremities carries a risk of peripheral nerve damage. Vascular surgeries, such as replacing sections of diseased peripheral arteries or inserting an arteriovenous graft, put the patient at risk for thrombus formation at the surgical site and subsequent ischemia of tissues distal to the thrombus. Assessment of *circulation, sensation, and mobility* (CSM) includes having the patient move the hand or foot distal to the surgical site through a full range of motion, assessing all surfaces for intact sensation, and assessing peripheral pulses and capillary refill. Refer to Table 39-3, Assessing for Peripheral Nerve Function, for specific nerve monitoring on page 1293. The nurse must be aware of any pertinent information from the patient's history that may be significant (e.g., patient is deaf or hard of hearing, has a history of seizures, has diabetes, is allergic to certain medications or to latex).

Maintaining a Patent Airway

The primary objective in the immediate postoperative period is to maintain pulmonary ventilation and thus prevent hypoxemia (reduced oxygen in the blood) and hypercapnia (excess carbon dioxide in the blood). Both can occur if the airway is obstructed and ventilation is reduced (hypoventilation). Besides checking the provider's orders for and administering supplemental oxygen, the nurse assesses respiratory rate and depth, ease of respirations, oxygen saturation, and breath sounds.

Patients who have experienced prolonged anesthesia usually are unconscious, with all muscles relaxed. This relaxation extends to the muscles of the pharynx. When the patient lies on their back, the lower jaw and the tongue fall backward and the air passages become obstructed (Fig. 4-6). This is called *hypopharyngeal obstruction.* Nursing actions can include stimulating the patient to take deep breaths, positioning the patient on their side, and providing supplemental oxygen if needed (Odom-Forren, 2023). If the patient remains unresponsive, the nurse may conduct the chin tilt or jaw thrust (refer to Chapter 55) to open the airway (Odom-Forren, 2023).

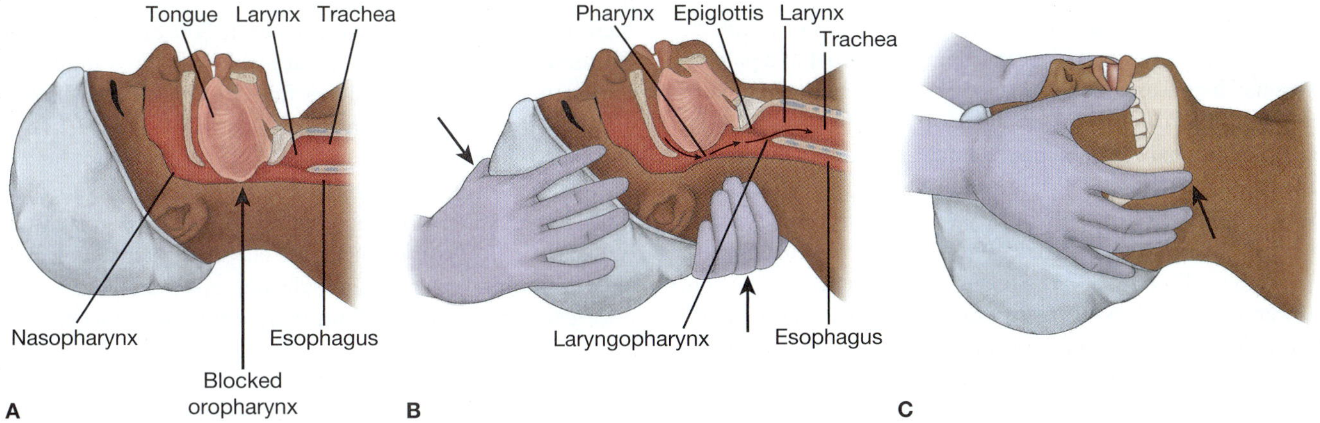

FIGURE 4-6 (A) A hypopharyngeal obstruction occurs when neck flexion permits the chin to drop toward the chest; obstruction almost always occurs when the head is in the midposition. (B) Tilting the head back to stretch the anterior neck structure lifts the base of the tongue off the posterior pharyngeal wall. The direction of the arrows indicates the pressure of the hands. (C) Opening the mouth is necessary to correct valve-like obstruction of the nasal passage during expiration, which occurs in about 30% of unconscious patients. Open the patient's mouth (separate lips and teeth) and move the lower jaw forward, so that the lower teeth are in front of the upper teeth. To regain backward tilt of the neck, lift with both hands at the ascending rami of the mandible.

Pearls for Practice

Signs of hypopharyngeal occlusion include choking; noisy and irregular respirations; decreased oxygen saturation; and, within minutes, a blue, dusky color (cyanosis) of the skin. Because movement of the thorax and the diaphragm does not necessarily indicate that the patient is breathing, the nurse needs to place their palm at the patient's nose and mouth to feel the exhaled breath.

The anesthesia provider may leave a hard rubber or plastic airway in the patient's mouth (oral airway is used with an unresponsive patient) or nares (nasal airway is better tolerated by an arousable or awake patient) to maintain a patent airway (Odom-Forren, 2023). Such a device should not be removed until signs such as gagging indicate that reflex action is returning. Alternatively, the patient may enter the PACU with an endotracheal tube still in place and may require continued mechanical ventilation. The nurse maintains the head of bed elevation at 30 degrees or greater while intubated (to decrease risk of aspiration) if not contraindicated, and assists in initiating the use of the ventilator and in the weaning and extubation processes. Some patients, particularly those who have had extensive or lengthy surgical procedures, may be transferred from the OR directly to the intensive care unit (ICU) or from the PACU to the ICU while still intubated and receiving mechanical ventilation.

Respiratory difficulty also can result from excessive secretion of mucus or aspiration of vomitus. Placing the patient on their side in the recovery position will allow the fluid to escape from the mouth. The head of the bed is elevated 15 to 30 degrees unless contraindicated, and the patient is closely monitored to maintain the airway as well as to minimize the risk of aspiration. If vomiting occurs, the patient is turned to the side to prevent aspiration, and the vomitus is collected in the emesis basin. Mucus or vomitus obstructing the pharynx or the trachea is suctioned with a pharyngeal suction tip or a nasal catheter introduced into the nasopharynx or oropharynx. Caution is necessary in suctioning the throat of a patient who has had a tonsillectomy or other oral or laryngeal surgery because of risk of bleeding and discomfort.

An additional common postoperative respiratory complication is laryngospasm, which is usually the result of an irritable airway or allergy in which the laryngeal muscles contract and the vocal chords either partially or completely obstruct the airway (Odom-Forrem, 2023). Symptoms may include wheezing (lower airway narrowing) or stridor (upper airway narrowing), flaring nostrils, accessory use of muscles, central cyanosis, decreased oxygen saturation, restlessness, hypoxemia, a rocking motion of the chest when attempting to breathe (O'Brien, 2018), and respiratory obstruction (Odom-Forrem, 2023). The nurse should hyperextend the patient's neck, coach the patient to take slow, deep breaths, administer humidified oxygen, and prepare to administer an aerosol with racemic epinephrine (an inhalation sympathomimetic bronchodilator agent) to decrease airway swelling, while offering reassurance since patients are often frightened (Odom-Forrem, 2023; Schick, 2021). Decadron may also be prescribed to reduce the inflammation. Since edema may recur, the patient is observed closely.

Maintaining Cardiovascular Stability

To monitor cardiovascular stability, the nurse assesses the patient's mental status; vital signs; cardiac rhythm; skin temperature, color, and moisture; and urine output. Central venous pressure, pulmonary artery pressure, and arterial lines are monitored if the patient's condition requires such assessment. The nurse also assesses the patency of all IV lines. The primary cardiovascular complications seen in the PACU include hypotension and shock, hemorrhage, hypertension, and arrhythmias.

Hypotension and Shock

Hypotension can result from blood loss, hypoventilation, position changes, pooling of blood in the extremities, or side effects of medications and anesthetics. The most common cause is loss of circulating volume through blood and plasma loss. If the amount of blood loss exceeds 500 mL (especially if the loss is rapid), replacement is usually indicated.

Fluid loss is a significant potential problem for surgical patients, owing to their preoperative NPO status, evaporation of fluid intraoperatively, and significant shifting of sodium-rich fluid from the intravascular space to the extracellular space because of inflammatory process, trauma, or infection. The fluid lost from the blood stream sequesters in the tissues or "third space," which may be noted by the presence of edema. It is important for the nurse to understand that, although the patient may clinically present with edema (often associated with fluid volume excess), a hypovolemia exists intravascularly that can progress to shock if fluids are not managed adequately. In addition, the nurse considers fluid loss related to evaporation in the OR. For example, it is estimated that, with surgery involving an open abdomen, insensible fluid losses can reach 500 to 1,000 mL/hr (Rothrock, 2019). When evaluating the patient's fluid volume status, the nurse considers fluid loss from the nasogastric tube, urinary output, drains, estimated blood loss (EBL), and evaporation.

Shock, one of the most serious postoperative complications, can result from hypovolemia and decreased intravascular volume. The types of shock are classified as hypovolemic, cardiogenic, neurogenic, anaphylactic, septic, distributive and obstructive. See Chapter 53 for more information on shock.

Hemorrhage

Hemorrhage is an uncommon yet serious complication of surgery that can result in death. It can present insidiously or emergently at any time in the immediate postoperative period or up to several days after surgery (Table 4-7). When blood loss is extreme, the patient is apprehensive, restless, agitated and thirsty; the skin is cold, moist, and pale. The pulse rate

TABLE **4-7 Classifications of Hemorrhage**

Classification	Defining Characteristic
Time Frame	
Primary	Hemorrhage occurs at the time of surgery.
Intermediary	Hemorrhage occurs during the first few hours after surgery when the rise of blood pressure to its normal level dislodges insecure clots from untied vessels.
Secondary	Hemorrhage may occur sometime after surgery if a suture slips because a blood vessel was not tied securely, became infected, or was eroded by a drainage tube.
Type of Vessel	
Capillary	Hemorrhage is characterized by a slow, general ooze.
Venous	Darkly colored blood bubbles out quickly.
Arterial	Blood is bright red and appears in spurts with each heartbeat.
Visibility	
Evident	Hemorrhage is on the surface and can be seen.
Concealed	Hemorrhage is in a body cavity and cannot be seen.

increases, the temperature falls, hypotension is seen with a narrowed pulse pressure (difference between systolic and diastolic pressure; normal pulse pressure is approximately 40 mm Hg), and respirations are rapid and deep, often of the gasping type spoken of as "air hunger." Capillary refill is prolonged (normal is less than 2 seconds), and there is diminished urine output. If hemorrhage progresses untreated, cardiac output decreases, arterial and venous blood pressure and hemoglobin levels fall rapidly, the lips and the conjunctivae become pale, and the patient grows weaker and obtunded but remains conscious until near death.

Pearls for Practice

The term obtunded comes from the root word, obtund, which means "dulled or less sharp," and is used to describe a patient who presents with less than full alertness (altered LOC). Rather than use broad terms like stuporous or obtunded, it is beneficial to describe the behavior in detail.

Pearls for Practice

When bleeding is present, the nurse recognizes that fluid replacement typically follows a "3 in 1" rule (depending on comorbidities), where 300 mL of an isotonic IV fluid is infused for every 100 mL shed blood (3:1), whereas replacement with blood products (e.g., packed red blood cells [PRBCs], fresh frozen plasma [FFP]) is calculated at a 1:1 ratio (100 mL blood loss with 100 mL of blood products) (Schick, 2021). In addition, the nurse may see a ratio where PRBCs, FFP, and platelets are infused at a ratio of 1:1:1 or 2:1:1. Research reveals that early resuscitation with a 1:1:1 ratio resulted in greater rates of achieving hemostasis and fewer deaths due to exsanguination at 24 hours (Moore & Raval, 2022, pp. 4–5).

The initial therapeutic measures are transfusing blood or blood products and determining the cause of hemorrhage. The surgical site and incision should always be inspected for bleeding. If bleeding is evident, a sterile gauze pad and a pressure dressing are applied to reinforce the original surgical dressing, and the site of the bleeding is elevated to heart level if possible. The patient is placed in the shock position (flat on back; legs elevated at a 20-degree angle; knees kept straight). If hemorrhage is suspected but cannot be visualized, the patient may be taken back to the OR for emergency exploration of the surgical site.

In addition, the nurse should be aware of any special considerations related to blood loss replacement. Some patients may decline blood transfusions for religious or cultural reasons and may identify this request on their advance directives or living will.

Pearls for Practice

*Always wear gloves when handling blood. To prevent warming of the blood, administration should begin within 30 minutes of retrieving the blood. If this is not possible, the blood should be returned to the blood bank. Baseline vital signs are obtained. Normal saline injection (0.9% sodium chloride) is used to initiate a transfusion of red blood cells (RBCs), whole blood, platelets, or leukocytes. Hypotonic or hypertonic solutions are **never used** because hemolysis of the RBCs occurs. No medications or other solutions except 0.9% sodium chloride should be added to or infused simultaneously through the same blood set. Refer to Chapter 19 for more details on blood transfusion.*

Pearls for Practice

Hemoglobin levels as low as 7 g/dL are generally tolerated by most asymptomatic patients; however, for patients with cardiopulmonary disease a goal of 9 to 10 g/dL may be appropriate for major surgery (Cohn, 2020). The nurse understands that the transfusion of 1 unit of packed RBCs should increase the hemoglobin level by 1 g/dL and the hematocrit by 3%.

Hypertension and Arrhythmias

Hypertension is common in the immediate postoperative period secondary to sympathetic nervous system stimulation from pain, hypoxia, or bladder distention. Arrhythmias are associated with electrolyte imbalance, altered respiratory function, pain, hypothermia, stress, and anesthetic agents. Both hypertension and arrhythmias are managed by treating the underlying causes.

Relieving Pain and Anxiety

IV opioid analgesics are administered judiciously and often in the PACU. IV opioids provide immediate pain relief and are short acting, thus minimizing the potential for drug interactions or prolonged respiratory depression while there are anesthetics still active in the patient's system. The PACU nurse monitors the patient's physiologic status, manages pain, and provides psychological support in an effort to relieve the patient's fears and concerns. The nurse checks the medical record for special needs and concerns of the patient. When the patient's condition permits, a close member of the family may visit in the PACU. This often decreases the family's anxiety and helps the patient feel more secure.

Controlling Nausea and Vomiting

Postoperative and postdischarge nausea and vomiting (PONV/PDNV) is one of the most commonly occurring postoperative complications, frequently resulting in prolonged postoperative stay, unanticipated admission, and increased health care costs. Postoperative nausea occurs with an incidence of approximately 40% to 50%, vomiting of 25% to 30%, and PONV of 30% (Gecit & Ozbayir, 2020, p. 625). Health care providers have yet to reach consensus regarding an evidence-based multidisciplinary, multimodel treatment approach to PONV/PDNV. The nurse should intervene at the patient's first report of nausea to control the problem rather than wait for it to progress to vomiting.

Many medications are available to control nausea and vomiting without oversedating the patient; they are commonly administered during surgery, as well as in the PACU. Medications such as metoclopramide, prochlorperazine, promethazine, dimenhydrinate, hydroxyzine, and scopolamine are commonly prescribed (Rothrock, 2019). Although it is costly, ondansetron is frequently used as an effective antiemetic with few side effects.

ASPAN has developed a practice guideline for nurses to treat this postoperative complication (Odom-Forren, 2021). It includes the identification of risk factors (e.g., for adults undergoing general inhaled anesthesia); risks include female sex, being a nonsmoker, young age, history of PONV or motion sickness, and the use of postoperative intravenous opioids and type of surgery (increased incidence in laparoscopic, bariatric, gynecologic surgery; and cholecystectomy; Gan et al., 2020). Recommended treatments can range from no prophylaxis treatment to several antiemetic combinations for patients at higher risk (Gan et al., 2020; Odom-Forren, 2021).

Preparing for Discharge from the PACU

A patient remains in the PACU until fully recovered from the anesthetic agent. Indicators of recovery include stable blood pressure, adequate respiratory function, adequate oxygen saturation level compared with baseline, and spontaneous movement or movement on command. Discharge criteria should be developed collaboratively with the anesthesia department using the standards below:

- Stable vital signs
- Return to baseline LOC
- Uncompromised pulmonary function and adequate airway
- Ability to cough and clear secretions
- Pulse oximetry readings indicating adequate blood oxygen saturation
- Adequate intake and output
- Nausea and vomiting absent or under control
- Acceptable pain level
- Stable sensory and motor function
- Satisfactory condition of surgical site; patent tubes, drains, IVs and catheters

Many hospitals use a scoring system (e.g., Aldrete score) to determine the patient's general condition and readiness for transfer from the PACU. Throughout the recovery period, the patient's physical signs are observed and evaluated by means of a scoring system based on a set of objective criteria (Aldrete & Wright, 1992; Cook, 2021) that includes consciousness, activity, breathing, pulse oximetry, and circulation. The patient is assessed at regular intervals (e.g., every 15 minutes), and a total score is calculated and recorded on the assessment record. Patients remain in the PACU until their condition improves or they can be transferred safely to an ICU or surgical unit or discharged (depending on their preoperative baseline score).

The patient is discharged from the phase I PACU by the anesthesia provider to the critical care unit, the medical-surgical unit, the phase II PACU, or home with a responsible family member.

Nursing Management of Direct Discharge Home

To ensure patient safety and recovery, expert patient teaching and discharge planning are necessary when a patient undergoes same-day or ambulatory surgery. Because anesthetics cloud memory for concurrent events, verbal and written instructions should be given to both the patient and the adult who will be accompanying the patient home. Alternative formats (e.g., large print, Braille) of instructions or use of a sign interpreter may be required to ensure patient and family understanding. A translator may be required if the patient and family members do not understand English.

The patient and caregiver (e.g., family member or friend) are informed about expected outcomes and immediate, anticipated postoperative changes. The nurse provides written instructions about wound care, activity and dietary recommendations, medications, and follow-up visits to the surgeon. The patient's caregiver at home is provided with verbal and written instructions about what to look for and about the actions to take if complications occur. Prescriptions and medication reconciliation are given to the patient and/or caregiver. The nurse's or surgeon's telephone number is provided, and the patient and caregiver are encouraged to call with questions and to schedule follow-up appointments.

Pearls for Practice

Medication reconciliation is the process of creating the most accurate list possible of all medications a patient is taking—including drug name, dosage, frequency, and route—and comparing that list against the provider's admission, transfer, and/or discharge orders, with the goal of providing correct medications to the patient at all transition points within the hospital (Institute for Healthcare Improvement [IHI], 2022).

Although recovery time varies depending on the type and extent of surgery and the patient's overall condition, instructions usually advise limited activity for 24 to 48 hours. During this time, the patient should not drive a vehicle, drink alcoholic beverages, or perform tasks that require energy or skill. Fluids may be consumed as desired, and smaller-than-normal amounts may be eaten at mealtime. Patients are cautioned not to make important decisions at this time, because the medications, anesthesia, and surgery may affect their decision-making ability.

Nursing Management of the Hospitalized Postoperative Patient

Given the complexities of patient care treatment and management, multisystem disease, and workplace demands, it is important that the traditional "nurse-to-nurse" patient handoff now be a comprehensive, thorough, and sophisticated account of patient information focusing on patient safety (Krenzischek, 2021). Hand-off communication must also allow opportunity for questions to be answered. The *SBAR* format is an increasingly popular approach to the standardization of relaying of this crucial information. SBAR is a mnemonic for:

Situation (What is happening at the present time?)
Background (What are the circumstances leading up to this situation?)
Assessment (What do I think the problem is?)
Recommendation (What should we do to correct the problem?) (IHI, n.d.).

Whatever approach is used in each institution, it is essential that the method is used by all staff members during all hand-offs across all phases of surgical patient care.

Receiving the Patient in the Clinical Unit

The patient's room is readied by assembling the necessary equipment and supplies: IV pole, drainage receptacle holder, suction equipment, oxygen, emesis basin, tissues, disposable pads, blankets, and postoperative documentation. When the call comes to the unit about the patient's transfer from the PACU, the need for any additional items should be communicated. The PACU nurse reports data about the patient to the receiving nurse. The report includes relevant demographic data, medical diagnosis, procedure performed, type of anesthesia, comorbid conditions, allergies, unexpected intraoperative events, EBL, types and amounts of fluids received, medications administered for pain, types of IV fluids or medications infused, whether the patient has voided, and information that the patient and family have received about the patient's condition. Usually, the surgeon speaks to the family after surgery and relays the general condition of the patient. The receiving nurse reviews the postoperative orders, admits the patient to the unit, performs an initial assessment, and attends to the patient's immediate needs.

Providing Care for the First 24 Hours After Surgery

During the first 24 hours after surgery, nursing care of the hospitalized patient on the general medical-surgical unit involves continuing to help the patient recover from the effects of anesthesia, frequently assessing the patient's physiologic status, monitoring for complications, managing pain, and implementing measures designed to achieve the long-range goals of independence with self-care, successful management of the therapeutic regimen, discharge to home, and full recovery. In the initial hours after admission to the clinical unit, primary concerns include adequate ventilation, hemodynamic stability, incisional pain, surgical site integrity, nausea and vomiting, neurologic status, and spontaneous voiding. The pulse rate, blood pressure, respiration rate, and oxygen saturation are recorded per institutional policy. Typically, vital signs are recorded frequently until stable and then regularly until the patient is discharged. Frequency of vital sign measurements will depend upon the nature of the operation and the clinical course. Thereafter, vital signs are measured less frequently if they remain stable.

Typically, patients begin to return to their usual state of health several hours after surgery or after waking up the next morning. Although pain may still be intense, many patients feel more alert, less nauseous, and less anxious. They have begun their breathing and leg exercises, and many will have dangled their legs over the edge of the bed, stood, and ambulated a few feet or been assisted out of bed to the chair at least once. Many will have tolerated a light meal and had IV fluids discontinued. The focus of care shifts from intense physiologic management and symptomatic relief of the adverse effects of anesthesia to regaining independence with self-care and preparing for discharge (all discussed in the following nursing process section).

NURSING PROCESS

The Hospitalized Patient Recovering from Surgery

ASSESSMENT

Assessment of the hospitalized postoperative patient includes monitoring vital signs, completing a review of the systems, and observing for potential postoperative complications on arrival of the patient to the clinical unit and at regular intervals thereafter.

Respiratory status is important because pulmonary complications are among the most frequent and serious problems encountered by the surgical patient. The nurse observes for airway patency, watching for laryngeal edema, which is often heralded by inspiratory stridor. The quality of respirations, including depth, rate, and sound, are assessed regularly. Chest auscultation verifies that breath sounds are normal (or abnormal) bilaterally, and the findings are documented as a baseline for later comparisons. Pulse oximetry is assessed to monitor respiratory status and end-tidal carbon dioxide, if appropriate. Often, because of the effects of analgesic and anesthetic medications, respirations are slow. Shallow and rapid respirations may be caused by pain, constricting dressings, gastric dilation, abdominal distention, or obesity. Noisy breathing may be due to obstruction by secretions or the tongue.

The nurse assesses the patient's pain level using a verbal or visual analog scale and assesses the characteristics of the pain. The patient's appearance, pulse, respirations, blood pressure, skin color (adequate or cyanotic), and skin temperature (cold and clammy, warm and moist, or warm and dry) are clues to cardiovascular function. When the patient arrives in the clinical unit, the surgical site is observed for bleeding, type and integrity of dressings, and functioning of all tubes and drains.

The nurse also assesses the patient's mental status and LOC, speech, and orientation, and compares them with the preoperative baseline. Although a change in mental status or postoperative restlessness may be related to anxiety, pain, or medications, it may also be a symptom of oxygen deficit, hypoglycemia, or hemorrhage. These serious causes must be investigated and excluded before other causes are pursued.

General discomfort resulting from lying in one position on the operating table, the surgeon's handling of tissues, the body's reaction to anesthesia, and anxiety are also common causes of restlessness. These discomforts may be relieved by administering the prescribed analgesics, changing the patient's position frequently, and assessing and alleviating the cause of anxiety. Drainage-soaked bandages may cause discomfort. The nurse reinforces or changes the dressing completely, as prescribed by the provider, which may make the patient more comfortable. The bladder is assessed for distention, because urinary retention can also cause restlessness.

DIAGNOSIS

Major nursing diagnoses may include the following:

- Ineffective airway clearance related to depressed respiratory function, pain, and bed rest
- Acute pain related to surgical incision
- Decreased cardiac output related to shock or hemorrhage
- Activity intolerance related to generalized weakness secondary to surgery
- Altered skin integrity related to surgical incision and drains
- Ineffective thermoregulation related to surgical environment and anesthetic agents
- Malnutrition risk, less than body requirements, related to decreased intake and increased need for nutrients secondary to surgery
- Constipation risk related to effects of medications, surgery, dietary change, and immobility
- Urinary retention
- Injury risk related to surgical procedure/positioning or anesthetic agents
- Anxiety related to surgical procedure
- Ineffective self-health management risk of therapeutic regimen related to wound care, dietary restrictions, activity recommendations, medications, follow-up care, or signs and symptoms of complications

PLANNING

The major goals for the patient include optimal respiratory function, relief of pain, optimal cardiovascular function, increased activity tolerance, unimpaired wound healing, maintenance of body temperature, and maintenance of nutritional balance. Further goals include resumption of usual pattern of bowel and bladder elimination, identification of any perioperative positioning injury, acquisition of sufficient knowledge to manage self-care after discharge, and absence of complications.

NURSING INTERVENTIONS

PROMOTING RESPIRATORY FUNCTION

Increasing age, smoking, COPD, long duration of surgery, and incisional site (chest and upper abdomen), as well as comorbidities, such as heart failure, arrhythmias, diabetes mellitus, and swallowing disorders, are associated with an increased risk for postoperative pulmonary complications. Respiratory depressive effects of opioid medications, decreased lung expansion secondary to pain, operative position that may have limited maximum respiratory function, impaired mucociliary clearance of secretions, and decreased mobility combine to put the patient at risk for common respiratory complications, particularly atelectasis (alveolar collapse; incomplete expansion of the alveoli), pneumonia, and hypoxemia (Marley, 2021). Atelectasis remains a risk for the patient who is not moving well or ambulating, who is not performing deep breathing or coughing out retained secretions, or who is not using an incentive spirometer. Signs and symptoms include decreased breath sounds over the affected area, crackles, and cough. Pneumonia is characterized by chills and fever, tachycardia, and tachypnea. Cough may or may not be present and may or may not be productive. Risk factors for postoperative pneumonia are patients with COPD, impaired cough, and acute bronchitis or lower airway infections.

Pearls for Practice

Hemoglobin (Hb), the main component of erythrocytes (red blood cells [RBCs]), provides the transportation of oxygen and carbon dioxide and a normal level is approximately 15 g of hemoglobin per 100 mL of blood. Cyanosis appears when a minimum of 5 g/dL of deoxyhemoglobin is present in the blood; thus, the nurse needs to recognize that cyanosis may be marked in those patients with polycythemia (increase in the number of RBCs) but very difficult to detect in patients with anemia (Marley, 2021).

The types of hypoxemia that can affect postoperative patients are subacute and episodic. Subacute hypoxemia is a constant low level of oxygen saturation, although breathing appears normal. Episodic hypoxemia develops suddenly, and the patient may be at risk for cerebral dysfunction, myocardial ischemia, and cardiac arrest. Risk for hypoxemia is present in patients who have undergone major surgery (particularly thoracic or abdominal), are obese, or have pre-existing pulmonary problems. Hypoxemia can be detected by pulse oximetry, which measures blood oxygen saturation. Factors that may affect the accuracy of pulse oximetry readings include cold extremities, tremors, atrial fibrillation, and acrylic nails. Research reveals that different colored nail polish demonstrated altered pulse oximetry readings in healthy subjects, for example, blue, green and black nail polish produces falsely low readings; thus, it seems reasonable that nail polish should be removed prior to SpO_2 (peripheral capillary oxygen saturation) determination to ensure accurate readings (Philips & Hornacky, 2021e). False high saturations may be seen in patients who have elevated carboxyhemoglobin levels (recall smokers have higher levels because of carbon monoxide [CO]); a high carbon monoxide level is also seen in smoke inhalation and carbon monoxide poisoning and with dark skin tones and pigmentation (O_2 saturation overestimated by ~2%; Torp et al., 2022). Carboxyhemoglobin closely resembles oxyhemoglobin and is perceived by the sensor to be oxygenated; thus, the reading may be falsely elevated (Philips & Hornacky, 2021e). The nurse recognizes that pulse oximeters typically are calibrated to a range of saturation from 70% to 100% with an accuracy of 2% to 4%, which means that saturations lower than 70%, may not be accurate compared with ABGs. Refer to Chapter 7 for more details on oxygen saturation.

Preventive measures and timely recognition of signs and symptoms help avert pulmonary complications. Strategies to prevent respiratory complications include use of an incentive spirometer and deep-breathing exercises and sitting in an upright position that is unrestricted, thus allowing for maximum pulmonary expansion (if not contraindicated). Mobilization of patients is an important nursing intervention that will assist in maximizing lung expansion and improving circulation, thus facilitating gas exchange while additionally decreasing the risk of DVT. Crackles indicate static pulmonary secretions that need to be mobilized by coughing retained secretions and deep-breathing exercises. When a mucus plug obstructs one of the bronchi entirely, the pulmonary tissue beyond the plug collapses, and massive atelectasis results. Thus, coughing is also encouraged to dislodge mucus plugs.

Pearls for Practice

It is important to consider that coughing is a forced expiratory maneuver; thus, the nurse should encourage the patient to use the incentive spirometer or take deep breaths after coughing to re-expand alveoli. A common recommendation for use of the incentive spirometer is 10 deep breaths every hour while awake.

To clear secretions and prevent pneumonia, the nurse encourages the patient to turn frequently (every 2 hours) and take deep breaths hourly. These pulmonary exercises should begin as soon as the patient arrives on the clinical unit and continue until the patient is discharged. Even if the patient is not fully awake from anesthesia, they can be asked to take several deep breaths. This helps expel residual anesthetic agents, mobilize secretions, and prevent alveolar collapse (atelectasis). Careful splinting of abdominal or thoracic incision sites helps the patient overcome the fear that the exertion of coughing might open the incision. Analgesic agents are administered to permit more effective coughing, and oxygen is administered as prescribed to prevent or relieve hypoxia. To encourage lung expansion, the patient is encouraged to yawn or take sustained maximal inspirations to create a negative intrathoracic pressure and expand lung volume to total capacity.

Pearls for Practice

Coughing is contraindicated in patients who have head injuries or who have undergone intracranial surgery (because of the risk for increasing intracranial pressure) and in patients who have undergone eye surgery (because of the risk for increasing intraocular pressure) or plastic surgery (because of the risk for increasing tension on delicate tissues).

RELIEVING PAIN

Most patients experience some pain after a surgical procedure. Many factors (motivational, affective, cognitive, and emotional) influence the pain experience. The degree and severity of postoperative pain and the patient's tolerance for pain depend on the incision site, the nature of the surgical procedure, the extent of surgical trauma, the type of anesthetic agent, and how the

(*continued on page 148*)

agent was administered. The Agency for Healthcare Research and Policy reports that the most reliable indicator of the existence and intensity of pain is the patient's self-report. As noted over two decades ago by McCaffery, pain is "whatever the person says it is, existing whenever the experiencing person says it does" (McCaffery & Pasero, 1999, p. 5). The definition highlights the subjective nature of pain and that patients are the best authority on the existence of pain. Therefore, it is important to complete a thorough preoperative pain evaluation and develop pain goals for the surgical patient. This preparation, which includes information such as what to expect, how the pain will be managed, how to report, and reassurance, can contribute to reducing anxiety and, possibly, the level of postoperative pain experienced. Refer to Chapter 6 for details on patient-controlled analgesia (PCA) and epidural infusions.

For pain that is difficult to control, a subcutaneous pain management system may be used. This is a silicone catheter that is inserted at the site of the affected area. The catheter is attached to a pump that delivers a continuous amount of local anesthetic at a specific amount determined and prescribed by the provider.

Complete absence of pain in the area of the surgical incision may not occur for a few weeks, depending on the site and nature of the surgery, but the intensity of postoperative pain gradually subsides on subsequent days. However, pain control continues to be an important concern for the patient and the nurse. Effective pain management allows the patient to participate in care, perform deep-breathing and leg exercises, and tolerate activity. Poor pain control contributes to postoperative complications and increased length of stay. The nurse continues to assess the pain level, the effectiveness of analgesic agents, and factors that influence pain tolerance (e.g., energy level, stress level, cultural background, meaning of pain to the patient). The nurse explains that taking an analgesic agent before the pain becomes intense is more effective and offers medication to the patient at appropriate intervals rather than waiting for the patient to request it. Nonpharmacologic pain relief measures, such as imagery, music, relaxation, massage, application of heat or cold (if prescribed), and distraction, are discussed in Chapter 6.

PROMOTING CARDIAC OUTPUT

If signs and symptoms of shock or hemorrhage occur, treatment and nursing care are implemented as described previously in the discussion of care in the PACU.

Although most patients do not hemorrhage or go into shock, changes in circulating volume, the stress of surgery, and the effects of medications and preoperative preparations all affect cardiovascular function. IV fluid replacement is standard for up to 24 hours after surgery or until the patient is stable and tolerating oral fluids. Close monitoring is indicated to detect and correct conditions such as fluid volume deficit, altered tissue perfusion, and decreased cardiac output, all of which can increase the patient's discomfort, place them at risk of complications, and prolong the hospital stay. Some patients are at risk of fluid volume excess secondary to existing cardiovascular or renal disease, advanced age, or the release of adrenocorticotropic hormone and antidiuretic hormone as a result of the stress of surgery (Rothrock, 2019). Consequently, fluid replacement must be managed carefully, and intake and output records must be accurate.

Nursing management includes assessing the patency of the IV lines and ensuring that the correct fluids are administered at the prescribed rate. Intake and output, including emesis and output from wound drainage systems, are recorded separately and totaled to determine fluid balance. If the patient has an indwelling urinary catheter, hourly outputs are monitored, and rates of less than 30 mL/hr (0.5–1 mL/kg/hr) are reported; if the patient is voiding, an output of less than 240 mL per 8-hour shift is reported. Levels of electrolytes, hemoglobin, and hematocrit are monitored. Decreased hemoglobin and hematocrit levels can indicate blood loss or dilution of circulating volume by IV fluids. Recall that the fluid changes associated with surgery cause fluid extravasation into the tissues. This "third-spaced" fluid usually returns to the intravascular space by postop day (POD) 2 or 3. At this time period, the nurse assesses for evidence of fluid volume excess. If hemodilution is contributing to the decreased hemoglobin and hematocrit levels, the nurse expects that, as the stress response abates and fluids are mobilized and excreted, the hemoglobin and hematocrit will rise.

Venous stasis from dehydration, immobility, and pressure on leg veins during surgery put the patient at risk for DVT. Leg exercises and frequent position changes are initiated early in the postoperative period to stimulate circulation. Patients should avoid positions that compromise venous return, such as raising the bed's knee gatch, placing a pillow under the knees, sitting for long periods, and dangling the legs with pressure at the back of the knees. Venous return is promoted by elastic compression stockings, sequential compression devices (SCDs), and early ambulation. Early ambulation has a significant effect on recovery and the prevention of complications and can begin, in many instances, on the evening of surgery. Postoperative activity orders are checked before the patient is assisted in getting out of bed. Sitting up at the edge of the bed for a few minutes may be all that the patient who has undergone a major surgical procedure can tolerate at first.

ENCOURAGING ACTIVITY

Most surgical patients are encouraged to be out of bed as soon as possible. Early ambulation reduces the incidence of postoperative complications, such as atelectasis, hypostatic pneumonia, GI discomfort, and circulatory problems. Ambulation improves ventilation and reduces the stasis of bronchial secretions in the lungs. It also reduces postoperative abdominal distention by increasing GI tract and abdominal wall tone and stimulating peristalsis. Early ambulation prevents stasis of blood by increasing the rate of circulation in the extremities; as a result, thrombophlebitis or phlebothrombosis occurs less frequently. Often, pain is decreased when early ambulation is possible, and the hospital stay is shorter and less costly, a further advantage to the patient and the hospital.

Despite the advantages of early ambulation, patients may be reluctant to get out of bed on the evening of surgery. Reminding them of the importance of early mobility in preventing complications may help patients overcome their fears. When a patient gets out of bed for the first time, orthostatic hypotension, also called postural hypotension, is a concern. Orthostatic hypotension is an abnormal drop in blood pressure that occurs as the patient changes from a supine to a standing position (refer to Chapter 11). It is common after surgery because of changes in circulating blood volume and bed rest. Approximately 500–700 mL of blood momentarily shifts to the lower body when changing position to standing from supine, resulting in decreased venous return (decreased preload) and arterial pressure. Signs and symptoms include an increase in heart rate of 15 beats per minute (bpm) with a decrease in systolic pressure of 20 mm Hg or a 10 mm Hg decrease in diastolic pressure with position change (typically within 3 minutes). Patients often also complain of weakness, dizziness, leg buckling, and visual blurring. Older adults are at increased risk for orthostatic hypotension secondary to age-related changes in vascular tone. Refer to Chapter 11 for details on assessing for orthostatic hypotension.

To assist the postoperative patient in getting out of bed for the first time after surgery, the nurse:

- Helps the patient move gradually from the lying position to the sitting position by raising the head of the bed, and encourages the patient to splint the incision when applicable. It may be easier for postoperative patients with abdominal incisions to roll on their side first with the head of the bed elevated. Once the patient is on their side, the nurse has the patient move their feet off the side of the bed and push off their elbow into a sitting position.
- Positions the patient completely upright (sitting) and turned, so that both legs are hanging over the edge of the bed. The nurse allows the patient to sit for a few minutes and assesses for dizziness and vital sign changes if indicated. If patient is asymptomatic, the nurse asks the patient to push down with their arms on the mattress and stand up.
- Helps the patient stand beside the bed

After becoming accustomed to the upright position, the patient may start to walk. The nurse should be at the patient's side to give physical support and encouragement. Care must be taken not to tire the patient; the extent of the first few periods of ambulation varies with the type of surgical procedure and the patient's physical condition and age.

Whether or not the patient can ambulate early in the postoperative period, bed exercises are encouraged to improve circulation. Unless contraindicated by the operative event, bed exercises consist of the following:

- Arm exercises (full range of motion, with specific attention to abduction and external rotation of the shoulder)
- Hand and finger exercises
- Foot exercises to prevent DVT, foot drop, and toe deformities, and to aid in maintaining good circulation
- Leg flexion and leg-lifting exercises to prepare the patient for ambulation
- Abdominal and gluteal contraction exercises

Hampered by pain, dressings, IV lines, or drains, many patients cannot engage in activity without assistance. Prolonged inactivity may lead to pressure ulcers, DVT, atelectasis, constipation, anorexia, and malaise. Helping the patient increase their activity level on the first postoperative day is an important nursing function. One way to increase the patient's activity is to have the patient perform as much routine hygiene care as possible. Setting up the patient to bathe with a bedside wash basin or, if possible, assisting the patient to the bathroom to sit in a chair at the sink not only gets the patient moving but also helps restore a sense of self-control and prepares the patient for discharge.

To be discharged safely to home, patients need to be able to ambulate a functional distance (e.g., length of the house or apartment), get in and out of bed unassisted, and be independent with toileting if possible. Patients can be asked to perform as much as they can and then to call for assistance. The patient and the nurse can collaborate on a schedule for progressive activity that includes ambulating in the room and hallway and sitting out of bed in the chair. Assessing the patient's vital signs and oxygen saturation before, during, and after a scheduled activity helps the nurse and patient determine the rate of progression. By providing physical support, the nurse maintains the patient's safety; by communicating a positive attitude about the patient's ability to perform the activity, the nurse promotes the patient's confidence. The nurse should make sure the patient continues to perform bed exercises, wears pneumatic compression or elastic compression stockings when in bed, and rests as needed. If the patient has had orthopedic surgery of the lower extremities or will require a mobility aid (e.g., walker, crutches) at home, a physical therapist may be involved the first time the patient gets out of bed to teach how to ambulate safely or to use the mobility aid correctly. If patients are required to climb steps at home, their ability to do so must be assessed before discharge.

PROMOTING WOUND HEALING

Ongoing assessment of the surgical site involves inspection for approximation of wound edges, integrity of sutures or staples, redness, discoloration, warmth, swelling, unusual tenderness, or drainage. The area around the wound should also be inspected for a reaction to tape or trauma from tight bandages.

Principles of Wound Healing

With shorter hospital stays, much of the healing takes place at home, and both the hospital and home care nurse should be informed about the principles of wound healing. Surgical wound healing occurs in three phases: inflammatory, proliferative, and maturation (Table 4-8). Wounds also heal by different mechanisms, depending on the condition of the wound. These mechanisms are first-, second-, and third-intention wound healing (Fig. 4-7) (Rothrock, 2019).

First-Intention Healing. Wounds made aseptically with a minimum of tissue destruction that are properly closed will heal with little tissue reaction by first intention (primary union). When wounds heal by **first-intention healing**, granulation tissue is not visible and scar formation is minimal. Postoperatively, many

(*continued on page 150*)

TABLE 4-8 **Phases of Wound Healing**

Phase	Duration	Events
Inflammatory (also called lag or exudative phase)	1–4 days	Blood clot forms Wound becomes edematous Debris of damaged tissue and blood clot are phagocytosed
Proliferative (also called fibroblastic or connective tissue phase)	5–20 days	Collagen produced Granulation tissue forms Wound tensile strength increases
Maturation (also called differentiation, resorptive, remodeling, or plateau phase)	21 days to months or even years	Fibroblasts leave wound Tensile strength increases Collagen fibers reorganize and tighten to reduce scar size

of these wounds are covered with a dry sterile dressing. If a cyanoacrylate tissue adhesive (LiquiBand) was used to close the incision without sutures, a dressing is contraindicated.

Second-Intention Healing. **Second-intention healing** (granulation) occurs in infected wounds (abscess) or in wounds in which the edges have not been approximated. When an abscess is incised, it collapses partly, but the dead and dying cells forming its walls are still being released into the cavity. For this reason, drainage tubes are or gauze packing is inserted into the abscess pocket to allow drainage to escape easily. Gradually, the necrotic material disintegrates and escapes, and the abscess cavity fills with a red, soft, sensitive tissue that bleeds easily. This tissue is composed of minute, thin-walled capillaries and buds that later form connective tissue. These buds, called *granulations,* enlarge until they fill the area left by the destroyed tissue. Healing is complete when skin cells (epithelium) grow over these granulations. This method of repair is called *healing by granulation,* and it takes place whenever pus is formed or when loss of tissue has occurred for any reason. When the postoperative wound is to be allowed to heal by secondary intention, it is usually packed with moist saline sterile dressings and covered with a dry sterile dressing.

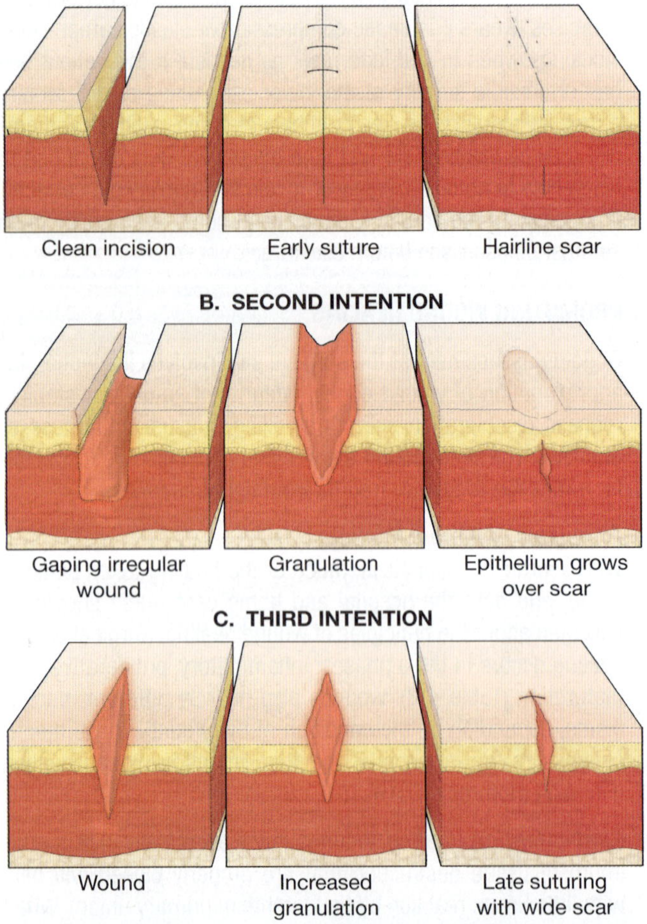

FIGURE 4-7 **Types of wound healing: first-intention healing, second-intention healing, and third-intention healing.**

Third-Intention Healing. **Third-intention healing** (secondary suture) is used for deep wounds that either have not been sutured early or break down and are resutured later, thus bringing together two opposing granulation surfaces. This results in a deeper and wider scar. These wounds are also packed postoperatively with moist gauze and covered with a dry sterile dressing.

Alternatively, wound vacuum-assisted closure (VAC) also known as *negative pressure wound therapy* may be used in the management of open wounds (Fig. 4-8). It applies subatmospheric pressure to the wound surface and consists of a foam dressing, semiocclusive adhesive cover, fluid collection system, and suction pump. The wound VAC removes exudates and reduces edema; it also has been shown to speed up the development of granulation tissue, increase angiogenesis, and reduce bacterial bioburden (Perry et al., 2022). Contraindications include wounds with necrotic tissue; malignancy within the wound; exposed arteries, veins, nerves, or vascular grafts; untreated osteomyelitis; and nonenteric and unexplored fistulas (Perry et al., 2022). The nurse follows institutional protocols regarding replacement of the vacuum dressings (variable, 3–7 days), and collaborates with wound care specialists as needed. Although continuous therapy is generally delivered

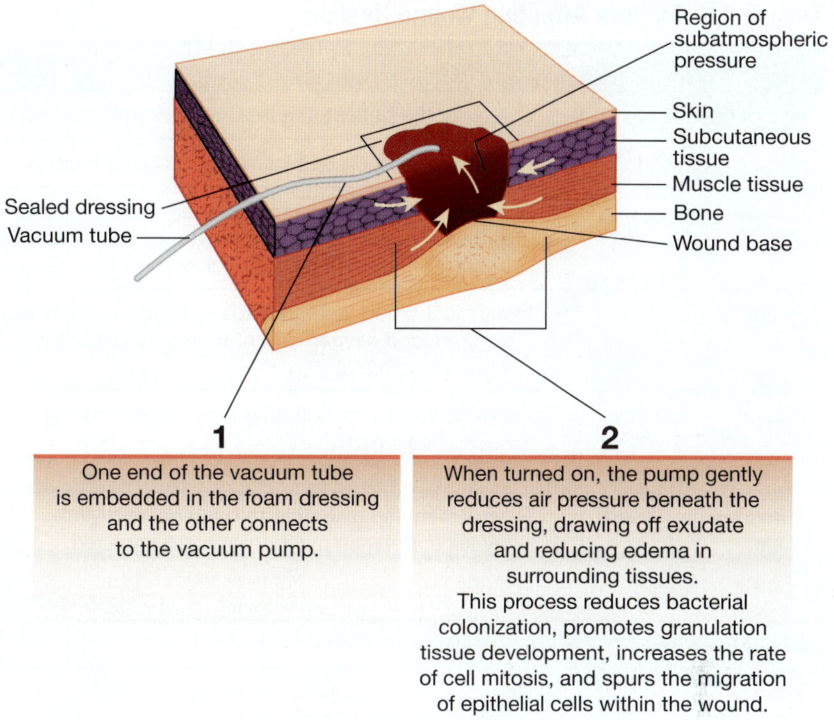

FIGURE 4-8 **Wound vacuum-assisted closure (VAC).**

at 125 mm Hg, lower levels of pressure (75–80 mm Hg) can be used to reduce pain without compromising effectiveness. Newer devices may be intermittent therapy and include the use of wound installation with topical solutions (NICE, 2021; Perry et al., 2022). The nurse follows the manufacturer's instructions for use (IFU), including the prescribed pressure ranges, and confers with the surgeon and wound care specialist with any concerns. In the event that brisk, bright-red bleeding is noted or there is evidence of evisceration or dehiscence, or possible wound infection, the provider is immediately notified (Perry et al., 2022).

As a wound heals, many factors, such as adequate nutrition, cleanliness, rest, and position determine how quickly healing occurs. Specific nursing assessments and interventions that address these factors and help promote wound healing are presented in Table 4-9. Management of surgical drains and dressings is discussed in more detail below.

Managing Drains

Wound drains are tubes that exit the peri-incisional area, either into a portable wound suction device (closed) or into the dressings (open). The principle involved is to allow the escape of blood and serous fluids that could otherwise serve as a culture medium for bacteria. In portable wound suction, the use of gentle, constant suction enhances drainage of these fluids and collapses the skin flaps against the underlying tissue, thus removing "dead space." Types of wound drains include the Penrose, Hemovac, and Jackson–Pratt drains (Fig. 4-9). Output from wound drainage systems and all new drainage is recorded. The amount of bloody drainage on the surgical dressing is assessed frequently. Spots of drainage on the dressings are outlined with a pen, and the date and time of the outline are recorded on the dressing, so that increased drainage can be seen easily. A certain amount of bloody drainage in a wound drainage system or on the dressing is expected, but excessive amounts should be reported to the surgeon. Increasing amounts of fresh blood on the dressing should be reported immediately. Some wounds are irrigated heavily before closure in the OR, and open drains exiting the wound may be embedded in the dressings. These wounds may drain large amounts of blood-tinged fluid that saturate the dressing. The dressing can be reinforced with sterile gauze bandages; the time at which they were reinforced should be documented. If drainage continues, the surgeon should be notified so that the dressing can be changed. Multiple similar drains are numbered or otherwise labeled (e.g., left lower quadrant, left upper quadrant), so that output measurements can be recorded reliably and consistently. Careful positioning and safeguarding that any drains are secure can prevent the dislodgment of nasogastric tubes, chest tubes, and the drains themselves.

Changing the Dressing

Although the first postoperative dressing is usually changed by a member of the surgical team, subsequent dressing changes in the immediate postoperative period are usually performed by the nurse. A dressing is applied to a wound for one or more of the following reasons: (1) to provide a proper environment for wound healing; (2) to absorb drainage; (3) to splint or immobilize the wound; (4) to protect the wound and new epithelial tissue from mechanical injury; (5) to protect the wound from bacterial contamination and from soiling by feces, vomitus, and urine; (6) to promote hemostasis, as in a pressure dressing; and (7) to provide mental and physical comfort for the patient.

The patient is told that the dressing is to be changed and that it is a simple procedure associated with little discomfort.

(*continued on page 153*)

TABLE **4-9 Factors Affecting Wound Healing**

Factors	Rationale	Nursing Interventions
Age of patient	The older the patient, the less resilient the tissues.	Handle all tissues gently.
Handling of tissues	Rough handling causes injury and delayed healing.	Handle tissues carefully and evenly.
Hemorrhage	Accumulation of blood creates dead spaces as well as dead cells that must be removed. The area becomes a growth medium for organisms.	Monitor vital signs. Observe incision site for evidence of bleeding and infection.
Hypovolemia	Insufficient blood volume leads to vasoconstriction and reduced oxygen and nutrients available for wound healing.	Monitor for volume-deficit (circulatory impairment). Correct by fluid replacement as prescribed.
Patient overactivity	Prevents approximation of wound edges; resting favors healing.	Use measures to keep wound edges approximated: taping, bandaging, splints. Encourage rest.
Immunosuppressed state	Patient is more vulnerable to bacterial and viral invasion; defense mechanisms are impaired.	Provide maximum protection to prevent infection. Restrict visitors with colds; institute mandatory hand hygiene by all staff.
Local Factors		
Edema	Reduces blood supply by exerting increased interstitial pressure on vessels	Elevate part; apply cool compresses.
Inadequate dressing technique		Follow guidelines for proper dressing technique.
Too small	Permits bacterial invasion and contamination	
Too tight	Reduces blood supply carrying nutrients and oxygen	
Nutritional deficits	Protein–calorie depletion may occur. Insulin secretion may be inhibited, causing blood glucose to rise.	Correct deficits; this may require parenteral nutritional therapy. Monitor blood glucose levels. Administer vitamin supplements as prescribed.
Foreign bodies	Foreign bodies retard healing.	Keep wounds free of dressing threads and talcum powder from gloves.
Oxygen deficit (tissue oxygenation insufficient)	Insufficient oxygen may be due to inadequate lung and cardiovascular function as well as localized vasoconstriction.	Encourage deep breathing, turning, controlled coughing, and supplemental oxygen as prescribed.
Drainage accumulation	Accumulated secretions hamper healing process.	Monitor closed drainage systems for proper functioning. Institute measures to remove accumulated secretions.
Medications		
Corticosteroids	May mask presence of infection by impairing normal inflammatory response	Be aware of action and effect of medications patient is receiving.
Anticoagulants	May cause hemorrhage	
Broad-spectrum and specific antibiotics	Effective if administered immediately before surgery for specific pathology or bacterial contamination. If administered after wound is closed, ineffective because of intravascular coagulation.	

Factors	Rationale	Nursing Interventions
Systemic Disorders		
Hemorrhagic shock Acidosis Hypoxia Kidney failure Hepatic disease Sepsis Smoking Immunodeficiency diseases; chemotherapy; radiation Poor nutrition Obesity Diabetes	Depress cell functions that directly affect wound healing	Be familiar with the nature of the specific disorder. Administer prescribed treatment. Cultures may be indicated to determine appropriate antibiotic.
Wound Stressors		
Vomiting Valsalva maneuver Heavy coughing Straining	Produce tension on wounds, particularly of the torso	Encourage frequent turning and ambulation and administer antiemetic medications as prescribed. Assist patient in splinting incision.

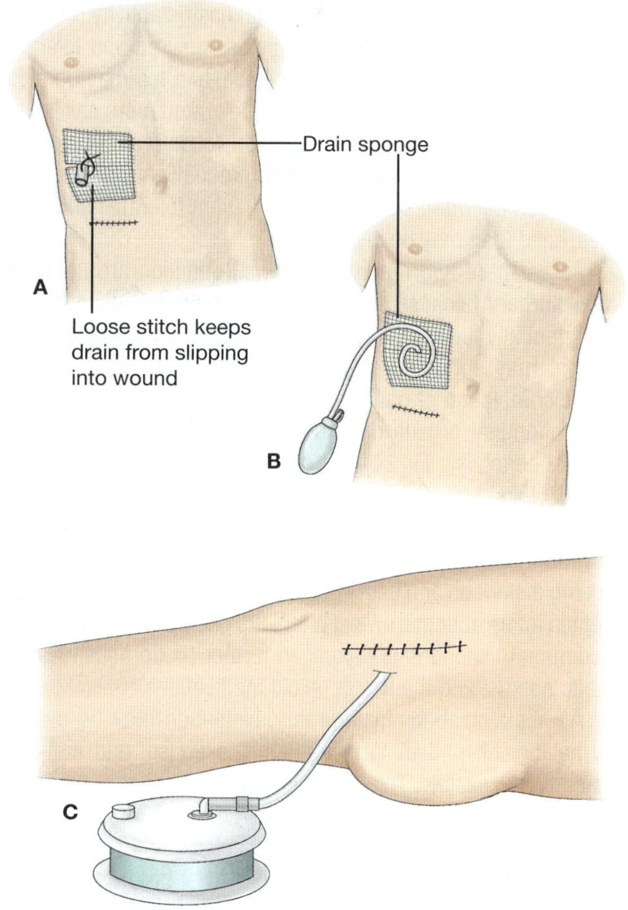

FIGURE 4-9 **Types of surgical drains: (A) Penrose, (B) Jackson-Pratt, (C) Hemovac.**

The dressing change is performed at a suitable time (e.g., not at mealtimes or when visitors are present). Privacy is provided, and the patient is not unduly exposed. The nurse should avoid referring to the incision as a scar because the term may have negative connotations for the patient. Assurance is given that the incision will shrink as it heals and that the redness will fade.

The nurse carries out hand hygiene before and after the dressing change and wears disposable gloves for the dressing change itself. The tape or adhesive portion of the dressing is removed by pulling it parallel with the skin surface and in the direction of hair growth, rather than at right angles. Nonirritating solvents aid in removing adhesive painlessly and quickly. The old dressing is removed and then deposited in a container designated for disposal of biomedical waste. In accordance with standard precautions, dressings are never touched by ungloved hands because of the danger of transmitting pathogenic organisms.

Pearls for Practice

There is a dearth of research regarding the influence of sterile or aseptic versus clean gloves and SSIs related to wound care. Therefore, the nurse will perform dressing changes depending upon institutional policy. However, the nurse should consider the patient's immune status and depth of a wound when selecting dressing technique of sterile versus clean technique. In addition, use of gloves does not preclude meticulous hand hygiene.

If the patient is sensitive to adhesive tape, the dressing may be held in place with hypoallergenic tape. Many tapes are

(*continued on page 154*)

porous to permit ventilation and prevent skin maceration. The correct way to apply tape is to place the tape at the center of the dressing and then press the tape down on both sides, applying tension evenly, away from the midline. The incorrect way to apply tape—to fix one end of the tape to the skin and to pull it tight over the dressing—often wrinkles and pulls the skin in the process. The resulting continuous and forceful traction produces a shearing effect, causing the epidermal layer to slip sideways and become separated from the deeper dermal layers. Some wounds become edematous after having been dressed, causing considerable tension on the tape. If the tape is not flexible, the stretching bandage will also cause a shear injury to the skin. This can result in denuded areas or large blisters and should be avoided. An elastic adhesive bandage (Elastoplast, 3M Microfoam) may be used to hold dressings in place over mobile areas, such as the neck or the extremities, or where pressure is required. A tubular band netting (which stretches and holds the dressing in place without tape) may also be considered.

While changing the dressing, the nurse has an opportunity to teach the patient how to care for the incision and change the dressings at home. The nurse observes for indicators of the patient's readiness to learn, such as looking at the incision, expressing interest, or assisting in the dressing change.

MAINTAINING NORMAL BODY TEMPERATURE

The patient is still at risk for MH and hypothermia in the postoperative period. Efforts are made to identify MH and to treat it early and promptly.

Patients who have been anesthetized are susceptible to chills and drafts. Attention to hypothermia management, begun in the intraoperative period, extends into the postoperative period to prevent significant nitrogen loss and catabolism. Signs of hypothermia are reported to the physician member of the surgical team. The room is maintained at a comfortable temperature, and blankets are provided to prevent chilling. Treatment includes oxygen administration, adequate hydration, and proper nutrition. The patient is also monitored for cardiac arrhythmias. The risk of hypothermia is greater in the older patient and in those who were in the cool OR environment for a prolonged period.

MANAGING GI FUNCTION AND RESUMING NUTRITION

GI discomfort (nausea, vomiting, hiccups) and resumption of oral intake are issues for both the patient and the nurse. Nausea and vomiting are common after anesthesia (Ward, 2023). They are more common in females, in obese people (fat cells act as reservoirs for the anesthetic), in patients prone to motion sickness, and in patients who have undergone lengthy surgical procedures. Other causes of postoperative vomiting include an accumulation of fluid in the stomach, inflation of the stomach, and the ingestion of food and fluid before peristalsis resumes.

If vomiting is likely because of the nature of surgery, a nasogastric tube is inserted intraoperatively and remains in place throughout the surgery and the immediate postoperative period. A nasogastric tube (NG tube) also may be inserted before surgery if postoperative distention is anticipated. In addition, an NG tube may be inserted if a patient who has food in the stomach requires emergency surgery. Refer to Chapter 21 for further details on NG tubes.

Hiccups, produced by intermittent spasms of the diaphragm secondary to irritation of the phrenic nerve, can occur after surgery. The irritation may be direct, such as from stimulation of the nerve by a distended stomach, subdiaphragmatic abscess, or abdominal distention; indirect, such as from toxemia or uremia that stimulates the nerve; or reflexive, such as irritation from a drainage tube or obstruction of the intestines. Usually, these occurrences are mild, transitory attacks that cease spontaneously. If hiccups persist, they may produce considerable distress and serious effects such as vomiting, exhaustion, and wound dehiscence. The provider may prescribe phenothiazine medications for intractable hiccups (Ferri, 2023b).

Once nausea and vomiting have subsided and the patient is fully awake and alert with the nurse having documented resumption of bowel sounds, the nurse should offer the patient something to drink or eat. The sooner the patient can tolerate a usual diet, the more quickly normal GI function will resume. Taking food by mouth stimulates digestive juices and promotes gastric function and intestinal peristalsis. The return to normal dietary intake should proceed at a pace set by the patient. Of course, the nature of the surgery and the type of anesthesia directly affect the rate at which normal gastric activity resumes. Liquids are typically the first substances desired and tolerated by the patient after surgery. Water, juice, and tea may be given in increasing amounts. Cool fluids are tolerated more easily than are those that are ice cold or hot. Soft foods (gelatin, custard, milk, and creamed soups) are added gradually after clear fluids have been tolerated. As soon as the patient tolerates soft foods well, solid food may be given.

Assessment and management of GI function are important after surgery because the GI tract is subject to uncomfortable or potentially life-threatening complications. Any postoperative patient may suffer from abdominal distention, resulting from the accumulation of gas in the intestinal tract. Manipulation of the abdominal organs during surgery may produce a loss of normal peristalsis for 24–48 hours, depending on the type and extent of surgery. Even though nothing is given by mouth, swallowed air and GI secretions enter the stomach and intestines; if not propelled by peristalsis, they collect in the intestines, producing distention and causing the patient to complain of fullness or pain in the abdomen. Most often, the gas collects in the colon. Abdominal distention is increased further by immobility, anesthetic agents, and the use of opioid medications.

After major abdominal surgery, distention may be avoided by having the patient turn frequently, exercise, and ambulate as early as possible. This also alleviates distention produced by swallowing air, which is common in anxious patients. An NG tube inserted before surgery may remain in place until full peristaltic activity (indicated by the passage of flatus) has resumed. The nurse can determine when peristaltic bowel sounds return by listening to the abdomen with a stethoscope (normal frequency of bowel sounds are 5–34 clicks and gurgles per minute). Bowel sounds are documented so that diet progression can occur.

Paralytic ileus (failure of forward movement of bowel contents; when due to paralysis of the intestinal muscles, also termed postoperative adynamic ileus) and intestinal obstruction are potential postoperative complications that occur more frequently in patients undergoing intestinal or abdominal surgery.

PROMOTING BOWEL FUNCTION

Constipation is common after surgery and can range from a minor to a serious complication. Decreased mobility, decreased oral intake, and opioid analgesics contribute to difficulty having a bowel movement. In addition, irritation and trauma to the bowel during surgery may inhibit intestinal movement for several days. The combined effect of early ambulation, improved dietary intake, and a stool softener (if prescribed) promotes bowel elimination. Until the patient reports return of normal bowel function, the nurse should assess the abdomen for distention and the presence and frequency of bowel sounds. If the abdomen is not distended and bowel sounds are normal, and if the patient does not have a bowel movement by the second or third postoperative day, the provider should be notified.

MANAGING VOIDING

Urinary retention after surgery can occur for various reasons. Anesthetics, anticholinergic agents, and opioids interfere with the perception of bladder fullness and the urge to void and inhibit the ability to initiate voiding and completely empty the bladder. Abdominal, pelvic, and hip surgery may increase the likelihood of retention secondary to pain. In addition, some patients find it difficult to use the bedpan or urinal in the recumbent position.

Bladder distention and the urge to void should be assessed at the time of the patient's arrival on the unit and frequently thereafter. The patient is expected to void within 6–8 hours after surgery (this includes time spent in the PACU). If the patient has an urge to void and cannot, or if the bladder is distended and no urge is felt or the patient cannot void, a portable ultrasound device (bladder scan) should be performed to assess degree of distention and possible need for urinary catheterization. All methods to encourage the patient to void should be tried (e.g., letting water run, applying heat to the perineum). The bedpan should be warm; a cold bedpan causes discomfort and automatic tightening of muscles (including the urethral sphincter). If the patient cannot void on a bedpan, it may be possible to use a commode rather than resorting to catheterization. Patients with a penis are often permitted to sit up or stand beside the bed to use the urinal, but safeguards should be taken to prevent the patient from falling or fainting due to loss of coordination from medications or orthostatic hypotension. If the patient cannot void in the specified time frame and a bladder scan verifies distention, the patient is catheterized and the catheter is removed after the bladder has emptied. Straight intermittent catheterization is preferred over indwelling catheterization, because the risk of infection is increased with an indwelling catheter.

Even if the patient voids, the bladder may not necessarily be empty. The nurse notes the amount of urine voided and uses the bladder scan to assess residual volume. If more than 200 mL of residual urine is seen on the bladder scanner, it is considered diagnostic of urinary retention. At present, there is no officially established volume that defines normal or impaired emptying. The Agency for Healthcare Policy and Research (AHCPR) suggests that a PVR less than 50 cc represents adequate emptying and a PVR greater than 200 cc represents inadequate emptying (Ballstaedt & Woodbury, 2022). If a bladder scan is not available in your institution, the nurse can palpate the suprapubic area for distention or tenderness after the patient urinates to assess for residual urine (normally the bladder is not palpated unless it is distended at which time, you will feel a smooth, round, tense mass at or above the suprapubic region) (Ball et al., 2023). Intermittent catheterization may be prescribed every 4–6 hours until the patient can void spontaneously and the postvoid residual is less than 200 mL.

MAINTAINING A SAFE ENVIRONMENT

During the immediate postoperative period, the patient recovering from anesthesia should have two side rails up, and the bed should be in the low position. The nurse assesses the patient's LOC and orientation and determines whether the patient needs their eyeglasses or hearing aid because impaired vision, inability to hear postoperative instructions, or inability to communicate verbally places the patient at risk for injury. All objects the patient may need should be within reach, especially the call light. Any immediate postoperative orders concerning special positioning, equipment, or interventions should be implemented as soon as possible. The patient is instructed to ask for assistance with any activity. Although restraints are occasionally necessary for the disoriented patient, they should be avoided if at all possible. Agency policy on the use of restraints must be consulted and followed.

PROVIDING EMOTIONAL SUPPORT TO THE PATIENT AND FAMILY

Although patients and families are undoubtedly relieved that surgery is over, anxiety levels may remain high in the immediate postoperative period. Many factors contribute to this anxiety: Pain, being in an unfamiliar environment, inability to control one's circumstances or care for oneself, fear of the long-term effects of surgery, fear of complications, fatigue, spiritual distress, altered role responsibilities, ineffective coping, and altered body image are all potential reactions to the surgical experience. The nurse helps the patient and family work through their anxieties by providing reassurance and information and by spending time listening to and addressing their concerns. The nurse describes hospital routines and what to expect in the ensuing hours and days until discharge and explains the purpose of nursing assessments and interventions. Informing patients when they will be able to drink fluids or eat, when they will be getting out of bed, and when tubes and drains will be

(*continued on page 156*)

removed helps them gain a sense of control and participation in recovery and engages them in the plan of care. Acknowledging family members' concerns and accepting and encouraging their participation in the patient's care assists them in feeling that they are helping their loved one. The nurse can modify the environment to enhance rest and relaxation by providing privacy, reducing noise, adjusting lighting, providing enough seating for family members, and encouraging a supportive atmosphere.

MANAGING POTENTIAL COMPLICATIONS

The RN must be alert for the development of additional postoperative complications that include cardiac complications, DVT and pulmonary embolism (PE), hematoma, wound infection, and/or wound dehiscence and evisceration. The following sections detail each of these complications.

Cardiac Complications

A postoperative cardiac complication is myocardial ischemia/infarction (MI). The nurse is aware that in the postoperative patient, clinical presentation is often subtle. Perioperative MIs are frequently silent or may present with dyspnea, hypotension, or atypical pain. If suspected, the nurse alerts the surgical team; obtains vital signs and oxygen saturation; performs a cardiac, peripheral vascular, pulmonary assessment, and electrocardiogram; and anticipates laboratory work to assess cardiac biomarkers will be obtained. Refer to Table 13-6 for cardiac laboratory tests on page 490.

As a result of excessive IV fluid administration intraoperatively, the nurse is alert for the development of heart failure (HF), which can present in the immediate postoperative period, or on POD 2–3 when fluid shifting causes increased intravascular volume. Daily weights are an important parameter for judging fluid balance. The nurse is aware that when calculating new gain or loss that 500 mL approximates 1 lb or 1,000 mL approximates 1 kg (2.2 lb). In addition, the nurse observes for jugular vein distention, crackles, dyspnea, wheezing, cough, and fatigue. Refer to Chapters 13 and 14 for details of care of the patient with MI and HF.

Deep Vein Thrombosis and Pulmonary Embolism

DVT and other complications, such as PE, are serious potential complications of surgery (Box 4-8). The stress response that is initiated by surgery inhibits the fibrinolytic system, resulting in blood hypercoagulability. Dehydration, low cardiac output, blood pooling in the extremities, and bed rest add to the risk of thrombosis formation. Although all postoperative patients are at some risk, factors such as a history of thrombosis, malignancy, trauma, obesity, indwelling venous catheters, and hormone use (e.g., estrogen) increase the risk. The first symptom of DVT may be swelling of the involved extremity, often accompanied by a low-grade fever. The edema is associated with impaired venous flow. Tenderness, which usually occurs later, is produced by inflammation of the vein wall, and firmness may be detected along the involved veins by gently palpating the affected extremity (palpated cord). Refer to Chapter 17 for details on DVT.

BOX 4-8

Risk Factors for Postoperative Deep Vein Thrombosis

- Orthopedic patients having hip surgery, knee reconstruction, and other lower extremity surgery
- Urologic patients having transurethral prostatectomy and older patients having urologic surgery
- General surgical patients older than 40 years of age; those who are obese; those with a malignancy; those who have had prior DVT or PE; and those undergoing extensive, complicated surgical procedures
- Gynecologic (and obstetric) patients older than 40 years of age with added risk factors (varicose veins, previous venous thrombosis, infection, malignancy, obesity)
- Neurosurgical patients, similar to other surgical high-risk groups (in patients with stroke, for instance, the risk of DVT in the paralyzed leg is as high as 75%)

Prophylactic treatment for postoperative patients at risk is common practice until the patient is ambulatory. External pneumatic compression may be used alone or in combination with elastic stockings and anticoagulation. The benefits of early ambulation and hourly leg exercises in preventing DVT cannot be overemphasized, and these activities are recommended for all patients, regardless of their risk. It is important to avoid the use of blanket rolls, pillow rolls, or any form of elevation that can constrict vessels under the knees. Even prolonged "dangling" (having the patient sit on the edge of the bed with legs hanging over the side) can be dangerous and is not recommended in susceptible patients because pressure under the knees can impede circulation. Adequate hydration is also encouraged; the patient can be offered juices and water throughout the day to avoid dehydration.

PE from DVT is a postoperative risk for patients owing to immobility, venous stasis, venous trauma, and hypercoagulability. Clinically, symptoms of PE include sudden onset of shortness of breath, tachypnea, tachycardia, low-grade temperature, chest pain (pleuritic in nature), and apprehension. Patients who have had major orthopedic surgery of a lower extremity, including hip or knee arthroplasty and hip fracture surgeries, as well as major trauma patients, are at high risk for PE. Some form of prophylactic therapy is expected in high-risk patients to reduce the risk of DVT and PE. Refer to Chapter 9 for more details on PE.

Hematoma

At times, concealed bleeding occurs beneath the skin at the surgical site. This hemorrhage usually stops spontaneously but results in clot (hematoma) formation within the wound. If the clot is small, it will be absorbed and need not be treated. If the clot is large, the wound usually bulges somewhat, and healing will be delayed unless the clot is removed. After several sutures are removed by a member of the surgical team, the clot is evacuated and the wound is packed lightly with gauze. Healing occurs usually by granulation, or a secondary closure may be performed.

TABLE **4-10 Wound Classification and Associated Surgical Site Infection Risk**

Surgical Category	Determinants of Category	Expected Risk of Postsurgical Infection (%)
Clean	Nontraumatic site Uninfected site No inflammation No break in aseptic technique No entry into respiratory, alimentary, genitourinary, or oropharyngeal tracts Clean wounds are primarily closed (Wolpert, 2023)	1–5
Clean-contaminated	Entry into respiratory, alimentary, genitourinary, or oropharyngeal tracts without unusual contamination Minor break in aseptic technique Mechanical drainage Includes the biliary tract, appendix, vagina, and oropharynx, provided no evidence of infection or major break in technique is encountered (Wolpert, 2023).	8–11
Contaminated	Open, newly experienced traumatic wounds Gross spillage from GI tract Major break in aseptic technique (e.g., open cardiac massage) Entry into genitourinary or biliary tract when urine or bile is infected	15–20
Dirty-Infected Wound	Traumatic wound with delayed repair, devitalized tissue, foreign bodies, or fecal contamination Acute inflammation and purulent drainage encountered during procedure Organisms causing postoperative infection were present in the operative field before the operation. Includes those with a foreign object lodged in the wound (such as a bullet or other debris; Talbot, 2021; Wilson, 2023; Wolpert, 2023)	27–40

Data from Wilson, J. (2019). Preventing wound infection. In Jennie Wilson (Ed.), *Infection control in clinical practice* (3rd ed., Chapter 8, pp. 279–306). Elsevier Inc.

Wolpert, M. (2023). Health care–associated infections (HAIs). In F. Ferri (Ed.), *Ferri's clinical advisor* (1st ed., p. 682). Elsevier Inc.

Talbot, T. (2020). Surgical site infections and antimicrobial prophylaxis. In J. Bennett (Ed.), *Mandell, Douglas, and Bennett's principles and practice of infectious diseases* (9th ed., Chapter 313, pp. 3743–3756). Elsevier Inc.

Infection (Wound Sepsis)

The creation of a surgical wound disrupts the integrity of the skin and its protective function. Exposure of deep body tissues to pathogens in the environment places the patient at risk for infection of the surgical site, a potentially life-threatening complication. Surgical site infection (SSI) increases hospital length of stay, costs of care, risk for further complications, and readmission to a hospital.

Multiple factors place the patient at risk for wound infection. One risk factor relates to the type of wound. Surgical wounds are classified according to the degree of contamination. Table 4-10 defines the terms used to describe surgical wounds and gives the expected rate of wound infection per category. Other risk factors include both patient-related factors and those associated with the surgical procedure. Factors related to the surgical procedure include the method of preoperative skin preparation, surgical attire of the team, method of sterile draping, duration of surgery, antimicrobial prophylaxis, aseptic technique, factors related to surgical technique, drains or foreign material, OR ventilation, length of procedure, and exogenous microorganisms. Efforts to prevent wound infection are directed at reducing these risks. Current guidelines to prevent SSIs suggest that an appropriate prophylactic antibiotic that is based on current recommendation be administered within 1 hour of surgical incision (2 hours are allowed for the administration of vancomycin and fluoroquinolones) and discontinuation of prophylactic antibiotics within 24 hours after surgery, owing to the link between the development of resistant organisms and excessive use of antibiotics. Discontinuation of the antibiotic is extended to within 48 hours for cardiothoracic procedures for adult patients. The Centers for Medicaid and Medicare Services introduced the program Surgical Care Improvement Project (SCIP), which is a national quality partnership of organizations interested in improving surgical care by significantly reducing surgical complications. They provide guidelines for antibiotic therapy throughout the patient's hospitalization, and the list of prevention measures can be found at www.jointcommission.org

(*continued on page 158*)

Wound infection may not be evident until at least POD 5. Most patients are discharged before that time, and more than half of wound infections are diagnosed after discharge, highlighting the importance of patient education regarding wound care. Risk factors for wound sepsis include wound contamination, foreign body, faulty suturing technique, devitalized tissue, hematoma, debilitation, dehydration, malnutrition, anemia, advanced age, extreme obesity, shock, length of preoperative hospitalization, duration of surgical procedure, and associated disorders (e.g., diabetes mellitus, immunosuppression). Signs and symptoms of wound infection include increased pulse rate and temperature; an elevated white blood cell count; wound swelling, warmth, tenderness, or discharge; and incisional pain. Local signs may be absent if the infection is deep. *Staphylococcus aureus* accounts for many postoperative wound infections. Other infections may result from *Escherichia coli, Proteus vulgaris, Aerobacter aerogenes, Pseudomonas aeruginosa,* and other organisms. Although they are rare, beta-hemolytic streptococcal or clostridial infections can develop rapidly and be deadly. If wound infection due to beta-hemolytic streptococcus or clostridium occurs, strict infection-control practices are needed to prevent the spread of infection to others. Intensive medical and nursing care is essential if the patient is to survive.

When a wound infection is diagnosed in a surgical incision, the surgeon may remove one or more sutures or staples and, using aseptic precautions, separate the wound edges with a pair of blunt scissors or a hemostat, opening the incision to allow for drainage. Another option is for the patient to be referred to interventional radiology for percutaneous drainage. Antimicrobial therapy and a wound care regimen are also initiated.

Wound Dehiscence and Evisceration

Wound **dehiscence** (disruption of surgical incision or wound) and **evisceration** (protrusion of wound contents) are serious surgical complications that usually occur between the 5th and 10th postoperative days (Phillips & Hornacky, 2021e) (Fig. 4-10). Dehiscence and evisceration are especially serious when they involve abdominal incisions or wounds. These complications result from sutures giving way, from infection, or, more frequently, from marked distention or strenuous cough. They may also occur because of increasing age; obesity; poor nutritional status (hypoproteinemia, hypoalbuminemia); steroid use or immunosuppression (cancer); previous radiation; the presence of diabetes, uremia, or sepsis; or pulmonary or cardiovascular disease in patients undergoing abdominal surgery. Local risk factors include inadequate closure, excessive tension on the wound edges, incisions longer than 18 cm, and improper surgical technique such as placing sutures too close to the wound edges or too close together, among other technical errors (DeVolder, 2023).

When the wound edges separate slowly, the intestines may protrude gradually or not at all, and the earliest sign may be a gush of bloody (serosanguineous) peritoneal fluid from the wound. When a wound ruptures suddenly, coils of intestine may push out of the abdomen. The patient may report that "something gave way." The evisceration causes pain and may be associated with vomiting.

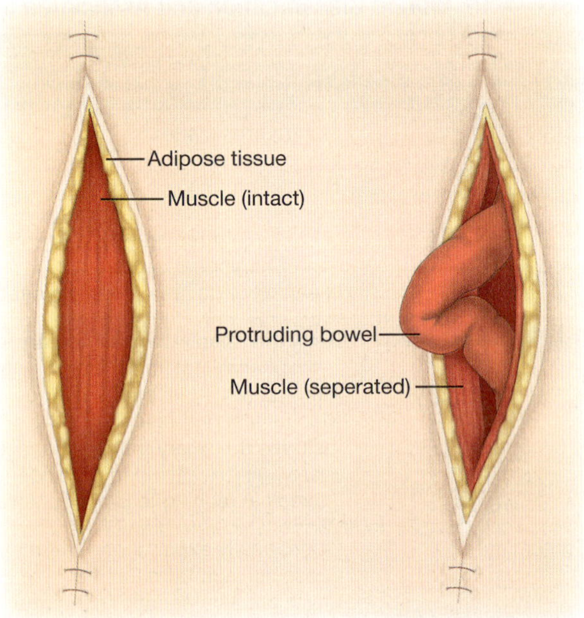

FIGURE 4-10 **(A) Wound dehiscence; (B) wound evisceration.**

An abdominal binder, properly applied, is a prophylactic measure against an evisceration and often is used along with the primary dressing, especially in patients with weak or pendulous abdominal walls or when rupture of a wound has occurred. If evisceration occurs, the nurse aseptically covers the abdominal contents with moist saline dressings to prevent drying of the bowel; notifies the surgical team immediately; and assesses the patient's vital signs, including oxygen saturation. The patient remains in bed with knees bent to reduce abdominal muscle tension. The patient should be NPO and an should be IV established for fluid management. After the patient returns from surgery, review splinting of the abdomen and anticipate the use of an abdominal binder.

PROVIDING DISCHARGE TEACHING

Patients have always required detailed discharge instructions to become proficient in special self-care needs after surgery; however, dramatically reduced hospital lengths of stay during the past decade have greatly increased the amount of information needed while reducing the amount of time in which to provide it. Box 4-9 provides patient education about wound care.

EVALUATION

Expected patient outcomes may include the following:

1. Maintains optimal respiratory function:
    a. Performs deep-breathing exercises
    b. Displays clear breath sounds
    c. Uses incentive spirometer as prescribed
    d. Splints incisional site when coughing to reduce pain
2. Indicates that pain is decreased in intensity or acceptable to patient

BOX 4-9

Patient Education

Wound Care Instructions

Until Sutures are Removed

1. Keep the wound dry and clean:
   - If there is no dressing, ask your nurse or provider if you can bathe or shower.
   - If a dressing or splint is in place, do not remove it unless it is wet or soiled.
   - If wet or soiled, change dressing yourself if you have been taught to do so; otherwise, call your nurse or provider for guidance.
   - If you have been taught, instruction might be as follows:
     - Cleanse area *gently* with sterile normal saline once or twice daily.
     - Cover with a sterile Telfa pad or gauze square large enough to cover the wound.
     - Apply hypoallergenic tape (Dermicel or paper). Adhesive is not recommended because it is difficult to remove without possible injury to the incisional site.
2. Immediately report any of these signs of infection:
   - Increasing redness, swelling, tenderness, pain, or increased warmth around the wound
   - Red streaks in the skin near the wound
   - Pus or discharge, foul odor
   - Chills or temperature higher than 37.7° C (100° F)
3. If soreness or pain causes discomfort, apply a dry cool pack (containing ice or cold water) or take prescribed acetaminophen tablets (2) every 4–6 hours. Avoid using aspirin without direction or instruction because bleeding can occur with its use.
4. Swelling after surgery is common. To help reduce swelling, elevate the affected part to the level of the heart:
   - Hand or arm:
     - Sleep: Elevate arm on pillow at side
     - Sitting: Place arm on pillow on adjacent table
     - Standing: Rest affected hand on opposite shoulder; support elbow with unaffected hand
   - Leg or foot:
     - Sitting: Place a pillow on a facing chair; provide support underneath the knee
     - Lying: Place a pillow under affected leg

After Sutures Are Removed

Although the wound appears to be healed when sutures are removed, it is still tender and will continue to heal and strengthen for several weeks.

1. Follow recommendations of your provider or nurse regarding extent of activity.
2. Keep the suture line clean; do not rub vigorously; pat dry. Wound edges may look red and may be slightly raised. This is normal.
3. If the site continues to be red, thick, and painful to pressure after 8 weeks, consult the health care provider. (This may be due to excessive collagen formation and should be checked.)

3. Increases activity as prescribed:
   a. Alternates periods of rest and activity
   b. Progressively increases ambulation
   c. Resumes normal activities within prescribed time frame
   d. Performs activities related to self-care
4. Wound heals without complication
5. Maintains body temperature within normal limits
6. Resumes oral intake:
   a. Reports absence of nausea and vomiting
   b. Eats at least 75% of usual diet
   c. Is free of abdominal distress and gas pains
   d. Exhibits normal bowel sounds
7. Reports resumption of usual bowel elimination pattern
8. Resumes usual voiding pattern
9. Is free of injury
10. Exhibits decreased anxiety
11. Acquires knowledge and skills necessary to manage therapeutic regimen
12. Experiences no complications

Gerontologic Considerations

Older patients recover more slowly, have longer hospital stays, and are at greater risk for the development of postoperative complications. Some of the major threats to recovery include pneumonia, decline in functional ability, exacerbation of comorbid conditions, pressure ulcers, decreased oral intake, GI disturbance, and falls. Expert nursing care can help the older adult avoid these complications or minimize their effects.

Postoperative delirium, characterized by confusion, perceptual and cognitive deficits, altered attention levels, disturbed sleep patterns, and impaired psychomotor skills, is a significant problem for older adults. Causes of delirium are multifactorial (refer to Box 4-10 for causes of delirium). Skilled and frequent assessment of mental status and of all physiologic factors influencing mental status helps the nurse plan care because delirium may be the initial or only early indicator of infection, fluid and electrolyte imbalance, or deterioration of respiratory or hemodynamic status in the aging patient.

Recognizing postoperative delirium and identifying and treating its underlying cause are the goals of care. Sometimes postoperative delirium is mistaken for pre-existing dementia or is attributed to age. In addition to monitoring and managing identifiable causes, the nurse implements supportive interventions. Keeping the patient in a well-lit room and close to the nurses' station can help with sensory deprivation. At the same time, distracting and unfamiliar noises should be minimized. Because pain can contribute

BOX 4-10

Causes of Postoperative Delirium

- Acid–base disturbances
- Age greater than 80 years
- Fluid and electrolyte imbalance
- Dehydration
- History of dementia-like symptoms
- Hypoxia
- Hypercarbia
- Infection (urinary tract, wound, respiratory)
- Medications (anticholinergics, benzodiazepines, central nervous system depressants)
- Blood loss
- Decreased cardiac output
- Cerebral hypoxia
- Heart failure
- Acute myocardial infarction
- Hypothermia or hyperthermia
- Unfamiliar surroundings and sensory deprivation
- Emergent surgery
- Alcohol withdrawal
- Urinary retention
- Fecal impaction
- Polypharmacy
- Presence of multiple diseases
- Sensory impairments
- High stress or anxiety levels
- Pain

to postoperative delirium, adequate pain control is essential. The nurse collaborates with the physician or geriatric nurse specialist and the patient to achieve pain relief without oversedation.

The patient is reoriented as often as necessary, and staff should introduce themselves each time they come in contact with the patient. Engaging the patient in conversation and care activities and placing a clock and calendar nearby may improve cognitive function. Physical activity should not be neglected while the patient is confused because physical deterioration can worsen delirium and place the patient at increased risk for other complications. Restraints should be avoided because they also can worsen confusion. If possible, a family member or staff member is asked to stay with the patient instead.

Other problems confronting the older postoperative patient, such as pneumonia, altered bowel function, DVT, weakness, and functional decline, often can be prevented by early and progressive ambulation. Ambulation means walking, not just getting out of bed and sitting in a chair. Prolonged sitting positions that promote venous stasis in the lower extremities should be avoided. Assistance with ambulation may be required to keep the patient from bumping into objects and falling. A physical therapy referral may be indicated to promote safe, regular exercise for the older adult.

Urinary incontinence can be prevented by providing easy access to the call bell and the commode and by prompting voiding. Early ambulation and familiarity with the room help the patient to become self-sufficient sooner.

Optimal nutritional status is important for wound healing, return of normal bowel function, and fluid and electrolyte balance. The nurse and patient can consult with the dietitian to plan appealing, high-protein meals that provide sufficient fiber, calories, and vitamins. Nutritional supplements may be recommended. Multivitamins, iron, and vitamin C supplements aid in tissue healing, formation of new RBCs, and overall nutritional status and are commonly prescribed postoperatively.

In addition to monitoring and managing physiologic recovery of the older adult, the nurse identifies and addresses psychosocial needs. The older adult may require much encouragement and support to resume activities, and the pace may be slow. Sensory deficits may require frequent repetition of instructions, and decreased physiologic reserve may necessitate frequent rest periods. The older adult may require extensive discharge planning to coordinate both professional and family care providers, and the nurse, social worker, or nurse case manager may institute the plan for continuing care.

CHAPTER REVIEW

NCLEX-Style Review Questions

1. A 70-year-old patient is admitted to the preoperative unit for a liver resection that is scheduled for 6 hours of surgery. What basic principles should guide the preoperative nurse's assessment? Select all that apply.
   a. Older patients do not experience as much preoperative anxiety as younger patients.
   b. The older patient has less physiologic reserve than the younger patient.
   c. Older patients experience less pain.
   d. Older patients have increased susceptibility to hypothermia.
   e. There is an increased vulnerability to changes in circulating volume and blood oxygen levels in the older patient.

2. A nurse is caring for a postoperative patient who had spinal anesthesia. The patient complains of headache. What actions should the nurse take? Select all that apply.
   a. Lower the head of the patient's bed.
   b. Maintain a quiet environment
   c. Encourage the patient to lay on their right side.
   d. Do nothing, as this is a normal response to the spinal anesthesia.
   e. Keep the patient hydrated.

3. A nurse is caring for a postoperative patient on POD 2. The patient had a large upper abdominal incision. While assessing the patient at the beginning of the shift, which of the following signs and symptoms suggest atelectasis? Select all that apply.
   a. Decreased breath sounds
   b. Productive cough of purulent sputum
   c. Crackles
   d. Restlessness
   e. Hyperresonance

4. The nurse would be alerted to the occurrence of malignant hyperthermia when the patient demonstrates what manifestation? Select all that apply.
   a. Tachycardia
   b. Bradypnea
   c. Hypercarbia
   d. Generalized muscle weakness
   e. Masseter muscle spasm

5. In the case above, select all appropriate treatment options for malignant hyperthermia.
   a. Decrease the anesthetic dose immediately.
   b. Administer 100 % oxygen.
   c. Begin active cooling measures.
   d. Continue cooling measures until temperature returns to 98.6.
   e. Administer dantrolene IV.

REFERENCES AND SELECTED READINGS

References and selected readings associated with this chapter can be found on the website that accompanies the book. Visit **http://thepoint.lww.com/Honan3e** to access the references and other additional resources associated with this chapter.

CHAPTER 5

Cancer Care

Kristen V. Roche

Learning Objectives

After reading this chapter, you will be able to:

1. Compare the structure and function of the normal cell and the cancer cell.
2. Differentiate between benign and malignant tumors.
3. Identify agents and factors that have been found to be carcinogenic.
4. Describe the significance of health education and preventive care in decreasing the incidence of cancer.
5. Differentiate among the various types of surgical procedures used in cancer treatment, diagnosis, prophylaxis, and palliation.
6. Describe the roles of surgery, radiation therapy, chemotherapy, targeted agents, and immunotherapy in treating cancer.
7. Describe the special nursing needs of patients receiving chemotherapy and immunotherapy.
8. Describe common nursing diagnoses and collaborative problems of patients with cancer.
9. Describe the concept of hospice in providing care for patients with advanced cancer.
10. Discuss the role of the nurse in assessment and management of common oncologic emergencies.

Cancer is not a single disease with a single cause; rather, it is a highly heterogeneous group of diseases with different causes, manifestations, treatments, and prognoses. Cancer nursing, also called **oncology** nursing, encompasses all age groups and nursing specialties, and is carried out in a variety of health care settings, including the home, community, acute care institutions, rehabilitation centers, and hospice. The scope, responsibilities, and goals of oncology nursing are as diverse and complex as those of any nursing specialty. Oncology nurses must be prepared to support patients and families through a wide range of physical, emotional, social, cultural, and spiritual experiences from diagnosis through end of life and survivorship.

EPIDEMIOLOGY OF CANCER

Although cancer affects people of all ages, most cancers occur in people older than 65 years of age. Overall, the incidence of cancer is higher in males than in females and is higher in industrialized nations.

From the latest annual cancer case report of 2020, the World Health Organization (WHO) estimated more than 19.2 million new cases being diagnosed worldwide (Hatta et al., 2021). In the United States, approximately 1.89 million cases will be diagnosed in 2021, the equivalent of 5,200 new cases each day (Siegel et al., 2021). Figure 5-1 depicts the most common cancers diagnosed in males and females in 2021. Prostate, lung, bronchus, and colorectal cancers (CRCs) account for 46% of all incident cases in males, with prostate cancer alone accounting for 26% of the diagnosis. For females, breast cancer, lung cancer, and CRCs account for 50% of all new diagnoses, with breast cancer alone accounting for 30% of female cancers (Siegel et al., 2021).

Cancer is the second leading cause of death after heart disease in both males and females nationally but is the leading cause of death in many states, and in people who are Hispanic, Asian American, or Alaska Native (Siegel et al., 2021). An estimated 608,570 Americans will die from cancer in 2021, corresponding to more than 1,600 deaths per day. The greatest number of deaths are from cancers of the lung, prostate, and colorectum in males, and cancers of

Estimated New Cases

Males			Females		
Prostate	248,530	26%	Breast	281,550	30%
Lung & bronchus	119,100	12%	Lung & bronchus	116,660	13%
Colon & rectum	79,520	8%	Colon & rectum	69,980	8%
Urinary bladder	64,280	7%	Uterine corpus	66,570	7%
Melanoma of the skin	62,260	6%	Melanoma of the skin	43,850	5%
Kidney & renal pelvis	48,780	5%	Non-Hodgkin lymphoma	35,930	4%
Non-Hodgkin lymphoma	45,630	5%	Thyroid	32,130	3%
Oral cavity & pharynx	38,800	4%	Pancreas	28,480	3%
Leukemia	35,530	4%	Kidney & renal pelvis	27,300	3%
Pancreas	31,950	3%	Leukemia	25,560	3%
All Sites	**970,250**	**100%**	**All Sites**	**927,910**	**100%**

Estimated Deaths

Males			Females		
Lung & bronchus	69,410	22%	Lung & bronchus	62,470	22%
Prostate	34,130	11%	Breast	43,600	15%
Colon & rectum	28,520	9%	Colon & rectum	24,460	8%
Pancreas	25,270	8%	Pancreas	22,950	8%
Liver & intrahepatic bile duct	20,300	6%	Ovary	13,770	5%
Leukemia	13,900	4%	Uterine corpus	12,940	4%
Esophagus	12,410	4%	Liver & intrahepatic bile duct	9,930	3%
Urinary bladder	12,260	4%	Leukemia	9,760	3%
Non-Hodgkin lymphoma	12,170	4%	Non-Hodgkin lymphoma	8,550	3%
Brain & other nervous system	10,500	3%	Brain & other nervous system	8,100	3%
All Sites	**319,420**	**100%**	**All Sites**	**289,150**	**100%**

FIGURE 5-1 Ten Leading Cancer Types for the Estimated New Cancer Cases and Deaths by Sex, United States, 2021. Estimates rounded to the nearest 10 and cases exclude basal cell and squamous cell cancers and in situ carcinoma except urinary bladder. (Adapted from Siegel, R. L., Miller, K. D., Fuchs, H. D., & Jemal, A. (2021). Cancer statistics, 2021. *CA: Cancer Journal for Clinicians*, *71*, 7–33.)

the lung, breast, and colorectum for females (see Fig. 5-1) (Siegel et al., 2021).

The 5-year relative survival rate for all cancers combined diagnosed during 2010 to 2016 was 67% overall, 68% in White individuals, and 63% in Black individuals (Siegel et al., 2021). Gains in survival have been especially rapid for hematopoietic (related to the formation of blood cells) and lymphoid (related to lymph or the lymphatic tissue where lymphocytes are formed) malignancies due to improvement in treatment protocols, including the development of targeted therapies. For example, the 5-year relative survival rate for chronic myeloid leukemia increased from 22% in the mid-1970s to 72% for those diagnosed during 2010 to 2016, and most patients treated with tyrosine kinase inhibitors experience near-normal life expectancy (Siegel et al., 2021).

Mortality rates are a better indicator of progress against cancer than incidence or survival because they are less affected by biases resulting from changes in detection practices. The cancer death rate rose during most of the 20th century, largely because of a rapid increase in lung cancer deaths among males because of the tobacco epidemic (Siegel et al., 2021). However, reduction in smoking as well as improvements in early detection and treatment for some cancers have resulted in a continuous decline in the cancer death rate since its peak of 215.1 (per 100,000) in 1991. The progress against cancer reflects large decreases in mortality for the four major sites (lung, breast, prostate, and colorectal) (Siegel et al., 2021).

Cancer occurrence and outcomes vary considerably between racial and ethnic groups, largely because of inequalities in wealth that lead to differences in risk factor exposures and barriers to high-quality cancer prevention, early detection, and treatment (Siegel et al., 2021). These inequalities ultimately stem from hundreds of years of structural racism, including residential, educational, and occupational segregation and discriminatory policies in criminal justice and housing that have altered the balance of prosperity, security, and health (Siegel et al., 2021).

Characteristics of Malignant Cells

The primary difference between malignant (cancerous) and benign cells is that malignant cells have abnormal regulation of growth. Cancer cells continue to grow, even at the expense of their host. They demonstrate uncontrolled cell growth that follows no physiologic demand.

Benign and malignant growths are classified and named by the tissue of origin. Benign and malignant cells differ in many cellular growth characteristics, including the method and rate of growth, ability to metastasize or spread, general effects, destruction of tissue, and ability to cause death. These differences are summarized in Table 5-1.

Despite their individual differences, all cancer cells share some common cellular characteristics in relation to the cell membrane, special proteins, the nuclei, chromosomal abnormalities, and the rate of mitosis and growth. Characteristics of cancer cells include:

- Pleomorphism: Cells vary in size and shape
- Polymorphism: Nucleus is enlarged and variable in shape
- Chromosomal mutations including translocations, deletions, amplification, and aneuploidy (abnormal number of chromosomes)
- Production of surface enzymes that aid in invasion and metastasis
- Loss of antigens that label the cell as "self"
- Production of new tumor-associated antigens that label the cell as "nonself"
- Increased rate of anaerobic (absence of free oxygen) metabolism
- Loss of contact inhibition, which normally halts cell division once cells are in contact with one another
- Defect in cell recognition and adhesion (cancer cells do not recognize and adhere to each other as normal cells do)
- Loss of control of proliferation
- Increased mitotic index: Tumors have a larger number of cells that are in mitosis
- Abnormal lifespan: Cancer cells tend to live longer than normal cells

Carcinogenesis

Carcinogenesis is a multistep process that refers to the transformation of a normal cell into a tumoral neoplastic cell. The etiology is complex, multifactorial, and can involve cellular, molecular, genetic, epigenic (how behaviors and environment can cause changes that affect the way your genes work), and environmental alterations (Moindjie et al., 2021). The result of these mutations is uncontrolled proliferation of abnormal cells.

Pearls for Practice: Pathophysiology

Although cancer originates from a single mutated cell (monoclonal origin), over time due to subsequent mutations, the tumor cells become heterogeneous in their cellular properties. In addition, cells within different regions of an established tumor may express different genes and different mutations (Harrington et al., 2021). Understanding the characteristics of the cancer cells assists in developing novel therapies to eliminate it.

The following cellular changes are essential to carcinogenesis:

- loss of sensitivity to growth inhibitory signals
- evasion of apoptosis (programmed cell death)
- limitless replicative potential
- angiogenesis (growth of new blood vessels)
- potential for metastatic/tissue invasion

TABLE **5-1 Characteristics of Benign and Malignant Neoplasms**

Characteristics	Benign Neoplasms	Malignant Neoplasms
Cell characteristics	Well-differentiated cells that resemble cells in the tissue of origin	Cells are undifferentiated, with anaplasia (loss of differentiation of cells) and atypical structure that often bear little resemblance to cells in the tissue of origin
Mode of growth	Grows by expansion without invading the surrounding tissues; usually encapsulated	Grows by invasion, sending out processes that infiltrate the surrounding tissues
Rate of growth	Usually progressive and slow; may come to a standstill or regress	Variable and depends on level of differentiation; the more undifferentiated the cells, the more rapid the rate of growth
Metastasis	Does not spread by metastasis	Gains access to the blood and lymph channels to metastasize to other areas of the body

Grossman, S., & Porth, C. (2014). *Pathophysiology: Concepts of altered health states* (9th ed.). Lippincott Williams & Wilkins.

Cells acquire these properties through genetic and epigenetic alterations (external modifications to DNA that turn genes "on" or "off" but do not change the DNA sequence itself) over time as a result of genomic instability, acquired and inherited mutations, changes in the microenvironment, cell selection, and clonal expansion (Grant, 2021).

Carcinogenesis has been described previously as a three-step process, including tumor initiation, promotion, and progression. *Initiation* is the process by which a carcinogenic agent interacts with DNA to produce damage that, if not repaired before the next cell division, could lead to error-prone DNA replication (Grant, 2021). Although initiation is irreversible, not all initiated cells will go on to become a tumor as many of these cells may die by apoptosis. *Promotion* involves the clonal expansion of the initiated cell, in which the initiated cell divides into other cells that now have the same alterations in DNA if not repaired in time (Grant, 2021). Initiated cells may have a selective growth advantage allowing the cells to divide and evade death, resulting in the proliferation and survival of premalignant cells and the formation of benign lesions like polyps. *Progression* is the stage in which benign lesions acquire the ability to proliferate and invade adjacent tissue and establish distant sites of metastasis through the acquisition of additional mutations (Grant, 2021). While this simplistic model has been used over time to understand the multistep process of carcinogenesis, we now understand that cancer is a complex result of multiple sequential mutations in combination with epigenetic changes and prolonged changes in the cellular microenvironment (Grant, 2021).

Mutations can be either germ-line mutations or somatic mutations. Germ-line mutations occur in the DNA of sperm or egg cells. These are inheritable mutations that can also be passed on to offspring. Somatic mutations are acquired mutations that occur in nongerm cells and cannot be inherited or passed on. Once DNA damage has occurred, there are two possible cellular outcomes. Most probable is repair of the damage. If DNA repair does not take place prior to the next cycle of DNA replication prior to cell division, three types of mutational events may occur: (a) error-prone replication; (b) frame-shift mutations (most commonly single-base deletions) that tend to occur when a carcinogen adduct is bound to a nucleotide base (DNA adduct is a segment of DNA bound to a cancer-causing chemical that can initiate carcinogenesis—when a chemical binds to DNA, it becomes damaged resulting in abnormal replication that could be the start of mutation and lead to cancer without proper DNA repair); and (c) DNA strand breaks (Grant, 2021).

Normal genes involved in cell growth are called proto-oncogenes, while tumor suppressor genes direct the programmed suppression of normal cell growth (Olsen et al., 2019). Proto-oncogenes are the first regulatory factors of this biologic process. They act in transmitting signals, resulting as growth factors. The activation process leading to proto-oncogenes are chromosomal translocation, point mutation, and gene amplification (Kontomanolis et al., 2020). Tumor-suppressor genes block the growth of cancer and contribute to the normal development of cells (Kontomanolis et al., 2020). Genetic mutations in proto-oncogenes and tumor suppressor genes disrupt normal cell processes, inhibiting apoptosis, disrupting DNA repair processes, and inducing immortality. **Apoptosis** is the innate cellular process of programmed cell death. Replication of the mutated genes allows for development of malignancy (Olsen et al., 2019).

The most extensively studied tumor-suppressor gene is the p53 transcription factor. In response to cellular stresses, a variety of mechanisms converge on p53 leading to its stabilization and accumulation (Dutt & Stambolic, 2021). Contingent on the nature of the stress and cellular context, p53 then activates the expression of genes leading to DNA repair and growth arrest on the one hand and apoptotic cell death on the other. In the absence of p53, cells are impaired in their ability to respond appropriately to oncogenic mutations and stresses, leading to proliferation, growth, and marked genetic instability. In addition, p53 is now understood to control the expression of sets of genes involved in other roles, including autophagy (the body's way of cleaning out damaged cells), metabolism, inflammation, and cell plasticity (Dutt & Stambolic, 2021).

Pearls for Practice: Pathophysiology

Carcinogenesis is the result of both genetic and epigenetic changes. The term epigenetics refers to heritable, reversible changes in gene expression that do not involve changes to the underlying DNA sequence (Boutros et al., 2021). Epigenetic changes can affect the efficacy of DNA repair genes, altering specific gene expression and disrupting normal expression of proto-oncogenes and tumor suppressor genes (Olsen et al., 2019).

All cells, both healthy and malignant, proliferate by way of the cell cycle (see Fig. 5-2). The cell cycle time is the time required for one cell to divide and reproduce two identical daughter cells. The cell cycle of any cell has four distinct phases, each with a vital underlying function:

1. G_1 phase: RNA and protein synthesis occur
2. S phase: DNA synthesis occurs
3. G_2 phase: premitotic phase; DNA synthesis is complete, mitotic spindle forms
4. Mitosis: cell division occurs

The G_0 phase, the resting or dormant phase of cells, can occur after mitosis and during the G_1 phase. In the G_0 phase, there are cells that are not actively dividing but have the potential to enter into the cell cycle. Mitosis (cell division) occurs more frequently in malignant cells than in normal cells. As the cells grow and divide, more glucose and oxygen are needed. If glucose and oxygen are unavailable, malignant cells use anaerobic metabolic channels to produce

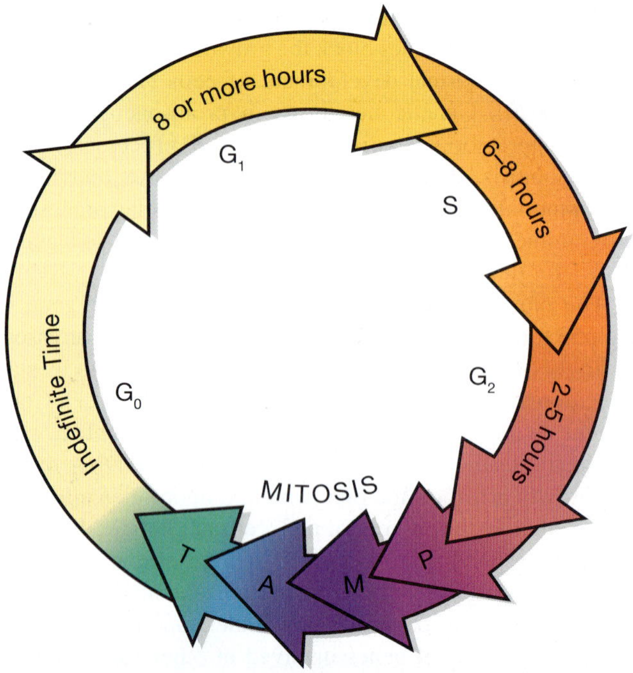

FIGURE 5-2 **Phases of the cell cycle extend over the interval between the midpoint of mitosis and the subsequent end point in mitosis in a daughter cell. G_0 is the resting, or dormant, phase of the cell cycle. G_1 is the postmitotic phase during which ribonucleic acid (RNA) and protein syntheses are increased and cell growth occurs. In the S phase, nucleic acids are synthesized and chromosomes are replicated in preparation for cell mitosis. During G_2, RNA and protein synthesis occur as in G_1. A, anaphase; M, metaphase; P, prophase; T, telophase. (Redrawn from Porth, C. M. (2002). *Pathophysiology: Concepts of altered health states* (6th ed.). Lippincott Williams & Wilkins.)**

energy, which makes the cells less dependent on the availability of a constant oxygen supply.

Proliferation through the cell cycle is controlled by a balance of positive and negative signals received from inside and outside of the cell (known as *signal-transduction pathway*) (Harrington et al., 2021). A decrease or increase in the cell's ability to respond to a signal may result in increased proliferation.

Thus, cancer development and progression are a result of a series of mutations over time that destabilize the genome and allow for uncontrolled cell growth. This makes the cells further susceptible to mutations and causes alterations in the surrounding tissue, favoring growth and invasion into surrounding tissue (Harrington et al., 2021).

Metastasis

Tumors also have the capacity to invade and spread from their original site to other organs in the body. This process is known as metastasis. Metastasis formation is the major cause of death in most patients with cancer. Despite extensive research, targeting metastatic seeding (referring to the ability of circulating tumor cells to move multidirectionally, rather than linearly as in one direction to the nearest regional lymph node) and colonization is still an unresolved challenge (Bergers & Fendt, 2021). Metastasis is a multistep process consisting of a series of sequential events: (1) local invasion into the tumor-associated stroma; (2) intravasation into hematopoietic, lymphatic systems or peritoneum; (3) survival in circulation; (4) extravasation into premetastatic niches at distant organs; and (5) colonization to form metastasis (Wei et al., 2020).

The most common sites of metastasis include the bones, lungs, liver, and central nervous system (CNS). The site of metastasis is influenced by the availability of a blood supply, cell receptors, and genes that may direct the malignant cell to travel to specific sites, and the presence of growth factors essential for metastatic growth that may be elicited only in selected organs.

Angiogenesis

Malignant cells require oxygen and nutrients to survive and proliferate, and therefore need to reside near blood vessels to access the blood circulation system (Lugano et al., 2019). Angiogenesis is a process whereby new vascular structures emerge from ones that have already been established in tissues or tumor masses (Rak & Emmenegger, 2021). Tumors can be vascularized either through co-option of the preexisting vasculature, or by inducing new blood vessel formation through a variety of molecular or cellular mechanisms. Vascular homeostasis is regulated by many pro- and anti-angiogenic factors (Lugano et al., 2019). Initiation of blood vessel formation is induced when pro-angiogenic signaling is dominating, a process that in tumors has been coined the "angiogenic switch." The angiogenic switch released tumors from dormancy and sparks rapid growth of malignant cells in association with new blood vessel formation (Lugano et al., 2019).

Lymphatic Spread

The transport of tumor cells through the lymphatic circulation is the most common mechanism of metastasis. Tumor emboli enter the lymph channels by way of the interstitial fluid, which communicates with lymphatic circulation. Malignant cells also may penetrate lymphatic vessels by invasion. After entering the lymphatic circulation, malignant cells either lodge in the lymph nodes or pass between the lymphatic and venous circulations. Tumors arising in areas of the body with rapid and extensive lymphatic circulation are at high risk for metastasis through lymphatic channels. Breast tumors frequently metastasize in this manner through axillary, clavicular, and thoracic lymph channels.

Hematogenous Spread

Hematogenous spread is the dissemination of malignant cells via the bloodstream and is directly related to the vascularity of the tumor. Malignant cells can travel through the bloodstream, attach to endothelium, and attract fibrin, platelets, and clotting factors to seal themselves from immune system surveillance. The endothelium retracts, allowing the malignant cells to enter the basement membrane and secrete lysosomal enzymes. These enzymes destroy surrounding body tissues and thereby allow implantation.

Etiology

At present, cancer is regarded as a genetic disease arising from numerous mutations in oncogenes and tumor suppressor genes. Are gene mutations in the cell nucleus the causal event in the origin of cancer, or is the damaged genetic material just the consequence and not the primary cause of cancer (Poljsak et al., 2019)? Expert panels have recommended that integrative transdisciplinary studies of modifiable exposures, tumor characteristics, and clinical outcomes are urgently needed to improve strategies for precision prevention and treatment (Ogino et al., 2019). Recently, other factors implicated in carcinogenesis include viruses and bacteria, physical agents, chemical agents, genetic or familial factors, dietary and lifestyle factors, and hormonal agents.

Viruses and Bacteria

Viruses are thought to incorporate themselves into the genetic structure of cells, thus altering future generations of that cell population—perhaps leading to cancer.

The human papillomaviruses (HPVs) are members of the Papillomaviridae (PV) family. To date, over 450 distinct types of HPV belong to this virus family. Most of these viruses are low risk, and are associated with benign lesions such as papillomas, warts, wedges, and Heck disease (focal epithelial hyperplasia). Malignant lesions by carcinogenic HPV are anal, genital (penile, vulval, vaginal, cervical), and some types of oral (Santacroce et al., 2021).

Hepatitis C virus (HCV) infects an estimated 170 million persons worldwide and thus represents a viral pandemic, one that is five times as widespread as infection with the human immunodeficiency virus type 1 (HIV-1) (Lauer & Walker, 2021). The institution of blood screening measures in developed countries has decreased the risk of transfusion-associated hepatitis to a negligible level, but new cases continue to occur mainly as a result of injection-drug use and, to a lesser degree, through other means of percutaneous or mucous-membrane exposure (Lauer & Walker, 2021). The natural history of HCV infection has been very difficult to assess, because of the usually silent onset of the acute phase as well as the frequent paucity of symptoms during the early stages of chronic infection (Lauer & Walker, 2021). Most chronic viral infections will lead to hepatitis and to some degree of fibrosis. Severe complications and death usually occur only in persons with cirrhosis, which is estimated to develop in 15% to 20% of those infected. Once cirrhosis is established, the risk of hepatocellular carcinoma is approximately 1% to 4% per year. Hepatocellular carcinoma can occur without cirrhosis but is rare (Lauer & Walker, 2021).

A few bacteria are associated with the development of cancer. An example is *Helicobacter pylori (H pylori)*, which is a powerful inducer of precancerous lesions and gastric cancer (Bakhti & Latifi-Navid, 2021). Because the inner layer of the stomach can also become inflamed and damaged, *H. pylori* can lead to cancer in the lower part of the stomach and is also associated with some types of stomach lymphoma.

Physical Agents

Physical factors associated with carcinogenesis include exposure to sunlight or radiation. Exposure to ionizing radiation can occur with repeated diagnostic x-ray procedures or with radiation therapy used to treat disease. Fortunately, improved x-ray equipment appropriately minimizes the risk to healthy tissue of extensive radiation exposure. Radiation therapy used in disease treatment and exposure to radioactive materials at nuclear weapon manufacturing sites or nuclear power plants are associated with a higher incidence of leukemias; multiple myeloma; and cancers of the lung, bone, breast, thyroid, and other tissues. Background radiation from the natural decay process produces radon that has also been associated with lung cancer.

Chemical Agents

Relative to normal cells, cancerous cells have impaired ability to control cell division, to age, and to undergo apoptotic (programmed) cell death. Any chemical agent that triggers or contributes to the impairment of these processes could promote progression to malignancy, tumor growth, and metastasis, especially with chronic exposure (Grant, 2021). Chemicals may also promote the growth of initiated cells indirectly, for example, by causing the death of nearby cells that triggers the establishment of a chronic tumor-promoting inflammatory environment (Grant, 2021).

Cigarette smoking increases the risk of several cancers, including those of the oral cavity and larynx, esophagus, pancreas, uterine cervix, kidney, bladder, stomach, colorectum, liver, and acute myeloid leukemia. Cigarette smoking is by far the most important risk factor for lung cancer, with approximately 80% of lung cancer deaths in the United States still caused by smoking (*Cancer Facts & Figures*, 2020).

Alcohol consumption is an established cause of at least seven types of cancer. In 1987, the International Agency for Research on Cancer first classified the consumption of alcoholic beverages as carcinogenic to humans (Rock et al., 2020). Broadly, the carcinogenic effects of ethanol found in alcoholic beverages and acetaldehyde involve DNA and protein damage and alterations, oxidative stress, inhibition of DNA repair and cell death, increased cell proliferation, nutritional malabsorption, changes in DNA methylation, and, for breast cancer, increased estrogen levels (Rock et al., 2020).

Many chemical substances found in the workplace have proved to be carcinogens or co-carcinogens. The extensive list of suspected chemical substances continues to grow and includes aromatic amines and aniline dyes; pesticides and formaldehydes; arsenic, soot, and tars; asbestos; benzene; betel nut and lime; cadmium; chromium compounds; nickel and zinc ores; wood dust; beryllium compounds; and polyvinyl chloride.

Genetics or Familial Factors

Observations over time have shown that cancers cluster in some families. This may be due to genetics, shared environments, cultural or lifestyle factors, or chance alone. Obtaining an accurate family history is essential in guiding referrals to genetic counseling and testing for hereditary cancer syndromes, such as hereditary breast and ovarian cancer syndrome (HBOC) and Lynch syndrome. *BRCA1* and *BRCA2* are the genes associated with hereditary breast and ovarian cancer syndrome, and *MLH1, MSH2, MSH6,* and *PMS2* are the genes associated with Lynch syndrome. Lynch syndrome, also known as *hereditary nonpolyposis colorectal cancer (HNPCC)*, is an inherited disorder that increases the risk of developing many other types of cancer, particularly colorectal cancer.

Technical advances in genome sequencing and the implementation of next-generation sequencing (NGS) in clinical oncology have paved the way for individualizing cancer patient therapy based on molecular profiles (Colomer et al., 2020). NGS is most appropriate for patients who have an advanced cancer in which there are several commonly identified molecular targets, particularly when they are useful at the initial therapy. Additionally, NGS testing can be helpful in navigating patients to clinical trials and can offer individual options in patients with rare cancers (Colomer et al., 2020). Clinical trials are showing that NGS testing can have an impact in the response rate and progression-free survival of patients and can therefore be a very useful strategy leading to new molecularly-targeted treatment decisions (Colomer et al., 2020).

The *BRCA1/2* genes account for approximately 25% of hereditary breast cancer cases. However, additional genes have been discovered that may contribute to hereditary breast cancer risk. Next-generation gene sequencing has the potential to detect these other lower penetrance genes that may be responsible for hereditary breast cancer. One commercially available targeted panel that tests for 17 of these genes is called Breast Next™ (Ambry Genetics Laboratories, n.d.).

Approximately 5% of cancers in adults display a familial predisposition. Key indicators of hereditary risk include:

- younger than usual age at time of diagnosis (e.g., colon cancer before age 50),
- multiple family members in one generation with cancer,
- multiple generations with cancer(s) associated with hereditary risk,
- presence of nonmalignant changes associated with hereditary risk (e.g., dysplastic nevi),
- presence of rare tumors commonly associated with hereditary risk (e.g., medullary thyroid cancer),
- any pattern of cancers associated with a hereditary cancer syndrome (e.g., Lynch syndrome),
- bilateral cancer in a paired organ (e.g., breast cancer in both breasts),
- multiple synchronous cancers (e.g., colon cancer with more than one tumor in the colon), or
- an individual with more than one primary cancer (based on information from Hampel et al., 2015; National Comprehensive Cancer Network, 2018; Pierle & Mahon, 2019).

Cancers associated with familial inheritance include retinoblastomas; nephroblastomas (kidney tumor); pheochromocytomas (adrenal medulla tumor); malignant neurofibromatosis (tumors of nerve tissue); and breast, ovarian, colorectal, stomach, prostate, and lung cancers.

Dietary and Lifestyle Factors

Since the early 1980s, the government and leading nonprofit health organizations, such as the American Cancer Society (ACS) and the World Cancer Research Fund/American Institute for Cancer Research (WCRF/AICR), have released cancer prevention guidelines and recommendations focused on weight management, physical activity, diet, and alcohol consumption (Rock et al., 2020). The combination of these risk factors accounted for at least 18.2% of cancer cases and 15.8% of cancer deaths in the United States in 2014, the second highest percentages for any risk factor (after cigarette smoking) in both males and females (Islami et al., 2018).

Prospective studies have shown that diets with higher intake of fruits, vegetables, and whole-grain foods, and lower intake of red and processed meats and salt, are related to reduced risks of cancer and death and that a healthy diet can improve overall survival after diagnosis of breast and CRCs. Although the relationship between vegetable and fruit intake with lowering cancer risk is weaker than previously believed, the 2018 WCRF/AICR report concluded that consuming nonstarchy vegetables and/or whole fruit "probably" protects against several aerodigestive cancers, including mouth, pharynx, larynx, nasopharynx, esophagus, lung, stomach, and CRCs (World Cancer Research Fund/American Institute for Cancer Research, 2019). There is ongoing research on the potential cancer chemopreventive properties of particular vegetables and fruits, or groups of those, including dark-green and orange vegetables, cruciferous vegetables (e.g., cabbage, broccoli, cauliflower, brussel sprouts), soy products, legumes, allium vegetables (onions and garlic), and tomato products. Evidence has shown that higher intake of red and processed meat is specifically associated with high risk or colorectal cancer; there is little evidence that meat intake is associated with risk of other cancers (Knuppel et al., 2020).

In 2018, both the WCRF/AICR and Physical Activity Guidelines Advisory Committee (PAGAC) reports concluded that there was sufficient and robust evidence establishing a link between physical activity and a lower risk of colon cancer. Beyond colon cancer, the strength of the evidence and/or the cancer types linked to physical inactivity is less consistent. The PAGAC concluded that there was strong evidence for six additional cancer types, including breast, kidney, endometrial, bladder, esophageal (adenocarcinoma), and stomach (cardia) cancers (Rock et al., 2020). It is estimated that 1.5% of all cancers diagnosed in the United States during 2014 in males and 4.4% of all cancers diagnosed in females are attributable to physical inactivity, as are 1.4% of all cancer deaths in males and 3.0% of all cancer deaths in females (Rock et al., 2020).

Hormonal Agents

Tumor growth may be promoted by disturbances in hormonal balance, including prolonged exposure to the hormone either by the body's own (endogenous) hormone production or by administration of exogenous hormones. Cancers of the breast and uterus (estrogen dependent) and prostate (androgen dependent) are thought to depend on endogenous hormonal levels for growth.

In general, most previous studies examining the relationship between breast cancer risk factors and tumor behavior have focused on the individual tumor characteristics, and not their constellation. Higher BMI, for instance, is reportedly associated with a higher grade or larger size tumors; nulliparity and menopausal hormone therapy use with highly proliferating and lobular carcinomas, respectively; and higher parity with p53 expressing tumors. In addition, lack of breast feeding and older age at first full-term pregnancy may also influence clinical outcomes following a breast cancer diagnosis (Abubakar et al., 2021).

Numerous studies have investigated the association between breastfeeding and ovarian cancer risk. Through a pooled analysis of over 9,000 females with ovarian cancer and controls from 13 case control studies participating in the Ovarian Cancer Associated Consortium from 1989 to 2009, breastfeeding was associated with a 24% reduced risk of invasive epithelial ovarian cancer (Babic et al., 2020). Independent of parity, ever having breastfed was associated with a reduction in risk of all invasive ovarian cancers, particularly high-grade serous and endometrioid cancers (Babic et al., 2020).

Conflicting literature exists regarding the relationship of combined oral contraceptives (COCs) and breast cancer risk. Although earlier studies demonstrated an association between the use of COCs and overall breast cancer risk in previous and current users, more recent research exhibits a small increased risk in current users only, with risk declining within 5 years after discontinuation. Furthermore, recent research demonstrates that COCs may protect against ovarian, endometrial, and colorectal cancer (Graafland et al., 2020).

Role of the Immune System

In humans, malignant cells can develop at any time in the lifespan. However, some evidence indicates that the immune system can detect the development of malignant cells and destroy them before cell growth becomes uncontrolled. When the immune system fails to identify and stop the growth of malignant cells, clinical cancer develops.

An intact immune system can combat cancer cells in several ways. Usually, the immune system recognizes as foreign certain antigens on the cell membranes of many cancer cells. These antigens, known as *tumor-associated antigens* (also called *tumor cell antigens*), can stimulate both cellular and humoral immune responses.

Along with the macrophages, T lymphocytes are responsible for recognizing tumor-associated antigens. When T lymphocytes, the soldiers of the cellular immune response, recognize tumor antigens, other T lymphocytes that are toxic to the tumor cells are stimulated. These lymphocytes proliferate and are released into the circulation. In addition to possessing cytotoxic (cell-killing) properties, T lymphocytes can stimulate other components of the immune system to rid the body of malignant cells.

A model has been proposed to describe the role of the immune response (immunoediting) during various stages of tumor progression, which includes three phases: elimination, equilibrium, and escape (Saibil et al., 2021). During the elimination phase, the immune system recognizes tumor cells and mounts a response to the tumor. During the equilibrium phase, the immune system and the tumor are in dynamic equilibrium, where the combination of the genomic instability of tumor cells and selective pressure exerted by the antitumor immune response results in editing of the tumor cell population (Saibil et al., 2021). During the escape phase, enough tumor cell variants arise that the tumor can escape elimination by the immune system (Saibil et al., 2021).

The failure of the immune system to respond promptly to the malignant cells allows the tumor to grow too large to be managed by normal immune mechanisms. Newer therapies are attempting to restore or stimulate the immune response to treat cancer (discussed later in the chapter).

Patients who are immunocompromised have been shown to have an increased incidence of cancer. Organ transplant recipients who receive immunosuppressive therapy to prevent organ rejection have an increased incidence of lymphoma, Kaposi sarcoma, squamous cell cancer of the skin, and cervical and anogenital cancers. Patients with immunodeficiency diseases, such as AIDS, have an increased incidence of Kaposi sarcoma, lymphoma, and rectal, head, and neck cancers.

Treatment with certain types of chemotherapy, including alkylating agents and topoisomerase II inhibitors can increase the risk of developing another malignancy over the course of a lifetime. Autoimmune diseases, such as rheumatoid arthritis and Sjogren syndrome, are associated with increased cancer development. Finally, age-related changes, such as declining organ function, increased incidence of chronic diseases, and diminished immunocompetence, may contribute to an increased incidence of cancer in older people.

PREVENTION

Nurses play a critical role in every level of prevention, including primary, secondary, and tertiary prevention. Primary prevention efforts focus on preventing or delaying onset of cancer, while secondary prevention focuses on the early detection of cancer with the goal of identifying cancer in early stages before symptoms develop. Tertiary prevention includes the management of the disease and prevention of progression to later stages. Primary prevention, screening and early diagnosis, multimodal treatment, and survivorship as well as palliative care represent first-line approaches to the increasing cancer incidence worldwide (Gillman et al., 2021). Beyond primary prevention, secondary and tertiary cancer prevention might also contribute to an overall reduction of cancer-related deaths by 70%. The adoption of economically affordable and feasible cancer control plans, specific vaccination policies, and cancer screening programs could be the most effective ways to provide social and economic benefices by reducing cancer incidence and cancer-related mortality rates (Gillman et al., 2021).

Primary Prevention

Primary prevention refers to avoiding an outcome by taking interventions against factors that are causal to that outcome (Gillman et al., 2021). Nurses play a critical role in educating the community about cancer prevention. Nurses can use their teaching and counseling skills to encourage participation in cancer prevention programs, minimize exposure to known carcinogens, and to adopt healthy lifestyles, including the avoidance of tobacco products, achieving and maintaining a healthy body weight, encouraging physical activity, following a healthy eating pattern at all ages (one that limits or does not include red and processed meats, sugar sweetened beverages, or highly processed foods and refined grain products), and avoiding alcohol intake (Rock et al., 2020; American Cancer Society, 2020). Vaccinations also fall under the umbrella of primary prevention. The ACS recommends routine HPV vaccination between ages 9 and 12 years to achieve higher ontime vaccination rates, which will lead to increased numbers of cancers prevented (Saslow et al., 2020; American Cancer Society, 2020).

For individuals at high risk for cancer, prevention should be undertaken by a multidisciplinary team and based on effective use of both surgical and preventive therapy interventions (Thorat & Balasubramanian, 2020). For example, bilateral risk-reducing mastectomy reduces the risk of developing breast cancer by 90% in high-risk females such as carriers of BRCA mutations. Additionally, selective estrogen receptor modulators (SERMs), like tamoxifen, and aromatase inhibitors (AIs) form the mainstay of endocrine treatment in breast cancer. Both these types of agents have shown efficacy as preventive therapies (Thorat & Balasubramanian, 2020).

Secondary Prevention

Nurses must be aware of factors such as race, cultural influences, access to care, provider–patient relationship, level of education, income, and age, which influence the knowledge, attitudes, and beliefs people have about cancer. These factors also may affect the health-promoting behaviors people practice.

Public awareness about health-promoting behaviors can be provided in a variety of ways, including health education and health maintenance programs. Although primary prevention programs may focus on the hazards of tobacco use or the importance of nutrition, secondary prevention programs focus on early detection. Nurses and providers must encourage people to comply with detection efforts as suggested by the ACS (Table 5-2). Many organizations conduct cancer-screening events that focus on cancers with the highest incidence rates or those that have improved survival rates if diagnosed early, such as breast cancer. These events offer education and examinations, such as mammograms, for minimal or no cost. Often these programs are targeted at people who lack access to health care or cannot afford to participate on their own. In developing these programs, nurses must use strategies that are culturally sensitive to foster participation.

Unfolding Patient Stories: D. B. • Part 1

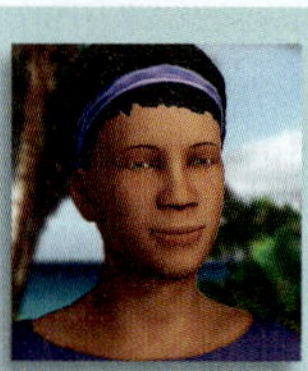

D. B., a 39-year-old cisgender woman diagnosed with uterine fibroids, dysmenorrhea, and menorrhagia, is scheduled for a total abdominal hysterectomy with bilateral salpingo-oophorectomy. D. B. has a family history of uterine and ovarian cancer. The patient asks the nurse what can be done to further reduce her and her family members' risk for cancer. What patient and family education should the nurse present on risk reduction strategies, health promotion, and cancer screening? (D. B.'s case continues in Chapter 32.)

Care for this and other patients in a realistic virtual environment: ***vSim** for Nursing* (thepoint.lww.com/vSimMedicalSurgical). Practice documenting these patients' care in DocuCare (thepoint.lww.com/DocuCareEHR).

DIAGNOSIS

A cancer diagnosis is based on an assessment of physiologic and functional changes and results of the diagnostic evaluation.

TABLE **5-2 American Cancer Society Recommendations for Early Detection of Cancer in Asymptomatic, Average Risk People**

Site	Gender	Age-Specific Evaluation and Frequency
Breast	F	**Females aged 40–44** should have the choice to start annual breast cancer screening with mammograms if they wish to do so. **Females aged 45–54** should get mammograms every year. **Females 55 and older** should switch to mammograms every 2 years or can continue yearly screening. Screening should continue as long as a female is in good health and is expected to live 10 more years or longer. **All females** should be familiar with the known benefits, limitations, and potential harms linked to breast cancer screening.
Colon/Rectum	F/M	For people at average risk for colorectal cancer, the ACS recommends starting regular screening at **age 45**. This can be done either with a sensitive test that looks for signs of cancer in a person's stool (a stool-based test), or with an examination that looks at the colon and rectum (a visual examination). If the person is in good health, they should continue regular screening through **age 75.** For people **aged 76 through 85**, it is recommended they talk with their health care provider about whether screening should continue. People **over 85** should no longer get colorectal cancer screening. Those who choose to be screened with a test other than colonoscopy, the recommendation states that any abnormal test result needs to be followed up with a colonoscopy.
Prostate	M	The ACS recommends that males make an informed decision with a health care provider about whether to be tested for prostate cancer. Starting at **age 50**, males should discuss with health care provider about the pros and cons of testing so they can decide if testing is the right choice for them. If the person is African American or has a father or brother who had prostate cancer before **age 65**, they should discuss this with their provider starting at **age 45**. If the individual decides to be tested, they should get a PSA blood test with or without a rectal examination.
Cervix	F	**Cervical cancer screening should start at age 25.** **People between the ages of 25 and 65** should get a primary human papillomavirus (HPV) test done every 5 years. If a primary HPV test is not available, a co-test (an HPV test with a Pap test) every 5 years or a Pap test every 3 years are still good options **People over age 65** who have had regular cervical cancer testing in the past 10 years with normal results should not be tested for cervical cancer. Those with a history of a serious cervical precancer should continue to be tested for at least 25 years after that diagnosis, even if testing goes past age 65 • **People whose cervix has been removed by surgery** for reasons not related to cervical cancer or serious precancer should not be tested. • **People who have been vaccinated against HPV** should still follow the screening recommendations for their age groups.
Endometrium	F	The ACS recommends that at the time of menopause, all females should be told about the risks and symptoms of endometrial cancer. Females should report any unexpected vaginal bleeding or spotting to their doctors. Some females, because of their history, may need to consider having a yearly endometrial biopsy.
Lung cancer	M/F	The ACS advises that health care providers, and people at increased risk for lung cancer, follow the recently updated recommendations for annual lung cancer screening from the U.S. Preventive Services Task Force (USPSTF), the American Academy of Family Physicians (AAFP), or the American College of Chest Physicians. These organizations recommend yearly lung cancer screening with LDCT scans for people who: are **50 to 80** years old and are in fairly good health **and** currently smoke or have quit in the past 15 years and have at least a 20 pack-year smoking history. In addition, it's important to screen patients regarding their smoking history and refer for counseling to quit smoking. Patients should be educated regarding the possible benefits, limits, and harms of screening with LDCT scans, and go to a center that has experience in lung cancer screening and treatment if they have a significant smoking history or are current smokers.

Adapted from Fontham, E. T. H., Wolf, A. M. D., Church, T. R., Etzioni, R., Flowers, C. R., Herzig, A., Guerra, C. E., Oeffinger, K. C., Shih, Y. T., Walter, L. C., Kim, J. J., Andrews, K. S., DeSantis, C. E., Fedewa, S. A., Manassaram-Baptiste, D., Saslow, D., Wender, R. C., Smith, R. A. (2020). Cervical cancer screening for individuals at average risk: 2020 guideline update from the American Cancer Society. *CA Cancer J Clin*, *70*(5), pp. 321–346. doi: 10.3322/caac.21628.

Diagnostic Evaluation

The diagnostic evaluation is guided by information obtained through a complete history and physical examination. Knowledge of suspicious symptoms and of the behavior of types of cancer assists in determining which diagnostic tests are most appropriate. Patients with suspected cancer undergo extensive testing to (1) determine the presence of a tumor and its extent, (2) identify possible spread (metastasis) of disease or invasion of other body tissues, (3) evaluate the function of involved and uninvolved body systems and organs, and (4) obtain tissue and cells for analysis to assist in the evaluation of tumor type, stage, grade, and molecular and genetic changes.

Patients undergoing extensive testing are usually fearful of the procedures and anxious about the possible test results. The nurse can help relieve the patient's fear and anxiety by explaining the tests to be performed, the sensations likely to be experienced, and the patient's role in the test procedures. The nurse encourages the patient and family to voice their fears about the test results, supports the patient and family throughout the test period, and reinforces and clarifies information conveyed by the primary care provider.

Tumor Staging and Grading

A complete diagnostic evaluation includes identifying the stage and grade of the tumor. This is accomplished before the treatment begins to provide baseline data for evaluating outcomes of therapy and to maintain a systematic and consistent approach to ongoing diagnosis and treatment. Treatment options and prognosis are based on the stage and grade of disease as well as the molecular and genetic profile.

Staging

Staging determines the size of the tumor and the extent of disease. Several systems exist for classifying the disease stage. The TNM system is frequently used for many solid tumor types. In this system, "T" is used to describe the size of the primary tumor and its invasion into adjacent tissues, "N" is used to describe regional lymph node involvement of a tumor, and "M" is used to identify the presence of distant metastases of the primary tumor (Box 5-1) (Rosen & Sapra, 2021). A variety of other staging systems are used to describe the extent of cancers that are not well described by the TNM system, such as CNS cancers, hematologic cancers, and malignant melanoma. Staging systems also provide a convenient shorthand notation that condenses lengthy descriptions into manageable terms for comparisons of treatments and prognoses.

Grading

Grading refers to the classification of the tumor cells. Grading systems seek to define the type of tissue from which the tumor originated and the degree to which the tumor cells retain the functional and histologic characteristics of the tissue of origin. Samples of cells to be used to establish the grade of a tumor may be obtained through cytology (examination of cells from tissue scrapings, body fluids, secretions, or washings), biopsy, or surgical excision.

This information helps the health care team predict the behavior and prognosis of various tumors. The tumor is assigned a numeric value ranging from I to IV (Box 5-2). Grade I tumors, also known as *well-differentiated tumors,* closely resemble the tissue of origin in structure and function. Tumors that do not clearly resemble the tissue of origin in structure or function are described as *poorly differentiated* or *undifferentiated* and are assigned grade IV. These tumors

BOX 5-1

TNM Classification System

T	The extent of the primary tumor.
N	The absence or presence and extent of regional lymph node metastasis.
M	The absence or presence of distant metastasis.

The use of numerical subsets of the TNM components indicates the progressive extent of the malignant disease.

Primary Tumor (T)

Tx	Primary tumor cannot be assessed.
T0	No evidence of primary tumor.
Tis	Carcinoma in situ.
T1, T2, T3, T4	Increasing size and/or local extent of the primary tumor.

Regional Lymph Nodes (N)

Nx	Regional lymph nodes cannot be assessed.
N0	No regional lymph node metastasis.
N1, N2, N3	Increasing involvement of regional lymph nodes.

Distant Metastasis (M)

M0	No distant metastasis
M	Distant metastasis

Data from Edge, S., Byrd, D. R., Compton, C. C., Fritz, A. G., Greene, F. L., & Trotti, A. (Eds.). (2010). *AJCC cancer staging manual* (7th ed.). Springer-Verlag.

BOX 5-2 **Grading**

GX	Grade cannot be assessed
G1	Well differentiated
G2	Moderately differentiated
G3	Poorly differentiated
G4	Undifferentiated

tend to be more aggressive and less responsive to treatment than are well-differentiated tumors.

Genetic Testing: Precision Medicine

Over the last decade, there has been a paradigm shift toward a more personalized approach to cancer treatment. Precision medicine, also known as personalized medicine, is a strategy that allows the selection of a treatment based on the patient's genetic makeup. In the case of cancer, the treatment is tailored to consider the genetic changes that may occur in an individual's tumor (Bashraheel et al., 2020).

Precision medicine emerged in oncology with the discovery of molecularly-targeted agents based on DNA molecular information of the patient's tumors. While traditional chemotherapy destroys rapidly dividing cells by interfering with DNA replication and cell division, molecularly-targeted agents alter the function of specific molecular targets in cell signaling, proliferation, apoptosis, angiogenesis, metabolism, migration, or invasion. Cancer precision medicine is defined as "the use of therapeutics that are expected to confer benefit to a subset of patients whose cancer displays specific molecular or cellular features (most commonly genomic changes and changes in gene or protein expression patterns)" (Malone et al., 2020, p. 1).

Precision medicine has already transformed cancer care—both common and rare malignancies can be targeted by specific therapies to improve clinical outcomes in patients (Malone et al., 2020). The expansion to other molecular characterization technologies beyond genomics, such as transcriptomics, epigenetics, and immunophenotyping, and to the evaluation of drug combinations beyond monotherapy approaches will hopefully increase the clinical utility and scope of precision medicine (Malone et al., 2020). Patients represent active key stakeholders in precision medicine initiatives; thus, resources must be deployed to optimize their education and engagement (Malone et al., 2020).

MANAGEMENT

The range of possible treatment goals may include cancer prevention, complete eradication of the malignant disease (**cure**), prolonged survival and prevention of progression (**control**), or relief of symptoms associated with the disease (**palliation**).

Several factors are considered when determining a treatment plan, including the tumor type, stage, and grade; functional or **performance status** (PS), a measure of how well a patient is able to perform ordinary tasks and carry out daily activities, of the patient; comorbidities; and organ function.

Despite the increasing sophistication and cost of contemporary cancer care, evaluation of PS—an integral aspect of treatment selection, toxicity monitoring, and clinical trial eligibility—has remained essentially unchanged since 1948 (Scott et al., 2020). Evaluation of PS was standardized using a physician-rated scale, now known as Karnofsky Performance Status (KPS), ranging from 0 (dead) to 100 (well-functioning) with 10-point increments. The simpler 6-point Eastern Cooperative Oncology Group (ECOG) PS scale (0 [fully active] to 5 [dead]) was introduced to evaluate patient reaction to chemotherapy, along with patient-reported pain, nausea, and appetite (Scott et al., 2020). Advances in health technology may provide unpresented opportunities to improve PS assessment in cancer.

A variety of approaches, including surgery, radiation therapy, chemotherapy, targeted therapy, and immunotherapy, may be used at various times throughout treatment. Understanding the principles of each treatment modality and how they interrelate is important in understanding the rationale and goals of treatment.

The health care team, the patient, and the patient's family must have a clear understanding of the treatment options, goals, and potential impact on quality of life. Open communication and support are vital as the patient and family periodically reassess treatment plans and goals when complications of therapy develop or disease progresses.

Surgery

Surgery is used for a variety of different reasons and at different times during the cancer trajectory. Surgery may be the primary method of treatment, or it may be prophylactic, palliative, or reconstructive. Diagnostic surgery is the definitive method for identifying the cellular characteristics of the tumor that influence all treatment decisions.

Diagnostic Surgery

Diagnostic surgery, such as a **biopsy**, must be performed to obtain a tissue sample for the analysis of cells suspected to be malignant. In most instances, the biopsy is taken from the actual tumor, but in some situations, it is necessary to biopsy lymph nodes near the suspicious tumor. Many cancers metastasize from the primary site to other areas of the body through the lymphatic circulation. Knowing whether adjacent lymph nodes contain tumor cells is critical to staging the cancer and will impact the need for systemic therapies instead of or in addition to surgery to combat tumor cells that have gone beyond the primary tumor site.

Surgery as Primary Treatment

When surgery is the primary approach in treating cancer, the goal is to remove the entire tumor or as much as is feasible (a procedure sometimes called *debulking*) and any involved surrounding tissue, including regional lymph nodes.

Two common surgical approaches used for treating primary tumors are local and wide excisions:

- A *local excision* is warranted when the mass is small. It includes removal of the mass and a small margin of normal tissue that is easily accessible.
- *Wide* or *radical excisions* (*en bloc dissections*) include removal of the primary tumor, lymph nodes, adjacent involved structures, and surrounding tissues that may be at high risk for tumor spread. This surgical method can result in disfigurement and altered functioning. However, wide excisions are considered if the tumor can be removed completely and the chances of cure or control are good.

Prophylactic Surgery

Prophylactic surgery involves removing nonvital tissues or organs that are likely to develop cancer. Several factors are considered when providers and patients discuss possible prophylactic surgery; these include family history and genetic predisposition, presence or absence of symptoms, potential risks and benefits, ability to detect cancer at an early stage, and the patient's acceptance of the postoperative outcome.

Colectomy (surgical resection of the colon), mastectomy (removal of breast), and oophorectomy (surgical procedure to remove one or both of the ovaries) are examples of prophylactic surgeries. Recent developments in the ability to identify genetic markers indicative of a predisposition to develop some types of cancer may play a role in decisions concerning prophylactic surgeries. Several factors are considered when deciding to proceed with a prophylactic mastectomy, including a strong family history of breast cancer; positive results in *BRCA1* or *BRCA2* testing; an abnormal physical finding on breast examination, such as progressive nodularity and cystic disease; a proven history of breast cancer in the opposite breast; abnormal mammography findings; and abnormal biopsy results.

Because the long-term physiologic and psychological effects are unknown, prophylactic surgery is offered selectively to patients with a thorough discussion of potential risks and benefits with patients and families. Preoperative teaching and counseling, as well as long-term follow-up, are provided.

Pearls for Practice

BRCA1 (breast cancer 1) *and* BRCA2 (breast cancer 2) *are clinical markers associated with the hereditary development of breast and ovarian cancer. Mutations of the* BRCA1 *and* BRCA2 *genes account for most inherited breast cancers. Studies have shown* BRCA1 *mutation carriers have a lifetime risk of approximately 57% to 72% for breast cancer and 39% to 44% for ovarian cancer, whereas* BRCA2 *mutation carriers have an estimated 45% to 69% risk of breast cancer and an 11% to 18% risk of ovarian cancer (Collins & Isaacs, 2020). Breast cancer risk-reducing recommendations, including surveillance, risk-reducing surgery, and/or chemoprevention, must consider a patient's personal preferences, quality of life, and life expectancy. Specific recommendations should also be followed for special* BRCA1/2 *carrier populations, such as pregnant or lactating patients and males (Collins & Isaacs, 2020).*

Palliative Surgery

When cure is not possible, the goals of treatment are to make the patient as comfortable as possible and to improve quality of life as defined by the patient. Palliative surgery is performed to relieve complications of cancer, such as ulcerations, obstructions, hemorrhage, pain, and malignant effusions. Honest and informative communication with the patient and family about the risks, benefits, and goals of surgery is essential.

Nursing Management in Cancer Surgery

A multidisciplinary approach to patient care is essential before, during, and after any type of surgery. The effects of surgery on the patient's body image, self-esteem, and functional abilities are addressed. If necessary, a plan for postoperative rehabilitation is made before the surgery is performed.

The nurse must complete a thorough preoperative assessment for factors that may affect the patient undergoing the surgical procedure, including medical history, prior cancer treatments, and any complications associated with those treatments. Another key aspect in the preoperative assessment in older patients is to define the treatment goal (Kenig, 2020). Cardiac risk factors that increase the risk for complications in noncardiac surgery include age, heart failure, valvular heart disease, myocardial infarction, and pulmonary vascular disease (Li et al., 2019). Preexisting pulmonary disease can increase the risk for postoperative pneumonia and pleural effusions. Patients with cancer may be at increased risk for bleeding (see Chapter 19) and may require additional tests prior to surgery to assess individual bleeding risk. For major or complex surgical procedures with a known high risk of significant blood loss (e.g., >500 to 1,000 mL), advanced discussions with the surgical team, a hemostasis expert, and/or the patient's primary clinician may identify opportunities to implement preoperative or intraoperative measures to avoid transfusion (Graetz et al., 2021).

Patients who are undergoing surgery for the diagnosis or treatment of cancer are often anxious about the surgical procedure, possible findings, postoperative limitations, changes in normal body functions, and prognosis. The patient and family require time, support, and assistance to deal with the possible changes and outcomes resulting from the surgery.

The nurse provides education and emotional support by assessing the needs of the patient and family and by discussing their fears and coping mechanisms with them. The nurse encourages the patient and family to take an active role in decision-making when possible. If the patient or family asks about the results of diagnostic testing and surgical procedures, the nurse's response is guided by the information the provider has previously conveyed to the patient and family. The patient and family may also ask the nurse to explain and clarify information that the provider initially gave but that they did not grasp because they were anxious at the time. It is important that the nurse communicate frequently with providers and other members of the health care team to be certain that the information provided is consistent.

After surgery, the nurse assesses the patient's responses to the surgery and monitors the patient for possible complications, such as infection, bleeding, thrombophlebitis, wound dehiscence, fluid and electrolyte imbalance, and organ dysfunction. The nurse also provides for the patient's comfort. Postoperative teaching addresses decreasing the risk for complications, including deep vein thrombosis (DVT) and pneumonia, as well as education on wound care, activity, nutrition, and medication information.

Patients undergoing surgery for cancer require general perioperative nursing care, as described in Chapter 4, along with specific care related to age, organ impairment, nutritional deficits, disorders of coagulation, and altered immunity that may increase the risk of postoperative complications. Combining other treatment methods, such as radiation and chemotherapy, with surgery also contributes to postoperative complications, such as infection, impaired wound healing, altered pulmonary or kidney function, and the development of venous thromboembolism (VTE), also known as DVT. The incidence of VTE in cancer patients is significantly increased to 4% to 20% compared with the normal population. Cancer patients with VTE have higher mortality rates than those without VTE, and VTE treatment can postpone or complicate cancer treatment (Weitz et al., 2020).

Pearls for Practice

Approximately 50% of patients with DVT are asymptomatic. The nurse should inquire about an ache or pain in the calf that is aggravated by standing or walking. In addition, it is important to assess for asymmetry of the limbs as slight swelling may be noted as well as erythema and warmth of the involved extremity. Venous distention in the affected limb that persists despite elevation of the extremity may be noted. Patients may also present with low-grade fever and tachycardia.

Plans for discharge, follow-up and home care, and treatment are initiated as early as possible to ensure continuity of care from hospital to home or from a cancer referral center to the patient's local hospital and health care provider. Patients and families are also encouraged to use community resources, such as the ACS, for support and information.

Radiation Therapy

In **radiation therapy**, ionizing radiation is used to interrupt cellular growth. More than half of patients with cancer receive a form of radiation therapy at some point during treatment. Radiation may be used to cure the cancer, as in head and neck, prostate, lung, and bladder cancers. A key goal and main challenge of radiation therapy is the elimination of tumors without any concurring damages of the surrounding healthy tissues and organs (Gregoire et al., 2020).

Palliative radiation therapy is used to relieve the symptoms of metastatic disease, especially when the cancer has spread to the brain, bone, or soft tissue, or to treat oncologic emergencies, such as superior vena cava syndrome (SVCS) or spinal cord compression.

Two types of ionizing radiation—electromagnetic rays (x-rays and gamma rays) and particles (electrons [beta particles], protons, neutrons, and alpha particles)—can lead to tissue disruption. Radiation disrupts malignant cell proliferation through the alteration in DNA structure. Ionizing radiation breaks the strands of the DNA helix, leading to cell death. Ionizing radiation can also ionize constituents of body fluids, especially water, leading to the formation of free radicals and irreversible DNA damage. If the DNA is incapable of repair, the cell may die immediately, or it may initiate apoptosis (Mcquestion et al., 2021; Iwamoto et al., 2012).

Cells are most vulnerable to the disruptive effects of radiation during DNA synthesis and mitosis. Therefore, those body tissues that undergo frequent cell division are most sensitive to radiation therapy. These radiosensitive tissues include bone marrow, lymphatic tissue, epithelium of the GI tract, hair cells, and gonads. Slower-growing tissues and tissues at rest are relatively radioresistant (less sensitive to the effects of radiation). Such tissues include muscle, cartilage, and connective tissues.

A radiosensitive tumor is one that can be destroyed by a dose of radiation that still allows for cell regeneration in the normal tissue. Tumors that are well oxygenated also appear to be more sensitive to radiation (Mcquestion et al., 2021). In theory, therefore, radiation therapy may be enhanced if more oxygen can be delivered to tumors. In addition, if the radiation is delivered when most tumor cells are cycling through the cell cycle, the number of cancer cells destroyed (cell kill) is maximal. Certain chemicals, including chemotherapy and some targeted agents (e.g., EGFR inhibitors) act as radiosensitizers and sensitize more hypoxic (oxygen-poor) tumors to the effects of radiation therapy (Mcquestion et al., 2021).

Radiation Delivery

Radiation is delivered to tumor sites by external or internal methods.

External Radiation

If external radiation therapy is used, one of several delivery methods may be chosen, depending on the depth of the tumor. Kilovoltage therapy devices deliver the maximal radiation dose to superficial lesions, such as lesions of the skin and breast. Conversely, linear accelerators and betatron machines produce higher-energy x-rays and deliver their dosage to deeper structures with less harm to the skin and less scattering of radiation within the body tissues.

Internal Radiation

Internal radiation implantation, or **brachytherapy**, delivers a high dose of radiation to a localized area. The specific radioisotope for implantation is selected based on its half-life, which is the time it takes for half of its radioactivity to decay. This internal radiation can be implanted by means of needles, seeds, beads, or catheters into body cavities (e.g., vagina, abdomen, pleura) or interstitial compartments (e.g., breast). With internal radiation therapy, the farther the tissue is from the radiation source, the lower the radiation exposure. This spares the noncancerous tissue from the radiation dose and toxicity. Brachytherapy may also be administered orally, as with the isotope iodine-131, which is used to treat thyroid carcinomas.

Intracavitary Radiation. Intracavitary radioisotopes are used frequently to treat gynecologic cancers. A bowel prep is administered and the patient is maintained on clear liquids the day before admission. In these malignancies, the radioisotopes are inserted into applicators specially positioned in the cervix and vagina, after the position is verified by x-ray. These radioisotopes remain in place for a prescribed time period (generally around 1 week) and then are removed. The patient is maintained on bed rest and carefully log-rolled to prevent displacement of the intracavitary delivery device. The head of the bed must not be elevated greater than 15 degrees due to the risk of perforating the uterus with the appliance. An indwelling urinary catheter is inserted to ensure that the bladder remains empty, which minimizes the exposure of the bladder to radiation. Low-residue diets and antidiarrheal agents, such as diphenoxylate, are provided to prevent bowel movements during therapy that might displace the radioisotopes. Pain management is also a priority for these patients as the presence of the appliance can be painful. Patient-controlled analgesia is a common method used for pain management in this population. Patients are also at risk for atelectasis, pressure ulcers, and DVT due to bed rest, so preventative measures, including incentive spirometry, a pressure-relieving mattress, sequential compression devices, and prophylactic anticoagulation, are essential to preventing these complications.

Safety. Because patients receiving internal radiation emit radiation while the implant is in place, contacts with the health care team are guided by principles of *time, distance,* and *shielding* to minimize exposure of personnel to radiation. As the amount of *time* with the patient increases, the nurse's exposure to radiation increases. The goal of nursing care for this population is to deliver safe and efficient care that meets the patient's needs in the shortest amount of time, in general, no more than 30 minutes per 8-hour shift. The principle of distance means that the closer you are to the patient, the greater the radiation exposure. When not providing direct care (e.g., when talking with the patient), stand at least 6 feet from the patient to minimize exposure. Organize activities outside the room when possible, for example, preparation of meals and medication. *Shielding* refers to the use of a lead shield to buffer the exposure to radiation. Often, the rooms that patients stay in may be lead-lined, or portable lead shields or aprons may be available to minimize exposure.

Other safety precautions used in caring for a patient receiving brachytherapy include assigning the patient to a private room, posting appropriate notices about radiation safety precautions, having staff members wear dosimeter badges (to track cumulative radiation exposure), ensuring that pregnant staff members are not assigned to the patient's care, prohibiting visits by children or pregnant visitors, limiting visits from others to 30 minutes daily, and seeing that visitors maintain a 6-foot distance from the radiation source.

Nurses must be prepared to respond to a radiation emergency. If the radiation implant becomes dislodged, the nurse's priority is to ensure the safety of the patient. Metal forceps and a lead-lined container should be available in the room. The nurse can use the forceps to pick up the radiation source and place the source into the lead-lined container. Once the source is contained, the radiation safety officer should be contacted immediately. Then the patient, nurse, and room will be monitored for radioactivity using a Geiger counter. The staff exposed should report to their occupational health department for an evaluation. Nurses should refer to their institution's radiation safety committee's guidelines for specific measures.

Radiation Dosage

The radiation dosage is dependent on the sensitivity of the target tissues to radiation and on the tumor size. The lethal tumor dose is defined as the dose that will eradicate 95% of the tumor while preserving normal tissue. With external radiation, the total radiation dose is delivered over several weeks to allow healthy tissue to repair and to achieve greater cell kill by exposing more cells to the radiation as they begin active cell division. Repeated radiation treatments over time (fractionated doses) also allow for the periphery of the tumor to be reoxygenated repeatedly because tumors shrink from the outside inward. This increases the radiosensitivity of the tumor, thereby increasing tumor cell death.

Toxicity

Toxicity of radiation therapy is localized to the region being irradiated. Toxicity may be increased if concomitant chemotherapy is administered. Acute local reactions occur when normal cells in the treatment area are also destroyed and cellular death exceeds cellular regeneration. Altered skin integrity is a common effect and can include **alopecia** (hair loss), erythema, and shedding of skin (desquamation). Re-epithelialization occurs after treatments have been completed; healing can take several weeks.

Alterations in oral mucosa secondary to radiation therapy include **stomatitis** (inflammation of the mucous membrane of the mouth), **xerostomia** (dryness of the mouth), change and loss of taste, and decreased salivation. The entire GI mucosa may be involved, possibly resulting in esophageal irritation with chest pain and dysphagia. Anorexia, nausea, vomiting, and diarrhea may occur if the stomach or colon is in the irradiated field. Symptoms subside and GI re-epithelialization occurs after treatments have been completed; however, it may take several weeks for stomatitis to resolve. Xerostomia and taste changes may never return to normal.

Bone marrow cells proliferate rapidly, and if sites containing bone marrow (e.g., the iliac crest, sternum) are included in the radiation field, anemia, leukopenia (decreased WBCs), and **thrombocytopenia** (a decrease in platelets) may result. The patient is then at increased risk for infection and bleeding until blood cell counts return to normal. Chronic anemia may occur commonly due to the cumulative effects of radiation and may be evidenced by shortness of breath, dizziness, fatigue, decreased oxygen saturation, and decreased activity tolerance.

Acute side effects to radiation therapy can occur within hours to days of receiving the first treatment. Bone marrow suppression, gonadal toxicity, skin changes, salivary changes, and GI side effects, such as nausea, may occur acutely.

Late effects from radiation are seen months to years after therapy even in the absence of acute symptoms. These effects can include changes to the CNS, head and neck, lungs, heart, liver, pancreas, gastrointestinal system, gynecologic organs, urinary tract and prostate, spleen and lymph nodes, and bone and soft tissues (Albano et al., 2021).

Nursing Management in Radiation Therapy

Providing Patient Education

Patient education is a continuous process throughout the cancer experience (Olsen et al., 2019). Patients receiving radiation therapy, and their families, often have questions and concerns about its safety. To answer questions and allay fears about the effects of radiation on the tumor and on the patient's normal tissues and organs, the nurse explains the procedure for delivering radiation and describes the equipment, the duration of the procedure (often minutes only), the methods for immobilizing the patient during the procedure, and the sensory experience, including the absence of pain, during the procedure.

If a radioactive implant is used, the nurse informs the patient and family about the restrictions placed on visitors and health care personnel and other radiation precautions. The patient also should understand their own role before, during, and after the procedure. Patients with seed implants may be able to return home because the radiation exposure to others is minimal. Information about any precautions, if needed, is provided to the patient and family members to ensure safety. See Chapters 32 and 33 for further discussion of radiation treatment for gynecologic cancers and prostatic cancer, respectively.

Protecting Skin and Oral Mucosa

The nurse regularly assesses the patient's skin, oral mucosa, nutritional status, and general feeling of well-being. As many as 95% of patients receiving radiation experience radiation dermatitis. A true collaboration between providers and patients is needed to alleviate radiation dermatitis symptoms, reduce the possibility of delaying radiation therapy, and provide the best possible quality of life while symptoms are acute (Pembroke & Nemeth, 2020).

The skin in the radiation field must be protected from irritation, and the patient is instructed to avoid using ointments, lotions, or powders on the treated area. The patient is instructed to gently cleanse the skin with lukewarm water and a mild, nondeodorant soap using the fingertips or a soft washcloth (no scrubbing) and then gently pat the area dry. If temporary skin markings were applied to facilitate external radiation treatments, warn the patient not to remove the markings. Avoid any perfumed lotion or powder; avoid applying makeup to the treatment field. Emollients such as Aquaphor® may be used as directed by the radiation oncologist to soothe and moisturize irritated skin. However, even approved emollients should not be used up to 4 hours before the treatment time. Lotions and emollients may amplify the effects of the radiation on the skin. Electric razors should be used for shaving, but aftershave products should be avoided. Patients should be instructed to avoid constrictive clothing that may irritate skin. Loose, cotton clothing is usually most comfortable. Other instructions include avoiding sun exposure, wind, extreme temperatures, heating lamps, heating pads, and ice packs to the area being treated—these are all potential sources of thermal injury. Avoid itching skin, and avoid applying tape to radiated areas to minimize trauma to the skin (Mcquestion et al., 2021).

Gentle oral hygiene is essential to remove debris, prevent irritation, and promote healing (see Box 5-3 for detailed instructions). If systemic symptoms, such as weakness and fatigue, occur, the patient may need assistance with activities of daily living and personal hygiene (see Nursing Process later in the chapter). In addition, the nurse offers reassurance by explaining that these symptoms are a result of the treatment and do not represent deterioration or progression of the disease.

Chemotherapy

In **chemotherapy**, antineoplastic agents are used in an attempt to destroy tumor cells by interfering with cellular

BOX 5-3

Patient Education: Mouth Care for Patients Receiving Head and Neck Radiation Therapy

- Use a bland mouth rinse (such as salt water or baking soda and water) often. Gently swish and gargle with this before and after meals and at bedtime. You may use it more often as needed to soothe a dry or sore mouth. To make the mouth rinse, mix 1 teaspoon of baking soda or 1 teaspoon of table salt with 16 oz of water.
- Use fluoride preparations daily as instructed by your dentist. Brush your teeth using a soft-bristled toothbrush three to four times a day. Floss your teeth daily.
- Dentures should be left out if they are irritating to the gums or are poorly fitting.
- Avoid alcoholic beverages, tobacco, highly spiced foods, and commercial mouthwashes containing alcohol.
- Once you begin to experience pain or sensitivity in your mouth, avoid foods and drinks that are too hot or too cold. Room temperature is best. Avoid carbonated drinks such as soda or sparkling water.
- Avoid acidic fruits and juices like tomato, orange, lemon, grapefruit, and pineapple. Avoid rough, crunchy foods such as pretzels, nuts, and chips.
- Inspect your mouth daily and report any changes to your nurse or doctor.
- For a dry mouth, drink 8 oz of water or other noncaffeinated beverage every 2 to 3 hours. Keep a cool mist humidifier running, especially at night.
- Moisturize lips frequently with water-based moisturizer (e.g., lanolin type product).
- Discuss with your provider the risks/benefits of utilizing pain medications premeals.

functions, including replication. Chemotherapy is used primarily to treat systemic disease rather than localized lesions that are amenable to surgery or radiation. Chemotherapy may also be used locally for instillations (e.g., bladder, peritoneum) or topical therapy; although chemotherapy may be used as single agents, more commonly, they are used in combination. Chemotherapy generally affects the cell cycle and cell kinetics and is associated with nonspecific cytotoxic effects on normal tissues. Chemotherapy includes alkylating agents, antimetabolites, antitumor antibiotics, nitrosoureas, and plant alkaloids (e.g., taxanes, vinca alkaloids, camptothecines) (Olsen et al., 2019). The goals of chemotherapy (cure, control, palliation) define the medications to be used and the aggressiveness of the treatment plan. Chemotherapy may also be delivered in the setting of a clinical trial (see Box 5-4).

Cell Kill and the Cell Cycle

Each time a tumor is exposed to a chemotherapeutic agent, a percentage of tumor cells (20% to 99%, depending on dosage) are destroyed. Repeated doses of chemotherapy are necessary over a prolonged period to achieve regression of the tumor. Eradication of 100% of the tumor is almost impossible. Instead, the goal of treatment is eradicating enough of the tumor so that the remaining tumor cells can be destroyed by the body's immune system.

Cells that are actively dividing within a tumor are the most sensitive to chemotherapeutic agents. Nondividing cells capable of future proliferation (cells in the G_0 phase, see Fig. 5-2) are the least sensitive to antineoplastic medications and, consequently, are potentially dangerous. However,

BOX 5-4

Investigational Antineoplastic Therapies and Clinical Trials

Evaluation of the effectiveness and toxic potential of promising new modalities for preventing, diagnosing, and treating cancer is accomplished through clinical trials. Before new therapies are approved for clinical use, they are subjected to rigorous and lengthy evaluations to identify beneficial effects, adverse effects, and safety.

- *Phase I* clinical trials determine optimal dosing, scheduling, toxicity, and pharmacokinetics. The goal is to determine a tolerable dose, mode, and schedule of administration.
- *Phase II* trials determine effectiveness with specific tumor types and further define toxicities. Phase I and II trials often involve small numbers of patients to help guide decisions about the utility of further research on a given agent. Participants in early trials are often those who have not responded to standard forms of treatment. Since the goals of Phase I and II trials are not focused on efficacy and extending survival, patients and families must be fully informed about the experimental nature and goal of the trial.
- *Phase III* clinical trials establish the effectiveness of new medications or procedures as compared with conventional approaches.
- *Phase IV* testing looks at long-term safety and efficacy. Phase IV trials occur after medication/procedure has been approved.

Nurses may assist in the recruitment, eligibility screening, consent, and education processes for patients who participate in clinical trials. In many cases, nurses are instrumental in monitoring and promoting adherence as well as documenting data describing patients' responses and adverse effects. The physical and emotional needs of patients in clinical trials are addressed in much the same way as those of patients who receive standard forms of cancer treatment.

Data from Clinical Trials Information for Patients and Caregivers, 2019.

the nondividing cells must also be destroyed to eradicate a cancer. As dividing cells are killed by chemotherapy, nondividing cells are recruited into the cell cycle to divide and replace the dying cells. Repeated cycles of chemotherapy must be used to kill these newly dividing cells.

Chemotherapy drugs are often given in combination (referred to as a *protocol* or *regimen*). Combinations of drugs or combination therapies (e.g., drug alone vs. drug plus radiation therapy) generally provide superior efficacy and a survival advantage over monotherapy in many tumor types and combination regimens, although the mechanism by which this occurs is not fully understood in some cases. Hypotheses include that one agent may potentiate the effect of another, or that the combined agent or therapies create effects that together are distinctly unique (Olsen et al., 2019). Tumor cell populations are heterogenous; therefore, a combination of agents or therapies with different mechanisms of action can increase the proportion of cells killed at any one time (Olsen et al., 2019).

Classification of Chemotherapeutic Agents

Chemotherapeutic agents may be classified by their relationship to the cell cycle. Certain chemotherapeutic agents that are specific to certain phases of the cell cycle are termed *cell-cycle–specific agents.* These agents destroy cells that are actively reproducing by means of the cell cycle; most affect cells in the S phase by interfering with DNA and RNA synthesis. Other agents, such as the vinca or plant alkaloids, are specific to the M phase, where they halt mitotic spindle formation. Chemotherapeutic agents that act independently of the cell cycle phases are termed *cell-cycle-nonspecific agents.* These agents usually have a prolonged effect on cells, leading to cellular damage or death. Not only can multiple agents be given that act on different phases of the cell cycle, but chemotherapy is administered using a variety of schedules and doses designed to achieve therapeutic goals, based on the principles of cellular kinetics (Olsen et al., 2019).

Chemotherapeutic agents are also classified by chemical group, each with a different mechanism of action. These include the alkylating agents, nitrosoureas, antimetabolites, antitumor antibiotics, plant alkaloids, hormonal agents, and miscellaneous agents. The classification, mechanism of action, common medications, and common side effects of selected antineoplastic agents are listed in Table 5-3.

Administration of Chemotherapeutic Agents

Chemotherapeutic agents may be administered in the hospital, clinic, or home setting by a variety of routes including topical, oral, IV, intramuscular, subcutaneous, arterial, intracavitary, and intrathecal routes. Intrathecal chemotherapy is the administration of medication into the cerebrospinal fluid. This can be accomplished through a lumbar puncture or through the placement of an intraventricular catheter with the tip lying in the fourth ventricle of the brain. This route is used to treat or prevent CNS metastasis. The route of administration usually depends on the type of agent; the required dose; and the type, location, and extent of tumor being treated. Guidelines for the administration of chemotherapy have been developed by the Oncology Nursing Society (ONS) (Olsen et al., 2019). The use of oral agents to treat cancer is increasing dramatically. Patient education and consistent monitoring of patient adherence is essential to maximize safety.

Dosage

Dosage of antineoplastic agents is based primarily on the patient's total body surface area, previous response to chemotherapy or radiation therapy, function of major organ systems, and performance status.

Pearls for Practice

Because of the high potential for error related to chemotherapy dosing, the standard expectation is that two nurses verify the chemotherapy doses to ensure accuracy. The Mosteller equation for calculation of body surface area is the most used formula in the United States:

$$\sqrt{\frac{\text{height (cm)} \times \text{weight (kg)}}{3600}}$$

Infusion-Related Events

Nurses administering chemotherapy must carefully assess the patient for infusion-related events, such as infusion reactions, hypersensitivity, and extravasation. Specific assessments vary based on the medication being administered (see Table 5-3).

Infusion Reaction. Reactions that occur during or shortly after drug infusion are described as infusion reactions. These reactions may be allergic or nonallergic in nature. Infusion reactions can often be anticipated when administering drugs such as monoclonal antibodies (mAbs), because of the antibody-antigen interactions that release cytokines, but the exact mechanism is unclear (Olsen et al., 2019). Although standard infusion reactions can affect any organ system in the body, the most common signs and symptoms are flushing, itching, change in heart rate and blood pressure, dyspnea, back pain, fever, chills, rash, throat tightening, hypoxia, seizures, and dizziness or syncope (Olsen et al., 2019). It is prudent to differentiate between infusion reactions and hypersensitivity reactions (HSRs), as the latter type of infusion reaction is characterized by an allergic component (Olsen et al., 2019).

Hypersensitivity. HSRs are unexpected, mediated by the immune system, and usually allergic in nature. Immediate HSRs can occur within 5 minutes after the start of infusion to as late as 6 hours after its completion (Olsen et al., 2019). Anaphylaxis is an HSR that is systemic and can be life

TABLE **5-3 Selected Antineoplastic Agents**

Drug Class and Examples	Mechanism of Action	Cell Cycle Specificity	Most Common Side Effects
Alkylating Agents			
Altretamine, bendamustine, busulfan, carboplatin, chlorambucil, cisplatin, cyclophosphamide, dacarbazine, ifosfamide, melphalan, nitrogen mustard, oxaliplatin, temozolomide, thiotepa	Break DNA helix strand, thereby interfering with DNA replication	Cell-cycle nonspecific	Bone marrow suppression, nausea, vomiting, cystitis (cyclophosphamide, ifosfamide), stomatitis, alopecia, gonadal suppression, renal toxicity (cisplatin)
Nitrosoureas			
Carmustine (BCNU), lomustine (CCNU), semustine (methyl CCNU), streptozocin	Break DNA helix, interfering with DNA replication; cross the blood–brain barrier	Cell-cycle nonspecific	Delayed and cumulative myelosuppression, especially thrombocytopenia; nausea, vomiting
Topoisomerase I Inhibitors			
Irinotecan, topotecan	Induce breaks in the DNA strand by binding to enzyme topoisomerase I, preventing cells from dividing	Cell-cycle specific (S phase)	Bone marrow suppression, diarrhea, nausea, vomiting, hepatotoxicity
Antimetabolites			
5-azacitidine, capecitabine, cladribine, clofarabine, cytarabine, decitabine, floxuridine, fludarabine, 5-fluorouracil (5-FU), gemcitabine, 6-mercaptopurine, methotrexate, nelarabine, pemetrexed, pentostatin, pralatrexate, 6-thioguanine	Interfere with the biosynthesis of metabolites or nucleic acids necessary for RNA and DNA synthesis	Cell-cycle specific (S phase)	Nausea, vomiting, diarrhea, bone marrow suppression, stomatitis, renal toxicity (methotrexate), hepatotoxicity
Antitumor Antibiotics			
Bleomycin, dactinomycin, daunorubicin, doxorubicin, epirubicin, idarubicin, mitomycin, mitoxantrone, valrubicin	Interfere with DNA synthesis by binding DNA, thereby preventing RNA synthesis	Cell-cycle nonspecific	Bone marrow suppression, nausea, vomiting, alopecia, anorexia, cardiac toxicity (doxorubicin, daunorubicin, idarubicin, mitoxantrone)
Mitotic Spindle Poisons			
Plant alkaloids: etoposide, teniposide, vinblastine, vincristine (VCR), vindesine, vinorelbine *Taxanes:* cabazitaxel, docetaxel, paclitaxel	Act in late G2 phase, blocking DNA production and in M phase preventing cell division Stabilize microtubules, inhibiting cell division	Cell-cycle specific (G2 and M phase) Cell-cycle specific (G2 and M phase)	Plant alkaloids: bone marrow suppression (mild with VCR), neuropathies (VCR), stomatitis Taxanes: alopecia, bone marrow suppression, bradycardia, hypersensitivity reactions, neuropathy
Hormonal Agents			
Androgens and antiandrogens, estrogens and antiestrogens, progestins and antiprogestins, aromatase inhibitors, luteinizing hormone–releasing hormone analogs, steroids	Bind to hormone receptor sites that alter cellular growth; block binding of estrogens to receptor sites (antiestrogens); inhibit RNA synthesis; suppress aromatase of P450 system, which decreases estrogen level	Cell-cycle nonspecific	Hypercalcemia, increased appetite, masculinization, feminization, sodium and fluid retention, nausea, vomiting, hot flashes, vaginal dryness
Miscellaneous Agents			
Arsenic trioxide, Asparaginase, hydroxyurea, mitotane, procarbazine Romidepsin Vorinostat	Unknown or too complex to categorize Inhibit histone deacetylase	Varies	Anorexia, nausea, vomiting, bone marrow suppression, hepatotoxicity, anaphylaxis, hypotension, altered glucose metabolism

Adapted from Olsen et al. (2019); Polovich et al. (2014).

threatening. Although uncommon with most antineoplastic agents, it is well established with platinum drugs and taxanes. HSRs with platinum agents do not usually occur until the patient has received several doses of the agent (generally after six to seven cycles) (Olsen et al., 2019). Common signs and symptoms of anaphylaxis caused by IV medications include flushing, itching, angioedema (face, eyelids or lips), cough, nasal congestion, shortness of breath, wheezing, sensation of choking, change in voice quality, tachycardia, fainting, hypo- or hypertension, loss of consciousness, nausea, vomiting, cramping/diarrhea, impending sense of doom, tunnel vision, and back, chest, or pelvic pain (Olsen et al., 2019). Response to HSRs includes stopping the infusion as soon as symptoms are observed, as well as staying with the patient; monitoring vital signs every 2 minutes until the patient is stable, then every 5 minutes for 30 minutes, then every 15 minutes; maintaining a patent airway; administering oxygen as needed; maintaining a patent IV with running normal saline; administering emergency medications such as antihistamines, epinephrine, bronchodilators, and corticosteroids as ordered; and providing emotional support to the patient. In mild reactions, re-initiation of the infusion at a slower rate may be considered. For patients with more severe reactions, additional considerations are required for retreatment, including premedication with steroids and antihistamines (H_1 and H_2 blockers). Rapid drug desensitization is cost effective and safe for allergic patients with cancer if the benefit of therapy outweighs any other risk (e.g., survival and quality of life) (Olsen et al., 2019).

Extravasation. Special care must be taken whenever IV vesicant agents are administered. **Vesicants** are agents that, if deposited into the subcutaneous tissue (**extravasation**), cause tissue ulceration and necrosis as well as damage to underlying tendons, nerves, and blood vessels. Although the complete mechanism of tissue destruction is unclear, it is known that the pH of many antineoplastic drugs is responsible for the severe inflammatory reaction as well as the ability of some of these drugs (e.g., anthracyclines) to bind to tissue DNA. Sloughing and ulceration of the tissue may be so severe that skin grafting may be necessary. The full extent of tissue damage may take several weeks to become apparent. Some examples of medications classified as vesicants include anthracyclines (daunorubicin, doxorubicin, epirubicin, idarubicin, dactinomycin, mitomycin, mitoxantrone, and trabectedin), plant alkaloids (vinblastine, vincristine, vindesine, vinorelbine), and taxanes (cabazitaxel, docetaxel, paclitaxel) (Olsen et al., 2019).

Pearls for Practice

Prior to administration of any anticancer agent, the nurse must be aware of a drug's vesicant potential. If frequent administration of antineoplastic vesicants is anticipated in a patient with poor veins, or if a vesicant agent requires administration over more than 1 hour, a central venous access device (CVAD) must be inserted to promote safety during medication administration. Complications associated with CVAD use include infection and thrombosis. Educating the patient about all risks associated with vesicant chemotherapy administration is critical.

Irritants are agents that may inflame and irritate peripheral veins, but do not cause tissue damage. Examples of irritants include bleomycin, carboplatin, and carmustine (Olsen et al., 2019).

Flare reactions are characterized by transient erythema along the vein above the peripheral IV site and may be accompanied by pruritus and urticaria; blood return is present. These types of reactions may be observed during peripheral administration of anthracyclines or mechlorethamine (Olsen et al., 2019).

Patients must understand the importance of prompt reporting of any signs and symptoms of extravasation. Risk factors for extravasation include small and/or fragile veins, lymphedema, obesity, impaired level of consciousness (LOC), history of multiple venipunctures, poor cannula size selection, and poor vein selection. Extravasation can occur because of accidental puncturing of the vein or with movement of the cannula itself due to patient activity or a poorly secured catheter. Prolonged peripheral IV infusions of vesicants carry an increased risk of extravasation; therefore, vesicant infusions lasting more than 1 hour should be administered through a CVAD (Figs. 5-3 and 5-4).

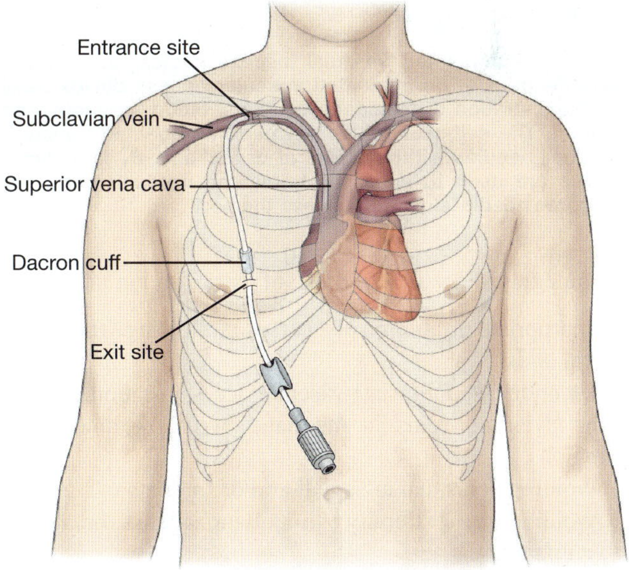

FIGURE 5-3 Central venous access device. The central venous catheter is inserted into the subclavian vein and advanced until its tip lies in the superior vena cava just above the right atrium. The proximal end is then tunneled from the entry site through the subcutaneous tissue of the chest wall and brought out through an exit site on the chest. The Dacron cuff anchors the catheter in place and serves as a barrier to infection.

A

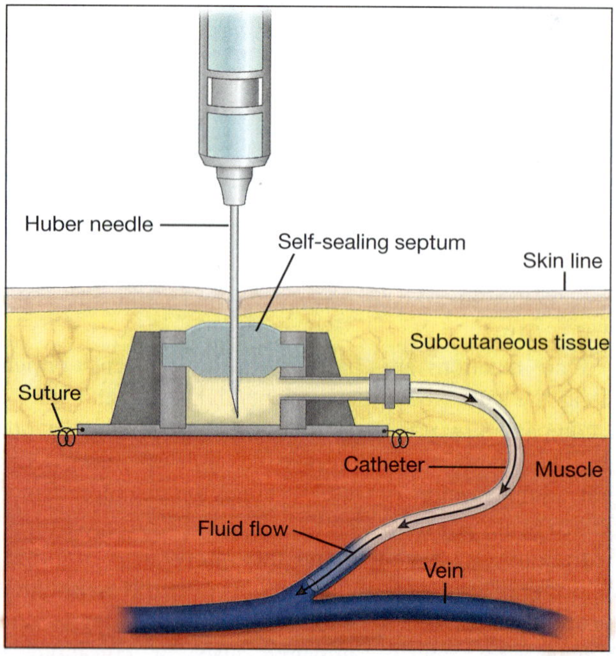

B

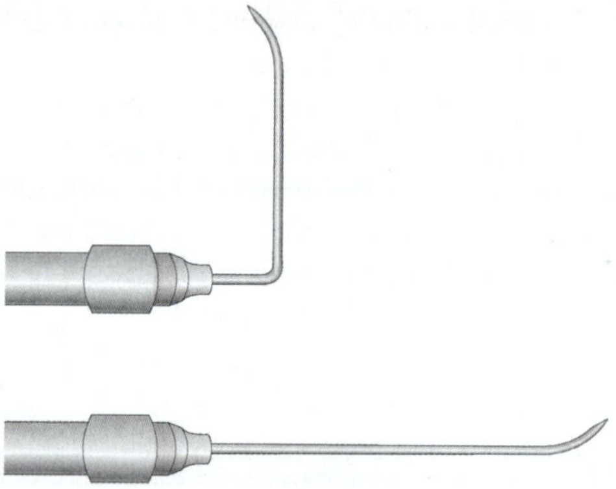

FIGURE 5-4 Implanted vascular access device. A. A schematic diagram of an implanted vascular access device used for administration of medications, fluids, blood products, and nutrition. The self-sealing septum permits repeated puncture by Huber needles without damage or leakage. B. Two Huber needles are used to enter the implanted vascular port. The 90-degree needle is used to access the port.

Strategies to decrease the risk of extravasation include:

- Appropriate training of nurses following the ONS standards
- Selection of appropriate vascular access location, including avoiding veins in the hand, wrist, or antecubital regions
- Avoiding veins that are small and/or fragile
- Avoiding an extremity with lymphedema or recent venipuncture
- Use of the smallest size of cannula in the largest available vein
- Use of a small-bore plastic cannula that is 1.2- to 1.5-cm long
- Use of a clear dressing
- Avoiding the use of a butterfly needle

Pearls for Practice

Indications of extravasation during administration of vesicant agents include:

- *Absence of blood return from the IV catheter*
- *Resistance to flow of IV fluid*
- *Leaking around the insertion site*
- *Swelling, pain, burning, or redness or blistering at the site, or if using a CVAD, pain in the upper arm, upper back, chest, neck, or jaw*
- *Some drugs (such as DNA-binding vesicants) can be retained and recirculated in the tissue for a long period of time, causing a late onset of symptoms (Olsen et al., 2019)*

If any one of the above signs is present, extravasation should be suspected. The medication administration should be stopped immediately. The nurse should attempt to aspirate any residual drug from the IV line. If an antidote is indicated, the nurse should administer it immediately (as ordered). Selection of the neutralizing solution or antidote depends on the extravasated agent.

Dexrazoxane is approved in the setting of anthracycline extravasation with efficacy rates as high as 98% in preventing tissue damage. It is recommended to initiate the first dexrazoxane infusion as soon as possible and within 6 hours of the anthracycline extravasation (Olsen et al., 2019).

Examples of neutralizing solutions include sodium thiosulfate, hyaluronidase, and sodium bicarbonate. Hyaluronidase is an enzyme administered as a subcutaneous injection into the extravasation site that degrades hyaluronic acid in tissues and promotes diffusion of the extravasated agent. It is recommended for extravasation of vinca alkaloids, etoposide and taxanes; however low levels of evidence support its use. Sodium thiosulfate, which neutralizes mechlorethamine (nitrogen mustard), is administered subcutaneously into the extravasation site (Olsen et al., 2019). It is essential for nurses to keep up with the research findings related to extravasation and to apply the evidence to clinical practice.

The involved extremity should be elevated for the first 48 hours. Ice is applied to the site (unless the extravasated vesicant is a vinca alkaloid, in which case warm compresses are used) four times a day for 20 minutes for the first 48 hours, and the patient is educated to avoid further trauma to the site (including heat, constrictive clothing, sunlight) and to report changes in the skin integrity and appearance of the extravasation site to the provider immediately. In collaboration with the provider, refer patients for specialized care when indicated (e.g., plastic or hand surgery consultation, physical therapy, pain management, rehabilitation services) (Olsen et al., 2019). Recommendations and guidelines for managing vesicant extravasation have been issued by individual medication manufacturers, pharmacies, and the ONS, and they differ for each medication.

Protecting Caregivers

Many drugs used in the treatment of cancer are hazardous to health care workers. In 1990, ASHP (then known as the American Society of Hospital Pharmacists) provided the first definition of hazardous drugs, which consisted of the following five characteristics: carcinogenicity, genotoxicity, teratogenicity, reproductive toxicity, and organ toxicity. A sixth characteristic, a new drug similar in structure or toxicity to drugs classified as hazardous using the preceding criteria, was added by NIOSH in 2016 (Olsen et al., 2019). In the United States, an estimated 8 million health care workers are potentially exposed to hazardous drugs or drug waste at their place of employment (Purdy, 2021). Those involved in handling chemotherapeutic agents may be exposed to low doses of the agents by direct contact, inhalation, or ingestion. Nurses who handle these agents must receive education on safe handling measures to minimize risks of exposure. Urinalyses of personnel repeatedly exposed to cytotoxic agents have demonstrated the presence of these agents. Although long-term studies of nurses who handle chemotherapeutic agents have not been conducted, chemotherapeutic agents are associated with secondary formation of cancers and chromosomal abnormalities. Additionally, acute symptoms such as hair loss, abdominal pain, fatigue, nausea, nasal irritation or sores, contact dermatitis, allergic reactions, skin injury, and eye injury can be found in exposed health care workers (Olsen et al., 2019). In an effort to minimize the exposure of health care workers to hazardous substances, the Occupational Safety and Health Administration (OSHA), ONS, hospitals, and other health care agencies have developed specific precautions for health care providers involved in the preparation and administration of chemotherapy (Box 5-5).

BOX 5-5

Safety in Administering Chemotherapy

Safety recommendations from the Occupational Safety and Health Administration (OSHA), Oncology Nursing Society (ONS), hospitals, and other health care agencies for the preparation and handling of antineoplastic agents include the following:

- Use a biologic safety cabinet for the preparation of all chemotherapy agents.
- Wear gloves that have been tested with chemotherapeutic agents when handling antineoplastic drugs and the excretions of patients who received chemotherapy.
- Wear disposable, nonabsorbent long-sleeved gowns with cuffs when preparing and administering chemotherapy agents.
- Use closed-system devices.
- Use Luer-Lok fittings on all IV tubing used to deliver chemotherapy.
- Prime the IV tubing with the diluent, not the medication.
- Work below eye level. Use eye protection if there is a risk of splashing.
- Do not open or crush oral medication.
- Dispose off all equipment used in chemotherapy preparation and administration in appropriate, leak-proof, and puncture-proof containers.
- Dispose off all chemotherapy wastes as hazardous materials.

When followed, these precautions greatly minimize the risk of exposure to chemotherapy agents.

Toxicity

Cells with rapid growth rates (e.g., epithelium, bone marrow, hair follicles, sperm) are most susceptible to the effects of chemotherapy.

GI System

Chemotherapy-induced nausea and vomiting (CINV) is a common and feared side effect of chemotherapy and may persist for as long as 24 to 48 hours after its administration. Delayed nausea and vomiting may persist for several days after chemotherapy. Delayed nausea and vomiting occur commonly with carboplatin, cisplatin, cyclophosphamide, and doxorubicin (Olsen et al., 2019). Anticipatory nausea occurs before chemotherapy administration; it is likely a conditioned response and therefore occurs after a previous experience with CINV. It may be triggered by a particular smell, taste, or sight (Olsen et al., 2019). The primary risk factor for CINV is the emetogenic potential of the agents being used (how likely the agents are to cause nausea and vomiting). Patient-specific risk factors include a history of CINV, female sex, under 50 years of age, and history of motion sickness. Patients who have a history of low or no alcohol consumption have more nausea and vomiting than patients with a history of high alcohol consumption (Olsen et al., 2019).

The vomiting response is coordinated by the vomiting center of the brain, located in the medulla oblongata. It integrates a variety of peripheral and central pathways and elicits the emetic reflex as a response. The peripheral pathway originates in the gastrointestinal tract, where stimuli such as pharyngeal stimulation or gastric/duodenal distention are transmitted via the abdominal vagal afferents. Abdominal vagal afferent fibers express a variety of receptors (e.g., 5–HT3, neurokinin (NK) 1, and cholecystokinin-1) that can trigger the emetic response when stimulated, with 5–HT3 being the main mediator (Gupta et al., 2021). In contrast, the central emesis pathway describes brain input to the vomiting center, eliciting an emetic response. The vomiting center receives direct cholinergic and histaminic input to induce vomiting in response to pain, vestibular perturbation, or emotional factors. The vomiting center also receives inputs from the chemoreceptor trigger zone (area postrema) in response to endogenous toxins and other chemical stimuli. Neurochemical mediators of the latter pathway include the neurotransmitter serotonin (5–HT3) and its receptors, substance P and the NK-1 receptor, and dopamine and its receptors (Gupta et al., 2021).

Chemotherapy drugs can activate neurotransmitter receptors in the postrema of the brain (medullary structure in the brain that controls vomiting) or stimulate vagal afferents near the enterochromaffin cells in the intestine (located in the epithelial layer of the entire gastrointestinal tract). The peripheral pathway is activated within 24 hours after initiation of chemotherapy by the oxidative action of free radicals generated by chemotherapeutic agents, which stimulate enterochromaffin cells in the gastrointestinal tract to release serotonin. Serotonin subsequently stimulates abdominal afferent vagal fibers as part of the peripheral emesis pathway and actives the emetic response via the vomiting center. Chemotherapy drugs can also elicit the release of substance P in both the central and peripheral nervous systems, resulting in NK-1–mediated vomiting (Gupta et al., 2021).

The goal of antiemetics is to prevent CINV. The nurse considers the level of emetogenicity based on the medication, route of administration, and dose administered. Choose the prophylactic antiemetic regimen based on the drug with the highest emetogenicity, while also considering patient-specific risk factors (Olsen et al., 2019). Corticosteroids have been used in CINV for decades and are a mainstay treatment for both acute and delayed CINV (Gupta et al., 2021). NK-1 receptor antagonists act peripherally and centrally by blocking the binding substance P at the NK-1 receptor and are typically administered in combination with a 5–HT3 antagonist and dexamethasone (Gupta et al., 2021). Patients should also have medication at home for as-needed use for breakthrough nausea and vomiting. Other agents used for the management of CINV include olanzapine and dopamine receptor antagonists, benzodiazepines, and cannabinoids (Gupta et al., 2021).

Delayed nausea is often more common and severe than acute nausea and is more difficult to treat. 5–HT3 receptor antagonists, although effective for the prevention of acute vomiting, are not as effective for delayed vomiting. Management includes daily dexamethasone and olanzapine, as well as a NK-1 receptor antagonist in combination with a 5–HT3 receptor antagonist and dexamethasone for patients receiving carboplatin (Olsen et al., 2019). Finally, in addition to pharmacologic management, behavioral interventions such as hypnosis, progressive muscle relaxation, biofeedback, yoga, systemic desensitization, music therapy, and acupuncture/acupressure can be used to manage anticipatory CINV (Olsen et al., 2019).

Hematopoietic System

Most chemotherapeutic agents cause **myelosuppression** (depression of bone marrow function), resulting in decreased production of blood cells. Myelosuppression decreases the number of WBCs (leukopenia), red blood cells (RBCs) (anemia), and platelets (thrombocytopenia) and increases the risk of infection and bleeding. Depression of these cells is a common reason for decreasing the dose of the chemotherapeutic agents. Monitoring blood cell counts frequently is essential because it allows strategies to be implemented to protect patients from infection and injury.

Other agents, called colony-stimulating factors (granulocyte colony-stimulating factor [G-CSF], granulocyte-macrophage colony-stimulating factor [GM-CSF], and erythropoietin [EPO]), can be administered after chemotherapy. G-CSF and GM-CSF stimulate the bone marrow to produce WBCs, including neutrophils, at an accelerated rate, thus decreasing the duration of **neutropenia** (low level of neutrophils, a type of white blood cell). G-CSF decreases the episodes of infection and reduces the need for antibiotics, allowing for timelier cycling of chemotherapy with less need for dose reductions.

Erythropoietin-stimulating agents (ESAs) stimulate RBC production, thus decreasing the symptoms of chronic anemia and reducing the need for blood transfusions, yet increasing the risk of thromboembolic events. Studies have also reported decreased survival, increased mortality during active study phase, and/or an increased risk of cancer progression or recurrence with the use of ESAs in patients with cancer (Bohlius et al., 2019). ESAs are currently indicated in patients with cancer who are receiving myelosuppressive chemotherapy with noncurative intent and anemia that cannot be adequately managed with transfusional support (Bohlius et al., 2019).

Reproductive System

Ovarian and testicular function can be affected by chemotherapeutic agents, resulting in possible sterility. Abnormal ovulation, early menopause, or permanent sterility may occur. In males, temporary or permanent azoospermia (absence of spermatozoa) may develop. Patients interested in exploring fertility preservation options should be referred to a reproductive specialist. In addition, referral to a psychologist may be appropriate for patients expressing distress related to potential or actual fertility (Olsen et al., 2019).

Prior to initiating treatment, patients and their partners need to be informed about potential changes in reproductive and sexual function resulting from chemotherapy. It is important to educate patients honestly and directly, utilizing an interprofessional approach. This is optimal, as these are complex ethical and psychological issues (Olsen et al., 2019). Patients should be advised to use reliable methods of birth control while receiving chemotherapy and not to assume that sterility has resulted.

Nursing Management in Chemotherapy

Nurses play an important role in assessing and managing many of the problems experienced by patients undergoing chemotherapy. Chemotherapeutic agents have systemic effects on normal cells as well as malignant ones, which means that these problems are often widespread, affecting many body systems. Nurses must recognize the potential side effects specific to the drug or drugs that the patient is receiving, and target assessments based on expected side effects. Common side effects seen with chemotherapy include myelosuppression, alopecia, nausea and vomiting, anorexia, and fatigue. The nursing care specific to these side effects is discussed in the nursing process section starting on page 192.

Targeted Therapies

Recent advances in the fields of molecular biology, biochemistry, immunology, and genetics have led to an improved understanding of cancer development. Traditional therapies such as chemotherapy and radiation are nonspecific, affecting all rapidly dividing cells. As a result, both healthy and malignant cells are subject to harmful systemic effects of treatment. **Targeted therapies** seek to minimize the negative effects on healthy tissues by disrupting specific cancer cell functions, such as malignant transformation, communication pathways (also called *cell signaling* or *signal transduction*), processes for growth and metastasis, as well as genetic coding. Targeted therapies can be divided into two categories: those with an extracellular target, such as receptors on the surface of the cells (e.g., mAbs), and those with an intracellular target (e.g., tyrosine kinase inhibitors).

Monoclonal antibodies have a specific target that may be unique to the tumor cell or may target proteins that support tumor growth. Monoclonal antibodies may inhibit the binding of growth factors to receptors on the cell surface, which shuts down the subsequent steps necessary for tumor cell division. Monoclonal antibodies also can act directly on the tumor cell to induce death. In addition, mAbs are involved in stimulating antibody-dependent cellular cytotoxicity (ADCC) in which the antibody binds to tumor cell antigen and natural killer (NK) cells recognize the antibody-covered cell, stimulating cytotoxic proteins to be released to destroy the tumor cell (Olsen et al., 2019). Monoclonal antibodies can be conjugated or unconjugated. Unconjugated mAbs kill tumor cells from the direct action of the antibody on the target (e.g., rituximab, which targets C20; trastuzumab, which targets HER2; cetuximab, which targets EGFR). Conjugated mAbs are antibodies attached to antitumor agents (radioisotopes, chemotherapy drugs, toxins). The mAb attaches to its target and releases the antitumor agent into the cell, stimulating cell death (e.g., brentuximab vedotin). Infusion reactions are common with mAbs and require careful monitoring (see section on infusion related events) (Olsen et al., 2019).

Drugs that target intercellular pathways include tyrosine kinase inhibitors, which direct many cellular functions, including cell signaling, growth, and division. Examples of tyrosine kinase targets include BCR-ABL, mTOR, and BRAF. Growth factors and growth factor receptors are also targets; examples of growth factors include EGFR and VEGF (Olsen et al., 2019). Many of the drugs targeting these kinases and growth factors are taken orally, and adherence is critical to response. See Tables 5-4 and 5-5 for examples of targeted therapies and approved cytokines.

Immunotherapy

As discussed earlier, the immune system is critical in preventing, controlling, and eliminating cancer. Malignancy develops because of multiple mechanisms of immune failure or suppression. Immune therapies, including cytokines, vaccines, and checkpoint inhibitors, were developed to restore or stimulate the body's own immune response to treat the cancer.

Cytokines, including interferon (IFN) alpha and interleukin-2 (IL-2), have been in use for many years in the treatment of melanoma. While the exact mechanisms are unknown, the cytokines cause induction of lymphokine-activated killer cells, NK cells, and IFN gamma production, as well as inhibits tumor growth by stimulating growth and activity of T cells and B lymphocytes (Olsen et al., 2019). Cytokine toxicities vary by agent, and use can potentially cause ongoing overstimulation of the immune system, which may require lifelong management (Olsen et al., 2019).

Checkpoint molecules contribute to the inhibition of T-cell immune responses. Cytotoxic T-lymphocyte antigen 4 (CTLA-4) binds to the antigen-presenting cells, downregulating T cell activity. CTLA-A expression decreases the activation of T cells, as well as sends inhibitory signals to the T cell. CTLA-4 is expressed by activated CD8+ cells, but the primary role of CTLA-4 is diminishing helper T-cell activity and enhancing immunosuppressive activity (Olsen et al., 2019). Programmed cell death protein 1 (PD-1) is an inhibitory receptor on T cells that interacts with its ligand, programmed cell death-ligand 1 (PD-L1) (Olsen et al., 2019). Ligands are small molecules that transmit signals in between or within cells. PD-1/PD-L1 interaction inhibits T-cell proliferation and cytotoxic function, induces T-cell regulatory function, and induces T-cell apoptosis. PD-L1 overexpression has been observed in several tumor types and is correlated with poor prognosis (Olsen et al., 2019). Indications for checkpoint inhibitors are rapidly expanding and include both solid tumor and hematologic malignancies.

Nursing Management in Immunotherapy

Patients receiving immunotherapy require careful monitoring and thorough patient education regarding reportable side effects and self-care. The nurse should be familiar with each agent given and its potential effects. Adverse effects, including flu-like symptoms such as fever, chills, myalgia (muscle pain), nausea, and vomiting, as seen with IFN therapy, may not be life threatening. However, the nurse must be aware of the impact of these side effects on the patient's quality of life and should implement supportive care measures, such as NSAIDs for flu-like symptoms and antiemetics for nausea and vomiting to relieve symptoms. Other life-threatening adverse effects (e.g., capillary leak syndrome, pulmonary edema, hypotension) may occur with IL-2 therapy, requiring aggressive fluid resuscitation and, at times, vasopressors (refer to Chapter 53 for details on managing shock). The

TABLE **5-4 Selected Food and Drug Administration–Approved Targeted Therapies**

Monoclonal Antibody	Indication	Target	Selected Side Effects
Alemtuzumab	Chronic lymphocytic leukemia	CD52, a marker on cell membrane of lymphocytes, monocytes, and macrophages	Infusion reactions; fever; chills; rash; hives; itching; decreased WBC, platelet, and RBC counts
Bevacizumab	Metastatic colorectal cancer	Vascular endothelial growth factor	Arterial and venous thrombosis, hypertension, hemorrhage, GI perforation, proteinuria, congestive heart failure
Cetuximab	Metastatic colorectal cancer	Epidermal growth factor	Infusion reactions, fever, chills, rash, hives, itching, acne-like rash, lung inflammation, kidney failure, diarrhea, nausea, abdominal pain, vomiting
Gemtuzumab ozogamicin	Acute leukemia	CD33, a marker on cell membrane of leukemic cells	Infusion reactions; fever; chills; weakness; headache; tachycardia; hemorrhage; local skin reaction; rash; stomatitis; decreased platelet, WBC, and RBC counts; increased liver function tests
Ibritumomab tiuxetan	Non-Hodgkin lymphoma	CD20, a marker on cell membrane of lymphocytes	Decreased platelets, WBC, and RBC counts; weakness; fever; chills
Ofatumumab	Non-Hodgkin lymphoma	CD20, a marker cell membrane of lymphocytes	Infusion reactions, neutropenia, thrombocytopenia, hepatitis B reactivation, intestinal obstruction
Panitumumab	EGFR + metastatic colorectal cancer	Binds to EGFR receptor	Acneform rash, paronychia, dry skin, fissures, fatigue, low magnesium, infusion reactions
Pertuzumab	HER2 + metastatic breast cancer	Targets extracellular domain for HER2	Cardiomyopathy, infusion reactions, peripheral edema, alopecia, rash, diarrhea, myelosuppression
Rituximab	Non-Hodgkin lymphoma	CD20, a marker on cell membrane of lymphocytes	Infusion reactions, fever, chills, back pain, night sweats, infection
Tositumomab	Non-Hodgkin lymphoma	CD20, a marker on cell membrane of lymphocytes	Infusion reactions, fever chills, rash, hives, itching, anemia, thrombocytopenia, decreased WBC count
Trastuzumab	Breast cancer	HER2, a growth factor protein on cell membrane	Infusion reactions, hypotension, fever, chills, heart failure
Small Molecule Inhibitors	**Indication**	**Target**	**Selected Side Effects**
Acalabrutinib	Mantle cell lymphoma	Inhibits Bruton tyrosine kinase	Hemorrhage, infections, anemia, neutropenia, thrombocytopenia, second primary malignancies, atrial fibrillation and flutter, headache, diarrhea, fatigue, myalgia, bruising
Axitinib	Advanced renal carcinoma	Inhibits VEGF	Hypertension, DVT/PE, bleeding, hypothyroidism, GI perforation, proteinuria, elevated LFTs
Belinostat	Relapsed or refractory peripheral T-cell lymphoma	Inhibits HDAC	Thrombocytopenia, leukopenia, anemia, infections, hepatotoxicity, TLS, nausea, fatigue, pyrexia, vomiting

Small Molecule Inhibitors	Indication	Target	Selected Side Effects
Bortezomib	Myeloma	Inhibits proteasome 26S	Peripheral neuropathy, hypotension, nausea, vomiting, diarrhea, constipation, fatigue, myelosuppression, reactivation of herpesvirus
Bosutinib	CML	Inhibits BCR-ABL	Diarrhea, nausea, vomiting, abdominal pain, myelosuppression, LFT elevation, rash, headache
Cabozantinib	Metastatic medullary thyroid cancer	Tyrosine kinase inhibitor	GI perforation, bleeding, DVT/PE, wound complications, hypertension, proteinuria, mucositis, abdominal pain, nausea vomiting, taste changes, myelosuppression
Carfilzomib	Myeloma	Inhibits proteasome 20S	CHF, MI, dyspnea, infusion reactions, myelosuppression, LFT elevation, renal toxicity, fatigue, peripheral edema, peripheral neuropathy, reactivation of herpesvirus
Crizotinib	ALK + NSCLC	Inhibits multiple kinases including ALK	LFT abnormalities, QT prolongation, pneumonitis, nausea, diarrhea, vomiting, edema, anorexia, fatigue, dyspnea, neutropenia
Dasatinib	CML	Inhibits BCR-ABL	Myelosuppression, fluid retention, pleural effusion, diarrhea, nausea, vomiting, bleeding, pulmonary hypertension
Erlotinib	NSCLC	Inhibits tyrosine kinase interfering with EGFR	Rash, diarrhea, anorexia, fatigue, dyspnea, GI bleeding, kidney and liver toxicity, MI, CVA, eye problems
Everolimus	ER + HER2neg breast cancer; metastatic neuroendocrine tumors; renal cell carcinoma	FKBP12 and mTOR	Pneumonitis, infections, mucositis, kidney failure, diarrhea, nausea, vomiting, fatigue, taste changes, headache, cough, dyspnea, myelosuppression, hyperglycemia
Ibrutinib	Mantle cell lymphoma, CLL/SLL with 17p deletion, Waldenstrom macroglobulinemia, marginal zone lymphoma, GVHD	Inhibits Bruton tyrosine kinase	Hemorrhage, infections (progressive multifocal leukoencephalopathy, PJP), thrombocytopenia, neutropenia, anemia, atrial fibrillation, hypertension, TLS, nausea, vomiting, rash, musculoskeletal pain
Imatinib	CML	BCR-ABL	Nausea, vomiting, myalgias, fluid retention, myelosuppression, hypothyroidism, rash
Lapatinib	Advanced HER2+ breast cancer	EGFR and HER2	Diarrhea, palmar-plantar erythrodysesthesia (hand-foot syndrome), nausea, vomiting, rash, fatigue, QT prolongation, cardiomyopathy, liver and lung toxicity
Nilotinib	CML	BCR ABL	Rash, headache, fatigue, nausea, vomiting, diarrhea, constipation, myelosuppression, liver toxicity, QT prolongation, lipase elevation

(continued)

TABLE 5-4 **Selected Food and Drug Administration–Approved Targeted Therapies (*continued*)**

Small Molecule Inhibitors	Indication	Target	Selected Side Effects
Olaparib	Ovarian, fallopian tube or primary peritoneal cancer, BRCA-mutated advanced ovarian cancer, BRCA-mutated HER2–negative metastatic breast cancer	Inhibits PARP enzymes	MDS/AML, pneumonitis, anemia, nausea, vomiting, diarrhea, fatigue, URI, arthralgia/musculoskeletal pain, dermatitis/rash
Pazopanib	Advanced renal cell carcinoma	VEGF	Liver toxicity, cardiomyopathy, DVT/PE, GI perforation, hypertension, hypothyroidism, proteinuria, infection, myelosuppression, low magnesium and phosphorous, headache, myalgias
Regorafenib	Metastatic colorectal cancer; locally advanced or unresectable gastrointestinal stromal tumors (GIST)	Inhibits multiple kinases	Liver toxicity, bleeding, skin reactions, hypertension, poor wound healing, asthenia, fatigue, anorexia, diarrhea, mucositis, infection, myelosuppression, low calcium/potassium/sodium/phosphorous, proteinuria
Romidepsin	Cutaneous T-cell lymphoma, peripheral T-cell lymphoma	Inhibits HDAC	Thrombocytopenia, leukopenia, anemia, infections, ECG changes (QT prolongation), TLS, nausea, fatigue, vomiting, anorexia
Romiplostim	Thrombocytopenia	Binds to and activates the TPO receptor	Progression to AML in patients with MDS, thrombotic/thromboembolic complications, arthralgia, dizziness, insomnia, pain in extremities, myalgia
Ruxolitinib	Myelofibrosis	JAK1 and JAK2	Myelosuppression, infection
Sorafenib	Unresectable hepatocellular carcinoma and advanced renal cell cancer	Multikinase inhibitor	Palmar plantar erythrodysesthesia (hand-foot syndrome) is erythema, edema, numbness, and desquamation (skin sloughing or peeling) on palms of the hands and soles of the feet (and occasionally elsewhere), rash, hypertension, MI, mucositis, dyspepsia, elevated lipase, diarrhea, nausea, vomiting, loss of appetite, QT prolongation, low phosphorous, myelosuppression
Sunitinib	GIST Advanced renal cell carcinoma Unresectable pancreatic neuroendocrine tumors	Tyrosine kinase inhibition	Myelosuppression, liver toxicity, decreased LVEF, hypothyroidism, diarrhea, constipation, nausea, vomiting, stomatitis, skin changes, fatigue, hypertension, QT prolongation, impaired wound healing, DVT/PE
Temsirolimus	Advanced renal cell carcinoma	FKBP12, mTOR inhibition	Rash; asthenia; mucositis; nausea; anorexia; myelosuppression; elevated blood sugar, lipids, and cholesterol; elevations in creatinine; low phosphorous; LFT abnormalities; infections

Small Molecule Inhibitors	Indication	Target	Selected Side Effects
Vandetanib	Unresectable, locally advanced or metastatic medullary thyroid cancer	VEGFR and EGFR inhibition	Skin changes, photosensitivity, QT prolongation, pneumonitis, ischemic cardiovascular events, diarrhea, hypothyroidism, hypertension, fatigue, nausea, anorexia, headache
Vemurafenib	Unresectable melanoma or melanoma with BRAF mutation	BRAF inhibition	Hypersensitivity, skin reactions, QT prolongation, liver toxicity, photosensitivity, eye changes, alopecia, itching, nausea, fatigue, headache, diarrhea
Vismodegib	Metastatic basal cell carcinoma	Hedgehog pathway inhibitor	Alopecia, taste changes, weight loss, fatigue, anorexia, nausea, vomiting, arthralgias
Ziv-aflibercept	Metastatic colorectal carcinoma	VEGF	Bleeding, impaired wound healing, GI perforation, hypertension, arterial thrombolic events, CVA, angina, proteinuria, nephrotic syndrome, myelosuppression, anorexia, diarrhea, fatigue, elevated LFTS

Adapted from Olsen et al. (2019).

nurse must work closely with providers to assess and manage potential toxicities of immunotherapy. The specific nursing care required will depend on the agent being administered.

The nurse teaches patients self-care and assists in providing for continuing care. Some cytokines, such as IFN, EPO, and G-CSF, can be administered by the patient or family members at home. As needed, the nurse teaches the patient and family how to administer these agents through subcutaneous injections. The nurse also provides instructions about side effects and helps the patient and family identify strategies to manage many of the common side effects of cytokine therapy, such as fatigue, anorexia, and flu-like symptoms.

Patients being treated with checkpoint inhibitor therapies must be monitored carefully over long periods of time for immune-related adverse effects (irAEs); monitoring should include complete blood counts, liver function tests (LFTs), metabolic panels, and thyroid function tests. Early recognition of irAEs is critical to safe and effective management,

TABLE **5-5 Selected Side Effects of Food and Drug Administration–Approved Cytokines**

Agent Cytokines	Selected Side Effects
Interferon alfa	Flu-like symptoms (fever, chills, weakness, muscle and joint pain, headaches); fatigue; anorexia; mental status changes; depression; irritability; insomnia; rash; pruritus; irritation at the injection site; decreased WBC, RBC, and platelet counts; abnormal liver function values
Interleukin-2	Flu-like symptoms (fever, chills, weakness, muscle and joint pain, headaches); fatigue, anorexia, nausea, vomiting, diarrhea, capillary leak syndrome, edema and fluid retention, hypotension, tachycardia, skin rash, erythema, desquamation
Filgrastim (granulocyte growth factor)	Bone pain, malaise, fever, fatigue, headache, skin rash
Sargramostim (granulocyte-macrophage growth factor)	Allergic/anaphylactic reaction with first dose, bone pain, fever, fatigue, headache, weakness, chills, skin rash, pruritis, infection
Epoetin alfa (erythrocyte growth factor)	Fever, fatigue, weakness, diarrhea, dizziness, edema, shortness of breath
Oprelvekin (platelet growth factor)	Edema, fever, headache, rash, chills, joint/muscle/bone pain, fatigue, nausea, vomiting, abdominal pain, constipation, rhinitis, cough, arrhythmia, skin discoloration, bleeding

Adapted from Olsen et al. (2019).

which may include the use of immunosuppressive agents. Patients and caregivers should be educated on irAEs, including signs, symptoms, and management (Olsen et al., 2019).

Referral for home care may be indicated to monitor the patient's responses to treatment and to continue to reinforce patient and family teaching. During home visits, the nurse assesses the patient's and family members' technique in administering medications. The nurse collaborates with providers, third-party payers, and pharmaceutical companies to help the patient obtain reimbursement for home administration of these therapies. The nurse also reminds the patient about the importance of keeping follow-up appointments with providers and assesses the patient's need for changes in care.

Hematopoietic Stem Cell Transplantation

Many malignancies exhibit a dose-related response to chemotherapy; by increasing the dose of chemotherapy, the number of malignant cells destroyed is increased. The dose of chemotherapy that is delivered is limited by the toxicity, specifically myelosuppression. Bone marrow transplant (hematopoietic stem cell transplant) (HPSCT) involves the administration of healthy hematopoietic stem cells in patients with dysfunctional or depleted marrow. This helps to augment bone marrow function and allows, depending on the disease being treated, to either destroy tumor cells with malignancy or to generate functional cells that can replace the dysfunctional ones in cases like immune deficiency syndromes, hemoglobinopathies, and other diseases (Khaddour et al., 2021).

The process of obtaining donor cells has evolved over the years. Traditionally, donor cells were obtained by harvesting large amounts of bone marrow tissue under general anesthesia in the operating room. Currently, a process referred to as *peripheral blood stem cell transplantation* (PBSCT) has gained widespread use. This method of collection uses apheresis methods to collect donor peripheral blood stem cells (PBSCs) for reinfusion. Apheresis is the removal of blood from the body by the withdrawal of blood, its separation into plasma and cells, and the reintroduction of the cells. For PBSCT, a growth factor medication is administered to the patient to increase the number of peripheral stem cells. The collected stem cells are frozen and stored until needed for the patient. This is a safer and more cost-effective means of collection, rather than the traditional harvesting of marrow.

Types of Stem Cell Transplantation

Types of stem cell transplantation (SCT) are based on the source of donor cells and include:

- Autologous (from patient)
- Allogeneic (from a donor other than the patient); either a related donor (i.e., family member) or a matched unrelated donor (national bone marrow registry, Cord Blood Registry)
- Syngeneic (from an identical twin)

Autologous hematopoietic SCT, or HSCT, is considered for patients with hematologic malignancies requiring treatment with myeloablative doses of chemotherapy (doses high enough to obliterate marrow function) to achieve cure or prolong survival. Autologous stem cell transplant accounts for most hematopoietic stem cell transplants in the United States in patients diagnosed with myeloma and cases of recurrent lymphomas (Khaddour et al., 2021). In autologous transplant, cells are collected from the patient and preserved for reinfusion at a later date. The preparative regimen consists of administration of chemotherapy with or without total body irradiation for the eradication of malignant cells and induction of immune tolerance for the transfused cells to engraft properly (Khaddour et al., 2021). Until engraftment (repopulation of the marrow with healthy cells) occurs in the bone marrow, there is a high risk of infection, sepsis, and bleeding. Acute toxicities from chemotherapy and radiation therapy may be severe, including mucositis (inflammation and ulceration of the mucous membranes lining the digestive tract), diarrhea, poor appetite, and myelosuppression. No immunosuppressant medications are necessary after autologous bone marrow transplant because the patient does not receive foreign cells. A disadvantage of autologous transplantation is the risk that viable tumor cells may remain despite high-dose chemotherapy.

Allogeneic stem cell transplant is used primarily for disease of the bone marrow, including acute and chronic leukemias, myelodysplastic syndrome, and aplastic anemia. Allogenic stem cell transplants depend on the availability of a human leukocyte antigen–matched donor, which could be a matched family member, unrelated match donor, or mismatched family donors (haploidentical) (Khaddour et al., 2021).

Allogeneic HSCT involves either myeloablative (high-dose) or nonmyeloablative (reduced-intensity) chemotherapy. In myeloablative allogeneic HSCT, the recipient must undergo high doses of chemotherapy and, in some cases, total body irradiation to destroy all existing bone marrow and residual malignant disease. The harvested donor marrow or PBSCs are infused intravenously, similar to a blood transfusion, into the recipient. The infused cells travel to the bone marrow, where the cells mature and proliferate. When the new bone marrow becomes functional, producing RBCs, WBCs, and platelets, engraftment is considered complete (2 to 4 weeks). An advantage of allogeneic HSCT is that the transplanted cells are immunologically intolerant of a patient's malignancy. The donor's healthy immune system can recognize the patient's malignancy as foreign and kill any remaining tumor cells. This is referred to as the **graft-versus-tumor effect**. However, patients can also experience graft versus host disease (GVHD) because of the donor's immune system (T cells) recognizing the recipient's tissues as foreign.

Syngeneic transplants use an identical twin as the donor. Syngeneic transplants result in less incidence of GVHD and graft rejection; however, there is also less graft-versus-tumor effect to fight the malignancy.

In nonmyeloablative allogeneic HSCT, the chemotherapy doses are lower and are aimed at suppressing the recipient's immune system to allow engraftment of donor bone marrow or PBSCs. The lower doses of chemotherapy create less organ toxicity and, thus, can be offered to older patients or those with underlying organ dysfunction, for whom high-dose chemotherapy would be prohibitive. Once the transplanted donor cells begin to grow and reproduce (referred to as *engraftment*), the donor's healthy immune system keeps the patient's cancer cells from growing.

Before engraftment, patients are at high risk for infection, sepsis, and bleeding. Side effects of the high-dose chemotherapy and total body irradiation can be acute and chronic. Acute side effects include alopecia, hemorrhagic cystitis (inflammation of the bladder), hepatic venous occlusive disease (VOD), nausea, vomiting, diarrhea, and severe stomatitis. Chronic complications include chronic GVHD, infection with encapsulated bacteria, and varicella zoster virus (Khaddour et al., 2021).

To prevent **GVHD**, patients receive immunosuppressant drugs, such as cyclosporine, tacrolimus, or sirolimus. In allogeneic transplant recipients, GVHD occurs when the T lymphocytes proliferating from the transplanted donor marrow or PBSCs become activated and mount an immune response against the recipient's tissues (skin, GI tract, liver). T lymphocytes respond in this manner because they view the recipient's tissue as "foreign," immunologically different from what they recognize as "self" in the donor. GVHD can be categorized into acute or chronic, which are both subcategorized into classic and late onset, classic, and chronic overlap. Acute GVHD usually develops within 3 months (Khaddour et al., 2021).

The first 100 days after allogeneic HSCT are crucial for patients; the immune system and blood-making capacity (hematopoiesis) must recover sufficiently to prevent infection and hemorrhage. Most acute side effects, such as nausea, vomiting, and mucositis, also resolve in the initial 100 days after transplantation. In addition to acute GVHD, patients are also at risk for hepatic VOD or hepatic sinusoidal obstruction syndrome (HSOS), a result of chemotherapy during preparative regimen that occurs within the first 6 weeks following a hematopoietic stem cell transplant. The agents most implicated in causing this syndrome are oral busulfan and cyclophosphamide. The pathophysiology consists of endothelial damage to the hepatic sinusoids leading to obstruction and necrosis of the centrilobular liver (Khaddour et al., 2021). VOD can lead to acute liver failure and death and presents as painful hepatomegaly (enlarged liver), elevated bilirubin levels, ascites, and weight gain in the absence of other causes. Coagulopathy and acute kidney failure can also accompany VOD. There are no standard treatments for VOD; defibrotide has shown promise with response rates of 30% to 60%. Ursodiol has shown some efficacy in the preventative setting and is initiated prior to transplant in some institutions. Fortunately, 70% of patients have resolution of VOD without intervention. Supportive care includes maintaining fluid balance through strict monitoring of I/O and twice-daily weights, pain management, monitoring for signs of bleeding and administering blood products as ordered, and ensuring patient safety.

Nursing Management in Stem Cell Transplantation

Providing Care During Treatment

Skilled nursing care is required during all phases of transplant. In the pretransplant phase, the nurse educates the patient about what to expect, pretransplant testing, and finding a donor. When the patient is admitted for high-dose chemotherapy with or without total body irradiation, the nurse educates the patient about expected side effects, expected onset and recovery, and critical self-care measures to decrease the risk of infection. The acute toxicities of nausea, vomiting, diarrhea, mucositis, myelosuppression, and hemorrhagic cystitis require close monitoring and constant attention by the nurse.

Nursing management during the bone marrow or stem cell infusions consists of monitoring the patient's vital signs and blood oxygen saturation; assessing for adverse effects, such as fever, chills, shortness of breath, chest pain, cutaneous reactions (hives), nausea, vomiting, hypotension or hypertension, tachycardia, anxiety, and taste changes; and providing ongoing support and patient teaching.

Throughout the period of bone marrow aplasia (inability to create new cells) until engraftment of the new marrow occurs, the patient is at high risk for death from sepsis and bleeding. The patient requires support with blood products and hematopoietic growth factors. Potential infections may be bacterial, viral, fungal, or protozoan in origin. Renal complications may arise from the nephrotoxic chemotherapy agents used in the conditioning regimen or those used to treat infection (amphotericin B, aminoglycosides). Tumor lysis syndrome (Box 5-6) is an uncommon occurrence with conditioning as most patients do not have a large disease burden at the time of transplant. Acute tubular necrosis is a risk following conditioning therapy (refer to Chapter 26 for details).

GVHD requires skillful nursing assessment to detect early effects on the skin, liver, and GI tract, including red maculopapular rash commonly found on the palms of the hands and soles of the feet, elevated LFTs, weight gain, jaundice, right upper quadrant pain, diffuse abdominal pain, early satiety, and diarrhea. Diarrhea resulting from GVHD may be of large volume; therefore, all stools must be measured and monitored for the presence of blood. VOD resulting from the conditioning regimens used in HSCT can result in fluid retention, jaundice, abdominal pain, ascites, tender and enlarged liver, and encephalopathy. Pulmonary complications, such as pulmonary edema, interstitial pneumonia, and other pneumonias, often complicate the recovery after

BOX 5-6

Focus on Pathophysiology

Tumor Lysis Syndrome

Malignant cells contain higher intracellular levels of potassium, phosphorous, and nucleic acids than do healthy cells. As the malignant cells are killed by chemotherapy, biotherapy, or corticosteroids, the intracellular contents are released into the bloodstream, leading to hyperkalemia, hyperphosphatemia, and hyperuricemia. The elevation in phosphorous results in an inverse decline in calcium levels. The crystallization of phosphates and uric acid salts in the kidneys can result in acute kidney injury, evidenced by an increase in serum creatinine and acidemia. The treatment plan includes aggressive hydration of 2 to 4 L/day, diuresis (once hydration has commenced), and administration of allopurinol or rasburicase. Additionally, timely management includes treatment of individual metabolic derangements (Brydges & Brydges, 2021). Nursing considerations include strict monitoring of urine output and intake, monitoring of weight changes, and assessment of signs and symptoms of electrolyte disturbances.

transplant. Immunosuppressive agents, including cyclosporine, tacrolimus, and rapamycin, require close monitoring of blood levels and kidney function; doses are adjusted based on blood levels. Physical therapy and occupational consults as well as endocrine consult for diabetic education need to be considered (Neumann, 2019).

Providing Post Transplantation Care

Ongoing nursing assessment and coordination of care in follow-up visits is essential to detect and manage late effects of therapy after HSCT, which occur 100 days or more after the procedure. Late effects include infections (e.g., varicella zoster infection), restrictive pulmonary abnormalities, and recurrent pneumonia. Sterility may result. Chronic GVHD involves the skin, liver, intestine, esophagus, eyes, lungs, joints, and oral and vaginal mucosa. Cataracts may also develop after total body irradiation.

Psychosocial assessments by nursing staff must be ongoing. Professional counseling can be helpful in coping with body image changes as well as the stress of treatment. Some of the stressors reported include fatigue, cognitive alteration, sleep disorder, anxiety disorder, depression, posttraumatic stress disorder, posttraumatic growth, and sexual dysfunction (Jacobs et al., 2019).

NURSING PROCESS
The Patient With Cancer

Nurses play a critical role in monitoring for changes over time; identifying problems and alterations in quality of life; and collaborating with patients, families, and members of the multidisciplinary team to optimize patient care. The nursing approach to the most common problems in patients with cancer will be discussed here. A plan of nursing care for a patient with cancer is available online at http://thepoint.lww.com/Honan3e.

ASSESSMENT

Individuals with cancer may experience a range of side effects with varying severity depending on the cancer type, tumor stage, and treatment modalities being used. Assessment of common problems is presented with related interventions below.

DIAGNOSIS

Appropriate nursing diagnoses of the patient with cancer may include:

- Impaired oral mucous membranes
- Impaired skin integrity
- Nausea
- Pain, acute
- Pain, chronic
- Imbalanced nutrition: less than body requirements
- Fatigue
- Activity intolerance
- Risk for infection
- Risk for bleeding
- Disturbed body image

Based on the assessment data, potential complications include the following:

- Infection and sepsis
- Hemorrhage
- SVCS
- Spinal cord compression
- Hypercalcemia
- Pericardial effusion
- Disseminated intravascular coagulation (DIC)
- Syndrome of inappropriate secretion of antidiuretic hormone (SIADH)
- Tumor lysis syndrome

See Table 5-6 for more information on oncologic emergencies.

PLANNING

The major goals for the patient may include relief of fatigue, absence of complications, management of stomatitis, maintenance of nutrition, body image, relief of pain, and effective progression through the grieving process.

NURSING INTERVENTIONS

PREVENTING/MINIMIZING FATIGUE

Fatigue in patients with cancer has been underreported, underdiagnosed, and undertreated. Fatigue is a common symptom in patients with cancer and is nearly universal in those receiving cytotoxic chemotherapy, radiation therapy, bone marrow transplantation, or treatment with biologic response

(*continued on page 198*)

TABLE **5-6 Oncologic Emergencies: Manifestations and Management**

Emergency	Diagnostic Approaches and Clinical Manifestations	Medical and Nursing Management

Superior Vena Cava Syndrome (SVCS)
Compression or invasion of the superior vena cava by tumor, enlarged lymph nodes, or intraluminal thrombus that obstructs venous circulation, or drainage of the head, neck, arms, and thorax. Compression of the SVC restricts venous return, decreasing cardiac output. Typically, SVCS is associated with bronchogenic cancer but can be associated with other cancers such as lymphoma. Internal occlusion can precipitate SVCS if a central vein catheter becomes occluded. If untreated, SVCS may lead to cerebral anoxia (due to cerebral edema), laryngeal edema, bronchial obstruction, and death.
	Diagnostic
	Diagnosis is confirmed by
	• clinical findings
	• CXR, chest CT with contrast (Azizi et al., 2020).
	• MRI
	• biopsy to obtain tissue diagnosis to determine cause is important in initiating treatment
	Clinical
	Gradually or suddenly impaired venous drainage giving rise to:
	• progressive dyspnea (most common symptom), cough, hoarseness, chest pain, and facial swelling, cyanosis, plethora (redness) of the face, complaints of difficulty buttoning shirt collars
	• engorged and distended jugular, temporal, and arm veins
	• dilated thoracic vessels causing prominent venous patterns on the chest wall
	Blood pressure that is falsely elevated in the upper extremities and low in the lower extremities
	Tachycardia
	Late signs: increased intracranial pressure, associated visual disturbances, headache, dizziness, confusion, syncope and altered mental status, irritability, lethargy, respiratory distress due to laryngeal edema (Klein-Weigel et al., 2020)
		Medical
		• The goal is control or cure of the underlying malignancy or cause by:
		  • radiation therapy to shrink tumor size, relieving symptoms
		  • chemotherapy for chemosensitive cancers (e.g., lymphoma, small cell lung cancer) or when the mediastinum has been irradiated to maximum tolerance
		  • anticoagulant or thrombolytic therapy for intraluminal thrombosis
		  • stent placement to restore blood flow
		• Supportive measures such as oxygen therapy, bronchodilators, corticosteroids, diuretics, and anxiolytics
		Nursing
		• Identify patients at risk for SVCS.
		• Monitor and report clinical manifestations of SVCS.
		• Monitor vital signs as well as cardiopulmonary and neurologic status.
		• Facilitate breathing by positioning the patient properly. Assist the patient to maintain an upright position (elevated 45 degrees). This helps to promote comfort and reduce anxiety; it also reduces intracranial pressure.
		• Remove rings and restrictive clothing.
		• Assist patient with ADLs to minimize energy expenditures.
		• Monitor the patient's fluid volume status; assess weights and I/Os regularly.
		• Ensure that the patient avoids the Valsalva maneuver, which may worsen symptoms, by providing cough suppressants and stool softeners as needed.

Spinal Cord Compression (SCC) Occurs when a malignant disease or a pathologically collapsed vertebrae compresses or displaces the thecal sac that contains the spinal cord, leading to neurologic impairment. The prognosis depends on the severity and rapidity of onset with median of 6 months survival from time of SCC diagnosis.	***Diagnostic*** • MRI or CT of the entire spine should be performed immediately when epidural spinal cord compression is suspected, not only to define the diagnosis, but also to determine the method of treatment (Chen et al., 2021). The sensitivity for MRI detection is 93%, specificity 97%, and overall accuracy 95% (Chen et al., 2021). ***Clinical*** • Percussion tenderness at the level of compression • Abnormal reflexes • Sensory (40–90%) and motor (60–85%) abnormalities • Local or radicular back or neck pain along the dermatomal areas innervated by the affected nerve root (e.g., thoracic radicular pain extends in a band around the chest or abdomen) • Pain exacerbated by movement, supine recumbent position, coughing, sneezing, or the Valsalva maneuver	***Medical*** • Radiation therapy is the initial treatment of choice for those with a radiosensitive tumor type who are not surgical candidates; radiation will reduce tumor size to halt progression. • Corticosteroid therapy at time of presentation to decrease inflammation and swelling at the compression site. • Surgery is only necessary if the spinal cord is unstable, or if the compression is caused by bone fragments from fracture of the vertebral body. Direct decompressive surgery combined with radiotherapy is superior to manage SCC caused by metastatic cancer, than radiotherapy alone (Chen et al., 2021). • Chemotherapy or hormonal therapy as adjuvant to radiation therapy. • *Note:* Despite treatment, patients with poor neurologic function before treatment are less likely to regain complete motor and sensory function; less than 30% of patients who lost the ability to walk before radiation regain the ability to ambulate. • Pain management is a priority.

(continued)

TABLE 5-6 **Oncologic Emergencies: Manifestations and Management (*continued*)**

Emergency	Diagnostic Approaches and Clinical Manifestations	Medical and Nursing Management
	• Back pain is the most common (83–95%) and often the first symptom preceding other symptoms by as much as 2 months • Neurologic dysfunction, and related motor and sensory deficits (numbness, tingling, feelings of coldness in the affected area, inability to detect vibration, loss of positional sense) • Motor loss ranging from subtle weakness to flaccid paralysis • Bladder and/or bowel dysfunction depending on level of compression (above S2, overflow incontinence; from S3 to S5, flaccid sphincter tone and bowel incontinence). These tend to be late symptoms (Chen et al., 2021)	***Nursing*** • Perform ongoing assessment of neurologic status, including motor and sensory function to identify existing and progressing dysfunction. • Control pain with pharmacologic and nonpharmacologic measures. • Prevent complications of immobility resulting from pain and decreased function (e.g., skin breakdown, urinary stasis, thrombophlebitis, decreased clearance of pulmonary secretions). • Maintain muscle tone by assisting with range-of-motion exercises in collaboration with physical and occupational therapists. • Institute intermittent urinary catheterization and bowel training programs for patients with bladder or bowel dysfunction. • Maintain safety by assisting the patient with ADLs and ambulation.
Hypercalcemia In patients with cancer, hypercalcemia is a potentially life-threatening metabolic abnormality resulting when the calcium released from the bones exceeds the amount that the kidneys have the ability to excrete or the bones can reabsorb. It may be the result of: • Bone destruction by tumor cells and subsequent release of calcium. • Production of prostaglandins and osteoclast-activating factors, which stimulate bone breakdown and calcium release. • Tumors that produce parathyroid-like substances that promote calcium release. • Overproduction of vitamin D analogues (calcitriol), seen most commonly in hematologic malignancies (Bassatne et al., 2021). • Most commonly seen in breast cancer, squamous cell carcinoma of the lung, head and neck cancers, and renal cell carcinoma (Bassatne et al., 2021).	***Diagnostic*** Serum calcium level exceeding 11 mg/dL (2.74 mmol/L) Moderate hypercalcemia: 12–14 mg/dL Severe hypercalcemia: greater than 14 mg/dL ***Clinical*** Early signs: fatigue, weakness, lethargy, irritability, cognitive changes, personality changes, confusion, decreased level of responsiveness, hyporeflexia, nausea, vomiting, constipation, anorexia, polyuria (excessive urination), polydipsia (excessive thirst), nocturia, dehydration Late signs: ataxia, stupor, seizures, coma, arrhythmias, ileus, kidney failure, heart block, cardiac arrest	***Medical*** See Chapters 3 and 30. ***Nursing*** • Identify patients at risk for hypercalcemia and assess for signs and symptoms of hypercalcemia. • Educate patient and family on prevention, including hydration and ambulation/weight-bearing activity. • Teach at-risk patients to recognize and report signs and symptoms of hypercalcemia promptly. • Ensure that patients consume (PO or IV) a total of 3 L of fluid daily unless contraindicated by existing kidney or cardiac disease. • Monitor I/O and daily weight. • Explain the use of dietary and pharmacologic interventions, such as stool softeners and laxatives for constipation. • Discuss antiemetic therapy if nausea and vomiting occur. • Advise patients to maintain nutritional intake without restricting normal calcium intake. • Implement safety measures, including fall and seizure precautions. • Promote mobilization by assisting with ambulation and providing active resistive exercises for patients on bed rest; emphasize the importance of mobility in preventing demineralization and breakdown of bones.

Emergency	Diagnostic Approaches and Clinical Manifestations	Medical and Nursing Management
Pericardial Effusion and Cardiac Tamponade Cardiac tamponade is an accumulation of fluid in the pericardial space. The fluid compresses the heart and thereby impedes expansion of the ventricles, limiting cardiac filling during diastole. As ventricular volume and cardiac output fall, the heart pump fails, and circulatory collapse develops. With gradual onset, fluid accumulates slowly, and the outer layer of the pericardial space stretches to compensate for rising pressure. Large amounts of fluid accumulate before symptoms of heart failure occur. With rapid onset, pressures rise too quickly for the pericardial space to compensate. Malignancies, particularly from adjacent thoracic tumors (lung, breast, lymphoma), and side effects of cancer treatment are the most common causes of cardiac tamponade. High doses of radiation to fields involving the heart also have been implicated in pericardial fibrosis, pericarditis, and resultant cardiac tamponade. Untreated pericardial effusion and cardiac tamponade lead to circulatory collapse and cardiac arrest. Patients with tamponade caused by malignant disease have death rates exceeding 75% within 12 months (Stashko & Meer, 2020).	***Diagnostic*** • Electrocardiography (ECG) • Echocardiogram is the preferred imaging modality (Stashko & Meer, 2020). • In small effusion, chest x-rays show small amounts of fluid in the pericardium; in large effusions, x-ray films disclose "water-bottle" heart (obliteration of vessel contour and cardiac chambers) • CT scans help diagnose pleural effusions and evaluate effect of treatment ***Clinical*** • Fatigue, dyspnea, orthopnea, nonproductive cough, dull or diffuse chest pain • Neck vein distention during inspiration (Kussmaul sign) • Pulsus paradoxus (systolic blood pressure decreases exceeding 10 mm Hg during inspiration; pulse gets stronger on expiration) • Distant heart sounds, rubs and gallops, cardiac dullness • Shifted point of maximal impulse (PMI) • Compensatory tachycardia (heart beats faster to compensate for decreased cardiac output) • Increased venous and vascular pressures • Narrow pulse pressure (the difference between systolic and diastolic blood pressure) • Shortness of breath and tachypnea • Weakness, chest pain, orthopnea, anxiety, diaphoresis, lethargy, and altered consciousness from decreased cerebral perfusion • Low-voltage QRS on EKG; electrical alternans	***Medical*** • Pericardiocentesis (the aspiration or withdrawal of pericardial fluid by a large-bore needle inserted into the pericardial space). In malignant effusions, pericardiocentesis provides only temporary relief; fluid usually reaccumulates. Windows or openings in the pericardium can be created surgically as a palliative measure to drain fluid into the pleural space. Catheters may also be placed in the pericardial space, and sclerosing agents (such as doxycycline, talc, bleomycin) are injected to prevent fluid from reaccumulating. • Radiation therapy; antineoplastic agents. In mild effusions, prednisone and diuretic medications may be used. ***Nursing*** • Monitor vital signs, oxygen saturation, cardiac and respiratory examination frequently. • Assess for pulsus paradoxus. • Monitor ECG tracings. • Assess heart and lung sounds, neck vein filling, level of consciousness, respiratory status, and skin color and temperature. • Monitor and record intake and output. • Review laboratory findings (e.g., arterial blood gas and electrolyte levels). • Elevate the head of the patient's bed to ease breathing. • Minimize patient's physical activity to reduce oxygen requirements; administer supplemental oxygen as prescribed. • Provide frequent oral hygiene. • Reposition and encourage the patient to cough, use pursed-lip breathing, and take deep breaths. Assist patient with ADLs to conserve energy. • Maintain oxygen saturation greater than 92%. • Administer analgesics and anxiolytics as ordered.
Disseminated Intravascular Coagulation (DIC, also called consumption coagulopathy) Complex disorder of coagulation and fibrinolysis (destruction of clots), which results in thrombosis and bleeding. DIC is most commonly associated with hematologic cancers (leukemia); cancer of prostate, GI tract, and lungs; chemotherapy (methotrexate, prednisone, L-asparaginase, vincristine, and 6-mercaptopurine); and disease processes such as sepsis, hepatic failure, and anaphylaxis.	***Diagnostic*** • Prolonged prothrombin time (PT or protime) • Prolonged international normalized ratio (INR) • Prolonged partial thromboplastin time (PTT) • Prolonged thrombin time (TT) • Decreased fibrinogen level • Decreased platelet level • Decrease in clotting factors • Decreased hemoglobin • Decreased Hct • Elevated fibrin split products (or fibrin degradation products) • Elevated D-dimer test • Positive protamine sulfate precipitation test (thrombin activation test)	***Medical*** The underlying cause of DIC must be treated. • Chemotherapy, biologic response modifier therapy, radiation therapy, or surgery is used to treat the underlying cancer. • Antibiotic therapy is used for sepsis. • Prophylactic anticoagulation therapy, such as heparin infusions, have not been shown to prevent thrombus in this population. Anticoagulants may be used if the patient develops venous thromboembolism (Smith, 2021). • Transfusions of fresh-frozen plasma (containing clotting factors) or cryoprecipitate (containing fibrinogen), packed RBCs and platelets may be used as replacement therapy in patients with evidence of bleeding.

(continued)

TABLE **5-6 Oncologic Emergencies: Manifestations and Management (*continued*)**

Emergency	Diagnostic Approaches and Clinical Manifestations	Medical and Nursing Management
Blood clots form when normal coagulation mechanisms are triggered. Once activated, the clotting cascade continues to consume clotting factors and platelets faster than the body can replace them, which can result in bleeding. Clots are deposited in the microvasculature, placing the patient at great risk for impaired circulation, tissue hypoxia, and necrosis. In addition, fibrinolysis occurs, breaking down clots and increasing the circulating levels of anticoagulant substances, thereby placing the patient at risk for hemorrhage. Mortality among patients affected by DIC can be as high as 80% (Smith, 2021).	***Clinical*** *Chronic DIC:* characterized by diffuse thrombosis or subacute bleeding. Few or no observable symptoms or easy bruising, prolonged bleeding from venipuncture and injection sites, bleeding of the gums, and slow GI bleeding *Acute DIC:* life-threatening hemorrhage and infarction; clinical symptoms of this syndrome are varied and depend on the organ system involved in thrombus and infarction or bleeding episodes. Bleeding can occur anywhere.	***Nursing*** • Monitor vital signs. • Measure and document intake and output. • Assess skin color and temperature; lung, heart, and bowel sounds; level of consciousness; headache; visual disturbances; chest pain; decreased urine output; and abdominal tenderness. • Inspect all body orifices, tube insertion sites, incisions, and bodily excretions for bleeding. • Review laboratory test results. • Minimize physical activity to decrease injury risks and oxygen requirements. • Prevent bleeding; apply pressure to all venipuncture sites, and avoid nonessential invasive procedures; avoid the use of tourniquets; provide electric rather than straight-edged razors; avoid tape on the skin and advise gentle but adequate oral hygiene with use of a soft toothbrush or toothette. • Assist the patient to turn, cough, and take deep breaths every 2 hours. • Reorient the patient, if needed; maintain a safe environment; and provide appropriate patient education and supportive measures.
Syndrome of Inappropriate Secretion of Antidiuretic Hormone (SIADH) SIADH is a result of the failure in the negative feedback mechanism that normally regulates the release of antidiuretic hormone (ADH). Some malignancies, such as small-cell lung cancer, inappropriately release ADH. The excessive release of ADH produced by tumor cells or by the abnormal stimulation of the hypothalamic–pituitary network leads to uncontrolled water reabsorption. The most common cause of SIADH is cancer, especially small cell cancer of the lung. Medications, including antineoplastics—vincristine, vinblastine, cisplatin, and cyclophosphamide—and morphine also stimulate ADH secretion (see Chapters 3 and 30 for details on SIADH).	***Diagnostic*** • Decreased serum sodium level • Decreased serum osmolality • Increased urine osmolality • Increased urinary sodium level • Increased urine specific gravity • Decreased blood urea nitrogen (BUN), creatinine, and serum albumin levels secondary to dilution • Abnormal water load test results ***Clinical*** *Mild SIADH:* serum sodium 125–134 mEq/L *Signs and symptoms include:* increased thirst, anorexia, nausea, fatigue, weakness, headache *Moderate SIADH:* serum sodium levels between 115 and 124 mEq/L (120 mmol/L) *Signs and symptoms include:* personality changes, irritability, nausea, anorexia, vomiting, weight gain, oliguria, fatigue, muscular pain (myalgia), headache, lethargy, and confusion *Severe SIADH:* serum sodium levels less than 115 mEq/L *Signs and symptoms include:* seizure, abnormal reflexes, delirium, ataxia, papilledema, coma, and death. Number and severity of symptoms depend on the rate of onset; the faster the onset of SIADH, the more symptomatic the patient may be. Signs and symptoms of fluid volume overload, including edema, are rare.	***Medical*** • The underlying cause of SIADH must be treated to effectively treat SIADH. • Discontinue the offending medication. • Fluid intake limited to 500–1,000 mL/day to increase the serum sodium level. If water restriction alone is not effective in correcting or controlling serum sodium levels, demeclocycline is often prescribed to inhibit ADH secretion and promote water excretion. • If neurologic symptoms are severe, parenteral sodium replacement and diuretic therapy are indicated. Electrolyte levels are monitored carefully to detect secondary magnesium, potassium, and calcium imbalances. • After the symptoms of SIADH are controlled, the underlying cancer is treated. If water excess continues despite treatment, pharmacologic intervention may be indicated. Fluid restriction; hypertonic (3%) saline may be administered. Tolvaptan (oral V2 receptor antagonist), salt tablets, and loop diuretics may also be utilized (Olsen et al., 2019). • The goal is to increase the serum sodium level slowly. Increasing the serum sodium level too quickly can cause intracellular dehydration, which may result in serious neurologic impairment. ***Nursing*** Early identification of at-risk patients is essential to promote early intervention. • Maintain intake and output measurements; assess urine specific gravity. • Assess level of consciousness, lung and heart sounds, vital signs, daily weight; also assess for nausea, vomiting, anorexia, edema, fatigue, and lethargy.

Emergency	Diagnostic Approaches and Clinical Manifestations	Medical and Nursing Management
		• Monitor laboratory test results—including serum electrolyte levels, osmolality, and BUN—creatinine, and urinary sodium levels. • Minimize the patient's activity, provide appropriate oral hygiene, maintain environmental safety, and restrict fluid intake if necessary. • Maintain safety: implement fall and seizure precautions for sodium levels below 120 mEq/L.
Tumor Lysis Syndrome (TLS) TLS is a rapidly developing oncologic emergency that results from the rapid release of intracellular contents as a result of radiation- or chemotherapy-induced cell destruction of large or rapidly growing cancers, such as leukemia, lymphoma, and small cell lung cancer. Cancer cells have an abnormally high amount of potassium, phosphate, and nucleic acids. The release of these intracellular contents from the tumor cells leads to electrolyte imbalances—hyperkalemia, hypocalcemia, hyperphosphatemia, and hyperuricemia—because the kidneys can no longer excrete large volumes of the released intracellular metabolites. These metabolic abnormalities may result in life-threatening arrhythmias, seizures, and kidney failure.	***Diagnostic*** Two or more of the following laboratory abnormalities within 3 days prior to and up to 7 days after initiation of cytotoxic therapy: • Uric acid greater than 8 mg/dL • Phosphorus greater than 4.5 mg/dL • Potassium greater than 6 mEq/L • Calcium less than 7 mg/dL • OR 25% change from baseline in any of the above analytes • (Puri et al., 2020) ***Clinical*** Clinical manifestations depend on the extent of metabolic abnormalities. • Neurologic: fatigue, weakness, memory loss, altered mental status, muscle cramps, irritability, paresthesias (numbness and tingling), tetany seizures • Cardiac: hypotension, peaked T waves, flattened P waves, widened QRS waves, ST depression, dysrhythmias, cardiac arrest • GI: anorexia, nausea, vomiting, abdominal cramps, diarrhea • Renal: flank pain, oliguria, anuria, kidney failure, hematuria, acidic urine pH	***Medical*** Prevention, early detection, and prompt management are critical in decreasing morbidity and mortality. • To prevent kidney failure and restore electrolyte balance, aggressive hydration (2–4 L/day) is initiated 48 hours before the initiation of cytotoxic therapy to increase urine volume and eliminate uric acid and electrolytes (Brydges & Brydges, 2021). • Following aggressive hydration, diuretic therapy may be used to increase electrolyte excretion (potassium, uric acid). • Allopurinol is the agent of choice in low risk patients, while Rasburicase is recommended for high-risk patients or patients with impaired renal function. Rasburicase converts uric acid into allantoin, which is a substance that is soluble in urine. It should be avoided in patients with glucose-6-phosphate dehydrogenase deficiency (Olsen et al., 219). • Administration of a cation-exchange resin, such as sodium polystyrene sulfonate (Kayexalate) to treat hyperkalemia by binding and eliminating potassium through the bowel. (Refer to Chapter 3 for treatment of hyperkalemia.) • Administration of hypertonic dextrose and regular insulin temporarily shifts potassium into cells and lowers serum potassium levels. • Administration of phosphate-binding gels, such as aluminum hydroxide, treats hyperphosphatemia by promoting phosphate excretion in the feces. • Hemodialysis is performed when patients have persistently elevated electrolytes with worsening kidney function or in patients with symptomatic electrolyte imbalances or fluid volume overload from TLS management. ***Nursing*** • Identify at-risk patients. • Institute essential preventive measures as described above. • Assess patient for signs and symptoms of electrolyte imbalances. • Monitor serum electrolyte and uric acid levels. • Assess for evidence of fluid volume overload secondary to aggressive hydration by monitoring I/O and daily weights. • Instruct patients to report symptoms indicating electrolyte disturbances.

modifiers (National Comprehensive Cancer Network [NCCN], 2021). Fatigue is a subjective symptom that must be assessed in a systematic way, similarly to pain, relying on the patient's self-report. The nurse should ask the patient to describe the severity of the fatigue. The patient can use a scale of 0 to 10, with 0 being no fatigue and 10 being severe fatigue, or patients can simply state none, mild, moderate, or severe. The nurse should also assess the onset of fatigue as well as aggravating and alleviating factors, including physiologic and psychological stressors that can contribute to fatigue, such as pain, nausea, dyspnea, constipation, fear, and anxiety. The nurse assesses for feelings of weariness, weakness, lack of energy, inability to carry out necessary and valued daily functions, lack of motivation, and inability to concentrate. The patient may become less verbal and may appear pale, with relaxed facial musculature. The nurse helps the patient and family understand that fatigue is an expected side effect of cancer and cancer treatment. Fatigue may be exacerbated by the stress of coping with cancer. It does not always signify that the cancer is advancing or that the treatment is failing.

Nursing strategies are implemented to minimize fatigue or to help the patient cope with existing fatigue. Educational interventions and cognitive behavioral therapies, including providing anticipatory guidance that fatigue is an expected side effect of cancer treatment, have been shown to reduce the severity of cancer-related fatigue (NCCN, 2021). Helping the patient identify sources of fatigue aids in selecting appropriate and individualized interventions.

Ways to conserve energy are developed to help the patient plan daily activities. Alternating periods of rest and activity are beneficial. Consider initiation and/or encourage maintenance of a physical activity/exercise program, as appropriate per health care provider, consisting of cardiovascular endurance (walking, jogging, or swimming) and resistance (weights) training (NCCN, 2021). The nurse assists in educating the patient on local resources for exercise and yoga. The nurse also counsels on sleep hygiene, including not staying in bed if the patient is not sleeping; going to bed only when sleepy and at the same time every night; using the bed only for sleep and sexual activity; avoiding daytime napping or, if needed, limiting naps to 30 minutes; avoiding caffeine, nicotine, and alcohol after noon; and using a relaxing routine within 2 hours of going to bed, such as a warm bath or shower, reading, or listening to music (NCCN, 2021).

The patient is encouraged to maintain as normal a lifestyle as possible by continuing with activities that they value and enjoy. Prioritizing necessary and valued activities can help the patient plan for each day. The patient and family are encouraged to plan to reallocate responsibilities, such as attending to childcare, cleaning, and preparing meals. Patients who are employed full-time may need to reduce the number of hours worked each day or week. The nurse helps the patient and family cope with these changing roles and responsibilities. The nurse also addresses factors that contribute to fatigue, such as poor nutrition, pain, nausea, and depression, and implements pharmacologic and nonpharmacologic strategies to manage these symptoms. The nurse provides nutrition counseling to patients who are not eating enough calories or protein. Small, frequent meals require less energy for digestion. The nurse monitors the patient for deficiencies in serum hemoglobin and Hct, and administers blood products or ESAs as prescribed. In addition, the nurse monitors the patient for alterations in oxygenation and electrolyte balances. Physical therapy and assistive devices are beneficial for patients with impaired mobility. Studies have evaluated the use of psychostimulants, such as methylphenidate and modafinil, for the treatment of fatigue with mixed results; more data are needed before these interventions can be recommended safely (NCCN, 2021).

MONITORING AND MANAGING INFECTION AND SEPSIS

Monitoring for Infection. For patients in all stages of cancer, the nurse assesses risk factors for infection and observes for clinical signs and symptoms, as infection is the leading cause of death in cancer patients. The nurse monitors laboratory studies to detect early changes in WBC counts. Common sites of infection, such as the oropharynx, skin, perianal area, urinary tract, GI tract, and respiratory tract, are assessed frequently. The typical signs of infection (swelling, erythema [redness], drainage, and pain) may not occur in immunosuppressed patients because of a diminished local inflammatory response. Fever or localized tenderness may be the only sign of infection. The nurse also monitors the patient for sepsis, particularly if invasive catheters or venous access devices are in place.

WBC function is often impaired in patients with cancer. There are two types of WBCs: granulocytes (neutrophils, eosinophils, basophils) and agranulocytes (lymphocytes, monocytes, macrophages). The neutrophils, totaling 60% to 70% of the body's total WBCs, play a major role in combating infection by engulfing and destroying microorganisms in a process called *phagocytosis.* Both the total WBC count and the number of neutrophils is important in determining the patient's ability to fight infection. A decrease in circulating WBCs is referred to as *leukopenia. Granulocytopenia* or *neutropenia* is a decrease in neutrophils (see Chapters 18 and 19).

A differential WBC count identifies the relative numbers of WBCs and permits tabulation of the absolute neutrophil count (ANC). The ANC includes the number of polymorphonuclear neutrophils (mature neutrophils, reported as "polys," PMNs, or "segs") and immature forms of neutrophils (reported as bands, metamyelocytes, and "stabs"). The ANC is calculated by the following formula:

$$\text{Total WBC} \times [\%\text{segs} + \%\text{bands}]$$

For example, if the total WBC count is 6,000 cells/mm^3, with segmented neutrophils 25% and bands 25%, the ANC is 3,000 cells/mm^3. That is $6{,}000 \times [0.25 + 0.25] = 6{,}000 \times 0.5 = 3{,}000$.

Neutropenia, an abnormally low ANC, is associated with an increased risk for infection. The risk for infection rises as the ANC decreases and persists. An ANC less than 500 cells/mm^3 reflects a severe risk of infection. **Nadir** is the lowest ANC after myelosuppressive chemotherapy or radiation therapy. Therapies that suppress bone marrow function are called *myelosuppressive.* Therapies that severely suppress bone marrow function are called *myeloablative.* The nadir is reached, on average, 7 to 10 days following chemotherapy treatment and takes an additional 7 to 14 days to recover. The patient is at increased risk for infection throughout the duration of neutropenia.

Gram-positive bacteria (*Streptococcus* and *Staphylococcus* species) and gram-negative organisms (*Escherichia coli, Klebsiella pneumoniae,* and *Pseudomonas aeruginosa*) are the most frequently isolated causes of infection. Fungal organisms, such as *Candida albicans,* also contribute to the incidence of serious infection. Viral infections in immunocompromised patients are caused most commonly by herpes viruses and respiratory viruses.

Pearls for Practice

For Black adults, normal levels are 3,200 to 10,000 cells/mm^3. For others, normal adult WBC levels are 4.5 to 10.5 $\times$ 10^3 cells/mm^3 or 4,500 to 10,500 cells/mm^3 (Fischbach et al., 2022). A WBC level (count) below 500 or above 30,000 is a critical value.

Managing Patients with Febrile Neutropenia. A fever in a patient with neutropenia is considered an emergency due to the high mortality rate associated with sepsis in neutropenic patients. Hospitalized patients who are neutropenic and become febrile are assessed immediately for infection. Cultures of blood, sputum, urine, stool, catheter, or wounds are obtained. In addition, a chest x-ray is often included to assess for pulmonary infections. If a patient is at home and develops neutropenic fever, the patient is instructed to notify their health care provider and seek medical attention immediately.

Pearls for Practice

Fever is often the only sign of infection in immunocompromised patients. Although fever may be related to a variety of noninfectious conditions, including the underlying cancer, any temperature of 38.3°C (100.9°F) or higher or a sustained temperature of 38.0°C (100.4°F) for 1 hour is reported and addressed promptly (NCCN, 2021).

Empiric antibiotics are initiated to treat infections immediately after cultures are obtained. The term *empiric antibiotics* refers to the use of broad-spectrum antibiotics used to treat infection before a definitive organism is identified. Often, Gram stains are ordered along with cultures to assist providers in identifying the most appropriate antibiotic. Empiric antibiotics have been employed due to the high incidence of mortality associated with untreated infection in neutropenic patients. Broad-spectrum antibiotic coverage or empiric therapy most often includes a combination of medications to defend the body against the major pathogenic organisms (both gram positive and gram negative). It is important for the nurse to administer these medications promptly, immediately after two sets of blood cultures are obtained, according to the prescribed schedule, to achieve adequate blood levels of the medications (NCCN, 2021).

Minimizing the Risk of Infection in Neutropenic Patients. Strict asepsis is essential when handling IV lines, catheters, and other invasive equipment. Patients are advised to minimize contact with anyone who might be sick and to avoid crowds. Patients with profound immunosuppression, such as allogeneic HSCT recipients or patients with acute leukemia, should be placed in single rooms where the air is filtered. To reduce the risk of foodborne illnesses, patients are educated to avoid raw meat, eggs, or fish; deli meats; unroasted raw nuts or nuts in the shell; miso products; raw grain products; unpasteurized milk products; and soft cheese, cheese with uncooked vegetables, or cheese with mold. Fruits and vegetables must be washed well, eliminating soft fruits such as berries that are difficult to wash.

Hand hygiene and appropriate general hygiene are critical to reduce exposure to potentially harmful bacteria and to eliminate environmental contaminants. Invasive procedures, such as injections, vaginal or rectal examinations, rectal temperatures, and surgery, are avoided. The patient is encouraged to cough and to perform deep-breathing exercises frequently to prevent atelectasis and other respiratory problems. Prophylactic antimicrobial therapy may be used for patients who are expected to be profoundly immunosuppressed and at risk for certain infections, such as patients undergoing autologous or allogeneic stem cell transplant and patients with acute leukemia. The nurse teaches the patient and family to recognize signs and symptoms of infection that should be reported, performs effective hand hygiene, uses antipyretics, maintains skin integrity, and administers hematopoietic growth factors when indicated.

MONITORING AND MANAGING BLEEDING AND HEMORRHAGE

The nurse assesses the patient with cancer for factors that may contribute to bleeding. Bleeding may result from a reduction in the quantity or quality of platelets, a decrease in clotting factors, or from DIC (see Chapter 19 for details on DIC). Treatment-related factors include bone marrow suppression from radiation, chemotherapy, and other medications that interfere with coagulation and platelet functioning, such as aspirin and other nonsteroidal anti-inflammatory medications, dipyridamole, heparin, or warfarin.

Thrombocytopenia often results from bone marrow depression after certain types of chemotherapy and radiation therapy. Tumor infiltration of the bone marrow can also impair the normal production of platelets. In some cases, platelet destruction is associated with an enlarged spleen (hypersplenism) and abnormal antibody function, which occur with leukemia and lymphoma. Chapter 18 details thrombocytopenia. Refer to Box 18-2 for thrombocytopenia precautions.

(continued on page 200)

Concept Mastery Alert

A nurse can best detect early signs and symptoms of thrombocytopenia by closely observing the client's skin for petechiae and bruising.

The nurse administers platelet transfusions as ordered and monitors for signs of transfusion reaction, including fever, chills, urticaria, and shortness of breath. In limited circumstances, the nurse may administer Interleukin (IL)-11, which has been approved by the U.S. Food and Drug Administration (FDA) to prevent severe thrombocytopenia and to reduce the need for platelet transfusions after myelosuppressive chemotherapy in patients with nonmyeloid malignancies. In some instances, the nurse teaches the patient or family members to administer IL-11 in the home.

When a hospitalized patient experiences bleeding, the nurse monitors blood pressure, pulse, and respiratory rates every 15 to 30 minutes. Serum hemoglobin and Hct are monitored carefully for changes indicating blood loss. The nurse tests all urine, stool, and emesis for occult blood. Neurologic assessments are performed to detect changes in orientation and behavior. Headaches reported by the patient or abnormal neurologic findings must be reported to the provider immediately as even subtle signs may indicate an intracranial hemorrhage. The nurse administers fluids and blood products as prescribed to replace any losses.

Pearls for Practice

One unit of platelets is approximately 50 to 70 mL; in general, four to six units are pooled for a platelet transfusion and infused according to the patient's tolerance. The platelet transfusion is anticipated to increase the platelet count 5,000 to 10,000/mL per unit.

ASSESSING AND MANAGING STOMATITIS

Mucositis is a potential complication of systemic cytotoxic therapy, epidermal growth factor receptor (EGFR) inhibitors, tyrosine kinase inhibitors, and radiation therapy that leads to inflammation and ulceration of any portion of the GI tract from the oral cavity throughout the alimentary canal. One form of mucositis, stomatitis, is an inflammatory response of the oral tissues that is characterized by mild erythema and edema or, if severe, by painful ulcerations, bleeding, and secondary infection. Stomatitis commonly develops 5 to 14 days after patients receive myelosuppressive chemotherapeutic agents and often coincides with the WBC nadir (lowest level). Prevalence and incidence are inconsistent because of the lack of standardized scoring criteria, tumor location, and different treatment regimens, as well as underreporting. Incidence in HSCT recipients varies between 47% and 100%. Intensity of the conditioning regimen, transplant type, and total body irradiation can influence incidence as well as severity (Olsen et al., 2019).

As a result of normal everyday wear and tear, the epithelial cells that line the oral cavity undergo rapid turnover and slough off routinely. Historically, oral mucositis was attributed to the direct effects of cytotoxic drugs. Poor oral hygiene, existing dental disease, use of other medications that dry mucous membranes, advanced age, smoking, previous cancer treatment, diminished kidney function, and impaired nutritional status all contribute to morbidity associated with stomatitis. Radiation-induced xerostomia (dry mouth) associated with decreased function of the salivary glands may contribute to stomatitis in patients who have received radiation to the head and neck.

Myelosuppression (bone marrow depression), resulting from underlying disease or its treatment, predisposes the patient to oral bleeding and infection. Severe pain associated with ulcerated oral tissues can significantly interfere with nutritional intake, speech, and a willingness to maintain oral hygiene. Severe stomatitis may cause or prolong hospitalizations. In addition, stomatitis may lead to interruptions in chemotherapy and radiation administration or decreases in the intended dosing until the inflammation subsides. Further, it may significantly reduce the patient's quality of life.

Nurses must perform routine oral assessments in patients at risk for developing stomatitis and in patients with established stomatitis. Utilizing a standardized assessment tool or scale when performing a physical examination will aide in considering the symptoms, signs, and functional disturbances associated with the mucositis/stomatitis (Olsen et al., 2019). The assessment should include the color and moisture of the lips and oral mucosa; presence of ulcerations; presence of edema of the lips, buccal mucosa, or tongue; and quantity and quality of saliva. Additionally, patient-reported outcome questionnaires are helpful in assessing symptom burden, functionality, and pain reduction (Olsen et al., 2019).

Although multiple studies on stomatitis have been published, the optimal prevention and treatment approaches have not been identified. Future studies will focus on addressing the cascade of inflammatory events and release of chemical substances that leads to the cellular and tissue destruction underlying stomatitis. Routine, good oral hygiene, including brushing, flossing, and rinsing, is necessary to minimize the risk of oral complications associated with cancer therapies. Soft-bristled toothbrushes and nonabrasive toothpaste prevent or reduce trauma to the oral mucosa. Oral swabs with sponge-like applicators may be used in place of a toothbrush for painful oral tissues. Flossing may be performed unless it causes pain or bleeding. Oral rinses with saline solution or tap water after meals and at bedtime may be necessary for patients who cannot tolerate tooth brushing. Products that irritate oral tissues or impair healing, such as alcohol-based mouth rinses, are avoided. Foods that are difficult to chew or that are hot or spicy are avoided to minimize further trauma. The patient's lips are lubricated to keep them from becoming dry and cracked. Topical anti-inflammatory and anesthetic agents may be prescribed to promote healing and minimize discomfort. Products that coat or protect oral mucosa, such as mucoadhesive hydrogel and calcium phosphate rinses, are used to promote comfort and prevent further trauma (Brown and Gupta, 2020). Patients who experience severe pain and discomfort with stomatitis may benefit from, and/or require systemic analgesic pre/post meals and around the clock as appropriate. The nurse should assess for dysphagia risk prior to premeal medication administration.

Adequate fluid and food intake is encouraged. In some instances, parenteral hydration and nutrition are necessary. Topical or systemic antifungal and antibiotic medications are prescribed to treat local or systemic infections.

Oral cryotherapy is recommended for patients receiving bolus 5-fluorouracil or high-dose melphalan with or without total body irradiation, a conditioning regimen (Olsen et al., 2019). Similarly, low-level laser therapy is recommended for patients receiving HSCT conditioned with high-dose chemotherapy with or without total body irradiation and patients receiving radiation therapy without concomitant chemotherapy for head and neck cancer (Olsen et al., 2019). In addition, the American Academy of Nursing recommends against the use of "magic mouthwash"—a mixed medication formulation that typically includes anticholinergic medications, an anaesthetic, and an antacid or mucosal coating agent—which has traditionally been prescribed as a treatment intervention since there is a lack of evidence supporting its ongoing use (Cullen et al., 2018).

Palifermin, a synthetic form of human keratinocyte growth factor, is an IV medication approved in 2005 by the FDA for treatment of mucositis in patients with hematologic malignancies who are undergoing high-dose chemotherapy or total body radiation prior to HCST. Palifermin appears to promote more rapid replacement of cells in the mouth and GI tract, decreasing the incidence and duration of severe mucositis. It has not yet been tested in other patients with cancer. Careful timing of administration and monitoring are essential for maximum effectiveness and to detect adverse effects (Olsen et al., 2019).

CARING FOR PATIENTS WITH NAUSEA AND VOMITING

Nausea is an unpleasant sensation experienced in the back of the throat, epigastrium, or stomach that may result in vomiting. Nausea is one of the most feared side effects of cancer treatment. The potential causes of nausea are numerous, and nurses should not assume that nausea is due to chemotherapy; all potential causes must be considered. Causes of nausea include primary or metastatic tumor involving the CNS; gastroparesis (slowed gastric emptying); obstruction in the GI tract; infection; hypercalcemia; kidney or liver dysfunction; hyponatremia; and side effects of medications including chemotherapy, morphine, and antibiotics. Risk factors for treatment-induced nausea include younger age, female sex, and a history of treatment-induced nausea and vomiting.

Nausea is a subjective phenomenon analogous to pain. Nausea is best assessed by eliciting the patient's self-report. The following components should be assessed: timing of nausea in relation to treatment, perceived meaning of nausea to the patient, onset, frequency, associated symptoms, precipitating and alleviating factors, and previous experiences with nausea. Physical assessment should include signs of sweating, tachycardia, dizziness, pallor, excessive salivation, weakness, gastric distention, abdominal tenderness, and evaluation of bowel sounds. Laboratory values including electrolytes and kidney function should be monitored.

The prevention of chemotherapy-induced nausea and vomiting is a priority (see earlier discussion). For nausea and vomiting unrelated to chemotherapy, medications including serotonin receptor antagonists (e.g., ondansetron), dopamine receptor antagonists (e.g., metoclopramide), phenothiazines (e.g., prochlorperazine), corticosteroids (e.g., dexamethasone), and cannabinoids (e.g., dronabinol) can be used. Antiemetics should be administered around the clock with breakthrough doses as needed. Nonpharmacologic interventions that have proven to be effective in decreasing nausea include relaxation, guided imagery, acupressure, acupuncture, deep breathing, and eliminating odors. Patients should be instructed to avoid reclining within the first 30 minutes after eating. Dietary interventions include eating small, frequent meals and eating bland, chilled foods.

MAINTAINING SKIN INTEGRITY

The nurse assesses the patient with cancer for any skin problems. Maintaining integrity of skin and tissue poses a problem for patients with cancer because of the effects of chemotherapy, radiation therapy, surgery, and invasive procedures carried out for diagnosis and therapy. Numerous cutaneous side effects have been reported from traditional chemotherapy drugs, including cytarabine, anthracyclines, 5-fluorouracil, capecitabine, taxanes, and methotrexate (Olsen et al., 2019). Cutaneous adverse events can affect the skin, hair, nails, and mucosa. Epidermal growth factor receptor (EGFR) inhibitors, which can include both targeted agents and monoclonal antibodies are associated with many cutaneous reactions. More than 80% of patients with have a cutaneous reaction (in the form of papulopustular rash) from treatments with EGFR inhibitors (Olsen et al., 2019).

As part of the assessment, the nurse assesses the patient for risk factors, including treatment type, nutritional deficits, bowel and bladder incontinence, immobility, immunosuppression, multiple skin folds, and changes related to aging. The nurse notes the presence of skin lesions, ulcers, rashes, or ulcerations secondary to the tumor or the effects of treatment.

Some of the most frequently encountered disturbances of tissue integrity, in addition to stomatitis, include skin and tissue reactions to radiation therapy, alopecia, and metastatic skin lesions. Patients with skin and tissue reactions to radiation therapy require careful skin care to prevent further skin irritation, drying, and damage. The skin over the affected area is handled gently, avoiding rubbing and use of hot or cold water, soaps, powders, lotions, and cosmetics. Patients may avoid tissue injury by wearing loose-fitting, cotton clothes and avoiding clothes that constrict, irritate, or rub the affected area. If blistering occurs, care is taken not to disrupt the blisters, thus reducing the risk of introducing bacteria. Moisture- and vapor-permeable dressings, such as hydrocolloids and hydrogels, are helpful in promoting healing and reducing pain. Aseptic wound care is indicated to minimize the risk for infection and sepsis. Topical antibiotics,

(continued on page 202)

such as 1% silver sulfadiazine cream, may be prescribed for use on areas of moist desquamation (painful, red, moist skin). Patients should apply sunscreen daily to exposed skin areas regardless of the season. Sunscreens with the following characteristics is recommended: hypoallergenic, high sun protection factor (at least 30), PABA free, UVA and UVB protection (broad spectrum), and containing zinc oxide or titanium dioxide (Olsen et al., 2019).

Helping Patients Cope with Alopecia. The nurse notes the presence of alopecia (hair loss), which is another form of tissue disruption common in patients with cancer who receive radiation therapy or chemotherapy. In addition, the nurse assesses the psychological impact of this side effect on the patient and family.

The temporary or permanent thinning or complete loss of hair is a potential adverse effect of various radiation therapies and chemotherapeutic agents. The extent of alopecia depends on the type, dose, and duration of therapy. Combination chemotherapy is more likely to cause complete hair loss than monotherapy. These treatments cause alopecia by damaging stem cells and hair follicles. As a result, the hair is brittle and may fall out or break off at the surface of the scalp. Hair loss may be patchy or total and involve scalp hair and body hair, although loss of body hair is less frequent (Olsen et al., 2019). Hair loss usually begins 2 to 3 weeks after the initiation of treatment; regrowth begins within 8 weeks after the last treatment and may take up to 6 months for complete regrowth. Some patients who undergo radiation to the head may sustain permanent hair loss. Many health care providers view hair loss as a minor problem when compared with the potentially life-threatening consequences of cancer. However, for many patients, hair loss is a major assault on body image, resulting in depression, anxiety, anger, rejection, and isolation. To patients and families, hair loss can serve as a constant reminder of the challenges cancer places on coping abilities, interpersonal relationships, and sexuality.

Scalp cooling has been shown to be effective in reducing chemotherapy-induced alopecia for certain chemotherapy-regimens (e.g., docetaxel-cyclophosphamide); however, its efficacy for many other chemotherapies is less established (Haque et al., 2020). Contraindications exist for scalp cooling and include patients with known hematologic malignancies because of reports of scalp metastasis and lack of safety data, as well as patients with cold sensitivity, cold agglutinin disease, cryoglobulinemia, and cryofibrinogenemia. Patients may experience headaches, excessive coldness, or feelings of claustrophobia (Olsen et al., 2019).

The nurse provides information about alopecia and supports the patient and family in coping with changes in body image. The patient is advised to use baby shampoo with neutral pH balance and to avoid using permanent waves, bleach, and coloring agents on hair, as well as vigorous brushing, hot rollers, and excessive heat with hair dryer use. Patients are advised to avoid excessive brushing or combing (Olsen et al., 2019). The patient is encouraged to acquire a wig or hairpiece before hair loss occurs, so that the replacement matches the patient's own hair. Use of attractive scarves and hats may make the patient feel less conspicuous. The nurse can refer the patient to supportive programs, such as "Look Good, Feel Better," offered by the ACS. The scalp should be protected from cold and sun with hats, scarves, wigs, and sunscreen (Olsen et al., 2019). Knowledge that hair usually begins to regrow after therapy is completed may comfort some patients, although patients must be prepared that the color and texture of the new hair may be different.

IMPROVING NUTRITIONAL STATUS

Assessment of the patient's nutritional status is an important nursing role. Impaired nutritional status may contribute to disease progression, decreased survival, immune incompetence, increased incidence of infection, delayed tissue repair, diminished functional ability, decreased capacity to continue antineoplastic therapy, increased length of hospital stays, and impaired psychosocial functioning. Altered nutritional status, weight loss, and cachexia (muscle wasting, emaciation) are complex states and may be secondary to decreased protein and caloric intake, metabolic or mechanical effects of the cancer, systemic disease, side effects of the treatment, or the patient's emotional status.

The nursing assessment of nutritional status includes monitoring the patient's weight and caloric intake consistently. Other information obtained by assessment includes diet history, any episodes of anorexia, changes in appetite, situations and foods that aggravate or relieve anorexia, and medication history. Difficulty in chewing or swallowing is identified, and the presence of nausea, vomiting, or diarrhea is noted. The patient should be screened for food insecurity, financial distress, and the ability to prepare food, and is referred to community resources if needed.

Clinical and laboratory data useful in assessing nutritional status include anthropometric measurements (triceps skin fold and middle-upper arm circumference), serum protein levels (albumin, prealbumin, and transferrin), serum electrolytes, lymphocyte count, hemoglobin levels, Hct, urinary creatinine levels, and serum iron levels.

Pearls for Practice

A normal serum albumin is 3.5 to 5.2 g/dL or 35 to 52 g/L and gives the clinician a quick assessment of protein stores. In a seminal study by Seltzer et al. (1979), a sixfold increase in mortality was seen with an albumin level of less than 35 g/L, while recent studies reveal that 1 g/dL lower baseline serum albumin concentration was associated with higher risk of both hospitalization and death (Shannon et al., 2021). Since albumin is degraded over 14 to 21 days, it is not a good measure for assessing recent nutritional deficits. Since prealbumin has a half-life of 2 days, it is a better measure of response to dietary treatments. The normal reference range for prealbumin in males is 19 to 37 mg/dL, and in females, 17 to 31 mg/dL.

Understanding Cancer-Related Causes of Malnutrition. Most patients with cancer experience some weight loss during their illness. Anorexia, malabsorption, and cachexia are examples of nutritional problems that commonly occur in patients with cancer; special attention is needed to prevent weight loss and promote nutrition.

Anorexia. Anorexia is defined as an involuntary loss of appetite. Among the many causes of anorexia in patients with cancer are alterations in taste, manifested by increased salty, sour, and metallic taste sensations, and altered responses to sweet and bitter flavors. These changes lead to decreased appetite, decreased nutritional intake, and protein–calorie malnutrition. Taste alterations may result from mineral (e.g., zinc) deficiencies, increases in circulating amino acids and cellular metabolites, or the administration of chemotherapeutic agents. Patients undergoing radiation therapy to the head and neck may experience "mouth blindness" (MacCarthy-Leventhal, 1959) which is a severe impairment of taste. Alterations in the sense of smell also alter taste; this is a common experience of patients with head and neck cancers.

Anorexia may occur because people feel full after eating only a small amount of food. This is referred to as *early satiety.* This sense of fullness occurs secondary to a decrease in digestive enzymes, abnormalities in the metabolism of glucose and triglycerides, and prolonged stimulation of gastric volume receptors, which convey the feeling of being full. Psychological distress (e.g., fear, pain, depression, and isolation) throughout illness may also have a negative impact on appetite. Patients may develop an aversion to food because of nausea and vomiting after treatment.

Cachexia. Cachexia is a multifactorial syndrome characterized by loss of appetite, weight, and skeletal muscle, leading to fatigue, functional impairment, increased treatment-related toxicity, poor quality of life, and reduced survival (Roeland et al., 2020). The onset of cachexia has been described as a weight loss in excess of 5% over the preceding 6 months, or a BMI <20 kg/m^2 with ongoing 2% weight loss, or depletion of muscle mass and $>2\%$ weight loss. Refractory cachexia has been conceptualized as a clinically resistant catabolic state characterized by poor performance status, progressive cancer, and a life expectancy <3 months; however, there are not yet consensus diagnostic criteria for refractory cachexia. Limitations of these definitions include the lack of inclusion of cancer stage and goal of treatment (i.e., curative vs. palliative) (Roeland et al., 2020).

Promoting Nutrition. Whenever possible, every effort is used to maintain adequate nutrition through the oral route. Strong evidence supports early nutritional counseling as beneficial for prevention and reduction of cachexia (Olsen et al., 2019). High calorie/high protein supplements should be encouraged. Food should be prepared in ways that make it appealing. Unpleasant smells are avoided. Family members are included in the plan of care to encourage adequate food intake. The patient's preferences, as well as physiologic and metabolic requirements, are considered when selecting foods. Small, frequent meals are provided with supplements between meals. Patients often tolerate larger amounts of food earlier in the day rather than later, so meals can be planned accordingly. To avoid early satiety, the patient should avoid drinking fluids while eating. Oral hygiene before mealtime often makes meals more pleasant. It is important to assess and manage pain, nausea, and other symptoms that may interfere with nutrition. Progestins and corticosteroids are the only two classes of drugs that have demonstrated effectiveness as appetite stimulants (Olsen et al., 2019).

If adequate nutrition cannot be maintained by oral intake, nutritional support via the enteral route may be necessary. Short-term nutritional supplementation may be provided through a nasogastric tube. However, if nutritional support is needed for longer than several weeks, a gastrostomy or jejunostomy tube may be inserted. The patient and family are taught to administer enteral nutrition in the home.

If malabsorption is a problem, enzyme and vitamin replacement may be instituted. Additional strategies include changing the feeding schedule, using simple diets, and relieving diarrhea. If malabsorption is severe, parenteral nutrition may be necessary. Parenteral nutrition can be administered in several ways: by a long-term venous access device (e.g., right atrial catheter), by an implanted venous port, or by a peripherally inserted central catheter (PICC) (Fig. 5-5). The nurse teaches the patient and family to care for venous access devices and to administer parenteral nutrition when appropriate. Home care nurses may assist with or supervise parenteral nutrition administration in the home.

Interventions to reduce cachexia usually do not prolong survival or improve nutritional status significantly. Optimal management of other symptoms that may be contributing, such as depression, anxiety, nausea, or xerostomia, is critical to promoting improved nutritional intake. Further study is needed to assess the effects of nutritional intervention on disease status and the patient's quality of life. Before invasive nutritional strategies are instituted, the nurse should assess the patient carefully and discuss goals of care and options with the patient and family.

(*continued on page 204*)

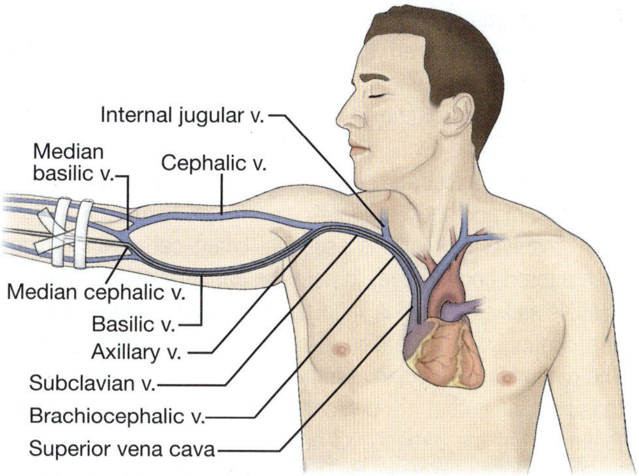

FIGURE 5-5 A peripherally inserted central catheter (PICC) is advanced through the cephalic or basilic vein to the axillary, subclavian, or brachiocephalic vein or the superior vena cava.

RELIEVING PAIN

The nurse assesses the patient with cancer for the source and site of pain. In cancer, pain and discomfort may be related to the underlying disease, pressure exerted by the tumor, diagnostic procedures, or the cancer treatment itself. As in any other situation involving pain, cancer pain is affected by both physical and psychosocial influences. A comprehensive pain assessment is completed including onset, duration, location, quality or characteristics, quantity, aggravating and alleviating factors, associated symptoms, and the treatments that the patient has used to relieve pain.

The nurse also assesses those factors that increase the patient's perception of pain, such as fear and apprehension, fatigue, anger, and social isolation. Pain assessment scales (see Chapter 6) are useful for assessing the patient's pain before pain-relieving interventions are instituted and for evaluating the effectiveness of these interventions.

Various pharmacologic and nonpharmacologic options are available for managing cancer pain. No reasonable approaches, even those that may be invasive, should be overlooked because of a poor or terminal prognosis. The nurse helps the patient and family take an active role in managing pain. The nurse provides education and support to correct fears and misconceptions about opioid use. Inadequate pain control leads to suffering, anxiety, fear, immobility, isolation, and depression. The goal, regardless of the patient's disease status, is to maximize quality of life and optimize functional ability by adequately managing pain. Refer to Chapter 6 for details on managing cancer pain.

IMPROVING BODY IMAGE

The nurse identifies potential threats to the patient's body image and assesses each individual's ability to cope with the many assaults to body image that may be experienced throughout the course of disease and treatment. Entry into the health care system is often accompanied by depersonalization. Threats to self-concept are enormous as the patient faces the realization of illness, disfigurement, possible disability, and possible death. To accommodate treatments or because of the disease, many patients with cancer are forced to alter their lifestyles. Priorities and values change when body image is threatened. Disfiguring surgery, hair loss, cachexia, skin changes, altered communication patterns, and sexual dysfunction are some of the devastating results of cancer and its treatment that threaten the patient's self-esteem and body image.

A positive approach is essential when caring for patients with altered body image. To help the patient retain control and positive self-esteem, it is important to encourage independence and continued participation in self-care and decision-making. The patient is assisted to assume those tasks and participate in those activities that are personally of most value. Any negative feelings that the patient has or threats to body image should be identified and discussed. The nurse serves as a listener and counselor to both the patient and the family. Referral to a support group can provide the patient with additional assistance in coping with the changes resulting from cancer or its treatment. In many cases, cosmetologists can provide ideas about hair or wig styling, makeup, and the use of scarves and other head coverings to help with body image concerns.

Patients who experience alterations in sexuality and sexual function are encouraged to discuss concerns openly with the health care team and with their partners. Alternative forms of sexual expression are explored with patients and their partners to promote positive self-worth and acceptance. Nurses who identify serious physiologic, psychological, or communication difficulties related to sexuality or sexual function are in a key position to help patients and partners seek further counseling if necessary.

TEACHING PATIENTS SELF-CARE

Many patients with cancer return home from acute-care facilities to receive treatment in the home or outpatient area. The shift from the acute care setting also shifts the responsibility for care to the patient and family. As a result, family members and friends must assume increased involvement in patient care, which requires teaching that enables them to provide quality care. Teaching initially focuses on providing information needed by the patient and family to address the most immediate care needs likely to be encountered at home.

Side effects of treatments and changes in the patient's status that should be reported are reviewed verbally and reinforced with written information. Strategies to deal with side effects of treatment are discussed with the patient and family. Other learning needs are identified based on the priorities conveyed by the patient and family as well as on the complexity of care provided in the home.

Technologic advancements allow home administration of chemotherapy, parenteral nutrition, blood products, parenteral antibiotics, and parenteral analgesics as well as management of symptoms and care of vascular access devices. Although home care nurses provide care and support for patients receiving this advanced technical care, patients and families need instruction and ongoing support that allow them to feel comfortable and proficient in managing these treatments at home. Follow-up visits and telephone calls from the nurse are often reassuring and increase the patient's and family's comfort in dealing with complex and new aspects of care. Continued contact facilitates evaluation of the patient's progress and assessment of the ongoing needs of the patient and family.

CONTINUING CARE

Referral for home care is often indicated for patients with cancer. The responsibilities of the home care nurse include assessing the home environment, suggesting modifications in the home or in care to help the patient and family address the patient's physical needs, providing physical care, and assessing the psychological and emotional impact of the illness on the patient and family.

Assessing changes in the patient's physical status and reporting relevant changes to the provider help ensure that appropriate and timely modifications in therapy are made. The home care nurse also assesses the adequacy of pain management and the effectiveness of other strategies to prevent or manage the side effects of treatment modalities.

It is necessary to assess the patient's and family's understanding of the treatment plan and management strategies and to reinforce previous teaching. The nurse often facilitates coordination of patient care by maintaining close communication with all involved health care providers. The nurse may make referrals and coordinate available community resources (e.g., local office of the ACS, home aides, church groups, parish nurses, support groups) to assist patients and caregivers.

EVALUATION

Nurses play an important role in evaluating the expected outcomes for patients with cancer. To maximize beneficial outcomes and intervene in the presence of potential complications, evaluation of the patient's and family's needs are assessed because cancer affects not only the patient but also the family members. In addition, with the shift away from inpatient care, many families are caring for patients at home and should be considered members of the health care team. The nurse can refer the patient and family to a variety of support groups sponsored by the ACS or available community resources. The nurse also collaborates with a variety of providers (e.g., physical and occupational therapists, wound and ostomy nurses, nutritionists, pharmacists, social workers, psychologists, and clergy or spiritual advisors) to help identify appropriate interventions that support the goal of regaining the highest level of function and independence possible for the patient.

Expected patient outcomes may include the following:

1. Maintains integrity of oral mucous membranes
2. Maintains adequate tissue integrity
3. Maintains adequate nutritional status
4. Achieves relief of pain and discomfort
5. Demonstrates increased activity tolerance and decreased fatigue
6. Exhibits improved body image and self-esteem
7. Progresses through the grieving process
8. Experiences no complications, such as infection, or sepsis, and no episodes of bleeding or hemorrhage

GERONTOLOGIC CONSIDERATIONS

As a result of an increased life expectancy and an increased risk of cancer with age, nurses are providing cancer-related care for growing numbers of older patients. About 60% of cancers occur in people 65 years of age or older. Adults who are 85 years and older, occasionally referred to as the "oldest old," are the fastest-growing age group in the United States, and are expected to nearly triple from 6.4 million in 2016 to 19.0 million by 2060 (DeSantis et al., 2019). This change is largely due to public health measures such as smoking cessation, improved screening, and medical advances. Nursing care of the older population requires addressing special needs, including physical, psychosocial, and financial concerns.

Oncology nurses working with the older population must understand the normal physiologic changes that occur with aging. These changes include decreased skin elasticity; decreased skeletal mass, structure, and strength; decreased organ function and structure; impaired immune system mechanisms; alterations in neurologic and sensory functions; and altered drug absorption, distribution, metabolism, and elimination. These changes ultimately influence the ability of older patients to tolerate cancer treatment. In addition, many older patients have other chronic diseases and associated treatments that may limit tolerance to cancer treatments. The reported prevalence of polypharmacy in the older population varies substantially, ranging from 10% to 96% (Shrestha et al., 2019). In the oncology setting, polypharmacy with inappropriate medications may contribute to the patient's worsened condition, frailty syndrome, poor physical function, poor survival, and a higher number of comorbidities (Shrestha et al., 2019).

Potential chemotherapy-related toxicities, such as renal impairment, myelosuppression, fatigue, and cardiomyopathy, may increase because of declining organ function and diminished physiologic reserves. The recovery of normal tissues after radiation therapy may be delayed, and older patients may experience more severe adverse effects, such as mucositis, nausea and vomiting, and myelosuppression. Because of decreased tissue-healing capacity and declining pulmonary and cardiovascular functioning, older patients are slower to recover from surgery. Older patients are also at increased risk for complications such as atelectasis, pneumonia, and wound infections.

Access to cancer care for older patients may be limited by discriminatory or fatalistic attitudes of health care providers, caregivers, and patients themselves. Issues such as the gradual loss of supportive resources, declining health or loss of a spouse, and unavailability of relatives or friends may result in limited access to care and unmet needs for assistance with activities of daily living. In addition, the economic impact of health care may be difficult for those living on fixed incomes.

Nurses must be aware of the special needs of the aging population. Nurses carefully monitor older patients receiving cancer treatments for signs and symptoms of adverse effects. In addition, older patients are instructed to report all symptoms to their provider. It is not uncommon for older patients to delay reporting symptoms, attributing them to "old age." Many older people do not want to report illness for fear of losing their independence or financial security. Sensory losses (e.g., hearing and visual losses) and memory deficits are considered when planning patient education because they may affect the patient's ability to process and retain information. In such cases, the nurse acts as a patient advocate, encouraging independence and identifying resources, such as home care, for support when indicated.

END-OF-LIFE CONSIDERATIONS

The needs of patients with terminal illnesses are best met by a comprehensive multidisciplinary program that focuses on quality of life, palliation of symptoms, and provision of psychosocial and spiritual support for patients and families when cure and control of the disease are no longer possible. Over the past five decades, palliative care has evolved from a philosophy of care that focuses on the last days of life to a professional specialty that delivers comprehensive supportive care to patients with advances illness throughout the disease trajectory (Hui & Bruera, 2020). Currently, the major service delivery models, including specialist palliative care, namely outpatient palliative care clinics, inpatient palliative care consultation teams, acute palliative care units, community based palliative care, and hospice care, complement one another to provide comprehensive supportive care from diagnosis to end of life (Hui & Bruera, 2020).

Hospice care is often delivered through coordination of services provided by hospitals and the community. Although providers, social workers, clergy, dietitians, pharmacists, physical therapists, and volunteers are involved in patient care, nurses are most often the coordinators of hospice activities. It is essential that home care and hospice nurses possess advanced skills in communication, assessing and managing pain, nutrition, dyspnea, bowel dysfunction, and skin impairments.

In addition, hospice programs facilitate clear communication among family members and health care providers. Most patients and families are informed of the prognosis and are encouraged to participate in decisions regarding pursuing or terminating cancer treatment. Through collaboration with other support disciplines, the nurse helps the patient and family cope with changes in role identity, family structure, grief, and loss. Hospice nurses are actively involved in bereavement counseling. In many instances, family support for survivors continues for approximately 1 year.

CHAPTER REVIEW

NCLEX-Style Review Questions

1. In assessing understanding of discharge education in a patient with neutropenia, which patient statements indicate awareness of appropriate actions? Select all that apply.
   a. "I should stay away from crowds and people who are sick."
   b. "I should wash my hands carefully after using the bathroom and before eating meals."
   c. "If I have a fever or chills, I should take acetaminophen immediately and recheck my temperature an hour later."
   d. "My WBC count should recover about 5 to 7 days after my treatment is completed."
   e. "If I shave, I will use an electric razor to prevent cuts so germs can't get in."

2. A nurse is caring for a patient receiving brachytherapy for cervical cancer. Which of the following statements regarding the nursing care of this patient is true? Select all that apply.
   a. The patient must be maintained on bed rest.
   b. The head of the bed must be elevated more than 30 degrees to decrease the risk of aspiration.
   c. Pain management is a priority.
   d. The patient will have an indwelling urinary catheter.
   e. A diet high in protein will be provided to prevent hypoalbuminemia.

3. A patient is receiving external beam radiation therapy for head and neck cancer. The patient reports moderate to severe pain to the tongue and buccal mucosa that is interfering with their ability to eat, sleep, and speak. Which of the following interventions would you recommended for this patient? Select all that apply.
   a. Take pain medication 30 minutes before meals.
   b. Avoid acidic, spicy, and sharp foods such as chips.
   c. Keep dentures out when not eating to promote healing.
   d. Rinse the oral mucosa regularly with an alcohol-based solution.
   e. Avoid brushing the teeth to prevent additional trauma to the oral mucosa.

4. As a nurse who provides care on an oncology unit, you are aware that many of your patients who undergo surgery during cancer treatment face a particularly high risk of deep vein thrombosis (DVT). In light of this risk, you should prioritize assessments of which of the following? Select all that apply.
   a. Erythema and warmth of the involved extremity
   b. Petechiae and hematomas on the lower extremities
   c. Lung sounds and O_2 saturation
   d. Limb symmetry and calf pain
   e. Low-grade temperature and tachycardia

5. A 54-year-old patient receiving monthly chemotherapy for colon cancer comes into your clinic after his fifth monthly dose. Which lab results do you report to the provider before administering the chemotherapy? Select all that apply.

a. Hemoglobin of 14.5 g/dL
b. Thrombocyte count of 42,000/mm^3
c. BUN of 12 mg/dL
d. White blood cell count of 2,400/mm^3
e. Temperature of 101.2°F
f. Urine specific gravity of 1.012

6. A patient with lung cancer is admitted to your unit with suspected superior vena cava syndrome (SVCS). List the signs and symptoms you are assessing for? Select all that apply.

a. Upper arm edema
b. Lower leg edema
c. Flat neck veins
d. Lying flat relieves symptoms
e. Complaints of tight shirt collar buttons
f. Plethora (erythema of the face)

REFERENCES AND SELECTED READINGS

References and selected readings associated with this chapter can be found on the website that accompanies the book. Visit **http://thepoint.lww.com/Honan3e** to access the references and other additional resources associated with this chapter.

CHAPTER 6

Pain Management

Elissa Mastrangelo • Mary Dudley

Learning Objectives

After reading this chapter, you will be able to:

1. Compare characteristics of acute pain, chronic pain, and cancer pain.
2. Describe the effects of acute and chronic pain.
3. Describe the pathophysiology of pain.
4. Describe factors that can alter the response to pain.
5. Demonstrate appropriate use of pain measurement instruments.
6. Explain the nursing role in multidisciplinary pain management.
7. Identify nonpharmacologic pain relief interventions for selected groups of patients.
8. Develop a plan to prevent and treat the adverse effects of analgesic agents.
9. Use the nursing process as a framework for the care of patients with pain.

The International Association for the Study of Pain (IASP) defines pain as "An unpleasant sensory and emotional experience associated with, or resembling that associated with, actual or potential tissue damage" (IASP, July 2020). Pain is the most common reason for seeking health care (Jameson et al., 2020). Pain is associated with many disorders, diagnostic tests, and treatments. Pain disables and distresses more people than any single disease, varies widely in intensity, and spares no age group. Because nurses spend more time with patients in pain than other health care providers, nurses need to understand the pathophysiology of pain, the physiologic and psychological consequences of acute and chronic (persistent) pain, and the methods used to treat pain. Nurses encounter patients in pain in a variety of settings, including acute care, outpatient, and long-term care settings, as well as in the home. Therefore, they must have the knowledge and skills to assess pain, implement pain relief strategies, and evaluate the effectiveness of these strategies, regardless of setting.

TYPES OF PAIN

Pain is categorized according to its duration, location, and etiology. In general, four basic categories of pain are recognized: acute pain, chronic (persistent, nonmalignant) pain, cancer-related pain, and acute-on-chronic pain.

Acute Pain

Usually of recent onset and commonly associated with a specific injury, trauma, or painful medical procedures, acute pain indicates that damage or injury has occurred. Pain is significant in that it draws attention to a threat and teaches people to avoid similar potentially painful situations. Thus, pain is both a sensation and a warning signal. If no lasting damage occurs and no systemic disease exists, acute pain usually decreases as healing occurs or as the underlying cause is treated. Acute pain can be an isolated one-time incident or recur at regular intervals, such as menstrual cramping, or sporadically, as with angina or migraine headaches. If untreated, acute pain may lead to chronic pain.

Chronic Pain

Chronic pain is a persistent or intermittent pain that lingers beyond the expected healing time (more than 3 months). It is associated with a variety of degenerative or traumatic conditions, such as arthritis, degenerative disc disease, and intervertebral disc herniation, but often a specific cause or injury for the chronic pain may not be found. It may have a poorly defined onset, and it is often difficult to treat because the cause or origin may be unclear. Although acute pain may be a useful signal that something is wrong, chronic or persistent pain may become a patient's primary disorder with symptoms of refractory pain (when pain cannot be adequately controlled despite aggressive measures), functional and psychological impairment, and disability (Majedi et al., 2020). Medical-surgical nurses care for patients with chronic pain when these patients are admitted to the hospital for management or when they develop other new etiologies.

Cancer-Related Pain

Pain associated with cancer may be acute or chronic. Pain resulting from cancer is so ubiquitous that when cancer patients are asked about the most feared consequences of cancer, pain is reported most frequently. Most patients with cancer experience pain; in a recent literature review, 35% to 96% of patients with advanced cancer experience pain (Henson et al., 2020). Pain in patients with cancer can be directly associated with the cancer (e.g., bony infiltration with tumor cells or nerve compression), a result of cancer treatment (e.g., surgery or radiation), or unrelated to the cancer (e.g., trauma). However, most pain associated with cancer is a direct result of tumor involvement. Although the pain may be acute, it is characterized more frequently as chronic. As in other situations involving pain, the experience of cancer pain is influenced by both physical and psychosocial factors.

Cancer can cause pain in various ways. Pain may be associated with various cancer treatments. Acute pain is linked with trauma from surgery. Occasionally, chronic pain syndromes, such as postsurgical neuropathies (pain related to nerve tissue injury), occur. Some chemotherapeutic agents cause tissue necrosis, peripheral neuropathies, and stomatitis—all potential sources of pain—whereas radiation therapy can cause pain secondary to skin or organ inflammation.

For some patients with advanced cancer, pain that continues to increase over time may be a sign that the tumor growth has progressed and that death is near. It is vital for the nurse to recognize the progression of symptoms correlating with the disease process so as to provide physical and emotional support to both the patient and loved ones. As patients anticipate the pain and their anxiety increases, pain perception heightens, producing fear and further pain. Chronic cancer pain, then, can be best described as a cycle progressing from pain to anxiety to fear and back to pain.

Acute-on-Chronic Pain

Many patients with chronic pain who are opioid dependent require surgery for an unrelated condition. An example would be a patient with chronic back pain who is scheduled for a total knee replacement. Ideally, this group of patients would be identified before surgery to facilitate a multimodal pain treatment plan. Typically, these patients exhibit increased opioid requirements after surgery. The addition of pain and interventional specialists to the care team should be employed when available.

EFFECTS OF PAIN

Regardless of its nature, pattern, or cause, pain that is inadequately treated has harmful effects beyond the suffering it causes.

Effects of Acute Pain

Unrelieved acute pain can affect the pulmonary, cardiovascular, gastrointestinal (GI), endocrine, and immune systems. The stress response (neuroendocrine response to stress) that occurs with trauma also occurs with severe pain. The widespread endocrine, immunologic, and inflammatory changes that occur with stress can have significant negative effects. This is particularly harmful in patients whose health is already compromised by age, illness, or injury.

The stress response generally consists of increased metabolic rate and cardiac output, impaired insulin response, increased production of cortisol, and increased retention of fluids. Box 6-1 discusses the physiologic impact of acute pain. The stress response may increase the risk of physiologic disorders (e.g., myocardial infarction, pulmonary infection,

BOX 6-1

Physiologic Response to Acute Pain

Endocrine and metabolic response	Activation of sympathetic nervous system and an increase in glucagon secretion, which causes hyperglycemia, increased lipolysis (fat breakdown), accelerated protein breakdown, and nitrogen loss. The stress response presents as hypertension, tachycardia, arrhythmias, myocardial ischemia, protein catabolism, immune system suppression, and impaired renal excretory function.
Pulmonary function	Decreased phrenic nerve activity and diaphragmatic dysfunction manifested as a decrease in functional residual capacity and a decrease in tidal volume.
GI motility	Decreased gastric motility, especially in the colon. The stomach and small intestines recover within 12 to 24 hours after abdominal surgery; however, the colon is inhibited for at least 48 to 72 hours.
Cardiovascular	Increased sympathetic tone, which causes an increase in heart rate and blood pressure as well as redistribution of blood to and within various organs. The redistribution predisposes patients to myocardial ischemia in the presence of coronary artery disease and may induce arrhythmias.
Immune system	Decreased responsiveness to antigens, delayed hypersensitivity, natural killer cell activity, and antibody response.

Adapted from American Society of Pain Management Nursing, *Core curriculum for pain management nursing*, 3rd ed.

thromboembolism, prolonged paralytic ileus). Patients with severe pain and associated stress may be unable to take deep breaths and may experience increased fatigue and decreased mobility. Although these effects may be tolerated by young, healthy people, they may hamper recovery in patients who are older, debilitated, or critically ill. Effective pain relief may result in faster recovery and improved outcomes.

Effects of Chronic Pain

Like acute pain, chronic pain also has adverse effects. Suppression of the immune function associated with chronic pain may promote tumor growth. In addition, chronic pain often results in anger, depression, anxiety, fatigue, and disability. Patients may be unable to continue the activities and interpersonal relationships that they had engaged in before the pain began, with resultant impact on their quality of life. Disabilities may range from curtailing participation in physical activities to being unable to take care of personal needs, such as dressing or eating. Regardless of how patients cope with persistent pain, disability can result if the pain persists for an extended period.

Nurses should understand the effects of chronic pain on patients and families and should be knowledgeable about pain relief strategies and appropriate resources to assist effectively with pain management. Chronic pain that has become refractory to conventional treatment modalities can predispose a patient to take large quantities of opioid medications. Health care providers face the challenge of uncontrolled pain despite continued opioid dose increases. In some cases, patients can become hyperalgesic or have opioid-induced hyperalgesia (OIH), which is defined as the state of nociceptive sensitization caused by long-term exposure to opioids. A patient will report more pain or uncontrolled pain despite an increase in opioid dose. It may be hard for the patient to understand that reducing opioids in the state of hyperalgesia will help with the reduction of pain. The general health care provider can seek referral to available pain resources, such as a consult from an existing pain service or an evaluation by a certified pain nurse specialist.

Effects of Cancer Pain

As noted above, cancer pain may have aspects that are both acute and chronic. In addition, patients with cancer often have multiple causes of pain (e.g., direct tumor involvement, tumor invasion of the nerve and hollow viscera) involving multiple sites (bone pain, pain from chemotherapy, radiation, surgery). There can be significant changes in the patient's personality (mood disturbances, anxiety, and depression), lifestyle (lack of confidence in ability to control pain, decreased social interactions), and functional ability. Given the multidimensional aspects of cancer pain, it follows that a multidimensional plan is needed to manage the challenging aspects of cancer pain effectively.

PATHOPHYSIOLOGY OF PAIN

The processing of noxious stimuli and the resulting perception of pain involve the peripheral nervous system and central nervous system (CNS). Various nerve mechanisms and structures are involved in the transmission of pain to and from the brain, including nociceptors, or pain receptors, and chemical mediators. **Nociceptors** are free nerve endings found in the skin. These receptors are preferentially sensitive to intense, potentially damaging mechanical, thermal, or chemical stimuli. Although the skin contains the highest density of nociceptors, they also are found in joints, connective tissues, blood vessels, periosteum, skeletal muscle, fascia, tendons, most visceral organs, and the corneas, and have the potential to respond to painful stimuli. When stimulated, nociceptors send signals to local blood vessels, mast cells, hair follicles, and sweat glands, often resulting in clinical findings associated with pain, such as vasomotor, autonomic, and visceral effects.

The nociceptors transmit information about the noxious, distressing, or damaging stimuli to neurons located in the spinal cord or brainstem, and this sensory information is integrated in the thalamus along with higher brain structures generating protective somatic and autonomic reflexes, endocrine actions, emotional responses, learning and memory about the event, and cortical awareness of pain (Kendroud et al., 2022).

Peripheral Nervous System Response

A number of **allogenic** (pain-causing) substances that enhance the sensitivity of nociceptors are released into the extracellular tissue as a result of tissue damage. Histamine, bradykinin, acetylcholine, serotonin (5-hydroxytryptamine or 5-HT), calcitonin gene-related peptide (CGRP), and substance P are chemicals that increase the transmission of pain (Ban et al., 2020). The injured tissue releases bradykinin and prostaglandins that sensitize or activate nociceptors, which, in turn, release substance P. Substance P acts on mast cells to release histamine and CGRP, which dilates the blood vessels, resulting in edema and an inflammatory process. Serotonin (5-HT) is released from platelets and activates nociceptors. **Prostaglandins** are chemical substances that are believed to increase the sensitivity of pain receptors by enhancing the pain-provoking effect of bradykinin. It is interesting to note that aspirin and other nonsteroidal anti-inflammatory drugs (NSAIDs) block the enzyme needed for prostaglandin synthesis, resulting in pain control. At the peripheral nervous system level, two main types of fibers are involved in **nociception** (the neurologic transmission of pain impulses). The larger, myelinated A delta fibers transmit the initial pain sensation rapidly, at a rate of 12 to 34 m/sec, to the brain (acute pain, or "fast pain"). This type of pain frequently is associated with mechanical or thermal stimuli. The smaller, unmyelinated C fibers transmit impulses at a rate of 0.5 to 2 m/sec (Tkacs et al., 2020). This is called "second pain" or "slow-wave pain" due to delayed onset and longer duration. It has dull, aching, diffuse, or burning qualities, which last longer than the initial fast pain. Chronic pain is believed to be associated with C-fiber stimulation.

If there is repeated C-fiber stimulation, there is a heightened response in spinal cord neurons, causing the person to perceive more pain. For this reason, it is important to treat patients with analgesic agents when they first feel pain. Patients require less medication and experience more effective pain relief if analgesia is administered before they become sensitized to the pain.

Central Nervous System Response

For pain to be consciously perceived, neurons in the ascending system must be activated. Activation occurs as a result of input from the nociceptors. After tissue injury occurs, nociception continues and relays the impulses to the dorsal horn of the spinal cord. Upon entering the spinal cord at the dorsal horn, the pain impulse crosses the spinal cord and passes upward to the brain by the anterolateral pathway to the thalamus. Then the pain signals are transmitted to other areas of the brain and sensory cortex where the conscious experience or perception of pain occurs. Figure 6-1 illustrates pain transmission.

Chemicals that reduce or inhibit the transmission or perception of pain include **endorphins, enkephalins, and dynorphins** (Tkacs et al., 2020). These chemical, morphine-like neurotransmitters are endogenous (produced by the body) and reduce nociceptive transmission.

Just as the ascending system relays signal up to the brain for interpretation, the descending control system is considered inhibitory. It is always somewhat active, and it prevents continuous transmission of painful stimuli, partly through the action of the endorphins. Cognitive processes may stimulate endorphin production in the descending control system. The effectiveness of this system is illustrated by the effects of distraction. The distractions of visitors or a favorite television show may increase activity in the descending control system. Therefore, patients who have visitors or who are engaged in a television program may not report pain because activation of the descending control system results in less noxious or painful information being transmitted to consciousness. In addition, tactile stimulation can modulate pain through a complex process of tactile information being transmitted by large and small fibers throughout the CNS (Norris, 2019).

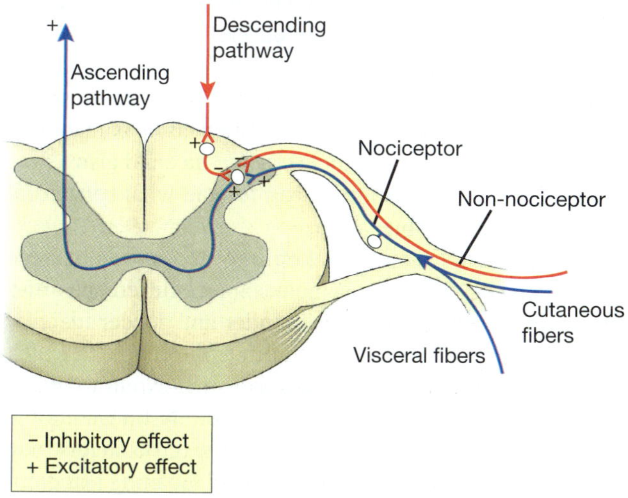

FIGURE 6-1 A schematic representation of aspects of nociceptive system.

The neuromatrix theory of pain proposed by Melzack (2001) provides a conceptual framework to examine chronic pain. It proposes that in response to injury, inflammation, disease, or chronic stress, the body–self neuromatrix activates perceptual, homeostatic, and behavioral responses. Endocrine, autonomic, immune, and opioid systems contribute to this interactive cognitive interpretation of pain. The pain experience is distinctive to each individual, shaped by sensory, psychosocial, and genetic factors, and modulated by various sensory inputs from the environment and by cognitive events, such as psychological stress (Mallick-Searle et al., 2021). Thus, pain occurs in response to a widely distributed neural network in the brain (sensory, affective, and cognitive dimensions) rather than only to the sensory input of injury, inflammation, or pathology.

Pearls for Practice

Large internal organs (viscera) have a low density of nociceptors; as a result, typically, visceral pain is poorly localized, nauseating, and frequently associated with diaphoresis and autonomic symptoms. Typically, pain originating in these large, internal organs results from intense stimulation of multipurpose receptors that respond to inflammation, stretching, ischemia, dilation, and spasm of the internal organs. An intense response in these fibers can cause severe pain.

FACTORS INFLUENCING PAIN RESPONSE

Several factors, including past experiences with pain, anxiety, culture, age, gender, genetics, and expectations about pain relief, influence a person's experience of pain. These factors may increase or decrease perception of pain, increase or decrease tolerance for pain, and affect responses to pain.

Past Experience

The way a person responds to pain is a result of many separate painful events during a lifetime. The nurse understands that a patient's pain history may provide vital information on how a person has been able to positively cope and manage their pain as well as what has hindered their physical and emotional well-being. This information will shape the patient's current expectation of pain and or pain

BOX 6-2

Common Concerns and Misconceptions About Pain and Analgesia

Misconception	Evidence
Patients with chronic pain have a higher tolerance to pain.	Patients with chronic pain have a decreased tolerance to pain associated with decreased endorphins, the effect of neurotransmitters, and physiologic responses. In patients with chronic pain, signals for pain and muscle spasm continue to be transmitted by the nervous system.
Chronic pain is due to psychological disturbance.	When unable to find a physiologic reason for pain, providers often attribute chronic pain to a psychological issue and, in addition, have demonstrated more positive responses to patients when pathology is found.
Chronic pain is caused by stress, and if the stress is relieved, pain abates.	Coping with chronic pain can be stressful, which can lead to suffering and depression.
Patients will exaggerate their pain in order to receive increased compensation payments.	No evidence exists that patients report increased pain when seeking compensation or litigation.
Patients in chronic pain demonstrate manipulative behavior.	It is rare for patients with chronic pain to misrepresent their symptoms. Rather, some patients may seek out a variety of providers to obtain relief.
Depression causes chronic pain.	There is a correlation between chronic pain and depression; however, it is more likely that the stress of managing the chronic pain leads to depression.
People will become addicted to pain medicine easily.	Research suggests a negligible risk of developing a substance use disorder (SUD) when patients are prescribed opioids for pain. Misconceptions are related to a lack of knowledge of tolerance, physical dependence, and addiction.
Often, patients are noncompliant and to blame for their physical symptoms.	Evidence shows that patients with chronic pain are generally compliant, and, if not, the reasons are attributed to treatment side effects or lack of treatment response.

Data from Sargent (2020). R6 student nurse attitudes and knowledge regarding chronic pain in the older adult. *Pain Management Nursing*, *21*(2), 220.

management. If pain is relieved promptly and adequately, the person may be less fearful of future pain and better able to tolerate it.

Anxiety and Depression

Although it is commonly believed that anxiety increases pain, this is not necessarily true (see Box 6-2 for common misconceptions about pain). However, anxiety that is associated with pain may increase the patient's perception of pain. For example, the patient who was treated 2 years ago for breast cancer and who now has hip pain may fear that the pain indicates metastasis. In this case, the patient's anxiety may result in increased pain. However, anxiety that is unrelated to the pain (e.g., anxiety about who is taking care of the pets while the patient is in the hospital) may distract the patient and may actually decrease the perception of pain.

Just as anxiety is associated with pain because of concerns and fears about an underlying disease, depression and chronic pain frequently coexist. The presence of depression with chronic pain varies widely, with studies reporting 10% to 100% (Tenti et al., 2021); therefore, screening for depression is important in patients with chronic pain due to the negative impact of depression on patients' lives.

The COVID-19 pandemic has impacted chronic pain patients, particularly those with neuropathy and chronic migraines. Social isolation and the inability to have in-office visits with health care providers contributed to patient reports of increasing pain and worsening of clinical conditions. Patients reported worsening agitation, anxiety, and sadness (Consonni et al., 2021). Thus, the nurse is aware that any health crisis has the potential to interfere with both physical and mental health of patients.

Culture

Beliefs about pain and how to respond to it differ from one culture to the next. Early in childhood, people learn from those around them what responses to pain are acceptable or unacceptable. For example, a child may learn that a sports injury is not expected to hurt as much as a comparable injury caused by a motor vehicle crash. The child also learns what stimuli are expected to be painful and what behavioral responses are acceptable.

Cultural factors must be taken into account to manage pain effectively. Factors that help explain differences in a cultural group include age, sex, gender and gender identity, education level, and income. In addition, the degree to which patients identify with culture influences the extent to which they will adopt new health behaviors or rely on traditional health beliefs and practices. A wide range of behaviors may be seen in response to pain, ranging from moaning and complaining about pain and describing pain as "unbearable" to behaving in a quiet, stoic manner rather than expressing the pain verbally. The nurse must respond to the person's perception of pain and assess the person's behavior, taking into consideration cultural influences. The nurse who recognizes cultural differences has insight into the impact of pain on the patient and is more accurate in assessing pain and in planning appropriate treatments to relieve pain.

The main issues to consider when caring for patients of a different culture are:

- What does the illness mean to the patient?
- Are there culturally based stigmas related to this illness or pain?
- What is the role of the family or significant others in the patient's health care decisions?
- Are traditional or customary pain relief remedies used?
- What is the role of stoicism in the patient's culture?
- Are there culturally determined ways of expressing and communicating pain?
- Does the patient have any fears about the pain?

The nurse should avoid bias and stereotyping the patient by culture and should provide individualized care rather than assuming that a patient of a specific culture will exhibit more or less pain. In addition to avoiding stereotyping, health care providers should individualize the amount of medications or therapy according to the information provided by the patient. The nurse should recognize that stereotypes exist and become sensitive to how they negatively affect care; refer to Box 6-2 for common misconceptions.

Pearls for Practice: Lifting the Lens

A contributor to health care disparities is implicit bias, which is defined as a form of bias that occurs automatically and unintentionally and that nevertheless affects clinical judgments, decisions, and behaviors (NIH, 2022). We must be cognizant of the fact that as humans, we hold attitudes about people based on race or ethnicity, gender, body weight, religion, and/or political views, among others. Unfortunately, many patients with chronic pain already feel stigmatized and marginalized, and Black, Indigenous, and People of Color (BIPOC) patients are particularly vulnerable (Ghoshal et al., 2020). Nurses need to be aware of bias and recognize that it can affect our professional perceptions, decisions, and actions. Specific behaviors that convey attentiveness and empathy could include focused eye contact with the patient, using a softer tone, gentle physical touch, actively listening to the patient, and allowing patients the time needed to voice their concerns. It will take the deliberate work of every nurse to begin to address the stigma that chronic pain patients experience—one patient at a time.

Age

Assessment and treatment of pain in older individuals poses many challenges. Older adults experience age-related physiologic changes in the peripheral nervous system and CNS. In addition, altered drug metabolism in the liver and decreased renal excretion can lead to adverse effects, particularly opioids from higher plasma concentrations. Thus, to avoid the risk of toxicity, dosages and/or interval modifications of medications may be necessary. Older adults with comorbid conditions may be prescribed multiple medications. Multiple drug classes may increase the risk of toxicity or reduce the efficacy of analgesics. Polypharmacy is common, and the nurse must recognize side effects of analgesic medications.

Adults with cognitive impairment require different approaches to pain assessment with a focus on functional ability. The increasing older adult population is at high risk for developing chronic pain conditions such as osteoarthritis, osteoporosis-related fractures, and diabetic and vascular neuropathies.

Persistent, unrelieved pain may have adverse consequences on an older adult's social, physical, and financial well-being. In addition, the cardiovascular, endocrine, neurologic, musculoskeletal, and immune systems are impacted. Pain in older individuals can lead to depression, decreased mobility, insomnia, confusion, and delirium. Older adults are often reluctant to voice concerns about pain. Some older patients feel pain is a normal part of aging. They may also fear new diagnostic tests and the addition of medications such as opioids and possible side effects such as constipation.

Nurses and health care providers need to utilize evidence-based pain assessment tools in the older population with a focus on function both at rest and with movement (Booker et al., 2020). An appropriate multimodal analgesic plan needs to be implemented using pharmacologic and nonpharmacologic modalities. Table 6-1 provides gerontologic considerations related to pain management.

Gender

Epidemiologic and clinical studies have established that females are more sensitive to pain, despite the same disease conditions (Kim & Kim, 2020). These conditions include musculoskeletal disorders, such as rheumatoid arthritis (RA) and osteoarthritis. There have been no significant sex-related differences found generally with low-back pain conditions, which may contribute to occupation factors. "Although, psychological factors, including coping with pain, mood, and sensitivity to pain, may play a role in mediating the sex-related differences in arthritis pain," the data suggest that molecular mechanisms, including variations in immune cell types and inflammatory cytokines, such as increased C-reactive protein (CRP), may explain the sex-related differences among arthritis-induced pain, as seen in animal models. Also, of note is a correlation to total fat mass and fat/muscle ratio in predicting musculoskeletal pain. It is suggested that decreases in estrogen levels as seen in postmenopausal females and an increase in fat

TABLE **6-1** **GERONTOLOGIC CONSIDERATIONS / For Pain Management**

Physiologic Changes Influencing Pain Response	Pain Management Interventions
• Higher incidence of chronic illnesses • Increased use of prescription and OTC medications • Sensitivity to medications and increased risk for drug toxicity • Changes in medication absorption and metabolism due to decreased function of the liver, kidney, and GI system • Altered distribution of medications due to changes in body weight, protein stores, and distribution of body fluid • Slowed metabolism of medications • Higher blood levels of medications • Susceptibility to depression of both the nervous and the respiratory systems; hypoxia and hypercarbia can worsen workload on the heart, resulting in myocardial ischemia	• Obtain a careful medication history to identify potential drug interactions. • Administer analgesic agents, keeping a balance between minimal side effects and effective pain relief. • Consider possible need for slightly smaller initial dose of analgesic medication than prescribed for younger patients. • Patient may need prolonged dosing interval for subsequent doses. • Refer to clinical practice guidelines for managing persistent pain as needed. • Perform frequent assessments and evaluation of patient responses to pain interventions.

OTC, over the counter.

mass may also cause a higher pain sensitivity (Kim & Kim, 2020).

Pearls for Practice

With regard to terminology, it is important for nurses to distinguish sex assigned at birth and gender. While sex refers to the classification of humans based on biology, anatomy, or chromosomes (generally, XX for female and XY for male), gender is more complex and refers to the person's self-representation, social, cultural, psychological, and/or emotional traits, often influenced by societal expectations. For example, an individual may identify their gender as male or female, corresponding with their sex at birth, which is termed cisgender. *An individual may identify differently from their sex assigned at birth, termed* transgender. *Some individuals are more fluid than binary labels and identify as* nonbinary. *Note that both sex and gender are distinct from a person's sexual orientation, which describes the emotional or physical attractions such as straight, lesbian, gay men or men who have sex with men (MSM), asexual/aromantice, bisexual, etc.*

PAIN ASSESSMENT

The role of primary health care providers is to assess and relieve pain by the administration of medications and other treatments. Nurses collaborate with other health care professionals while administering most pain relief interventions, evaluating their effectiveness, and serving as patient advocates when the intervention is ineffective. In addition, nurses serve as educators to patients and families, teaching them to manage the pain relief regimen themselves when appropriate.

The definition of pain forwarded by the IASP identified at the beginning of this chapter encompasses the multidimensional nature of pain. An early broad definition of pain by McCaffery is, "whatever the person says it is, existing whenever the experiencing person says it does" (McCaffery & Pasero, 1999, p. 5). This definition emphasizes the highly subjective nature of pain and pain management. Patients are the best authority on the existence of pain. In patients unable to self-report pain, appropriate pain assessment tools should be used.

Pain assessment is one core element of patient care that requires ongoing surveillance. Self-report of pain intensity and distress should be used whenever possible. Regular assessment and documentation of pain, including the patient's functional ability, help monitor the efficacy of analgesic modalities.

Although it is important to believe patients who report pain, it is equally important to be alert to patients who deny pain in situations where pain would be expected. A nurse who suspects pain in a patient who denies it should explore with the patient the reason for suspecting pain, such as discussing the fact that the disorder or procedure is painful for most people or pointing out that the patient grimaces when moving or avoids movement. It also may be helpful to explore why the patient may be denying pain. Some people deny pain because they fear the treatment that may result if they report or admit pain. Others deny pain for fear of becoming addicted to **opioids** (previously referred to as narcotics) if these medications are prescribed. The American Pain Foundation developed the Pain Care Bill of Rights, which addresses the importance of pain management (Box 6-3).

The highly subjective nature of pain means that pain assessment and management present challenges for all clinicians. The report of pain is a social transaction; that is, the assessment and management of pain will require the establishment of rapport and trust with the person in pain. In assessing a patient with pain, the nurse reviews the patient's description of the pain and other factors that may influence pain (e.g., previous experience, anxiety, age) as well as the patient's response to pain relief strategies. Documentation of the pain level as rated on a pain scale becomes part of the

BOX 6-3

Pain Care Bill of Rights

Patient Bill of Rights

U.S. PAIN FOUNDATION WANTS YOU TO KNOW: AS A PERSON WITH PAIN, YOU HAVE MANY RIGHTS.

1. Patients have the right to care from the health care provider of their choice.
2. Patients have the right to ask questions about a health care provider's education, licensure, and experience.
3. Patients have the right to care that is respectful, objective, and nondiscriminatory.
4. Patients have the right to have their pain effectively and safely managed.
5. Patients have the right to ask for and receive a referral to a pain management specialist.
6. Patients have the right to have their pain examined regularly and their treatments adjusted for continued or improved pain management.
7. Patients have the right to receive clear, accurate information about all treatment options available, including the risks and benefits of each option.
8. Patients have the right to refuse suggested methods of pain treatment.
9. Patients have the right to a second opinion.
10. Patients have the right to participate in their pain treatment decisions. If patients cannot fully participate in their treatment decisions, patients have the right to be represented by family members and/or guardians.
11. Patients have the right to have costs explained to them before proceeding with care and have the right to have medical bills explained after care is delivered.
12. Patients have the right to read and make copies of their health information and relevant records.
13. Patients have the right to ask their health care provider to amend or correct any information in their health records.
14. Patients have the right to speak confidentially with their health care providers.
15. Patients have the right to complain about or appeal issues related to treatment, health plans, health care personnel, and health care facilities.

If you feel your rights have been violated, please contact U.S. Pain Foundation at contact@uspainfoundation.org.

Courtesy of the U.S. Pain Foundation, 2021.

patient's medical record, as does the record of the pain relief obtained from interventions.

Pain assessment includes determining what level of pain relief the patient with acute illness believes is needed to recover quickly or improve function, or what level of relief the patient with chronic or terminal illness requires to maintain comfort. Part of a thorough pain assessment is understanding the patient's expectations and misconceptions about pain, which may include the notion that pain is a normal experience, that pain builds character, that pain medication side effects are worse than the pain, and the fear of becoming addicted to opioids. People who understand that pain relief not only contributes to comfort but also hastens recovery are more likely to request or self-administer treatment appropriately.

Pearls for Practice

The Joint Commission for accreditation of hospitals published new and revised pain management standards effective January, 2019. The overall goal of these standards is to improve pain assessment and pain management and ensure safe opioid-prescribing practices (The Joint Commission Perspectives, 2022). Every patient is screened/assessed for pain on admission to a hospital and at each office/clinic visit. The nurse will evaluate the patient's pain using evidence-based scales that are clinically and developmentally appropriate. Pain is reassessed and documented after any intervention and with a change in a patient's condition. The nurse will set an acceptable pain goal with input from the patient and family when appropriate. An individualized pain management plan is developed by the provider using pharmacologic and nonpharmacologic modalities. The intent of this chapter is to present the scope of pain assessment and interventions available for the RN.

Characteristics of Pain

The factors to consider in a complete pain assessment are the intensity, timing, location, quality, and personal meaning of pain; aggravating and alleviating factors; and pain behaviors. Pain assessment begins by careful patient observation, noting overall posture and presence or absence of overt pain behaviors. In addition, it is essential to ask the patient to describe the specifics of the pain. The words used to describe the pain may point toward the cause. A detailed history should follow the initial description of pain.

Intensity

The intensity of pain ranges from none to mild discomfort to excruciating. There is no correlation between reported intensity and the stimulus that produced it. The reported intensity is influenced by the person's **pain threshold** and **pain tolerance**. Pain threshold is the smallest stimulus for which a person reports pain, and pain tolerance is the maximum amount of pain a person can tolerate. To understand variations, the nurse can ask about the present pain intensity as well as the least and the worst pain intensity. Various scales and surveys are helpful to patients trying to describe pain intensity; see the later discussion of Instruments for Assessing the Perception of Pain on page 217.

Timing

Sometimes, the cause of pain can be determined when its temporal aspects are known. Therefore, the nurse inquires about the onset and duration of pain, the relationship between time and intensity (e.g., at what time is the pain worst), and changes in rhythmic patterns. The patient is asked if the pain began suddenly or increased gradually. Sudden pain that rapidly reaches maximum intensity is indicative of tissue rupture; thus, immediate assessment and intervention is necessary. Pain from chronic ischemia gradually increases and becomes intense over a longer time. The chronic (or persistent) pain of arthritis illustrates the usefulness of determining the relationship between time and intensity because people with arthritis usually report that pain is worse in the morning.

Location

The location of pain is best determined by having the patient point to the area of the body involved. Some general assessment forms include drawings of human figures, on which the patient is asked to shade in the area involved. This is especially helpful if the pain radiates (**referred pain**). The shaded figures are helpful in determining the effectiveness of treatment or change in the location of pain over time.

Pearls for Practice

Patients with irritation of a visceral organ frequently complain of pain that is referred—that is, pain is sensed not at that site but a distance away. A factor associated with this finding is that structures develop from the same embryonic segment or dermatome. Thus, since the heart and the arm have the same segmental origin, chest pain may be referred to the arm, and since the testicle migrated from where the kidney and ureter also developed, ureter distension may cause testicular pain. In addition, irritation under the diaphragm may be referred to the shoulder. Common sites of pain referral assist the clinician in considering sources for the patient's complaints. See Figure 6-2.

Quality

The nurse asks the patient to describe the pain without offering clues. For example, the nurse asks the patient to describe what the pain feels like. The nurse must give the patient sufficient time to describe the pain and then record all words in the answer. If the patient cannot describe the quality of the pain, the nurse can suggest words such as burning, aching, throbbing, or stabbing. It is important to document the exact words used by the patient to describe the pain and which words were suggested by the nurse conducting the assessment.

Personal Meaning

Pain means different things to different people; as a result, patients experience pain differently. The meaning of the pain experience helps the clinician understand how the patient is affected and assists in planning treatment. It is important to ask how the pain impacts the person's daily life. Some people with pain can continue to work or study, whereas others may be disabled by their pain, which may affect family finances. For some patients, the recurrence of pain may mean worsening of disease, such as the spread of cancer.

Aggravating and Alleviating Factors

The nurse asks the patient what, if anything, makes the pain worse, what makes it feel better, and asks specifically about the relationship between activity and pain. This helps detect factors associated with pain. For example, in a patient with advanced metastatic cancer, pain with coughing may signal spinal cord compression. The nurse also ascertains whether environmental factors influence pain because they may be modified more easily than other factors. For example, making the room warmer may aid in patient relaxation, which

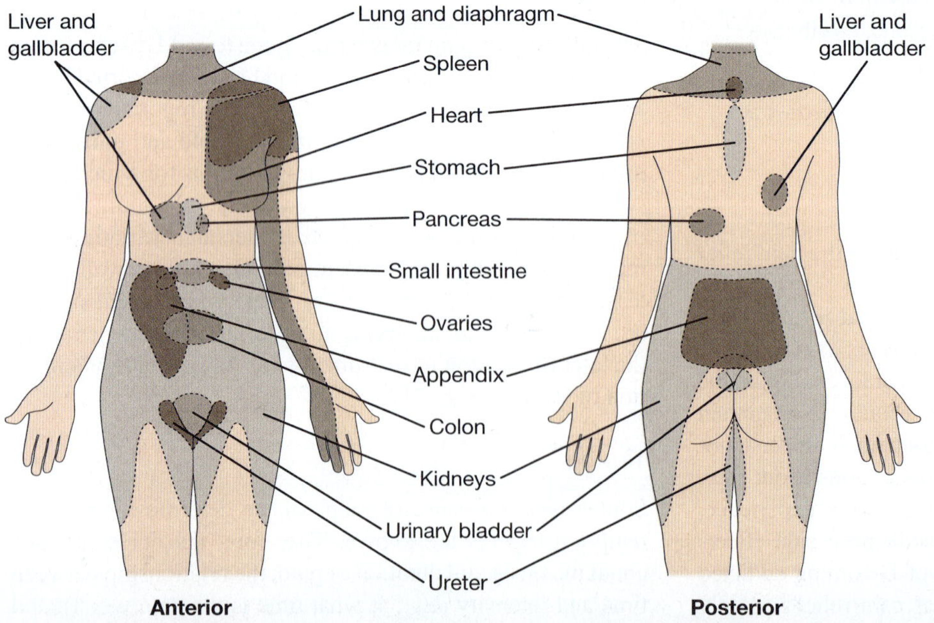

FIGURE 6-2 **Referred pain. Certain visceral organs can refer pain to specific cutaneous areas. If all special tests are negative yet the individual continues to feel pain at a specific site, it may be referred pain. (From Anderson, M. K. (2012). *Foundations of athletic training: Prevention, assessment, and management* (5th ed.). Wolters Kluwer Health.)**

may decrease the person's pain. Finally, the nurse asks the patient whether the pain is influenced by or affects the quality of sleep or anxiety. Both can significantly influence pain intensity and the quality of life.

Knowledge of alleviating factors assists the nurse in developing a treatment plan. Therefore, it is important to ask about the patient's use of medications (prescribed and over-the-counter [OTC]), including amount and frequency. In addition, the nurse asks if herbal remedies, nonpharmacologic interventions, or alternative therapies have been used with success. This information assists the nurse in determining teaching needs.

Pain Behaviors

When experiencing pain, people express pain through many different behaviors. Nonverbal and behavioral expressions of pain can be useful indicators of the quality or intensity of pain. A patient may grimace, cry, rub the affected area, guard the affected area, or immobilize it. Others may moan, groan, grunt, or sigh. Not all patients exhibit the same behaviors, and different meanings may be associated with the same behavior.

Sometimes, in nonverbal patients, pain behaviors are used as a proxy to assess pain. It is unwise to make judgments and formulate treatment plans based on behaviors that may or may not indicate pain. In unconscious patients, pain should be assumed to be present and treated. All patients have a right to adequate pain management.

Physiologic responses to acute pain, such as tachycardia, hypertension, tachypnea, pallor, diaphoresis, mydriasis (pupillary dilatation), hypervigilance, and increased muscle tone, are related to stimulation of the autonomic nervous system. These responses are short-lived as the body adapts to the stress. These physiologic signs could be the result of a change in the patient's condition, such as the onset of hypovolemia. Use of physiologic signs to indicate pain is unreliable. Although it is important to observe for any and all pain behaviors, the absence of these behaviors does not indicate an absence of pain.

Instruments for Assessing the Perception of Pain

Only the patient can describe and assess the individual pain experience accurately. Therefore, a number of pain assessment tools have been developed to assist in the assessment of the patient's perception of pain. Such tools may be used to document the need for intervention, to evaluate the effectiveness of the intervention, and to identify the need for alternative or additional interventions if the initial intervention is ineffective in relieving the pain. For a pain assessment tool to be useful, it must require little effort on the part of the patient, be easy to understand and use, be easily scored, and be sensitive to small changes in the characteristic being measured. Figure 6-3 shows a pain assessment pathway that can be used at the time of assessment to direct clinical decisions for pain management.

Pearls for Practice

The Numeric Pain Scale is the most commonly used scale when a patient is able to self-report. The scale is based on a 0 to 10 numeric rating with 0 being "no pain" and 10 being "the worst pain imaginable." Pain scores represent an important component of pain management. However, other assessments can provide objective information on a patient's pain, such as consideration of functional ability, psychological and emotional states, satisfaction ratings with their current treatment, and inquiring about any adverse treatment effects.

Visual Analog Scales

Visual analog scales (VAS) are useful in assessing the intensity of pain (Fig. 6-4). One version of the scale includes a horizontal 10-cm line, with anchors (ends) indicating the extremes of pain. The patient is asked to place a mark indicating where the current pain lies on the line. The left anchor usually represents "none" or "no pain," whereas the right anchor usually represents "severe" or "worst possible pain." To score the results, a ruler is placed along the line, and the distance the patient marked from the left or low end is measured and reported in millimeters or centimeters.

Some patients (e.g., children, older adults, patients with visual or cognitive impairment) may find it difficult to use an unmarked VAS. In those circumstances, ordinal scales, such as a simple descriptive pain intensity scale or a 0 to 10 numeric pain intensity scale, may be used.

Faces Pain Scale—Revised

The Wong–Baker Faces pain scale uses six facial expressions that range from content to obvious distress (Fig. 6-5). The patient is asked to point to the face that most closely resembles the experienced pain intensity. It is used for individuals 3 years of age and older and is not limited to children.

Guidelines for Using Pain Assessment Scales

Using a written scale to assess pain may not be possible if a person is seriously ill, is in severe pain, or has just returned from surgery. In these cases, the nurse can ask the patient, "On a scale of 0 to 10, 0 being no pain and 10 being the worse pain that you can ever imagine, how bad is your pain?" For patients who have difficulty with a 0 to 10 scale, a 0 to 5 scale may be tried. Whichever scale is used, it should be used consistently. Most patients usually can respond without difficulty. Ideally, the nurse teaches the patient how to use the pain scale before the pain occurs (e.g., before surgery). The nurse can integrate function into the pain scale and explain "pain that is a 5 or 6" is pain that can interrupt focus or concentration. This means the patient has difficulty

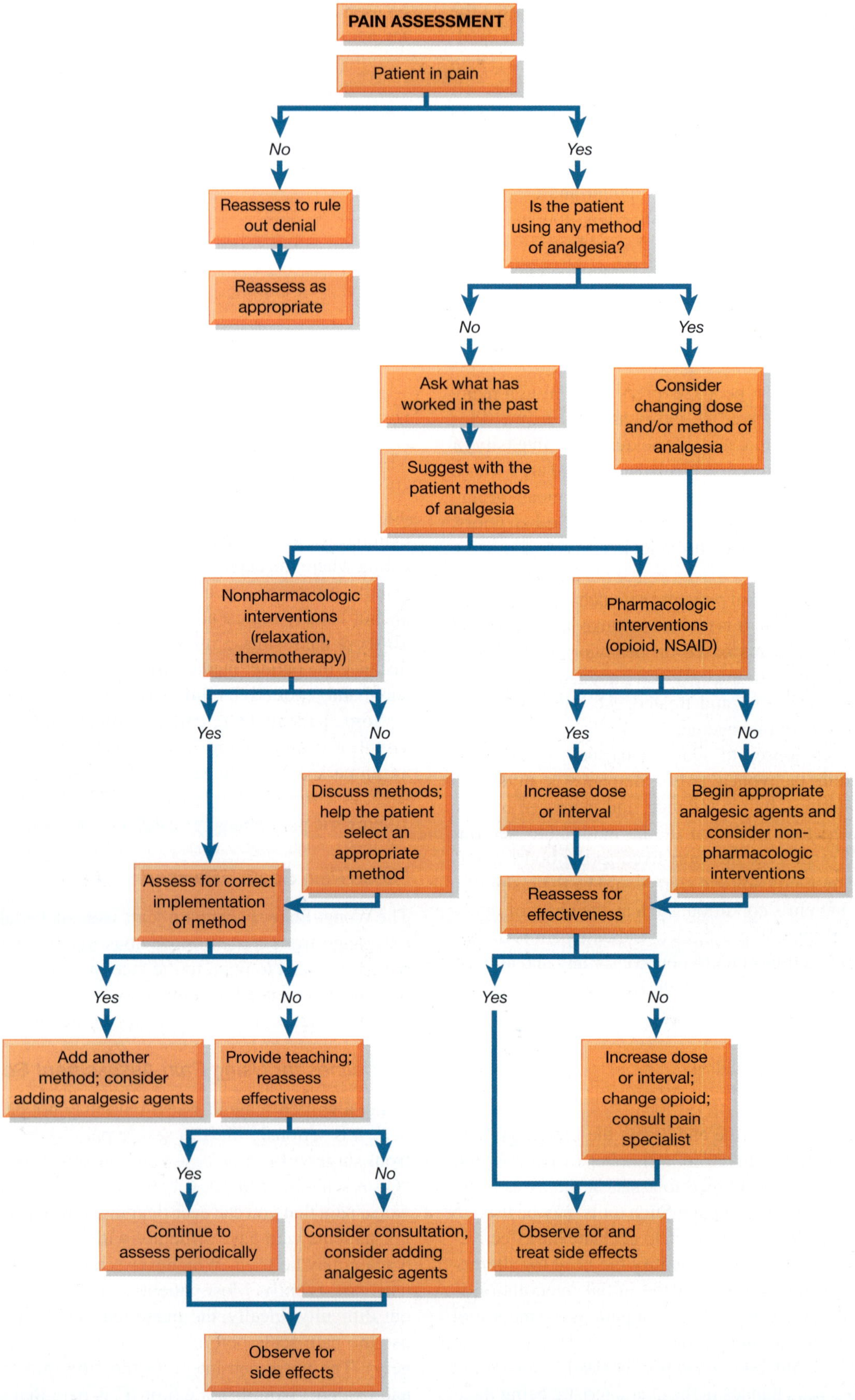

FIGURE 6-3 **Pain assessment pathway.**

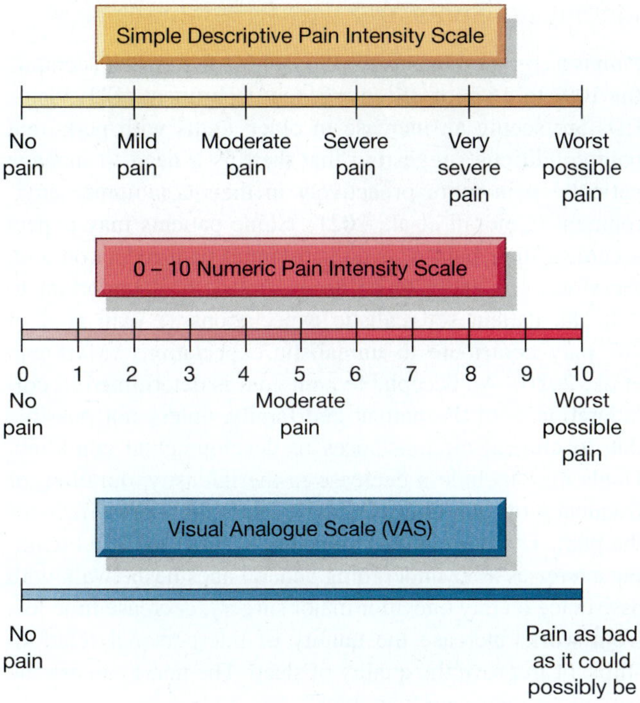

FIGURE 6-4 **Examples of pain intensity scales.**

reading a book or watching TV because the pain can be disruptive intermittently. Pain that is higher than "7 or 8" may cause the patient to think or focus only on pain. A "pain that is a 9 or 10" can mean the patient cannot even think clearly or do anything because the pain is the worst pain imaginable. The patient's numerical rating is documented and used to assess the effectiveness of pain relief interventions.

If a particular patient does not speak English or cannot clearly communicate information needed to manage pain, an interpreter/translator and/or caregivers familiar with the person's method of communication should be consulted and a method established for pain assessment. Often, a chart can be constructed with English words on one side and the patient's language on the other. Then the patient can point to the corresponding word to tell the nurse about the pain.

When people with pain are cared for at home by family caregivers or home care nurses, a pain scale may help assess the effectiveness of the interventions if the scale is used before and after the interventions are implemented. Scales that address the location and pattern of pain may be useful in identifying new sources or sites of pain in patients who are chronically or terminally ill and in monitoring changes in the patient's level of pain. For example, a home care nurse who sees a patient only at intervals may benefit from consulting the patient's or family's written record of pain scores to evaluate how effective the pain management strategies have been over time.

Guidelines for Assessing Pain in Patients With Disabilities

Alternative forms of communication may be necessary for people with sensory impairments or other disabilities.

- For people who are blind and who know how to read Braille, pain assessment instruments can be obtained in Braille. In addition, computer software is available that allows written documents to be scanned and converted into Braille. If these programs are not available, agencies that provide services for people who are blind may be able to assist in developing Braille versions.
- For people who are deaf or hard of hearing, outside interpreters (i.e., not family members) should be used. Other

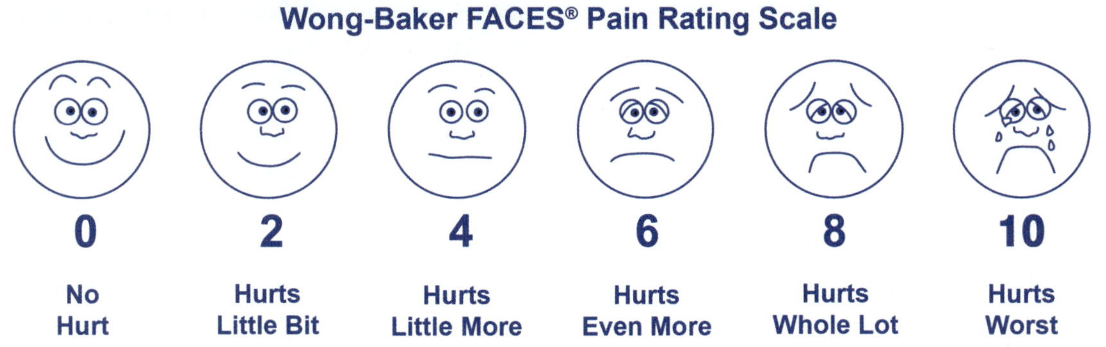

FIGURE 6-5 **Wong-Baker FACES Pain Rating Scale. This pain scale is especially suited for helping children describe pain. Instructions for using this scale follow: "These faces show how much something can hurt. This face (*point to left-most face*) shows *no pain.* The faces show more and more pain (*point to each from left to right*) up to this one (*point to right-most face*). It shows *very much pain.* Point to the face that shows how much you hurt (right now)." Score the chosen face 0, 2, 4, 6, 8, or 10, counting left to right, so 0 = no pain and 10 = very much pain. Do not use words like "happy" or "sad." This scale is intended to measure how children feel inside, not how their face looks. (Wong-Baker FACES Foundation (2020). Wong-Baker FACES® Pain Rating Scale. Retrieved September 9, 2022, from http://www.WongBakerFACES.org, with permission. Originally published in *Whaley & Wong's Nursing Care of Infants and Children*. © Elsevier Inc.)**

useful communication strategies may include sign language, written notes, or pictures. When writing notes on a "magic slate" or making written notes, it is necessary to make every effort to guard the patient's privacy and confidentiality.
- For people with disabilities that result in communication impairment, computer-generated speech may be useful.

Pearls for Practice

For people with cognitive impairment, a triangulated approach may be useful, which includes self-report, caregiver report, and direct observation. For acute pain, behaviors that are suggestive of pain may include sympathetic nerve stimulation (increased heart rate, dilated pupils, diaphoresis, hypertension), grimacing, frowning, changes in sleep patterns and nutritional intake, vocalizations (noisy respirations, moaning), changes in mental status (confusion, irritability), guarding, bracing, and behavioral changes (aggressive, disruptive, social withdrawal) (Resnick et al., 2021). The nurse is aware that chronic pain is usually not associated with autonomic activation that causes the vital sign changes noted above. The PAINADD (pain assessment in advanced dementia) is a behavioral pain assessment tool used in adults with moderate to severe dementia and in nonverbal adults. It is a five-item tool used by the nurse to observe patient's breathing, negative vocalization, facial expression, body language, and consolability. Each item is scored on a 0 to 2 range, with a maximum score of 10 indicating severe pain (Natavio et al., 2020).

THE NURSE'S ROLE IN PAIN MANAGEMENT

The nurse helps relieve pain by administering pain-relieving interventions (including both pharmacologic and nonpharmacologic approaches), assessing the effectiveness of those interventions, monitoring for adverse effects, and serving as an advocate for the patient when the prescribed intervention is ineffective in relieving pain. It is important to assess the patient's medical history and family history for response to analgesics (e.g., codeine). For example, the metabolism of codeine differs because of individual genetic variations in drug-metabolizing enzymes. Thus, some patients are poor metabolizers of codeine with no pain relief from administration and others who are ultra-rapid metabolizers are at risk for toxicity (Magarbeh et al., 2021). When assessing a patient's lack of response to codeine, or untoward response, it may be appropriate to consider a genetic cause and obtain a prescription for a different opioid. In addition, the nurse provides education to the patient and family to enable them to manage the prescribed intervention themselves when appropriate.

Identifying Goals for Pain Management

Pain is a common reason most people seek care and accounts for 10% to 15% of all emergency department (ED) visits. EDs are seeing an increase in older adults with persistent pain conditions suggesting that there is a need to manage patients' pain more proactively in their community environment (Colorafi et al., 2021). Some patients may expect a cure of their pain or even substantial pain reduction and, therefore, are likely to be disappointed. It is important to help the patient set realistic expectations. A pain goal of "0" may contribute to unrealistic expectations (Markman et al., 2020). An acceptable pain goal is determined in collaboration with the patient and family, unless not possible due to clinical circumstances or developmental condition. Goals may include a decrease in the intensity, duration, or frequency of pain and a decrease in the negative effects of the pain. Therefore, goals might be to perform deep breathing exercises after undergoing general anesthesia, walk with assistance on day one after major surgery, decrease time lost from work, increase the quality of interpersonal relationships, or improve the quality of sleep. The nurse can ask the patient "is your pain tolerable?"

To determine the goal, a number of factors are considered. The first factor is the severity of the pain as judged by the patient. A patient with chronic pain may report the pain at 8 out of 10 on a daily basis; the patient may want the pain to be more tolerable and strive for a comfort score of 5 out of 10. Each patient is different in what that comfort score may be; therefore, this assessment is important to tailor each treatment plan accordingly. The second factor is the anticipated harmful effects of pain. Patients with other serious health issues are at much greater risk for harmful effects of pain than are young, healthy patients (e.g., older patients with unrelieved pain who have contributing comorbidities and are on chronic pain-relieving medications may be at higher risk for falls). The third factor is the anticipated duration of the pain. In patients with pain from a disease such as cancer, the pain may be prolonged, possibly for the remainder of the patient's life. Therefore, interventions will be needed for some time and should not detract from the patient's quality of life. In the acute stages of illness, the patient may be unable to participate actively in relief measures, but when the patient has sufficient mental and physical energy, the patient may learn self-management techniques to relieve the pain. Therefore, as the patient progresses through the stages of recovery, increased patient use of self-management of pain relief measures may be a goal.

Patients who receive palliative care for pain when they are conscious should continue to receive pain treatment when they cannot communicate. It should be assumed that the pain persists even if the patient is unconscious. Family members often can be taught what unique behaviors to look for to assess for pain: a furrowed brow, stiffening of a part of the body, or moaning (refer to Chapter 2 for more details on palliative care). The goals for pain treatment include not simply pain reduction but also improved functional ability, sleep, psychological well-being, and social interaction.

Providing Patient Education

Patient education is extremely important since the patient or family or close relationships may be responsible for managing the pain at home and preventing or managing side effects. Teaching about pain and strategies to relieve it may reduce the threat of the pain and, thus, the pain itself, in the absence of other relief measures and may enhance the effectiveness of the pain relief measures used.

The nurse also provides information by explaining how pain can be controlled. For example, the patient should be informed that pain should be reported in the early stages. When the patient waits too long to report pain, **sensitization** may occur, and the pain may become so intense that it is difficult to relieve. Sensitization results from a heightened nervous system response after exposure to a noxious (pain) stimulus. This results in an increased and prolonged pain experience. When health care providers assess and treat pain before it becomes severe, sensitization is diminished or avoided, and less medication is needed.

Providing Physical Care

Patients in pain may be unable to participate in the usual activities of daily living or to perform usual self-care and may need assistance to carry out these activities. Usually patients are more comfortable when physical and self-care needs have been met and efforts have been made to ensure the patient is in as comfortable a position as possible. A fresh gown and change of bed linens, along with efforts to make the person feel refreshed (e.g., brushing teeth, combing hair), often increase the level of comfort and improve the effectiveness of the pain relief measures.

In acute, long-term, and home settings, the nurse who provides physical care to patients also has the opportunity to perform complete assessments and to identify problems that may contribute to the patient's discomfort and pain. Appropriate and gentle physical touch during care may be reassuring and comforting. If transdermal treatments such as fentanyl (an opioid analgesic) patches or intravenous (IV) or epidural catheters are used, the skin around the patch or catheter should be assessed for integrity during physical care.

Managing Anxiety Related to Pain

Anxiety may affect the patient's response to pain. A patient who anticipates pain may become increasingly anxious. Anticipatory guidance about the nature of the impending painful experience and the ways to reduce pain often decreases anxiety. Pain relief measures should be used *before* pain becomes severe. It is important to explain to all patients that pain relief or control is more successful if such measures begin before the pain becomes unbearable. Administering medications early before an expected painful procedure or activity will lessen pain more effectively and allow the patient to meet goals of care. A patient who experiences nausea after pain medication may feel compelled to pass on subsequent pain medication dosing, causing anxiety and pain to build. Premedicating with antiemetics or changing to a different pain medication is recommended to mitigate the side effects of the pain medications. The nurse is aware that, often, people who experience pain use previously learned strategies; therefore, it is important to teach the patient about measures to relieve pain. This nursing action may lessen the threat of pain and give the patient a sense of control. The patient's anxiety may be reduced by explanations that point out the degree of pain relief that can be expected from each measure. For example, a patient who is informed that an intervention may not eliminate pain completely is less likely to become anxious when a certain amount of pain persists. A positive nurse–patient relationship characterized by trust is essential. Acknowledging to the patient, "I know that you have pain," often has positive impact on the patient's psychological state. Occasionally, patients who fear that no one believes their pain feel relieved to know that the nurse believes that the pain exists.

A patient who is anxious about pain may be less tolerant of the pain, which, in turn, may increase anxiety levels. To prevent the pain and anxiety from escalating, the anxiety-producing cycle must be interrupted. An anxiety disorder that is not under control will have an effect on the patient's pain perception. Pain intensity is heightened, and the response to pain may cause more undue stress.

PAIN MANAGEMENT STRATEGIES

Reducing the patient's pain to a "tolerable or comfortable" level with minimal side effects is considered the goal of pain management. Looking further, even patients who have described pain relief as adequate often report disturbed sleep and marked distress because of pain. In view of the harmful effects of pain and inadequate pain management, the goal of the nurse is to relieve pain. Pain management strategies include both pharmacologic and nonpharmacologic approaches. These approaches are selected on the basis of the requirements and goals of particular patients.

Pearls for Practice

Analgesic medications are appropriate when patients are in pain. These agents are not considered a last resort to be used only when other pain relief measures fail. Any intervention is most successful if it is initiated before pain sensitization occurs, and usually, the greatest success is achieved if several interventions are applied simultaneously. Nonpharmacologic interventions include efforts to create a quiet environment, comfort measures (e.g., backrub, change of position, use of heat or cold compresses), use of relaxation exercises (e.g., focused breathing, visualization, guided imagery), and diversional or distraction activities (Andrew-Cooper & Kozachik, 2019).

Pharmacologic Interventions

Pharmacologic management of pain is accomplished in collaboration and communication with health care providers, patients, and, often, families. A physician, nurse practitioner, or physician assistant prescribes specific multimodal medications for pain. The nurse may insert an IV line for administration of analgesic medications. Alternatively, an anesthesiologist or nurse anesthetist may insert an epidural catheter for administration of such analgesic agents. However, it is the nurse who maintains the analgesia, assesses its effectiveness, and reports whether the intervention is ineffective or produces side effects.

There are two general categories of analgesic agents: opioids and nonopioids. These agents work by different mechanisms on the pain pathways. Nonopioid agents have analgesic, antipyretic, and anti-inflammatory actions which help relieve pain. Examples may include NSAIDs, acetaminophen, and corticosteroids. For chronic pain, antidepressant and antiseizure medications, local anesthetics, topical agents, baclofen, and N-methyl-D-aspartate (NMDA) receptor antagonists also may be used.

Opioid Analgesic Agents

The goal of administering opioids is to relieve pain and improve quality of life; therefore, the route of administration, dose, and frequency of administration are determined on an individual basis. Factors that are considered in determining the route, dose, and frequency of medication include the characteristics of the pain (e.g., its expected duration and severity), the overall status of the patient (e.g., NPO [nil per os, or nothing by mouth] status), the patient's response to analgesic medications, and the patient's report of pain. Opioids can be administered by various routes—oral, IV, subcutaneous (SC), intraspinal, intranasal, buccal mucosa, rectal, and transdermal. Although the oral route is usually preferred for opioid administration, oral opioids must be given frequently enough to be effective. Opioid analgesic agents given orally may provide a more consistent serum level than those given intravenously.

Pearls for Practice

The nurse recognizes that the route of administration determines response time to the medication. IV medications are the most direct route, and responses are expected in the shortest time frame. The nurse also recognizes that when intramuscular (IM) or SC routes are selected, there will be variable responses depending on blood flow to the extremity.

If the patient is expected to require opioid analgesic agents at home, the clinician should consider the ability of the patient and family to administer opioids as prescribed at the planning stages and should take steps to ensure that the required medications will be available to the patient. Many pharmacies, especially those in smaller rural areas or inner cities, may be reluctant to stock large amounts of opioids. Therefore, arrangements must be made ahead of time for obtaining these prescription medications.

Side Effects

With the administration of opioids by any route, side effects must be considered and anticipated. Clinicians who take steps to minimize the side effects increase the likelihood that the patient will receive adequate pain relief without interrupting therapy to treat the effects.

Respiratory Depression and Sedation. Respiratory depression is the most serious adverse effect of opioid analgesic agents administered orally, intravenously, subcutaneously, intrathecally (delivered between the tissue in the spinal canal), or by an epidural (outside the dura mater layer) route. The risk of respiratory depression increases with age and with the concomitant use of other opioids or other CNS depressants.

A patient who receives opioids by any route must be assessed frequently for changes in respiratory status (see Box 6-6). Specific notable changes are shallow respirations, decreasing respiratory rate, hypercarbia (increased carbon dioxide in blood), and decreasing oxygen saturation. Sedation is one of the first signs of impending respiratory depression and may occur with any route of administration.

The nurse is aware that when opioid doses are increased, or concomitant administration of sedating medications occurs, the risk of respiratory depression increases. There is strong evidence that opioid-induced respiratory depression is highest within the first 24 hours postoperatively (Jungquist et al., 2020). Patients often develop tolerance so that, in time, they are no longer sedated by the dose that had caused sedation initially. Increasing the time between doses or reducing the dose temporarily, as prescribed, usually prevents deep sedation from occurring. The institution of a continuous pulse oximetry and/or end tidal CO_2 monitoring may be initiated by the nurse for closer monitoring for patients at risk for respiratory depression. Patients at risk for sedation (e.g., individuals with obesity, older individuals, individuals who smoke, and patients with impaired renal or hepatic function) must be monitored closely for changes in respiratory status. Patients are also at risk for problems associated with sedation and immobility. The nurse must initiate strategies to prevent problems, such as skin breakdown. All patients receiving opioids should be screened for sedation prior to and after administration of the opioid using the Pasero Opioid-Induced Sedation Scale (POSS) (Box 6-4).

Nausea and Vomiting. Nausea and vomiting frequently occur with opioid use. Usually, these effects can occur immediately

BOX 6-4

Pasero Opioid-Induced Sedation Scale (POSS)

S = Sleep, easy to arouse
Acceptable; no action necessary; may increase opioid dose if needed

1 = Awake and alert
Acceptable; no action necessary; may increase opioid dose if needed

2 = Slightly drowsy, easily aroused
Acceptable; no action necessary; may increase opioid dose if needed

3 = Frequently drowsy, arousable, drifts off to sleep during conversation
Unacceptable; monitor respiratory status and sedation level closely until sedation level is stable at less than 3 and respiratory status is satisfactory; decrease opioid dose 25% to 50% or notify prescriber or anesthesiologist for orders; consider administering a nonsedating, opioid-sparing nonopioid, such as acetaminophen or an NSAID, if not contraindicated.

4 = Somnolent, minimal or no response to verbal and physical stimulation
Unacceptable; stop opioid; consider administering naloxone; notify prescriber or anesthesiologist; monitor respiratory status and sedation level closely until sedation level is stable at less than 3 and respiratory status is satisfactory.

or hours after initial administration. Patients, especially postoperative patients, may not think to tell the nurse that they are nauseated, particularly if the nausea is mild. However, a patient receiving opioids should be assessed for nausea and vomiting, which may be triggered by a position change and may be prevented by having the patient change positions slowly. Adequate hydration and the administration of antiemetic agents may also decrease the incidence of nausea. Opioid-induced nausea and vomiting often subside within a few days. Patients may be sensitive to a particular opioid and may benefit from decreasing the dose, switching to a different opioid, and the addition of a nonopioid pain medication.

Constipation. Constipation, a common side effect of opioid use, can occur in patients after surgery and in patients receiving opioids. Preventing constipation must be a high priority in all patients receiving opioids, and an effective bowel program is needed. Whenever a patient receives opioids, a bowel regimen should begin at the same time. Tolerance to this side effect does not occur; rather, constipation persists even with long-term use of opioids.

Several strategies may help prevent and treat opioid-related constipation. Mild laxatives and a high intake of fluid and fiber may be effective in managing mild constipation. Unless contraindicated, a mild laxative and a stool softener should be administered on a regular schedule. However, continued severe constipation often requires the use of a stimulating cathartic agent, such as senna derivatives or bisacodyl. Additional laxatives used include suppositories, enemas, and lactulose, along with diet modification and increased intake of fluid and fiber (Saha et al., 2020). If appropriate, a moderate amount of physical activity (30 to 60 min/day) has demonstrated improvement in the consistency of stools (Mesía et al., 2020).

The Oncology Nursing Society (ONS) Guidelines panel suggests treatment with a peripherally acting mu-opioid receptor antagonist (PAMORA) (i.e., methylnaltrexone, alvimopan, naloxegol, and naldemedine) in addition to the existing bowel regimen (LeFebvre et al., 2020). PAMORAs are effective in countering the gastric peristaltic effects of morphine without a significant affecting central analgesia (Daniali et al., 2020). Of note, the PAMORA alvimopan is approved for the treatment or prevention of postoperative ileus since research reveals improved GI recovery after surgery and reduced length of hospital stay (Chamie et al., 2021).

Pruritus and Urinary Retention. When asked about drug allergies, patients with previous hospital experience (especially for surgery) may report that they are "allergic" to morphine. This report should be investigated thoroughly. Commonly, this allergy is described as itching only. Pruritus (itching) is a frequent side effect of opioids administered by any route, but it is not an allergic reaction. It can be relieved by administering prescribed antihistamines. It is important to assess patients for drowsiness when antihistamines are administered. Epidural (discussed later in this chapter) or continuous IV administration of opioids also may cause urinary retention. The patient should be monitored and may require urinary catheterization. A weight-based low-dose naloxone infusion may be prescribed to relieve problems of nausea, vomiting, itching, urinary retention, and ileus in patients who are receiving continuous opioids for the relief of acute postoperative pain.

Endocrine Deficiencies. The nurse understands that chronic use of opioids is associated with decreased testosterone levels, leading to hypogonadism, sexual dysfunction, infertility, and accelerated osteoporosis (exact mechanism for osteopenia and osteoporosis is not known). Opioid-induced hypogonadism is treatable with appropriate hormone replacement therapy. Screening should be considered for osteoporosis for patients on chronic opioid medication. Refer to Chapter 40 for details on osteoporosis.

Inadequate Pain Relief

One factor commonly associated with ineffective pain relief is an inadequate dose of opioids. This is most likely to occur when the caregiver underestimates the patient's pain or fails to consider differences in absorption and action after a change in the route of administration. Consequently, the patient receives doses that are too small to be effective and, possibly, too infrequent to relieve pain. For example, if opioid delivery is changed from the IV route to the oral route, the oral dose must be approximately three times greater than that given parenterally to provide relief. Because of differences in absorption of orally administered opioids among individuals, patients must be assessed carefully to ensure that the pain is relieved.

Table 6-2 lists opioids and dosages that are equivalent to morphine; Table 6-3 is an equianalgesic table that

TABLE **6-2 Selected Opioid Analgesic Agents Commonly Used for Moderate and Severe Pain in Adults**

	Starting Dose (milligrams)			
Name	**Moderate Pain**	**Severe Pain**	**Comments**	**Precautions and Contraindications**
Morphine	—	30–60 (oral) 10 (parenteral)	Binds to opioid receptors in the CNS to produce analgesia, euphoria, and sedation. May be administered orally, parenterally, epidural and intrathecal.	Use with caution, especially in older patients, very ill patients, and those with respiratory impairment. Major risks include respiratory depression, apnea, circulatory depression, respiratory arrest, shock, and cardiac arrest. Obtain history of hypersensitivity to opioids. Monitor patient closely. If prescribed in correct dose, oral preparations are effective in treating moderate and severe pain. Care should be exercised in using morphine in patients with renal insufficiency, due to accumulation of morphine metabolites.
Codeine	15–30 (oral)	60 (oral) up to 360/24 hrs	Binds to opioid receptors in the CNS to produce analgesia, euphoria, and sedation. Is also an antitussive. 10% of people lack the enzyme needed to make codeine active and therefore may not achieve adequate analgesia. Ultra-rapid metabolizers have an enzyme that converts codeine to morphine at a more rapid rate and may reach toxicity levels faster than the general population. Codeine may cause more nausea and constipation per unit of analgesia than other mu-agonist opioids.	Many preparations of codeine and the other opioids in this table are combinations with nonopioid analgesics. Caution must be used in patients with impaired ventilation, bronchial asthma, increased intracranial pressure, or impaired liver and renal function and in older and very ill patients. Due to potential for breathing difficulties, misuse and addiction, the Food and Drug Administration (FDA) recommends against the use of codeine or combination products for children under 18 years of age.
Oxycodone (OxyContin™)	5 (oral)	10–20 (oral)	Binds to specific opioid receptors in the CNS to produce analgesia, euphoria, and sedation	Caution must be used in patients with impaired ventilation, bronchial asthma, increased intracranial pressure, or impaired liver function and in older and very ill patients.
Hydrocodone (Vicodin™)	5–10 (oral)	—	—	Most preparations are combined with nonopioid analgesics. Adjustment of dosage is needed in patients with renal and liver disease
Tramadol (Ultram™)	50–100 (oral)	—	Binds to opioid receptors and inhibits reuptake of norepinephrine and serotin.	Most common side effects are dizziness, nausea, constipation, and somnolence. Lowers seizure threshold.

CNS, central nervous system; MAO, monoamine oxidase.

Adapted from Nursing Drug Handbook 2022.

TABLE **6-3 Approximate Dose Equivalents for Opioid Analgesics**[a]

Drug	Oral Dose (mg)	Parenteral Dose[b]
Morphine[c]	30	10 mg
Codeine[d]	200	100–120 mg
Fentanyl[e,f]	NA	100 μg or 0.1 mg
Hydrocodone (Vicodin)	30–45	NA
Hydromorphone (Dilaudid)[c]	7.5	1.5 mg
Levorphanol	4	1 mg
Methadone[g,h]	The conversion ratio of methadone is variable. Please refer to specific conversion tables based upon single-opioid or multiple-opioid regimens.	
Oxycodone (OxyContin)[d]	20	Only available orally (tablet and liquid), not available parenterally
Oxymorphone (Opana, Opana ER, and OpanaIV[c])	10	1 mg
Buprenorphine	NA	0.4 mg

IV, IV; NA, not available.

[a]Published tables vary in the suggested doses that are equianalgesic to morphine. Many of these doses are based on clinical consensus rather than well-controlled trials. Clinical response is the criterion that must be applied for each patient; titration to clinical response is necessary. Because there is not complete cross-tolerance among these drugs, usually it is necessary to use a lower-than-equianalgesic dose when changing drugs and reiterate according to response.

[b]Parenteral dosing includes IV and subcutaneous administration. Onset and duration may vary slightly between these routes; however, doses remain approximately equal. The intramuscular route is not recommended because of variability in uptake of the drug and painful injection.

[c]Caution: For morphine, hydromorphone, and oxymorphone, rectal administration is an alternate route for patients unable to take oral medications. Equianalgesic doses may differ from oral to parenteral doses because of pharmacokinetic differences. Note: A short-acting opioid normally should be used for initial therapy of moderate to severe pain.

[d]Caution: Doses of aspirin and acetaminophen in combination opioid/NSAID preparations must be adjusted to the patient's body weight.

[e]Transdermal fentanyl is an alternative. Transdermal fentanyl dosage is not calculated as equianalgesic to a single morphine dosage but is calculated based on a 24-hour opioid dose. See package insert for dosing calculations. Transdermal fentanyl should not be used in opioid-naïve patients.

[f]Transmucosal and buccal fentanyl are also available and indicated for breakthrough pain, although they are not bioequivalent. Titration of either should be conducted gradually; neither should be used in opioid-naïve patients.

[g]Caution: Methadone is much more potent than indicated in older published literature.

Potency varies and is not linear—it is noted to be between two and ten times as potent as morphine—depending on opiate history. When morphine at lower doses (e.g., 30–60 mg/day orally) is switched to methadone, the potency may be three to five times; when switched from high doses (e.g., more than 300 mg/day orally), the potency may be 12 times or even higher.

[h]Caution: The oral-to-IV dose ratio of methadone is not well established. The IV route is used very seldom except in cancer centers with a pain service that is familiar with parenteral methadone. IV use of methadone is associated with QTc wave prolongation.

providers may use when changing routes of administration (e.g., from IV to oral medications in preparation for patient discharge). These tables serve only as a guide; the doses listed are not necessarily the most appropriate doses for all patients. However, the tables do give clinicians some idea of equivalency.

After administering the first dose of an opioid, the nurse should perform a complete pain assessment to determine the efficacy of that dose. The time, date, patient's pain rating (scale of 0 to 10), analgesic agent, other pain relief measures, side effects, and patient activity are recorded. If the pain has not decreased in 30 minutes (sooner if an IV route is used) and the patient is reasonably alert and has a satisfactory respiratory status, blood pressure, and pulse rate, then some change in analgesia is indicated. In general, calculate the equianalgesic dose of the new opioid, and then reduce the dose by 50% to avoid potential cross-tolerance (Bhatnagar & Pruskowski, 2022).

Cross-tolerance is a phenomenon that occurs when a patient who is tolerant to the effects of a certain pharmaceutical agent also develops a tolerance to another agent. From here, the dose can be adjusted to each individual response. Although extended-release agents come in the same dosage form and contain the same drug, they are not considered therapeutically equivalent because they use different release mechanisms. Patients who need to change brands should be monitored carefully both for overdose and for inadequate pain relief.

Because of the fear of promoting addiction or causing respiratory depression, health care providers tend to prescribe and administer inadequate dosages of opioid agents to treat acute pain or persistent pain, particularly in patients who are terminally ill. Long-term use of opioids can lead to dependence and a substance use disorder (SUD) (Umberger & Gaggis, 2020). In the past decade, there has been a dramatic increase in opioid prescriptions, which is associated with increased opioid misuse, overdose, and accidental deaths. Currently, there is a general agreement that opioids are overprescribed and that education regarding management of acute and chronic pain by health care providers is inadequate yet essential. Efforts must be made to educate future health care professionals to treat patients in pain and mitigate risk of overdose, opioid misuse, opioid use disorder (OUD), and related deaths (Aronowitz et al., 2021).

Genetic factors play a role in the varied patient responses to NSAIDs and opioids. The most **extensively** studied genetic variation related to pain in humans is in the metabolism of codeine. Drug metabolism involves genetically controlled enzyme activity for absorption, distribution, inactivation, and excretion. In studies of both experimental and clinical pain, multiple polymorphisms (DNA proteins with variant alleles) result both in poor metabolism and poor analgesic efficacy, leading to changes in drug absorption, distribution, and elimination (Hindmarsh et al., 2021). Currently, there is no practical lab test for evaluating genetic variations of drug metabolism; thus, the nurse collaborates with the pain specialist and pharmacist for a multidisciplinary approach to pain management to ensure optimal patient safety and outcomes.

Pearls for Practice

Conversion tables available for the transdermal systems should be used only to establish the initial dose of the transdermal fentanyl or buprenorphine when patients switch from oral morphine to the transdermal route of delivery (and not vice versa). If these tables are used inappropriately to determine the dosages of oral morphine for patients who have been receiving transdermal fentanyl or buprenorphine, many patients will not achieve satisfactory analgesia and will require an increase in their opioid dose to treat breakthrough pain.

Pearls for Practice

If the conversion table or equation is used incorrectly to calculate a morphine dose, there is a risk of overdose. If a patient requires a change from transdermal fentanyl or buprenorphine back to oral or IV morphine (as in the case of surgery), the patch should be removed and IV morphine administered on an as-needed basis. Before a new patch is applied, the patient should be checked carefully for any older, forgotten patches, which should be removed and discarded. Patches should be replaced every 72 hours.

Opioid Use With Selected Conditions and Medications

A number of factors may influence the safety and effectiveness of opioid administration. Opioid analgesic agents are primarily metabolized by the liver and excreted by the kidney. Therefore, metabolism and excretion of analgesic medications are impaired in patients with liver or kidney disease, increasing the risk of cumulative or toxic effects.

Patients with untreated hypothyroidism are more susceptible to the analgesic effects and side effects of opioids. In contrast, patients with hyperthyroidism may require larger doses for pain relief. Patients with a decreased respiratory reserve from disease or aging may be more susceptible to the depressant effects of opioids and must be monitored carefully for respiratory depression.

Patients who are dehydrated are at increased risk for the hypotensive effects of opioids. Patients who become hypotensive after the administration of an opioid should be kept recumbent and rehydrated unless fluids are contraindicated. Patients who are dehydrated also are more likely to experience nausea and vomiting with opioid use. Rehydration usually relieves these symptoms.

Patients receiving certain other medications, such as monoamine oxidase (MAO) inhibitors, phenothiazines, or tricyclic antidepressants, may have an exaggerated response to the depressant effects of opioids. Patients taking these medications should receive small doses of opioids and must be monitored closely. Continued pain in these patients indicates that a therapeutic level of the analgesic has not been achieved. Patients must be monitored for sedation even if an analgesic effect has not been obtained.

Tolerance and Addiction

There is no maximum safe dosage of opioids, nor is there any easily identifiable therapeutic serum level. Both the maximal safe dosage and the therapeutic serum level are relative and individual.

Tolerance (the need for increasing doses of opioids to achieve the same therapeutic effect) develops in almost all patients taking opioids for extended periods. Patients requiring opioids over a long term, especially cancer patients, need increasing dosages to relieve pain, although after the first few weeks of therapy, the progressively increasing dosages may no longer be required and the patient can be placed on maintenance dosages. Patients who become tolerant to the analgesic effects of large doses of morphine may obtain pain relief by changing to a different opioid. Symptoms of physical dependence may occur when the opioids are discontinued; dependence often occurs with opioid tolerance and does not indicate a SUD. It is an expected physiologic response that will occur in all people exposed to continuous opioid administration (Umberger & Gaddis, 2020).

Pearls for Practice

Although patients may need increasing levels of opioids, they are not developing a SUD. Physical tolerance usually occurs with increasing dosages. Tolerance to opioids is common and becomes a problem primarily in terms of delivering or administering the medication.

SUD is a DSM5 diagnosis that occurs when an individual who uses substances experiences loss of control, continued use despite negative consequences, and physiologic manifestations. The terms "addict," "drug abuser," or "user" perpetuate stigma and bias among health care providers toward patients and should be avoided. Fear that patients will develop OUD has contributed to inadequate treatment of pain. This fear is commonly expressed by health care providers as well as patients and results from lack of knowledge about the risk. In addition, providers may misinterpret the sole findings of tolerance and withdrawal, which are known effects of opioids, as an SUD. Current research suggests that patients with a history of other substance use are at higher risk for OUD (St. Marie & Broglio, 2019). Health care providers should be discouraged from withholding opioid analgesics for patients in acute pain because of concerns about SUD. Providers should adopt a multimodal approach to pain management in all patients (St. Marie & Broglio, 2019). Medications to treat OUD include methadone, which in the outpatient setting can only be dispensed in federally regulated opioid treatment programs, buprenorphine, and naltrexone.

Currently, over 19.3 million adults in the United States are dealing with OUD; thus, it is likely that nurses in acute care will encounter patients with a history of SUD seeking care for acute or chronic pain (Kaye et al., 2020). Nurses should consider that each individual person has the right to be treated for pain. Opioid-tolerant patients are defined as patients using >60 mg equivalent dose of morphine per 24 hours. The use of multimodal analgesia is a treatment strategy in opioid-tolerant patients. Opioid-sparing techniques include the use of NSAIDs, acetaminophen, gabapentin, duloxetine, regional blocks, and local infiltration of anesthetics (Kaye et al., 2020). If prescribed, the opioids should be tapered slowly to prevent withdrawal symptoms; the use of a mutually agreeable pain contract should be considered. The use of complementary therapies is suggested and is described later in the chapter.

Pearls for Practice

Patients admitted to the hospital suffering from an acute illness who have a history of substance use and are currently on methadone maintenance treatment (MMT) should have their methadone dose continued or an equivalent opioid given to prevent craving. Also, the patient's methadone treatment facility should be consulted. Additional opioids can be prescribed on an as-needed basis if indicated while applying the same monitoring guidelines for potential opioid-induced side effects. Patients may also be taking sublingual buprenorphine for the treatment of both pain and OUD. This drug may be continued in the perioperative and postoperative period, utilizing services of a multidisciplinary team (Li et al., 2020).

Pearls for Practice

Patients may be monitored during opioid therapy with urine toxicology studies. They should be informed to avoid eating poppy seeds, which can make a urine drug screen (UDS) positive for opiates, depending on where the threshold for opioid screening is set.

NSAIDs

NSAIDs are thought to decrease pain by inhibiting cyclooxygenase (COX), the enzyme involved in the production of prostaglandin (which is believed to increase the sensitivity of pain receptors) from traumatized or inflamed tissues. There are two types of COX: COX-1 and COX-2.

COX-1 mediates prostaglandin formation involved in the maintenance of physiologic functions, such as platelet aggregation, which prevents ischemia and promotes mucosal integrity. Inhibition of COX-1 may result in gastric ulceration, bleeding, and kidney damage.

COX-2 mediates prostaglandin formation that results in symptoms of pain, inflammation, and fever. Therefore, inhibition of COX-2 is desirable. Celecoxib is an example of a COX-2 inhibitor. There is evidence of increased cardiovascular risk associated with COX-2 inhibitors. Ibuprofen, another NSAID, blocks both COX-1 and COX-2. It is effective in relieving mild to moderate pain and has a low incidence of adverse effects. Aspirin, the oldest NSAID, also blocks COX-1 as well as COX-2; however, because it causes frequent and severe side effects, aspirin is used infrequently to treat significant acute or persistent pain.

NSAIDs are very helpful in treating arthritic diseases and may be especially powerful in treating cancer-related bone pain. They have been combined effectively with opioids to treat pain and decrease the incidence of opioid-related adverse effects. A regimen of a fixed-dose, time-contingent NSAID (e.g., every 6 hours) and a separately administered fluctuating dose of opioid may be effective in managing moderate to severe cancer pain. In more severe pain, the opioid dose is also fixed, with an additional fluctuating dose as needed for **breakthrough pain** (a sudden increase in pain despite the administration of pain-relieving medications). Most patients tolerate NSAIDs well. However, those with impaired kidney function may require a smaller dose and must be monitored closely for side effects. Patients taking

NSAIDs may bruise easily because these drugs inhibit platelet aggregation. Furthermore, NSAIDs may displace other medications, such as warfarin, from serum proteins and increase their effects. Thus, high doses or prolonged use can irritate the stomach and, in some cases, result in gastric ulcers and GI bleeding as well. For this reason, the use of NSAIDs is dependent on the individual patient's risk factors. If administered, monitoring for GI bleeding is indicated, and gastroprotective agents should be considered to prevent this complication (Sherman et al., 2020).

Drug Alert

Cardiovascular risks of NSAIDs: NSAIDs, especially COX-2 inhibitors, should be avoided or used with caution in patients with a cardiac history. The use of COX-2 inhibitors may decrease prostacyclin levels, which may lead to increased thrombotic risk (Sherman et al., 2020). In addition, NSAIDs may exacerbate hypertension and heart failure as well as impair kidney function.

Local Anesthetic Agents

Local anesthetics work by blocking nerve conduction when applied directly to the nerve fibers. They can be applied directly to the site of injury (e.g., a topical anesthetic spray for sunburn) or directly to nerve fibers by injection or at the time of surgery. Also, they can be administered through an epidural catheter (see later discussion of Intraspinal and Epidural Administration).

Local anesthetic agents have been successful in reducing the pain associated with thoracic, abdominal, and upper and lower extremity surgical procedures. Local anesthetics may be injected by the surgeon during the procedure or by the anesthesiologist preoperatively as a peripheral nerve blockade. Local anesthetic agents are rapidly absorbed into the bloodstream, resulting in decreased availability at the surgical or injury site and an increased anesthetic level in the blood, increasing the risk of toxicity.

A topical anesthetic agent known as *eutectic mixture* (emulsion of local anesthetics), or EMLA cream, has been effective in preventing the pain associated with invasive procedures, such as lumbar puncture or the insertion of IV lines. To be effective, EMLA must be applied to the site 60 minutes before the procedure.

A lidocaine 5% patch acts locally by targeting damaged nerves responsible for discharging pain impulses and is approved for limited use. The lidocaine 5% patch provides sufficient medication for anesthetic effect but not enough to cause total sensory block in the area of application, so it has a wide margin of safety. The recommended dose is one to three patches at a time applied over the affected area for 12 hours daily.

Topical NSAIDs also have been beneficial in randomized controlled studies for patients with rheumatologic disorders and have demonstrated comparable efficacy for regional pain conditions but with fewer adverse effects than systemic NSAIDs (Cohen & Raja, 2016; Thorfinnson et al., 2021).

Antidepressant and Antiseizure Medications

Pain of neurologic origin (e.g., causalgia [intense burning pain and sensitivity to the slightest vibration or touch]), tumor impingement on a nerve, postherpetic neuralgia) is difficult to treat and, in general, is not responsive to opioid therapy. If these pain syndromes are accompanied by dysesthesia (burning or cutting pain), then they may be responsive to serotonin–norepinephrine reuptake inhibitors (SNRIs), tricyclic antidepressants, or neuropathic agents. Duloxetine is prescribed for pain resulting from diabetic neuropathy, fibromyalgia, and chronic musculoskeletal pain. When indicated, tricyclic antidepressant agents, such as amitriptyline or imipramine, are prescribed in doses considerably smaller than those generally used for depression. Since antidepressants have the FDA warnings of worsening mood and suicidal ideations, patients should be informed about side effects before beginning this treatment (Thour & Marwaha, 2022). Patients also need to know that a therapeutic effect may not occur until they have taken the medication for 4 weeks.

Another class of drugs, gabapentinoids were originally developed as anticonvulsant agents. Pregabalin and gabapentin are recommended for neuropathic pain. The Neuropathic Pain Interest Group of the IASP recommends pregablin as the drug of choice for neuropathic pain. Nurses should be aware that the most common side effects of pregabalin are somnolence and dizziness. Initial therapy is begun at a low dose with careful titration to achieve therapeutic response and minimize side effects (Freynhagen et al., 2021).

Antiseizure medications, such as phenytoin or carbamazepine, may be used in doses lower than those prescribed for seizure disorders. They may be beneficial in patients with neuropathic pain who do not respond to antidepressants; however, they also have the FDA warnings of mood changes, worsening depression, and suicidal ideation, predominantly in adolescents and young adults (Bailly & Belaid, 2021). Because a variety of medications can be tried, nurses should be familiar with the possible side effects of each and should teach patients and families how to recognize these effects.

Approaches to Using Analgesic Agents

The nurse obtains the patient's medication history (e.g., current, usual, or recent use of prescription or OTC medications or herbal agents), along with a history of health disorders and allergies. Certain medications or conditions may affect the analgesic medication's effectiveness or its metabolism and excretion. Before administering analgesic agents, the nurse should assess the patient's pain status, including the intensity of current pain, changes in pain intensity after the previous dose of medication, and side effects of the medication. Medications are most effective when the dose and interval between doses are individualized to meet the needs of a particular patient.

Balanced Analgesia

Pharmacologic interventions are most effective when a multimodal, or balanced, analgesia approach is used. Multimodal analgesia combines two or more analgesic agents or techniques that act by different mechanisms to provide analgesia with better pain relief and less opioid side effects. Using two or three types of agents simultaneously can maximize pain relief while minimizing the potentially toxic effects of any one agent (Sherman et al., 2020). When one agent is used alone, it usually must be used in a higher dose to be effective.

Treating Cancer Pain

Different kinds of pain are treated with different medications. Multimodal analgesia is the use of opioids, nonopioid analgesics, and adjuvant agents together to maximize the efficacy and minimize side effects from one analgesic (mainly opioids).

The World Health Organization (WHO) introduced a three-step analgesic ladder approach to pain management in 1986. Since its adoption, there has been an increased awareness of opioid misuse contributing to the current opioid epidemic. A fourth step has been adopted by interventional pain specialists for management of chronic noncancer pain (Fig. 6-6). Analgesics are administered based on the patient's level of pain and functional ability.

In step one, nonopioid analgesics (e.g., acetaminophen and NSAIDs) are used for mild pain; step two recommends weak opioid analgesics (e.g., codeine, tramadol) for moderate pain. As pain increases in severity, step three suggests the use of strong opioid analgesics (e.g., morphine, hydromorphone, oxycodone, fentanyl, etc.) for severe pain. Also, adjuvant medications are administered to enhance the effectiveness of analgesics. Examples of adjuvant medications include antidepressants, antiseizure agents, antispasmodics, local anesthetics, radiopharmaceuticals (radioactive agents that may be used to treat painful bone tumors), and corticosteroids. Step four is utilized by interventional pain specialists with a wide variety of techniques including peripheral nerve blocks, epidurals, spinal cord stimulators, and neurolytic blocks. Nurses should be aware that these modalities may decrease the potential side effects of excessive opioid exposure such as sedation and cognitive decline (Yang et al., 2020). Currently, according to Yang et al. (2020) and current literature, the integrative medicine therapies can be adopted to each step for decreasing or eliminating the use of analgesics in the chronic noncancer pain management. These interventions are utilized for disorders such as degenerative, musculoskeletal, and neuropathic disorders.

Preventing and reducing pain help to decrease anxiety and break the pain cycle. This can be accomplished best by administering analgesics on a regularly scheduled basis as prescribed (the preventive, preferred approach to pain management), with additional analgesics administered for breakthrough pain as needed and as prescribed (Yang et al., 2020).

Preventive Approach

With the preventive approach, analgesic agents are administered at set intervals so that the medication acts before

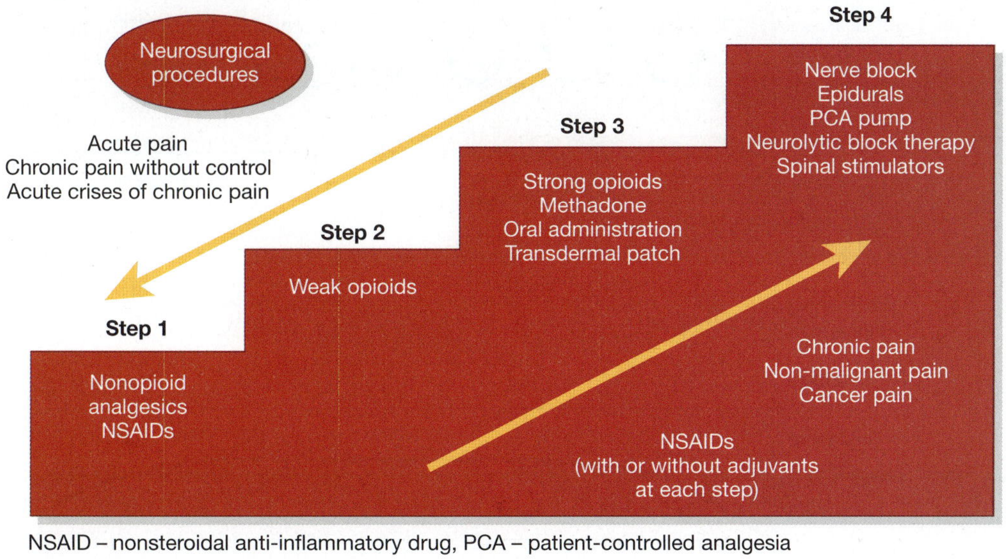

FIGURE 6-6 Adaptation of the analgesia ladder using the World Health Organization (WHO) model. It integrates a fourth step that includes neurosurgical procedures such as spinal cord stimulators and invasive techniques such as nerve blocks NSAID—nonsteroidal anti-inflammatory drug, PCA—patient-controlled analgesia. (Reprinted with permission from Vargas-Schaffer, G. [2010]. Is the WHO analgesic ladder still valid? *Can Fam Physician*, *56*[6], 514–517; originally adapted from World Health Organization. Traitement de la douleur cancéreuse. Geneva, Switzerland: World Health Organization, 1987.)

the pain becomes severe and before the serum opioid level decreases to a subtherapeutic level. For example, a patient takes prescribed morphine or a prescribed NSAID every 4 to 6 hours rather than waiting until the pain is severe. If the pain is likely to occur around the clock or for a substantial portion of a 24-hour period, a regular around-the-clock schedule of administering analgesia may be indicated. Even if the analgesic is prescribed *pro re nata* (PRN), or "as needed," it can be administered on a preventive basis before the patient is in severe pain as long as the prescribed interval between doses is observed. The preventive approach reduces the peaks and troughs in the serum level and provides more pain relief with fewer adverse effects.

Smaller doses of medication are needed with the preventive approach because the pain does not escalate to a level of severe intensity. Therefore, a preventive approach may result in the administration of less medication over a 24-hour period, helping prevent tolerance to analgesic agents and decreasing the severity of side effects (e.g., sedation, constipation). Better pain control can be achieved with a preventive approach, reducing the amount of time patients are in pain.

In using the preventive approach, the nurse assesses the patient for sedation before administering the next dose. It is not safe to medicate the patient with opioids repeatedly if the patient is sedated or not in pain. Appropriate pain and sedation scales approved for use by the institution should be utilized.

Individualized Dosage

The dosage and the interval between doses should be based on the patient's requirements rather than on an inflexible standard or routine. As noted earlier, metabolism and absorption of medications are highly variable. Therefore, a certain dose of an opioid medication given at specified intervals may be effective for one patient but ineffective for another.

As in the preventive approach discussed above, the nurse does not wait for the patient to complain of pain and then administer analgesia. To receive pain relief from an opioid analgesic, the serum level of that opioid must be maintained at a minimum therapeutic level (Fig. 6-7). The lower the serum opioid level, the more difficult it is to achieve the therapeutic level with the next dose. If pain is reported to be continuous, then a long-acting or around-the-clock administration of an opioid needs to be considered.

Routes of Administration

The route selected for administration of an analgesic agent (Table 6-4) depends on the condition of the individual patient and the desired effect of the medication. Analgesic agents can be administered by parenteral, oral, rectal, transdermal (skin patch), transmucosal, intraspinal, or epidural routes. Each method of administration has advantages and disadvantages. The route chosen should be based on patient need. Box 6-5 discusses the safe use of transdermal fentanyl administration.

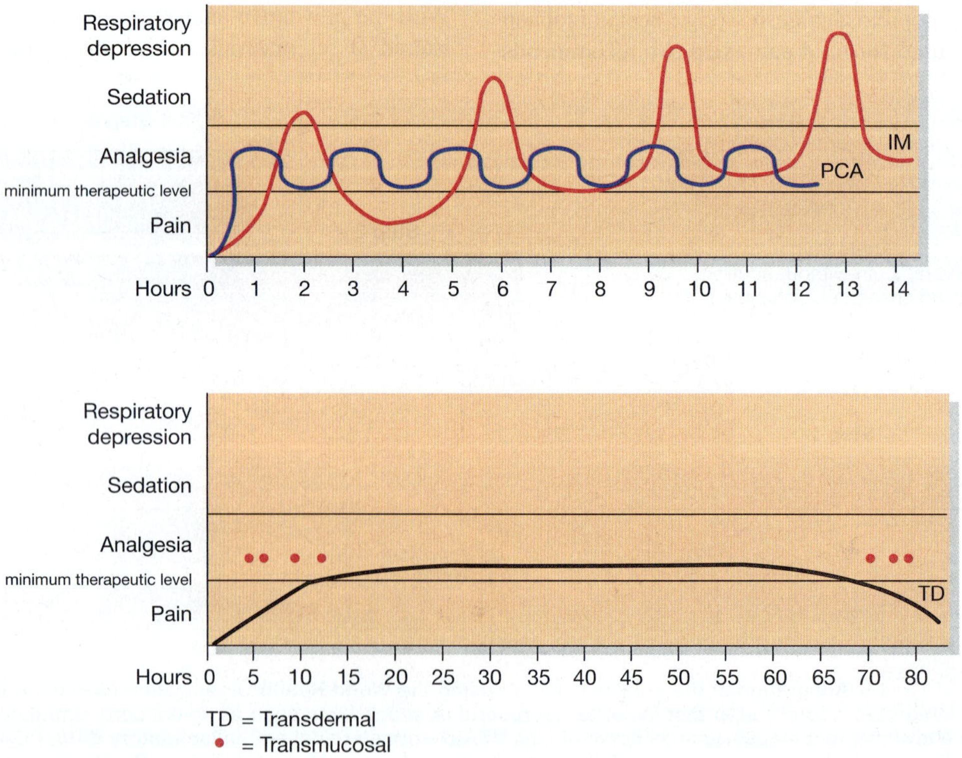

FIGURE 6-7 Relationship of mode of delivery of analgesia to serum analgesic level. *Top:* Intramuscular (IM) and IV patient-controlled analgesia (PCA). *Bottom:* Transdermal (TD) and transmucosal (•) delivery.

TABLE **6-4 Administration Routes for Analgesics**

Route	Patient Factors	Advantages	Disadvantages
IV	Can be used if patient has had nothing by mouth. Side effects are nausea, vomiting.	Rapid, reliable effect, helps make patient feel more comfortable; may be administered by push or slow push (e.g., over a 5- to 10-minute period); may be administered by continuous infusion with a pump. Continuous infusion provides a steady level of analgesia over 24-hour period.	Short duration; careful calculation of dosage needed. Possible respiratory depression.
Intramuscular	Can be used if patient has had nothing by mouth. Side effects are nausea, vomiting.	Limited to emergency setting where no IV access can be obtained or patient preference.	Slower entry into bloodstream; slow metabolism. Absorption depends on site selected and amount of body fat.
Subcutaneous	Use if patient is in severe pain or had limited IV sites. Use for home pain management.	Effective, convenient.	Limited to small volume that can be administered at one time into the subcutaneous tissue.
Oral	Preferred over parenteral administration if patient can take medication by mouth.	Easy, noninvasive, not painful. Severe pain can be relieved with oral opioids if dose is high enough. Gradual dose increase provides additional pain relief without producing respiratory depression or sedation.	Increased doses needed as the disease progresses; tolerance may develop to the medication. Change from parenteral to oral route requires equianalgesic dosing to avoid withdrawal reaction and recurrence of pain.
Rectal	Use if patient is unable to take medications by any other route. Side effects include bleeding problems.	Prolonged duration of action	Onset of action unclear; delayed absorption compared with other routes of administration.
Transdermal	Use for home pain management or hospice care in patients currently taking oral sustained-release opioid.	Consistent opioid serum level; slightly less constipation than oral opioids; less costly than parenteral route.	Delay in effect while the dermal layer is saturated. Increased absorption in febrile patients. Require short-acting opioids for breakthrough pain; more expensive than sustained-release opioids.
Transmucosal	Use in patients on sustained-release opioid who experience breakthrough pain.	Rapid onset of action in nasal sprays allows analgesia to be achieved within 5–10 minutes; significant decreases in pain intensity; high patient satisfaction.	This route promotes rapid absorption and high bioavailability as a result of a highly vascularized oral mucosa entering systemic circulation directly and bypassing the GI tract and first-pass effect in the liver.

Patient-Controlled Analgesia

Used to manage postoperative pain as well as persistent pain in hospitals or home settings, **patient-controlled analgesia** (PCA) allows patients to control the administration of their own medication within predetermined safety limits.

The PCA pump is a device that lets the patient self-administer a predetermined amount of medication safely (demand dose) with episodes of increased pain or painful activities.

The patient presses a button at a preset interval to deliver a dose. Patients are encouraged to press the button in anticipation of pain, for example, before getting out of bed following abdominal surgery. A PCA pump is electronically controlled by a timing device. To ensure safety, the prescriber will order time intervals for demand dosing and maximum dose limits. Routes of administration include IV, SC, epidural, or peripheral nerve.

BOX 6-5

Safe Use of Transdermal Fentanyl

In 2018, The Institute for Safe Medical Practices (ISMP) called for the elimination of prescribing fentanyl patches for opioid-naive patients and/or patients with acute pain. This recommendation was incorporated into the 2020 Best Practices for Hospitals.

- Patients should be cautioned that a sudden and possibly dangerous rise in the level of fentanyl in their blood can occur with use of alcohol or other medications that affect brain function, an increase in body temperature or exposure to heat, or use of other medicines that affect the metabolism of fentanyl.
- Patients should be informed about signs and symptoms of fentanyl overdose (i.e., shallow or difficult breathing; fatigue, extreme sleepiness, or sedation; inability to think, talk, or walk normally; and feeling faint, dizzy, or confused).

The PCA pump also can be programmed to deliver a constant, background infusion of medication (or basal rate) and still allow the patient to administer additional bolus doses as needed. The nurse also can administer clinician doses, which typically are higher doses than the demand dose. The timer can be programmed to prevent additional doses from being administered until a specified time period has elapsed (lock-out time) and until the first dose has had time to exert its maximal effect. Even if the patient pushes the button multiple times in rapid succession, no additional doses are released. If another dose is required at the end of the delay period, the button must be pushed again for the dose to be delivered. Patients who are controlling their own opioid administration usually become sedated and stop pushing the button before any significant respiratory depression occurs. Nevertheless, assessment of respiratory status remains a major nursing role.

Pain should be brought under control before a PCA is started with the use of IV pain medication. Then, after control is achieved, the pump is programmed to deliver small doses of medication at a time. If a patient with severe pain has a low serum level of opioid analgesic, it is difficult to regain control with the small doses available by pump. The patient is instructed not to wait until the pain is severe before pushing the button to obtain a bolus dose. Since the patient can maintain a near-constant level of medication, the periods of severe pain and sedation that occur with the traditional PRN regimen are avoided. If PCA is to be used in the patient's home, the patient and family are taught about the operation of the pump as well as about the side effects of the medication and strategies to manage them.

Pearls for Practice

Family members are cautioned not to push the button for a patient, especially if the patient is asleep, because this overrides some of the safety features of the PCA system.

Intrathecal and Epidural Administration

Infusion of opioids or local anesthetic agents into the intrathecal space or epidural space has been used for effective control of pain in postoperative patients and those with chronic pain unrelieved by other methods. A catheter is inserted into the epidural space at the thoracic or lumbar level for administration of opioid or anesthetic agents (Fig. 6-8). With intrathecal administration, medications infuse directly into the subarachnoid space and cerebrospinal fluid, which surrounds the spinal cord. With epidural administration, medication is deposited in the epidural space of the spinal canal and diffuses into the subarachnoid space. It is believed that pain relief from intrathecal administration of opioids is based on the existence of opioid receptors in the spinal cord.

A low concentration of a local anesthetic agent, often in combination with an opioid, can be administered continuously in low doses, intermittently on a schedule, or on demand as the patient requires it. Research studies have shown a reduction in pain scores in postlaparotomy patients on day 1 when local anesthetics are combined with opioids in the epidural infusion (Mariano, 2021). Epidural anesthesia provides an effective analgesic modality for labor. In addition, epidural analgesia for thoracic surgery provides

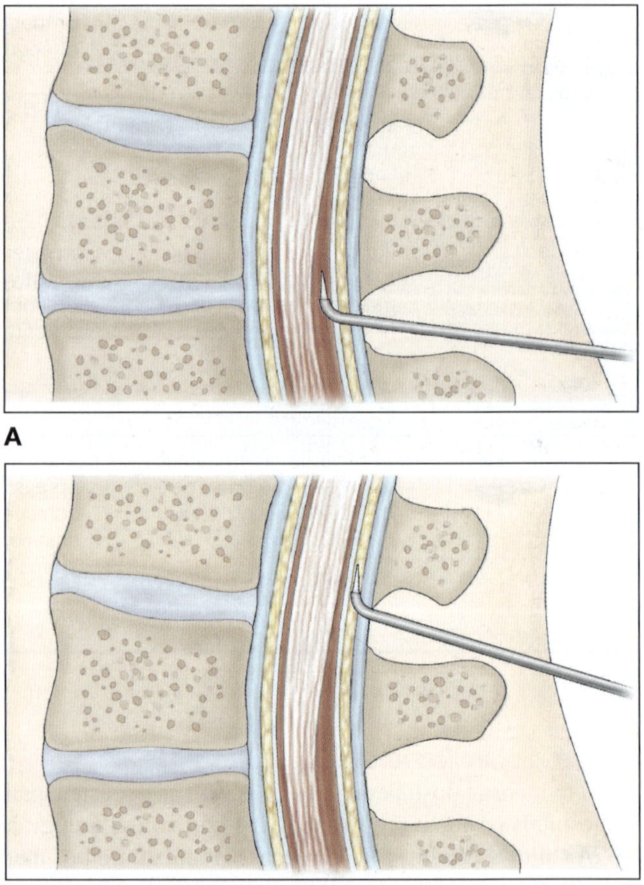

A

B

FIGURE 6-8 Placement of intraspinal catheters for administration of analgesic medications: (A) intrathecal route; (B) epidural route.

superior pain control, less sedation, and better pulmonary function than parenteral opiates (Razi et al., 2021).

For patients who have persistent, severe pain that fails to respond to other treatments or for those who obtain pain relief only with the risk of serious side effects, medication administered by a long-term intrathecal or epidural catheter may be effective.

Pearls for Practice

Epidural catheters inserted for pain control are usually managed by nurses. Baseline information necessary to provide safe and effective pain control includes the level or site of catheter insertion, the medications (e.g., local anesthetic agents, opioids) that have been administered, and the medications anticipated in the future. Sensory deficits can occur with the use of local anesthetics, and patients must be assessed frequently. An infusion with a lower concentration of local anesthetic allows for administration of a greater concentration of opioid with a lower risk of sensory deficits. The nurse should notify the provider for inadequate analgesia, sedation, motor and sensory deficits, back pain, headache, and temperature >101°F.

Adverse effects associated with intrathecal administration include postdural puncture headache resulting from loss of spinal fluid when the dura is punctured. The dura must be punctured with the intrathecal route, and dural puncture may occur inadvertently with the epidural route. If dural puncture occurs inadvertently, spinal fluid seeps out of the spinal canal.

Headache resulting from spinal fluid loss may be delayed. Therefore, the nurse needs to assess regularly for headache after either type of catheter is placed. If headache develops, the patient should remain flat in bed, consume large amounts of fluids (provided the medical condition allows), caffeinated drinks, and acetaminophen and/or NSAIDs, if there are no contraindications. An epidural blood patch may be performed to reduce leakage of spinal fluid (typically if the headache does not resolve) (Azzi et al., 2021). Refer to Chapter 42 for more details on spinal headaches.

Respiratory depression generally peaks 6 to 12 hours after epidural opioids are administered, but it can occur earlier or up to 24 hours after the first injection. It is important for the nurse to monitor the patient closely during the postoperative period with particular attention to sedation and oxygen saturation. Depending on the lipophilicity (affinity for body fat) of the opioid injected, the time frame for respiratory depression can be short or long. Morphine is hydrophilic (it has an affinity to water), and the time for peak effect is longer than that of fentanyl, which is lipophilic. The nurse must assess and record respiratory status and sedation levels using a sedation scale according to agency policy. The health care provider will need to be notified if the patient has a sedation scale of less than 3 on the Pasero Opioid-Induced Sedation Scale (POSS) (Junquist et al., 2020). The POSS evaluates the patient's level of consciousness since sedation precedes respiratory depression (Boxes 6-4 and 6-6 [research brief]). The patient should be easily aroused if slightly drowsy, and should be able to remain awake during conversation. Opioid antagonist agents such as naloxone must be available for IV use if respiratory depression occurs (see Box 6-7).

Cardiovascular effects (hypotension) may result from relaxation of the vasculature in the lower extremities. However, bradycardia may occur with placement of a high thoracic epidural affecting the cardiac accelerator nerves. Therefore, the nurse should assess frequently for decreases in blood pressure, pulse rate, and urine output.

Urinary retention and pruritus may develop, and the health care provider may prescribe IV infusion of low-dose naloxone to combat these effects. The nurse administers doses that are small enough to reverse the side effects of the opioids without reversing the analgesic effects. Diphenhydramine or low-dose IV infusion of naloxone also may be used to relieve opioid-related pruritus.

Precautions must be taken to avoid infection at the catheter site and catheter displacement. The epidural catheter insertion site should be inspected routinely for any signs of infection or drainage. Only medications without preservatives should be administered into the subarachnoid or epidural space because of the potential neurotoxic effects of preservatives.

BOX 6-6

Nursing Research

Bridging the Gap to Evidence-Based Practice

From Kaiser, J. (2020). Nurses' knowledge of opioids: Foundations for clinical practice. *Journal of Nursing Care Quality, 35*(4), 348–352.

ABSTRACT

Background: The opioid crisis has influenced practice changes to mitigate risks to patients receiving opioids. It is essential that nurses understand contemporary guidelines to provide safe patient care for patients receiving opioids.

Purpose: This study was designed to assess general knowledge of opioids among nurses in nonprescribing patient care roles.

Methods: A survey was developed, validated, and deployed to 564 nurses in a large hospital system.

Results: Nurses had strong knowledge of basic pharmacology, the conjunctive use of nonopioids for pain relief, and differences in analgesia for chronic versus acute pain. Opportunity for education included risk factors for opioid-related adverse events, medication combinations, differences in opioid-tolerant and opioid-naive patients, and recognition and management of overdose.

Conclusions: Results of this study can be used to guide continuing education and academic curricula to ensure nurses are equipped with the key knowledge to provide safe quality clinical care.

BOX 6-7

Opioid Analgesic Orders: General Considerations for the Nurse

A. Opioid analgesic orders or a hospital protocol should include the expectation that a nurse will hold the opioid dose if a patient is sedated excessively and notify the provider. The nurse documents the rationale for holding the dose, utilizing the POSS sedation scale. The nurse recognizes that a fall in oxygen saturation can represent a critical level of respiratory depression and the need for immediate intervention to prevent life-threatening hypoxemia.

B. In the event of oversedation or life-threatening respiratory depression, the hospital protocol should include that naloxone should be available for the nurse. In general, 0.1 to 0.4 mg of naloxone and 9 mL of normal saline are mixed in a syringe, and this dilute solution is administered very slowly (e.g., 1 mL or 0.04 mg over 1 minute) while observing the patient's response (titrate to effect). Patients should be monitored after being recovered with naloxone because the patient can fall back into unresponsiveness as the half-life of naloxone is only about 30 minutes before wearing off.

C. The nurse is aware that naloxone is administered incrementally in order to improve respiratory function but not reverse all analgesia, to avoid recurrence of severe pain.

D. When naloxone is administered in excessive doses, excitement, blood pressure lability, pulmonary edema, ventricular tachycardia and fibrillation, and seizures may be caused in postoperative patients (Jordan & Morrison-ponce, 2022).

Adapted from Pasero, C., Portenoy, R. K., & McCaffery, M. (1999). Opioid analgesics. In Pain: Clinical manual (2nd ed.). Mosby, p. 267; American Pain Society (APS). (2003). *Principles of analgesic use in the treatment of acute pain and chronic cancer pain* (5th ed.). American Pain Society.

Pearls for Practice

Patients managed with epidural catheters who are also receiving antithrombotic therapy are at an increased risk for the development of an epidural hematoma.

The nurse should be aware that symptoms of an epidural hematoma include back pain, sensory and motor dysfunction of the lower limbs, and bladder and bowel abnormalities (Vo et al., 2020). The American Society of Regional Anesthesia (ASRA) and Pain Medicine have evidence-based guidelines for regional and epidural anesthesia in patients receiving antithrombotic or thrombolytic therapy. These guidelines include timing of needle placement between last dose of anticoagulant and spinal injection or catheter placement, use of antithrombotic agents in patients with indwelling spinal or epidural catheters, and minimum time between catheter removal and next dose of anticoagulant. Timing of catheter insertion and removal is dependent upon prophylaxis or therapeutic prescribing of the antithrombotic therapy. The nurse is aware that reversal agents are available for some anticoagulants (e.g., vitamin K for warfarin, or protamine sulfate for heparin), but the only reversal for antiplatelet medications is that of a platelet transfusion.

Placebo Effect

A **placebo effect** occurs when a person responds to the medication or other treatment because of an expectation that the treatment will work rather than because it actually does so. The American Society for Pain Management Nurses contends that placebos (tablets or injections with no active ingredients) should not be used to assess or manage pain in any patient, regardless of age or diagnosis (Fernandez-Castro et al., 2021). Furthermore, the group recommends that all health care institutions have policies in place prohibiting the use of placebos for this purpose. Educational programs should be conducted to educate nurses and other health care providers about effective pain management, and ethics committees should assist in developing and disseminating these policies.

Nonpharmacologic Interventions

Analgesic medication is the most powerful tool for pain relief that is available, but it is not the only one. Nonpharmacologic nursing interventions can assist in pain relief, usually with low risk to the patient. Although such measures are not a substitute for medication, they may be all that is necessary or appropriate to relieve episodes of pain lasting only seconds or minutes. In instances of severe pain that lasts for hours or days, combining nonpharmacologic interventions with medications may be the most effective way to relieve pain.

Cutaneous Stimulation and Massage

Nurses can be proactive in providing pain relief options and comfort measures to improve daily function and mood levels among the older patients with chronic pain conditions as well as in pediatric settings during painful procedures such as in heel sticks or venipuncture. One holistic approach seen within complementary and alternative medicine (CAM) is massage therapy (MT). MT is a common nonpharmacologic pain multimodality and has been shown to be effective in acute and chronic conditions. The mechanism of action of MT with respect to pain is not well understood. Some of the theories suggest that MT may stimulate large nerve fibers that inhibit input from the smaller nerve fibers that act as pain receptors, therefore diminishing pain perception. MT may also release biochemical reactions seen in soft tissues (e.g., endorphins, serotonin) that can improve oxygenation and blood flow (Berstein & Karkhaneh, 2021). Some examples of MT include "*a patterned and purposeful soft-tissue manipulation accomplished by use of digits, hands, forearms, elbows, knees and/or without the use emollients, liniments, heat and cold, hand-held tools or external apparatus, for the intent of therapeutic change*" (Johnson & Booker, 2021).

Thermal Therapies

Ice and heat therapies may be effective pain relief strategies in some circumstances; however, their effectiveness and mechanisms of action need further study. Proponents believe that ice and heat stimulate the nonpain receptors in the same receptor field as the injury. Both ice and heat therapy must be applied carefully and monitored closely to avoid injuring the skin. Neither therapy should be applied to areas with impaired circulation or used in patients with impaired sensation.

For greatest effect, ice should be placed on the injury site immediately after injury or surgery. Ice therapy after joint surgery can significantly reduce the amount of analgesic medication required. Ice therapy also may relieve pain if applied later. Care must be taken to assess the skin before treatment and to protect the skin from direct application of the ice. Ice should be applied to an area for no longer than 15 to 20 minutes at a time and should be avoided in patients with compromised circulation (Moon et al., 2020). Prolonged applications of ice may result in frostbite or nerve injury. Application of heat increases blood flow to an area and may contribute to pain reduction and promote muscle relaxation. Both dry and moist heat may provide some analgesia, but their mechanisms of action are not well understood.

Pearls for Practice

Heat should not be applied to a painful area that is the site of acute, untreated infection (e.g., mastitis, tooth abscess) because it may cause increased pain with increased blood flow to the site.

Transcutaneous Electrical Nerve Stimulation

Transcutaneous electrical nerve stimulation (TENS) is a noninvasive treatment modality to promote analgesia in acute and chronic pain conditions. The device uses a battery-operated unit with electrodes applied to the skin to produce an electrical current such as a tingling, vibrating, or buzzing sensation in the area of pain. Research studies have demonstrated that TENS therapy is most beneficial in patients with greater hypersensitivity as seen with fibromyalgia conditions. A study sample of patients with fibromyalgia conditions showed a 30% decrease in pain and a 20% decrease in fatigue with TENS therapy (Vance & Zimmerman, 2021). The literature suggested that neuronal networks may activate descending inhibitory systems, resulting in a decrease in hyperalgesia through sensitized central pain mechanisms. This inhibitory mechanism affects pain perception to the brain. TENS units can be adjustable to low and high frequency and as well as in intensities. It is used as a "counter irritant" in targeting large A delta fibers which are activated by mechanical and thermal stimuli. This mechanism blocks the transmission of pain by releasing endogenous endorphins that provide pain relief via opioid receptors (Crumble, 2021).

Distraction

Distraction helps relieve both acute and chronic pain (Alsabri et al., 2021). Distraction, which involves focusing the patient's attention on something other than the pain, may be the mechanism responsible for other effective cognitive techniques. Distraction is thought to reduce the perception of pain by stimulating the descending control system, resulting in fewer painful stimuli being transmitted to the brain. The effectiveness of distraction depends on the patient's ability to receive and create sensory input other than pain. Distraction techniques may range from simple activities, such as watching television or listening to music, to highly complex physical and mental exercises. Pain relief generally increases in direct proportion to the patient's active participation, the number of sensory modalities used, and interest in the stimuli. Therefore, the stimulation of sight, sound, and touch is likely to be more effective in reducing pain than is the stimulation of only a single sense.

Visits from family and friends are effective in relieving pain. Watching an action-packed movie on a large screen with "surround sound" through headphones may be effective (provided the patient finds it acceptable). Others may benefit from games and activities (e.g., chess, crossword puzzles) that require concentration. Not all patients obtain pain relief with distraction, especially those in severe pain. Severe pain may prevent patients from concentrating well enough to participate in complex physical or mental activities.

Relaxation Techniques/Meditation

Skeletal muscle relaxation is believed to reduce pain by relaxing tense muscles that contribute to the pain. A simple relaxation technique consists of abdominal breathing at a slow, rhythmic rate. The patient may close both eyes and breathe slowly and comfortably. A constant rhythm can be maintained by counting silently and slowly with each inhalation ("in, two, three") and exhalation ("out, two, three"). When teaching this technique, the nurse may count out loud with the patient at first. Slow, rhythmic breathing may also be used as a distraction technique. Relaxation techniques, as well as other noninvasive pain relief measures, may require practice before the patient becomes skilled in using them. Patients who already know a relaxation technique may need to be reminded to use it to reduce or prevent increased pain. Almost all people with persistent pain can benefit from some method of relaxation. Meditation has demonstrated impact on lowering of blood pressure and heart rate, increased cerebral blood flow, and decreased levels of hormones associated with stress (Alsabri et al., 2021). Regular relaxation periods may help combat the fatigue and muscle tension that occur with and increase chronic pain.

Guided Imagery

Guided imagery is using one's imagination in a special way to achieve a specific positive effect. Guided imagery for relaxation and pain relief may consist of combining slow, rhythmic breathing with a mental image of relaxation and comfort. The nurse instructs the patient to close the eyes and breathe slowly in and out. With each slowly exhaled breath, the patient imagines muscle tension and discomfort being breathed out, carrying away pain and tension and leaving behind a relaxed and comfortable body. With each inhaled breath, the patient imagines healing energy flowing to the area of discomfort.

If guided imagery is to be effective, it requires a considerable amount of time to explain the technique and time for the patient to practice it. Usually, the patient is asked to practice guided imagery for approximately 5 minutes, three times per day. Several days of practice may be needed before the intensity of pain is reduced. Many patients begin to experience the relaxing effects of guided imagery the first time they try it. Pain relief can continue for hours after the imagery is used. Patients should be informed that guided imagery may work only for some people. Guided imagery should be used only in combination with all other forms of treatment that have demonstrated effectiveness.

Hypnosis

Hypnosis, which has been effective in relieving pain or decreasing the amount of analgesic agents required in patients with acute and chronic pain, may promote pain relief in particularly difficult situations (e.g., burns). The mechanism by which hypnosis acts is unclear. Its effectiveness depends on the hypnotic susceptibility of the individual (Alsabri et al., 2021). In some cases, hypnosis may be effective in the first session, with effectiveness increasing in additional sessions. In other cases, hypnosis does not work at all. Usually, hypnosis must be induced by specially skilled people (a psychologist or a nurse with specialized training in hypnosis). Some patients may learn to perform self-hypnosis.

Music Therapy

Music therapy is an inexpensive and effective therapy for the reduction of pain and anxiety in some patient populations. Research has shown that it reduces postoperative pain, fatigue, and anxiety (Bojorquez et al., 2020). Music therapy was also found to decrease pain in persons with chronic pain including fibromyalgia and chronic osteoarthritis (Brubaker et al., 2020). More research needs to be done to determine the mechanism by which music exerts its positive effect on pain relief.

Acupuncture

The insertion of the needles is intended to stimulate or improve the balance of the flow of "life energy" or *qi* (pronounced chi), whereas a blockage of flow or imbalance of *qi* is associated with patient complaints or disease. Although very different from a Western medical view of pathophysiology, acupuncture has been shown to have various physiologic effects on the body, including stimulation of endorphins (Huang et al., 2020). Research suggests that acupuncture may be beneficial for pain associated with fibromyalgia, headache, and chronic pain and has been used with varied conditions such as stroke, analgesia during childbirth, and infertility treatment. In addition, acupuncture is potentially effective in reducing postoperative nausea and vomiting and chemotherapy-induced nausea and vomiting (Huang et al., 2020).

Movement Therapy

Physical movement, such as yoga and tai chi, to restore balance to the body has gained popularity and had positive health benefits in patients with low back pain and back-related disabilities. In addition, often tai chi can be used by patients with a variety of conditions including chronic low back pain, connective tissue disorders, and hypertension (Huang et al., 2021).

Alternative Therapies

The National Institutes of Health has established the National Council for Complementary and Alternative Medicine (NCCAM) to examine the effectiveness of complementary and alternative therapies (CAM). The new field of integrative medicine allows for a combination of mainstream medicine and alternative therapies that enhance effectiveness and safety for patients seeking CAM therapies for pain and other disorders. The use of CAM has increased in the United States, and patients with cancer or rheumatologic conditions use CAM at a higher rate than the general population. Studies show the use of CAM in cancer patients was reported by 40% to 85% of patients (Ng & Sharma, 2020).

When caring for patients who are using or considering using untested therapies, it is imperative for the nurse not to diminish the patient's hope. This must be weighed against the nurse's responsibility to protect the patient from costly and potentially harmful and dangerous therapies that the patient is not in a position to evaluate scientifically. The nurse encourages the patient to assess the effectiveness of the therapy continually using standard pain assessment techniques. All use of alternative and complementary therapies needs to be discussed with the patient's health care provider.

Herbal Therapies

The use of herbal supplements is a popular therapy in the United States. In 2019, it is estimated that sale of dietary supplements exceeded 10 billion dollars. These products do not undergo the same scrutiny by the FDA as do conventional drugs. There are potential adverse effects of taking an herbal supplement along with an analgesic medication. For example, case reports show that taking ibuprofen and ginkgo increase the risk of bleeding. CAM therapies are used widely by patients receiving treatment for cancer. Nurses should have open nonjudgmental communication with their patients to inquire about the use of herbal therapies. Many sites are available on the Internet to assess for drug–herb interactions (Babos et al., 2021).

Neurologic and Neurosurgical Approaches to Pain Management

In some situations, especially with long-term and severe intractable pain, usual pharmacologic and nonpharmacologic methods of pain relief are ineffective. In those situations, neurologic and neurosurgical approaches to pain management may be considered. *Intractable pain* refers to pain that cannot be relieved satisfactorily by the usual approaches, including medications. Such pain often is the result of malignancy (especially of the cervix, bladder, prostate, and lower bowel), but it may occur in other conditions, such as postherpetic neuralgia, trigeminal neuralgia, spinal cord arachnoiditis, and uncontrollable ischemia and other forms of tissue destruction.

Neurologic and neurosurgical methods available for pain relief include (1) stimulation procedures (intermittent electrical stimulation of a tract or center to inhibit the transmission of pain impulses), (2) administration of intraspinal opioids (see previous discussion), and (3) interruption of the tracts conducting the pain impulse from the periphery to cerebral integration centers. Stimulation of nerves with minute amounts of electricity is used if other pharmacologic and nonpharmacologic treatments fail to provide adequate relief. These treatments are reversible. If they need to be discontinued, the nervous system continues to function. However, methods that involve interruption of the tracts are destructive or ablative procedures. They are used only after other methods of pain relief have failed because their effects are permanent.

Stimulation Procedures

Electrical stimulation, or neuromodulation, is a method of suppressing pain by applying controlled low-voltage electrical pulses to the different parts of the nervous system. Electrical stimulation is thought to relieve pain by blocking painful stimuli. This pain-modulating technique is administered by many modes. TENS (discussed earlier) and dorsal spinal cord stimulation are the most common types of electrical stimulation used. There are also brain-stimulating techniques in which electrodes are implanted in the periventricular area of the posterior third ventricle, allowing the patient to stimulate this area to produce analgesia.

Spinal cord stimulation is a technique used for the relief of persistent, intractable pain, ischemic pain, spinal stenosis pain, pain from angina, and other neuropathic pain syndromes. A surgically implanted device allows the patient to apply pulsed electrical stimulation to the dorsal aspect of the spinal cord to block pain impulses (the largest accumulation of afferent fibers is found in the dorsal column of the spinal cord) (Joosten and Franken, 2020). The dorsal column stimulation unit consists of a radiofrequency stimulation transmitter, a transmitter antenna, a radiofrequency receiver, and a stimulation electrode. The battery-powered transmitter and antenna are worn externally; the receiver and electrode are implanted. A laminectomy is performed above the highest level of pain input, and the electrode is placed in the epidural space over the posterior column of the spinal cord. The placement of the stimulating systems varies. An SC pocket is created over the clavicular area or at some other site for placement of the receiver. The two are connected through an SC tunnel. As implantable devices carry higher risks than conservative nonoperative approaches, this treatment is generally reserved for patients who have exhausted more conservative options (Joosten and Franken, 2020).

Deep brain stimulation is performed in patients with special pain problems if there is no response to the usual techniques of pain control. Under local anesthesia, electrodes are introduced through a burr hole in the skull and inserted into a selected site in the brain, depending on the location or type of pain. After the effectiveness of stimulation is confirmed, the implanted electrode is connected to a radiofrequency device or pulse-generator system operated by external telemetry. It is used in patients with neuropathic pain that may be caused by damage or injury from a stroke, chronic cluster headaches, brain or spinal cord injuries, or Parkinson disease.

Interruption of Pain Pathways

Pain-conducting fibers can be interrupted at any point from their origin to the cerebral cortex. In doing so, some part of the nervous system is destroyed, resulting in varying amounts of neurologic deficit and incapacity. For example, a radiofrequency ablation procedure of the dorsal root uses thermal energy to selectively destroy neurons located in the posterolateral spinal cord where sensory fibers enter into the spinal cord. Ablation procedures may be used in neuropathic pain, phantom limb pain, and traumatic brachial and lumbosacral plexus avulsion injuries.

Unfolding Patient Stories: S.C. • Part 1

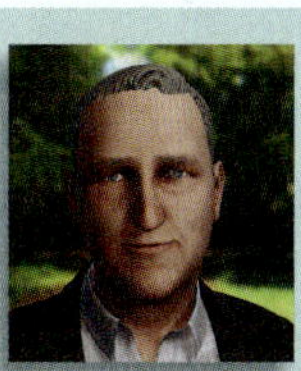

A 52-year-old patient arrives in the ED with severe abdominal pain. The provider has ordered buprenorphine 0.3 mg IV push for pain. Explain the assessments performed by the nurse prior to, during, and following the administration of the medication. Also, consider nonpharmacologic interventions the nurse can incorporate to assist with pain relief. (This story continues in Chapter 23.)

Care for patients in a realistic virtual environment: ***vSim** for Nursing* (thepoint.lww.com/vSimMedicalSurgical). Practice documenting these patients' care in DocuCare (thepoint.lww.com/DocuCareEHR).

BOX 6-8

Pearls for Assessing Response to Therapeutic Interventions

The nurse will:

- Obtain baseline pain and functional assessment.
- Administer analgesic therapy, both pharmacologic and nonpharmacologic.
- Reassess after the intervention has reached peak effect.
- Document the patient reports of ability to meet desired goal as evidenced by a functional assessment (e.g., drinking fluids, coughing, ambulating).
- Documents patient participation in activities important to self and to family (e.g., family activities, interpersonal relationships, parenting, social interaction, recreation, work).
- Documents patient's report of adequate sleep.
- Notify the health care provider if pain is unrelieved.

The patient or family will:

- State correct dose(s) of medication.
- Administer correct dose(s) using correct procedure.
- Identify side effects of medication(s).
- Describe actions taken to prevent or correct side effects.
- Report practice of nonpharmacologic strategies to the provider.
- Describe expected outcomes of nonpharmacologic strategies.

BOX 6-9

Resources for Nurses Caring for Patients in Pain

The American Society for Pain Management Nursing (ASPMN) is an "organization of nurses dedicated to promoting and providing optimal care of individuals with pain, including the management of its sequelae." The organization has established evidence-based consensus statements on nursing pain management practices. Examples of the consensus guidelines include the following:

- Monitoring for Opioid-Induced Advancing Sedation and Respiratory Depression
- Pain Assessment in the Patient Unable to Self-Report
- Prescribing and Administering Opioid Doses Based Solely on Pain Intensity
- Authorized Agent-Controlled Analgesia
- Pain Management at End of Life
- Registered Nurse Management and Monitoring of Analgesia By Catheter Technique

ASPMN offers national Pain Management Nursing Certification to RNs who met the eligibility criteria to become certified. Refer to this link for further details: https://www.painmanagementnursing.org

EVALUATING PAIN MANAGEMENT STRATEGIES

An important aspect of caring for patients in pain is reassessing the pain after the intervention has been implemented. The measure's effectiveness is based on the patient's assessment of pain and functional ability as reflected in pain assessment tools. If the intervention was ineffective, the nurse should consider other measures. If these are ineffective, pain relief goals need to be reassessed in collaboration with the primary care provider and/or interdisciplinary team. The nurse serves as the patient's advocate in obtaining additional pain relief.

After interventions have had a chance to work, the nurse asks the patient to rate the intensity of pain. The nurse repeats this assessment at appropriate intervals after the intervention and compares the result with the previous rating. In addition, functional assessments should be carried out to assess the effectiveness of the pain relief measures and provide a basis for continuing or modifying the plan of care. A plan of nursing care for a patient with pain is available at http://thepoint.lww.com/Honan3e. Expected patient outcomes are given in Box 6-8, and resources for nurses caring for patients in pain are provided in Box 6-9.

CHAPTER REVIEW

NCLEX-Style Review Questions

1. The nurse is managing an epidural catheter for a patient diagnosed with lung cancer. The patient now complains of a headache. Which of the following interventions should the nurse perform? Select all that apply.
  a. Increase the dosage of anesthetic.
  b. Place in semi-Fowler position.
  c. Reassess the patient's vital signs and O_2 sat.
  d. Initiate administration of prescribed fluids.
  e. Lower the head of the bed
  f. Assess neurologic status

2. The nurse is caring for an 80-year-old patient following right hip surgery. When administering pain medication to this patient, what is important for the nurse to remember? Select all that apply.
  a. Older patients have a faster metabolism than their younger counterparts.
  b. Altered drug metabolism in the liver and decreased renal excretion can lead to adverse effects.
  c. Older patients have a lower incidence of chronic illness.
  d. Older patients infrequently use OTC medications.
  e. Polypharmacy is common in older patients.
  f. Older patients have an increased risk for drug toxicity.

3. A patient who was diagnosed with a pancreatic tumor is receiving morphine 2 mg subcutaneously every 3 to 4 hours for treatment of pain associated with the tumor. After 2 days of receiving this dose every 4 hours, the patient tells the nurse that the medication is needed more frequently to control their pain. What is the nurse's best response to this situation?
   a. The patient is becoming addicted to the morphine.
   b. A tolerance to the morphine is developing.
   c. Administering the morphine every 3 hours will increase the patient's physical dependence on the drug.
   d. Physical dependence should be avoided at all costs, and the drug should continue to be administered every 4 hours.
   e. The medication should be administered at a shorter interval than every 4 hours.
   f. The dose of medication and/or route may need to be adjusted.
4. A patient who had abdominal surgery 5 days ago complains of sharp, throbbing abdominal pain that ranks 8 on a scale of 0 (no pain) to 10 (worst pain). The patient's pain rating has averaged at a 3/10 for the first 5 days postoperatively on epidural administration of hydromorphone. However, opioid administration via epidural catheter was discontinued earlier this morning. Which of the following would be the nurse's priority actions?
   a. Obtain an order to restart the epidural opioid administration.
   b. Assess the patient's vital signs and O_2 sat.
   c. Check the patient's chart to determine what additional pain medications can be administered.
   d. Explain to the patient that their pain should not be this severe 5 days postoperatively.
   e. Perform a GI assessment: note distention, presence or absence of bowel sounds, presence of flatus, last BM.
   f. Evaluate the abdominal wound: note wound approximation, healing ridge (POD 5), presence of drainage, erythema, tenderness
5. What instruction should the nurse stress when teaching the preoperative patient about correct use of the PCA device?
   a. Push the button when you feel the pain beginning rather than waiting until the pain is at its worst.
   b. Push the button every 15 minutes whether you feel pain at that time or not.
   c. Instruct your family or visitors to press the button for you when you are sleeping.
   d. Try to go as long as you possibly can before you press the button.
   e. Notify the nurse if you do not feel any effect within 15 minutes.
   f. Press the button in anticipation of pain, for example, before getting out of bed following abdominal surgery.

REFERENCES AND SELECTED READINGS

References and selected readings associated with this chapter can be found on the website that accompanies the book. Visit **http://thepoint.lww.com/Honan3e** to access the references and other additional resources associated with this chapter.

Problems Related to Gas Exchange and Respiratory Function

A 43-year-old patient diagnosed with laryngeal cancer will undergo a total laryngectomy. The patient is very anxious about how to manage postoperative care once discharged. How can the nurse address the patient's fears?

- **Discuss potential complications that may arise following a total laryngectomy.**
- **Discuss areas to be included in teaching the patient self-care.**
- **Discuss area support groups for laryngectomy patients.**

CHAPTER 7

Nursing Assessment: Respiratory Function

Linda Honan

Learning Objectives

After reading this chapter, you will be able to:

1. Describe the structures and functions of the upper and lower respiratory tracts.
2. Define ventilation, perfusion, diffusion, and shunting.
3. Explain the use of inspection, palpation, percussion, and auscultation for respiratory assessment.
4. Discriminate between normal and abnormal breath sounds.
5. Use assessment parameters appropriate for determining the characteristics and severity of the major symptoms of respiratory dysfunction.
6. Identify the nursing implications of the various procedures used for diagnostic evaluation of respiratory function.

Disorders of the respiratory system are commonly encountered by nurses in every setting from the community to the intensive care unit. Expert assessment skills must be developed and used when caring for patients with acute and chronic respiratory problems. In addition, an understanding of respiratory function and the significance of abnormal diagnostic test results is essential.

ANATOMY AND PHYSIOLOGY OVERVIEW

The respiratory system is composed of the upper and lower respiratory tracts, blood vessels, thoracic cage (spine, ribs, and sternum) and respiratory muscles, chiefly the diaphragm (Fig. 7-1). Respiration requires **ventilation** (movement of air from the atmosphere to the alveoli [the functional unit of the lung]), **diffusion** (exchange of oxygen [O_2] and carbon dioxide [CO_2] at the alveolar–capillary membrane), and perfusion (blood flow). In addition, innervations of the respiratory system are controlled by the neurologic system (medulla, pons, spinal nerves), muscular system (diaphragm, intercostal muscles), and chemical regulation.

Anatomy of the Upper Respiratory Tract

Upper airway structures consist of the nose, sinuses and nasal passages, pharynx, tonsils and adenoids, and larynx, which warm, humidify, and filter atmospheric air.

Nose

The anterior nares (nostrils) are the external openings of the nasal cavities. The internal portion of the nose is divided into two by a narrow vertical divider, the *septum*, which is richly supplied with sensory nerves and blood vessels. Each nasal cavity is divided into three passageways by the projection of the turbinates (also called conchae), which are highly sensitive. The middle passageway, or meatus, lies under the middle turbinate and contains the ostia (openings) of three of the paranasal sinuses (discussed below) that drain into this area. The nasal cavities are lined with highly vascular ciliated mucous membranes (nasal mucosa). Mucus, secreted continuously by goblet cells, covers the surface of the nasal mucosa and is moved back to the nasopharynx by the action of the **cilia** (fine hairs).

Pearls for Practice

The nurse considers that prolonged obstruction of the ostia (as with a nasotracheal tube or nasogastric [NG] tube) is associated with sinusitis (Stacy, 2022). Patients with endotracheal intubation are also at risk for nosocomial sinusitis because of pooling of nasopharyngeal secretions.

Paranasal Sinuses

The paranasal sinuses include four pairs of bony cavities or air spaces that drain into the nasal cavity and lighten the

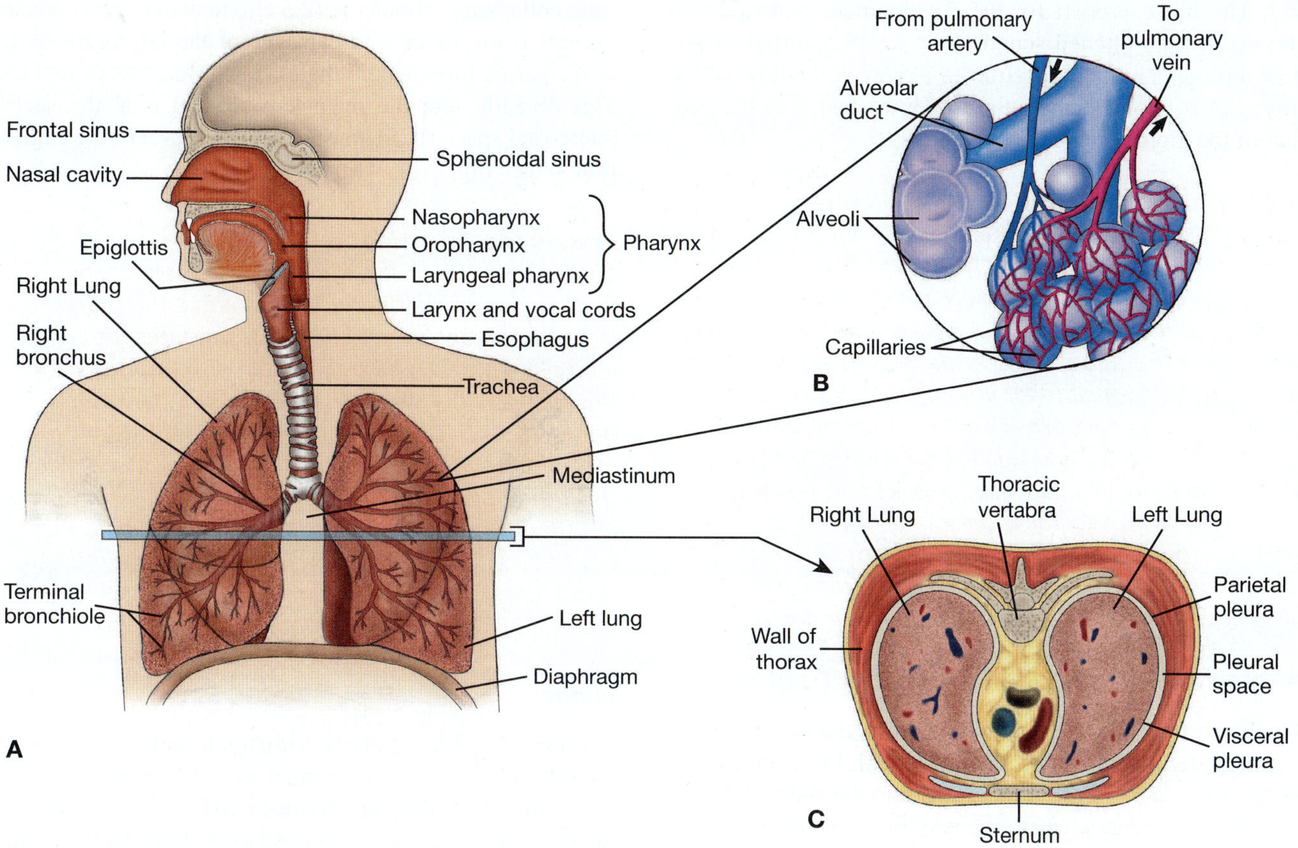

FIGURE 7-1 The respiratory system. A. Upper respiratory structures and the structures of the thorax. B. Alveoli. C. A horizontal cross-section of the lungs.

weight of the skull. The sinuses are named by their location: frontal (above the eyebrows), ethmoidal (between the eyes and behind the nose), sphenoidal (behind the ethmoid sinuses), and maxillary (located on the cheeks below the eyes). They serve as a resonating chamber in speech and are a common site of infection.

Pharynx, Tonsils, and Adenoids

The pharynx, or throat, is a tube-like structure that connects the nasal and oral cavities to the larynx and is a passageway for the respiratory and digestive tracts. It is divided into three regions: nasal, oral, and laryngeal. The nasopharynx is located posterior to the nose and above the soft palate. The adenoids, or pharyngeal tonsils, are located in the roof of the nasopharynx. Air entering reaches the nasopharynx, where it contacts sensitive nerves. Some of these nerves detect odors; others provoke sneezing to expel irritating dust. The eustachian tubes are also located here, they connect the middle ear to the nasopharynx and function to drain mucus and equalize pressures. The oropharynx houses the faucial, or palatine tonsils. The tonsils, the adenoids, and other lymphoid tissue encircle the throat. These structures are important links in the chain of lymph nodes guarding the body from invasion by organisms entering the nose and the throat. The laryngopharynx extends from the hyoid bone to the cricoid cartilage.

Larynx

The larynx, or voice organ, connects the pharynx and the trachea. The major function of the larynx is vocalization. It also protects the lower airway from foreign substances and facilitates coughing. It is frequently referred to as the voice box and consists of the following:

- *Epiglottis:* A valve flap of cartilage (lid-like structure) that covers the entrance to the larynx during swallowing; it is essential to prevent aspiration (inhalation of food or fluid into the lungs)
- *Glottis:* The opening between the vocal cords in the larynx
- *Thyroid cartilage:* The largest of the cartilage structures; it can be felt anteriorly as the “Adam’s apple”
- *Cricoid cartilage:* The only complete cartilaginous ring in the larynx (located below the thyroid cartilage)
- *Arytenoid cartilages:* Used in vocal cord movement with the thyroid cartilage
- *Vocal cords:* Ligaments controlled by muscular movements that produce sounds; located in the lumen of the larynx

During expiration, the vocal cords vibrate to produce high or low sounds. High sounds are associated with a taut glottis, whereas low sounds are associated with a more relaxed one. The nurse is alert for the development of stridor, an abnormal, high-pitched sound, as it signifies turbulent airflow through a partially obstructed airway at the level of the supraglottis, glottis, subglottis, and/or trachea. Any obstruction of the glottis area can be fatal.

Pearls for Practice

Any artificial airway bypasses the normal protective function of warming, humidifying, and filtering the air. Although, O_2 can be humidified and warmed, it cannot be filtered; thus, any artificial airway is a risk factor for infection. In addition, since artificial airways bypass the larynx (responsible for voice), communication is a priority nursing concern. The upper airway also serves as a conduit for air to reach the lungs. The nurse is alert for any obstruction—such as a foreign body; the tongue; swelling secondary to allergic reaction, infection, or trauma; or neurologic impairment in which nerves or muscles may be impaired—that predisposes the patient to airway obstruction.

Anatomy of the Lower Respiratory Tract

The lower respiratory tract consists of the trachea, right and left mainstem bronchi, secondary bronchi, bronchioles, and lungs, and can be further subdivided into the conducting airways and the acinus, where the respiratory bronchioles and alveoli (functional unit of the lung) are located.

Trachea

The trachea, or windpipe, is composed of smooth muscle with C-shaped rings of cartilage at regular intervals. The cartilaginous rings are incomplete on the posterior surface and give firmness to the wall of the trachea, preventing it from collapsing. About 1 in (2.5 cm) in diameter, the trachea extends from the cricoid cartilage of the larynx to the top of the carina (area where the trachea bifurcates or divides). This division into the mainstem bronchi is at the second intercostal space (ICS) anteriorly (at the level of the angle of Louis) (see Fig. 7-2).

Pearls for Practice

*The angle of Louis is a significant anatomical landmark that has implications for cardiac and pulmonary assessment as well as clinical procedures (i.e., EKG lead placement). Since the angle of Louis relates to the second rib, the nurse understands the ICS directly **below** this rib is the second ICS. The aortic valve is auscultated at the second ICS right sternal border (SB); the pulmonary valve is heard at the second ICS, left SB. The angle of Louis is also anatomically where the trachea bifurcates into the left and right mainstem bronchus. The angle of Louis is also referred to as the sternal angle or the manubriosternal junction.*

Lungs

The lungs are paired elastic structures enclosed in the thoracic cage, which is an airtight chamber with distensible walls (Fig. 7-3). They are divided into lobes by fissures. The lungs are separated into upper and lower lobes by the oblique or major fissures that begin at T3 posteriorly and terminate at the sixth rib in the midclavicular line (MCL) bilaterally. To find T3, the nurse asks the patient to flex the neck forward; the most protruding spinous process is C7. The nurse palpates below this process from here to T1, T2, and T3. An additional horizontal fissure produces the middle lobe of the right lung. It begins anteriorly at approximately the fourth

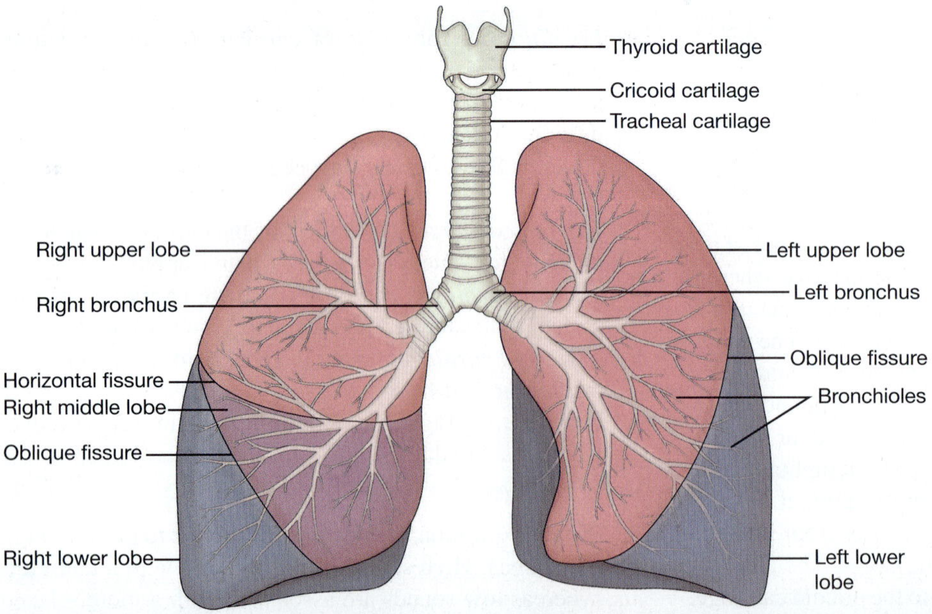

FIGURE 7-2 Anterior view of the lungs. The lungs consist of five lobes. The right lung has three lobes (upper, middle, lower); the left has two (upper and lower). The lobes are further subdivided by fissures. The bronchial tree, another lung structure, inflates with air to fill the lobes.

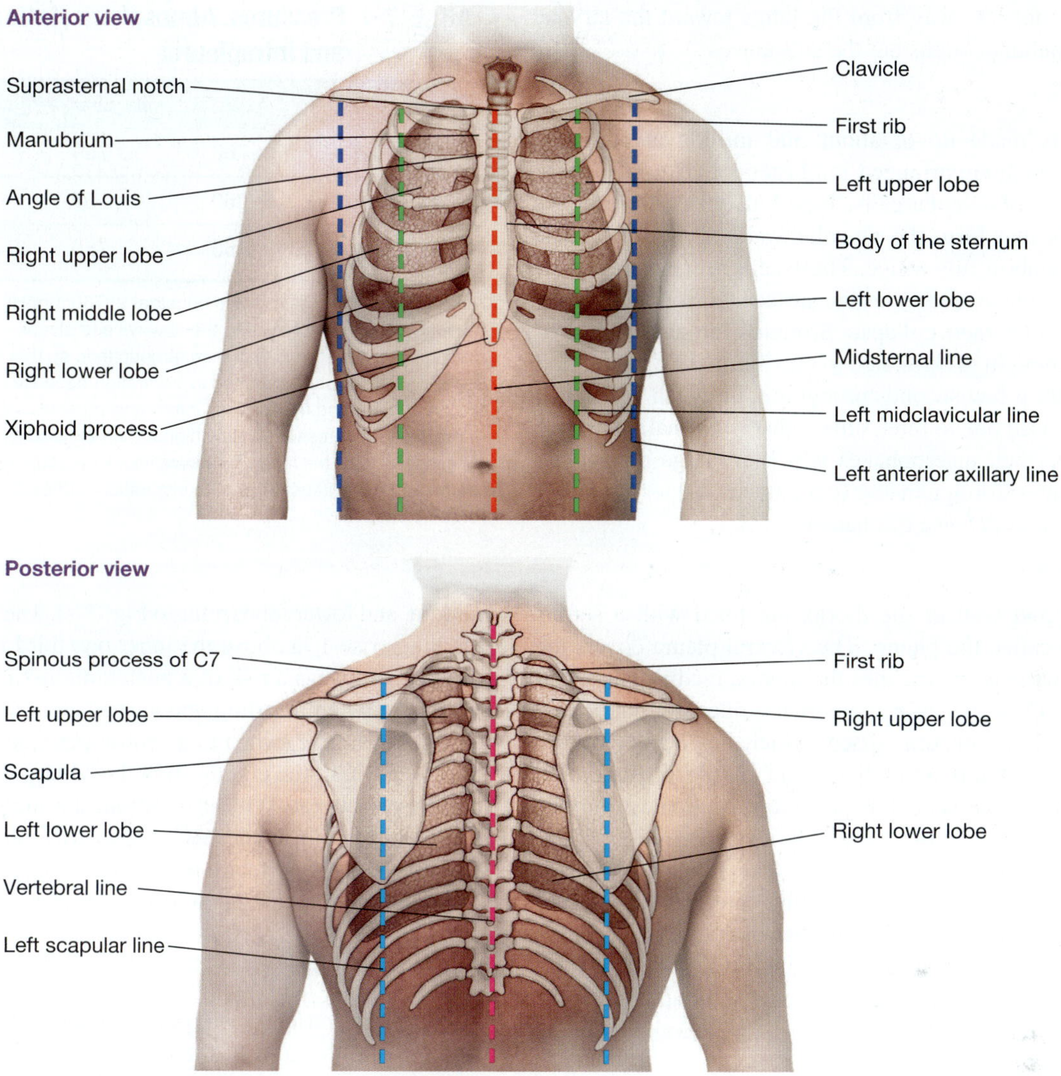

FIGURE 7-3 Landmarks in respiratory assessment.

rib at the right SB and extends to the fifth rib in the midaxillary line (MAL). It is essential for nurses to understand that the right middle lobe can be auscultated only anteriorly (see later discussion and Box 7-6 on page 257).

Bronchi and Bronchioles

The bronchi begin at the carina. The right main bronchus, which provides air to the right lung, is wider, shorter (about 2.5 cm long), and more vertical in direction than the left main bronchus, which supplies the left lung. Because of the anatomical structure, aspiration of material tends to occur in the right lung. The mainstem bronchi divide into five lobar bronchi: three in the right lung and two in the left lung, to correspond with each respective lobe of the lung. The lobar bronchi enter the lung at the hilum (a fissure or opening) along with blood vessels, nerves, and lymphatics. The lobar bronchi branch into segmental bronchi (10 on the right and 9 on the left). They are the structures identified when choosing the most effective postural drainage position for a given patient. The segmental bronchi further subdivide until they branch into bronchioles. Bronchioles have no cartilage in their walls, so patency depends entirely on the elastic recoil of the surrounding smooth muscle and on the alveolar pressure. Bronchioles then become respiratory bronchioles with actual alveolar sacs imbedded in their walls, which allow gas exchange to occur. Up until this point, the exchange of O_2 and CO_2 has not occurred, so this area is termed *anatomical dead space*. It is calculated to be 2 mL/kg of body weight and comprises one third of the tidal volume (TV) in a healthy adult patient; thus, a full one third of TV is rebreathed due to dead space (Quinn et al., 2021). TV is the amount of air that moves in or out of the lungs with each respiratory cycle; a normal TV is approximately 500 mL.

There are characteristics common to most of the conducting airways: the production of mucus, the presence of serous glands that secrete a watery substance containing antibacterial enzymes, and surfaces covered with cilia. These cilia create a constant whipping motion that propels mucus and foreign substances away from the lungs toward the larynx, where the patient coughs out the substances.

Alveoli

The lung is made up of about 300 million alveoli (see Fig. 7-1), which are arranged in clusters of 15 to 20. There are two types of alveolar cells. Type I alveolar cells are epithelial cells that form the alveolar walls. Type II alveolar cells are metabolically active. These cells secrete surfactant, a phospholipid that decreases the surface tension in the alveoli and prevents their collapse. Stimulus for surfactant production is thought to be related to maximum deep inspiration sustained for a few seconds or sighing, in which a person's TV is increased one to three times what is normal. There are also alveolar cell macrophages which are large phagocytic cells that ingest foreign matter (e.g., mucus, bacteria) and act as an important defense mechanism.

Pleura

The lungs and wall of the thorax are lined with a serous membrane called the pleura. The visceral pleura covers the lungs; the parietal pleura lines the thorax, mediastinum, and diaphragm. Only the parietal pleura has fibers for pain transmission. The intrapleural space, which lies between these two layers, contains a small amount of pleural fluid (0.1 to 0.3 mL/kg) that serves to provide a frictionless surface between the two pleura in response to changes in respiration (Krishna & Rudrappa, 2021). The intrapleural space is negative, with the average resting interpleural pressure –4 cm H_2O, that is 4 cm of water, below that of atmospheric pressure at rest, and remains so during inspiration and expiration. Thus, under normal conditions, the intrapleural space is always negative. Refer to Table 7-1 for pleural pressures.

Pearls for Practice

The pleural cavity is a "potential" space, that is a place where fluid can accumulate (between the visceral and parietal pleura) up to 20 mL. Fluid collection is seen in infection, malignancy, or inflammatory conditions as well as illnesses that alter the hydrostatic or oncotic pressures in the pleural space like heart failure, nephrotic syndrome, liver cirrhosis, and hypoalbuminemia. This abnormal collection of fluid or exudate is termed a pleural effusion. Patients would present with shortness of breath but may be asymptomatic depending on the size of the effusion.

Mediastinum

The mediastinum is in the middle of the thorax, between the pleural sacs. It contains the great vessels of the heart, the heart, esophagus, trachea, thoracic duct, thymus, and lymph nodes, as well as the vagus, cardiac, and phrenic nerves.

Lobes

Each lung is divided into lobes. The left lung consists of an upper and lower lobe, whereas the right lung has an upper, middle, and lower lobe (refer to Fig. 7-2). The upper lobes of the lungs rise 1 in above the inner one third of the clavicle, so there is always a risk of a pneumothorax (air in the pleural space) when inserting venous catheters in the neck. The base of each lung (when in a neutral position) is at the sixth rib in the MCL, the eighth rib in the MAL, and the tenth rib posteriorly at rest. With inspiration, the lungs can descend to the eighth rib in the MCL, tenth rib in the MAL, and twelfth rib at the vertebral border. Use Figure 7-3 to find the common landmarks used in respiratory assessment.

TABLE 7-1 Pressures: Atmospheric, Intrapulmonary, and Intrapleural

Pressure	At Rest	Inspiratory	Expiratory
Atmospheric	760	760	760
Intrapulmonary	760	757	763
Intrapleural	756	750	756

Atmospheric pressure remains constant at 760 mm Hg. For air to enter the lungs, the pressure within the airways and alveoli (intrapulmonary pressure) must become less than atmospheric so that the air can be pulled in. This is accomplished in inspiration because of the action of the diaphragm and the external intercostal muscles. At expiration, the intrapulmonary pressure is now higher than atmospheric pressure and air escapes from the lungs. The intrapleural pressure (pressure within the pleural cavity) fluctuates with inspiration and expiration but always remain negative.

Thoracic Cage

The 12 ribs, costal cartilages (cartilages that connect the sternum and the ends of the ribs; termed the *costochondral junction*), manubrium, sternum, xiphoid process, and vertebral column provide the structure that supports and protects the lung. The notch on the top of the manubrium may be referred to as the *suprasternal notch, sternal notch,* or *jugular notch.* Seven ribs and their costal cartilages articulate directly to the body of the sternum; ribs 8 to 10 attach to cartilage of the seventh rib. Ribs 11 and 12 do not have an anterior attachment and are sometimes referred to as "floating ribs." Posteriorly, each rib attaches to a vertebra. An important landmark for nurses to use when counting ribs is the angle of Louis, which is where the manubrium (top of sternum, approximately 4 cm long) and the body of the sternum meet at the second rib. This area is also termed the manubriosternal junction and can be palpable as a transverse ridge in most patients. The second costal cartilages articulate with the sternum here at the angle of Louis; the ICS below the angle is the second ICS.

It is important to recognize that any alteration in the bony structure of the thorax affects the ability of the lungs to function. The costal angle (lower parts of the anterior rib cage near the xiphoid process) normally is about 90 degrees.

Respiratory Muscles

Ventilation requires movement of the walls of the thoracic cage and of its floor, the *diaphragm.* The diaphragm is a dome-shaped muscle that, when contracted (during inspiration), pulls the lungs in a downward and forward direction; the abdomen appears to enlarge because the abdominal contents are being compressed by the diaphragm. With inspiration, the diaphragmatic pull elongates the chest cavity, and the external intercostal muscles (located between and along the lower borders of the ribs) contract to raise the ribs, which expands the anteroposterior (AP) diameter of the thorax. The effect of these movements is to decrease the intrapulmonary pressure (pressure within the lung) to less than atmospheric pressure, which causes air to rush into the lung (see Table 7-1). With expiration, the diaphragm and intercostals recoil, which increases the intrapulmonary pressure over atmospheric pressure so that gases are expelled from the lung. While inspiration is an active process, expiration is passive. In respiratory diseases, such as chronic obstructive pulmonary disease (COPD), the act of breathing becomes work requiring energy.

Additional accessory muscles of inspiration, including the scalene (elevates the first two ribs), sternocleidomastoid (raise the sternum), and the alae nasi (flaring of nostrils), may be called upon to assist with inspiration when exercising, while the abdominal and internal intercostal muscles may be used to increase expiration.

Pearls for Practice

The diaphragm is innervated by the phrenic nerve, which exits the spinal column at the level of C3 to C5. Any fracture at or above this level will cause respiratory paralysis. Thus, in any condition where the spine is potentially injured, early immobilization with a cervical collar (c-collar) must be applied and the patient log rolled until diagnostic testing confirms no fracture of the cervical spine.

Neuroanatomy Related to Respiration

The rhythm of breathing is controlled by the medulla oblongata and pons. In addition, central chemoreceptors located in the medulla respond to changes in PCO_2 and pH levels in the cerebrospinal fluid and alter the depth and then the rate of ventilation to correct an imbalance. In addition, peripheral chemoreceptors are located in the aortic arch and the carotid arteries that respond first to changes in PaO_2 (less than 60 mm Hg) and then to $PaCO_2$ and pH by altering the depth and rate of respiration. These chemoreceptors no longer respond to $PaCO_2$ or pH in patients with COPD because of the persistently high levels of $PaCO_2$ that exist with this disorder. Thus, the primary drive to breathe comes from a low O_2 level rather than a high CO_2 level. If O_2 is administered at a high enough rate to raise the PaO_2 to normal, there is a risk of obliterating the hypoxic drive. Therefore, low-flow O_2 is administered to a patient with COPD while the nurse carefully assesses for complications.

A final reflex to consider is the Hering–Breuer reflex that prevents the overinflation of the lungs. It is activated by stretch receptors located within the smooth muscle of large and small airways that inhibit further inspiration.

Function of the Respiratory System

The cells of the body require O_2. Certain vital tissues, such as the brain and the heart, cannot survive for long without a continuous supply. However, as a result of oxidation in the body tissues, CO_2 is produced and must be removed from the cells to prevent the buildup of acid waste products. The respiratory system performs this life-sustaining function of gas exchange.

Respiration

The process of **respiration** requires gas exchange both in the lungs, termed *external or pulmonary respiration,* and, ultimately, in the tissues, termed *internal or cellular respiration.* External respiration requires three processes: (1) *ventilation,* the act of breathing (inspiration and expiration); (2) *perfusion,* blood flow to the alveoli, so that gases can be exchanged; and (3) *diffusion,* movement of gases from a higher area of concentration to a lower area across the alveolar–capillary membrane. Within the lungs, oxygen is in high concentration within the alveoli and lower in the pulmonary capillaries. This concentration difference exerts the driving pressure for the movement of oxygen (via diffusion) from the alveoli into the pulmonary capillaries. Conversely, carbon dioxide has a higher concentration in the blood than in the alveoli, and it diffuses from the blood into the alveoli to be exhaled from the body. The end result is O_2-rich blood leaving the pulmonary veins (the only veins other than the umbilical vein to carry oxygenated blood) to systemic circulation. Internal respiration refers to the process by which O_2 is supplied to, and CO_2 is removed from, the body cells by way of the circulating blood. Cells are in close contact with capillaries, the thin walls of which permit easy passage or exchange of O_2 and CO_2. Oxygen diffuses from the capillaries through the capillary walls to the interstitial fluid. At this point, O_2 diffuses through the membrane of tissue cells, where it is used by mitochondria for cellular respiration. The movement of CO_2 occurs by diffusion in the opposite direction—from cell to blood. These processes are critical for survival.

Ventilation

During inspiration, air flows from the environment into the trachea, bronchi, bronchioles, and alveoli. During expiration, alveolar gas travels the same route in reverse.

Physical factors that govern air flow in and out of the lungs are collectively referred to as the *mechanics of ventilation* and include air pressure variances, resistance to air flow (the narrower the airway, the greater the resistance to flow),

BOX 7-1

Causes of Increased Airway Resistance

Common phenomena that may alter bronchial diameter, which affects airway resistance, include the following:

- Contraction of bronchial smooth muscle—as in asthma
- Thickening of bronchial mucosa—as in chronic bronchitis
- Obstruction of the airway—by mucus, a tumor, or a foreign body
- Loss of lung elasticity—as in emphysema, which is characterized by connective tissue encircling the airways, thereby keeping them open during both inspiration and expiration

and lung compliance (the dispensability of the lung, or how well the lung stretches).

Airway Resistance

Resistance is determined chiefly by the radius or size of the airway through which the air is flowing. Any process that changes the bronchial diameter or width affects airway resistance and alters the rate of air flow for a given pressure gradient during respiration (Box 7-1). With increased resistance, greater-than-normal respiratory effort is required to achieve normal levels of ventilation.

Compliance

Compliance is a measure of the elasticity, expandability, and distensibility of the lungs and thoracic structures. Consider an elastic band: When it is stretched, it easily returns to its normal shape; so too should the lungs. Factors that determine lung compliance are the surface tension of the alveoli (normally low with the presence of surfactant) and the connective tissue (i.e., collagen and elastin) of the lungs.

Compliance is normal if the lungs and thorax easily stretch and distend when pressure is applied. High or increased compliance occurs if the lungs have lost their elasticity (cannot return to normal state) and the thorax is overdistended (i.e., in emphysema). Low or decreased compliance occurs if the lungs and thorax are "stiff" (difficult to stretch). Conditions associated with decreased compliance include pneumothorax, hemothorax, pleural effusion, pulmonary edema, atelectasis, pulmonary fibrosis, and acute respiratory distress syndrome (ARDS), all of which are discussed in later chapters in this unit.

Lung Volumes and Capacities

Lung function, which reflects the mechanics of ventilation, is viewed in terms of lung volumes and lung capacities. These terms are described in Table 7-2 and illustrated in Figure 7-4. Three common measurements that the medical-surgical nurse should understand are TV, minute ventilation, and vital capacity. The volume of each breath is referred to as the *TV* and can be measured by a bedside spirometer. If the patient is breathing through an endotracheal tube or tracheostomy, the spirometer is attached directly to it, and the exhaled volume is obtained from the reading on the gauge. In other patients, the spirometer is attached to a face mask or a mouthpiece positioned so that it is airtight, and the exhaled volume is measured.

The TV may vary from breath to breath. To ensure that the measurement is reliable, it is important to measure the volumes of several breaths and to note the range of TVs, together with the average TV. But measurements like respiratory rates and TV alone are unreliable indicators of adequate ventilation because both can vary widely from breath to breath. However, together the TV and respiratory rate are important because the minute ventilation is useful in detecting respiratory failure.

Minute ventilation is the volume of air expired per minute. It is equal to the product of the TV in liters multiplied by the respiratory rate or frequency. In practice, the minute ventilation is not calculated but is measured directly using a spirometer. Minute ventilation may be decreased by a variety of conditions that result in hypoventilation. When the minute ventilation falls, alveolar ventilation in the lungs also decreases, and the $PaCO_2$ increases.

Forced vital capacity requires having the patient take in a maximal breath and exhale fully and forcefully. Most patients can exhale at least 80% of their vital capacity in 1 second (forced expiratory volume in 1 second, or FEV_1) and almost all of it in 3 seconds (FEV_3). A reduction in FEV_1 (ability to get the air OUT of the lung) suggests abnormal pulmonary air flow. If the patient's FEV_1 and forced vital capacity are reduced proportionately, maximal lung expansion is restricted in some way. If the reduction in FEV_1 greatly exceeds the reduction in forced vital capacity, the patient may have some degree of airway obstruction. Often forced vital capacity is reduced in COPD because of air trapping, and a decreased FEV is a valuable clue to the severity of the expiratory airway obstruction.

Thus, pulmonary function tests (PFTs) can aid in diagnosing restrictive or obstructive pulmonary disorders. Restrictive disorders are ones that make the lungs stiff; they decrease the total volume of air the lungs can hold. This is typically due to a decrease in the elasticity of the lungs or the inability of the chest wall to expand during inhalation. Examples of restrictive lung diseases are asbestosis, sarcoidosis, and pulmonary fibrosis. Obstructive disorders cause a narrowing or blockage in exhaled airflow and are commonly associated with COPD (discussed in Chapter 10).

Diffusion and Perfusion

Diffusion is the process by which O_2 and CO_2 are exchanged at the air–blood interface. The alveolar–capillary membrane is ideal for diffusion because of its thinness and large surface area. In the normal, healthy adult, O_2 and CO_2 travel across the alveolar–capillary membrane without difficulty as a result of differences in gas concentrations in the alveoli and capillaries.

TABLE **7-2 Lung Volumes and Lung Capacities**

Term	Symbol	Description	Normal Value[a]	Significance
Lung Volumes				
Tidal volume	VT or TV	The volume of air inhaled and exhaled with each breath	500 mL or 5–10 mL/kg	The tidal volume may not vary, even with severe disease.
Inspiratory reserve volume	IRV	The maximum volume of air that can be inhaled after a normal inhalation	3,100 mL	Inspiratory reserve volume is decreased in obstructive lung disorders.
Expiratory reserve volume	ERV	The maximum volume of air that can be exhaled forcibly after a normal exhalation	1,200 mL	Expiratory reserve volume is decreased with restrictive conditions, such as obesity, ascites, or pregnancy.
Residual volume	RV	The volume of air remaining in the lungs after a maximum exhalation	1,200 mL	Residual volume may be increased with obstructive disease.
Lung Capacities				
Vital capacity	VC	The maximum volume of air exhaled from the point of maximum inspiration VC = TV + IRV + ERV	4,800 mL	A decrease in vital capacity may be found in neuromuscular disease, generalized fatigue, atelectasis, pulmonary edema, and COPD.
Inspiratory capacity	IC	The maximum volume of air inhaled after normal expiration IC = TV + IRV	3,600 mL	A decrease in inspiratory capacity may indicate restrictive disease; may also be decreased in obesity.
Functional residual capacity	FRC	The volume of air remaining in the lungs after a normal expiration FRV = ERV + RV	2,400 mL	Functional residual capacity may be increased with COPD and decreased in ARDS.
Total lung capacity	TLC	The volume of air in the lungs after a maximum inspiration TLC = TV + IRV + ERV + RV	6,000 mL	Total lung capacity may be decreased with restrictive disease (atelectasis, pneumonia) and increased in COPD.

[a]Values for healthy males; females are 20–25% less.
ARDS, acute respiratory distress syndrome; COPD, chronic obstructed pulmonary disease.

Pulmonary perfusion is the actual blood flow through the pulmonary circulation. The blood is pumped into the lungs by the right ventricle (RV) through the pulmonary artery. The pulmonary artery divides into the right and left branches to supply both lungs. These two branches divide further to supply all parts of each lung, and continues until it forms the capillaries that surround the alveoli. Normally, about 2% of the blood pumped by the RV does not perfuse the alveolar capillaries. This "shunted" or diverted blood drains into the left side of the heart without participating in

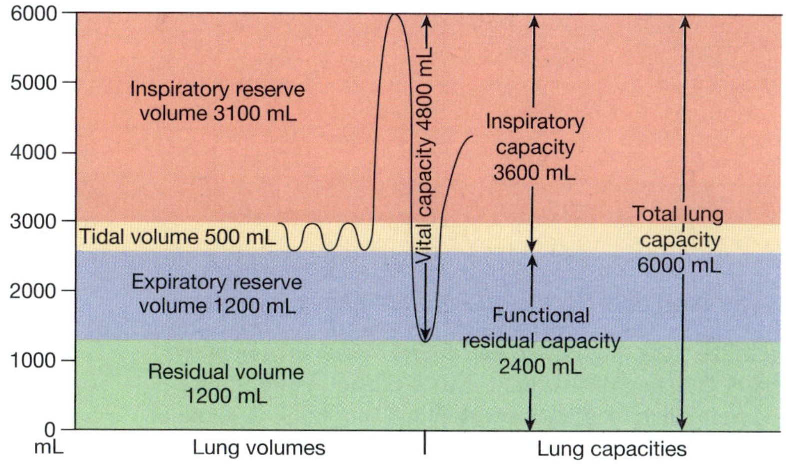

FIGURE 7-4 **Spirometry recordings of respiratory volumes (*left*) and diagram of lung capacities (*right*). The tidal volume (TV, *yellow*) is the amount of air inhaled and exhaled during normal breathing; the inspiratory reserve volume (IRV, *pink*) is the maximal amount of air in excess of the tidal volume that can be forcefully inhaled; the maximal expiratory reserve (ERV, *blue*) is the maximal amount of air that can be exhaled in excess of tidal volume; and the residual volume (RV, *green*) is the air that continues to remain in the lung after maximal expiratory effort. The functional residual capacity (FRC) is the sum of the ERV and the RV. The vital capacity is the sum of IRV, TV, and ERV. (From Porth, C. M. [2015]. *Essentials of pathophysiology* [4th ed.]. Lippincott Williams & Wilkins.)**

alveolar gas exchange. After gas exchange occurs, the oxygenated blood returns to the left side of the heart through the pulmonary veins.

The pulmonary circulation is considered a low-pressure system because the systolic blood pressure in the pulmonary artery is typically 25 mm Hg and the diastolic pressure is 8 mm Hg with a mean of 15 mm Hg which is six times lower than systemic arterial circulation (Mccormack & West, 2022). Because of right-sided low pressures, the pulmonary vasculature normally can vary its capacity to accommodate the blood flow it receives. However, pulmonary blood flow is also not consistent. Regardless of body position, the lower (dependent) areas of the lung receive greater blood flow than upper (nondependent) areas due to gravity pulling blood down toward the base (Powers & Dhamoon, 2021). When a person is in an upright position, the pulmonary artery pressure is not great enough to supply blood to the apex (or top) of the lung against the force of gravity. Thus, when a person is upright, the lung may be considered to be divided into three sections: an upper part with poor blood supply, a lower part with maximal blood supply, and a section between the two with an intermediate supply of blood. When a person that is supine (lying on their back) turns to one side, more blood passes to the dependent lung (the part of the lung that is now lowest). Thus, the nurse should consider that the dependent lung, regardless of position, is better perfused. Of note, recently the prone position (or lying face down) has been used effectively with patients with ARDS associated with COVID-19 (discussed later in this unit). The proposed rationale behind the use of the prone position is that it allows for improved expansion of the dorsal (or back/posterior) lung regions, thus improving ventilation of the this section of the lung and improving ventilation/perfusion ($\dot{V}/\dot{Q}$) matching, enhancing removal of secretions, and improving diaphragmatic excursion, which may ultimately improve oxygenation by increasing $\dot{V}/\dot{Q}$ matching (Sinha et al., 2022; Villar et al., 2021). See Box 7-2.

BOX 7-2

Nursing Research

Bridging the Gap to Evidence-Based Practice

Ryan, P., Fine, C., & DeForge, C. (2021). An evidence-based protocol for manual prone positioning of patients with ARDS. *Critical Care Nurse, 41*(6), 55–60. https://doi.org/10.4037/ccn2021900

Purpose: Manual prone positioning has been shown to reduce mortality among patients with moderate-to-severe acute respiratory distress syndrome (ARDS), but it is associated with a high incidence of pressure injuries and unplanned extubations. This study investigated the feasibility of safely implementing a manual prone positioning protocol that uses a dedicated device.

Design: An existing safe patient-handling device was modified to enable staff to safely perform manual prone positioning with few complications for patients receiving mechanical ventilation. All staff received training on the protocol and use of the device before implementation. This study included 36 consecutive patients who were admitted to the medical intensive care unit at a large academic medical center because of hypoxemic respiratory failure/ARDS and received mechanical ventilation and prone positioning. Data were collected on clinical presentation, interventions, and complications.

Findings: Using the robust protocol and the low-cost device, staff can safely perform a low-volume, high-risk maneuver. This method provides cost savings compared with other prone positioning methods.

Nursing Implications: This article revealed that when faced with limited experience in new procedures such as proning, this team of researchers recognized that resources were needed to help educate the staff, manage the complex patient population, and limit potential risks associated with the prone position such as airway complications (e.g., unplanned extubation) and pressure injuries. Their work may serve as a guide to other health care institutions when instituting proning protocols.

Pearls for Practice

Perfusion is also influenced by alveolar pressure. The pulmonary capillaries are sandwiched between adjacent alveoli. If the alveolar pressure is sufficiently high, the capillaries are squeezed. Depending on the pressure, some capillaries completely collapse, whereas others only narrow.

Pulmonary artery pressure, gravity, and alveolar pressure determine the patterns of perfusion. In lung disease, these factors vary, and the perfusion of the lung may become very abnormal.

Ventilation and Perfusion Balance and Imbalance

Ventilation is the flow of gas in and out of the lungs (normally at a rate of 4 L/min), and perfusion is the filling of the pulmonary capillaries with blood (normally at a rate of 5 L/min). Thus, the alveolar (ventilation) to capillary (perfusion) ratio is 4:5 or 0.8. Adequate gas exchange depends on an adequate $\dot{V}/\dot{Q}$ ratio.

$\dot{V}/\dot{Q}$ imbalance occurs as a result of inadequate ventilation, inadequate perfusion, or both. There are four possible $\dot{V}/\dot{Q}$ states in the lung: normal $\dot{V}/\dot{Q}$ ratio, low $\dot{V}/\dot{Q}$ ratio (shunt), high $\dot{V}/\dot{Q}$ ratio (dead space), and absence of ventilation and perfusion (silent unit) (Box 7-3).

Shunting is the term used to describe conditions in which ventilation is impaired and perfusion is adequate. Normal shunting is about 2%; severe **hypoxia** can result when significant shunting occurs secondary to airway obstruction such as a mucus plug, atelectasis, infective process, or tumor, since in these conditions blood is bypassing the alveoli without gas exchange. However, adequate ventilation but impaired perfusion (as in pulmonary emboli, which is a blood clot in pulmonary vessels), termed *increased dead space*, also causes hypoxia. In this situation, the alveolus has inadequate perfusion, and gas exchange does not occur. As noted, both conditions result in **hypoxia** (low levels of

BOX 7-3

Understanding Ventilation and Perfusion

Normal Ventilation and Perfusion

When ventilation and perfusion ($\dot{V}/\dot{Q}$) are matched, unoxygenated blood from the venous system returns to the right side of the heart through the pulmonary arteries to the lungs, carrying carbon dioxide (CO_2). The arteries branch into alveolar capillaries. Gas exchange takes place in the alveolar capillaries. Normal ventilation is 4 L/min, and perfusion is normally at a rate of 5 L/min. Thus, the alveolar (ventilation) to capillary (perfusion) ratio is 4:5 or 0.8.

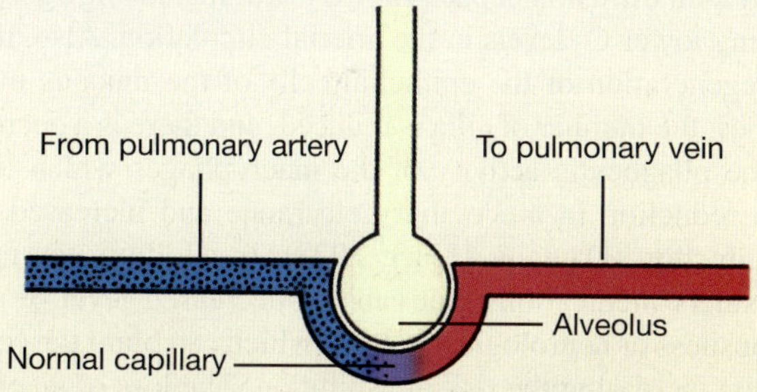

Ventilation and Perfusion Mismatch

Conditions that may produce a $\dot{V}/\dot{Q}$ mismatch include the following:

1. Shunting (reduced ventilation to a lung unit) causes unoxygenated blood to move from the right side of the heart to the left side and into systemic circulation; it may result from physical defects or airway obstruction, such as with pneumonia, atelectasis, tumor, or a mucus plug. When the $\dot{V}/\dot{Q}$ ratio is low, pulmonary circulation is adequate, but not enough oxygen (O_2) is available to the alveoli for normal diffusion. To illustrate, assume the ventilation is now 2 L/min versus a perfusion of 5 L/min. The ratio is now 2:5 or reduced to 0.4. A portion of the blood flowing through the pulmonary vessels doesn't become oxygenated.

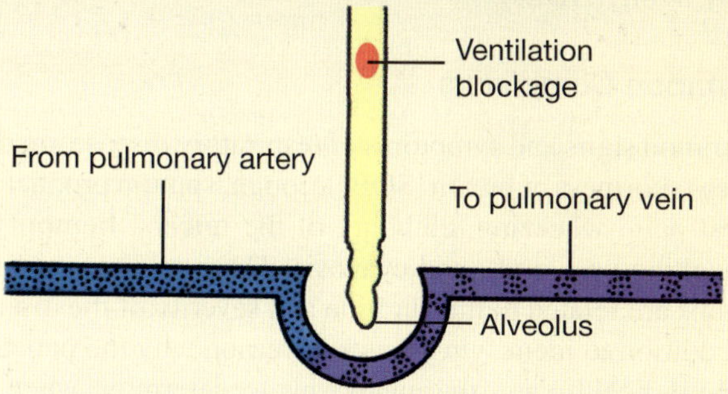

2. Dead-space ventilation (reduced perfusion to a lung unit) occurs when alveoli do not have adequate blood supply for gas exchange to occur, such as with pulmonary emboli (PE) and pulmonary infarction. When the $\dot{V}/\dot{Q}$ ratio is high, as shown here, ventilation is normal, but alveolar perfusion is reduced or absent. Note the narrowed capillary, indicating poor perfusion. This commonly occurs from a perfusion defect, such as PE, or a disorder that decreases cardiac output (cardiogenic shock). In this situation, assume the ventilation is normal at 4 L/min but perfusion is reduced to 3 L/min; thus, the ratio is 4:3 or increased to 1.3.

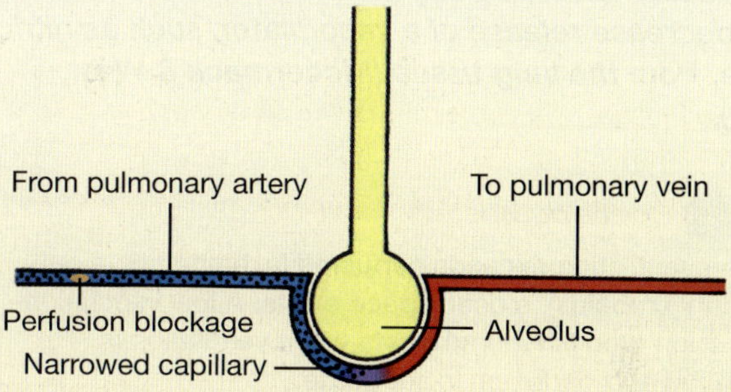

3. A silent unit (a combination of shunting and dead-space ventilation) occurs when little or no ventilation and perfusion are present, such as in acute respiratory distress syndrome. The silent unit indicates an absence of ventilation and perfusion to the lung area.

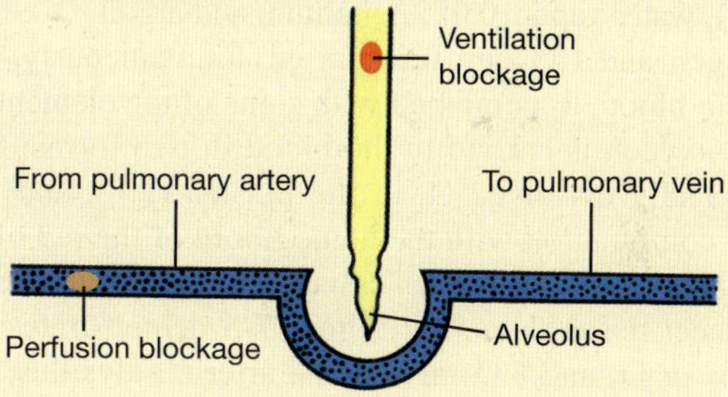

Key to the figures: Blue, blood with CO_2; red, blood rich in O_2; purple, blood with CO_2 and O_2.
Adapted from Knapp, R. (2020). *Hemodynamic monitoring made incredibly visual* (4th ed.). Lippincott Williams & Wilkins.

cellular O_2). Supplemental O_2 is of use in conditions causing an increase in dead space, as long as the impaired perfusion is not massive; supplemental O_2 may not improve **hypoxemia** in shunting, however, as the O_2 does not come in contact with alveoli (areas of diffusion). In fact, a reduced response to oxygen therapy differentiates shunting from other mechanisms of hypoxemia (Tkacs, 2021).

Pearls for Practice: Physiology

The nurse understands that when alveolar oxygen levels drop below 60 mm Hg, the adjacent blood vessels constrict, with resulting increased vascular resistance (Norris, 2019). The lower the O_2 level, the higher the pulmonary vasoconstriction, which, in turn, causes strain on the RV. Recall the RV must

push blood through this increased resistance, leading to RV strain. This effect is opposite to the effect observed in systemic vessels, which dilate rather than constrict in response to low O_2 levels. The pathophysiology of hypoxia-induced vasoconstriction is complex and, although not completely understood, is thought to be related to factors such as an increased intracellular calcium ion concentration of pulmonary vascular smooth muscle cells; pulmonary artery behavior itself which constricts with low O_2 concentration; vasoconstrictor peptides, known as endothelin's that are released by pulmonary vascular endothelial cells resulting in vasoconstriction; and/ or a decrease release of a vasodilator, such as nitric oxide, from the lung tissue (Mccormack & West, 2022).

Concept Mastery Alert

When ventilation exceeds perfusion (exhibited by a pulmonary embolus), a dead space exists. A low ventilation–perfusion ratio (shunting) exists when ventilation is impaired and perfusion is adequate.

Gas Exchange

The air we breathe is a gaseous mixture consisting mainly of nitrogen (78.62%) and O_2 (20.84%), with traces of CO_2 (0.04%), water vapor (0.05%), helium, and argon.

Oxygen and CO_2 are transported simultaneously, dissolved in blood, or combined with some of the elements of blood. Oxygen is carried in the blood in two forms: first, as physically dissolved O_2 in the plasma (2%), and second, in combination with the hemoglobin of the red blood cells (98%). Hemoglobin is essential to supply sufficient O_2 to meet tissue demands. Figure 7-5 demonstrates differences in O_2 and CO_2 in venous, arterial, alveolus, and atmosphere.

Pearls for Practice

Hemoglobin rapidly combines reversibly with O_2; that is, it allows O_2 to be released quickly to the tissues to satisfy metabolic needs. Some hemoglobin exists in forms such as methemoglobin (commonly seen in drug reaction) or is combined with carbon monoxide (as in smoke inhalation), in which case the hemoglobin cannot bind O_2, resulting in tissue hypoxia and lactic acidosis. Thus, the nurse is aware that O_2 delivery to tissues is dependent upon hemoglobin, O_2 content, and cardiac output. While a healthy heart generally can increase cardiac output to compensate for diseased lungs or a low hemoglobin level, a diseased heart may be unable to. It is important for the nurse to consider that a combination of poor oxygenation, low hemoglobin level, and low cardiac output may be rapidly fatal.

Gerontologic Considerations

A gradual decline in respiratory function begins in early to middle adulthood and affects the structure and function of the respiratory system. With aging (age 40 years and above), changes occur in the alveoli that reduce the surface area available for the exchange of O_2 and CO_2. At approximately 50 years of age, the alveoli begin to lose elasticity. A decrease in vital capacity occurs with loss of chest wall mobility, which restricts the tidal flow of air. The amount of respiratory dead space increases with age. These changes result in a decreased diffusion capacity for O_2 with increasing age, producing lower O_2 levels in the arterial circulation. Also, there is degeneration of the epithelial cells of the mucous membranes, the number of cilia is reduced, and there is a decrease in the phagocytic activity of the macrophages which leads to a reduction in mucociliary clearance and increased risk of infection (Davis & Heuer, 2022). In addition, the nurse considers medications that cause a decreased level of consciousness or neurologic disorders which can blunt the cough reflex, increasing the risk of aspiration. The loss of an effective cough reflex contributes to the increased susceptibility of older patients to lung infections. Gerontologic changes in the respiratory system are summarized in Table 7-3.

ASSESSMENT OF THE RESPIRATORY SYSTEM

Health History

The health history focuses on the physical and functional problems of the patient and the effects of these problems on the patient, including their ability to carry out activities of daily living (ADLs).

Common Complaints

Common signs and symptoms of respiratory disease are **dyspnea** (shortness of breath [SOB]), cough, sputum production, chest pain, wheezing, clubbing of the fingers, **hemoptysis** (coughing up blood), and cyanosis. These clinical manifestations are related to the duration and severity of the disease. In addition to identifying the chief reason why the patient is seeking health care, the nurse tries to determine when the health problem or symptom started, how long it has lasted, if it was relieved at any time, and how relief was obtained. The nurse obtains information about precipitating factors, duration, severity, and any associated factors or symptoms.

Dyspnea

Dyspnea is the subjective experience of "shortness of breath (SOB)" (Norris, 2019). Dyspnea (difficult or labored breathing, breathlessness, SOB) is a symptom common in life-threatening conditions such as pulmonary embolism (PE), pulmonary edema, acute airway obstruction from

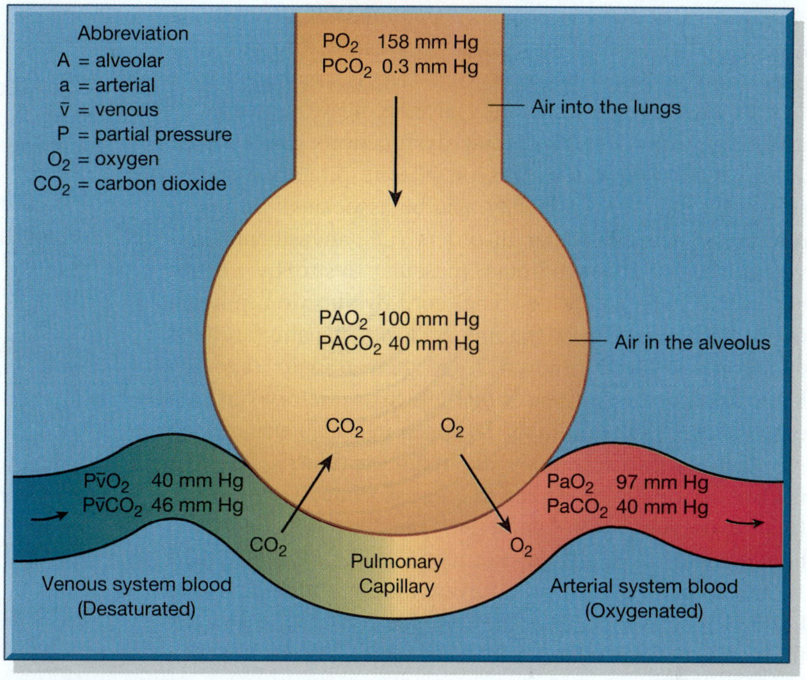

FIGURE 7-5 **Changes occur in the partial pressure of gases during respiration. These values vary as a result of the exchange of O_2 and CO_2 as well as the changes that occur in their partial pressures as venous blood flows through the lungs.**

TABLE 7-3 Age-Related Changes in the Respiratory System

Component	Structural Changes	Functional Changes	History and Physical Findings
Defense mechanisms (respiratory and nonrespiratory)	↓ Number of cilia and ↓ mucus; ↓ thirst response ↓ Cough and gag reflex Loss of surface area of the capillary membrane Lack of a uniform or consistent ventilation and/or blood flow	↓ Protection against foreign particles; may have less moisture within the mucous membranes of the upper and lower respiratory tracts ↓ Protection against aspiration ↓ Antibody response to antigens ↓ Response to hypoxia and hypercapnia (chemoreceptors)	Thickened mucus, cough reflex may be reduced ↑ Infection rate History of respiratory infections, COPD, pneumonia Risk factors: smoking, environmental exposure, TB exposure
Lung	↓ Size of airway ↑ Diameter of alveolar ducts ↑ Collagen of alveolar walls ↑ Thickness of alveolar membranes ↓ Elasticity of alveolar sacs	↑ Airway resistance ↑ Pulmonary compliance ↓ Expiratory flow rate ↓ Oxygen diffusion capacity ↑ Dead space Premature closure of airways ↑ Air trapping ↓ Expiratory flow rates Ventilation–perfusion mismatch ↓ Exercise capacity ↑ Anteroposterior (AP) diameter	Unchanged total lung capacity (TLC) ↑ Residual volume (RV) ↓ Inspiratory reserve volume (IRV) ↓ Expiratory reserve volume (ERV) ↓ Forced vital capacity (FVC) and vital capacity (VC) ↑ Functional residual capacity (FRC) ↓ PaO_2 ↑ CO_2
Chest wall and muscles	Calcification of intercostal cartilages Arthritis of costovertebral joints ↓ Continuity of diaphragm ↓ Muscle mass Muscle atrophy	↑ Rigidity and stiffness of thoracic cage ↓ Respiratory muscle strength ↑ Work of breathing ↓ Capacity for exercise ↓ Peripheral chemosensitivity ↑ Risk for inspiratory muscle fatigue	Barrel chest ↑ AP diameter Shortness of breath ↑ Abdominal and diaphragmatic breathing ↓ Maximum expiratory flow rates
Skeletal changes	↑ dorsal curve of the thoracic spine Osteoclastic activity is greater than osteoblastic activity	↑AP/lateral chest diameter Enlargement of the cancellous bone spaces and a thinning of the trabeculae	Kyphosis; loss of height; ↑ AP/lateral chest diameter; skeletal changes also contribute to a decrease in vital capacity ↑ Risk of osteoporosis

↑, increased; ↓, decreased.

anaphylaxis or foreign bodies, pneumothorax, pneumonia, myocardial infarction, or cardiac tamponade. Chronic dyspnea (longer than 4 weeks in duration) is associated with COPD, asthma, interstitial lung disease, heart failure (HF), cardiomyopathy or myocardial dysfunction, gastroesophageal reflux disease (GERD), or other respiratory diseases (Hashmi et al., 2021). It may also be associated with neurologic or neuromuscular disorders (i.e., myasthenia gravis, Guillain–Barré syndrome, muscular dystrophy, central nervous system [CNS] or spinal cord dysfunction, phrenic nerve paralysis), kidney (failure, acidosis), hepatic (ascites), endocrine (hyperthyroidism), and hematologic (anemia, hemoglobinopathy) diseases that affect respiratory function or physical deconditioning. Dyspnea can also occur after physical exercise in people without disease (Norris, 2019). It is also a symptom at the end of life, associated with anxiety (with hyperventilation), depression, and fear in patients and helplessness in caregivers (Batra et al., 2021; Celik, 2022). If the patient is experiencing severe dyspnea, the nurse may need to modify or abbreviate the questions asked and the timing of the health history to avoid increasing the patient's breathlessness and anxiety.

Clinical Significance. In general, acute diseases of the lungs produce a more severe grade of dyspnea than do chronic diseases. Sudden dyspnea in a healthy person may indicate pneumothorax (air in the pleural space), acute respiratory obstruction, or ARDS. In immobilized patients, sudden dyspnea may denote PE. *Orthopnea* (inability to breathe unless sitting or standing) may be found in patients with heart disease and occasionally in patients with COPD; dyspnea with an expiratory **wheeze** occurs with COPD. Noisy breathing may result from a narrowing of the airway or localized obstruction of a major bronchus by a tumor or foreign body. The presence of both inspiratory and expiratory wheezing usually signifies asthma if the patient does not have HF. The nurse asks about indigestion or difficulty swallowing (dysphagia), which is associated with GERD or gastric secretion aspiration in the lungs (Hashmi et al., 2021). Thus, dyspnea occurs with a variety of disorders, requiring a thorough health history.

The circumstance that produces the dyspnea must be determined; it is important to ask the patient the following questions:

- How much exertion triggers SOB?
- Is there an associated cough?
- Is the SOB related to other symptoms, such as diaphoresis, cough, hemoptysis, chest discomfort, wheeze, orthopnea, stridor, edema, or sinusitis?
- Was the onset of SOB sudden or gradual?
- At what time of day or night does the SOB occur?
- Is the SOB worse when the patient is flat in bed?
- Does the SOB occur at rest? With exercise? Running? Climbing stairs?
- Is the SOB worse while walking? If so, when walking how far? How fast?

BOX 7-4

Grading Dyspnea

To assess **dyspnea** as objectively as possible, ask the patient to briefly describe how various activities affect their breathing. Then document their response using this grading system:

- *Grade 0:* Not troubled by breathlessness except with strenuous exercise
- *Grade 1:* Troubled by shortness of breath when hurrying on a level path or walking up a slight hill
- *Grade 2:* Walks more slowly on a level path because of breathlessness than do people of the same age or has to stop to breathe when walking on a level path at their own pace
- *Grade 3:* Stops to breathe after walking about 100 yards (91 m) on a level path
- *Grade 4:* Too breathless to leave the house or breathless when dressing or undressing

- How many level blocks can you walk without becoming short of breath?
- How many level blocks could you walk 6 months ago?
- What makes the SOB worse? What relieves it?

Other issues that are important in the assessment of dyspnea include: the patient's rating of the intensity of breathlessness, the effort required to breathe, and the severity of the breathlessness or dyspnea. Patients use a variety of terms and phrases to describe breathlessness, such as "can't get enough air," "hard to breath," "feeling tight," and the nurse needs to clarify what terms are most familiar to the patient and what these terms mean. Several scales are available to assess the severity of dyspnea, including visual analog scales similar to pain scales, where one side denotes no dyspnea and the extreme is maximal dyspnea. These scales can be used to assess changes in the severity of dyspnea over time (Norris, 2019). Box 7-4 illustrates one such scale.

Relief Measures. The management of dyspnea is aimed at identifying and correcting its cause. Relief of the symptom sometimes is achieved by placing the patient at rest with the head elevated (semi- to high Fowler position), encouraging the patient to lean forward with arms and upper body supported on a table (orthopneic position), and using pursed-lip breathing (i.e., breathing in through the mouth and exhaling slowly through pursed lips to facilitate exhalation of air). Medical and nursing intervention in the presence of acute dyspnea will include intravenous (IV) access, cardiac and pulse oximetry monitoring, O_2 administration in patients with hypoxemia (low O_2 saturation), and airway management equipment at the bedside. Specific treatment will depend on the cause of the dyspnea (i.e., chest tube insertion for pneumothorax, diuretics for HF). For COPD, pulmonary rehabilitation is helpful to improve exercise tolerance (see Chapter 10 for interventions for COPD) (Jameson et al., 2020).

Cough

A cough is one of the most common reasons for seeking heath care in the United States (Sharma, 2021). Involuntary coughing can be initiated by a variety of nerve receptors in the oropharynx, larynx, and tracheobronchial tree that can be stimulated by irritation (airborne irritants such as smoke, smog, perfume, powders, or dust), excess secretions, or a foreign body. These signals are transmitted to the vagus nerve and to the cough center (medulla). Although the cough is a reflex that protects the lungs from the accumulation of secretions or the inhalation of foreign bodies, it can also be a symptom of a number of disorders of the pulmonary system, or it can be suppressed in other disorders. Duration is an important factor to determine; a cough is considered acute if present for less than 3 weeks, persistent if between 3 and 8 weeks (termed subacute), and chronic if greater than 8 weeks.

An acute cough may indicate serious pulmonary disease, pulmonary infection, or inflammatory and neoplastic conditions, but they may be caused by a variety of other problems, including cardiac disease, medications (e.g., ACE inhibitors), smoking, aspiration, and many extrapulmonary conditions. Most commonly, an acute cough is due to an acute viral upper respiratory infection, also known as the common cold, and acute bronchitis (Sharma et al., 2021). A subacute cough frequently occurs after a respiratory infection due to continued irritation of cough receptors via ongoing or resolving bronchial or sinus inflammation (Sharma et al., 2021). A chronic cough is >8 weeks and is frequently associated with postnasal drip, asthma, and GERD (Goggins, 2022).

Pearls for Practice

A "dry" cough associated with ACE inhibitors occurs in 2% to 33% of patients (Chung & Mazzone, 2022). It is often associated with a sensation of a "tickle" in the throat, and may occur within a few hours of taking the medication or weeks to months after initiating therapy. The cough disappears within days or weeks after the medication is discontinued.

It is important to consider that the cough reflex may be impaired by weakness or paralysis of the respiratory or abdominal muscles. Risk factors include prolonged inactivity, surgery, the presence of an NG tube (may prevent closure of the glottis), or depressed function of the medullary centers in the brain (e.g., anesthesia, drugs that depress the cough center, brain disorders) predisposing the patient to pulmonary problems (Norris, 2019).

The nurse is aware that a persistent and frequent cough can be exhausting and have significant impact on the patient's lifestyle and sense of well-being. Coughs can be significant enough to cause incontinence, vomiting, rib fractures, cervical disc prolapse, pain, petechiae, and syncope.

Clinical Significance. To help determine the cause of the cough, the nurse needs the patient to describe the characteristics of the cough. A dry, irritative cough is a feature of an upper respiratory tract infection of viral origin, or a side effect of ACE inhibitor therapy. Laryngotracheitis causes an irritative, high-pitched cough. Tracheal lesions produce a brassy cough. Pertussis has a characteristic long, strident inspiratory noise (a whoop) before the cough. A hacking cough may be suggestive of pneumonia. A severe or changing cough may indicate bronchogenic carcinoma. Pleuritic chest pain that accompanies coughing may indicate pleural or chest wall (musculoskeletal) involvement.

The time of coughing is also noted. Coughing at night may herald the onset of left-sided HF or bronchial asthma. A cough in the morning with sputum production may indicate bronchitis. A cough that worsens when the patient is supine suggests postnasal drip (sinusitis) or reflux (spill-over of gastric contents into the larynx). Coughing after food intake may indicate aspiration of material into the tracheobronchial tree. A cough of recent onset is usually from a viral or upper respiratory tract infection.

Pearls for Practice

Coughs are not localized only to a pulmonary problem. For example, chronic cough without heartburn is seen in 75% of patients with GERD (Sharma et al., 2021). Common conditions associated with 90% of cases of chronic cough are postnasal drip, asthma, GERD, and the use of ACE inhibitors (even several months before the onset of cough) (Suneja et al., 2020).

Relief Measures. Treatment depends on the cause of the cough. Treatment may include cautious use of cough suppressants because, while they may relieve the cough, they do not address the etiology of the cough. Other treatments are antihistamines, decongestants, or nasal corticosteroids if the etiology of the cough is postnasal drip, or H_2-blockers or PPIs when cough is associated with GERD. If the cough is a result of irritation, smoking cessation strategies are indicated. Drinking warm beverages may relieve cough caused by throat irritation, and honey can provide symptomatic relief (Chung & Mazzone, 2022).

Sputum Production

Mucous membranes line the internal walls of the respiratory tract. Mucus maintains a moist internal environment that traps particles for removal. It is difficult to quantify normal sputum production since airway mucus is normally swallowed upon reaching the throat. Once coughed or spit out (expectorated), it is called sputum. A patient who coughs long enough almost invariably produces sputum. Sputum production is the reaction of the lungs to any constantly recurring irritant. It also may be associated with a nasal discharge.

Clinical Significance. The nature of the sputum is indicative of the causal condition. The nurse asks about the amount, frequency, color, consistency, and odor of sputum production. Since sputum production is unnoticed and swallowed, any complaint of sputum needs to be investigated. To help quantify the amount of sputum production, patients are asked to describe the volume of sputum production in terms of teaspoon (~5 mL) to cupful (~240 mL); however, this is difficult to calculate because of how much sputum may have been swallowed by the patient. When asking about frequency, the nurse consider sputum production during meals or with fluids which may suggest dysphagia and aspiration.

A profuse amount of purulent sputum (thick and yellow or green) is a common sign of bacterial infection, lung abscess, or bronchiectasis. However, colored sputum does not always indicate bacterial infection, since white cells in inflammatory processes affect sputum color (Goggins et al., 2022). A small amount of purulent sputum is associated with acute bronchitis, pneumonia during resolution, small tuberculous cavities, or lung abscess. Sputum that looks like currant jelly is associated with *Klebsiella pneumoniae.* Purulent rust-colored sputum suggests *pneumococcal pneumonia.* A gradual increase of sputum over time may indicate the presence of chronic bronchitis, which is defined as a productive cough for >3 months or bronchiectasis. Asthma patients also may have a productive cough due to excess mucus production. Expectorated blood-stained sputum tends to be a complaint of patients with bronchogenic carcinoma, PE, pulmonary arteriovenous malformations, bronchiectasis, bleeding disorders, and TB (Goggins et al., 2022). Profuse, frothy, white or pink material, often welling up into the throat, may indicate pulmonary edema. Foul-smelling sputum and bad breath point to the presence of a lung abscess, bronchiectasis, or an infection caused by anaerobic organisms. A musty odor may indicate pseudomonas infection, and foul-smelling sputum is noted in lung abscess or bronchiectasis (Gupta, 2019). In addition, in patients that are dehydrated, have altered consciousness, or have a weak cough, the nurse needs to be concerned about the potential for sputum retention.

Relief Measures. If the sputum is too thick for the patient to expectorate, it is necessary to decrease the sputum's viscosity by increasing its water content through adequate hydration (drinking water) and inhalation of aerosolized solutions, which may be delivered by any type of nebulizer. Unless contraindicated due to cardiac, liver, or kidney disease, an intake of 2,500 mL per day is suggested to decrease the viscosity of secretions and improve ciliary action in removing secretions (Haugen & Galura, 2020).

Smoking is contraindicated with excessive sputum production because it interferes with ciliary action, increases bronchial secretions, causes inflammation and hyperplasia of the mucous membranes, and reduces production of surfactant. When a person stops smoking, sputum volume decreases and resistance to bronchial infections increases.

The patient's appetite may decrease because of the odor of the sputum or the taste it leaves in the mouth. The nurse encourages adequate oral hygiene and wise selection of food, measures that stimulate the appetite.

Hemoptysis

Hemoptysis (bloody sputum) is a symptom of both pulmonary and cardiac disorders. The onset of hemoptysis is usually sudden, and it may be intermittent or continuous. Signs vary from blood-stained or steaked sputum to a large sudden life-threatening hemorrhage. Frank bloody sputum (obvious, visible presence of blood) may indicate a PE, bronchogenic carcinoma, or erosion of a bronchial artery by cavitary tuberculosis, whereas blood-stained sputum (streaks of blood) may indicate inflammation in the nose, nasopharynx, gums, larynx, or bronchi, or airway trauma from severe coughing, and is usually associated with smoking (Swartz, 2021). The amount of blood produced is not always proportional to the seriousness of the cause. Iatrogenic causes may include transbronchial lung biopsies, anticoagulation, or pulmonary artery rupture due to distal placement of a balloon-tipped catheter (Nadler & Gonzales, 2022). It is important to determine the presence of a respiratory infection and past or current tobacco use, and the nurse must exclude the bleeding is not hematemesis (vomiting blood) or epistaxis (nose bleed).

Pearls for Practice

Blood from the lung is usually bright red, frothy, and mixed with sputum. Initial symptoms include a tickling sensation in the throat, a salty taste, a burning or bubbling sensation in the chest, and perhaps chest pain, in which case the patient tends to splint the bleeding side. The nurse asks about any sensation of warmth in the chest which may indicated the location from which the hemoptysis originated (Swartz, 2021).

If the hemorrhage is in the stomach, the blood is vomited (hematemesis) rather than coughed up. Blood that has been in contact with gastric juice is sometimes so dark that it is referred to as "coffee grounds" and may be mixed with food. This blood generally has an acid pH.

Chest Pain

Chest pain or discomfort may be associated with pulmonary or cardiac disease. Chest pain associated with pulmonary conditions may be sharp, stabbing, and intermittent, or it may be dull, aching, and persistent. The pain usually is felt on the side where the pathologic process is located, but it may be referred elsewhere—for example, to the neck, back, or abdomen.

Clinical Significance. Chest pain may occur with pneumonia, PE with lung infarction, and pleurisy. Chest pain also may be a late symptom of bronchogenic carcinoma. In carcinoma, the pain may be dull and persistent because the cancer has invaded the chest wall, mediastinum, or spine.

Lung disease does not always cause thoracic pain because the lungs and the visceral pleura lack sensory nerves and are insensitive to pain stimuli. However, the parietal pleura has a rich supply of sensory nerves that are stimulated by inflammation and stretching of the membrane. Pleuritic pain from irritation of the parietal pleura is sharp and seems to "catch" on inspiration; patients often describe it as "like the stabbing of a knife." The nurse assesses the quality, intensity, and radiation of pain and identifies and explores precipitating factors and their relationship to the patient's position. In addition, it is important to assess the relationship of pain to the inspiratory and expiratory phases of respiration.

Relief Measures. Analgesic medications may be effective in relieving chest pain, but care must be taken not to depress the respiratory center or a productive cough, if present. Nonsteroidal anti-inflammatory drugs (NSAIDs) achieve this goal and, therefore, are used for pleuritic pain. A regional anesthetic block may be performed to relieve extreme pain. Patients may be more comfortable when they lie on the affected side because this splints the chest wall, limits expansion and contraction of the lung, and reduces the friction between the injured or diseased pleura on that side. Pain associated with cough, deep breathing, or changing position may be reduced manually by splinting the rib cage with hands or pillows.

Wheezing

Wheezing is often the major finding in a patient with bronchoconstriction, edema or secretions and is associated with partially obstructed airway. It is heard with or without a stethoscope, depending on its location. Wheezing is a high-pitched, musical sound heard mainly on expiration; however, it may be heard on both inspiration and expiration. Wheezing is associated with a variety of clinical conditions other than asthma such as a foreign body, HF, or acute bronchitis. The nurse needs to assess for all possible etiologies (discussed later in this chapter). Oral or inhalant bronchodilator medications reverse wheezing in most instances.

Pearls for Practice

If a patient has severe bronchospasm, there may be an absence of wheezing or gas movement. Thus, a "quiet" chest is a "scary" chest.

Patient and Family History

The nurse also assesses for risk factors and genetics factors that may contribute to the patient's lung condition (Boxes 7-5 and 7-6).

BOX 7-5 Risk Factors for Respiratory Disease

- Smoking (the single most important contributor to lung disease)
- Exposure to secondhand smoke
- Personal or family history of lung disease
- Genetic makeup
- Allergens and environmental pollutants
- Recreational and occupational exposure

BOX 7-6 Risk Factors for Hypoventilation

- Limited neurologic impulses transmitted from the brain to the respiratory muscles, as in spinal cord trauma, cerebrovascular accidents, tumors, myasthenia gravis, Guillain–Barré syndrome, polio, and drug overdose
- Depressed respiratory centers in the medulla, as with anesthesia, sedation, and drug overdose
- Limited thoracic movement (e.g., kyphoscoliosis), limited lung movement (e.g., pleural effusion, pneumothorax), or reduced functional lung tissue (e.g., chronic pulmonary diseases, severe pulmonary edema, decreased lung volumes with obesity)

Social History

The nurse inquires about current or past smoking and calculates pack/year history. This is calculated by the number of packs smoked per day times the number of years the patient has smoked. Thus, 2 packs per day times 20 years equals a 40-pack/year history.

The impact of signs and symptoms on the patient's ability to perform ADLs and to participate in usual work and family activities is assessed. Questions related to sleep–rest patterns should include asking about nocturnal dyspnea (waking up with SOB) or orthopnea as well as quantifying the number of pillows used at night. In addition, psychosocial factors that may affect the patient are explored. These factors include anxiety, role changes, family relationships, financial problems, employment status, and the strategies the patient uses to cope with them. It is also important to ask questions concerning immunizations, medications, exposure to environmental hazards, use of O_2, hospitalizations, and medical and surgical history. Many respiratory diseases are chronic and progressively debilitating and disabling. Therefore, ongoing assessment of the patient's physical abilities, psychosocial supports, and quality of life is needed to plan appropriate interventions. It is important that the patient with a respiratory disorder understand the condition and be familiar with necessary self-care interventions. The nurse evaluates these factors over time and provides education as needed.

Physical Assessment

Complete respiratory assessment includes assessment of the integument and upper and lower respiratory structures. The nurse also observes the work of breathing (e.g., nasal flaring, mouth breathing, use of accessory muscles, splinting).

Pearls for Practice

Before entering the room, the nurse can begin a pulmonary assessment by observing the patient's position and ease of breathing. Use of accessory muscles, an open mouth, nasal flaring, suprasternal, substernal or intercostal retractions, and an inability to lie flat in the bed are observed, as is the number of pillows used for comfort. The nurse asks the patient how many pillows they use at night to obtain relief from SOB (described as orthopnea) and notes on the EMR the number of pillows required for patient relief (e.g., two- or three-pillow orthopnea). The nurse also assesses for paroxysmal nocturnal dyspnea, which is commonly associated with left-sided heart failure (see Chapter 11).

Assessment of the Integumentary System

Respiratory conditions may have skin and nail manifestations.

Inspection of Color

Cyanosis, a bluish coloring of the skin, is a very late indicator of hypoxia. The presence or absence of cyanosis is determined by the amount of unoxygenated hemoglobin in the blood. Cyanosis appears when there is at least 5 g/dL of unoxygenated hemoglobin (normal hemoglobin is approximately 15 g/dL). Thus, a full one third of the hemoglobin is deoxygenated before cyanosis is observed. In addition, a patient with anemia rarely manifests cyanosis, and a patient with polycythemia may appear cyanotic even if adequately oxygenated. Thus, cyanosis is *not* a reliable sign of hypoxia.

Assessment of cyanosis is affected by room lighting, the thickness of the patients skin, the amount of melanin in the patient's skin, and the distance of the blood vessels from the surface of the skin. Cheeks, nose, ears, and oral mucosa are the best areas to assess cyanosis as the skin in these areas is thin, and blood supply is generous (Pahal & Goyal, 2022). Central cyanosis (tongue and lips), often associated with clubbing of the fingers and toes, indicates inadequate oxygenation of blood, whereas peripheral cyanosis (nailbeds) results from vasoconstriction or diminished peripheral blood flow in the distal extremities from a variety of causes and does not necessarily indicate a central systemic problem. In addition, the two may coexist. In people with melanin-rich skin, the nurse assesses for central cyanosis by examining for dull, dark color in the buccal mucosa (inside of the cheek) and hard palate (roof of the mouth).

Inspection for Clubbing of the Fingers

Clubbing of the fingers is found in patients with chronic hypoxic conditions, chronic lung and pleural infections, or malignancies of the lung and pleural. It is also associated with cyanotic congenital heart disease, infective endocarditis, GI disease, and chronic hepatic fibrosis (Swartz, 2021; Burcovschii & Aboeed, 2021). It is painless, usually bilateral, and may be reversed if the causative factor is removed (Suneja et al., 2020). This finding may be manifested initially as sponginess of the nail bed and loss of the nail bed angle, resulting in a bulbous enlargement of the distal segments of the fingers and toes (see Chapter 50, Box 50-4). It may be related to vascular endothelial growth factor (VEGF), which leads to increased vascularity, permeability, and ultimately connective tissue changes (Burcovschii & Aboeed, 2021).

Assessment of Upper Respiratory Structures

For a routine examination of the upper airway, only a simple light source, such as a penlight, is necessary.

Inspection and Palpation of Nose and Sinuses

The nurse inspects the external nose for lesions, asymmetry, or inflammation and then asks the patient to tilt the head backward. Gently pushing the tip of the nose upward, the nurse examines the internal structures of the nose, inspecting the mucosa and septum for color, swelling, exudate, or bleeding. The nasal mucosa is normally redder than the oral mucosa. It may appear swollen and hyperemic if the patient has a common cold, but in allergic rhinitis, the mucosa appears pale and swollen. Most people have a slight degree of septal deviation, but actual displacement of the cartilage into either the right or left side of the nose may produce nasal obstruction. Such deviation usually causes no symptoms. Observation of nasal flaring and mouth breathing suggests respiratory distress. Next, the nurse may palpate the frontal and maxillary sinuses for tenderness, which suggests inflammation. Using the thumbs, gentle pressure is applied in an upward fashion at the supraorbital ridges (frontal sinuses) and in the cheek area adjacent to the nose (maxillary sinuses) (Fig. 7-6).

Inspection of Pharynx and Mouth

The mouth and pharynx are assessed by asking the patient to open the mouth wide and take a deep breath. Usually, this flattens the posterior tongue and briefly allows a full view of the anterior and posterior pillars, tonsils, uvula, and posterior pharynx (Fig. 7-7). These structures are inspected for color, symmetry, and evidence of exudate, ulceration, or enlargement. If a tongue blade is needed to depress the tongue to visualize the pharynx, it is pressed firmly down on the midpoint of the arched tongue to avoid a gagging reflex (Bickley, 2021).

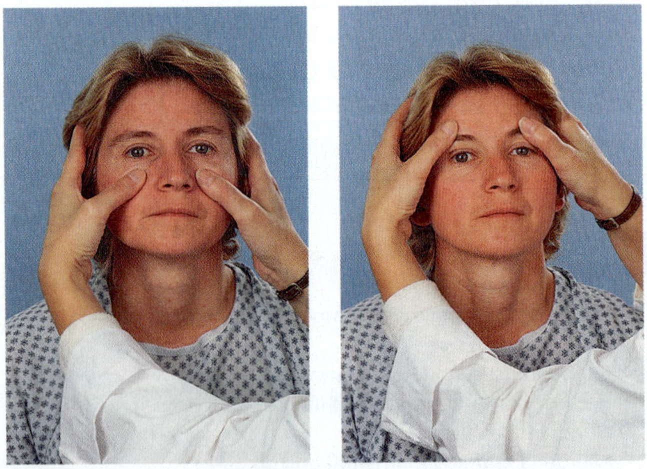

FIGURE 7-6 Technique for palpating the frontal sinuses at left and the maxillary sinuses at right.

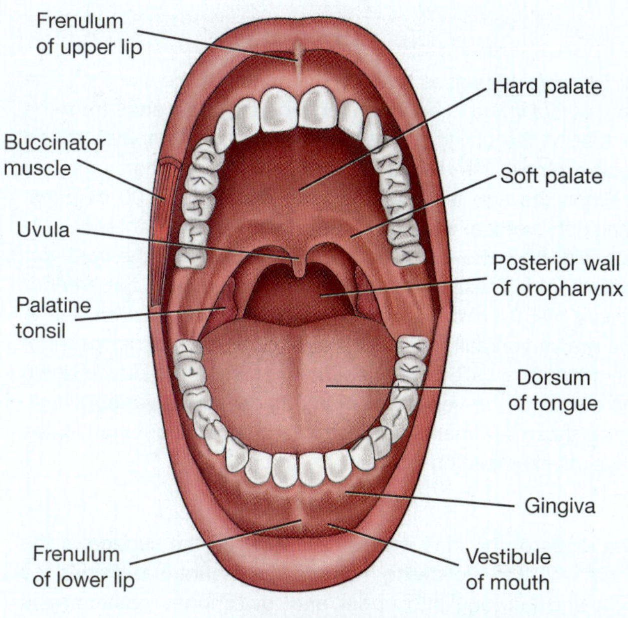

FIGURE 7-7 The pharynx and other oral structures—pillars, tonsils, uvula, hard and soft palates, posterior pharynx, and tongue—are easily seen when the mouth is open.

Palpation of the Trachea

The position and mobility of the trachea are noted by placing the thumb and index finger of one hand on either side of the trachea just above the sternal notch. The trachea is highly sensitive, and palpating too firmly may trigger a coughing or gagging response. The trachea is normally in the midline as it enters the thoracic inlet behind the sternum, but it may be deviated by masses in the neck or mediastinum. The trachea may deviate away from a life-threatening tension pneumothorax and toward an atelectasis or fibrosis of the lung (Suneja et al., 2020).

Physical Assessment of the Lower Respiratory Structures and Breathing

Lower respiratory assessment consists of four areas: inspection, palpation, percussion, and auscultation. The patient should be positioned upright, if possible, to assess the posterior thorax and lungs, and supine to assess the anterior chest and lung with chest exposed. The patient should be draped to protect privacy and facilitate patient comfort during the exam.

Thoracic Inspection

The nurse observes the skin over the thorax for color and turgor and for evidence of loss of subcutaneous tissue. In recording or reporting the findings, anatomic landmarks are used as points of reference (Box 7-7). Normally, there is symmetry in chest movement. It is important to note asymmetry, if present. In thin people, it is quite normal to note a slight retraction of the ICSs during quiet breathing. Bulging of the ICSs during expiration implies obstruction of expiratory airflow, as in emphysema. Marked retraction on inspiration, particularly if asymmetric, implies blockage of a branch of the respiratory tree. Asymmetric bulging of the ICSs, on one side or the other, is created by an increase in pressure within the hemithorax. This may be a result of air trapped under pressure within the pleural cavity, where it is not normally present (pneumothorax), or the pressure of fluid within the pleural space (pleural effusion).

Pearls for Practice

Frequently, patients with COPD are found to have cachexia and muscle dysfunction. These patients should be screened for malnutrition and referred to a nutrition practitioner when there is diminished nutritional intake or weight loss (Haugen & Galura, 2020).

Chest Configuration. Normally, the ratio of the AP diameter to the lateral diameter is 1:2. However, four main deformities of the chest are associated with respiratory disease that alter this relationship: barrel chest, funnel chest (pectus excavatum), pigeon chest (pectus carinatum), and kyphoscoliosis (see Fig. 7-8).

Barrel chest occurs as a result of lung hyperinflation, as in emphysema. There is an increase in the AP diameter of the thorax so that it approximates a 1:1 ratio. In a patient with emphysema, note the costal angle will also be greater than 90 degrees.

Funnel chest or pectus excavatum is the most common developmental chest wall deformity. It is a depression in the lower portion of the sternum, so that the sternum appears "bowl-like," and the AP ratio may be less than 1:2. It may be symmetrical or asymmetrical to the midline of the sternum. Most patients are asymptomatic but if the depression is marked, patients may have restriction on PFTs and obstructive or restrictive lung disease with aging; thus, medical-surgical nurses should assess these patients' pulmonary function thoroughly and encourage the use of the incentive spirometer (IS) (Sharma & Carter, 2021). In addition, abnormalities of the mitral valve, especially mitral valve prolapse (MVP), arrhythmias, and conduction defects may be seen with this deformity; thus, an electrocardiogram, and echocardiogram are performed to evaluate cardiac function (Swartz, 2021). Refer to a pediatric resource for further details.

Pectus carinatum is also a congenital structural abnormality in which the sternum is displaced anteriorly, increasing the AP diameter. For some patients, this deformity is associated with a rigid chest wall in which the AP diameter is almost fixed in full inspiration. In some patients, reduced pulmonary endurance is seen (McHam & Winkler, 2022).

A *kyphoscoliosis* is characterized by elevation of the scapula and a corresponding S-shaped spine. This deformity limits lung expansion within the thorax. It may occur with osteoporosis and other skeletal disorders that affect the thorax.

BOX 7-7

Locating Thoracic Landmarks

With respect to the thorax, location is defined both horizontally and vertically. With respect to the lungs, location is defined by lobe.

Horizontal Reference Points

Horizontally, thoracic locations are identified according to their proximity to the rib or the intercostal space under the examiner's fingers. On the anterior surface, identification of a specific rib is facilitated by first locating the angle of Louis. This is where the manubrium joins the body of the sternum in the midline. The second rib joins the sternum at this prominent landmark.

Other ribs may be identified by counting down from the second rib. The intercostal spaces are referred to in terms of the rib immediately above the intercostal space; for example, the fifth intercostal space is directly below the fifth rib.

Locating ribs on the posterior surface of the thorax is more difficult. The first step is to identify the spinous process. This is accomplished by finding the seventh cervical vertebra (*vertebra prominens*), which is the most prominent spinous process. When the neck is slightly flexed, the seventh cervical spinous process stands out. Other vertebrae are then identified by counting downward.

Vertical Reference Points

Several imaginary lines are used as vertical referents or landmarks to identify the location of thoracic findings. The *midsternal line* passes through the center of the sternum. The *midclavicular line* is an imaginary line that descends from the middle of the clavicle. The *point of maximal impulse* of the heart normally lies medial to this line on the left thorax.

When the arm is abducted from the body at 90 degrees, imaginary vertical lines may be drawn from the anterior axillary fold, from the middle of the axilla, and from the posterior axillary fold. These lines are called, respectively, the *anterior axillary line*, the *midaxillary line*, and the *posterior axillary line*. A line drawn vertically through the superior and inferior poles of the scapula is called the *scapular line*, and a line drawn down the center of the vertebral column is called the *vertebral line*. Using these landmarks, for example, the nurse communicates physical examination findings.

Lobes of the Lungs

The lobes of the lung may be mapped on the surface of the chest wall in the following manner. The fissure that divides the right and left lung into upper and lower lobes posteriorly is termed the oblique fissure. It begins at T3 (spinous process) and obliquely to sixth rib in the midclavicular line (MCL) bilaterally. The right lung is further divided anteriorly by the horizontal fissure, which runs close to the fourth rib at the sternal border (SB) to the fifth rib in the midaxillary line (MAL). There is no presentation of the right middle lobe on the posterior surface of the chest.

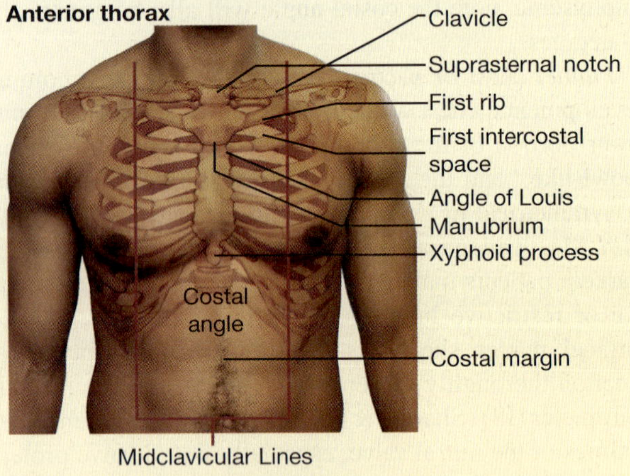

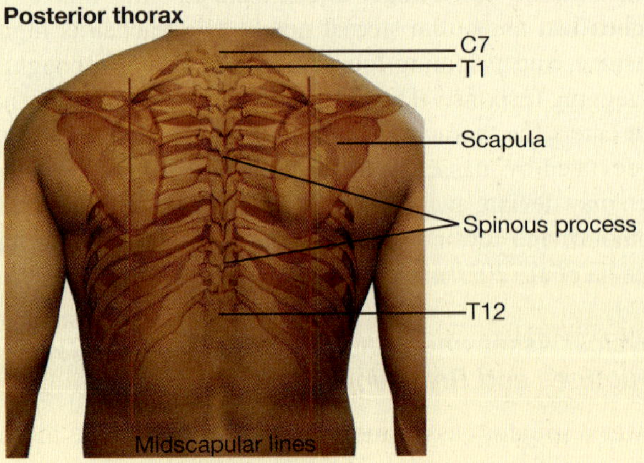

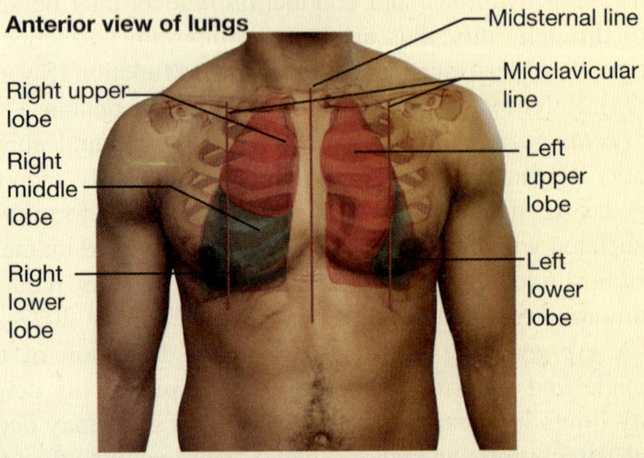

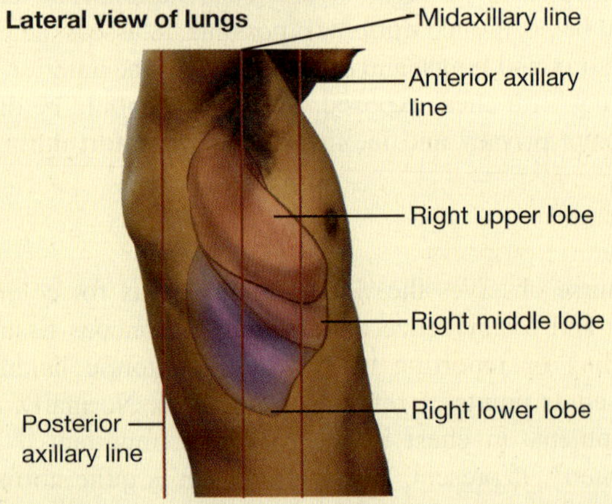

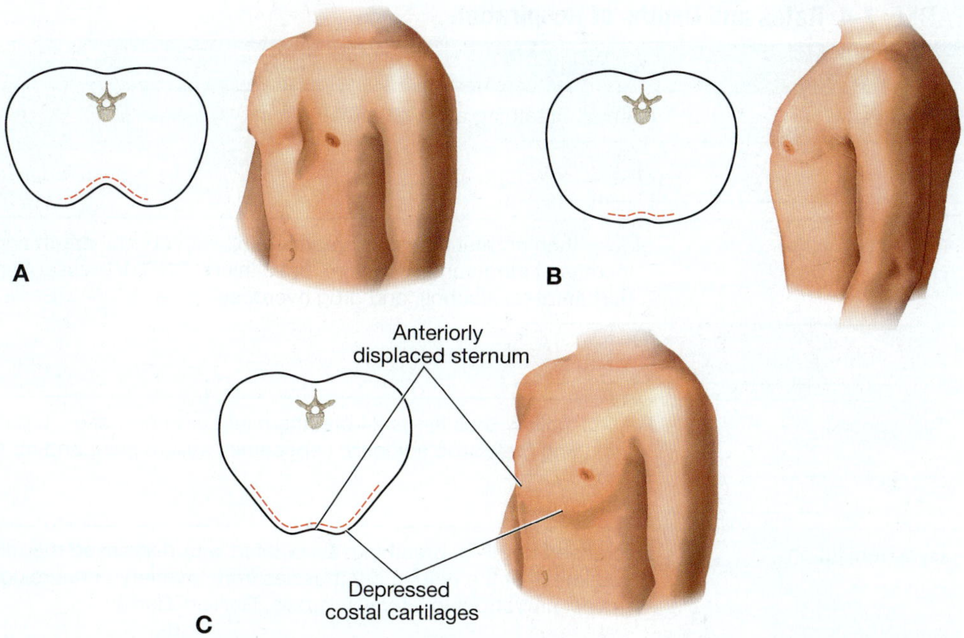

FIGURE 7-8 Deformities of the thoracic wall. (A) Funnel chest (pectus excavatum); (B) Barrel chest; (C) Pigeon chest (pectus carinatum).

In addition, the nurse notes the presence of paradoxical chest movements known as a *flail chest*, which occurs with multiple ipsilateral (same side) rib fractures. In this condition, asymmetrical chest movements are observed; during inspiration, the unstable chest wall collapses inward and then bulges outward with expiration. It is associated with respiratory distress and crepitus (see later discussion). The priorities for a flail chest include maintaining adequate ventilation (which can include intubation and ventilator management), fluid management, pain control, and management of the unstable chest wall, which may include surgical stabilization of the fractures (Perera & King, 2022).

Breathing Patterns and Respiratory Rates. Observing the rate and depth of respiration is a simple but important aspect of assessment. The normal adult who is resting comfortably takes 12 to 20 breaths per minute. Except for occasional sighs, respirations are regular in depth and rhythm. This normal pattern is described as *eupnea.*

Certain patterns of respiration are characteristic of specific disease states. Respiratory rhythms and their deviation from normal are important observations that the nurse reports and documents. The rates and depths of various patterns of respiration are presented in Table 7-4.

Pearls for Practice

One should not rely on only visual inspection of the rate and depth of a patient's respiratory excursions to determine the adequacy of ventilation. Respiratory excursions may appear normal or exaggerated due to an increased work of breathing, but actually the patient may be moving only enough air to ventilate the dead space. If there is any question regarding adequacy of ventilation, auscultation or pulse oximetry (or both) should be used for additional assessment of respiratory status.

Thoracic Palpation

The nurse palpates the thorax for tenderness, masses, lesions, respiratory excursion, vocal fremitus, and crepitus.

Respiratory Excursion. Respiratory excursion is an estimation of thoracic range and expansion and may disclose significant information about thoracic movement during breathing. The patient is instructed to inhale deeply while the movement of the nurse's thumbs is observed (placed along the costal margin on the anterior chest wall) during inspiration and expiration. This movement is normally symmetric.

Posterior assessment is performed by placing the thumbs adjacent to the spinal column at the level of the tenth rib (Fig. 7-9). The hands lightly grasp the lateral rib cage. Sliding the thumbs medially about 2.5 cm (1 in) raises a small skinfold between the thumbs. The patient is instructed to take a full inspiration and to exhale fully. The nurse observes for normal flattening of the skinfold and feels the symmetric movement of the thorax.

Asymmetric excursion may be due to a localized problem in the underlying chest wall, pleura, or lung; causes include pain (fractured ribs, trauma, splinting secondary to pleurisy or incisional pain), fibrosis, consolidation (lobar pneumonia), pleural effusion, or unilateral bronchial obstruction (Bickley, 2021). Equal but diminished expansion is seen in neurologic disease and emphysema.

Tactile Fremitus. The detection of palpable sound vibration transmitted to the chest wall as the patient speaks is

TABLE **7-4 Rates and Depths of Respiration**

	Definition
Eupnea 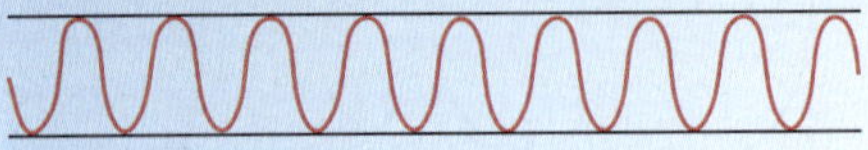	Normal, breathing at 12–20 breaths/min
Bradypnea 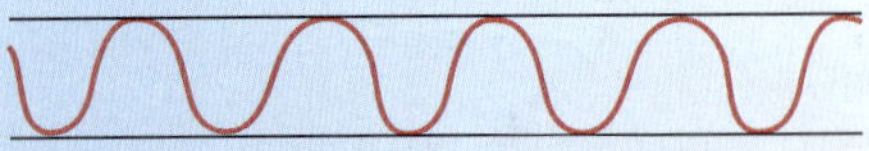	Slower than normal rate (<10 breaths/min), with normal depth and regular rhythm; associated with increased intracranial pressure, brain injury, CNS depressants (e.g., opiates, benzodiazepines, barbiturates, alcohol), and drug overdose
Tachypnea 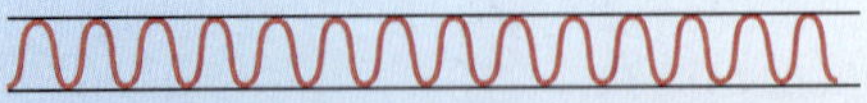	Rapid, shallow breathing >24 breaths/min; commonly seen in patients with a number of causes including metabolic acidosis, septicemia, severe pain, and rib fracture
Hypoventilation 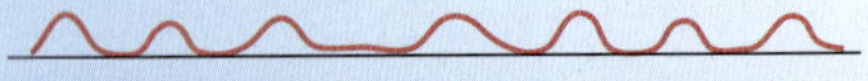	Decreased depth of breathing; associated with decreased medullary respiratory center drive, weakness of the respiratory muscles from a variety of neurologic disorders (e.g., myasthenia gravis, amyotrophic lateral sclerosis, Guillain–Barré)
Hyperventilation 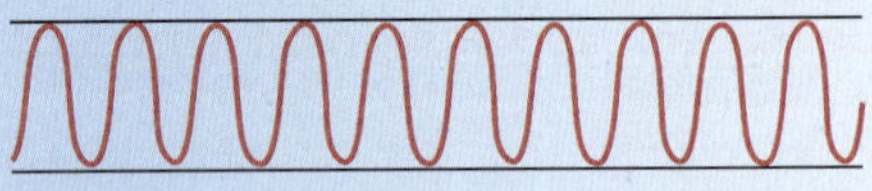	Increased rate and depth of breathing associated with severe acidosis of diabetic or renal origin and hypoxemia. *Kussmaul respiration* if caused by diabetic ketoacidosis is increased depth of breathing, however the respiratory rate may be fast, normal, or slow (Bickley et al., 2021).
Apnea 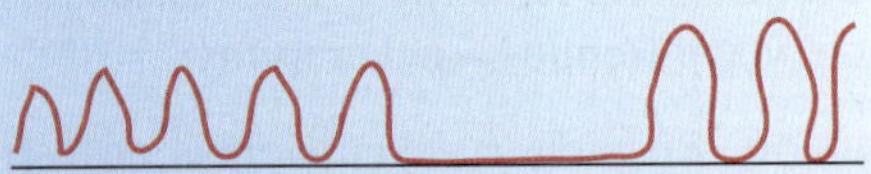	Period of cessation of breathing. Time duration varies; apnea may occur briefly during other breathing disorders, such as with sleep apnea. Life-threatening if sustained.
Cheyne–Stokes 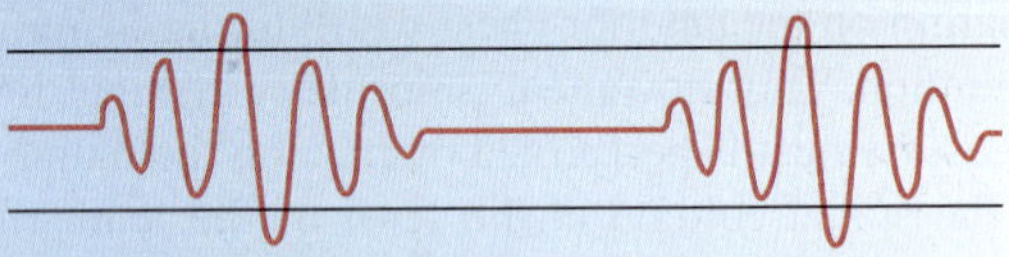	Regular cycle in which the rate and depth of breathing increase and then decrease until apnea (usually about 20 seconds) occurs. It may be seen during the sleep of normal children and the aged, also associated with heart failure and damage to the respiratory center (drug-induced, tumor, trauma).
Biot respiration 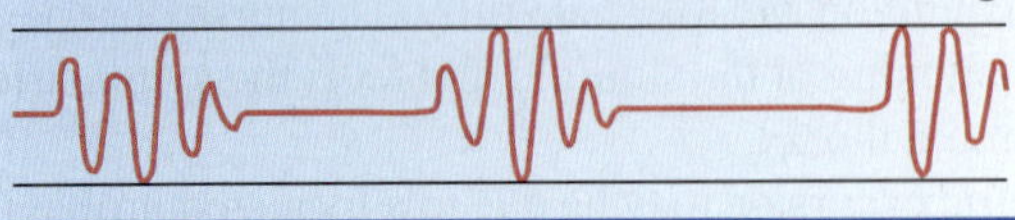	Irregular pattern, with periods of normal breathing (3–4 breaths) followed by a varying period of apnea (usually 10–60 seconds). Uncommon, but associated with some central nervous system disorders, meningitis, brain injury at the medullary level (Bickley et al, 2021).

called *tactile fremitus.* Thus, the sound that is started at the larynx moves down through the bronchial tree to the lung parenchyma and is then transmitted out to the chest wall. It provides useful information about the density of the underlying lung tissue (Swartz, 2021). Normal fremitus is widely varied. It is influenced by thickness of the chest wall, especially with an increase in subcutaneous tissue associated with obesity, and pitch (lower-pitched sounds travel better and produce greater vibration of the chest wall). Vibrations are felt easier with a thin patient and more difficult with a muscular or obese patient. Fremitus is most pronounced in the second ICS lateral to the sternum and medial to the scapula, the level of the bronchus. Therefore, it is most palpable in the upper thorax, anteriorly and posteriorly.

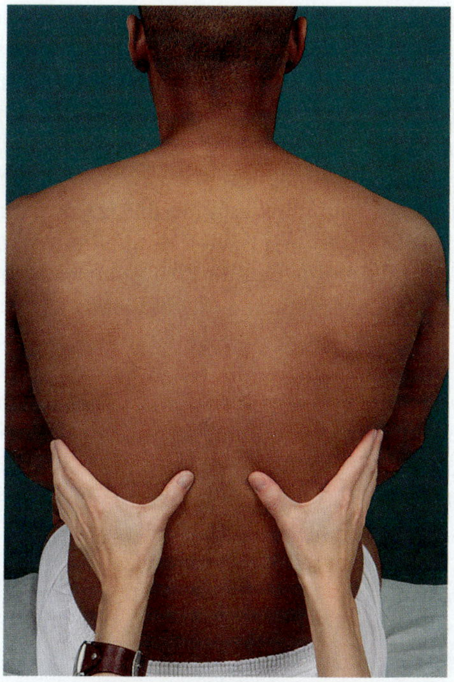

FIGURE 7-9 **Method for assessing posterior respiratory excursion. Place both hands posteriorly at the level of T9 or T10. Slide hands medially to pinch a small amount of skin between your thumbs. Observe for symmetry as the patient exhales fully following a deep inspiration.**

The patient is asked to fold their arms across the chest wall touching the opposite shoulder to displace both scapulae and to repeat "99" or "1, 2, 3" as the nurse's hands move down the patient's thorax comparing vibrations from similar areas (Fig. 7-10). Firm pressure is important to detect vibratory sensations effectively (Teall et al., 2021). Some clinicians test for fremitus using both hands simultaneously to compare the two sides, whereas others prefer a systematic survey of the chest wall with one hand. The vibrations are detected with the palmar surfaces of the fingers and hands, or the ulnar aspect of the extended hands, on the thorax. Bony areas are not tested.

Air does not conduct sound well, but a solid substance such as fluid that increases the density of the lung that occurs in pneumonia, does. Therefore, an increase in solid tissue of the normally air-filled lung enhances fremitus, and conversely, an increase of air of the lung impedes sound. Patients with emphysema, which results in trapping of air, exhibit almost no tactile fremitus. A patient with consolidation of a lobe of the lung from pneumonia has increased tactile fremitus over that lobe. Air in the pleural space does not conduct sound; thus, a pneumothorax will have absent fremitus (Bickley, 2021). In the case of pleural effusion, decreased fremitus is noted at the effusion; however, the lung above the effusion may reveal increased fremitus as the fluid compresses the lung.

Crepitus. Crepitus or subcutaneous emphysema is indicated by the presence of air bubbles in the subcutaneous tissues or underlying muscle; upon palpation, the sensation of bubbles under the fingers can be felt and, occasionally, crackling can be heard. Crepitus is not painful. The gas bubbles move with palpation. It is associated with pneumothorax, trauma (e.g., fractured rib piercing the lung), surgical wounds, or gas gangrene.

Thoracic Percussion

Percussion sets the chest wall and underlying structures in motion, producing audible and tactile vibrations. It helps to determine whether underlying tissues are filled with air, fluid, or solid material and is used to estimate diaphragmatic excursion. If possible, the patient is positioned in a sitting

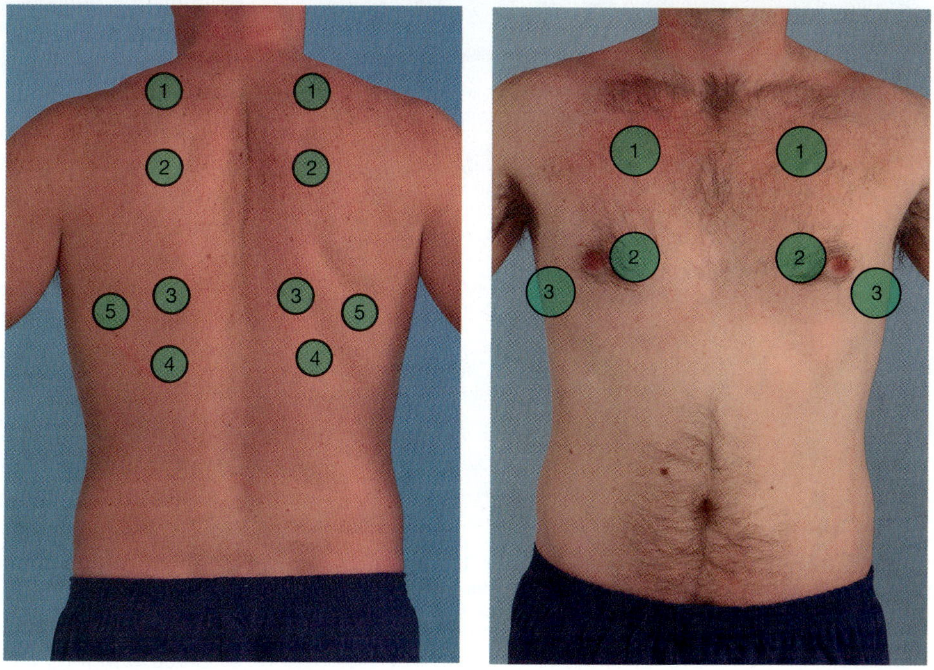

FIGURE 7-10 **The palpation sequence for tactile fremitus.**

position with the head flexed forward and the arms crossed in front of the chest touching the opposite shoulder, which exposes more lung area for assessment by separating the scapulae widely. The nurse maintains a position to the side of the patient in order to comfortably and firmly hyperextend the middle finger of the nondominant hand (pleximeter finger) in the ICSs, being careful to avoid contact with any other finger on the chest wall as sound will be dampened. Bony structures (scapulae or ribs) are not percussed. While the middle finger is positioned firmly against the chest wall in the ICS, the middle finger of the opposite hand strikes the pleximeter finger in a quick and sharp manner. The striking finger aims for the distal interphalangeal joint (below the nail and above the distal joint). The term to describe the sound heard over a normal lung is resonant. Normally dullness is heard over bone; thus, if this sound is noted over lung tissue, it is associated with consolidation, such as from pneumonia or a tumor. Hyperresonant sounds, which are louder and lower-pitched sounds, are associated with COPD or pneumothorax. It takes practice to develop comfort striking the finger with a quick, sharp but relaxed wrist motion and training to distinguish dullness, resonance, and hyperresonance. The sound will penetrate only 5 to 7 cm, so any density below this depth will not be discovered. The nurse proceeds down the posterior thorax, percussing in symmetric areas on each side at intervals of 5 to 6 cm (2 to 2.5 in) from the apex to the base (Fig. 7-11). Dullness over the lung occurs when air-filled lung tissue is replaced by fluid or solid tissue.

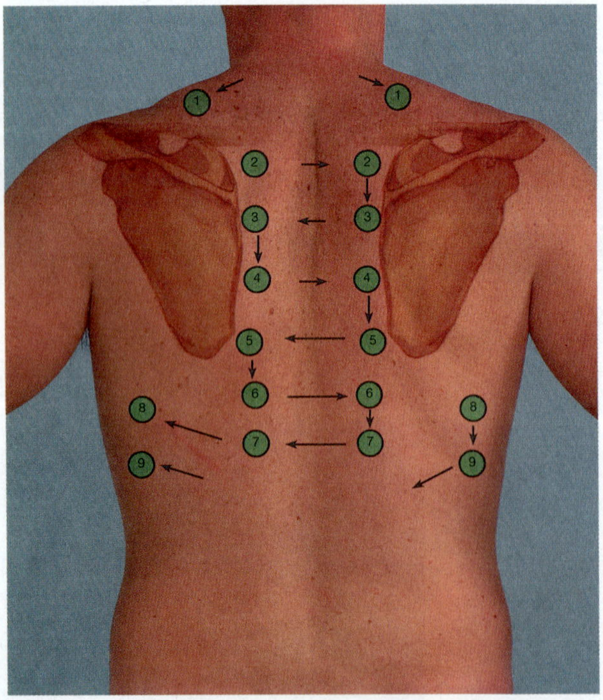

FIGURE 7-11 Percussion of the posterior thorax. With the patient in a sitting position, symmetric areas of the lungs are percussed at 5-cm intervals. This progression starts at the apex of each lung and concludes with percussion of each lateral chest wall.

Diaphragmatic Excursion. The normal resonance of the lung stops at the diaphragm. The position of the diaphragm is different during inspiration and expiration. Initially, the nurse determines the change from resonance (normal lung) to dullness (structures below the diaphragm) during normal breathing. Posteriorly, the lung normally ends at the tenth ICS with quiet respiration, and the diaphragm is generally two interspaces below this level. The point on the midscapular line at which the percussion changes from resonance to dullness is marked with a pen. An additional area medial or lateral to this area should be assessed to confirm the change to dullness. Then the patient is instructed to inhale fully and hold it while the nurse again percusses downward from the marked area to the new level of dullness of the diaphragm. With deep inspiration, the diaphragm descends. This point is also marked. The distance between the two markings indicates the range of motion of the diaphragm. The new position for the transition between resonance and dullness is 5 to 6 cm lower in healthy adults as their diaphragms descend with deeper breaths (Suneja et al., 2020). Decreased diaphragmatic excursion may occur with pleural effusion, a paralyzed hemidiaphragm, and emphysema.

Thoracic Auscultation

Auscultation is useful in assessing the flow of air through the bronchial tree and in evaluating the presence of fluid or solid obstruction in the lung. The nurse places the ear tips of the stethoscope with the ear pieces facing forward (in the same direction as your ear canal). Many stethoscopes come with a variety of ear tips. Choose the ones that create the best seal. Following hand hygiene, the nurse warms the stethoscope in their hands before applying directly to the patient's skin.

The nurse auscultates for normal breath sounds, adventitious (additional or abnormal) sounds, and voice sounds. Examination includes auscultation of the anterior, posterior, and lateral thorax and is performed as follows. The nurse places the diaphragm of the stethoscope firmly against the chest wall as the patient breathes slowly and deeply through an open mouth. Corresponding areas of the chest are auscultated in a systematic fashion from the apices to the bases (anteriorly, and posteriorly) and along MALs (lateral). The sequence of auscultation and the positioning of the patient are similar to those used for percussion. Often it is necessary to listen to two full inspirations and expirations at each anatomic location for valid interpretation of the sound heard. Repeated deep breaths may result in symptoms of hyperventilation (e.g., lightheadedness); this is avoided by having the patient rest and breathe normally periodically during the examination.

Breath Sounds. The diaphragm of the stethoscope is used to assess for lung sounds. Normal breath sounds are distinguished by their location over a specific area of the lung and are identified as bronchial (tubular), which may possibly be heard over the manubrium; bronchovesicular, which are heard at the first and second ICS, at approximately the angle of Louis anteriorly and between the scapula posteriorly; and vesicular (dominant sound over the remaining lung) breath sounds. In bronchial breath sounds, the inspiration phase is shorter than expiration; in bronchovesicular sounds, inspiration and expiration phases are equal; and with vesicular sounds, inspiration is longer than expiration.

The location, quality, and intensity of breath sounds are determined during auscultation. As the nurse moves down the chest wall, the sounds decrease. When airflow is decreased by fluid (pleural effusion) or tissue (obesity), breath sounds may be diminished or absent. For example, the breath sounds of the patient with emphysema are faint or often completely inaudible. Bronchial and bronchovesicular sounds that are audible anywhere except over the main bronchus in the lungs signify pathology, usually indicating consolidation in the lung (e.g., pneumonia). This finding requires further evaluation.

Adventitious Sounds. An abnormal condition that affects the bronchial tree and alveoli may produce adventitious sounds that are superimposed over usual breath sounds. Adventitious sounds include discrete, noncontinuous sounds (**crackles**); continuous musical sounds (wheezes); low-pitched rattling sounds (rhonchi); loud and high-pitched sound (stridor); and a creaking or grating sound (pleural friction rub) (Table 7-5).

TABLE **7-5 Abnormal (Adventitious) Breath Sounds**

Breath Sound	Description	Etiology
Crackles		
Crackles in general	Soft, high-pitched, discontinuous popping sounds that occur during inspiration; sounds like several hairs rubbing together between the thumb and index finger	Secondary to fluid in the airways or alveoli or to opening of collapsed alveoli; when present in patients without lung disease, crackles (formerly termed rales) are specific for heart failure (HF).
Coarse crackles	Discontinuous popping sounds heard in early inspiration and may last throughout expiration; harsh, louder, lower-pitched sound originating in the large bronchi	Associated with obstructive pulmonary disease, asthma, pneumonia
Fine crackles	Discontinuous high-pitched popping sounds heard in mid- late inspiration especially in dependent areas of the lung; originates in the alveoli	Associated with interstitial pneumonia, restrictive pulmonary disease (e.g., fibrosis), atelectasis, HF. In HF, crackles may be heard widely over both lung fields (typically beginning at the bases) and may be accompanied by expiratory wheezing (cardiac asthma).
Wheezes		
Wheezes	Musical sound, usually heard on expiration but may be heard on inspiration or both phases, can be low pitched or high	Associated with turbulent airflow and small airway vibration in which there is partial obstruction, commonly seen with COPD, asthma, and bronchitis
Rhonchi	Coarse, discontinuous, low-pitched rumbling sounds that are heard more pronounced during expiration; caused by air moving through an airway obstructed by thick secretions, muscular spasm, tumor, or external pressure (Ball et al., 2023)	Secretions within the larger airways that clear or change significantly after an effective cough; heard in a wide variety of pathologies, any of which cause increased secretions (e.g., cystic fibrosis, pneumonia, bronchitis or emphysema)
Stridor	Loud, rough, continuous, high-pitched sound that is pronounced during inspiration; it indicates proximal airway obstruction.	Turbulent air flowing through a narrowed trachea or larynx; loudest over the trachea. Commonly a medical emergency that needs to be recognized early. Diagnoses include epiglottitis, vocal cord dysfunction, croup, fixed obstruction, and airway edema (which could be secondary to trauma or an allergic reaction)
Friction Rubs		
Pleural friction rub	Harsh, crackling sound, like two pieces of leather being rubbed together. Heard during inspiration alone or during both inspiration and expiration. May subside when patient holds breath. Coughing will not clear sound. Auscultate in the region where patient complains of pleuritic pain.	Secondary to inflammation and loss of lubricating pleural fluid

Crackles (formerly referred to as *rales*) are discrete, noncontinuous sounds that result from delayed reopening of deflated airways or air bubbling through small fluid-filled distal airway as in HF (Suneja et al., 2020). The sound resembles hairs being rubbed together. They may be classified as fine or coarse. Fine crackles are noncontinuous high-pitched sounds that have a popping quality, usually heard during inspiratory. Coarse crackles are a lower pitch and louder. It will take time for the nurse to identify the discrete differences. Crackles may or may not be cleared by coughing depending on the etiology. They reflect underlying inflammation or congestion and often are present in such conditions as pneumonia, bronchitis, HF, bronchiectasis, atelectasis, and pulmonary fibrosis. Usually crackles are heard on inspiration, but they also may be heard on expiration.

Wheezes are associated with bronchial wall oscillation and changes in airway diameter. Although usually heard on expiration, wheezes may be heard on inspiration, or both phases. They are commonly heard in patients with asthma, chronic bronchitis, or bronchiectasis.

Rhonchi are low-pitched gurgling sounds produced by secretions within the larger airways. Rhonchi clear or change significantly after an effective cough. Rhonchi is associated with pneumonia, COPD, bronchiectasis, chronic bronchitis, or cystic fibrosis (Teall et al., 2021).

Stridor, a high-pitched, "crowing" harsh inspiratory sound associated with partial obstruction of the larynx or trachea that demands immediate attention since it may signal impending airway closure and asphyxiation (Suneja et al., 2020).

Pleural friction rubs result from inflammation of the pleural surfaces that induces a creaking, grating sound usually heard in inspiration and expiration (late in inspiration and early in expiration) (Teall et al., 2021). This sound can be enhanced by applying pressure to the chest wall with the diaphragm of the stethoscope. A pleural friction rub can be heard in pleuritis (inflammation of the pleural) or pleural effusion (Adderley & Sharma, 2022). Pleural fluid can accumulate in the pleural space because of a variety of etiologies, including transudation of fluid from the pleural and pulmonary vessels (increased venous hydrostatic pressure, decreased oncotic pressure, capillary leak); increased production of pleural fluid (inflamed pleura or pleural neoplasm); decreased pleural absorption of fluid (lymphatic obstruction, systemic venous hypertension); or by bleeding into the pleural space (Fitzpatrick et al., 2022). Pleural fluid dampens vibrations from the bronchotrachea so vocal fremitus, breath sounds, and whispered and spoken voice are decreased (see below), and dullness is noted on percussion in the area of fluid accumulation.

Voice Sounds. The sound heard through the stethoscope as the patient speaks is known as *vocal resonance*. The vibrations produced in the larynx are transmitted to the chest wall as they pass through the bronchi and alveolar tissue. During the process, the sounds are diminished in intensity and altered so that syllables are not distinguishable. Voice sounds are usually assessed by having the patient repeat "99" or "eee" while the nurse listens with the stethoscope in corresponding areas of the chest, from the apices to the bases.

Bronchophony describes vocal resonance that is more intense and clearer than normal. *Egophony* describes voice sounds that are distorted and is best appreciated by having the patient repeat the letter E. The distortion produced by consolidation transforms the sound into a clearly heard "A" rather than "E." Bronchophony and egophony have precisely the same significance as bronchial breathing with an increase in tactile fremitus. When an abnormality is detected, it should be confirmed using more than one assessment method. A change in tactile fremitus is more subtle and can be missed, but bronchial breathing and bronchophony can be noted loudly and clearly.

Whispered pectoriloquy is a very subtle finding which is heard only in the presence of rather dense consolidation of the lungs. Transmission of the high-frequency components of sound is so enhanced by the consolidated tissue that even whispered words are heard, a circumstance not noted in normal physiology. The significance is the same as that of bronchophony (Bickley, 2021).

The physical findings for the most common respiratory diseases are summarized in Table 7-6.

Diagnostic Evaluation

A wide range of diagnostic studies, described in the following sections, may be performed to aid in diagnosing or monitoring patients with a variety of respiratory conditions.

Pulmonary Function Tests

PFTs are used routinely in patients with chronic respiratory disorders. These tests are performed to assess respiratory function and to determine the extent of dysfunction. PFTs are useful in screening patients for major surgery, monitoring the course of a patient with an established respiratory disease, and assessing the response to therapy. They are useful as screening tests in potentially hazardous industries, such as coal mining and those that involve exposure to asbestos and other noxious fumes, dusts, or gases.

PFTs generally are performed by a technician using a spirometer that has a volume-collecting device attached to a recorder that demonstrates volume and time simultaneously. A number of tests are carried out because no single measurement provides a complete picture of pulmonary function.

PFT results are interpreted on the basis of the degree of deviation from normal, taking into consideration the patient's height, weight, age, and gender. Because there is a wide range of normal values, PFTs may not detect early localized changes.

TABLE 7-6 **Assessment Findings in Common Respiratory Disorders**

Disorder	Tactile Fremitus	Percussion	Auscultation
Consolidation (e.g., pneumonia)	Increased	Dull	Bronchial breath sounds, crackles, bronchophony, egophony, whispered pectoriloquy
Bronchitis	Normal	Resonant	Normal to decreased breath sounds, coarse crackles, wheezes, rhonchi
Emphysema	Decreased	Diffusely hyperresonant	Decreased intensity of breath sounds, usually with prolonged expiration, wheezes and rhonchi of associated bronchitis
Asthma (severe attack)	Normal to decreased	Resonant	Wheezes
Pulmonary edema	Normal	Resonant	Crackles at lung bases, possibly wheezes
Pleural effusion	Decreased to absent but may be increased toward the top of a large pleural effusion	Dull	Decreased to absent breath sounds, friction rub, bronchial breath sounds and bronchophony, egophony, and whispered pectoriloquy above the effusion over the area of compressed lung
Pneumothorax	Decreased to absent over the pneumothorax	Hyperresonant	Absent breath sounds
Atelectasis	Decreased fremitus	Dull (if large)	Decreased to absent breath sounds, fine crackles; trachea may be deviated toward the affected side

Patients with respiratory disorders may be taught how to measure their peak flow rate (which reflects maximal expiratory flow) at home using a spirometer to monitor progress of therapy, assess effect of alteration of medications, and use as a guide for when to notify the health care provider.

Arterial Blood Gas Studies

Measurements of blood pH and of arterial O_2 and CO_2 tensions are obtained when managing patients with respiratory problems and adjusting O_2 therapy as needed. The arterial O_2 tension (PaO_2) indicates the degree of oxygenation of the blood, and the arterial CO_2 tension ($PaCO_2$) indicates the adequacy of alveolar ventilation (i.e., how effectively CO_2 is exhaled from the body). Arterial blood gas (ABG) studies aid in assessing the ability of the lungs to provide adequate O_2 and remove CO_2 as well as the ability of the kidneys to reabsorb or excrete bicarbonate ions to maintain normal body pH. ABG levels are obtained through an arterial puncture at the radial, brachial, or femoral artery or through an indwelling arterial catheter. Before obtaining an ABG from the radial artery, it is necessary to test the patency of the ulnar artery by performing the Allen test (refer to Chapter 11 for details).

Pulse Oximetry

Pulse oximetry is a noninvasive method of continuously monitoring the O_2 saturation of hemoglobin (SaO_2). When O_2 saturation is measured with pulse oximetry, it is referred to as SpO_2. Although pulse oximetry does not replace ABG measurement, it is an effective tool (with some caveats discussed below) to monitor for subtle or sudden changes in O_2 saturation as this measurement is available in real time.

A probe or sensor is attached to a well-perfused fingertip (Fig. 7-12), forehead, earlobe, or bridge of the nose. The sensor detects changes in O_2 saturation levels by monitoring light signals (one red and one infrared) generated by the oximeter and reflected by blood pulsing through the tissue at the probe. Normal SpO_2 values are 95% to 100%. Values of less than 90% imply inadequate oxygenation, and further evaluation is needed. SpO_2 values obtained by pulse oximetry are unreliable in cardiac arrest and shock (decreased pulsatile force of blood), if dyes (i.e., methylene blue) or vasoconstrictor medications have been used or if the patient has severe anemia. Furthermore, they are not reliable detectors of hypoventilation or rising CO_2 which leads to respiratory acidosis. False high saturations may be seen in patients who have elevated carboxyhemoglobin levels, a high carbon monoxide level (smoke inhalation and carbon monoxide poisoning), and dark skin tones and pigmentation (O_2 saturation overestimated by ~2%) (Torp et al., 2021). Also it is important to understand that the pulse oximeters typically are calibrated to a range of saturation from 70% to 100% with an accuracy of 2% to 4%, which means that saturations lower than 70%, may not be accurate compared with ABGs.

Pearls for Practice: Lifting the Lens

Recently, it was learned that at least one medical device nurses use daily to monitor our patient may be biased. The device is the pulse oximeter, which is used for warning of low blood oxygenation and is frequently considered the fifth vital sign. Research reveals that

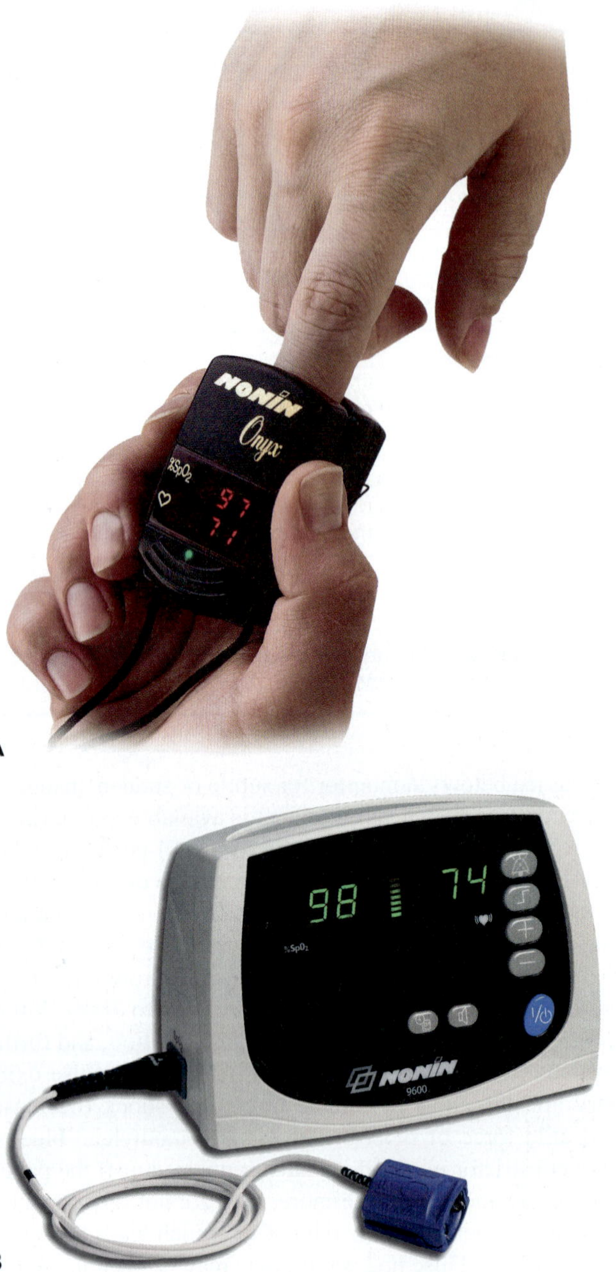

FIGURE 7-12 **Measuring blood oxygenation with pulse oximetry reduces the need for invasive procedures, such as drawing blood for analysis of O_2 levels. A. Self-contained digital fingertip pulse oximeter, which incorporates the sensor and display into one unit. B. Table top model with sensor attached. Memory permits tracking heart rate and O_2 saturation over time.**

the device may be missing three times as many cases of occult hypoxemia, defined as a significant difference between concurrently drawn ABGs and SpO_2 (i.e., an arterial oxygen saturation of <88% despite an oxygen saturation of 92% to 96% on pulse oximetry), in Black patients, since dark skin tones respond differently to these wavelengths of light, particularly visible light (Sjoding et al., 2020; Kadambi, 2021). In fact, in a more recent study, hidden hypoxemia was noted in 6.8% of Black patients, 6.0% in Hispanic patients, 4.8% of Asian patients, and 4.9% of White patients, resulting in higher rates of mortality and future organ dysfunction (Wong et al., 2021). Authors call for mitigating bias by ensuring that companies become race-aware (and gender-aware) when developing new technology to explicitly avoid bias, and bedside nurses should have a seat at the table with device manufacturers to advocate for representation of all demographic groups to minimize health inequity (Kadambi, 2021).

End Tidal CO_2

End-tidal CO_2 ($ETCO_2$) is a continuous recording of the concentration of CO_2 at the end of expiration. It is also known as capnography. An $ETCO_2$ monitor may be a separate monitor or part of the patient's bedside hemodynamic monitoring system. In a healthy patient, because the end-tidal gas is primarily alveolar gas and is virtually identical to $PaCO_2$ (arterial partial pressure of CO_2), $ETCO_2$ is used clinically as an estimate of $PaCO_2$.

In addition, it is used to (1) ensure that airway adjuncts (such as endotracheal tubes) are placed correctly in the trachea (and not in the esophagus) of a mechanically ventilated patient, (2) assess the effectiveness of interventions related to mechanical ventilation, such as weaning from the ventilator, neuromuscular blockade used with mechanical ventilation, and changing body positioning, and (3) assess the adequacy of chest compressions during cardiopulmonary resuscitation. Normally, $ETCO_2$ is 1 to 5 mm Hg lower than arterial CO_2 pressure so the typical range is 30 to 40 mm Hg versus 35 to 45 mm Hg for arterial CO_2 (Stacy, 2022). An early sign of malignant hyperthermia is a rapidly rising $ETCO_2$ especially if it is unresponsive to hyperventilation (refer to Chapter 4).

Pearls for Practice

The nurse should alert the provider when there is any significant change in the $ETCO_2$ waveform since it can indicate a change in the patients pulmonary status and loss of the waveform herald a loss of effective respirations (Stacy, 2022).

Sputum Studies

Sputum is obtained for analysis to identify pathogenic organisms and to determine whether malignant cells are present. It also may be used to assess for hypersensitivity states (in which there is an increase in eosinophils). In general, sputum cultures are used in diagnosis, for drug sensitivity testing, and to guide treatment.

Expectoration is the usual method for collecting a sputum specimen. The patient is instructed to clear the nose and throat and rinse the mouth to decrease contamination of the sputum. After taking a few deep breaths, the patient coughs forcefully on exhalation (rather than spits), using the diaphragm, and expectorates into a sterile container. An early morning specimen is best because a greater volume of secretions is present as a result of nighttime pooling; 2 to 3 mL is generally a sufficient amount (Stacy, 2022).

If the sputum cannot be raised spontaneously, respiratory therapy personnel may assist the patient in obtaining an "aerosol-induced" specimen with an ultrasonic nebulizer until a strong cough reflex is initiated. The specimen is labeled as being aerosol induced. Other methods of collecting sputum specimens include chest physiotherapy, nasotracheal or tracheal suctioning, and bronchoscopy.

Pearls for Practice

A sputum specimen is sealed in a sterile container and placed in a leak-proof biohazard bag. The specimen is sent as soon as possible to the laboratory after being labeled properly within 2 hours. Usually sputum specimens are not refrigerated; however, if there is a delay > 2 hours then the specimen should be refrigerated (Blakeborough & Watson, 2019). Allowing the specimen to stand for several hours in a warm room results in the overgrowth of contaminant organisms and may make it difficult to identify the pathogenic organisms (especially Mycobacterium tuberculosis).

Pearls for Practice

The nurse understands that a specimen will be sent to the lab for a stat gram stain and a culture and sensitivity (C&S). The gram stain will differentiate between different types of bacteria based on the biochemical properties of their cell walls (i.e., gram negative or gram positive), which will guide clinicians on prescribing initial antibiotic treatment. The nurse will see this described as "empiric" antibiotic, while the C&S will specify the specific bacteria in the specimen and which medications work best (sensitivities to a variety of antibiotics). The C&S will typically require 48 hours; thus, the gram stain allows the clinician to begin clinical management while awaiting the C&S results, at which time the antibiotic treatment may be altered.

Imaging Studies

Imaging studies, including x-rays, computed tomography (CT), magnetic resonance imaging (MRI), contrast studies, and radioisotope diagnostic scans may be part of any diagnostic workup, ranging from a determination of the extent of infection in sinusitis to tumor growth in cancer.

Chest X-Ray

Normal pulmonary tissue is radiolucent; therefore, densities produced by fluid, tumors, foreign bodies, and other pathologic conditions can be detected by x-ray examination. The routine chest x-ray consists of two views—a frontal view (posterior to anterior) and lateral view. Usually chest x-rays are taken after full inspiration (a deep breath) because the lungs are best visualized when they are well aerated. Also, the diaphragm is at its lowest level, and the largest expanse of lung is visible. The chest x-ray is the most frequently requested x-ray as it is used to assess for disorders of the lung, mediastinum, and bony thorax (Fischbach, 2022), and often used determine the anatomical position of central lines, chest tubes, and nasogastric (NG) tubes.

Computed Tomography

CT is an imaging method in which the lungs are scanned in successive layers by a narrow-beam x-ray. The images produced provide a cross-sectional view of the chest. CT can distinguish fine tissue density. It may be used to define pulmonary nodules and small tumors adjacent to pleural surfaces that are not visible on routine chest x-rays as well as to demonstrate mediastinal abnormalities and hilar adenopathy, which are difficult to visualize with other techniques. Contrast agents are useful when evaluating the mediastinum and its contents. Computed tomography pulmonary angiography (CTPA), which uses the injection of contrast media, has become the standard imaging technique for diagnosing PE rather than a $\dot{V}/\dot{Q}$ lung scan because of its wide availability, the rapid results, and its sensitivity and specificity (Weitz & Ginsberg, 2020).

Magnetic Resonance Imaging

MRI is similar to CT except that with MRI, magnetic fields and radiofrequency signals are used instead of a narrow-beam x-ray. MRI yields a much more detailed diagnostic image than CT. MRI is used to characterize pulmonary nodules, to help stage bronchogenic carcinoma (assessment of chest wall invasion), and to evaluate inflammatory activity in interstitial lung disease, acute PE, and chronic thrombolytic pulmonary hypertension.

Positron Emission Tomography

Positron emission tomography (PET) imaging involves the combined use of positron-emitting radionuclides and emission CT. PET generates high-resolution images of body function and metabolism; thus, PET provides physiologic, anatomic, and biochemical data. PET images include glucose metabolism, O_2 utilization, blood flow, and tissue perfusion. Clinical PET is useful for aiding in diagnosis of many disease states, primarily in oncology, neurology, and cardiology.

Fluoroscopic Studies

Fluoroscopy shows a continuous x-ray image that is used to assist with invasive procedures, such as a chest needle biopsy or transbronchial biopsy, that are performed to identify lesions. It also may be used to study the movement of the chest wall, mediastinum, heart, and diaphragm; to detect diaphragm paralysis; and to locate lung masses.

Pulmonary Angiography

Pulmonary angiography (also known as angiogram) involves the rapid injection of a radiopaque agent into the vasculature of the lungs for radiographic study of the pulmonary vessels. Pulmonary angiography is not without complications; mortality rate associated with pulmonary angiography is 0.2%, with deaths usually occurring in patients with hemodynamic compromise or respiratory failure (Weitz & Ginsberg, 2020). Because of its associated risks and due to introduction of CTPA, pulmonary angiography is used infrequently.

Radioisotope Diagnostic Procedures (Lung Scans)

Several types of lung scans—V/Q scan, gallium scan, and PET—are used to assess normal lung functioning, pulmonary vascular supply, and gas exchange.

A V/Q lung scan is performed by injecting a radioactive agent into a peripheral vein and then obtaining a scan of the chest to detect radiation. The isotope particles pass through the right side of the heart and are distributed into the lungs in proportion to the regional blood flow, making it possible to trace and measure blood perfusion through the lung. This procedure is used clinically to measure the integrity of the pulmonary vessels relative to blood flow and to evaluate blood flow abnormalities, as seen in pulmonary emboli. The imaging time is 20 to 40 minutes, during which the patient lies under the camera with a mask fitted over the nose and mouth. This is followed by the ventilation component of the scan. The patient takes a deep breath of a mixture of O_2 and radioactive gas, which diffuses throughout the lungs. A scan is performed to detect ventilation abnormalities in patients who have regional differences in ventilation. Ventilation without perfusion is seen with pulmonary emboli. V/Q scanning has been replaced by CTPA and currently is considered a second-line modality in the diagnosis of PE. However, V/Q scan remains a valuable tool in the diagnosis of acute PE in patients with a normal chest x-ray or patients who cannot undergo CTPA (history of angiographic contrast media allergy, renal impairment, or females younger than 40 years to reduce radiation exposure to the breasts) (Weitz & Ginsberg, 2020). In pregnant patients, lung scanning produces less maternal and fetal radiation exposure and is sometimes preferred over CTPA (Weitz & Ginsberg, 2020).

A gallium scan is a radioisotope lung scan used to detect inflammatory conditions, abscesses, adhesions, and the presence, location, and size of tumors. It is used to stage bronchogenic cancer, Hodgkin lymphomas, and non-Hodgkin lymphomas and document tumor regression after chemotherapy or radiation (Fischbach, 2022). Gallium is injected intravenously, and scans are taken at intervals (e.g., between 6 hours and 48 hours) to evaluate gallium uptake by the pulmonary tissues. Although gallium is radioactive, the risk of radiation exposure is lower than x-ray or CT scan. PET scans (discussed previously) have replaced gallium scans for the identification of malignancy (Pagana, 2021).

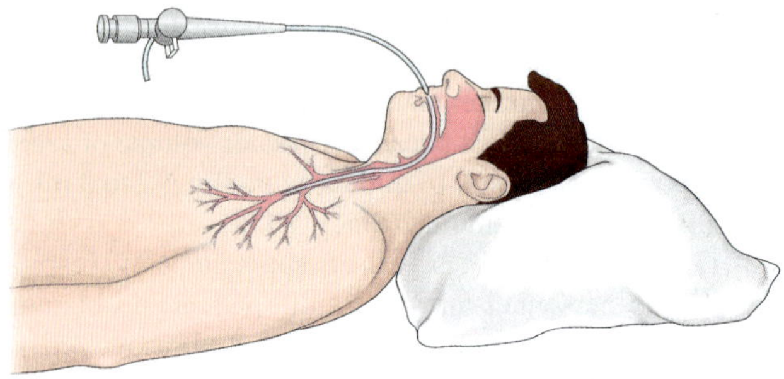

Fiberoptic bronchoscopy

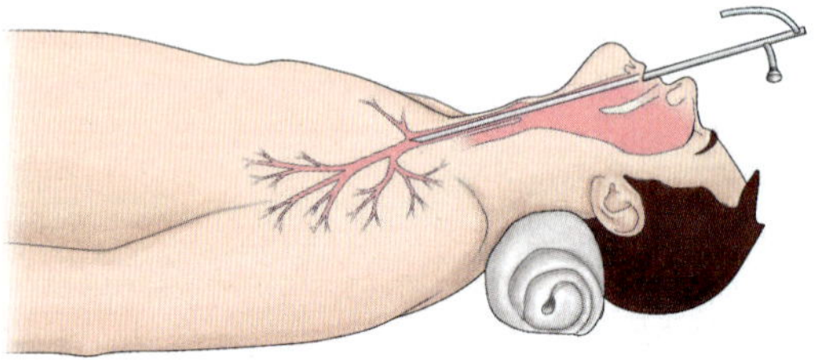

Rigid bronchoscopy

FIGURE 7-13 Endoscopic bronchoscopy permits visualization of bronchial structures. The bronchoscope is advanced into bronchial structures orally. Bronchoscopy permits the provider not only to diagnose but also to treat various lung problems.

Endoscopic Procedures

Bronchoscopy

Bronchoscopy is the direct inspection and examination of the larynx, trachea, and bronchi for diagnosis of infectious, inflammatory, and malignant disease of the chest through a flexible (commonly) or rigid (less frequently) fiberoptic bronchoscope (Fig. 7-13).

Therapeutic bronchoscopy is used to (1) obtain biopsy specimens, (2) remove foreign bodies from the tracheobronchial tree, (3) perform difficult endotracheal intubations, (4) remove secretions obstructing the tracheobronchial tree when the patient cannot clear them, (5) diagnose lung infection, inflammation, and interstitial diseases, (6) destroy and excise lesions, (7) place endobronchial radiation therapy (brachytherapy) and laser therapy of obstructive airway lesions, (8) stent obstructing endobronchial lesions, and (9) dilate stenotic airways.

Possible complications of bronchoscopy include a reaction to the local anesthetic, infection, aspiration, bronchospasm, **hypoxemia** (low blood O_2 level), pneumothorax, bleeding, and perforation.

Before the procedure, a signed consent form is obtained from the patient. Food and fluids are withheld for 8 hours before the test to reduce the risk of aspiration when the cough reflex is blocked by anesthesia. The nurse explains the procedure to the patient to reduce fear and decrease anxiety and administers preoperative medications if required.

The patient must remove dentures and other oral prostheses. Usually the examination is performed under local anesthesia or moderate sedation. A topical anesthetic such as lidocaine may be sprayed on the pharynx or dropped on the epiglottis and vocal cords and into the trachea to suppress the cough reflex and minimize discomfort. Sedatives (usually diazepam or midazolam) are administered intravenously as prescribed to provide moderate sedation (Fischbach, 2022). Resuscitative and suctioning equipment should be available.

After the procedure, it is important that the patient takes nothing by mouth until the cough reflex returns, because the preoperative sedation and local anesthesia impair the protective laryngeal reflex and swallowing for several hours. The patient is instructed to spit out saliva rather than swallow it until the gag reflex returns. Once the patient demonstrates a cough reflex, the nurse may offer ice chips and, eventually, fluids. The nurse also monitors the patient's respiratory status and observes for hypoxia, hypotension, tachycardia, arrhythmias, hemoptysis, subcutaneous air or crepitus, stridor, or dyspnea. Any abnormality is reported promptly. The patient is not discharged from the recovery area until adequate cough reflex and respiratory status are present. The nurse instructs the patient and family caregivers to report any SOB or bleeding immediately.

Pearls for Practice

Anesthesia can temporarily impair the pharyngeal reflex (ninth, tenth, CN), which is responsible for the gag reflex and swallowing; to prevent aspiration, before refeeding the patient, the nurse must reassess return of this reflex (refer to Chapter 42 for details on assessment).

Thoracentesis

A thoracentesis (aspiration of fluid or air from the pleural space) is performed on patients with various clinical problems. As a diagnostic or therapeutic procedure, thoracentesis may be used for removal of fluid and air from the pleural cavity, aspiration of pleural fluid for analysis, pleural biopsy, or instillation of medication into the pleural space. Care of the patient undergoing thoracentesis is discussed in Box 7-8. A needle biopsy of the pleura may be performed at the same time. Studies of pleural fluid include gram stain culture and sensitivity, acid-fast staining and culture, differential cell count, cytology, pH, specific gravity, total protein, glucose, lactic dehydrogenase (LDH) and carcinoembryonic antigen (CEA) (Pagana et al., 2021).

BOX 7-8

GUIDELINES FOR NURSING CARE

Assisting the Patient Undergoing Thoracentesis

Equipment

- Thoracentesis tray
- Local anesthetic
- Sterile gloves
- Sterile collection bottles
- Germicide solution

Implementation

ACTIONS	RATIONALE
1. Ascertain in advance that a chest x-ray and ultrasound (if available) have been ordered and completed and the consent form has been signed. The nurse also anticipates that coagulation studies are evaluated and any coagulopathy corrected before the procedure.	1. Posterior-anterior (PA view) and lateral decubitus chest x-ray films are obtained before the procedure and ultrasound if available to determine optimal site for thoracentesis. When thoracentesis is performed under ultrasound guidance, it has a lower rate of complications than when it is performed without ultrasound guidance, including a decrease in postprocedure pneumothorax, less accidental organ puncture, and improved site selection. If fluid is loculated (isolated in a pocket of pleural fluid), ultrasound scans are performed to help select the best site for needle aspiration. Correction of coagulopathy may be necessary to decrease the bleeding risk with this procedure.
2. Assess the patient for allergy to the local anesthetic to be used.	2. If the patient is allergic to the anesthetic prescribed initially, then assessment findings provide an opportunity to use a safer anesthetic. Local anesthetic minimizes patient's discomfort during thoracentesis needle insertion.

(*continued on page 272*)

BOX 7-8

GUIDELINES FOR NURSING CARE (*continued*)

Assisting the Patient Undergoing Thoracentesis (*continued*)

ACTIONS	RATIONALE
3. Administer sedation if prescribed.	3. Sedation enables the patient to cooperate with the procedure and promotes relaxation.
4. Inform the patient about the nature of the procedure and: a. The importance of remaining immobile b. Pressure sensations to be experienced c. That minimal discomfort is anticipated after the procedure	4. An explanation helps to orient the patient to the procedure, provides anticipatory guidance, and provides an opportunity to ask questions and verbalize anxiety.
5. Position the patient comfortably with adequate supports. If possible, place the patient upright or in one of the following positions: a. Sitting on the edge of the bed with the feet supported and arms and head on a padded over-the-bed table b. Straddling a chair with arms and head resting on the back of the chair c. If the patient's condition precludes sitting, the side-lying position with patient's back flush with the edge of the bed and the affected side down can be used (Stacy, 2022).	5. The upright position facilitates the removal of fluid that usually localizes at the base of the thorax. A position of comfort helps the patient to relax.
6. Support and reassure the patient during the procedure: a. Prepare the patient for the cold sensation of skin germicide solution and for a pressure sensation from infiltration of local anesthetic agent. b. Encourage the patient to refrain from coughing.	6. Sudden and unexpected movement, such as coughing, by the patient can traumatize the visceral pleura and lung.
7. Expose the entire chest. The site for aspiration is visualized by chest x-ray, ultrasound, and percussion (with attention to the site of maximal dullness on percussion).	7. If air is in the pleural cavity, the thoracentesis site is usually in the second or third intercostal space in the midclavicular line because air rises in the thorax.
8. The procedure is performed under aseptic conditions. After the skin is cleansed, the provider uses a small-caliber needle to inject a local anesthetic slowly into the intercostal space.	8. An intradermal wheal is raised slowly; rapid injection causes pain. The parietal pleura is very sensitive and should be well infiltrated with anesthetic before the physician passes the thoracentesis needle through it.
9. The provider advances the thoracentesis needle with the syringe attached. When the pleural space is reached, suction may be applied with the syringe:	9. Use of thoracentesis needle allows proper insertion:
a. A 20-mL syringe with a three-way stopcock is attached to the needle (one end of the adapter is attached to the needle and the other to the tubing leading to a receptacle that receives the fluid being aspirated).	a. When a large quantity of fluid is withdrawn, a three-way stopcock serves to keep air from entering the pleural cavity.
b. If a considerable quantity of fluid is removed, the needle is held in place on the chest wall with a small hemostat.	b. The hemostat steadies the needle on the chest wall. Sudden pleuritic chest pain or shoulder pain may indicate that the needle point is irritating the visceral or the diaphragmatic pleura.
c. The nurse should anticipate that no more than 1 L will be removed from the chest. Amounts greater than 1 to 1.5 L can result in re-expansion pulmonary edema (Fischbach, 2022), with symptoms that are severe coughing and shortness of breath (Stacy, 2022).	c. To prevent re-expansion pulmonary edema. If the patient has these symptoms (coughing and SOB), it is an indication to discontinue the procedure (Stacy, 2022).
10. After the needle is withdrawn, pressure is applied over the puncture site and a small, airtight, sterile dressing is fixed in place.	10. Pressure helps to stop bleeding, and the airtight dressing protects the site and prevents air from entering the pleural cavity.
11. Advise the patient that they will be on bed rest and a chest x-ray will be obtained after thoracentesis.	11. A chest x-ray verifies that there is no pneumothorax.
12. Record the total amount of fluid withdrawn from the procedure and document the nature of the fluid, its color, and its viscosity. If indicated, prepare samples of fluid for laboratory evaluation. A specimen container with formalin may be needed for a pleural biopsy.	12. The fluid may be clear, serous, bloody, purulent, etc.

ACTIONS	RATIONALE
13. Monitor the patient at intervals for increasing respiratory rate; increased dyspnea; asymmetry in respiratory movement; faintness; vertigo; tightness in chest; uncontrollable cough; blood-tinged, frothy mucus; a rapid pulse; and signs of hypoxemia.	13. Pneumothorax, tension pneumothorax, subcutaneous emphysema, and pyrogenic infection are complications of a thoracentesis. Pulmonary edema or cardiac distress can occur after a sudden shift in mediastinal contents when large amounts of fluid are aspirated.

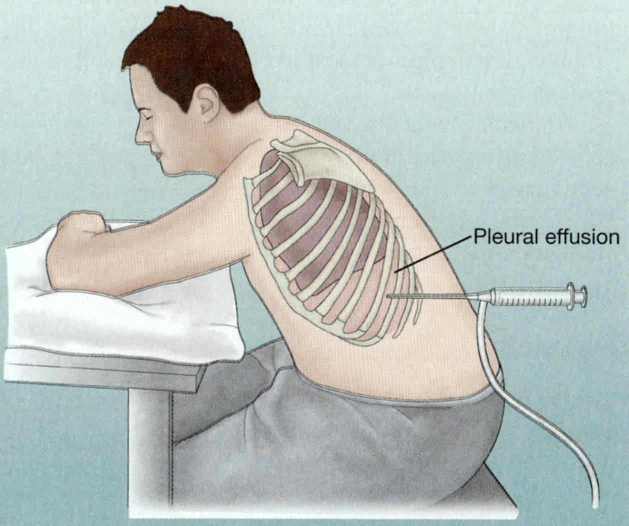

CHAPTER REVIEW

NCLEX-Style Review Questions

1. The patient is admitted with hypoxemia and fever, expectorating green sputum, and chest film reveals right middle and lower lobe pneumonia. The oxygen saturation is 89% and the patient complains of shortness of breath (SOB). What physical examinations findings are associated with this condition? Select all that apply.
   a. Whispered pectoriloquy
   b. Bronchial breath sounds
   c. Eupnea
   d. Stridor
   e. Dull percussion on right middle and lower lobe
2. In the case above, which interventions are appropriate for this patient? Select all that apply.
   a. Maintain the head of bed less than 30 degrees
   b. Administer oxygen via nasal cannula
   c. Turn the patient on the left side to prevent hypoxemia
   d. Prepare for intubation
   e. Turn the patient on the right side to prevent hypoxemia
3. You are working the emergency room (ER) and a patient is en route after sustaining a traumatic injury while diving. A cervical collar was applied and oxygen was administered. The patient is moving all limbs and asking that the C-collar be removed. Which of the following assessments are the priority tasks when the patient arrives? Select all that apply.
   a. Assess vital signs
   b. Remove the C-collar
   c. Insert intravenous catheter(s)
   d. Apply pulse oximetry monitoring
   e. Log roll the patient if needed
4. A patient is admitted to the ICU after falling from a roof and sustaining fractures of the first three ribs on the right side. The patient is dyspneic, and crepitus (subcutaneous emphysema) can be palpated. The chest x-ray reveals a pneumothorax. What physical examination finding are associated with pneumothorax? Select all that apply.
   a. Dullness to percussion on the right
   b. Increased fremitus on the right
   c. Decreased or absent breath sounds on auscultation of the right
   d. Hyperresonance on the right
   e. Egophony on the right

5. A patient is admitted to the ER after hitting the steering wheel in a motor vehicle crash. The patient is alert, restless, complaining of chest and back pain, and skin is cool and slightly clammy. Breath sounds are diminished over the left side. An upright chest x-ray reveals fractures of the left 5th through 7th ribs and a 25% left hemothorax. Pertinent data are: B/P is 80/50; HR is 125; RR is 28 and slightly labored. O_2 sat is 93% on room air. Which of the following measures is most likely to be included in this patient's initial care?

a. Immediate endotracheal intubation
b. Chest tube insertion
c. Oxygen administration
d. IV at a keep-vein-open rate
e. Pericardiocentesis

REFERENCES AND SELECTED READINGS

References and selected readings associated with this chapter can be found on the website that accompanies the book. Visit **http://thepoint.lww.com/Honan3e** to access the references and other additional resources associated with this chapter.

CHAPTER 8

Nursing Management: Patients With Upper Respiratory Tract Disorders

Kelly Martinez

Learning Objectives

After reading this chapter, you will be able to:

1. Compare and contrast the upper respiratory tract infections with regard to cause, incidence, clinical manifestations, management, and the significance of preventive health care.
2. Use the nursing process as a framework for care of patients with upper airway infection.
3. Describe the nursing management of the patient with obstructive sleep apnea.
4. Describe the nursing management for patients receiving continuous positive-pressure (CPAP) or bi-level (BiPAP) breathing.
5. Describe nursing management of the patient with epistaxis.
6. Describe nursing management of patients undergoing laryngectomy.
7. Describe the nursing care for a patient with an endotracheal tube or a tracheostomy.
8. Demonstrate the procedure of tracheal suctioning.

Many upper airway disorders are relatively minor, and their effects are limited to mild and temporary discomfort for the patient. Others may be acute, severe, and life-threatening and may require permanent alterations in breathing and speaking. The nurse must have expert assessment skills, an understanding of the wide variety of disorders that may affect the upper airway, and an awareness of the impact of these alterations on patients.

UPPER AIRWAY INFECTIONS

Upper airway infections, also known as upper respiratory tract infections (URIs), are the most common cause of illness, and affect most people on occasion. URIs are usually caused by viruses, affect the upper respiratory passages, and lead to mucous membrane inflammation. However, they are self-limited. URIs affect the nasal cavity, sinuses, pharynx, larynx, and large airways (Hinkle et al., 2022; Thomas & Bomar, 2021). There are many causative organisms, and people are susceptible throughout their lives.

Some infections are acute, with symptoms that last several days, while others are chronic, with symptoms that last a long time or recur. Patients with these conditions seldom require hospitalization. URIs affect the nasal cavity; ethmoidal air cells; and frontal, maxillary, and sphenoid sinuses (see Fig. 8-1), as well as the larynx and trachea. About 90% of upper respiratory disorders stem from a viral infection of the upper respiratory passages and subsequent mucous membrane inflammation.

RHINITIS

Rhinitis is a group of disorders characterized by inflammation and irritation of the mucous membranes of the nose, nasal congestion, rhinorrhea (inflammation of mucous membranes lining the nose), sneezing, itching, and other symptoms (Dykewicz et al., 2020). Rhinitis may be acute or chronic, nonallergic or allergic (see Chapter 37 for information about allergic rhinitis).

Pearls for Practice

The term rhinorrhea refers to the free discharge of nasal mucus, whereas cerebrospinal fluid rhinorrhea is the discharge of cerebrospinal fluid through the nose, typically due to a skull fracture (see Chapter 44).

Viral rhinitis is the most frequent viral infection in the United States and is referred to as the "common cold." On average, adults have two to four colds a year, and children average more (ALA, 2020; CDC, 2021A; Sexton & McClain, 2022).

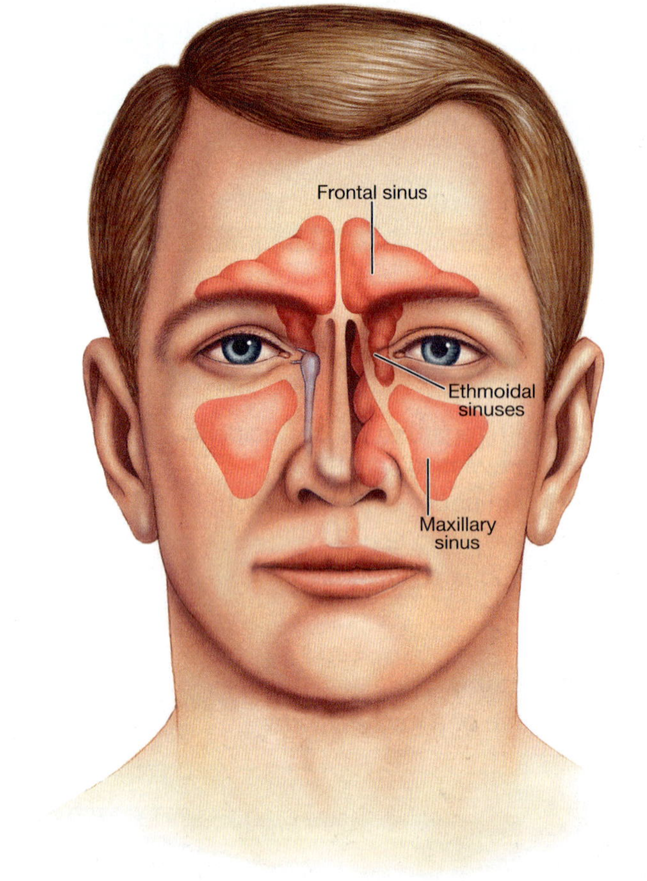

FIGURE 8-1 **Sinuses are air-filled cavities in your head. This image details the sphenoid sinuses, frontal sinuses, and ethmoid sinuses. (From Anatomical Chart Company.)**

TABLE 8-1 Causes of Rhinitis

Category	Causes
Allergic	Seasonal (pollens) Perennial (dust/mold)
Vasomotor	Idiopathic Abuse of nasal decongestants (rhinitis medicamentosa) Drugs (ACE inhibitors, phosphodiesterase-5 selective inhibitors, alpha-receptor antagonists, phentolamine, cocaine use) Psychological stimulation (anger, sexual arousal) Irritants (smoke, air pollution, exhaust fumes, cocaine)
Mechanical	Tumor Deviated septum Septal perforation Foreign body Cerebrospinal fluid leak
Chronic inflammatory	Polyps Sarcoidosis Wegener granulomatosis Vasculitis
Infectious	Acute viral infection Acute or chronic sinusitis
Hormonal	Pregnancy Use of oral contraceptives

Adapted from Takashima and Ahmed (2022).

Pathophysiology

Nonallergic rhinitis may be caused by a variety of factors, including environmental factors such as changes in temperature or humidity, odors, or foods; infection; age; systemic disease; illegal drugs (e.g., cocaine); over-the-counter (OTC) and prescribed nasal decongestants; and the presence of a foreign body.

The most common cause of nonallergic rhinitis is the common cold. Colds are believed to be caused by as many as 200 different viruses. Rhinovirus is the most common cause, accounting for 10% to 40% of colds. Other common cold viruses include coronavirus, influenza virus, parainfluenza virus and respiratory syncytial virus (RSV) (American Lung Association, 2020). Each virus may have multiple strains. Because of this diversity of causes, development of a vaccine is almost impossible. Immunity after recovery is variable and depends on many factors, including a person's natural host resistance and the specific virus that caused the cold. Drug-induced rhinitis is associated with antihypertensive agents (e.g., angiotensin-converting enzyme [ACE] inhibitors and beta-blockers), aspirin and nonsteroidal anti-inflammatory (NSAIDs), lipid-lowering medications (statins, also known as HMG-CoA reductase inhibitors, such as atorvastatin and simvastatin), oral contraceptives, psychotropic agents (some antidepressants, antipsychotics, antianxiety medications), withdrawal of alpha-adrenergic agonists (e.g., clonidine), and chronic use of nasal decongestants (Hinkle et al., 2022). Other causes of rhinitis are identified in Table 8-1. Figure 8-2 shows the pathologic processes involved in rhinitis and sinusitis.

Risk Factors

Colds are highly contagious and are spread through droplets either touched or inhaled (American Lung Association, 2020). The viruses that cause the cold may live on the skin for up to 2 hours and can shed for about 2 days before the symptoms appear and during the first part of the symptomatic phase. The risk of person-to-person transfer is based on the time spent with that individual, the proximity to one another, and the amount of virus that is shed (Edwards, 2019). Viral rhinitis is mostly seen between September and May.

In the United States, adults generally have two to four colds per year, while children have an average of six to eight times a year between September and May (American Lung Association,

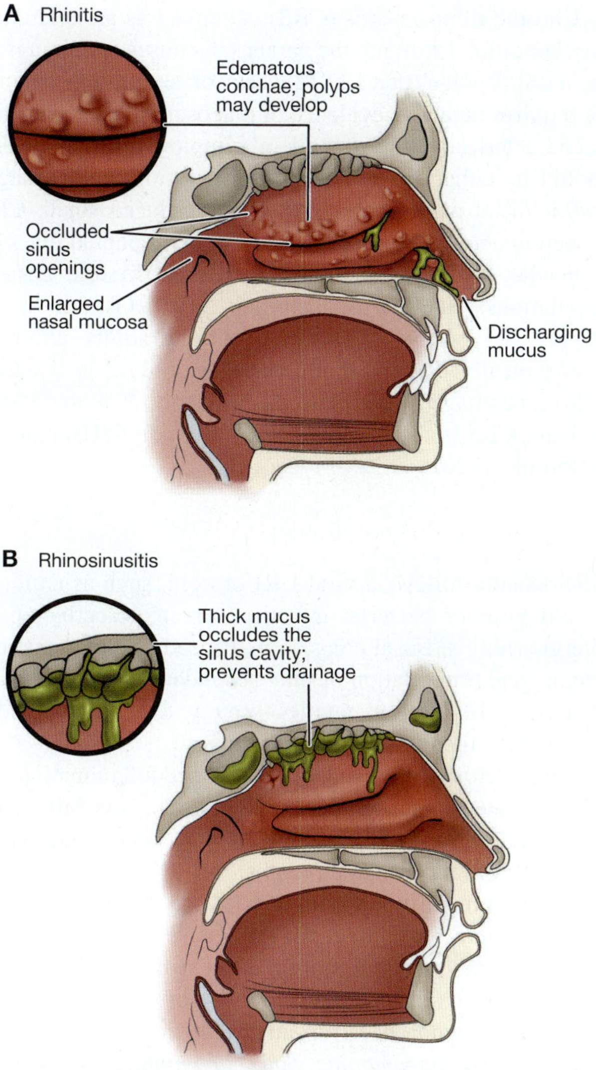

FIGURE 8-2 **Pathophysiologic processes in rhinitis and rhinosinusitis. Although pathophysiologic processes are similar in rhinitis and sinusitis, they affect different structures. In rhinitis (A), the mucous membranes lining the nasal passages become inflamed, congested, and edematous. The swollen nasal conchae block the sinus openings, and mucus is discharged from the nostrils. Rhinosinusitis (B) is also marked by inflammation and congestion, with thickened mucous secretions filling the sinus cavities and occluding the openings.**

2020). Adult females are more susceptible than adult males. Viral rhinitis can occur at any time of the year, but three time periods account for the epidemics in the United States: in September, just after the opening of school; in late January; and toward the end of April. Risk factors for the common cold include exposure to children in day care, at-home caregivers, stress, and sleep disturbances. Contrary to popular belief, cold temperatures and exposure to cold, rainy weather do not increase the incidence or severity of the common cold (Sexton et al., 2019).

Clinical Manifestations and Assessment

The signs and symptoms of nonallergic rhinitis may vary from patient to patient and may depend on age, underlying illness, chronic illnesses, and causative infectious agent. Common signs and symptoms include rhinitis (excessive nasal drainage, runny nose), nasal congestion, nasal discharge (purulent with bacterial rhinitis), sore throat, a dry or "scratchy throat," conjunctivitis (inflammation of the conjunctiva, typically marked by pinkness or redness of the sclera and by itching, burning, irritation, etc.), sneezing, malaise, and a cough that appears after the onset of nasal discharge. Fever is uncommon in adults with a cold but may be present in children. Many patients complain of sneezing, malaise, headache, and pressure or discomfort in their face particularly if sinusitis is also present (Sexton et al., 2019). In addition to the above symptoms, viral rhinitis may present with sore throat, general malaise, low-grade fever, chills, and muscle aches. As the illness progresses, cough usually appears. In some people, the virus exacerbates herpes simplex, commonly called a "cold sore." The symptoms of viral rhinitis may last from 1 to 2 weeks.

Medical and Nursing Management

Management consists of symptomatic therapy. Medication therapy for allergic and nonallergic rhinitis focuses on symptom relief. The choice of medications depends on the symptoms, adverse reactions, adherence factors, risk of drug interactions, and cost to the patient.

Analgesics, such as acetaminophen and NSAIDs, are effective in relieving cold symptoms, such as headache, ear pain, muscle and joint pains, malaise, and sneezing, and short courses of standard doses in this setting are generally safe and well tolerated (Sexton et al., 2019). The four major categories of medications used to manage cold symptoms are antihistamines, decongestants, antitussives, and expectorants. Antihistamines remain the most common treatment and are administered for sneezing, nasal congestion, pruritus, and rhinorrhea, but appear to be more beneficial when used in combination with other agents, such as decongestants and analgesics. The most common adverse effects of antihistamines are sedation, dry mouth, gastrointestinal (GI) upset, and cardiac arrhythmias (George et al., 2018; Sexton et al., 2019). Antihistamines have been show to aggravate certain conditions and should be used with caution in patients with asthma, urinary retention, hypertension, open-angle glaucoma, and prostatic hypertrophy (George et al., 2018). Topical nasal decongestants should be used with caution. Topical therapy delivers medication directly to the nasal mucosa, but its overuse can produce *rhinitis medicamentosa* (an increase in the severity or duration of rhinitis that results from prolonged use of decongestant nasal spray) or rebound rhinitis (Green et al., 2020).

A topical or oral decongestant may be used if the patient is experiencing nasal congestion. Decongestants cause vasoconstriction, leading to a decrease in sinusoid engorgement and mucosal edema (George et al., 2018). The use of saline nasal spray can act as a mild decongestant and can liquefy mucus to prevent crusting. Antitussives can be used to suppress coughing. Expectorants are available without a prescription and are used to reduce the viscosity and volume of sputum produced and therefore promote removal of secretions (George et al., 2018). Several antiviral medications are available by prescription. Antimicrobial agents (antibiotics) should not be used because they do not affect the virus or reduce the incidence of bacterial complications, and they have been implicated in development of organisms resistant to therapy.

Herbal medicines (e.g., echinacea, zinc lozenges, zinc nasal spray) are used frequently to treat the common cold; however, evidence regarding their effectiveness in shortening the symptomatic phase is questionable (American Lung Association, 2020). The inhalation of steam or heated, humidified air has been a mainstay of home remedies for common cold sufferers, but the value of this therapy has not been demonstrated.

If symptoms suggest a bacterial infection, an antimicrobial agent will be used. Other treatment measures include adequate fluid intake, adequate rest, prevention of chilling, and warm saltwater gargles to soothe the sore throat. Patients with nasal septal deformities or nasal polyps may be referred to an ear, nose, and throat (ENT) specialist.

RHINOSINUSITIS

Rhinosinusitis, formerly called *sinusitis*, is an inflammatory process involving the paranasal sinuses and nasal cavity (Patel et al., 2020). The clinical practice guideline for adult rhinosinusitis released by the American Academy of Otolaryngology–Head and Neck Surgery Foundation recommends use of the term *rhinosinusitis* because sinusitis is almost always accompanied by inflammation of the nasal mucosa (American Academy of Otolaryngology–Head and Neck Surgery Foundation, 2018). In the United States, rhinosinusitis affects 1 out of every 7 adults, and more than 30 million are diagnosed each year. Rhinosinusitis also accounts for 16 million office visits per year. According to the National Ambulatory Medical Care Survey (NAMCS), approximately 14% of adults report having an episode of rhinosinusitis each year. Incidence is higher in females than males and is highest in those between the ages of 45 and 64 years (Brook et al., 2021).

Uncomplicated rhinosinusitis does not extend beyond the paranasal sinuses and nasal cavity. Rhinosinusitis is classified by duration of symptoms as acute (less than 4 weeks), subacute (4 to 12 weeks), and chronic (more than 12 weeks) with or without acute exacerbations (Patel & Hwang, 2021a). Rhinosinusitis can be further classified as an **acute bacterial rhinosinusitis** (ABRS) or **acute viral rhinosinusitis** (AVRS) (Brook et al., 2021). Recurrent acute rhinosinusitis (ARS) is characterized by three or more acute episodes of ABRS per year without symptoms of rhinosinusitis between episodes (Patel & Hwang, 2021a).

Chronic rhinosinusitis (CRS) is defined as an inflammatory condition involving the paranasal sinuses and linings of the nasal passages that last 12 weeks or longer. The diagnosis requires objective evidence of mucosal inflammation and is characterized by two or more symptoms, one of which should be either nasal blockage, congestion, or discharge, and/or facial pain or pressure, and/or reduced smell. CRS is seen in about 5% and 12% of the general population with somewhat higher estimations reported in Middle Eastern populations (Hamilos & Holbrook, 2020; Ostovar et al., 2019). CRS occurs in both children and adults, although it is typically diagnosed in young or middle-aged adults with a mean age of 39 years old. In about 20% to 33% of patients, CRS is accompanied with nasal polyps (Hamilos & Holbrook, 2020).

Pathophysiology

ARS usually follows a viral URI or cold, such as an unresolved viral or bacterial infection, or an exacerbation of allergic rhinitis. Nasal congestion, caused by inflammation, edema, and transudation of fluid secondary to URI, leads to obstruction of the sinus cavities (see Fig. 8-2). This provides an excellent medium for bacterial growth.

CRS occurs with episodes of prolonged inflammation and with repeated or inadequate treatment of acute infections. Irreversible damage to the mucosa may occur, and symptoms last for longer than 3 months.

The vast majority of cases of ARS are due to viral infection. Common viral infections that cause ARS are rhinovirus, influenza virus, and parainfluenza virus. Acute bacterial infection occurs in only 0.5% to 2.0% of episodes of ARS. The most common bacterial infections that cause ARS are *Streptococcus pneumoniae* and *Haemophilus influenzae*. Less common are *Staphylococcus aureus* and *Moraxella catarrhalis* (Patel & Hwang, 2021a). Other organisms that are occasionally isolated include *Chlamydia pneumoniae, Streptococcus pyogenes,* viruses, and fungi (*Aspergillus fumigatus*). Immunodeficiency should be considered in patients with CRS or acute recurrent rhinosinusitis. Acute fulminant/invasive sinusitis is a life-threatening illness and is commonly attributed to *Aspergillus*.

Risk Factors

Some people are more prone to rhinosinusitis because of chronic inflammation of the nasal passages due to exposure to environmental hazards, such as paint, sawdust, and chemicals. If sinus drainage is obstructed by a deviated septum or by hypertrophied turbinates, spurs, or nasal polyps or tumors, sinus infection may persist as a smoldering (persistent) secondary infection or progress to an acute suppurative process (causing purulent discharge). Other conditions that can block the normal flow of sinus secretions include abnormal structures of the nose, enlarged adenoids, diving and swimming, tooth infection, trauma to the nose, tumors, and the pressure of foreign objects. Immunocompromised patients are at increased risk for the development of fungal sinusitis. Fungal sinusitis in immunocompromised patients can be divided into three categories: (1) fungus ball, (2) chronic erosive (noninvasive) sinusitis, and (3) allergic fungal sinusitis. *A. fumigatus* is the most common organism associated with fungal sinusitis. The fungus ball is usually a brown or greenish-black material with the consistency of peanut butter or cottage cheese.

Clinical Manifestations and Assessment

Symptoms of ABRS include nasal congestion, purulent nasal drainage accompanied by nasal obstruction or a combination of facial pain, pressure, or a sense of fullness (referred to collectively as facial pain–pressure–fullness), or a combination. The facial pain–pressure–fullness may involve the anterior face or the periorbital region. The patient may also report fever, fatigue, cough, cloudy or colored nasal discharge, congestion, blockage, or stuffiness, as well as a localized or diffuse headache. The occurrence of symptoms for 10 days or more after the initial onset of upper respiratory symptoms indicates ABRS (Patel & Hwang, 2021a).

The symptoms of AVRS are similar to those of ABRS with the exception of the duration of symptoms. Symptoms of AVRS occur for less than 10 days after the onset of upper respiratory symptoms and do not worsen (Patel & Hwang, 2021a).

Clinical manifestations of CRS are similar to ABRS and include mucopurulent drainage, nasal obstruction, cough, chronic hoarseness, chronic headaches in the periorbital area, facial pain or pressure, and **hyposmia** (decreased sense of smell) (Hamilos & Holbrook, 2020). As a result of chronic nasal congestion, the patient is usually required to breathe through the mouth. Snoring, sore throat, and, in some situations, adenoidal hypertrophy may also occur. In general, these symptoms are most pronounced on awakening in the morning.

To diagnose the rhinosinusitis, a careful history and physical examination are performed. It is essential to obtain any history of comorbid conditions, including asthma, and history of tobacco use. A history of fever, fatigue, previous episodes and treatments, and previous response to therapies are also obtained.

The head and neck, particularly the nose, ears, teeth, sinuses, pharynx, and chest, are examined. The physical assessment includes examination of the external nose for evidence of anatomical abnormality. Nasal mucous membranes are assessed for erythema, pallor, atrophy, edema, crusting, discharge, polyps, erosions, and septal perforations or deviations. There may be tenderness to palpation over the infected sinus area.

Diagnostic imaging (x-ray, computed tomography [CT], magnetic resonance imaging [MRI]) is not recommended for the diagnosis of ARS if the patient meets clinical diagnostic criteria (Patel & Hwang, 2021a). Diagnostic testing may be required to rule out other local or systemic disorders, such as tumor, fistula, and allergy for the patient with CRS. Nasal endoscopy may be indicated to rule out underlying diseases, tumors, and sinus mycetomas (fungus balls).

Medical and Nursing Management

Treatment of acute and chronic rhinosinusitis depends on the cause. The goals of treatment of ARS are to treat the infection, shrink the nasal mucosa, and relieve pain. General measures include adequate hydration, saline sprays, and steam inhalation as it may provide some relief from congestion (Patel & Hwang, 2021b). Patients are instructed to sleep with the head of the bed elevated and to avoid exposure to cigarette smoke and fumes. Patients are cautioned to avoid caffeine and alcohol, which can lead to dehydration.

Treatment of acute and chronic rhinosinusitis typically involves sterile intranasal saline spray and decongestants (Tewfik, 2018). Decongestants or nasal saline spray can improve patency of the ostiomeatal unit (area where the frontal and maxillary sinuses normally drain into the nasal cavity) and improve drainage of the sinuses. Topical decongestants are used only in adults and should not be used for longer than 3 consecutive days. Oral decongestants must be used short term for 3 to 5 days and must be used cautiously in patients with hypertension. OTC antihistamines and prescription antihistamines are used if an allergic component is suspected. Patients with AVRS should be managed with supportive care. Patients with ABRS should be observed for the possible need for antibiotics (Patel & Hwang, 2021b). Observation without the use of antibiotics is an option for some patients with uncomplicated ABRS (mild pain, temperature of less than 38.3 °C [101 °F]). Follow-up is essential. Studies suggest that most patients will improve spontaneously. Antibiotics can be started if the patient is unlikely to follow-up or if the patient's symptoms worsen or fail to improve within the 7- to 10-day observation period (Patel & Hwang, 2021b). The recommended first-line drug for both children and adults is amoxicillin-clavulanate. Doxycycline may be used as an alternative for patients who cannot tolerate amoxicillin-clavulanate. For patients with a penicillin allergy, doxycycline or a respiratory fluoroquinolone such as levofloxacin or moxifloxacin is recommended (CDC, 2017; Patel & Hwang, 2021b). Prescribed medications may be required for a period of 3 to 4 weeks for CRS and recurrent ARS. Other antibiotics such as cephalosporins, macrolides, and trimethoprim–sulfamethoxazole are no longer recommended because they are not effective in treating antibiotic-resistant organisms that are commonly associated with ABRS (Tewfik, 2018).

For patients with concomitant asthma, leukotriene inhibitors may be used. Leukotriene inhibitors block the binding of *leukotrienes,* which are inflammatory mediators (Massoth et al., 2019). If allergies are a possible cause of CRS, oral antihistamines or nasal corticosteroids may be prescribed (Eguiluz-Gracia et al., 2019). The use of intranasal inhalations has been associated with a significant improvement of symptoms of CRS and a reduction in nasal bacteria (Vathanophas et al., 2019). Intranasal corticosteroids have been shown to produce complete or marked improvement in acute symptoms of CRS, with or without the presence of nasal polyps (Macias-Valle & Psaltis, 2021; Segboer et al., 2019).

If standard medical therapy fails to treat CRS and symptoms persist, endoscopic sinus surgery (ESS) may be indicated to correct structural deformities that obstruct the ostia (openings) of the sinuses (Alanin & Hopkins, 2020). Patients undergoing ESS report a reduction of all symptoms (Veloso-Teles & Cerejeira, 2017). Excising and cauterizing nasal polyps, correcting a deviated septum, incising and draining the sinuses, aerating the sinuses, and removing tumors are some of the specific procedures performed. If sinusitis is caused by a fungal infection, surgery is required to excise both the fungus ball and necrotic tissue and drain the sinuses. Antimicrobial agents are administered before and after surgery. Some patients with severe chronic sinusitis obtain relief only by relocating to a dry climate.

Complications

If untreated, ARS may lead to severe complications. Complications occur when the infection spreads beyond the paranasal sinuses and nasal cavity and enters the central nervous system, orbit, or surrounding tissues. These complications include periorbital cellulitis, orbital cellulitis, osteomyelitis of the sinus bones, meningitis, intracranial abscess, and septic cavernous sinus thrombosis (Patel & Hwang, 2021a). These complications require prompt treatment, some including prolonged use of antibiotics. Complications of CRS, although uncommon, include severe orbital cellulitis, subperiosteal abscess, cavernous sinus thrombosis, meningitis, encephalitis, and ischemic infarction. CRS can also lead to intracranial infection.

PHARYNGITIS

Acute **pharyngitis** is a sudden inflammation of the pharynx involving the back portion of the tongue, soft palate, and tonsils. Chronic pharyngitis is a persistent inflammation of the pharynx and is commonly referred to as a sore throat. Approximately 12 million health care visits in the United States are due to acute pharyngitis each year (Chow & Doron, 2018; Hinkle et al., 2022).

Pathophysiology

Most cases of acute pharyngitis are caused by viral infection. Responsible viruses include the adenovirus, influenza virus, Epstein–Barr virus, and herpes simplex virus. Bacterial organisms account for the remainder of the cases. Ten percent of adults with pharyngitis have group A beta-hemolytic streptococcus, more commonly known as group A streptococcus (GAS), streptococcal pharyngitis, or "strep throat." Other bacterial organisms found in acute pharyngitis include *Mycoplasma pneumoniae, Neisseria gonorrhoeae,* and *H. influenzae* type B. All patients with acute pharyngitis should be tested for COVID-19 with a sensitive reverse-transcriptase polymerase chain reaction (PCR) test. This should be done to identify those with the illness, isolate them, perform contact tracing, and quarantine those who have been exposed (Chow & Doron, 2020).

Risk Factors

According to the Centers for Disease Control and Prevention (CDC, 2021b), the risk factors for acute pharyngitis include close contact with another person with group A strep pharyngitis. Other risk factors are being a parent of a school-aged child and being in crowded areas. Acute pharyngitis is most common in children 5 to 15 years of age; however, anyone can contract it at any age (CDC, 2021b). Chronic pharyngitis is common in adults who work or live in dusty surroundings, use their voice to excess, suffer from chronic cough, or habitually use alcohol and tobacco.

Clinical Manifestations and Assessment

The signs and symptoms of acute pharyngitis include a fiery-red pharyngeal membrane and tonsils, lymphoid follicles that are swollen and flecked with white-purple exudate, enlarged and tender cervical lymph nodes, and no cough (Fig. 8-3). Creamy exudates may be present in

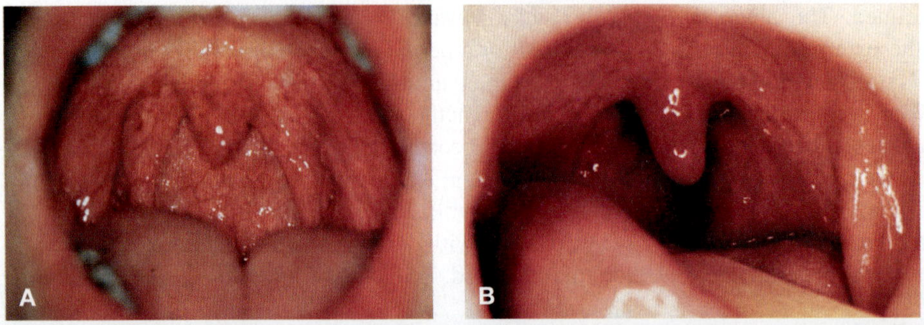

FIGURE 8-3 Pharyngitis, inflammation without exudate. A. Redness and vascularity of the pillars and uvula are mild to moderate. B. Redness is diffuse and intense. Each patient would probably complain of a sore throat. (From Bickley, L. S., & Szilagyi, P. G. [2013]. *Bates' guide to physical examination and history taking* [9th ed.]. Lippincott Williams & Wilkins.)

the tonsillar pillars. A fever greater than 100.4 °F (38 °C), malaise, and sore throat also may be present. Patients with GAS pharyngitis may exhibit vomiting, anorexia, and a characteristic scarlatina-form rash of the skin and tongue (strawberry or raspberry tongue) with urticaria known as *scarlet fever.*

Patients with chronic pharyngitis complain of a constant sense of irritation or fullness in the throat, mucus that collects in the throat and can be expelled by coughing, and difficulty swallowing. A sore throat that is worse with swallowing in the absence of pharyngitis suggests the possibility of thyroiditis and should be referred for evaluation.

Accurate diagnosis of pharyngitis is essential to determine the causative organism and to initiate treatment early. Rapid antigen detection testing (RADT) strep test and strep culture (sometimes referred to as STCX) should be used and require proper collection technique because improper collection reduces the accuracy of the test (Ackley et al., 2022; Chow & Doron, 2020).

Medical and Nursing Management

Viral pharyngitis is treated with supportive measures. Antibiotics will have no effect on the organism. Oral corticosteroids do not affect the clinical course but have been shown to reduce odynophagia (painful swallowing). Benzocaine or lidocaine mouth rinses also provide mild pain relief to the oropharynx. Patients can use nonsteroidal anti-inflammatory drugs and acetaminophen to help reduce pain and fever if present.

For bacterial pharyngitis treatments focus on the eradication of GAS. The recommended treatment is a 6- to 10-day course of amoxicillin. A single intramuscular dose of benzathine penicillin G can be administered if patient adherence is in question. When a bacterial cause is suggested or demonstrated, penicillin is usually the treatment of choice in acute pharyngitis. As noted with GAS, if patient compliance is a concern, then the patient may receive a one-time intramuscular dose of benzathine penicillin G. Patients who have a penicillin or amoxicillin allergy should receive cephalexin, clindamycin, or clarithromycin (Sykes et al., 2020). Nasal congestion may be relieved by short-term use of nasal sprays or medications containing ephedrine sulfate or phenylephrine hydrochloride. For a patient with a history of allergy, one of the antihistamine decongestant medications is prescribed orally every 4 to 6 hours. Supportive care for all types of pharyngitis includes analgesics, antipyretics, warm or cold fluids, soft foods, and avoidance of irritants (e.g., smoking).

Treatment of chronic pharyngitis is based on relieving symptoms, avoiding exposure to irritants, and correcting any upper respiratory, pulmonary, or cardiac condition that might cause a chronic cough. For adults with chronic pharyngitis, tonsillectomy is an effective option.

Complications

Uncomplicated viral infections usually subside promptly, within 3 to 10 days after the onset. However, pharyngitis caused by more virulent bacteria, such as GAS, is a more severe illness. If left untreated, the complications can be severe and life-threatening. Complications include rhinosinusitis, otitis media, peritonsillar abscess, mastoiditis, and cervical adenitis (inflammation of lymph nodes in the neck). In rare cases, the infection may lead to bacteremia, pneumonia, meningitis, rheumatic fever, rheumatic heart disease, or glomerulonephritis. Acute poststreptococcal glomerulonephritis (APSGN) is a complication that follows roughly 10 days after the onset of streptococcal infection and results in temporary or persistent kidney failure (<1% of children, up to 10% of adults) (Clinical Overview, 2022). APSGN is characterized by the rapid onset of gross hematuria, edema (leading to respiratory distress and pulmonary edema), and hypertension, and is usually preceded by an episode of GAS pharyngitis or pyoderma (skin infection with pustules) (Chaturvedi et al., 2018).

LARYNGITIS

Laryngitis is inflammation of the larynx that is primarily due to an acute viral infection, which is typically mild and self-limiting, lasting for 3 to 7 days (Gupta & Mahajan, 2022). Secondary causes are due to bacteria. Laryngitis can also be caused by overuse of voice, exposures to irritants, or as an URI symptom.

Pathophysiology

Laryngitis can be due to infectious or noninfectious causes. Common viral infections include rhinovirus, parainfluenza virus, RSV, coronavirus, adenovirus, and influenza. It also may be caused by an infection involving the vocal cords. Noninfectious causative factors include voice abuse or exposure to dust, chemicals, smoke, and other pollutants. Laryngitis is also associated with GERD (referred to as reflux laryngitis), allergic rhinitis, and pharyngitis (Hinkle et al., 2022). Bacterial invasion may be secondary. Asthma may contribute to laryngitis as the chemicals from inhalers create irritation, and long-term use of steroid inhalers use can predispose a patient to fungal laryngitis (Gupta & Mahajan, 2022). The onset of infection may be associated with exposure to sudden temperature changes, dietary deficiencies, malnutrition, or an immunosuppressed state. Viral laryngitis is common in the winter and is easily transmitted to others.

Clinical Manifestations and Assessment

Signs of acute laryngitis include hoarseness or **aphonia** (complete loss of voice) and severe cough. Other signs of acute laryngitis include sudden onset aggravated by cold dry wind. The throat feels worse in the morning and improves when the patient is indoors in a warmer climate. At times, the patient presents with a dry cough and a dry, sore throat that worsens in the evening hours. If allergies are present, the uvula will be visibly edematous. Many patients also complain of a "tickle" in the throat that is made worse by cold air or cold liquids. Chronic laryngitis is marked by persistent hoarseness.

Medical and Nursing Management

Management of acute or chronic laryngitis includes resting the voice, avoiding irritants (including smoking), getting enough rest, drinking additional fluids, and inhaling cool steam or an aerosol. Dietary modifications and restrictions are recommended for patients with GERD. Decongestants should be avoided due to their drying effects. In addition, alcohol and caffeine should be avoided because of their diuretic effects (Gupta & Mahajan, 2022). The majority of patients recover with conservative treatment; however, laryngitis tends to be more severe in older adults and may be complicated by pneumonia.

Antibiotics should not be used in a healthy individual with acute laryngitis. Antibiotics may be used in high-risk patients and patients with severe symptoms (Gupta & Mahajan, 2022). For chronic laryngitis, the use of topical corticosteroids may be given by inhalation. These preparations have few systemic or long-lasting effects and may reduce local inflammatory reactions. Treatment for reflux laryngitis typically involves use of proton pump inhibitors (PPIs) given once daily.

NURSING PROCESS
The Patient With Upper Airway Infection

ASSESSMENT

A health history may reveal signs and symptoms of headache, sore throat, pain around the eyes and on either side of the nose, difficulty in swallowing, cough, hoarseness, fever, stuffiness, and generalized discomfort and fatigue. Determining when the symptoms began, what precipitated them, what (if anything) relieves them, and what aggravates them is part of the assessment. Inspection may reveal swelling, lesions, or asymmetry of the nose, as well as bleeding or discharge. The nurse inspects the nasal mucosa for abnormal findings such as increased redness, swelling, exudate, and nasal polyps, which may develop in chronic rhinitis. The mucosa of the nasal turbinates may also be swollen (boggy) and pale, bluish-gray. The nurse palpates the frontal and maxillary sinuses for tenderness, which suggests inflammation, and then inspects the throat by having the patient open the mouth wide and take a deep breath. The tonsils and pharynx are inspected for abnormal findings such as redness, asymmetry, or evidence of drainage, ulceration, or enlargement. The nurse also palpates the trachea to determine the midline position in the neck and to detect any masses or deformities. The neck lymph nodes are palpated for enlargement and tenderness.

DIAGNOSIS

Appropriate nursing diagnoses may include:

- Ineffective airway clearance related to excessive mucus production secondary to retained secretions and inflammation.
- Acute pain related to upper airway irritation secondary to an infection.
- Verbal impairment related to physiologic changes and upper airway irritation secondary to infection, swelling, hoarseness, or loss of speech.
- Fluid volume deficit risk related to decreased fluid intake and increased fluid loss secondary to diaphoresis associated with a fever.
- Knowledge deficiency regarding prevention of URIs, treatment regimen, surgical procedure, or postoperative care.

PLANNING

The major goals for the patient may include maintenance of a patent airway, relief of pain, maintenance of effective means of communication, normal hydration, knowledge of how to prevent upper airway infections, and absence of complications.

NURSING INTERVENTIONS

MAINTAINING A PATENT AIRWAY

An accumulation of secretions can block the airway in patients with URI. As a result, changes in the respiratory pattern occur, and the work of breathing increases to compensate for the blockage. The nurse can implement several measures to loosen thick secretions or to keep the secretions moist so that they can be expectorated easily. Increasing fluid intake helps thin the mucus. Use of room vaporizers or steam inhalation may also loosen secretions and reduces inflammation of the mucous membranes. To enhance drainage from the sinuses, the nurse instructs the patient about the best position to assume; this depends on the location of the infection or inflammation.

PROMOTING COMFORT

URIs usually produce localized discomfort. The nurse encourages the patient to take analgesics as prescribed. Other helpful measures include topical anesthetic agents for symptomatic relief of herpes simplex blisters and sore throats, hot packs to relieve the congestion of rhinosinusitis and promote drainage, and warm-water gargles or irrigations to relieve the pain of a sore throat. The benefits of this treatment depend on the degree of heat that is applied. The nurse encourages rest to relieve the generalized discomfort and fever that accompany many upper URIs.

PROMOTING COMMUNICATION

URIs may result in hoarseness or loss of speech. The nurse instructs the patient to refrain from speaking as much as possible.

Additional strain on the vocal cords may delay full return of the voice. The nurse encourages the patient and family to use alternative forms of communication, such as a memo pad.

ENCOURAGING FLUID INTAKE

In URIs, the work of breathing and the respiratory rate increase as inflammation and secretions develop. This may increase insensible fluid loss. Fever further increases the metabolic rate, diaphoresis, and fluid loss. Sore throat, malaise, and fever may interfere with a patient's willingness to eat and drink. The nurse provides a list of easily ingested foods to increase caloric intake during the acute phase of illness. These include soups, pudding, yogurt, cottage cheese, high-protein drinks, and popsicles. The nurse encourages the patient to drink 2 to 3 L of fluid per day during the acute stage of airway infection, unless contraindicated, to thin the secretions and promote drainage. Liquids (hot or cold) may be soothing, depending on the disorder. In severe situations, IV fluids may be needed.

PREVENTING INFECTION

Prevention of most URIs is difficult because of the many potential causes. But because most URIs are transmitted by hand-to-hand contact, the nurse teaches the patient and family techniques to minimize the spread of infection to others, including frequent handwashing. The nurse advises the patient to avoid exposure to people who are at risk for serious illness including older adults, immunosuppressed people, and those with chronic health problems. The nurse may advise patients and those at increased risk from a respiratory infection to consider an annual influenza and pneumococcal vaccine as recommended by the primary care provider (PCP). A follow-up appointment with the PCP may be indicated for patients with compromised health status to ensure that the respiratory infection has resolved.

MONITORING AND MANAGING POTENTIAL COMPLICATIONS

Because most patients with URIs are managed at home, patients and their families must be instructed to monitor for signs and symptoms and to seek immediate medical care if the patient's condition does not improve or if the patient's physical status appears to be worsening. Symptoms that require further attention include persistent or high fever, increasing shortness of breath, confusion, and increasing weakness and malaise. Potential complications include sepsis, meningitis or brain abscess, and peritonsillar abscess, otitis media, or rhinosinusitis.

Sepsis and meningitis may occur in patients with compromised immune status or in those with an overwhelming bacterial infection. The nurse explains to the patient that fever, severe headache, and **nuchal rigidity** (stiffness of the neck/inability to bend the neck) are signs of potential complications. The patient with sepsis requires expert care to treat the infection, stabilize vital signs, and prevent or treat septicemia and shock. Deterioration of the patient's condition necessitates intensive care measures (e.g., hemodynamic monitoring and administration of vasoactive medications, IV fluids, nutritional support, corticosteroids) to monitor the patient's status and to support the patient's vital signs. High doses of antibiotics may be administered to treat the causative organism. The nurse's role is to monitor the patient's vital signs, hemodynamic status, and laboratory values; administer needed treatment; alleviate the patient's physical discomfort; and provide explanations, teaching, and emotional support to the patient and family. Refer to Chapter 53 for management of septic shock.

The patient and family are instructed about the signs and symptoms of otitis media and rhinosinusitis (periorbital edema, severe facial pain on palpation) and about the importance of follow-up with the PCP to ensure adequate evaluation and treatment of these conditions.

Potential for airway compromise is possible in severe pharyngitis. Symptoms that require provider referral include dyspnea, drooling, inability to swallow, and inability to fully open the mouth. The skin should be examined for possible rash because acute pharyngitis may precede some other communicable diseases (e.g., rubella). For the patient with laryngitis, the signs and symptoms that require contacting the health care provider include loss of voice with sore throat that makes swallowing saliva difficult, hemoptysis, and noisy respirations.

EVALUATION

Expected outcomes include:

1. Maintains a patent airway by managing secretions:
   a. Reports decreased congestion.
   b. Assumes best position to facilitate drainage of secretions.
   c. Uses self-care measures appropriately and consistently to manage secretions during the acute phase of illness.
2. Reports relief of pain and discomfort using pain intensity scale:
   a. Uses comfort measures: Analgesics, hot packs, gargles, rest.
   b. Demonstrates adequate oral hygiene.
   c. Free of pain in ears, sinuses, and throat.
3. Demonstrates ability to communicate needs, wants, level of comfort.
4. Maintains adequate fluid and nutrition intake.
5. Utilizes strategies to prevent upper airway infections:
   a. Demonstrates hand hygiene technique.
   b. Identifies the value of the influenza and pneumococcal vaccines.
6. Absence of complications:
   a. No signs of sepsis: Fever, hypotension, deterioration of cognitive status.
   b. Vital signs and hemodynamic status normal.
   c. No evidence of neurologic involvement.
   d. No signs of development of brain abscess.
   e. Resolution of URI without development of otitis media or rhinosinusitis.

OBSTRUCTION AND TRAUMA OF THE UPPER RESPIRATORY AIRWAY

OBSTRUCTION DURING SLEEP

Obstructive sleep apnea syndrome (OSAS) is a disorder characterized by recurrent episodes of upper airway obstruction and a reduction in ventilation. OSAS interferes with the person's ability to obtain adequate sleep, which can lead to decreased energy, cognitive deficits, mood changes, excessive sleepiness, and effects on work performance and activities of daily living. In the United States, OSAS affects 26% of individuals between 30 and 70 years (Kline, 2022; Santilli et al., 2021; Stepnowsky et al., 2019).

Various definitions of OSAS—also referred to as obstructive sleep apnea/hypopnea syndrome (OSAHS) or upper respiratory resistance syndrome (UARS)—exist, leading to overestimation of the prevalence of this syndrome.

Pathophysiology

OSAS is a disorder characterized by recurrent episodes of upper airway obstruction, causing a reduction in ventilation followed by frequent arousals and periodic oxyhemoglobin desaturations during sleep (Santilli et al., 2021; Temirbekov et al., 2018). OSAS is characterized by complete (apnea) or partial (hypopnea) obstruction of the upper airway. These obstruction episodes will be more than 5 per hour and last at least 10 seconds (Santilli et al., 2021). Repetitive apneic events result in hypoxia and hypercapnia (abnormal level of carbon dioxide in the blood), which trigger a sympathetic response (increased heart rate and increased tone and contractility of smooth muscle). An obstruction may be caused by mechanical factors such as a reduced diameter of the upper airway or dynamic changes in the upper airway during sleep.

Patients with OSAS have a higher prevalence of cardiovascular diseases, metabolic disorders, depression, and hypertension and an increased risk of myocardial infarction, stroke, and death (Baran et al., 2021; Stepnowsky et al., 2019). Patients with underlying cardiovascular disease may find the nocturnal **hypoxemia** may predispose them to arrhythmias. A high percentage of the morbidity and mortality related to OSAS is related to cardiovascular disease and cardiac rhythm disorders (Laczay & Faulx 2021). Obstructive and nocturnal hypoxemias are also associated with an increased risk of lung cancer (Seijo et al., 2019). OSAS can also increase insulin resistance and other metabolic changes that can increase the risk of vascular disease (Song et al., 2019).

Risk Factors

Sleep apnea is more prevalent in males, especially those who are older and overweight. However, postmenopausal and obese females are at increased risk of developing OSAS as well. The major risk factor for OSAS is obesity around the neck that narrows and compresses the upper airway. Older adults have a higher prevalence of OSAS. Other associated factors include alteration in the upper airway, such as structural changes (e.g., tonsillar hypertrophy, abnormal posterior positioning of one or both jaws, excessive fat deposits in the lateral walls of the pharynx, and craniofacial structural abnormalities) that contribute to the collapsibility of the airway and increase the risk of sleep apnea (Kline et al., 2020; Oliven et al., 2018). Other risk factors of OSAS include smoking, having a family history of snoring or OSAS, and nasal congestion. OSAS is also linked to substances and medications, including alcohol, benzodiazepines, narcotics, and possibly gabapentinoids, such as gabapentin (Kline et al., 2020).

Clinical Manifestations and Assessment

OSAS is characterized by frequent and loud snoring with breathing cessation for 10 seconds or longer, for at least five episodes per hour, followed by awakening abruptly with a loud snort as the blood oxygen level drops. Classic signs and symptoms of OSAS are presented in Box 8-1. Symptoms typically progress with increases in weight and aging as well as during the transition to menopause (Kline et al., 2020; Santilli et al., 2021).

Several screening tools/questionnaires are available to assess the frequency and severity of symptoms (Bazemore et al., 2019). The gold standard for diagnosis of sleep apnea is based on clinical symptoms plus polysomnographic findings (sleep study). This overnight sleep study measures multiple physiologic signals related to sleep (electroencephalogram [EEG], electrocardiogram [ECG], and airflow), in order to gauge oxyhemoglobin saturation, brain activity, eye movement, thoracic muscle activity, body position, respiratory rate, heart rate, cardiac arrhythmias, chest impedance, and airflow (Santilli et al., 2021; Kline et al., 2020).

Medical Management

Treatments are varied but include weight loss and avoidance of alcohol, hypnotic medications, positional therapy, and

BOX 8-1 **Focused Assessment**

Obstructive Sleep Apnea Syndrome (OSAS)

Be alert for the following signs and symptoms:

- Excessive daytime sleepiness
- Frequent nocturnal awakening
- Insomnia
- Loud snoring
- Morning headaches
- Intellectual deterioration
- Personality changes, irritability
- Impotence
- Systemic hypertension
- Arrhythmias
- Pulmonary hypertension, cor pulmonale
- Polycythemia
- Enuresis

mandibular advancement devices (MADs) (American Sleep Apnea Association, 2019). Weight loss reduces the number of apneas and hypopneas per hour of total sleep time as measured by the apnea–hypopnea index (AHI). Oral appliances designed to reposition the mandible or tongue may be useful in select patients. These devices are not very beneficial in some older adults, as full dentition is required (Gottlieb & Punjabi, 2020).

Noninvasive Positive-Pressure Ventilation

In more severe cases of OSAS involving hypoxemia with severe carbon dioxide retention (hypercapnia), the treatment includes continuous positive airway pressure (CPAP) or bilevel positive airway pressure (BiPAP) therapy with supplemental oxygen. Patients are considered candidates for noninvasive ventilation if they have acute or chronic respiratory failure, acute pulmonary edema, chronic obstructive pulmonary disease (COPD), chronic heart failure, or OSAS. The device also may be used at home to improve tissue oxygenation and to rest the respiratory muscles while the patient sleeps at night (Gottlieb & Punjabi, 2020; Seyfi et al., 2019; Suen et al., 2020).

CPAP provides positive pressure to the airways throughout the respiratory cycle, preventing collapse (Gottlieb & Punjabi, 2020). A CPAP delivery system is comprised of an air pump that is connected to a nasal, oral, or combined mask by a flexible tube. The air pump extracts external filtered air to deliver the pressurized airflow that can be adjusted. The leak-proof mask keeps the alveoli open, thereby preventing respiratory failure. CPAP is the most effective treatment for OSAS because the positive pressure acts as a splint, keeping the upper airway and trachea open during sleep. To use CPAP, the patient must be breathing independently (Gottlieb & Punjabi, 2020; Marin-Oto et al., 2019; Morton & Fontaine, 2018; Patil et al., 2019).

BiPAP helps to make breathing easier and results in a lower average airway pressure and offers independent control of inspiratory and expiratory pressures while providing pressure-support ventilation. It delivers two levels of positive airway pressure via a nasal or oral mask, nasal pillow, or mouthpiece with a tight seal and a portable ventilator. Each inspiration can be initiated either by the patient or by the machine (programmed backup rate). The backup rate ensures that the patient will receive a set number of breaths per minute. BiPAP is most often used for patients who require ventilatory assistance at night, such as those with severe COPD or sleep apnea. Tolerance is variable; BiPAP usually is most successful with highly motivated patients (Morton & Fontaine, 2018; Patil et al., 2019).

Problems with CPAP or BiPAP therapy are common. Commonly reported adverse effects of CPAP include skin irritations, pain, rash, or breakdown at the mask contact points (usually the bridge of the nose) (Alqahtani et al., 2018). Dryness or irritation of the nasal and pharyngeal membranes, nasal congestion, and eye irritation from leakage from the mask are also reported (Volsko, 2019). Gastrointestinal bloating secondary to air swallowing is another common side effect (Basner, 2016; Pan et al., 2020). Proper fitting of the mask should allow for therapy to continue. Although these treatments are effective in managing OSAS, patient compliance with treatment continues to be a major concern (Seo & Lee, 2020).

Surgical Management

Surgical procedures (e.g., tonsillectomy or **uvulopalatopharyngoplasty** [termed UPPP, the surgical resection of pharyngeal soft tissue and uvula]) may be performed to correct the obstruction if the airway is in jeopardy or the patient has been unsuccessful with CPAP therapy.

The most effective surgical treatment for OSAS is maxillomandibular advancement surgery (MMA). This procedure has a success rate of 75% to 100%. Some researchers now consider MMA the gold standard for treatment because the procedure enlarges the upper airway (Chang et al., 2020). Nasal septoplasty may be performed for anatomic nasal septal deformities (Dizdar et al., 2019). In 2014, the U.S. Food and Drug Administration approved hypoglossal nerve stimulation as an approach to treat OSAS. This treatment involves neurostimulation by surgically implanting an upper airway stimulation device. This is an alternative for patients who have difficulty tolerating or who are not adherent with CPAP therapy (Chang et al., 2020).

Tracheostomy relieves upper airway obstruction but has many adverse effects, including speech difficulties and increased risk of infections. These procedures, as well as other maxillofacial surgeries, are reserved for patients with life-threatening arrhythmias or severe disabilities who have not responded to conventional therapy (Chang et al., 2020).

Pharmacologic Therapy

Although medications are not generally recommended for OSAS, modafinil has been shown to reduce daytime sleepiness (Greenblatt & Adams, 2022). Some patients report better results with intranasal mometasone furoate as this medication decreases nasal congestion and increases the size of the airway (Greenblatt & Adams, 2022). With protriptyline, patients report improvements in daytime sleepiness and have been shown to have an increase in oxygen saturation (Arredondo et al., 2022). Other medications have been investigated in trials to treat OSAS. Some of these medications include theophylline and acetazolamide, which stimulates the respiratory drive, or drugs that reduce upper airways from collapsing (e.g., desipramine), antimuscarinics (e.g., oxybutynin), or noradrenergic agents (e.g., atomoxetine). Although these drugs have shown to aid in some improvements, their use is controversial and no pharmacologic agent has proven to be sufficiently effective (Kryger & Malhotra, 2022). Patients must understand that medications are not a substitute for CPAP or BiPAP therapy. Administration of low-flow nasal oxygen at night can help relieve hypoxemia in some patients but has little effect on the frequency or severity of apnea. Further study on the effectiveness of pharmacologic therapy is needed.

Nursing Management

The patient with OSAS may not recognize the potential consequences of the disorder. The nurse explains the disorder and relates symptoms (daytime sleepiness, morning headaches, heartburn, insomnia, snoring) to the underlying disorder. The nurse also instructs the patient and family about treatments, including weight loss, avoiding alcohol and sedative medications, and the correct and safe use of prescribed therapies such as CPAP, BiPAP, and oxygen therapy. The nurse encourages the patient regarding weight loss since evidence exists that it reduces the severity of OSAS, and if significant, may potentially allow some patients to discontinue CPAP therapy (Paul & Hayes, 2022).

EPISTAXIS (NOSEBLEED)

Epistaxis, a hemorrhage from the nose, is caused by the rupture of tiny, distended vessels in the mucous membrane of any area of the nose. Most commonly, the site is the anterior septum, where three major blood vessels enter the nasal cavity. Several risk factors may be associated with epistaxis and are described in Box 8-2.

Males experience more nosebleeds than females. Nosebleeds may occur either in the anterior portion (>80%) of the nose (anterior epistaxis) or posterior portion (~5%) of the nose (posterior epistaxis) (Ali, 2023). Anterior epistaxis causes include, antiplatelet or anticoagulant medications, drying of the nasal passages, trauma, and inhaled drugs and/or chemicals. Posterior epistaxis causes include hypertension, diabetes, and trauma (Hogan, 2019). However, ~90% of epistaxis events are idiopathic (Ali, 2023). Commonly used products that increase the risk for epistaxis are cocaine and OTC nasal steroid sprays (Buttaravoli et al., 2022).

BOX 8-2 Risk Factors for Epistaxis

- Local infections/inflammation (vestibulitis, rhinitis, rhinosinusitis, sinusitis, nasal polyps)
- Systemic infections (scarlet fever, malaria)
- Drying of nasal mucous membranes (cold, dry environment); overuse of decongestant nasal sprays
- Structural deformities (deviated septum, chronic perforations)
- Nasal inhalation of illicit drugs (e.g., cocaine), irritants
- Trauma (digital trauma as in picking the nose; blunt trauma; fracture; forceful nose-blowing)
- Nasal or facial surgery
- Arteriosclerosis
- Hypertension
- Tumor (sinus or nasopharynx)
- Coagulopathy (thrombocytopenia, hemophilia, von Willebrand disease)
- Drugs: Use of aspirin, nonsteroidal anti-inflammatory drugs (NSAIDs), warfarin
- Liver disease
- Osler–Weber–Rendu (hereditary hemorrhagic telangiectasia)
- Foreign bodies in the nasal cavity

Medical Management

Management of epistaxis depends on its cause and the location of the bleeding site. Initial treatment includes applying direct pressure. The patient sits upright with the head tilted forward to prevent swallowing and aspiration of blood and is directed to pinch the soft outer portion of the nose against the midline septum for 5 or 10 minutes continuously. Swallowed blood may act as an irritant causing the patient to vomit. Ice may be applied to the bridge of the nose to help constrict blood vessels (Khan et al., 2017). If sustained pressure is unsuccessful, the nose must be examined using good illumination and suction to determine the site of bleeding (Cash et al., 2020; Smith et al., 2019). Cotton applicators soaked in a topical vasoconstrictor such as phenylephrine or oxymetazoline may be inserted into the nose to reduce the blood flow (Cash et al., 2020). Visible bleeding sites may be cauterized with silver nitrate or electrocautery (high-frequency electrical current). A sterile oxidized regenerated cellulose supplemental patch (Surgicel) may be used (Cash et al., 2020). If the origin of the bleeding cannot be identified, the nose may be packed with gauze impregnated with petroleum jelly or antibiotic ointment. The packing may remain in place for 48 hours or up to 5 or 6 days if necessary to control bleeding. Antibiotics may be prescribed because of the risk of iatrogenic sinusitis and toxic shock syndrome.

Nursing Management

The nurse monitors the patient's vital signs, assists in the control of bleeding, and provides tissues and an emesis basin to allow the patient to expectorate any excess blood. The nurse continuously assesses the patient's airway and breathing, as well as vital signs. On rare occasions, a patient with significant hemorrhage requires IV infusions of crystalloid solutions (normal saline or lactated Ringer's) as well as cardiac and pulse oximetry monitoring.

Once the bleeding is controlled, the nurse instructs the patient to avoid vigorous exercise for several days and to avoid hot or spicy foods and tobacco, as they may cause vasodilation and an increased risk of rebleeding. Discharge teaching includes reviewing ways to prevent epistaxis: avoiding forceful nose-blowing, straining, high altitudes, and nasal trauma. Adequate humidification may prevent drying of the nasal passages. The nurse instructs the patient how to apply direct pressure to the nose in case of a recurrent nosebleed. If recurrent bleeding cannot be stopped, the patient is instructed to seek additional medical attention.

NASAL OBSTRUCTION

The passage of air through the nostrils is frequently obstructed by a deviation of the nasal septum, hypertrophy of the turbinate bones, or the presence of nasal polyps. Chronic nasal congestion forces the patient to breathe through the mouth, producing dryness of the oral mucosa and other problems including persistent dry, cracked lips. Patients with chronic nasal congestion often suffer from sleep deprivation due to difficulty maintaining an adequate airway while lying flat during sleep.

Medical Management

The treatment of nasal obstruction requires the removal of the obstruction, followed by measures to treat chronic infection. Measures to reduce or alleviate nasal obstruction include nonsurgical as well as surgical techniques. Commonly used medications include nasal corticosteroids. Treatment with nasal corticosteroids for 1 to 3 months is beneficial in treatment of small polyps, avoiding surgical intervention. Additional medications may include antibiotics for the treatment of underlying infection or antihistamines for management of allergies. Hypertrophied turbinates may be treated by applying an astringent agent to shrink them. A more aggressive approach in treating nasal obstruction caused by turbinate hypertrophy involves surgical reduction of the hypertrophy, a procedure known as functional rhinoplasty.

Nursing Management

Most of these surgical procedures are performed on an outpatient basis. Postoperatively, the nurse elevates the head of the bed to promote drainage and to alleviate discomfort from edema. Frequent oral hygiene is encouraged to overcome dryness caused by breathing through the mouth. Before discharge, the patient is instructed to avoid blowing the nose with force during the postoperative recovery period. The patient is also instructed about the signs and symptoms of bleeding and infection and when to contact the provider.

FRACTURES OF THE NOSE

Nasal fracture is the most common fracture involving the face. Fractures of the nose usually result from a direct assault. Nasal fractures may affect the ascending process of the maxilla and the septum. The torn mucous membrane results in a nosebleed. In a series of complications, the patient could ultimately experience a hematoma, infection, abscess, and a vascular/septic necrosis. However, serious consequences usually do not occur.

Clinical Manifestations and Assessment

The signs and symptoms of a nasal fracture are pain, bleeding from the nose externally and internally into the pharynx, swelling of the soft tissues adjacent to the nose, periorbital ecchymosis, nasal obstruction, and deformity. The patient's nose may have an asymmetric appearance that may not be obvious until the edema subsides.

The nose is examined internally to rule out the possibility that the injury may be complicated by a fracture of the nasal septum and a submucosal septal hematoma (Papadakis et al., 2019). Clear fluid draining from either nostril suggests a fracture of the cribriform plate with leakage of cerebrospinal fluid (CSF). Because CSF contains glucose, it can readily be differentiated from nasal mucus by means of a dipstick. Refer to Chapter 44 for details of CSF leaks.

Pearls for Practice

If CSF is suspected, the patient is instructed not to cough or blow the nose. If the patient has to sneeze, do so with an open mouth. The head of bed should be elevated, and nothing should be inserted into the nares. The primary concern of CSF rhinorrhea (leakage of CSF via the nares) is the complication of meningitis.

Careful inspection or palpation discloses any deviations of the bone or disruptions of the nasal cartilages. An x-ray may reveal displacement of the fractured bones and may help rule out extension of the fracture into the skull.

Medical Management

Any bleeding is controlled with the use of packing. For the patient who has sustained traumatic force to break the nose or any facial bone, the possibility of a cervical spine fracture must be considered. If suspected, stabilize the cervical spine and log roll the patient if turning is required. Uncomplicated nasal fractures may be treated initially with analgesic agents, use of ice to reduce swelling, and ENT follow-up.

Treatment of nasal fractures is aimed at restoring nasal function and returning the aesthetic appearance of the nose to baseline. Reduction of the fracture is performed as soon as possible. If edema is too severe to reduce the fraction immediately, reduction is performed within 3 to 7 days. Fractures that heal but are misaligned may require surgical intervention, such as rhinoplasty, to reshape the external appearance of the nose. In patients who develop a septal hematoma, the provider will drain the hematoma through a small incision. Antibiotic coverage is expected after septal hematoma evacuation. A septal hematoma that is not drained can lead to permanent deformity of the nose.

Nursing Management

Immediately after the fracture, the nurse applies ice and encourages the patient to keep the head elevated. The nurse instructs the patient to apply ice packs to the nose for 20 minutes, four times each day, to decrease swelling. The packing inserted to stop the bleeding may be uncomfortable and unpleasant, and obstruction of the nasal passages by the packing forces the patient to breathe through the mouth. This, in turn, causes the oral mucous membranes to become dry. Mouth rinses help to moisten the mucous membranes and to reduce the odor and taste of dried blood in the oropharynx and nasopharynx. Use of analgesic agents, such as acetaminophen, is preferred initially over NSAIDs, such as ibuprofen or naproxen, in the first 2 days to avoid increasing the risk of bleeding. The nurse reminds the patient to avoid sports activities, especially contact sports, for 6 weeks.

LARYNGEAL OBSTRUCTION

Laryngeal obstruction is characterized by an obstruction in airflow within the larynx. It is an umbrella term for anything that may obstruct the supraglottic and/or the glottic level of the larynx (Lee et al., 2018). Obstruction of the larynx caused by edema is a serious, often fatal, condition. The larynx contains a narrow space between the vocal cords (glottis), through which air must pass. Swelling of the laryngeal mucous membranes may close off the opening tightly, leading to life-threatening hypoxia or suffocation.

Pathophysiology

Edema of the glottis occurs rarely in patients with acute laryngitis, occasionally in patients with urticaria, and more frequently in patients with severe inflammation of the throat, as in scarlet fever. It is an occasional but usually preventable cause of death in severe anaphylaxis (angioedema). Hereditary angioedema (HAE) is also characterized by episodes of life-threatening laryngeal edema. Laryngeal edema in people with HAE can occur at any age, although young adults are at greatest risk. Laryngospasm, a severe form of airway obstruction, may be triggered by mechanical stimulation of the larynx or by cord irritation due to aspiration of oral secretions, blood, or vomitus (Bork et al., 2020; Lee et al., 2018).

Risk Factors

Risk factors for laryngeal obstruction are provided in Box 8-3. Foreign bodies frequently are aspirated into the pharynx, the larynx, or the trachea.

Clinical Manifestations and Assessment

The foreign objects obstruct the air passages and cause difficulty in breathing, hoarseness, and stridor, which may lead to asphyxia; and later, the obstructing objects may be drawn farther down, entering the bronchi or a bronchial branch and causing symptoms of irritation, such as a croup (barking) cough, expectoration of blood or mucus, or labored breathing. The patient may demonstrate lowered oxygen saturation; however, normal oxygen saturation should not be interpreted as a sign that the obstruction is not significant. Use of accessory muscles to maximize airflow may occur and is often manifested by retractions in the neck or abdomen during inspirations. Patients who demonstrate these symptoms may need ventilatory support (i.e., mechanical ventilation or positive-pressure ventilation).

A thorough history can be very useful to the health care team in diagnosing and treating the patient with a laryngeal obstruction. The nurse obtains a history from the patient or family about alcohol or tobacco consumption, current medications, family history of airway problems, recent infections, pain or fever, dental pain or poor dentition, and any previous surgeries or trauma. Emergency measures to secure the patient's airway should not be delayed to obtain a history or perform tests. The patient's clinical presentation and x-ray findings confirm the diagnosis of laryngeal obstruction.

BOX 8-3 Risk Factors for Laryngeal Obstruction

- History of allergies that may result in anaphylaxis
- Inhalation/ingestion of foreign body (balloon fragments, chewing gum, drug packets)
- Heavy alcohol consumption or tobacco use (causing a tumor)
- Family history of airway problems (suggests angioedema)
- Use of ACE inhibitors
- Recent throat pain or fever (suggests infectious process)
- History of surgery or previous tracheostomy (suggests possible subglottic stenosis)

Medical and Nursing Management

Medical management is based on the initial evaluation of the patient and the need to ensure a patent airway. If the airway is obstructed by a foreign body and signs of asphyxia are apparent, immediate treatment is necessary. Frequently, if the foreign body has lodged in the pharynx and can be visualized, the finger can dislodge it. If the obstruction is in the larynx or the trachea, the clinician or other rescuer tries the subdiaphragmatic abdominal thrust (Heimlich) maneuver. If all efforts are unsuccessful, an immediate tracheotomy is necessary. If the obstruction is caused by edema resulting from an allergic reaction, treatment may include administration of subcutaneous epinephrine and a corticosteroid (see Chapter 37). Continuous pulse oximetry is essential. Box 8-4 describes nursing management of an upper airway obstruction.

CANCER OF THE LARYNX

Laryngeal cancer accounts for 1% of all cancers in the United States. Cancer of the larynx is a malignancy in and around the larynx (voice box). Squamous cell carcinoma is the most common form of cancer of the larynx, although small cell carcinomas also occur. Carcinoma of the glottis is more common than that of the supraglottic areas, whereas tumors of the subglottic area are rare (Huether & McCance, 2019).

Carcinogens associated with laryngeal cancer include tobacco (smoke, smokeless) and alcohol and their combined effects. Occupational or environmental exposure to asbestos, wood dust, coal dust, steel dust, cement dust, tar products,

BOX 8-4

Management of Upper Airway Obstruction

Adequate ventilation is dependent on free movement of air through the upper and lower airways. Maintaining a patent (open) airway is achieved through meticulous airway management, whether in an emergency situation, such as airway obstruction, or in long-term management, as in caring for a patient with an endotracheal or a tracheostomy tube. The patient with an altered level of consciousness from any cause is at risk for upper airway obstruction because of loss of the protective reflexes (cough and swallowing) and loss of the tone of the pharyngeal muscles, which causes the tongue to fall back and block the airway.

The nurse makes rapid observations to assess for signs and symptoms of upper airway obstruction: assessing the patient's level of consciousness (LOC), inspecting the chest for movement and use or retraction of accessory muscles, and noting skin color and any obvious signs of deformity or obstruction of the airway (trauma, food, teeth, tongue, vomitus). The nurse should palpate the trachea for midline location and look for any specific areas of tenderness, fracture, or subcutaneous emphysema (crepitus). Auscultation is performed to assess for audible air movement, stridor (inspiratory crowing sound), or wheezing (high-pitched musical sound) that may be present over the lower trachea and bilaterally in all lobes. As soon as an upper airway obstruction is identified, the nurse takes the following emergency measures:

Clearing the Airway

- Hyperextend the patient's neck by placing one hand on the forehead and placing the fingers of the other hand underneath the jaw and lifting upward and forward. This action pulls the tongue away from the back of the pharynx. Note that this position is used only if the cervical spine is free of injury.

  Assess the patient by observing the chest and listening and feeling for the movement of air.

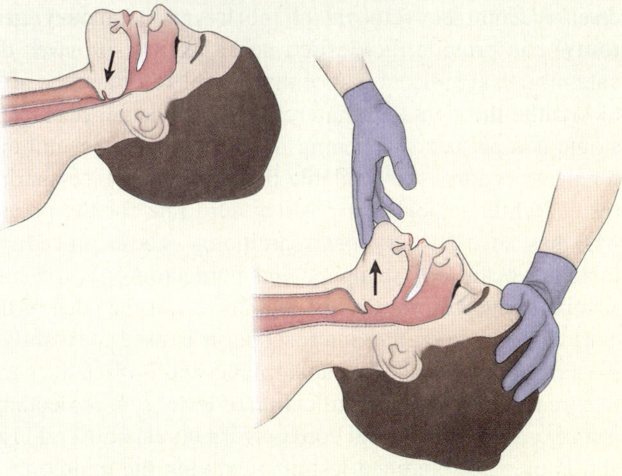

- Use a cross-finger technique to open the mouth and observe for obvious obstructions, such as secretions, blood clots, or food particles.
- If no passage of air is detected, apply five quick sharp abdominal thrusts just below the xiphoid process to expel the obstruction. Repeat this procedure until the obstruction is expelled.

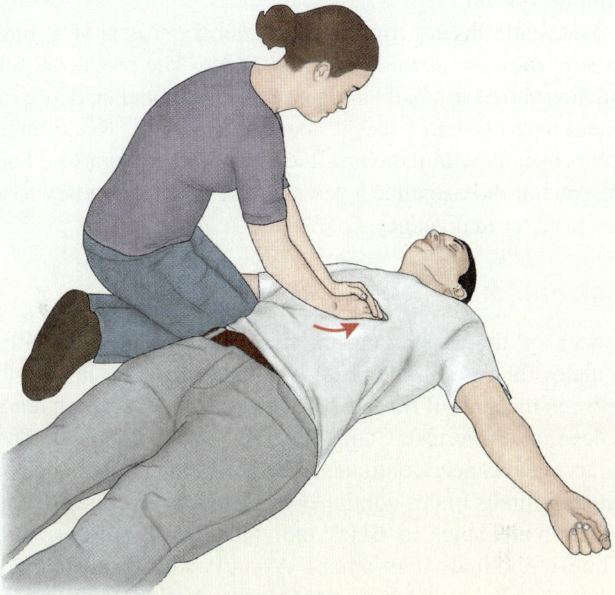

- After the obstruction is expelled, roll the patient as a unit onto the side for recovery.
- When the obstruction is relieved, if the patient can breathe spontaneously but not cough, swallow, or gag, insert an oral or nasopharyngeal airway.

Bag and Mask Resuscitation

- Use a resuscitation bag and mask if assisted ventilation is required.
- Apply the mask to the patient's face and create a seal by pressing the thumb of the nondominant hand on the bridge of the nose and the index finger on the chin. Using the rest of the fingers on that hand, pull on the chin and the angle of the mandible to maintain the head in extension. Use the dominant hand to inflate the lungs by squeezing the bag to its full volume.

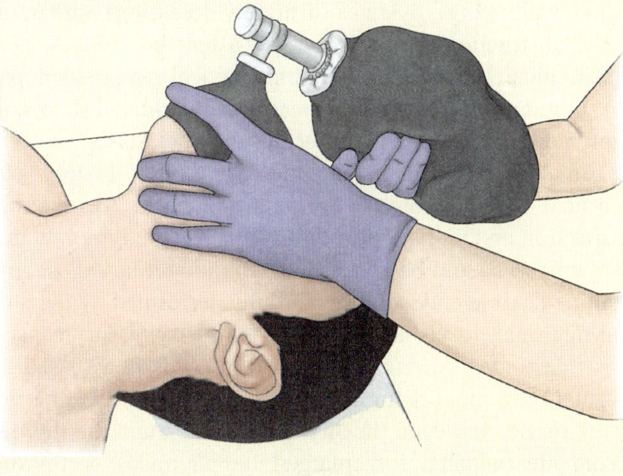

leather, formaldehyde, and iron compounds and fumes have also been implicated. Other contributing factors include straining the voice, chronic laryngitis, nutritional deficiencies (riboflavin), family predisposition, and a weakened immune system.

Metastatic disease from the true vocal cords is very rare because they are devoid of lymph nodes. The prognosis for patients who have small laryngeal cancers without evidence of spread to the lymph nodes is about 75% to 95%. Recurrence occurs usually within the first 2 to 3 years after diagnosis. The presence of disease after 5 years is very often secondary to a new primary malignancy.

Risk Factors

Cancer of the larynx occurs five times more frequently in males than in females, and it is most common in people between the ages of 60 and 70 years, as it takes several years to develop (American Cancer Society, 2020). The incidence of laryngeal cancer continues to decline, but the incidence in females versus males continues to increase. The disease has a higher incidence in Black individuals and non-Hispanic White individuals than among Asian/Pacific Islander individuals and American Indian/Alaska Native individuals. Other risk factors for cancer of the larynx are tobacco smoke and products, alcohol use, being overweight, human papillomavirus (HPV), genetics, and workplace exposures (American Cancer Society, 2020).

Clinical Manifestations and Assessment

Hoarseness of more than 2 weeks duration occurs in the patient with cancer in the glottic area because the tumor impedes the action of the vocal cords during speech. The voice may sound harsh, raspy, and lower in pitch. Affected voice sounds are not early signs of subglottic or supraglottic cancer. The patient may complain of a persistent cough or sore throat and pain and burning in the throat, especially when consuming hot liquids or citrus juices. A lump may be felt in the neck. Later symptoms include **dysphagia** (difficulty swallowing), dyspnea (difficulty breathing), unilateral nasal obstruction or discharge, persistent hoarseness, persistent ulceration, and foul breath. Cervical lymph adenopathy, unintentional weight loss, a general debilitated state, and pain radiating to the ear may occur with metastasis.

An initial assessment includes a complete history and physical examination of the head and neck. An external inspection and palpation of the larynx and the lymph nodes in the neck should be performed. An indirect laryngoscopy, using a flexible endoscope, is initially performed by the otolaryngologist to visually evaluate the pharynx, larynx, and possible tumor. Mobility of the vocal cords is assessed; if normal movement is limited, the growth may affect muscle, other tissue, and even the airway. The neck and the thyroid gland are palpated for enlarged lymph nodes or thyroid gland.

Diagnostic procedures that may be utilized include endoscopy, optical imaging, and CT scans. A direct laryngoscopic examination performed under local or general anesthesia may be required to evaluate all areas of the larynx. Direct visualization and palpation of the vocal folds may yield a more accurate diagnosis.

CT and MRI are used to assess regional adenopathy and soft tissue and to help stage and determine the extent of a tumor. MRI is also helpful in posttreatment follow-up to detect a recurrence. Positron emission tomography (PET) scanning may also be used to detect recurrence of a laryngeal tumor after treatment.

Medical Management

The goals of treatment of laryngeal cancer include cure; preservation of safe, effective swallowing; preservation of useful voice; and avoidance of permanent tracheostomy (Mannelli et al., 2018; Tamaki et al., 2018). Treatment options include surgery, radiation therapy, and chemotherapy. The prognosis depends on a variety of factors: tumor stage, the patient's gender and age, and pathologic features of the tumor, including the grade and depth of infiltration. The treatment plan also depends on whether this is an initial diagnosis or a recurrence.

Surgery and radiation therapy are both effective methods in the early stages of cancer of the larynx. Chemotherapy traditionally has been used for recurrence or metastatic disease. It has also been used more recently in conjunction with radiation therapy, to avoid a total laryngectomy, or preoperatively, to shrink a tumor before surgery.

Surgical Management

Surgical management depends largely on the stage of the disease. Complete removal of the larynx (total **laryngectomy**) can provide the desired cure, but it also leaves the patient with significant loss of the natural voice and the need to breathe through a stoma created in the lower neck. The stoma is a permanent opening into the trachea. Several different procedures are available that can offer voice-sparing results while achieving a positive cure rate for the patient who has an early laryngeal carcinoma. These procedures include vocal cord stripping and cordectomy. Vocal cord stripping involves removal of the mucosa of the edge of the cord using an operating microscope. It is used to treat dysplasia, hyperkeratosis, and leukoplakia and is often the curative treatment for this classification of lesions. A cordectomy is an excision of the vocal cord performed via transoral laser and is used for confined lesions involving the middle third of the vocal cord. The probability of poor voice quality is related to the extent of tissue removed.

These partial resections are increasingly common surgical procedures, using total laryngectomy as salvage therapy for recurrences (Patel et al., 2019). Several different types of laryngectomy are considered for patients with more extensive involvement. These include partial laryngectomy, supraglottic laryngectomy, hemilaryngectomy, or total laryngectomy.

- *Partial laryngectomy* (laryngofissure–thyrotomy): A portion of the larynx is removed, along with one vocal cord and the tumor; all other structures remain. The airway remains intact, and the patient is expected to have no difficulty swallowing. The voice quality may change, or the patient may sound hoarse. It is associated with a high cure rate.
- *Supraglottic laryngectomy:* The hyoid bone, glottis, and false cords are removed in a voice-sparing operation. The true vocal cords, cricoid cartilage, and trachea remain intact. A tracheostomy is left in place until the glottic airway is established. Postoperative irradiation may be indicated. The quality of the voice may change.
- *Hemilaryngectomy:* The thyroid cartilage of the larynx is split in the midline of the neck, and the portion of the vocal cord (one true cord and one false cord) is removed with the tumor. Some change may occur in the voice quality. The voice may be rough, raspy, and hoarse and have limited projection. The airway and swallowing remain intact.
- *Total laryngectomy:* The larynx is completely removed, including the hyoid bone, epiglottis, cricoid cartilage, and two or three rings of the trachea. The tongue, pharyngeal walls, and trachea are preserved. This procedure is performed for advanced laryngeal cancer and results in permanent loss of the voice and a change in the airway (Cancer Treatment Centers of America, 2022).

Surgery for laryngeal cancer is more difficult when the lesion involves the midline structures or both vocal cords. With or without neck dissection, a total laryngectomy requires a permanent tracheal stoma (Fig. 8-4) because the larynx that provides the protective sphincter is no longer present. The tracheal stoma prevents the aspiration of food and fluid into the lower respiratory tract since the pharyngeal opening to the trachea is now closed, leaving the pharynx open only to the esophagus. The patient will have no voice but will have normal swallowing. A total laryngectomy changes the manner in which airflow is used for breathing and speaking, as depicted in Figure 8-5. Patients who have this procedure require alternatives to normal speech.

Complications that may occur include death, a salivary leak, wound infection from the development of a pharyngocutaneous fistula, dysphagia, cellulitis, neck abscess, incisional dehiscence, hematoma, chyle leak, pneumonia, and cervical esophageal stricture. Some patients develop complications

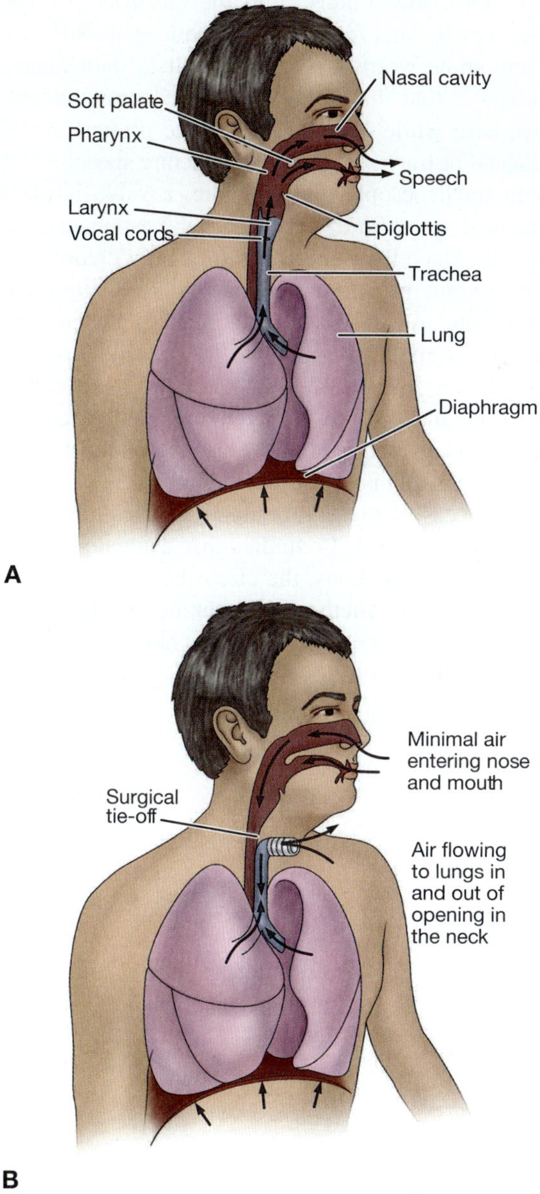

FIGURE 8-4 **Total laryngectomy produces a change in airflow for breathing and speaking. A. Normal airflow. B. Airflow after total laryngectomy.**

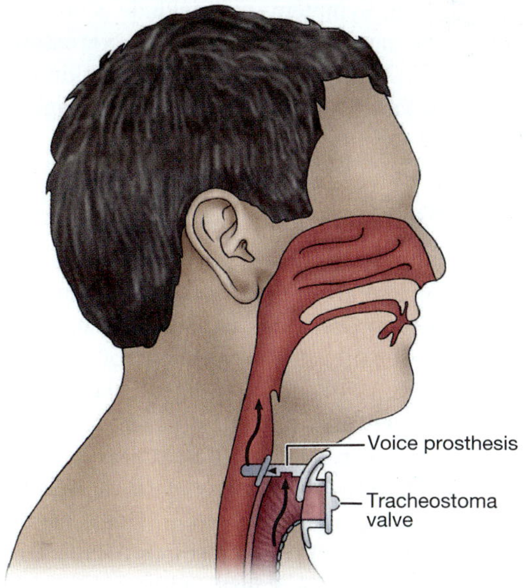

FIGURE 8-5 **Schematic representation of tracheoesophageal puncture speech (TEP). Air travels from the lung through a puncture in the posterior wall of the trachea into the esophagus and out the mouth. A voice prosthesis is fitted over the puncture site.**

after leaving the hospital setting, requiring readmission. Advances in surgical techniques for treating laryngeal cancer may minimize the cosmetic and functional deficits previously seen with total laryngectomy. Some microlaryngeal surgery can be performed endoscopically. Many patients who have undergone a total laryngectomy report a good quality of life overall (Boyapati et al., 2022; Goepfert et al., 2017; Kallappa & Kallavalappil, 2021). For more details refer to Chapter 21.

Radiation Therapy

The goal of radiation therapy is to eradicate the cancer and preserve the function of the larynx. The decision to use radiation therapy is based on several factors, including the staging of the tumor and the patient's overall health status, lifestyle (including occupation), and personal preference. Early-stage vocal cord tumors are treated initially with irradiation. One of the benefits of radiation therapy is that patients retain a near-normal voice. A few develop chondritis (inflammation of the cartilage) or stenosis; a small number may require laryngectomy later. Radiation therapy may also be used preoperatively to reduce the tumor size. Radiation therapy is combined with surgery in advanced laryngeal cancer as adjunctive therapy to surgery or chemotherapy and as a palliative measure.

When laryngeal cancer is diagnosed in the early stages, chemotherapy and radiation therapy together can result in a cure and have shown good results with more advanced stages when used in combination with surgeries (Huether & McCance, 2019). Complications from radiation therapy are a result of external radiation to the head and neck area, which may also include the parotid gland, which is responsible for mucus production. Symptoms may include acute mucositis, ulceration of the mucous membranes, pain, **xerostomia** (dry mouth), loss of taste, dysphasia, fatigue, and skin reactions. Complications occurring later may include laryngeal necrosis, edema, and fibrosis.

Speech Therapy

The patient who undergoes a laryngectomy faces potentially complex and frustrating communication problems. These are related to alterations in communication methods, perceived voice quality, and perceptions of quality of life related to communication, disfigurement, and socialization. To minimize anxiety and frustration for the patient and family, the nurse discusses the loss or alteration of speech with the patient and family before surgery, and the speech therapist conducts a preoperative evaluation. The nurse discusses with the patient and family those methods of communication that will be available in the immediate postoperative period. These include writing, lip speaking, and communication or word boards. A system of communication is established with the patient, family, nurse, and provider, and is implemented consistently after surgery.

In addition, a long-term postoperative communication plan for **alaryngeal communication** is developed. The three most common techniques of alaryngeal communication are esophageal speech, artificial larynx (electrolarynx), and tracheoesophageal puncture.

With esophageal speech, patients compress air into the esophagus and expel it, setting off a vibration of the pharyngeal esophageal segment. The technique can be taught once the patient begins oral feedings after surgery. The patient learns to belch and use this action to transform simple explosions of air from the esophagus to sound for speech purposes. The speech therapist continues to work with the patient to make speech intelligible. The success rate is low.

With the electrolarynx, a battery-powered apparatus projects sound into the oral cavity. When the mouth forms words (articulation), the sounds from the electrolarynx become audible words. The voice that is produced sounds mechanical, and some words may be difficult to understand. The advantage is that the patient is able to communicate with relative ease while working to become proficient at either esophageal or tracheoesophageal puncture speech.

With tracheoesophageal puncture, a valve is placed in the tracheal stoma to divert air into the esophagus and out the mouth. Once the puncture is surgically created and has healed, a voice prosthesis (Blom-Singer) is fitted over the puncture site. A speech therapist teaches the patient how to produce sounds. Moving the tongue and lips to form the sound into words produces speech. To prevent airway obstruction, the prosthesis is removed and cleaned when mucus builds up (see Fig. 8-5). This method most resembles normal speech and is easily learned.

The success of these various approaches to preserve or restore speech varies. In studies that evaluated the effectiveness of these methods, the electrolarynx was used more often than the other methods of speaking, and tracheoesophageal speech was preferred over esophageal speech (Apert et al., 2022; Huether & McCance, 2019; Zenga et al., 2018).

Pearls for Practice

Following a total laryngectomy, the patient may lose the ability to speak, which may lead to a decrease in a patient's quality of life (Tsao et al., 2022). The reconstructive goals are restoring the pharynx and possibly the voice. Mainly three methods may be able to restore the patient's voice: by esophageal speech (ES), by using external voice devices such as an electrolarynx (EL), or with a tracheoesophageal puncture (TEP) with the placement of artificial valves (voice prostheses).

Nursing Management

Teaching the Patient Preoperatively

The nurse reinforces information related to diagnosis and treatment options given to the patient and family by the provider and clarifies any misconceptions. Informational materials (written and audiovisual) about the surgery are given to the patient and family for review and reinforcement. If a complete laryngectomy is planned, the patient must understand that the natural voice will be lost but that special training can provide a means for communicating. The patient needs to know that temporarily communication will be possible by writing or by using a special communication board. The patient's ability to sing, laugh, and whistle will be lost.

The nurse reviews equipment and treatments for postoperative care with the patient and family, teaches important coughing and deep-breathing exercises, and assists the patient to perform return demonstrations. The nurse clarifies the patient's role in the postoperative and rehabilitation periods.

Reducing Anxiety and Depression

Patients undergoing surgery for laryngeal cancer may have many fears. These fears may relate to the diagnosis of cancer and the possibility of permanent loss of the voice and disfigurement. The nurse provides the patient and family with opportunities to ask questions, verbalize feelings, and discuss perceptions. The nurse should address any questions and misconceptions the patient and family have. During the preoperative or postoperative period, a visit from someone who has had a laryngectomy may reassure the patient that people are available to assist with rehabilitation.

In the immediate postoperative period, the nurse spends time with the patient, focusing on building trust and reducing the patient's anxiety. Clear instructions and explanations are given to the patient and family in a calm, reassuring manner before and during each contact with the patient. The nurse seeks to learn from the patient what activities promote feelings of comfort and assists the patient in such activities (e.g., listening to music, reading). Relaxation techniques, such as guided imagery and meditation, are often helpful.

Maintaining a Patent Airway

The nurse promotes a patent airway by positioning the patient in the semi-Fowler or Fowler position after recovery from anesthesia. This position decreases surgical edema and promotes lung expansion. Observing the patient for restlessness, labored breathing, apprehension, and increased pulse rate helps to identify possible respiratory or circulatory problems. The nurse assesses the patient's lung sounds and reports changes that may indicate impending complications. Medications that depress respiration, particularly opioids, should be used cautiously. Adequate use of analgesic medications is essential for pain relief, as postoperative pain can result in shallow breathing and an ineffective cough. The nurse encourages the patient to turn, cough, and take deep breaths. If needed, suctioning may be performed to remove secretions, but the nurse must avoid disruption of suture lines. The nurse also encourages and assists the patient with early ambulation to prevent atelectasis, pneumonia, and deep vein thrombosis. Pulse oximetry is used to monitor the patient's oxygen saturation level.

If a total laryngectomy was performed, a laryngectomy tube may not be used; in others, it is used temporarily; and in many, it is used permanently. The laryngectomy tube, which is shorter than a tracheostomy tube but has a larger diameter, is the patient's only airway. The care of this tube is the same as for a tracheostomy tube (see discussion later in the chapter). If a tracheostomy tube without an inner cannula is used, humidification and suctioning of this tube are essential to prevent formation of mucous plugs.

Frequently, the patient coughs up large amounts of mucus through this opening. Because air passes directly into the trachea without being warmed and moistened by the upper respiratory mucosa, the tracheobronchial tree compensates by secreting excessive amounts of mucus. The patient will have frequent coughing episodes and may develop a brassy-sounding, mucus-producing cough. The nurse reassures the patient that these problems will diminish in time, as the tracheobronchial mucosa adapts to the altered physiology.

After the patient coughs, the tracheostomy opening must be wiped clean and clear of mucus. A simple gauze dressing, washcloth, or even paper towel (because of its size and absorbency) worn below the tracheostomy may serve as a barrier to protect the clothing from the copious mucus that the patient may expel initially.

One of the most important factors in decreasing cough, mucus production, and crusting around the stoma is adequate humidification of the environment. Mechanical humidifiers and aerosol generators (nebulizers) increase the humidity and are important for the patient's comfort. The laryngectomy tube may be removed when the stoma is well healed, within 3 to 6 weeks after surgery. The nurse teaches the patient how to clean and change the tube and remove secretions.

Wound drains, inserted during surgery, may be in place to assist in removal of fluid and air from the surgical site. Suction also may be used, but cautiously, to avoid trauma to the surgical site and incision. The nurse observes, measures, and records drainage. When drainage is less than 30 mL/day for 2 consecutive days, a member of the surgical team usually removes the drains.

Promoting Alternative Communication Methods

Establishing an effective means of communication is the primary goal in the rehabilitation of the patient with a laryngectomy. To understand and anticipate the patient's postoperative needs, the nurse works with the patient, speech therapist, and family to encourage use of alternative communication methods. These means of communication are established preoperatively and must be used consistently by all personnel who come in contact with the patient. The patient is unable to use an intercom system. A call bell or hand bell must be placed within easy reach of the patient. A reusable writing board often is used for communication, so the nurse documents which hand the patient uses for writing so that the opposite arm can be used for IV infusions. To ensure the patient's privacy, the nurse discards any old notes used for communication. If the patient cannot write, a picture–word–phrase board or hand signals can be used. Writing everything or communicating through gestures can be very time-consuming and frustrating. The patient must be given adequate time to communicate their needs. The patient may become impatient and angry when not understood.

Promoting Adequate Nutrition and Hydration

Postoperatively, the patient may not be permitted to eat or drink for several days. Alternative sources of nutrition and hydration include IV fluids, enteral feedings through a nasogastric or gastrostomy tube, and parenteral nutrition.

When the patient is ready to start oral feedings, a speech therapist or radiologist may conduct a swallow study to evaluate the patient's risk for aspiration. Once the patient is cleared for oral feedings, the nurse explains that thick liquids will be used first because they are easy to swallow. Different swallowing maneuvers are attempted with various food consistencies. Once the patient is cleared for food intake, the nurse stays with the patient during initial oral feedings and keeps a suction setup at the bedside for needed suctioning. The nurse observes the patient for any difficulty swallowing, particularly when eating resumes, and reports its occurrence to the provider.

The nurse instructs the patient to avoid sweet foods, which increase salivation and suppress the appetite. Solid foods are introduced as tolerated. The patient is instructed to rinse the mouth with warm water or mouthwash after oral feedings and to brush the teeth frequently.

Because taste and smell are so closely related, taste sensations are altered for a while after surgery because inhaled air passes directly into the trachea, bypassing the nose and the olfactory end organs. Over time, the patient usually accommodates to this change and olfactory sensation adapts, often with return of interest in eating. The patient's weight and laboratory data are monitored to ensure that nutritional and fluid intake are adequate. Skin turgor and vital signs are assessed for signs of decreased fluid volume.

Promoting Positive Body Image and Self-Esteem

The majority of adults who undergo reconstructive surgery due to cancer develop a level of body image dissatisfaction. The reaction of family members and friends is a major concern for the patient. Therefore, nurses and other members of the multidisciplinary team need to recognize and address any body image dissatisfaction as well as the emotional and behavioral consequences associated with it. This is why the nurse needs to encourage the patient to express feelings about the changes brought about by surgery, particularly feelings related to fear, anger, depression, and isolation (Williams, 2021). Encouraging use of previous effective coping strategies may be helpful. Referral to a support group, such as the International Association of Laryngectomees (IAL) and I Can Cope (American Cancer Society), may help the patient and family deal with the changes in their lives. In addition to its work through support groups, the IAL encourages an exchange of ideas and methods for teaching and learning alaryngeal methods of communication.

Promoting Self-Care

A positive approach is important when caring for the patient and includes promotion of self-care activities. The patient and family should begin participating in self-care activities as soon as possible. The nurse assesses the patient's readiness for decision-making and encourages the patient to participate actively in performing care. The nurse needs to support the patient and the family, especially when explaining the tubes, dressings, and drains that are in place postoperatively.

Monitoring and Managing Potential Complications

The potential complications after laryngectomy include respiratory distress and hypoxia, infection, wound breakdown, and tracheostomal stenosis. Refer to Chapter 21: Nursing Process: The Patient Undergoing a Neck Dissection for additional complications of hemorrhage, aspiration, chyle fistula, and nerve injury.

Respiratory Distress and Hypoxia

The nurse monitors the patient for signs and symptoms of respiratory distress and hypoxia, particularly restlessness, irritation, agitation, confusion, tachypnea, use of accessory muscles, and decreased oxygen saturation on pulse oximetry (SpO_2). Any change in respiratory status requires immediate intervention. Hypoxia may cause restlessness and an initial rise in blood pressure; this is followed by hypotension and somnolence. Cyanosis is a late sign of hypoxia. Obstruction needs to be ruled out immediately by suctioning and by having the patient cough and breathe deeply. Hypoxia and airway obstruction, if not immediately treated, are life-threatening.

Other nursing measures include repositioning of the patient to ensure an open airway and administering oxygen as prescribed. Oxygen should be used with caution in patients with chronic obstructive pulmonary disease (see Chapter 10).

Pearls for Practice

Adequate oxygenation is important in the management of hypoxia and should never be withheld. Monitoring and assessment are key in the care of patients with COPD on supplemental oxygen is with the goal of achieving and maintaining an oxygen saturation of greater than or equal to 90%.

Pulse oximetry is helpful in assessing response to therapy. The nurse considers patency of the airway, protective reflexes, inspired oxygen concentration, and respiratory drive when assessing adequacy of the airway.

The nurse should always be prepared for possible intubation and mechanical ventilation. The nurse must be knowledgeable about the hospital's emergency code protocols and skilled in use of emergency equipment. The nurse must remain with the patient at all times during respiratory distress. The emergency call bell and telephone should be used to initiate a code, call for further assistance, and summon the provider immediately if nursing measures do not improve the patient's respiratory status.

Pearls for Practice

After a total laryngectomy, it is advisable to have a properly sized replacement laryngectomy tube and an appropriately sized replacement cuffed tracheostomy tube at the bedside should the treatment of the patient's respiratory distress require placement on a mechanical ventilator. If the patient suffers a respiratory arrest, the nurse is aware that the naso/oro pharynx is now distinct from the tracheal bronchial tree, meaning the patient CANNOT be intubated orally. The airway must be managed via a laryngectomy tube or tracheostomy tube, allowing for rescue breathing via mouth-to-neck or bag-valve mask with supplemental oxygen delivery.

Infection

The nurse monitors the patient for signs of postoperative infection. These include an increase in temperature and pulse, a change in the type of wound drainage, and increased areas of redness or tenderness at the surgical site. Other signs include purulent drainage, odor, and increased wound drainage. The nurse monitors the patient's white blood cell (WBC) count. An elevation in WBCs (leukocytosis) may indicate the body's effort to combat infection. In older adults, infection can be present without an increase in the patient's WBC count. WBCs will be suppressed in the patient with decreased immune function (e.g., patients with HIV infection or those receiving chemotherapy or radiation therapy); this predisposes the patient to a severe infection and sepsis. Antimicrobial (antibiotic) medications must be administered as scheduled. All suspicious drainage is cultured, and the patient may be placed in isolation as indicated. The nurse reports any significant change in the patient's status to the surgeon.

Wound Breakdown

Wound breakdown caused by infection, poor wound healing, development of a fistula, radiation therapy, or tumor growth can create a life-threatening emergency. The carotid artery, which is close to the stoma, may rupture from erosion if the wound does not heal properly. This is referred to as carotid blowout syndrome and is reviewed in Chapter 21. The nurse observes the stoma area for wound breakdown, hematoma, and bleeding and reports this to the surgeon. If wound breakdown occurs, the patient must be monitored carefully and identified as being at high risk for carotid hemorrhage.

Tracheostomal Stenosis

Tracheostomal stenosis is an abnormal narrowing of the trachea or the tracheostomy stoma. Infection at the stoma site, excessive traction on the tracheostomy tube by the connecting tubing, and persistent high tracheostomy cuff pressure are risk factors for tracheostomal stenosis. The maximum cuff pressures should be 25 mm Hg, as this is considered as a safe upper limit with a range of 20 to 25 mm Hg being recommended (Patton, 2019). The incidence of this condition varies widely and is often preventable. The nurse assesses the patient's stoma for signs and symptoms of infection and immediately reports any evidence of this to the provider. Tracheostomy care is performed routinely. The nurse assesses the connecting tubing (e.g., ventilation tubing) and secures the tubing to avoid excessive traction on the patient's tracheostomy. The nurse ensures that, for the patient who is breathing independently (without ventilator), the tracheostomy cuff is deflated (for a patient with a cuffed tube).

Pearls for Practice

An inflated tracheostomy cuff will not prevent aspiration. For some patients, deflation of the tracheostomy tube allows the larynx to elevate, which improves swallowing. For others, inflating the cuff may avoid aspiration (Hudson & Carr, 2020), but it interferes with the swallow mechanism. Goff and Patterson (2019) analyzed multiple studies and concluded that the research to date has not reached a consensus in order to establish a standard of care for tracheostomy and cuff management as they relate to swallowing. The nurse recognizes that the act of swallowing requires exquisite coordination between 26 muscles and 6 cranial nerves; thus, the decision to administer medications or food by mouth in a patient with a tracheostomy should be made as a team, which should include a formal swallowing evaluation, consideration of the patient's medical and psychological status (Hudson & Carr, 2020), and patient-specific recommendations for inflating or deflating the cuff. Until then, enteral feedings will be needed to maintain nutritional needs.

Teaching Patients Self-Care

In preparing the patient to go home, the nurse assesses the patient's readiness to learn and the level of knowledge about self-care management. The patient will need to learn a variety of self-care behaviors, including tracheostomy and stoma care (described later in the chapter), wound care, and oral hygiene. The nurse also instructs the patient about the need for adequate dietary intake, safe hygiene, and recreational activities.

Special precautions are needed in the shower to prevent water from entering the stoma. Wearing a loose-fitting plastic bib over the tracheostomy or simply holding a hand over the opening is effective. Swimming is not recommended because a person with a laryngectomy can drown without submerging their face. Hair sprays, loose hair, and powder should not get near the stoma, because they can block or irritate the trachea and possibly cause infection.

The nurse teaches the patient and caregiver the signs and symptoms of infection and identifies indications that require contacting the provider after discharge. The nurse teaches the patient and family to wash their hands before and after caring for the tracheostomy, to use tissue to remove mucus, and to dispose of soiled dressings and equipment properly. If the patient's surgery included cervical lymph node dissection, the nurse teaches the patient exercises for strengthening the shoulder and neck muscles.

Recreation and exercise are important for the patient's well-being and quality of life, and all but very strenuous exercise can be enjoyed safely. Avoidance of strenuous exercise and fatigue is important because the patient will have more difficulty speaking when tired, which can be discouraging. Additional safety points to address include the need for the patient to wear or carry medical identification—such as a bracelet or card—to alert medical personnel to the special requirements for resuscitation should this need arise. If resuscitation is needed, direct mouth-to-stoma ventilation should be performed. For home emergency situations, pre-recorded emergency messages for police, the fire department, or other rescue services can be kept near the phone to be used quickly.

The nurse instructs and encourages the patient to perform oral care on a regular basis to prevent halitosis and infection. Brushing the teeth or dentures and rinsing the mouth several times a day will assist in maintaining proper oral hygiene. If the patient is receiving radiation therapy, synthetic saliva may be required because of decreased saliva production. The nurse instructs the patient to drink water or sugar-free liquids throughout the day and to use a humidifier at home.

It is important that the person who has had a laryngectomy have regular physical examinations and seek advice concerning any problems related to recovery and rehabilitation. The patient is also reminded to participate in health promotion activities and health screening as well as about the importance of keeping scheduled appointments with the provider, speech therapist, and other health care providers.

ARTIFICIAL AIRWAYS

The patient with an airway disorder such as a laryngeal obstruction or cancer may require the use of a temporary or, in some cases, a permanent artificial airway. Two types of artificial airways that may be used include an endotracheal tube (ETT) or a tracheostomy tube. General recommendations are to favor a tracheostomy tube rather than ETT when a patient requires long-term mechanical ventilation, to prevent the complications of endotracheal intubation, for example, tracheal stenosis and vocal cord paralysis. Past recommendations were to move from an ETT to a tracheostomy after 11 to 21 days on the ventilator. The current recommendations are to provide a tracheostomy as early as 72 hours in certain cases to promote earlier weaning, especially if the patient has other medical complications, has had difficulty weaning, or has trauma accompanied with the prolonged need for an artificial airway (Morton et al., 2018). To provide for adequate ventilation, mechanical ventilation may be required to ensure adequate oxygenation.

ETT and tracheostomy tubes have several disadvantages. The tubes cause discomfort, the cough reflex is depressed because closure of the glottis is hindered, and secretions tend to become thicker because the warming and humidifying effect of the upper respiratory tract has been bypassed. The swallowing reflexes are depressed because of prolonged disuse and the mechanical trauma produced by the endotracheal or tracheostomy tube, thus increasing the risk of aspiration. In addition, ulceration and stricture of the larynx or trachea may develop. Of great concern to the patient is the inability to talk and to communicate needs.

ENDOTRACHEAL INTUBATION

Endotracheal intubation is a temporary means of providing an airway for patients who cannot maintain an adequate airway on their own (e.g., comatose patients, patients with upper airway obstruction), for patients needing mechanical ventilation, and for suctioning secretions from the pulmonary tree.

Pearls for Practice

For any patient with an artificial airway, a self-inflating bag-valve mask device or Ambu bag must be at the bedside as well as suction catheters and suctions source.

Endotracheal intubation involves passing an ETT through the mouth or nose into the trachea (Fig. 8-6) with the aid of a laryngoscope or illuminated glidescope by specifically trained personnel. It is the method of choice in emergency care. Once the tube is inserted, a cuff is inflated to prevent air from leaking around the outer part of the tube, to minimize the possibility of subsequent aspiration, and to prevent movement of the tube. The nurse listens for bilateral breath sounds and observes for chest movement. Lack of breath sounds is associated with esophageal intubation, while breath sounds heard in only one lung suggest placement in mainstem bronchus rather than approximately 3 to 4 cm above the carina to allow for bilateral lung expansion.

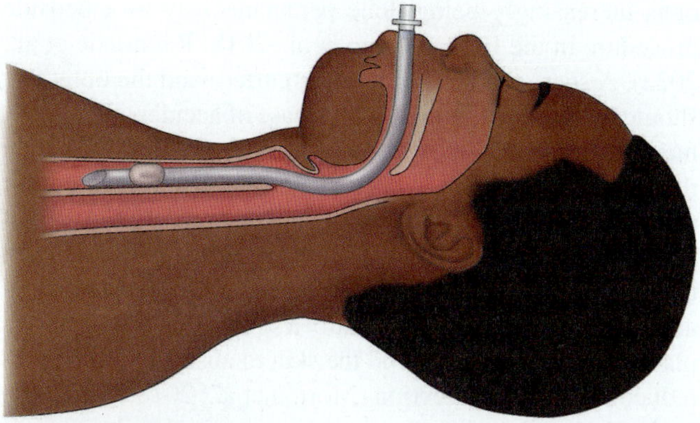

FIGURE 8-6 Endotracheal tube in place. The tube has been inserted using the oral route. The cuff has been inflated to maintain the tube's position and to minimize the risk of aspiration.

A chest x-ray is obtained to confirm placement. After placement is confirmed, the nurse notes placement by recording the level of insertion (marked in centimeters on the side of the tube) at the teeth or nares (if inserted nasally) and secures the tube with tape or a commercial tube holder to prevent movement and potential dislodgment (Stacy, 2022).

The nurse should be aware that complications could occur from pressure exerted by the cuff on the wall of the trachea. Low cuff pressure can increase the risk for aspiration pneumonia. High cuff pressure can cause tracheal bleeding, ischemia, and pressure necrosis. The cuff should be inflated between 20 and 25 mm Hg. Routine deflation of the cuff is not recommended because of the increased risk for aspiration and hypoxia. The cuff must be deflated before the ETT is removed. Tracheobronchial secretions are suctioned through the tube (see description in Tracheostomy section). Because mechanical ventilation bypasses the upper airway, the body's protective mechanism for humidifying and warming inspired air is not possible. These two processes must be added to the ventilator circuit in the form of a humidifier with temperature control (Morton et al., 2018). Warmed, humidified oxygen should always be introduced through the tube, whether the patient is breathing spontaneously or is receiving ventilatory support. Endotracheal intubation should be used until a time when it is prudent to consider a tracheostomy to decrease oropharyngeal irritation and trauma to the tracheal lining, to reduce the incidence of vocal cord paralysis (secondary to laryngeal nerve damage), and to decrease the work of breathing.

Pearls for Practice

A type of hospital-acquired pneumonia is VAP, which is defined as pneumonia occurring in a patient who is being mechanically ventilated within 48 hours or more after intubation. Since ETTs facilitate the migration of organisms into the lower respiratory tract, an evidence-based group of interventions (termed a bundle) have been developed to decrease the incidence. One intervention is the use of a contemporary ETT that contains a port that can be connected for subglottic suctioning. An analysis of research studies found that the use of subglottic secretion drainage is an effective measure to reduce VAP incidence, but did not impact the duration of mechanical ventilation or length of stay (Pozuelo-Carrascosa et al., 2020) (Fig. 8-7). For more details on VAP see Chapter 54.

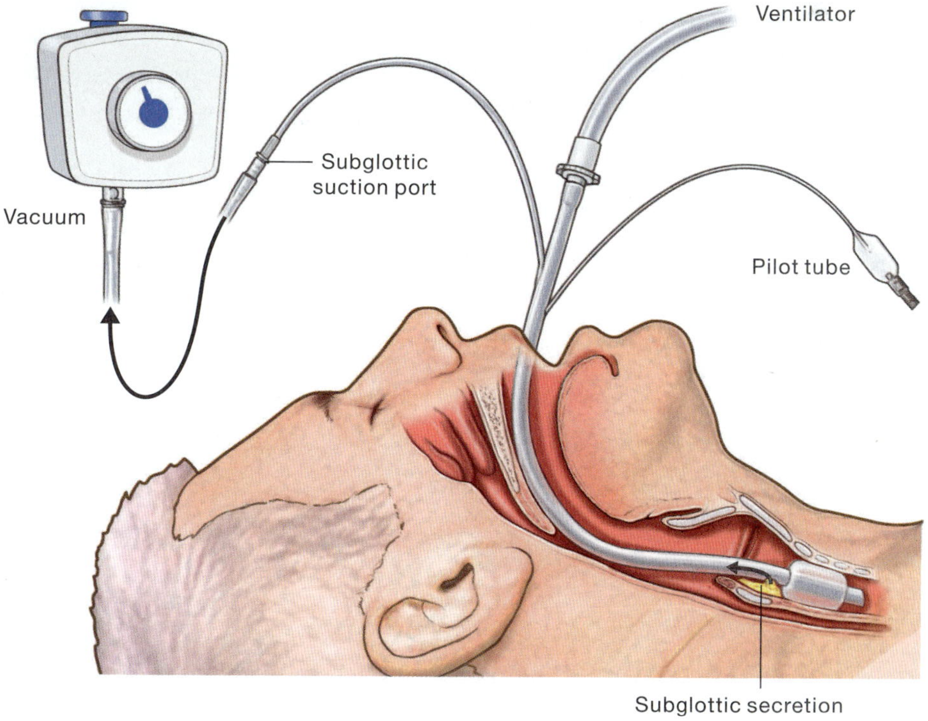

FIGURE 8-7 Endotracheal tube with subglottic suction port placed posteriorly and above the cuff for drainage of pooled secretion in the semi-recumbent position. (From Gregory, D., Stephens, T., Raymond-Seniuk, C., & Patrick, L. [2019]. *Fundamentals: Perspectives on the art and science of Canadian nursing* [2nd ed., Fig. 33-23]. Lippincott Williams & Wilkins.)

Unintentional or premature removal of the tube is a potentially life-threatening complication of endotracheal intubation that is a frequent problem in intensive care units and occurs mainly during nursing care or by the patient.

TRACHEOSTOMY

A **tracheotomy** is a surgical procedure in which an opening is made into the trachea. The indwelling tube inserted into the trachea is called a **tracheostomy tube**. A tracheostomy may be either temporary or permanent.

A tracheostomy is used to bypass the mouth, upper airway, and glottis, and this decreases problems of airway resistance and occlusion, and allows for the removal of tracheobronchial secretions, to permit the long-term use of mechanical ventilation, to prevent aspiration of oral or gastric secretions in the unconscious or paralyzed patient (by closing off the trachea from the esophagus), and to replace an ETT. Many disease processes and emergency conditions make a tracheostomy necessary, including total laryngectomy.

Procedure

A surgical opening is made between the second and third tracheal rings. After the trachea is exposed, an obturator guides insertion of the cuffed tracheostomy tube by creating a pathway for the tracheostomy tube. The obturator is removed immediately after the tracheostomy tube is in place. This procedure can be done in the Operating Room or is increasingly being done percutaneously as a bedside procedure in the ICU (Morton et al., 2018; Raimonde et al., 2022). A spare tracheostomy tube (cuffed) and the obturator should be available in the room in case of accidental dislodgment of the tracheostomy tube. The cuff is inflated to occlude the space between the tracheal walls and the tube, to permit effective mechanical ventilation, and to decrease the risk of aspiration. The tracheostomy tube is held in place by twill tape or a cloth neckband with velcro band fasteners placed around the patient's neck. Usually a square of sterile gauze is placed between the tube and the skin to absorb drainage and reduce the risk for infection (Morton et al., 2018; Raimonde et al., 2022). The nurse should refer to institutional protocols regarding tracheostomy management.

Tube Types

Types of tracheostomy tubes include (Fig. 8-8):

- *Cuffed tracheostomy tube:* This is required when placing a patient on a ventilator because the balloon prevents air from being diverted out to the upper airway (Fig. 8-8A).
- *Fenestrated tube:* This tube allows some air flow up to the larynx, which allows for vocalization (Fig. 8-8B).
- *Uncuffed (cuffless) tube:* This tube does not permit ventilator management but will allow talking if the airway is not edematous and the patient covers or "buttons" the end of the tube. This allows air to flow from the nose and mouth past the larynx and vocalization (Fig. 8-8C).

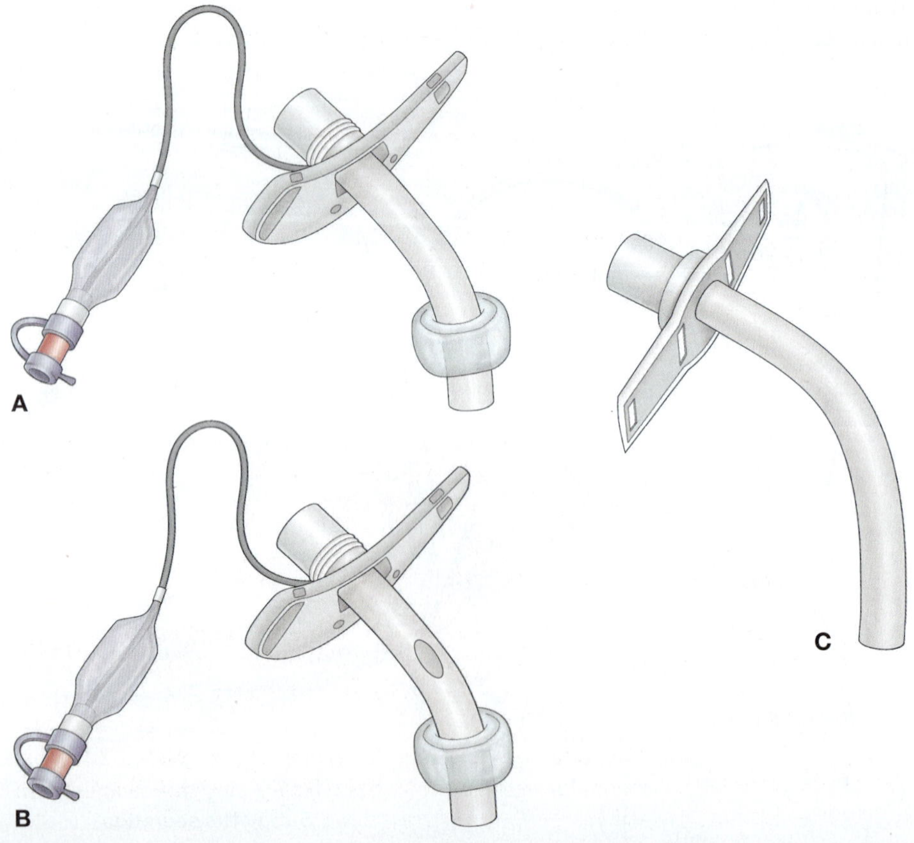

FIGURE 8-8 Tracheostomy tubes. A. Cuffed tracheostomy tube; used for patients on mechanical ventilation. B. Cuffed fenestrated tube; allows the patient to talk. C. Uncuffed tracheostomy tube; not used for adult patients on mechanical ventilation; often used for permanent tracheostomy patients who are not ventilator dependent.

Pearls for Practice

In an emergency, if an Ambu bag or ventilator was used on a cuffless tube, then the nurse needs to understand that air will follow the path of least resistance, out the nose and mouth rather than into the lungs. Therefore, any patient who has a cuffless tracheostomy must have the exact size tracheostomy tube at the bedside with a cuff. In an emergency, the provider will change the cuffless tube to a cuffed tube and inflate the balloon, allowing for ventilation with an Ambu bag or ventilator.

Pearls for Practice

Tracheostomy tubes are most often made of materials such as polyvinyl chloride or silicone-based plastics; occasionally, you may care for patients who have a stainless steel or metal tube. Stainless steel or metal tubes are rarely used today because of their increased costs, rigidity, and lack of a cuff, which prevents mechanical ventilation in an emergency (Perry et al., 2022). The nurse understands that these types of tubes are sensitive to temperature and need to be protected from extreme heat and cold to prevent tissue injury (Perry et al., 2022). In addition, they contain an inner cannula that is cleaned and replaced routinely or for secretion removal, and a cuffed tube of the same size is needed at the bedside in case emergency ventilation is required.

Complications

Complications may occur early or late in the course of tracheostomy tube management. Early complications include bleeding, pneumothorax, air embolism, aspiration, subcutaneous or mediastinal emphysema, recurrent laryngeal nerve damage, and posterior tracheal wall penetration. Long-term complications include airway obstruction from accumulation of secretions or protrusion of the cuff over the opening of the tube, infection, rupture of the innominate artery, dysphagia, tracheoesophageal fistula, tracheal dilation, and tracheal ischemia and necrosis. Tracheal stenosis may develop after the tube is removed. Box 8-5 provides information about preventing complications.

Nursing Management

The patient with an artificial airway requires continuous monitoring and assessment. The airway must be kept patent by proper suctioning of secretions. After the vital signs are stable, the patient is placed in a semi-Fowler position to facilitate ventilation, promote drainage, minimize edema, and prevent strain on the suture lines. Analgesia and sedative agents must be administered with caution because of the risk of suppressing the cough reflex.

Major objectives of nursing care are to alleviate the patient's apprehension, provide an effective means of communication, and prevent infection. The nurse keeps paper and pencil or a reusable writing board and the call light within the patient's reach at all times to ensure a means of communication. The care of the patient with a tracheostomy tube is summarized in Box 8-6.

For the patient with a tracheostomy tube, a Passy-Muir Valve (PMV) allows the patient to speak. The device is a positive-closure, one-way speaking valve. The PMV opens upon inspiration to allow the patient to inspire through the tracheostomy tube and then closes after inspiration, redirecting the exhaled air around the tube, through the vocal cords, and out of the mouth. The tracheostomy cuff must be deflated completely before the PMV is placed.

BOX 8-5

Preventing Complications Associated With Endotracheal and Tracheostomy Tubes

- Administer adequate warmed humidity.
- Maintain cuff pressure at appropriate level.
- Suction as needed per assessment findings.
- Maintain skin integrity. Change tape and dressing as needed or per protocol.
- Auscultate lung sounds.
- Monitor for signs and symptoms of infection, including temperature and white blood cell count.
- Administer prescribed oxygen and monitor oxygen saturation.
- Monitor for cyanosis.
- Maintain adequate hydration of the patient.
- Use sterile technique when suctioning and performing tracheostomy care.
- For ETT, verify position of the ETT by noting the placement of the ETT in centimeters at the teeth or nares and compare it with the desired placement

Suctioning the Tracheal Tube (Tracheostomy or Endotracheal Tube)

When a tracheostomy or ETT is in place, it is necessary to suction the patient's secretions because of the decreased effectiveness of the cough mechanism. Tracheal suctioning is performed when adventitious breath sounds are detected or whenever secretions are obviously present. Unnecessary suctioning can initiate bronchospasm and cause mechanical trauma to the tracheal mucosa.

All equipment that comes into direct contact with the patient's lower airway must be sterile to prevent pulmonary and systemic infections. The procedure for suctioning a tracheostomy is presented in Box 8-7. Recent research analysis suggests using minimally invasive endotracheal suctioning, in which the suction catheter is inserted to the length of the ETT or tracheostomy tube only, results in less effect on physiologic indices and thus fewer adverse effects than routine endotracheal suctioning. Specifically, a significant drop in peripheral O_2 saturation and increase in systolic and diastolic

BOX 8-6

GUIDELINES FOR NURSING CARE

Providing Care for a Patient With a Tracheostomy Tube

Equipment

- Sterile gloves
- Goggles, mask, or face shield
- Sterile cotton-tipped applicators
- Disposable inner cannula, size for patient
- Sterile dressing
- Twill tape or commercially prepared tracheostomy holder
- Normal saline solution or sterile water
- Person to assist with changing the tracheostomy tie/holder
- Additional personal protective equipment (PPE), such as a: gown if concern regarding contact with secretions

Implementation

ACTIONS	RATIONALE
1. Gather the needed equipment.	1. Everything needed to care for a tracheostomy should be readily on hand for the most effective care. Having necessary supplies and equipment readily available allows the procedure to be completed efficiently.
2. Provide patient and family instruction on the key points for tracheostomy care; inspect the tracheostomy dressing for moisture or drainage.	2. The tracheostomy dressing is changed as needed to keep the skin clean and dry. To prevent potential breakdown, moist or soiled dressings should not remain on the skin.
3. Perform hand hygiene.	3. Hand hygiene reduces bacteria on hands.
4. Explain procedure to patient and family.	4. A patient with a tracheostomy is apprehensive and requires ongoing assurance and support.
5. Put on clean gloves; remove and discard the soiled dressing in an appropriate container. Discard gloves.	5. Observing body substance isolation reduces cross-contamination from soiled dressings.
6. Prepare sterile supplies, including normal saline solution or sterile water, cotton-tipped applicators, dressing, and tape.	6. Sterile equipment minimizes transmission of surface flora to the sterile respiratory tract.
7. Put on sterile gloves. (Some providers approve clean technique for long-term tracheostomy patients in the home.)	7. Clean technique may be used in the home because of decreased exposure to potential pathogens.
8. Cleanse the wound and the plate of the tracheostomy tube with sterile cotton-tipped applicators moistened with sterile saline solution.	8. Rinsing prevents retention of residue.
9. Soak inner cannula in sterile saline; rinse with saline solution; inspect to be sure all dried secretions have been removed. Dry and reinsert inner cannula or replace with a new disposable inner cannula.	9. Soaking loosens and removes secretions from the inner lumen of the tracheostomy tube. Retained secretions could harbor bacteria, leading to infection. Some plastic tracheostomy tubes may be damaged by using peroxide.
10. Observe skin around tracheal stoma, under TT flange, and under tracheal ties for pressure injury: blistering, erythema, drainage, foul odor, bleeding, or other discoloration.	10. The nurse observes for signs of infection, skin breakdown and pressure injuries, and signs of granuloma formation which are complications associated with a tracheostomy.
11. Place clean twill tape in position to secure the tracheostomy tube by inserting one end of the tape through the side opening of the outer cannula. Take the tape around the back of the patient's neck and thread it through the opposite opening of the outer cannula. Bring both ends around, so that they meet on one side of the neck. Tighten the tape until only two fingers can be inserted comfortably under it. Secure with a knot. For a new tracheostomy, two people should assist with tape changes. Remove soiled twill tape after the new tape is in place. In place of twill tape, a commercially prepared tracheostomy tube holder may be used.	11. This taping technique provides a double thickness of tape around the neck, which is needed because the tracheostomy tube can be dislodged by movement or by a forceful cough if left unsecured. However, it cannot be so tight that it causes constriction of the jugular vein. Therefore, changing ties should always be a two-person task. A dislodged tracheostomy tube is difficult to reinsert, and respiratory distress may occur. Dislodgment of a new tracheostomy is a medical emergency.
12. Remove old tapes and discard in a waste container after the new tape is in place.	12. Tapes with old secretions may harbor bacteria.

ACTIONS	RATIONALE
13. Although some long-term tracheostomies with healed stomas may not require a dressing, other tracheostomies do. Use a sterile tracheostomy dressing, fitting it securely under the twill tape and flange of tracheostomy tube, so that the incision is covered, as shown below. A sterile pre-cut "drain" sponge may be available also.	13. Healed tracheostomies with minimal secretions do not need a dressing. Dressings that will shred are not used around a tracheostomy because of the risk that pieces of material, lint, or thread may get into the tube and eventually into the trachea, causing obstruction or abscess formation.
14. Dispose of all used equipment in waste receptacle, remove and discard gloves, and perform hand hygiene.	14. Disposing of all used equipment, cleaning agents, and gloves prevents the spread of contaminants/bacteria. Performing hand hygiene prevents the spread of infection.

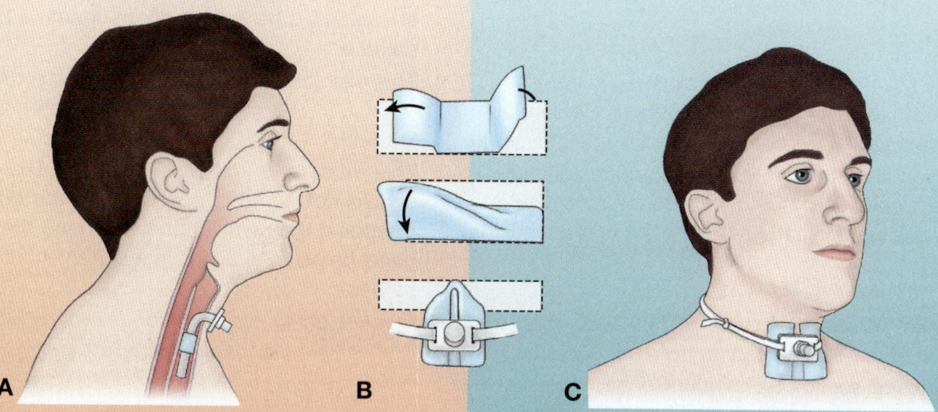

(A) The cuff of the tracheostomy tube fits smoothly and snugly in the trachea in a way that promotes circulation but seals off the escape of secretions and air surrounding the tube. **(B)** For a dressing change, a specially designed drain sponge or a 4 × 4-in gauze pad may be folded (cutting would promote shredding, placing the patient at risk for aspiration) around the tracheostomy tube and **(C)** stabilized by slipping the neck tape ties through the neck plate slots of the tracheostomy tube. The ties may be fastened to the side of the neck to eliminate the discomfort of lying on the knot.

BOX 8-7

GUIDELINES FOR NURSING CARE

Performing Tracheal Suction

Equipment

- Suction catheters, may be available in a commercially prepared kit
- Gloves (sterile and nonsterile), mask, and goggles. Additional PPE, such as a gown, as required.
- Basin for sterile normal saline solution for irrigation
- Manual resuscitation bag with supplemental oxygen
- Portable or wall suction unit with tubing

Implementation

ACTIONS	RATIONALE
1. Explain the procedure to the patient before beginning, and offer reassurance during suctioning. Unless contraindicated, elevate the head of the patient's bed; semi-Fowler position is preferred. Monitor the patient's cardiopulmonary status before, during, and after the suctioning period. If possible, continuous pulse oximetry and cardiac monitoring should be initiated before the procedure.	1. Patients are apprehensive and require ongoing assurance and support. Elevation of bed maximizes diaphragmatic excursion. Cardiopulmonary instability, particularly arrhythmias or arterial desaturation, hypertension or hypotension will necessitate immediate termination of the suctioning procedure
2. Perform hand hygiene. Put on nonsterile gloves, goggles, gown, and mask.	2. Hand hygiene reduces transmission of microorganisms and body secretions; donning PPE follows standard precautions.
3. Secure the end of the suction tubing to the suction device. Place the open end within reach in preparation for connecting to the suction catheter. Turn on suction source (pressure should not exceed 120 mm Hg) (Brinton, 2019).	3. High vacuum pressures are associated with mucosal injury.

(continued on page 302)

BOX 8-7

GUIDELINES FOR NURSING CARE (*continued*)

Performing Tracheal Suction (*continued*)

ACTIONS	RATIONALE
4. To perform open-suction technique: Open-suction catheter kit on a clean surface, using the inside of the wrapping as a sterile field. Suction catheter should be less than half of the internal lumen of the endotracheal tube or tracheostomy.	4. If the catheter is too small, it will not adequately remove secretions, and if it is too large, it will obstruct airflow around the catheter during insertion. To calculate the catheter size needed, note the interior diameter (ID) of the tracheostomy tube, divide by two, and then multiply by three to obtain the French size. For example, a size 8 tracheostomy tube would accommodate a 12-French suction catheter.
Set up a sterile solution container. Fill basin with approximately 100 mL of sterile normal saline or water. Be careful not to touch the inside of the container. Don sterile gloves.	This maintains sterility and follows standard precautions.
Pick up suction catheter; avoid touching nonsterile surfaces. With the nondominant hand, pick up the connecting tubing. Secure the suction catheter to the suction tubing.	This maintains catheter security. The dominant hand should not come in contact with the connecting tubing. Wrapping the sterile catheter around the sterile dominant hand helps to prevent inadvertent contamination of the catheter.
Check equipment for proper functioning by suctioning a small amount of sterile saline solution from the container.	Ensures equipment function.
To perform closed-suction technique: Connect the suction tubing to the closed system suction port, according to the manufacturer's guidelines. The sterile suction catheter is in a clear plastic sleeve (see illustration). This system allows the patient to remain connected to the ventilator during suctioning.	

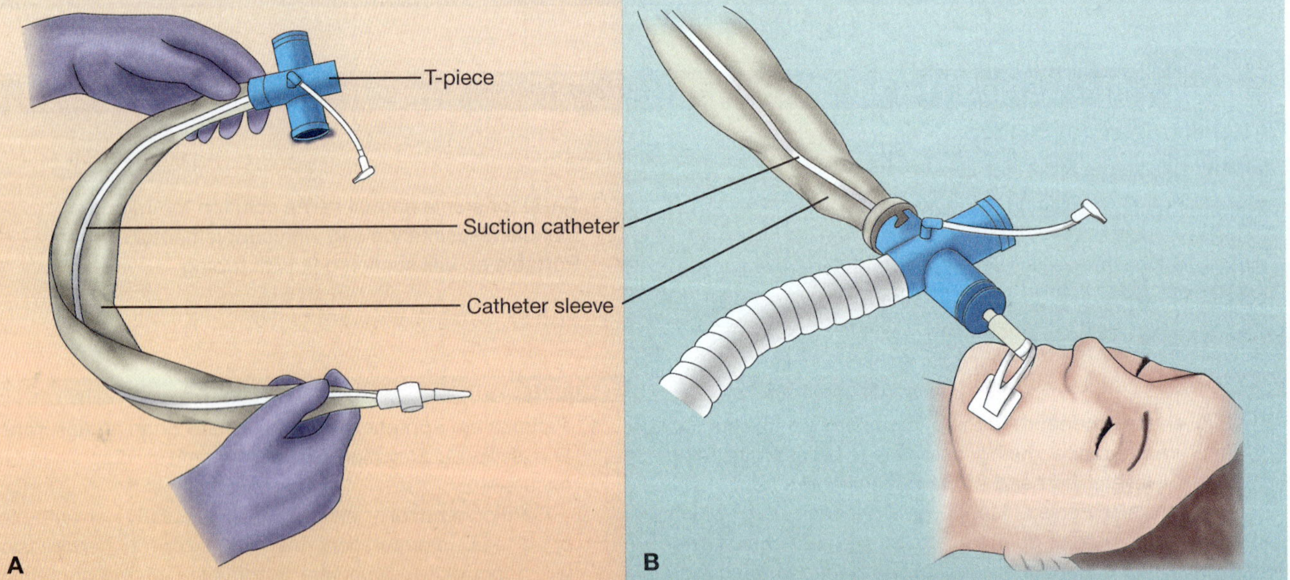

Closed airway suction system. **(A)** Closed tracheal suction system. **(B)** Closed system connected by a T-piece to the endotracheal tube and ventilator.

ACTIONS	RATIONALE
5. Follow institution guidelines related to hyperoxygenating the patient's lungs before suctioning. In general, for the nonventilator-dependent patient, humidified oxygen via a tracheostomy mask is placed over the tracheostomy for several deep breaths (5–6) before suctioning, or if on a ventilator, preoxygenate the patient with 100% oxygen for at least 30 seconds prior to and after suctioning. Return to the previous oxygen setting after suctioning is completed	5. Routine use of hyperinflation is not recommended due to the risk of barotrauma (damage to the lung from rapid or excessive pressure changes) from large volumes, high peak pressures, and patient discomfort. Hyperoxygenation with 100% oxygen is used to prevent a decrease in arterial oxygen levels during the suctioning procedures. Press the suction hyperoxygenation button on the ventilator with the nondominant hand.

ACTIONS	RATIONALE
OR Increase the baseline fraction of inspired oxygen (FiO_2) level on the mechanical ventilator. Return to the previous oxygen setting after suctioning is completed	
Disconnect the ventilator or gas delivery tubing from the end of the endotracheal or tracheostomy tube, attach the manual resuscitation bag (MRB) to the tube with the nondominant hand, and administer five to six breaths. Attach a PEEP valve to the MRB for patients on more than 5 cm H_2O PEEP (refer to Chapter 54). Verify 100% oxygen delivery capabilities of MRB.	Using this added valve increases the amount of air left in the lungs at the end of exhalation, increasing functional residual capacity.
6. With the suction off, gently and quickly insert the catheter with the dominant hand into the artificial airway to the extent of the tracheostomy or ETT (not to pass beyond the tip of the tubes), which can be measured. Other researchers suggest passing the catheter to the carina (strong cough reflex or where resistance is felt), then pull back 1 to 2 cm before suctioning is performed; this is termed *minimally invasive suctioning.* Deeper suctioning may be necessary in patients with large amounts of secretions in the lower airways, since minimally invasive suctioning removes secretions from central airways only.	6. Suction should be applied only as needed to remove secretions and for as short a time as possible to minimize decreases in arterial oxygen levels.
7. Place the nondominant thumb over the control vent of the suction catheter, and apply continuous or intermittent suction. Rotate the catheter 360 degrees between the dominant thumb and forefinger as you withdraw the catheter in the sterile catheter sleeve (closed-suction technique) or out of the open airway (open-suction technique). The suctioning procedure should take no more than 15 seconds, waiting at least 1 minute between suctioning events.	7. Tracheal damage from suctioning is similar with intermittent or continuous suction. Decreases in arterial oxygen levels during suctioning can be kept to a minimum with brief suction periods.
8. After suctioning, hyperoxgenate the patient for at least 1 minute as described earlier. Inflate the patient's lungs for several breaths. Assess oxygen saturation and evidence of bradycardia and arrhythmias (particularly if deep suctioning was required).	8. Arterial oxygen desaturation and cardiopulmonary complications increase with each successive pass.
9. Repeat steps until the airway is clear.	9. The number of suction passes should be based on patient assessment and presence of secretions (Perry et al., 2022).
10. Rinse catheter by suctioning a few milliliters of sterile saline solution from the basin between suction attempts.	10. Removes the buildup of secretions in the connecting tubing and/or the inline suction catheter.
11. When the lower airway has been adequately cleared of secretions, suction the nasal or oropharyngeal cavity.	11. Prevents contamination of the lower airways with upper airway organisms.
12. Rinse suction tubing.	12. Removes contaminates from tubing
13. Discard catheter, gloves, and basin appropriately. If using the open-suction technique, wrap the catheter around the dominant hand. Pull glove off inside out. Catheter remains in the glove. Pull other glove off in the same manner. Discard both gloves, and turn off suction device.	13. Reduces transmission of microorganisms. Solutions and catheters that come in direct contact with the lower airways during suctioning must be kept sterile to decrease the risk of nosocomial pneumonia.
14. Perform hand hygiene.	

blood pressure and mean arterial pressure (MAP) occurred with routine suctioning when compared to the minimally invasive group (Shamali et al., 2019). In minimally invasive endotracheal suctioning the suction catheter is inserted to the carina and then retracted 1 to 2 cm before suctioning is performed; an alternative option is to measure the length of the suction catheter estimated by measuring an identical ETT (Blakeman et al., 2022). However, deep suctioning may be necessary in patients with large amounts of secretions in the lower airways, since minimally invasive suctioning removes secretions from central airways only. Deep suctioning may lead to episodes of bradycardia due to stimulation of the vagus nerve. As research data are analyzed, best practice related to suctioning practices will be established.

In mechanically ventilated patients, an inline suction catheter may be used to allow rapid suction when needed and to minimize cross-contamination by airborne pathogens. An inline suction device allows the patient to be suctioned without being disconnected from the ventilator circuit.

Pearls for Practice

The instillation of normal saline into an artificial airway (tracheostomy tube or ETT) "should not be routinely instilled in the airway prior to airway suctioning" (van der Lee et al., 2019, p. 243). However, in a recent international research study with an expert panel, clinicians noted the instillation of saline is used "only when secretions are very tenacious and unable to be cleared using other techniques" (van der Lee et al., 2019, p. 239). Yet, the practice of saline instillation is known to cause severe coughing episodes, hypoxemia, hypertension, bronchospasm, and dislodgment of bacterial biofilm colonized in the ETT into the lower airway which can lead to VAP (Dexter & Scott, 2019). To date, no studies demonstrate any benefit of normal saline instillation during suctioning (Caparros & Forbes, 2014). This practice appears to be a tradition-based practice without evidence to support its ongoing use. Many researchers suggest that additional well-designed studies are urgently needed as a way to cease this practice or verify its efficacy (see Box 8-8).

Managing the Cuff

For the patient being supported with a mechanical ventilator, the cuff on the endotracheal or tracheostomy tube must be inflated. The pressure within the cuff should be the lowest possible pressure that allows delivery of adequate tidal volumes. Cuff pressure must be monitored at least every 8 hours by attaching a handheld pressure gauge to the pilot balloon of the tube or by using the minimal leak volume or minimal occlusion volume technique. Usually the pressure is maintained at less than 25 cm H_2O to prevent injury; when cuff pressure exceeds capillary perfusion pressure, necrosis of the tracheal wall, ischemia, and stenosis can occur.

BOX 8-8

Nursing Research

Bridging the Gap to Evidence-Based Practice

Bourgault, A. M., & Upvall, M. J. (2019). De-implementation of tradition-based practices in critical care: A qualitative study. *International Journal of Nursing Practice*. 25(2), e12723. https://doi.org/10.1111/ijn.12723

Purpose

The purpose of this study was to explore the process of tradition-based practice (TBP) de-implementation by critical care nurses. Ritualistic and routine practices have been described as sacred cows or TBPs. Many clinical practices have insufficient or no evidence and may lead to poor patient outcomes. De-implementation (termination) of potentially harmful, ineffective, or non–cost-effective TBP is necessary to facilitate evidence-based practice (EBP) in the clinical setting.

Design

Descriptive qualitative inquiry guided this study. This approach lends itself to obtaining details, leading to a deeper understanding of commonplace events or occurrences by those with experience in the field. Twenty-two critical care nurses from an acute care hospital in central Florida participated. Individual and focus group interviews were performed from March to July 2016 and analyzed using thematic analysis.

Findings

Three themes were identified: (a) uncertainty—participants were unsure if practices were based on tradition or research evidence. All participants were aware of EBP, yet most were unable to describe or identify a TBP; (b) desire to know—despite the inability to differentiate between nursing practices guided by tradition versus evidence, there was a genuine desire to optimize patient outcomes based on current nursing practice; and (c) preparing for practice change—participants acknowledged that practice change is a frequent occurrence. Despite this, they expressed an attitude of *business as usual* to maintain current practice unless there was a clear indication for change. Daily nursing practice is complex, and nurses appeared to find comfort in routines. There was a risk for nurses to feel overwhelmed if too many changes were implemented simultaneously. In summary, nurses were uncertain about the scientific underpinnings of everyday clinical practices and had difficulty differentiating TBP from EBP. De-implementation processes and strategies appeared to replicate implementation processes.

Nursing Implications

The authors' findings suggest that nurses with a positive attitude toward EBP and readiness for practice change may be lacking fundamental skills to assess clinical practices for empirical evidence. Nurses should be supported to disclose knowledge gaps and develop EBP knowledge, including de-implementation. Nurses are encouraged to question the scientific underpinnings of clinical practices and seek information as needed. Nurses also raised concerns about their capacity to manage multiple concurrent or consecutive practice changes to avoid confusion and frustration, but the ideal number of changes is unknown. More research is needed to evaluate de-implementation processes and strategies used for de-implementation. An emphasis should be placed on ensuring that nurses are knowledgeable about fundamental EBP skills to encourage assessment of clinical practices for supporting research evidence. Awareness and understanding of TBPs will facilitate a more comprehensive approach toward achieving the gold standard of EBP.

Clinical Judgment Case

A 76-year-old patient comes into the emergency room (ER) after aspirating fluids. The patient has an extensive medical history that includes diabetes mellitus type 2, aortic valve disease, myocardial infarction (15 years ago), and gastroparesis. Vital signs are as follows: 100.4 °F, 122 bpm and regular, 28 respiratory rate (RR) with an oxygen saturation of 85% on room air with a blood pressure of 128/68 mm Hg. Heart sounds are S1, S2 with grade 3/6 systolic murmur that radiates to the right neck, without gallop; the point of maximum impulse (PMI) is nondisplaced (5th intercostal space [ICS], midclavicular line). On pulmonary exam, you hear crackles bibasilar (both lung bases) and scattered wheezing; there is dyspnea, nasal flaring, mouth breathing, and intercostal retractions. Cough is productive, clear sputum. Abdomen is soft, nondistended, nontender. Normoactive bowel sounds are present in all four quadrants, denies nausea, vomiting, or diarrhea. Skin is warm and moist, capillary refill is 2 seconds and pedal and posterior tibial pulses are 3+. The patient is anxious and becoming increasingly restless. Stat laboratory testing included a complete blood count (CBC), coagulation studies, lactate level, and chemistry (including electrolytes, glucose, and BUN and creatinine) that is sent to the lab and an IV is inserted. You are awaiting the laboratory results. An IV is started for medication and fluid administration. A decision is made to intubate the patient with an endotracheal tube (ETT) by the ER provider, midazolam is administered IV since it provides anxiolysis and some amnesia, facilitating endotracheal intubation; the fraction of inspired oxygen (FiO_2) is initiated at 50%, the crash cart is brought to the bedside, and the oxygen saturation is currently 96%. You have listened to lung sounds and hear breath sounds in both left and right lung fields and observe symmetrical chest expansion. A stat portable chest film is ordered to confirm placement of the ETT, and arterial blood gases (ABGs) are to be obtained in 20 minutes.

Step One: Recognize cues where relevant and important information is identified from different sources, such as medical history or vital signs.

Answer: Pulmonary aspiration of fluid with signs and symptoms of dyspnea, intercostal retractions, nasal flaring, mouth breathing, clear sputum, positive cough, anxiety, and restlessness. Physical exam findings of grade 3/6 systolic murmur, bibasilar crackles, diffuse wheezing, and moist skin. Vital signs of concern are tachycardia (122), tachypnea (28), oxygen saturation of 85% on room air and temperature of 100.4°F. An extensive medical history that includes diabetes mellitus type 2, aortic valve disease, myocardial infarction (15 years ago), and gastroparesis. Patient was just intubated and placed on mechanical ventilation with 50% FiO_2; the oxygen saturation is currently 96%. You auscultated bilateral breath sounds and observed bilateral chest movement. Chest film and ABGs ordered, awaiting laboratory results.

Step Two: Analyze cues, which is organizing and linking the recognized cues to the patient's clinical presentation.

Answer: You cluster the dyspnea, intercostal retractions, nasal flaring, mouth breathing, clear sputum, positive cough, bibasilar crackles, diffuse wheezing, tachycardia (122), tachypnea (28) and temperature of 100.4 °F with pulmonary aspiration. You cluster the anxiety, restlessness, oxygen saturation of 85% on room air, tachycardia and tachypnea with hypoxemia. The grade 3/6 systolic murmur is associated with aortic valve disease. You recognize that moist skin can be associated with fever, anxiety and hypoglycemia (history includes diabetes mellitus type 2). Previous history of myocardial infarction (15 years ago) is a risk factor for future cardiovascular events. Gastroparesis is a risk factor for aspiration as is ETT intubation. Patient was just intubated and placed on 50% FiO_2, with oxygen saturation of 96% however x-ray has not confirmed placement as yet. ABGs will assess efficacy of FiO_2 of 50%.

Step Three: Prioritize hypotheses, where hypotheses are evaluated and ranked according to priority. This can include urgency, likelihood, risk, difficulty, and/or time. In this phase you cluster your findings, to arrive at a list of problems (actual and/or potential problems) you believe the patient is experiencing and determine the importance or urgency. What do you think is of greatest concern?

Answer: The potential hypothesis includes (1) airway management (promoting gas exchange, supporting tissue oxygenation); (2) preventing ETT complications such as ventilator-acquired pneumonia (VAP) related to intubation; (3) potential for cardiac event and hemodynamic instability related to history of MI and current stressor; (4) potential for acute respiratory distress syndrome (ARDS) related to aspiration; and (5) potential for stress hyperglycemia related to aspiration. In the moment, you prioritize airway management.

Step Four: Generate solutions, which is identifying expected outcomes and using hypotheses to define a set of interventions for the expected outcomes.

Answer: You recall the priority of airway, breathing and circulation (ABC), so the urgency is deemed to confirm placement of the ETT. Once the chest x-ray verifies placement, you will note placement by recording the level of insertion (marked in centimeters on the side of the tube) at the teeth or nares (if inserted nasally) and secure the tube with tape or a commercial tube holder to prevent movement and potential dislodgment. A self-inflating bag-valve mask device or Ambu bag must be at the bedside along with suction catheters and a suction source. You are also aware that complications could occur from pressure exerted by the cuff on the wall of the trachea and that low cuff pressure can increase the risk for aspiration pneumonia, while high cuff pressure can cause tracheal bleeding, ischemia, and pressure necrosis. Respiratory therapy typically measures the cuff pressures, which should be <25 mm Hg. In addition, although the patient's current diagnosis is aspiration, you know that all intubated patients are at risk for a type of hospital-acquired pneumonia termed VAP, which is defined as pneumonia occurring in a patient who is being mechanically ventilated within 48 hours or more after intubation. Since ETTs facilitate the migration of organisms into the lower respiratory tract, an evidence-based group of interventions (termed a bundle) have been developed to decrease the incidence. The VAP recommendations include elevating the head of bed 30 to 45 degrees, drainage of secretions collected above the cuff of the ETT, maintaining endotracheal cuff pressures, weaning from the ventilator as soon as possible, brushing teeth every 12 hours to reduce pathogen load, and employing safe suctioning techniques. You will want to place the patient on cardiac monitor and evaluate the ECG for ischemic changes or arrhythmias and monitor the oxygen saturation continuously. You assess for any changes in your cardiopulmonary assessment that suggest hemodynamic instability (decreasing BP, decreasing mean arterial pressure [MAP], decreasing urinary output [<.5 mL/Kg/hr], presence of S3 [heart failure], S4 [MI], edema, jugular vein distention (JVD)—right-sided HF or increasing dyspnea, hypoxemia, and increases crackles with left-sided HF). You will monitor blood sugar and assess for hypoglycemia (which may be related to the diaphoresis) or hyperglycemia (which may be related to the stress of the situation activating the sympathetic nervous system, which increases catecholamines, hepatic glycogenolysis, and the release of large quantities of glucose into the bloodstream while inhibiting the release of insulin). In addition, you are aware that hyperglycemia is also a risk factor for aspiration since it is associated with delayed gastric emptying by disrupting postprandial (after a meal) stomach contractions; thus, discharge planning will need to include diabetes prevention strategies. You are also aware that aspiration of liquids (or foods) into the lungs can cause ARDS (30% of cases are associated with aspiration), which is a noncardiac pulmonary edema (the alveolar–capillary membrane is disrupted as a result of aspiration).

Step Five: Take action, where the solutions that address the highest priorities are implemented.

Answer: The chest film confirms placement, and you record the level of insertion (marked in centimeters on the side of the tube) at the teeth and secure the ETT. The Ambu bag and suction equipment are brought to the bedside, the patient is placed on cardiac monitor, and the oxygen saturation is continuously monitored. ABGs on FiO_2 of 50% revealed pH 7.37, pCO_2 of 38 mm Hg, pO_2 of 118 mm Hg, HCO_3 of 24 mEq/L and saturation of 98%. The FiO_2 was decreased to 40%, and ABGs will be repeated in 2 hours. You are aware that when lungs are damaged, FiO_2 that is >50% may result in a toxic alveolar O_2 concentration. In general, durations of FiO_2 >50% for >24 have resulted in oxygen toxicity, but it has occurred in as short as 6 hours. Also, excessive O_2 concentrations have been associated with ARDS. The most important intervention for infection control to prevent VAP is handwashing and hand rubbing with alcohol-based solutions. To minimize VAP, you will brush the patient's teeth, elevate the head of bed (HOB) 30 to 45 degrees, use sedatives as sparingly as feasible, maintain ETT cuff pressures at an appropriate level (<25 mm Hg), ensure that secretions are cleared from above the cuff before it is deflated, avoid saline instillation with suctioning, turn the patient at least every 2 hours, and change ventilator circuit when it is contaminated. You will confer with the providers about early enteral nutrition and early tracheostomy (within 7 days of intubation) if patient is unable to be extubated from ETT. In addition, you will also monitor for high- and low-pressure alarms. A low-pressure alarm may indicate disconnection from the machine, ventilator circuit leak, endotracheal tube (ETT) cuff leakage, or migration of the ETT into the upper airway (the nurse assesses previous documented ETT placement marking at the lip or nares). Conversely, a high-pressure alarm usually indicates resistance to or obstruction of airflow from biting on the ETT, a kink in the tubing, build-up of secretions, patient coughing, or something as severe as bronchospasm or pneumothorax. You will monitor the patient's blood sugar and treat hyperglycemia or hypoglycemia as prescribed. Symptoms you are alert for related to ARDS include increasing respiratory distress (dyspnea, air hunger, and hypoxemia); anxiety and agitation; sputum that is foamy; frothy and often blood-tinged or pink secretions; confusion; crackles in the lung bases (especially in the dependent lung areas) that rapidly progress toward the apices of the lungs; wheezing; tachycardia; chest x-ray revealing increased bilateral interstitial markings, often in a patchy appearance; and ABG analysis demonstrating worsening hypoxemia. You want to minimize noise and establish a method of communication with the patient (white board, paper and pen, word boards) since stress will increase patient's oxygen needs. In addition, it is important to provide the patient with explanations of what is happening. To minimize hazards of immobility, active range-of-motion of extremities and out-bed (OOB) to the chair activities are performed. DVT prophylaxis includes anticoagulants and sequential compression devices (SCDs), range-of-motion (ROM) activity.

Step Six: Evaluate outcomes, which is comparing observed outcomes against expected outcomes.

Answer: The patient is extubated within 48 hours and is currently preparing for discharge. No oxygen has been required for 16 hours, and the oxygen saturation is 95%. The patient has not required insulin, is currently receiving metformin, and glucose levels have ranged from 102 to 118 mg/dL. A swallow study was performed and revealed no problems with the oral, pharyngeal, and esophageal stages of swallowing. However, the patient was diagnosed with diabetic gastroparesis, which was a significant risk factor for the aspiration, and is following up with endocrinology and has scheduled an upper GI endoscopy. This was your first experience with an intubated patient, and you provided the most current evidence-based care for a patient with an ETT, but you were also alert to the many potential problems that could have occurred (hemodynamic instability, VAP, ARDS, DVT, hazards of immobility, hyper/hypoglycemia). In addition, you provided important psychological support, recognizing that communication and development of a therapeutic relationship were important aspects of your care and part of the healing process. While treatment plans are complex and potential complications are around every corner, never forget the "care" that is essential to nursing.

CHAPTER REVIEW

NCLEX-Style Review Questions

1. A patient who has just had a total laryngectomy for cancer is being discharged. Which statement indicates the patient needs further teaching on care of the tracheostomy? Select all that apply.

a. "I must avoid getting any objects in the stoma."
b. "I can take a shower when I get home."
c. "I know it's really important to keep my scheduled appointments with the surgeon and my speech therapist."
d. "I need to clean around the stoma once a week."
e. "I will wash my hands before and after caring for the tracheostomy."

2. The nurse assesses the patient with acute pharyngitis for what signs and symptoms that indicate a complication of group A streptococcus (GAS) pharyngitis? Select all that apply.

a. Pain and spasm of the lower leg muscles
b. Rapid onset of gross hematuria
c. Reduced visual fields, blurred vision, and insomnia
d. Heartburn and abdominal distention
e. Edema and hypertension

3. For a patient who comes in to the emergency room with an epistaxis, which interventions will you implement? Select all that apply.
   a. Apply ice to the back of the neck
   b. Pinch the nares against the midline septum for 5 or 10 minutes
   c. Encourage them to blow their nose vigorously
   d. Use high Fowler with the head tilted forward
   e. Encourage the patient to swallow the blood

4. A patient who was involved in a motor vehicle accident and was admitted with maxillofacial injuries is currently postop day 2 from undergoing nasal surgical fracture repair with posterior packing in place. Which symptoms would alert the nurse to the possibility of continued active bleeding? Select all that apply.
   a. Black, tarry stools
   b. Raccoon eyes
   c. Mean arterial pressure of 65 mm Hg
   d. Friction rub
   e. Tachycardia

5. A patient had a respiratory arrest requiring emergency intubation with an endotracheal tube (ETT). Which nursing interventions are appropriate after the provider places the ETT? Select all that apply.
   a. Auscultate for bilateral breath sounds
   b. Ensure STAT chest x-ray confirms placement
   c. Ensure that the ETT is secured with either waterproof medical tape or ETT holder
   d. Ensure the exact size cuffed tracheostomy is at the bedside
   e. An obturator should be available in the room in case of accidental dislodgment

REFERENCES AND SELECTED READINGS

References and selected readings associated with this chapter can be found on the website that accompanies the book. Visit **http://thepoint.lww.com/Honan3e** to access the references and other additional resources associated with this chapter.

CHAPTER 9

Nursing Management: Patients With Chest and Lower Respiratory Tract Disorders

Laura Kierol Andrews

Learning Objectives

After reading this chapter, you will be able to:

1. Identify patients at risk for atelectasis and describe nursing interventions related to its prevention and management.
2. Compare and contrast the various pulmonary infections with regard to causes, clinical manifestations, nursing management, complications, and prevention.
3. Use the nursing process as a framework for care of the patient with pneumonia.
4. Describe the nursing management for patients receiving oxygen therapy, mini-nebulizer therapy, incentive spirometry, chest physiotherapy, and breathing retraining.
5. Relate pleurisy, pleural effusion, and empyema to pulmonary infection.
6. Relate the therapeutic management techniques of acute respiratory distress syndrome (ARDS) to the underlying pathophysiology of the syndrome.
7. Describe risk factors and measures appropriate for prevention and management of pulmonary embolism (PE).
8. Describe risk factors for the development of occupational lung disease.
9. Discuss the modes of therapy and related nursing management for patients with lung cancer.
10. Describe the complications of chest trauma and their clinical manifestations and nursing management.
11. Describe nursing measures to prevent aspiration.
12. Explain the principles of chest drainage and the nursing responsibilities related to the care of the patient with a chest drainage system.

It is common for patients in medical and surgical areas to have lower respiratory tract conditions. The care of these patients requires judicious assessment and management skills as these conditions are often serious and life-threatening and have a significant impact on activities of daily living and quality of life.

ATELECTASIS

Atelectasis is the collapse of alveoli, leading to the loss of lung volume. It is classified by its cause (absorptive, obstructive, or compressive) and can affect subsegmental, segmental, lobar, or whole lung areas. The diagnosis of atelectasis is based on both clinical and radiologic findings.

Pathophysiology

Absorptive atelectasis occurs by surfactant inactivation or when less than normal levels of inhaled nitrogen (*nitrogen wash-out*) are present in the alveoli. The most common condition that causes an inactivation of surfactant is acute respiratory distress syndrome (ARDS), in which pulmonary edema fluid dilutes and/or reduces surfactant production. The loss of surfactant causes a reduction in alveoli surface tension and leads to their collapse. Nitrogen wash-out is a condition that occurs when high levels of inhaled oxygen (FiO_2 greater than 60%) lessen the amount of nitrogen gas needed to stent open alveoli. In addition, the use of some general anesthetics can cause an absorptive atelectasis.

Compressive atelectasis occurs as a result of external forces compressing pleural and/or lung tissues. Common

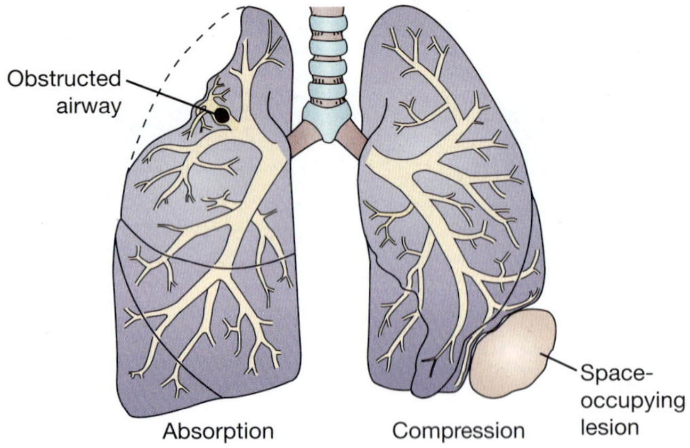

FIGURE 9-1 **Atelectasis caused by airway obstruction and absorption of air from the involved lung area (*left*) and by compression of the lung tissue (*right*). (From Grossman, S., & Porth, C. M. [2014]. *Pathophysiology: Concepts of altered health states* [9th ed.]. Lippincott Williams & Wilkins.)**

causes of this type of atelectasis are pleural effusions, lung tumors, pneumothoraces (air in the pleural space), hemothoraces (blood in the pleural space), and abdominal distention.

Obstructive atelectasis occurs when there is a mechanical obstruction of airways (secretions, mucous plugs, airway tumors, peribronchial lymph node enlargement, foreign bodies) or from low-tidal-volume breathing (which results in hypoventilation of alveoli and then absorption of alveolar gases), causing lung tissue collapse (Fig. 9-1).

Each type of atelectasis can cause a mismatching of lung ventilation in relation to perfusion that results in deoxygenated blood reaching systemic circulation and lowering oxygen supply to tissues. The most common cause of atelectasis is the obstruction of airways by secretions, mucus, foreign bodies, bronchial tumors, and oxygen toxicity.

Risk Factors

Postoperative patients, especially those who undergo abdominal and/or thoracic procedures, are at risk to develop atelectasis due to anesthetic- and/or narcotic-induced hypoventilation, incisional pain, abdominal distention, and immobility, all of which impair the ability to breathe deeply (expand lung volume) and cough (expel secretions). Additional risk factors for developing atelectasis include chronic lung disease, morbid obesity, opioid administration, blood transfusions, tobacco use, anesthesia time greater than 4 hours, prior cerebrovascular accident (CVA), lung cancer, pleural effusions, and nasogastric tube placement (Lagier et al., 2022).

Clinical Manifestations and Assessment

Signs and symptoms include dyspnea, cough, leukocytosis (elevated white blood cell [WBC] count), diminished breath sounds, and sputum production. Fever is often cited as a clinical sign of atelectasis, but there is no correlation between the severity of atelectasis on chest radiology and the presence of fever. However, atelectasis should be suspected in postoperative patients with low-grade temperature (Crompton et al., 2019). Physical examination findings relate to the severity of collapse. For a small atelectatic area, findings include crackles, decreased breath sounds, and decreased tactile fremitus over the affected lung area(s). For a large atelectatic area, findings include tracheal deviation toward the atelectatic area, decreased fremitus, bronchial breath sounds, egophony (secondary to lobar or lung collapse), and asymmetry of the chest.

If obstruction by an airway tumor or foreign body is the cause, wheezing and stridor can occur. Patients with acute atelectasis or atelectasis involving large areas, such as segments, lobes, or whole lung areas, can develop significant respiratory distress manifested by dyspnea, tachycardia, tachypnea, anxiety, restlessness, pleural pain, and hypoxemia. They may also have paroxysmal breathing, retractions, and use of accessory muscles. Chronic atelectasis has manifestations similar to those of acute atelectasis, and chronic patients are at risk of developing a postobstructive pneumonia.

Atelectasis is diagnosed by radiologic studies such as chest x-ray, computed tomography (CT) scanning, or ultrasound. Radiologic findings of atelectasis may reveal opacity or patchy infiltrates underlying the affected tissue. Larger areas of collapse can reveal shifting of the heart border, hilar vessels, and hemidiaphragm toward the affected sections. Ultrasound can detect several lung pathologies, is portable, and does not expose patients to radiation (Lagier et al., 2022).

Hypoxemia can be detected by arterial blood gas (ABG) analysis, which shows a decreased PaO_2 and oxygen saturation. Noninvasive pulse oximetry (POX) can be used to detect hypoxemia (SpO_2 less than 90%), but ABGs are the gold standard.

Medical and Nursing Management

The prevention of atelectasis is the primary management goal in at-risk patients (Box 9-1). Patients need to be educated and able to perform maneuvers that can improve ventilation and remove secretions. Immobile patients should be turned frequently, and all patients should be ambulated as soon as possible to improve lung expansion and mobilization of secretions. Lung volume expansion maneuvers, such as controlled deep breathing, coughing exercises (if secretions are present), and use of incentive spirometry (IS), should be initiated early in the postoperative period (Pastene et al., 2022). Patients who have asthma, chronic obstructive pulmonary disease (COPD), lung cancer, and thoracic or abdominal surgeries are at very high risk for developing atelectasis. These patients require additional interventions to prevent atelectasis. The use of aerosolized (nebulized) bronchodilators and/or mucolytics, followed by chest physiotherapy (CPT) (chest percussion and postural drainage), and positive expiratory pressure (PEP) therapy (Acapella®, Aerobika®, MetaNeb®) may be instituted.

BOX 9-1 **Health Promotion**

Preventing Atelectasis

- Change patient's position frequently, especially from supine to upright position, to promote ventilation and prevent secretions from accumulating.
- Match ventilation to perfusion: blood flow is greater in the dependent area, so when the "good lung" is also dependent, a match exists between best ventilation and best perfusion. A mismatch occurs when the affected lung is positioned down because of the increase in blood flow to an area with less ventilation capacity. Although you need to turn the patient every 2 hours to promote secretion removal, the affected lung should be dependent for the least amount of time possible and POX should be monitored.
- Encourage early mobilization from bed to chair, followed by early ambulation.
- Encourage appropriate deep breathing and coughing to mobilize secretions and prevent them from accumulating.
- Teach/reinforce appropriate technique for incentive spirometry.
- Administer prescribed opioids and sedatives judiciously to prevent respiratory depression.
- Perform postural drainage and chest percussion, if indicated.
- Institute suctioning to remove tracheobronchial secretions, if indicated.

Incentive Spirometry

Incentive spirometry (IS) is a method of deep breathing that provides visual feedback to encourage the patient to inhale slowly and deeply via a handheld spirometer. This prevents or reduces atelectasis by stimulating alveolar cells to secrete surfactant, which decreases the surface tension in the alveoli and improves inspiratory muscle performance. The use of IS is discussed in Box 9-2.

BOX 9-2 **Patient Education**

Using an Incentive Spirometer

The inhalation of air, in a slow and controlled manner, helps inflate the lungs. The marker within the spirometer will measure the depth of each breath.

- Assume an upright position if possible (sitting or semi-Fowler).
- Breathe using your diaphragm.
- Place mouthpiece firmly in the mouth, and breathe in deeply and slowly, holding each breath in for 3–4 seconds and exhaling slowly.
- Repeat 6–10 times per session.
- Use spirometer every hour while awake (keep it within reach).
- If secretions are present, try coughing, with splinting of incision, after each use.

Pearls for Practice

Surfactant, which decreases the surface tension in the alveoli, thus reducing their risk of collapse, needs to be replaced continuously. One stimulus for replacement is maximum deep inhalation that is sustained for a few seconds. Adults sigh or deep breathe at one and a half to two times their normal tidal volume (~500 mL) six to eight times every hour. Any etiology that results in monotonous hypoventilation will lead to atelectasis. IS encourages the patient to sigh or deep breathe. The IS is typically graduated to 1.5 L and allows the user to see the depth of their breath by the rise of the three balls inside. Coughing is a forced expiratory maneuver that can "squeeze" alveoli. If coughing is needed to expel secretions, the nurse should follow the coughing maneuvers with the use of IS to reexpand the alveoli and encourage surfactant replacement. Assisting a patient to splint incisions will help improve the efficacy of coughing.

Nebulizer Therapy

Nebulizer therapy dispenses aerosolized medications to a patient's lungs via handheld or face mask devices. The medication is inhaled with a flow of compressed air or oxygen, producing a visible mist. The patient breaths through the mouth, taking slow, deep breaths, and then holds the breath for a few seconds. The patient is encouraged to cough during the treatment, which assists in increasing intrathoracic pressure and promoting secretion expectoration. Antibiotics, bronchodilators, and mucolytic medications can be nebulized.

Chest Physiotherapy

Chest physiotherapy (CPT), with or without nebulizer medications, also can be used to prevent or treat atelectasis, bronchial obstructions, and pneumonias. CPT includes **postural drainage**, **chest percussion**, vibration, and breathing retraining. The goals of CPT are to remove bronchial secretions, improve ventilation, and increase the efficiency of the respiratory muscles. In addition, teaching the patient effective coughing technique is an important part of CPT.

Postural drainage uses specific positions that allow gravity to aid in the removal of pulmonary secretions. Patients who lie supine will have secretions accumulate in the posterior lung sections, whereas upright patients will pool secretions in their lower lobes. By having the patient change positions (Fig. 9-2), secretions can drain from the affected bronchioles into the bronchi and trachea and then be removed by coughing or suctioning. Postural drainage is usually performed two to four times daily, prior to meals (to prevent nausea, vomiting, or aspiration) and at bedtime. Prescribed nebulizer therapy should be given prior to postural drainage to dilate the bronchioles, reduce bronchospasm, and thin secretions. The patient is instructed to remain in each position for 10 to

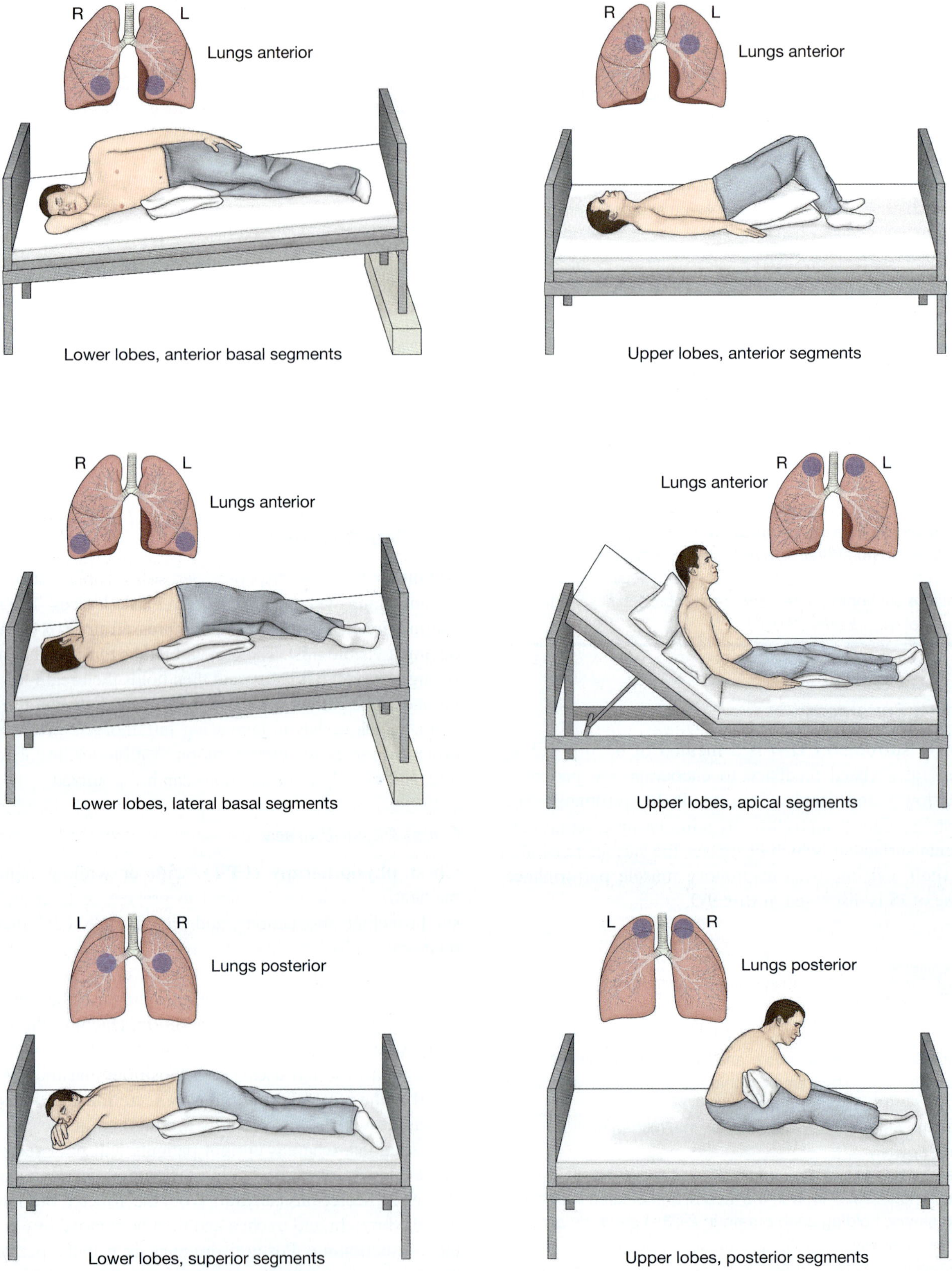

FIGURE 9-2 Positions used in lung drainage.

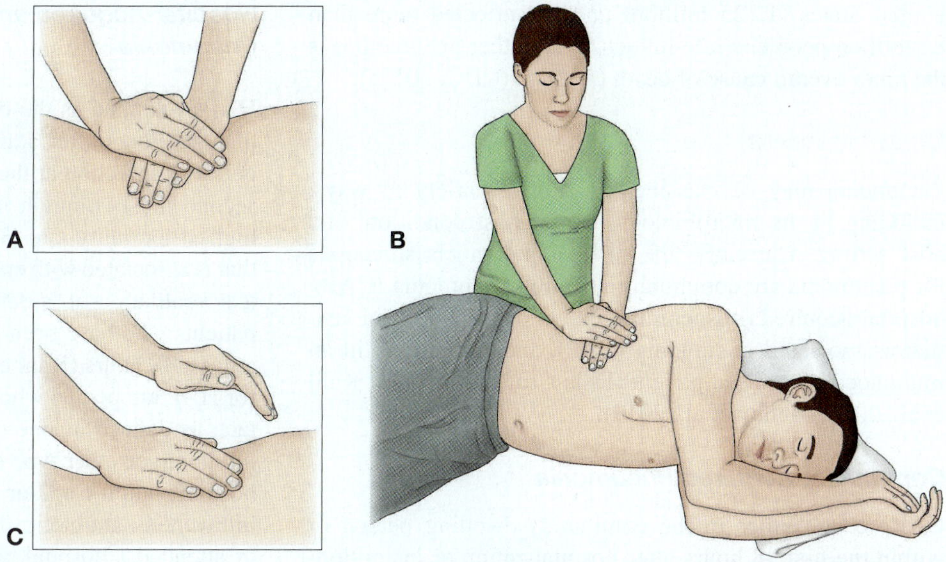

FIGURE 9-3 Percussion and vibration. A. Proper hand position for vibration. B. Proper technique for vibration. The wrists and elbows remain stiff; the vibrating motion is produced by the shoulder muscles. C. Proper hand position for percussion.

15 minutes, inhaling slowly through the nose and exhaling slowly through pursed lips. If the patient cannot tolerate a position, the nurse modifies it for comfort. When changing positions, the patient should be instructed to take a deep breath and cough out secretions, or the nurse may have to suction if the patient is unable to cough.

Chest percussion and vibration can be used in each position to loosen secretions (Fig. 9-3). Percussion is performed by the nurse or respiratory therapist by rapidly "clapping" their cupped hands over the affected lung lobe. This is done for 1 to 2 minutes in each postural area. Commercial percussion vests and beds are also available for use. Vibration is performed either manually or with a mechanical device. The nurse places their hands over the affected area and rapidly contracts the arms and shoulders while the patient exhales. This maneuver is done for 5 to 10 breaths over each lung area.

Other Treatments

If the cause of atelectasis is bronchial obstruction from secretions, the secretions must be removed by forceful coughing or suctioning to allow air to reenter that portion of the lung. Mucolytic agents such as acetylcysteine (Mucomyst), hypertonic saline (3%, 6%) or dornase alfa can be added to loosen and thin tenacious mucus (Bradley et al., 2019). If intensive pulmonary toilet maneuvers and nebulizers fail to remove the obstructive mucus, a bronchoscopy can be performed. A bronchoscopy can also be used to remove foreign bodies from airways. Patients with airways tumors also may undergo biopsy for diagnostic purposes, cryotherapy (cold therapy), or laser therapy via bronchoscopy. Additional therapies for these patients include airway stents or radiation and chemotherapy.

If the cause of atelectasis is compression of lung tissue, the goal is to decrease or remove the compression. Large pleural effusions that collapse lung tissue can be removed by **thoracentesis** (removal of fluid by needle aspiration) or chest tube insertion (thoracostomy). A **hemothorax** or **pneumothorax** usually is treated by inserting a chest tube to drain the blood or air that is collapsing the lung. No matter what the cause of atelectasis, in patients with significant hypoxemia, intubation and mechanical ventilation with **positive end-expiratory pressure (PEEP)** may be necessary to provide adequate ventilation and oxygenation.

Complications

Usually mild atelectasis can be managed with lung expansion maneuvers, CPT, and mobilization of the patient, but in some cases patients can develop severe hypoxia, respiratory distress, or pneumonia. Mortality is highest in patients who require intubation and mechanical intubation, especially for more than 48 hours. Complications also can occur from treatments used to treat atelectasis, such as bronchoscopy, thoracentesis, and thoracostomy, all of which place the patient at risk for infection, bleeding, and pneumothorax.

RESPIRATORY INFECTIONS

PNEUMONIA

Pneumonia is the infection of the lower respiratory tract caused by a variety of microorganisms, including bacteria, viruses, fungi, protozoa, and parasites. Pneumonia is common, affecting 1% of the population. Pneumonia causes more than 1.5 million hospitalizations annually and is associated with considerable mortality and morbidity (CDC, 2022a, 2022e, 2022j). Pneumonia caused by COVID-19 is the leading cause of death by infectious source in the

United States (1.125 million) and has affected more than 82 million people, while influenza and other pneumonias is the ninth overall cause of death (52,544) (CDC, 2022a).

Classifications

Pneumonia may be classified in a wide variety of ways, including by its microbiologic cause, host condition, and host setting. Currently, the most common classifications for pneumonia are community-acquired pneumonia (CAP), hospital-acquired (**nosocomial**) pneumonia (HAP) and ventilator-associated pneumonia (VAP), and pneumonia in an immunocompromised patient (Dela Cruz et al., 2021; Kalil et al., 2016; Metlay et al., 2019).

Community-Acquired Pneumonia

CAP occurs either in the community-dwelling person or within the first 48 hours after hospitalization or institutionalization. Most cases of CAP occur in the winter and early spring months, and prevalence rates are higher in older people. Each year approximately 2,000 admissions per 100,000 people in the United States required hospitalization for CAP (McLaughlin et al., 2020); these patients have a mortality rate of 1% to 23%, with ICU patients having the highest rates of death (Regunath & Oba, 2022). The need for hospitalization for CAP depends on the severity of the pneumonia, which is assessed by factors such as

- altered mental status,
- azotemia (higher than normal blood levels of urea or other nitrogen-containing compounds),
- respiratory rate greater than or equal to 30 breaths per minute (BPM),
- low blood pressure (BP) (systolic BP less than 90 or diastolic BP less than 60),
- tachycardia (HR greater than 125 bpm),
- high fever (temperature greater than 104°F) or afebrile,
- age 65 years or older
- arterial pH <7.35
- poor oxygenation (PaO_2 less than 70 mm Hg if less than 50 years old, PaO_2 less than 60 mm Hg if over 50 years old)
- inability to reliably take medications or $PaO_2/FiO_2 \leq 250$ (Metlay et al., 2019) (P/F ratio is discussed on page 337),
- septic shock,
- respiratory failure requiring oxygen therapy or mechanical ventilation.

In addition, people of advanced age with at least one comorbid disorder are at higher risk for needing hospitalization (McLaughlin et al., 2020). The most common causative microbe of CAP is the gram-positive *Streptococcus pneumoniae* (pneumococcus); however, that causative agent is identified definitively in less than 50% to 60% of CAP cases (Kim et al., 2022). Other causative agents are *Haemophilus influenzae, Staphylococcus aureus, Moraxella catarrhalis, Legionella* spp., and viruses.

Hospital-Acquired and Ventilator-Associated Pneumonia

HAP is defined as the onset of pneumonia symptoms more than 48 hours after admission in patients who had no evidence of infection at the time of hospitalization. HAP is the second most common nosocomial infection but carries the highest mortality rate (33% to 50%). VAP is a type of HAP that is associated with **endotracheal intubation** and mechanical ventilation; it is defined as pneumonia that develops in patients who have been receiving mechanical ventilation for at least 48 hours (Kalil et al., 2016). Other associated factors for HAP are people who have had extensive health care contact, as defined as one of the following: resident of a nursing home or other type of long-term care facility, acute care hospitalization for 2 or more days within the last 90 days, intravenous antibiotic therapy, wound care, chemotherapy, or attended a hospital or hemodialysis clinic within the last 30 days. It is reported that HAP accounts for 25% of intensive care unit infections and causes increased length of stay, leading to greater costs of care ($40,000 per case) (Kalil et al., 2016). In some studies, VAP carries a mortality rate of 20% to 50%, but recent data show a decline in this number to 13% (Kalil et al., 2016). It can be even higher when lung infection is caused by high-risk pathogens such as COVID-19 (Alotaibi et al., 2022; CDC, 2022a). Refer to Figure 9-4 or pathogenesis of VAP. Recommendations to prevent VAP include elevating the head of bed 30 to 45 degrees, drainage of secretions collected above the cuff of the ETT, maintaining endotracheal cuff pressures, weaning from the ventilator as soon as possible, brushing teeth every 12 hours to reduce pathogen load, considering initiation of enteral feeding within 48 hours to prevent translocation of intestinal flora to the lungs by stimulating effective intestinal functioning, employing safe suctioning techniques (see Chapter 8, Box 8-7), and using a new ventilator circuit for each patient, changing the circuit only if soiled or damaged (Isac et al., 2021).

HAP occurs when at least one of three conditions exists: host defenses are impaired, microorganisms reach the lower respiratory tract (usually by microaspiration of oropharyngeal microorganisms), or a highly virulent organism is present. Certain factors may predispose patients to HAP because of impaired host defenses (e.g., severe acute or chronic illness), a variety of comorbid conditions, supine positioning, aspiration, altered mental status, malnutrition, prolonged hospitalization, hypotension, and metabolic disorders. Hospitalized patients are also exposed to potential bacteria from other sources (e.g., transmission of pathogens from health care workers' hands, respiratory devices, and water reservoirs that are contaminated). Numerous intervention-related factors also may play a role in the development of HAP (e.g., therapeutic agents that cause central nervous system [CNS] depression with hypoventilation, endotracheal intubation, or inappropriate use of antibiotics). Alterations in the gastric pH due to illness and medications can disrupt the stomach

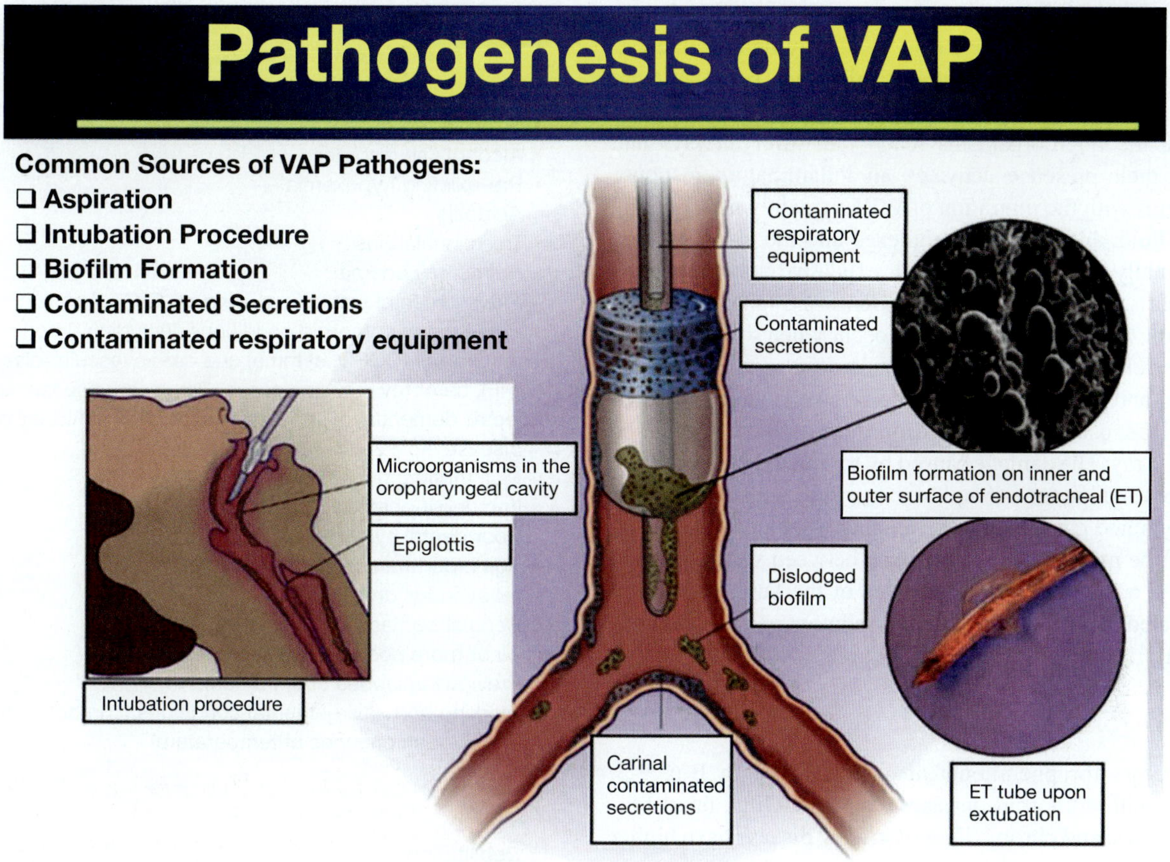

FIGURE 9-4 **Pathogenesis of VAP. (From Sachdev, G., & Napolitano, L. M. [2012]. Postoperative pulmonary complications: pneumonia and acute respiratory failure. *Surgical Clinics of North America*, *92*[2], 321–344.)**

lining, exposing patients to enteric bacteria. The mortality of HAP is related to the virulence of the organisms, their resistance to antibiotics, and the patient's underlying condition. The common organisms responsible for HAP and VAP include gram-negative bacilli and gram-positive cocci. Gram-negative organisms include *Pseudomonas aeruginosa, Escherichia coli, Klebsiella pneumoniae, Acinetobacter* spp., *Serratia* spp., *Stenotrophomonas maltophilia,* and *H. influenzae.* Gram-positive organisms include *S. aureus* (MSSA and MRSA) and *S. pneumoniae.* Viruses (except the COVID-19 virus) or fungi are less common causative agents, except in the immunocompromised patient.

Pneumonia in the Immunocompromised Hosts

Pneumonia in the immunocompromised hosts includes *Pneumocystis jirovecii* pneumonia (PJP), fungal pneumonias, and *Mycobacterium tuberculosis.* Pneumonia in the immunocompromised hosts occurs with use of corticosteroids or other immunosuppressive agents, chemotherapy, nutritional depletion, use of broad-spectrum antimicrobial agents, acquired immunodeficiency syndrome (AIDS), genetic immune disorders, and long-term life-support technology (mechanical ventilation). In addition, increasing numbers of patients with impaired defenses develop HAP from gram-negative bacilli, which poses difficulty in providing coverage. In addition, the combination of an immunocompromised patient and some gram-negative bacilli impacts the incidence of mortality.

Pneumonia in immunocompromised hosts may be caused by the organisms also observed in CAP or HAP. PCP is rarely observed in immunocompetent hosts and is often an initial AIDS-defining complication. Whether patients are immunocompromised or immunocompetent, the clinical presentation of pneumonia is similar, but PCP has a subtle onset, with progressive dyspnea, fever, and a nonproductive cough. Refer to Chapter 36 for more information about PJP and HIV.

Pathophysiology

Pneumonia can arise from several vectors: from normal flora present in patients whose resistance has been altered; aspiration of flora present in the nasopharynx or oropharynx; the inhalation of airborne microorganisms from other people (sneezing, coughing, or talking); contaminated water sources or respiratory equipment; or blood-borne organisms that enter the pulmonary circulation (hematogenous spread) and become trapped in the pulmonary capillary beds.

Normal host defenses (cough, ciliary clearance, and alveolar macrophages) and intact upper airway defense mechanisms usually prevent potentially infectious particles from reaching the sterile lower respiratory tract.

Once the microorganisms reach the lower airways and alveoli, their presence activates an inflammatory response that begins with the migration of WBCs (mainly neutrophils), plasma fluid, and immune complexes into the alveoli, filling the normally air-filled spaces with exudative liquids and cellular debris. This causes alveolar edema and lung tissue consolidation. Additional damage can occur when some microorganisms release toxins that further damage respiratory cells. Alveolar and bronchial tissues become swollen and infiltrated with WBCs, causing **consolidation** of lung tissue that can be seen on x-ray. The damage caused by toxins and inflammatory mediators and immune complexes interferes with the diffusion of oxygen and carbon dioxide, leading to clinical manifestations of the pneumonia. A mismatch between ventilation and perfusion occurs in the affected area of the lung, and poorly oxygenated blood returns from the pulmonary vasculature to the heart, resulting in arterial hypoxemia.

Risk Factors

Risk factors for pneumonia are summarized in Box 9-3. Patients with comorbid diseases such as COPD, heart failure, diabetes, and chronic liver or kidney disease have higher mortality rates than those without comorbid diseases. In addition, in conditions with impaired swallowing and altered mental status there is increased risk related to chronic aspiration of oropharyngeal secretions (Stacy, 2022). Lifestyle factors associated with an increased risk of pneumonia include cigarette smoking, alcohol use, contact with children and pets, and living in a household with more than 10 people (Daly & Ellison, 2020).

BOX 9-3

Risk Factors for Pneumonia

Community-Acquired Pneumonia (CAP)

- Smoking
- Alcohol use disorder
- Pre-existing hypoxemia
- Acidosis
- Toxic inhalations
- Pulmonary edema
- Altered mental status (e.g., seizure, CVA)
- Presence of comorbid conditions, including chronic respiratory (COPD, asthma) and cardiovascular diseases (HF), cerebrovascular disease, Parkinson disease, epilepsy, dementia, dysphagia, HIV, or chronic kidney or liver disease
- Malnutrition; underweight
- Immunosuppressive therapies
- Poor dental hygiene
- Age older than 65 years
- Intravenous drug use
- Regular contact with children
- 10 or more people living in a household
- Previous episodes of pneumonia
- Working and environmental conditions (contact with dust and sudden changes of temperature)

Hospital-Acquired Pneumonia (HAP) and Ventilator-Associated Pneumonia (VAP)

- Debilitation
- Malnutrition
- Altered mental status
- Previous exposure to antibiotics (within the last 90 days)
- Hospital stays of 5 days or longer
- High rates of antibiotic resistance (hospital or unit-specific)
- Immunosuppressive therapies or diseases
- Prolonged (greater than 48 hours) intubation or a tracheostomy
- Male biologic sex
- Treatment related, e.g., mechanical ventilation, unintentional extubation, upper abdominal surgery, thoracic surgery
- Supine position

Clinical Manifestations and Assessment

Pneumonia varies in its signs and symptoms depending on the causal organism and the presence of underlying disease; however, it is not possible to diagnose a specific type of pneumonia by clinical manifestations alone. The classic clinical manifestations of pneumonia are fever, cough (productive or nonproductive), dyspnea, and leukocytosis. Patients can also present with rigors (shaking chills), pleuritic chest pain (sudden, intense, and described as sharp, stabbing, or burning), tachypnea, use of accessory muscles, tachycardia, fatigue, and anorexia. Some patients initially exhibit an upper respiratory tract infection (nasal congestion, sore throat), and the onset of symptoms of pneumonia is gradual and nonspecific. Then the predominant symptoms may be headache, low-grade fever, pleuritic pain, myalgia (muscle pain), rash, and pharyngitis.

Physical examination findings may reveal bronchial breath sounds over consolidated lung areas, crackles, increased tactile fremitus (vocal vibration detected on palpation), percussion dullness, egophony ("E" to "A"), and whispered pectoriloquy (whispered sounds are easily auscultated through the chest wall). These changes occur because sound is transmitted better through solid or dense tissue (consolidation) than through normal air-filled tissue. **Purulent** sputum or slight changes in respiratory symptoms may be the only sign of pneumonia in patients with COPD. It may be difficult to determine whether an increase in symptoms is an exacerbation or an infectious process.

The diagnosis of pneumonia is made by history (particularly of a recent respiratory tract infection), physical examination, chest x-ray, blood culture (bloodstream invasion, called *bacteremia*, occurs frequently), sputum examination (gram stain and culture), and rapid bacterial antigen testing of urine or oropharyngeal swabs. A urine test may be ordered when pneumococcal pneumonia is suspected since the enzyme-linked immunosorbent assay (ELISA) can detect pneumococcal cell wall or capsular polysaccharide in the urine of 80% of patients with bacteremic pneumococcal pneumonia (Kim et al., 2022). In addition, a urinary antigen test can be obtained to assess for *Legionella pneumophila* if suspected.

The sputum sample is obtained by having patients do the following: (1) rinse the mouth with water to minimize contamination by normal oral flora, (2) breathe deeply several times, (3) cough deeply, and (4) expectorate the raised sputum into a sterile container. The best time to collect the sputum culture is in the morning because the sputum is more concentrated and less likely to be contaminated with saliva and nasopharyngeal secretions. More invasive procedures may be used to collect sputum specimens (nasotracheal or orotracheal suctioning or bronchioalveolar lavage via bronchoscopy).

Pearls for Practice

Since timely initiation of antibiotic treatment is important, the nurse understands that a STAT sputum gram stain may be obtained. The gram stain will inform the provider whether the organisms are gram positive (thick cell walls) or gram negative (thin cell walls). Since results are available rapidly, the provider can prescribe an antibiotic with efficacy to the identified bacteria (positive, negative) and fungi (yeasts, molds), but not viruses. Thus, the nurse understands the difference between empiric coverage and culture documented. Culture documented will name the specific organism and antibiotics that are sensitive or resistant to the specified organism.

Chest x-ray findings associated with pneumonia vary depending upon microbial causes, but a new pulmonary infiltrate or consolidation is often seen within 48 hours of onset of symptoms. Infiltrates can involve segments or lobes, or be multilobar.

Unfolding Patient Stories: K.B. • Part 1

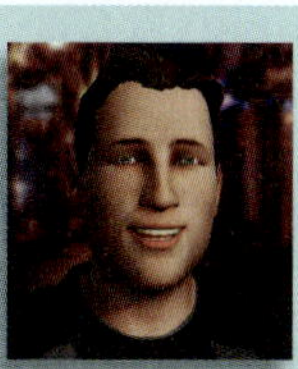

K.B., a 27-year-old, has a history of fatigue, high fever, and a productive cough for a week and arrives in the emergency department with difficulty breathing. A chest x-ray reveals a right lower lobe pneumonia. What are the clinical manifestations and assessment findings associated with a right lower lobe pneumonia that the nurse should investigate when evaluating the patient? (K.B.'s case continues in Chapter 16.)

Care for K.B. and other patients in a realistic virtual environment: ***vSim** for Nursing* (thepoint.lww.com/vSimMedicalSurgical). Practice documenting these patients' care in DocuCare (thepoint.lww.com/DocuCareEHR).

Medical and Nursing Management

Pharmacologic Therapy

The treatment of pneumonia includes administration of the appropriate antibiotic. The choice of antibiotic is determined by the classification of pneumonia (i.e., CAP vs. HAP), results of Gram stains, culture sensitivities, antigen testing, and patient's comorbid conditions. Initial treatment for CAP is empiric unless sputum culture and sensitivity results are available. Empiric therapy for non-CAP is usually initiated with a broad-spectrum IV antibiotic and may be monotherapy or combination therapy. The choice of antibiotics is based on assessment of risk of multidrug resistance (MDR) pathogens and early versus late onset of HAP or VAP symptoms (Table 9-1). Once the microbacterial cultures and sensitivities are available, therapy should be narrowed to avoid emergence of drug-resistant pathogens. Box 9-4 depicts the risk factors for developing MDR pathogens.

Prompt administration of antibiotics in patients is a key treatment measure. If specific pathogens responsible for the

TABLE **9-1** **Empiric Antibiotic Therapy for Hospital-Acquired or Ventilator-Associated Pneumonia**

Type	Drugs
Early onset (less than 5 days), with no risk factors for multidrug-resistant pathogens	Ampicillin-sulbactam OR Ceftriaxone OR Levofloxacin, moxifloxacin, or ciprofloxacin OR Ertapenem
Late onset (5 days or more) or risk factors for multidrug-resistant pathogens	Cefepime or ceftazidime OR Imipenem or meropenem OR Piperacillin-tazobactam AND Ciprofloxacin or levofloxacin OR Amikacin, gentamicin, or tobramycin AND Linezolid or vancomycin (MRSA)

Data from Metlay, J. P., Waterer, G. W., Long, A. C., Anzueto, A., Brozek, J., Crothers, K., Cooley, L. A., Dean, N. C., Fine, M. J., Flanders, S. A., Griffin, M. R., Metersky, M. L., Musher, D. M., Restrepo, M. I., & Whitney, C. G. (2019). Diagnosis and treatment of adults with community-acquired pneumonia. *American Journal of Respiratory and Critical Care Medicine*, *200*(7), e45–e67; American Thoracic Society; Infectious Diseases Society of America. (2005). Guidelines for management of adults with hospital-acquired ventilator associated, and healthcare-associated pneumonia. *American Journal of Respiratory and Critical Care Medicine*, *171*, 388–416; Musher, D. (2020). Overview of pneumonia. In L. Goldman & A. Schafter (Eds.), *Goldman-Cecil medicine* (26th ed.). Elsevier, Saunders.

BOX 9-4

Risk Factors for the Development of Multidrug-Resistant Pathogens

- Antibiotic use in preceding 90 days
- Current hospitalization 5 days or longer
- Immunocompromised (by disease or therapies)
- Increased frequency of drug resistance in the community or hospital unit
- Presence of risk factors for HAP, VAP, CAP

pneumonia are identified, more specific, less broad-spectrum agents should be used. The recommended duration of treatment for CAP is a minimum of 5 days. Patients should be afebrile for at least 2 days before antibiotics are discontinued. Patients with nosocomial pneumonias are treated for 7 to 10 days, as long as the patient is showing signs of clinical improvement. Emerging data are demonstrating that shorter durations of antibiotic use are producing good clinical responses and fewer emergences of MDR pathogens (Kalil et al., 2019).

Antibiotics are ineffective in viral pneumonia, and their use may be associated with adverse effects (superinfections, MDR pathogens). Patients who develop pneumonia or who are at risk for influenza can be treated with antiviral agents. The CDC (2016b) recommends early initiation of antiviral therapy (within 48 hours of symptoms onset) for people with suspected or confirmed influenza who are severely ill or hospitalized or are at risk for complications.

Oxygen Inhalation Therapy

Oxygen inhalation therapy is the administration of oxygen at a concentration greater than that found in the environmental atmosphere. At sea level, the concentration of oxygen in room air is 21% and has a relative humidity of 50% under normal circumstances; the lungs contribute about 250 mL of H_2O per day to maximally saturate inspired air. The goal of using oxygen therapy is to prevent or correct tissue hypoxia, which is decreased oxygen supply to the tissues (Box 9-5). Hypoxia is often confused with hypoxemia. Hypoxemia is a decrease in the arterial oxygen content or arterial oxygen tension (partial pressure of oxygen, PaO_2) and is measured by ABG or POX. Hypoxemia is defined as a PaO_2 level of less than 60 mm Hg and/or a POX level of less than 90%. When administering oxygen to a patient, a nurse must keep in mind that oxygen transport to the tissues is dependent not only on the arterial oxygen content but also on cardiac output, hemoglobin concentration, and metabolic requirements.

Indications for Oxygen Therapy

The use of oxygen to *treat* patients with hypoxia is based on clinical indicators such as subjective information (dyspnea, chest pain), ABG analysis, POX, and physical examination findings. A change in respiratory rate or pattern (e.g., bradypnea, tachypnea, Cheyne–Stokes breathing), change in mental status (agitation, anxiety, disorientation, confusion, lethargy, coma), change in BP, change in heart rate (bradycardia or tachycardia), development of arrhythmias, cyanosis (late sign), diaphoresis, or cool extremities are signs of hypoxia. The development of these signs and symptoms depends on how suddenly the hypoxia develops. Acute onset tends to show signs of neurologic and cardiovascular impairment, while with chronic onset, patients complain of fatigue, drowsiness, dyspnea on exertion (DOE), and inattentiveness.

The administration of oxygen to *prevent* hypoxemia in high-risk patients who do not have clinical indicators of hypoxia is common in hospitals, but should only be initiated based on pulse oximetry (POX 94% or less)

BOX 9-5

Types of Hypoxia

Hypoxia can occur from either severe pulmonary disease (inadequate oxygen supply) or from extrapulmonary disease (inadequate oxygen delivery) affecting gas exchange at the cellular level. The four general types of hypoxia are hypoxemic hypoxia, circulatory hypoxia, anemic hypoxia, and histotoxic hypoxia.

Hypoxemic Hypoxia

Hypoxemic hypoxia is a decreased oxygen level in the blood resulting in decreased oxygen diffusion into the tissues. It may be caused by hypoventilation, high altitudes, ventilation–perfusion mismatch (as in pulmonary embolism), shunts in which the alveoli are collapsed and cannot provide oxygen to the blood (commonly caused by atelectasis), and pulmonary diffusion defects. It is corrected by increasing alveolar ventilation or providing supplemental oxygen.

Circulatory Hypoxia

Circulatory hypoxia results from inadequate capillary circulation. It may be caused by decreased cardiac output, local vascular obstruction, low-flow states such as shock, or cardiac arrest. Although tissue partial pressure of oxygen (PO_2) is reduced, arterial oxygen (PaO_2) remains normal. Circulatory hypoxia is corrected by identifying and treating the underlying cause.

Anemic Hypoxia

Anemic hypoxia is a result of decreased effective hemoglobin concentration, which causes a decrease in the oxygen-carrying capacity of the blood. It is rarely accompanied by hypoxemia. Carbon monoxide poisoning, because it reduces the oxygen-carrying capacity of hemoglobin, produces similar effects but is not strictly anemic hypoxia because hemoglobin levels may be normal.

Histotoxic Hypoxia

Histotoxic hypoxia occurs when a toxic substance, such as cyanide, interferes with the ability of tissues to use available oxygen.

(O'Driscoll et al., 2017). High-risk patients are those who are at risk of rapidly developing hypoxemia or who will not tolerate even mild hypoxemia. Patients with pneumonia, PE, suspected myocardial injury or infarction, and head trauma or injury are just a few examples.

Methods of Oxygen Administration

Oxygen is dispensed from a cylinder or a piped-in system, and a flow meter regulates the flow of oxygen in liters per minute. A variety of oxygen delivery systems are available (Table 9-2). Each system and oxygen flow rate is designed to provide a specific **fraction of inspired oxygen** (FiO_2), percentage of oxygen, or liters per minute (L/min). The appropriate form of oxygen therapy is best determined by ABG levels, which indicate the patient's oxygenation status (POX and/or PaO_2).

Oxygen delivery systems are classified as low-flow or high-flow. Low-flow systems contribute partially to the inspired gas the patient breathes, which means that the patient breathes some room air along with the oxygen. These systems do not provide a constant or known concentration of inspired oxygen. The amount of inspired oxygen changes as the patient's breathing changes. Examples of low-flow systems include nasal cannula, simple mask, partial-rebreather, and nonrebreather masks. In contrast, high-flow systems provide the total amount of inspired air. A specific percentage of oxygen is delivered independent of the patient's breathing. High-flow systems are indicated for patients who require a constant and precise amount of oxygen. Examples of such systems include transtracheal catheters, Venturi masks, aerosol masks, tracheostomy collars, high-flow nasal cannula (HFNCs), and face tents.

TABLE **9-2 Oxygen Administration Devices**

Device	Suggested Flow Rate (L/min)	O_2 Percentage Setting	Advantages	Disadvantages
Low-Flow Systems				
Cannula	1–2 3–5 6	23–30 30–40 42	Lightweight, comfortable, inexpensive, continuous use with meals and activity	Nasal mucosal drying, variable FiO_2, nasal polyps or a deviated septum may impede flow
Oropharyngeal catheter	1–6	23–42	Inexpensive, does not require a tracheostomy	Nasal mucosa irritation; catheter should be changed frequently to alternate nostril
Mask, simple	6–8	40–60	Simple to use, inexpensive	Poorly fitting, variable FiO_2, must remove to eat
Mask, partial rebreather	8–11	50–75	Moderate O_2 concentration	Warm, poorly fitting, must remove to eat
Mask, nonrebreather	12	80–100	High O_2 concentration	Poorly fitting
High-Flow Systems				
Transtracheal catheter	¼–4	60–100	More comfortable, concealed by clothing, less oxygen liters per minute needed than nasal cannula	Requires frequent and regular cleaning, requires surgical intervention
Mask, Venturi	4–6	24, 26, 28	Provides low levels of supplemental O_2	Must remove to eat
	6–8	30, 35, 40, 50	Precise FiO_2, additional humidity available	
Mask, aerosol	8–10	30–100	Good humidity, accurate FiO_2	Uncomfortable for some
Tracheostomy collar	8–10	30–100	Good humidity, comfortable, fairly accurate FiO_2	
Face tent	8–10	30–100	Good humidity, fairly accurate FiO_2	Bulky and cumbersome
Oxygen-Conserving Devices				
Pulse dose (or demand)	10–40 mL/breath		Deliver O_2 only on inspiration, conserve 50–75% of O_2 used	Must carefully evaluate function individually

Concept Mastery Alert

For patients fitted with partial rebreathing masks, the masks should always be filled, whether the patient is inhaling or exhaling.

A nasal cannula is used when the patient requires a low to medium concentration of oxygen for which precise accuracy is not essential. This method is relatively simple and allows the patient to move about in bed, talk, cough, and eat without interrupting oxygen flow. Flow rates in excess of 6 to 8 L/min may lead to swallowing of air or may cause irritation and drying of the nasal and pharyngeal mucosa, and if the patient has nasal polyps or a deviated septum, oxygen flow may be blocked (Stacy, 2022). When oxygen is administered via cannula, the percentage of oxygen reaching the lungs varies with the depth and rate of respirations, particularly if the nasal mucosa is swollen or if the patient is a mouth breather.

Pearls for Practice

The nurse is aware that patients with nasal cannula often develop irritation and erythema on their ears and cheeks due to pressure of the cannula tubing. Gauze or protective devices that pad the pressure points may be used around the cheeks and ears during prolonged use.

Oxygen masks come in several forms (Fig. 9-5). Each is used for different purposes. *Simple masks* are used to administer low to moderate concentrations of oxygen. The body of the mask itself gathers and stores oxygen between breaths. The patient exhales directly through openings or ports in the body of the mask. If oxygen flow ceases, the patient can draw air in through these openings around the mask edges. Although widely used, these masks cannot be used for controlled oxygen concentrations and must be adjusted for proper fit. They should not press too tightly against the skin because this can cause a sense of claustrophobia as well as skin breakdown; adjustable elastic bands are provided to ensure comfort and security.

Partial-rebreathing masks have a reservoir bag that must remain inflated during both inspiration and expiration. The nurse adjusts the oxygen flow to ensure that the bag does not collapse during inhalation. A high concentration of oxygen can be delivered because both the mask and the bag serve as reservoirs for oxygen. Oxygen enters the mask through small-bore tubing that connects at the junction of the mask and bag. As the patient inhales, gas is drawn from the mask, from the bag, and potentially from room air through the exhalation ports. As the patient exhales, the first third of the exhalation fills the reservoir bag. This is mainly dead space and does not participate in gas exchange in the lungs. Therefore, it has a high oxygen concentration. The remainder of the exhaled gas is vented through the exhalation ports. The actual percentage of oxygen delivered is influenced by the patient's ventilatory pattern.

Nonrebreathing masks are similar in design to partial-rebreathing masks except that they have additional valves. A one-way valve located between the reservoir bag and the base of the mask allows gas from the reservoir bag to enter the mask on inhalation but prevents gas in the mask from flowing back into the reservoir bag during exhalation. One-way valves located at the exhalation ports prevent room air

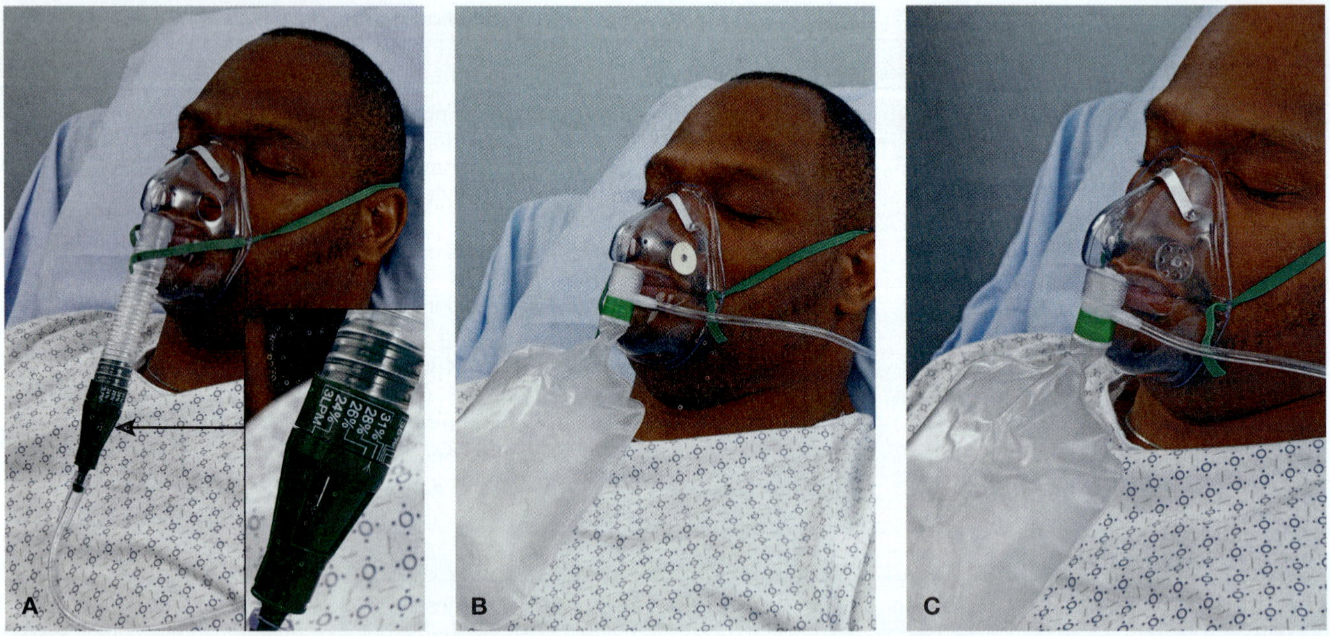

FIGURE 9-5 **Types of oxygen masks used to deliver varying concentrations of oxygen. A. Venturi mask. B. Nonrebreather. C. Partial rebreather.**

from entering the mask during inhalation. They also allow the patient's exhaled gases to exit the mask on exhalation. As with the partial-rebreathing mask, it is important to adjust the oxygen flow so that the reservoir bag does not completely collapse on inspiration. In theory, if the nonrebreathing mask fits the patient snugly, and both side exhalation ports have one-way valves, it is possible for the patient to receive 100% oxygen, making the nonrebreathing mask a high-flow oxygen system. However, because it is difficult to get an exact fit from the mask on every patient, and some nonrebreathing masks have only one one-way exhalation valve, it is almost impossible to ensure 100% oxygen delivery, thus making it a low-flow oxygen system.

The *Venturi mask* is the most reliable and accurate method for delivering precise concentrations of oxygen through noninvasive means. The mask is constructed in a way that allows a constant flow of room air blended with a fixed flow of oxygen. It is used primarily for patients with COPD because it can accurately provide appropriate levels of supplemental oxygen, thus avoiding the risk of suppressing the hypoxic drive (refer to Chapter 10 for further details).

Pearls for Practice

The nurse is aware that patients with severe COPD characteristically have a chronically elevated $PaCO_2$, a normal pH, an elevated HCO_3, and a PaO_2 level that usually is less than 60 mm Hg. As a result, the chemoreceptors in the aortic and carotid bodies are desensitized to the ventilatory stimulation from an increased $PaCO_2$ level but instead remain sensitive to PaO_2. Thus, the goal of oxygen therapy is to raise the oxygen level to the patient's chronic baseline level (or a POX of 88% to 92%), not above it.

The Venturi mask uses the Bernoulli principle of air entrainment (trapping the air like a vacuum), which provides a high air flow with controlled oxygen enrichment. For each liter of oxygen that passes through a jet orifice, a fixed proportion of room air is drawn in. A precise volume of oxygen can be delivered by varying the size of the jet orifice and adjusting the flow of oxygen. As the percent of inspired oxygen increases using a Venturi mask, the room air-to-oxygen ratio decreases, causing the maximum concentration of oxygen to be around 40% (Weekley & Bland, 2022). A disadvantage to Venturi masks (as well as other masks) is the inability of the patient to eat, drink, or easily communicate while wearing the device. Excess gas leaves the mask through the two exhalation ports, carrying with it the exhaled carbon dioxide. This method allows a constant oxygen concentration to be inhaled regardless of the depth or rate of respiration.

The mask should fit snugly enough to prevent oxygen from flowing into the patient's eyes. The nurse checks the patient's skin for irritation. It is necessary to remove the mask so that the patient can eat, drink, and take medications, at which time supplemental oxygen is provided through a nasal cannula.

BOX 9-6

Approximate FiO_2 of Nasal Cannula Flow Rates

Each liter (L) of flow is approximately an addition of 4% FiO_2

- 1 L/min = 24% FiO_2
- 2 L/min = 28% FiO_2
- 3 L/min = 32% FiO_2
- 4 L/min = 36% FiO_2
- 5 L/min = 40% FiO_2
- 6 L/min = 44% FiO_2

Data from Tokrczyk et al. (2013).

The nurse must understand how to convert percentage of oxygen with a mask to liters per minute for a nasal cannula (Box 9-6).

HFNCs are a less invasive oxygen delivery system that consists of an air-oxygen blender, humidification source, and heater that can deliver FiO_2 ranges of 21% to 100% oxygen, at flow rates up to 60 L/min, through a large diameter nasal cannula (Nishimura, 2019) (Fig. 9-6). HFNCs have an advantage over face mask systems as patients find them less cumbersome to wear and less confining than tight face masks, and patients are able to eat, drink, and speak without obstruction. HFNCs are used for patients with acute hypoxic respiratory failure (pneumonia, ARDS), postextubation support needs, cardiogenic pulmonary edema, and heart failure (Lodeserto et al., 2018).

The *transtracheal oxygen catheter* is inserted directly into the trachea and is indicated for patients with chronic oxygen therapy needs. These catheters are more comfortable, less dependent on breathing patterns, and less obvious than other oxygen delivery methods. Because no oxygen is lost into the surrounding environment, the patient achieves adequate oxygenation at lower rates, making this method less expensive and more efficient.

Other oxygen devices include *aerosol masks, tracheostomy collars*, and *face tents*, all of which are used with aerosol devices (nebulizers) that can be adjusted for oxygen concentrations from 27% to 100% (0.27 to 1.00). If the gas mixture flow falls below patient demand, room air is pulled in, diluting the concentration. The aerosol mist delivered by the nebulizer must be available for the patient during the entire inspiratory phase. The nurse notifies the respiratory therapist if the nebulizer is not functioning properly.

Hyperbaric oxygen therapy is the administration of oxygen at pressures greater than 1 atmosphere. As a result, the amount of oxygen dissolved in plasma is increased, which increases oxygen levels in the tissues. During therapy, the patient is placed in a small (single patient use) or large (multiple patient use) cylindrical chamber. Hyperbaric oxygen therapy is used to treat conditions such as air embolism, carbon monoxide poisoning, gangrene, tissue necrosis, and hemorrhage. Potential side effects include ear trauma, CNS disorders, and oxygen toxicity.

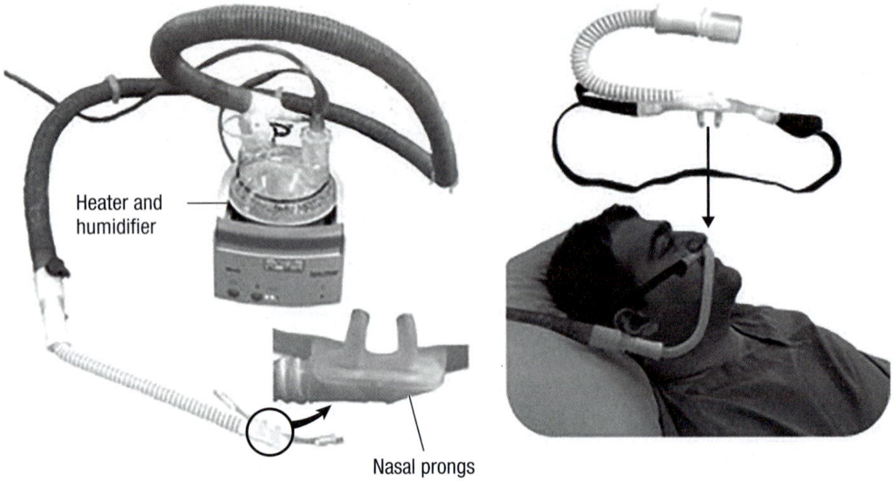

FIGURE 9-6 **High-flow nasal cannula. The high-flow nasal cannula helps with severe breathing problems. (From Marini J. J., & Dries, D. J. [2018]. In *Critical care medicine: The essentials and more* [5th ed., Chapter 7, Fig. 12.]. Lippincott, Williams & Wilkins.)**

Complications

Oxygen, like other medications, should be administered with caution and a careful assessment of patient response. A high concentration of oxygen is contraindicated in the patient with COPD because it may worsen alveolar ventilation by decreasing the patient's ventilatory drive, leading to further respiratory decompensation.

When oxygen is metabolized, it produces free radicals that can cause cellular damage. This side effect of oxygen therapy is called *oxygen toxicity.* Although healthy lungs may be able to tolerate FiO_2 levels of less than 60%, when lungs are damaged FiO_2 over 50% may result in a toxic alveolar O_2 concentration and absorptive atelectasis (Stacy, 2022). Toxic levels of oxygen are reached when FiO_2 levels are greater than 50% for >24 to 48 hours, but it has occurred in as short as 6 hours (Christiani, 2020; Hochberg et al., 2021; Stacy, 2022). Signs and symptoms of oxygen toxicity include chest pain, paresthesias (a burning or prickling sensation), dyspnea, restlessness, fatigue, malaise, progressive respiratory distress, atelectasis, pulmonary infiltrates, and fibrosis. The prevention of oxygen toxicity is achieved by using the lowest level of oxygen needed clinically. If a patient remains hypoxemic on toxic levels of oxygen, additional measures should be instituted, such as intubation and mechanical ventilation.

Oxygen supports combustion; therefore, its use is a fire hazard. No smoking or open flames should be allowed near oxygen use. In addition, the risk of cross-contamination of oxygen supplies (mask, tubing, cannulas) should be addressed and equipment changed per infection control policy.

Supportive Care

Supportive care for pneumonia includes hydration to combat insensible fluid losses from fever and tachypnea. Antipyretics may be used to treat headache, aches, and fever. Warm, moist inhalations are helpful in relieving bronchial irritation.

Additional therapies must be considered for the hospitalized patient with pneumonia. Nutritional assessment and support, deep vein thrombosis prophylaxis, nebulized bronchodilators or mucolytics, and comfort care measures should be individualized for each patient (Box 9-7).

Prevention

Pneumococcal disease is more prevalent in people with alcohol use disorder, chronic diseases (heart, lung, renal and liver), diabetes, and sickle cell anemia, as well a those who are immunocompromised (HIV, steroids, chemotherapy,

BOX 9-7 **Highlighting Gerontology**

Pneumonia in older patients may occur as a primary diagnosis or as a complication of a chronic disease process. Pulmonary infections in older people frequently are difficult to treat and result in a higher mortality rate than in younger people. General deterioration, weakness, abdominal symptoms, incontinence, anorexia, confusion, tachycardia, and tachypnea may signal the onset of pneumonia. The diagnosis of pneumonia may be missed because the classic symptoms of cough, chest pain, and sputum production may be absent or masked in older patients. Fever as a symptom can be missed as well because 30% to 40% of older patients are afebrile. Also, the presence of some signs may be misleading. Abnormal breath sounds, for example, may be caused by atelectasis that occurs as a result of decreased mobility, decreased lung volumes, or other respiratory function changes. It may be necessary to obtain chest x-rays to differentiate chronic heart failure, which is often seen in older individuals, from pneumonia as the cause of clinical signs and symptoms.

Supportive treatment includes hydration (with caution and with frequent assessment because of the risk of fluid overload in older people), supplemental oxygen therapy, and assistance with deep breathing, coughing, frequent position changes, and early ambulation. All of these are particularly important in the care of older patients with pneumonia. To reduce or prevent serious complications of pneumonia in older individuals, vaccination against pneumococcal and influenza infections is recommended.

cancer), smoke, or are asplenic (absence of spleen). Pneumococcal vaccinations (PCV13, PCV15, PCV20, and PPSV23) have been demonstrated to prevent pneumonia in otherwise healthy populations by 90%. The vaccine provides specific prevention against pneumococcal pneumonia and other infections caused by *S. pneumoniae* (otitis media, other upper respiratory tract infections). Vaccines should be avoided during the first trimester of pregnancy (CDC, 2022g, 2022j).

To reduce or prevent serious complications of CAP in high-risk groups, vaccination against pneumococcal infection is advised for people 2 to 64 years of age with chronic illnesses or who are immunocompromised or asplenic, as well as for anyone 65 years or older. People who smoke or those with asthma between the ages of 19 and 64 should get vaccinated. If the vaccine was given prior to age 65, it should be repeated once after 5 years. If a patient is initially vaccinated with PCV15, a follow-up dose of PPSV23 should be administered (CDC, 2022g).

NURSING PROCESS
The Patient With Pneumonia

ASSESSMENT

Nursing assessment is critical in detecting pneumonia. Patients with fever, chills, dyspnea, and cough should alert the nurse to the possibility of pneumonia. Respiratory assessment further identifies the clinical manifestations of pneumonia: pleuritic-type pain, fatigue, tachypnea, use of accessory muscles for breathing, tachycardia, coughing, and purulent sputum. The nurse monitors the patient for the following:

- Changes in temperature and pulse
- Amount, odor, consistency, and color of secretions
- Frequency and severity of cough
- Degree of tachypnea or shortness of breath
- Pulse oximetry
- Changes in physical assessment findings (primarily assessed by inspecting and auscultating the chest)
- Changes in the chest x-ray findings
- Changes in WBCs; a normal WBC or leukocyte count does not exclude infection. Pneumonia may be associated with leukocytosis or leukopenia; lymphopenia (a type of WBC) is associated with COVID-19 (Lee et al., 2021).

In addition, it is important to assess patients, especially older patients, for unusual behavior, altered mental status, dysphagia, dehydration, excessive fatigue, and concomitant heart failure.

DIAGNOSIS

Appropriate nursing diagnoses may include:

- Ineffective airway clearance related to copious tracheobronchial secretions
- Impaired gas exchange
- Activity intolerance related to impaired respiratory function
- Risk for deficient fluid volume related to fever, a rapid respiratory rate, and sepsis
- Malnutrition risk for less than body requirements
- Knowledge deficiency about the treatment regimen and preventive health measures

Collaborative problems or potential complications that may occur include the following:

- Continuing symptoms after initiation of therapy
- Shock
- Respiratory failure
- Atelectasis
- Pleural effusion
- Confusion
- Superinfection

PLANNING

The major goals may include improved airway patency, rest to conserve energy, maintenance of proper fluid volume, maintenance of adequate nutrition, an understanding of the treatment protocol and preventive measures, and absence of complications.

NURSING INTERVENTIONS

IMPROVING AIRWAY PATENCY

Removing secretions is important because retained secretions interfere with gas exchange and may slow recovery. The nurse encourages hydration (2 to 3 L/day) because adequate hydration thins and loosens pulmonary secretions. Hydration must be achieved more slowly and with careful monitoring in patients with pre-existing conditions, such as heart or kidney failure. Humidification may be used to loosen secretions and improve ventilation. A high-humidity face mask (using either compressed air or oxygen) delivers warm, humidified air to the tracheobronchial tree and helps to liquefy secretion. Coughing can be initiated either voluntarily or by reflex. Lung expansion maneuvers, such as deep breathing with an incentive spirometer, may induce a cough. A directed cough may be necessary to improve airway patency. The nurse encourages the patient to perform an effective, directed cough, which includes correct positioning, a deep inspiratory maneuver, glottic closure, contraction of the expiratory muscles against the closed glottis, sudden glottic opening, and an explosive expiration.

Pearls for Practice

In general, the dependent lung is associated with improved perfusion. If the goal is to match ventilation with perfusion, the "good lung down" is a position that will facilitate this. However, any position for a prolonged period of time is associated with stagnation of secretions and pressure on the dependent lung, increasing the risk of atelectasis in the dependent lung. Therefore, the nurse turns the patient at regular intervals. The nurse is aware that

(continued on page 324)

when the affected lung is positioned dependently, the oxygen saturation should be assessed to note the impact of this position on oxygen level. In addition, the nurse is aware that in the case of unilateral (one lung) pulmonary hemorrhage or pulmonary abscess, "good lung down" is contraindicated to prevent blood or infected material from draining into the good lung.

CPT is important in loosening and mobilizing secretions. Indications for CPT include sputum retention not responsive to spontaneous or directed cough, a history of pulmonary problems previously treated with CPT, continued evidence of retained secretions (decreased or abnormal breath sounds, change in vital signs), abnormal chest x-ray findings consistent with atelectasis or infiltrates, and deterioration in oxygenation.

The nurse may consult the respiratory therapy department for volume-expansion protocols and secretion-management protocols that help direct the respiratory care of the patient and match the patient's needs with appropriate treatment schedules.

After each position change, the nurse encourages the patient to breathe deeply and cough. If the patient is too weak to cough effectively, the nurse may need to remove the mucus by nasotracheal suctioning. It may take time for secretions to mobilize and move into the central airways for expectoration. Therefore, it is important for the nurse to monitor the patient for cough and sputum production after the completion of CPT.

The nurse also administers and titrates oxygen therapy as prescribed or via protocols. The effectiveness of oxygen therapy is monitored by improvement in clinical signs and symptoms, patient comfort, and adequate oxygenation values as measured by POX or ABG analysis.

PROMOTING REST AND CONSERVING ENERGY

The nurse encourages the debilitated patient to rest and avoid overexertion and possible exacerbation of symptoms. The patient should assume a comfortable position to promote rest and breathing (e.g., semi-Fowler position) and should change positions frequently to enhance secretion clearance as well as ventilation and perfusion in the lungs. It is important to instruct outpatients not to overexert themselves and to engage in only moderate activity during the initial phases of treatment.

PROMOTING FLUID INTAKE

The respiratory rate of patients with pneumonia increases because of the increased workload imposed by labored breathing and fever. An increased respiratory rate leads to an increase in insensible fluid loss during exhalation and can lead to dehydration. Therefore, it is important to encourage increased fluid intake (at least 2 L/day), unless contraindicated.

MAINTAINING NUTRITION

Many patients with shortness of breath and fatigue have a decreased appetite and consume only fluids. Fluids with electrolytes and protein-supplementation drinks can be prescribed to patients. In addition, IV fluids and nutrients may be administered if necessary.

PROMOTING PATIENT KNOWLEDGE

The patient and family are instructed about the cause of pneumonia, management of symptoms of pneumonia, signs and symptoms that should be reported to the health care provider or nurse, and the need for follow-up. The patient also needs information about factors (both patient risk factors and external factors) that may have contributed to development of pneumonia and strategies to promote recovery and prevent recurrence. If the patient is hospitalized, they are instructed about the purpose and importance of management strategies that have been implemented and about the importance of adhering to them during and after the hospital stay. Explanations should be given in simple and clear language that the patient can understand. If possible, written instructions and information should be provided, with alternative formats available for patients with hearing or vision loss, if necessary. Because of the severity of symptoms, the patient may require that instructions and explanations be repeated several times.

MONITORING AND MANAGING POTENTIAL COMPLICATIONS

Continuing Symptoms after Initiation of Therapy. The patient is observed for response to antibiotic therapy; patients usually begin to respond to treatment within 24 to 48 hours after antibiotic therapy is initiated. If the patient started taking antibiotics before evaluation by culture and sensitivity of the causative organisms, antibiotics may need to be changed once the results are available. The patient is monitored for changes in physical status (deterioration of condition or resolution of symptoms) and for persistent or recurrent fever, which may be a result of medication allergy (signaled possibly by a rash); medication resistance or slow response (greater than 48 hours) of the susceptible organism to therapy; superinfection; pleural effusion; or pneumonia caused by an unusual organism, such as *P. jirovecii* or *Aspergillus fumigatus*, or multidrug resistant organisms (MRSA, VRE, ESBL *E. coli*). Failure of the pneumonia to resolve or persistence of symptoms despite improvement on the chest x-ray raises the suspicion of other underlying disorders, such as lung cancer or lung abscess. As previously described, lung cancers may invade or compress airways, causing an obstructive atelectasis that may lead to pneumonia.

In addition to monitoring for continuing symptoms of pneumonia, the nurse also monitors for other complications, such as shock and multisystem failure and atelectasis, which may develop during the first few days of antibiotic treatment.

Shock and Respiratory Failure. Severe complications of pneumonia include sepsis and septic shock as well as respiratory failure. These complications are encountered primarily in patients who have received nonspecific, inadequate, or delayed treatment in combination with particularly virulent pathogens. These complications are also encountered when the infecting organism is resistant to therapy, when a comorbid disease complicates the pneumonia, or when the patient is immunocompromised.

Severe sepsis is defined as a systemic inflammatory response related to an infection such as pneumonia, with dysfunction or failure of one or more organs (e.g., acute kidney injury [AKI], ARDS, or disseminated intravascular coagulation). *Septic shock* occurs when severe sepsis is accompanied by hypotension that is refractory to the infusion of IV fluids. Severe sepsis and septic shock can lead to multiorgan dysfunction and carry a high mortality rate.

If the patient is seriously ill, aggressive therapy may include hemodynamic and ventilator support to combat peripheral vascular collapse, maintain arterial blood pressure, and provide adequate oxygenation. A vasopressor agent may be administered by continuous IV infusion and at a rate adjusted in accordance with the blood pressure response. Corticosteroids may be administered parenterally to combat shock and toxicity in patients who are extremely ill with pneumonia and at apparent risk for death from the infection, or who have adrenal insufficiency. However, whether corticosteroids are beneficial in patients with pneumonia remains uncertain (Evans et al., 2021). Patients may require endotracheal intubation and mechanical ventilation. Heart failure, cardiac arrhythmias, pericarditis, and myocarditis also are complications of pneumonia that may lead to shock.

The nurse assesses for signs and symptoms of shock and respiratory failure by evaluating the patient's vital signs, POX values, and hemodynamic monitoring parameters. The nurse reports signs of deteriorating patient status and assists in administering IV fluids and medications prescribed to combat shock. Intubation and mechanical ventilation may be required if respiratory failure occurs.

Atelectasis and Pleural Effusion. Atelectasis (from obstruction of a bronchus or small airways by accumulated secretions) may occur at any stage of acute pneumonia. Parapneumonic **pleural effusions** occur in at least 40% of bacterial pneumonias. A parapneumonic effusion is any pleural effusion associated with bacterial pneumonia, lung abscess, or bronchiectasis. After the pleural effusion is detected on a chest x-ray or CT scan, a thoracentesis may be performed to remove the fluid. The fluid is sent to the laboratory for analysis. There are three stages of parapneumonic pleural effusions based on pathogenesis: uncomplicated, complicated, and empyema. An **empyema** occurs when thick, purulent fluid accumulates within the **pleural space**, often with fibrin development and a loculated (walled-off) area where the infection is located (see later discussion). A chest tube may be inserted to treat pleural infection by establishing proper drainage of the empyema. Sterilization of the empyema cavity usually requires 4 to 6 weeks of antibiotics, but sometimes surgical management is required.

The patient is assessed for atelectasis, and preventive measures are initiated to prevent its development. If pleural effusion develops and thoracentesis is performed to remove fluid, the nurse assists in the procedure and explains it to the patient. After thoracentesis, the nurse monitors the patient for pneumothorax or recurrence of pleural effusion. If a chest tube needs to be inserted, the nurse monitors the patient's respiratory status and assesses functioning of the chest drainage system (see later discussion).

Superinfection. Superinfections may occur with the administration of any antibiotic but are more common with the use of high-dose, broad-spectrum, and multiple antibiotics. Superinfections are the overgrowth of endogenous flora. Common superinfections are oral yeast (thrush), vaginal candidiasis, and *Clostridium difficile* colitis (pseudomembranous colitis). The patient is monitored for manifestations of superinfection (i.e., white coating of tongue or oral mucosa, vaginal discharge, and diarrhea). These signs are reported, and the nurse assists in implementing therapy to treat superinfection.

Confusion. A patient with pneumonia is assessed for confusion (metabolic encephalopathy) and other more subtle changes in cognitive status. Confusion and changes in cognitive status resulting from pneumonia are poor prognostic signs. Confusion may be related to hypoxemia, fever, dehydration, sleep deprivation, or developing sepsis. Also the patient's underlying comorbid conditions may play a part in the development of confusion. Addressing the underlying factors and ensuring patient safety are important nursing interventions.

PROMOTING HEALTH

The nurse encourages the patient to stop smoking. Smoking inhibits tracheobronchial ciliary action, which is the first line of defense of the lower respiratory tract. Smoking also irritates the mucous cells of the bronchi and inhibits the function of alveolar macrophage (scavenger) cells. The patient is instructed to avoid stress, fatigue, sudden changes in temperature, and excessive alcohol intake, all of which lower resistance to pneumonia. The nurse reviews with the patient the principles of adequate nutrition and rest because one episode of pneumonia may make a patient susceptible to recurring respiratory tract infections.

EVALUATION

Expected patient outcomes may include the following:

1. Demonstrates improved airway patency, as evidenced by adequate oxygenation by POX or ABG analysis, normal temperature, normal breath sounds, and effective coughing
2. Rests and conserves energy by limiting activities and remaining in bed while symptomatic and then slowly increasing activities
3. Maintains adequate hydration, as evidenced by an adequate fluid intake and urine output as well as normal skin turgor
4. Consumes adequate dietary intake, as evidenced by maintenance or increase in body weight without excess fluid gain
5. States explanation for management strategies
6. Complies with management strategies
7. Exhibits no complications:
   - Exhibits acceptable vital signs, POX, and ABG measurements
   - Reports productive cough that diminishes over time

(continued on page 326)

- Has absence of signs or symptoms of shock, respiratory failure, or pleural effusion
- Remains oriented and aware of surroundings
- Maintains or increases weight
- Complies with treatment protocol and prevention strategies

PULMONARY TUBERCULOSIS

Tuberculosis (TB) is an infectious disease that primarily affects the lung parenchyma. The primary infectious agent, *M. tuberculosis*, is an acid-fast aerobic bacilli that grows slowly and is sensitive to heat and ultraviolet light. It is a resistant bacterium that can persist in calcified and necrotic lesions and remain able to reinitiate growth.

TB is a worldwide public health problem, and mortality and morbidity rates continue to rise. *M. tuberculosis* infects an estimated one third of the world's population and is the second leading cause of death from infectious disease in the world (COVID-19 being the first) (WHO [World Health Organization], 2022), although cases in the United States have declined slightly. TB is closely associated with poverty, malnutrition, overcrowding, substandard housing, and inadequate health care (CDC, 2020b, 2022, 2022b; Nahid et al., 2019).

Pathophysiology

TB spreads from person to person by airborne transmission. An infected person releases droplet nuclei (usually particles 1 to 5 μm in diameter) through talking, coughing, sneezing, laughing, or singing. Larger droplets settle; smaller droplets remain suspended in the air and are inhaled. Several factors determine the transmission of *M. tuberculosis* and include characteristics of the source case, exposed person, and exposure, and the virulence of the *M. tuberculosis* strain. Box 9-8 depicts risk factors for TB.

TB begins when a susceptible person inhales mycobacteria and the bacteria are transmitted through the airways to the alveoli, where macrophages ingest the bacilli. If the bacilli escape the antimicrobial activities of the macrophages, an infection begins. This stage, called *primary TB*, usually is clinically silent and is due to the chronic inflammatory response that the bacterium provokes. The bacilli may be transported via the lymph system and bloodstream to other parts of the body (kidneys, bones, cerebral cortex) and other areas of the lungs (upper lobes). The spreading of TB via lymphatics and blood is called *miliary TB*. The body's immune system responds by initiating an inflammatory reaction. Phagocytes (neutrophils and macrophages) engulf many of the bacteria, and TB-specific lymphocytes destroy the bacilli along with normal tissue. This tissue reaction results in the accumulation of exudate in the alveoli, causing bronchopneumonia. The initial infection usually occurs 2 to 10 weeks after exposure.

Granulomas, new tissue masses of live and dead bacilli, are surrounded by macrophages, which form a protective wall. Then they are transformed to a fibrous tissue mass, the central portion of which is called a Ghon tubercle. The material (bacteria and macrophages) becomes necrotic, forming a cheesy mass. This mass may become calcified and form a collagenous scar. At this point, the bacteria become dormant, and there is no further progression of active disease. Most individuals who acquire TB will eliminate or contain the infection, which is termed *latent TB infection*, where a skin test or blood test is usually positive, but there is no evidence of clinical disease. Thus, the patient has the infection but not the disease; the disease cannot be spread because although the bacteria are alive in their body it is inactive. Approximately 10% (range 5% to 15%) of those with latent infection can progress to active disease within years to

BOX 9-8

Risk Factors for Tuberculosis (TB)

- Being born in foreign countries with high prevalence of TB
- Being medically underserved and/or with low income Populations include:
  - Unhoused
  - Medically underserved populations
- Underrepresented groups particularly children under age of 15 years and people between 15 and 44 years (e.g., rate in Native American individuals was nine times higher than in White individuals; U.S.-born Black people was seven times higher than in non-Hispanic U.S.-born White individuals (Fitzgerald et al., 2020)
- Individuals emigrated from developing countries
- Those living in overcrowded, substandard housing
- Being a resident or employee of correction centers, homeless shelters, long-term care facilities
- Being a health care worker caring for high-risk patients
- Being a health care worker performing high-risk activities:
  - Administration of aerosolized medications
  - Sputum-induction procedures, including suctioning and coughing procedures
  - Bronchoscopy
  - Intubations
- Unprotected exposure to TB patients
- Advanced age
- Traveling abroad to work in endemic areas (Southeastern Asia, Africa, Latin America, Caribbean)
- Infants and children exposed to high-risk patients
- Substance use disorder (IV/injection drug use and alcoholism)
- Immunocompromise:
  - Human immunodeficiency virus (HIV) infections
  - Malignancies: Head, neck, lung, hematologic
  - Long-term corticosteroid use
  - Immunosuppressive drug therapies
  - Organ transplantation
- Comorbidities:
  - Malnutrition
  - Diabetes
  - Silicosis
  - Chronic kidney disease
  - Gastric or intestinal bypass surgery

decades following initial infection (Bouton & Fort, 2023; Jilani et al., 2022).

After initial exposure and infection, *active disease* may develop by primary infection (discussed earlier) or as a reactivation of latent TB because of a compromised or inadequate immune system response. The term reactivation TB is used to describe when TB develops from a breakdown of the host defenses (months to years after primary infection). It most commonly occurs in the lungs, preferentially involving the apical (upper) or posterior segments of the upper lobes or the superior segments of the lower lobes. In this case, the Ghon tubercle ulcerates, releasing the cheesy material into the bronchi. Then the bacteria become airborne, resulting in further spread of the disease. The ulcerated tubercle heals and forms scar tissue. This causes the infected lung to become more inflamed, resulting in further development of bronchopneumonia and tubercle formation. Unless the process is arrested, it spreads slowly downward to the hilum of the lungs and later extends to adjacent lobes. The process may be prolonged and is characterized by long remissions when the disease is arrested, followed by periods of renewed activity.

Clinical Manifestations and Assessment

The signs and symptoms of pulmonary TB are insidious. Most patients have a low-grade fever, cough, night sweats, fatigue, and weight loss. Initially the cough is nonproductive but progresses to be mucopurulent. Dyspnea, chest pain, and **hemoptysis** (bloody sputum) occur as the disease progresses. Both the systemic and the pulmonary symptoms are chronic and may have been present for weeks to months. Older patients usually present with less pronounced symptoms than younger patients (Box 9-9). Extrapulmonary disease occurs in up to 16% of cases in the United States. In immunocompromised patients (e.g., AIDS), extrapulmonary disease is more prevalent and is manifested by neurologic deficits, bone pain, meningitis symptoms (stiff neck, headache, fever, confusion, and seizures), and urinary tract symptoms (dysuria).

A complete history, physical examination, tuberculin skin test or blood test such as QuantiFERON-TB Gold, chest x-ray, acid-fast bacilli (AFB) smear, and sputum culture are used to diagnose TB (Bouton & Fort, 2023; Lewinsohn et al., 2017). If the patient is infected with TB, the chest x-ray usually reveals lesions in the upper lobes, and the AFB smear contains mycobacteria.

BOX 9-9 **Highlighting Gerontology**

TB may have atypical manifestations in older patients, whose symptoms may include unusual behavior and altered mental status, fever, anorexia, and weight loss. In many older patients, the tuberculin skin test produces no reaction (loss of immunologic memory) or delayed reactivity for up to 1 week (recall phenomenon). A second skin test is performed in 1 to 2 weeks.

Tuberculin Skin Test

The Mantoux test is used to determine whether a person has been infected with the TB bacillus. The Mantoux test is a standardized procedure and should be performed only by those trained in its administration and reading (Fig. 9-7). Tubercle bacillus extract (tuberculin), purified protein derivative (PPD), is injected into the intradermal layer of the inner aspect of the forearm, approximately 4 in below the elbow. Intermediate-strength PPD, in a tuberculin syringe with a 0.5-in 26- or 27-gauge needle, is used. The needle, with the bevel facing up, is inserted beneath the skin. Then, 0.1 mL of PPD is injected, creating an elevation in the skin, a *wheal* or *bleb.* The site, antigen name, strength, lot number, date, and time of the test are recorded. The test result is read 48 to 72 hours after injection. Tests read after 72 hours tend to underestimate the true size of **induration** (hardening).

A reaction occurs when an induration at the injection site is present. After the area is inspected for induration, it is lightly palpated across the injection site, from the area of normal skin to the margins of the induration. The diameter of the induration (not erythema) is measured in millimeters at its widest part, and the size of the induration is documented. Erythema without induration is not considered significant. The size of the induration determines the significance of the reaction. A reaction of 0 to 4 mm is considered not significant; a reaction of 5 mm or greater may be significant in people who are considered to be at risk (discussed shortly). An induration of 10 mm or greater is usually considered

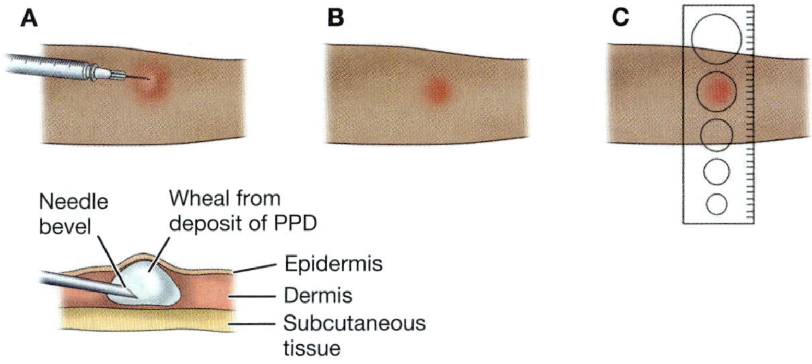

FIGURE 9-7 The Mantoux test for tuberculosis. A. Correct technique for inserting the needle involves depositing the purified protein derivative (PPD) intradermally with the needle bevel facing upward. B. The reaction to the Mantoux test usually consists of a *wheal,* a hive-like, firm welt. C. To determine the extent of the reaction, the wheal is measured using a commercially prepared gauge. Interpretation of the Mantoux test is discussed on this page.

significant in people who have normal or mildly impaired immunity. A significant reaction indicates past exposure to *M. tuberculosis* or vaccination with Bacille Calmette–Guérin (BCG) vaccine. The BCG vaccine is used in Europe and Latin America but not routinely in the United States.

Pearls for Practice

Ambiguity exists in interpretation of the tuberculin skin test (TST) when patients were vaccinated with BCG because of its low specificity and poor ability to identify those likely to develop active disease (Muñoz et al., 2017). Recall that specificity of a laboratory test reveals how often the test is negative in patients who do not have the disease, e.g., 100% specificity correctly identifies a person who does not have the disease. QuantiFERON-TB Gold and the T-spot (referred to as Interferon Gamma Release Assays [IGRA]) test may be considered for screening in a patient with prior BCG immunization because of the lack of cross-reactivity with antigens (since TB skin testing results may be falsely positive, especially if done within 10 years of vaccination) (Clinical Overview, 2022; de Lima Corvino et al., 2021).

A reaction of 5 mm or greater is defined as positive in patients who are HIV positive or have HIV risk factors and are of unknown HIV status, in those who are close contacts of someone with active TB, in those who are undergoing immunosuppressive therapy, and in those who have chest x-ray results consistent with TB. Patients with HIV are at risk for developing cutaneous anergy (absence of normal immune response) from impaired cellular immunity and may have a false-negative reaction to PPD skin testing. These patients may undergo Mantoux-method skin testing with mumps and candida antigens to assess for anergy. A positive test result is an induration of 5 mm or greater, meaning the patient has relatively intact cell-mediated immunity and can mount a reaction to PPD testing (Chapter 35 details anergy further).

A significant (positive) reaction does not necessarily mean that active disease is present in the body. More than 90% of people who are tuberculin-significant reactors do not develop clinical TB. However, all significant reactors are candidates for active TB. In addition, a nonsignificant (negative) skin test does not exclude TB infection or disease because patients who are immunosuppressed cannot develop an immune response that is adequate to produce a positive skin test.

TB Blood Testing

There are two FDA-approved blood tests for the detection of TB by interferon-gamma release assay, the QuantiFERON-TB Gold and the T-spot. A positive test indicates that the person has been infected with TB and further testing is needed to determine latency versus active disease. These blood tests are recommended over the Mantoux test when a person has received the BCG vaccine or when it is impractical to return for a second visit to read a TST (CDC, 2022h; de Lima Corvino et al., 2021; Lewinsohn & Daley, 2019).

Classification

Data from the history, physical examination, TB test, chest x-ray, and microbiologic studies are used to classify TB into one of five classes. A classification scheme provides public health officials with a systematic way to monitor epidemiology and treatment of the disease (American Thoracic Society & Centers for Disease Control and Prevention [ATS & CDC], 2000; WHO, 2021):

- Class 0: No exposure; not infected
- Class 1: Exposure; no evidence of infection
- Class 2: Latent infection; no disease (e.g., positive PPD reaction but no clinical evidence of active TB)
- Class 3: Disease; clinically active
- Class 4: Previous disease; not clinically active
- Class 5: Suspected disease; diagnosis pending

Medical and Nursing Management

Pharmacologic Therapy

Pulmonary TB is treated primarily with anti-TB agents, as either active disease treatment or prophylactic treatment for people exposed and at risk for developing the disease. A prolonged treatment duration is necessary to ensure eradication of the organisms and to prevent relapse. The continuing (since the 1950s) and increasing resistance of *M. tuberculosis* to TB medications is a worldwide concern and challenge in TB therapy. Several types of drug resistance must be considered when planning effective therapy:

- *Primary drug resistance:* Resistance to one of the first-line anti-TB agents in people who have not had previous treatment
- *Secondary or acquired drug resistance:* Resistance to one or more anti-TB agents in patients undergoing therapy
- *MDR:* Resistance to two agents, isoniazid (INH) and rifampin. The populations at greatest risk for MDR are those who are living with HIV, living in an institutional setting, or unhoused.

The increasing prevalence of drug resistance points out the need to begin TB treatment with three or more medications to ensure completion of therapy and to develop and evaluate new anti-TB medications.

Treatment Regimens

Monotherapy is never used for the active disease to reduce the risk of the mycobacterium developing antibiotic resistance (Jilani et al., 2022). In current TB therapy, four first-line medications are used: INH, rifampin, pyrazinamide, and ethambutol. Combination medications, such as INH and rifampin

(Rifamate) or INH, pyrazinamide, and rifampin (Rifater), and other medications administered twice a week (e.g., rifapentine) are available to help improve patient adherence. Capreomycin, ethionamide, para-aminosalicylate sodium, and cycloserine are second-line medications. Additional potentially effective medications include other aminoglycosides, quinolones, rifabutin, clofazimine, and combinations of medications (Lewinshon et al., 2017; National Institute of Diabetes and Digestive and Kidney Diseases [NIDDKD], 2021).

Recommended treatment guidelines for newly diagnosed cases of presumably drug-susceptible active pulmonary TB have two parts: an initial treatment phase and a continuation phase. The initial phase consists of multiple medications (INH, rifampin, pyrazinamide, and ethambutol) and multiple dosing regimen choices of these four medications. This initial intensive treatment regimen is administered for 8 weeks and has 4 dosing options that range from daily to 2 or 5 times per week. Then the regimen may be decreased to INH and rifampin, depending, for example, on the HIV treatment status, extent of disease, regimen used, and treatment response (Bouton & Fort, 2023). The continuation phase of treatment varies and can last for an additional 18 or 31 weeks. The 18-week period is used for the majority of patients. The 31-week period is recommended for patients with cavitary pulmonary TB whose sputum culture after the initial 2 months of treatment is positive; those whose initial phase of treatment did not include pyrazinamide (PZA); and those being treated once weekly with INH and rifapentine whose sputum culture is positive at the end of the initial phase of treatment. In general, people are considered noninfectious after 2 to 3 weeks of continuous medication therapy. Usually vitamin B6 (pyridoxine) is administered with INH to prevent INH-associated peripheral neuropathy. The total number of doses taken, not simply the duration of treatment, more accurately determines whether a course of therapy has been completed (Nahid et al., 2016).

Several types of drug-resistant TB have emerged over the last two decades. Multidrug resistant and extensively drug resistant TB are identified by sputum culture and sensitivity, but it may take weeks for results to be available. Nucleic acid amplification testing (NAAT) for the TB complex is performed on respiratory specimens (it is also used to diagnose COVID-19 with test results within 48 hours compared with more than 7 to 10 days for AFB culture). Treatment for resistant TB requires an infectious disease expert referral to prevent treatment failure and additional drug resistance (Clinical Overview, 2022). The nurse anticipates that additional antimicrobial agents (up to six) may be prescribed for a longer duration (Nahid et al., 2019).

INH also may be used as a prophylactic (preventive) measure for people who are at risk for significant disease, including:

- Household family members of patients with active disease
- Patients with HIV infection who have a PPD test reaction with 5 mm of induration or greater
- Patients with fibrotic lesions suggestive of old TB detected on a chest x-ray and a PPD reaction with 5 mm of induration or greater
- Patients whose current PPD test results show a change from former test results, suggesting recent exposure to TB and possible infection (skin test converters)
- Users of IV/injection drugs who have PPD test results with 10 mm of induration or greater
- Patients with high-risk comorbid conditions and a PPD result with 10 mm of induration or greater

Other candidates for preventive INH therapy are those 35 years or younger who have PPD test results with 10 mm of induration or more and one of the following criteria:

- Foreign-born individuals from countries with a high prevalence of TB
- High-risk, medically underserved populations
- Patients living in an institutional setting

Prophylactic INH treatment involves taking daily doses for 6 to 12 months. Liver enzymes, blood urea nitrogen (BUN), and creatinine levels are monitored monthly to detect changes in liver and kidney function. Sputum culture results are monitored for AFB to evaluate the effectiveness of treatment and the patient's adherence to the treatment regimen.

Side Effects of Medication Therapy

It is important to assess medication side effects, because often they are a reason why patients fail to adhere to the prescribed medication regimen. Efforts are made to reduce the side effects and to motivate the patient to take the medications as prescribed.

The nurse instructs the patient to take the medication either on an empty stomach or at least 1 hour before meals because food interferes with medication absorption (although taking medications on an empty stomach frequently results in gastrointestinal upset). Patients taking INH should avoid foods that contain tyramine and histamine (tuna, aged cheese, red wine, soy sauce, yeast extracts) because eating them while taking INH may result in headache, flushing, hypotension, lightheadedness, palpitations, and diaphoresis.

In addition, rifampin can increase the metabolism of certain other medications, making them less effective. These medications include beta-blockers, oral anticoagulants such as warfarin, digoxin, quinidine, corticosteroids, oral hypoglycemic agents, oral contraceptives, theophylline, and verapamil. This issue should be discussed with the prescriber and pharmacist so that medication dosages can be adjusted accordingly. The nurse informs the patient that rifampin may discolor contact lenses and that the patient may want to wear eyeglasses during treatment. The nurse monitors for other side effects of anti-TB medications, including hepatitis, neurologic changes (hearing loss, neuritis, visual changes, neuropathy), and rash. Renal and hepatic function tests as well as sputum AFB results are monitored closely. The nurse carefully monitors vital signs and observes for spikes in temperature or changes in the patient's clinical status. Changes in the patient's respiratory status are reported to the primary health care provider. The nurse instructs the patient about the risk of drug resistance if the medication regimen is not followed strictly and continuously.

The strict adherence to complex medication regimens is an important area of education of the TB patient. Drugs must be taken exactly as prescribed, and noncompliance can lead to continued infection and drug resistance. Directly observed therapy (DOT) can be implemented to ensure that patients are compliant with medications regimens. In DOT, a trained health care provider administers each dose of anti-TB medication. DOT can be prescribed by a health care provider such as a physician, nurse practitioner, or a local board of health.

Patient Teaching

The care of patients with TB involves education related to halting the spread of the infection and its complex drug regimens. Patients should be instructed to cover their mouth and nose when they cough or sneeze, dispose of facial tissues in plastic bags, and wear a mask when in public until sputum samples are documented as free of AFB. Patients in hospital settings will be placed on airborne precautions, including staying in a negative-pressure room that vents air to the outside, and staff must wear fitted filtration masks (N95 or high-efficiency particulate air respirators) when in the room. It is recommended that the patient be maintained on airborne precautions until three consecutive negative AFB sputum specimens (obtained at least 8 hours apart with one obtained as an early-morning specimen) have been demonstrated (CDC, n.d.). Health care providers who have the potential to be in contact with TB patients must be fit tested at least yearly and when their weight changes or if they have respiratory disorders such as asthma. Also patients must wear surgical masks when outside of the negative-pressure rooms.

Malnutrition may be a consequence of the patient's lifestyle, lack of knowledge about adequate nutrition and its role in health maintenance, lack of resources, fatigue, or lack of appetite because of coughing and mucus production and medication side effects. To counter the effects of these factors, the nurse collaborates with the dietitian, provider, social worker, family, and patient to identify strategies to ensure an adequate nutritional intake and the availability of nutritious food. Identifying facilities (e.g., shelters, soup kitchens, Meals on Wheels) that provide meals in the patient's neighborhood may increase the likelihood that the patient with limited resources and energy will have access to a more nutritious intake. High-calorie nutritional supplements may be suggested as a strategy for increasing dietary intake using food products normally found in the home. Purchasing food supplements may be beyond the patient's budget, but dietitians can help develop recipes to increase caloric intake despite minimal resources.

PULMONARY EDEMA

Pulmonary edema is defined as abnormal accumulation of fluid within the lung tissue, the alveolar space, or both. Acute pulmonary edema, often called "flash" pulmonary edema, is a severe, life-threatening condition. Classification of pulmonary edema is based on its causative origin: cardiogenic or noncardiogenic. Noncardiogenic pulmonary edema includes ARDS, neurogenic, reexpansion, and negative-pressure pulmonary edema. ARDS will be discussed later in this chapter, and cardiogenic pulmonary edema is discussed in Chapter 14.

Pathophysiology

In each type of pulmonary edema, capillary fluid leaks or is forced by high capillary hydrostatic pressure into alveolar spaces. The edematous alveoli are unable to participate in gas exchange, causing intrapulmonary shunting of blood and hypoxemia. The pathophysiology of cardiogenic pulmonary edema is discussed in Chapter 14. The most common form of noncardiogenic pulmonary is ARDS, a form of acute lung injury (ALI) in which a precipitating injury (direct or indirect) to the lung triggers a systemic inflammatory response that causes pulmonary capillaries to leak fluid into the alveoli. Neurogenic pulmonary edema can occur after epileptic seizures or injuries to the head, brain, or spine. It is theorized to occur as the result of the massive surge of central sympathetic output, which increases blood flow to pulmonary vasculature. The vasoconstriction causes elevations in hydrostatic pressure, which results in extravasation of fluid into the pulmonary interstitium. Reexpansion pulmonary edema may result from a rapid reinflation of the lung after removal of air from a pneumothorax or evacuation of fluid from a large pleural effusion or hemothorax. This rapid negative-pressure change within the lungs causes capillary fluid to be pulled into the alveolar spaces. This is similar to negative-pressure pulmonary edema, in which an obstruction in the trachea or large bronchi causes a person to attempt to forcefully inhale against a closed glottis or airway. This pulls fluid into the alveolar spaces. Common causes of this type of edema are choking, angioedema, and manual strangulation.

Clinical Manifestations and Assessment

Increasing respiratory distress, characterized by dyspnea, air hunger, and hypoxemia is present. Usually patients are very anxious and often agitated. As the fluid leaks into the alveoli and mixes with air, a foam or froth is formed (more common in cardiogenic edema). The patient coughs up (or the nurse suctions out) these foamy, frothy, and often blood-tinged or pink secretions. The patient experiences acute respiratory distress and may become confused or stuporous.

Auscultation reveals crackles in the lung bases (especially in the dependent lung areas) that rapidly progress toward the apices of the lungs. These crackles are caused by the movement of air through the alveolar fluid. Also patients may present with wheezing. The chest x-ray reveals increased bilateral interstitial markings, often in a patchy appearance, with or without cardiomegaly. The patient may have tachycardia. Pulse oximetry values begin to fall, and ABG analysis demonstrates worsening hypoxemia.

Medical Management

Management focuses on correcting the underlying disorder. If the pulmonary edema is cardiac in origin, then improvement in left ventricular function is the goal (see Chapter 14). Oxygen is administered to correct the hypoxemia; in some circumstances, intubation and mechanical ventilation are necessary. Noncardiogenic pulmonary edema treatment is aimed at treating the underlying cause of the ALI (i.e., infection, massive blood transfusions, pancreatitis), removing obstructions causing negative-pressure edema, and providing supportive care such as oxygen, mechanical ventilation, and judicious IV fluids.

Nursing Management

Nursing management includes assisting with administration of oxygen and intubation and mechanical ventilation if respiratory failure occurs. The nurse also administers medications (e.g., morphine, vasodilators, inotropic medications, diuretics, and pre- and afterload agents) as prescribed, and monitors the patient's responses.

PLEURAL CONDITIONS

Pleural conditions are disorders that involve the membranes covering the lungs (visceral pleura) and the surface of the chest wall (parietal pleura) or disorders affecting the pleural space. The most common pleural conditions are pleurisy, pleural effusions, and empyemas.

PLEURISY

Pathophysiology

Pleurisy (pleuritis) refers to inflammation of both layers of the pleurae (parietal and visceral). Pleurisy may develop in conjunction with pneumonia or an upper respiratory tract infection, TB, or collagen diseases; after trauma to the chest, pulmonary infarction, or PE; in patients with primary or metastatic cancer; and after **thoracotomy**. The parietal pleura has nerve endings; the visceral pleura does not. When the inflamed pleural membranes rub together during respiration (intensified on inspiration), the result is severe, sharp, knifelike pain.

Clinical Manifestations and Assessment

The key characteristic of pleuritic pain is its relationship to respiratory movement: Taking a deep breath, coughing, or sneezing worsens the pain as does movement of the chest or trunk. Pleuritic pain is limited in distribution rather than diffuse; it usually occurs only on one side. The pain is typically described as sharp or stabbing, but also may be dull, burning pain, or a "catch" while breathing (Leard, 2023). The pain may become minimal or absent when the breath is held, leading to rapid shallow breathing. It may be localized or may refer to the same side shoulder or neck. Patients often prefer the body position that minimizes the motion of the affected region, often lying on the affected side, which limits its expansion of the chest wall (Leard, 2023; Polgar-Bailey, 2021). Later, as pleural fluid accumulates, the pain decreases. A pleural friction rub may be heard on auscultation.

Medical and Nursing Management

The objectives of treatment are to discover the underlying condition causing the pleurisy and to relieve the pain. As the underlying disease (e.g., pneumonia, infection, pneumothorax, PE, chest trauma, malignancy, TB) is treated, the pleuritic inflammation usually resolves. At the same time, it is necessary to monitor for signs and symptoms of pleural effusion, such as shortness of breath, pain (typically sharp and worsens with inspiration), assumption of a position that decreases pain, decreased chest wall excursion, dullness to percussion in the area of the effusion, along with diminished breath sounds and absent tactile fremitus.

Prescribed analgesics and topical applications of heat or cold or lidocaine patches provide symptomatic relief. Nonsteroidal anti-inflammatory drugs (NSAIDs) may provide pain relief while allowing the patient to take deep breaths and cough more effectively. If the pain is severe, a narcotic or an intercostal or erector spinae nerve block (provides anesthesia to the anterior, posterior and lateral thoracic wall) may be required.

PLEURAL EFFUSION AND EMPYEMA

Pleural effusion, a collection of fluid in the pleural space, is rarely a primary disease process but usually occurs secondary to other diseases (Fig. 9-8). Normally, the pleural space contains a small amount of fluid (20 to 25 cc), which acts as a lubricant that allows the pleural surfaces to move without friction. Pleural effusion may be a complication of heart failure, TB, pneumonia, pulmonary infections (particularly viral infections), nephrotic syndrome, connective tissue disease, pulmonary embolus, and neoplastic tumors. In addition, abdominal processes such as pancreatitis or cirrhosis with ascites can cause pleural effusions. The most common malignancies associated with a pleural effusion are bronchogenic carcinoma and breast cancer. An empyema is an accumulation of thick, purulent fluid (pus) within the pleural space and is a type of pleural effusion.

Pathophysiology

In certain disorders, fluid may accumulate in the pleural space to a point at which it becomes clinically evident. This

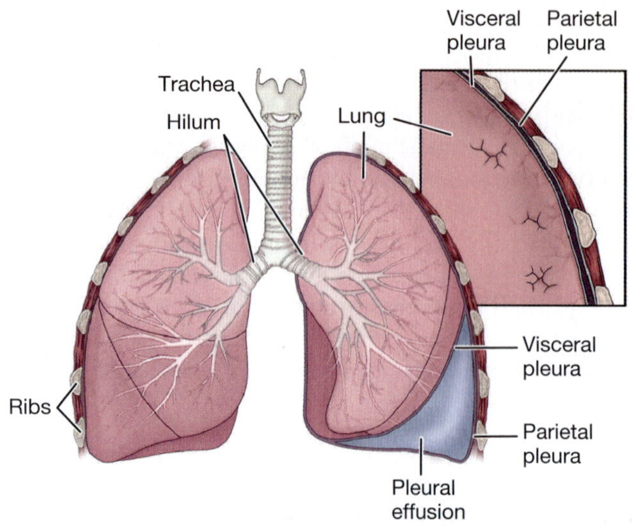

FIGURE 9-8 In pleural effusion, an abnormal volume of fluid collects in the pleural space, causing pain and shortness of breath. Pleural effusion is usually secondary to other disease processes.

almost always has pathologic significance. A pleural effusion can be composed of a relatively clear fluid or it can be bloody or purulent. An effusion of clear fluid may be a transudate or an exudate. A transudate (filtrate of plasma that moves across intact capillary walls) occurs when factors influencing the formation and reabsorption of pleural fluid are altered, usually by imbalances in hydrostatic (as in heart failure) or oncotic pressures (as in hypoalbuminemia). The finding of a transudative effusion generally implies that the pleural membranes are not diseased. A transudative effusion most commonly results from heart failure or volume resuscitation causing volume overload. An exudate (extravasation of fluid into tissues or a cavity) usually results from inflammation by bacterial products or tumors involving the lungs or pleural surfaces. Empyemas are exudative pleural effusions by definition.

Most empyemas occur as complications of bacterial pneumonia or lung abscess, with *Streptococcus pneumonia* being the most common causative microbe. They also result from penetrating chest trauma, hematogenous infection of the pleural space, nonbacterial infections, and iatrogenic causes (after thoracic surgery or thoracentesis). At first, the pleural fluid is thin, with a low leukocyte count, but it frequently progresses to a fibropurulent stage and, finally, to a stage at which it encloses the lung within a thick exudative membrane ("peel"). A chest x-ray, CT scan, or ultrasound determines whether fluid is free flowing or loculated (fixed pocket[s]).

Clinical Manifestations and Assessment

Usually, the clinical manifestations are caused by the underlying disease. Pneumonia causes fever, chills, and pleuritic chest pain, whereas a malignant effusion may result in dyspnea, difficulty lying flat (orthopnea), and coughing. The severity of symptoms is determined by the size of the effusion, the speed of its formation, whether it is a transudate or exudate, and the underlying lung disease. A large pleural effusion causes dyspnea. A small to moderate pleural effusion usually causes minimal or no dyspnea. Patients with empyemas tend to be acutely ill, with more severe inflammatory symptoms (fever, chills, pain, cough, dyspnea, and tachycardia).

Assessment of the area of the pleural effusion reveals decreased or absent breath sounds, decreased fremitus, and a dull, flat sound on percussion. In the case of an extremely large or rapidly accumulating pleural effusion, the assessment reveals a patient in acute respiratory distress. The patient may have tracheal deviation away from the affected side, hypoxemia (SpO_2 less than 90%), hypotension, and tachycardia.

Physical examination, chest x-ray, chest CT, ultrasound, and thoracentesis confirm the presence of fluid. In some instances, a lateral decubitus x-ray is obtained. For this x-ray, the patient lies on the unaffected side in a side-lying position. A pleural effusion can be diagnosed because this position allows for the "layering out" of the fluid, and an air-fluid line is visible.

Pleural fluid is analyzed by bacterial culture, gram stain, AFB stain (for TB), red blood cell and WBC counts and differential, chemistry studies (glucose, amylase, lactic dehydrogenase, protein), cytologic analysis for malignant cells, and pH. A pleural biopsy also may be performed as a diagnostic tool.

Medical Management

The objectives of treatment are to discover the underlying cause of the pleural effusion; to prevent reaccumulation of fluid; and to relieve discomfort, dyspnea, and respiratory compromise. Specific treatment is directed at the underlying cause (e.g., heart failure, pneumonia, cirrhosis). If the pleural fluid is an exudate, more extensive diagnostic procedures are performed to determine the cause. Treatment for the primary cause is then instituted.

Thoracentesis is performed to remove fluid, to obtain a specimen for analysis, and to relieve dyspnea and respiratory compromise (Fig. 9-9). Thoracentesis may be performed under ultrasound guidance or blindly. Depending on the size of the pleural effusion, the patient may be treated by removing the fluid during the thoracentesis procedure or by inserting a chest tube connected to a water-seal drainage system or suction to evacuate the pleural space and reexpand the lung. In general, no more than 1,000 to 1,500 mL of fluid should be removed during a single thoracentesis due to the potential complication of reexpansion pulmonary edema and to avoid symptomatic hypovolemia (Krishna & Rudrappa, 2021; Park & Mallema, 2022). If the empyema is loculated, fibrinolytic agents, such as tissue plasminogen activator (tPA) and tPA-deoxyribonuclease (DNase), can be instilled via a chest tube to dissolve fibrinous septations and improve

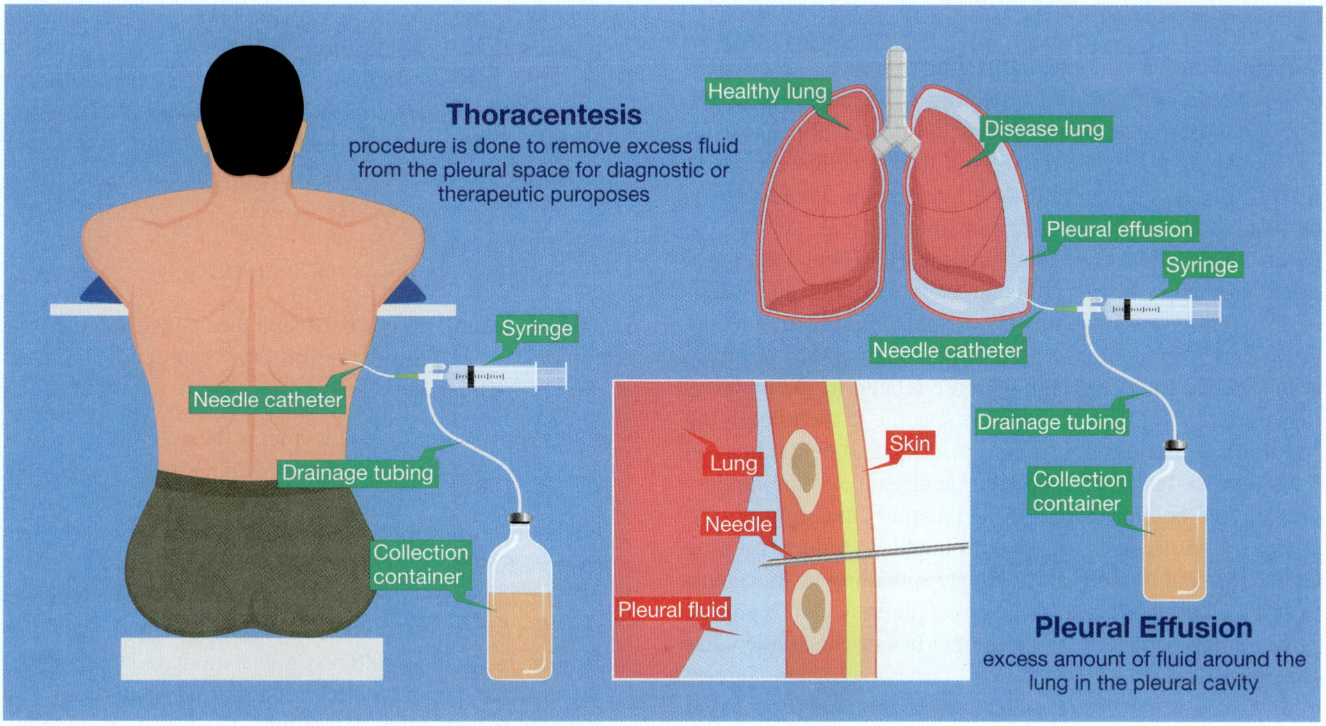

FIGURE 9-9 **Thoracentesis. (Shutterstock.com/Pepermpron.)**

drainage (Chan, 2022). Often surgical management via thoracotomy or video-assisted thoracoscopic surgery (VATS) with lung decortication is required for patients with acute respiratory compromise, sepsis, or hemodynamic instability (Dhanasopon et al., 2022). Decortication is the surgical removal of fibrous tissue in the pleural space; this procedure is called a *pleural peel.*

Pearls for Practice

When a large amount of effusion fluid (approximately 1,000 to 1,500 mL) is removed from the pleural space, the negative intrapleural pressure increases, which can lead to edema when the lung does not reexpand to fill the space. Symptoms of severe coughing and shortness of breath are cues that the nurse should be alert for and if present indicate that the procedure should be discontinued (Stacy, 2022).

However, if the underlying cause is a malignancy, the effusion tends to recur within a few days or weeks. Repeated thoracenteses result in pain, depletion of protein and electrolytes, and sometimes pneumothorax. Once the pleural space is drained adequately, a chemical pleurodesis may be performed to obliterate the pleural space and prevent reaccumulation of fluid. Pleurodesis may be performed using either a VATS or a chest tube. A chemically irritating agent (e.g., talc, bleomycin, doxycycline, minocycline) is instilled into the pleural space (Ali & Surani, 2022; Bashour et al., 2022). With the chest tube approach, after the agent is instilled, the chest tube is clamped for 60 to 90 minutes, and the patient is assisted to assume various positions to promote uniform distribution of the agent and to maximize its contact with the pleural surfaces. The tube is unclamped as prescribed, and chest drainage may be continued several days longer to prevent reaccumulation of fluid and to promote the formation of adhesions between the visceral and parietal pleurae.

Other treatments for malignant pleural effusions include repeated needle thoracentesis, tube thoracostomy, chemical pleurodesis, surgical pleurectomy and decortication, pleuroperitoneal shunt, and tunneled pleural catheters (TPCs). Pleuracotomy involves the insertion of a small catheter attached to a drainage bottle for outpatient management (PleurX catheter [Denver Biomedical]), or implantation of a pleuroperitoneal shunt. A pleuroperitoneal shunt consists of two catheters connected by a pump chamber containing two one-way valves. Fluid moves from the pleural space to the pump chamber and then to the peritoneal cavity. The patient manually pumps on the reservoir daily to move fluid from the pleural space to the peritoneal space. Because pleuroperitoneal shunts have a median length of patency of 2.5 months due to clotting of the shunt (25% of the time), risk of shunt infection, and need for manual operation, pleuroperitoneal shunts have largely been replaced with TPCs (Park & Mallemat, 2022; Reddy et al., 2019). The TPC catheter is a soft silicone tube inserted percutaneously as an outpatient using ultrasound, allowing the patient to return home with minimum sedation and less time spent in the hospital. Patients manage their catheter drainage in their homes. After the thoracentesis a chest x-ray is obtained to determine residual fluid and presence of a pneumothorax (Krishna & Rudrappa, 2021).

Nursing Management

The nurse's role in the care of patients with a pleural effusion or empyema includes implementing the medical regimen. The nurse prepares and positions the patient for thoracentesis and offers support throughout the procedure. Refer to Box 7-8 for Assisting the Patient Undergoing Thoracentesis on page 271. The nurse is responsible for making sure the thoracentesis fluid amount is recorded and sent for appropriate laboratory testing. If a chest tube drainage and water-seal system is used, the nurse is responsible for monitoring the system's function and recording the amount of drainage at prescribed intervals. Nursing care related to the underlying cause of the pleural effusion is specific to the underlying condition. Pain management is a priority, and premedication for the procedure with a narcotic analgesic and antianxiety drug should be considered. If the patient is undergoing tPA/DNase or pleurodesis, the patient requires frequent turning and movement to facilitate adequate spreading of the agents over the pleural surface. Treatment of pleurisy pain is similar to the care of patients with chest tubes because the patient has considerable pain on inspiration. The nurse offers suggestions to enhance comfort, such as turning frequently onto the affected side to splint the chest wall and reduce the stretching of the pleurae. The nurse also teaches the patient to use the hands or a pillow to splint the rib cage while coughing. Administration and assessment of the effects of narcotics or NSAIDs is necessary.

ACUTE RESPIRATORY FAILURE

Acute respiratory failure (ARF) is a sudden and life-threatening deterioration of the gas exchange function of the lung. It occurs in approximately 56% of patients admitted to critical care unit, making it the most frequent type of organ failure (Stacy, 2022). It exists when the exchange of oxygen for carbon dioxide in the lungs cannot keep up with the rate of oxygen consumption and carbon dioxide production by the cells of the body. ARF is classified as hypoxemic (decrease in arterial oxygen tension [PaO_2] to less than 50 mm Hg on room air) and/or hypercapnic (increase in arterial carbon dioxide tension [$PaCO_2$] to greater than 50 mm Hg with an arterial pH of less than 7.35).

It is important to distinguish between ARF and chronic respiratory failure. Chronic respiratory failure is defined as deterioration in the gas exchange function of the lung that has developed insidiously or has persisted for a long period. The absence of acute symptoms and the presence of a chronic respiratory acidosis (elevated $PaCO_2$ and bicarbonate, and hypoxemia) suggest the chronicity of the respiratory failure. Two causes of chronic respiratory failure are COPD (discussed in Chapter 10) and neuromuscular diseases (discussed in Chapter 45). Patients with these disorders develop a tolerance to the gradually worsening hypoxemia and hypercapnia (excess CO_2 in the blood, also known as hypercarbia). However, patients with chronic respiratory failure can develop ARF. For example, a patient with COPD may develop an exacerbation or infection that causes additional deterioration of gas exchange. The principles of management of acute versus chronic respiratory failure are different; the following discussion is limited to ARF.

Pathophysiology

In ARF, the ventilation or perfusion mechanisms in the lung are impaired. Impaired respiratory system mechanisms leading to ARF include:

- *Alveolar hypoventilation,* which is the inability to deliver oxygen to the alveoli and remove CO_2 from the alveoli, may be due to a variety of causes including obesity, chest wall deformities, neuromuscular disorders, CNS depression, or COPD.
- *Diffusion abnormalities* are related to problems with gas transfer across the alveolar–capillary membrane, which may be due to increased resistance, increased thickness of the alveolar–capillary membrane, or any pathology that impacts the alveolar epithelium, the capillary endothelium, or the interstitial space between them.
- *Ventilation–perfusion mismatching.* Alveolar ventilation brings oxygen to the lung and removes the alveolar CO_2 (ventilation), while blood brings CO_2 to the alveoli and takes up the O_2 from the alveoli (perfusion). Thus, the O_2 and CO_2 levels are determined by the matching of ventilation with perfusion.
- *Shunting* occurs when perfusion is adequate to the lung but ventilation is impaired; thus, deoxygenated blood continues to the left side of the heart. (Conditions associated with this include right-to-left shunts with cardiac abnormalities such as septal defects, or pulmonary diseases such as pneumonia, ARDS, or pulmonary edema, in which the alveoli are affected and unable to be ventilated.)
- *Increased physiologic dead space* describes situations in which ventilation of the lung is adequate but perfusion is impaired, as with PE. This mismatch also results in impaired gas exchange.

Common causes of ARF can be classified into four categories: decreased respiratory drive, dysfunction of the chest wall, dysfunction of the lung parenchyma, and other causes.

Decreased Respiratory Drive

Decreased respiratory drive may occur with severe brain injury with increased intracranial pressure, lesions or trauma of the brainstem (multiple sclerosis, tumor, or herniation), use of sedative medications, and metabolic disorders such as severe hypothyroidism. These disorders impair the response of chemoreceptors in the brain to normal respiratory stimulation.

Dysfunction of the Chest Wall

The impulses arise in the respiratory center and travel through nerves that extend from the brainstem down the spinal cord to receptors in the muscles of respiration. Any disease or disorder of the nerves, spinal cord, muscles, or neuromuscular junction involved in respiration seriously affects ventilation and may ultimately lead to ARF. These include musculoskeletal disorders (muscular dystrophy, polymyositis, chest wall trauma), neuromuscular junction disorders (myasthenia gravis, poliomyelitis), some peripheral nerve disorders, and spinal cord disorders (amyotrophic lateral sclerosis, Guillain–Barré syndrome). In cervical spinal cord injury (C 1–5) loss of spontaneous respirations will occur because of paralysis of the diaphragm. Chest wall trauma, such a flail chest, can cause instability of the thorax and impair ventilation.

Pearls for Practice

With cervical spinal injuries, the rigid cervical collar is left in place until the provider confirms stability of the C spine. The nurse is aware that any fracture above the C5 level risks respiratory paralysis since motor innervations to the diaphragm from the phrenic nerve are at the C3–C5 level.

Dysfunction of Lung Parenchyma

Pleural effusion, hemothorax, pneumothorax, and airway obstruction are conditions that interfere with ventilation by preventing expansion of the lung. These conditions, which may cause respiratory failure, usually are produced by an underlying lung disease, pleural disease, or trauma and injury. Other diseases and conditions of lung parenchyma that lead to ARF include pneumonia, pulmonary contusions, status asthmaticus, atelectasis, PE, exacerbation of COPD, ARDS, and pulmonary edema.

Other Causes

In the postoperative period, especially after major thoracic or abdominal surgery, inadequate ventilation and respiratory failure may occur because of several factors. During this period, for example, ARF may be caused by the effects of anesthetic agents, analgesics, and sedatives, which may depress respiration (as described earlier) or enhance the effects of opioids and lead to hypoventilation. Pain may interfere with deep breathing and coughing.

Clinical Manifestations and Assessment

Early signs are those associated with impaired oxygenation and may include restlessness, fatigue, headache, dyspnea, air hunger, mild tachycardia and tachypnea, and increased BP. As the hypoxia progresses, more obvious signs may be present, including confusion, lethargy, increasing tachycardia, tachypnea, **central cyanosis**, diaphoresis, and finally respiratory arrest. Physical findings are those of acute respiratory distress, including use of accessory muscles, decreased breath sounds if the patient cannot adequately ventilate, and other findings related specifically to the underlying disease process and cause of ARF. The nurse recognizes that the clinical manifestations are usually related to hypoxemia, hypercapnia, and acidosis.

Medical Management

The objectives of treatment are to correct the underlying cause and to restore adequate gas exchange in the lungs. Supplemental oxygen administration is used to improve hypoxemia. If narcotics are thought to be the cause of hypoventilation, reversal agents, such as naloxone (for opiates) or flumazenil (for benzodiazepines) can be administered. Depending on the cause of ARF, positive pressure may be used to open collapsed or fluid-filled alveoli and facilitate their participation in gas exchange, or high-flow oxygen therapy or mechanical ventilation may be required to maintain adequate ventilation and oxygenation while the underlying cause is corrected (Stacy, 2022). Medications that facilitate dilation of the airways (bronchodilators) may be beneficial, and steroids may be administered to decrease airway inflammation. Sedation may be necessary for patient comfort and to decrease the work of breathing, particularly if mechanical, ventilation is initiated. In some patient's neuromuscular paralysis may be required to facilitate optimal ventilation and decrease oxygen consumption (Stacy, 2022).

Nursing Management

Nursing management of patients with ARF includes assisting with intubation and maintaining mechanical ventilation. Usually patients are managed in the ICU. The nurse assesses the patient's respiratory status by monitoring the level of responsiveness, ABG levels, POX, and vital signs. In addition, the nurse assesses the entire respiratory system and implements strategies (e.g., turning schedule, mouth care, skin care, range-of-motion exercises for the extremities) to prevent complications. Related to positioning, the nurse recognizes that the most dependent lung is better perfused. Thus, when turning patients, the least affected lung is positioned down; however, the patient is turned every 2 hours, and the POX is continuously monitored for signs of oxygen desaturation. The nurse also assesses the patient's understanding of the management strategies that are used and initiates some form of communication to enable the patient to express concerns and needs to the health care team.

Finally, the nurse addresses the problems that led to the ARF. As the patient's status improves, the nurse assesses the patient's knowledge of the underlying disorder and provides teaching as appropriate to address the disorder.

ACUTE RESPIRATORY DISTRESS SYNDROME

Acute respiratory distress syndrome (ARDS) (previously called adult respiratory distress syndrome) is a severe form of **acute lung injury** (ALI) that affects over 200,000 people each year. This clinical syndrome is characterized by a sudden and progressive pulmonary edema, increasing bilateral infiltrates on chest x-ray, hypoxemia refractory to supplemental oxygen, and reduced lung compliance. These signs occur in the absence of left-sided heart failure. Patients with ARDS usually require mechanical ventilation with a higher-than-normal airway pressure. ARDS has been associated with a mortality rate as high as 36% to 47% (Qadir et al., 2021). The major cause of death in ARDS is multisystem organ failure.

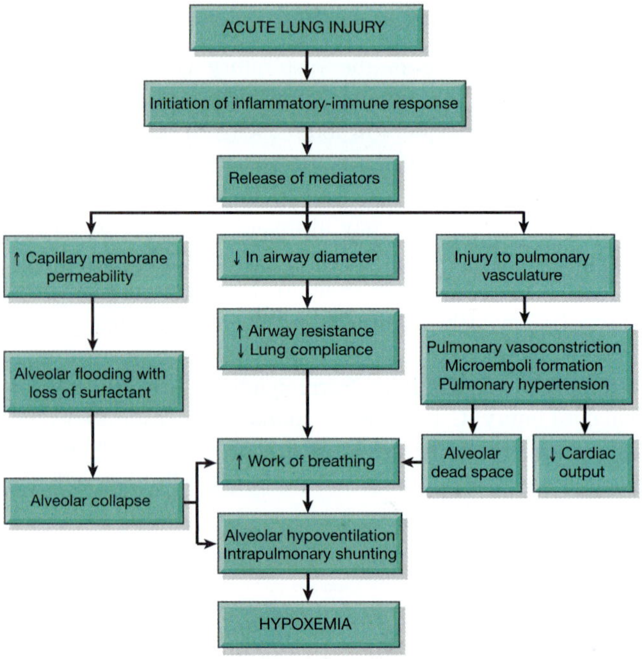

FIGURE 9-10 Pathogenesis of acute respiratory distress syndrome (ARDS).

Pathophysiology

ARDS occurs as a result of an inflammatory trigger that initiates the release of cellular and chemical mediators, causing diffuse epithelial cell injury to the alveolar capillary membrane. This leads to leakage of protein-rich fluid and blood cells into the alveolar interstitial spaces and alterations in the capillary bed.

Severe ventilation–perfusion mismatching occurs in ARDS. Alveoli collapse because of the inflammatory infiltrate, blood, fluid, and surfactant dysfunction. Small airways are narrowed because of interstitial fluid and bronchial obstruction. Lung compliance becomes markedly decreased (stiff lungs), and the result is a characteristic decrease in functional residual capacity (FRC) and severe hypoxemia. The blood returning to the lung for gas exchange is pumped through the nonventilated, nonfunctioning areas of the lung, causing shunting. This means that blood is interfacing with nonfunctioning alveoli, and gas exchange is markedly impaired, resulting in severe, refractory hypoxemia. Figure 9-10 shows the sequence of pathophysiologic events leading to ARDS.

Risk Factors

A wide range of factors are associated with the development of ARDS, including direct injury to the lungs (e.g., smoke inhalation, nonfatal drowning) or indirect insult to the lungs (e.g., septic shock, massive fluid resuscitation) (see Box 9-10 for risk factors). Transfusion-related acute lung injury (TRALI) and transfusion-associated circulatory overload (TACO) are two forms of ALI that result from transfusion of blood products. TRALI is an immune reaction that causes an increase in pulmonary vascular permeability, and TACO causes an increase in hydrostatic pressure, both causing pulmonary edema (refer to Chapter 19 for details on TRALI and TACO). Most recently, an increase in ARDS is related to COVID-19 (Xu et al., 2020).

BOX 9-10 Risk Factors for Acute Respiratory Distress Syndrome (ARDS)

- Systemic sepsis (40%)
- Aspiration: nonfatal drowning, aspiration of gastric contents (more than 30% of cases)
- Trauma (more than 20% of cases)
- Multiple transfusions, blood products
- Drugs (overdose of morphine, methadone, heroin; reaction to nitrofurantoin)
- Hematologic disorders (e.g., disseminated intravascular coagulopathy, massive transfusions, cardiopulmonary bypass)
- Noxious inhalation (high concentrations of oxygen; chlorine gas)
- Postresuscitation
- Localized infection
- Burns
- Metabolic disorders (pancreatitis, uremia)
- Shock
- Major surgery
- Fat or air embolism
- History of chronic alcohol use disorder in patients with critical illness
- Pneumonia (aspiration of gastric contents and sepsis together account for more than 85% of cases of ARDS in recent clinical trials)
- COVID-19

Data from Mercado (2022). Acute respiratory distress syndrome In F. Ferri (Ed), *Ferri's clinical advisor 2022* (pp. 81–85). Elsevier Inc.

Pearls for Practice

The name COVID-19 derives from "corona" (CO), "virus" (VI), "disease" (D), and the year it was discovered—2019. You know it as the highly infectious disease that was the most consequential global health crisis since the influenza pandemic of 1918, resulting in nearly 7 million deaths globally as of November of 2022 (Cascella et al., 2022; Worldometer, 2022). "Coronavirus" is a general term that includes a large family of viruses that range from the common cold to severe acute respiratory syndrome coronavirus 2 or SARS-CoV-2, which is the virus that causes COVID-19. SARS-CoV-2 causes interstitial pneumonia and progressive hypoxemic respiratory failure that can be mild, but approximately 17% of patients progress to ARDS (Chen et al., 2020). Clearly the principal target for SARS-CoV-2 is the respiratory system; however, it affects neurologic, cardiovascular, and gastrointestinal systems by direct viral toxicity; ischemic injury caused by vasculitis, thrombosis, or thromboinflammation; immune dysregulation; and renin-angiotensin-aldosterone system (RAAS) dysregulation (Coopersmith et al., 2021).

Clinical Manifestations and Assessment

Clinically, the acute phase of ARDS is marked by a rapid onset of severe dyspnea that usually occurs 12 to 48 hours after the initiating event. A characteristic feature is arterial hypoxemia that does not respond to supplemental oxygen. On chest x-ray, the findings are similar to those seen with cardiogenic pulmonary edema and appear as bilateral, patchy infiltrates that quickly worsen. On chest CT, bilateral, patchy infiltrates with consolidation are usually more pronounced in the dependent (posterior) lung areas. The ALI then progresses to fibrosing alveolitis with persistent, severe hypoxemia. The patient also has increased alveolar dead space (ventilation to nonperfused alveoli) and decreased pulmonary compliance ("stiff lungs," which are difficult to ventilate). Clinically, the patient is thought to be in the recovery phase if the hypoxemia begins to resolve, the chest x-ray improves, and the lungs become more compliant.

The primary symptom is dyspnea, and the increased work of breathing is reflected by tachypnea, nasal flaring, intercostal retractions, and use of accessory muscles, and crackles are auscultated as the fluid begins to leak into the alveolar interstitial space (Storzer, 2023). Pink frothy sputum may be present. ABGs are analyzed to assess the severity of hypoxemia, which is the hallmark of ARDS (Storzer, 2023). A diagnosis of ARDS may be made based on the following criteria: a history of systemic or pulmonary risk factors, acute onset of respiratory distress, bilateral pulmonary infiltrates, clinical absence of left-sided heart failure, and a ratio of PaO_2 to FiO_2 of less than 300 mm Hg (severe refractory hypoxemia). The normal ratio of PaO_2 to FiO_2 is over 300 mm Hg. Severity of ARDS is measured by calculation of PaO_2/FiO_2 ratio. A ratio of 200 to 300 is mild, 100 to 199 is moderate, and less than or equal to 100 is severe (Fan et al., 2018).

Pearls for Practice

A quick calculation the nurse can perform to assess the patient's pulmonary status is the ratio of the patient's arterial oxygen level (PaO_2) obtained from ABGs and the amount of oxygen inspired (FiO_2). This is also known as the P/F ratio. If the patient's PaO_2 is 75 mm Hg on 45% FiO_2, then the nurse converts the FiO_2 to a percentage. Thus, an FiO_2 of 45% become 0.45. The simple calculation is 75/0.45, which equals a P/F ratio of 167, suggesting a moderate ARDS. To illustrate a patient with normal pulmonary function, an ABG may reveal a PaO_2 of 100 mm Hg on room air (FiO_2 of 21%); therefore, the patient's P/F ratio would be 100/0.21 = 476.

Medical Management

The primary focus in the management of ARDS includes identification and treatment of the underlying causative condition. Aggressive, supportive care must be provided to compensate for the severe respiratory dysfunction. This supportive therapy almost always includes intubation and mechanical ventilation. In addition, circulatory support, adequate fluid volume, and nutritional support are important. Supplemental oxygen is used as the patient begins the initial spiral of hypoxemia. As the hypoxemia progresses, intubation and mechanical ventilation are instituted. The concentration of oxygen and ventilator settings and modes are determined by the patient's status. This is monitored by ABG analysis, POX, and bedside pulmonary compliance testing.

Positive End-Expiratory Pressure

PEEP is a critical part of the treatment of ARDS. Use of PEEP helps increase FRC and reverse alveolar collapse by keeping the alveoli open, resulting in improved arterial oxygenation and a reduction in the severity of the ventilation–perfusion imbalance. Also, the use of PEEP can allow for the use of lower, safer FiO_2 levels (60% or less FiO_2). The goal is a PaO_2 of greater than 60 mm Hg or an oxygen saturation level of greater than 90% at the lowest possible FiO_2. Evidence suggests that ARDS should be managed with a low tidal volume (6 cc/kg of ideal body weight), pressure-limited approach (plateau pressure of 30 mm Hg or less) with low or moderately high PEEP. Although the optimal level of PEEP has not been established, higher levels of PEEP may be beneficial for moderate to severe ARDS (Fan et al., 2018; Matthay & Slutsky, 2020).

The use of positive-pressure ventilation (as opposed to normal negative-pressure breathing) increases intrathoracic pressure and causes a decrease in preload to the heart. This drop in preload can result in decreased cardiac output and hypotension. Systemic hypotension also may occur in ARDS as a result of hypovolemia secondary to leakage of fluid into the interstitial spaces. Hypovolemia must be treated carefully without causing further fluid overload. IV crystalloid or colloid solutions are administered with careful monitoring of pulmonary status. Inotropic (e.g., dobutamine) or vasopressor agents (e.g., norepinephrine, dopamine, and epinephrine) may be required. Central venous catheters and, occasionally, pulmonary artery pressure catheters may be used to monitor the patient's fluid status and the severe and progressive pulmonary hypertension sometimes observed in ARDS. Arterial catheterization is required as patients with ARDS need frequent blood gas analysis. Additional details on PEEP are found in Chapter 54.

Pharmacologic Therapy

Numerous pharmacologic treatments are under investigation to stop the cascade of events leading to ARDS; however, the mainstay of treatment is related to improving oxygenation and preventing complications. Thus, prophylaxis for prevention of DVT and stress ulcer is common.

ARDS patients often require IV sedation and pain medication to combat anxiety and agitation from hypoxemia and intubation. In extreme cases, patients may require chemical paralysis with neuromuscular blockers in order to adequately ventilate and oxygenate them.

Nutritional Therapy

Adequate nutritional support is vital in the treatment of ARDS. Patients with ARDS require 12 to 25 kcal/kg/day to meet caloric requirements. Enteral feeding is the first consideration; however, parenteral nutrition also may be required (Compher et al., 2022).

Nursing Management

General Measures

A patient with ARDS is critically ill and requires close monitoring in the intensive care unit. Many different respiratory modalities can be used in this situation (oxygen administration, nebulizer therapy, CPT, endotracheal intubation or tracheostomy, mechanical ventilation, PEEP, suctioning, bronchoscopy). Frequent assessment of the patient's status is necessary to evaluate the effectiveness of treatment.

In addition to implementing the medical plan of care, the nurse considers other patient needs. Positioning is important. The nurse turns the patient frequently to improve ventilation and perfusion in the lungs and enhance secretion drainage. However, the nurse must monitor the patient closely for deterioration in oxygenation with changes in position. Oxygenation in patients with ARDS is sometimes improved in the prone position, and data indicate this position reduces mortality in patients with moderate to severe ARDS (initial P/F less than 150 mm Hg) (Fan et al., 2018; Matthay & Slutsky, 2020; Walter, 2022). This position may be evaluated for improvement in oxygenation and used in special circumstances. Devices and specialty beds are available to assist the nurse in placing the patient in a prone position.

Pearls for Practice

Recall that previous discussion about matching ventilation with perfusion. In ARDS, the dependent areas of the lung are more heavily damaged (whereas it was previously believed that diffuse damage existed), and turning a patient to the prone position (patient is lying face down onto their anterior chest and abdomen) improves perfusion to less damaged parts of lungs, improving ventilation/perfusion matching (Stacy, 2022). In addition, this position redistributes the weight of the heart, improving alveolar recruitment and decreasing pulmonary vascular resistance (Morata et al., 2021). Prone positioning appears to be more effective when initiated during the early phases of ARDS and applied for at least 12 hours a day (Apte et al., 2021; Reece-Anthony et al., 2022). It is contraindicated in patients with increased intracranial pressure, recent tracheal surgery, hemodynamic instability, spinal instability, unstable fractures, burns, pregnancy, or some abdominal surgeries (Reece-Anthony et al., 2022; Stacy, 2022). Nurses must be familiar with the protocol for turning to the prone position (typically "proning teams" are created) that require a minimum of five practitioners, including an airway-trained practitioner (Reece-Anthony et al., 2022). Complications include airway obstruction, endotracheal tube dislodgement, hypotension, arrhythmias, loss of venous access, facial and airway edema, a greater need for sedation, and increased risk of pressure injuries (Reece-Anthony et al., 2022; Stacy, 2022).

The patient can be extremely anxious and agitated because of the increasing hypoxemia, dyspnea, and intubation. The nurse explains all procedures and provides care in a calm, reassuring manner. It is important to reduce the patient's anxiety, because anxiety increases oxygen expenditure by preventing rest. Rest is essential to limit oxygen consumption and reduce oxygen needs.

Ventilator Considerations

If the patient is intubated and receiving mechanical ventilation with PEEP, several considerations must be addressed. PEEP is an unnatural pattern of breathing that feels strange to patients. The patient may be anxious and "fight" or "buck" the ventilator (ventilator dysynchrony). It is important for the nurse to assess for problems with ventilation that may be causing the anxiety reaction: tube blockage by kinking or retained secretions, other acute respiratory problems (e.g., pneumothorax, pain), a sudden decrease in the oxygen level, the level of dyspnea, or ventilator malfunction. In most cases, sedation may be required to decrease the patient's oxygen consumption, allow the ventilator to provide full support of ventilation, and decrease the patient's anxiety. Sedatives that may be used are lorazepam, midazolam, ketamine, dexmedetomidine, and propofol. Judicious use of sedatives is necessary to prevent or reduce ICU delirium (Heim et al., 2019).

If satisfactory oxygen levels cannot be maintained despite the use of sedatives, neuromuscular blocking agents, such as pancuronium, vecuronium, atracurium, or rocuronium, may be administered to paralyze the patient. These agents paralyze skeletal muscles, including respiratory muscles, leading to respiratory arrest if the patient is not intubated and on adequate ventilator settings. With paralysis, the patient appears to be unconscious, loses motor function, and cannot breathe, talk, or blink independently. However, the patient retains sensation and is awake and able to hear and these agents do not affect smooth muscles (pupillary response, uterine contractions). Paralytic agents should be used only by personnel who are trained in airway and ventilator management. The nurse must reassure the patient that the paralysis is a result of the medication and is temporary. Paralysis should be used for the shortest possible time and never without adequate sedation and pain management.

Use of paralytic agents has many dangers and side effects. The nurse must be sure the patient does not become disconnected from the ventilator because respiratory muscles are paralyzed and the patient will be apneic. Consequently, the nurse ensures that the patient is closely monitored, and all ventilator and patient alarms must be on at all times. Eye care is important as well, because the patient cannot blink, thus increasing the risk of corneal abrasions (eye care is described in Chapter 45). Neuromuscular blockers predispose the patient to deep venous thrombosis (DVT), muscle atrophy, and skin breakdown; therefore, passive range-of-motion exercises and skin assessment are important nursing actions.

Pearls for Practice

If a patient is on concurrent administration of aminoglycosides and/or steroids, this increases the chance of the chemically paralyzed patient developing critical illness polyneuropathy. This is a severe form of muscle atrophy and deconditioning that can occur within 24 hours; it requires intensive physical therapy to correct, increases the patient's risks of developing complications, and prolongs hospital lengths of stay.

The patient may have discomfort or pain but cannot communicate these sensations. Signs of pain, such as tachycardia, diaphoresis, and hypertension, must be assessed for and treated. Analgesia **must** be administered concurrently with neuromuscular blocking agents. The nurse must anticipate the patient's needs regarding pain and comfort. The nurse checks the patient's position to ensure it is comfortable and in normal body alignment.

The nurse talks to, and not about, the patient while in the patient's presence; remember the patient is awake and able to hear. In addition, it is important for the nurse to describe the purpose and effects of the paralytic agents to the patient's family. If family members are unaware that these agents have been administered, they may become distressed by the change in the patient's status.

PULMONARY ARTERIAL HYPERTENSION

Pulmonary circulation is a low-pressure system intended to accommodate high blood flow from the right ventricle. The pulmonary vasculature is compliant and thin walled in order to facilitate gas exchange. The normal mean pulmonary pressure is 12 to 15 mm Hg with the capacity to dilate and constrict as needed. Pulmonary arterial hypertension (PAH) exists when the mean pulmonary artery pressure exceeds 25 mm Hg at rest or 30 mm Hg with activities. Unlike systemic BP, these pressures cannot be measured indirectly; instead, they must be measured via right-sided heart catheterization (see Chapter 14) with a pulmonary artery catheter or estimated with an echocardiogram. In the absence of these measurements, clinical recognition becomes the only indicator for the presence of pulmonary hypertension; however, PAH is a condition that is not clinically evident until late in its progression.

There are two types of PAH: idiopathic PAH (formerly known as primary) and secondary PAH due to a known cause. The World Health Organization and New York Heart Association further classify PAH into five categories (see Box 9-11). Idiopathic PAH is a very uncommon disease. It occurs most often in females 20 to 40 years of age, either sporadically or in patients with a family history, and is usually fatal within 5 years of diagnosis. There are several possible causes, but the exact cause is unknown (Fitzpatrick et al., 2022b; Hoeper et al., 2022).

In contrast, secondary PAH due to a known cause is more common and results from existing cardiac (left ventricular failure, mitral stenosis) or pulmonary disease (emphysema, pulmonary fibrosis, or thromboembolism). The prognosis

BOX 9-11 Classifications of Pulmonary Hypertension

Group 1	Pulmonary HTN
Group 2	Pulmonary venous HTN
Group 3	Pulmonary HTN due to lung disease or hypoxemia
Group 4	Pulmonary HTN due to pulmonary obstruction
Group 5	Pulmonary HTN secondary to unclear or multifactorial

BOX 9-12

Causes of Pulmonary Arterial Hypertension (PAH)

- Collagen vascular diseases
- Congenital systemic-to-pulmonary shunts
- Portal hypertension
- Altered immune mechanisms (HIV infection)
- Diseases associated with significant venous or capillary involvement
- Chronic thrombotic or embolic disease
- Pulmonary venous hypertension
- Pulmonary vasoconstriction due to hypoxemia
- Chronic obstructive pulmonary disease (COPD), interstitial lung disease, sleep-disordered breathing
- Drug and toxin-induced (e.g., methamphetamines, dasatinib, and toxic rapeseed oil)
- Miscellaneous causes: Sarcoidosis, histiocytosis, compression of pulmonary vessels

depends on the severity of the underlying disorder and the changes in the pulmonary vascular bed. A common cause of PAH is pulmonary artery constriction due to chronic hypoxemia and hypercapnia from COPD (Box 9-12) (Fitzpatrick et al., 2022). Conditions such as collagen vascular disease, congenital heart disease, portal hypertension, and HIV infection increase the risk for PAH in susceptible patients.

Pathophysiology

In patients with PAH, the pulmonary vasculature is injured, which leads to endothelial and smooth muscle thickening and hypertrophy, leading to noncompliant and narrowed vessels. Normally, the pulmonary vascular bed can handle the blood volume delivered by the right ventricle. It has a low resistance to blood flow and compensates for increased blood volume by dilation of the vessels in the pulmonary circulation. However, if the pulmonary vascular bed is destroyed or obstructed, the ability to handle whatever flow or volume of blood it receives is impaired, and the increased blood flow then increases the pulmonary artery pressure. As the pulmonary arterial pressure increases, the pulmonary vascular resistance also increases. This increased workload affects right ventricular function. The myocardium ultimately cannot meet the increasing demands imposed on it, leading to right ventricular hypertrophy (enlargement and dilation) and failure (cor pulmonale).

Clinical Manifestations and Assessment

Dyspnea, the main symptom of both types of PAH, occurs at first with exertion and eventually at rest. Other signs and symptoms include chest pain, weakness, fatigue, syncope, occasional hemoptysis, and signs of right-sided heart failure (peripheral edema, ascites, distended neck veins, hepatomegaly, and right ventricular third heart sound [S3], heart murmur, splitting of second heart sound).

Diagnosis of idiopathic PAH is made by exclusion of secondary causes such as COPD, PE, HIV, and cardiac disease. Several tests are used to determine whether there is a known cause for the pulmonary hypertension. Complete diagnostic evaluation includes a history, physical examination, chest x-ray, pulmonary function studies, electrocardiogram (ECG), echocardiogram, ventilation–perfusion scan ($\dot{V}/\dot{Q}$ scan), CT or magnetic resonance (MR) angiography, sleep studies, autoantibody tests (to identify diseases of collagen vascular origin), HIV tests, liver function testing, hypercoagulation studies, and cardiac catheterization. Pulmonary function studies may be normal or show a slight decrease in vital capacity and lung compliance with a mild decrease in the diffusing capacity. The PaO_2 also is decreased (hypoxemia). Complete blood count is usually normal but may show polycythemia (Hct of more than 54% in males or 51% in females). The ECG reveals right atrial enlargement (and tall peaked P waves in inferior leads); right-axis deviation, right ventricular hypertrophy (tall R waves in V_2 and tall R waves in V_5); and ST-segment depression, T-wave inversion, or both in V_{1-4}. An echocardiogram can assess the progression of the disease and rule out other conditions with similar signs and symptoms. A $\dot{V}/\dot{Q}$ scan or pulmonary CT or MR angiography detects defects in pulmonary vasculature, such as PE. Cardiac catheterization of the right side of the heart reveals elevated pulmonary arterial pressure and determines whether there is a vasoactive component to the pulmonary hypertension. Acute vasodilator testing can be performed with the right heart catheterization to determine if there is a reduction in mean pulmonary artery pressure when a short-acting vasodilator (adenosine, epoprostenol, or inhaled nitric oxide) is administered. A positive response is a decrease in the mean pulmonary artery pressure of more than 10 mm Hg to a value of less than 40 mm Hg, with increased or unchanged cardiac output (Fitzpatrick et al., 2022). Fewer than 10% of patients are responsive in idiopathic PAH, but these patients benefit from calcium-channel blockers.

Medical Management

The goal of treatment is to manage the underlying condition related to PAH of known cause. Hypoxemia, at rest or during exertion, should be treated with supplemental oxygen. Appropriate oxygen therapy can reverse the vasoconstrictive effect and reduce the pulmonary hypertension. Pharmacologic agents such as diuretics, digoxin, anticoagulant therapy (increased incidence of clots in pulmonary system), and calcium-channel blockers (nifedipine, diltiazem) (if they responded to the vasodilator testing described above) may be prescribed. Because calcium-channel blockers are effective in only a small percentage of patients, other treatment options, including prostacyclin, which acts as a potent vasodilator of pulmonary arteries and inhibitor of platelet aggregation, are often necessary (Fitzpatrick et al., 2022).

Vasodilating agents can be used to improve exercise tolerance and hemodynamic function as well as extend survival.

Oral phosphodiesterase inhibitors (sildenafil, tadalafil) can be used alone or in combination with endothelin receptor antagonists (bosentan, ambrisentan, macitentan). Epoprostenol is given by continuous infusion, treprostinil by subcutaneous injection, bosentan and sildenafil by mouth, and iloprost by inhalation. Current therapies are not curative, have considerable side effects, and are often quite expensive. Lung or heart–lung transplantation is reserved for patients who have advanced disease despite maximal medical therapy (Fitzpatrick et al., 2022b).

Nursing Management

The major nursing goal is to identify patients at high risk for PAH, such as those with COPD, PE, congenital heart disease, and mitral valve disease. The nurse also must be alert for signs and symptoms of deterioration such as worsening dyspnea, hypoxemia, and right ventricular failure. Oxygen therapy is administered as ordered, and the patient and family are instructed about the use of home oxygen supplementation. In patients treated with prostacyclin (i.e., epoprostenol or treprostinil), education about the need for central venous access (epoprostenol), or subcutaneous infusion (treprostinil) is discussed. In addition, the nurse reviews proper administration and dosing of the medication, usual side effects such as pain at the injection site, and potential severe side effects of hypotension, flushing of skin, bradycardia, and headache associated with IV administration. Emotional and psychosocial aspects of this disease must be addressed.

PULMONARY EMBOLISM

Pulmonary embolism (PE) refers to the obstruction of the pulmonary artery or one of its branches by a thrombus (or thrombi) that originates somewhere in the venous system or right side of the heart. Hospitalized patients are at a high risk for PE; it is estimated that more than 900,000 people suffer from DVT/PE, and almost 100,000 deaths are attributed to PE annually (CDC, 2022f). It is the third leading cause of death in hospitalized patients and the leading cause of preventable hospital deaths; it is often not diagnosed until autopsy (CDC, 2022c, 2022f). PE is a common disorder and often is associated with trauma, arrhythmia (atrial fibrillation), surgery (orthopedic, major abdominal, pelvic, gynecologic), pregnancy, heart failure, malignancies, age greater than 50 years, hypercoagulable states, and prolonged immobility. It also may occur in apparently healthy people. Risk factors for thromboembolism are identified in Box 9-13.

BOX 9-13

Risk Factors for Thromboembolism

- Acute medical illness (CVA, acute MI, heart failure, neuromuscular diseases)
- Major surgery (abdominal, orthopedic, gynecologic, urologic, neurosurgical, oncologic)
- Trauma (multisystem trauma, spinal cord injury or fracture, hip or pelvic fractures)
- Cancer (localized or metastatic) receiving chemotherapy or radiation therapy
- History of thromboembolism
- Obesity
- Immobility for more than 2 days
- Age older than 40 years (risk doubles with each subsequent decade)
- Hypercoagulable conditions
- Prolonged mechanical ventilation
- Neuromuscular paralytic use
- Central venous catheters
- Severe sepsis
- Heparin-induced thrombocytopenia (HIT)

Pathophysiology

Most commonly, PE is due to a blood clot or thrombus. However, there are other types of emboli: air, fat, amniotic fluid, tumor cells, intravenously injected particulates, and septic (from bacterial invasion of the thrombus). Although most thrombi originate in the deep veins of the legs, other sites include the pelvic veins and the right atrium of the heart. In addition, with the increased use of central venous catheters, upper extremity DVT is increasing in incidence and currently represents about 5% of PE (Storzer, 2023). Venous thrombosis can result from Virchow's triad which includes three factors: (1) the slowing of blood flow (or venous stasis), (2) blood vessel wall injury (particularly the endothelial lining), and (3) hypercoagulability. In atrial fibrillation, blood stagnates in the fibrillating atria, and stagnant blood forms clots. These clots can travel into the pulmonary circulation.

When a thrombus completely or partially obstructs a pulmonary artery or its branches, the alveolar dead space is increased. Alveolar dead space is an area that is ventilated but receives little or no blood flow. Therefore, gas exchange is impaired or absent in this area. In addition, various vasoactive substances are released from the clot and surrounding area, and these cause regional blood vessels and bronchioles to constrict. The reflex bronchoconstriction and vasoconstriction causes impaired gas exchange and the loss of alveolar surfactant, which results in atelectasis and hypoxemia. The hemodynamic consequences are increased pulmonary vascular resistance and pulmonary artery pressures, which put a strain on the right ventricle. When the work requirements of the right ventricle exceed its capacity, right ventricular failure occurs, leading to a decrease in cardiac output followed by a decrease in systemic blood pressure and the development of shock. PE is categorized as *low risk* (no hemodynamic instability), *submassive* (right ventricular strain or hypokinesis [abnormally decreased muscle movement] on echocardiogram or evidence of myocardial necrosis), or *massive* (sustained hypotension [systolic BP <90 mm Hg] for >15 minutes, or signs of shock or hypoxia).

Clinical Manifestations and Assessment

Symptoms depend on the size of the thrombus and the area of the pulmonary artery occluded by the thrombus. Acute onset of dyspnea is the most frequent symptom, followed by pleuritic chest pain, cough, hemoptysis, and palpitations. The most common signs found on physical assessment are tachypnea, crackles, tachycardia, and presence of an S_4 heart sound and split S_2. DVT is closely associated with development of PE. Typically, these patients report sudden onset of pain and/or swelling and warmth of the proximal or distal extremity, skin discoloration (red or dusky blue in color), and superficial vein distention.

Shock can develop with massive PEs or in patients with pre-existing heart failure. Pronounced dyspnea, sudden substernal pain, rapid and weak pulse, hypotension, syncope, and sudden death can occur. Multiple small emboli can lodge in the terminal pulmonary arterioles, producing multiple small infarctions of the lungs. A pulmonary infarction causes necrosis of an area of the lung. The clinical picture may mimic that of bronchopneumonia or heart failure. In atypical instances, PE causes few signs and symptoms, whereas in other instances it mimics various other cardiopulmonary disorders.

Death from PE commonly occurs within hours of the onset of symptoms; therefore, early recognition and diagnosis are priorities. Because the symptoms of PE can vary from mild to severe, a diagnostic workup is performed to rule out other diseases. The initial diagnostic workup includes chest x-ray, ECG, peripheral vascular studies (duplex ultrasound, venogram), ABG analysis, and D-dimer.

The chest x-ray is most helpful in excluding other possible causes such as pneumonia, COPD, and pulmonary edema due to heart failure. ABG analysis may show hypoxemia and hypocapnia (from tachypnea); however, ABG measurements may be normal even in the presence of PE. The classic ECG pattern associated with PE, although rare, is S_1, Q_3, T_3, meaning a deep S wave in lead I, a Q wave in lead III and an inverted T wave in lead III. More common ECG findings are sinus tachycardia, PR-interval depression, and nonspecific T-wave changes. Peripheral vascular studies used to diagnose a DVT may include impedance plethysmography, Doppler ultrasonography, or venography. If a DVT is present with the associated signs and symptoms of PE, the patient is treated for both. The D-dimer assay is used to evaluate patients with possible PE. Emergency departments in particular have used this as a rapid, cost-effective test. D-dimer is a protein fragment that is produced when forming or breaking down blood clots (fibrin degradation) (fibrin lysis); blood clots generally break down slowly after they are formed, releasing D-dimer into the blood. D-dimer is used only to rule out a PE; as a negative result, it has a 95% predictive ability, meaning 95% of patients with PE have an elevated D-dimer. If the D-dimer is negative, the diagnosis of PE is excluded, whereas a positive test generally prompts a computed tomographic pulmonary angiography (CTPA). For most patients with suspected PE, CTPA is the first-choice diagnostic imaging modality because it is sensitive and specific for the diagnosis of PE (Fu, 2020; Thompson et al., 2022).

Pearls for Practice

The nurse understands that there is a higher rate of false-positive D-dimers in patients with acute illness, those over 50 years, pregnant females, and those with kidney disease (Thompson et al., 2022).

If a facility does not have access to a CTPA, a $\dot{V}/\dot{Q}$ scan is ordered. The $\dot{V}/\dot{Q}$ scan was once the second choice for diagnosis of a PE (with pulmonary angiogram [discussed below] considered the best diagnostic procedure). It is minimally invasive, involving the administration of a radioactive agent (both IV and inhaled). This scan evaluates different regions of the lung (upper, middle, lower) and allows comparisons of the percentage of ventilation and perfusion in each area. This test has a high sensitivity but can be more cumbersome than a CT scan and is not as accurate as a pulmonary angiogram. Patients who have an underlying lung disease, such as COPD or pneumonia, often have inconclusive $\dot{V}/\dot{Q}$ scan results; also patients who are mechanically ventilated cannot undergo this test (see Chapter 7 for more details).

Contrast angiogram CT scan has gained popularity for use in the diagnosis of PE. Limitations to the use of CT scanning are that patients must be cooperative and able to have IV contrast (no contrast allergies, normal renal function), and it is less sensitive than a pulmonary angiogram. Pulmonary angiography allows for the visualization of the pulmonary vasculature under fluoroscopy with IV contrast. It requires interventional radiologists to perform the test with specific equipment and personnel that may not be available in many hospitals, and the test is costly.

Prevention

For patients at risk for PE, the most effective approach for prevention is to prevent DVT. General preventive measures include active leg exercises to avoid venous stasis, early ambulation (Anderson et al., 2019; Fernando et al., 2022), use of elastic compression stockings, and intermittent pneumatic compression (IPC) devices. The use of elastic compression stockings and mechanical devices (e.g., IPC or sequential compression devices [SCD]) has recently been called into question since elastic compression stockings are associated with pressure injuries, particularly in patients with critical illness, postoperative patients with fluid overload, and those that are confused or sedated since they cannot report pain or discomfort associated with the elastic stockings (Siby, 2021). In a recent study, discontinuation of graduated compression stockings use while maintaining mechanical devices eliminated the risk of associated pressure injuries without putting patients at a greater risk for DVT (Siby, 2021). In addition, the American Society of Hematology's (ASH) recent guidelines for prevention of DVT for hospitalized surgical patients includes using mechanical devices over graduated compression stockings, but they note additional research is important to strengthen or adapt their recommendation (Anderson et al., 2019). What is clear is that prevention of DVT decreases the risk of PE and that the nurse should follow institutional protocol for DVT prevention.

The mechanical devices (IPCs or SCDs) are used to prevent venous stasis through compression and relaxation of the calf muscles, similar to the effect of muscle contraction. They have effectively reduced the risk of DVT and have been shown to be an effective primary therapy for patients who are unable to receive anticoagulation therapy, but a combination of pharmacologic agents with mechanical devices is more effective (Insin et al., 2021). Several types are available, such as foot, calf, and thigh-high compression as well as graduated, asymmetric, and circumferential compression. There is little evidence favoring any particular type of compression. Graduated compression involves the sequential movement of air in the sleeve up the leg, followed by relaxation of the sleeve. The advantage of this therapy is the extended duration of compression compared with standard inflation. Asymmetric compression involves inflating only the area on the back of the leg or foot, whereas circumferential compression involves even compression of the entire leg. Assessment of the patient's skin is an important nursing function when mechanical devices are in use. IPCs or SCDs need to be used for at least 16 hours per day to be effective.

Prophylactic anticoagulation therapy is prescribed based on assessment of a patient's risk level. Table 9-3 illustrates the risk stratification and recommended prophylaxis. Prophylactic anticoagulant therapy may include low-dose or adjusted-dose heparin, low–molecular-weight heparin (LMWH), or oral anticoagulants.

Pearls for Practice

Low doses of heparin may be administered before surgery to reduce the risk of postoperative DVT and PE. Heparin should be administered subcutaneously 2 hours before surgery (and continued every 8 to 12 hours until the patient is discharged). Low-dose heparin is thought to enhance the activity of antithrombin III, a major plasma inhibitor of clotting factor X. This regimen is not recommended for patients with an active thrombotic process or for those undergoing major orthopedic surgery, open prostatectomy, or surgery on the eye or brain.

Medical Management

There is a wide spectrum of clinical presentation in PE depending on the size of the emboli, ranging from incidental finding to sudden circulatory collapse and shock. Because PE is often a medical emergency, emergency management is of primary concern. After emergency measures have been initiated and the patient is stabilized, the treatment goal is to dissolve (lyse) the existing emboli and prevent new ones from forming. Treatment may include a variety of modalities:

- General measures to improve respiratory and vascular status
- Anticoagulation therapy
- Thrombolytic therapy
- Surgical intervention

TABLE **9-3 Recommended Deep Vein Thrombosis Prophylaxis**

Risk Level	Recommended Prophylaxis
Low risk:	Early mobilization, mechanical aid (intermittent pneumatic compression devices) until ambulatory (>300 feet/day)
Minor surgery + age under 40 years and no additional DVT risk factors	Mechanical aid (intermittent pneumatic compression devices) until ambulatory
Moderate risk:	Mechanical aid (intermittent pneumatic) until ambulatory >300 feet per day OR
Major surgery + age over 40 years and no additional DVT risk factors	Heparin: 5,000 units SC q12h (start 2 hours prior to surgery) or Enoxaparin 40 mg. SC daily or Dalteparin 5,000 units SC daily (Bouton & Fort, 2023)
High risk:	Mechanical aid (intermittent pneumatic compression or graded compression stockings) AND
Major surgery + age over 40 years and/or other DVT risk factors	Heparin 5,000 units SC q8h (start 2 hours prior to surgery) or Enoxaparin 40 mg SC daily or Dalteparin 5,000 units SC daily
Hip arthroplasty	Enoxaparin 30 mg SC q 12 hours × 10–14 days Fondaparinux 2.5 mg SC daily × 10–14 days Dabigatran 220 mg PO daily × 28–35 days Warfarin (INR 2.0–3.0) for 14–21 days
Knee arthroplasty	Enoxaparin 30 mg SC q 12 hours × 10–14 days Apixaban 2.5 mg PO BID × 12 days Rivaroxaban 10 mg PO daily × 12 days Warfarin (target INR 2.0–3.0) for 14–21 days

Emergency Management

Current recommendations suggest that pulmonary embolism response teams (PERT) that include cardiology, critical care specialists, emergency medicine specialists, and health care team members provide rapid coordination, assessment, and treatment for patients with the greatest risk of mortality from PE (Hussey & Conway, 2020). Massive PE is a life-threatening emergency. The immediate objective is to stabilize the cardiopulmonary system. A sudden increase in pulmonary resistance increases the work of the right ventricle, which can cause acute right-sided heart failure with cardiogenic shock. Emergency management consists of the following actions:

- Oxygen is administered immediately to relieve hypoxemia, respiratory distress, and central cyanosis. If severe hypoxia exists, intubation and ventilator management is required.
- Intravenous infusion lines are inserted to establish routes for medications or fluids that will be needed. If hypotensive, normal saline will be administered (Hussey & Conway, 2020). However, the patient is monitored closely, because if the right ventricle is stressed and the patient receives too much fluid, more dysfunction can result (Hussey & Conway, 2020).
- A perfusion scan, hemodynamic measurements, and ABG determinations are performed. CT angiogram or pulmonary angiography may be performed.
- An echocardiogram can be done at the bedside to assess right ventricular function.
- Hypotension is treated with IV fluid resuscitation (as noted above); however, with right ventricular dysfunction pharmacotherapeutics are needed and may take the form of vasopressors (dopamine, norepinephrine, epinephrine) or inotropic support (dobutamine).
- The ECG is monitored continuously for arrhythmias and right ventricular failure, which may occur suddenly.
- Digitalis glycosides, IV diuretics, and antiarrhythmic agents are administered when appropriate.
- Blood is drawn for serum electrolytes, complete blood count, and coagulation studies (PT, international normalized ratio [INR], partial thromboplastin time [PTT], D-dimer, anti-Xa activity, cardiac biomarkers [troponin, BNP], lactate, type and screen). ABGs will be analyzed.
- If the patient has suffered massive embolism and is hypotensive, an indwelling urinary catheter is inserted to monitor urinary output.
- Small doses of IV morphine or sedatives are administered to relieve patient anxiety, to alleviate chest discomfort, to improve tolerance of the endotracheal tube, and to ease adaptation to the mechanical ventilator.
- IV thrombolytic agents (tPA [Alteplase, Reteplase]) may be used in patients who are hemodynamically unstable (hypotension, ECG strain patterns or echocardiographic evidence of right ventricular strain or failure) to lyse the clot(s).
- Catheter-directed ultrasound thrombolytic therapy may be used for patients with submassive or massive PE, but specialized equipment and personnel are needed for this therapy (Khan et al., 2019).
- Initiation of low–molecular-weight heparins (SC route), direct oral anticoagulants (DOACs) (apixaban, rivaroxaban), or IV heparin should be considered.
- Placement of an inferior vena cava (IVC) filter is considered if anticoagulation is contraindicated (head, ocular or spinal surgery/trauma, hemorrhagic stroke, severe thrombocytopenia [platelets <50,000], concurrent bleeding [GI]).

Pharmacologic Therapy

Anticoagulation Therapy

Anticoagulant therapy (unfractionated or low–molecular-weight heparins) is traditionally the primary method for managing acute DVT and PE. Refer to Figure 9-11 for Risk and Treatment Algorithm for Pulmonary Embolism. Heparin is used to prevent recurrence of emboli but has no effect on emboli that are already present. Heparin is generally recommended for all patients who have been diagnosed with PE and should be administered by continuous intravenous infusion and dosed using weight-based nomograms. In general, a therapeutic heparin dose is administered as a one-time 80 units/kg bolus, and then a continuous IV infusion (18 units/kg/hr) is started to maintain the PTT at 1.5 to 2.5 times the normal level or anti-Xa level of 0.3–0.7 units/mL (Lexicomp, 2022b). Rapid achievement and maintenance of a therapeutic PTT or anti-Xa are important to reduce the risk for recurrent PE. In addition to examining the PTT or anti-Xa, a complete blood count is monitored, generally a minimum of two to three times per week due to the risk for bleeding and heparin-induced thrombocytopenia (HIT), discussed in Chapter 13. Enoxaparin, a low–molecular-weight heparin, is administered subcutaneously at 1 mg/kg every 12 hours or 1.5 mg/kg daily. This should be reserved for hemodynamically stable patients in order to ensure that the drug is being absorbed into the vasculature. Enoxaparin has an advantage over heparin as its levels do not need to be monitored in most cases and IV access is not an issue. People who are pregnant, have a BMI ≥30 kg/m^2, or weigh less than 45 kg (female) or 57 kg (male) should have anti-Xa peak levels monitored (drawn 4 to 6 hours after third dose administered) (Lexicomp, 2022a).

Therapy may be changed to an oral regimen, such as warfarin, as soon as the patient is able to take oral medications. Heparin must be continued until the INR is within a therapeutic range, typically 2 to 3 (Lexicomp, 2022b). Once the patient starts an oral regimen, it is important that they continue to take the same brand of warfarin because the bioavailability may vary greatly among brands.

High doses of subcutaneous low-molecular-weight heparin or heparinoids may also be used to maintain a therapeutic PTT or anti-Xa level while oral anticoagulation therapy is being adjusted. Argatroban and bivalirudin are

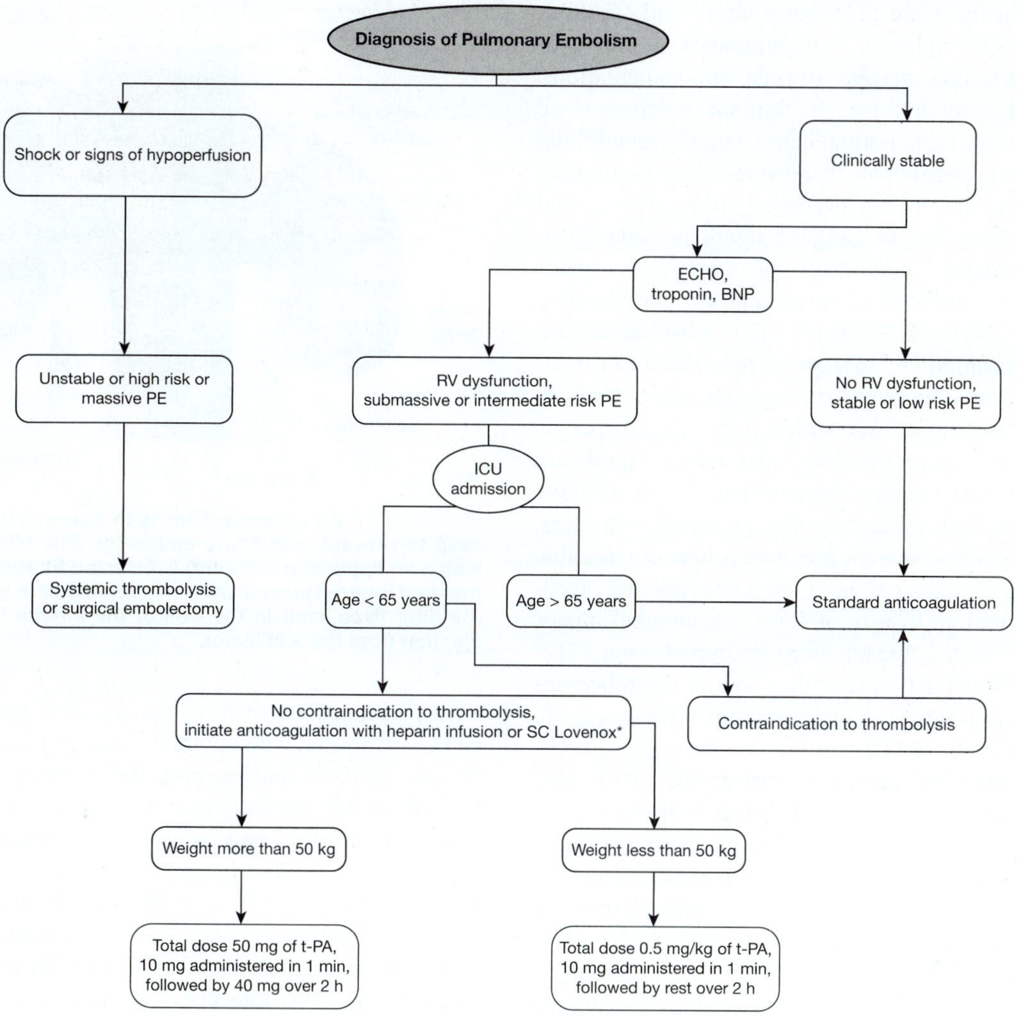

* If no renal dysfunction, use enoxaparin 1 mg/kg SC, maximum dose to not exceed 80 mg BID. If renal dysfunction, use IV heparin infusion with initial bolus at 70 mg/kg, max dose not to exceed 6,000 Units. During t-PA Infusion and 3 hours after infusion, heparin infusion was dosed at 10 U/kg/h or a maximum of 1,000 U/hr. Subsequent dose titrated to 1.5–2 times aPTT with initial maintenance of 18 U/kg/h.

Doses adapted from the MOPETT trial.

FIGURE 9-11 Decision-making algorithm for pulmonary embolism. (Mattu, A., Chanmugam, A. S., Swadron, S. P., Woolridge, D., & Winters, M. [2017]. ***Avoiding common errors in the emergency department*** **[2nd ed., Fig. 238-1]. Wolters Kluwer. Used with permission.)**

alternatives for patients in whom heparin or heparinoids are contraindicated (e.g., patients with HIT). These agents are direct thrombin inhibitors; therefore, they require less frequent monitoring and dose adjustment. Both medications have contraindications and side effects that the nurse must be aware of before administration. Heparins, argatroban, and bivalirudin are all contraindicated in patients with overt major bleeding and in patients who are hypersensitive to these agents or at high risk for bleeding (e.g., recent CVA), anomaly of vessels or organs, recent major surgery, recent puncture of large vessels, or organ biopsy. Major side effects are bleeding anywhere in the body and anaphylactic reaction resulting in shock or death. Other side effects include fever, abnormal liver function, and allergic skin reaction. Patients must continue to take some form of anticoagulation for at least 3 to 6 months after the embolic event.

Novel oral anticoagulants such as apixaban and rivaroxaban (factor Xa inhibitors) are now approved for the initial treatment of DVT and PE. Dabigatran (direct thrombin inhibitor) and edoxaban (factor Xa inhibitor) are approved for treatment or DVT and PE after initial therapy with parenteral anticoagulation is used (Bikdeli et al., 2022). These agents have the advantage of not requiring monitoring of INR or PTT levels, but renal function must be assessed during therapy (refer to Chapter 17 for more details on DVT).

Thrombolytic Therapy

Thrombolytic therapy (urokinase, streptokinase, tPA) also may be used in treating PE, particularly for patients who are severely compromised (e.g., those who are hypotensive or have RV dysfunction, patent foramen ovale, large or saddle embolism [this term refers to a relatively large clot that is lodged within the main pulmonary artery and straddles [extends into] both right and left pulmonary arteries], or significant hypoxemia despite oxygen supplementation). Thrombolytic therapy dissolves the thrombi or emboli more quickly and restores more normal hemodynamic functioning of the pulmonary circulation, thereby reducing pulmonary hypertension and improving perfusion, oxygenation, and cardiac output. However, bleeding is a significant side effect, up to 13% of patients who undergo this therapy experience a major bleed, and the rate of intracranial or fatal bleeding can reach 1.8% (Weitz & Ginsberg, 2020). Absolute contraindications to thrombolytic therapy include history of hemorrhagic CVA, active intracranial neoplasm, recent brain or spinal surgery, ischemic CVA within 3 months, suspected aortic dissection, active bleeding, and recent significant closed head or facial trauma (Sherman et al., 2023). Relative contraindications for thrombolytic therapy are age >75 years, current use of anticoagulation, pregnancy, noncompressible vascular punctures, CPR >10 minutes, recent internal bleeding, dementia, remote history of CVA (<3 months), major surgery within 3 weeks, and uncontrolled hypertension (SBP greater than 180 or DBP greater than 110 or thrombocytopenia of less than 100,000 platelets per mm^3) (Powers et al., 2019; Sherman et al., 2023).

Before thrombolytic therapy is started, INR, PTT, Hct, and platelet counts are obtained. Heparin is stopped prior to administration of a thrombolytic agent. During therapy, all but essential invasive procedures are avoided because of potential bleeding. If necessary, packed red cells, cryoprecipitate, or frozen plasma is administered to replace blood loss and reverse the bleeding tendency. After the thrombolytic infusion is completed (which varies in duration according to the agent used and the condition being treated), anticoagulant therapy is initiated.

Surgical Management

A surgical embolectomy is rarely performed but may be indicated if the patient has a massive PE or hemodynamic instability and must have the clot removed to help reduce right-sided heart failure, or if there are contraindications to thrombolytic therapy. This invasive procedure involves removal of the actual clot and must be performed by a cardiovascular surgical team with the patient on cardiopulmonary bypass. The procedure has a high intraoperative mortality rate and has typical postoperative complications.

Venous catheter embolectomy via rheolytic (injection of pressured saline or TPA) or rotating blades can be used to break up clots in the pulmonary vasculature. These catheters are placed via the femoral vein, threaded through the right heart, and up to the clot. An IVC filter is usually inserted at the time of surgery to protect against a recurrence.

IVC filters are mesh-like devices used to trap thrombi from the pelvic and lower extremities to prevent them from traveling to the lungs. The IVC filters can be either permanent or retrievable. Research reveals that the filters do not have prolonged survival, in part because permanent filters can be associated with complications such as IVC occlusion because of clots, and recurrent DVT. Alternatively, retrievable filters have recently been noted for problems of device migration or thrombosis in up to 10% of patients. Thus the insertion of IVC filters generally is restricted to patients who have high risk for recurrent PE and an absolute contraindication for anticoagulation, experience significant bleeding while on anticoagulation, or recurrent PE despite adequate treatment. The IVC filters (e.g., Greenfield filter) are inserted via the femoral or internal jugular vein (Fig. 9-12). This filter is advanced into the IVC, where it is opened.

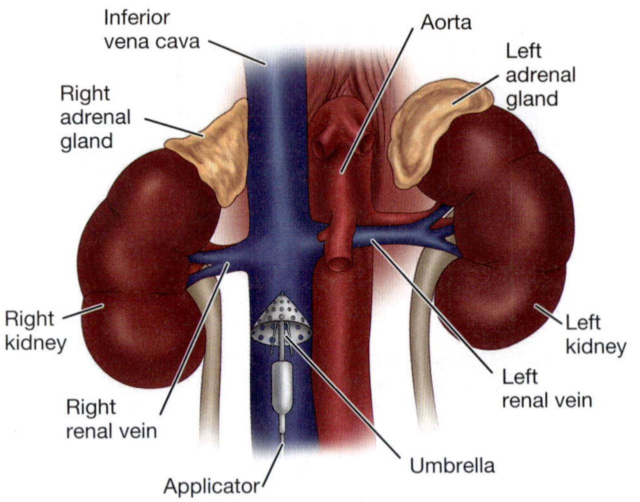

FIGURE 9-12 An umbrella filter is in place in the inferior vena cava to prevent pulmonary embolism. The filter (compressed within an applicator catheter) is inserted through an incision in the right internal jugular vein. The applicator is withdrawn when the filter fixes itself to the wall of the inferior vena cava after ejection from the applicator.

Nursing Management

Minimizing the Risk of Pulmonary Embolism

A key role of the nurse is to identify the patient at high risk for PE and to minimize the risk of PE in all patients. The nurse must have a high degree of suspicion for PE in all patients but particularly in those with conditions predisposed to a slowing of venous return.

Preventing Thrombus Formation

Preventing thrombus formation is a major nursing responsibility. The nurse encourages ambulation and active and passive leg exercises to prevent venous stasis in patients who are prescribed bed rest. The nurse instructs the patient to move the legs in a "pumping" exercise so that the leg muscles can help increase venous flow. The nurse also advises the patient not to sit or lie in bed for prolonged periods, not to cross the legs, and not to wear constrictive clothing. Legs should not be dangled or feet placed in a dependent position while the patient sits on the edge of the bed; instead, feet should rest on the floor or on a chair. In addition, IV catheters (for parenteral therapy or measurements of central venous pressure [CVP]) should not be left in place for prolonged periods.

Assessing Potential for Pulmonary Embolism

All patients are evaluated for risk factors for thrombus formation and PE. The nurse does a careful assessment of the patient's health history, family history, and medication record. On a daily basis, the patient is asked about pain or discomfort in the extremities. In addition, the extremities are evaluated for unilateral leg warmth, redness, and inflammation.

Monitoring Thrombolytic Therapy

The nurse is responsible for monitoring thrombolytic and anticoagulant therapy. Thrombolytic therapy (streptokinase, urokinase, tPA) causes lysis of deep vein thrombi and PE, which helps dissolve the clots. During thrombolytic infusion, while the patient remains on bed rest, vital signs are assessed every 15 minutes for 2 hours, then every 2 hours for 4 hours, and invasive procedures are avoided. PTT testing should be performed every 6 hours after thrombolytics are started.

Pearls for Practice

The activated PTT (aPTT) and anti-factor Xa are more sensitive tests than the PTT for the monitoring of heparin therapy. A normal APTT is 21 to 35 seconds and anti-factor Xa activity <0.30. The goal of heparin therapy is to extend the aPTT to 1.5 or 2.5 the normal level and anti-factor Xa activity to 0.5 to 1 (low–molecular weight heparin) and 0.3 to 0.7 (heparin). The nurse is aware that when the aPTT is over 70 seconds or anti-factor Xa activity >1, the risk for spontaneous bleeding increases. Many institutions have protocols for increasing or decreasing the heparin dosage depending on the aPTT or anti-factor Xa activity. If no protocols are available, the nurse contacts the provider immediately with aPTTs of greater than 90 seconds.

The INR was developed as a consistent way of monitoring prothrombin times, which are used for monitoring warfarin therapy. A normal INR is about 1. The goal of warfarin therapy is to extend the INR to 2 to 3, depending on the reason the patient is anticoagulated. The higher the number, the longer the blood takes to clot. A patient with atrial fibrillation may have a goal INR of 2.5, whereas a patient with a mechanical heart valve may have a maximum goal of an INR of 3.5. Any INR over 3.6 is a critical value that necessitates notification of the patient's provider. With an elevated aPTT and/or INR, the nurse observes the patient for hematuria, hematemesis, melena, petechiae, unusual bruising, and any evidence of bleeding (hypotension, tachycardia, dyspnea, etc.).

Managing Pain

Chest pain, if present, is usually pleuritic rather than cardiac in origin. A semi-Fowler position provides a more comfortable position for breathing. It is important to continue to turn patients frequently and reposition them to improve the **ventilation–perfusion ratio** in the lung. The nurse administers opioid analgesics as prescribed for severe pain.

Managing Oxygen Therapy

It is important to ensure that the patient understands the need for continuous oxygen therapy. The nurse assesses the patient frequently for signs of hypoxemia and monitors the POX values to evaluate the effectiveness of the oxygen therapy. Deep breathing and IS are indicated for all patients to minimize or prevent atelectasis and improve ventilation. Nebulizer therapy or percussion and postural drainage may be used for management of secretions.

Relieving Anxiety

The nurse encourages the stabilized patient to talk about any fears or concerns related to this frightening episode, answers the patient's and family's questions concisely and accurately, explains the therapy, and describes how to recognize untoward effects early.

Monitoring for Complications

When caring for a patient who has had PE, the nurse must be alert for the potential complication of cardiogenic shock or right ventricular failure subsequent to the effect of PE on the cardiovascular system.

Providing Postoperative Care

The nurse measures the patient's pulmonary arterial pressure or CVP, and urinary output. The nurse also assesses the insertion site of the arterial catheter for hematoma formation and infection. It is important to maintain the BP at a level that supports perfusion of vital organs. To prevent peripheral venous stasis and edema of the lower extremities, the nurse encourages isometric exercises, use of mechanical devices, elastic compression stockings (depending on institutional protocol), and walking when the patient is permitted out of bed. Sitting is discouraged, because hip flexion compresses the large veins in the legs.

Pearls for Practice

The nurse is aware that a mean arterial pressure (MAP) of 65 mm Hg is recommended to maintain adequate tissue perfusion.

OCCUPATIONAL LUNG DISEASES

Diseases of the lungs occur in numerous occupations as a result of exposure to several different types of agents.

Examples include mineral dusts (asbestos, silica, coal), metal dusts, biologic dusts (spores, mycelia, bird droppings), manufactured fibers (glass or ceramic fibers), and toxic fumes (nitrogen dioxide, sulfur dioxide, chlorine, ammonia). One category of occupational lung disease that causes chronic fibrotic lung disease is pneumoconiosis, which is caused by the inhalation of inert, inorganic, or silicate dusts. The effects of inhaling these materials depend on the composition of the substance, its concentration, its ability to initiate an immune response, its irritating properties, the duration of exposure, and the individual's response or susceptibility to the irritant. The most common types of pneumoconiosis are coal worker's pneumoconiosis, silicosis, and **asbestosis**. Smoking may compound the problem and may increase the risk of lung cancers in people exposed to the mineral asbestos and other potential carcinogens. Many people with early pneumoconiosis are asymptomatic, but advanced disease often is accompanied by disability and premature death. Between 1996 and 2005, pneumoconiosis was cited as the cause of death of 9,646 people in the United States (CDC, 2011, 2022L).

Silicosis is a chronic fibrotic pulmonary disease caused by inhalation of silica dust (silicon dioxide). Exposure to silica and silicates occurs in almost all mining, quarrying, and tunneling operations. Glass manufacturing, stone-cutting, manufacturing of abrasives and pottery, and foundry work are other occupations with exposure hazards. Finely ground silica, such as that found in soaps, polishes, and filters, is extremely dangerous (Fitzpatrick et al., 2022a).

Asbestosis is a disease characterized by diffuse nodular interstitial fibrosis from the inhalation of asbestos dust. Current laws restrict the use of asbestos, but many industries used it in the past. Therefore, exposure occurred, and may still occur, in people in numerous occupations, including asbestos mining and manufacturing, shipbuilding, demolition of structures containing asbestos, and roofing. Materials such as shingles, cement, vinyl asbestos tile, fireproof paint and clothing, brake linings, and filters all contained asbestos at one time, and many of these materials are still in existence. Chronic exposure may also occur by washing clothes that have been in contact with asbestos. Additional diseases related to asbestos exposure include lung cancer, mesothelioma, and asbestos-related pleural effusion (Fitzpatrick et al., 2022a).

Coal worker's pneumoconiosis ("black lung disease") includes a variety of respiratory diseases found in coal workers who have inhaled coal dust over the years. Coal miners are exposed to dusts that are mixtures of coal, kaolin, mica, and silica (Fitzpatrick et al., 2022a).

Pathophysiology

The pathophysiology of each type of pneumoconiosis (any chronic lung disease caused by the inhalation of particles) begins with the inhalation and deposition of industrial dusts or particles in the lungs. In silicosis, the inhaled silica particles form nodular lesions throughout the lungs. With the passage of time and further exposure, the nodules enlarge and coalesce. Dense masses form in the upper portion of the lungs, resulting in the loss of pulmonary volume. **Restrictive lung disease** (disease of the lungs that limits their ability to expand fully) and obstructive lung disease from secondary emphysema result. Cavities can form as a result of superimposed TB. Exposure of 15 to 20 years is usually required before the onset of the disease and shortness of breath occurs. Fibrotic destruction of pulmonary tissue can lead to emphysema, pulmonary hypertension, and cor pulmonale (right ventricular failure).

In asbestosis, inhaled asbestos fibers enter the alveoli, where they are surrounded by fibrous tissue. The fibrous tissue eventually obliterates the alveoli. Fibrous changes also affect the pleura, which thickens and develops plaque. The result of these physiologic changes is a restrictive lung disease, with a decrease in lung volume, diminished exchange of oxygen and carbon dioxide, and hypoxemia.

When coal dust is deposited in the alveoli and respiratory bronchioles, macrophages engulf the particles (by phagocytosis) and transport them to the terminal bronchioles, where they are removed by mucociliary action. In time, the clearance mechanisms cannot handle the excessive dust load, and the macrophages aggregate in the respiratory bronchioles and alveoli. Fibroblasts appear and a network of reticulin (similar in composition to collagen) is laid down surrounding the dust-laden macrophages. The bronchioles and the alveoli become clogged with coal dust, dying macrophages, and fibroblasts. This leads to the formation of the coal macule, the primary lesion of the disorder. Macules appear as blackish dots on the lungs. Fibrotic lesions develop and, as the macules enlarge, the weakening bronchioles dilate, with subsequent development of localized emphysema. The disease begins in the upper lobes of the lungs but may progress to the lower lobes.

Clinical Manifestations and Assessment

Patients with acute silicosis present with dyspnea, fever, cough, and weight loss, and progression of the disease is rapid. Symptoms are more severe in patients whose disease is complicated by progressive massive fibrosis. More commonly, this disease is a chronic problem with a long latency period. In patients with asbestosis, the onset of the disease is insidious, and patients have progressive dyspnea, persistent, dry cough, mild to moderate chest pain, anorexia, weight loss, and malaise. Early physical findings include bibasilar fine, end-inspiratory crackles, and, in more advanced cases, clubbing of the fingers. Patients with coal miner's disease usually present with a chronic cough and sputum production, similar to the signs encountered in chronic bronchitis. As the disease progresses, patients develop dyspnea and cough up large amounts of sputum with varying amounts of black fluid (melanoptysis), particularly if they are smokers.

As each of these diseases progresses, worsening dyspnea and hypoxemia occur. Eventually, patients develop respiratory failure and cor pulmonale. A high proportion of workers who have been exposed to asbestos dust, especially those who smoke or have a history of smoking, die of lung cancer. Malignant mesothelioma, a rare cancer of the pleura or peritoneum that is strongly associated with asbestos exposure, may also occur.

Medical Management

The medical treatment for these specific pneumoconioses is limited to supportive care, as the fibrotic process is irreversible. Oxygen therapy, diuretics, inhaled beta-adrenergic agonists, anticholinergics, and bronchodilator therapy can be used to maximize pulmonary and cardiac function and preserve activity tolerance. It is imperative that patients avoid any additional environmental exposures and stop smoking. There is a higher incidence of TB in patients with silicosis; therefore, they should have a tuberculin skin test and chest radiograph. Preventing this disease is key because there is no effective treatment. Instead, treatment focuses on early diagnosis and management of complications.

CHEST TUMORS

Tumors of the lung may be benign or malignant. A malignant chest tumor can be primary, arising within the lung, chest wall, or mediastinum, or it can be a metastasis from a primary tumor site elsewhere in the body. Metastatic lung tumors occur frequently because the bloodstream transports cancer cells from primary cancers elsewhere in the body to the lungs.

LUNG CANCER (BRONCHOGENIC CARCINOMA)

Lung cancer is the leading cancer killer among males and females in the United States. In 2019, 221,097 people in the United States were diagnosed with lung cancer. That same year, 139,601 people died of the disease. There has been a statistical decrease in the incidence of lung cancer in both males and females (except American Indian, Alaska Native, and Asian/Pacific Islander women) in the years between 2002 and 2019 (CDC, 2022d). In approximately 70% of patients with lung cancer, the disease has spread to regional lymphatics and other sites by the time of diagnosis. As a result, the long-term survival rate is low.

Pathophysiology

Eighty percent of lung cancer in females and 90% in males are caused by cigarette smoking, with the remainder being attributed to other carcinogens, including radon gas and occupational and environmental agents (CDC, 2021).

Classification and Staging

For purposes of staging and treatment, most lung cancers are classified into one of two major categories: small cell lung cancer (25% of lung cancers) and nonsmall cell lung cancer (75% of lung cancers) (Table 9-4). In nonsmall cell lung carcinoma (NSCLC), the cell types include squamous cell carcinoma (20% to 30%), large cell carcinoma (10%), and

TABLE **9-4 Lung Cancer Types and Characteristics**

Tumor Classification	Growth Rate	Clinical Manifestations	Treatment	Metastasis
Nonsmall Cell Lung Cancer (NSCLC)				
Squamous cell	Slow	Cough, hemoptysis, pneumonia, atelectasis, chest pain (late sign), unexplained weight loss	Surgical resection, adjunctive chemotherapy	Late: Brain, liver, bones, adrenals
Adenocarcinoma	Moderate	Dyspnea, pleuritic chest pain, pleural effusions, unexplained weight loss	Surgical resection, adjunctive chemotherapy	Early: Liver, brain, bones, kidneys, adrenals
Large cell (undifferentiated)	Rapid	Chest wall pain, cough, sputum production, hemoptysis, pleural effusion, pneumonia, unexplained weight loss	Surgical resection	Early: Brain, liver, bones, adrenals
Small Cell Lung Cancer (SCLC)				
Oat cell and intermediate cell type	Very rapid	Cough, unexplained weight loss, dyspnea, airway obstruction, hilar mass on x-ray, pneumonia, paraneoplastic syndromes (SIADH, hypercalcemia, Cushing's, myopathies)	Chemotherapy, radiation therapy	Early: Liver, bone, bone marrow, brain, adrenals

SIADH, syndrome of inappropriate antidiuretic hormone secretion.

adenocarcinoma (30% to 40%), including bronchoalveolar carcinoma. Most small cell carcinomas arise in the major bronchi and spread by infiltration along the bronchial wall.

In addition to classification according to cell type, lung cancers are staged. The stage of the tumor refers to the size of the tumor, its location, whether lymph nodes are involved, and whether the cancer has metastasized, referred to as the TNM ("T" refers to the extent of the primary tumor, "N" refers to lymph node involvement, and "M" refers to the extent of metastasis) (Archer et al., 2022). NSCLC is staged as I to IV. Stage I is the earliest stage and has the highest cure rates, whereas stage IV designates metastatic spread. Small cell lung cancers are classified as limited or extensive. Diagnostic tools and further information on staging were described in Chapter 5.

Risk Factors

Various factors have been associated with the development of lung cancer (Box 9-14). Other factors that have been associated with lung cancer include genetic predisposition and underlying respiratory diseases, such as COPD and TB. Since tobacco smoking is the most important risk factor, the U.S. Preventive Services Task Force recommends that smokers with a 20-pack year smoking history be screened annually with low-dose CT (USPSTF, 2021).

Clinical Manifestations and Assessment

Often, lung cancer develops insidiously and is asymptomatic until late in its course. The signs and symptoms depend on the location and size of the tumor, the degree of obstruction, and the existence of metastases to regional or distant sites. The most frequent symptom of lung cancer is cough or change in a chronic cough. The cough starts as a dry, persistent cough, without sputum production. When obstruction of airways occurs, the cough may become productive due to infection.

Dyspnea occurs in many patients. Hemoptysis or blood-tinged sputum may be expectorated. Chest or shoulder pain may indicate chest wall or pleural involvement by a tumor. Pain also is a late manifestation and may be related to metastasis to the bone.

BOX 9-14 Risk Factors Associated With Lung Cancer

- Tobacco smoking: Assess pack/year history (number of packs smoked per day × years of smoking)
- Passive smoking
- Secondhand smoke (closed areas; home, building, automobile)
- Environmental and occupational exposure (vehicle emissions, pollutants, urban areas, radon gas, arsenic, asbestos, chromates, coal fumes, radiation)
- Family history (close relative with lung cancer)
- Low intake of fruits and vegetables

In some patients, a recurring fever is an early symptom in response to a persistent infection in an area distal to the tumor. In fact, cancer of the lung should be suspected in people with repeated unresolved upper respiratory tract infections. If the tumor spreads to adjacent structures and regional lymph nodes, the patient may present with chest pain and tightness, hoarseness (involving the recurrent laryngeal nerve), dysphagia, head and neck edema, and symptoms of pleural or pericardial effusion. The most common sites of metastases are lymph nodes, bone, brain, contralateral lung, adrenal glands, and liver. Nonspecific symptoms of weakness, anorexia, and weight loss also may be present.

If pulmonary symptoms occur in smokers, cancer of the lung should always be considered. A chest x-ray is performed to search for pulmonary densities, pulmonary nodules, atelectasis, and infection. CT scans of the chest are used to identify small nodules not easily visualized on the chest x-ray and also to examine areas for lymphadenopathy.

Fiberoptic bronchoscopy provides a detailed study of the tracheobronchial tree and allows for brushings, washings, and biopsies of suspicious areas. For peripheral lesions not amenable to bronchoscopic biopsy, a transthoracic **fine-needle aspiration** may be performed under CT guidance to aspirate cells from a suspicious area. In some circumstances, an endoscopy with esophageal ultrasound may be used to obtain a transesophageal biopsy of enlarged subcarinal (below the carina) lymph nodes that are not easily accessible by other means.

A variety of scans may be used to assess for metastasis of the cancer. These may include bone scans, abdominal scans, positron emission tomography (PET) scans, and liver ultrasound. CT of the brain, magnetic resonance imaging (MRI), and other neurologic diagnostic procedures are used to detect CNS metastases. Mediastinoscopy or mediastinotomy may be used to obtain biopsy samples from lymph nodes in the mediastinum.

If surgery is a potential treatment, the patient is evaluated to determine whether the tumor is resectable and whether the patient can tolerate the physiologic impairment resulting from such surgery. Pulmonary function tests, ABG analysis, $\dot{V}/\dot{Q}$ scans, and exercise testing may all be used as part of the preoperative assessment.

Medical Management

The objective of management is to provide a cure, if possible. Treatment depends on the cell type, the stage of the disease, and the patient's physiologic status (particularly cardiac and pulmonary status). In general, treatment may involve surgery, radiation therapy (XRT), or chemotherapy—or a combination of these. Newer and more specific therapies to modulate the immune system (gene therapy, therapy with defined tumor antigens) are under study.

Surgical Management

Surgical resection is the preferred method of treating patients with localized nonsmall cell tumors, no evidence of metastatic spread, and adequate cardiopulmonary function. The cure rate of surgical resection depends on the type and stage of the cancer. Surgery is primarily used for NSCLCs because small cell cancer of the lung grows rapidly and metastasizes early and extensively. Lesions of many patients with bronchogenic cancer are inoperable at the time of diagnosis.

Several different types of lung resection may be performed. The most common surgical procedure for a small, apparently curable tumor of the lung is lobectomy (removal of a lobe of the lung). In some cases, an entire lung may be removed (pneumonectomy).

Radiation Therapy

XRT may offer cure in a small percentage of patients. It is useful in controlling neoplasms that cannot be surgically resected but are responsive to radiation. Irradiation also may be used to reduce the size of a tumor, to make an inoperable tumor operable, or to relieve the pressure of the tumor on vital structures. It can reduce symptoms of spinal cord metastasis and superior vena caval compression. Also, XRT is used to treat metastases to the brain. XRT may help relieve cough, chest pain, dyspnea, hemoptysis, and bone and liver pain. Relief of symptoms may last from a few weeks to many months and is important in improving the quality of the remaining period of life. Radiofrequency ablation and cryoablation are two types of nonsurgical therapies that have been used to treat lung tumors.

Chemotherapy, Targeted Therapy, and Immunotherapy

Chemotherapy is used to alter tumor growth patterns, to treat distant metastases or small cell cancer of the lung, and as an adjunct to surgery or XRT. Chemotherapy may provide relief, especially of pain, but it does not usually cure the disease or prolong life to any great degree. Chemotherapy is also accompanied by side effects. It is valuable in reducing pressure symptoms of lung cancer and in treating brain, spinal cord, and pericardial metastases. Targeted therapy (TT) targets specific proteins, genes and tissue to block the growth and spread of cancer cells (afatinib, dacomitinib, getitnib). Immunotherapy (IT) enhances natural immune defenses against cancer cell pathways (PD-1, PD-PL1, CTLA-4 pathways) (ipilimumab, pembrolizumab, nivolumab) (ASCO, 2022). The choice of agent depends on the growth of the tumor cell and the specific phase of the cell cycle that the medication affects. In combination, TT and IT with surgery, chemotherapy may be administered before surgery (neoadjuvant therapy) or after surgery (adjuvant therapy). Combinations of two or more medications may be more beneficial than single-dose regimens.

Palliative Therapy

Palliative therapy may include XRT or chemotherapy to shrink the tumor to provide pain relief, a variety of bronchoscopic interventions to open a narrowed bronchus or airway, and pain management and other comfort measures. Evaluation and referral for hospice care are important in planning for comfortable and dignified end-of-life care for the patient and family (refer to Chapter 2).

Treatment-Related Complications

A variety of complications may occur as a result of treatment for lung cancer. Surgical resection may result in respiratory failure, particularly if the cardiopulmonary system is compromised before surgery. Surgical complications and prolonged mechanical ventilation are potential outcomes. XRT may result in diminished cardiopulmonary function and other complications, such as pulmonary fibrosis, pericarditis, myelitis, and cor pulmonale. Chemotherapy, particularly in combination with XRT, can cause pneumonitis. TT and IT can cause dizziness, nausea, fatigue, diarrhea, and skin rashes. Pulmonary and systemic toxicity is a potential side effect of chemotherapy, IT, and TT.

Nursing Management

Nursing care of patients with lung cancer is similar to that for other patients with cancer and addresses the physiologic and psychological needs of the patient. The physiologic problems are primarily due to the respiratory manifestations of the disease. Nursing care includes strategies to ensure relief of pain and discomfort and to prevent complications.

Managing Symptoms

The nurse instructs the patient and family about the potential side effects of the specific treatment and strategies to manage them. Strategies for managing such symptoms as dyspnea, fatigue, nausea and vomiting, anorexia, and fatigue help the patient and family cope with therapeutic measures. See Chapter 5.

Relieving Breathing Problems

Airway clearance techniques are key to maintaining airway patency through the removal of excess secretions. This may be accomplished through deep-breathing exercises, CPT, directed cough, suctioning, and, in some instances, bronchoscopy. Bronchodilator medications may be prescribed to promote bronchial dilation. As the tumor enlarges or spreads, it may compress a bronchus or involve a large area of lung tissue, resulting in an impaired breathing pattern and poor gas exchange. At some stage of the disease, supplemental oxygen will probably be necessary.

Nursing measures focus on decreasing dyspnea by encouraging the patient to assume positions that promote lung expansion and to perform breathing exercises for lung expansion and relaxation. Patient education about energy conservation and airway clearance techniques is also necessary. Many of the techniques used in pulmonary rehabilitation can be applied to patients with lung cancer. Depending

BOX 9-15 **Highlighting Gerontology**

At the time of diagnosis of lung cancer, most patients are older than 65 years of age and have stage III or IV disease (CDC, 2022d). Although age is not a significant prognostic factor for overall survival and response to treatment for either NSCLC or small cell lung cancer, older patients have specific needs. Depending on the comorbidities and functional status of older patients, chemotherapy agents, doses, and cycles may need to be adjusted to maintain quality of life. Issues that must be considered in the care of older patients with lung cancer include functional status, comorbid conditions, nutritional status, cognition, concomitant medications, and psychological and social support.

on the severity of disease and the patient's wishes, a referral to a pulmonary rehabilitation program may be helpful in managing respiratory symptoms.

Providing Psychological Support

Another important part of the nursing care of patients with lung cancer is provision of psychological support and identification of potential resources for the patient and family (Box 9-15). Refer to Chapter 5.

TUMORS OF THE MEDIASTINUM

Tumors of the mediastinum include neurogenic tumors, tumors of the thymus, lymphomas, germ cell tumors, cysts, and mesenchymal tumors. These tumors may be malignant or benign. They are usually described in relation to location: anterior, middle, or posterior masses or tumors.

Clinical Manifestations and Assessment

Nearly all symptoms of mediastinal tumors result from the pressure of the mass against important intrathoracic organs. Symptoms may include cough, wheezing, dyspnea, anterior chest or neck pain, bulging of the chest wall, heart palpitations, angina, other circulatory disturbances, central cyanosis, superior vena cava syndrome (i.e., swelling of the face, neck, and upper extremities; Fig. 9-13), marked distention of the veins of the neck and the chest wall (evidence of the obstruction of large veins of the mediastinum by extravascular compression or intravascular invasion), and dysphagia and weight loss from pressure or invasion into the esophagus.

Most often, chest x-rays are used to diagnose mediastinal tumors and cysts. CT is the standard diagnostic test for assessment of the mediastinum and surrounding structures. MRI, as well as PET, may be used in some circumstances.

Medical and Nursing Management

If the tumor is malignant and has infiltrated the surrounding tissue and complete surgical removal is not feasible, XRT, chemotherapy, or both are used.

Many mediastinal tumors are benign and operable. The location of the tumor (anterior, middle, or posterior compartment) in the mediastinum dictates the type of incision. The common incision used is a median sternotomy; however, a thoracotomy may be used, depending on the location of the tumor. Additional approaches include a bilateral anterior thoracotomy (clamshell incision) and VATS. The care is the same as for any patient undergoing thoracic surgery. Major complications include hemorrhage, injury to the phrenic or laryngeal nerve, and infection.

CHEST TRAUMA

Major chest trauma may occur alone or in combination with multiple other injuries. Chest trauma is classified as either blunt or penetrating. Blunt chest trauma results from rapid deceleration injury (e.g., motor vehicle accident [MVA], falls) or direct injury (abuse, crushing, and explosions). Penetrating trauma occurs when a foreign object penetrates the chest wall (stabbing, gunshot wounds, and shrapnel).

BLUNT TRAUMA AND PENETRATING TRAUMA

Blunt thoracic injures are responsible for majority of trauma deaths (Dogrul et al., 2020). It is often difficult to identify the extent of the damage because the symptoms may be occult and vague.

Pathophysiology

The most common causes of blunt chest trauma are MVAs (trauma from steering wheel, seat belt), falls, and bicycle crashes (trauma from handlebars) (Sayed et al., 2022). Mechanisms of blunt chest trauma include acceleration (moving object hitting the chest or patient being thrown into an object), deceleration (sudden decrease in rate of speed or velocity, such as an MVA), shearing (stretching forces to areas of the chest causing tears, ruptures, or dissections), and compression (direct blow to the chest, such as a crush injury or explosion). Injuries to the chest are often life-threatening and result in one or more of the following pathologic states:

- Hypoxemia from disruption of the airway; injury to the lung parenchyma, rib cage, and respiratory musculature; massive hemorrhage; collapsed lung; pulmonary contusion and pneumothorax
- Hypovolemia from massive fluid loss from the great vessels, cardiac rupture, or hemothorax
- Cardiac failure from cardiac tamponade, cardiac contusion, or increased intrathoracic pressure

These pathologic states frequently result in impaired ventilation and perfusion leading to ARF, hypovolemic shock, and death.

Gunshot and stab wounds are the most common causes of penetrating chest trauma. These wounds are classified

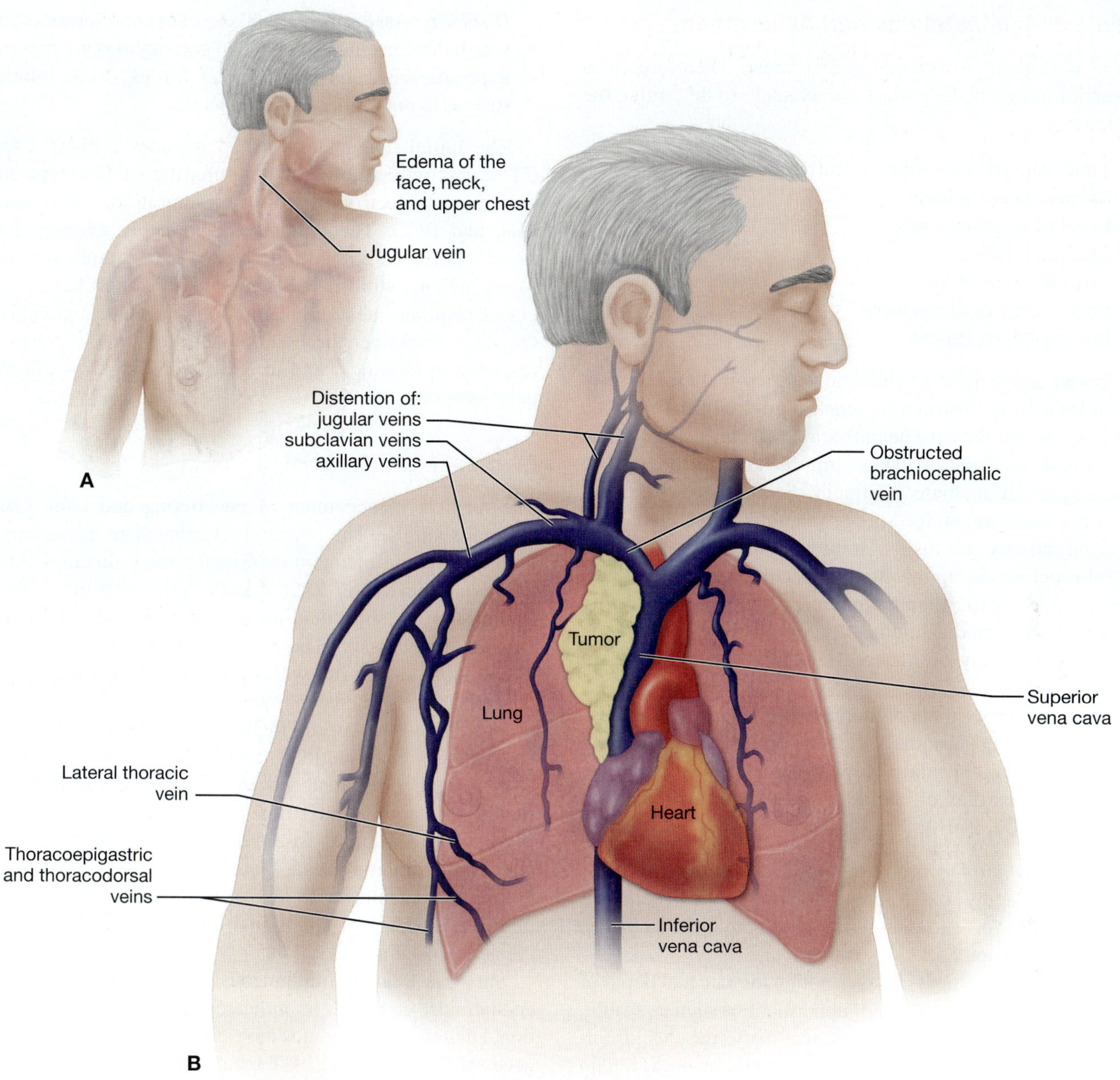

FIGURE 9-13 Clinical signs of the superior vena cava syndrome. (A) Shows facial edema, plethora, jugular venous distention, and prominent superficial vessels in the neck and upper chest. (B) Depicts the vascular anatomy and collateral vessel formation in a patient with superior vena cava syndrome. (DeVita, V. T., Jr., Lawrence, T. S., & Rosenberg, S. A. [2016]. ***DeVita, Hellman, and Rosenberg's cancer, principles and practice of oncology: Review*** **[10th ed.]. Wolters Kluwer. Used with permission.)**

according to their velocity. In general, stab wounds are considered low-velocity trauma because the weapon destroys a small area around the wound. The appearance of the external wound may be very deceptive because pneumothorax, hemothorax, lung contusion, and cardiac tamponade, along with severe and continuing hemorrhage, can occur from any small wound, even one caused by a small-diameter instrument such as an ice pick.

Gunshot wounds may be classified as low-, medium-, or high-velocity. The factors that determine the velocity and resulting extent of damage include the distance from which the gun was fired, the caliber of the gun, and the construction and size of the bullet. A bullet can cause damage at the site of penetration and along its pathway, and a gunshot wound to the chest can produce a variety of pathophysiologic changes. The bullet may ricochet off bony structures and damage the chest organs and great vessels or can travel into the abdomen. If the diaphragm is involved in a gunshot wound or a stab wound, injury to the chest cavity must be considered.

Clinical Manifestations and Assessment

Time is critical in treating chest trauma. Therefore, it is essential to assess the patient immediately to determine the following:

- Time elapsed since injury occurred
- Mechanism of injury
- Level of responsiveness
- Specific injuries
- Estimated blood loss
- Recent drug or alcohol use
- Prehospital treatment

Initial assessment of thoracic injuries includes assessment for airway obstruction, **tension pneumothorax**, open pneumothorax, massive hemothorax, flail chest, and cardiac tamponade and rupture. These injuries are life-threatening and require immediate treatment. Secondary assessment includes assessment for simple pneumothorax, hemothorax, pulmonary contusion, traumatic aortic rupture, tracheobronchial disruption, sternal fracture, esophageal perforation, traumatic diaphragmatic injury, and penetrating wounds to the mediastinum. Although listed as secondary, these injuries may be life-threatening as well (Gao et al., 2022).

The rapid assessment of thoracic injuries involves the use of the Advanced Trauma Life Support (ATLS) algorithm of "**C**atastrophic bleeding, **A**irway, **B**reathing, **C**irculation, **D**isability (neurologic), and **E**xposure/Environmental control" (ACSCOT, 2018):

- *Catastrophic bleeding:* Assess for life-threatening hemorrhage, apply direct pressure compression bandage; tourniquet for extremity bleeding (note time applied). Refer to Chapter 55.
- *Airway:* Assessment includes noting the rate and depth of breathing and observing for abnormalities such as stridor, cyanosis, nasal flaring, use of accessory muscles, drooling, and overt trauma to the face, mouth, or neck; obtain POX. Use cervical immobilization, avoiding excessive movement if spinal injury is suspected, and apply cervical collar.
- *Breathing:* Assess the chest for symmetric movement, symmetry of breath sounds, open chest wounds, entrance or exit wounds, impaled objects, distended neck veins, and paradoxical chest wall motion. Palpate the thorax for tenderness and crepitus (subcutaneous emphysema), and assess the position of the trachea. In addition, assess the chest wall for bruising, petechiae, lacerations, and burns. Note mental status to support airway protection.
- *Circulation:* Assess vital signs (quality of pulse, pulse pressure, BP, MAP), cardiac rhythm, and skin color, temperature, capillary refill; note evidence of shock (increased HR, increased RR, decreased BP, narrow PP, decreased MAP, delayed capillary refill, cool extremities, mottled skin, etc.).
- *Disability:* Assess the patient's level of consciousness and note if concurrent head or spinal cord injuries are present.
- *Exposure/Environmental:* Assess for exposure injuries such as hypothermia or hyperthermia.

The initial diagnostic workup includes a chest x-ray, CT scan, complete blood count, clotting studies, type and crossmatch, electrolytes, oxygen saturation, ABG analysis, and ECG. The patient is completely undressed to avoid missing additional injuries that may complicate care. Many patients with injuries involving the chest have associated head and abdominal injuries that require attention. Ongoing assessment is essential to monitor the patient's response to treatment and to detect early signs of clinical deterioration.

Medical Management

The medical management of penetrating and blunt chest trauma is similar. The objective of immediate management is to restore and maintain cardiopulmonary function. After an adequate airway is ensured and ventilation is established, examination for shock and intrathoracic and intra-abdominal injuries is necessary. There is a high risk for associated intra-abdominal injuries with stab wounds below the level of the fifth anterior intercostal space (ICS).

The diagnostic workup includes a chest x-ray, chemistry profile, ABG analysis, POX, and ECG. The patient's blood is typed and cross-matched in case blood transfusion is required. After the status of the peripheral pulses is assessed, a large-bore IV line is inserted. An indwelling catheter is inserted to monitor urinary output. A nasogastric tube is inserted and connected to low suction to prevent aspiration, minimize leakage of abdominal contents, and decompress the gastrointestinal tract.

Shock is treated simultaneously with colloid solutions, crystalloids, or blood, as indicated by the patient's condition. Diagnostic procedures are carried out as dictated by the needs of the patient (e.g., CT scans of chest or abdomen, flat plate x-ray of the abdomen, abdominal ultrasound to check for bleeding).

A chest tube is inserted into the pleural space in most patients with penetrating wounds of the chest to achieve rapid and continuing reexpansion of the lungs, especially in wounds above the fifth ICS (nipple line). The insertion of the chest tube frequently results in a complete evacuation of the blood and air. The chest tube also allows early recognition of continuing intrathoracic bleeding, which would make surgical exploration necessary. If the patient has a penetrating wound of the heart or great vessels, the esophagus, or the tracheobronchial tree, surgical intervention is required.

Patients with penetrating chest wound usually require exploratory surgery. In extreme cases, an emergency thoracotomy may be performed in the trauma room to access bleeding from large vessels such as the aorta, pulmonary artery, or heart.

Pearls for Practice

Cues that suggest a chest tube may be required include dyspnea, tachypnea, decreased or absent breath sounds on the affected side, decreased POX, tachycardia, crepitus, hyperresonance on the affected side, tracheal deviation (to unaffected side), anxiety, restlessness, nasal flaring, mouth breathing, and use of accessory muscle.

Chest Tubes

Chest tubes may be inserted to drain fluid or air from any of the three compartments of the thorax (the right and left pleural spaces and the mediastinum). The pleural space, located between the visceral and parietal pleura, normally contains 25 mL or less of fluid, which helps lubricate the visceral and parietal pleura. Surgical incision of the chest wall almost always causes some degree of pneumothorax (air accumulating in the pleural space) or hemothorax (buildup of serous fluid or blood in the pleural space). Air and fluid collect in the pleural space, restricting lung expansion and reducing gas exchange. Placement of a chest tube in the pleural space restores the normal negative intrathoracic pressure needed for lung reexpansion after surgery or trauma.

The mediastinal space is an extrapleural space that lies between the right and left thoracic cavities and contains the large blood vessels, heart, mainstem bronchus, and thymus gland. If fluid accumulates here, the heart can become compressed and stop beating, causing death. Mediastinal chest tubes can be inserted either anteriorly or posteriorly to the heart to drain blood after surgery.

Catheters

There are two types of chest tubes: small-bore or "pigtail catheters" and large-bore catheters. Small-bore catheters (7 to 14 Fr) can be inserted through a small skin incision and are connected to a chest drainage system. Large-bore catheters, which range in size up to 40 Fr, are also usually connected to a **chest drainage system** (Fig. 9-14) to collect any pleural fluid and monitor for air leaks. The nurse is aware that chest tubes are placed around

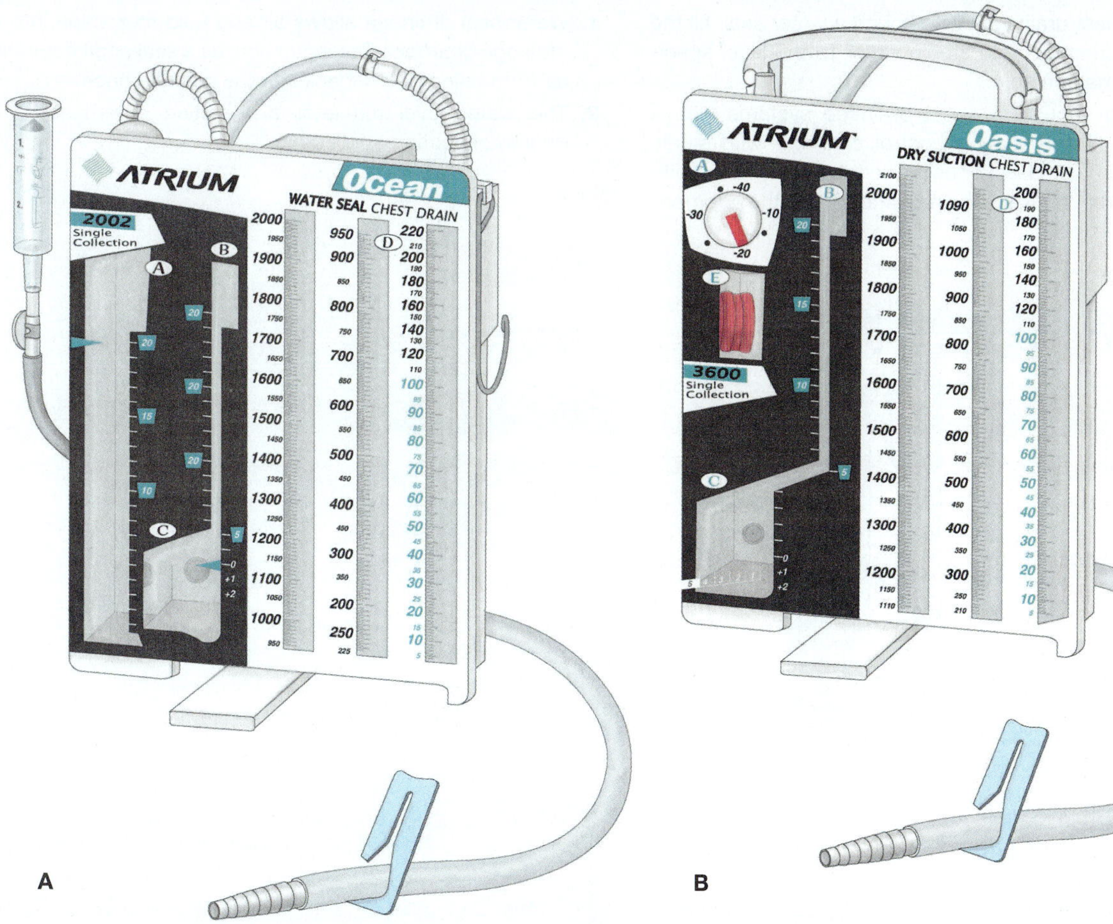

FIGURE 9-14 Chest drainage systems. **A.** The Atrium Ocean is an example of a water-seal chest drain system composed of a drainage chamber and water-seal chamber. The suction control is determined by the height of the water column in that chamber (usually 20 cm). *A*, suction control chamber; *B*, water-seal chamber; *C*, air leak zone; *D*, collection chamber. **B.** The Atrium Oasis is an example of a dry suction water-seal system that uses a mechanical regulator for vacuum control, a water-seal chamber, and a drainage chamber. *A*, dry suction regulator; *B*, water-seal chamber; *C*, air leak monitor; *D*, collection chamber; *E*, suction monitor bellows. (Art redrawn with permission from Atrium Medical Corporation, Hudson, New Hampshire.)

second or third ICS for pneumothorax (air rises) and around the fifth or sixth ICS for fluid (e.g., hemothorax, pleural effusion, postoperatively). After the chest tube is positioned, it is sutured to the skin and connected to a drainage apparatus to remove the residual air and fluid from the pleural or mediastinal space. This results in the reexpansion of remaining lung tissue.

Chest Drainage Systems

Chest drainage systems have a suction source, a collection chamber for pleural drainage, and a mechanism to prevent air from reentering the chest with inhalation. Various types of chest drainage systems are available for use in removal of air and fluid from the pleural space and reexpansion of the lungs. Chest drainage systems come with either wet (water-filled suction chamber) or dry suction control. In wet suction systems, the amount of suction is determined by the amount of water instilled in the suction chamber. Wet systems use a water seal to prevent air from moving back into the chest on inspiration. Dry systems use a one-way valve, have a water-seal chamber and may have a suction control dial in place of the water. Both systems can operate by gravity drainage, without a suction source (Fig. 9-14; Box 9-16).

BOX 9-16

GUIDELINES FOR NURSING CARE

Managing Chest Drainage Systems

Equipment

- Chest drainage system
- Dressings
- Sterile water
- Tape
- Marker

ACTION	RATIONALE
1. If using a chest drainage system with a water seal, fill the water-seal chamber with sterile water to the level specified by the manufacturer.	1. Water-seal drainage allows air and fluid to escape into a drainage chamber. The water acts as a seal and keeps the air from being drawn back into the pleural space.
2. When using suction in chest drainage systems with a water seal, fill the suction control chamber with sterile water to the 20 cm level or as prescribed. In systems with dry suction regulator, set the regulator dial at the appropriate suction level. 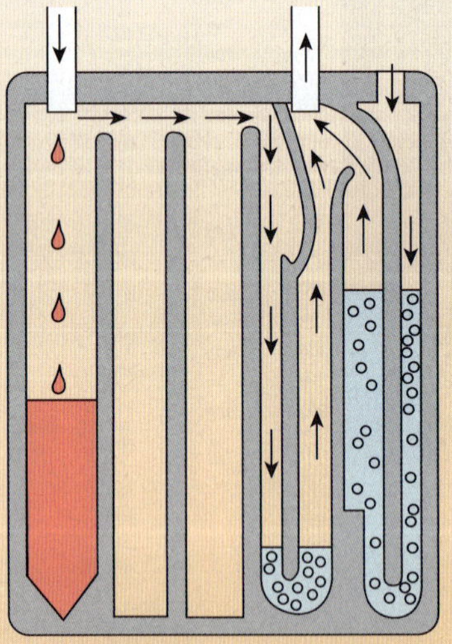 Pleur-evac system.	2. The water level regulator dial setting determines the degree of suction applied.
3. Attach the drainage catheter exiting the thoracic cavity to the tubing coming from the collection chamber. Tape securely with adhesive tape.	3. In chest drainage units, the system is closed.
4. If suction is used, connect the suction control chamber tubing to the suction unit. If using a wet suction system, turn on the suction unit and increase pressure until slow but steady bubbling appears in the suction control chamber. If using a chest drainage system with a dry suction control chamber, turn the regulator dial to 20 cm H_2O.	4. With a wet suction system, the degree of suction is determined by the amount of water in the suction control chamber and is not dependent on the rate of bubbling or the pressure gauge setting on the suction unit. With a dry suction control chamber, the regulator dial replaces the water.

ACTION	RATIONALE
5. Mark the drainage from the collection chamber with tape on the outside of the drainage unit. Mark hourly/daily increments (date and time) at the drainage level. Be familiar with what the expected color of chest drainage should be.	5. This marking shows the amount of fluid loss and how fast fluid is collecting in the drainage chamber. It serves as a basis for determining the need for blood replacement, if the fluid is blood. Visibly bloody drainage will appear in the chamber in the immediate postoperative period but should gradually become serous. Notify the health care provider when there is a sudden increase of more than 100 mL of drainage over 1 hour, or according to the health care provider order, which can indicate fresh bleeding. A reoperation or autotransfusion may be needed. Drainage of 200 mL/hr is usually associated with bleeding complications. Usually, drainage decreases progressively in the first 24 hours. A sudden decrease in the amount of chest tube drainage suggests a possible clot or obstruction in the chest tube (Perry et al., 2022). Recent open-chest surgery drainage is initially bright red and gradually becomes serosanguinous. Blood-tinged fluid is expected from a malignancy, pulmonary infarction, or severe inflammation. Frank blood is expected from a hemothorax. Purulent drainage is expected with an empyema (Perry et al., 2022).
6. Ensure that the drainage tubing does not kink, loop, or interfere with the patient's movements.	6. Kinking, looping, or pressure on the drainage tubing can produce back pressure, which may force fluid back into the pleural space or impede its drainage.
7. Encourage the patient to assume a comfortable position with good body alignment. With the lateral position, make sure that the patient's body does not compress the tubing. The patient should be turned and repositioned every 1.5 to 2 hours. Provide adequate analgesia.	7. Frequent position changes promote drainage, and good body alignment helps prevent postural deformities and contractures. Proper positioning also helps breathing and promotes better air exchange. Analgesics may be needed to promote comfort.
8. Assist the patient with range-of-motion exercises for the affected arm and shoulder several times daily. Provide adequate analgesia.	8. Exercise helps to prevent ankyloses (abnormal stiffening and immobility of a joint) of the shoulder and to reduce postoperative pain and discomfort. Analgesics may be needed to relieve pain.
9. If the drainage is bloody, gently drain the tubing in the direction of the drainage chamber. Gentle "milking" may be warranted if allowed according to institutional policy in cases of active bleeding to prevent obstruction in the tubing. If "gentle milking" is allowed, *do not compress the tubing completely*. In general, the prevention of dependent loops, laying of the tubing horizontally across the bed that then drops vertically into the chest drainage system is sufficient for fluid drainage.	9. Gentle "milking" may prevent the tubing from becoming obstructed by clots and fibrin. Constant attention to maintaining the patency of the tube facilitates prompt expansion of the lung and minimizes complications. However, compressing the tubing may cause high negative pressure in the pleural space and lung entrapment, so routine "milking" is discouraged.
10. Make sure there is fluctuation ("tidaling") of the fluid level in the water-seal chamber (in wet systems), or check the air leak indicator for leaks (in dry systems with a one-way valve). *Note:* Fluid fluctuations in the water-seal chamber or air leak indicator area will stop when: • The lung has reexpanded • The tubing is obstructed by blood clots, fibrin, or kinks • A loop of tubing hangs below the rest of the tubing • Suction motor or wall suction is not working properly	10. Fluctuation of the water level in the water seal shows effective connection between the pleural cavity and the drainage chamber and indicates that the drainage system remains patent. Fluctuation is also a gauge of intrapleural pressure in systems with a water seal (wet and dry, but not with the one-way valve).

(*continued on page 358*)

BOX 9-16

GUIDELINES FOR NURSING CARE (*continued*)

Managing Chest Drainage Systems (*continued*)

ACTION	RATIONALE
11. With a dry system, assess for the presence of the indicator (bellows or float device) when setting the regulator dial to the desired level of suction.	11. An air leak indicator shows changes in intrathoracic pressure in dry systems with a one-way valve. Bubbles will appear if a leak is present. The air leak indicator takes the place of fluid fluctuations in the water-seal chamber. The indicator shows that the vacuum is adequate to maintain the desired level of suction.
12. Observe for air leaks in the drainage system; they are indicated by constant bubbling in the water-seal chamber. Also assess the chest tube system for correctable external leaks. Notify the provider immediately of excessive bubbling in the water-seal chamber not due to external leaks.	12. Leaking and trapping of air in the pleural space can result in tension pneumothorax.
13. When turning down the dry suction, depress the manual high-negativity vent, and assess for a rise in the water level of the water-seal chamber.	13. A rise in the water level of the water-seal chamber indicates high negative pressure in the system that could lead to increased intrathoracic pressure.
14. Observe and immediately report rapid and shallow breathing, cyanosis, pressure in the chest, subcutaneous emphysema, symptoms of hemorrhage, or significant changes in vital signs.	14. Many clinical conditions can cause these signs and symptoms, including tension pneumothorax, mediastinal shift, hemorrhage, severe incisional pain, pulmonary embolus, and cardiac tamponade. Surgical intervention may be necessary.
15. Encourage the patient to breathe deeply and cough at frequent intervals. Provide adequate analgesia. If needed, request an order for patient-controlled analgesia. Also teach the patient how to perform incentive spirometry.	15. Deep breathing and coughing help to raise the intrapleural pressure, which promotes drainage of accumulated fluid in the pleural space. Deep breathing and coughing also promote removal of secretions from the tracheobronchial tree, which, in turn, promotes lung expansion and prevents atelectasis (alveolar collapse).
16. If the patient is lying on a stretcher and must be transported to another area, place the drainage system below the chest level. Do *not* clamp the chest tube during transport. In the event of a chest tube disconnection and risk of contamination, submerge the tube 2 to 4 cm (1 to 2 inches) below the surface of a 250-mL bottle of sterile water or NS until a new chest tube unit can be set up (Perry et al., 2022).	16. The drainage apparatus must be kept at a level lower than the patient's chest to prevent fluid from flowing backward into the pleural space. Clamping can result in a tension pneumothorax.
17. When assisting in the chest tube's removal, instruct the patient to perform a gentle Valsalva maneuver or to breathe quietly. Then the chest tube is clamped and removed quickly. Simultaneously, a small bandage is applied and made airtight with petrolatum gauze covered by a 4 × 4-inch gauze pad and thoroughly covered and secured in position with wide tape.	17. The chest tube is removed as directed when the lung is reexpanded (usually within 24 hours to several days), depending on the cause of the pneumothorax. During tube removal, the chief priorities are preventing air from entering the pleural cavity as the tube is withdrawn and preventing infection.

Water-Seal Systems. The traditional water-seal system (or wet suction) for chest drainage has three chambers: a collection chamber, a water-seal chamber, and a wet suction control chamber. The collection chamber acts as a reservoir for fluid draining from the chest tube. It is graduated to permit easy measurement of drainage. Suction may be added to create negative pressure and promote drainage of fluid and removal of air. The suction control chamber regulates the amount of negative pressure applied to the chest and is determined by the water level which is usually set at –20 cm H_2O; adding more fluid results in more suction. After attaching wall suction to the suction control chamber, the nurse turns the wall suction on and bubbling appears in the suction chamber. Despite how vigorously the suction chamber is bubbling, the nurse is aware that suction is maintained by the water level (usually –20 cm H_2O); thus, suction is applied to the suction control chamber until gentle bubbling is seen. A positive-pressure valve is located at the top of the suction chamber that automatically opens with increases in positive pressure within the system. Air is automatically released through a positive-pressure relief valve if the suction tubing is inadvertently clamped or kinked.

The water-seal chamber has a one-way valve or water seal that prevents air from moving back into the chest when the patient inhales. There is an increase in the water level with inspiration and a return to the baseline level during exhalation; this is referred to as *tidaling*. If bubbling is present, either intermittent or continuous, an air leak is present within the system or the patient. The nurse must investigate the system for loose connections. Bubbling and tidaling do not occur when the tube is placed in the mediastinal space; however, fluid may pulsate with the patient's heartbeat. If the chest tube is connected to gravity drainage only, suction is not used. Two-chamber chest drainage systems (water-seal chamber and collection chamber) are available for use with patients who need only gravity drainage.

The water level in the water-seal chamber reflects the negative pressure presents in the intrathoracic cavity. A rise in the water level of the water-seal chamber indicates negative pressure in the pleural or mediastinal space. Excessive negative pressure can cause trauma to tissue. Most chest drainage systems have an automatic means to prevent excessive negative pressure. By pressing and holding a manual high-negativity vent (usually located on the top of the chest drainage system) until the water level in the water-seal chamber returns to the 2-cm mark, excessive negative pressure is avoided, thus preventing damage to tissue.

Pearls for Practice

The water column of the chest drainage system has a large arm and a small arm of the water seal; when a patient breathes spontaneously the water level in the water-seal chamber rises in the large arm, and falls with exhalation. Bubbling in the small arm of the water seal on exhalation indicates an air leak. The nurse understands that if a patient is on a mechanical ventilator, the opposite happens; that is, the water level in the water-seal chamber decreases on inhalation in the large arm and rises with exhalation. When there is no movement in the water column (absence of tidaling), the nurse observes for kinked tubing or a clamped tube but also understands that when the lung has completely reexpanded (no fluid or air remains in the intrapleural space) tidaling ceases.

Dry Suction Water-Seal Systems. Dry suction water-seal systems, also referred to as dry suction, have a collection chamber for drainage, a water-seal chamber, and a dry suction control chamber. The water-seal chamber is filled with water to the 2-cm level. Bubbling in this area can indicate an air leak. The dry suction control chamber contains a regulator dial that regulates vacuum to the chest drain. Water is not needed for suction in these systems. Without the bubbling in the suction chamber, the system is quieter. However, if the container is knocked over, the water seal may be lost.

Once the tube is connected to the suction source, the regulator dial allows the desired level of suction to be dialed in; the suction is increased until an indicator appears. The indicator has the same function as the bubbling in the traditional water-seal system; that is, it indicates that the vacuum is adequate to maintain the desired level of suction. Some drainage systems use a bellows (a chamber that can be expanded or contracted) or an orange-colored float device as an indicator of when the suction control regulator is set.

When the water in the water seal rises above the 2-cm level, intrathoracic pressure increases. Dry suction water-seal systems have a manual high-negativity vent located on top of the drain. The manual high-negativity vent is pressed until the indicator appears (either a float device or bellows) and the water level in the water seal returns to the desired level, indicating that the intrathoracic pressure is decreased.

Dry Suction Systems With a One-Way Valve. A third type of chest drainage system is dry suction with a one-way mechanical valve. This system has a collection chamber, a one-way mechanical valve, and a dry suction control chamber. The valve permits air and fluid to leave the chest but prevents their movement back into the pleural space. This model lacks a water-seal chamber and therefore can be set up quickly in emergency situations, and the dry control drain still works even if it is knocked over. This makes the dry suction systems useful for the patient who is ambulating or being transported. However, without the water-seal chamber, there is no way to tell by inspection whether the pressure in the chest has changed, even though an air leak indicator is present so that the system can be checked. If an air leak is suspected, 30 mL of water is injected into the air leak indicator or the container is tipped so that fluid enters the air leak detection chamber. Bubbles will appear if a leak is present.

If the chest tube has been inserted to reexpand a lung after pneumothorax, or if very little fluid drainage is expected, a one-way "flutter" valve (Heimlich valve) may be connected to the chest tube (Fig. 9-15). When the patient inhales, the flutter valve collapses on itself (preventing air from being drawn into the intrapleural space), and on exhalation, the positive pressure generated by the air leaving the intrapleural space causes the valve to open so air is released. This valve is attached to a collection bag. It is not used when patients need fluid drained (e.g., a hemothorax or a pleural effusion) (Perry et al., 2022).

Pearls for Practice

If the chest tube becomes dislodged, the nurse will immediately cover the exit site with petrolatum gauze covered by a 4- × 4-inch gauze pad, secure it in place with wide tape, and notify the provider. If an air leak is present, the chest dressing is taped only on two or three sides to allow air to escape the chest wall opening and prevent tension pneumothorax.

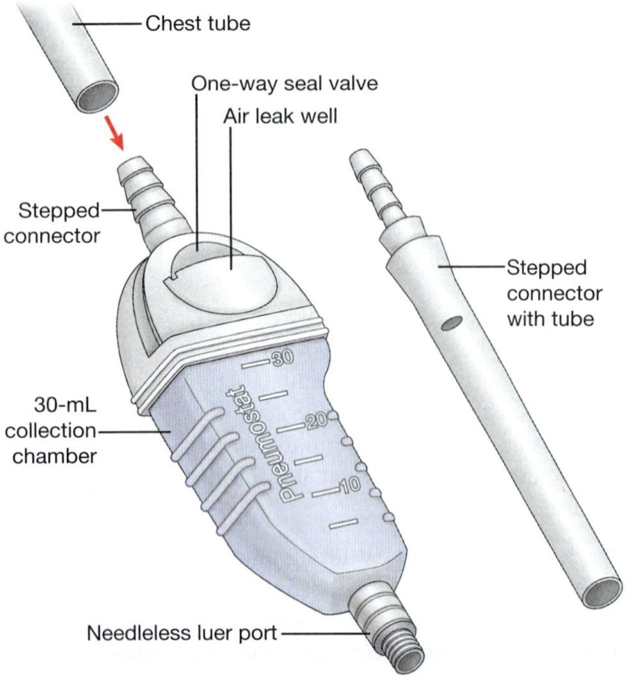

FIGURE 9-15 **One-way (Heimlich) valve, a disposable, single-use chest drainage system with 30-mL collection volume. Used when minimal volume of chest drainage is expected.**

STERNAL AND RIB FRACTURES

Sternal fractures are most common in MVAs, caused by a direct blow to the sternum via the steering wheel. Rib fractures are the most common type of chest trauma, occurring in more than 10% of patients admitted with blunt chest injury (Nelson et al., 2022). Most rib fractures are benign and are treated conservatively, but mortality increases with the number of ribs fractured and age (Bass et al., 2022). Fractures of the first three ribs are rare but can result in a high mortality rate because they are associated with laceration of the subclavian artery or vein. The fifth through ninth ribs are the most common sites of fractures. Fractures of the lower ribs are associated with injury to the spleen and liver, which may be lacerated by fragmented sections of the rib.

Clinical Manifestations and Assessment

Patients with sternal fractures have anterior chest pain, overlying tenderness, ecchymosis, crepitus, swelling, and possible chest wall deformity. For patients with rib fractures, clinical manifestations are similar: severe pain, point tenderness, and muscle spasm over the area of the fracture that is aggravated by coughing, deep breathing, and movement. The area around the fracture may be bruised. To reduce the pain, the patient splints the chest by breathing in a shallow manner and avoids sighs, deep breaths, coughing, and movement. This reluctance to move or breathe deeply results in diminished ventilation, atelectasis (collapse of unaerated alveoli), pneumonitis, and hypoxemia. Respiratory insufficiency and failure can be the outcomes of such a cycle.

The patient must be evaluated closely for underlying cardiac or abdominal injuries. A crackling, grating sound in the thorax (subcutaneous crepitus) may be detected with auscultation or felt with palpation. The diagnostic workup may include a chest x-ray, thoracic CT scan, rib films of a specific area, ECG, continuous POX, and ABG analysis.

Medical and Nursing Management

Medical management is directed toward relieving pain, avoiding excessive activity, and treating any associated injuries. Surgical fixation is rarely necessary unless fragments are grossly displaced and pose a potential for further injury.

The goals of treatment for rib fractures are to control pain and to detect and treat the injury. Narcotics are most often used to relieve pain and to allow deep breathing and coughing. Care must be taken to avoid oversedation and suppression of respiratory drive. Alternative strategies to relieve pain include an intercostal or erector spinae nerve blocks and ice or lidocaine patches over the fracture site. External splints are not recommended, since they limit chest wall expansion and increase the risk of developing atelectasis (Mondor, 2022). Usually the pain abates in 5 to 7 days, and discomfort can be relieved with epidural analgesia, patient-controlled analgesia, or nonopioid analgesia (NSAIDs). Most rib fractures heal in 3 to 6 weeks.

FLAIL CHEST

Flail chest is frequently a complication of blunt chest trauma from a steering wheel injury. It usually occurs when three or more adjacent ribs (multiple contiguous ribs) are fractured at two or more sites, resulting in free-floating rib segments. It may also result as a combination fracture of ribs and costal cartilages or sternum (Fig. 9-16). As a result, the chest wall loses stability, causing respiratory impairment and usually severe respiratory distress. In addition, due to the force needed to break ribs or the sternum, often an underlying pulmonary or cardiac contusion is present.

Pathophysiology

During inspiration, as the chest expands, the detached part of the rib segment (flail segment) moves in a paradoxical manner (pendelluft movement) in that it is pulled inward during inspiration, reducing the amount of air that can be drawn into the lungs. On expiration, because the intrathoracic pressure exceeds atmospheric pressure, the flail segment bulges outward, impairing the patient's ability to exhale. The mediastinum then shifts back to the affected side. This paradoxical action results in increased dead space, a reduction in alveolar ventilation, and decreased compliance. Retained airway secretions and atelectasis frequently accompany flail chest. On palpation of the chest wall, crepitus may be felt and tenderness the near fractured ribs is expected (Mondor, 2022). The patient has

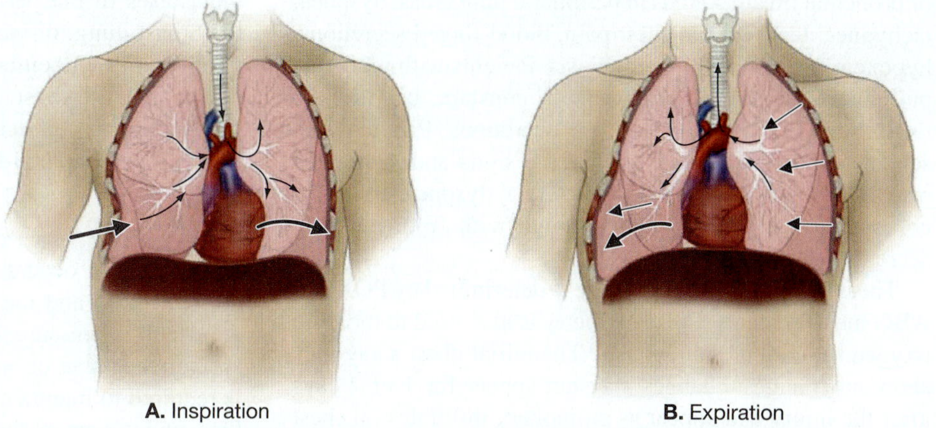

FIGURE 9-16 **Flail chest is caused by a free-floating segment of rib cage resulting from multiple rib fractures. A. Paradoxical movement on inspiration occurs when the flail rib segment is sucked inward and the mediastinal structures shift to the unaffected side. The amount of air drawn into the affected lung is reduced. B. On expiration, the flail segment bulges outward, and the mediastinal structures shift back to the affected side.**

hypoxemia, and if gas exchange is greatly compromised, respiratory acidosis develops as a result of carbon dioxide retention. Hypotension, inadequate tissue perfusion, and metabolic acidosis often follow as the paradoxical motion of the mediastinum decreases cardiac output

Medical and Nursing Management

As with rib fracture, treatment of flail chest is usually supportive. Management includes providing ventilatory support, clearing secretions from the lungs, and controlling pain. Specific management depends on the degree of respiratory dysfunction. If only a small segment of the chest is involved, the objectives are to clear the airway through positioning, coughing, deep breathing, and suctioning to aid in the expansion of the lung, and to relieve pain by intercostal nerve blocks, high thoracic epidural blocks, or cautious use of IV opioids.

For mild to moderate flail chest injuries, the underlying pulmonary contusion is treated by monitoring fluid intake and appropriate fluid replacement while relieving chest pain. Pulmonary physiotherapy focusing on lung volume expansion includes deep breathing exercises, IS, and nebulized bronchodilators and mucolytics.

For severe flail chest injuries, endotracheal intubation and mechanical ventilation are required to provide internal pneumatic stabilization of the flail chest and to correct abnormalities in gas exchange. This helps treat the underlying pulmonary contusion, serves to stabilize the thoracic cage to allow the fractures to heal, and improves alveolar ventilation and intrathoracic volume by decreasing the work of breathing. In rare circumstances, surgery may be required to more quickly stabilize the flail segment.

Regardless of the type of treatment, the patient is carefully monitored by serial chest x-rays, ABG analysis, POX, and bedside pulmonary function monitoring. Pain management is key to successful treatment. Patient-controlled analgesia, intercostal nerve blocks, epidural analgesia, and intrapleural administration of opioids may be used to relieve or manage thoracic pain.

PULMONARY CONTUSION

Pulmonary contusion is a common thoracic injury and is frequently associated with blunt trauma often associated with a traffic accident or an injury due to high pressure affecting the chest (Rendeki & Molnár, 2019). It is defined as damage to the lung tissues resulting in hemorrhage and localized edema (i.e., bruised lung). Pulmonary contusion represents a spectrum of lung injury characterized by the development of infiltrates and various degrees of respiratory dysfunction and sometimes respiratory failure. A contusion is sustained in up to 50% of patients who experience blunt force trauma (Zingg et al., 2022). Pulmonary contusion may not be evident initially on examination but develops in the posttraumatic period; it may involve a small portion of one lung, a massive section of a lung, one entire lung, or both lungs. The contusion may cause minimal respiratory distress, however, can progress into a rapidly manifesting ARDS and pneumonia (Rendeki & Molnar, 2019).

Pathophysiology

The primary pathologic defect is an abnormal accumulation of fluid in the interstitial and intra-alveolar spaces. It is thought that injury to the lung parenchyma and its capillary network results in a leakage of serum protein and plasma. The leaking serum protein exerts an osmotic pressure that enhances loss of fluid from the capillaries. Blood, edema, and cellular debris (from cellular response to injury) enter the lung and accumulate in the bronchioles and alveoli, where they interfere with gas exchange. The patient has hypoxemia and carbon dioxide retention. Occasionally, a contused lung occurs on the other side of the point of body impact; this is called a *contrecoup contusion.*

Clinical Manifestations and Assessment

The clinical manifestations of pulmonary contusions can vary based on the severity of bruising and parenchymal involvement (Rendeki & Molnár, 2019). The most common signs and symptoms are crackles, decreased breath sounds, or bronchial breath sounds in peripheral lung areas, dyspnea, tachypnea, tachycardia, chest pain, blood-tinged secretions, hypoxemia, and respiratory acidosis. Patients with moderate pulmonary contusions often have a constant, but ineffective, cough and cannot clear their secretions. Patients with severe pulmonary contusion have the signs and symptoms of ARDS; these may include hypoxemia, dyspnea, agitation, combativeness, and productive cough with frothy, bloody secretions.

The efficiency of gas exchange is determined by POX and ABG measurements. Pulse oximetry is also used to measure oxygen saturation continuously. The initial chest x-ray may show no changes; changes may not appear for 1 or 2 days after the injury and appear as pulmonary infiltrates on chest x-ray.

Medical and Nursing Management

Treatment priorities include maintaining the airway, providing adequate oxygenation, and controlling pain. In mild pulmonary contusion, judicious hydration via IV fluids and oral intake is important to mobilize secretions. However, fluid intake must be monitored closely to avoid hypervolemia, which can increase the risk of pulmonary edema and consequently aggravates gas exchange. Volume expansion techniques, postural drainage, physiotherapy including coughing, and endotracheal suctioning are used to remove the secretions. Pain is managed by intercostal nerve blocks or by opioids via patient-controlled analgesia or other methods. Usually supplemental oxygen is given by mask or cannula for hypoxemia (saturation less than 90%).

In patients with moderate pulmonary contusions, bronchoscopy may be required to remove secretions. Intubation and mechanical ventilation with PEEP may also be necessary to maintain the pressure and keep the lungs inflated. In patients with severe contusion, who may develop respiratory failure, aggressive treatment with endotracheal intubation and ventilatory support, diuretics, and fluid restriction may be necessary.

Antimicrobial medications may be prescribed for the treatment of pulmonary infection. This is a common complication of pulmonary contusion because the fluid and blood that extravasates into the alveolar and interstitial spaces serve as an excellent culture medium.

CARDIAC TAMPONADE

Cardiac tamponade is compression of the heart resulting from fluid or blood within the pericardial sac. It usually is caused by blunt or penetrating trauma to the chest. A penetrating wound of the heart is associated with a high mortality rate. Cardiac tamponade also may follow diagnostic cardiac catheterization, angiographic procedures, and pacemaker insertion, which can produce perforations of the heart and great vessels. Pericardial effusion with fluid compressing the heart also may develop from metastases to the pericardium from malignant tumors of the breast, lung, or mediastinum and may occur with lymphomas and leukemias, renal failure, TB, and high-dose radiation to the chest. It can progress to cardiogenic shock, cardiac arrest, and death. Cardiac tamponade is discussed in detail in Chapter 14.

PNEUMOTHORAX

Pneumothorax occurs when the parietal or visceral pleura are punctured and the pleural space is exposed to positive atmospheric pressure. Normally, the pressure in the pleural space is negative or subatmospheric; this negative pressure is required to maintain lung inflation. When either pleura is breached, air enters the pleural space, and the lung or a portion of it collapses.

Types of Pneumothorax

Types of pneumothorax include simple, traumatic, and tension pneumothorax (Fig. 9-17).

Simple Pneumothorax

A simple, or spontaneous, pneumothorax most commonly occurs as air enters the pleural space through the rupture of a bleb or a bronchopleural fistula. A spontaneous pneumothorax may occur in an apparently healthy person (most commonly in young males) in the absence of trauma due to rupture of an air-filled bleb, or blister, on the surface of the lung, allowing air from the airways to enter the pleural cavity. It may also be associated with bullous lung diseases such as emphysema or pulmonary fibrosis. The severity of pneumothorax is graded on the degree of collapse: 15% or less—small, 5 to 15%—moderate, and >60%—large; treatment is determined by the size and cause of injury and may include catheter aspiration or tube thoracostomy (Heiner, 2023).

Traumatic Pneumothorax

A traumatic pneumothorax occurs when air escapes from a laceration in the lung itself and enters the pleural space or enters the pleural space through a wound in the chest wall. It may result from blunt trauma, penetrating chest or abdominal trauma, or diaphragmatic tears. Traumatic pneumothorax may occur during invasive thoracic procedures (i.e., thoracentesis, transbronchial lung biopsy, insertion of a subclavian line) in which the pleura is punctured inadvertently or with barotrauma (trauma caused by rapid or extreme changes in air pressure) from mechanical ventilation. A traumatic pneumothorax resulting from major trauma to the chest is often accompanied by a hemothorax (collection of blood in the pleural space resulting from torn intercostal vessels, lacerations of the great vessels, or lacerations of the lungs). Often both blood and air are found in the chest cavity (hemopneumothorax) after major trauma.

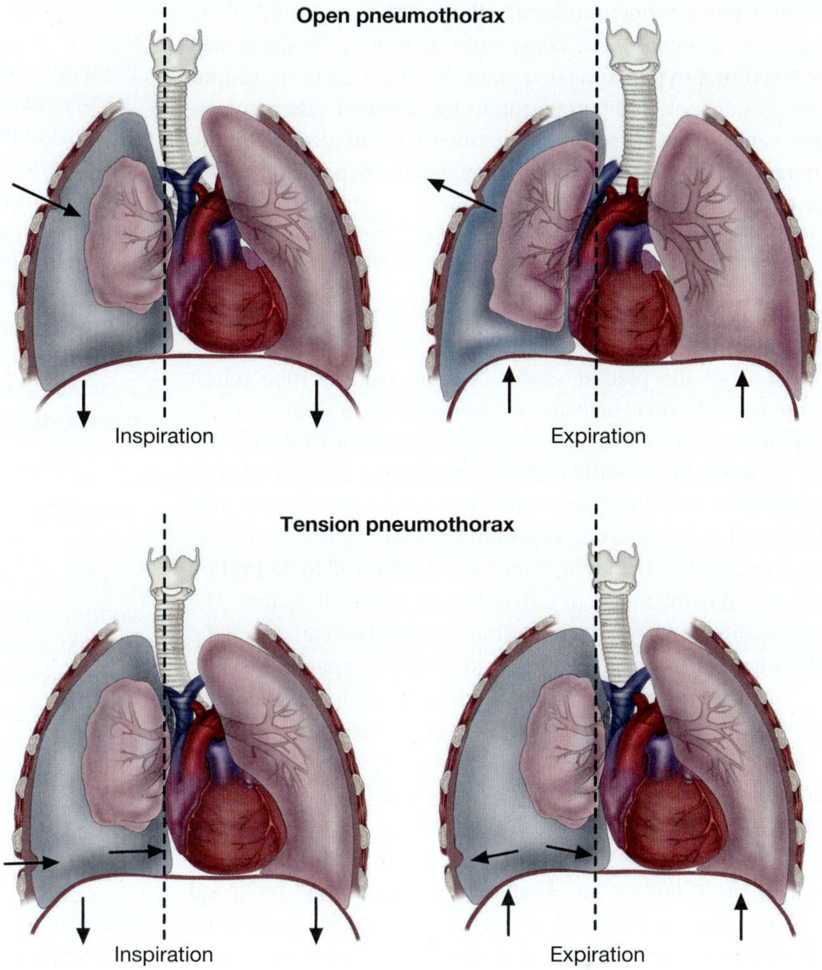

FIGURE 9-17 **Open and tension pneumothorax.**

Open pneumothorax is one form of traumatic pneumothorax. It occurs when a wound in the chest wall is large enough to allow air to pass freely in and out of the thoracic cavity with each attempted respiration. Because the rush of air through the wound in the chest wall produces a sucking sound, such injuries are termed *sucking chest wounds.*

Tension Pneumothorax

A tension pneumothorax occurs when air is drawn into the pleural space from a lacerated lung or through a small opening or wound in the chest wall. It may be a complication of other types of pneumothorax. In contrast to open pneumothorax, the air that enters the chest cavity with each inspiration is trapped; it cannot be expelled during expiration through the air passages or the opening in the chest wall. In effect, a one-way valve or ball valve mechanism occurs, where air enters the pleural space but cannot escape. With each breath, tension (positive pressure) is increased within the affected pleural space. This causes the lung to collapse and the heart, the great vessels, and the trachea to shift toward the unaffected side of the chest (mediastinal shift). Both respiration and circulatory function are compromised because of the increased intrathoracic pressure, which decreases venous return to the heart, causing decreased cardiac output and impairment of peripheral circulation. In extreme cases, cardiac arrest can occur.

Clinical Manifestations

The signs and symptoms associated with pneumothorax depend on its size and cause. Usually pain is sudden and may be pleuritic. The patient may have only minimal respiratory distress with slight chest discomfort and tachypnea with a small simple or uncomplicated pneumothorax. If the pneumothorax is large and the lung collapses totally, acute respiratory distress occurs. The patient is anxious, has dyspnea and air hunger, has increased use of the accessory muscles, and may develop severe hypoxemia. In assessing the chest for any type of pneumothorax, the nurse assesses tracheal alignment, expansion of the chest, and breath sounds, and percusses the chest. In a simple pneumothorax, the trachea is midline, expansion of the chest is decreased, breath sounds may be diminished, and percussion of the chest may reveal normal sounds or hyperresonance depending on the size of the pneumothorax. The nurse assesses the affected lung for crepitus or subcutaneous emphysema and notes the extent of it in the patient's record.

In a tension pneumothorax, the trachea may shift away from the affected side, chest expansion may be decreased or fixed in a hyperexpansion state, breath sounds are diminished or absent, and percussion to the affected side is hyperresonant. The clinical picture is one of air hunger, agitation, increasing hypoxemia, central cyanosis, hypotension, and tachycardia.

Medical and Nursing Management

Medical management of pneumothorax depends on its cause and severity. The goal of treatment is to evacuate the air or blood from the pleural space. A thoracostomy tube (chest tube) is used to evacuate any accumulated air or fluid. A small, simple pneumothorax is treated with a small chest tube (20-Fr, or 10- to 14-Fr "pigtail" catheter) inserted at the second ICS, at the midclavicular line or fifth ICS at the midaxillary line. Larger pneumothoraxes, especially if there is fluid or blood present, are managed with larger-sized tubes (32 to 36 Fr) that are placed in the fourth or fifth ICS at the midaxillary line. The tube is directed posteriorly to drain the fluid and air. Once the chest tube or tubes are inserted and suction is applied (usually to –20 mm Hg suction), effective decompression of the pleural cavity (drainage of blood and/or air) occurs.

The severity of open pneumothorax depends on the amount and rate of thoracic bleeding and the amount of air in the pleural space. The pleural cavity can be decompressed by needle aspiration (thoracentesis) or by chest tube drainage of the blood or air. Then the lung is able to reexpand and resume the function of gas exchange. As a rule, the chest wall is opened surgically (thoracotomy) if more than 1,500 mL of blood is aspirated initially by thoracentesis (or is the initial chest tube output) or if chest tube output continues at greater than 200 mL/hr. The urgency with which the blood must be removed is determined by the degree of respiratory compromise. An emergency thoracotomy may also be performed in the emergency department if a cardiovascular injury secondary to penetrating trauma is suspected. The patient with a possible tension pneumothorax should be given a high concentration of supplemental oxygen immediately to treat the hypoxemia, and POX should be used to monitor oxygen saturation.

In an emergency situation, a tension pneumothorax can be decompressed or quickly converted to a simple pneumothorax by inserting a large-bore needle (14-gauge) at the second ICS, midclavicular line on the affected side (needle thoracostomy). This relieves the pressure and vents the positive pressure to the external environment. A chest tube is then inserted and connected to suction to remove the remaining air and fluid, reestablish the negative pressure, and reexpand the lung. If the lung reexpands and air leakage from the lung parenchyma stops, further drainage may be unnecessary. If a prolonged air leak continues despite chest tube drainage to underwater seal, surgery may be necessary to close the leak. A plan of nursing care for the patient after thoracotomy is available online at http://thepoint.lww.com/Honan3e.

SUBCUTANEOUS EMPHYSEMA

No matter what kind of chest trauma a patient has, when the lung or the air passages are injured, air may enter the tissue planes and pass for some distance under the skin (e.g., neck, chest). The tissues give a crackling sensation when palpated, and the subcutaneous air produces an alarming appearance as the face, neck, body, and scrotum become misshapen by subcutaneous air. Fortunately, subcutaneous emphysema in and of itself usually is not a serious complication. The subcutaneous air is absorbed spontaneously if the underlying air leak is treated or stops spontaneously. In severe cases, in which there is widespread subcutaneous emphysema, a tracheostomy is indicated if airway patency is threatened.

ASPIRATION

Aspiration of stomach contents into the lungs is a serious complication that can cause pneumonia and result in the clinical picture of coughing, wheezing, crackles, cyanosis, tachycardia, tachypnea, dyspnea, hypoxemia, hypertension or hypotension, fever, and, finally, death. Copious amounts of sputum are produced as alveolar edema develops (Stacy, 2022). It can occur when the protective airway reflexes are decreased or absent due to a variety of factors

Pathophysiology

The primary factors responsible for death and complications after aspiration of gastric contents are the volume and character of the aspirated gastric contents. For example, a small, localized aspiration from regurgitation can cause pneumonia and acute respiratory distress; a massive aspiration is usually fatal. Factors that increase the risk of aspiration are discussed in Box 9-17.

A full stomach contains food particles. If these are aspirated, the problem then becomes one of mechanical blockage of the airways and secondary infection or chemical pneumonitis. During periods of fasting, the stomach contains acidic gastric juice, which, if aspirated, can be very destructive to the alveoli and capillaries. Fecal contamination (more likely seen in intestinal obstruction) increases the likelihood of death because the endotoxins produced by intestinal organisms may be absorbed systemically, or the thick proteinaceous material found in the intestinal contents may obstruct the airway, leading to atelectasis and secondary bacterial invasion.

Aspiration pneumonitis may develop from aspiration of gastric contents, which can also cause a chemical burn of the tracheobronchial tree and pulmonary parenchyma. An ensuing inflammatory response occurs. This results in the destruction of alveolar–capillary endothelial cells, with a consequent outpouring of protein-rich fluids into the interstitial and intra-alveolar spaces. As a result, surfactant is lost, which, in turn, causes the airways to close and the alveoli

BOX 9-17

Risk Factors for Aspiration

- Altered level of consciousness (cerebrovascular accident, head trauma, intracranial mass/tumor, drug overdose, alcohol intoxication, seizures, oversedation)
- Neurologic disorders (Parkinson disease, myasthenia gravis, multiple sclerosis, amyotrophic lateral sclerosis)
- Dysphagia (esophageal stricture, diverticula or neoplasm, tracheoesophageal fistula, cardiac sphincter incompetence, achalasia [lack of the lower esophageal sphincter to relax, preventing food from passing into the stomach])
- Altered airway or oropharyngeal anatomy (head and neck malignancy, surgery and/or radiation therapy to head and neck)
- Disruption via mechanical instruments (endotracheal intubation, tracheostomy, naso-/orogastric tube [any size], bronchoscopy, laryngoscopy, upper GI endoscopy)
- Recumbent position
- Protracted vomiting
- Nasogastric feeding
- Gastric outlet obstruction

to collapse. Finally, the impaired exchange of oxygen and carbon dioxide causes respiratory failure.

Aspiration pneumonia develops after inhalation of colonized oropharyngeal material. The pathologic process involves an acute inflammatory response to bacteria and bacterial products. Most commonly, the bacteriologic findings include gram-positive cocci, gram-negative rods, and, occasionally, anaerobic bacteria.

Prevention

Prevention is the primary goal when caring for patients at risk for aspiration. Examples of risk factors for aspiration include decreased level of consciousness, supine positioning, presence of a nasogastric tube, tracheal intubation and mechanical ventilation, and advanced age (Yanagita et al., 2022). Hyperglycemia is also a risk factor for aspiration since it is associated with delayed gastric emptying by disrupting postprandial (after a meal) stomach contractions (Stacy, 2022). Evidence confirms that one of the main preventive measures for aspiration is placing at-risk patients in a semirecumbent position (elevation of the head of the bed to a 30- to 45-degree angle) (American Association of Critical Care Nurses [AACN], 2016; Güner & Kutlutürkan, 2021).

Compensating for Absent Reflexes

Aspiration may occur if the patient cannot adequately coordinate protective glottic, laryngeal, and cough reflexes. This hazard is increased if the patient has a distended abdomen, is supine, has the upper extremities immobilized by IV infusions or hand restraints, receives local anesthetics to the oropharyngeal or laryngeal area for diagnostic procedures, has been sedated, or has had long-term intubation.

When vomiting, people can normally protect their airway by sitting up or turning on the side and coordinating breathing, coughing, gag, and glottic reflexes. If these reflexes are active, an oral airway should not be inserted. If an airway is in place, it should be pulled out the moment the patient gags so as not to stimulate the pharyngeal gag reflex and promote vomiting and aspiration. Suctioning of oral secretions with a catheter should be performed with minimal pharyngeal stimulation.

In addition, using the smallest effective level of sedation is prudent in patients at risk for aspiration.

Assessing Feeding Tube Placement

When a patient is intubated, aspiration may occur even with a nasogastric tube in place and may result in nosocomial pneumonia. Assessment of nasogastric tube placement is key to the prevention of aspiration. The best method for determining tube placement is via an x-ray taken immediately after an enteral feeding tube is placed and prior to beginning feeds. Nurses should mark the place where the tube exits the nares or lips and note this in the patient's chart. This marking should be assessed whenever medication is administered via the tube or at least every 4 hours. A combination of methods is recommended to assess tube placement, including assessment of the patient's tolerance to medication and feeding administration (noting abdominal distention and complaints of abdominal pain, observing for passage of flatus and stool) as well as measurement of tube length, visual assessment of aspirate, or testing the pH measurement of aspirate which remains an area where further research is warranted. None of these methods has been shown to accurately assess the placement of the tube (Bloom & Seckel, 2021). It is important for the nurse to understand that where research is ongoing, they should follow institutional procedures. Refer to the AACN Prevention of Aspiration Practice Alert (https://www.aacn.org/clinical-resources/practice-alerts/initial-and-ongoing-verification-of-feeding-tube-placement-in-adults).

Patients who receive continuous or timed-interval tube feedings must be positioned properly. Patients receiving continuous infusions are given small volumes under low pressure in an upright position, which helps prevent aspiration. Patients receiving tube feedings at timed intervals are maintained in an upright or semirecumbent position (elevation of the head of the bed to a 30- to 45-degree angle) during the feeding and for a minimum of 30 minutes afterward to allow the stomach to empty partially. Because there is controversy over the assessment of gastric residual volume (GRV) and research does not demonstrate prevention of early detection of feeding intolerance or aspiration (Bloom & Seckel, 2021), the nurse should follow institutional procedures related to GRV. Tube feedings must be given only when it is certain that the feeding tube is positioned correctly in the stomach or in the small bowel. Many patients today receive enteral feeding directly into the small intestine through a small-bore flexible feeding tube or surgically implanted tube. Feedings are given slowly and are regulated by a feeding pump (refer to Chapter 21 for more details). The nurse should be aware that the results of routine chest and abdominal x-ray will report tube location.

Clinical Judgment Case

Your patient is 66 years old and is 5 days postlaryngeal surgery for cancer, where a partial laryngectomy was performed (a portion of the larynx was removed, along with one vocal cord and the tumor; all other structures remain). Medical history includes hypertension, chronic obstructive pulmonary disorder (COPD) with a 30-pack year smoking history (1 pack per day [PPD] × 30 years), and type 2 diabetes; home medications include hydrochlorothiazide, metformin, and albuterol. The patient rang the call bell stating, "I think I choked on my tea. I can't breathe." Upon walking in the room, you find the patient leaning forward on the edge of the bed and note respiratory distress, characterized by dyspnea, use of accessory muscles, intercostal retractions, nasal flaring, mouth breathing, coughing of tea colored fluid followed by frothy secretions. You hear crackles in the right lower lobe (RLL) and scattered rhonchi and wheezing throughout. The patient's skin is warm and dry with delayed skin turgor and vital signs are as follows: 100.7°F, HR 112 and regular, 28 RR with an oxygen saturation of 90% on room air, and blood pressure 132/78 mm Hg. Heart sounds are S1 S2 without murmur, gallop or rub; neck veins are flat. There is no peripheral edema, capillary refill is 2 seconds, and dorsalis pedis and posterior tibial pulses are 2+ to 3+ bil. The patient is anxious and restless.

Step One: Recognize cues where relevant and identify important information from different sources, such as medical history or vital signs.

Answer: Postop Day (POD) 5 after partial laryngectomy, a 66-year-old with sudden onset shortness of breath (SOB), dyspnea, use of accessory muscles, intercostal retractions, nasal flaring, mouth breathing, coughing of tea colored fluid followed by frothy secretions, tachycardia (112), tachypnea (28), crackles in RLL and scattered rhonchi and wheezing throughout, O_2 sat of 90% on room air (RA), delayed skin turgor, flat neck veins, temp 100.7°F, patient stated that they "choked," displays anxiety and restlessness. Medical history of hypertension, COPD, 30-pack year smoking history, and type 2 diabetes.

Step Two: Analyze cues, which is organizing and linking the recognized cues to the patient's clinical presentation.

Answer: You have clustered the symptoms to be associated with aspiration; symptoms which suggest aspiration of oropharyngeal contents (food or fluids into the lung) include cough (productive), tachypnea, dyspnea, hypoxemia, tachycardia, fever and the lung exam which includes diffuse wheezing, and rhonchi, and crackles in the RLL. You are also concerned about the development of aspiration pneumonia (cues are fever, respiratory distress [use of accessory muscles, intercostal retractions, nasal flaring, mouth breathing], cough, and RLL crackles) or chemical pneumonitis (aspiration of highly acidic gastric juices results in edema, collapse of alveoli, ventilation–perfusion mismatch), and hypoxemia (O_2 sat of 90%, diffuse wheezing and rhonchi) and acute respiratory distress syndrome (ARDS) (cues are frothy sputum, crackles, respiratory distress) related to the aspiration which triggers a systemic inflammatory response that causes pulmonary capillaries to leak fluid into the alveoli. You cluster POD 5 after laryngeal surgery as a risk for impaired swallowing (dysphagia). Signs of fluid volume deficit include tachycardia, delayed skin turgor, and flat neck veins. You also link the age, COPD history, and smoking history with potential for pneumonia. You cluster the rhonchi with COPD and smoking history.

Step Three: Prioritize hypotheses, where hypotheses are evaluated and ranked according to priority. This can include urgency, likelihood, risk, difficulty, and/or time. In this phase, you cluster your findings to arrive at a list of problems (actual and/or potential) you believe the patient is experiencing and determine the importance or urgency. What do you think is of greatest concern?

Answer: You prioritize hypoxemia as the greatest risk of injury to this patient, requiring removal of as much aspirate as possible, limiting the spread of what is left in the lung, and prevention of further aspiration.

Step Four: Generate solutions, which is identifying expected outcomes and using hypotheses to define a set of interventions for the expected outcomes.

Answer: Since hypoxemia exists (O_2 sat is 90%) oxygen needs to be administered, and the head of the bed (HOB) should be raised to high Fowler position. You are aware that in the majority of cases severe hypoxemia occurs rapidly within the first 30–60 minutes after aspiration. Suctioning may be necessary to remove the aspirate from the lungs, but given the recent laryngeal surgery (POD 5), a flexible bronchoscopy will avoid blind insertion and potential damage to the new surgical site. Close monitoring of the patient's oxygen saturation is important, and immediate intubation with mechanical ventilation should be provided if hypoxia worsens. The crash cart should be brought near the bed in case of further decompensation of the patient. You anticipate a stat chest x-ray will be done and nebulized albuterol may be used to treat wheezing. You anticipate that ARDS may be occurring if the hypoxemia does not respond to oxygen therapy. Early signs of ARDS will be increased pH and a decreased $PaCO_2$, secondary to an increased respiratory rate with progression to respiratory acidosis with hypercapnia, and chest x-ray findings of increased bilateral interstitial markings, often in a patchy appearance. If present, you anticipate transfer to the intensive care unit since ventilatory support with the use of positive end-expiratory pressure (PEEP) is the treatment of choice. In addition, you anticipate that hypotension may occur if ARDS develops as a result of hypovolemia secondary to leakage of fluid into the interstitial spaces. You will repeat vital signs every 15 minutes. If hypotension exists, it must be treated carefully without causing further fluid overload, so you will carefully monitor the patient's cardiopulmonary status (heart and lung sounds, O_2 sat, RR, jugular vein distention [JVD], peripheral edema). Your patient is anxious and agitated, which can worsen the hypoxemia and dyspnea. It will be important to explain all procedures and provide care in a calm, reassuring manner, to reduce your patient's anxiety, because anxiety increases oxygen expenditure. Rest is essential to limit oxygen consumption and reduce oxygen needs.

Step Five: Take action, where the solutions that address the highest priorities are implemented.

Answer: You elevate the HOB to high Fowler position, ask the patient to cough to clear secretions, and place the patient on low flow oxygen at 2 L via nasal cannula but anticipate that the provider may change it to a higher concentration of oxygen such as high-flow nasal cannulas (HFNCs). You are aware that oxygen ranges can be from 21% to 100% with HFNC. Although the patient has a history of COPD, which characteristically is associated with chronically elevated $PaCO_2$, a normal pH, an elevated HCO_3, and a PaO_2 level that usually is less than 60 mm Hg, the goal of oxygen therapy is to raise the oxygen level to 92%, not above it. However, in this situation the priority is in the management of hypoxia, and oxygen should never be withheld! You flush the peripheral IV with to ensure access is available, place the patient on a cardiac monitor, note the development of any arrhythmias, and monitor the oxygen saturation continuously. You repeat the vital signs and reassess the patient's pulmonary exam and cardiovascular status. You are alert to increasing dyspnea, falling oxygen saturation, and unstable vital signs. The crash cart is placed outside the patient's room. You also orient the patient to the treatment plan since you are aware that stress increases the hypoxemia. You page respiratory therapy to offer an albuterol nebulizer treatment and notify the provider of the change in the patient's condition. The provider orders a stat chest film and ABGs.

Step Six: Evaluate outcomes, which is comparing observed outcomes against expected outcomes.

Answer: You continue to evaluate vital signs and physical examination findings. The patient was placed on 40% FiO_2 and the oxygen saturation continued to deteriorate necessitating intubation and transfer to the ICU for ventilator management. The patient did indeed aspirate, resulting in a right lower lobe aspiration pneumonia. The patient was treated with antibiotics, bronchodilators and ultimately was extubated and is currently on 2 L nasal cannula. The patient is transferring back to your unit today. Their first words to you were, "Thank you for responding so quickly when I was in trouble." Your quick action of elevating the HOB, applying oxygen, ensuring the patient had IV access, placing the patient on the cardiac monitor and continuous O_2 saturation monitoring did not prevent the aspiration pneumonia, but because of your quick action, the patient had a bronchoscopy at the bedside which removed much of the aspiration and prevented the development of ARDS. Positioning (HOB up), clearing secretions (coughing and bronchoscopy), and administering oxygen helped prevent potential ARDS. A swallow study will be performed this afternoon to assess future risk for aspiration, in which case thickened liquids or pureed diets and dietary consult will help with the postoperative dysphagia. There is no doubt that this was a stressful situation, but you remained calm and remembered that hypoxemia was the greatest risk of injury to this patient.

CHAPTER REVIEW

NCLEX-Style Review Questions

1. The nurse is caring for a client diagnosed with ARDS. In evaluating the use of PEEP, what outcome would the nurse expect to find? Select all that apply.
  a. Increased ventilation–perfusion mismatch
  b. Increased FRC
  c. Decreased intrathoracic pressure
  d. Hypertension
  e. Decrease in preload

2. In a client with pulmonary artery hypertension (PAH), which sign(s) should lead the nurse to suspect right-sided heart failure (cor pulmonale)? Select all that apply.
  a. Jugular vein distention
  b. Productive cough
  c. Leg edema
  d. Hepatosplenomegaly
  e. Bilateral crackles

3. A patient with a suspected pulmonary embolus is brought to the emergency department complaining of shortness of breath and chest pain. Which of the following additional signs and symptoms would the nurse expect to assess in this patient? Select all that apply.
  a. Tachypnea
  b. Thick green sputum
  c. Bradycardia
  d. Hyperresonance
  e. Tachycardia
  f. Blood-tinged sputum

4. A patient is admitted to the ICU after hitting the steering wheel in a motor vehicle crash. The patient is alert, restless, complaining of chest and back pain, and skin is cold and slightly clammy. Breath sounds are diminished over the left side. An upright chest x-ray reveals fractures of the left fifth through seventh ribs and a 25% left hemothorax. Pertinent data are: BP is 80/50; HR is 125; RR is 28 and slightly labored. O_2 sat is 93% on room air. Which of the following measures is most likely to be included in this patient's initial care? Select all that apply.
  a. Immediate endotracheal intubation
  b. Chest tube insertion
  c. Oxygen administration
  d. IV fluid bolus
  e. Pericardiocentesis

5. Early signs of respiratory failure include which of the following? Select all that apply.
  a. Restlessness
  b. Tachycardia
  c. Cyanosis
  d. Tachypnea
  e. Respiratory arrest

REFERENCES AND SELECTED READINGS

References and selected readings associated with this chapter can be found on the website that accompanies the book. Visit **http://thepoint.lww.com/Honan3e** to access the references and other additional resources associated with this chapter.

CHAPTER 10

Nursing Management of Patients Diagnosed With Chronic Obstructive Pulmonary Disease and Asthma

Linda Honan • Lauren Collin

Learning Objectives

After reading this chapter, you will be able to:

1. Describe the pathophysiology of chronic obstructive pulmonary disease (COPD).
2. Discuss the major risk factors for developing COPD and interventions used to minimize or prevent these risk factors.
3. Use the nursing process as a framework for care of patients with COPD.
4. Develop a teaching plan for patients with COPD.
5. Describe the pathophysiology of asthma.
6. Discuss the medications used in asthma management.
7. Describe asthma self-management strategies.

Chronic obstructive pulmonary disease (COPD) and asthma are the most common chronic pulmonary disorders. Nurses working with patients with these chronic pulmonary diseases care for them across the spectrum of care, from outpatient and home care to emergency, inpatient, critical care and, finally, in the hospice setting. Patients with COPD (also may be referred to as chronic obstructive lung disease or COLD) and asthma need care from nurses who not only have astute assessment and clinical management skills but who also understand how these disorders can affect quality of life. In addition, the nurse's knowledge of palliative and end-of-life care is important for affected patients (refer to Chapter 2). Patient, family, and other caregivers require teaching to enhance self-management with any chronic pulmonary disorder.

COPD

A new proposed definition of **chronic obstructive pulmonary disease (COPD)** is a "heterogeneous (diverse) lung condition characterized by chronic respiratory symptoms (dyspnea, cough, sputum production, exacerbations), due to abnormalities in the airway (bronchitis, bronchiolitis), and/or alveoli (emphysema) that cause persistent, often progressive airflow obstruction" (GOLD, 2023, p. 5).

An estimated 15.7 million Americans have the diagnosis of COPD (CDC, 2022a). The actual incidence of COPD is thought to be much higher as many cases are undiagnosed. Worldwide, COPD is the third leading cause of death and it is the fourth leading cause of death in the United States (Jain, 2023; WHO, 2022). In addition, COPD is a major cause of morbidity and accounts for an annual cost estimated to be $32 billion, including health care expenditures, mortality costs, lost workdays, and other indirect costs (Vega-Olivia et al., 2022). The nurse also recognizes that COPD contributes to other leading causes of death, including COVID-19, pneumonia, cardiovascular diseases, stroke, and lung cancer (Lee & Sin, 2022).

Pathophysiology

Recently, the global initiative for chronic obstructive lung disease, which provides evidence-based reference tools and represents the current best practices for the care of patients with COPD emphasized a more holistic strategy to approaching this disorder. They call on clinicians and researchers to consider all gene–environment interactions that a person might encounter through the lifespan (referred to as the time axis or T) to better understand the roles of genes (G) and environmental exposures (E) in development of COPD (Agusti et al., 2022; GOLD, 2023). The pathologic changes that characterize COPD are complex and include interactions between genes (G) and environment (E) over a lifetime (T) of the individual (termed GETomics) that results in damage to the lung airways, parenchyma, and pulmonary vasculature (GOLD, 2023). Increased inflammatory cells in the airways, lung parenchyma and pulmonary vessels and high levels of proinflammatory cytokines results in inflammatory and structural changes in the lungs leading to a loss of pulmonary function, specifically FEV_1 (forced expired volume in 1 second). Destruction of the lung parenchyma also can result in emphysematous changes which further contributes to airflow limitation and impaired gas exchange.

Pearls for Practice

Normally, ~80% or more of the expiratory volume can be expelled in 1 second. Obstructive lung disease is defined as a postbronchodilator FEV_1/FVC (forced expired volume in 1 second as a ratio of forced vital capacity [volume of lungs from full inspiration to forced maximal expiration that is expressed as a percentage of the predicted normal for a person]) ratio of less than 70%. The patient demonstrates a degree of reversibility if the pulmonary function values improve significantly (more than 12% and 200 mL in either FEV_1 or FVC) after administration of the bronchodilator. Usually, patients who demonstrate complete reversibility to normal values are diagnosed with asthma. Patients who demonstrate some reversibility that does not reach normal values may be diagnosed with COPD with some reversible component or overlap of COPD and asthma. However, it is important to consider that PFTs become abnormal ONLY when lung damage exceeds 30% and small airway obstruction exceeds 75%, making the diagnosis of early COPD challenging (Şerifoğlu & Ulubay, 2019).

Emphysema is a pathologic condition that is characterized by loss of lung elasticity, abnormal enlargement of the airspaces beyond the terminal bronchioles with destruction of the walls of the alveoli (parenchymal destruction) (Fig. 10-1). **Chronic bronchitis** is a disease of the small airways, and has the hallmark feature of a productive cough for at least 3 months per year over 2 consecutive years (in the absence of any other explanation for the symptoms). Chronic mucus hypersecretion has been implicated as a cause of lung function decline, exacerbations, and infections. Thickening of the epithelium, smooth muscle hypertrophy, and airway

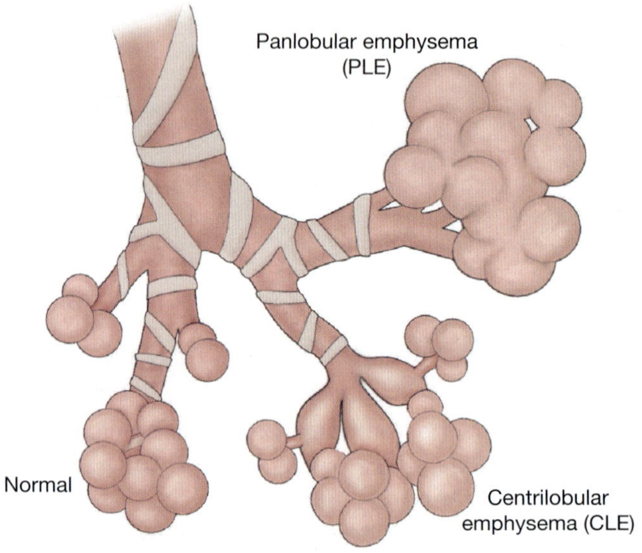

FIGURE 10-1 Changes in the alveolar structure in centrilobular and panlobular emphysema. In panlobular emphysema, the bronchioles, alveolar ducts, and alveoli are destroyed, and the airspaces within the lobule are enlarged. On centrilobular emphysema, the pathologic changes occur in the lobule, whereas the peripheral portions of the acinus are preserved.

inflammation are implicated in remodeling of the airways (Fig. 10-2). Although COPD is usually divided into two subtypes: chronic bronchitis and emphysema, patients with COPD often have overlapping features of both disorders (see Box 10-1). In addition, there are patients that have respiratory symptoms and/or structural changes but normal spirometry. New terminology to describe this population is "pre-COPD" (GOLD, 2023). Not all pre-COPD patients will go on to develop the disease, the challenge is the current lack of evidence on best practices for these patients.

In the later stages of COPD, gas exchange is often impaired. As the alveolar walls continue to break down, the pulmonary capillary bed is reduced in size. Resistance to pulmonary blood flow is increased, forcing the right ventricle to maintain a higher and higher pressure in the pulmonary artery. Chronic hypoxemia (low oxygen) increases pulmonary artery pressures and can lead to pulmonary hypertension

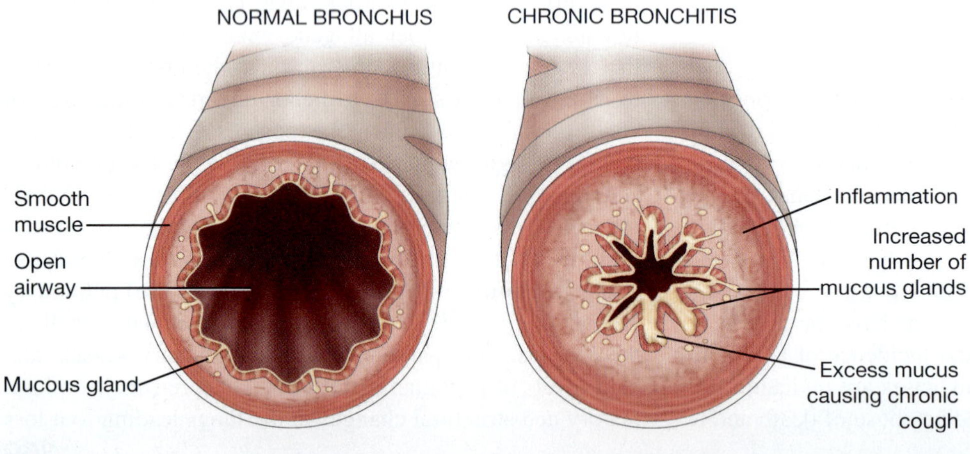

FIGURE 10-2 Pathophysiology of chronic bronchitis as compared to a normal bronchus. The bronchus in chronic bronchitis is narrowed and has impaired air flow due to multiple mechanisms: inflammation, excess mucus production, and potential smooth muscle constriction (bronchospasm).

BOX 10-1

Two Prototypes of COPD; Clinical Features

Emphysema

Characterized by the destruction of lung parenchyma leading to the loss of surface area, elastic recoil of the lungs, and structural support that maintains a patient airway.

Abnormal permanent dilatation of distal airways (respiratory bronchioles, alveolar ducts, and alveolar sacs) accompanied by destructive changes in the alveolar walls.

Increased dyspnea and work of breathing

Air trapping is increased because of the loss of elastic recoil in airway support structures (causes increased A-P diameter). Hyperinflated lungs flattens the diaphragm.

Air sacs are replaced by bullae and capillary area is proportionately diminished.

Impaired gas exchange leads to hypoxemia and hypercapnia, which can lead to respiratory failure

Ventilation/perfusion changes results in increased Functional Residual Capacity (FRC).

*Genetic factors, including alpha-1 anti-trypsin (AAT) deficiency, an autosomal recessive disease, is a cause, particularly in younger age, and primarily involves the lower lobes of the lungs

Chronic Bronchitis

Characterized by narrowing of small airways, inflammation, and mucous production. Chronic cough with sputum production on a daily basis for a minimum of 3 months a year for 2 consecutive years.

Hypersecretion of mucus and impaired cilia lead to a chronic productive cough.

Increase in bronchial wall thickness with progressive obstruction to airflow (chronic obstructive bronchitis)

Exacerbations are usually associated with infection.

Increased ventilation/perfusion abnormalities, increases hypoxemia, CO_2 retention, and acidemia.

Hypoxemia increases pulmonary vascular constriction, raising pulmonary artery pressures leading to right-sided heart failure (cor pulmonale).

Data from Devasahayam, J., LaFreniere, K., & Naik, R. (2022). Chronic emphysema. In *StatPearls [Internet]*. StatPearls Publishing. https://www.ncbi.nlm.nih.gov/books/NBK539910/
Storzer, D. (2023). Pulmonary system. In T. Hartjes (Ed.), *AACN core curriculum for progressive and critical care nursing* (8th ed., Chapter 3, pp. 63–175). Elsevier Inc.

(recall that hypoxemia is associated with pulmonary vascular bed *vasoconstriction*). This higher pressure in the pulmonary artery results in right ventricular hypertrophy. Ultimately, cor pulmonale, or right ventricular failure, can occur. In addition, decreased carbon dioxide elimination results in increased carbon dioxide tension in arterial blood (hypercapnia or hypercarbia) and leads to respiratory acidosis and chronic respiratory failure. In acute illness, worsening hypercapnia can lead to acute respiratory failure. COPD is considered a systemic disease and may affect skeletal muscle as well as the functioning of the cardiovascular, neurologic, psychiatric, and endocrine systems.

Risk Factors

The risk factors for the development for COPD are outlined in Box 10-2. The most important risk factor is tobacco smoking (cigarettes, pipes, cigars, water pipes, marijuana). Environmental tobacco smoke (ETS), also known as secondhand smoke, is also a risk factor for the development of COPD. The effects of cigarette smoke are complex and lead to the development of COPD in <50% of smokers (GOLD, 2023). Tobacco smoke irritates the airways and, in susceptible individuals, results in mucus hypersecretion and airway inflammation.

Aging is often listed as a risk factor for COPD due to the physiologic decline in pulmonary function often seen in older patients, however, it is unclear if healthy aging leads to COPD or if it is the sum of cumulative effects of exposure over a lifetime (GOLD, 2023). Fetuses exposed to maternal smoking in utero have altered lung growth and development and may have epigenic changes (the process where gene activity is altered without changing the DNA sequence) in the immune system; this is an example of where GETomics research is needed (Christenson et al., 2022; GOLD, 2023). Household air pollution exposure in the form of biomass (open fire) cooking and heating in poorly ventilated areas is a risk factor for the development of COPD in resource-limited nations; more research is needed on household air pollution related COPD and the evaluation of interventions to decrease that risk (GOLD, 2023). Other factors that put people at risk for COPD include prolonged and intense exposure

BOX 10-2

Known Risk Factors for Chronic Obstructive Pulmonary Disease

- Tobacco smoke (cigarette, pipe, cigar, water pipe, marijuana)
- Environmental tobacco smoke
- Genetic factors (e.g., severe inherited alpha-1 antitrypsin deficiency)
- Occupational exposure to chemical agents and fumes (GOLD, 2023)
- Exposure to particles: organic and inorganic dusts, open fires from wood, animal dung, crop residue, and coal
- Air pollution (GOLD, 2023)
- Biomass cooking in poorly ventilated areas

Possible Risk Factors

- Economically marginalized
- Asthma/bronchial hyperreactivity
- Chronic bronchitis/mucus hypersecretion
- Severe respiratory infections in childhood

to occupational dusts, fumes, and chemicals, inhalation of pesticides, history of previous lung infections including tuberculosis and outdoor air pollution (Christenson et al., 2022; GOLD, 2023). These exposures likely contribute to and accelerate the development of COPD among smokers, and interact with host susceptibility factors, "ultimately resulting in COPD pathogenesis and progression" (Christenson et al., 2022, p. 2227).

Pearls for Practice

The use of electronic nicotine device systems (vaping), which delivers an aerosol of nicotine by heating a liquid, has been promoted as an alternative to smoking, however, research findings reveal increased respiratory symptoms, incident airway disease, and decline of lung function with use. Not only does it potentially increase a person's exposure risk, but it has also been associated with decreased rates of smoking cessation (Bhatta & Glantz, 2020; Christenson et al., 2022). Further research is needed to determine the long-term benefit versus risks for use in smoking cessation.

A host risk factor for COPD (and also hepatic cirrhosis) is a deficiency of an enzyme inhibitor that is an inherited mutation in the *SERPINA1* gene (previously known as *PI* gene) that protects the lung parenchyma from injury: alpha$_1$-antitrypsin. **Alpha$_1$-antitrypsin deficiency** accounts for 1% to 5% of cases of COPD in the United States but it is important to recognize that not all alpha-1-antitrypsin deficient individuals will develop lung disease (Minami & Diaz, 2023). Genetically susceptible people are more sensitive to environmental factors (e.g., smoking, air pollution, infectious agents, allergens) and have a higher risk of developing chronic obstructive symptoms. As noted earlier, not all smokers get COPD, but it does occur more frequently in families. Studies to identify other genetic factors associated with COPD, such as accelerated lung aging (lungs normally grow and matures until age 25 [earlier in females]) are new areas of research (GOLD, 2023).

Pearls for Practice

The nurse considers that worldwide one third of patients with COPD never smoked, and many smokers never develop this disorder (with the exception of patients with α1-antitrypsin deficiency), thus the traditional view that this disorder is self-inflicted is questioned (Agusti et al., 2022). Clearly, there is an interplay occurring and the new strategy of considering the interaction between genetics and environment over the course of a lifetime offers the potential to "develop a new understanding of underlying pathogenic mechanisms over the lifespan—could enable identification of novel targets for the prevention and early treatment of COPD" (Agusti et al., 2022, p. 515).

Clinical Manifestations and Assessment

COPD is characterized by the primary symptoms of dyspnea, chronic cough, sputum production, and exacerbations (acute respiratory events characterized by increased respiratory symptoms). Dyspnea is defined as an awareness of uncomfortable breathing that may vary in intensity. It often starts as mild and is noticed only with vigorous activities, such as stair-climbing and playing sports. As the disease progresses, dyspnea may become severe and often interferes with the person's activities of daily living. In more severe cases of COPD, dyspnea can occur at rest. Chronic cough and sputum production often precede the development of airflow limitation by many years. In early-stage disease, the person may note an early morning cough productive of a small to moderate amount of white to clear sputum. During exacerbations, which are complex inflammatory events, often sparked by viral or bacterial infections or by environmental impacts such as pollution, an increase in the amount and viscosity of sputum may occur, and the sputum may change color. Exacerbations are associated with increased airway inflammation, mucus production, and air trapping which results in worsening of airflow limitation and dynamic lung hyperinflation causing dyspnea (Vega-Olio et al., 2022). Of note, at present there are "no clinical, physiologic, radiologic, or biologic marker that can predict exacerbation onset" (Christenson et al., 2022, p. 2023).

COPD is diagnosed based on history, physical examination, and pulmonary function testing. A positive history of progressive dyspnea and/or a productive cough in a cigarette smoker leads to a suspicion of COPD. Smoking history is usually expressed as "pack/years": the number of packs smoked per day times the number of years of smoking. A person who has smoked an average of 2 packs per day for 20 years has a smoking history of 40 pack/years.

Physical examination findings may be near normal in those with beginning and sometimes moderate disease. Findings consistent with more advanced COPD may include signs of hyperinflation: an increased anterior to posterior diameter of the chest, referred to as "barrel chest"; bilateral intercostal retractions at the posterior axillary line; horizontal fixation of the ribs in the inspiratory position; and hyperresonance to percussion, particularly in thin individuals. Breath sounds may be diminished; prolonged exhalation (bronchovesicular breath sounds) is usually heard throughout the chest; often adventitious sounds (coarse crackles and wheezes) are heard when the patient has increased secretions or bronchial hyperreactivity as well as during an exacerbation. Clubbing is associated with significant cardiopulmonary disease including chronic hypoxic conditions, chronic lung and pleural infections, or malignancies of the lung and pleural as well as cyanotic congenital heart disease, infective endocarditis, but it is also associated with GI disease and chronic hepatic fibrosis. While the exact mechanism is unknown, clubbing may be related to vascular endothelial growth factor (VEGF), which leads to increased vascularity, permeability, and ultimately connective tissue changes (Burcovschii & Aboeed, 2021). Refer to Box 50-4 and Figure 50-5.

Pulmonary function studies are used to help confirm the diagnosis, determine disease severity, and monitor disease progression, thus both pulmonary function tests, which are breathing tests that assess how well the lungs work by measuring lung volume, capacity, rates of flow, and gas exchange, as well as symptom assessment are crucial when diagnosing COPD. **Spirometry** is used to evaluate airflow obstruction. Spirometry results are expressed as an absolute value and as a percentage of the predicted value using appropriate normal values for gender, race, age, weight, and height. With obstruction, the patient has difficulty exhaling or cannot forcibly exhale air from the lungs, reducing the **FEV_1**. Obstructive lung disease is defined as a postbronchodilator FEV_1/FVC ratio of less than 70%. The lower the FEV_1, the more severe the disease process.

Bronchodilator reversibility testing may be performed to rule out asthma and to guide initial treatment. Spirometry is first obtained; the patient is given an inhaled bronchodilator and spirometry is repeated. The patient demonstrates a degree of reversibility if the pulmonary function values improve significantly (more than 12% and 200 mL of the baseline value) after administration of the bronchodilator. Usually, patients who demonstrate complete reversibility to normal values are diagnosed with asthma. Patients who demonstrate some reversibility that does not reach normal values may be diagnosed with COPD with some reversible component or an overlap of COPD and asthma. Patients who do not show a significant response to a bronchodilator test still may be given a trial of bronchodilator treatment to determine if it helps relieve symptoms. Additional tests of pulmonary function include total lung capacity (TLC) and diffusion capacity. These tests are used to diagnose coexisting restrictive disease, in which the lung is restricted from filling to its normal capacity of air, and to help predict the contribution of emphysematous changes in the diagnosis.

Arterial blood gas (ABG) measurements may be obtained to assess baseline oxygenation and gas exchange and are especially important in advanced COPD. In addition, a chest x-ray may be obtained to establish the patient's baseline and to exclude alternative diagnoses. A chest x-ray is seldom diagnostic in COPD unless obvious bullous disease or severe hyperinflation is present. Chest x-rays are more commonly used in exacerbations to determine if the patient has an infiltrate or a concomitant lung mass. A computed tomography (CT) scan is not routinely obtained in the diagnosis of COPD, but a high-resolution CT scan may help in the differential diagnosis or to evaluate patients for surgical procedures such as bullectomy or lung-volume reduction surgery (LVRS). Screening for $alpha_1$-antitrypsin deficiency is recommended for symptomatic patients younger than 45 years, those with a strong family history of COPD, and every patient with a diagnosis of COPD (GOLD, 2023; Minami & Diaz, 2023).

Different methods are used to classify COPD by stages depending on severity. The updated GOLD guidelines include lung function measurement and exacerbation history to stage patients. Staging is used to determine prognosis, guide therapy, and to develop research protocols. In mild disease, the patient may be asymptomatic. As lung function (FEV_1/FVC%) declines, symptoms start to appear. The more severe the decline in lung function is, the more severe the COPD. The GOLD guidelines classify airflow limitation severity using spirometric cutoff points ranging from stage 1 (mild; FEV_1 ≥80% of predicted values) to GOLD stage 4 (very severe; FEV_1 <30% of predicted values) (GOLD, 2023). Other factors that determine prognosis include history of cigarette smoking in terms of pack/years, continued cigarette smoking, passive smoke exposure, age, rate of decline of FEV_1, hypoxemia, pulmonary artery pressure, resting heart rate, weight loss, number of exacerbations, and reversibility of airflow obstruction. Staging severity serves as a guideline to treatment protocols, but variation occurs depending on the patient characteristics, comorbid conditions, and response to interventions.

The differential diagnosis of COPD includes: asthma, heart failure, bronchiectasis (abnormal widening of the bronchi or their branches, causing a risk of infection), tuberculosis, lung cancer, and bronchiolitis (inflammation of the bronchioles) (Heiner, 2023). Many patients with COPD have at least one comorbidity which commonly includes cardiac disease (HF, arrhythmias [atrial fibrillation is associated with a low FEV_1]), peripheral atherosclerosis, hypertension, stroke, diabetes mellitus, arthritis, lung cancer, osteoporosis, obstructive sleep apnea (OSA), muscle weakness, cachexia, anxiety, anemia, polycythemia, periodontitis, cognitive impairment, and depression (GOLD, 2023; Vega-Olivo et al., 2022). The aforementioned comorbidities are associated with adverse symptoms and exacerbations (Christenson et al., 2022).

In the past overlap syndromes such as asthma and COPD were described, however, recent guidelines suggest they be considered as separate disorders that may share some clinical features but should be treated according to each specific guideline (i.e., asthma guidelines along with pharmacologic and nonpharmacologic treatment for COPD) (GOLD, 2023).

Pearls for Practice

Early research finding on the relationship between SARS-CoV-2 revealed increased adverse effects when patients with COPD were infected with COVID-19 such as more frequent hospital admission, increased ICU admission, higher readmission rates, increased need for mechanical ventilation, more frequent cardiovascular events and higher mortality. While the mechanisms for the heightened morbidity and mortality are unknown, suggested theories include ACE2 receptors are increased in the small airways of patients with COPD and this is where SARS-CoV-2 binds, or that a proinflammatory state exists in patients with COPD and is associated with increasing age, "which could provide a lung environment more prone to severe COVID-19 disease" (Christenson et al., 2022, p. 2235; GOLD, 2023).

Medical Management

The goals of medical therapy are to prevent, stabilize, manage, and monitor the disease; reduce symptoms; assess and reduce exacerbation risk and rate; promote maximal functional ability; prevent premature disability; assist the individual to adapt to the handicap caused by the disorder and limit adverse prognosis as the disease progresses. The management of the patient depends on the severity of the COPD. In early-stage disease, clinical strategies are aimed at maximizing pulmonary function, keeping the patient active, preventing exacerbations, and engaging the patient in self-management. In progressive stages, more intensive therapies are added. In very late-stage disease, palliative care should be considered (see Fig. 10-3).

Stabilizing Disease Progression

Smoking cessation slows the accelerated decline in lung function and the progression of COPD (GOLD, 2023). Greater than 80% of tobacco users in the United States use combustible products, primarily in the form of cigarettes but also cigars, pipes, and waterpipes (hookah), and 19% of tobacco smokers reported using multiple tobacco products (Cornelius et al., 2022). Factors associated with continued smoking vary among patients and may include the strength of the nicotine addiction, continued exposure to smoking-associated stimuli (at work or in social settings), stress, anxiety/depression, and habit. Nicotine binds to receptors in the brain that release neurotransmitters, such as dopamine resulting in rewarding effects that relieve stress or negative emotions and in addition smoking becomes associated with specific circumstances or behaviors; the addictive potential depends on the speed of nicotine delivery to the brain (most rapid with inhalation) and on nicotine dose (Cornelius et al., 2022).

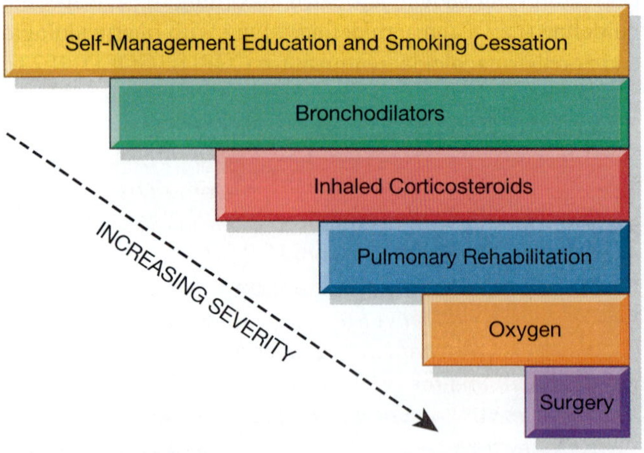

FIGURE 10-3 Treatment options for COPD. (Redrawn from *Breathing better with a COPD diagnosis,* U.S. Department of Health and Human Services, NIH publication No. 07–5841.)

Because multiple factors are associated with continued smoking, successful cessation often requires multiple strategies. Health care providers should promote cessation by explaining the risks of smoking and personalize the "at-risk" message to the patient. Encouraging the patient to set a definite "quit date" is associated with more successful smoking cessation. Brief counseling may work for many smokers; referral to a smoking cessation program may be helpful for those unable to quit on their own. Follow-up from the nurse within a few days after the established "quit date" is associated with an increased rate of success; the nurse can review progress and address any problems with the patient. The nurse educates the patient about withdrawal symptoms from nicotine which include "cigarette craving and nonspecific symptoms such as irritability, restlessness, difficulty concentrating, anxiety, and anhedonia (reduced ability to feel pleasure)" as well as increased appetite and insomnia (Bassil et al., 2022; Cornelius et al., 2022, p. 567). Patients attempting to quit smoking often do not recognize that these symptoms represent withdrawal. Continued reinforcement with telephone calls or clinic visits is beneficial. Relapses should be analyzed (on average six attempts are made to quit before achieving long-term tobacco abstinence), and the patient and health care provider should jointly identify possible solutions to prevent future backsliding (Cornelius et al., 2022). In addition, it is important to provide hope to patients that their efforts can be successful, as an example, more than 61% of former smokers have quit successfully (Creamer et al., 2019).

Pharmacotherapy increases long-term smoking abstinence rates when used in conjunction with smoking cessation counseling. Nicotine replacement (gum, inhaler, nasal spray, transdermal patch, sublingual tablet, or lozenges) reliably increases long-term abstinence rates and may be used as a single agent or in combination with other pharmacologic agents. Varenicline, bupropion SR and nortriptyline also have been shown to increase long-term quit rates. Bupropion is particularly useful in those concerned with weight gain during smoking abstinence as it may result in weight loss. Varenicline reduces nicotine withdrawal symptoms and has been associated with increased quit rates. Recent research reveals that among all monotherapies, varenicline showed a higher level of evidence of smoking cessation (Shang et al., 2022). In addition, combination treatments, such as varenicline plus bupropion and nicotine replacement therapy have a higher probability of being the best smoking cessation interventions (Shang et al., 2022).

Drug Alert
Bupropion is contraindicated in patients with a history of seizures as it may lower the seizure threshold.

Electronic cigarettes, or "e-cigarettes, produced by a variety of manufacturers are usually battery-operated devices that vaporize a mist of nicotine to the user. The use of e-cigarettes as a cessation aid is controversial because of the small number of high-quality randomized trials, limited evidence on current devices, and lack of longitudinal data (Rigotti et al., 2022). It is important to recognize that the FDA regulates e-cigarettes as tobacco products, not as medical products and has not evaluated them for medical use as a cessation aid. Heated tobacco products (HTPs) are designed to heat tobacco to a high enough temperature to release aerosol, without burning it or producing smoke. They differ from e-cigarettes because they heat tobacco leaf/sheet rather than a liquid. Both have been used by some smokers when trying to quit. A recent Cochran review noted that heated tobacco users have lower exposure to toxicants/carcinogens than cigarette smokers, however the effectiveness of heated tobacco on cigarette smoking cessation remains uncertain (Tattan-Birch et al., 2022). Further research on the effectiveness and safety of HTPs is needed.

Recent public health efforts nationally includes *Tobacco 21* legislation which increased the federal minimum age for sale of tobacco products from 18 to 21 years in 2019, and the U.S. Food and Drug Administration policy prioritizing enforcement against flavored electronic cigarette products, such as fruit and mint flavors in January of 2020.

Smoking cessation can begin in a variety of health care settings: outpatient clinics, pulmonary rehabilitation, community health programs, and hospitals as well as in the home. Regardless of the setting, nurses have the opportunity to teach patients about the risks of smoking and the benefits of smoking cessation. Various materials, resources, and programs developed by several organizations (e.g., Agency for Health Care Research and Quality, U.S. Public Health Service, CDC, National Cancer Institute, American Lung Association, American Thoracic Society, American Cancer Society) are available to assist with this effort. Online programs may be useful to some smokers. One such program is "the ex" plan, which can be found at BecomeAnEX.org (https://www.becomeanex.org/). Box 10-3 outlines a smoking cessation approach that incorporates the current concepts in a concise outline. Refer to Chapter 1, Box 1-8 about the stages of change related to health teaching.

BOX 10-3

Health Promotion

The Clinician Uses 5-Step Model for Smoking Cessation

1. **Ask** about tobacco-use status at every visit to identify smokers and document findings
2. **Advise** Urge every patient to quit in clear, strong, and personalized manner; even brief advice can improve quit rates compared with patients who receive no advice. For the ex-tobacco user, how recent did they quit and are there any challenges to remaining abstinent?
3. **Assess** the willingness of the patient to quit (within 30 days)
4. **Assist** in developing a plan, examples can include counseling, smoking cessation programs, and pharmacotherapy to help the patient quit. Note AHRQ tearsheets for patient education are available at https://www.ahrq.gov/prevention/guidelines/tobacco/clinicians/tearsheets/index.html
5. **Arrange** a follow-up visit by phone or in person

Quitting Smoking: Help for the Smoker

Cigarette smoking has long been known to damage the heart, lungs, and other organs of the body. Cancer, problems with circulation, and premature wrinkling are among its other effects. Cigar, pipe, and marijuana smoke are also known to be harmful. Smoking is the single most preventable cause of premature death and disability. Quitting smoking increases your chance of living a longer, healthier life. Here are some tips for helping you quit.

- *Determine your readiness to quit: how motivated are you?*
  - Have you set a date to quit? A willingness to set a quit-date within 2 weeks indicates good motivation for quitting.
  - Can you list your reasons for wanting to quit? Health, saving money, feeling control over your habits, smelling better, and setting an example for others are some reasons for quitting. Make your reasons for quitting personal.
  - What obstacles do you anticipate?
  - Have you prepared for quitting?
    - Throw away all smoking-related materials: cigarettes, ashtrays, lighters
    - Make a plan for dealing with smoking urges
- *Develop an action plan.*
  - For immediate urges to smoke: practice the "4 Ds"
    - ***Delay:*** the urge to smoke will lessen in 3 minutes whether or not you have a cigarette
    - ***Deep breathe:*** take several deep breaths when the urge strikes to help take the edge off
    - ***Drink water:*** it helps to clear out the nicotine faster
    - ***Do something else:*** distraction helps you ignore the urges to smoke
  - Change your Thinking: remind yourself that you are choosing to become a nonsmoker and that it takes active work to do so
  - Reward Yourself for Not Smoking: set aside the money you would have spent on cigarettes and buy yourself something as a reward
- *Discuss the need for nicotine replacement or other medications.*
  - Many smokers are much more successful in quitting with the assistance of medications like bupropion, varenicline, and/or one of the nicotine replacement products (patch, gum, inhaler, nasal spray, or lozenge). Discuss this with your health care provider.
- *Don't give up if you have a slip or relapse.*
  - Many people need several tries at quitting before they are successful. Keep at it, and you will be successful.
- *Seek help if trying to quit on your own hasn't worked.*
  - Find a local stop smoking program in your area. Your primary provider, local hospital, visiting nurse, or lung association may know of a local program.

Adapted from the Norwalk Hospital Patient Education Guidelines.

Pharmacologic Therapy

Pharmacologic agents are an important part of the treatment of COPD that will vary based upon the patient condition (e.g., stable vs. exacerbated state) and fall into several categories.

Bronchodilators

Bronchodilators relieve bronchospasm, reduce airway obstruction, and aid in secretion clearance. The most frequently used classes of bronchodilators include sympathomimetics, also called beta adrenergic or beta$_2$ agonists (both short and long acting); anticholinergics, also called muscarinic antagonists (both short and long term), or a combination of the two agents. Methylxanthines, for example, theophylline-like medications, are used less frequently than in the past but may still be useful for some patients. The methylxanthines that are currently available have a narrow therapeutic range and have serious side effects. They are often used as a third-line agent when other bronchodilators don't completely control symptoms.

Bronchodilators are usually delivered by the inhaled route (metered-dose inhalers, dry powder inhalers [DPIs], or by nebulization). Oral forms of bronchodilators are rarely given because of side effects. Long-acting sympathomimetics (also known as long-acting beta adrenergics **[LABAs]**) and anticholinergic bronchodilators (also known as long-acting muscarinic antagonists **[LAMAs]**) are considered maintenance medications and are usually administered on a regular basis. Short-acting sympathomimetics (also known as short-acting beta adrenergics **[SABAs]**) are most often used on an as-needed basis to help with dyspnea and secretion clearance. SABAs may be used prophylactically before the patient participates in dyspnea-producing activity, such as eating or walking. Short-acting muscarinic antagonists (**SAMAs**) are sometimes used for quick relief.

Corticosteroids

Inhaled and systemic corticosteroids (oral or intravenous) may also be used in COPD. Systemic steroids are usually reserved for acute exacerbations and for those with severe symptoms that do not respond adequately to bronchodilators. Long-term treatment with oral corticosteroids is associated with an increased incidence of side effects, some of which are serious (hyperglycemia, osteoporosis, cataracts, hypertension, peptic ulcers, psychic disorders, masking of infections, weight gain, and cushingoid effects) (Boardman, 2021). Inhaled corticosteroids may be used alone by inhaler devices or in combination with LABAs and/or LAMAs. Recent GOLD recommendations (2023) de-emphasize the use of inhaled steroids and emphasize the use of long-acting bronchodilators. Side effects of inhaled steroids include hoarseness, dry mouth, and oral fungal infections. Patients should be instructed to rinse and gargle after using inhaled steroid preparations to decrease the risk of oral thrush. An association between regular use of inhaled corticosteroids in those with severe disease and pneumonia has been shown (GOLD, 2023). Most providers reserve their use for those with more severe diseases or for patients who have a history of exacerbation and have elevated serum eosinophils (which play a key role in inflammation; GOLD, 2023).

Medication regimens used to manage the symptoms of COPD are based on disease, symptom severity, and risk for exacerbation. For mild COPD, a short-acting bronchodilator is usually prescribed for symptom relief. For moderate to severe COPD, a short-acting bronchodilator along with regular treatment with a LABA, a LABA/steroid combination, and/or a LAMA may be used. For severe or very severe COPD, medication therapy includes regular treatment with one or more bronchodilators and may include a methylxanthine and inhaled or systemic corticosteroids (GOLD, 2023). Recently triple therapy has been studied in patients with moderate-to-severe COPD, in which inhaled corticosteroid, long-acting β2 agonists (LABAs), and long-acting muscarinic antagonists (LAMAs) are combined into a single inhaler. Triple therapy was associated with exacerbation reduction, particularly in individuals with elevated eosinophil counts, and a moderate mortality benefit in secondary analyses; however, further studies are needed to assess benefit versus risk (GOLD, 2023).

A **metered-dose inhaler** (MDI) is a pressurized device that contains an aerosolized suspension of medication. A measured amount of medication is released with each activation of the canister. Patients must be instructed on the correct use of inhalers. With the correct technique, 20% of the dose of medication is inhaled into the lung. However, research continues to reveal that poor technique when using MDI is a persistent problem. A recent study noted critical errors were observed in 39.3% of stable patients with COPD (Duarte-de-Araújo et al., 2019). Proper technique is important to ensure adequate deposition into the airways. Common mistakes made by patients using MDIs include having difficulty coordinating actuation with inhalation, breathing in too quickly, not breath-holding after inhalation, forgetting to exhale completely before each dose, not shaking the canister before each dose, and aiming the inhaler at the roof of the mouth or tongue rather than the throat.

A spacer (holding chamber) may also be used for patients who have difficulty coordinating activation of the MDI with inspiration. They are particularly useful for MDI steroids as less medication is deposited in the oropharynx, decreasing inhaled steroid side effects. Spacers come in several designs, but all are attached to the MDI and have a mouthpiece on the opposite end. Once the canister is activated, the aerosol particles stay suspended in the chamber for several seconds, allowing the patient to inhale after actuating the inhaler. Box 10-4 outlines the important steps for using an MDI and spacer correctly. Patients need a periodic review of the correct inhaler technique to increase optimal therapeutic effect. DPIs include a variety of medications and devices. Specific

BOX 10-4

Patient Education

Using Inhalers Correctly

Many medicines taken for breathing are given by the inhaled method. Inhaled medicine goes directly to the lungs. But you need to learn to use inhalers correctly. With perfect technique, you get about 20% (Newman, 2017) of the medication in your lungs. So, **good** technique is very important.

Correct Technique for Using Metered-Dose Inhalers

- Remove the cap from the mouthpiece of the inhaler.
- Shake your inhaler for 5–6 seconds.
- Place the mouthpiece of the inhaler in your mouth with your tongue and teeth out of the way.
- As you depress the inhaler take a deep breath with your mouth wide open. Inhale for 5–6 seconds if you can. *Slow is the way to go.* The more slowly you breathe in, the deeper the medicine gets.
- At the end of the deep breath, hold your breath for at least 3–10 seconds.
- Exhale through pursed lips.
- If more than one puff is prescribed, repeat the above steps.
- After your last puff, rinse your mouth with mouthwash or water to help prevent dryness. If you are using inhaled steroids, rinse, gargle, and spit out the water or mouthwash.
- Rinse the mouthpiece thoroughly with warm water at least once a day. Let it air dry before assembling and storing it.

Other points: Do not use your inhaler more often than your health care provider recommends. An occasional extra puff or treatment of your quick-acting bronchodilator is ok, but if you find yourself using your inhaler more frequently than usual, that may be a sign that you're getting ill and need to contact your provider.

Other inhaled medicines, e.g., those obtained without a prescription, should not be used unless approved by your primary provider. Mixing certain medicatons can cause serious side effects.

Spacer Devices

Spacer devices are used with inhalers when:

- You have a hard time using your inhaler correctly
- When the taste of the propellant in the inhaler is disturbing
- When you are using inhaled steroids and have problems with yeast infections in your mouth

Here is the technique for using an inhaler with a spacer:

- Take the cap off the inhaler and the spacer.
- Place the inhaler mouthpiece in the end of the spacer.
- Shake your inhaler for 5–6 seconds.
- Place the spacer mouthpiece in your mouth.
- Depress the inhaler into the spacer.
- Inhale slowly for 5–6 seconds.
- Hold your breath for about 10 seconds.
- Repeat the steps for each puff of medication.

package insert information on the use of these inhalers is available from the manufacturer. The most common medications administered by metered dose or DPIs used for both COPD and asthma are shown in Table 10-1. Nebulized medications (aerosolization of medication via a jet nebulizer and an air compressor) may also be effective in patients who cannot use an MDI properly or who prefer this method of administration. Several formulations of medications are available for nebulization. Patients need to learn proper technique for administration by nebulizers. Disinfection of the medication cup needs to be performed on a regular basis to avoid bacterial growth and inhalation by the patient.

Other Medications

Vaccinations (e.g., influenza, pneumococcus, pertussis, SARS-CoV-2, and shingles) reduce the incidence of pneumonia, hospitalizations for cardiac conditions, and deaths in the general older population (Christenson et al., 2022). Patients should receive a yearly influenza vaccine. The CDC currently recommends one dose of 20-valent pneumococcal conjugate vaccine (PCV20) or one dose of 15-valent pneumococcal conjugate vaccine (PCV15), followed by 23 valent pneumococcal polysaccharide vaccine (PPSV23) for patients with COPD. A one-time booster of pertussis (TDAP-tetanus, diphtheria, and pertussis), as well as routine shingles vaccines and COVID-19 vaccinations, are also recommended (CDC, 2021, 2022b).

Oral phosphodiesterase 4 (PDE_4) inhibitors (e.g., roflumilast) may be used to reduce the airway inflammation seen in COPD; it is contraindicated in moderate to severe liver disease (Crocetti et al., 2022). Side effects include severe nausea, diarrhea, weight loss, headache, sleep disturbances, and mood disturbances; these may limit its usefulness in some patients.

Other pharmacologic treatments that may be used for COPD include alpha1-antitrypsin augmentation therapy for those with a diagnosed deficiency, antibiotic agents for acute infection, and mucolytic agents for help with secretion clearance. No evidence exists regarding the use of antitussives in COPD (GOLD, 2023).

Pharmacologic treatment of COPD poses many challenges for patients. Multiple drugs and drug classes are included in treatment regimens, and many drugs go by multiple names. In addition, multiple delivery methods, poly-pharmacy particularly with other comorbid conditions, expense, and side effects can contribute to poor adherence. Patients often confuse the concepts of maintenance medications and "quick-relief" medications and may not use them correctly. Repeated patient education is important.

Exacerbations and Complications

Exacerbations of COPD are complex inflammatory events, that represent an acute worsening of the patient's symptoms that necessitates a change in treatment (GOLD, 2023). Exacerbations of COPD are associated with disease progression

TABLE **10-1 Common Inhaled Medications Used in COPD and Asthma**

Medication Class	Generic Name (Trade Name)	
Short-acting beta-adrenergic (SABA) aka beta2 agonist	**albuterol solution for nebs** *(comes in three strengths)* **albuterol sulfate HFA** **levalbuterol HFA**	• Used “as-needed for quick relief” or on a timed basis • MDIs generally given as two puffs as needed or four times a day • May or may not need a spacer with MDI for good technique • MDIs now come with a dose counter • ProAir also available in RespiClick device
Short-acting muscarinic antagonist (SAMA) aka short-acting anticholinergic	**ipratropium HFA**	• Used as a timed medication or as alternative for “quick relief” • Generally given as two puffs four times a day (up to 12 puffs in 24 hours)
SAMA/SABA combination	**ipratropium/albuterol**	• May be used as first-line therapy or quick relief • Combivent generally administered four times a day by Respimat device
Long-acting muscarinic antagonist (LAMA) aka LA anticholinergic	**tiotropium** **aclidinium** **umeclidinium**	• First-line therapy for moderate to severe disease (in COPD) • Tiotropium given once a day; aclidinium given twice a day • Tiotropium approved for reducing COPD exacerbations • Tiotropium also available in Respimat device • Each medication comes with its own delivery device
Long-acting beta adrenergic (LABA) aka LA beta2 agonist	**arformoterol tartrate solution** **salmeterol DPI** **formoterol DPI** **indacaterol**	• Used in moderate to severe COPD often in combination with corticosteroids • Each medication comes with its own delivery device • Not for acute symptoms • Salmeterol and formoterol both one puff twice a day, indacaterol once daily • This class not used as monotherapy in asthma
Combinations of long-acting: LAMA/LABA	**umeclidinium/vilanterol** **tiotropium/olodaterol**	• Used for moderate to severe COPD • Given one puff once daily for umeclidinium/vilanterol • Tiotropium bromide and olodaterol are given two actuations once a day by Respimat
Inhaled glucocorticosteroids (ICS)	**ciclesonide HFA** **mometasone** **fluticasone HFA** **budesonide DPI** **beclomethasone**	• Generally used in persistent asthma/later stages of COPD • Patients need to rinse out their mouths to prevent oral thrush • Spacers are also useful to help prevent thrush • All devices have counters beclomethasone (QVAR) • All come in two strengths except for Flovent, which comes in three • Are maintenance or controller medications in both asthma and COPD, not to be used as needed • Most are given twice a day, strength varies based on patient's severity of illness and history of recent exacerbation
Combinations of long acting: LABA/Corticosteroid combination	**fluticasone/salmeterol** **budesonide/formoterol** **mometasone/formoterol** **fluticasone/vilanterol**	• Used in moderate to severe COPD and asthma • Patients need to rinse out their mouths to prevent oral thrush • Each drug has its own delivery device and technique • Fluticasone/vilanterol (Breo Elipta) given once daily, others every 12 hours

HFA, hydrofluoroalkane used as propellant; DPI, dry powder inhaler.

and an accelerated decline in pulmonary function. Signs and symptoms may include increased dyspnea, cough with or without increased sputum production and purulence, respiratory failure, changes in mental status, or worsening blood gas abnormalities. The primary causes of acute exacerbations include infection (bacterial [40% to 60%], viral [30%] and atypical bacteria [5% to 10%]), response to pollutants and allergens, nonadherence to treatment, and associated comorbidities (Hogea et al., 2020). The best predictor for an exacerbation is a previous history of one (GOLD, 2023). Severe exacerbations requiring hospitalization are associated with an increase in mortality.

Prevention of exacerbations is associated with preservation of pulmonary function and a decrease in hospitalizations. Smoking cessation; COVID-19, influenza, and pneumococcal vaccines; inhaled drugs (LABAs, LAMAs with or without corticosteroids); and phosphodiesterase inhibitors have been associated with a prolonged time between exacerbations (GOLD, 2023). For the prevention of exacerbations, azithromycin is associated with improved quality of life and a decrease in exacerbations, and roflumilast has demonstrated decreased incidence of exacerbation in patients with symptoms of chronic bronchitis (GOLD, 2023).

During an exacerbation, optimization of bronchodilator medications, inhaled or systemic corticosteroids, antibiotic agents, oxygen therapy, and intensive respiratory interventions may also be used. Early treatment with antibiotics in patients needing hospitalization for an acute exacerbation may result in improved outcomes. The use of noninvasive ventilation is recommended initially since it has been shown to reduce intubation risk, length of hospital stay, and mortality in respiratory failure due to COPD exacerbations (GOLD, 2023). For patients who are experiencing exacerbation while on dual therapy, the GOLD (2023) recommendations include escalating to triple therapy to decrease future exacerbations.

Indications for hospitalization for an acute exacerbation of COPD include severe COPD, marked increase in intensity of symptoms that does not respond adequately to initial therapy, inadequate home support, confusion or lethargy, respiratory muscle fatigue, paradoxical chest wall movement, peripheral edema, worsening or new onset of central cyanosis, persistent or worsening hypoxemia, and the need for noninvasive or invasive assisted mechanical ventilation (GOLD, 2023). The risk of death from an exacerbation of COPD is closely related to the development of respiratory acidosis (10% mortality); the presence of significant comorbidities; the need for noninvasive or invasive positive-pressure ventilatory support (mortality rate nearly reaches 40% if patient is intubated); and a high DECAF score, which includes **D**yspnea, **E**osinopenia, **C**onsolidation, **A**cidemia and **A**trial **F**ibrillation, at the time of hospital admission (Bansal & Gaude, 2020).

Respiratory insufficiency and failure are major life-threatening complications of COPD. The acuity of the onset and the severity of respiratory failure depend on baseline pulmonary function, pulse oximetry or ABG values, comorbid conditions, and the severity of other complications of COPD. Respiratory insufficiency and failure may be chronic (with severe COPD) or acute (with a severe exacerbation or pneumonia in a patient with COPD). Acute respiratory insufficiency and failure may necessitate ventilatory support until the underlying cause, such as infection, can be treated. Management of the patient requiring ventilatory support is discussed in Chapter 54.

Other complications of COPD include pneumonia, atelectasis, pneumothorax, and pulmonary arterial hypertension. Pulmonary hypertension is more common in patients with chronic hypoxemia and severe disease and is associated with decreased survival. The diagnosis of pulmonary hypertension associated with COPD is suspected in patients complaining of dyspnea and fatigue that appear to be disproportionate to pulmonary function abnormalities. Enlargement of the central pulmonary arteries on chest radiograph and an echocardiogram suggestive of right ventricular enlargement and elevated plasma brain natriuretic peptide (BNP) may be present. Medical management of pulmonary hypertension associated with COPD includes stabilization of the underlying lung disease, administration of long-term supplemental oxygen, and diuretics. During acute episodes, treatment may include positive-pressure ventilation.

Pearls for Practice: Pathophysiology

Brain Natriuretic Peptide (BNP) is secreted from the overdistended cardiac chambers. High BNP levels (greater than 100 pg/mL) indicate abnormal ventricular function or symptomatic heart failure. BNP levels are useful for diagnosing heart failure. The higher the BNP level, the more severe the heart failure.

Pneumothorax is a less common complication of COPD but can be life-threatening in patients who have minimal pulmonary reserve. Patients with severe emphysematous changes can develop large bullae, which may rupture and cause a pneumothorax. Development of a pneumothorax may be spontaneous or related to an activity such as severe coughing or large intrathoracic pressure changes. Signs and symptoms of a pneumothorax include sudden chest pain that is sharp and abrupt, a significant and sudden increase in severe shortness of breath, asymmetry of chest movement, unilateral retractions, hyperresonance on percussion (excessive air trapped in the pleural space), crepitus (cracking sensation when touching affected area), bilateral differences in breath sounds, and/or oxygen desaturation. Pneumothorax in a patient with underlying lung disease is a medical emergency. Rapid response teams or emergency services should be initiated (refer to Chapter 9).

The clinical and economic impact of frequent readmissions has prompted an examination of factors that contribute to frequent hospitalizations. Patients with comorbidities, a history of prior exacerbations, individual patient and caregiver factors, and lack of integration of inpatient and outpatient care are suggested as possible contributing factors. It is important to emphasize that pulmonary rehabilitation programs have demonstrated decreased mortality rates and should be encouraged by nurses for our patients. However, access can be limited given relatively small numbers of pulmonary rehab programs compared to the number of patients with COPD (GOLD, 2023).

Oxygen Therapy

Oxygen therapy may be administered during an acute exacerbation, as long-term continuous therapy for severe chronic resting hypoxemia (PaO_2 <55 mm Hg, or <60 mm Hg if cor pulmonale or secondary polycythemia is present), and during exercise and sleep for selected patients. The goal of oxygen therapy is to maintain tissue oxygenation and decrease the work of the cardiopulmonary system (GOLD, 2023). Oxygen is generally administered to acutely ill COPD patients when their room air oxygen saturation is less than 88% or if they are showing signs of increased cardiopulmonary work: increased shortness of breath, increased work of breathing (use of accessory muscles, retractions, nasal flaring, etc.), tachypnea, tachycardia, or elevated blood pressure. Oxygen is administered to maintain a target oxygen saturation of 88% to 92% (GOLD, 2023). Recall that when the O_2 saturation is measured with pulse oximetry, it is referred to as SpO_2.

Pearls for Practice

Due to the imperfect correlation between oxygen saturation via pulse oximeter (SpO_2) and arterial blood gases (ABGs), and the realization that the O_2 sat does not provide information regarding pH or $PaCO_2$ (degree of acidosis), the nurse recognizes that when concerned about the patient's status, the provider will be notified regarding the need for ABGs. Recent GOLD recommendations (2023) include drawing ABGs when the SpO_2 is below 92%. In addition, the nurse is aware that oxygen is a drug and therefore has side effects. Hyperoxygenation (PaO_2 >100 mm Hg) is to be avoided. In general, for patients at risk for oxygen-induced hypercapnia (e.g., COPD, asthma, and obesity-associated hypoventilation), oxygen therapy should be started when SpO_2 is ≤88% and stopped when it is >92%, and for those patients without risk factors, oxygen therapy should be started when SpO_2 is ≤92% and stopped when it is >96% (Allardet-Servent et al., 2019). However, there is no set standard; thus, the nurse should confer with the provider to discuss what the lower limit of the SpO_2 should be for their patient before initiating oxygen administration (and at what FiO_2), what the target therapeutic SpO_2 is, and the upper limit of SpO_2 at which the nurse will stop the oxygen in order to prevent hyperoxemia.

Pearls for Practice: Pathophysiology

When the PaO_2 is >100 mm Hg, cardiovascular and pulmonary effects include a 10% decrease in cardiac output and heart rate, vasoconstriction that decreases regional blood flow (~20%) to the brain, heart (coronary vasoconstriction and reduced coronary arterial blood flow), skin, skeletal muscle, and hypercapnia (increased CO_2); thus, hyperoxygenation is to be avoided (Allardet-Servent et al., 2019).

A small subset of COPD patients with chronic hypercapnia (elevated $PaCO_2$ levels) may be at some risk for respiratory failure should they receive too high an oxygen concentration. Concern persists that such patients would lose their "drive to breathe," also called "hypoxic drive." However, over-concern may lead patients to receive too little oxygen, resulting in hypoxemia. While hypercapnic patients are at increased risk for respiratory failure, the risk is related to the severity of their COPD. Adequate oxygenation is important in their management and should never be withheld. Key in the care of patients with COPD on supplemental oxygen is monitoring and assessment. Pulse oximetry is helpful in assessing response to therapy. ABGs are needed to assess $PaCO_2$ levels. Adequate oxygenation of patients (keeping the oxygen saturation *at or above* 90%) is important to prevent vital organ damage while monitoring for any possible complications of oxygen supplementation. Alternative delivery devices such as Venturi masks or ventilatory support (noninvasive by mask [noninvasive positive-pressure ventilation (NPPV)] or by intubation) may be necessary during acute exacerbations to ensure adequate gas exchange.

Pearls for Practice: Pathophysiology

What does hypoxic drive mean? Recall that central chemoreceptors (located in the medulla) respond to changes in PCO_2 and pH and alter the depth and rate of ventilation as needed. There are also peripheral chemoreceptors (located in the aortic arch and the carotid arteries) that respond first to changes in PaO_2 (less than 60 mm Hg) and then to $PaCO_2$ and pH by altering the depth and rate of respiration. In COPD, the chemoreceptors no longer respond to $PaCO_2$ or pH because of the persistent hypercarbia; thus, the primary drive to breathe comes from a low O_2 level. If O_2 is administered at a high enough rate to raise the PaO_2 to a normal level, there is a risk of obliterating the hypoxic drive. That is why low-flow O_2 is administered to a patient with COPD while the nurse carefully assesses for complications. However, as noted, if higher flow is needed, oxygen is never withheld and the nurse is aware that intubation or noninvasive positive-pressure ventilation (NPPV) may be required.

Two seminal landmark studies showed the value of long-term supplemental oxygen in patients who are chronically hypoxemic (British Medical Research Working Party, 1981; Nocturnal Oxygen Therapy Trial Group, 1980). Long-term oxygen therapy (worn more than 15 hours per day) was associated with increased survival, improved quality of life, a modest reduction in pulmonary arterial pressure, and decreased dyspnea. Long-term oxygen therapy is usually introduced in severe COPD with chronic resting hypoxemia. Indications generally include a PaO_2 of 55 mm Hg or less, or <60 mm Hg if right ventricular failure or secondary polycythemia is present; or an oxygen saturation of 88% or less. Evidence of tissue hypoxia and organ damage such as pulmonary hypertension, secondary polycythemia, edema from right-sided heart failure, or impaired mental status indicates a need for long-term oxygen therapy. For patients with exercise-induced hypoxemia, oxygen supplementation during exercise may improve performance; however, long-term oxygen therapy is not routinely recommended (GOLD, 2023). Patients who are hypoxemic while awake are likely to be so during sleep. Therefore, nighttime oxygen therapy may be recommended; the prescription for oxygen therapy is for continuous 24-hour use. Intermittent oxygen therapy is indicated for patients who desaturate only during exercise or sleep. Oxygen may also be prescribed in patients who become hypoxemic at high-altitude situations, for example, during air travel and high-altitude environments. Specialized studies done in a pulmonary function laboratory can determine which patients may need oxygen at high altitude.

Home oxygen is usually supplied by several different methods, including oxygen concentrators, compressed gas cylinders, liquid oxygen, or some combination of these. Newer concentrator/compressors allow appropriate patients to fill their own gas cylinders. Demand portable oxygen systems (liquid and gas systems) and small portable oxygen concentrators have allowed many patients to have more freedom and time away from their stationary systems. Patients need to be evaluated with the chosen system to ensure adequate oxygen saturation. Also, COPD patients should be evaluated for OSA since clear benefits have been demonstrated with the use of continuous positive airway pressure (CPAP) for patients with COPD and OSA.

Surgical Treatments

Bullae are enlarged airspaces that do not contribute to ventilation but occupy space in the thorax. Bullae may compress areas of healthier lung tissue and impair gas exchange. If they are limited in number, bullae may be surgically excised. A bullectomy (surgical excision of the bullae) may help reduce dyspnea and improve lung function. It can be performed thoracoscopically (with a video-assisted thoracoscope), via bronchoscopy (highly selected subgroup) or via a limited thoracotomy incision (GOLD, 2023).

Lung volume reduction surgery (LVRS) is an option for a subset of patients with severe emphysema. Patients with predominately upper lobe disease benefit the most. LVRS involves the removal of a portion of the diseased lung parenchyma. Successful LVRS results in reduced hyperinflation and improvement in the elastic recoil and diaphragmatic mechanics. LVRS is not curative but may decrease dyspnea, improve lung function, and improve the patient's overall quality of life. Careful selection of patients for LVRS is essential to decrease morbidity and mortality. The National Emphysema Treatment Trial found that the addition of LVRS to optimal medical management and rehabilitation led to overall improvement in exercise tolerance and survival in a subgroup of patients with predominantly upper lobe disease (GOLD, 2023).

Lung transplantation is an alternative surgical treatment for end-stage COPD that is considered when life expectancy is no more than 36 months despite maximum medical management with persistent disease symptoms (Williams-Taylor et al., 2022). Annually, >1,000 lung transplants are conducted and, while improved quality of life and functional capacity is seen in a selected group of patients with COPD, survival is variable, with 2/5 patients surviving 2 years post-transplant (GOLD, 2023). Over 70% of lung transplants in patients with COPD are double lung transplants, and 30% are single-lung; the median survival post lung transplant is 5.9 years (GOLD, 2023). Specific criteria exist for referral for lung transplantation. Patients are prioritized based on the severity of their disease, age, and prognosis. Limited organ availability is a concern and may limit transplantation as an option. Patients who have had a lung transplant need special care when hospitalized. Transplanted patients are on multiple medications to prevent organ rejection and are at markedly increased risk for infection. Coordination of care with the transplant center should be done when patients require hospitalization.

Pulmonary Rehabilitation

Pulmonary rehabilitation for patients with COPD is well established and widely accepted as a means to alleviate symptoms and optimize functional status. It is now considered part of the recommended treatment for symptomatic COPD. The primary goals of rehabilitation are to reduce symptoms, improve quality of life, and increase participation in everyday activities (GOLD, 2023). Pulmonary rehabilitation services are multidisciplinary and include assessment, education, physical reconditioning, skills training, and psychological support. Patients are taught methods to alleviate symptoms through breathing exercises and learning how to pace activities. Physical conditioning through endurance and strength training is an essential component of rehabilitation. Energy conservation skills are used to improve functional status and decrease dyspnea and fatigue. Nutritional counseling and medication education are other important components of rehabilitation.

The demonstrated benefits of pulmonary rehabilitation include improvement in symptoms and exercise tolerance, improved quality of life, and a reduction in hospitalizations. It is particularly effective after exacerbations in patients with COPD and exercise limitations (GOLD, 2023). Selection of a program depends on the patient's physical, functional, and psychosocial status; insurance coverage; geographic location; and preference. Barriers include scarcities of programs, social isolation, cost, transportation access, and mobility; however, new research on the benefit of virtual rehabilitation programs developed during the COVID-19 pandemic offers promising future directions (GOLD, 2023). Patients with moderate to severe lung disease may benefit the most from pulmonary rehabilitation. Patients with very severe disease may also benefit.

Nursing Management

Nurses play a key role in the care of the patient with COPD. In an office setting, nurses may assist in the assessment of patients suspected of having COPD or help manage patients with known COPD, teach techniques for managing the common problems associated with living with COPD, and review the use of prescribed medications. In acute care settings, nursing care focuses on assessing patients for problems with dyspnea, gas exchange, and secretion clearance. In addition, nurses assess for and help manage respiratory failure, administer medications and treatments to support the cardiopulmonary system, assist the patient to recover from an acute exacerbation, and help prepare patients for discharge. Nursing care in extended-care facilities and home care focuses on helping patients maintain disease stability, improve functional capacity, and learn self-management strategies. Nursing care of patients with very severe and end-stage disease focuses on palliative measures aimed at symptom relief and helping the patient and family cope with limited prognosis.

In addition, nurses may identify potential candidates for pulmonary rehabilitation and reinforce the material learned in the rehabilitation program. Not all patients have access to a formal rehabilitation program. Nurses can teach patients and families rehabilitation concepts as well as facilitate specific services: respiratory therapy for equipment and oxygenation needs, physical therapy for exercise and breathing retraining, occupational therapy for conserving energy during activities of daily living, psychosocial therapy, and nutritional counseling. Numerous educational materials are available to assist nurses in teaching patients with COPD. Potential resources include organizations such as the American Lung Association, the American Association of Cardiovascular and Pulmonary Rehabilitation, the American Thoracic Society, the American College of Chest Physicians, and the American Association for Respiratory Care. Online information is also available through these organizations (see resource list at the end of the chapter).

Assessing the Patient

Assessment includes obtaining information about current symptoms as well as previous disease manifestations. In addition to the questions obtained in a basic health history, key questions should focus on the main symptoms of COPD: shortness of breath (dyspnea), cough, sputum production, and recent exacerbations. Patients with moderate to severe COPD may always have some symptoms. It is helpful to ask patients how their current symptoms compare to their usual amount of shortness of breath, cough, and sputum. When quantifying dyspnea, it can be helpful to use a numeric scale based on 0 to 10, with 0 being no shortness of breath and 10 being the worst. For example, if the patient's usual rating of shortness of breath is a 4 and is now a 7, a significant change has occurred. A change in sputum color, quantity, or thickness is also significant. Additional symptoms of a change in condition may include increased fatigue and a decreased ability to perform one's usual activities. The Medical Research Council created a dyspnea or breathlessness scale (see Fig. 10-4) that includes description of degrees of activity when a patient becomes breathless (such as "with strenuous exercise") or limits what a person can do (such as "too breathless to leave the house") using a scale of 0–4 (Yorke et al., 2022).

Other assessment questions may include the presence of other medical problems (cardiovascular, diabetes, stroke, history of pneumonia, cancer), allergies, history of smoking in pack-years, current smoking, a history of past exacerbations and pulmonary hospitalizations including a history of intubations, a description of how the patient spends a usual day, sleep quality and amount, problems with mood (anxiety and/or depression), and what self-care measures the patient is currently using.

Physical examination should focus on observing the patient's breathing pattern and body position. Accessory muscle use, shoulder elevation, and the tripod position (leaning forward with the arms braced on the knees) are associated with increased respiratory distress. A change in respiratory rate is also a significant examination finding. A normal resting respiratory rate is 8 to 16 breaths per minute (a respiratory rate of 20 is considered the upper limit of normal by some sources). Many patients with COPD will have respiratory rates of 20 to 24 at baseline. When the respiratory rate is greater than the patient's baseline, it may signal an acute problem. It is helpful to ask patients if they are aware of their increased respiratory rate. They may relate this to a recent exacerbation of symptoms. Assessment of breath sounds should include quality (good aeration or diminished), the presence of adventitious sounds (crackles or wheezes), and whether the adventitious sounds clear with cough. Patient assessment is aided by a review of laboratory data, including pulmonary function tests, tests of oxygenation, and radiologic studies.

A systematic assessment of the patient helps the nurse determine if the patient is stable, becoming acutely ill and needs medical intervention, or becoming more severely ill and needs emergency medical attention.

Common Problems

COPD is a chronic illness and by its definition is not curable. Several common problems of COPD are amenable to treatment and nursing interventions. Table 10-2 lists the most

MODIFIED MRC DYSPNEA SCALE[a]

PLEASE TICK IN THE BOX THAT APPLIES TO YOU | ONE BOX ONLY | Grades 0 - 4

mMRC Grade 0.	I only get breathless with strenuous exercise.	☐
mMRC Grade 1.	I get short of breath when hurrying on the level or walking up a slight hill.	☐
mMRC Grade 2.	I walk slower than people of the same age on the level because of breathlessness, or I have to stop for breath when walking on my own pace on the level.	☐
mMRC Grade 3.	I stop for breath after walking about 100 meters or after a few minutes on the level.	☐
mMRC Grade 4.	I am too breathless to leave the house or I am breathless when dressing or undressing.	☐

[a] Fletcher CM. BMJ 1960; 2: 1662.

FIGURE 10-4 The Medical Research Council (MRC) dyspnea or breathlessness scale. (Used with permission from Global Initiative for Chronic Obstructive Lung Disease (GOLD), available from www.goldcopd.org, published in Fontana, WI, USA.)

common problems associated with a diagnosis of COPD. The nursing goals for patients are compatible with other members of the health care team and may include smoking cessation, improved dyspnea, improved gas exchange, more effective airway clearance, decreased incidence of exacerbations, increased exercise tolerance, maintaining ideal body weight, increased self-management, improved coping ability, adherence to the therapeutic program including medications and oxygen, home care, and absence of complications.

Nursing Interventions

Smoking

Although many patients believe that smoking cessation is futile, continued smoking does increase the rate of lung function decline and disabling symptoms. Even brief counseling by nurses and other health professionals about the hazards of smoking can be beneficial. Hospitalized smokers may present a "teachable moment." Relating the cause of the hospitalization to smoking behavior personalizes the message to the patient. Administering and teaching patients about pharmacologic agents that increase the likelihood of a successful quit attempt is an additional nursing intervention. Refer to the previous discussion and Box 10-3 on page 375 for more information on helping smokers to quit.

TABLE 10-2 Common Problems Associated with COPD

- Continued smoking
- Dyspnea
- Impaired gas exchange
- Cough and ineffective airway clearance
- Fatigue
- Decreased exercise tolerance
- Decreased functional capacity
- Deficient knowledge of self-care strategies to be performed at home
- Anxiety
- Depression
- Limited prognosis in severe disease
- Potential complications:
  - Respiratory insufficiency or failure
  - Pulmonary infection and pneumonia
  - Pulmonary hypertension
  - Cor pulmonale (right-sided heart failure)

Chronic Dyspnea

Chronic dyspnea is one of the most common problems among patients with moderate to severe COPD. Dyspnea or shortness of breath is an uncomfortable awareness of breathing that is often described by patients as an inability to get enough air into the lungs. Acute dyspnea occurs during an exacerbation, with increased activity, from anxiety and panic, and because of acute coexisting medical conditions (e.g., anemia, heart failure, pneumonia). Chronic dyspnea is different from acute dyspnea in that the patient may exhibit no visible signs of distress. Analogous to pain, dyspnea occurs "when the patient says it does" and feels like "the patient says it does."

The management of dyspnea focuses on assessing the underlying causes and administering therapies to reduce the symptoms. Nursing management includes administering bronchodilators to increase airway patency, assisting acutely ill patients with activities of daily living to decrease the work of breathing, administering oxygen therapy when hypoxemia contributes to dyspnea, and teaching strategies for relieving increased shortness of breath and for limiting future episodes.

BOX 10-5 **Patient Education**

Managing an Acute Episode of Shortness of Breath

(Use this method to control your breathing when you become more short of breath from overexertion or anxiety and to help you avoid panic.)

Step One: Position *(find the most comfortable position to allow the air to move in and out of your lungs). Maintaining the head of the bed elevated 30–45 degrees unless medically contraindicated improves ventilation and prevents aspiration (Storzer, 2023). An overbed table may be helpful for those patients with emphysema.*

- Leaning forward with your back straight
- Leaning over a table with your arms resting on the table
- Placing pillows under your arms and keeping them supported and relaxed

Step Two: Breathing *(begin to control your breathing)*

- Breathe out through pursed or slightly puckered lips
- Breathe in through your mouth if you are very short of breath
- It may help to puff your cheeks out as you breathe out
- Breathe out longer and longer each breath until it starts to feel more comfortable
- As your breathing gets more comfortable, breathe in through your nose and out through pursed lips

Step 3: Relaxation *(once your breathing starts to slow down)*

- Relax your neck and shoulders
- Allow your arms to become limp
- Close your eyes if that helps you to relax

Additional Points

- When your breathing is in control, resume your previous activity at a slower pace.
- It may help to use your "quick-relief" medication in addition to pursed-lip breathing.
- Breathe out for the hardest part of the exertion.
  Example: While climbing stairs, breathe in while standing still; breathe out while climbing one or more steps. Pause again to breathe in; breathe out while you climb.
- Practice **position, breathing, and relaxation** when you are not short of breath to help you avoid panic.
- **If your shortness of breath continues or gets worse, call your primary provider.**

Ineffective breathing patterns and shortness of breath are partially due to the ineffective respiratory mechanics of the chest wall, lungs, and diaphragm; airway obstruction; the metabolic cost of breathing; and stress. Breathing retraining may help improve breathing patterns. Pursed-lip breathing helps slow exhalation and is thought to prevent the collapse of the small airways, effectively allowing more air to be exhaled and decreasing hyperinflation. A simple explanation to patients is that pursed-lip breathing makes "more room to breathe." It may promote relaxation and reduce feelings of panic, allowing patients to gain control of their breathing. Box 10-5 provides a patient handout and method of helping patients deal with an acute episode of their chronic dyspnea.

Pearls for Practice

The nurse uses the skill of inspection in detecting deterioration in patients with pulmonary disorders such as observing the breathing pattern (i.e., rapid and shallow or slow and deep), use of accessory muscles (open mouth, intercostal or neck muscle use, retractions), diaphoresis, body position (i.e., upright, leaning forward to optimize breathing mechanics, also known as tripoding), inability to speak in full sentences, central cyanosis (blue/gray tone of the tongue and mucous membranes; recall that in people with melanin-rich skin you will observe for dull, dark color in the buccal mucosa [inside of the cheek] and hard palate [roof of the mouth]), and deterioration in the patient's level of consciousness. It is important not to underestimate the value of inspection when assessing patients and to not privilege technology over your observation. If concerned, notify the provider.

An additional patient teaching strategy is to advise the use of a small handheld fan and let the air flow on the cheek (refer to Box 10-6). Patients frequently report that cool, moving air reduces their sensation of dyspnea. Relaxation techniques such as progressive muscle relaxation may also be useful.

Diaphragmatic breathing has long been taught to patients with COPD; it involves breathing in slowly and deeply through the nose using the diaphragm with minimum movement of the chest, with one hand placed on the chest and the other on the belly (Hamasaki, 2020). The diaphragmatic breathing technique is not standardized; for example, the optimal posture when performing it has not been elucidated (e.g., supine, semi recumbent, or seated position), and the length of inspiration to expiration varies from 4 to 8 seconds (Hamasaki, 2020). The technique can be difficult for patients to learn; however, when combined with pursed lip breathing, research reveals improved pulmonary function and exercise capacity in patients with COPD (GOLD, 2023; Yang et al., 2020). Patients with milder disease and those with voice or woodwind musical training may feel the technique to be beneficial, but those with more severe disease may find diaphragm breathing too difficult to do. Inspiratory muscle training (IMT) involves having the patient train against a resistive load. Several commercial devices are available for use. IMT improves inspiratory muscle strength and endurance, which may be of benefit in some patients, but it is not currently recommended as standard care (Barman et al., 2022; GOLD, 2023).

Limiting future episodes of shortness of breath include exercise training to improve endurance, teaching patients how to pace their activities with their breathing, and helping

BOX 10-6

Nursing Research

Bridging the Gap to Evidence-Based Practice

Luckett, T., Roberts, M., Smith, T., Garcia, M., Dunn, S., Swan, F., Ferguson, C., Kochovska, S., Phillips, J. L., Pearson, M., Currow, D. C., & Johnson, M. J. (2022). Implementing the battery-operated handheld fan as an evidence-based, non-pharmacological intervention for chronic breathlessness in patients with chronic obstructive pulmonary disease (COPD): A qualitative study of the views of specialist respiratory clinicians. *BMC Pulmonary Medicine*, *22*(1), 129. https://doi.org/10.1186/s12890-022-01925-z.

Purpose

The battery-operated handheld fan ("fan") is an inexpensive and portable nonpharmacologic intervention for chronic breathlessness. Evidence from randomized controlled trials suggests the fan reduces breathlessness intensity and improves physical activity in patients with a range of advanced chronic conditions. Qualitative data from these trials suggests the fan may also reduce anxiety and improve daily functioning for many patients. This study aimed to explore barriers and facilitators to the fan's implementation in specialist respiratory care as a nonpharmacologic intervention for chronic breathlessness in patients with chronic obstructive pulmonary disease (COPD).

Design

A qualitative approach was taken, using focus groups. Participants were clinicians from any discipline working in specialist respiratory care at two hospitals. Questions were asked about current fan-related practice and perceptions regarding benefits, harms and mechanisms, and factors influencing its implementation. Analysis used a mixed inductive/deductive approach.

Forty-nine participants from nursing (n = 30), medical (n = 13), and allied health (n = 6) disciplines participated across nine focus groups. The most influential facilitator was a belief that the fan's benefits outweighed disadvantages. Clinicians' beliefs about the fan's mechanisms determined which patient subgroups they targeted, for example anxious or palliative/end-stage patients. Barriers to implementation included a lack of clarity about whose role it was to implement the fan, what advice to provide patients, and limited access to fans in hospitals. Few clinicians implemented the fan for acute-on-chronic breathlessness or in combination with other interventions.

Findings

Implementation of the fan in specialist respiratory care may require service- and clinician-level interventions to ensure it is routinely recommended as a first-line intervention for chronic breathlessness in patients for whom this symptom is of concern, regardless of COPD stage.

Nursing Implications

Service- and clinician-level interventions are needed to implement handheld fans in specialist respiratory services for chronic breathlessness in patients with COPD. Behavior change strategies are needed to increase clinician capability, opportunity, and motivation to recommend the fan as a first-line intervention for breathlessness (rather than reserving it for patients who are anxious or palliative/end-stage) and integrating it with other strategies. Making fans available and incorporated into routine care in hospitals will overcome the main environmental barrier to implementation and is likely to be cost-effective. Educational efforts should focus on persuading clinicians to recommend the fan to any patient with COPD for whom breathlessness impacts daily life, regardless of anxiety and disease stage, and further research is required to identify the optimal approach to training patients in using the fan.

patients anticipate dyspnea-producing activities and plan how they will keep their dyspnea at a manageable level. For example, if a patient is short of breath when climbing stairs, climbing more slowly and only during exhalation may help keep dyspnea at a manageable level. A simple teaching strategy is "pause, breathe in, exhale, and climb one to two steps."

In very severe COPD, simple tasks may cause severe dyspnea that is not adequately responsive to medications and breathing techniques. The administration of opioids may be effective in relieving dyspnea but must be used with caution because of respiratory depressant side effects. In addition, it is important to recognize that while opioids may be beneficial in relief of dyspnea, there will be no concomitant benefit in oxygenation (Murphy & Wagner, 2021). Patients and families need to be taught how to use opioids effectively. Concerns over physical dependence, addiction, and respiratory depression need to be addressed, but opioids should not be withheld in very severe patients for whom palliative care is the goal. Noninvasive positive-pressure ventilation (NPPV) also has been used for treatment of dyspnea in patients with severe COPD (see Chapter 54).

Pearls for Practice

The use of NPPV received increased attention during the COVID-19 pandemic. NPPV is providing positive pressure via a variety of interfaces (full or partial face masks, nasal masks, hoods, and helmets) to the patient's upper airway, typically with the supplemental oxygen ranging from 21% to 100% (Roberts, 2021). The two modalities include continuous positive airway pressure (CPAP) and bilevel positive airway pressure (BiPAP). In BiPAP inspiratory positive airway pressure (IPAP) forces air into the lungs, which increases the patient's tidal volume (the amount of air moved into and out of the lungs in one inspiration and expiration; normal is 500 mL), and positive end expiratory pressure or PEEP, which keeps the alveoli open during expiration. The positive pressure is maintained using a tight-fitting interface (e.g., mask) to lessen loss of pressure, which can be uncomfortable and claustrophobic for patients, and nursing plays an important role in explaining the treatment and offering support. PEEP prevents complete exhalation of a patient's breath; the higher the PEEP, the more air remains in the patient's lungs at the end of expiration, which prevents the alveoli from collapsing and therefore facilitates gas exchange and thus tissue oxygenation. PEEP also decreases the work of breathing, "since inflating a partially open alveoli requires significantly less energy and effort than inflating a completely collapsed alveoli, much in the same way that blowing up a balloon that already contains air is significantly less challenging than blowing up a balloon that is completely empty" (Roberts, 2021, p. 3). Side effects of positive pressure ventilation include barotrauma (damage to the lung caused by pressure changes), malnutrition (as patients cannot eat while using these devices), skin pressure damage from the interface use, nausea and/or vomiting, and decreased cardiac output (since the positive intrathoracic pressure reduces blood returning to the heart or preload and thus cardiac output; Roberts, 2021).

Impaired Gas Exchange

Patients with more severe disease and those experiencing an exacerbation are at increased risk for hypoxemia, oxygen desaturation, and hypercapnia. Nursing care includes monitoring the patient for hypoxemia by oximetry and ABG measurements and administering supplemental oxygen. As mentioned under Medical Management, over-concern about hypercapnia should never result in under treating the patient. Adequate oxygenation (keeping the oxygen saturation *at or above* 88%) is important to protect vital organ function.

Pearls for Practice

Nurses are aware that a contraindication to oxygen therapy is when patients are active smokers because of the fire risk. In addition, open flames in the home (gas stoves, kerosene space heaters, or open fires) may also present a risk (McDonald, 2022). Additional issues of concern are decreased mobility with oxygen use and nasal irritation. Patient teaching should also include patient understanding that oxygen is a drug and is not adjusted without consultation with the provider (McDonald, 2022). An "Oxygen in Use" sign should be posted on the doors of the home.

Patients requiring oxygen therapy need to be taught the importance of adhering to the oxygen prescription. Patients often think they can tell when they need oxygen by their symptoms. The presence or absence of dyspnea is unreliable in detecting the need for supplemental oxygen. Many hypoxemic patients do not feel dyspnea. In addition, many patients who are dyspneic do not have significant hypoxemia or oxygen desaturation.

The pulmonary arteries respond to hypoxemia by constricting, causing increased pressure to occur. Pulmonary hypertension and right ventricular hypertrophy and failure may occur as a result of chronic, untreated hypoxemia. Chronic hypoxemia affects the function of other vital organs. Cognitive impairment is greater in hypoxemic patients. Long-term oxygen is the prescribed treatment. Teaching patients who need home oxygen should include an explanation of supplemental oxygen's effect on improved cardiac and cognitive function as well as improved prognosis. The teaching plan should include the number of hours per day to wear oxygen, the dose of oxygen (usually given as number of liters per minute), and special instructions for using oxygen for sleep and exercise. Home care companies supplying oxygen to patients usually employ respiratory therapists and/or nurses. Home care professionals help patients use their oxygen more effectively, identify special equipment needs, troubleshoot equipment, and explore the use of oxygen for work and travel.

Pearls for Practice

The nurse is aware that Medicare criteria for home supplemental oxygen are a PaO_2 of 55 mm Hg or below and an oxygen saturation of 88% or less while breathing room air at rest. The threshold for patients with cor pulmonale, heart failure (HF), or erythrocytosis (hematocrit >55%) is slightly higher at a PaO_2 of 56 to 59 mm Hg to qualify for supplemental O_2 (CMS, 2021). In addition, patients who do not have hypoxemia at rest but desaturate (defined as an arterial PO_2 at or below 55 mm Hg or an arterial oxygen saturation at or below 88%) during exercise (defined as either the functional performance of the patient or a formal exercise test), supplemental oxygen is provided for use during exercise if the use of oxygen improves the hypoxemia that was demonstrated during exercise when the patient was breathing room air (CMS, 2021).

Cough and Ineffective Airway Clearance Risk

Patients with mucus hypersecretion or a comorbidity of bronchiectasis as well as those experiencing an acute exacerbation may have increased sputum quantity and viscosity. In addition, many patients are too weak or fatigued to clear secretions effectively.

Diminishing the quantity and viscosity of sputum can help clear the airways and improve pulmonary ventilation and gas exchange. Pulmonary irritants should be eliminated or reduced, particularly cigarette smoking, secondhand smoke, aerosol cleaning and household products, cooking that produces fumes, and powders used when bathing patients. Nursing interventions include instruction on directed or controlled coughing and drinking enough fluid to prevent dehydration. Box 10-7 can be used to teach patients effective coughing and how to deal with uncontrolled coughing spasms.

Some patients require more intense secretion-clearance techniques. Chest physiotherapy with postural drainage and/or

BOX 10-7

Patient Education

Controlled Cough

An effective cough moves secretions (also called sputum, phlegm, or mucus) out of the smaller airways of the lungs. An effective cough should use just enough effort to remove secretions but not so much as to cause pain, coughing spasms, or exhaustion.

One Coughing Technique

- Sit up leaning slightly forward with your back straight and your head tilted down.
- Take 2 slow deep breaths and exhale through pursed lips.
- Take another deep breath in, and hold your breath for 2–3 seconds.
- Open your mouth so that your lips are slightly parted. Cough, cough, cough from your stomach without breathing in (coughing the air out of your lungs with little coughs).
- If coughing from the stomach is too hard, try: huff, huff, huffing the air out.
- Finish exhaling through pursed lips.
- Breathe in slowly through your nose and exhale through pursed lips 2–3 times. Then try clearing your throat or coughing the secretions out of your mouth.
- Repeat if necessary.
- Check your sputum for color, quantity, and consistency.

If you don't cough out any sputum after 2–3 controlled coughs, wait 15–20 minutes and try again. Avoid continuous coughs to minimize your risk of injury or fatigue. Try using your inhaled bronchodilator before coughing to make it easier to get results.

Controlling Coughing Spasms

If you go into a coughing spasm:

- Take several short sniffs of air in through your nose to help cut down on the irritation.
- Avoid inhaling quickly through your mouth as it may make you cough more; breathe out through pursed lips and relax your shoulders.

It may take a few breaths to control the coughing spasm, so be patient and keep trying.

Once you get the cough under control and after resting a few minutes, try the controlled cough.

mechanical percussion and vibration, the use of positive expiratory pressure devices (PEP therapy) using devices such flutter, acapella, cornet, and the active cycle of breathing technique (ACBT) (see Box 10-8), and suctioning may be needed for patients who are unable to cough sputum out effectively. These therapeutic modalities may decrease the frequency of infections, prevent airway deterioration, and reduce, to some extent, the progression of lung disease (Zisi et al., 2022). Patients receiving one or more of these more intense techniques need to be monitored for their response to treatment. Very frail patients may experience too much fatigue, pain, or dyspnea. Respiratory therapists are often consulted when these more intense forms of secretion clearance are needed.

Decreased Exercise Tolerance

Patients with advanced COPD experience progressive intolerance and disability during activity and exercise. Exacerbations and hospitalizations add to decreased activity, muscle weakness, and fatigue. Interventions used during acute exacerbations may weaken the patient further; for example, systemic corticosteroids are associated with myopathy (muscle weakness), particularly in the leg muscles.

Nursing interventions focus on therapies to help the patient recover from the effects of an acute exacerbation, maintain or regain independence in ambulation and performing activities of daily living, and improve stamina and strength. Early mobilization in patients experiencing an acute exacerbation, including those in intensive care, is associated with improvements in exercise tolerance and may help patients recover more quickly. Box 10-8 provides information to use with patients.

Interventions preparing the patient for discharge or work with outpatients may include teaching alternating high-energy with low-energy activities throughout the day to better manage energy expenditure. The patient may benefit from exercise training to strengthen the muscles of the upper and lower extremities and to improve exercise tolerance and endurance. Use of walking aids may be recommended to improve activity levels, balance, and ambulation. Pulmonary rehabilitation staff, occupational therapists, and physical therapists can be consulted to assist patients with improving exercise tolerance and self-care.

Nutrition

Patients with COPD may have a number of issues related to nutrition. Some individuals become underweight and have difficulty consuming enough calories to meet their body's metabolic requirements. Weight loss is worsened by exacerbations, dyspnea, coughing, sputum production, or anorexia from medications (e.g., bronchodilators, steroids, antibiotics), oxygen use ("oxygen by nasal cannula disturbs the sense of smell and therefore taste because olfaction plays a dominant role in the taste of foods") or emotional issues (Boardman, 2021; Ziegler & Reid-Hector, 2022, p. 389). A reduction in body mass index is a risk factor for pneumonia in COPD patients (GOLD, 2023). Emphysema is more commonly associated with a low BMI because it produces a catabolic state; patients appear thin and many times cachectic (physical wasting, nutritionally depleted), whereas chronic bronchitis is associated with normal or high BMI (Ziegler & Reid-Hector, 2022). Some patients may be overweight because of increased fat mass or increased fluid retention. Overweight patients may need the help of

BOX 10-8 **Patient Education**

Exercises to Do in Bed or in a Chair When You Are in the Hospital or Recovering from Being Sick

Deep Breathing

Every hour you are awake, take **10 slow, deep breaths.** Exhale through pursed lips.

If you get tired after five breaths, rest a minute or two and do the second set of five.

Moving in Bed

Roll from side to side in the bed at least every hour. This helps your breathing, circulation, and skin.

Leg Work to Keep Your Muscles from Getting Too Weak

Ankle Pumps: Flex your ankles and point your toes toward your head, and then point your toes down.

Quad Sets: Tighten your knee and press it into the bed or chair for a count of 5.

Buttocks Squeeze: Squeeze your buttocks together for a count of 5.

Leg Lifts: Bend your knee and bring your leg up toward your chest. Lower your knee slowly back down on the bed. You can also try lifting your leg up and down slowly with your knee in the straight position.

Arm Work

Raise your arms above your head as you breathe in, and then lower them back down to your sides as you breathe out.

Additional Points

- ***Remember to breathe as you do the exercises.*** Avoid holding your breath.
- Try doing five of each arm or leg exercise every 2–3 hours.
- ***As soon as you can, get out of bed to a chair.*** Get up several times a day for short periods to improve your stamina and avoid too much fatigue.
- ***Take short walks.*** Walk with your nurse if you feel unsure of your balance.
- Wear your oxygen for activity if your provider prescribes it.

nutrition education by a dietician to help them lose weight safely. Exercise should be encouraged to help them increase muscle mass.

Hospitalized patients may have difficulty eating because the act of eating may cause increased dyspnea. Oral nutritional supplements are useful for increasing body weight and respiratory function. Weight gain in underweight patients results in improved exercise capacity and quality of life. However, some patients negate the effectiveness of the supplements by using them as meal substitutes.

Therapy is aimed at assessing the nutritional status of the patient, treating the underlying cause, and stabilizing weight and body composition. Nursing interventions include:

- timing bronchodilator therapy before meals
- assisting severely dyspneic patients during mealtimes to minimize energy spent eating
- teaching patients to eat small, frequent meals to help them avoid becoming too full; large meals affect abdominal distention, which impairs diaphragmatic function (Boardman, 2021)
- encouraging choices of calorie-rich foods and providing patients with oral supplements
- referring patients to dieticians
- encouraging progressive periods of exercise aimed at increased muscle mass

Enhancing Self-Care Strategies

Self-management strategies are aimed at involving the patient in the decision-making process and goal formation. It is important for patients to participate in setting and accepting realistic short- and long-term goals. If COPD is mild or moderate, the goals may be to increase exercise tolerance and prevent further loss of pulmonary function. In severe disease, the goals are to preserve current pulmonary function, increase activity tolerance, and relieve symptoms as much as possible. In very severe disease, the goals may shift to relief of severe dyspnea and preparing for a peaceful death. As severity increases, goals and expectations may change.

Examples of patient goals compatible with the concept of self-care include learning to balance diminished exercise tolerance with the desire to maintain participation in important activities; recognizing the effect that environmental factors have on breathing and dealing with respiratory irritants; preventing and recognizing the signs and symptoms of exacerbations and complications; learning how to handle an exacerbation and/or complication; managing a complex medical regimen that includes medication, exercise, oxygen, nutrition, and other medical conditions; and deciding on the course of treatment in very severe disease.

Interventions that help patients plan participation in favorite activities with less shortness of breath can be very helpful. For example, attendance at a special event such as a wedding or graduation may be very tiring for patients with more severe disease, yet they still may wish to participate. Strategies to minimize stress and shortness of breath may include using quick-relief medications prior to the event; planning to attend part of the event such as only the ceremony or reception to minimize fatigue; using an assistive device during the event; and maintaining the prescribed medications, oxygen, and exercise program to maximize physical health. Helping patients delineate and decide on possible strategies may allow participation and enhance self-efficacy.

Many patients with COPD are sensitive to changes in air quality, fluctuations in temperature and humidity, and respiratory irritants in the environment. Nursing interventions include teaching patients to check local weather conditions and air alerts for extremes of temperature and humidity and for poor air quality. Teaching patients to create "transitions zones" when they go from one extreme temperature to another can be useful. For example, during hot, humid weather, patients can be taught to turn the air-conditioning off in the car and crack the window to allow the outside air to gradually mix with the inside air. The more gradual transition to hotter, more humid air may make breathing easier for many patients.

Prevention and early recognition of exacerbations of COPD are important self-care measures for patients to learn. Preventative measures include handwashing to minimize the transmission of infectious agents; avoiding or minimizing contact with sick individuals; and receiving immunizations against influenza, pneumococcal pneumonia, and COVID-19. Patients should be taught to report signs of infection, including increased dyspnea as well as fever or change in sputum color, character, consistency, or amount. Any marked worsening of symptoms (chest tightness, dyspnea, and fatigue) also suggests infection and should be reported by patients to their primary provider. Viral infections may make patients more susceptible to more serious bacterial infections.

Pearls for Practice

High fevers of 102 °F or greater accompanied by shaking chills are signs of a more serious infection such as pneumonia. Patients should be instructed to go to the nearest emergency room as soon as possible.

Patients with more severe diseases often have significant variation in daily symptoms and may have difficulty determining if they are becoming acutely ill. A change in typical routines, increased activity, family and caregiver events, increased stress; and fatigue are some of the causes of "bad-breathing days." A knowledge of the patient's past response to "bad-breathing" days can help guide patient teaching. For example, a patient with moderate disease may note a slight increase in sputum volume, no change in sputum color, and a slight increase in usual dyspnea (from a 4 out of 10 to a 5) and deny fever or chills. Instruction might include using prescribed quick-relief medication (usually a SABA), using pursed-lip breathing and cough techniques, monitoring for increased symptoms, and contacting the primary provider should symptoms worsen or persist. Conversely, a patient with similar symptoms but a history of requiring more intensive intervention such as systemic corticosteroids, antibiotics, emergency room visits, or hospitalizations may be instructed to contact their provider more quickly.

Respiratory Failure

Patients with severe and very severe COPD and those with hypercapnia are at increased risk for acute respiratory failure. Nursing interventions of hospitalized patients include frequent monitoring for signs and symptoms of impending respiratory failure, more intensive treatments aimed at clearing the airways, and frequent communication and coordination of care with other members of the health care team, for example, internists, hospitalists, pulmonologists, and respiratory therapists.

Pearls for Practice

Signs of impending respiratory failure and need for intensive care:

- *Severe dyspnea not responding to treatment*
- *Tachypnea alternating with bradypnea (slow respiratory rate below 8 breaths per minute) and apnea as fatigue ensues*
- *Hyperventilation that may deteriorate to rapid and shallow breathing*
- *Anxiety*
- *Change in mental status*
- *Worsening hypoxemia that is unresponsive to oxygen therapy*
- *Worsening hypercapnia*
- *Worsening acidosis*
- *Evidence of respiratory muscle fatigue: increased use of accessory muscles, paroxysmal respiratory movement (inward movement of abdomen on inspiration)*

Patients who show signs and symptoms of impending acute respiratory failure must be monitored more closely until transfer to an intensive care can be accomplished. Interventions include providing adequate oxygenation, administration of medications to maximize bronchodilatation, and close monitoring of mental status until more intensive therapy can be initiated. In addition, NPPV may be needed. Patients not responding to NPPV may require intubation and invasive ventilatory support. Chapter 54 covers these therapies in more detail. Patients transferred to a medical unit following an acute episode of respiratory failure require the same close monitoring to avoid another episode.

Enhancing Individual Coping Strategies

COPD and its progression promote a cycle of physical, social, and psychological consequences, all of which are interrelated. Research reveals that an estimated 33% of patients with COPD have co-morbidities of anxiety and/or depression (Fogh-Andersen et al., 2021). Management of these comorbid conditions is important in maintaining COPD disease stability. Nursing interventions include assessing patients for anxiety and depression and promoting interventions to maximize physical functioning, psychological and emotional stability, and social support. After the initial assessment of the patient, the nurse may provide referrals to psychiatric and social services, pulmonary rehabilitation, pastoral care, and home care.

Pearls for Practice

Anxiety may be a sign of worsening respiratory status and impending respiratory failure. Anxiety should not be attributed to psychological causes until the patient

is assessed for vital sign changes, tests of oxygenation, and mental status changes. Anxiolytics are generally contraindicated in patients with impending acute respiratory failure. Certain medications, in particular high-dose systemic corticosteroids, also can make patients feel extremely anxious and should be considered as a possible cause.

Any factor that interferes with normal breathing may induce anxiety, depression, and changes in behavior. Fatigue is a major symptom in many patients with COPD. Restricted activity, reversal of family roles due to loss of employment, the frustration of having to work to breathe, and the realization that the disease is prolonged and unrelenting may cause the patient to become angry, depressed, and demanding. Sexual function may be compromised, which also diminishes self-esteem. Nursing interventions include discussions with patients and families about the chronic nature of lung disease, support as roles change and spouses or significant others assume responsibilities once managed by the patient, and palliative and hospice care when patients near end-stage disease (refer to Chapter 2). Patients with severe anxiety and depression may need a referral to a mental health specialist. Many areas have support groups for patients with chronic lung disease that are usually administered by local pulmonary rehabilitation programs or local chapters of the American Lung Association. Participation in support groups may help many patients discuss common problems with professionals and patients with similar issues.

Continuing Care

Nursing interventions include assessment for and referral to community resources when hospitalized patients are nearing discharge. Nurses caring for outpatients with COPD may also identify community care needs as patients become more disabled. Referral to an inpatient pulmonary rehabilitation program or extended-care facility may be needed for patients who have had prolonged hospital stays and are severely disabled. Home care through a nursing agency may be appropriate for many patients. Home visits provide a more accurate assessment of the patient's daily life, physical and psychological status, and adherence to the prescribed regimen. Home care visits by physical and occupational therapists may help the patient gain endurance and strength enough to attend an outpatient pulmonary rehabilitation program. Strategies that may help with the dyspnea include fans, oxygen and opiates (Christenson et al., 2022). Refer to Box 10-6.

As patients become more severely ill, medical therapy may not adequately relieve symptoms. Discussions about prognosis and end of life are difficult for many patients, families, and professionals. Fears of suffering, a desire to stay alive as long as possible, and depression are some of the factors that may interfere with discussions about the end of life. Areas identified as being of major importance for patients with end-stage COPD include adequate symptom management (particularly avoiding severe, uncontrolled dyspnea); psychological, emotional, and spiritual needs; and privacy and dignity. Assurances that patients and families will not be abandoned as the disease progresses and making every effort to help the patient avoid suffering are important parts of caring.

Advanced care planning includes discussing patients' wishes should the need for more invasive procedures arise such as intubation, acute and long-term mechanical ventilation, feeding tubes, and placement of a tracheostomy tube. Nursing interventions include participation in these discussions with patients and families and providing support to them as they struggle with decision-making. Chapter 2 presents a more thorough discussion of end-of-life care.

ASTHMA

Asthma is a common heterogeneous disease of the airways that is complex and characterized by recurring and variable symptoms, expiratory airflow limitation, and usually bronchial hyperresponsiveness. Inflammation is the key underlying feature and leads to recurrent episodes of asthma symptoms: cough, chest tightness, wheeze, and dyspnea. Symptoms' occurrence and severity may vary over time.

An estimated 24.8 million persons (7.7% of the population) have asthma (CDC, 2022). Asthma accounts for 1.6 million emergency room visits, approximately 183,000 hospitalizations, and 4,145 deaths per year (CDC, 2022).

The U.S. National Heart Lung and Blood Institute Expert Panel Guidelines (first produced in 1997 and updated most recently in 2020) provide evidence-based information to assist in the diagnosis and management of patients with asthma. A portion of the guidelines "Asthma and Treatment Action Plan" was updated in 2022. Multinational guidelines known as the Global Strategy for Asthma Management and Prevention (GINA) were updated in 2021.

Just as with COPD, recent efforts recognize the complex gene–environment interactions that modulate the immune responses and, although not fully understood, are risk factors for the development of asthma. A number of studies have classified patients with asthma into "phenotypes," (set of observable characteristics of an individual resulting from the interaction of its genotype with the environment that is shared by some but not all patients with asthma); thus, "asthma is not one disease, but it is a syndrome composed of multiple phenotypes (Cloutier et al., 2020, p. X1V). Common phenotypes include allergic asthma, nonallergic asthma, adult onset or late-onset asthma, asthma with persistent airflow limitation, and asthma with obesity (GINA, 2021). While some phenotype-guided treatments are available, further research is needed to understand the clinical utility of phenotyping in asthma (GINA, 2021).

Atopy, the genetic predisposition for the development of an IgE-mediated (antibody associated with allergic reaction and inflammation) response to allergens, is the strongest predisposing factor for allergic asthma. Chronic exposure to airway allergens may sensitize IgE antibodies and the cells of the airway. Common allergens can be seasonal (grass, tree, and weed pollens) or perennial (e.g., mold, dust, roaches, animal dander). Atopy may also occur in the absence of asthma.

A variety of nonallergen triggers such as exercise, stress, extreme heat or cold, and viral respiratory infections may also cause asthma symptoms and exacerbation. Eosinophilic asthma is an example of nonatopic or intrinsic asthma that develops in adulthood and accounts for fewer than 5% of cases of asthma (Drazen & Bel, 2020). It is not associated with allergies and is often accompanied by chronic rhinosinusitis and nasal polyposis. The eosinophilic airway inflammation observed in this type of asthma is not dependent on adaptive immunity, so there is not an associated IgE response (Drazen & Bel, 2020). Patients with this type of asthma often have a severe form with elevated eosinophil counts in peripheral blood and generally require high doses of systemic glucocorticoids (it is poorly responsive to inhaled glucocorticoids). Recently, injectable biologic treatments that target this eosinophilic phenotype are prescribed, such as mepolizumab, reslizumab, or reslizumab, which are humanized monoclonal antibodies that reduce eosinophil counts (Clinical Overview, 2022). These medications inhibit interleukin (IL)-5, which reduces blood and bronchoalveolar eosinophilia; the medications are expensive, and most insurance companies require specific clearance before the drugs can be administered (Drazen & Bel, 2020; Sharma et al., 2022).

Most people with asthma are sensitive to a variety of triggers, both allergens and nonallergens. Asthma symptoms and severity may vary in an individual person at different points in time. The dose and response to environmental exposures, activities engaged in, the particular asthma control measures used, the frequency of exacerbations, and other factors all influence the disease course in a given individual. Risk factors for exacerbations include a history of ≥1 exacerbation per year, socioeconomic problems, poor medication adherence, incorrect inhaler technique, low FEV_1, smoking, and blood eosinophilia (GINA, 2022, p. 2).

Although asthma is typically diagnosed in childhood, it can develop at any age. To illustrate, the incidence of first asthma diagnosis for those older than 65 years of age is 3.1% per year compared to 4.0% annually for those between 18 and 34 years. Risk factors for adult-onset asthma include prematurity history, early lung infections, rhinitis, smoking, and obesity (Wu et al., 2019). In addition, late-onset asthma is less frequently associated with allergy and often more severe than childhood-onset asthma (Hammad & Lambrecht, 2021).

Pathophysiology

The underlying pathology in asthma is reversible and diffuse airway inflammation and an exaggerated hyperresponsiveness (respond to stimuli in an exaggerated manner) to a variety of stimuli (Norris & Tuan, 2020). Acute inflammation

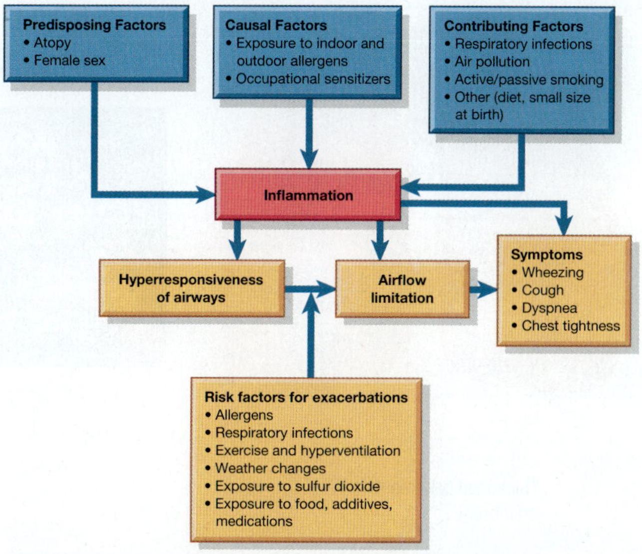

FIGURE 10-5 Pathophysiology of asthma. (Adapted from material developed for the Global Initiative for Asthma (GINA). http://www.ginasthma.org)

leads to airflow limitation and changes in the airways. Bronchoconstriction, the contraction of the smooth muscle of the airways, occurs in response to a variety of allergens and irritants. Airway edema (swelling of the membranes that line the airways) becomes more progressive as asthma severity increases. Mucus hypersecretion and mucus plugs can occur. The airways of some asthmatics may undergo "remodeling," which includes persistent changes in airway structure (airway smooth muscle hyperplasia, goblet cell metaplasia, and exaggerated subepithelial collagen deposition), in which case the airflow limitations may only be partially reversible (Hammad & Lambrecht, 2021; Norris & Tuan, 2020). Figure 10-5 depicts some of the pathophysiologic features of asthma.

Many cells and cellular elements play a role in the inflammation of asthma. Mast cells, neutrophils, eosinophils, and T lymphocytes cause epithelial injury. Mast cells, when activated, release several chemicals called mediators, which include histamine, bradykinin, prostaglandins, interleukins, and leukotrienes. Their actions immediately cause bronchoconstriction (Rosenthal & Rosenjack Burchum, 2021). Leukotrienes increase mucus secretion that frequently obstructs the airway further and causes additional release of histamine from the mast cells; histamine will also contribute to bronchoconstriction and plasma leakage from nearby vessels (Tan, 2023). These mediators perpetuate the inflammatory response, which produces a state of *bronchial hyperreactivity* (Norris & Tuan, 2020). Regulation of these chemicals is the aim of much of the current research regarding pharmacologic therapy for asthma. Refer to Figure 10-6.

Clinical Manifestations and Assessment

Asthma is diagnosed based on history, physical examination, and spirometry. Symptoms often occur at night or early in

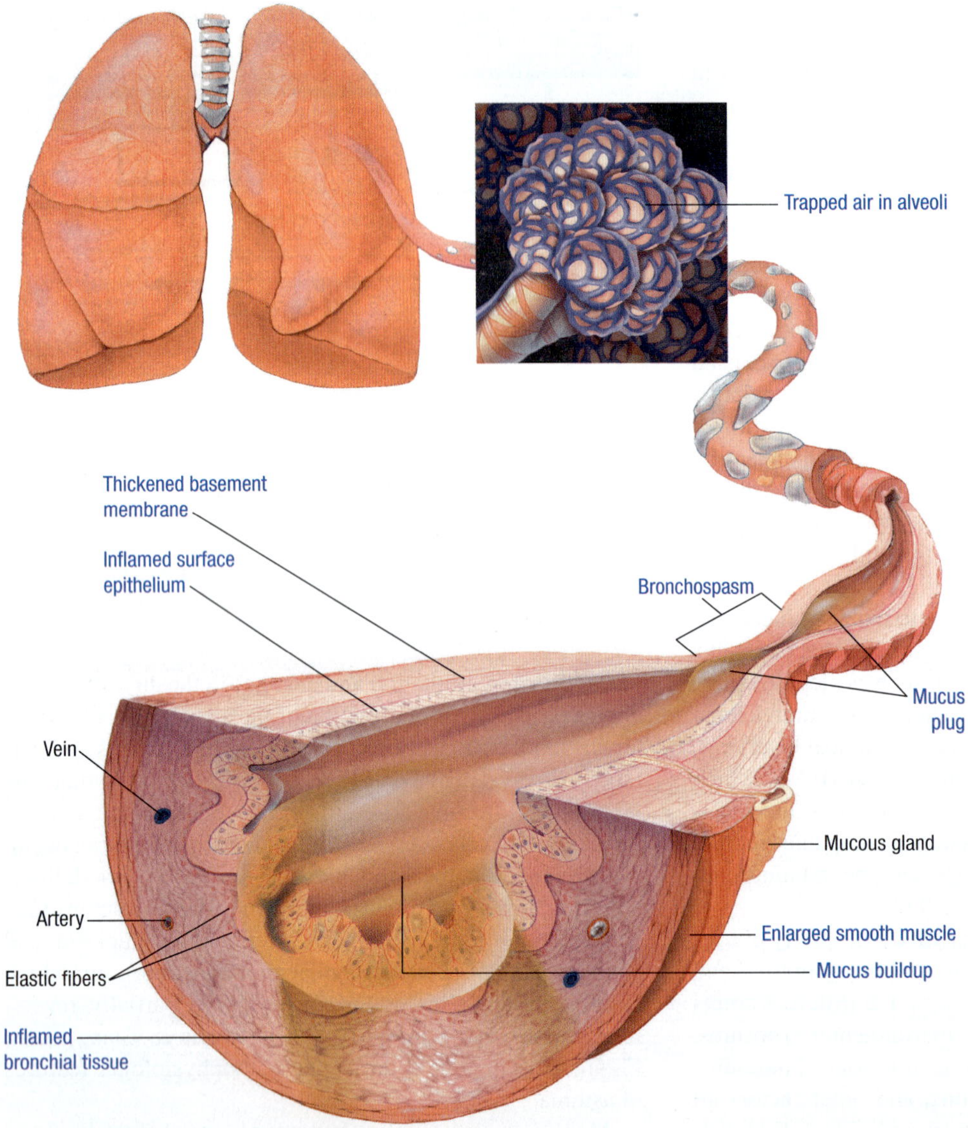

FIGURE 10-6 **In asthma, inflammation and smooth muscle spasms severely constrict the airways. Released histamine stimulates the mucous membranes to secrete excessive mucus, further narrowing the bronchial lumen. On inhalation, the narrowed bronchial lumen can still expand slightly, allowing air to reach the alveoli. On exhalation, increased intrathoracic pressure may close the bronchial lumen. Mucus fills the lung bases, inhibiting alveolar ventilation. (Figure courtesy of the Anatomical Chart Company.)**

the morning and may awaken patients. Asthma symptoms may occur suddenly or develop over several hours or days. Asthma is categorized according to symptoms and objective measures of airflow obstruction.

A complete family, environmental, and occupational history helps establish the diagnosis. A history of cough, especially at night, recurrent wheeze, chest tightness, and/or difficulty breathing may indicate the presence of asthma. A report of symptoms that occur or worsen with exercise, exposure to allergens, irritants, occupational irritants, weather changes, stress, menstrual cycles, or strong expression of emotions such as hard laughing or crying increase the suspicion. Table 10-3 lists common allergens and irritants that may trigger an asthma episode. Cough, with or without mucus production, may be the only symptom reported by some patients. Exercise-induced asthma is common and is defined as symptoms occurring during or soon after stopping exercise. Occupational asthma is worse on workdays and improved on days off. Many patients develop chronic asthma after years of exposure to an occupational trigger and may have persistent asthma even when not working.

Physical examination findings may reveal generalized wheezing initially heard during expiration. In between asthma episodes, physical examination findings may be normal.

Pearls for Practice

The occurrence of a severe, continuous reaction referred to as acute severe asthma (formerly known as status asthmaticus) is considered life-threatening. In more severe episodes, diaphoresis, tachypnea, tachycardia, restlessness, an inability to speak complete sentences, use of accessory muscles, and a refusal to recline are seen along with hypoxemia and hypercarbia. The presence of wheezing is unreliable because if the airflow is so significantly impaired a wheeze cannot be produced. When airflow rates are very low, the "quiet chest" with minimal air movement may signal impending respiratory failure.

TABLE **10-3 Common Asthma Triggers**

Antigens
• Pollens: tree, grass, ragweed • Molds: indoor (basements, bathrooms, wet rugs) and/or outdoor (spring/fall) • House dust mite • Cockroaches • Animal dander: cats, dogs, guinea pigs, birds • Foods: peanuts, strawberries, shellfish • Occupational exposures: animals, baking products, toluene, chemical fumes • Drugs: aspirin sensitivity, noncardioselective beta blockers
Irritants
• Viral respiratory infections • Occupational irritants: dust, fumes • Gastroesophageal reflux disease • Sinus infection and postnasal drip • Cigarette smoke and odor: primary and secondhand • Forceful respiratory maneuvers: hard laughing, crying, yelling • Cold, dry air • Foods, food additives, and preservatives • Vapors, gases, aerosols • Endocrine factors: menses, pregnancy, thyroid disease • Exercise • Air pollution, smog • Scented products • Emotions and stress • Obesity

Adapted from Hashmi, M. F., Tariq, M., & Cataletto, M. E. (2022). Asthma. In *StatPearls [Internet]*. StatPearls Publishing. https://www.ncbi.nlm.nih.gov/books/NBK430901

Spirometry may reveal an obstructive pattern (FEV_1/FVC% less than 70%). Reversibility, defined as a 12% or 200 mL increase of FEV_1, FVC, or both suggests asthma. Spirometry may be normal if the patient is between asthma episodes. Special pulmonary function tests, such as methacholine challenge, exercise challenge, or the administration of cold air to induce symptoms, may be used to diagnose asthma when simple spirometry is normal and asthma is suspected.

Other laboratory tests that are done less often may include CBC count with differential to evaluate for eosinophilia, serum immunoglobulin E, allergy testing, chest x-rays to exclude alternative diagnoses, and blood gases when patients experience symptoms of a severe exacerbation. The most common differential diagnoses in adults include vocal cord dysfunction; foreign-body obstruction; heart failure; pulmonary embolism; cough secondary to drugs, for example, angiotensin-converting enzyme (ACE) inhibitors; benign or malignant tumors obstructing airways; eosinophilic pneumonia; interstitial lung disease; bronchiectasis; bronchiolitis obliterans; sarcoidosis; and COPD (Schoettler & Strek, 2020). In addition to being part of the differential diagnosis, COPD and asthma can coexist (GINA, 2021; GOLD, 2023). Figure 10-7 is an example of a tool that can be used to evaluate patients with asthma and reminds providers and patients of the risk factors associated with exacerbation (GINA, 2021).

Medical Management

The overall goals of management are to reduce impairment, exacerbations, and the risk of adverse outcomes. Reducing impairment includes freedom from symptoms (including no nighttime awakenings), minimal need of inhaled short-acting beta agonist (SABA) (two or fewer times a week), morning peak expiratory flow (PEF) ≥80% predicted every day (discussed shortly), and satisfaction with care. The goals of reducing risk include preventing recurrent exacerbations, providing optimal pharmacotherapy with minimal side effects, and preventing loss of function. The components of management include assessment and monitoring, patient education, environmental control and management of comorbid conditions, and pharmacologic therapy. Refer to Figure 10-8 for initial treatment recommendations for adults with asthma based on the stepwise approach to the pharmacologic management of asthma; the treatment can progress upward if needed to achieve asthma symptom control and reduce the risk of exacerbations or step down when symptom control is achieved (GINA, 2021).

Assessment and Monitoring

Once asthma is diagnosed and disease severity is determined, ongoing assessment and monitoring begins, which includes a determination of how well the asthma is controlled and how responsive it is to treatment. A determination of potential risk for exacerbations is also useful. Monitoring adverse reactions from treatment may guide changes in treatment. Measures used to periodically assess established asthma include written or verbal reports of symptoms and symptom relief (asthma diaries), the frequency of the use of quick-relief medications, the individual's ability to participate in normal activities, the frequency of exacerbations, and monitoring of pulmonary function by periodic spirometry or home PEF monitoring.

Home PEF monitoring may be useful in some patients with asthma. A PEF meter is a small handheld device that measures the fastest flow the patient can generate after taking a deep breath in and blowing out as hard and fast as possible. PEF monitoring is used for different reasons: to establish the diagnosis in symptomatic patients with normal spirometry, to monitor disease in patients with more severe disease or a history of frequent exacerbations, or in patients who have difficulty perceiving an asthma exacerbation until it becomes severe. Proper technique is essential to make peak-flow monitoring useful (see Box 10-9). Once the baseline or personal best PEF is determined, changes can be used to determine the need to adjust medication protocols. Written asthma action plans based on fluctuations in PEF and/or symptoms are useful for many patients.

Newer forms of assessment may include analysis of expectorated sputum for eosinophilia and exhaled nitric

A. Asthma symptom control		Level of asthma symptom control		
In the past 4 weeks, has the patient had:		**Well controlled**	**Partly controlled**	**Uncontrolled**
• Daytime asthma symptoms more than twice/week?	Yes☐ No☐	None of these	1–2 of these	3–4 of these
• Any night waking due to asthma?	Yes☐ No☐			
• SABA reliever for symptoms more than twice/week?*	Yes☐ No☐			
• Any activity limitation due to asthma?	Yes☐ No☐			

B. Risk factors for poor asthma outcomes

Assess risk factors at diagnosis and periodically, particularly for patients experiencing exacerbations.

Measure FEV_1 at start of treatment, after 3–6 months of controller treatment to record the patient's personal best lung function, then periodically for ongoing risk assessment.

Having uncontrolled asthma symptoms is an important risk factor for exacerbations.[95]

Additional **potentially modifiable risk factors for flare-ups (exacerbations)**, even in patients with few symptoms† include:

- ***Medications***: high SABA use (≥3 x 200-dose canisters/year associated with increased risk of exacerbations;[123,96] increased mortality particularly if ≥1 canister per month[71,97]); inadequate ICS: not prescribed ICS; poor adherence;[98] incorrect inhaler technique[99]
- ***Other medical conditions***: obesity;[100,101] chronic rhinosinusitis;[101] GERD;[101] confirmed food allergy;[102] pregnancy[103]
- ***Exposures***: smoking;[104] e-cigarettes;[105] allergen exposure if sensitized;[104] air pollution[106-108]
- ***Context***: major psychological or socioeconomic problems[109]
- ***Lung function***: low FEV_1, especially <60% predicted;[104,110] high BD responsiveness[101,111,112]
- ***Type 2 inflammatory markers***: higher blood eosinophils;[101,113,114] elevated FeNO (in adults with allergic asthma taking ICS)[115]

Other major independent risk factors for flare-ups (exacerbations)

- Ever intubated or in intensive care unit for asthma[116]
- ≥1 severe exacerbation in last 12 months[117,118]

Having any of these risk factors increases the patient's risk of exacerbations *even if they have few asthma symptoms*

Risk factors for developing persistent airflow limitation

- History: preterm birth, low birth weight and greater infant weight gain;[119] chronic mucus hypersecretion[120,121]
- Medications: lack of ICS treatment in patients who had a severe exacerbation[122]
- Exposures: tobacco smoke;[120] noxious chemicals; occupational exposures[44]
- Investigations: low initial FEV_1;[121] sputum or blood eosinophilia[121]

Risk factors for medication side-effects

- Systemic: frequent OCS; long-term, high dose and/or potent ICS; also taking P450 inhibitors[123]
- Local: high dose or potent ICS;[123,124] poor inhaler technique[125]

BD: bronchodilator; FEV_1: forced expiratory volume in 1 second; ICS: inhaled corticosteroid; OCS: oral corticosteroid; P450 inhibitors: cytochrome P450 inhibitors such as ritonavir, ketoconazole, itraconazole; SABA: short-acting beta$_2$-agonist. *Based on SABA (as-needed ICS-formoterol reliever not included); excludes reliever taken before exercise. For children 6–11 years, also refer to Box 2-3, p.37. See Box 3-8, p.76 for specific risk reduction strategies. †'Independent' risk factors are those that are significant after adjustment for the level of symptom control.

FIGURE 10-7 **Global Initiative for Asthma 2022 assessment of asthma symptom control and future risk. FeNO, fractional exhaled nitric oxide. (From Global Initiative for Asthma, Global Strategy for Asthma Management and Prevention, 2022. Box 2-2, reprinted with permission. www.ginasthma.org)**

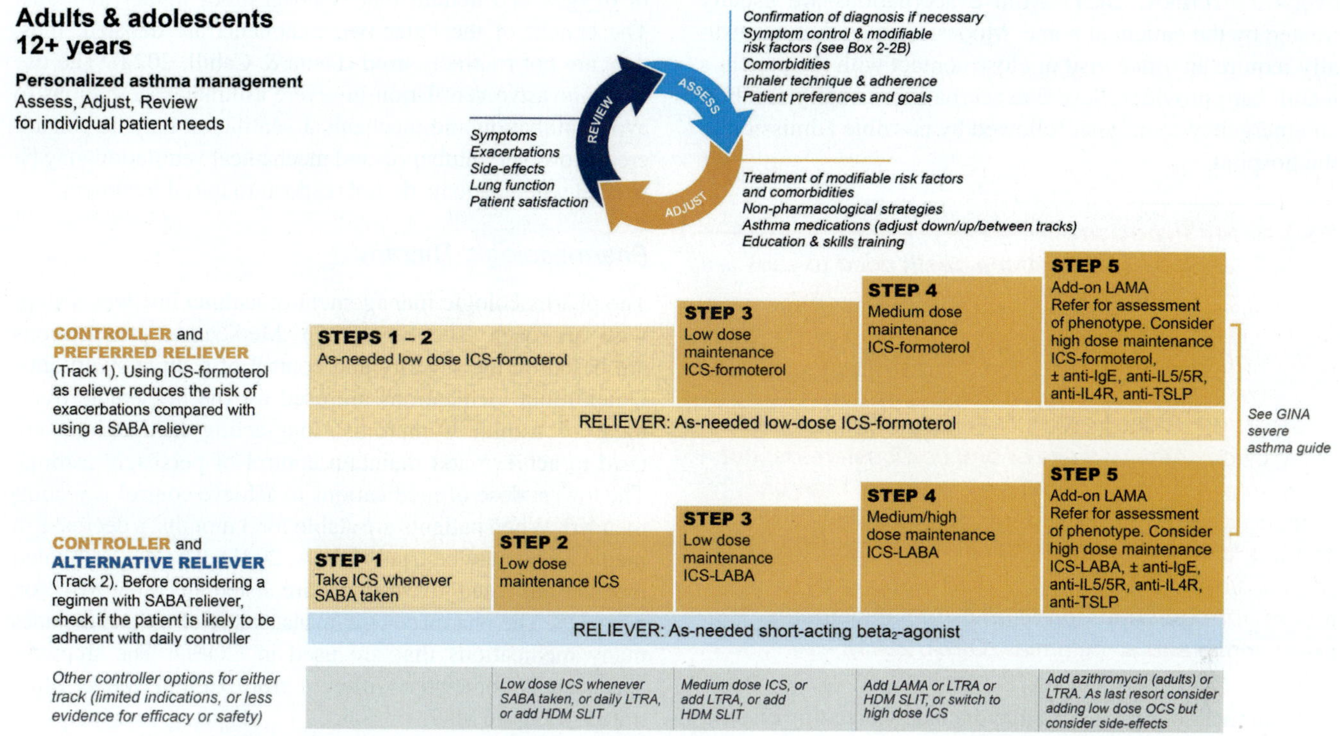

FIGURE 10-8 Personalized management for adults and adolescents to control symptoms and minimize future risk. (© 2020 Global Initiative for Asthma, reprinted with permission. www.ginasthma.org.)

oxide (NO). Recall that eosinophils generate inflammatory enzymes and release leukotrienes and many proinflammatory enzymes (Norris & Tuan, 2020). NO exhaled in breath is a method used to measure airway inflammation, as there is a highly significant relationship between exhaled NO levels and the extent of eosinophilia in the airway. In addition, there is an equally important relationship between eosinophilic airway inflammation and steroid responsiveness, thus it is a tool that allows one to assess active airways disease and better direct targeted treatments (e.g., increasing ICS, adding systemic steroids or using adjunctive medications aimed to treat eosinophilic asthma; Antus & Barta, 2022).

BOX 10-9 Patient Teaching

How to Use a Peak Flow Meter

- Stand or sit up straight.
- Put the marker on the peak-flow meter at zero.
- Take a full, deep breath in.
- Place the meter in your mouth with your tongue and teeth out of the way and seal your lips around the meter.
- Blow out as hard and fast as possible.
- Repeat the procedure two more times.
- Write down the highest reading.

Use your peak flow meter at the same time of day for 2 weeks to establish your "personal best." Work with your primary provider nurse, or asthma educator to help you use your peak flow numbers to help you control your asthma better and help you decide when to call your provider or go to the emergency room.

Note: Your peak flow score is also called your peak expiratory flow (PEF).

Patient Education

Asthma is a chronic illness and requires lifelong management by patients and providers to achieve the goals of therapy. The concept of partnership is one in which the provider and patient work together to establish mutually agreed upon goals and treatments. Patients need to learn and manage multiple areas, for example, identification and management of triggers, monitoring for early warning signs of an acute episode, and taking prescribed medications correctly. Comorbid conditions, side effects, financial issues, living conditions, different beliefs about asthma, and other factors may influence the patient's adherence to the asthma management plan. Involving the patient in the decision-making process may increase adherence and positively affect outcomes.

Exacerbations and Complications

An asthma exacerbation is an acute or subacute episode of worsening shortness of breath, cough, wheeze, and/or chest tightness. Asthma exacerbations are classified by the severity of symptoms, the response to treatment, and PEF measurements. When considering the patient's personal best PEF, an exacerbation is considered severe when the PEF is ≤50% predicted or a moderate exacerbation if the PEF is >50% but <70% (Fanta & Cahill, 2022). The standard classifications of mild, moderate, or severe disease is determined after the patient has been on treatment for a number of months. It is not a static classification and will change over time (GINA, 2021). Mild exacerbations are usually treated by the patient at home. Moderate exacerbations usually require an office visit or close contact with the patient's health care provider. Severe exacerbations usually result in an emergency room visit followed by possible admission to the hospital.

Pearls for Practice

Patients at high risk for asthma death need to seek medical care early during an exacerbation. Risk factors that place the patient at high risk include a history of a previous severe exacerbation requiring intensive care and/or intubation; a hospitalization or emergency room visit in the past year; current or recently discontinued use of oral corticosteroids; not using inhaled corticosteroids; using more than one canister of a SABA per month; poor adherence to medications and/or action plan; food allergy; history of psychiatric disease or psychosocial problems; and major comorbid conditions such as diabetes, pneumonia, and arrhythmias (GINA, 2021).

Complications of asthma may include worsening disease, acute severe asthma (status asthmaticus), and respiratory failure. Airway obstruction, particularly during acute asthmatic episodes, often results in hypoxemia, requiring the administration of oxygen and the monitoring of pulse oximetry and ABGs. Antibiotics are rarely needed but may be used for concomitant pneumonia or bacterial sinusitis.

Acute severe asthma or ***status asthmaticus*** is a severe asthma episode that is refractory to initial therapy. It is a medical emergency. Symptoms include tachypnea (>30 breaths/min), tachycardia (>120 beats/min), use of accessory muscles, diaphoresis, inability to speak in full sentences or phrases, inability to lie supine due to breathlessness, and pulsus paradoxus (i.e., a fall in systolic blood pressure of more than 12 mmHg during inspiration; Fanta & Cahill, 2022). Not all patients present with these manifestations; the measurement of PEF is an objective assessment of the severity of an asthma attack. However, if impending respiratory failure is suspected, this should be deferred (Fanta & Cahill, 2022). In general, a PEF below 200 L/min indicates severe obstruction for most adults except for the older patient (>65), or those with short height (Fanta & Cahill, 2022).

Status asthmaticus may occur following a viral respiratory infection, allergen exposure, outdoor air pollution, seasonal change, or poor adherence to controller medications (GINA, 2021). It may also occur with little or no warning and can progress rapidly to severe obstruction.

Patients must be monitored closely in the emergency room or intensive care unit. Oxygen, adequate hydration, frequent or continuous nebulization of SABAs, inhaled ipratropium, and systemic corticosteroids are frequently used to manage this condition. Other treatments that have been tried include intravenous magnesium sulfate and inhaled heliox (a mixture of oxygen and helium that is seven times lighter than air). The benefit of the latter two treatments are debated; thus, they are not routinely used (Fanta & Cahill, 2022). The use of noninvasive ventilation in severe asthma exacerbations to avoid intubation and mechanical ventilation may be considered. However, intubation and mechanical ventilation may be needed when patients do not respond to initial treatment.

Pharmacologic Therapy

The pharmacologic management of asthma involves a stepwise approach (see Fig. 10-7). Medication prescriptions are based on the severity and control of asthma symptoms. Quick-relief medications are used for the immediate treatment of asthma symptoms; long-acting medications are used to achieve and maintain control of persistent asthma. The lowest dose of medications to achieve control is recommended. When patients are stable for 3 months, a decrease in medications may be tried (GINA, 2021). The major inhaled medications used for asthma are listed in Table 10-1 on page 378. The pharmacologic management of asthma includes many medications that are used in COPD. The stepwise approach is somewhat different from COPD and is illustrated in Figure 10-7.

Pearls for Practice

The nurse teaches patients and families that there are two components of asthma care: controller pharmacologic treatments that are used daily to prevent symptoms, reduce exacerbations, and improve lung function regardless of symptoms; and the use of acute relievers, also known as rescue medications (e.g., SABAs such as albuterol), to relieve acute symptoms.

For patients with mild intermittent disease, a SABA administered by MDI may be all that is needed. Control of persistent asthma is accomplished primarily with regular use of anti-inflammatory medications. Inhaled corticosteroids are the treatment of choice. The dose of inhaled corticosteroids is adjusted based on patient symptoms and asthma control. A spacer should be used with inhaled corticosteroids; patients should gargle and spit out water after administration to prevent thrush, a troublesome complication associated with the use of inhaled corticosteroids. Inhaled corticosteroids may be used alone or in combination with LABAs.

Drug Alert

A black box warning has been issued for a LABA for patients with asthma. One large clinical trial found an increase in asthma deaths and exacerbations in patient using a LABA. The current guidelines recommend using LABAs only in combination with inhaled corticosteroids (FDA Drug Safety Communication, 2018).

Leukotriene modifiers (inhibitors), or antileukotrienes, are a class of medications that include montelukast (Singulair, zafirlukast [Accolate]), and zileuton (Zyflo). Leukotriene inhibitors act either by interfering with leukotriene synthesis or by blocking the receptors where leukotrienes exert their action. Leukotrienes promote smooth muscle constriction, blood vessel permeability, and inflammatory responses; thus, leukotriene inhibitors can decrease bronchoconstriction and inflammatory responses of edema and mucus secretion (Rosenthal & Rosenjack Burchum, 2021). They may provide an alternative to inhaled corticosteroids for mild persistent asthma, or they may be added to a regimen of inhaled corticosteroids in more severe asthma to improve control. Adverse effects include depression, aggression, and suicidal behavior (Gold Standard, 2022; Rosenthal & Rosenjack Burchum, 2021). Careful monitoring of liver function is recommended for patients taking zileuton.

Cromolyn sodium, also known as cromoglycates, stabilize mast cells. They are used primarily for mild persistent asthma as an alternative medication in patients not tolerating inhaled corticosteroids or as a preventive treatment for exercise asthma.

Omalizumab (anti-IgE) is used as an additional therapy for patients with severe, persistent asthma who have sensitivity to specific allergens, for example, cats, dogs, and cockroaches. Omalizumab is administered by subcutaneous injection. Because of the potential for serious allergic reactions during administration, careful monitoring and possible treatment for anaphylaxis is required.

Pearls for Practice

It is important for the nurse to recognize an anaphylactic reaction and initiate prompt emergency interventions. Signs and symptoms include urticaria (hives); angioedema; bronchoconstriction; cough; stridor; cardiac arrhythmias; hypotension; and GI symptoms of nausea, vomiting, and diarrhea. Assessment of the patient's airway and cardiovascular status is essential. Supplemental oxygen therapy is administered, and endotracheal intubation may be required to provide sufficient oxygenation.

Other occasionally useful medications include methylxanthines and anticholinergics. Methylxanthines, sustained-release theophylline medications, are mild to moderate bronchodilators. They are mainly used as an adjunct when long-term controllers fail to achieve relief of nighttime symptoms. They are usually administered by mouth but may also be administered intravenously (Rosenthal & Rosenjack Burchum, 2021). Methylxanthines have a narrow therapeutic range that necessitates monitoring of the serum theophylline level. Traditionally, dosages are adjusted to maintain theophylline levels between 10 and 20 μg/mL; however, dosages are based on patient response. Many will improve at levels of 5 μg/mL, and, "as a rule, there is little benefit to increasing levels to greater than 15 μg/mL; therefore, levels between 5 and 15 μg/mL are appropriate for most patients (Rosenthal & Rosenjack Burchum, 2021, p. 570)." The anticholinergic ipratropium may be used as an alternative quick-relief medication when the patient cannot tolerate SABAs.

Oral corticosteroids are used to gain quick control of asthma and during acute exacerbations. Patients with severe persistent asthma that is not adequately controlled may need long-term oral corticosteroids.

A new class of therapies for patients with severe persistent asthma, frequent exacerbations, and an eosinophilic phenotype despite guideline-based therapy, are biologics as an additional therapy. Examples include anti–interleukin (IL)-5 antibodies, mepolizumab, reslizumab, benralizumab, or anti-IL4α receptor antibody dupilumab (Tan, 2023). They are administered subcutaneously with the exception of Reslizumab, which is administered intravenously.

Environmental Control and Management of Triggers and Comorbid Conditions

Reducing exposure to asthma triggers may reduce asthma symptoms, inflammation, and the need for higher doses of medications. Skin testing is useful in some patients to identify specific allergens and in patients who may be candidates for immunotherapy. Effective allergen and trigger avoidance may be complicated when the patient's asthma is triggered by multiple allergens and irritants. Ongoing education and prioritizing the contribution of specific triggers in individuals may be needed. When patients have many triggers, specific trigger management may need to be designed to stress the management of the most troublesome triggers first and manage less troublesome triggers later. For example, if a patient has a severe reaction to cockroach antigen and less of a reaction to dust mites, initial efforts should be directed at cockroach control.

Drug Alert

Patients with persistent asthma, nasal polyps, and sensitivity to aspirin or nonsteroidal anti-inflammatory drugs (NSAIDs) need to avoid using these drugs because of the risk of severe or even fatal reactions. Hypersensitivity to aspirin or NSAIDs is among the most common causes of drug-induced hypersensitivity resulting in a wide spectrum of immunologic and inflammatory processes. The incidence of aspirin-exacerbated respiratory disease among adults with asthma is 7.2% but is up to 14.9% among those with severe asthma (Ferri, 2022).

Asthma management is complicated by comorbid conditions, particularly COPD, allergic bronchopulmonary aspergillosis (aspergillosis, commonly found in soil, is a fungi to which patients with asthma or cystic fibrosis may have an allergic or hypersensitive reaction), gastroesophageal reflux disease (GERD), obesity, OSA, rhinitis, sinusitis, stress, and depression. Adequately treating these conditions may improve the control of asthma. Most patients with comorbid conditions should be referred to a pulmonary or asthma specialist.

Nursing Management

Nursing care of patients with asthma depends on the setting the nurse works in and on the severity of the patient's disease. Patients may be treated successfully as outpatients if asthma symptoms are relatively mild or may require hospitalization and intensive care if symptoms are acute and severe. Asthma episodes may be frightening to patients and families. Reassurance and a calm approach are important aspects of care.

Nursing assessment includes taking a history of the patient's symptoms, self-care measures used, sequence of the current asthma episode, and response to medication and treatments used. A history of allergic reactions to medications, current prescription and nonprescription medications (including complementary and alternative therapy [CAM]), recent exposure to allergens and triggers, previous hospitalizations, emergency room visits, intensive care unit admissions, intubations for asthma, and the patient's perception of asthma severity are additional elements to include in a nursing assessment. Physical examination is similar to that used with COPD. Peak-flow measurements and pulse oximetry are additional assessment measures.

Nursing interventions for patients admitted for an asthma exacerbation include administering medications and treatments as prescribed; monitoring patients' response; preparing patients for discharge; educating patients about treatment, medication administration, identification, and management of asthma triggers; prevention and treatment of future exacerbations; and medical follow-up.

The main focus of nursing management of patients with acute severe asthma is to actively assess the patient's airway and the response to treatment. Nursing care includes frequent monitoring of the patient's vital signs, oxygen saturation, and cardiac rhythm until status asthmaticus is under control; assessing for signs of dehydration and managing fluid intake; administering systemic corticosteroids, bronchodilators, and other medications as ordered (often given as continuous therapy); assisting patients with daily activity to help them conserve energy; and providing a quiet environment that is free of respiratory irritants including flowers, perfumes, powders, or odors of cleaning agents. The administration of heliox and magnesium sulfate are additional interventions that may be used and require close monitoring.

Patients with acute severe asthma or *status asthmaticus* who are not responding adequately to treatment and patients with severe comorbidities may need to be transferred to intensive care. Intubation and mechanical ventilation may also be needed. Frequent communication and consultation with physicians, respiratory therapists, and rapid response teams is important in any patient hospitalized for asthma. Discharge criteria include an FEV_1 or peak flow *measurement of* 70% or higher predicted (good response) or a *measurement of* 50% to 70% predicted in some patients (moderate response), a sustained response to bronchodilator treatment, no or mild distress, and the absence of hypoxemia. Patients being discharged from an emergency room or hospital may benefit from referral to an asthma clinic, asthma or pulmonary specialist, and/or visiting nurse agency. Home visits may be particularly useful for patients with recurrent exacerbations and emergency room visits. The home visit may give a more accurate picture of the individual's allergens and triggers.

Patient Teaching

Patient teaching is a critical component of the nursing care of patients with asthma. Complex treatment regimens, including multiple and different types of inhalers, monitoring of asthma control, antiallergy therapy, therapy for comorbid conditions, identification of early warning signs, and recognition and avoidance of triggers are essential for long-term control. Patient education may include the nature of asthma as a chronic inflammatory disease, the definition of inflammation and bronchoconstriction, the goals of asthma control, the purpose and action of each medication (quick-relief medications and controllers), triggers to avoid and how to do so, proper inhalation technique, performance and recording of PEF, implementation of an action plan designed with their health care provider, and recognition of the signs and symptoms indicating the need for prompt medical assistance.

An assortment of excellent educational material is available from the NHLBI and other sources. The choice of educational materials used should be based on the patient's diagnosis, causative factors, educational and reading level, and cultural background.

Unfolding Patient Stories: J.H. • Part 1

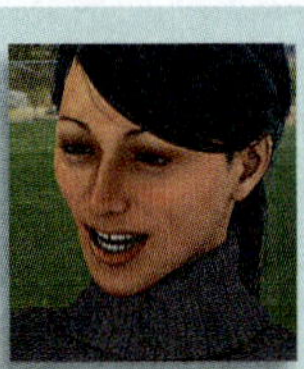

J.H. is 33 years old and was diagnosed with asthma in childhood. The patient has come to the clinic multiple times over the last 2 months complaining of continued symptoms. The asthma action plan was adjusted by the primary provider last month. What measures can the nurse take to determine areas needing education reinforcement? How can the nurse ensure that J.H. is accurately following the prescribed asthma regimen and monitoring medication effectiveness? (J.H.'s story continues in Chapter 37.)

Care for J.H. and other patients in a realistic virtual environment: ***vSim** for Nursing* (thepoint.lww.com/vSimMedicalSurgical). Practice documenting these patients' care in DocuCare (thepoint.lww.com/DocuCareEHR).

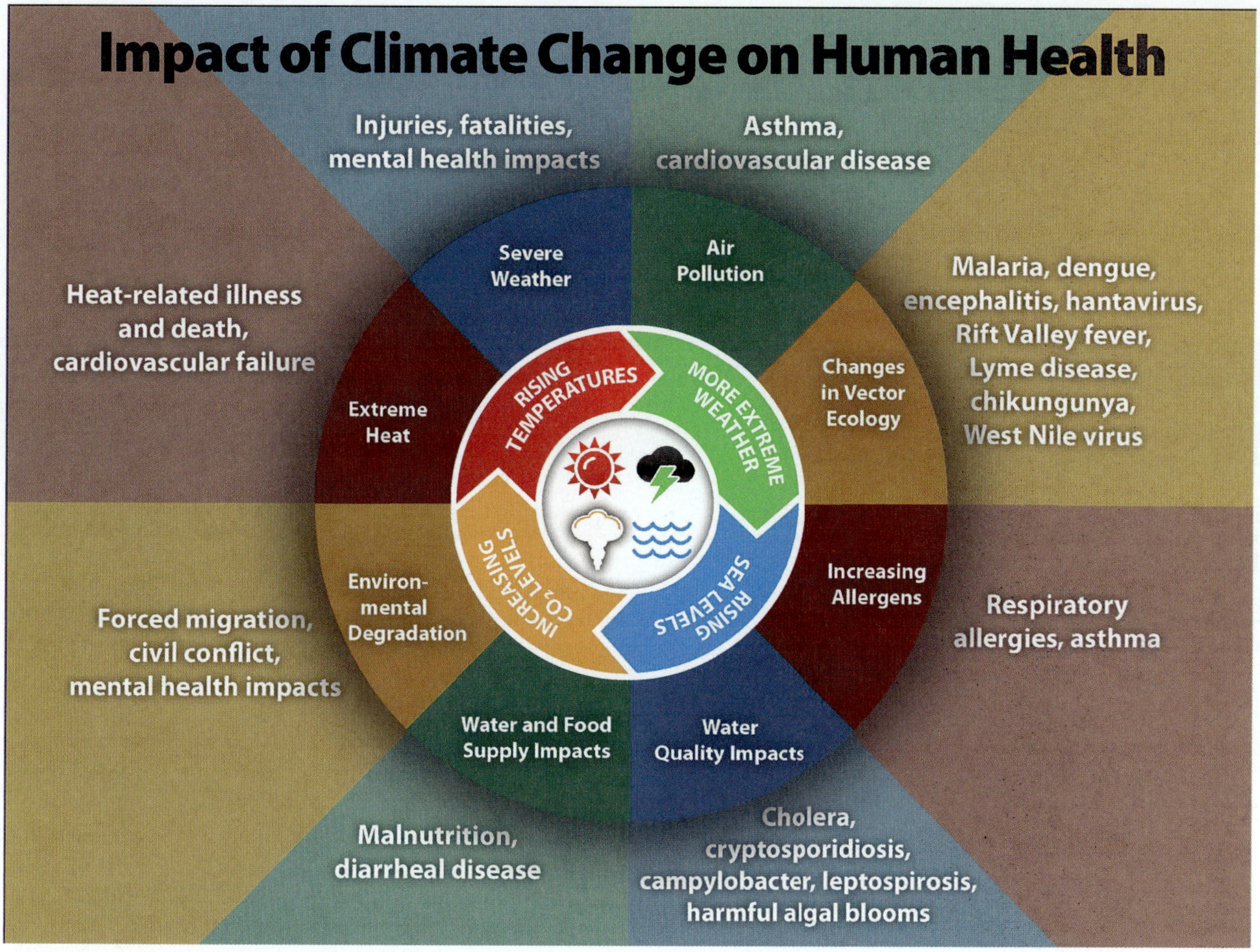

Pearls for Practice: Lifting the Lens

Note in the image above the impact of climate change on health. Rising temperatures worsen air quality (increases respiratory difficulty), increase pollen count (increases allergic reactions and asthma attacks in some), and increase ground-level ozone pollution (particularly in heavily populated urban areas) that reduces lung function, and increase the risk of asthma attacks and exacerbation of other chronic lung diseases (Anderko & Pennea, 2022; CDC, 2022c). An additional threat is wildfires that reduce air quality, both locally and in areas downwind of fires (CDC, 2022c). Nurses will need to educate patients about preventive measures in extreme heat; such measures include increasing hydration, use of electric fans and/or air conditioning, staying indoors and avoiding outdoor activities where possible, and wearing cool and sun-protective clothing (Liu et al., 2021). The nurse offers resources to patients and families related to air pollution and health.

Here are resources for patients and families:

Air Quality

Check air quality (www.airnow.gov/sites/default/files/2018-06/aqi-forecasts.pdf)

Exercise early in morning or on days with low ozone levels

Avoid outdoor activities during extreme heat days

Check pollen levels (www.pollen.com)

Stay indoors when pollen levels are high and close windows

Purchase an air filter for your home

During pollen season, change clothes and remove shoes when coming indoors

Shower and shampoo at night before bed

Be alert to local air quality reports during fire season (www.airnow.gov)

Check updated recommendations for keeping children safe during wildfires, including mask wearing (www.pehsu.net)

Develop an evacuation plan if you live in an area threatened by wildfires

Extreme Heat

Limit physical exertion outdoors; stay in the shade

Drink water more often than usual to prevent dehydration

Take cool showers and baths

Eat lightly; avoid using stoves or ovens to heat food

Properly refrigerate food to avoid food spoiling in high temperatures with the potential for food poisoning
Store water and nonperishable food in case of power outage
Close curtains and blinds to keep out sunlight
Use air-conditioning when available, or identify location of and transportation to local cooling centers or move to lower floors in home
Dress in loose, lightweight, and light-colored clothing
Know the warning signs of heat exhaustion and heat stroke (www.cdc.gov/disasters/extremeheat/pdf/Heat_Related_Illness.pdf)

CHAPTER REVIEW

NCLEX-Style Review Questions

1. During morning rounds on a medical floor, the nurse assesses a patient admitted the previous evening with an exacerbation of COPD. The patient is complaining of increased dyspnea and is sitting on the side of the bed with their arms braced against their knees. The respiratory rate was 20 on admission and is now 28. Breath sounds are diminished with coarse crackles heard throughout. The oxygen saturation is 93% on 2 L/min of supplemental oxygen. The nurse would perform which of the following? Select all that apply.
   a. Administer albuterol using a spacer that has been ordered "as needed."
   b. Switch the patient's oxygen to a Venturi mask at 32%.
   c. Instruct the patient to begin pursed-lip breathing.
   d. Instruct the patient in controlled cough.
   e. Observe for signs and symptoms of further deterioration.

2. The following day the patient's symptoms are improving. There is less dyspnea, and the patient is able to walk to the bathroom with minimal assistance. In preparing for discharge, a home oxygen assessment is ordered. The patient's room air oxygen saturation is 88% at rest and 86% with exertion. Oxygen administered by nasal cannula at 2 L/min raises the oxygen saturation to 94% at rest and 92% when walking. Home oxygen is ordered as 2 L/min 24 hours a day. Teaching about home oxygen would include which of the following? Select all that apply.
   a. Oxygen improves cardiac and cognitive function and improves prognosis.
   b. Oxygen needs to be worn only when the patient is short of breath.
   c. Oxygen improves cardiac and cognitive function but does not improve prognosis.
   d. Home oxygen must be kept away from open flames.
   e. "Oxygen in Use" signs should be posted on the doors of the home.

3. A 62-year-old patient is being seen at the health care provider's office for an initial evaluation of symptoms of shortness of breath, cough, and sputum production. Spirometry reveals an FEV_1 of 65% predicted. The FVC is 90%, and FEV_1/FVC is 60%. The patient is diagnosed with COPD. The patient's history includes smoking for over 35 years. The patient smokes 10 cigarettes a day and has tried to quit several times; they were able to quit for 1 week a few years ago. Concerns include weight gain once they quit smoking. The provider gave a prescription for bupropion and nicotine nasal spray. The nurse is asked to review an approach to smoking cessation. What should be included in the teaching plan? Select all that apply.
   a. Bupropion and nicotine replacement can assist in the quitting process.
   b. Successful smoking cessation includes multiple approaches.
   c. Dealing with the habit of smoking is important to success.
   d. Quitting smoking once COPD is diagnosed has no effect on lung function.
   e. Smoking cessation does not impact the progression of COPD.

4. A hospital conducts an outpatient clinic for patients with asthma. The nurse working in the clinic is responsible for teaching patients about their medications. Which is true about inhaled medications? Select all that apply.
   a. All inhalers must be given with a spacer device.
   b. Inhaled corticosteroids are used on an as-needed basis for quick relief.
   c. Long-acting beta adrenergics (LABAs) can be used as monotherapy to control asthma.
   d. LABAs and inhaled corticosteroids are used as controllers in the management of asthma.
   e. Rinse and gargle after using inhaled steroid preparations to decrease the risk of oral thrush.

5. An asthma educator is teaching a new patient with asthma and their family about the use of a peak flow meter. What is included in the teaching? Select all that apply.

a. Teach that the meter is measuring the highest airflow during a forced inspiration.
b. Teach that the meter is measuring the highest airflow during a forced expiration.
c. Teach the patient to stand or sit up straight and put the marker on the meter at zero.
d. Teach the patient to place the meter in their mouth with their tongue and teeth out of the way, seal their lips around the meter, and inhale as hard and fast as possible.
e. Teach the patient to place the meter in their mouth with their tongue and teeth out of the way, seal their lips around the meter, and exhale as hard and fast as possible.

REFERENCES AND SELECTED READINGS

References and selected readings associated with this chapter can be found on the website that accompanies the book. Visit **http://thepoint.lww.com/Honan3e** to access the references and other additional resources associated with this chapter.

Resources

American Thoracic Society
www.thoracic.org/patients
www.livebetter.org (Live Better with Pulmonary Rehab)

COPD Foundation
http://www.copdfoundation.org/What-is-COPD/Understanding-COPD/What-is-COPD.aspx

National Heart Lung & Blood Institute
http://www.nhlbi.nih.gov/health/health-topics/topics/copd/

American Lung Association
http://www.lung.org/lung-disease/copd/about-copd/understanding-copd.html

The Pulmonary Education and Research Foundation: PERF
https://perf2ndwind.org/

Problems Related to Cardiovascular and Circulatory Function

The nurse is caring for a 60-year-old patient who is being seen in the cardiology clinic for evaluation and treatment of hypertension. The current blood pressure is 180/90 mm Hg. This patient has a history of heart failure (HF) and has not followed up with a provider for 3 years. There are concerns about the patient's adherence to the medication regimen. In addition, the patient currently smokes and has a history of two packs of cigarettes per day for 15 years. The patient's body mass index (BMI) is 35.1.

- **Identify factors in this case that are significant for cardiovascular disease.**
- **Discuss factors that can influence a patient's nonadherence to a medication regimen.**
- **What areas of teaching would be important to emphasize with this patient?**
- **Discuss target organs that may be affected by the patient's history of hypertension and HF.**

CHAPTER 11

Nursing Assessment: Cardiovascular and Circulatory Function

Linda Honan

Learning Objectives

After reading this chapter, you will be able to:

1. Describe the relationship between the anatomic structures and physiologic functions of the heart and peripheral circulation.
2. Discuss the significance of the health history and physical assessment to the diagnosis of cardiovascular disorders.
3. Discuss the clinical indications, patient preparation, and other related nursing implications for common tests and procedures used to assess cardiovascular and circulatory function.
4. Compare the various methods of hemodynamic monitoring (e.g., central venous pressure, pulmonary artery pressure, and arterial pressure monitoring) with regard to indications for use, potential complications, and nursing responsibilities.

Cardiovascular disease (CVD) refers to diseases involving the heart and blood vessels. CVD is the top cause of death worldwide for adults; it claims the life of one person every 37 seconds (Virani et al., 2021; American Heart Association [AHA], 2021). Given the prevalence of CVD, nurses practicing in most settings will be assessing and managing patients with one or more disorders associated with the heart or blood vessels. An understanding of the structure and function of the cardiovascular system in health and disease is essential to the development of cardiovascular assessment skills.

ANATOMY AND PHYSIOLOGY OVERVIEW

The unique function of the cardiovascular system is to circulate blood through a network of blood vessels (arteries, capillaries, and veins) via two interdependent circulatory systems called the *pulmonary circulatory system* (right heart) and *systemic circulatory system* (left heart) (Fig. 11-1). The *lymphatic system* complements the function of the circulatory system by draining excessive interstitial fluid from the tissues and returning it into the bloodstream via the internal jugular and subclavian veins.

Anatomy and Physiology of the Vascular System

The vascular system is composed of blood vessels that circulate blood throughout the body and back to the heart. There are several types of blood vessels, including arteries, arterioles, capillaries, venules, and veins.

Arteries and Arterioles

Arteries are thick-walled structures that transport blood containing oxygen and nutrients from the heart to the tissues of the body. The aorta, the largest artery, has a diameter of approximately 25 mm (1 in) in the average-sized adult (Upchurch & Perry, 2019). It has numerous branches that continue to divide into progressively smaller arteries and eventually become *arterioles*, which are embedded within the tissues. The diameter of arterioles and small arteries ranges from 20 to 130 μm, and due to the small lumen size, these blood vessels can be closed down to generate high resistance to blood flow (Kierszenbaum & Tres, 2020).

The walls of the arteries and arterioles are composed of the *intima*, a thin, smooth endothelial cell layer; the *media*, the middle layer of smooth muscles and elastic fibers; and the *adventitia*, a protective layer of connective tissue that anchors these vessels to surrounding structures. The media is well developed in the arteries, whereas in smaller arteries and arterioles, there is much less elastic tissue.

Capillaries

Capillaries are narrow vessels (5 to 10 μm) formed by a single layer of endothelial cells that permit continuous movement of fluid and exchange of oxygen and nutrients to the cells and removal of carbon dioxide and other metabolic

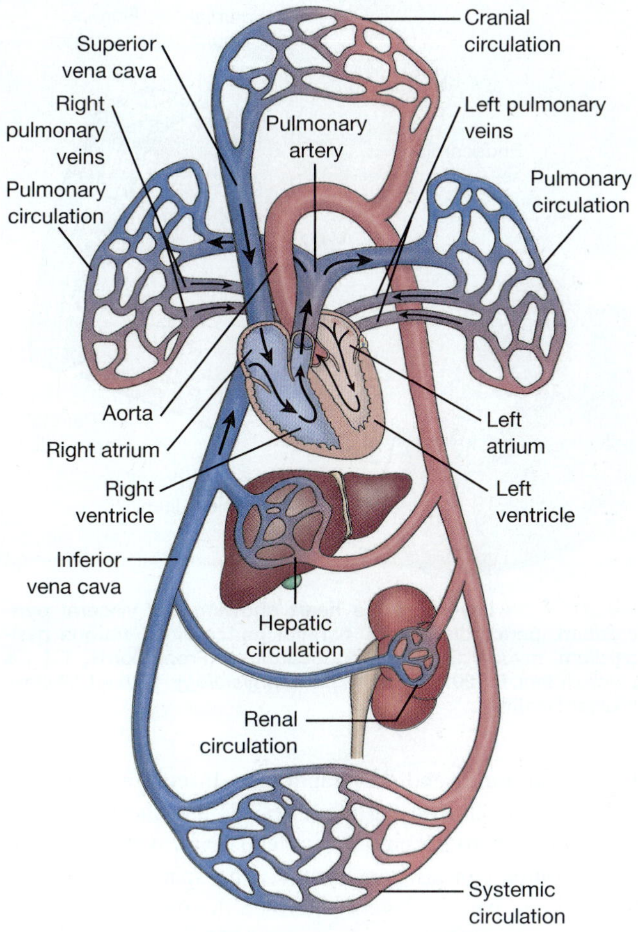

FIGURE 11-1 Pulmonary and systemic circulation. Oxygen-rich blood from the pulmonary circulation is pumped from the left side of the heart into the aorta and the systemic arteries to the capillaries, where the exchange of nutrients and waste products takes place. The deoxygenated blood returns to the right side of the heart by way of the systemic veins and is pumped into the pulmonary circulation. *Arrows* represent the direction of blood flow through the great vessels and chambers of the heart. The *blue shading* represents venous blood and the *red shading* represents arterial blood.

wastes. The small size of the capillaries is still large enough to accommodate one red blood cell but thin enough for gas diffusion (Kierszenbaum & Tres, 2020). The amount of oxygen extracted differs by tissue type. For example, the heart has large metabolic requirements, extracting approximately 70% to 80% of the oxygen delivered, whereas other organs extract about 20%. Thus, the oxygen extraction rate will vary depending on specific tissue type or how hard it is working.

Capillary membrane permeability and hydrostatic and osmotic pressures are the primary controls for the amount and direction of fluid filtering across the capillary membrane into the interstitium (space around the cells). Under normal conditions, capillary permeability remains constant. Hydrostatic pressure is generated by the blood pressure (BP) which "pushes" the fluid out of the capillary during systole. It is fluid, not blood; because the capillary is so small, only fluid is allowed to escape and enter the interstitial space. Osmotic pressure is created by plasma proteins (primarily albumin), which are not allowed under normal circumstances to filter out of the capillary, so these proteins remain in the capillary. It is the concentration of the plasma proteins that "pulls" the water from the interstitial space back into the venous end of the capillary (Fig. 11-2). The excess interstitial fluid that is not reabsorbed into the venous end of the capillary enters the lymphatic system. These processes—filtration, reabsorption, and lymph formation—aid in maintaining tissue fluid volume and removing tissue waste and debris.

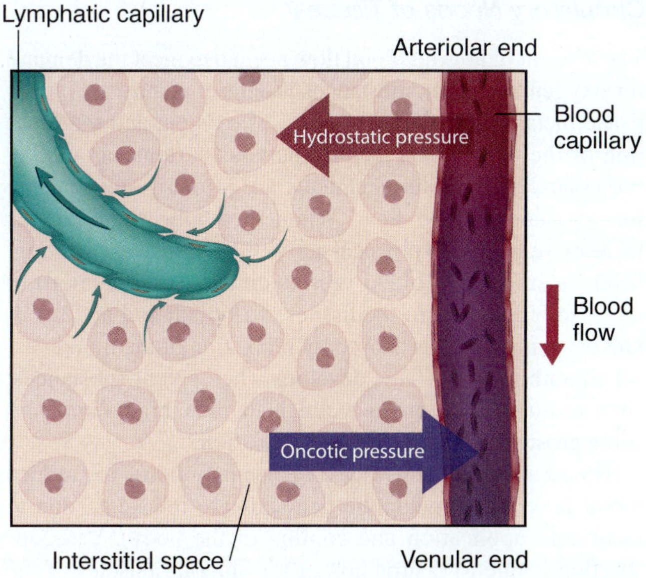

FIGURE 11-2 Hydrostatic and osmotic pressure and lymphatic drainage. (Shutterstock/Alila Medical Media.)

Tissue *edema*, an accumulation of excessive interstitial fluid, occurs for a variety of reasons including conditions that obstruct lymph drainage (e.g., cancer that is affecting the lymphatic system); increased capillary membrane permeability (e.g., septicemia); significantly elevated venous pressure (e.g., deep vein thrombosis); and decreased osmotic force generated by the plasma proteins (e.g., hypoalbuminemia in liver failure).

Venules and Veins

The venous system has venules and veins, which are responsible for returning blood to the heart after cellular exchange of oxygen, nutrients, and metabolic waste products. The return of blood to the heart begins as capillaries merge to form thin-walled vessels called *venules* that merge to form larger vessels or veins. The veins contain approximately 75% of total blood volume. Compared with arteries, veins have three thin, less muscular layers. Thus, veins readily distend, permitting large volumes of blood to accumulate in these blood vessels under low pressure. Transport of venous blood back to the right side of the heart is facilitated by the pumping action of the skeletal muscles and the presence of one-way valves, which prevent backward blood flow and enhance the pumping action of skeletal muscles.

Circulatory Needs of Tissues

The amount of arterial blood flow needed to meet the demand for oxygen and other substances is determined by the rate of tissue metabolism, the availability of oxygen, and the function of the tissues. The central nervous system, circulating hormones, and certain chemicals are primarily responsible for regulating blood flow. When metabolic requirements increase (e.g., due to physical activity, local heat application, fever, or infection), blood vessels dilate (vasodilatation) to increase blood flow to the tissues. Vasodilatation and resultant lowering of BP is caused by relaxation of the blood vessel smooth muscles. This develops when potent substances, such as nitric oxide, prostacyclin, histamine, bradykinin, and some prostaglandins, enter the circulation.

Blood vessels constrict (vasoconstriction) to reduce blood flow when metabolic demands are low (e.g., due to local cold application and cooling of the body). Vasoconstriction is due to contraction of the smooth muscles of the arteries, arterioles, and veins. This action causes narrowing of the lumen of the blood vessels and an elevation in BP. It is stimulated by the release of norepinephrine from the sympathetic nervous system, epinephrine from the adrenal medulla, and angiotensin II. Angiotensin II is the end result of a series of interactions beginning with renin (synthesized by the kidney) and angiotensinogen, a circulating serum protein produced by the liver, which forms angiotensin I. An enzyme (angiotensin-converting enzyme) secreted by the pulmonary vasculature converts angiotensin I into angiotensin II (a potent vasoconstrictor).

Anatomy and Physiology of the Heart

The heart is a hollow, muscular organ located in the center of the thorax, where it occupies the space between the lungs (mediastinum) and rests on the diaphragm. It weighs approximately 300 g (10.6 oz) and is about the size of a clenched fist, though size varies based on age, gender, body stature, physical condition, and presence of CVD.

The walls of the heart are made up of three layers (Fig. 11-3). The inner layer, or *endocardium*, consists of endothelial tissue and lines the inside of the heart and valves. The middle layer, or myocardium, forms an interconnected network of muscle fibers, which encircles the heart in a figure-eight pattern. During myocardial contraction, this configuration facilitates a twisting and compressive movement beginning from the top to the bottom of the heart. The exterior layer of the heart is called the *epicardium.*

The heart is encased in a tough fibrous sac called the *pericardium*, which is composed of two layers (see Fig. 11-3), the fibrous pericardium (outer layer) and the thin serous layer (inner layer). This inner layer, termed the epicardium, is further subdivided into the visceral and parietal layers. The tough, outer, fibrous layer holds the heart in place and is attached to the great vessels of the heart (the superior and inferior vena cava, pulmonary artery [PA], pulmonary veins, and aorta) and the diaphragm. In contrast, the thin visceral layer lies on the great vessels and the heart itself and folds over to become the parietal layer, which lines the tough, outer, fibrous pericardium. The space between the visceral and parietal layers is termed the pericardial space, and under normal circumstances, it holds approximately 30 to 50 mL of fluid, which lubricates the surface of the heart and reduces friction during systole (Norris, 2019). The *base* and *apex* are common terms used to describe the top and bottom of the heart. The base of the heart is the upper portion, where the great vessels enter and exit the heart. The lowest aspect of the heart is called the apex or the point of maximal impulse (PMI), where the pulsation caused by contraction of the heart can be palpated. The apex of the heart is located in the midclavicular line (MCL) of the chest wall at the fifth intercostal space (ICS) or 7 to 9 cm from the left sternal border.

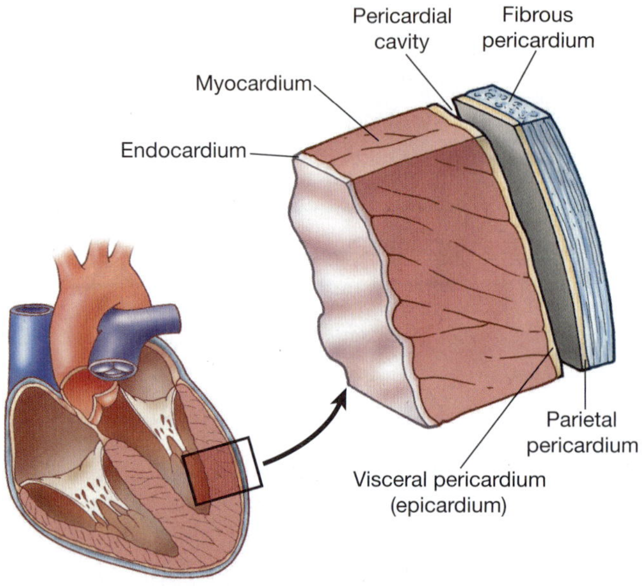

FIGURE 11-3 Layers of the heart showing the visceral pericardium, pericardial cavity, parietal pericardium, fibrous pericardium, myocardium, and endocardium. (From Norris, T. L., & Lalchandani, R. [2019]. *Porth's pathophysiology*. 10th ed. Wolters Kluwer Health.)

Coronary Arteries

The coronary arteries, originating from the aorta just above the aortic valve, supply arterial blood to the heart (Fig. 11-4). The coronary arteries, which feed the heart muscle, receive most of the blood during diastole, when the aortic valve closes. The left coronary, often referred to as the *left main coronary artery,* bifurcates into the left anterior descending artery (LAD) that supplies the anterior wall of the heart and the *circumflex artery* that circles to the left side, feeding the lateral wall of the heart.

The right side of the heart is supplied by the right coronary artery (RCA), which progresses around to the bottom or inferior wall of the left ventricle. The RCA branches into

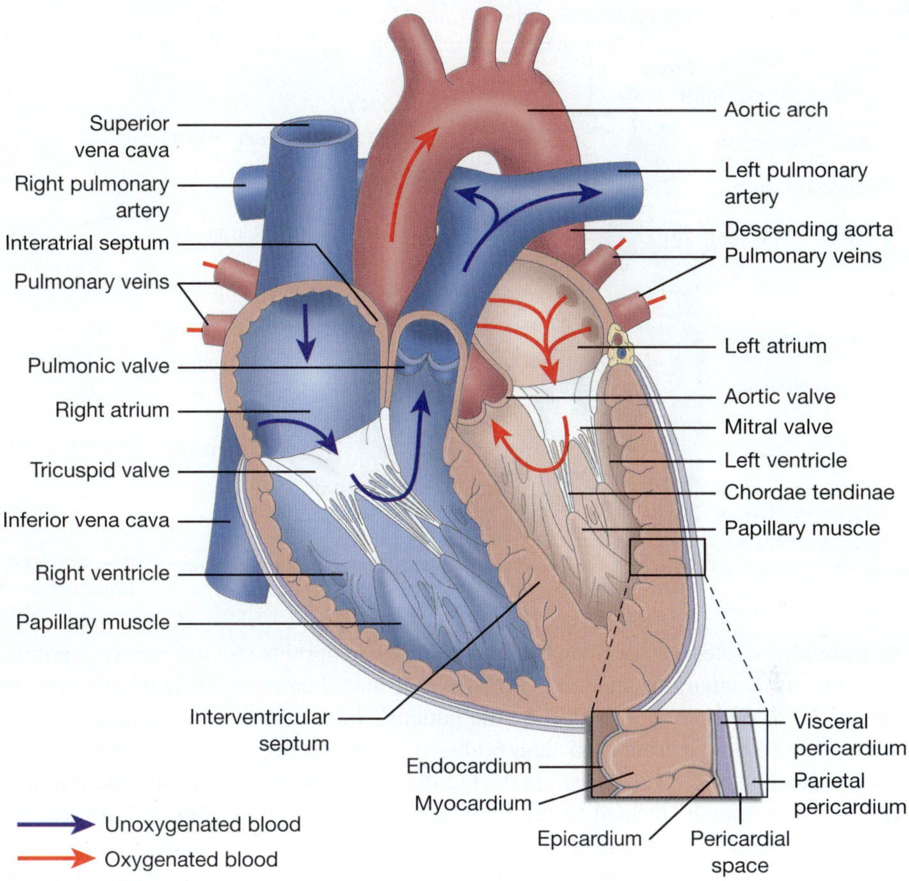

FIGURE 11-4 Anatomy of the heart. *Arrows* represent blood flow through the chambers of the heart.

the posterior descending artery, which supplies the posterior wall of the left ventricle. The blood supply to the sinoatrial (SA) node is most often (70% of the time) derived from the RCA. However, in 25% of normal hearts, the SA nodal artery arises from the circumflex artery, and in 5% of cases, both the RCA and the circumflex artery contribute to this vessel (Durresi et al., 2021). The RCA usually supplies the atrioventricular (AV) nodal artery and the LAD supplies the bundle of His. Superficial to the coronary arteries are the coronary veins. Venous blood from these veins returns to the heart primarily through the coronary sinus, which is located in the posterior wall of the right atrium.

Heart Chambers, Valves, and Great Vessels

The right and left sides of the heart each have an upper chamber, or atrium, that collects blood and a larger lower pumping chamber, called a *ventricle* (Fig. 11-5). Blood flows into the right atrium from the superior and inferior vena cava and passes through the tricuspid valve to the right ventricle. The right ventricle pumps the blood in need of oxygenation across the pulmonary valve into the PA. The PA is the only artery carrying deoxygenated blood (other than the umbilical arteries in the fetus). Oxygenated blood returns to the left atrium via the pulmonary veins. The left atrium contracts, and blood flows through the mitral valve to the left ventricle. The left ventricle pumps the blood through the aortic valve into systemic circulation. Thus, two sets of valves are located within the right and left heart that provide one-way blood flow through these chambers. Valves separating the atria from the ventricles are termed *AV valves*, whereas valves located between the right and left ventricles and their respective great vessels (PA and aorta) are called *semilunar valves* because they are shaped like half-moons.

Cardiac Conduction System

The cardiac conduction system is composed of specialized cells that are capable of spontaneously initiating an electrical impulse (automaticity), responding to an electrical impulse (excitability), and propagating these impulses from one cell to another (conductivity) (Fig. 11-6). The **SA node**, the primary pacemaker of the heart, initiates electrical impulses at an inherent rate of 60 to 100 beats per minute (bpm). Note, this is the same as a normal pulse rate because the SA node is pacing the heart. These impulses move across the atria via internodal pathways causing the atria to contract and then move onto the AV node that is located low in the atrial septum. At the AV node, a slight delay occurs, which synchronizes atrial and ventricular activity and permits adequate time for the ventricles to fill. If the SA node fails in

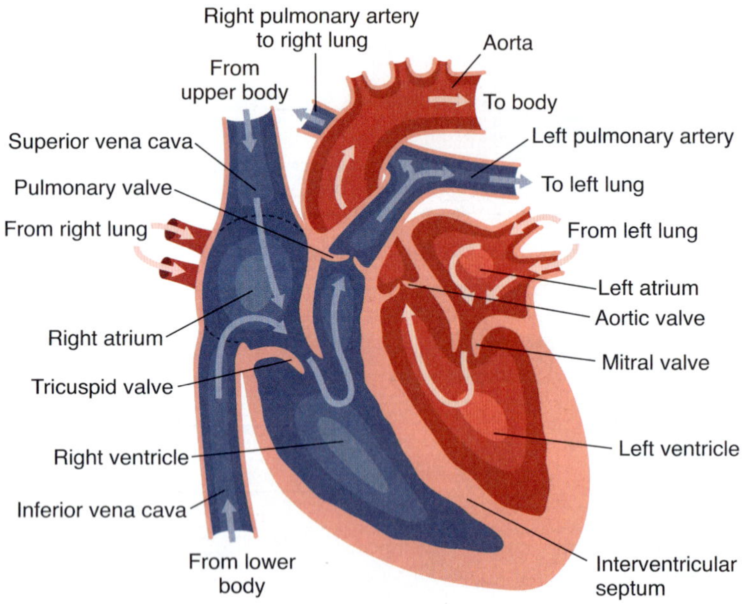

FIGURE 11-5 Circulation of blood through the heart. (Image from Shutterstock.com.)

its pacemaker role, the AV node is capable of assuming this function by discharging electrical impulses at an inherent rate of 40 to 60 bpm. If this occurs, the patient's heart rate is considered bradycardic (less than 60 bpm). Impulses are then conducted to the ventricles via the bundle of His, to the right bundle branch (located in the right ventricle) and left bundle branches (located in the left ventricle), and finally to the Purkinje fibers, the point at which the ventricles are stimulated to contract (ventricular systole). The conduction tissue in the ventricles has an inherent rate of 30 to 40 bpm, which will assume the pacemaker role should the SA and AV nodes fail to provide electrical impulses.

At the cellular level, the electrical activity of the heart is due to the exchange of electrically charged particles, called *ions*, across channels located in the cellular membranes. These channels regulate the movement and speed of ions, specifically sodium and potassium. When the cell is in its resting or polarized state, sodium is the primary extracellular ion, whereas potassium is the primary intracellular ion. This difference in ion concentration causes the inside of the cell to have a negative charge compared with the positive charge on the outside. A reversal of these charges occurs during electrical stimulation of the myocardial cells as sodium ions move into the cell and potassium ions exit. This exchange of ions characterizes the period known as **depolarization**, which is followed rapidly by the contraction of the stimulated myocardium. Once depolarization is complete, the exchange of ions reverts back to its polarized state. This period is known as **repolarization**. It is analogous to a rest period that allows the myocardial cells to prepare for the next depolarization and subsequent contraction.

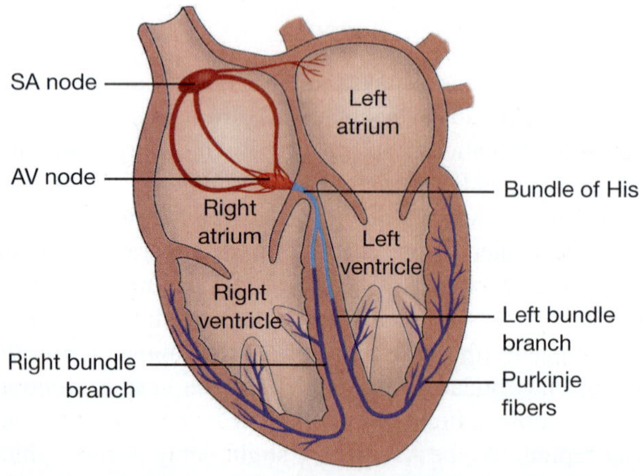

FIGURE 11-6 Cardiac conduction system. AV, atrioventricular; SA, sinoatrial.

Cardiac Hemodynamics

Cardiac hemodynamics describes the pumping forces or pressure required by the heart to maintain blood flow throughout the cardiovascular system. An important determinant of blood flow is the principle that fluid flows from a region of higher pressure to one of lower pressure. The pressures responsible for blood flow are generated during systole and diastole. Figure 11-7 identifies the pressures in the great vessels and heart chambers during systole and diastole.

Cardiac Cycle

The cardiac cycle is the term used to describe the events that occur in the heart from the beginning of one heartbeat to the beginning of the subsequent one. Therefore, the number of cardiac cycles completed in a minute is dependent on the heart rate. Each cardiac cycle has three major sequential events, which include **diastole** (resting and filling), atrial **systole** (contracting), and ventricular systole (contracting). Diastole is the period in which the atria and ventricles are in a relaxed state, allowing the ventricles to fill with blood. Systole refers to the period of myocardial contraction. Note that there is

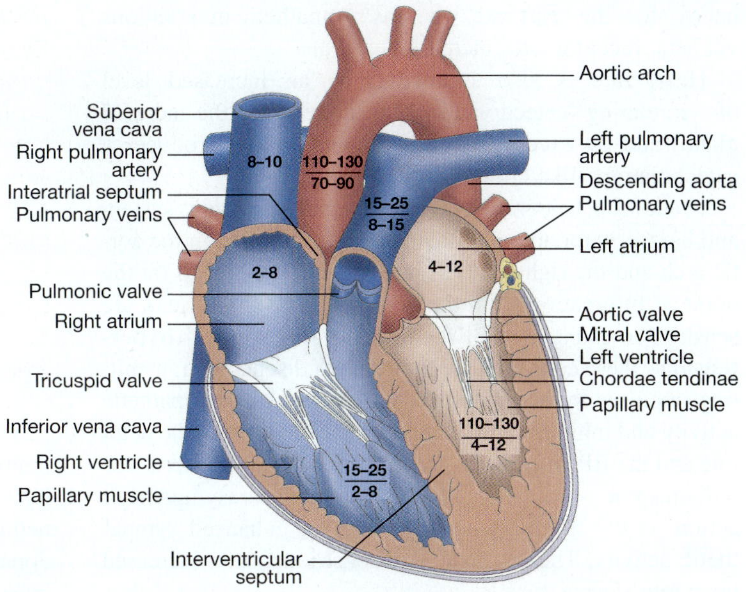

FIGURE 11-7 Great vessel and chamber pressures. Pressures are identified in mm Hg as mean pressure or systolic over diastolic pressure.

atrial contraction, which fills the ventricles with blood, and ventricular contraction, which sends the blood to the lung (from the right ventricle) and body (from the left ventricle).

Deoxygenated blood (venous blood) from the tissues enters the pulmonary circulation by flowing into the right atrium via the superior vena cava (head, neck, and upper extremities), inferior vena cava (trunk and lower extremities), and coronary sinus (heart). On the left side of the heart, oxygenated blood from the pulmonary circulation returns to the left atrium via the four pulmonary veins. Note that the pulmonary veins are carrying oxygenated blood.

During diastole, the pressure in the ventricles is reduced, allowing the AV valves (tricuspid valve in the right heart and mitral valve in the left heart) to open. Blood flows freely from both atria into the ventricles. At the end of diastole, the atria contract (atrial systole), forcing the remaining blood into the ventricles. Atrial systole, better known as the "atrial kick," is an important event because it augments ventricular blood volume by 15% in those without disease to up to 40% in patients with stiff, noncompliant ventricles (Zimetbaum, 2020).

Pearls for Practice

Loss of the atrial kick decreases cardiac output, leading to the development of symptoms in the patient such as dizziness, lightheadedness, syncope, decreased activity tolerance, and hypotension. Atrial fibrillation is an arrhythmia that is known to be associated with the loss of the atrial kick. Loss of coordinated atrial contraction into the ventricle will decrease the left ventricular preload (volume) and therefore significantly lower cardiac output.

During ventricular systole, rising pressure in the ventricles closes the AV valves, preventing the regurgitation of blood back into the atria, and forces the semilunar valves (pulmonic valve in the right side of the heart and aortic valve in the left side of the heart) to open. The structures attached to the AV valves (chordae tendineae and papillary muscles) keep the valve leaflets closed, preventing regurgitation of blood into the atria. This function permits the one-way flow of blood from the right ventricle into the PA and into the lungs for oxygenation (pulmonary circulation) and from the left ventricle into the aorta and out into the remainder of the body via the systemic circulation.

Cardiac Output

Cardiac output refers to the amount of blood pumped by each ventricle in liters per minute (L/min). In an adult at rest, the cardiac output is about 4 to 6 L/min but varies greatly depending on the metabolic needs of the body.

Cardiac output is a function of the **stroke volume** and the heart rate. Stroke volume is the amount of blood ejected with each heartbeat and includes both the contractility of the heart (stroke) and the amount of blood (volume). The average resting stroke volume is about 70 mL. Each time the heart beats, only a fraction of the blood present in the ventricles is ejected, which is referred to as the **ejection fraction** (EF). The EF of the left ventricle (normally 50% to 70%) is commonly assessed because it is an important noninvasive measure of myocardial contractility: the EF is lower in conditions that depress myocardial contractility (e.g., myocardial infarction [MI] and heart failure [HF]).

Effect of Heart Rate on Cardiac Output. Cardiac output meets the metabolic demands of the tissues in part by changes in heart rate. For example, the heart rate increases during periods of high oxygen demand, such as physical activity, and returns to baseline heart rate at rest. Changes in heart rate are accomplished by inhibition or stimulation of the SA node through the parasympathetic and sympathetic divisions of the autonomic nervous system. The parasympathetic impulses, which travel to the SA node via the vagus nerve, slow the heart rate, whereas sympathetic innervations via $beta_1$ receptor sites increase heart rate.

Heart rate is also stimulated by an increased level of circulating catecholamines (secreted by the adrenal gland) and by excess thyroid hormone, which produces a catecholamine-like effect.

In addition, heart rate is affected by central nervous system and baroreceptor activity. **Baroreceptors**, located in the aortic arch and the right and left internal carotid arteries (at the point of bifurcation from the common carotid arteries), are sensitive to changes in BP. During elevations in BP (**hypertension**), these cells increase their rate of discharge, transmitting impulses to the medulla. This initiates parasympathetic activity and inhibits sympathetic response, lowering the heart rate and the BP. In contrast, low BP (hypotension) exerts less baroreceptor stimulation, decreasing the parasympathetic action on the SA node and allowing for enhanced sympathetic activity. The resultant vasoconstriction and increased heart rate elevate the BP.

Effect of Stroke Volume on Cardiac Output. Stroke volume is a major determinant of cardiac output and is influenced by three interdependent factors: preload, afterload, and contractility.

Preload refers to the pressure generated in the ventricles at the end of diastole (filling with blood) and the resultant stretching of the muscle fibers. A direct relationship exists between end-diastolic blood volume and the degree of stretch. As the volume of blood increases, the degree of stretch increases, resulting in stronger contraction and a greater stroke volume. This relationship, called the Frank–Starling (or Starling) law of the heart, is maintained until the physiologic limit of the muscle is reached.

Preload is decreased by a reduction in the volume of blood returning to the ventricles. Vasodilatation and loss of fluid volume from bleeding, diuresis, vomiting, diarrhea, or excessive diaphoresis reduce preload. Preload is increased by increasing the return of circulating blood volume to the ventricles. Controlling the loss of blood or body fluids and replacing fluids (i.e., blood transfusions and intravenous [IV] fluid administration) are examples of ways to increase preload.

Afterload, the amount of resistance to ejection of blood from the ventricle, is the second determinant of stroke volume. The right side of the heart collects venous blood, which has a very low pressure and is met with little resistance as blood is ejected into the pulmonary vascular system, better known as **pulmonary vascular resistance (PVR)**. On the other hand, the left side of the heart requires significantly higher pressures to overcome resistance created by the arteries in the systemic circulation. This resistance is called **systemic vascular resistance (SVR)**.

An inverse relationship exists between afterload and stroke volume. For example, afterload is increased by arterial vasoconstriction, which leads to decreased stroke volume. The opposite is true with arterial vasodilation, a situation that reduces afterload and improves stroke volume.

Pearls for Practice

Preload reflects the volume of blood returning to the right and left ventricles at the end of diastole. Central venous pressure (CVP) monitoring measures right heart preload, whereas PA monitoring measures left ventricular preload.

Afterload is directly affected by arterial vascular tone. Afterload is increased as SVR increases due to vasoconstriction of the aorta and arteries. The opposite effect occurs with arterial vasodilatation. SVR greater than 1,200 dynes implies vasoconstriction, whereas SVR less than 900 dynes implies vasodilation.

Contractility refers to the force generated by the contracting myocardium under any given condition. Contractility is enhanced by circulating catecholamines, sympathetic neuronal activity, and certain medications (e.g., digoxin, IV dopamine, dobutamine). Increased contractility results in increased stroke volume. Contractility is depressed by hypoxemia, acidosis, and certain medications (e.g., beta-adrenergic blocking medications).

Anatomy and Physiology of the Lymphatic System

The lymphatic system and the cardiovascular system are closely linked. The lymphatic system is formed by lymph, lymph vessels, and lymph nodes. This system collects interstitial fluid, called lymph, and returns it to the cardiovascular system, thus helping maintain preload. The lymphatic system plays an important role in the immune system as well by producing lymphocytes (a white blood cell [WBC]), which defend the body against disease.

Lymph is a fluid similar to plasma that contains plasma proteins, lymphocytes, and other factors. It is formed by the filtration of interstitial fluid into the lymph vessels. Lymph vessels are a complex network of thin-walled vessels that resemble veins with a few exceptions; lymph vessels have thinner walls, more valves, and lymph nodes. Lymph readily filters into these vessels because they are very permeable and not pressurized.

Lymph nodes, small, bean-shaped structures, filter lymph and provide an environment for lymphocytes to perform their immune function after exposure to foreign antigens, such as bacteria or viruses. Lymph nodes are located in clusters throughout the trunk and neck. Enlarged nodes may be palpated in the neck, axilla, and groin. As lymph circulates through these vessels, it passes through one or more lymph nodes before it is returned to the venous blood via the superior vena cava.

The lymphatic vessels converge into two main structures: the thoracic duct and the right lymphatic duct. The thoracic duct drains the entire body except the right sides of the head, neck, thorax, and upper extremity, which drain into the right lymphatic duct. The right lymphatic duct drains into the right subclavian vein, and the larger thoracic duct drains into the junction of the left subclavian vein and the left internal jugular vein, where it reenters the systemic venous circulation. The lymphatic vessels rely on one-way valves, arterial pulsations, and contraction of the lymphatic walls and adjacent skeletal muscle to propel lymph toward the venous drainage points in the subclavian veins. Approximately 2 to 3 L of lymph is transported daily.

Gerontologic Considerations

As people age, myocardial muscle mass shrinks (atrophy) and its walls thicken (hypertrophy). The aging process also results in decreased elasticity and widening of the aorta, calcification and stiffening of the blood vessels, thickening and increased rigidity of the cardiac valves, and increased connective tissue in the cardiac conduction system. Turbulent blood flow may produce murmurs, many benign (Gawlik et al., 2020). A decrease in the number of pacemaker cells occurs and the SA node may become thicker, predisposing older adults to arrhythmias (McGowan, 2020). The heart rate and contractile responses to sympathetic signals are reduced and lead to a diminished ability to respond to acute conditions (Marks, 2020). These changes lead to decreased cardiac output and impaired blood flow to the tissues. As a result, the aging heart has limited ability to respond to increased demands for oxygen and nutrients caused by physical or emotional stress and disease states. These age-associated changes place older adults at risk for the development of serious symptoms, including fatigue, shortness of breath, angina, palpitations, leg pain, dizziness, and syncope. Age-related changes of the cardiovascular system are summarized in Table 11-1.

Gender Considerations

The female heart is smaller and weighs less when compared to the male heart. Coronary arteries of the female heart are smaller and thus occlude from **atherosclerosis** more easily, making procedures such as cardiac catheterization and percutaneous coronary interventions (PCIs) technically more difficult with a higher incidence of postprocedural complications. In addition, the resting heart rate, stroke volume, and EF of a female heart are higher than those of a male heart. The first onset of coronary artery disease (CAD) in females is almost a decade later than in their male counterparts. These sex-based differences in disease presentation previously attributed to the premenopausal protection of circulating estrogen are currently under investigation since

TABLE **11-1** **GERONTOLOGIC CONSIDERATIONS / Age-Related Changes in the Cardiovascular System**

Cardiovascular System Component	Structural Changes	Functional Changes	History and Physical Examination Findings
Ventricular myocardium	Hypertrophy and thickening of the left ventricular (LV) wall	Stiff, noncompliant ventricles Decrease in cardiac output	Fatigue, ↓ exercise tolerance HF or arrhythmia signs/symptoms PMI palpated lateral to midclavicular line Auscultation reveals S_4
Valves	Calcification of AV valves	Turbulent blood flow across valves	Murmurs and thrills
Conduction system	Deposits of connective tissue	↓ SA node rate and ↓ speed of conduction	Bradycardia Heart block
Sympathetic nervous system	↓ Response to beta-adrenergic stimulation	↓ HR and contractility "in" response "to" exercise ↑ Time for HR to return to baseline	Fatigue and ↓ exercise tolerance
Aorta and arteries	Calcification and stiffening of the blood vessels ↓ Elasticity and widening of aorta	Left ventricular hypertrophy	Progressive ↑ systolic BP; ↑ diastolic BP Widening pulse pressure
Baroreceptor response	↓ Baroceptor sensitivity to episodes of hypertension and hypotension	Baroreceptors fail to regulate HR and vascular tone, causing a slow response to postural changes	Postural hypotension, dizziness, or syncope when sitting or standing up

AV, atrioventricular; BP, blood pressure; HF, heart failure; HR, heart rate; PMI, point of maximal impulse; SA, sinoatrial; ↓, decreased; ↑, increased.

associations cannot be inferred to be causation (Mauvais-Jarvis et al., 2020).

Male sex is considered a risk factor for CVD; however, since similar numbers of males and females die from CVD annually in the United States, nurses should consider anyone at risk for CVD regardless of sex. Because of differences in onset and hormonal factors, all patients should be monitored related to lipids, BP, weight, and insulin resistance.

Research on cardiovascular risks of transgender people is limited, but data suggest that hormone therapy for transgender women either decreases the risk for MI or is neutral. However, there is an increased incidence of venous thromboembolism (VTE) in patients taking estradiol (Seal, 2019). As with all patients with possible increased risk of CVD, nurses should counsel transgender people on lifestyle modifications related to body mass index (BMI), smoking cessation, cholesterol, or anything else relevant to the individual.

ASSESSMENT OF THE CARDIOVASCULAR SYSTEM

The frequency and extent of the nursing assessment of the cardiovascular system are based on several factors, including the severity of the patient's symptoms, the presence of risk factors, the practice setting, and the purpose of the assessment. Although the key components of the cardiovascular assessment remain the same, the assessment priorities vary according to the needs of the patient. For example, an emergency department nurse caring for a patient who is admitted with symptoms associated with acute coronary syndrome (ACS) (a term used for any condition brought on by a sudden blockage of blood flow to the heart) performs a rapid and focused assessment because treatment of ACS is time dependent since time is muscle!

Pearls for Practice: Pathophysiology

ACS evolves from inflammation, rupture, or erosion of atheromatous plaque within the coronary arteries. Platelet activation results in aggregation of the platelets and interruption of coronary blood flow (Foley & Sweet, 2020). When flow is interrupted, ischemia of the tissues ensues. Without reestablishment of blood flow, tissue death or infarction of the tissue (MI) occurs. The role of inflammation in the pathophysiology of atherosclerosis has garnered significant research attention. Current understanding is that the immune responses of monocytes, macrophages, neutrophils, T lymphocytes, and B lymphocytes are initiators and expanders of atherosclerosis. "Inflammatory biomarkers such as high-sensitivity C-reactive protein and interleukin-6 are known to predict future cardiovascular events, as well as conventional low-density or high-density lipoprotein cholesterol" (Moriya, 2019, p. 22).

Inflammation is not only a risk factor for CVD, it has a central role in the development of disease and is therefore a treatable component in patient care. Prevention and treatment of CVD includes management of both lipids and inflammation. Statins have anti-inflammatory properties, and monoclonal antibodies that decrease the inflammatory response have significantly reduced cardiovascular events and are currently indicated for cardiovascular event prevention.

Health History

Nurses practicing in settings where patients with CVD are seen must be experts at recognizing cardiac symptoms as well as expediting timely and often lifesaving care. Likewise, patients must be able to recognize when they are experiencing these symptoms and know how to manage them. All too often, patients fail to appreciate the significance of new or worsening cardiac symptoms. This problem results in prolonged delays in seeking treatment. Major barriers to seeking prompt lifesaving care include lack of knowledge about personal risk and symptoms of heart disease, lack of access to medical care, and reluctance to seek care for milder symptoms that may be dismissed or initially self-managed, among others (Stain et al., 2020). Box 11-1 discusses the impact of nursing staffing levels on survival of patients who experienced in-hospital cardiac arrest. As a patient advocate, nurses recognize that structural variables such as staffing ratios impact outcome measures.

Common Complaints

Common CVD signs and symptoms with related medical diagnoses in parentheses include the following:

- Chest pain or discomfort (ACS that includes unstable angina and acute MI, arrhythmias, valvular heart disease, thoracic aortic aneurysm, aortic dissection)
- Pain or discomfort in other areas of the upper body, including one or both arms, the back, neck, jaw, shoulder, or stomach (ACS, thoracic aneurysm)
- Dizziness, syncope, or changes in level of consciousness (ACS, cardiogenic shock, cerebrovascular disorders, arrhythmias, hypotension, postural hypotension, vasovagal episode, aortic aneurysm)
- **Intermittent claudication** or rest pain in lower extremities, especially at night (peripheral arterial disease [PAD])
- Palpitations or tachycardia (ACS, caffeine or other stimulants, electrolyte imbalances, HF, stress, valvular heart disease, ventricular aneurysm, hypovolemia)
- Peripheral edema (HF, PVD), weight gain (HF), or ascites and abdominal distension due to enlarged liver and spleen (HF)
- Shortness of breath (SOB) or dyspnea with or without chest pain (ACS, cardiogenic shock, HF, pulmonary edema, valvular heart disease, low Hct, low total protein

BOX 11-1

Nursing Research

Bridging the Gap to Evidence-Based Practice

Carthon, M. B., Brom, H., McHugh, M., et al. (2021). Better nurse staffing is associated with survival for Black patients and diminishes racial disparities in survival after in-hospital cardiac arrests. *Medical Care, 59*(2), 169–176.

Background: Racial disparities in survival among patients who had an in-hospital cardiac arrest (IHCA) have been linked to hospital-level factors.

Objectives: To determine whether nurse staffing is associated with survival disparities after IHCA.

Research Design: Cross-sectional data from (1) the American Heart Association's Get With the Guidelines-Resuscitation database; (2) the University of Pennsylvania Multi-State Nursing Care and Patient Safety Survey; and (3) The American Hospital Association annual survey. Risk-adjusted logistic regression models that took account of the hospital and patient characteristics were used to determine the association of nurse staffing and survival to discharge for Black and White patients.

Subjects: A total of 14,132 adult patients aged 18 and older between 2004 and 2010 in 75 hospitals in four states.

Results: In models that accounted for hospital and patient characteristics, the odds of survival to discharge was lower for Black patients than for White patients (odds ratio [OR] = 0.70; 95% confidence interval [CI], 0.61–0.82). A significant interaction was found between race and medical-surgical nurse staffing for survival to discharge, such that each additional patient per nurse lowered the odds of survival for Black patients (OR = 0.92; 95% CI, 0.87–0.97) more than for White patients (OR = 0.97; 95% CI, 0.93–1.00).

Conclusions: The findings suggest that disparities in IHCA survival rates between Black and White patients may be linked to the level of medical-surgical nurse staffing in the hospitals in which they receive care. The benefit of being admitted to hospitals with better staffing may be especially pronounced for Black patients.

Nursing Implications: It is important for nurses to recognize that structural variables such as staffing ratios influence patient outcome measures, and this article provides evidence of the impact of nurse staffing and patient survivability. Current research is analyzing the influence of changes in nurse staffing levels on patient outcomes. The authors hypothesize that differences between Black and White patients in the likelihood of survival to discharge after an IHCA would be at least partly attributable to Black patients being disproportionately cared for in hospitals with poorer nurse staffing. Nurses will need to stay current to the research and advocate for the profession with the awareness that the downstream impact of better staffing will be seen in improved patient outcomes.

and albumin, low EF, pericardial tamponade, valvular heart defect, pulmonary hypertension, cardiac arrhythmia, intracardiac shunting); orthopnea (breathlessness while lying flat); paroxysmal nocturnal dyspnea (PND) (waking at night with sudden onset of shortness of breath); wheezing (high-pitched, musical breath on inspiration, expiration, or both; HF; pulmonary edema; low EF)

- Cough (left-sided HF, ACS, valvular heart disease)
- Unusual fatigue characterized by feeling more tired or fatigued than usual (early warning symptom of ACS, HF, valvular heart disease)
- Cyanosis (poor oxygenation related to arterial desaturation or presence of abnormal hemoglobin).

Chest Pain

Chest pain and chest discomfort are common symptoms caused by a number of cardiac and noncardiac problems. Table 11-2 identifies the characteristics of common causes of chest pain. To differentiate among these causes of pain, the nurse asks the patient to identify the quantity (0 = no pain to 10 = worst pain), location, and quality of pain. It is important to identify the events that precipitated symptom onset, the duration of the symptom, measures that aggravate or relieve the symptom, and associated signs and symptoms, such as diaphoresis or nausea. The nurse should keep the following points in mind when assessing patients with chest pain or discomfort:

- The severity and duration of chest pain or discomfort do not predict the seriousness of its cause. For example, a patient experiencing esophageal spasm may rate chest pain as a "10/10," whereas a patient experiencing an acute MI may report only mild to moderate chest pressure.
- More than one cardiac condition may occur simultaneously. During an acute MI, patients may report chest pain from myocardial **ischemia** (inadequate oxygen supply to the tissues), shortness of breath from HF, and palpitations from arrhythmias. Both HF and arrhythmias are complications of an acute MI.

Symptoms of Acute Coronary Syndrome

Nurses must take complaints of patients with cardiac symptoms seriously until the cause is determined. Because CAD is so prevalent, all patients reporting new or worsening cardiac symptoms, particularly those at risk for CAD or who have a history of CAD, should be evaluated initially for ACS. There are several distinct characteristics of ACS symptoms that need to be kept in mind during assessment:

- Many patients with ACS experience prodromal symptoms prior to developing the acute event. Prodromal symptoms include unusual fatigue, shortness of breath, orthopnea, sleep disturbances, pain or discomfort in the chest, heart racing, diaphoresis, vomiting, numbness or burning, and aching or discomfort in the arms (Heidarzadeh et al.,

TABLE 11-2 Characteristics of Cardiac and Noncardiac Causes of Chest Pain

Location	Character	Duration	Precipitating Events and Aggravating Factors	Alleviating Factors
Angina pectoris Acute coronary syndrome (ACS) (ST-elevation myocardial infarction [STEMI] and non–ST-elevation myocardial infarction [NSTEMI] or unstable angina) 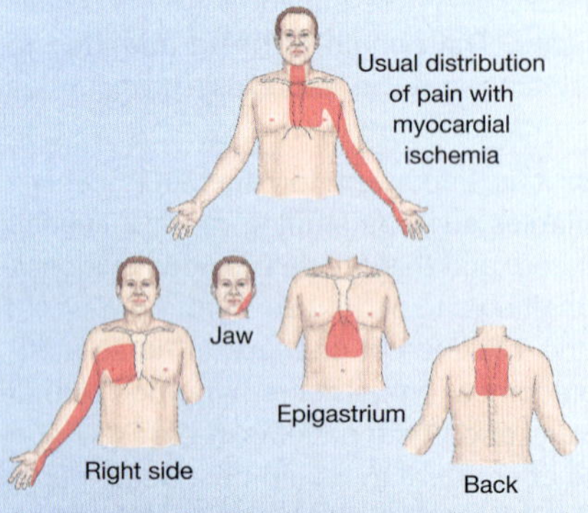 Less common sites of pain with myocardial ischemia	Angina: Uncomfortable pressure, squeezing, or fullness in substernal chest area Can radiate across chest to the medial aspect of one or both arms and hands, jaw, shoulders, upper back, or epigastrium Radiation to arms and hands, described as numbness, tingling, or aching ACS: Same as angina pectoris Pain or discomfort ranges from mild to severe Associated with shortness of breath, diaphoresis, palpitations, unusual fatigue, and nausea or vomiting	Angina: 5–15 minutes ACS: 15 min or more	Angina: Physical exertion, emotional upset, eating large meal, or exposure to extremes in temperature ACS: Emotional upset or unusual physical exertion occurring within 24 hours of symptom onset Can occur at rest or while asleep	Angina: Rest, nitroglycerin, oxygen ACS: Morphine, reperfusion of coronary artery with thrombolytic agent or percutaneous coronary intervention
Pericarditis 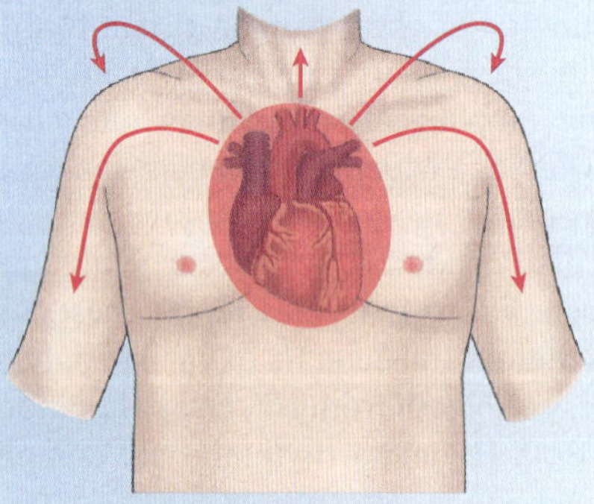	Sharp, severe substernal or epigastric pain Can radiate to neck, arms, and back Associated symptoms include fever, malaise, dyspnea, cough, nausea, dizziness, and palpitations	Intermittent	Sudden onset Pain increases with inspiration, swallowing, coughing, and rotation of trunk	Sitting upright and leaning forward, analgesia, anti-inflammatory medications
Pulmonary disorders (pneumonia, pulmonary embolism) 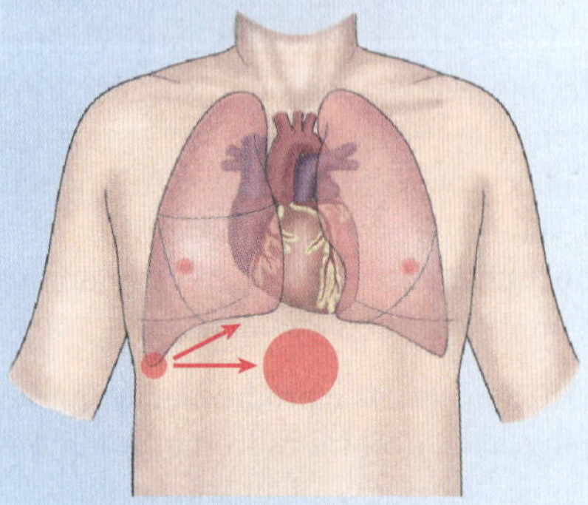	Sharp, severe substernal or epigastric pain arising from inferior portion of pleura (referred to as pleuritic pain). Patient may be able to localize the pain.	30 minutes or more	Follows an infectious or noninfectious process (MI, cardiac surgery, cancer, immune disorders, uremia) Pleuritic pain increases with inspiration, coughing, movement, and supine positioning Occurs in conjunction with community-acquired or nosocomial lung infections (pneumonia) or deep vein thrombosis (pulmonary embolism)	Treatment of underlying cause

Location	Character	Duration	Precipitating Events and Aggravating Factors	Alleviating Factors
Esophageal disorders (hiatal hernia, reflux esophagitis or spasm) 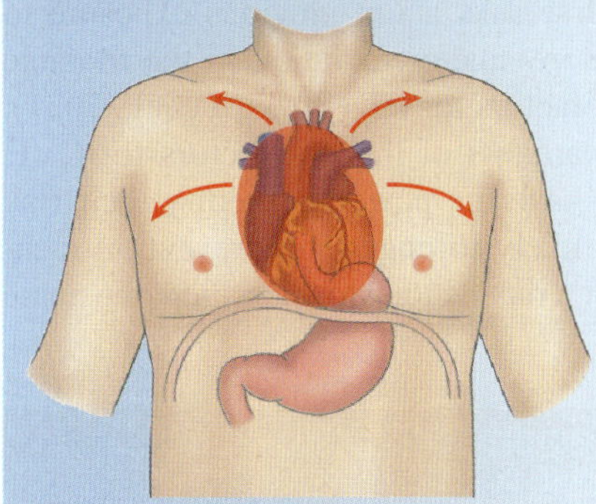	Substernal pain described as sharp, burning, or heavy Often mimics cardiac pain Can radiate to neck, arm, or shoulders	5–60 minutes	Recumbency, cold liquids, exercise	Food or antacid
Anxiety and panic disorders 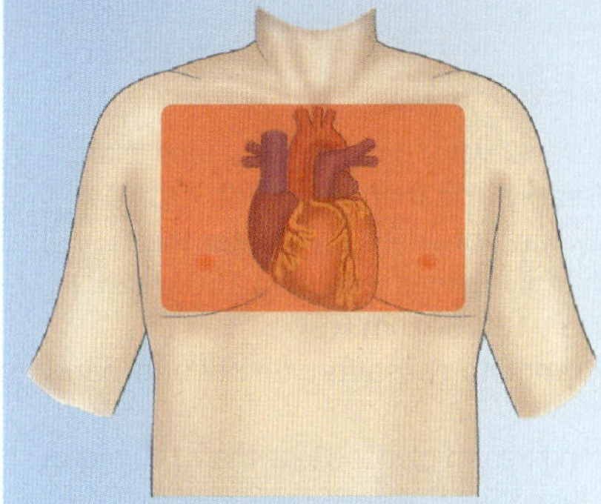	Pain described as stabbing to dull ache Associated with diaphoresis, palpitations, shortness of breath, tingling of hands or mouth, feeling of unreality, or fear of losing control	Peaks in 10 minutes	Can occur at any time, including during sleep Can be associated with a specific trigger	Removal of stimulus, relaxation, medications to treat anxiety or underlying disorder
Musculoskeletal disorders (costochondritis) 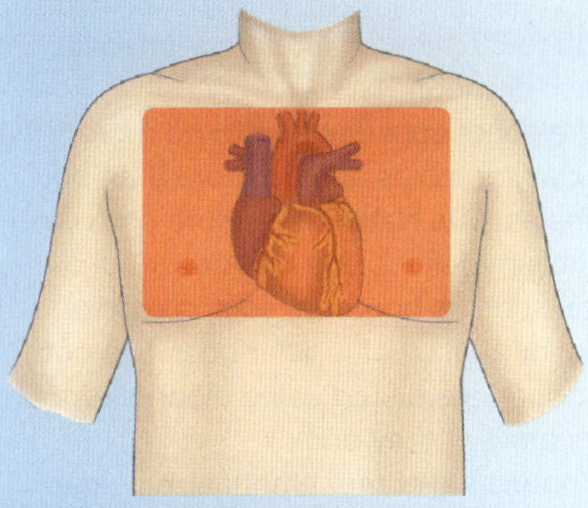	Sharp or stabbing pain localized in anterior chest Most often unilateral Can radiate across chest to epigastrium or back	Hours to days	Most often follows respiratory tract infection with significant coughing, vigorous exercise, or posttrauma Some cases are idiopathic Exacerbated by deep inspiration, coughing, sneezing, and movement of upper torso or arms	Rest, ice, or heat Analgesic or anti-inflammatory medications
Dissecting aorta	Severe, persistent tearing pain in anterior chest/back Radiates to shoulders, epigastrium or abdomen Associated with diaphoresis and tachycardia	Sudden onset	Hypertension, blunt chest trauma, or cocaine use	Medical or surgical interventions

2021). In a recent study, female patients were more likely than male patients to report back pain, pain or discomfort between or under the shoulder blade, sleep disturbances, anxiousness, or heart racing. Generalized chest pain and loss of appetite were more frequently reported by male patients than female patients (Shi et al., 2020). Because these symptoms are less severe than what is experienced during ACS, patients often attribute them to a benign problem, such as stress, and fail to seek medical care. Only 41% of patients attributed their prodromal symptoms to the heart (Shi et al., 2020). Nurses should include a question regarding presence of prodromal symptoms when assessing patients with cardiac symptoms.

- In general, patients with ACS experience signs and symptoms of myocardial ischemia either at rest or with minimal exertion. The symptoms may be similar to those of chronic angina and include substernal chest pain or discomfort that may radiate to the jaw, one or both arms, the back, neck, shoulder, or stomach. The pain and discomfort associated with an ACS event is often diffuse rather than localized. It is often associated with diaphoresis (Ferri, 2022). However, dyspnea, nausea, diaphoresis, hiccups (if the phrenic nerve is stimulated), or syncope may be the only symptoms of ACS, so nurses must always have a high degree of suspicion for any patient who manifests these symptoms (Bashore et al., 2022; Ferri, 2022; Foley & Sweet, 2020). Approximately one third of patients diagnosed with MI have no chest pain (Bashore et al., 2022; Ferri, 2022). Risk factors for silent ACS include female sex, those with a history of diabetes, patients that are in surgery (perioperative MI) particularly in the older population, and those who have obstructive sleep apnea (OSA) (Gul & Makaryus, 2022; Bashore et al., 2022). Also, patients who have had heart transplants do not experience chest pain because pain receptors are denervated during the transplant procedure (Foley & Sweet, 2020). In addition, 10% of patients with ACS present in heart failure, and these patients have a higher mortality rate (Bashore et al., 2022).
- Neuropathies in older adult patients and those with diabetes may prevent these patients from experiencing pain or discomfort associated with myocardial ischemia. Instead, they may report unusual fatigue or shortness of breath (McGarry & Shenvi, 2021).
- A 12-lead electrocardiogram (ECG) and serum laboratory analysis of cardiac biomarkers are necessary to determine if the patient with ACS symptoms is experiencing unstable angina or acute MI.

History

Epidemiologic studies show that certain conditions or behaviors (i.e., risk factors) are associated with a greater incidence of CAD, cerebrovascular disease, and PAD. The nurse might ask:

- How is your health? Have you noticed any changes from last year? From 5 years ago?
- Do you have a cardiologist or primary health care provider? How often do you go for checkups?
- What are your risk factors for heart disease? What do you do to reduce these risk factors? Box 11-2 lists risk factors for CVD and treatment goals.

In addition, the nurse asks about previous exposure to cardiotoxic chemotherapy and/or radiation to the thoracic region, which are risk factors for HF (Bozkurt et al., 2021). Patients who have awareness of the risk factors for CVD and believe that they have the power to modify their risk factors may be more likely to engage in prevention measures. Once the patient's risk factors are identified, the nurse

BOX 11-2 **Risk Factors for Cardiovascular Diseases**

Nonmodifiable Risk Factors

- Older age
- Male sex (earlier than in females)
- Heredity

Modifiable Risk Factors and Treatment Goals[a]

- Hyperlipidemia (low-density lipoprotein [LDL] less than 100 mg/dL and preferably less than 70 mg/dL if CAD present; high-density lipoprotein [HDL] greater than 60 mg/dL is optimal; triglycerides less than 150 mg/dL)
- Hypertension (less than 130/80 mm Hg)[b]
- Cigarette smoking (complete cessation, no second-hand tobacco exposure)[b]
- Diabetes mellitus (fasting serum glucose less than 110 mg/dL and hemoglobin A_{1c} less than 7%)[b]
- Obesity and overweight (BMI 18.5 to 24.9 kg/m^2; waist circumference: male 40 inches or less, female 35 inches or less)
- Physical inactivity (30 to 60 minutes moderate-intensity aerobic activity 5 days or more)
- Alcohol intake (Limit alcohol consumption to no more than two drinks per day for males and no more than one drink per day for females. The National Institute on Alcohol Abuse and Alcoholism defines one drink as 1.5 fl oz of 80-proof spirits, such as bourbon, scotch, vodka, or gin; 5 fl oz of wine; or 12 fl oz of regular beer. It is not recommended that nondrinkers start using alcohol or that drinkers increase the amount they drink.)
- Diet and nutrition (Choose a diet that emphasizes vegetables, fruits, and whole grains. A heart-healthy diet also includes low-fat dairy products, poultry, fish, legumes, nuts, and nontropical vegetable oils. Limit the intake of sweets, sugar-sweetened beverages, and red meats.)
- Stress (Recommend stress reduction.)
- The clustering of risk factors can lead to synergistic increases in the risk for events.

[a]American Heart Association-recommended goals are given in parentheses.

[b]Modifiable risk factors of hypertension, diabetes, and cigarette smoking have recently declined, although hyperlipidemia has shown no significant change, and obesity has steadily increased (Gola, 2022).

determines if patients have a plan for making necessary lifestyle changes and if assistance is needed to support these changes.

Pearls for Practice: Pathophysiology

Metabolic syndrome exists if the patient has any three of the following findings:

- *Increased waist circumference by ethnically appropriate cut points*
- *Elevated triglycerides 150 mg/dL or greater (nonfasting)*
- *Reduced HDL cholesterol less than 40 mg/dL in males or less than 50 mg/dL in females*
- *Elevated fasting glucose of 100 mg/dL or greater*
- *Blood pressure values of systolic 130 mm Hg or higher and/or diastolic 85 mm Hg or higher*

This syndrome increases the risk of both CVD and diabetes (Swarup et al., 2021).

Family History

The nurse inquires about a history of cardiac disease in the patient's family, including the following:

- A history of sudden death (younger than age 60) in family members with or without symptoms or known CAD (Bickley et al., 2021)
- A history of CAD, coronary artery bypass graft (CABG) surgery, PCI, atrial or ventricular arrhythmias, and/or conduction system disease (Bozkurt et al., 2021)
- A family member with a biochemical or neuromuscular condition (e.g., hemochromatosis [excessive iron retention in the body] or muscular dystrophy)
- DNA mutation or other genetic testing performed on any family member, such as genetic variant for cardiomyopathy or hereditary amyloidosis, often affecting the liver, nerves, heart, and kidney (Bozkurt et al., 2021)
- Additional genetic abnormalities associated with cardiovascular disorders, including familial hypercholesterolemia, hypertrophic cardiomyopathy, long QT syndrome, and elevated homocysteine levels (discussed later in this chapter)
- Any family history of hypertension, stroke, diabetes, and obesity (Bickley et al., 2021)

The family history can include important risk factors independent of other measurable risk factors. BP and lipid levels are influenced by genetics. However, research reveals the heritability of ideal cardiovascular health is less than 20%, suggesting strong environmental and behavioral influences on the development of CVD (Lloyd-Jones, 2020). In fact, the AHA and the American College of Cardiology (ACC) recognize that social determinants of health (SDOHs) are strong contributors to the risk for CVD and should be evaluated for each individual patient in order to target preventative strategies (Arnett et al., 2019; Mannoh et al., 2021). For example, the nurse considers the impact of environment such as neighborhood safety, lack of safe places to exercise outdoors, lack of healthy food availability, and transportation challenges to clinic visits as risk factors for disease.

Lifting the Lens

A recent study evaluated the SDOHs including education (less than high school); annual household income (less than $35,000); race; living in a zip code with high poverty rates (more than 25% of residents living below the federal poverty line); residence in states with the most limited public health infrastructure; not seeing close friends or family in the past month; and lack of health insurance. Patients with three or more of these SDOHs were 67% more likely to have a fatal coronary heart disease event (Safford et al., 2021). Thus, nurses know our lens must focus not just on the patient but also on the environment where the patient lives and the health care institutions where we work.

Social History

Medications

Nurses collaborate with other health care providers to obtain a complete list of the patient's medications, including dose and frequency. Vitamins, herbal supplements, and over-the-counter medications are included on this list. Over-the-counter and prescription medications that have been reported to result in cardiotoxicity with excessive and prolonged use or misuse include amphetamine/dextroamphetamine, anabolic steroids, decongestants, ephedrine, ephedra (herb banned in the United States), and nonsteroidal anti-inflammatory drugs (NSAIDs) (Bozkurt et al., 2021). During this aspect of the health assessment, the nurse asks questions to determine if patients are taking their medications safely and effectively. A careful medication history often uncovers common medication errors and causes for nonadherence to the medication regimen. The nurse considers the following areas:

- Is the patient independent in taking medications?
- Are the medications taken as prescribed?
- Does the patient know what side effects to report to the prescriber if they experience them?
- Does the patient understand why the medication regimen is important?
- Are doses ever forgotten or skipped, or does the patient ever decide to stop taking a medication without consulting a provider?

Sample questions may include the following:

- "What medications do you currently take (name, dose, times per day, years on the medication)?"
- "What other inhalers, drops, creams, or injections do you take regularly?"
- "What medications do you buy in the drug store, pharmacy, or online?"
- "What herbal or vitamin products do you take regularly?"

- "Do you ever forget to take a medication? If so, what do you do?"
- "Are there any of your medications that you think have negative effects for you?"
- "Do any of the medications you take get in the way of what is important to you?"

Nutrition and Metabolism

Dietary modifications, exercise, weight loss, and careful monitoring are important strategies for managing cardiovascular risk factors such as hyperlipidemia, hypertension, and diabetes mellitus. Diets that are restricted in sodium, fat, cholesterol, and/or calories are commonly prescribed. The nurse obtains the following information:

- How often the patient self-monitors BP, blood glucose, and weight as appropriate to their medical diagnoses
- The patient's knowledge regarding target goals for each of the risk factors and any problems achieving or maintaining these goals
- What the patient normally eats and drinks in a typical day and any food preferences (including cultural or ethnic preferences)
- Eating habits (canned or commercially prepared foods vs. fresh foods; restaurant cooking vs. home cooking; assessing for high-sodium foods, dietary intake of fats)
- Who shops for groceries and prepares meals
- Access to fresh fruits and vegetables
- Nearby parks, recreational facilities, and transportation resources (Mannoh et al., 2021)
- Access to a scale for daily weighing
- Sodium intake via the salt shaker or salt substitutes at the table or in cooking

Pearls for Practice

The nurse instructs the patient with a cardiac history to call their provider if they experience weight gain of 3 lb (1.4 kg) in 2 days or 5 lb (1.4 to 2.3 kg) in a week since this is an indication that a change in medical management is needed. A 3-lb gain represents approximately 1,500 mL of extra fluid (500 mL = 1 lb). The nurse asks about the presence of peripheral edema and SOB, which suggests HF.

Elimination

Typical bowel and bladder habits need to be identified. Nocturia (awakening at night to urinate) is common in patients with HF. Fluid collected in the dependent tissues (extremities) during the day redistributes into the circulatory system once the patient is recumbent at night. The increased circulatory volume is excreted by the kidneys (increased urine production).

Pearls for Practice

When straining during defecation, the patient bears down (the Valsalva maneuver), which momentarily increases pressure on the baroreceptors. This triggers a vagal response, causing the heart rate to slow, which may lead to syncope (fainting) in some patients. Thus, patients with cardiac disease are placed on stool softeners to prevent the Valsalva sequela of reduced preload to the heart, syncope, bradycardia, and/or arrhythmias. Straining during urination can produce the same response.

Because many cardiac medications can cause gastrointestinal side effects or bleeding, the nurse asks about bloating, diarrhea, constipation, stomach upset, heartburn, loss of appetite, nausea, and vomiting. Patients taking platelet-inhibiting medications such as aspirin, platelet aggregation inhibitors, IV anticoagulants, or oral anticoagulants are screened for bloody urine (hematuria) or stools (red, black, or tarry), epistaxis (nosebleed), or unusual bruising.

Activity and Exercise

Changes in a patient's activity tolerance may be gradual and go unnoticed. The nurse determines if there are recent changes by comparing the patient's current activity level with that performed in the past 6 to 12 months. New symptoms or a change in the usual symptoms during activity is a significant finding. Activity-induced angina or SOB may indicate CAD, which requires medical attention. Arterial insufficiency is suspected if the patient experiences intermittent claudication, described as a muscular, cramping pain in the lower extremities that occurs with activity and is relieved by rest. Angina and intermittent claudication occur when there is tissue ischemia or inadequate arterial blood supply in the setting of increased demand (e.g., exercise, stress, or anemia). As the tissues are forced to function without adequate nutrients and oxygen, muscle metabolites and lactic acid are produced. Pain is experienced as the metabolites aggravate the nerve endings of the surrounding tissue. **Rest pain** is a persistent pain in the anterior portion of the foot at rest that can worsen at night and indicates significant arterial insufficiency and a critical state of ischemia.

Fatigue, which is the subjective experience of persistent and extreme tiredness and mental and physical exhaustion, is associated with a CAD after ACS, low left ventricular EF (less than 50%), and certain medications (e.g., beta-adrenergic blocking agents), and it can result in activity intolerance. Patients with fatigue may benefit from having their medications adjusted and learning energy-conservation techniques. Additional areas to explore include the presence of architectural barriers in the home (stairs, multilevel home), the patient's involvement in cardiac rehabilitation, and the patient's typical exercise pattern, including intensity, frequency, and duration.

Sleep and Rest

Clues to worsening cardiac disease, especially HF, can be revealed by sleep-related events. Determining where the patient sleeps or rests and any recent changes in sleep habits is important. Worsening HF is characterized by pulmonary congestion resulting in dyspnea at rest or when lying down. *Orthopnea* is the term used to indicate dyspnea that occurs in the recumbent position. The nurse asks the patient if they have an inability to sleep in a bed and instead prefer a chair. The nurse may also ask about the number of pillows required to sleep at night to avoid SOB. The nurse would record this, for example, as "2 pillow orthopnea." Orthopnea is a specific symptom of HF that correlates with the severity of pulmonary congestion (Rogers & O'Connor, 2020). Bendopnea, or SOB on bending down, has been reported in 28% of patients with HF (Greenberg et al., 2020). Patients with worsening HF may report that they sleep upright in a chair instead of in bed; increase the number of pillows used; awaken from sleep with sudden onset of dyspnea called PND, often associated with coughing, wheezing, and a sense of impending doom; or awaken with angina (nocturnal angina). PND occurs at night usually within 1 hour after going to bed and is relieved after sitting up or standing for 15 to 30 minutes; it may be associated with coughing (Rogers & O'Connor, 2020). It tends to recur nightly at a relatively constant time after the patient lies down (Greenberg et al., 2020). Multiple theories of the cause of PND include the reabsorption of fluid from dependent areas of the body (arms and legs) back into the circulatory system within hours of lying in bed. This sudden fluid shift increases preload and places too great a demand on the heart of patients with HF, causing sudden pulmonary congestion, or the increased venous return (preload) puts pressure on the bronchial arteries, resulting in a mechanical obstruction to the airways, causing sudden SOB. Finally, another proposed etiology is associated with the natural decrease in the adrenal activity of the heart at hour of sleep (HS), so there is decreased inotropic (contraction) and decreased chronotropic (heart rate), resulting in the sudden SOB.

Mounting evidence points to the cardiac consequences associated with sleep-disordered breathing (SDB). SDB can be categorized as OSA, with which there is cessation of airflow due to mechanical obstruction causing apnea and hypopnea (shallow respirations), or as central sleep apnea (CSA), with which there is an absence of respiratory effort and airflow during sleep (Dubrock et al., 2020). OSA is highly prevalent and associated with obesity, while CSA is most often associated with HF. These abnormal sleep events cause frequent recurring hypoxemia and hypercapnia (excessive carbon dioxide in the bloodstream), sympathetic nervous system activation with subsequent vasoconstriction, and increased intrathoracic pressure that puts mechanical stress on the heart and large artery walls.

Untreated SDB has been linked to CAD, hypertension, HF, and arrhythmias. SDB is treated with the use of continuous positive airway pressure (CPAP) and mandibular advancement devices (MADs). These devices maintain an open airway during sleep, preventing hypoxemia and resulting abnormal elevations in BP. Many patients are unaware they have SDB. The cardinal signs of SBD are loud, disruptive snoring and apnea lasting 10 seconds or more. Obesity and large neck circumference are two important risk factors for SDB. For example, a neck circumference greater than 43 cm (17 in) in males and greater than 37 cm (15 in) in females is associated with OSA and a 10% increase in weight predicts a sixfold increase in the likelihood of developing clinically significant OSA (Paul & Hayes, 2022). During the health history, the nurse assesses for SDB by asking high-risk patients if they snore loudly, have frequent bouts of awakening from sleep, waking with a headache, or experience severe daytime sleepiness (hypersomnolence). For patients with a diagnosis of SDB, the nurse determines if the patient has been prescribed CPAP or an MAD and the frequency of its use. Patients who are being admitted to the hospital or going for an ambulatory surgical procedure should be instructed to bring their sleep aid devices with them.

Cognition and Perception

Evaluating cognitive ability helps determine whether the patient has the capacity to manage safe and effective self-care independently. Is the patient's short-term memory intact? Is there any history of dementia? Is there evidence of depression or anxiety? Can the patient read? Can the patient read English? What is the patient's reading level? What is the patient's preferred learning style? What information does the patient perceive as important? Providing the patient with written information can be a valuable part of patient education but only if the patient can read and comprehend the information.

Related assessments include possible hearing or visual impairments. If vision is impaired, patients with HF may not be able to weigh themselves independently or keep records of weight, BP, pulse, or other data requested by the health care team.

Self-Perception and Self-Concept

Self-perception and self-concept are related to the cognitive and emotional processes that people use to formulate their beliefs and feelings about themselves. It is important for the nurse to understand patients' beliefs and feelings about their health, as these concepts are key determinants of patients' adherence to new medical regimens and lifestyle changes (e.g., smoking cessation, weight reduction, exercise), which are necessary for effective self-management after an acute cardiac event. Patients who have misperceptions about the health consequences of their cardiac illness are at risk for nonadherence to their treatment plans. Responses of patients to the following questions will guide the nurse in planning interventions to ensure that patients are prepared to manage their illness and that adequate services are in place to support the patient's recovery and self-management needs.

- What is your cardiac problem, and what do you think has contributed to this problem?

- What consequences do you think this illness will have on your current lifestyle (leisure and physical activities, work, role in the family, social relationships)?
- How much of an influence do you think you have on controlling this illness?

Sexuality and Reproduction

A common problem for patients with cardiac diseases, including hypertension, CAD, and HF, is a decrease in frequency of and satisfaction with sexual activity. These changes are associated with inadequate information, depression, and fear of having a cardiac event (e.g., acute MI, sudden death) or development of bothersome symptoms (e.g., chest discomfort, SOB, palpitations). In male patients, impotence may develop as a side effect of cardiac medications (e.g., beta-blockers); some will stop taking their medication as a result. Other medications may be substituted, so patients should be encouraged to discuss these problems with their health care providers.

Patients and their partners may not have adequate information about the physical demands related to sexual activity and ways in which these demands can be modified. The physiologic demands are greatest during orgasm, reaching three to five metabolic equivalents (METs) between partners with a long-standing relationship; alternately, sex outside of a committed relationship can lead to higher energy demands (Davis, 2019). Patients should be reassured that in general, sexual activity typically can be resumed, and the timing depends on the type of heart procedure or cardiac event. Patients recovering from MI may be able to have sex after 2 weeks, but those recovering from cardiac surgery or complicated cardiac events may have to wait up to 8 weeks (NICE, 2020; Elsevier Patient Education, 2021). Sharing this information may make the patient and their partner more comfortable about resuming sexual activity. Patients with implantable cardioverter defibrillators (ICDs) often have fears about the perceived strain of sexual activity on the heart and the risk of an ICD shock. However, the absolute risk associated with sexual activity is considered to be extremely low, since for most patients, sex represents only moderate stress on the heart (Pedretti et al., 2021). In addition, erectile dysfunction medications should be avoided for patients using nitrates for angina due to CAD (Davis, 2019).

A reproductive history is necessary for those of childbearing age, particularly those with seriously compromised cardiac function. Some patients may be advised by their health care providers not to become pregnant. The reproductive history includes information about previous pregnancies, plans for future pregnancies, oral contraceptive use (especially in those older than 35 years of age who smoke), menopausal status, and use of hormone therapy.

Coping and Stress Tolerance

Anxiety, depression, social isolation, hostility, acute and chronic stress, and low social support are known to influence both the development of and recovery from CAD and HF (Albus et al., 2019). High levels of anxiety are associated with an increased incidence of CAD and in-hospital complications after MI. In addition, acute, high-stress situations can lead to plaque ruptures via the acute response of stress hormones, and the immune and coagulation systems and can trigger an acute MI (Albus et al., 2019). For example, the risk of a MI in a bereaved person who experienced the stress of losing a loved one is 21 times higher in the first 24 hours of the stressor (Albus et al., 2019, pp. 1178–1179). In contrast, social support can provide protective factors and reduce the risk of illness and mortality from CVD.

Patients with a diagnosis of acute MI and depression have an increased risk of rehospitalization and death, more frequent angina, more physical limitations, and poorer quality of life compared to patients without depression. People experiencing depression are less motivated to adhere to the recommended lifestyle changes and medical regimens necessary to prevent future cardiac events. In fact, depression, anxiety, and stress were the main predictors of level of adherence to medications in a recent study of patients with CVD (Malak et al., 2021). In addition, recent research reveals that patients with CVD and major depressive disorder are more likely to experience a cardiovascular complication requiring intervention than those without depression (Subramaniapillai et al., 2021). Nurses should assess patients with CVD for depression by asking them if they are feeling sad, if they have lost interest in things they usually enjoy, or if they have thoughts about death or suicide. Other indications of depression include feelings of worthlessness or guilt, problems falling asleep or staying asleep, having difficulty concentrating, restlessness, and recent changes in appetite or weight. Antidepressant use is associated with reduced in-hospital mortality (Subramaniapillai et al., 2021).

Stress initiates a variety of physiologic responses, including increased levels of catecholamines and cortisol, and it has been strongly linked to cardiovascular events. The stability, affordability, accessibility, quality, and safety of the patient's living environment are important factors that can increase or decrease stress and influence CVD, so the nurse must assess the housing and living situation (Sims et al., 2020). In summary, patients need to be assessed for sources of stress, previously used coping styles and effectiveness, perception of their current mood and coping ability, and SDOH. Consultation with a psychiatric advanced practice nurse, psychologist, psychiatrist, and/or social worker or community support group is indicated for anxious or depressed patients or those patients with limited social supports. It is also helpful for those having difficulty coping with their cardiac illness.

Roles and Relationships

Patients with CVD are being managed with complex medical regimens and sophisticated technology, such as ICDs and left ventricular assist devices. Hospital stays for cardiac disorders have shortened, and many invasive diagnostic cardiac procedures, such as cardiac catheterization, are being performed in the ambulatory setting. Therefore, social support is often necessary to facilitate patient's self-management of cardiac illnesses. Patients with lower levels of social support have been shown to have an increased risk for cardiac-related mortality compared with others who have higher levels of support. In fact, the effect of loneliness on mortality is comparable to that of smoking as heavy as 15 cigarettes per day (Albus et al., 2019).

To assess a patient's role in the family and their relationships, both components of social support, the nurse asks the patient: With whom do you live? Who is your primary caregiver at home? Who helps you manage your health? The nurse also assesses for any significant effects that the cardiac illness has had on the patient's role in the family. Does the family have adequate finances and health insurance? The answers to these questions help the nurse determine if consultation with social services or others is necessary to tailor the plan of care to meet the patient's self-care needs.

Physical Assessment

During the physical assessment, the nurse is evaluating the cardiovascular system for any deviations from normal regarding the following (examples of abnormalities are in parentheses):

- The heart as a pump (reduced pulse pressure, gallop sounds, murmurs, displaced PMI)
- Atrial and ventricular filling volumes and pressures (elevated jugular venous distension [JVD], peripheral edema, ascites, crackles, postural changes in BP)
- Cardiac output (reduced pulse pressure, hypotension, tachycardia, reduced urine output, or decreased level of consciousness)
- Compensatory mechanisms (peripheral vasoconstriction, tachycardia)
- Peripheral vascular system (reduced or absent peripheral pulses; pallor or rubor; cool temperature; presence of ulcers; edema [pitting or nonpitting], trophic changes of hair loss, brittle nails, and muscle atrophy; claudication; abnormal ankle–brachial index [ABI]; sensory and motor deficits; presence of a limb bruit)

Assessment of General Appearance and Cognition

The nurse notes signs of distress, which may include pain or discomfort, SOB, or anxiety. The patient's height and weight are measured to calculate BMI (weight in kilograms/square of the height in meters), as well as the waist circumference. These measures are used to determine if obesity (BMI greater than 30 kg/m^2) and abdominal fat (in males, a waist circumference greater than 40 in; in females, a waist circumference greater than 35 in) are placing the patient at risk for CAD.

To assess cognition, the nurse evaluates the patient's level of consciousness (alert, lethargic, stuporous, comatose) and mental status (oriented to person, place, time; coherence). Changes in level of consciousness and mental status may be attributed to inadequate perfusion of the brain from a compromised cardiac output or thromboembolic event (stroke).

Inspection and Palpation of the Skin

The signs and symptoms of an acute obstruction of arterial blood flow in the extremities are referred to as the six *P*s, which are *p*ain (out of proportion to examination); *p*allor; diminished or absent *p*ulses; *p*aresthesia; *p*oikilothermia (coldness); and *p*aralysis. Additional changes resulting from a chronically reduced supply of oxygen and nutrients to the skin include hair loss, brittle nails, dry or scaling skin, atrophy, skin color changes, and ulcerations. Table 11-3 summarizes common skin findings in patients with CVD.

The nurse assesses capillary refill time, which indicates the adequacy of arterial perfusion to the extremities. To perform this test, the nurse compresses the nail bed for 5 seconds to occlude perfusion (the nail bed blanches). Then, the nurse releases pressure and determines the time it takes to restore perfusion. Normally, reperfusion occurs within 2 seconds as evidenced by the return of color to the nail bed. Prolonged capillary refill time indicates compromised arterial perfusion, a problem associated with PAD, cardiogenic shock, and HF. The nurse records the patient's bilateral capillary refill in seconds. It is important to recognize that three signs of reduced peripheral perfusion are cool limbs, capillary refill time of more than 5 seconds, and mottling of the skin; these signs increase the probability of poor perfusion and adverse outcome (McGee, 2022).

Peripheral edema, or fluid accumulation in dependent areas of the body (feet, legs, and sacrum in the bedridden patient), is a common finding in patients with CVD. Edema does not become clinically apparent until the interstitial volume has increased by 2.5 to 3 L (Goyal et al., 2021). The nurse assesses the patient for pitting edema (a depression over an area of pressure) by using the thumb to place firm pressure over the dorsum of each foot, behind each medial malleolus, and over the shins or sacral area for at least 2 seconds. The depression created by this pressure is graded as absent or present on a scale from slight (1+) to very marked (4+). Scales may measure the degree of pitting edema based on a clinician's judgment of the depth of edema (in mm or in) or of the time the indentation remains after release of pressure (termed "pit to recovery time"). In general, in adults, about 4.5 kg (10 lb) of fluid accumulates before pitting edema is detectable (Suneja et al., 2020). It is important that clinicians use a consistent scale in order to ensure reliable clinical measurements and management. Peripheral edema is observed in patients with HF and peripheral vascular diseases, such as deep vein thrombosis or chronic venous insufficiency. The nurse notes whether the edema is generalized (related to systemic causes such as HF, kidney disease, cirrhosis, hypoalbuminemia, sepsis) or localized (related to one limb and may be associated with deep vein thrombosis, lymphatic obstruction, or an IV infiltration).

TABLE **11-3 Common Skin Findings Associated With Cardiovascular Diseases**

Findings	Associated Causes and Conditions
Clubbing of the fingers or toes (thickening of the skin under the fingers or toes)	Chronic hemoglobin desaturation most often due to congenital heart disease, advanced pulmonary diseases and lung cancer; also associated with malignancies and inflammatory bowel disease
Cool/cold skin and diaphoresis	Low cardiac output (e.g., cardiogenic shock, AMI) causing sympathetic nervous system stimulation with resultant vasoconstriction
Cold, pain, pallor of the fingertips or toes	Intermittent arteriolar vasoconstriction (Raynaud disease). Skin may change in color from white, to blue and red accompanied by numbness, tingling, and burning pain.
Cyanosis, central (a bluish tinge observed in the lips, tongue, and buccal mucosa)	Serious cardiac disorders (pulmonary edema, cardiogenic shock, congenital heart disease) as venous blood passes through the pulmonary circulation without being oxygenated
Cyanosis, peripheral (a bluish tinge, most often of the nails and extremities)	Peripheral vasoconstriction, allowing more time for the hemoglobin molecules to become desaturated. It can be caused by exposure to cold environment, anxiety, or ↓ cardiac output.
Ecchymosis or bruising (a purplish-blue color fading to green, yellow, or brown)	Blood leaking outside of the blood vessels Excessive bruising is a risk for patients on anticoagulants or platelet-inhibiting medications; coagulopathies, trauma
Edema, lower extremities (collection of fluid in the interstitial spaces of the tissues)	HF and vascular problems (PAD, chronic venous insufficiency, DVT, thrombophlebitis)
Hematoma (localized collection of clotted blood in the tissue)	Bleeding after catheter removal/tissue injury in patients on anticoagulant/antithrombotic agents.
Pallor (↓ skin color in fingernails, lips, oral mucosa and lower extremities)	Anemia or ↓ arterial perfusion. Suspect PAD if feet develop pallor after elevating legs 60 degrees from a supine position. Normally there is a return of color to the skin in about 10 seconds or less, and veins of the feet fill in 15 seconds. There will be a delay in patients with PAD.
Rubor (a reddish-blue discoloration of the legs, seen within 20 seconds to 2 minutes after placing the patient in a dependent position)	Filling of dilated capillaries with deoxygenated blood, indicative of PAD
Ulcers, feet and ankles (superficial, irregular ulcers at medial malleolus; red to yellow granulation tissue) Painful, deep, round ulcers on feet or from exposure to pressure; pale to black wound base	Rupture of small skin capillaries from chronic venous insufficiency Prolonged ischemia to tissues due to PAD; can lead to gangrene
Thinning of skin around a pacemaker or an implantable cardioverter defibrillator	Erosion of the device through the skin
Xanthelasma (yellowish, raised plaques observed along nasal portion of eyelids)	Elevated cholesterol levels (hypercholesterolemia)
Osler nodes (acutely painful purplish nodules on the palms of the hands and the soles of the feet)	Infective endocarditis
Splinter hemorrhages are small, linear hemorrhages of the finger or toenail that are frequently due to trauma but also seen in infective endocarditis.	Frequently due to trauma but also seen in infective endocarditis
Janeway lesions are irregular, non-tender, erythematous, or hemorrhagic macules or papules commonly found on the palm and soles, lasting days to weeks.	Acute infective endocarditis

AMI, acute myocardial infarction; DVT, deep vein thrombosis; HF, heart failure; PAD, peripheral arterial disease.

Data from Bickley, L., Szilagyi, P., Hoffman, R., & Sorino, R. (2021). *Bates' guide to physical examination and history taking* (13th ed.). Lippincott/Williams & Wilkins.

Bunce, N., Ray, R., & Patel, H. (2021). Cardiology. In: *Kumar and Clark's clinical medicine* (10th ed., ch. 30, pp. 1019–1132). Elsevier and Sustersic, K. (2021). *Evidence-based physical examination: Best practices for health & well-being assessment.* Springer Publishing Co. ProQuest Ebook Central, http://ebookcentral.proquest.com/lib/yale-ebooks/detail.action?docID=6165608.

Swartz, M. (2021). The Heart. In Swartz, M. (Ed.), *Textbook of physical diagnosis: History and examination* (8th ed.). Elsevier Inc.

In addition, the nurse inspects the patient for scars that may be associated with prior cardiac surgery or an implanted cardiac pacemaker or defibrillator; heaves; lifts; and abnormal pulsations, which will be discussed shortly.

Assessment of Blood Pressure

Systemic arterial BP is the pressure exerted on the walls of the arteries during ventricular systole and diastole. It is affected by factors such as cardiac output; distention of the arteries; intimal thickening; aortic compliance; and the volume, velocity, and viscosity of the blood. The definition of ideal BP continues to evolve; the current recommendation is that the systolic pressure should be 120 mm Hg or lower and diastolic pressure 80 mm Hg or lower. Table 11-4 details current standards, the threshold of hypertension, and the target of BP control. A BP of less than 90/60 mm Hg is termed *hypotension;* it is an ominous finding in hospitalized patients, predicting increased mortality and adverse outcome (McGee, 2022). The nurse evaluates the patient for hypotension, taking into account new relatively low levels of BP in the light of past readings and the patient's clinical state (Bickley et al., 2021).

During the first encounter with a new patient, BP measurements should be obtained in both arms. There may be a 5- to 10-mm Hg difference in pressure between extremities. A BP difference greater than 10 mm Hg may be indicative of arterial obstruction (on the limb with lower pressure, such as subclavian artery obstruction) or aortic dissection and requires further evaluation. See Chapter 12 for more information on BP.

TABLE **11-4 Blood Pressure Classifications**

American College of Cardiology/American Heart Association Classifications		
Classification	**Systolic Pressure (mm Hg)**	**Diastolic Pressure (mm Hg)**
Normal	<120	<80
Elevated	120–129	<80
Hypertension		
Stage 1	130–139	80–90
Stage 2	≥140	≥90

Data from Whelton, P. K., Carey, R. M., Aronow, W. S., Casey, D. E. Jr., Collins, K. J., Dennison Himmelfarb, C., DePalma, S. M., Gidding, S., Jamerson, K. A., Jones, D. W., MacLaughlin, E. J., Muntner, P., Ovbiagele, B., Smith, S. C. Jr., Spencer, C. C., Stafford, R. S., Taler, S. J., Thomas, R. J., Williams, K. A. Sr., ..., Wright, J. T. Jr. (2018). 2017 ACC/AHA/AAPA/ABC/ACPM/AGS/APhA/ASH/ASPC/NMA/PCNA guideline for the prevention, detection, evaluation, and management of high blood pressure in adults: A report of the American College of Cardiology/American Heart Association Task Force on clinical practice guidelines. *Journal of the American College of Cardiology*, *71*(19), e127–e248. doi: 10.1016/j.jacc.2017.11.006

The Mean Arterial Pressure

A useful measurement is the mean arterial pressure (MAP), which is calculated by adding the systolic BP plus two times the diastolic pressure divided by three. This is in recognition of the different durations of systole and diastole (with diastole being twice as long as systole), thus contributing unequally to average BP values (Mangione et al., 2021). As an example, if the blood pressure is 120/66 mm Hg, the MAP would be $120 + (2 \times 66) \div 3 = 252 \div 3 = 84$. The MAP is used to reflect the perfusion pressure to major organs. The cardiac monitor automatically makes the calculation, or if the BP is taken by cuff pressure, it can be calculated manually. Major organs require a MAP of at least 65 mm Hg for perfusion (the normal range is 70 to 110 mm Hg). If MAP drops below this point for an extended period, end-organ ischemia and infarction can occur. A MAP of at least 60 mm Hg is needed to perfuse the coronary arteries. If the MAP drops below 60 mm Hg, blood will not be able to perfuse cerebral tissues as well, leading to a loss of consciousness and quickly ensuing neuronal death (Lough et al., 2022).

Pulse Pressure

Pulse pressure is the difference between the systolic and the diastolic pressures, which is normally 40 mm Hg. It indicates how well the body is maintaining cardiac output.

Pearls for Practice

A pulse pressure lower than 30 mm Hg signifies a serious reduction in cardiac output and requires further evaluation.

Postural Blood Pressure Changes

Postural (orthostatic) hypotension is a significant decrease in BP with a change in body position from supine to sitting or standing or from sitting to standing. It may be accompanied by dizziness, lightheadedness, or syncope.

The most common cause of postural hypotension in patients with CVD is due to a reduction in preload from overdiuresis or severe blood loss, dehydration, or use of medications that causes vasodilatation (nitrates and antihypertensive agents) as well as diseases of the autonomic nervous system. The following recommendations are important when assessing the patient for postural changes in BP:

- The patient is positioned supine for 3 to 10 minutes before obtaining the initial BP and heart rate.
- After obtaining supine measurements, the patient is positioned on the side of the bed with feet dangling, then, if appropriate, with the patient standing at the side of the bed.
- Wait 1 to 3 minutes after each position change before obtaining the BP and heart rate.
- Return the patient to a supine position if dizziness or lightheadedness is reported after the patient sits or stands.
- Record heart rate and BP in each position and any symptoms that accompany the postural change.

Normal postural responses that occur when a person moves from a lying to a sitting or standing position include (1) a heart rate increase of 5 to 20 bpm above the resting rate (to offset reduced stroke volume and maintain cardiac output); (2) a decrease of 10 mm Hg or less in systolic pressure; and (3) a slight increase of 5 mm Hg in diastolic pressure. An increase in heart rate of 15 bpm and/or at least a 20 mm Hg decrease in systolic pressure or a 10 mm Hg decrease in diastolic pressure within 3 minutes are abnormal findings and require further evaluation to determine etiology (Bickley et al., 2021; Suneja et al., 2020). Of note, postural dizziness (severe enough to stop the test) or an increase in heart rate of at least 30 bpm has sensitivity of 97% and specificity of 96% for blood loss of at least 630 mL (Mangione et al., 2021).

Palpation of Arterial Pulses

The examination of arterial pulses involves assessment of the pulse rate, rhythm, and quality.

Pulse Rate

The normal pulse rate varies from a low of 50 bpm in healthy, athletic young adults to rates well in excess of 100 bpm after exercise or during times of excitement. Anxiety frequently raises the pulse rate during the physical examination. If the rate is higher than expected, the nurse should reassess the pulse at the end of the physical examination when the patient may be more relaxed. A heart rate lower than 60 is termed bradycardia, whereas a heart rate greater than 100 is termed tachycardia. Shock can be indicated with a rapid, thready, or weak pulse. Of note, a palpable radial pulse is estimated to approximate a systolic BP of 80 mm Hg; if the nurse cannot palpate the radial pulse, the femoral pulse is evaluated. A palpable femoral pulse is associated with a systolic pressure of 70 mm Hg (Swartz & Phrampus, 2021).

Pulse Rhythm

The rhythm of the pulse is normally regular, though slight irregularities in rhythm can occur due to changes in vagal tone during the respiratory cycle (pulse rate accelerates with inspiration and slows with expiration). This phenomenon, called *sinus arrhythmia,* normally occurs in children and young adults.

During the initial cardiac examination, or if the pulse rhythm is irregular, the nurse assesses pulse rate for a *pulse deficit*, defined as the difference between the apical (apex of the heart, apical impulse is visible in 20% of normal people) and the peripheral pulse rates (Suneja et al., 2020). The pulse deficit is ascertained by simultaneously auscultating the apical pulse and palpating the radial pulse for 1 minute. The nurse should anticipate finding a pulse deficit in patients with arrhythmias, especially atrial fibrillation, atrial flutter, and ventricular arrhythmias. Some of the ventricular systoles generated by these arrhythmias may be much weaker than others; therefore, they are heard during auscultation but do not produce a palpable pulse.

Pulse Quality

The pulse quality or amplitude is indicative of the BP in the artery and is used to assess peripheral arterial circulation. The right and left temporal, common carotid, brachial, radial, and lower extremity arteries are palpated, one side at a time, and compared for symmetry in quality. Light palpation is essential as firm finger pressure can obliterate the temporal, dorsalis pedis, and posterior tibial arteries.

The quality of each of the pulses is reported by using descriptors (absent, diminished, normal, or bounding) or the following 0-to-4 scale:

0: Pulse not palpable or absent
+1: Weak, thready pulse; difficult to palpate; obliterated with pressure
+2: Diminished pulse; cannot be obliterated
+3: Easy to palpate, full pulse; cannot be obliterated
+4: Strong, bounding pulse; may be abnormal

When documenting the pulse quality, specify the artery location and scale range (e.g., "left radial +3/+4"). Other pulse scales exist; the nurse uses the institution's scale to ensure consistent clinical measurements and management.

Inspection of Jugular Venous Pulsations

Right-sided heart function can be estimated by observing the pulsations of the jugular veins of the neck, which reflects the CVP (right ventricular end-diastolic pressure or right ventricular preload). If internal jugular vein pulsations are difficult to visualize, the external jugular veins are used because they are more superficial and visible right above the clavicles, adjacent to the sternocleidomastoid muscles. In the supine position, the patient's external jugular veins are quite visible but disappear as the head is elevated greater than 30 degrees. The nurse assesses the right internal jugular vein rather than the left because it is anatomically straighter. To assess the jugular venous pressure (JVP), the nurse uses the angle of Louis, or the sternal angle, as a reference point (Fig. 11-8). The patient is positioned between 30 and 60 degrees, wherever the top of the venous pulsation can be seen in a good light (Bunce et al., 2021). A ruler is placed on the sternal angle vertically, and another straight edge is used as the horizontal reference line. Place the straight edge perpendicular to the ruler across the highest point of the internal jugular pulsation or the point just above where the external jugular appears to collapse. A measurement of 3 cm above the sternal angle indicates an elevated JVP (Sustersic, 2020).

Obvious distention of the jugular veins with the patient's head elevated to 90 degrees indicates an abnormal increase in the CVP. This occurs with right-sided HF, cardiac tamponade (see Chapter 14), and less commonly with obstruction of blood flow in the superior vena cava. If JVD is noticed, the nurse assesses for facial edema and dilated collateral vessels on the anterior chest and back, which is indicative of central venous obstruction and superior vena cava syndrome (see Chapter 5) (Suneja et al., 2020).

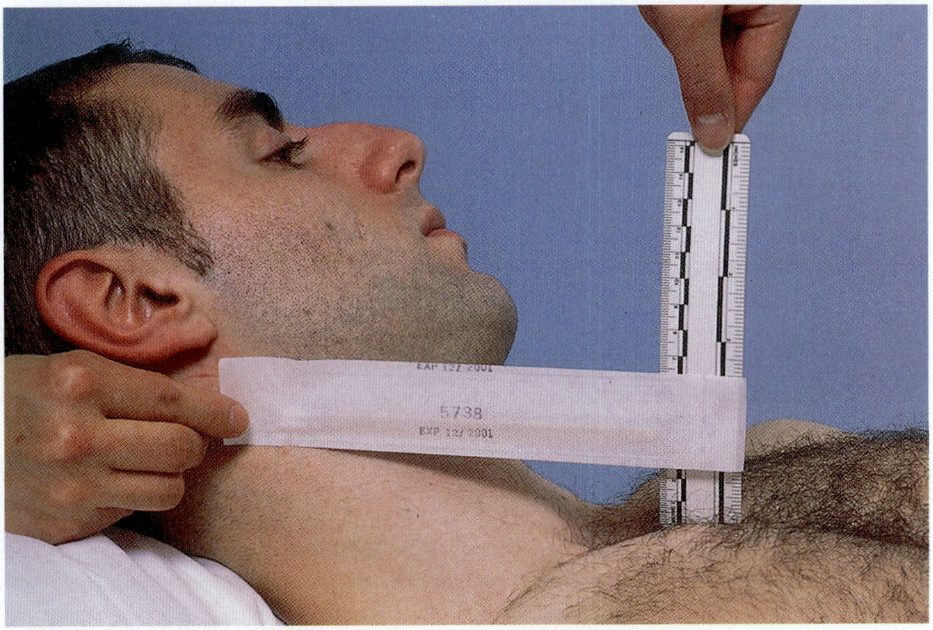

FIGURE 11-8 Measuring the JVP with a horizontal card and vertical ruler. (From Bickley, L. S., Szilagyi, P. G., Hoffman, R. M., & Soriano, R. P. [2021]. *Bates' guide to physical examination and history taking*. 13th ed. Wolters Kluwer Health.)

Inspection and Palpation of the Heart

The heart is examined by inspection, palpation, and auscultation of the precordium or anterior chest wall that covers the heart and lower thorax. A systematic approach is used to examine the precordium in the following areas (Fig. 11-9):

1. *Aortic area:* Second ICS to the right of the sternum. To determine the correct ICS, the nurse first finds the angle of Louis by locating the bony ridge at the junction of the body of the sternum and the manubrium. From this angle, the second ICS is located by sliding one finger to the right of the sternum. Subsequent ICSs are located from this reference point by palpating down the rib cage.
2. *Pulmonic area:* Second ICS, left sternal border (LSB)
3. *Erb point:* Third ICS, LSB
4. *Tricuspid area:* Fourth and fifth ICSs, LSB
5. *Mitral (apical area):* Left fifth ICS space at the MCL

For most of the examination, the patient lies supine with the head of the bed slightly elevated. A right-handed examiner stands at the right side of the patient, a left-handed examiner at the left side.

Each area of the precordium is inspected for abnormal pulsations. A subtle pulsation located over the apical area, called the **apical impulse** or PMI, is a normal finding observed in young patients and adults who have thin chest walls. The nurse uses the palm of the hand to locate the apical impulse initially and the fingerpads to assess its size and quality. Palpation of the apical impulse may be facilitated by placing the patient in the left lateral position as this position brings the heart into closer contact with the chest wall (see Fig. 11-10).

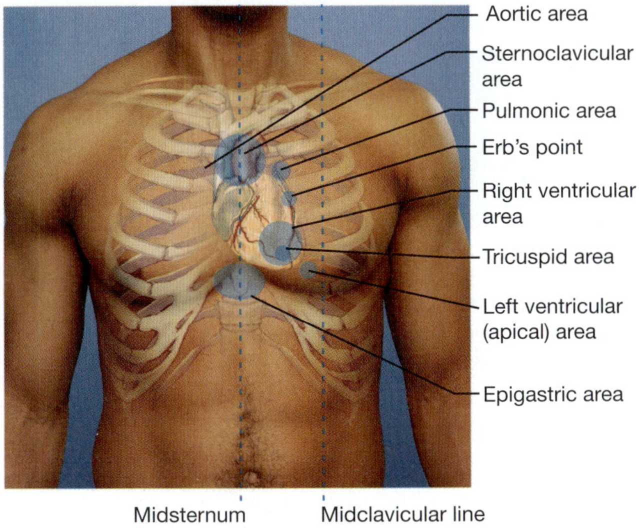

FIGURE 11-9 Areas of the precordium to be assessed when evaluating heart function.

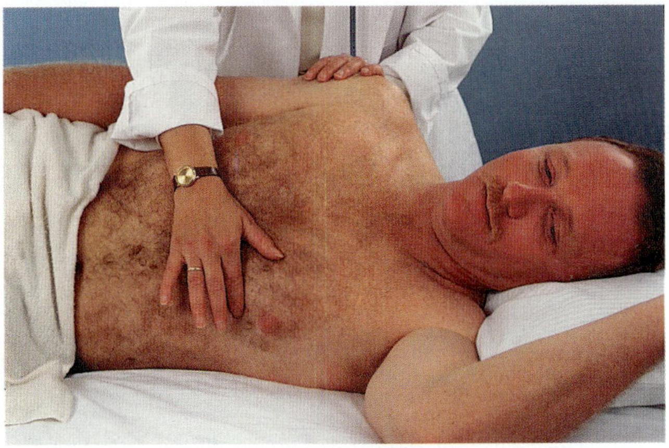

FIGURE 11-10 Locating and palpating the apical impulse, also called the point of maximal impulse (PMI), in the left lateral position. The apical pulse is normally located at the fifth intercostal space to the left of the sternum at the midclavicular line. The nurse locates the impulse with the palm of the hand and palpates with the fingerpads. (© B. Proud.)

Normally, the apical impulse is palpable 7 to 9 cm from the left sternal border in the fifth ICS and is no larger than 2 cm in diameter. Feeling the impulse in two or more adjacent ICSs indicates left ventricular hypertrophy or cardiac enlargement. A vibration or purring sensation felt over any of the precordial areas indicates abnormal, turbulent blood flow. It is best detected by using the palm of the hand. This vibration is called a *thrill*, which is associated with a loud murmur (Grades 4 to 6, Box 11-3). Depending on the location of the thrill, it may be indicative of serious valvular heart disease or a defect (abnormal opening) in the septum of the atria or ventricles. Thrills that are palpated over blood vessels are associated with significant obstruction of a large artery, such as the carotid artery.

Auscultation of the Heart

A stethoscope is used to auscultate each of the locations identified in Figure 11-9, to assess heart rate and rhythm, and to evaluate heart sounds. The apical area is auscultated for 1 minute to determine the apical pulse rate and the regularity of the heartbeat.

Heart Sounds

Normal Heart Sounds. Normal heart sounds, referred to as S_1 and S_2, are produced by closure of the AV valves and the semilunar valves, respectively. The period between S_1 and S_2 corresponds with ventricular systole (Fig. 11-11). When the heart rate is within the normal range, diastole (period between S_2 and S_1) is twice as long as systole. However, as the heart rate increases, diastole shortens.

S_1—First Heart Sound. Tricuspid and mitral valve closure creates the first heart sound (S_1). The word "lub" is used to replicate its sound. S_1 is usually heard the loudest at the apical area (fifth ICS, left MCL, or mitral area). S_1 is easily identifiable and serves as the point of reference for the remainder of the cardiac cycle. If you are having difficulty determining S_1 from S_2, simply palpate the pulse since ventricular systole or contraction results in the palpated pulse; this will cue you into the S_1.

BOX 11-3

Characteristics of Heart Murmurs

The following characteristics provide information needed to determine the cause and clinical significance of heart murmurs.

Location: Pinpoints where the murmur is heard the loudest to identify the involved underlying structures (see Fig. 11-9)

Timing: Describes when the murmur is heard (systole, diastole, or both)

Intensity: A grading system is used to describe the intensity or loudness of a murmur:

- Grade 1: Very faint and difficult for the inexperienced clinician to hear
- Grade 2: Quiet, but readily perceived by the experienced clinician
- Grade 3: Easily heard, no palpable thrill
- Grade 4: Loud and may be associated with a thrill (a thrill feels like a purring cat under the area)
- Grade 5: Very loud; heard when stethoscope is partially off the chest; associated with a thrill
- Grade 6: Extremely loud; detected with the stethoscope off the chest; associated with a thrill

Pitch: Describes the sound frequency ranging from high to medium to low

Quality: Describes the sound that the murmur resembles (rumbling, blowing, whistling)

Radiation: Identifies if the sound of the murmur is transmitted to other precordial areas

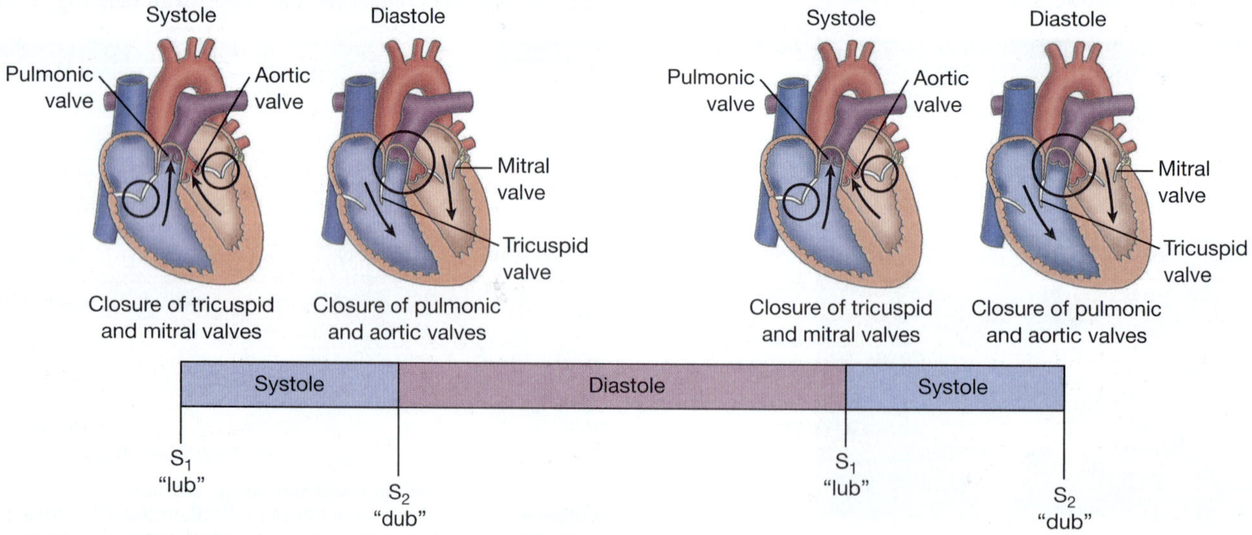

FIGURE 11-11 Normal heart sounds. The first heart sound (S_1) is produced by closure of the mitral and tricuspid valves ("lub"). The second heart sound (S_2) is produced by closure of the aortic and pulmonic valves ("dub"). *Arrows* represent the direction of blood flow during systole and diastole.

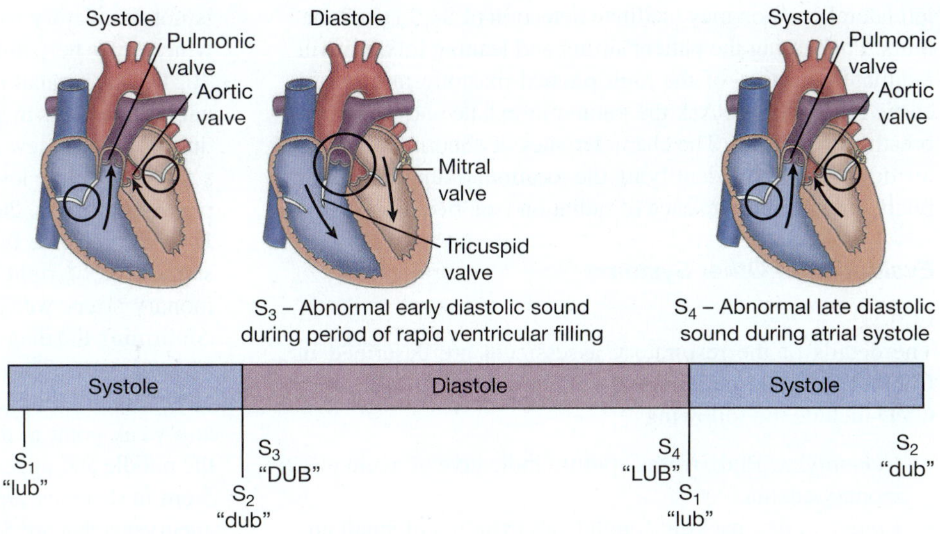

FIGURE 11-12 Gallop sounds. An S_3 ("DUB") is an abnormal sound heard early in diastole, immediately following S_2 (closure of the semilunar valves). This sound is generated very early in diastole as blood flowing into the right or left ventricle is met with resistance. S_4 ("LUB") is an abnormal sound created during atrial systole as blood flowing into the right or left ventricle is met with resistance. *Arrows* show the direction of blood flow.

S_2—Second Heart Sound. Closure of the pulmonic and aortic valves produces the second heart sound (S_2), commonly referred to as the "dub" sound. S_2 is heard the loudest over the aortic (second ICS, right sternal border) and pulmonic areas (second ICS, LSB).

Abnormal Heart Sounds. Abnormal sounds develop during systole or diastole when structural or functional heart problems are present. High-pitched heart sounds are heard best with the diaphragm of the stethoscope (e.g., aortic, pulmonic, tricuspid and mitral valve closure, and regurgitant murmurs), whereas low-pitched sounds (e.g., gallop rhythms or mitral stenosis) are better heard with the bell.

S_3—Third Heart Sound. An S_3 is an abnormal sound heard early in diastole as blood flows from the atrium into a noncompliant ventricle. It is heard immediately after S_2. "Lub-dub-DUB" is used to imitate the abnormal sound of a beating heart when an S_3 (DUB) is present. It represents a normal finding in children and young adults, up to 35 or 40 years of age. In these cases, it is called a *physiologic S_3* (Fig. 11-12). In adults, S_3 is a significant finding, suggesting HF. The S_3 often disappears after the patient is treated with diuretic medications or dialysis (McGee, 2022). It is heard best by using the bell of the stethoscope at the cardiac apex with the patient in the left lateral position.

S_4—Fourth Heart Sound. S_4 occurs late in diastole (see Fig. 11-12). S_4, heard just before S_1, is generated during atrial contraction as blood forcefully enters a noncompliant ventricle. This resistance to blood flow is due to ventricular hypertrophy caused by ischemic, hypertensive, or hypertrophic cardiomyopathy. The mnemonic used to imitate this gallop sound is "LUB-lub-dub." S_4 (LUB) is auscultated using the bell of the stethoscope over the apical area with the patient in the left lateral position. Since an S_4 requires an effective atrial contraction, it does not occur in patients with atrial fibrillation. There are times when both S_3 and S_4 are present, creating a quadruple rhythm, which sounds like "LUB lub-dub DUB." During a tachycardia, all four sounds combine into a loud sound, referred to as a summation gallop.

Clicks and Snaps. Opening and closing of diseased valve leaflets create abnormal sounds, called clicks and snaps. Clicks are heard during S_1 or systole. They are brief and high-pitched, heard early in systole as ridged, calcified semilunar valves are forced open during ventricular contraction. Opening snaps are high-pitched diastolic sounds, therefore heard during S2, as stenotic AV valves are forced open. These sounds are the loudest in the areas directly over the diseased valve.

Murmurs. These are a result of turbulent blood flow across rigid, calcified valves; leaky valves that allow backward blood flow (regurgitation); defects (abnormal openings) in the septum, aorta, or PA; or abnormally high velocity of blood flow through a normal structure (e.g., with fever, pregnancy, hyperthyroidism). Murmurs are described by several characteristics (see Box 11-3) that are used to determine the cause and clinical significance.

Friction Rub. A harsh, grating sound that can be heard in both systole and diastole is called a friction rub. It was thought to be caused by abrasion of the inflamed pericardial surfaces from pericarditis, but newer theories indicate the movement of fibrin strands caused by inflammation since the rub is also associated with pericardial effusions (Chahine & Siddiqui, 2021). A pericardial friction rub can be heard best using the diaphragm of the stethoscope over the LSB; it is generally louder on inspiration with the patient sitting up and leaning forward (Chahine & Siddiqui, 2021).

Auscultative Procedure

During auscultation, the patient remains supine. Using the diaphragm of the stethoscope, the nurse auscultates the precordium to identify S_1 and S_2 and then listens for abnormal systolic or diastolic sounds. Repositioning the patient into the left lateral position may facilitate detection of S_3, S_4, and murmurs. Positioning the patient sitting and leaning forward will facilitate detection of the high-pitched diastolic murmur of aortic regurgitation. Ask the patient to exhale and hold their breath as you listen. The characteristics of abnormal findings are documented by identifying the location, timing, intensity, pitch, quality, and presence of radiation (see Box 11-3).

Evaluation of Other Systems

Lungs

The details of the respiratory assessment are described in Chapter 7. Abnormal findings exhibited by patients with CVD include the following:

- *Hemoptysis:* Pink, frothy sputum indicative of acute pulmonary edema
- *Cough:* A dry, hacking cough from irritation of small airways from pulmonary congestion associated with HF
- *Crackles:* Typically, first noted at the bases (due to the effect of gravity on fluid accumulation and decreased ventilation of basilar tissue). Crackles may progress to all portions of the lung fields as a result of worsening HF or atelectasis associated with bed rest; splinting from ischemic pain; or the effects of analgesics, sedatives, or anesthetic agents.
- *Wheezes:* Compression of the small airways by interstitial pulmonary edema may cause wheezing. Beta-adrenergic blocking agents (beta-blockers), such as propranolol (Inderal), may cause airway narrowing, especially in patients with underlying pulmonary disease.

Abdomen

The abdomen is assessed for distention and ascites, hepatojugular reflux, and pulsatile mass.

- *Abdominal distension:* A protuberant abdomen with bulging flanks indicates ascites. Ascites develops in the late stages of HF as abnormally high pressures in the right side of the heart impede the return of venous blood. As a result, the liver and spleen become engorged with excessive venous blood (hepatosplenomegaly). As pressure in the portal system rises, fluid shifts from the vascular bed into the abdominal cavity. Ascitic fluid, found in the dependent or lowest points in the abdomen, will shift with position changes.
- *Hepatojugular reflux:* This test is performed when right ventricular or biventricular HF is suspected. The patient is semirecumbent with the head of bed elevated 30 to 45 degrees and the head turned so that the jugular venous pulse is visible in the lower part of the neck. The patient is instructed to breathe with their mouth open to prevent a Valsalva maneuver (Swartz, 2021). While observing the jugular venous pulse, steady pressure of around 20 to 35 mm Hg is applied over the abdomen for at least 10 seconds (see Chapter 14 for further details). The site of compression does not significantly alter the test, so it is not mandatory to apply pressure directly on the liver, which may be painful for some patients (Vaidya et al., 2021). The normal response is for the internal and external jugular veins to show a transient increase in distention during the first few cardiac cycles, which is followed by a fall to baseline levels during the latter part of the compression (Swartz, 2021). An increase of 3 cm or more in JVP is indicative of a positive hepatojugular reflux and suggestive of right ventricular failure or elevated pulmonary artery wedge pressure. This positive test aids in confirming the diagnosis of HF.
- *Pulsatile mass:* The most important diagnostic indication of an abdominal aortic **aneurysm** (a localized dilation formed at a weak point in the arterial wall) is a pulsatile mass in the middle and upper abdomen. Aneurysms between 3 and 5 cm in diameter are difficult to detect, but about 80% of aneurysms that are 5 cm or larger can be palpated (McGee, 2021). The nurse is aware that the aorta is retroperitoneal and that in overweight patients, there may be no overt signs. A systolic **bruit** (abnormal sound associated with turbulent blood flow in an artery) may be heard over the mass.

Gerontologic Considerations

The incidence of atherosclerosis, HF, and CAD increases with advancing age. Peripheral pulses of older adult patients are readily palpable because of decreased elasticity of the arteries and a loss of adjacent connective tissue. In older patients, symptoms of PAD may be more pronounced than in younger patients. The classic symptom of intermittent claudication may occur after walking only a few blocks or after walking up a slight incline. Prolonged pressure exerted on areas of the toes or feet further compromises arterial perfusion, which can lead to ulceration, infection, and gangrene. The nurse screens the older adult patient for risk factors of CVD, including smoking, diabetes, hypertension, hyperlipidemia, and family history, and counsels the patient accordingly on lifestyle modifications and risk reduction.

Isolated systolic hypertension, associated with significant cardiovascular morbidity and mortality, is a common finding in older adults. There is a higher risk for postural hypotension as well, reflecting a decrease in the sensitivity of the postural reflexes; this must be considered prior to prescribing new cardiovascular medications. In addition, many older adult patients are on numerous medications; the use of five or more medications is termed polypharmacy and is associated with falls, frailty, disability, and mortality in older adults (Varghese et al., 2021).

Diagnostic Evaluation

Diagnostic tests and procedures are used to confirm the data obtained by the history and physical assessment. Some tests are easy to interpret, but others must be interpreted by expert clinicians. All tests should be explained to the patient. Some necessitate special preparation before they are performed and special monitoring by the nurse after the procedure.

Laboratory Tests

Laboratory tests may be performed for the following reasons:

- To assist in identifying the cause of cardiovascular signs and symptoms
- To identify abnormalities in the blood that affect the prognosis of a patient with CVD
- To assess the degree of inflammation
- To screen for risk factors associated with CAD
- To determine baseline values before initiating therapeutic interventions
- To ensure that therapeutic levels of medications (e.g., antiarrhythmic agents, warfarin) are maintained
- To assess the effects of medications (e.g., the effects of diuretics on serum potassium levels)

Because different laboratories use various types of equipment and methods of measurements, normal test values may vary depending on the laboratory and the health care institution.

Cardiac Biomarker Analysis

Plasma levels of cardiac biomarkers are used to diagnose acute MI in conjunction with the history, physical examination, and ECG. These substances leak into the bloodstream after injured myocardial cells rupture their cell membranes. Biomarkers have a specific timeline for when they first rise, peak, and then return to normal. This timeline helps the clinician decide which test to order, based on the timing of patient's symptom onset.

- *Creatine kinase (CK)/creatine kinase–myoglobin binding (CK-MB):* CK is released from three types of damaged tissue (myocardium, skeletal muscle, and other organs, including the brain, uterus, and small intestine). CK-MB is the cardiac-specific isoenzyme that rises within 4 to 8 hours after myocardial injury, peaks in 12 to 24 hours, and returns to normal within 3 to 4 days.
- *Myoglobin:* This heme protein transports oxygen to cardiac and skeletal muscle cells. Its small molecular structure allows it to be released rapidly from damaged myocardial tissue and accounts for its early rise. Myoglobin is not used alone to diagnose MI because elevations can also occur in patients with kidney or musculoskeletal disease. However, negative results are helpful in ruling out acute MI. Myoglobin rises within 1 to 3 hours of tissue injury, peaks in 6 to 9 hours, and returns to normal in 24 hours (Fischbach et al., 2021).

Troponin T and I: Cardiac troponin is unique to the heart muscle, is highly concentrated in cardiomyocytes, and is the preferred test to diagnose MI (Fischbach et al., 2022). These heme proteins regulate the contractile function of the myocardium. After very small areas of myocardial injury, these biomarkers rise early (within 1 to 3 hours), peak in 12 hours, and return to normal within 3 to 10 days. Troponin T is sensitive but less specific since it is also positive with angina at rest, so troponin I is assessed for an MI. Serial sampling of troponin is assessed at 0, 4, 8, and 12 hours after chest pain to rule out acute MI. A normal troponin I is 0 to 0.4 ng/mL, and a normal troponin T is less than 0.01 ng/mL. A critical troponin I is higher than 1.5 ng/mL and needs to be reported to the provider immediately.

Blood Chemistry, Hematology, and Coagulation Studies

Table 11-5 provides information about common serum laboratory tests and the implications for patients with CVD.

Lipid Profile. The lipid profile helps evaluate a person's risk for atherosclerosis, myocardial occlusion, and coronary arterial occlusion, or to diagnose a specific lipoprotein abnormality, such as hereditary hyperlipoproteinemias. The profile (cholesterol, triglycerides, LDL, and HDL levels) is also frequently a part of thyroid, liver, and kidney function and diabetes studies. In addition, they are used to monitor effectiveness of diet, medications, lifestyle changes (e.g., exercise), and stress management (Fischbach et al., 2022). The blood specimen for the lipid profile should be obtained after a 12-hour fast, though nonfasting specimens may be taken. Pretest, the patient is instructed that dietary intake at least 2 weeks before testing will affect results, and it is recommended that the patient abstains from alcohol for 24 hours before testing.

Cholesterol Levels. Cholesterol is a lipid required for hormone synthesis and cell membrane formation. It comes from the diet (animal products) and the liver, where cholesterol is synthesized. Factors that contribute to variations in cholesterol levels include age, sex, diet, exercise patterns, genetics, tobacco use, and stress levels. A normal level is less than 200 mg/dL.

LDL is the primary transporter of cholesterol and triglycerides into the cell. One harmful effect of LDL is the deposition of these substances into the walls of arteries. Elevated LDL levels are associated with a greater incidence of atherosclerosis and CAD (Norris & Tuan, 2020). A normal level is less than 130 mg/dL; however, the LDL level should be less than 70 mg/dL in patients at high risk for heart disease. For patients at moderately high risk, the LDL should be less than or equal to 100 mg/dL (depending on other cardiac risk factors) (Pagana et al., 2021).

In contrast, HDL has a protective action by transporting cholesterol away from the arterial wall to the liver for excretion. A normal level is 45 mg/dL or higher for males and 55 mg/dL or higher for females (Pagana et al., 2021). Factors associated with lowering HDL levels are smoking, diabetes, obesity, and physical inactivity. Total HDL cholesterol is an independent, inverse risk factor for CAD. Whereas low levels (less than 35 mg/dL) are believed to increase a person's risk for CAD, high levels (higher than 60 mg/dL) are considered protective (Pagana et al., 2021).

Triglycerides. Triglycerides, composed of free fatty acids and glycerol, are stored in the adipose tissue and are a source of

TABLE **11-5 Common Serum Laboratory Tests and Implications for Patients With Cardiovascular Disease**

Laboratory Test/Reference Range	Implications
Blood Chemistries	
Sodium (Na^+) 135–145 mEq/L	*Hyponatremia:* ↓ Na levels can be due to thiazide diuretics or from fluid excess, as seen in HF. *Hypernatremia:* ↑ Na levels indicate fluid deficits and can result from ↓ water intake or hypovolemia.
Potassium (K^+) 3.5–5 mEq/L	*Hypokalemia:* ↓ K levels often due to use of K-excreting diuretics, which can cause ventricular tachycardia and fibrillation and predispose digitalis toxicity in patients taking digoxin. Earliest ECG change is often PVCs, which can deteriorate into ventricular tachycardia (VT) or ventricular fibrillation (VF) without appropriate treatment. *Hyperkalemia:* ↑ K levels due to ↑ intake of foods high in K or overuse of K supplements; ↓ renal excretion of K; use of K-sparing diuretics (e.g., spironolactone); or use of angiotensin-converting enzyme (ACE) inhibitors, and angiotensin-receptor blockers (ARBs); kidney failure; extensive skeletal muscle destruction (rhabdomyolysis); tumor lysis syndrome Can cause heart block, asystole, and ventricular arrhythmias
Calcium (Ca^{++}) 8.5–10.5 mg/dL	Necessary for blood coagulability, neuromuscular activity, and automaticity of the sinoatrial and atrioventricular nodes. *Hypocalcemia:* ↓ calcium levels slow nodal function and decrease myocardial contractility resulting in ↓ CO and hypotension. Latter effect ↑ risk of HF. Rhythm disturbances are variable, ranging from bradycardia, a prolonged QTc interval, VT and asystole. *Hypercalcemia:* ↑ Ca levels are associated with use of thiazide diuretics that ↓ renal excretion of Ca. Hypercalcemia potentiates digitalis toxicity, causes ↑ myocardial contractility, and shortening ventricular repolarization (shortened Q-Tc). Rhythm disturbances may include bradycardia and ↑ risk of heart block and hypertension
Magnesium (Mg^{++}) 1.3–2.4 mEq/L	Needed to absorb Ca, maintain K stores, metabolize adenosine triphosphate, synthesize protein and carbohydrate, maintain muscular contraction, and help control atrioventricular node conduction. *Hypomagnesemia:* ↓ Mg levels are due to enhanced renal excretion of Mg from loop diuretics or digitalis therapy. ECG changes are similar to those in hypokalemia and hypocalcemia: prolonged PR and QTc intervals, presence of U waves, T wave flattening, and widened QRS complex. ↓ Mg levels predispose patients to atrial or ventricular tachycardias including torsades de pointes *Hypermagnesemia:* Rare, ↑ magnesium levels are caused by use of cathartics or antacids containing Mg, kidney failure, and tumor lysis syndrome (TLS). ↑ Mg levels depress myocardial contractility and excitability heart block or asystole.
Blood urea nitrogen (BUN) 6–20 mg/dL Creatinine Males: 0.9–1.3 mg/dL Females: 0.6–1.1 mg/dL	End products of protein metabolism excreted by the kidneys End product of muscle metabolism excreted by the kidneys Renal impairment is detected by an ↑ in BUN and creatinine. A normal creatinine level and an ↑ BUN detect an intravascular fluid volume deficit, bleeding, or increased protein intake.
Glucose (fasting): 65–110 mg/dL	↑ Glucose levels result from stress as endogenous epinephrine is mobilized to convert liver glycogen to glucose; diabetes
Hemoglobin A1c (HbA_{1c}) <5.6	Monitored in people with diabetes, as it reflects blood glucose levels over 2–3 months. Goal: hemoglobin A_{1c} less than 7%.
Coagulation Studies	
Activated partial thromboplastin time (aPTT) 21–35 seconds	Used to monitor patient's response to unfractionated heparin. Heparin dose is adjusted to maintain a therapeutic range of 1.5–2.5 times baseline values. aPTT is a more sensitive version of partial thromboplastin time (PTT) used to monitor heparin therapy.
Prothrombin time (PT) 11–13 seconds	Measures the activity of five factors in the blood clotting pathway (prothrombin, fibrinogen, factors V, VII, X). Used to monitor patients on warfarin therapy. Therapeutic range is 1.5–2 times normal.

Laboratory Test/Reference Range	Implications
International normalized ratio (INR) 0.8–1.2 normal	Standardized method for monitoring prothrombin levels in patients receiving warfarin therapy. Therapeutic range 2–3.5, depending upon diagnosis.
Hematologic Studies	
Complete blood count (CBC)	Identifies the total number of white and red blood cells and platelets, and measures hemoglobin and Hct.
White blood cell (WBC) count 4,500–10,500/mm^3	WBC counts are monitored in immunocompromised patients (e.g., post heart transplant) or those at risk for infection (e.g., after invasive procedures or surgery).
Red blood cell (RBC) count Normal range males: 4.5–5.5 million cells/mm^3 Nonpregnant females: 4.0–5.0 million cells/mm^3	RBCs, also called erythrocytes, are primarily composed of hemoglobin needed for oxygen transport from the lungs to the tissues.
Hct Males: 41–53% Females: 36–46% Hemoglobin Males: 13.5–18 g/100 mL Females: 12–16 g/100 mL	Represents the percentage of RBCs found in 100 mL of whole blood. The RBCs contain hemoglobin, which transports oxygen to the cells. Low hemoglobin and Hct levels can cause more frequent angina episodes or acute MI in patients with cardiovascular diseases.
Platelets 140,000–400,000/mm^3	Initiate thrombus formation by clumping together at sites of vessel wall injury. Monitor for thrombocytopenia if aspirin, clopidogrel, eptifibatide, or tirofiban is prescribed.

Normal values vary by laboratory; the nurse follows institutional levels. Refer to Table 13-5 for cardiac biomarkers.

Data from Fischbach, F. T., Fischbach, M. A., & Stout, K. (2022). *A manual of laboratory and diagnostic tests* (11th ed.). Lippincott/Williams & Wilkins.

energy. A normal level is 40 to 160 mg/dL for males and 35 to 135 mg/dL for females (Pagana et al., 2021). Triglyceride levels increase after meals and are affected by stress. Diabetes, alcohol use disorder, and obesity can elevate triglyceride levels. Triglyceride levels greater than 150 mg/dL are another risk factor for cardiac disease (Pagana et al., 2021).

Atrial Natriuretic Peptide. Atrial natriuretic peptide (ANP) is a hormone secreted from the cardiomyocytes (muscle cells in the heart) in the right atrium, it elevates in response to atrial stretch from hypervolemia as well as in response to hypertension (Sandefur & Jialal, 2021). Although it is not routinely measured, a normal ANP is 22 to 77 pg/mL. The brain (B-type) natriuretic peptide (BNP) that is discussed next is the preferred peptide test for the diagnosis and management of heart failure.

Brain (B-Type) Natriuretic Peptide. BNP, secreted from the ventricles, is a neurohormone that responds to volume overload in the heart by acting as a diuretic and vasodilator. BNP levels are useful for the prompt diagnosis of HF, since it correlates to left ventricular pressures. A BNP level of 100 to 300 pg/mL indicates HF is present, and the higher the BNP level, the more severe the HF (Pagana et al., 2021). This test may be evaluated in patients experiencing SOB, particularly if the patient also has chronic obstructive pulmonary disease (COPD). If BNP is elevated, the SOB is related to HF. If BNP levels are normal, the SOB is associated with a pulmonary etiology rather than a cardiac one.

C-Reactive Protein. C-reactive protein (CRP) is produced by the liver in response to systemic inflammation. Inflammation is thought to play a role in the development and progression of atherosclerosis. Persistently elevated CRP levels can be seen in chronic inflammatory conditions such as chronic infections or inflammatory joint disorders like rheumatoid arthritis. A normal level is less than 1.0 mg/dL; levels of higher than 3.0 mg/dL are associated with high cardiac risk and are used as an adjunct to other tests to predict CAD risk. However, given the poor specificity of CRP to CAD risk, the test is currently undergoing more evaluation (Nehring et al., 2021).

Homocysteine. Homocysteine, an amino acid, can damage the endothelial lining of arteries and promote thrombus formation. Elevated levels are linked to the development of atherosclerosis and an increased risk for CAD, stroke, venous thrombosis, and peripheral vascular disease. Elevated homocysteine levels are associated with genetic factors and a diet low in folic acid and vitamin B_{12}. A 10- to 12-hour fast is necessary prior to obtaining the blood sample. Test results are interpreted as normal if they are between 4 and 14 μmol/L, borderline if they are between 12 and 15 μmol/L, and high risk for vascular disease if they are greater than 15 μmol/L (Pagana et al., 2021).

Electrocardiogram

The ECG is a graphic recording of the electrical activity of the heart. The ECG is obtained by placing disposable electrodes in standard positions on the skin of the chest wall and extremities. The standard 12-lead ECG records electrical impulses of the heart on special graph paper from 12 different reference points referred to as *leads*. It is used to diagnose arrhythmias, conduction abnormalities, enlarged heart chambers, and myocardial ischemia or infarction.

The cardiac rhythm is observed continuously by placing the patient on a bedside (hardwire) monitor or **telemetry** (battery-operated transmitting device worn by the patient), both of which transmit to a central bank of monitors. The telemetry system is wireless and allows patients to be monitored while ambulating. These forms of monitoring have graded visual and audible alarms that sound when an arrhythmia is detected. However, many of the alarms can be false alarms, caused by artifacts that mimic an arrhythmia. Common causes of false alarms include patient movement, incorrect alarm parameter settings, bathing or turning, improper skin preparation or ECG electrode placement, and faulty connections of leads or electrodes.

Nurses dealing with excessive alarms may become desensitized to these sounds and develop alarm fatigue. Alarm fatigue delays the nurse's response time or results in missed alarms of undetected arrhythmias leading to serious adverse events (Leigher et al., 2020). Nursing interventions that facilitate acquisition of accurate data, reduce risk of alarm fatigue, and ensure patient safety when using various forms of cardiac monitoring include customization of clinical alarms according to the patient's condition, provision of staff education on alarm customization, troubleshooting, proper electrode placement and skin preparation, the creation of an alarm committee that includes multidisciplinary members, assessing the appropriateness of physiologic monitoring for each patient, and reviewing criteria for the discontinuation of monitors (Fujita & Choi, 2020). Key to the elimination of artifacts is using proper skin preparation before applying electrodes and changing the electrode every 24 hours. Continuous ECG monitoring is discussed in Chapter 16.

Patients requiring ECG monitoring need to be informed of the purpose of the monitoring and cautioned that it does not detect symptoms such as dyspnea or chest pain. Therefore, patients need to be advised to report symptoms to the nurse whenever they occur.

Pearls for Practice

In emergencies, the nurse assesses patients for the "ABCs" of resuscitation—airway, breathing, circulation—and intervenes as appropriate. If the patient is experiencing hemodynamic compromise, the nurse will initiate monitoring of the cardiac rhythm (hardwire) and also obtain a 12-lead ECG. The patient will remain on the cardiac monitor to allow for evaluation of patient's response to treatment. With hardwire monitoring, the patient's cardiac rhythm can be viewed at the bedside, whereas telemetry transmits the patient's rhythm to a central monitoring system removed from the bedside.

Stress Testing

Stress testing is used to evaluate the response of the cardiovascular system to increased demands for oxygen and nutrients. This noninvasive test is used to determine the (1) presence of atherosclerosis in the arteries of the heart and lower extremities, (2) functional capacity of the heart after an MI or heart surgery, (3) effectiveness of the medical regimen, and (4) extent of cardiac symptoms such as angina, arrhythmias, inordinate blood pressure elevations, and functionally incompetent heart valves. The stress test is usually combined with a radionuclide imaging technique or echocardiogram to examine myocardial function during exercise and at rest.

Procedure

During an exercise stress test, the patient walks on a treadmill (most common) or pedals a stationary bicycle while the ECG, heart rate, and BP are monitored. Exercise intensity progresses according to established protocols in which the speed and grade of the treadmill are increased every few minutes. The usual goal of exercise stress testing is to increase the heart rate to just below maximal levels or to the target heart rate (Pagana et al., 2021). In general, the target heart rate is 80% to 90% of the maximal heart rate, which is determined by a chart using the patient's age and sex (the target rate is about 220 minus the patient's age).

If the patient is unable to exercise, a pharmacologic stress test is performed. Patients undergoing a pharmacologic stress test with radionuclide imaging will receive an infusion of a coronary vasodilator, such as dipyridamole adenosine or regadenoson. If one coronary artery is significantly occluded, the coronary blood flow is diverted to the opened vessels (Pagana et al., 2021). Dobutamine is another chemical that can stress the heart with its positive inotropic effect (increased strength of contraction), mimicking the physiologic effects of exercise.

Throughout the test, the patient is assessed for signs and symptoms of myocardial or leg ischemia (claudication) by monitoring the ECG, BP, physical appearance, perceived exertion, and symptoms, including chest pain; tachycardia; cardiac arrhythmias; increasing premature ventricular contractions; ECG changes (e.g., ST-segment variance greater than 1 mm, ST-segment depression greater than 0.2 mm); dyspnea; dizziness; leg cramping; and fatigue. The stress test is said to be positive if evidence of myocardial ischemia is detected by changes in the patient's ECG or claudication is validated by a decrease in ankle pressure. A test is negative when the patient does not exhibit significant symptoms, arrhythmias, or other ECG abnormalities at 85% of maximum heart rate predicted for age and sex (Fischbach et al., 2022). A positive stress test is an indication for additional testing.

Nursing Interventions

Patients are instructed to fast for 4 hours before the test, avoiding tobacco, caffeine, and other stimulants. Medications may be taken with sips of water. Clothes and rubber-soled shoes suitable for exercising should be worn. The nurse describes the monitoring equipment and symptoms to report and reviews the exercise protocol and the need for the patient to put forth their best efforts to complete the test. The test usually takes approximately 45 minutes. If vasodilating agents are used, patients are informed that they may have transient flushing or nausea. If the stress test is to be combined with imaging techniques, information related to these techniques is also reviewed. After the test, patients are monitored for 10 to 15 minutes or until stable, and then patients may resume their usual activities.

Radionuclide Imaging

Radionuclide imaging studies involve the use of radioisotopes to evaluate coronary artery perfusion noninvasively, to detect myocardial ischemia and infarction, and to assess left ventricular function. Radioisotopes are atoms in an unstable form that give off small amounts of energy in the form of gamma rays as they decay. When radioisotopes are injected into the bloodstream, the energy emitted can be detected by a gamma scintillation camera positioned over the body. These radioisotopes are called tracers. Pregnancy is a contraindication for most nuclear imaging.

Myocardial Perfusion Imaging

Myocardial perfusion imaging is performed using two types of techniques—single-photon emission computed tomography (SPECT) or positron emission tomography (PET). It is commonly performed after an acute MI to determine if arterial perfusion to the heart is compromised during activity and to evaluate the extent of myocardial damage. It is also used to evaluate if myocardial ischemia from CAD is the cause of chest pain or other CAD-related symptoms.

These imaging techniques are performed in combination with stress testing to compare images obtained when the heart is resting to images of the heart in a stressed state resulting from exercise or medications. An area of the myocardium that shows no perfusion or reduced perfusion is said to have a “defect” present. Comparing resting images with images taken after the stress test helps differentiate ischemic myocardium from infarct-related myocardium. A defect that does not change in size before and after stress is called a fixed defect. Fixed defects indicate that there is no perfusion in that area of the myocardium, which is the case after an MI. Defects that appear or that get larger after the stress test images are taken indicate reduced perfusion to that area of the heart. Because the defect disappears with rest, it is called a reversible defect. Reversible defects constitute positive stress test findings. Typically, cardiac catheterization is recommended after a positive test result to determine the severity of obstructions to blood flow caused by CAD.

SPECT is a painless, noninvasive procedure that involves the injection of a radiopharmaceutical tracer. The patient is positioned supine on the table, and the gamma camera circles around the chest area converting the signals from the traces into pictures of the heart. The procedure takes approximately 30 minutes. The second scan is repeated following the exercise or pharmacologic stress test. SPECT imaging is often combined with CT scans. The radioactivity decays over time and is eliminated in urine, feces, and other body fluids. The half-life of the tracer ranges from 6 hours to 8 days depending on the radiopharmaceutical agent used (Fischbach et al., 2022).

PET provides physiologic, anatomic, and biochemical data and is useful for measuring myocardial blood flow and perfusion as well as detecting CAD (Fischbach et al., 2022). During PET, tracers are administered IV; one compound is used to determine blood flow in the myocardium, and another determines the metabolic function. The radionuclides used in PET scans have very short half-lives (2 minutes to 2 hours) (Fischbach et al., 2022). The PET camera provides detailed three-dimensional images of the distributed compounds. The viability of the myocardium is determined by comparing the extent of glucose metabolism in the myocardium to the degree of blood flow. For example, ischemic but viable tissue will show decreased blood flow and elevated metabolism. For a patient with this finding, revascularization through surgery or PCIs will probably be indicated to improve heart function. Restrictions of food intake before the test vary among institutions, but because PET evaluates glucose metabolism, the patient’s blood glucose level should be within the normal range before testing. It is recommended that the patient fasts for 6 hours before the scan. The procedure requires the patient to lie still during the PET scan. PET imaging is often combined with computed tomography (CT) scans (PET/CT).

The patient undergoing nuclear imaging techniques with stress testing should be prepared for the type of stressor to be used (exercise or drug) and the type of imaging technique (SPECT or PET). The patient may be concerned about receiving a radioactive substance and needs to be reassured that these tracers are safe—the radiation exposure is similar to that of other diagnostic x-ray studies. No postprocedure radiation precautions are necessary.

Test of Ventricular Function and Wall Motion

Equilibrium radionuclide angiocardiography (ERNA), also known as multiple-gated acquisition (MUGA) scanning, is a noninvasive technique that uses a radioactive isotope tracer and a conventional scintillation camera interfaced with a computer to record images of the heart during several hundred heartbeats. The computer processes the data and allows for sequential images of the functioning heart. These images are analyzed to evaluate left ventricular function, wall motion, and EF. This scanning procedure can be used to assess for differences in left ventricular function during rest and exercise. The patient is reassured that the radiation exposure is minimal and is instructed to remain motionless during the scan. It is recommended that the patient fast for 3 to 4 hours before the scan (Fischbach et al., 2022). The duration of the examination is approximately 30 to 45 minutes.

Echocardiography

Traditional Echocardiography

Echocardiography, a noninvasive ultrasound test, is used to examine cardiac structures and function, including the size of the chambers, the thickness of the ventricular walls, and any structural abnormalities. It also allows for an assessment of contractility and left ventricular EF (Fischbach et al., 2022).

Procedure. A handheld transducer generates high-frequency sound waves through the chest wall into the heart and records the return signals for display on an oscilloscope and recording on a videotape. An ECG is recorded simultaneously to assist with interpreting the echocardiogram.

It is often combined with Doppler ultrasound and color Doppler to evaluate the direction and velocity across the heart's valves. Three-dimensional echocardiography is a newer technique that allows for the assessment of chamber volumes, valvular abnormalities, and other structural pathologies (Fischbach et al., 2022).

Nursing Interventions. The nurse prepares the patient for the test by explaining that it is a painless procedure and that the transducer emits sound waves as it is moved across the surface of the chest wall. Gel applied to the skin helps transmit the sound waves. Periodically, the patient is asked to turn onto the left side or hold a breath. The test takes about 30 to 45 minutes.

Transesophageal Echocardiography

Procedure. Transesophageal echocardiography (TEE) involves threading a small transducer through the mouth and into the esophagus via an endoscope. This technique provides clearer images than other ultrasound methods because ultrasound waves are passed through less dense tissue. It is an important diagnostic tool for determining if atrial or ventricular thrombi are present in patients with HF, valvular heart disease, and arrhythmias. It is also useful to assess function of prosthetic valves, diagnose endocarditis, evaluate valvular regurgitation and congenital abnormalities, and examine the aorta for dissecting aneurysms.

Typically, a topical anesthetic is sprayed onto the pharynx and IV sedation is used during a TEE because of the discomfort associated with the positioning of the transducer. Once the patient is sedated, the transducer is inserted into the mouth and the patient is asked to swallow several times until it is positioned in the esophagus.

Complications are uncommon during TEE, but if they do occur, they are serious. These complications are caused by sedation and impaired swallowing resulting from the topical anesthesia (respiratory depression and aspiration) and by insertion and manipulation of the transducer into the esophagus and stomach (vasovagal response or esophageal perforation). The patient must be assessed before TEE for a history of dysphagia (difficulty swallowing) or radiation therapy to the chest, which increases the risk of complications.

Nursing Interventions. Prior to the test, the nurse provides preprocedural education and ensures that patients have a clear understanding of what the test entails and why it is being performed. Patients are instructed not to eat or drink anything for 4 to 6 hours before the study; that an IV will be inserted to administer medications, including a sedative to keep the patient comfortable; and that after the removal of dentures, a topical anesthetic agent is used to numb the throat. After the procedure, the nurse informs patients that they will remain in bed with the head of the bed elevated to 45 degrees and will be offered something to drink as soon as they recover from the sedation and swallow, cough, and gag reflexes have returned. Patients are reminded that a sore throat may be present for the next 24 hours. They are to report the presence of a persistent sore throat, SOB, or difficulty swallowing. If the procedure is performed in an outpatient setting, patients must have someone transport them home.

The nurse follows the organization's moderate sedation policy. During the test, the nurse provides emotional support and monitors the patient's comfort level, level of consciousness, BP, ECG, respiration, and oxygen saturation (SpO_2). Liquids and food are withheld until patients are fully alert and the effect of the topical anesthetic agent is reversed; swallowing reflexes may be diminished for several hours. Once the patient begins taking liquids, the patient should be assessed for dysphagia.

Cardiac Catheterization

This invasive diagnostic procedure uses fluoroscopy (an imaging technique that visualizes the heart on an x-ray screen) to guide catheter placement into the heart to view the chambers and coronary arteries. This procedure is usually performed in the outpatient setting, unless the condition of the patient is serious enough to require hospitalization, such as HF or acute MI. There are no absolute definitive contraindications for cardiac catheterization (Manda & Baradhi, 2021).

Cardiac catheterization is the gold standard for diagnosing CAD and quantifying the extent of coronary artery obstruction (reported as a percentage). Cardiac catheterization is also used to diagnose pulmonary hypertension and valvular heart disease. Results of this procedure are used to determine if revascularization procedures (PCI or coronary artery bypass surgery) or valve replacement/repair are indicated. In preparation for the procedure, patients have blood tests performed to evaluate metabolic function (electrolytes and glucose) and renal function (blood urea nitrogen and creatinine levels). Baseline coagulation studies (activated thromboplastin time, international normalized ratio (INR), and prothrombin time) are obtained to guide dosing of anticoagulation during the procedure. An ECG and chest x-ray are also obtained. Because bleeding and hematoma formation are procedure risks, a complete blood cell count (Hct, hemoglobin, platelets) is necessary to establish baseline values. Later, these results are compared with postprocedure results to monitor for blood loss. Routine, scheduled medications, such as cardiac drugs or insulin, are administered before the procedure unless directed otherwise. Patients who are managed on warfarin are informed to discontinue the medication 1 to 2 days before the procedure (depending on renal function). Patients will have their INR evaluated preprocedure. If the radial site is selected for the test, the target INR range of 2.0 to 2.5 may be recommended the morning of the procedure, whereas if the femoral artery is selected, the target range of the INR may be below 2 (Holmes & Sarafoff, 2022). For patients with diabetes, metformin is discontinued 2 to 3 days before the cardiac catheterization because of the potential development of lactic acidosis; normal renal function should be confirmed before the medication is restarted after the procedure. In addition, it is important that the nurse documents the neurovascular status of both upper and lower extremities so that a baseline assessment is available for comparison postprocedure. Patients are on nothing-by-mouth (NPO) orders for at least 6 hours, and an IV is established for sedation, fluids, heparin, and other medications. BP and multiple ECG leads are monitored to observe for hemodynamic instability and arrhythmias, and pulse oximetry is used to monitor respiratory status.

Prior to the procedure, patients having experienced a reaction to contrast agents are premedicated with antihistamines and steroids. Contrast agents can induce contrast-induced nephropathy (CIN), a form of acute kidney injury (AKI) in patients who have diabetes, HF, renal insufficiency or renal disease, hypotension, dehydration, left ventricular dysfunction, and anemia. It is the third leading cause of iatrogenic AKI (Modi et al., 2022). Patients at risk for CIN-AKI receive pre- and postprocedure preventive strategies. IV hydration increases vascular volume and facilitates removal of contrast from the kidneys. Administration of sodium bicarbonate aids in protecting the renal tubules from an acidic environment by alkalinizing the renal tubular fluid; it may be administered before and during the procedure (Modi et al., 2022). Advise the patient that they may feel a pumping sensation, feel warmth or hot flash for 30 to 60 seconds, and have a metallic taste for a few seconds during injection of contrast medium (Fischbach et al., 2022). Angina may occur when the contrast agent is injected. In addition, an important role of the nurse is to prepare the patient and family for the cardiac catheterization. Box 11-4 outlines the information that should be reviewed prior to the procedure.

BOX 11-4 **Patient Education**

Preparing for a Cardiac Catheterization

Goal: To ensure adequate preparation for the procedure

- Ask patients about any concerns or fears they have about the procedure.
- Remind patients to fast for at least 6 hours before the procedure.
- Understand the procedure involves lying on a hard table for about an hour.
- Assure patient that medications will be given to maintain comfort.
- Tell patients that they may experience palpitations due to extra heartbeats that can occur as the catheter is advanced through the heart. Flushing and a sensation similar to the need to void may occur after injection of the contrast agent, which subsides in 1 minute or less.

Procedure

Right-Heart Catheterization. Right-heart catheterization is performed to evaluate pressures and oxygen saturations in the chambers of the right side of the heart and the function of the tricuspid and pulmonary valves. Since it is evaluating the right side of the heart, venous access is needed. It involves the passage of a catheter from the medial cubital, brachial, or femoral vein into the right atrium, right ventricle, and PA. Complications, though rare, include arrhythmias, infection, and perforation of the septum or chamber wall.

Left-Heart Catheterization. Left-heart catheterization is performed to evaluate the patency of the coronary arteries and the function of the left ventricle and the mitral and aortic valves. It is performed by the insertion of a catheter into the radial or femoral artery that is advanced into the aorta, left ventricle, and coronary arteries. If the radial artery approach is selected, the Allen test is performed to confirm adequate collateral circulation to the hand (discussed later in this chapter). The radial artery approach is associated with reduction in major bleeding, access-related complications, mortality, and major adverse cardiac events (Manda & Baradhi, 2021). Rare complications include arrhythmias, acute MI, perforation of the heart or great vessels, and systemic embolization.

Angiography. Angiography involves the injection of a contrast agent into the vascular system to visualize the heart and blood vessels. *Coronary angiography* is produced through the injection of the contrast agent into the coronary arteries to determine patency. An *aortogram* is produced through the injection of the contrast agent to highlight the aorta and its major arteries.

Arterial Hemostasis. Once the arterial catheter is removed, either manual pressure or vascular closure devices such as self-absorbing sutures or hemostasis-promoting pads or patches are used to achieve hemostasis. Major benefits of the vascular closure devices include immediate hemostasis, less pressure, and a shorter time on bed rest. Rare complications associated with these devices include bleeding around the closure device, infection, and arterial obstruction.

Nursing Interventions

After cardiac catheterization, the nurse:

- Assesses the catheter access site frequently for bleeding or hematoma formation. The incidence of this complication is significantly reduced if radial access was selected. If femoral artery access was used, the nurse should suspect retroperitoneal bleeding if there is a sudden change in the patient's hemodynamic status (significant change in vital signs) with or without back pain. The nurse is aware that in some patients, there may not be any visible swelling in the groin. If hematoma develops, notify the provider and apply direct pressure to the site. Many patients are treated with a reversal of anticoagulation, application of manual compression and volume resuscitation, and observation. Some patients need coiling of the bleeding vessel, balloon angioplasty, or covered stents for bleeding from larger vessels (Manda & Baradhi, 2021). Assess for a pulsatile mass at the site selected for the procedure and a new bruit, which indicates turbulent blood flow and is associated with a pseudoaneurysm; this happens when the hematoma maintains continuity with the lumen of the artery. Ultrasound Doppler imaging or CT angiography diagnoses a pseudoaneurysm. If it is less than 2 to 3 cm in size, it may heal spontaneously (Manda & Baradhi, 2021).

- Assesses for arrhythmias using cardiac monitoring or by assessing the apical and peripheral pulses for a pulse deficit. The nurse observes for ventricular arrhythmias, which may be related to irritation or ischemia of the myocardium by the procedure; these are treated with antiarrhythmic drugs. In addition, a vagal response, causing bradycardia and hypotension, can be triggered by discomfort from manual pressure used to obtain hemostasis as the arterial or venous catheter is removed. It is reversed by infusing IV fluid and administering IV atropine to treat the bradycardia as prescribed.
- Maintains the patient on bed rest after the procedure until hemostasis of the involved blood vessels is achieved, which is based upon variables such as catheter insertion site, size of the catheter used, anticoagulation status of the patient, and other patient variables (e.g., advanced age, obesity, bleeding disorder). Variations exist in time on bed rest and range from 2 to 8 hours. If the femoral artery was accessed, bed rest is maintained for up to 6 hours with the affected leg straight and the head elevated to 30 degrees. The head is not elevated more than 30 degrees to prevent undue strain on the insertion site (Fischbach et al., 2022). For comfort, the patient may be turned from side to side with the affected extremity straight. If a percutaneous closure device or patch was deployed, the nurse reviews local nursing care standards and anticipates that the patient will have fewer activity restrictions. Analgesic medication is administered for discomfort.
- Instructs the patient to report chest pain and bleeding or sudden discomfort from the catheter insertion sites immediately.
- Assesses for CIN-AKI by monitoring for an increase in creatinine levels. An increase of serum creatinine of at least 0.5 mg/dL or a 25% increase from baseline within 48 to 72 hours after contrast exposure is considered CIN. In CIN, the creatinine usually begins to rise within 24 hours after the administration of contrast agent, peaks between 3 and 5 days, and returns to baseline in 7 to 10 days (Modi et al., 2022). The nurse maintains IV fluid and bicarbonate administration as prescribed, and accurate intake and output are recorded.
- Assesses peripheral perfusion of the involved limb, including peripheral pulses, capillary refill, and neurovascular status per institution policy until discharge, as embolization is infrequent but can cause limb or end-organ ischemia. Any change in peripheral perfusion is reported immediately as indicated during assessment of color, motion, sensation, capillary refill times, temperature, and pulse quality.
- Ensures patient safety by instructing the patient to ask for help when getting out of bed the first time. The patient is assessed for bleeding from the catheter access site and for orthostatic hypotension.
- Provides patients with additional instructions at time of discharge (Box 11-5).

Hemodynamic Monitoring

Hemodynamic monitoring continuously assesses the cardiovascular function of patients who are critically ill. It requires a special catheter and pressure monitoring system composed of a continuous flushing device to maintain catheter patency, a transducer to convert the pressure coming from the artery or

BOX 11-5 **Patient Education**

Self-Management After Cardiac Catheterization

Goal: To ensure that patients have information they need to reduce the risk of postprocedure complications and to understand their treatment plan.

- For the next 24 hours, do not bend at the waist, strain, or lift heavy objects.
- If the radial artery was used, avoid sleeping on the affected arm for 24 hours and refrain from repetitive movement of the affected extremity for 24 to 48 hours.
- Avoid tub baths, but shower as desired.
- Ask your provider about when you may resume your usual activities.
- Call your provider if you have any bleeding, swelling, new bruising, or pain from your procedure puncture site, or a temperature of 101.5°F (38.6°C) or more.
- Talk with your provider about getting assistance with lifestyle changes to reduce your risk for future heart problems. If test results show that you have CAD, ask your provider to refer you to a local cardiac rehabilitation program.
- Your provider may prescribe new medications. If you suspect that any of these are causing side effects, call your provider immediately. Do not stop taking any medications before talking to your provider.

heart chamber into an electrical signal, and a monitor, which displays the pressure waveform on a bedside oscilloscope.

Procedure

Central Venous Pressure Monitoring. CVP is measured by positioning a catheter in the vena cava (superior or inferior) or right atrium. It reflects right ventricle preload because pressure in the vena cava, right atrium, and right ventricle are all equal at the end of diastole. Normal CVP is 2 to 8 mm Hg. A CVP of greater than 8 mm Hg indicates hypervolemia (excessive fluid circulating in the body) or right-sided HF. On the contrary, a CVP of less than 2 mm Hg indicates a reduction in preload or hypovolemia. Complications of CVP monitoring are infection, pneumothorax, and air embolism.

Pulmonary Artery Pressure Monitoring. PA pressure monitoring involves the use of a balloon-tipped catheter that is inserted through a large vein (subclavian, jugular, or femoral) and connected to the pressure monitoring system (Fig. 11-13). The catheter is threaded through the right side of the heart

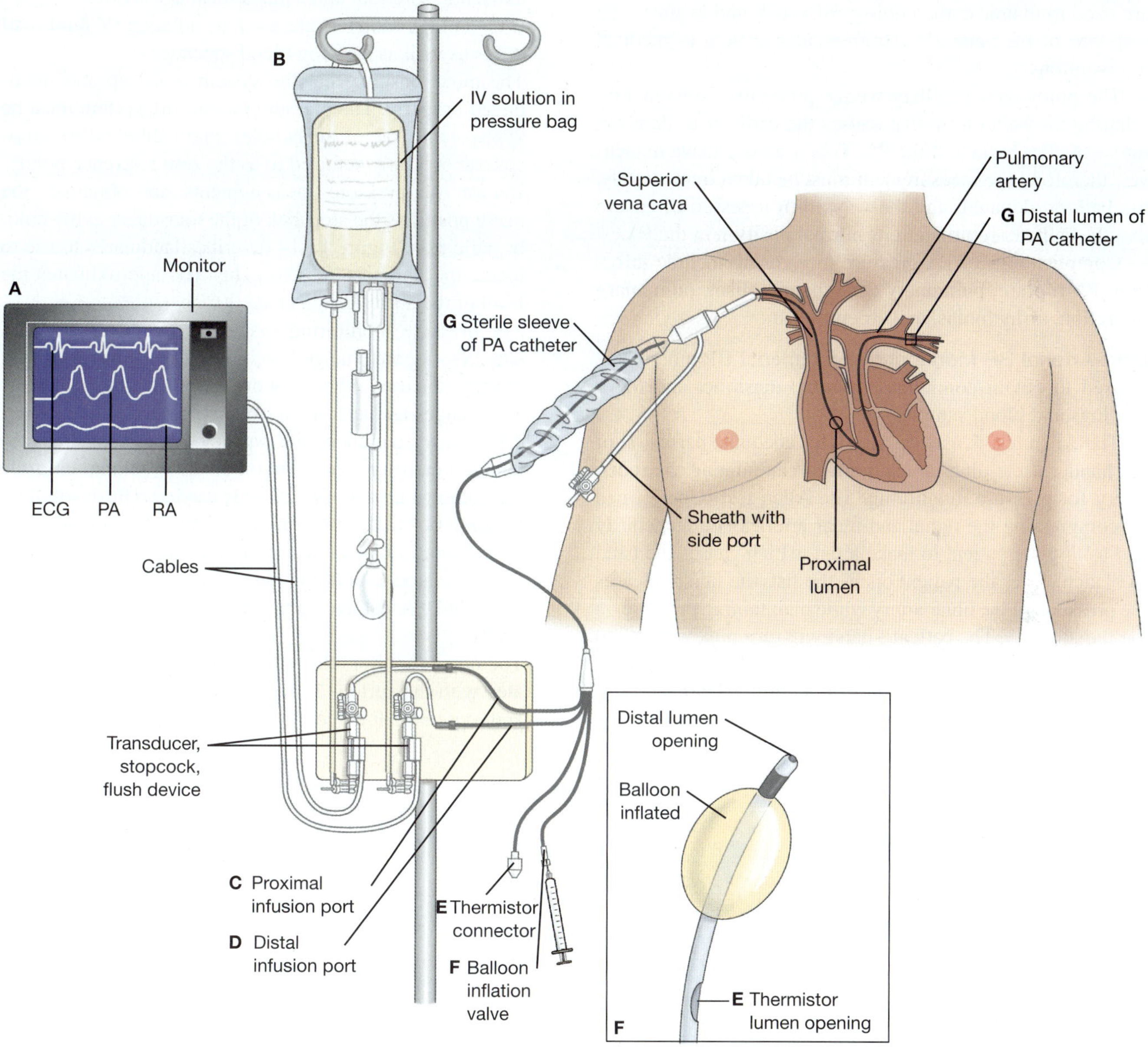

FIGURE 11-13 **Pulmonary artery (PA) catheter and pressure monitoring systems. A. Bedside monitor that connects with cables to (B) the pressure monitoring systems (includes IV solution in a pressure bag, IV tubing, and two transducers with stopcocks and flush devices). This system connects to (C) the proximal infusion port that opens in the right atria and is used to infuse fluids or medications and monitor central venous pressures and (D) the distal infusion port. This port opens in the PA and is used to monitor PA pressures. E. The thermistor connector is attached to the bedside cardiac monitor to obtain cardiac output. F. An air-filled syringe is attached to the balloon inflation valve during catheter insertion and measurement of PA wedge pressure. G. PA catheter positioned in the PA. Note the sterile sleeve over the PA catheter. The PA catheter is threaded through the sheath until it reaches the desired position in the PA. The side port on the sheath is used to infuse medications or fluids. ECG, electrocardiogram; RA, right atrium.**

into the PA. It is used in patients who are critically ill to measure the cardiac output as well as the right atrial, PA systolic and diastolic, and pulmonary capillary wedge pressures (see Fig. 11-7 for normal pressures).

The PA diastolic and PA wedge pressures are used most often because they reflect left ventricular preload. These readings are possible because at the end of diastole, when the ventricle is completely filled and the mitral valve is open, there is equalization of pressure within all left heart chambers and vessels (left ventricle and atrium, pulmonary veins and arteries). The PA diastolic and PA wedge pressures are used to diagnose the etiology of shock and evaluate the response of the patient's cardiovascular system to medical interventions.

The pulmonary capillary wedge pressure is obtained by inflating the balloon tip that causes the catheter to float out into a smaller branch of the PA. This is an occlusive maneuver; therefore, the measurement must be taken immediately, the balloon deflated, and the waveform assessed to ensure that the catheter returned to its normal position in the PA.

Complications of PA pressure monitoring include infection, PA rupture, pulmonary thromboembolism, pulmonary infarction, arrhythmias, and air embolism.

Intra-Arterial BP Monitoring. Intra-arterial BP monitoring is used to obtain continuous systolic, diastolic, and MAP readings and blood samples.

The Allen test is used to assess for adequate perfusion of the hand via the ulnar artery prior to cannulating the radial artery for pressure monitoring. The Allen test is performed by compressing the radial and ulnar arteries simultaneously and asking the patient to make a fist, which causes the hand to blanch. After the patient opens the fist, the nurse releases the pressure on the ulnar artery while maintaining pressure on the radial artery. The patient's hand will turn pink within 3 to 5 seconds if the ulnar artery is patent (Bickley et al., 2021). If other arteries are selected for cannulation, a Doppler ultrasound is used to assess perfusion to the involved limb.

Complications associated with arterial monitoring include arterial obstruction with distal ischemia, hemorrhage, air embolism, arteriospasm, and infection.

Nursing Interventions

Nurses receive comprehensive training prior to using hemodynamic monitoring technologies. The following guidelines are used to ensure safe and effective care:

- The insertion site is prepared following hospital policy, which includes clipping excessive hair, cleansing with an antiseptic solution, and using a local anesthetic.
- CVP and PA catheters are used for infusing IV fluids and drugs as well as drawing blood specimens.
- The nurse ensures that the system is set up and maintained properly. The pressure monitoring system must be kept patent, free of air bubbles, and calibrated to atmospheric pressure (referred to as the zero reference point).
- Before the pressure measurements are obtained, the nurse positions the stopcock of the transducer at the phlebostatic axis. Figure 11-14 describes landmarks to use to locate the phlebostatic axis. This axis approximates the level of the atria (Lough et al., 2022).
- The pressure monitoring system and catheter insertion site dressing are changed according to hospital policy. In general, the dressing is kept dry and air-occlusive. Dressing changes are performed using sterile technique.
- The flush system maintains patency of the fluid-filled system and catheter. The solution of 0.9% sodium chloride (also known as *normal saline*) is used as a flush solution. In some hospitals, heparin is added as an anticoagulant. A pressure infusion cuff covers the bag of flush solution and is inflated to 300 mm Hg.
- CVP and PA catheter placement is confirmed by chest x-ray.
- The nurse monitors the patient for complications associated with the various forms of hemodynamic monitoring and reports findings immediately.

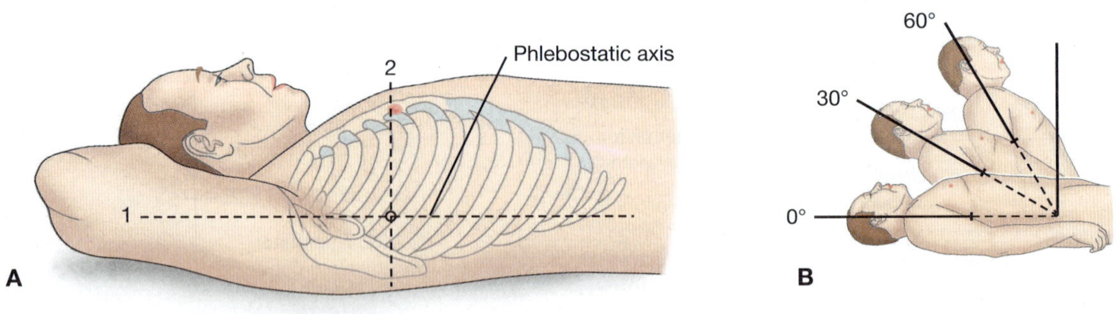

FIGURE 11-14 **A. The phlebostatic axis is the reference point for the atrium when the patient is in supine position. It is the intersection of two lines on the left chest wall: (1) the midaxillary line drawn between the anterior and posterior surfaces of the chest and (2) the line drawn through the fourth intercostal space. Its location is identified with a skin marker. The stopcock of the transducer used in hemodynamic monitoring is "leveled" at this mark prior to obtaining pressure measurements. B. Measurements can be taken with the head of the bed (HOB) elevated to 60 degrees. Note the phlebostatic axis changes as the HOB is elevated so that the stopcock and the transducer must be repositioned after each position change.**

Doppler Ultrasound Flow Studies

Doppler ultrasound studies are most often used to detect obstruction of blood flow to the extremities or head due to a thrombus and determine if atherosclerosis is present in the lower extremities in patients with intermittent claudication. This technology uses a handheld device, called a *transducer*, which sends and receives sound waves that "echo" or bounce off blood cells. The transducer is placed in contact with the skin over the blood vessel being examined. Normally, the transducer detects rhythmic changes in the sound waves that are generated as blood cells flow through patent blood vessels. Obstruction to blood flow is evidenced by no change in sound waves.

Standard Doppler ultrasound studies are combined with computer technology to provide additional information about blood flow. Duplex Doppler ultrasound provides a picture of the blood vessel and a graph describing the speed and direction of blood flow, and color Doppler ultrasound produces colors to visualize these dimensions of blood flow.

When the nurse has difficulty finding a pulse, the continuous wave Doppler, a portable device, can be used. This device is used to hear, rather than feel the pulse. Box 11-6 describes how to use the continuous wave Doppler to evaluate pulses in the lower extremities.

The continuous wave Doppler is also used to obtain systolic BPs in the extremities to calculate the **ankle-brachial index (ABI)**. This ratio compares the ankle-to-arm systolic BPs and is an indicator of perfusion to the lower extremities. It is recommended that the ABI be measured in those who smoke and are over 50 years old, patients with diabetes over age 50, and anyone older than 70. The patient should rest supine for 10 to 20 minutes before the procedure. Place the ankle blood pressure cuff just above the malleoli (immediately above the ankle). Locate the posterior tibial pulse with the Doppler, and inflate the cuff 20 to 30 mm Hg above the number at which the pulse is last heard. Slowly release the pressure until the pulse is heard. This is the systolic pressure. Repeat the procedure using the dorsalis pedis pulse (Bickley et al., 2021). An ABI is calculated for each leg. The ABI for each lower extremity is calculated by selecting the higher of the two ankle systolic pressures (obtained from both the posterior tibial and dorsalis pedis arteries) and dividing it by the higher of the right and left brachial systolic pressures (Stanford Medicine 25, 2021). For example, the patient's right brachial systolic pressure is 160 mm Hg, and the right posterior tibial systolic pressure is 80 mm Hg. Therefore, 80/160 = 0.5 ABI.

$$\text{Right ABI} = \frac{\text{Highest Pressure in Right Foot}}{\text{Highest Pressure in Both Arms}}$$

The ankle systolic pressure is normally the same or slightly higher than the brachial systolic pressure, resulting in an ABI of 1 to 1.4. An ABI greater than 1.4 suggests a noncompressible calcified vessel, whereas an ABI lower than 0.9 is considered diagnostic of PAD. As PAD progresses, the systolic BP in the ankle of the affected extremity decreases. An ABI of 0.8 to 0.99 indicates mild PAD; 0.5 to 0.8 indicates moderate PAD (claudication present); and less than 0.5 indicates severe PAD (pain at rest).

BOX 11-6

Evaluating Lower Extremity Pulse Using a Continuous Wave Doppler

The patient is placed in a supine position for 10 minutes with the head of the bed elevated to 20 to 30 degrees; the legs are externally rotated to permit adequate access to the medial malleolus. Acoustic gel is applied to the skin to permit uniform transmission of the ultrasound wave (do not use ECG gel). The tip of the Doppler transducer is positioned at a 45- to 60-degree angle over the expected location of the artery and angled slowly to identify arterial blood flow. Avoid using excessive pressure as diseased arteries can collapse if too much pressure is applied over the artery.

CHAPTER REVIEW

NCLEX-Style Review Questions

1. A patient who was admitted with heart failure exhibits these hemodynamic parameters: CVP 15 mm Hg; BP 90/50 mm Hg; pulse 132 bpm; respirations 36 breaths per minute. What are the therapy goals for this patient? Select all that apply.
   a. To decrease myocardial workload
   b. To decrease preload
   c. To increase myocardial contractility
   d. To increase myocardial workload
   e. To increase preload
   f. To decrease myocardial contractility

2. A patient has 4+ pitting edema of the lower extremities and sacral area. Select all the possible reasons for this excess accumulation of interstitial fluid.
   a. IV infiltration
   b. Septicemia
   c. Deep vein thrombosis (DVT)
   d. Liver failure
   e. HF
   f. Hypoalbuminemia

3. A patient calls the visiting nurse complaining of a 4-lb weight gain in the past 48 hours despite maintaining their typical daily diet. Select the symptoms that you will inquire about that suggest HF.

a. Dyspnea
b. Constipation
c. Shoes or rings that are tight
d. No difficulty in the supine position
e. Fatigue
f. Paroxysmal nocturnal dyspnea

4. A 45-year-old patient with a history of diabetes, hypertension, and cigarette smoking comes into the emergency department via ambulance. From the table below, select the top three patient findings that require follow-up, the condition that would be the primary concern, and the immediate nursing interventions.

Patient Findings	Condition Patient is Most Likely Experiencing	Nursing Actions to Take
Diaphoresis	Acute coronary syndrome (ACS)	Repeat vital signs including SpO_2
SOB	Community-acquired pneumonia	Connect to hardwire cardiac monitor.
BP of 118/76 mm Hg	Aortic dissection	Insert a Foley catheter for output measurement.
Capillary refill of 2 seconds	Gastroesophageal reflux disease (GERD)	Obtain a 12-lead ECG.
Irregular pulse of 110 bpm		Expect to draw a stat myoglobin level.

5. A patient has just undergone a cardiac catheterization using the right radial artery. The patient is entering the recovery area and you are the nurse accepting this patient. Select the patient findings that are of concern to you, the condition you believe the patient is experiencing, and the action(s) you are expected to take.

Patient Findings	Condition Patient is Most Likely Experiencing	Nursing Actions to Take
Positive history of renal insufficiency	Pseudoaneurysm of radial artery	Strict intake and output
Baseline creatinine of 1.2 mg/dL	Pulmonary emboli	Monitor for elevation of creatinine by 0.2 mg/dL in 24 hours
Urinary output of <0.5 mL/kg/hr	Contrast-induced nephropathy (CIN)	IV hydration with normal saline (0.9% NaCl)
Blood glucose of 101 mg/dL	Chronic kidney disease	Obtain stat 12-lead ECG
Hypotension during the cardiac catheterization		Sodium bicarbonate administration

REFERENCES AND SELECTED READINGS

References and selected readings associated with this chapter can be found on the website that accompanies the book. Visit **http://thepoint.lww.com/Honan3e** to access the references and other additional resources associated with this chapter.

CHAPTER 12

Nursing Management: Patients With Hypertension

Carol Ann Wetmore

Learning Objectives

After reading this chapter, you will be able to:

1. Compare and contrast the continuum of normotension, hypertension, and hypertensive urgency and hypertensive emergency.
2. Assess for risk factors for primary and secondary hypertension.
3. Correlate pathophysiology of hypertension to complications in target organs.
4. Identify nursing management of patients with hypertension risk factors and hypertension, including lifestyle changes and pharmacologic therapy.
5. Summarize management of the patient experiencing hypertensive emergency.
6. Incorporate current evidence when caring for the patient with hypertension risk factors and hypertension.

Hypertension, or elevated blood pressure (BP), is a serious medical condition that significantly increases the risks of heart, brain, kidney, and other diseases. An estimated 1.28 billion adults aged 30 to 79 years worldwide have hypertension, and it is also increasingly a problem of older school-aged children and adolescents that has increased in prevalence in parallel with the obesity epidemic (Al Kibria et al., 2019; Macumber & Flynn, 2020; World Health Organization [WHO], n.d.). An estimated 46% of adults with hypertension are unaware that they have the condition and fewer than half of adults (42%) with hypertension are diagnosed and treated (Centers for Disease Control and Prevention [CDC], 2021). Even fewer, approximately one in five, adults (21%) with hypertension have it under control (WHO, n.d.). High BP was a primary or contributing cause of death for more than 670,000 deaths in the United States in 2020 (CDC, 2022a). Hypertension remains one of the most important public health problems in the United States, affecting 46% of adults with increased risk for progressive vascular and renal damage, which increases the risk of cardiovascular diseases (CVDs), such as ischemic and hemorrhagic stroke (Leite et al., 2022; Rodríguez-Lesmes, 2021). High BP costs the United States about $131 billion each year (Kirkland et al., 2018). Worldwide, controlling BP levels is one of the most cost-effective methods for reducing premature mortality. The importance of preventive care, consistent screening, and careful management for improving BP management by primary providers cannot be overstated (Rodríguez-Lesmes, 2021).

High BP is often called the "silent killer" because it usually has no warning signs or symptoms, and many people do not know they have it (American Heart Association [AHA], n.d.). Most people with high BP have no signs or symptoms, even if BP readings reach dangerously high levels. A few people with high BP may have headaches, shortness of breath, or nosebleeds (epistaxis), but these signs and symptoms are not specific and usually do not occur until high BP has reached a severe or life-threatening stage (Wenzel et al., 2020). Undiagnosed, untreated, or undertreated hypertension may lead to target organ damage causing myocardial infarction (MI), heart failure, damaged and narrowed arteries, aneurysms, kidney damage or failure, stroke, dementia, and hypertensive retinopathy (Cameron, 2019) (National Heart, Lung, and Blood Institute [NHLBI], 2022).

Pearls for Practice

The nurse understands that target organ or end-organ damage refers to the changes to organs that are dependent on the circulatory system, such as the heart, kidneys, brain, and eyes. Target organ or end-organ damage can result in coronary heart disease/myocardial infarction and heart failure (heart); proteinuria and renal failure (kidneys); vascular and hemorrhagic stroke (brain); retinopathy (eyes); and, in the vasculature, atherosclerotic changes in the blood vessels including the development of stenoses and aneurysms. This damage is associated with uncontrolled hypertension but can also be related to hypotension or hypovolemia, when limited blood flow damages the organs.

Pearls for Practice

Every 10 years, the U.S. Department of Health and Human Services (USDHHS) provides scientific insights and lessons from the decade, along with new knowledge from current data, trends, and innovations. Healthy People 2030 reflects assessments of major risks to health and wellness, changing public priorities, and emerging issues related to national preparedness and prevention (Office of Disease Prevention and Health Promotion [ODPHP], 2020).

HYPERTENSION

The AHA and American College of Cardiology (ACC) published the latest standards regarding hypertension guidelines that cover aspects of the diagnosis, evaluation, monitoring, secondary causes, and drug and nondrug treatment of hypertension. In particular, emphasis was made on strategies for accurate measurement of BP in all settings where valid BP measurements are desired (Flack & Adekola, 2020). In 2017, the ACC/AHA published guidelines for prevention, detection, evaluation, and management of high BP in adults, and the criteria for hypertension diagnosis based on office BP was modified to a systolic BP ≥130 mm Hg and diastolic BP ≥80 mm Hg (compared to the previous threshold of ≥140/90 mm Hg); in 2019, the ACC/AHA issued guidelines on primary prevention of CVD—they recommend a BP target of lower than 130/80 mm Hg for most patients (Flack & Adekola, 2020). The BP categories are detailed in Table 12-1. It is important to remember that these categories should not be based on BP readings at a single point in time but rather should be confirmed by two or more readings (averaged) made on at least two separate occasions. Individuals are classified according to their highest systolic or diastolic BP category, and if a difference of >10 mm Hg between the limbs exists, the higher pressure limb reading is used. In particular, BP readings should also be documented in out-of-office settings, like the home or via ambulatory BP monitoring, for comparison with office BP readings (Flack & Adekola, 2020). There is evidence that a patient's visit-to-visit blood pressure variability (BPV) is an independent risk factor for hypertensive target organ damage and cardiovascular events. It is unclear whether the excess cardiovascular risk associated with BPV is a direct result of the mechanical effect of BP variations or merely reflects the fact that the abnormal cardiovascular regulatory mechanisms that lead to higher visit-to-visit BPV also cause higher CV event rates (McAlister et al., 2021). Repeat readings and at-home or community monitoring of BP is important for these patients. It is important that the patient's cuff is checked for accuracy and cuff size (discussed later in this chapter).

Pathophysiology

The arterial BP is the force that moves blood through the arterial system, reflecting the intermittent contraction and relaxation of the left ventricle. It is determined by factors including blood volume, elastic properties of the blood vessels, cardiac output (CO), and peripheral vascular resistance (PVR; Norris, 2019).

The arterial BP represents the force that distributes blood throughout the body. The highest arterial pressure is the systolic pressure (corresponding with ventricular contraction), and the lowest is the diastolic pressure (corresponding with ventricular relaxation and filling). The systolic BP reflects the combined factors of the volume of blood ejected from the ventricles with each beat (stroke volume [SV]); the rate and force with which the blood is ejected; and the elasticity, or compliance, of the aorta and large arteries. The diastolic

TABLE **12-1 Classification of Blood Pressure (BP) in Adults**

BP Category	Systolic BP (mm Hg)		Diastolic BP (mm Hg)
Normal	Less than 120	and	Less than 80
Elevated	120–129	or	Less than 80
Hypertension			
Stage 1	130–139	or	80–89
Stage 2	140 or higher	or	90 or higher
Hypertensive urgency	>180	or	120 without signs and symptoms of end-organ damage
Hypertensive emergency	>180	or	120 mm Hg and objective findings of acute end-organ dysfunction (usually of the heart, kidneys, or brain).

Individuals with SBP and DBP in 2 categories should be designated to the higher BP category.

BP indicates blood pressure based on an average of ≥2 careful readings obtained on ≥2 occasions; DBP, diastolic blood pressure; SBP, systolic blood pressure (Carey & Whelton, 2018; Whelton et al., 2018).

BP reflects the combined factors of the closure of the aortic valve, the energy that has been stored in the elastic fibers of the large arteries during systole, and the resistance to flow through arterioles into the capillaries. Closure of the aortic valve at the onset of diastole and recoil of the elastic fibers in the aorta and large arteries continue to drive the blood forward, even though the ventricles are not contracting. These effects, in the elastic vessels, convert the pulsatile systolic flow in the ascending aorta into a continuous, nonpulsating flow in the peripheral arteries and arterioles (Norris, 2019).

Pearls for Practice

The systolic pressure is the peak pressure that occurs with ventricular contraction forcing blood under high pressure into the aorta and to the arteries that feed the body. Diastolic pressure occurs with relaxation of the ventricles; it is the pressure of the remaining blood (at rest) exerting pressure against the arterial walls.

For hypertension to develop, there must be a change in one or more factors affecting PVR or CO, and there must also be a problem with the body's control systems that monitor or regulate pressure. An elevation in BP increases the workload of the left ventricle by increasing the pressure against which the heart must pump as it ejects blood into the systemic circulation. This increased pressure increases the workload of the heart and, over time, the left ventricular wall remodels (changes) and hypertrophies (becomes thicker) to compensate for the increased work. This left ventricular hypertrophy is a major risk factor for coronary heart disease, cardiac arrhythmias, sudden death, and heart failure because it cannot pump efficiently (Norris, 2019). Management of hypertension aims to decrease PVR or blood volume, or the strength, force, and rate of myocardial contraction.

BP has circadian variations and tends to be highest shortly after awakening and then decreases throughout the day, reaching the lowest point between 2 AM and 5 AM. Nocturnal BP tends to decline by 10% to 20%. Decreases in nocturnal dipping of BP have been shown to be a useful predictor of the likelihood of adverse cardiovascular events. A decline in nocturnal BP dipping, such as what occurs in people who repetitively have shortened sleep periods or people who do not get adequate sleep, serves as a stronger predictor of adverse cardiac effects than daytime BP levels (Cheng et al., 2021; Norris, 2019; Ogugu et al., 2022). Methods to evaluate the BP include ambulatory blood pressure monitoring (ABPM), which involves wearing a BP cuff on the arm that is attached to a small recording device and is worn for 24 hours, allowing measurements during a variety of activities, and has been associated with temporary sleep disturbance and extremity bruising (Guirguis-Blake et al., 2021). Home blood pressure monitoring (HBPM) is when patients monitor their own BP episodically while in their own home, typically using an electronic BP device.

Hypertension falls into two categories: primary hypertension, which is high BP from an unidentified cause (Carey & Whelton, 2018; McAlister et al., 2021; Mwansa & Mazimba, 2018; Norris, 2019); and secondary hypertension, which is high BP related to an identified cause. These causes include narrowing of the renal arteries or renal artery stenosis, kidney disease, hyperaldosteronism (mineralocorticoid hypertension), medications, pregnancy, and coarctation of the aorta (Carey & Whelton, 2018; McAlister et al., 2021; Mwansa & Mazimba, 2018; Norris, 2019).

Pearls for Practice: Pathophysiology

Coarctation of the aorta is a congenital condition in which there is a narrowing in the area of the arch of the aorta. The aortic narrowing increases the resistance to blood flow, causing the left ventricle to increase pressure in the attempt to overcome the resistance. For adults under 30 years of age with elevated brachial BP, a thigh BP measurement is indicated; if the thigh measurement is lower than arm pressures, a diagnosis of coarctation of the aorta should be considered. Coarctation can be surgically repaired to remove the restriction to flow through the aorta and normalize blood pressure, although recurrence of the narrowing postsurgical correction is common (Carey & Whelton, 2018; Norris, 2019).

White coat hypertension is characterized by an elevated BP in the provider's office but normal readings when measured outside the office with either ABPM or HBPM. The patient's basic instructions for ABPM include not removing the cuff, avoiding strenuous activity, and trying to relax when the device is taking a reading. The monitor is programmed to take a BP reading automatically at desired intervals such as every 30 minutes throughout the 24-hour period (Wühl, 2022). The prevalence of white coat hypertension is higher with increasing age, among females, and with routine office measurement of BP by clinician observers versus unattended BP measurements (Carey & Whelton, 2018). As long as there is no target organ damage despite high office BP readings (which is assumed to be caused by a transient sympathetic response), the cardiovascular complication risk of white coat hypertension has been considered minimal, and most guidelines do not recommend pharmacologic treatment of white coat hypertension. However, recent research reveals that white coat hypertension is associated with "an unfavorable metabolic risk factor profile, a more frequent asymptomatic organ damage, and a greater risk of future progression to high cardiovascular risk conditions and cardiovascular morbid and fatal events" leading to a revised conclusion that it is not clinically innocent (Mancia et al., 2020, p. 1677). The nurse should continue to monitor revised guidelines as evidence accumulates.

In contrast, masked hypertension is characterized by office readings suggesting normal BP but out-of-office

(ABPM/HBPM) readings that are consistently above normal (Carey & Whelton, 2018). The prevalence of masked hypertension varies from 10% to 26% (mean 13%) in population-based surveys and from 14% to 30% in normotensive clinic populations. The risk of cardiovascular complications and all-cause mortality in persons with masked hypertension is similar to that noted in those with sustained hypertension and about twice as high as the corresponding risk in normotensive patients (Carey & Whelton, 2018; Holanger et al., 2020).

In several studies, the association between cardiovascular risk and BP was strongest for systolic readings taken at nighttime, an observation that usually resulted in patients being diagnosed with hypertension or referred for ambulatory BP monitoring. The addition of BP readings via automated office machines has been introduced as an alternative to ambulatory monitoring, although 24-hour and nighttime BP continue to be considered the optimal measurements for estimating cardiovascular risk (Yang et al., 2019).

Risk Factors

In the 1940s, I. H. Page recognized that it was unlikely that all types of hypertension and arteriosclerosis would be explained by single mechanisms. Page noted that the nature of circulation, the problem of getting the right amount of blood to the right part of the body at the right time, is an amazingly complicated and difficult one. He proposed the mosaic theory of hypertension as a causal framework (Page, 1960). The mosaic theory has been revisited through the years, and there is continued evidence to support each of the mechanisms theorized that mediate BP and hypertension. The physiologic mechanisms in this theory include the vasculature, kidneys, sympathetic nervous system, baroreceptors, renin–angiotensin–aldosterone system, and insulin resistance. These mechanisms interact with one another in sometimes complex ways to cause elevated BP levels (Hengel et al., 2022). Figure 12-1 details the revised Mosaic Theory incorporating new understanding of cellular, environmental, and genetic mechanisms (Harrison et al., 2021; Page, 1982).

No precise cause can be identified for most cases of hypertension; as suggested by the mosaic theory, hypertension is a multifactorial condition. Risk factors are often categorized as being modifiable versus relatively nonmodifiable. Modifiable risk factors include dyslipidemia, obesity (body mass index [BMI] ≥30 kg/m^2), diabetes mellitus, active or passive cigarette smoking, and physical inactivity. Nonmodifiable factors include advancing age, family history, male biologic sex, low social economic status, psychosocial stress, chronic kidney disease (CKD), and obstructive sleep apnea (Mwansa & Mazimba, 2018).

Poor diet, physical inactivity, and excess intake of alcohol, alone or in combination, are the underlying causes of hypertension. Some of the diet-related factors associated with high BP include a BMI ≥25 (overweight) and a BMI ≥30

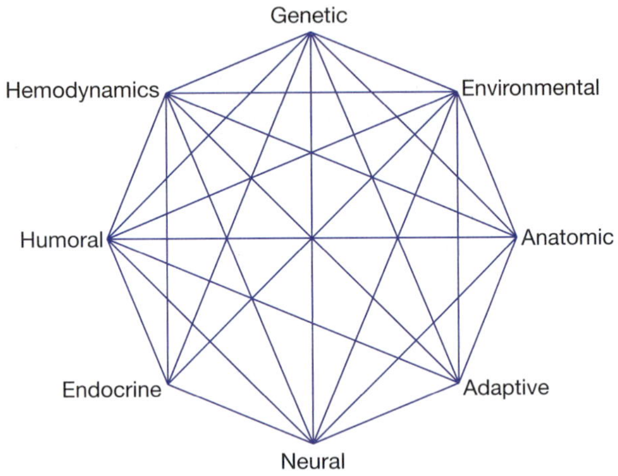

FIGURE 12-1 A revised mosaic theory incorporating new understanding of cellular, environmental, and genetic mechanisms. (Reprinted with permission from Harrison, D. G., Coffman, T., & Wilcox, C. S. [2021]. Pathophysiology of hypertension the mosaic theory and beyond. *Circulation Research*, *128*, 847–863. https://doi.org/doi:10.1161/CIRCRESAHA.121.318082)

(obesity); excess intake of sodium; and insufficient intake of potassium, calcium, magnesium, protein (especially from vegetables), fiber, and fish fats (Carey & Whelton, 2018; Clinical Overview, 2022).

Gut microbiota have also been linked to hypertension (Carey & Whelton, 2018; Durgan, 2019; Pestana-Oliveira et al., 2021). Increasing evidence indicates that hypertension and hypertensive end-organ damage are not only mediated by hemodynamic injury but that inflammation also plays an important role. The complement system protects the host from a hostile microbial environment and maintains tissue and cell integrity through the elimination of altered or dead cells. Activation of the complement system may drive the pathology of hypertension through its effects on innate and adaptive immune responses, in addition to the direct effects on the vasculature. Recent experimental data strongly support a role for complement in all stages of arterial hypertension (Wenzel et al., 2020). Other studies have compared the gut microbiota of pre- and hypertensive patients. While the gut microbiota of normotensives and hypertensives were statistically distinct from one another, there was no distinguishable difference between pre- and hypertensive patients. These studies indicate that gut dysbiosis precedes and contributes to the development of hypertension in various animal models and patients (Durgan, 2019; Li et al., 2017; Pestana-Oliveira et al., 2021; Toral et al., 2019).

Renal function and vasculature can influence BP, leading to hypertension. The kidney has at least four major roles in BP levels and the development of hypertension. One is the production of renin that cleaves angiotensinogen to angiotensin I, which in turn is acted on by the angiotensin-converting enzyme (ACE) to generate angiotensin II. A second major role of the kidney in hypertension is to reset or alter the pressure via diuresis and natriuresis (excretion of sodium in the urine). A rise in BP causes brisk diuresis and natriuresis, thereby returning BP toward normal values (Harrison et al., 2021). A third, recently recognized, role of the kidney in hypertension is to modulate systemic sympathetic tone. Renal efferent nerves regulate renal blood flow, glomerular filtration rate, tubular reabsorption of sodium and water, and release of renin and prostaglandins, all of which contribute to cardiovascular and renal regulation. Renal afferent nerves complete the feedback loop via central autonomic nuclei where the signals are integrated and modulate central sympathetic outflow. Renal sympathetic nerve activity (RSNA) is commonly increased in pathophysiologic conditions such as hypertension and chronic- and end-stage kidney disease (Sata et al., 2018). A fourth important role of the kidney in hypertension is to serve as a site of immune activation (Harrison et al., 2021).

Resistance to insulin may be a common factor linking hypertension, type 2 diabetes mellitus, hypertriglyceridemia, obesity, and glucose intolerance. Metabolic syndrome can be diagnosed if patients present with three or more of the following conditions: abdominal obesity, hypertension, elevated blood sugar levels, high blood triglycerides, and low–high-density lipoprotein (HDL) cholesterol.

Some cardiovascular changes that are attributed to age are the result of pathologic conditions. There is a slight left ventricular hypertrophy with age, and the aorta becomes dilated and elongated. Another age-related physiologic change in the cardiovascular system is that throughout the adult years, the heart muscle loses its efficiency and contractile strength, resulting in reduced CO under conditions of physiologic stress. SV decreases by 1% per year (Eliopoulos, 2022) (see Fig. 12-2).

The prevalence of hypertension increases with aging. The majority of individuals over age 60 years have hypertension. The incidence of hypertension increases with advancing age and is the most prevalent CVD of older adults (Norris, 2019). Hypertension is common in older adults in the United States, with an estimated prevalence of 76% among adults aged 65 to 74 years and 82% of adults aged ≥75 years (Clark et al., 2020). Elevated BP and older age are associated with similar changes in brain structure and function. The parallel brain changes associated with increasing age and BP include neuropsychological function, regional cerebral blood flow responses to cognitive and metabolic challenges, white matter disruptions, gray matter volume, cortical thinning, and neurovascular coupling. Treatment of hypertension helps many of these changes but fails to reverse them (Jennings et al., 2020). Systolic BP continues to rise throughout life; while diastolic pressure rises until approximately 50 years old, it tends to level off over the next decade and may remain the same or fall later in life (Jennings et al., 2020). Females show somewhat lower systolic BP prior to menopause and then surpass males after menopause. Ultimately, 59% of males and 67% of females over the age of 60 have hypertension (Norris, 2019).

High BP is more common in non-Hispanic Black adults (56%) than in non-Hispanic White adults (48%), non-Hispanic Asian adults (46%), or Hispanic adults (39%; CDC, 2022b). Studies also indicate that Black populations tend to develop hypertension at an earlier age than other populations (Norris, 2019). Among those recommended to take BP medication, BP control is higher among non-Hispanic White adults (32%) than in non-Hispanic Black adults (25%), non-Hispanic Asian adults (19%), or Hispanic adults (25%; CDC, 2022b). Also, non-Hispanic Black adults with diabetes, hypertension, or a family history of CKD have a two- to fourfold greater incidence of ESKD or death than nonunderrepresented counterparts with similar CKD risk factors (Brown, 2021).

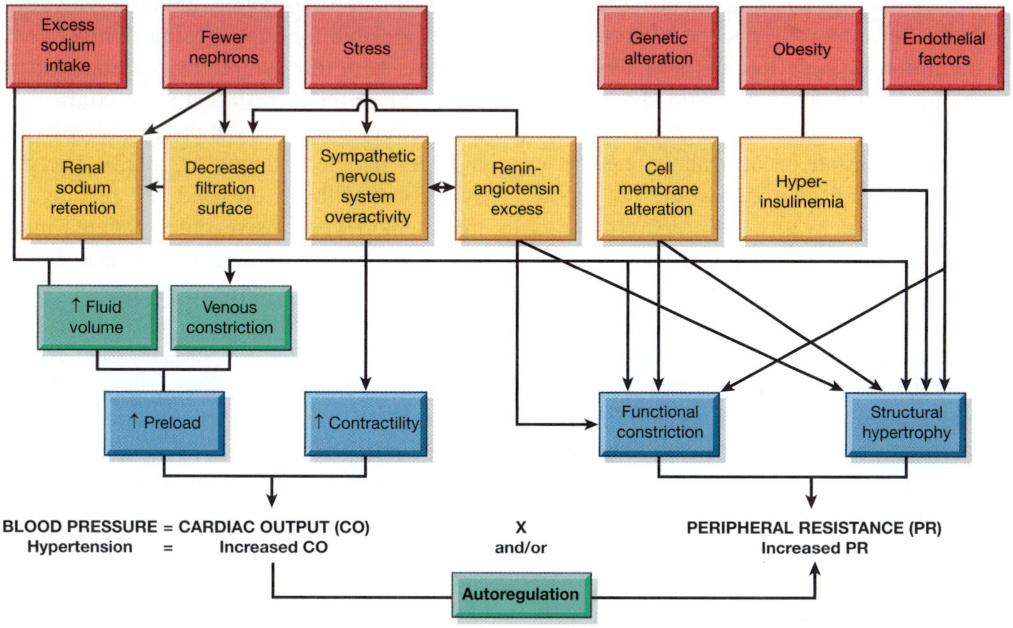

FIGURE 12-2 **Factors involved in control of BP. (Adapted from Kaplan, N. M., Lieberman, E., & Neal, W. [2014].** ***Kaplan's clinical hypertension*** **[11th ed.]. Lippincott Williams & Wilkins.)**

Pearls for Practice: Lifting the Lens

Health care providers are increasingly aware of how the intersection of structural and social determinants of health (SSDOH) impacts patients' well-being; it is understood that disparities in the ability to control hypertension contribute to higher cardiovascular morbidity and mortality among underresourced and low socioeconomic groups (Razon et al., 2021). A recent review of clinical guidelines for adult hypertension management revealed that 72% recommend activities related to SSDOH, with the majority focusing on financial security. Examples of strategies when cost is a barrier to medication adherence (and thus control) are prescribing generic medications, altering daily dosages, using combination medications, and reduced copayments. However, Razon et al. (2021) argue that "existing guidelines fail to provide clinicians and health care systems with comprehensive, actionable, evidence-based guidance on how to integrate our growing knowledge about SDH into patient care (p. 1128)." For example, they suggest "research that will help answer [the patient's] questions about whether spending money to buy this medication was more important than buying the healthy foods which is also recommended (p. 1128)?" What is needed are guidelines that are evidence-based on how we can intervene on social determinants to improve hypertension management. As this evidence grows, health care providers will need to incorporate these research-based interventions that address SSDOH into their care.

High BP is more common in some areas of the United States than in others. Self-reported rate of hypertension by state (using a definition of hypertension as a BP ≥140/≥90 mm Hg) can be more than 50% higher in some states versus others. However, this likely underreports the true effect of hypertension in each state because about one in five adults with high BP is unaware of it and would not report having it (CDC, 2022b).

Epidemiologic studies have identified a direct relationship between BMI and BP that is continuous and almost linear (Carey & Whelton, 2018). The relationship between obesity at a young age and change in obesity status over time is strongly related to future risk of hypertension. Of particular note though, becoming normal weight reduces the risk of developing hypertension to a level similar to those who had never been obese; the patient can expect about 1 mm Hg reduction in BP for every 1-kg reduction in body weight) (Carey & Whelton, 2018; Whelton et al., 2018).

In the United States, approximately 25% of females of reproductive age have hypertension. Of these, fewer than half are aware of their diagnosis and, when diagnosed, only 10% have their BP controlled. Further, racial differences exist, with more than half of Black females aged 20 years or older having hypertension (Virani et al., 2020; Basile Ibrahim et al., 2021). Selecting the appropriate hormonal contraception in females with hypertension is important because females with established hypertension who use combined oral contraceptives (COCs) are at higher risk of stroke and MI than normotensive nonusers. However, the absolute risk is relatively low among females of reproductive age (Shufelt & LeVee, 2020).

Gerontologic Considerations

The U.S. Census Bureau projects that there will be a substantial increase in the number of individuals over age 65 between 2010 and 2030 due to the impact of the baby boomers, who began to enter this group in 2011. In 2030, it is projected that this group will represent nearly 20% of the total U.S. population. The growth of the older adult population is due in part to increasing life expectancy. Advancements in disease control and health technology, lower infant and child mortality rates, improved sanitation, and better living conditions have increased life expectancy for most Americans. Not only are more people reaching old age, but they are living longer once they do; the number of people in their 70s and 80s has been steadily increasing and is expected to continue to increase (Eliopoulos, 2022).

Throughout the adult years, the heart muscle loses its efficiency and contractile strength, resulting in reduced CO especially under conditions of physiologic stress (Eliopoulos, 2022). The incidence of hypertension increases with advancing age and is the most prevalent CVD of older adults. Many older individuals have high BP arising from the vasoconstriction associated with aging, which produces peripheral resistance. Hyperthyroidism, parkinsonism, Paget disease (see Chapter 40), anemia, and thiamine deficiency can also be responsible for hypertension. While hypertension overall presents with few symptoms, waking with a dull headache, impaired memory, disorientation, confusion, epistaxis, and a slow tremor may be symptoms of hypertension, especially in older people (Eliopoulos, 2022). The presence of these symptoms with an elevated BP reading usually warrants treatment. Hypertensive older patients may be advised to rest; reduce their sodium intake; and, if necessary, reduce their weight as a first line of treatment.

The average older American is at risk for polypharmacy. Most older people use at least one drug regularly, with the median being seven prescribed medications (Williams et al., 2019). Being prescribed five or more medications is considered polypharmacy. Not all medications they take are for high BP, but many interact with antihypertensive medications, such as tricyclic antidepressants, nonsteroidal anti-inflammatories, antidiabetics, antianxiety medications, antidepressants, sedatives, nasal decongestants, and thiazide diuretics (Burchum & Rosenthal, 2021). The drug regimen of an elderly patient with hypertension should be reviewed carefully at every visit.

An orthostatic decline in BP accompanies advanced age and contributes to potential adverse effects with some antihypertensive drugs. Orthostatic or postural hypotension is defined as a decline in SBP >20 mm Hg or DBP >10 mm Hg after 1 to 3 minutes on movement from supine to standing position (Hogan-Quigley & Palm, 2021; Mwansa & Mazimba, 2018). Caution is especially advisable when initiating pharmacotherapy with two antihypertensive drugs in older patients because there is an increased potential for hypotension or orthostatic hypotension in some patients (Carey & Whelton, 2018).

Pearls for Practice

During the initial treatment of hypertension, the nurse monitors the blood pressure to evaluate response to the treatment. It is important to recognize that if the mean BP is lowered more than 40% in the initial 24 hours, then symptoms of cerebral hypoperfusion may occur, which may present as a sudden onset of lightheadedness or syncope (Ferri, 2022).

Pearls for Practice

The difference between systolic and diastolic pressures is known as the pulse pressure. The normal pulse pressure is approximately 40 mm Hg (Hogan-Quigley & Palm, 2021). A diminished pulse pressure may be caused by decreased stroke volume, as in heart failure, hypovolemia, and severe aortic stenosis; and increased peripheral resistance, as in exposure to cold and severe heart failure. Causes of increased pulse pressure include increased stroke volume, decreased peripheral resistance, or both, as in fever, anemia, hyperthyroidism, aortic regurgitation, arteriovenous fistulas, and patent ductus arteriosus; increased stroke volume related to slow heart rates, as in bradycardia and complete heart block; and decreased compliance (increased stiffness) of the aortic walls, as in aging or atherosclerosis (Hogan-Quigley & Palm, 2021).

To reduce the cardiovascular and cerebrovascular risks, older adults should begin treatment with lifestyle modifications and nonpharmacologic interventions (Carey & Whelton, 2018; Flack & Adekola, 2020). The recommended interventions include weight loss to achieve ideal body weight but aim for at least a 1-kg reduction in body weight for most adults who are overweight. Dietary changes include consuming a diet rich in fruits, vegetables, whole grains, and low-fat dairy products, with reduced content of saturated and total fat. This is known as the Dietary Approaches to Stop Hypertension (DASH) diet plan. Reducing intake of dietary sodium is important. The target of no more than 2,300 mg a day has been further reduced to an ideal limit of no more than 1,500 mg per day for most adults (AHA, 2021). Patients are taught to avoid prepared foods, to not add salt to foods, and to increase intake of dietary potassium to 3,500 to 5,000 mg/day, preferably by eating a diet rich in potassium (Carreira-Míguez et al., 2022; Flack & Adekola, 2020; Hiremath et al., 2022; Mayo Clinic, n.d.). Physical activity in three different forms is recommended: aerobic exercise for 90 to 150 minutes per week, dynamic resistance exercise 90 to 150 minutes per week with six exercises, three sets/exercise, 10 repetitions/set; and isometric hand grip resistance exercises, four times for 2 minutes with 1 minute between exercises sets (Bennie et al., 2019; Carey & Whelton, 2018; Punia & Kulandaivelan, 2019). Finally, moderating alcohol consumption for those who consume alcohol is another lifestyle change recommendation. Males should drink two drinks or fewer daily and females one drink or less daily (Carey & Whelton, 2018). Each of these interventions has accompanying evidence of decrease in BP without pharmacologic intervention (Islam et al., 2021).

If medications are needed to achieve the BP goal, the starting dose should be half that used in younger patients and increased slowly. Many practitioners advocate for "start low and go slow" with medication regimens in the older population. Adherence may be more difficult for the elderly when memory impairment exists or due to the expense of treatment plans. The nurse should ensure that the patient understands the regimen and can see and read instructions, open the medication container, and get the prescription refilled. Family or caregivers should be included in the teaching program so that they can assist with the regimen as necessary, encourage adherence to the treatment plan, and know when and whom to call for questions or problems.

Pearls for Practice

The older population is more sensitive to volume depletion caused by diuretics and to sympathetic inhibition caused by adrenergic antagonists. Teach patients to change positions slowly when moving from a lying or sitting position to a standing position and to use supportive devices, such as handrails and walkers, to prevent falls that could result from dizziness.

Blood Pressure Assessment and Measurement

For diagnosis and management of high BP, proper methods for accurate measurement and documentation of BP are critical (see Box 12-1). The AHA/ACC (Carey & Whelton, 2018) provides clear documentation of the method recommended for accurate measurement of BP. The patient's preparation and comfort are just the beginning. The patient should be instructed to avoid caffeine, exercise, and smoking for at least 30 minutes before their appointment and measurement of BP. Prior to the measurement, the patient should be asked to empty their bladder and then be relaxed, sitting in a chair (feet on floor, back supported) for at least 5 minutes. Measurements made while the patient is sitting or lying

BOX 12-1

GUIDELINES FOR NURSING CARE

Measuring BP

Assessment is based on the average of at least two readings. (If two readings differ by more than 5 mm Hg, additional readings are taken and an average reading is calculated from the results.)

Equipment

- Recently calibrated aneroid manometer, or validated electronic device
- Cuff
- Stethoscope

Implementation

NURSING ACTION	RATIONALE
1. Instruct the patient to: • Avoid smoking cigarettes or ingesting nicotine, exercising, or drinking caffeine for 30 minutes before BP is measured. • Sit quietly for 5 minutes before the measurement, without talking or moving around before recording blood pressure. • Sit comfortably with the forearm supported at heart level on a firm surface, palm up, both feet firmly on the ground, back supported; avoid talking while the measurement is being taken. The selected arm should be bare to the shoulder, and if the garment sleeve is raised, it should be loose so blood flow is not impinged.	1. Listening carefully helps ensure an accurate measurement is taken. Stimuli such as food, alcohol, caffeine, nicotine, and exercise within 30 minutes before blood pressure measurement may affect the reading. Crossing legs, talking, and doing mental tasks while the BP is measured increase blood pressure.
2. Select the size of the cuff based upon the size of the patient. (The cuff size should have a bladder width of at least 40% of limb circumference and length at least 80% of limb circumference.) The average adult cuff is 12–14 cm wide and 30-cm long.	2. Using a cuff that is too small will give a higher BP measurement, and using a cuff that is too large results in a lower BP measurement compared to one taken with a properly sized cuff.
3. Wrap the cuff firmly around the arm (half the distance between the acromion [bony process on the shoulder blade] and the olecranon [elbow] is used to determine the midpoint of the arm). Center the cuff bladder approximately 2 cm (~1 in) above the elbow crease, with the midline of the bladder directly over the brachial artery. One finger should fit between the cuff and the patient's arm.	3. Proper setup is required for accurate reading. If the cuff is too loose, a false high reading occurs; if it is too tight, a false low reading occurs.
4. Position the patient's arm at the level of the heart, preferably by resting the arm on a firm surface such as the examination table.	4. Positioning the arm above heart level will give a falsely low reading; a reading when the patient's arm is below heart level will be falsely elevated.
5. Palpate the systolic pressure before auscultating, using the radial or brachial artery (inflate the cuff until the pulse disappears; then deflate the cuff and note the pressure at which the pulse reappears. This is the systolic pressure by palpation).	5. This technique prevents the risks of overinflation, undue patient discomfort, and/or underestimation of systolic blood pressure. It also helps to detect the presence of an auscultatory gap more readily; an auscultatory gap is present when there is intermittent disappearance of the initial Korotkoff sounds after their first appearance (associated with older patients with hypertension), leading to underestimation of systolic blood pressure.
6. Ask the patient to sit quietly while the BP is measured.	6. BP can increase when the patient is engaged in conversation.
7. The nurse positions themself so that the manometer is at the eye level. Tighten the thumbscrew of the pressure bulb and rapidly inflate the cuff to 30 mm Hg above the palpated systolic pressure. Slowly loosen the thumbscrew to deflate the cuff of the sphygmomanometer, releasing the pressure at 2 mm Hg per second. Listen carefully. Note the pressure at which the first sound is auscultated. This is the systolic reading. Continue to listen to the Korotkoff sounds. Determine the pressure when the pulsations disappear completely; this is the diastolic reading.	7. Misalignment between the eye and the mercury meniscus or aneroid manometer may cause the meniscus to be read as higher or lower than the actual position. Listening carefully ensures an accurate measurement.

NURSING ACTION	RATIONALE
8. Initially, record BP results of both arms and take subsequent measurements from the arm with the higher BP.	8. A difference of 10–15 mm Hg may indicate arterial obstruction on the side with the lower value.
9. Record the site where the BP was measured and the position of the patient (e.g., right arm).	9. This is especially important when assessing for orthostatic changes.
10. Inform the patient of their BP value and what it means. Emphasize the need for periodic reassessment, and encourage patients who measure BP at home to keep a written record of readings.	10. This engages the patient in the teaching process and correlates diet and medication adherence with BP.

Data from Carey and Whelton (2018) and Hogan-Quigley and Palm (2021).

on an examining table are not appropriate. The patient and staff should not talk or move around during measurement (Muntner et al., 2019). All clothing should be removed from the arm being used for measurement. The BP device used should be validated and calibrated regularly. The patient's arm should be supported at the level of the right atrium, referred to as the phlebostatic axis, which approximates the level of the atrium; it is located at the intersection of the fourth intercostal space and mid-chest level (halfway between the anterior and posterior chest surfaces or the midaxillary line) (see Fig. 11-14). Correct cuff size is also important; the bladder must encircle 80% of the arm and is placed no less than 2.5 cm (~1 in) from the antecubital fossa (Efre, 2023). BP should be recorded in both arms for the first visit, and the arm yielding the higher reading should be used in subsequent assessments. If a repeat assessment is necessary on the same arm, wait 1 to 2 minutes before repeating the reading. For auscultatory readings, SBP should be initially estimated by radial pulse obliteration, then inflate the cuff 20 to 30 mm Hg above this level for the auscultatory reading. Deflate the cuff pressure 2 mm Hg per second, listening carefully for Korotkoff sounds (Carey & Whelton, 2018; Hogan-Quigley & Palm, 2021). An alternative placement is the use of a large thigh cuff applied to the mid-thigh area, using the popliteal pulse, which is audible with a stethoscope at the popliteal space (Kallenbach, 2021). In addition, the BP can be monitored directly and continuously with an invasive "arterial line" requiring the insertion of a thin catheter into an artery and electronic monitoring equipment, typically in an intensive care unit (see Chapter 54).

Pearls for Practice

BP cuffs should never be placed on an extremity with deep vein thrombosis, grafts, ischemic changes, an arteriovenous (AV) fistula or graft, or breast or axillary surgery on that side (Kallenbach, 2021; Perry et al., 2022).

Pearls for Practice

False low readings are found if the arm is above the level of the heart, and when using a cuff that is too large. False high readings are found if the arm is below the level of the heart, the cuff is too small, or the arm is not supported (Perry et al., 2022).

Self-monitoring of BP or HBPM refers to the regular measurement of BP by an individual at home or elsewhere outside the clinical setting. Among individuals with hypertension, self-monitoring of BP, without other interventions, has shown limited evidence for treatment-related BP reduction and achievement of BP control. However, with the increased recognition of inconsistencies between office and out-of-office BPs and greater reduction in BP being recommended for hypertension control, increased attention is being paid to out-of-office BP readings. Although ABPM is generally accepted as the best out-of-office measurement method since it records the BP variations over 24 hours, HBPM is often a more practical approach in clinical practice. Studies have shown that when consistently higher 24-hour and nighttime BPs are documented by HBPM and ABPM, those readings were associated with greater risk of mortality and poor cardiovascular outcomes. Therefore, the HBPM and ABPM may be considered optimal measurements for estimating CV risk (Yang et al., 2019).

Pearls for Practice

Normally, the BP should vary by no more than 5 mm Hg between arms. If there is a difference, record both initially. Later, record the higher number. A difference of 10 mm Hg or more between the patient's arms is found in approximately 5% of the population and may indicate thoracic outlet syndrome or arterial obstruction on the side with the lower value (Lough, 2022).

Pearls for Practice: Pathophysiology

Thoracic outlet syndrome is a condition where upper extremity symptoms are believed to result from neurovascular compression at the thoracic outlet. Compression may occur in three anatomic structures: arteries, veins, and nerves (Ferri, 2022). If arterial compression is present, the involved extremity will be cool with a weak or absent pulse. A decrease in blood pressure (on the involved limb) greater than 20 mm Hg compared with the opposite arm is sometimes noted.

Clinical Manifestations and Assessment

Because there are typically no symptoms of hypertension, physical examination may be unremarkable, other than elevated BP. Many symptoms are associated with target or end-organ damage. The nurse should question the patient about anginal pain; shortness of breath; alterations in speech, vision, or balance; epistaxis; headaches; dizziness; or nocturia. Further assessment includes asking about personal, social, or financial factors; or unacceptable pharmaceutical side effects that may interfere with the patient's ability to adhere to the medication regimen (Carey & Whelton, 2018; Hogan-Quigley & Palm, 2021). Laboratory testing is also important when assessing patients for hypertension; tests typically include fasting blood glucose (including hemoglobin A_{1c}), complete blood count, lipid profile, serum creatinine with estimated glomerular filtration rate (eGFR), serum sodium, potassium, calcium, thyroid-stimulating hormone, urinalysis, and electrocardiogram (Cameron, 2019; Carey & Whelton, 2018; Clark et al., 2020).

Hypertension may be asymptomatic and remain so for many years; however, when signs and symptoms appear, target organ damage of the brain, heart, kidneys, and the eyes presents as focal neurologic deficits, dyspnea, chest pain, headache, and loss of vision (Vinayak et al., 2020). Patients with poorly managed hypertension or hypertensive emergencies (discussed shortly) most often present to the emergency department with acute heart failure with pulmonary edema, acute coronary syndrome, acute aortic syndrome including acute aortic dissection, hypertensive encephalopathy, or ischemic or hemorrhagic stroke (Vinayak et al., 2020). Coronary artery disease with angina or MI is a common consequence of hypertension. Left ventricular hypertrophy occurs in response to the increased workload placed on the ventricle as it contracts against higher systemic pressure. When heart damage is extensive, heart failure follows (Norris, 2019). Pathologic changes in the kidneys, indicated by microalbuminuria, increased blood urea nitrogen (BUN) and serum creatinine levels, and nocturia result (Unger et al., 2020). Cerebrovascular involvement may lead to stroke or transient ischemic attack (TIA), manifested by alterations in vision or speech, dizziness, weakness, a sudden fall, or hemiplegia. Occasionally, retinal changes such as hemorrhages, arteriolar narrowing, and cotton-wool spots (small infarctions) occur. In severe hypertension, papilledema (swelling of the optic disc) may be seen. A risk factor assessment is needed to classify and guide the treatment of the hypertensive individual at risk for cardiovascular damage (Vinayak et al., 2020). Risk factors and cardiovascular problems related to hypertension are presented in Box 12-2.

BOX 12-2

Risk Factors for Cardiovascular Problems in Hypertensive Patients

Major Risk Factors (in Addition to Hypertension)

- Smoking
- Dyslipidemia (elevated LDL [or total] cholesterol and/or low HDL cholesterol)[a]
- Diabetes mellitus[a]
- Impaired renal function (GFR less than 60 mL/min and/or microalbuminuria)
- Obesity (body mass index [BMI] of 30 kg/m^2 or higher)[a]
- Physical inactivity
- Age (over 55 years for males, 65 years for females)
- Alcohol use
- Family history of cardiovascular disease (in female relative under 65 years or male relative under 55 years)

Target Organ Damage or Clinical Cardiovascular Disease

- Heart disease (left ventricular hypertrophy, angina, or previous MI, previous coronary revascularization, heart failure)
- Stroke or TIA
- Chronic kidney disease
- Peripheral arterial disease
- Retinopathy

Norris (2019).

[a]These risk factors plus hypertension, elevated triglyceride levels, and abdominal obesity are components of metabolic syndrome.

Medical and Nursing Management

While the BP threshold for specific hypertension diagnosis varies, the treated BP targets for patients with hypertension are consistent for all; BP should be less than 130/80. Patients with elevated BP are encouraged to make the lifestyle changes that have been previously described; once a patient is diagnosed with either Stage 1 or Stage 2 hypertension, pharmacotherapeutics will be added to the lifestyle change recommendations (Carey & Whelton, 2018).

Patient engagement and participation in self-care, patient-centered care, self-management support, and shared decision-making are important primary health care and health policy issues. Given the heavy reliance on lifestyle changes to help control BP, follow through and adherence are very important to therapeutic success (Dineen-Griffin et al., 2019; Tusa et al., 2021).While it is called self-management, the best success comes with structured patient–provider support that can include one-on-one patient–provider consultation, ongoing follow-up, and provision of education materials (Box 12-3). Interventions should be tailored to the patient's specific needs and may include combinations of strategies to improve a patient's disease or treatment knowledge, independent monitoring of symptoms, encouraging self-treatment through a personalized action plan in response worsening symptoms or exacerbations, psychological coping and stress management strategies, and enhancing responsibility in medication adherence and lifestyle choices. Follow-up may include tailored feedback, monitoring of progress with respect to patient-set health

BOX 12-3

Nursing Research

Bridging the Gap to Evidence-Based Practice

Helping Patients Help Themselves: A Systematic Review of Self-Management Support Strategies in Primary Health Care Practice

Dineen-Griffin, S., Garcia-Cardenas, V., Williams, K., & Benrimoj, S. I. (2019). Helping patients help themselves: A systematic review of self-management support strategies in primary health care practice. *PLoS One*, *14*(8), e0220116. https://doi.org/10.1371/journal.pone.0220116

Purpose

To examine self-management support interventions in primary care on health outcomes and to identify effective strategies that facilitate positive clinical and humanistic outcomes.

Design

A systematic review of randomized controlled trials evaluating self-management support interventions was conducted; eligible studies assessed the effectiveness of individualized interventions with follow-up delivered face-to-face to adult patients with any condition in primary care, compared with usual standard of care. Matrices were developed that mapped the evidence and components for each intervention. The methodologic quality of included studies was appraised.

Findings

Findings reveal a structured patient–provider exchange is required in primary care, including a one-on-one patient–provider consultation, ongoing follow-up and provision of self-help materials. Interventions should be tailored to patient needs and may include combinations of strategies to improve a patient's disease or treatment knowledge, independent monitoring of symptoms, encouraging self-treatment through a personalized action plan in response to worsening symptoms or exacerbations, psychological coping and stress management strategies, and enhancing responsibility in medication adherence and lifestyle choices. Follow-up may include tailored feedback, monitoring of progress with respect to patient-set health care goals, or honing problem-solving and decision-making skills. Theoretical models provided a strong base for effective self-management support (SMS) interventions. Positive outcomes for effective SMS included improvements in clinical indicators, health-related quality of life, self-efficacy (confidence to self-manage), disease knowledge, and control. An SMS model has been developed that sets the foundation for the design and evaluation of practical strategies for the construct of self-management support interventions in primary health care practice.

Nursing Implications

Primary care professionals now have evidence-based strategies and structure to deliver SMS in practice. For this collaborative partnership approach to be more widely applied, future research should build on these findings for optimal SMS service design and upskilling health care providers to effectively support patients in this collaborative process.

care goals, or honing problem-solving and decision-making skills (Dineen-Griffin et al., 2019).

The nurse encourages self-management, which may include self BP monitoring, and education to initiate and maintain lifestyle changes. Self-management and education empower patients to ask questions and voice concerns. These individuals are less likely to be hospitalized, have fewer emergency department and unscheduled medical visits, and have fewer days off from work.

The nurse should routinely ask whether patients take herbal supplements or over-the-counter (OTC) medications that may increase BP. These include caffeine and ephedra, which are stimulants; licorice, which has an aldosterone-like effect; and acetaminophen and NSAIDs, which may lead to fluid retention (Carey & Whelton, 2018).

Lifestyle Changes

Table 12-2 summarizes recommended lifestyle modifications. Research findings demonstrate that weight loss, reduced alcohol and sodium intake, and regular physical activity for 30 minutes on most days are effective lifestyle adaptations to reduce BP. Counsel the patient that smoking cessation will decrease the risk for heart disease. Treatment of sleep apnea and underlying thyroid disorders and management of blood glucose are also recommended (Bennie et al., 2019; Carey & Whelton, 2018). The nurse should emphasize the concept of lifelong BP control and adherence to treatment rather than cure and absolute compliance.

Every patient with hypertension should be offered information regarding lifestyle modifications to reduce BP (Tusa et al., 2021). Specific information regarding diet, exercise, avoidance of salt/sodium intake and alcohol, and smoking cessation should be included. Adhering to the American Heart Association's Dietary Approaches to Stop Hypertension (DASH) approach helps decrease BP and lower lipid levels, reducing the risk of CVDs; for example, research revealed that by following this diet the systolic BP decreases by about 6 to 11 mm Hg in hypertensive as well as normotensive people (Challa et al., 2022; NHLBI, 2021). Refer to Table 12-3 for details on DASH diet.

DASH is low in saturated and trans fats and rich in potassium, calcium, magnesium, fiber, and protein and helps lower blood glucose levels, triglycerides, LDL-C, and insulin resistance (Challa et al., 2022). Further, the DASH approach emphasizes vegetables, fruits, and fat-free or low-fat dairy products. It includes whole grains, fish, poultry, beans, seeds, nuts, and vegetable oils and limits sodium, sweets, sugary beverages, and red meats; this not only lowers BP but also prevent CVD (NHLBI, 2021). Consistent with the DASH approach, the target sodium intake of 2,300 mg daily (1 teaspoon), has been limited further to 1,500 mg

TABLE **12-2 Lifestyle Modifications to Prevent and Manage Hypertension**[a]

Modification	Recommendation	Goal of SBP[b] Reduction (Range)[c]
Weight reduction	Maintain normal body weight (body mass index 18.5–24.9 kg/m^2).	5–20 mm Hg/10 kg
Adopt DASH eating plan	Consume a diet rich in fruits, vegetables, fiber, potassium, and low-fat dairy products; reduce consumption of animal protein, fat, and saturated fat.	8–14 mm Hg
Dietary sodium reduction	Reduce dietary sodium intake to 2,300 mg (2.4 g) sodium; may need to decrease to 1,500 mg daily.	2–8 mm Hg
Physical activity	Engage in regular aerobic physical activity such as 30 minutes of brisk walking 3–5 days per week.	4–9 mm Hg
Moderation of alcohol consumption	Limit consumption to no more than two drinks (e.g., 24-oz beer, 10-oz wine, or 3-oz 80-proof whiskey) per day in most males and to no more than one drink per day in females and people weighing less than average.	2–4 mm Hg

[a]For overall cardiovascular risk reduction, stop smoking.

[b]SBP, systolic BP.

[c]The effects of implementing these modifications are dose- and time-dependent and could be greater for some individuals.

Data from Bennie et al. (2019), Carey and Whelton (2018), Punia and Kulandaivelan (2019).

daily (Wong Berta, 2022). Studies have demonstrated that increased sodium intake is particularly detrimental and is associated with higher risk of hypertension in patients with elevated triglycerides (Choi et al., 2020).

A diet high in fruits and vegetables is associated with lower systolic and diastolic BP. Maintaining or attaining normal weight is advised. Obesity may increase the risk of hypertension through overactivation of the sympathetic nervous system, activation of the renin–angiotensin–aldosterone system, sodium retention, and increased HR. The role of increased inflammatory markers, such as C-reactive protein, is becoming increasing clear as a risk factor for CVD and an outcome predictor. Inflammation leads to endothelial dysfunction and abnormal lipid levels (Kaura et al., 2022; Ratkovic et al., 2022). Regular exercise is associated with lower BP regardless of BMI. Exercise may improve inflammatory markers and cause an increase in endothelial nitric oxide synthase, a potent vasodilator (Carey & Whelton, 2018).

TABLE **12-3 The Dietary Approaches to Stop Hypertension (DASH) Diet**

Food Group	Number of Servings Per Day
Grains	6–8
Meat, fish, and poultry	6 or less
Vegetables	4 to 5
Fruits	4 to 5
Low-fat or fat-free dairy foods	2 to 3
Sodium	2,300 mg/day[a]
Fats and oils	2–3
Nuts, seeds, peas, and dry beans	4 or 5 weekly
Sweets	5 or fewer weekly

[a]1,500 mg sodium lowers blood pressure even further than 2,300 mg sodium daily.

When following the DASH eating plan, it is important to choose foods that are low in saturated and trans fats; rich in potassium, calcium, magnesium, fiber, and protein; and lower in sodium.

From https://www.nhlbi.nih.gov/education/dash-eating-plan. Updated December 21, 2021.

Pearls for Practice

Reducing table salt to about 1 teaspoon per day, or ~2,300 to 2,400 mg of sodium, can reduce systolic BP by 2 to 8 mm Hg.

Alternate Therapies

Complementary and alternative therapies can have significant impact on improving BP levels. There are other complementary interventions that aid in complying with antihypertensive therapies (Moore & Mary, 2020). Biofeedback-assisted home-based breathing relaxation intervention (BAHRI), a complementary therapy that included a simple abdominal breathing exercise practiced by patients at home, resulted in significant reduction in systolic and diastolic BP. The patients who participated in the BAHRI also decreased their medication doses because of reduced BP as well. Telephonic reminders boosted the adherence to the therapeutic measures and optimized BP control (Elavally et al., 2020). Qigong is a traditional fitness method that originated from China. It has the elements of body movement, mind guidance, and breath control, and the combination of these elements has the effect of lowering BP and reducing mortality (Dong et al., 2021).

Blood Pressure Monitoring

The nurse must ensure that follow-up is provided for any person identified as having an elevated BP level. Each person should be given a written record of their BP at the screening. The AHA and the NHLBI provide printed and electronic patient education materials (see reference resources, web addresses). Continuity of care has been described as a multifaceted concept that includes informational continuity (the sharing of information among professionals about the patient), longitudinal continuity (a patient is seen by the same practitioner for the entire course of treatment), and interpersonal continuity (ongoing therapeutic relationship between a patient and one or more providers). Continuity of care is associated with better quality of care because deterioration in patients' conditions could be less likely to go undetected or untreated. Moreover, continuity of care improves patient satisfaction, facilitates higher patient self-care behaviors, and improves adherence to providers' recommendations and regimens (Chan et al., 2021). Providing patients with the right information at the right time is important to tailoring health messages and making communication relevant for patients (Cappelletti et al., 2020).

Pharmacologic Therapy

The ideal characteristics of drug treatment for hypertension include treatments that are evidence-based in relation to morbidity/mortality prevention, have a once-daily regimen which provides 24-hour BP control, are affordable and/or cost-effective relative to other agents, and are well tolerated (Unger et al., 2020). Medication adherence is influenced by multiple factors such as the disease itself, perceived health status, medication knowledge, patient–nurse interaction, economic status, and the level of health literacy (Kilic & Dag, 2020). The teach-back method has demonstrated effectiveness in a broad spectrum of medical outcomes, evidencing better outcomes in disease-specific knowledge, adherence, and self-efficacy (Parra et al., 2021).

The recommended systolic pressure of 130 mm Hg is the upper limit of normal at all ages (Carey & Whelton, 2018). Pharmacologic agents, in addition to lifestyle modifications, provide the primary basis for treatment of hypertension. The initial antihypertensive treatment should include a thiazide or thiazide-like diuretic, angiotensin-converting enzyme inhibitor (ACEI), angiotensin-receptor blocker (ARB), or calcium-channel blocker (CCB). Refer to Figure 12-3 for recommendations for treatment and follow-up of hypertension. Table 12-4 and Figure 12-4 detail a variety of pharmacologic agents for hypertension. Many patients can be started on a single agent. Considerations to determine the best plan of care, especially starting a regimen of two drugs from different classes, include patients with stage 2 hypertension, age, cardiac risk stratification, concurrent medications, drug adherence, drug interactions, the overall treatment regimen, out-of-pocket costs, and comorbidities. Importantly, engaging the patient in shared decision-making, along with the provider's judgment, should be a critical influencer regarding the choice of antihypertensive agents (Carey & Whelton, 2018).

Drug Alert

The nurse understands that patients receiving angiotensin-converting enzyme inhibitors (ACEIs) can develop angioedema, usually within hours to 1 week after starting therapy. However, it can also occur months or years later. It is the number one cause of acute angioedema in some hospitals and occurs in 0.1% to 2.2% of patients receiving an ACEI (Dinulos, 2021).

Drug Alert

Aspirin, ibuprofen, and other nonsteroidal anti-inflammatory drugs (NSAIDs) may reduce the antihypertensive effects of ACE inhibitors due to prostaglandin inhibition, which causes vasoconstriction of the afferent arteriole, decreasing blood flow to the kidneys and increasing the risk of acute kidney injury and reduced renal function (Shaddock et al., 2020). It is important for the nurse to consider that NSAIDs are available over the counter and patients need to be educated in avoiding their use, especially in those with reduced renal function. Patients should be counseled to use the shortest duration of therapy as possible, to consider substituting with acetaminophen (Tylenol), and the importance of staying hydrated during NSAID therapy (Shaddock et al., 2020).

Patient Education and Counseling

Every adult with hypertension should have a clear, detailed, and current evidence-based plan of care that ensures the achievement of treatment and self-management goals and encourages effective management of comorbid conditions as well as timely follow-up with the health care team (Carey & Whelton, 2018). Patient education should be offered in many forms to maximize impact on the patient and patient success and should be team based, taking advantage of interprofessional skill sets, knowledge, and strengths (Cappelletti et al., 2020; Carey & Whelton, 2018; Singh et al., 2021). Communicating alternative behaviors that support self-management of healthy BP in addition to medication adherence is important. This should be done both verbally and in writing (Cote et al., 2021). After the provider's visit, if the patient has a mobile phone, medical information and

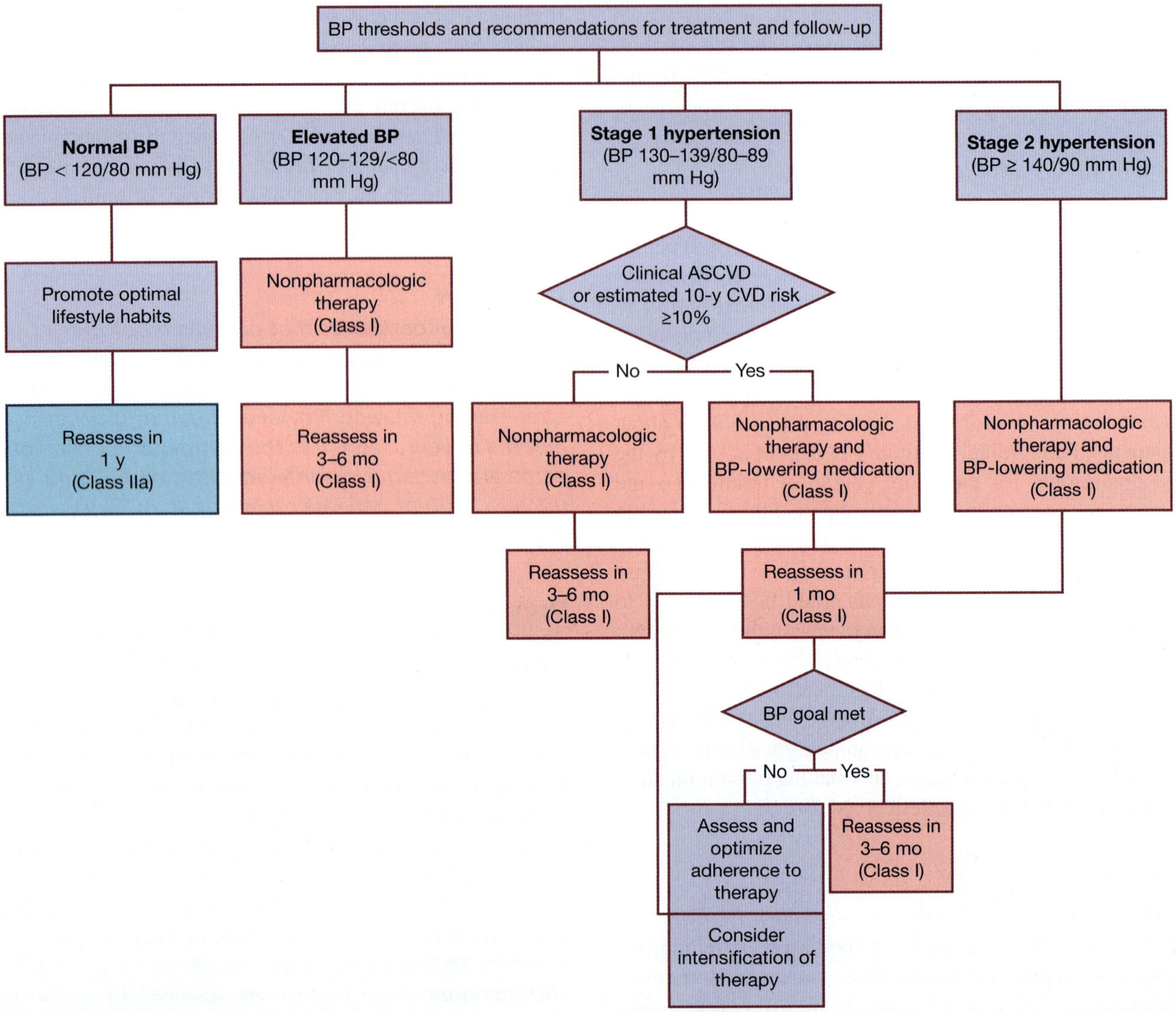

FIGURE 12-3 Algorithm for the treatment of hypertension. (From Whelton, P. K., Carey, R. M., Aronow, W. S., Casey, D. E. Jr., Collins, K. J., Dennison Himmelfarb, C., DePalma, S. M., Gidding, S., Jamerson, K. A., Jones, D. W., MacLaughlin, E. J., Muntner, P., Ovbiagele, B., Smith, S.C. Jr., Spencer, C. C., Stafford, R. S., Taler, S. J., Thomas, R. J., Williams, K. A. Sr.,...Wright, J. T. Jr. [2018]. 2017 ACC/AHA/AAPA/ABC/ACPM/AGS/APhA/ASH/ASPC/NMA/PCNA guideline for the prevention, detection, evaluation, and management of high blood pressure in adults: A report of the American College of Cardiology/American Heart Association Task Force on Clinical Practice Guidelines. *Hypertension*, *71*(6), e13–e115 with permission of American Heart Association. https://www.ahajournals.org/doi/pdf/10.1161/HYP.0000000000000066)

patient instruction can be sent via the phone as an additional level of communication. Inclusion of a family member or friend who can help clarify and encourage self-management treatment goals is suggested when appropriate (Cappelletti et al., 2020; Gamage et al., 2020; Kilic & Dag, 2020; Singh et al., 2021).

Once a patient begins pharmacologic therapy, regardless of how well they feel, they must be cautioned to not make medication changes without consulting their prescriptive provider. Given that HTN causes structural changes in the cardiovascular system, reduction of the types and doses of medication a patient takes should be done with caution. About 25% of patients can withdraw antihypertension medication without a return of hypertension for two or more years (Jennings, 2017; van der Wardt et al., 2017). Patients who have achieved key lifestyle modifications such as sustained weight loss have the highest incidence of success with stopping antihypertensive medications.

Complications

Prolonged BP elevation damages blood vessels, particularly in target organs such as the heart, kidneys, brain, and eyes. The consequences of prolonged, uncontrolled hypertension are MI, heart failure, left ventricular hypertrophy, kidney failure, stroke, TIA, and impaired vision. An acute elevation in BP associated with end-organ damage is termed *hypertensive emergency.* It was formerly referred to as hypertensive

TABLE **12-4 Medication Therapy for Hypertension**

Medication	Major Action	Considerations
Primary Agents		
Diuretics (thiazide or thiazide-type)		
Chlorthalidone, hydrochlorothiazide, indapamide, metolazone	Decrease blood volume, renal blood flow, and cardiac output Natriuresis, negative sodium balance Directly affect vascular smooth muscle	Side effects: Dry mouth, thirst, nausea, weakness, drowsiness, postural hypotension Considerations: Monitor for signs of sodium, potassium, and magnesium imbalance
Angiotensin-Converting Enzyme (ACE) Inhibitors		
Captopril, enalaprilat/enalapril, fosinopril, lisinopril, quinapril, ramipril	Inhibit conversion of angiotensin I to angiotensin II; reduce peripheral resistance	Side effects: Hypotension, tachycardia, hyperkalemia, azotemia, angioedema (rare but life threatening) Contraindications: Pregnancy
Angiotensin II Receptor Blockers (ARBs)		
Candesartan, irbesartan, losartan olmesartan, telmisartan, valsartan	Block the effects of angiotensin II at the receptor; reduce peripheral resistance	Side effects: Hypotension, hyperkalemia Contraindications: Pregnancy
Calcium-Channel Blockers		
Nondihydropyridines Diltiazem, verapamil **Dihydropyridines** Amlodipine, felodipine, isradipine, nifedipine	Nondihydropyridines: Agents that affect the heart and blood vessels Inhibit calcium ion influx; reduce cardiac afterload, workload Dihydropyridine: Agent that acts mainly on blood vessels	Do not discontinue suddenly. Side effects: Hypotension, bradycardia, HF dizziness, edema Contraindications: Sick sinus syndrome, heart blocks
Secondary Agents		
Diuretics—loop		
Bumetanide, furosemide, toresemide	Inhibit sodium chloride transport in the ascending limbs of the loop, resulting in natriuresis (excretion of sodium in the urine) and diuresis	
Diuretics—potassium sparing		
Amiloride, triamterene, spironolactone	Act on the distal convoluted tubule and on aldosterone to increase urinary output without potassium loss	Avoid use if hyperkalemia or severe kidney dysfunction Monitor K^+ and kidney function; consider risk vs. benefit if combined with ACEI, ARB, K^+ sparing diuretic, or K^+ supplement
Beta Blockers		
Atenolol, propranolol, metoprolol, nadolol, timolol	Block beta-adrenergic receptors of sympathetic nervous system, causing vasodilation, decreased cardiac output, and heart rate	Side effects: Hypotension, bradycardia, heart failure, fatigue, depression, weakness, impotence, rebound hypertension, hypoglycemia Contraindications: Asthma, COPD
Alpha Blockers		
Doxazosin, prazosin hydrochloride, terazosin	Peripherally acting vasodilator	Side effects: Vomiting and diarrhea, urinary frequency, and tachycardia if not controlled with beta blocker; drowsiness
Combined Alpha and Beta Blockers		
Carvedilol, labetalol hydrochloride	Block alpha- and beta-adrenergic receptors; cause peripheral dilation and decrease peripheral vascular resistance	Side effects: Orthostatic hypotension, tachycardia or bradycardia Contraindications: Asthma and COPD

(*continued*)

TABLE **12-4 Medication Therapy for Hypertension (*continued*)**

Medication	Major Action	Considerations
Direct Renin Inhibitor (DRI)		
Aliskiren	Blocks the conversion of pro-renin to renin, thereby blocking renin-angiotensin system activation at its origin	Side effects: Diarrhea, cough, flulike symptoms, and rash. DRI aliskiren can injure or be fatal to the developing fetus.
Vasodilators		
Hydralazine, Minoxidil	Direct-acting arterial vasodilators decrease peripheral resistance; concurrently elevate cardiac output; act directly on smooth muscle of blood vessels	Side effects: Headache, tachycardia, flushing, and dyspnea, lupus erythematosus–like syndrome, hirsutism, dizziness, headache, nausea, edema, tachycardia, profound hypotension, thiocyanate toxicity
Sodium nitroprusside	Peripheral vasodilation by relaxation of smooth muscle	Side effects: Hypotension, tachycardia, flushing, headache. Protect bag and lines from light (Efre & Boling, 2023). Concern exists related to potential lethal complications from cyanide toxicity in both birthing parent and fetus; "administered only for pregnant females with life-threatening severe hypertension" (Dugal, 2020, p. 2850)

Data from Carey and Whelton (2018), Department of Veterans Affairs (VA) and Department of Defense (DoD, 2020), Flack and Adekola (2020), and Sharma et al. (2021).

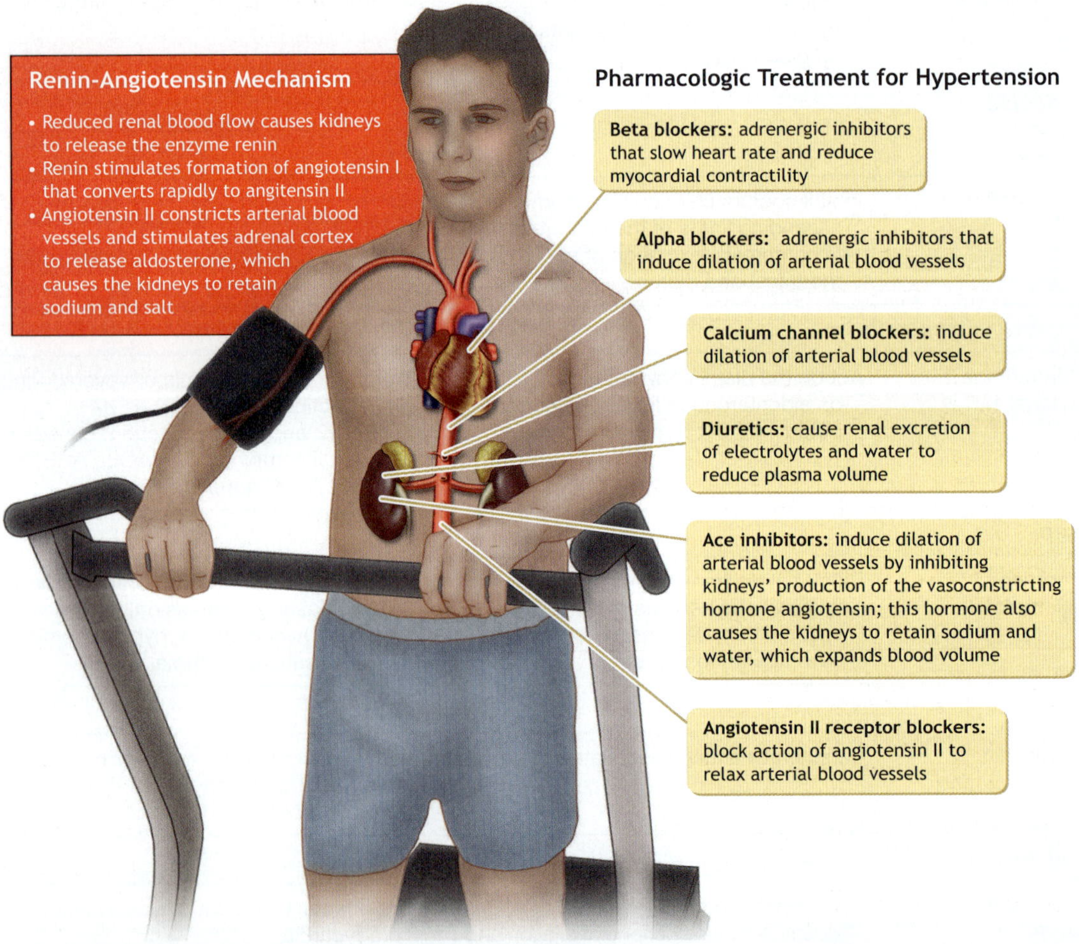

FIGURE 12-4 **Pharmacologic treatment for hypertension. (Reproduced with permission from McArdle, W. D., Katch, F. I., & Katch, V. L. [2014]. *Exercise physiology* [8th ed., Fig. 15.10]. Wolters Kluwer Health.)**

crisis or malignant hypertension (Haynes & Henry, 2022). In contrast, hypertensive urgencies are situations associated with severe BP elevation in otherwise stable patients without acute or impending change in target organ damage or dysfunction. Many of these patients have withdrawn from or are nonadherent to antihypertensive therapy and do not have clinical or laboratory evidence of acute target organ damage. These patients should not be considered as having a hypertensive emergency and instead are treated by reinstitution or intensification of antihypertensive drug therapy, often with rapid-acting oral antihypertensive agents (Haynes & Henry, 2022) and treatment of anxiety as applicable. Oral doses of fast-acting agents are recommended for the treatment of hypertensive urgencies (see Table 12-4). If severe hypertension is present but does not yet pose an immediate threat of organ damage, reducing BP over 24 to 48 hours is preferable since rapid reductions can cause cerebral ischemia, MI, and acute kidney injury; thus, pressure should be reduced gradually when possible (Rosenthal & Burchum, 2021).

HYPERTENSIVE EMERGENCY

Hypertensive emergency is an acute complication of HTN, defined as a severe increase in BP (commonly above 180/120 mm Hg) associated with potentially life-threatening target organ damage such as MI, ischemic stroke, hemorrhagic stroke, or pulmonary edema (Waldron et al., 2019). It occurs in less than 1% of patients with hypertension but when present is life threatening, necessitating early recognition and treatment to reduce morbidity and mortality (Haynes & Henry, 2022). The 1-year death rate associated with hypertensive emergencies is >79%, and the median survival is 10.4 months if the emergency is left untreated (Whelton et al., 2017). It can be precipitated by nonadherence or an inadequate treatment plan for hypertension. For those patients without a history of hypertension who develop hypertensive emergency, etiologies include acute kidney failure, acute CNS events (subarachnoid hemorrhage, intracerebral hemorrhage, or stroke), acute aortic dissection, pregnancy-induced eclampsia, hyperthyroidism, pheochromocytoma (a tumor of the adrenal medulla that causes excess secretion of catecholamines, refer to Chapter 30), substance use disorder (cocaine or amphetamines), and medication–food interactions such as tyramine-containing foods or beverages (beer or aged cheese; Haynes & Henry, 2022; Mathews et al., 2021; Sharma et al., 2021). Risk factors for hypertensive emergency include female biologic sex, obesity, presence of hypertensive or coronary heart disease, a higher number of prescribed antihypertensive drugs, and nonadherence to medication (Sharma et al., 2021). The common acute target organ damage among patients with HTN emergencies include acute or worsening heart failure, MI (both ST elevation and non-ST elevation), aortic dissection, ischemic stroke, hemorrhagic stroke, and HTN encephalopathy (Carey & Whelton, 2018; Waldron et al., 2019).

Pearls for Practice

In hypertensive emergency, commonly reported symptoms by patients included chest pain (89%), visual disturbances (89.8%), dyspnea (82.7%), headache (82.1%), dizziness (52%), conjunctival hemorrhages (41.5%), tinnitus (38.2%), and epistaxis (34.4%) in an international research study (Saladini et al., 2020). The nurse recognizes these symptoms and immediately assesses the blood pressure when a patient presents with any of the complaints described.

Management of Hypertensive Crises

In adults with a hypertensive emergency, admission to an intensive care unit is recommended for continuous monitoring of BP with an arterial line whenever possible, for assessment of target organ damage, and for parenteral administration of an appropriate medication (Carey & Whelton, 2018). However, insertion of an arterial line should not delay treatment (Mathews et al., 2020). For adults with a compelling condition such as aortic dissection, severe preeclampsia or eclampsia, or pheochromocytoma crisis, the SBP should be reduced to less than 140 mm Hg during the first hour and to less than 120 mm Hg in aortic dissection, which is a cardiac surgical emergency if it involves the ascending aorta (see Chapter 17). For adults without a compelling condition, SBP should be reduced by no more than 25% within the first hour; then, if stable, to 160/100 mm Hg within the next 2 to 6 hours; and then cautiously to normal during the following 24 to 48 hours (Carey & Whelton, 2018).

The medications used to manage hypertensive emergencies are best administered in continuous IV infusions of a short-acting titratable antihypertensive agent using an infusion pump, and BP should be monitored continuously (Rosenthal & Burchum, 2021). The nurse avoids the sublingual and IM routes, as their absorption and dynamics are unpredictable. Medications may include clevidipine hydrochloride, enalaprilat, esmolol, fenoldopam, hydralazine, labetalol, nicardipine, or sodium nitroprusside, which have immediate, short-lived actions. Sodium nitroprusside is unsuitable for long-term use because of development of a metabolite that causes cyanide-like toxicity (blurred vision, confusion, tinnitus, seizures); the risk peaks within 48 to 72 hours of therapy or with renal insufficiency (Efre & Boling, 2023; Haynes & Henry, 2022). The thiocyanate blood level should be measured at 48 hours, and levels should not exceed 1.7 mmol/L (Efre & Boling, 2023). For those with severe preeclampsia or eclampsia, hydralazine and *labetalol* have been widely used (Elliot, 2022). If the patient is pregnant, fetal movements, baseline fetal heart rate, and variability should be monitored. Once the BP is controlled, medications can be switched to oral formulations (Sharma et al., 2021). For more information about these medications, see Table 12-4.

The nurse observes the patient closely for evidence of end-organ dysfunction and recognizes that treatment within an hour is necessary to prevent end-organ damage; accurate vital sign measurements must be performed (Aquilina et al., 2019). Related to neurologic compromise, the nurse is alert to changes in the level of consciousness, new complaint of headache, blurred vision, mental confusion, nausea/vomiting, stupor, seizures, coma, or changes in the cranial nerve assessment. Strict intake and output measurement is expected, and the provider is alerted if the hourly output is <0.5 mL/Kg/hr or there is a sudden absence of urine output (anuria). Any alteration in the patient's baseline blood chemistry, BUN, and serum creatinine values is evaluated to assess for renal compromise. In addition, cardiac compromise can present with arrhythmias, ECG changes, complaints of chest pain, or "tearing" sensation, a significant difference of BP measurement in both arms consistent with dissecting aneurysm, shortness of breath, jugular vein distention (JVD), change in pulmonary (crackles) and/or cardiac exam (e.g., new murmur, S3, S4) consistent with MI or HF.

Drug Alert

ACEIs and ARBs block aldosterone and may cause hyperkalemia when used with potassium-sparing diuretics or salt substitutes that contain potassium. The nurse should monitor the potassium level and teach the patient to avoid salt substitutes.

The nurse follows up with teaching about a hypertensive emergency and encourages the patient to take charge of managing hypertension.

Clinical Judgment Case

A 42-year-old patient comes into the emergency room (ER) complaining of sudden onset of severe midsternal chest pain; the patient states "the pain feels like it is going right through to my back." The patient's skin is cool, and vital signs are as follows: 98.7°F, heart rate 118 and regular, 24 respiratory rate (RR) with an oxygen saturation of 93% on room air, and blood pressure 192/124 mm Hg. Heart Sounds are S1, S2 with grade 3/6 blowing diastolic murmur noted in second intercostal space (ICS), right sternal border (RSB) radiating down the left sternal border; the point of maximum impulse (PMI) is nondisplaced (fifth intercostal space [ICS], midclavicular line); there is no S3 but S4 is noted in mitral area. When you ask the patient if any provider ever noted a heart murmur, the patient replies "no, never." Crackles are heard at bases bilaterally, no jugular vein distention (JVD). Abdomen is soft, nondistended, nontender, bowel sounds are present in all 4 quadrants. Capillary refill is 4 seconds bilaterally and dorsalis pedis and posterior tibial pulses are 1+ bilaterally; there is delayed skin turgor, no peripheral edema. The patient's history includes appendectomy as a child and no medical history. The patient is anxious and restless.

Step One: Recognize cues where relevant and important information is identified from different sources, such as medical history or vital signs.

Answer: Significant cues include severe sudden onset midsternal chest pain that "feels like it is going right through to my back." New onset of grade 3/6 blowing diastolic murmur noted in second intercostal space (ICS), right sternal border (RSB) radiating down the left sternal border, S4, and bibasilar crackles. The patient's skin is cool, capillary refill of 4 seconds and pedal and posterior tibial pulses are 1+; delayed skin turgor. The patient is anxious and restless. Significant vital signs are heart rate of 118 and regular, 24 RR with an oxygen saturation of 93% on room air and blood pressure of 192/124 mm Hg.

Step Two: Analyze cues, which is organizing and linking the recognized cues to the patient's clinical presentation.

Answer: You have clustered the patient's symptoms to be associated with a hypertensive emergency, which you know is a systolic pressure >180 mm Hg, or diastolic pressure >120 mm Hg with signs of end-organ damage. You associate the chest pain, bibasilar crackles, tachypnea (RR 24), and decreased oxygen saturation (93% on room air) with a potential new diagnosis of myocardial infarction (MI) and/or left-sided heart failure (HF) and end-organ damage due to hypertensive emergency. The S4 is associated with hypertension or MI. You also cluster the new-onset chest pain that radiates to the back, new-onset diastolic murmur that is heard along the left sternal border with aortic regurgitation, and hypertension with potential ascending aortic dissection. You recall the murmurs radiate in the direction of flow and the aortic valve, which is normally closed in diastole, is now allowing blood to flow retrograde into the left ventricle. You cluster the cool skin, capillary refill of 4 seconds and pedal and posterior tibial pulses of 1+ bil, and delayed skin turgor with potential for limb ischemia related to a potential aortic dissection. You recall that in aortic dissection, the blood is entering a false lumen between the intima [inner layer] and media [middle layer] of the arterial wall; the extension of this lumen can occlude blood flow to the "true" aortic lumen and patients can present with a variety of symptoms depending on which arteries are not receiving blood flow; in this case, you consider the *dissection is causing impaired blood flow to the lower extremity*. The patient is anxious and restless related to decreased oxygen saturation and/or aortic dissection. The tachycardia may be related to the potential aortic dissection, potential myocardial infarction and or left sided HF.

Step Three: Prioritize hypotheses, where hypotheses are evaluated and ranked according to priority. This can include urgency, likelihood, risk, difficulty and/or time. In this phase you cluster your findings to arrive at a list of problems (actual and or potential problems) you believe the patient is experiencing and determine the importance or urgency. What do you think is of greatest concern?

Answer: The potential hypothesis includes (1) hypertensive emergency; (2) poor peripheral perfusion r/t potential aortic dissection; (3) potential myocardial infarction; (4) potential left sided HF; (5) hemodynamic instability; and (6) potential end target organ damage which may also include the kidneys, brain, and eyes. In the moment, you prioritize the hypertensive emergency as the greatest risk of injury to this patient.

Step Four: Generate solutions, which is identifying expected outcomes and using hypotheses to define a set of interventions for the expected outcomes.

Answer: Since hypertensive emergency is present, you recognize the need to place the patient on a cardiac monitor and start two large-gauge IVs for emergency intravenous medications. You will want to administer oxygen to improve the oxygen saturation, which on admission was 93% on room air. You will monitor the oxygen saturation continuously and vital signs every 15 minutes at a minimum. Since you are concerned about a potential aortic dissection, which results from the creation of a false lumen between the intima (inner layer) and media (middle layer) of the arterial wall, you want to assess the BP in both arms to evaluate for significant deviations and are aware that a difference of more than 20 mm Hg in blood pressure between the arms should raise suspicion of ascending aortic dissection. You also want to inquire what that pain feels like; if the patient describes "tearing sensation," you recognize this as a symptom of an aortic dissection. You expect an emergency transthoracic echocardiography (TTE), which is an echocardiogram that is done by holding a probe (transducer) over the patient's chest, and computed tomography (CT) of the chest and abdomen with intravenous contrast will be ordered because rapid visualization of the thoracic structures can be seen. A chest radiograph may be diagnostically helpful if it shows the mediastinum is already widened. Stat laboratory testing that will evaluate the patient's baseline will include: complete blood count (CBC), type and cross-match of the blood in anticipation of blood transfusions (blood products may need to be administered, particularly if the aorta ruptures), coagulation studies, lactate level (to assess for acidemia), BNP (to assess for HF), troponin (to assess for MI), renal function (to assess renal compromise), and chemistry.

Step Five: Take action, where the solutions that address the highest priorities are implemented.

Answer: Although you are not aware of the precipitating event, the patient has a hypertensive emergency and the priority is to decrease the blood pressure. You place the patient in a semi-fowler position and maintain a calm, reassuring environment since anxiety will elevate the HR and BP further. You assess the BP in both arms, and you note a difference of >26 mm Hg. You ask the patient to describe the pain, which they describe as "ripping or tearing." You notify the provider of these findings. You start two large -gauge IV lines to establish access for medication administration and potential need for fluid replacement if the BP drops. You place the patient on a cardiac monitor, evaluate the electrocardiogram (ECG) for ischemic changes or arrhythmias, and monitor the oxygen saturation continuously. You administer oxygen at 2 liters via nasal cannula. You also ask the patient about the use of any illicit drugs and find that the patient used cocaine before the chest pain. You are aware that cocaine can cause an abrupt, transient, severe increase in blood pressure, which is a risk factor for nontraumatic aortic dissection. You are aware that the brain can also be affected by the hypertensive emergency, so you perform a neurologic assessment noting any visual field deficit, weakness or numbness, pupils, complaints of headache, and any language deficit. You prepare for an arterial line which will be placed since BP monitoring occurs frequently (often every 2–3 minutes) until target BP and HR are reached. You also prepare the likely prescribed medications that will include morphine, which decreases sympathetic nervous system stimulation and relieves pain; and sodium nitroprusside, which is a peripheral vasodilatory of arterial and venous smooth muscle, which decreases the afterload lowering the BP. This is the medication of choice with dissecting aneurysms. It is typically prescribed initially at 0.25 to 0.5 mcg/kg/min IV. You calculate the patient's weight, which is 198 lb. You convert this to kg: 2.2 lb = 1 kg;

therefore, the patient weights 90 kg. The nitroprusside medication works in 1 to 2 minutes and lasts 1 to 10 minutes, which is why it is administered as a continuous infusion; it is reversed by stopping the infusion. The provider orders 0.5 mcg/kg/min continuous IV infusion; the medicine comes prepared from pharmacy 50 mg in 250 mL D5W, which means 0.2 mg = 1 mL. You now need to convert milligrams to micrograms (1 *milligram* [*mg*] is equal to 1,000 *micrograms* [μg]), which means you multiply 0.2 × 1,000 = 200 mcg/mL. If the patient is to receive 0.5 mcg × 90 kg, that equals 45 mcg in 1 minute. You multiply 45 mcg × 60 (because 60 minutes = 1 hour) = 2,700 mcg. Your prepared solution is 200 mcg/mL, so divide 2,700 mcg by 200 (mcg/mL), and you will set the pump at a rate of 13.5 ml/hr. NOTE: Always verify your calculation with another nurse or provider or pharmacist. In addition, with nitroprusside, the bag and IV line must be protected from light (it is light sensitive, and this prevents drug degradation). You will titrate (increasing or decreasing an infusion for therapeutic effect) the medication based upon the BP every 5 to 10 minutes to the desired BP range, which the provider has set as a systolic pressure of <120 mm Hg. You will observe for signs of cyanide toxicity (blurred vision, seizures, tinnitus), particularly after 48 hours of infusion. Each institution will have policies and procedures to follow with IV drips, and you should know that if you have any doubt about the medication, you should consult with your pharmacist. An indwelling catheter will be inserted since monitoring the hourly urine output is important. You expect a minimum urinary output of 0.5 mL/kg/hr which in this patient is 45 mL/hr. You also monitor for any changes in peripheral perfusion since aortic rupture can occur. You assess for any changes in cardiopulmonary assessment and neurovascular status (including assessing for pain, pallor, poikilothermia [cool limbs] paresthesia, paralysis, and movement of the limb) and alert the provider with any changes since severe chest pain, hypotension, and hemorrhagic shock suggest aortic rupture.

Step Six: Evaluate outcomes, which is comparing observed outcomes against expected outcomes.

Answer: The TTE and CT scan revealed an ascending aortic dissection, and the patient was immediately transferred to the operating room for a thoracic endovascular aortic repair (TEVAR), which is a minimally invasive technique that has largely replaced traditional open surgical repair. The troponin and BNP were within normal limits; therefore, your patient did not have an MI or HF. The patient subsequently recovered and was discharged home. When the patient presented with a hypertensive emergency, you cast the net wide in considering precipitating events, such as MI or left-sided heart failure, but did not consider cocaine as a possibility. With each clinical experience you will add to your database; in the future, because of your experience with this patient, you will always assess the BP in both arms and perform a neurologic assessment since target organs can include more than the heart (brain, eyes, kidneys, etc.). In addition, you now recognize the importance of math calculations and the reason your nursing program focused on them. Your confidence and knowledge will grow with your efforts.

CHAPTER REVIEW

NCLEX-Style Review Questions

1. You are working in a primary care clinic and are evaluating a patient for hypertension. Place the actions in the correct order.

a. Inform the patient to not talk during the reading.
b. Bring the patient into the room but wait 5 minutes before auscultating the blood pressure.
c. Sit the patient in chair with back supported and legs firmly on the floor.
d. Record the point on the manometer when you hear the first clear sound that reflects the systolic BP and the point at which the sound disappears (diastolic BP).
e. Deflate the cuff pressure 2 mm of Hg per second.
f. Place the cuff no less than 1 in from the antecubital fossa.

2. A patient is admitted with aortic dissection and hypertensive emergency. On admission, the BP is 240/120. The nurse recognizes which of the following is consistent with current BP management strategies? Select all that apply.
   a. Treatment in the first hour is important to prevent end-organ damage.
   b. In 1 hour, the patient's target SBP should be less than 120 mm Hg.
   c. The blood pressure can be monitored on a medical unit every 15 minutes.
   d. The nurse should anticipate using oral medications for hypertensive emergency.
   e. The nurse should anticipate the administration of a continuous IV infusion of short-acting titratable antihypertensive agent.

3. The nurse is teaching a patient about BP self-monitoring. What direction should be included in the plan of care? Select all that apply.
   a. You may sit or stand when taking your BP.
   b. Do not eat or drink for at least 2 hours before measuring your BP.
   c. Make sure the cuff is loose enough to avoid squeezing your arm too tightly.
   d. Keep your arm at heart level.
   e. Avoid talking during BP measurement.

4. Which of the symptoms below suggest acute end-organ dysfunction seen in hypertensive emergency? Select all that apply.
   a. Polyuria
   b. Chest pain
   c. Pulse pressure of 40 mm Hg
   d. Seizures
   e. Oliguria

5. Which of the following conditions would prevent you from using the left limb for a blood pressure reading? Select all that apply.
   a. DVT in the left limb
   b. Postbilateral lymph node dissection
   c. Cast on the right limb
   d. Arteriovenous (AV) fistula right limb
   e. Postleft axillary vascular repair

REFERENCES AND SELECTED READINGS

References and selected readings associated with this chapter can be found on the website that accompanies the book. Visit **http://thepoint.lww.com/Honan3e** to access the references and other additional resources associated with this chapter.

CHAPTER 13

Nursing Management: Patients With Coronary Vascular Disorders

Jose Chavez

Learning Objectives

After reading this chapter, you will be able to:

1. Summarize the pathophysiology, risk factors, clinical manifestations, and treatment of coronary atherosclerosis.
2. Summarize the pathophysiology, clinical manifestations, and treatment of angina pectoris.
3. Describe percutaneous coronary intervention (PCI) and coronary artery revascularization procedures.
4. Explain the nursing care of a patient who has had a PCI procedure for treatment of coronary artery disease.
5. Describe the nursing care of a patient who has undergone cardiac surgery.
6. Summarize the pathophysiology, clinical manifestations, and treatment of myocardial infarction.

Cardiovascular disease (CVD) is the leading cause of death in the United States and globally, and accounts for more than 17.9 million deaths per year, a number that is expected to increase to more than 23.6 million by 2030 (World Health Organization [WHO], 2021). About one of every three deaths in America and 32% of all deaths globally can be attributed to CVD, affecting all segments of the population. Coronary artery disease (CAD) is the most prevalent type of CVD in adults. For this reason, it is important for nurses to become familiar with various manifestations of coronary artery conditions and methods for assessing, preventing, and treating these disorders medically and surgically.

CORONARY ATHEROSCLEROSIS

The most common cause of CVD in the United States is **atherosclerosis**, an abnormal accumulation of lipid or fatty substances and fibrous tissue in the lining of arterial blood vessel walls. These substances create blockages and narrow the coronary vessels in a way that reduces blood flow to the myocardium. It is now known that atherosclerosis involves a repetitious inflammatory response to injury to the artery wall and subsequent alteration in the structural and biochemical properties of the arterial walls.

Pathophysiology

Atherosclerosis begins as fatty streaks of lipids that are deposited in the intima of the arterial wall. These lesions commonly begin early in life, perhaps even in childhood. Not all fatty streaks develop into more advanced lesions later. Genetics and environmental factors influence the progression of these lesions. The continued development of atherosclerosis involves an inflammatory response, which begins with injury to the vascular endothelium. The injury may be initiated by smoking, hypertension (HTN), and other factors. The presence of inflammation has multiple effects on the arterial wall, including the attraction of inflammatory cells (including macrophages or monocytes, white blood cells [WBCs]) (Prado & Napierkowski, 2020). The macrophages infiltrate the injured vascular endothelium and ingest lipids, which turn them into what are called "foam cells." These foam cells are present in all stages of atherosclerotic plaque formation (Porth, 2019). Activated macrophages also release biochemical substances that can further damage the endothelium, attracting platelets, and initiating clotting.

Smooth muscle cells within the vessel wall subsequently proliferate and form a fibrous cap over a center that is filled with lipid and inflammatory infiltrate. These deposits, called **atheromas** or plaques, protrude into the lumen of the vessel, narrowing it, and obstructing blood flow (Fig. 13-1). If the

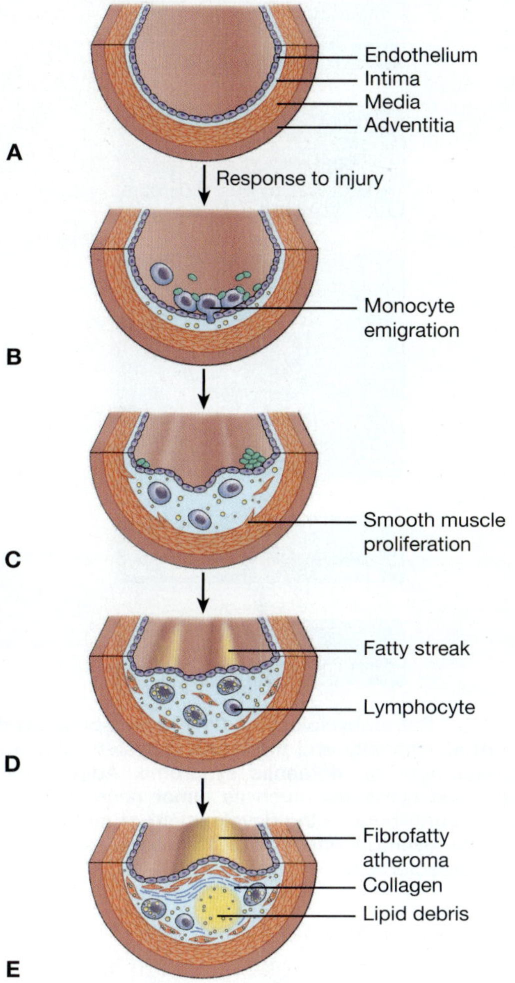

FIGURE 13-1 Atherosclerosis begins as monocytes and lipids enter the intima of an injured vessel (A, B). Smooth muscle cells proliferate within the vessel wall (C) contributing to the development of fatty accumulations and atheroma (D). As the plaque enlarges, the vessel narrows and blood flow decreases (E). The plaque may rupture and a thrombus might form, obstructing blood flow.

fibrous cap of the plaque is thick and the lipid pool remains relatively stable, it can resist the stress from blood flow and vessel movement. If the cap is thin and inflammation is ongoing, the lipid core may grow, causing it to rupture, and this ruptured plaque is a focus for thrombus formation. Then the thrombus may obstruct blood flow, leading to sudden cardiac death or an acute **myocardial infarction (MI)**, which is the death of a portion of the heart muscle. Thus, atherosclerosis can produce narrowing of the lumen of a blood vessel, sudden obstruction of a blood vessel due to plaque rupture, and weakening of a blood vessel, resulting in aneurysm formation or emboli formation because of direct damage to the endothelium.

The anatomic structure of the coronary arteries makes them particularly susceptible to the mechanisms of atherosclerosis. There are three major coronary arteries and they have multiple branches; atherosclerotic lesions most often form where the vessels branch (Fig. 13-2). Although heart disease is most often caused by atherosclerosis of the coronary arteries, other phenomena may also decrease blood flow to the heart. Examples include vasospasm (sudden constriction or narrowing) of a coronary artery, myocardial trauma from internal or external forces, structural disease, congenital anomalies, decreased oxygen supply (e.g., from acute blood loss, anemia, or low blood pressure), and increased oxygen demand (e.g., from rapid heart rate, thyrotoxicosis, or use of cocaine).

Risk Factors

Epidemiologic studies point to several factors that increase the probability that CAD will develop in a person. Some risk factors are uncontrollable, including:

- Age (males over 45 years old, postmenopausal people)
- Sex (in people less than 55 years of age, males are at a greater risk; after 55 years of age, males and females have

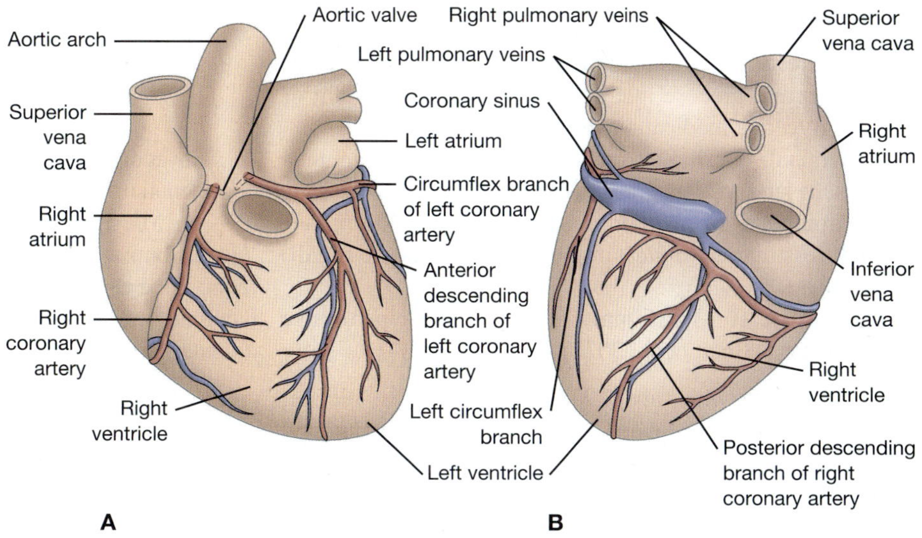

FIGURE 13-2 The coronary arteries supply the heart muscle with oxygenated blood, adjusting the flow according to metabolic needs: (A) anterior view and (B) posterior view of heart.

the same risk; or people under 55 years of age who have premature menopause without estrogen replacement therapy)
- Ethnicity (African American, Mexican American, Native American, and some Asian American populations demonstrate increased risk)
- Family history of first-degree relative with premature diagnosis of heart disease

Known modifiable risk factors include diabetes mellitus (DM) and pre-diabetes, HTN, smoking, obesity, physical inactivity, high blood cholesterol, unhealthy diet, alcohol use and stress (Brown et al., 2022).

Risk factors identified more recently include sleep apnea, metabolic syndrome (discussed below), increased body mass index (BMI), chronic kidney disease, chronic infections (Bonsignore et al., 2019), nonalcoholic fatty liver disease (NAFLD) (Sheth & Chopra, 2021), and influenza; additional risk factors may include conditions thought to be proinflammatory (e.g., rheumatoid arthritis) (Yedlapati et al., 2021; Wilson, 2022).

Pearls for Practice

Obesity (BMI of 35% or higher) in and of itself is associated with all-cause mortality regardless of level of physical activity. Questions exist regarding whether obesity itself is a risk factor for CAD or cardiovascular events, or if it is the relationship of obesity to glucose intolerance, insulin resistance, HTN, physical inactivity, and dyslipidemia that increases risk. Given the significant risk that DM, HTN, and hyperlipidemia impose on coronary disease, nurses need to make efforts toward increasing awareness of the crucial role that these disorders have on cardiovascular mortality and morbidity.

A cluster of metabolic abnormalities now known as **metabolic syndrome** is known to be a major risk factor for CAD (Fig. 13-3). A diagnosis of this syndrome includes any combination of three of the following conditions:

- Insulin resistance (fasting glucose greater than 100 mg/dL or abnormal glucose tolerance test) or taking insulin or hypoglycemic medication (Bhatt et al., 2022)
- Abdominal obesity (waist circumference greater than 35 inches in females, greater than 40 inches in males)
- Dyslipidemia (triglycerides greater than 150 mg/dL; HDL less than 50 mg/dL in females, less than 40 mg/dL in males)
- HTN (at least 130/85 mm Hg) or on antihypertensive medication (Bhatt et al., 2022)

Many people with type 2 DM fit this clinical picture. Measurement of lipoprotein, homocysteine (an amino acid associated with cardiac disease), and CRP may also be appropriate in people who are identified as being at risk (Bouzidi et al., 2020).

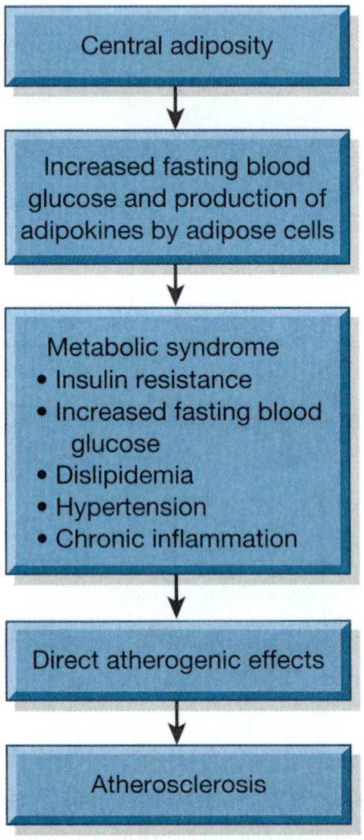

FIGURE 13-3 **Pathophysiology of CVD in metabolic syndrome. Both central adiposity and the immune system play a role in the development of metabolic syndrome. Adipokines (such as leptin) and cytokines (such as tumor necrosis factor) are thought to contribute to the development of metabolic abnormalities. The eventual effect of these processes is the promotion of atherosclerosis.**

Pearls for Practice

CRP is a protein that is released in the blood during inflammatory states. It is virtually absent in the blood of healthy people. There are two types of CRP assays. The first measures CRP (normal typically 0.3 to 20 mg/dL) and is typically used to assess inflammatory disease, detect infections postoperatively, detect transplant rejection, and monitor inflammatory processes. The second is the high-sensitivity CRP (hs-CRP) that is useful in assessing the risk of a cardiac event (Fischbach et al., 2022). A normal level is less than 0.1 mg/dL or less than 1 mg/L, respectively (Fischbach et al., 2022).

In addition, a risk equivalent is a condition that places patients at high risk for experiencing a cardiac event, such as an MI. Having one or more of the conditions listed as contributing to metabolic syndrome may place patients at the same risk of having a cardiac event as someone who has already experienced one (Powers et al., 2019). Risk equivalents for cardiac events are detailed in Box 13-1.

Clinical Manifestations and Assessment

Coronary atherosclerosis produces symptoms and complications according to the location and degree of narrowing of the arterial lumen, thrombus formation, and obstruction of

BOX 13-1

Coronary Artery Disease Risk Equivalents

Individuals at highest risk for a cardiac event within 10 years are those with known existing coronary artery disease (CAD) who have experienced a cardiac event, and those without a known history of cardiac event but have any one or more of the following diseases, which are called CAD risk equivalents (Powers et al., 2019). Risk equivalents are essentially disease processes that involve atherosclerotic disease.

- Diabetes mellitus
- Peripheral arterial disease
- Abdominal aortic aneurysm
- Carotid artery disease
- Chronic kidney disease (CKD)
- Large vessel atherosclerotic ischemic stroke

blood flow to the myocardium. This impediment to blood flow is usually progressive, causing an inadequate blood supply that deprives the cardiac muscle cells of oxygen needed for their survival. The condition is known as **ischemia**. **Angina pectoris** refers to chest pain that is brought about by myocardial ischemia. If the decrease in blood supply is significant enough, of long enough duration, or both, death of myocardial cells, or MI, may result. Over time, irreversibly damaged myocardium undergoes degeneration and is replaced by scar tissue, causing various degrees of myocardial dysfunction. Significant myocardial damage may result in persistently low cardiac output (CO), and if the heart cannot support the body's needs for oxygenated blood, the result is heart failure. Myocardial hypoxia due to CAD may also lead to lethal cardiac rhythm disturbances that may result in sudden cardiac death.

Pearls for Practice

Classic signs and symptoms of myocardial ischemia include acute onset of chest pain (often described as crushing pain, usually substernal but may be in other areas of the chest, jaw, back, or arms). Some patients present with "atypical" symptoms, such as shortness of breath (SOB) (dyspnea [particularly in older individuals]), extreme fatigue, palpitations, diaphoresis, and nausea and vomiting. The pain of an MI may be differentiated from angina by persistence of the pain despite rest and nitroglycerine. Females often complain of atypical chest pain and nonspecific signs and symptoms. The older population in particular may present with dizziness, or syncope (Golla & Satya, 2022). Thus, the nurse is alert to both typical and atypical signs associated with cardiac disease.

In older individuals, sometimes there will not be a classic presentation of symptoms (referred to as "silent" ischemia), making recognition and diagnosis a clinical challenge. Older patients should be encouraged to recognize their chest pain–like symptoms (anginal equivalent), for example, weakness, as an indication that they should rest or take prescribed medications and contact their provider with concerns. Pharmacologic stress testing may be used to diagnose CAD in older patients or those who have a limited ability to exercise because of other conditions (e.g., peripheral vascular disease, arthritis, degenerative disk disease, physical disability, foot problems).

Prevention and Medical and Nursing Management

Controlling cholesterol, treating hyperlipidemia, and managing HTN and DM are discussed here; additional medical and nursing management is discussed under angina.

Controlling Cholesterol Abnormalities

The association of a high blood cholesterol level with CAD is well established. The metabolism of fats is an important contributor to the development of CAD. Fats, which are insoluble in water, are encased in water-soluble lipoproteins that allow them to be transported within the circulatory system. The various lipoproteins are categorized by their protein content, which is measured in density. The density increases when more protein is present. Four elements of fat metabolism—total cholesterol, LDL, HDL, and triglycerides—affect the development of heart disease. Cholesterol is processed by the GI tract into lipoprotein globules called *chylomicrons*. These are reprocessed by the liver as lipoproteins (Fig. 13-4). This is a physiologic process necessary for the formation of lipoprotein-based cell membranes and other important metabolic processes. When an excess of LDL is produced, LDL particles adhere to vulnerable points in the arterial endothelium. Here, macrophages ingest them, leading to the formation of foam cells and the beginning of plaque formation.

All adults 20 years of age or older should have a fasting lipid profile (total cholesterol, LDL, HDL, and triglyceride) performed at least once every 5 years and more often if the profile is abnormal. Patients younger than 20 years of age with a known family history of hyperlipidemia and/or vascular disease should probably be tested earlier. Patients who have had an acute event (e.g., MI), a **percutaneous coronary intervention (PCI)**, or a **coronary artery bypass graft (CABG)** require assessment of the LDL cholesterol level within a few months of the event or procedure because LDL levels may be low immediately after the acute event or procedure. Subsequently, lipids should be monitored regularly until the desired level is achieved.

LDL exerts a harmful effect on the coronary vasculature because the small LDL particles can be transported easily into the vessel lining. In contrast, HDL promotes the use of total cholesterol by transporting LDL to the liver, where it is biodegraded and then excreted. The level of HDL should exceed 40 mg/dL and ideally should be more than 60 mg/dL. A high HDL level is a strong negative risk factor for heart

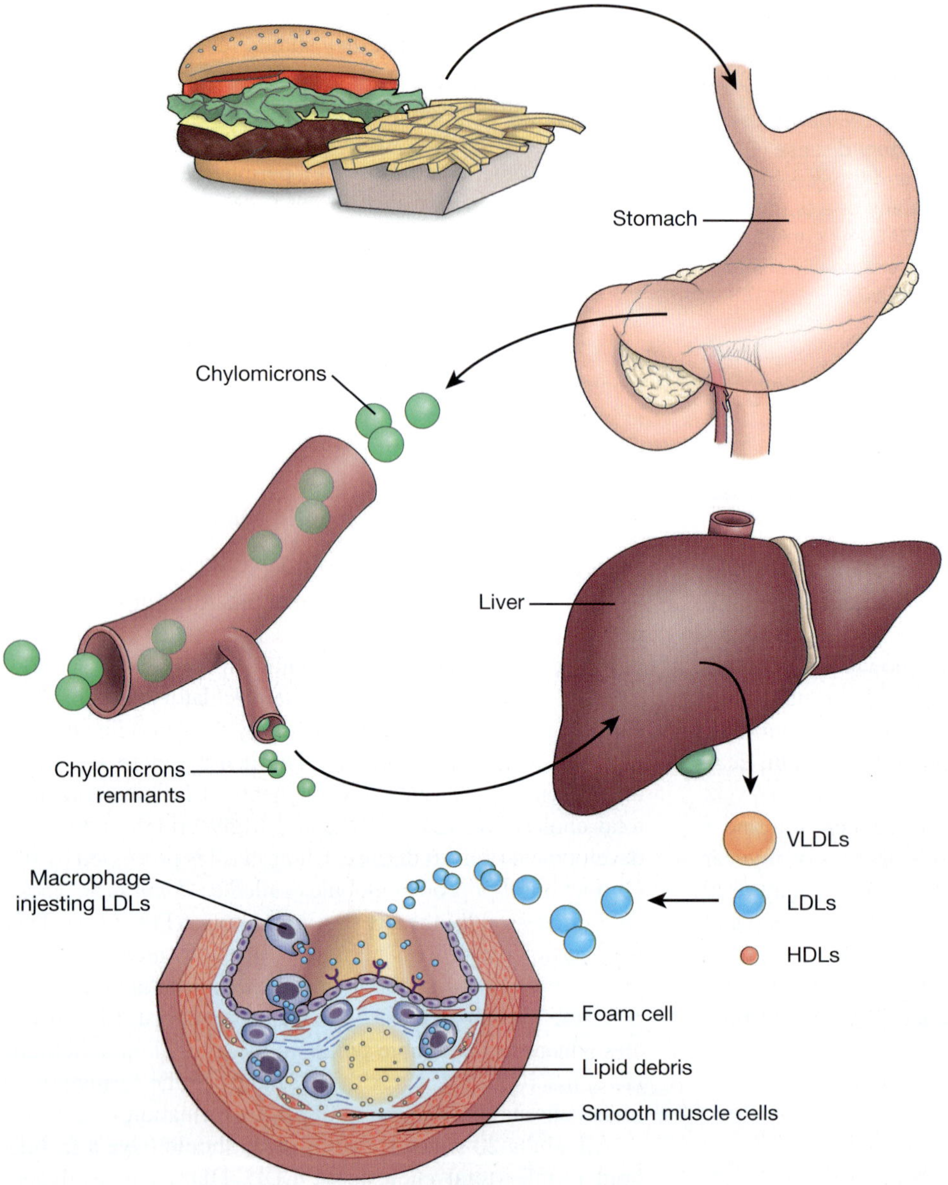

FIGURE 13-4 **Lipoproteins and the development of atherosclerosis. As dietary cholesterol and saturated fat are processed by the GI tract, chylomicrons enter the blood. They are broken down into chylomicron remnants in the capillaries. The liver processes them into lipoproteins. When these are released into the circulation, excess low-density lipoproteins (LDLs) adhere to receptors on the intimal wall. Macrophages also ingest LDLs and transport them into the vessel wall, beginning the process of plaque formation. HDLs, high-density lipoproteins; VLDL, very–low-density lipoprotein.**

disease (i.e., it protects against disease). In 2018, the guidelines for the treatment of high blood cholesterol levels were updated by the American College of Cardiology and the American Heart Association (ACC-AHA) Task Force on Practice Guidelines. The guidelines emphasize pharmacologic treatment to include those without any history of heart disease and includes guidance to population subgroups (younger age groups, racial and ethnic groups), and the initiation or addition of newer nonstatin agents, such as PCSK9 inhibitors and cholesterol absorption inhibitors (Khera, 2018; DePhillips et al., 2021).

Those who would benefit from statin therapy (cholesterol-lowering medications) are those:

1. With clinically evident atherosclerotic CVD
2. With primary low-density lipoprotein (LDL) cholesterol levels of at least 190 mg/dL
3. With type 1 or type 2 DM (ages 40 to 75 years) and an LDL cholesterol level of 70 mg/dL or higher, without clinically evident atherosclerotic CVD
4. Without clinically evident atherosclerotic CVD or DM with an LDL cholesterol level range of 70 to 189 mg/dL and an estimated 10-year risk of atherosclerotic CVD of at least 7.5% (Note: Web-based calculators are available at https://www.cvriskcalculator.com/ and https://tools.acc.org/ascvd-risk-estimator-plus/#!/calculate/estimate/).

In these patient groups, high-intensity statin therapy (designed to reduce LDL cholesterol levels by as much as 50% or more) is generally recommended; it is believed that the benefit outweighs the risk. Research has demonstrated that primary prevention with statins reduces total mortality as well as nonfatal atherosclerotic cardiovascular events (see Table 13-1 for commonly prescribed medications affecting lipoprotein metabolism).

TABLE **13-1 Medications Affecting Lipoprotein Metabolism**

Medication	Lipid/Lipoprotein Effects	Side Effects	Contraindications
HMG-CoA Reductase Inhibitors (Statins)			
Lovastatin Pravastatin Simvastatin Fluvastatin Atorvastatin[a] Rosuvastatin[a] Pitavastatin	LDL ↓ 18–55% HDL ↑ 5–15% TG ↓ 7–30%	Myopathy, myalgias, increased liver enzyme levels, ↑ blood sugar	**Absolute:** Active liver disease, pregnancy, lactation **Relative:** Drug–drug interactions can increase the risk of adverse events—refer to pharmacist
Nicotinic Acid			
Niacin Immediate-release nicotinic acid Extended-release nicotinic acid Sustained-release nicotinic acid	LDL ↓ 5–25% HDL ↑ 15–35% TG ↓ 20–50%	Flushing, hyperglycemia, hyperuricemia (or gout), upper GI distress, hepatotoxicity	**Absolute:** Chronic liver disease, severe gout **Relative:** Diabetes, hyperuricemia, peptic ulcer disease
Fibric Acids			
Fenofibrate Gemfibrozil Fenofibric acid	LDL ↓ 5–20% (may be increased in patients with high TG) HDL ↑ 10–20% TG ↓ 20–50%	Dyspepsia, rash, pruritis, gallstones, myopathy, unexplained non-CHD deaths	**Absolute:** Severe kidney disease, severe liver disease
Bile Acid Sequestrants			
Cholestyramine Colesevelam Colestipol HCl	LDL ↓ 15–30% TG no change or increase	GI distress, constipation, vitamin K deficiency, Decreased uptake of fat-soluble vitamins, drug interactions (binds to other drugs and prevents absorption)	**Absolute:** dysbetalipoproteinemia, TG >400 mg/dL, bowel obstruction, TG-induced pancreatitis **Relative:** TG >200 mg/dL
Omega-3 Fatty Acids *Eicosapentaenoic acid/docosahexaenoic acid (EPA/DHA)*	TG ↓ 25–30% LDL ↑ 5–10% (with dose of 4 g/day)	Flushing, elevated liver enzymes, bleeding risk eructation, and gastric irritation (taste perversion, dyspepsia) and allergic reactions (fish) When used in amounts greater than 3 g/day, EPA is POSSIBLY UNSAFE, and can thin the blood and increase the risk for bleeding	**Absolute:** hypersensitivity to any component of this medication Use caution if hypersensitivity to fish/shellfish, bleeding risk, active liver disease
PCSK9 Inhibitor Evolocumab Alirocumab (self-injected under the skin with a pre-filled, single-use SureClick Autoinjector)	↓ LDL 58–71%	Allergic reaction; flu-like symptoms; back pain; redness, pain, or bruising at the injection site	**Absolute:** hypersensitivity reaction to evolocumab
Cholesterol Absorption Inhibitor Ezetimibe	↓ LDL (~18%), ↑ HDL 1–4%, ↓ TG 5–10%	Allergic reaction, arthralgia, diarrhea, back pain, stomach or abdominal pain, fever, sore throat	Allergy to ezetimibe; active liver disease

Note: Statin therapy are considered first-line agents; the other agents listed below are generally reserved for patients with tolerability issues or hypertriglyceridemia.

HMG-CoA, 3-hydroxy-3-methylglutaryl coenzyme A; LDL, low-density lipoprotein; HDL, high-density lipoprotein; TG, triglycerides; ↓, decrease; ↑, increase; CHD, coronary heart disease.

[a]Atorvastatin and rosuvastatin are both "high-intensity statins," high-intensity statins daily dose lowers LDL-C by approx. ≥50% and are the most commonly prescribed (Skeik et al., 2021).

Moderate-intensity statin therapy (aims for a reduction of 30% to less than 49% in LDL cholesterol levels) is recommended for patients who cannot tolerate high-intensity treatment or patients with DM and a 10-year risk of atherosclerotic CVD of less than 7.5%. People receiving statin therapy should be monitored for muscle and hepatic injury and new-onset DM.

Serum cholesterol and LDL levels often can also be influenced by diet and physical activity. Depending on the patient's LDL level and risk of CAD, medication to treat hyperlipidemia may also be prescribed. Medication should be used in conjunction with a heart-healthy diet and an exercise program since even modest lifestyle changes in diet and exercise can significantly reduce cardiovascular risk markers, such as lipid profiles, inflammatory risk markers, and total body weight (DePhillips et al., 2021). Refer to Table 13-1.

Treating Hyperlipidemia

Lipid-lowering medications can reduce CAD mortality in patients with elevated lipid levels and at-risk patients with normal lipid levels. Patients with elevated cholesterol levels should be monitored for adherence to the therapeutic plan, the effect of cholesterol-lowering medications, and the development of side effects. Based on high-quality randomized controlled trials (RCTs), fasting lipid measurement should be repeated 4 to 12 weeks after starting the statin or after dose adjustment to assess adherence and response to LDL-cholesterol–lowering medications and lifestyle changes. Following that, lipid measurement should be repeated every 3 to 12 months as needed (Hoover, 2019).

Lifestyle changes need to be incorporated into any treatment regimen and include:

- Dietary measures include a heart-healthy diet (monitor and treat hyperlipidemia if dietary control is not enough).
- Increase physical activity: When adults do the equivalent of at least 150 minutes of moderate-intensity aerobic activity each week, the benefits are substantial. As a person moves from 150 minutes a week toward 300 minutes a week, the health benefits become more extensive. Research studies consistently show that activity performed on at least 3 days a week produces health benefits (Department of Health and Human Services, 2018; Kondamudi, 2021)
- Smoking cessation (people who stop smoking reduce their risk of heart disease 30% to 50% within the first year, and the risk continues to decline thereafter): One year after stopping smoking, the risk of dying from coronary heart disease is reduced by about one-half and continues to decline over time (Rigotti, 2021)
- Stress management
- HTN management
- DM management

Managing Hypertension

The risk of CVD increases as blood pressure increases. Elevated blood pressure may result in increased stiffness of the vessel walls, leading to vessel injury and a resulting inflammatory response within the intima. Inflammatory mediators then lead to the release of growth-promoting factors that cause vessel hypertrophy and hyperresponsiveness. These changes result in acceleration and aggravation of atherosclerosis. HTN also increases the work of the left ventricle, which must pump harder to eject blood into the arteries. Over time, the increased workload causes the heart to enlarge and thicken and may, eventually, lead to cardiac failure.

Early detection of high blood pressure and adherence to a therapeutic regimen can prevent the serious consequences associated with untreated elevated blood pressure. HTN is discussed in detail in Chapter 12.

Controlling Diabetes Mellitus

The relationship between DM and heart disease has been confirmed. Patients with diabetes are two- to threefold more likely than nondiabetic patients to experience the development of CVD (Brownlee et al., 2020), and diabetes is considered equivalent to existing CAD as a risk factor for a secondary cardiac event (Powers et al., 2019). The nurse considers that the presence of HTN *OR* DM increases the risk of atherosclerosis by twofold; when combined (HTN *AND* DM), the risk increases eightfold. If hyperlipidemia is added, the risk increases 20-fold (Norris, 2019). It is understood that accelerated CVD is the leading cause of death in people with both type 1 and type 2 DM.

Hyperglycemia fosters dyslipidemia, increased platelet aggregation, and altered red blood cell function, which can lead to thrombus formation. Control of diabetes is essential in preventing or modulating the development of CAD. Unfortunately, tight control of glucose levels in people with DM has not been associated consistently with significant reductions in risk for macrovascular cardiovascular disease; however, treatment of type 2 DM with sodium-glucose cotransporter-2 inhibitors or glucagon-like peptide-1 receptor agonists can reduce the risk of cardiovascular events (Rigato et al.,

Unfolding Patient Stories: C.S. • Part 1

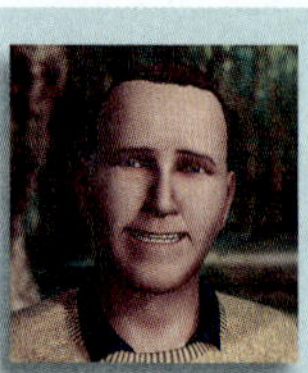

C.S., who has a family history of atherosclerotic CVD, is diagnosed with HTN and hyperlipidemia during a routine visit to the primary provider. The patient is overweight, smokes a half pack of cigarettes per day, and describes a stressful work situation. What questions can the nurse ask C.S. to help develop a plan for patient education? What topics are important for the nurse to address, and how can the information be presented? (C.S.'s story continues in Chapter 55.)

Care for C.S. and other patients in a realistic virtual environment: ***vSim*** *for Nursing* (thepoint.lww.com/vSimMedicalSurgical). Practice documenting these patients' care in DocuCare (thepoint.lww.com/DocuCareEHR).

2020). The American Diabetes Association and the European Association for the Study of Diabetes recommend lowering A1c to 7.0% to reduce the risk of microvascular complications, but this target is not universally valid for all patients (Rigato et al., 2020). Diabetes is discussed in detail in Chapter 29.

ANGINA PECTORIS

Angina pectoris is a clinical syndrome usually characterized by episodes of paroxysms of pain, pressure, or discomfort in the chest, jaw, shoulder, back, or arm that is caused by myocardial ischemia (Golla, 2022). The cause is insufficient coronary blood flow (usually caused by atherosclerotic disease), resulting in a decreased oxygen supply when there is increased myocardial demand for oxygen in response to physical exertion or emotional stress. In other words, oxygen demand exceeds the supply. The severity of angina is based on the precipitating activity and its effect on activities of daily living. Types of angina are listed in Box 13-2.

Pathophysiology

Angina is usually caused by atherosclerotic disease. Almost invariably, angina is associated with significant obstruction of a major coronary artery. Normally, the myocardium extracts a large amount of oxygen from the coronary circulation to meet its continuous demands. When there is an increase in demand, flow through the coronary arteries needs to be increased. When there is a blockage in a coronary artery, flow cannot be increased, and ischemia results. Because angina is a symptom of coronary atherosclerosis, the risk factors are the same.

BOX 13-2

Types of Angina

- *Stable angina:* Predictable and consistent pain that occurs on exertion and is relieved by rest
- *Unstable angina* (also called preinfarction angina or crescendo angina): Symptoms occur more frequently and last longer than in stable angina. The threshold for pain is lower, and pain may occur at rest.
- *Intractable or refractory angina:* Severe incapacitating chest pain
- *Variant angina* (also called **Prinzmetal angina**): Pain at rest with reversible ST-segment elevation; thought to be caused by coronary artery vasospasm
- *Silent ischemia:* Objective evidence of ischemia (such as electrocardiogram changes with a stress test), but patient reports no symptoms

Clinical Manifestations and Assessment

Ischemia of the heart muscle may produce pain or other symptoms, varying in severity from mild indigestion to a choking or heavy sensation in the upper chest that ranges from discomfort to agonizing pain accompanied by severe apprehension and a feeling of impending death. Typically, the pain or discomfort is poorly localized and may radiate to the neck, jaw, shoulders, and inner aspects of the upper arms, usually the left arm. The patient often feels tightness or a heavy, choking, or strangling sensation that has a vise-like, insistent quality. The patient with DM may not have severe pain with angina because diabetic neuropathy can dull the perception of pain. A female may have different symptoms than a male because coronary disease in females tends to be more diffuse and affects long segments of the artery rather than discrete segments. Table 13-2 discusses anginal pain.

TABLE **13-2 Assessing Angina**

Acronym	Factors about Pain that Need to Be Assessed	Assessment Questions
P	Position/Location Provocation/Palliation	"Where is the pain? Can you point to it?" "What were you doing when the pain began?" "What makes it worse?" "What makes it better?"
Q	Quality Quantity	"How would you describe the pain?" "Is it like any pain you had before?" "Has the pain been constant?"
R	Radiation	"Can you feel the pain anywhere else?"
S	Severity Symptoms	"How would you rate the pain on a 0–10 scale, with 0 being no pain and 10 being the most amount of pain?" (or use visual analog scale or adjective rating scale) "Did you notice any other symptoms with the pain?" (such as nausea, vomiting, diaphoresis)
T	Timing	"How long ago did the pain start?"

Adapted from Bickley, L. S., Szilagyi, P. G., Hoffmann, R. M., & Sorino, R. P. (2021). *Bates' guide to physical examination and history taking* (13th ed.). Lippincott Williams & Wilkins.

The nurse is alert for complaints of unusual fatigue; weakness or numbness in the arms, wrists, and hands; SOB; pallor; diaphoresis; anxiety; dizziness or lightheadedness; and nausea and vomiting that may accompany the pain (called *associated signs and symptoms*). Angina may subside with rest or nitroglycerin. In many patients, anginal symptoms follow a stable, predictable pattern.

The diagnosis of angina begins with the patient's history related to the clinical manifestations of ischemia. A 12-lead electrocardiogram (ECG) and blood laboratory biomarker values help in making the diagnosis. The patient may undergo an exercise or pharmacologic stress test in which the heart is monitored by ECG, echocardiogram, or both. The patient may also be referred for a nuclear scan or invasive procedure (e.g., cardiac catheterization, coronary artery angiography).

Medical Management

The objectives of the medical management of CAD and angina are to decrease the oxygen demand of the myocardium and to increase the oxygen supply. Medically, these objectives are met through pharmacologic therapy and control of risk factors. Alternatively, reperfusion procedures may be used to restore the blood supply to the myocardium. These include PCI procedures (e.g., percutaneous transluminal coronary angioplasty [PTCA] with intracoronary stent placement, atherectomy) and CABG. PCI is currently the preferred method of treatment for patients with simple coronary artery lesions, and recent advancements in PCI techniques have allowed for its use in difficult lesions (Iftikhar & Hu, 2021).

Pharmacologic Therapy

Several types of drugs are used to treat coronary vascular disease:

- *Positive inotrope:* A medication that increases myocardial contractility (force of contraction)
- *Negative inotrope:* A medication that decreases myocardial contractility
- *Positive chronotrope:* A medication that increases heart rate
- *Negative chronotrope:* A medication that decreases heart rate

Nitrates

Nitrates remain the mainstay treatment of coronary ischemia. A vasoactive agent (e.g., nitroglycerin) is administered to reduce myocardial oxygen consumption, which decreases ischemia and relieves pain. Nitroglycerin dilates primarily the veins and, in higher doses, also the arteries. Dilation of the veins causes venous pooling of blood throughout the body. As a result, less blood returns to the heart, and filling pressure (preload) is reduced. If the patient is hypovolemic (does not have adequate circulating blood volume), the decrease in filling pressure can cause a significant decrease in CO and blood pressure; thus, it is important for the nurse to monitor the patient's response to nitrates. Nitrates also relax the systemic arteriolar bed and increase oxygen supply, bringing about a more favorable balance between supply and demand.

Pearls for Practice

The nurse must evaluate for hypotension before administering nitrates. Once hypotension is excluded, a sublingual nitroglycerin tablet is administered. Vital signs are monitored while evaluating for resolution of symptoms since even small doses can produce sudden hypotension and bradycardia. Usually, this reaction can be reversed with intravenous atropine (Mega & Morrow, 2019).

When nitroglycerin is administered sublingually (SL), the patient's response is assessed (relief of chest pain and effect on blood pressure and heart rate). If the chest pain is unchanged or is lessened but still present, nitroglycerin SL administration is repeated up to a total of three doses. Each time, blood pressure, heart rate, and the ST segment (if the patient is on a monitor with ST-segment monitoring capability) are assessed. If the pain is significant and continues after these interventions, the patient is evaluated further for acute MI and further intervention is necessary.

Pearls for Practice

As with any medication, the nurse should always check the expiration dates on the bottle of nitroglycerin tablets.

Most patients with angina pectoris must self-administer nitroglycerin on an as-needed basis. A key nursing role in such cases is educating patients about the medication and how to take it (Box 13-3). SL nitroglycerin comes in tablet and spray forms.

Beta-Adrenergic Blocking Agents

Beta-blockers, such as metoprolol and atenolol, reduce myocardial oxygen consumption by blocking beta-adrenergic sympathetic stimulation to the heart. The result is a reduction in heart rate, slowed conduction of impulses through the conduction system, decreased blood pressure, and reduced myocardial **contractility** (negative chronotrope [rate] and negative inotrope [strength or force]) to balance the myocardial oxygen needs (demands) and the amount of oxygen available (supply). This helps control chest pain and delays the onset of ischemia during work or exercise. Beta-blockers reduce the incidence of recurrent angina, infarction, and cardiac mortality. Patients taking beta-blockers are cautioned not to stop taking them abruptly because angina may worsen and MI may develop.

Calcium-Channel Blocking Agents

Calcium-channel blockers have a variety of effects. These agents decrease sinoatrial node automaticity and atrioventricular node

BOX 13-3 **Patient Education**

Self-Administration of Nitroglycerin

- Instruct the patient to make sure the mouth is moist, the tongue is still, and saliva is not swallowed until the nitroglycerin tablet dissolves. Place the tablet under the tongue or between the cheek and gum, and let it dissolve.
- Advise the patient to carry the medication at all times as a precaution. However, because nitroglycerin is very unstable, it should be carried securely in its original container (e.g., capped, dark, glass bottle); tablets should never be removed and stored in metal or plastic pillboxes.
- Explain that nitroglycerin is volatile and is inactivated by heat, moisture, air, light, and time. Instruct the patient to renew the nitroglycerin supply every 6 months.
- Inform the patient that the medication should be taken in anticipation of any activity that may produce pain. Because nitroglycerin increases tolerance for exercise and stress when taken prophylactically (i.e., before angina-producing activity, such as exercise, stair-climbing, or sexual intercourse), it is best taken before pain develops.
- Recommend that the patient note how long it takes for the nitroglycerin to relieve the discomfort. Advise the patient that if pain persists after taking three sublingual tablets at 5-minute intervals, emergency medical services should be called.
- Discuss possible side effects of nitroglycerin, including flushing, throbbing headache, hypotension, and tachycardia.
- Advise the patient to sit down for a few minutes when taking nitroglycerin to avoid hypotension and syncope.

conduction, resulting in a slower heart rate and a decrease in the strength of the heart muscle contraction (negative inotropic and negative chronotropic effects). These effects decrease the workload of the heart. Calcium-channel blockers also relax the blood vessels, causing a decrease in blood pressure and an increase in coronary artery perfusion. Calcium-channel blockers increase myocardial oxygen supply by dilating the smooth muscle wall of the coronary arterioles; they decrease myocardial oxygen demand by reducing systemic arterial pressure and the workload of the left ventricle. They may be prescribed to prevent and treat vasospasm (as in variant angina). The calcium-channel blockers most commonly used are amlodipine and diltiazem.

Antiplatelet and Anticoagulant Medications

Antiplatelet medications are administered to prevent platelet aggregation and subsequent thrombosis, which impedes blood flow. The patient receiving anticoagulation therapy should be monitored for signs and symptoms of external and internal bleeding, such as low blood pressure, increased heart rate, and decreased serum hemoglobin and hematocrit. The patient should be placed on bleeding precautions, which include:

- Applying pressure to the site of any needle puncture for a longer time than usual
- Avoiding intramuscular (IM) injections
- Avoiding tissue injury and bruising from trauma or use of constrictive devices (e.g., continuous use of an automatic blood pressure cuff)

Examples of antiplatelet and anticoagulant medications include aspirin, clopidogrel, heparin, glycoprotein, and IIb/IIIa inhibitors. Aspirin prevents platelet activation and reduces the incidence of MI and death in patients with CAD.

Clopidogrel or ticlopidine is given to patients who are allergic to aspirin or is given in addition to aspirin in patients at high risk for MI. Unlike aspirin, these medications take a few days to achieve their antiplatelet effect. They also may cause GI upset.

IV unfractionated heparin (UFH) prevents the formation of new blood clots. Treating patients with unstable angina with heparin reduces the occurrence of MI. A decrease in platelet count or evidence of thrombosis may indicate a serious complication called *heparin-induced thrombocytopenia* (HIT), an antibody-mediated reaction to heparin that may result in thrombosis. Patients who have received heparin within the past 3 months and those who have been receiving UFH for 5 to 15 days are at high risk for HIT.

Pearls for Practice

HIT is a complication of anticoagulation with UFH or low–molecular-weight heparin (LMWH). It is an immune-mediated disorder in which antibodies form against the heparin-platelet factor 4 complex. The antibody complex attaches to the platelet, causing its aggregation. The reticuloendothelial system destroys activated platelets, thus resulting in decreased platelet counts. Frequently, procoagulants are also generated, resulting in thrombosis. A complication of HIT is heparin-associated thrombocytopenia and thrombosis (HITT). In the presence of unexplained thrombocytopenia or venous or arterial thrombosis associated with thrombocytopenia, HIT should be considered. Discontinuation of heparin as soon as the diagnosis is suspected is warranted (Crowther, 2022).

IV administration of glycoprotein (*GP*) *IIb/IIIa agents* (abciximab, tirofiban, and eptifibatide) is indicated for hospitalized patients with unstable angina and as an adjunct therapy for PCI. These agents prevent platelet aggregation by blocking the GPIIb/IIIa receptors on the platelets, preventing adhesion of fibrinogen and other factors that cross-link platelets to each other and thereby would normally allow platelets to form a thrombus (clot). As with heparin, bleeding is the major side effect, and bleeding precautions should be initiated.

Oxygen Administration

Oxygen therapy is usually initiated at the onset of chest pain in an attempt to increase the amount of oxygen delivered to the myocardium and to decrease pain. Blood oxygen saturation is monitored by pulse oximetry; the normal oxygen saturation (SpO_2) level is greater than 95%.

Percutaneous Coronary Interventions

PCIs to treat angina and CAD most commonly include balloon angioplasty with intracoronary stent implantation. The patient in whom an acute MI is suspected may be referred for an immediate intervention, in which case the occluded coronary artery is opened and reperfusion to the area that had been deprived of oxygen is reestablished. The duration of oxygen deprivation is directly related to the number of cells that die; therefore, the time from the patient's arrival in the emergency department to the time PCI is performed is critical and should be less than 90 minutes (time is muscle!). This is frequently referred to as *door-to-balloon time,* "*DTB,*" or "*time to device.*" A cardiac catheterization laboratory and staff must be available 24 hours a day, 7 days a week if an emergent PCI is to be performed within this short time.

Pearls for Practice

An accurate assessment of a patient's peripheral vascular system must be documented preprocedure. This data will be used to evaluate postoperative vascular status. The assessment should include extremities color, sensation, temperature, capillary refill, and peripheral perfusion using the grading scale common to the nurse's institution. The affected extremity is assessed every 15 minutes for the first hour and then according to hospital protocol.

Diagnostic Cardiac Catheterization and Percutaneous Coronary Intervention

Cardiac catheterization is a diagnostic procedure carried out in the cardiac catheterization laboratory where a vascular catheter is inserted in an artery (mostly radial or femoral) and threaded through the blood vessels to the heart; dye that is seen on fluoroscopy (x-ray) is then injected, and the structures of the heart and the patency of the coronary arteries are visualized. Coronary vessels with blockages are definitively identified and, often during the same procedure, are opened by a PCI. During PCI, the vascular catheter that is balloon-tipped is used to open blocked coronary arteries. Most often a stent is then deployed to maintain patency of the artery. PCI is used in patients with angina and as an intervention for acute MI. Catheter-based interventions can also be used to open blocked CABGs.

PCI is used more often now than ever before; it is the fifth most common procedure carried out yearly in the United States (Agency for Healthcare Research and Quality [AHRQ], 2021). Hollow catheters called *sheaths* are inserted usually via the radial or femoral artery and occasionally the brachial artery. Catheters are then threaded through the sheaths, up through the aorta, and into the coronary arteries. Angiography is performed using injected radiopaque contrast agents (commonly called *dye*) to identify the location and extent of the blockage. A balloon-tipped dilation catheter is passed through the sheath and positioned over the lesion. The physician determines the catheter position by examining markers on the balloon that can be seen with fluoroscopy. When the catheter is positioned properly, the balloon is inflated with high pressure for several seconds and then deflated. The pressure compresses and possibly "cracks" the atheroma (Fig. 13-5). The media and adventitia of the coronary artery are also stretched. The appropriate stent is then put into place to keep the artery open (see Fig. 13-6).

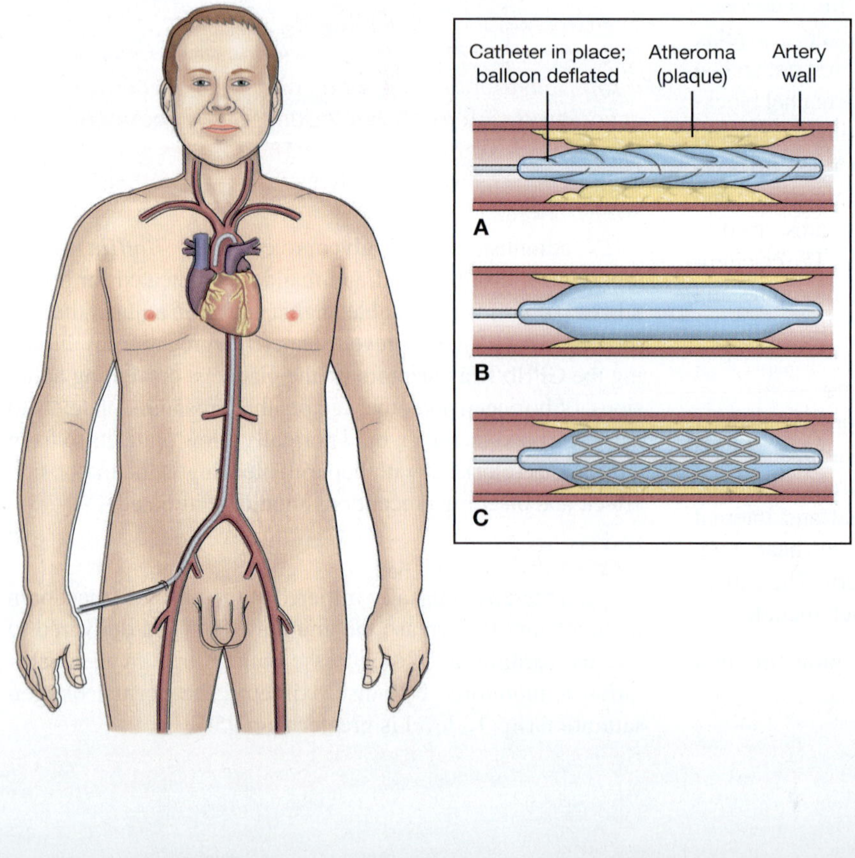

FIGURE 13-5 **Percutaneous coronary intervention. A. A balloon-tipped catheter is passed into the affected coronary artery and placed across the area of the atheroma (plaque). B. The balloon is then rapidly inflated and deflated with controlled pressure. C. A stent is placed to maintain patency of the artery, and the balloon is removed.**

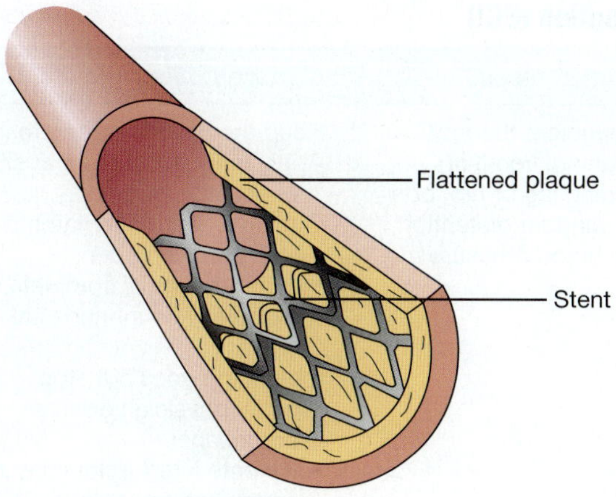

FIGURE 13-6 **Vascular stent.**

Pearls for Practice

It is critical that an "Allen's test" is assessed preintervention to ensure ulnar arterial flow to the hand since adequacy will permit a radial artery approach for a PCI procedure (refer to Chapter 11). The radial approach provides direct access to the ascending aorta and allows for immediate mobilization following PCI.

Several inflations and several balloon sizes may be required to achieve the goal, usually defined as an improvement in blood flow and residual stenosis of less than 20%. Other measures of the success of a PCI are an increase in the artery's lumen, a difference of less than 20 mm Hg in blood pressure from one side of the lesion to the other, and no clinically obvious arterial trauma. Because the blood supply to the coronary artery decreases while the balloon is inflated, the patient may complain of chest pain and the ECG may display significant ST-segment changes. Intracoronary stents are usually positioned in the intima of the vessel to maintain patency after the balloon is withdrawn. PCI procedures have a success rate of greater than 95%; the only exception is a chronic total coronary (100%) obstruction of the lumen, where the ability to negotiate a guidewire through the blockage is only about 50% to 90% (and varies substantially with the operator's expertise) (Teirstein & Lytle, 2020). Refer to Table 13-3 for complications after PCI.

Coronary Artery Stent

After PCI, the area that has been treated may potentially close off partially or completely, a process called *restenosis.* The intima of the coronary artery has been injured and responds by initiating an acute inflammatory process. This process may include the release of mediators that lead to vasoconstriction, clotting, and scar tissue formation. A coronary artery stent is placed to overcome these risks. Restenosis happens in 10% to 50% of patients with PCI after balloon angioplasty *without* stenting, usually within 6 months (Teirstein & Lytle, 2020). A **stent** is a metal mesh that provides structural support to a vessel at risk of acute closure. Either bare metal or "drug-eluting" stents are used; there are guidelines in place to aid in determining which the cardiologist should choose. The stent is positioned over the angioplasty balloon. When the balloon is inflated, the mesh expands and presses against the vessel wall, holding the artery open. The balloon is withdrawn, but the stent is left permanently in place within the artery; eventually, endothelium covers the stent, and it is incorporated into the vessel wall. Stents have been shown to improve long-term outcomes of PCI (Pearce et al., 2019). However, about 10% of PCIs are performed for in-stent restenosis (ISR), which generally occurs within 12 months after stent placement (Levin & Cutlip, 2020). The rate of ISR has remained relatively unchanged even with the introduction of drug-eluting stents (Shlofmitz et al., 2019). Because of the risk of thrombus formation in the stent, the patient receives antiplatelet medications (e.g., clopidogrel and aspirin). These medications are routinely continued for at least 3 to 6 months to decrease the risk of thrombus formation.

Complications that can occur during a PCI procedure include dissection, perforation, abrupt closure, or vasospasm of the coronary artery; acute MI; acute arrhythmias (e.g., ventricular tachycardia); and cardiac arrest. These may require emergency surgical treatment. Complications after the procedure may include abrupt closure of the coronary artery and vascular complications, such as bleeding at the insertion site, retroperitoneal bleeding, hematoma, pseudoaneurysm, arteriovenous fistula, or arterial thrombosis and distal embolization, as well as acute kidney injury. Risk factors for the aforementioned complications include older age, female sex, larger vascular sheath size, low BMI, renal insufficiency, and degree of anticoagulation during the procedure (Mauri & Bhatt, 2019).

Pearls for Practice

Transradial artery access (TRA) for percutaneous coronary intervention (PCI) is associated with lower bleeding and vascular complications than transfemoral artery access (TFA), especially in patients with acute coronary syndromes (ACS). Use of TRA for coronary angiography and PCI may also be associated with improved measures of quality of life and reduced costs compared with TFA (Mason et al., 2018). Femoral access is still required for those with small or tortuous radial vessels or for interventional procedures that are high risk and may require large-bore catheters (Lough et al., 2022).

Pearls for Practice

Kidney failure is associated with post-PCI procedural mortality and is directly related to the extent of the patient's baseline kidney disease (Mauri & Bhatt, 2019). Patients admitted with mild kidney dysfunction are at a higher risk for kidney failure and more adverse cardiac events (MACE) after PCI; therefore,

TABLE **13-3 Complications after Percutaneous Coronary Intervention (PCI)**

Complication	Signs and Symptoms	Possible Causes	Nursing Actions
Bleeding or hematoma	Expanding mass surrounding puncture site; hard lump or bluish tinge at sheath insertion site	Anticoagulant therapy, coughing, vomiting, bending leg or hip, obesity, bladder distention, high blood pressure	Keep the patient on bed rest. Apply manual pressure at site of sheath insertion. Outline extent of hematoma with a marking pen. Monitor results of complete blood cell count and vital signs. If bleeding does not stop, notify physician or nurse practitioner. Anticipate interruption of anticoagulant and antiplatelet therapies. Blood transfusion may be indicated.
Lost or weakened pulse distal to sheath insertion site	Extremity cool, cyanotic, pale, or painful	Arterial thrombus or embolus	Assess peripheral circulation by comparing bilateral pulses; note temperature, capillary refill, sensation, and movement, as well as color of the affected extremity. Notify physician or nurse practitioner. Anticipate surgery and anticoagulation or thrombolytic therapy.
Pseudoaneurysm and arteriovenous fistula; if they rupture, sudden massive swelling and severe pain will be seen.	A large painful pulsatile mass felt or bruit heard near sheath insertion site	Vessel trauma during procedure	Notify physician or nurse practitioner. Anticipate ultrasound-guided compression. If the pseudoaneurysm is small (less than 2 cm), it may be observed and monitored clinically. Assess circulation, sensation, and motility of involved extremity. Prepare patient for surgery to close fistula if indicated.
Retroperitoneal bleeding (blood collecting in the retroperitoneal space may not produce obvious swelling or skin color changes)	Back or flank pain Unexplained hypotension Tachycardia Restlessness and agitation Decreased hemoglobin/hematocrit Cullen sign (bluish to purplish periumbilical discoloration) and Grey Turner sign (flank discoloration) may be noted with retroperitoneal bleed (see Fig. 26-10 on page 923).	Arterial tear causing bleeding into flank area	Notify physician or nurse practitioner immediately. Stop any anticoagulation medication. Anticipate need for IV fluids and/or administration of blood.
Acute kidney injury	Decreased urine output, elevated blood urea nitrogen (BUN), creatinine	Nephrotoxic contrast agent	Provide hydration to promote excretion of contrast material. Monitor urine output. Monitor BUN and creatinine. Administer renal protective agents (e.g., acetylcysteine before and after procedure as prescribed).

Complication	Signs and Symptoms	Possible Causes	Nursing Actions
Allergic reaction	Urticaria, hives, sneezing, and bronchospasm	Allergic reaction to dye is higher in patients allergic to penicillin and in those with known prior reaction to contrast material.	Anticipate administering prednisone, antihistamines, and H_2 blockers before the coronary procedure for patients with known prior reaction to contrast material. If anaphylaxis occurs, the nurse anticipates administering epinephrine and IV saline for hydration.
Cardiac tamponade	Tachypnea, tachycardia, hypotension, jugular venous distention, and muffled heart sounds; cool extremities from hypoperfusion in some patients	Most common cause is perforation due to rupture of a coronary artery.	Anticipate a pericardiocentesis in patients with compromised hemodynamic status.
Chest pain/acute ischemic event/spasm	Complaints of chest pain	Benign stent sensation, acute stent thrombosis, abrupt vessel closure, transient coronary spasms, side branch occlusion, and distal embolization of debris	Notify the provider when patient complains of chest pain. Monitor vital signs, O_2 sat, and lung and cardiac sounds. Assess peripheral perfusion. Monitor electrocardiogram (ECG). Perform serial tests for cardiac markers. Measure troponin. Obtain a 12-lead ECG with any episodes of chest pain.

Data from Gomes, B. B. (2015). Care of the patient undergoing radial approach heart catheterization: Implications for medical-surgical nurses. *Medsurg Nursing*, *24*(3), 173–176; Agency for Healthcare Research and Quality. (2021). HCUP fast stats—Most common operations during inpatient stays. https://www.hcup-us.ahrq.gov/faststats/NationalProceduresServlet?year1=2018&characteristic1=0&included1=1&year2=2005&characteristic2=0&included2=1&expansionInfoState=hide&dataTablesState=hide&definitionsState=hide&exportState=hide; and Mullin, M. (2014). Transradial approach versus transfemoral approach for coronary angiography and coronary angioplasty. *Critical Care Nursing Quarterly*, *37*(2), 159–169.

monitoring of urinary output and renal function tests is particularly critical in this patient population. There is a 20% higher risk for death at 1 year following PCI than in those with preserved renal function (Mauri & Bhatt, 2019). The risk for nephropathy is dependent on the dose of contrast dye used and the level of hydration. Ensuring adequate intravenous hydration surrounding the procedure can help protect against renal compromise.

Postprocedure Care

Patient care is similar to that for a cardiac catheterization. Many patients are admitted to the hospital the day of the PCI and discharged the next day; increasingly selected patients are treated as outpatients and released 6 to 12 hours after the procedure without an overnight stay (Teirstein & Lytle, 2020). When the PCI is performed emergently to relieve acute coronary syndrome (ACS), the patient will usually go to a critical care unit to be monitored closely for a slightly longer period of time. During the PCI, patients receive IV heparin and are monitored for signs of bleeding. Most bleeding occurs within the first 2 to 3 hours after the procedure; therefore, it is imperative that the site is checked frequently for evidence of bleeding or hematoma (Lough et al., 2022). Patients may also receive a GPIIb/IIIa agent (e.g., eptifibatide) for several hours following the PCI to prevent platelet aggregation and thrombus formation in the coronary artery and stent. Hemostasis at the access site is achieved, and sheaths may be removed at the end of the procedure by using a vascular closure device (e.g., Angio-Seal, VasoSeal) or a device that sutures the vessels. Hemostasis after sheath removal may also be achieved by direct manual pressure, a mechanical compression device (e.g., C-shaped clamp), or a pneumatic compression device (e.g., FemoStop or TR band).

Occasionally, the patient may return to the nursing unit with the femoral or brachial vascular access sheaths in place. This may happen if there is a planned trip back to the catheterization lab or if the activated clotting time (ACT) is too high to remove the sheath safely. The sheaths are removed when blood studies (e.g., ACT) indicate that the heparin is no longer active and the clotting time is within an acceptable range. This usually takes a few hours, depending on the amount of heparin given during the procedure. As long as a sheath is in place, the patient must remain in bed and avoid bending the affected limb. The head of the bed (HOB) is not elevated beyond 30 degrees if there is a femoral sheath

BOX 13-4

Nursing Care after Cardiac Cath/PCI via Radial Approach

Assessment

- Monitor vital signs (including pulse oximetry[a]), neurovascular checks,[b] site and limb assessment per policy and/or provider's order (expect Q15 minutes x4, Q30 minutes x4, Q1 hour x4, and then Q4 hours or routine).
- Observe site for any bleeding, ecchymosis, or hematoma. Observe appearance of skin under and around the compression device (i.e., TR band).
- Avoid use of affected arm for blood pressure and blood draws for 24 hours.
- After a diagnostic cardiac catheterization, the TR band is likely to remain in place for a minimum of 1 hour (follow provider's order).
- After an interventional procedure (angioplasty with stent placement), the TR band is likely to remain in place for a minimum of 2 hours (follow provider's order).

Activity

- The patient may be out of bed with assistance (per provider's order) while the radial artery compression device is in place. Typically there is no restriction on head of bed elevation; the affected arm is kept straight and no pressure is applied to the limb. An ace wrap or an arm board can be applied to prevent wrist flexing. As noted above, avoid blood pressures and blood draws from the procedural arm for 24 hours.
- When removing the Radial compression device, the nurse should position the patient either in a bed or stretcher or in a chair that allows for elevation of legs in the event of a vagal response (drop in blood pressure and/or heart rate).

Reportable to the Provider

- Changes in sensation or pain in affected extremity, hematoma, bleeding, ecchymosis, blistering of the skin, appearance of mottling, absence of radial or ulnar pulse
- Any variance of the patient's vital signs

Patient and Family Education

- Report any symptoms of pain, numbness, or tingling in the affected extremity, as well as redness or streaking, swelling, and discharge from the site.
- For 24 hours after procedure, minimize manipulation of the affected wrist (no flexing), including no weight-bearing on wrist when rising from bed/chair. Elevating the affected arm and applying ice will promote comfort and decrease swelling.
- Do not drive.
- Remove occlusive dressing after 24 hours and leave open to air. If minor oozing occurs, apply dressing for 12 more hours; the site may be washed with mild soap and water. Avoid excess moisture to the access site, especially submerging the hand in water and flexing the wrist for 72 hours after procedure.
- If bleeding should occur: sit down and hold pressure at the site for 10 minutes. If bleeding stops, sit with the wrist straight for 2 hours and notify the provider. If bleeding does not stop after 10 minutes or a large amount of bleeding is noted, call 911 and lie down. DO NOT drive yourself to the hospital.
- Avoid heavy lifting (over 5 lb).
- Do not operate heavy equipment.
- Avoid excessive wrist movement.
- Avoid vigorous exercise using arm.
- Plan for a follow-up appointment within 1–2 weeks; use the call-back number with 24-hour service if needed.

[a]The Pulse oximetry probe should be on either the thumb or index finger of the affected hand because impaired radial artery circulation will be revealed in these digits.

[b]Neurovascular checks include color, temperature, sensation (presence or absence of numbness and tingling), pulses (radial and ulnar of the affected limb), and capillary refill.

Data from Gomes, B. B. (2015). Care of the patient undergoing radial approach heart catheterization: Implications for medical-surgical nurses. *Medsurg Nursing, 24*(3), 173–176; Agency for Healthcare Research and Quality (AHRQ). (2021). HCUP fast stats—Most common operations during inpatient stays. https://www.hcup-us.ahrq.gov/faststats/NationalProceduresServlet?year1=2018&characteristic1=0&included1=1&year2=2005&characteristic2=0&included2=1&expansionInfoState=hide&dataTablesState=hide&definitionsState=hide&exportState=hide; and Mullin, M. (2014). Transradial approach versus transfemoral approach for coronary angiography and coronary angioplasty. *Critical Care Nursing Quarterly, 37*(2), 159–169.

in place. After the sheath removal, the patient maintains bed rest for 3 to 6 hours according to the hospital's policy. Sheath removal and the application of pressure on the vessel insertion site may cause the heart rate to slow and the blood pressure to decrease (vasovagal response). An IV bolus of atropine is usually given to treat this response. If the radial approach was used, the patient will have fewer restrictions on mobility but should not bend or put pressure on the affected area; the nurse should follow the institutional policy for specific restrictions. Refer to Box 13-4 for the care of the patient after radial artery approach.

Some patients with unstable lesions and at high risk for abrupt vessel closure are restarted on heparin after sheath removal, or they receive an IV infusion of a GPIIb/IIIa inhibitor. These patients are monitored more closely and may recover more slowly.

Pearls for Practice

Post PCI, IV fluids may be administered to promote excretion of the contrast medium. The nurse is alert for signs of fluid volume excess that may include complaints of SOB at rest or with exertion, orthopnea, paroxysmal nocturnal dyspnea, cough, development or increased crackles in the lungs, S_3 gallop, jugular vein distention (JVD), and pulsus alternans (characterized by alternating strong and weak peripheral pulses). Changes in vital signs will vary depending on whether CO is increased [HTN] or reduced (hypotension).

After hemostasis is achieved, a pressure dressing is applied to the site. Patients resume self-care and ambulate unassisted within a few hours of the procedure. The duration of immobilization depends on the size and location of the sheath inserted, the amount of anticoagulant administered, the method of hemostasis, the patient's underlying condition, and the physician's preference. On the day after the procedure, the site is inspected and the dressing replaced with an adhesive bandage. The nurse teaches the patient to monitor the site for bleeding or the development of a hard mass indicative of hematoma. On discharge, heavy lifting is discouraged for several days if the femoral artery was used, and intense aerobic exercise is typically discouraged for 2 to 4 weeks (especially after stent implantation). There is usually no driving for 24 hours due to the use of sedating agents used for the procedure (Teirstein & Lytle, 2020).

Surgical Procedures: Coronary Artery Revascularization

Advances in diagnostics, medical management, and surgical and anesthesia techniques, as well as the care provided in critical care and surgical units, home care, and rehabilitation programs, have continued to make surgery a viable treatment option for patients with CAD. CABG has been done for over 60 years now, with techniques ever-evolving and improving. CABG is a surgical procedure in which a blood vessel is grafted to the occluded coronary artery so that blood can flow beyond the occlusion; it is also called a bypass graft.

Major indications for CABG include:

- Alleviation of angina that cannot be controlled with medication or PCI
- Treatment of multivessel CAD and complicated lesions
- Prevention and treatment of MI, arrhythmias, or heart failure
- Treatment for complications from an unsuccessful PCI

The recommendation for CABG is determined by several factors, including the number of diseased coronary vessels, the location complexity of the lesions (blockages), the degree of left ventricular dysfunction, the presence of comorbidities, the patient's symptoms, and any previous treatment. CABG surgery remains the standard of care for patients with complex CAD, although technologic advancements in both PCI and in CABG surgery make it difficult to compare these interventions historically. Cardiologists and cardiac surgeons work together to determine the most appropriate treatment for an individual patient (Iftikhar & Hu, 2021).

For a patient to be considered for CABG, the coronary arteries to be bypassed must have approximately a 70% occlusion (50% if in the left main coronary artery). If a significant blockage is not present, the flow through the artery will compete with the flow through the bypass, and circulation to the ischemic area of the myocardium may not be improved. It is also necessary that the artery be patent beyond the area of blockage or the flow through the bypass will be impeded.

Vessels commonly used for CABG are the greater saphenous vein, followed by the lesser saphenous vein (other veins may also be used) as well as the internal thoracic arteries (Fig. 13-7). If a vein is to be used, it is removed from its original location and grafted to the ascending aorta and the coronary artery distal to the lesion. The saphenous veins are used in emergency CABG procedures because they can be obtained quickly by one surgeon while another performs the chest surgery. A common adverse effect of vein removal is edema in the extremity from which the vein was taken. The degree of edema varies and usually diminishes over time. Within 5 to 10 years, atherosclerotic changes often develop in saphenous vein grafts.

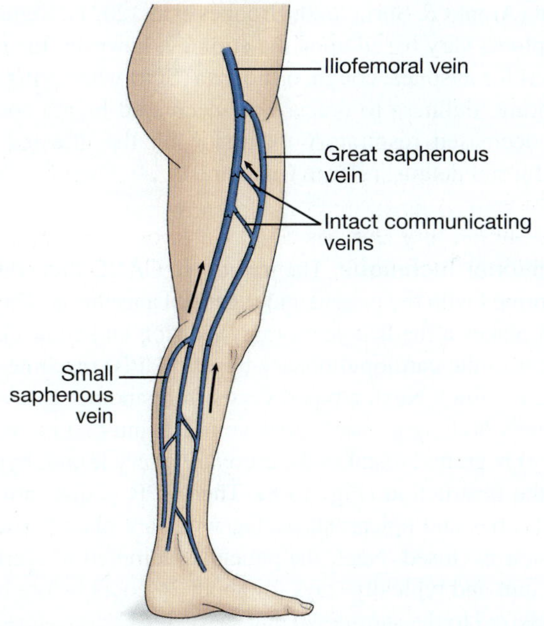

FIGURE 13-7 **The greater and lesser saphenous veins are commonly used in bypass graft procedures.**

The right and left internal mammary arteries and, less frequently, the radial arteries are also used for CABG. Arterial grafts are preferred to venous grafts because they do not develop atherosclerotic changes as quickly and remain patent longer. The surgeon leaves the proximal end of the mammary artery intact and detaches the distal end of the artery from the chest wall. This end of the artery is then grafted to the coronary artery distal to the occlusion. The internal mammary arteries may not be long enough to use for multiple bypasses. Because of this, many CABG procedures are performed with a combination of venous (reversed segments of veins [reversed because of venous valves]) and arterial grafts.

After CABG, up to 90% of patients develop pleural effusions (fluid collection within the pleural space) in the immediate postoperative period, which is associated with a variety of etiologies, including accumulation of pleural fluid because of heart failure (HF), surgical tissue trauma, hemorrhage from harvesting of the IMA, longer period of intubation (postoperative intubation greater than 24 hours), postoperative atelectasis and diaphragmatic dysfunction, or chylothorax (lymphatic fluid in the pleural space) because of unintended thoracic duct injury during the operative event (Aranki & Suri, 2020; Brookes et al., 2021). Signs and symptoms vary based upon the etiology; however, the nurse is alert for dyspnea, cough, orthopnea (SOB when lying flat), splinting, dullness to percussion, decreased breath sounds, and decreased respiratory excursion on the affected side (for further details, refer to Chapter 9).

Coronary Artery Bypass Graft Surgery

Traditional Technique. The traditional CABG procedure is performed with the patient under general anesthesia. The surgeon makes a median sternotomy incision and connects the patient to the cardiopulmonary bypass (CPB) machine (discussed below). Next, a blood vessel from another part of the patient's body (e.g., saphenous vein, left internal mammary artery) is grafted distal to the coronary artery lesion, bypassing the obstruction (Fig. 13-8). Then CPB is discontinued, chest tubes and epicardial pacing wires are placed, and the incision is closed. Next, the patient is admitted to a critical care unit and typically stays for about 24 hours before being transferred to the step-down unit.

Many cardiac surgical procedures are possible because of CPB (i.e., extracorporeal circulation) (Fig. 13-9). The procedure mechanically circulates and oxygenates blood for the body while bypassing the heart and lungs. CPB maintains perfusion to body organs and tissues and allows the surgeon to complete the anastomoses in a motionless, bloodless surgical field.

CPB is accomplished by placing a cannula in the right atrium, vena cava, or femoral vein to withdraw blood from the body. The cannula is connected to tubing filled with an isotonic crystalloid solution (usually 5% dextrose in lactated Ringer solution). Venous blood removed from the body by the cannula is filtered, oxygenated, cooled or warmed by the machine, and then returned to the body. The cannula used to return the oxygenated blood is usually inserted in the ascending aorta, or it may be inserted in the femoral artery.

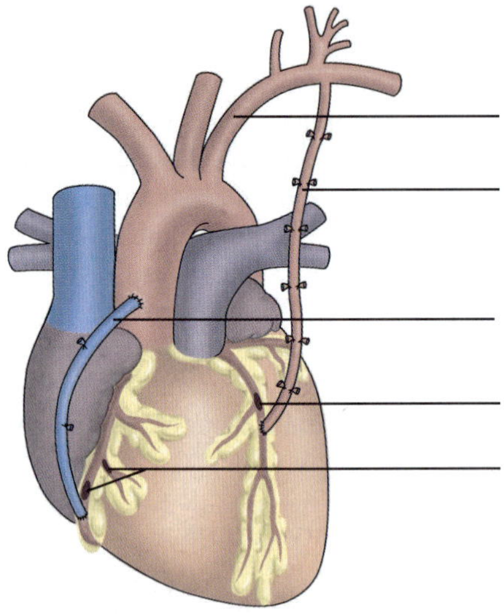

FIGURE 13-8 **Coronary artery bypass grafts. One or more procedures may be performed using various veins and arteries. A. Left internal mammary artery, used frequently because of its functional longevity. B. Saphenous vein, also used as bypass graft.**

The heart is stopped by the injection of cardioplegia solution, which is high in potassium, into the coronary arteries. The patient receives heparin to prevent clotting and thrombus formation in the bypass circuit when blood comes in contact with the foreign surfaces of the tubing. At the end of the procedure, when the patient is disconnected from the bypass machine, protamine sulfate is administered to reverse the effects of heparin.

During the procedure, hypothermia is maintained, usually 28° to 32°C (82.4° to 89.6°F). The blood is cooled during CPB and returned to the body. The cooled blood slows the body's basal metabolic rate, thereby decreasing the oxygen demand. Cooled blood usually has a higher viscosity, but the crystalloid solution used to prime the bypass tubing dilutes the blood. When the surgical procedure is completed,

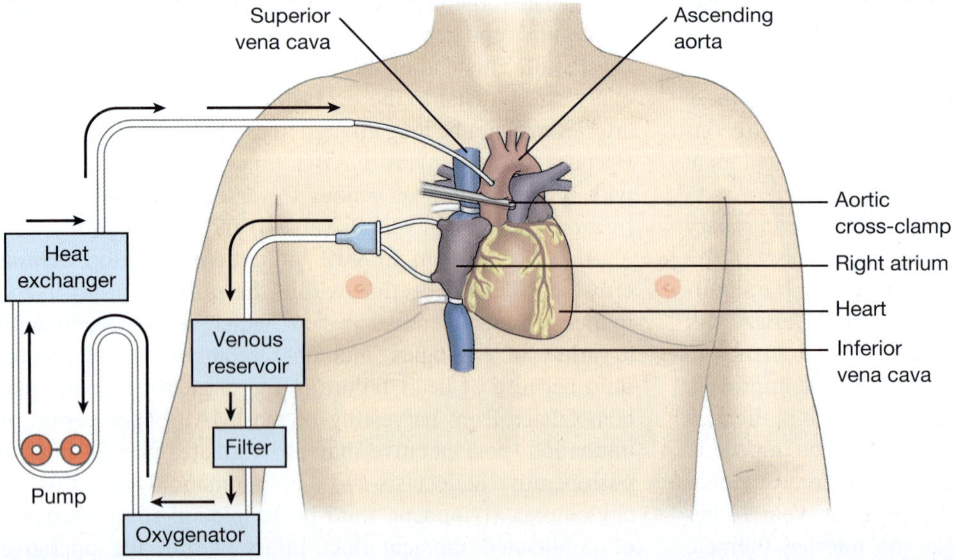

FIGURE 13-9 **The cardiopulmonary bypass (CPB) system, in which cannulas are placed through the right atrium into the superior and inferior vena cavae to divert blood from the body and into the bypass system. The pump system creates a vacuum, pulling blood into the venous reservoir. The blood is cleared of air bubbles, clots, and particulates by the filter and then is passed through the oxygenator, releasing carbon dioxide and obtaining oxygen. Next, the blood is pulled to the pump and pushed out to the heat exchanger, where its temperature is regulated. Then the blood is returned to the body via the ascending aorta.**

the blood is rewarmed as it passes through the CPB circuit. Urine output, arterial blood gases (ABGs), electrolytes, and coagulation studies are monitored to assess the patient's status during CPB.

Alternate Technique. Another type of CABG procedure often done today is the "off pump" CABG or "OPCAB." The potential benefits of OPCAB include a decrease in the incidence of stroke and other neurologic complications, reduced blood usage, less kidney injury, and fewer cardiac rhythm disturbances. Also done today is the "MIDCAB," or minimally invasive coronary artery bypass surgery. The MIDCAB is performed on a beating heart via a thoracotomy incision and is only suitable for certain lesions that are located in the arteries on the anterior portions of the heart. Patients undergoing any type of CABG surgery will go to the intensive care unit for approximately 24 hours, and then transfer to the step-down unit. The average overall hospital stay for CABG surgery is anticipated at 5 days.

Complications of Coronary Artery Bypass Graft

CABG may result in complications such as MI, arrhythmias, hemorrhage, and kidney dysfunction. Table 13-4 presents an overview of the potential complications in the postoperative cardiac surgical patient. Although most patients improve symptomatically following surgery, CABG is not a cure for CAD, and angina, exercise intolerance, or other symptoms experienced before CABG may recur. Medications required before surgery may need to be continued. Lifestyle modifications recommended before surgery remain important to treat the underlying CAD and for the continued viability of the newly implanted grafts.

TABLE 13-4 **Potential Complications of Cardiac Surgery**

Complication	Description	Assessment and Management
Cardiac Complications *Decreased Cardiac Output*		
Hypovolemia (most common cause of decreased cardiac output after cardiac surgery)	• Net loss of blood and intravascular volume • Surgical hypothermia (as the reduced body temperature rises after surgery, blood vessels dilate and more volume is needed to fill the vessels). • IV fluid loss to the interstitial spaces because surgery and anesthesia make capillary beds more permeable. • Increased heart rate, arterial hypotension, low pulmonary artery wedge pressure (PAWP), and low central venous pressures (CVP) often are seen.	• Fluid replacement may be prescribed. Replacement fluids include: Colloid (albumin, heta-starch), packed red blood cells, or crystalloid solution (normal saline, lactated Ringer solution).
Persistent bleeding	• Cardiopulmonary bypass may cause platelet dysfunction, and hypothermia alters clotting mechanisms. • Surgical trauma causing tissues and blood vessels to ooze bloody drainage. • Intraoperative anticoagulant (heparin) therapy • Postoperative coagulopathy may also result from liver dysfunction and depletion of clotting components.	• Accurate measurement of wound bleeding and chest tube blood is essential. Bloody drainage should not exceed 200 mL/hr for the first 4–6 hours. Drainage should decrease and stop within a few days, while progressing from sanguineous to serosanguineous and serous drainage. • Protamine sulfate may be administered to neutralize unfractionated heparin; vitamin K and blood products may be used to treat hematologic deficiencies. • If bleeding persists, the patient may return to the operating room.
Cardiac tamponade	• Fluid and clots accumulate in the pericardial sac, which compresses the heart, preventing blood from filling the ventricles. • Signs and symptoms include arterial hypotension, tachycardia, muffled heart sounds, decreasing urine output, and ↑ CVP. Additional signs and symptoms: arterial pressure waveform demonstrating a pulsus paradoxus (decrease of more than 10 mm Hg during inspiration) and decreased chest tube drainage (suggesting that the drainage is trapped or clotted in the mediastinum).	• The chest drainage system is checked to eliminate possible kinks or obstructions in the tubing. • Patency of the tubing in the chest drainage system must be maintained, the nurse can facilitate movement of the fluid by adjusting the position of the tubing therefore helping with forward flow. • Chest x-ray may show a widening mediastinum. • Emergency medical management is required; may include pericardiocentesis or return to surgery.

(continued)

TABLE **13-4 Potential Complications of Cardiac Surgery (*continued*)**

Complication	Description	Assessment and Management
Fluid overload	• High PAWP, CVP, and pulmonary artery diastolic pressures, as well as crackles indicate fluid overload.	• Diuretics are prescribed and the rate of IV fluid administration is reduced. • Alternative treatments include continuous renal replacement therapy and dialysis.
Hypothermia	• Low body temperature leads to vasoconstriction, shivering, and arterial hypertension.	• Patient is rewarmed gradually after surgery, decreasing vasoconstriction.
Hypertension	• Results from postoperative vasoconstriction. It may stretch suture lines and cause postoperative bleeding. The condition may be transient.	• Vasodilators (nitroglycerin nitroprusside may be used to treat hypertension. Administer cautiously to avoid hypotension.
Tachyarrhythmias	• Increased heart rate is common with perioperative volume changes. Uncontrolled atrial fibrillation commonly occurs during the first few days postoperatively.	• If a tachyarrhythmia is the primary problem, the heart rhythm is assessed and medications (e.g., adenosine, amiodarone, digoxin, diltiazem, esmolol, lidocaine, procainamide), may be prescribed. Patients may be prescribed antiarrhythmics before coronary artery bypass graft (CABG) to minimize the risk of postoperative tachyarrhythmias. • Carotid massage may be performed by a provider to assist with diagnosing or treating the arrhythmia. • Cardioversion and defibrillation are alternatives for symptomatic tachyarrhythmias. • For patients who cannot attain normal sinus rhythm, an alternate goal may be to establish a stable rhythm that produces a sufficient cardiac output.
Bradycardias	• Decreased heart rate	• Many postoperative patients will have temporary pacer wires that can be attached to a pulse generator (pacemaker) to stimulate the heart to beat faster. Less commonly, atropine, epinephrine, or isoproterenol may be used to increase heart rate.
Cardiac failure (decreased cardiac output)	• Myocardial contractility may be decreased perioperatively.	• The nurse observes for and reports falling mean arterial pressure; rising PAWP, pulmonary artery diastolic pressure, and CVP; increasing tachycardia; restlessness and agitation; peripheral cyanosis; venous distention; labored respirations; and edema. • Medical management includes diuretics, digoxin, and IV inotropic agents.
MI (may occur intraoperatively or postoperatively)	• Portion of the cardiac muscle dies; therefore, contractility decreases. Impaired ventricular wall motion further decreases cardiac output. Symptoms may be masked by the postoperative surgical discomfort or the anesthesia–analgesia regimen.	• Careful assessment to determine the type of pain the patient is experiencing; myocardial infarction (MI) suspected if the mean blood pressure is low with normal preload. • Serial electrocardiograms (ECGs) and cardiac biomarkers assist in making the diagnosis (alterations may be due to the surgical intervention). Analgesics are prescribed in small amounts while the patient's blood pressure and respiratory rate are monitored (because vasodilation secondary to analgesics or decreasing pain may occur and compound the hypotension). • Activity progression depends on the patient's activity tolerance.
Pulmonary Complications		
Impaired gas exchange	• During and after anesthesia, patients require mechanical assistance to breathe. • Potential exists for postoperative atelectasis. • Anesthetic agents stimulate production of mucus, and chest incision pain may decrease the effectiveness of ventilation.	• Pulmonary complications are often detected during assessment of breath sounds, oxygen saturation levels, arterial blood gases, and when monitoring peak pressure and exhaled tidal volumes on the ventilator. • Extended periods of mechanical ventilation may be required while complications are treated.

Complication	Description	Assessment and Management
Fluid Volume Complications		
Hemorrhage	• Untoward and excessive bleeding may be life-threatening.	• Serial hemoglobin, hematocrit, and coagulation studies are performed to guide therapy. • Administration of fluids, colloids, and blood products: packed red blood cells, fresh frozen plasma, platelet concentrate. • Administration of aprotinin perioperatively to reduce blood transfusion needs. • Administration of desmopressin acetate (DDAVP) to enhance platelet function.
Neurologic Complications		
Neurologic changes; stroke	• Inability to follow simple commands within 6 hours of recovery from anesthetic; different capabilities on right or left side of body	• Neurologically, most patients begin to recover from anesthesia in the operating room. • Patients who are older or who have kidney or hepatic failure may take longer to recover. • Patient should be evaluated for stroke when neurologic changes are evident.
Kidney Failure and Electrolyte Imbalance		
Kidney failure	• Usually acute and resolves within 3 months but may become chronic and require ongoing dialysis	• May respond to diuretics or may require continuous renal replacement therapy (CRRT) or dialysis
Acute kidney Injury	• Often results from hypoperfusion of the kidneys or from injury to the renal tubules by nephrotoxic medications	• Fluids, electrolytes, BUN, creatinine, and urine output are monitored frequently. Follow your medical center's protocol for postprocedure hydration
Electrolyte imbalance	• Postoperative imbalances in potassium, magnesium, sodium, calcium, and blood glucose are related to surgical losses, metabolic changes, and the administration of medications and IV fluids.	• Monitor electrolytes and basic metabolic studies frequently. • Implement treatment to correct electrolyte imbalance promptly
Other Complications		
Hepatic failure	• Most common in patients with cirrhosis, hepatitis, or prolonged right-sided heart failure	• Use of medications metabolized by the liver must be minimized. • Bilirubin, albumin, and amylase levels are monitored, and nutritional support must be provided.
Infection	• Surgery and anesthesia alter the patient's immune system. Many invasive devices are used to monitor and support the patient's recovery and may serve as a source of infection.	• The following must be monitored to detect signs of possible infection: body temperature, white blood cell (WBC) counts and differential counts, incision and puncture sites, cardiac output and systemic vascular resistance, urine (clarity, color, and odor), bilateral breath sounds, sputum (color, odor, amount), as well as nasogastric secretions. • Antibiotic therapy may be expanded or modified as necessary. • Invasive devices must be discontinued as soon as they are no longer required. Institutional protocols for maintaining and replacing invasive lines and devices must be followed to minimize the patient's risk for infection.

Note: The patient may require interventions for more than one complication at a time. Collaboration among nurses, physicians, pharmacists, respiratory therapists, and dietitians is necessary to achieve the desired patient outcomes.

NURSING PROCESS
The Postoperative Cardiac Surgery Patient

Initial postoperative care focuses on achieving or maintaining hemodynamic stability and recovery from general anesthesia. Care will be provided in the PACU or intensive care unit, with the patient transferred to the step-down or progressive care unit usually within 24 hours. Care focuses on the monitoring of cardiopulmonary status, pain management, wound care, progressive activity, and nutrition. Education about medications and risk factor modification is emphasized. Discharge from the hospital may occur 3 to 5 days after CABG in patients without complications.

The immediate postoperative period for the patient who has undergone cardiac surgery presents many challenges to the health care team. Specific information about the surgical procedure and important factors about postoperative management are communicated by the surgical team and anesthesia personnel to the critical care nurse, who then assumes responsibility for the patient's care. A plan of nursing care for the patient after cardiac surgery is available online at http://thepoint.lww.com/Honan3e.

ASSESSMENT

In the critical care environment, a complete assessment of all systems is performed hourly for at least 12 hours to determine the postoperative status of the patient compared with the preoperative baseline and to identify anticipated changes since surgery. The following parameters are assessed:

- *Neurologic status:* Level of responsiveness, pupil size and reaction to light, reflexes, facial symmetry, movement and strength of upper and lower extremities
- *Cardiac/hemodynamic status:* Heart rate and rhythm, heart sounds, pacemaker status, arterial blood pressure, central venous pressure (CVP), pulmonary artery pressure, pulmonary artery wedge pressure (PAWP), waveforms from the invasive blood pressure lines, CO or index, systemic and pulmonary vascular resistance, pulmonary artery oxygen saturation (SvO_2), bleeding (from mediastinal chest tubes), trending of CBC. Refer to Chapter 54 for a detailed description of hemodynamic monitoring.
- *Respiratory status:* Chest movement, breath sounds, ventilator settings, respiratory rate, peak inspiratory pressure, arterial oxygen saturation (SaO_2), percutaneous oxygen saturation (SpO_2), end-tidal CO_2, ABGs
- *Peripheral vascular status:* Peripheral pulses; color of skin, nail beds, mucosa, lips, and earlobes; skin temperature; capillary refill, edema (pitting or non); condition of dressings and invasive lines
- *Kidney function:* Urinary output; urine specific gravity and osmolality may be assessed, trending of serum blood urea nitrogen (BUN) and creatinine
- *Fluid and electrolyte status:* Intake, output from all drainage tubes, all CO parameters, mucous membranes, skin turgor, presence of edema, and analysis of laboratory values including electrolytes, calcium, and magnesium
- *Pain:* Nature, type, location, and duration (incisional pain must be differentiated from anginal pain); apprehension; response to analgesics

The assessment also includes observing all equipment and tubes to determine whether they are functioning properly (Fig. 13-10).

As the patient regains consciousness and progresses through the postoperative period, the nurse also assesses indicators of psychological and emotional status. The patient may exhibit behavior that reflects denial or depression or may experience postcardiotomy delirium. Characteristic signs of delirium include transient perceptual illusions, visual and auditory hallucinations, disorientation, and paranoid delusions.

DIAGNOSIS

Appropriate nursing diagnoses of the patient recovering from cardiac surgery may include:

- Decreased CO/tissue perfusion
- Fluid volume and electrolyte imbalance
- Impaired gas exchange
- Alteration in cerebral circulation
- Pain

PLANNING

The goal after CABG surgery is to maintain hemodynamic stability, adequate gas exchange, fluid volume balance, and cerebral perfusion. As the patient progresses toward hospital discharge, patient education and activity progression must be included in the plan of care.

NURSING INTERVENTIONS

RESTORING CARDIAC OUTPUT

To evaluate the patient's cardiac status, the nurse primarily determines the effectiveness of the CO through clinical observations and routine measurements: serial readings of blood pressure, heart rate, CVP, arterial pressure, and pulmonary artery pressures.

Kidney function is related to cardiac function as blood pressure and heart rate drive glomerular filtration; therefore, the urinary output is measured and recorded. Urine output of less than 30 mL/hr or 0.5 mL/kg/hr may indicate a decrease in CO. Body tissues depend on adequate CO to provide a continuous supply of oxygenated blood to meet the changing demands of the organs and body systems. Because the buccal mucosa, nail beds, lips, and earlobes are sites with rich capillary beds, they should be observed for cyanosis or duskiness as possible signs of reduced CO. The nurse notes distention of the neck veins along with an elevated CVP, signaling right-sided heart failure. In general, if the CO has decreased, the skin becomes cool, moist, and cyanotic or mottled.

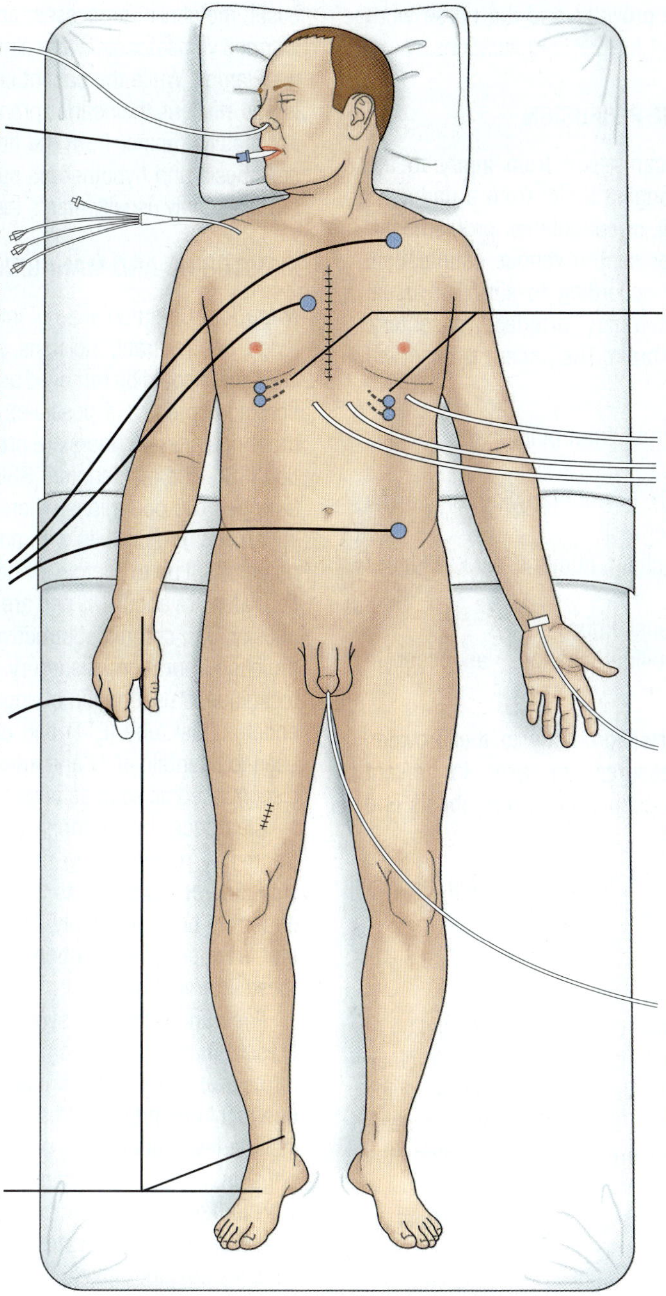

FIGURE 13-10 **Postoperative care of the cardiac surgical patient requires the nurse to be proficient in interpreting hemodynamics, correlating physical assessments with laboratory results, sequencing interventions, and evaluating progress toward desired outcomes.**

Arrhythmias may develop when perfusion of the heart is poor. Common arrhythmias encountered during the postoperative period are atrial fibrillation (Afib), bradycardias, tachycardias, and ectopic beats. Afib is one of the most frequently encountered arrhythmias of CABG, occurring in up to 50% of patients, typically within 5 days (Ata & Abanoz, 2021; Bachar & Manna, 2021). Afib increases the risk of clot formation and embolization (two- to threefold increase in the incidence of postoperative stroke), and some studies have shown that POAF (postoperative Afib) is associated with an increased long-term risk for death and thromboembolic complications (Taha et al., 2020). Therefore, patients at risk for this arrhythmia may be prescribed prophylactic beta-blocking agents preoperatively (Bachar & Manna, 2021). Risk factors for developing postoperative Afib are older, hypertensive, previous Afib, and heart failure. Epicardial pacing wires are typically placed during the surgery, and the nurse and provider work collaboratively if pacing is needed postoperatively to stabilize a rhythm. Continuous observation of the cardiac monitor for arrhythmias is essential.

Any indications of decreased CO are reported promptly to the provider. These assessment data and results of diagnostic tests are used to determine the cause of the problem. After

(*continued on page 484*)

a diagnosis has been made, the provider and the nurse work together to restore CO and prevent further complications.

MAINTAINING ADEQUATE TISSUE PERFUSION

Thromboemboli formation also can result from injury to the intima of the blood vessels, dislodging a clot from a damaged valve, loosening of mural thrombi, or coagulation problems. Air embolism can result from CPB or central venous cannulation. Symptoms of embolization vary according to site. The usual embolic sites are the lungs, coronary arteries, mesentery, spleen, extremities, kidneys, and brain. The patient is observed for the onset of the following:

- Chest pain and respiratory distress from pulmonary embolus or MI
- Severe abdominal or back pain, bowel emptying, or nausea and vomiting from mesenteric emboli
- Pain, cessation of pulses, blanching, numbness, or coldness in an extremity
- Decreased urine output from renal emboli
- One-sided weakness and pupillary changes, as occur in stroke

All such symptoms are reported promptly to the provider. After surgery, the following measures are taken to prevent venous stasis, which can cause deep venous thrombosis and subsequent pulmonary embolism:

- Applying elastic bandage wraps, elastic stocking, and/or sequential pneumatic compression wraps
- Discouraging crossing of legs
- Early and frequent ambulation

Inadequate kidney perfusion can occur as a complication of cardiac surgery. One possible cause is low CO. Trauma to blood cells during CPB can cause hemolysis of red blood cells, which then occlude the renal glomeruli. In addition, the use of vasopressor agents to increase blood pressure may constrict the renal arterioles and reduce blood flow to the kidneys.

Nursing management includes accurate measurement of urine output. An output of less than 30 mL/hr or 0.5 mL/kg/hr may indicate hypovolemia or renal insufficiency. Fluids may be prescribed to increase CO and renal blood flow. IV diuretics may be administered to increase urine output. The nurse should be aware of the patient's BUN, serum creatinine, and urine and serum electrolyte levels. Abnormal levels are reported promptly because it may be necessary to adjust fluids and the dose or type of medication administered. If efforts to maintain kidney perfusion are ineffective, the patient may require continuous renal replacement therapy (CRRT) or dialysis (refer to Chapter 26).

MAINTAINING NORMAL BODY TEMPERATURE

Patients are usually hypothermic when admitted to the critical care unit following the cardiac surgical procedure if their surgery was done using CPB. The patient must be warmed to a normal temperature gradually. This is accomplished partially by the patient's basal metabolic processes and often with the assistance of warmed ventilator air, warm air via a warming system, blankets, or heat lamps. While the patient is hypothermic, the clotting process is less efficient, the heart is prone to arrhythmias, and oxygen does not readily transfer from the hemoglobin to the tissues. Because anesthesia and hypothermia suppress normal basal metabolism, oxygen supply usually meets the cellular demand.

MONITORING AND MANAGING POTENTIAL COMPLICATIONS

Infection. Common sites of infection postoperatively include the lungs, urinary tract, incisions, and intravascular catheters. Foley catheters should be removed as early as possible to prevent infection (postop day 1 if possible). There is no evidence that wound dressings after 48 hours are protective against surgical site infection (SSI). The incidence of SSIs post-CABG ranges from 0.35 to 8.49 per 100 operations where the majority of the infections are superficial. Prophylaxis with an antimicrobial reduces the occurrence of SSI up to fivefold (Anderson, 2019). Sternal wound infection rates are about 1% and are dependent on risk factors such as obesity, DM, chronic obstructive pulmonary disease (COPD), and prolonged duration of surgery (Bachar & Manna, 2021). Aseptic technique is used when changing dressings and when providing endotracheal tube (ETT) and catheter care. Closed systems are used to maintain all IV and arterial lines. All invasive equipment is discontinued as soon as possible after surgery.

Clearance of pulmonary secretions is accomplished by frequently repositioning the patient, suctioning, chest percussion, and/or vibration, as well as teaching and encouraging the patient to breathe deeply, cough, and use the incentive spirometer frequently. Prevention of atelectasis is achieved through these interventions.

Postpericardiotomy syndrome (PPS), has a variable clinical presentation ranging from mild forms of the disease to severe forms presenting with cardiac tamponade or respiratory distress due to a large pleural effusion (Maranta et al., 2022). Symptoms include fever, pericardial pain, pleural pain, dyspnea, pericardial effusion, pericardial friction rub, and arthralgia, in combination with leukocytosis (elevated WBCs) and elevation of the erythrocyte sedimentation rate and CRP. PPS occurs between 1 and 6 weeks postoperatively, with nearly 80% to 85% of the patients developing PPS within the first month after surgery and up to 20% of patients later (13% in the second and 7% in the third month) (Maranta et al., 2022). The incidence is near 10% of patients undergoing cardiac surgery, but varies among different studies and registries (2% to 30%), as well as according to the type of cardiac surgery performed (Gabaldo et al., 2019). Although the pathogenesis of this syndrome is unknown, it is thought to be related to the release of antigens in the pericardial and pleural sac with an autoinflammatory response in some predisposed patients (younger age and females appear to be at higher risk), while others suggest the production of anti-heart antibodies in response to myocardial injury (Maranta et al., 2022). Since PPS is one of the most common complications of cardiac surgery in the late postoperative period, after discharge from the hospital, postoperative instructions will include instruction that the surgeon should be notified if symptoms appear. Anti-inflammatory agents (NSAIDs) often produce a dramatic improvement in symptoms within 48 hours, and 95% resolve without sequelae (Maranta et al., 2022).

Fluid Volume and Electrolyte Imbalance. Fluid and electrolyte imbalance may occur after cardiac surgery. Nursing assessment includes monitoring of intake and output, weight, hemodynamic parameters, hematocrit levels, distention of neck veins, edema, breath sounds, and electrolyte levels. Changes in serum electrolytes are reported promptly so that treatment can be instituted. Especially important are high or low levels of potassium, magnesium, sodium, and calcium. Elevated blood glucose levels are common in the postoperative period. Administration of insulin may be required in patients both with and without DM to achieve the glycemic control necessary for promoting wound healing.

Impaired Gas Exchange. Impaired gas exchange is another possible complication after cardiac surgery. All body tissues require an adequate supply of oxygen for survival. To achieve this after surgery, an ETT with ventilator assistance will be needed initially postop (for an average of about 6 hours). The assisted ventilation is continued until the patient's blood gas measurements are acceptable and the patient demonstrates the ability to breathe independently. To ensure adequate gas exchange, the nurse assesses and maintains the patency of the ETT. The patient is suctioned when necessary. Because a patent airway is essential for oxygen and carbon dioxide exchange, the ETT must be secured to prevent it from slipping into the right mainstem bronchus or accidental dislodgment. The patient is weaned from the ventilator and extubated as soon as possible, usually within 6 hours of CABG. Physical assessment and ABG results guide the process. Before being extubated, the patient should have cough and gag reflexes and stable vital signs; be able to lift the head off the bed or give firm hand grasps; have adequate vital capacity, negative inspiratory force, and minute volume appropriate for body size; and have acceptable ABG levels while breathing without the assistance of the ventilator. Refer to Chapter 54 for additional information related to ventilators and weaning.

During this time, the nurse assists with the weaning process and eventually with the removal of the ETT. Deep breathing and coughing are encouraged at least every 1 to 2 hours after extubation (removal of the endotracheal tube [ETT]) to open the alveolar sacs and provide for increased ventilation as well as to clear secretions (preventing atelectasis).

The patient is assessed continuously for signs of impaired gas exchange: restlessness, anxiety, cyanosis of mucous membranes and peripheral tissues, and tachycardia. Breath sounds are assessed frequently, as well as ABGs, oxygen saturation, and end-tidal CO_2. Following extubation, aggressive pulmonary interventions, such as turning, coughing of secretions, using incentive spirometer, and deep breathing, are necessary to prevent atelectasis and pneumonia.

When the patient's condition stabilizes, body position is changed every 1 to 2 hours. Frequent changes of patient position provide for optimal pulmonary ventilation and perfusion by allowing the lungs to expand more fully.

Alteration in Cerebral Circulation. Brain function depends on a continuous supply of oxygenated blood. The brain does not have the capacity to store oxygen and must rely on adequate continuous perfusion by the heart. Hypoperfusion or microemboli may produce central nervous system injury after cardiac surgery. Approximately 0.5% to 3.5% of patients experience seizures after CABG. Causes include hypoxemia, metabolic disturbances (e.g., hyponatremia, hypoglycemia), drug toxicity (e.g., lidocaine, procainamide), and structural brain injury such as stroke (McGarvey et al., 2021).

It is important to observe the patient for any symptoms of hypoxia: restlessness, headache, confusion, dyspnea, hypotension, and cyanosis. An assessment of the patient's neurologic status includes the level of consciousness (LOC), response to verbal commands and painful stimuli, pupil size and reaction to light, facial symmetry, movement of the extremities, and handgrip strength. Any indication of a change in status is immediately reported to the provider and documented in the medical record.

MINIMIZING SENSORY-PERCEPTION IMBALANCE

Some patients exhibit abnormal behaviors that occur with varying intensity and duration. In the early years of cardiac surgery, this phenomenon occurred more frequently than it does today. Advances in surgical techniques and the delivery of anesthetic agents have significantly decreased the incidence of postoperative delirium. However, incident rates of 3% to 32% of delirium after cardiac surgery are seen in those with pre-existing organic mental disorders (e.g., stroke, dementia), significant prior alcohol consumption, advanced age, or intracranial cerebral artery disease (McGarvey et al., 2021). In those without the aforementioned risk factors, the nurse should consider etiologies of anxiety, sleep deprivation, increased sensory input, medications, and physiologic problems such as hypoxemia. Delirium may appear after a 2- to 5-day stay in an intensive care environment and is associated with increased morbidity and mortality, including postoperative complications of respiratory insufficiency and sternal instability, prolonged length of stay, increased need for skilled nursing facility placement, and reduced cognitive and functional recovery, making early recognition and response crucial. Treatment of postoperative delirium requires an assessment for the etiology and correction of potentially reversible causes (McGarvey et al., 2021).

Careful explanations of all procedures and the need for cooperation help keep the patient oriented throughout the postoperative course. Continuity of care is desirable; a familiar face and a nursing staff with a consistent approach help the patient feel safe. The patient's family should be welcomed at the bedside. Some patients have difficulty learning and retaining information after cardiac surgery. Many patients have difficulties in cognitive function after cardiac surgery, a phenomenon that does not occur after other types of major surgery. The patient may experience recent memory loss, short attention span, difficulty with simple math, poor handwriting, and visual disturbances.

(continued on page 486)

Patients with these difficulties often become frustrated when they try to resume normal activities and learn how to care for themselves at home. The patient and family are reassured that the difficulty usually resolves gradually and most patients will return to their preoperative baseline by 3 to 12 months after surgery (McGarvey et al., 2021). A well-designed plan of nursing care can assist the nursing team in coordinating their efforts for the emotional well-being of the patient.

RELIEVING PAIN

Deep pain may not be felt in the peri-incisional area but may occur in a broader, more diffuse area. Patients who have had cardiac surgery experience pain caused by the interruption of intercostal nerves along the incision route and irritation of the pleura by the chest catheters. Incisional pain may also be experienced from peripheral vein or artery graft harvest sites. Multimodal pain management is utilized through all stages (pre-, intra-, post-op) in order to mitigate the use of opioids post-op and post-hospitalization. Most commonly, scheduled acetaminophen and gabapentinoids are administered around the clock, reserving opioids for severe or breakthrough pain (Perry & Grant, 2020). NSAIDs are generally avoided since the Food and Drug Administration (FDA) issued a boxed warning against their use after CABG surgery because of cardiovascular safety concerns.

Patients report the most pain during coughing, turning, and moving. Physical support of the incision with a folded bath blanket or small pillow during deep breathing and coughing helps to minimize pain (often referred to as "splinting"). Then the patient should be able to participate in respiratory exercises and increase self-care progressively. Patient comfort improves after the removal of the chest tubes. The patient is observed for any adverse effects of opioids, which may include respiratory depression, hypotension, ileus, or urinary retention. If serious side effects occur, an opioid antagonist (e.g., naloxone) may be used.

EVALUATION

Expected patient outcomes may include:

- Maintains adequate CO
- Maintains adequate gas exchange
- Maintains fluid and electrolyte balance
- Experiences decreased symptoms of sensory-perception disturbances
- Experiences relief of pain
- Maintains adequate tissue perfusion
- Maintains normal body temperature
- Incisions are well healed
- Performs self-care activities
- Engages in follow-up care with health care providers and cardiac rehabilitation services
- Adheres to recommendations for diet and lifestyle changes to maintain optimal future health
- Exhibits no complications

MYOCARDIAL INFARCTION (MI)

Coronary occlusion, heart attack, and **MI** are terms used synonymously, but the preferred term is **MI**.

Pathophysiology

In an MI, an area of the myocardium is permanently destroyed. MI is usually caused by reduced blood flow in a coronary artery due to the rupture of an atherosclerotic plaque and subsequent occlusion of the artery by a thrombus. In unstable angina, the plaque ruptures, but the artery is not completely occluded. Because unstable angina and acute MI are considered to be the same process but occurring at different points along a continuum, the term **acute coronary syndrome (ACS)** may be used in lieu of these diagnoses. Other causes of MI include vasospasm (sudden constriction or narrowing) of a coronary artery, decreased oxygen supply (e.g., from acute blood loss, anemia, or low blood pressure), and increased demand for oxygen (e.g., from a rapid heart rate, thyrotoxicosis, or ingestion of cocaine). In each case, a profound imbalance exists between myocardial oxygen supply and demand.

The area of infarction develops over minutes to hours. As the cells are deprived of oxygen, ischemia develops, cellular injury occurs, and the lack of oxygen results in infarction, or the death of cells. The expression "time is muscle" reflects the urgency of appropriate treatment to improve patient outcomes. Each year in the United States, more than 1,500,000 people die from acute MIs; it is the most common cause of death in those over 40 years (Golla & Satya, 2022). Nearly every 34 seconds, one American has a coronary event, and every 1 minute 24 seconds, an American will die of one (Golla & Satya, 2022).

Various descriptions are used to further identify an MI: the type of MI (ST-segment elevation, non–ST-segment elevation), the location of the injury to the ventricular wall (anterior, inferior, posterior, or lateral wall), the point in time within the process of infarction (acute, evolving, or old), and the extent of the damage to the myocardium caused by the MI (partial or full thickness). Partial infarcts are associated with severely narrow coronary arteries and present as non–ST-segment elevation, while full-thickness infarcts commonly occur with obstruction of a single coronary artery and present as ST elevation on ECG readings (Porth, 2019).

The ECG usually identifies the type and location, and other ECG indicators such as a Q wave and patient history identify the timing. Regardless of the location of the infarction of cardiac muscle, the goal of medical therapy is to prevent or minimize myocardial tissue death and to prevent complications.

Risk Factors

Risk factors for MI are the same as those described for atherosclerosis and angina.

BOX 13-5 **Focused Assessment**

Acute Myocardial Infarction (MI) or Acute Coronary Syndrome (ACS)

Be alert for the following signs and symptoms:

Cardiovascular
- Chest pain or discomfort, palpitations
- S_3, S_4, and new onset of a murmur
- Increased jugular venous distention (may be seen if the MI has caused heart failure)
- Elevated blood pressure (because of sympathetic stimulation) or decreased blood pressure (because of decreased contractility, impending cardiogenic shock, or medications)
- Pulse deficit, indicating atrial fibrillation
- In addition to ST-segment and T-wave changes, tachycardia, bradycardia, or arrhythmias on electrocardiogram (ECG)

Respiratory
- Shortness of breath, dyspnea, tachypnea, and crackles if MI has caused pulmonary congestion
- Pulmonary edema

Gastrointestinal
- Nausea and vomiting

Genitourinary
- Decreased urinary output (may indicate cardiogenic shock)

Skin
- Cool, clammy, diaphoretic, and pale appearance (due to sympathetic stimulation, may indicate cardiogenic shock)

Neurologic
- Anxiety, restlessness, and lightheadedness (may indicate increased sympathetic stimulation or a decrease in contractility and cerebral oxygenation or cardiogenic shock)

Psychological
- Fear with feeling of impending doom
- Denial

Clinical Manifestations and Assessment

Chest pain that occurs suddenly and continues despite rest and medication is the presenting symptom in most patients with an MI. However, up to 25% of patients with an MI are asymptomatic during the acute event (Berg et al., 2021). In particular, patients with diabetic neuropathy may not experience chest pain; a high degree of suspicion must be maintained for an MI in diabetic patients admitted with associated symptoms of dyspnea, syncope, fatigue, diaphoresis, or lightheadedness. Physical examination findings depend on the location and extent of the MI and can include S4 gallop; an S3, JVD, crackles on pulmonary examination and peripheral edema if HF is present. Up to 30% of patients with ST elevation myocardial infarction (STEMI) have prodromal (early nonspecific) symptoms. Box 13-5 discusses assessment parameters. In many cases, the signs and symptoms of MI cannot be distinguished from those of unstable angina. The diagnosis of MI is generally based on the presenting symptoms, physical findings, ECG, and laboratory test results (e.g., serial cardiac biomarker values). The prognosis depends on the severity of coronary artery obstruction and the extent of myocardial damage.

Pearls for Practice

The nurse recognizes that other conditions that may be confused with an MI include: angina, pericarditis, aortic dissection, pulmonary emboli, pneumonia, pneumothorax, esophageal disorders, or costochondritis (refer to Table 11-2 for differentiation).

Pearls for Practice

Females often present with symptoms different from those seen in males; in fact, 50% of females with an MI do not complain of chest pain (Pagidipati & Douglas, 2019). Therefore, a high level of suspicion is associated with vague complaints such as fatigue, shoulder blade discomfort, and/or SOB (Pagidipati & Douglas, 2019). In addition, females experience more lethal and severe first acute MIs than males regardless of comorbidity (mortality rates for females after an acute MI are 26% compared with 14.9% for males), have longer reperfusion times (females have smaller coronary arteries), and have higher risk of bleeding with antithrombotic therapy (Golla & Satya, 2022).

Patient History

The patient history has two parts: the description of the presenting symptom(s) (e.g., pain) and the history of previous illnesses and family history of heart disease. The patient's risk factors for heart disease should also be evaluated.

Electrocardiogram

The ECG provides information that assists in diagnosing acute MI. It should be obtained within 10 minutes from the time a patient reports pain or arrives in the emergency department. By monitoring serial ECG changes over time, the location, evolution, and resolution of an MI can be identified and monitored. The ECG changes that occur with an MI are seen in the leads that view the involved surface of the heart. The extent of ischemia and resultant injury through the various layers of the heart determines the type of ECG changes seen. The classic ECG changes are T-wave inversion, ST-segment elevation, and development of an abnormal Q wave (Fig. 13-11). The first ECG signs of an acute MI occur as a result of myocardial ischemia and injury. As the area becomes ischemic, myocardial repolarization is delayed, causing the T wave (representing ventricular depolarization) to invert.

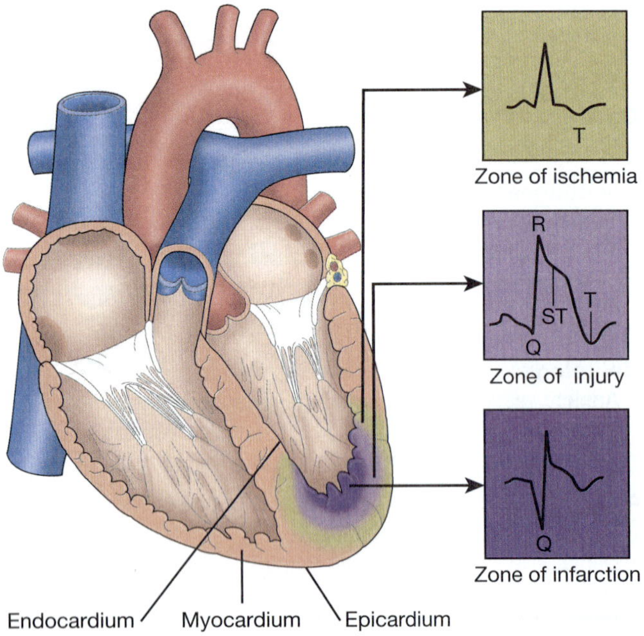

FIGURE 13-11 Effects of ischemia, injury, and infarction on an electrocardiogram (ECG) recording. Ischemia causes inversion of the T wave because of altered repolarization. Cardiac muscle injury causes elevation of the ST segment and tall, symmetrical T waves. Later, Q waves develop because of the absence of depolarization current from the necrotic tissue and opposing currents from other parts of the heart.

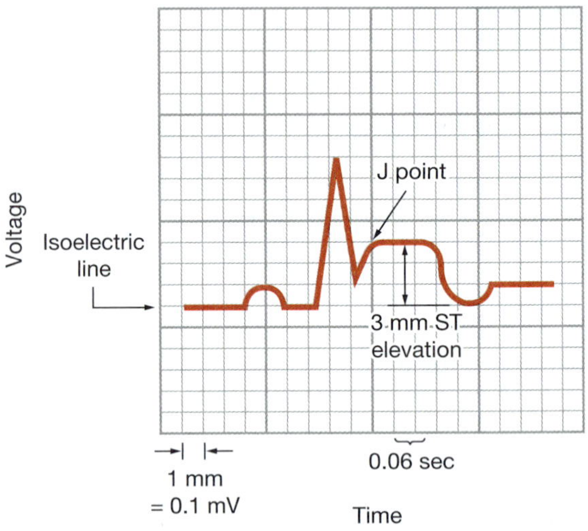

FIGURE 13-12 Using the electrocardiogram (ECG) to diagnose acute myocardial infarction (MI). (ST-segment elevation is measured 0.06 to 0.08 seconds after the J point. An elevation of more than 1 mm in contiguous leads is indicative of acute MI.)

The ischemic region may remain depolarized while adjacent areas of the myocardium return to the resting state. As ischemia progresses to injury, the T wave becomes enlarged and symmetric. Myocardial injury also causes ST-segment changes. The ST segment may rise at least 1 mm above the isoelectric line (area between the T wave and the next P wave is used as the reference for the isoelectric line), or there may be non–ST-segment elevation. Remember that there may be a combination of ischemia, injury, and infarction occurring simultaneously, thus resulting in mixed ECG patterns.

Pearls for Practice

Because lethal arrhythmias can appear suddenly in patients with MIs (most deaths with STEMI occur within the first hour of its onset and usually result from ventricular fibrillation [Mega & Morrow, 2019]), all patients should have bedside monitoring of the ECG and intravenous access!

The beginning of the ST segment is usually identified by a change in the thickness or angle of the terminal portion of the QRS complex and is called the *J point* (Fig. 13-12). The J point is the end of ventricular depolarization (QRS) and the beginning of the ventricular repolarization (ST segment) and is identified by a change from an essentially vertical angle (QRS) to a more horizontal angle (ST segment). This J point is normally on the baseline, and elevation in the ST segment in two contiguous leads is a key diagnostic indicator for MI. The nurse assesses for ST elevation, as it relates to the isoelectric line, at a point 0.08 seconds past the J point.

The appearance of abnormal Q waves is another indication of MI. A Q wave is a negative deflection that signals the beginning of ventricular depolarization; however, abnormal Q waves represent myocardial necrosis and can develop within 1 to 3 days of an MI. A pathologic Q wave is identified by an abnormal depth and duration of the Q wave or the appearance of "new" Q waves not previously seen in ECG tracings. The pathologic Q wave, therefore, reflects the conduction from other parts of the heart because of necrotic tissue. An abnormal Q wave is 0.04 seconds or longer, 25% of the R-wave depth (provided the R wave exceeds a depth of 5 mm), or did not exist before the event. An acute MI may also cause a significant decrease in the height of the R wave. During an acute MI, injury and ischemic changes are usually present. An abnormal Q wave may be present without ST-segment and T-wave changes, which indicates an old, not acute, MI. For some patients, there are no persistent ECG changes, and the MI is diagnosed by blood levels of cardiac biomarkers.

Using the above information, patients are diagnosed with one of the following forms of ACS:

- *Unstable angina:* The patient has clinical manifestations of coronary ischemia, but ECG or cardiac biomarkers show no evidence of acute MI.
- *STEMI:* The patient has ECG evidence of acute MI with characteristic changes in two contiguous leads on a 12-lead ECG. In this type of MI, significant damage to the myocardium occurs.
- *Non-STEMI:* The patient has elevated cardiac biomarkers but no definite ECG evidence of acute MI.

Table 13-5 details the distinguishing features of unstable angina, STEMI and non-STEMI. During recovery from an

TABLE 13-5 **Distinguishing Features of Acute Coronary Syndromes**

		Myocardial Infarction	
Feature	**Unstable Angina**	**NSTEMI**	**STEMI**
Typical symptoms	Crescendo, rest, or new-onset severe angina	Prolonged "crushing" chest pain, more severe and wider radiation than usual angina	
Serum biomarkers	No	Yes	Yes
Electrocardiogram initial findings	ST depression and/or T-wave inversion	ST depression and/or T-wave inversion	ST elevation (and Q waves later)

Reproduced with permission from Lilly, L. S. (2020). *Pathophysiology of heart disease: An introduction to cardiovascular medicine* (7th ed. Table 7-6). Wolters Kluwer Health.

MI, the ST segment often is the first ECG indicator to return to normal (in 1 to 6 weeks). The T wave becomes large and symmetric for 24 hours, and it then inverts within 1 to 3 days for 1 to 2 weeks (Fig. 13-13). Q-wave alterations are usually permanent. An old ST-segment elevation MI is usually indicated by an abnormal Q wave or decreased height of the R wave without ST-segment and T-wave changes.

Echocardiogram

The echocardiogram is used to evaluate ventricular function. It may be used to assist in diagnosing an MI, especially when the ECG is nondiagnostic. The echocardiogram can detect hypokinetic and akinetic wall motion, can determine the ejection fraction, and can also assess valvular function.

Laboratory Tests

Laboratory tests called *cardiac biomarkers* are used to diagnose an MI (Table 13-6). The nurse understands that with damage of the myocardial tissue, the intracellular contents leak out of the cardiac muscle and ultimately are detected in the bloodstream. Newer laboratory tests with faster results, and thus producing earlier diagnosis, include troponin analysis. These tests are based on the release of cellular contents into the circulation when myocardial cells die.

Creatinine Kinase and Its Isoenzymes

Creatinine kinase–myocardial band (CK-MB) is the cardiac-specific isoenzyme; CK-MB is found mainly in cardiac cells and, therefore, increases only when there has been damage to these cells. Elevated CK-MB assessed by mass assay is an indicator of acute MI; its level begins to increase within a few hours, peaks within 24 hours of an MI and returns to normal within 48 to 72 hours. A normal CK-MB is 0 to 3 ng/mL or 1 to 3 μg/L. If the patient has cardiac complaints and negative CK-MB for more than 48 hours, then etiologies for the symptoms outside of an MI will be assessed.

Myoglobin

Myoglobin is a hemeprotein that helps transport oxygen. Like the CK-MB enzyme, myoglobin is found in cardiac and skeletal muscle. A normal level is 5 to 70 ng/mL or 5 to 70 μg/L. The myoglobin level starts to increase within 1 to 3 hours and peaks within 12 hours after the onset of symptoms. An increase in myoglobin is not very specific in indicating an acute cardiac event; however, negative results are an excellent parameter for ruling out an acute MI. Although troponins have largely replaced myoglobin in the detection of acute MI, myoglobin remains valuable in the evaluation of skeletal muscle injury due to rhabdomyolysis (see Box 41-9) (Patibandla et al., 2021).

Troponin

Troponin, a protein found in the myocardium, regulates the myocardial contractile process. The newer-generation "high-sensitivity" troponin assays are able to reliably detect the most minor serum elevations in cardiac troponin. There are three isomers of troponin: C, I, and T. Troponin C binds

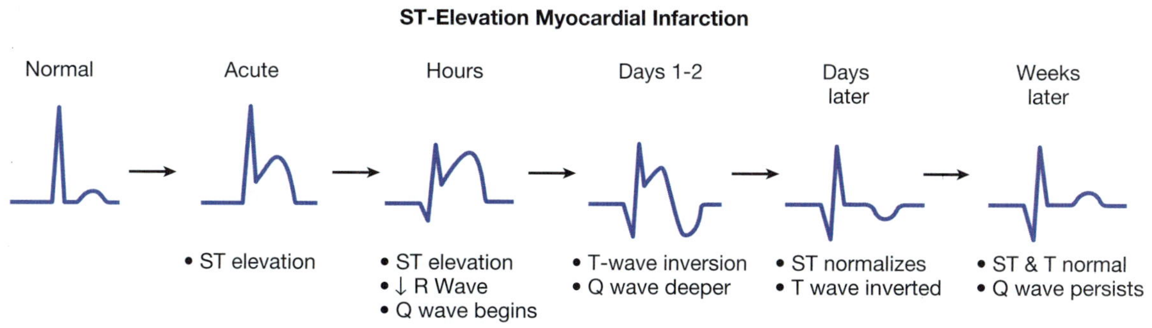

FIGURE 13-13 **ECG evolution during ST-segment-elevation myocardial infarction. (Reproduced with permission from Lilly, L. S. [2020].** ***Pathophysiology of heart disease: An introduction to cardiovascular medicine*** **[7th ed.]. Figure 7-7. Wolters Kluwer Health.)**

TABLE **13-6 Biomarkers of Acute Myocardial Infarction**

Serum Test	Earliest Increase (hours)	Test Running Time (minutes)	Peak (hours)	Return to Normal
Total creatinine kinase (CK)	3–6	30–60	24–36	3 days
CK-MB:isoenzyme	4–8	30–60	12–24	3–4 days
Mass assay	2–3	30–60	10–18	3–4 days
Myoglobin	1–3	30–60	4–12	12 hours
Troponin T or I	3–4	30–60	4–24	1–3 weeks

calcium to activate muscle contraction, while troponins I and T are specific for cardiac muscle, and are currently recognized as reliable and critical biomarkers of myocardial injury. A normal troponin I level is less than 0.5 ng/mL. An increase in the level of troponin in the serum can be detected within a few hours during acute MI. It remains elevated for a long period, often as long as 3 weeks, and it, therefore, can be used to detect recent myocardial damage. Elevated levels should always be assumed to be the result of myocardial damage; however, due to the sensitivity of troponin, small serum elevations also can be detected in conditions other than MI, such as acute cardiac strain or inflammation (e.g., in heart failure, myocarditis, hypertensive crises, or pulmonary embolism [due to right ventricular strain]) (Berg et al., 2021). If the initial troponin level is less than 0.4 ng/mL, but suspicion remains for an MI, the level should be repeated in 5 to 6 hours (Ferri, 2022).

Pearls for Practice: Pathophysiology

A negative level of Troponin I normal level is less than 0 to 0.4 ng/mL. If there is clinical suspicion of an evolving acute MI or ischemic episode, repeat testing in 5 to 6 hours is recommended (Ferri, 2022). An indeterminate level is if the troponin is between 0.05 and 0.49 ng/mL, whereas strong probability of acute MI is associated with a level ≥0.05 ng/mL. Levels greater than 1.5 ng/mL are critical.

Pearls for Practice

The United States Food and Drug Administration (USFDA) released an updated safety warning that biotin (vitamin B7), that is found in multivitamins and in hair, skin, and nail supplements, could interfere with some laboratory tests, causing incorrect results that could go undetected (USFDA, 2019). The daily recommended allowance for biotin is 0.03 mg and that amount does not typically cause interference in lab tests; however, many supplements contain 20 mg of biotin, and some containing up to 100 mg per pill, with recommendations to take multiple pills per day. Specifically, biotin has been associated with a falsely low cardiac troponin test results, causing missed or delayed diagnosis. The nurse asks about all supplement use and alerts the provider and lab when a troponin level is drawn. Both the provider and the laboratory should be made aware because some laboratories may be using assays with biotin technology. In addition, a daily dose of 10 mg of biotin was shown to interfere thyroid-stimulating hormone (TSH) assays (Ylli et al., 2021).

Medical Management

The goals of medical management are to minimize myocardial damage, preserve myocardial function, and prevent complications. These goals are facilitated by the use of guidelines developed by the American College of Cardiology and the American Heart Association (Box 13-6). They may be achieved by reperfusing the area with the emergency PCI or the use of thrombolytic medications in a medical center not capable of doing a PCI. Minimizing myocardial damage is

BOX 13-6 **Medical Treatment Guidelines for Acute Myocardial Infarction**

Use rapid transit to the hospital.
Obtain 12-lead electrocardiogram (ECG) to be read within 10 minutes.
Obtain laboratory blood specimens of cardiac biomarkers, including troponin.
Obtain other diagnostics to clarify the diagnosis.
Begin routine medical interventions:

- Supplemental oxygen
- Nitroglycerin
- Morphine
- Aspirin 162–325 mg
- Beta blocker
- Angiotensin-converting enzyme inhibitor or angiotensin-receptor blocker within 24 hours

Evaluate for indications for reperfusion therapy:

- Percutaneous coronary intervention
- Thrombolytic therapy

Continue therapy as indicated:

- IV heparin or low–molecular-weight heparin
- Clopidogrel or antiplatelet-like agent
- Glycoprotein IIb/IIIa inhibitor

also accomplished by reducing myocardial oxygen demand and increasing oxygen supply with medications, oxygen administration, and bed rest. The resolution of pain and ECG changes indicate that demand and supply are in equilibrium; they may also indicate reperfusion. Visualization of blood flow through an open vessel in the catheterization laboratory is evidence of reperfusion.

Pearls for Practice

The nurse is aware that the mean arterial pressure or MAP is calculated as systolic BP + (diastolic BP ×'s 2)/3. A normal MAP is 70 to 105 mm Hg, and a MAP >60 mm Hg is necessary to perfuse the coronary arteries. A MAP of <65 mm Hg for an extended period can result in end organ ischemia. A MAP between 70 and 90 mm Hg is preferable for a patient with heart disease to decrease left ventricular (LV) workload (Lough et al., 2022).

Pharmacologic Therapy

The patient with suspected MI is given aspirin, nitroglycerin, morphine, a beta blocker, and other medications as indicated, while the diagnosis is being confirmed. Patients should receive a beta blocker initially, throughout the hospitalization, and upon discharge. Also on discharge, there needs to be documentation that the patient was discharged on a statin, an **angiotensin-converting enzyme (ACE)** inhibitor, or an **angiotensin-receptor blocking agent (ARB)**, and aspirin. These are "quality indicators" for ACS treatment and are now publicly reported measures. Remember **SAAB:** *s*tatin, *a*ce or arb, *a*spirin, *b*eta-blockers. If any of these are not prescribed, clear documentation as to why not must be provided.

Thrombolytics

In non–PCI-capable hospitals, initial assessment of patients should include evaluation of the contraindications to administration of a thrombolytic agent. The purpose of **thrombolytics** is to dissolve and lyse the thrombus in a coronary artery (thrombolysis), allowing blood to flow through the coronary artery again (reperfusion), minimizing the size of the infarction, and preserving ventricular function. Hospitals monitor their ability to administer these medications **within 30 minutes** from the time the patient arrives in the emergency department. This is called *door-to-needle time* or "*time to needle.*" The thrombolytic agents used most often are alteplase (t-PA, Activase) and reteplase (r-PA, TNKase). Box 13-7 discusses the administration of and contraindications for thrombolytic therapy.

Analgesics

The analgesic of choice for acute MI is morphine sulfate administered in IV boluses to reduce pain and anxiety. It reduces preload and afterload (peripheral arterial and venous dilation), which decreases the workload of the heart. Morphine also relaxes bronchioles to enhance oxygenation. The

BOX 13-7

Administration of Thrombolytic Therapy

Indications

- No PCI-capable center available in the next 120 minutes (Berg et al., 2021)
- Chest pain for longer than 20 minutes, unrelieved by nitroglycerin
- ST-segment elevation in at least two leads that face the same area of the heart
- Less than 6 hours from onset of pain

Absolute Contraindications

- Active bleeding (excluding menses)
- Known bleeding disorder
- History of hemorrhagic stroke
- History of intracranial vessel malformation
- Known malignant intracranial neoplasm
- Ischemic stroke within 3 months (except acute ischemic stroke within 4.5 hours)
- Recent major surgery or trauma
- Uncontrolled hypertension
- Suspected aortic dissection
- Pregnancy

Nursing Considerations

- Minimize the number of times the patient's skin is punctured.
- Avoid intramuscular injections.
- Draw blood for laboratory tests when starting the IV line.
- Start IV lines before thrombolytic therapy; designate one line to use for blood draws.
- Avoid continual use of noninvasive blood pressure cuff.
- Monitor for acute arrhythmias and hypotension.
- Monitor for reperfusion; resolution of angina or acute ST-segment changes on the ECG.
- Check for signs and symptoms of bleeding: decrease in hematocrit and hemoglobin values, decrease in blood pressure, increase in heart rate, oozing or bulging at sites of invasive procedure, back pain, muscle weakness, changes in level of consciousness, complaints of headache.
- Treat major bleeding by discontinuing thrombolytic therapy and any anticoagulants; apply direct pressure and notify the provider immediately.
- Treat minor bleeding by applying direct pressure if accessible and appropriate; continue to monitor for bleeding.

Note: If possible, a patient should always be transferred to a hospital with PCI capability within 2 hours.

Data from O'Gara, P. T., Kushner, F. G., Ascheim, D. D., Casey, D. E., Jr, Chung, M. K., de Lemos, J. A., Ettinger, S. M., Fang, J. C., Fesmire, F. M., Franklin, B. A., Granger, C. B., Krumholz, H. M., Linderbaum, J. A., Morrow, D. A., Newby, L. K., Ornato, J. P., Ou, N., Radford, M. J., Tamis-Holland, J. E.,… Zhao, D. X. (2013). ACCF/AHA guideline for the management of ST-elevation myocardial infarction: A report of the American College of Cardiology Foundation/American Heart Association Task Force on Practice Guidelines. *Journal of the American College of Cardiology*, *61*, e78.

cardiovascular response to morphine is monitored carefully, particularly the blood pressure, which can decrease, and the respiratory rate, which can be depressed. Because morphine decreases the sensation of pain, ST-segment monitoring may be a better indicator of subsequent ischemia than assessment of pain.

Pearls for Practice

Maintaining the patient in a supine position and elevating the lower extremities if blood pressure falls can minimize hypotension following the administration of nitroglycerin and morphine. Such positioning is undesirable in patients with pulmonary edema, but morphine rarely produces hypotension in these circumstances (Mega & Morrow, 2019).

Angiotensin-Converting Enzyme Inhibitors

ACE inhibitors prevent the conversion of angiotensin I to angiotensin II. In the absence of angiotensin II, the blood pressure decreases, and the kidneys excrete sodium and fluid (diuresis), decreasing the oxygen demand of the heart. The use of ACE inhibitors in patients after MI decreases mortality rates and prevents remodeling of myocardial cells, which is associated with the onset of heart failure. It is important to ensure that the patient is not hypotensive, hyponatremic, hypovolemic, or hyperkalemic before administering ACE inhibitors. Blood pressure; urine output; and levels of serum sodium, potassium, and creatinine need to be monitored closely. An ARB can be used in place of an ACE inhibitor.

Pearls for Practice

The nurse remembers the mnemonic MONA when treating potential MI patients: morphine, oxygen, nitrates, and aspirin. However, there are always caveats! Morphine will provide analgesia but also may induce vasodilation and decreased preload, and should be avoided in patients with right ventricular (RV) involvement who usually present with bradycardia and hypotension. Oxygen is administered at 2 to 4 L/min by nasal cannula or face mask if hypoxemia exists (SaO_2 <90%), but if the saturation is normal, then administration of oxygen may promote coronary vasoconstriction and generate toxic O_2 metabolites. Nitrates facilitate coronary vasodilation, however should not be administered if the systolic BP is <90 mm Hg or ≥30 mm Hg below baseline or there is severe bradycardia with HR <50 beats/min), tachycardia (>100 beats/min), or an RV infarction is suspected (Lee, 2021). Also, nitrates should not be administered to patients who have received a phosphodiesterase inhibitor for erectile dysfunction within the last 24 hours (48 hours for tadalafil). Finally, the nurse knows that aspirin inhibits platelet activation but must first be crushed and chewed to enhance drug absorption and delivery.

Reperfusion Procedures

Reperfusion procedures may be used to restore the blood supply to the myocardium. These include PCI procedures (e.g., intracoronary stents, atherectomy), and CABG. See discussion under "angina pectoris" section for detailed descriptions.

Cardiac Rehabilitation

After the MI patient is free of symptoms, an active rehabilitation program is initiated. Cardiac rehabilitation is a program that targets risk reduction through education, individual and group support, and physical activity. Most insurance programs, including Medicare, cover the cost of cardiac rehabilitation. The nurse needs to encourage the patient and ensure that referral from the hospital for outpatient cardiac rehabilitation is accomplished.

Cardiac rehabilitation is categorized into three phases. Phase I begins with the diagnosis of atherosclerosis, which may occur when the patient is admitted to the hospital for ACS (e.g., unstable angina or acute MI). It includes any post-procedural activity that occurs during the hospitalization. Phase I consists of low-level activities and initial education for the patient and family.

Phase II occurs after the patient has been discharged. It usually lasts for 4 to 6 weeks but may extend to 6 months. This outpatient program consists of supervised, often ECG-monitored, exercise training that is individualized based on the results of an exercise stress test.

Phase III focuses on maintaining cardiovascular stability and long-term conditioning. The patient is usually self-directed during this phase and does not require a supervised program, although it may be offered. The goals of each phase build on the accomplishments of the previous phase. Health promotion is discussed in Box 13-8.

Nursing Management

Relieving Pain and Other Signs and Symptoms of Ischemia

Balancing myocardial oxygen supply with demand (e.g., as evidenced by the relief of chest pain) is the top priority in the care of the patient with an acute MI. Although medication therapy is required to accomplish this goal, nursing interventions are also important.

The recommended treatment for acute MI is reperfusion with thrombolytic therapy (*time to needle*) or emergent PCI (*time to device*) for patients who present to the health care facility immediately and who have no major contraindications. These therapies are important because, in addition to relieving symptoms, they aid in minimizing or avoiding permanent injury to the myocardium. With or without reperfusion, administration of aspirin, an IV beta blocker, and nitroglycerin is indicated. Use of a GPIIb/IIIa agent or heparin may also be indicated. Aspirin (300 mg) should be administered unless already given (e.g., by emergency

BOX 13-8
Health Promotion

Promoting Health after Myocardial Infarction and Other Acute Coronary Syndromes

To extend and improve the quality of life, a patient who has had an MI must learn to adjust their lifestyle to promote heart-healthy living. With this in mind, the nurse and patient develop a program to help the patient achieve desired outcomes.

Changing Lifestyle During Convalescence and Healing

Adaptation to an MI is an ongoing process and usually requires some modification of lifestyle. Some specific modifications include:

- Avoiding any activity that produces chest pain, extreme dyspnea, or undue fatigue
- Avoiding extremes of heat and cold and walking against the wind
- Losing weight, if indicated
- Stopping smoking and use of tobacco; avoiding second-hand smoke
- Using personal strengths to support lifestyle changes
- Developing heart-healthy eating patterns, including avoiding large meals and hurrying while eating
- Modifying meals to align with the Therapeutic Lifestyle Changes (TLCs) or the Dietary Approaches to Stopping Hypertension (DASH) diet
- Adhering to medical regimen, especially in taking medications
- Following recommendations that ensure blood pressure and blood glucose are in control
- Pursuing activities that relieve and reduce stress

Adopting an Activity Program

In addition, the patient needs to undertake an *orderly* program of increasing activity and exercise for long-term rehabilitation as follows:

- Engaging in a regimen of physical conditioning with a gradual increase in activity duration and then a gradual increase in activity intensity
- Walking daily, increasing distance and time as prescribed
- Monitoring pulse rate during physical activity until the maximum level of activity is attained
- Avoiding activities that tense the muscles: isometric exercise, weight-lifting, any activity that requires sudden bursts of energy
- Avoiding physical exercise immediately after a meal
- Alternating activity with rest periods (some fatigue is normal and expected during convalescence)
- Participating in a daily program of exercise that develops into a program of regular exercise for a lifetime

Managing Symptoms

The patient must learn to recognize and take appropriate action for possible recurrences of symptoms as follows:

- Call 911 if chest pressure or pain (or anginal equivalent) is not relieved in 15 minutes by nitroglycerin.
- Contact the provider if any of the following occur: shortness of breath, fainting, slow or rapid heartbeat, swelling of feet and ankles.

services or home treatment) or contraindicated (known allergy). A previous history of gastritis or indigestion is not a contraindication to the use of aspirin in ACS (Bossard et al., 2021). Since the goal is rapid therapeutic aspirin level in the blood, the patient should chew the tablet to promote buccal absorption rather than absorption through the gastric mucosa (Mega & Morrow, 2019). The nurse administers morphine to relieve pain and anxiety and to promote vasodilation, reducing preload and afterload.

Pearls for Practice

Bleeding complications are most common after thrombolytic therapy, and intracranial hemorrhage is the most serious complication (frequency is generally less than 1%); therefore, any change in the LOC, cranial nerve changes, motor weakness, etc. is reported immediately to the provider.

Oxygen should be administered along with medication therapy to assist with the relief of symptoms. Administration of oxygen, even in low doses, raises the circulating level of oxygen to reduce pain associated with low levels of myocardial oxygen. The route of administration, usually by nasal cannula, and the oxygen flow rate are documented. A flow rate of 2 to 4 L/min is usually adequate to maintain oxygen saturation levels of 96% to 100% if no other disease is present. It should be noted that no benefit has been demonstrated to administering supplemental oxygen in patients with normal SaO_2 (Golla & Satya, 2022).

Vital signs are assessed frequently as long as the patient is experiencing pain and other signs or symptoms of acute ischemia. Physical rest in bed with the backrest elevated (semi-Fowler position) helps decrease chest discomfort and dyspnea. Elevation of the head and torso is beneficial for the following reasons:

- Tidal volume improves because of reduced pressure from abdominal contents on the diaphragm and better lung expansion and gas exchange.
- Drainage of the upper lung lobes improves.
- Venous return to the heart (preload) decreases, reducing the work of the heart.

Pearls for Practice

HOB elevation is beneficial for patients with cardiac disease; however, if the patient becomes hypotensive, the patient may be placed in the supine position with legs elevated to increase venous return.

Improving Respiratory Function

Regular and careful assessment of respiratory function can help the nurse detect early signs of pulmonary complications. Scrupulous attention to fluid volume status prevents overloading the heart and lungs.

Promoting Adequate Tissue Perfusion

Limiting the patient to bed or chair rest during the initial phase of treatment is particularly helpful in reducing myocardial oxygen consumption. This limitation should remain until the patient is pain-free and hemodynamically stable. Checking skin temperature, capillary refill, and peripheral pulses frequently is important in monitoring tissue perfusion. Pulse oximetry should be in use, and efforts toward minimizing myocardial oxygen consumption should be in place. Maintaining the patient at rest both physically and emotionally by providing a quiet atmosphere and mild anxiolytic medications may be considered in some cases.

Reducing Anxiety

Alleviating anxiety and decreasing fear are important nursing functions that reduce the sympathetic stress response. Decreased sympathetic stimulation decreases the workload of the heart, which may relieve pain and other signs and symptoms of ischemia.

Monitoring and Managing Potential Complications

Complications that can occur after acute MI are caused by the damage that occurs to the myocardium and the conduction system as a result of the reduced coronary blood flow. Because these complications can be life-threatening, close monitoring for and early identification of their signs and symptoms is critical. Refer to Chapter 53 for details of cardiogenic shock.

The nurse closely monitors and reports changes in cardiac rate/rhythm, heart and lung sounds, blood pressure, pain, respiratory status, urinary output, skin color/temperature, LOC, ECG changes, and laboratory values. Also, stool softeners should be considered to prevent constipation and straining. The nurse institutes emergency measures when necessary.

CHAPTER REVIEW

NCLEX-Style Review Questions

1. A patient arrives in the emergency room from an ambulance complaining of nausea, diaphoresis, SOB, and squeezing substernal chest pain that radiates to the left shoulder and jaw. Enroute vital signs were as follows: 98.8°F, heart rate 92 and regular, 18, and 110/70. The O_2 sat was 89%. The nurse should perform which interventions? Select all that apply.
   a. Complete admission registration, alert the catheter laboratory team, establish an IV access, and record all vital signs
   b. Alert the catheter laboratory team, administer oxygen, obtain blood work, and notify the health care provider
   c. Establish an IV, give sublingual nitroglycerin as ordered, insert a Foley catheter, and alert the catheter laboratory team
   d. Administer oxygen, apply a cardiac monitor, record patient's vital signs, and give sublingual nitroglycerin as ordered
   e. Reassess vital signs immediately, apply a cardiac monitor, administer oxygen (2–4 LPM), start an IV, and prepare to administer morphine and nitrates

2. What does the nurse recognize as an absolute contraindication for thrombolytic therapy? Select all that apply.
   a. Active bleeding
   b. Current anticoagulant therapy
   c. Over age 75
   d. Severe hepatic disease
   e. History of hemorrhagic stroke

3. The nurse is caring for a nonsmoking female patient with the diagnosis of coronary atherosclerosis who has been admitted to the hospital with angina. The patient states that they never experience chest pain going down the arm or in the middle of the chest. The nurse is not surprised at this statement and explains to the patient that:
   a. Females who have ischemia are usually totally asymptomatic.
   b. Females have been found to have more atypical symptoms such as dyspnea and nausea.
   c. Chest pain occurs only with strenuous exercise.
   d. Cigarette smoking is usually the contributing factor to chest pain.
   e. Symptoms such as fatigue and indigestion may be reported by females.

4. Two hours after cardiac catheterization that was accessed via the right femoral artery route, an adult client complains of numbness and pain in the right foot. What action should the nurse take immediately? Select all that apply.
   a. Call the provider immediately.
   b. Check the client's peripheral pulses (pedal/posterior tibial).
   c. Take the client's blood pressure.
   d. Recognize that this is an expected response and reassess the patient in 1 hour.
   e. Compare the baseline assessment to current findings

5. A 54-year-old patient comes to triage complaining of severe, left-sided, pressure-like chest pain, and left arm

numbness. The pain began 2 hours ago and is unrelieved by rest. The patient is anxious, diaphoretic, and complaining of nausea. Cardiac monitoring is begun, and oxygen is given at 2 L/min. An intermittent infusion device (IID) is in place, and vital signs are as follows: BP of 128/68 mm Hg; pulse, 76 beats/min; respirations easy and regular at 20 breaths/min. ECG reveals normal sinus rhythm with occasional unifocal premature ventricular contractions (PVCs). The nurse suspects an MI based on an elevation in the which lab study? Select all that apply.

a. CK-MB
b. LDH
c. Troponin I
d. SGPT
e. Myoglobin

REFERENCES AND SELECTED READINGS

References and selected readings associated with this chapter can be found on the website that accompanies the book. Visit **http://thepoint.lww.com/Honan3e** to access the references and other additional resources associated with this chapter.

CHAPTER 14

Nursing Management: Patients With Complications From Heart Disease

Margaret T. Bowers

Learning Objectives

After reading this chapter, you will be able to:

1. Compare and contrast heart failure (HF) with preserved ejection fraction and reduced ejection fraction, including pathophysiology and clinical manifestations.
2. Describe the management of patients with HF.
3. Develop a teaching plan for patients with HF.
4. Describe the assessment and management of patients with pulmonary edema.
5. Describe the management of patients with cardiogenic shock.
6. Describe the management of patients with pericardial effusion.
7. Describe emergency management of patients with cardiac arrest.

Today, patients with heart disease can be assisted to live longer and achieve a higher quality of life than they could even a decade ago. Through advances in diagnostic procedures that allow earlier and more accurate diagnoses, treatment can begin well before significant debilitation occurs. Newer treatments, technologies, and pharmacotherapies are being developed rapidly. However, heart disease remains a chronic condition, and complications may develop. This chapter presents the complications most often resulting from heart diseases and the treatments provided by the health care team for these complications.

HEART FAILURE

Heart failure (HF) is a clinical syndrome which results from functional and/or structural changes in the heart. It may be associated with pulmonary or systemic congestion, which is verified by elevated natriuretic peptide levels (Bozkurt et al, 2021). Fluid overload and decreased tissue perfusion result when the heart cannot generate a cardiac output (CO) sufficient to meet the body's demands. (See Chapter 11 for a review of cardiac hemodynamics.) The term *HF* indicates myocardial disease in which there is a problem with contraction of the heart resulting in a reduced ejection fraction (EF) or difficulty filling of the heart with preserved EF that may or may not cause pulmonary or systemic congestion. Some cases of HF are reversible, depending on the cause. Most often, HF is a progressive, lifelong diagnosis that is managed with lifestyle changes and medications to prevent acute congestive episodes.

Pearls for Practice: Terminology

Previously, the term diastolic HF was used when describing HF with a preserved or near-normal EF, which is found more commonly in female and older adult patients, whereas the term systolic HF referenced those with reduced EF (Contrera et al., 2023).

CHRONIC HEART FAILURE

As with coronary artery disease (CAD), the incidence of chronic HF increases with age. The nature of chronic HF can be either reduced or preserved EF with reduced EF being the most common (Bozkurt et al., 2021). In the United States, the lifetime risk of developing HF is 20% for those who are 40 years and older. Currently, over 6.2 million people aged 20 years or older in the United States have HF, and 650,000 new cases are diagnosed each year (Virani et al., 2021). Although HF can affect people of all ages, the incidence increases from approximately 20 per 1,000 individuals 65 to 69 years of age to more than 80 per 1,000 among those aged 85 years or older. HF is the most common reason for hospitalization of people older than 65 years of age and the second most common reason for visits to a health care provider. The rate of hospital readmission remains staggeringly high. The economic burden caused by HF is estimated to rise from $30.7 billion in 2012 to $69.8 billion in 2030 (Virani et al., 2021).

The increase in the incidence of HF reflects the increased number of older adults and improvements in treatment of cardiac diseases, resulting in increased survival rates. Many hospitalizations could be prevented by appropriate outpatient care. Prevention and early intervention to arrest the progression of HF are major health initiatives in the United States.

Types and Classification

An assessment of the **EF** is performed to assist in determining the type of HF. EF, an indication of the volume of blood ejected with each contraction, is calculated by subtracting the amount of blood at the end of systole from the amount at the end of diastole and calculating the percentage of blood that is ejected. A normal EF is 50% to 70% of the ventricular volume; the ventricle does not empty completely between contractions. There are four types of HF, which are identified by assessment of left ventricular functioning, usually by echocardiogram. The most common type is an alteration in ventricular contraction called HF with reduced EF ≤40%, which is characterized by a weakened heart muscle. HF with preserved EF ≥50% is characterized by a stiff and noncompliant heart muscle, making it difficult for the ventricle to fill. Between these two ends of the spectrum include HF with mildly reduced EF, between 41% and 49% and HF with improved EF where EF was ≤40% at baseline with a ≥10% improvement to >40% (Bozkurt, 2021).

Pearls for Practice: Pathophysiology

In HF with preserved EF, there is a normal EF; therefore, a normal EF does not mean or equate to normal CO. A normal EF is not a reliable gauge of normal CO. The nurse is aware that a low CO is the fundamental pathophysiologic abnormality of all HF.

Although a low EF is a hallmark of HF, the severity of HF is frequently classified according to the patient's symptoms. The American College of Cardiology and the American Heart Association developed a classification system for HF that incorporates a patient's clinical status and pathophysiology of the disease in its classification. Stages of HF (A–D) were defined for use in understanding and managing the progression of HF, including risk factors for HF and primary prevention strategies; the stage classifications continue to be used today (Bozkurt, 2021). In addition, Figure 14-1 considers the natural history and progressive nature of HF. Treatment guidelines have been developed for each stage.

Pathophysiology

HF results from a variety of cardiovascular (CV) conditions (including chronic hypertension [HTN], CAD, valvular disease, congenital heart defects, and arrhythmias) as well as from conditions such as diabetes mellitus, fever, infection, thyrotoxicosis, iron overload, hypoxia, anemia, and pulmonary embolus (Schwinger, 2021). Significant myocardial dysfunction most often occurs before the patient experiences signs and symptoms of HF, such as shortness of breath (SOB), edema, or fatigue.

As HF develops, the body activates neurohormonal compensatory mechanisms. These mechanisms represent the body's attempt to cope with the HF and are responsible for the signs and symptoms that eventually develop. Understanding these mechanisms is important because the treatment of HF is aimed at relieving them (Fig. 14-2).

The sympathetic nervous system is stimulated to release epinephrine and norepinephrine. The purpose of this initial response is to increase heart rate and **contractility** and support the failing myocardium, but the continued response has multiple negative effects. Sympathetic stimulation causes vasoconstriction of the skin, gastrointestinal (GI) tract, and kidneys. A decrease in renal perfusion due to low CO and vasoconstriction then causes the release of renin by the kidney. Renin promotes the formation of angiotensin I, a benign, inactive substance. Angiotensin-converting enzyme (ACE) in the lumen of pulmonary blood vessels converts angiotensin I to angiotensin II, a potent vasoconstrictor, which then increases the blood pressure and **afterload** (see ***Pearls for Practice*** below). Angiotensin II also stimulates the release of aldosterone from the adrenal cortex, resulting in retention of sodium and fluid, excretion of potassium (K^+) by the renal tubules, and stimulation of the thirst center. This leads to the fluid volume overload commonly seen in HF. Angiotensin, aldosterone, and other neurohormones (e.g., endothelin, prostacyclin) lead to an increase in **preload** (see ***Pearls for Practice*** below) and afterload, which increases stress on the ventricular wall, causing an increase in the workload of the heart. In addition, the combination of medication treatments for HF coupled with the release of aldosterone predisposes patients with HF to hypokalemia. A counter-regulatory mechanism is attempted through the release of natriuretic peptides. Atrial natriuretic peptide (ANP) and B-type natriuretic peptide (BNP) are released from the overdistended cardiac chambers (Fig. 14-3). These substances promote vasodilation and diuresis. However, their effect is usually not strong enough to overcome the negative effects of the other mechanisms.

Pearls for Practice

Preload is the stretching of the cardiac muscle prior to contraction. Ventricular preload is determined by the volume of blood in the ventricle prior to the onset of systole and is a function of both venous return and end-systolic volume of the chamber. For example, when venous return or volume of blood entering the heart is increased, preload increases. In contrast, if there is a loss of blood due to hemorrhage, less

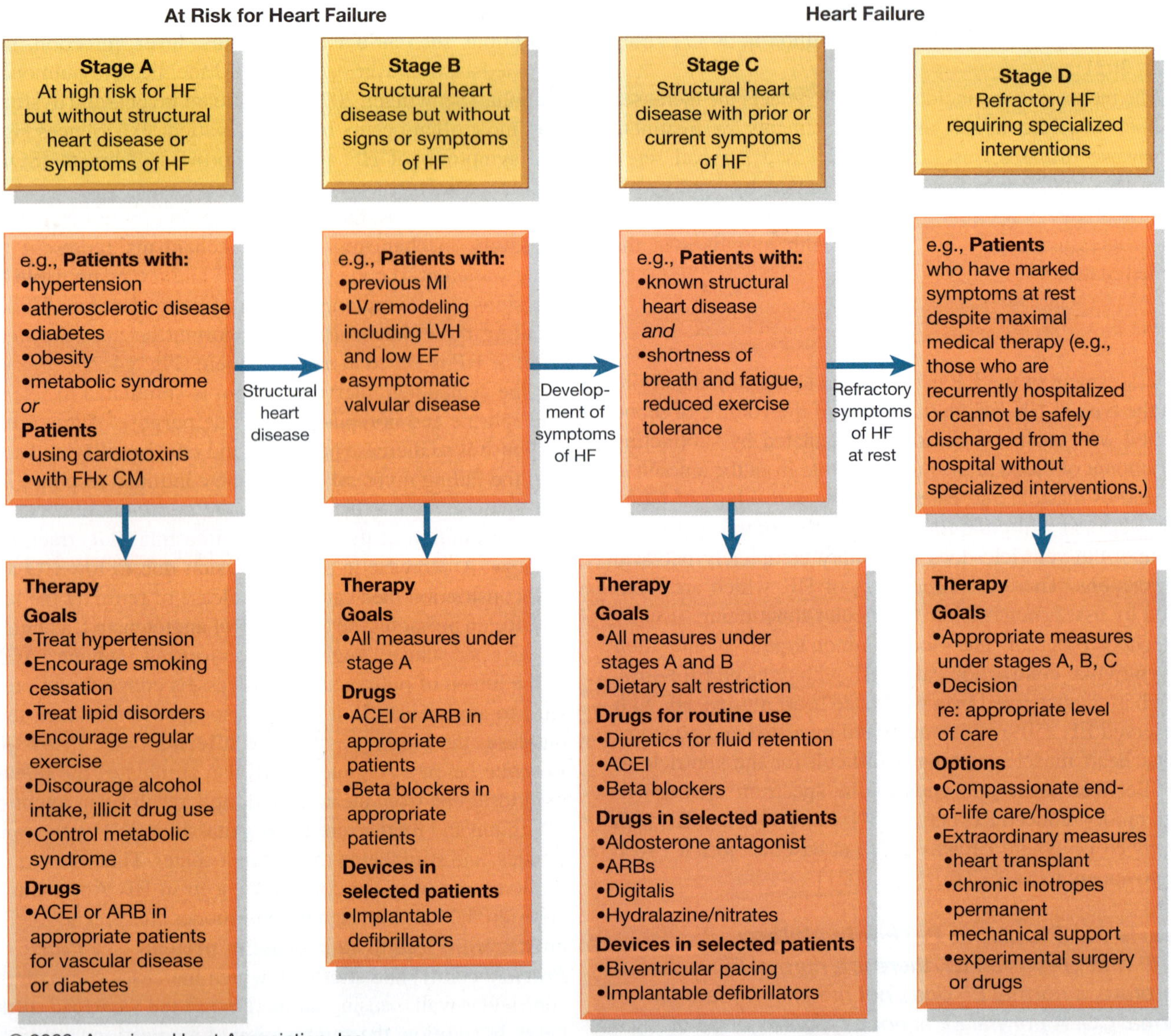

FIGURE 14-1 Stages in the development of heart failure. ACEI, angiotensin-converting enzyme inhibitor; ARB, angiotensin receptor blocker; EF, ejection fraction; FHx CM, family history of cardiomyopathy; LV, left ventricle; LVH, left ventricular hypertrophy; MI, myocardial infarction. (From American Heart Association [AHA]. [2009]. 2009 focused update: ACCF/AHA guidelines for the diagnosis and management of heart failure in adults. *Circulation*, *119*, 1977–2016. Reprinted with permission.)

blood returns to the atria and this leads to decreased ventricular filling and reduced preload. Regardless of the chamber (atria or ventricle), preload is related to the volume just prior to contraction. Afterload is resistance to flow (the pressure gradient that the ventricles must overcome to pump blood out of the ventricles to either the lungs or systemic circulation).

As the heart's workload increases, contractility of the myocardial muscle fibers decreases. Decreased contractility results in an increase in end-diastolic blood volume (preload) in the ventricle, stretching the myocardial muscle fibers and increasing the size of the ventricle (ventricular dilation). The increased size of the ventricle further increases the stress on the ventricular wall, adding to the workload of the heart. One way the heart compensates for the increased workload is to increase the thickness of the heart muscle (ventricular hypertrophy). However, hypertrophy results in an abnormal proliferation of myocardial cells, a process known as *ventricular remodeling*. Under the influence of neurohormones (e.g., angiotensin II), large myocardial cells are produced that are dysfunctional and die early, leaving the other normal myocardial cells to struggle to maintain CO (Schwinger, 2021). The heart does not pump sufficient blood to the body, which causes the body to stimulate the heart to work harder; the heart cannot respond, and failure becomes worse. This cycle repeats itself, thus contributing to an ongoing process of further cardiac decline.

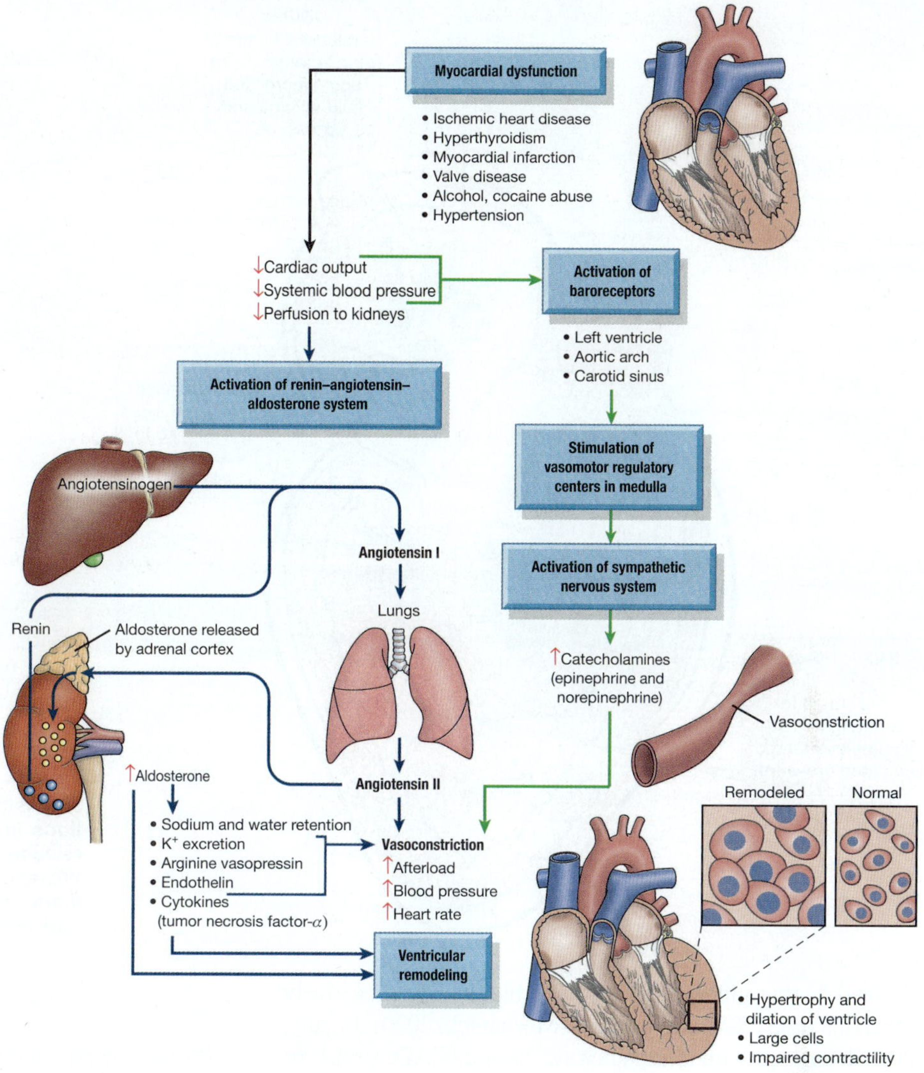

FIGURE 14-2 The pathophysiology of heart failure. A decrease in cardiac output activates multiple neurohormonal mechanisms that ultimately result in the signs and symptoms of HF.

HF with preserved EF develops because of continued increased workload on the heart, which responds by increasing the number and size of myocardial cells (i.e., ventricular hypertrophy and altered cellular functioning). These responses cause resistance to ventricular filling, which increases ventricular filling pressures despite a normal or reduced blood volume. Less blood in the ventricles causes decreased CO. The low CO and high ventricular filling pressures can cause the same neurohormonal responses as described for systolic HF. Table 14-1 provides a comparison of the stages of HF from at-risk to symptomatic HF (Bozkurt, 2021). Table 14-2 articulates the pathophysiologic changes associated with HF.

Risk Factors

There are important risk factors for HF that can be modified before actual structural heart disease occurs. Early identification and treatment of these risk factors or comorbidities may prevent or decrease the occurrence of the onset of HF. Risk factors that are asymptomatic for HF are included in stage A HF.

An example of such an HF risk factor is HTN. HTN is a risk for both males and females, but it is more profound in females. In fact, it is the primary etiology of HF in females. The incidence of HF increases as blood pressure increases, duration increases, and the patient's age increases. Long-term treatment of HTN reduces the risk by 50% (Ahmad, 2016). It has been estimated that the lifetime risk of HTN in the United States is more than 75%. It is, therefore, an important risk factor to treat early, and patients should be encouraged to maintain their blood pressure below 140/90 mm Hg consistently in patients without comorbidities and below 130/80 mm Hg in patients with comorbidities (Al-Makki et al., 2021).

Those with diabetes mellitus or cardiometabolic syndrome are at greater risk of HF. Cardiometabolic syndrome is confirmed in patients who have any three of the following: abdominal obesity, elevated triglyceride levels (over 150 mg/dL), decreased high-density lipoprotein (HDL) (<40 mg/dL for males, <50 mg/dL for females), HTN, and

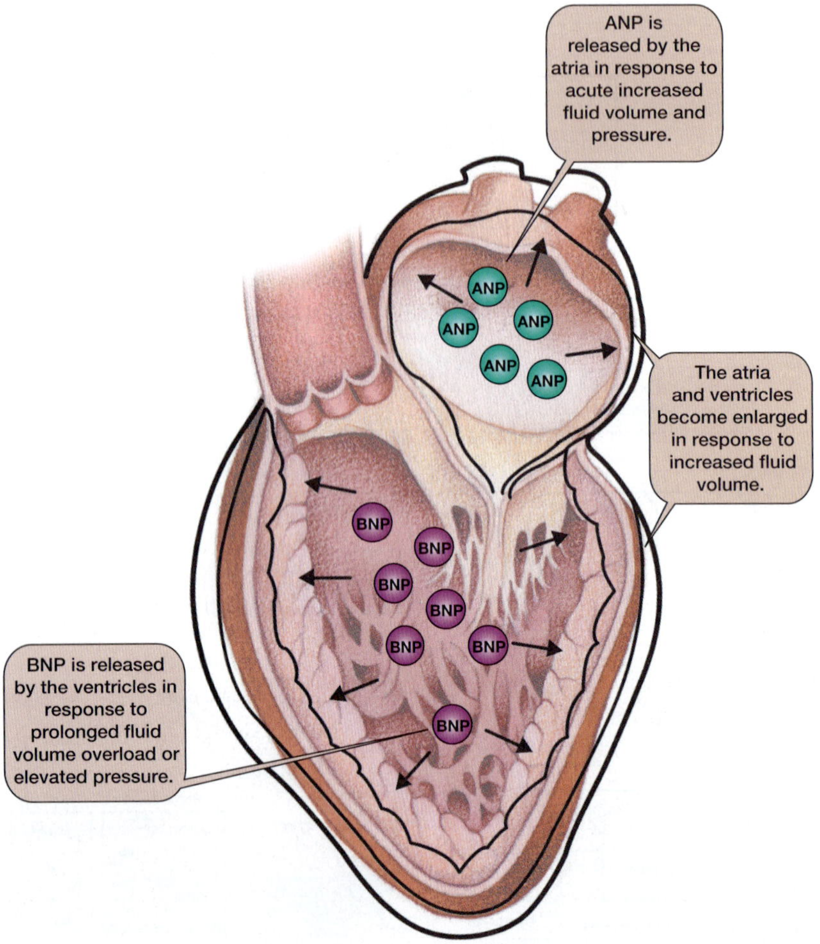

FIGURE 14-3 A-type natriuretic peptide (ANP) and B-type natriuretic peptide (BNP). Disruptions in intravascular fluid balance trigger the release of ANP and BNP. (From Lippincott Williams & Wilkins. [2010]. ***Cardiovascular care made incredibly visual*** **[2nd ed., p. 50]. Lippincott Williams & Wilkins.)**

elevated fasting glucose. These comorbidities also negatively affect outcomes for those with HF (Mechanick, 2020). Finally, those diagnosed with atherosclerotic disease (CAD, stroke, or peripheral vascular disease) are likely to develop HF without adequate control of CV risk. It is important to note that the primary cause of HF in males is CAD (Schwinger, 2021).

Clinical Manifestations and Assessment

All types of HF share similar clinical findings. Overt signs of HF include resting dyspnea, bendopnea (SOB within 30 seconds of bending over at the waist [due to fluid or pressure changes in the abdomen]), cyanosis, and cachexia

TABLE 14-1 Comparison of Systolic and Diastolic Heart Failure

	HF With Reduced Ejection Fraction	HF With Preserved Ejection Fraction
Pathophysiology	• Impaired ventricular pumping of blood during systole • Characterized by reduced stroke volume, incomplete ventricular emptying, cardiac dilation, and elevated left ventricular diastolic pressure • Reduced cardiac output evokes compensatory neurohormonal responses that increase heart rate, sodium and water retention, and vasoconstriction	• Impaired ventricular relaxation filling during diastole • Characterized by a stiffened left ventricle that cannot relax and fill sufficiently at normal diastolic pressure • The result is either decreased left ventricular end-diastolic volume (leading to decreased cardiac output) or a compensatory rise in left ventricular filling pressure, which can lead to pulmonary venous hypertension
Causes/etiology	• Usually caused by ischemic or idiopathic dilated cardiomyopathy, when the left ventricle cannot adequately contract or squeeze out its contents, so that preload increases and stroke volume decreases	• Usually caused by hypertensive, hypertrophic, or restrictive cardiomyopathy

HF, heart failure.

TABLE **14-2 Symptom Comparison of Left- Versus Right-Sided Heart Failure**

	Left-Sided HF	Right-Sided HF
Pathophysiology	• Pulmonary congestion from impaired left ventricle (LV) function • LV cannot pump blood out of the ventricle effectively into the aorta and the systemic circulation • Pulmonary venous blood volume and pressure increase, forcing fluid from the pulmonary capillaries into the pulmonary tissues and alveoli, causing pulmonary interstitial edema and impaired gas exchange	• Right ventricle pump failure leading to congestion in the peripheral tissues and the viscera (peripheral edema, sacral edema, ascites, hepatomegaly [enlarged liver]; see Box 14-1) • Right side of the heart cannot eject blood and cannot accommodate all the blood that normally returns to it from the venous circulation • Increased venous pressure leads to jugular vein distension (JVD) and increased hydrostatic pressure throughout the venous system. Normal central venous pressure (CVP) is 2–8 mm Hg. A CVP greater than 8 mm Hg associated with hypervolemia (excessive fluid circulating in the body) or right-sided HF

HF, heart failure.

(physical wasting), peripheral edema resulting from long-standing heart disease. A baseline height and weight should be documented on admission and weight rechecked each morning. Obtaining daily weights and tracking trends in weight, along with an accurate intake and output log, provide an easy and accurate way to monitor fluid balance. Documenting fluid balance is an important surveillance strategy in controlling HF symptoms.

Pearls for Practice

Daily weights should be at the same time, on the same scale, and with the patient wearing the same clothes for accuracy. The nurse is aware that when calculating new gain or loss that 500 mL approximates 1 lb, or 1,000 mL approximates 1 kg (2.2 lb).

A thorough CV assessment is performed, which includes blood pressure measurement in both sitting and standing positions in order to detect orthostatic hypotension (sustained reduction in systolic blood pressure of at least 20 mm Hg or diastolic blood pressure of 10 mm Hg; see Chapter 11).

Tachycardia (heart rate over 120 bpm) may signal worsening HF. When the heart rate is rapid, the stroke volume (SV) decreases because the ventricle has less time to fill. This, in turn, produces increased pressure in the atria and, eventually, in the pulmonary vascular bed. A weak, thready pulse and *pulsus alternans* (pulse is regular but force of amplitude varies with alternating beats from large to small) are signs of decreased left ventricular function.

Left ventricular hypertrophy (LVH) may displace the apical pulse left and downward toward the axilla from its normal location at the fifth intercostal space, medial to the midclavicular line. Right-sided HF may present with an elevation in jugular venous pressure greater than 4 cm above the sternal angle. This is an estimate, not a precise measurement, of central venous pressure (CVP).

An S_3 heart sound is a sign that the heart is beginning to fail and that increased blood volume is filling the ventricle with each beat. Other sounds may include mitral and tricuspid regurgitation murmurs. The nurse may detect an S_4 sound if the patient has increased resistance to ventricular filling because of increased stiffness of the ventricular myocardium.

The nurse auscultates the lungs for crackles (formerly called rales) which are discrete, discontinuous crackling sounds heard at the end of inspiration. They are produced by alveolar fluid accumulation and are not cleared with coughing. It is recommended that the nurse begins auscultation at the base of the lungs to detect crackles in HF patients and notes the extension; typically crackles start at the lung bases (bibasilar) and are heard progressively higher in the lungs as HF worsens. Wheezing may also be heard in some patients. The rate and depth of respirations are also documented. Dullness to percussion may indicate pleural effusions which occur due to the movement of fluid and impaired lymphatic drainage as a result of elevated systemic venous pressure in HF.

The nurse assesses dependent parts of the patient's body for perfusion and edema. With significant decreases in SV, there is a decrease in perfusion to the periphery, causing the skin to feel cool and to appear pale or cyanotic. If the patient is sitting upright, the feet and lower legs are examined for edema; if the patient is supine in bed, the sacrum and back are also assessed for edema. Fingers and hands may also become edematous. The nurse notes the location and extent of the edema and assesses for evidence of pitting edema (refer to Chapter 11).

Hepatomegaly, hepatojugular reflux, and ascites can occur with venous congestion due to right-sided HF. Recall with right-sided HF, there is accumulation of fluid in the systemic venous circulation. To assess for hepatojugular reflux, the patient is positioned in bed so that the nurse can observe the blood column of the jugular veins above the clavicle. The patient is asked to breathe normally while manual pressure is applied over the right upper quadrant of the abdomen for at least 5 seconds (Thibodeau & Drazner, 2018). If the top of the jugular venous column in the neck rises at least 3 to 4 cm, and persists as long as the abdominal pressure is continued, it is considered positive hepatojugular reflux, which indicates that the right ventricle cannot accommodate the additional volume of displaced blood; when the right ventricle cannot

BOX 14-1 **Focus on Assessment**

Left-Sided Versus Right-Sided HF

Be alert for the following signs and symptoms:

Left-Sided HF

- Dyspnea, orthopnea, paroxysmal nocturnal dyspnea (PND)
- Cough
- Pulmonary crackles (rales)
- Decrease O_2 saturation levels
- S_3 ventricular gallop
- Oliguria, if kidney perfusion is diminished (Note: Nocturia may occur when perfusion improves with sleeping due to improved perfusion at rest.)
- Decreased perfusion to other systemic organs (advanced failure):
  - Sluggish GI motility
  - Dizziness, lightheadedness, confusion, restlessness
  - Anxiety
  - Skin cool and clammy
  - Decrease in EF
  - Tachycardia and/or weak/thready pulse
  - Fatigue or activity intolerance

Right-Sided HF

- Lower extremity dependent edema (dependent edema is swelling that follows the position of the body):
  - Legs and feet
  - May progress to thighs, external genitalia, lower trunk, abdomen, and sacral edema (in a bedbound patient)
  - Pitting edema (indentations in the skin remain even after slight compression with the fingertips)
- Hepatomegaly (enlargement of the liver)
- Ascites (accumulation of fluid in the peritoneal cavity)
- Anorexia and nausea
- Weight gain due to retention of fluid
- Weakness/fatigue from reduced CO and impaired cognition
- Decreased perfusion to other systemic organs (advanced failure)

accommodate this additional volume, an increase in jugular venous pressure is seen (Ball et al., 2023). A positive hepatojugular reflux is associated with right HF and constrictive pericarditis.

Sensorium and level of consciousness must be evaluated. As the volume of blood ejected by the heart decreases, so does the amount of oxygen transported to the brain. Patients may complain of dizziness or lightheadedness. Box 14-1 compares and contrasts assessment findings in left- and right-sided HF.

Diagnostic evaluation includes the following:

- A chest x-ray to determine the presence and extent of cardiac enlargement or pulmonary congestion and to help identify pulmonary disease. Cardiomegaly may indicate reduced EF; whereas a normal heart size suggests preserved EF.
- A 12-lead electrocardiogram (ECG) to determine the presence of cardiac arrhythmias, LVH, and previous or current myocardial infarction (MI). If the patient has left ventricular dysfunction, the ECG usually indicates a left ventricular electrical abnormality specific to ventricular dilation or hypertrophy.
- A two-dimensional (2D) echocardiogram with Doppler flow study is a noninvasive test to look for structural cardiac abnormalities to measure the EF.
- A three-dimensional (3D) echocardiogram with strain measurements is quickly replacing the 2D mode due to greater accuracy (Baldea et al., 2020).
- Cardiac magnetic resonance testing (now considered the gold standard for assessing cardiac function) to detect pathologic involvement which is useful in determining prognosis (Elmadi, 2022). It is a more expensive test than both the 2D and 3D with strain and may only be available at large or regional medical facilities.
- Laboratory tests to help diagnose HF include complete blood cell count, electrolyte levels (including calcium and magnesium), blood urea nitrogen, creatinine, serum glucose, serum albumin, liver function tests, thyroid-stimulating hormone, urinalysis, and BNP levels. High BNP levels (greater than 100 pg/mL) indicate abnormal ventricular function or symptomatic HF. The higher the BNP level, the more severe the CHF (Pagana et al., 2021).
- A right-sided heart catheterization may be performed to determine the heart's preload pressures and pulmonary pressures to determine the degree of HF and the need for further intervention. A patient with angina who is a candidate for coronary revascularization may undergo a left heart cardiac catheterization with coronary arteriography.

Pearls for Practice

A right heart catheterization involves inserting a catheter (typically a thermodilution pulmonary artery [PA] catheter; see Chapter 54) via the brachial, internal jugular, or femoral vein and threading the catheter through the superior vena cava (or inferior vena cava if the femoral vein is used) to the right heart chambers and into the PA. Pressure readings are obtained from the right atrium, the right ventricle, the PA, the PA occlusion wedge position, and CO. Whereas in a left-sided heart catheterization, a catheter is inserted into the arterial system (typically using the radial, brachial, or femoral artery) and threaded upward (to the left heart) recording pressure measurements in the aortic root, the left ventricle, and the left atrium. The coronary arteries are also visualized and the data obtained also calculates the left ventricular EF.

Medical Management

Treatment begins with prevention. Identifying patients at risk is the first step in the care and treatment of HF.

The overall goals of management of HF are to relieve patient symptoms, improve functional status and quality of life, and extend survival. Treatment is based on the type, severity, and cause of HF. Specific objectives include the following:

- Eliminate or reduce any etiologic contributory factors, especially those that may be reversible (e.g., atrial fibrillation, excessive alcohol ingestion, uncontrolled HTN).
- Reduce the workload on the heart by reducing afterload and preload.
- Optimize all therapeutic regimens.
- Prevent exacerbations of HF.

Treatment options vary according to the severity of the patient's condition (see Fig. 14-1).

Lifestyle Changes

Managing the patient with HF includes providing general education and counseling to the patient and family. It is important that the patient and family understand the nature of HF and the importance of their participation in the treatment regimen. Lifestyle recommendations include restriction of dietary sodium; avoidance of excessive fluid intake, alcohol, and smoking; weight reduction when indicated; and regular exercise. The patient must know how to recognize signs and symptoms that need to be reported to the health care professional such as weight gain, increasing SOB, worsening **orthopnea** (SOB when lying flat), fatigue, and edema.

Pharmacologic Therapy

Several medications (Table 14-3) are prescribed routinely for HF with reduced EF (HFrEF), including angiotensin receptor blocker/neprilysin inhibitor, ACE inhibitors, beta blockers, diuretics, mineralocorticoid receptor antagonist, and sodium-glucose co-transporter-2 inhibitors. Medications for HF with preserved EF (HFpEF) depend on the underlying condition, such as HTN or valvular dysfunction.

TABLE **14-3 Pharmacologic Treatment of Heart Failure**

Drug Class	Pharmacokinetics	Indications and Nursing Implications
Diuretics	Diuretics prompt the kidneys to excrete sodium, chloride, and water, reducing fluid volume. They reduce preload.	• Diuretics should never be used alone to treat HF because they don't prevent further myocardial damage and are used to improve symptoms. • Loop diuretics, such as furosemide, bumetanide, and torsemide, are the preferred first-line diuretics because of their efficacy in patients with and without kidney impairment. • Spironolactone should be added to a patient's regimen if they have HFrEF with recurrent symptoms at rest despite therapy with either neprilysin inhibitor, angiotensin-converting enzyme (ACE) inhibitor or angiotensin receptor blocker (ARB), and beta blockers, and diuretics.
Inotropes	Inotropes affect the force of myocardial contraction. Positive inotropes increase force of myocardial contraction and also increase workload of heart and oxygen demand. Negative inotropes decrease force of myocardial contraction and decrease workload of heart and oxygen demand.	• Digoxin is a weak inotrope and increases the heart's ability to contract and improves HF symptoms and exercise tolerance in patients with mild to moderate HF. • Major adverse reactions to positive inotropes include arrhythmias; gastrointestinal problems, such as anorexia; and neurologic symptoms, such as confusion (Bistola, 2019). • Intravenous (IV) inotropes, such as dobutamine, dopamine, and milrinone, can also be used for long-term support (e.g., patients awaiting cardiac transplant) via a tunneled central venous catheter or peripherally inserted central catheter.
Neprilysin inhibitor	Neprilysin inhibitors, such as sacubitril, break down a variety of vasoactive peptides resulting in both diuresis and natriuresis, vasodilation, reduction in cardiac fibrosis, and hypertrophy (Docherty et al., 2020).	• Neprilysin inhibitors are used in combination with an ARB and the most common adverse reactions include hypotension, worsening kidney function, and potassium retention. Improves quality of life in patients with chronic HF and decreases hospitalizations.
ACE inhibitors	ACE inhibitors, such as captopril and ramipril, block the conversion of angiotensin I to angiotensin II, a vasoconstrictor that can raise blood pressure. These drugs alleviate HF symptoms by causing vasodilation and decreasing myocardial workload. They are preload and afterload reducers that provide renal protection.	• The most common adverse reaction to ACE inhibitors is a dry cough. Other adverse reactions include angioedema, hypotension, worsening kidney function, and potassium retention.

(continued)

TABLE **14-3 Pharmacologic Treatment of Heart Failure (*continued*)**

Drug Class	Pharmacokinetics	Indications and Nursing Implications
Angiotensin II receptor blockers	Angiotensin II receptor antagonists selectively block the binding of angiotensin II to specific tissue receptors in vascular smooth muscle and the adrenal glands. Overall effects include blocking the vasoconstricting effect of the renin–angiotensin system and blocking aldosterone release, leading to a reduction in sodium and water retention. They have little effect on potassium. They are preload and afterload reducers.	• Patients who cannot take ACE inhibitors may be prescribed ARBs instead. Angiotensin receptor antagonists are similar to ACE inhibitors for nursing implications. Evidence suggests patients may not exhibit the side effect of a cough as they do with ACE inhibitors.
Aldosterone receptor antagonists	Aldosterone receptor antagonists, such as eplerenone, block aldosterone from binding to receptors in the kidneys. This allows the kidneys to eliminate excess sodium and water. They are a preload reducer.	• This therapy reduces the effects of sodium and water retention, vasoconstriction, and myocardial remodeling. • Since these medications are potassium sparing, nursing care should include guidance about potassium-containing salt substitutes and foods high in potassium.
Beta blockers	Beta-adrenergic blockers, such as bisoprolol, metoprolol, and carvedilol, block the effects of catecholamines, resulting in reduction of heart rate, decreased peripheral vasoconstriction, and decreased myocardial demand. Beta blockers can interfere with the passage of air into the lungs. However, selective beta blockers avoid this problem. They are a negative inotrope.	• Long-term therapy reduces HF symptoms and improves the patient's functional status.
Vasodilators/ nitrates	Vasodilators/nitrates are used for arterial and venous smooth muscle relaxation. They are preload and afterload reducers.	• The combination of hydralazine and nitrates is recommended to improve outcomes for patients self-described as African American (Khazanie et al., 2016) with moderate to severe HF symptoms who are on optimal ACE inhibitors, beta blockers, and diuretics.

HF, heart failure; HFrEF, heart failure with reduced ejection fraction.

Additional Therapies

Additional therapy and surgical treatment are described in Table 14-4. Box 14-2 discusses the psychological impact of these therapies.

Nursing Management

Despite advances in medical and surgical approaches to HF, mortality remains high. Nurses can make a major difference in promoting positive outcomes. Caring for patients with HF requires a collaborative, interdisciplinary team approach. Nurses play a pivotal role in the care and ongoing teaching of this patient population (Rice et al., 2018).

Assessing the Patient

The nursing assessment for the patient with HF focuses on observing for effectiveness of therapy and for the patient's ability to understand and implement self-management strategies. Signs and symptoms of pulmonary and systemic fluid overload are recorded and reported immediately so that adjustments can be made in therapy. The nurse also explores the patient's emotional response to the diagnosis of HF, a chronic and often progressive condition.

The health history focuses on the signs and symptoms of HF, such as fatigue, SOB, **dyspnea on exertion (DOE)** (SOB that occurs with exertion), and cough. Sleep disturbances, particularly sleep suddenly interrupted by acute, severe SOB termed PND, may be reported. PND is noted after lying in recumbent position (usually within 1 hour), and relieved by sitting or standing. The nurse also asks about the number of pillows needed for sleep (an indication of orthopnea) and bendopnea (SOB when bending over), edema, abdominal symptoms, altered mental status, activities of daily living, daily weight, and the activities that cause fatigue. The nurse explores the patient's understanding of HF, self-management strategies, and the desire to adhere to those strategies. The nurse helps patients identify the impact the illness has had on their quality of life and successful coping skills that they have used. Often family and significant others are included in these discussions.

Monitoring Intake and Output

If the patient is hospitalized, the nurse measures output carefully to establish a baseline against which to assess the effectiveness of diuretic therapy. Intake and output records are rigorously maintained. It is important to know whether the

TABLE **14-4 Modalities for Treatment of Heart Failure**

Modality	Indications	Description/Procedure
Ultrafiltration (UF)	Eases symptoms for patients in decompensated HF and can help some patients to respond again to conventional drug therapy; it is a low-volume extracorporeal process that removes fluid from the intravascular compartment. Currently, UF may be used to remove excess volume from patients with acute decompensated heart failure when the kidneys are unresponsive to diuretics (Lough, 2022).	• Uses a mechanical pump and a hemofilter to remove a specified amount of fluid with each treatment, alleviating the patient's symptoms. • Treatment time varies depending on patient needs. • During treatment, the intravascular fluid volume remains stable, since fluid shifts from the interstitial space to replace fluid lost in treatment, which reduces edema and third-spacing. However, as with diuretic therapy, the patient's volume status needs to be monitored very closely, because effective intravascular volume depletion can be detrimental in those with cardiac disease (Hatamizadeh, 2021).
Cardiac resynchronization therapy (CRT)	In the patient with HF who does not improve with standard therapy, CRT may be beneficial. CRT involves the use of a biventricular pacemaker to treat electrical conduction defects. Left bundle branch block is a feature of delayed conduction that is frequently seen in patients with HF that results in dyssynchronous conduction and contraction of the right and left ventricles, which can further decrease EF (Glickson et al., 2022).	• Use of a pacing device with leads placed in the right atrium, right ventricle, and left ventricular can synchronize the contractions of the right and left ventricles. This intervention has been shown to improve cardiac output, optimize myocardial energy consumption, reduce mitral regurgitation, and slow the ventricular remodeling process. For selected patients, this results in fewer symptoms and increased functional status (Glickson et al., 2022). For patients who require CRT and an implantable cardiac defibrillator (ICD), combination devices are available.
Implantable cardiac defibrillators (ICDs)	Patients with HF are at high risk for arrhythmias. In patients with life-threatening arrhythmias, placement of an ICD can prevent sudden cardiac death and extend survival.	• ICDs can provide a range of therapies that include cardioversion, defibrillation, and pacing. A lead or leads are placed in the appropriate chamber's endocardium and attached to a generator box that can be implanted in the right or left side of the chest, under the clavicle. • Wearable cardioverter defibrillators can be used as a bridge to implantable defibrillators (Cheung et al., 2021).
Ventricular access devices/destination therapy	Patients with end-stage HF may require a ventricular assist device (VAD) for greater support for the failing ventricle(s). A VAD can reduce myocardial ischemia and workload, limit permanent cardiac damage, and restore adequate organ perfusion. Indications for use include the following: as a bridge to myocardial recovery in acute ventricular failure (e.g., shock, acute MI, etc.), as a bridge to heart transplantation in chronic ventricular failure, and for permanent therapy for end-stage chronic HF. VADs are also known as *destination therapy.*	• VADs are mechanical blood pumps that work by augmenting or replacing the function of either the left or right ventricle. 1. There are a variety of FDA-approved devices that are used as bridges to transplantation in adults. These devices are either pulsatile or continuous flow (Stelik & Kirklin, 2021). • All VADs share a common problem with infectious complications, risk for thromboembolic complications, and possibility of mechanical failure common to any machine.
Heart transplant	For some patients with end-stage HF, cardiac transplantation is the only option for long-term survival. Some of these patients require mechanical circulatory assistance with an implanted ventricular assist device as a bridge therapy to cardiac transplantation. Research continues toward perfection of a totally implantable artificial heart that may be used as an alternative to transplantation.	Heart transplantation involves replacing a person's diseased heart with a donor heart. This is an option for advanced HF patients when all other therapies have failed (Tong & Khush, 2021).

HF, heart failure.

BOX 14-2

Nursing Research

Bridging the Gap to Evidence-Based Practice

Foster, M. (2018). A mobile application for patients with heart failure: Theory- and evidence-based design and testing. *Computers, Informatics, Nursing: CIN*, *36*(11), 540–549. https://doi.org/10.1097/CIN.0000000000000465

What are the evidence-based approaches and key factors associated with successful outcomes in teaching patients with HF? (Foster, 2018)

Purpose

To provide supporting evidence associated with successful educational approaches for patients with HF using a mobile application.

Design

This small study beta tested a mobile application intervention to support self-care and increase symptom awareness in community-dwelling patients with heart failure. Participants entered physiologic data, answered qualitative questions about symptoms, and reviewed heart failure education within the HF App daily. Two validated instruments, the Self-care of Heart Failure Index and Heart Failure Somatic Awareness Scale, were administered both before and after the intervention, and results were compared using t tests.

Results

Results indicated that there were clinically significant changes from preintervention to postintervention in self-care scores in each subscale, with a statistically significant difference in the confidence subscale scores ($P = .037$). These results indicate that incorporating mobile applications that comprise symptom monitoring, reminders, education, and the ability to track trends in physiologic data is most useful to assist individuals with heart failure to perform effective self-care.

Nursing Implications

The nurse's approach to teaching self-care measures to HF patients should be guideline directed and evidence based. It should include the following:

- Early instruction reinforced through the hospital stay and at discharge (Charais, 2020)
- Assessment of patient's health literacy, educational preferences, and knowledge of HF tailored to the patient's needs, including preferred language and learning style (visual, verbal, and/or multimedia)
- Teach-back methods (Charais, 2020)
- Family and caregivers (Kitko et al., 2020)
- Evidence-based and novel teaching techniques to enhance knowledge as well as build skills and confidence (Kitko et al., 2020)
- Clarification with patient of who will be providing posthospitalization management and then communication of the plan to that provider in order to coordinate care, reduce polypharmacy, and reduce readmissions
- Assessment of learning after discharge through telephone follow-up and repeating information at each outpatient visit (Charais, 2020)
- Assessment of patient's adherence with self-care monitoring at each outpatient visit and addressing factors that limit adherence
- Community-based classes, groups, or other creative programming

patient has ingested more fluid than they have excreted (positive fluid balance), which then is correlated with a gain in weight. The patient must be monitored for **oliguria** (diminished urine output, less than 400 mL/24 hours) or anuria (urine output less than 100 mL/24 hours).

The patient is weighed daily in the hospital or at home, at the same time of day, with the same type of clothing, and on the same scale after voiding. If there is a significant change in weight (i.e., 2 to 3 lb increase in a day or 5 lb increase in a week), the patient is instructed to notify their provider or to adjust the medications (e.g., increase the diuretic dose) per the provider's directions.

ACUTE HEART FAILURE AND PULMONARY EDEMA

Pulmonary edema is the abnormal accumulation of fluid in the lungs. The fluid may accumulate in the interstitial spaces and in the alveoli. Pulmonary edema can be categorized into two subsets, depending on the etiology: cardiogenic and noncardiogenic (Dobbe et al., 2019).

Pathophysiology

Cardiogenic pulmonary edema is an acute event that results from HF. It can occur acutely, such as with MI, or it can occur as an exacerbation of chronic HF. Myocardial scarring as a result of ischemia can limit the distensibility of the ventricle and render it vulnerable to a sudden increase in workload. With increased resistance to left ventricular filling, blood backs up into the pulmonary circulation. The patient quickly develops pulmonary edema, sometimes called *flash pulmonary edema,* from the blood volume overload in the lungs. Pulmonary edema can also be caused by noncardiac disorders, such as kidney failure, liver failure, and oncologic conditions that cause the body to retain fluid. The pathophysiology is similar to that seen in HF, in that the left ventricle cannot handle the volume overload, and blood volume and pressure buildup in the left atrium. The rapid increase in atrial pressure results in an acute increase in pulmonary venous pressure, which produces an increase in hydrostatic pressure that forces fluid out of the pulmonary capillaries into the interstitial spaces and alveoli.

Impaired lymphatic drainage also contributes to the accumulation of fluid in the lung tissues. The fluid within the alveoli mixes with air, creating "bubbles" that are expelled from the mouth and nose, producing the classic symptom of pulmonary edema: frothy sputum and the flooding of the alveoli with fluid from the capillaries, producing thin secretions containing air bubbles that frequently are colored with hemoglobin (Dobbe et al., 2019; Simko & Culleiton, 2020). Because of the fluid within the alveoli, air cannot enter, and gas exchange is impaired. The result is hypoxemia, which is often severe. The onset may be preceded by premonitory symptoms of pulmonary congestion, but it also may develop quickly in the patient with a ventricle that has little reserve to meet increased oxygen needs.

Clinical Manifestations and Assessment

As a result of decreased cerebral oxygenation, the patient becomes increasingly restless and anxious. Clinical manifestations include a sudden onset of breathlessness, sense of suffocation, cough that produces a large amount of frothy sputum (which may be blood tinged), cold and moist skin, cyanotic (bluish) nail beds, a weak and rapid pulse, pulmonary crackles, expiratory wheezing.

In addition, oxygen demand increases, yet oxygen saturation is significantly decreased. The patient, nearly suffocated by the blood-tinged, frothy fluid filling the alveoli, is literally drowning in secretions. The situation demands immediate action.

Medical and Nursing Management

Although the etiology of pulmonary edema may vary, management of symptoms follows the similar clinical management plan for treating acute decompensated HF (oxygen, diuretics, pharmacologic preload [volume] and afterload [resistance to flow] reduction, and, possibly, hemodynamic monitoring). Additional therapies may include early rescue with noninvasive mask ventilation and bronchodilator therapy with select beta$_2$-agonist medications like albuterol (Simko & Culleiton, 2020).

CARDIOGENIC SHOCK

Cardiogenic shock occurs when decreased CO leads to inadequate tissue perfusion and initiation of the shock syndrome. Cardiogenic shock may occur following MI, when a large area of myocardium becomes ischemic, necrotic, and hypokinetic (slow or diminished muscle motion). It also can occur as a result of end-stage HF, cardiac tamponade, pulmonary embolism (PE), cardiomyopathy, and arrhythmias. Cardiogenic shock is a life-threatening condition with a high mortality rate.

Pathophysiology

The signs and symptoms of cardiogenic shock reflect the circular nature of the pathophysiology of HF. The degree of shock is proportional to the extent of left ventricular dysfunction. The heart muscle loses its contractile power, resulting in a marked reduction in SV and CO. The decreased CO, in turn, reduces arterial blood pressure and tissue perfusion in the vital organs (heart, brain, lung, kidneys). Flow to the coronary arteries is reduced, resulting in decreased oxygen supply to the myocardium, which increases ischemia and further reduces the heart's ability to pump. Inadequate emptying of the ventricle also leads to increased pulmonary pressures, pulmonary congestion, and pulmonary edema, exacerbating the hypoxia, causing ischemia of vital organs, and setting a vicious cycle in motion.

Clinical Manifestations and Assessment

The classic signs of cardiogenic shock are those of tissue hypoperfusion and result from HF and the overall shock state. They include cerebral hypoxia (restlessness, confusion, agitation), low blood pressure, rapid and weak pulse, cold and clammy skin, tachypnea with respiratory crackles, and decreased urinary output. Initially, arterial blood gas (ABG) analysis may show respiratory alkalosis related to the tachypnea; however, metabolic acidosis will develop due to accumulation of lactic acid related to anaerobic metabolism (discussed shortly). Ventricular arrhythmias are common and result from myocardial ischemia.

The patient with cardiogenic shock is managed in an intensive care unit. A PA catheter may be inserted to measure CO and other hemodynamic parameters that are used to assess the severity of the problem and to guide patient management. The PA wedge pressure (indirect estimate of left atrial pressure or left ventricular preload) is elevated and the CO is decreased as the left ventricle loses its ability to pump. The systemic vascular resistance (SVR) is elevated because of the sympathetic nervous system stimulation that occurs as a compensatory response to the decrease in blood pressure. The decreased blood flow to the kidneys causes a hormonal response (i.e., activation of the renin–angiotensin–aldosterone system) that causes fluid retention and further vasoconstriction. Tachycardia, increases in circulating volume, and vasoconstriction occur to maintain circulation to the brain, heart, kidneys, and lungs but at a cost: an increase in the workload of the heart.

Pearls for Practice

The nurse is aware that hemodynamic findings include decreased CO or cardiac index (CI), increased PA wedge pressure (also known as PA occlusion pressure) or CVP (or both), and increased SVR.

The reduction in blood volume delivered to the tissues results in an increase in the amount of oxygen extracted from the blood that is delivered to the tissues (to try to meet the cellular demand for oxygen). The increased systemic oxygen extraction results in decreased venous (mixed and central) oxygen saturation. When the cellular oxygen needs cannot be met, anaerobic metabolism and buildup of lactic acid occur. As a result, ABGs would reveal metabolic acidosis. Continuous central venous oximetry and measurement of blood lactic acid levels may help assess the severity of the shock as well as the effectiveness of treatment. Refer to Chapter 54 for further discussion on lactic acid levels.

Continued cellular hypoperfusion eventually results in organ failure. The patient becomes unresponsive, severe hypotension ensues, and the patient develops shallow respirations and cold, cyanotic, or mottled skin. Laboratory test results indicate organ dysfunction.

Medical Management

The most important approach to treating cardiogenic shock is to correct the underlying problem, reduce any further demand on the heart, improve oxygenation, and restore tissue perfusion. For example, if the ventricular failure is the result of an acute MI, emergency percutaneous coronary intervention may be indicated. Major arrhythmias are corrected because they may have caused or contributed to the shock. If the patient has hypervolemia, diuresis is indicated. Diuretics, vasodilators, and mechanical therapies, such as continuous renal replacement therapy, have been used to reduce the circulating blood volume. If hypovolemia (low intravascular volume) is suspected or detected through hemodynamic pressure readings, the patient is given IV volume expanders (e.g., normal saline solution, lactated Ringer solution, albumin) to increase the amount of circulating fluid. The patient is placed on strict bed rest to conserve energy. If the patient has hypoxemia, as detected by pulse oximetry or ABG analysis, oxygen administration is increased, often under positive pressure when regular flow is insufficient to meet tissue demands. Intubation and sedation may be necessary to maintain oxygenation. The settings for mechanical ventilation are adjusted according to the patient's oxygenation status and the need for conserving energy. Ventilator management is discussed in Chapter 54.

PERICARDIAL EFFUSION AND CARDIAC TAMPONADE

Pericardial effusion (accumulation of fluid in the pericardial sac) may accompany pericarditis, advanced HF, metastatic carcinoma, chemotherapy, cardiac surgery, or trauma.

Pathophysiology

Normally, the pericardial sac contains less than 50 mL of fluid, which is needed to decrease friction for the beating heart. An increase in pericardial fluid raises the pressure within the pericardial sac and compresses the heart. This has the following effects:

- Increased right ventricular end-diastolic pressure (RVEDP) and left ventricular end-diastolic pressure (LVEDP)
- Decreased venous return
- Inability of the ventricles to distend and fill adequately

Pericardial fluid may accumulate slowly without causing noticeable symptoms until a large amount accumulates. However, a rapidly developing effusion can stretch the pericardium to its maximum size and, because of increased pericardial pressure, venous return to the heart is obstructed and the amount of blood pumped out with each contraction is reduced, which decreases CO. The result is cardiac tamponade (i.e., compression of the heart).

Clinical Manifestations and Assessment

The patient may report a feeling of fullness within the chest or may have substantial or ill-defined pain. The feeling of pressure in the chest may result from stretching of the pericardial sac. Because of increased pressure within the pericardium, venous pressure tends to increase, as evidenced by engorged neck veins during inspiration. This rise in venous pressure and vein distension during inspiration is known as Kussmaul sign (Shako et al., 2022). If hemodynamic pressures are monitored, the nurse will note equivalent diastolic pressures in all chambers, so that right and left atrial pressures, RVEDP, LVEDP, and PA diastolic pressures become equal or nearly equal (a difference of less than 3 to 5 mm Hg) (Alerhand, 2022). Other signs include dyspnea, cough, and labile or low blood pressure. Systolic blood pressure that is markedly lower during inhalation is called **pulsus paradoxus**. The difference in systolic pressure between the point that is heard during exhalation and the point that is heard during inhalation is measured. Pulsus paradoxus exceeding 10 mm Hg is abnormal. A pericardial friction rub may be heard. The cardinal signs of cardiac tamponade are falling systolic blood pressure, narrowing pulse pressure (difference between the systolic and diastolic pressure should normally be above 40 mm Hg), rising venous pressure (increased JVD) during inspiration, and distant (muffled) heart sounds (Fig. 14-4). If untreated, shock and death can result.

Pearls for Practice

Classic cues associated with cardiac tamponade include the presence of elevated CVP (with neck vein distention), muffled heart sounds, and hypotension, which is termed Beck triad.

A chest x-ray shows a large pericardial effusion. A transthoracic echocardiogram is performed to confirm the diagnosis.

Medical and Nursing Management

Pericardiocentesis

If cardiac function becomes seriously impaired as a result of pericardial effusion, **pericardiocentesis** (puncture of the pericardial sac to aspirate pericardial fluid) is performed to remove fluid from the pericardial sac (Fig. 14-5). The major goal of this procedure is to prevent cardiac tamponade, which restricts normal heart filling and contraction.

During the procedure, vital signs, oxygen saturation, ECG, and, if applicable, hemodynamic pressures are measured. Emergency resuscitation equipment should be readily available. The head of the bed is elevated to 45 to 60 degrees, placing the heart in proximity to the chest wall so that the

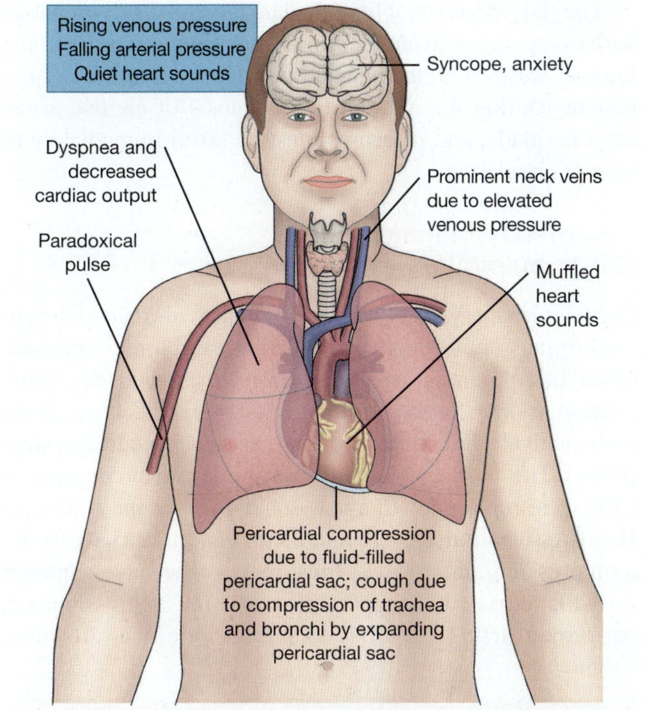

FIGURE 14-4 **Assessment findings in cardiac tamponade resulting from pericardial effusion include feelings of faintness, shortness of breath, and anxiety from decreased cardiac output; cough from pressure created in the trachea from swelling of the pericardial sac; distended neck veins from rising venous pressure; Kussmaul sign; paradoxical pulse; and muffled or distant heart sounds.**

needle can be inserted into the pericardial sac more easily. If a peripheral IV line is not already in place, one is inserted, and a slow IV infusion is started in case it becomes necessary to administer emergency medications or blood products.

The pericardial aspiration needle is attached to a 50-mL syringe by a three-way stopcock. Several possible sites are used for pericardial aspiration. Typically, ultrasound imaging is used to guide placement of the needle into the pericardial space. The needle is advanced slowly until it has entered the pericardium and fluid is obtained.

A resulting decrease in CVP and an associated increase in blood pressure after withdrawal of pericardial fluid indicate that the cardiac tamponade has been relieved. The patient almost always feels immediate relief. If there is a substantial amount of pericardial fluid, a small catheter may be left in place to drain recurrent accumulation of blood or fluid. Pericardial fluid is sent to the laboratory for examination for tumor cells, bacterial culture, chemical and serologic analysis, and differential blood cell count.

Complications of pericardiocentesis include ventricular or coronary artery puncture, arrhythmias, pleural laceration, gastric puncture, and myocardial trauma. After pericardiocentesis, the patient's heart rhythm, blood pressure, venous pressure, and heart sounds are monitored to detect possible recurrence of cardiac tamponade. If it recurs, repeated aspiration is necessary. Cardiac tamponade may require surgical treatment by open pericardial drainage called a pericardiotomy.

Pericardiotomy

Recurrent pericardial effusions, usually associated with neoplastic disease, may be treated by a **pericardiotomy** (pericardial window). Under general anesthesia, a portion of the pericardium is excised to permit the pericardial fluid to drain continuously into the mediastinum and is reabsorbed via lymphatics (Selvakumar, 2022). The nursing care is the same as that for other cardiac surgery (see Chapter 13).

CARDIAC ARREST

Cardiac arrest occurs when the heart ceases to produce an effective pulse and circulate blood.

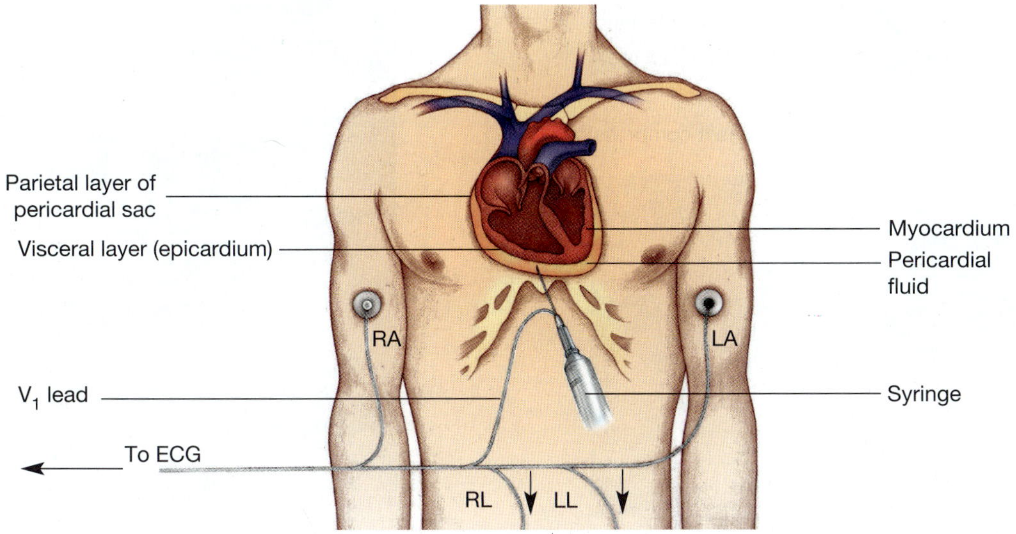

FIGURE 14-5 **Pericardiocentesis. (From Lippincott Williams & Wilkins. [2010].** ***Cardiovascular care made incredibly visual*** **[2nd ed., p. 231]. Lippincott Williams & Wilkins.)**

Pathophysiology

Cardiac arrest may be caused by a cardiac electrical event such as ventricular fibrillation, progressive profound bradycardia, or when there is no heart rhythm at all (asystole). Cardiac arrest may follow respiratory arrest; it may also occur when electrical activity is present but there is ineffective cardiac contraction or circulating volume, which is called **pulseless electrical activity (PEA)**. PEA can be caused by hypovolemia (e.g., with excessive bleeding), hypoxia, hypothermia, hyperkalemia, massive PE, MI, and medication overdose (e.g., beta blockers, calcium-channel blockers) or toxins. In the absence of hypovolemia and tension pneumothorax, PEA strongly suggests cardiac tamponade (Mondor, 2022).

Clinical Manifestations and Assessment

In cardiac arrest, consciousness, pulse, and blood pressure are lost immediately. Ineffective respiratory gasping may occur. The pupils of the eyes begin dilating within 45 seconds. Seizures may or may not occur.

The risk of irreversible brain damage and death increases with every minute from the time that circulation ceases. The interval varies with the age and underlying condition of the patient. During this period, the diagnosis of cardiac arrest must be made, and measures must be taken immediately to restore circulation.

Emergency Management: Cardiopulmonary Resuscitation

Cardiopulmonary resuscitation (CPR) provides blood flow to vital organs until effective circulation can be reestablished. Once loss of consciousness has been established, the resuscitation priority for the adult in most cases is placing a phone call to activate the code team or the emergency medical system (EMS). The "A-B-Cs" (airway, breathing, and circulation) of CPR were replaced with a new standard from the American Heart Association in 2010 and continued in 2015. "C-A-B" (compression, airway, and breathing) is the new sequence for CPR in basic life support (Box 14-3). Compressions are performed first. Exceptions to this include near-drowning

BOX 14-3 Performing One-Person CPR

1. Establish unresponsiveness by asking, "Are you okay?" Tap or gently shake the patient along with determining if patient is not breathing or not breathing normally (i.e., only gasping).
2. After initiating the emergency response team or calling for a defibrillator when a patient is unresponsive, position the patient supine on a hard surface.

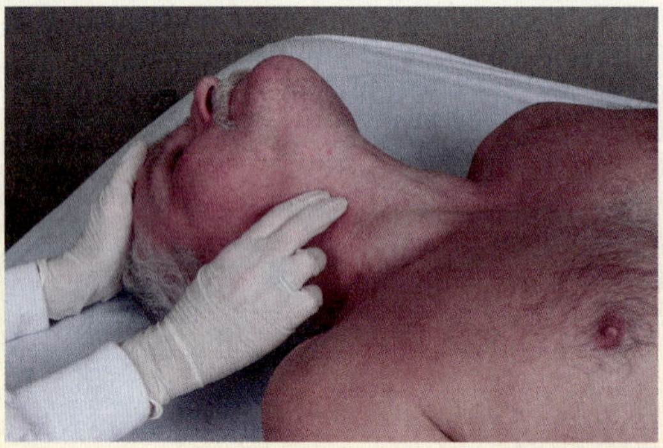

Unless a definite pulse is felt, initiate chest compressions.

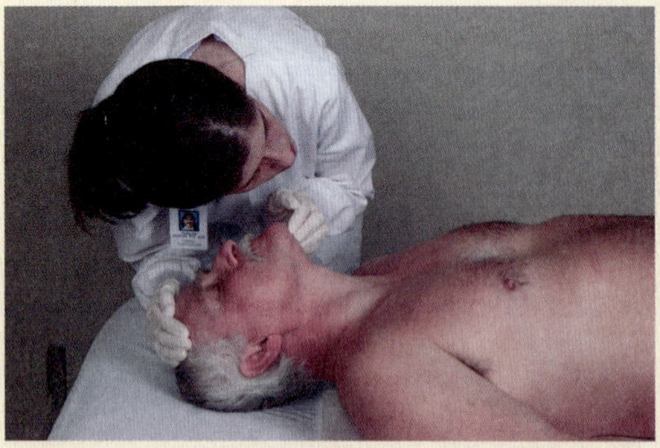

3. Place one hand on top of the other on the lower half of the sternum between the nipples, with elbows locked. Compress the chest 2 in (or one third the depth of the chest) at a rate of 100 to 120 compressions per minute, keeping your hands on the chest. Allow equal time for compressions and full chest recoil. Continue for 30 compressions, then give two ventilations and resume compressions quickly for five cycles (2 minutes) before rechecking the pulse.

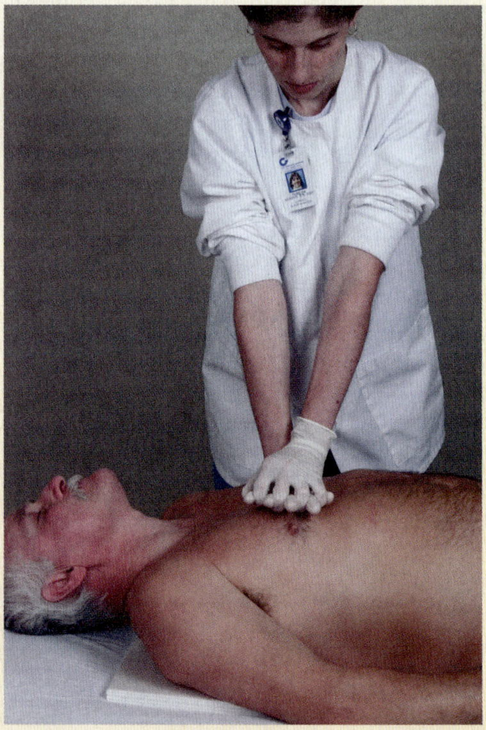

and respiratory arrest situations for which 2 minutes of conventional CPR (A-B-C) with rescue breathing should be performed before activating the EMS (Kleinman, 2018).

Resuscitation of adults consists of the following steps:

1. Establish unresponsiveness: no breathing or no normal breathing (gasping). Activate EMS and get defibrillator or automatic external defibrillator (AED).
2. Check pulse at carotid artery for no more than 10 seconds.
3. Perform chest compressions to a depth of at least 2 in for 30 times, allowing for chest recoil after each compression.
4. Airway/breathing: Open airway, give two quick breaths followed by 30 compressions.
5. Defibrillation: Shock with standard defibrillator or AED for ventricular tachycardia and ventricular fibrillation.

If the patient is already being monitored or is immediately placed on the monitor using the multifunction pads or the quick-look paddles (found on most defibrillators) and the ECG shows ventricular tachycardia or ventricular fibrillation, immediate defibrillation rather than CPR is the treatment of choice (Panchal et al., 2020). Survival from pulseless ventricular tachycardia or ventricular fibrillation is inversely related to the time interval between its onset and termination. Optimization occurs with CPR and advanced cardiac life support, including defibrillation and drug therapy, if they are provided at the earliest opportunity (Panchal et al., 2020). If the patient has not been defibrillated within 10 minutes, the chance of survival is close to zero. Refer to Chapter 16 for more details on defibrillation.

Recent research on CPR performed in the field for persons in out-of-hospital cardiac arrest by bystanders supports eliminating mouth-to-mouth or rescue breathing and using "hands-only" cardiac compression only. No differences in patient survival were seen when bystanders received emergency dispatcher instructions for compression-only versus compression-plus rescue breathing CPR (Panchal et al., 2020).

Clinical Judgment Case

A 72-year-old patient comes into the emergency room (ER) complaining of significant SOB and increased weight (5 lb gain in 72 hours). The patient's skin is moist, there is 3+ pitting edema of lower extremities, jugular vein distention (JVD), and vital signs are as follows: 98.7°F, heart rate (HR) 116 and regular, 24 RR with an oxygen saturation of 94% on room air and the blood pressure is 100/46. The patient denies pain in the chest, jaw, back, or arms. Heart sounds are S1, S2, and S3; the point of maximum impulse (PMI) is displaced laterally to the anterior axillary line. Pulmonary examination reveals crackles 1/2 up the lung fields bilaterally. The patient denies nausea or vomiting. Abdomen is soft, nondistended, nontender, last BM was yesterday, formed brown stool, no evidence of bleeding. Capillary refill is 4 seconds and pedal and posterior tibial pulses are 1+ bil. The patient's history included diabetes type 2 (40-year history), hyperlipidemia, HFrEF, and hypothyroidism. The patient states that they were just discharged 72 hours ago. The patient's discharge medications included an ACE inhibitor, beta blocker, and diuretic as well as a statin, Synthroid, and metformin.

Step One: Recognize cues where relevant and identify important information from different sources, such as medical history or vital signs.

Answer: History of HF (reduced ejection fraction), diabetes for >40 years, and hyperlipidemia. Complaints of SOB, and weight gain and an inability to breathe laying down (orthopnea). Physical examination findings of full neck veins, S3, displaced PMI, bilateral crackles to the mid and capillary refill of 4 seconds, diminished peripheral pulses, moist skin, and 3+ pitting edema. Cues of concern related to vital signs: HR of 116 and regular, 24 RR, O_2 saturation of 94% and blood pressure is 100/46.

Step Two: Analyze cues by organizing and linking the recognized cues to the patient's clinical presentation.

Answer: You have clustered the patient's symptoms to be associated with decompensated HF progressing to cardiogenic shock. Specially, signs of fluid volume excess include JVD, 3+ pitting edema, bilateral crackles, decreased O_2 saturation, S3 gallop rhythm, orthopnea, and weight gain. You recognize that the symptoms of JVD and 3 + pitting edema are associated with right ventricular failure whereas the crackles, decreased O_2 sat, dyspnea, orthopnea, tachycardia, moist skin, and S3 are associated with left ventricular failure. You associate the tachycardia with the body's attempt to increase the CO. The blood pressure of 100/46 is hypotensive and you calculate the mean arterial pressure (MAP) which is systolic pressure (100 mm Hg), plus the diastolic pressure (46 mm Hg) x's 2/3 (100 + 92 = 192/3 = 64 mm Hg). Since the MAP reflects perfusion to major organs, you are aware that an MAP below 65 mm Hg, for an extended period, can cause end-organ ischemia and infarction can occur. You are concerned that the decreased CO will lead to inadequate tissue perfusion and initiation of cardiogenic shock. You are also aware that this patient was discharged 72 hours ago and potential etiologies of the acute rapid decompensation (e.g., new MI, PE, arrhythmias, hypothyroidism, adherence/understanding of patient's medication administration, dietary habits) need to be investigated to determine the cause of the acute decompensation.

Step Three: Prioritize hypotheses, where hypotheses are evaluated and ranked according to priority. This can include urgency, likelihood, risk, difficulty, and/or time. In this phase, you cluster your findings to arrive at a list of problems (actual and/or potential problems) you believe the patient is experiencing and determine the importance or urgency. What do you think is of greatest concern?

Answer: The potential hypotheses include (1) decompensated HF; etiologies for the decompensated HF include myocardial infarction, pulmonary edema, anemia, renal insufficiency, arrhythmia, hypothyroidism (2) potential for cardiogenic shock, and (3) potential deficient knowledge regarding medication administration and/or dietary restriction. At the moment, you prioritize cardiogenic shock as the greatest risk of injury to this patient.

Step Four: Generate solutions, which involves identifying expected outcomes and using hypotheses to define a set of interventions for the expected outcomes.

Answer: Since a cardiac event is suspected, you recognize the need to place the patient on a cardiac monitor and start an IV for emergency medication administration. Given the patient is demonstrating fluid volume excess, you anticipate that IV fluids will not be administered. You elevate the head of the bed to decrease patient's orthopnea and administer low-flow oxygen to improve the oxygen saturation which on admission was 94% on room air. You will monitor the oxygen saturation continuously and vital signs every 15 minutes. You recognize that while elevation of the head of bed (HOB) will help relieve the SOB, the B/P may decline further risking the MAP, so monitoring of the vital signs is important. You recognize that an ECG will help identify the presence of arrhythmia or ECG changes associated with an MI. You expect laboratory testing that will evaluate potential causes (anemia [Hgb], renal insufficiency [BUN/creatinine], MI [cardiac biomarkers], hypothyroidism [TSH, free T4]) and the BNP will reflect the ventricular volume expansion. You anticipate that hemodilution will be seen (e.g., decreased Hct, decreased sodium, potassium, and BUN [see Chapter 3]). An echocardiogram may be ordered to evaluate structural changes such as LVH (suggested by the displaced PMI), and the ejection fraction (EF).

Step Five: Take action, where the solutions that address the highest priorities are implemented.

Answer: You start the IV, place the patient on a cardiac monitor and move the 12-lead ECG machine to the bedside as the provider comes in to assess the patient. The oxygen saturation is also monitored continuously and currently, oxygen is administered at 1 L. A 12-lead ECG is ordered as is a bedside echocardiogram. The diuretic furosemide 20 mg is ordered IV and you assess the K^+ before administering (K^+ was 4.1 mEq/L) IV. You are aware that diuretics are administered to decrease the preload. Nitrates are also administered which will also decrease the preload and vasodilate the coronary arteries. You are aware that vasodilators such as nitroglycerin affect venous dilation which decreases the preload (the more the vein dilates the less volume returned to the heart) but arterial dilation also occurs which decreases the afterload or SVR and therefore, the CO increases. However, the risk of decreasing the afterload is significant hypotension; thus, the BP is strictly monitored as is intake and output. You repeat the vital signs while observing the cardiac rhythm and oxygen saturation.

Step Six: Evaluate outcomes, which involves comparing observed outcomes against expected outcomes.

Answer: The troponin I level comes back as 0.2 which is normal, there is no evidence of anemia (Hgb is 15 g), the BUN/Cr are within normal limits and there is evidence of hemodilution with HCT of 31% and hyponatremia (Na-131 mEq/l), the ECG reveals sinus tachycardia with no ST changes. The TSH is high and the free T4 is low, representing hypothyroidism. The urinary output increases significantly and the patient has voided over 1 L in the last hour. VS repeated are now HR of 92 and regular, RR 16, oxygen saturation of 97% on 1 L, and BP is now 126/72. An echocardiogram reveals LVH and an ejection fraction of 35% associated with HF. On discussion with the patient regarding their thyroid medication, they stated that they ran out of thyroid medication and have not taken any since they were hospitalized. Thus, you recognize the impact of the thyroid on the heart, specifically its effect on left ventricular function, and now add thyroid disease as a risk factor for cardiac disease. You are learning to interrelate content from one body system (endocrine) to another (cardiac). Each day, you will connect content more and more. Keep going.

CHAPTER REVIEW

NCLEX-Style Review Questions

1. Which outcome measures demonstrate the effectiveness of treatment for a patient with right ventricular failure? Select all that apply.
   a. Clear breath sounds
   b. Decreasing peripheral edema
   c. Tachypnea
   d. Central venous pressure (CVP) of 4 mm Hg
   e. Hepatomegaly

2. The nurse is caring for a patient with right ventricular failure. What symptom will the patient most likely exhibit? Select all that apply.
   a. Crackles on auscultation
   b. Jugular vein distention
   c. Pulmonary edema
   d. CVP of 6 mm Hg
   e. Pitting edema

3. Which parameters listed below indicate that diuretic therapy has been effective in a patient with heart failure?
   a. Dyspnea decreases
   b. Jugular vein distention (JVD) increases
   c. Urinary output increases
   d. Serum osmolality decreases
   e. Serum osmolality increases

4. Which signs and symptoms are associated with cardiac tamponade and are collectively termed Beck triad? Select all that apply.
   a. Jugular venous distention
   b. Peripheral edema
   c. Muffled heart sounds
   d. Hypotension
   e. Frothy sputum

5. Your patient K. L. has mild heart failure (HF) with a serum sodium of 129 mEq/L, pitting edema of the ankles and crackles are heard in bilateral lung bases. You expect that K. L would benefit most from which treatment? Select all that apply.
   a. Hypertonic saline infusion
   b. Administration of 5% dextrose in water (D5W)
   c. Vasopressin (ADH)
   d. Furosemide (Diuretic)
   e. Fluid restriction

REFERENCES AND SELECTED READINGS

References and selected readings associated with this chapter can be found on the website that accompanies the book. Visit **http://thepoint.lww.com/Honan3e** to access the references and other additional resources associated with this chapter.

CHAPTER 15

Nursing Management: Patients With Structural, Inflammatory and Infectious Cardiac Disorders

Leonie L. Rose Bovino • Jeanine L. May

Learning Objectives

After reading this chapter, you will be able to:

1. Define valvular disorders of the heart and describe the pathophysiology, clinical manifestations, and management of patients with mitral and aortic regurgitation and/or stenosis.
2. Describe types of cardiac valve repair and replacement procedures used to treat valvular problems and the care needed by patients who undergo these procedures.
3. Describe the pathophysiology, clinical manifestations, and management of patients with intracardiac septal defects.
4. Describe the pathophysiology, clinical manifestations, and management of patients with cardiomyopathy.
5. Describe the pathophysiology, clinical manifestations, and management of patients with infections of the heart.
6. Describe the rationale for prophylactic antibiotic therapy for patients with valvular heart disease, rheumatic heart disease, and infective endocarditis.

Structural disorders of the heart present many challenges for the patient, family, and health care team. Dysfunctional heart valves, intracardiac septal defects, cardiomyopathies, and inflammatory and infectious diseases of the heart muscle alter cardiac output (CO) and interfere with the heart's ability to pump blood sufficiently to meet the body's demand for oxygen. Nursing care for patients with these disorders requires an understanding of cardiac anatomy; structure and physiology (function) of heart valves, pericardium, myocardium, and endocardium; and knowledge of the causes and management of each disorder. Noninvasive and invasive treatments include medication management, supportive care, valve repair or replacement, septal repair, mechanical circulatory assist devices, and cardiac transplantation. Nurses play an integral role in caring for patients with structural, infectious, and inflammatory cardiac conditions.

VALVULAR DISEASE

Properly functioning heart valves allow blood to flow in one direction through the heart and vasculature. Blood flow becomes turbulent when heart valves do not close or open properly. The turbulent flow of blood through the heart valve results in a murmur, as in Table 15-1. Acquired valvular heart disease is a progressive disorder that develops slowly, although it can occur acutely in certain conditions. Common causes include degenerative disease, rheumatic heart disease (RHD), and infective endocarditis (IE) (inflammation of the inner lining of the heart, the endocardium, which is discussed later in this chapter). Compensatory mechanisms can maintain equilibrium for an extended period, and it may be years before the disease progresses, causes the patient become symptomatic, and requires treatment.

Progression of valvular heart disease can result in heart failure, arrhythmias, stroke, and sudden death. The aim of interventions for managing and treating acquired valvular heart disease is to prevent the sequelae of atrial fibrillation (AF), thromboembolism, pulmonary artery hypertension, and heart failure. Clinician scientists have significantly improved treatment and outcomes over the past several decades. These advances are primarily due to the development of management guidelines, improvements in noninvasive monitoring of cardiac function, advancements in valvular reconstruction procedures, and improved prosthetic valves.

A detailed review of normal cardiac valvular anatomy is found in Chapter 11 and shown in Figure 15-1. **Stenosis** or narrowing of the opening of the valve occurs when leaflets fail to open correctly, reducing the forward flow of blood through the valve, as shown in Figure 15-2A. The volume

TABLE **15-1 Heart Murmurs**

Murmur	Timing	Description	Auscultation Site
Mitral stenosis	Diastole (S2)	Low-pitched, rumbling, decrescendo	Apex
Mitral regurgitation	Systole (S1)	High-pitched, loud, rumbling	Apex
Aortic stenosis	Midsystolic (S1)	Loud, crescendo–decrescendo	2nd ICS right sternal border; may radiate into the neck
Aortic regurgitation	Early Diastole (S2)	High-pitched blowing sound, decrescendo	Left sternal border, at the 3rd ICS

of blood in the chamber increases, forcing the heart to work harder to eject blood through the narrowed valve opening. The heart's afterload (force the heart exerts to pump blood) increases, leading to decreased CO. Refer to Figure 15-3 for the pathophysiology of heart failure related to valvular heart disease.

Regurgitation, or valvular insufficiency, occurs when valves do not close completely, and blood flows backward through the valve, as shown in Figure 15-2. If the aortic valve is affected, blood will flow backward into the left ventricle (LV) during diastole. If the mitral valve is affected, blood will flow back into the left atrium (LA) during systole. Preload, the stretch of the cardiac muscle at the end of diastole, is increased. Mitral valve **prolapse** (MVP) occurs when the **mitral valve** does not close properly and the valve leaflets balloon back into the LA during systole. Understanding the structure and function of heart valves, and pathophysiology (functional changes) from valvular disorders, as shown in Figures 15-2 and 15-3, is necessary to provide appropriate nursing care for patients with valvular heart disease. Valvular

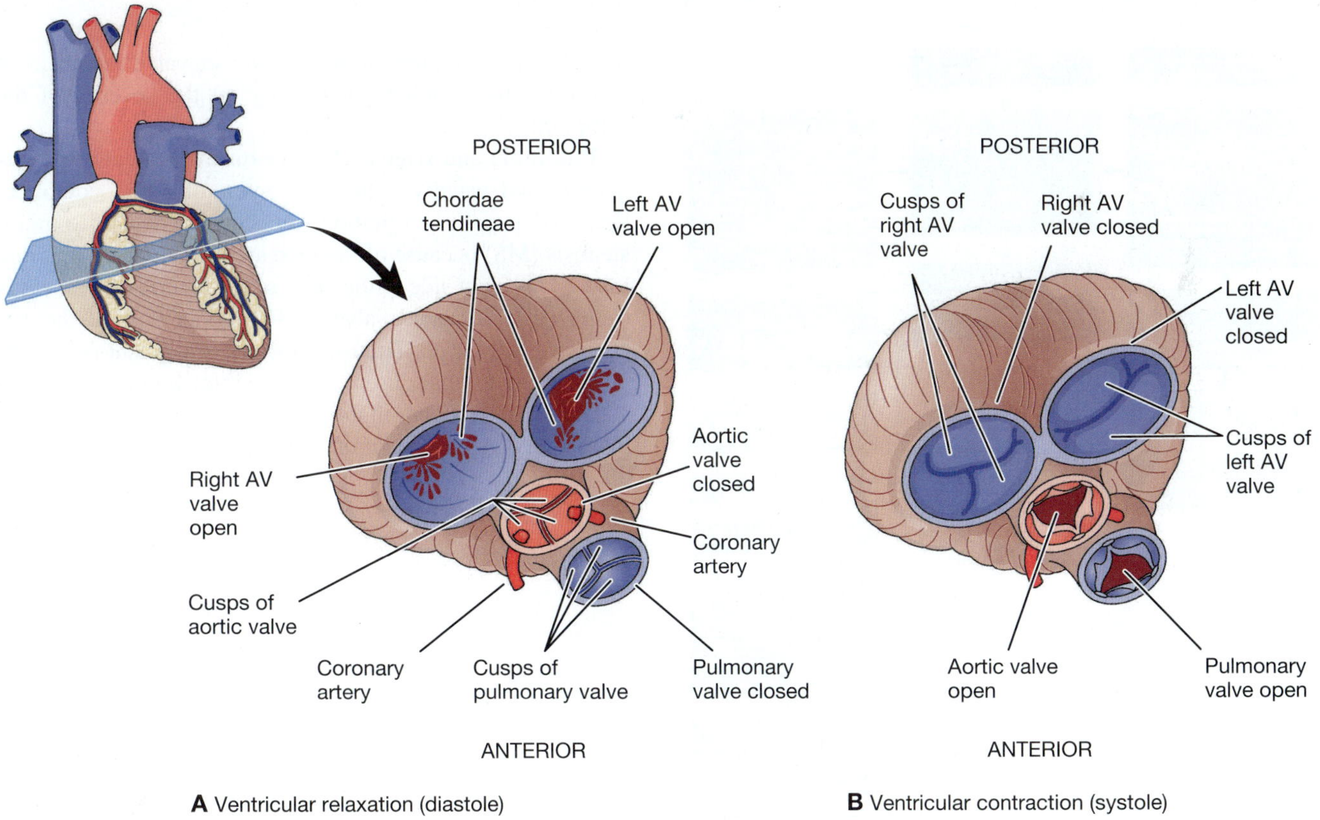

FIGURE 15-1 **Heart valves (superior view from anterior, atria removed). Valves keep blood flowing in a forward direction through the heart. A. When the heart is relaxed (diastole), the AV valves are open and blood flows freely from the atria to the ventricles. The pulmonary and aortic valves are closed. B. When the ventricles contract (systole), the AV valves close and blood pumped out of the ventricles opens the pulmonary and aortic valves. Zooming in: How many cusps does the right AV valve have? The left? Answer: the right AV valve has three cusps (Tricuspid valve) versus two on the left or mitral valve.**

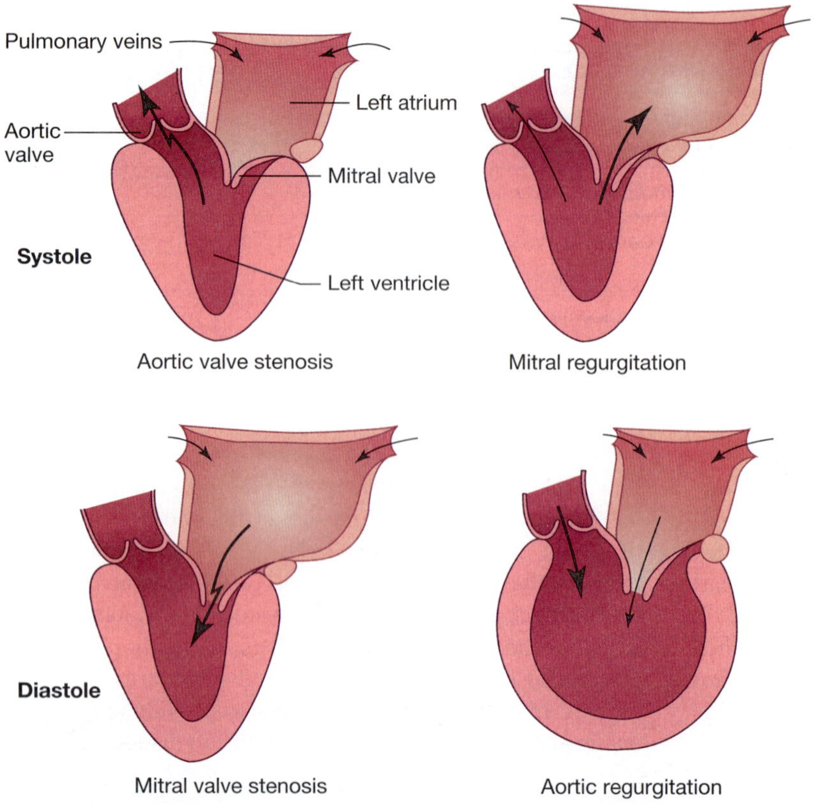

FIGURE 15-2 **Alterations in hemodynamic function that accompany aortic valve stenosis, mitral valve regurgitation, mitral valve stenosis, and aortic valve regurgitation. The *thin arrows* indicate the direction of normal flow, and *thick arrows* show the direction of abnormal flow.**

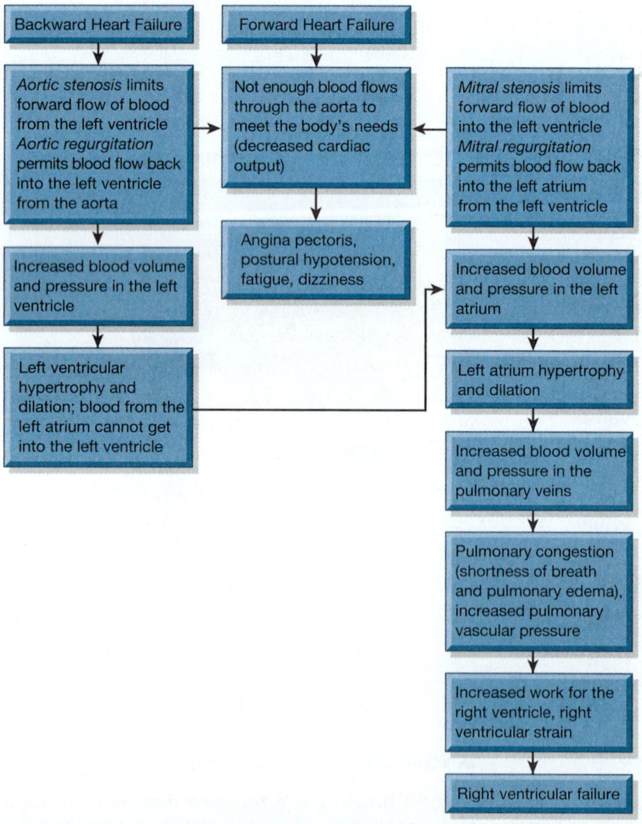

FIGURE 15-3 **Pathophysiology: Left-sided heart failure as a result of aortic and mitral valvular heart disease and the development of right ventricular failure.**

disorders may require surgical repair or valve replacement to correct the problem, depending on the severity of the symptoms.

Pulmonic and **tricuspid valve** disorders occur less frequently and usually with fewer symptoms and complications. Tricuspid regurgitation can occur secondary to mitral stenosis (MS) because of the increased volume and pressure load on the right side of the heart and infection of the heart's lining (IE). Tricuspid valve repair is only done if there is severe regurgitation. Tricuspid valve replacement is uncommon. Multivalvular disease is possible: regurgitation and stenosis may co-occur in the same or different valves, or one disease may occur in two or more valves.

Pearls for Practice

Stenosis restricts blood flow from the heart because the valves do not open properly and fully; regurgitation causes blood to flow backward into the heart. Blood volume and pressures are increased behind the affected valve and reduced in front of the affected valve.

MITRAL STENOSIS

In MS, the valve opening is narrowed, and blood flow from the LA into the LV is slowed during diastole. MS is slow and progressive. Symptoms may take decades to appear, eventually culminating in heart failure.

Pathophysiology

The mitral valve opening area is normally 4 to 6 cm^2, but over time as fibrous tissue replaces normal valve tissue, the leaflets begin to thicken and fuse. In significant stenosis the opening narrows to 1 cm^2 or less, and left atrial pressure increases because of the resistance caused by slowed blood flow through the narrowed orifice. The LA dilates and hypertrophies because of the increased blood volume. Sluggish atrial blood flow can lead to clot formation and thromboembolism. Because there is no functional valve to protect the pulmonary veins from the backward flow of blood from the atrium, pulmonary venous pressure rises, and the pulmonary circulation becomes congested. As a result, the right ventricle (RV) must contract against abnormally high pulmonary pressure. Pulmonary hypertension increases the work of the RV, which causes the RV and right atrium to enlarge. Eventually, this results in right-sided heart failure.

Risk Factors

MS is often caused by rheumatic fever (RF) or endocarditis. These two conditions gradually cause the mitral valve leaflets to thicken, potentially producing leaflet fusion. Typically MS occurs 20 to 40 years after RF, and symptoms do not develop for another 10 years. Although rheumatic disease is rare in developed countries, MS is still prevalent in developing nations where RF is common (Carabello, 2020). Radiation therapy to the chest area also can result in MS. It is more common in females than in males. Rarely it can result from a congenital defect.

Clinical Manifestations and Assessment

Although patients with MS can remain asymptomatic, symptoms usually develop when the pressure in the LA becomes greater than that of the LV after the valve opening is reduced by one-third to one-half its usual size. Dyspnea on exertion (DOE) results from pulmonary congestion. Patients become progressively fatigued due to low CO. Palpitations, chest pain, and paroxysmal nocturnal dyspnea (PND) can occur. As the LA becomes more distended, palpitations, premature beats, AF, and paroxysmal atrial tachycardia may occur. AF is common in people with symptomatic MS, and AF increases the risk of developing a stroke. Dyspnea at rest is likely with severe MS. Other symptoms include cough, sometimes with hemoptysis from ruptured pulmonary veins, hoarseness from the dilated atrium impinging on the left recurrent laryngeal nerve, palpitations, orthopnea, and recurrent respiratory infections. Later, symptoms of right heart failure, including peripheral edema and ascites, occur.

A loud S1 and an opening snap can be heard because of the elevated left atrial pressure. The opening snap is a high-pitched sound heard in early diastole (S2) by the opening of a stenotic valve. The murmur is caused by turbulent blood flow through the abnormally narrow valve opening from the LA into the LV. Due to the increased blood volume and pressure, the atrium dilates and becomes electrically unstable, leading to atrial arrhythmias. The pulse can be irregular because of AF. Echocardiography is the most sensitive and specific noninvasive method to diagnose MS and is used to evaluate valve morphology and measure cardiac pressures. Cardiac catheterization is not indicated unless clinical findings and echo results are discordant.

MITRAL VALVE PROLAPSE (MVP)

MVP is the most common mitral valve abnormality, affecting 2% to 3% of the population, and has a familial trend and a wide range of causes and presentations. In MVP, a portion of one or both mitral valve leaflets bulge back into the LA during systole, with or without mitral regurgitation (MR). MVP is the most common cause of chronic primary MR in high-income countries.

Pathophysiology

There are two subgroups of MVP. Younger populations, <50 years of age, often females, present with myxomatous degeneration (pathologic weakening of connective tissue), which can cause one or both valve leaflets to become enlarged and floppy (Barlow disease) (Basso et al., 2019). Barlow disease may be associated with connective tissue disorders (e.g., Marfan syndrome [see Chapter 17]). Over time, as the leaflets prolapse, they can stretch to a degree where the leaflet edges do not fully coapt or close, resulting in MR.

Risk Factors

Assigned females at birth and family history are associated with MVP. It often occurs in people with Marfan syndrome, a connective tissue disorder.

Clinical Manifestations and Assessment

MVP is commonly asymptomatic. However, fatigue, dyspnea, palpitations, and chest pain may develop over time. Atypical chest pain is unrelated to activity and may be caused by abnormal stress on the chordae tendineae and papillary muscles. Shortness of breath (SOB) is not correlated with activity levels or pulmonary function.

Echocardiography is used to diagnose and monitor the progression of MVP. Cardiac auscultation may reveal a mitral mid-systolic click, indicating that a valve leaflet is ballooning into the LA. A late systolic murmur may be heard if progressive valve leaflet stretching and regurgitation have occurred.

MITRAL REGURGITATION

MR, also termed *mitral insufficiency*, is the backward flow of blood from the LV into the LA during systole because the valve fails to close completely. Disease processes, including MVP, that alter valve leaflets, mitral annulus, chordae tendineae, and the papillary muscle may result in MR.

Pathophysiology

When the mitral valve leaflets thicken, fibrose, and contract, they cannot close completely. Consequently, blood is forced back into the LA causing left atrial pressure to rise. The LA stretches to accommodate the increased volume, and left atrial dilation occurs. In addition, during diastole, regurgitant blood from the LV increases the volume load in the LA. These hemodynamic changes occur slowly in chronic MR. Over time, compensatory left ventricular dilation and hypertrophy occur to maintain a normal CO. Eventually this leads to left ventricular failure. The backward flow of blood from the LV increases pulmonary venous pressure. Pulmonary congestion elevates pulmonary artery pressure; this further strains the RV, causing enlargement and RV failure.

Risk Factors

MR is more common in older adults and can result over time from normal aging. Primary MR is a disease of the mitral leaflets or chords, versus secondary MR, which results from disease of the LV or LA. The most common causes of primary MR are MVP, IE, RHD, and collagen vascular disease. RHD can permanently damage the heart valves and result in a thick, rigid mitral valve that does not open and close completely, leading to MR. Secondary MR can result from myocardial infarction (MI) and dilated cardiomyopathy (DCM).

Clinical Manifestations and Assessment

Acute MR (discussed shortly) manifests as severe left-sided heart failure. Patients with acute MR may report a sudden inability to breathe accompanied by chest pain. In contrast, patients with chronic MR can remain asymptomatic for years as symptoms develop gradually. Chronic MR commonly leads to LV dysfunction. As the LV becomes progressively impaired, and CO diminishes, fatigue, tachycardia, and weakness can occur. Increased left atrial pressure leads to increased pulmonary congestion, resulting in orthopnea, DOE, PND, and peripheral edema. Progressive LA dilatation increases the risk of AF. In acute MR, the murmur may be soft or even absent due to equalization of pressure in the LA and ventricle, and the absence of a systolic murmur often leads to misdiagnosis of MR as severe respiratory distress (Watanabe, 2019).

Physical examination may reveal a hyperdynamic point of maximal impulse, displaced leftward and downward because of the hypertrophied LV. Approximately 30% of patients with acute MR have no murmur. For others, a holosystolic (pansystolic) murmur is heard as a high-pitched, blowing sound at the apex; radiation to the axilla is possible (Watanabe, 2019). An S3 may be present because of increased blood flow into the ventricle during diastole.

A chest radiograph may reveal left ventricular and left atrial enlargement. An echocardiogram provides information regarding left ventricular size and function, left atrial size, and pulmonary artery pressures as well as the anatomy of the valve. Also, echocardiography is used to monitor the severity and progression of MR. Cardiac catheterization may be used if there is a discrepancy between clinical and noninvasive findings to determine the severity of MR.

ACUTE MITRAL REGURGITATION

Acute MR is a cardiac emergency because of sudden and severe hemodynamic compromise. It is almost always symptomatic. The causes of acute MR are diverse but can commonly result from papillary muscle rupture as a complication of MI, rupture of the chordae tendineae from IE, or trauma.

Pathophysiology

An acute MI can damage the ventricular wall and disrupt the attachment of the papillary muscle or the chordae tendineae. Without a normally functioning valve to direct the flow of blood forward, a large amount of blood from the LV flows backward into the LA, increasing left atrial pressure and forcing blood back into the pulmonary circulation. The lack of forward flow diminishes the CO, leading to hypotension and cardiogenic shock. Compensatory mechanisms lead to an increase in systemic vascular resistance (SVR), which can worsen regurgitation.

Clinical Manifestations and Assessment

Acute MR manifests as signs of left- and right-sided heart failure. The patient may present with severe SOB, dyspnea on exertion, hypotension, tachycardia, peripheral edema, ascites, and jugular venous distention (JVD). There may be evidence of poor tissue perfusion with peripheral vasoconstriction, pallor, and diaphoresis.

Rapid assessment with an echocardiogram is necessary to establish a diagnosis. Often the LA and ventricle are normal in size, and systolic function can be hyperdynamic or normal; flail leaflet may also be seen.

AORTIC STENOSIS

Aortic stenosis (AS) is a narrowing of the valve opening between the LV and the aorta, resulting in obstruction of blood flow across the valve.

Pathophysiology

Progressive narrowing of the valve orifice develops gradually over several years to several decades, increasing afterload. Because the narrowing occurs slowly, the LV can adapt by contracting more slowly and forcibly than usual, squeezing the blood through the smaller opening. Normal blood volume in the LV is maintained for a while, but, eventually, LV pressure increases, causing the ventricular wall to hypertrophy to maintain CO. Diastolic dysfunction leads to increased work of the heart, which results in left ventricular failure. This results in elevated left atrial pressure, pulmonary congestion, and heart failure.

Risk Factors

The buildup of calcium deposits on heart valves is the most common cause of AS. As calcification progresses, valve leaflets become more rigid and outflow from the LV becomes obstructed. Another risk factor is a congenital malformation, such as a bicuspid aortic valve which affects males more frequently than females and typically manifests after age 40 years (Clinical Overview, 2022a). Acquired AS is common in those over 70 years of age; prevalence ranges from 9% to 45% in patients with a mean age of 54 to 81 years, and AS increases with age and affects genders equally (Clinical Overview, 2022a; Pujari & Agasthi, 2022). Besides degeneration of the valve, RHD also can lead to AS.

Clinical Manifestations and Assessment

Since it develops slowly, and the LV can compensate, AS can be asymptomatic for decades. Exertional dyspnea or decreased exercise tolerance can be early signs. The triad of symptoms associated with AS includes angina due to LV hypertrophy and diminished coronary blood flow; dyspnea due to increased pulmonary venous pressure from LV failure; and syncope, usually with exertion, due to a reduction in cerebral blood flow that occurs when vasodilation leads to a decrease in arterial pressure in the setting of fixed CO. With AS, the heart rate will increase in an attempt to increase the CO. Symptomatic AS has a poor prognosis if untreated.

Pearls for Practice

Patients with AS have SAD symptoms: syncope, angina, and dyspnea.

With AS, a systolic murmur may be heard on auscultation over the aortic area (second intercostal space [ICS], right sternal border) and may radiate into the neck. (A systolic murmur occurs between S1 and S2, representing the closure of the mitral and tricuspid valves and the opening of the aortic and pulmonary valves, respectively.) The AS murmur results from blood flowing through the narrowed opening of the stenotic aortic valve. The nurse should instruct the patient to lean forward during auscultation to accentuate the murmur. The murmur gets louder with exhalation. In severe AS, radiation of the murmur to the carotid arteries may result in a palpable thrill or a vibration. The vibration is caused by turbulent blood flow across the narrowed valve orifice. An S4 gallop may be heard.

Echocardiography is used to diagnose and monitor the progression of AS. It will demonstrate calcification of the valve or decreased mobility of valve cusps, as well as the size and function of LV. Cardiac catheterization can measure the severity of AS when noninvasive testing is inconclusive.

AORTIC REGURGITATION

Aortic regurgitation (AR), also referred to as aortic insufficiency, is the backward flow of blood into the LV from the aorta during diastole. AR occurs when the valve leaflets do not close completely or from dilatation of the ascending aorta (ascending aortic aneurysm, aortic dissection). Leaflet abnormalities causing AR include bicuspid aortic valves, calcific degeneration, endocarditis, and RHD. Diseases of the aorta or trauma can also cause incomplete aortic valve closure resulting in retrograde blood flow from the aorta to the LV during diastole in addition to the blood delivered by the LA.

Pathophysiology

Acute AR

If AR is acute, the LV lacks time to dilate in response to the additional volume load. As a result, LV end-diastolic pressure increases rapidly, resulting in backflow to the LA and pulmonary veins and decreased blood flow to the coronary arteries. Reduced blood flow to the coronary arteries may lead to myocardial ischemia. The patient develops pulmonary edema, which may progress to heart failure and cardiogenic shock.

Chronic AR

In chronic AR, the LV undergoes dilatation of the LV chamber (eccentric hypertrophy) to accommodate blood volume overload and pump a greater stroke volume. The entire stroke volume is ejected into the aorta, increasing systolic blood pressure and afterload. Afterload excess leads to increased LV wall thickness (concentric hypertrophy). During the early phases of chronic AR, ejection fraction (EF) is normal or even increased but eventually falls to subnormal levels. The arteries attempt to compensate for the higher pressures by reflex vasodilation; the peripheral arterioles relax, reducing peripheral resistance and diastolic blood pressure. Although compensatory mechanisms allow patients to remain asymptomatic despite pressure and volume overload, symptoms typically occur when left ventricular dysfunction develops.

Risk Factors

AR can occur from valve leaflet or aortic root abnormalities. Common valve leaflet abnormalities include calcific valve disease and congenital causes (e.g., unicuspid, bicuspid, and quadricuspid aortic valves). Because they affect the valve leaflets, RHD and IE can cause AR. Disorders affecting the aortic root, such as Marfan syndrome and dissecting aortic aneurysms, can lead to AR, as can chronic hypertension (Otto et al., 2021a, 2021b).

Clinical Manifestations and Assessment

AR may be asymptomatic for years, but as the disease progresses, symptoms related to increased stroke volume become apparent. Palpitations, particularly when lying down, and visible neck vein pulsations result from the increased force and volume of the blood ejected from the hypertrophied LV. Later symptoms, including dyspnea, fatigue, angina, orthopnea, and pulmonary congestion, signify decreased cardiac reserve and LV failure.

Pulse pressure, the difference between systolic and diastolic pressures, widens, resulting in high systolic and low diastolic blood pressure. Systolic blood pressure in the lower extremities is higher than in the upper extremities. Another characteristic sign of AR is the water-hammer pulse, in which the pulse has a rapid upstroke and collapses. A decrescendo diastolic murmur is heard as a high-pitched blowing sound at the 3rd or 4th ICS at the left sternal border with the patient sitting up and leaning forward. If the AR is severe, the murmur may be holodiastolic (heard throughout S2) and radiate widely along the left sternal border.

Echocardiography is a diagnostic tool for diagnosing and determining the etiology and severity of AR, valve morphology, and degree of LV hypertrophy. Patients with symptoms usually have echocardiograms every 4 to 6 months, and those without symptoms have annual echocardiograms. Cardiac catheterization is not necessary for most patients with AR. Exercise stress testing will assess functional capacity and symptom response.

MEDICAL AND NURSING MANAGEMENT OF VALVULAR DISORDERS

The valvular diseases discussed thus far in the chapter share some commonalities in their medical and nursing management. No treatment is required for asymptomatic patients with valvular pathology. The goal of medical therapy is not curative; it is symptom relief. The definitive treatment for a valvular problem is the mechanical restoration of valve function. Management is aimed at the specific valvular problem, that is, decreasing regurgitant volume, improving CO, and reducing pulmonary congestion. The American Heart Association/American College of Cardiology (AHA/ACC) recommends anticoagulation for AF irrespective of whether the AF pattern is paroxysmal, persistent, or permanent (January et al., 2019). Diuretics, vasodilators, and sodium restriction may be used to reduce preload and pulmonary congestion.

Medication Therapy

AS

Hypertension is commonly associated with AS. The AHA/ACC recommends treatment with an angiotensin-converting enzyme (ACE) inhibitor or angiotensin receptor blocker (ARB), starting at a low dose and titrating upward to achieve blood pressure control. Coronary artery disease is also commonly associated with AS. Patients should be screened and treated for hyperlipidemia (Otto et al., 2021a).

AR

Clinicians should treat hypertension in asymptomatic patients with chronic AR. The ACC/AHA recommends treatment with ACE inhibitors, ARB, or sacubitril/valsartan for patients with symptomatic, severe AR or LV systolic dysfunction who are not candidates for surgery.

MS

Anticoagulation decreases the risk of thromboembolic events in patients with rheumatic MS (the most common cause of MS worldwide) and AF. In patients with MS who are in normal sinus rhythm and tachycardia, the ACC/AHA guideline recommends heart rate control with beta-blockers (BBs), calcium channel blockers (CCBs), or ivabradine (Otto et al., 2021a).

MR

Vasodilator therapy appears effective in acute severe symptomatic MR but does not improve the severity in patients with chronic primary MR if the patient is normotensive. For patients with LV dysfunction, the standard HF regimen, including beta-adrenergic blockade, ACE inhibitors or ARBs, and possibly aldosterone antagonists, may improve function.

Pearls for Practice

Venous dilation resulting from nitroglycerin decreases blood return to the heart, thus decreasing CO and increasing the risk of syncope and coronary artery blood flow. The nurse teaches the patient the importance of relieving chest pain with rest before taking nitroglycerin and anticipating the potential adverse effects (orthostatic hypotension and syncope).

Pearls for Practice

The treatment for symptomatic AS is valve repair or replacement. Angiotensin-converting enzyme inhibitors and angiotensin receptor blockers are vasodilators that are a cornerstone of heart failure therapy. However, their use may reduce pressure distal to the stenotic valve without increasing CO, which can cause syncope. Nitrates may be used cautiously to treat angina, and diuretics to decrease pulmonary congestion. The risk associated with nitrates and diuretics is that preload and systemic arterial blood pressure can be critically reduced. The nurse must be aware that patients with AS depend on the end-diastolic or blood volume in the ventricles before systole (preload). Close monitoring for hypotension is necessary when administering both.

Symptoms may appear or worsen when the heart rate increases, such as during exercise, and may be triggered by pregnancy or additional stress on the body, such as a pulmonary infection. Valvular problems increase the patient's risk of developing bacterial endocarditis. Thrombi may occur on the valve leaflets and can embolize to cause transient ischemic attacks (TIAs). The AHA/American Stroke Association recommends daily aspirin for people with documented TIA, even in sinus rhythm (Kleindorfer et al., 2021). Eliminating caffeine and alcohol may control or reduce symptoms. The nurse encourages the patient to read labels on over-the-counter products, such as cough medicine, because these products may contain alcohol, caffeine, ephedrine, and epinephrine, which may produce arrhythmias.

Treatment of arrhythmias, heart failure, or other complications is described in Chapters 14 and 16. If symptoms develop on optimal medical therapy, surgical repair with valvuloplasty or valve replacement should be considered before ventricular dysfunction worsens. Intra-aortic balloon counterpulsation may be considered as it aids afterload reduction until surgery is performed; however, it is contraindicated in AR because it increases regurgitation.

Assessing Valvular Heart Disorders

The nurse assesses the patient with valvular heart disease for signs and symptoms of heart failure, arrhythmias, and other symptoms such as dizziness, syncope, weakness, or chest pain. Heart and lung sounds are auscultated, and peripheral pulses are palpated. The nurse teaches the patient about the diagnosis, the progressive nature of valvular disease, and treatment. The nurse instructs the patient to report new symptoms or changes to the health care provider. Treatment is not required until the patient becomes symptomatic. Management should include cardiovascular risk reduction of hyperlipidemia, hypertension, tobacco use, physical inactivity, and weight. The nurse should monitor patients for activity intolerance, fatigue, palpitations, diaphoresis, pallor, dyspnea, and tachycardia.

Pearls for Practice

Evaluating the patient's response to physical activity is essential because a decrease in activity tolerance may indicate deterioration in cardiac function, which may signify that the heart can no longer increase CO sufficiently to meet the oxygen demands associated with exercise.

VALVE REPAIR AND REPLACEMENT PROCEDURES

Most patients with valvular heart disease are medically managed until symptoms become unmanageable, or the ventricles begin to fail. However, medication cannot cure valve disease. If the condition worsens, or drugs fail to control symptoms, a percutaneous transcatheter intervention or surgery is indicated to repair or replace diseased heart valves. Compared to more invasive surgical procedures, a percutaneous transcatheter approach avoids the risks associated with cardiopulmonary bypass and median sternotomy (procedure to separate the sternum). It is associated with less pain and a shorter recovery time. It is essential to employ a shared decision-making process with the patient regarding their preferences before deciding on a transcatheter versus open surgical approach and valve repair or replacement. The nurse should ensure the patient is aware of the risks associated with each procedure and the use of anticoagulant therapy.

Valvotomy, also called valvulotomy, refers to the incision of a valve. Valvuloplasty, the repair of a cardiac valve, can be done percutaneously or surgically. Percutaneous balloon dilatation of stenotic valves is an appropriate alternative to surgical valve replacement or repair in some patients with valvular heart disease. In general, patients do not require continuous anticoagulation when they undergo valvuloplasty.

Balloon aortic valvuloplasty (BAV), called percutaneous balloon aortic valvotomy, is infrequently done as a bridge to aortic valve replacement (AVR) in hemodynamically unstable patients. BAV has a short duration of benefit and minimal prolongation of survival. In percutaneous balloon valvotomy, a balloon is inflated across the stenotic (narrowed) aortic valve to open the commissures, the site of the junction between adjacent cusps of the heart valves. Valvular stenosis occurs when the valves become stiffened or fused. Balloon valvuloplasty makes the valve more flexible and can lessen the severity of the stenosis. As the balloon inflates, the calcified leaflets are cracked and split open, and the valve ring stretches. It is typically performed in the cardiac catheterization laboratory. Potential complications include AR, emboli, stroke, ventricular perforation, rupture of the aortic valve annulus, ventricular arrhythmias, mitral valve damage, and bleeding from the catheter insertion sites. The procedure is only palliative and is ineffective long-term in improving aortic flow. When performed in patients with calcified aortic valves, calcium regrows, leading to the recurrence of AS within 6 to 12 months (Hanna, 2017). Surgical or transcutaneous AVR should be performed after the patient is stabilized. Balloon valvuloplasty may be performed as long-term therapy in children and young adults whose valves are not calcified when leaflet fusion is the cause of stenosis. Most children eventually require AVR later in adulthood. In a percutaneous balloon mitral valvotomy, a guidewire is advanced percutaneously from the femoral vein to the RA, through a puncture in the septum to the mitral valve, as shown in Figure 15-4. A balloon catheter is placed over the guidewire so the balloon tip is directly inside the narrowed valve. The balloon is inflated and deflated several times to widen the valve opening. During the procedure, an echocardiogram may be done to determine the valve leaflets' mobility and function. Percutaneous balloon mitral valvotomy is contraindicated for patients with heavily calcified valves, left atrial thrombus, or moderate to severe coexisting MR. Patients may have some MR after the procedure. Other potential complications include left-to-right atrial shunts through an atrial septal defect (ASD) caused by the procedure and emboli from dislodged left atrial thrombus.

Concept Mastery Alert

Commissurotomy is the splitting or separating of fused cardiac valve leaflets. Valvuloplasty is a general term for repairing a stenosed or regurgitant cardiac valve by commissurotomy, annuloplasty (repair of a cardiac valve's outer ring), leaflet repair, or chordoplasty (repair or restoration of chordae tendinae, the fibrous connections between the valve leaflets and the papillary muscles).

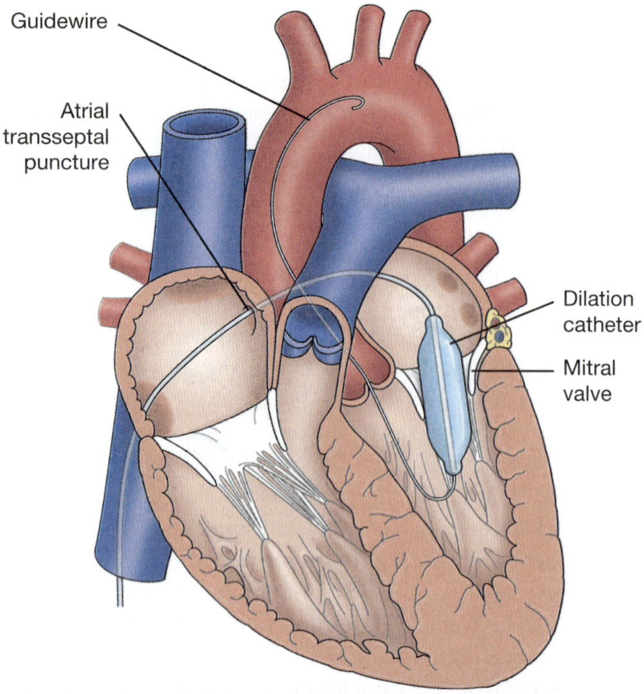

FIGURE 15-4 Balloon valvuloplasty: Cross section of heart illustrating the guidewire and dilation catheter placed through an atrial transseptal puncture and across the mitral valve. The guidewire is extended out from the aortic valve into the aorta for catheter support.

Regurgitation can be treated surgically by **annuloplasty** (repair of a cardiac valve's outer ring) (see Fig. 15-5), valve **leaflet** repair (see Fig. 15-6), and **chordoplasty** (repair of the tendinous fibers that connect the edges of the atrioventricular valve leaflets to the papillary muscles). Mitral annuloplasty narrows the diameter of the valve's orifice to treat valvular regurgitation. An annuloplasty ring prosthesis is sutured to the annulus and leaflets, creating an annulus of the desired size, as shown in Figure 15-5.

As shown in Figure 15-5, leaflet repair includes removing excess leaflet tissue and the repair of leaflet damage from stretching or tearing using pericardial or synthetic patches.

Stretched chordae tendineae can be shortened, lengthened, or replaced with synthetic chordae. Torn chordae can be reattached to the leaflet.

Patients with severe degenerative MR who are not candidates for surgery and who are older, symptomatic, and very high risk or not surgical candidates may benefit from transcatheter mitral valve repair. The FDA approved the MitraClip, to treat high-risk patients with MR. A small clip is attached to the leaky mitral valve, allowing it to close more completely. The clip approximates the edges of both mitral valve leaflets, creating a double mitral opening (edge-to-edge-repair). Sometimes two clips are needed (approximately 40% of cases). The MitraClip is delivered percutaneously through a small surgical passage through the wall of the right and left atrium. A transcatheter aortic valve replacement (TAVR) or transcatheter aortic valve implantation (TAVI) is a minimally invasive procedure for inserting a new valve without removing the old valve in treating aortic valve pathology. A collapsible artificial valve is inserted into the stenotic aortic valve through a catheter inserted either into the femoral artery (transcatheter) or through a small incision in the chest wall allowing insertion through the LV (transapical). Then the replacement valve is positioned in the damaged valve, and as it expands, it pushes the damaged valve leaflets aside and becomes the functional valve. TAVR procedures eliminate the need for general anesthesia and are performed under local anesthesia with mild to moderate sedation.

Surgical valve replacement is the definitive treatment for symptomatic AS. Surgical procedures include an open commissurotomy (splitting or separating fused cardiac valve leaflets) to increase the size of the specific valve orifice when the valve is not calcified. Although some valves can be repaired by commissurotomy, most require replacement because of significant calcification or regurgitation. However, surgical valve replacement for MS is indicated when the valvular problem is not amenable to a percutaneous procedure, percutaneous valvotomy failed, or when there is another indication for surgery, such as coronary artery disease, aortic valve disease, or concomitant mitral or tricuspid regurgitation (Otto et al., 2021a, 2021b).

When surgical **valve replacement** is indicated, a decision must be made to use either a mechanical or a bioprosthetic (tissue, biologic) valve. Consideration must be given to durability, risk of thrombosis, survival rates, and technical issues. Figure 15-7 shows a prosthetic valve replacement surgery.

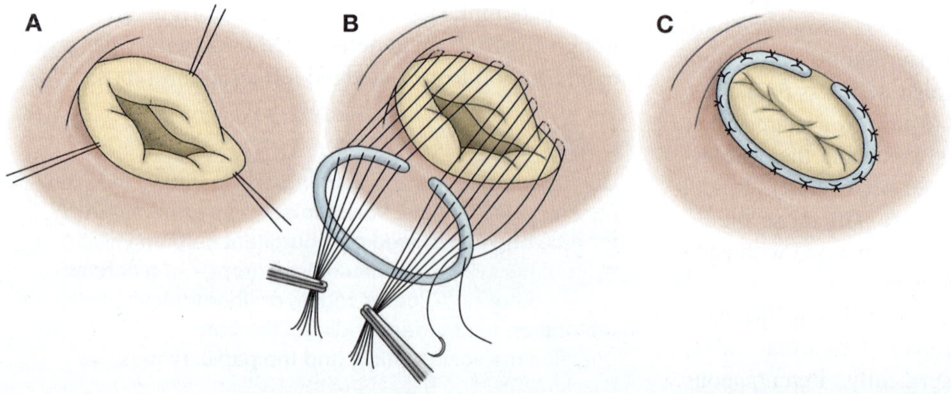

FIGURE 15-5 Annuloplasty ring insertion. A. Mitral valve regurgitation; leaflets do not close. B. Insertion of an annuloplasty ring. C. Completed valvuloplasty; leaflets close.

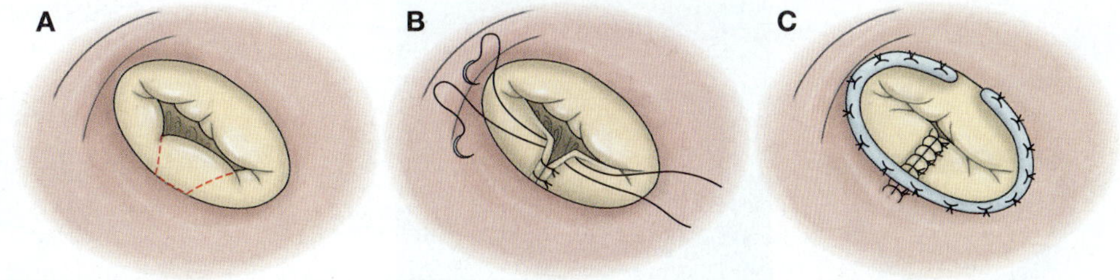

FIGURE 15-6 **Valve leaflet resection and repair with a ring annuloplasty. A. Mitral valve regurgitation; the section indicated by *dashed lines* is excised. B. Approximation of edges and suturing. C. Completed valvuloplasty, leaflet repair, and annuloplasty ring.**

Types of Valve Prostheses

Two types of valve prostheses are available: mechanical and bioprosthetic (tissue, biologic) and are depicted in Figure 15-8. The advantage of a mechanical valve is its durability. The major disadvantage is the need for anticoagulation. Bioprosthetic valves have the advantage that they do not require anticoagulation; however, they are less durable. Age, lifestyle, medical history, and valve location determine whether a mechanical or bioprosthetic valve is used.

Mechanical Valves

Three major types of mechanical valves exist: (a) bi-leaflet valve, (b) tilting disk, and (c) caged-ball. The bi-leaflet valve, manufactured by St. Jude, CarboMedics, and On-X, and the single-tilting disc valve (e.g., Medtronic Hall) are used today; the caged-ball valve (Starr-Edwards) is no longer used because of the higher risk of thromboembolism associated with it.

The age and life expectancy of the patient determine the need for the durability of a bioprosthetic valve. Mechanical valves are more durable than bioprosthetic valves and may be more likely to be used in younger patients. However, patients with mechanical valves require lifelong anticoagulation due to the risk of thromboembolism and valve thrombosis, and with this comes the additional risk of bleeding complications.

Bioprosthetic Valves

Bioprosthetic valves are less durable than mechanical valves because of the structural degeneration that occurs over time, leading to the need for reoperation. The major disadvantage of tissue valves is that they lack longevity. In general, older patients have shorter anticipated survival, so the risk of reoperation is less than it would be for a younger person. Because long-term anticoagulation generally is not recommended for bioprosthetic valves after the first 3 months of implantation, these valves are the valves of choice when anticoagulation is contraindicated or should be avoided, such as in females of childbearing age, patients who are nonadherent with medications and follow-up, patients with a history of bleeding disorders, and others who cannot tolerate long-term anticoagulation.

Types of bioprosthetic valves include **homograft** (preserved human cadaver), pericardial, and **xenograft** (bovine, porcine, or equine). In general, homografts are used for the treatment of valve endocarditis. Newer tissue valves demonstrate improved hemodynamics compared with older models. Refer to Figure 15-8 for additional images of bioprosthetic valves.

Nursing Management: Valvuloplasty and Replacement

Before surgery, compensatory mechanisms allowed the heart to adjust gradually to the valvular pathology; surgery abruptly "corrects" blood flow through the heart. Complications unique to valve replacement are related to sudden changes in intracardiac blood pressure. Valve replacement for a stenotic valve improves blood flow through the heart. Symptoms of heart failure resolve in hours to days. With

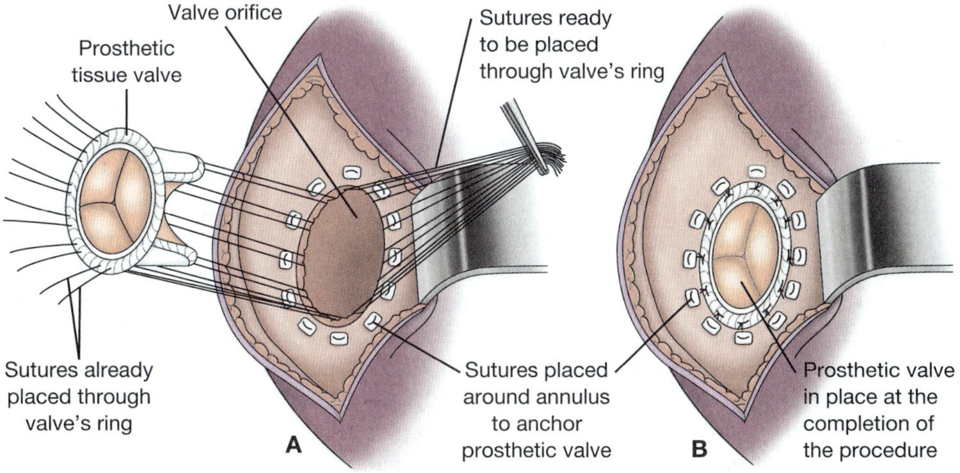

FIGURE 15-7 **Valve replacement. A. The native valve is trimmed, and the prosthetic valve is sutured in place. B. Once all sutures are placed through the ring, the surgeon slides the prosthetic valve down the sutures and into the natural orifice. The sutures are then tied off and trimmed.**

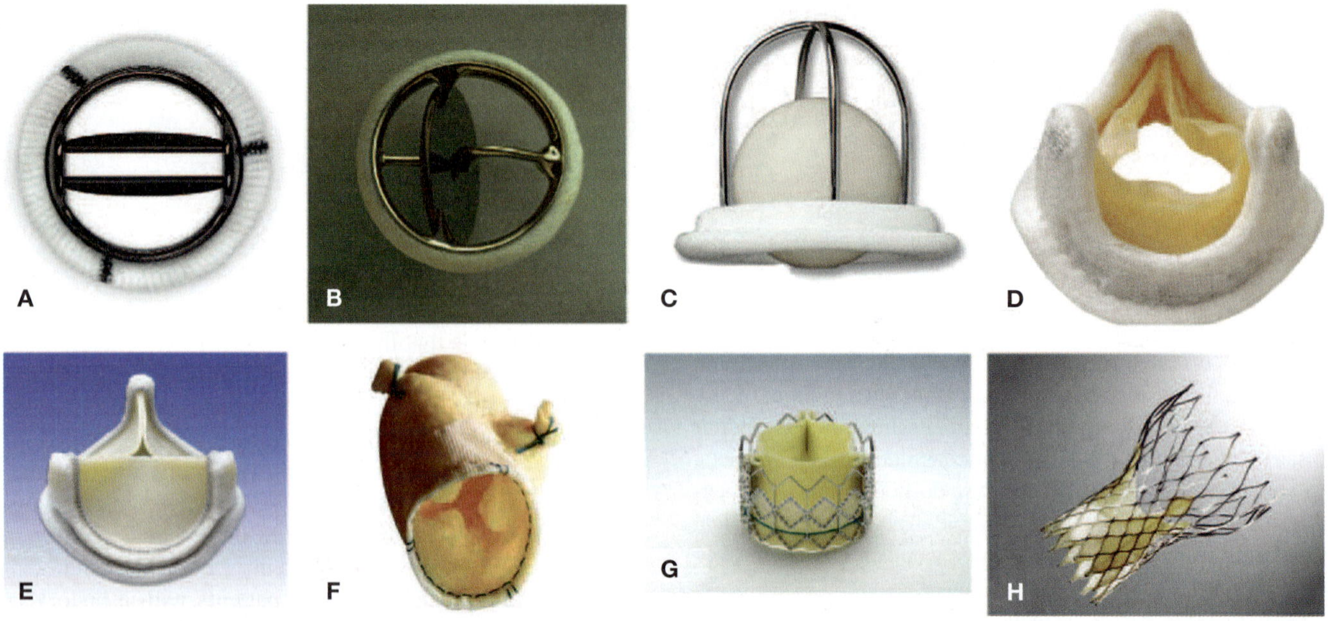

FIGURE 15-8 Common mechanical and tissue valve replacements. Different types of prosthetic heart valves. A. Bileaflet mechanical valve (St. Jude's); this is the most commonly used prosthetic valve, which consists of two semicircular leaflets that pivot on hinges. The leaflets swing partially open and are designed to close so that an acceptable amount of regurgitant blood flow is permitted. B. Monoleaflet, tilting disk mechanical valve (Medtronic Hall). C. Caged ball valve (Starr-Edwards); this valve was discontinued in 2007; however, you may care for patients who had this valve implanted. D. Stented porcine bioprosthesis (Medtronic Mosaic). E. Stented pericardial bioprosthesis (Carpentier-Edwards Magna). F. Stentless porcine bioprosthesis (Medtronic Freestyle). G. Percutaneous bioprosthesis expanded over a balloon (Edwards Sapien). H. Self-expandable percutaneous bioprosthesis (CoreValve).

valve replacement for a regurgitant valve, it may take months for the chamber into which blood had been regurgitating to achieve its optimal postoperative function. Signs and symptoms of heart failure resolve as heart function improves.

The nurse should assess patients with percutaneous valvuloplasty procedures for signs and symptoms of emboli and heart failure. Postprocedure care is the same for patients with percutaneous coronary intervention, as discussed in Chapter 13.

Patient care following valve repair or replacement is similar to that of a patient recovering from coronary artery bypass surgery, as discussed in Chapter 13. In the immediate postoperative phase, the nurse should focus on hemodynamic stabilization: augmenting preload, reducing afterload, and enhancing contractility, recognizing that the heart is adjusting to improved function. Patients are at risk for postoperative complications, including thromboembolism, bleeding, IE, arrhythmias, structural deterioration (bioprosthetic valves), and hemolytic anemia.

Thromboembolism is the most common complication of prosthetic valves and can lead to hemodynamic compromise by occluding the valve orifice. Long-term anticoagulation with warfarin, a vitamin K antagonist, is indicated after mechanical valve replacement. Heparin is used as a "bridge" until an acceptable level of anticoagulation with warfarin is evident. Frequently low-dose aspirin is used with warfarin in patients with an indication for antiplatelet therapy when there is a low risk of bleeding. Newer oral anticoagulants, such as dabigatran, rivaroxaban, and apixaban, are not recommended (Otto et al., 2021a, 2021b).

The risk of thromboembolism is lower in patients with bioprosthetic valves. The ACC/AHA guideline recommends low-dose (75 to 100 mg daily) aspirin, provided there are no other indications for oral anticoagulants. For patients with additional thrombotic risk factors, such as concurrent AF, anticoagulation with warfarin generally is prescribed for 3 months postoperatively. The nurse educates the patient about long-term anticoagulant therapy, including its risks and the need for frequent follow-up appointments and blood laboratory studies. Patients receiving warfarin will have individualized target international normalized ratios (INRs), typically between 2 and 3.5 seconds, and will vary based on the type of valve.

Prosthetic valve endocarditis occurs more often with tissue valves. It can occur early, within the first 60 days after surgery, or later. Signs include fever, heart failure, embolic events, and new murmur. In general, for a patient with a prosthetic heart valve, if the temperature is higher than 100°F, endocarditis must be excluded by blood culture. In contrast, broad-spectrum antibiotics must be begun while awaiting culture results (Carabello, 2020). Hemolytic anemia may result from the destruction of red blood cells by the movement of the prosthetic valve disk or caged ball.

Conduction disturbances and atrial arrhythmias frequently occur following valve surgery, likely due to circulating catecholamines, myocardial inflammation, and electrolyte imbalances. Digoxin, BBs, and CCBs may be used to treat arrhythmias.

The nurse provides teaching about all prescribed medications. Patients with prosthetic valves require education to prevent IE with antibiotic prophylaxis. The AHA/ACC recommends antibiotic prophylaxis for dental procedures that involve manipulation of gingival tissue, the periapical region of teeth, or perforation of the oral mucosa, not for routine cleaning (Otto et al., 2021a, 2021b).

INTRACARDIAC SEPTAL DEFECTS AND REPAIR

The atrial or ventricular septum can have an abnormal opening between the right and left sides of the heart, causing oxygenated blood to be shunted from the left side of the heart, which is under greater pressure, to the right, and mixing of oxygenated and deoxygenated blood occurs. A small septal defect will be asymptomatic and have minimal effect on heart function, but larger ones may require repair to prevent problems related to excess blood volume in the right side of the heart. Over time, a large defect can cause pulmonary congestion, which can cause elevated right heart pressure; eventually this may cause right heart failure and pulmonary hypertension.

Most large septal defects are repaired during infancy or childhood to prevent later problems. A patent foramen ovale (PFO) is a small ASD that is typically asymptomatic until adulthood and may not be detected until the patient presents with symptoms of a TIA or a stroke. Other symptoms can include exercise intolerance, fatigue, and dyspnea, and these can be mild and are often ignored. Larger ASDs can lead to more severe symptoms. Echocardiography is used to detect the presence and type of ASD (refer to Fig. 15-9).

Normally thrombi are filtered out of the blood by the lungs. With an ASD, however, there is a risk that the clot could bypass the lungs and travel directly to the brain, causing a TIA or stroke. AF is common in patients with ASDs and further increases risk of stroke. Closure of the PFO is usually a percutaneous procedure to implant a device to plug the opening. Often anticoagulation with aspirin is prescribed. Small ventricular septal defects (VSDs) are rarely closed in adults unless there is evidence of endocarditis or if valve function is compromised due to the location of the defect. A stitch or pericardial or synthetic patch is used to

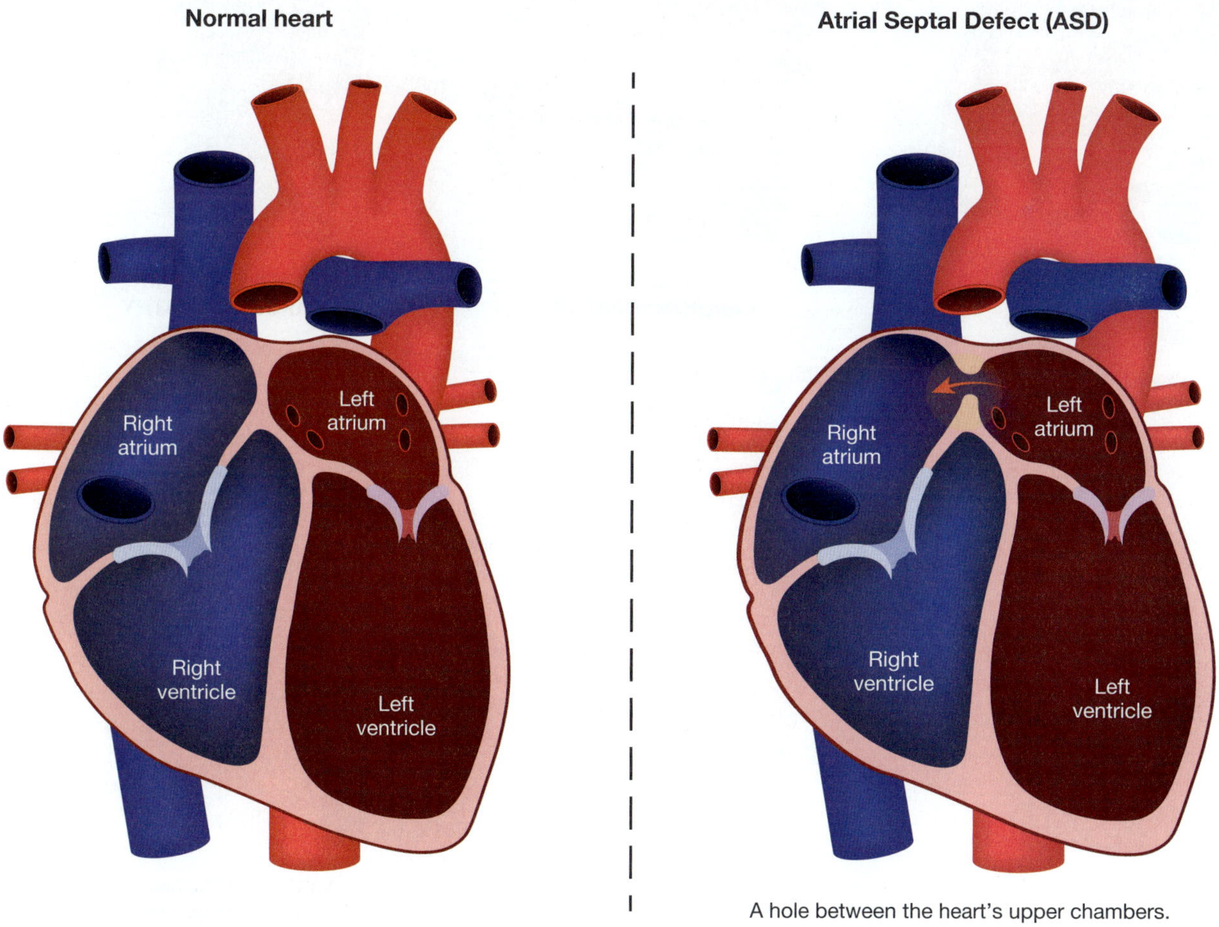

FIGURE 15-9 **Normal heart versus atrial septal defect. (From Shutterstock, ID: 2158273205.)**

close the opening. ASD repairs have low morbidity and mortality rates. Patients should be taught the importance of IE antibiotic prophylaxis for 6 months after the repair.

CARDIOMYOPATHY

Cardiomyopathy is a disorder of the myocardium (heart muscle) distinguished by structural abnormalities, mechanical and electrical dysfunction, and the absence of associated valvular disease, coronary artery disease, or congenital heart disease. In 2006, the AHA classified the condition into primary cardiomyopathies (genetic, acquired, or mixed in etiology) in which the disease process is largely confined to the heart; and secondary cardiomyopathies, those that occur as part of a systemic condition. Most cardiomyopathy is inherited or genetic, but other etiologies include inflammation (e.g., connective tissue diseases), toxins (e.g., excessive alcohol intake, chemotherapy), infection (e.g., Epstein-Barr virus, RF), and other (e.g., pregnancy-induced, stress-induced). Regardless of cause, cardiomyopathy results in impaired CO. Cardiomyopathy is characterized by abnormal hypertrophy or dilation of the ventricles that leads to decreased exercise tolerance, arrhythmias, and heart failure (refer to Fig. 15-10). Decreased stroke volume stimulates the sympathetic nervous system and the renin–angiotensin–aldosterone

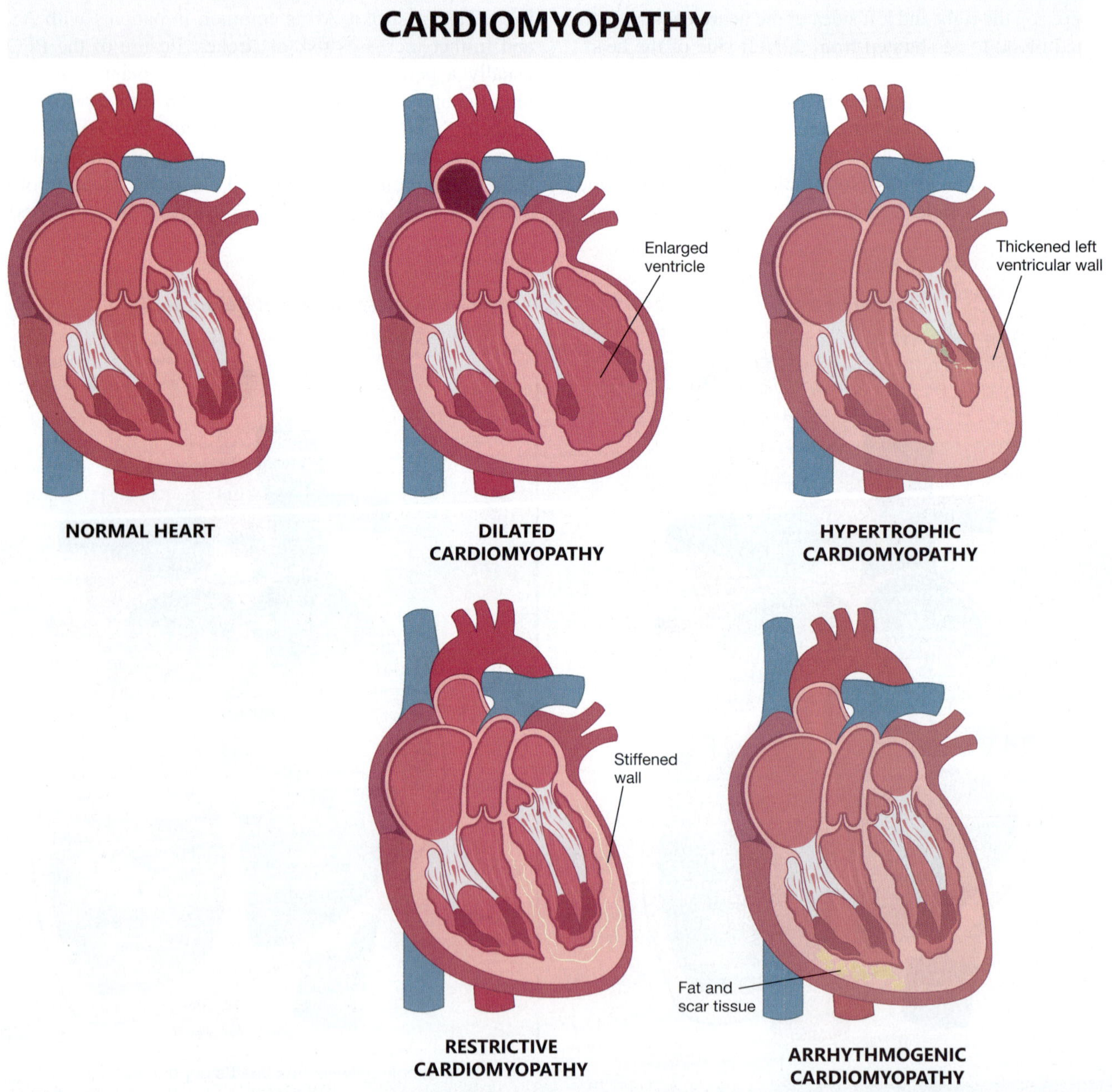

FIGURE 15-10 **Types of cardiomyopathies. (From Shutterstock, ID: 2150215157.)**

response, resulting in increased SVR and increased sodium and fluid retention, which places an increased workload on the heart. These alterations lead to severe heart failure, lethal arrhythmias, myocardial tissue destruction, and death.

DILATED CARDIOMYOPATHY

DCM is the most common cardiomyopathy and is distinguished by significant irreversible dilation of the left or both ventricles and systolic dysfunction without a known condition affecting preload, such as hypertension or valve disease. It is a common cause of heart failure, with prevalence estimated to be 1 in 1:2,500 in the general population, but this ratio may be an underestimation and the major reason for cardiac transplantation (Orphanou et al., 2022). Most DCM is caused by a genetic abnormality, or a viral infection and it is generally not diagnosed until symptoms appear.

Pathophysiology

Systolic dysfunction, ventricular remodeling, and fibrosis are characteristics of DCM. Initially, reduced contractility increases ventricular volumes to maintain CO, producing a thin-walled and dilated LV. Over time, this compensatory mechanism fails. The structural change in the LV (ventricular dilation) and excessive pressure and volume impair contraction, decreasing the amount of blood ejected from the ventricle with systole and increasing the amount of blood remaining in the ventricle after contraction. Subsequently, less blood is able to enter the ventricle during diastole. Abnormal hemodynamics result in further LV remodeling and continuing reduced contractility leads to a decreased LV ejection fraction (LVEF) and heart failure.

Clinical Manifestations and Assessment

Initial clinical presentation is usually with heart failure; symptoms of dyspnea, fatigue, bendopnea, orthopnea, exercise intolerance, and volume overload are most common and are progressive. Arrhythmias and SCD frequently occur. Altered valve function, usually mitral and tricuspid regurgitation, can result from a thinned, stretched ventricle, and this can further reduce LVEF. Physical assessment findings are consistent with fluid overload: crackles, JVD, displacement of PMI laterally, and peripheral edema. Chest auscultation may reveal an S3 gallop or a holosystolic murmur if severe MR is present. Echocardiography has a critical role in the diagnosis of DCM, as it can evaluate LV function and size, as well as valvular abnormalities, including the detection of reduced LVEF dilatation of the LV and impaired contractility Angiography may be used to exclude coronary artery disease and an electrocardiogram (ECG) will assess for conduction abnormalities or arrhythmias.

HYPERTROPHIC CARDIOMYOPATHY

Hypertrophic cardiomyopathy (HCM) is characterized by a hypertrophied, nondilated LV that can lead to obstruction of left ventricular outflow in approximately 75% of cases (Ommen et al., 2020). HCM is an autosomal dominant heart muscle disorder and is one of the most common types of inherited cardiomyopathy, occurring in 1 out of 500 people (0.20%) (Ommen et al., 2020). It is the most common cause of SCD in young people.

Pathophysiology

At the cellular level, cardiac muscle cells normally lay parallel to and end-to-end with each other. However, in HCM, the myocytes are hypertrophied and disorganized, and interstitial fibrosis is present. Over time, the heart muscle enlarges and asymmetrically thickens, especially along the septum. The increased thickness of the heart muscle reduces the size of the ventricles, making it more difficult to pump blood. The LV walls stiffen, preventing it from properly relaxing and filling with blood resulting in diastolic dysfunction. The stiffer, smaller-than-normal ventricular chamber creates a higher-velocity flow of blood out of the LV into the aorta. Left ventricular outflow tract (LVOT) obstruction occurs if the mitral valve presses on the septum and blocks blood flow. This causes high systolic pressure in the LV that leads to prolonged ventricular relaxation and diminished CO, resulting in diastolic dysfunction. This decreases the effectiveness of contractions and increases the risk of ventricular arrhythmias.

Clinical Manifestations and Assessment

Clinical presentation varies widely: Many patients with HCM remain asymptomatic or experience only minor symptoms. Others may exhibit dyspnea with exercise or at rest, fatigue, chest pain, palpitations, dizziness, or presyncope and syncope. AF is common and results from atrial enlargement. Initial presentation may be with ventricular arrhythmias, SCD, or end-stage heart failure that requires mechanical circulatory support (MCS) or cardiac transplantation. Patients with HCM may have systolic ejection murmurs that become more pronounced when the patient moves from standing to a squatting position. Mitral murmurs occur because of regurgitation. Echocardiography is used to detect HCM; a hypertrophied LV confirms diagnosis when other causes are excluded. Current treatments for HCM (medication, myectomy, and alcohol septal ablation) are geared toward slowing down the disease progression and symptom relief. An implanted cardioverter defibrillator (ICD) may be inserted to prevent SCD.

RESTRICTIVE CARDIOMYOPATHY

Restrictive cardiomyopathy (RCM) is characterized by diastolic dysfunction and impaired ventricular filling during diastole. RCM is rare, accounting for 5% of all cardiomyopathy, and frequently idiopathic (Brown et al., 2022). Other causes of RCM are infiltrative diseases such as amyloidosis or sarcoidosis, storage diseases, for example, hemochromatosis, and radiation fibrosis. RCM can occur after a heart transplant.

Abnormal myocardial relaxation with interstitial fibrosis and calcifications are the primary abnormalities of RCM.

Pathophysiology

Abnormally rigid ventricular walls result in poor ventricular compliance. Stiff ventricular walls lack ventricular stretch, or flexibility, to expand as they fill with blood. Typically, ventricular wall thickness is normal and the ventricular chambers are not dilated. Systolic function (contractility) is normal or near normal. Atrial enlargement may be present. Impaired diastolic filling occurs because the rigid ventricular walls do not relax and fill with normal blood volume. Blood volume ejected from the LV is less than normal. CO can be increased by an increase in heart rate but, eventually, becomes ineffective due to shortened filling time. As the disease progresses, heart failure with preserved EF occurs.

Clinical Manifestations and Assessment

Signs and symptoms of RCM are similar to constrictive pericarditis: dyspnea, orthopnea, nonproductive cough, PND, fatigue and decreased exercise tolerance. Peripheral edema, JVD, and hepatomegaly may be present on physical examination, and an S4 may be heard with auscultation. Echocardiography typically demonstrates normal ventricular dimensions with normal or nearly normal systolic function. With disease progression, edema worsens, and ascites, anasarca, or pulmonary edema may develop. Signs and symptoms of worsening heart failure appear.

ARRHYTHMOGENIC CARDIOMYOPATHY

Arrhythmogenic cardiomyopathy (ACM) is an inherited cardiomyopathy affecting the RV or LV, or both. It is characterized by ventricular dysplasia, arrhythmias (mainly ventricular tachycardia) and heart failure. Although it is a rare cardiomyopathy, occurring in approximately 1:2,000 to 1:5,000 (0.0005% to 0.0002%) cases of CM, ACM accounts for up to 11% of all SCD cases, primarily in young healthy adults and athletes (Shah et al., 2022).

Presenting symptoms range from palpitations and syncope to arrhythmias and SCD. The main clinical feature of ACM is myocardial electrical instability with ventricular ectopy and ventricular tachycardia commonly occurring. Biventricular or RV failure is less common and observed mainly in patients with long-term disease protected from SCD by ICD implantation.

Pathophysiology

ACM occurs when the RV is progressively infiltrated and replaced with fibrous scar and fatty tissue. This results from a defect in proteins connecting the myocytes. Loss of adhesion between myocytes can lead to detachment. This can be exacerbated by exercise (thus explaining why this is the most common cause of SCD in athletes). Initially, localized areas of the RV are affected, but, as the disease progresses, both ventricles can be affected. When the ventricular myocardium is replaced with fibrofatty tissue, arrhythmias often develop, increasing the risk of SCD. Over time, myocardial contractility weakens and progresses to heart failure.

Clinical Manifestations and Assessment

ACM is often clinically underrecognized. Usually presentation is in early adulthood, with ventricular arrhythmias. Cardiac arrest or SCD may be the initial presentation. Symptoms, including lightheadedness, fatigue, palpitations, and syncope (often during exercise) are related to the arrhythmia. Ventricular tachycardia with left bundle branch block morphology is the classic presentation. ACM should be suspected in patients with palpitations, syncope, ventricular tachycardia, or SCD, especially among previously symptom-free athletes. Family history, ECG, and a history of arrhythmias can help establish a diagnosis of ACM.

STRESS (TAKOTSUBO) CARDIOMYOPATHY

Stress (Takotsubo, broken-heart syndrome) cardiomyopathy is a syndrome of transient LV dysfunction that causes rapid but reversible myocardial weakness. Presentation mimics MI; however, there is no evidence of coronary artery blockage with angiography. Ventricular function fully returns within several days to several months. LV morphology, as seen with echocardiography or ventriculogram, demonstrates apical and midventricular contractile abnormalities (hypokinesis or akinesis) with sparing of the base as well as resultant ballooning of the ventricle that is seen with angiography (refer to Fig. 15-11). Stress cardiomyopathy is frequently, but not always, precipitated by profound emotional, psychological, or physical distress. It occurs predominantly in postmenopausal females, and patients with neurologic or psychiatric disorders may be predisposed.

Pearls for Practice

The name Takotsubo refers to a type of ceramic jar used by the Japanese to catch octopus; it has a narrow opening and neck, with a much wider body and base which resembles the heart's condition in stress or Takotsubo cardiomyopathy which is similar to echocardiogram findings in 75% of cases (an apical ballooning involving LV) (Amin et al., 2020).

Pathophysiology

The pathophysiology of stress cardiomyopathy is not completely understood. Catecholamine release triggered by activation of the sympathetic system during sudden stress may cause myocardial toxicity or induce microvascular spasm that can stun the myocardium.

Clinical Manifestations and Assessment

Clinical presentation of stress-induced cardiomyopathy is similar to that of ST-segment elevation MI (STEMI).

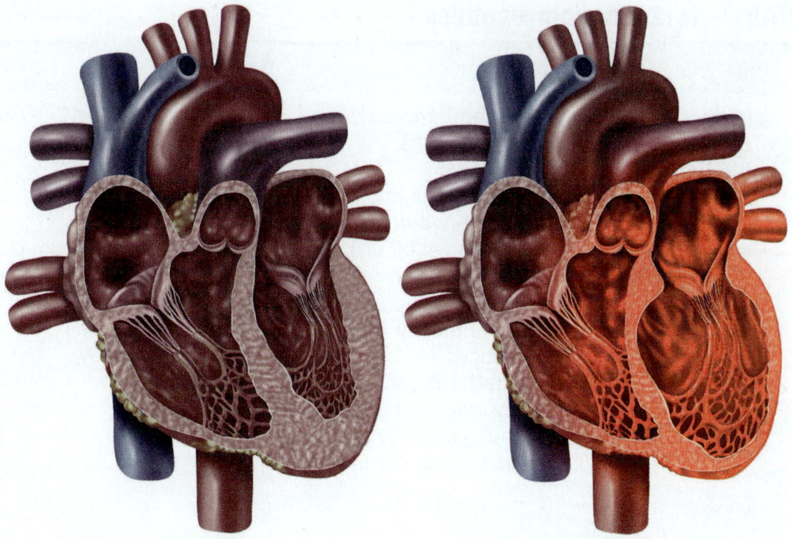

FIGURE 15-11 **Takotsubo cardiomyopathy. Apical ballooning effect from Takotsubo cardiomyopathy (right) versus normal heart. (From Shutterstock, ID: 2233171505.)**

Presenting symptoms typically include acute substernal chest pain, dyspnea, and syncope following an emotionally or physically stressful trigger. In some cases, these symptoms may be severe and can include hypotension, arrhythmias, heart failure, and cardiogenic shock. ST-segment elevation may be present on ECG. Cardiac troponin levels are elevated and creatine kinase may be normal or mildly elevated, although in lower levels than seen with acute MI. Conversely, serum brain natriuretic peptide (BNP) is elevated. Stress cardiomyopathy should be suspected in postmenopausal females with a suspected acute coronary syndrome (ACS), acute heart failure or cardiogenic shock following an emotionally or physically stressful event. Typically, patients are treated as if they are having ACS and undergo urgent cardiac catheterization. An absence of significant coronary artery disease with ballooning of the LV seen during ventriculography, with rapid and complete recovery, is the hallmark feature of stress-induced cardiomyopathy. See Table 15-2.

Pearls for Practice

DCM is a floppy heart; HCM is an enlarged, thickened heart; RCM is a stiff, rigid heart; ACM is an arrhythmia-prone heart; and stress cardiomyopathy is a stressed heart.

MEDICAL AND NURSING MANAGEMENT OF CARDIOMYOPATHY

Cardiomyopathy is diagnosed by obtaining a thorough health history including a family history to assess for the presence of cardiomyopathy, heart failure, or cardiac arrest in relatives; physical examination; and with the use of diagnostic tests and procedures. Physical examination may reveal the presence of a heart murmur, and if there is fluid overload, crackles, JVD, and lower extremity edema may be present.

The ECG can detect arrhythmias (irregular heart rhythms) and abnormal conduction (heart blocks). Echocardiography is the primary tool used to evaluate cardiomyopathy because it assesses both the structure (shape and size) and function (pumping action) of the ventricles, including valvular abnormalities and EF. A chest x-ray can identify the extent of cardiac enlargement and the presence of pulmonary congestion. Other tests that may be done include event monitors to record the heart's electrical activity over a 24- to 72-hour period to detect the presence of intermittent arrhythmias, or a stress test to evaluate the heart during increasing amounts of work (or stress). When physical activity is not tolerated, medication is administered to simulate exertion. Cardiac catheterization is done to measure pressure and blood flow in the heart and can detect the presence of coronary artery disease. Endomyocardial biopsy may be performed; analysis of myocardial tissue may be used to guide therapy or to establish a precipitating cause, if unknown. Genetic testing is done to determine if cardiomyopathy is inherited and whether gene mutations are present. Screening of asymptomatic family members should be arranged if cardiomyopathy is suspected because of family history, and genetic testing may be offered to first-degree blood relatives (e.g., parents, siblings, and children). If a genetic mutation is suspected or discovered for HCM, DCM, and ACM, additional screening of family members with echocardiography (echo), and ECG should be considered, as early diagnosis and treatment can prevent or delay significant symptoms and SCD.

HCM

Risk factors for SCD should be assessed. Patients with (a) a history of SCD, (b) a first-degree relative with SCD, (c) a history of ventricular tachycardia or ventricular fibrillation, (d) unexplained syncope, (e) LV hypertrophy >30 mm, or (f) an abnormal response to exercise should be referred for an ICD.

TABLE **15-2 Cardiomyopathies**

Type	Description	Etiology	Pathophysiology	Clinical Manifestations
Dilated cardiomyopathy (DCM) 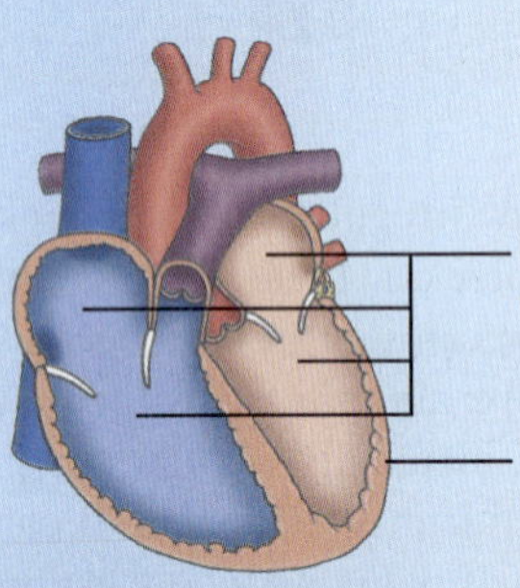 	Significant, irreversible dilation of the ventricles Systolic dysfunction without hypertrophy Increased ventricular systolic and diastolic volumes with decreased left ventricular (LV) function Impaired contractility may result in HF, ventricular arrhythmias, and sudden cardiac death.	It occurs most often in adults in a wide range of ages; in adults, commonly manifests in the third or fourth decade of life, and males are affected more than females (Clinical Overview, 2022b).	Reduced ventricular wall thickness and increased myocardial mass result in poor systolic function. Decreased blood volume ejected from the ventricle during systole increases blood volume remaining in the ventricle after contraction. Then less blood is able to enter the ventricle during diastole, increasing end-diastolic pressure and, eventually, increasing pulmonary and systemic venous pressures. Valvular regurgitation can result from an enlarged stretched ventricle. Poor blood flow through the ventricle may cause ventricular or atrial thrombi, which may embolize to other locations in the body.	Symptoms are progressive and include dyspnea, fatigue, volume overload, weight gain, chest pain due to coronary artery disease or pulmonary embolism, or abdominal discomfort from hepatomegaly. Signs include: holosystolic murmur (heard on S1) due to MR, thromboembolism, ventricular arrhythmias, and sudden cardiac death. HF may be the initial presentation.
Hypertrophic cardiomyopathy (HCM) 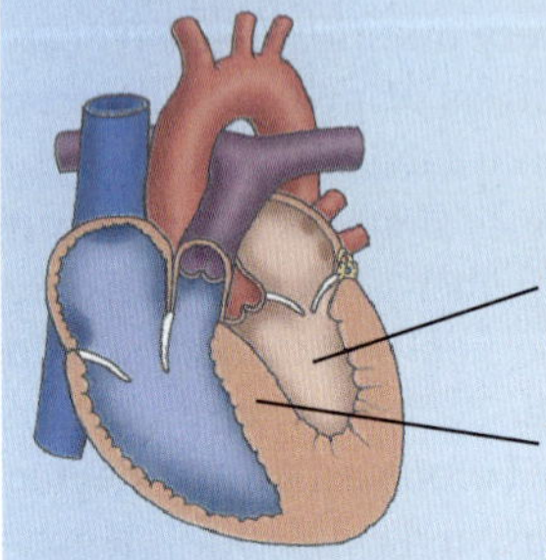 	Hypertrophied, nondilated LV leads to obstruction of left ventricular outflow, without cardiac or systemic disease	HCM is an inherited autosomal dominant heart muscle disorder and one of the most common types of cardiomyopathies. It is the most common cause of sudden cardiac death (SCD) in young athletes.	Heart muscle asymmetrically increases in mass, especially along the septum, and increased thickness reduces the size of the ventricular cavities, taking longer to relax after systole. During diastole, ventricular filling is impaired; atrial contraction at the end of diastole becomes critical for filling and systolic contraction. Smaller-than-normal LV cavity creates high-velocity blood flow from the LV into the aorta. Left ventricular outflow tract obstruction causes high systolic pressure in the LV that leads to prolonged ventricular relaxation and diminished cardiac output, resulting in diastolic dysfunction. Systolic function is normal or high, resulting in an above-normal ejection fraction.	Most patients with HCM are asymptomatic, but some present with ventricular arrhythmias, SCD, or other symptoms: syncope, dyspnea, or chest pain. Atrial fibrillation commonly occurs from atrial enlargement. Systolic ejection murmurs (heard on S1) do not radiate to the neck. Mitral murmurs result from regurgitation.

Type	Description	Etiology	Pathophysiology	Clinical Manifestations
Restrictive cardiomyopathy (RCM) 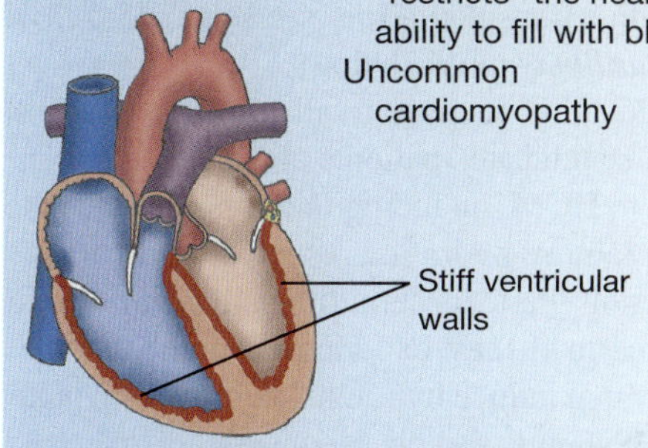 	Characterized by diastolic dysfunction that negatively affects or "restricts" the heart's ability to fill with blood Uncommon cardiomyopathy	Frequently idiopathic Associated with amyloidosis and endomyocardial fibrosis (scarring of the heart) Often occurs after a heart transplant	Stiff ventricular walls lack ventricular stretch (flexibility to expand as they fill with blood). This impairs diastolic filling, resulting in diastolic HF. Normal, or slightly increased, ventricular wall thickness and atrial enlargement with normal systolic function are characteristic. Atrioventricular block and symptomatic bradycardia can occur.	Symptoms are similar to constrictive pericarditis: dyspnea, nonproductive cough, chest pain, and exercise intolerance. Signs may include jugular venous distention, edema, ascites, anasarca, pulmonary edema, and an S3 and S4 can be heard with auscultation.
Arrhythmogenic right ventricular cardiomyopathy/ dysplasia (ARVC/D) 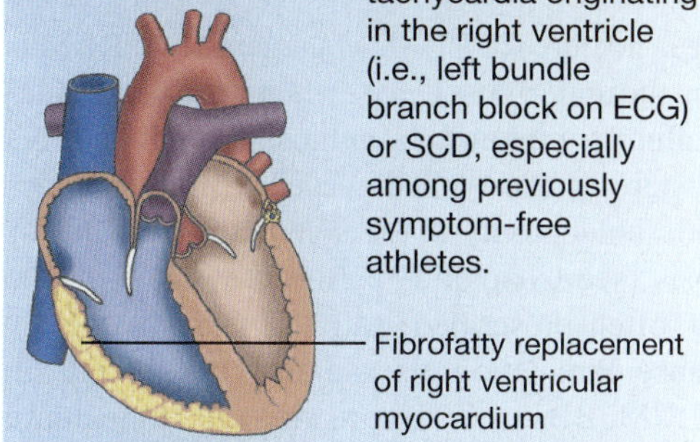 	Rare but increasingly recognized condition ARVC/D should be suspected in patients with ventricular tachycardia originating in the right ventricle (i.e., left bundle branch block on ECG) or SCD, especially among previously symptom-free athletes.	Familial in more than 50% of patients and usually occurs in early adulthood (Wylie, 2022)	ARVC/D occurs when the right ventricle is progressively infiltrated and replaced with fibrous scar and adipose tissue. Initially, only localized areas of the right ventricle are affected, but, as the disease progresses, the entire heart is affected. Eventually, the right ventricle dilates and develops poor contractility, and arrhythmias occur.	Symptoms are consistent with right HF. Supraventricular arrhythmias may occur. Ventricular arrhythmias and SCD may be the initial presentation, and often diagnosis is made postmortem. Family history, ECG, and a history of arrhythmias can help establish a diagnosis of ARVC/D.
Stress-induced (Takotsubo) cardiomyopathy 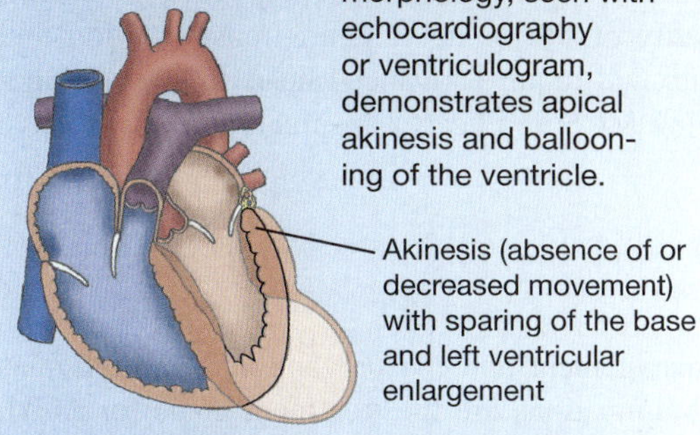 	Syndrome of transient LV dysfunction. Ventricular function fully returns within weeks. LV morphology, seen with echocardiography or ventriculogram, demonstrates apical akinesis and ballooning of the ventricle. It has been identified predominantly in white, postmenopausal females. Noncardiac comorbidities, such as anxiety, chronic pulmonary disease, and thyroid disease are associated.	Precipitated by emotional or physical distress	The pathophysiology of stress-induced cardiomyopathy remains unclear. One theory gaining acceptance is catecholamine excess triggered by activation of the sympathetic system.	Clinical presentation is identical to that of acute ST-segment elevation MI: acute substernal pain and shortness of breath following an emotionally or physically stressful trigger. ST-segment elevation may be present on ECG, and cardiac enzymes may be mildly elevated, disproportionate to levels seen with acute MI. Acute presentation may be severe; arrhythmias, HF, pulmonary edema, and cardiogenic shock have been reported in the absence of significant coronary artery disease. Ballooning of the LV, with rapid and complete recovery, is the hallmark feature.

BBs (e.g., atenolol) decrease heart rate and may prevent arrhythmias. A faster heart rate can worsen LVOT obstruction and reduce CO. A slower heart rate increases diastolic time which improves filling of the LV. A slower rate will also decrease myocardial oxygen demand. This can prevent or decrease angina resulting from poor coronary artery perfusion. Nondihydropyridine CCBs (e.g., verapamil and diltiazem) improve ventricular filling and may help reduce chest pain, DOE, and arrhythmias. Antiarrhythmics (e.g., disopyramide) may be initiated to maintain or restore normal heart rhythm, treat arrhythmias, and prevent SCD. In 2022, the FDA approved a new drug, mavacamten, for the treatment of adults with symptomatic obstructive HCM. Mavacamten is a cardiac myosin inhibitor that improves functional capacity and symptoms by decreasing excessive contractility. It has been shown to reduce the need for septal myomectomy (Desai et al., 2022). Because it can cause heart failure due to systolic dysfunction, it is available only through a restricted program. Mavacamten must be slowly uptitrated with regular echocardiographic assessment of cardiac function. Systemic anticoagulation may be needed to prevent thromboembolic events.

Drug Alert

Mavacamten reduces LVEF and can cause heart failure due to systolic dysfunction. Echocardiogram assessments of LVEF are required prior to and during treatment. Initiation of mavacamten in patients with LVEF <55% is not recommended. Interrupt mavacamten if LVEF is <50% at any visit or if the patient experiences heart failure symptoms or worsening clinical status.

Certain medications are contraindicated with HCM, particularly in patients with LVOT obstruction. Vasodilators (e.g., nitroglycerin, ACE-I), dihydropyridine CCBs (e.g., amlodipine and nifedipine), and angiotensin II receptor blockers (ARBs) can cause hypotension and worsen heart failure symptoms. Diuretics should be avoided because they reduce preload, resulting in less LV filling and greater LVOT obstruction. Vasodilatory and diuretic medications may decrease CO in patients with HCM because they tend to be dependent upon preload.

Drug Alert

Dihydropyridine calcium channel blockers (DHP CCBs) tend to be more potent vasodilators than nondihydropyridine drugs and are not recommended to treat HCM because they can cause hypotension that reduces CO. Nondihydropyridine calcium channel blockers (non-DHP CCBs) act mainly on the heart and are less potent vasodilators. They exhibit negative inotropic effects that reduce myocardial conduction and contractility to improve LV filling.

When medication therapy fails to significantly improve a patient's signs and symptoms, procedures and surgical options are considered, including septal myectomy (removal of hypertrophied portion of the septum that is obstructing the flow of blood from the LV to the aorta), alcohol septal ablation, MCS, and cardiac transplantation (see section *Surgical Interventions for Cardiomyopathy* below).

In addition to education relevant to all cardiomyopathies (see below), the nurse educates patients about lifestyle considerations specific to HCM, including the importance of the importance of maintaining hydration, especially in patients with LVOT obstruction. Patients should be advised to avoid the use of nitroglycerin if they experience angina, as well vasodilators, as they can induce hypotension or worsen heart failure symptoms. Patients should be instructed to avoid competitive sports and high-intensity or sustained activities to reduce the risk of SCD.

RCM

Currently, there is no cure for RCM. Management of RCM is aimed at treating the underlying cause, when known, and alleviating heart failure symptoms. Immunosuppressive agents such as corticosteroids are typically used to treat sarcoidosis. Therapeutic phlebotomy is the standard treatment for hemochromatosis (see Chapter 19). Antiarrhythmics, BBs, and CCBs may often prescribed, and ICDs are frequently implanted because conduction disease and arrhythmias are common with RCM. BBs or CCBs are also used to increase filling time. Diuretics can reduce volume overload but require close monitoring to prevent excessive diuresis as patients with RCM rely on high filling pressures to maintain CO. AF is common, and patients may require anticoagulation. RCM is progressive and proper management may prolong survival, improve quality of life or delay heart transplantation, but many patients will require advanced heart failure management including MCS and heart transplantation or palliative care.

ACM

Symptom management and the prevention of arrhythmias and other complications are the treatment goals for ACM. ACE-I or ARBs reduce the workload of the heart. BBs decrease heart rate and contractility to improve CO and prevent arrhythmias and may also be prescribed to reduce or prevent inappropriate ICD shocks. Antiarrhythmics also control heart rate and rhythm. Procedures such as cardioversion (delivering a shock to restore a normal rhythm), and catheter (radiofrequency) ablation that uses energy to destroy abnormal electrical pathways causing arrhythmias (refer to Chapter 16) may be considered. Pacemakers or ICDs are recommended to prevent arrhythmias in patients with ACM, and MCS and cardiac transplant may be considered for uncontrolled heart failure symptoms or refractory ventricular arrhythmias.

Stress Cardiomyopathy

For stress cardiomyopathy, accurate diagnosis and differentiation from STEMI is critical to avoid unnecessary treatments, such as administration of thrombolytics, which can harm the patient. Because stress cardiomyopathy is difficult to differentiate from ACSs without coronary angiography, the patient should be prepared for cardiac catheterization to assess for coronary artery blockages and left ventriculogram to evaluate the LV for apical ballooning.

When the diagnosis of stress cardiomyopathy has been established medication therapy is aimed at reducing myocardial workload. In contrast to other types of cardiomyopathy, ACE-I or ARBs are generally used for only a few months, until LV function is restored. BBs are used initially to inhibit the effects of catecholamines and also to reduce the heart's workload during recovery. Anxiolytics may be prescribed to mitigate the effects of stress hormones.

Psychological care and support is necessary, and the nurse may initiate consultation with or referral to a social worker, counselor or support group to assist the patient with coping skills, stress management, and addressing specific life changes or stressors.

Medication reconciliation is key to preventing drug–drug interactions, prescription cascade, and polypharmacy. Teach patients and caregivers how to accurately monitor blood pressure and heart rate at home.

Cardiomyopathy can be asymptomatic, but over time as compensatory mechanisms fail, symptoms worsen and lead to heart failure, regardless of the type of cardiomyopathy. Treatment is supportive and in addition to symptom relief, priorities are prevention of complications, including prevention of ventricular arrhythmias to reduce the risk of SCD. Underlying causes should be treated if known.

Supportive care with standard heart failure medication therapy, including ACE inhibitors, aldosterone receptor antagonists (ARBs), angiotensin receptor-neprilysin inhibitors (ARNIs), BBs, and diuretics, may be prescribed. BBs reduce catecholamine response, decrease heart rate, and have been shown to reduce mortality.

Pacemakers are used to correct conduction abnormalities and control heart rate when tachyarrhythmias or bradyarrhythmias are present. ICDs are recommended when there is a high risk for life-threatening arrhythmias, particularly for ACM. Unstable patients may require positive inotropic medications, vasopressors, and intra-aortic balloon pumps (IABPs), implantable devices, or surgery. IABP (described in Chapter 54), septal myectomy or alcohol septal ablation, left ventricular assist devices (VADs), and heart transplantation may be necessary in the most severe cases.

Nursing management of all cardiomyopathies includes careful cardiovascular assessment for signs of worsening symptoms of fluid overload and heart failure, including dyspnea, the presence of crackles during auscultation of lungs, worsening hypoxia, the presence of an S3 gallop during auscultation of the heart and peripheral edema. The nurse should be alert to changes in mental status, tachycardia, change in cardiac rhythm or decreased urinary output despite diuretics. The nurse provides patient education including the importance of self-monitoring for symptoms, medication compliance, sodium and fluid restriction, stress-management techniques, adequate rest, and gradual increases in physical activity (Malik et al., 2022). The nurse helps the patient to understand doses and explains how each medication helps to maintain cardiac function. The nurse instructs the patient about potential drug–drug interaction side effects and to report any adverse reaction. The nurse can help the patient to understand procedures and test results, including genetic testing and risk.

Arrhythmias occur frequently; continuous cardiac monitoring is recommended with personnel and equipment readily available to treat life-threatening arrhythmias. Bedrest is initially recommended to decrease cardiac workload. Physical activity is increased slowly, and the patient is asked to report symptoms that occur with increasing activity. For patients who receive an implantable cardiac device, the nurse provides education about signs and symptoms of infection, avoidance of heavy lifting, and the need for regular cardiology follow-up care. The nurse instructs patients with an ICD defibrillator to notify their cardiology provider if a shock is delivered. The nurse teaches the patient that changes in signs and symptoms, such as syncope or weight gain should be reported immediately. The nurse should provide education to patients with cardiomyopathy regarding lifestyle that includes eating a healthy diet limited in sodium and processed foods, smoking cessation, and stress reduction. The safest type and amount of physical activity should be reviewed and weight loss should be encouraged if patients are overweight to decrease the heart's oxygen demand.

SURGICAL INTERVENTIONS FOR CARDIOMYOPATHY

When cardiomyopathy symptoms worsen and heart failure progresses, lifestyle and medications become insufficient to manage the disease. When medical treatment is no longer effective, surgical intervention, including cardiac transplantation, is considered.

Septal Myectomy and Alcohol (Ethanol) Septal Ablation

People with HCM who have LVOT obstruction often experience severe symptoms and functional limitation. Two established procedures, septal myectomy and alcohol septal ablation, can significantly relieve the obstruction, resulting in clinical improvement of signs and symptoms. A septal myectomy is open-heart surgery in which a part of the thickened septum that bulges into the LV is removed. This increases LV outflow and decreases force on the mitral valve to improve blood flow through the heart and out to the body. Mitral valve intervention may be beneficial if the mitral valve leaflet is interfering with the outflow of blood to the aorta; if needed this procedure is often performed at the same time as the septal myectomy.

Septal ablation is the destruction of the hypertrophied septum caused by injecting alcohol into the artery that supplies blood to that area. The alcohol is toxic and causes myocytes to shrink and die. The myocardial scar tissue remaining is thinner than the heart muscle and improves blood flow through the heart. Alcohol septal ablation improves symptoms, but a possible complication with this procedure is permanent heart block, which can occur when the conduction system is damaged by the ablation. This occurs in as many as 10% of the cases and requires implantation of a pacemaker. A 2020 meta-analysis of septal myectomy and alcohol septal ablation found that younger patients may benefit from septal myectomy while older adults with comorbidities and higher surgical risk may benefit from septal ablation (Bytyçi et al., 2020).

Mechanical Circulatory Support

MCS has evolved greatly, and its use has increased dramatically since the late 1960s when a VAD was first used for postcardiotomy shock. MCS has three main functions: (a) reduce or assume the workload of the heart, (b) support systemic circulation, completely or partially, and (c) improve myocardial oxygenation. Patients who cannot be weaned from cardiopulmonary bypass and patients in cardiogenic shock may benefit from short-term (hours to days) MCS for the management of hemodynamically unstable acute, decompensated heart failure while the patient's own heart recovers. Typically, an IABP, described in Chapter 54, or an extracorporeal membrane oxygenator (ECMO) is used to provide support in these cases.

Intra-Aortic Balloon Pump

The IABP decreases the workload of the heart. Deflation of the balloon just before systole reduces LV afterload, which decreases myocardial oxygen consumption and increases CO. Diastolic augmentation during balloon inflation improves coronary artery blood flow by increasing coronary artery perfusion pressure and improving blood flow to peripheral organs. The IABP is used pre- and postoperatively in patients with severely compromised left ventricular function, in patients with myocardial ischemia undergoing complex percutaneous coronary interventions, and for patients with complications resulting from acute MI, such as papillary muscle rupture, awaiting surgical repair. Bleeding, limb ischemia, infection, and vascular injury are potential complications of IABP, and monitoring the patient for compromised circulation and hemodynamic instability is a priority for nursing management.

Extracorporeal Membrane Oxygenator

ECMO uses a pump to circulate blood through an oxygenator outside the body to provide both cardiac and respiratory support by artificially removing the carbon dioxide and reoxygenating red blood cells. Blood is rewarmed and returned to the body. The purpose of ECMO is to allow for recovery of the lungs and heart and it is typically used for a few days to several weeks. Refer to Chapter 54 for additional details. A standard cardiopulmonary bypass machine is used for a matter of hours to provide support during open-heart cardiac surgical procedures.

Ventricular Assist Devices

Increasingly, MCS is used long-term (months to years) for the management of advanced heart failure from causes including cardiomyopathy (heart failure is described in detail in Chapter 14). VADs support a failing heart by generating blood flow to the systemic circulation and unloading the ventricle. Most patients receive a left VAD, but some may receive a biventricular device (BiVAD) or a total artificial heart (TAH). Historically, this therapy was used temporarily for patients with difficulty weaning from cardiopulmonary bypass following cardiothoracic surgery as a bridge to recovery. Nondurable (temporary) support indications include cardiogenic shock, acute myocarditis (discussed shortly), and acute, reversible heart failure. Another nondurable indication is the use of a VAD as a bridge to the decision (BTD) to allow time to evaluate whether a transplant or other treatment is best suited to a patient. A bridge-to-bridge (BTB) VAD is used when emergent stabilization is necessary, with a plan to transition to a longer-term device when the patient becomes more clinically stable.

Durable or long-term indications for VADs include the bridge to transplant (BTT), in patients failing on maximal medical therapy to sustain life until a donor's heart becomes available, or as destination therapy (DT) in patients with end-stage heart failure who are not transplant candidates and for whom ventricular recovery is not possible. Increasingly, VADs are being used as DT. See Figure 15-12 for an example of long-term use of VAD.

VADs have pumps that are outside the body (extracorporeal) and can be broadly classified as pulsatile volume displacement or continuous flow (axial flow, centrifugal). Most are surgically inserted via sternotomy, but some short-term use VADs can be inserted percutaneously. First-generation volume-displacement pumps developed in the 1970s provided good hemodynamic support but were limited by a lack of long-term durability, an extensive surgical procedure for insertion, and a large external driveline that was prone to infection. First-generation implantable pulsatile pumps

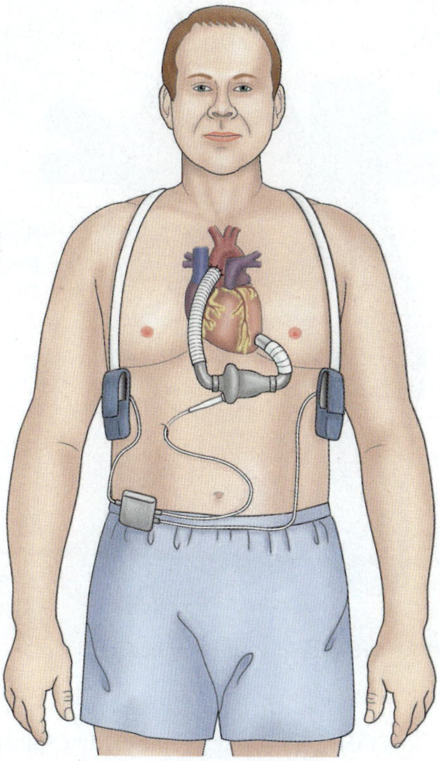

FIGURE 15-12 Left ventricular assist device.

are no longer available and extracorporeal first-generation pumps are rarely implanted today.

Second- and third-generation LVADs are continuous flow pumps and have only one moving part, making them more durable. Because they have smaller drivelines, the risk of infection and surgical trauma is reduced. Second-generation axial flow pumps contain an impeller that generates a continuous, nonpulsatile flow by a rotor spinning around a central shaft and returning blood to the aorta at a constant rate. Third-generation VADs generate centrifugal force from a spinning rotor, resulting in a nonpulsatile flow of blood and have been designed for long-term use (estimated durability of 10 years). Compared with earlier LVADs, the third-generation VADs optimize blood flow to reduce the risk of thrombus formation and are smaller in size to facilitate surgical implantation. Newer VADs provide patients with a better quality of life, including improved mobility and restoration of end-organ function.

Contraindications to VADs include an inability to tolerate anticoagulation, an abdominal aortic aneurysm greater than 5 cm, active systemic infection or high chronic risk of infection, although the decision to insert a VAD will often involve a cumulative assessment of several relative contraindications and the associated overall risk (Kirklin et al., 2020; Shen & Andrawes, 2019).

Pearls for Practice

The nurse understands that there is no palpable pulse or measurable "normal" systolic or diastolic blood pressure in patients with continuous flow LVADs where the majority of blood flow is through the LVAD. The nurse auscultates below the heart to hear the hum of the device running. The gold standard to measure the blood pressure is insertion of an arterial line in the hospitalized patient (Agarwal, 2022). If an arterial line is not in place the best reflection of the MAP (mean arterial pressure) is to use a manual blood pressure cuff and Doppler at the brachial artery (Dirks & Waters, 2022). The nurse refers to their health care facility's target MAP; current guidelines recommend a MAP of 80 mm Hg or lower (Agarwal, 2022). The nurse evaluates level of consciousness, skin color, respiratory rate, urine output and temperature to determine whether the patient is receiving adequate support, and assesses the system controller, observes the driveline, being careful not to put undue stress on it. For patients that will be discharged with a VAD, patient education focuses on contingency plans, including uninterrupted electrical access, access to a telephone for emergencies, and understanding the limitations of battery life.

Total Artificial Hearts

TAHs are designed to replace both ventricles. SynCardia Total Artificial Heart is the only biventricular MCS device approved for BTT by the U.S. Food and Drug Administration (FDA) for people with end-stage irreversible heart failure who are candidates for heart transplant. Made of a biocompatible plastic, it has two ventricles and four valves that use a pulsatile flow to circulate blood throughout the body. More than 1,100 have been implanted.

Complications

Complications of VADs and TAHs include infection, ventricular arrhythmias, thrombus, thromboemboli, hemolysis, hemorrhage, right heart failure, multisystem failure, and mechanical failure of the device. Anticoagulation to reduce the risk of thrombus formation and thromboembolism, while avoiding the risk of bleeding, is challenging, and anticoagulation therapy depends on device type, patient history, and platelet responsiveness. Infection is another major complication, particularly with extracorporeal devices as the percutaneous driveline exit site commonly becomes infected. Infection at this site can spread quickly through the entire system causing sepsis, a systemic infection.

Nursing care for patients with mechanical assist devices (MADs) focuses on the assessment of and minimization of complications as well as providing emotional support and education about the MAD and the underlying cardiac disease. If a durable VAD is being considered, the patient's ability to manage the VAD should be assessed. When assessing the patient with a VAD, it is important to remember that there may not be any palpable pulse because blood flow throughout the cardiac cycle is continuous, not pulsatile.

Pulse oximetry may be unmeasurable or unreliable, and obtaining VAD pressure may be difficult or not possible. It is recommended that a Doppler ultrasound be used with a sphygmomanometer to obtain a VAD pressure.

Heart Transplantation

Heart transplantation is considered for eligible patients with end-stage heart failure who are receiving optimized medical therapy but remain symptomatic. Heart transplant procedures, medications and survival have advanced and continue to improve since the first human-to-human heart transplant was performed in 1967. The discovery in the 1980s and 1990s of cyclosporine and tacrolimus, immunosuppressants that significantly decrease the body's rejection of transplanted organs, advanced heart transplantation and survival.

Typical transplant candidates have advanced heart failure, severe symptoms, and functional limitations uncontrolled by medical therapy, no other surgical options, and a poor life expectancy from heart disease. As discussed earlier, VADs serve as a "BTT" for patients waiting for a heart transplant, and approximately 50% of heart recipients receive MCS before transplant. A multidisciplinary team screens the candidate before recommending the transplantation procedure. A primary factor to be considered is the candidate's prognosis after transplantation.

Transplant candidates cannot have any systemic illness with a life expectancy <2 years despite heart transplantation, or multisystem disease with severe organ dysfunction. Irreversible pulmonary hypertension is contraindicated because this would lead to right ventricular failure of the transplanted heart. Other contraindications include substance use disorder (current), severe symptomatic cerebrovascular disease, inability to adhere to drug therapy regimen, as well as active malignancy and active infection, as both of these can worsen as a result of the antirejection medications.

In addition to having severely compromised physical health, patients also struggle with psychosocial issues. Waiting for a donor heart is stressful for the patient and family. Much unpredictability and uncertainty exist regarding when or whether a donor heart will become available.

Orthotopic Transplantation

Orthotopic transplantation, as depicted in Figure 15-13, is the most common surgical procedure for cardiac transplantation. The recipient's heart is removed, leaving a portion of the recipient's atria with the vena cava and pulmonary veins in place. The donor heart, which usually has been preserved in ice, is prepared for implant by cutting away a small section of the atria that corresponds with the sections of the recipient's heart that were left in place. The donor heart is implanted by suturing the donor atria to the residual atrial tissue of the recipient's heart. After the venous or atrial anastomoses are complete, the recipient's pulmonary artery and aorta are sutured to those of the donor heart.

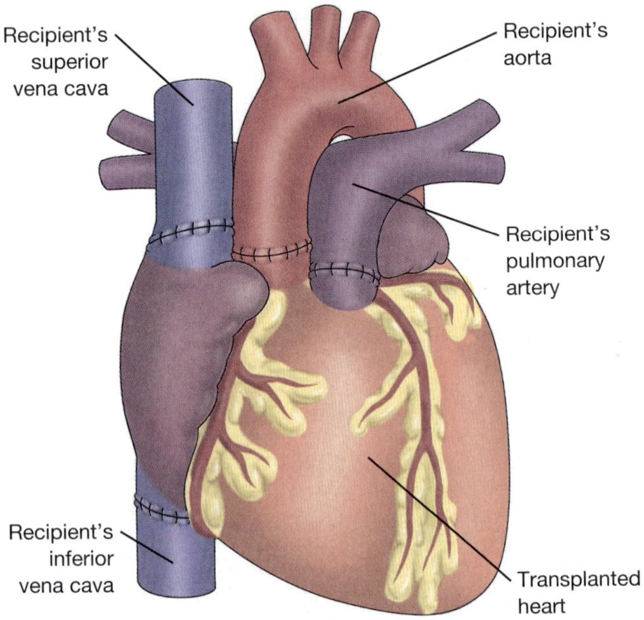

FIGURE 15-13 **Orthotopic method of heart transplantation.**

Rarely (less than 1%), a heterotopic cardiac transplant may be performed because of significant pulmonary hypertension, small donor heart, or expected poor function of the donor heart. In this case, the recipient's heart is left in place and the donor heart is placed next to it and they are joined together.

Postoperative Course

Heart transplant recipients constantly balance the risk of rejection with the risk of infection. They must adhere to a complex regimen of diet, medications, activity, follow-up laboratory studies, biopsies of the transplanted heart (to diagnose rejection), and clinic visits. Commonly, patients receive cyclosporine or tacrolimus, azathioprine or mycophenolate mofetil, and corticosteroids to minimize rejection.

The transplanted heart is denervated; it has no nerve connections to the recipient's body, and the sympathetic and vagus nerves do not affect the transplanted heart. The resting rate of the transplanted heart is approximately 70 to 90 beats/min, but it increases gradually if catecholamines are in the circulation. Patients must gradually increase and decrease their exercise (i.e., extended warm-up and cool-down periods), because 20 to 30 minutes may be required to achieve the desired heart rate. Atropine does not increase the heart rate of transplanted hearts.

Rejection is most common in the first 3 to 6 months following transplant, although the risk of infection continues to be a significant risk even after the first year because of the immunosuppressant medications. In addition to rejection and infection, other complications include posttransplant lymphoproliferative disease and the development of allograft vasculopathy or rapidly progressing atherosclerosis in the arteries of the transplanted heart. Osteoporosis frequently occurs as a side effect of the antirejection medications and pretransplantation dietary insufficiency and long-term sedentary lifestyle. Immunosuppressants and corticosteroids can cause weight gain, diabetes, dyslipidemia, kidney failure, and disturbances of the central nervous and gastrointestinal systems, and toxicity from immunosuppressants can occur.

Transplant recipients face a number of stressors, including (a) coping with complications such as graft rejection; (b) managing a complex posttransplant regimen consisting of multiple medications; exercise and dietary prescriptions; regular medical follow-up evaluations and laboratory tests; lifestyle restrictions related to smoking, alcohol, and other potentially harmful substances; (c) transitioning from their roles as patients who are critically ill or at end of life to roles and lifestyles that are less illness-focused; (d) psychological acceptance of the transplant and the fact that someone else lost their life when the patient regained theirs; and (e) coping with financial issues, such as the cost of surgery and medications.

INFLAMMATORY DISEASES OF THE HEART

Any of the heart's three layers can become inflamed or affected by a variety of causes including infections (viral, bacterial, fungal), inflammatory disorders (autoimmune diseases, connective tissue disorders, inflammatory bowel disease, drug-induced, postoperative (heart and lung surgeries), or idiopathic (no specific cause can be found). The diseases are named for the layer of the heart most involved in the infectious process: endocarditis (endocardium), myocarditis (myocardium), and pericarditis (pericardium) (see Fig. 15-14). These diseases may damage heart muscle, valves, or pericardium and impact cardiac function and, indirectly, quality of life. The ideal management for all infectious diseases is prevention.

ACUTE RHEUMATIC FEVER AND RHEUMATIC HEART DISEASE

Acute RF is a systemic inflammatory condition that is a complication of pharyngitis caused by Group A beta-hemolytic streptococcal (GAS), also called *Streptococcus pyogenes* and commonly known as strep throat. Acute RF almost always occurs in children or adolescents; however, because suspected strep throat is treated swiftly with antibiotics, it now occurs rarely in the United States.

Pathophysiology

Acute RF results in damage to connective tissues, especially in the heart, brain, joints, and skin. It is triggered by the body's immune response to GAS bacteria. It is thought that the immune system is unable to distinguish between

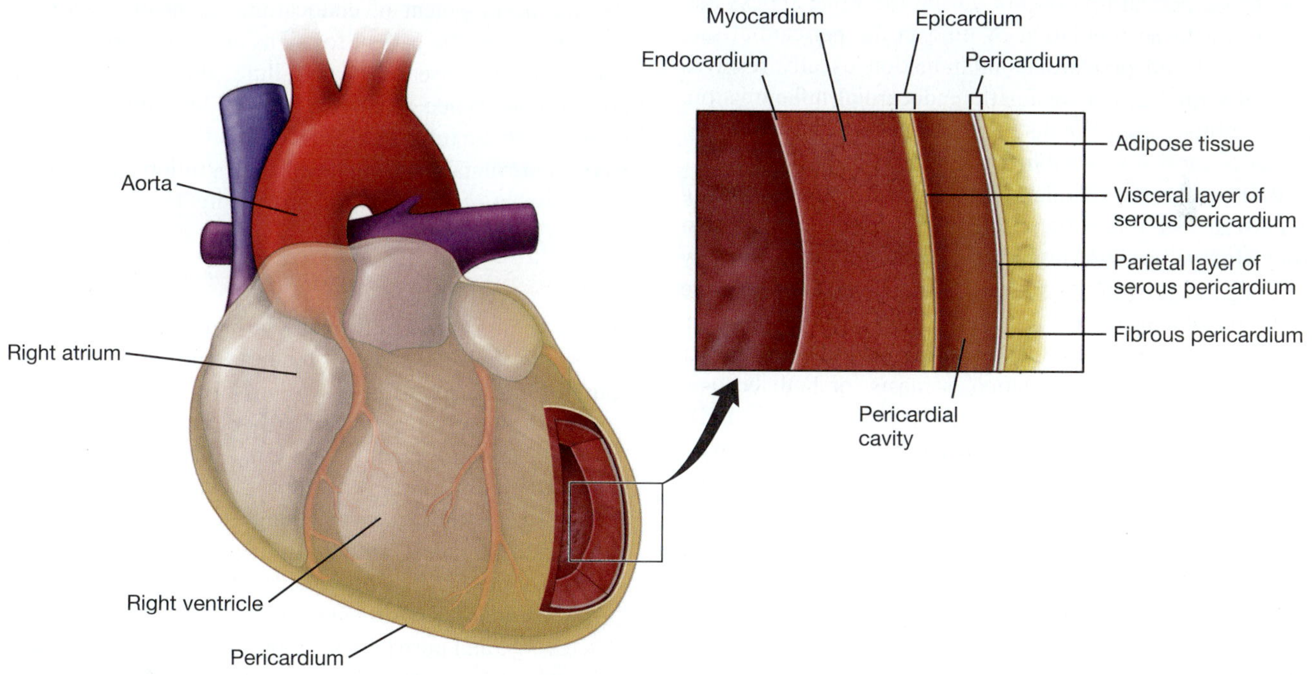

FIGURE 15-14 The layers of the heart. Layers of the heart and pericardium. This schematic diagram shows the anatomic relationship between the layers of the heart. In the middle mediastinum, the heart and roots of the great vessels are surrounded by the pericardium, which is often covered by highly variable amounts of adipose tissue. The pericardium has two layers: a tough external fibrous layer called the fibrous pericardium and a parietal layer of serous pericardium that lines its inner surface. The parietal layer of the serous pericardium is reflected back at the great vessels entering and leaving the heart as the visceral layer of the serous pericardium or epicardium. The epicardium lines the outer surface of the heart. The pericardial cavity is a space between the visceral and parietal layers of the serous pericardium, and it is lined by the mesothelial cells. Deep within the epicardium is the myocardium, which consists of cardiac muscle. Note the small amount of adipose tissue of the epicardium, which contains the coronary arteries and cardiac veins. The inner layer of the myocardium is called the endocardium, which is lined by the mesothelium with an underlying thin layer of connective tissue.

the invading bacteria and its own host tissues, resulting in inflammation and tissue damage. RHD is a condition in which permanent damage to the heart valves occurs from a prior episode of RF.

Clinical Manifestations and Assessment

Early symptoms include acute febrile illness accompanied by sore throat, and swollen glands. Two to four weeks later, polyarthritis and other manifestations including carditis, valvulitis, chorea, and subcutaneous nodules and erythema marginatum often develop. Polyarthritis occurs in 60% to 80% of cases, and swollen, tender, painful joints can persist for up to 4 weeks (Steer & Gibofsky, 2022). Erythema marginatum is a non-itchy macular rash on the trunk and proximal extremities that blanches with pressure, is not indurated, and does not scar. It often occurs with subcutaneous nodules: round, firm, painless bumps beneath the skin that usually disappear after 1 to 2 weeks. Patients also may develop chorea, which is characterized by spontaneous, purposeless movements of the trunk and extremities. Outbursts of crying or inappropriate laughing may also occur. Typically self-limiting, chorea can last for weeks to months.

Rheumatic carditis is inflammation of the pericardium, myocardium, or endocardium, separately or in combination. Rheumatic myocarditis can temporarily weaken the pumping ability of the heart and cause conduction abnormalities. Rheumatic pericarditis occurs during the acute illness and may result in accumulation of fluid in the pericardial sac. Myocardial and pericardial inflammation usually resolves without sequelae, but rheumatic endocardial inflammation, or valvulitis, often results in permanent adverse effects, primarily cardiac valve abnormalities.

RHD is chronic valvular disease caused by RF following an untreated strep infection. Progressive valvular dysfunction from RF develops into chronic valve disease in approximately 60% of patients with RF (Antunes, 2020). Stenosis of the valve causes blood to be forced through the valve at higher pressure, thus increasing the heart's workload. Heart murmurs characteristic of valvular regurgitation, stenosis, or both become audible on auscultation. Since most patients with RHD develop mitral insufficiency, a blowing, high-pitched holosystolic murmur is frequently heard. Diastolic murmurs are heard if AR occurs. Heart valve leaflets can thicken, causing them to shorten and preventing them from closing completely. This results in regurgitation of blood backward through the valve. Most commonly, this affects the mitral valve, although any of the heart valves may be affected. The myocardium compensates for some time, but as the valvular pathology progresses, compensatory mechanisms fail, and heart failure results.

Medical and Nursing Management

Throat cultures are necessary to diagnose the presence of a streptococcal infection. Secondary prevention of RHD occurs when strep throat is rapidly diagnosed and treated with antibiotics. If group A beta-hemolytic streptococcus is identified, aggressive treatment with penicillin for a 10-day course of therapy is prescribed. Clarithromycin or clindamycin may be prescribed for patients who are penicillin-allergic. Aspirin, or other anti-inflammatory medicines, is usually prescribed.

The revised Jones criteria help standardize the diagnosis of RF by classifying the signs of RF into major and minor categories. Having two major (e.g., polyarthritis, carditis, subcutaneous nodules, erythema marginata, or chorea) or one major and two minor (e.g., fever, elevated erythrocyte sedimentation rate [ESR] or serum C-reactive protein [CRP] level) clinical findings and a throat culture indicating recent infection with GAS pharyngitis indicate a high probability of RF.

Long-term antibiotic prophylaxis against group A strep is indicated in cases of known RF. People who have recovered from RF should have annual cardiac evaluations to identify the presence of new heart murmurs, which suggest the presence of RHD. The existence and extent of cardiac damage may not be fully apparent during the acute phase of RF but manifests later in life as RHD.

The diagnosis of RHD is typically confirmed by an echocardiogram which assesses the type and severity of valve dysfunction (regurgitation and/or stenosis), as well as size and function of the left and right ventricles. Trace or mild MR should be distinguished from pathologic (severe) regurgitation, as patients with mild valvular dysfunction may not require further treatment. However, there is risk of recurrent RF, the development of endocarditis or heart failure. The nurse monitors the patient for signs and symptoms of worsening valvular disease, heart failure, thromboemboli, and arrhythmias. When a new murmur is detected in a patient with a systemic infection, endocarditis should be suspected. RHD is preventable through early recognition and appropriate treatment of streptococcal pharyngitis to prevent RF.

INFECTIVE ENDOCARDITIS

IE is an inflammation of the endocardium, the membrane that lines the interior chambers of the heart and forms the valves, caused by a bacterial or less commonly, a fungal infection. Rarely, massive bacteremia or particularly virulent microorganisms cause endocarditis on normal valves, but usually the bacteria affix to a heart valve that is abnormal or damaged. Factors such as the presence of a prosthetic heart valve, a congenital cardiac defect, an intracardiac device, RHD or a previous episode of endocarditis, account for the majority of IE. Other conditions, such as intravenous substance use, immunosuppression, and nosocomial exposures, such as the presence of an indwelling central venous catheter, predispose the patient to IE because they can introduce bacteria into the bloodstream.

Pathophysiology

Eighty to 90% of IE is caused by gram-positive staphylococci, streptococci, and enterococci, bacteria that are commonly found on the skin and mouth. IE also can be fungal.

Systemic infection can result in IE, but pathogens also can enter the bloodstream because of surgical or dental procedures or through direct contamination, when a person who injects drugs (PWID) reuses a needle. Although constant blood flow in the heart prevents bacteria and fungi from adhering to endocardial surfaces, with IE the microbes colonize at and "stick" to the site of an abnormality or injury of the endocardium, such as a prolapsed mitral valve, a prosthetic valve, or an implanted device such as a pacemaker. Inflammation and infection result in endothelial damage; platelets, fibrin, blood cells, and the pathogens cluster as vegetations on the endocardium, commonly on heart valves. The vegetations are friable and fragments can break off, move through the bloodstream, and cause systemic or pulmonary embolization. Untreated, IE may erode through the endocardium into the underlying structures (e.g., valve leaflets), causing tears or deformities of valve leaflets, dehiscence of prosthetic valves, deformity of the chordae tendineae, or paravalvular abscesses (see Fig. 15-15).

IE is classified as acute or subacute. Acute IE has a rapid onset, occurring within days to weeks, and is characterized by high fever and chills. It can rapidly damage cardiac valves. Subacute IE occurs gradually, progresses slowly, and its course is prolonged. Often, the onset of IE is insidious, and signs and symptoms slowly develop from inflammation, destruction of the heart valves, and embolization of the vegetative growths on the heart.

Risk Factors

Pre-existing heart disease, including congenital heart defects such as a bicuspid aortic valve, a structural abnormality such as MVP, RHD, and age-related, degenerative valvular changes, increases the risk of developing IE. A cardiac valve with epithelial damage will attract bacteria to its surface, leading to endocardial infection. Central venous access devices and long-term indwelling catheters, such as those used for hemodialysis, are associated with the hospital-acquired IE. Intravenous substance use and body piercing are risk factors for IE (see Box 15-1).

Clinical Manifestations and Assessment

The clinical presentation of IE is variable, and symptoms are often vague and insidious. Fever over 38.0°C (100.4°F) is

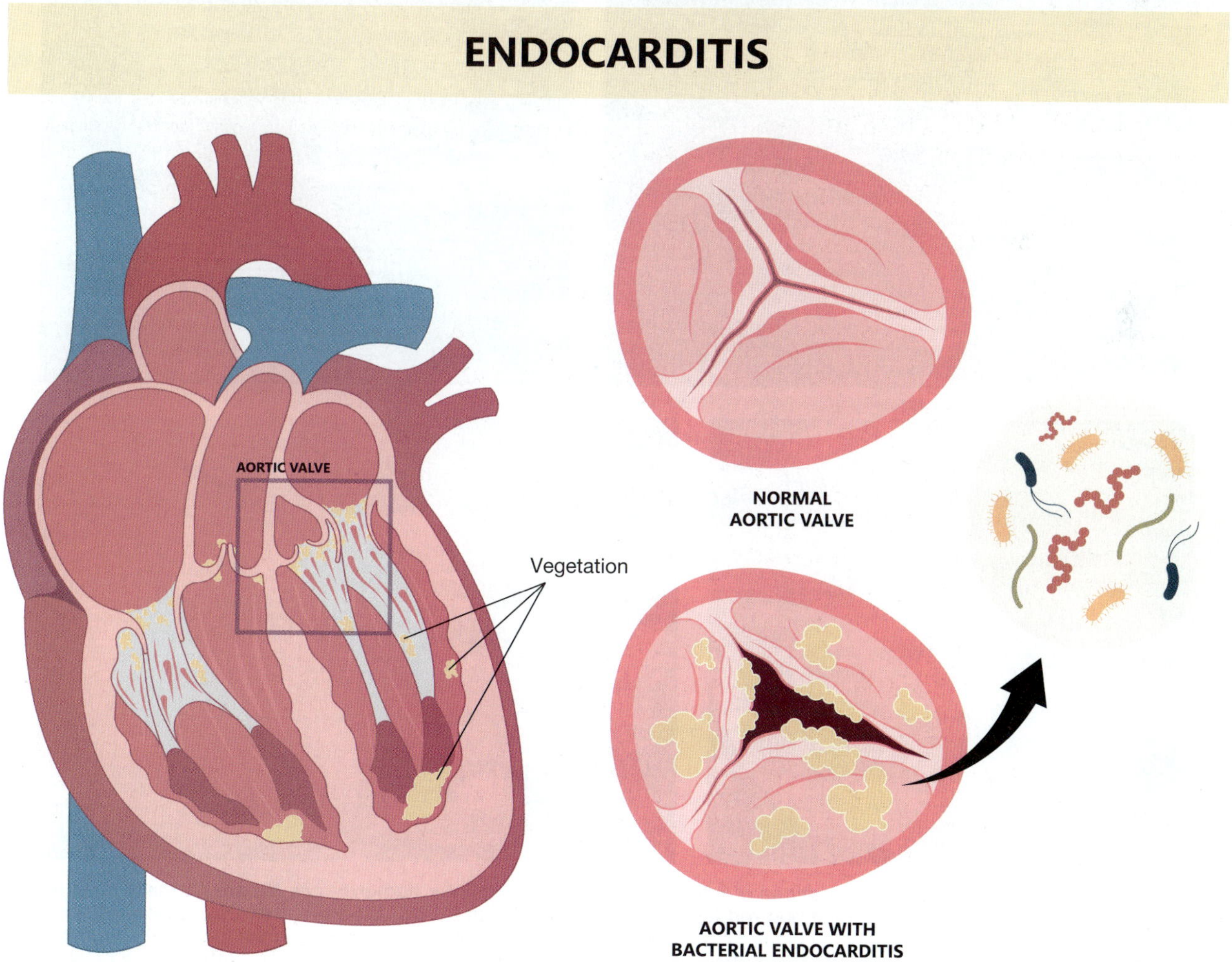

FIGURE 15-15 **Endocarditis. (From Shutterstock, ID: 2147874475.)**

BOX 15-1
Risk Factors for Infective Endocarditis

- Acquired valvular dysfunction
- Age over 60 years
- Body piercing
- Congenital heart disease
- History of infective endocarditis
- Indwelling, long-term use catheters, including parenteral nutrition lines, IV lines into the right atrium, hemodialysis catheters
- Intravenous drug use
- Prosthetic heart valves

the most common symptom, occurring in >90% of IE cases, but may be intermittent or absent, especially in patients who are receiving antibiotics, antipyretics or corticosteroids, or who are immunocompromised (Yallowitz & Decker, 2022). It can be associated with chills, anorexia, weight loss, dyspnea, myalgias, arthralgias, and night sweats. A heart murmur may be absent initially but develops in almost all patients. Murmurs that worsen over time are indicative of progressive damage from vegetations, and valve dysfunction can lead to heart failure. In fact, heart failure is the most frequent complication, occurring in up to 70% of patients (Philip & Bond, 2022).

In addition to fever and heart murmur, cutaneous signs may be present. Splinter hemorrhages may be seen under the fingernails and toenails, and petechiae may appear on the neck, chest, abdomen, conjunctiva, and mucous membranes. Osler nodes, Janeway lesions, and Roth spots are distinguishing signs of IE, and are the result of microembolization (see Fig. 15-16). Osler nodes are painful, erythematous nodules present on the pads of fingers or toes. Janeway lesions are painless, red or purple macules found on the palms and soles. Roth spots, seen on fundoscopic exam, are oval retinal hemorrhages with pale centers. Due to earlier diagnosis and improved treatment, these classic signs of IE are seen in less than 10% of patients with IE (Yallowitz & Decker, 2022). Central nervous system manifestations of IE include headache, transient cerebral ischemia, and strokes, caused by

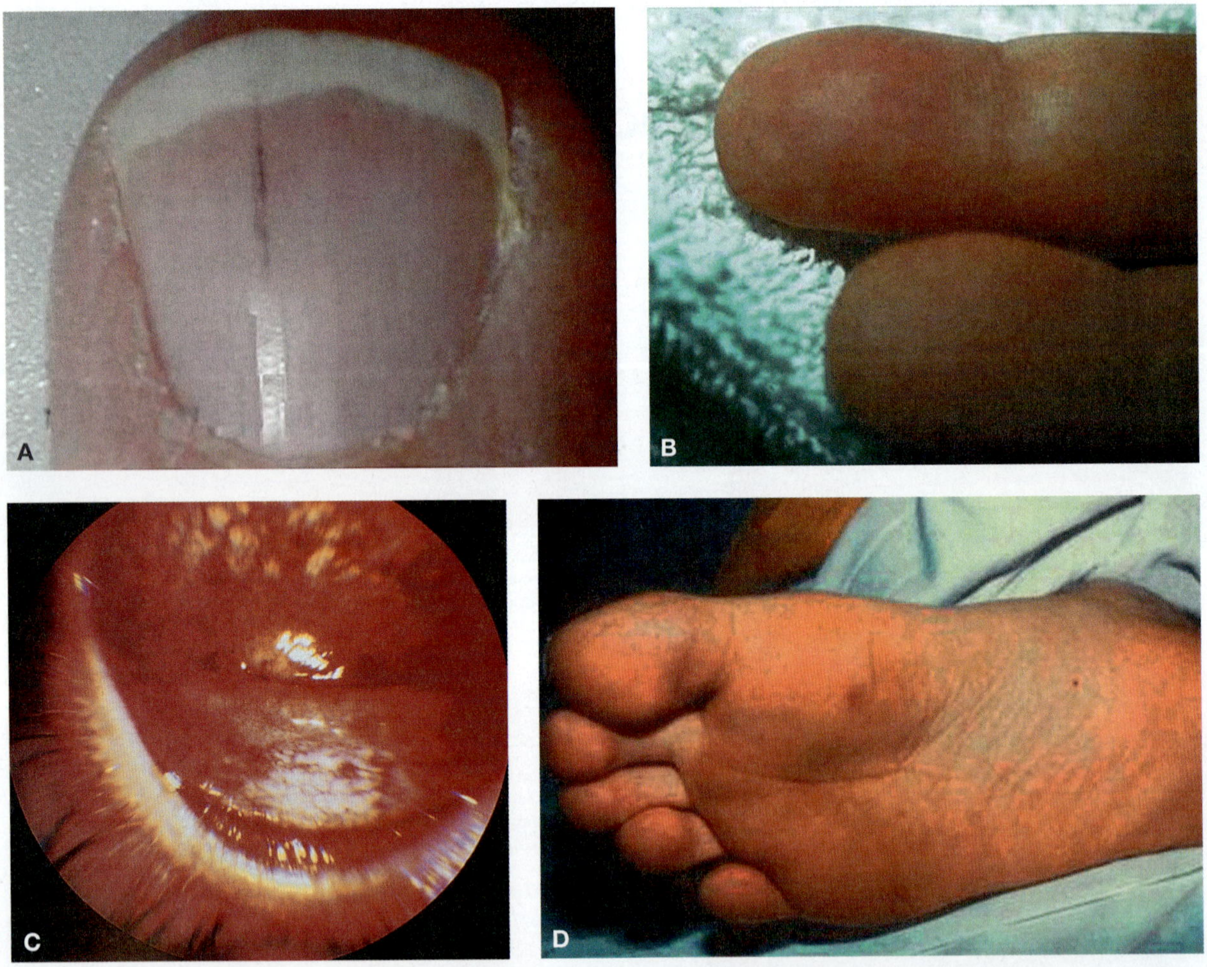

FIGURE 15-16 Common peripheral manifestations of infective endocarditis. Splinter hemorrhages **(A)** are normally seen under the fingernails or toenails. They are usually linear and red for the first 2 to 3 days and brownish thereafter. Osler's nodes **(B)** are tender subcutaneous nodules, often in the pulp of the digits or the thenar eminence (the fleshy prominence at the base of the thumb). **C.** Conjunctival petechiae. Janeway's lesions **(D)** are nontender erythematous, hemorrhagic, or pustular lesions, often on the palms or soles. (From Mylonakis, E., & Calderwood, S. B. [2001]. Infective endocarditis in adults. *New England Journal of Medicine, 345*, 1318–1330.)

emboli to the cerebral arteries. Embolization may be a presenting symptom; it may occur at any time and may involve other organ systems.

Positive blood cultures are highly sensitive for diagnosis; however, negative blood cultures do not definitely rule out IE, especially if a patient has received antibiotics or if slow-growing bacteria are present. The modified Duke Criteria are used to aid in the diagnosis of IE using physical examination findings, blood culture results and echocardiographic findings. Major clinical criteria are positive blood cultures and evidence of endocardial involvement. When these are supplemented by minor clinical criteria, such as predisposing cardiac conditions or IV substance use disorder, persistent fever without an alternative cause, systemic or pulmonary embolism, Osler nodes, or Roth spots, a diagnosis of IE can be made. A diagnosis of IE is established with two major criteria or one major and three minor criteria, or five minor criteria. A possible diagnosis of IE is made when one major and one minor or three minor criteria are present (Philip & Bond, 2022).

Echocardiography can detect the presence of vegetations or abscesses, prosthetic valve dehiscence, new regurgitation, or heart failure, and is recommended for all patients with suspected IE. Other abnormal findings include anemia, elevated white blood cell (WBC) count, elevated sedimentation rate (ESR), and elevated CRP. Abnormal ECG findings include atrioventricular blocks, bundle branch blocks, and fascicular blocks.

Medical and Nursing Management

Treatment of IE focuses on eliminating the infection and preventing complications. A prompt diagnosis followed by immediate institution of antibiotic therapy can reduce the risk of complications and the need for surgery. Antibiotics are initiated after blood cultures have been obtained. Treatment with a prolonged course of intravenous antibiotic therapy is targeted to the pathogen identified by the blood cultures; however, presumptive antibiotic treatment may be initiated while awaiting the blood culture results. Antibiotic therapy is administered for 6 weeks or more, particularly in cases involving a prosthetic valve, to ensure eradication of the infection. Many patients have peripherally inserted central catheters (PICCs) or other long-term IV access. Nursing management of patients with endocarditis includes prevention of the complications of long-term IV therapy. Invasive lines and wounds must be assessed for erythema (redness), tenderness, warmth, swelling, drainage, or other signs of infection. Blood cultures are taken periodically to monitor the effect of therapy, and serum levels of the selected antibiotic may be monitored. Despite advances in treatment, morbidity and mortality remain high (Rajani & Klein, 2020). Nurses should monitor vital signs and be alert for signs and symptoms that can indicate complications such as persistent infection, heart failure, kidney failure, or emboli. A new or worsening murmur may indicate dehiscence of a prosthetic valve, rupture of an abscess, or injury to valve leaflets. When IE is complicated by life-threatening conditions such as persistent or recurrent infection, cardiac failure, hemodynamic instability, large vegetations or emboli, myocardial abscess, or fungal endocarditis, surgical intervention is indicated. Most patients who have prosthetic valve endocarditis require valve replacement. If the patient has undergone surgical treatment, the nurse provides postoperative care and instructions. Patients with IV substance use pose additional challenges, as mortality is higher than in the general IE population and their care should be managed by a multidisciplinary care team that includes addiction specialists in addition to cardiac, cardiothoracic, and infectious diseases. Refer to Box 15-2.

The patient should be taught to recognize the symptoms of endocarditis and to seek medical assistance should symptoms recur. The patient and family should be instructed about medications as well as signs and symptoms of infection. The nurse provides the patient and family with emotional support and facilitates coping strategies during the prolonged course of the infection and antibiotic treatment. The nurse instructs all patients with IE about the importance of excellent daily dental hygiene and the highest-risk patients about the need for prophylactic antibiotic use before certain dental procedures.

Infectious Endocarditis Prophylaxis

Prevention of IE is important, and antibiotic prophylaxis is recommended prior to certain dental procedures for a subset of patients who are at highest risk of adverse outcomes. For patients with (1) a prosthetic cardiac valve or previous valve repair, (2) history of IE, (3) congenital heart disease with persistent risk of IE, and (4) heart transplantation with valvular disease, antibiotic prophylaxis is warranted for dental procedures that involve manipulation of gingival tissue, the periapical region of teeth, or perforation of the oral mucosa (Ferri, 2023). Antibiotic prophylaxis is ***not*** recommended for (1) routine anesthetic injections through noninfected tissue, (2) taking dental radiographs, or (3) placement or adjustment of removable prosthodontic or orthodontic appliances or for respiratory, gastrointestinal, urogenital, or skin/soft tissue procedures (Philip & Bond, 2022). The reasons for the changes in prophylaxis are related to the low incidence associated with the aforementioned procedures and the risk of the emergence of resistant organisms. Refer to Box 15-3 for indications for antibiotic prophylaxis.

MYOCARDITIS

Myocarditis is an inflammation of the heart muscle (myocardium), resulting from infectious and noninfectious sources. Viral infection, including SARS-CoV-2, is the most common cause, and bacterial infections, parasites, drug hypersensitivity reactions, environmental toxins, autoimmune responses, and peripartum cardiomyopathy also can

BOX 15-2

Nursing Research

Ray, V., Waite, M. R., Spexarth, F. C., Korman, S., Berget, S., Kodali, S., Kress, D., Guenther, N., & Murthy, V. S. (2020). Addiction management in hospitalized patients with intravenous drug use-associated infective endocarditis. *Psychosomatics*, *61*(6), 678–687. https://doi.org/10.1016/j.psym.2020.06.019

Purpose

Infections related to intravenous drug use and opioid use disorders (OUDs) are increasing nationwide. Endocarditis is a recognized complication of intravenous drug use, and inpatient treatment typically focuses on infection management without attention to underlying addiction.

Design

A comprehensive intervention for inpatients with infective endocarditis and intravenous drug use was implemented by a multidisciplinary team at a large midwestern hospital. The team included behavioral health/addiction medicine, infectious disease, pain medicine, cardiothoracic surgery, pharmacy, and nursing to address the OUD while managing the infection. The intervention was assessed by measuring the initiation of medication-assisted treatment and endocarditis-related readmissions. Patients were identified from the medical records using discharge diagnosis codes for OUDs and infective endocarditis. In addition to medical management of infective endocarditis, the multidisciplinary intervention included early involvement of addiction medicine and the pain management at the time of admission. Patient interventions included education, motivational interviewing, behavioral health engagement, collaborative pain management, individual/family therapy, medication evaluation, and initiation of medication-assisted treatment. Caregivers were also educated on OUDs and ways to support patients undergoing interventions.

Findings

Both the historical control group (N = 37) and the intervention group (N = 33) were comparable in age, gender, race, marital status, psychiatric history, and smoking but differed by employment status, religious affiliation, and use of psychiatric medications. At discharge, 18.9% of the control group and 54.5% in the intervention group were initiated on medication-assisted treatment for OUDs. No differences in readmission rates were found.

Nursing Implications

Multidisciplinary teams for treating inpatients with intravenous drug use and infective endocarditis are feasible and can increase the uptake of OUD-specific treatment.

lead to myocarditis. In some cases the cause is unknown, or idiopathic. Myocarditis can be fulminant, acute, subacute, or chronic. Mild cases of myocarditis with few symptoms are often self-limited and resolve without treatment, while more serious cases result in persistent cardiac dysfunction, cardiomyopathy or cardiogenic shock and death.

Pathophysiology

An immune-mediated process is initiated by cardiac tissue injury that results in cardiac inflammation. This leads to myocyte degeneration or necrosis (e.g., cardiac cell death). Myocyte damage causes the acute release of myocyte antigens and cytokines. Subsequently, T and B lymphocytes infiltrate the myocardium, and clear the virus. The immune response continues, and infected myocytes are lysed. Inflammation from an inappropriate immune response can cause myocyte necrosis that destroys heart muscle acutely. When inflammation and myocardial injury persist due to an autoimmune reaction, it can result in fibrosis and subsequent cardiac remodeling and can lead to DCM, heart failure, ventricular arrhythmias, and death (Cooper & Knowlton, 2021).

BOX 15-3

Indications for Infective Endocarditis Antibiotic Prophylaxis

- Prosthetic heart valve or previous heart valve repair
- Previous infective endocarditis
- Cardiac transplant recipients with a structurally abnormal valve with regurgitation
- Congenital heart disease with persistent risk of IE:
  - Unrepaired cyanotic congenital abnormalities
    - Completely repaired congenital defects with prosthetic material, during first 6 months after surgery
- Repaired congenital defects with residual defect adjacent to prosthetic material

Clinical Manifestations and Assessment

Clinical presentation can vary widely; symptoms can range from mild systemic findings of fever, myalgias, fatigue, cough, chest pain, palpitations and dyspnea to ventricular arrhythmias, heart failure, cardiogenic shock, DCM, and sudden cardiac death (SCD). Patients may report a history of recent respiratory infection or of rash following administration of a new drug or vaccine may be reported. Signs may be consistent with fluid overload: S3 gallop, JVD, peripheral edema, orthopnea, and tachycardia. Crackles (rales) may be detected with auscultation of lung fields. Hepatomegaly can occur when fluid overload backs up to the liver. There is evidence of poor perfusion including hypotension, altered mental status, and end-organ dysfunction in more severe presentations. Fulminant myocarditis is typically preceded by a viral syndrome and presents with sudden-onset signs and symptoms consistent with impending cardiogenic shock.

Serum B-type natriuretic peptide (BNP) and troponin levels are commonly elevated. CRP and ESR may be elevated and eosinophilia may be seen on the WBC count. Echocardiography is used to determine the presence and degree of LV dysfunction when myocarditis is suspected and may show nonspecific findings or demonstrate impaired heart muscle function or pericardial effusion. Chest radiography may reveal cardiomegaly (enlarged heart) and evidence of pulmonary congestion. Arrhythmias and LV hypertrophy may be detected by an ECG. Endomyocardial biopsy can be used to confirm diagnosis; however, because of significant risks to the patient with obtaining a myocardial tissue sample, this should only be utilized in certain cases when a confirmatory diagnosis is needed to guide the appropriate selection of treatment.

Medical and Nursing Management

For patients with myocarditis, supportive care is of primary importance with a goal of maintaining hemodynamic stability and improving symptoms. Treatment is directed at the cause, when known. ACE-Is, ARBs, BBs, and diuretics are prescribed to treat heart failure symptoms when present. If an autoimmune process is suspected, steroids or immune globulin may be prescribed to reduce inflammation. Severe cases will require hemodynamic support with inotropic medications. Surgical options, such as the placement of a VAD or TAH or heart transplantation, should be considered when there is no improvement in symptoms or hemodynamic status despite maximal medical therapy.

Nursing care of the patient with myocarditis focuses on limiting myocardial oxygen demand. Bedrest and supplemental oxygen may be indicated to decrease the heart's workload. Physical assessment should focus on the early identification of worsening signs and symptoms of heart failure. In addition to monitoring vital signs, oxygenation, heart and lung sounds, peripheral perfusion, and fluid status. The nurse must assess for the development of arrhythmias and hemodynamic compromise and be prepared to use emergency equipment as there is a high risk for life-threatening ventricular arrhythmias. The nurse must also provide emotional support to the patient and family; myocarditis can be particularly stressful due to its variable presentation and course. In more severe cases, nurses should educate and prepare the patient for VADs. Prior to discharge, patients should be advised of any activity restrictions, taught to recognize signs and symptoms of heart failure and instructed to contact 911 for worsening symptoms.

PERICARDITIS

Pericarditis is an inflammation of the pericardium, the membranous sac surrounding the heart. The pericardium holds the heart in place, prevents it from overexpanding if blood volume increases, reduces friction between the heart and surrounding tissues, and protects the heart from infection and malignancy (see Figs. 15-14 and 15-17). Pericarditis can be infectious (viral, bacterial, or fungal) or noninfectious. Most pericarditis is idiopathic and assumed to be caused by viral infection (Dababneh & Siddique, 2022). Causes of the less common, noninfectious pericarditis include acute MI, chest trauma or cardiac surgery, autoimmune disorders, medications (e.g., isoniazid, hydralazine), and malignancy. A list of the most frequently occurring causes of pericarditis is provided in Box 15-4.

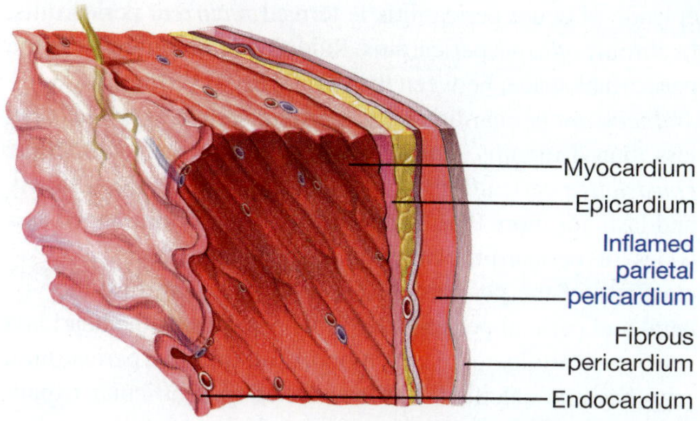

FIGURE 15-17 **Tissue changes in pericarditis. Normally, the epicardium and pericardium slide over each other easily because they are lubricated by a small amount of fluid. Thicker material replaces this fluid in pericarditis.**

Pathophysiology

The pericardial sac consists of two layers, the parietal (outer) layer and the visceral (inner) layer that is affixed to the heart. A small amount of fluid (15 to 50 mL) separates the layers. Acute pericarditis develops rapidly, occurring when the pericardial sac becomes inflamed. Pericarditis may lead to *pericardial effusion*, an accumulation of fluid in the pericardial space. This may result in increased pressure on the heart, leading to cardiac tamponade (refer to Chapter 14).

Acute pericarditis is the first episode of pericardial inflammation, and pericarditis that reappears 4 to 6 weeks after an

BOX 15-4 Causes of Pericarditis

- Acute myocardial infarction (MI)
- Bacterial infection (e.g., streptococci, staphylococci, meningococci)
- Cancer, particularly metastasis to the heart from lung or breast tumors or lymphoma
- Chest trauma: chest injury, invasive cardiac procedures, such as implantation of pacemaker or defibrillator (ICD) or cardiac surgery,
- Disorders of adjacent structures: dissecting aneurysm, pulmonary disease (e.g., pneumonia)
- Fungal infection (e.g., *Aspergillus, Candida, Histoplasma*)
- Idiopathic
- Medications (e.g., procainamide, hydralyzine, and isoniazid)
- Metabolic disorders, primarily kidney failure and uremia
- Radiation therapy of chest and upper torso, especially for breast cancer, lung cancer, or lymphoma (peak occurrence 5–9 months after treatment)
- Rheumatic diseases (systemic lupus erythematosus, rheumatoid arthritis, and mixed connective tissue disease)
- Viral infection (e.g., coxsackie, hepatitis B, influenza, mononucleosis, mumps, varicella)

episode of acute pericarditis is termed *recurrent* pericarditis. In chronic *effusive* pericarditis, fluid slowly accumulates in the pericardial space, between the two layers of the pericardium.

Incessant pericarditis lasts approximately 4 to 6 weeks but less than 3 months. The symptoms are continuous. Chronic *constrictive* pericarditis is rare and typically develops slowly and lasts for more than 3 months. Frequent or prolonged episodes of pericarditis can lead to thickening and decreased elasticity of the pericardium, and scarring may fuse the visceral and parietal pericardium. This compresses the heart and restricts its ability to fill with blood. Over time, the pericardium may become calcified, further restricting ventricular expansion during diastole. With less filling, the ventricles pump less blood, leading to decreased CO and signs and symptoms of heart failure. Because higher pressure is required to fill the compressed heart, pressure increases in the veins that return blood to the heart. This increased systemic venous pressure will lead to peripheral edema and liver failure.

Clinical Manifestations and Assessment

Chest pain, frequently severe, is the most common symptom of acute pericarditis. Dyspnea unrelated to exertion is typical of pericarditis; SOB occurs as a result of pericardial compression from cardiac tamponade. Irritation of the pericardium causes pain that is typically persistent, sharp, pleuritic, and retrosternal. Although usually felt in the midchest, it may be localized to the left anterior chest, radiate to the neck, shoulders, or arms. In contrast to myocardial ischemic pain, the discomfort is pleuritic, and worsens with deep inspiration, coughing, lying down, or turning. It is characteristically relieved by leaning forward or sitting because that position reduces pressure on the parietal pericardium. Although not heard in all patients with pericarditis, a common finding in approximately 35% to 85% of cases, is a creaky or scratchy friction rub (Dababneh & Siddique, 2022). Fever and a nonproductive cough may be present.

Pearls for Practice

A pericardial friction rub is diagnostic of pericarditis. It has a creaky, grating, or scratchy sound, is louder at the end of exhalation. Nurses can assess for the presence of a pericardial friction rub by placing the diaphragm of the stethoscope tightly against the thorax and auscultating the left lower sternal border (LLSB) in the fourth intercostal space, the site where the pericardium comes into contact with the left chest wall. The rub is best heard when the patient is sitting and leaning forward. The friction rub is caused by the inflamed layers of the pericardium rubbing against each other and is often intermittent.

A diagnosis of acute pericarditis is made if at least two of the following are present: pleuritic chest pain, pericardial friction rub, 12-lead ECG demonstrating widespread ST elevation without reciprocal changes or T-wave inversion, and a new or worsening pericardial effusion. Chest radiograph (CXR) may reveal enlargement of the cardiac silhouette (Ridley, 2019) and echocardiography is done to assess for pericardial effusion or tamponade, but the absence of effusion does not exclude pericarditis. Elevated WBC count, ESR, and CRP are laboratory signs of inflammation, but they are not sensitive or specific for acute pericarditis. Troponin may be used to rule out myocarditis.

Medical and Nursing Management

The goals of management are to provide symptom relief, reduce inflammation, prevent recurrence and detect signs and symptoms of cardiac tamponade. If the underlying cause is known, it should be treated; however, typically it is not necessary to confirm the etiology as most pericarditis is viral, resolves without sequelae, and may be managed in the outpatient setting. Patients with any high-risk feature, including fever >38°C, subacute onset, large pericardial effusion or tamponade, lack of response to anti-inflammatory therapy after 1 week of treatment, or evidence of myocardial involvement should be admitted to the hospital for treatment. Additional predictors of elevated risk include immunosuppression, oral anticoagulation, and trauma. Nonsteroidal anti-inflammatory medications (NSAIDs) and aspirin constitute first-line treatment for acute pericarditis. In addition, a 3-month course of colchicine (with weight-adjusted dosing) is recommended to reduce the risk of recurrent pericarditis. Strenuous activity should be avoided. Corticosteroids can be prescribed when the patient does not respond to NSAIDs and colchicine, but corticosteroids may prolong the course of recovery or can increase the risk of a recurrent pericarditis, so they are not typically used for initial management of acute pericarditis. Rarely, in some cases of constrictive pericarditis, surgical removal of the pericardium (pericardiectomy) may be necessary to provide relief from restrictive inflammation and scarring and to prevent impaired diastolic filling and subsequent severe heart failure with preserved EF.

In addition to pain management, patients with acute pericarditis benefit from positioning: sitting upright and leaning forward will relieve pressure on the pericardium. Patients with chest pain often benefit from psychological support, and reassurance that the chest pain they are experiencing is not a heart attack. The nurse educates patients about the importance of adherence to their prescribed medications to reduce the risk of recurrent and incessant pericarditis, possible side effects of medications and when to seek emergent care.

Pearls for Practice

The mnemonic "CUPS" reminds the nurse of the four potential pharmacologic therapies and management approaches in pericarditis where C refers to Colchicine, U refers to treating Underlying causes, P refers to pain relievers in the form of nonsteroidal anti-inflammatory drugs (NSAIDs) as well as proton pump inhibitors to serve as gastric protection with the use of NSAIDs, and S refers to potential use of steroids (El Hussein & Ha, 2021).

Complications

Nurses caring for patients with pericarditis must be aware of the potential of serious complications. The two major complications of pericarditis are pericardial effusion, the accumulation of fluid in the pericardial sac, and cardiac tamponade, compression of the heart from excessive fluid buildup (refer to Chapter 14).

NURSING PROCESS
The Patient With Pericarditis

ASSESSMENT

Pain is the primary symptom of the patient with pericarditis, and it is assessed while repositioning the patient. The nurse tries to identify whether the pain is influenced by inspiration or expiration; breath holding; flexion, extension, or rotation of the spine and neck; by movements of the shoulders and arms; and by coughing or swallowing. Recognizing that deep inspiration or coughing intensifies pain may help to differentiate the pain of pericarditis from the pain of MI. To distinguish a pericardial friction rub from a pleural friction rub, the patient is asked to hold their breath; a pericardial friction rub will continue. A pericardial friction rub occurs when the pericardial surfaces lose their lubricating fluid because of inflammation. The rub is audible on auscultation and is synchronous with the heartbeat but is often intermittent and does not always occur. The patient's temperature is monitored frequently. Pericarditis may cause an abrupt onset of fever in a patient who has been afebrile.

DIAGNOSIS

Based on the assessment data, a major nursing diagnosis may be:

- Acute pain related to inflammation of the pericardium

PLANNING

The nursing plan focuses on two goals: pain relief and absence of complications.

NURSING INTERVENTIONS

PAIN RELIEF

Relief of pain is achieved by chair rest because sitting upright and leaning forward is the posture that tends to relieve pain. It is important to instruct the patient to restrict activity until the pain subsides. As the chest pain and friction rub abate, activities of daily living may be resumed gradually. If the patient is taking analgesics or colchicine for the pericarditis, their responses are monitored and recorded. Patients taking NSAIDs are assessed for gastrointestinal adverse effects. If chest pain and friction rub recur, bed rest or chair rest is resumed.

MONITORING AND MANAGING POTENTIAL COMPLICATIONS

Pericardial Effusion. Fluid that accumulates between the pericardial linings or in the pericardial sac is called *pericardial effusion* (see Chapter 14). The fluid can constrict the myocardium and impair its ability to pump. CO declines with each contraction. Failure to identify and treat this problem can lead to cardiac tamponade and possible sudden death.

Cardiac Tamponade. The first symptoms of cardiac tamponade are often SOB, chest tightness, dizziness, or restlessness. Assessment of blood pressure may reveal a pulsus paradoxus, a decrease of 10 mm Hg or more in the systolic blood pressure during inspiration. Usually, the systolic pressure decreases and the diastolic pressure remains stable; hence, pulse pressure narrows. The patient may have tachycardia, and the ECG voltage may be decreased or the QRS complexes may alternate in height (electrical alternans). Heart sounds may progress from distant to imperceptible. Neck vein distention and other signs of rising central venous pressure develop. These signs occur as the fluid-filled pericardial sac compresses the myocardium. Blood continues to return to the heart from the periphery but cannot flow into the heart to be pumped back into the circulation. The nurse notifies the provider immediately and prepares to assist with diagnostic echocardiography and pericardiocentesis (see Chapter 14). The nurse stays with the patient and continues to assess and record signs and symptoms while intervening to decrease patient anxiety.

EVALUATION

Expected patient outcomes include:

1. Freedom from pain
   a. Performs activities of daily living without pain, fatigue, or SOB
   b. Temperature returns to normal range
   c. Exhibits no pericardial friction rub
2. Absence of complications
   a. Sustains blood pressure in normal range
   b. Has heart sounds that are strong and can be auscultated
   c. No evidence of effusion or tamponade

CHAPTER REVIEW

NCLEX-Style Review Questions

1. Severe aortic stenosis is associated with which of the following findings? Select all that apply.
   a. Pulmonary edema
   b. Increased CO
   c. Decreased left ventricular pressure
   d. Left ventricular hypertrophy
   e. Elevated left atrial pressures

2. Which of the following are symptoms associated with AS? Select all that apply.
   a. Dyspnea
   b. Diastolic murmur
   c. Syncope
   d. Angina
   e. Seizures

3. Management of patients with cardiomyopathy is directed at preventing and treating heart failure. The treatment of heart failure includes which of the following? Select all that apply.
   a. Reducing circulating blood volume
   b. Reducing myocardial oxygen needs
   c. Increasing CO by improving contractility or reducing peripheral resistance
   d. Increasing preload
   e. Increasing myocardial oxygen needs

4. Which of the following are indications for a ventricular assist device (VAD) as a bridge to recovery. Select all that apply.
   a. Acute myocarditis
   b. Cardiogenic shock following an acute myocardial infarction
   c. End-stage heart failure
   d. Failure to wean from cardiopulmonary bypass following cardiac surgery
   e. An inability to tolerate anticoagulation

5. A patient presents with chest pain. Acute myocardial infarction is excluded and the patient is diagnosed with pericarditis. Which of the following medications would the provider be most likely to prescribe initially? Select all that apply.
   a. Acetaminophen (Tylenol)
   b. Ibuprofen (Motrin)
   c. Colchicine
   d. Broad-spectrum antibiotic
   e. Coumadin (Warfarin)

REFERENCES AND SELECTED READINGS

References and selected readings associated with this chapter can be found on the website that accompanies the book. Visit **http://thepoint.lww.com/Honan3e** to access the references and other additional resources associated with this chapter.

CHAPTER 16

Nursing Management: Patients With Arrhythmias and Conduction Problems

Catherine G. Winkler

Learning Objectives

After reading this chapter, you will be able to:

1. Describe methods to monitor, diagnose, and treat arrhythmias.
2. Analyze elements of an electrocardiogram (ECG) rhythm strip: atrial and ventricular rate, atrial and ventricular rhythm, P wave and shape, PR interval, the QRS complex and shape, QRS duration and QT interval, and the ST interval.
3. Identify the ECG criteria, causes, and management of several arrhythmias, including conduction disturbances.
4. Use the nursing process as a framework for care of patients with arrhythmias.
5. Compare and contrast the different types of electrical therapies, their uses, possible complications, and nursing implications.
6. Describe the key points of using a defibrillator and the associated waveforms.
7. Identify the clinical indications for pacemakers and implantable cardioverter defibrillators (ICDs).
8. Identify the electrophysiology diagnostic studies and interventional procedures that patients undergo to treat arrhythmias (e.g., catheter ablation).
9. Identify the transcatheter structural interventions where postprocedural monitoring is recommended.
10. Describe the patient education that is indicated for patients who experience arrhythmias.
11. Consider the importance of the ethical implications of deactivation of cardiovascular implantable electronic devices (CIEDs) at end of life.
12. Describe the impact of COVID-19 on the conduction system and the management of arrhythmias.

Arrhythmias (also called *dysrhythmias*) are disorders of the electrical impulse within the heart that cause disturbances of heart rate, heart rhythm, or both. Without a normal rate and regular rhythm, the heart does not perform efficiently as a pump to circulate oxygenated blood. Arrhythmias may initially produce symptoms related to the hemodynamic effect they cause, such as a decrease in cardiac output. Refer to Table 16-1 for signs and symptoms of a decreased cardiac output. In addition to decreasing the cardiac output, some arrhythmias increase the risk of clot formation within the chambers of the heart. Arrhythmias are usually named according to the site of origin of the impulse (e.g., atria or ventricle) and the mechanism of formation or conduction involved (bradycardia [too slow], tachycardia [too fast], premature [early], etc.) and syndromes associated with it. Arrhythmias confirmed by an electrocardiogram (ECG) can be paroxysmal in nature and occur without signs or symptoms leading to a difficulty in estimating prevalence. The presence of an arrhythmia is confirmed by ECG and it can be associated with a higher morbidity and mortality (Desai & Hajouli, 2022).

THE ELECTROCARDIOGRAM

The electrical impulse that travels through the heart can be viewed by means of an ECG. Each phase of the cardiac cycle is reflected by specific waveforms (discussed later in the chapter). The number and placement of the electrodes used depend on the type of ECG needed. The electrodes record waveforms that appear on the paper or monitor and represent the electrical current in relation to the two electrodes (Fig. 16-1). Heart rate and rhythm may be monitored

TABLE **16-1 Signs and Symptoms of Decreased Cardiac Output**

System	Signs and Symptoms of Decreased Cardiac Output
Respiratory	Tachypnea, shortness of breath (SOB), orthopnea, dyspnea on exertion (DOE), hypoxemia, crackles on lung auscultation, wheeze, dry or productive cough
Cardiac and peripheral vascular	Edema, jugular vein distention (JVD), displaced point of maximum impulse (PMI), S_3 gallop rhythm, tricuspid and/or mitral regurgitation murmurs, hypotension, decreased mean arterial pressure (MAP), narrow pulse pressure, cool skin and extremities, delayed capillary refill, tachycardia
Renal	Decreased urinary output, oliguria, rising creatinine
Gastrointestinal	Abdominal distention, ascites, liver engorgement, positive abdominojugular reflex
Central nervous	Dizziness, decreased sensorium, syncope, fatigue
Behavioral/emotional	Anxiety, restlessness

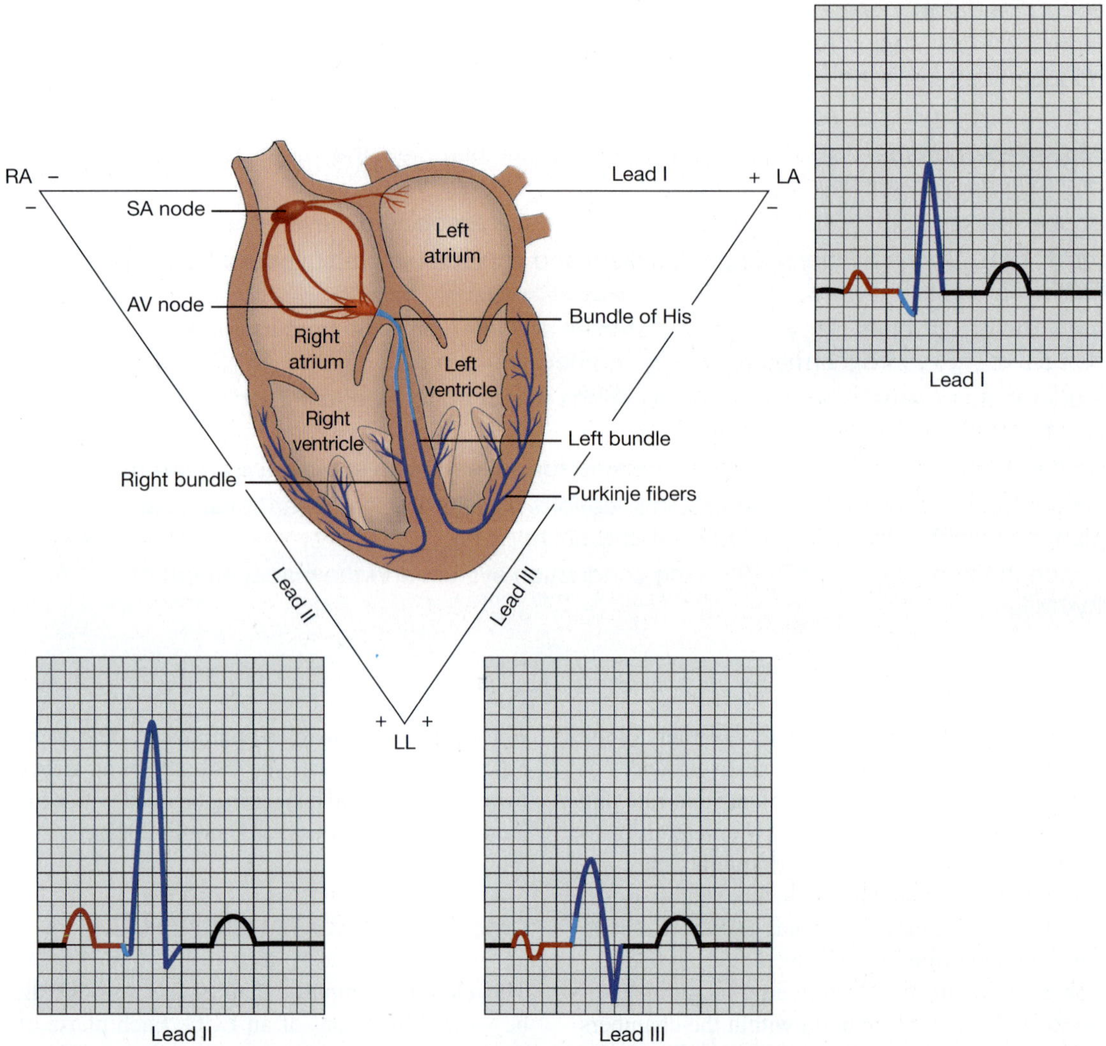

FIGURE 16-1 **Relationship of electrocardiogram (ECG) complex, lead system, and electrical impulse. The heart conducts electrical activity, which the ECG measures and records. The configurations of electrical activity displayed on the ECG vary depending on the lead (or view) of the ECG and on the rhythm of the heart. Therefore, the configuration of a normal rhythm tracing from lead I will differ from the configuration of a normal rhythm tracing from lead II, lead II will differ from lead III, and so on. The same is true for abnormal rhythms and cardiac disorders. To make an accurate assessment of the heart's electrical activity or to identify where, when, and what abnormalities occur, the ECG needs to be evaluated from every lead, not just from lead II. Here the different areas of electrical activity are identified by color. RA, right arm; LA, left arm; SA, sinoatrial; AV, atrioventricular; LL, left leg.**

BOX 16-1

Understanding Electrodes, Wires, and Leads

Electrodes

Electrodes are electrical contacts that are placed on the patient's skin. They come in various shapes. Today's electrodes are disposable for single patient use. They all contain conductive gel and a connector for a wire.

Wires

The electrode is connected to a recording device by a set of wires or cables. The wires are color coded, although the coding system is not internationally consistent. For 12-lead ECGs, there are 10 wires, one for each electrode. For continuous monitoring, there may be anywhere from three to five wires. Three- and four-wire systems allow monitoring of limb leads only, whereas five-wire systems allow monitoring of limb leads plus a chest lead. Some wires come preattached to the electrodes and are disposable; others need to be attached to the electrode and are reusable.

Leads

Leads are the images the nurse sees on the paper or monitor. They represent an examination of the heart from a specific viewpoint. The direction of the ECG complex varies depending on which lead is viewed. The direction of the electric current determines how the waveforms appear on paper.

effectively through only two electrodes; however, the use of 10 electrodes (resulting in 12 leads) provides more detailed information and is the basis for understanding other types of electrocardiographic monitoring. The difference between electrodes, wires, and leads is described in Box 16-1.

THE 12-LEAD ELECTROCARDIOGRAM

An ECG contains information about the contraction and relaxation of heart chambers. This diagnostic information could vary over time because of changes in the patients' condition that are associated with either the resolution of or the addition of a new cardiac problem. The 12-lead ECG is a diagnostic tool that uses 10 electrodes: one placed on each limb and six placed on the chest (precordial). In combination, these 10 electrodes produce 12 different waveforms (or leads). These 12 leads include three bipolar leads (I, II, III) and nine unipolar leads (aVR, aVL, aVF, V_1–V_6). Bipolar leads measure electrical activity traveling between a positive and negative electrode, while unipolar leads record electrical activity from a single reference point. Together, the 12 leads show electrical activity in both a frontal plane and a transverse plane. When viewed together, these two planes provide important diagnostic information beyond heart rate and rhythm, including conduction abnormalities such as bundle branch block (BBB), heart chamber enlargement, localization of ischemia or infarction, and even noncardiac conditions. These noncardiac conditions include but are not limited to electrolyte imbalances, postconscious sedation, a neurologic event, drugs, toxins, or hypothermia (Sandau et al., 2017; Lough et al., 2022). The 12-lead ECG produces an image of the entire heart, whereas particular leads view specific areas of the heart.

Electrode placement for a 12-lead ECG must be accurate and consistent as misplacement can result in altered waveforms, which can lead to an inaccurate diagnosis and treatment. Electrode placement is important in arrhythmia identification and is crucial in identifying changes related to ischemia (decreased blood flow often due to atherosclerosis), infarction (cellular damage or death because of limited blood supply), and many arrhythmias. In addition, electrode placement is important for customization to the patient to ensure that clinically relevant data are obtained through placing electrodes strategically on the person to capture and view the best clinical ECG data.

The four limb electrodes are placed on the lower legs, near the ankles, and on the arms, near the wrists. The remaining six electrodes are placed across the left side of the chest. Locating the specific anatomical landmark is critical for correct chest electrode placement (Box 16-2). Further, if the patient needs a series of ECGs, consistency of electrode placement is key for the analysis of the ECG over time. In some cases, the chest electrodes are left in place, or the correct location is marked with an indelible pen to ensure the identical placement for follow-up ECGs.

The specific locations for electrode placement are shown in Figure 16-2.

- V_1 Right side of the sternum, fourth intercostal space
- V_2 Left side of the sternum, fourth intercostal space
- V_3 Midway between V_2 and V_4
- V_4 Midclavicular line, fifth intercostal space (under the breast in females)
- V_5 Left anterior axillary line, same level as V_4
- V_6 Left midaxillary line, same level as V_4.

BOX 16-2

Correct Electrode Placement

Too often, arbitrary markings are used to determine rib positions, such as the areola of the breast. Valid ECG monitoring requires counting ribs for correct placement of electrodes. Begin by finding the sternal notch and slowly move your finger down the manubrium, until a rise is noted. Next, move your hand laterally from the rise until you note the rib at the sternal margin; this is the second rib. Underneath this rib is the second intercostal space (ICS). Count down two more ribs to the fourth ICS and place V_1 electrode on right side of sternum and V_2 on left side of sternum. V_3 electrode will be placed midway between V_2 and V_4. The V_4 electrode is placed at the fifth ICS at the midclavicular line. The V_5 electrode is placed at the same level of V_4 at the left anterior axillary line, and the V_6 electrode is at same level as V_4 and V_5 at the left midaxillary line. It may be helpful to mark this placement for consistent ECG placements in the future.

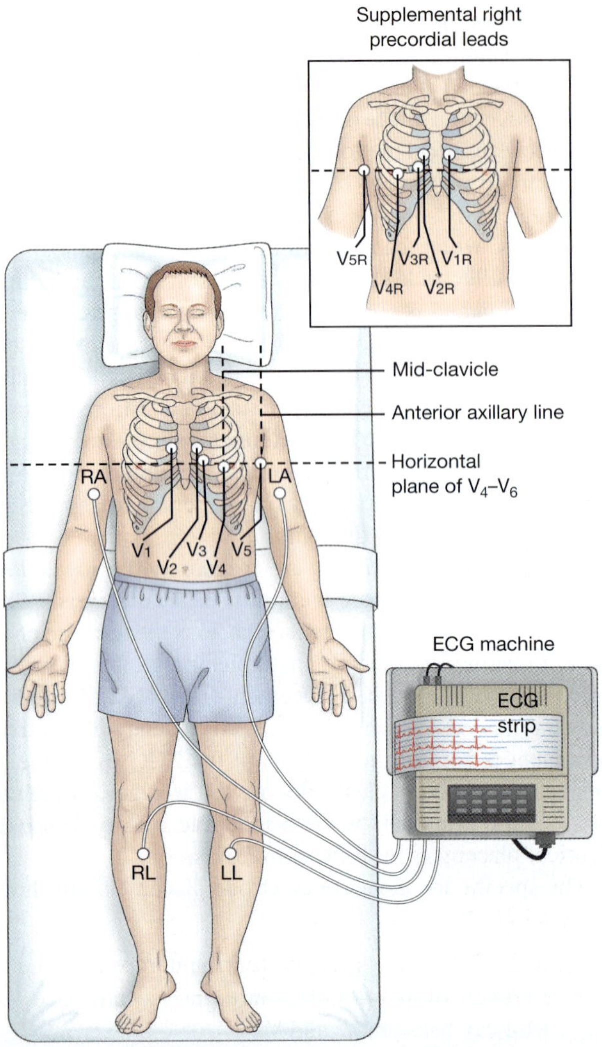

FIGURE 16-2 **ECG electrode placement. The standard left precordial leads are V_1—fourth intercostal space, right sternal border; V_2—fourth intercostal space, left sternal border; V_3—diagonally between V_2 and V_4; V_4—fifth intercostal space, left midclavicular line; V_5—same level as V_4, anterior axillary line; V_6 (not illustrated)—same level as V_4 and V_5, midaxillary line. The right precordial leads, placed across the right side of the chest, are the mirror opposite of the left leads. RA, right arm; LA, left arm; RL, right leg; LL, left leg. (Adapted from Molle, E. A., Kronenberger, J., West-Stack, C., & Durham, L. S. [2005].** ***Lippincott Williams & Wilkins' pocket guide to medical assisting*** **[2nd ed.]. Lippincott Williams & Wilkins.)**

The precordial (anterior surface over the heart) leads reflect the electrical activity primarily in the left ventricle. In some circumstances, an alternative electrode placement may be required. For example, in patients with suspected right-sided heart damage, right-sided chest leads are required to evaluate the right ventricle (see Fig. 16-2). Electrodes for V_1R (R refers to the right side of the chest) through V_6R are placed in the mirror image of the electrodes on the left side of the chest as detailed here:

V_1R	Left side of the sternum, fourth intercostal space
V_2R	Right side of the sternum, fourth intercostal space
V_3R	Midway between V_2 and V_4
V_4R	Midclavicular line, fifth intercostal space (under the breast in females)
V_5R	Right anterior axillary line, same level as V_4
V_6R	Right midaxillary line, same level as V_4

CONTINUOUS MONITORING

Targeted or patient-centric ECG monitoring is best applied when an immediate assessment of the patient can be made to determine the optimal monitoring level. Based on the admission diagnosis and changes in the clinical course during hospitalization, ongoing medical decisions are predicated on the goals of care and specific interventions. Patients are monitored for a variety of reasons: to detect changes in the patient's clinical condition, to diagnose a problem, to assess a response to an intervention, to prevent an undesirable event, for surveillance before and after cardiac surgery and transcatheter aortic valve replacement (TAVR), and for the presence of medication-induced changes to the ECG such as Q-T interval lengthening. Specifically, the goals of electrocardiographic monitoring have grown from just heart rate and rhythm determination to the diagnosis of complex arrhythmias, silent myocardial ischemia, and drug-induced QT interval prolongation (Sandau et al., 2017).

The American Heart Association (AHA) practice standards for ECG monitoring in the hospital setting were last published in 2017 by Sandau and colleagues and provide direction in deciding which patients are best served by cardiac monitoring during an episode of illness. Significant changes have occurred from the 2004 practice guidelines (Drew et al., 2004) with the original AHA (Sandau et al., 2017) and current standards that address the newer concern of overuse and underuse of ECG monitoring with the problem of alarm fatigue. The practice standards group recommendations were based upon levels of evidence by estimate of treatment effect (level A—multiple populations evaluated through level C—limited populations evaluated) and size of treatment effect (class I where benefit exceeds risk through class III—no benefit and maybe harm) (Sandau et al., 2017).

- Class I: Benefit exceeds risk. Procedure /treatment should be performed/administered.
- Class IIa and IIb: Benefit exceeds risk. Procedure/treatment are reasonable to administer for IIa and may be considered for IIb.
- Class III: No benefit and possible harm.

The practice standards above by Sandau and colleagues (2017) refer to only hospitalized patients. After a decision is made regarding the benefit of ECG monitoring and the intensity that is required for the patient, the specific inpatient setting and the timeframe for monitoring are selected. Monitoring is an important diagnostic tool for heart disease and changes in health status. Important clinical decisions are made based on the data, to include medication therapy, device (pacemaker, ICD) adjustments, further diagnostic testing, referral for cardiac consultation, unit transfers, and length of stay. The decision to provide electrocardiographic monitoring of the patient requires ongoing assessment of the continued need with health care team to include physicians, nurses, nurse practitioners, and if applicable, designated monitor watchers. Some hospitals have dedicated monitor watchers when a central bank of monitors is used on step-down medical-surgical floors (Funk et al., 2021).

Further, as important as understanding when a patient does require ECG monitoring is recognizing when the patient does not need cardiac monitoring. Unnecessary monitoring increases health care costs, diverts nursing and medical staff from other important work, and may give the patient an incorrect message about their own cardiac health (i.e., that the patient is more ill than they actually are). In addition, the ubiquitous nature of alarms in hospitals has been associated with compromised patient safety to such an extent that the Joint Commission has deemed alarm management a National Patient Safety Goal 2022 (The Joint Commission, 2021). This safety goal has remained on the National Patient Safety Goal list for least 10 years. New safety issues were further identified in the 2017 practice standards for electrocardiographic monitoring of patients in the inpatient setting with expert opinion used or an interdisciplinary committee to decide on monitoring specific patient populations and alarm management if clinical trial data are not available to guide recommendations (Sandau et al., 2017).

Accordingly, ECG monitoring with human oversight of the patient remains indispensable but needs to be evaluated continuously because the standard of care changes over time and the aim needs to be to deliver the right "type" and "dose" of cardiac monitoring to meet the patient's clinical care needs. Through an understanding of the patient's underlying condition and the pathology, the nurse can select the leads that will supply the most clinically significant information based on the capability of the electrocardiographic monitoring technology used within an organization. The AHA practice standards for ECG monitoring along with interprofessional guidance and communication are important to assure that the standard of care is met with the goal of using hospital order sets.

ECG monitoring systems vary in sophistication but, in general, can do the following:

- Monitor one limb lead or one limb lead plus one chest lead
- Monitor ST segments (ST-segment depression is a marker of myocardial ischemia; ST-segment elevation provides evidence of an evolving MI)
- Monitor QT segments for prolongation
- Provide graded visual and audible alarms (based on priority, ventricular fibrillation [VF] would be highest)
- Provide computerized rhythm monitoring (arrhythmias are interpreted and stored in the memory of the monitoring system)
- Produce a graphical recording
- Interface with the electronic medical record (as applicable)

BOX 16-3

Helpful Hits for Applying Electrodes

These guidelines optimize skin adherence and the conduction of electrical currents.

- Have the patient positioned supine with the head of the bed at an angle of 30–40 degrees. This will make it easier to find the intercostal spaces for electrode placement. Provide as much privacy for the patient as possible.
- Débride the skin surface of dead cells with soap and water, and dry well. This decreases skin impedance and increases conductivity.
- Clip (do not shave) hair from around the electrode site if needed.
- If the patient is diaphoretic, apply a small amount of benzoin to the skin or wipe with alcohol, avoiding the area under the center of the electrode. (These are controversial recommendations. Benzoin, like alcohol, may increase the risk of burns if the patient requires cardioversion or defibrillation.)
- Check the electrodes for expiration date before applying them to the patient and inspect the package. If the package has been opened or the product is passed the expiration date the electrodes may be dried out and will not work properly.
- Connect the electrodes to the lead wires prior to placing them on the chest; peel the backing off the electrode and make sure the center is moist with electrode gel.
- Locate the landmarks for lead placement and use light, consistent pressure to secure the electrode.
- Change the electrodes every 24–48 hours (or as recommended by the manufacturer), examine the skin for irritation, and apply the electrodes to different locations. This, too, is debatable although evidence suggests that changing the electrodes daily decreases the number of "false alarms" according to the AACN Practice Alert on Alarm Management (2019).
- If the patient is sensitive to the electrodes, use hypoallergenic electrodes.

Continuous monitoring systems have anywhere from three to five electrodes with capability of viewing two to ten leads. Box 16-3 provides helpful hints on how to apply these electrodes. In continuous monitoring, although limb electrodes are still used, they are positioned on the torso as opposed to the lower legs and arms, as in a 12-lead ECG. This allows for greater patient movement and comfort and reduced interference from skeletal muscle artifact. The four disposable electrodes are positioned in specific locations on the patient's chest, and a cable is connected to the monitor or telemetry device in the following arrangement: the right arm (RA) electrode placed on the right upper chest (below the clavicle) and the RA wire (usually white) attached; the left arm (LA) electrode placed on the left upper chest (below the clavicle) and the LA wire (usually black) attached; the left leg (LL) electrode placed on the left torso below the rib cage and on the left side of the abdomen and the LL wire (usually red) attached; the right leg (RL) electrode placed on the right torso and the RL wire (usually green) attached. A maxim used to recall placement is "white on right (snow over grass [green]) and smoke (black) over fire (red)." The color-coding of wires is not an international standard; therefore, this maxim may not be applicable to electrode placement at your organization. To reduce interference from skeletal muscle when placing electrodes, it is helpful to avoid bony prominences or areas that have significant movement. It is also important to ensure that the electrodes have not expired (expiration date on package) and, if the package has been opened, that the electrodes have not dried out. In addition, the electrodes need to be applied properly to the skin by prepping the skin (cleansing and wiping it dry) according to manufacturer's directions and removing excessive chest hair (Sandau et al., 2017). Expert opinion and research support proper skin preparation to reduce the number of false alarms because it optimizes signal transmission. The study by Leigher and colleagues (2020) found that two nursing actions, preparing the skin for monitoring and changing the electrodes daily resulted in a decreased number of alarms in the intensive care unit. Among patients in the PULSE trial, correct placement of the precordial lead occurred only 20% of the time at baseline but improved right away after interactive online education to 59% (Funk et al., 2017). Then, once electrodes are secure and leads attached the signals are transmitted directly to a bedside monitor (hardwire) or more commonly by radio waves from a small transmitter box to a central monitoring station (telemetry). The most basic monitoring system uses three electrodes to allow monitoring in one of three bipolar limb leads. Leads that can be monitored are lead I (positive electrode on the LA, negative electrode on the RA), lead II (positive electrode on the LL and negative electrode on the RA), and lead III (positive electrode on the LL and negative electrode on the LA). These are useful for heart rate and basic rhythm recognition. They are inadequate for accurately identifying many arrhythmias, especially tachycardias (increased heart rate) with a wide QRS. Bipolar limb lead monitoring systems are often found on portable monitors, defibrillators, and some telemetry ECG devices.

Five-electrode monitoring systems use four electrodes placed as above, in the LA, RA, LL, and RL positions, as well as one chest electrode that can be placed in any one of the precordial locations (V_1–V_6). Monitoring systems with five electrodes permit the nurse to decide which leads will be monitored based on the patient's diagnosis and condition. Five-electrode systems have a display that allows two leads to be monitored simultaneously; typically, the nurse chooses one limb lead and one precordial lead to be viewed. The ability to monitor a limb lead and precordial lead simultaneously is often necessary for accurate identification of many arrhythmias, including arrhythmias with a wide QRS complex (BBBs, ventricular pacemaker rhythms, and wide QRS tachycardias). Two leads commonly used for continuous monitoring are leads II and V_1. Lead II provides the best visualization of atrial depolarization (represented by the P wave) and is preferred for monitoring atrial activity and heart rate. Lead V_1 best records ventricular depolarization and is most helpful when monitoring the patient for tachycardias. The updated AHA Practice Standards for ECG monitoring in hospitals (Sandau et al., 2017) recommend V_1 as the preferred lead to monitor for wide QRS complex tachycardia and to distinguish V1 and aberrancy (unusual conduction). The next best lead is V_6. Monitoring for ST-segment changes is also important in terms of detecting ischemia. If the patient's history is known, it is best to monitor the patient in a more directed way using the leads that reflect the vessels involved in the ischemic event. Refer to the monitoring recommendations in Table 16-2 when the patient's history is known.

TABLE **16-2 Monitoring Recommendations, Vessels, and Recommended Leads**

Type of Monitoring	Coronary Vessel Involved	Lead Selection
Arrhythmia monitoring Primary lead	LAD	V_1—intraventricular septum
Arrhythmia monitoring Secondary lead	Left circumflex	V_6—lateral wall
Ischemia monitoring	LAD	V_3—anterior wall V_1, V_2, V_4
Ischemia monitoring	RCA	III—inferior wall II, aVF
Ischemia monitoring	Left circumflex	V_5 and V_6—lateral wall I, aVL—sometimes no change V_1, V_2, or V_3 for reciprocal changes posterior wall
If ischemic footprint unknown	LAD and RCA	V_3 and III—anterior and inferior leads
Demand ischemia	Left circumflex	V_5—lateral wall
QT-interval monitoring	N/A	Monitor in the lead with best defined T wave

LAD, left anterior descending; RCA, right coronary artery.

Further, patients who have or are at risk for prolongation of the QT interval should also be monitored. Prolongation of the QT interval can occur because of a genetic predisposition or through acquired abnormalities such as kidney failure, hypokalemia, and acute pancreatitis. However, in the acute care setting, QT prolongation is often due to medications, to include many drug categories such as antibiotics, antipsychotics, antiarrhythmics, antidepressants, and antiemetics (Farzam & Tivakaran, 2021). The corrected QT (QTc) is considered prolonged when it is above 0.47 second in males and 0.48 second in females (Berul, 2020). If the QTc is above 0.50 second in anyone, it can be associated with a higher risk of torsade de pointes (TdP) which is discussed later in this chapter. In a case study article by Klotzbaugh and colleagues (2020) the authors point out that the QTc serves as a biomarker of sorts that should be reviewed when prescribing medications that have a propensity for proarrhythmic activity.

Ambulatory Electrocardiography

Ambulatory ECG is a continuous form of monitoring used in the outpatient setting to identify the etiology of distressing symptoms (pre-syncope, syncope, palpitations) that may be caused by arrhythmias, myocardial ischemia, or pacemaker dysfunction. In addition to monitoring for arrhythmias and evaluation of silent ischemia, ambulatory monitoring is used to evaluate arrhythmia and device therapy as well as prognosis and risk stratification of various cardiac populations. Ambulatory ECG monitoring to include insertable cardiac monitors (defibrillator, pacemaker, or ECG monitoring [smaller than an AAA battery] that continuously and wirelessly monitor the patient's cardiac rhythm) may also be used in patients who have had a cryptogenic stroke (strokes that cannot be attributable to any specific cause) where paroxysmal AF is suspected. In a study by Bernstein and colleagues (2021) using long-term continuous monitoring resulted in atrial fibrillation (AF) detected in 12.1% of patients compared with the usual care group 1.8%. The authors recommend additional research to be conducted to better determine if this finding is of clinical significance. Ambulatory monitoring may also be used to monitor patients who have hypertrophic cardiomyopathy, or in patients with variant angina. The patient wears a portable recording device (i.e., Holter monitor) that is connected to the chest by electrodes and lead wires. The patient keeps a diary while wearing this device, noting the type and time of symptoms or performance of unusual activities. The patient may also wear an event loop monitor or an implantable loop recorder, which are categorized as intermittent recorders and selected when patients have infrequent symptoms. The monitoring period may be as short as 24 to 48 hours or as long as several months.

Transtelephonic Monitoring

Transtelephonic monitoring (TTM), a form of outpatient ECG monitoring, transmits ECG signals via the telephone. Chest electrodes are connected to a transmitter box. To send the ECG, the telephone mouthpiece is placed over the transmitter box, and the ECG is evaluated at another location. This method is used for diagnosing arrhythmias and evaluating permanent cardiac pacemakers. It is a patient-activated recording that can be sent directly over the phone line and captures data when symptoms present during activities of daily living.

Wireless Mobile Cardiac Monitoring Systems

This outpatient monitoring system, mobile cardiac telemetry (MCT), uses a small sensing device worn by the patient; it transmits the ECG signal to a monitor. When an arrhythmia is detected, the system transmits the ECG to a monitoring center via a telephone line or a wireless communication system. This system enhances detection and early treatment of arrhythmias since data are sent in real time with no delays in contrast to devices where the recording is gathered, stored, and retrieved for interpretation at a later time. Accordingly, the intensity and timeliness of the data are dictated by the device's technology and/or the policies and procedures of the organization.

INTERPRETING THE ELECTROCARDIOGRAM

ECG waveforms are printed on graph paper that is divided by light and dark vertical and horizontal lines at standard intervals (Fig. 16-3). Time and rate are measured on the horizontal axis of the graph, and amplitude or voltage is measured on the vertical axis. Each small block on the graph paper equals 0.04 second, and five small blocks form a large block, which equals 0.2 second. When an ECG waveform moves toward the top of the paper, it is called a *positive deflection.* When it moves toward the bottom of the paper, it is called a *negative deflection.*

The ECG is composed of waveforms (including the P wave, the QRS complex, the T wave, and possibly a U wave) and of segments or intervals (PR interval, the ST segment, and the QT interval) (see Fig. 16-3).

The **P wave** represents the electrical impulse starting in the sinus node and spreading through the atria (atrial **depolarization** leading to atrial contraction).

The **PR interval** is measured from the beginning of the P wave to the beginning of the QRS complex and represents the time needed for sinus node stimulation, atrial depolarization, and conduction through the AV node before ventricular depolarization. In adults, the normal range for the PR is 0.12 to 0.20 second.

The **QRS complex** represents ventricular depolarization. Not all QRS complexes have all three waveforms. The Q wave is the first negative deflection after the P wave. The R wave is the first positive deflection after the P wave, and the S wave is the first negative deflection after the R wave. The

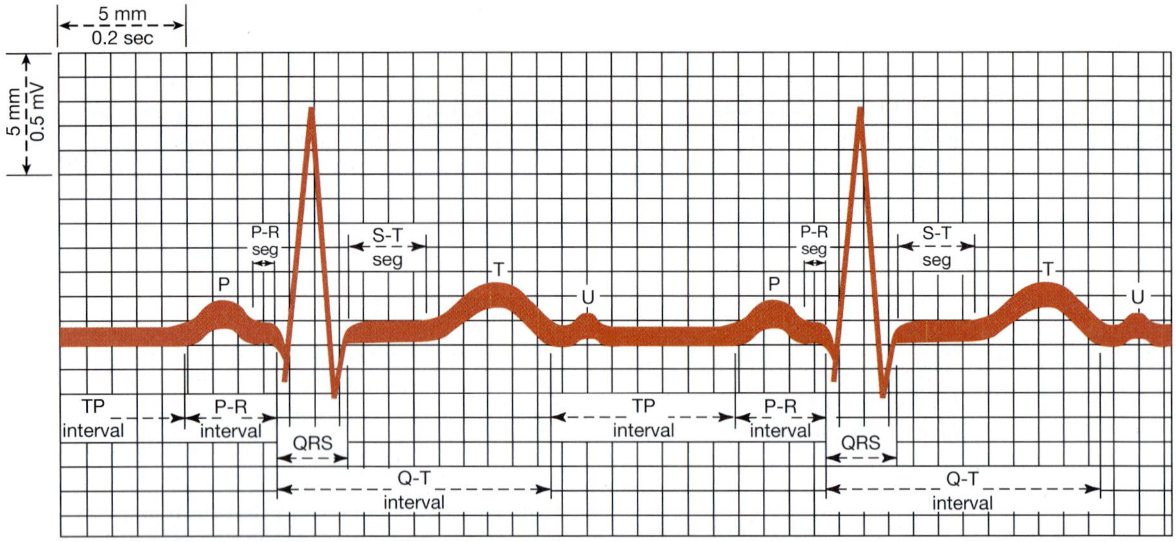

FIGURE 16-3 **ECG and commonly measured components. Each small box represents 0.04 second on the horizontal axis and 1 mm or 0.1 millivolt on the vertical axis. The PR interval is measured from the beginning of the P wave to the beginning of the QRS complex; the QRS complex is measured from the beginning of the Q wave to the end of the S wave; the QT interval is measured from the beginning of the Q wave to the end of the T wave; and the TP interval is measured from the end of the T wave to the beginning of the next P wave.**

QRS complex is normally less than 0.10 second in duration (2.5 small boxes).

The **T wave** represents ventricular repolarization or electrical recovery. It follows the QRS complex and is usually in the same direction as the QRS complex. Atrial repolarization also occurs but is not visible on the ECG because it occurs at the same time as the QRS.

The **U wave** may or may not be present and is thought to represent repolarization of the Purkinje fibers; it is, however, sometimes seen in patients with hypokalemia (low potassium levels), hypertension, or heart disease. If present, the U wave follows the T wave and is usually smaller than the P wave. If tall, it may be mistaken for an extra P wave.

The **ST segment**, which represents early ventricular repolarization, lasts from the end of the QRS complex to the beginning of the T wave. The beginning of the ST segment is usually identified by a change in the thickness or angle of the terminal portion of the QRS complex and is called the *J point*. The end of the ST segment may be more difficult to identify because it merges into the T wave. The ST segment is analyzed to identify whether it is above or below the **isoelectric line**, which may be, among other signs and symptoms, a sign of cardiac ischemia.

Pearls for Practice

Nurses should note ST-segment changes and obtain a 12-lead ECG because:

- *ST-segment depression is seen with ischemia*
- *ST-segment elevation is seen with injury*
- *Q waves are seen with necrosis and infarction*
- *Patients sometimes have silent myocardial ischemia with no associated symptoms such as chest pain. Often silent ischemia occurs in patients with diabetes. Therefore, ST-segment changes viewed on an ECG may be the only way to know that there is a significant cardiac problem. Further, females often experience atypical symptoms of ischemia such as profound fatigue and nausea that are not readily recognized as ischemia. Therefore, like silent ischemia the ECG may be the only indicator of a serious cardiac occurrence.*

The **QT interval**, which represents the total time for ventricular depolarization and repolarization, is measured from the beginning of the QRS complex to the end of the T wave. The QT interval varies with heart rate, gender, and age. If the QT interval becomes prolonged, the patient may be at risk for a lethal ventricular arrhythmia called *torsade de pointes*. The QTc is calculated based on heart rate and is a determinant of risk for TdP arrhythmia. The nurse should measure the QT interval every 8 to 12 hours and calculate the QTc on printouts of rhythm strips from the bedside or telemetry monitor for patients at risk for TdP. An alternative is to use the cardiac monitoring system QT measurement if your hospital system has it as a feature. As referenced earlier, QTc greater than 0.47 second for males or greater than 0.48 second for females is indicative of increased risk of TdP, and a QTc of more than 0.50 second is considered dangerously prolonged.

Pearls for Practice

The QT interval (QTc) using the Bazett formula: QT interval divided by the square root of the RR interval. The RR interval is measured from one R wave to the next R wave that comes before the QT interval being measured (Bazett, 1920).

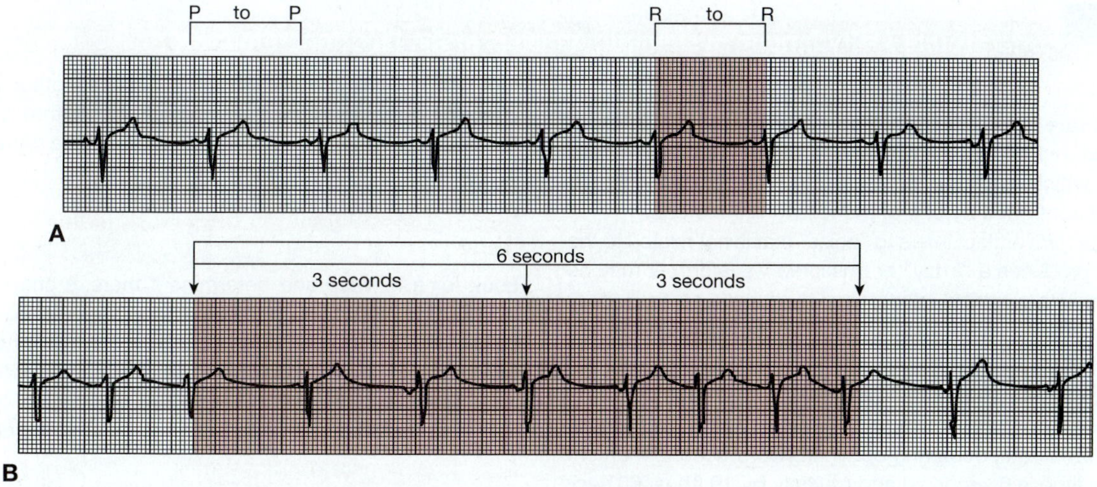

FIGURE 16-4 **A. Ventricular and atrial heart rate determination with a regular rhythm: 1,500 divided by the number of small boxes between two P waves (atrial rate) or between two R waves (ventricular rate). In this example, there are 25 small boxes between both the R waves and the P waves, so the heart rate is 60 bpm. B. Heart rate determination if the rhythm is irregular. There are approximately 7 RR intervals in 6 seconds, so there are about 70 RR intervals in 60 seconds (7 × 10 = 70). The ventricular heart rate is 70 bpm.**

The **PP and RR intervals** are measured from the beginning of one P or R wave to the beginning of the next P or R wave. The PP interval is used to determine atrial rate and rhythm. The RR interval is measured from one QRS complex to the next QRS complex. The RR interval is used to determine ventricular rate and rhythm (Fig. 16-4).

A systemic approach to the diagnosis of an arrhythmia is the best method. In the text by B. G. Petty (2020) the recommendation is to ask yourself three important questions: is the rhythm too fast or too slow, is it supraventricular (that is does the electrical impulse comes from a focus above the atrioventricular node [AV node]) or is it ventricular in etiology (below the A-V node), and is it regular or irregular? The first question would define the arrhythmia as too fast if over 100 beats per minute (bpm) and too slow if under 60 bpm. The second question would be determined by the presence or absence of P waves and the duration of the QRS complex. If the QRS complex is <0.12 second, then it is considered supraventricular. However, if the QRS is ≥0.12 second it could still be supraventricular if there is a conduction defect such as a BBB (which will be described shortly) or the arrhythmia is ventricular in origin (Petty, 2020). The third question refers to the regularity of the R-R interval. Of note, a small variation in the ventricular depolarization is normal.

ANALYZING THE ELECTROCARDIOGRAM RHYTHM STRIP

The ECG must be analyzed in a systematic manner to determine the patient's cardiac rhythm and to detect arrhythmias and conduction disorders. If continuous ST-segment monitoring is in use, evidence of myocardial ischemia, injury, and infarction may also be detected.

Box 16-4 is an example of a method that can be used to analyze the patient's rhythm.

Normal **sinus rhythm** (NSR) occurs when the electrical impulse starts at the sinus node and travels through the normal conduction pathway. NSR serves as a baseline for comparison in identifying all other arrhythmias.

ECG characteristics are:

Rate: 60 to 100 in the adult
Rhythm: Regular
P wave: Normal and consistent shape; always in front of the QRS
PR interval: Consistent interval between 0.12 and 0.20 second
QRS duration: Less than 0.10 second

See Figure 16-5.

ARRHYTHMIAS

As our population grows older, where we now define older groups who range from youngest old (65 to 74 years of age) to elite old (centenarians), the normative aging processes coupled with high incidences of heart disease and polypharmacy with frequent drug–drug interactions demonstrate that arrhythmias will continue to be a growing health care concern requiring monitoring, ongoing assessment, and treatment. Nurses are in a unique position to be the ones who first discover the arrhythmia and, then later, to educate the patient on the management of this condition to preserve and support a good quality of life.

SINUS NODE ARRHYTHMIAS

SINUS ARRHYTHMIA

Sinus arrhythmia occurs when the sinus node creates an impulse at an irregular rhythm. Sometimes the irregularity

BOX 16-4

Interpreting Arrhythmias: Systematic Analysis of the Electrocardiogram

Step 1: Determine the Heart Rate

The heart rate is usually visible on the monitor display or on the printed rhythm strip. However, the monitor will also record "artifact," which may alter the heart rate. The heart rate should always be confirmed by one of the following methods.

Note: the term artifact refers to "noise" that is not related to the heart and produces a "fuzzy" or obscured waveform. It may be associated with electrical interference by outside sources, poor electrode contact, patient tremors, and malfunction of equipment.

Six-second Method

Locate the 3-second markers along the top or bottom of the ECG paper. Count the number of R waves (ventricular rate) or P waves (atrial rate) occurring between two 3-second markers (thus total time is 6 seconds) and multiply by 10 (thus, 60 seconds or 1 minute).

Large-box Method

Count the number of large boxes between two consecutive R waves (ventricular rate) or P waves (atrial rate) and divide into 300. If, for example, there are four large boxes between two R waves, the heart rate is 300/4, or 75.

Small-box Method

Count the number of small boxes between two consecutive R (ventricular rate) or P waves (atrial rate) waves and divide into 1,500. If, for example, there are 10 small boxes between two R waves, the heart rate is 1500/10, or 150 (see Fig. 16-4).

The normal heart rate is between 60 and 100. The term *bradycardia* is used when the heart rate is below 60, whereas *tachycardia* refers to rates above 100.

Step 2: Determine the Rhythm Regularity

Measure the distance between two consecutive R waves (ventricular regularity) or between two consecutive P waves (atrial regularity). Compare the distance between other RR or PP intervals. If the distance is consistent, the rhythm is regular; if the distance varies, the rhythm is irregular. The normal rhythm is regular.

Step 3: Determine if the Rhythm Originated in the SA Node

Look for a P wave and determine if there is one P wave for every QRS. Determine if the size and shape of the P wave is consistent. The normal rhythm has one P wave for every QRS complex. Because P waves represent the contraction across both atria, irregularities in shape are noted with conduction defect within the atrium, atrial enlargement, or hypertrophy.

Step 4: Evaluate Conduction

Measure the PR interval and the QRS duration. The normal PR interval is between 0.12 (three small boxes) and 0.20 (five small boxes) second. The normal QRS interval is less than 0.10 second (2.5 small boxes). QRS duration of more than 0.10 is termed "wide QRS" and is indicative of abnormal ventricular conduction, such as BBBs or ventricular tachycardia.

Step 5: Evaluate the Appearance of the Rhythm

Look for premature beats or elevated or depressed ST segments. ST elevation/depression is associated with ventricular injury/ischemia.

Step 6: Interpret the Rhythm

Compare the findings to the defining characteristics of specified arrhythmias.

Step 7: If a change is noted from the patient's baseline, evaluate the patient, consider obtaining a 12-lead ECG, and report the change to the provider as appropriate

is associated with the respiratory cycle. The rate increases with inspiration and decreases with expiration because the SA node fires more quickly with inspiration. Sinus arrhythmia does not cause any significant hemodynamic effect and is not clinically significant. It occurs frequently in the young and decreases in frequency with age.

SINUS BRADYCARDIA

Pathophysiology

Sinus bradycardia occurs when the sinus node creates an impulse at a slower-than-normal rate (40 to 60 beats/minute). The causes include lower metabolic needs (e.g., sleep,

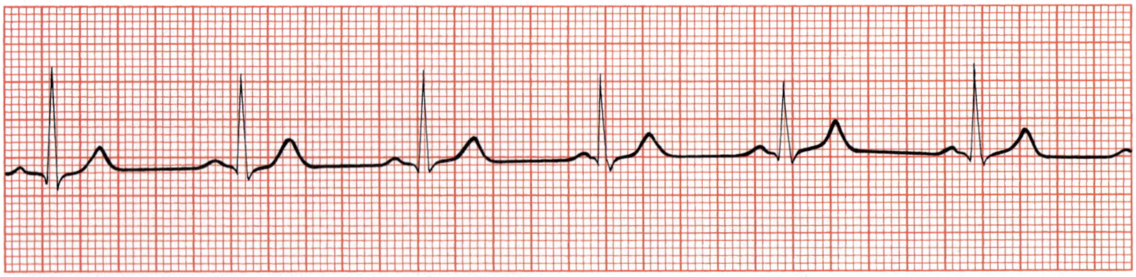

FIGURE 16-5 A typical rhythm strip. It can be as short or as long as you need to decipher the rhythm. This particular strip represents a continuous recording of lead II in a patient with normal sinus rhythm, the normal rhythm of the heart.

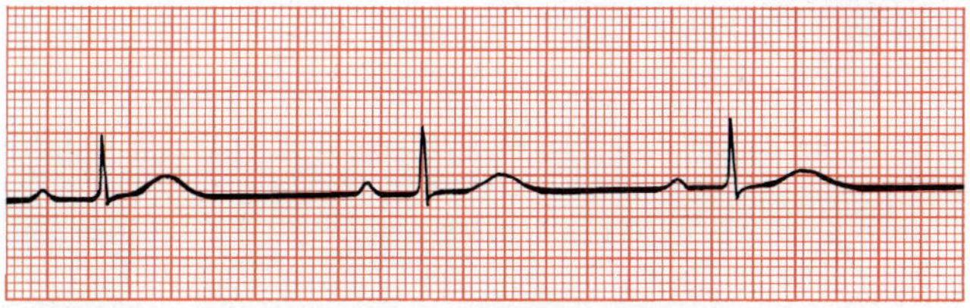

FIGURE 16-6 Sinus bradycardia. More than seven large squares separate each beat, and the rate is 40 to 45 beats per minute.

athletic training, hypothyroidism), vagal stimulation (e.g., from vomiting, suctioning, severe pain, extreme emotions), medications (e.g., calcium-channel blockers, amiodarone, beta blockers), increased intracranial pressure (ICP), and myocardial infarction (MI) or with hypoxemia or obstructive sleep apnea.

Clinical Manifestations and Assessment

Sinus bradycardia often does not cause symptoms though the context or etiology may be important to treat. The patient is assessed to determine the hemodynamic effect, if any, and the possible cause of the arrhythmia.

ECG characteristics are:

Rate: Less than 60 bpm
Rhythm: Regular
P wave: Present before each QRS and consistent in size and shape
PR interval: Normal
QRS duration: Normal

See Figure 16-6.

Medical and Nursing Management

Only bradycardias that cause serious signs and symptoms (altered mental status, ongoing chest pain, hypotension, or shock) require immediate treatment. Treatment of symptomatic bradycardia includes transcutaneous pacing and atropine (decreases parasympathetic tone). If pacing is unavailable or ineffective, a dopamine or epinephrine infusion may be considered. If significant bradycardia is due to medications, the medications should be withheld while their necessity is re-evaluated. For chronic symptomatic bradycardia, permanent pacing may be clinically indicated.

Pearls for Practice

For new-onset syncope (fainting or passing out) and bradycardia, the nurse asks the patient about recent medications during patient admission history, since medications are the cause of most cases of symptomatic bradycardia. Consider a wide variety of medications, including beta-adrenergic blocking eye drops for the treatment of glaucoma. Recall that if the puncta is not occluded with administration, the medication can drain into tear ducts and be systemically absorbed, resulting in syncope secondary to bradycardia and further, that there may be a need to discontinue eye drops according to Wang et al. (2019).

SINUS TACHYCARDIA

Pathophysiology

Sinus tachycardia occurs when the sinus node creates an impulse at a faster-than-normal rate. Causes may include the following:

- Physiologic or psychological stress (e.g., acute blood loss, anemia, shock, hypervolemia, hypovolemia, heart failure (HF), pain, pulmonary emboli, hypermetabolic states, fever, exercise, anxiety)
- Medications that stimulate the sympathetic response (e.g., catecholamines, aminophylline, atropine, thyroid medications), stimulants (e.g., caffeine, alcohol, nicotine), and illicit drugs (e.g., amphetamines, cocaine, ecstasy)

Clinical Manifestations and Assessment

Sinus tachycardia often does not cause symptoms like bradycardia, the context is important to determine if an intervention is clinically indicated. As the heart rate increases, the diastolic filling time decreases, possibly resulting in reduced cardiac output and associated symptoms (refer to Table 16-1). If the rapid rate persists and the heart can no longer compensate for the decreased ventricular filling, the patient may develop acute pulmonary edema or cardiac ischemia.

ECG characteristics are:

Rate: Greater than 100 bpm
Rhythm: Regular
P wave: Present before each QRS and consistent in size and shape
PR interval: Normal
QRS duration: Normal

See Figure 16-7.

Medical and Nursing Management

Treatment of sinus tachycardia is usually determined by the severity of symptoms and directed at identifying and treating its cause. For example, tachycardia caused by acute blood loss would be treated with intravenous (IV) fluid replacement and blood transfusion. Common causes of sinus tachycardia in hospitalized patients include agitation, hemorrhage, or sepsis; in outpatient settings consider hyperthyroidism, anemia, infection or inflammation, and hypovolemia.

Pearls for Practice

There are some early cues to be alert for in patients with cardiac conditions. The nurse understands that the faster the heart rate, the less filling time for the ventricles. Recall CO = SV × HR, and with a decreased SV (less filling time), despite an increased HR, the CO will decrease. In addition, the tachycardia puts a strain on the heart that can result in a mismatch between

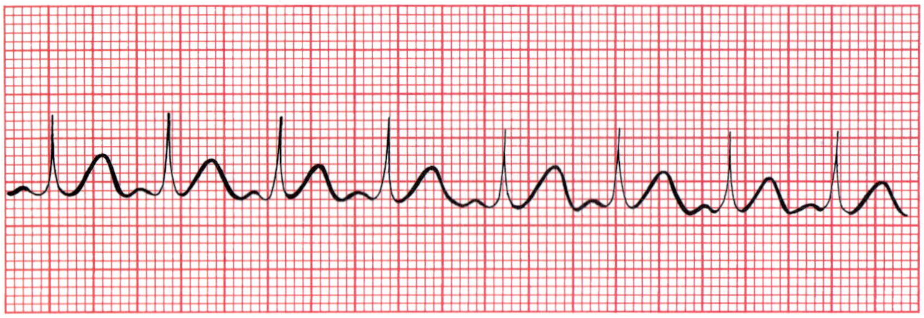

FIGURE 16-7 **Sinus tachycardia. Each beat is separated by two and one half large squares for a rate of 120 beats per minute.**

myocardial supply and demand. The heart rate is putting additional demands on the coronary arteries, and you cannot be assured the supply will reciprocate, and if prolonged myocardial ischemia can progress to necrosis or cell death. Thus, the nurse will consider tachycardia as an important cue seen in the early stages of clinical deterioration of patients with cardiac conditions (White et al., 2021). In addition, tachypnea which is a respiratory rate >20 is seen in the early stages of clinical deterioration that occurs because of the altered myocardial oxygen supply and demand resulting in anaerobic metabolism and metabolic acidosis (White et al., 2021).

ATRIAL ARRHYTHMIAS

PREMATURE ATRIAL COMPLEX

Pathophysiology

A premature atrial complex (PAC) is a single ECG complex that occurs when an electrical impulse starts in the atrium before the next normal impulse of the sinus node. The PAC may be caused by caffeine, alcohol, nicotine, stretched atrial myocardium (e.g., as in hypervolemia), anxiety, hypokalemia (low potassium level), hypermetabolic states (e.g., with pregnancy), hypoxemia, or atrial ischemia, injury, or infarction.

Clinical Manifestations and Assessment

Premature atrial contractions s are common ECG findings, often found without cardiac pathology. The patient may report, "My heart skipped a beat"; however, many times the patient is asymptomatic.

ECG characteristics are:

Rate: Depends on the underlying rhythm
Rhythm: Irregular
P wave: Size and shape of the P wave associated with the premature beat is different from sinus node–generated P wave
PR interval: The PR interval of the premature beat is greater than 0.12 second but shorter than the sinus generated PR interval
QRS duration: Normal

See Figure 16-8.

Medical and Nursing Management

If PACs are infrequent, no treatment is necessary since hemodynamic stability is maintained. If they are frequent (more than six per minute), this may be a sign of a worsening condition or the onset of more serious arrhythmias, such as AF, and further work-up is clinically indicated.

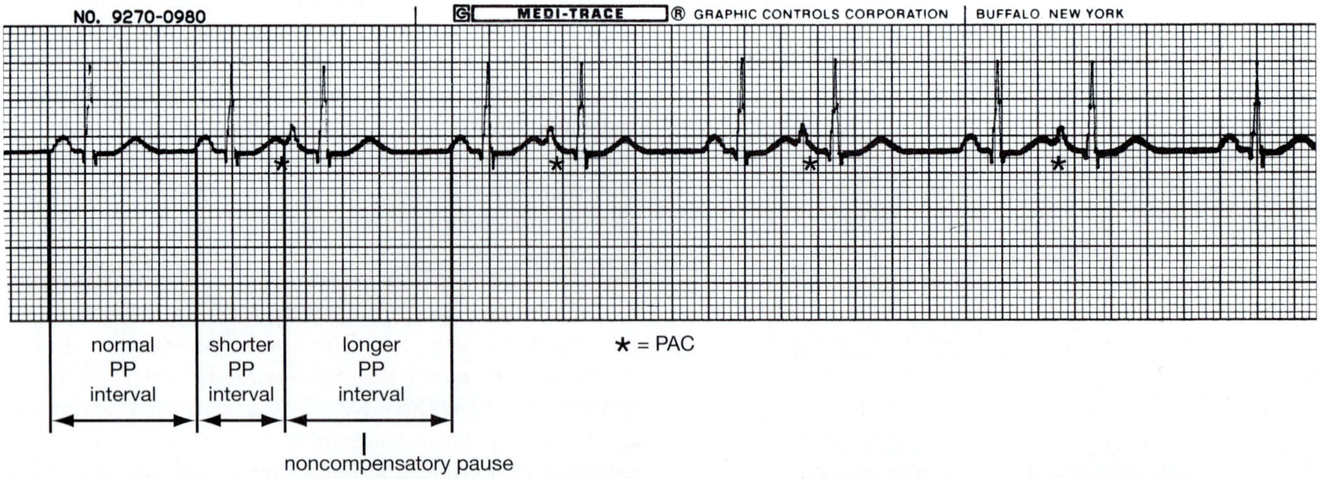

FIGURE 16-8 **Premature atrial complex (PAC). Normal sinus rhythm with one premature atrial contraction (PAC).**

ATRIAL FLUTTER

Pathophysiology

Atrial flutter occurs in the atrium and creates impulses at a rapid but regular atrial rate between 220 and 350 times per minute. Because the atrial rate is faster than the AV node can conduct, not all atrial impulses are conducted into the ventricle. This is an important feature of this arrhythmia because if all atrial impulses were conducted to the ventricle, the ventricular rate would also be 220 to 350, which would result in a life-threatening arrhythmia. Atrial flutter is a macro-reentrant tachycardia that originates in the right atrium at the level of the tricuspid valve annulus (ring of tough fibrous tissue that is attached to and supports the leaflets of the heart valve) (Ziccardi et al., 2021). Re-entry refers to the fact that the impulse can get caught up in a loop where it begins spinning around over and over again, resulting in additional atrial or flutter waves. Causes include coronary artery disease (CAD), hypertension, mitral or tricuspid valve disease, hyperthyroidism or thyrotoxicosis, chronic lung disease, cor pulmonale (right ventricular failure), pulmonary emboli, previous extensive atrial ablation, and cardiomyopathy. Atrial flutter occurs more frequently in males and aging is a significant risk factor for its development (Ziccardi et al., 2021). In addition, a clinical relationship between atrial flutter and AF can be appreciated often in the same patient post open heart surgery. Also of note, postoperative AF or flutter occurred in 12.3% of patients who had surgical or transcatheter valve replacement for severe aortic stenosis, with a significantly higher incidence in the surgical group, both in the early and late phase of recovery (Shahim et al., 2021).

Clinical Manifestations and Assessment

Patients who have atrial flutter may be asymptomatic. More often, atrial flutter causes serious signs and symptoms, such as fatigue, lightheadedness, syncope, chest pain, shortness of breath, and low blood pressure. The risk of mural (wall) emboli forming in the atria increases with this arrhythmia because without a strong atrial contraction, stasis of blood occurs; therefore, the nurse remains alert for signs of pulmonary or systemic emboli. In addition, atrial flutter can increase the risk of decompensated HF, induced cardiomyopathy, and embolic stroke.

ECG characteristics are:

Rate: Atrial rate ranges between 220 and 350 bpm; ventricular rate usually ranges between 75 and 150 depending on AV node conduction

Rhythm: Usually regular but may be irregular because of a change in the AV conduction

P wave: Flutter waves in a characteristic "sawtooth" pattern

PR interval: Not measurable

QRS duration: Normal

See Figure 16-9.

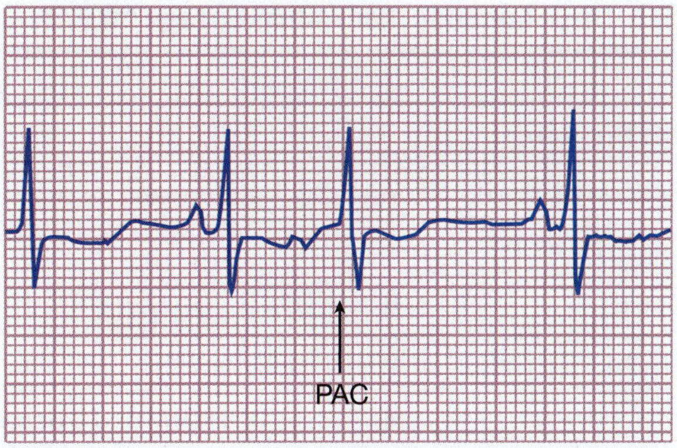

FIGURE 16-9 The classic saw-toothed pattern of atrial flutter.

Medical and Nursing Management

The initial evaluation of atrial flutter is to determine the cause of the arrhythmia through diagnostic testing to include an ECG, echocardiogram, and bloodwork. After confirming the rhythm with a 12-lead ECG, the echocardiogram will determine if the etiology of the rhythm is from structural heart disease, and/or a low ejection fraction (Ziccardi et al., 2021). Further, the echocardiogram would evaluate the presence of atrial or ventricular thrombus in advance of cardioversion which is important to treat to avoid the clot breaking loose resulting in a cerebrovascular accident. A TEE or transesophageal echo is the type of echo that would be done to visualize the atrium which is where the thrombus is more often located (January et al., 2019). Lab work is important to determine if there are any triggers for Aflutter such as an electrolyte disturbance, abnormal thyroid function, infection, anemia, or hypoxia (Ziccardi et al., 2021). These conditions would be important to treat to then lower the threshold of ongoing AFlutter. Management involves rhythm and rate control along with anticoagulation due to embolization risk. It is essential to manage this rhythm because if left untreated remodeling of the atrium results making it more difficult to manage and maintain a sinus rhythm (Ziccardi et al., 2021). The initial treatment for atrial flutter commonly is pharmacologic or electrical cardioversion, ultimately followed by ablation (discussed later in this chapter) to terminate it and restore NSR (January et al., 2019).

If the patient is unstable, urgent electrical **cardioversion** is usually indicated (discussed later in this chapter). For patients who have atrial flutter, antithrombotic therapy is recommended per the same risk profile used for AF (January et al., 2019). In addition, antiarrhythmics such as amiodarone, flecainide, and propafenone are useful for pharmacologic cardioversion of AF or atrial flutter, provided there are no contraindications to the selected medication along with the use of beta blockers (metoprolol, carvedilol) and calcium channel blockers (verapamil, diltiazem) (Ziccardi et al., 2021). Refer to Table 16-3 for medication management of AF.

TABLE **16-3 Common Medication Dosage for Rate Control of AF**

	Intravenous Administration	Usual Oral Maintenance Dose
Beta Blockers		
Metoprolol tartrate	2.5–5.0 mg IV bolus over 2 minutes; up to 3 doses	25–100 mg BID
Metoprolol XL	N/A	50–400 mg QD
Atenolol	N/A	25–100 mg QD
Esmolol	500 mcg/kg IV bolus over 1 minute, then 50–300 mcg/kg/min IV	N/A
Propranolol	1 mg IV over 1 minute, up to 3 doses at 2-minute intervals	10–40 mg TID or QID
Nadolol	N/A	10–240 mg QD
Carvedilol	N/A	3.125–25 mg BID
Bisoprolol	N/A	2.5–10 mg QD
Nondihydropyridine Calcium Channel Antagonists		
Verapamil	0.075–0.15 mg/kg IV bolus over 2 minutes; may give an additional 10.0 mg after 30 minutes if no response, then 0.005 mg/kg/min infusion	180–480 mg QD (ER)
Diltiazem	0.25 mg/kg IV bolus over 2 minutes, then 5–15 mg/hr	120–360 mg QD (ER)
Digitalis Glycosides		
Digoxin	0.25 mg IV with repeat dosing to a maximum of 1.5 mg over 24 hours	0.125–0.25 mg QD
Others		
Amiodarone[a]	300 mg IV over 1 hour, then 10–50 mg/hr over 24 hours	100–200 mg QD

[a]Multiple dosing schemes exist for the use of amiodarone.

AF, atrial fibrillation; BID, twice daily; ER, extended release; IV, intravenous; N/A, not applicable, QD, once daily; QID, 4 times a day; TID, 3 times a day.

Data from January, C. T., Wann, L. S., Alpert, J. S., Calkins, H., Cigarroa, J. E., Cleveland, J. C., Conti, J. B., Ellinor, P. T., Ezekowitz, M. D., Field, M. E., Murray, K. T., Sacco, R. L., Stevenson, W. G., Tchou, P. J., Tracy, C. M., & Yancy, C. W. (2014). 2014 AHA/ACC/HRS Guideline for the Management of Patients with Atrial Fibrillation: Executive Summary. *Circulation*, *130*, 2071–2104.

American Heart Association (AHA). (2020). Guidelines for Cardiopulmonary Resuscitation and Emergency Cardiovascular Care. https://cpr.heart.org/en/resuscitation-science/cpr-and-ecc-guidelines/adult-basic-and-advanced-life-support/iv-medications-commonly-used-for-acute-rate-control-in-atrial-fibrillation-and-atrial-flutter

ATRIAL FIBRILLATION

Pathophysiology

AF is a common arrhythmia according to the Centers for Disease Control and Prevention (CDC, 2022). It is estimated that the number of people with AF may reach 12.1 million in the United States by 2030 (CDC, 2022). Further, White people of European descent are more likely to develop AF than Black individuals, and females with a longer lifespan than males will experience AF more often than males (CDC, 2022). AF causes rapid, disorganized, and uncoordinated electrical activity within the atria. AF may be transient, starting and stopping suddenly and occurring for a very short time (paroxysmal), or it may be persistent, requiring treatment to terminate the rhythm or to control the ventricular rate. Further, AF may be described in terms of duration of episodes, such as long-standing, permanent, or nonvalvular AF. Long-standing persistent AF is continuous or AF lasting longer than 12 months in duration; permanent AF is used when the physician and patient together decide to stop further attempts to restore and maintain NSR. Finally, the term nonvalvular AF is used when AF exists in the absence of rheumatic mitral stenosis, a mechanical or bioprosthetic heart valve, or mitral valve repair. The erratic atrial contraction promotes formation of thrombi within the atria, increasing the risk for an embolic event such as stroke (brain attack). In fact, patients with AF have a four- to fivefold increase in the risk for stroke according to Alberts and colleagues (2020) and a twofold increase in mortality (Alberts et al., 2020). As mentioned above, AF is usually associated with increasing age, European ancestry along with valvular heart disease, CAD, hypertension, HF, cardiomyopathy, diabetes, obstructive sleep apnea, obesity, hyperthyroidism, pulmonary disease, chronic lung disease, chronic kidney disease, and after surgery (especially open-heart surgery) (CDC, 2022). Physiologic stressors, such as hypoxia, infection, and hypoglycemia; as well as the use of caffeine, alcohol, or sympathomimetic drugs; and smoking are also associated with AF. Psoriasis was thought to be a potential risk factor for AF possibly related to an inflammatory process. However, a retrospective review and analysis of data from the National Inpatient Sample by Edigin and colleagues (2020) determined that psoriasis does not worsen outcomes of patients admitted to the hospital with AF.

Clinical Manifestations and Assessment

Some people with AF may be asymptomatic. However, when there is a rapid ventricular response, which reduces the time for ventricular filling, the result is a smaller stroke volume and likely symptoms such as shortness of breath, fatigue, palpitations, lightheadedness, and even hypotension (Desai & Hajouli, 2021). In addition, loss of the atrial contraction (sometimes referred to as *atrial kick*) reduces ventricular filling volume and decreases cardiac output by 25%. This often leads to symptoms of fatigue and malaise. The shorter time in diastole reduces the time available for coronary artery perfusion, thereby increasing the risk for myocardial ischemia. Approximately 10% to 21% of patients with AF also have acute coronary syndrome (Jacek, 2021). In addition, patients are at risk for the development of HF and impaired end-organ perfusion (Jacek, 2021).

ECG characteristics are:

Rate: Atrial rate is 300 to 400, with a variable ventricular response rate (typically rapid)
Rhythm: Irregular
P wave: No discernible P waves; irregular undulating waves may be seen and are referred to as *fibrillatory waves*
PR interval: Not measurable
QRS duration: Normal

See Figure 16-10.

Pearls for Practice

The three cornerstones of AF management include rate control, rhythm control, and prevention of thromboembolism.

Medical and Nursing Management

Treatment of AF depends on its cause and duration and the patient's symptoms, age, and comorbidities. Once the pattern, clinical history, and symptoms are established, it is important to then assess for the presence of structural heart disease and identification of any correctable secondary causes, such as sleep apnea or substance abuse. The clinical work up of AF is often the same as what is done in the context of atrial flutter as discussed earlier in this chapter. The management of AF includes controlling the ventricular rate and achieving rhythm conversion to sinus rhythm if possible. Cardioversion of AF can be done either by medication or an electrical shock. Direct-current cardioversion is more effective than pharmacologic cardioversion (however, it is important to consider that when AF onset is more recent, then pharmacologic cardioversion will be more effective). Still, electrical cardioversion is indicated when a patient with new-onset AF is hemodynamically unstable and should be repeated if sinus rhythm cannot be maintained for a clinically meaningful time between procedures (Weant et al., 2020). Shocks are delivered in sync with the QRS wave. Biphasic defibrillators are used more often with less energy required (150 to 200 joules [unit of energy]) than when using the older, monophasic defibrillators with higher-energy settings. Pharmacologic cardioversion is done with IV medications to control rate such as a beta blocker, metoprolol, and a calcium channel blocker such as diltiazem. Rhythm control agents include ibutilide and amiodarone (prolongs action potential in cardiac cells), and procainamide, flecainide, and propafenone (blocks sodium channels) (Weant et al., 2020). Commonly used oral medications include flecainide and propafenone. For ventricular rate control, the medications that are used are beta blockers and calcium channel antagonists along with Digoxin (reserved for those patients who are sedentary or with systolic HF). In addition, magnesium is used adjunctively for AF since it reduces conduction through the AV node (Weant et al., 2020).

Pearls for Practice

For a patient with new-onset AF for over 48 hours, or when the onset is unknown, the nurse is aware that a transesophageal echocardiography (TEE) should be performed before cardioversion to rule out a left atrial thrombus. The rationale behind this is that with cardioversion, if the patient converts to a sinus rhythm, the risk increases for embolization of the clot resulting in a potential cerebral vascular accident (CVA). If no thrombi are present, then cardioversion can be performed safely; however, the patient needs to be educated that 4 weeks of anticoagulation will be maintained after cardioversion to prevent thromboembolism (January et al., 2019).

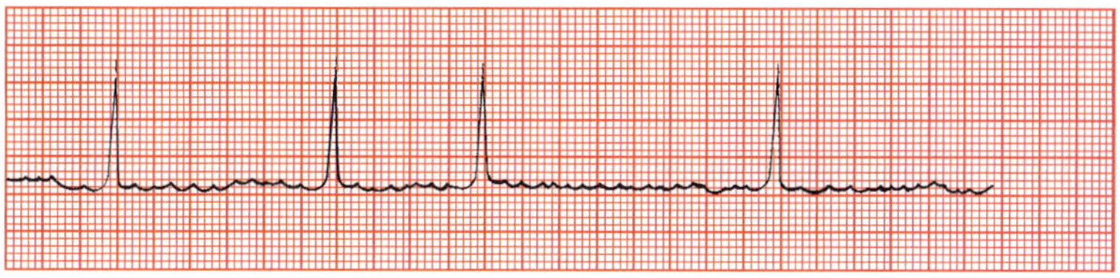

FIGURE 16-10 **Atrial fibrillation with a slow, irregular ventricular rate.**

If delayed cardioversion is selected rather than emergent cardioversion, then the patient typically receives 3 weeks of therapeutic anticoagulation to prevent a thrombus and a TEE should be performed prior to cardioversion. Accordingly, all patients with AF, regardless of whether a rhythm or rate control plan is chosen, should be treated with antithrombotic therapy.

If the QRS is wide and the ventricular rhythm is irregular, AF with an accessory pathway, such as Wolff–Parkinson–White syndrome, should be suspected. Medications that block atrial-ventricular (AV) conduction (e.g., adenosine, digoxin, diltiazem, and verapamil) should be avoided because they may actually cause an increase in ventricular rate given that conduction is via an alternative pathway rather than via the AV node. Expert consultation will be required to determine appropriate treatment.

Antithrombotic therapy prevents thromboembolism, and long-term anticoagulant therapy is prescribed using warfarin, or warfarin alternatives—factor Xa inhibitor (rivaroxaban or apixaban) or direct thrombin inhibitor (dabigatran). These therapies are indicated if the patient with AF is at high risk for stroke using the CHADS2DS-VASc scoring system (i.e., over 75 years of age or has hypertension, female gender, diabetes, HF, or history of stroke). There are no effective reversal agents for these warfarin-alternative agents; therefore, they should not be used in patients who have severe hepatic dysfunction due to coagulopathies and impaired pharmacokinetics (Jacek, 2021). However, as an alternative non–vitamin K oral anticoagulants or direct oral anticoagulants are safe and are of equivalent value in reducing incidence of stroke and embolic events (January et al., 2019). If immediate anticoagulation is necessary, the patient may be placed on heparin until the warfarin level is therapeutic (January et al., 2019).

Pearls for Practice

No therapy, cardiac medications or cardioversion may be used to convert lone AF (also referred to as idiopathic AF [where there is no clear cause for the rhythm]) for patients over 65 years of age without heart disease. If there are no contraindications, anticoagulation therapy may be started without direct treatment of arrhythmia itself. If warfarin is used, the international normalized ratio (INR) should be 2.0 to 3.0 with a target of 2.5. An INR below 2.0 is not effective at preventing strokes. If the patient has a mechanical valve, then the target INR should also be 2.5 to 3 depending on risk factors (Huda et al., 2021).

Pacemaker implantation or catheter ablation is sometimes indicated for patients who are unresponsive to medications. Catheter ablation is a minimally invasive procedure during which high-frequency radio waves are applied to destroy the tissue at the site of the arrhythmia. Ablation procedures are usually performed in electrophysiology (EP) laboratories and are similar to other types of heart catheterization procedures in that a catheter is used. However, the differences include longer procedure times (approximately 6 to 8 hours) for ablation, the catheter delivers high energy to stop an arrhythmia, and it is indicated for conduction diagnosis and treatment alone—not for diagnosis and treatment of disease in the coronary arteries. During a catheter ablation, long, thin, flexible tubes are placed in the heart via the vascular system. A diagnostic catheter determines where the abnormal tissue that is causing the arrhythmia is located. High-frequency energy is sent into the tissue, creating a lesion or scar. The area is now ablated (destroyed), thus facilitating normal electrical conduction. Cryoballoon ablation is a newer procedure that has been effective in preventing paroxysmal AF in patients who were unable to be medically managed with antiarrhythmic medications. Pulmonary vein isolation using cryoablation can be achieved in most people with shorter procedure time with a lower incidence of pericardial effusion and cardiac tamponade (Penela & Cappato, 2021). However, the potential complications of this procedure include phrenic nerve injury, although the incidence is only 1% to 2% (Penela & Cappato, 2021). There have been many improvements in existing ablation techniques and tools have increased the efficacy and safety of catheter AF ablation (Kotalczyk et al., 2021). A recent trial revealed that an early rhythm control strategy (associated with standard of care) reduced the composite endpoint of cardiovascular-related death, stroke, or hospitalization in patients with newly diagnosed AF (Kirchhof et al., 2020).

A few approaches are effective in preventing the occurrence of postoperative AF, including preoperative administration of a beta blocker or immediate postoperative administration of IV amiodarone.

SUPRAVENTRICULAR TACHYCARDIA

Pathophysiology

Supraventricular tachycardia (SVT) is a broad term used to describe tachycardias where the atrial and/or the ventricular rates exceed 100 bpm at rest. The mechanism involves an electrical impulse originating above the ventricles, commonly from tissue at the HIS bundle and above (AV node). The heart rate is increased by an abnormal electrical impulse starting in the atria, and the ventricular rate follows the atrial impulse resulting in this "tachy" arrhythmia. Broadly, SVT includes sinus tachycardia, focal and multifocal (having different points or origin) atrial tachycardias, junctional tachycardias, AV nodal re-entry tachycardia (AVNRT), and various other accessory pathway-mediated reentrant tachycardias. Technically, AF is an SVT, but it is not grouped this way in the AHA guidelines (2020) and was addressed separately. Supraventricular ventricular tachycardias even without AF included in the group are among the most common arrhythmias that require treatment. Conduction abnormalities may occur because of aberrant conduction, a pre-existing BBB, or an accessory pathway that results in pre-excitation.

Further, the presence of AV dissociation (where the ventricular rate is faster than the atrial rate or in other cases where fusion complexes occur that represent the dissociation of supraventricular impulses from ventricular) provides assistance with diagnosis of ventricular tachycardia (VT) versus SVT. It is sometimes difficult to differentiate between the two arrhythmias without a 12-lead ECG.

Clinical Manifestation

SVT's effect on a patient's quality of life varies; the degree of impact is often affected by the frequency of episodes, the duration, and the timing of the SVT (whether with exercise or also at rest). Symptoms vary depending on the rhythm and the patient, with reports of palpitations, chest pain, shortness of breath, dizziness, and syncope, along with panic and anxiety, which heighten the degree of symptoms and confounds the diagnosis of SVT.

ECG characteristics are:

Rate: over 100 bpm
Rhythm: Regular
P wave: If visible, inverted P waves sometimes seen after the QRS
PR interval: Not measurable
QRS duration: In paroxysmal SVT, the QRS is normal

See Figure 16-11.

Medical and Nursing Management

Treatment of atrial SVT depends on its cause and duration and the patient's symptoms, age, and comorbidities. Vagal maneuvers are recommended as a first step to discontinue the rhythm in patients who are hemodynamically stable. Often this intervention does not work or only works for a short duration. Medical management in the short term in a patient who is stable with a regular SVT is with adenosine (Brugada et al., 2020). If the patient becomes hemodynamically unstable, cannot be rate controlled with medication or it is ineffective, the treatment recommendation is synchronized cardioversion. IV beta blockers, IV diltiazem, or IV verapamil (class IIa) can also be used to convert the patient's rhythm to NSR (Brugada et al., 2020).

For ongoing management, patients are placed on oral beta blockers, diltiazem, or verapamil and sometimes taught how to do the vasovagal maneuver. The vasovagal maneuver where a person bares down to slow their rate is occasionally used to slow a rhythm in the inpatient setting but isn't used as often for ongoing management. Antiarrhythmic medications do carry the potential for adverse side effects. Therefore, due to the potential side effects, today more often patients are referred for catheter ablation with a high degree of success and low rate of complications (Brugada et al., 2020).

JUNCTIONAL ARRHYTHMIAS

JUNCTION RHYTHM

Pathophysiology

Junctional rhythm occurs when the AV node, instead of the sinus node, becomes the pacemaker of the heart. When the sinus node slows (e.g., from increased vagal tone) or when the impulse cannot be conducted through the AV node (e.g., because of complete heart block), the AV node automatically discharges an impulse. Junctional escape rhythm may be caused by acute coronary syndromes; valvular disease; hypoxia; increased parasympathetic tone; or the effects of medication, including digoxin, beta blockers, and calcium channel blockers.

Clinical Manifestations and Assessment

The patient may be asymptomatic, or experience signs and symptoms associated with a decreased cardiac output.

ECG characteristics are:

Rate: 40 to 60 bpm
Rhythm: Regular
P wave: If visible, may be before, during, or after the QRS

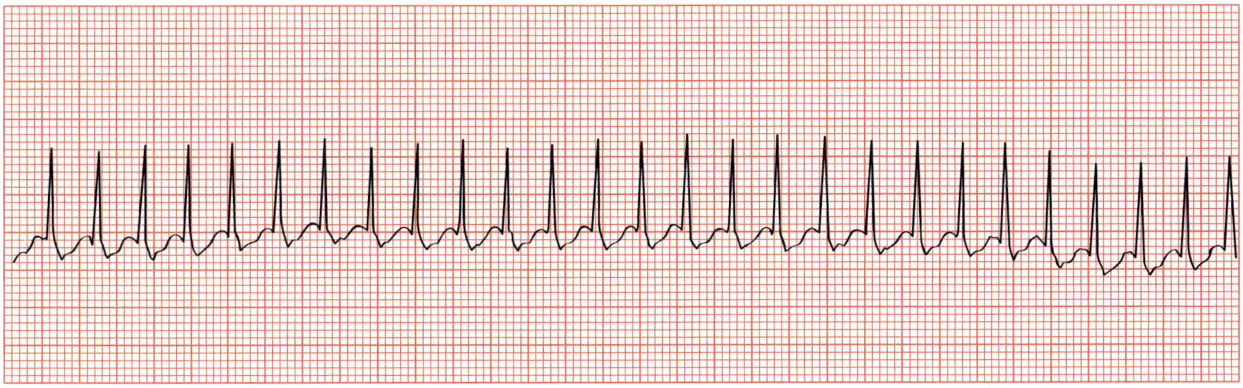

FIGURE 16-11 **Supraventricular tachycardia: note rate above 220, abnormal P waves, no beat-to-beat variability.**

A

B

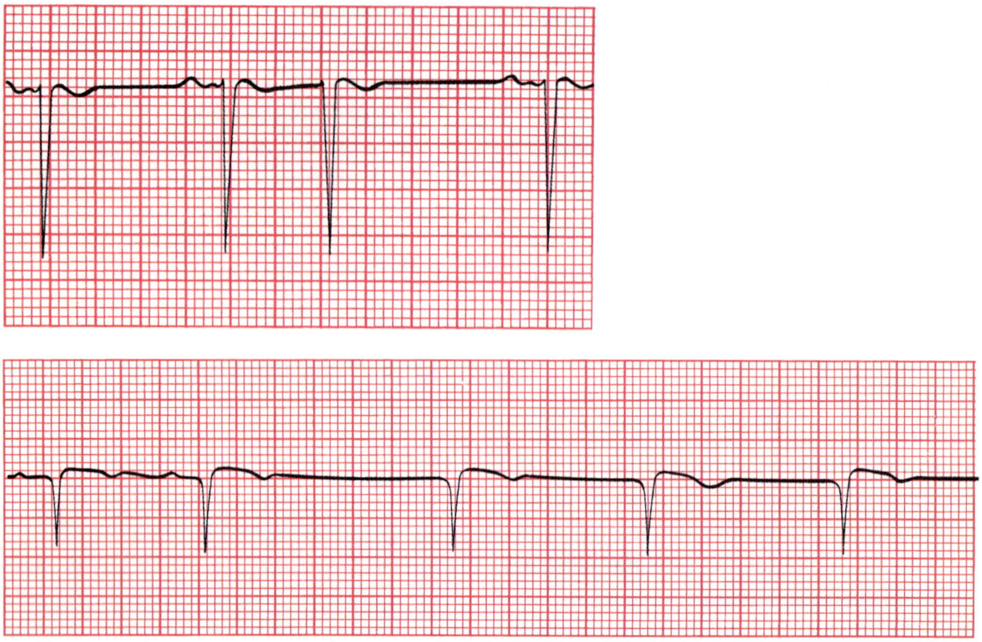

FIGURE 16-12 **Junctional rhythm note short PR intervals. A. A junctional premature beat. The third beat is obviously premature, and there is no P wave preceding the QRS complex. B. The third beat is a junctional escape beat, establishing a sustained junctional rhythm. It looks just like a junctional premature beat, but it occurs late, following a prolonged pause, rather than prematurely.**

PR interval: If a P wave is visible, less than 0.12 second
QRS duration: Normal

See Figure 16-12.

Medical and Nursing Management

If the patient is symptomatic, the treatment is the same as for bradycardia; the patient may be paced (temporary or permanent) or is given IV atropine or epinephrine to treat the rhythm acutely. Later, the patient is managed with a permanent pacemaker if the underlying cause of the junctional rhythm cannot be resolved.

VENTRICULAR ARRHYTHMIAS

ABNORMAL VENTRICULAR CONDUCTION (BBB)

Pathophysiology

If there is a delay or defect in the conduction system within the ventricles (right and left bundle branches), the QRS complex will be prolonged or widened (greater than 0.12 second). A BBB may be described as right or left and complete or incomplete. They may occasionally be present in otherwise healthy individuals; however, they may also be caused by ventricular enlargement (ventricular hypertrophy or cardiomyopathy) or anteroseptal myocardial ischemia or infarction. A BBB may be clinically insignificant, though it can be serious when associated with an acute MI.

Medical and Nursing Management

The goal is to treat the underlying cause of the BBB when possible, such as by maximizing medical management of CAD or cardiomyopathy. However, in the presence of an acute MI, BBB may progress to complete heart block, which may require temporary pacing during the acute phase of illness.

PREMATURE VENTRICULAR COMPLEX

Pathophysiology

A premature ventricular complex (PVC) is an impulse that starts in a ventricle and is conducted through the ventricles before the next normal sinus impulse. Premature ventricular contractions can occur in healthy people and are likely common. Potential mechanisms for PVCs include triggered activity, automaticity, and reentry (Marcus, 2020). Premature ventricular contractions are commonly asymptomatic but can also result in palpitations (irregular heartbeats), dyspnea (shortness of breath), presyncope, and fatigue (Marcus, 2020). Increasing age, a taller height, a higher blood pressure, a history of heart disease, performance of less physical activity, and smoking each predict a greater PVC frequency (Marcus, 2020). Premature ventricular contractions are also caused by cardiac ischemia or infarction, increased workload on the heart (e.g., exercise, fever, hypervolemia, HF, tachycardia), digitalis toxicity, hypoxia, acidosis, or electrolyte imbalances, especially hypokalemia. Research suggests that PVCs may be an early marker for the development of HF. Most patients with PVCs may require only reassurance, treatment is generally reserved for either symptomatic PVCs or concern for PVC-induced cardiomyopathy. Premature ventricular contraction burden remains the most reliable PVC-associated predictor of HF. Further research is needed to better understand the clinical relevance of PVCs in the development of HF. A higher frequency of PVCs was associated with a decrease in left ventricular ejection fraction (LVEF), which is the amount of blood ejected out of the left ventricle per each ventricular contraction, an increase in HF, and an increase mortality. Of note, the terms congestive heart failure (CHF) and HF are used interchangeable. In addition, a reduced LVEF, and other underlying pathology such as structural heart disease that may either contribute to the cause of the PVCs or render them more symptomatic (Marcus, 2020). Data regarding caffeine consumption are conflicting and not strong enough to support a broad recommendation against caffeine consumption in general (Marcus, 2020). Beta blockers, calcium channel blockers, or catheter ablation are each reasonable first-line strategies to treat PVCs, with the final decision driven by the specific patient characteristics and preferences (Marcus, 2020).

Clinical Manifestations and Assessment

The patient may be asymptomatic or complain that their heart "skipped a beat." The effect of a PVC depends on its timing in the cardiac cycle and how much blood was in the ventricles when they contracted. *Bigeminy* is a rhythm in which every other complex is a PVC. In *trigeminy,* every third complex is a PVC, and in *quadrigeminy*, every fourth complex is a PVC. Premature ventricular contractions may present singly or in pairs (often referred to as couplets). Three or more successive PVCs are termed *ventricular tachycardia* (VT) (discussed next). Multifocal PVCs are ones that originate from different parts of the ventricles resulting in different complexes.

ECG characteristics are:

Rate: Depends on the underlying rhythm
Rhythm: Regular
P wave: Visibility of P wave depends on the timing of the PVC; may be absent (hidden in the QRS or T wave) or in front of the QRS. If the P wave follows the QRS, the shape of the P wave may be different
PR interval: If the P wave is in front of the QRS, the PR interval is less than 0.12 second
QRS duration: Duration of the QRS in a PVC is 0.12 second or longer (wide); shape is bizarre and abnormal

See Figure 16-13.

Medical and Nursing Management

Initial treatment is aimed at correcting the cause of the arrhythmia (e.g., treat hypokalemia). Long-term pharmacotherapy for PVCs is not indicated unless the patient is symptomatic. In the absence of disease, PVCs usually are not serious. In the patient with an acute MI or in the context of HF, PVCs may be more frequent and reflect underlying heart disease or represent an early modifiable risk factor for HF. As referenced earlier in the chapter, if PVCs are significant enough to cause symptoms, then catheter ablation and/or medical management may be necessary.

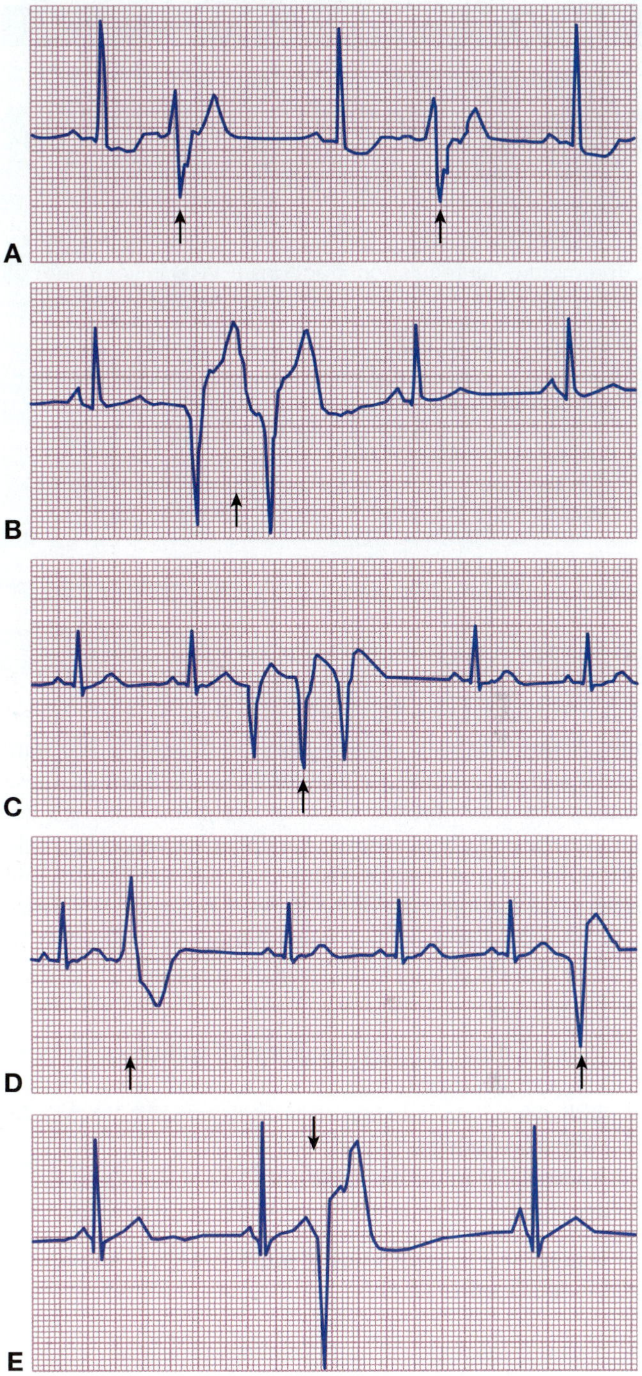

FIGURE 16-13 Dangerous forms of premature ventricular contractions (PVCs): (A) bigeminy, (B) couplets, (C) run, (D) multifocal, and (E) R-on-T phenomenon.

Unfolding Patient Stories: KB • Part 2

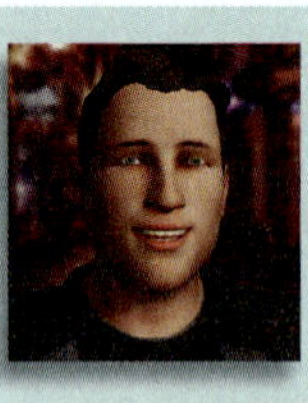

Recall from Chapter 9 KB, who came to the emergency department with difficulty breathing after a week of flu-like symptoms, productive cough, and high fever, was diagnosed with a right lower lobe pneumonia. Sinus tachycardia with occasional unifocal premature ventricular contractions (PVCs) is seen on the cardiac monitor. What are potential causes for the tachycardia and PVCs that the nurse should investigate when considering the patient's age of 27 years, symptoms experienced over the last week, and the clinical manifestations associated with his diagnosis?

Care for KB and other patients in a realistic virtual environment: ***vSim** for Nursing* (thepoint.lww.com/vSimMedicalSurgical). Practice documenting these patients' care in (thepoint.lww.com/DocuCareEHR).

VENTRICULAR TACHYCARDIA

Pathophysiology

Ventricular tachycardia is defined as three or more consecutive ventricular beats occurring at a rate exceeding 100 bpm. The causes are similar to those of PVCs. Ultimately, those causes will determine the course of treatment with consideration to the underlying disease; the projected, associated risk; the period of time that the risk exists; and the benefits and risks as well as tolerance of the planned treatment. VT is usually associated with acute coronary artery syndrome (ACS) but can also occur in specific clinical conditions:

- after an MI,
- with inherited primary arrhythmia syndromes, such as long QT syndrome,
- with electrolyte imbalances,
- cardiomyopathies,
- structural heart disease, and
- due to proarrhythmic medications that may precede VF.

Untreated VT can deteriorate into VF, a lethal arrhythmia and sudden cardiac death.

Clinical Manifestations and Assessment

The patient can experience a range of symptoms related to decreased cardiac output, such as hypotension or syncope, pulselessness, and unresponsiveness. In contrast, some patients may be initially asymptomatic but usually will decompensate hemodynamically.

ECG characteristics are:

Rate: 100 to 250 bpm
Rhythm: Regular
P wave: Usually not visible; if visible are not associated with the QRS complex (called *dissociation*)
PR interval: None
QRS duration: Greater than 0.12 second

See Figure 16-14.

Medical and Nursing Management

The patient's tolerance for this rapid rhythm depends on the ventricular rate and underlying disease. Several factors together with the ventricular rate and the etiology determine the initial treatment, including the following: identifying the rhythm as monomorphic (having a consistent QRS shape and rate) or polymorphic (having varied QRS shapes and rhythms); determining the existence of a prolonged QT interval before the initiation of VT; and ascertaining the patient's heart function. If the patient is stable, continuing the assessment, especially obtaining a 12-lead ECG, may be the only action necessary.

Vasopressin with epinephrine is no longer administered to patients in cardiac arrest because it was determined that there was no added benefit to using vasopressin (Panchal et al., 2020). However, per these guidelines, epinephrine alone should be considered if the patient's rhythm is a pulseless ventricular tachycardia to establish a rhythm that can be treated by defibrillation. Whereas, amiodarone (administered IV) is often the antiarrhythmic medication of choice for a stable patient with VT. Cardioversion is the treatment of choice for monophasic VT in a symptomatic patient. However, many antiarrhythmic drugs other than beta blockers have not been shown to be effective in the treatment of primary ventricular arrhythmia or in sudden cardiac

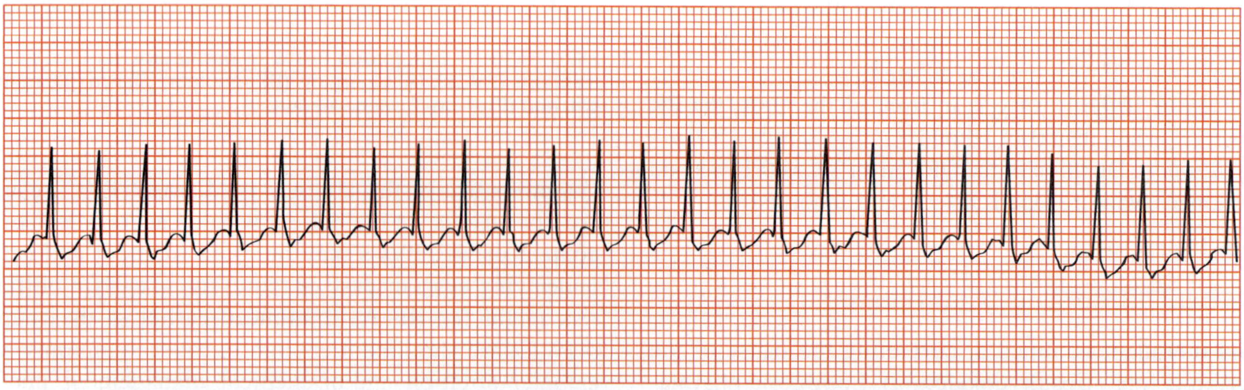

FIGURE 16-14 **Ventricular tachycardia: rapid and regular rhythm, wide QRS complex without P waves.**

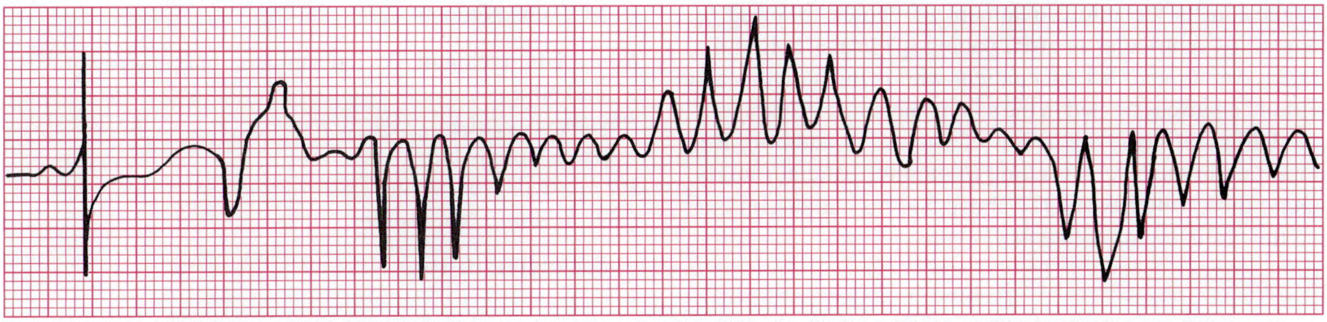

FIGURE 16-15 **Torsades de pointes. (From Lippincott. [2005].** ***Just the facts: ECG interpretation*****. Lippincott Williams & Wilkins.)**

death prevention but may be helpful as an adjunct therapy in management of patients who are arrhythmia prone (Panchal et al., 2020). Importantly, AF should be suspected as the cause of a wide, complex tachycardia with an irregular rhythm, and it should be treated appropriately.

Pearls for Practice

The nurse observes the patient's response hemodynamically to the VT. Obtain vital signs, auscultate lungs and heart, monitor urine output, and assess the patient's level of consciousness. If a patient demonstrates hypotension, shock, angina, symptoms of congestive heart failure (crackles, decreasing oxygen saturation, shortness of breath [left-sided HF] or edema, jugular vein distention [right-sided HF]), or symptoms of cerebral hypoperfusion, the nurse prepares for cardioversion.

TdP (Fig. 16-15) is a polymorphic VT usually preceded by a prolonged QT interval that can be congenital or acquired and is relatively uncommon. Acquired torsades is frequently associated with drug therapy, hypokalemia, or hypomagnesemia, and risk factors such as older than 65 years old, female sex, bradycardia, heart disease, and diuretic use (Cohagan & Brandis, 2021). The vulnerable period for TdP in hospitalized patients occurs during initiation, increasing the dose or overdose of QT-prolonging medications (Sandau et al., 2017). Additional risk factors for TdP are described in Box 16-5 which includes some of the QT-prolonging medications. Since QT-prolonging agents can be found in all classes of medications, a website has been established for patients and health care professionals (www.QTdrugs.org). Up-to-date information is provided at this site regarding QT-prolonging medications and drug-to-drug interactions that can also affect the QT interval. Because this rhythm is likely to cause the patient to deteriorate and become pulseless, immediate treatment is usually required. Standard antiarrhythmic agents may be administered with temporary pacing, but treatment will depend on the cause of torsades and management should focus on removing the etiology of this arrhythmia. For example, in acquired torsades, IV

BOX 16-5

Risk Factors for Torsade de Pointes

1. QT interval prolongation
2. Advanced age in hospitalized patient
3. Female sex
   a. Risk increased two- to threefold
4. Electrolyte imbalance
   a. Primarily hypokalemia
   b. Hypocalcemia
   c. Hypomagnesemia
5. Structural heart disease
   a. Ischemic heart disease
   b. Cardiomyopathy
6. Metabolic syndromes
   a. Hypothyroidism
   b. Anorexia
7. Pharmacologic factors
   a. Antiarrhythmic medications—most potent QT interval prolonging
      i. Class Ia—quinidine and procainamide
      ii. Class III—dofetilide, ibutilide, sotalol, and amiodarone
         • More than 80 medications are noted to pose a moderate to high risk for prolonging the QT interval
   b. Other medications with ability to prolong QT have been found in almost every other class of therapeutic agent.
8. Congenital
   a. Congenital severe bradycardia (long QT syndrome)
   b. Autosomal-dominant syndromes
   c. Autosomal-recessive cases
9. Other
   a. Intracranial events (e.g., subarachnoid hemorrhage) may be as high as 8% if associated with hypokalemia
   b. Cocaine
   c. Hypothermia
   d. HIV infection
   e. Myocardial ischemia
   f. Impaired hepatic or renal function
   g. Hypothermia

Data from Ferri, F. (2019). Torsade de pointes. In: *Ferri clinical advisor*. Elsevier, Inc.; UpToDate (2022). Retrieved April 8, 2022, from https://www.uptodate.com/contents/image?imageKey=CARD%2F57431; Khatib, R., Sabir, F. R. N., Omari, C., Pepper, C., & Tayebjee, M. H. (2021). Managing drug-induced QT prolongation in clinical practice. *Postgraduate medical journal*, *97*(1149), 452–458.

magnesium is the initial treatment of choice followed by temporary ventricular or atrial pacing (Cohagan & Brandis, 2021). Any type of VT in a patient who is unconscious and without a pulse is treated in the same manner as VF: immediate **defibrillation** is the action of choice. In addition, it is important in the hospital setting to monitor patients closely, noting those who have a QTc above 500 ms and discontinuing the offending medications.

Pearls for Practice

When caring for a patient experiencing an emergent cardiac arrhythmia, consider the following.

1. *Assess the patient's condition.*
2. *If patient has a loss of respirations, a loss of pulse, a decrease in level of consciousness, or significant change in blood pressure or oxygen saturation, call a cardiac arrest code. If the patient is alert without a significant change in vital signs, call for a rapid response team (RRT) or alert the provider stat to the patient's change in condition. Speak with the patient as it applies to keep the patient informed and calm.*
3. *While awaiting arrival of the medical team, continue to assess the patient, apply supplemental oxygen, ensure adequate IV access, and bring emergency equipment and a bedside monitor to the patient's room.*

VENTRICULAR FIBRILLATION

Pathophysiology

VF is a rapid, disorganized ventricular rhythm that causes ineffective quivering of the ventricles. No atrial activity is seen on the ECG. Causes of VF are the same as for VT; it may also result from untreated or unsuccessfully treated VT.

Clinical Manifestations and Assessment

Clinical manifestations include absence of an audible heartbeat, a palpable pulse, and respirations. Cardiac arrest and death are imminent.

ECG characteristics are:

Rate: Often cannot be determined, but is greater than 220 bpm
Rhythm: Irregular
P wave: Not visible
PR interval: Not visible
QRS duration: Not visible

See Figure 16-16.

Medical and Nursing Management

Treatment of choice is immediate defibrillation if available, immediate cardiopulmonary resuscitation (CPR), and activation of emergency services. After the initial defibrillation, five cycles of CPR, alternating with a rhythm check and defibrillation, are used to convert VF to an electrical rhythm that produces a pulse (AHA, 2020). Vasoactive medications (epinephrine) should be administered as soon as possible after the second rhythm check (immediately before or after the second defibrillation). Often antiarrhythmic medications (amiodarone, lidocaine, or possibly magnesium) will be administered though there is lack of evidence to support their routine use after a cardiac arrest (AHA, 2020). Once the patient is intubated, CPR should be administered continuously with one breath every 6 seconds and a compression rate of 100 to 120 per minute. In addition, underlying and contributing factors are identified and eliminated throughout the event.

IDIOVENTRICULAR RHYTHM

Pathophysiology

Idioventricular rhythm, also called *ventricular escape rhythm*, occurs when the impulse starts in the conduction system below the AV node. When the sinus node fails to create an impulse (e.g., from increased vagal tone) or when the impulse is created but cannot be conducted through the AV node (e.g., due to complete AV block), the Purkinje fibers automatically discharge an impulse.

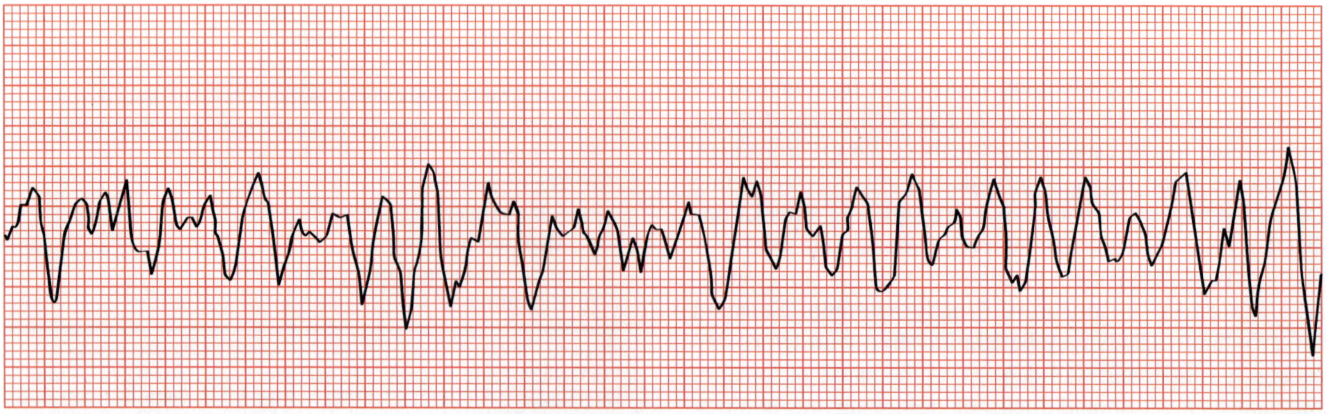

FIGURE 16-16 **Coarse ventricular fibrillation: Chaotic electrical activity.**

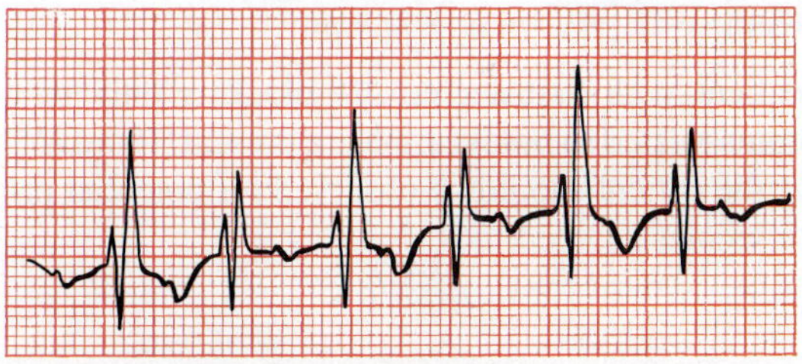

FIGURE 16-17 Idioventricular rhythm. There are no P waves, the QRS complexes are wide, and the rate is about 75 beats per minute.

Clinical Manifestations and Assessment

Idioventricular rhythm commonly causes the patient to lose consciousness and experience other signs and symptoms of reduced cardiac output.

ECG characteristics are:

Rate: 20 to 40; if the rate exceeds 40, the rhythm is known as *accelerated idioventricular rhythm* (AIVR)
Rhythm: Regular
P wave: Not visible
PR interval: Not visible
QRS duration: Duration is 0.12 second or more

See Figure 16-17.

Medical and Nursing Management

If the patient is in cardiac arrest, treatment is the same as for asystole (absence of electrical activity and pulse); if the patient is not in cardiac arrest, treatment is the same as for bradycardia. Interventions include identifying the underlying cause, administering IV epinephrine (repeating every 3 to 5 minutes as needed), and vasopressor medications, CPR, and initiating emergency pacing (Jordan et al., 2021). Asystole is a nonshockable rhythm. In some cases, idioventricular rhythm may cause no symptoms of reduced cardiac output.

VENTRICULAR ASYSTOLE

Pathophysiology

Commonly called *flatline*, ventricular asystole is characterized by absent QRS complexes confirmed in two different leads. Asystole is seen in the absence of cardiac electrical activity; because there is no contraction, there is no perfusion.

Clinical Manifestations and Assessment

There is no heartbeat, no palpable pulse, and no respiration. Without immediate treatment, ventricular asystole is fatal.

ECG characteristics are:

Rate: Not measurable
Rhythm: Not measurable
P wave: Usually not visible
PR interval: Not measurable
QRS duration: Absent

See Figure 16-18.

Medical and Nursing Management

Asystole is treated by focusing on high-quality CPR with minimal interruptions and identifying underlying and contributing factors. A mnemonic taught in Advanced Cardiac Life Support (ACLS) for the reversible causes of cardiac arrest involves the Hs & Ts. The Hs include hypovolemia, hypoxia, hydrogen ion (acidosis), hypo/hyperkalemia, and hypothermia. The Ts include tension pneumothorax, tamponade-cardiac, toxins, and thrombosis (both pulmonary and coronary) (Jordan et al., 2021).

Because of the poor prognosis associated with asystole, if the patient does not respond to CPR, medical management, and other interventions aimed at correcting underlying causes, resuscitation efforts are usually ended ("the code is called") unless special circumstances (e.g., hypothermia, transportation to a hospital is required) exist. Patients who are victims of cardiac arrest have a very poor prognosis with asystole representing the terminal rhythm (Jordan et al., 2021).

PULSELESS ELECTRICAL ACTIVITY

In some situations, the patient may have an organized electrical rhythm visible on the monitor display but is unresponsive, not breathing, and pulseless. This is termed *pulseless electrical activity* (PEA) and is considered a cardiac arrest. The patient should receive immediate CPR and life support.

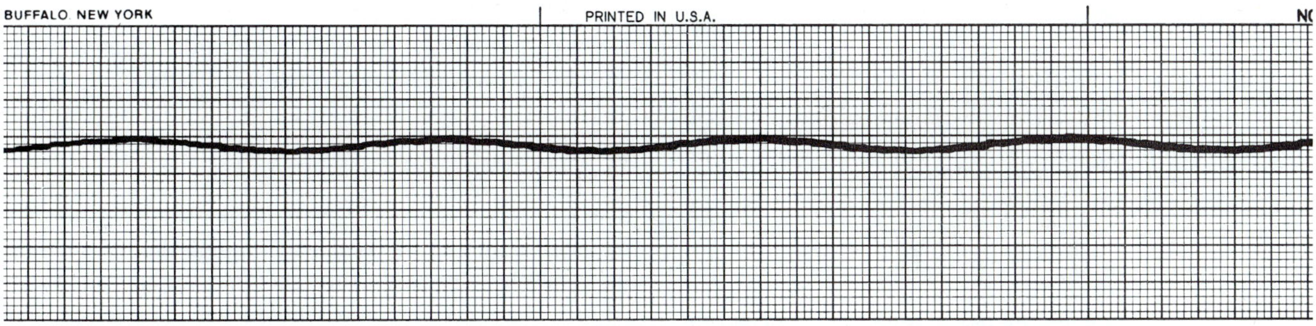

FIGURE 16-18 Asystole. Always check two different leads to confirm rhythm.

CONDUCTION ABNORMALITIES

AV blocks occur when the conduction of the impulse through the AV nodal area is decreased or stopped. These blocks can be caused by medications (e.g., digitalis, calcium channel blockers, beta blockers), myocardial ischemia and infarction, valvular disorders, myocarditis often caused by a virus or with a bacterial infection such as in Lyme Disease.

The clinical signs and symptoms of a heart block vary with the ventricular rate and the severity of any underlying disease processes. Whereas first-degree AV block rarely causes any hemodynamic effect, the other blocks may result in decreased heart rate, causing a reduction in perfusion to vital organs, such as the brain, heart, kidneys, lungs, and skin. A patient with third-degree AV block caused by digitalis toxicity may be stable; another patient with the same rhythm caused by acute MI may be unstable. Therefore, the context and general condition of the patient are factors. Health care providers must always keep in mind the need to treat the patient, not the rhythm. The treatment is based on the hemodynamic effect of the rhythm.

FIRST-DEGREE ATRIOVENTRICULAR BLOCK

First-degree AV block occurs when atrial conduction is delayed through the AV node, resulting in a prolonged PR interval.

Pathophysiology

First-degree block may occur without an underlying pathophysiology or may be the result of medications such as beta blockers, calcium channel blockers, or digoxin. It can also result from conditions that increase parasympathetic (vagal) tone, such as vomiting or Valsalva maneuver.

Clinical Manifestations and Assessment

The patient is usually asymptomatic.

ECG characteristics are:

Rate: Depends on underlying rhythm
Rhythm: Regular
P wave: Present before each QRS and consistent in size and shape
PR interval: Greater than 0.20 second
QRS duration: Normal

See Figure 16-19.

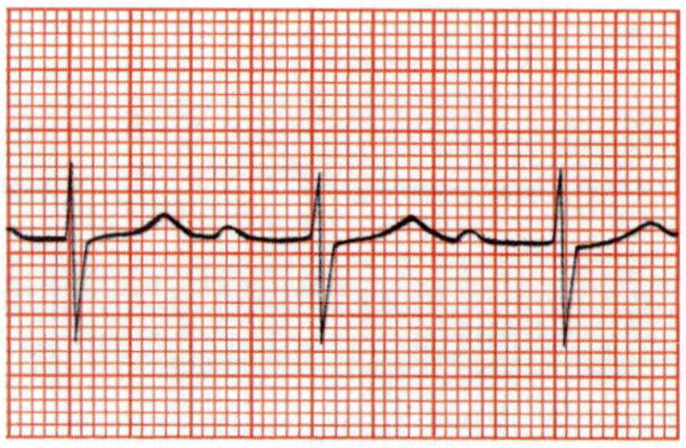

FIGURE 16-19 First-degree AV block. Note the prolonged PR interval.

Medical and Nursing Management

The patient with first-degree AV block is only treated if symptoms related to bradycardia are present. If the AV block is new, the patient should be observed for potential progression to second-degree block.

SECOND-DEGREE ATRIOVENTRICULAR BLOCK, TYPE I (WENCKEBACH)

Second-degree AV block, type I, occurs when there is a repeating pattern in which all but one of a series of atrial impulses are conducted through the AV node into the ventricles (e.g., every four of five atrial impulses are not conducted). Each atrial impulse takes a longer time for conduction than the one before, until one impulse is fully blocked, thus an increasing PR interval is seen with each successive beat until a P wave is seen without a resulting QRS. Because the AV node is not depolarized by the blocked atrial impulse, the AV node has time to fully repolarize so that the next atrial impulse can be conducted within the shortest amount of time.

Pathophysiology

Second-degree AV block, type I, is caused by a gradual and progressive conduction delay through the AV node. It may be related to increased parasympathetic (vagal) tone, ischemia, or medications that slow conduction, such as beta blockers, calcium channel blockers, and digoxin.

Clinical Manifestations and Assessment

Signs and symptoms are related to bradycardia and may include chest discomfort, dyspnea, and hypotension.

ECG characteristics are:

Rate: Atrial rate faster than ventricular rate
Rhythm: The atrial rhythm is usually regular; the ventricular rhythm is usually irregular
P wave: Size and shape normal
PR interval: PR interval becomes longer with each succeeding ECG complex until there is a P wave not followed by a QRS
QRS duration: Normal

See Figure 16-20.

Medical and Nursing Management

If the patient has symptomatic bradycardia, treatment with atropine or transcutaneous pacing is indicated.

SECOND-DEGREE ATRIOVENTRICULAR BLOCK, TYPE II

Second-degree AV block, type II, occurs when only some of the atrial impulses are conducted through the AV node into the ventricles. The ECG will reveal P waves not followed by a QRS. It is less common but more severe as it can progress to complete third-degree heart block.

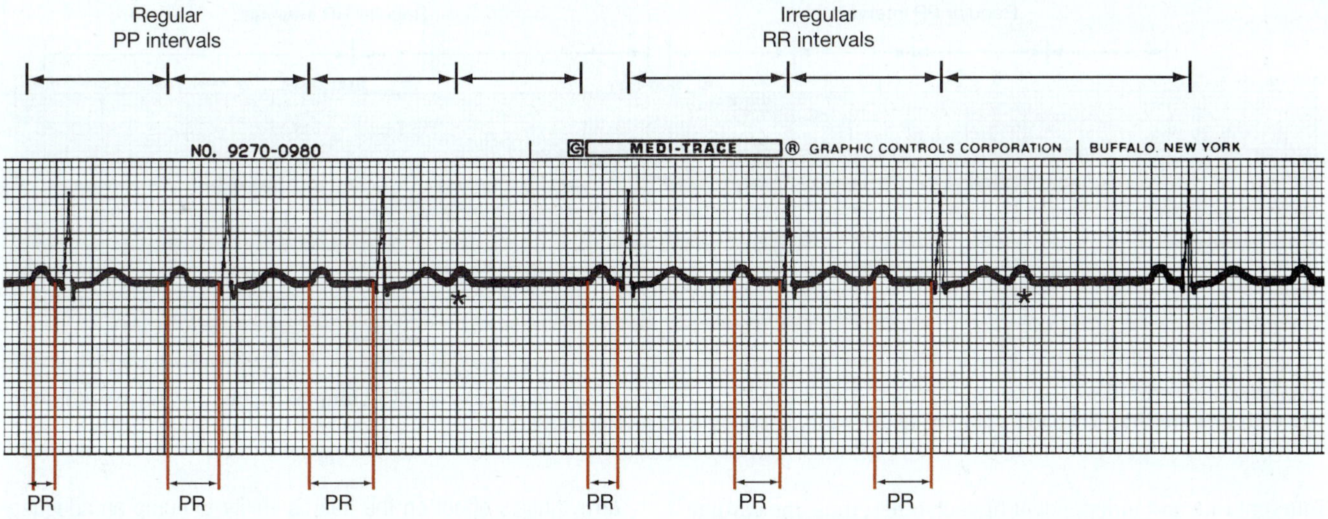

FIGURE 16-20 **Mobitz type I second-degree AV block (Wenckebach block). The PR intervals become progressively longer until one QRS complex is dropped.**

Pathophysiology

Conduction is blocked below the AV node. It is caused by ischemia, usually due to blockage of the left coronary artery.

Clinical Manifestations and Assessment

Signs and symptoms are related to bradycardia and may include chest discomfort, dyspnea, and hypotension.

ECG characteristics are:

Rate: Atrial rate 60 to 100 bpm; ventricular rate less than atrial rate

Rhythm: Atrial rhythm is regular (constant PP interval); ventricular rhythm is irregular

P wave: Normal

PR interval: Constant, no progressive prolongation with conducted beats

QRS duration: Normal or wide depending on the location of the block relative to the AV node

See Figure 16-21.

Medical and Nursing Management

If the patient has symptomatic bradycardia, treatment with atropine or pacing is indicated.

THIRD-DEGREE ATRIOVENTRICULAR BLOCK

Third-degree AV block occurs when no atrial impulse is conducted through the AV node into the ventricles. In third-degree AV block, two separate impulses stimulate the heart: one stimulates the atria, represented by the P wave, and one stimulates the ventricles, represented by the QRS complex, but there is no relationship or synchrony between the atrial and the ventricular contraction. Each is beating at its own

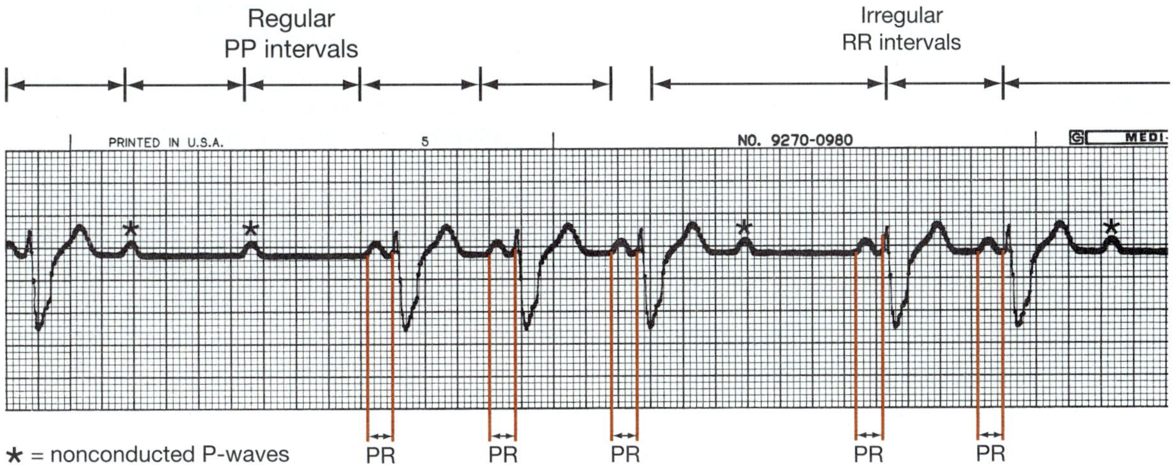

FIGURE 16-21 **Mobitz type II second-degree AV block. On this ECG, each third P wave is not followed by a QRS complex (dropped beat).**

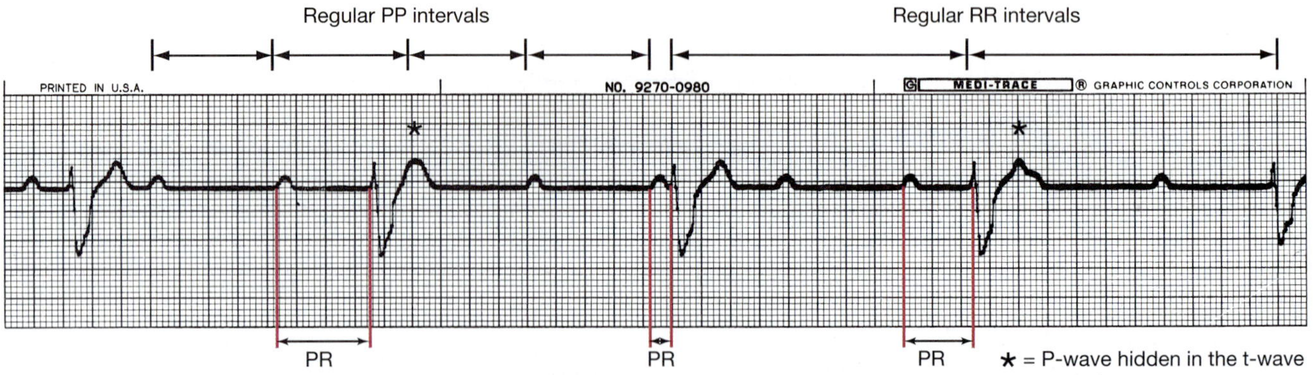

FIGURE 16-22 **Third-degree AV block. The P waves appear at regular intervals, as do the QRS complexes, but they have nothing to do with one another. The QRS complexes are wide, implying a ventricular origin.**

inherent rate and independent of each other; thus, the cardiac output is affected. P waves may be seen, but the atrial electrical activity is not conducted down into the ventricles. This is called AV dissociation.

Pathophysiology

Complete heart block is caused by injury to the conduction system so that there is no conduction between the atria and the ventricles.

Clinical Manifestations and Assessment

Signs and symptoms are related to bradycardia and may include syncope, chest discomfort, angina, dyspnea, and hypotension.

ECG characteristics are:

Rate: Atrial rate 60 to 100 bpm, ventricular rate 20 to 40 bpm

Rhythm: Atrial and ventricular rhythms are both regular but independent of each other

P wave: Normal, more P waves than QRS complexes

PR interval: Not present; no relationship between the P wave and the R wave

QRS duration: Normal or wide depending on the location of the block relative to the AV node

See Figure 16-22.

Medical and Nursing Management

If the patient has symptomatic bradycardia, treatment with atropine or pacing is indicated.

NURSING PROCESS
The Patient With an Arrhythmia

ASSESSMENT

Major areas of assessment include possible causes of the arrhythmia, contributing factors, the associated risks, and the arrhythmia's effect on the heart's ability to pump an adequate blood volume.

A health history is obtained to identify any previous occurrences of possible decreased cardiac output, such as near-syncope or syncope (fainting), lightheadedness, dizziness, nausea, fatigue, chest discomfort, shortness of breath, and/or palpitations. Comorbidities or coexisting conditions that could be a possible cause of the arrhythmia (e.g., heart disease, chronic obstructive pulmonary disease, severe pre-existing thyroid disease, sarcoidosis, some neuromuscular diseases, COVID-19, or Lyme disease) may also be identified. All medications, prescribed and over the counter, are reviewed. Laboratory results are reviewed to assess levels of medications, as well as factors that could contribute to the arrhythmia (e.g., anemia, hypokalemia, hypomagnesemia). A psychosocial assessment is performed to identify the possible effects of the arrhythmia, the patient's perception of the arrhythmia, and whether anxiety is a significant contributing factor.

During physical assessment, the nurse assesses the patient's skin, which may be pale and cool. Signs of fluid retention, such as neck vein distention and crackles and wheezes auscultated in the lungs, may be detected. The presence of peripheral edema is assessed as well as its extent and whether it is pitting or not. The rate and rhythm of apical and peripheral pulses are also assessed, and any pulse deficit (see Chapter 11) is noted. The nurse auscultates for extra heart sounds (especially S_3 and S_4) and for heart murmurs, evaluates blood pressure, and assesses the patient's usual versus current weight.

Pearls for Practice

Cardiac output is calculated as heart rate (HR) × stroke volume (SV). Stroke volume is the amount of blood ejected by the left ventricle with each contraction. If an arrhythmia occurs, the HR and SV can be affected, decreasing the filling times for the ventricle and, ultimately, causing a decreased cardiac output. The nurse is alert for patient complaints of dizziness, syncope, shortness of breath, peripheral edema, weight gain, crackles, fatigue, chest pain, or discomfort.

DIAGNOSIS

Appropriate nursing diagnoses of the patient with an arrhythmia may include:

- Cardiac output, decreased
- Anxiety related to fear of the unknown
- Knowledge deficit regarding the arrhythmia and its treatment

Potential complications may include the following:

- Cardiac arrest (see Chapter 13)
- Heart failure (see Chapter 14)
- Thromboembolic event, especially with AF (see Chapters 9 and 46)

PLANNING

The major goals for the patient would include eliminating or decreasing the occurrence of the arrhythmia, minimizing anxiety, and acquiring knowledge about the arrhythmia and its treatment.

NURSING INTERVENTIONS

MONITORING AND MANAGING THE ARRHYTHMIA

The nurse regularly evaluates the patient's blood pressure, pulse rate and rhythm, rate and depth of respirations, breath sounds, oxygen saturation levels, and daily weights. The nurse also asks the patient about episodes of chest pain, syncope, lightheadedness, dizziness, or fainting as part of the ongoing assessment as well as frequency of palpitations and overall level of fatigue. If a patient with an arrhythmia is hospitalized, the nurse may obtain a 12-lead ECG, continuously monitor the patient, and analyze rhythm strips to track and trend the arrhythmia. The patient should have vascular access and supplemental oxygen at the bedside.

The nurse assesses and observes for the beneficial and adverse effects of each antiarrhythmic medication. The nurse also manages medication administration carefully so that a constant serum blood level of the medication is maintained.

In addition to medication, the nurse assesses for factors that contribute to the arrhythmia, such as too much caffeine and stress, smoking, drinking alcohol, prescriptive and nonprescriptive medications and assists the patient in developing a plan to make lifestyle changes that eliminate or reduce these factors.

MINIMIZING ANXIETY

When the patient experiences episodes of arrhythmia, the nurse maintains a calm and reassuring attitude. This assists in reducing anxiety (reducing the sympathetic response) and fosters a trusting relationship with the patient. In addition, the nurse can help the patient develop a system to identify possible causative, influencing, and alleviating factors (e.g., keeping a diary). The nursing goal is to maximize the patient's control and to make the episode less threatening. In addition, involving family members can also be beneficial for the patient; the family can be involved in providing an educated support system and a plan of action if the patient experiences a hemodynamically unstable rhythm.

TEACHING PATIENTS SELF-CARE

The nurse explains the importance of maintaining therapeutic serum levels of antiarrhythmic medications so that the patient understands why medications should be taken regularly each day. If the patient has a potentially lethal arrhythmia, it is also important to establish with the patient and family a plan of action to take in case of an emergency. Family members should be encouraged to learn CPR as well as how to use an automated external defibrillator (AED). Occasionally patients wear a defibrillator vest to manage arrhythmias in the short term while allowing time to determine if the patient's cardiac output will improve post-MI or while trying to diagnose the cause of a clinically significant arrhythmia. This wearable defibrillator is worn only for a period of a few weeks to months, and then, depending on the patient's progress, the device is discontinued with no further device used or a permanent ICD is placed (discussed shortly) (Figs. 16-23 and 16-24). The patient and family should also be taught about potential effects or presentation of the arrhythmia and the signs and symptoms. This information allows the patient and family to feel more in control and better prepared for possible events.

CONTINUING CARE

Home care is warranted if the patient has significant comorbidities, socioeconomic issues, or limited self-management skills

(continued on page 574)

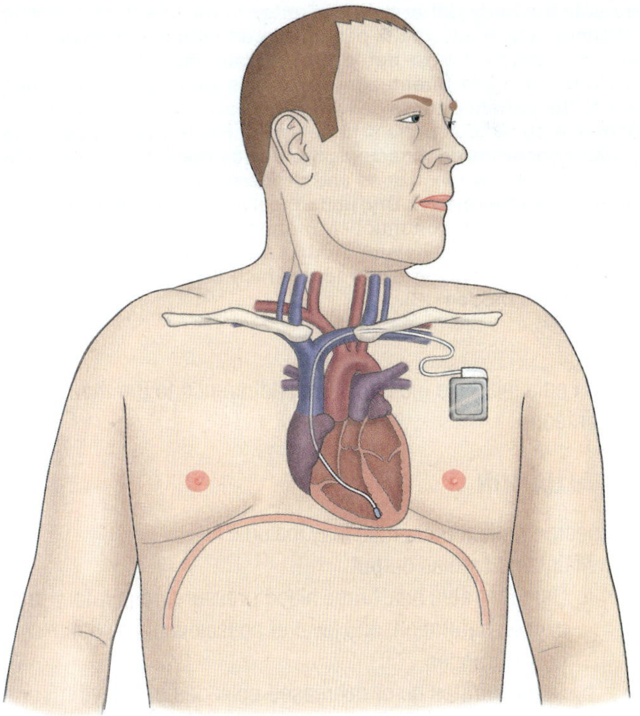

FIGURE 16-23 **The implantable cardioverter defibrillator (ICD) consists of a generator and a sensing/pacing/defibrillating electrode.**

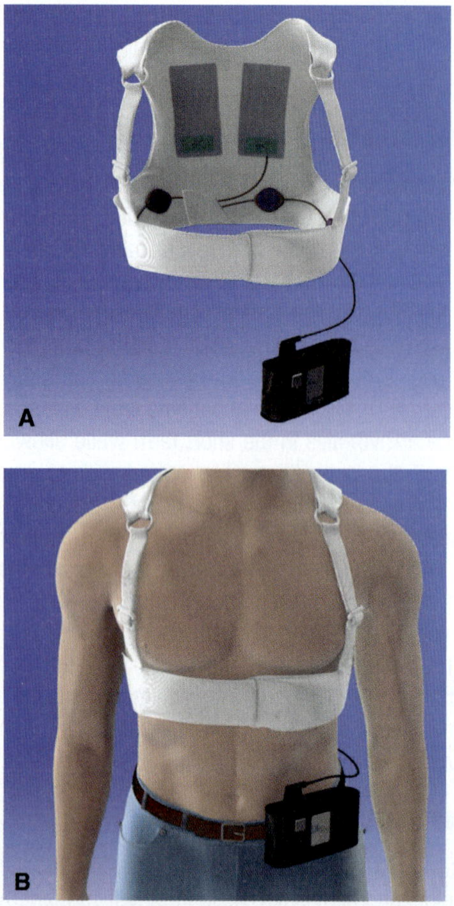

FIGURE 16-24 **The LifeVest is a wearable defibrillator. Unlike an implantable cardioverter defibrillator (ICD), the LifeVest is worn outside the body rather than implanted in the chest. This device continuously monitors the patient's heart with dry, nonadhesive sensing electrodes to detect life-threatening abnormal heart rhythms. If a life-threatening rhythm is detected, the device alerts the patient prior to delivering a treatment shock, and thus allows a conscious patient to delay the treatment shock. If the patient becomes unconscious, the device releases a Blue™ gel over the therapy electrodes and delivers an electrical shock to restore normal rhythm. Dry, nonadhesive sensing electrodes on this electrode belt continuously monitor patient's heart (A). This monitor is worn in a holster around the waist and collects ECG data from the sensing electrodes which can later be sent to a provider via modem (B).**

that could increase the risk for nonadherence to the therapeutic regimen.

EVALUATION

Expected patient outcomes may include:

1. Maintains cardiac output:
   a. Demonstrates heart rate, blood pressure, respiratory rate, oxygen saturation, and level of consciousness within normal ranges
   b. Demonstrates no or decreased episodes of arrhythmia
2. Experiences reduced anxiety:
   a. Expresses a positive attitude about living with the arrhythmia
   b. Expresses confidence in ability to take appropriate actions in an emergency
3. Expresses understanding of the arrhythmia and its treatment:
   a. Explains the arrhythmia and its effects
   b. Describes the medication regimen and its rationale
   c. Explains the need to maintain a therapeutic serum level of the medication
   d. Describes a plan to eliminate or limit factors that contribute to the arrhythmia
   e. States actions to take in the event of an emergency

ADJUNCTIVE MODALITIES AND MANAGEMENT

Acute arrhythmias may be treated with medications or with electrical therapy (emergency defibrillation, cardioversion, or pacing), or, in many cases, both are used concurrently and sequentially to prevent the occurrence of arrhythmias. Many antiarrhythmic medications are used to treat atrial and ventricular tachyarrhythmias. The choice of medication depends on the specific arrhythmia and its duration, the presence of HF and other diseases, and the patient's response to previous treatment. Electrical therapies include cardioversion and defibrillation for acute tachyarrhythmia, and implantable devices (pacemakers for bradycardias and implantable cardioverter defibrillator [ICD] for chronic tachyarrhythmias). These devices are often referred to as cardiovascular implantable electronic devices (CIEDs). Catheter ablation is also available depending on the type of arrhythmia. The nurse is responsible for assessing the patient's understanding of and response to therapy, as well as the patient's self-management abilities.

CARDIOVERSION AND DEFIBRILLATION

Cardioversion and defibrillation are used to treat tachyarrhythmias by delivering an electrical current that depolarizes a critical mass of myocardial cells. When the cells repolarize, the sinus node is usually able to recapture its role as the heart's pacemaker. One major difference between cardioversion and defibrillation is the timing of the delivery of electrical current. In cardioversion, the delivery of the electrical current is synchronized with the patient's intrinsic rhythm; in defibrillation, the delivery of the current is unsynchronized or delivered independent of the patient's intrinsic rhythm.

The electrical current may be delivered externally through the skin with the use of paddles or with electrode pads, or it may be delivered internally as part of open-heart surgery. The paddles or pads may be placed on the front of the chest (Fig. 16-25) (standard paddle placement), or one paddle may be placed on the front of the chest and the other connected to an adapter with a long handle and placed under

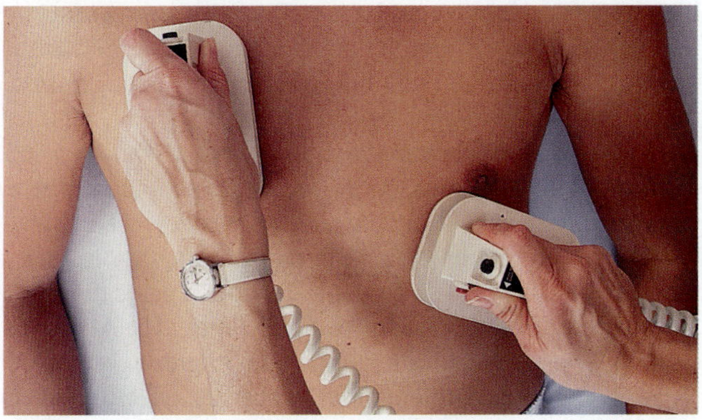

FIGURE 16-25 **Standard paddle placement for defibrillation and for pads. One pad goes to the upper chest just right of the sternum and the other at the apex of the heart on the patient's left lateral chest, under the left breast.**

the patient's back (anteroposterior placement) (Fig. 16-26). Whether using pads or paddles, the nurse must observe two safety measures. First, good contact must be maintained between the pads or paddles and the patient's skin (with a conductive medium in between them) to prevent electrical current from leaking into the air (arcing) when the defibrillator is discharged. Second, no one is to be in contact with the patient or with anything that is touching the patient when the defibrillator is discharged, to minimize the chance that electrical current will be conducted to anyone other than the patient. Box 16-6 lists key points for assisting with cardioversion or defibrillation.

Pearls for Practice

Two types of defibrillators are used today for external cardioversion and defibrillation: the older, monophasic sinusoidal waveform and the newer, biphasic truncated waveform. The new biphasic defibrillators use less energy to convert arrhythmias to normal sinus rhythm, which is a benefit. These defibrillators work through automatically adjusting to the patient's transthoracic impedance. The nurse understands that the amount of energy delivered to the heart is inversely related to transthoracic resistance so lowering the resistance helps to deliver optimal current to "shock" the heart. Of note, the trend is toward the use of the biphasic defibrillator, manufacturers no longer make the monophasic defibrillator though you may still come across them in hospitals. Refer to recommendations in Box 16-6 for further details.

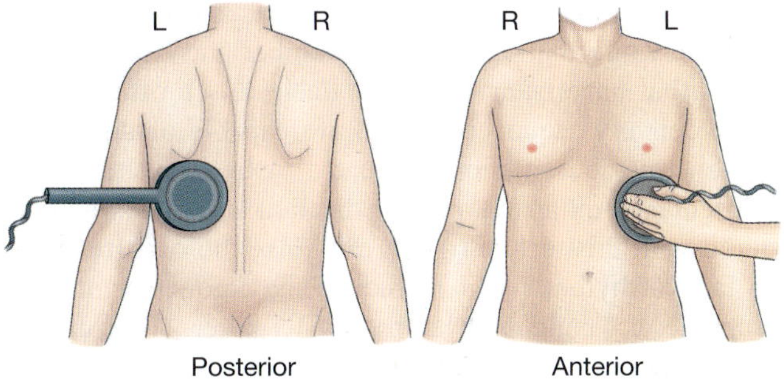

FIGURE 16-26 **Anteroposterior paddle placement for defibrillation.**

BOX 16-6

Assisting With External Cardioversion or Defibrillation

When assisting with external cardioversion or defibrillation, the nurse should remember these key points:

- Use multifunction conductor pads or paddles with a conducting medium between the paddles and the skin (the conducting medium is available as a sheet, gel, or paste). Do not use gels or pastes with poor electrical conductivity (e.g., ultrasound gel). Conductive electrode gel has been noted to reduce the transthoracic impedance (TTI) and without the use of a gel or paste there could be an increase in TTI of more than 100% (Heyer et al., 2022). Further, it is important for the nurse to consider that TTI is influenced by factors such as electronic configurations (waveforms), electrode/tissue interface (gels) and patient properties such as age and body measurements that separately and together will affect defibrillation (Heyer et al., 2022).
- Place paddles or pads so that they do not touch the patient's clothing or bed linen and are not near medication patches or direct oxygen flow.
- If using paddles, exert 20–25 lb of pressure to ensure good skin contact. This lowers the transthoracic resistance.
- Before pressing the discharge button, call "Clear!" three times. Ensure that you and everyone else are not touching the patient, bed, or equipment. Perform a final visual check to ensure that you, and everyone else, are clear of the patient and anything touching the patient.
- Record the delivered energy.
- After the event is complete, inspect the skin under the pads or paddles for burns; if any are detected, consult with the physician or a wound care nurse about treatment.
- If cardioverting, ensure that the monitor leads are attached to the patient and that the defibrillator is in the synchronized mode ("sync"). If defibrillating, ensure that the defibrillator is not in the synchronized mode (most machines default to the "not-sync" mode).

Electrical Cardioversion

Electrical cardioversion involves the delivery of a "timed" electrical current to terminate a tachyarrhythmia. In cardioversion, the defibrillator is set to synchronize with the ECG on a cardiac monitor so that the electrical impulse discharges during ventricular depolarization (QRS complex). The synchronization prevents the discharge from occurring during the vulnerable period of repolarization (T wave), which could result in VT or VF. When the synchronizer is on, no electrical current is delivered if the defibrillator does not discern a QRS complex. Because there may be a short delay until recognition of the QRS, the discharge buttons of an external defibrillator must be held down until the shock has been delivered.

If the cardioversion is elective and the arrhythmia has lasted longer than 48 hours, anticoagulation for a few weeks before cardioversion may be indicated. Digoxin is usually withheld for 48 hours before cardioversion to ensure the resumption of sinus rhythm with normal conduction. The patient is instructed not to eat or drink for at least 4 hours before the procedure. Before cardioversion, the patient receives IV moderate sedation as well as an analgesic medication or anesthesia. The amount of voltage used varies, depending on the defibrillator's technology and the type of arrhythmia.

Pearls for Practice

When the heart returns to a normal sinus rhythm after cardioversion, the atria beat forcefully. If a clot has formed in the atria, systemic emboli may result, thus anticoagulation is needed if the arrhythmia has lasted over 48 hours. The nurse is alert for systemic signs of embolization, such as sudden onset shortness of breath or chest pain with pulmonary emboli or neurologic changes (visual, motor, sensory, headache, etc.; refer to Chapter 46) with cerebral emboli.

Defibrillation

Defibrillation is used in emergency situations as the treatment of choice for VF and pulseless VT. Defibrillation is not used on patients who are conscious or have a pulse. About half of all sudden deaths occur in the pre-hospital setting; of these, about 75% happen in the home, and 50% of these are unwitnessed. In the adult patient, VF is the most common cause of sudden cardiac arrest. The definitive treatment for VF is to perform electrical defibrillation. When defibrillation is delayed, effectiveness is reduced by almost 10% per minute.

VF is the leading cause of cardiac arrest, and defibrillation is the best treatment option for terminating VF. External defibrillation when used within minutes of the onset of VF can save lives (Goyal et al., 2022).

The electrical voltage required to defibrillate the heart is usually greater than that required for cardioversion and may cause more myocardial damage. Defibrillators are classified as monophasic or biphasic as discussed in the Pearls for Practice. Monophasic defibrillators deliver current in only one direction and require increased energy loads; they are rarely used today. Newer biphasic defibrillators deliver the electrical charge to the positive paddle, which then reverses back to the originating paddle. The recommended energy levels for defibrillation vary according to the type of waveform and the manufacturer of the defibrillator. Following defibrillation, CPR is initiated immediately if a rhythm resulted that did not resume perfusion, and other advanced life support treatments are begun. This treatment with continuous CPR, medication administration, and defibrillation continues until a stable rhythm resumes or it is determined that the patient cannot be revived.

Often automated external defibrillators (AEDs) are used today by both laypersons and health care providers where the device once attached to the patient interprets the rhythm. Based on an algorithm when the patient's rhythm is determined to be "shockable," the defibrillator will guide the operator's or rescuer's action to discharge a shock. The AEDs are commonly placed in locations where large groups of people meet and/or in remote locations. They are often found in schools, airports, stadiums, on board aircraft, and in hospitals. The assignment of AEDs in the hospital setting makes sense to facilitate early rescue by providers who—although they are clinically oriented—are not necessarily proficient in interpreting arrhythmias due to infrequent occurrences of lethal arrhythmias, such as on a maternal child health unit.

Implantable Cardioverter Defibrillator

Often patients will have ICD/pacemaker devices placed if they have tachyarrhythmias to manage both the rapid and slow rates. The ICD is a device that detects and terminates life-threatening episodes of tachycardia or fibrillation. ICDs are used for patients who have survived sudden cardiac death syndrome, usually caused by VF, or have experienced symptomatic VT. Other people at risk of sudden cardiac death include those with dilated cardiomyopathy, hypertrophic cardiomyopathy, arrhythmogenic (capable of inducing an arrhythmia) right ventricular dysfunction, and prolonged QT syndrome. In addition, patients with moderate to severe left ventricular dysfunction, with a low ejection fraction (less than 30%), or with or without nonsustained VT are at high risk for cardiac arrest; therefore, prophylactic implantation may be indicated. ICDs may also be implanted in patients with symptomatic, recurrent, medication-refractory AF.

An ICD consists of a generator and at least one lead that can sense intrinsic electrical activity and deliver an electrical impulse. The device is usually implanted much like a pacemaker (Fig. 16-23). ICDs are designed to respond to two criteria: a rate that exceeds a predetermined level, and a change in the isoelectric line segments. When an arrhythmia occurs, the device automatically charges and delivers the programmed charge through the lead to the heart. ICD surveillance is similar to that of the pacemaker; however, it includes information about the number and frequency of shocks that have been delivered. Each device offers a different delivery sequence, but all are capable of delivering high-energy defibrillation to treat a tachycardia (atrial or ventricular). Antiarrhythmic medication usually is administered with this technology to minimize the occurrence of the tachyarrhythmia and to reduce the frequency of ICD discharge. In patients who have SVT, there is a choice between a single- and dual-chamber (DC) ICD dependent on the patient's clinical condition. The DC algorithm senses and interprets data from the atrium and ventricle to classify the rhythm and treat. In a retrospective cohort study of the National Cardiovascular Data Registry, a total of 3,100 older patients (Standard deviation was 76.3 years) were included with 80.6% male with first-time implantation of a cardiac resynchronization therapy (CRT) defibrillator or DC device placed between 2010 and 2016 to review outcomes (Borne et al., 2020). The results indicated that in the cohort of older patients having an ICD implanted with bradycardia but without a class 1 or strong indication for CRT, CRT-D (defibrillator) was associated with better outcomes compared with DC devices (Borne et al., 2020). Better outcomes that were measured were all-cause mortality and HF hospitalization. The findings were in the context of variation in device type and with the rate of CRT increasing over time (Borne et al., 2020).

Some ICDs can respond with antitachycardia pacing or overdrive, in which the device delivers electrical impulses at a fast rate in an attempt to disrupt the tachycardia or by low-energy (low-intensity) cardioversion or by defibrillation. Antitachycardia pacing is used to terminate tachycardias caused by a conduction disturbance called *re-entry*. Some ICDs also have pacemaker capability if the patient develops bradycardia, which sometimes occurs after treatment of the tachycardia. In addition, many ICDs have other functions, such as storage of detected arrhythmias and the ability to perform electrophysiologic testing.

Pearls for Practice

Patients who have ICDs must take care when coming into contact with devices that have strong magnetic fields. These devices may interfere with ICD function especially with prolonged exposure. It is important for the nurse to refer the patient to the AHA website: http://www.heart.org/ or to the ICD manufacturer webpage to learn more about the potential environmental issues associated with ICDs so that the patient can take the necessary precautions. Further, the overall risk of clinically significant adverse events related to electrical magnetic interference (EMI) in recipients of CIEDs is very low. Therefore, no special precautions are needed when household appliances are used in close proximity to the ICD. Environmental and industrial sources of EMI are relatively safe when the exposure time is limited and distance from the CIEDs is maximized. The risk of EMI-induced events is highest within the hospital environment. Physician awareness of the possible interactions and methods to minimize them is warranted (Link, 2021).

Complications associated with the ICD implantation can be divided into surgical and long-term risks. In the category of surgical risks, the problems that can occur include infection, bleeding, dislodgment of lead, cardiac perforation, and lung collapse. All of these risks are very rare (Knight et al., 2021). In terms of longer-term complications, possible issues include infection or erosion of the device and problems associated with the technical aspects of the equipment, such as premature battery depletion and dislodged or fractured leads (Knight et al., 2021). In a cross-sectional survey of 434 ICD patients who had a primary indication for the device, almost 10% of ICD recipients regretted their decision after implantation. Predictors included younger age, higher education levels, complicated perioperative period, and lack of preoperative information (Varghese et al., 2020). Accordingly, the literature also suggests that more research and work need to be done in the area of communication with the patient about the ICD prior to implantation. Pederson who conducted the Defib-Women trial in 2016 and was cited in an article by Antipolis in 2021 stated, "Most patients adapt well to living with an ICD. For others it completely changes their life, with worries about shocks from the device, body image, and livelihood as some need to change their job." Therefore, there is a need for the nurse to assess the patient to determine the best follow-up especially since this procedure may be done in 1-day surgery with minimal time to teach and provide education and emotional support. Schulz and colleagues (2020) designed a web-based structured intervention that included 6 weeks of group and individual support and education for 118 patients who had ICDs placed. Although the primary outcome of improving psychological well-being associated with the ICD was neutral, the researchers believed there were benefits in terms of a reduction in depression and an improvement in self-management. Nurses should advocate for patients and their families to ensure that informed consent is achieved before implantation of an ICD.

Newer features in modern ICDs (e.g., antitachycardia pacing therapy) coupled with the broad goals of both preventing inappropriate shocks and delivering shocks for symptomatic ventricular arrhythmias are offering advances in providing medical devices safely to such patients (Knight et al., 2021). Patients who have ICDs are clinically monitored, and their devices can be interrogated remotely and in-person to program them to meet the specific clinical indications; often hospitals or cardiologists offices will have an arrhythmia clinic associated with it.

Deactivation of the ICD at End of Life

When a patient is in the terminal phases of illness, the ICD is no longer an appropriate intervention in the management of clinical care, and thoughtful consideration is required of the deactivation plan. Ideally, the conversation regarding the ICD and the possible need to deactivate it in a terminal illness should be discussed before the device is even implanted in the patient. Guidelines or protocols are needed in the United States to provide both patients and providers with direction for management of this lifesaving device in the context of life-ending disease along with ethical and legal implications. Further, both pacemakers and ICDs should be considered fully as they relate to the end of life to then estimate the potential benefits and harm associated with the device while allowing death with dignity. Pacemakers are not as controversial because in contrast with the ICD, there are no associated painful discharges of shocks to treat an arrhythmia in a patient who is dying. Deactivation of an ICD would not cause the death of a patient; rather this will allow a natural death to occur. Nurses, along with the interdisciplinary team, will need to collaborate to address the ethical challenges associated with withdrawal of life-sustaining treatments and should conduct advance care planning conversations to prepare the patient and family for defibrillator deactivation (Stoevelaar et al., 2020).

PACEMAKER THERAPY

A pacemaker is an electronic device that delivers electrical stimulation to the heart to regulate the heart rate when a patient has a slower-than-normal heart rate or conduction disturbance. They may also be used to control some tachyarrhythmias or to treat advanced HF that does not respond to medication. Pacemakers may be temporary or permanent. Temporary pacemakers may be transvenous, transcutaneous, or epicardial.

Pacemaker Design and Types

Pacemakers consist of two components: an electronic pulse generator and pacemaker electrodes or leads. The generator contains the energy source that determines the rate (measured in bpm) and the strength or output (measured in milliamperes [mA]) of the electrical stimulus delivered to the heart. The generator can be programmed to detect the heart's intrinsic electrical activity and to cause an appropriate response; this component of pacing is called *sensitivity* and is measured in millivolts (mV). Leads can be threaded through a major vein into the right ventricle (endocardial leads), or they can be lightly sutured onto the outside of the heart and brought through the chest wall during open heart surgery (epicardial wires). The endocardial leads may be placed temporarily with catheters through a great vessel (transvenous wires), usually guided by fluoroscopy. The endocardial and epicardial wires are connected to a temporary external generator.

Endocardial leads may also be placed permanently, usually through the external jugular vein, and connected to a permanent generator. The generator is implanted in a subcutaneous pocket created in the pectoral region below the clavicle (Fig. 16-27), may be implanted on the nondominant side. The procedure usually takes about 1 hour, and it is performed in a cardiac catheterization or EP lab using a local anesthetic. Batteries need replacement after approximately 10 years; and battery replacement is usually performed using a local anesthetic.

If a patient suddenly develops a symptomatic bradycardia, emergency pacing may be started with transcutaneous pacing. Large-pacing ECG electrodes (pads) are placed on the patient's chest and back. The electrodes are connected to the temporary pacemaker generator (Fig. 16-28). Because the impulse must travel through the patient's skin and tissue before reaching the heart, transcutaneous pacing can cause significant discomfort and is intended to be used only in emergencies. If the patient is alert, sedation and analgesia may be administered.

When pacing is initiated, the ECG tracing will display a straight vertical line, called a *pacemaker spike*, with each pacemaker impulse. The appropriate ECG complex should immediately follow the pacing spike; therefore, a P wave should follow an atrial pacing spike and a QRS complex should follow a ventricular pacing spike. Because the impulse starts in a different place than the patient's normal rhythm, the QRS complex or P wave that responds to pacing looks different from the patient's normal ECG complex. *Capture* is

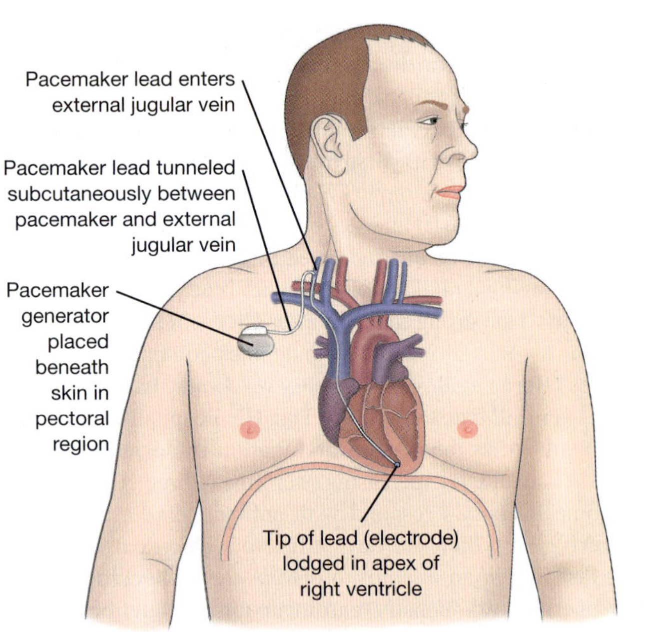

FIGURE 16-27 **Implanted transvenous pacing lead (with electrode) and pacemaker generator.**

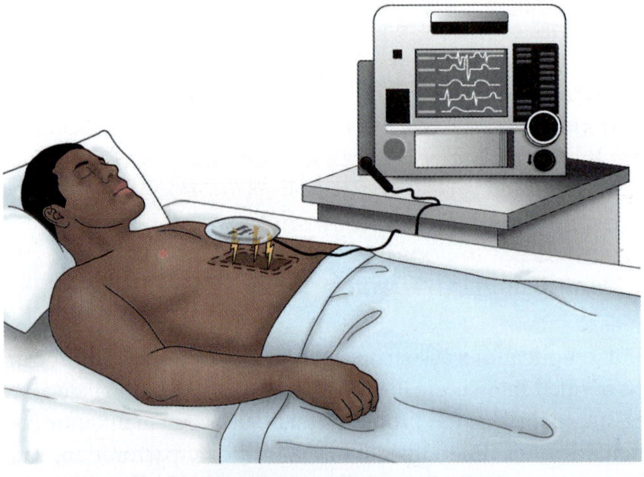

FIGURE 16-28 **Transcutaneous pacemaker with electrode pads connected to the anterior and posterior chest walls.**

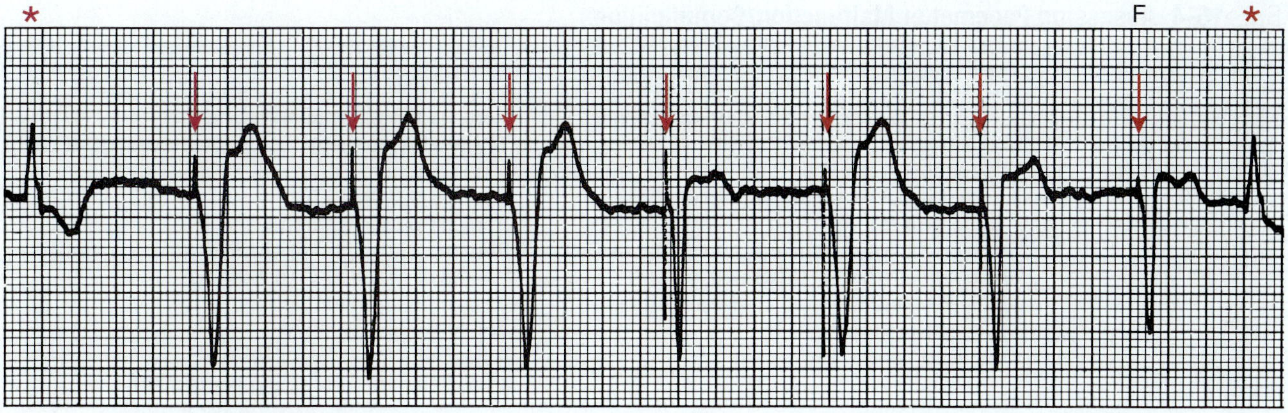

FIGURE 16-29 **Pacing with appropriate sensing (on-demand pacing) in lead V_1. *Arrows* denote pacing spike. *Asterisk* (*) denotes intrinsic (patient's own) beats, therefore no pacing.**

a term used to denote that the appropriate complex followed the pacing spike (Fig. 16-29). *Synchronized biventricular pacing*, also called *cardiac resynchronized therapy* (CRT), has been found to modify the intraventricular, interventricular, and atrial-ventricular conduction defects identified with symptomatic moderate to severe (New York Heart Association Functional Class III and IV) left ventricular dysfunction and HF. The generator for biventricular pacing has three leads: one for the right atrium; one for the right ventricle, as with most standard pacemaker generators; and one for the left ventricle, usually placed in the left lateral wall. Studies have shown that this therapy improves cardiac function, resulting in decreased HF symptoms and an improved quality of life. The American College of Cardiology Foundation and the AHA developed four stages for HF, and it is at the level of stage B that a pacemaker or, in many cases, an ICD is recommended to prevent sudden cardiac death (Chapter 14 reviews the stages for HF).

Complications of Pacemaker Use

Complications associated with pacemakers relate to their presence within the body and improper functioning. The following complications may arise from a pacemaker:

- Local infection
- Bleeding and hematoma
- Hemothorax
- Ventricular ectopy and tachycardia
- Movement or dislocation of the lead placed
- Phrenic nerve stimulation (hiccuping may be a sign)
- Rarely, cardiac tamponade

In the initial hours after a temporary or permanent pacemaker is inserted, the most common complication is dislodgment of the pacing electrode. Minimizing patient activity can help prevent this complication. If a temporary electrode is in place, the extremity through which the catheter has been advanced is immobilized. With a permanent pacemaker, the patient is instructed initially to restrict strenuous activity on the side of the implantation for 2 weeks.

The ECG is monitored very carefully to detect pacemaker malfunction. Improper pacemaker function, which can arise from failure in one or more components of the pacing system, is outlined in Table 16-4. Pacemaker settings (e.g., rate, energy output [mA], sensitivity [mV], and duration of interval between atrial and ventricular impulses [AV delay]) should be noted in the patient's record.

A patient experiencing pacemaker malfunction may develop bradycardia as well as signs and symptoms of decreased cardiac output. The degree to which these symptoms become apparent depends on the severity of the malfunction, the patient's level of dependency on the pacemaker, and the patient's underlying condition. Pacemaker malfunction is diagnosed by analyzing the ECG and through *interrogation* of the pacemaker's stored bank of activity, performed by trained personnel.

Inhibition of permanent pacemakers or reversion to asynchronous fixed rate pacing can occur with exposure to strong electromagnetic fields (electromagnetic interference [EMI]). However, recent pacemaker technology allows patients to safely use most household electronic appliances and devices (e.g., microwave ovens, electric tools). Objects that contain magnets (e.g., the earpiece of a phone; large stereo speakers; portable media players; magnet therapy products, such as mattresses, jewelry, and wraps) should not be near the generator for longer than a few seconds. Patients are advised to keep digital cellular phones at least 6 to 12 in away from (or on the side opposite of) the pacemaker generator and not to carry them in a shirt pocket.

Pacemaker Surveillance

Pacemaker clinics have been established to monitor patients and to test pulse generators for impending pacemaker battery failure. A computerized device is held over the generator to interrogate it with painless radio signals; it detects the generator's settings, battery status, pacing threshold, sensing function, lead integrity, and other stored information. Several factors, such as lead fracture, muscle inhibition, and insulation disruption, also may be assessed. If indicated, the pacemaker is turned off for a few seconds, using a

TABLE **16-4 Assessing Pacemaker Malfunction/Complications**

Problem	Possible Cause	Intervention
Failure to pace; the pacemaker fails to deliver the correct number of electrical stimuli per minute	Output failure—oversensing and undersensing Battery failure Loose connection between lead wire and generator Fracture or displacement of pacing lead wire Pulse generator failure Electromagnetic interference (potential causes of EMI include use of the TENS unit, electroconvulsive therapy, and monopolar electrocautery) Sensitivity setting too high Lead displacement	Replace the pulse generator battery Tighten the connections between pacing lead and pulse generator Replace the lead wire Replace pulse generator unit Remove the source of electromagnetic interference or moderate it if possible. Check with pacemaker manufacturer. Adjust sensitivity setting Adjust lead May require programming adjustment
Failure to capture; the pacemaker does not depolarize the heart	Battery failure Fracture or displacement of pacing lead wire Perforation of the myocardium by the lead wire Scar tissue or edema formation at lead tip Energy output (mA) too low Increase in stimulation threshold due to medication Electrolyte imbalance Myocardial Infarction	Replace battery Reposition patient; replace the lead wire Surgical repair Replace pacing lead Increase the output (mA) Increase the output (mA) Correct electrolyte imbalances May require programming adjustment

EMI, electromechanical interference; TENS, transcutaneous electrical nerve stimulation; mA, miliamperage.

Data from Neelankavil et al., 2013; Liaquat, M. T., Ahmed, I., & Alzahrani, T. (2022). Pacemaker malfunction. In *StatPearls* [Internet]. Treasure Island (FL): StatPearls Publishing; 2022 Jan.

magnet or a programmer, while the ECG is recorded to assess the patient's underlying cardiac rhythm. Changes may be made in the programming of the pacemaker or ICD prior to surgery or procedures where the device may need to be adjusted. Therefore, it is very important that the perioperative team is made aware of the device that the patient has implanted. In addition, it is important to have a list of manufacturer contacts should there be an emergent need requiring technical support. Transtelephonic transmission of the generator's information is another follow-up method. Special equipment is used to transmit information about the patient's pacemaker over the telephone to a receiving system at a pacemaker clinic. The information is converted into tones; equipment at the clinic converts these tones to an electronic signal and records them on an ECG strip. The pacemaker rate and other data concerning pacemaker function are obtained and evaluated by a cardiologist. This simplifies the diagnosis of a failing generator, reassures the patient, and improves management when the patient is physically remote from pacemaker testing facilities.

ELECTROPHYSIOLOGIC STUDIES

An EP study is a minimally invasive procedure used to evaluate and treat significant arrhythmias. It also is indicated for patients with symptoms that suggest an arrhythmia that has gone undetected and undiagnosed by other methods. An EP study is used to do the following:

- Identify the impulse formation and propagation through the cardiac electrical conduction system
- Assess the function or dysfunction of the SA and AV nodal areas
- Identify the location (called *mapping*) and mechanism of dysrhythmogenic foci (where the arrhythmia is originating)
- Assess the effectiveness of antiarrhythmic medications and devices for the patient with an arrhythmia
- Treat certain arrhythmias through the destruction of the causative cells (**ablation**)

An EP procedure is a type of cardiac catheterization that is performed in a specially equipped cardiac catheterization laboratory by an electrophysiologist. One of the main purposes of programmed stimulation is to assess the ability of the area of the myocardium to cause an arrhythmia. If the arrhythmia can be reproduced by programmed stimulation, it is called *inducible.* Once an arrhythmia is induced, a treatment plan is determined and implemented. If, on the follow-up EP study, the tachyarrhythmia cannot be induced, then the treatment is determined to be effective. Different medications may be administered and combined with electrical devices (pacemaker, ICD) to determine the most effective treatment to suppress the arrhythmia.

Patient care, patient teaching, and associated complications of an EP study are the same as those associated with cardiac catheterization (see Chapter 13). The study is usually about 2 hours in length; however, if the electrophysiologist conducts not only a diagnostic procedure but also treatment, the study can take up to 8 hours.

Patients who are to undergo an EP study may be anxious about the procedure and its outcome. Before the procedure, the patient should receive instructions, including its usual duration, the environment where the procedure is performed, and what to expect. Although an EP study is not painful, it does cause discomfort and can be tiring. It may also cause feelings that were experienced when the arrhythmia occurred in the past. In addition, the nurse should prepare the patient for the procedure and what will be expected (lying very still during the procedure, reporting symptoms or concerns, etc.).

The patient should also know that the arrhythmia may occur during the procedure. It often stops on its own; if it does not, treatment is given to restore the patient's normal rhythm. The arrhythmia may have to be terminated using cardioversion or defibrillation, but this is performed under more controlled circumstances than if performed in an emergency. Postprocedural care is similar to that for cardiac catheterization.

CARDIAC CONDUCTION SURGERY

Atrial tachycardias and VTs that do not respond to medications and are not suitable for antitachycardia pacing may be treated by methods that include a maze procedure and ablation. The *maze procedure* is an open-heart surgical procedure for refractory AF. Sometimes, it is referred to as a Cox procedure or a mini-maze. The surgeon will ablate and/or use small incisions to create nonconducting scar tissue to stop the arrhythmia. This procedure is sometimes done together with an EP procedure or done when a patient is having another surgery such as a CABG or with valve replacement.

Catheter ablation done by radiofrequency destroys specific cells that are the cause or central conduction route of a tachyarrhythmia. It is performed with or after an EP study. Usual indications for ablation are recurrent atrial arrhythmias or VT unresponsive to previous therapy (or for which the therapy produced significant side effects). In addition to the standard catheter radiofrequency ablation, as mentioned earlier in the chapter, cryoablation is a newer type of treatment where the cardiac tissue is frozen, usually in the area of the pulmonary arteries. It often can be done faster since the tissue is frozen in a circle with the end of the catheter all at one time, discontinuing the arrhythmia. This is becoming a safe and effective alternative to radiofrequency ablation.

ARRHYTHMIAS IN THE CONTEXT OF COVID-19 INFECTION

COVID-19 or SARS-COV-2 infection is caused by a very infectious pathogen that has over the course of the pandemic led to a high mortality rate globally with death rates still increasing at the time of this publication. Further, COVID-19 has caused many complex symptoms characterized by respiratory involvement, systemic inflammatory responses, and in some cases, cardiac involvement (Mountantonakis et al., 2021). In a review of the literature by Veer et al. (2020) cardiac arrhythmias were found to be fairly common. In a cohort of 138 hospitalized patients with COVID-19, 16.7% of the patients had arrhythmias and as expected the incidence was higher in ICU than non-ICU patients (44.4% vs. 6.9%). According to the researchers, Lazzerini, Boutjdir, and Capecchi (2020), arrhythmias occurred most often in the context of myocarditis, cytokine storm, electrolyte abnormalities, hypoxia, shock, and myocardial injury.

AF was the most frequently encountered arrhythmia in patients hospitalized with COVID-19 with 17.6% experiencing this arrhythmia in a chart review of 9,564 patients. Of those, 65.7% or 1,109 patients had new-onset AF (Mountantonakis et al., 2020). As also referenced in the article by Mountantonakis and colleagues (2020), AF caused adverse hemodynamic effects that led to patient decline along with a hypercoagulable state that can occur with severe acute respiratory infection further influencing thromboembolic events. Accordingly, any occurrence of AF and in particular new-onset AF was associated with a significantly higher risk of mortality (Mountantonakis et al., 2020). Into the future as the pandemic becomes endemic, AF will need to be considered and then if it occurs monitored and treated in patients who develop COVID-19 infection.

Clinical Judgment Case

The scenario is as follows. You are working in the Emergency Room (ER) and a patient arrives complaining of nausea, indigestion, fatigue, and some chest discomfort. As you take vital signs, you notice the patient is diaphoretic (sweating). Vitals are as follows: T 98.7, heart rate of 104 and irregular, respiratory rate of 24 with a saturation of 94% on room air, and blood pressure is 102/40. Lungs are clear to auscultation, heart sounds are S1, S2, and S4, without murmur or rub. Neck veins are flat. Abdomen is soft, nondistended, nontender and bowel sounds are present in all four quadrants. Pedal, posterior tibial and radial pulses are 2+ bilaterally and capillary refill is <2 seconds, no peripheral edema. The patient has not voided as yet. The patient denies any cardiac history, has never smoked, and only medications include daily vitamins. The patient's age is 67 and is menopausal.

Step One: Recognize cues where relevant, and important information is identified from different sources, such as medical history or vital signs.

Answer: Although the patient has a negative cardiac history you are concerned because of age, sex, and patient's concerns which include nausea, fatigue, indigestion, chest discomfort, diaphoresis, and S4 gallop. Vitals that are of concern include tachycardia with heart rate of 104 and irregular nature of the pulse, tachypnea with a respiratory rate of 24 with a saturation of 94% on room air and blood pressure of 102/40.

Step Two: Analyze cues, which is organizing and linking the recognized cues to the patient's clinical presentation.

Answer: You have linked the presenting symptoms with age and sex and are aware that females often experience atypical symptoms of ischemia such as profound fatigue and nausea that are not readily recognized as ischemia. You are also linking the tachycardia as an important cue that often presents in the early stages of clinical deterioration of patients with cardiac conditions. You are also aware that tachycardia alone can result in decreased stroke volume and adds stress to the coronary arteries because the demand for coronary blood to perfuse the heart is increased with an elevated heart rate. In addition, you recognize that an S4 gallop is associated with stiffness of the ventricle and is frequently heard in those with hypertension or myocardial infarction. The patient is not hypertensive and in fact the BP is low. You quickly calculate the mean arterial pressure which is the systolic blood pressure (102) + the diastolic blood pressure of 40 mm Hg ×'s 2 which + 102 + 80 or 182 divided by 3 or 60.66 mm Hg. You are aware a normal MAP is between 70 and 105 mm Hg, and that this is an excellent measure of perfusion pressure of the body, and that a MAP >60 mm Hg is necessary to perfuse the coronary arteries. You are concerned about the effect of decreased perfusion on the patient's kidneys and the patient has not voided yet. In addition, the tachypnea and the oxygen saturation concern you because it is below normal values and the patient has no history of smoking. You realize tachypnea is a cue to clinical deterioration in patients with cardiac conditions and may be related to mismatch between myocardial supply and demand resulting in anaerobic metabolism and metabolic acidosis.

Step Three: Prioritize hypotheses, where hypotheses are evaluated and ranked according to priority. This can include urgency, likelihood, risk, difficulty, and/or time. In this phase you cluster your findings, to arrive at a list of problems (actual and/or potential problems) you believe the patient is experiencing and determine the importance or urgency. What do you think is the greatest concern?

Answer: Your greatest concern is that your patient is having a cardiac event such as a myocardial infarction, you are also concerned about a cardiac arrhythmia. The pulse is irregular and "tachy" and you are concerned about the decreased MAP and lack of perfusion to the coronary arteries, kidneys, and brain and the tachypnea with potential metabolic acidosis.

Step Four: Generate solutions, which is identifying expected outcomes and using hypotheses to define a set of interventions for the expected outcomes.

Answer: You need to see what the patient's cardiac rhythm is and will want to place the patient on a cardiac monitor as well as obtain a 12-lead ECG. You want to observe the patient's rhythm in real time and the 12-lead ECG although essential in this case will not allow you to view the patient's heart rate and rhythm continuously. You anticipate that you will draw cardiac biomarkers along with CBC, chemistry studies which will include electrolytes and BUN and creatinine to assess renal function, and coagulation studies (e.g., before PCI). Based on the ECG findings, and blood work you may want to alert the cardiac catheterization department. You are aware that the time from the patient's arrival in the emergency department to the time that Percutaneous Coronary Interventions (PCIs) are performed is critical and should be less than 90 minutes (time is muscle!). You also want to place the patient on low-flow oxygen to increase myocardial oxygenation. You are also aware that IV access is critical, for if the patient does deteriorate, medications will need to be administered urgently. You are also awaiting orders and anticipate that aspirin will be ordered and will be chewed by patient for rapid buccal absorption. You also recognize that you will need to repeat vital signs and reassess the patient for additional physical examination findings.

Step Five: Take action, where the solutions that address the highest priorities are implemented.

Answer: In this situation, you have decided your priority action is to alert the attending provider and oxygen is administered at 2 L via nasal cannula and you obtain the 12-lead ECG, lab work, and place the patient on the cardiac monitor with continuous oxygen saturation measurement. Repeat vital signs reveal tachycardia persists, the oxygen saturation is now 98% and the respiratory rate is 20, the BP is 108/40 with a MAP of 62.6 which is still <65 mm Hg (a MAP of <65 mm Hg for an extended period can result in end-organ ischemia) and there are no changes related to physical examination findings. A peripheral IV is inserted and flushed with normal saline (known as saline lock or an intermittent infusion device [IID]). The ECG reveals sinus tachycardia and PVCs. You notice ST elevation in leads V3–V5 (precordial area) and alert the provider. The lab calls and alerts you that the troponin in elevated. A normal troponin I level is less than 0.5 ng/mL and this patient's level is 0.8 ng/mL. The provider calls the cardiac cath team to alert them of patient in the ED with new MI.

Step Six: Evaluate outcomes, which is comparing observed outcomes against expected outcomes.

Answer: Because of your astute care, you recognized that females often experience atypical symptoms of ischemia, and you alerted the ED team to this possibility resulting in superb care and immediate intervention by the cardiac catheter team where the occluded coronary artery was opened and reperfusion to the area that had been deprived of oxygen was re-established. You are aware that the duration of oxygen deprivation is directly related to the number of cells that die; therefore, the time from the patient's arrival in the emergency department to the time PCI is performed is critical. Congratulate yourself, you recognized subtle cues and responded preventing delays in this patient's treatment!

CHAPTER REVIEW

NCLEX-Style Review Questions

1. The nurse entering the patient's medical-surgical room finds the patient in cardiac arrest. Cardiopulmonary resuscitation (CPR) is initiated, and the code team is alerted. Upon arrival of the code team and placement of the patient on a cardiac monitor, the electrocardiogram reveals this rhythm:

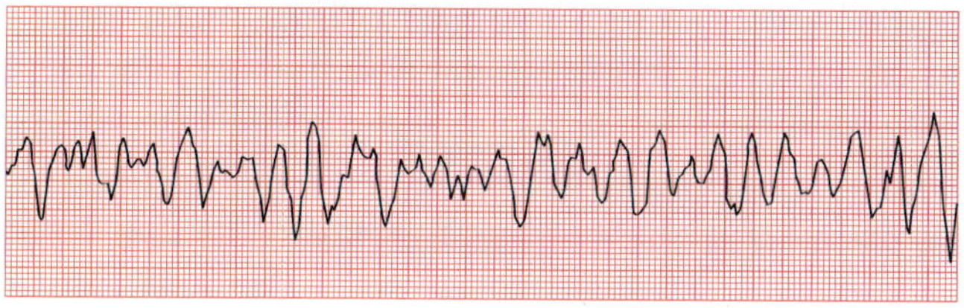

The next step in prioritizing the management of this patient will include which of the following?

1. Cardiopulmonary resuscitation
2. Defibrillation
3. Immediate transfer to the intensive care unit
4. Obtain ABGs

a. 1 + 4
b. 2 + 3
c. 1 + 2
d. 1 + 3

2. A patient on the cardiac telemetry unit unexpectedly goes into ventricular fibrillation. The advanced cardiac life support team prepares to defibrillate. Which of the following choices indicates the correct placement of the conductive gel pads? Select all that apply.

a. Anteroposterior placement with a pad on the front of the chest and the other placed under the patient's back
b. One pad on the right side below the bottom rib and the other on the left shoulder
c. The left and right upper halves of the sternum
d. The right side of the sternum just below the clavicle and left of the precordium
e. The right clavicle and right lower sternum

3. The health care provider is caring for a patient admitted to the cardiac care unit. The patient's electrocardiogram (ECG) has the following characteristics:

- Atrial rate = 64 beats/minute and regular
- Ventricular rate = 38 beats/minute and regular
- No relationship between P waves and QRS complexes
- P-R interval not measured
- QRS complex = 0.14 second

Based on these findings, the nurse interprets this arrhythmia as which from column 1? Which intervention do you anticipate from column 2?

Column 1	Column 2
a. Ventricular fibrillation	a. Pacemaker insertion
b. Third-degree heart block	b. Cardiac catheterization
c. Mobitz type II second-degree AV block	c. Immediate defibrillation
d. Atrial fibrillation	d. Thrombolytic therapy

4. Which ECG strip is associated with an embolic stroke?

a.

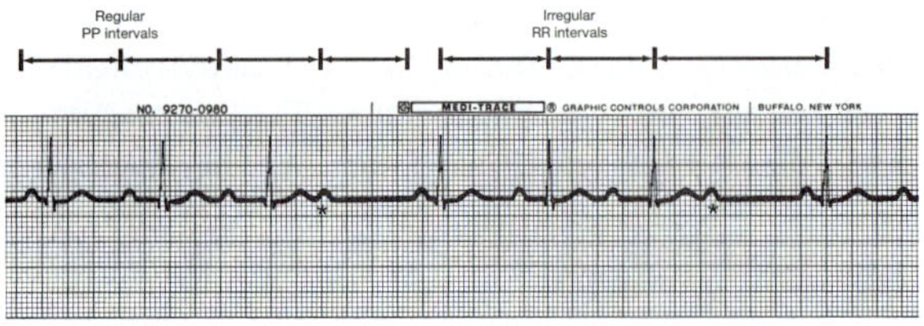

b.

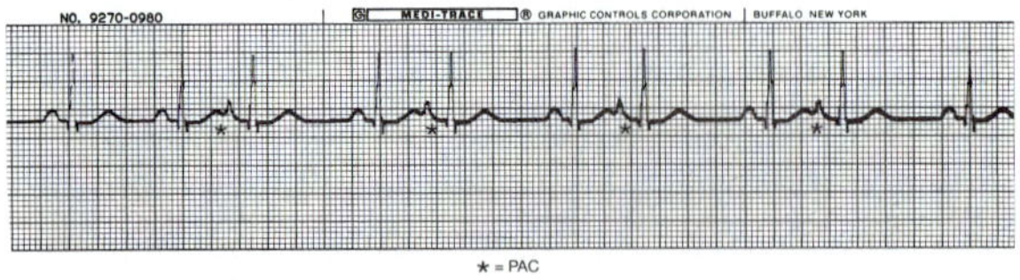

c.

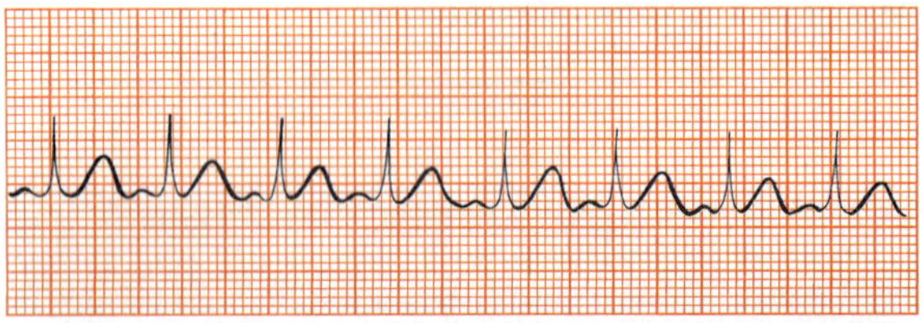

d.

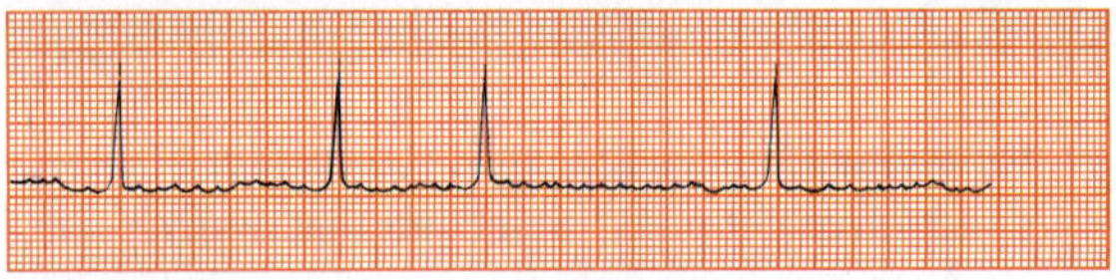

5. Which of the following cues should alert you to a potential deterioration of the patient's condition? Select all that apply.

a. Tachycardia
b. New development of an arrhythmia
c. Mean arterial pressure (MAP) of 70 mm Hg
d. Hourly urinary output of 1 mL/kg/hr
e. Oxygen saturation of 93% on room air

REFERENCES AND SELECTED READINGS

References and selected readings associated with this chapter can be found on the website that accompanies the book. Visit **http://thepoint.lww.com/Honan3e** to access the references and other additional resources associated with this chapter.

CHAPTER 17

Nursing Management: Patients With Vascular Disorders and Problems of Peripheral Circulation

Patricia Aguinaldo

Learning Objectives

After reading this chapter, you will be able to:

1. Identify factors that affect peripheral blood flow and tissue oxygenation.
2. Recognize clinical manifestations, management, and prevention of arterial disorders.
3. Describe the prevention and management of deep venous thrombosis.
4. Define medical and nursing management of venous and arterial ulcers.
5. Describe nursing management of lymphedema.

Conditions of the vascular system include arterial disorders, venous disorders, lymphatic disorders, and cellulitis. Nursing management depends on an understanding of the structure and function of the vascular and lymphatic systems.

Intact, patent, and responsive blood vessels are necessary to deliver adequate oxygen to tissues and remove metabolic wastes. Reduced blood flow through blood vessels characterizes all peripheral vascular diseases (PVDs). Perfusion is about supply versus demand. Even modestly reduced blood flow may be inadequate to maintain tissue integrity if tissue requirements are high. When arterial blood flow decreases, ischemia follows, and tissues become malnourished and ultimately die, unless blood flow is restored. Thus, the effect of decreased blood flow depends on the extent to which tissue demands exceed the supply of oxygen.

Nurses are in key positions to help patients with vascular disorders learn about the disease and their risk factors. Learning to modify the risk factors and manage their disorders may increase the lifespan of patients with vascular disorders.

ARTERIAL DISORDERS

Arteries become damaged or obstructed as a result of atherosclerotic plaque, thromboemboli, chemical or mechanical trauma, infections or inflammatory processes, vasospastic disorders, and congenital malformations. A sudden arterial occlusion causes profound and often irreversible tissue ischemia and tissue death. When arterial occlusions develop gradually, there is less risk of sudden tissue death because **collateral** circulation may develop (the rerouting of blood vessels, in which new blood vessels join to take over some of the circulation of blocked vessels), giving that tissue the opportunity to adapt to gradually decreased blood flow. However, continued decreased perfusion results in ischemia and tissue death.

PERIPHERAL ARTERIAL DISEASE

Peripheral artery disease (PAD) refers to any disease process that affects the arteries. Various PADs result in ischemia and produce the signs and symptoms described in Box 17-1. The type and severity of symptoms depends partly on the type, stage, and extent of the disease process and on the speed with which the disorder develops. Arterial insufficiency of the extremities is a common cause of disability. Frequently the legs are affected more than the upper extremities.

Clinical recognition of PAD varies in individuals; it is a slow process that begins in early adulthood and increases with age. PAD is one manifestation of **atherosclerosis**; thus systemic diseases that affect arteries of the brain, heart, kidneys, mesentery, and limbs should be suspected. Approximately 40% to 60% of patients with PAD also have significant coronary disease, and up to 30% have carotid artery disease (Aboyans & Criqui, 2020). Patients with PAD have an increased risk of mortality, myocardial infarction (MI), and cerebrovascular disease. Many patients with PAD are not receiving any treatment for their disease because they do not realize they have the condition (Zemaitis et al., 2022).

Pathophysiology

As the lumen narrows and blood flow decreases, ischemia occurs, which progresses to infarction in the distal tissues. In PAD, obstructive lesions are predominantly confined to

BOX 17-1 **Focused Assessment**

Lower Extremity Peripheral Arterial Disease

Be alert for the following signs and symptoms:

- Structural changes, resulting from chronic lack of oxygen and nutrient delivery to the tissues:
  - Hair loss distal to the occlusion
  - Thick, opaque nails; shiny, dry skin
  - Skeletal muscle atrophy
- Skin color changes:
  - Elevational pallor
  - Dependent rubor (red color when limb dependent from dilated damaged vessels)
- Pulse changes:
  - Pulses diminished or absent below area of stenosis/obstruction-pedal, posterior tibial, popliteal, femoral
  - Cool extremity distal to occlusion
- Sensation changes:
  - Paresthesias
  - Numbness
  - Tingling of extremities
- Ulcers or gangrene (traumatic or spontaneous on onset) located at tips of toes, between toes, over areas of pressure, such as the heel, or areas susceptible to trauma like the shin; defined punched out (circular), necrotic/yellow ulcer base, dry, pale in appearance; usually very painful; poor healing of injuries on the extremities
- Edema, although frequently absent, may be present and related to dependency

segments of the arterial system extending from the aorta below the renal arteries to the popliteal artery. Most distal occlusive disease is frequently seen in patients with diabetes mellitus (DM) and older individuals.

Arteriosclerosis is the most common disease of the arteries. It is a diffuse process whereby muscle fibers and endothelial linings of the walls of small arteries and arterioles become thickened. Atherosclerosis involves changes of the intima consisting of an accumulation of lipids, calcium, blood components, complex carbohydrates, and fibrous tissue, referred to as *atheromas* or *plaques*. Atherosclerosis causes arterial **stenosis**, obstruction by thrombosis, **aneurysm**, ulceration, and vessel rupture.

Arterial bifurcations are more vulnerable to atherosclerosis than other areas of the arteries (Fig. 17-1). These include the distal abdominal aorta, the common iliac arteries, the orifice of the superficial femoral, *profunda femoris* arteries, the superficial femoral artery in the adductor canal (which is particularly narrow), and anywhere along the arteries distal to the knee. The gradual narrowing of the arterial lumen stimulates the development of collateral circulation (Fig. 17-2) from pre-existing vessels.

Risk Factors

Risk factors for developing PAD are similar to those for developing coronary artery disease (Haynes & Henry, 2022) (Box 17-2). The age of onset and disease severity is influenced by the type and number of atherosclerotic risk factors. Risk factors include modifiable (e.g., diet, smoking) and nonmodifiable (e.g., race and age) factors. Evidence indicates that modification may slow the disease process. Of those that can be modified, tobacco use is one of the most important in atherosclerotic lesion development (Campia et al., 2019). Nicotine decreases blood flow, increases heart rate (HR) and blood pressure (BP), and increases the risk for clot formation by increasing platelet aggregation. According to research findings (Aboyans & Criqui, 2020), smokers have a three-fold increased risk of developing PAD compared to nonsmokers. Body mass index (BMI) of 30 kg/m^2 or greater, stress, and lack of exercise also have been identified as contributing to the disease process.

Hypertension accelerates the rate at which atherosclerotic lesions form in high-pressure vessels and, therefore, is a major PAD risk factor. In addition, approximately 21% of patients with DM have PAD (Liao et al., 2019), and about 7 to 15 times the amputation rate of those without DM. Tight control of diabetes is essential; the risk of developing PAD increases by 28% for every 1% increase in glycosylated hemoglobin (Azzopardi et al., 2019). Higher total cholesterol is associated with increased risk of PAD, whereas higher high-density lipoprotein (HDL) cholesterol is associated with decreased risk (Campia et al., 2019).

Homocysteine is a protein that promotes coagulation, and is clearly associated with elevated thrombotic risk; however, elevated levels of homocysteine have only weakly predicted cardiovascular risk (Libby, 2021). It is associated with genetic factors and a diet low in folic acid, vitamin B_6, and vitamin B_{12}. Randomized trials using vitamin treatments to lower homocysteine levels have not documented improvements in cardiovascular outcomes (Libby, 2021). The enrichment of cereals and flour with folate in the United States has been thought to have improved its dietary intake and should lower blood homocysteine levels in the American population (Libby, 2021). In addition, since inflammation plays a fundamental role in the development and progression of atherosclerosis, elevated C-reactive protein (CRP) levels are strongly associated with the development of PAD.

Clinical Manifestations and Assessment

Most patients with PAD are initially asymptomatic. However, studies have demonstrated that for every patient who has symptomatic disease, approximately three times more patients have no symptoms (Ferri, 2022).

Approximately 1% to 5% of patients with PAD have **critical limb ischemia** (CLI) with chronic ischemic pain at rest (rest pain), nonhealing, ulcers, or gangrene. A small number of patients with PAD have **acute limb ischemia** (ALI), a sudden decrease in limb perfusion, most commonly caused by either thrombosis or embolism, that produces new or worsening symptoms that may threaten limb viability. Other potential causes of acute arterial occlusion include

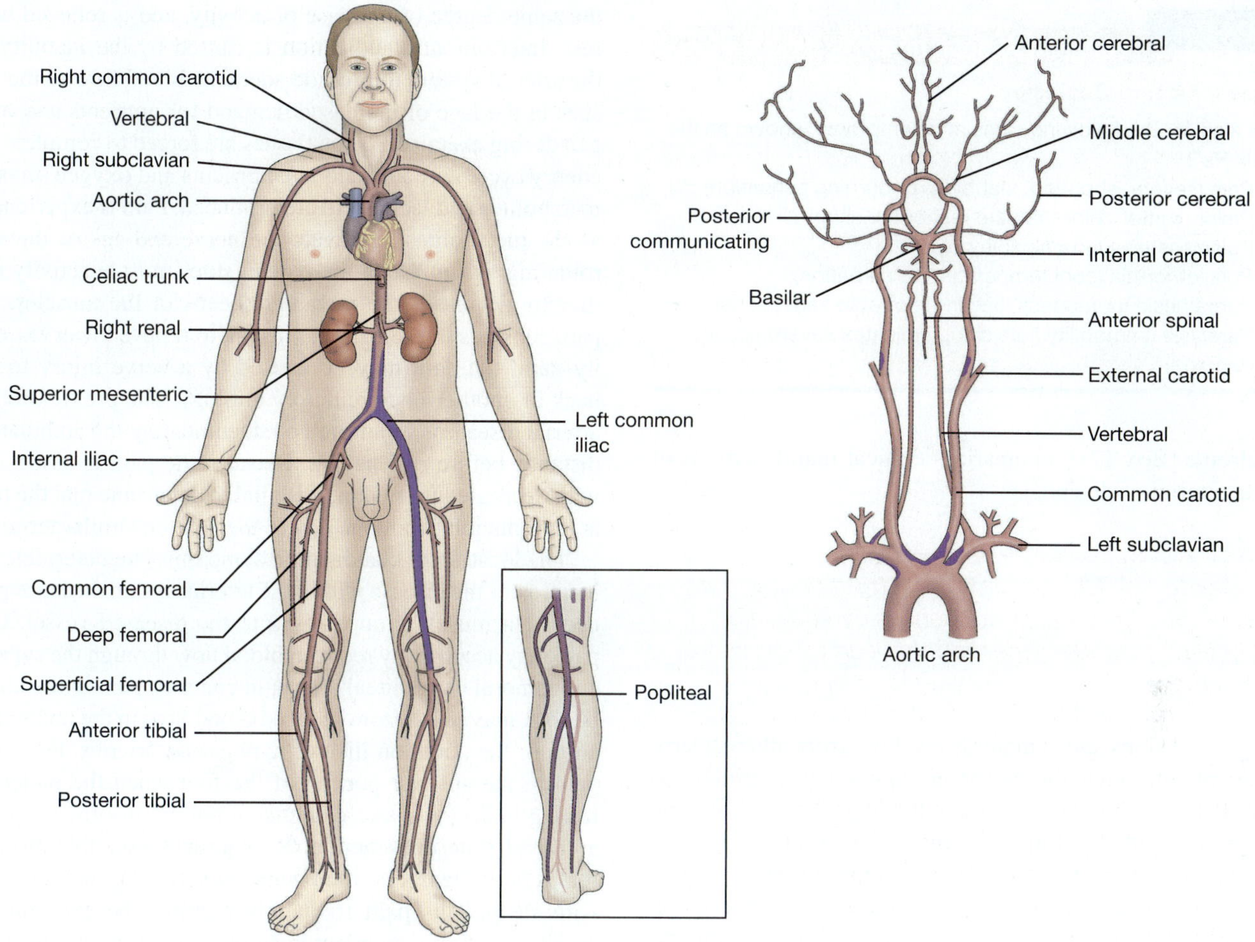

FIGURE 17-1 Common sites of atherosclerotic obstruction in major arteries.

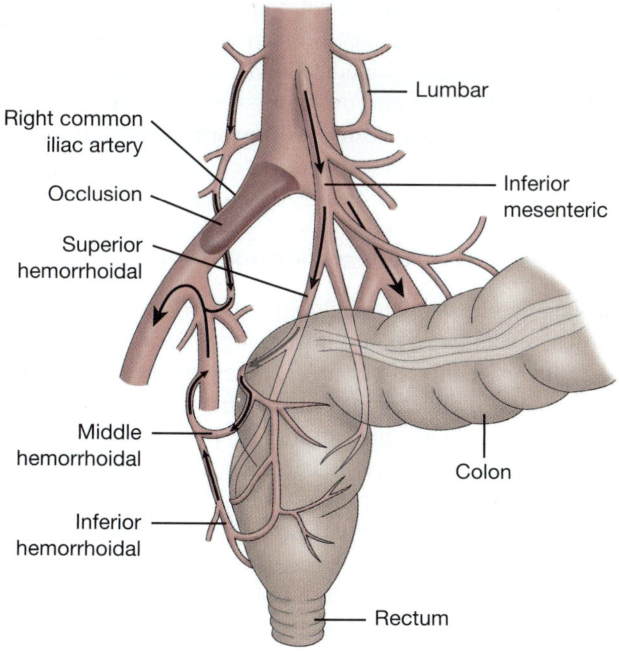

FIGURE 17-2 Development of channels for collateral blood flow in response to occlusion of the right common iliac artery and the terminal aortic bifurcation.

atherosclerotic stenosis, aneurysm, arterial dissection, arterial embolization, cardiac embolization, trauma (blunt injuries, fractures), tumor compression, graft thrombosis, drug use disorder, low cardiac output, phlegmasia cerulea dolens (massive iliofemoral venous thrombosis), and compartment

BOX 17-2

Risk Factors for Peripheral Arterial Disease (PAD)

- Family history
- Age (risk increases with age, especially after age 65 years)
- Smoking (3–4 times more common than nonsmokers)
- Pre-existing health conditions:
  - Coronary artery disease
  - Cerebral artery disease
  - Diabetes mellitus (every 1% elevation in hemoglobin A1c is associated with a 30% increase PAD risk)
  - Hypertension (increases risk by about threefold)
  - Dyslipidemia (fasting total cholesterol above 270 mg/dL is associated with a twofold increase in PAD)
  - Clotting disorders
  - Hyperhomocysteinemia is associated with a twofold risk of PAD (Clinical Overview, 2021)

BOX 17-3 **Focused Assessment**

Acute Arterial Occlusion

Be alert for the following signs and symptoms, known as the "Six Ps":

- Pain (severe, shooting, stabbing, or burning sensation)
- Pallor (lighter color than the rest of the skin)
- Pulselessness (no palpable pulse)
- Poikilothermia (cool temperature to palpation)
- Paresthesia (numbness, tingling, hot/cold sensations)
- Paralysis (immobility [late sign], indicates severe tissue damage)

syndrome. Box 17-3 summarizes clinical manifestations of acute arterial occlusion.

Pearls for Practice

In patients with CLI, minor trauma from poorly fitting shoes or carelessly clipped toenails can cause a nonhealing wound or infection that can progress to amputation.

Clinical signs and symptoms resulting from atherosclerosis are manifested in the end-organ supplied by arterial blood flow. Patients complain of pain in the fingers or feet or muscle groups with use (not the joints). For example, walking causes pain in the leg muscles, and upper extremity physical activity causes pain in the arm muscles. A description of pain and its precipitating factors, skin color and temperature assessment, and peripheral pulse presence and character are important assessment parameters diagnosing arterial disorders.

Pain

The hallmark symptom for PAD in the lower extremity is **intermittent claudication** (Box 17-4). This pain may be described as aching or cramping in a muscle that occurs with the same degree of exercise or activity, and is relieved with rest. Intermittent claudication is caused by the inability of the arterial system to provide adequate blood flow to the tissues in the face of increased demand for nutrients and oxygen during exercise. As the tissues are forced to complete the energy cycle without adequate nutrients and oxygen, muscle metabolites and lactic acid are produced. Pain is experienced as the metabolites aggravate the nerve endings of the surrounding tissue. When the patient stops muscle activity and thereby decreases the metabolic needs of the muscles, the pain subsides. If the patient must sit to relieve lower extremity pain, the pain may be caused by a nerve injury to the back or another noncirculatory etiology. The progression of arterial disease is monitored by documenting the ambulatory distance before pain is felt. Because the pain is associated with decreased perfusion, it is vital to determine that the pain is reproducible from one day to the next on similar terrain.

The location of claudication symptoms can determine the location of the disease within the arterial system because pain occurs in muscle groups distal to the diseased vessel. Calf pain may accompany reduced blood flow through the superficial femoral or popliteal artery; in contrast, pain in the hip or buttock may result from reduced blood flow in the abdominal aorta or the common iliac or hypogastric arteries. Persistent pain in the anterior portion of the foot when the patient is resting indicates a severe degree of arterial insufficiency and a critical state of ischemia. **Rest pain** is how this discomfort is described; it is often worse at night and may interfere with sleep. This pain frequently requires the extremity to be lowered to a dependent position to improve perfusion to the distal tissues. The dependent position of the lower extremity may cause edema in the leg and foot; thus edema may be associated with PAD. Rest pain is also associated with limb-threatening ischemia. Refer to Table 17-1 for information on differentiating claudication from other causes.

Upper extremity atherosclerotic stenosis may cause arm fatigue and pain with exercise (forearm claudication) and inability to hold or grasp objects (e.g., painting, combing hair, placing objects on shelves above the head).

BOX 17-4 **Intermittent Claudication (IC)**

- Cramp-like pain in a muscle
- Consistently reproduced with the same degree of exercise or activity
- Relieved by stopping muscle use
- Caused by inability of the arterial system to provide blood flow that keeps up with increased demand
- Site of arterial disease can be determined by the location of claudication
- Pain occurs in muscle groups distal to the diseased vessel
- 70–80% of patients do not have worsening symptoms
- <10% of individuals with claudication will progress to critical limb ischemia (CLI) with 5% requiring amputation) (Aboyans & Criqui, 2020)
- Dependent position reduces pain

Changes in Skin Appearance and Temperature

Inadequate blood flow results in cool and pale extremities. Further reduction of blood flow to the tissues, which occurs when the extremity is elevated, results in an even whiter or more blanched appearance to the skin compared to the contralateral limb. When the extremity is placed in a dependent position after elevation, it becomes a reddish-blue color called **rubor**. This color change suggests severe peripheral arterial damage, in which vessels that are unable to constrict eventually remain dilated. *Cyanosis*, a bluish tint of the skin, is manifested when the amount of oxygenated hemoglobin contained in the blood is reduced. Skin color changes may be more subtle in darkly pigmented individuals. Comparing the contralateral limb is the best way to discern color changes. Capillary refill time (CRT) is frequently used as

TABLE **17-1 Differentiation of Claudication from Other Disorders in the Lower Extremities**

	Intermittent Claudication	Spinal Stenosis	Arthritis	Venous Congestion	Compartment Syndrome
Character	Aching, cramping	Same as claudication or tingling, weakness, clumsiness	Aching	Tightness	Tightness, tense
Location	Dependent on area of obstruction: buttock, hip, thigh, calf, foot	Buttock, hip, thigh	Hip, thigh, knee	Groin, thigh	Dependent on area of high pressure; frequently the tibia, however can occur in foot, thigh, gluteal region
Response to exercise	Yes	Variable	Variable	After walking	Can occur because of inordinate stress or exercise
Response to walking	Reproducible	Variable	Variable	Variable	Excessive exercise
Relief of discomfort	Relief with cessation of muscle activity	Relief with sitting or changing position	Slow relief with avoidance of weight bearing	Slow relief with leg elevation	Unrelieved
Other	Associated with atherosclerosis and decreased pulses	History of back problems	Discomfort at the joints	History of deep vein thrombosis, signs of venous congestion; edema	Seen in athletes. May occur with trauma

Adapted from White, C. J. (2016). Atherosclerotic peripheral arterial disease. In L. Goldman & A. I. Schafer (Eds.), *Goldman-Cecil medicine* (25th ed.). Elsevier, Saunders.

an assessment of peripheral perfusion. The nurse depresses the nail bed of the finger or toe between their fingers until it blanches. After releasing the pressure, the skin color in normal tissue is expected to return in fewer than 2 seconds. However, recent research findings question the efficacy of this test in assessing circulatory volume because of poor agreement among observers. Therefore, the nurse considers this test not as a definitive marker for impaired perfusion but rather as an adjunctive tool to consider when clustering other manifestations of peripheral perfusion.

Additional changes that result from a chronically reduced nutrient supply include loss of hair; brittle nails; dry, shiny, or scaling skin; atrophy; and ulcerations. Skin and nail changes, ulcers, gangrene, and muscle atrophy may be evident in chronic arterial disease but cannot be relied to diagnose acute arterial insufficiency.

Pulses

Unequal pulses between extremities or the absence of an ordinarily palpable pulse is a sign of PAD. Palpation of pulses (Fig. 17-3) is subjective. Box 17-5 provides tips for palpating pulses. The presence of foot pulses does not exclude the possibility of PAD, and further investigation is required in the presence of leg pain. After exercise, the pulses may not be palpable; this is known as "disappearing pulses" and is caused by the increased need for blood flow in the working muscle, which the arteries cannot provide. The change in pulses should be reproducible and is consistent with the distance the patient walks before experiencing claudication. **Bruits** may be auscultated with a stethoscope just distal to arterial stenosis, indicating turbulent blood flow with vessel stenosis. Complete occlusion of a vessel should make bruits disappear (McGee, 2022).

Ankle-Brachial Index

The presence of PAD is defined as an ankle-brachial index (ABI) of less than 0.90. ABI is calculated as the ratio of the systolic blood pressure (SBP) in the ankle divided by the higher of the two brachial SBPs (see Chapter 11).

Sensory Changes

Numbness, paresthesias, and motor deficits indicate tissue anoxia. Motor deficits typically progress from distal to proximal; therefore, the nurse assesses initially for the weakness of the foot muscles. In contrast, paresthesia denotes ischemia that threatens limb survival.

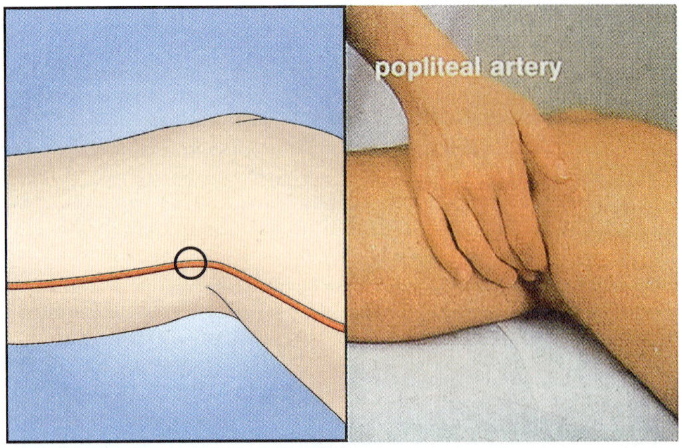

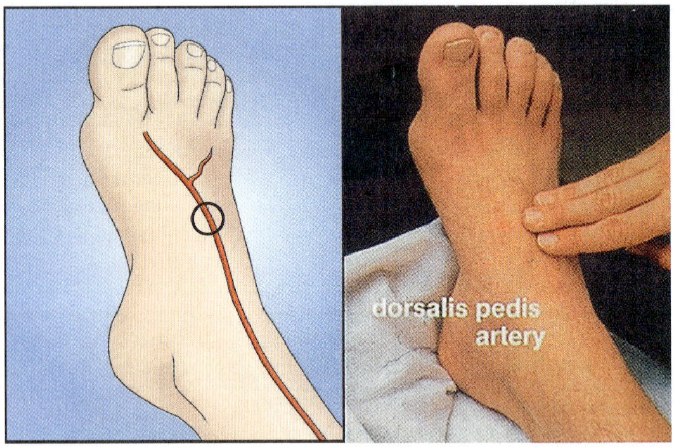

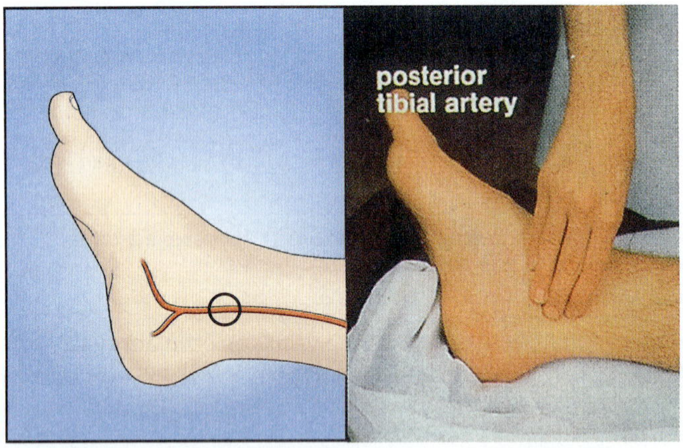

FIGURE 17-3 **Assessing peripheral pulses. (*Left*) Popliteal pulse. (*Right*) Dorsalis pedis pulse. (*Bottom*) Posterior tibial pulse.**

Pearls for Practice

The nurse is aware that in the event of acute occlusion of arterial circulation, symptoms will include pain, pallor, poikilothermia (coldness), paresthesias, delayed capillary refill, cyanosis, and decreased or absent pulses. The nurse expects to see hair loss, thickened nails, muscle atrophy, and smooth and shiny skin with chronic arterial disease.

Diagnostic Tests

Various noninvasive and invasive tests are performed to diagnose abnormalities that affect the arteries. When pulses cannot be palpated reliably, a handheld continuous wave (CW) Doppler ultrasound device may be used to hear (*insonate*) signals in the vessels (Fig. 17-4). The Doppler emits a signal through the tissues, which is reflected off the moving blood cells and returned to the device. Then the filtered output Doppler signal is transmitted to a loudspeaker or headphones, where it can be heard for interpretation. Doppler studies are more useful when combined with the **ankle-brachial index (ABI)**.

BOX 17-5 **Tips for Palpating Peripheral Pulses**

- Use tips of fingers to palpate. To avoid mistaking your own pulse for that of the patient, use light touch and avoid using only the index finger for palpation because this finger has the strongest arterial pulsation of all the fingers. The thumb should not be used for the same reason.
- Palpate bilaterally and simultaneously.
- Compare both sides for symmetry in rate, rhythm, and quality (the nurse should grade according to the institution's/facility's scale).
- Document as present, absent, or bounding (e.g., aneurysm).

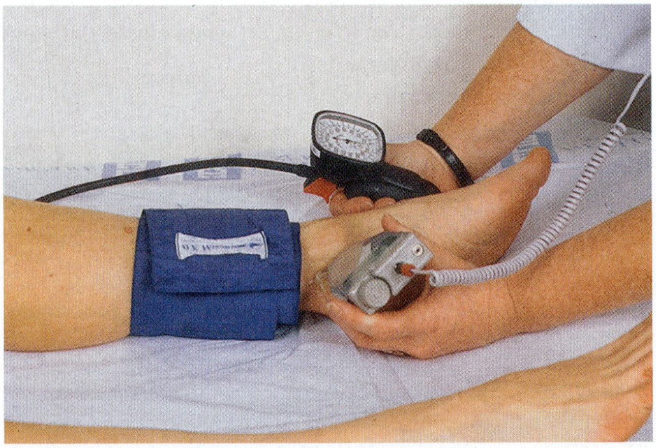

FIGURE 17-4 **Continuous-wave (CW) Doppler ultrasound detects blood flow in peripheral vessels (demonstrated in obtaining ABI).**

TABLE **17-2 Noninvasive and Invasive Vascular Tests**

Test	Purpose
Doppler Ultrasound Flow Studies	Evaluation of arterial signals Blood pressure measurement in the limbs Assessment of vessel size and compressibility Assessment for presence of thrombus Assessment of valve function
Exercise Testing	Assessment of ankle systolic blood pressure in response to walking on treadmill (normal response is little or no drop in ankle systolic pressure after exercise) Assessment for claudication (a drop in ankle pressure correlates with claudication distance reported by the patient)
Duplex Ultrasonography	Localization of vascular obstruction Evaluation of stenosis Assessment for vascular reflux Provides both image and audible signal
Computed Tomography Angiography (CTA) (spiral or helical CT that provides a series of images in continuous spiral)	Demonstration of cross-sectional images of soft tissue Diagnoses of abdominal aneurysms, graft infections or occlusions, hemorrhage
Magnetic Resonance Angiography (MRA) (standard magnetic resonance imaging [MRI] scanner with software programmed to isolate blood vessels and reassemble images in three dimensions)	Detection of changes, aneurysms, DVT Useful in poor kidney function or contrast agent allergy
Air Plethysmography	Measurement of volume, ejection fraction, and residual volume Quantification of venous reflux and calf muscle pump ejection
Venous Duplex	Assessment of venous reflux Manual compression of the veins
Angiography	Confirmation of occlusive arterial disease when considering interventions Patient may report the sensation of warmth during injection and may have immediate or delayed allergic reaction to the iodine in the contrast agent Digital subtraction angiography (DSA) has bony structures removed from the image
Venography	Radiopaque contrast agent injected into the venous system produces an image showing an unfilled segment of vein Used to outline vein for thrombolytic therapy Infrequently used (duplex ultrasound is standard for diagnosing venous thrombosis)
Vascular Endoscopy (Angioscopy)	Use of fiber optics to visualize the vessel lumen Used to identify plaque, thrombus, hemorrhage, ulcers Used to remove debris or remove venous valves

(Chapter 11 provides a detailed discussion of Doppler, ultrasound, and ABI.) The "gold standard" for diagnosis and evaluation of PAD is invasive digital angiography where the location and severity of vascular occlusion is defined; however, it is typically reserved for patients who also need concomitant endovascular revascularization (discussed shortly) (Firnhaber & Powell, 2019; Tran, 2021). Additional diagnostic tools are discussed in Table 17-2.

Medical Management

Medical management is aimed at reducing the patient's risk for life-threatening complications of atherosclerosis. Improving walking distance and salvaging the limb includes the use of exercise, pharmacologic treatment, risk factor modification (control of hypertension, hypercholesterolemia, and DM, and cessation of smoking), and invasive options. Revascularization is recommended if there is a reasonable likelihood of symptomatic improvement and an inadequate response to pharmacologic or exercise therapy. Invasive methods include surgery and percutaneous endoscopic procedures.

Management of Intermittent Claudication

Treatment goals for patients with intermittent claudication are to relieve symptoms, improve exercise performance, and improve functional abilities. In general, patients with intermittent claudication feel better when in an exercise program; therefore, initial treatment should be focused on a structured exercise program and pharmacotherapy. Patients are advised to "walk into the pain" of claudication, pause until the pain subsides, and continue walking. If this program is combined with weight reduction and tobacco cessation, patients may improve their activity tolerance and experience pain relief without further intervention.

Pharmacologic Therapy

Cilostazol is a phosphodiesterase III inhibitor that is a vasodilator and interferes with platelet aggregation. It is prescribed in combination with an exercise program to improve walking distance (Ferri, 2022). Guidelines recommend a 3- to 6-month course of cilostazol as first-line pharmacotherapy treatment for patients with intermittent claudication to evaluate the efficacy (Kherallah et al, 2021). The usefulness of the drug is limited, however, by its adverse effect profile (e.g., dizziness, gastrointestinal symptoms) and its contraindication for use in patients with heart failure (Ferri, 2022; Firnhaber & Powell, 2019).

Antiplatelet agents, such as aspirin or clopidogrel, help prevent the formation of thromboemboli, which can lead to MI and stroke. Aspirin (usually 75 to 325 mg/day) is shown to reduce the risk of MI, stroke, and death in patients with vascular disease. Clopidogrel is also indicated to prevent cardiovascular ischemic events in patients with PAD (Kherallah et al., 2021). Other pharmacologic agents include statin medications for patients with PAD and antihypertensive therapy to patients with hypertension (HTN) and PAD to decrease the risk of MI, stroke, heart failure, and cardiovascular death (Ferri, 2022). ACE inhibitor (ACEI) has demonstrated a reduction in mortality in both symptomatic and asymptomatic patients with PAD in the heart outcomes prevention evaluation study (Tran, 2021).

Thrombolysis

Thrombotic stenosis or occlusion may be treated by **thrombolysis**. After catheter insertion into the affected vessel, the thrombolytic agent is injected directly into the thrombus. It will lyse the thrombus (clot). The patient is admitted to a special or critical care unit for continuous monitoring. Vital signs are taken frequently, according to the facility's protocol. The patient is monitored closely for any signs of bleeding, as this is the most common side effect of thrombolytic therapy. The nurse minimizes the number of punctures for IV lines and obtaining blood samples, avoids intramuscular injections, prevents tissue trauma, and applies pressure at least twice as long as usual after any puncture is performed. Patients will have follow-up images to determine treatment effectiveness. Refer to Table 17-2 for discussion of thrombolytic agents.

Pearls for Practice

To monitor patients post-intervention, it is essential that a baseline assessment of the extremity is documented so that the nurse can determine changes in perfusion of the extremity post-instrumentation.

Surgical Management

Disabling claudication or risk for amputation indicates surgical or percutaneous intervention. Percutaneous, catheter-based endovascular treatments with or without stenting are seen increasingly over open surgical approaches because of the relative safety, success, and durability, but will be dependent on the anatomic complexity of occlusion, patient's surgical risk, and expertise of the provider (Tran, 2021). The initial treatment goals for ALI are to prevent worsening ischemia and thrombus propagation, manage pain, and preserve tissue. Anticoagulation is started immediately upon recognizing the acute ischemia. Revascularization or **arterial bypass** is the first-line intervention used in ALI treatment. Vascular surgical procedures are divided into two groups: inflow procedures, which improve blood supply from the aorta into the femoral artery, and outflow procedures, which provide blood supply to vessels below the femoral artery. The procedure performed depends on the degree and location of the stenosis or occlusion. When the diffuse disease is present, an inflow procedure is performed first. The restoration of arterial flow may be sufficient after this procedure so that other procedures may not be needed. The patient's overall health and ability to tolerate a procedure factors into the decision as to what approach is best for each patient. For some patients who are at high risk or in a life-threatening situation, primary amputation may be the best choice.

Bypass grafts are placed to reroute blood flow around the stenosis or occlusion. Grafts below the knee require the use of native vein (i.e., autologous; the patient's own vein) to ensure patency; however, synthetic grafts may be used for bypass procedures on larger vessels above the knee. Several synthetic materials are available for peripheral bypass grafting. Cryopreserved saphenous and umbilical veins are also available but usually do not last as long as native veins or synthetic grafts. Graft patency is determined by the graft size, graft type, and location. Great care is taken to prevent graft infection as the graft must be removed if infected. Vein grafts are reversed before creating the graft conduit to prevent the valves from causing an occlusion, or they are left in place (in situ), and the valves are removed with a unique instrument (valvulotome).

Doppler evaluation of the graft and the proximal vessels beyond the graft is usually performed for postprocedural vascular patients. In addition, patients may have arterial studies, ABI, and arterial waveform analysis performed in the vascular laboratory after arterial reconstructive procedures and prior to discharge. The disappearance of a pulse or a Doppler signal that was previously present may indicate an occluded graft and requires notification of the surgeon.

Endovascular Intervention

Several percutaneous interventional techniques are available to remove plaque and dilate vessels. **Angioplasty**, also called percutaneous transluminal **balloon angioplasty**

(PTA), may be performed with or without a **stent**. Balloons are inserted into the vessels via a catheter and expanded at the stenotic site within the vessel. The expanding balloon cracks the atherosclerotic plaque and opens the vascular lumen. Stents may be inserted to support the vessel wall and maintain patency. Complications from PTA include hematoma, embolization, dissection of the vessel, bleeding, intimal damage (dissection), and stent migration. The advantage of angioplasty, stents, and **stent-grafts** compared to open surgical procedures is the decreased length of hospital stay required for the treatment and more minor physical trauma to the patient than open surgical procedures. Percutaneous catheter procedures may be performed in an outpatient setting, depending on the patient condition.

Nursing Management

Providing Postoperative Care

In the postoperative period, the nurse collaborates with the surgeon about the patient's appropriate activity level based on the patient's condition. In general, patients are encouraged to move the involved extremity and be active. The primary objective in the postprocedural period is to maintain adequate circulation. Anticoagulant therapy may be continued after surgery to prevent thrombosis of the graft. Metabolic abnormalities, kidney failure, and **compartment syndrome** are potential complications after arterial occlusions or operations (refer to Chapter 41 for details of compartment syndrome). The nurse assesses for evidence of local complications, such as hemorrhage or thrombosis, by performing neurovascular checks of the limb and systemic complications, by monitoring vital signs, intake and output, physical assessment parameters (e.g., pulmonary, cardiac, PV, GI, mental status), and laboratory data. Any evidence of deterioration is reported to the surgical team immediately (cool; dusky; weakened pulses; delayed capillary refill; decreased sensory/motor function; progressive, unrelieved pain).

Providing Pain Relief

Often narcotics are needed to manage rest pain until circulation can be restored. After interventions, pain management is similar to other postoperative patient care, keeping in mind that the patient may have been taking large doses of narcotics preoperatively and may need more pain medication than expected to relieve symptoms.

Maintaining Tissue Integrity

Poorly perfused tissues are susceptible to damage and infection. When lesions develop, healing may be delayed or inhibited because of the poor blood supply to the area. Infected, nonhealing ulcers of the extremities can be debilitating and may require prolonged, often expensive treatments and run the risk of potential limb loss; therefore, measures to prevent tissue loss and amputation are a high priority. Patients must be taught to avoid trauma; wear sturdy, well-fitting shoes or slippers; and use neutral soaps and body lotions. Patients with vascular disease are taught the same precautions that patients with DM are taught for foot care (see Chapter 29, Box 29-8). Patients with open arterial or venous ulcers are given detailed wound care instructions. Risk factor modification is the most effective intervention for preventing the progression of vascular disease (e.g., maintaining A1c within a target range for patients with DM).

Patients and their families are educated on environmental and behavioral risk factors associated with ischemia. For example, excess heat may increase the metabolic rate of the extremities and increase the need for oxygen beyond that provided by the reduced arterial flow through the diseased artery. Cold temperature is associated with vasoconstriction, which decreases perfusion to the extremities. Nicotine from tobacco products causes vasospasm and dramatically reduces circulation to the extremities. Tobacco smoke also impairs oxygen transport and cellular use and increases blood viscosity. Patients with arterial insufficiency who use tobacco must be fully informed of the effects of nicotine on circulation and encouraged to stop using tobacco. Second-hand smoke is also harmful to the vascular system.

Emotional upsets cause vasoconstriction by stimulating the sympathetic nervous system. This can be minimized by avoiding stressful situations or by following a stress-management program. Counseling services or relaxation training may be indicated for people who cannot cope effectively with situational stressors.

Constrictive clothing and accessories are avoided, as are heating pads and hot water bottles. The temperature of bathwater should also be evaluated, and the overall water temperature in the home decreased to prevent scalding. Tight socks, panty girdles, belts, and shoelaces are discouraged because they may impede arterial circulation to the extremities and promote venous congestion and edema.

Pearls for Practice

Lower extremity elevation is associated with decreased arterial flow, which lessens tissue perfusion and increases pain. A dependent position improves flow and decreases pain.

UPPER EXTREMITY ARTERIAL OCCLUSIVE DISEASE

Arterial occlusions from atherosclerosis occur less frequently in the upper extremities than in the legs.

Pathophysiology

Upper extremity arterial symptoms and occlusive disease are more likely caused by vasospasm, trauma, or constrictive arterial disorders than by atherosclerosis.

Stenosis may occur at the origin of the subclavian artery proximal to the vertebral artery. Arterial blood flows to the brain via the carotid and vertebral arteries. If there is diminished flow to the arm from the subclavian artery due to the stenosis, there will be preferential reverse flow down the vertebral artery to the arm while being used. This is called *subclavian steal syndrome* as the arm is "stealing" blood from the brain.

Clinical Manifestations and Assessment

The patient may complain of arm fatigue and pain when using the arm to paint or comb hair and occasionally report difficulty when driving. Patients also report dizziness, vertigo, ataxia, syncope, or bilateral visual changes when using the arm.

Assessment findings in the ischemic upper extremity may include coolness and pallor of the affected extremity, decreased capillary refill, a decreased amplitude and delay in radial artery pulse on the affected side, and a difference in arm BPs of at least 15 mm Hg (affected limb pressure is lower) (Shankar Kikkeri & Nagalli, 2021). Noninvasive studies performed to evaluate for upper extremity arterial occlusions include upper and forearm BP determinations and duplex ultrasound to identify the anatomic location of the lesion and to evaluate the hemodynamics of the blood flow.

Medical and Nursing Management

Surgical bypass or a PTA procedure may be indicated. If the stenosis involves the subclavian artery with siphoning of blood from the intracranial circulation to the arm, a carotid-to-subclavian artery bypass or reimplantation of the subclavian to the carotid artery may be performed.

INFLAMMATORY DISORDERS

Various inflammatory diseases affect the arterial system. Examples are Takayasu arteritis, Behçet disease, and giant cell arteritis. The inflammatory response creates granuloma formation and causes vessel destruction. Initial treatment for active vascular inflammatory diseases is high-dose corticosteroids. Revascularization, if indicated, is delayed until the inflammatory process in under control.

RAYNAUD DISEASE AND RAYNAUD PHENOMENON

Primary *Raynaud disease* (primary Raynaud phenomenon or idiopathic Raynaud phenomenon) refers to vasospasm that occurs with cold or stress. Patients with scleroderma or systemic lupus erythematosus may have the same signs and symptoms. This is called *secondary Raynaud phenomenon.*

Pathophysiology

Raynaud disease is of unknown etiology. While its exact cause is unknown, it may be associated with immunologic disorders. Emotional factors or cold may trigger episodes.

Raynaud disease usually occurs in females between 16 and 40 years of age, and it occurs more frequently in cold climates and during the winter (Casanegra & Shepherd, 2021). It may cause skin and muscle atrophy.

The prognosis varies; patients may slowly improve, become progressively worse, or show no change.

Clinical Manifestations and Assessment

The patient's skin becomes cyanotic due to vasospasm, and then vasodilation causes redness (rubor). Numbness, tingling, and burning pain occurs. Although typically the fingers are involved, the toes may also be affected (Musa & Qurie, 2021). Typically, the radial, ulnar, and pedal pulses are normal; fingers and toes may be cool between attacks and may perspire excessively.

Medical and Nursing Management

The disorder is generally benign and self-limiting with appropriate patient teaching and lifestyle modifications. The patient is instructed to avoid the stimuli (e.g., cold, tobacco) that provoke vasoconstriction. Patients are encouraged to dress warmly; wear gloves and mittens; and protect the trunk, head, and feet with warm clothing to prevent cold-induced reflex vasoconstriction. Tobacco use is contraindicated. The patient may be prescribed calcium-channel blockers to relieve symptoms. Digital sympathectomy (interrupting the sympathetic nerves) may help some patients.

Pearls for Practice

Remember the red, white, and blue of Raynaud! The intense spasm of the digital arteries produces initial pallor (white), followed over minutes by capillary dilation and filling with deoxygenated venous blood, resulting in cyanosis (blue). On relaxation of the arterial spasm, the circulation improves (warm red digits).

THROMBOANGIITIS OBLITERANS (BUERGER DISEASE)

Buerger disease is characterized by recurring inflammation of the intermediate and small arteries and veins, resulting in thrombus formation and vessel occlusion. It occurs in both the upper and lower extremities. It is differentiated from vessel diseases by microscopic appearance.

Buerger disease is an autoimmune disease. While its etiology is unknown, it is believed to be an autoimmune **vasculitis** (inflammation of a blood vessel). It most often occurs in males between 25 and 45 years of age (with one report suggesting a median age at diagnosis of 38.5) and is reported in all races; however, prevalence of is as high as 45% to 63% in India, 16% to 66% in Korea and Japan, and as high as 80% among Ashkenazi Jewish individuals (Patel & Wang, 2023; Vu & Patel, 2022). Tobacco use is a causative factor, and continued use interferes with healing. Pain is generally bilateral and symmetric with focal lesions.

Treatment is essentially the same as for atherosclerotic PAD; sympathetic block may dilate vessels and increase blood flow. Again, tobacco cessation is mandatory for healing to occur.

ANEURYSMS

An aneurysm is a localized out-pouching, sac, or dilation formed at a weak point in the artery wall (Fig. 17-5). Its shape or form classifies it. The most common forms of aneurysms are saccular and fusiform. A *saccular aneurysm* projects from one side of the vessel only. If an entire arterial segment becomes dilated, a *fusiform aneurysm* develops. Very small aneurysms due to localized infection are called *mycotic aneurysms. Aortic aneurysms* occur in the abdominal and thoracic aorta and are characterized by disruption and loss of elastic fibers, resulting in degeneration of the medial vessel wall. It is thought to be an inflammatory process.

ABDOMINAL AORTIC ANEURYSM

The cause of abdominal aortic aneurysm (AAA), the most common type of degenerative aneurysm, has historically been attributed to atherosclerotic changes in the aorta. The etiology is unknown and is likely multifactorial including genetic, environmental, hemodynamic, and immunologic factors, with the most common association being atherosclerosis (Ferri, 2022). It is unclear whether atherosclerosis causes or results from AAA. Most AAAs are asymptomatic and are found on routine examinations or during a workup for another condition. The U.S. Preventive Services Task Force recommends one-time ultrasound screening for males 65 to 75 years of age who have ever smoked (Ferri, 2022). Aneurysms are serious because they can rupture, leading to hemorrhage and death. If the AAA ruptures, mortality rates as high as 95% are seen, because most patients do not reach the hospital in time for surgical repair. Of those who reach the hospital, the mortality rate is still 50%, compared with the 1% to 4% mortality rate for elective repair of a nonruptured AAA (Ferri, 2022).

Pathophysiology

All aneurysms involve a damaged media layer of the vessel. This may be caused by congenital weakness, trauma, or disease. The degradation of the medial elastin fibers and collagen (which gives the vessel strength) leads to the weakening and dilation of the aorta and the development of an aneurysm. After an aneurysm develops, it tends to enlarge, growing at a rate of 0.2 to 0.3 cm/yr for small AAA (3 to 5 cm) and 0.3 to 0.5 cm/year for those >5 cm on average; however, there is no predictable pattern (Shaw et al., 2021).

Risk Factors

Risk factors include age (over 50), male biologic sex, tobacco use, family history, occlusive atherosclerotic disease, and hypertension. Many types of aneurysms have a genetic basis. Patient education includes advising biologic family members to be evaluated for aneurysms.

Clinical Manifestations and Assessment

Nearly 75% of patients with AAA are asymptomatic, and the disorder is discovered on routine examination or when ordering studies for other complaints (Ferri, 2022). Some patients may note that they can feel their heart beating in their abdomen when lying down, or they may say they feel an abdominal mass or abdominal throbbing. A major vessel may be occluded if the AAA is associated with thrombus, or smaller distal occlusions may result from emboli. Small **cholesterol**, platelet, or fibrin emboli may lodge in the digital arteries, causing cyanosis and mottling of the toes.

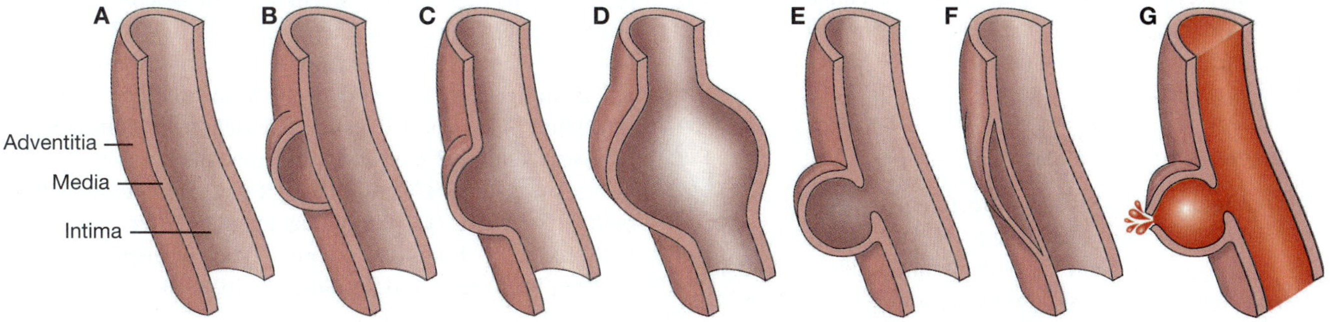

FIGURE 17-5 **Characteristics of arterial aneurysm. (A) Normal artery. (B) False aneurysm (pseudoaneurysm); actually a pulsating hematoma. The clot and connective tissue are outside the arterial wall. (C) True aneurysm. One, two, or all three layers of the artery may be involved. (D) Fusiform aneurysm; symmetric, spindle-shaped expansion of entire circumference of involved vessel. (E) Saccular aneurysm; a bulbous protrusion of one side of the arterial wall. (F) Dissecting aneurysm; this usually is a hematoma that splits the layers of the arterial wall. (G) Ruptured aneurysm.**

Signs of impending aneurysm rupture include severe back or abdominal pain, which may be persistent or intermittent (recall the aorta is in the retroperitoneal space). Abdominal pain is often localized in the middle or lower abdomen to the left of the midline. Low back pain may be present because of the pressure of the aneurysm on the lumbar nerves. This is a significant symptom, usually indicating that the aneurysm is expanding rapidly and is about to rupture. Indications of a rupturing AAA include constant, intense back pain; falling BP; and decreasing hematocrit. Rupture into the peritoneal cavity is rapidly fatal, and surgical repair is the only chance for survival. A retroperitoneal rupture of an aneurysm may result in hematomas in the scrotum, perineum, flank, or penis. Cullen sign (bluish to purplish periumbilical discoloration) and Grey Turner sign (flank discoloration) may be noted with retroperitoneal blood from leaking or ruptured AAA (see Fig. 26-10 on page 923). Symptoms of abdominal distention, constipation, or urinary retention may be caused by a hematoma that compresses the bowel or the urinary tract or by impaired blood supply to these organs (Shaw et al., 2021).

The most important diagnostic indication of an AAA is a pulsatile mass in the abdomen. These aneurysms can be palpated if the patient is not obese. Physical examination has a sensitivity of 76% for detecting AAAs >5 cm but only 29% for AAAs 3.0 to 3.9 cm (Ferri, 2022). The aorta is slightly left of midline, measures approximately 2 cm, and is palpated a few centimeters above the umbilicus (level of bifurcation to the iliac arteries). The aortic width is measured using both hands by noting the width of the pulsations, not the intensity. A systolic bruit may be heard over the mass. Duplex ultrasonography or computed tomography (CT) is used to determine the aneurysm's size, length, and location. An aorta that is 3 cm or greater in width is indicative of an AAA.

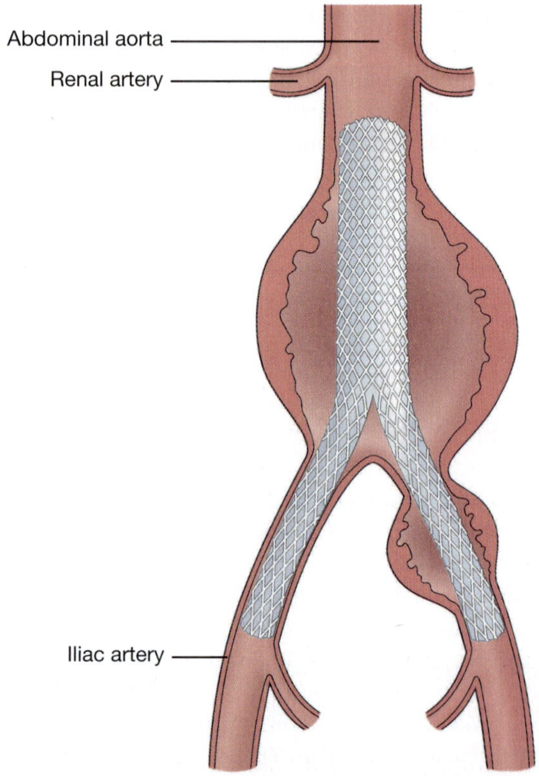

FIGURE 17-6 **AneuRx Endograft repair of an abdominal aortic aneurysm (Medtronic).**

Medical Management

Screening intervals are proposed based on the size of the aneurysm. When the aneurysm is small (3.0 to 3.9 cm), ultrasonography is conducted at 3-year intervals, whereas an AAA greater than 4.5 cm is evaluated annually (Ferri, 2022). Some aneurysms remain stable over many years of observation; however, elective repair should be considered when the AAA exceeds 5 to 5.5 cm, is demonstrated as rapidly enlarging >0.5 cm over 6 months, or becomes symptomatic (Shaw et al., 2021).

Pharmacologic Therapy

The optimal medical therapy treatment for AAA is called anti-impulse therapy, which consists of slowing down the HR and decreasing the BP with antihypertensive medications to reduce the stress against the aortic wall. Guidelines recommend a target HR <60, and SBP of 100 to 120 mm Hg (Azizzadeh & Arbabi, 2022). The HR and BP are closely monitored over time if an aneurysm is stable in size based on serial duplex ultrasound scans. There is an association between increased diastolic BP, size increase, and rupture; therefore, antihypertensive agents, including diuretics, beta-blockers, angiotensin-converting enzyme (ACE) inhibitors, angiotensin II receptor antagonists, and calcium-channel blockers, may be prescribed to maintain the patient BP within acceptable limits.

Surgical Management

An expanding or enlarging AAA is likely to rupture or dissect. Surgery is the treatment of choice for AAAs more than 5.5 cm wide or those that are enlarging (Shaw et al., 2021). An alternative for treating an infrarenal (below the renal arteries) AAA is endovascular grafting, which involves percutaneous transluminal placement and attaching an aortic graft prosthesis across the aneurysm (Fig. 17-6). This procedure is performed under local or regional anesthesia. Potential complications are similar to those of other endograft procedures (discussed later). It is essential to consider that the overall surgical mortality rate associated with a ruptured aneurysm is up to 95%; therefore, early intervention is warranted (Ferri, 2022). Nursing management after surgery can be found after discussing of other types of aneurysms (see Nursing Management After Surgical Interventions, p. 14).

THORACIC AORTIC ANEURYSM

Approximately 85% of all cases of thoracic aortic aneurysms are caused by atherosclerosis. Ascending thoracic aortic aneurysms are often associated with genetic mutations such as Marfan syndrome. They occur most frequently in males between 40 and 70 years of age. The thoracic area is the most common site for a dissecting aneurysm. About one third of patients with thoracic aneurysms die of rupture of the aneurysm.

Pearls for Practice: Pathophysiology
Marfan Syndrome

Marfan syndrome is an inherited disorder (autosomal dominant) of fibrous connective tissue with prominent features affecting the skeleton, heart, great vessels, and eye. Classically, the patient is very tall with extremely long limbs and digits, along with joint hypermobility. Other bony changes are anterior chest deformity (pectus), scoliosis, thoracic lordosis, high-arched palate with crowded teeth, and some ligamentous laxity (Geiger et al., 2022). Ocular problems include myopia and retinal detachment. The major life-threatening problem is aortic aneurysm or dissection; aortic and mitral valves can also be affected. The label MASS syndrome is sometimes used when describing some of the features of Marfan syndrome referring to mitral valve, aorta, skeletal, and skin involvement. Medical care consists of cardiac and aorta monitoring by physical examination and echocardiography (Ferri, 2022). Surgical repair of the dilated aortic root/ascending aorta is repaired as described previously (>5 cm).

Clinical Manifestations and Assessment

More than 95% of thoracic aortic aneurysms are asymptomatic until the point of dissection or rupture (Misra & Henkin, 2021). Symptoms depend on how rapidly the aneurysm dilates and how the pulsating mass affects surrounding intrathoracic structures. In most cases, pain is the most prominent symptom. The pain is usually constant and of boring quality, but it may occur only when the person is supine. Other symptoms are dyspnea, the result of the pressure of the aneurysm sac against the trachea, the main bronchus, or the lung itself; cough, frequently paroxysmal and with a brassy quality; hoarseness, stridor, or weakness or complete loss of the voice (aphonia), resulting from pressure against the laryngeal nerve; and dysphagia (difficulty in swallowing) due to impingement on the esophagus by the aneurysm (Misra & Henkins, 2021).

When the aneurysm compresses large veins in the chest the superficial veins of the chest, neck, or arms become dilated; edematous areas on the chest wall and cyanosis are often evident. Pressure against the cervical sympathetic chain can result in unequal pupils. Diagnosis of a thoracic aortic aneurysm is principally made by chest x-ray, transesophageal echocardiography (TEE), and CT.

Medical Management

As previously stated, aneurysms are sometimes managed medically with risk factor modification, especially BP control, pain management, and close monitoring of symptoms. However, if there is rapid TAA growth rate (>0.5 cm in 6 months or >1 cm in 1 year) prophylactic repair is warranted (Misra & Henkin, 2021). An aneurysm is treated by open surgical method or an endovascular procedure in most cases. General measures such as controlling BP and correcting risk factors are important. Although the optimal BP target for patients with TAA remains unclear, many aim for systolic pressure less than 120 mm Hg with antihypertensive medications or a beta blocker (Misra & Henkins, 2021). In addition, smoking cessation is extremely important for all patients with TAA since the rate of thoracic aneurysm expansion is nearly double in active smokers (Misra & Henkin, 2021). The goal of surgery is to repair the aneurysm and restore vascular continuity with a vascular graft. Intensive monitoring is usually required after an open surgical procedure, and the patient is cared for in the critical care unit. Open surgical repair is the gold standard for TAA of the ascending aorta and aortic arch, but thoracic endovascular aortic repair (TEVAR) is now preferred for TAA of the descending aorta in the absence of inherited connective tissue disease, such as Marfan syndrome (Misra & Henkins, 2021). TEVAR of unruptured thoracic aneurysms decreases postoperative recovery time and decreases complications compared with traditional surgical techniques; however in aneurysms of >6.0 cm, open surgical replacement was preferred in the arch, except in older individuals or high-risk patients (Sharples et al., 2022). One-year overall survival was 82.5% after endovascular stent grafting and 79.3% after open surgical replacement and the variables that affected survival were related to the site of the aneurysm, the patient's age, stage of the disease and time waiting for procedure (Sharples et al., 2022). These endovascular grafts are inserted into the thoracic aorta via various vascular access routes, including the femoral or iliac artery.

The immediate concern is BP control and a device-related complication termed an *endoleak* from the endovascular graft. An endoleak is a persistent leaking of blood from the graft and into the aneurysm sac. Early leaks have the potential to rupture within the first 30 postoperative days (primary endoleaks), but late endoleaks (secondary endoleaks) can occur as late as 7 years after the procedure. An endoleak is screened by CT scanning and duplex ultrasound. The nurse considers that during the operative procedure, necessary vessel clamping can have a profound effect on the mesentery circulation (gut), renal circulation (kidneys), and artery of Adamkiewicz (supplies the lower two thirds of the spinal cord). Postoperatively, regardless of type of procedure performed, the patient is assessed for changes in mentation, vision, speech, or motor strength, as well as pain in the abdomen or flank, vomiting, or bloody diarrhea, which may indicate embolization to cerebral, mesentery circulation or other organs and should be reported to the surgeon immediately. In addition, depending on the length of time the aorta was clamped during the surgery, concerns include spinal cord ischemia with resultant paraplegia and renal insufficiency. Thus, both kidney function and sensory/motor function are assessed postoperatively. Patients undergoing open surgical procedures go to the intensive care unit and typically are on mechanical ventilation postoperatively. Endovascular procedures may not require intensive care unit monitoring postprocedure.

PERIPHERAL ANEURYSMS

Aneurysms may also arise in the peripheral vessels, most often as a result of atherosclerosis. These may involve the renal artery, femoral artery, or (most frequently) popliteal artery. Between 50% and 60% of popliteal aneurysms are bilateral and may be associated with AAAs.

The aneurysm produces a pulsating mass and disturbs peripheral circulation distal to it. Pain and swelling develop because of pressure on adjacent nerves and veins. Diagnosis is made by duplex ultrasonography and CT to determine the size, length, and extent of the aneurysm. Arteriography may be performed to evaluate the level of proximal and distal involvement.

DISSECTING ANEURYSM

Occasionally, in an aorta diseased by arteriosclerosis, a tear develops in the intima or the media degenerates, resulting in a dissection (a false lumen that communicates with the true lumen) (refer to Fig. 17-5). Dissections may be treated medically or surgically.

Pathophysiology

Arterial dissections are commonly associated with poorly controlled hypertension, blunt force chest trauma, and cocaine use. Dissection is caused by a rupture in the intimal layer. A rupture may occur through adventitia or into the lumen through the intima, allowing blood to reenter the main channel, resulting in chronic dissection or occlusion of branches of the aorta. As the separation progresses, the arteries branching from the involved area of the aorta shear and occlude. The tear occurs most commonly in the aortic arch region, with the highest mortality rate associated with ascending aortic dissection. The dissection of the aorta may progress toward the heart, obstructing the orifices of the coronary arteries, producing hemopericardium (effusion of blood into the pericardial sac), or aortic insufficiency, or it may extend distally, occluding the arteries supplying the GI tract, kidneys, spinal cord, and legs. Without treatment, nearly 75% of patients with ascending aortic dissections can be expected to die within 2 weeks, and 90% of all patients with untreated dissections will die within a year (Bautz & Schneider, 2020).

Clinical Manifestations and Assessment

The onset of symptoms is usually sudden. Severe and persistent pain, described as tearing or ripping, may be reported. The pain is in the anterior chest or back and extends to the shoulders, epigastric area, or abdomen. Aortic dissection may be mistaken for an acute MI, confusing the clinical picture and initial treatment. Cardiovascular, neurologic, and GI symptoms are responsible for other clinical manifestations, depending on the location and extent of the dissection. For example, if the dissection extends to the renal arteries, patients can present with acute kidney failure (AKF); with mesentery involvement, abdominal pain and bloody diarrhea may be seen; and lower extremity ischemia can be seen with iliac involvement. The patient may appear pale. Diaphoresis and tachycardia may be detected. BP may be elevated or markedly different from one arm to the other if dissection involves the orifice of the subclavian artery on one side. Early diagnosis is difficult because of the variable clinical picture associated with this condition.

Nursing Management after Surgical Interventions

Surgical repair of the aorta is performed for dissection, rupture, and aneurysm. General postoperative nursing assessment involves frequent vital signs; recording of intake and output; assessing oxygen saturation; bilateral comparison of upper arm BPs and peripheral pulses; and assessing motor and sensory function, temperature of extremities, color changes, and capillary refill. According to a protocol, the patient who has had an endovascular repair must lie supine. The patient needs to use a bedpan or urinal while on bed rest. The access site (usually the femoral or iliac artery) is assessed when monitoring vital signs and pulses. The nurse assesses for bleeding, pulsation, swelling, pain, and hematoma formation. In addition, the patient is monitored for signs of embolization to the lower extremities; therefore, skin changes of the lumbar area, buttocks, and lower extremity (plantar area of the feet or toes is often affected) are assessed for extremely tender, irregularly shaped, cyanotic areas.

The patient's temperature should be monitored according to a protocol, and any signs of the postimplantation syndrome should be reported. Postimplantation syndrome typically begins within 24 hours of stent-graft placement and consists of a spontaneously occurring fever, leukocytosis, and, occasionally, transient thrombocytopenia. The exact etiology is unknown, but the symptoms are thought to be related to the activation of cytokines, which results from thrombosis in the repaired aneurysm that occurs because of the release of coagulation proteins and platelets. These symptoms can be managed with mild analgesics or anti-inflammatory agents, such as acetaminophen or ibuprofen, and usually subside within a week.

Because of the increased risk for hemorrhage, the surgeon is notified of persistent coughing, sneezing, vomiting, or SBP greater than 180 mm Hg. Most patients can resume their preprocedure diet and are encouraged to drink fluids. An IV infusion may be continued until the patient can drink normally. Fluids are important to maintain blood flow through the arterial repair site and to assist kidneys with excreting

IV contrast agents and other medications used during the procedure. According to a protocol, after a procedure that involves a catheter in the groin, the patient may be able to roll from side to side and may be able to ambulate with assistance to the bathroom. After the patient can take adequate fluids orally, the IV infusion may be discontinued and the IV access converted to a saline lock. Postoperative care requires intense pulmonary, cardiovascular, renal, and neurologic status monitoring. Pulmonary complications include the potential development of acute respiratory distress syndrome (ARDS), particularly if large quantities of blood were required intraoperatively (refer to Chapter 9 for discussion of ARDS). MI and arrhythmias are potential cardiac complications and are discussed in Chapters 13 and 16, respectively. GI complications include a risk for ischemic colitis, and symptoms include bloody diarrhea, abdominal distention, leukocytosis, fever, and abdominal pain. Because AKF is a potential complication, urine output is monitored hourly, and laboratory parameters are observed (blood urea nitrogen [BUN] and creatinine values) for significant changes. Potential injury to the spinal cord with resultant paraplegia requires that the nurse assess the patient's sensory/motor function postoperatively. In addition, since it is important that perfusion to the spinal cord must be maintained, the nurse frequently assesses BP measurements, and the surgeon is alerted upon evidence of decreasing parameters.

Before discharge, the patient is assisted in developing and implementing a plan to stop using tobacco and to manage pain. The patient may need to be encouraged to make the lifestyle changes necessary to adequately manage a chronic disease, including modifications in diet, activity, and hygiene. The nurse assesses the patient's resources, including family and friends, to assist as needed. The nurse ensures that the patient has the knowledge and ability to assess for disease progression and postoperative complications as needed.

VENOUS DISORDERS

Venous blood flow is reduced by a thrombus or **embolus** obstructing a vein, by incompetent venous valves, or by a reduction of the pumping action effectiveness of surrounding muscles. Decreased venous blood flow causes increased venous pressure, which increases capillary hydrostatic pressure, facilitating filtration of fluid out of the capillaries into the interstitial space, resulting in development of tissue edema. In addition, edematous tissue does not receive adequate nutrition from the blood and is more susceptible to breakdown, injury, and infection. Thus, the nurse is aware that edematous tissue is fragile tissue.

VENOUS THROMBOSIS

The terms *venous thrombosis, deep vein thrombosis* (DVT), *thrombophlebitis, venous thromboembolism (VTE)*, and *phlebothrombosis* do not necessarily reflect identical disease processes, but they are grouped for clinical purposes.

BOX 17-6

Virchow Triad

1. *Stasis of blood:* Caused by immobility (bed rest, long plane/car/train rides, BMI > 35 kg/m^2 constrictive devices, paralysis, paresis, recent surgery, varicose veins, pregnancy) (Conway, 2020).
2. *Vessel wall injury:* Caused by trauma (fractures, contusions), central venous catheterization, vascular devices (PICC, central lines, pacemaker wires), IV medications, cancer therapy (hormonal, chemotherapy, or radiotherapy)
3. *Altered coagulation:* Caused by estrogen-containing oral contraception or hormone replacement, cancer (secretes procoagulants), smoking, dehydration, hypercoagulable states, late pregnancy, and the postpartum period

Pathophysiology

The exact cause of venous thrombosis remains unclear. Three factors, known as *Virchow triad* (Box 17-6), are believed to play a significant role in the development of venous thrombosis. This hypercoagulability has been recently seen in COVID-19, secondary to acute inflammatory changes. In patients with COVID-19, the risk is increased for VTE (Teuwen et al., 2020). Hypercoagulable states are hereditary, such as Factor V Leiden mutation. Patients with these states should have a hematology consult.

Upper extremity venous thrombosis is not as common as lower extremity thrombosis. However, it may occur in patients with IV catheters (IV lines or wires from pacemaker leads, chemotherapy ports, dialysis catheters, or parenteral nutrition lines) or in patients with an underlying hypercoagulation disorder. Effort thrombosis is caused by repetitive motion (as in competitive swimmers, tennis players, and construction workers) that irritates the vessel wall, causing inflammation and subsequent thrombosis.

Venous thrombi are aggregates of platelets attached to the vein wall with a tail-like appendage containing fibrin, white blood cells, and many red blood cells. The thrombus can propagate as successive layers of thrombus form. A propagating venous thrombosis is dangerous because it is often the source of a pulmonary embolism (PE). Thrombus fragmentation can occur spontaneously or in association with elevated venous pressure, as when a person stands suddenly or engages in muscular activity after prolonged inactivity. After an episode of acute DVT, recanalization of the lumen of the vessel occurs. However, the venous valves remain open and are ineffective. Reverse venous flow contributes to chronic venous insufficiency. Over time, postphlebitic syndrome (Box 17-7) occurs, manifested by the skin and tissue changes.

Clinical Manifestations and Assessment

A major problem associated with recognizing DVT is that the signs and symptoms are nonspecific. The exception is

BOX 17-7 **Focus on Pathophysiology**

Postphlebitic Syndrome

Postphlebitic syndrome develops as follows:

1. Venous valve injury results in an incompetent valve and reverse venous flow.
2. Fluid, plasma, and red blood cells leak into the interstitial tissue.
3. Edema forms around ankles and/or lower legs.
4. Staining of skin occurs as red blood cells break down, releasing hemosiderin.
5. Subcutaneous tissue becomes firm and fibrotic.
6. Loss of elasticity in the skin and subcutaneous tissue results.
7. Tissue becomes vulnerable to trauma and ulcer formation.

phlegmasia cerulea dolens (massive iliofemoral venous thrombosis). The entire extremity becomes massively swollen, tense, and painful, with arterial ischemia (bluish color) and potential loss of distal pulses. Despite this variability, clinical signs should always be investigated.

Deep venous obstruction is associated with edema of the extremity due to inhibition of venous outflow. The nurse should note any differences in leg circumference bilaterally from thigh to ankle; increase in the leg's surface temperature, particularly the calf or ankle; and areas of tenderness or superficial thrombosis. Swelling can be measured by obtaining the circumference of the affected extremity at specific levels and comparing one extremity with the other at the same level. Asymmetry of extremities (calf swelling at least 3 cm larger than asymptomatic leg), measured 10 cm below the tibial tuberosity, should alert the nurse to a potential DVT. In addition, the nurse should assess for the presence of a low-grade fever.

Tenderness, which usually occurs later, is produced by inflammation of the vein wall, and firmness may be detected along the involved veins by gently palpating the affected extremity (palpated cord). *Homan sign* (pain in the calf after the foot is sharply dorsiflexed) used to be considered a sign of DVT, but it is not reliable and is not used anymore. Dilation and prominence of the superficial veins may be noted. In some cases, signs and symptoms of a PE are the first indications of DVT.

Superficial vein thrombosis produces pain or tenderness, redness, and warmth in the involved area. Many of these thromboses dissolve spontaneously. This condition can be treated at home with bed rest, limb elevation, analgesics, and anti-inflammatory medication. It should be noted that while nonsteroidal anti-inflammatory drugs (NSAIDs) provide analgesia, they are associated with an increase in VTE, caused by an embolism breaking off and lodging in a smaller vein (Cumhur Cure et al., 2020).

Careful assessment is the key in detecting early signs of lower extremity venous disorders. Patients with a history of varicose veins, hypercoagulation in COVID-19, active cancer, cardiovascular disease, or recent major surgery or injury are at high risk. Other patients at high risk include those who are experiencing obesity (BMI> 35 kg/m^2), immobility, or older individuals, and females taking oral contraceptives or hormone replacement therapy (HRT).

Pearls for Practice

The D-dimer blood assay is a marker of coagulation activity. When a clot lyses, fibrin degradation occurs, and a D-dimer is positive. When positive, it is associated with clot breakdowns, such as the presence of DVT or PE. However, it is also associated with a variety of nonthrombotic disorders, including recent surgery, hemorrhage, trauma, cancer, MI, pneumonia, and sepsis. Thus, D-dimers are frequently elevated due to some systemic illness; however, a negative D-dimer decreases the likelihood of a DVT or PE.

Prevention

Preventive measures should be instituted for patients at risk for DVT. These might include physical interventions, such as elastic compression stockings, intermittent pneumatic compression devices, and body positioning and exercise. Medications to prevent thrombosis include anticoagulant therapy, such as subcutaneous unfractionated or low–molecular-weight heparin (LMWH). Studies are ongoing as to which prevention method works best with which patient population. Guidelines for intervention are continuously evolving, as seen in the recent pandemic with COVID-19. It is up to the practitioner to keep up with the research findings and apply the evidence to clinical practice.

Medical Management

The treatment objectives for DVT are to prevent the thrombus from growing and fragmenting (risking PE) and to prevent recurrent thromboemboli. Interventions to prevent thrombus formation are indicated in patients with thrombophlebitis, recurrent embolus formation, persistent leg edema from heart failure, and in any patients who may require lengthy immobilization. This is especially the case for patients hospitalized with COVID-19, which should receive prophylaxis, unless contraindicated by increased bleeding risk.

Pharmacologic Therapy

Heparin

Anticoagulant therapy is effective prophylaxis; however, anticoagulants do not dissolve a thrombus that has already formed.

Unfractionated Heparin. Unfractionated heparin is administered subcutaneously to prevent development of DVT. In the event of a DVT, although heparin can be administered subcutaneously, common practice is to administer heparin via an IV drip to prevent the extension of a thrombus and the development of new thrombi. IV heparin produces an immediate anticoagulant effect, and, therefore, is used when rapid anticoagulant effects are desired. Unfractionated heparin is administered via an infusion pump to control the rate carefully. Dosage is based on the patient's weight, and a pretreatment clotting profile detects any possible bleeding tendencies. If renal insufficiency exists, lower doses of heparin are required. Periodic coagulation tests and hematocrit levels are obtained. Heparin is in the effective or therapeutic range when the activated partial thromboplastin time (aPTT) is 1.5 to 2.5 times the baseline control. Anti-factor Xa level is another functional assay commonly used in institutions to measure therapeutic unfractionated heparin levels; the nurse should be informed of what protocol is used in their institution. Normal aPTT level is 21 to 35 seconds (Fischbach et al., 2022). This closely corresponds to a 0.3 to 0.7 anti-factor Xa units/mL (Teien & Lie, 1977; Warnock & Huang, 2022). If the PTT is greater than 100 seconds, the risk for hemorrhage is significant! Typically, the PTT or anti-factor Xa level is measured 6 hours after therapy is started. The nurse is aware that heparin has a half-life of about 60 minutes; therefore, in an emergency, the heparin is discontinued for at least 1 hour.

Warfarin, an oral anticoagulant, is administered soon after initiating heparin therapy since warfarin may require 3 to 5 days to achieve a therapeutic effect. Both medications are administered concurrently until a therapeutic international normalized ratio (INR) is achieved. Medication dosage is regulated by monitoring the aPTT for heparin, the INR for warfarin, and the platelet count, to assess for potential complications of heparin therapy (discussed later in this chapter).

Low–Molecular-Weight Heparin. Subcutaneous LMWH is an effective treatment for some cases of DVT. These agents have longer half-lives than unfractionated heparin so doses can be given in one or two subcutaneous injections each day. Doses are adjusted according to patient weight. LMWH prevents the extension of a thrombus and development of new thrombi, and they are associated with fewer bleeding complications and lower risks of heparin-induced thrombocytopenia (HIT) than is unfractionated heparin. Because there are several preparations, the dosing schedule must be based on the product used and the protocol at each institution. Because LMWH is cleared almost entirely by the kidneys, clearance can be variable in patients with renal insufficiency. Thus, a longer half-life may be expected. The cost of LMWH is higher than that of unfractionated heparin; however, another benefit is that LMWH may be used safely in pregnant patients.

Pearls for Practice

Heparin-induced thrombocytopenia or HIT is a complication associated with the anticoagulant heparin (unfractionated heparin [UFH] and low–molecular-weight heparin). There are two types of HIT: type one is common (occurring in 10% to 20% of patients receiving heparin), appearing 1 to 4 days after exposure to heparin, is mild (platelet count decreases to a low of 100,000/μL), and transient (Crowther, 2022; Suarez, 2022). It is not associated with thromboemboli or hemorrhage, and management consists of observing the patient and platelet count, without discontinuing the heparin (Crowther, 2022). Whereas type 2 HIT is an autoimmune response to the administration of heparin that happens 5 to 10 days after the start of heparin. It occurs in 1% to 3% of patients receiving heparin but is more severe with platelet counts decreasing (thrombocytopenia) usually >20,000/μL; the median nadir 60,000/μL (Crowther, 2022; Suarez, 2022). In addition, 30% to 80% of patients will develop thromboemboli in which case the term HITT is used, referring to Heparin-Induced Thrombocytopenia and Thrombosis; and rarely hemorrhage can occur. Treatment consists of stopping the heparin and administering alternative nonheparin anticoagulation such as direct thrombin inhibitor (DTI) to prevent thrombosis (Crowther, 2022; Suarez, 2022). UpToDate has a calculator for calculating the pretest probability of heparin-induced thrombocytopenia (HIT) which can be accessed at https://www.uptodate.com/contents/calculator-4-ts-score-for-calculating-the-pretest-probability-of-heparin-induced-thrombocytopenia-hit.

Direct Thrombin Inhibitor. Thrombin's role in clot formation is to convert soluble fibrinogen to insoluble fibrin while stimulating platelet activation; thus, direct thrombin inhibitors (DTIs) impede this process. In addition, DTIs have a more predictable anticoagulant effect than heparin and do not cause an immune-mediated thrombocytopenia. Two parenteral DTIs are approved for use as anticoagulants in the United States: bivalirudin and argatroban. Desirudin and lepirudin have been discontinued. There is no specific antidote to reverse the effects of parenteral DTIs. Thus, the nurse observes for evidence of bleeding and reports to the provider any concerns. There is one oral DTI that is available: dabigatran. Currently, reversal of dabigatran's anticoagulant effects can be achieved in emergencies with the use of idarucizumab.

In addition to parenterally administered heparins, oral direct factor Xa inhibitors can be utilized, although clinical applications differ. Oral direct factor Xa inhibitors include rivaroxaban, apixaban, and edoxaban. They are at least as effective and safe as warfarin. Their ability to be administered in fixed doses without routine coagulation monitoring has led to an increase in their use. However, it has yet to be determined if the reduced need for monitoring overrides the increase in cost. Additionally, the absence of an easy antidote when patients have major bleeding is a current concern.

Thrombolytic Therapy

Unlike heparin, thrombolytic (fibrinolytic) therapy lyses and dissolves thrombi. Therefore, there is an increase in bleeding complications with thrombolytics compared with heparin.

TABLE **17-3 Arterial and Venous Thrombolysis**

Indications (Arterial and Venous)	Drug	Advantages (All Drugs in Arterial and Venous Thrombosis)	Disadvantages (All Drugs in Arterial and Venous Thrombosis)
In situ thrombosis of less than 14 days	Alteplase	Clot lysis between 6 and 72 hours Preferred choice for clot removal if no contraindications Avoidance of invasive surgical operations May be repeated if needed.	Limited in DVT lysis by long infusion times and risks of hemorrhagic complications associated with large doses
Nonlife-threatening limb ischemia (arterial)	Reteplase	Superior thrombus penetration	Risk factors for hemorrhagic complications: older age, lower body weight, elevated pulse pressure, uncontrolled hypertension, recent stroke, recent operation, bleeding disorder, congestive heart failure

Please refer to the latest guidelines from the manufacturer for indications, dosages, general warnings, and precautions. Currently complications (among others) associated with thrombolysis include (1) increased risk of bleeding, (2) orolingual angioedema, (3) cholesterol embolism, and (4) reembolization from the lysis.

Data from Alteplase (Activase) (2016). www.Activase.com. Genentech Inc.; Reteplase (Reteplase) (2015). Chiesi, Cary, NC; Sobieszcyk, P. S. (2013). Acute arterial occlusion. In M. A. Creager, J. A. Beckman, J. Loscalzo (Eds.), *Vascular medicine: A companion to Braunwald's heart disease*. Elsevier Saunders.

Since thrombolytics have not decreased the incidence of post-thrombotic syndrome or pulmonary emboli, this therapy is generally reserved for patients with life-threatening limb ischemia due to massive thrombosis. If bleeding occurs, the thrombolytic agent is discontinued. See Table 17-3 for thrombolytic therapy.

Oral Anticoagulants

Warfarin is a vitamin K antagonist (VKA) that is frequently used for extended anticoagulant therapy. Routine coagulation monitoring is essential to ensure that therapeutic response is obtained and maintained over time. Interactions with a range of other medications and various foods with vitamin K can reduce or enhance the anticoagulant effects of warfarin. Warfarin has a narrow therapeutic window, and there is a slow onset of action. The INR monitors oral anticoagulants, such as warfarin. Because the full anticoagulant effect of warfarin is delayed for 3 to 5 days, treatment is initially supported with concomitant parenteral anticoagulation with heparin until the warfarin demonstrates anticoagulant effectiveness; then the heparin can be discontinued and the patient maintained on oral warfarin. A normal INR is approximately 1. The target INR depends on why the person is being anticoagulated. If, for example, anticoagulation is related to atrial fibrillation or DVT, the INR range will be 2 to 3, with a goal of 2.5. Once INR is stable, levels are checked weekly for 2 to 4 weeks, progressing monthly thereafter. Refer to Table 17-4 for a list of therapeutic goals for INR.

Surgical Management

Surgery is necessary for DVT when anticoagulant or thrombolytic therapy is contraindicated, the danger of PE is likely, or the venous drainage is so severely compromised that permanent damage to the extremity is likely. A thrombectomy (removal of the thrombosis) is the procedure of choice. A vena cava filter may be placed at the time of the thrombectomy; this filter traps large emboli and prevents PE (see Chapter 9, Fig. 9-8). Research notes that an inferior vena cava (IVC) filter is associated with a reduction in the risk of recurrent PE; however, this is balanced against the risk of thrombosis, filter migration, recurrent DVT (Weitz & Ginsberg, 2020). In addition, IVC filter does not alter mortality. However, a vena cava filter may be indicated if there is a contraindication to or complication of anticoagulation therapy (e.g., hemorrhagic

TABLE **17-4 Therapeutic Context**

	INR	Target
Non–hip surgery	1.5–2.5	2.0
Hip surgery	2.0–3.0	2.5
Primary and secondary prevention of deep vein thrombosis	2.0–3.0	2.5
Prevention of systemic embolism in patients with atrial fibrillation	2.0–3.0	2.5
Recurrent systemic embolism	3.0–4.5	3.5
Prevention of recurrent deep vein thrombosis (two or more episodes)	2.5–4.0	3.0
Cardiac stents	3.0–4.5	3.5
Prevention of arterial thrombosis, including patients with mechanical heart valves	2.5–3.5	3.0

Reproduced from Fischbach, F. T., Fischbach, M. A., & Stout, K. (2022). *A manual of laboratory and diagnostic tests* (11th ed., Table 2.10). Lippincott Williams & Wilkins.

stroke, active internal bleeding, pregnancy) and should be removed as soon as anticoagulation can be safely started (Kaatz, 2021). It is important to recognize that a filter does not prevent other thrombi from forming. Balloon angioplasty and stent placement are used in the iliac veins of patients with acute and chronic venous disease.

Nursing Management

Monitoring Drug Therapy

When the patient is receiving anticoagulant therapy, the nurse frequently monitors the aPTT, prothrombin time (PT), INR, activated coagulation time (ACT), hemoglobin and hematocrit values, platelet count, and fibrinogen level, depending on which medication is given.

Nurses must watch for potential complications; the principal one is spontaneous bleeding anywhere in the body. Bleeding from the kidneys is detected by microscopic urine examination and is often the first sign of excessive dosage. Bruises, nosebleeds, and bleeding gums are also early signs. To promptly reverse the effects of heparin, protamine sulfate is administered. Risks of protamine administration include bradycardia and hypotension, which is minimized by slow administration. Protamine sulfate is available for use in patients receiving LMWH, but it is less effective with LMWH than with unfractionated heparin. Reversing the anticoagulation effects of warfarin is more complex, but effective measures may include administration of vitamin K and/or infusion of fresh-frozen plasma or prothrombin concentrate. Oral vitamin K significantly reduces the INR within 24 hours. Low-dose IV vitamin K is also effective.

HIT may be another complication of therapy, which is defined as a sudden decrease in the platelet count by at least 30% of baseline levels in patients receiving heparin.

Pearls for Practice

An average adult platelet count is 140 to 400 × 10^3/mm^3. A platelet count of more than 50 × 10^3/mm^3 is generally not associated with spontaneous bleeding. However, a platelet count of less than 20 × 10^3/mm^3 is associated with bleeding from gums and injection sites; epistaxis (nose bleed), ecchymoses (bruising), and petechiae may be noted. When the platelet count drops to less than 10 × 10^3/mm^3, spontaneous intracranial hemorrhage becomes a significant risk (Fischbach et al., 2022). Bleeding precautions are recommended for patients with a platelet count of less than 50,000/mm^3.

Patients at greatest risk for bleeding are those who receive unfractionated heparin for an extended period of time (i.e., several days or weeks). Therefore, it is preferable not to anticoagulate patients with unfractionated heparin over the long term. Beginning warfarin concomitantly with heparin can provide a stable INR by day 5 of heparin treatment, at which time the heparin is discontinued.

The administration of LMWH is less frequently associated with HIT. The thrombocytopenia results from an autoimmune mechanism that destroys platelets. If the process is not stopped, platelets may aggregate, initiating inappropriate clotting, and thrombosis may occur. This severe complication results in thromboembolic manifestations throughout the body, and the prognosis is highly guarded.

Prevention of thrombocytopenia depends on regular monitoring of platelet counts. Early signs of complications associated with anticoagulants include a decreasing platelet count, the need for increasing doses of heparin to maintain the therapeutic level, and thromboembolic or hemorrhagic complications, such as skin necrosis at the injection site and at distal sites of thromboses, and skin discoloration consisting of hemorrhagic areas, hematomas, purpura, and blistering. If thrombocytopenia does occur, platelet aggregation studies are conducted, the heparin is discontinued, and alternative anticoagulant therapy is initiated rapidly because the continued prothrombotic state poses an ongoing threat of continuous clot development.

Bivalirudin and argatroban are intravenous DTIs approved for the treatment of HIT. Bivalirudin has a half-life of 25 minutes (in those with normal kidney function), is metabolized by the kidneys and liver, and can be monitored using the activated clotting time (ACT) and aPTT (Drug Monograph, 2022). An initial IV bolus infusion followed by a continuous infusion with subsequent adjustments to maintain the aPTT between 1.5 and 2.5 times baseline is recommended. The anticoagulant effect is immediate and coagulation times return to baseline approximately 1 hour after completion of infusion (Collins, 2022). Argatroban has a half-life of 30 to 45 minutes, is metabolized by the liver, and is unaffected by kidney function. The anticoagulant effect of argatroban is predictable, with low variability between patients, but it is dose-dependent and requires monitoring with either the aPTT or ACT. There is no safe, rapidly acting antidote if the patient develops bleeding complications from DTIs. There are new medications being tested for long-term anticoagulation, but the guidelines have weak recommendations for their use and further research is warranted. The clinician is responsible to keep up with the current research and recommendations for all interventions.

Pearls for Practice

In the event of that life-threatening bleeding complications occurs with IV argatroban (a direct thrombin inhibitor), the infusion will be discontinued. The nurse expects to obtain aPTT and hemoglobin and hematocrit and prepare for blood transfusion(s). The aPTT should return to baseline within 2 to 4 hours after the medication is stopped but may be slower if the patient has liver disease (Crowther, 2022). In the event of hypovolemic shock, fluids, vasopressors, supine position with legs elevated may be considered to increase venous pressure, and plasma expanders

such as albumin may be used while waiting for blood products. The nurse is alert to signs and symptoms of hypovolemic shock such as decreasing urine output (<0.5 mL/Kg/hr), oliguria, hypotension, decreased mean arterial pressure (MAP), decreased pulse pressure, flat neck veins, altered mental status (anxiety may be earliest symptom), delayed capillary refill, pallor, cool extremities, tachycardia, and tachypnea. Recall that hypotension may not be seen until there is 30% loss of the patient's total blood volume.

Because oral anticoagulants interact with many other medications and herbal and nutritional supplements, close monitoring of the patient's medication schedule is necessary. Many medications and supplements potentiate or inhibit oral anticoagulants; it is always wise to check to see if any medications or supplements the patient is taking are contraindicated with warfarin. In general, 3 months of therapy is expected (Weitz & Ginsberg, 2020).

Providing Comfort

Elevation of the affected extremity, elastic compression stockings, and analgesics for pain relief are adjuncts to therapy. They help improve circulation and increase comfort.

Warm, moist packs applied to the affected extremity reduce the discomfort associated with DVT, as do mild analgesics prescribed for pain control. When the patient begins to ambulate, elastic compression stockings are used. Walking is better than standing or sitting for long periods. The patient is advised to elevate the legs when not ambulating.

Pearls for Practice

Does research show that bed rest or ambulation is best for a patient with a DVT? The believe that ambulation may dislodge thrombi in the legs, precipitating a pulmonary emboli (PE), is unfounded (Ferri, 2022; Lipp & Hull, 2022); however, there are several methodologic differences noted in current research studies indicating the need for further research. For example, the risk of PE during more aggressive forms of exercise, physical therapy, or rehabilitation is unknown (Lipp & Hull, 2022). What is known is that existing research shows evidence that bed rest is an important risk factor for DVT and is physically, emotionally, and socially distressing that simultaneously affects QOL of our patients (Gong et al., 2020). Until evidenced based research is compelling, the issue of bed rest versus activity in patients with DVT continues as an institutional protocol. The nurse should follow the facility's protocol but be cognizant of the findings described here.

Applying Compression Therapy

Increased venous pressure causes the long-term adverse effects of venous disease. Treatment for venous insufficiency is external compression, which counteracts this pressure and protects the tissues from further damage.

Elastic compression stockings are prescribed for patients with chronic venous insufficiency. These stockings exert a sustained, graduated compression over the extremity, compressing the superficial veins, minimizing venous blood pooling, and resulting in an increased flow toward the deep veins. They also prevent the sequelae of a postphlebitic syndrome (fibrosis, ulceration). Stockings are available in knee-high, thigh-high, or waist-high lengths.

Short stretch elastic wraps may be applied from the toes to the knee in a 50% spiral overlap. These wraps are available in two-, three-, or four-layer systems, including an inner layer of soft padding. Other types of compression include the Unna boot, which consists of a gauze roll impregnated with glycerin, gelatin, and sometimes zinc oxide or calamine. It is applied without tension in a circular, angular fashion from the base of the toes to the tibial tuberosity with a 50% spiral overlap. This compression type may remain in place for as long as one week. Other manufactured rigid dressings are available to augment the calf muscle pump during ambulation effectively. Patients may find these dressings easier to wear than the Unna boot or a compression stocking.

Intermittent pneumatic compression devices can be used with elastic compression stockings to prevent DVT and reduce edema. They consist of an electric motor attached to plastic knee-high or thigh-high sleeves, with single-chamber or multiple sequential chamber air bladders. These devices mimic muscle contraction and apply pressure to the veins, increasing blood velocity during bed rest.

Body Positioning and Exercise

When the patient is on bed rest, the feet and lower legs should be elevated periodically above the level of the heart. This position allows the veins to empty rapidly. Active and passive leg exercises, particularly those involving calf muscles, should be performed to increase venous flow. Early ambulation is most effective in preventing venous stasis. Deep-breathing exercises produce increased negative pressure in the thorax, which assists in emptying the large veins. The ambulatory patient is instructed to avoid sitting for more than 2 hours at a time and to perform active and passive leg exercises during long car, train, and plane trips when ambulation is not possible.

VARICOSE VEINS

Varicose veins (varicosities) are abnormally dilated, tortuous, superficial veins caused by incompetent venous valves. They occur more frequently in the lower extremities, the saphenous veins, or the lower trunk, but they can occur elsewhere in the body.

Pathophysiology

Varicose veins may be primary (without the involvement of deep veins) or secondary (resulting from obstruction of deep veins). Reflux of venous blood in the veins results in venous stasis. If the superficial veins are affected without deep vein involvement, the patient may be asymptomatic but may be troubled by the appearance of the distended veins.

Risk Factors

The prevalence of varicose veins varies widely, which is reported in 1% to 73% of females and 2% to 56% of males (Alsaigh & Fukaya, 2021). A hereditary weakness of the vein wall may contribute to the development of varicosities, and it commonly occurs in several members of the same family. Varicose veins are rare before puberty. Pregnancy may cause varicosities secondary to hormonal effects related to venous distensibility, increased pressure by the gravid uterus, and increased blood volume. Additional risk factors include previous DVT, increasing age, BMI >30 kg/m^2, and multiple pregnancies (Clinical Overview, 2022; Fort, 2023).

Clinical Manifestations and Assessment

Symptoms, if present, may include dull aches, muscle cramps, increased muscle fatigue in the lower legs, ankle edema, and a feeling of heaviness of the legs. Nocturnal cramps are common. When deep venous obstruction results in varicose veins, the patient develops the signs and symptoms of chronic venous insufficiency: edema, pain, pigmentation changes, and ulcers. Susceptibility to injury and infection increases.

Diagnostic tests for varicose veins include the duplex scan, which documents the anatomic site of reflux and provides a quantitative measure of the severity of valvular reflux. Air plethysmography measures the changes in venous blood volume. Venography is not routinely performed to evaluate for valvular reflux.

Prevention

The patient should avoid activities that increase venous hypertension, such as wearing constricting clothing, crossing the legs at the thighs, and sitting or standing for long periods. Changing position frequently, elevating the legs when tired, and getting up to walk for several minutes of every hour promote circulation. The patient is encouraged to walk 1 or 2 miles each day if there are no contraindications. Walking up the stairs rather than using the elevator or escalator is helpful, and swimming is good exercise. Walking must incorporate the heel-toe step rather than a shuffle to elicit the calf muscle pump effect. Patients who are overweight should be encouraged to begin a weight-reduction plan.

Surgical Management

Ligation and Stripping

Surgery for varicose veins requires that the deep veins be patent and functional. The saphenous vein is ligated and divided. The vein is ligated high in the groin, where the saphenous vein meets the femoral vein. Pressure and elevation minimize bleeding during surgery. Vein stripping, which used to be a standard surgical procedure, has been replaced by the venous ablation techniques.

Ablation Procedures

Thermal ablation is a nonsurgical approach using thermal energy. Radiofrequency ablation uses an electrical contact inside the vein. As the device is withdrawn, the vein is sealed. Laser ablation uses a laser fiber tip that seals the vein (decompresses it). Topical gel may be used first to numb the skin along the course of the saphenous vein. To protect the surrounding tissue, a series of small punctures are made along the vein, and 100 to 200 mL of dilute lidocaine is delivered to the perivenous space using ultrasound guidance. The goal of this tumescent anesthesia (i.e., anesthesia that causes localized swelling) is to provide analgesia, thermal protection (the cuff of fluid surrounds the veins and accompanying nerves), and extrinsic compression of the vein. The saphenous vein is entered percutaneously near the knee using ultrasound guidance. The device is then activated and withdrawn, sealing the vein. Small bandages and compression stockings are applied after the procedure. The patient is asked not to remove the stockings for at least 48 hours. After this time, the patient rewraps the legs and wears compression stockings while ambulatory for a period of time. Patients must be ambulatory prior to being discharged from the outpatient facility and have no activity restrictions, except that swimming is discouraged for 3 weeks. NSAIDs, such as ibuprofen or acetaminophen, are used as needed for pain. The patient is informed that bruising along the course of the vein, leg cramps (for a few days), and difficulty straightening the knees (for up to 1.5 weeks) may be experienced post procedure.

Sclerotherapy

Sclerotherapy involves the injection of an irritating chemical into a vein to produce localized phlebitis and fibrosis, thereby obliterating the lumen of the vein. This treatment may be performed alone for small varicosities or may follow vein ablation or ligation. Sclerosing is palliative rather than curative. Sclerotherapy is typically performed in an examination or procedure room and does not require any sedation. After the sclerosing agent is injected, elastic compression bandages are applied to the leg and are worn according to a protocol, followed by elastic compression stockings. Walking activities are encouraged to maintain blood flow and to dilute the sclerosing agent within the deep venous system.

Postprocedure Nursing Management

After venous ablation procedures, bed rest is discouraged; the nurse encourages the patient to become ambulatory as soon as sedation has worn off. The patient should walk according to an individualized protocol and to increase walking and activity as tolerated. Elastic compression stockings may be worn continuously or just when awake and upright (depending on the individual care provider's protocol) for 1 to 2 weeks after vein procedures. The nurse assists the patient in performing exercises and moving the legs. The foot of the bed should be elevated. Standing and sitting are discouraged. Jogging and hard-impact exercises should be avoided.

Analgesics are prescribed to help the patient move the affected extremities more comfortably. Dressings are inspected for bleeding and signs of infections, particularly at the groin, where the risk of bleeding is most common. The nurse is alert for reports of the sensation of "pins and needles" as sensation is regained. Hypersensitivity to touch in the involved extremity may indicate a temporary or permanent nerve injury from the procedure because the saphenous vein and nerve are close to each other in the leg.

Usually, the patient may shower after the first 24 hours. The patient is given instructions to dry the incisions well with a clean towel, using a patting technique rather than rubbing. Application of skin lotion is avoided until the incisions are completely healed to avoid infection. The patient is also instructed to apply sunscreen or zinc oxide to the incision area prior to sun exposure for 6 months; otherwise, hyperpigmentation of the incision, scarring, or both may occur. The nurse encourages the use of a mild analgesic as prescribed and regular short walking to provide relief.

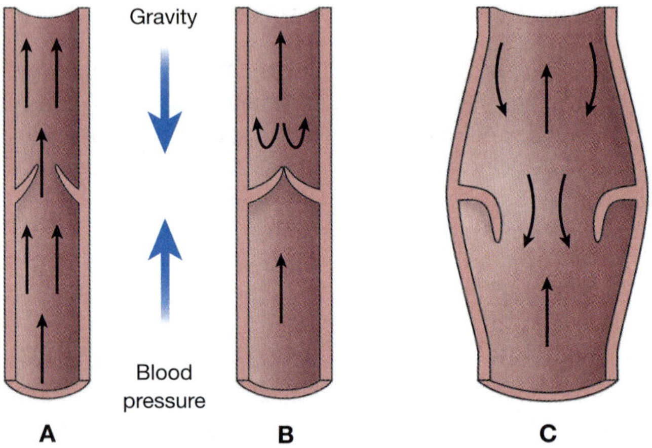

FIGURE 17-7 **Competent valves showing blood flow patterns when the valve is open (A) and closed (B), allowing blood to flow against gravity. (C) With faulty or incompetent valves, the blood cannot move toward the heart.**

CHRONIC VENOUS INSUFFICIENCY

Venous insufficiency results from obstruction of the venous valves in the legs and a reflux of blood. Both superficial and deep leg veins can be involved. A prolonged increase in venous pressure causes venous hypertension. Because the walls of veins are thinner and more elastic than arterial walls, they distend readily when venous pressure is elevated consistently. In this state, leaflets of the venous valves are stretched and prevented from closing completely, allowing a backflow or reflux of blood in the veins (Fig. 17-7). Duplex ultrasound confirms the obstruction and identifies incompetent venous valves.

Clinical Manifestations and Assessment

Classic signs of venous disease are edema and increased skin pigmentation, termed *hemosiderosis.* Because of the poor venous return, there is extravasation of red blood cells, which break down and deposit hemosiderin (a pigment that gives red blood cells their color), staining the skin a gray-brown. Varicosities and telangiectasias are also commonly noted. The extremity is warm, and pulses are present (assuming no concomitant arterial disease) but may be difficult to feel due to the extensive edema.

Postthrombotic syndrome is the long-term result of an incompetent venous system and venous hypertension. Venous obstruction, poor calf muscle pumping, and valvular reflux also contributes to the development of severe postthrombotic syndrome. It is characterized by chronic edema, altered pigmentation, pain, and stasis dermatitis, which is also known as *dermatosclerosis.* The patient may notice aching and heaviness less in the morning after rest and elevation and more in the evening. The disorder is longstanding, challenging to treat, and often disabling.

Medical and Nursing Management

Management of patients with venous insufficiency is directed at reducing venous stasis and preventing ulcers (see additional discussion below). Measures that increase venous blood flow are antigravity activities, such as elevating the leg, and compressing superficial veins with elastic compression stockings.

Elevating the legs decreases edema, promotes venous return, and provides symptomatic relief; therefore, the legs should be elevated frequently throughout the day. At night, the patient should sleep with the foot of the bed elevated. Prolonged sitting or standing in one position is detrimental; walking should be encouraged.

VASCULAR ULCERS

Vascular ulcers include ischemic arterial ulcers, venous ulcers, and ulcers on the lymphatic limb (Table 17-5). Treatment is different for each of these ulcers because treatment is determined on the basis of etiology, which varies for each type of ulcer. Ulcers are not likely on lymphatic limbs.

TABLE **17-5 Arterial and Venous Ulcer Characteristics**

	Arterial	Venous
Location	Distal to arterial stenosis, heels, toes, over bony prominences, metatarsals, malleoli, between toes, trauma points	Around ankle, lower third of leg, more often on medial side
Ulcer base	Dry, pale gray or yellow; may be necrotic	Generally shallow but may be deep. Pink, but may be beefy red with granulation tissue. Ulcer bed usually moist. May have copious drainage
Shape	Border regular and well demarcated	Irregular border
Surrounding tissue	Pale; cooler than other skin areas. In longstanding insufficiency, skin is thin.	Darkened color in gaiter area. Temperature higher than other skin areas. Brawny edema. Skin may be thick and fibrotic (woody). May be oozing and crusted
Edema	Minimal unless leg is dependent often	May be severe
Pain	Claudication. Rest pain; continuous pain worsens with elevation and eases with dependency.	Aching, throbbing, heaviness. Superficial stinging when open to air during dressing changes
Pulses	May be absent or diminished; often disappears with exercise	Usually present with only venous etiology but may be difficult to palpate with edema
ABI	Less than 0.90	Greater than 0.90
Wound treatment	Moist wound healing after revascularization. Monitor for infection. Keep dry gangrene dry.	Compression. Elevation above heart. Absorptive dressings
Operative procedures	Arterial bypass. Angioplasty. Stent placement	Vein ligation/stripping. Valve grafts. Sclerotherapy. Laser or radiofrequency ablation

Usually, associated venous disease or trauma to the already compromised tissue is present when they occur.

Pathophysiology

Venous ulceration is the most severe complication of chronic venous insufficiency and can be associated with other conditions affecting the circulation of the lower extremities. Cellulitis or dermatitis may complicate the care of chronic venous insufficiency and venous ulcer. Venous ulcers develop as a result of increased venous pressure or external trauma.

Atherosclerosis, the most common cause of peripheral arterial occlusive disease, primarily affects the superficial femoral and popliteal vessels, reducing blood flow to the lower extremities. Ulceration develops as a result of ischemia.

Clinical Manifestations and Assessment

Venous ulcers occur in the lower part of the extremity, in the area of the medial malleolus of the ankle, called the *gaiter area.* They range from small to large, are superficial, irregular in shape, highly exudative, and associated with peri-ulcer hemosiderin staining of the skin. The skin becomes dry, cracked, and pruritic; subcutaneous tissues fibrose and atrophy. As a result, the risk for injury and infection of the extremities is increased.

Typically, arterial ulcers are small lesions on the tips of toes or in the web spaces between the toes. Ulcers often occur on the medial side of the hallux or lateral fifth toe and may be caused by a combination of ischemia and pressure. Arterial insufficiency may result in gangrene of the toe (digital gangrene), which may be precipitated by trauma (Box 17-8).

Medical and Nursing Management

Patients with ulcers can be effectively managed by advanced practice nurses or wound-ostomy-continence nurses in collaboration with health care providers. It is the nurse's duty to be aware that all ulcers have the potential to become infected.

Pharmacologic Therapy

Superficial bacteria colonize all ulcers. Most leg ulcers do not need antibiotics. Directed antibiotic therapy is prescribed when the ulcer is infected, with the specific antibiotic agent based on culture and sensitivity test results. When indicated, oral or intravenous antibiotics are usually prescribed because topical antibiotics have not proven to be effective for leg ulcers.

Wound Cleansing and Debridement

As a general rule, arterial ulcers are kept dry, and necrotic tissue is not debrided until revascularization procedures are

BOX 17-8
Gangrene of the Toe

Gangrene of the toes, resulting from severe arterial ischemia, causes the digits to turn black. Debridement is contraindicated in these instances. Although the toes are gangrenous, this is the dry form of gangrene. Managing dry gangrene is preferable to debriding and creating an open wound that will not heal because of insufficient circulation. A distal amputation requires adequate circulation to heal. Without it, further amputation, such as below the knee or above the knee may be necessary. A higher-level amputation in an older person often results in loss of independence and possibly the need for institutional care. Dry gangrene of the toe(s) in an older person with poor circulation, who is asymptomatic, is usually left undisturbed. The toes are kept clean and dry until they separate from the viable tissue. Soaking is avoided.

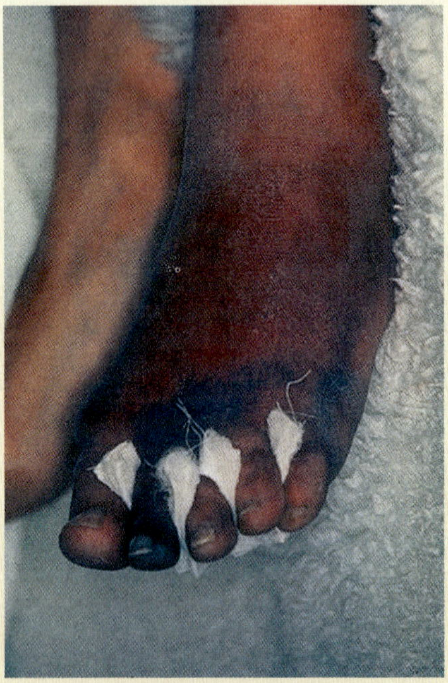

performed due to the risk of infection and likelihood of non-healing associated with poor peripheral perfusion.

Venous ulcers with necrotic tissue should be debrided. The wound is kept clean of drainage to promote healing. The wound is cleansed using normal saline solution or a noncytotoxic wound-cleansing agent with each dressing change. The cleansing agent should be applied to the wound with enough force to wash the surface debris away. If there is necrotic tissue at the base of the venous wound, debridement or removal of nonviable tissue may be necessary. Removing the dead tissue is vital in promoting wound healing. There are several methods of debridement, which are the following:

- *Surgical debridement:* This is the fastest method and can be performed by a physician, skilled advanced practice nurse, or wound-ostomy-continence nurse in collaboration with the physician.
- *Wet to dry or nonselective debridement:* This method can be accomplished by applying saline-impregnated gauze to the ulcer. When the dressing dries, it is removed, along with the debris adhering to the gauze. Pain management is usually necessary.
- *Enzymatic debridement:* This method involves the application of enzyme ointments prescribed to treat the ulcer. The ointment is applied to the lesion but not to normal, healthy surrounding skin. Most enzymatic ointments are covered with saline-soaked gauze that has been thoroughly wrung out. Then a dry gauze dressing and a loose bandage are applied. The enzymatic ointment is discontinued when the necrotic tissue has been debrided, and an appropriate wound dressing is applied.
- *Autolytic debridement:* With this method, an occlusive absorptive dressing, such as a hydrocolloid, is placed over the wound and left in place for a few (3 to 7) days to allow enzymes from the body to liquefy the necrotic tissue and separate it from the viable tissue. These dressings maintain or create a moist wound environment which assists with the removal of necrotic tissue while preserving viable tissue (Zaratkiewicz et al., 2020). A variety of dressing types that can facilitate autolysis, including foam, hydrofibers, alginates, and hydrocolloids. The wound is irrigated copiously during dressing changes to cleanse away the necrotic tissue.

Wound Dressings

After the circulatory status is assessed and determined to be adequate for healing, surgical dressings are used to promote a moist environment. The simplest method is to use a wound contact material next to the wound bed and cover it with gauze. Other available options that promote the growth of granulation tissue and reepithelialization include *hydrocolloids.* These materials also provide a barrier for protection because they adhere to the wound bed and surrounding tissue. However, these dressings may not be effective treatment for deep wounds and infected wounds; therefore, patient and family education is necessary before beginning and throughout the wound care program. See Chapter 51 for further information about wound care.

Stimulated Healing

Tissue-engineered human skin equivalent is a skin product cultured from human dermal fibroblasts and keratinocytes used in combination with therapeutic compression. When applied, it seems to react to factors in the wound and may interact with the patient's cells to stimulate the production of growth factors. Application is not difficult, no suturing is involved, and the procedure is painless.

Hyperbaric Oxygenation

Hyperbaric oxygenation (HBO) may be beneficial to wound healing as an adjunct treatment in patients with DM who evidence no signs of skin healing after standard wound treatment. HBO is accomplished by placing the patient into a chamber that increases barometric pressure while breathing 100% oxygen. The process by which HBO works involves several factors. The edema in the wound area is decreased as high oxygen tension facilitates vasoconstriction and enhances the ability of leukocytes to phagocytize and kill bacteria. In addition, HBO is thought to increase the diffusion of oxygen to the hypoxic wound, thereby enhancing epithelial migration and improving collagen production.

Compression

Leg elevation helps to promote edema reduction. Venous ulcers require external compression. The *Unna boot* or commercial two- and three-layer compression bandages are available for this treatment. An *Unna boot* is a gauze dressing impregnated with a paste combined of glycerin, zinc oxide, and, sometimes, calamine. It is layered on the leg like a cast, from the tips of the toes to just below the knee. Extra padding is used if there is copious wound drainage, and an elastic bandage is placed over the dressing. Once the dressing dries, it becomes rigid. The boot is changed weekly. Its effectiveness depends on healthy calf muscle and the ability to ambulate.

LYMPHATIC DISORDERS

The lymphatic system consists of a set of vessels that start as lymph capillaries, which drain unabsorbed plasma from the interstitial spaces (spaces between the cells). The lymphatic capillaries unite to form the lymph vessels, which pass through the lymph nodes and then empty into progressively larger channels, most of which drain into the thoracic duct that joins the jugular vein on the left side of the neck.

Fluid drained from the interstitial space by the lymphatic system is called *lymphatic drainage.* Lymph flow depends on the intrinsic contractions of the lymph vessels, the contraction of muscles, respiratory movements, and gravity. The lymphatic vessels of the extremities empty into nodes of the axillae and the groin. Under certain abnormal conditions, the fluid filtered out of the capillaries may greatly exceed the amounts reabsorbed and carried away by the lymphatic vessels. This imbalance results from various etiologies, including damage to capillary walls and subsequently increased permeability, obstruction of lymphatic drainage, the elevation of venous pressure, or decrease in plasma protein osmotic force. Accumulation of excess interstitial fluid that results from these processes is known as lymphedema. In general, the nurse is aware that edema usually represents an accumulation of 2.5 to 3 L of interstitial fluid. If the edema is *pitting*—that is, when the nurse presses the thumb into the edematous area for 5 seconds, an imprint of the finger is noted—it is estimated that approximately 4.5 kg (10 lb) of fluid has accumulated (Suneja et al., 2020). Refer to Chapter 11 for more details on assessing pitting edema.

Lymphangiography and lymphoscintigraphy are two diagnostic tests to assess lymphatic function. Lymphangiography involves injecting a contrast agent into a lymphatic vessel in each foot (or hand), followed by taking a series of x-rays after the injection, 24 hours later, and periodically thereafter. A diagnosis of lymphedema is confirmed by the failure to identify subcutaneous lymphatic collection of contrast agent and the persistence of contrast agent in the tissue for days afterward.

Lymphoscintigraphy is a reliable alternative to lymphangiography. A radioactively labeled colloid is injected subcutaneously in the second interdigital space. The extremity is then exercised to facilitate the uptake of the colloid by the lymphatic system, and serial images are obtained at preset intervals.

LYMPHANGITIS AND LYMPHADENITIS

Lymphangitis is an acute inflammation of the lymphatic channels. It arises most commonly from an infection in an extremity. Usually, the infectious organism is a hemolytic streptococcus. The characteristic red streaks that extend up the arm or the leg from an infected wound outline the course of the lymphatic vessels as they drain.

The lymph nodes located along the course of the lymphatic channels also become enlarged, red, and tender (acute lymphadenitis). They can also become necrotic and form an abscess (suppurative lymphadenitis). The nodes involved most often are those in the groin, axilla, or cervical region. Because these infections are nearly always caused by organisms sensitive to antibiotics, it is unusual to see abscess formation. Recurrent episodes of lymphangitis are often associated with progressive lymphedema. After acute attacks, and if the edema has subsided, an elastic compression stocking or sleeve should be worn on the affected extremity for several months to prevent long-term edema.

LYMPHEDEMA AND ELEPHANTIASIS

Lymphedema is swelling in the extremities due to an accumulation of lymphatic drainage from blocked lymphatic vessels.

Pathophysiology

Lymphedemas are classified as primary (congenital malformations) or secondary (acquired obstructions). Tissue swelling occurs in the extremities because of an increased quantity of lymph that results from obstruction of lymphatic vessels. It is especially marked when the extremity is in a dependent position. Initially, the edema is soft and pitting. As the condition progresses, the edema becomes firm, nonpitting, and less responsive to treatment. The most common type is congenital lymphedema (*lymphedema praecox*), which is caused by hypoplasia (underdevelopment) of the lymphatic system of the lower extremity.

The obstruction may be in the lymph nodes and the lymphatic vessels. Sometimes, it is seen in the arm after an axillary node dissection (e.g., for breast cancer) and associated with varicose veins or chronic thrombophlebitis. In the latter case, the lymphatic obstruction usually is caused by chronic lymphangitis. Lymphatic obstruction caused by a parasite (filaria) is seen frequently in patients in the tropics and is the most common cause of lymphedema worldwide. When chronic swelling is present, there may be frequent bouts of acute infection characterized by high fever and chills and increased residual edema after the inflammation has resolved. These lead to chronic fibrosis, thickening of the subcutaneous tissues, and hypertrophy of the skin. This condition, in which chronic swelling of the extremity recedes only slightly with elevation, is referred to as *elephantiasis*.

Clinical Manifestations and Assessment

The diagnosis of lymphedema is made by clinical evaluation and exclusion of other causes of edema. In the early stages, the tissue is soft and pliable, but in advanced lymphedema, the tissue becomes firm and thick, often with overlapping folds of tissue. Early diagnosis is essential to prevent tissue destruction. In the lower extremities, the toes are squared, and there is an inability to pick up or pinch a fold of skin at the base of the second toe or finger (called Stemmer sign) (Ferri, 2022).

Medical Management

Treatment focuses on reducing the edema and preventing increased edema, infections, and tissue damage. Treatment may consist of comprehensive decongestive therapy provided by a certified lymphedema therapist, use of a pump to reduce the edema, and elastic and nonelastic compression wraps or garments to maintain the edema reduction.

Care must be taken to avoid any break in the skin that would allow bacteria to enter the tissue. If the etiology is due to a lymphatic filarial parasite, then patients are treated with an antifilarial medication (Diemert, 2020). If the patient is returning to endemic areas, then repeated treatments may be attempted. Antibiotics used to be prescribed frequently for prophylaxis because chronic infections were common in some individuals. They are very selectively prescribed now because of the rise in antibiotic-resistant infections. Patients need support and must be taught that lymphedema requires lifelong vigilance. The patient needs to learn about the condition and how to manage it (Box 17-9). The nurse provides access to resources available, both in the local area and credible online references. Certified therapists are located by accessing http://www.lymphnet.org.

Pharmacologic Therapy

In the past, the diuretic, furosemide was prescribed as initial therapy to prevent fluid overload while the extracellular fluid was mobilized. However, diuretics should be *avoided* since they have not been found to be effective in removing proteins from lymphedematous quadrants and may promote the development of volume depletion (Ferri, 2022; Jameson et al., 2020). No pharmacologic therapy has been shown to be beneficial in the treatment of lymphedema. It is important that the patient maintains proper moisturized skin care with the use of diuretics.

BOX 17-9 Patient Education for Lymphedema

- Keep skin clean and dry.
- Wear compression support garments as prescribed.
- Avoid blood pressure cuffs, needle sticks, injections, or procedures on the affected limb.
- Report new swelling, redness, pain, heat, rash, blisters, or fever to the provider/nurse.
- Avoid tight clothing.
- Check feet with a mirror for sores, rashes, or cracks in the skin.
- Avoid trauma: Pet scratches, insect bites, burns, sports injuries, bruising.
- Clean cuts or insect bites with soap and water and apply antibiotic ointment.
- Elevate the affected limb whenever possible.

Exercise and Compression

Active and passive exercises assist in moving lymphatic fluid into the bloodstream. External compression devices move the fluid proximally from the foot to the hip or from the hand to the axilla. When the patient is ambulatory and the limb is reduced to an acceptable size, custom-fitted elastic compression stockings or sleeves are placed; those with the highest compression strength, 30 to 40 mm Hg, may be required. When the leg is affected, continuous bed rest with the leg elevated for a limited time may aid in mobilizing the fluids. *Manual lymphatic drainage* is a highly specialized massage technique designed to direct or shift the congested lymph through functioning lymphatics with preserved drainage capacity. *Manual lymphatic drainage* used in combination with compression bandages, exercises, skin care, pressure gradient sleeves, and, sometimes, pneumatic pumps, depending on the severity and stage of the lymphedema. If the patient is in the hospital and in bed, there may be a reduction of the size of the limb in 24 hours. In this case, a compression garment is placed to maintain the reduction. If the patient is at home, it is impractical to expect a 24-hour bed rest; therefore, the patient may be advised to sit with the legs elevated for 20 minutes three to four times a day. The nurse recognizes there are complications associated with prolonged bed rest, so the plan must be individualized for each person and agreed upon between the patient and the practitioner.

Surgical Management

Surgery is performed if the edema is severe and uncontrolled by medical therapy, if mobility is severely compromised, or if infection persists. One surgical approach involves the excision of the affected subcutaneous tissue and fascia, followed by skin grafting to cover the defect. Copious amounts of lymphatic fluid may make skin grafts nonadherent. Another procedure involves the surgical relocation of superficial lymphatic vessels into the deep lymphatic system by means of a buried dermal flap to provide a conduit for lymphatic drainage. This procedure has had limited success. Surgery is rarely performed in these patients in most hospitals. Patients who would benefit from surgery must be referred to specialized centers.

Nursing Management

After surgery, the management of skin grafts and flaps is the same as when these therapies are used for other conditions. Antibiotics are prescribed. Constant elevation of the affected extremity and observation for complications is essential. Complications may include flap necrosis, hematoma or abscess under the flap, and cellulitis. The nurse instructs the patient or caregiver to inspect the dressing daily. Unusual drainage or any inflammation around the wound margin suggests infection and should be reported to the surgeon. The patient is informed that there may be a loss of sensation in the skin graft area. The patient is also instructed to avoid the application of heating pads or exposure to the sun to prevent burns or trauma to the area. The patient is taught to inspect the skin for evidence of infection.

CELLULITIS

Cellulitis is the most common infection of the skin and subcutaneous tissue that causes limb swelling. Cellulitis occurs as a single isolated event or a series of recurrent events. It is often misdiagnosed, usually as recurrent thrombophlebitis or chronic venous insufficiency. It occurs when an entry point through normal skin barriers allows bacteria to enter. Cellulitis occurs most frequently in patients with DM, those who are immunosuppressed, and in patients with venous and lymphatic compromise (Ferri, 2022). It is also diagnosed in otherwise healthy tissue.

Pathophysiology

Cellulitis occurs when there is an entry point through the normal skin barrier. This allows bacteria to enter the subcutaneous tissue.

Clinical Manifestations and Assessment

The acute onset of swelling, localized redness, and pain is frequently associated with systemic signs of fever, chills, and sweating. The redness may not be uniform and often skips areas. Dimpling in the skin is seen when the edema surrounds hair follicles. Regional lymph nodes may also be tender and enlarged.

Medical Management

Mild cases of cellulitis are treated on an outpatient basis with oral antibiotic therapy. If the cellulitis is severe, the patient is treated with IV antibiotics. The key to preventing recurrent episodes of cellulitis is directed in adequate antibiotic therapy for the initial event and in identifying the site of bacterial entry. The most commonly overlooked areas are the cracks and fissures that occur in the skin between the toes. Other possible locations are drug-use injection sites, contusions, abrasions, ulcerations, ingrown toenails, and hangnails.

Nursing Management

The patient is instructed to elevate the affected area above heart level and apply warm, moist packs to the site. Patients with sensory and circulatory deficits, such as those caused by DM and paralysis, should use caution when applying warm packs because burns may occur; it is advisable to use a thermometer or have a caregiver ensure that the temperature is not more than lukewarm. Patient education should focus on preventing recurrent episodes. The patient with PVD or DM should receive education or reinforcement about skin and foot care.

Clinical Judgment Case

A 67-year-old patient was discharged home 5 days ago after an open reduction and internal fixation (ORIF) of a left femur fracture and now presents to the Emergency Room (ER) with complaints of swelling of the left lower extremity (LLE). Medical history includes hypertension, chronic bronchitis, current cigarette smoker with a 30-pack year smoking history (1pack per day [PPD] × 30 years), type 2 diabetes, and recent COVID-19 infection; home medications include hydrochlorothiazide, metformin, albuterol and aspirin (as an anticoagulant after orthopedic surgery). The patient also informs you that the prescribed pain medication (patient cannot recall the discharge medication name) causes nausea, so the patient has been taking ibuprofen 400 mg every 4–6 hours for the past 2 days for pain. The patient's body mass index is >35 kg/m^2, skin is warm and dry with delayed skin turgor, dry mucous membranes, and vital signs are as follows: 99.8°F, HR 92 and regular, 20 RR with an oxygen saturation of 96% on room air and the blood pressure is 122/78 mm Hg. Heart sounds are S1, S2 without murmur, gallop or rub; neck veins are flat; scattered rhonchi are noted on pulmonary exam, cough is nonproductive, abdomen is soft, nondistended and nontender, bowel sounds are present in all 4 quadrants, + flatus, no BM today. There is pedal edema of LLE extending to the hip (nonpitting), capillary refill is 2 seconds and dorsalis pedis and posterior tibial pulses are 2+ to 3+ bil. There is no erythema of the LLE, but the LLE is warm to touch, left hip dressing is intact, and the patient is complaining of "fullness" of the LLE.

Step One: Recognize cues where relevant and important information is identified from different sources, such as medical history or vital signs

Answer: Post-op day (POD) 5 after ORIF left femur fracture; medical history of hypertension, chronic bronchitis, current smoker, 30-pack year smoking history, type 2 diabetes, and recent COVID-19 infection. In addition, the patient's BMI > 35 kg/m^2, delayed skin turgor, dry mucous membranes, scattered rhonchi, and nonproductive cough on pulmonary exam are concerning. Significant vital signs include low-grade temperature of 99.8°F, pedal edema extending to the hip (nonpitting), warmth and feeling of "fullness" of LLE. Left hip dressing intact. Nausea from pain medication (cannot recall the medication name); patient has been taking ibuprofen 400 mg every 4–6 hours for pain.

Step Two: Analyze cues, which is organizing and linking the recognized cues to the patient's clinical presentation.

Answer: You have clustered the patients BMI, post-op day 5 from ORIF left femur fracture, current smoker, post COVID-19 infection (associated with hypercoagulability) as risk factors for DVT, and the signs and symptoms of edema, warmth and fullness of the LLE, and low-grade temperature to be associated with DVT; you have clustered dry mucous membranes, delayed skin turgor, flat neck veins, and low-grade temp with fluid volume deficit. You also cluster the low-grade temperature with rhonchi and nonproductive cough and are concerned about the potential of atelectasis versus pulmonary infection (given extensive smoking history). In addition, you consider UTI as potential cause of the low-grade temperature if the patient was catheterized during the ORIF procedure. You also recognize that asymmetry of the limbs could be associated with the surgical procedure itself (there is no erythema, tenderness, or superficial veins).

Step Three: Prioritize hypotheses, where hypotheses are evaluated and ranked according to priority. This can include urgency, likelihood, risk, difficulty, and/or time. In this phase you cluster your findings, to arrive at a list of problems (actual and or potential problems) you believe the patient is experiencing and determine the importance or urgency. What do you think is of greatest concern?

Answer: You prioritize evaluation for DVT since you are aware that a DVT is significant risk factor for pulmonary emboli. You are also concerned about potential fluid-volume deficit, etiology of the low-grade temperature, and discharge medication plan (patient self-medicating with NSAID in the event a DVT is present).

Step Four: Generate solutions, which are identifying expected outcomes and using hypotheses to define a set of interventions for the expected outcomes.

Answer: You are aware that DVT commonly occurs at least 2–5 days after surgery, and this is POD 5 from left femur fracture ORIF. In addition, you know that hypercoagulation is associated with COVID-19, and the recent major surgery, a BMI >35 kg/m^2, and older individuals are all risk factors for DVT. Although you note asymmetry of the lower extremities you will want to measure the circumference of the extremities 10 cm below the tibial tuberosity since you are aware that a difference in circumference of the calves of 3 cm or more is suspicious for a DVT. You are also aware that ibuprofen, which is a nonsteroidal anti-inflammatory drug (NSAID) provides analgesia, but might increase the risk of venous thromboembolism (VTE). You anticipate a chest film and urine specimen may be part of the screening tests pursued.

Step Five: Take action, where the solutions that address the highest priorities are implemented.

Answer: You ask the patient about other symptoms of a UTI such as dysuria, frequency, urgency, nocturia, and incontinence. You also ask the patient about their ambulation at home since you are aware the risk for DVT increases in patients unable or reluctant to ambulate. You compare the patient's lower extremities using 10 cm below the tibial tuberosity to ensure measuring at the same level and note there is asymmetry—the LLE is 4 cm larger than the RLE which you suspect is a potential DVT. You notify the ER provider of your findings, and a D-dimer level and compression ultrasonography are ordered as well as a CBC, coagulation studies, electrolytes, BUN/Cr, glucose, urinalysis, and chest x-ray. You will closely monitor for signs of PE and report immediately any chest pain, dyspnea, hemoptysis, or tachypnea. You apply external pneumatic compression device to the right lower extremity and start an IV in case emergency fluids and medications are required. You repeat the vital signs and reassess the limb.

Step Six: Evaluate outcomes, which is comparing observed outcomes against expected outcomes.

Answer: The ultrasonography is negative for DVT. The D-dimer is elevated; however, the recent surgery can be responsible for this finding. The urinalysis and chest film are negative. The orthopedic surgeon visits the patient in the ER and is confident there is no DVT and that the LLE edema is expected postoperatively. The surgical dressing is changed and there is no evidence of a surgical site infection. The patient is to be discharged home; however, blood work revealed hemoconcentration (the sodium, BUN, and Hct are elevated slightly above normal) and the patient was educated on the importance of increasing fluid intake. You also took the time to re-educate the patient on the importance of leg exercises, early ambulation, avoiding prolonged periods of inactivity or sitting for extended periods of time and sitting with knees bent or crossed for long periods. The patient is to be maintained on aspirin for a minimum of 30 days and the patient was educated not to take ibuprofen since both medications are NSAIDs, and instead acetaminophen should be used for pain. This is one of those situations where the patient did not suffer a complication but this case should impress on you the importance of all members of the health care team educating the patient about expectations once they are discharged home. Without proper patient education, it is difficult for patients to understand and manage their care, and nurses are well placed to deliver this education.

CHAPTER REVIEW

NCLEX-Style Review Questions

1. The nurse is caring for a patient diagnosed with peripheral arterial disease. Based on assessment, which clinical manifestation would be consistent with acute arterial occlusion? Select all that apply.
   a. Pallor
   b. Paresthesia
   c. Hyperthermia
   d. Poikilothermia
   e. Loss of toe hairs

2. A new postsurgical patient has been prescribed unfractionated heparin to prevent DVT. What is a true statement regarding the use of heparin? Select all that apply.
   a. Heparin has a half-life of approximately 60 minutes.
   b. Therapeutic PT level is 1.5 to 2.5 times the baseline control.
   c. Vitamin K interferes with the action of heparin.
   d. Heparin is administered by gravity drip.
   f. Therapeutic aPTT level is 1.5 to 2.5 times the baseline control.

3. The nurse is using a hydrocolloid dressing for a patient who is undergoing autolytic debridement of a necrotic venous ulcer. What is characteristic of this type of debridement? Select all that apply.
   a. Accomplished by applying enzymatic ointment to the lesion
   b. Left in place for 3 to 7 days
   c. The fastest method of debridement
   d. Accomplished by applying saline impregnated gauze to the ulcer
   f. Assists with the removal of necrotic tissue while preserving viable tissue

4. Which of the following findings are associated with a possible DVT? Select all that apply.
   a. Calf tenderness
   b. Unilateral limb edema
   c. 1+ pedal pulse
   d. Cool limb
   e. Atrophy of the limb

5. Which characteristic is consistent with an arterial ulcer? Select all that apply.

a. Pink or beefy red appearance with granulation tissue
b. May have severe edema
c. Darkened color tissue in gaiter area
d. Pale and cool extremity
e. Pale wound base

REFERENCES AND SELECTED READINGS

References and selected readings associated with this chapter can be found on the website that accompanies the book. Visit **http://thepoint.lww.com/Honan3e** to access the references and other additional resources associated with this chapter.

UNIT FIVE

Problems Related to Hematologic Function

A 65-year-old individual has been diagnosed with chronic myeloid leukemia (CML). The patient is complaining of fatigue, a 10-lb weight loss in the past month, and anxiety about starting chemotherapy.

- **What is the only curative treatment for CML?**
- **Discuss the three phases of the disease.**
- **Discuss important nursing considerations of the patient undergoing treatment for CML (imatinib).**

CHAPTER 18

Nursing Assessment: Hematologic Function

Kristen V. Roche

Learning Objectives

After reading this chapter, you will be able to:

1. Describe the structure and function of the hematologic system.
2. Describe the process of hematopoiesis.
3. Differentiate types of blood cells and their function.
4. Describe the processes involved in maintaining hemostasis.
5. Differentiate between normal and abnormal hematologic laboratory values.
6. Describe the pertinent components of nursing assessment based on abnormal hematologic laboratory values.
7. Describe the procedure and patient preparation for a bone marrow biopsy.

Unlike many other body systems, the hematologic system truly encompasses the entire human body. Patients with hematologic disorders often have significant abnormalities in blood tests but few or no symptoms. Therefore, the nurse must have an understanding of the pathophysiology of the patient's condition and the ability to make a thorough assessment that relies heavily on the interpretation of laboratory tests. It is equally important for the nurse to anticipate potential patient needs and to target nursing interventions accordingly. A basic appreciation of blood cells and bone marrow function is critical to the understanding of hematologic diseases.

ANATOMY AND PHYSIOLOGY OVERVIEW

The hematologic system consists of the blood and the sites where blood is produced, including the bone marrow and the **reticuloendothelial system** (RES). Blood is a specialized organ that differs from other organs in that it exists in a fluid state. Blood is composed of plasma and various types of cells. **Plasma** is the fluid portion of blood; it is thin and colorless and contains various proteins, such as albumin, globulin, **fibrinogen**, and other factors necessary for clotting, as well as electrolytes, waste products, and nutrients. Approximately 55% of blood volume is plasma, and 45% consists of various cellular components.

Blood

The cellular component of blood consists of three primary cell types (Table 18-1): **erythrocytes** (**red blood cells [RBCs]**), **leukocytes** (**white blood cells [WBCs]**), and **thrombocytes** (**platelets**). As noted above, these cellular components of blood normally make up approximately 45% of the blood volume. Because most blood cells have a short lifespan, the need for the body to replenish its supply of cells is continuous; this process is termed **hematopoiesis** (the formation and production of blood cells). RBCs generally live for 120 days, WBCs live from days to years depending on the type, and platelets live for 7 to 10 days. Hematopoiesis usually occurs in the bone marrow in adults, and when it takes place in sites outside of the bone marrow, it is termed *extramedullary hematopoiesis*. These sites are usually found in organs that are vigorously involved in fetal hematopoiesis, including the liver, spleen, and lymph nodes (Kapatia et al., 2019).

Under normal conditions, adult bone marrow produces approximately 175 billion erythrocytes, 70 billion **neutrophils** (a mature type of WBC), and 175 billion platelets each day. When a body requires more blood cells due to an infection (when neutrophils are needed to fight the invading pathogen) or while bleeding (when more RBCs and platelets are needed), the marrow increases its production of the cells required. Thus, under normal conditions, the marrow responds to increased demand and releases adequate numbers of cells into the circulation.

TABLE 18-1 **Blood Cells**

Cell Type	Major Function
WBC (Leukocyte)	Fights infection
Neutrophil	Essential in preventing or limiting bacterial infection via phagocytosis
Monocyte	Enters tissue as macrophage; highly phagocytic, especially against fungus
Eosinophil	Involved in allergic reactions (neutralizes histamine); digests foreign proteins
Basophil	Contains histamine; integral part of hypersensitivity reactions
Lymphocyte	Integral component of immune system
T lymphocyte	Responsible for cell-mediated immunity; recognizes material as "foreign"
B lymphocyte	Responsible for humoral immunity; many mature into plasma cells to form antibodies
Plasma cell	Secretes immunoglobulin (Ig, antibody); most mature form of B lymphocyte
RBC (Erythrocyte)	Carries hemoglobin to provide oxygen to tissues; average lifespan is 120 days
Platelet (Thrombocyte)	Fragment of megakaryocyte; provides basis for coagulation to occur; maintains hemostasis; average lifespan is 7 days

Blood makes up approximately 7% to 10% of the normal body weight and amounts to 5 to 6 L of volume. Blood circulates through the vascular system carrying oxygen and nutrients to the various cells throughout the body to promote cell growth and function. Blood also carries proteins such as hormones, antibodies, and other substances to their sites of action or use. In addition, blood carries waste products produced by cellular metabolism to the lungs, skin, liver, and kidneys for elimination.

To prevent blood loss following trauma or injury, an intricate clotting mechanism is activated to seal any leak in the blood vessels. Excessive clotting is equally as dangerous as excessive blood loss because it can obstruct blood flow to vital tissues. To prevent this, the body has a fibrinolytic (clot-disrupting) mechanism that eventually dissolves clots (**thrombi**) formed within blood vessels. The balance between these two systems, clot formation and clot dissolution, or **fibrinolysis**, is called **hemostasis**.

Bone Marrow

The bone marrow is the site of hematopoiesis, or blood cell formation (Fig. 18-1). In children, blood formation involves all skeletal bones, but with aging, marrow activity is usually limited to the pelvis, ribs, vertebrae, and sternum.

Marrow, which accounts for up to 4% to 5% of total body weight, consists of islands of cellular components (red marrow) separated by fat (yellow marrow). As the adult ages, the proportion of active marrow is gradually replaced by fat; however, in the healthy person, the fat can again be replaced by active marrow when more blood cell production is required. In adults with disease that causes marrow destruction, fibrosis, or scarring, the liver and spleen can also resume production of blood cells.

The marrow is highly vascular. Within it are primitive cells called **stem cells**, which can self-replicate, thereby ensuring a continuous supply of stem cells throughout the life cycle. When stimulated, stem cells can begin a process of **differentiation** into either **myeloid** or **lymphoid** stem cells. Lymphoid stem cells produce either T or B **lymphocytes**, whereas myeloid stem cells differentiate into three broad cell types: erythrocytes, leukocytes, and platelets. With the exception of lymphocytes, all blood cells are derived from myeloid

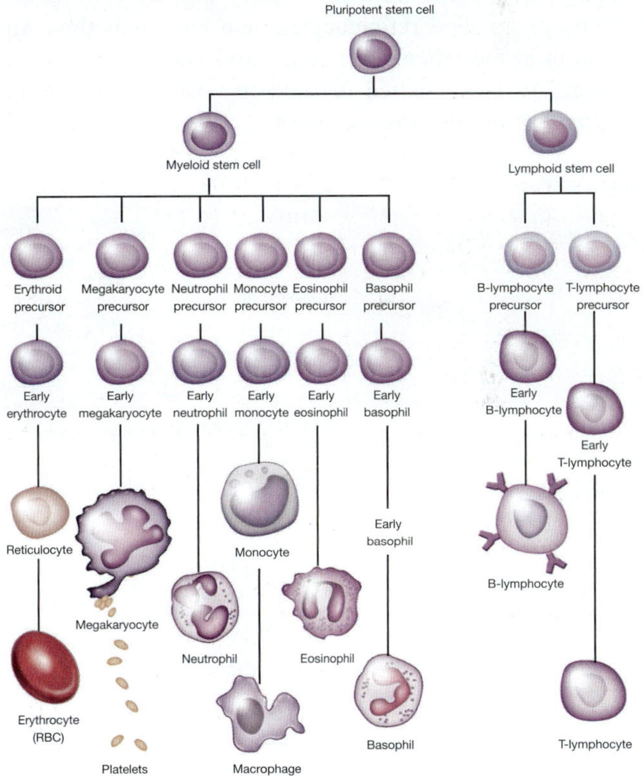

FIGURE 18-1 Hematopoiesis. Uncommitted (pluripotent) stem cells can differentiate into myeloid or lymphoid stem cells. These stem cells then undergo a complex process of differentiation and maturation into normal cells that are released into the circulation. The myeloid stem cell is responsible not only for all nonlymphoid white blood cells (WBCs) but also for the production of red blood cells (RBCs) and platelets. Each step of the differentiation process depends in part on the presence of specific growth factors for each cell type. When the stem cells are dysfunctional, they may respond inadequately to the need for more cells, or they may respond excessively, sometimes uncontrollably, as in leukemia.

stem cells. A defect in a myeloid stem cell can cause problems with erythrocyte, leukocyte, and platelet production. Many complex mechanisms are involved in hematopoiesis, most at the molecular level.

Erythrocytes (Red Blood Cells)

The normal erythrocyte has a biconcave disk shape (Fig. 18-2). It has a diameter of approximately 8 μm and is so flexible that it can pass easily through capillaries that may be as small as 2.8 μm in diameter. The membrane of the red cell is very thin so that gases, such as oxygen and carbon dioxide, can easily diffuse across it; the disk shape provides a large surface area that facilitates the absorption and release of oxygen molecules.

Mature erythrocytes consist primarily of **hemoglobin (Hgb)**, which contains iron and makes up 95% of the cell mass. Mature erythrocytes have no nuclei, and they have many fewer metabolic enzymes than do most other cells. The presence of a large amount of Hgb enables the red cell to perform its principal function of oxygen transport. Occasionally, the marrow releases slightly immature forms of erythrocytes, called **reticulocytes**, into the circulation. An elevation in the reticulocyte count may occur as a normal response to an increased demand for erythrocytes (as in bleeding) or in some disease states.

The oxygen-carrying Hgb molecule is made up of four subunits, each containing a heme portion attached to a globin chain. Iron is present in the heme component of the molecule. An important property of heme is its ability to bind to oxygen loosely and reversibly. Oxygen readily binds to Hgb in the lungs and is carried as **oxyhemoglobin** in arterial blood. Oxyhemoglobin is a brighter red than Hgb; Hgb that contains lesser amounts of oxygen (reduced Hgb) is darker; this is why arterial blood is a brighter red than venous blood. The oxygen readily dissociates (detaches) from Hgb in the tissues, where the oxygen is needed for cellular metabolism. In venous blood, Hgb combines with hydrogen ions produced by cellular metabolism and thus buffers excessive acid. Whole blood normally contains approximately 15 g of Hgb per 100 mL of blood.

Erythropoiesis

Erythroblasts arise from the primitive myeloid stem cells in bone marrow. The erythroblast is an immature nucleated cell that accumulates Hgb and then gradually loses its nucleus. At this stage, the cell is known as a *reticulocyte*. Further maturation into an erythrocyte entails the loss of the dark-staining material within the cell and slight shrinkage. Then the mature erythrocyte is released into the circulation.

Differentiation of the primitive myeloid stem cell of the marrow into an erythroblast is stimulated by **erythropoietin**,

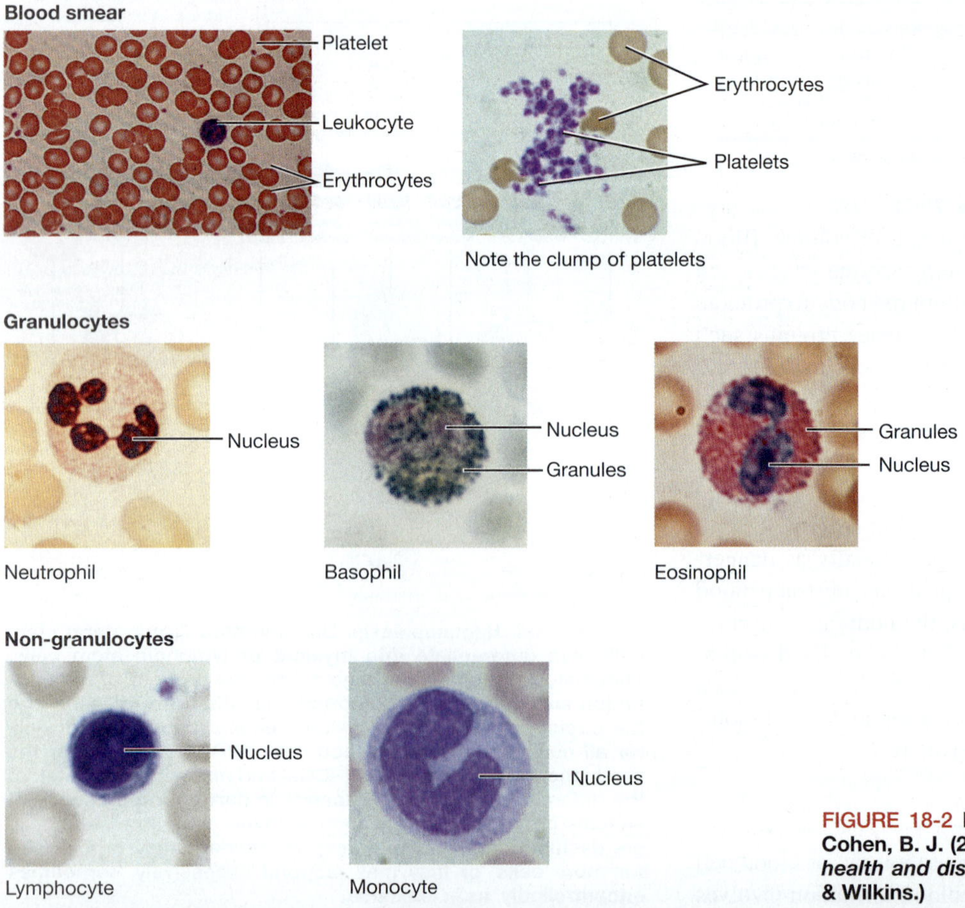

FIGURE 18-2 Normal types of blood cells. (From Cohen, B. J. (2016). *Memmler's the human body in health and disease* (12th ed.). Lippincott Williams & Wilkins.)

a hormone produced primarily by the kidney. If the kidney detects low levels of oxygen (as would occur in **anemia**, in which fewer red cells are available to bind to oxygen, or with people living at high altitudes), the release of erythropoietin is stimulated. The increase in erythropoietin production then stimulates the marrow to increase production of erythrocytes. The entire process typically takes 5 days.

For normal erythrocyte production, the bone marrow also requires iron, vitamin B_{12}, folic acid, pyridoxine (vitamin B_6), protein, and other factors. A deficiency in any one of these factors during erythropoiesis can result in decreased red cell production and anemia.

Iron Stores and Metabolism. The average daily diet in the United States contains 10 to 15 mg of elemental iron, but only 0.5 to 1 mg of ingested iron is normally absorbed from the small intestine daily. The rate of iron absorption is regulated by the amount of iron already stored in the body and by the rate of erythrocyte production. Additional amounts of iron, up to 2 mg daily, must be absorbed by menstruating individuals to replace that lost during menstruation. Total body iron content in the average adult is approximately 3 to 4 g. Iron utilization occurs within the mitochondria, cytoplasm, and nucleus. Iron is required in the mitochondria for synthesis of heme. Outside of its role in the mitochondria, iron acts as an essential cofactor for the activity of many enzymes. When levels exceed ferritin storage capacity, iron is stored in the form of hemosiderin, a complex of ferritin aggregates, denatured proteins, and lipids. Hemosiderin deposits are most commonly observed in macrophages (a type of WBC), particularly in the liver and spleen, sites that are important for maintaining iron homeostasis, and following hemorrhage, suggesting that its formation may be related to the breakdown of RBCs and Hgb (Brown et al., 2020).

The concentration of iron in blood is normally about 75 to 175 μg/dL (13 to 31 μmol/L) for males and 65 to 165 μg/dL (11 to 29 μmol/L) for females. With iron deficiency, bone marrow iron stores are depleted rapidly; Hgb synthesis is depressed, and the erythrocytes produced by the marrow are small and low in Hgb. This is known as *microcytic anemia* (characterized by small RBCs). Part of a standard complete blood count (CBC) includes the mean corpuscular volume (MCV), which measures the size of the RBCs. In microcytic anemia, a small (less than 82 μm^3) MCV is seen. This is the most common form of anemia, both in childhood and adulthood. Microcytic anemias are highly heterogeneous (diverse), and they may either be acquired (mostly due to iron deficiency) or inherited. Inherited forms may be present at or around birth. Of note, MCV is lower in childhood than in adulthood, and a nutritional iron deficiency may account for the appearance of congenital microcytic anemia that can be misdiagnosed as an inherited form of microcytic anemia. Inherited microcytic anemias make up a wide spectrum of conditions associated with different pathogenic mechanisms that are broadly classified into three subgroups: (1) defects in globin chains (hemoglobinopathies and thalassemias); (2) defects in heme synthesis (protoporphyrin IX deficiency); and (3) defects in iron availability or iron acquisition by the erythroid precursors (Cappellini et al., 2020). Iron deficiency in the adult can indicate that blood has been lost from the body (e.g., most commonly from bleeding in the gastrointestinal [GI] tract or heavy menstrual flow). The source of iron deficiency should be investigated promptly because iron deficiency in an adult may be a sign of bleeding in the GI tract or colon cancer.

Vitamin B_{12} and Folic Acid Metabolism. Vitamin B_{12} and folic acid are required for the synthesis of DNA in many tissues. Deficiencies of either of these vitamins have a significant impact on erythropoiesis. Both vitamin B_{12} and folic acid are derived from the diet and depend on a functioning intestinal mucosa for absorption. Vitamin B_{12} combines with intrinsic factor produced in the stomach and is absorbed in the distal ileum.

Pearls for Practice

It is important for nurses to recall that patients who have had a partial or total gastrectomy may have limited amounts of intrinsic factor; therefore, the absorption of vitamin B_{12} may be diminished, leading to anemia. The effects of either decreased absorption or decreased intake of vitamin B_{12} may not be apparent for 2 to 4 years.

Red Blood Cell Destruction

Aged erythrocytes lose their elasticity and become trapped in small blood vessels and the spleen. They are removed from the blood by the reticuloendothelial cells, particularly in the liver and the spleen. As the erythrocytes are destroyed, most of their Hgb is recycled. Some Hgb also breaks down to form bilirubin and is secreted in the bile. Most of the iron is recycled to form new Hgb molecules within the bone marrow; small amounts are lost daily in the feces and urine and monthly in the menstrual flow.

Leukocytes (White Blood Cells)

Leukocytes are divided into two general categories: granulocytes and agranulocytes. In normal blood, the total leukocyte count is 5,000 to 10,000 cells/mm^3. Of these, approximately 60% to 70% are granulocytes, and 30% to 40% are lymphocytes. Both types of leukocytes protect the body against infection and tissue injury.

Granulocytes

Granulocytes are defined by the presence of granules in the cytoplasm of the cell. Granulocytes are divided into three main subgroups (see Fig. 18-2): eosinophils, basophils, and neutrophils. **Neutrophils** are the most numerous cells of this class. Neutrophils are also called *polymorphonuclear neutrophils* (PMNs or polys) or *segmented neutrophils* (segs).

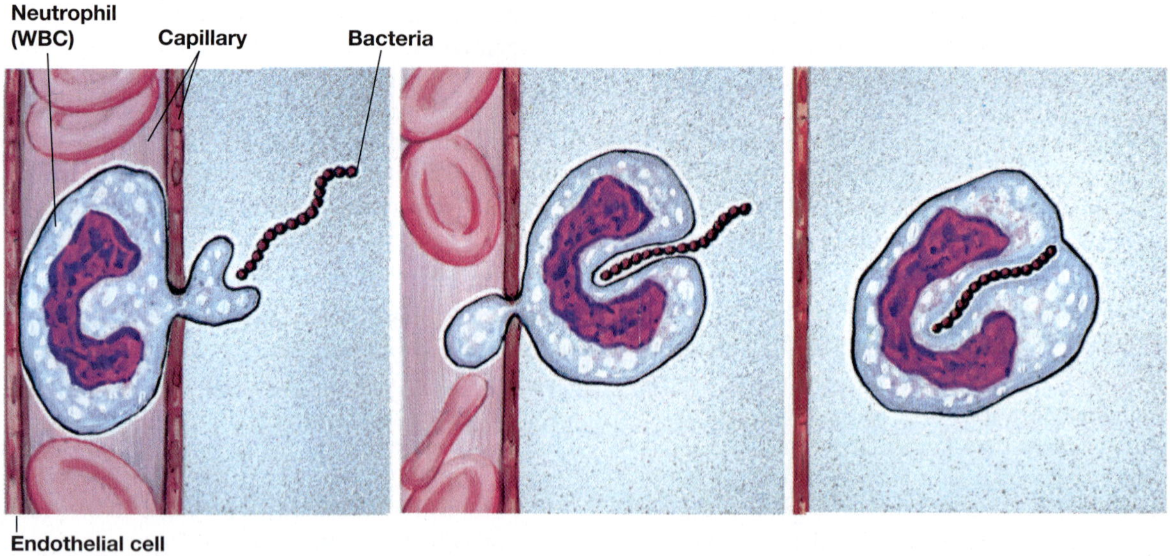

FIGURE 18-3 **Phagocytosis. In order for phagocytosis to occur, a foreign body (such as bacteria, parasites, or cellular debris) must adhere to the cell wall of the phagocyte. The phagocyte then extends around the foreign body by projecting out pseudopods, engulfing the foreign body. Once inside the phagocyte, the engulfed material is left in a vacuole, where enzymes within the cell destroy the foreign material.**

The nucleus of the mature neutrophil has multiple lobes (usually two to five), or a "segmented" nucleus. Immature neutrophils are referred to as "stabs" or "bands." The immature granulocyte has a single-lobed, elongated nucleus and is called a **band cell**. Ordinarily, band cells account for only a small percentage of circulating granulocytes, though their percentage can increase greatly under conditions in which neutrophil demand increases, such as infection. An increased number of band cells is sometimes called **bandemia**. A patient with bandemia should be evaluated thoroughly for infection.

Fully mature neutrophils result from the gradual differentiation of myeloid stem cells, specifically myeloid **blast cells**. The process, called **myelopoiesis**, takes an average of 10 days (see Fig. 18-1). Once the neutrophil is released into the circulation from the marrow, it stays there for only about 6 hours before it migrates into the body tissues to perform its function of **phagocytosis** (ingestion and digestion of bacteria and particles; Fig. 18-3). Here, neutrophils survive no more than 1 to 2 days before they die.

Eosinophils play a key role in response to parasitic and allergic diseases. The presence of certain microbes (such as parasites) results in the release of the granular contents of the eosinophil, allowing for destruction and phagocytosis of the organism.

Basophils are the least numerous of the circulating leukocytes and have characteristically large, dark-purple granules. The granules contain heparin and histamine and are released in response to exposure to allergens.

The number of circulating granulocytes found in the healthy person is relatively constant. An elevation in the total number of WBCs may indicate infection, trauma, tissue injury, or malignancy (such as leukemia), or it may be a side effect of certain medications, such as corticosteroids. A WBC count that is below normal may be related to viral infections, the result of side effects from medications such as antiviral medications, or an indication of a more serious condition, such as leukemia or myelodysplastic syndrome (MDS).

Agranulocytes

Monocytes and lymphocytes are leukocytes with granule-free cytoplasm—hence the term *agranulocyte* (see Fig. 18-2).

Monocytes. Monocytes (also called *mononuclear leukocytes*) have a single-lobed nucleus. They are the largest of the leukocytes. In normal adult blood, monocytes account for approximately 5% of the total leukocyte count. When released from the marrow, monocytes spend a short time in the circulation (approximately 24 hours) and then enter the body tissues. Within the tissues, the monocytes continue to differentiate into **macrophages**, which can survive for months. Macrophages are particularly active in the spleen, liver, peritoneum, and alveoli; they remove debris from these areas and phagocytize bacteria within the tissues (see the "Reticuloendothelial System" section).

Lymphocytes. Mature lymphocytes are small cells with scanty cytoplasms (see Fig. 18-2). Immature lymphocytes are produced in the marrow from the lymphoid stem cells. A second major source of production is the cortex of the thymus. Cells derived from the thymus are known as T lymphocytes (or T cells); those derived from the marrow can also be T cells but are more commonly B lymphocytes (or B cells). Lymphocytes complete their differentiation and maturation primarily in the lymph nodes and in the lymphoid tissue of the intestine and spleen after exposure to a specific antigen. Mature lymphocytes are the principal cells of the immune system, producing antibodies and identifying other cells and organisms as foreign.

Function of Leukocytes

Granulocytes protect the body from invasion by bacteria and other foreign entities. Neutrophils arrive at a given site within 1 hour after the onset of an inflammatory reaction and initiate phagocytosis, but they are short lived. An influx of monocytes follows; these cells continue their phagocytic activities for long periods as macrophages. This process constitutes a second line of defense for the body against inflammation and infection. Although neutrophils often can work adequately against bacteria without the help of macrophages, macrophages are particularly effective against fungi and viruses.

The primary function of lymphocytes is to produce substances that aid in attacking foreign material. T lymphocytes kill foreign cells directly or release a variety of *lymphokines*, substances that enhance the activity of phagocytic cells. T lymphocytes are responsible for delayed allergic reactions, rejection of foreign tissue (e.g., transplanted organs), and destruction of tumor cells. This process is known as *cellular immunity*. The main mechanism of the B lymphocyte response is the secretion of antibodies (immunoglobulins), which are a specialized class of circulating glycoproteins that bind antigen on pathogens or toxins with high specificity. Immunoglobulin M (IgM) is the first secreted antibody of the immune response and can be expressed by some B cells even in the absence of antigen exposure, contributing to natural *humoral immunity*. Another name for humoral immunity is "antibody-mediated immunity," and this physiologic mechanism protects the body from pathogens and foreign substances. In some cases, when the antigen is repetitive in nature, the B cell receives a strong enough signal to be activated without any T-cell help. In most cases though, B cells require help from T cells to be fully activated (Kirman & Ghittoni, 2020).

Eosinophils have a critical role in allergy and hypersensitivity reactions because they tend to participate in the late phase of allergic responses. In asthma, eosinophils in the lung contribute to airway hyperresponsiveness, mucus production, tissue damage, and airway remodeling. Basophils and mast cells contain granules of proinflammatory chemicals such as histamine. Immediately after tissue injury or during the early phase of an allergic response, these cells degranulate (release cellular content), releasing histamine, a potent mediator of vasodilation. In an allergic response, prompt antihistamine administration can counteract the action of basophils and mast cells and reduce the systemic allergic reaction (Kirman & Ghittoni, 2020).

Platelets (Thrombocytes)

Platelets, or thrombocytes, are not technically cells; rather, they are granular fragments of giant cells in the bone marrow, called *megakaryocytes*. Platelet production in the marrow is regulated in part by the hormone thrombopoietin, which stimulates the production and differentiation of megakaryocytes from the myeloid stem cell.

Platelets play an essential role in the control of bleeding (hemostasis). They circulate freely in the blood in an inactive state, where they nurture the endothelium of the blood vessels, maintaining the integrity of the vessel. When vascular injury occurs, platelets collect at the site and are activated. They adhere to the site of injury and to each other, forming a platelet plug that temporarily stops bleeding. Substances released from platelet granules activate coagulation factors in the blood plasma and initiate the formation of a stable clot composed of **fibrin**, a filamentous protein.

Plasma and Plasma Proteins

After cellular elements are removed from blood, the remaining liquid portion is called *plasma*. More than 90% of plasma is water. The remainder consists primarily of plasma proteins, clotting factors (particularly fibrinogen), and small amounts of other substances such as nutrients, enzymes, waste products, and gases. If plasma is allowed to clot, the remaining fluid is called **serum**. Serum has essentially the same composition as plasma, except that fibrinogen and several clotting factors have been removed in the clotting process.

Plasma proteins consist primarily of albumin and the globulins. The globulins can be separated into three main fractions (alpha, beta, and gamma), each of which consists of distinct proteins that have different functions. Important proteins in the alpha and beta fractions are the transport globulins and the clotting factors that are made in the liver. The transport globulins carry various substances in bound form in the circulation. For example, thyroid-binding globulin carries thyroxin, and transferrin carries iron. The clotting factors, including fibrinogen, remain in an inactive form in the blood plasma until activated by the clotting cascade. The gamma globulin fraction refers to the immunoglobulins, or antibodies. These proteins are produced by the well-differentiated lymphocytes and plasma cells. The actual fractionation of the globulins can be measured on a specific laboratory test (serum protein electrophoresis, or SPEP).

Albumin is particularly important for the maintenance of fluid balance within the vascular system. Capillary walls are impermeable to albumin, so its presence in the plasma creates an osmotic force that keeps fluid within the vascular space. Albumin, which is produced by the liver, has the capacity to bind to several substances that are transported in plasma (e.g., certain medications, calcium, bilirubin, and some hormones). People with poor liver function may have low concentrations of albumin with a resultant decrease in osmotic pressure and the development of edema.

Reticuloendothelial System

The RES (also called the *mononuclear phagocytic system*) is a system of phagocytic cells, including monocytes and macrophages. The RES is divided into the primary and secondary lymphoid systems. The primary lymphoid system is the site of RES cell production and includes the bone marrow and thymus. The secondary lymphoid system is the site of RES cell function and includes the liver, spleen, and lymph nodes. In the liver, spleen, lymph nodes, and other areas throughout the body, these cells function to recognize foreign cells and trigger an immune response.

The spleen has multiple functions, including recycling of iron, pooling of platelets, and blood volume regulation. It also acts as a filter for bacteria. In addition, the spleen is a major source of fetal hematopoiesis. It can resume hematopoiesis later in adulthood if necessary, particularly when marrow function is compromised (e.g., in bone marrow fibrosis, also known as myelofibrosis).

Hemostasis

Hemostasis refers to prevention of blood loss from intact vessels as well as the termination of bleeding when blood vessels are damaged. The prevention of blood loss from intact vessels requires adequate numbers of functional platelets. Platelets nurture the endothelium and thereby maintain the structural integrity of the vessel wall. Two processes are involved in arresting bleeding: primary hemostasis and secondary hemostasis (Fig. 18-4).

Primary hemostasis is an aggregation of platelets forming a plug at the damaged side of exposed endothelial cells (Chaudhry & Babiker, 2019). Damage to the blood vessel exposes collagen, which reacts with and binds to a large protein complex known as von Willebrand factor (vWf) (DeLoughery, 2019). The vWf attaches to the platelet receptor glycoprotein (GPIb); this binding leads to physiologic changes called platelet activation. In addition, vWf carries factor VIII to the vessel, which assists in fibrin clot formation (DeLoughery, 2019).

For the coagulation process to be activated correctly, circulating inactive coagulation factors must be converted to active forms. This process occurs on the surface of the aggregated platelets at the site of vessel injury. Secondary hemostasis includes the two main coagulation pathways, intrinsic and extrinsic, that meet up at a point to form the common pathway. Clotting by the intrinsic pathway is activated when the collagen that lines blood vessels is exposed. As with the extrinsic pathway, clotting factors are activated sequentially until fibrin is ultimately formed. These fibrin subunits have an affinity for each other and combine into fibrin strands that bond the platelets together, stabilizing the platelet plug (Chaudhry & Babiker, 2019).

As the injured vessel is repaired and again covered with endothelial cells, the fibrin clot is no longer needed. The fibrin is digested via two systems: the plasma fibrinolytic system and the cellular fibrinolytic system. The substance **plasminogen** is required to lyse (break down) the fibrin. Plasminogen, which is present in all body fluids, circulates with fibrinogen and is incorporated into the fibrin clot as it forms. When the clot is no longer needed (e.g., after an injured blood vessel has healed), the plasminogen is activated to form plasmin. Plasmin digests the fibrinogen and fibrin. The byproducts of clot digestion, called *fibrin degradation products*, are released into the circulation. Through this system, clots are dissolved as tissue is repaired, and the vascular system returns to its normal baseline state.

Gerontologic Considerations

In older adult patients, the bone marrow's ability to respond to the body's need for blood cells (erythrocytes, leukocytes, and platelets) may be decreased. This decreased ability is a result of many factors, including diminished production of the growth factors necessary for hematopoiesis by stromal cells (cells that can differentiate) within the marrow or a diminished response to growth factors (in the case of erythropoietin). In addition, in older adult patients, the bone marrow may be more susceptible to the myelosuppressive effects of medications. As a result of these factors, when an older person needs more blood cells (e.g., leukocytes in infection, erythrocytes in anemia), the bone marrow may not be able to increase production of these cells adequately. **Leukopenia** (a decreased number of circulating leukocytes), thrombocytopenia (a decrease in the platelet count), and/or anemia can result.

Anemia is the most common hematologic condition affecting older patients; with each successive decade of life, the incidence of anemia increases. Anemia frequently results from iron deficiency (in the case of blood loss) or from a nutritional deficiency, particularly folate or vitamin B_{12} deficiency or protein–calorie malnutrition; it may also result from inflammation, chronic disease such as an underlying malignancy, or alcohol use disorder. Management of the disorder varies, depending on the etiology. Therefore, it is important to identify the cause of the anemia rather than to consider it an inevitable consequence of aging. Older people with concurrent cardiac or pulmonary problems may not tolerate anemia well, and a prompt, thorough evaluation is always warranted.

ASSESSMENT AND DIAGNOSTIC EVALUATION

Most hematologic diseases reflect a defect in the hematopoietic or hemostatic systems, or in the RES. The defect can be quantitative (e.g., increased or decreased production of cells), qualitative (e.g., the cells that are produced are not functioning normally), or both.

Many hematologic conditions lack symptoms initially. Therefore, an extensive history and laboratory tests are used to determine a diagnosis. For many hematologic conditions, continued monitoring of laboratory results over time is essential to establish trends. Trends help establish the acuity of the condition, and they facilitate evaluation of the response to interventions.

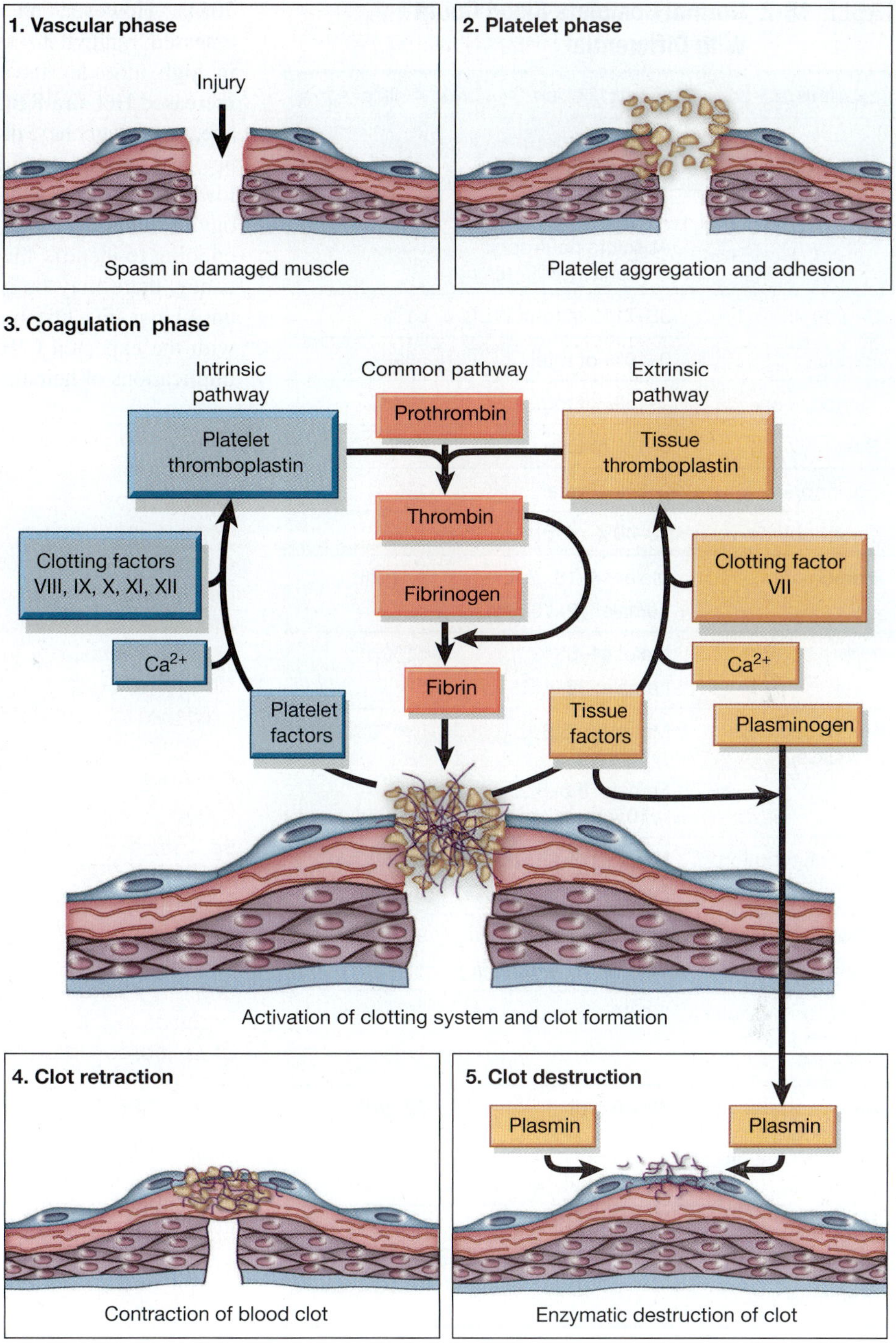

FIGURE 18-4 **Hemostasis. When the endothelial surface of a blood vessel is injured, several processes occur. In primary hemostasis, platelets within the circulation are attracted to the exposed layer of collagen at the site of injury. They adhere to the site of injury, releasing factors that stimulate other platelets to aggregate at the site, forming an unstable platelet plug. In secondary hemostasis, based on the type of stimulus, one of two clotting pathways is initiated—the intrinsic or extrinsic pathway—and the clotting factors within that pathway are activated. The end result from either pathway is the conversion of prothrombin to thrombin. Thrombin is necessary for fibrinogen to be converted into fibrin, the stabilizing protein that anchors the fragile platelet plug to the site of injury to prevent further bleeding and permit the injured vessel or site to heal. (Modified from www.irving-crowley.com/cls/clotting.gif.)**

Hematologic Studies

The most common tests used to assess bone marrow function are the CBC and the peripheral blood smear (PBS). Blood for both the CBC and PBS is typically obtained by venipuncture. The CBC measures the total number of blood cells (leukocytes, erythrocytes, and platelets) as well as the Hgb, **hematocrit** (Hct) (percentage of blood volume consisting of erythrocytes), and RBC indices (Table 18-2). Because cellular morphology (shape and appearance of the cells) is particularly important in most hematologic disorders, the blood cells involved must be examined. This process is referred to as the *manual examination of the peripheral smear*. In this test, a drop of blood is spread on a glass slide, stained, and examined under a microscope. Visualizing the shape and size of the leukocytes, erythrocytes, and platelets provides useful information in identifying hematologic conditions. Increases or decreases in any one parameter of the

TABLE 18-2 Normal Complete Blood Count With Differential

Example: 42-Year-Old White[a] Patient Assigned Male at Birth		
Tests	**Normal Reference Range**	**Case Example**
WBC	5,000–10,000/μL Absolute neutrophil count >1,800/μL	5,300/μL
Segments	38–71% of total WBC	61%
Bands	0–10% of total	5%
Monocytes	2–15% of total	11%
Basophils	0–1% of total	0%
Eosinophils	0–5% of total	1%
Lymphocytes	20–40% of total	22%
Hemoglobin	Male: 14–18 g/dL Female: 12–16 g/dL	17 g/dL
Hct	Male: 41–53% Female: 36–46%	51%
Red blood cells (RBCs)	Male: 4.5–5.5 × 10^6/mm^3 Female: 3.8–5.2 × 10^6/mm^3	5 × 10^6/mm^3
RBC distribution width (%)	Male: 11.8–15.6% Female: 11.9–15.5%	12%
Mean corpuscular volume (MCV)	Male: 81–101.4 (fL) Female: 81.1–99.8 (fL)	90 fL
Mean corpuscular hemoglobin (MCH)	28–34 pg/cell	30 pg/cell
Mean corpuscular hemoglobin concentration (MCHC)	32–36 g/dL	32 g/dL
Platelets	150–400,000/mm^3	200,000/mm^3
Mean platelet volume	7.4–10.3 fL	8 fL

[a]People of African ancestry may have lower WBC, neutrophil, and platelet counts.

RBC, red blood cell; WBC, white blood cell.

Adapted from Fischbach, F. T., Fischbach, M. A., & Stout, K. (2021). *Fischbach's A manual of laboratory and diagnostic tests* (11th ed). Wolters Kluwer.

CBC may indicate a hematologic disorder and indicate the need for further testing (refer to Chapter 19).

Results of lab tests can provide valuable information regarding the overall health of the patient and the patient's response to disease and treatment (Van Leeuwen & Bladh, 2021). However, an abnormal CBC should always be assessed relative to the patient's baseline. People living in high altitudes have increased Hgb values, as well as increased Hct and RBC count. Physiologic variants such as age, sex, pregnancy, drugs, and race can also affect lab values. For example, individuals of African descent may have lower Hgb, WBC, neutrophil, and platelet counts. The etiology of this differentiation remains unknown, but research is ongoing to identify the responsible genetic variant. In pregnancy, there may be a progressive decrease in neutrophils until labor (Fischbach et al., 2021). Nurses must be familiar with the expected CBC parameters and aware of potential implications of hematologic alterations.

Pearls for Practice

A falsely elevated Hct is noted if blood is drawn from a capillary puncture and a microhematocrit is done, (Fischbach et al., 2021), or more commonly in conditions of fluid volume loss (such as dehydration). Since no single test confirms hemoconcentration, the nurse must assess for signs of fluid deficit, such as weight loss, dry mucous membranes, delayed skin turgor, orthostatic hypotension, decreased pulse pressure (the difference between the systolic and diastolic pressure), decreasing urinary output with elevated urine specific gravity, and vital sign changes (increasing heart rate and decreasing blood pressure as volume is lost). Regardless of the etiology, an Hct of greater than 60% is associated with spontaneous clotting of blood (Fischbach et al., 2021). Likewise, in times of hemodilution (i.e., fluid gain), a falsely lower Hct is noted. The nurse assesses for weight gain, moist mucous membranes, edema, hypertension, crackles in the lung fields, an S_3 gallop over the mitral area, increased urinary output with decreased specific gravity, and distended neck veins.

As noted earlier, results should be assessed relative to an individual's baseline. There is a tendency toward lower Hct values in people older than 60 years of age, corresponding to lower RBC count values in this age group (e.g., 38% to 49% in males and 34% to 45% in females) (Elsevier Patient Education, 2022). In addition, the Hct slightly decreases in the physiologic hemodilution of pregnancy, termed "hydremia." Clinically, decreased Hct values are an indicator of anemia, a condition in which there is a reduction in the packed cell volume (PCV). An Hct less than 30% means that the patient is moderately to severely anemic; an Hct of less than 20% can lead to cardiac failure and death (Fischbach et al., 2021).

Assessing the Patient With Low Hemoglobin and Hct

Patients with mildly to moderately lowered Hgb and Hct levels may be asymptomatic due to effective compensatory mechanisms. However, a careful history may uncover the following: progressive fatigue, poor activity tolerance, headaches, dizziness, irritability, difficulty sleeping or concentrating, tinnitus, anorexia, dyspnea, palpitations, chest pain, indigestion, abnormal menstruation, impotence, and loss of libido. On physical examination, pallor is the most common and obvious sign of anemia. Pallor can be most easily assessed in the oral mucous membranes, nail beds, conjunctiva, and creases of the palms. Other findings may include tachypnea, tachycardia and flow murmurs, and hypotension. Tachypnea and tachycardia may be seen with activity. Patients with hemolytic anemia may exhibit jaundice and splenomegaly.

Pearls for Practice

The nurse needs to establish each patient's baseline skin color in order to assess for changes such as pallor or cyanosis. The skin surfaces that have the least amount of pigmentation include the palms of the hands, soles of the feet, abdomen, and buttocks. The nurse observes for an underlying reddish tone; regardless of skin color, this is typical of all healthy skin (Giger & Haddad, 2021). An absence of a reddish tone may result in pallor. In addition, the nurse assesses the conjunctivae which will reflect the color changes of cyanosis or pallor.

BOX 18-1

Calculating the Absolute Neutrophil Count

Normally, the neutrophil count is greater than 2,000/mm^3. The ANC is calculated using this formula:

$$(\text{Total WBC} \times [\% \text{ segs} + \% \text{ bands}]) \div 100 = \text{ANC}$$

For example, if the total WBC count is 3,000/mm^3 with 72% neutrophils and 3% bands, the ANC would be calculated as follows:

$$3{,}000 \times [72\% + 3\%] = 225{,}000$$

$$225{,}000 \div 100 = 2{,}250/\text{mm}^3$$

This result is not indicative of neutropenia because the ANC is greater than 1,000/mm^3 despite the low total WBC count (3,000/mm^3).

Conversely, in the following example, neutropenia is evident despite a normal WBC count (5,500/mm^3) with 8% neutrophils and 0% bands:

$$5{,}500 \times (8\% + 0\%) = 440/\text{mm}^3 \text{ should be}$$
$$5{,}500 \times 8 = 44{,}000 \div 100 = 440/\text{mm}^3$$

Here, the ANC is severely low (440/mm^3) despite the normal total WBC count (5,500/mm^3).

When evaluating neutropenia, it is important to calculate the ANC and to not rely solely on the total WBCs and percentage of neutrophils alone.

Assessing the Patient With a Low White Blood Cell Count

When assessing a patient with low WBC count, the nurse must examine the WBC differential to see which type of WBC is low. The myeloid and/or lymphoid lines may be low. However, the most critical factors influencing an individual's risk for infection are the severity and duration of neutropenia. Nurses caring for a patient with a low WBC count should calculate the absolute neutrophil count (ANC; Box 18-1). Neutropenia severity is classified using the following guidelines:

- ANC of 1,500 to 1,000/mm^3 indicates mild neutropenia.
- ANC of 999 to 500/mm^3 indicates moderate neutropenia.
- ANC of less than 500/mm^3 indicates severe neutropenia.

Patients with severe neutropenia are at significantly increased risk for developing opportunistic infections and sepsis. The nurse is aware that the usual signs and symptoms of infection (e.g., erythema, pain, drainage, pyuria) are muted and therefore not usually present in the patient with severe neutropenia since the usual inflammatory findings of leukocytosis (increased WBCs) or WBCs in the urine or at the infection site depend on neutrophils. Common sites of infection leading to sepsis are the lung (64% of cases), abdominal sites (20%), the bloodstream (15%), and the genitourinary system (14%) (Tavakoli & Carannante, 2021). Thus, patients with neutropenia must be assessed carefully:

- *Skin*: Check for tenderness, erythema, edema, breaks in skin integrity, moisture, drainage, lesions (especially under breasts, axillae, groin, skin folds, bony prominences, perineum, and perirectum); check all puncture sites (e.g., IV sites) and central venous access device sites for erythema, tenderness, induration, and drainage.
- *Oral mucosa*: Check for moisture, lesions, color (check palate, tongue, buccal mucosa, gums, lips, oropharynx); assess level of pain and taste changes, which may precede objective signs of mucosal damage by 3 to 5 days.
- *Respiratory*: Check for presence of cough, sore throat, tachypnea, pain on inspiration; auscultate breath sounds. Note color, amount, and consistency of sputum.
- *Gastrointestinal*: Check for abdominal discomfort and distention by palpating the abdomen; assess for nausea, change in bowel pattern; auscultate bowel sounds.
- *Genitourinary*: Check for dysuria, urgency, frequency; check urine for color, clarity, and odor.
- *Neurologic*: Ask about headache, neck stiffness, visual disturbances; assess level of consciousness, orientation, and behavior.
- *Temperature*: Check for elevation (greater than 38°C [100.4°F]).

The nurse is aware that patients with neutropenia often do not manifest the classic signs of infection, such as pus, because pus is composed of WBCs. Signs of infection may be subtle; therefore, the presence of fever may be the only sign that the patient has an infection and should be addressed immediately.

Pearls for Practice

Bacteremia, which is the presence of bacteria in the blood, may be the only evidence of infection in a patient with neutropenia. It occurs in 10% to 25% of patients with neutropenic fever, a temperature higher than 38°C (100.4°F) for at least an hour or a single oral temperature of 38.3°C (101°F) or higher. The presence of febrile neutropenia is a medical emergency that often results in hospitalization. Recently, an epidemiologic shift has occurred, with gram-positive organisms such as Staphylococcus species now being more common than gram-negative infections such as Pseudomonas aeruginosa. Community-acquired respiratory viral infections as well as reactive viral infections such as herpes simplex and varicella zoster are common in high-risk patients with prolonged neutropenia and/or those taking long-term high-dose steroids. Invasive fungal infections, such as those caused by Candida and Aspergillus, are also more common in high-risk patients with neutropenia and should be considered in patients with persistent fevers after the first week of neutropenia (McGrath et al., 2020).

Pearls for Practice

Agranulocytosis or marked neutropenia and leukopenia place a patient at significant risk for infection. These patients are best managed by an interprofessional team that includes practitioners, nurses, and pharmacists. Nurses should provide thorough education about what signs and symptoms to monitor for and when to call the provider. Education should be provided as to when to avoid large crowds and the utilization of a face mask. Ongoing education about the importance of handwashing is also crucial (Justiz Vaillant & Zito, 2020). Refer to Chapter 5 for further discussion.

Assessing the Patient at Risk for Bleeding

Assessment of bleeding history should include asking about prior bleeding events over time, such as bleeding during infancy and childhood, or any bleeds severe enough to require surgical intervention, nasal packing, or cautery; a visit to the emergency room; or a transfusion. Additional questioning should include outcomes of bleeding events, such as severity, length of time, character of bleeding (e.g., diffuse oozing, bleeding from a specific source), and history of poor wound healing (Ma, 2021). An isolated history of easy bruising requires further questioning, as this common report lacks sensitivity and specificity and may be a sign of trauma or skin fragility rather than a true bleeding disorder (Ma, 2021).

If the individual has a menstrual history and/or has been pregnant, assess for history of menorrhagia, duration of menses, bleeding with delivery, postpartum bleeding, and early pregnancy loss (Ma, 2021). Excessive menstrual bleeding can be due to many causes (e.g., anatomic lesions, hormonal factors, impaired hemostasis). A bleeding disorder is found in as many as 10% to 30% of people who have histories of excessive menstrual bleeding (Ma, 2021).

Sites and character of bleeding may help distinguish disorders of primary hemostasis (platelet function) from secondary hemostasis (coagulation factor function). Platelet and vascular disorders are generally characterized by mucosal bleeding (e.g., of the mouth, nose, urinary tract, GI tract) (Ma, 2021). Epistaxis may be a presenting finding in von Willebrand or hereditary hemorrhagic telangiectasia. Coagulation factor disorders are generally characterized by bleeding into muscles and joints and delayed bleeding after a bleeding challenge (Ma, 2021).

A family history of bleeding should be obtained to help determine the likelihood of an inherited condition. Some individuals may be aware of a specific diagnosis from a first- or second-degree relative; others may report a family history of severe bleeding requiring medical interventions. While a positive family history increases the likelihood of an inherited bleeding disorder, lack of a family history does not eliminate the possibility. As many as 30% to 40% of individuals with hemophilia A have a *de novo* (new) germline mutation and have a negative family history (Ma, 2021).

Laboratory Tests to Assess Type of Bleeding Defect

Hemostasis and coagulation tests are generally done for patients with bleeding disorders, vascular injury or trauma, or coagulopathies. These include the CBC, PBS, prothrombin time and international normalized ratio (PT/INR), and partial thromboplastin time (PTT). PT measures the function of second-stage clotting factors, while PTT determines the overall capability of the blood to clot. Factor assays are definitive coagulation studies of a specific clotting factor (e.g., VII for hemophilia) (Fischbach et al., 2021).

A CBC and PBS are performed to assess platelet count, size, and shape. The presence of schistocytes (irregularly contracted, fragmented cells) can suggest a multitude of diagnoses, such as disseminated intravascular coagulation (DIC), thrombocytopenia purpura, and other microangiopathic anemias (Fischbach et al., 2021). These must be ruled out, as they require prompt intervention.

Pseudothrombocytopenia (PTCP), a relatively common finding in clinical laboratories, can lead to diagnostic errors, overtreatment, and further (even invasive) unnecessary testing. Clinical consequences with potential life-threatening events (e.g., unnecessary platelet transfusion, inappropriate treatment including splenectomy or corticosteroids) are still observed when PTCP is not readily detected (Lardinois et al., 2021). The incidence of PTCP is higher in patients with identified risk factors, including male sex, underlying diseases, or therapy with drugs such as low-molecular-weight heparin. New technologies such as fluorescence or optical platelet counting should be implemented in clinical

BOX 18-2

Nursing Interventions for Patients With Thrombocytopenia (Platelet Count Below 50,000/mm^3)

Prevent Complications: Implement Bleeding Precautions

- Avoid giving aspirin and aspirin-containing medications or other medications known to inhibit platelet function, like nonsteroidal anti-inflammatory drugs, if possible.
- Assess for use of herbal medications, such as *Ginkgo biloba*, which can predispose the patient to bleeding.
- Do not administer intramuscular injections.
- Do not insert indwelling catheters.
- Do not use the rectal route for taking temperatures or administering medications.
- Use stool softeners and oral laxatives to prevent constipation.
- Use the smallest possible needles when performing venipuncture.
- Apply pressure to venipuncture sites for 5 minutes or until bleeding has stopped.
- Use only soft-bristled toothbrushes for mouth care.
- Do not permit wearing of restrictive clothing; avoid tourniquets or overinflation of blood pressure cuffs.
- Lubricate lips with water-soluble lubricant every 2 hours while the patient is awake.
- Avoid suctioning if possible; if unavoidable, use only gentle suctioning.
- Discourage vigorous coughing or blowing of the nose.
- Use only an electric razor for shaving.
- Pad side rails as needed.
- Prevent falls by ambulating with the patient as necessary and keeping the environment safe.
- Teach the patient to avoid contact sports and sports with risk for falling or injury (such as biking or rollerblading).
- Teach the patient to avoid sexual intercourse (both vaginal and anal) until platelet count is over 50,000/mm^3.
- Hematest secretions and excretions for occult blood for early identification of internal bleeding.

Control Bleeding

- Apply direct pressure by compression or pinching of the lower soft cartilaginous part of the nose for 10 minutes (Ferri, 2022).
- Use manual pressure with gauze over the source of bleeding.
- For epistaxis, position the patient in a high Fowler position with the body tilted forward and the mouth open so that the blood can be spit out instead of swallowed; apply an ice pack to the bridge of the nose to cause a vasoconstrictive effect.
- Hemostatic agents such as thromboplastin, absorbable gelatin, fibrin sealants, collagen, and alginate can be used for hemostasis at wound sites and central venous access device sites that are bleeding.
- Notify the health care provider for prolonged bleeding (e.g., unable to stop within 10 minutes).
- Administer platelets, fresh-frozen plasma, and/or packed RBCs as prescribed.

Adapted from Doenges, M. E., Moorhouse, M. F., & Murr, A. C. (2019). *Nurse's pocket guide: Diagnoses, prioritized interventions, and rationales* (15th ed.). F.A. Davis Company.

laboratories, as they will provide a valuable and suitable support for correcting spuriously low platelet count. Alternative anticoagulants to ethylenediaminetetraacetic acid (EDTA) (e.g., magnesium sulfate) should now be reconsidered in blood samples when there is clear evidence of PTCP. Finally, the counting method should always be reported (Lardinois et al., 2021).

There are several congenital and acquired disorders affecting platelet number, platelet function, or both. Testing is challenging because some tests are highly operator dependent, many tests are poorly standardized and poorly reproducible, and no test is able to assay all aspects of platelet function (Ma, 2021). When platelet function testing is indicated, it is generally performed by the hematology consult and/or in specialized laboratories with expertise in their methods and interpretation (Ma, 2021). These include platelet aggregation studies, the platelet function analyzer (PFA-100), genetic testing, and electron microscopy.

Thrombocytopenia severity can be described as follows: excess bleeding that may occur as a result of injury, trauma, or surgery with a platelet count of 50,000 to 100,000/mm^3; platelet counts of 20,000/mm^3 or less increase the risk for spontaneous bleeding; and platelet counts of 10,000/mm^3 or less are associated with serious episodes of spontaneous bleeding, including intracranial hemorrhage. Bleeding precautions are recommended for patients with a platelet count of less than 50,000/mm^3. The nursing care and patient education required to safely care for patients with thrombocytopenia are outlined in Box 18-2.

PT directly measures a potential defect in stage II of the clotting mechanism (extrinsic coagulation system) through analysis of the clotting ability of five plasma coagulation factors (i.e., prothrombin, fibrinogen, factor V, factor VII, and factor X). In addition to screening for deficiency of prothrombin, PT is used to evaluate dysfibrinogenemia, the heparin effect and coumadin effect, liver failure, and vitamin K deficiency (Fischbach et al., 2021). The INR is a comparative ratio of PT ratios (Fischbach et al., 2021). This is calculated by dividing the PT by the control and then applying the International Sensitivity Index.

PTT can detect deficiencies of the intrinsic thromboplastin system and also reveal defects in the extrinsic coagulation mechanism pathway (Fischbach et al., 2021). Prolongation of both the PT and PTT may indicate a deficiency of factor I, II, V, or X. Used together, PTT and PT will detect approximately 95% of coagulation defects (Fischbach et al., 2021).

A thorough physical examination can be useful in determining the source of the hemostatic defect. Abnormalities of the vascular system give rise to local bleeding, usually into the skin. Because platelets are primarily responsible for

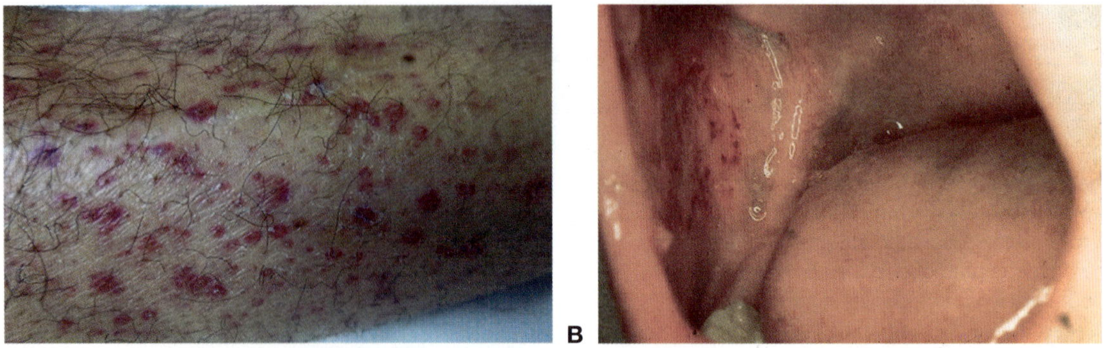

A B

FIGURE 18-5 **Petechiae of limb and oral cavity. (Reproduced with permission from Council, L. M., Sheinbein, D. M., & Cornelius, L. A. (2016).** ***The Washington manual of dermatology diagnostics.*** **Wolters Kluwer Health.)**

hemostasis in small vessels, patients with platelet defects develop petechiae (Fig. 18-5), often in clusters; these are most often seen first on the extremities and then the mucous membranes. With prolonged thrombocytopenia, petechiae may also be seen on the trunk.

Other pertinent assessment findings include ecchymoses or hematomas, conjunctival hemorrhages, bleeding gums, bleeding at puncture sites (venipuncture); hypotension, tachycardia, dizziness, epistaxis (nosebleed); respiratory distress, tachypnea, hemoptysis (coughing of blood); abdominal or back pain, hematemesis (vomiting blood), abdominal distention, rectal bleeding; vaginal or urethral bleeding; and headache, blurred vision, and mental status changes.

Pearls for Practice

Because of the risk of spontaneous intracranial bleeding, patients with very severe thrombocytopenia (platelet count below 10,000/mm^3) must be monitored closely for subtle changes in mental status, including irritability and restlessness, and educated to report even mild headaches immediately.

In contrast to platelet defects, coagulation factor defects do not tend to cause superficial bleeding because the primary hemostatic mechanisms are still intact. Instead, bleeding occurs deeper within the body (e.g., subcutaneous or intramuscular hematomas, hemorrhage into joint spaces). Because of this bleeding, the patient may report joint pain.

External bleeding diminishes very slowly when local pressure is applied; it often recurs several hours after pressure is removed. For example, severe bleeding may start several hours after a tooth extraction.

Bone Marrow Aspiration and Biopsy

A bone marrow examination is important in the evaluation of several hematologic disorders and infectious diseases (Fischbach et al., 2021). The decision to perform a bone marrow evaluation is made after the critical assessment of pertinent information available from the history, physical examination, and laboratory studies, including a review of the CBC and examination of the PBS (Zehnder, 2020).

Indications for bone marrow aspiration include evaluation of unexplained anemia, leukopenia, thrombocytopenia, or pancytopenia; evaluation of unexplained elevations in peripheral blood counts; diagnosis and staging of leukemia, lymphoma, or solid tumors; evaluation of iron metabolism and stores; evaluation of suspected deposition and storage diseases (e.g., amyloidosis, Gaucher disease); evaluation of fever of undetermined origin; evaluation of unexplained splenomegaly; or confirmation that the bone marrow is normal in a potential allogeneic hematopoietic cell donor (a donor that is not the patient) in select patients (Zehnder, 2020).

For example, a patient with an abnormal CBC undergoes a bone marrow biopsy and aspirate with results revealing acute myeloid leukemia. After receiving chemotherapy to treat the leukemia, another bone marrow aspirate and biopsy are done to assess response to treatment; if the treatment was effective, no leukemia cells should be seen in the biopsy or aspirate specimens.

Normal bone marrow is in a semifluid state and can be aspirated through a special hollow core, large-bore needle. In adults, bone marrow is usually aspirated from the posterior iliac crest. The aspirate provides a sample of cells. Aspirate alone may be adequate for evaluating certain conditions, such as anemia. However, in most cases, a biopsy is also performed. Biopsy samples are taken from the posterior iliac crest; occasionally, an anterior iliac approach is required. The sternum can be used to obtain an aspirate but should not be used to obtain a biopsy because of its proximity to vital organs. A bone marrow biopsy shows the architecture of the bone marrow as well as its degree of cellularity.

The first step in the procedure is obtaining informed consent. Informed consent is obtained by the physician, nurse practitioner, or physician's assistant performing the procedure and includes the reason the procedure is being performed, alternatives, and risks of the procedure. Risks include infection, bleeding, and pain. The risk for bleeding is somewhat increased if the patient's platelet count is low (less than 20/mm^3) or if the patient has been taking a medication (e.g., aspirin) that alters platelet function. Complications following bone marrow aspiration and biopsy are rare (Stensby et al., 2020). Postoperative bleeding is common due to the high vascularity of the sampled tissue. Rarely, retroperitoneal or gluteal hemorrhage can occur, typically due to injury of the internal iliac artery or superior gluteal artery. Hemorrhage, cardiac tamponade, and death can occur if a needle is misplaced during sternal aspiration, and extreme caution should be exercised if this site is chosen for sampling. Infection is a risk of any invasive procedure and can be minimized with proper sterile technique (Rindy & Chambers, 2021).

Most adult patients need no more preparation than a careful explanation of the procedure and the sensations they will experience, but for some anxious patients, administration of an antianxiety agent, such as lorazepam, may be useful. Pediatric patients usually require deeper sedation. Though this procedure is potentially painful, generous local anesthesia and a skilled operator minimize the risk for discomfort.

After informed consent is obtained, the patient is assisted to either a prone or lateral decubitus position. The skin is cleansed using aseptic technique and either a chlorhexidine-based solution or povidone-iodine. A sterile drape is applied; then the skin is numbed using a 1% to 2% lidocaine solution. It is essential to anesthetize the periosteum broadly due to the high sensitivity of this structure (Rindy & Chambers, 2021). The bone itself cannot be numbed. An aspirate needle is inserted with a stylet in place through the numbed skin into the cortical bone through to the marrow; when the needle is felt to go through the outer cortex of bone and into the marrow cavity, the stylet is removed, a syringe is attached, and a small volume (1 to 3 mL) of marrow fluid is aspirated (this is often referred to as the aspirate sample) (Fischbach et al., 2021).

Patients typically feel a sensation of pressure as the needle is advanced into position. The aspiration of fluid causes a sudden and sharp but brief pain resulting from the suction exerted as the marrow is aspirated into the syringe; the patient should be warned about this. Taking deep breaths or using relaxation techniques often helps ease the discomfort. Once the aspirate sample is obtained, the aspirate needle is removed and a longer hollow-core needle with stylet is inserted through the same hole in the skin. At this point, if computed tomography (CT) guidance is being utilized, the region of interest should be scanned in the axial plane to determine needle trajectory (Rindy & Chambers, 2021). Once the proper angulation has been achieved, the needle can be advanced and anchored into the cortical bone (Rindy & Chambers, 2021). Once the bone marrow cavity has been entered, the stylet can be removed. Next, the needle is turned clockwise and then counterclockwise several times to help loosen the specimen; the needle is carefully removed, revealing a solid core specimen of bone and bone marrow inside the hollow needle. A probe is used to gently push the specimen out of the needle and into a specimen container. During the biopsy, the patient may feel pressure but should not feel pain; if the patient experiences pain radiating down the leg, repositioning of the needle may be necessary. After the marrow sample is obtained, apply pressure to the puncture site until bleeding ceases; this can take several minutes (Fischbach et al., 2021). Apply a sterile dressing to the site. Most patients have no discomfort after a bone marrow aspiration, but the site of a biopsy may ache for 3 or 4 days. Patients should be instructed not to submerge in a bath for 24 hours, until the site heals. A mild analgesic (e.g., acetaminophen) may be useful. Aspirin-containing analgesics should be avoided because of the increased risk of bleeding.

The nurse should understand the importance and necessity of education both before and after the procedure as well as emotional support during it. The nurse should review instructions about postprocedure care, such as vital sign monitoring, site care, and when to call the health care provider (signs and symptoms of infection and bleeding should be reviewed). Soreness over the puncture site as previously described following the procedure is normal, whereas continued or severe pain may indicate fracture and should be evaluated (Fischbach et al., 2021).

The bone marrow aspirate and biopsy samples are evaluated by a pathologist who ultimately provides a summary of findings. The aspirate provides information on the cell type, size, shape, and number present in the marrow and also allows for specialized tests, including flow cytometry, cytogenetic studies, and molecular studies to be conducted, all of which help classify the bone marrow disorder. The bone marrow biopsy provides information on the cellularity of the marrow as well as the severity of disease or dysfunction; normal cellularity can be estimated based on subtracting the patient's age from 100. For example, a 30-year-old female should have a cellularity of 70%. Fewer cells than expected is referred to as "hypocellular"; more cells than expected is called "hypercellular."

Unfolding Patient Stories: L.B. • Part 1

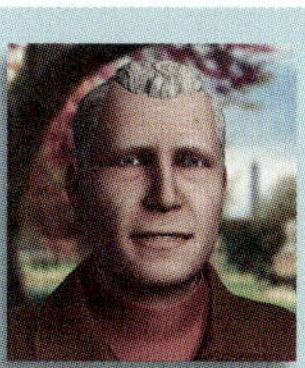

L.B. is a 76-year-old patient fell while working outdoors presents to the emergency department with a hip fracture. What physical assessment and laboratory data can assist the nurse in evaluating for actual or potential internal blood loss from the fracture? What laboratory data suggests that the patient is at higher risk of bleeding? (L.B.'s story continues in Chapter 25.)

Care for L.B. and other patients in a realistic virtual environment: ***vSim** for Nursing* (thepoint.lww.com/vSimMedicalSurgical). Practice documenting these patients' care in DocuCare (thepoint.lww.com/DocuCareEHR).

CHAPTER REVIEW

NCLEX-Style Review Questions

1. A nurse is caring for a patient who is 73 years old with a platelet count of 5,000/mm^3 resulting from myelodysplastic syndrome. At 10 pm, the patient complains of a headache. Which actions should the nurse take immediately? Select all that apply.

a. Administer aspirin per as-needed (PRN) order.
b. Obtain vital signs including oxygen saturation.
c. Administer acetaminophen per PRN order.
d. Assess neurologic status, including orientation and cranial nerves, motor, and sensory function.
e. Notify the health care provider.
f. Administer oxygen at 2 L/min via nasal cannula.

2. A patient presents to their primary care provider with a complaint of a "cold that just won't go away." They have a CBC drawn, revealing the following: WBC 4.5: segs 5, bands 0, lymphs 45, eosinophils 5, basophils 5, monocytes 5, blasts 35. What is the patient's absolute neutrophil count (ANC)?

a. 500
b. 250
c. 225
d. 2,250

3. Which signs and symptoms are associated with anemia? Select all that apply.

a. Dyspnea
b. Bradycardia
c. Pallor
d. Constipation
e. Fatigue
f. Weakness

4. A patient with thrombocytopenia due to chemotherapy develops a nosebleed (epistaxis). What is the nurse's expected response?

a. Apply ice to the back of the neck
b. Apply direct pressure to the bleeding nares
c. Ask the patient to blow the nose vigorously as the nurse applies firm pressure to the nares
d. Apply ice to the bridge of the nose
e. Place the patient in a supine position, leaning on their side
f. Position the patient in a high Fowler position, leaning slightly forward

5. A 42-year-old patient was admitted to your unit for chemotherapy. The patient received a third dose of chemotherapy yesterday. The lab called and reported that your patient's platelet count is 19,000 cells/mm^3. What interventions are appropriate based on this lab value? Select all that apply.

a. Place the patient in a private room.
b. Take a rectal temperature every 4 hours.
c. Check the patient's stool for melena or occult blood.
d. Remove all plants from the patient's room.
e. Observe the patient for petechiae or ecchymoses.
f. Avoid overinflation of blood pressure cuffs.

REFERENCES AND SELECTED READINGS

References and selected readings associated with this chapter can be found on the website that accompanies the book. Visit **http://thepoint.lww.com/Honan3e** to access the references and other additional resources associated with this chapter.

CHAPTER 19

Nursing Management: Patients With Hematologic Disorders

Naomi Cazeau

Learning Objectives

After reading this chapter, you will be able to:

1. Differentiate between the different types of anemias and compare and contrast the physiologic mechanisms, clinical manifestations, medical management, and nursing interventions for each.
2. Compare the leukemia types in terms of incidence, physiologic alterations, clinical manifestations, management, and prognosis.
3. Discuss physiologic mechanisms, clinical manifestations, medical management, and nursing interventions for myelodysplastic syndromes.
4. Discuss nursing management of patients with lymphoma and multiple myeloma.
5. Discuss nursing management of patients with bleeding or thrombotic disorders.
6. Identify therapies for blood disorders, including the nursing implications for the administration of blood components.

Hematologic disorders include both benign and malignant conditions. These disorders can impact every system in the body. Nursing care of these patients requires an understanding of the anatomy and physiology of hematopoiesis and immunology, as well as astute assessment skills.

RED BLOOD CELL DISORDERS

Anemia

Anemia, a condition in which the **hemoglobin** concentration is lower than normal, reflects the presence of fewer than normal **erythrocytes** (red blood cells [RBCs]) within the circulation. As a result, the amount of oxygen delivered to body tissues is also diminished. Anemia is not a specific disease state per se but a sign of an underlying disorder. It is among the most common hematologic conditions, affecting nearly one fourth of the world's population (Gardner & Kassebaum, 2020). Anemia is a common occurrence among all age groups, with prevalence highest among children less than 5 years old (Gardner & Kassebaum, 2020). The treatment varies based on the cause. The different classifications of anemia, as well as the nursing management of each, will be discussed here.

Classification of Anemias

Anemia can be classified by cellular morphology (shape) or by physiologic process. Morphologic classification is the most common approach and includes the cell size, color, and shape. Changes in the size of the RBC are described as normocytic (normal or average size), macrocytic (larger than normal), or microcytic (smaller than normal). Changes in the color of the RBC are described as **normochromic** (normal in color), hyperchromic (darker cellular contents), or hypochromic (pale or lighter cellular contents) (see Table 19-1). A physiologic approach (see Table 19-2) classifies anemia according to whether the deficiency in erythrocytes is caused by a defect in their production (hypoproliferative anemia), by their destruction (hemolytic anemia), or by their loss (e.g., bleeding) (Fig. 19-1).

To determine whether the presence of anemia in a given patient is caused by destruction or by inadequate production of erythrocytes, consider the following factors:

- The marrow's ability to respond to decreased erythrocytes (as evidenced by an increased reticulocyte count (immature RBCs) in the circulating blood)
- The degree to which young erythrocytes (**nucleated RBCs**) proliferate in the bone marrow and the manner in which they mature (as observed on bone marrow biopsy). Unlike most of the cells in your body, RBCs lack nuclei once matured; thus, if nucleated, the nurse recognizes that this suggests a high demand for the bone marrow to produce RBCs
- The presence or absence of end products of erythrocyte destruction within the circulation (e.g., increased bilirubin

TABLE **19-1 Classification of Anemia by Morphology**

Type of Anemia	Morphology	Examples	Laboratory Values Expected
Normocytic (MCV 80–100 fL), normochromic	Cells of normal size with normal Hgb content	Aplastic anemia Acute blood loss Hemolytic anemia Anemia of chronic disease Sickle cell anemia	Normal MCV Normal MCHC ↓ Hgb ↓ Hct
Microcytic (MCV less than 80 fL), hypochromic	Small, reduced amount of Hgb	Iron deficiency anemia Sideroblastic anemia Thalassemia	↓ MCV ↓ MCHC ↓ Hgb ↓ Hct
Macrocytic (MCV greater than 100 fL), normochromic	Large in size, thickness, and volume	Folic acid deficiency Vitamin B_{12} deficiency Alcohol abuse Medications (e.g., hydroxyurea)	↑ MCV Normal MCHC ↓ Hgb ↓ Hct

MCV, mean corpuscular volume; MCHC, mean corpuscular hemoglobin concentration; Hgb, hemoglobin; Hct, hematocrit.

level, decreased haptoglobin [a protein produced by the liver] level)

Hypoproliferative Anemias

In hypoproliferative anemias, the marrow cannot produce adequate numbers of erythrocytes. The reticulocyte count reflects bone marrow production of RBCs. In anemia due to blood loss, a healthy bone marrow compensates for losses and increases RBC production, reflected as an increased reticulocyte count. In hypoproliferative anemias, the bone marrow cannot mount an adequate response to anemia, and this lack of RBC production is reflected as a low reticulocyte count.

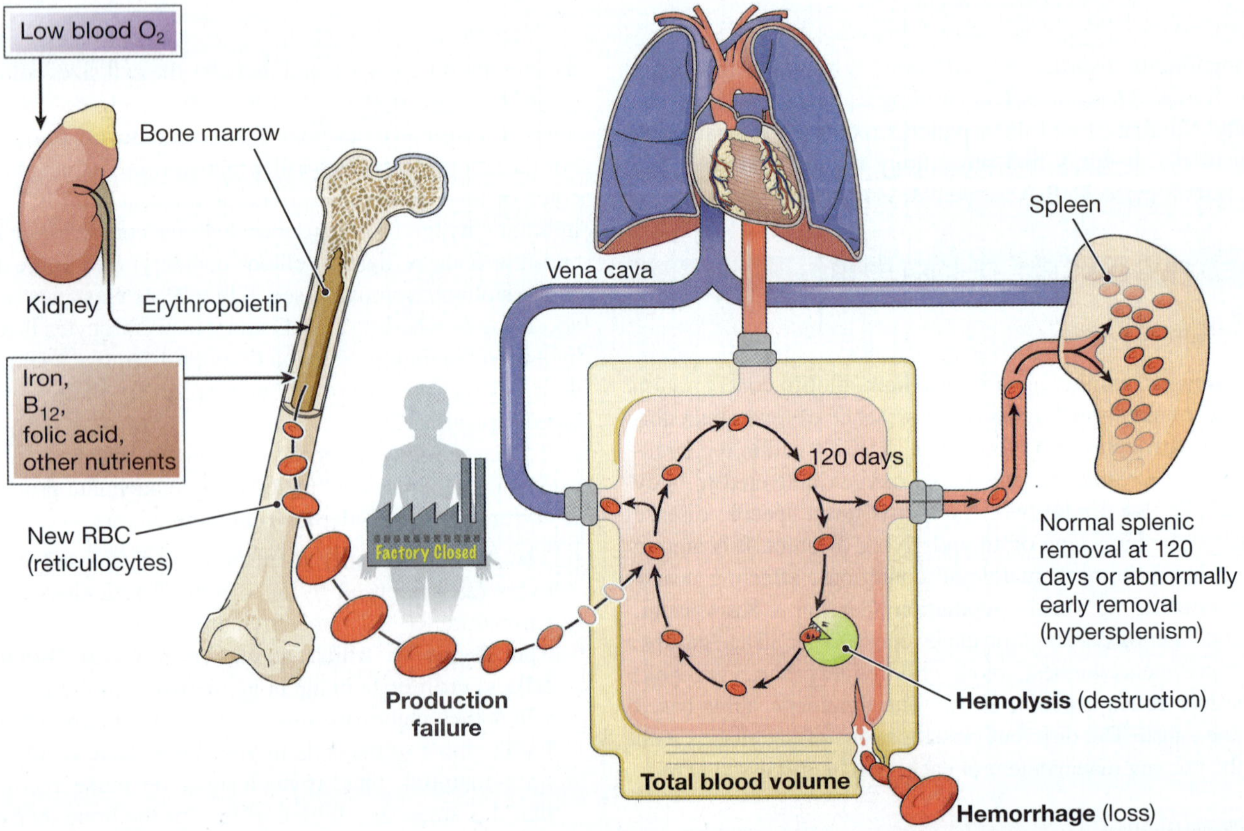

FIGURE 19-1 **Production, circulation, and death of red blood cells. Every anemia is caused by at least one of three problems: (1) decreased red cell production, (2) loss of red cells by hemorrhage, or (3) early death (destruction) of RBCs. (From McConnell, T. H. [2007].** ***The nature of disease pathology for the health professions*****. Lippincott Williams & Wilkins.)**

TABLE **19-2 Anemia Classification by Etiology**

Type of Anemia	Pathophysiology	Laboratory Findings	Treatment
Hypoproliferative (Decreased Production)			
Pernicious, megaloblastic	Vitamin B_{12} deficiency; lack of intrinsic factor required for B_{12} absorption	Decreased vitamin B_{12} level; increased MCV Elevated methylmalonic acid and homocysteine levels Low reticulocyte count	B_{12} replacement Cyanocobalamin 1,000 µg IM monthly
Folate deficiency	Decreased folic acid intake; impaired absorption; alcohol impairs folate metabolism in the liver, causing a significant depletion in folate reserves Decreases in folate impair DNA synthesis and increase erythroblast cell deaths	Decreased folate levels Increased MCV	Oral folic acid 1–5 mg/day PO
Iron deficiency	Chronic blood loss, failure to recapture iron from recycled RBCs Demands for iron exceed iron intake. Decreased iron intake results in use and depletion of iron stores, resulting in decreased Hgb production	Decreased reticulocytes, iron, ferritin, iron saturation, MCV Increased TIBC	Iron replacement therapy: ferrous sulfate 325 mg PO t.i.d. Parenteral iron therapy reserved for those who cannot take oral replacement due to intolerance, poor enteral absorption, or continued blood loss IV iron therapy requires careful monitoring for signs of hypersensitivity
Decreased erythropoietin production	Kidney disease can impair erythropoietin production (due to renal disease, malignancy), which, in turn, decreases RBC production	Decreased erythropoietin level; normal MCV and MCH; increased creatinine level	Erythropoietin replacement
Anemia of chronic disease (seen in AIDS, malignancy, SLE, chronic kidney disease, chronic liver disease, rheumatoid arthritis)	Marked by three defects: Decreased erythrocyte lifespan, ineffective bone marrow response to erythropoietin, altered iron metabolism	Normal MCV and MCHC Low serum iron Low or normal TIBC Normal or high ferritin	Primary treatment is to treat the underlying cause
Aplastic anemia	An immune response mediated by cytotoxic T cells; targets the cells in the bone marrow, causing cell death and bone marrow failure Hereditary or acquired (exposure to benzene, pesticides)	Decreased reticulocyte count Decreased white blood cells, Hgb, Hct, and platelets	Immunosuppressive therapy (e.g., cyclosporine, corticosteroids, antithymocyte globulin) Stem cell transplant
Blood Loss			
Bleeding	Bleeding from gastrointestinal tract, menorrhagia (excessive menstrual flow), epistaxis (nosebleed), trauma results in decrease in circulating blood volume and decreased Hgb and Hct	Increased reticulocyte level Normal Hgb and Hct if measured soon after bleeding starts, but levels decrease thereafter Normal MCV initially but later decreases Decreased ferritin and iron levels (later)	Packed RBC transfusions Identify and control source of blood loss

(*continued*)

TABLE **19-2 Anemia Classification by Etiology (*continued*)**

Type of Anemia	Pathophysiology	Laboratory Findings	Treatment
Hemolysis (Destruction of RBCs)			
Autoimmune hemolytic anemia Acquired; caused by extrinsic insults such as infection, medications, venom, trauma	Both inherited and acquired forms result in hemolysis within blood vessels and/or lymphoid tissue	Presence of schistocytes Increased spherocyte level Increased reticulocytes	Immunosuppressive therapy (i.e., corticosteroids) Acquired: remove insult, treat underlying disorder
Thalassemias A group of inherited forms of autoimmune hemolytic anemia	Caused by cellular abnormalities of the Hgb structure, marked by an imbalance between the beta chain and alpha chain of Hgb, resulting in RBC membrane damage, ineffective RBC production, and hemolysis	Decreased MCV; fragmented RBCs Increased reticulocyte level	Transfusion therapy with PRBCs Monitor ferritin regularly to assess for iron overload
Sickle cell disease	Inherited disorder in which abnormal hemoglobin (HbS) polymerizes when deoxygenated, creating a semisolid gel that makes an RBC rigid with a distorted shape (sickle cell) that leads to hemolytic anemia, pain (stasis of RBCs in capillaries), and organ failure	Anemia (resulting from chronic hemolysis), reticulocytosis, leukocytosis, and thrombocytosis are common. Elevations of bilirubin and lactate dehydrogenase are also common. Peripheral blood smear may reveal sickle cells	Transfusion therapy with PRBCs Monitor ferritin regularly to assess for iron overload Hydroxyurea

MCV, mean corpuscular volume; MCHC, mean corpuscular hemoglobin concentration; TIBC, total iron binding capacity; Hgb, hemoglobin; Hct, hematocrit; AIDS, acquired immune deficiency syndrome; SLE, systemic lupus erythematosus; RBCs, red blood cells; PRBCs, packed RBCs.

Inadequate production of erythrocytes may result from marrow damage due to medications (e.g., chloramphenicol) or chemicals (e.g., benzene) or from a lack of essential factors (e.g., iron, vitamin B_{12}, folic acid, **erythropoietin**) necessary for erythrocyte formation.

Iron Deficiency Anemia

The development of iron deficiency anemia occurs when the body's iron stores are depleted and there is no iron available for hemoglobin synthesis. The volume of individual iron stores is dependent upon sex, age, rate of growth, and the balance between dietary iron absorption and losses. Iron is stored primarily in the liver, spleen, and bone marrow. The remainder of iron exists as hemoglobin and proteins. Iron deficiency anemia is diagnosed based on the presence of a microcytic anemia, low serum iron level, low transferrin saturation percentage, and low ferritin level (Elstrott et al., 2020).

Iron deficiency anemia is the most common type of anemia in all age groups, and it is the most common anemia in the world. It is particularly prevalent in developing countries, where inadequate iron stores can result from inadequate intake of iron (seen with vegetarian diets) or from blood loss (e.g., from intestinal hookworm). Iron deficiency is also common in the United States. In children, adolescents, and pregnant females, the cause is typically inadequate iron in the diet to keep up with increased growth. However, for most adults with iron deficiency anemia, the cause is blood loss. In fact, in adults, the cause of iron deficiency anemia should be considered to be bleeding until proven otherwise. Patients with chronic alcohol use disorder often have chronic blood loss from the GI tract, which causes iron loss and eventual anemia. Other causes include iron malabsorption, as is seen after gastrectomy or with celiac disease.

Medical Management

Except in the case of pregnancy, the cause of iron deficiency should be investigated. Anemia may be a sign of a curable GI cancer or of uterine fibroid tumors. Stool specimens should be tested for occult blood and *H. pylori* infection. Blood samples should be sent for celiac serology and antiparietal cell antibodies (to rule out pernicious anemia). In the presence of iron deficiency, the American Gastroenterological Association (AGA) also recommends esophagogastroduodenoscopy (EGD) and colonoscopy on asymptomatic pre- and postmenopausal females and all asymptomatic males who have no other clear explanation for the iron deficiency anemia (i.e., vegan diet, nongastrointestinal blood loss) (Ko et al., 2020).

Iron replacement therapy is available via both oral and intravenous routes. The oral route is generally preferred given its wide availability, low cost, and safety (Auerbach, 2021). Several oral iron preparations are available for treating iron deficiency anemia. GI side effects, including nausea and epigastric discomfort, occur in up to 70% of patients taking oral iron (Auerbach, 2021).

Vitamin C facilitates the absorption of iron. Therefore, oral iron should be taken with a glass of orange juice or a vitamin C tablet on an empty stomach to maximize absorption. However, taking iron on an empty stomach and taking iron with vitamin C can increase GI side effects; therefore, patients should be monitored closely. In addition, calcium supplements can decrease iron absorption; therefore, administration of these two medications should be staggered (Auerbach, 2021).

The hemoglobin level should begin to rise after 1 week of replacement and should increase by 1 to 2 g/dL within 4 to 8 weeks. If hemoglobin levels fail to improve within this time frame, adherence to the regimen should be assessed and IV iron replacement should be considered. If the patient has been adherent to the prescribed regimen, then assess for absorption problems, continued blood loss, concomitant deficiencies (folate, B_{12}, copper), and drug interactions. Diet has been implicated when large quantities of phytates from cereals or tannate from teas inhibit iron absorption (Auerbach, 2021). In addition, iron absorption is impaired by conditions that affect the duodenum's ability to absorb iron, as in extensive gastric surgery, generalized intestinal malabsorption, atrophic gastritis, as well as long-term use of proton pump inhibitors (PPIs) or histamine 2 receptor blockers (H_2) (Auerbach et al., 2020; Hamano et al., 2020). Iron store repletion can necessitate iron replacement therapy for as long as 3 to 6 months (Ning & Zeller, 2019).

In some cases, oral iron is poorly absorbed or poorly tolerated, or iron supplementation is needed in large amounts. In these situations, IV administration of iron may be needed. There are currently six available intravenous iron preparations:

- low–molecular-weight heparin [LMWH] iron dextran,
- ferric gluconate,
- iron sucrose,
- ferumoxytol,
- ferric derisomaltose, and
- ferric carboxymaltose.

All IV iron preparations carry some risk for hypersensitivity. LMWH iron dextran is the only formulation that requires a test dose due to the risk of hypersensitivity. This medication also allows the delivery of higher doses of iron (1,000 mg) over 1 hour. Ferric gluconate and iron sucrose must be given in smaller doses, whereas ferumoxytol, ferric derisomaltose and ferric carboxymaltose allow higher doses to be given over shorter periods of time (15 minutes) (Auerbach, 2021). In most cases, multiple doses of IV iron replacement are required to replace the patient's iron stores.

Nursing Management

Preventive education is important, because iron deficiency anemia is common in menstruating and pregnant females. Food sources high in iron include organ meats (beef or calf's liver, chicken liver), other red meats, beans (black, pinto, and garbanzo), leafy green vegetables, raisins, and molasses. Taking iron-rich foods with a source of vitamin C (e.g., orange juice) enhances the absorption of iron.

The nurse helps the patient select a healthy diet and refers the patient to a registered dietitian as appropriate. Nutritional counseling can be provided for those whose usual diet is inadequate. Patients with a history of eating fad diets or strict vegetarian diets are counseled that such diets often contain inadequate amounts of absorbable iron. The nurse encourages the patient to continue iron therapy as long as it is prescribed, even if the symptoms of anemia resolve. The nurse helps to assess and manage side effects of oral iron replacement.

Because iron is best absorbed on an empty stomach, the patient is instructed to take the supplement an hour before meals. Many patients have difficulty tolerating iron supplements because of GI side effects (diarrhea, constipation, epigastric discomfort, nausea, and vomiting). Some iron formulations are designed to limit GI side effects by the addition of a stool softener or use of sustained-release formulations to limit nausea or gastritis. While enteric-coated formulations (i.e., iron protein or ferrous glycine sulfate) have lower frequencies of adverse effects, they may be absorbed poorly and should be avoided (Auerbach, 2021). Specific patient teaching aids (Box 19-1) can assist patients with the use of iron supplements.

IV supplementation may be used when the patient's iron stores are completely depleted, if the patient has impaired

BOX 19-1 **Patient Education**

Taking Oral Iron Supplements

- Take iron on an empty stomach (1 hour before or 2 hours after a meal). Because iron absorption is reduced with food, especially dairy products and antacids, avoid taking iron with these items.
- To prevent gastrointestinal distress, the following schedule may work better if more than one tablet a day is prescribed: Start with only one tablet per day for a few days, then increase to two tablets per day, and then three tablets per day. This method permits the body to adjust gradually to the iron.
- Increase the intake of vitamin C (citrus fruits and juices, strawberries, tomatoes, broccoli), to enhance iron absorption.
- Eat foods high in fiber to minimize problems with constipation.
- Remember that stools will become dark in color.
- To prevent staining the teeth with a liquid preparation, use a straw or place a spoon at the back of the mouth to take the supplement. Rinse the mouth thoroughly afterward.

iron absorption, or the patient cannot tolerate oral forms of iron supplementation. Due to the risk for hypersensitivity reactions with parenteral iron formulations, the patient should be monitored closely during and shortly after the infusion; vital signs should be monitored carefully per institution guidelines.

Megaloblastic Anemias

In the anemias caused by deficiencies of either vitamin B_{12} or folic acid, identical bone marrow and peripheral blood changes occur because both vitamins are essential for normal DNA synthesis. In either anemia, the erythrocytes that are produced are abnormally large and are called *megaloblastic red cells*; therefore, the mean corpuscular volume (MCV) is elevated. Other cells derived from the **myeloid** (bone marrow) stem cell are also abnormal, resulting in low leukocyte and platelet counts in advanced stages of disease. A bone marrow analysis reveals **hyperplasia** (abnormal increase in the number of cells), and the precursor erythroid and myeloid cells are large and atypical in appearance.

Pathophysiology

Folic Acid Deficiency. Folic acid is stored as compounds referred to as *folates*. The folate stores in the body are much smaller than those of vitamin B_{12}, and they are quickly depleted when the dietary intake of folate is deficient (within 4 months). Folate is found in green leafy vegetables, legumes, egg yolks, fortified foods like cereal and liver (Wusigale & Liang, 2020). Folate deficiency occurs in people who rarely eat uncooked vegetables. Alcohol increases folic acid requirements; patients with alcohol use disorder (sometimes referred to as "alcoholism") usually have a diet that is deficient in the vitamin. Folic acid requirements are also increased in patients with chronic hemolytic anemias and in females who are pregnant because the need for erythrocyte production is increased in these conditions. Folate is absorbed in the upper small intestine; therefore, some patients with malabsorptive diseases of the small bowel, such as celiac sprue, may not absorb folic acid normally (Montoro-Huguet et al., 2021).

Vitamin B_{12} Deficiency. A deficiency of vitamin B_{12} can occur in several ways. Inadequate dietary intake is rare but can develop in strict vegans (who consume no meat or dairy products). Faulty absorption from the GI tract is a more common cause. This occurs in conditions such as Crohn disease, or after ileal resection, bariatric gastric bypass surgery, or gastrectomy. Even if adequate vitamin B_{12} and intrinsic factor are present, a deficiency may occur if disease involving the ileum or pancreas impairs absorption. Another cause is the absence of intrinsic factor, as in pernicious anemia. Intrinsic factor is normally secreted by cells within the gastric mucosa and under normal circumstances binds with the dietary vitamin B_{12} and travels with it to the ileum, where the vitamin is absorbed. Without intrinsic factor, orally consumed vitamin B_{12} cannot be absorbed, and eventually erythrocyte production is diminished. Pernicious anemia, which tends to run in families, is primarily a disorder of adults, particularly older adults. Pernicious anemia is an autoimmune disorder involving autoantibodies to intrinsic factor and parietal cells resulting in poor absorption of B_{12} (Means & Fairfield, 2021). For unknown reasons, patients with pernicious anemia have a higher incidence of gastric cancer, adenocarcinomas, and other cancers compared to the general population (Ammouri et al., 2020). Though routine screening for this population has not yet been recommended, these patients should understand their risks and be educated on reporting any new symptoms promptly to health care providers. It is recommended that patients with newly diagnosed pernicious anemia or any patient with pernicious anemia and GI symptoms undergo screening endoscopy (Chan & Wong, 2021). The body normally has large stores of vitamin B_{12} so years may pass before the deficiency results in anemia. Because the body compensates so well, the anemia can be severe before the patient becomes symptomatic.

Clinical Manifestations and Assessment

People with vitamin B and/or folic acid deficiency may present with nonspecific symptoms including fatigue, mood changes, memory difficulty, and weakness (Means & Fairfield, 2021). Assessment of patients who have or are at risk of megaloblastic anemia includes inspection of the skin and mucous membranes. Mild jaundice may be apparent and is best seen in the sclera without using fluorescent lights. Vitiligo (patchy loss of skin pigmentation) and premature graying of the hair are often seen in patients with pernicious anemia. The tongue is smooth, red, and sore (referred to as glossitis).

Symptoms of folic acid and vitamin B_{12} deficiencies are similar, and the two anemias may coexist. However, the neurologic manifestations of vitamin B_{12} deficiency do not occur with folic acid deficiency, and they persist if vitamin B_{12} is not replaced. Therefore, careful distinction between the two anemias must be made. Serum levels of both vitamins can be measured. In the case of folic acid deficiency, even small amounts of folate increase the serum folate level. Therefore, measuring the amount of folate within the red cell itself (red cell folate) is a more sensitive test in determining true folate deficiency (Means & Fairfield, 2021).

Neurologic symptoms are seen in severe vitamin B_{12} deficiency and pernicious anemia and include psychiatric symptoms and peripheral neuropathy (Means & Fairfield, 2021). This presentation happens infrequently due to earlier diagnosis.

After the body's stores of vitamin B_{12} are depleted, the patient may begin to show signs and symptoms of the anemia. However, because the onset and progression of the anemia are so gradual, the body can compensate very well until the anemia is severe so that the typical manifestations of anemia (weakness, listlessness, fatigue) may not be apparent

BOX 19-2

Focused Assessment

Anemia

Be alert for the following signs and symptoms:

- General:
  - Weakness, fatigue
  - Dizziness
  - Pica (craving unusual items including: ice, starch, or dirt)
- Neurologic[a]:
  - Numbness and tingling (paresthesias), irritability
  - Weakness
  - Headache
  - Poor coordination, confusion
  - Gait disturbances
  - Reflex abnormalities
  - Loss of position (proprioception) and vibration sense
  - Spasticity
  - Roaring, rushing, ringing, or pounding sensation in the ears
- Integumentary:
  - Pallor of the skin and mucous membranes
  - Jaundice (hemolytic anemia)
  - Brittle, ridged, concave nails
  - Impaired wound healing
  - Loss of elasticity
  - Early thinning and graying of hair
  - Dry skin
  - Painful mouth sores
  - Beefy red, sore tongue (megaloblastic anemia)
  - Smooth and red tongue (iron deficiency anemia)
  - Ulcerated corners of the mouth (angular cheilitis)
- Cardiovascular:
  - Palpitations
  - Chest pain
  - Tachycardia
  - Hypotension
  - Peripheral edema
  - Murmurs
- Respiratory:
  - Dyspnea
  - Orthopnea
  - Tachypnea
- Gastrointestinal:
  - Anorexia, nausea, vomiting
  - Dysphagia
  - Abdominal pain
  - Flatulence
  - Diarrhea
  - Hepatomegaly
  - Splenomegaly
- Musculoskeletal:
  - Muscle pain (claudication)

[a]Neurologic signs and symptoms are most commonly seen in pernicious anemia.

initially. The hematologic effects of deficiency are accompanied by effects on other organ systems, particularly the GI tract and nervous system (Box 19-2). These symptoms are progressive, although the course of illness may be marked by spontaneous partial remissions and exacerbations. Without treatment, patients can die after several years, usually from heart failure secondary to anemia.

Medical Management

Underlying causes for vitamin B_{12} and folate deficiency should be investigated and treated. Dietary counseling should include discussion on increasing dietary sources of folic acid. Supplemental oral folic acid should be administered at a dosage of 1 to 5 mg daily until recovery (Khan & Jialal, 2021). Patients with malabsorption will need to continue folic acid supplements over the long term. Pregnant patients should take folic acid (0.4 to 0.8 mg daily) when planning for pregnancy as well as throughout the course of pregnancy (Orabona et al., 2020).

Vitamin B_{12} deficiency is treated by vitamin B_{12} replacement. Vegetarians can prevent or treat deficiency with oral supplements, vitamins, or fortified soy milk. When the deficiency is due to the more common defect in absorption or the absence of intrinsic factor, replacement by intramuscular (IM) injections of vitamin B_{12} is necessary. The replacement schedule includes daily or every other day administration of 1 mg (1,000 μg) of cyanocobalamin IM for 1 week, followed by weekly administration for 1 to 2 months and then monthly through the remainder of the patient's life (Sanz-Cuesta et al., 2020).

As vitamin B_{12} is replaced, the reticulocyte count rises within 1 week, and in several weeks all the blood counts should improve to normal. The characteristic beefy red, sore tongue feels better and appears less red in several days. However, the neurologic manifestations require more time for recovery; if there is severe neuropathy, the patient may never recover fully. To prevent recurrence of pernicious anemia, vitamin B_{12} therapy must be continued for life.

Pearls for Practice

Even when the megaloblastic anemia is severe, RBC transfusions may not be used because the patient's body has compensated over time by expanding the total blood volume. Administration of blood transfusions to such patients, particularly older adults or those who have cardiac dysfunction, can precipitate pulmonary edema. If transfusions are required, the RBCs should be transfused slowly, with careful attention to signs and symptoms of fluid overload.

Nursing Management

In the setting of peripheral neuropathy, the nurse needs to pay particular attention to ambulation and should assess the patient's gait and stability as well as the need for assistive devices (e.g., canes, walkers) and for assistance in managing daily activities. Of particular concern is ensuring safety when position sense, coordination, and gait are affected. Physical and occupational therapy referrals may be needed. If sensation is altered, the patient needs to be instructed to avoid excessive heat and cold.

Because mouth and tongue soreness may restrict nutritional intake, the nurse advises the patient to eat small amounts of bland, soft foods frequently and educates the patient on routine mouth care. The nurse also may explain that other nutritional deficiencies, such as alcohol-induced anemia, can induce neurologic problems.

Anemia in Kidney Disease

The degree of anemia in patients with end-stage kidney disease (ESKD) varies greatly, but in general patients do not become significantly anemic until the serum creatinine level exceeds 3 mg/dL.

Pathophysiology

This anemia is caused by both a mild shortening of erythrocyte lifespan and a deficiency of erythropoietin (necessary for **erythropoiesis**). As kidney function decreases, erythropoietin, which is produced by the kidney, also decreases. Because erythropoietin is also produced outside the kidney, some erythropoiesis continues, even in patients whose kidneys have been removed. However, the number of RBCs produced is small and the degree of erythropoiesis is inadequate.

Patients undergoing long-term hemodialysis lose blood into the dialyzer and, therefore, may become iron deficient. Folic acid deficiency develops because this vitamin passes into the dialysate. Therefore, patients who receive hemodialysis and who have anemia should be evaluated for iron and folate deficiency and treated appropriately.

Clinical Manifestations and Assessment

For patients with ESKD, the symptoms of anemia, including fatigue and decreased activity tolerance, are often the most disturbing. If untreated, the hematocrit may fall to between 20% and 30%, although in rare cases it may fall to less than 15%. The erythrocytes appear normal in shape, size, and color on the peripheral smear.

Medical and Nursing Management

The availability of recombinant erythropoietin (also referred to as erythropoiesis stimulating agents or ESAs) (epoetin alfa, darbepoetin alfa) has dramatically altered the management of anemia in ESKD by decreasing the need for RBC transfusion, with its associated risks. Adequate iron stores are essential for optimal response to erythropoietin. Iron stores, including transferrin saturation and ferritin, must be measured prior to starting ESAs, and iron replacement should be initiated in patients with a ferritin of less than 100 ng/mL. Erythropoietin, in combination with oral iron supplements, can raise and maintain hematocrit levels to between 33% and 38%. This treatment has been successful with dialysis patients. ESAs carry an increased risk of death and cardiovascular events, including stroke, venous thromboembolism (VTE), and myocardial infarction (MI) when hemoglobin targets exceed 11 g/dL; therefore, the lowest dose required to reduce transfusion requirements is recommended (Patel & Patel, 2021).

Hypertension is also seen in this patient population when the hematocrit rapidly increases to a high level. Therefore, the hemoglobin and blood pressure should be checked frequently when a patient with kidney disease begins erythropoietin therapy. The dose of erythropoietin should be titrated to the goal hemoglobin based on available guidelines (Patel & Patel, 2021). Some patients may require initiation of antihypertensive therapy.

Anemia of Chronic Disease

The term "anemia of chronic disease" is a misnomer in that only the chronic diseases of inflammation, infection, and malignancy cause this type of anemia. Many chronic inflammatory diseases are associated with a **normochromic, normocytic** anemia (i.e., the erythrocytes are normal in color and size). These disorders include rheumatoid arthritis; severe, chronic infections; and many cancers. It is, therefore, imperative that the "chronic disease" be diagnosed when this form of anemia is identified so that it can be managed appropriately.

The anemia is usually mild to moderate and nonprogressive. It develops gradually over 6 to 8 weeks and then stabilizes at a hematocrit seldom less than 25%. The hemoglobin level rarely falls below 9 g/dL, and the bone marrow has normal cellularity with increased stores of iron as the iron is diverted from the serum.

Most of these patients have few symptoms and do not require treatment for the anemia. With successful treatment of the underlying disorder, the bone marrow iron is used to make erythrocytes and the hemoglobin level rises.

Hemolytic Anemias

In hemolytic anemias, premature destruction of erythrocytes results in the liberation of hemoglobin from the erythrocytes into the plasma. The increased erythrocyte destruction leads to tissue hypoxia, which, in turn, stimulates erythropoietin production. This increased production is reflected in an increased reticulocyte count as the bone marrow responds to the destruction of erythrocytes. The released hemoglobin is converted in large part to bilirubin; therefore, the bilirubin concentration rises. **Hemolysis** can result from an abnormality within the erythrocyte itself (e.g., sickle cell anemia, glucose-6-phosphate dehydrogenase [G-6-PD] deficiency) or within the plasma (e.g., immune hemolytic anemias), or from direct injury to the erythrocyte within the circulation (e.g., hemolysis caused by mechanical heart valve).

In hemolytic anemias, the erythrocytes have a shortened lifespan; thus, their number in the circulation is reduced. Fewer erythrocytes result in decreased available oxygen, causing hypoxia, which, in turn, stimulates an increase in erythropoietin release from the kidney. The erythropoietin stimulates the bone marrow to compensate by producing new erythrocytes and releasing some of them into the circulation somewhat prematurely as reticulocytes. If the red cell destruction persists, the hemoglobin is broken down excessively; about 80% of the heme is converted to bilirubin, conjugated in the liver, and excreted in the bile.

The mechanism of erythrocyte destruction varies, but all types of hemolytic anemia share certain laboratory features: the reticulocyte count is elevated, the fraction of indirect (unconjugated) bilirubin is increased, and the supply of haptoglobin (a binding protein for free hemoglobin) is depleted as more hemoglobin is released. As a result, the plasma haptoglobin level is low. The severity of anemia will increase if the marrow does not compensate by replacing the hemolyzed erythrocytes (poor response indicated by a decreased reticulocyte count). Causes of hemolytic anemia are discussed in Box 19-3.

BOX 19-3

Causes of Hemolytic Anemias

Inherited Hemolytic Anemia

- Abnormal hemoglobin:
  - Sickle cell anemia
  - Thalassemia
- RBC membrane abnormality:
  - Hereditary spherocytosis
  - Hereditary elliptocytosis
  - Acanthocytosis
  - Stomatocytosis
- Enzyme deficiencies:
  - Glucose-6-phosphate dehydrogenase (G-6-PD) deficiency

Acquired Hemolytic Anemia

- Antibody-related:
  - Iso-antibody/transfusion reaction
  - Autoimmune hemolytic anemia (AIHA)
  - Cold agglutinin disease
- Not antibody-related:
  - RBC membrane defects
  - Paroxysmal nocturnal hemoglobinuria (PNH)
  - Liver disease
  - Uremia
  - Trauma
  - Mechanical heart valve
  - Microangiopathic hemolytic anemia
  - Infection
  - Bacterial
  - Parasitic
  - Disseminated intravascular coagulation (DIC)
  - Toxins
  - Hypersplenism

Autoimmune Hemolytic Anemia

Autoimmune hemolytic anemia (AIHA) results when the patient's own immune system hemolyzes RBCs (Berensten & Barcellini, 2021). Hemolysis results from antibodies directed against surface antigens on the erythrocyte (Berensten & Barcellini, 2021). The term AIHA is used to describe a group of pathologies that each differ in terms of their pathophysiology and clinical presentation (Berensten & Barcellini, 2021); these pathologies include warm AIHA, cold agglutinin disease/syndrome, and drug-induced AIHA (Berensten & Barcellini, 2021).

Warm AIHA

Pathophysiology

The pathophysiology of warm AIHA is complex. It involves the activation of the mononuclear phagocytic system, T-lymphocyte system, and, in 50% of cases, the complement system. In warm AIHA, antibodies bind to erythrocytes most actively at temperatures of 37° C (98.6° F) (Berensten & Barcellini, 2021). While 50% of cases of warm AIHA are due to unknown cause, common underlying etiologies include immunologic or lymphoproliferative disorders such as chronic lymphocytic leukemia (CLL) or systemic lupus erythematosus (SLE) (Berensten & Barcellini, 2021). COVID-19 has also been associated with warm AIHA (Berensten & Barcellini, 2021).

Medical Management

In warm AIHA, the treatment includes high doses of corticosteroids, which decrease the macrophage's ability to clear the antibody-coated erythrocytes. If the hemoglobin level returns to normal, usually after several weeks, the corticosteroid dose can be lowered or, in some cases, tapered and discontinued. However, corticosteroids rarely produce a lasting remission. Additional immunosuppressive agents used in the treatment of warm AIHA include the monoclonal antibody rituximab, azathioprine, cyclophosphamide, cyclosporine, mycophenolate mofetil, bortezomib, and intravenous immunoglobulin (Berensten & Barcellini, 2021). Splenectomy (removal of the spleen) removes the major site of erythrocyte destruction; therefore, splenectomy may be performed if medications do not produce a remission (Berensten & Barcellini, 2021). Transfusions may be necessary if the anemia is severe; it may be extremely difficult to cross-match samples of available units of packed red blood cells (PRBCs) with that of the patient.

Cold Agglutinin Disease

Pathophysiology

Cold agglutinin disease is a rare AIHA in which cold-reactive antibodies, or autoantibodies that bind to antigens on erythrocytes at temperatures below 37° C (<98.6° F), cause erythrocyte agglutination or clumping (Berensten &

Barcellini, 2021; Roth et al., 2021). Like warm AIHA, the hemolysis in cold agglutinin disease is also driven by activation of the complement system, which leads to erythrocyte phagocytosis by the mononuclear phagocytic system in the liver (Berensten & Barcellini, 2021; Roth et al., 2021). Erythrocyte agglutination from this disease can lead to impaired circulation and acrocyanosis (cyanosis of the hands and feet caused by slow circulation), which can cause cold-induced circulatory disorders such as Raynaud-like phenomena (Berensten & Barcellini, 2021). Cold agglutinin disease is a low-grade, clonal, lymphoproliferative bone marrow disorder, whereas cold-agglutinin syndrome is a transient disorder caused by infections (i.e., influenza, COVID-19), malignancy, and autoimmune disorders (Jensen et al., 2020; Roth et al., 2021).

Medical Management

There is no approved treatment for cold-agglutinin disease. High-dose corticosteroids should not be used to treat this disorder given poor response rates with this treatment (Berensten & Barcellini, 2021). Rituximab is an effective treatment, though relapse commonly occurs within 1 year (Roth et al., 2020). Eculizumab is another monoclonal antibody that reduces the need for transfusion (Roth et al., 2020). Additional treatments include cytotoxic agents such as fludarabine and bendamustine (Roth et al., 2020). Treatment of the underlying disorder may improve cold agglutinin syndrome (Berensten & Barcellini, 2021).

Drug-Induced Hemolytic Anemia

Drug-induced hemolytic anemia is an immunologically mediated hemolytic anemia induced by medications (Berensten & Barcellini, 2021). There are two subtypes, drug-dependent, which relies on the presence of the offending agent, and drug-independent which persists even in the absence of the medication. A number of medications have the potential to induce drug-induced hemolytic anemia. Common medications include antibiotics (i.e., ceftriaxone, cephalosporins, and piperacillin), nonsteroidal anti-inflammatory medications, fludarabine, bendamustine, and checkpoint inhibitors (Berensten & Barcellini, 2021). Medical management includes discontinuance of the offending agent (Berensten & Barcellini, 2021).

Nursing Management

Patients may have great difficulty understanding the pathologic mechanisms underlying the disease and may need repeated explanations in terms they can understand. Patients who have had a splenectomy should be vaccinated against pneumococcal and encapsulated bacterial infections (e.g., Pneumovax) and informed that they are permanently at greater risk for infection. Patients receiving long-term corticosteroid therapy, particularly those with concurrent diabetes mellitus (DM) or hypertension (HTN), need careful monitoring of blood sugar and blood pressure. They must understand the need for adherence to the medication and the importance of never abruptly discontinuing it. A written explanation and a tapering schedule should be provided, and needed adjustments based on hemoglobin levels should be emphasized. Similar teaching should be provided when immunosuppressive agents are used. Corticosteroid therapy is not without significant risk, and patients need to be monitored closely for complications. The nurse also educates patients with cold agglutinin disease/syndrome to avoid cold temperatures and reinforces the need for thermal protection (Berensten & Barcellini, 2021).

Pearls for Practice

The spleen plays a major role in preventing infection against different organisms, including Streptococcus, Neisseria, and Haemophilus (Mondor, 2022). Patients who have a splenectomy are at risk for overwhelming postsplenectomy infection (OPSI); the risk is greatest in the first 2 years after removal (Ferri, 2022). In fact, patients without a spleen (asplenic) have a two- to threefold increase of sepsis and infection-related mortality (Aulakh, 2022). The common organism S. pneumoniae is responsible for 50% to 90% of all cases. Currently the standard of care includes immunization with pneumococcal, meningococcal, and Haemophilus influenzae type B vaccines within 2 weeks of splenectomy if the patient was not immunized prior to splenectomy. The rates of OPSI are reported to be less than 3% after routine immunization (Villamizar, 2021).

Thalassemia

The thalassemias are a group of hereditary anemias characterized by **hypochromia** (an abnormal decrease in the hemoglobin content of erythrocytes), extreme **microcytosis** (smaller-than-normal erythrocytes), destruction of blood elements (hemolysis), and variable degrees of anemia due to impaired hemoglobin production and ineffective RBC production (Taher et al., 2021). The thalassemias occur worldwide, but the highest prevalence is found in people of Mediterranean, African, and Southeast Asian ancestry.

Thalassemias are classified into two major groups according to which hemoglobin chain is diminished: alpha or beta. The alpha thalassemias occur mainly in people with Asian and Middle Eastern ancestry, and the beta thalassemias are most prevalent in people with ancestry from Mediterranean regions but also occur in those with Middle Eastern or Asian ancestry. The alpha thalassemias are milder than the beta forms and often occur without symptoms; the erythrocytes are extremely microcytic, but the anemia, if present, is mild.

The severity of beta thalassemia varies depending on the extent to which the hemoglobin chains are affected. Patients with mild forms have a microcytosis and mild anemia. If left untreated, severe beta thalassemia (*thalassemia major*, or *Cooley anemia*) can be fatal within the first few years of life. Peripheral blood stem cell transplant (PBSCT) offers a chance of cure, but when this is not possible, the disease is usually treated with transfusion of PRBCs. Complications related to lifelong transfusions include the development of anti-RBC antibodies, transfusion-associated infections, and iron overload. Transfusional iron overload is the primary cause of death in patients with thalassemia (90% of deaths). In the 1980s, life expectancy was not expected to exceed the third decade of life. However, with improvements in methods to measure iron overload as well as treatments for iron overload, life expectancy has improved (Taher et al., 2021).

Patient teaching during the reproductive years should include preconception counseling about the risk of thalassemia major.

Treatment of iron overload involves the use of chelating agents. Deferoxamine (given IV or SQ), deferasirox (oral), and deferiprone (oral) are used alone or in combination to treat iron overload. Each medication requires monitoring for toxicity, including agranulocytosis (deficiency of granulocytes in the blood, causing increased vulnerability to infection), neutropenia (deferiprone), liver function abnormalities (deferasirox), annual eye and hearing examinations (due to risk for ocular toxicity and ototoxicity) (all) (Taher et al., 2021). Side effects of the oral agents include nausea, vomiting, diarrhea, and abdominal pain and may contribute to interruptions in therapy. Adherence with these agents is essential to response; therefore, nursing education should focus on necessary monitoring parameters and the importance of taking agents as directed.

SECONDARY POLYCYTHEMIA

Polycythemia, literally meaning "too many cells in the blood," refers to an increased number of erythrocytes. It is a term used when the hematocrit is elevated (to greater than 55% in males, greater than 50% in females). Polycythemia is classified as either primary or secondary (Tefferi, 2020). Primary polycythemia, also known as polycythemia vera (PV) is a malignant condition that will be described later in the chapter; secondary polycythemia is a benign condition, discussed below.

Pathophysiology

Secondary polycythemia is caused by excessive production of erythropoietin. This may occur in response to a reduced amount of oxygen, which acts as a hypoxic stimulus, as in cigarette smoking, obstructive sleep apnea, chronic obstructive pulmonary disease (COPD), or cyanotic heart disease, or in nonpathologic conditions, such as living at a high altitude. It can also result from certain hemoglobinopathies (e.g., hemoglobin Chesapeake), in which the hemoglobin has an abnormally high affinity for oxygen. Secondary polycythemia can also occur from neoplasms (e.g., renal cell carcinoma) that stimulate erythropoietin production.

Medical and Nursing Management

Management of secondary polycythemia generally involves treatment of the underlying primary conditions. If the cause cannot be corrected (e.g., by treating the renal cell carcinoma or improving pulmonary function), therapeutic phlebotomy may be necessary in symptomatic patients to reduce blood viscosity and volume. Iron replacement may be necessary to avoid further production of microcytic hypochromic erythrocytes (Tefferi, 2022).

CLINICAL MANIFESTATIONS AND ASSESSMENT OF ANEMIA

Aside from the severity of the anemia itself, several factors influence the development of anemia-associated symptoms:

- The rapidity with which the anemia has developed
- The duration of the anemia (i.e., chronicity)
- The metabolic requirements of the patient
- Other concurrent disorders or disabilities (e.g., cardiopulmonary disease)

In general, the more rapidly an anemia develops, the more severe its symptoms. An otherwise healthy person can often tolerate as much as a 50% gradual reduction in hemoglobin without pronounced symptoms or significant incapacity, whereas the rapid loss of as little as 30% may precipitate profound vascular collapse in the same person. A person who has become gradually anemic, with hemoglobin levels between 9 and 11 g/dL, may have few or no symptoms other than mild tachycardia on exertion and fatigue.

People who usually are very active or who have significant demands on their lives are more likely to experience symptoms. Patients with hypothyroidism with decreased oxygen needs may be completely asymptomatic, without tachycardia or increased cardiac output, at a hemoglobin level of 10 g/dL. Similarly, patients with coexistent cardiac, vascular, or pulmonary disease may develop more pronounced symptoms of anemia (e.g., dyspnea, chest pain, muscle pain or cramping) at a higher hemoglobin level than those without these concurrent health problems.

The most common signs and symptoms of anemia are discussed in Box 19-2. A careful and thorough assessment is essential in identifying potential complications and targeting nursing interventions.

A variety of hematologic studies are performed to determine the type and cause of the anemia (see Chapter 18 for a detailed overview). In an initial evaluation, the hemoglobin, **hematocrit**, reticulocyte count, and RBC indices, particularly the MCV and red cell distribution width (RDW), are particularly useful. Iron studies (serum iron level, total iron-binding capacity [TIBC], % saturation, and ferritin), as well as serum vitamin B_{12} and folate levels are also frequently obtained. Other tests include haptoglobin (if hemolysis is suspected) and erythropoietin levels. The remaining complete blood count (CBC) values are useful in determining whether the anemia is an isolated problem or part of another hematologic condition, such as **leukemia** or myelodysplastic syndrome (MDS) (a group of disorders where the bone marrow does not produce enough healthy blood cells). Bone marrow aspiration and biopsy may be performed. In addition, other diagnostic studies, including endoscopy and colonoscopy, may be performed to determine the presence of underlying chronic illness, such as malignancy, or the source of any blood loss, such as polyps or ulcers within the gastrointestinal (GI) tract.

NURSING MANAGEMENT

Managing Fatigue

The most common symptom and complication of anemia is fatigue. This distressing symptom is too often minimized by health care providers. Fatigue is often the symptom that has the greatest negative impact on a patient's level of functioning and consequent quality of life. Patients often describe the fatigue from anemia as oppressive. Fatigue can interfere with a person's ability to work, both inside and outside the home. It can disrupt relationships with family and friends. Patients often lose interest in hobbies and activities, including sexual activity. The severity of distress from fatigue is often related to a person's responsibilities and life demands as well as the amount of assistance and support received from others.

Other factors that may be contributing to fatigue should also be assessed and managed including pain, emotional distress, sleep disturbances, comorbidities, physical deconditioning, and nutritional deficiencies (National Comprehensive Cancer Network [NCCN], 2023).

Nursing interventions can focus on assisting the patient to prioritize activities and to establish a balance between activity and rest that is realistic and feasible from the patient's perspective. Patients with chronic anemia need to maintain some physical activity and exercise to prevent the deconditioning that results from inactivity. Short periods of daily exercise can also decrease the severity of fatigue (Brennan-Cook, 2020).

Maintaining Adequate Nutrition

Inadequate intake of essential nutrients, such as iron, vitamin B_{12}, and folic acid can cause anemia. The symptoms associated with anemia (e.g., fatigue, anorexia) can, in turn, interfere with maintaining adequate nutrition. A healthy diet should be encouraged. The nurse may inform the patient that alcohol interferes with the utilization of essential nutrients and should advise the patient to avoid alcoholic beverages or to limit intake. Dietary teaching sessions should be individualized and culturally sensitive to food preferences and food preparation. The involvement of family members enhances compliance with dietary recommendations. Dietary supplements (e.g., vitamins, iron, folate, protein) may be prescribed as well depending on the results of testing.

Equally important, the patient and family must understand the underlying cause of the anemia because many forms of anemia are not the result of a nutritional deficiency. In such cases, even an excessive intake of nutritional supplements will not improve the anemia. A potential problem in patients with chronic transfusion requirements occurs with the indiscriminate use of iron supplements. These individuals are at risk for iron overload from their transfusions. The addition of an iron supplement will only increase their iron burden, contributing to risk for end-organ damage.

Maintaining Adequate Perfusion

Patients with acute blood loss or severe hemolysis may have decreased tissue perfusion from decreased blood volume or reduced circulating erythrocytes (decreased hematocrit). Lost volume is replaced with transfusions or IV fluids, based on the symptoms and the laboratory test results. Supplemental oxygen may be necessary, but it is rarely needed on a long-term basis unless there is underlying severe cardiac or pulmonary disease. The nurse monitors the patient's vital signs and pulse oximetry readings closely; other medications, such as antihypertensive agents, may need to be adjusted or withheld.

Complications

General complications of severe anemia include heart failure, paresthesias (abnormal sensation of pricking, tingling, numbness, burning, etc.), and confusion. At any given level of anemia, patients with underlying heart disease are far more likely to have angina or symptoms of heart failure than those without heart disease.

PLATELET DISORDERS

Thrombocythemia

Thrombocythemia is the overproduction of platelets. There are two types with very different etiologies and treatment approaches: primary or essential (a malignant condition described later in the chapter) and secondary (a benign condition discussed here). Refer to Chapter 18 for discussion of bleeding disorders.

SECONDARY THROMBOCYTOSIS

Increased platelet production is the primary mechanism of secondary, or reactive, **thrombocytosis**. The platelet count is above normal, but, in contrast to primary thrombocythemia, an increase to more than 1 million/mm^3 is rare. Platelet function is normal; the platelet survival time is normal or decreased. Consequently, symptoms associated with hemorrhage or thrombosis are rare. Many disorders or conditions can cause a reactive increase in platelets, including infection, chronic inflammatory disorders, iron deficiency, malignant disease, acute hemorrhage, and splenectomy (see later discussion of primary thrombocythemia). Treatment is aimed at the underlying disorder. With successful management, the platelet count usually returns to normal.

THROMBOCYTOPENIA

Thrombocytopenia (low platelet level) can result from various factors: decreased production of platelets within the bone marrow, increased destruction of platelets, or increased consumption of platelets. There are numerous causes of thrombocytopenia, including malignancy, infection, medications, autoimmunity immune thrombocytopenia purpura (ITP), and disseminated intravascular coagulation (DIC). The primary strategy for managing thrombocytopenia is correction or treatment of the underlying cause or removal of the offending agent.

Clinical Manifestations and Assessment

Bleeding and petechiae usually do not occur with platelet counts greater than 50,000/mm^3, although excessive bleeding can follow surgery or trauma. When the platelet count drops to less than 20,000/mm^3, petechiae can appear, along with spontaneous nasal and gingival bleeding, excessive menstrual bleeding, and excessive bleeding after surgery or dental extractions. When the platelet count is less than 10,000/mm^3, spontaneous, potentially fatal CNS or GI hemorrhage can occur. If the platelets are dysfunctional due to disease (e.g., MDS) or medications (e.g., aspirin), the risk for bleeding may be much greater even when the actual platelet count is not significantly reduced.

A platelet deficiency that results from decreased production (e.g., leukemia, MDS) is diagnosed by examining the bone marrow via aspiration and biopsy. Infections, either viral or bacterial, as well as alcohol can suppress platelet production. Therefore, laboratory tests should include testing for HIV and hepatitis B and C.

When platelet destruction is the cause of thrombocytopenia, the marrow shows increased megakaryocytes (the cells from which the platelets originate) and normal or even increased platelet production as the body attempts to compensate for the decreased platelets in circulation. Another cause of thrombocytopenia is sequestration. Approximately one third of the circulating platelets are within the spleen, and a greatly enlarged spleen results in increased sequestration of platelets.

Many medications (e.g., sulfa drugs, methotrexate) can either decrease platelet production or shorten their lifespan. Numerous genetic causes of thrombocytopenia have been discovered, including autosomal dominant, autosomal recessive, and X-linked mutations (Maida, 2021).

An important cause to exclude is *pseudothrombocytopenia*. Here, platelets aggregate and clump in the presence of ethylenediamine tetra-acetic acid (EDTA), the anticoagulant present in the tube used for CBC collection. This clumping accounts for up to 30% of instances of isolated thrombocytopenia (Scavone et al., 2021). A manual examination of the peripheral smear can easily determine platelet clumping as the cause of thrombocytopenia; newer cell counter machines can also detect this.

Medical Management

The management of thrombocytopenia is usually treatment of the underlying cause. If the platelet count is low due to medications, removal of the offending agent may improve the platelet count. Medications strongly associated with thrombocytopenia include antibiotics (quinine, quinidine, penicillin, cephalosporin, vancomycin, trimethoprim-sulfamethoxazole, sulfonamides, and sulfonylureas), cardiovascular medications (digoxin, salicylates, and abciximab), and some miscellaneous agents (cimetidine, famotidine, ranitidine, valproate, and interferon) (Arnold & Cuker, 2021). When the platelet count is predictably lowered as a result of chemotherapy treatment, platelet transfusions may be needed to support the patient and prevent bleeding.

In hospitalized patients with chemotherapy-induced thrombocytopenia, platelets should be transfused to maintain a platelet count of more than 10,000/mm^3 to reduce the risk for spontaneous bleeding (Khan & Anwer, 2021). Outpatients may be transfused more liberally (e.g., a platelet count less than 20,000/mm^3) because they may not be able to get daily transfusions due to logistical constraints (e.g., transportation availability). See Table 19-6 for further information on platelet transfusion parameters.

If excessive platelet destruction occurs, transfused platelets are also destroyed, and the platelet count does not increase. The most common cause of excessive platelet destruction is immune thrombocytopenia purpura (ITP) (see the following discussion). In some instances, splenectomy can be a useful therapeutic intervention, but often it is not an option; for example, in patients in whom the spleen is enlarged due to portal hypertension related to cirrhosis, splenectomy may cause more bleeding disorders.

Nursing Management

Nursing interventions for patients with thrombocytopenia are listed in Chapter 18, Box 18-3.

IMMUNE THROMBOCYTOPENIA PURPURA (ITP)

ITP is a hematologic disorder that is characterized by autoimmune destruction of platelets that results in thrombocytopenia (platelet count $<100 \times 10^9$ /L) as well as bleeding and/or bruising (Singh et al., 2021). Historically, this disorder was referred to as "idiopathic" thrombocytopenia purpura because in many cases the underlying causes were unknown. In recent years, scientists have uncovered a number of etiologies leading to our current understanding of ITP as an autoimmune process, thus leading to the change in terminology from *idiopathic* to *immune* (Song & Al-Samkari, 2021). There are two forms of ITP: primary and secondary. Primary ITP is the presence of thrombocytopenia in the absence of potential cause (i.e., infection, cancer). Secondary ITP is thrombocytopenia that results from a condition (i.e., SLE), disorder, or medication, such as sulfa drugs (Song & Al-Samkari, 2021).

Pathophysiology

Although the precise cause of ITP remains unknown, the platelet count is decreased by a combination of T-cell dysregulation, antibody-mediated platelet destruction, and impaired platelet production secondary to antiplatelet antibodies produced by B cells (Sing et al., 2021). In addition, there is an inappropriately low rise in serum thrombopoietin, a hormone that stimulates platelet production (Kuter, 2021). Antiplatelet antibodies may also be present in the blood (Kuter, 2021).

Clinical Manifestations and Assessment

Many patients have no symptoms, and the low platelet count is an incidental finding. Common physical manifestations are easy bruising, heavy menses, and petechiae on the extremities or trunk. Patients with simple bruising or petechiae, termed "dry purpura," tend to have fewer complications from bleeding than do those with bleeding from mucosal surfaces, such as the GI tract (including the mouth) and pulmonary system (e.g., hemoptysis), termed "wet purpura." Patients with wet purpura have a greater risk of intracranial bleeding than do those with dry purpura.

Severe bleeding is rare in patients with platelet counts exceeding 30,000/mm^3 (Kuter, 2021). Despite low platelet quantity, the platelets are young and very functional. They adhere to endothelial surfaces and to one another so that spontaneous bleeding does not always occur. Thus, treatment may not be initiated unless bleeding becomes severe or life-threatening, the platelet count is extremely low (less than 10,000/mm^3), or in those with risk factors for bleeding, such as uncontrolled hypertension or peptic ulcer disease (Kuter, 2021).

Medical Management

The primary goal of treatment is a "safe" platelet count. Because the risk for bleeding typically does not increase until the platelet count is less than 10,000/mm^3, a patient whose count exceeds 30,000/mm^3 to 50,000/mm^3 may be carefully observed without additional intervention. However, if the count is less than 30,000/mm^3 or if bleeding occurs, corticosteroids are the standard first-line treatment (Kuter, 2021). Corticosteroids moderate immune function and impair macrophage recognition of auto-antibody–coated platelets (Singh et al., 2021). Second-line therapies for patients who do not improve on steroids or whose platelet count drops after cessation of steroids include splenectomy, rituximab, and thrombopoietin receptor antagonists (TPO-RAs) (Neunert et al., 2019).

Splenectomy removes the mechanism for platelet destruction (Singh et al., 2021). Patients who have undergone splenectomy are permanently at risk for sepsis, most commonly caused by pneumococcus or encapsulated bacteria. Though the incidence of sepsis in asplenia is relatively rare, when sepsis does develop in asplenic patients, there is a mortality rate of up to 50% (Bayrhuber et al., 2020). Prevention of fatal infection depends on comprehensive patient education, vaccination, and early antibiotic initiation in the onset of fever (Tahir et al., 2020). Prior to splenectomy, these patients should receive pneumococci (Pneumovax), *Haemophilus influenzae* type B, influenza virus, and meningococcal vaccines. PCV13 followed by PPSV23 8 weeks later is recommended for the prevention of pneumococcal infection; the series should be completed at least 2 weeks before splenectomy. A second dose of PPSV23 should be repeated in 5 years. Boosters of the meningococcal vaccine must be given every 5 years, and influenza vaccines should be given every year (Tahir et al., 2020). If an asplenic patient has a fever, antibiotics should be administered immediately. For this reason, asplenic patients are often given prescriptions for antibiotics such as amoxicillin or levofloxacin so that they always have antibiotics on hand.

Rituximab, a monoclonal antibody that targets the CD 20 marker on B cells, has been used successfully to treat ITP following treatment with steroids. Rituximab depletes the B cells that produce platelet-destroying autoantibodies, effectively increasing the platelet count. Although rituximab has not been approved by the U.S. Food and Drug Administration (FDA) for the treatment of ITP, it is widely used in clinical practice. Studies have demonstrated a response rate between 40% and 70%; however, when used in combination with dexamethasone, higher response rates have been seen (Song & Al-Samkari, 2021). Rituximab is well tolerated and has few side effects. Immunosuppression is an important consideration particularly given the recent COVID-19 pandemic. The B-cell depletion effect of rituximab may impair response to vaccinations, such as the COVID-19 vaccine, for 6 months or greater after treatment (Song & Al-Samkari, 2021).

Romiplostim and eltrombopag are thrombopoietin receptor agonists (TPO-Ras) that promote platelet production by stimulating proliferation and differentiation of platelet precursors (Song & Al-Samkari, 2021). Romiplostim is administered weekly via subcutaneous injection, and eltrombopag is a pill given once daily. These drugs are not currently considered curative, and most patients require continuation of therapy to maintain response (Kuter, 2021).

Despite the extremely low platelet count, platelet transfusions are usually avoided. Transfusions tend to be ineffective because the patient's antiplatelet antibodies bind with the transfused platelets, causing them to be destroyed. Platelet counts can actually drop after platelet transfusion. Occasionally, transfusion of platelets may protect against catastrophic bleeding in patients with severe wet purpura.

Nursing Management

Nursing care includes an assessment of the patient's lifestyle to determine the risk of bleeding from activity. Also a careful medication history is obtained, including use of over-the-counter medications, herbs, and nutritional supplements. The nurse must be alert for sulfa-containing medications and others that alter platelet function (e.g., aspirin-based or other nonsteroidal anti-inflammatory drugs [NSAIDs]) (see Box 19-4). The nurse assesses for any history of recent viral illness and for risk factors for hepatitis and HIV. Reports of headache or visual disturbances should be reported to the licensed provider immediately as these symptoms can signal intracranial bleeding. Patients who are admitted to the hospital with wet purpura and low platelet counts should have a neurologic assessment incorporated into their routine vital sign measurements. All IM injections and rectal medications should be avoided, and rectal temperature measurements should not be performed because they can stimulate bleeding.

Patient teaching addresses signs of exacerbation of disease (petechiae, ecchymoses, wet purpura), how to contact appropriate health care personnel, the name and type of medication inducing ITP (if appropriate), current medical treatment (medications, tapering schedule if relevant, side effects), and the frequency of monitoring the platelet count. The patient is instructed to avoid all agents that interfere with platelet function (see Box 19-4). The patient should avoid constipation, as well as the Valsalva maneuver (straining to have a bowel movement). Electric razors should be used for shaving, and soft-bristled toothbrushes should replace stiff-bristled ones. The patient is also counseled to refrain from sexual intercourse when the platelet count is less than 50,000/mm^3. Patients who are receiving corticosteroids long term are at risk for complications, including osteoporosis, proximal muscle wasting, cataract formation, and dental caries. Bone mineral density should be monitored, and these patients may benefit from calcium and vitamin D supplementation and bisphosphonate therapy to prevent significant bone disease.

BOX 19-4

Medications and Substances that Impair Platelet Function

- Anesthetic agents:
  - Local anesthetics
  - Halothane
- Antibiotics:
  - Beta-lactam antibiotics
  - Penicillins
  - Cephalosporins
  - Nitrofurantoin
  - Sulfonamides
- Anticoagulation agents:
  - Heparin
  - Fibrinolytic agents
- Anti-inflammatory agents (Nonsteroidal):
  - Aspirin
  - Ibuprofen
  - Naproxen
- Antineoplastic agents:
  - Carmustine
  - Daunorubicin
  - Mithramycin
- Cardiovascular drugs:
  - Beta blockers
  - Calcium-channel blockers
  - Isosorbide
  - Nitroglycerine
  - Nitroprusside
  - Quinidine
- Medications that increase platelet cAMP:
  - Dipyridamole
  - Prostacyclin
  - Theophylline
- Food and food additives:
  - Caffeine
  - Chinese black tree fungus
  - Clove
  - Cumin
  - Ethanol
  - Fish oils
  - Garlic
  - Onion extract
  - Turmeric
- Plasma expanders:
  - Dextrans
  - Hydroxyethyl starch
- Psychotropic agents:
  - Tricyclic antidepressants
  - Phenothiazines
- Miscellaneous:
  - Antihistamines
  - Clofibrate
  - Furosemide
  - Heroin
  - Contrast agents
  - Ticlopidine
  - Vitamin E
- Herbal supplements:
  - Feverfew
  - Ginger
  - Gingko
  - Ginseng
  - Kava

PLATELET DEFECTS

Quantitative platelet defects are relatively common (thrombocytopenia), but qualitative defects can occur also. With qualitative defects, the number of platelets may be normal, but the platelets do not function normally. See Chapter 18 for an outline of testing for platelet defects.

An important functional platelet disorder is that induced by aspirin. Even small amounts of aspirin reduce normal platelet aggregation, and the prolonged bleeding time lasts for several days after aspirin ingestion. Although this does not cause bleeding in most people, patients with a coagulation disorder (e.g., hemophilia) or thrombocytopenia can have significant bleeding after taking aspirin, particularly if invasive procedures or trauma has occurred.

NSAIDs can also inhibit platelet function, but the effect is not as prolonged as with aspirin (about 5 days vs. 7 to 10 days). Other causes of platelet dysfunction include possibly metabolic products affecting platelet function, MDS, multiple myeloma (MM) (due to abnormal proteins interfering with platelet function), cardiopulmonary bypass, and other medications (see Box 19-4).

Clinical Manifestations and Assessment

Bleeding may be mild or severe. The extent is not necessarily correlated with the platelet count or with tests that measure coagulation (prothrombin time [PT], partial thromboplastin time [PTT]). Ecchymoses are common, particularly on the extremities. Patients with platelet dysfunction may be at risk for significant bleeding after trauma or invasive procedures (e.g., biopsy, dental extraction).

Medical Management

If the platelet dysfunction is caused by medication, use of the offending medication should be stopped, if possible, particularly when bleeding occurs or prior to an invasive procedure. If platelet dysfunction is marked, bleeding often can be prevented by transfusion of normal platelets before or during invasive procedures. Aminocaproic acid, an antifibrinolytic agent, may be required to prevent significant bleeding after such procedures.

Nursing Management

Patients with significant platelet dysfunction need to be instructed to avoid substances that can diminish platelet function, such as certain over-the-counter medications, herbs, nutritional supplements, and alcohol. They also need to serve as their own advocates and inform their health care providers (including dentists) of the underlying condition before any invasive procedure is performed so that appropriate steps can be initiated to diminish the risk of bleeding. Bleeding precautions should be initiated as appropriate (see Chapter 18, Box 18-2).

BLEEDING DISORDERS

Von Willebrand Disease

Von Willebrand disease (vWD) is the most common inherited bleeding disorder in humans (Rick, 2021). The disease is a result of deficiency, dysfunction, or absence of von Willebrand Factor (vWF) (Rick, 2021). vWF is necessary for factor VIII activity and is essential for platelet adhesion at the site of vascular injury. Although synthesis of factor VIII is normal in vWD, its half-life is shortened; therefore, factor VIII levels are mildly low (15% to 50% of normal).

There are three types of vWD. Type 1, the most common, is a quantitative defect in vWF and is inherited in an autosomal dominant pattern (Rick, 2021). Type 2 shows variable qualitative defects based on the specific vWF subtype involved (with subtypes 2A, 2B, 2M, and 2N). Type 3 is very rare and is characterized by a severe vWF deficiency as well as by a significant deficiency of factor VIII.

Clinical Manifestations and Assessment

The history should include questions related to bleeding following a procedure, such as a dental procedure; need for blood transfusions following surgery or childbirth; history of heavy menses; and easy bruising (Rick, 2021). Patients commonly have mucocutaneous bleeding, including nosebleeds and large bruises (Rick, 2021). Females may report heavy menses. Bleeding with minor surgery may also be seen. Joint bleeding is uncommon (Rick, 2021).

Laboratory test results show a normal platelet count but a prolonged bleeding time and a normal or slightly prolonged PTT. These defects are not static, and laboratory test results can vary widely within the same patient over time. As the laboratory values can vary over time so can the history and extent of bleeding. For example, a careful history of prior bleeding may show little problem with postoperative bleeding on one occasion but significant bleeding from a dental extraction at another time. Laboratory tests required to diagnose vWD include the vWF ristocetin cofactor activity, vWF antigen, factor VIII activity, and, for patients with suspected type 2 defects, vWF multimers (Rick, 2021).

Medical Management

The goal of treatment is to replace the deficient protein (e.g., vWF or factor VIII) at the time of spontaneous bleeding or prior to an invasive procedure to minimize postprocedural bleeding. There are two general strategies to meet this goal. For types 1 and 1A, the first line of treatment is administration of a synthetic form of the hormone vasopressin, called desmopressin (DDAVP). Desmopressin causes the release of vWF stored within the endothelium, resulting in a temporary increase in circulating vWF and factor VIII (Rick, 2021). Desmopressin can be administered intranasally or intravenously. With major surgery or invasive procedures, IV administration is preferable. DDAVP is contraindicated in patients with unstable coronary artery disease because it can induce platelet aggregation and can cause an MI. Side effects include headache, facial flushing, tachycardia, hyponatremia from free water retention, and, rarely, seizures. DDAVP should be used with caution in type 2B vWD because of risk of thrombocytopenia and has no efficacy for type 3 vWD (Rick, 2021).

The second strategy is the administration of concentrates of vWF and factor VIII (Rick, 2021). Administration of these agents shortens bleeding time through normalization of multimer patterns (Rick, 2021). Replacement continues for several days to ensure correction of the factor VIII deficiency. The dosage and frequency of administration depend on factor VIII levels; doses may need regular adjustment based on trough levels. Antibody (inhibitor) formation is usually seen only in patients with type 3 vWD when large amounts of replacement products have been administered.

Other agents may be effective in reducing the bleeding. Aminocaproic acid is useful in managing mild forms of mucosal bleeding, for example, prior to dental work (Rick, 2021). Hormonal contraceptives, such as the levonorgestrel-releasing intrauterine device, have demonstrated efficacy in reducing menorrhagia in females with bleeding disorders (Rick, 2021). Platelet transfusions may be useful when significant bleeding is present.

Pearls for Practice

Avoidance of aspirin and other NSAIDs is important nursing education to share with patients who have vWD.

ACQUIRED COAGULATION DISORDERS

The most common causes of acquired coagulation disorders include liver disease, vitamin K deficiency, and DIC, all of which can result in abnormal bleeding.

LIVER DISEASE

With the exception of factor VIII, most blood coagulation factors are synthesized in the liver. Therefore, liver dysfunction (due to cirrhosis, tumor, or hepatitis; see Chapter 24) can result in diminished amounts of the factors needed to maintain coagulation and hemostasis. Prolongation of the PT, unless it is caused by vitamin K deficiency, may indicate severe liver dysfunction. Although minor bleeding is common (e.g., ecchymoses), these patients are also at risk for significant bleeding, related especially to trauma or surgery. Transfusion of fresh-frozen plasma may be required to replace clotting factors and to prevent or stop bleeding. Patients may also have life-threatening hemorrhage from peptic ulcers or esophageal varices. In these cases, replacement with fresh-frozen plasma, PRBCs, and platelets is usually required.

VITAMIN K DEFICIENCY

The synthesis of many coagulation factors depends on vitamin K. Vitamin K deficiency is common in malnourished patients, and some antibiotics decrease the intestinal flora that produce vitamin K, depleting vitamin K stores. Administration of vitamin K (phytonadione), either orally or as a subcutaneous injection, can correct the deficiency quickly; adequate synthesis of coagulation factors is reflected by normalization of the PT.

COMPLICATIONS OF ANTICOAGULANT THERAPY

Anticoagulants are used in the treatment or prevention of thrombosis. These agents, particularly warfarin or heparin, can cause bleeding. If the PT or PTT is longer than desired, and bleeding has not occurred, the medication can be stopped or the dose decreased. Vitamin K is administered as an antidote for warfarin toxicity. Protamine sulfate is rarely needed for heparin toxicity because the half-life of heparin is very short. The half-life of the anticoagulant effect of heparin is ~1.5 hours and does not increase with dose (Collins, 2022). With significant bleeding, fresh-frozen plasma is needed to replace the vitamin K–dependent coagulation factors.

DISSEMINATED INTRAVASCULAR COAGULATION (DIC)

DIC is not a disease but a sign of an underlying condition. DIC may be triggered by sepsis, trauma, cancer, shock, abruptio placentae, toxins, or allergic reactions. The severity of DIC is variable, but it is potentially life-threatening. Identification of patients who are at risk for DIC and recognition of the early clinical manifestations of this syndrome can result in earlier medical intervention, which may improve the prognosis. However, the primary prognostic factor is the ability to treat the precipitating underlying condition.

Pathophysiology

Normal hemostatic mechanisms are altered in DIC so that a massive amount of tiny clots form in the microcirculation. Initially, the coagulation time is normal. However, as the platelets and clotting factors are consumed to form the microthrombi, coagulation fails. Thus, the paradoxical result of excessive clotting is bleeding. The clinical manifestations of DIC are reflected in the organs, which are affected either by excessive clot formation (with resultant ischemia to all or part of the organ) or by bleeding. The excessive clotting triggers the fibrinolytic system to release fibrin degradation products, potent anticoagulants, which exacerbates the bleeding. The bleeding is characterized by consumption of platelets and clotting factors, thus precipitating low platelet and fibrinogen levels (due to the consumption of fibrinogen); prolonged PT, PTT, and **thrombin** time; and elevated fibrin degradation products (**D-dimers**) (see Table 19-3 for an overview of laboratory values commonly found in DIC).

TABLE **19-3 Laboratory Values Commonly Found in Disseminated Intravascular Coagulation (DIC)**[a]

Test	Function Evaluated	Normal Range	Changes in DIC
Platelet count	Platelet number	150,000–450,000/mm^3	↓
Prothrombin time (PT)	Extrinsic pathway	11–13 seconds	↑
Partial thromboplastin time (PTT)	Intrinsic pathway	23–35 seconds	↑
Activated partial thromboplastin time (aPTT)	Intrinsic pathway	21–35 seconds	↑
Thrombin time (TT)	Clot formation	12–19 seconds	↑
Fibrinogen	Amount available for coagulation	200–400 mg/dL	↓
D-dimer	Local fibrinolysis	0–250 ng/mL	↑
Fibrin degradation products (FDPs) or fibrin split products (FSPs)	Fibrinolysis	0–5 µg/mL	↑
Euglobulin clot lysis	Fibrinolytic activity	2 or more hours	1 hour or less

[a]Because DIC is a dynamic condition, the laboratory values measured will change over time. Therefore, a progressive increase or decrease in a given laboratory value is likely to be more important than the actual value of a test at a single point in time. Note values can vary by laboratory.

Clinical Manifestations and Assessment

Patients with frank DIC may bleed from mucous membranes, venipuncture sites, and the GI and urinary tracts. The bleeding can range from minimal occult internal bleeding to profuse hemorrhage from all orifices. The patient may also develop organ dysfunction, such as kidney failure and pulmonary and multifocal CNS infarctions, as a result of microthromboses, macrothromboses, or hemorrhages.

During the initial process of DIC, the patient may have no new symptoms, the only manifestation being a progressive decrease in the platelet count. As the thrombosis becomes more extensive, the patient exhibits signs and symptoms of thrombosis in the organs involved. Then, as the clotting factors and platelets are consumed to form these thrombi, bleeding occurs. Initially, the bleeding is subtle, but it can develop into frank hemorrhage. Signs and symptoms, which depend on the organs involved, are listed in Table 19-4.

Medical Management

The most important management factors in DIC are early recognition and treatment of the underlying cause; until the cause is controlled, the DIC will persist (Adelborg et al., 2020). Correcting the secondary effects of tissue ischemia by improving oxygenation, replacing fluids, correcting electrolyte imbalances, and administering vasopressor medications is also important.

Blood product support includes platelets, fresh-frozen plasma, and cryoprecipitate (to replace fibrinogen). The decision to transfuse should be based on laboratory trends and the patient's condition. FFP should be given in the presence of bleeding and prolonged PT/PTT; platelets are transfused if the platelet count is less than 50,000/mm^3; cryoprecipitate is considered in patients with a fibrinogen below 1.5 g/L (less than 150 mg/dL) (Adelborg et al., 2020).

A controversial treatment strategy is to interrupt thrombosis through the use of heparin infusion. Heparin may inhibit the activation of the coagulation pathway in sepsis, inhibiting microthrombi formation and thereby correcting perfusion of the organs. However, a beneficial effect of heparin on outcomes in patients with DIC has never been demonstrated in controlled trials and may increase the incidence and risk for bleeding in patients with DIC. Heparin is indicated only in patients with clinically evident thromboembolism in a large blood vessel or with evidence of tissue damage secondary to thromboemboli; extreme caution must be used due to the high risk for bleeding (Adelborg et al., 2020). There is a recent trend toward using LMWH due to decreased bleeding risks and predictable half-life (Adelborg et al., 2020).

Antithrombin (AT) infusions can also be used for their anticoagulant and anti-inflammatory properties. Bleeding can be significant, particularly when administered in association with heparin. Use of AT has yet to demonstrate a survival advantage and needs further study (Adelborg et al., 2020).

Nursing Management

Nurses need to be aware of which patients are at risk of DIC. Sepsis and acute promyelocytic leukemia (APML) are the most common causes of DIC. Patients need to be assessed thoroughly and frequently for signs and symptoms of thrombi and bleeding and monitored for any

TABLE **19-4 Assessing for Thrombosis and Bleeding in Disseminated Intravascular Coagulation (DIC)**[a]

System	Signs and Symptoms of Microvascular Thrombosis	Signs and Symptoms of Microvascular and Frank Bleeding
Integumentary system (skin)	↓ Temperature and sensation; ↑ pain; cyanosis in extremities, nose, earlobes; focal ischemia, superficial gangrene	Petechiae, including oral mucosa; bleeding: gums, oozing from wounds, previous injection sites, around catheters (IV or Foley); tracheostomies; epistaxis; diffuse ecchymoses; subcutaneous hemorrhage; joint pain
Circulatory system	↓ Pulses; capillary filling time greater than 3 seconds	Tachycardia
Respiratory system	Hypoxia (secondary to clot in lung); dyspnea; chest pain with deep inspiration; ↓ breath sounds over areas of large embolism	High-pitched bronchial breath sounds; tachypnea; ↑ consolidation; signs and symptoms of acute respiratory distress syndrome
Gastrointestinal system	Gastric pain; "heartburn"	Hematemesis (heme⊕ NG output) melena (heme⊕ stools → tarry stools → bright-red blood from rectum) retroperitoneal bleeding (abdomen firm and tender to palpation; distended; ↑ abdominal girth; back pain)
Kidney system	↓ Urine output; ↑ creatinine, ↑ blood urea nitrogen	Hematuria
Neurologic system	↓ Alertness and orientation; ↓ pupillary reaction; ↓ response to commands; ↓ strength and movement ability	Anxiety; restlessness; ↓ mentation, altered level of consciousness; headache; visual disturbances; conjunctival hemorrhage

heme⊕, positive for hemoglobin.
[a]Signs of microvascular thrombosis are the result of an inappropriate activation of the coagulation system, causing thrombotic occlusion of small vessels within all body organs. As the clotting factors and platelets are consumed, signs of microvascular bleeding appear. This bleeding can quickly extend into frank hemorrhage. Treatment must be aimed at the disorder underlying the DIC; otherwise, the stimulus for the syndrome will persist.

progression of these signs. Timely recognition of symptoms and prompt reporting to the medical team can help facilitate early intervention and improve outcomes (see Table 19-4).

In addition, the nurse monitors and manages potential complications. Assessment and interventions should target potential sites of end-organ damage (see Table 19-4). As organs are inadequately perfused because of occlusion by microthrombi, organ function diminishes; the kidneys, lungs, brain, and skin are particularly vulnerable, and kidney dysfunction is common. Lack of renal perfusion may result in acute kidney injury (AKI) and kidney failure, sometimes requiring dialysis. Placement of a large-bore dialysis catheter is extremely hazardous for this patient population and should be accompanied by adequate platelet and plasma transfusions. Liver dysfunction is also relatively common, reflected in altered liver function tests, depleted albumin stores, and diminished synthesis of clotting factors. Respiratory function warrants careful monitoring and aggressive measures to diminish alveolar compromise, such as incentive spirometry. Suctioning (if required) should be performed as gently as possible to diminish the risk for additional bleeding. CNS involvement can be manifested as headache, visual changes, and alteration in level of consciousness. A plan of nursing care for the patient with DIC is available online at http://thepoint.lww.com/Honan3e.

Pearls for Practice

The nurse understands that perfusion must be maintained to all organs, and when there is uncontrolled hypertension, or hypotension or hypovolemia, the heart, kidneys, brain, and eyes can sustain damage. With hypotension and hypovolemia, the lack of perfusion of blood results in end-organ ischemia. However, in uncontrolled hypertension, a number of factors are implicated including the sympathetic nervous system stimulation (increased vasoconstriction), the renin–angiotensin system, metabolic and inflammatory factors and endothelial (inner lining of blood vessels) dysfunction and remodeling of the small and large arteries leading to a reduced dilation capability which are associated with cardiac (left ventricular hypertrophy, coronary heart disease, angina, myocardial infarction, heart failure), kidneys (proteinuria, AKI, chronic kidney failure), brain (vascular and hemorrhagic stroke) and eyes (retinopathy) (Naranjo et al., 2021; Marini et al., 2021).

THROMBOTIC DISORDERS

Several conditions can alter the balance within the normal hemostatic process and cause excessive thrombosis. Abnormalities that predispose a person to thrombotic events include decreased clotting inhibitors within the circulation (which enhances coagulation), altered liver function (which may decrease production of clotting factors or clearance of activated coagulation factors), lack of fibrinolytic enzymes, and tortuous vessels (which promote platelet aggregation). Thrombosis can be caused by more than one predisposing factor. Several conditions can result from thrombosis, such as MI (see Chapter 13), cerebral vascular accident (CVA) (brain attack or stroke; see Chapter 46), and peripheral arterial occlusion (see Chapter 17). Several inherited or acquired deficiency conditions, including hyperhomocysteinemia, AT III deficiency, protein C deficiency, APC resistance, factor V Leiden, and protein S deficiency, can predispose a patient to repeated episodes of thrombosis; these are referred to as hypercoagulable states or thrombophilia. Table 19-5 lists these disorders, their abnormal laboratory values, and the need for family testing.

Thrombosis requires anticoagulation therapy. The duration of therapy varies with the location and extent of the thrombosis, precipitating events (e.g., trauma, immobilization), and concurrent risk factors (e.g., use of oral contraceptives, tortuous blood vessels, history of thrombotic events). With some conditions, lifelong anticoagulant therapy is necessary. Refer to Chapter 17 for details on anticoagulation.

TABLE **19-5 Hypercoagulable States**

Disorder	Abnormal Laboratory Value[a]
Inherited Disorders (Family Testing Necessary)	
Hyperhomocysteinemia	Homocysteine ↑ after methionine load
Antithrombin III (AT III) deficiency	AT III ↓
Protein C deficiency	Protein C activity ↓ (must be measured off warfarin [Coumadin])
Activated protein C (APC) resistance	Must be measured off anticoagulant; less than 2× prolongation of PTT when APC added. Patients with APC resistance have a smaller increase in clotting time than normal (i.e., the prolongation of clotting time is less than normal).
Factor V Leiden	Positive
Protein S deficiency	Protein S activity ↓; must be measured off warfarin (Coumadin)
Dysfibrinogenemia	↑ thrombin time; ↑ reptilase time; ↓ functional fibrinogen; often requires special fibrinogen assays
Acquired Disorders (Family Testing Unnecessary)	
Anticardiolipin antibody	Positive
Cancer	Varied, depending on disorder
Lupus anticoagulant	Positive
Hyperhomocysteinemia	Homocysteine ↑ after methionine load
AT III deficiency	AT III ↓
Paroxysmal nocturnal hemoglobinuria	+ Hamm test; acid hemolysis
Myeloproliferative disorders	Varied, depending on disorder
Nephrotic syndrome	Varied, depending on disorder
Cancer chemotherapy	Varied, depending on specific agent

[a]Protein C and protein S are vitamin K–dependent proteins. Warfarin (Coumadin) interferes with the hepatic synthesis of vitamin K–dependent factors, which may decrease levels of protein C or protein S; therefore, protein C and protein S should be measured while the patient is off warfarin.

MALIGNANT HEMATOLOGIC CONDITIONS

Myeloproliferative Neoplasms

Myeloproliferative neoplasms (MPNs) are a group of myeloid malignancies with varying clinical presentation, disease course, treatment, and prognosis. In 2016, the World Health Organization (WHO) updated their classification of MPNs, which now include: PV, essential thrombocythemia (ET), primary myelofibrosis (PMF), chronic myelogenous leukemia (CML), chronic neutrophilic leukemia (CNL), chronic eosinophilic leukemia, and MPN-unclassifiable (MPN-U) (Barbui et al., 2018; Thapa et al, 2022). Here we will focus on the most common MPNs: PV, ET, and CML.

POLYCYTHEMIA VERA

PV is a clonal myeloproliferative disorder that is characterized by increased hemoglobin and hematocrit levels in the setting of a mutation of the JAK-2 gene, which regulates cell growth (Tefferi et al., 2021). The bone marrow is hypercellular, and, though the erythrocyte elevation is predominant, the leukocyte and platelet counts are also elevated. The incidence of polycythemia has been estimated at 1 per 100,000 people. The median age at onset is 60 years, occurring most commonly in patients 50 to 75 years of age; males are affected more than females (Tefferri, 2022). PV is not curable. However, with treatment, survival can be more than a decade (Tefferi, 2022).

Pathophysiology

PV requires the presence of an elevated Hgb (greater than 18.5 g/dL in males and greater than 16.5 g/dL in females) or evidence of increased RBC mass (over 56% in males; over 50% in females) and the presence of a JAK2 genetic mutation. Additional criteria include a hypercellular bone marrow and low serum erythropoietin levels (Tefferi, 2020).

Clinical Manifestations and Assessment

Patients may present with a ruddy complexion (referred to as plethora) and complaints related to splenomegaly, including left upper quadrant pain and early satiety. Symptoms result from increased blood volume (headache, dizziness, tinnitus, fatigue, paresthesias, and blurred vision) or from increased blood viscosity (angina, claudication, dyspnea, and thrombophlebitis), particularly if the patient has atherosclerotic blood vessels. For this reason, blood pressure is often elevated. Uric acid may be elevated, resulting in gout and kidney stone formation. Another common and bothersome problem is generalized pruritus, which may be caused by histamine release due to the increased number of basophils. A hallmark feature of PV is severe and painful itching that is triggered by exposure to water (referred to as aquagenic pruritus) (Tefferri, 2020). Erythromelalgia a syndrome of painful burning, warmth, and redness in a localized distal area of the extremities; it most commonly occurs in the fingers and toes and is only partially relieved by cooling.

Complications

Patients with PV are at increased risk for thromboses, including cerebrovascular accident (CVA or stroke), MI, and deep vein thrombosis (DVT); thrombotic complications are the most common cause of death. Risk factors for thrombosis in PV include age over 60 years, a history of vascular events, and smoking (Christensen et al., 2021; Greisshammer et al., 2019). Bleeding is also a complication in the setting of extremely high platelet counts (exceeding 1.5 million) and associated acquired vWD (Tefferi, 2022). The bleeding can be significant and can occur in the form of nosebleeds, ulcers, frank GI bleeding, hematuria, and intracranial hemorrhage.

Medical Management

The goals of therapy include preventing thrombosis, palliating disease-associated symptoms, and delaying progression of disease to myelofibrosis or AML (Tefferri, 2022). Treatment strategies to achieve these goals include phlebotomy to reduce the hematocrit, antiplatelet therapy to reduce thrombosis risk, cytoreduction to control the blood counts, and modification of cardiovascular risk factors (Christensen et al., 2021; Tefferri et al., 2021).

Phlebotomy is a critical part of therapy to lower the hematocrit and is the only treatment that has demonstrated improved survival (Tefferri et al., 2021). It involves removing enough blood (initially 500 mL once or twice weekly) to diminish the blood viscosity and then intermittently to maintain the hematocrit below 45%. Many patients are managed by routine phlebotomy on an intermittent basis.

Additional therapy may be indicated based on the individual risk for thrombosis (high risk vs. low risk). Risk factors for high-risk disease include a history of thrombosis or age over 60 years with a JAK2 mutation. Patients with high-risk disease with a history of venous thrombosis are treated with hydroxyurea and systemic anticoagulation; patients with high-risk disease and a history of arterial thrombosis are treated with hydroxyurea and once-daily low-dose aspirin (40 to 100 mg once or twice daily (Bharti, 2022; Freeman, 2023; Tefferri et al., 2021). High-risk patients with additional cardiovascular risk factors and a history of arterial thrombosis should be advised to take aspirin twice a day; if they are high risk with additional CV risk factors and a history of venous thrombosis, once-daily aspirin may be added to systemic anticoagulation (Tefferri et al., 2021). Patients with very low risk (no history of thrombosis, age under 60 years, and no JAK2 mutation) and low-risk disease (no risk of thrombosis, age under 60 years, JAK2 mutation present) may be managed with aspirin alone (Tefferi et al., 2021).

Randomized studies have demonstrated the value of low-dose aspirin (40 to 100 mg/day) and should be administered in the absence of contraindications (i.e., history of GI bleeding, hemorrhagic stroke). Aspirin is also effective in alleviating vasomotor symptoms, including painful erythromelalgia (a symptom that affects the extremities causing redness, warmth, and burning pain), headaches, pruritus, lightheadedness, tinnitus, paresthesias, and chest pain (Tefferi, 2022). Aspirin must be used with caution in patients with platelet counts exceeding 1 million/mm^3 given the risks for acquired vWD and associated bleeding risk.

Patients receiving hydroxyurea appear to have a lower incidence of thrombotic complications than do those treated by phlebotomy alone; this may result from a more effectively controlled platelet count. Patients on hydroxyurea must be counseled on avoiding pregnancy. Other side effects include mouth sores, skin (leg) ulcers, and nail changes (Tefferi, 2022).

For patients unable to tolerate or who are resistant to hydroxyurea, interferon alpha-2b is also an effective treatment for cytoreduction (Tefferi, 2022). Interferon alpha is also effective in alleviating the pruritus associated with PV (Tefferi, 2022) but may be difficult for patients to tolerate because of its frequent side effects (e.g., flu-like syndrome, depression).

Ruxolitinib, an oral JAK1-2 inhibitor that targets the JAK mutation, may also be used to treat hydroxyurea-resistant or hydroxyurea-intolerant patients (Tefferi, 2022). Studies have demonstrated that ruxolitinib lowers hematocrit to target goals, reduces spleen size, reduces thrombotic risk and PV-related symptoms. However, there is no evidence that ruxolinitib reduces the malignant JAK2 mutation or reduces PV transformation (i.e., leukemia or myelofibrosis) (Tefferi, 2022).

Busulfan, an alkylating agent, is also used to treat hydroxyurea-resistant PV. However, the medication's side-effect profile, which includes cytopenias and secondary leukemias, has made it a less attractive option. It is generally used among older adults (>65) (Tefferi et al., 2021).

Patients with PV who smoke must be counseled on smoking cessation. Other modifiable cardiovascular risk factors, including obesity, hypertension, and DM, should also be addressed (Christensen et al., 2021).

Nursing Management

The nurse's role is primarily that of educator. Risk factors for thrombotic complications, particularly smoking, obesity, and poorly controlled HTN, should be assessed, and the patient should be instructed about risk reduction as well as the signs and symptoms of thrombosis. To reduce the likelihood of DVT, activity should be promoted, and crossing the legs and use of restrictive clothing should be avoided. The nurse instructs patients to walk around frequently on long flights. Patients with a history of bleeding are usually advised to avoid aspirin and aspirin-containing medications because these medications alter platelet function. The nurse encourages minimizing alcohol intake to further diminish the risk of bleeding. The patient needs to be instructed to avoid iron supplements, including those within multivitamin supplements, because the iron can further stimulate RBC production. For pruritus, the nurse may recommend bathing in tepid or cool water (hot water can exacerbate the symptom), limiting bathing time to 30 minutes or extending to every other day, and avoiding vigorous toweling-off after bathing. Use of mild soaps, application of emollient lotions, adding colloidal oatmeal treatment to bath water, use of cotton blankets and clothing, and washing sheets, clothing, and undergarments with baby detergent may also decrease pruritus.

ESSENTIAL THROMBOCYTHEMIA

ET (primary thrombocythemia) is a chronic, clonal, MPN characterized by a sustained increase in platelet count or **thrombocytosis**. The incidence of ET is estimated at 1 to 3 per 100,000 per year (Tefferi & Pardanni, 2019). The median age at onset is 60. It is more common among females. Twenty percent of ET patients are under 40 years of age. Patients with ET generally have a near normal life expectancy (Kvasnicka, 2020).

Pathophysiology

Similar to PV, most cases of ET are driven by acquired mutations in *JAK2* (60% of ET cases); the remainder of patients will have mutations in either *CALR* or *MPL* genes (Kvasnicka, 2020). The criteria proposed in 2015 by WHO for diagnosis of ET include: a platelet count of $450/mm^3$ or higher; a bone marrow biopsy with increased numbers of large, mature megakaryocytes and no significant increase in neutrophil granulopoiesis or erythropoiesis; not meeting WHO criteria for CML, PV, PMF, MDS, or other myeloid neoplasm; and/or presence of a clonal marker (such as *JAK2, MPL*, or *CALR* mutation) (Kvasnicka, 2020).

Clinical Manifestations and Assessment

The diagnosis of ET is made by ruling out secondary causes of thrombocytosis (see earlier discussion). Iron deficiency should be excluded because a reactive increase in the platelet count often accompanies this deficiency. Occult malignancy should be excluded. The CBC shows markedly large and abnormal platelets. CBC, bone marrow aspiration and biopsy, and mutational testing for *JAK2, MPL*, and *CALR* are the cornerstones of diagnostic evaluation for ET (Tefferi & Pardanani, 2019).

Many patients with ET are asymptomatic; the illness is diagnosed as the result of finding an elevated platelet count on a CBC. Symptoms, when they do occur, result primarily from hemorrhage or vaso-occlusion in the microvasculature. Symptoms occur most often when the platelet count exceeds 1 $million/mm^3$. However, symptoms do not always correlate with the extent to which the platelet count is elevated. Thrombosis is common and can be either arterial or venous (Tefferi & Barbui, 2020). Vasomotor symptoms are not infrequent complaints and can include visual disturbances, lightheadedness, headaches, palpitations, atypical chest pain, and distal paresthesias (Tefferi & Pardanani, 2019). Headache is the most common neurologic complication, followed by transient ischemic attacks, dizziness, syncope, and seizures. More common forms of venous thrombosis include DVT and pulmonary embolism; less commonly, stroke and MI occur. Small vessel vaso-occlusive manifestations cause symptoms of erythromelalgia (described earlier).

Because these platelets can be dysfunctional, minor or major hemorrhage can also occur. The GI tract is the most common site of bleeding, followed by the skin, eyes, urinary tract, tooth socket and gums, joints, or brain. Bleeding typically does not occur unless the platelet count exceeds 1 $million/mm^3$. The spleen may be enlarged but usually not to a clinically significant extent.

Risk stratification for thrombosis and bleeding in ET includes four categories: very low-risk (no thrombosis history, ≤60 years, no JAK2 mutation); low-risk (no thrombosis history, ≤60 years, JAK2 mutation); intermediate-risk (no history of thrombosis, ≥60 years, no JAK2 mutation), and high-risk (history of thrombosis or >60 years with JAK2 mutation) (Tefferi & Barbui, 2020).

Medical Management

Treatment for ET is guided by thrombotic risk with a primary goal of preventing vascular complications (Tefferi & Pardanani, 2019).

Very low-risk patients who do not have cardiovascular risk factors can be monitored without the addition of therapy Tefferi & Barbui, 2020). Very low-risk patients with cardiovascular risk factors and low-risk patients are managed with aspirin (81 mg either once or twice daily) (Tefferi & Pardanani, 2019). Intermediate- and high-risk patients are also managed with aspirin plus hydroxyurea (Tefferi & Barbui, 2020). High-risk patients who have history of venous thrombosis are managed with hydroxyurea plus systemic anticoagulation (Tefferi & Barbui, 2020). Patients resistant to or intolerant of hydroxyurea may be treated with pegylated interferon alpha, busulfan, and, more rarely, anagrelide or ruxolitinib (Tefferi & Barbui, 2020; Tefferi & Pardanani, 2019). Interferon alpha has been associated with high hematologic response rates for ET, but its use is limited by side effects, including cytopenias, flu-like symptoms, and fatigue, contributing to discontinuation in up to 20% of patients (Tefferi & Pardanani, 2019). As in PV, in the setting of very high platelet counts, acquired vWD can occur. Such patients may be tested for von Willebrand factor, and avoid use of aspirin if factor levels are less than 30% (Tefferi & Pardanani, 2019).

Rarely, the occlusive symptoms of ET are so great that the platelet count must be reduced immediately. When necessary, plateletpheresis (see later discussion) can reduce the amount of circulating platelets but only transiently. The extent to which symptoms and complications (e.g., thromboses) are reduced by pheresis remains unclear.

Nursing Management

Patients with ET need to be instructed about the accompanying risks of hemorrhage and thrombosis. The patient is informed about signs and symptoms of thrombosis, particularly the neurologic manifestations, such as visual changes, numbness, tingling, and weakness as well as chest pain, and extremity swelling, redness, or pain. Risk factors for thrombosis are assessed, and measures to diminish risk factors (particularly cessation of tobacco use and weight management) are encouraged.

Patients receiving aspirin therapy should be informed about the increased risk of bleeding. Patients who are at risk for bleeding should be instructed about medications (e.g., aspirin, NSAIDs) and other substances (e.g., alcohol) that can alter platelet function and, therefore, should be avoided. Patients receiving interferon therapy are taught to self-administer the medication and manage any side effects promptly (primarily fatigue, flu-like symptoms, and depression).

CHRONIC MYELOID LEUKEMIA (CML)

Pathophysiology

CML is a clonal myeloid MPN marked by the proliferation of stem cells with the presence of the Philadelphia chromosome (a balanced mutation of chromosomes 9 and 22 [t9;22]) resulting in the production of the bcr/abl kinase protein, which is responsible for aberrant cell growth.

CML involves an overproduction of myeloid blood cells. This disease typically presents with an elevated WBC (leukocytosis), mild anemia, and thrombocytopenia (Kreipe, 2020). Because there is an uncontrolled proliferation of cells, the marrow expands into the cavities of long bones (e.g., the femur), resulting in bone pain, and myeloid cells may also be produced in the liver and spleen (extramedullary hematopoiesis), resulting in enlargement of these organs that is sometimes painful.

There are three phases of the disease: the chronic phase, where most of the leukocytes produced are mature and retain some ability to function normally; the accelerated phase, in which the numbers of abnormal cells are being produced at a faster rate; and blast crisis, in which the predominant cell type is immature. Most patients are diagnosed in the chronic phase. Untreated CML will progress to advanced phases in 3 to 5 years (Kreipe, 2020). Once the disease transforms to the acute phase (blast crisis), the overall survival rarely exceeds several months.

Epidemiology

The incidence of CML is estimated at 1.75 per 100,000 individuals in the United States (Hoglund et al., 2021). CML may be seen at any age, but is uncommon in children and adolescents (Hoglund et al., 2021). The incidence of CML increases with age, with the median age at diagnosis being 66 years (Hoglund et al., 2021). Thus, the prevalence of CML is predicted to increase because of demographics (aging population), and the acknowledgment that because of highly effective therapies for CML, there will be an increased number of those living with the disease. CML is slightly more common in males (Hoglund et al., 2021).

Clinical Manifestations and Assessment

The clinical picture of CML varies based on the phase of the disease. During the chronic phase, 30% to 50% of patients are asymptomatic, and so the diagnosis may be detected based on abnormal blood work. The most common symptoms include fatigue, night sweats, abdominal pain, early satiety, and weight loss (Sampaio et al., 2021).

Patients with extremely high leukocyte counts (over $100{,}000/mm^3$) may exhibit signs of leukostasis (the excessive volume of leukocytes slows and inhibits blood flow through the capillaries via increased viscosity) including confusion, vision changes, shortness of breath, or chest pain due to decreased capillary perfusion to the brain, eyes, and lungs. The patient may have an enlarged, tender spleen. The liver may also be enlarged.

Medical Management

Advances in understanding of the pathology of CML at a molecular level have led to dramatic changes in its treatment. The development of drugs that target and inhibit the bcr/abl tyrosine kinase protein (called tyrosine kinase inhibitors or

TKIs) have significantly extended survival for patients with CML and have shifted the paradigm of CML management to that of a chronic disease.

Therapy depends on the stage of disease. In the chronic phase, the expected outcome is correction of the chromosomal abnormality (i.e., conversion of the malignant stem cell population back to normal), and the standard therapy is a TKI. TKIs approved for the front-line setting include imatinib, nilotinib, and dasatinib. TKIs approved in the second-line setting include dasatinib, nilotinib, and bosutinib (Sampaio et al., 2021). Initial response to therapy is measured through monitoring of the CBC with expected normalization of blood counts within the first 4 to 6 weeks, called a complete hematologic response. Subsequent response to TKI therapy using blood measurement of bcr/abl quantity (molecular testing) is done every 3 months with the goal of reaching major molecular response. Achievement and maintenance of early major molecular response is predictive of longer survival (Sampaio et al., 2021). There are established goals for molecular response at set time points, including 3 months, 6 months, 12 months, etc. (Deininger et al., 2020). If patients do not meet established milestones, assessment of adherence must be performed as well as resistance testing. There is a blood test to assess for the development of mutational resistance to TKIs. The test will alert the provider if the patient has developed resistance to a particular TKI and will direct the provider to TKIs to which the disease remains sensitive. Adherence to prescribed therapy is essential to response; when adherence falls below 90%, response to therapy declines.

During the initial phase of treatment, if there is significant leukocytosis (elevated WBCs), the WBC needs to be reduced quickly to minimize complications from leukostasis. This goal can be achieved by using drugs like hydroxyurea in conjunction with initiation of TKI therapy. In the case of an extreme leukocytosis at diagnosis (e.g., leukocyte count greater than 300,000/mm^3), a more emergent treatment may be required. In this instance, *leukapheresis* (in which the patient's blood is removed and separated, with the leukocytes withdrawn, and the remaining blood returned to the patient) can reduce the number of leukocytes temporarily.

The treatment of CML in the accelerated and blast phases is more challenging, as many patients in advanced stages of disease have developed resistance to TKIs. There is no consensus on optimal treatment of patients with advanced CML (Deininger et al., 2020). Options for treatment include clinical trials, second-line TKIs based upon mutation analysis or allogeneic hematopoietic stem cell transplantation (AHSCT) (discussed in Chapter 5) (Deininger et al., 2020). Prognosis at time to progression is 7 to 11 months (Lauseker et al., 2019).

The accelerated or transformation phase can be insidious or rapid. In the accelerated phase, the patient may complain of bone pain and may report fevers (without any obvious sign of infection), night sweats, and weight loss. Even with treatment, the spleen may continue to enlarge. The patient may become more anemic and thrombocytopenic.

In the acute form of CML (blast crisis), the disease progresses to either acute lymphocytic leukemia (ALL) or acute myeloid leukemia (AML) blast phase, and treatment is targeted to the specific type. Patients whose disease evolves into a "lymphoid" blast crisis are more likely to reenter a chronic phase after ALL induction therapy. For those whose disease evolves into AML, therapy is largely ineffective in achieving a second chronic phase. Life-threatening infections and bleeding occur frequently in this phase.

Allogeneic stem cell transplantation remains the only curative treatment for CML. However, the efficacy of imatinib in first-line treatment and the treatment-related mortality of stem cell transplant limit the use of transplant to patients with high risk or relapsed disease or in those patients who are resistant to TKI therapy (Sampaio, 2021).

Nursing Management

The nurse must educate the patient on proper administration of TKI therapy. Some TKIs require timing around meals (nilotinib), and patients may need assistance with optimal scheduling. Antacids, PPIs, and grapefruit juice may interfere with drug absorption, and patients must be counseled to avoid these while on TKI therapy. There are a number of other drug interactions with TKIs, and nurses should collaborate with the pharmacist to review the patient's drug list for potential interactions. Most patients will require lifetime therapy with TKIs. Each TKI has a specific side-effect profile that may interfere with adherence and tolerance. For example, GI side effects and fluid retention are common with some of the TKIs. Patients must be counseled on the individual side-effect profile of the drug and be instructed to notify their health care team promptly with any new symptoms. The nurse's role in side-effect anticipation and management is critical. The nurse also plays an active role in the assessment and promotion of adherence to TKI therapy. Counseling on the importance of medication adherence and use of supportive tools such as mobile reminder applications may help to promote adherence (Cazeau, 2021).

BONE MARROW FAILURE SYNDROMES

Bone marrow failure syndrome is the term for a classification that includes aplastic anemia (AA), paroxysmal nocturnal hemoglobinuria (PNH), and MDS.

APLASTIC ANEMIA (AA)

AA is a rare disease caused by a decrease in or damage to bone marrow stem cells, damage to the microenvironment within the marrow, and replacement of the marrow with fat, resulting in cytopenias (reduction in number of blood cells). This disease occurs equally in males and females and is often a disease of the young, with peak incidence occurring in childhood and between the ages of 20 to 25 years (Moore & Krishnan, 2021).

Pathophysiology

While AA is most often idiopathic (without clear cause), immune effects on marrow function (e.g., viral infection, idiosyncratic drug reactions, direct stem cell toxicity [radiation, chemotherapy]) have also been implicated as an underlying etiology (Moore & Krishnan, 2021). The most common hereditary cause for AA is Fanconi anemia (Moore & Krishnan, 2021). PNH has also been associated with the development of AA (Menter & Tzankov, 2020).

Agents that regularly produce marrow aplasia include benzene and benzene derivatives (e.g., airplane glue). Certain toxic materials, such as inorganic arsenic and several pesticides (including dichlorodiphenyltrichloroethane [DDT], which is no longer used or available in the United States), have also been implicated as potential causes. Other possible origins include cytotoxic agents used in cancer chemotherapy: alkylating agents (busulfan, cyclophosphamide), antimetabolites (antifolic compounds), antimitotics (vincristine, vinblastine, colchicine), and some antibiotics (daunorubicin, doxorubicin) (Menter & Tzankov, 2020). Pregnancy has also been associated with AA, and while the causal relationship is unknown, it may reflect a high level of immunologic activation during pregnancy; the prognosis is poor and associated with bleeding complications (Jaime-Pérez & Gómez-Almaguer, 2021).

Clinical Manifestations and Assessment

The manifestations of AA are often insidious. Patients may present with symptoms of anemia or bleeding. Symptoms of anemia, including fatigue, shortness of breath, and decreased activity tolerance, are usually present at the time of diagnosis. Symptoms related to leukopenia and thrombocytopenia may include fevers, minor infections, petechia or ecchymosis (Moore & Krishnan, 2021). CBC may reveal neutropenia, anemia, and/or thrombocytopenia. The MCV is usually elevated. A bone marrow aspirate and biopsy provides the most sensitive evidence for AA. There is an absence of dysplasia, which helps to distinguish between AA and MDS (which is marked by dysplasia) (Menter & Tzankov, 2020).

Medical Management

Severe AA, defined by the degree of cytopenias, must be treated quickly. Symptomatic anemia and thrombocytopenia can be supported with transfusions of irradiated blood and platelets, respectively. In patients with an absolute neutrophil count (ANC) below 500/μL, prophylactic antibiotics should be considered, and in the presence of fever, empiric antibiotics must be started promptly (Moore & Krishnan, 2021).

In patients under 40 years of age who have a matched sibling donor, stem cell transplant is the definitive treatment and is considered curative (Moore & Krishnan, 2021). In patients over 40 years of age or those with no matched sibling, immunosuppressive therapy (IST) is the primary treatment. A combination of antithymocyte globulin (ATG) (a purified gamma globulin solution, is obtained from horses or rabbits immunized with human T lymphocytes) and cyclosporine (a calcineurin inhibitor) is employed. Complete response to IST (development of normal blood counts) occurs in up to 70% of young adults; however, relapse is common after treatment withdrawal (Menter & Tzankov, 2020). If relapse occurs following treatment with IST (i.e., the patient becomes pancytopenic [reduction of RBCs, WBCs, and platelets] again), reinstitution of the same immunologic agents may induce another remission. Corticosteroids are useful as immunosuppressive agents; however, they have significant side effects, including bone complications (i.e., avascular necrosis) and life-threatening infections. For this reason, long-term use of steroids is not recommended.

In patients who do not respond to IST, matched unrelated stem cell transplant should be considered; however, the mortality rate is higher (Menter & Tzankov, 2020). Frail older adult patients or those with significant comorbidities may be poor candidates for IST, and alternative therapies, such as androgens or supportive care, should be considered.

Supportive therapy plays a major role in the management of AA. Blood-product support with irradiated products is recommended (Moore & Krishnan, 2021). In patients with a low neutrophil count (below 500) and receiving IST, prolonged neutropenia increases the risk for mold infections; these types of infections are associated with high mortality rates. Therefore, antifungal prophylaxis with agents such as voriconazole or posaconazole is recommended for patients with severe AA and should continue as long as the patient is neutropenic. There remains some controversy related to antibacterial prophylaxis due to concerns for antimicrobial resistance. Patients at highest risk for bacterial sepsis are patients with severe AA, and antibiotic prophylaxis in this case may be considered (Moore & Krishnan, 2021). Prophylaxis with an antipneumocystis agent (such as aerosolized pentamidine) is essential. Antiviral prophylaxis is routinely recommended for transplant recipients and, in many centers, also considered for those treated with IST (Moore & Krishnan, 2021).

Death in this population is most commonly caused by hemorrhage or infection.

Nursing Management

Patients with AA are vulnerable to problems related to erythrocyte (RBC), leukocyte (WBC), and platelet deficiencies. They should be assessed carefully for signs of infection and bleeding. Specific nursing interventions are outlined in the sections on neutropenia and thrombocytopenia.

Patients receiving ATG must be educated to promptly report signs and symptoms of hypersensitivity reactions and should be reassured that the nurses who administer ATG are properly trained to respond to these reactions. Nurses should educate patients taking cyclosporine regarding the importance of taking the medication as directed and monitoring drug levels and blood pressure as well as reporting signs and symptoms of high blood pressure. The nurse provides anticipatory guidance regarding hirsutism and gingival hyperplasia as these side effects may significantly impact body image and coping.

MYELODYSPLASTIC SYNDROMES (MDSs)

MDS represents a group of heterogeneous diseases with highly variable disease courses, prognoses, treatment strategies, and risk for leukemic transformation. It is characterized by abnormal and ineffective cell growth (Buckstein, 2020). Accurate diagnosis is essential for guiding discussion regarding treatment options and prognosis.

MDS is rare in children, and incidence increases with age. Median age at diagnosis is 71 years; peak incidence is in the seventh and eighth decades of life (Buckstein, 2020). Incidence in the United States has been estimated at 13,000 new cases a year as of 2015 (Buckstein, 2020).

Pathophysiology

MDS is a group of diseases characterized by ineffective hematopoiesis, dysplasia in at least one cell line (RBC, platelet, or WBC), progressive bone marrow failure, and variable risk for progression to leukemia (Buckstein, 2020).

Clinical Manifestations and Assessment

The majority of symptoms and clinical complications in this population result from cytopenias and the risk for leukemic progression (Buckstein, 2020). Thirty percent of patients with MDS will progress to AML (Hospital & Vey, 2020). The risk for leukemia progression varies with the percentage of blasts in the bone marrow, the number and depth of cytopenias, and the presence of high-risk cytogenetic abnormalities and other genetic mutations such as tp53 (Hospital & Vey, 2020). Patients may present with fatigue, dyspnea, activity intolerance, unexplained bruising or bleeding, or recurrent infections. However, many patients are asymptomatic at the time of diagnosis, and in these cases, the diagnosis is suspected based on routine bloodwork alone (Buckstein, 2020).

Diagnosis includes a review of the CBC as well as bone marrow biopsy and aspirate. CBC is evaluated for cytopenias, peripheral blasts, and morphologic abnormalities. The reticulocyte count helps assess the bone marrow response to anemia. Other causes of anemia are ruled out. Serum EPO (erythropoietin) levels are checked to determine the potential role of ESAs in the management of MDS. Aspirate is sent for flow cytometry, cytogenetics, and assessment of genetic mutations. Aspirate is evaluated for evidence of dysplasia, blast count, number of monocytes, ringed sideroblasts, and megakaryocytes, which helps to classify the MDS subtype. The biopsy is evaluated for cellularity and the presence of blasts. Cytogenetics are critical to the prognostic classification of MDS. Favorable cytogenetic abnormalities include deletion of 11q, loss of chromosome Y, or deletion of 5q. Poor cytogenetic abnormalities include a complex karyotype (three or more cytogenetic abnormalities) (Bewersdorf & Zeidan, 2020).

Testing for mutations in specific genes has also become important in predicting prognosis in MDS. For example, mutation in TP53 is an independent predictor of poor prognosis in MDS (Bewersdorf & Zeidan, 2020).

The WHO provides diagnostic categorization of MDS based on morphology and blast percentage. The International Prognostic Scoring System (IPSS) helps to provide prognostic data using number of cytopenias, cytogenetics, and blast percentage, which helped to predict overall survival and risk for transformation to leukemia (Bewersdorf & Zeidan, 2020).

Medical Management

Treatment strategies depend on the risk category (low risk vs. high risk), performance status, quality of life, and presence of comorbidities (Fenaux & Ades, 2020). Strategies for treatment of low-risk MDS focus on minimizing the symptoms associated with cytopenias and minimizing transfusion requirements, whereas in high-risk disease, immediate treatment is indicated to improve overall survival since the life expectancy is less than 2 years (Fenaux & Ades, 2020). The initial approach to treatment may be to treat symptomatically and monitor the counts over time to assess how quickly the cytopenias progress (Fenaux & Ades, 2020).

For symptomatic anemia, transfusions of PRBCs are the mainstay of treatment (Fennaux & Andes, 2020). Long-term transfusion dependence is associated with iron overload so attempts to decrease transfusion requirements with use of other therapies may be considered. Platelet transfusions may be considered in the setting of bleeding (Hambley & DeZern, 2020). Granulocyte-colony stimulating factor (G-CSF) may be considered in neutropenic patients with recurrent infections. ESAs may be considered in transfusion-dependent patients with a serum EPO less than 500 mU/mL (Hambley & DeZern, 2020).

Lenalidomide is an oral angiogenesis inhibitor that is indicated in patients with transfusion-dependent MDS who have low-risk disease and a deletion 5q cytogenetic abnormality with or without other cytogenetic abnormalities. For further discussion of lenalidomide, refer to section on myeloma.

Patients with high-risk disease are at higher risk for transformation to leukemia; decision to treat must consider the patient's performance status and presence of comorbidities in order to predict treatment tolerance. The only cure for MDS is allogeneic stem cell transplant. Many patients may not be eligible due to advanced age, comorbidities, and lack of a suitable donor (Hambley & DeZern, 2020).

Azacitidine is a hypomethylating agent approved in the United States for the treatment of MDS with studies demonstrating improved blood counts, prolonged overall survival, prolonged time to progression to AML, and improved quality of life (Hambley & DeZern, 2020). Response to treatment can take 4 to 6 months of therapy; providing patients anticipatory guidance and setting realistic expectations around this is critical (Hambley &DeZern, 2020).

High-intensity therapy includes chemotherapy similar to that used in the treatment of AML, and stem cell transplant. The morbidity and mortality of high-intensity therapies is high. Therefore, high-intensity therapy is generally reserved for younger patients with no comorbidities. The goal of high-intensity therapy is to induce a remission prior to stem cell transplant (Hambley & DeZern, 2020).

Nursing Management

It is critical that the nurse provides patient education about the disease and management of symptoms, including reportable signs and symptoms of anemia, thrombocytopenia, and infection. The nurse helps the patient to track and trend blood counts and monitor transfusion requirements. The nurse helps the patient understand treatment options and have realistic expectations about timing of response. The majority of care for MDS is provided in the outpatient setting with the patient and family having primary responsibility for care at home. The nurse helps the patient and family with self-care needs and identifies needs for visiting nurse services.

ACUTE LEUKEMIA

Acute leukemias are aggressive forms of hematologic malignancies that are characterized by a rapid, continuous turnover of immature, dysfunctional cells. Normally, production of specific blood cells from their stem cell precursors is regulated carefully according to the body's needs. If the mechanisms that control the production of these cells are disrupted as a result of mutations, the cells proliferate excessively and mature abnormally.

Often hematopoietic malignancies are classified by the cells involved. **Leukemia**, literally "white blood," is a term used to describe neoplastic proliferation of one particular hematopoietic cell type (**granulocytes**, **monocytes**, lymphocytes, or, infrequently, erythrocytes or megakaryocytes). The defect originates from the hematopoietic stem cell, in either the myeloid or **lymphoid** stem cell lineage. Preferential proliferation of leukemia cells leads to decreased production of normal hematopoietic cells (Jäger et al., 2021).

Thus the common feature of acute leukemias is an unregulated proliferation of leukocytes in the bone marrow and a suppression of other blood cells, including RBCs and platelets. The bone marrow becomes packed with abnormal cells and ultimately begins to release these cells into the circulation prematurely. The increase in the number of leukocytes in the circulation is referred to as *leukocytosis*. Typically, only one specific type of leukocyte is increased, most commonly either the neutrophils (myeloblast) or the lymphocytes (lymphoblast). Extramedullary hematopoiesis is also seen with resultant splenomegaly. With acute leukemias, there can be infiltration of other organs, such as the meninges, lymph nodes, gums, and skin (leukemia cutis).

The cause of leukemia is not fully known, but there is some evidence that genetic influences and viral pathogenesis may be involved. Bone marrow damage from radiation exposure or from chemicals benzene, topoisomerase II inhibitors (such as etoposide) and alkylating agents (e.g., cyclophosphamide [Cytoxan], melphalan [Alkeran]) can cause leukemia.

The leukemias are commonly classified according to the stem cell line involved, either lymphoid or myeloid. They are also classified as either acute or chronic based on the phase of cell development that is halted, with few leukocytes differentiating beyond that phase.

In acute leukemia, the onset of symptoms is abrupt, often occurring within a few weeks. Leukocyte development is halted at the blast phase so that most leukocytes are undifferentiated, immature cells (blasts). Acute leukemia progresses very rapidly; death can occur within weeks to months without aggressive treatment.

In chronic leukemia, symptoms evolve over a period of months to years. Most of the leukocytes produced are mature and retain some ability to function normally. Chronic leukemia progresses more slowly; the disease trajectory can extend for years.

ACUTE MYELOID LEUKEMIA

AML results from a defect in the hematopoietic stem cell that differentiates into all myeloid cells: monocytes, granulocytes (neutrophils, basophils, eosinophils), erythrocytes, and platelets. All age groups are affected; the incidence rises with age, with a peak incidence at age 60 years. Median age of diagnosis is 65 years (Sweet & Asghari, 2021). AML accounts for 80% of acute leukemias in adults and 18% of leukemias in children (Jain & Rampal, 2021; Sweet & Asghari, 2021).

AML represents a heterogeneous group of clonal myeloid malignancies marked by an excess of myeloid blast cells (greater than 20%). Classification of AML has evolved from a morphologic classification to one based on cytogenetic and molecular abnormalities. The French American British system classifies AML based primarily on morphology and stage of maturation arrest, with eight subtypes. The more recent classification system is that of the WHO, which incorporates cytogenetic and molecular abnormalities, allowing for improved prognostication (Sweet & Asghari, 2021). There are cytogenetic abnormalities that may be considered favorable (translocation 15;17, translocation 8;21, and inversion 16), whereas survival is poor in instances of unfavorable cytogenetic abnormalities (deletions of chromosome 5 or

7 and patients with more than three abnormalities [referred to as a complex karyotype]) (Sweet & Asghari, 2021). The identification of molecular mutations has further complicated the classification of AML. Mutations in NPM1, FLT3, and CEBPA genes have resulted in the identification of four groups with very different prognoses, with mutations in NPM1 or CEBPA being favorable while mutations in FLT3-ITD are unfavorable (Sweet & Asghari, 2021).

The prognosis of AML is highly variable and related to patient age, performance status, and cytogenetic and molecular characteristics of their disease (Sweet & Asghari, 2021). The strongest risk factors for resistant disease, early relapse, and decreased survival include advanced age, poor functional status, and complex cytogenetic abnormalities. Patients over 65 years of age have a poorer response to treatment and a worse prognosis than younger patients. Those who have leukemia stemming from pre-existing MDS or who previously received alkylating agents or topoisomerase II inhibitors for cancer (secondary AML) have a much worse prognosis; the leukemia tends to be more resistant to treatment, resulting in a much shorter duration of remission. With treatment, patients with secondary AML survive an average of less than 1 year, with death usually a result of infection or hemorrhage. Patients receiving supportive care also usually survive less than 1 year, dying of infection or bleeding.

Clinical Manifestations and Assessment

Most signs and symptoms of AML result from insufficient production of normal blood cells. Fever and infection result from neutropenia, weakness and fatigue from anemia, and bleeding tendencies from thrombocytopenia. The proliferation of leukemic cells within organs leads to a variety of additional symptoms: pain from an enlarged liver or spleen, hyperplasia of the gums, and bone pain from expansion of the bone marrow.

AML develops without warning, with symptoms occurring over a period of weeks to months. The CBC may show a decrease in both erythrocytes and platelets. Although the total leukocyte count can be low, normal, or high, usually the percentage of normal cells is vastly decreased. The differential may reveal the presence of circulating blasts and a decreased neutrophil count.

Diagnosis is established with bone marrow aspirate and biopsy with biopsy revealing more than 20% myeloblasts. Aspirate samples are sent for flow cytometry, analysis of cytogenetic abnormalities, and genetic mutations.

Complications

Complications of AML include bleeding and infection, the major causes of death. The risk of bleeding correlates with the severity of thrombocytopenia. The low platelet count can result in **ecchymoses** (bruises) and **petechiae** (pinpoint red or purple hemorrhagic spots on the skin) (Fig. 19-2). Major spontaneous hemorrhages also may develop when the platelet count drops to less than 10,000/mm^3. The most common sites of bleeding are GI, pulmonary, and intracranial. Fever increases platelet consumption and, therefore, may increase the likelihood of bleeding.

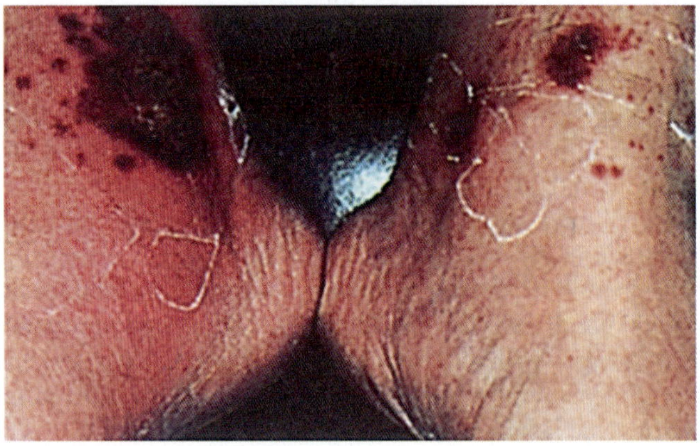

FIGURE 19-2 Petechia and purpura. (From Bickley, L. S. [2013]. *Bates' guide to physical examination* [11th ed.]. Lippincott Williams & Wilkins.)

Because of the lack of mature and normal granulocytes, infection is the most common cause of death in patients with acute leukemia. The likelihood of infection increases with the degree and duration of neutropenia; neutrophil counts that persist at less than 100/mm^3 for prolonged periods make the likelihood of systemic infection extremely high. As the duration of severe neutropenia increases, the patient's risk of developing fungal infection also increases (see Chapter 5 for calculation of the Absolute Neutrophil Count [ANC]).

Medical Management

When considering approaches to therapy for AML, the first determination is if the patient would be a candidate for allogeneic stem cell transplant. In general, patients who are considered transplant candidates will be treated with an aggressive approach. Patients who are not transplant candidates due to poor performance status, advanced age, or significant comorbidity would be treated with a less aggressive approach focused on optimizing quality of life.

The initial objective of treatment is to achieve complete remission, in which there is no evidence of residual leukemia in the bone marrow. For patients with a good performance status and absence of comorbidities, attempts are made to achieve remission by the aggressive administration of chemotherapy, called *induction therapy*, which usually requires hospitalization for several weeks. Induction therapy typically involves IV administration of cytarabine and an anthracycline, such as idarubicin or daunorubicin. The choice of agents is based on the patient's performance status and history of prior antineoplastic treatment. For older patients or patients with poor performance status and comorbidities, less aggressive approaches may be used. Enrollment in clinical trials is always encouraged.

The aim of induction therapy is to eradicate the leukemic cells, but this is often accompanied by the eradication of normal types of myeloid cells. Thus, the patient becomes severely pancytopenic. During this time, the patient is hospitalized due to high risk for life-threatening complications. Common complications include bacterial, fungal, and, occasionally, viral infections; bleeding; and severe mucositis, which can cause mouth pain and diarrhea as well as a marked decline in the ability to eat and meet nutritional demands. Supportive care consists of administering blood products (PRBCs and platelets) and promptly treating infections.

Response to treatment is assessed using bone marrow aspirate and biopsy after induction when blood counts are recovering. The expected result is an absence of leukemic blasts and recovery of normal marrow function. When the patient has recovered from the induction therapy (i.e., the neutrophil and platelet counts have returned to normal and any infection has resolved) and response to induction has been assessed, they typically receive *consolidation therapy* (additional postremission chemotherapy) to eliminate any residual leukemia cells that are not clinically detectable and to reduce the chance for recurrence. Multiple treatment cycles of various agents are used, with most regimens using high-dose cytarabine.

Following consolidation therapy, the next step is determined based on the patient's risk for recurrence. Patients with low- or intermediate-risk leukemia may not require further treatment after they complete consolidation therapy. Patients with high-risk leukemia, or patients who have been treated for a relapse, may be candidates for PBSCT. When a suitable donor is identified (either a sibling or unrelated donor identified in the national registry), the patient embarks on an even more aggressive regimen of chemotherapy (sometimes in combination with total body radiation therapy), with the treatment goal of destroying the hematopoietic function of the patient's bone marrow. The patient is then "rescued" with the infusion of the donor stem cells to reinitiate hematopoiesis. In addition to providing a "rescue" and a healthy source of hematopoiesis, infusion of donor cells also provides protection against disease recurrence. The healthy immune system of the donor kills residual cancer cells and prevents cancer recurrence; this is known as the *graft versus leukemia* effect. Patients who undergo PBSCT have a significant risk for infection, graft-versus-host disease (GVHD, in which the donor's lymphocytes [graft] recognize the patient's body as "foreign" and attack the "foreign" host), and other complications. Refer to Chapter 5 for a detailed discussion of PBSCT. For patients who are not candidates for transplant, less aggressive approaches to therapy with drugs like hypomethylating agents (decitabine or azacitidine) may be considered (Jammal et al., 2021).

Another important option for the patient to consider is supportive care alone. In fact, supportive care may be the only option if the patient has significant comorbidity, such as extremely poor cardiac, pulmonary, kidney, or liver function; advanced age; or poor performance status. In such cases, aggressive antileukemia therapy is not used; occasionally, hydroxyurea may be used to control the WBC count and prevent the potential sequelae of leukocytosis. Patients are supported with antimicrobial therapy and transfusions as needed. This treatment approach provides the patient with some additional time at home; however, death frequently occurs within months, typically from infection or bleeding. (Refer to Chapter 2 for a discussion of end-of-life care.)

Treatment of relapsed AML may involve different combinations of chemotherapy if the patient is in good physical condition, or less aggressive therapies or supportive care alone may be used. Clinical trials may also be considered. Relapsed AML is often difficult to treat and overall survival rate is low.

Nursing Management

The priority nursing interventions for the patient with AML include infection prevention, bleeding prevention, promoting comfort, and patient education. Nursing care to prevent infection and bleeding are discussed in detail in Chapters 5 and 18. Patients with a new diagnosis of AML are experiencing a crisis and require an overwhelming amount of education about their disease, self-care, and treatment strategies. The role of the nurse is critical in alleviating anxiety by providing information tailored to the patient's readiness and educational level.

The nurse also assesses for complications of treatment. Massive leukemic cell destruction from chemotherapy results in the release of intracellular electrolytes and fluids into the systemic circulation. Increases in uric acid levels, potassium, and phosphate are seen; this process is referred to as **tumor lysis** syndrome (see Chapter 5). Patients require a high fluid intake and prophylaxis with allopurinol to prevent crystallization of uric acid and subsequent stone formation. Anorexia, nausea, vomiting, diarrhea, and severe mucositis are common.

ACUTE PROMYELOCYTIC LEUKEMIA (APML)

APML is a subtype of AML that is characterized by the cytogenetic abnormality of translocation 15;17, which results in the PML-RARα protein. APML, unlike most other types of AML, is highly curable. APML is often associated with life-threatening DIC, and once the diagnosis is presumed, treatment must start emergently. Diagnosis is established through the detection of the PML-RARα protein, which can be detected in the blood. A bone marrow aspirate and biopsy is also done to establish the diagnosis though detection of PML-RARα protein justifies initiation of treatment. Treatment includes all-trans-retinoic acid (ATRA), an oral agent that stimulates differentiation of the promyelocytes into mature neutrophils. Aggressive supportive care to manage DIC in the initial stages of the disease is critical. Platelets and cryoprecipitate are used to minimize bleeding risk. ATRA has also been shown to decrease the risk of coagulopathy, which is the leading cause of death in APML (Sanz & Barragan, 2021). One fourth of patients treated with ATRA will experience differentiation syndrome in the first 21 days of induction treatment with ATRA. The symptoms include weight gain, shortness of breath, fever, hypotension, effusions, and liver and kidney dysfunction. Risk for differentiation syndrome is increased when the WBC count is over 30,000/microL. Often steroids are used to prevent and treat this syndrome. Diuretics also may be used to manage volume overload. ATRA may be used in combination with chemotherapy or arsenic trioxide, which is also a differentiating agent (Sanz & Barragan, 2021).

Response to treatment is assessed through measurement of PML-RARα protein levels in the blood and bone marrow.

The nursing role in APML is critical; astute assessment skills should be focused on identifying early signs and symptoms of DIC and differentiation syndrome. Daily weights and strict I/Os are important data points in assessing for differentiation syndrome. The nurse also counsels the patient on the importance of adherence to ATRA therapy. For patients on arsenic therapy, monitoring of ECG for prolongation of the QT interval is essential. Other drugs that prolong the QT interval should be minimized (refer to Chapter 16 for drugs associated with prolonged QT).

ACUTE LYMPHOCYTIC LEUKEMIA

ALL results from an uncontrolled proliferation of immature lymphoid cells (lymphoblasts) derived from the lymphoid stem cell. The cell of origin is the precursor to the B lymphocyte in approximately 85% of ALL cases; T-lymphocyte ALL occurs in approximately 15% to 20% of ALL cases. The *BCR-ABL* translocation or Philadelphia chromosome (see earlier CML discussion) is found in 20% of ALL blast cells. ALL is most common in young children, with boys affected more often than girls. ALL accounts for up to 80% of pediatric leukemias and 20% of adult leukemias (Gurbuxani et al., 2021). The peak incidence is 4 years of age. After 15 years of age, ALL incidence decreases with a second peak occurring after age 50 (Brown et al., 2021).

Clinical Manifestations and Assessment

Immature lymphocytes proliferate in the marrow and impede the development of normal myeloid cells. As a result, normal hematopoiesis is inhibited, resulting in reduced numbers of leukocytes, erythrocytes, and platelets. Leukocyte counts may be either low or high, but there is always a high proportion of immature cells. Manifestations of leukemic cell infiltration into other organs are more common with ALL than with other forms of leukemia and include pain from an enlarged liver or spleen and bone pain. The testes and central nervous system (CNS) are sanctuary sites where leukemic cells may infiltrate. The patient may exhibit testicular swelling or discomfort, or headache, visual changes, vomiting, and neurologic deficits from CNS invasion. Children are more likely to report musculoskeletal symptoms, including bone and joint pain (Gurbuxani et al., 2021).

Diagnosis is established with bone marrow aspirate and biopsy, with bone marrow biopsy demonstrating lymphoblasts at 20% or higher. Aspirate samples are evaluated for flow cytometry as well as cytogenetic and molecular abnormalities. Due to the high incidence of CNS involvement, diagnostic lumbar puncture is also performed. Typically chemotherapy is given into the intrathecal space at the time of initial lumbar puncture to treat or provide prophylaxis for ALL in the CNS (Mackey et al., 2021).

Males should have a testicular examination, and abnormalities on examination warrant evaluation with ultrasound as the testes are a sanctuary site for ALL.

Medical and Nursing Management

The expected outcome of treatment is complete remission. Lymphoid blast cells are typically very sensitive to corticosteroids and to vinca alkaloids; therefore, these medications are an integral part of the initial induction therapy. Because ALL frequently invades the CNS, prophylaxis with cranial irradiation or intrathecal (injection of medications into the subarachnoid space [cerebral spinal fluid]) chemotherapy (e.g., methotrexate), or both is also a key part of the treatment plan (Mackey, 2021).

Treatment protocols for ALL tend to be complex, using a wide variety of chemotherapeutic agents given over a protracted period of time. Treatment includes an induction phase, followed by a consolidation phase, followed by a maintenance phase, when lower doses of medications are given for up to 3 years. Despite the complexity, treatment can often be provided in the outpatient setting.

Tyrosine kinase inhibitors in combination with chemotherapy are the standard frontline treatment for patients with Philadelphia chromosome–positive ALL (Brown et al., 2021). Patients with Philadelphia chromosome-negative disease, multiagent chemotherapy is the standard frontline therapy (Brown et al., 2021). Monoclonal antibodies, in which the antibody specific for the antigens expressed on the ALL blast cell are a type of targeted therapy also used to treat ALL (Brown et al., 2021). Allogeneic hematopoietic stem cell transplantation (ASCT) is also used in the treatment of ALL (Brown et al., 2021).

Infections, especially viral infections, are common. The use of corticosteroids to treat ALL increases the patient's susceptibility to infection. Patients with ALL often require prophylactic antimicrobials to decrease the risk of certain types of infection. Patients with ALL tend to have a better response to treatment than do patients with AML. ASCT offers a chance for prolonged remission, or even cure, if the illness recurs after therapy.

Nursing Management for Acute Myeloid Leukemia and Acute Lymphocytic Leukemia

Nursing management of the patient with ALL is similar to the care of patients with AML. The nursing priorities include the prevention of infection and bleeding as well as management of symptoms, such as nausea and pain, often resulting from mucositis. As ALL is a disease that most commonly affects children and young adults, fertility preservation should be discussed prior to the initiation of treatment.

Although the clinical picture varies with the type of leukemia as well as the treatment implemented, the health history may reveal a range of subtle symptoms reported by the patient before the problem is detectable on physical examination. Weakness and fatigue are common manifestations, not only of the leukemia but also of the resulting complications of anemia and infection. If the patient is hospitalized, the assessments should be performed daily or more frequently as warranted. Because the physical findings may be subtle initially, a thorough, systematic assessment incorporating all body systems is essential. For example, a dry cough, mild dyspnea, and diminished breath sounds may indicate a pulmonary infection. However, the infection may not be seen initially on the chest x-ray; the absence of neutrophils delays the inflammatory response against the pulmonary infection, and it is the inflammatory response that produces the x-ray changes. The platelet count can become dangerously low, leaving the patient at risk for significant bleeding. The specific body system assessments are delineated in the neutropenic precautions and bleeding precautions found in Chapters 5 and 18, respectively. When serial assessments are performed, current findings are compared with previous findings to evaluate the patient's condition for improvement or worsening.

The nurse also must monitor the results of laboratory studies closely. It is particularly important to trend the leukocyte count, ANC, hematocrit, platelet, creatinine and electrolyte levels, and liver function tests. During initial treatment for acute leukemia, the ANC often drops below 100/mm^3, placing the patient at very high risk for infection (Mackey et al., 2021). Empiric antibiotics are used to treat infection preemptively when the patient has a fever of **100.4°F** or greater. Culture results need to be reported immediately so that antimicrobial therapy can be modified appropriately based on microbial sensitivity.

LYMPHOMA

The lymphomas are neoplasms (abnormal growth of tissue) of lymphoid tissue, usually derived from B lymphocytes. These tumors usually start in lymph nodes but can involve lymphoid tissue in the spleen, the GI tract (e.g., the wall of the stomach), the liver, or the bone marrow. Often they are classified according to the degree of cell differentiation and the origin of the predominant malignant cell. Lymphomas can be classified into two broad categories: Hodgkin lymphoma and non-Hodgkin lymphoma (NHL). NHLs can be furthered characterized into low grade and high grade.

HODGKIN LYMPHOMA

Hodgkin lymphoma is a relatively rare malignancy that has an impressive cure rate. In 2018, nearly 80,000 individuals were diagnosed with Hodgkin lymphoma, with more cases in males than females (Hjalgrim & Jarrett, 2020).

Pathophysiology

Unlike other lymphomas, Hodgkin lymphoma is unicentric in origin in that it initiates in a single node. The disease spreads by contiguous extension along the lymphatic system. The malignant cell of Hodgkin lymphoma is the Reed–Sternberg cell, a large tumor cell that is morphologically unique and is thought to be of immature lymphoid origin. It is the pathologic hallmark and essential diagnostic criterion for Hodgkin disease. However, the tumor is very heterogeneous and actually may contain few Reed–Sternberg cells. Repeated biopsies may be required to establish the diagnosis.

The cause of Hodgkin lymphoma is unknown, but a viral etiology is suspected. In fact, several classic Hodgkin lymphoma subtypes have been associated with the Epstein–Barr virus (Visser et al., 2020).

The WHO classifies Hodgkin lymphoma into two groups: classic Hodgkin lymphoma (92% to 97% of cases), which has four main histologic subtypes based on the number of lymphocytes, Reed–Sternberg cells, and the presence of fibrous tissue; and nodular lymphocyte-predominant Hodgkin lymphoma (3% to 8% of cases) (Hjalgrim & Jarrett, 2020).

Risk Factors

Hodgkin lymphoma is somewhat more common in males than females and has two peaks of incidence: one in the early 20s and the other after 50 years of age. Disease occurrence has a familial pattern: first-degree relatives have a higher-than-normal frequency of disease, but the actual incidence of this pattern is low. Hodgkin lymphoma is seen more commonly in patients receiving chronic IST (e.g., for kidney transplant) and in woodworkers. Also it is seen in veterans of the military who were exposed to the herbicide Agent Orange.

Clinical Manifestations and Assessment

Hodgkin lymphoma usually begins as a painless enlargement of one or more lymph nodes above the diaphragm (most commonly in the cervical or supraclavicular region) (Armitage & Friedberg, 2020). The individual nodes are painless and rubbery or firm but not hard. A mediastinal mass may be seen on chest x-ray; occasionally, the mass is large enough to compress the trachea and cause dyspnea and cough. Pruritus is common; it can be extremely distressing, and the cause is unknown. Rarely patients experience brief but severe pain after drinking alcohol, usually at the site of the tumor (Armitage & Friedberg, 2020). Again, the cause of this is unknown.

All organs are vulnerable to invasion by Hodgkin lymphoma. The symptoms result from compression of organs by the tumor, such as cough and pulmonary effusion (from pulmonary infiltrates), jaundice (from hepatic involvement or bile duct obstruction), abdominal pain (from splenomegaly or retroperitoneal adenopathy), or bone pain (from skeletal involvement). Herpes zoster infections are common. A cluster of constitutional symptoms have important prognostic implications. Referred to as "B symptoms," they include fever (without chills), drenching sweats (particularly at night), and unintentional weight loss of more than 10%. B symptoms are found in 40% of patients and are more common in advanced disease. An elevated **erythrocyte sedimentation rate** (ESR) represents a poor prognostic indicator (Armitage & Friedberg, 2020).

Pearls for Practice

The erythrocyte sedimentation rate (ESR, also known as the sed rate) is a common blood test that increases with inflammatory activity, which can be caused by autoimmune disease, infections or tumors. It is not specific for any one disease but is used to assess for the presence of increased inflammatory activity. It measures the rate at which the RBCs fall to the bottom of the test tube. Those with inflammatory disorders have an increase in the number of proteins in the blood which increases their sticking together or clumping of RBCs and they fall at a faster rate, thus a higher sed rate is seen (Tishkowski & Gupta, 2021). A normal sed rate for adult males is 0 to 15 mm/hr, and females are 0 to 20 mm/hr (Fischbach et al., 2022).

A mild anemia is the most common hematologic finding. The leukocyte count may be elevated or decreased. The platelet count is typically normal unless the tumor has invaded the bone marrow, suppressing hematopoiesis. Patients with Hodgkin lymphoma have impaired cellular immunity as evidenced by an absent or decreased reaction to skin sensitivity tests (e.g., *Candida,* mumps).

Because many manifestations are similar to those occurring with infection, diagnostic studies are performed to rule out an infectious origin for the disease. The diagnosis is made by means of an excisional lymph node biopsy and the finding of the Reed–Sternberg cell. Once the diagnosis is confirmed and the histologic type is established, it is necessary to assess the extent of the disease, a process referred to as *staging*. See Chapter 5 for discussion of staging.

In addition to a careful physical examination, a chest x-ray; computed tomography (CT) scan of the chest, abdomen, and pelvis; and a positron emission tomography (PET) scan are all obtained to assist with staging. The PET scan may be the most sensitive imaging test in identifying residual disease. Laboratory tests include CBC, platelet count, ESR, lactate dehydrogenase (LDH), and liver and kidney function studies. A bone marrow biopsy is performed if there are signs of marrow involvement, and some physicians routinely perform bilateral biopsies. Bone scans may be performed to identify any involvement in these areas.

Medical Management

The general goal in treatment of Hodgkin lymphoma, regardless of stage, is cure. Overall, cure rates for Hodgkin lymphoma are high (80% to 85%) (Parsons et al., 2020). Treatment is determined primarily by the stage of the disease, not the histologic type; however, extensive research is ongoing to target treatment regimens to histologic subtypes or prognostic features. Traditionally, early Hodgkin disease was treated by a staging laparotomy followed by radiation therapy. This treatment method has been replaced by a short course (2 to 4 months) of chemotherapy followed by radiation therapy in early-stage disease (I and II). Advanced-stage disease is often treated with chemotherapy alone as the role of radiation in advanced disease has not been demonstrated in clinical trials (Hoppe et al., 2020). For advanced-stage classical Hodgkin lymphoma, front-line treatment includes combination chemotherapy, such as ABVD (doxorubicin, bleomycin, vinblastine, and dacarbazine), BEACOPP (bleomycin, etoposide, doxorubicin, cyclophosphamide, vincristine, procarbazine, and prednisone) or the Stanford V regimen (doxorubicin, vinblastine, mechlorethamine, vincristine, bleomycin, etoposide, and prednisone) (Hoppe et al., 2020).

Even when Hodgkin lymphoma does recur, the use of high doses of chemotherapeutic agents, followed by autologous PBSCT, can be effective in controlling the disease and extending survival time (Hoppe et al., 2020).

Newer therapies for Hodgkin lymphoma have emerged, including monoclonal antibodies, antibody–drug conjugates (brentuximab vedotin), and checkpoint inhibitors (nivolumab and pembrolizumab). These new agents offer promising potential alternatives to classical chemotherapy but are currently limited to the relapsed/refractory setting (Hoppe et al., 2020).

Nursing management is similar to that of NHL and is discussed in that section.

Long-Term Complications of Therapy

Much is now known about the long-term effects of chemotherapy and radiation therapy, primarily from the large numbers of people who were cured of Hodgkin lymphoma by these treatments. Long-term complications include hypothyroidism, immune dysfunction, dental caries, cardiomyopathy, infertility, and secondary malignancies. The incidence of late effects increases over time (Yahalom et al., 2020). Patients should be followed carefully for late effects, including surveillance for and assessment of risk factors for secondary cancers. Lung cancer and breast cancer are the most common type of secondary malignancy in patients with

Hodgkin disease, particularly following combination chemotherapy and radiation (Plattel & Lugtenberg, 2020).

Secondary cancers, including lung, breast, lymphoma, and leukemia, as well as cardiovascular disease, including heart failure, valvular disease, coronary artery disease, and MI, are late effects of treatment for Hodgkin lymphoma (Engert & Younes, 2020). Secondary cancers are the leading cause of death in survivors of Hodgkin lymphoma. Among female survivors of childhood Hodgkin lymphoma, breast cancer is the most common secondary cancer. There are many contributing risk factors for secondary breast cancer, with age at time of chest radiation being the most important risk factor (Schaapveld et al., 2020). For survivors of Hodgkin lymphoma who were treated with radiation to the chest, screening for breast cancer using mammography is recommended beginning 8 years from the time of radiation to the chest or beginning at age 40, whichever comes first (Schaapveld et al., 2020). Breast MRI in addition to mammogram is recommended for females treated with radiation to the chest between 10 and 30 years of age (Schaapveld et al., 2020). It is critical that survivors of Hodgkin lymphoma are counseled on their risk for secondary cancers and cardiovascular risk and that the recommended screening tests are adhered to throughout the patient's lifetime (Aleman & Cutter, 2020; Schaapveld et al., 2020).

Patients should be encouraged to reduce other factors that increase the risk of developing secondary cancers and cardiovascular disease, such as use of tobacco and alcohol and exposure to environmental carcinogens, as well as maintaining an exercise regimen and healthy weight. Revised treatment approaches are under investigation with the goal of minimizing the risk for complications (secondary malignancy and cardiovascular disease) without sacrificing the potential for cure.

NON-HODGKIN LYMPHOMAS

The NHLs are a heterogeneous group of cancers that originate from the neoplastic growth of lymphoid tissue. As in CLL, the neoplastic cells are thought to arise from a single clone of lymphocytes; however, in NHL, the cells may vary morphologically. Most NHLs involve malignant B lymphocytes; about 10% involve T lymphocytes and natural killer (NK) cells (Abramson, 2020). In contrast to Hodgkin lymphoma, the lymphoid tissues involved in NHL are largely infiltrated with malignant cells. The spread of these malignant lymphoid cells occurs unpredictably, and true localized disease is uncommon. Lymph nodes from multiple sites may be infiltrated as may sites outside the lymphoid system (extranodal tissue).

Pearls for Practice

Natural Killer (NK) cells are the third lymphocyte (WBC), after T and B cells, and they play essential roles in the frontline's defense of the innate immune system (Rahman & Bordoni, 2022). These cells, as the name suggests, can kill the target cells, such as tumor cells or cells infected with a virus, without prestimulation, whereas other immune cells demand time to induce their cytolytic activity. That is why NK cells are an attractive target for cancer immunotherapies and some therapeutic monoclonal antibodies rely on NK cell killing; they are the ready to perform machinery of the immune system (Eismann, n.d.).

There are an estimated 72,000 new cases of NHL diagnosed yearly, making it the most common hematologic malignancy and the seventh most common malignancy in the United States (Abramson, 2020). The incidence increases with each decade of life, is higher in whites than other ethnic groups, and is diagnosed in patients with an average age of 50 to 60 years. Although no common etiologic factor has been identified, the incidence of NHL has increased in people with immunodeficiencies or autoimmune disorders; treatment with immunosuppressive medications; prior treatment for cancer; prior organ transplant; viral infections (including EBV and HIV); and exposure to pesticides, solvents, dyes, or defoliating agents, including Agent Orange. In addition, some cases may be explained by improved pathology techniques (Abramson, 2020). Prognosis varies greatly among the various types of NHL. NHL can be further characterized as low grade or high grade. The most common types of low-grade lymphomas include CLL and follicular lymphoma. High-grade lymphomas include diffuse large B-cell lymphoma, peripheral T-cell lymphomas, and Burkitt lymphoma.

Long-term survival (over 10 years) is commonly achieved in low-grade, localized lymphomas. Even with aggressive disease forms, cure is possible in at least one third of patients who receive aggressive treatment.

Clinical Manifestations and Assessment

Symptoms are highly variable, reflecting the diverse nature of the NHLs. Lymphadenopathy is most common; however, in more indolent (less aggressive) types of lymphomas, the lymphadenopathy can wax and wane. With early-stage disease or with the types that are considered more indolent, there may be no symptoms, and the illness typically is not diagnosed until it progresses to a later stage, when the patient becomes symptomatic. At these stages (III or IV), lymphadenopathy is prominent. One third of patients with NHLs have "B symptoms" (recurrent fever, drenching night sweats, and unintentional weight loss of 10% or more). Lymphomatous masses can compromise organ function. For example, a mass in the mediastinum can cause respiratory distress; abdominal masses can compromise the ureters, leading to kidney dysfunction; and splenomegaly can cause abdominal discomfort, nausea, early satiety, anorexia, and weight loss. Less than 10% of patients will experience CNS involvement at some point in their disease. Certain populations have higher rates of CNS involvement, including patients with HIV or those with testicular, breast, epidural, or sinus involvement.

The actual diagnosis of NHL is categorized into a highly complex classification system based on histopathology, immunophenotyping, and cytogenetic analyses of the malignant cells. The specific histopathologic type of the disease has important prognostic implications. Treatment also varies and is based on these features. Staging, also an important factor, is typically based on data obtained from CT and PET scans, bone marrow biopsy, and, occasionally, cerebrospinal fluid analysis. The stage is based on the site of disease and its spread to other sites. For example, in stage I disease, only one area of involvement is detected; thus, stage I disease is highly localized and may respond well to localized therapy (e.g., radiation therapy). In contrast, in stage IV disease, at least one extranodal site is detected.

Medical Management

Treatment is based on the classification of disease, the stage of disease, prior treatment (if any), and the patient's ability to tolerate therapy. If the disease is not an aggressive form and is truly localized, radiation alone may be the treatment of choice.

Low-grade lymphomas may not require treatment until the disease progresses to a later stage, but historically they have been relatively unresponsive to treatment, and, in most cases, use of therapeutic modalities did not improve overall survival. More aggressive types of NHL (e.g., lymphoblastic lymphoma, Burkitt lymphoma) require prompt initiation of combination chemotherapy; however, these types tend to be more responsive to treatment. CNS involvement may occur with some aggressive forms of NHL; in this situation, intrathecal (spinal thecal or the space under the arachnoid membrane of the brain or spinal cord) chemotherapy is used in addition to systemic chemotherapy. Radiation may also be used for palliation of symptoms.

With aggressive types of NHL, aggressive combinations of chemotherapeutic agents are given even in early stages. More intermediate forms are commonly treated with combination chemotherapy and radiation therapy for stage I and II diseases. The advent of the monoclonal antibody, rituximab, which targets the CD20 antigen on the surface of B cells, has improved survival in patients with NHL significantly. The combination of rituximab with conventional chemotherapy (cytoxan, doxorubicin, vincristine, and prednisone [CHOP]) is now considered standard treatment for common, aggressive B-cell lymphomas (Abramson, 2020). Unfortunately, more than 30% of patients with diffuse large B-cell NHL will experience a relapse. Treatment for relapsed disease includes rituximab and combination chemotherapy followed by high-dose chemotherapy with stem cell support, which offers the best chance for response. For patients who are not eligible for transplant, chemotherapy may be used alone (Abramson, 2020). A number of novel therapies are under investigation in an attempt to enhance the efficacy of frontline therapy and improve outcomes in patients with relapsed or refractory disease. Chimeric antigen receptor engineered T cells (CAR-T) are a recently approved novel treatment for relapsed NHL (DLBL and MCL). CAR-T cells are autologous T cells collected from a patient and modified in a lab to target antigens present on cancer cells (Abramson, 2020). CAR-T cell therapy can cause potentially life-threatening inflammatory responses called cytokine release syndrome (CRS) and immune effector cell–associated neurotoxicity syndrome (ICANS) (Freyer & Porter, 2020). CRS can lead to DIC and/or capillary leak syndrome (Freyer & Porter, 2020). Patients who develop ICANS may have confusion, aphasia, obtundation, or seizures (Freyer & Porter, 2020). ICANS is treated with corticosteroids. CRS is generally managed with an IL-6 receptor antagonist (tocilizumab) and possibly the addition of corticosteroids (Freyer & Porter, 2020).

Nursing Management

Lymphoma is a highly complex constellation of diseases. When caring for patients with lymphoma, it is extremely important to know the specific disease type, stage of disease, treatment history, and current treatment plan. Most of the care for patients with Hodgkin lymphoma or NHL takes place in the outpatient setting, unless complications occur (e.g., infection, respiratory compromise due to mediastinal mass). The most commonly used treatment methods are chemotherapy and radiation therapy. Chemotherapy causes systemic side effects (e.g., myelosuppression, nausea, hair loss, risk of infection), whereas radiation therapy causes specific effects that are limited to the area being irradiated. For example, patients receiving abdominal radiation therapy may experience nausea and diarrhea but not hair loss. Regardless of the type of treatment, all patients experience fatigue. The nurse caring for patients receiving CAR-T therapy monitors the patient's neurologic status closely with routine neurologic assessments at baseline as well as post-therapy. Patients are also closely monitored for signs of inflammation by close assessment of vital signs and lab work.

The risk for infection is significant for these patients, not only from treatment-related myelosuppression but also from the defective immune response that results from the disease itself. Patients need to be taught to minimize the risks of infection, to recognize signs of possible infection, and to contact the health care professional should such signs develop (see Chapters 5 and 18). Additional complications depend on the location of the lymphoma. Therefore, it is important for the nurse to know the tumor location so that assessments can be targeted appropriately. For example, patients with lymphomatous masses in the upper chest should be assessed for superior vena cava obstruction or airway obstruction if the mass is near the bronchus or trachea.

Many lymphomas can be cured with current treatments. However, as survival rates increase, the incidence of secondary malignancies, particularly AML or MDS, also increases. Therefore, survivors should be screened regularly for the development of second malignancies.

CHRONIC LYMPHOCYTIC LEUKEMIA (CLL)

CLL is classified as a type of low-grade lymphoma as it is a disease that encompasses both CLL and small lymphocytic lymphoma (SLL). It is the most frequent form of leukemia in Western countries (Moia et al., 2021). It is a common malignancy of older adults with a mean age at diagnosis of 70 to 75 years (Catovsky et al., 2019). Prognosis for CLL is highly variable, ranging from 2 to 20 years (Rai & Stilgenbauer, 2022a).

Pathophysiology

CLL is typically derived from a malignant clone of B lymphocytes (T-lymphocyte CLL is rare). In contrast to the acute forms of leukemia, most of the leukemia cells in CLL are fully mature. It appears that these cells can escape **apoptosis** (programmed cell death), resulting in an excessive accumulation of the cells in the marrow and circulation. The antigen CD52 is prevalent on the surface of many of these leukemic B cells.

Two classification systems are in regular use to stage CLL; the disease is classified into three (Binet system; stage A, B, C) or five stages (Rai system; stage 0–IV). Both staging systems help to estimate prognosis and assist with treatment stratification (Catovsky et al., 2019). In the early stage, an elevated lymphocyte count is seen; it can exceed $100,000/mm^3$. Because the lymphocytes are small, they can travel easily through the small capillaries within the circulation, and the pulmonary and cerebral complications of leukocytosis (as seen with myeloid leukemias) typically are not found in CLL.

Lymphadenopathy occurs as the lymphocytes are trapped within the lymph nodes. The nodes can become very large and are sometimes painful. Hepatomegaly and splenomegaly then develop.

In later stages, anemia and thrombocytopenia may develop. Typically treatment is initiated in the later stages; earlier treatment does not appear to increase survival so treatment for limited-stage disease is employed only if the patient is symptomatic (Rai & Stilgenbauer, 2022a). Autoimmune complications also can occur at any stage as either AIHA or ITP.

Clinical Manifestations and Assessment

Many patients are asymptomatic and are diagnosed incidentally during routine physical examinations or during treatment for another disease. At the time of diagnosis, lymphadenopathy is seen in 50% to 90% of patients and splenomegaly in 25% to 55% of patients (Rai et al., 2021). An increased lymphocyte count (lymphocytosis) is always present. The erythrocyte and platelet counts may be normal or, in later stages of the illness, decreased.

Approximately 5% to 10% of patients with CLL present with "B symptoms," a constellation of symptoms including fevers, fatigue, drenching sweats (especially at night), and unintentional weight loss (Rai et al., 2021). Patients with CLL have defects in their humoral and cell-mediated immune systems; therefore, infections are common. The defect in cellular immunity is evidenced by an absent or decreased reaction to skin sensitivity tests (e.g., *Candida*, mumps), which is known as **anergy**. Life-threatening infections are common. Viral infections, such as herpes zoster, can become widely disseminated.

Medical Management

In early stages, CLL may require no treatment. The decision to treat is triggered by symptom progression, including drenching night sweats, fatigue, weight loss, painful lymphadenopathy or progressive cytopenias, or the development of an associated autoimmune disorder (such as AIHI or ITP) (Rai & Stilgenbauer, 2022b). The period of observation can be as long as several years. Treatment options are selected based on the patient's age, performance status, comorbidities, and risk factors (deletion of chromosome 17 predicts poor response to therapy) (Rai & Stilgenbauer, 2022b). Five to 10% of patients will experience a transformation from CLL to a more aggressive form of lymphoma. The median survival in this population is 5 months, and often aggressive therapy is employed.

The combination of FCR (fludarabine, cyclophosphamide, and rituxan) is an acceptable treatment option for young patients who have a good performance status and do not have the TP53 or del17p disease mutations (Rai & Stilgenbauer, 2022b). Given the major side effects associated with FCR (i.e., prolonged bone marrow suppression manifested by prolonged periods of neutropenia, lymphopenia, and thrombocytopenia), preference is now given to targeted therapies such as acalabrutinib (kinase inhibitor), venetoclax (BCL-2 inhibitor), and ibrutinib (tyrosine kinase inhibitor) (Rai & Stilgenbauer, 2022b). Bacterial infections are common in patients with CLL, and treatment with IV immunoglobulin (IVIG) may be given to selected patients with low immunoglobulin levels to decrease the risk for infection.

MULTIPLE MYELOMA (MM)

MM is a malignant disease of the plasma cell; it is the second most common hematologic cancer in high-income countries (van de Donk et al., 2021). Plasma cells are mature B cells that secrete immunoglobulins, proteins necessary for antibody production (IgG, IgA, IgM, IgD, IgE) to fight infection. Myeloma results in the production of monoclonal antibody proteins (M protein). Median age at diagnosis is 60 years with the majority of patients over 70 years of age (van de Donk et al., 2021). The incidence rate is more than twice as high in the Black population as compared to White populations (Marinac et al., 2020). Most patients develop resistance to treatment over time (van de Donk et al., 2021). The overall survival of MM is estimated at 10 years for patients who receive stem cell transplant and 4 to 5 years for those ineligible for transplant (van de Donk et al., 2021).

Pathophysiology

Clonal plasma cells develop as a result of a series of acquired genetic mutations and alterations in the bone marrow microenvironment that create an environment favorable to myeloma cell growth (van de Donk et al., 2021). Myeloma cells grow and accumulate in the bone marrow, resulting in bone lesions and bone marrow failure (van de Donk et al., 2021). In MM, the malignant plasma cells produce an increased amount of a specific immunoglobulin that is nonfunctional. Functional types of immunoglobulin are still produced by nonmalignant plasma cells but in lower-than-normal quantity. The nonfunctional, specific immunoglobulin secreted by the myeloma cells is detectable in the blood and/or urine and is referred to as the *monoclonal protein*, or *M protein*. This protein serves as a useful marker to monitor the extent of disease and the patient's response to therapy. In addition, the presence of light chains (antibodies are made up of light chains and heavy chains) in the urine (sometimes referred to as *Bence–Jones protein*) is considered to be a major criterion in the diagnosis of MM. The monoclonal protein is commonly measured by serum or urine protein electrophoresis. Moreover, the patient's total protein level is typically elevated, again due to the production of M protein.

To establish a diagnosis of myeloma, there must be a measurable M protein in the serum and/or urine; in the absence of measurable M protein, an abnormal serum free light chain ratio may substitute for this criteria. Bone marrow aspirate and biopsy are performed; the presence of more than 10% plasma cells in the bone marrow is another hallmark diagnostic criterion. The diagnosis of myeloma also requires evidence of end-organ damage, including: anemia, hypercalcemia, kidney dysfunction, or bone destruction (van de Donk et al., 2021). Testing for end-organ damage includes serum creatinine, hemoglobin/hematocrit, calcium, and x-rays of the axial skeleton to detect lytic lesions.

Malignant plasma cells also secrete certain substances to stimulate the creation of new blood vessels to enhance the growth of these clusters of plasma cells; this process is referred to as **angiogenesis**. Occasionally, the plasma cells infiltrate other tissue, in which case they are referred to as *plasmacytomas*. Plasmacytomas can occur in the sinuses, spinal cord, and soft tissues.

Clinical Manifestations and Assessment

As many as 90% of patients with MM develop bone lesions. Although patients can have asymptomatic bone involvement, the most common presenting symptom of MM is bone pain, usually in the back or ribs. Unlike arthritic pain, the bone pain associated with myeloma increases with movement and decreases with rest; patients may report that they have less pain on awakening, but the pain intensity increases during the day. In myeloma, a substance secreted by the plasma cells, osteoclast-activating factor, and other substances (e.g., interleukin-6 [IL-6]) are involved in stimulating osteoclasts. Both mechanisms appear to be involved in the process of bone breakdown. Thus, lytic lesions as well as osteoporosis may be seen on bone x-rays (they are not well visualized on bone scans). The bone destruction can be severe enough to cause vertebral collapse and fractures, including spinal fractures, which can impinge on the spinal cord and result in spinal cord compression. It is this bone destruction that causes significant pain.

If the bone destruction is fairly extensive, excessive ionized calcium is lost from the bone and enters the serum; therefore, hypercalcemia may develop (frequently manifested by excessive thirst, dehydration, constipation, altered mental status, confusion, and, rarely, coma). Kidney failure may also occur; the configuration of the circulating immunoglobulin molecule (particularly the shape of lambda light chains) can damage the renal tubules.

As more and more malignant plasma cells are produced, the marrow has less space for erythrocyte production, and anemia may develop. This anemia is also caused to a great extent by a diminished production of erythropoietin by the kidney. The patient may complain of fatigue and weakness due to the anemia. In the late stage of the disease, a reduced number of leukocytes and platelets may also be seen because the bone marrow is infiltrated by malignant plasma cells.

Pearls for Practice

Any older patient whose chief complaint is back pain and who has an elevated total protein level should be evaluated for possible myeloma. Older patients with anemia should also have myeloma on the list of differential diagnoses.

Medical Management

There is no cure for MM. Even autologous PBSCT is considered to extend remission rather than provide a cure. However, for many patients, it is possible to control the illness and maintain their level of functioning quite well for several years. Initial treatment is dictated by risk level and transplant eligibility. Patients who are transplant eligible are treated with combination therapy, including a proteasome inhibitor (bortezomib in low- and intermediate-risk patients and carfilzomib in high-risk patients), lenalidomide, and dexamethasone for four cycles followed by autologous transplant and maintenance therapy with either lenalidomide (low-risk patients) or a proteasome inhibitor (high-risk patients) (Kumar et al., 2020). Patients who are not eligible for transplant are treated with bortezomib, lenalidomide, and dexamethasone for several cycles followed by maintenance therapy with a proteasome inhibitor for intermediate- and high-risk patients. Frail older adult patients may be treated with lenalidomide and dexamethasone (Kumar, 2020).

Recent advances in the understanding of the process of angiogenesis have resulted in new therapeutic options. The sedative thalidomide, initially used as an antiemetic, and the newer agents, lenalidomide, and pomalidomide, have significant antimyeloma effects. These agents inhibit the cytokines necessary for new vascular generation, such as vascular endothelial growth factor, and for myeloma cell growth and survival, such as IL-6 and tumor necrosis factor, by boosting the body's immune response against the tumor and by creating favorable conditions for apoptosis (programmed cell death) of the myeloma cells. Thalidomide, lenalidomide, and pomalidomide are not typical chemotherapeutic agents and have unique side-effect profiles. Thalidomide commonly causes fatigue, dizziness, constipation, rash, and peripheral neuropathy. Lenalidomide and pomalidomide side-effect profiles are quite different from that of thalidomide: myelosuppression and infections such as pneumonia are more common, whereas sedation, neuropathy, and constipation are not (Kumar et al., 2020). Patients who have progressed on thalidomide still can be treated with lenalidomide; lenalidomide is thought to exhibit more antimyeloma activity than thalidomide. Often lenalidomide is used in combination with bortezomib; together, the two drugs are synergistic and may improve outcomes.

Thalidomide, lenalidomide, and pomalidomide are contraindicated in pregnancy because of associated severe birth defects. In addition, due to the risks for birth defects, use of either agent requires registry into a monitoring program that ensures routine pregnancy testing, contraception, and control of drug distribution. Patients must be counseled monthly and agree to use approved methods of birth control prior to taking these drugs.

Newer agents recently approved for the treatment of myeloma include the monoclonal antibodies (MoAb), elotuzumab and daratumumab. Elotuzumab is a humanized MoAb that targets the CS-1 antigen that is expressed in 97% of cases of myeloma. CS-1 stimulates tumor growth and cell adhesion through interaction with the bone marrow microenvironment; elotuzumab interferes with the activity of CS-1. Elotuzumab, in combination with immunomodulatory drugs and dexamethasone, has been shown to be very effective in the relapsed/refractory setting (Trudel et al., 2019).

Radiation therapy is very useful in strengthening the bone at a specific lesion, particularly one at risk for bone fracture or spinal cord compression. It is also useful in relieving bone pain and reducing the size of plasma cell tumors that occur outside the skeletal system. However, because it is a nonsystemic form of treatment, it does not diminish the source of the bone conditions (i.e., the production of malignant plasma cells). Therefore, typically radiation therapy is used in combination with systemic treatment such as chemotherapy.

When lytic lesions result in vertebral compression fractures, vertebroplasty is often performed. This procedure is performed under fluoroscopy. A hollow needle is positioned within the fractured vertebra, and when the precise location is confirmed, an orthopedic cement is injected into the vertebra to stabilize the fracture and strengthen the vertebra. For most patients, relief from pain is almost immediate. This procedure has been enhanced by concomitant kyphoplasty, the use of a special inflatable balloon inserted into the vertebra to increase the height of the vertebra prior to injecting the cement.

All patients with myeloma are at risk for skeletal-related events (SREs), including pathologic fractures and spinal cord compression. Bisphosphonate therapy has been shown to decrease the risk of SREs in patients with and without bone involvement (Mukkamalla & Malipeddi, 2021). As a result of this data, all patients with symptomatic myeloma should receive bisphosphonate therapy with either pamidronate or zoledronic acid, as an adjunct to their antimyeloma therapy (Kumar, 2020). Pamidronate and zoledronic acid have been shown to strengthen bone in MM by diminishing the secretion of osteoclast-activating factor, thus controlling bone pain and potentially preventing bone fracture. These agents are also effective in managing and preventing hypercalcemia. However, a complication associated with IV bisphosphonates is osteonecrosis of the jaw, which can result in intractable pain, swallowing difficulty, sinusitis, soft-tissue abscesses, and extraoral fistulas (a permanent abnormal passageway between the mouth and exterior of the body). Zoledronic acid has a higher incidence of osteonecrosis of the jaw compared with pamidronate (Mukkamalla & Malipeddi, 2021). Patients should receive a comprehensive dental examination and appropriate dental interventions as needed prior to initiation of bisphosphonate therapy. Throughout the duration of treatment, careful assessment for this complication should be performed.

Hyperviscosity may result from elevations in the M protein levels. When patients have signs and symptoms of hyperviscosity, such as mental status changes or blurred vision, plasmapheresis may be used to lower the immunoglobulin level. Symptoms may be more useful than serum viscosity levels in determining the need for this intervention.

MM increases the risk for the development of VTE. Drugs such as thalidomide, lenalidomide, and pomalidomide are also thrombogenic; the risk for VTE increases when these agents are used in combination with dexamethasone. To minimize the risk for VTE, patients are educated to maintain an active lifestyle including daily exercise. In addition, prophylaxis with aspirin is recommended unless contraindicated.

Nursing Management

Pain management is very important in patients with MM. NSAIDs can be very useful for mild pain or can be administered in combination with opioid analgesics. Because NSAIDs can cause gastritis and kidney dysfunction, kidney function must be monitored carefully. The patient needs to be educated about activity restrictions (e.g., lifting no more than 10 lb, use of proper body mechanics). Braces are needed occasionally to support the spinal column. Patients must understand the importance of reporting any new pain promptly as there is risk for spontaneous pathologic fractures that require prompt intervention to minimize morbidity.

Peripheral neuropathy is a common side effect of the immunomodulatory agents used to treat MM, occurring in as many as 80% of patients. Peripheral neuropathy can significantly impact the patient's quality of life and ability to perform activities of daily living (ADLs). The physical examination should include an assessment of neuropathy using a neurotoxicity assessment tool as well as a subjective assessment of the patient's discomfort. Management of peripheral neuropathy may include decreasing drug doses, holding therapy, treating discomfort with medications such as gabapentin, and involving other disciplines such as occupational and physical therapy to maximize and restore function.

The patient also needs to be instructed about the signs and symptoms of hypercalcemia. Maintaining mobility and hydration is important to minimize risk of exacerbations of this complication; however, the primary cause is the disease itself. Also kidney function should be monitored closely. Kidney failure can become severe, and dialysis may be needed. Maintaining high urine output with aggressive hydration (3 L/day) can be very useful in preventing or limiting this complication.

Because antibody production is impaired, infections, particularly bacterial infections, are common and can be life-threatening. The patient needs to be instructed in appropriate infection-prevention measures, such as hand hygiene and avoiding sick individuals, and should be advised to contact the health care provider immediately if they have a fever or other signs and symptoms of infection. The patient should receive vaccines for pneumonia (Pneumovax) and influenza. Patients with MM may have a poor response to vaccination for COVID-19 due to their disease process as well as the B-cell–directed therapies they often receive; close monitoring for vaccination response and additional vaccination doses may be warranted (Ludwig et al., 2021). Sometimes prophylactic antibiotics are used. IVIG can be useful for patients with recurrent infections and low levels of immunoglobulins.

Many patients with MM are treated with high doses of corticosteroids for protracted periods of time. Patients must be monitored for potential short- and long-term effects of steroids, including hyperglycemia and insomnia (short term), and osteopenia, osteoporosis, cataracts, and diabetes (long term).

Gerontologic Considerations

The incidence of MM increases with age; the disease is less common in patients younger than 40 years of age. Due in part to the aging population, incidence is rising. Back pain, which is often a presenting symptom in this disease, should be investigated closely in older patients. In addition, any patient over 40 years of age presenting with anemia should undergo a workup for myeloma, primarily through an evaluation of the serum protein electrophoresis (SPEP). Autologous PBSCT is an option that can prolong remission and potentially cure some patients, but it is unavailable to many older people because of age limitations, poor performance status, and comorbidities.

THERAPIES FOR BLOOD DISORDERS

Splenectomy

Each year 25,000 splenectomies are performed in the United States with the estimated prevalence of asplenic patients reaching 1 million (Cardoso et al., 2018; Lee, 2020). Removal may be an emergency, in the case of trauma or rupture, or elective in the case of treating selected hematologic disorders. Because the spleen is very vascular, severe hemorrhage can result if the spleen is ruptured. Under such circumstances, splenectomy becomes an emergency procedure.

Splenectomy is also a possible treatment for other hematologic disorders. For example, an enlarged spleen may be the site of excessive destruction of blood cells. If the destruction is life-threatening, surgery may be life-saving. This is the case in AIHA and ITP when these disorders do not respond to more conservative measures, such as corticosteroid therapy. Some patients with grossly enlarged spleens develop severe thrombocytopenia due to the platelets being sequestered in the spleen; splenectomy removes the "trap," and platelet counts may normalize over time.

In general, the mortality rate after splenectomy is low. Laparoscopic splenectomy can be performed in selected patients, with a resultant decrease in postoperative morbidity. The most common complications in patients following splenectomy include infection, thrombosis, and bleeding (Malato et al., 2020). Although young children are at the highest risk after splenectomy, all age groups are vulnerable to overwhelming, lethal infections and should receive recommended vaccinations and be treated promptly for fever or signs of infection (see earlier detailed discussion about splenectomy care in ITP section).

Often, patients with high platelet counts have even higher counts after splenectomy (over 1 million/mm^3), which can predispose them to serious thrombotic or hemorrhagic problems. However, this increase is transient and usually does not warrant additional treatment.

THERAPEUTIC APHERESIS

Apheresis is a Greek word meaning separation. In therapeutic apheresis (or pheresis), blood is taken from the patient and passed through a centrifuge, in which a specific component is separated from the blood and removed. Then the remaining blood is returned to the patient.

The most common apheresis modalities used include therapeutic plasma exchange (e.g., used to treat hyperviscosity in plasma cell disorders), leukocytopheresis (used to treat symptomatic leukocytosis in patients with leukemia), extracorporeal photopheresis (ECP) (used to treat cutaneous T-cell lymphoma, Sezary syndrome, and GVHD), thrombocytopheresis (used to treat symptomatic thrombocytosis with MPNs), and erythrocytapheresis (used in selected cases of PV or ET) (Fridey & Kaplan, 2021).

The entire system is closed so the risk of bacterial contamination is extremely low. When platelets or leukocytes are removed, the decrease in these cells within the circulation is temporary. However, the temporary decrease provides a window of time until suppressive medications (e.g., chemotherapy) can have therapeutic effects. Sometimes plasma is removed rather than blood cells—typically so that specific, abnormal proteins within the plasma are lowered transiently until a long-term therapy can be initiated.

Also apheresis is used to obtain larger amounts of platelets from a donor than can be provided from a single unit of whole blood. A unit of platelets obtained in this way is equivalent to six to eight units of platelets obtained from six to eight separate donors via standard blood donation methods. Platelet donors can have their platelets apheresed as often as every 14 days.

Leukocytes can be obtained similarly, typically after the donor has received growth factors (G-CSF, GM-CSF) to stimulate the formation of additional leukocytes and thereby increase the leukocyte count. The use of these growth factors also stimulates the release of stem cells within the circulation. Apheresis is used to harvest these stem cells (typically over a period of several days) for use in PBSCT.

THERAPEUTIC PHLEBOTOMY

Therapeutic phlebotomy is the removal of a certain amount of blood under controlled conditions. Usually patients with elevated hematocrits (e.g., those with PV) or excessive iron absorption (e.g., hemochromatosis) can be managed by periodically removing 1 unit (about 500 mL) of whole blood; however, a smaller volume may be indicated for older adults, those with low body mass, comorbidities, or females (Tefferi, 2022). Eventually, this process can produce iron deficiency, leaving the patient unable to produce as many erythrocytes. The actual procedure for therapeutic phlebotomy is similar to that for blood donation (see later discussion).

BLOOD COMPONENT THERAPY

A single unit of whole blood contains 450 mL of blood and 50 mL of an anticoagulant. A unit of whole blood can be processed and dispensed for administration. However, it is more appropriate, economical, and practical to separate that unit of whole blood into its primary components: erythrocytes, platelets, and plasma (leukocytes are rarely used; see later discussion). Because the plasma is removed, a unit of PRBCs is very concentrated (hematocrit approximately 70%). Each component must be processed and stored differently to maximize the longevity of the viable cells and factors within it; each individual blood component has a different storage life. PRBCs are stored at 4° C. With special preservatives, they can be stored safely for up to 42 days before they must be discarded. In contrast, platelets must be stored at room temperature because they cannot withstand cold temperatures, and they last for only 5 days before they must be discarded. To prevent clumping, platelets are agitated gently while stored. Plasma is frozen immediately to maintain the activity of the clotting factors within; it lasts for 1 year if it remains frozen. Alternatively, plasma can be further pooled and processed into blood derivatives, such as albumin, immune globulin, factor VIII, and factor IX. Table 19-6 describes each blood component and how each is commonly used.

Blood transfusion is discussed in detail on page 676.

Special Preparations

Factor VIII concentrate (antihemophilic factor) is a lyophilized (to dry by freezing in a high vacuum) or freeze-dried concentrate of pooled fractionated human plasma. It is used in treating hemophilia A. Factor IX concentrate (prothrombin complex) is prepared similarly and contains factors II, VII, IX, and X. It is used primarily for treatment of factor IX deficiency (hemophilia B). Factor IX concentrate is also useful in treating congenital factor VII and factor X deficiencies. Recombinant forms of factor VIII, such as Humate-P or Alphanate, are also useful. Because they contain vWF, these agents are used in vWD as well as in hemophilia A, particularly when patients develop acquired factor VIII inhibitors (e.g., antibodies).

Plasma albumin is a large protein molecule that usually stays within vessels and is a major contributor to plasma oncotic pressure. This protein is used to expand the blood volume of patients in hypovolemic shock and, rarely, to increase the concentration of circulating albumin in patients with hypoalbuminemia. There are two formulations available that differ on the albumin concentration: albumin 5% and 25%.

Pearls for Practice

Albumin is administered as 5% or 25%. The 5% is classified as iso-oncotic and increases intravascular fluid volume by the amount administered, whereas the 25% solution is hyperoncotic and increases plasma volume at a 4:1 ratio, that is for every mL administered, 400% will be pulled into the intravascular space or bloodstream (Barlow et al.,

TABLE **19-6 Blood and Blood Components Commonly Used in Transfusion Therapy**[a]

	Composition	Indications and Considerations
Whole blood	Cells and plasma, hematocrit about 40%	Volume replacement and oxygen-carrying capacity; usually used only in significant bleeding (more than 25% blood volume lost)
Packed red blood cells (PRBCs)	RBCs with little plasma (hematocrit about 70%); some platelets and WBCs remain. Platelets in the unit are not functional; WBCs in the unit may cause reaction and are not functional.	Hemoglobin less than 7–8 g/dL; symptomatic anemia
Platelets—random	Platelets (5.5×10^{10} platelets/unit) Plasma; some RBCs, WBCs survival ↓ in presence of fever, chills, infection Repeated treatment leads to ↓ transfused platelet survival due to alloimmunization	To prevent bleeding in patients with a platelet count below 10,000/mm^3 To prevent bleeding in patients with fever or sepsis and platelet count below 20,000/mm^3 Prior to major surgery or invasive procedure when platelet count *is less than or equal to* 50,000/mm^3 Prior to ocular surgery or neurosurgery when platelet count is *less than or equal to* 100,000/mm^3
Platelets—single donor	Platelets (3×10^{11} platelets/unit) 1 unit is equivalent to 6–8 units of random platelets	Used to decrease alloimmunization risk by limiting exposure to multiple donors Preferred for patients who will require repeated transfusions over time
Plasma or fresh-frozen plasma (FFP)	Plasma; all coagulation factors Complement	Bleeding in patients with coagulation factor deficiencies To reverse the effects of warfarin in presence of major bleeding
Granulocytes	Neutrophils (greater than 1×10^{10}/unit); lymphocytes; some RBCs and platelets	Severe neutropenia in selected patients; controversial, rarely used
Donor lymphocytes (white blood cells [WBCs])	Lymphocytes (number varies) taken from a donor and infused into a recipient	Stimulate graft-versus-disease effect in a patient who has undergone prior allogeneic stem cell transplant
Cryoprecipitate	Fibrinogen 150 or greater mg/bag, contains high concentrations of factor VIII and fibrinogen; AHF (VIII:C) 80–110 units/bag	von Willebrand disease Hypofibrinogenemia Hemophilia A
Antihemophilic factor (AHF)	Factor VIII	Hemophilia A
Factor IX concentrate	Factor IX	Hemophilia B (Christmas disease)
Factor IX complex	Factors II, VII, IX, X	Hereditary factors VII, IX, X deficiency Hemophilia A with factor VII inhibitors
Albumin	Albumin 5%, 25%	Hypoproteinemia Burns Volume expansion by 5% to ↑ intravascular volume; 25% → ↑ intravascular volume which ↓'s hematocrit due to hemodilution
IV gamma globulin (IVIG)	IgG antibodies	Hypogammaglobulinemia (in CLL, recurrent infections) ITP Primary immunodeficiency states
Antithrombin III concentrate (AT III)	AT III (trace amounts of other plasma proteins)	AT III deficiency with or at risk for thrombosis

AHF, antihemophilic factor; CLL, chronic lymphocytic leukemia; ITP, immune thrombocytopenic purpura.

[a]The composition of each type of blood component is described, as well as the most common indications for using a given blood component.

2020). The nurse understands that by administering a colloid like albumin, a high oncotic pressure gradient is created which will pull or draw fluid from the interstitial space into the intravascular space, in an attempt to restore fluid balance.

Immunoglobulin is a concentrated solution of the antibody IgG; it contains very little IgA or IgM. It is prepared from large pools of plasma. The IV form (IVIG) is used in various clinical situations to replace inadequate amounts of IgG in patients who have experienced recurrent bacterial infection (e.g., those with CLL, BMT or PBSCT recipients) to reduce the risk for future infection. It is also used in certain autoimmune disorders, such as ITP. IVIG, in contrast to all other fractions of human blood, cells, or plasma, can survive being subjected to heating at 60° C (140° F) for 10 hours to free it of the viral contaminants that may be present.

PHARMACOLOGIC ALTERNATIVES TO BLOOD TRANSFUSIONS

Pharmacologic agents that stimulate production of one or more types of blood cells by the marrow are commonly used (Box 19-5).

Manufacturing artificial blood is problematic, given the myriad functions of blood components. Research has focused on the role of blood in oxygen transport or its role as an oxygen carrier and the manufacturing of a suitable RBC substitute. The substitutes can be classified as perfluorocarbon emulsions that have a high gas-dissolving capacity for oxygen and hemoglobin-based oxygen carriers (Fridey, 2021). Current artificial RBC products have distinct advantages and disadvantages compared with human RBCs. These products can be rendered essentially sterile, resulting in fewer immune-related transfusion problems. They require

BOX 19-5 Pharmacologic Alternatives to Blood Transfusions

Growth Factors

Recombinant technology has provided a means to produce hematopoietic growth factors necessary for the production of blood cells within the bone marrow. By increasing the body's production of blood cells, transfusions and complications resulting from diminished blood cells (e.g., infection from neutropenia or transfusions) may be avoided. However, the successful use of growth factors requires functional bone marrow.

Erythropoietin

Erythropoietin (epoetin alpha/EPO) is an effective alternative treatment for patients with chronic anemia secondary to diminished levels of erythropoietin, as in chronic kidney disease. This medication stimulates erythropoiesis. It also has been used for patients who are anemic from chemotherapy or zidovudine (AZT) therapy and for those who have diseases involving bone marrow suppression, such as myelodysplastic syndrome (MDS). Recent studies have shown that exceeding the recommended Hgb goal of 11 g/dL results in increased risk for cardiovascular events, including stroke and MI. In addition, use of erythropoietin has been associated with decreased survival in certain types of cancer. EPO has been used safely in the preoperative setting to decrease the need for allogeneic blood transfusions. In this setting, erythropoietin also can enable a patient to donate several units of blood for future use (e.g., preoperative autologous donation). The medication can be administered intravenously or subcutaneously, although plasma levels are better sustained with the subcutaneous route. Side effects are rare, but erythropoietin can cause or exacerbate hypertension. If the anemia is corrected too quickly or is overcorrected, the elevated hematocrit can cause headache, hypertension, and, potentially, seizures. These adverse effects are rare except for in patients with kidney failure. Serial CBCs should be performed to evaluate the response to the medication. The dose and frequency of administration are titrated to the hematocrit.

Granulocyte-Colony Stimulating Factor (G-CSF)

G-CSF (filgrastim) is a cytokine that stimulates the proliferation and differentiation of myeloid stem cells; a rapid increase in neutrophils is seen within the circulation. G-CSF is effective in improving transient but severe neutropenia after chemotherapy or in some MDS subtypes. It is particularly useful in preventing bacterial infections that would be likely to occur with neutropenia. G-CSF is administered subcutaneously on a daily basis. The primary side effect is bone pain; this probably reflects the increase in hematopoiesis within the marrow. Serial CBCs should be performed to evaluate the response to the medication and to ensure that the rise in white blood cells is not excessive. The effect of G-CSF on myelopoiesis is short; the neutrophil count drops once the medication is stopped. There is a long-active formulation, Pegfilgrastim that is given once per chemotherapy cycle to decrease the risk for infection.

Granulocyte-Macrophage Colony Stimulating Factor (GM-CSF)

GM-CSF (sargramostim) is a cytokine that is naturally produced by a variety of cells, including monocytes and endothelial cells. It works either directly or synergistically with other growth factors to stimulate myelopoiesis. GM-CSF is not as specific to neutrophils as is G-CSF; thus, an increase in erythroid (RBC) and megakaryocytic (platelet) production also may be seen. GM-CSF serves the same purpose as G-CSF. However, it may have a greater effect on macrophage function and, therefore, may be more useful against fungal infections, whereas G-CSF may be better used to fight bacterial infections. GM-CSF is also administered subcutaneously. Side effects include bone pain, fevers, and myalgias.

no refrigeration, have possible unlimited availability, long storage life, and require no cross-matching (Fridey, 2021). Potential problems associated with these products include low concentrations of 2,3-DPG, the shifting of the oxyhemoglobin dissociation curve to the left, and a decrease in the off-loading of oxygen at the tissue level. Because the substitutes are also nitric oxide scavengers, vasoconstriction may occur, risking pulmonary hypertension and myocardial ischemia (Fridey, 2021). Finally, the solutions may also result in platelet activation (Fridey, 2021). Thus, further study is needed to establish safety and efficacy.

PROCURING BLOOD, BLOOD PRODUCTS, AND BLOOD TRANSFUSIONS

Blood Donation

To protect both the donor and the recipients, all prospective donors are examined and interviewed before they are allowed to donate their blood. The intent of the interview is to assess the general health status of the donor and to identify risk factors that might harm a recipient of the donor's blood. Donors should be in good health and meet a number of specific criteria (Box 19-6).

Potential donors should be asked whether they have consumed any aspirin or aspirin-containing medications within the past 3 days. Although aspirin use does not render the donor ineligible, the platelets obtained would be dysfunctional and therefore not useful; aspirin usage within 48 to 72 hours contraindicates platelet donation. Aspirin does not affect the erythrocytes or plasma obtained from the donor.

Directed Donation

At times, friends and family of a patient wish to donate blood specifically for that person. These blood donations are termed *directed donations*. These donations are not particularly safer than those provided by random donors.

Standard Donation

Phlebotomy consists of venipuncture and blood withdrawal. Standard precautions are used. Donors are placed in a semi-recumbent position, and venipuncture with a large bore IV is performed. Withdrawal of 450 mL of blood usually takes less than 15 minutes. After the needle is removed, donors are asked to hold the involved arm straight up, and firm pressure is applied with sterile gauze for 2 to 3 minutes or until bleeding stops. Then a firm bandage is applied. The donor remains recumbent until they feel able to sit up, usually within a few minutes.

The donor is instructed to:

- leave the dressing on for a few hours
- avoid heavy lifting or vigorous exercise for the rest of the day

BOX 19-6

Eligibility Requirements for Blood Donation

All donors are expected to meet the following minimum requirements:

- Be healthy and feeling well
- Be at least 17 years old in most states
- Body weight should exceed 50 kg (110 lb) for a standard 450-mL donation.
- Males must be at least 5′1″ tall; females must be at least 5′5″
- No fever or signs/symptoms of infection.
- Blood pressure less than 180/100 at least 90/50
- The hemoglobin level should be at least 12.5 g/dL for females, 13.0 g/dL for males. For all donors, the hemoglobin level can be no greater than 20 g/d.
- Wait at least 8 weeks between whole blood (standard) donations.

Contraindications to Blood Donation

- A history of viral hepatitis at any time in the past. If the donor lives with or has had sexual contact with a person who has hepatitis, the donor must wait 12 months after the last contact to donate
- A history of untreated malaria because malaria can be transmitted by transfusion even years later
- A history of syphilis or gonorrhea; acceptable if it has been more than 3 months since donor completed treatment for syphilis or gonorrhea
- A history or evidence of IV drug use, must wait 3 months after using IV drugs
- A history of possible exposure to HIV
- A recent tattoo within the last 3 months because of the risk of blood-borne infections (e.g., hepatitis, HIV)
- Recent immunizations (exception: influenza, pneumonia, tetanus, or meningitis, provided that the donor is symptom free and afebrile)
- Pregnancy, because of the nutritional demands of pregnancy on the mother
- A diagnosis of leukemia or lymphoma, including Hodgkin disease and other cancers of the blood, hemochromatosis, sickle cell disease, or active skin infections at the venipuncture site
- A history of bleeding problems or use of "blood thinner" such as fondaparinux, warfarin, apixaban, dalteparin, heparin, enoxaparin, dabigatran, edoxaban, and rivaroxaban
- Wait for 3 months after receiving a blood transfusion from another person in the United States. Cannot donate if blood transfusion was received since 1980 in France, Ireland, England, Wales, Scotland, Northern Ireland, Channel Islands, Isle of Man, Gibraltar or Falkland Islands, related to concerns about variant CJD, or "mad cow" disease

For a detailed list of eligibility criteria by topic, visit the American Red Cross website: https://www.redcrossblood.org/donate-blood/how-to-donate/eligibility-requirements.html.

- increase fluid intake by drinking an extra four 8-oz glasses of fluid and avoid alcoholic beverages over the next 24 hours

Specimens from this donated blood are tested to detect infections and to identify the specific blood type (see later discussion).

Autologous Donation

A patient's own blood may be collected for future transfusion; this method is useful for many elective surgeries in which the potential need for transfusion is high (e.g., orthopedic surgery). Preoperative donations are ideally collected 4 to 6 weeks before surgery. Iron supplements are prescribed during this period to prevent depletion of iron stores. Occasionally, erythropoietin (epoetin-alfa) is given to stimulate erythropoiesis, so that the donor's hematocrit remains high enough to be eligible for donation. Typically, one unit of blood is drawn each week; the number of units obtained varies with the type of surgical procedure to be performed (i.e., the amount of blood anticipated to be transfused). Phlebotomies are not performed within 72 hours of surgery.

The primary advantage of autologous transfusions is the prevention of viral infections from another person's blood. It is the policy of the American Red Cross that autologous blood be transfused only to the donor. If the blood is not required, it can be frozen until the donor needs it in the future (for up to 10 years). The blood is never returned to the general donor supply of blood products to be used by another person.

The disadvantage of autologous donation is that it may be performed even when the likelihood is small that the anticipated procedure will necessitate a transfusion. Needless autologous donation is expensive, takes time, and uses resources inappropriately. Furthermore, although autologous transfusion can eliminate the risk of viral contamination, the risk for bacterial contamination is the same as that in transfusion from random donors.

Contraindications to donation of blood for autologous transfusion are acute infection, severely debilitating chronic disease, hemoglobin level of less than 12.5 g/dL, hematocrit less than 38%, unstable angina, and acute cardiovascular or cerebrovascular disease.

Intraoperative Blood Salvage

This transfusion method provides replacement for patients who cannot donate before surgery and for those undergoing vascular, orthopedic, or thoracic surgery. During a surgical procedure, blood lost into a sterile cavity (e.g., hip joint) is suctioned into a cell-saver machine. The whole blood or PRBCs are washed, often with saline solution, filtered, and then returned to the patient as an IV infusion. The goal of intraoperative salvage is to reduce the need for allogeneic blood transfusions. Devices that collect blood for reinfusion allow for either washing or not washing prior to transfusion. If the blood is washed (with normal saline) to remove lysed RBC debris and contaminants, it can be stored up to **4 hours** at room temperature after processing. However, unwashed products must be filtered to remove clots and tissue debris and must be infused within **6 hours** from the start of collection due to the risk from other contaminants (Heath & Shander, 2022). Autologous blood is not collected from patients with known systemic infections (Phillips & Hornacky, 2021; Waters, 2021). Early research on the use of intraoperative blood salvage in those at high risk of postpartum hemorrhage undergoing cesarean sections demonstrate lower incidence of transfusion-related adverse events and shorter hospital stay among other findings (Obore et al., 2022). Thus, nurses may use cell salvage in a variety of settings.

Hemodilution

This transfusion method may be initiated before or after induction of anesthesia. About one to two units of blood are removed from the patient through a venous or arterial line and simultaneously replaced with a colloid or crystalloid solution. Then the blood that is obtained is reinfused after surgery. The advantage of this method is that the patient loses fewer erythrocytes during surgery because the added IV solutions dilute the concentration of erythrocytes and lower the hematocrit. However, patients who are at risk of myocardial injury should not be further stressed by hemodilution.

Complications of Blood Donation

The overall incidence of complications secondary to blood donation is very low (2% to 5%) (Kleinman, 2022). The most common complications include bleeding secondary to needle injury (such as hematoma formation) and vasovagal reactions. Excessive bleeding at the donor's venipuncture site is sometimes caused by a bleeding disorder in the donor but more often results from a technique error: laceration of the vein, excessive tourniquet pressure, or failure to apply enough pressure after the needle is withdrawn. A donor who appears pale or complains of faintness should immediately lie down or sit with the head lowered below the knees. They should be observed for another 30 minutes.

BLOOD PROCESSING

Samples of the unit of blood are always taken immediately after donation so that the blood can be typed and tested. Each donation is tested for antibodies to HIV 1 and 2, hepatitis B core antibody (anti-HBc), hepatitis C virus (HCV), West Nile virus, and human T-cell lymphotropic virus type I (anti–HTLV-I/II). The blood is also tested for hepatitis B, hepatitis C virus, and pallidum (syphilis) (Kleinman, 2022). Negative reactions are required for the blood to be used, and each unit of blood is labeled to certify the results. Blood is also screened for Cytomegalovirus (CMV); if it tests positive for CMV, it still can be used except in recipients who are negative for CMV and who are immunocompromised (e.g., BMT or PBSCT recipients).

Equally important to viral testing is accurate determination of the blood type. More than 200 antigens have been identified on the surface of RBC membranes. Of these, the most important for safe transfusion are the ABO and Rh systems. The ABO system identifies which antigens are present on the membrane of a person's erythrocytes: A, B, both A and B, or neither A nor B (type O). Individuals have antibodies in their plasma that are directed against blood group antigens that their RBCs do not express. For example, a person with type A blood expresses the A antigen on the RBC membrane and has anti-B antibodies. To prevent a significant reaction, the same type of PRBCs should be transfused. In an emergency situation in which the patient's blood type is not known, type O blood may be transfused safely.

The Rh antigen (also called D) is present on the surface of erythrocytes in 85% of the population (Rh-positive). Those who lack the D antigen are called Rh-negative. PRBCs are routinely tested for the D antigen as well as ABO. Patients with Rh-positive blood can receive Rh-negative blood; however, patients who are Rh negative should only receive Rh-negative blood.

The majority of transfusion reactions (other than those due to procedural error) are due to the presence of donor leukocytes within the blood component unit (PRBCs or platelets); the recipient may form antibodies to the antigens present on these leukocytes. PRBC components typically have 1 to 3×10^9 leukocytes remaining in each unit. Leukocytes from the blood product are frequently filtered to diminish the likelihood of developing reactions and refractoriness to transfusions, particularly in patients who have chronic transfusion needs. Filtration can occur at the time the unit is collected from the donor and processed, which achieves better results but is more expensive, or at the time the blood component is transfused by attaching a leukocyte filter to the blood administration tubing. Many centers advocate routinely using leukopoor filtered blood components for people who have or are likely to develop chronic transfusion requirements.

When a patient is extremely immunocompromised, as in the case of bone marrow or stem cell transplant, any donor lymphocytes must be removed from the blood components. In this situation, the blood component is exposed to low amounts of radiation (25 Gy) that kill any lymphocytes within the blood component. Irradiated blood products are highly effective in preventing transfusion-associated GVHD, which is fatal in most cases. Irradiated blood products have a shorter shelf life.

TRANSFUSION

Administration of blood and blood components requires knowledge of correct administration techniques and possible complications. It is very important to be familiar with the facility's policies and procedures for transfusion therapy.

Setting

Although most blood transfusions are performed in the acute care setting, patients with chronic transfusion requirements often can receive transfusions in other settings, including free-standing infusion centers, ambulatory care clinics, providers' offices, and, occasionally, even patients' homes. Typically, patients who need chronic transfusions but are otherwise stable physically are appropriate candidates for outpatient therapy. Verification and administration of the blood product are performed as in a hospital setting.

Method

Transfusing blood components are presented in Box 19-7.

Nursing Management

Nursing responsibilities include pretransfusion and post-transfusion assessment.

Pretransfusion Assessment

Patient history is an important component of the pretransfusion assessment to determine the history of previous transfusions as well as previous reactions to transfusion. The history should include the type of reaction, its manifestations, the interventions required, and whether any preventive interventions were used in subsequent transfusions. It is important to assess the number of pregnancies a patient has had because a high number can increase their risk for reaction due to antibodies developed from exposure to fetal circulation. Patients with blood disorders, such as sickle cell anemia or CLL, and patients who have received a stem cell transplant also may be at increased risk for transfusion reactions based on the number of previous transfusions. Other concurrent health problems should be noted, with careful attention to cardiac (particularly heart failure with a decreased left ventricular ejection fraction), pulmonary, and vascular disease.

A systematic physical assessment and measurement of baseline vital signs are important before transfusing any blood product. The respiratory system should be assessed, including careful auscultation of the lungs and the patient's use of accessory muscles. Cardiac system assessment should include careful inspection for any edema as well as other signs of cardiac failure (e.g., jugular venous distention). The skin should be observed for rashes, petechiae, and ecchymoses. The sclera should be examined for icterus. In the event of a transfusion reaction, a comparison of findings can help differentiate between types of reactions.

Pearls for Practice

To evaluate a patient's response to therapy, the nurse is aware that when administering PRBCs it is expected that one unit of PRBCs will raise the hemoglobin by 1 g and Hct by 3%, if the patient is not bleeding or

BOX 19-7

Transfusion of Packed Red Blood Cells (PRBCs)

Preprocedure

- Confirm that the transfusion has been prescribed.
- Confirm that a current type and screen of the patient's blood is on file per institution policy.
- Check that patient's blood has been typed and cross-matched.
- Verify that patient has been provided informed consent per institution or agency policy.
- Explain the procedure to the patient. Instruct the patient in signs and symptoms of transfusion reaction (itching, hives, swelling, shortness of breath, fever, chills).
- Take the patient's temperature, pulse, respiration, oxygen saturation, and blood pressure to establish a baseline for comparing vital signs during transfusion.
- Perform hand hygiene and wear gloves in accordance with standard precautions.
- Use a 20-gauge or larger needle for insertion in a large vein. Use special tubing that contains a blood filter to screen out fibrin clots and other particulate matter. Do not vent the blood container.

Procedure

- Obtain the PRBCs from the blood bank *after* the IV line is started and vital signs are assessed. (Institution policy may limit release to only one unit at a time.)
- Double-check the labels with another licensed provider (nurse, advanced practice provider, or physician) to make sure that the ABO group and Rh type agree with the compatibility record. Check to see that the number and type on the donor blood label and on the patient's chart are correct. Check the patient's identification by using two forms of identification (can include the patient's name, date of birth, and medical record number) comparing the blood product label to the patient identification bracelet. Also ask the patient to confirm their name and date of birth.
- Check the blood for gas bubbles and any unusual color or cloudiness. (Gas bubbles may indicate bacterial growth. Abnormal color or cloudiness may be a sign of hemolysis.)
- Make sure PRBC transfusion is initiated within 30 minutes after removal of the PRBCs from the blood bank refrigerator.
- For the first 15 minutes, run the transfusion slowly—no faster than 5 mL/min. Observe the patient carefully for adverse effects. If no adverse effects occur during the first 15 minutes, then increase the flow rate unless the patient is at high risk for circulatory overload.
- Monitor the patient closely for 15–30 minutes to detect signs of reaction. Monitor vital signs at regular intervals per institution or agency policy; compare the results with baseline measurements. Increase frequency of measurements based on the patient's condition. Observe the patient frequently throughout the transfusion for any signs of adverse reaction, including restlessness, hives, nausea, vomiting, torso or back pain, shortness of breath, flushing, hematuria, fever, or chills. Should any adverse reaction occur, stop infusion immediately, notify the health care provider, and follow the agency's transfusion reaction policy.
- Note that administration time does not exceed 4 hours because of the increased risk for bacterial growth.
- Be alert for signs of adverse reactions: circulatory overload, sepsis, febrile reaction, allergic reaction, and acute hemolytic reaction.
- Change blood tubing after every 2 units transfused to decrease the chance of bacterial contamination.

Postprocedure

- Obtain vital signs and compare them with baseline measurements.
- Dispose of used materials properly.
- Document the procedure in the patient's medical record, including patient assessment findings and tolerance to procedure.
- Monitor the patient for response to and effectiveness of the procedure.

Note: Never add medications to blood or blood products; if blood is too thick to run freely, normal saline may be added to the unit. If blood must be warmed, use an in-line blood warmer with a temperature monitoring system.

Note: Fresh-frozen platelets (FFPs) require ABO but not Rh compatibility. Typically platelets are not cross-matched for ABO compatibility. Never add medications to blood or blood products. Both platelets and FFPs can be infused as rapidly as the patient can tolerate, based on fluid status and cardiac function.

hemolyzing. If administering platelets (which generally consists of six units of pooled platelets from random donors [random donor platelets or RDP]), the count should increase by approximately 30,000 mm^3 in an adult of average size (Yuan, 2021).

Providing Patient Teaching

Reviewing the signs and symptoms of a transfusion reaction is crucial for patients who have not received a transfusion before. Even for patients who have received prior transfusions, a brief review of the signs and symptoms of transfusion reactions is essential. Signs and symptoms of a reaction include fever, chills, itching, hives, respiratory distress, low back pain, nausea, pain at the IV site, or anything "unusual." Although a thorough review is very important, it is also important to reassure the patient that the blood is tested carefully against the patient's own blood (cross-matched) to diminish the likelihood of any adverse reaction. Such assurance can be extremely beneficial in allaying anxiety.

Monitoring and Managing Potential Complications

Any patient who receives a blood transfusion may develop complications from that transfusion. When explaining the reasons for the transfusion, it is important to include the risks and benefits and what to expect during and after the transfusion. Patients must be informed that the supply

BOX 19-8

Diseases Transmitted by Blood Transfusion

Hepatitis (Viral Hepatitis B, C)

- Greater risk from pooled blood products and blood of paid donors than from volunteer donors
- Screening test detects most hepatitis B and C
- Since 1972, the blood supply has been screened for hepatitis B in the United States, making the risk of transfusion-transmitted HBV extremely rare (CDC, 2019)
- Since 1992, the blood supply has been screened for hepatitis C in the United States, making the risk of transfusion-transmitted HCV extremely rare (CDC, 2019)

HIV and HTLV

- Donated blood screened for antibodies to HIV
- Transmittal risk estimated at 1 in 1.4 million to 1 in 1.8 million units (del Rio et al., 2020).
- People with high-risk behaviors (multiple sex partners, anal sex, IV/injection drug use) and people with signs and symptoms that suggest AIDS should not donate blood

Cytomegalovirus (CMV)

- Transmittal risk greater for premature newborns with CMV antibody-negative mothers and for immunocompromised recipients who are CMV negative (e.g., those with acute leukemia, organ or tissue transplant recipients)
- Blood products rendered "leukocyte-reduced" help reduce the transmission of virus

Graft-Versus-Host Disease (GVHD)

- Occurs only in severely immunocompromised recipients (e.g., leukemia, bone marrow, and stem cell transplantation)
- Transfused lymphocytes engraft in the recipient and attack host lymphocytes or body tissues; signs and symptoms are fever, diffuse reddened skin rash, nausea, vomiting, diarrhea
- Preventive measures include irradiating blood products to inactivate donor lymphocytes (no known radiation risks to transfusion recipient) and processing donor blood with leukocyte-reduction filters

Creutzfeldt–Jakob Disease (CJD)

- Rare, fatal disease causing irreversible brain damage
- No evidence of transmittal by transfusion, but hemophiliacs and others are concerned that transmittal is possible
- All blood donors must be screened for positive family history of CJD. Those with a blood relative with CJD are not eligible to donate blood
- Potential donors who spent 6 months or more in the United Kingdom (or Europe) from 1980 to 1996 cannot donate blood; blood products from a donor who develops CJD are recalled

For more detailed guidelines regarding travel, CJD, and blood donations, please visit the American Red Cross website: http://www.redcrossblood.org/donating-blood/eligibility-requirements

of blood is not completely risk-free, although it has been tested carefully (Box 19-8). Nursing management is directed toward preventing complications, promptly recognizing complications if they develop, and promptly initiating measures to control complications. The following sections describe the most common or potentially severe transfusion-related complications. Table 19-7 summarizes potential long-term complications.

Febrile Nonhemolytic Transfusion Reaction (FNHTR)

A febrile nonhemolytic transfusion reaction is defined by a temperature of 100.4° F or a 1° C (1.8° F) increase in temperature with or without chills during or within 6 hours following completion of a transfusion (Silvergleid, 2021). An FNHTR is caused by antibodies to donor leukocytes that remain in the unit of blood or blood component; it is the most common type of transfusion reaction, accounting for more

TABLE 19-7 Common Complications Resulting from Long-Term Packed Red Blood Cell (PRBC) Transfusion Therapy[a]

	Manifestation	Management
Infection	Hepatitis (B, C) Cytomegalovirus (CMV)	May immunize against hepatitis B; give alpha-interferon for hepatitis C; monitor liver function Use WBC filters to protect against CMV
Iron overload	Heart failure Endocrine failure (diabetes, hypothyroidism, hypoparathyroidism, hypogonadism)	Prevent or treat using iron chelation therapy
Transfusion reaction	Sensitization Febrile reactions	Diminish by RBC phenotyping, using WBC-filtered, leukocyte-reduced, or irradiated products

WBC, white blood cell; RBC, red blood cell.

[a]Patients with long-term transfusion therapy requirements are at risk not only for the transfusion reactions discussed in the text but also for the complications noted above. In many cases, the use of WBC-filtered (e.g., leukocyte-poor) blood products is standard for patients who receive long-term PRBC transfusion therapy. Blood product irradiation, which more effectively reduces the leukocytes in the product, is reserved for patients at highest risk for infection, alloimmunization, and GVHD. Iron chelation may be used in select populations to reduce iron burden.

than 90% of reactions. It occurs more frequently in patients who have had previous transfusions (exposure to multiple antigens from previous blood products) and in Rh-negative people who have borne Rh-positive children (exposure to an Rh-positive fetus raises antibody levels in the mother). These reactions occur in 1% of PRBC transfusions and 20% of platelet transfusions. Rates have declined since the standardization of leukocyte reduction, which significantly decreases the number of leukocytes in a transfused product, thus decreasing the risk of an antibody–antigen reaction (Silvergleid, 2021). More than 10% of patients with chronic transfusion requirements develop this type of reaction.

The diagnosis of a febrile nonhemolytic reaction is made by excluding other potential causes, such as a hemolytic reaction, sepsis, or bacterial contamination of the blood product. The signs and symptoms of a febrile nonhemolytic transfusion reaction are chills (minimal to severe) followed by fever. The fever typically begins within 2 hours after the transfusion is begun. Although the reaction is not life-threatening, the fever, and particularly the chills and muscle stiffness, can be frightening to the patient.

This reaction can be diminished, even prevented, by further depleting the blood component of donor leukocyte through filtration. Antipyretics can be given to prevent fever, but routine premedication is not advised because it can mask the beginning of a more serious transfusion reaction. For recurrent FNHTRs despite leukoreduction, washed PRBCs may be indicated (Kleinman, 2022).

Acute Hemolytic Reaction

The most dangerous, and potentially life-threatening, type of transfusion reaction occurs when the donor blood is incompatible with that of the recipient. Antibodies already present in the recipient's plasma rapidly combine with antigens on donor erythrocytes, and the erythrocytes are hemolyzed (destroyed) in the circulation (intravascular hemolysis). The most rapid hemolysis occurs in ABO incompatibility. This reaction can occur after transfusion of as little as 10 mL of PRBCs. Rh incompatibility often causes a less severe reaction. The most common causes of acute hemolytic reaction are errors in blood component labeling and patient misidentification that result in the administration of an ABO-incompatible transfusion (Tobian, 2022a).

Symptoms consist of fever, chills, nausea, vomiting, chest tightness, dyspnea, hypotension, flank pain, hematuria, oliguria, bleeding, and anxiety (Tobian, 2022a). As the erythrocytes are destroyed, the hemoglobin is released from the cells and excreted by the kidneys; therefore, hemoglobin appears in the urine (hemoglobinuria). Hypotension, bronchospasm, and vascular collapse may result. Diminished renal perfusion results in acute kidney injury, and DIC also may occur.

The reaction must be recognized promptly and the transfusion discontinued immediately. Blood and urine specimens must be obtained and analyzed for evidence of hemolysis, including DAT testing, haptoglobin, LDH, bilirubin, creatinine, PT/PTT, and fibrinogen. Treatment goals include maintaining blood volume and renal perfusion and preventing and managing DIC if needed. Acute hemolytic transfusion reactions are preventable. Meticulous attention to detail in labeling blood samples and blood components and accurately identifying the recipient cannot be overemphasized.

Delayed Hemolytic Reaction

Delayed hemolytic reactions usually occur within 14 days after transfusion, when the level of antibody has been increased to the extent that a reaction can occur. The hemolysis of the erythrocytes is extravascular via the reticuloendothelial system (RES) and occurs gradually.

Signs and symptoms of a delayed hemolytic reaction are fever, anemia, increased bilirubin level, decreased or absent haptoglobin, and possibly jaundice. Rarely is there hemoglobinuria. In general, these reactions are not dangerous, but it is useful to recognize them because subsequent transfusions with blood products containing these antibodies may cause a more severe hemolytic reaction. However, recognition is also difficult because the patient may not be in a health care setting to be tested for this reaction, and even if the patient is hospitalized, the reaction may be too mild to be recognized clinically. Because the amount of antibody present can be too low to detect, it is difficult to prevent delayed hemolytic reactions. Fortunately, the reaction is usually mild and requires no intervention.

Allergic Reaction

Allergic reactions occur in 1% to 3% of transfusions. An allergic reaction is marked by the development of urticaria (hives) or generalized itching, rash, or wheezing during a transfusion (Tobian, 2022b). The cause of these reactions is thought to be a sensitivity reaction to a plasma protein within the blood component being transfused. The reactions are usually mild and respond to antihistamines. If the symptoms resolve after administration of an antihistamine (e.g., diphenhydramine), the transfusion may be resumed. Rarely, the allergic reaction is severe, with bronchospasm, laryngeal edema, and shock. These reactions are managed with epinephrine, corticosteroids, and pressor support, if necessary.

Giving the patient antihistamines before the transfusion may prevent future reactions. For severe reactions, future blood components are washed to remove any remaining plasma proteins. Leukocyte filters are not useful to prevent such reactions because the offending plasma proteins can pass through the filter.

Transfusion-Related Acute Lung Injury

Transfusion-related acute lung injury (TRALI) is defined as new-onset lung injury within 6 hours of transfusion with an oxygen saturation of at least 90% on room air and bilateral infiltrates on chest x-ray (Kleinman & Kor, 2021). TRALI is caused by neutrophil sequestration and priming in the lungs along with activation of the recipient's neutrophils as a result of transfused blood product (Kleinman & Kor, 2021). Signs of TRALI include an onset of symptoms within 6 hours of transfusion; symptoms include dyspnea, cyanosis, hypotension, fever, chills, hypoxia, and/or pulmonary artery pressure at or below 18 mm Hg (and/or no evidence of circulatory overload/left atrial hypertension) (Kleinman & Kor, 2021). TRALI is often a diagnosis of exclusion because symptoms overlap with other transfusion reaction types (e.g., transfusion-associated circulatory overload [TACO] and FNHTR). Workup should include exclusion of hemolysis, CBC (leukopenia may be seen with TRALI), and chest x-ray, which may reveal bilateral infiltrates. Treatment consists of respiratory support and pressors. Treatment with steroids has not been shown to provide benefits to the patient.

Transfusion-Associated Circulatory Overload

TACO is among the leading causes of transfusion-related mortality (Tobian, 2022c). If too much blood is infused too quickly, hypervolemia can occur. Risk factors include older age (>70), the number of units infused, history of HF, valvular heart disease, cardiomegaly, recent MI (past 30 days), COPD, renal dysfunction, or anemia (Tobian, 2022c; Graham et al., 2021). Careful transfusion of blood products plays a major role in reducing the risk of TACO. If the administration rate is sufficiently slow, circulatory overload may be prevented. Concurrent intravenous fluid administration should be avoided. Patients at risk must be monitored carefully. For patients who are at risk of, or already in, circulatory overload, diuretics are administered after the transfusion or between units of products (Tobian, 2022c).

Pearls for Practice

When administering blood products in patients at risk for TACO, the nurse considers all infusing IV solutions and informs the provider so that IV rates can be altered to lower rates while blood is infusing.

Signs of circulatory overload include dyspnea, orthopnea (shortness of breath [SOB] on lying down), tachycardia, and sudden anxiety. Jugular vein distention, an S3 gallop, crackles at the base of the lungs, and an increase in blood pressure can also occur. If the transfusion is continued, pulmonary edema can develop, as manifested by severe dyspnea and coughing up of pink, frothy sputum. These signs and symptoms usually present within 2 hours of initiation of transfusion but may take as long as 6 hours to manifest (Tobian, 2022c).

If fluid overload is mild, often the transfusion can be continued after slowing the rate of infusion and administering diuretics. However, if the overload is severe, the patient is placed in an upright position with the feet in a dependent position, the transfusion is discontinued, and the provider is notified. The IV line is kept patent with a very slow infusion of normal saline solution or a saline or heparin lock device to maintain access to the vein in case IV medications are necessary. Supplementary oxygen may be needed to treat severe dyspnea, particularly if the oxygen saturation is <90 mm Hg. Oxygen is titrated to maintain adequate oxygenation while other interventions are addressed (Tobian, 2022c).

Bacterial Contamination

The incidence of bacterial contamination of blood components is very low; however, administration of contaminated products puts the patient at great risk. Gram-negative bacteria, including *Pseudomonas*, *Yersinia*, and *Enterobacter*, are the most common organism found in contaminated RBC products, but *Serratia* can be present also (Spelman & MacLaren, 2020). Contamination can occur at any point during procurement or processing but is usually due to organisms on the donor's skin (Spelman & MacLaren, 2022). Many bacteria cannot survive in the cold temperatures used to store PRBCs, although some organisms can survive cold temperatures. Parasites that infect RBCs, such as *Babesia* or other species of malaria, are more likely to cause infection from RBCs (Spelman & MacLaren, 2022). Platelets are at greater risk of contamination because they are stored at room temperature. Since 2004, blood centers have developed rapid methods of culturing the platelet unit to decrease the risk of using a contaminated platelet unit for transfusion. Despite bacterial testing, this complication has not been eradicated, thus mandating that nurses remain vigilant for this complication.

Preventive measures include meticulous care in the procurement and processing of blood components. When PRBCs or whole blood is transfused, it should be administered within a **4-hour** period because warm room temperatures promote bacterial growth. A contaminated unit of blood product may appear normal, or it may have an abnormal color.

The signs of bacterial contamination are fever, chills, and hypotension, which most commonly occur during the transfusion. Occasionally, the signs of a reaction may occur hours after the transfusion is complete. If the condition is not recognized and treated immediately with fluids and broad-spectrum antibiotics, shock can occur. While these reactions are rare, they can be fatal (Spelman & MacLaren, 2022). The median interval between completion of transfusion and appearance of symptoms is 30 minutes (range 0 to 5 hours) (Spelman & MacLaren, 2022). Patient education must include prompt reporting of any signs of transfusion reaction at home and need for emergent evaluation.

The following steps are taken to determine the type and severity of the reaction:

- Stop the transfusion. Maintain the IV line with normal saline solution through new IV tubing, administered at a slow rate.
- Assess the patient carefully. Compare the vital signs with baseline. Assess the patient's respiratory status carefully. Note the presence of adventitious breath sounds, use of accessory muscles, extent of dyspnea, changes in mental status including anxiety and confusion, and changes in

oxygen saturation. Note any chills, diaphoresis, jugular vein distention, and reports of back pain or urticaria.

- Notify the health care provider of the assessment findings, and implement any treatments prescribed. Continue to monitor the patient's vital signs and respiratory, cardiovascular, and renal status.
- Notify the blood bank that a suspected transfusion reaction has occurred.
- Send the blood container and tubing to the blood bank for repeat typing and culture. The identifying tags and numbers are verified.

If a hemolytic transfusion reaction or bacterial infection is suspected, the nurse does the following:

- Obtain appropriate blood specimens from the patient (this usually includes blood cultures, a CBC and a type and screen, LDH, DAT, haptoglobin).
- Collect a urine sample as soon as possible for a hemoglobin determination.
- Document the reaction according to the institution's policy.

CHAPTER REVIEW

NCLEX-Style Review Questions

1. The nurse is explaining the potential signs and symptoms of a transfusion reaction to a patient who is receiving a blood transfusion for the first time. How will the nurse ensure safe blood product administration? Select all that apply.
   a. Check ABO compatibility by comparing the blood product label to the patient's medical record.
   b. Use two patient identifiers, such as the patient's date of birth and name, to verify the blood product.
   c. Administer the blood product slowly for the first 15 minutes.
   d. Administer acetaminophen and diphenhydramine, which are standard premedications used in all transfused patients.
   e. Obtain baseline vital signs before the transfusion is administered.

2. A patient is being treated for sepsis. On the second day of receiving care, the patient experiences epistaxis and persistent bleeding from a venipuncture site. The nurse suspects DIC. Which laboratory result supports the nurse's suspicion? Select all that apply.
   a. Increased fibrinogen, decreased PTT, decreased platelets
   b. Decreased fibrinogen, increased PTT, increased platelets
   c. Decreased fibrinogen, increased PTT, decreased platelets
   d. Increased fibrinogen, increased PTT, increased platelets
   e. Increased fibrin split products, increased PT, increased D-dimer

3. The nurse provides patient education related to the management of iron deficiency anemia. Which statement made by the patient signifies understanding of the education provided? Select all that apply.
   a. "I should take my iron pills with a glass of orange juice."
   b. "I should take my iron pills with breakfast to decrease stomach upset."
   c. "Iron pills often cause constipation so I should decrease my fluid and fiber intake."
   d. "I will need to take these pills for only a few days, and then my problem will be fixed."
   e. "I will take my iron pills 1 hour before a meal or 2 hours after a meal"

4. A 83-year-old patient was admitted to the hospital with GI bleeding. After receiving a unit of packed cells, the patient is complaining of increasing shortness of breath and anxiety. Which of the variables in column one are you concerned about? Select all that apply. In column two select the one condition the patient may be experiencing, and in column three select all actions to address the patient's needs.

Variables of concern	Condition the patient may be experiencing	Expected nursing actions
99.0°F temperature	TACO	Monitor vital signs
HR 122 and irregular	Hemolytic reaction	Assess lung sounds
Crackles at the lung bases	Allergic reaction	Maintain IV rate as ordered, while blood is administered
O_2 saturation of 90%	Febrile nonhemolytic transfusion reaction	Elevate the HOB with feet dependent
UO of 1 mL/kg/h		Oxygen at low flow
Jugular vein distension (JVD)		Insert Foley catheter to monitor urine output

5. Which of the following variables are risk factors for transfusion associated circulatory overload (TACO)? Select all that apply.

a. Blood that is infused too quickly
b. Number of units infused
c. History of GI bleeding
d. History of asthma
e. History of heart failure

REFERENCES AND SELECTED READINGS

References and selected readings associated with this chapter can be found on the website that accompanies the book. Visit **http://thepoint.lww.com/Honan3e** to access the references and other additional resources associated with this chapter.

Problems Related to Digestive, Gastrointestinal, and Metabolic Function

A 55-year-old patient is undergoing bariatric surgery to treat morbid obesity. The Patient is 120 lb over the ideal body weight and has comorbidities of diabetes and hypertension.

- **Discuss patient selection for bariatric surgery.**
- **What lifestyles changes might the patient expect?**
- **What complications should the patient be aware of regarding the surgical procedure?**

CHAPTER 20

Nursing Assessment: Digestive, Gastrointestinal, and Metabolic Function

Deborah Bain Fahs

Learning Objectives

After reading this chapter, you will be able to:

1. Describe the anatomy and physiology of the gastrointestinal (GI) tract.
2. Identify the metabolic functions of the liver.
3. Discuss important physical assessment findings of the GI tract.
4. Identify the assessment parameters used to determine the status of the upper and lower GI tract.

The gastrointestinal (GI) system performs the functions of ingestion, digestion, and elimination. Its major organs include the esophagus, stomach, small intestines, large intestines, pancreas, gallbladder, spleen, and liver (a most complex organ) (Norris, 2019). An understanding of the structure and function of the GI system, biliary tract, and pancreas is essential to providing clinical care. Interruption of any of these functions can quickly affect the patient nutritionally and cause a myriad of fluid, electrolyte, and acid–base imbalances. When performing the GI assessment, the nurse must remember that many people have pre-existing conditions which may be exacerbated or new conditions can develop when illness in another system(s) occurs.

ANATOMIC AND PHYSIOLOGIC OVERVIEW OF THE DIGESTIVE SYSTEM

Anatomy of the Gastrointestinal Tract

The GI tract extends from the **mouth** to the esophagus, stomach, small and large intestines, and rectum, to the terminal structure, the **anus** (Fig. 20-1). The oral mucosa is lined by keratinized or a hardened outer layer of cells located on the superior section of the tongue and hard palate as well as nonkeratinized cells or epithelial or surface living cells found in the cheeks, lips, and inferior portion of the tongue which do not absorb molecules with the exception of the mucosa inferior to tongue. The tongue facilitates chewing, tasting, and preparing food for swallowing (Norris, 2019; Ogobuiro et al., 2021). The three pairs of salivary glands, parotid, sublingual and submandibular secrete buffers, glycoproteins or mucins, and salivary amylase, lubricate the mouth, moisten food to assist in swallowing, and begin the process of lipid and carbohydrate digestion. The teeth help to break down food and the pharynx serves as a conduit for food traveling to the esophagus (Ogobuiro et al., 2021). The **esophagus** is a straight, hollow tube approximately 25 cm (10 in) long which is located anterior to the spine and posterior to the trachea and heart (Muller, 2019). Its function is to serve as a passageway for food to advance from the pharynx to sphincters in the lower and upper esophageal sphincters. The lower esophageal sphincter passes through the diaphragm via an opening or hiatus and is joined with the stomach (Norris, 2019).

The **stomach** is situated in the left upper portion of the abdomen under the left lobe of the liver and the diaphragm, overlaying most of the pancreas (see Fig. 20-1). A hollow muscular organ, the stomach stores food during eating, secretes digestive fluids, and propels the partially digested food into the small intestine. The gastroesophageal junction is the inlet to the stomach. The stomach has four anatomic regions: the cardia (entrance), fundus, body, and pylorus (outlet). Circular smooth muscle in the wall of the pylorus forms the pyloric sphincter and controls the opening between the stomach and the small intestine, allowing for both stomach emptying and prevention of regurgitation of intestinal contents back into the stomach (Muller, 2019; Norris, 2019).

The **small intestine** or middle section of the GI tract, is divided into three segments: the duodenum, the jejunum, and the ileum. The duodenum is approximately 25 cm (10 in) in length and accommodates the opening of the common bile and pancreatic duct where bile and pancreatic juices enter the intestines. Food is digested and absorbed in the middle segment of the small intestine which is the jejunum and the distal segment of the ileum; together they measure 3 m (~10 ft)

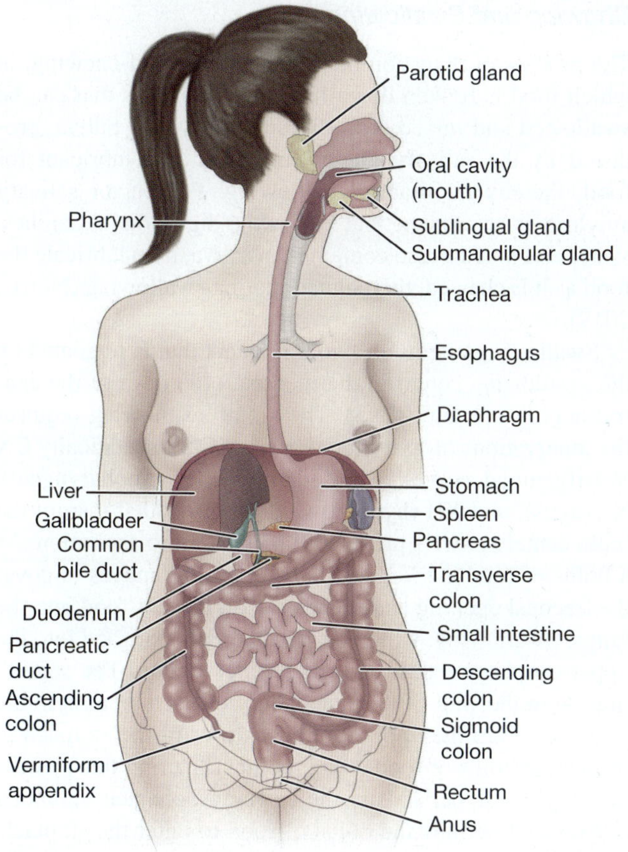

FIGURE 20-1 **Organs of the digestive system and associated structures.**

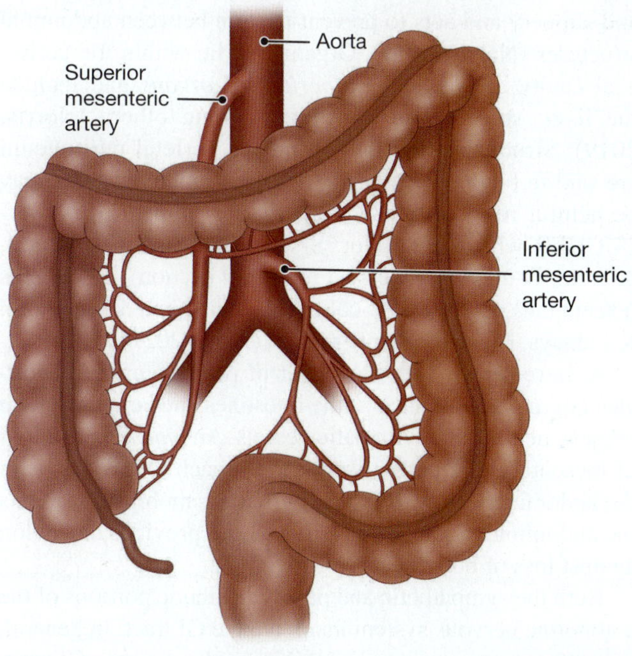

FIGURE 20-2 **Anatomy and blood supply of the large intestine.**

with a diameter of approximately 2.5 cm (~1 in) (Muller, 2019; Norris, 2019). The ileocecal valve is the sphincter that separates the small intestine and the large intestine. It controls the movement of digested food from the ileum into the cecal portion of the large intestine and prevents the backward flow of feces from the cecum into the small intestine. The appendix is attached to the cecum approximately 2.5 cm (1 in) from the ileocecal valve (Norris, 2019).

The **large intestine** is estimated to be 1.5 m (~5 ft) in length with a diameter of 7.6 cm (~3 in). It consists of an ascending segment on the right side of the abdomen, a transverse segment that extends from right to left in the upper abdomen, and a descending segment on the left side of the abdomen. The large intestine aids in water, mineral, salt, and vitamin absorption. Completing the terminal portion of the large intestine are the sigmoid colon, the rectum, and the anus. Regulating the anal outlet is a network of striated muscle, which forms both the internal and the external anal sphincters (Muller, 2019; Norris, 2019).

Pearls for Practice

Since the sigmoid colon lies on the left side of the lower abdomen, the nurse understands that the best position for administration of an enema is left lateral position.

Various sources describe the blood supply to the stomach, duodenum, spleen, and pancreas as simple and fairly uniform; however vascular patterns can be inconsistent and arbitrary. Most of blood supply to the liver, gallbladder, stomach, duodenum, pancreas, and spleen originates from the celiac artery with the superior mesenteric artery, inferior pancreoduodenal branch providing a significantly smaller amount (Fig. 20-2). There are variations, however, in that in 55% of individuals, the celiac artery extends into three subdivisions: hepatic, splenic, and left gastric comprising a truncated tripod shape, while 45% of individuals exhibit multiple variations, posing potential challenges for endoscopists attempting to identify the source of a bleed (Floch, 2019). GI venous drainage system consists of the celiac vein which drains the second section of the duodenum. The third section of the duodenum and the beginning two thirds of the transverse colon is drained by the superior mesenteric vein and the remaining transverse colon and rectum is drained by the mesenteric vein. These veins nourish the liver with 75% of its blood supply in addition to draining nutrients and toxins from the digestive tract. The remaining blood supply arises from the hepatic artery. Blood flow to the liver alone is approximately 25% of the total cardiac output (Harkins & Ahmad, 2021).

The internal abdominal cavity is lined with peritoneum, which is the largest serous membrane in the body having a surface area similar to that of skin. The peritoneum is a single sheet that has visceral and parietal components. The visceral peritoneum covers the abdominal organs, and the parietal peritoneum lines the walls of the abdominal pelvic cavity. Between these two layers is a potential space containing fluid secreted by the serous membranes. This fluid is wet and slippery and acts to prevent friction between abdominal structures (Norris, 2019). Organs that lie within the peritoneal cavity are called *intraperitoneal organs* and include the liver, spleen, and appendix, among others (Norris, 2019). Structures that lie behind the parietal peritoneum are said to be *retroperitoneal*. A useful mnemonic that may be helpful in identifying retroperitoneal structures is SAD PUCKER which stands for: S-suprarenal (adrenal) glands, A-aorta, D-duodenal (second and third section), P-pancreas (except tail), U-ureters, C-colon (ascending and descending), K-kidneys, E-esophagus, R-rectum (Kang, 2021).

A *mesentery* is a double layer of peritoneum that encircles internal organs such as the intestines and contains blood vessels, nerves, and lymphatic vessels. An *omentum* is a fold of mesentery that passes from the stomach to the organs in the abdominal cavity. It is a sheet that has mobility, cushions the abdominal organs against injury, and provides insulation against loss of body heat (Norris, 2019).

Both the sympathetic and parasympathetic portions of the autonomic nervous system innervate the GI tract. In general, sympathetic nerves exert an inhibitory effect on the GI tract, whereas parasympathetic nerve stimulation causes peristalsis and increases secretory activities. The sphincters relax under the influence of parasympathetic stimulation except for the sphincter of the upper esophagus and the external anal sphincter, which are under voluntary control (Norris, 2019).

Pearls for Practice

The nurse is aware that the vagus nerve (cranial nerve [CN] X) surrounds the anus and can be stimulated with rectal temperatures or bearing down forcefully, which causes a parasympathetic response of decreased heart rate and blood pressure. Thus, contraindications to rectal temperatures include cardiac conditions, such as myocardial infarction (MI), because of the risk of bradycardia and arrhythmias. In addition, recent rectal, anal, vaginal, and prostate surgeries would prohibit rectal temperatures because of proximity to the surgical site.

Function of the Digestive System

All cells of the body require nutrients. These nutrients are derived from the diet and need the GI system for digestion, absorption via blood or lymphatic channels, and elimination. Primary functions of the GI tract are the following:

- The breakdown of food particles into the molecular form for **digestion**
- The absorption into the bloodstream of small nutrient molecules produced by digestion
- The **elimination** of undigested unabsorbed foodstuffs and other waste products

After food is ingested, it is propelled through the GI tract, coming into contact with a wide variety of secretions that aid in its digestion, absorption, or elimination (Norris, 2019).

Chewing and Swallowing

The process of digestion begins with the act of chewing, in which food is broken down into small particles that can be swallowed and mixed with digestive enzymes. Saliva, produced by the salivary glands functions as a lubricant for food, thereby facilitating swallowing. Ptyalin, or salivary amylase, is an enzyme that begins the digestion of starches. Water and mucus, also contained in saliva, help lubricate the food as it is chewed, thereby facilitating swallowing (Norris, 2019).

Swallowing begins as a voluntary act that is regulated by the swallowing center in the medulla oblongata of the central nervous system (CNS). The act of swallowing requires the innervations of five cranial nerves (CN), specifically CN V (trigeminal nerve), VII (facial), IX (glossopharyngeal), X (vagus), and XII (hypoglossal). Diseases that disrupt the brain centers or CNs predispose the patient to aspiration. As a bolus of food is swallowed, the epiglottis moves to cover the tracheal opening and prevents aspiration of food into the lungs. Swallowing, which propels the bolus of food into the upper esophagus, thus ends as a reflex action. The smooth muscle in the wall of the esophagus contracts in a rhythmic sequence from the upper esophagus toward the stomach to propel the bolus of food along the tract. During this process of esophageal peristalsis, the lower esophageal sphincter relaxes and permits the bolus of food to enter the stomach. Subsequently, the lower esophageal sphincter closes tightly, preventing reflux of stomach contents into the esophagus (Norris, 2019).

Gastric Function

The stomach, which stores and mixes food with secretions, secretes a highly acidic fluid in response to the presence or anticipated **ingestion** of food. This fluid, which can total over 2 L/day, derives its acidity from **hydrochloric acid** (HCl) secreted by the glands of the stomach. The function of this gastric secretion is twofold: to break down food into more absorbable components and to aid in the destruction of most ingested bacteria. **Pepsin**, an important enzyme for protein digestion, is the end product of the conversion of pepsinogen from the chief cells (Table 20-1). **Intrinsic factor**, also secreted by the gastric mucosa, combines with dietary vitamin B_{12} so that the vitamin can be absorbed in the ileum. In the absence of intrinsic factor, vitamin B_{12} cannot be absorbed and pernicious anemia results (Muller, 2019; Norris, 2019).

Pearls for Practice

The nurse is aware that patients with critical illness may develop bleeding caused by stress ulceration. Thus, it is common prophylactic practice to prescribe medications to suppress acid production of the stomach for patients at risk of stress ulcer bleeding (see Chapters 22 and 52 for Curling ulcer).

TABLE **20-1 The Major Digestive Enzymes and Secretions**

Enzyme/Secretion	Enzyme Source	Digestive Action
Action of Enzymes That Digest Carbohydrates		
Ptyalin (salivary amylase)	Salivary glands	Starch → dextrin, maltose, glucose
Amylase	Pancreas and intestinal mucosa	Starch → dextrin, maltose, glucose Dextrin → maltose, glucose
Maltase	Intestinal mucosa	Maltose → glucose
Sucrase	Intestinal mucosa	Sucrose → glucose, fructose
Lactase	Intestinal mucosa	Lactose → glucose, galactose
Action of Enzymes/Secretions That Digest Protein		
Pepsin	Gastric mucosa	Protein → polypeptides
Trypsin	Pancreas	Proteins and polypeptides → polypeptides, dipeptides, amino acids
Aminopeptidase	Intestinal mucosa	Polypeptides → dipeptides, amino acids
Dipeptidase	Intestinal mucosa	Dipeptides → amino acids
Hydrochloric acid	Gastric mucosa	Protein → polypeptides, amino acids
Action of Enzymes Secretions That Digest Fat (Triglyceride)		
Lingual lipase	Lingual glands in the mouth	Small amount of triglycerides (<10%)
Pancreatic lipase	Pancreas	Triglycerides → fatty acids, monoglycerides
Bile	Liver and gallbladder	Fat emulsification

Peristaltic contractions in the stomach propel the stomach's contents toward the pylorus. Because large food particles cannot pass through the pyloric sphincter, they are churned back into the body of the stomach. In this way, food in the stomach is agitated mechanically and broken down into smaller particles. Peristalsis in the stomach and contractions of the pyloric sphincter allow the partially digested food to enter the small intestine at a rate that permits efficient absorption of nutrients. This partially digested food mixed with gastric secretions is called **chyme**. Hormones, neuroregulators, and local regulators found in the gastric secretions control the rate of gastric secretions and influence gastric motility (Table 20-2) (Norris, 2019).

Small Intestine Function

The digestive process continues in the duodenum. Duodenal secretions come from the accessory digestive organs—the pancreas and liver—and the glands in the wall of the intestine itself. These secretions contain digestive enzymes: amylase, lipase, and bile. Pancreatic secretions have an alkaline pH due to their high concentration of bicarbonate. This alkalinity neutralizes the acid entering the duodenum from the stomach. Digestive enzymes secreted by the pancreas include **trypsin**, which aids in digesting protein; **amylase**, which aids in digesting starch; and **lipase**, which aids in digesting fats. These secretions drain into the pancreatic duct, which empties into the duodenum along with the common bile duct at a short, dilated tube called the *hepatopancreatic ampulla*, or ampulla of Vater. Bile, secreted by the liver and stored in the gallbladder, aids in emulsifying ingested fats, making them easier to digest and absorb. The sphincter of Oddi (muscle tissue at the confluence of the common bile duct and the duodenum) controls the flow of bile. When this sphincter is closed, bile will move back into the common bile duct and gallbladder. Hormones, neuroregulators, and local regulators found in these intestinal secretions control the rate of intestinal secretions and also influence GI motility. Intestinal secretions total approximately 1 L/day of pancreatic juice, 700 mL/day of bile, and 2 L/day of secretions from the glands of the small intestine. Tables 20-1 and 20-2 give further information about the actions of digestive enzymes and GI regulatory substances (Norris, 2019).

Two types of contractions occur regularly in the small intestine: segmentation contractions and intestinal peristalsis. *Segmentation contractions* produce mixing waves that move the intestinal contents back and forth in a churning motion. *Intestinal peristalsis* propels the contents of the small

TABLE 20-2 **The Major Gastrointestinal Regulatory Substances**

Substance	Stimulus for Production	Target Tissue	Effect on Secretions	Effect on Motility
Neuroregulators				
Acetylcholine (main parasympathetic neurotransmitter)	Sight, smell, chewing food, stomach distention	Gastric glands, other secretory glands, gastric and intestinal muscle	Increased gastric acid	Generally increased; decreased sphincter tone
Norepinephrine (secreted by sympathetic nerve endings)	Stress, other various stimuli	Secretory glands, gastric and intestinal muscle	Generally inhibitory	Generally decreased; increased sphincter tone
Hormonal Regulators				
Gastrin	Stomach distention with food	Gastric glands	Increased secretion of gastric juice, which is rich in HCl	Increased motility of stomach, decreased time required for gastric emptying Relaxation of ileocecal sphincter Excitation of colon Constriction of gastroesophageal sphincter
Cholecystokinin	Fat in duodenum	Gallbladder Pancreas Stomach	Release of bile into duodenum Increased production of enzyme-rich pancreatic secretions Inhibits gastric secretion somewhat	Delays gastric emptying
Secretin	pH of chyme in duodenum below 4–5	Stomach Pancreas	Inhibits gastric secretion somewhat Increased production of bicarbonate-rich pancreatic juice	Inhibits stomach contractions
Local Regulator				
Histamine	Unclear; substances in food	Gastric glands	Increased gastric acid production	Increased bowel peristalsis

Adapted from Morris, A. L., & Mohiuddin, S. S. Biochemistry, nutrients. Updated May 12, 2021; Norris, 2019; Prosapio et al., 2021.

intestine toward the colon. Both movements are stimulated by the presence of chyme (Norris, 2019).

Food, initially ingested in the form of fats, proteins, and carbohydrates, is broken down into absorbable particles (constituent nutrients) by the process of digestion. Carbohydrates are broken down into disaccharides (e.g., sucrose, maltose, and galactose) and monosaccharides (e.g., glucose and fructose). Glucose is the major carbohydrate that tissue cells use as fuel. Proteins are a source of energy after they are broken down into amino acids and peptides. Ingested fats become monoglycerides and fatty acid by the process of emulsification, which makes them smaller and, therefore, easier to absorb. Chyme in the small intestine allows for continued breakdown and absorption of nutrients (Norris, 2019).

Small, finger-like projections called villi are present throughout the entire intestine and function to produce digestive enzymes as well as to absorb nutrients. Absorption is the primary function of the small intestine. Water must be secreted into the GI tract on a daily basis in order for hydrolysis, a breakdown of compounds involving water, to occur. Because the intestinal mucosa cannot absorb large molecules such as fats, proteins and carbohydrates, they must be broken down so that absorption can take place. Digestion of carbohydrates and proteins begins in the stomach but the majority of digestion occurs in the small intestines. Fat absorption takes place only in the small intestines. The liver which produces bile and the pancreas which produces digestive enzymes facilitate the digestive process. Nutrients enter the lumen of the GI tract and are absorbed through active transport and diffusion. The large intestine plays a larger role in osmosis or water reabsorption. Vitamin B_{12} relies on a particular carrier transport system and is not absorbed without the presence of the intrinsic factor, secreted by the stomach parietal cells. Amino acids and glucose are transported in the presence of sodium and are absorbed via an osmotic gradient (Floch, 2019; Norris, 2019).

Colon Function

After eating, residual waste material passes into the terminal ileum and slowly into the proximal portion of the right colon through the ileocecal valve. With each peristaltic wave of the small intestine, the valve opens briefly and permits some of the contents to pass into the colon. It is estimated that there are 300 to 500 different species of intestinal bacteria in the large intestine, the vast majority being anaerobic bacteria. This intestinal flora also provides a critical resistance to potential invading pathogens. The nurse is aware that broad-spectrum antibiotics have the potential to disrupt this normal intestinal flora and place the patient at risk for overgrowth of pathogens, such as *Clostridium difficile*. Probiotics, such as lactobacilli, are live organisms considered healthy for the host organisms and often are administered to restore the microbial balance in the intestines (Norris, 2019).

The ~5-foot-long large intestine or large bowel includes the cecum (most proximal part of the large intestine), ascending, transverse, descending and sigmoid colon. The terminal part of the intestine consists of the rectum and anal canal (most distal part of the large intestine). The large intestine is wider and shorter than the small intestine and its main purpose is the efficient reabsorption of water and electrolytes and to rid the body of undigested and residual food in the form of feces. In general, the large intestine secretes mostly mucus which is influenced by the autonomic nervous system. Mucus secretions increase when extreme parasympathetic stimulation occurs resulting in large amounts of mucus in the stool. The bowel does not secrete water or electrolytes; however, both are lost when the bowel becomes inflamed or irritated (Norris, 2019).

Pearls for Practice

Approximately 9 L of fluid are sent through the GI tract daily, and all but 100 mL are reabsorbed; thus the nurse is aware that any process or pathology that increases peristalsis will result in decreased fluid, nutrient, and electrolyte reabsorption, resulting in malnutrition, profound dehydration, and electrolyte depletion.

Waste Products of Digestion

Of the 7,000 mL of fluid secreted into the GI tract, about 100 to 200 mL exit the body as part of the stool. The rest of this fluid is reabsorbed in the small and large intestines. Although the majority of this fluid consists of water it also contains sodium and potassium, much like extracellular fluid. Feces consist of undigested food, inorganic materials, water, and bacteria (Ogobuiro et al., 2021). Fecal matter is approximately 75% water. Stool consistency depends upon the proportion of solid to liquid matter as well as rapid or slow colonic transit time. Stool volume is increased with diarrhea-related illnesses such as cholera. Dietary intake plays a role in stool composition and bowel functioning and medications with anticholinergic properties are linked to constipation (Heltmann et al., 2021). The relationship between exercise and bowel function is undetermined (Heltmann et al., 2021; Mawer & Alhawaj, 2020). The brown color of the feces results from the breakdown of bile by the intestinal bacteria (Norris, 2019).

Elimination of stool begins with distention of the rectum, which reflexively initiates contractions of the rectal musculature and relaxes the normally closed internal anal sphincter. The internal sphincter is controlled by the autonomic nervous system; the external sphincter is under the conscious control of the cerebral cortex. During defecation, the external anal sphincter voluntarily relaxes to allow colonic contents to be expelled. Normally, the external anal sphincter is maintained in a state of tonic contraction. Thus, defecation is seen to be a spinal reflex (involving the parasympathetic nerve fibers) that can be inhibited voluntarily by keeping the external anal sphincter closed. Contracting the abdominal muscles (straining) facilitates emptying of the colon. The frequency of defecation in humans within a 24-hour period varies and is influenced by the person's age and diet; however the majority of individuals have a bowel movement once a day (Mawer & Alhawaj, 2020; Norris, 2019).

ACCESSORY DIGESTIVE ORGANS

Liver

The liver weighing approximately 1.3 kg (3 lb) is located in the right upper quadrant and is the largest visceral organ of the body. It can be considered a chemical factory that manufactures, stores, alters, and excretes a large number of substances involved in metabolism. The location of the liver is essential in this function because it receives nutrient-rich blood directly from the GI tract and then either stores or transforms these nutrients into chemicals that are used elsewhere in the body for metabolic needs (Norris, 2019; Small et al., 2020). The liver is especially important in the synthesis of glucose, protein, and blood-clotting factors (Norris, 2019).

An important and unique characteristic of the liver is its ability to regenerate. The normal liver maintains a constant mass regulated by the metabolic needs and size of the person. After removal or injury of liver tissue, hepatocytes proliferate to replace the mass of the liver to its original size, although this is generally as a result of tissue injury rather than during homeostasis. This physiologic feature is important in the event of liver transplant. Thus, the liver displays an extraordinary ability to regenerate cells through matrix remodeling; however, chronic damage results in depletion of this cell pool and subsequent liver failure (Codero-Espinoza et al., 2021).

The major functions of the liver include glucose metabolism, conversion of ammonia to urea, protein metabolism, fat metabolism, vitamin and iron storage, drug metabolism, bile formation, and bilirubin excretion (Norris, 2019; Small et al., 2020).

Bile, which is manufactured by the liver and plays a major role in the digestion and absorption of fats in the GI tract, is stored temporarily in the gallbladder until it is needed for digestion, at which time the gallbladder empties and bile enters the intestine (Fig. 20-3). Waste products removed by the liver are secreted into bile. The smallest bile ducts, called *canaliculi*, are located between the lobules of the liver. The canaliculi receive secretions from the hepatocytes and carry them to larger bile ducts, which eventually form the hepatic duct. The hepatic duct from the liver and the cystic duct from the gallbladder join to form the common bile duct, which empties into the small intestine. The sphincter of Oddi, located at the junction where the common bile duct enters the duodenum, controls the flow of bile into the intestine (Norris, 2019).

The liver is located behind the ribs in the upper right portion of the abdominal cavity and below the diaphragm and under normal conditions cannot be palpated as it lies within the rib cage. It is enclosed by a fibrous capsule and is divided into two large lobes and two smaller lobes. It spans from 2 to 6 in or 6 to 15 cm but averages about 4 to 5 in or 11 to 12 cm (Small et al., 2020) and weighs approximately 1.3 kg or 3 lb (Norris, 2019).

The circulation of the blood into and out of the liver is of major importance to liver function. The blood that perfuses the liver comes from two sources. Approximately 75% of the blood supply comes from the portal vein, which drains the GI tract and is rich in nutrients. The remainder of the blood supply enters by way of the hepatic artery and is rich in oxygen. Terminal branches of these two blood vessels join to form common capillary beds, which constitute the sinusoids of the liver (Fig. 20-4). Thus, a mixture of venous and arterial blood bathes the liver cells (hepatocytes). The sinusoids empty into venules that occupy the center of each liver lobule and are called the *central veins*. The central veins join to form the hepatic vein, which constitutes the venous drainage from the liver and empties into the inferior vena cava, close to the diaphragm. Thus, there are two sources of blood flowing into the liver and only one exit pathway. Because of the pressure differences between the hepatic and portal veins, the liver normally stores approximately 500 to 1,000 mL of blood, which can be available in times of hypovolemia. However, in conditions such as right heart failure, in which blood flows back into the vena cava, additional blood accumulates in the liver (Norris, 2019).

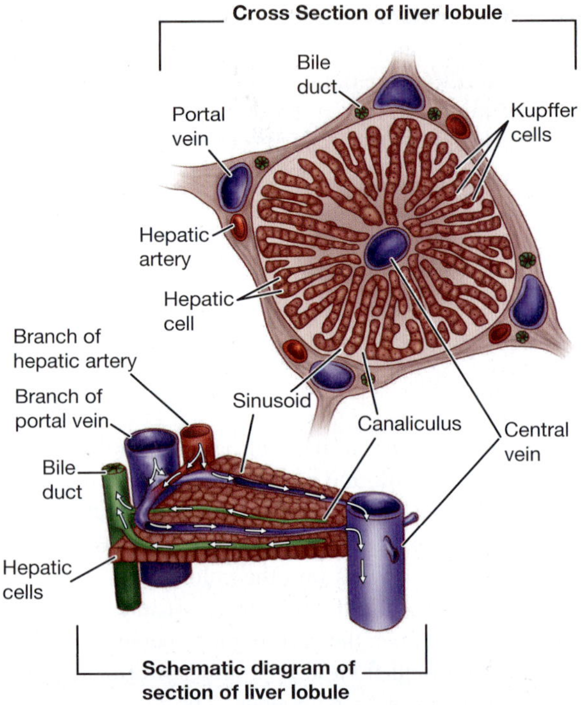

FIGURE 20-4 **A section of liver lobule showing the location of hepatic veins, hepatic cells, liver sinusoids, and branches of the portal vein and hepatic artery.**

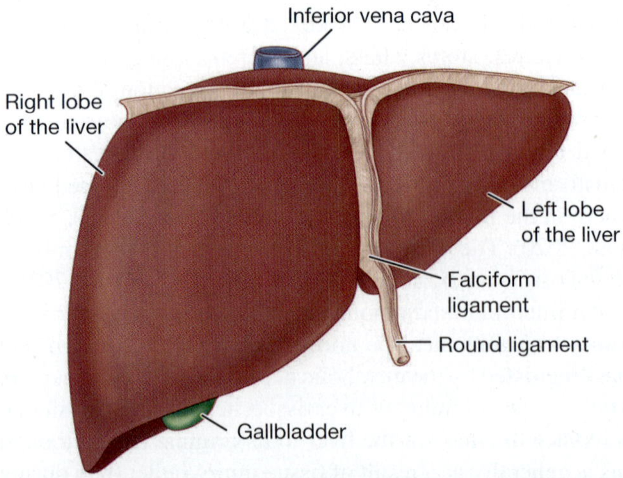

FIGURE 20-3 **The liver and biliary system.**

In addition to hepatocytes, phagocytic cells belonging to the reticuloendothelial system (RES) are present in the liver. Other organs that contain reticuloendothelial cells are the spleen, bone marrow, lymph nodes, and lungs. In the liver, these cells are called *Kupffer cells*. As the most common phagocyte in the human body, their main function is to engulf particulate matter (e.g., bacteria) that enters the liver through the portal blood (Norris, 2019).

The Gallbladder

The gallbladder, a pear-shaped, hollow, saclike organ, is approximately 10 cm or 4 in long and lies in a shallow depression on the inferior surface of the liver, to which it is

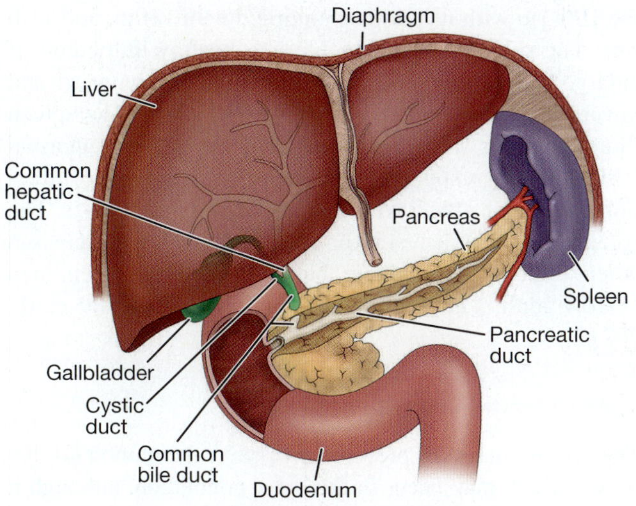

FIGURE 20-5 **The liver, biliary system, and pancreas.**

attached by loose connective tissue. The capacity of the gallbladder is 30 to 60 mL of bile. Its wall is composed largely of smooth muscle. The gallbladder is connected to the common bile duct by the cystic duct (Pitchumani, 2019) (Fig. 20-5).

The gallbladder functions as a storage area for bile. Between meals, when the sphincter of Oddi is closed, bile produced by the hepatocytes enters the gallbladder. During storage, a large portion of the water in bile is absorbed through the walls of the gallbladder so that gallbladder bile is five to ten times more concentrated than that originally secreted by the liver. When food enters the duodenum, the gallbladder contracts and the sphincter of Oddi relaxes, which allows the bile to enter the intestine. This response is mediated by secretion of the hormone **cholecystokinin (CCK)** from the intestinal wall (in the presence of partially digested fats and proteins in the lumen of the duodenum) and by neurons from the enteric nervous system (Pitchumani, 2019).

Bile is composed of water, bile salts (which are important in digestion), bilirubin, cholesterol as well as some byproducts of metabolism. The bile ducts secrete sodium, chloride, bicarbonate, and potassium which are also components in bile. The bile salts, together with cholesterol, assist in emulsification of fats in the distal ileum. Then they are reabsorbed into the portal blood for return to the liver, after which they are excreted into the bile once again. Because of the enterohepatic circulation, only a small fraction of the bile salts that enter the intestine are excreted in the feces. This decreases the need for active synthesis of bile salts by the liver cells. Approximately half of the bilirubin, a pigment derived from the breakdown of red blood cells (RBCs), is converted by the intestinal flora into urobilinogen, a highly soluble substance. Urobilinogen is either excreted in the feces and urine or returned to the portal circulation, where it is re-excreted into the bile (Norris, 2019).

Jaundice or a yellowish discoloration of the skin, occurs with excessive levels of bilirubin in the blood. It becomes noticeable when serum bilirubin levels exceed 2 to 2.5 mg/dL. Prehepatic jaundice, in most cases, occurs with excessive hemolysis of RBCs in which RBCs are destroyed so rapidly that the liver is unable to remove the excess bilirubin. This occurs following a hemolytic blood transfusion reaction or in spherocytosis, an inherited disorder in which RBC membranes are abnormal. Another cause of prehepatic jaundice is neonatal hyperbilirubinemia which may occur during the first 14 days of life resulting from an increased production of bilirubin and the limited ability to effectively excrete it. Intrahepatic jaundice, also called hepatocellular jaundice, occurs when the liver is directly affected and is unable to eliminate bilirubin from the blood or unable to effectively conjugate bilirubin. Gilbert disease, an inherited and benign disorder affecting 8% of people, impairs the removal of bilirubin from the blood. The most common causes of intrahepatic jaundice are diseases of the liver such as hepatitis and/or cirrhosis. Other causes may be drugs such as oral contraceptives, estrogen, anabolic steroid, isoniazid, rifampin, chlorpromazine, and halothane (Norris, 2019). If the flow of bile is impeded (e.g., by gallstones in the bile ducts), bilirubin does not enter the intestine. As a result, blood levels of bilirubin increase and cause jaundice which may involve yellowing of the sclera, termed *icterus*. Increased levels of bilirubin cause increased renal excretion of urobilinogen, resulting in dark-colored urine, which, since bile is a soap, will be frothy when agitated. If the bile is prevented from entering the small intestine, clay-colored stool will be noted. Bile salts are also irritating to the skin; thus, the nurse is alert for complaints of itchy skin or pruritus. These changes produce many of the signs and symptoms seen in gallbladder disorders (Norris, 2019; Small et al., 2020).

The Pancreas

The pancreas is approximately 6 in in length and is located in the posterior region of the upper abdomen just behind the stomach. It has **endocrine** as well as **exocrine** functions (see Fig. 20-5). The exocrine functions include secretion of pancreatic enzymes into the GI tract through the pancreatic duct. It also functions as an endocrine gland in that it manufacturers and releases insulin into the bloodstream (Small et al., 2020).

The Exocrine Pancreas

The secretions of the exocrine portion of the pancreas are collected in the pancreatic duct, which joins the common bile duct and enters the duodenum at the ampulla of Vater. Surrounding the ampulla is the sphincter of Oddi, which partially controls the rate at which secretions from the pancreas and the gallbladder enter the duodenum (Norris, 2019).

The secretions of the exocrine pancreas are digestive enzymes high in protein content and an electrolyte-rich fluid; they include amylase, trypsin, and lipase. The pancreatic enzymes are inactive when secreted and only become activated when entering the intestine. This concept is important since if secreted in the active form they would digest the pancreas. Hormones originating in the GI tract stimulate the secretion of these exocrine pancreatic juices. The hormone **secretin** is the major stimulus for increased bicarbonate secretion from the pancreas (Engjom et al., 2020).

The Endocrine Pancreas

The islets of Langerhans, the endocrine part of the pancreas, are collections of cells embedded in the pancreatic tissue. They are composed of alpha, beta, and delta cells. The hormone produced by the beta cells is called *insulin*. The alpha cells secrete glucagon, and the delta cells secrete somatostatin. Refer to Chapter 29 for details on insulin and glucagon secretion. Somatostatin is a hormone secreted in the pancreas, the stomach, and the small intestine. It decreases GI activity after ingestion of food and also acts in the islets of Langerhans to inhibit the release of insulin and glucagon. By decreasing the transit time and inhibiting insulin and glucagon, it is proposed that absorption of foodstuffs and nutrients is enhanced (Norris, 2019).

Spleen

The spleen is a lymphoid organ located high in the left upper abdominal cavity, left mid axillary line, and is parallel to the 10th rib with its width spanning the 9th, 10th, and 11th ribs. The spleen is not palpable in a healthy individual; if enlarged, its lower pole can be palpated downward and toward the midline (Jarvis & Eckhardt, 2020). The spleen filters antigens from the blood, removes old or abnormal RBCs, and is responsible for immune response to infection because it is rich with B- and T-cell lymphocytes. The spleen serves as a reservoir for blood which is released when there is appreciable blood loss. The spleen in a healthy adult is approximately 4 in in length (Crane et al., 2021).

Gerontologic Considerations

There is an increased prevalence of several common GI disorders which may occur in the older population, although it appears the effects are less prevalent in comparison with other bodily systems. Thus, aging per se appears to have minimal direct effect on most GI functions, in large part because of the functional reserve of the GI tract (Table 20-3). Common problems in the older adult range from a decrease in taste buds resulting in less enjoyment while eating, constipation secondary to decreased bowel motility or acid reflux due to a delay in gastric emptying, which may lead to challenges with

TABLE **20-3 GERONTOLOGIC CONSIDERATIONS / Age-Related Changes of the Gastrointestinal System**

Component	Structural Changes	Implications
Oral Cavity and Pharynx	• Injury/loss or decay of teeth • Atrophy of taste buds • Decreased saliva production • Reduced ptyalin and amylase in saliva • Atrophy of gingival tissue	Difficulty chewing and swallowing
Esophagus	• Decreased motility and emptying • Weakened gag reflex • Decreased resting pressure of lower esophageal sphincter • Decreased muscle tone and weakness in lower esophageal sphincter	Reflux and heartburn Dysphagia (difficulty swallowing) Dyspepsia (indigestion)
Stomach	• Degeneration and atrophy of gastric mucosal surfaces with decreased production of HCl • Decreased secretion of gastric acids and most digestive enzymes • Decreased motility and emptying	Delayed gastric emptying Food intolerances Malabsorption Decrease in absorption of iron and vitamin B_{12} Anorexia Anemia
Small Intestine	• Atrophy of muscle and mucosal surfaces • Thinning of villi and epithelial cells	Decreased motility and transit time, which lead to complaints of indigestion and constipation
Large Intestine	• Decrease in mucus secretion • Decrease in elasticity of rectal wall • Decreased tone of internal anal sphincter • Slower and duller nerve impulses in rectal area	Decreased absorption of nutrients (dextrose, fats, calcium, and iron), leading to decreased sensation to defecate and increased constipation Fecal incontinence from decrease or loss of sphincter control
Liver	• Decrease in size and weight • Decrease in total hepatic blood flow • Decreased drug metabolism	Decreases in size proportional to decreases in body size and weight Increased incidence of drug toxicity

the older adult meeting nutritional needs. The liver decreases in size as individuals age; however, in general, the liver cells appear to be quite well preserved because of the regenerative capability of hepatocytes. There appears to be reduced hepatic clearance of drugs in the older adult secondary to changes in liver perfusion and endothelial cell functioning, as well as the ability of drug-binding power to proteins; however this is variable among individuals (Papadakis et al., 2022).

ASSESSMENT

Health History

A focused GI assessment begins with a complete history. Information about abdominal pain, appetite changes, dysphagia, unintentional weight loss, excessive gas or heartburn, jaundice, change in bowel movements, presence of black, tarry stool, rectal bleeding, persistent nausea, vomiting, diarrhea, constipation, oral ulcerations, bilious vomit, unexplained fever, and previous personal or family history of GI disease is investigated. Past and current medication use and any previous diagnostic studies such as colonoscopy, treatments, and past surgeries are noted (Bickley et al., 2021; Small et al., 2020).

The initial presentation of a patient with liver disease varies greatly and can range from elevated liver enzymes on routine screening with no clinical signs or symptoms of disease to the patient who presents in liver failure with jaundice, hepatitis, or GI bleeding. A comprehensive and complete health history is critical to determine exposure to hepatotoxic substances (including alcohol) or infectious agents causing liver dysfunction (Bickley et al., 2021; Jarvis & Eckhardt, 2020).

Current History

One of the crucial factors in providing quality health care is establishing a trusting relationship between the health care provider and the patient which includes active listening and developing an awareness and understanding of the patient's culture and belief system (Jarvis & Ekchardt, 2020). Social determinants of health are important to understand when obtaining a patient's health history as it can be influenced by a number of factors including access to and quality of health care and education, social and community context, economic stability, and neighborhood environment (U.S. Department of Health and Human Services, Office of Disease Prevention and Health Promotion, 2021). The nurse must be cognizant of any number of social, environmental, and economic disparities that have the potential to negatively impact health status based on race or ethnicity, religion, socioeconomic status, age, gender, sexual orientation or gender identity, geographic or living condition, mental health status, cognitive, sensory or physical disabilities, among others (Jarvis & Eckhardt, 2020). This includes mode of transportation, housing situation, access to quality education, clean water and air, and access to nutritious food (Jarvis & Eckhardt, 2020). It is crucial that the nurse explores any of these obstacles affecting the patient's health status or care while establishing a thorough health history. The visit continues as a complete metabolic panel, including liver function studies and complete blood count (CBC) are obtained and in selective case, hemoccult stool tests, erythrocyte sedimentation rate, hepatitis panel, urinalysis, urine culture, and lipase which may be necessary in determining the diagnosis. Imaging studies may include endoscopy with biopsy, abdominal imaging such as x-ray, ultrasound, CT scan or hepatobiliary scans with nuclear tracers and colonoscopy (Small et al., 2020).

Questions are raised about the use of tobacco and alcohol and include the need for detailed answers about type, amount, length of use, and the date of discontinuation, if any. The amount and type of alcohol consumption are identified using screening questionnaires that have been developed for this purpose (Bickley et al., 2021; Small et al., 2020). One such questionnaire is the Alcohol Use Disorders Identification Test-Concise (AUDIT-C). This questionnaire is considered succinct as well as reliable in recognizing patients who may have alcohol use disorder or those who may be dependent (Bickley et al., 2021). As in any health history, it is important to include questions about psychosocial, spiritual, or cultural factors that may be affecting the patient (Bickley et al., 2021; Jarvis & Eckhardt, 2020).

Lifestyle behaviors that increase the risk for exposure to infectious agents and potential toxins are identified. The patient's history of alcohol and drug use, including but not limited to the use of IV injection drugs, provides additional information about exposure to toxins and infectious agents impacting an individual's health (Bickley et al., 2021; Jarvis & Eckhardt, 2020; Small et al., 2020). The patient's occupational, recreational, and travel history may assist in identifying exposure to hepatotoxins (e.g., industrial chemicals, other toxins) (Bickley et al., 2021). The nurse should be aware of all prescribed as well as "over-the-counter" medications the patient is taking. Drug-induced liver injury accounts for more than 50% of all liver failure cases in the United States and this type of injury may be quite severe. Acute liver injury may occur secondary to acetaminophen, antimicrobials, lipid-lowering drugs, psychotropic agents, and nonsteroidal and other anti-inflammatory medications (Norris, 2019). Inflammation of the liver can also be caused by hepatotropic viruses which affect hepatocytes. These include Epstein–Barr virus, cytomegalovirus, herpes viruses, enteroviruses, and hepatitis A (HAV), hepatitis B (HBV), hepatitis C (HCV), hepatitis D (HDV) (which is associated with HBV), and hepatitis E (HEV). Hepatitis G (HGV) has been discovered in 2% of blood donors in the United States however is not linked to liver disease (Norris, 2019). Hepatitis A is transmitted primarily via the fecal–oral route by ingesting contaminated milk, water, or shellfish from infected water. Patients should be asked about traveling to countries and communities with high rates of infection and the hepatitis A vaccine is advised. Hepatitis B is transmitted by exposure via inoculation with infected blood or serum as well as through body secretions. This virus can produce acute or chronic hepatitis which may progress to cirrhosis, fulminant hepatitis, and massive necrosis. There is also a carrier state. Globally, 350 million people have been infected long-term with HBV, but acute infection rates in the United States have declined since 1990 secondary to vaccinations. The patient should be asked about risk factors which include injection drug use, heterosexuals with multiple sex partners, men who have sex with men, health care workers who may have bloodborne exposure, accidental needle sticks or risk for mucosal exposures from infected patients, pregnant people positive for HBV (the risk to the fetus is 10% to 15%) and patients who have had blood transfusions, although routine screening has markedly reduced the risk. The patient should be educated that the hepatitis B vaccine produces long-term protection. HCV has infected 3 to 4 million people worldwide, and more than 350,000 deaths occur from hepatitis C–associated diseases. Currently, the most prevalent form of transmission in the United States and in Canada results from recreational injection drug use. Patients should also be asked about high-risk sexual practices defined as sex with multiple partners or sex with a person who is HCV infected. The nurse should also obtain a health history from pregnant people who are HCV ribonucleic acid (RNA) positive as the transmission rate to the infant is 4.6% to 10%. Health care workers should be asked about needlestick injuries. Individuals who have had tattoos, acupuncture, or body piercings may also be at risk for HCV infection via transmission of small droplets of blood. Hepatitis D virus may occur in patients infected with hepatitis B as it requires HBV to replicate. Hepatitis E virus (HEV) is transmitted by the fecal–oral route and symptoms are similar to HAV. Travel to locations endemic to hepatitis E place patients at risk for this form of viral hepatitis. Chronic HEV infection has been associated with genotype 3 (the most common genotype [strain of the virus] linked to HEV in Europe and the United States) as well as those undergoing chemotherapy or those who have had solid organ transplants. While HEV infrequently develops into acute or severe cases, it is fatal in 2% of all HEV infections, and immunocompromised patients have considerable mortality rates (Norris, 2019). A thorough medication history to assess liver dysfunction should address all current and past prescription medications, over-the-counter medications, herbal remedies, and dietary supplements. The patient should be advised that acetaminophen, a component in many cold remedies, may cause liver injury if the patient doubles or triples the maximum daily dose (Jarvis & Eckhardt, 2020).

Past History

The history also includes an evaluation of the client's medical history to identify risk factors for liver disease. Current and past medical conditions, including those of a psychological or psychiatric nature, are identified. The family history includes questions about familial liver disorders that may have their origin in alcohol use disorder or gallstone disease as well as other familial or genetic diseases, such as hemochromatosis, an inherited disorder manifested by increased intestinal absorption of iron in the liver, pancreas, heart, and other organs; Wilson disease, an autosomal recessive disorder of the liver resulting from excessive copper deposits; or alpha$_1$-antitrypsin disease, an autosomal recessive disorder causing damage to the liver and lungs (Bosch et al., 2022). A positive family history of hepatitis B may indicate vertical transmission (infection transmitted from mother to child [embryo, fetus, or baby] during pregnancy or childbirth) (Norris, 2019).

Common Complaints

Pain

Pain can be a major symptom of GI disease, and a thorough patient history can lead to an accurate diagnosis in 76% of cases. Pain may be described as visceral; that is, nociceptors (sensory receptors that are activated by noxious stimuli) in the abdominal organs are stimulated. This type of pain occurs when the intestines or biliary tree are distended or stretched and is often described by patients as cramping, aching, squeezing, or colicky, and it may be difficult for patient's to pinpoint the exact location. Examples are periumbilical pain which patients experience in early appendicitis or when the liver becomes distended in its capsule as in hepatitis. Parietal pain occurs when the parietal peritoneum is inflamed, as in peritonitis. It is a steady, severe pain that may be localized. Coughing or moving typically worsens the pain. Referred pain is pain that travels to a more distant site, where it localizes or presents. Such pain may occur when a patient is experiencing a myocardial infarction and describes pain in the mid-epigastric region or a patient with pancreatic or duodenal disorders describing pain in their back. The character, duration, pattern, frequency, location, and distribution of referred pain (Fig. 20-6) vary greatly depending on the underlying cause. Other factors such as meals, rest, activity, and defecation patterns may directly affect this pain (Bickley et al., 2021).

Pearls for Practice

The pain of appendicitis initially presents as vague discomfort in the periumbilical area. As the inflammatory process progresses to involve the parietal peritoneum, the pain localizes to the right lower quadrant. The nurse maintains a high degree of suspicion of appendicitis for patients complaining of abdominal pain, nausea, anorexia, and "migratory" pain.

Dyspepsia

Dyspepsia, which is upper abdominal discomfort or distress associated with eating (commonly called *indigestion*)

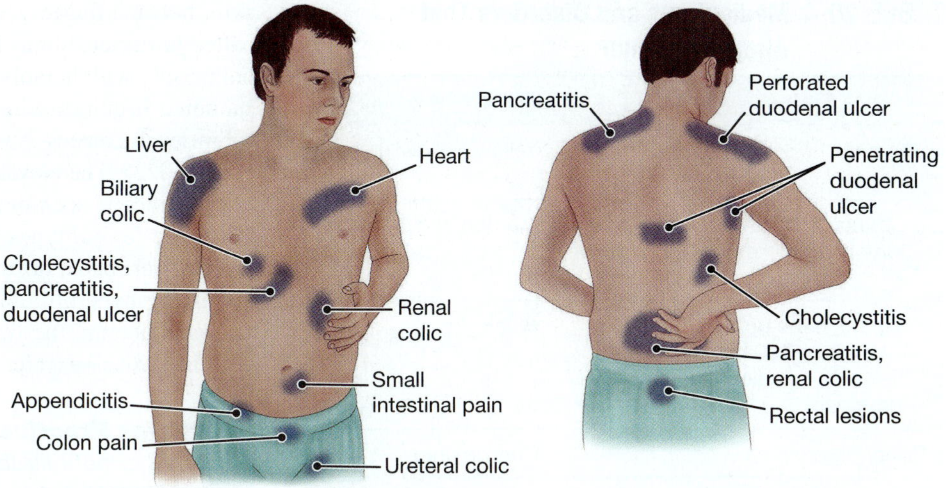

FIGURE 20-6 Common sites of referred abdominal pain.

is the most common symptom of clients with GI dysfunction. Indigestion is an imprecise term that refers to a host of upper abdominal or epigastric symptoms, such as pain, discomfort, nausea, fullness after eating, bloating, early satiety, belching, heartburn, and regurgitation (Bickley et al., 2021; McQuaid, 2022). Typically, fatty foods cause the most discomfort because they remain in the stomach for digestion longer than proteins or carbohydrates. Patients are generally advised to avoid caffeine, alcohol, chocolate, and tobacco as these substances relax the lower esophageal sphincter resulting in acid reflux. The patient is advised to avoid snacks before bedtime and to elevate the head of the bed prior to sleep (Jameson et al., 2020; Papadakis et al., 2022). A food diary, where the patient documents their food intake, symptoms, and daily events, may reveal precipitants of pain (McQuaid, 2022).

Intestinal Gas

The accumulation of gas in the GI tract may result in belching (expulsion of gas from the stomach through the mouth) or flatulence (expulsion of gas from the rectum). Usually, gases in the small intestine pass into the colon and are released as flatus. Patients often complain of bloating, distention, or feeling "full of gas," with excessive flatulence as a symptom of food intolerance or irritable bowel syndrome (Bickley et al., 2021; Jameson et al., 2020).

Nausea and Vomiting

Nausea is a vague, intensely unsettling sensation of sickness or "queasiness" that may or may not be followed by vomiting. It can be triggered by odors, activity, medications, or food intake. The emesis, or vomitus, may vary in color and content and may contain undigested food particles, blood (hematemesis), or bilious material mixed with gastric juices. The causes of nausea and vomiting are many. Nausea and vomiting may be symptomatic of a benign condition but depending on associated signs and symptoms, the nurse must also consider uremia, liver disease, hypercalcemia, adrenal insufficiency, diabetic ketoacidosis, bulimia, drug reactions, and emotional distress as possible causes (Bickley et al., 2021).

Change in Bowel Habits and Stool Characteristics

Diarrhea and constipation are quite common occurrences, and more than 1 billion worldwide experience diarrhea at least once a year (Jameson et al., 2020). Most cases are mild and self-limiting. Acute infectious diarrhea, however, is a common cause of death in developing nations. Changes in bowel habits may signal colonic dysfunction or disease. Diarrhea, an abnormal increase in the frequency of bowel movements and liquidity of the stool or in daily stool weight or volume, commonly occurs when the contents move so rapidly through the intestine and colon that there may be inadequate time for the GI secretions and oral contents to be absorbed. Typically, this physiologic function is associated with abdominal pain or cramping and nausea or vomiting (Bickley et al., 2021; Jameson et al., 2020). Diarrhea is considered "acute" when lasting less than 14 days and persistent when occurring for 14 to 30 days. It is considered chronic if lasting longer than 30 days. The nurse should question the patient concerning the characteristics of the stool; for example, volume, frequency, consistency, the appearance of mucus, oily substances or blood and the time of day, for example if diarrhea occurs only during the daytime hours or if it awakens the patient at night (Bickley et al., 2021). Possible causes of diarrhea include infection, foodborne illnesses, nosocomial infections, such as clostridium difficile, inflammatory bowel disease, antibiotics, food allergies, colorectal cancer, or thyroid disorders (Bickley et al., 2021; Jameson et al., 2020). Constipation, a decrease in the frequency of bowel movements, is described as stools that are hard, dry, and of smaller volume than normal and may be associated with abdominal fullness and incomplete defecation and straining (Jameson et al., 2020). Because elimination patterns vary widely from person to person, constipation can be difficult to define.

TABLE 20-4 Medications and Disorders That Alter Stool Color

Disease States	Color
Diarrhea	Yellow, yellow-green, green
Bleeding of the lower GI tract from tumors, hemorrhoids, fissures, or an inflammatory process	Maroon, red
Bleeding in the upper GI tract (more than 100 mL blood), bismuth, iron, licorice, and charcoal	Black
Biliary obstruction	Clay colored
Pancreatic disorder causing malabsorption of fat	Pale, with a greasy consistency

Adapted from Fischbach, F. T., Fischbach, M. A., & Stout, K., (2022). *Fischbach's a manual of laboratory and diagnostic tests* (11th ed.). Lippincott/Williams & Wilkins.

Constipation is common and rarely associated with death. The characteristics of the stool can vary greatly. Stool is normally light to dark brown; however, specific disease processes and ingestion of certain foods and medications may change the appearance of stool such as black with iron or bismuth administration (Table 20-4). Blood in the stool can present in various ways and must be investigated. If blood is shed in sufficient quantities (100 mL of blood) into the upper GI tract, it produces a tarry-black color (melena), whereas blood entering the lower portion of the GI tract called hematochezia, may appear bright or dark red. Lower rectal or anal bleeding is suspected if there is streaking of blood on the surface of the stool or if blood is noted on toilet tissue (Bickley et al., 2021). Constipation associated with rectal bleeding, weight loss or anemia, deserves further investigation (Jameson et al., 2018).

Pearls for Practice

Melena, or black "tarry" stools, occurs in association with upper GI bleeding from the esophagus, stomach, duodenum, or small intestine. Melena can result after blood loss in an amount as small as 60 mL and is caused by stomach acid (hydrochloric acid) or intestinal bacterial conversion of hemoglobin to the black pigment hematin. Pseudomelena, or false melena, is associated with ingestion of iron. The term hematochezia refers to stools that are maroon or bright red in color, signifying a bleeding below the ligament of Treitz (duodenum level) but may be associated with a rapid upper GI bleed.

Jaundice

When the bilirubin concentration in the blood is elevated abnormally, all the body tissues, including the sclerae and the skin, become tinged yellow or greenish yellow, a condition called **jaundice**. It may be present due to liver disease or less commonly with hemolytic disorders (Jameson et al., 2020). Jaundice becomes clinically evident when the serum bilirubin level exceeds 2.5 mg/dL (>41.6 mmol/L) (Fischbach et al., 2022). The elevated bilirubin stains tissues and fluid, but jaundice is seen most frequently in the sclera (icterus). There are several types of jaundice: hemolytic, hepatocellular or intrahepatic, obstructive jaundice, and jaundice due to hereditary hyperbilirubinemia. Hepatocellular and obstructive jaundice are the two types most commonly associated with liver disease (refer to Chapter 24) (Norris, 2019).

Pearls for Practice: Pathophysiology

A normal direct bilirubin is 0.0 to 0.3 mg/dL (Fischbach et al., 2022). Bilirubin, which gives bile its color, may be reported as direct (conjugated or combined in a molecule similar to glucose) or indirect (termed free or unconjugated). The direct bilirubin reflects bilirubin excreted by the GI tract, whereas indirect bilirubin reflects what normally circulates in the bloodstream (Fischbach et al., 2022). Both are elevated in a variety of disorders since bilirubin is produced in the liver, spleen, and bone marrow.

Ascites

Ascites is an increased accumulation of peritoneal fluid in the abdomen caused by a variety of disorders associated with the liver. One factor associated with development of ascites is portal hypertension and the resulting increase in capillary pressure and obstruction of venous blood flow through the damaged liver. **Portal hypertension** causes an increased pressure gradient (a difference in pressure between the portal vein and the hepatic veins), facilitating fluid accumulation in the peritoneal cavity. Another factor is the decreased synthesis of albumin in liver disease. The hypoalbuminemia results in decreased plasma oncotic pressure, which facilitates fluid accumulation in the abdominal cavity (Jameson et al., 2020; Norris, 2019). An obstruction of the normal lymphatic drainage can cause fluid accumulation in the peritoneum, as can cancers or inflammatory processes that stimulate increased production of peritoneal fluid. Ascites also can be associated with nonhepatic etiologies, such as kidney failure and heart failure. Spontaneous bacterial peritonitis can arise as a complication of cirrhosis-induced ascites which may lead to death (Jameson et al., 2020).

Pearls for Practice

To provide consistent measurements, the nurse marks the patient's abdomen above and below where they will measure (typically at the level of the umbilicus). A tape measure is placed between the upper and lower line and the measurements are obtained at the same time each day and before meals. The nurse records the measurement in the patient record.

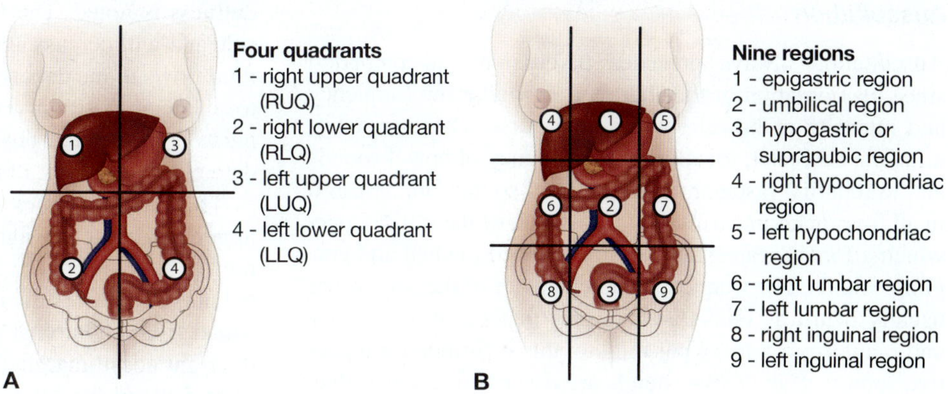

FIGURE 20-7 Division of the abdomen into (A) four quadrants or (B) nine regions.

Engorged Veins

Under normal conditions, the veins in the abdominal wall are barely noted unless the skin and subcutaneous fat are thin. When venous pressure increases as a result of obstruction, as in portal hypertension, vessels distal to the inferior vena cava engorge, and distended veins can be seen on the abdomen, chest, and extremities (Bickley et al., 2021; Norris, 2019; Small et al., 2020).

Physical Examination

For the purposes of examination and documentation, the abdomen can be divided into either four quadrants or nine regions (Fig. 20-7). The nurse must know the physical proximity of the organs and blood vessels to these quadrants or regions. Choosing one of these mapping methods and using it consistently will ensure a thorough evaluation of the abdomen and appropriate corresponding documentation (Bickley et al., 2021). The physical examination includes assessment of the mouth, abdomen, and rectum. Good lighting is necessary, as is full exposure of the abdomen. The patient should be comfortable and relaxed, with an empty bladder (Small et al., 2020). The patient lies supine with knees flexed slightly for inspection, auscultation, palpation, and percussion of the abdomen. Arms should not be raised over the head because the abdominal muscles tense in this position. A small pillow may be placed behind the patient's head for comfort. The patient's breasts are covered with a gown, and sheets are rolled down to above the symphysis pubis. Examination of the abdomen is performed with the nurse standing on the patient's right side (Bickley et al., 2021; Small et al., 2020).

Inspection

The mouth, tongue, buccal mucosa, teeth, and gums are inspected, noting any ulcers, nodules, swelling, discoloration, or inflammation. Dentures should be removed to allow for proper visualization of the entire oral cavity (Jarvis & Eckhardt, 2020).

The nurse inspects the abdominal skin for nodules, lesions, masses, scarring, discolorations, inflammation, bruising, increased vascularity of the abdominal skin, and striae (stretch marks). In the presence of liver disease, the nurse inspects the skin, mucosa, and sclera for jaundice (Bickley et al., 2021; Small et al., 2020). The extremities are assessed for muscle atrophy, edema, and skin excoriation secondary to scratching. The nurse observes the skin for petechiae or ecchymotic areas (bruises), spider angiomas, and palmar erythema, which is diffuse reddening of the palm associated with chronic liver disease (Bickley et al., 2021; Norris, 2019; Small et al., 2020). In addition, a male patient is assessed for unilateral or bilateral gynecomastia and testicular atrophy due to hormonal changes associated with liver disease (Norris, 2019). The patient's cognitive status (recall, memory, abstract thinking) and neurologic status are assessed. The nurse observes for general tremor, asterixis (flapping of the hands when wrists dorsiflexed), weakness, and slurred speech related to elevated ammonia levels secondary to liver failure; the nurse notes the patient's breath for **hepatic fetor**, a sweet, mildly fecal breath odor associated with encephalopathy (Norris, 2019). The contour and symmetry of the abdomen are noted, and any localized bulging, distention, or peristaltic waves are identified (Bickley et al., 2021). Expected contours of the anterior abdominal wall can be described as flat, rounded, or scaphoid (hollowed or shaped like a boat). The umbilicus is assessed for color, position, and shape. The umbilicus may be everted with increased intra-abdominal pressure. Ecchymoses around the umbilical area is termed *Cullen sign* and is associated with a retroperitoneal bleed due to any cause. Ecchymoses noted on either flank, the groin, or the abdomen, termed *Grey–Turner sign*, is also associated with a retroperitoneal bleed (see Chapter 26, Fig. 26-12). A hernia is a protrusion on the abdominal wall and may be noted anywhere in the abdomen. If ascites is suspected, the nurse notes bulging flanks when the patient is in the supine position as the weight of the fluid flows dependently to the sides (Bickley et al., 2021; Small et al., 2020).

Pearls for Practice

If abdominal distention is noted, the nurse assesses for common causes described as the 6 F's: fetus (pregnancy), feces (constipation), flatus, fat (obesity), fluid (ascites), and fibroids or "fatal growth" (often a neoplasm) (Barlotta et al., 2021).

Auscultation

Auscultation always precedes percussion and palpation since manipulation of the abdomen may alter the frequency and intensity of bowel sounds. The nurse listens to determine the character, location, and frequency of bowel sounds and to identify vascular sounds. Bowel sounds are assessed in all four quadrants using the diaphragm of the stethoscope, which affords greatest auscultation of high-pitched and gurgling sounds. The frequency and character of the sounds are usually heard as clicks and gurgles that occur irregularly and range from 5 to 34 per minute; this is termed normoactive sounds. *Hypoactive* sounds are described as fewer than 5 clicks or gurgles per minute, and *hyperactive* sounds are described as more than 34 per minute (Bickley et al., 2021). Hyperperistaltic sounds or gurgling is called borborygmic. High-pitched, high-frequency bowel sounds and abdominal cramping are suggestive of a partial intestinal obstruction (Suneja et al., 2020). The nurse should auscultate for bowel sounds for a maximum of 5 minutes before noting absent bowel sounds. Interpreting bowel sounds among various clinicians is subjective; therefore, its usefulness in the clinical setting has recently been questioned (Bickley et al., 2021; Jarvis & Echardt, 2020; Small et al., 2020). Listening for vascular sounds or bruits in the aortic, renal, iliac, and femoral arteries are noted using the bell of the stethoscope. Approximately 4% to 20% of individuals have systolic bruits heard in the epigastric region which are considered a normal finding; however, continuous bruits spanning across systole and diastole or a bruit auscultated away from the midline should be investigated (Bickley et al., 2021; Small et al., 2020). Bruits are associated with turbulent blood flow in an artery. Friction rubs are high-pitched grating sounds heard over the liver or spleen during respiration. These are rare findings but are associated with inflammation of the peritoneal surface secondary to a mass, gonococcal infection or splenic infarction (Bickley et al., 2021; Small et al., 2020).

Percussion

Percussion is used to assess the size and density of the abdominal organs and to detect the presence of air-filled, fluid-filled, or solid masses. It is used to estimate the size of the liver and spleen (Small et al., 2020). All quadrants are percussed for a sense of overall tympany and dullness. Tympany is the predominant sound that results from the presence of air in the stomach and intestines; dullness is heard over organs and solid masses. A tympanic sound audible throughout a protuberant abdomen may indicate an intestinal obstruction or paralytic ileus. Dullness auscultated in both flanks suggests ascites. If ascites is suspected, the nurse can test for shifting dullness, which may help confirm the presence of ascites. This is performed through percussion with the patient in supine position. In this position, the nurse percusses the top of the abdomen and notes tympany; however, when the abdomen in percussed laterally, the sound of dullness is noted. The nurse then rolls the patient on their side and will percuss again. Shifting dullness is noted as the fluid flows to the dependent regions when the patient moves to a lateral position (Bickley et al., 2021). However, the nurse is aware that physical examination is insensitive for detecting <1,500 mL of ascites fluid (Papadakis et al., 2022).

The nurse estimates the size of the liver by percussing its upper border at the right midclavicular line (MCL) beginning at lung resonance and changing to liver dullness; then the nurse percusses the lower border by noting the change in sound from abdominal tympany to liver dullness usually at the right costal margin. The normal liver span is 6 to 12 cm (2 to 5 in) in the MCL (Small et al., 2020). It is estimated that 60% to 70% of liver percussion correlates with the true measurement of the liver. A full bladder (400 to 600 mL) elicits dullness above the suprapubic area, whereas abdominal distention increases the area of tympany (Bickley et al., 2021). Splenic dullness may be audible from the sixth to the tenth rib at the left midaxillary line (Small et al., 2020).

Palpation

If a patient complains of abdominal pain, it is important to assess the area of tenderness last. Use of light palpation is appropriate for identifying areas of tenderness or muscular resistance, and deep palpation is used to identify masses. If a mass is noted, the nurse assesses its size, shape, location, consistency, pulsatility, mobility, and tenderness (Bickley et al., 2021; Small et al., 2020).

A palpable liver has a firm, sharp ridge, and a smooth surface (Fig. 20-8). If the liver is palpable, the examiner notes and records its size, its consistency, any tenderness, and whether its outline is regular or irregular. If the liver is enlarged, the degree to which it descends below the right

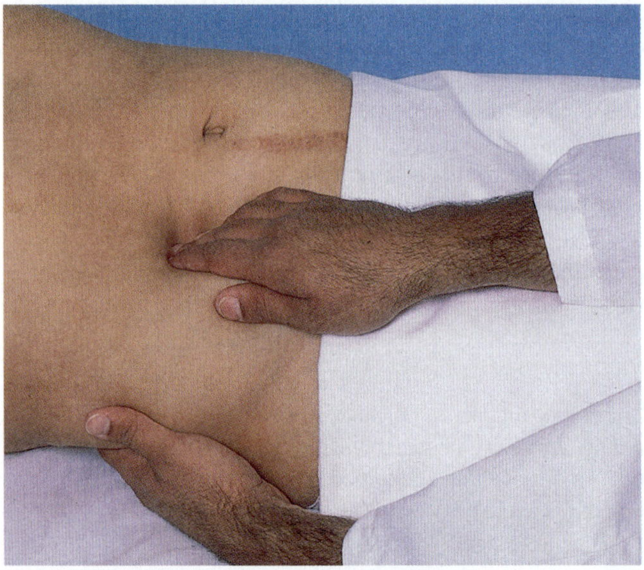

FIGURE 20-8 Technique for palpating the liver. The examiner places one hand under the right lower rib cage and presses downward with light pressure with the other hand.

costal margin is recorded to provide some indication of its size; however, it does not accurately indicate hepatomegaly (Bickley et al., 2021; Jarvis & Eckhardt, 2020; Small et al., 2020). The nurse determines whether the liver's edge is sharp and smooth or blunt or whether the enlarged liver is nodular or smooth. A cirrhotic liver may be palpated as firm but with a nontender edge; it may be fibrotic and contracted. Disorders with similar findings are hemochromatosis, amyloidosis, and lymphoma. A liver with a smooth but tender edge may indicate inflammation such as hepatitis or suggests venous congestion resulting from right sided heart failure (Bickley et al., 2021). The nurse suspects hepatocellular carcinoma when palpating a hard liver with an irregular surface; one or more nodules may be present, and the liver can be either tender or nontender (Bickley et al., 2021). The fluid wave test can be conducted if ascites is suspected. A fluid wave can be demonstrated by tapping the patient's flank sharply with one hand while the other hand receives the impulse against the opposite flank. There is a perceptible time lag between the tap and reception of the impulse. Since mesentery fat may produce a similar wave, the patient or an assistant presses the ulnar surface of their hand into the midline of the abdomen. A wave passing this hand barrier is usually caused by free fluid (Bickley et al., 2021; Jarvis & Eckhardt, 2020). This finding may be negative until ascites is visibly obvious and may be positive in patients without ascites, as for example in patients with large ovarian cysts filling the abdomen (Bickley et al., 2021; Suneja et al., 2020).

Cholecystitis, acute inflammation of the gallbladder, causes pain and tenderness making it difficult for the nurse to palpate and percuss the abdomen. The nurse should observe for Murphy sign (the patient's inability to take a deep breath or abruptly ceases breathing when the examiner's fingers are pressed below the right costal margin) (Bickley et al., 2021; Jarvis & Eckhardt, 2020; Small et al., 2020). Cholecystitis is three times as likely when the patient has a positive response to Murphy sign (Bickley et al., 2021); however it is a less reliable assessment finding in those 60 years and older (Jarvis & Eckhardt, 2020).

Pain anywhere near the right lower quadrant or the right flank region may indicate appendicitis. Testing for rebound tenderness is performed by applying steady pressure to McBurney's point which is an imaginary line approximately 1.5 to 2 in or one third of the way from the anterior iliac spine to the umbilicus (Bickley et al., 2021) and then releasing the pressure, termed *Blumberg's sign* (Small et al., 2020). If testing for rebound tenderness is undertaken, it is done at the end of the examination since the patient's pain will interfere with the remaining examination (Jarvis & Eckhardt, 2020; Small et al., 2020).

Pearls for Practice

Guarding, rigidity, and rebound tenderness (Blumberg sign) are reliable indicators of peritonitis, which is inflammation of the peritoneum. Peritonitis can be caused by bacterial invasion (i.e., ruptured appendix, perforated diverticulum), chemical irritation (i.e., perforated ulcer), abdominal trauma, and wounds.

Rectal Examination

The final part of the physical examination is evaluation of the terminal portions of the GI tract, the rectum, perianal region, and anus (Small et al., 2020). It would be prudent to have a chaperone present during these examinations (Suneja et al., 2020). The anal canal is approximately 3.8 cm in length in the adult. It has no hair or sebaceous glands and joins with the rectal mucosa at the anorectal junction. Concentric rings of muscle, the internal and external sphincters, normally keep the anal canal closed securely (Jarvis & Eckhardt, 2020). Latex free gloves, water-soluble lubrication, a penlight, fecal occult blood testing (FOBT) kit and drapes are necessary tools for the evaluation (Jarvis & Eckhardt, 2020). The nurse is aware that the rectal examination is generally uncomfortable and often embarrassing for the patient, thus offers emotional support if performed. A rectal examination should not be performed if the patient is neutropenic without specific indications (Suneja et al., 2020). For females, the rectal examination may be part of the gynecologic examination and the patient may assume the lithotomy, left lateral, or knee chest position. If examining the rectum only, the patient is asked to assume the left lateral position (Bickley et al., 2021). Male patients may be examined in the lateral decubitus position, standing with the elbows supported on the examination table or in lithotomy position. The patient's buttocks are carefully spread and visually inspected until the patient has relaxed the external sphincter control. The anal area should be examined for skin tags, fissures, hemorrhoids, or irritation (Gawlik et al., 2020). The internal examination is performed with a lubricated index finger inserted into the anal canal and rectum while the clinician assesses for tenderness, mass, strictures or spasms. The prostate and rectal wall should be examined and assessed for tenderness or nodules in the male patient, and a retroverted uterus in females may be felt (Gawlik et al., 2020; Jarvis & Eckhardt, 2020). The tone of the sphincter and the length of the anal canal should be noted. Sphincter tone is assessed by asking the patient to tighten the sphincter and the nurse should feel a gripping around the entire finger circumference. The nurse should note any blood on the examining glove and utilize the test kit for occult blood (Jarvis & Eckhardt, 2020). The patient is encouraged to focus on deep breathing during the brief examination (Jarvis & Eckhardt, 2020).

Pearls for Practice: Pathophysiology COVID-19 Effects on the Gastrointestinal System

Early in the COVID-19 pandemic, the great majority of research focused on respiratory inflammation, presentation, symptoms, and management; however, more recently it has been found that 33.7% of

COVID-19 positive patients also suffer from gastrointestinal symptoms with diarrhea being the most common symptom. In addition to diarrhea, the disease may also present with nausea, vomiting, and abdominal pain which at times appeared to precede respiratory sequela and ultimately may present as the only symptom or set of symptoms. Longevity of these symptoms appeared to last for some 1 to 14 days postacute symptom onset; however, the FAIR Health study which researched 2 million COVID-19 positive patients, found COVID-19 has long-range manifestations with 23.2% suffering from at least one post COVID-19 malady. This included both individuals with severe disease presentation as well as those who were asymptomatic, and with continued follow-up, these "long-haul" or persistent symptoms included gastrointestinal disorders. Although the pathophysiology remains unclear, many gastrointestinal-related complaints seen by various health providers may, in fact, be related to COVID-19. It is believed that the mechanism behind COVID-19 gastrointestinal-related manifestations may be caused by inflammatory reactions of goblet and intestinal epithelial cells which are protective of infection and external harm. Cytokines may play a role; however, other researchers biopsied human intestinal tissue from COVID-19 positive patients suffering from gastrointestinal symptoms and found the absence of proinflammatory GI response in the GI tract, despite COVID-19 being detected in the GI tissue samples. COVID-19 can infiltrate various other GI tissues such as the liver and biliary tree which may lead to months of GI manifestations including the loss of taste and smell impacting on patient's quality of life. It appears the relationship between COVID-19 and the GI system is both complicated and multifaceted, and further research is imperative both as it relates to acute illness and long-haul syndrome. In the meantime, vaccination remains the most rational solution to these sequential and concerning effects (Houston et al., 2021).

Diagnostic Evaluation

Initial diagnostic tests begin with serum laboratory studies, including but not limited to CBC, a complete metabolic panel, prothrombin time/partial thromboplastin time (PT/PTT), triglycerides, liver function tests, amylase, and lipase (Jameson et al., 2020; Papadakis et al., 2022) with the possibility of more specific studies, such as tumor markers which are used for early detection of cancer, to measure tumor aggression, response to therapy or to detect reoccurrence of cancer. Some tumor markers are carcinoembryonic antigen (CEA), cancer antigen (CA) 19-9, and alpha-fetoprotein, indicating sensitivity and specificity for colorectal and hepatocellular carcinomas, respectively. CEA is a protein that normally is not detected in the blood of a healthy person; therefore, when detected, it indicates that cancer is present but not what type of cancer is present. Practitioners can use CEA results to determine extent of the disease and the prognosis for patients with cancer, especially colorectal and other GI tumors and breast cancer. CA 19-9 is also a protein that exists on the surface of certain cells and is shed by tumor cells, making it useful as a tumor marker to follow the course of the cancer. CA 19-9 levels are elevated in most patients with advanced pancreatic cancer, but it also may be elevated in other conditions, such as biliary and stomach cancers (Pagana et al., 2021).

Many other modalities are available for diagnostic assessment of the GI tract. Table 20-5 identifies various procedures and their diagnostic uses.

The majority of these tests and procedures are performed on an outpatient basis in special settings designed for this purpose (e.g., endoscopy suite or GI laboratory). In the past, patients who required such tests were typically older adults; however, in recent years, partly due to heightened media exposure on the subject of early diagnosis of colorectal cancer, procedures such as colonoscopies are being performed in middle-aged adults (U.S. Prevention Services Task Force, 2021). From 1996 to 2010, colorectal mortality rates decreased 46%, and in 2020 there were an estimated 147,950 cases of colorectal cancer with 53,200 deaths. Results from a 2015 study conducted by the National Health Institute Survey found that 62% of the adults in the United States were screened for colon cancer. New cases have decreased by 3.2% every year for the past 10 years (Papadakis et al., 2022). Preparation for many of these studies such as the colonoscopy includes clear liquid diets, fasting, ingestion of a liquid bowel preparation, the use of laxatives or enemas, and ingestion or injection of a contrast agent or a radiopaque dye (Van Leeuwen & Bladh, 2019). If further assessment or treatment is needed after any outpatient procedure, the patient may be admitted to the hospital. Specific interventions for each diagnostic test are listed in Table 20-6.

General nursing interventions for the patient who is undergoing a GI diagnostic evaluation include:

- Providing needed information about the test and the activities required of the patient
- Providing instructions about postprocedure care and activity restrictions
- Providing health information and procedural teaching to patients and significant others
- Informing the physician or nurse practitioner of known medical conditions or abnormal laboratory values that may affect the procedure
- Assessing for adequate hydration before, during, and immediately after the procedure, and providing education about maintenance of hydration (Van Leeuwen & Bladh, 2019).

TABLE **20-5 Additional Laboratory Studies for Digestive, Gastrointestinal, and Metabolic Function**

Study	Clinical Functions
Abdominal x-ray	To determine gross liver size, assess for intestinal obstruction and/or fecal impaction, mechanical obstruction, intraabdominal mass, paralytic ileus; identification of free air under either diaphragm, which is associated with a perforation (usually in the GI tract).
Angiography	To visualize liver circulation and detect presence and nature of liver masses
Barium study of esophagus	To identify varices, which indicate increased portal blood pressure
Mesenteric arteriography	To visualize the mesenteric vessels. Note this has been largely replaced by multidetector computed tomographic angiography (MDCTA)
Cholecystogram and cholangiogram	To visualize gallbladder and bile duct
Cholesterol levels	Elevated in biliary obstruction; decreased in parenchymal liver disease
Computed tomography (CT) scan	To detect hepatic neoplasms; diagnose cysts, abscesses, and hematomas; and distinguish between obstructive and nonobstructive jaundice
Multidetector computed tomographic angiography (MDCTA)	Combines a CT scan with an injection of a special dye to produce pictures of blood vessels and tissues; to visualize the abdominal and mesenteric vessels
Electroencephalogram	To detect abnormalities that occur with hepatic coma
Endoscopic retrograde cholangiopancreatography (ERCP)	To visualize biliary structures and pancreas via endoscopy
Esophagoscopy/endoscopy	To search for esophageal varices and other abnormalities
Gamma-glutamyl transferase (GGT), gamma-glutamyl transpeptidase (GGTP), lactate dehydrogenase (LDH)	Markers for biliary stasis; also elevated alcoholism
Laparoscopy	To directly visualize the anterior surface of liver, gallbladder, and mesentery through a trocar
Liver biopsy (percutaneous or transjugular)	To determine anatomic changes in liver tissue
Liver scan with radio-tagged technetium	To show size and shape of liver; to show replacement of liver tissue with scars, cysts, or tumor
Magnetic resonance imaging (MRI)	To detect hepatic neoplasms; diagnose cysts, abscesses, and hematomas. Detects cerebral atrophy in encephalopathy
Serum alkaline phosphatase	In absence of bone disease, to measure biliary tract obstruction
Splenoportogram (splenic portal venography)	To determine adequacy of portal blood flow
Ultrasonography	To show size of abdominal organs and presence of masses

Stool Tests

Basic examination of the stool includes inspecting the specimen for consistency, color, and occult (not visible) blood. Additional studies, including fecal urobilinogen, fecal fat, nitrogen, *Clostridium difficile*, fecal leukocytes, parasites, pathogens, food residues, and other substances, require laboratory evaluation (Fischbach et al., 2021).

Usually stool samples are collected on a random basis unless a quantitative study (e.g., fecal fat, urobilinogen) is to be performed. Random specimens should be sent promptly to the laboratory for analysis; however, depending on the examination, the nurse should follow detailed laboratory instructions specific to each stool specimen until transported to the laboratory. Some stool collections require the patient to follow

TABLE **20-6 Gastrointestinal Laboratory Tests**

Test	Nursing Implications
Abdominal ultrasonography	• The patient is instructed to fast for 8–12 hours before the test to decrease the amount of gas in the bowel. • If barium studies are to be performed, they should be scheduled after ultrasonography; otherwise, the barium could interfere with the transmission of the sound waves. • Fasting and fluid restriction is required 8 hours prior to ultrasound of the abdomen, liver, biliary system, pancreas and spleen (Van Leeuwen & Bladh, 2019). • During the procedure, the patient is lying down. The patient may be asked to change position so that the health care provider can examine different areas. • The patient also may be asked to hold their breath for short periods of time during the examination.
Anoscopy, proctoscopy, and sigmoidoscopy	• Preparation varies according to providers. Patients may receive an enema until the returns are clear. • During the procedure, the nurse monitors vital signs, skin color and temperature, pain tolerance, and vagal response. • After the procedure, the nurse monitors the patient for rectal bleeding and signs of intestinal perforation (i.e., fever, rectal drainage, abdominal distention, and pain). On completion of the examination, the patient can resume regular activities and diet.
Breath tests	• The patient ingests a capsule of carbon-labeled urea, and a breath sample is obtained 10–20 minutes later. Because *Helicobacter pylori* metabolizes urea rapidly, the carbon is absorbed quickly; then it can be measured as carbon dioxide in the expired breath to determine whether *H. pylori* is present. • The patient is instructed to avoid antibiotics and loperamide for 1 month before the test; sucralfate and omeprazole for 1 week before the test; and cimetidine, famotidine, and ranitidine for 24 hours before the test.
Blood chemistry	• Many electrolytes are altered in GI dysfunction. Calcium is absorbed in the GI tract and may be measured to detect malabsorption. Excessive vomiting or diarrhea causes electrolyte depletion, thus requiring replacement. • Assays of serum enzymes are important in the evaluation of liver damage. AST and ALT are two enzymes found in most patients' livers and other organs. These enzymes are elevated in most liver disorders, but they are highest in conditions that cause necrosis (viral hepatitis). • Conjugated (direct) and unconjugated (indirect) bilirubin are important measurements in the diagnosis of jaundice. • Serum ammonia level is measured to evaluate liver function. • CA 19-9 and CEA are evaluated to diagnose, monitor the success of cancer therapy, and assess for the recurrence of cancer in the GI tract.
Cholangiography percutaneous transhepatic	• Assess biliary ducts for obstruction or jaundice in patient with persistent abdominal pain following cholecystectomy • Restrict fluids and fast 4–6 hours before procedure for better visualization • Contrast media injected via needle is introduced into liver capsule under fluoroscopy to visualize intra- and extrahepatic bile ducts to visualize possible obstruction caused by tumors, cysts, strictures, or stones may be followed by the placement of a drain, stent, or other interventions. • Patients are asked if they have an iodine allergy. In the past, nurses asked about shellfish allergy, however the nurse is cognizant that the reaction is caused by tropomyosin, a muscle protein, which is unrelated to the contrast used. However, in the case of an allergy to iodated contrast, the reaction is secondary to the contrast molecule. A true iodine allergy (although rare), would be problematic since iodine is necessary for thyroid hormone synthesis. • Patients are monitored post procedure for signs and symptoms of bleeding such as tachycardia, hypotension, confusion, restlessness, pallor, or shortness of breath.
CT	• CT may be performed with or without an oral or IV contrast agent, but the study is far superior with the administration of a contrast agent. • Any allergies to contrast agents, or iodine; the patient's current serum creatinine level; and urine levels of human chorionic gonadotropin must be determined before administration of a contrast agent. Patients allergic to the contrast agent may be premedicated with steroids and antihistamines before the scan. • In the case that a patient is taking metformin and iodinated contrast is to be used, metformin may be discontinued the day of the test and 48 hours afterward (Van Leeuwen & Bladh, 2019).

Test	Nursing Implications
Endoscopy through ostomy stoma	• Nursing interventions are similar to those for other endoscopic procedures.
ERCP	• Before the procedure, the patient is given an explanation of the procedure and their role in it. • The patient is NPO for several hours before the procedure. • Moderate sedation is used, and the sedated patient must be monitored closely. • The nurse observes closely for signs of respiratory and CNS depression, hypotension, oversedation, and vomiting. • During the procedure, the nurse monitors IV fluids, administers medications, and positions the patient. • After the procedure, the nurse monitors the patient's condition, observing vital signs and monitoring for signs of perforation, hemorrhage, or infection. • The nurse monitors the patient for side effects of any medications received during the procedure and for return of the gag and cough reflexes after the use of local anesthetics.
Fiberoptic colonoscopy	• Adequate colon cleansing provides optimal visualization and decreases the time needed for the procedure. The physician may prescribe a laxative for two nights before the examination and a Fleet's or saline enema until the return is clear the morning of the test. More commonly, polyethylene glycol electrolyte lavage solutions or Miralax/oral laxative solutions are used as intestinal lavages for effective cleansing of the bowel. • The patient maintains a clear liquid diet starting at noon the day before the procedure. Then the patient ingests the lavage solution orally at intervals over 3–4 hours. If necessary, the nurse can give the solution through a feeding tube if the patient cannot swallow. • Patients with a colostomy receive this same bowel preparation. • The use of lavage solutions is contraindicated in patients with intestinal obstruction, diverticulitis or recent bowel resection. • Side effects of the electrolyte solutions include nausea, bloating, cramping or abdominal fullness, and fluid and electrolyte imbalance.
Gastric analysis, gastric acid stimulation test	• The patient is asked to fast after the evening meal the night prior to the test and should not drink water 1 hour before the test begins. • Any medications that affect gastric secretions are withheld for 72 hours before the test; however this time frame varies with facility protocols. • Tobacco and chewing gum are not allowed 12 hours prior to the test because they increase gastric secretions.
Laparoscopy (peritoneoscopy)	• The patient is NPO 12 hours prior to the procedure. An empty stomach lowers the chance of vomiting during or after the procedure. • An enema may be prescribed the day before or several hours prior to the procedure to empty the colon. • The patient should ask the primary care provider if daily medicines should be taken the day of the laparoscopy. The patient may experience subcostal or shoulder discomfort following the procedure secondary to pneumoperitoneum secondary to the introduction of CO_2.
Lower GI series (barium enema)	• Preparation includes emptying and cleansing the lower bowel. This often necessitates a low-residue diet 1–2 days before the test, a clear liquid diet and a laxative the evening before, NPO after midnight, and cleansing enemas until returns are clear the following morning. • The nurse makes sure that barium enemas are scheduled before any upper GI studies. • Barium enemas are contraindicated in patients with megacolon, diverticulitis and acute ulcerative colitis. Barium enemas are contraindicated in patients with signs of perforation or obstruction; instead, a water-soluble contrast study may be performed. • Postprocedural patient education includes information about increasing fluid intake and may be given a laxative to expel barium contents. • The older adult may have reduced muscle tone, therefore making it difficult to retain the barium. • Inform the patient the stools may be white/light colored for 2–3 days following the procedure.

(*continued*)

TABLE **20-6 Gastrointestinal Laboratory Tests (*continued*)**

Test	Nursing Implications
MRI	• The patient should be NPO 6–8 hours before the study depending on the facility. • Any ferromagnetic objects (metals that contain iron) can be attracted to the magnet and cause injury. Items that can be problematic or dangerous include jewelry, pacemakers, dental implants, paperclips, pens, keys, IV poles, clips on patient gowns, and oxygen tanks. • The patient and family are informed that the study may take 60 minutes or longer; during this time, the technician will instruct the patient to take deep breaths at specific intervals. • The close-fitting scanners used in many MRI facilities may induce feelings of claustrophobia, and the machine will make a knocking sound during the procedure. Patients may choose to wear earplugs or a headset and listen to music or to wear a blindfold during the procedure. Open MRIs that are less close-fitting eliminate the claustrophobia that many patients experience. • MRI is contraindicated for patients with permanent pacemakers, artificial heart valves and defibrillators, implanted insulin pumps, or implanted transcutaneous electrical nerve stimulation devices because the magnetic field could cause malfunction of the device. • MRI is also contraindicated for patients with internal metal devices (e.g., aneurysm clips) or intraocular metallic fragments. Foil-backed skin patches (e.g., NicoDerm, nitroglycerine [Transderm-Nitro], scopolamine [Transderm-Scop]), clonidine transdermal patch should be removed before an MRI because of the risk of burns; however, the patient's physician should be consulted before the patch is removed to determine whether an alternative form of the medication should be provided.
PET	• The patient should be NPO for 4 hours on the day of the test. • The patient should refrain from alcohol, caffeine, and tobacco for 24 hours. • Diabetic patients should take their pretest dose of insulin with a meal 3–4 hours before the test. • The patient should be informed that an IV line may be inserted. • After the PET, the patient should change position slowly from lying to standing to avoid postural hypotension. • The patient should be encouraged to drink fluids and urinate frequently to aid in the removal of the radioisotope from the bladder.
pH monitoring	• The patient is NPO for 6 hours before the test. • Withholding PPIs prior to the test is dependent on the diagnosis being sought. If the patient has been unresponsive to PPI therapy and a weak or non-acid reflux diagnosis is being considered, PPI therapy should continue. If it is not clear whether or not the patient has GERD, PPI therapy is discontinued prior to the test (Butt & Kasmin, 2021).
Small-bowel enteroscopy with capsule endoscope (CE)	• The patient must be NPO approximately 8–10 hours before the test with only an occasional sip of water (Van Leeuwen & Bladh, 2019). • The patient should be instructed to discontinue medications with coating properties such as sucralfate and Pepto-Bismol 72 hours prior to the test and to refrain from tobacco products 24 hours before testing (Van Leeuwen & Bladh, 2019). • The patient wears an abdominal belt that houses a recorder to capture the transmitted images. • After the capsule is taken with a glass of water, the patient may return to normal activity for the remainder of the study. The patient can resume a normal diet 4 hours after the ingestion of the capsule. • At the end of the procedure the patient returns to the facility with the receiver for downloading to a central computer. • The procedure lasts approximately 8 hours. • The capsule endoscopy is a single-use device that is propelled through the GI tract by peristalsis and excreted naturally. The patient should be informed that the capsule will be excreted in the stool.

Test	Nursing Implications
Stool test for occult blood	• Should not be performed if there is hemorrhoidal bleeding. • Careful assessment of the patient's diet and medication regimen is essential to avoid incorrect interpretation of results. Red meats, fish, turnips, horseradish, and NSAIDs should be avoided for 72 hours prior to the study because they may cause a false-positive result. Ingestion of vitamin C from supplements or foods can cause a false-negative result. • A small amount of the specimen is applied to the guaiac-impregnated paper slide. If the test is performed at home, then the patient mails the slide to the health care provider or laboratory in an envelope provided for that purpose.
Upper GI fibroscopy/esophagogastroduodenoscopy	• The patient should be NPO for 6–8 hours prior to the examination. • A sedative that provides moderate sedation and relieves anxiety during the procedure may be administered at the initiation of the study. • Before the introduction of the endoscope, the patient is given a local anesthetic gargle or spray. • The patient is placed in the left lateral position with the neck tilted forward to facilitate clearance of pulmonary secretions and provide smooth entry of the scope. • After gastroscopy, assessment includes assessing level of consciousness, vital signs, oxygen saturation, pain level, and monitoring for signs of perforation (i.e., pain, bleeding, unusual difficulty swallowing, and rapidly elevated temperature). • After the patient's gag reflex has returned, lozenges, saline gargle, and oral analgesics may be offered to relieve minor throat discomfort. • Inform patients post procedure that they may experience belching, bloating and excess flatus secondary to insufflation.
Upper GI series (barium swallow)	• The patient is instructed to fast after midnight the day before the test. • Since the barium contrast material is swallowed, assess the patient's swallowing ability prior to the test. • The patient is asked to turn in various positions to facilitate adequate visualization of the esophagus. • Follow-up care is provided after the upper GI procedure to ensure that the patient has eliminated most of the ingested barium. Fluids may be increased to facilitate evacuation of stool and barium.
Urine tests	• Amylase can be detected in the urine. There is an increased renal clearance of amylase in patients with acute pancreatitis. Amylase levels in the urine remain high even after serum levels return to normal. Amylase may be present in the urine in nonpancreatic etiology. • Urine urobilinogen is a form of bilirubin that is converted by the intestinal flora and excreted in the urine. Its measurement is useful in the evaluation of liver and biliary obstruction. The presence of bilirubin in urine often precedes the development of jaundice.

ALT, alanine aminotransferase; AST, aspartate aminotransferase; CA 19-9, carbohydrate antigen 19-9; CEA, carcinoembryonic antigen; CT, computed tomography; ERCP, endoscopic retrograde cholangiopancreatography; GI, gastrointestinal tract; IV, intravenous; MRI, magnetic resonance imaging; NSAIDs, nonsteroidal anti-inflammatory drugs; NPO (nil per os), nothing by mouth; PET, positron emission tomography.

Adapted from Van Leeuwen, A. M., & Bladh, M. L. (2019). *Davis's comprehensive manual of laboratory and diagnostic tests with nursing implications* (8th ed.). F.A. Davis.

a specific diet or refrain from taking certain medications before the collection. Thorough and accurate patient education regarding a specific stool study prior to collection greatly increases the accuracy of study results (Fischbach et al., 2021).

Helicobacter pylori is a bacteria that can live in the mucosal lining of the stomach, which may cause peptic ulcer disease. The stool antigen test is a noninvasive, simple procedure for determining the presence of monoclonal antibodies specific to *H. pylori*, which places the patient at risk for peptic ulcer disease. It confirms the diagnosis as well as monitors if *H. pylori* has been eradicated following antibiotic treatment. This test may be performed in the laboratory or, most recently, in the office during a clinic visit. The patient may be asked to avoid proton pump inhibitors, antacids, oral bismuth subsalicylate or antibiotics prior to testing (Van Leeuwen & Bladh, 2019).

FOBT is one of the most commonly performed stool tests. It can be useful in initial screening for several disorders, although it is used most frequently in early cancer detection programs. FOBT can be performed at the bedside, in the laboratory, or at home. The nurse is aware that ingestion of red meat within 3 days before testing and ingestion of peroxidase-rich fruits and vegetables (turnips, artichokes, mushrooms, radishes, horse radishes, broccoli, bean sprouts, cauliflower, oranges, bananas, cantaloupes, and grapes) may cause false-positive results (Pagana et al., 2021). False-negative tests occur in the presence of large amounts of vitamin C and other antioxidants (Siddiqi et al., 2022). Due to the high number of false-positive and false-negative results, immunochemical fecal occult blood (iFOB) tests may be ordered. In this test, the stool is evaluated for human hemoglobin protein, which is not affected by diet, animal hemoglobin, human myoglobin, or peroxidase; thus, food restrictions are not necessary (Siddiqi et al., 2022). However, this test is only useful in screening for blood of the lower intestinal tract because in an upper GI bleed, the globin is destroyed before it reaches the rectum. According to the latest research, studies have shown that DNA testing is more sensitive than FOBT in detecting invasive cancers (Fischbach et al., 2021).

Breath Tests

The urea breath test is a noninvasive procedure used to detect *H. pylori*. After administering a carbon-labeled urea by mouth, the urea is absorbed through the gastric mucosa. In the presence of *H. pylori*, the urea is converted to CO_2 which is delivered to the lungs and exhaled. A mass spectrometer or gas chromatography measures the exhaled carbon. Currently, this test has been simplified to two breath samples collected before administration of the urea and 30 minutes after ingestion of the carbon-labeled urea (Pagana et al., 2021). This test provides reliable diagnostic information and is becoming increasingly popular because of its safety since it is a nonradioactive isotope (Pagana et al., 2021). As with the stool antigen test, antacids, proton pump inhibitors, and bismuth may interfere with obtaining accurate results.

Abdominal Ultrasonography

Ultrasonography is a noninvasive diagnostic technique used to view soft tissue structures in which high-frequency, inaudible sound waves are passed into internal body structures and the ultrasonic echoes are recorded on an oscilloscope as they strike tissues of different densities. A clear, water-based conducting gel is applied to the skin over the abdomen, which helps with the transmission of the sound waves. Then a handheld probe, called a transducer, is moved over the abdomen. Ultrasonography is particularly useful in the detection of an enlarged gallbladder or pancreas, the presence of gallstones, an enlarged ovary, an ectopic pregnancy, or appendicitis. Most recently this technique has proved useful in diagnosing acute colonic diverticulitis (Fischbach et al., 2021; Van Leeuwen & Bladh, 2019).

Ultrasonography is the diagnostic procedure of choice for gallbladder disease because it is rapid and accurate and can be used in patients with liver dysfunction and jaundice. It does not expose patients to ionizing radiation. The procedure is most accurate if the patient fasts for hours prior to the procedure so that the gallbladder is distended (Ferri, 2019). Ultrasound studies are based on analysis of reflected sound waves. Ultrasound findings include bile duct abnormalities, dilatation or obstruction, stones, acute cholecystitis, tumors, cysts, renal calculi, splenomegaly, pancreatitis, pseudocysts, cirrhosis, and ascites (Fischbach et al., 2021; Van Leeuwen & Bladh, 2019).

Cholescintigraphy (a nuclear medicine test also known as HIDA [hepatobiliary iminodiacetic acid]) or gallbladder scan helps determine if obstruction of the cystic duct is the underlying cause of cholecystitis. It is also used to differentiate obstructive versus nonobstructive jaundice, determine the cause of upper abdominal pain, and investigate biliary atresia. The patient is injected intravenously with a radionuclide and imaging begins immediately after injection. Images are taken at 5-minute intervals until the gallbladder and small intestines are visualized. A rapid flow of radionuclide through the liver cells and into the biliary tract within 15 to 30 minutes generally denotes a normally functioning gallbladder and, in most cases, rules out cholecystitis. The test is not as definitive for those patients with a bilirubin level greater than 10 mg/dL (Fischbach et al., 2021).

Endoscopic ultrasonography (EUS) is a specialized enteroscopic procedure that aids in the diagnosis of GI disorders by providing direct imaging of a target area. A small, high-frequency ultrasonic transducer is mounted at the tip of the fiberoptic scope, which displays an image that enables tumor staging and visualization of marginal structures. This procedure delivers results with higher-quality resolution and definition in comparison with regular ultrasonic imaging. EUS may be used for evaluating submucosal lesions, specifically determining their location and depth of penetration. In addition, EUS may aid in the evaluation of portal hypertension, pancreatitis, suspected pancreatic neoplasm, biliary tract disease, staging esophageal cancer, and to evaluate Barrett esophagitis (Chandrasekhara et al., 2019; Jameson et al., 2020).

Imaging Studies

Many minimally invasive and noninvasive imaging studies, including x-ray and contrast studies, computed tomography (CT), magnetic resonance imaging (MRI), positron emission tomography (PET), and virtual endoscopy, are available today to aid in the accurate assessment of the many possible causes of GI abnormalities.

Upper Gastrointestinal Tract Study

An upper GI study also called barium swallow or esophagram delineates the entire GI tract after the introduction of a contrast agent including the esophagus, stomach, duodenum, and the upper portion of the jejunum. A radiopaque liquid, the most commonly used is barium sulfate; however, diatrizoate meglumine may also be used. The nurse must ascertain the patient has no allergies to either contrast agent prior to administration. The GI series enables the examiner to gather information about the size, contour, stomach and peristaltic motility, and organ structures. This study may detect foreign bodies, hiatal hernias, pyloric stenosis, diverticulitis of the stomach, undigested food, stomach inflammation, gastric ulcers, tumors, volvulus, reflux, stomach polyps, and congenital anomalies. As the barium descends into the stomach, the position, patency, and caliber of the esophagus are visualized, enabling the examiner to detect or exclude any anatomic or functional derangement of that organ.

Fluoroscopic examination next extends to the stomach as its lumen fills with barium, allowing observation of stomach motility, thickness of the gastric wall, the mucosal pattern, patency of the pyloric valve, and the anatomy of the duodenum. Small-bowel x-rays taken while the barium is passing through that area allow for observation of the motility of the small bowel. Obstructions, ileitis, and diverticula can be detected if present (Fischbach et al., 2021; Pagana et al., 2021; Van Leeuwen & Bladh, 2019).

CT enteroclysis is an imaging study considered superior to conventional CT scanning and/or small-bowel examination. It involves a detailed, double-contrast hybrid, imaging study accomplished by infusing 1 to 2 L of an oral, neutral contrast agent via a nasojejunal tube to examine the entire small bowel. Abdominal CT imaging is also performed using an 18-gauge cannula to administer IV contrast solution. Because lesions may be obscured by a collapsed bowel, a key factor essential to bowel imaging involves luminal distention, and CT enteroclysis provides for optimal distention. This imaging study is used to detect inflammatory bowel disease, malabsorptive disorders, GI bleeding, and neoplasms. The study is an invasive procedure and increases the patient's exposure to radiation (Erturk et al., 2021).

Lower Gastrointestinal Tract Study

Visualization of the lower GI tract is obtained after rectal instillation of barium. The barium enema can be used to detect the presence of polyps, tumors, diverticulitis, colitis, obstructions, active bleeding or anatomic abnormalities contributing to a malfunctioning of the bowel. After proper preparation and evacuation of the entire colon, each portion of the colon may be readily observed. The procedure usually takes about 15 to 30 minutes, during which time x-ray images are obtained. The radiologist may encounter difficulty visualizing the lower GI tract if there has not been adequate bowel evacuation (Fischbach et al., 2021).

Other means for visualizing the colon include double-contrast studies and a water-soluble contrast study. A double-contrast, or air-contrast, barium enema involves the instillation of a thicker barium solution, followed by the instillation of air. The patient may feel some cramping or discomfort during this process. This test provides a contrast between the air-filled lumen and the barium-coated mucosa, allowing easier detection of smaller lesions (Fischbach et al., 2021).

Computed Tomography

CT provides cross-sectional images of abdominal organs and structures. Multiple x-ray images are taken from numerous angles, digitized in a computer, reconstructed, and then viewed on a computer monitor. The procedure is completely painless, but radiation doses are considerable. New continuous motion (helical or spiral), three-dimensional CT, which provides very detailed pictures of the GI organs and vasculature, has been developed (Fischbach et al., 2021).

Magnetic Resonance Imaging

MRI or magnetic resonance imaging is used in gastroenterology to supplement ultrasonography and CT. This noninvasive technique uses magnetic fields and radio waves to produce an image of the area being studied. While MRI can be performed with or without contrast, the use of oral contrast agents is used to enhance the image and has increased the application of this technique for the diagnosis of GI diseases. It is useful in evaluating the cause of abdominal pain, examining abdominal soft tissues, blood vessels, pancreatitis, gallstones, neoplasms, and sources of bleeding (Van Leeuwen & Bladh, 2019).

Positron Emission Tomography

Positron emission tomography, better known as PET scanning, integrates the use of positive emitting radionuclides to produce high-resolution body images and metabolic activity to detect abnormal cell functioning. Images generated include oxygen usage, blood and tissue perfusion, and glucose metabolism. The radioactive substances are injected into the body intravenously and usually are tagged with a radioactive atom (carbon 11, oxygen 15, or nitrogen 13 or fluorine) and images are displayed on a computer. It is useful in diagnosing, staging, and monitoring of therapy and in preoperative cancer staging in the lung, liver, colon, head and neck, breast as well as lymphomas and melanomas. PET scanning is also useful in differentiating pancreatitis masses from pancreatic cancer. The atoms decay quickly, do not harm the body and have lower radiation levels than a typical x-ray or CT scan (Fischbach et al., 2021; Van Leeuwen & Bladh, 2019). The scanner essentially "captures" where the radioactive substances are in the body, transmits information to a scanner, and produces a scan with "hot spots" for evaluation by the radiologist or oncologist (Van Leeuwen & Bladh, 2019).

Endoscopy Procedures

Endoscopy procedures are performed for a variety of reasons and are associated with a variety of psychological reactions from the patients. Many patients avoid the recommended endoscopies out of fear of the procedure or what the procedure may find. In recent years, propofol has been used increasingly during endoscopy procedures instead of sedation with the combination of an opiate and benzodiazepine.

Upper Gastrointestinal Fibroscopy/Esophagogastroduodenoscopy

Fibroscopy of the upper GI tract allows direct visualization of the esophageal, gastric, and duodenal mucosa through a lighted endoscope (Fig. 20-9). Esophagogastroduodenoscopy (EGD) is especially valuable when esophageal, gastric, or duodenal abnormalities such as bleeding, inflammatory processes, tumors, or neoplasms are suspected. This procedure can also be used to collect and evaluate secretions and tissue specimens for further analysis and to aspirate fluid,

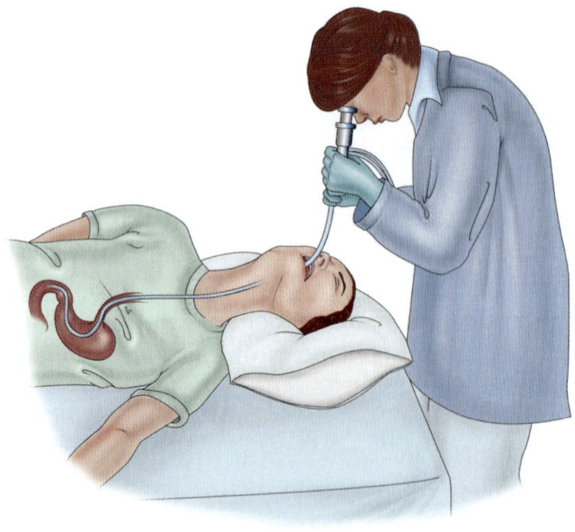

FIGURE 20-9 **Patient undergoing gastroscopy (fibroscopy of the upper GI tract).**

remove foreign bodies and/or abnormal tissue and to control bleeding. Currently, it is used more often than upper GI series (Van Leeuwen & Bladh, 2019). In EGD, the gastroenterologist views the GI tract through a viewing lens and can take still or video photographs through the scope to document findings. Electronic video endoscopes also are available that attach directly to a video processor, converting the electronic signals into pictures on a television screen. This allows larger and continuous viewing capabilities, as well as the simultaneous recording of the procedure. Therapeutic endoscopy can be used to dilate strictures, diagnose and treat hernias and to remove foreign objects. It is also used to place percutaneous gastric or duodenal feeding tubes (Pagana et al., 2021).

Side-viewing flexible scopes are used to visualize the common bile duct and the pancreatic and hepatic ducts through the ampulla of Vater in the duodenum. This procedure, called **endoscopic retrograde cholangiopancreatography (ERCP)**, uses the endoscope in combination with x-ray techniques to view the ductal structures of the biliary tract. ERCP is helpful in detecting and treating bile duct stones, bile duct strictures, pancreatic duct disruption, and sphincter of Oddi dysfunction. It should be used with caution in patients diagnosed with acute pancreatitis as it may worsen the severity of the condition (Van Leeuwen & Bladh, 2019). It is also useful in determining the cause of jaundice, persistent abdominal pain and to detect pancreatic tumors, malformations and pancreatitis, however, is contraindicated in patients with acute pancreatitis. ERCP manometry can be performed to measure pressure in the bile, pancreatic, and sphincter of Oddi ducts. Sedatives and analgesic agents (conscious sedation) are administered via IV prior to the procedure. In some instances, general anesthesia may be used. The examination of the hepatobiliary system is carried out via a side viewing flexible fiberoptic endoscope inserted through the esophagus to the descending duodenum

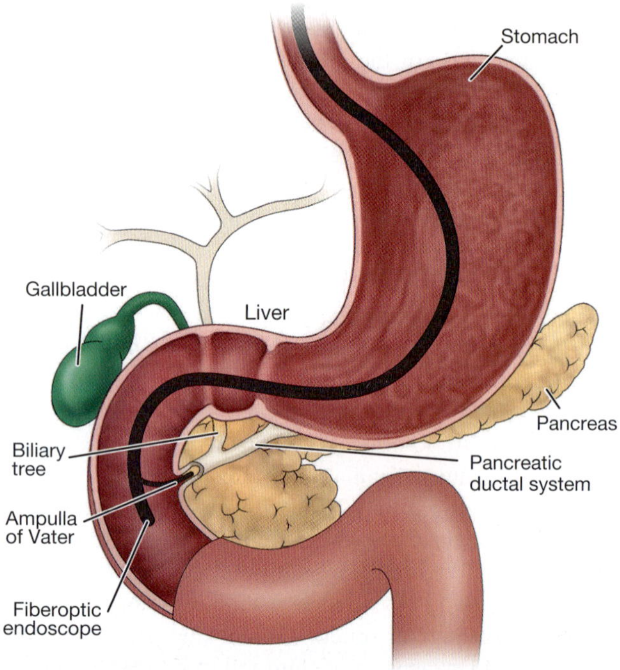

FIGURE 20-10 **Endoscopic retrograde cholangiopancreatography (ERCP). A fiberoptic duodenoscope, with side-viewing apparatus, is inserted into the duodenum. The ampulla of Vater is catheterized, and the biliary tree is injected with contrast agent. The pancreatic ductal system is also assessed, if indicated. This procedure is of special value in visualizing neoplasms of the ampulla area and extracting a biopsy specimen.**

(Fig. 20-10). To improve visualization of the ampulla of Vater, glucagon or anticholinergic agents may be administered intravenously to minimize the spasm of the duodenum (Pagana et al., 2021). The patient is initially placed in a left side-lying position with the knees flexed; however, once the endoscope is placed into the duodenum, the patient may be positioned in a prone, or semi-prone position. Biopsies specimens or cytology brushings are taken before removing the scope. The patient may experience abdominal discomfort for a few hours following the procedure. Possible complications include pancreatitis, sepsis, hemorrhage, perforation respiratory arrest, and aspiration (Fischbach et al., 2021).

Fiberoptic Colonoscopy

Direct visual inspection of the large intestine (anus, rectum, sigmoid, transcending and ascending colon) is possible by means of a flexible fiberoptic colonoscope (Fig. 20-11). These scopes have the same capabilities as those used for EGD but are larger in diameter and longer. Still and video recordings can be used to document the procedure and findings (Fischbach et al., 2021). This procedure is commonly used as a diagnostic aid and screening device. It is most frequently used for cancer screening (Box 20-1) and for surveillance in patients with previous colon cancer or polyps. In addition, tissue biopsies can be obtained as needed, and

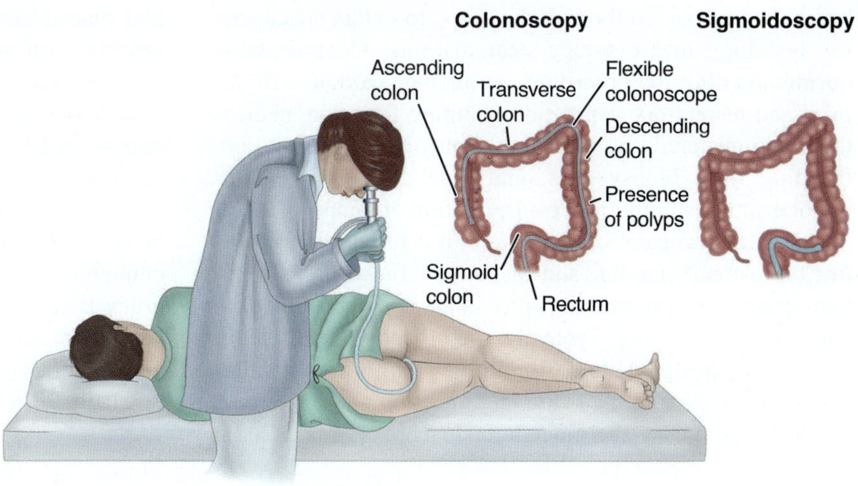

FIGURE 20-11 Colonoscopy. The flexible scope is passed through the rectum and sigmoid colon into the descending, transverse, and ascending colon.

polyps can be removed and evaluated. Other uses of colonoscopy include the evaluation of patients with change in bowel habits, occult bleeding, or anemia, to detect strictures, Hirschsprung disease, volvulus, and intussusception, and to diagnose and determine the extent of inflammatory or other bowel disease (Van Leeuwen & Bladh, 2019).

Therapeutically, the procedure can be used to remove all visible polyps with a special snare and cautery through the colonoscope. Many colon cancers begin with adenomatous polyps of the colon; therefore, one goal of colonoscopic polypectomy is early detection and prevention of colorectal cancer. This procedure also can be used to treat areas of bleeding or stricture. Bowel decompression (removal of intestinal contents to prevent gas and fluid from distending the coils of the intestine) also can be completed during the procedure. The patient should be advised to avoid or reduce the dosage of any medication or substance containing anticoagulant, thrombolytic, or antiplatelet properties as ordered by the health care provider. Interfering factors include gas and feces secondary to incomplete bowel cleansing, severe GI bleed and clotting, and colonic spasms (Van Leeuwen & Bladh, 2019).

Colonoscopy is performed while the patient is lying on the left side with the legs drawn up toward the chest. The patient's position may be changed during the test to facilitate advancement of the scope. Biopsy forceps or a cytology

BOX 20-1

Health Promotion

Guidelines for Colon and Rectal Cancer Screening

- Data from the U.S. Prevention Services Task Force (USPSTF) indicates with a high degree of certainty there is "substantial net benefit" for screening individuals ages 50–75 for colorectal cancer (American Medical Association, 2021, p. 1966) and moderate certainty that net benefits are moderate in screening for colorectal cancer in the 45–49 age group. This younger age group has recently been expanded for screening as previous guidelines recommended screening for ages 50 and over. It was also concluded with moderate certainty that while screening individuals ages 76–85 who have previously been screened yields small net benefits, but that individuals who have never undergone colorectal screening are more apt to benefit from screening. The assessment of net benefit relates to high sensitivity colonoscopy, computed tomography colonography, and flexible sigmoidoscopy. When selecting the method of colorectal cancer screening, the clinician must consider multiple factors according to the individual's risk factors which include type and frequency of screening. Recommended screening strategies are:
  - Annual high sensitivity guaiac (HSg) fecal occult blood test (FOBT) or fecal immunochemical test (FIT)
  - Stool DNA-FIT test every 1–3 years
  - CT colonography every 5 years
    - Flexible sigmoidoscopy every 5 years
  - Flexible sigmoidoscopy every 10 years + annual FIT
  - Colonoscopy every 10 years

For individuals 76–85 years of age, the clinician should consider the patient's overall health status including life expectancy, comorbid conditions, previous screening history and preferences.

All tests with positive results should be followed up with colonoscopy.

Individuals should talk to their providers about starting colorectal cancer screening earlier and/or undergoing screening more often if they have any of the following risk factors for colorectal cancer:

- A personal history of colorectal cancer or adenomatous polyps
- A family history of colorectal cancer
- A personal history of chronic inflammatory bowel disease
- A family history of a hereditary colorectal cancer syndrome such as familial adenomatous polyposis or hereditary nonpolyposis colon cancer

Data from the U.S. Prevention Services Task Force Recommendation Statement (August 24, 2021).

brush may be passed through the scope to obtain specimens for histology and cytology examinations. Complications during and after the procedure can include cardiac arrhythmias and respiratory depression resulting from the medications administered, vasovagal reactions, bowel perforation, bleeding from biopsy sites, and circulatory overload or hypotension resulting from overhydration or underhydration during bowel preparation. Therefore, it is important to monitor the patient's cardiac and respiratory function and oxygen saturation continuously, providing supplemental oxygen used as necessary. Typically, the procedure takes about 1 hour, and postprocedure discomfort results from instillation of air to expand the colon and insertion and movement of the scope during the procedure (Fischbach et al., 2021; Van Leeuwen & Bladh, 2019).

Virtual Colonoscopy

Historically, direct visualization of the bowel was the only means to evaluate the colon, but virtual colonoscopy (also known as CT colonography) has brought a more patient-friendly approach to this study. Virtual colonoscopy provides a computer-simulated endoluminal perspective of the air-filled distended colon using conventional spiral or helical CT scanning. In general, it is used to detect polyps or skin growths which may pose an increased colon cancer risk particularly if there are multiple polyps; however, it is less effective in detecting polyps less than 5 mm in size. Because it is less invasive and poses few complications, it can be used in patients unable to tolerate conventional colonoscopy secondary to heart, lung, or bleeding disorders or those patients unable to withstand sedation. No contrast medium is injected; however, if suspicious areas are visualized, the series may be repeated to include IV contrast. Polyp biopsy and removal cannot be performed using virtual colonoscopy; therefore, if polyps are visualized, the patient must be prepared to undergo conventional colonoscopy using the typical prep procedure (Van Leeuwen & Bladh, 2019).

Anoscopy, Proctoscopy, and Sigmoidoscopy

Endoscopic examination of the anus, rectum, and sigmoid and descending colon is used to evaluate chronic diarrhea, inflammation, diverticular disease, pain upon defecation, rectal itching or burning, the cause of pus, blood, or mucus in the stool, to detect volvulus in the sigmoid colon, and to observe for ulceration, fissures, abscesses, tumors, polyps, and other pathologic processes (Van Leeuwen & Bladh, 2019).

Flexible scopes have largely replaced the rigid scopes used in the past for routine examinations. The flexible fiberoptic sigmoidoscope (see Fig. 20-11) permits the colon to be examined up to 60 cm (~24 in) from the anus. It has many of the same capabilities as the scopes used for the upper GI study, including the use of still or video images to document findings (Van Leeuwen & Bladh, 2019).

For flexible scope procedures, the patient assumes a comfortable position on the left side with the right leg bent and placed anteriorly. It is important to keep the patient informed throughout the examination and to explain the sensations associated with the examination. In addition to visualizing the mucosal lining of the colon, the procedure allows for fluid removal, obtaining tissue for biopsy, polypectomies, hemorrhoidectomies, foreign-body removal, and to reduce volvulus. As with colonoscopy, the patient should be advised to avoid or reduce the dosage of any medication containing anticoagulant, thrombolytic or antiplatelet properties as ordered by the health care provider. Monitoring the patient for early signs of cardiac arrhythmias, perforation, and hemorrhage are important considerations (Van Leeuwen & Bladh, 2019).

Endoscopy for Esophageal Varices

Esophageal varices are varicosities that develop from elevated pressure in the veins that drain into the portal system. Varices are associated with cirrhosis of the liver. They are prone to rupture and often are the source of massive and sometimes fatal hemorrhage from the upper GI tract. Acute hemorrhage includes the administration of octreotide or vasopressin to decrease portal pressure. Balloon tamponade, endoscopic injection sclerotherapy, and vessel ligation are other treatments to control bleeding. Esophageal varices occur in at least 30% of patients during the course of their illness and despite improved treatment, the mortality rate is as high as 20% within 6 weeks of the bleeding event (Norris, 2019). Nursing support can be effective in relieving anxiety during this stressful experience.

Laparoscopy (Peritoneoscopy)

With the tremendous advances in minimally invasive surgery, diagnostic laparoscopy is efficient, cost-effective, and useful in the diagnosis of GI disease. After creating a pneumoperitoneum (gas, usually carbon dioxide, is insufflated into the peritoneal cavity to separate the intestines from the pelvic organs, creating a working space for visualization), a small incision, approximately 1 to 2 cm, is made through the abdomen allowing for the insertion of the fiberoptic laparoscope. This allows direct access to the organs and structures within the abdomen, permitting visualization and identification of any growths, anomalies, and inflammatory processes. In addition, biopsy samples can be taken from the structures and organs as necessary and some tumors can be resected. Depending on the severity of the infection, cholecystectomy, appendectomy as well as hernia repair, can also be performed via laparoscopy. This procedure can be used to evaluate peritoneal disease, abdominal masses, and gallbladder, splenic and liver disease. However, laparoscopy has not become an important diagnostic modality in patients with acute abdominal pain because less invasive tools (i.e., CT and MRI) are readily available. Laparoscopy usually requires general anesthesia and sometimes requires that the stomach and bowel be decompressed. Patient complaints of shoulder and abdominal pain may occur for 1 to 2 days following the procedure secondary to residual carbon dioxide effects. Postprocedure standard protocol for postoperative care is followed (see Chapter 4) (Van Leeuwen & Bladh, 2019).

Small-Bowel Enteroscopy

Capsule endoscopy or wireless endoscopy is a noninvasive enteroscopy that visualizes the entire small bowel, including the distal ileum. It is used to evaluate the source of GI bleeding, lesions, and inflammation (Chandrasekhara et al., 2019; Van Leeuwen & Bladh, 2019). Prior to the development of the capsule endoscopy, visualization of the small intestine was inadequate and providers relied primarily on barium x-rays for diagnosing disorders of the small intestine. The technique consists of the patient swallowing a capsule approximately the size of a vitamin pill that has embedded within it wireless miniature cameras that takes photographs at two frames per second as it passes through the GI tract. The digital storage device is worn by the patient around their waist for ~8 hours, after which the device is removed. The patient proceeds with their usual activities during the test. The camera takes photographs and transmits images of the esophageal and intestinal mucosa to detect inflammation or tumors. Photographs are downloaded to a computer and projected onto a monitor. The capsule endoscopy does not require sedation and is a more comfortable procedure for the patient. Randomized trials have shown that wireless capsule endoscopy has demonstrated superior results as compared to traditional push enteroscopy in that it identified lesions in the small intestine more accurately. This procedure has the ability to investigate the etiology of abdominal pain, detect ulcers, hiatal hernias, stenosis, strictures, esophageal injuries, obstructions, inflammatory bowel diseases as well as other malabsorptive disorders and to determine the location of a GI bleed (Van Leeuwen & Bladh, 2019). Colonoscopy may be used to follow up on any abnormal finding.

Another procedure used to visualize the entire mucosa of the small bowel, as well as to enable diagnostic and therapeutic interventions, is double balloon enteroscopy (DBE) used with a push and pull method. This endoscope has two balloons, one attached to the distal end of the scope and the other attached to the transparent overtube that slides over the endoscope. The endoscope is advanced using a push-and-pull technique that involves inflating and deflating the balloons alternatively. This process causes the telescoping of the small intestine onto the overtube, which enables the endoscope to visualize much more of the small intestine than the length of the scope itself. DBE is indicated in patients with inflammatory bowel disease, obstruction, neoplastic diseases, hemorrhagic disorders, bile/pancreatic diseases, and for the removal of foreign bodies (Chandrasekhara et al., 2019; Otani et al., 2018).

Endoscopy through Ostomy

Endoscopy using a flexible endoscope through an ostomy stoma is useful for visualizing a segment of the small or large intestine and may be indicated to evaluate the anastomosis for recurrent disease or to visualize and treat bleeding in a segment of the bowel (Devolder, 2019).

Gastric Analysis, Gastric Acid Stimulation Test, and pH Monitoring

Analysis of the gastric juice yields information about the secretory activity of the gastric mucosa and the presence or degree of gastric retention in patients thought to have pyloric or duodenal obstruction. It evaluates the gastric fluid for pH, color, presence of mucus, blood, abnormal cells, and microorganisms. It is also useful for diagnosing cancers, duodenal and peptic ulcers, pernicious anemia, **Zollinger–Ellison syndrome**, or atrophic gastritis (Van Leeuwen & Bladh, 2019).

The patient is positioned either sitting or reclining on the left side and a small nasogastric tube with a catheter tip marked at various points is inserted through the nose. Radiopaque dye is infused into the gastric tube and an x-ray is performed prior to beginning the study to confirm accurate placement. The entire stomach contents are aspirated by gentle suction into a syringe (Van Leeuwen & Bladh, 2019).

The gastric acid stimulation test usually is performed in conjunction with gastric analysis. Histamine or pentagastrin is administered subcutaneously to stimulate gastric secretions. It is important to inform the patient that this injection may produce a flushed feeling. The nurse monitors the patient's blood pressure and pulse frequently to detect hypotension. Gastric specimens are collected after the injection every 15 minutes for 1 hour and are labeled to indicate the time of specimen collection after histamine injection. The volume and pH of the specimen are measured (Van Leeuwen & Bladh, 2019).

One method of diagnosing reflux disease is through ambulatory pH monitoring, considered a valuable method for diagnosing gastroesophageal disease. This may be accomplished by attaching a transmitter sensitive to pH measurement to the esophagus or by inserting a catheter containing a probe through the nose and ending in the distal part of the esophagus to measure pH. These measurements are taken while the patient is ambulatory and are measured over 24 to 48 hours. A data logger is attached to the catheter and pH levels are recorded for a 24-hour time frame while the patient documents symptoms, bodily position (sitting or recumbent), and meals.

A more accurate method of evaluating pH is the Bravo method in which a wireless pH probe capsule (the size of a gel cap), temporarily attached to esophageal tissue measures pH data for 48 hours. It offers the advantage of pH monitoring of the esophagus without the transnasal catheter. The Bravo pH capsule transmits readings of the esophageal pH via radio telemetry to the pager-sized receiver worn on the patient's belt or waistband. The patient is able to eat and drink as per usual during the 24- to-48-hour monitoring time frame. The patient is instructed to push a button at the onset of symptoms, which then are associated with the presence or absence of acid reflux. Data are collected for up to 48 hours and then downloaded and analyzed. Within a few days after insertion, the capsule is shed from the esophagus and is eliminated through the patient's GI tract (Pagana et al., 2021). Monitoring of pH data should be implemented prior to surgical intervention as well as in cases in which patients are unresponsive to PPI therapy (Sitaraman & Friedman, 2018).

A Bernstein test may be performed to evaluate esophageal functioning by introducing an HCl solution into the esophagus to reproduce heartburn. It is used to detect/evaluate gastroesophageal reflux disease or esophagitis and is generally performed in conjunction with other tests measuring esophageal functioning. A catheter is introduced into the nose and into the esophagus where HCl is instilled through a small feeding tube positioned in the esophagus to try to elicit the reported chest pain or feelings of heartburn. The patient may experience a sore throat or hoarseness following the test and the nurse must be aware that aspirational pneumonia may occur as a complication (Pagana et al., 2021; Van Leeuwen & Bladh, 2019).

Esophageal Manometry

Esophageal manometry is a group of studies used to detect esophageal muscle functioning and structure. They are used to measure esophageal pressure, the presence of gastric acid in the esophagus, lower esophageal functioning and esophageal motility. A catheter is placed through the nose and into the esophagus and stomach. A small transducer is attached to the end of the tube so that lower esophageal pressure and peristaltic contractions can be measured while the patient swallows water or gelatin. It is used to detect motility abnormalities, such as achalasia (failure of the smooth muscle in the lower esophagus to relax which prevents food from passing into the stomach), esophageal spasms, esophagitis, difficulty swallowing, vomiting, regurgitation, or scleroderma (Van Leeuwen & Bladh, 2019).

Liver Function Tests

Early recognition and assessment of liver dysfunction is critical to provide timely and appropriate care for the patient with acute or chronic liver disease. More than 70% of the parenchyma of the liver may be damaged before liver function test results become abnormal. Liver function tests include alanine aminotransferase (ALT), aspartate aminotransferase (AST), albumin, alkaline phosphatase (ALP), direct and total bilirubin and total protein level. However, the nature and extent of liver dysfunction cannot be determined by these tests alone because other disorders can affect test results (Van Leeuwen & Bladh, 2019).

Serum aminotransferases (also called transaminases) are enzymes that reflect varying degrees of hepatocellular injury or inflammation of the liver and are useful in detecting acute liver disease, such as hepatitis. ALT, AST, and gamma-glutamyl transferase (GGT; also called G-glutamyl transpeptidase) are the most frequently used tests for liver damage. ALT levels increase primarily in liver disorders and may be used to monitor the course of hepatitis or cirrhosis or the effects of treatments that may be toxic to the liver (Norris, 2019; Van Leeuwen & Bladh, 2019). AST is present in tissues that have high metabolic activity; therefore, the level may be increased if there is damage to or death of tissues of organs such as the heart, liver, skeletal muscle, and kidney. Although not specific to liver disease, levels of AST may be increased in cirrhosis, hepatitis, and liver cancer. Abnormal aminotransferases may occur in the absence of any clinical indication of liver disease, and this finding requires further investigation to determine if it is incidental or if hepatic injury is present. In the majority of patients with liver disease, ALT levels are higher than AST with the exception of alcoholic hepatitis where the mitochondrial damage results in an increased release of mitochondrial AST in the bloodstream, as well as in cases of cirrhosis and hepatocellular carcinoma (Norris, 2019).

Increased GGT levels measure hepatic excretory function and are associated with cholestasis but also can be due to alcoholic liver disease. GGT is also present in the renal tubules, pancreas, prostate, brain, and heart. Elevations in ALP, also a measurement of hepatic excretory function, may indicate injury to the biliary tree (i.e., biliary obstruction), presence of tumors, primary biliary cirrhosis, and primary sclerosing cholangitis (Van Leeuwen & Bladh, 2019). Elevations of both ALP and GGT indicate disease of the liver or biliary system. Elevation of ALP with normal GGT levels should initiate evaluation for possible bone disease, as this enzyme is also present in bone tissue (Pagana et al., 2021).

Other important tests to determine the extent of liver dysfunction are serum bilirubin, a byproduct of heme metabolism and mostly produced in the liver and spleen, serum albumin which is synthesized in the liver, and prothrombin time, a protein made by the liver and reliant on vitamin K for production which is measured by the international normalized ratio (INR) (Van Leeuwen & Bladh, 2019). Common liver function tests are summarized in Table 20-7.

Liver Biopsy

Liver biopsy is considered a valuable and safe method in the diagnosis of liver disease. It is an essential diagnostic procedure in patients presenting with cirrhosis who do not have a history of alcohol ingestion, termed non-alcoholic fatty liver disease (NAFLD), the most frequently occurring type of chronic liver disease in the United States (Norris, 2019). It is useful in determining the unexplained cause of hepatomegaly, jaundice, suspected hepatitis, the diagnosis of primary or secondary liver tumors, and the persistent elevation of liver function tests (Pagana et al., 2021; Van Leeuwen & Bladh, 2019). A small sample of liver tissue is obtained, usually through needle aspiration, for microscopic evaluation of liver cells and architecture. The most common indication is to evaluate diffuse disorders of the parenchyma and to diagnose space-occupying lesions. Liver biopsy is especially useful

TABLE **20-7 Common Laboratory Tests to Assess Liver Function**

Test	Normal	Clinical Functions
Pigment Studies		
Serum bilirubin, direct	0–0.3 mg/dL (0–5.1 μmol/L)	These studies measure the ability of the liver to conjugate and excrete bilirubin. Results are abnormal in liver and biliary tract diseases and are associated with jaundice clinically (Van Leeuwen & Bladh, 2019).
Serum bilirubin, total	0–0.9 mg/dL (1.7–20.5 μmol/L)	
Urine bilirubin	0 (0)	
Urine urobilinogen	0.05–2.5 mg/24 hr (0.09–4. Ehrlich U/24 hr)	
Fecal urobilinogen (infrequently used)	50–300 mg/24 hr (100–400. Ehrlich U/100 g)	
Protein Studies		
Total serum protein	7.0–7.5 g/dL (70–75 g/L)	Proteins are components of muscles, enzymes, hormones, hemoglobin and serve as transport vehicles. They are foundational to the functioning of the body and the liver is a key organ in manufacturing plasma protein. Proteins play a significant role in maintaining osmotic pressure within the vascular space.
Serum albumin	4.0–5.5 g/dL (40–55 g/L)	Albumin is a protein made in the liver, thus is an important measurement of liver function. Their levels may be affected in a variety of liver impairments: albumin is affected in cirrhosis, chronic hepatitis; globulins are affected in cirrhosis, liver disease, chronic obstructive jaundice, and viral hepatitis.
Serum globulin	1.7–3.3 g/dL (17–33 g/L)	A/G ratio is reversed in chronic liver disease (decreased albumin and increased globulin).
Serum protein electrophoresis		
Albumin	4.0–5.5 g/dL (40–55 g/L)	
Alpha$_1$-globulin	0.15–0.25 g/dL (1.5–2.5 g/L)	
Alpha$_2$-globulin	0.43–0.75 g/dL (4.3–7.5 g/L)	
Beta-globulin	0.5–1.0 g/dL (5–10 g/L)	
Gamma-globulin	0.6–1.3 g/dL (6–13 g/L)	
Albumin/globulin (A/G) ratio	A > G or 1.5:1–2.5:1	
Prothrombin time	100% or 12–16 seconds	Prothrombin time may be prolonged in liver disease. It will not return to normal with vitamin K in severe liver cell damage.
Serum alkaline phosphatase	Varies with method: 2–5 Bodansky units 30–50 U/L at 34°C (17–142 U/L at 30°C) (20–90 U/L at 30°C)	Serum alkaline phosphatase is manufactured in bones, liver, kidneys, and intestine and excreted through biliary tract. In the absence of bone disease, it is a sensitive measure of biliary tract obstruction.
Serum aminotransferase studies		The studies are based on release of enzymes from damaged liver cells. These enzymes are elevated in liver cell damage.
AST	10–40 units (4.8–19 U/L)	
ALT	5–35 units (2.4–17 U/L)	
GGT, GGTP	10–48 IU/L	Elevated with alcohol use disorder. Marker for biliary cholestasis.
LDH	Adults: 140–280 U/L or 2.34–4.68 μkat/L	
Ammonia (plasma)	15–45 μg/dL (11–32 μmol/L)	Liver converts ammonia to urea. Ammonia level rises in liver failure.
Cholesterol		
HDL (high-density lipoprotein)	HDL Male: 35–70 mg/dL, Female: 35–85 mg/dL	Cholesterol levels are elevated in biliary obstruction and decreased in parenchymal liver disease.
LDL (low-density lipoprotein)	LDL <130 μg/dL	

when clinical findings and laboratory tests are not diagnostic. Bleeding and bile peritonitis after liver biopsy are the major complications; therefore, coagulation studies are obtained, their values are noted, and abnormal results are treated before liver biopsy is performed. A liver biopsy can be performed percutaneously with guided CT, MRI, ultrasound, or laparoscopy in the event of diffuse liver disease. "Direct" biopsy is a procedure targeting a focal area of the liver such as a suspected tumor (Pagana et al., 2021). Guidelines for assisting with a liver biopsy are found in Box 20-2.

BOX 20-2

GUIDELINES FOR NURSING CARE

Assisting With Percutaneous Liver Biopsy

Equipment

- Liver biopsy tray (contains needles, scalpel, specimen tubes, etc.)
- Sterile gloves
- Antiseptic solution
- Local anesthetic
- Sterile dressing
- Sphygmomanometer to monitor BP

Implementation

NURSING ACTION	RATIONALE
Preprocedure	
1. Ascertain that results of coagulation tests (prothrombin time, partial thromboplastin time, and platelet count) are available and that compatible donor blood is available.	1. Many patients with liver disease have clotting defects and are at risk for bleeding.
2. Check for signed consent; confirm that informed consent has been provided.	2. Ensure that the patient consents to this invasive procedure.
3. Measure and record the patient's pulse, respirations, and blood pressure immediately before biopsy.	3. Prebiopsy values provide a basis on which to compare the patient's vital signs and evaluate status after the procedure.
4. Describe to the patient in advance: steps of the procedure, sensations expected, after-effects anticipated, restrictions of activity, and monitoring procedures to follow.	4. Explanations allay fears and ensure cooperation.
During Procedure	
1. Support the patient during the procedure.	1. Encouragement and support of the nurse enhance comfort and promote a sense of security.
2. Expose the right side of the patient's upper abdomen (right hypochondriac).	2. The skin at the site of penetration will be cleansed and a local anesthetic will be infiltrated.
3. Instruct the patient to inhale and exhale deeply several times, finally to exhale, and to hold breath at the end of expiration. The provider promptly introduces the biopsy needle by way of the transthoracic (intercostal) or transabdominal (subcostal) route, penetrates the liver, aspirates, and withdraws.	3. Holding the breath immobilizes the chest wall and the diaphragm; penetration of the diaphragm thereby is avoided, and the risk of lacerating the liver is minimized.
4. Instruct the patient to resume breathing.	4. The patient often continues holding their breath because of anxiety.

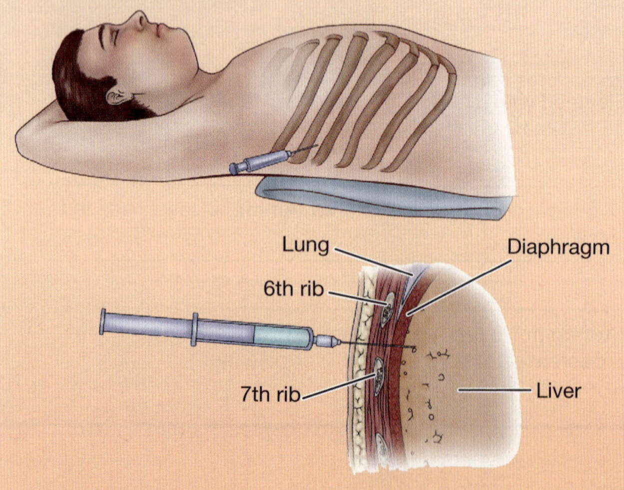

NURSING ACTION	RATIONALE
Postprocedure	
1. Immediately after the biopsy, some providers may suggest the patient turn onto the right side with a small pillow under the costal margin (provides extra pressure), and caution the patient to remain in this position, recumbent and immobile, for 2 hours. Instruct the patient to avoid coughing or straining.	1. In this position, the liver capsule at the site of penetration is compressed against the chest wall, and the escape of blood or bile through the perforation is prevented.

NURSING ACTION	RATIONALE
2. Measure and record the patient's pulse, respiratory rate, and blood pressure at 10- to 15-minute intervals for the first hour, then every 30 minutes for the next 1–2 hours or until the patient's condition stabilizes.	2. Changes in vital signs may indicate bleeding, severe hemorrhage, or bile peritonitis, rare but serious complications of liver biopsy.
3. If the patient is discharged after the procedure, instruct the patient to avoid heavy lifting (not > 10 lb) (4.5 kg), and strenuous activity for 1–2 weeks.	3. Activity restriction reduces the risk of bleeding at the biopsy puncture site.

Paracentesis

Although the development of ascites is not well understood, it is thought that portal hypertension is causative. Ascites is generally treated by dietary restriction of sodium and water as well as by initiating diuretic therapy, however, another means for the removal of large amounts of fluid (ascites) from the peritoneal cavity is paracentesis which involves a puncture or a small surgical incision through the abdominal wall under sterile conditions (Rodrigues et al., 2021). Paracentesis may be used for therapeutic reasons (removal of more than 5 L of fluid) to decrease intra-abdominal pressure resulting in dyspnea, abdominal pain, and abdominal fullness (Norris, 2019) or for therapeutic or diagnostic purposes (Norris, 2019; Pagana et al., 2021). Paracentesis can be performed at the bedside using anatomical markings and physical examination techniques to guide needle insertion; however more recently, point-of-care ultrasound technology has been implemented at the bedside to improve safety (Rodrigues et al., 2021). Paracentesis is contraindicated in patients with coagulopathy abnormalities, for those at high risk for bleeding or those who have had extensive, past abdominal surgeries. The ascitic fluid is evaluated for RBCs, white blood cells, protein, glucose, amylase, ammonia, ALP, lactic dehydrogenase, CEA) levels, cytology, bacteria, and fungi (Pagana et al., 2021). Volume expanders such as albumin may be administered concurrently to maintain sufficient circulatory volume caused by the removal of fluid resulting in decreased vascular volume and increased plasma renin production (Norris, 2019). Therapeutic paracentesis provides only temporary removal of fluid; ascites rapidly recur, necessitating repeated fluid removal (Pagana et al., 2021). Guidelines for assisting with paracentesis are found in Box 20-3.

BOX 20-3

GUIDELINES FOR NURSING CARE

Assisting With a Paracentesis

Equipment

- Paracentesis tray (contains trocar, syringe, needles, drainage tube)
- Sterile gloves
- Antiseptic solution
- Local anesthetic
- Sterile dressing
- Drainage collection bottles, receptacles
- Sphygmomanometer to monitor BP

Implementation

NURSING ACTION	RATIONALE
Preprocedure	
1. Check for signed consent form.	1. Ensure that patient has agreed to procedure.
2. Prepare the patient by providing the necessary information and instructions and by offering reassurance.	2. Having information increases the patient's understanding of the procedure and the reason for it.
3. Instruct the patient to void.	3. An empty bladder minimizes the risk of inadvertent puncture of the bladder and minimizes discomfort from a full bladder.
4. Gather appropriate sterile equipment and collection receptacles.	4. Sterility of equipment is essential to minimize risk of infection; having equipment available enables the procedure to be performed smoothly.
5. Place the patient in an upright position on the edge of the bed or in a chair with feet supported on a stool. Fowler position should be used by the patient confined to bed.	5. An upright position results in movement of the peritoneal fluid close to the abdominal wall and promotes easier puncture and removal of fluid.
6. Place the sphygmomanometer cuff around the patient's arm.	6. This allows the nurse to monitor the patient's blood pressure during procedure.
During Procedure	
1. The provider, using aseptic technique, inserts the trocar through a puncture below the umbilicus. The trocar, or needle, is connected to a drainage tube, the end of which is inserted into a collecting receptacle. (see the figure next page)	1. Sterile technique minimizes the risk of infection. Bleeding at the puncture site is minimal at this location. The fluid drains by gravity or mild siphon into the container.

(*continued on page 714*)

BOX 20-3

GUIDELINES FOR NURSING CARE (*continued*)

Assisting With a Paracentesis (*continued*)

NURSING ACTION	RATIONALE
2. Help the patient maintain position throughout the procedure.	2. The patient who is fatigued or weak may have difficulty maintaining an optimal position for drainage of fluid.

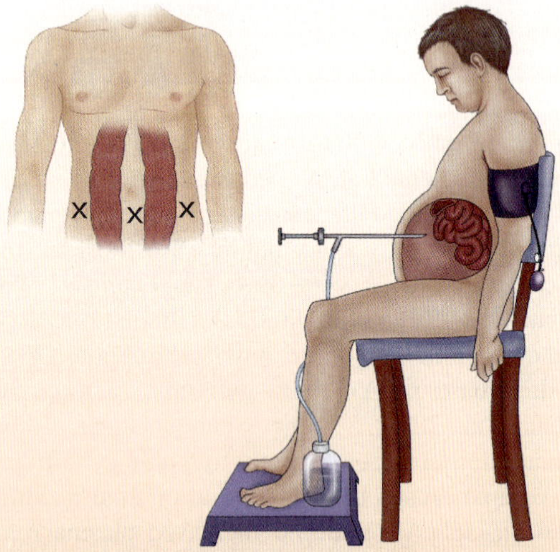

Figure on left shows possible sites for insertion of trocar.

NURSING ACTION	RATIONALE
3. Measure and record blood pressure at frequent intervals throughout the procedure.	3. Decreased blood pressure may occur with vascular collapse, which can result from removal of the fluid from the peritoneal cavity and fluid shifts.
4. Monitor the patient closely for signs of vascular collapse: pallor, increased pulse rate, or decreased blood pressure.	4. Vascular collapse (hypovolemia) may occur as fluid moves from the vascular system to replace fluid drained from peritoneal cavity.
Postprocedure	
1. Return the patient to bed or to a comfortable sitting position.	1. The weak or fatigued patient may have difficulty resuming a comfortable position without assistance.
2. Measure, describe, and record the fluid collected.	2. The volume of fluid removed may range from small to very large, and its removal may affect fluid and vascular status; volume should be included in input and output records. The characteristics of the fluid (clear vs. cloudy, red vs. colorless) may be helpful in diagnostic evaluation.
3. Label samples of fluid and send to laboratory.	3. Peritoneal fluid is analyzed as part of the diagnostic workup.
4. Monitor vital signs every 15 minutes for 1 hour, every 30 minutes for 2 hours, every hour for 2 hours, and then every 4 hours.	4. Vital signs (blood pressure, pulse rate) may change as fluid shifts occur after removal of fluid, especially if a large volume of fluid was removed.
5. Measure the patient's temperature.	5. An elevated temperature is a sign of infection and should be reported to the patient's provider.
6. Assess for hypovolemia, electrolyte shifts, changes in mental status, and encephalopathy.	6. Changes in fluid and electrolyte status and mental and cognitive status may occur with removal of fluid and fluid shifts and should be reported.
7. When taking vital signs, check puncture site for leakage or bleeding.	7. Leakage of fluid may occur because of changes in abdominal pressure and may contribute to further loss of fluid if undetected. Leakage suggests a possible site for infection, and bleeding may occur in patients with altered clotting secondary to liver disease.
8. Provide patient teaching regarding the need to monitor for bleeding or excessive drainage from the puncture site, the importance of avoiding heavy lifting or straining, the need to change position slowly, and frequency of monitoring for fever.	8. The patient (or family members) needs to monitor the patient overall and especially the puncture site for bleeding and excessive drainage if the patient is discharged home after the procedure. Heavy lifting or straining is avoided to enable the puncture site to close. Slow changes in position are recommended because of the risk of hypovolemia related to fluid removal. Monitoring for fever is needed to detect infection.

Transjugular Intrahepatic Portosystemic Shunt

One of the most valuable improvements in treating patients with refractory ascites who are diuretic resistant or to prevent reoccurrence of hemorrhage is by placement of a transjugular intrahepatic portosystemic shunt (TIPS) (Norris, 2019; Vizzutti et al., 2020). It is also used in those patients with persistent bleeding or rebleeding episodes when diuretic therapy and endoscopic procedures have been ineffective (Vizzutti et al., 2020). This shunt is surgically inserted under radiologic guidance through the internal jugular vein, creating a shunt or opening between the portal and hepatic veins in order to decrease portal pressure. IV albumin is administered to decrease the possibility of "post paracentesis circulatory dysfunction" and death. The nurse should monitor the patient for hepatic encephalopathy, a complication associated with the TIPS (Jameson et al., 2020; Norris, 2019). This complication is likely caused by the inability of ammonia and other toxic substances in the gut to pass through the liver (Norris, 2019).

CHAPTER REVIEW

NCLEX-Style Review Questions

1. Which of the following symptoms would be suspicious of appendicitis? Select all that apply.
   a. Right lower quadrant pain
   b. Periumbilical pain
   c. Anorexia
   d. Nausea
   e. Hypothermia
   f. Projectile vomiting

2. Which of the following foods could give a false-positive result on the fecal occult blood test (FOBT)? Select all that apply.
   a. Red meats
   b. Pasta
   c. Turnips
   d. Fish
   e. Whole-grain bread

3. Which question will best assist the nurse in the assessment of a patient with acute diarrhea? Select all that apply.
   a. "Have you had a colonoscopy in the last 3 months?"
   b. "Have you traveled outside the country recently?"
   c. "Do you have any trouble swallowing?"
   d. "Do you have hypertension?"
   e. "Have you recently been treated with antibiotics?"
   f. "Do you have hyperthyroidism?"

4. Your patient is scheduled for a liver biopsy. Which of the following laboratory tests would the nurse report to the provider urgently? Select all that apply.
   a. A prothrombin time (PT) of 30 seconds
   b. An activated partial thromboplastin time (aPTT) of 24 seconds
   c. An Hbg of 14 g/100 mL
   d. A platelet count of 49, 000 mm^3
   e. An Hct of 43%
   f. An INR of 2.5

5. When performing an abdominal assessment on a patient with suspected cholecystitis, how does the nurse palpate the patient's abdomen and what findings may be expected? Select all that apply.
   a. Palpate the right lower quadrant only
   b. Palpate the upper quadrants only
   c. Defer palpation and use percussion only
   d. Palpate the right upper quadrant last
   e. Positive rebound tenderness at McBurney's point
   f. Positive Murphy's sign

REFERENCES AND SELECTED READINGS

References and selected readings associated with this chapter can be found on the website that accompanies the book. Visit **http://thepoint.lww.com/Honan3e** to access the references and other additional resources associated with this chapter.

CHAPTER 21

Nursing Management: Patients With Oral and Esophageal Disorders and Patients Receiving Gastrointestinal Intubation, Enteral, and Parenteral Nutrition

Zachary R. Krom

Learning Objectives

After reading this chapter, you will be able to:

1. Describe nursing management of patients with conditions of the oral cavity.
2. Use the nursing process as a framework for care of patients undergoing neck dissection.
3. Describe the various conditions of the esophagus and their clinical manifestations and management.
4. Describe the purposes and types of gastrointestinal intubation.
5. Discuss nursing management of the patient who has a nasogastric or nasoenteric tube.
6. Identify the purposes and uses of parenteral nutrition.

Digestion begins in the mouth. Adequate nutrition is closely related to good dental health and the general condition of the mouth. Any discomfort or adverse condition in the oral cavity can affect a person's nutritional status, influencing the type and amount of food ingested and which food particles are exposed to salivary enzymes. Given the close relationship between adequate dietary intake and the upper gastrointestinal (GI) tract (lips, mouth, teeth, pharynx, esophagus), nursing assessment and health teaching related to food and fluid intake, general nutritional health, speech, and self-image is warranted. In some patients, specific pathologies impede the function of the GI system, and artificial devices must be placed to support nutritional intake. The nurse needs to be familiar with how to place these devices, manage them, and complications that can occur. These devices are associated with patients receiving supplemental enteral (involving or passing through the intestine, e.g., tube feeding) or parenteral (not involving the GI tract, typically intravenous, e.g., peripheral parenteral nutrition [PPN]) nutrition.

ORAL DISORDERS

Oral Care

The nurse understands that oral health is an essential component of a person's physical and psychological well-being; common oral problems include dental plaque and caries. Healthy teeth must be cleaned conscientiously and effectively daily. Brushing and flossing are particularly effective in mechanically breaking up the bacterial plaque that collects around teeth. The level of mouth care performed on or by patients depends upon patient condition and tolerance of the procedure. The ideal situation is when patients can brush and floss their teeth as they usually would at home. The American Dental Society recommends brushing twice a day and flossing once a day (2021). The primary focus of mouth care is to lessen the amount of bacterial film that accumulates on teeth, around gums, and in saliva (Box 21-1). Normal mastication (chewing) and the normal saliva flow also greatly aid in keeping the teeth clean. Because many ill patients do not eat adequate amounts of food, they produce less saliva, which, in turn, reduces this natural tooth-cleaning process. The nurse may need to assume the responsibility for brushing the patient's teeth. A soft-bristled toothbrush is more effective than a sponge or foam stick. If brushing is not possible, the nurse should wipe the teeth with a gauze pad and then have the patient swish an antiseptic mouthwash several times before expectorating into an emesis basin. To prevent drying, the nurse can coat the patient's lips with a water-based gel.

Not only is the bacterial film detrimental to the tooth surface and gums, but it also can potentially create problems in the respiratory system. This film can translocate to the lungs and cause an infection. A recent study found oropharyngeal colonization was significantly decreased in ventilated patients who received an oral solution of 0.12% chlorhexidine (Kes et al., 2021). Toothbrushing twice a day, oral moistening and suctioning every 2 to 4 hours is recommended for ventilated and nonventilated patients to reduce the incidence of pneumonia (Collins et al., 2020). For more information on VAP, refer to Chapter 9.

BOX 21-1
Health Promotion

Preventive Oral Hygiene

Instruct patients to:

- Brush teeth using a soft toothbrush at least twice daily. Hold toothbrush at a 45-degree angle against the gums and teeth. A small brush is better than a large brush. In addition to the teeth, the gums and tongue surface should be brushed.
- Floss at least once daily.
- Use an antiplaque mouth rinse.
- Visit a dentist at least every 6 months or when you have a chipped tooth, a lost filling, an oral sore that persists longer than 2 weeks, or a toothache.
- Avoid alcohol and tobacco products, including smokeless tobacco.
- Maintain adequate nutrition and avoid sweets.
- Replace your toothbrush at the first sign of wear, usually every 2 months.

Temporomandibular Joint Disorders

Temporomandibular joint (TMJ) disorders can originate within the joint capsule or involve the muscle tissue surrounding and supporting the joint. Osteoarthritis, rheumatoid arthritis, and disruption of the joint structures, such as dislocation or disc displacement, occur within the joint.

Clinical Manifestations and Assessment

Pain with mastication and pain in the joint are the two most common manifestations of TMJ disorder. Patients have pain ranging from a dull ache to throbbing, debilitating pain radiating to the ears, teeth, neck muscles, and facial sinuses. They often have restricted jaw motion and locking of the jaw. There also may be a sudden change in the way the upper and lower teeth fit together. The patient may hear clicking and grating noises, and chewing and swallowing may be difficult (National Institute of Dental and Craniofacial Research, 2018).

Diagnosis is based on the patient's report of pain, limitations in range of motion (ROM), dysphagia, difficulty chewing, speaking, or hearing. Magnetic resonance imaging (MRI), x-ray studies, and an arthrogram may be performed.

Medical Management

Conservative and reversible treatment is recommended. If irreversible surgical options are recommended, the patient is encouraged to seek a second opinion.

Nonsurgical Management

Although some practitioners think the role of stress in TMJ disorders is overrated, it is seen as an exacerbating factor rather than the primary cause of temporomandibular disorders, patient education in stress management may be helpful (to reduce grinding and clenching of teeth) (Dimitroulis, 2018). Occlusal guards can be used in conjunction with stress management to prevent further deterioration of the tooth surface and irritation of the joint. The patient may also benefit from ROM exercises without overextension of the joint. Pain management measures can include nonsteroidal anti-inflammatory drugs (NSAIDs) with the possible addition of opioids, muscle relaxants, or mild antidepressants. Occasionally, intraoral orthotics (a plastic guard worn over the upper and lower teeth) may be worn to reposition the condyle head in the joint space to a more normal position, which, in turn, relieves the stress and pressure of the joint on the tissues. This approach allows the tissues to heal.

Surgical Management

Correction of mandibular structural abnormalities may require surgery involving repositioning or reconstruction of the jaw. Simple fractures of the mandible without displacement, jaw repositioning (orthognathic) surgical correction to remedy cosmetic and functional jaw problems, may require surgery. Jaw reconstruction may also be necessary following severe facial trauma or due to facial reconstruction due to cancer surgery.

Most mandibular fractures are closed fractures. Intermaxillary fixation is the common method for fixing mandible fractures, which can involve wiring, arch bars, and splinting depending on the severity of injury (Grant & Manson, 2020). In some instances, the fracture repair involves wiring the patient's jaw shut for several weeks. Very rare circumstances require bone grafting. This procedure is often avoided due to the infection risk posed by the mouth and the complex vascularity of the face (Perez & Ellis, 2020).

Nursing Management

The patient who has had rigid fixation should be instructed not to chew food in the first 1 to 4 weeks after surgery. A liquid diet is recommended, and dietary counseling should be obtained to ensure optimal caloric and protein intake. To prevent aspiration, these patients should have wire cutters (for rigid fixation) or scissors (for rubber band fixation) at the bedside to release the jaw if the patient begins to vomit. The patient and family members should be instructed before discharge by the surgeon on where and how to cut the wires or rubber bands in an emergency before the patient is discharged. Rigid fixation remains for approximately 6 weeks depending upon the age of the patient, condition of the bone, and the extent of the mandible injury.

The patient needs specific guidelines for mouth care and feeding. Any irritated areas in the mouth should be reported to the surgeon. Emphasis is placed on the importance of keeping scheduled appointments to assess the stability of the fixation appliance.

Consultation with a dietitian may be indicated so that the patient and family can learn about foods high in essential nutrients and how they can be prepared to be consumed through a straw or spoon while remaining palatable. Nutritional supplements may also be recommended.

Disorders of the Salivary Glands

About 1,200 mL of saliva is produced daily and swallowed. The three primary functions of saliva are lubrication, protection against harmful bacteria, and digestion. The glands that can be affected include the parotids, the submandibular, and the sublingual.

Sialadenitis refers to the bacterial or viral infection of the salivary glands. The condition may be caused by dehydration, radiation therapy, stress, malnutrition, salivary gland calculi (stones), or improper oral hygiene. Patients with a bacterial infection have significant inflammation, pain, swelling, and purulent discharge. Treatment includes antibiotics, massage, hydration, warm compresses, and corticosteroids. Chronic sialadenitis with uncontrolled pain is treated by surgical drainage or excision of the gland and ducts.

Parotitis (inflammation of the parotid gland) is the most common inflammatory condition of the salivary glands. The parotids are the largest of the salivary glands. Mumps (epidemic parotitis), a communicable disease caused by a viral infection and most commonly affecting children, is an inflammation of a salivary gland, usually the parotid.

People who are older, acutely ill, or debilitated with decreased salivary flow from general dehydration or medications are at high risk for parotitis. The infecting organisms travel from the mouth through the salivary duct. The organism is usually *Staphylococcus aureus* (except in mumps). The onset of this complication is sudden, with an exacerbation of both the fever and the symptoms of the primary condition. The gland swells and becomes tense and tender (see Fig. 21-1). The patient feels pain in the ear, and swollen glands interfere with swallowing. The swelling increases rapidly, and the overlying skin soon becomes red and shiny. The patient may have purulent drainage from the site as well.

Medical management includes maintaining adequate nutritional and fluid intake, good oral hygiene, and discontinuing medications (e.g., tranquilizers, diuretics) that diminish salivation. Antibiotic therapy is necessary, and analgesics may be prescribed to control pain. If antibiotic treatment is ineffective, the gland may need to be drained by extraoral pressure applied to the area or by surgical removal via parotidectomy. Also, surgery may be necessary to treat chronic parotitis. The patient is advised to have any necessary dental work performed before surgery.

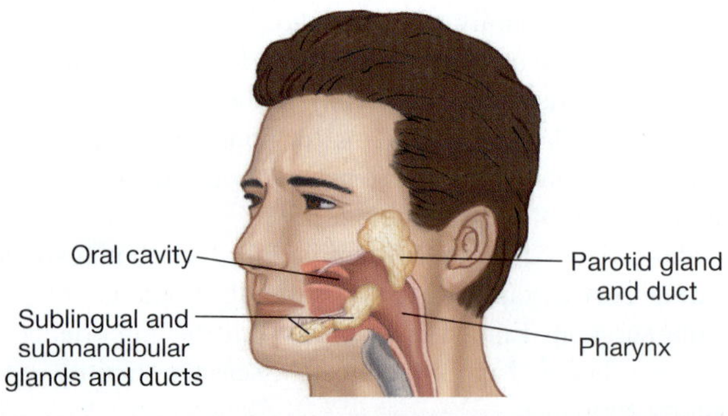

FIGURE 21-1 Parotid gland and duct. (Reprinted from Porth, C. M. [201]). *Essentials of pathophysiology: Concepts of altered states* [4th ed.]. Wolters Kluwer.)

Oral and Oropharyngeal Cancer

Cancers of the oral cavity, which can occur in any part of the mouth or throat, are curable if discovered early. 54,000 people were diagnosed with oral cancer in 2021, and approximately 11% died from the disease (American Cancer Society, 2021). These cancers are more prevalent in Whites than Blacks, and males have twice the risk of females being diagnosed (American Cancer Society, 2021).

Pathophysiology

Malignancies of the oral cavity are usually squamous cell cancers. Any area of the oropharynx can be a site of malignant growths, but the lips, the lateral aspects of the tongue, and the floor of the mouth are most commonly affected.

Risk Factors

Oral cancers are often associated with alcohol and all types of tobacco products, which, if used together, have a synergistic carcinogenic effect. Other factors include dietary deficiency, smoked meat ingestion, and prolonged exposure to sun and wind for lip cancer.

Cancer of the oral cavity affects males more often than females; however, the incidence of oral cancer in females increases, possibly because of increased use of tobacco and alcohol. Cancers of the oral cavity and oropharynx have a higher early incidence in the 50- to 60-year age group in the U.S. Black males, but with increasing age, White males predominate (Ritesh, 2022).

Clinical Manifestations and Assessment

Many oral cancers produce few or no symptoms in the early stages. Later, the most frequent sign is a painless sore or mass that will not heal. A typical lesion in oral cancer is a painless indurated (hardened) ulcer with raised edges. Tissue from any oral cavity ulcer that does not heal in 2 weeks should be examined through biopsy. As cancer progresses, the patient may complain of tenderness; difficulty in chewing, swallowing, or speaking; coughing of blood-tinged sputum; or enlarged cervical lymph nodes.

The diagnostic evaluation consists of an oral examination and assessing the cervical lymph nodes to detect possible metastases. Biopsies are performed on suspicious lesions (those that have not healed in 2 weeks). High-risk areas include the buccal mucosa and gingiva in people who use snuff or smoke cigars or pipes. For those who smoke cigarettes and drink alcohol, high-risk areas include the floor of the mouth, the ventrolateral tongue, and the soft palate complex (soft palate, anterior and posterior tonsillar area, uvula, and the area behind the molar and tongue junction).

Medical Management

Management varies with the nature of the lesion, the preference of the surgeon, and patient choice. Surgical resection, radiation therapy, chemotherapy, or a combination of these therapies may be adequate.

In cancer of the lip, usually, small lesions are excised liberally. Radiation therapy may be more appropriate for larger lesions involving more than one-third of the lip because of superior cosmetic results. The choice depends on the extent of the lesion and what is necessary to cure the patient while preserving the best appearance. Tumors larger than 4 cm often recur.

In cancer of the tongue, treatment with radiation therapy and chemotherapy may preserve organ function and maintain quality of life. A combination of radioactive interstitial implants (surgical implantation of a radioactive source into the tissue adjacent to or at the tumor site) and external beam radiation may be used. Surgical procedures include hemiglossectomy (surgical removal of half of the tongue) and total glossectomy (removal of the tongue).

Neck Dissection

Often cancer of the oral cavity has metastasized through the extensive lymphatic channel in the neck region (Fig. 21-2), requiring a neck dissection and reconstructive surgery of the oral cavity. Surgical treatment often is performed shortly after the completion of radiation or chemoradiation therapy. Other head and neck malignancies that may metastasize into the lymphatic channel include the oropharynx, hypopharynx, nasopharynx, nasal cavity, paranasal sinus, and larynx (Fig. 21-3). There are various types of neck dissection and they refer to how many of the neck levels and sublevels that are removed during the procedure. The Committee for Neck Dissection Classification from the Society of Head and Neck recommends providers include detailed descriptions of the procedure when using the terms radical, modified, comprehensive, full, and selective when referring to neck dissections to decrease confusion; patients need to be prepared for their surgery, treatment period and recovery (Robbins et al., 2008; Rosengren & Koinberg, 2021). A radical neck dissection involves removing all cervical lymph nodes from the mandible to the clavicle and removing the sternocleidomastoid muscle (SCM), internal jugular vein (IJV), and spinal accessory nerve (CN XI) on one side of the neck. The associated complications include shoulder drop and poor cosmesis (visible neck depression). Modified radical neck dissection, which preserves one or more nonlymphatic structures (SCM, IJV, or CN XI), is used more often. A selective node dissection (in comparison with a radical dissection) preserves one or more of the lymph node groups, the IJV, the SCM, and the spinal accessory nerve (Fig. 21-4).

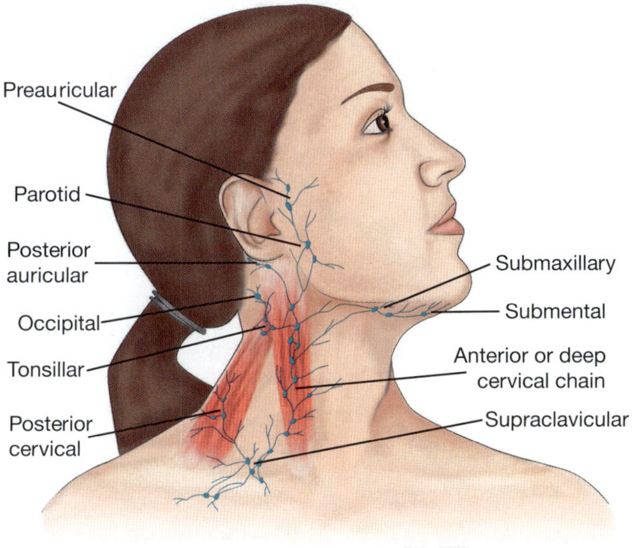

FIGURE 21-2 Lymphatic drainage of the head and neck.

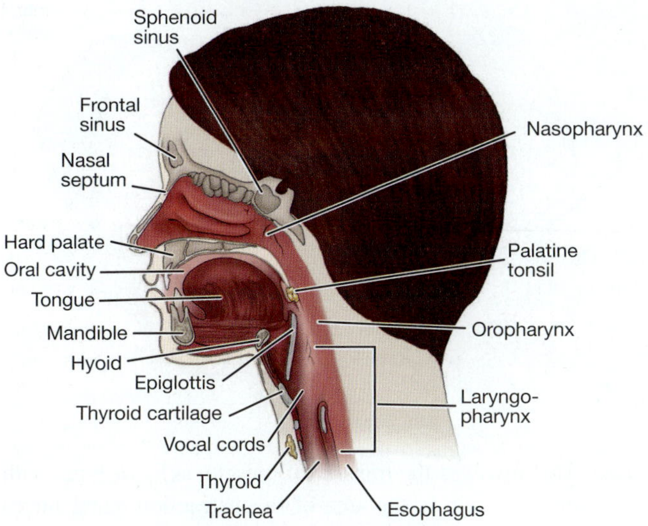

FIGURE 21-3 Anatomy of the head and neck.

Pearls for Practice

The nurse recognizes that when a laryngectomy (removal of the larynx) is performed, the patient will have a permanent laryngeal stoma (an artificial opening leading to the trachea) (Fig. 21-5). Nursing issues relate to airway management, communication, nutritional and emotional support.

Reconstructive techniques may be performed with a variety of grafts (Fig. 21-6). A cutaneous flap (skin and subcutaneous tissue), such as the deltopectoral flap, may be used. A myocutaneous flap (subcutaneous tissue, muscle, and skin) is a graft that is used more frequently; the pectoralis major muscle is also used. For large grafts, a microvascular-free flap may be

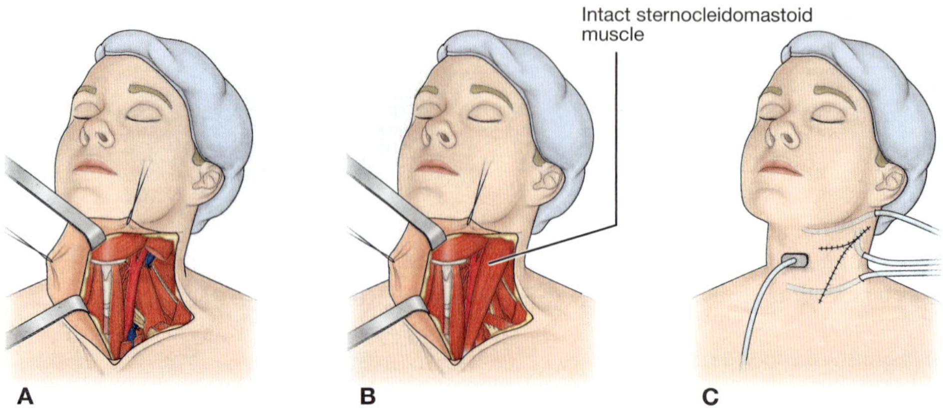

FIGURE 21-4 **(A) A classic radical neck dissection removes the sternocleidomastoid and smaller muscles. All tissue is removed from the ramus of the jaw to the clavicle. The jugular vein has also been removed. (B) The selective neck dissection is similar but preserves the sternocleidomastoid muscle, internal jugular vein, and spinal accessory nerve. The wound is closed (C), and portable suction drainage tubes are in place.**

used. This involves the transfer of muscle, skin, or bone with an artery and vein to the area of reconstruction using micro instrumentation. Areas used for a free flap include the scapula, the radial area of the forearm, or the fibula. The fibula, which provides a larger bone area, may be used if mandibular reconstruction is involved. Neck dissection is discussed in more detail in the nursing process section that follows.

Nursing Management

The nurse assesses the patient's nutritional status preoperatively, and a dietary consultation may be necessary. The patient may require enteral or parenteral feedings before and after surgery to maintain adequate nutrition. If a radial graft is to be performed, an Allen test on the donor's arm must be performed to ensure that the ulnar artery is patent. Refer to Chapter 11 for details on the Allen test.

Postoperatively, the nurse monitors the patient's ability to protect the airway by assessing the ability to swallow and manage oral secretions. Suctioning of oral secretions may be necessary, and the patient can be instructed to use a Yankauer suction device (tonsil tip suction) to remove oral secretions if appropriate. If grafting is part of the surgery, suctioning must be performed with care to prevent damage to the graft. The graft is assessed postoperatively for viability. Although color should be evaluated (white may indicate arterial occlusion, and blue mottling may indicate venous congestion), it can be challenging to assess the graft by looking into the mouth. An intermittent Doppler ultrasound device or fiberoptic monitoring device (producing a continuous audible pulse of the graft site) may be used to assess the graft perfusion.

Xerostomia, dryness of the mouth, is a frequent sequela of oral cancer, particularly when the salivary glands have been exposed to radiation or major surgery. Also, xerostomia

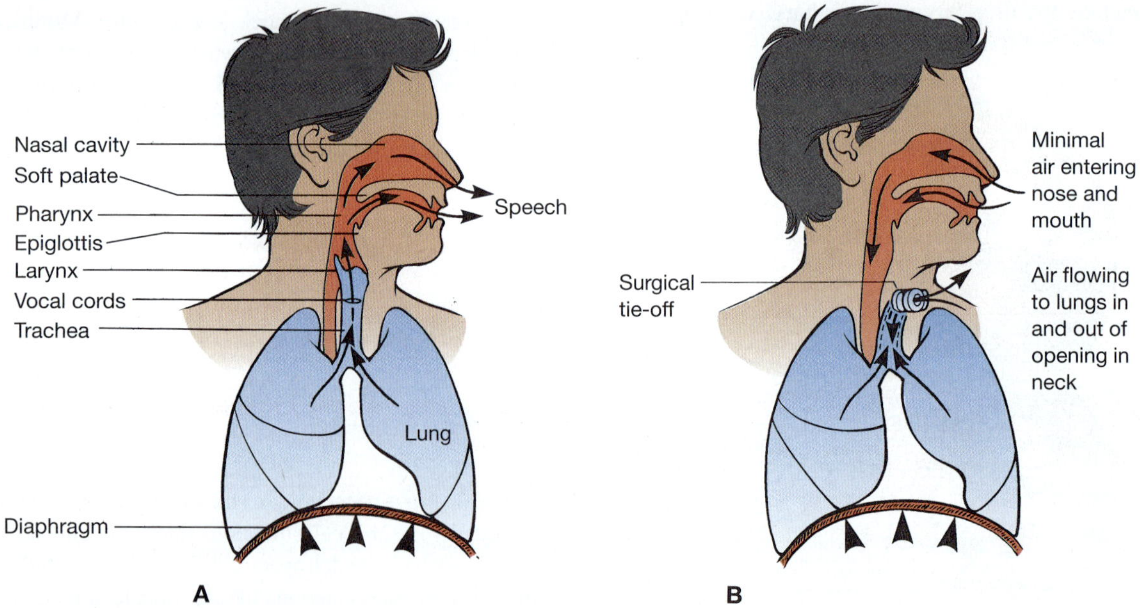

FIGURE 21-5 **Airflow after total laryngectomy. After a total laryngectomy, the patient breathes through a stoma. A. Normal airflow. B. Airflow after a total laryngectomy.**

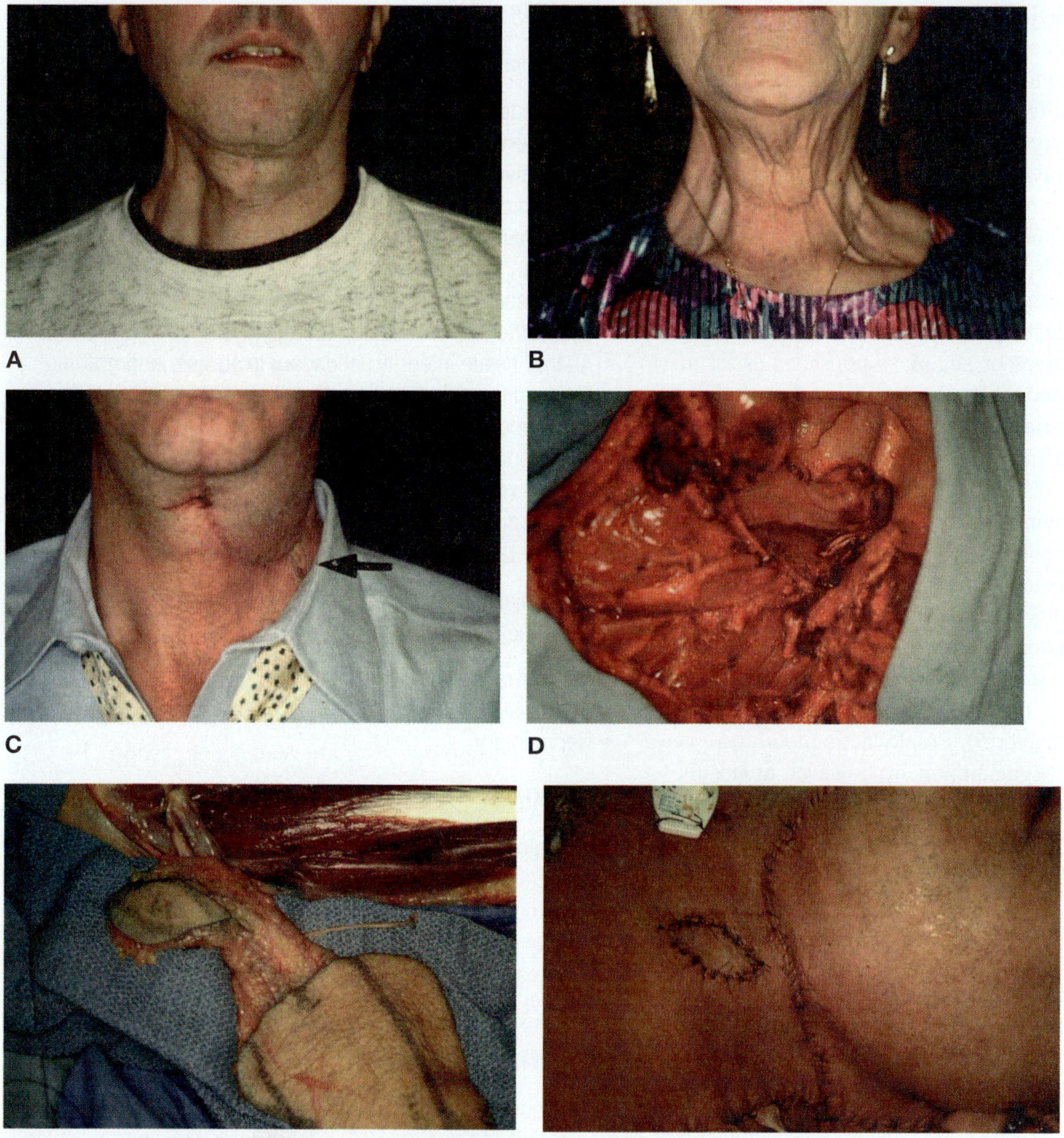

A B C D E F

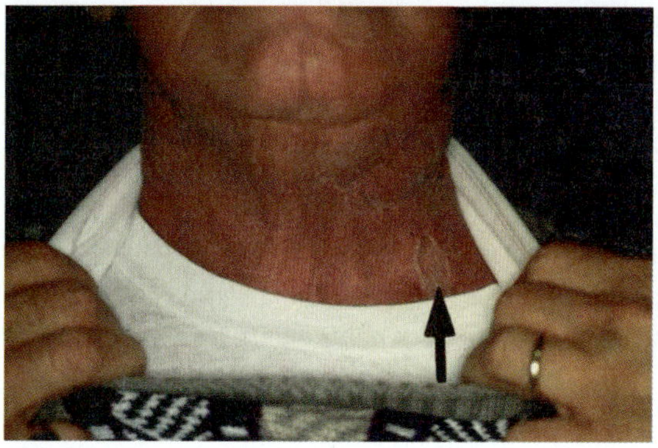

G

FIGURE 21-6 The impact of radical neck dissection on the appearance of the neck is evident in (A) and (B). The underlying structures are located immediately deep into the skin and are readily visible. The hollowed appearance of the contour of the neck serves as a constant reminder of the patient's disease. The effect of adjuvant radiation on the neck's soft tissues produces further fibrosis and contraction, leading to severe scarring and worsening the contour deformity. The placement of a soft tissue flap deep into the skin helps to ameliorate the usual concave appearance following a radical neck dissection (C). The photos that follow demonstrate the technique and the postoperative impact of using a radial forearm free flap with a proximal monitor paddle located in a window created in the caudal portion of the neck (D, E, F). The intent is to orient the proximal soft tissue flap in the direction of the sternocleidomastoid muscle to achieve symmetry with the nonoperative side. The intervening soft tissue helps provide durable improvement in the soft tissue contour and added vascularity to the overlying skin when the procedure is being performed in a patient with prior radiation (G). The skin monitor, used to assess the vascularity of the deep portion of the flap, is placed into the lower neck (G, *arrow*). In the latter setting, when removal of the sternocleidomastoid muscle is required, the added soft tissue helps protect the carotid artery and the microvascular pedicle.

is seen in patients receiving psychopharmacologic agents, patients with HIV infection, patients who cannot close the mouth, patients with endotracheal or tracheostomy tubes, and those with poor oral food intake.

The patient's mouth appears red, dry, and tender to palpation. Cracks in the dry oral mucosa may occur in which infection could develop. To minimize this problem, the patient is advised to avoid dry, crunchy, spicy, acidic, hard food, and irritating foods and fluids, as well as alcohol and tobacco. Also, the patient is encouraged to increase their intake of fluids (when not contraindicated) and to use a humidifier during sleep. Sucking on ice cubes or sugarless popsicles assist in keeping the mouth cool and moist. The use of synthetic saliva, a moisturizing, antibacterial gel, or a saliva-production stimulant, such as pilocarpine may be helpful, however would be contraindicated in patients with chronic cardiovascular or pulmonary disease, uncontrolled asthma, narrow-angle glaucoma, or those taking beta blockers (Wickham, 2020).

Stomatitis, or mucositis, which involves inflammation and breakdown of the oral mucosa, is often a side effect of chemotherapy or radiation therapy. Mucositis results in decreased oral intake and resultant malnutrition; therefore, the nurse performs routine oral assessments and follows treatment approaches (see Chapter 5). Prophylactic mouth care is started when the patient begins treatment; however, mucositis may become so severe that a break in treatment is necessary. Often if a patient receiving radiation therapy has poor dentition, extraction of the teeth before radiation treatment in the oral cavity is performed to prevent infection. As a result, many radiation therapy centers recommend fluoride treatments for patients receiving radiation to the head and neck.

People with cancer of the head and neck frequently have used alcohol or tobacco before surgery; postoperatively, the patient is encouraged to abstain from these substances. Treatment to decrease the likelihood of alcohol and nicotine withdrawal is recommended. Depression and anxiety are also common in this patient population. A recent study found that 19.4% of patients were diagnosed with an anxiety disorder within 2 weeks of their head and neck cancer diagnosis (Henry et al., 2021).

NURSING PROCESS
The Patient Undergoing a Neck Dissection

ASSESSMENT

Preoperatively, the patient's physical and psychological preparation for major surgery is assessed along with their knowledge of the preoperative and postoperative procedures. Postoperatively, the patient is assessed for complications, such as altered respiratory status, wound infection, and hemorrhage. As healing occurs, neck ROM is assessed to determine whether there has been a decrease in ROM due to nerve or muscle damage. A plan of nursing care for a patient who has undergone a neck dissection is available online at http://thepoint.lww.com/Honan3e.

DIAGNOSIS

Nursing diagnoses may include the following:

- Knowledge deficiency about preoperative and postoperative procedures
- Ineffective airway clearance related to obstruction by mucus, hemorrhage, or edema
- Acute pain related to surgical incision
- Infection risk related to surgical intervention secondary to decreased nutritional status, or immunosuppression from chemotherapy or radiation therapy
- Altered tissue integrity secondary to surgery and grafting
- Malnutrition risk, less than body requirements, related to disease process or treatment
- Situational low self-esteem related to diagnosis or prognosis
- Altered verbal communication secondary to surgical resection
- Impaired physical mobility secondary to nerve injury
- Anxiety related to cancer diagnosis and surgical dissection

Potential postoperative complications that may develop include the following:

- Hemorrhage
- Chyle fistula
- Nerve injury

PLANNING

The major goals for the patient include participation in the treatment plan, maintenance of respiratory status, attainment of comfort, absence of infection, viability of the graft, maintenance of adequate intake of food and fluids, effective coping strategies, effective communication, maintenance of shoulder and neck motion, and absence of complications.

NURSING INTERVENTIONS

Before surgery, the patient should be informed about the nature and extent of the surgery and the expectations and milestones in the postoperative period (see Chapter 4 for preoperative education). Methods for communication that will be used postoperatively will be determined preoperatively, examples are paper and pencil, magic slate, picture board, nonverbal cues, electronic communication board or device (Hudson & Carr, 2020).

For the patient who has had extensive neck surgery, specific postoperative interventions include maintenance of a patent airway and continuous assessment of respiratory status, wound care and oral hygiene, maintenance of adequate nutrition, and observation for hemorrhage or nerve injury.

MAINTAINING THE AIRWAY

After the endotracheal tube or airway has been removed and the effects of the anesthesia have worn off, the patient may be placed in Fowler position to facilitate breathing and promote comfort. This position also increases lymphatic and venous drainage, facilitates swallowing, and decreases venous pressure on the skin flaps.

In the immediate postoperative period, the nurse assesses for stridor (coarse, high-pitched sound on inspiration) by listening over the trachea with a stethoscope. This finding must be reported immediately because it indicates partial obstruction of the airway. Signs of respiratory distress, such as dyspnea, cyanosis, changes in mental status, and changes in vital signs, are assessed because they may suggest edema, hemorrhage, inadequate oxygenation, or inadequate drainage. The nurse understands that the oxygen saturation must be at or greater than 90% at a minimum and reports any deviation from the patient's baseline (Flanagan, 2019).

Pneumonia may occur in the postoperative phase if pulmonary secretions are not managed. To aid in the removal of secretions, coughing and deep breathing are encouraged. The patient should assume a sitting position, with the nurse supporting the neck so that the patient can bring up excessive secretions. If this is ineffective, the patient's respiratory tract may have to be suctioned. Care is taken to protect the suture lines during suctioning.

If the patient has had a laryngectomy performed their upper airway is altered so that the trachea brought to the level of the skin in the neck as a stoma. This section of the airway is no longer in continuity with the oropharyngeal cavity or the esophagus. The pharyngeal opening to the trachea is closed, resulting in the pharynx opening only to the esophagus. A laryngectomy tube is placed in the stoma until the patient has recovered. Suctioning is performed through the tube. In the event of an emergency, the nurse understands that resuscitation occurs through the stoma only. The size of the stoma is recorded in the medical record in case a tube is needed to be inserted via the stoma (Phillips & Hornacky, 2021). Humidified oxygen or room air is administered to decrease the viscosity of secretions and provide moisture since thick tenacious secretions are difficult to expectorate (Hudson & Carr, 2020). Patients and family members are instructed to use a cool mist vaporizer or humidified air compressor to decrease secretion viscosity upon discharge and also should be instructed on care of the stoma and suctioning of the airway. The patient also may be instructed on the use of the Yankauer suction to remove oral secretions. The nurse should not take the patient's temperature orally.

Before a patient takes food or fluid orally, the patient's swallowing function is evaluated to assess for dysphagia; it is important to determine the presence or absence of aspiration, any voice impairment, ease of movement of the larynx, any evidence of gurgling with respiration, pulmonary secretions, lung sounds, and oxygen saturation. As many as 20% to 25% of patients with chronic dysphagia (which ~60% of patients with head and neck cancer identify as the most troubling symptom after treatment) develop aspiration pneumonia (Yang et al., 2021). Many techniques may be considered to decrease dysphagia and the risk of aspiration, they include supraglottic swallowing, mendelson maneuver (a technique used to increase laryngeal elevation to improve clearing of the pharynx), and the shaker exercise (also known as the head lift) by the speech pathologist (Ferri, 2022). Seeking the guidance of a speech pathologist is recommended when considering aspiration prevention techniques such as these.

Pearls for Practice: Cues for Aspiration
Cues for Aspiration

The nurse is alert for the following symptoms which suggest aspiration of oropharyngeal or upper gastrointestinal contents, including food or fluids into the lungs: cough (productive), tachypnea, dyspnea, hypoxia, tachycardia, fever, and the lung examination may reveal diffuse wheezing, crackles or rhonchi; however, symptoms may be minimal in older patients and in those recently extubated. For example, postextubation dysphagia has been shown to occur in 41% of critically ill patients requiring endotracheal intubation, and one third of these patients experienced silent aspiration (McIntyre et al., 2022). Frequently, mental status changes are the earliest of aspiration pneumonia in older patients (Clinical Overview, 2022). Therefore, the nurse keeps a high degree of suspicion of aspiration in all patients with dysphagia.

Pearls for Practice

Failure to assess for dysphagia in the patient following postoperative neck dissection may result in severe respiratory compromise, prolonged mechanical ventilation, and aspiration pneumonia.

RELIEVING PAIN

Pain and the patient's fear of pain are assessed and managed. Patients with head and neck cancer often report less pain than do patients with other types of cancer; however, the nurse needs to be aware that each person's pain experience is individual. The nurse administers analgesics as prescribed and assesses their effectiveness.

PROVIDING WOUND CARE

Wound drainage tubes usually are inserted during surgery to prevent the subcutaneous collection of fluid. The drainage tubes are connected to a portable suction device (e.g., Jackson-Pratt) (see Box 32-4), and the container is emptied periodically. Between 80 and 120 mL of serosanguineous secretions may drain over the first 24 hours. Excessive drainage may be indicative of a chyle fistula or hemorrhage (see later discussion). If dressings are present, they may need to be reinforced periodically. Dressings are observed for evidence of hemorrhage and constriction, which impairs respiration and perfusion of the graft. A graft, if present, is assessed for color and temperature and for the presence of a pulse if applicable, to determine viability. The graft should be pale pink and warm to the touch. If lymphatic drainage is obstructed, then edema may develop. The surgical incisions are also assessed for infection, which is reported immediately. Prophylactic antibiotics may be prescribed.

(*continued on page 724*)

MAINTAINING ADEQUATE NUTRITION

Nutritional status is assessed preoperatively; early intervention to correct nutritional imbalances may decrease the risk of postoperative complications. Frequently, nutrition is less than optimal because of inadequate intake, and the patient often requires enteral or parenteral supplements preoperatively and postoperatively to attain and maintain a positive nitrogen balance.

The patient who can chew may take food by mouth; the level of the patient's chewing ability determines whether some diet modification (e.g., soft, puréed, or liquid foods) is necessary. Also food preferences should be discussed with the patient. Oral care before eating may enhance the patient's appetite, and oral care after eating is important to prevent infection and dental caries.

SUPPORTING COPING MEASURES

Preoperatively, information about the planned surgery is given to the patient and family. Postoperatively, psychological nursing interventions are aimed at supporting the patient who has had a change in body image or who has major concerns regarding the prognosis. The patient may have difficulty communicating and may be concerned about their ability to breathe and swallow normally. The nurse supports the patient's family and friends in encouraging and reassuring the patient that adjusting to the results of this surgery will take time.

The person who has had extensive neck surgery often is sensitive about their appearance. This can occur when the operative area is covered by bulky dressings, when the incision line is visible, or later after healing has occurred and the appearance of the neck, and possibly the lower face, has been altered significantly. If the nurse accepts the patient's appearance and expresses a positive, optimistic attitude, then the patient is more likely to be encouraged. The patient also needs an opportunity to express concerns regarding the success of the surgery and the prognosis. The American Cancer Society may be a resource to provide a volunteer to meet with the patient either preoperatively or postoperatively.

PROMOTING EFFECTIVE COMMUNICATION

If a laryngectomy was performed, the nurse explores other methods of communicating with the patient and obtains a consultation with a speech/language therapist. Alternatives to verbal communication may include use of a pencil and paper or pointing to needed items on a picture pad. Alternative speech techniques, such as an electrolarynx (a mechanical device held against the neck) or esophageal speech, may be taught by a speech/language therapist.

MAINTAINING PHYSICAL MOBILITY

Excision of muscles and nerves results in weakness at the shoulder that can cause shoulder drop, a forward curvature of the shoulder. Many problems can be avoided with a conscientious exercise program. Usually these exercises are begun after the drains have been removed and the neck incision is healed sufficiently. Physical therapists and occupational therapists can assist patients in performing these exercises.

Additionally because lymph node removal can cause nerve damage, and the sternocleidomastoid muscle may have been removed, neck mobility is impaired, thus the neck is supported by the nurse when getting the patient out of bed. Physical therapy can assist with developing a plan for neck and shoulder rehabilitation.

MONITORING AND MANAGING POTENTIAL COMPLICATIONS

Hemorrhage. Hemorrhage may occur from rupture of the carotid artery as a result of necrosis of the graft or damage to the artery itself from tumor or infection. It is also known as carotid blowout syndrome and is a medical emergency with a prevalence of 3.9% in patients with head and neck cancer. Mortality rates of 40% are seen and neurologic morbidity of 60% (Zhao et al., 2021). Emergency surgery using traditional arterial ligation or endovascular therapy is required (Zhao et al., 2021). The following measures are indicated:

- Vital signs are assessed. Tachycardia, tachypnea, and hypotension may indicate hemorrhage and impending hypovolemic shock.
- The patient is instructed to avoid the Valsalva maneuver (bearing-down activities such as having a bowel movement) to prevent stress on the graft and carotid artery.
- Signs of impending rupture, such as high epigastric pain or discomfort, are reported.
- Dressings and wound drainage are observed for excessive bleeding.
- If hemorrhage occurs, assistance is summoned immediately.
- Hemorrhage requires the continuous application of pressure to the bleeding site or major associated vessel.
- Close assessment must occur when changing the patient's position to assist in maintaining blood pressure yet minimizing the risk of aspiration and potentially losing airway patency.
- The nurse should maintain a controlled, calm manner to help allay the patient's anxiety.
- The surgeon is notified immediately because a vascular or ligature tear requires surgical intervention or endovascular therapy.

Chyle Fistula. A chyle fistula (milk-like lymphatic drainage from the thoracic duct into the thoracic cavity) may develop as a result of damage to the lymphatic thoracic duct during surgery. The nurse notes the color of the drainage from the neck drains and notifies the surgeon if milky, odorless discharge is seen since this is suspicious for a chyle leak. The diagnosis is made if the drainage has a triglyceride level greater than 110 mg/dL, a fat content of 0.4–4.0 g/dL, a protein content of 3 g/dL, and a specific gravity of 1.010 or greater. Treatment of a small leak (up to 500 mL or less) includes application of a pressure dressing and a diet of medium-chain fatty acids or parenteral nutrition (PN). Surgical intervention to repair the damaged duct is necessary for larger leaks.

Nerve Injury. Nerve injury can occur during a neck dissection procedure due to the location of multiple nerve pathways in and around muscle, lymphatic, and vascular structures.

Damage to the accessory nerve can result in shoulder pain and potential dysfunction. The facial nerve can also be damaged which would manifest as poor lower lip function. Tongue movement can be affected with injury to the hypoglossal nerve. If a patient has limited mobility of the arm in the postoperative period a brachial plexus injury is suspected. Damage to the phrenic nerve can affect the respiratory system and the patient's voice can be changed due to injury to the vagus nerve. The nurse assesses the functioning of the anatomic structures mentioned with the knowledge of the corresponding nerve pathways to the appropriate health care provider, such as the surgeon, physical therapist or speech pathologist and recommend interventions.

TEACHING PATIENTS SELF-CARE

The patient and caregiver require instructions about management of the wound, the dressing, and any drains that remain in place. Stoma covers may be suggested by the surgeon as it is worn over the patient's stoma to warm, moisten, and filter air. Patients who require oral suctioning or who have a tracheostomy may be very anxious about their care at home; the transition to home can be eased if the caregiver is given several opportunities to demonstrate the ability to meet the patient's needs. Also the patient and caregiver are instructed about possible complications, such as bleeding and respiratory distress, and when to notify the health care provider of signs and symptoms of these complications. In addition, patients are instructed not to shower until the health care provider approves and when allowed, they must use a waterproof cover over the stoma that will still allow them to breathe.

If the patient cannot take food by mouth, detailed instructions and demonstration of enteral or parenteral feedings will be required. Education in techniques of effective oral hygiene is also important.

A referral for home care nursing may be necessary in the early period after discharge. The nurse assesses healing, ensures that feedings are being administered properly, and monitors for any complications. The home care nurse assesses the patient's adjustment to changes in physical appearance and status as well as the patient's ability to communicate and to eat normally. Physical and speech therapy also may be continued at home.

The patient is given information regarding local support groups. The local chapter of the American Cancer Society may be contacted for information and equipment needed; there are additional patient resources on the web, for example, the American Head and Neck Society (https://www.ahns.info/for-patients/).

EVALUATION

Expected patient outcomes may include:

1. Discusses expected course of treatment
2. Demonstrates good respiratory exchange:
   a. Lungs are clear to auscultation
   b. Breathes easily with no shortness of breath
   c. Demonstrates ability to use suction effectively
3. Remains free of infection:
   a. Maintains normal laboratory values
   b. Normothermic
4. Graft is pink and warm to touch
5. Maintains adequate intake of foods and fluids:
   a. Accepts altered route of feeding
   b. Adequate fluid volume status
   c. Maintains or gains weight
6. Demonstrates ability to cope:
   a. Discusses emotional responses to the diagnosis
   b. Attends support group meetings
7. Verbalizes comfort
8. Attains maximal mobility:
   a. Adheres to physical therapy exercises
   b. Attains maximal ROM
9. Exhibits no complications:
   a. Vital signs stable
   b. No excessive bleeding or discharge
   c. Able to move muscles of lower face

DISORDERS OF THE ESOPHAGUS

The esophagus is a mucus-lined, muscular tube that carries food from the mouth to the stomach. It begins at the base of the pharynx and ends about 4 cm below the diaphragm. Two sphincters facilitate its ability to transport food and fluid. The upper esophageal sphincter, also called the *hypopharyngeal sphincter*, is located at the junction of the pharynx and the esophagus. The lower esophageal sphincter also called the *gastroesophageal sphincter* or *cardiac sphincter*, is located at the corner of the esophagus and the stomach. The lower esophageal sphincter prevents reflux (backward flow) of gastric contents. There is no serosal layer of the esophagus; therefore, it is more challenging to perform suturing or anastomosis if surgery is necessary.

Disorders of the esophagus include motility disorders, achalasia (muscles of the lower part of the esophagus fail to relax), hiatal hernias, diverticula, perforation, esophageal obstruction due to swallowed foreign bodies, chemical burns, gastroesophageal reflux disease, Barrett esophagus, and carcinoma. **Dysphagia** (difficulty swallowing), the most common symptom of esophageal disease, may vary from an uncomfortable feeling that a bolus of food is caught in the upper esophagus to acute pain on swallowing (**odynophagia**). Obstruction of food (solid and soft) and even liquids may occur anywhere along the esophagus. Often, the patient indicates that the problem is located in the upper, middle, or lower third of the esophagus.

Achalasia

Achalasia is absent or ineffective **peristalsis** of the distal esophagus, accompanied by failure of the esophageal sphincter to relax in response to swallowing. Narrowing

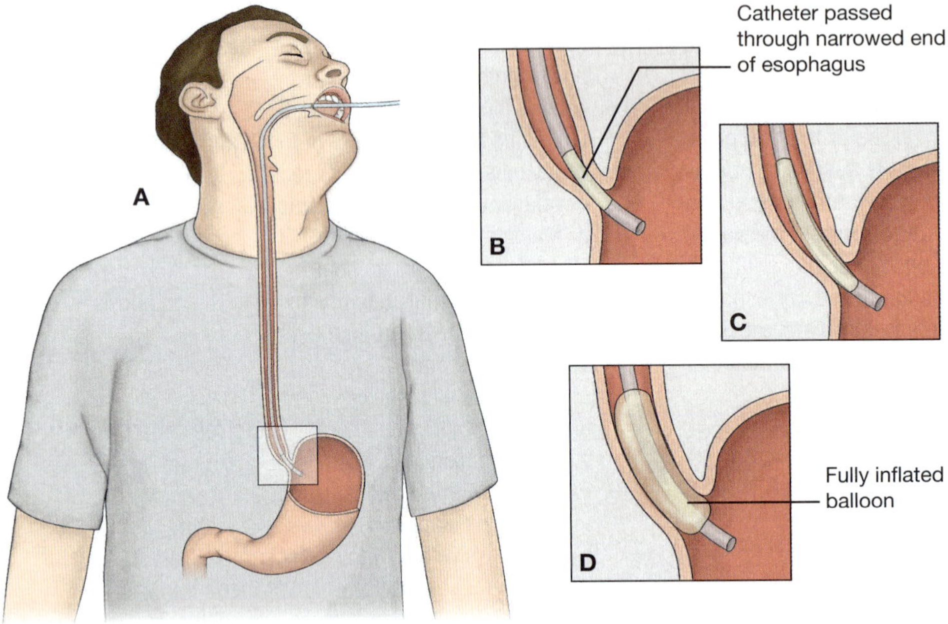

FIGURE 21-7 **Treatment of achalasia by pneumatic dilation. A–C. The dilator is passed, guided by a previously inserted guidewire. D. When the balloon is in the proper position, it is distended by pressure sufficient to dilate the narrowed area of the esophagus.**

of the esophagus just above the stomach results in a gradually increasing dilation of the esophagus in the upper chest. Achalasia may progress slowly and occurs most often in people 40 years or older.

Clinical Manifestations and Assessment

The primary symptom is difficulty in swallowing both liquids and solids. The patient has a sensation of food lodged in the lower portion of the esophagus. As the condition progresses, food is regurgitated either spontaneously or intentionally by the patient to relieve the discomfort produced by prolonged distention of the esophagus by food that will not pass into the stomach. The patient may also report chest pain and heartburn (**pyrosis**) that may or may not be associated with eating. Secondary pulmonary complications may result from aspiration of gastric contents.

X-ray studies show esophageal dilation above the narrowing at the gastroesophageal junction. Barium swallow, computed tomography (CT) of the chest, and endoscopy may be used for diagnosis; however, high-resolution *manometry*, a process in which a radiologist or gastroenterologist measures the esophageal pressure, confirms the diagnosis (Reider et al., 2020).

Medical and Nursing Management

The patient is instructed to eat slowly and to drink fluids with meals. As a temporary measure, calcium channel blockers and nitrates have decreased esophageal pressure and improved swallowing. Injection of botulinum toxin (Botox) to quadrants of the esophagus via endoscopy has been helpful because it inhibits smooth muscle contraction. Periodic injections are required to maintain remission.

Achalasia may be treated conservatively by pneumatic dilation to stretch the narrowed area of the esophagus (Fig. 21-7). Pneumatic dilation (forcefully dilating the lower esophagus by a balloon) has a high success rate. Although perforation is a potential complication, its incidence is low. The procedure can be painful; therefore, moderate sedation in the form of an analgesic or tranquilizer, or both, is administered for the treatment. The patient is monitored for perforation. Abdominal tenderness and fever may indicate perforation (see later discussion).

Achalasia may be treated surgically by esophagostomy. Usually, the procedure is performed laparoscopically, starting with a complete lower esophageal sphincter myotomy (cutting of muscle) and possibly including an antireflux procedure. The esophageal muscle fibers are separated to relieve the lower esophageal stricture.

Hiatal Hernia

In the condition known as hiatus (or hiatal) **hernia**, the opening in the diaphragm through which the esophagus passes becomes enlarged, and part of the upper stomach tends to move up into the lower portion of the thorax. A hiatal hernia occurs more often in females than in males. The most common type is type I or sliding (Falk & Katzka, 2020). It occurs when the upper stomach and the gastroesophageal junction are displaced upward and slide in and out of the thorax (Fig. 21-8A). A sliding hernia is the most commonly diagnosed of the four types. A rolling or paraesophageal hernia occurs when all or part of the stomach pushes through the diaphragm beside the esophagus (see Fig. 21-8B). In a type II hernia, the fundus and the greater curvature of the stomach is next to the esophagus, above the gastroesophageal junction. The mixed hernia, or type III, is characterized by the cardia and fundus being displaced upward.

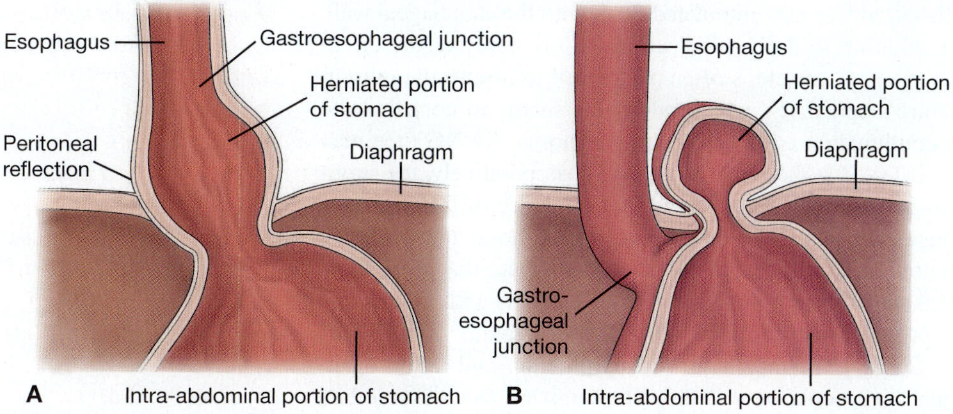

FIGURE 21-8 **A. Sliding esophageal hernia. The upper stomach and gastroesophageal junction have moved upward and slide in and out of the thorax. B. Paraesophageal hernia. All or part of the stomach pushes through the diaphragm next to the gastroesophageal junction.**

Clinical Manifestations and Assessment

The patient with a sliding hernia may have heartburn, regurgitation, and dysphagia, although many patients are asymptomatic. Often sliding hiatal hernia is implicated in reflux. The patient with a paraesophageal hernia usually feels an uncomfortable sense of fullness after eating or chest pain, or there may be no symptoms. Reflux usually does not occur because the gastroesophageal sphincter is intact. Hemorrhage, obstruction, and strangulation can occur with any hernia.

Diagnosis is confirmed by x-ray studies, barium swallow, and fluoroscopy.

Medical and Nursing Management

Management for a sliding hernia includes frequent, small feedings that can pass easily through the esophagus. The patient is advised not to recline for 1 hour after eating to prevent reflux or movement of the hernia and to elevate the head of the bed on 4- to 8-in (10- to 20-cm) blocks to prevent the hernia from sliding upward. Surgery is indicated when a patient has a significant esophageal injury or does not respond to medical management. Medical and surgical management of a paraesophageal hernia is similar to that for gastroesophageal reflux (see Chapter 22); however, people with paraesophageal hernias may require emergency surgery to correct torsion (twisting) of the stomach that can lead to restriction of blood flow to the area.

Diverticulum

A diverticulum is an outpouching of mucosa and submucosa that protrudes through a weak portion of the musculature that can occur at any location in the esophagus.

The most common type of esophageal diverticulum, which is found three times more frequently in males than in females, is the *Zenker diverticulum* (also known as pharyngoesophageal pulsion diverticulum or a pharyngeal pouch). It occurs posteriorly through the cricopharyngeal muscle in the midline of the neck. Usually, it is seen in people older than 60 years of age. Other types of diverticula include mid esophageal (rare), epiphrenic (large), and intramural diverticula (numerous and small; related to stricture).

Clinical Manifestations and Assessment

Symptoms experienced by the patient with a pharyngoesophageal pulsion diverticulum include difficulty swallowing, fullness in the neck, belching, regurgitation of undigested food, and gurgling noises after eating. The diverticulum, or pouch, becomes filled with food or liquid. When the patient assumes a recumbent position, undigested food is regurgitated, and coughing may be caused by irritation of the trachea. Also, halitosis and a sour taste in the mouth are common because of the decomposition of food retained in the diverticulum.

Symptoms produced by mid-esophageal diverticula are less acute. Due to the difficulty these patients have with food passing through their upper GI tract, they often have chest pain and difficulty swallowing. Some patients experience regurgitation of undigested food, and some do not experience any symptoms at all.

A barium swallow may determine the exact nature and location of a diverticulum. Often pressure studies are performed for patients with epiphrenic diverticula (occur in the distal 10 cm of the esophagus, most commonly 4 to 8 cm above the gastric cardia) to rule out a motility disorder (Bennett & Akhondi, 2022). Esophagoscopy usually is contraindicated because of the danger of perforation of the diverticulum.

Pearls for Practice

Blind insertion of NG tubes should be avoided in patients with esophageal diverticulum, esophageal varices, postgastric bypass, and lap banding procedures due to the potential of causing esophageal rupture or surgical site perforation.

Medical and Nursing Management

Because pharyngoesophageal pulsion diverticulum is progressive, the only means of cure is the surgical removal of the diverticulum. During surgery, care is taken to avoid trauma to the common carotid artery and IJVs. The sac is dissected free and amputated flush with the esophageal wall. In addition to a diverticulectomy, a myotomy of the cricopharyngeal muscle is often performed to relieve the musculature's spasticity, which otherwise seems to contribute to a continuation of the previous symptoms. An NG tube may be inserted at the time of surgery. Postoperatively, the surgical incision must be observed for evidence of leakage from the esophagus and a developing fistula. Food and fluids are withheld until radiographic studies indicate that there is no leakage at the surgical site. The diet begins with liquids and is progressively returned to solids as tolerated.

Surgery is indicated for epiphrenic and midesophageal diverticula only if the symptoms are troublesome and becoming worse. Treatment consists of a diverticulectomy and long myotomy. Intramural diverticula usually regress after the esophageal stricture is dilated.

Perforation

The esophagus is a common site of injury. Perforation may result from stab or bullet wounds of the neck or chest, trauma from a motor vehicle crash, caustic damage from a chemical burn, inadvertent puncture during a surgical procedure, or esophageal dilatation, or severe retching or vomiting (Boerhaave syndrome which is also known as spontaneous esophageal perforation or Mallory–Weiss syndrome [longitudinal superficial mucosal lacerations known as Mallory–Weiss tears]). Mortality rates of 40% are associated with Boerhaave syndrome, which is one of the most lethal GI tract disorders found (Turner & Turner, 2022). Both Boerhaave syndrome and Mallory–Weiss tear are associated with forceful retching and vomiting following excessive alcohol intake (Rawla & Devasahayam, 2022).

Clinical Manifestations and Assessment

The patient with a perforated esophagus has persistent pain, followed by dysphagia, fever, leukocytosis (elevated white blood cells). Other symptoms that may present depending on the extent of the tear include hematemesis (vomiting blood), subcutaneous emphysema, and severe hypotension. Clinical presentation will depend on the level of the perforation, the degree of leakage, and the time since the onset of the injury (Turner & Turner, 2022). In general, pain will be present and relate to the perforation site (e.g., neck, chest, epigastric region, or upper abdomen). In some instances, signs of pneumothorax are observed. Diagnostic studies include CT scan, if available, due to its higher sensitivity and more detailed assessment of the involved organs and to identify the injury site; esophagogram using a water-soluble contrast agent such as gastrografin which will reveal the extravasation of contrast material at the site of the perforation, or upper GI endoscopy. However, in the case of a suspected Boerhaave syndrome caution is used with endoscopy due to the risk of further esophageal perforation (Rawla & Devasahayam, 2022; Turner & Turner, 2022).

Pearls for Practice

Subcutaneous emphysema is air that is trapped underneath the dermal layers of skin and is palpated as crepitus or popping, crackling, or crunching sensation that is felt when pushing on the soft tissue in the affected area. In addition, the nurse should observe for swelling of the affected area. It is found in a variety of conditions such as pneumothorax (collapsed lung). In the presence of esophageal rupture, the air that is present in the esophagus escapes through the tear and is trapped in the dermal layer of the skin. Subcutaneous emphysema is a symptom of an underlying problem that needs to be investigated.

Medical and Nursing Management

Because of the high risk of infection, broad-spectrum antibiotic therapy is initiated. If the perforation is small enough and without symptoms, medical intervention may not be necessary. Nothing is given orally; nutrition is administered into the intestine, bypassing the stomach, or by the parenteral route. The type of nutritional support depends on the location and the extent of the injury. The enteral or parenteral nutrition lasts for at least 1 month to give the esophagus a chance to heal. After reevaluation of the esophageal tear, if there is no evidence of perforation, foods are reintroduced, beginning with liquids and then slowly progressing to solids as tolerated.

In cases where there is severe bleeding, the nurse monitors the patients for symptoms of hypovolemic shock (e.g., increased HR and RR, hypotension, decreased MAP, pulse is weak and thready, reduced skin turgor, delayed capillary filling time (>2 seconds) and intervenes immediately (see Chapter 53). Immediate IV fluid replacement in those with significant blood loss and blood replacement therapy with packed RBC may be required if the hemoglobin level is less than 8 g/dL (Rawla & Devasahayam, 2022). Surgery that includes primary esophageal repair through open thoracotomy versus video-assisted thoracotomy surgery (VATS) with fundic reinforcement, which is the gold standard within the first 24 hours; in such cases, postoperative nutritional support becomes a primary concern (Turner & Turner, 2022). Depending on the incision site and the nature of the surgery, the postoperative nursing management is similar to that for patients who have had thoracic or abdominal surgery.

Foreign Bodies

Many swallowed foreign bodies pass through the GI tract without the need for medical intervention. However, some swallowed foreign bodies (e.g., dentures, fish bones, pins, small batteries, items containing mercury or lead) may cause trauma to the esophagus or obstruct its lumen and must be removed. Pain and dysphagia may be present, and dyspnea may occur due to pressure on the trachea. The foreign body may be identified by x-ray. Perforation may have happened (see earlier discussion).

Glucagon, because of its relaxing effect on the esophageal muscle, may be injected intramuscularly. An endoscope (with a covered hood or overtube) may be used to remove the impacted food or object from the esophagus. Sodium bicarbonate and the tartaric acid mixture may be prescribed to increase intraluminal pressure by forming a gas, which works to dislodge the foreign body. Caution must be used with this treatment because there is a risk of perforation.

Chemical Burns

The severity of chemical burns to the esophagus depends on the characteristics of the substance: pH, concentration, volume, and duration of contact with the mucosa.

Clinical Manifestations and Assessment

Ingestion of the substance can be intentional or unintentional, which is essential to consider when assessing the patient or reviewing their history. Strongly alkaline substances are more damaging to the esophagus due to causing liquefactive necrosis when they contact the mucosa. Alkalis include lye, chemical strippers, and drain cleaners. In addition, chemical burns of the esophagus also may be caused by undissolved medications in the esophagus. An acute chemical burn of the esophagus may be accompanied by severe burns of the lips, mouth, and pharynx, resulting in airway compromise due to edema or excessive mucus production. Also, the patient may experience pain when swallowing.

Medical and Nursing Management

The patient's airway is prioritized, and they are treated for pain and possible shock. The patient's injury is evaluated using esophagoscopy. Vomiting and gastric lavage are avoided to prevent further exposure of the esophagus to the caustic agent. The patient is given nothing by mouth (NPO status), and IV fluids are administered. The medical team may insert an NG tube. There is no consensus on the use of corticosteroids to reduce inflammation and minimize scarring and stricture formation at this time.

After the acute phase has subsided, the patient may need nutritional support via enteral or parenteral feedings. The patient may require further treatment to prevent or manage strictures of the esophagus. Strictures are repeatedly dilated with progressively larger cylindrical rubber tubes or bougies. For strictures that do not respond to dilation, surgical management is necessary. Reconstruction may be accomplished by esophagectomy and colon interposition to replace the portion of the esophagus removed.

Barrett Esophagus

Barrett esophagus is a condition in which the lining of the esophageal mucosa is altered. The tissue at the gastroesophageal junction changes from the squamous epithelium (flat) to columnar epithelium (elongated). Barrett esophagus is sometimes found in patients being evaluated with a history of chronic regurgitation or heartburn (see Chapter 22). The disease may lead to esophageal cancer in some patients.

Clinical Manifestations and Assessment

The patient with Barrett esophagus complains of symptoms of GERD, notably frequent heartburn. The patient may also complain of symptoms related to peptic ulcers or esophageal stricture, or both.

An **esophagogastroduodenoscopy (EGD)** is performed. This usually reveals an esophageal lining that is red rather than pink, indicating the cellular change in tissue. With a biopsy, cellular changes and goblet cells (mucus-producing) are seen.

Medical and Nursing Management

Monitoring for Barrett esophagus varies depending on the extent of cell changes. Some providers recommend a repeat EGD in 6 to 12 months if the cellular changes are minor.

Photodynamic therapy (PDT) may be an alternative for the patient who is considered an operative risk (e.g., at least 70 years of age or older, significant cardiac risk). PDT is a laser thermal ablation of the esophageal mucosa that destroys the metaplastic cells once the patient has received a photosensitizing agent, such as sodium porfimer. PDT has been well documented in the literature as a safe and effective treatment.

Ablative techniques including radiofrequency, thermal, and argon plasma coagulation are commonly used with acid suppression treatment. In the past, esophagectomy was the standard of treatment for these patients. Early detection of precancerous changes and the occurrence of high complication rates for surgery have left esophagectomy for the treatment of advanced cases.

Cancer of the Esophagus

The American Cancer Society estimates that 19,260 esophageal cancer diagnoses were made in 2021 (2021). In the United States, esophageal cancer continues to represent 1% of all cancers diagnosed (American Cancer Society, 2021).

Pathophysiology

Esophageal cancer can be of two cell types: adenocarcinoma and squamous cell carcinoma. The rate of adenocarcinoma is rapidly increasing in the United States as well as in other Western countries. Adenocarcinoma is found in gland cells and is not common to the esophagus except in patients having Barrett esophagus, as described previously. As a result, patients with GERD and Barrett esophagus are at greater risk for developing esophageal cancer.

Tumor cells of adenocarcinoma and squamous cell carcinoma may spread beneath the esophageal mucosa or directly into, through, and beyond the muscle layers into the lymphatics. In the latter stages, obstruction of the esophagus is noted, with possible perforation into the mediastinum and erosion into the great vessels.

Risk Factors

Chronic irritation is a risk factor for esophageal cancer. In the United States, cancer of the esophagus has been associated with ingestion of alcohol and tobacco use. Additional risk factors for squamous cell carcinoma of the esophagus include chronic ingestion of hot liquids or foods, nutritional deficiencies, poor oral hygiene, exposure to nitrosamines in the environment or food, and some esophageal medical conditions, such as caustic injury. Nitrosamines are found in rubber products, cured meats, beer, and pesticides.

Clinical Manifestations and Assessment

Many patients have an advanced ulcerated lesion of the esophagus before symptoms are manifested. Symptoms include dysphagia, initially with solid foods and eventually with liquids; a sensation of a mass in the throat; painful swallowing; substernal pain or fullness; and, later, regurgitation of undigested food with foul breath and hiccups. The patient first becomes aware of intermittent and increasing difficulty in swallowing. As the tumor grows and the obstruction becomes nearly complete, liquids cannot pass into the stomach. Regurgitation of food and saliva occurs, hemorrhage may occur, and progressive loss of weight and strength occurs from starvation. Later symptoms include substernal pain, persistent hiccup, respiratory difficulty, and foul breath.

The delay between early symptoms and when the patient seeks medical advice is often 12 to 18 months. Any person having swallowing difficulties should be encouraged to consult a provider immediately.

Currently, diagnosis is often confirmed by endoscopy with biopsy (Rajaram et al., 2022). The biopsy can be used to determine the presence of disease and cell differentiation. At presentation, most patients have moderately differentiated tumors.

Several imaging techniques may provide valuable diagnostic information, such as CT, MRI, endoscopic ultrasound, and positron emission tomography (PET). Endoscopic ultrasound is also helpful in determining whether cancer has spread to the lymph nodes and other mediastinal structures. PET specifically assesses the metabolism of the cells being imaged so that malignant cells can be identified.

Medical Management

If esophageal cancer is detected early, treatment goals may be directed toward a cure; however, it is often seen in late stages, making relief of symptoms the only useful purpose of therapy. Treatment may include surgery, radiation, chemotherapy, or a combination of these modalities, depending on the type of cell, the extent of the disease, and the patient's condition. A standard treatment plan for a person who is newly diagnosed with esophageal cancer includes the following: preoperative combination chemotherapy/RT for 4 to 6 weeks (neoadjuvant chemoradiation), followed by a period of no medical intervention for 4 weeks, and, last, surgical resection of the esophagus.

Standard surgical management includes a total resection of the esophagus (esophagectomy), removing the tumor plus a wide tumor-free margin of the esophagus and the lymph nodes in the area. The surgical approach may be through the thorax or the abdomen, depending on the tumor's location. When tumors occur in the cervical or upper thoracic area, esophageal continuity may be maintained by a free jejunal graft transfer. The cancer is removed, and the area is replaced with a portion of the jejunum (Fig. 21-9). A segment of the colon may be used, or the stomach can be elevated into the chest and the proximal section of the esophagus anastomosed to the stomach.

Tumors of the lower thoracic esophagus are more amenable to surgery than are tumors located higher in the esophagus. GI tract integrity is maintained by anastomosing the lower esophagus to the stomach.

Surgical resection of the esophagus has a relatively high mortality rate because of infection, pulmonary complications, or leakage through the anastomosis. Postoperatively, the patient has an NG tube in place that should not be manipulated. The patient is NPO until x-ray studies confirm that the anastomosis is free from an esophageal leak, there is no obstruction, and there is no evidence of pulmonary aspiration.

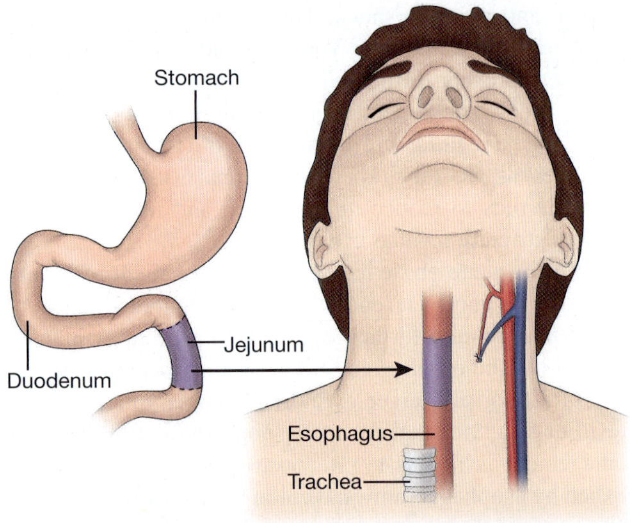

FIGURE 21-9 Esophageal reconstruction with free jejunal transfer. A portion of the jejunum is grafted between the esophagus and pharynx to replace the abnormal portion of the esophagus. The vascular structures are also anastomosed. A portion of the graft may be externalized through the neck wound to evaluate graft viability.

Palliative treatment may be necessary to keep the esophagus open, assist with nutrition, and control saliva. Palliation may be accomplished with dilation of the esophagus, laser therapy, placement of an endoprosthesis (stent), radiation, or chemotherapy.

Nursing Management

Intervention is directed toward improving the patient's nutritional and physical status in preparation for surgery, RT, or chemotherapy. A program to promote weight gain based on a high-calorie and high-protein diet, in liquid or soft form, is provided if adequate food can be taken by mouth. If this is not possible, parenteral or enteral nutrition is initiated. Nutritional status is monitored throughout treatment. The patient is informed about the nature of the postoperative equipment used, including that required for closed chest drainage, NG suction, parenteral fluid therapy, and gastric intubation.

Immediate postoperative care is similar to that provided for patients undergoing thoracic surgery. It is not uncommon for patients to be placed in an intensive care unit or step-down unit. After recovering from the effects of anesthesia, the patient is placed in a low Fowler position and later in a Fowler position to help prevent reflux of gastric secretions. The patient is observed for regurgitation and dyspnea. A common postoperative complication is aspiration pneumonia. Therefore, the patient is placed on a vigorous pulmonary plan of care that includes incentive spirometry (IS), sitting up in a chair, and, if necessary, nebulizer treatments. Chest physiotherapy is avoided due to the risk of aspiration. The patient's temperature is monitored to detect any elevation that may indicate aspiration or seepage of fluid through the operative site into the mediastinum or pleural cavity (depending on the surgeon's approach), which would mean an esophageal leak. Drainage from the cervical neck wound, usually saliva, is evidence of an early esophageal leak. Typically, no treatment other than NPO and parenteral or enteral support is warranted.

Cardiac complications include atrial fibrillation, which occurs due to irritation of the vagus nerve at the time of surgery. Typical medical management includes digitalization or beta blockade, depending on the patient's response. Cardioversion may be used on rare occasions.

During surgery, an NG tube is inserted and taped or sutured in place. It is connected to low suction.

Pearls for Practice

The NG tube is not manipulated; if displacement occurs, it is not likely to be replaced unless by the surgeon because damage to the anastomosis may occur.

The NG tube is commonly removed 5 to 7 days after surgery. Then a fiberoptic scope is often used by a speech pathologist to evaluate the patient's ability to swallow and rule out possible aspiration before the patient has a Gastrografin study to assess for an anastomotic leak. If a leak into the mediastinum or pleural cavity is visualized, the analysis is stopped immediately, the patient returns to being NPO, and the provider is notified.

If the patient completes both procedures successfully, they are advanced to a regular diet. Small, frequent feedings (6 to 8 per day) are recommended because large quantities of food overload the stomach and promote gastric reflux. When the patient can increase their food and fluid intake to an adequate amount, parenteral fluids are discontinued. After each meal, the patient remains upright for at least 2 hours to allow the food to move through the GI tract. It is a challenge to encourage the patient to eat because the appetite is usually poor. Family involvement and home-cooked favorite foods may help the patient to eat. Antacids may help patients with gastric distress. Metoclopramide helps promote gastric motility. Daily assessment of weight and nutritional intake is essential.

If chemotherapy and radiation are part of the therapy, the patient's appetite will be depressed further, and esophagitis may occur, causing pain when food is eaten. Liquid supplements may be tolerated more easily. However, supplements such as Boost and Ensure should be avoided because they promote *dumping syndrome* when large amounts of osmotically active solids and liquids rapidly "dump" into the duodenum. DS involves nausea and diarrhea that can result in symptoms of dehydration affecting the cardiac and respiratory systems. It can occur with each meal or approximately 20 minutes to 2 hours after eating, and although it can be quite disabling, it typically resolves without incident. (Dumping syndrome is discussed in detail later in this chapter.)

When the patient is ready to go home, the family is instructed about promoting nutrition, what observations to make, what measures to take if complications occur, how to keep the patient comfortable, and how to obtain needed physical and emotional support.

GASTROINTESTINAL INTUBATION

GI intubation involves inserting a tube into the stomach or past the stomach into the duodenum or jejunum. The insertion point can be at the patient's nose, mouth, or abdominal wall.

Clinical Indications

GI intubation can decompress (remove) stomach fluid or air, lavage the stomach in suspected poisonings or drug overdoses, prevent vomiting or aspiration, remove toxins, administer medications and nutrition, and treat an obstruction. The size and type of tube used are determined by its purpose.

Pearls for Practice

When you hear the term "decompression" related to the insertion of an NG tube, you understand that there are conditions that cause a delay or cessation of intestinal peristalsis which would result in gastric distention (since fluid and air would not continue into the intestine) and vomiting and abdominal distention can occur. The temporary insertion of a nasogastric (NG) tube that is connected to suction will empty the gastric contents and keep it empty until peristalsis returns, thus preventing vomiting. This is termed decompression of the stomach.

Tubes

Nasogastric and Orogastric Tubes

Often these types of tubes are used to decompress a stomach distended due to air or fluid. These tubes are of large bore and may be single or double lumen. The Levin tube is a single-lumen tube, ranging from 14 to 18 French (Fr) in size and is made of plastic or rubber with multiple distal openings or "eyes" near its tip (1 Fr equals one third of 1 mm; thus an 18 Fr is 6 mm in diameter). Circular markings at specific points on the tube serve as guides for insertion. The Levin tube is connected to low *intermittent* suction (30 to 40 mm Hg) to avoid erosion of gastric mucosa. The Salem sump tube (SST; discussed shortly) is connected to low continuous suction. Occasionally the tube is placed to gravity, and sometimes it is clamped to assess patient tolerance if the NG tube is withdrawn and minimize the need for reinsertion (Close, 2021; Hodin & Bordejanou, 2022).

Pearls for Practice

If a Levine tube is used, it must be on intermittent low wall suction (30 to 40 mm Hg) to prevent gastric erosion or tearing of the stomach lining (which can result after the stomach contents have been drained from suction, and continuous suction causes invagination of the mucosal lining of the stomach into the "eyes" of the tube).

The smaller the French size, the smaller the lumen of the tube. Contraindications to the placement of NG tubes include facial and head trauma, significant coagulopathies, deviated septum, esophageal trauma or obstruction (Sigmon et al., 2021). Caution is used when inserting NG tubes in patients with esophageal varices as well as postgastric bypass and lap-banding procedures (Koo & Walsh, 2019).

A gastric or SST is a double-lumen tube available in 12 to 18 Fr (although typically a 16 to 18 Fr is used for adults); it is marked from the distal end at particular distances indicated by the manufacturer. The larger main lumen tube is intended for suction, and the smaller lumen or *pigtail*, which is typically blue in color, is termed the *venting port.* The venting port ensures that the suction at the distal end of the tube is maintained at a safe level to preserve the stomach's mucosa by allowing atmospheric air to enter the blue lumen to prevent invagination of the stomach into the multiple distal openings. The blue venting port is never connected to suction or used for irrigation. You can hear a slight whistling from the blue venting port which will indicate the tube is drawing air. An **antireflux valve** can be placed in the venting port of the tube if gastric fluid leaks through the air vent. The venting tube (blue pigtail) must be higher than the stomach level to prevent the siphoning out of gastric contents via this lumen. If leakage has occurred via the air vent lumen (blue port), the larger lumen (one connected to suction) is irrigated with 30 mL of normal saline. Air is injected into the blue port to reestablish a buffer of air between the lumens, and an antireflux valve is applied to the venting lumen. The antireflux valve is a one-way valve that prevents gastric fluid from exiting the SST via the vent lumen (Fig. 21-10). As noted earlier, if an SST is used, it must be on continuous low suction.

Depending on the size of the SST, if gastric decompression is no longer needed, intermittent medications, intermittent liquid feedings, or continuous liquid feedings can be administered via the SST. However, to do so, the venting tube must be plugged to prevent the instilled fluid from leaking out via this lumen. A recent review of this practice offered three reasons why SSTs are not the best choice for tube feedings and they are: (1) a 16-Fr SST diameter is actually much smaller because of the diameter of the air vent lumen (blue port) and is approximately the size of a 12-Fr tube; (2) their study suggested an increased likelihood of tube obstruction due to the multiple distal drainage holes in an SST that cause accumulation of unwashable formula that is difficult to cleanse by flushing; and (3) additionally, "the multiple drainage holes at the distal end of the tube....must be inserted below the gastroesophageal junction, increasing the likelihood of serious injury, which is most likely when tubes are reinserted" (Smith et al., 2021, p. 565). The nurse is aware that replacing the NG tube is distressing for patients and to minimize their discomfort the SST has been used for tube feedings when suction is no longer needed. While research is ongoing, the nurse should follow institutional practices and recognize the balance between benefit versus risk. Residual volumes of stomach are discussed later in the chapter.

Postpyloric Tubes

Tubes that continue past the stomach and enter the duodenum and jejunum are longer, smaller-bore, single-lumen tubes. Duodenal and jejunal tubes are commonly 8 to 10 Fr and 110 to 140 cm long. Most often, postpyloric tubes are inserted into the nares and are designed primarily for continuous feeding into the small intestine when gastric feeding is not desired. Examples of contraindications for gastric feedings include patients with a high risk of aspiration and those undergoing gastric surgery. Patients having pancreatitis or pancreatic surgery may have jejunal tubes placed to rest the pancreas by bypassing the hepatopancreatic ampulla, thereby avoiding the release of digestive enzymes into the duodenum.

Postpyloric tubes can be inserted before or during surgery by interventional radiologists assisted by fluoroscopy or by a trained nurse or health care provider at the bedside.

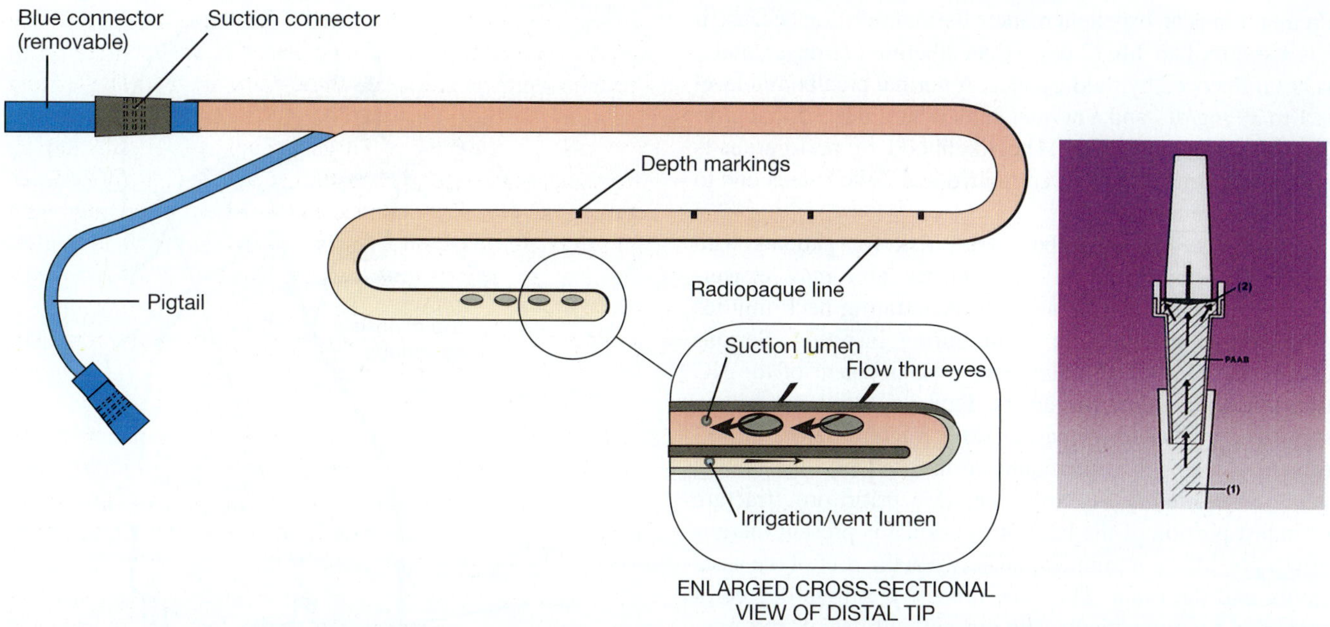

FIGURE 21-10 **Gastric sump tube (Salem) equipped with a one-way valve that allows air to enter and can prevent reflux of gastric contents. The antireflux valve is designed with a pressure-activated air buffer (PAAB). The buffer is activated (1) and the valve closes (2) when pressure from gastric contents enters the tubing. (Courtesy of Lippincott's Nursing Procedures and Skills.)**

At the bedside, the tube is advanced past the stomach actively, using a combination of air bolusing and peristalsis-enhancing medications such as metoclopramide, a gastric motility agent. Another method involves electromagnetic tube placement. In addition, self-advancing systems are available, which use a stylet inside the feeding tube that communicates with a receiver outside the patient's body to indicate the position of the tube tip in the patient's GI tract (see Fig. 21-11). A trained nurse or physician can determine where the tube terminates in the small intestine. This insertion method has been found to decrease the time between placement and initiation of feedings, decrease the number of x-rays, and decrease instances of misplacement and pneumothorax (Smithard et al., 2015).

Passive advancement involves waiting for the stomach and intestine's peristaltic movement to facilitate the tube's migration into the small intestine. Placing the patient on their right side may help advance the tube because gravity may assist the tube in passing through the pyloric sphincter and into the small intestine.

Nursing Management

Assessing the Patient before Tube Placement

When gastric or enteric/postpyloric intubation is ordered for a patient, the nurse needs to review the patient's history to check for contraindications for tube placement. Examples of contraindications include oral or nasal surgery, esophageal varices, esophageal diverticula, and esophageal or gastric surgery, such as a gastric pull-up or gastric bypass in which case, NG tubes should be placed under endoscopy (Sigmon, 2022). Such patients would have a greater risk for perforation, and altered anatomy would make tube placement difficult if the procedure details were unknown. It is also essential to consider the patient's nutritional status before a tube is inserted into their GI tract; serum albumin levels should be assessed.

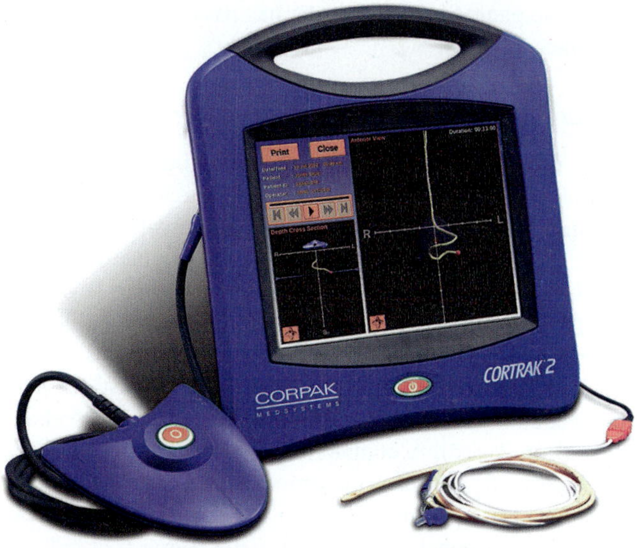

FIGURE 21-11 **All-in-one monitor with integrated visual display terminal, touch screen, and embedded computing system. The stylet tip contains an electromagnetic transmitter that generates a real-time signal as the feeding tube is inserted and advanced to the desired placement. The signal from the transmitting stylet is tracked throughout the placement procedure via a lightweight smart receiver unit (SRU) placed on the patient's xiphoid process. The real-time tube tip tracking aids confident, safe placement. The all-in-one monitor triangulates the signal from the SRU and displays a real-time representation of the feeding tube tip's passage as it proceeds down the esophagus and into the preferred placement position.**

Prealbumin is an excellent marker for malnutrition because it has a shorter half-life (2 days) than albumin (21 days), and it is not influenced by fluid balance. A normal prealbumin level is 1 to 39 mg/dL, and a normal adult albumin is 3.5–5.2 g/dL (Fischbach et al., 2022). The likelihood of perforation is higher in patients with severe nutritional deficiencies due to poor tissue integrity.

Passage of an NG tube carries risk for patients with known or suspected cervical injuries and may exacerbate hemorrhage in patients with penetrating neck injuries if coughing and gagging occur during insertion. Serious complications include pulmonary misplacement of the NG tube and intracranial placement. Patients with head trauma should be evaluated for basilar skull fracture before an NG tube is placed. The tube could be inserted into the cranial vault inadvertently, for example, if a cribriform fracture (thinnest portion of the base of the skull) is present there is now a potential communication between the roof of the nasal cavity and the brain. Thus, the nurse has a high degree of suspicion for any patients who present with facial fractures.

Preparing the Patient

Before the patient is intubated, the nurse explains the purpose of the tube; this information may assist the patient in being cooperative and tolerant of what is often an unpleasant procedure. Then the general activities related to inserting the tube are reviewed, including the fact that the patient may have to breathe through the mouth and that the procedure may cause gagging until the tube has passed the area of the gag reflex.

Inserting the Tube

Before inserting the tube, the nurse determines the length of tubing that will be needed to reach the stomach or the small intestine. A mark is made on the tube to indicate the desired length. There are several methods to estimate the depth that the tube should be placed, however all have some degree of error (Sigmon, 2022). One method to determine the length is by measuring the distance from the tip of the **n**ose to the **e**arlobe and from the earlobe to the **x**iphoid process for gastric placement and adding 10 cm (Taylor, 2020: Torsy et al., 2018) (Fig. 21-12). A common error in inserting NG tubes is to incorrectly estimate the proper length of the tube that should be inserted. Thus, NG tubes may be inserted too short (in the lower esophagus) or coiled in the stomach.

Inserting the tube is not a sterile procedure; the nurse and other staff involved should follow Universal Precautions procedures designated by their facility (gloves, gown, and face mask are recommended). While the tube is being inserted, the patient usually sits upright with a towel or some type of protective barrier spread bib-fashion over the chest. Tissue wipes are made available. Privacy and adequate light are provided. The provider may swab the nostril and spray the oropharynx with tetracaine/benzocaine at least 5 minutes before the procedure to numb the nasal passage and suppress the gag reflex. This makes the entire process more tolerable. Having the patient gargle with a liquid anesthetic or hold ice chips in the mouth for a few minutes can have a similar effect. Encouraging the patient to breathe through the mouth or pant often helps, as does swallowing water, if permitted.

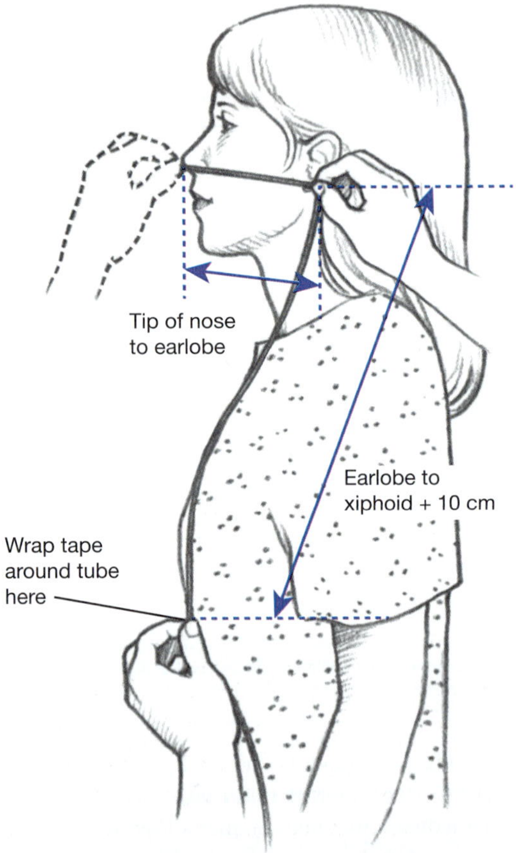

FIGURE 21-12 Measuring the length of the nasogastric tube for placement into the stomach. To determine how long the NG tube must be to reach the stomach, hold the end of the tube at the tip of the patient's nose. Extend the tube to the patient's earlobe and then down to the xiphoid process, + 10 cm (as shown above). (Reprinted with permission from *Nursing Procedures* [4th ed.]. Lippincott Williams & Wilkins, 2004.)

A polyurethane tube may need to be warmed to make it more pliable. To make the tube easier to insert, it should be lubricated with a water-soluble lubricant unless it has a hydrophilic coating.

The patient is placed in the Fowler position, and the nostrils are inspected for any obstruction. The more patent nostril is selected for use. The tip of the patient's nose is tilted up, and the tube is aligned to enter the nostril, following the floor of the nose (under the inferior turbinate), not upward toward the nasal bridge. The tube is advanced slowly to avoid pressure on the nasal turbinates until the posterior pharynx is reached. If significant resistance is encountered, the other nostril is tried rather than forcing the tube (Sigmon, 2022). When the tube reaches the posterior pharynx, the patient can rest for a few minutes before proceeding. Unless contraindicated, the patient is instructed to flex the neck to facilitate passage into the esophagus and to begin to swallow as the tube is advanced to the predetermined depth. The patient may also sip water through a straw to facilitate the advancement of the tube unless drinking is contraindicated. The oropharynx is inspected to ensure that the tube has not been coiled in the pharynx or mouth.

Confirming Placement

To ensure patient safety, it is essential to confirm that the tube has been placed correctly: the tube may be inserted into the lungs inadvertently, and this may go undetected in high-risk patients (e.g., those with decreased levels of consciousness, confused mental states, poor or absent cough and gag reflexes, or agitation during insertion). The gold standard for verifying placement of a blindly inserted tube is the radiographic or x-ray confirmation (Ecklund, 2017; Sigmon, 2022). X-ray confirmation of the lower chest/upper abdomen (abdominal radiograph) is necessary if the patient will be receiving feedings or medications through the tube. Once the x-ray confirms appropriate placement, the nurse notes the mark where the tube exits the nares or mouth (when the NG tube is placed orally) and document the incremental length (the number found on the tube in centimeters) and also the centimeter mark at the nares or mouth (Judd, 2020). If there is any change in the length of the external portion of the tube, the nurse is aware that tube migration may have occurred (Judd, 2020). When a tube is used to remove air or fluid and not instillation, the nurse can use a combination of visually assessing the aspirate, testing its pH, and using capnographic devices to determine placement. Visual assessment of the color of the aspirate may help identify tube placement. The gastric aspirate is most frequently cloudy and green, tan or off-white, or bloody or brown. The intestinal aspirate is primarily clear and yellow to bile-colored. The pleural fluid is usually pale yellow and serous, and tracheobronchial secretions usually consist of tan or off-white mucus. The appearance of the aspirate may help distinguish between gastric and intestinal placement but is of little value in ruling out respiratory placement.

Determining the pH of the tube aspirate is a more accurate method of confirming tube placement than is maintaining tube length or visually assessing tube aspirate. The pH method also can be used to monitor the advancement of the tube into the small intestine. The pH of gastric aspirate is acidic (1 to 5), typically less than 4. The pH of intestinal aspirate is approximately 6 or higher, and the pH of respiratory aspirate is more alkaline (greater than 6).

Patients receiving histamine 2 (H_2)-receptor antagonists or PPIs may demonstrate pH ranges from 0 to 6, which can affect pH by medications or formulas. This alkaline aspirate similar to the pH of pulmonary secretions could lead to malpositioned feeding tube (Methany et al., 2019). Therefore, testing the pH remains an area where further research is warranted. Capnography involves detecting carbon dioxide at the external end of the NG tubes which suggests placement in the tracheobronchial tree rather than the stomach. However, capnography cannot distinguish between placement in the esophagus and the stomach which can occur if the tube migrates into the esophagus which increases the risk for aspiration (Judd, 2020). In a recent systematic review involving 16 studies looking at the placement of feeding tubes in the lungs versus the GI tract found the effectiveness of capnographic methods to have a low to very low certainty of evidence (Chau et al., 2021). More recently, point-of-care ultrasound (POCUS) by nonradiologist is being investigated to confirm NGT insertion, and may show promise in the future (McMullen et al., 2022).

Placement also must be ensured at regular intervals once the device is placed. These times include when medications or fluids are given and every 4 hours for patients receiving continuous tube feedings. The traditional method was to inject air through the tube while auscultating the epigastric area with a stethoscope to detect air insufflation. However, research reveals that distinguishing variations in the sound of the air bubble entering the lungs, esophagus, stomach, or small intestine is not possible, thus this method is not accurate to determine placement (AACN, 2018; Judd, 2020). Instead of the auscultation method, a combination of four methods is recommended: assessing the patient's tolerance to medication and feeding administration, measurement of tube length, visual assessment of aspirate, and evaluate the pH measurement of aspirate.

To determine the feeding tolerance to ascertain placement, the nurse assesses the patient's respiratory status. Coughing, gagging, and decreased pulse oximetry could indicate that the tube has migrated. The nurse also inspects the oral cavity to visualize the tube in the back of the patient's throat. A patient can regurgitate the tube into the mouth with frequent gagging and coughing.

The nurse measures the exposed tube length every 4 hours and before administering enteral feeding or medications and compares it with the original measurement (Judd, 2020). An increase in the length of the exposed tube may indicate dislodgment.

Securing the Tube

After the correct position of the tip of the tube has been confirmed, the NG tube is secured to the nose (Fig. 21-13). A liquid skin barrier can be applied to the skin where the NG tube will be secured. The prepared area is covered with a strip of hypoallergenic tape, and then the tube is placed over the tape and secured with a second piece of tape. Instead of tape, several companies have feeding tube device holders that can be utilized. A nasal bridle can be used in patients in multiple levels of care who have a history of tube dislodgment due, for example, to impaired mental status related to dementia or traumatic brain injury. Bridling (Fig. 21-14) involves the insertion of a loop of strong but flexible material through the naris, around the nasal septum, and out the other

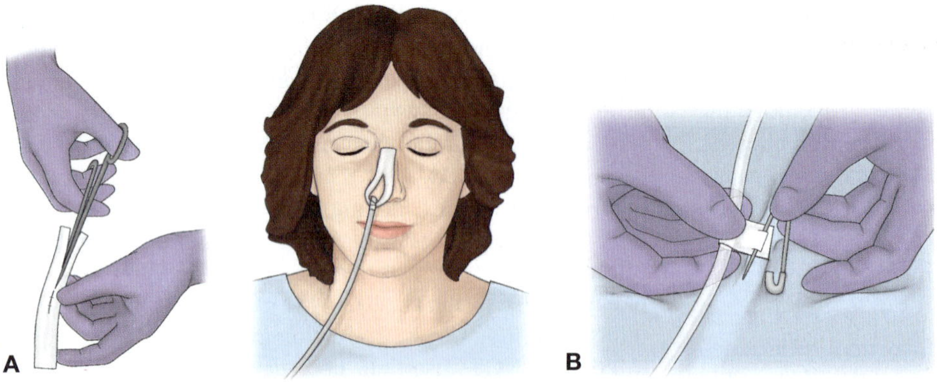

FIGURE 21-13 **Securing nasogastric (NG) tubes. A. The NG tube is secured to the nose with tape to prevent injury to the nasopharyngeal passages. B. The tubing is secured to the patient's gown with tape attached to a safety pin to avoid tension on the line.**

nare as a "bridle" to which the nasoenteric tube is secured. A recent meta-analysis involving 15 studies found no major nasal injuries associated with bridle usage, minor epistaxis, and minor ulcerations were reported (Lynch et al., 2018). In addition, it is wise to secure the NG tube to the patient's gown or pajamas with an elastic band and safety pin or with adhesive tape loops so that a tug on the tube will not pull on the nares. The NG tube must be secured without putting undue pressure on the medial or lateral nares to prevent tissue necrosis. In addition, the tape securing the tube should be changed daily, and the nares should be inspected for complications such as erosion (Baranoski & Ayello, 2020). The tube must be looped loosely to prevent tension and dislodgment.

Pearls for Practice

If the patient is ambulatory and has an SST, the blue pigtail must be above the stomach level to prevent gastric fluid from leaking out via this port. The pigtail can be fitted into the larger suction lumen to seal the NG tube while the patient is ambulating.

Monitoring the Patient and Maintaining Tube Function

It is essential to keep an accurate record of all fluid intake, feedings, and irrigation. When the NG tube is maintained to suction, the tube is irrigated every 4 to 6 hours with normal saline to avoid electrolyte loss through gastric drainage to maintain patency. The nurse records the amount, color, and type of all drainage every 8 hours.

When double- or triple-lumen tubes are used, each lumen is labeled according to its intended use: aspiration, feeding, or balloon inflation (refer to Sengstaken-Blakemore tube in Chapter 24).

When feedings or medications are ordered for administration through a GI tube, the nurse's responsibility is to maintain the patency and assess the patient's tolerance of the feeding or meds. Liquid nutritional solutions are commonly administered continuously via a programmable electronic pump or by syringe in intermittent boluses. The nurse needs to assess the feed volume in the bag to ensure it does not run dry with continuous feedings.

Administering Medication

When medications are administered through GI tubes, flushing the tube with 30 to 50 mL of (sterile) water and 15 mL after administration may decrease the risk of tube occlusion (Boullata et al., 2017; Cleary, 2022). With NG tubes and small-diameter nasoenteric tubes, complete crushing of medications in pill form is a necessity. Medications are not added to the nutrition formula since drug interactions may occur. If possible, a nurse should collaborate with the medical team and pharmacy to convert medications to liquid forms. Also, the nurse should be aware that administering extended-release tablets that would require crushing through such tubes is prohibited since overdosage can result.

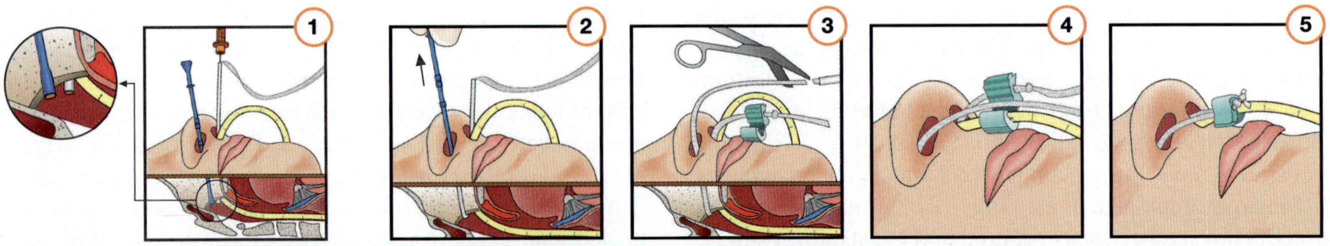

FIGURE 21-14 **A bridle nasal tube retaining system. The placement entails: (1) Advance catheter stylet and blue probe in opposite nares until magnets connect. Remove the orange stylet from the catheter. (2) Slowly remove the blue probe, drawing the white catheter around the vomer bone and out the opposite nare. (3) Cut the catheter off and discard. (4) Place tube and umbilical tape in clip. (5) Securely close clip 1 cm below the nose. Tie two to three knots and cut off the excess. (Reprinted with permission from AMT Bridle Nasal Tube Retaining System from Applied Medical Technology, Inc.)**

TABLE **21-1 Preparing Medication for Delivery by Feeding Tube**

Medication Form	Preparation
Liquid	None
Simple compressed tablets	Crush and dissolve in water
Buccal or sublingual tablets	Administer as prescribed
Soft gelatin capsules filled with liquid	Make an opening in the capsule and squeeze the contents out into water to dissolve
Enteric-coated tablets	Do not crush; change in form is required; consult pharmacy department as needed
Timed-release tablets	Do not crush tablets because doing so may release too much drug too quickly (overdose); check with pharmacist for alternative formulation
Timed-release capsules or sustained-release capsules	Some can be opened and contents added to tube-feeding formula; *always* check with pharmacist before doing this

However, occasionally, time-released capsules are permitted to be opened (not crushed) and administered. Pharmacy staff should be consulted if any questions or concerns exist about whether medications can be crushed or opened. The medical team should be notified to have the medications changed to liquid form whenever possible. Table 21-1 discusses administering medications.

Unclogging Tubes

When a tube becomes clogged with feedings or medications, several methods can be used to reestablish the patency of the tube without having to replace it. Smaller-diameter postpyloric tubes can clog if feedings are stopped and the tube is not flushed correctly. Warm water can be administered through the tube with caution using varying syringes; smaller syringes have a greater force to dislodge the clog. Cola and cranberry juice have historically been recommended as an effective, noninvasive means of unclogging tubes; however, a more consistently effective method involves instilling a mixture of pancreatic enzymes and sodium bicarbonate into the tube for 20 minutes to digest the clog. The nurse is aware that correct NG tube placement must be confirmed before any mixture is injected to unclog the tube.

Providing Oral and Nasal Hygiene

Regular and conscientious oral and nasal hygiene is vital for patient care because the tube causes discomfort and pressure and may be in place for several days. Moistened cotton-tipped swabs can be used to clean the nose, followed by cleansing with a water-soluble lubricant. Frequent mouth care is comforting for the patient. The nasal tape is changed daily, and the nose is inspected for skin irritation. If the nasal and pharyngeal mucosa is excessively dry, steam or cool vapor inhalations may be beneficial. Throat lozenges, an ice collar, chewing gum, or sucking on hard candies (if permitted) as well as limiting talking also assist in relieving patient discomfort. These activities keep the mucous membranes moist and help prevent inflammation of the parotid glands.

Monitoring and Managing Potential Complications

Problems associated with nasoenteric intubation include fluid volume deficit (FVD), pulmonary complications, and tube-related irritations. These potential complications require careful ongoing assessment.

Symptoms of FVD include dry skin and mucous membranes, decreased urinary output, increased urine specific gravity, lethargy, orthostatic hypotension, and increased heart rate. Also, a nurse can calculate the patient's pulse pressure (systolic blood pressure minus diastolic blood pressure) to predict the patient's volume status. A pulse pressure of less than 30 mm Hg is indicative of FVD. Assessment of FVD involves maintaining an accurate record of intake and output. This includes measuring NG or nasointestinal (NI) drainage, fluid instilled by irrigation of the NG/NI tube, water taken by mouth, vomitus, water administered with tube feedings, and IV fluids. Laboratory values, particularly electrolytes and blood urea nitrogen and creatinine, are monitored. The nurse assesses 24-hour fluid balance and reports negative fluid balance, increased NG output, interruption of IV therapy, or any other disturbance in fluid intake or output and weight.

Pulmonary complications from NG intubation occur because coughing and clearing of the pharynx are impaired, because gas buildup can irritate the phrenic nerve, and because tubes may become dislodged, retracting the distal end above the esophagogastric sphincter (which places the patient at risk for aspiration or breathing fluids or foods into the trachea and lungs). Medications such as metoclopramide can be administered to decrease potential problems. Signs and symptoms of complications include coughing during the administration of foods or medications, difficulty clearing the airway, tachypnea, and fever. Assessment includes regular auscultation of lung sounds and routine inspection of vital signs. It is essential to encourage the patient to cough and to take deep breaths regularly. The nurse also carefully confirms the proper placement of the tube by assessing tube length before instilling any fluids or medications.

Irritation of the mucous membranes is a common complication of NG/NI intubation. The nostrils, oral mucosa, esophagus, and trachea are susceptible to irritation and necrosis. Visible areas are inspected frequently, and the adequacy of hydration is assessed. When providing oral hygiene, the nurse carefully checks the mucous membranes for signs of irritation or excessive dryness. The nurse palpates the area around the parotid glands to detect any tenderness or enlarged nodes, indicating parotitis, and observes for any irritation or skin breakdown at the insertion site (e.g., nares) or of the mucous membranes. To preserve the skin integrity of the nares, the nurse should rotate the position of the tube on the wall of the nares once every 24 hours. In addition, it is crucial to assess the patient for esophagitis and tracheitis; symptoms include sore throat and hoarseness.

Pearls for Practice

The nurse alerts the health provider when new frank bleeding is noted in the NG tube drainage or if "coffee-ground material" is noted because it may indicate bleeding. Gastroccult testing is available to assess the presence of blood in gastric drainage. The nurse is aware that hemoccult test for stool cannot be used for evaluation of gastric drainage.

Removing the Tube

Before removing a tube, the nurse may clamp and unclamp it intermittently for a trial period of several hours to ensure that the patient does not experience nausea, vomiting, or distention. Before the tube is removed, it is flushed with 10 mL of water or normal saline to ensure it is free of debris and away from the gastric lining. Gloves are worn to remove the tube, and a towel or disposable pad is placed on the patient's chest. The tape or tube fixation device is removed from the nares and the tube is unsecured from the patient's gown. The tube is withdrawn gently and slowly for 15 to 20 cm (6 to 8 in) until the tip reaches the esophagus; the remainder is removed rapidly from the nostril. If the tube does not come out quickly, force should not be used, and the problem should be reported to the provider. As the tube is withdrawn, it is concealed in the disposable pad or towel to prevent secretions from soiling the patient or nurse. After the tube is removed, the nurse provides oral hygiene.

Administering Tube Feedings With Nasogastric and Nasoenteric Devices

Enteral nutrition feedings are given to meet nutritional requirements when oral intake is inadequate or impossible, and the GI tract is functioning normally. Tube feedings have several advantages over PN: they are low in cost, safe, well tolerated by the patient, and easy to use both in extended-care facilities and the patient's home. Other advantages include:

- Preserving GI integrity by delivery of nutrients and medications intraluminally
- Preserving the typical sequence of intestinal and hepatic metabolism
- Maintaining fat metabolism and lipoprotein synthesis
- Maintaining normal insulin/glucagon ratios

Tube feedings are delivered to the stomach (in the case of NG intubation or gastrostomy) or the distal duodenum or proximal jejunum (in the case of **nasoduodenal** or **nasojejunal tube** feeding). Nasoduodenal or nasojejunal feeding is indicated when the esophagus and stomach need to be bypassed or when the patient is at risk for aspiration. For long-term feedings (longer than 4 weeks), gastrostomy or jejunostomy tubes are preferred to administer medications or food. The numerous conditions requiring enteral nutrition are summarized in Table 21-2.

TABLE 21-2 Conditions Requiring Enteral Therapy

Condition or Need	Examples
GI problems	Fistula, short-bowel syndrome, mild pancreatitis, Crohn disease, ulcerative colitis, nonspecific maldigestion or malabsorption
Cancer therapy	Radiation, chemotherapy
Convalescent care	Surgery, injury, severe illness
Coma, semiconsciousness[a]	Stroke, head injury, neurologic disorder, neoplasm
Hypermetabolic conditions	Burns, trauma, multiple fractures, sepsis, AIDS, organ transplantation
Chronic illness, psychiatric or neurologic disorder	Alcohol use disorder, chronic depression, anorexia nervosa[a]
Debilitation[a]	Disease or injury
Maxillofacial or cervical surgery	Disease or injury, wired jaw, spinal cord injury
Oropharyngeal or esophageal paralysis[a]	Disease or injury, neoplasm, inflammation, trauma, respiratory failure

[a]Because some of these patients are at risk for regurgitating or vomiting and aspirating administered formula, each condition must be considered individually.

Reducing the Risk of Aspiration

To decrease the risk of aspiration and subsequent pneumonia, the head of the bed must remain elevated to 30 to 45 degrees at all times if appropriate for the patient's condition (AACN, 2018; Perry et al., 2022a). An elevated head of bed may not be suitable for some patients, such as those with spinal injuries or mobility restrictions, due to interventional procedures involving the vasculature of the groin. In these cases, it may be appropriate to adjust the hospital bed to a reverse Trendelenburg position per health care provider's order to decrease aspiration risk. If the patient is on bed rest, the tube feeding must be shut off when bed making, bathing, or anytime the head of the bed must be lowered to below 30 degrees. In the event that the tube feeding is shut off for an extended period of time, the tube-feeding rate is not adjusted to "catch up"; the rate is maintained as ordered (Perry et al., 2022a).

Residual Assessment

Patient tolerance of liquid enteral nutrition is determined by residual measurement, the presence or absence of nausea and vomiting, and increasing abdominal distention. Residual measurement or volume of aspiration is most easily assessed with large-bore GI tubes. Smaller-diameter nasojejunal tubes and duodenal tubes often collapse when suction is applied. The volume of aspirate indicates the rate at which the patient is digesting the feedings and how quickly the chyme is passing into the small intestine. The stomach volume is approximately 1 L, with an ability to stretch with increased intake depending on the size of the patient.

A 60-mL syringe is used to measure volumes from feeding tubes every 4 hours to assess gastric residuals. The nurse slowly applies steady pressure on the plunger and aspirates the residual volume until no more fluid can be withdrawn into the syringe. Policies vary according to institutions, and the nurse should follow unit guidelines. The American Society of Parenteral and Enteral Nutrition recommends that if gastric residual volumes are measured in ICU patients, feedings should be held for volumes over 500 mL (Boullata et al., 2017). The relationship between gastric residual volume on complications such as vomiting, pneumonia, aspiration, and increased mortality is unclear (Yasuda et al., 2021). Because individual procedures vary widely, and uncertainty exists regarding the assessment and treatment in high residual volumes, it is essential to follow institutional guidelines closely and hold feedings as indicated.

Osmosis, Osmolality, and Dumping Syndrome

Osmolality is an essential consideration for patients receiving tube feedings through the duodenum or jejunum. Feeding formulas with a high osmolality may lead to undesirable effects, such as dumping syndrome.

Fluid balance is maintained by **osmosis**, the process by which water moves through membranes from a dilute solution of lower **osmolality** (ionic concentration) to a more concentrated solution of higher osmolality until both solutions are of nearly equal osmolality. The osmolality of normal body fluids is approximately 300 mOsm/kg. The body attempts to keep the osmolality of the contents of the stomach and intestines at roughly this level.

Highly concentrated solutions and certain foods can upset the normal fluid balance in the body. Individual amino acids and carbohydrates are tiny particles that have a significant osmotic effect. Electrolytes, such as sodium and potassium, are comparatively small particles; they significantly affect osmolality and, consequently, the patient's ability to tolerate a given solution.

When a concentrated solution of high osmolality is administered in large amounts, water moves to the stomach and intestines from fluid surrounding the organs and the vascular compartment. The patient has a feeling of fullness, nausea, and diarrhea; this causes dehydration, hypotension, and tachycardia, collectively termed **dumping syndrome**. Patients vary in the degree to which they tolerate the effects of high osmolality; usually, debilitated patients are less tolerant. The nurse needs to be knowledgeable about the osmolality of the patient's formula and needs to observe for and take steps to prevent undesired effects. The following interventions can prevent dumping syndrome: using room-temperature feedings (gastric emptying will be faster if the temperature of the fluid is too hot or too cold), changing from **bolus** to continuous feedings if appropriate, having the patient remain in a semi-Fowler position for 1 hour after eating to allow the feedings to pass into the intestine gradually, and slowing the rate of feedings to allow more time for digestion.

Suppose a tube feeding uses a high-osmolality formula, in this case, the nurse observes the patient's sodium level and expects free water to be ordered by diluting the tube feeding or by periodic instillation of water by the health care team if rising sodium levels are seen. Response to the free water (either dilution of tube feeding or tap water instilled via the NG/NI tube) is assessed with subsequent electrolyte levels.

Pearls for Practice

The nurse understands that administering medication via an enteral tube is not the same as PO (per os or by mouth). For example, liquid antibiotics, laxatives, and vitamin and electrolyte solutions far exceed the osmolality of GI secretions (approximately 300 mOsm/kg). The practice of crushing multiple tablets and mixing powders together before administration is an unsafe habit. Mixing drugs together, whether solid or liquid, creates an unknown substance with an unpredictable mechanism of release and bioavailability. Proper flushing of the tube before, between, and after ***each*** *drug is recommended. Also, enteral feeding needs to be stopped and the feeding tube needs to be flushed before medication is administered. The pharmacist should be consulted regarding medication administration. Refer to the do not crush list at http://www.ismp.org/tools/donotcrush.pdf for specific information.*

Tube-Feeding Formulas

The choice of formula to be delivered by tube feeding is influenced by the GI tract's status and the patient's nutritional needs. Dietitians collaborate with providers and nurses to determine the best formula for the individual patient. The formula characteristics considered before selection include the chemical composition of the nutrient source (protein, carbohydrates, fat), caloric density, osmolality, residue, bacteriologic safety, vitamins, minerals, and cost.

Various major formula types for tube feedings are available commercially. Commercially prepared polymeric formulas (formulas with high molecular weight) are composed of protein, carbohydrates, and fats in a high–molecular-weight form (e.g., Boost Plus, TwoCal HN, Isosource). Chemically defined tube-feeding formulas (e.g., Peptamen 1.5 or Vivonex) contain predigested and easy-to-absorb nutrients. Modular products have only one major nutrient, such as protein (Beneprotein). Disease-specific formulas are available for various conditions. For patients with kidney failure, a formula such as Nepro, high in calories and low in electrolytes, is ideal because it is formulated to maintain electrolyte and fluid balance. For patients with severe chronic obstructive pulmonary disease, a formula such as Pulmocare may be selected because it is high in fat and low in carbohydrates, has a high density (1.5 calories/mL) that helps maintain fluid restriction and reduces carbon dioxide production. Excess carbohydrates may increase the production of CO_2, and this negatively impacts respiratory status. Fiber is added to some formulas (e.g., Jevity) to decrease the occurrence of diarrhea in some at-risk patients. Blenderized formulas also can be used. They can be made by the patient's family or obtained in a ready-to-use form that is carefully prepared according to directions. Some feedings are given as supplements, and others are designed to meet the patient's total nutritional needs.

Administration Methods and Frequency

The tube feeding and administration method frequency depend on the tube's location in the GI tract, patient tolerance, convenience, and cost. Intermittent bolus feedings are administered into the stomach (usually by gastrostomy tube) in large amounts at designated intervals and may be given four to eight times per day. The intermittent gravity drip, another method for administering tube feedings into the stomach, is commonly used when the patient is at home. In this instance, the tube feeding is administered over 30 minutes at designated intervals. Both of these tube-feeding methods are practical and inexpensive. However, the feedings delivered at variable rates may be poorly tolerated and time-consuming.

Often the continuous infusion method is used when feedings are administered into the small intestine. This method is preferred for patients at risk for aspiration or who tolerate tube feedings poorly (Heuschkel & Duggan, 2019). The feedings are given continuously at a constant rate using a pump. This method decreases abdominal distention, gastric residuals, and the risk of aspiration. However, pumps are expensive, and they allow the patient less flexibility than intermittent feedings.

An alternative to the continuous infusion method is **cyclic feeding**. The infusion is administered at a higher hourly volume over 8- to 12-hour intervals to meet the prescribed calories and macronutrients for 24 hours. Feedings may be infused at night to avoid interrupting the patient's lifestyle. Cyclic continuous infusions may be appropriate for patients being weaned from tube feedings to an oral diet, as supplements for patients who cannot eat enough, and for patients at home who need daytime hours free from the pump. Whichever method is chosen, the head of the bed must be maintained at a minimum of 30 degrees to decrease the risk of aspiration. A wide variety of containers, feeding tubes and catheters, delivery systems, and pumps are available for use with tube feedings. For patients who require long-term tube feedings resources such as the Oley Foundation are available for education, outreach, and networking (https://oley.org/) (Perry et al., 2022a).

Complications of Tube Feedings

Diarrhea, the most common complication associated with liquid feedings, is commonly due to the hyperosmolality of the feedings and the decreased serum osmolality of the patient's serum. Changing the concentration or type of formula often reduces or stops this complication.

Aspiration pneumonia is an essential mechanical complication. Aspiration can occur due to improperly placed tubes or when the patient vomits the formula into the airway. When aspiration occurs or is suspected, the nurse needs to stop the feeding, suction the pharynx and trachea, and closely assess the patient's respiratory status while contacting the provider. Aspiration prevention involves keeping the patient's head of the bed elevated to at least 30 degrees, verifying the tube placement on insertion, before food or medication administration, and periodically throughout a 24-hour shift.

Patients may have increased blood glucose as a metabolic complication of tube feedings. Carbohydrate content varies between the different types of the formula used and should be considered if the patient is hyperglycemic. The nurse should assess the patient's blood sugar frequently, especially when initiating a tube feeding. Additional complications of enteral therapy can be found in Table 21-3.

GASTROSTOMY

A **gastrostomy** is a surgical procedure in which an opening is created into the stomach to administer foods and fluids via a feeding tube.

Clinical Indications

Gastrostomy is preferred for prolonged enteral nutrition support when the patient's diagnosis makes it difficult to support the nutritional requirements, such as in patients with traumatic brain injury and neurodegenerative diseases (Alzheimer disease). Gastrostomy is also preferred over NG feedings in the comatose patient because the gastroesophageal sphincter remains intact. Regurgitation and aspiration are less likely to occur with a gastrostomy than with NG feedings.

Types

Different types of feeding gastrostomies may be used, including the Stamm (temporary and permanent), Janeway (permanent), and **percutaneous endoscopic gastrostomy (PEG)** tube (temporary) systems. The Stamm and Janeway gastrostomies require either an upper abdominal midline

TABLE **21-3 Complications of Enteral Therapy**

Complications	Causes	Selected Nursing Interventions: Treatment	Selected Nursing Interventions: Prevention
Gastrointestinal			
Diarrhea (most common)	Hyperosmolar feedings Rapid infusion/bolus feedings Bacteria-contaminated feedings Lactase deficiency Medications/antibiotic therapy Decreased serum osmolality level Food allergies Cold formula	Assess fluid balance and electrolyte levels; report findings Implement changes in tube-feeding formula or rate	Assess rate of infusion and temperature of formula Replace formula every 4 hours; change tube-feeding container and tubing daily
Nausea/vomiting	Change in formula or rate Hyperosmolar formula Inadequate gastric emptying	Review medications	Check residuals; if >200 mL consider promotility medications, if >500 mL, check with provider. (because individual procedures vary widely, it is important to follow institutional procedures closely and to hold feedings as indicated)
Gas/bloating/cramping	Air in tube	Notify provider if persistent	Keep tubing free of air
Dumping syndrome	Bolus feedings/rapid rate Cold formula	Check fiber and water content; report findings Check rate and temperature of formula	Avoid rapid infusion of feeding Administer feeding at or near room temperature
Constipation	High milk (lactose) content Lack of fiber Inadequate fluid intake/dehydration Opioid use	Check fiber and water content; report findings	Administer adequate amount of hydration as flushes
Mechanical			
Aspiration pneumonia	Improper tube placement Vomiting with aspiration of tube feeding Flat in bed Use of large tube	Assess respiratory status and notify provider	Implement reliable method for checking small-bore enteral tube placement (i.e., measuring length of exposed tube) Keep head of bed elevated 30–45 degrees continuously
Tube displacement	Excessive coughing/vomitus Tension on the tube or unsecured tube Tracheal suctioning Airway intubation	Stop feeding and notify provider	Check tube placement before administering feeding
Tube obstruction	Inadequate flushing/formula rate/inadequate medication crushing	Follow policy for declogging feeding tubes	Obtain liquid medications when possible, flush tube and medications adequately
Residue	Inadequate crushing of medications and flushing after administration		Flush tube and crush medications adequately
Nasopharyngeal irritation	Tube position/improper taping Use of large tubes	Assess nasopharyngeal mucous membranes every 4 hours	Tape tube to prevent pressure on nares

(*continued*)

TABLE 21-3 **Complications of Enteral Therapy (*continued*)**

		Selected Nursing Interventions	
Complications	**Causes**	**Treatment**	**Prevention**
Metabolic			
Hyperglycemia	Glucose intolerance High carbohydrate content of the feeding	Check blood glucose levels periodically Request dietary consult to reevaluate choice of feeding product	Collaborate with dietician for potential solution changes
Dehydration and azotemia (excessive urea in the blood)	Hyperosmolar feedings with insufficient fluid intake	Report signs and symptoms of dehydration Implement changes in tube-feeding formula, rate, or ratio to water	Provide adequate hydration through flushes or dilution of tube feeding

incision or a left upper quadrant transverse incision. The Stamm procedure involves using concentric pursestring sutures to secure the tube to the anterior gastric wall. To create the gastrostomy, an exit wound is made in the left upper abdomen. The Janeway procedure necessitates the creation of a tunnel (called a *gastric tube*) that is brought out through the abdomen to form a permanent **stoma**.

Insertion of a PEG requires the services of two physicians (or a physician and a nurse with specialty skills). After administering a local anesthetic, one health care provider inserts a cannula into the stomach through an abdominal incision and then threads a nonabsorbable suture through the cannula; the second provider inserts an endoscope via the patient's upper GI tract and uses the endoscopic snare to grasp the end of the suture and guide it up through the patient's mouth. The suture is knotted to the dilator tip at the end of the PEG tube. Then the provider who inserted the endoscope advances the dilator tip through the patient's mouth while the first provider pulls the suture through the cannula site. The attached PEG tube is guided down the esophagus, into the stomach, and out through the abdominal incision (Fig. 21-15). The mushroom catheter tip and internal crossbar secure the tube against the stomach wall. An external crossbar or bumper keeps the catheter in place. A tubing adaptor is in place between feedings, and a clamp or plug is used to close or open the tubing.

The initial PEG device can be removed and replaced once the tract is well established (10 to 14 days after insertion). Replacement of the PEG device is indicated to provide long-term nutritional support, replace a clogged or migrated tube, or enhance patient comfort. The PEG replacement device should be fitted securely to the stoma to prevent leakage of gastric acid and is maintained in place through traction between the internal and anchoring devices.

An alternative to the PEG device is a **low-profile gastrostomy device (LPGD)** (see Fig. 21-15). The LPGD may be inserted 3 to 6 months after initial gastrostomy tube placement. These devices are inserted flush with the skin; they

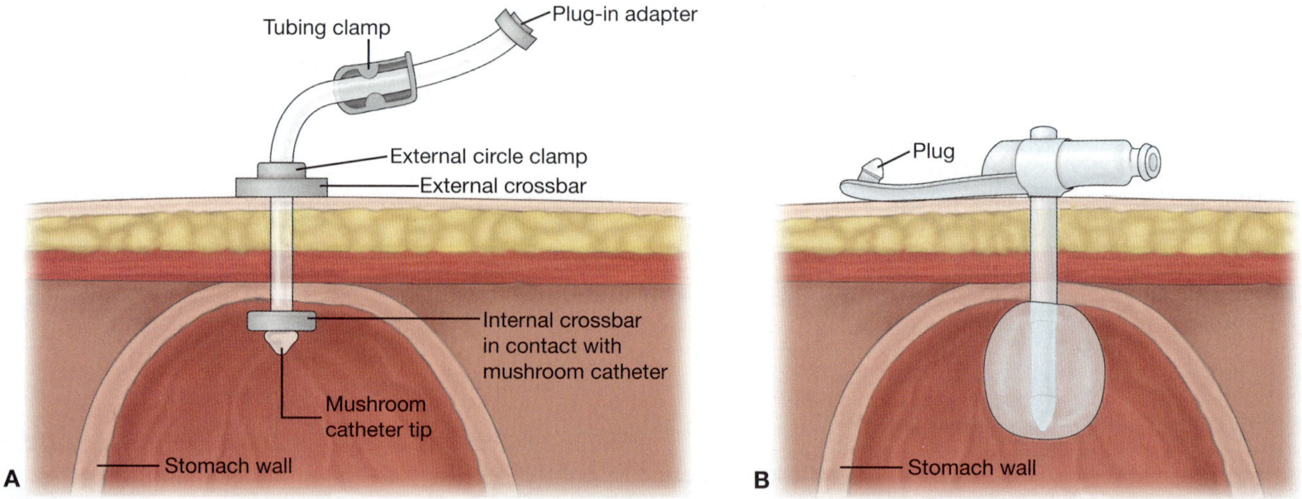

FIGURE 21-15 **A. A detail of the abdomen and the percutaneous endoscopic gastrostomy (PEG) tube, showing catheter fixation. B. A detail of the abdomen and the nonobturated low-profile gastrostomy device (LPGD) showing balloon fixation.**

eliminate the possibility of tube migration and obstruction and have antireflux valves to prevent gastric reflux. Two types of devices may be used—obturated or nonobturated. The obturated devices (G-button) have a dome tip that acts as an internal stabilizer. Only a physician may obturate (insert a tube that is larger than the actual stoma). The nonobturated device (MIC-KEY) has an external skin disk inserted into the stoma without force; a balloon is inflated to secure placement. A nurse in the home setting may insert these nonobturated devices. The drawbacks of both types of LPGDs are the inability to assess residual volumes (one-way valve) and the need for a special adaptor to connect the device to the feeding container.

Complications

Reflux from stomach feedings can result in aspiration pneumonia. Therefore, patients at risk for aspiration pneumonia are not ideal candidates for a gastrostomy. A jejunostomy is preferred, or jejunal feeding through a nasojejunal tube may be recommended.

Other complications of gastrostomy tube placement include premature removal, infection, and leakage around the insertion site. A loosely taped dressing can be placed over the top of the tube flange to prevent early removal. A fenestrated drape (split dressing) often used for tracheotomy care works well. In addition, a tube-securing device can be placed on the patient's abdomen or flank to decrease the tension on the insertion site further. These devices use adhesives and Velcro to fix the gastrostomy tube to the patient's skin temporarily. The nurse should educate the patient on how much mobility they have with the gastrostomy tube to prevent tension on the device (excessive movement is considered more than ¼ in [6 mm]) of the tube in or out of the stomach (Perry et al., 2022a). If the tube is removed inadvertently, the nurse should clean the site, place a dressing, and notify the provider as soon as possible.

Infection is prevented by assessing and cleansing the site daily. Soap and water can be used around the general area. To remove hardened feedings that may accumulate around the insertion site, the nurse can use normal saline. The area should be dried before a dressing is reapplied. If needed, a thin layer of protective skin barrier can be applied to the exit site if indicated (e.g., site excoriated) (Perry et al., 2022a). Redness, tenderness, leakage, swelling, bleeding, and skin breakdown should be documented, and the provider notified.

PARENTERAL NUTRITION

Parenteral nutrition (PN) provides nutrients to the body by a peripheral or central IV route. The solution is composed of a very complex admixture containing proteins, carbohydrates, fats, electrolytes, vitamins, trace minerals, and sterile water in a single container. The goals of PN are to improve nutritional status, establish a positive nitrogen balance (Box 21-2), maintain muscle mass, promote weight maintenance or gain, and support the healing process.

BOX 21-2

Establishing Positive Nitrogen Balance

The nitrogen balance is determined by how much nitrogen is taken into the body versus how much is excreted. Urine contains 90% of the excreted nitrogen, while the remaining 10% exits the body through sweat, hair, and stool (Dominiczak & Logue, 2019). When a patient's intake of protein and nutrients is significantly less than that the body requires to meet energy expenditures, a state of negative nitrogen balance results. In response, the body begins to convert the protein found in muscles into carbohydrates to meet energy needs. The result is muscle wasting, weight loss, fatigue, and, if left uncorrected, death.

The suggested daily protein intake for an average adult is 1.0–1.2 g of protein/kg of body weight (Dominiczak & Logue, 2019). Traditional IV fluids do not provide sufficient calories or nitrogen to meet the body's daily requirements. PN solutions, which supply nutrients such as dextrose, amino acids, electrolytes, vitamins, minerals, and fat emulsions, provide enough calories and nitrogen to meet the patient's daily nutritional needs. In general, PN usually provides 25–35 kcal/kg of ideal body weight and 1.0–1.5 g of protein/kg.

Fever, trauma, burns, major surgery, or hypermetabolic disease requires additional daily calories. The fluid volume necessary to provide these calories would surpass fluid tolerance and lead to pulmonary edema or heart failure. To provide the required calories in a small volume, it is necessary to increase the concentration of nutrients and use a route of administration (i.e., a large, high-flow vein, such as the subclavian) that rapidly dilutes incoming nutrients to the proper levels of body tolerance.

When highly concentrated dextrose is administered, caloric requirements are satisfied and the body uses amino acids for protein synthesis rather than for energy. Additional potassium is added to the solution to maintain proper electrolyte balance and to transport glucose and amino acids across cell membranes. To prevent deficiencies and fulfill requirements for tissue synthesis, other elements, such as calcium, phosphorus, magnesium, and sodium chloride, are added.

Clinical Indications

In both the home and hospital settings, PN is indicated in the following situations:

- The patient's intake is insufficient to maintain an anabolic state (e.g., severe burns, malnutrition, short bowel syndrome, AIDS, sepsis, cancer).
- The patient's ability to ingest food orally or by tube is impaired (e.g., paralytic ileus, Crohn disease with obstruction, postradiation enteritis, severe hyperemesis gravidarum in pregnancy).
- The patient is unwilling or unable to ingest adequate nutrients (e.g., anorexia nervosa, postoperative older patients).

- The underlying medical condition precludes being fed orally or tube (e.g., acute pancreatitis, high enterocutaneous fistula).
- Preoperative and postoperative nutritional needs are prolonged (e.g., extensive bowel surgery).

Pearls for Practice

Cues to malnutrition in patients include a prealbumin level that is less than 16 mg/dL, albumin that is less than 3.5 mg/dL, unintentional weight loss of 10% in 6 months or 5% in 3 months, or a body mass index (BMI) below 18.5. A BMI of less than 20 places a patient at risk for malnutrition (NHS, 2020).

PN therapy is recommended for 7 to 14 days preceding surgery with the goal of repleting protein, electrolyte, and micronutrients (Lakananurak & Gramlich, 2020).

Parenteral Formulas

A total of 2 to 3 L of the solution is administered over 24 hours using a filter (1.2-micron particulate filter). Before administration, the PN infusion must be inspected for clarity and any precipitate. The label is compared with the provider's order, noting the expiration date. **IV fat emulsions** (IVFEs, Intralipids) may be infused simultaneously with PN through a Y-connector close to the infusion site and *should not* be filtered. Before administration, the IVFE is inspected for frothiness, separation, or oily appearance. If any of these are present, the solution is not used. Usually, 500 mL of a 10% emulsion or 250 mL of 20% emulsion is administered over 6 to 12 hours, one to three times a week. IVFEs can provide up to 30% of the total daily calorie intake.

IVFEs can be admixed with other components of PN to create a "three-in-one formulation," commonly called a **total nutrient admixture** (TNA). All the parenteral nutrient components are mixed in one container and administered to the patient over a 24-hour period. A special final filter (1.5-micron filter) is used with this solution. Before administration, the solution is observed for oil droplets that have separated from the solution, forming a noticeable layer (referred to as cracking or oiling out); such a solution should be discarded.

Initiating Therapy

PN solutions have a higher glucose concentration than do regular IV fluids. As a result, PN is a medium in which bacteria can thrive. In fact, catheter-related bloodstream infection (CRBSI) is the most frequent complication found in both hospitalized patients and those with PN at home (Perry et al., 2022b). The nurse needs to use an aseptic technique when assessing the catheter port for the PN. The ports should be prepped with an antiseptic wipe. If the PN bag does not come with pre-primed tubing from the pharmacy, the nurse must take great care not to contaminate the bag or tubing. Also, the dressing on the catheter should be changed following the institution's policy to prevent infection at the insertion site. The nurse observes the patient for fever, chills, malaise, and elevated white blood cell count and alerts the provider as needed (Perry et al., 2022b). PN solutions are initiated slowly and advanced each day gradually to the desired rate as the patient's fluid and glucose tolerance permits. If the solution is administered too rapidly, the patient could become fluid overloaded. If this occurs, the rate should be decreased, and the patient's respiratory status should be monitored. The patient's laboratory test results and response to PN therapy are monitored on an ongoing basis by the provider and licensed nutrition provider. Standing orders are initiated for weighing the patient; monitoring intake, output, and blood glucose; and baseline and periodic monitoring of complete blood count, platelet count, and chemistry panel, including serum carbon dioxide, magnesium, phosphorus, triglycerides, and prealbumin. The blood glucose is typically measured every 6 hours until within normal limits for 48 hours; then daily while maintained on PN (Perry et al., 2022b). A 24-hour urine nitrogen determination may be performed for analysis of nitrogen balance. In most hospitals, the provider prescribes PN solutions on a daily standard PN order form. The formulation of the PN solutions is carefully calculated each day to meet the individual patient's complete nutritional needs.

Administration Methods

Peripheral Method

A peripheral parenteral nutrition (PPN) formula is prescribed when a patient's oral intake requires supplementation. This type of solution is not as hypertonic as PN or total parenteral nutrition (TPN), so it can be administered peripherally. PPN formulas are not nutritionally complete: there is typically less dextrose content.

Pearls for Practice

Any formula with a dextrose concentration of more than 10% should not be administered through peripheral veins because they irritate the intima (innermost walls) of small veins, causing a chemical phlebitis.

Lipids are administered simultaneously to buffer the PPN and to protect the peripheral vein from irritation. For PPN solutions, peripheral access is changed approximately every 3 days to decrease the likelihood of infiltration. These solutions use a *dedicated line*; no other medication or IV solution can be infused other than the PPN solution through this peripheral IV.

Central Method

Because TPN solutions have five or six times the solute concentration of blood (and exert an osmotic pressure of about 2,000 mOsm/L), they are injurious to the intima of peripheral veins. Therefore, to prevent phlebitis and other venous complications, these solutions are administered into the vascular system through a catheter inserted into a high-flow, large blood vessel, such as the subclavian vein. Then concentrated solutions are very rapidly diluted to isotonic levels by the blood in this vessel.

Four types of **central venous access devices (CVADs)** can be used to administer TPN: nontunneled (or percutaneous) central catheters, peripherally inserted central catheters (PICCs), tunneled catheters, and implanted ports. Whenever one of these catheters is inserted, catheter tip placement should be confirmed by x-ray studies before PN therapy is initiated. The optimal position is the mid proximal third of the superior vena cava at the right atrial junction.

Nontunneled Central Catheters

Nontunneled central catheters are used for short-term IV therapy (less than 6 weeks) in acute-care, long-term care, and home-care settings. The provider inserts these catheters. Examples of nontunneled central catheters are Vas-Cath, percutaneous subclavian Arrow, and Hohn catheters. The subclavian vein is the most common vessel used because the subclavian area provides a stable insertion site to which the catheter can be anchored, allows the patient freedom of movement, and offers easy access to the dressing site. The jugular vein should be avoided and only be considered for cannulation if the patient has no other access points. Jugular access should be used only temporarily for approximately 1 to 2 days.

A triple-lumen subclavian catheter can be used to ensure accessibility in a patient with limited IV access because it offers three ports for various uses (Fig. 21-16). Blood sampling and administration are commonly done through the distal port. All three ports can be used for medication administration. The nurse may stop an IV solution or medication drip temporarily (if warranted—some solutions cannot be stopped even for brief periods, such as a nitroglycerine drip with an acute MI patient) when drawing blood from another lumen on the triple-lumen catheter. Otherwise, these infusions can contaminate the studies ordered and alter the results. The nurse may also waste 5 to 10 cc of blood from the patient before drawing the actual specimen for analysis as an additional method for obtaining a clean sample.

If a single-lumen central catheter is used for administering TPN, various restrictions apply:

- Blood cannot be drawn from the catheter, and transfusions of blood products cannot be given through the main line because red blood cells may coat the lumen of the catheter, thereby reducing the flow of the nutritional solution.
- Medications cannot be administered because the drug may be incompatible with the solution's components (insulin is an exception). If medications must be given, they must be infused through a separate peripheral IV line, not by piggyback into the TPN line.

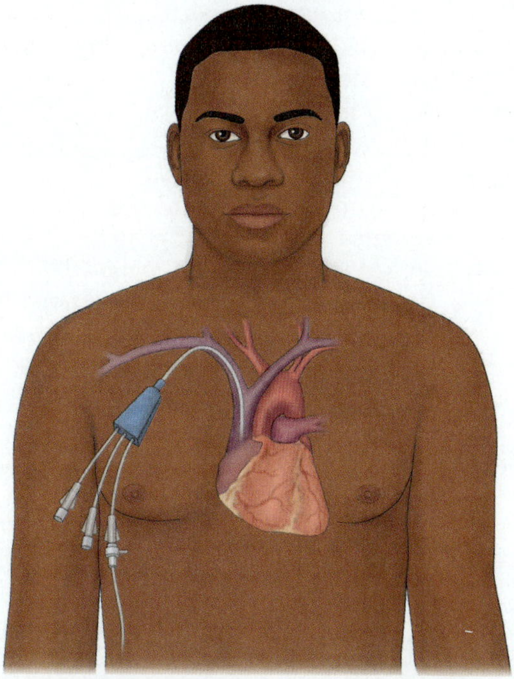

FIGURE 21-16 Subclavian triple-lumen catheter used for parenteral nutrition and other adjunctive therapy. The catheter is threaded through the subclavian vein into the vena cava. Each lumen is an avenue for solution administration. The lumens are secured with threaded needleless adapters or Luer-Lok–type caps when the device is not in use.

Once the catheter's position is confirmed, the prescribed TPN solution is started. The initial infusion rate is usually 50 mL/hr, and the rate is increased gradually to the maintenance rate or predetermined dose (e.g., 100 to 125 mL/hr). An infusion pump is always used for the administration of TPN.

Pearls for Practice

If, for any reason, there is a delay in the infusion rate, this solution is never increased beyond the hourly ordered rate. There is no "playing catch up" with TPN (Perry et al., 2022b). If the PN solution is terminated abruptly, a 5% or a 10% dextrose solution is administered for a period of hours to protect against rebound hypoglycemia. Specifically, a 5% solution is administered for PPN, while a 10% solution is administered for TPN at the same rate, owing to the approximate glucose concentration in the two solutions.

Pearls for Practice

Be alert for "refeeding syndrome" in the severely malnourished patient who begins enteral or parenteral nutrition. Refeeding syndrome is the potentially fatal fluids and electrolytes shift that may occur in malnourished patients receiving aggressive nutritional treatment in the form of enteral or parenteral nutrition. Risk factors include patients with conditions such as eating disorders, alcohol use disorder, malabsorptive conditions like inflammatory bowel disease, chronic malnutrition, poorly controlled diabetes, oncologic conditions, and postoperative state (Persaud-Sharma et al., 2021). A marker for refeeding syndrome is new onset of hypophosphatemia within 72 hours of the starting nutrition (Ben-Tovim & Theilla, 2021). It is also associated with hypokalemia and hypomagnesemia resulting in cardiac and respiratory failure, lethargy, confusion, coma, and even death (Cleary, 2022). That is why, international guidelines recommend that enteral nutrition be gradually increased over 24 to 48 hours in patients who are at high nutrition risk or severely malnourished (Ben-Tovim & Theilla, 2021) and monitoring of electrolytes--particularly serum phosphorus, potassium, and/or magnesium levels occur daily during the first week of replenishment and then three times in the following week (Persaud-Sharma et al., 2021).

An injection site cap is attached to the end of each central catheter lumen, creating a closed system. IV infusion tubing is connected to the insertion site cap of the central catheter with a threaded needleless adapter or Luer-Lok device. The manufacturer labels each lumen according to location (proximal, middle, and distal). To ensure patency, all lumens are flushed initially, daily when not in use, after each intermittent infusion, after blood drawing, and whenever an infusion is disconnected. The use of heparin when flushing central lines provides few benefits over the use of normal saline, to result in recommending its routine use (Sharma et al., 2019). Force is never used for flushing the catheter, as it can result in dislodging clots or fibrin that may accumulate around the lumens of the catheter. If resistance is met, aspiration may restore lumen patency. If this technique is ineffective the provider should be notified. A low-dose tissue plasminogen activator may be prescribed to dissolve a clot or fibrin sheath. If attempts to clear the lumen are ineffective, the lumen is labeled "clotted off" and not used again.

Peripherally Inserted Central Catheters

Peripherally inserted central catheters (PICCs) are used for intermediate-term (several days to months) IV therapy in the hospital, long-term care, or home setting. A specially trained nurse may insert these catheters at the bedside or in the outpatient setting. They also can be inserted using fluoroscopy by an interventional radiologist. PICC lines are placed in the arm, precisely the basilic or cephalic vein, via the antecubital space. Then the catheter is threaded to a designated location, depending on the type of solution to be infused (superior vena cava for TPN, which allows dilution of this hypertonic solution). Blood drawing and blood pressure measurement are avoided in the accessed arm. Additional details on PICC lines can be found in Chapter 3.

Tunneled Central Catheters

Tunneled central catheters are for long-term use and may remain in place for many years. These catheters are cuffed and can have single or double lumens; examples are the Hickman, Groshong, and PermCath. These catheters are inserted surgically. They are threaded under the skin (reducing the risk of ascending infection) to the subclavian vein, and the distal end of the catheter is advanced into the superior vena cava.

Implanted Ports

Implanted ports also are used for long-term home IV therapy; examples include the Port-A-Cath, Mediport, Hickman Port, and P.A.S. Port. Instead of exiting from the skin, as do the Hickman and Groshong catheters, the end of the catheter is attached to a small chamber that is placed in a subcutaneous pocket, either on the anterior chest wall or on the forearm. The subcutaneous port requires minimal care and allows complete patient freedom of activity. Implanted ports are more expensive than the external catheters, and access requires passing a special noncoring needle (Huber-tipped) through the skin into the chamber to initiate IV therapy.

Discontinuing Parenteral Nutrition

The PN solution is discontinued gradually to allow the patient to adjust to decreased levels of glucose. A patient's blood sugar must be followed closely when weaning a patient off PN, while on a continuous insulin infusion, or increasing enteral feedings concurrently. Providing oral carbohydrates can shorten the tapering time. Specific symptoms of rebound hypoglycemia include weakness, faintness, diaphoresis, shakiness, feeling cold, confusion, and increased heart rate. Once all IV therapy is completed, the nontunneled central venous catheter or PICC can be removed, and an occlusive dressing is applied to the exit site. Once a decision is made to discontinue the line, physicians or nurses who have been deemed competent in the removal procedure and are aware of the potential complications may remove central and PICC lines. Tunneled catheters and implanted ports are removed only by the physician.

Clinical Judgment Case

A 42-year-old patient who was admitted to the hospital for insertion of a port-A-Cath for chemotherapy 48 hours ago. The patient tolerated the procedure well and their first dose of chemotherapy. The patient is complaining of nausea and has had episodes of repeated retching and vomiting of clear liquids this morning. This afternoon, the patient begins retching violently and vomits a moderate amount of bright red blood. The patient's skin is dry, there is delayed skin turgor, jugular veins are flat, and vital signs are as follows: 98.7 F, HR is 112 and irregular, RR 24, with an oxygen saturation of 95% on room air and the blood pressure is 100/52. The patient is complaining of pain in the chest, however denies jaw, back, or arm pain. Heart sounds are S1 S2, without gallop or murmur; the point of maximum impulse (PMI) is nondisplaced. Lungs are clear. Abdomen is soft, nondistended, nontender, last BM was yesterday, formed brown stool, denies melena. Capillary refill is 2 seconds and pedal and posterior tibial pulses are 3+ bil. The patient's history included asthma, that is treated with albuterol prn and atrial fibrillation treated with warfarin.

Step One: Recognize cues where relevant and important information is identified from different sources, such as medical history or vital sign.

Answer: History of asthma, atrial fibrillation, cancer, post chemotherapy infusion, post insertion of port-A-Cath; warfarin therapy, vomiting, hematemesis. Complaints of chest pain, nausea; physical examination findings of flat neck veins and delayed skin turgor. Cues of concern related to vital signs: HR of 112 and irregular, 24 RR, and blood pressure is 100/52.

Step Two: Analyze cues, which is organizing and linking the recognized cues to the patient's clinical presentation.

Answer: You have clustered the hematemesis, hypotension, tachycardia, tachypnea, no melena, abdomen that is soft, nondistended, nontender with normal bowel sounds with an acute upper GI bleed (of unknown etiology) and risk of hypovolemia. Specifically, signs of fluid volume deficit include flat neck veins, delayed skin turgor tachycardia, tachypnea, and hypotension. The blood pressure of 100/52 is hypotensive and you calculate the mean arterial pressure (MAP) which is systolic pressure (100 mm Hg), plus the diastolic pressure (52 mm Hg) ×'s 2/3 (100 + 104 = 204/3 = 68 mm Hg). You associate the irregular HR with history of atrial fibrillation and the patient is treated with warfarin; you are concerned that the GI bleeding may be associated with abnormal bleeding times associated with the anticoagulant, or is related to new-onset disorder such as stress ulcer, or *Mallory–Weiss tear due to violent retching. You are also concerned that the chest pain may be associated with a cardiac event.*

Step Three: Prioritize hypotheses, where hypotheses are evaluated and ranked according to priority. This can include urgency, likelihood, risk, difficulty and/or time. In this phase you cluster your findings, to arrive at a list of problems (actual and or potential problems) you believe the patient is experiencing and determine the importance or urgency. What do you think is of greatest concern?

Answer: The potential hypothesis include: (1) myocardial infarction (MI) given patient complaint of chest pain, (2) upper GI bleed with potential for hypovolemic shock, and (3) potential cause of bleeding is abnormal International normalized ratio (INR) or prothrombin time (PT) related to warfarin administration versus new cause of acute upper GI bleeding. In the moment, you prioritize evaluation of MI (the MAP >65 mm Hg and you are aware that a MAP below 65 mm Hg, for an extended period, can cause end-organ ischemia and infarction can occur), over the potential for hypovolemic shock, but will continue to monitor the vital signs, O_2 saturation and physical examination findings. If significant blood loss occurs you will monitor for HR and RR elevation, decreased BP, decreased MAP, decreased pulse pressure, decreased peripheral perfusion, decreased urinary output, restlessness, delayed capillary refill, etc.

Step Four: Generate solutions, which is identifying expected outcomes and using hypotheses to define a set of interventions for the expected outcomes.

Answer: Since the priority is hemodynamic stability, with unknown cause of the GI bleeding, and you suspect a cardiac event, you place the patient on a cardiac monitor and are aware that an IV is necessary for emergency medication administration. The patient has a functioning port-A-Cath as well as a peripheral IV. Given the patient is demonstrating fluid volume deficit, you anticipate that IV fluids will be administered. You will monitor the oxygen saturation continuously and vital signs every 15 minutes. You recognize that an ECG will identify the presence of arrhythmia (recall this patient has a history of atrial fibrillation) or ECG changes associated with an MI. You expect laboratory testing that will evaluate for an MI (cardiac biomarkers) and evaluate blood loss with a stat H&H as well as STAT INR, PT (to assess for coagulopathy). You will check the medical record to verify that a blood type and crossmatch was performed as you are aware that GI hemorrhage is a potentially life-threatening emergency. You are also aware that in this situation the STAT H&H is a poor indicator of the severity of blood loss since as whole blood is lost, the plasma and red blood cells are lost in the same proportion, thus it may take several hours before the patient's H&H decreases. You also anticipate that once the patient is hemodynamically stable, controlling the bleeding will be the next priority and you expect that an emergency fiberoptic endoscopy will assess the cause of the bleeding.

Step Five: Take action, where the solutions that address the highest priorities are implemented.

Answer: You place the patient on a cardiac monitor and move the 12-lead ECG machine to the bedside as you alert the provider of the change in patient condition. The oxygen saturation is also monitored continuously and supplemental oxygen is supplemental oxygen is available if needed. A 12-lead ECG is ordered and stat blood work is drawn. Fluid resuscitation (IV solution of normal saline or lactated Ringer solution), is needed to achieve hemodynamic stability with the potential need for blood and if there is coagulopathy (you are awaiting the INR results) blood products (fresh frozen plasma, platelets). Finally, you anticipate diagnostic procedures to determine the exact cause of the bleeding. You will hold the warfarin dose which was due this hour due to the sudden GI bleeding and note the rationale in the medical record.

Step Six: Evaluate outcomes, which is comparing observed outcomes against expected outcomes.

Answer: The troponin I level comes back as 0.1 which is normal level, the ECG reveals rapid atrial fibrillation with no ST changes. The hematocrit has not changed and remains at 42%, the INR is 2.2. The patient has received 1 L of normal saline and an emergency endoscopy revealed a Mallory–Weiss tear due to retching that was treated with electrocoagulation. VS repeated are now HR of 90 and regular, RR 18, oxygen saturation of 97% on RA, and BP is now 122/68. The oncology team is notified and the patient is placed on an antiemetic regimen. The endoscopist has prescribed restarting warfarin this evening.

It is understandable that this was a scary situation but you have learned there are a variety of potential causes of hemodynamic instability and you cast the net wide in this situation (new MI, abnormal INR, stress ulcer), only to realize that regardless of the cause the lack of adequate circulating volume can lead to decreased tissue perfusion and hypovolemic shock. Because of your quick response in alerting the team, your patient is now stable. And you learning that retching and vomiting can lead to significant problems for your patients.

CHAPTER REVIEW

NCLEX-Style Review Questions

1. A patient has an NG tube inserted and placement is confirmed by x-ray. Select from the list below, appropriate options to verify the NG tube placement is maintained. Select all that apply.
   a. Air insufflation into NG tube and listening for air bubble
   b. Reassessing the marking at the nares or mouth and length of the external portion of the tube in centimeters
   c. Testing the NG tube drainage pH
   d. Using capnographic devices to determine placement
   e. Visually assessing the aspirate

2. A patient was admitted with hematemesis and diagnosed with esophageal rupture. Which of the following cues alert you to potential for hypovolemic shock. Select all that apply.
   a. Bradycardia
   b. Pulse pressure of 28 mm Hg
   c. Tachypnea
   d. MAP <65 mm Hg
   e. Capillary refill of 2 seconds

3. A nurse is caring for a patient on strict bowel rest and will need IV nutrition. The nurse knows the following devices are appropriate for TPN. Select all that apply.
   a. PICC line
   b. Triple-lumen catheter
   c. Large-bore IV line
   d. Implantable venous assess device (Port-A-Cath)
   e. Arterial line

4. A nurse receives report on a patient experiencing dumping syndrome. What symptoms would the patient be displaying 30 minutes after eating? Select all that apply.
a. Difficulty swallowing
b. Heartburn
c. Constipation
d. Cramping in the abdomen
e. Diarrhea

5. The nurse recognizes which of the following is a cause of xerostomia? Select all that apply.
a. HIV infection
b. Oral hypoglycemic medications
c. Tracheostomy tube
d. Inability to close the mouth
e. Kidney failure

REFERENCES AND SELECTED READINGS

References and selected readings associated with this chapter can be found on the website that accompanies the book. Visit **http://thepoint.lww.com/Honan3e** to access the references and other additional resources related to this chapter.

CHAPTER 22

Nursing Management: Patients With Gastric and Duodenal Disorders

Gwen M. Cassidy

Learning Objectives

After reading this chapter, you will be able to:

1. Describe the diagnosis and management of gastroesophageal reflux disease (GERD).
2. Compare and contrast the etiology, clinical manifestations, and management of acute gastritis, chronic gastritis, and peptic ulcer.
3. Describe the management of the patient with gastritis.
4. Describe the dietary, pharmacologic, and surgical treatment of peptic ulcer.
5. Describe the nursing management of patients who undergo surgical procedures to treat obesity.
6. Use the nursing process as a framework for care of patients undergoing gastric surgery.
7. Identify the complications of gastric surgery and their prevention and management.
8. Describe the clinical manifestations of severe acute respiratory syndrome *coronavirus 1* (SARS-CoV-1) virus in the gastrointestinal (GI) tract.

A person's nutritional status depends not only on the type and amount of intake but also on the functioning of the gastric and intestinal portions of the gastrointestinal (GI) system. This chapter describes disorders of the stomach and duodenum as well as their treatment and related nursing care.

GASTROESOPHAGEAL REFLUX DISEASE

Gastroesophageal reflux disease (GERD) is a common condition, affecting 15% to 20% of the worldwide population (Chapelle et al., 2020). GERD is a chronic disease. Considering the prevalence, it is importance for nurses to understand GERD and the treatment options available.

GERD is a condition where stomach contents will flow back into the esophagus (Fig. 22-1). There are multiple phenotypes, but the three most common are: nonerosive reflux disease (NERD), erosive esophagitis (EE), and Barrett esophagus (BE). NERD is the most common phenotype, seen in 60% to 70% of patients (Atunes et al., 2021). Most common manifestations of the disease are heartburn and regurgitation (Katz et al., 2022).

Pathophysiology

The pathophysiology of GERD is multifactorial, and treatment will be based on the specific cause of a patient's reflux.

The **lower esophageal sphincter (LES)** is a tonically contracted segment of smooth muscle that serves as the barrier between the stomach and esophagus. Along with the crural diaphragm (tendinous structures that form a tether for muscular contraction), this creates the esophagogastric junction (EGJ). Typically, this junction maintains a high-pressure zone which keeps the stomach contents from backflowing into the esophagus. There are transient LES relaxations (TLESRs) that respond to the stimulus of food in healthy individuals. Patients with GERD will have pathologic TLESRs that are not triggered by swallowing. This then allows the contents of the stomach to back up into the esophagus. Alcohol use, smoking, caffeine, and pregnancy are risk factors. Frequent TLESRs occur in 48% to 73% of reflux patients (Atunes et al., 2021).

Hiatal hernia is another cause of GERD. The stomach is dislocated through the diaphragm into the chest—separating the crural diaphragm from the LES and disrupting that pressure gradient. Many hiatal hernias are benign and are found incidentally. Larger hiatal hernias are found to be associated with increased GERD as well as EE, up to 94% in one study (Atunes et al., 2021).

Other pathophysiology includes ineffective esophageal motility and impaired mucosal defense. BMI >25 has an increased risk for GERD, especially patients with BMI >30.

Heartburn affects two thirds of pregnant females (Katz et al., 2022). Lifestyle modifications are the first-line treatment,

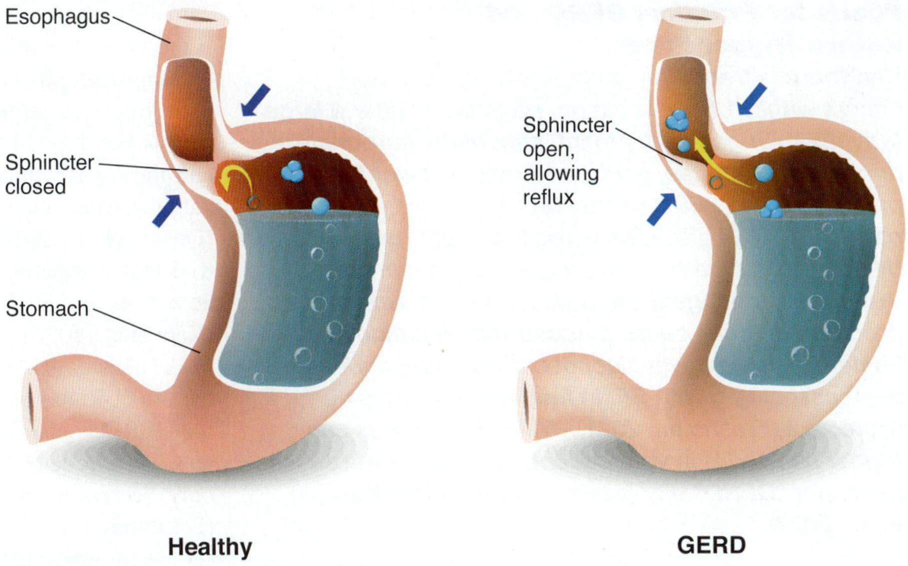

FIGURE 22-1 Heartburn and gastroesophageal reflux disease (GERD). If the esophageal sphincter does not close tight enough, stomach acid seep back into the esophagus, damaging it and causing the heartburn. (*Source:* Shutterstock.com.)

followed by antacids. Histamine H_2-receptor antagonists (blockers) (H2RA) and protein pump inhibitors (PPIs) are safe in pregnancy when clinically indicated. H2RA and PPI are all pregnancy category B (considered safe to use), except omeprazole, which is C (has *not* been shown to be harmful to fetuses, however concerns exist) (Katz et al., 2022).

Clinical Manifestations and Assessment

Heartburn and regurgitation are the most common symptoms of acid reflux. Heartburn is retrosternal burning sensation. Patients' description of this symptom can widely vary. Regurgitation is retrograde migration of stomach contents into the esophagus that can be with gastric contents alone or with food. Both symptoms can worsen with reclining (Katz et al., 2022).

Chest pain can be a symptom of GERD and it is considered an alarm symptom. It is important to exclude cardiac causes when a patient complains of chest pain. Other symptoms include dysphagia (difficulty swallowing or food getting stuck), odynophagia (pain with swallowing), belching and epigastric pain (dyspepsia). Cough, dysphonia (hoarse or abnormal voice), and dental erosions can also be indicative for GERD. Worth noting that cough is often multifactorial and further investigation is recommended for that symptom (Katz et al., 2022). Nausea is not commonly seen in GERD but can be in some cases.

The American College of Gastroenterology guidelines suggest an 8-week trial of PPIs for patients who have classic GERD symptoms (heartburn and regurgitation) with no alarm symptoms (Katz et al., 2022). If patient fails to improve or is unable discontinue the medication during that time, further testing is warranted.

Pearls for Practice

Optimal use of PPI medication is 30 to 60 minutes before a meal.

Esophagogastroduodenoscopy (EGD) is the next step to evaluate GERD. EGD is also important in the evaluation of patients with alarm symptoms (Katz et al., 2022). EGD can rule in or out inflammation of the esophagus (erosive esophagitis aka EE), BE, hiatal hernia (HH), esophageal cancer, and alternative causes for symptoms that are not reflux-related. EE is classified into four categories using the Los Angeles (LA) Classification of Gastroesophageal Reflux Disease Grade A-D with A being most mild and D severe. If GERD is suspected, but endoscopy is unrevealing, further investigation with pH testing is indicated (Katz et al., 2022). This is either done with a capsule that clips on to the esophagus or a catheter that is inserted transnasally. These tests can assess pathologic acid exposure as well as note correlation between symptoms and acid events (Fass et al., 2021). GERD is often misdiagnosed, and these tests are important in distinguishing true refractory GERD from other syndromes. Reflux monitoring is not recommended with patients with LA Grade C or D esophagitis or BE (Katz et al., 2022).

Medical Management

A combination of both lifestyle modifications and medications is the gold standard for treating pathologic acid reflux.

Lifestyle modifications are key to controlling acid reflux. If patient has BMI of >25, weight loss is recommended. Elevating head of the bed is also recommended, especially if patient complains of nocturnal symptoms. Patients should elevate with a wedge pillow or raising entire head of bed. Simply elevating with pillows does not improve posture and will be ineffective at improving reflux. Patients should also refrain from eating 3 hours prior to bedtime (Fass et al., 2021; Katz et al., 2022). "GERD" diets are not recommended as they are quite restrictive. Patients can complete a food log to identify specific trigger foods to avoid.

Pearls for Practice: GERD and Known Trigger Foods

Heartburn is frequently precipitated by food and occurs within 1 hour of eating, particularly after a large fatty meal. Sugar, peppermint, chocolate, carbonated drinks, citrus, coffee, garlic, and onions lower the pressure in the LES and may be triggers for your patient. Alcohol also effects the lower LES pressure, by decreasing the smooth muscle contractility of the lower esophageal and reduces gastric acid production. It can cause mucosal inflammation and hemorrhage, however alcohol has not independently been associated with BE; in fact, red wine may be protective (Freshman, 2021). While these foods can trigger heartburn in your patient, eliminating all of them in a "GERD" diet is not recommended (Katz et al., 2022).

PPIs are the first-line medication (Table 22-1). They are recommended both for symptom control, healing, and maintenance of EE (Katz et al., 2022). In cases of BE, EE, or symptom recurrence, maintenance PPI is recommended at lowest dose possible. In instances where patient does not have EE or BE and symptoms resolve with PPI, it is recommended to discontinue PPI and use only on-demand (Katz et al., 2022). H_2 receptor agonists (H2RA) (Table 22-1) can be given if no erosive disease is found on endoscopy. Tachyphylaxis which is a rapidly diminishing response to successive doses of a drug, rendering it less effective, is common when using H2RA chronically, so it is best used on as needed basis.

Pearls for Practice

Potassium-competitive acid blockers (PCABs) are emerging as a new class of acid suppressants and might serve as an alternative to PPI in the future.

Surgical Management

For patients who are unable to control their reflux with medications, surgical options will be considered. Criteria for surgical treatment can include uncontrolled esophagitis and positive pH testing. These procedures should be performed by a surgeon experienced in antireflux procedures.

Procedures

Laparoscopic Nissen fundoplication is considered the surgery of choice for uncontrolled GERD. In this procedure the gastric fundus is wrapped around the lower esophageal sphincter in the abdomen encircling the esophagus, thus creating a tight juncture. It has an overall effective quality-of-life (QOL) improvement of 67% to 83% (Alemenno et al., 2021) and 80% of patients were able to avoid resuming their PPI medications (Katz et al., 2022). The thoracic approach is called the Belsey Mark IV and can be recommended for patients with poor esophageal motility. The Hill Gastropexy is the stomach partially wrapped around the stomach.

Magnetic sphincter augmentation (MSA) is a small magnetic ring that surgically encircles the esophagus. The surgery is performed laparoscopically. It was approved in 2012 and the 6-year outcome data have been favorable; 79% of patients were able to stop their acid-reducing medication (Ferrari et al., 2020). Although there is not a randomized trial that compares the two surgeries, MSA was found to be a "safe and effective" alternative to laparoscopic Nissen (Katz et al., 2022).

As obesity is increasing in the United States and beyond, the use of Roux-en-Y gastric bypass (RYGB) as a treatment for GERD is also on the rise (discussed later in this chapter). Current data show that it is an effective surgery in not only decreasing acid exposure, but also remission of BE (Felsenreich et al., 2020). Roux-en Y is a recommended procedure for obese patients if they are able to adapt to the diet and lifestyle modifications as described later in the bariatric surgery section (Katz et al., 2022).

Dysphagia is the most common complication after these surgeries. Patients will sometimes have to be endoscopically dilated. Gas bloat due to inability to belch can also be a complication of the surgeries. Roux complications will be discussed in the lifestyle management section.

GASTRITIS

Gastritis (inflammation of the **gastric** or stomach mucosa) is a common GI problem. Gastritis may be acute, lasting several hours to a few days, or chronic, resulting from repeated exposure to irritating agents or recurring episodes of acute gastritis.

Acute gastritis is often caused by dietary indiscretion—the person eats food that is irritating, too highly seasoned, or contaminated with disease-causing microorganisms. Other causes of acute gastritis include overuse of aspirin and other nonsteroidal anti-inflammatory drugs (NSAIDs), excessive alcohol intake, bile reflux, and radiation therapy (RT). A more severe form of acute gastritis is caused by the ingestion of strong acid or alkali, which may cause the mucosa to become gangrenous or to perforate. Scarring can occur, resulting in **pyloric stenosis** or obstruction. Acute gastritis also may develop in acute illnesses, especially when the patient has had major traumatic injuries; burns; severe infection; liver, kidney, or respiratory failure; or major surgery. Gastritis may be the first sign of an acute systemic infection.

Chronic gastritis and prolonged inflammation of the stomach may be caused either by benign or malignant ulcers of the stomach or by the bacteria ***Helicobacter pylori* (*H. pylori*)** (Saleem & Howden, 2020). Also, chronic gastritis is sometimes associated with autoimmune diseases, such as pernicious anemia (Shah et al., 2021); dietary factors, such as caffeine; the use of medications such as NSAIDs,

TABLE **22-1 Pharmacotherapy for Gastritis and Peptic Ulcer Disease**

Pharmacologic Agent	Major Action	Nursing Considerations
Antibiotics		
Amoxicillin	A bactericidal antibiotic that assists with eradicating *H. pylori* bacteria in the gastric mucosa	• May cause diarrhea • Should not be used in patients allergic to penicillin
Clarithromycin	Exerts bactericidal effects to eradicate *H. pylori* bacteria in the gastric mucosa	• May cause gastrointestinal (GI) upset, headache, altered taste • Many drug–drug interactions (e.g., cisapride, colchicine, lovastatin, warfarin) • Question use of macrolides due to concern for clarithromycin resistance
Metronidazole	A synthetic antibacterial and antiprotozoal agent that assists with eradicating *H. pylori* bacteria in the gastric mucosa when administered with other antibiotics and proton pump inhibitors	• Should be administered with meals to decrease GI upset; may cause anorexia and metallic taste • Patient should avoid alcohol; Flagyl increases blood-thinning effects of warfarin (Coumadin)
Tetracycline	Exerts bacteriostatic effects to eradicate *H. pylori* bacteria in the gastric mucosa	• May cause photosensitivity reaction; warn patient to use sunscreen • May cause GI upset • Must be used with caution in patients with kidney or liver impairment • Milk or dairy products may reduce effectiveness
Rifabutin	Inhibits DNA-dependent RNA polymerase at the beta subunit which prevents chain initiation	• May cause severe cutaneous adverse reactions such as Stevens–Johnson syndrome • May cause GI upset • Must be used with caution in patients with liver impairment • May cause neutropenia or thrombocytopenia
Antidiarrheal		
Bismuth subsalicylate	Suppresses *H. pylori* bacteria in the gastric mucosa and assists with healing of mucosal ulcers	• Given concurrently with antibiotics to eradicate *H. pylori* infection • Should be taken on empty stomach
Histamine-2 (H_2) Receptor Antagonists		
Cimetidine	Decreases amount of HCl produced by stomach by blocking action of histamine on histamine receptors of parietal cells in the stomach	• May cause confusion, agitation, or coma in older individuals or those with kidney or liver insufficiency • Long-term use may cause diarrhea, dizziness, gynecomastia • Many drug–drug interactions (e.g., amiodarone, amitriptyline, benzodiazepines, metoprolol, nifedipine, phenytoin, warfarin [Coumadin])
Famotidine	Same as for cimetidine	• Best choice for critically ill patients because it is known to have the least risk of drug–drug interactions; does not alter liver metabolism • Prolonged half-life in patients with kidney insufficiency • Short-term relief for GERD
Nizatidine	Same as for cimetidine	• Recalled in due to concerns of *N*-Nitrosodimethylamine (NDMA), which has carcinogenic properties, contamination in the product
Ranitidine	Same as for cimetidine	• Recalled in 2020 due to concerns of *N*-Nitrosodimethylamine (NDMA), which has carcinogenic properties, contamination in the product

(*continued*)

TABLE 22-1 **Pharmacotherapy for Gastritis and Peptic Ulcer Disease (*continued*)**

Pharmacologic Agent	Major Action	Nursing Considerations
Roxatidine	Same as for cimetidine	• Prolonged half-life in patients with kidney and liver insufficiency • Single bedtime dose in combination with PPI to reduce nocturnal acid reflux • May cause headache, dizziness, constipation, nausea and vomiting, or abdominal discomfort • Not approved in the United States
Proton Pump Inhibitors of Gastric Acid (PPIs)		
Esomeprazole (Nexium)	Decreases gastric acid secretion by slowing the hydrogen–potassium adenosine triphosphatase (H^+, K^+-ATPase) pump on the surface of the parietal cells of the stomach	• Used mainly for treatment of duodenal ulcer disease and *H. pylori* infection • A delayed-release capsule that is to be swallowed whole and taken before meals—the capsule cannot be crushed or chewed • May increase **phenytoin, warfarin** levels. Food decreases absorption by up to 35%. • Most common side effects are headache, diarrhea, nausea, gas, abdominal pain constipation or dry mouth
Lansoprazole	Decreases gastric acid secretion by slowing the H^+, K^+-ATPase pump on the surface of the parietal cells	• A delayed-release capsule that is to be swallowed whole and taken before meals—the capsule cannot be crushed or chewed • May decrease **theophylline** levels • Side effects include confusion, dizziness, fast or irregular heart rate, jerky muscle movements, muscle cramps or weakness, bloody diarrhea, cough, or seizure
Omeprazole	Decreases gastric acid secretion by slowing the H^+, K^+-ATPase pump on the surface of the parietal cells	• A delayed-release capsule that is to be swallowed whole and taken before meals • May cause diarrhea, nausea and vomiting, constipation, abdominal pain, headache, or dizziness
Pantoprazole	Decreases gastric acid secretion by slowing the H^+, K^+-ATPase pump on the surface of the parietal cells	• A delayed-release capsule that is to be swallowed whole and taken before meals • May cause diarrhea and hyperglycemia, headache, abdominal pain, and abnormal liver function tests
Rabeprazole	Decreases gastric acid secretion by slowing the H^+, K^+-ATPase pump on the surface of the parietal cells	• A delayed-release tablet to be swallowed whole • May cause abdominal pain, diarrhea, nausea, and headache • Drug–drug interactions with digoxin, iron, and warfarin (Coumadin)
Prostaglandin E_1 analog		
Misoprostol	Synthetic prostaglandin; protects the gastric mucosa from agents that cause ulcers; also increases mucus production and bicarbonate levels	• Used to prevent ulceration in patients using NSAIDs • Administer with food • May cause diarrhea and cramping (including uterine cramping)
Sucralfate	Creates a viscous substance in the presence of gastric acid that forms a protective barrier, binding to the surface of the ulcer, and prevents digestion by pepsin	• Used mainly for the treatment of duodenal ulcers • Should be taken without food but with water • Other medications should be taken 2 hours before or after this medication • May cause constipation or nausea
Potassium-Competitive Acid Blockers		
Vonoprazan	Competes for K on luminal side of parietal cell, which causes inhibition of pumps and reduces acid	• Not yet available in the United States

GERD, gastroesophageal reflux disease; NSAID, nonsteroidal anti-inflammatory drug.

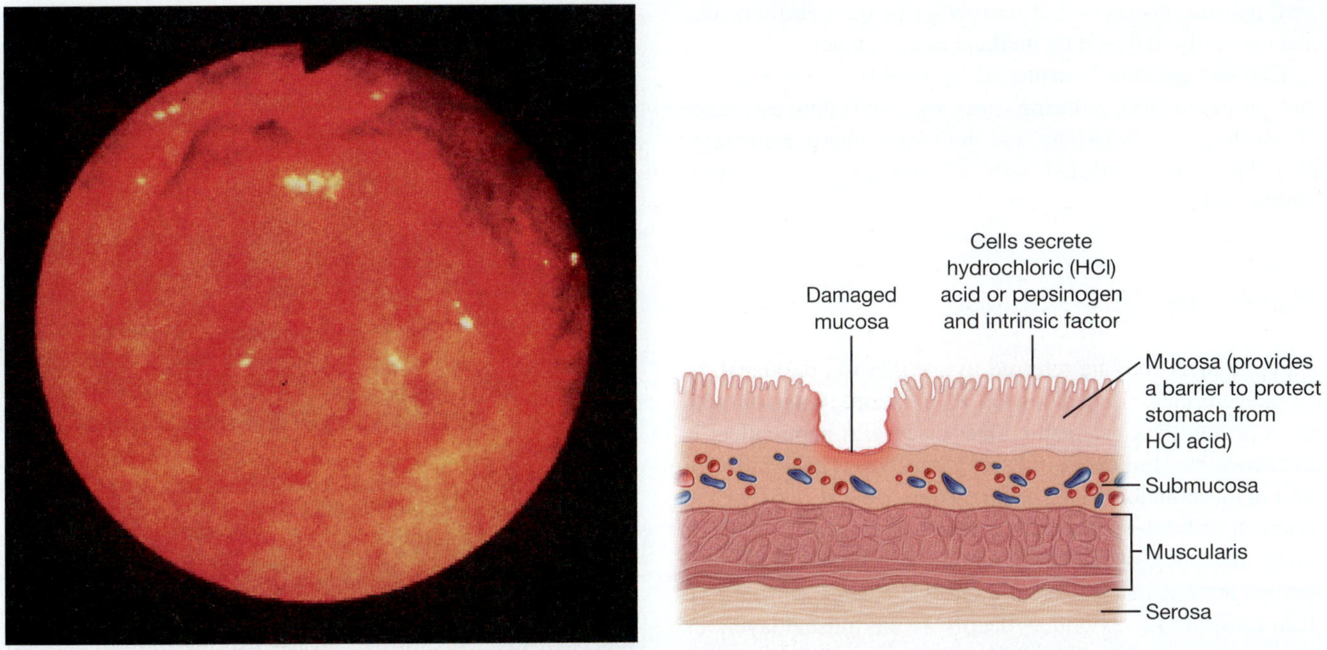

FIGURE 22-2 **Endoscopic view of erosive gastritis (*left*). Damage from irritants (*right*) results in increased intracellular pH, impaired enzyme function, disrupted cellular structures, ischemia, vascular stasis, and tissue death. (Grossman, S., & Porth, C. M. [2014]. *Porth's pathophysiology: Concepts of altered health states* [9th ed.]. Wolters Kluwer Health/Lippincott Williams & Wilkins.)**

bisphosphonate (e.g., alendronate, risedronate) or ibandronate; alcohol; smoking; or chronic reflux of pancreatic secretions and bile into the stomach.

Pathophysiology

In gastritis, the gastric mucous membrane becomes edematous and hyperemic (congested with fluid and blood) and undergoes superficial erosion (Fig. 22-2). It secretes a scanty amount of gastric juice, containing very little acid but much mucus. Superficial ulceration may occur and can lead to hemorrhage.

Clinical Manifestations and Assessment

The patient with acute gastritis may have a rapid onset of symptoms, such as abdominal discomfort, headache, lassitude, nausea, anorexia, vomiting, and hiccupping, which can last from a few hours to a few days. The patient with chronic gastritis may complain of anorexia, heartburn after eating, belching, a sour taste in the mouth, or nausea and vomiting. Some patients may have only mild epigastric discomfort or report intolerance to spicy or fatty foods or slight pain that is relieved by eating. Patients with chronic gastritis from vitamin deficiency usually have evidence of malabsorption of vitamin B_{12} caused by the production of antibodies that interfere with the binding of vitamin B_{12} to intrinsic factor. However, some patients with chronic gastritis have no symptoms.

Gastritis is sometimes associated with **achlorhydria** or hypochlorhydria (absence or low levels of hydrochloric acid [HCl]) or with hyperchlorhydria (high levels of HCl). Diagnosis can be determined by an upper GI x-ray series or endoscopy and histologic examination of a tissue specimen obtained by biopsy. Diagnostic measures for detecting *H. pylori* infection may be used and are discussed in the section on peptic ulcers.

Medical and Nursing Management

The gastric mucosa is capable of repairing itself after a bout of gastritis. As a rule, the patient recovers in about 1 day, although the appetite may be diminished for an additional 2 or 3 days. Acute gastritis is also managed by instructing the patient to refrain from alcohol and food until symptoms subside. When the patient can take nourishment by mouth, a nonirritating diet (such as the BRAT diet [Bananas, Rice, Applesauce, Toast]) is recommended. If the symptoms persist, IV fluids may need to be administered. If bleeding is present, management is similar to the procedures used to control upper GI tract hemorrhage, discussed later in this chapter.

If gastritis is caused by ingestion of strong acids or alkalis, emergency treatment consists of diluting and neutralizing the offending agent. To neutralize acids, common antacids are used; to neutralize an alkali, diluted lemon juice or diluted vinegar is used. If corrosion is extensive or severe, emetics and lavage are avoided because of the danger of perforation and damage to the esophagus.

Therapy is supportive and may include nasogastric (NG) intubation (see Chapter 21), analgesic agents and sedatives, antacids, and IV fluids. Fiberoptic endoscopy may be necessary. In extreme cases, emergency surgery may be required to remove gangrenous or perforated tissue. A gastric resection or a gastrojejunostomy (anastomosis of jejunum to stomach to detour around the pylorus) may be necessary to treat pyloric obstruction, a narrowing of the pyloric orifice that cannot be relieved by medical management.

Chronic gastritis is managed by modifying the patient's diet, promoting rest, reducing stress, recommending avoidance of alcohol and NSAIDs, and initiating pharmacotherapy. *H. pylori* may be treated with selected drug combinations (Table 22-1).

PEPTIC ULCER DISEASE

A peptic ulcer may be referred to as a gastric, duodenal, or esophageal ulcer, depending on its location. A person who has a peptic ulcer has peptic ulcer disease. A peptic ulcer is an excavation (hollowed-out area) that forms in the mucosal wall of the stomach, in the **pylorus** (the opening between the stomach and duodenum), in the **duodenum** (the first part of small intestine), or in the esophagus. Erosion of a circumscribed area of mucous membrane is the cause (Fig. 22-3). This erosion may extend as deeply as the muscle layers or through the muscle to the **peritoneum.**

Peptic ulcers are more likely to be in the duodenum than in the stomach. As a rule, they occur alone, but they may occur in multiples. Chronic gastric ulcers tend to occur in the lesser curvature of the stomach, near the pylorus. Table 22-2 compares the features of gastric and duodenal ulcers. Esophageal ulcers occur because of GERD.

Pathophysiology

Peptic ulcers occur mainly in the gastroduodenal mucosa because this tissue cannot withstand the digestive action of gastric acid (HCl) and pepsin. The erosion is caused by the increased concentration or activity of acid–pepsin or by decreased resistance of the mucosa. A damaged mucosa cannot

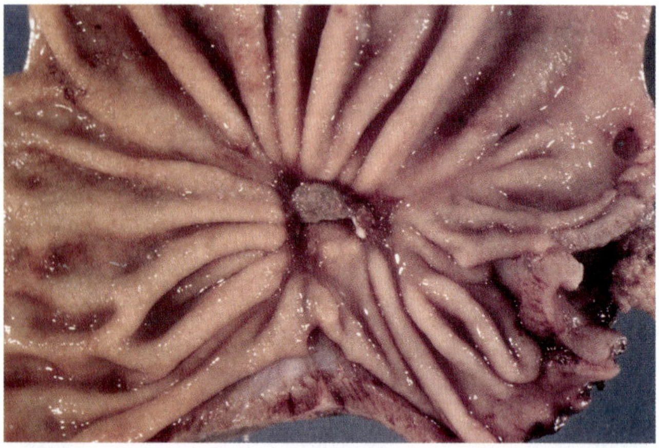

FIGURE 22-3 **Deep peptic ulcer. (Strayer, D., & Rubin, E. [2015]. *Rubin's pathology: Clinicopathologic foundations of medicine* [7th ed.]. Wolters Kluwer Health.)**

secrete enough mucus to act as a barrier against HCl. The use of NSAIDs inhibits the secretion of mucus that protects the mucosa. Adherence of the pill itself to the mucosa can also cause ulceration. Patients with duodenal ulcer disease secrete more acid than normal, whereas patients with gastric ulcer tend to secrete normal or decreased levels of acid. Damage to the gastroduodenal mucosa allows for decreased resistance to bacteria, and, thus, infection from *H. pylori* bacteria may occur.

Zollinger–Ellison syndrome (ZES) is suspected when a patient has several peptic ulcers or an ulcer that is resistant to standard medical therapy (Cho & Kasi, 2021). ZES is identified by the hypersecretion of gastric juice, duodenal ulcers, and gastrinomas (Islet cell tumors) in the pancreas. Ninety percent of tumors are found in the "gastric triangle," which encompasses the cystic and common bile ducts, the second and third portions of the duodenum, and the junction of the head and body of the pancreas. Approximately one third of

TABLE **22-2 Comparison of Duodenal and Gastric Ulcers**

Feature	Duodenal Ulcer	Gastric Ulcer
Incidence	30–60 years of age Male:female = 2:1 or 3:1 80% of peptic ulcers are duodenal	Usually 50 years of age or older Male: female = 1:1 15% of peptic ulcers are gastric
Symptoms and Clinical Findings	Hypersecretion of stomach acid (HCl) May have weight gain Pain occurs 2–3 hours after a meal; often awakened around 1 or 2 AM; ingestion of food relieves pain Vomiting uncommon Hemorrhage less likely than with gastric ulcer, but if present, melena more common than hematemesis More likely to perforate than gastric ulcers	Normal to hyposecretion of stomach acid (HCl) Weight loss may occur Pain occurs ½–1 hour after a meal; rarely occurs at night; may be relieved by vomiting; ingestion of food does not help, sometimes increases pain Vomiting common Hemorrhage more likely to occur than with duodenal ulcer; hematemesis more common than melena
Malignancy Possibility	Rare	Occasionally
Risk Factors	*H. pylori*, alcohol, smoking, cirrhosis, stress	*H. pylori*, gastritis, alcohol, smoking, use of nonsteroidal anti-inflammatory drugs (NSAIDs), stress

gastrinomas are malignant. Diarrhea and steatorrhea (unabsorbed fat in the stool) may be evident. The patient may have coexisting parathyroid adenomas (benign tumor of glandular origin) or hyperplasia and, therefore, may exhibit signs of hypercalcemia. The most common symptom is epigastric pain. *H. pylori* is not a risk factor for ZES.

Stress-related mucosal disease (SRMD) is a broad term used to describe the phenomenon of injury to the lining of the stomach and the duodenum during conditions of physiologic stress. Other terms commonly used include *stress erosion, stress ulcer, stress gastritis, erosive gastritis,* and *hemorrhagic gastritis*. These terms also have been given to the acute mucosal ulceration of the duodenal or gastric area that occurs after physiologically stressful events, such as burns, shock, severe sepsis, and multiple organ traumas. These ulcers, which are clinically different from peptic ulcers, are most common in ventilator-dependent patients after trauma or surgery (Vazin et al., 2021). Fiberoptic endoscopy within 24 hours of trauma or surgery reveals shallow erosions of the stomach wall; by 72 hours, multiple gastric erosions are observed. The prevalence of SRMD has been reported to be as high as 74% to 100% in critically ill patients (Wang et al., 2020). As the stressful condition continues, the ulcers spread. When the patient recovers, the lesions are reversed. This pattern is typical of stress ulceration.

Differences of opinion exist as to the actual cause of mucosal ulceration in stress ulcers, but the etiology is thought to be multifactorial. Usually, the ulceration is preceded by a shock state; often involving hypovolemia and hypoperfusion; leading to decreased gastric mucosal blood flow and gastric ischemia. This hypoperfusion triggers the body's protective mechanisms of activation of the sympathetic nervous system, increased catecholamine release causing further vasoconstriction, and reduced gastric blood flow. Gastric hypoperfusion leads to decreased gastric motility, decreased capacity to neutralize hydrogen ions, and the reflux of duodenal contents into the stomach. In addition, large quantities of pepsin are released. The combination of ischemia, acid, and pepsin creates an ideal climate for ulceration. A small study showed that serum levels of malondialdyde and superoxide dismutase (biomarkers of stress) were elevated in patients with SRMD, suggesting oxidative stress (Wang et al., 2020).

Stress ulcers should be distinguished from Cushing ulcers and Curling ulcers, two other types of gastric ulcers. Cushing ulcers are common in patients with head injury and brain trauma. They may occur in the esophagus, stomach, or duodenum and usually are deeper and more penetrating than stress ulcers. Curling ulcer is frequently observed about 72 hours after extensive burns and involves the antrum of the stomach or the duodenum.

Risk Factors

Peptic ulcer disease occurs with the greatest frequency in people between 40 and 60 years of age. It is relatively uncommon in females of childbearing age, but it has been observed in children and even in infants. After menopause, the incidence of peptic ulcers in females is almost equal to that in males. Peptic ulcers in the body of the stomach can occur without excessive acid secretion.

In the past, stress and anxiety were thought to be causes of ulcers, but research has documented that peptic ulcers result from infection with the gram-negative bacteria *H. pylori*, which may be acquired through ingestion of food and water. Person-to-person transmission of the bacteria also occurs through close contact and exposure to emesis. Although *H. pylori* infection is common in the United States, 80% to 90% of people do not develop ulcers or other complications of *H. pylori*. It is not known why *H. pylori* infection does not cause ulcers in all people, but several theories have been posited such as climate, gut microbiota (the microorganisms that colonize our digestive tract), diet, and education (Alexander et al., 2020).

In addition, excessive secretion of HCl in the stomach may contribute to the formation of peptic ulcers, and stress may be associated with its increased secretion. The ingestion of milk and caffeinated beverages, smoking, and alcohol also may increase HCl secretion. Stress and eating spicy foods may make peptic ulcers worse. Also it is worth noting that although stress does not cause peptic ulcers, it can increase the perceived symptoms such as dyspepsia.

Familial tendency also may be a significant predisposing factor. People with blood type O are more susceptible to peptic ulcers than are those with blood type A, B, or AB (Alexander et al., 2020). There also is an association between peptic ulcers and chronic pulmonary disease or chronic kidney disease. Other predisposing factors associated with peptic ulcer include chronic use of NSAIDs, alcohol ingestion, and excessive smoking.

Peptic ulcers are found in rare cases in patients with tumors that cause secretion of excessive amounts of the hormone gastrin. ZES consists of severe peptic ulcers, extreme gastric hyperacidity, and gastrin-secreting benign or malignant tumors of the pancreas.

Clinical Manifestations and Assessment

Symptoms of an ulcer may last for a few days, weeks, or months and may disappear only to reappear, often without an identifiable cause. Many people with ulcers have no symptoms, and perforation or hemorrhage may occur in 20% to 30% of patients who had no preceding manifestations.

As a rule, the patient with an ulcer complains of dull, gnawing pain or a burning sensation in the midepigastrium or in the back. It is believed that the pain occurs when the increased acid content of the stomach and duodenum erodes the lesion and stimulates the exposed nerve endings. Another theory suggests that contact of the lesion with acid stimulates a local reflex mechanism that initiates contraction of the adjacent smooth muscle. Pain is usually relieved by eating because food neutralizes the acid or by taking alkali; however, once the stomach has emptied or the alkali's effect has decreased, the pain returns. Sharply localized tenderness can be elicited by applying gentle pressure to the epigastrium at or slightly to the right of the midline.

Other symptoms include **pyrosis** (heartburn), vomiting, constipation or diarrhea, and bleeding. Pyrosis is a burning sensation in the esophagus and stomach that moves up to the mouth. Often heartburn is accompanied by sour eructation, or burping, which is common when the patient's stomach is empty.

Although vomiting is rare in uncomplicated duodenal ulcer, it may be a symptom of a complication of an ulcer. It results from obstruction of the pyloric orifice caused by either muscular spasm of the pylorus or mechanical obstruction from scarring or acute swelling of the inflamed mucous membrane adjacent to the ulcer. Vomiting may or may not be preceded by nausea; usually, it follows a bout of severe pain and bloating, which is relieved by vomiting the gastric contents. Emesis often contains undigested food eaten many hours earlier. Constipation or diarrhea may occur, probably as a result of diet and medications.

Fifteen percent of patients with peptic ulcer experience bleeding. The two most relevant risk factors for stress-related GI bleeding include prolonged mechanical ventilation and coagulopathy in the critically ill patient. Bleeding is considered a significant risk factor of morbidity/mortality for patients in the ICU (Vazin et al., 2020). Patients may present with GI bleeding as evidenced by the passage of **melena** (tarry stools). A small portion of patients who bleed from an acute ulcer have only very mild symptoms or none at all.

A physical examination may reveal pain, epigastric tenderness, or abdominal distention. A barium study of the upper GI tract may show an ulcer; however, endoscopy is the preferred diagnostic procedure because it allows direct visualization of inflammatory changes, ulcers, and lesions. Through endoscopy, a biopsy of the gastric mucosa and of any suspicious lesions can be obtained. Endoscopy may reveal lesions that, because of their size or location, are not evident on x-ray studies.

Stools may be tested periodically until they are negative for occult blood. Gastric secretory studies are of value in diagnosing achlorhydria and ZES. *H. pylori* infection may be determined by endoscopic and histologic examination of a tissue specimen obtained by biopsy or by a rapid urease test of the biopsy specimen. Other less invasive diagnostic measures for detecting *H. pylori* include serologic testing for antibodies against the *H. pylori* antigen, stool antigen test, and urea breath test (Mounsey & Leonard, 2019).

Medical and Nursing Management

Once the diagnosis is established, the patient is informed that the condition can be controlled. Recurrence may develop; however, peptic ulcers treated with antibiotics to eradicate *H. pylori* have a lower recurrence rate than those not treated with antibiotics. The goals are to eradicate *H. pylori* and to manage gastric acidity. Methods used include medications, lifestyle changes, and surgical intervention. The nurse instructs the patient about the factors that will relieve and those that will aggravate the peptic ulcer disease.

Pharmacologic Therapy

Currently, the most commonly used therapy for peptic ulcers is a combination of antibiotics, PPIs, and bismuth salts that suppress or eradicate *H. pylori* (see Table 22-1). This is, however, easier said than done. Only a few antibiotics (amoxicillin, clarithromycin, metronidazole, tetracycline, levofloxacin, and rifabutin) have been found to be effective and monotherapy does not reach sufficient efficacy (Tshibangu-Kabamba & Yamaoka, 2021). The most common cause of refractory *H. pylori* is antibiotic resistance, especially in the case of clarithromycin (Shah et al., 2021). It is important that the patient is asked prior to starting the first regimen if they have had any antibiotic exposure in the past. In cases where a patient has been exposed to a macrolide, clarithromycin is not recommended. Recommended therapy for 10 to 14 days includes triple therapy with two antibiotics (e.g., metronidazole or amoxicillin and clarithromycin) plus a PPI (e.g., lansoprazole, omeprazole, or rabeprazole), or quadruple therapy with two antibiotics (metronidazole and tetracycline) plus a PPI and bismuth salts. Longer treatment durations do lead to higher success in eradication (Shah et al., 2021). Ineffective acid suppression is also associated with failure. High-dose potent PPI or potassium-competitive acid blockers (PCAB [once available]) therapy should be considered for higher success rates (Shah et al., 2021).

One of the most common reasons for refractory *H.* pylori infections is failure to comply with medication regimens (Shah et al., 2021). The medication regimens are complicated and often not well understood by patients. The nurse is key in educating the patient regarding the importance of adhering to the prescribed medication. The nurse should identify barriers to adherence such as polypharmacy and work with patients to overcome them. The nurse should clearly explain potential adverse events and side effects of the medication. Rationale for prescribing such regimens should be described to patients to promote adherence (Shah et al., 2021). **Histamine-2 (H_2) receptor antagonists** (H_2 blockers) and PPIs are used to treat NSAID-induced ulcers and other ulcers not associated with *H. pylori* infection. One study notes that oral PPI use can be as effective as IV in duodenal ulcer healing (Csiki et al., 2021). Misoprostol (a mucosal protective drug) has similar effects as H_2 blockers in preventing ulcers when given in full doses, but its usefulness is limited due to GI side effects. It is not given to pregnant females because it can cause abortion, premature birth, or birth defects. Table 22-3 provides information about the drug regimens used for peptic ulcer disease.

Pearls for Practice

For patients with peptic ulcer disease who are taking NSAIDs or aspirin, the first step is to ensure the patient understands the need to stop such therapy.

TABLE **22-3 Drug Regimens for Peptic Ulcer Disease**

Indications	Drug Regimen	Comments
Ulcer healing	**H_2-receptor antagonists** Cimetidine 400 mg b.i.d. or 800 mg at bedtime Famotidine 20 mg b.i.d. or 40 mg at bedtime **Proton pump inhibitors (PPIs)** Omeprazole—40 mg daily Lansoprazole—30 mg daily Rabeprazole—20 mg daily Pantoprazole—40 mg daily Esomeprazole—40 mg daily	Should be used for 6 weeks for duodenal ulcer; 8 weeks for gastric ulcer Should be used for 4 weeks for duodenal ulcer and 6 weeks for gastric ulcer Healing occurs in 90% of patients who are compliant with therapy
Initial *Helicobacter pylori* therapy	**"Triple therapy"** PPI standard dose b.i.d. plus clarithromycin 500 mg b.i.d. plus amoxicillin 1,000 mg b.i.d. *or* metronidazole 500 mg t.i.d. for 10–14 days **"Quadruple therapy"** Bismuth Salt compound 2 tabs q.i.d. plus tetracycline 500 mg q.i.d. plus metronidazole 250 mg q.i.d. PPI standard dose b.i.d. daily for 14 days	Efficacy of therapy is approximately 85% q.i.d. dosing may decrease compliance Only in regions where *H. pylori* resistance is <15% and in patients with no history of macrolide exposure Can be used as second-line therapy if triple therapy fails
Therapy for retreatment of *H. pylori* therapy failure	Levofloxcacin 500 mg b.i.d. plus amoxicillin 750 mg t.i.d. PPI standard dose b.i.d. daily for 14 days Rifabutin 300 mg q.d. plus amoxicillin 750 mg t.i.d. PPI standard dose b.i.d. daily for 14 days Four (4) omeprazole-amoxicillin-rifabutin combination capsules (each capsule contains 10/250/12.5 mg) Amoxicillin 750 mg q.i.d. PPI standard dose b.i.d. daily for 14 days	PCN testing is recommended in the absence of anaphylaxis for patients labeled as having an allergy
Prophylactic therapy for NSAID ulcers	Peptic ulcer healing doses of PPIs (above) Misoprostol 200 μg q.i.d.	Prevents recurrent ulceration in approximately 80–90% of patients

NSAID, nonsteroidal anti-inflammatory drug.
Data from Shah et al. (2021).

For patients with ZES, hypersecretion of acid may be controlled with high doses of H2RA. These patients may require twice the normal dose, and dosages usually need to be increased with prolonged use. Octreotide, a medication that suppresses gastrin levels, also may be prescribed.

Patients at risk for stress ulcers (e.g., patients with head injury or extensive burns) may be treated prophylactically with IV H2RA and cytoprotective agents (e.g., misoprostol, sucralfate) because of the risk for upper GI tract hemorrhage.

Lifestyle Changes

Lifestyle changes include stress reduction, smoking cessation, and dietary modifications. Reducing environmental stress requires physical and psychological modifications on the patient's part as well as the aid and cooperation of family members and significant others. The nurse assists the patient to identify situations that are stressful or exhausting. A hectic lifestyle and an irregular schedule may aggravate symptoms and interfere with regular meals taken in relaxed settings along with the regular administration of medications. The patient may benefit from regular rest periods during the day, at least during the acute phase of the disease. Biofeedback, hypnosis, behavior modification, massage, or acupuncture may be helpful.

Studies have shown that smoking decreases the secretion of bicarbonate from the pancreas into the duodenum, resulting in increased acidity of the duodenum. Smoking is a known risk factor for PUD and continued smoking may significantly inhibit ulcer repair (Yim et al., 2021). Therefore, the patient is strongly encouraged to stop smoking. Smoking cessation support groups and other smoking cessation approaches should be offered to patients.

The intent of dietary modification for patients with peptic ulcers is to avoid oversecretion of acid and hypermotility in the GI tract. These can be minimized by avoiding extremes of temperature of food and beverage and overstimulation from consumption of meat extracts, alcohol, coffee (including decaffeinated coffee, which also stimulates acid secretion) and other caffeinated beverages, and diets rich in milk and cream (which stimulate acid secretion). In addition, an effort is made to neutralize acid by eating three regular meals a day. Small, frequent feedings are not necessary as long as an antacid or a histamine blocker is taken. Diet compatibility becomes an individual matter: the patient eats foods that are tolerated and avoids those that produce pain.

Surgical Management

The introduction of antibiotics to eradicate *H. pylori* and of H2RA as treatment for ulcers has greatly reduced the need for surgical intervention. However, surgery usually is recommended for patients with intractable ulcers (those that fail to heal after 12 to 16 weeks of medical treatment), life-threatening hemorrhage, perforation, or obstruction, and for those with ZES not responding to medications (Tarasconi et al., 2020). Surgical procedures include vagotomy, with or without **pyloroplasty** (transecting nerves that stimulate acid secretion and opening the pylorus) and **antrectomy**, which is removal of the pyloric (antrum) portion of the stomach with anastomosis to either the duodenum (gastroduodenostomy or Billroth I) or jejunum (gastrojejunostomy or Billroth II) procedure (see Table 22-4 and the section on Gastric Surgery).

Patients who require surgery may have had a long illness. They may be discouraged and have had interruptions

TABLE 22-4 **Surgical Procedures for Peptic Ulcer Disease**

Operation	Description	Comments
Vagotomy 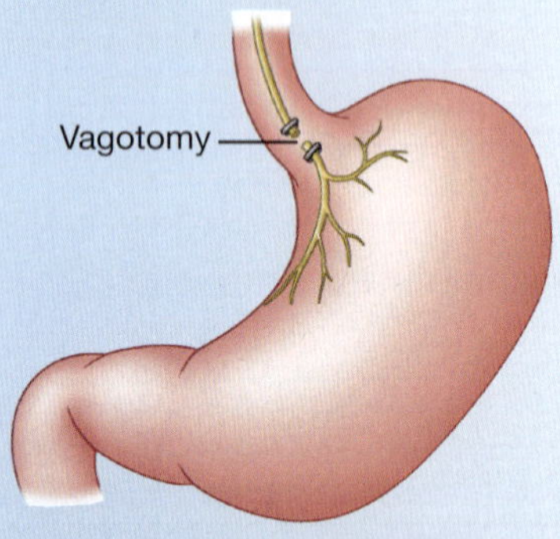	Severing of the vagus nerve. Decreases gastric acid by diminishing cholinergic stimulation to the parietal cells, making them less responsive to gastrin. May be performed via open surgical approach, laparoscopy, or thoracoscopy	May be performed to reduce gastric acid secretion. A drainage type of procedure (see pyloroplasty) is usually performed to assist with gastric emptying (because there is total denervation of the stomach). Some patients experience problems with feeling of fullness, dumping syndrome, diarrhea, and gastritis
Truncal Vagotomy	Severs the right and left vagus nerves as they enter the stomach at the distal part of the esophagus	This type of vagotomy is most commonly used to decrease acid secretions and reduce gastric and intestinal motility. Recurrence rate of ulcer is 10–15%.
Selective Vagotomy	Severs vagal innervation to the stomach but maintains innervation to the rest of the abdominal organs	With the availability of excellent acid secretion control with H_2-receptor antagonists and proton pump inhibitors, the need for surgical management of PUD has greatly decreased
Proximal (Parietal Cell) Gastric Vagotomy without Drainage	Denervates acid-secreting parietal cells but preserves vagal innervation to the gastric antrum and pylorus	No dumping syndrome. No need for drainage procedure. Recurrence rate of ulcer is 10–15%
Pyloroplasty 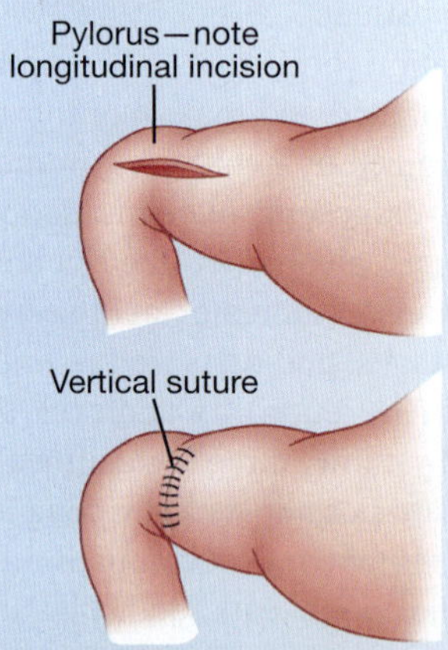	Longitudinal incision is made into the pylorus and transversely sutured closed to enlarge the outlet and relax the muscle	Usually accompanies truncal and selective vagotomies, which produce delayed gastric emptying due to decreased innervation

Operation	Description	Comments
Antrectomy		
Billroth I (Gastroduodenostomy) 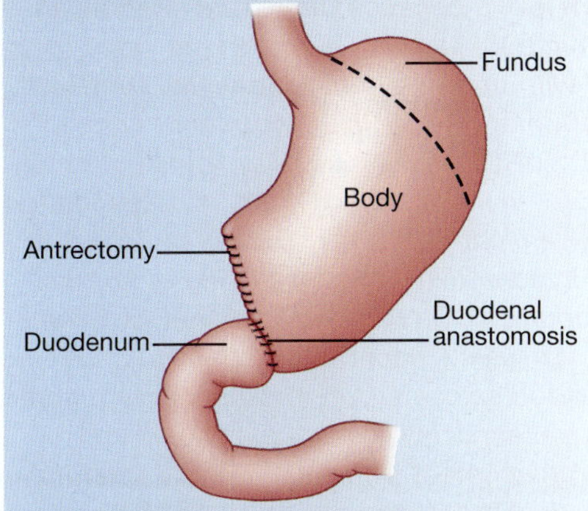	Removal of the lower portion of the antrum of the stomach (which contains the cells that secrete gastrin) as well as a small portion of the duodenum and pylorus. The remaining segment is anastomosed to the duodenum	May be performed in conjunction with a truncal vagotomy. The patient may have problems with feeling of fullness, dumping syndrome, and diarrhea. Recurrence rate of ulcer is 1%
Billroth II (Gastrojejunostomy) 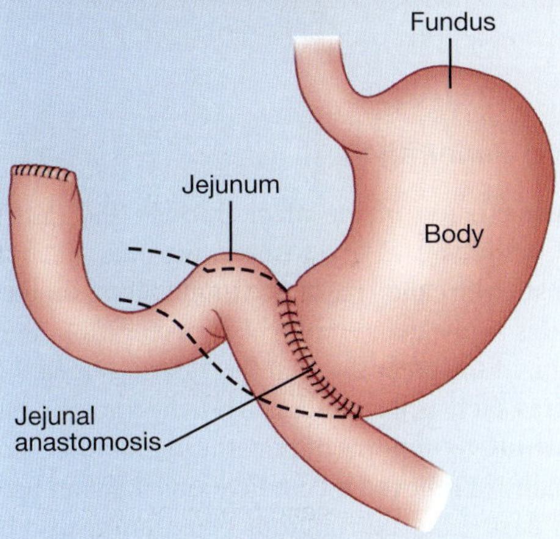	Removal of lower portion (antrum) of stomach with anastomosis to jejunum. Dotted lines show portion removed (antrectomy). A duodenal stump remains and is oversewn	Dumping syndrome, anemia, malabsorption, weight loss. Recurrence rate of ulcer is 10–15%

in their work role and pressures in their family life that affect their outlook on surgery and resolution of their disease. The nurse provides emotional support regarding the patient and family members altered role and additional responsibilities, and encourages them to express feelings, and ask questions. Referral to support groups or other services may be indicated.

Complications

Several complications may occur for the patient with peptic ulcer disease, including hemorrhage, perforation and penetration, and pyloric obstruction.

Pearls for Practice

The nurse reviews with the patient and family the signs and symptoms of complications to be reported. These complications include hemorrhage (cool skin, confusion, increased heart rate, labored breathing, and blood in the stool), penetration and perforation (severe abdominal pain, rigid and tender abdomen, vomiting, elevated temperature, and increased heart rate), and pyloric obstruction (nausea, vomiting, distended abdomen, and abdominal pain).

Hemorrhage

Gastritis and hemorrhage from peptic ulcer are the two most common causes of upper GI tract bleeding (which may also occur with esophageal varices, as discussed in Chapter 21). Hemorrhage, the most common complication, occurs in 28% to 59% of patients with peptic ulcers. Bleeding may be manifested by hematemesis (vomiting blood) or melena (Tarasconi et al., 2021). The vomited blood can be bright red, or it can have a dark "coffee grounds" appearance from the oxidation of hemoglobin to methemoglobin. When the hemorrhage is large (2,000 to 3,000 mL), most of the blood is vomited. Because large quantities of blood may be lost quickly, immediate correction of blood loss may be required to prevent hemorrhagic shock (Tarasconi et al., 2021). When the hemorrhage is small, much or all of the blood is passed in the stools, which appear tarry black because of the digested hemoglobin. Management depends on the amount of blood lost and the rate of bleeding.

The nurse assesses the patient for faintness or dizziness and nausea, which may precede or accompany bleeding. It is important to monitor vital signs frequently and to evaluate the patient for tachycardia, hypotension, and tachypnea. Other nursing interventions include monitoring the hemoglobin and Hct, testing the stool for gross or occult blood, and recording hourly urinary output to detect anuria or oliguria (absence of or decreased urine production).

Many times, the bleeding from a peptic ulcer stops spontaneously; however, the incidence of recurrent bleeding is high. Because bleeding can be fatal, the cause and severity of the hemorrhage must be identified quickly and the blood loss treated to prevent hemorrhagic shock.

If bleeding cannot be managed by medical therapies (IV infusion of crystalloids and colloids, gastric lavage, and pharmacologic agents), other treatment modalities may be used. Transendoscopic coagulation by laser, heat probe, medication, a sclerosing agent, or a combination of these therapies can halt bleeding and avert surgical intervention. There is debate regarding how soon endoscopy should be performed. Some clinicians believe endoscopy should be performed within the first 24 hours after hemorrhage has been stabilized. Others believe endoscopy may be performed during acute bleeding, as long as the esophageal or gastric area can be visualized (blood may decrease visibility).

For patients who are unable to undergo surgery, such as older patients with multiple comorbid conditions, selective embolization may be used (Kaminskis et al., 2019). This procedure involves forcing emboli of autologous blood clots with or without Gelfoam (absorbable gelatin sponge) through a catheter in the artery to a point above the bleeding lesion. This procedure is performed by an interventional radiologist.

Rebleeding may occur and often warrants surgical intervention. The nurse monitors the patient carefully so that bleeding can be detected quickly. Signs of bleeding include tachycardia, tachypnea, hypotension, mental confusion, thirst, and oliguria. If bleeding recurs within 48 hours after medical therapy has been initiated, or more than 6 to 10 units of blood are required within 24 hours to maintain blood volume, the patient may require surgery. Surgery may be recommended if the patient has three or more bleeding episodes. Other indications for surgery are the patient's age (massive hemorrhage is three times more likely to be fatal in people over 60 years of age), a history of chronic duodenal ulcer, and a coincidental gastric ulcer. The area of the ulcer is removed or the bleeding vessels are ligated. Many patients undergo procedures (e.g., vagotomy and pyloroplasty, gastrectomy) aimed at controlling the underlying cause of the ulcers (see Table 22-4).

Pearls for Practice

The nurse is aware that transfusions of blood lowers serum calcium levels because the citrate used as an anticoagulant in banked blood binds to the calcium. It is associated with massive transfusions (MT) defined as administration of greater than 10 units of packed red blood cells (pRBCs) in 24 hours or transfusion of 4 units of pRBCs in the first 30 minutes of resuscitation (D'Amore & Swaminathan, 2020). The nurse is alert to symptoms of hyperactive reflexes, tingling of fingers and around mouth, ECG changes, positive Chvostek or Trousseau sign (see Chapter 26 for details) and monitoring ionized calcium is important. Management of hypocalcemia, especially when ionized calcium is low, involves replacement with infusion of IV calcium. The nurse is aware that blood transfusions also put patients at risk for the development of transfusion-related acute lung injury (TRALI) and transfusion-associated circulatory overload (TACO). Refer to Chapter 19.

Perforation and Penetration

Perforation is the erosion of the ulcer through the gastric **serosa** into the peritoneal cavity without warning. It is an abdominal catastrophe and requires immediate surgery. Box 22-1 provides signs and symptoms of perforation. Penetration is erosion of the ulcer through the gastric serosa into adjacent structures such as the pancreas, biliary tract, or gastrohepatic **omentum**. Symptoms of penetration include back and epigastric pain not relieved by medications that had been effective in the past. Like perforation, penetration usually requires surgical intervention.

Because chemical peritonitis develops within a few hours after perforation and is followed by bacterial peritonitis, the perforation must be closed as quickly as possible and the abdominal cavity lavaged of stomach or intestinal contents. In select patients, it may be safe and advisable to perform

BOX 22-1 Focused Assessment

Perforation

Be alert for the following signs and symptoms:

- Sudden, severe upper abdominal pain (persisting and increasing in intensity); pain may be referred to the shoulders, especially the right shoulder, because of irritation of the phrenic nerve in the diaphragm
- Vomiting
- Collapse (fainting)
- Extremely tender and rigid (board like) abdomen
- Hypotension and tachycardia, indicating shock

surgery to treat the ulcer disease in addition to suturing the perforation.

During surgery and postoperatively, the stomach contents are drained by means of an NG tube. The nurse monitors fluid and electrolyte balance and assesses the patient for localized infection or peritonitis (increased temperature, abdominal pain, paralytic ileus, increased or absent bowel sounds, abdominal distention). Antibiotic therapy is administered parenterally as prescribed.

Pearls for Practice

Hematemesis (bright red or brown), "coffee grounds" vomiting (emesis), note the color will be dependent on the amount of gastric contents at the time of bleeding and the length of time the blood has been in contact with gastric secretions (Close, 2022). Hematochezia is the term for bright red stools, and melena refers to black, tarry, or dark red stools. Melena follows the digestion of blood from an upper GI bleed and may take several days to clear after the bleeding has stopped. Typically, blood in the GI tract results in increased peristalsis and diarrhea.

Pyloric Obstruction

Pyloric obstruction, also called **gastric outlet obstruction** (GOO), occurs when the area distal to the pyloric sphincter becomes scarred and stenosed from spasm or edema or from scar tissue that forms when an ulcer allternatively heals and breaks down. More than 95% of benign GOO is associated with peptic ulcer disease (duodenal or pyloric) (Jeong & Lee, 2020). The patient may have nausea and vomiting, constipation, epigastric fullness, anorexia, and, later, weight loss. On physical examination, abdominal distension may be noted with tympanic left upper quadrant.

In treating the patient with pyloric obstruction, the first consideration is to insert an NG tube to decompress the stomach. Usually, an upper GI study or endoscopy is performed to confirm pyloric obstruction. Decompression of the stomach and management of extracellular fluid volume and electrolyte balances may improve the patient's condition and avert the need for surgical intervention. A balloon dilation of the pylorus via endoscopy may be beneficial (Jeong & Lee, 2020). If the obstruction is unrelieved by medical management, surgery (in the form of a vagotomy and **antrectomy** or gastrojejunostomy and vagotomy) may be required. Recently, stent placement has been introduced as an alternative to surgical intervention with initial clinical success but may present problems with recurrent obstruction in patients with malignant gastric outlet obstruction (Jeong & Lee, 2020).

MORBID OBESITY

Morbid obesity is a term applied to people who are more than two times their ideal body weight or whose body mass index (BMI) exceeds 30 kg/m^2. Obesity is then classified into three additional categories: class 1 (BMI 30.0–34.9), class 2 (BMI 35.0–39.9) and class 3 (BMI >40) (Lin & Li, 2021). Some guidelines suggest measuring waist circumference to assess for abdominal obesity. Abdominal obesity is associated with increased health risks (Lin & Li, 2021). For example, waist circumference—more than 40 inches for males or more than 35 inches for females are considered as large waist circumferences (Haynes & Henry, 2022). While BMI is the gold standard for assessment for obesity, it only takes into account excess weight, but not necessarily excess fat. In cases where patients have lost weight but remain obese, BMI does not take into account the health benefits of weight loss. In the United States, where morbid obesity is a rapidly growing problem, 41.9% of adults are obese, and 9.2% are extremely obese (Center for Disease Control and Prevention [CDC], 2022). In addition, risk for diabetes mellitus (DM) has only been found to be accurate in white populations (Caleyachetty et al., 2021), which highlights the need to advocate for screening efforts, prevention and educational programs to end health disparities in high-risk and vulnerable populations.

Obesity is considered a chronic disease with multiple contributing factors. It is recognized that the main driving factor is abnormal satiety and feeding signaling. Other factors are genetic, behavior, cultural, and environmental (Kushner et al., 2020).

Patients with morbid obesity are at higher risk for health complications, such as DMs, heart disease, stroke, hypertension, gallbladder disease, osteoarthritis, sleep apnea and other breathing problems, and some forms of cancer (uterine, breast, colorectal, kidney, and gallbladder). They frequently suffer from low self-esteem, impaired body image, and depression. Patients with obesity are also at higher risk for complications with COVID-19 as outlined in the COVID-19 section below.

Medical Management

Conservative management of obesity consists of placing the person on a weight loss diet in conjunction with behavioral modification and exercise; however, dietary and behavioral approaches to obesity have had limited success. Dietician and behavioral health services can improve the efficacy of these interventions.

Pharmacologic Management

Pharmacologic management is recommended for patients with BMI >30 or >27 with comorbid conditions. Several medications are approved for treatment of obesity that work as an appetite reduction or inhibition of pancreatic lipase, which results in fat maldigestion. Examples include orlistat, liraglutide, and phentermine-topiramate (Lin & Lee, 2021). Orlistat, available by prescription and over the counter as Alli, reduces caloric intake by binding to gastric and pancreatic lipase to prevent digestion of fats. Side effects of orlistat may include increased frequency of bowel movements, increased gas with oily discharge, decreased food absorption, decreased bile flow, and decreased absorption of some vitamins. A multivitamin is usually recommended for patients taking orlistat. These medications are not recommended for pregnant females or those planning to become pregnant as weight loss offers no potential benefit during pregnancy. In addition, they have moderate efficacy as defined as <10% of body mass lost.

The newest medication to be approved is semaglutide. This medication was initially approved for type 2 DM. It is a GLP-1 analog that increases satiety and reduces hunger (Kushner et al., 2020). Semaglutide has been found effective in both weight loss and in reducing hemoglobin A1c.

Lorcaserin has been voluntarily removed from the U.S. market due to an increased safety risk of cancer (FDA, 2020). Sibutramine HCL was recently pulled from the European and U.S. markets because of the increased risk of heart attack and stroke associated with this medication. Rimonabant was pulled from the European markets and has not been approved for use in the United States due to concerns of neurologic and psychiatric side effects (FDA, 2022).

Surgical Management

Bariatric surgery, or surgery for morbid obesity, is performed only after other nonsurgical attempts at weight control have failed. There was a 10.8% increase of bariatric surgeries from 2017 to 2018 in the United States (English et al., 2020). Since 2011, there has been a 60% increase of bariatric procedures (English et al., 2020). Bariatric surgical procedures work by restricting a patient's ability to eat (restrictive procedure), interfering with ingested nutrient absorption (malabsorptive procedures), or both.

Different bariatric surgical procedures entail different lifestyle modifications, and patients must be well informed about the specific lifestyle changes, eating habits, and bowel habits that may result from a particular procedure. Studies have shown that the average weight loss after bariatric surgery in the majority of patients is approximately 61% of previous body weight; comorbid conditions such as DM, hypertension, and sleep apnea resolve; and dyslipidemia improves (Mechanick et al., 2020).

Patient selection is critical, and the preliminary process may necessitate 6 to 12 months of counseling, education, and evaluation by a multidisciplinary team, including social workers, dietitians, a nurse counselor, and a psychologist or psychiatrist, as well as a surgeon (Table 22-5) (Mechanick et al., 2020).

Because bariatric surgery involves such a drastic change in the functioning of the digestive system, body image, and lifestyle adjustments, patients need extensive counseling before and after the surgery (Mechanick et al., 2020). Guidelines have been developed to assist physicians and nurses in the care of patients having bariatric surgery (Mechanick et al., 2020). After bariatric surgery, all patients require lifelong monitoring of weight loss, comorbidities, metabolic and nutritional status, and dietary and activity behaviors because they are at risk for developing malnutrition or weight gain (Mechanick et al., 2019). Females of childbearing age who have bariatric surgery are advised to use contraceptives for approximately 12 to 18 months after surgery to avoid pregnancy until their weight stabilizes. Weight loss

TABLE **22-5 Selection Criteria for Bariatric Surgery**

Factor	Criteria
Weight (Adults)	• Body mass index (BMI) of at least 40 kg/m^2 with no comorbidities and procedures would not cause excessive risk • BMI of at least 35 kg/m^2 with obesity-associated comorbidity (e.g., severe sleep apnea, hypertension, cardiomyopathy related to obesity, severe diabetes mellitus; serious musculoskeletal or neurologic disorders) • BMI of 30–34.9 and type 2 diabetes mellitus with inadequate glycemic control despite optimal medication and lifestyle • BMI criteria should be adjusted for ethnicity (>25 for Asians)
Weight loss history	• Failure of previous nonsurgical attempts at weight reduction, including commercial programs (e.g., Weight Watchers, Inc.)
Commitment	• Expectation that patient will adhere to postoperative care • Follow-up visits with provider(s) and team members • Recommended medical management, including the use of dietary supplements • Instructions regarding any recommended procedures or tests • Culturally and educationally appropriate materials are recommended
Exclusions	• Reversible endocrine or other disorders that can cause obesity • Current drug or alcohol usage • Uncontrolled, severe psychiatric illness • Lack of comprehension of risks, benefits, expected outcomes, alternatives, and lifestyle changes required with bariatric surgery

Data from Mechanick, J. I., Apovian, C., Brethauer, S., Garvey, W. T., Joffe, A. M., Kim, J., Kushner, R. F., Lindquist, R., Pessah-Pollack, R., Seger, J., Urman, R. D., Adams, S., Cleek, J. B., Correa, R., Figaro, M. K., Flanders, K., Grams, J., Hurley, D. L., Kothari, S., Seger, M. V., & Still, C. D. (2020). AACE/TOS/ASMBS: Clinical practice guidelines for the perioperative nutritional, metabolic, and nonsurgical support of the bariatric surgery patient—2019 update. *Surgery for Obesity & Related Diseases*, *16*(2):175–247.

surgery has a positive correlation to fertility (Mechanick et al., 2019).

Procedures

The first surgical procedure used to treat morbid obesity was jejunoileal bypass. This procedure, which resulted in significant complications, has been largely replaced by gastric restriction procedures. RYGB, gastric banding, vertical banded gastroplasty, laparoscopic sleeve gastrectomy (SG), and biliopancreatic diversion with duodenal switch are the current procedures of choice. These procedures may be performed by laparoscopy or by an open surgical technique. Currently, 90% of all bariatric surgeries are done laparoscopically (Mechanick et al., 2020).

Gastric restrictive procedures, such as adjustable gastric banding (AGB), vertical banded gastroplasty and SG, cause early satiety during meals by decreasing the volume of the stomach. Laparoscopic AGB has replaced the vertical gastric banding (VGB) as the favored restrictive procedure. Malabsorptive procedures, such as biliopancreatic diversion with or without duodenal switch (BPD/DS), rely on bypassing various lengths of the small intestine, reducing nutrient absorption. Mixed procedures such as the RYGB combine gastric restriction with bypass of a short segment of the small intestine.

The RYGB is recommended for long-term weight loss. It is a combined restrictive and malabsorptive procedure. Biliopancreatic diversion with duodenal switch combines gastric restriction with intestinal malabsorption. See Figure 22-4A–E for additional details about these procedures. After weight loss, the patient may need surgical intervention for body contouring. This may include lipoplasty to remove fat deposits or a panniculectomy to remove excess abdominal skinfolds.

Complications

Bariatric surgical procedures have their own unique complications in addition to those associated with any major abdominal surgery. The most common complications are bleeding, blood clots, bowel obstruction, incisional or ventral hernias, and infection from a leak at the anastomosis. Prevention of complications is critical. Other postoperative problems that may occur include nausea, usually as a result of overfilling the stomach pouch or improper chewing; dumping syndrome associated with the consumption of simple sugars; and changes in bowel function, including diarrhea and constipation. Long-term complications that are related to nutritional deficiency may occur.

Nursing Management

Nursing management focuses on care of the patient after surgery. General postoperative nursing care is similar to that for a patient recovering from a gastric resection but with great attention given to the risks of complications associated with morbid obesity. Complications that may occur in the immediate postoperative period include peritonitis, stomal obstruction, stomal ulcers, atelectasis and pneumonia, thromboembolism, and metabolic imbalances resulting from prolonged vomiting and diarrhea or altered GI function. After bowel sounds have returned and oral intake is resumed, six small feedings consisting of a total of 600 to 800 calories per day are provided, and fluids are encouraged to prevent dehydration.

The patient is usually discharged in 4 days (23 to 72 hours for patients who have had laparoscopic procedures) with detailed dietary instructions (Box 22-2). The nurse instructs the patient to report excessive thirst or concentrated urine, both of which are indications of dehydration. Psychosocial interventions are also essential for these patients. Efforts are directed at helping them modify their eating behaviors and cope with changes in body image. The nurse explains that noncompliance by eating too much or too fast or eating high-calorie liquids and soft foods results in vomiting and painful esophageal distention. The nurse discusses dietary instructions before discharge and emphasizes the importance of routine follow-up outpatient appointments. Long-term side effects may include increased risk of gallstones, nutritional deficiencies (Table 22-6), and potential to regain weight. Factors integral to postsurgical weight loss success include dietary counseling; medication instruction on the importance of taking supplemental vitamin B_{12}, iron, and calcium as well as a standard multivitamin; cognitive-behavioral therapy; and support groups. Obese patients are at risk for vitamin and nutrient deficiencies (Mechanick et al., 2020). Nutritional deficits tend to stabilize by 2 years postprocedure and do not seem to be affected by type of gastric bypass procedure (Mechanick et al., 2020).

ESOPHAGEAL CANCER

Esophageal cancer is the eighth most common cancer worldwide and the sixth most common cause of death worldwide. In the United States, it is estimated that 18,440 new cases will occur each year. Esophageal cancer is highly lethal with 16,170 deaths from the disease (Siegel et al., 2020).

Pathophysiology

There are two types of malignant tumors that account for 95% of esophageal tumors—squamous cell (SCC) and adenocarcinoma (AC). SCC is found most predominately in the "esophageal cancer belt"—a region that spans both Africa and Asia. AC now accounts for the majority of tumors in Western countries (Table 22-7).

Pathogenesis of SCC is epithelial dysplasia that eventually leads to carcinoma in situ and invasive carcinoma. Precursor to AC is intestinal metaplasia. The metaplastic cells hyperproliferate and become dysplastic, which leads to malignancy.

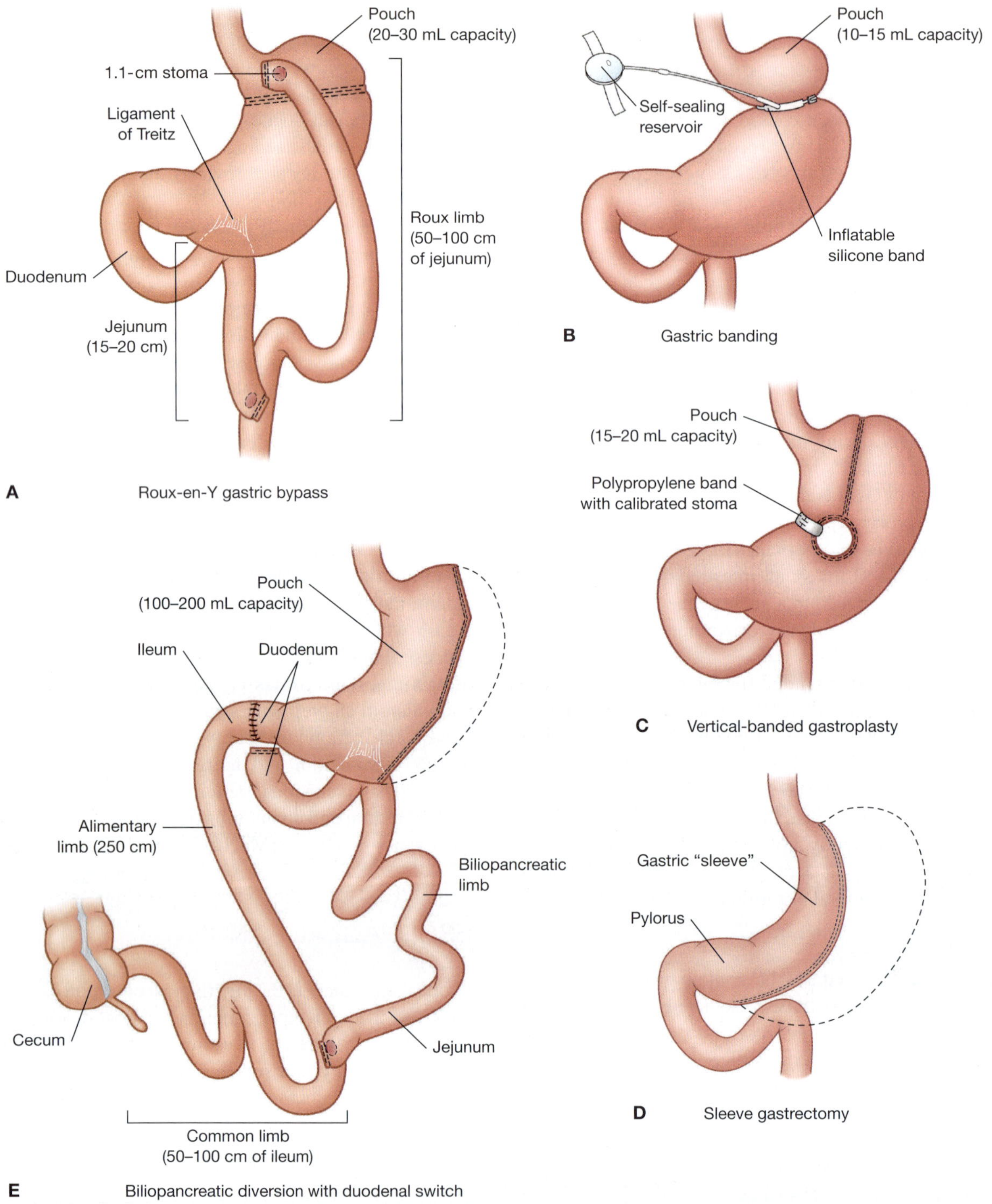

FIGURE 22-4 Surgical procedures for morbid obesity. A. Roux-en-Y gastric bypass. A horizontal row of staples across the fundus of the stomach creates a pouch with a capacity of 20 to 30 mL. The jejunum is divided distal to the ligament of Treitz, and the distal end is anastomosed to the new pouch. The proximal segment is anastomosed to the jejunum. B. Gastric banding. A prosthetic device is used to restrict oral intake by creating a small pouch of 10 to 15 mL that empties through the narrow outlet into the remainder of the stomach. C. Vertical-banded gastroplasty. A vertical row of staples along the lesser curvature of the stomach creates a new, smaller stomach pouch of 10 to 15 mL. D. Sleeve gastrectomy. The stomach is incised vertically and up to 85% of the stomach is surgically removed, leaving a "sleeve"-shaped tube that retains intact nervous innervation and does not obstruct or decrease the size of the gastric outlet. The tubular stomach has a limited gastric volume of 60 to 100 mL. E. Biliopancreatic diversion with duodenal switch. Half of the stomach is removed, leaving a small area that holds about 60 mL. The entire jejunum is excluded from the rest of the gastrointestinal tract. The duodenum is disconnected and sealed off. The ileum is divided above the ileocecal junction, and the distal end of the jejunum is anastomosed to the first portion of the duodenum. The distal end of the biliopancreatic limb is anastomosed to the ileum. (Reprinted with permission from Hinkle, J. L., & Cheever, K. H. [2013]. *Brunner & Suddarth's textbook of medical-surgical nursing* [13th ed.]. Lippincott, Wolters Kluwer Health.)

BOX 22-2

Patient Education

Dietary Guidelines for the Patient Who Has Had Bariatric Surgery

Nutrition:

- Eat six small meals per day (containing protein and fiber), and chew small bites of food thoroughly.
- Consume five daily servings of fresh fruits and vegetables.
- Include two protein snacks per day for a minimum protein intake of 60 g/d.
- Restrict total meal size to less than 1 cup.
- Eat only foods packed with nutrients (e.g., peanut butter, cheese, chicken, fish, beans).
- Do not eat and drink at the same time. Fluids should be consumed slowly.
- Concentrated sweets should be eliminated from the diet to avoid dumping syndrome.

Hydration:

- Fluids should be consumed slowly.
- Drink plenty of water, from 30 minutes after each meal to 15 minutes before the next meal.
- Avoid liquid calories, such as alcoholic beverages, fruit drinks, and regular soda (cola).

Supplements:

- Take 2 chewable multivitamin plus mineral (iron, folic acid, thiamine, copper, zinc) supplements daily.
- Diet/supplements should include 1,200–1,500 mg of elemental calcium.
- Diet/supplements should include:
  - 3,000 IU of vitamin D daily
  - Vitamin B12—1,000 ug/day
- Crushed or liquid rapid-release medications should be used instead of extended-release to maximize absorption.

Exercise:

- Walk for at least 30 minutes per day, minimum of 150 minutes (2½ hours) per week to a goal of 300 minutes (5 hours) per week, supplemented by strength training two to three times per week.

Data from Mechanick, J, I., Apovian, C., Brethauer, S., Garvey, W. T., Joffe, A. M., Kim, J., Kushner, R. F., Lindquist, R., Pessah-Pollack, R., Seger, J., Urman, R. D., Adams, S., Cleek, J. B., Correa, R., Figaro, M. K., Flanders, K., Grams, J., Hurley, D. L., Kothari, S., Seger, M. V., & Still, C. D. (2020). AACE/TOS/ASMBS: Clinical practice guidelines for the perioperative nutritional, metabolic, and nonsurgical support of the bariatric surgery patient–2019 update. *Surgery for Obesity & Related Diseases*, *16*(2):175–247.

Risk Factors

Common risk factors between the cancer types are male gender and smoking. It is not well understood why SCC is so prevalent in the esophageal cancer belt, but the working theory is that it is a combination of smoking, alcohol intake, a diet low in fruit and vegetables and drinking beverages at high temperatures (Yang et al., 2020). The most common additional risk factors for AC are GERD/BE and obesity. It is thought that the increase of obesity in Western countries is also leading to increase in esophageal cancer.

Clinical Manifestations and Assessment

Both types of tumor have similar clinical presentation. Dysphagia is the most common symptom and is classified as progressive with accompanying weight loss. Unfortunately, dysphagia commonly occurs when the luminal diameter is

TABLE **22-6 Nutritional Deficiencies After Bariatric Surgery**

Deficiency	Signs and Symptoms
Decreased hemoglobin	Anemia
Decreased ferritin	Anemia
Decreased iron	Fatigue, anemia, lethargy, pallor, and loss of hair
Decreased vitamin B_{12}	Macrocytic anemia, pernicious anemia, leukopenia, thrombocytopenia, paresthesia, neuropathy, muscular pains, weakness, fatigue, dizziness, and brittle nails
Decreased vitamin D_3	Symptoms may include osteopenia, muscle pain, bone fractures
Decreased β-carotene	Reducing the fat-soluble antioxidant capacity, neuropathy
Decreased calcium	Osteopenia, bone fractures
Decreased magnesium	Muscle cramps, muscle pain, constipation, headaches, insomnia, anxiety, hyperactivity
Decreased zinc	Delayed wound healing, altered immune function, mental lethargy, perhaps association with alopecia

Data from Gletsu-Miller, N., & Wright, B. (2013). Mineral malnutrition following bariatric surgery. *Advances in Nutrition*, *4*, 506–517.

TABLE 22-7 **Comparison of Squamous Cell and Adenocarcinoma Tumors**

Feature	Squamous Cell	Adenocarcinoma
Predominance	Was the most predominant of the 20th century Still the most prominent worldwide	Increasing in prevalence in Western countries >60% of tumors in Western countries
Pathophysiology	Precursor is epithelial dysplasia Leads to carcinoma in situ and eventually invasive carcinoma Generally, arises 10 years prior to adenocarcinoma Perioperative mortality higher	Precursor is intestinal metaplasia Metaplastic cells hyperproliferate As they acquire DNA damage, becomes dysplastic and eventually malignant Many (but not all) data support better prognosis
Risk Factors	Male gender (2.5:1) African American ethnicity (4:1) Middle esophagus Smoking Alcohol	Male gender (2.5:1) White ethnicity (4:1) Distal esophagus Smoking GERD/Barrett esophagus Obesity

<13 mm (normal is approximately 20 mm). Odynophagia or painful swallowing also occurs in about 20% of cases. Less common manifestations are regurgitation, anemia, TE fistula, and signs/symptoms of metastatic disease.

Endoscopy with biopsy is the diagnostic study of choice. Biopsy will confirm the diagnosis in 90% of cases with an accuracy of 98% if seven or greater biopsies are taken. Appropriate TNM staging (see Chapter 5) is critical as it directly impacts management. Endoscopic ultrasound plays a key role in locoregional staging (restricted to a localized region), but there is discussion in the role for determining surgical treatment.

Medical and Nursing Management

Small lesions (<2 cm) limited to the mucosa of the esophagus may be successfully resected via endoscopy. For larger lesions or more complex cancers, a multimodal approach is recommended. Tumor resection or esophagectomy will be considered. An esophagectomy is the surgical procedure that removes some or all of the esophagus and reconstructs it using part of an organ, usually the stomach. The two primary chemotherapy recommendations are low-dose weekly carboplatin plus paclitaxel regimen or fluorouracil, leucovorin, oxaliplatin, and docetaxel (FLOT) which is a combination of chemotherapy drugs (Demarest & Chang, 2021). FLOT therapy is preferred in AC. For both types of tumor, chemoradiotherapy (CRT) can be used even if patients are not surgical candidates. The CROSS trial, which is the standard of practice, shows significant survival benefit with CRT versus RT or surgery alone. This was validated at the 10-year mark (Eyck et al., 2020).

For patients with advanced and inoperable tumors, treatment will be RT with chemotherapy. The majority of patients will not benefit from an esophagectomy. Brachytherapy can be a more durable therapy than an esophageal stent (a stent can help reopen a blocked esophagus and ease symptoms), but is limited to patients with <6 months life expectancy. There is a risk of esophageal fistula formation with the use of stents.

For survivors of esophageal cancer, follow-up is key. The majority of recurrences will occur in the first year. Surveillance with history/physical, CBC, imaging, EGD/dilation, and nutrition is the recommended follow-up (NCCN guidelines, 2019).

Pearls for Practice

GERD is a main risk factor for AC. Education on GERD management is critical to avoid complications and even esophageal cancer for patients.

GASTRIC CANCER

The incidence of gastric or stomach cancer continues to decrease in the United States; however, it still accounts for more than 11,000 deaths annually (American Cancer Society, 2022). The prognosis is generally poor: usually the diagnosis is made late because most patients are asymptomatic during the early stages of the disease. Gastric cancer found before the age of 45 is called "early-onset gastric cancer (GC)," while cancer found after is called "conventional GC."

Pathophysiology

Most gastric cancers are ACs; they can occur anywhere in the stomach. The Lauren classification divides the cancers into two subtypes—intestinal and diffuse. Intestinal shows visible connections between the tumor cells, where the diffuse has no cohesion (Machlowska et al., 2020). The tumor infiltrates the surrounding mucosa, penetrating the wall of the stomach and adjacent organs and structures. Often the liver, pancreas, esophagus, and duodenum are affected at the time of diagnosis. Metastasis through lymph to the peritoneal cavity occurs later in the disease.

GI lymphoma represents a second classification, differing in pathogenesis, treatment, and prognosis. Gastric MALT (**m**ucosa-**a**ssociated **l**ymphoid **t**issue) lymphoma is the most common entity with *H. pylori* as the decisive pathogenic factor (Holmes et al., 2021). MALT is acquired as a secondary process against *H. pylori*. The bacterium is the cause of chronic gastritis and leads to the formation of intramucosal lymph follicles (Holmes et al., 2021). Eradication of the bacteria results in regression of the lymphoma in 77.5% of Stage I tumors. The nurse should discuss the risk of gastric MALT and the importance of *H. pylori* eradication. Chemotherapy or radiation may be required for patients with Stage II disease (Holmes et al., 2021).

Risk Factors

The typical patient with gastric cancer is between 55 and 84 years, with peak diagnosis at age 68 years, but gastric cancer can rarely occur in people younger than 40 years of age, then, incidence gradually increases (Clinical Overview, 2022). Males have a higher incidence of gastric cancer than do females. Native Americans, Hispanic American people, and Black individuals are twice as likely as White American individuals to develop gastric cancer (Jameson et al., 2020; NCI, 2020). The incidence of gastric cancer is much greater in Japan, which has instituted mass screening programs for earlier diagnosis. Diet appears to be a significant factor: a diet high in smoked, salted, or pickled foods and low in fruits and vegetables may increase the risk of gastric cancer. Other factors related to the incidence of gastric cancer include chronic inflammation of the stomach, *H. pylori* infection, Epstein–Barr virus, pernicious anemia, smoking, achlorhydria, gastric ulcers, previous subtotal gastrectomy (more than 20 years ago), and genetics.

Clinical Manifestations and Assessment

Symptoms of early disease, such as pain relieved by antacids, resemble those of benign ulcers and are seldom definitive because most gastric tumors begin on the lesser curvature of the stomach, where they cause little disturbance of gastric function. Symptoms of progressive disease include dyspepsia (indigestion), early satiety, weight loss, abdominal pain just above the umbilicus, loss or decrease in appetite, bloating after meals, nausea and vomiting, and symptoms similar to those of peptic ulcer disease.

The physical examination is usually not helpful in detecting the cancer because most early gastric tumors are not palpable. Advanced gastric cancer may be palpable as a mass. Ascites, hepatomegaly (enlarged liver), and jaundice may be apparent if the cancer cells have metastasized to the liver. Palpable nodules around the umbilicus, called Sister Mary Joseph's nodules, are a sign of a GI malignancy, usually a gastric cancer. Patients appear cachectic. Esophagogastroduodenoscopy for biopsy and cytologic washings is the diagnostic study of choice, and a barium x-ray examination of the upper GI tract also may be performed. Endoscopic ultrasound is an important tool to assess tumor depth and any lymph node involvement. Computed tomography (CT) completes the diagnostic studies, particularly to assess for surgical resectability of the tumor before surgery is scheduled. CT of the chest, abdomen, and pelvis is valuable in staging gastric cancer.

Medical and Nursing Management

There is no successful treatment for gastric carcinoma except removal of the tumor. If the tumor can be removed while it is still localized to the stomach, the patient may be cured. If the tumor has spread beyond the area that can be excised, cure is less likely. In many patients, effective palliation to prevent discomfort caused by obstruction or dysphagia may be obtained by resection of the tumor (see Gastric Surgery). A diagnostic laparoscopy may be the initial surgical approach to evaluate the gastric tumor, obtain tissue for pathologic diagnosis, and detect metastasis. The patient with a tumor that is deemed resectable undergoes an open surgical procedure to resect the tumor and appropriate lymph nodes. The patient with an unresectable tumor and advanced disease would undergo chemotherapy.

A total gastrectomy may be performed for a resectable cancer in the midportion or body of the stomach. The entire stomach is removed, along with duodenum, the section of esophagus attached to the stomach, supporting mesentery, and lymph nodes. Reconstruction of the GI tract is performed by anastomosing the end of the jejunum to the end of the esophagus, a procedure called an *esophagojejunostomy*.

A radical subtotal gastrectomy is performed for a resectable tumor in the middle and distal portions of the stomach. A Billroth I or Billroth II operation (see Table 22-4) is performed. The Billroth I involves a limited resection and offers a lower cure rate than the Billroth II. The Billroth II procedure is a wider resection that involves removing approximately 75% of the stomach and decreases the possibility of lymph node spread or metastatic recurrence.

A proximal subtotal gastrectomy may be performed for a resectable tumor located in the proximal portion of the stomach or cardia. A total gastrectomy or an esophagogastrectomy is usually performed in place of this procedure to achieve a more extensive resection. A palliative surgical procedure may be required for patients with gastric cancer to achieve a better QOL.

Common problems of advanced gastric cancer that often require surgery include pyloric obstruction, bleeding, and severe pain. Gastric perforation is an emergency situation requiring surgical intervention. A gastric resection may be the most effective palliative procedure for advanced gastric cancer. Palliative procedures, such as gastric or esophageal bypass, gastrostomy, or jejunostomy, may alleviate symptoms such as nausea and vomiting temporarily. Palliative rather than radical surgery may be performed if there is metastasis to other vital organs, such as the liver, or to achieve a better QOL. Patients often report a decrease in QOL when the symptom burden of the cancer is prevalent.

Symptoms include fatigue, pain, worry, irritability, lack of energy, and difficulty sleeping (Machlowska et al., 2020).

If surgical treatment does not offer cure, treatment with chemotherapy may offer further control of the disease or palliation (Machlowska et al., 2020). No consistent outcomes have been observed, however these therapies are generally proven to increase survivorship at around 50% (Machlowska et al., 2020). Commonly used chemotherapeutic agents used unaccompanied or in combination include (5-fluorouracil, epirubicin, cisplatin, irinotecan, capecitabine, docetaxel, oxaliplatin, doxorubicin, etoposide, and mitomycin-C). For improved response rates, it is more common to administer combination therapy, primarily 5-fluorouracil–based therapy, with other agents. Studies are being conducted to assess the use of chemotherapy before surgery. RT is used mainly for palliation in patients with obstruction, GI bleeding secondary to tumor, and significant pain. In addition, immunotherapy may be used in gastric carcinoma (Rodrigues & Figueiredo, 2022) (see Chapter 5). Assessment of tumor markers (blood analysis for antigens indicative of cancer), such as carcinoembryonic antigen (CEA), carbohydrate antigen (CA 19-9), and CA 50, may help determine the effectiveness of treatment. If these values were elevated before treatment, they should decrease if the tumor is responding to the treatment (Krasnick et al., 2022). Meticulous attention to nutrition (jejunal enteral feedings or total parenteral nutrition [TPN]) is an essential aspect of patient management.

GASTRIC SURGERY

Gastric surgery may be performed on patients with peptic ulcers who have life-threatening hemorrhage, obstruction, perforation, or penetration, or whose condition does not respond to medication. It also may be indicated for patients with gastric cancer or trauma. Surgical procedures include a vagotomy and **pyloroplasty** (transecting nerves that stimulate acid secretion and opening the pylorus), a partial gastrectomy, or a total gastrectomy (see Table 22-4).

NURSING PROCESS
The Patient Undergoing Gastric Surgery

ASSESSMENT

Before surgery, the nurse assesses the patient's and family's knowledge of pre- and postoperative surgical routines and the rationale for surgery. The nurse also assesses the patient's nutritional status: Has the patient lost weight? How much? Over how much time? The nurse is aware that a 5% weight loss in 30 days, a 7.5% weight loss in 90 days, or a greater than 10% weight loss in 180 days is associated with significant health risks (MedlinePlus, 2022). Does the patient have nausea and vomiting? Has the patient had hematemesis? The nurse assesses for the presence of bowel sounds and palpates the abdomen to detect masses or tenderness.

After surgery, the nurse assesses the patient for complications secondary to the surgical intervention, such as hemorrhage, infection, abdominal distention, atelectasis, or impaired nutritional status.

DIAGNOSIS

Nursing diagnoses may include the following:

- Anxiety related to surgical intervention
- Acute pain related to surgical incision
- Deficient knowledge about surgical procedure and postoperative course
- Imbalanced nutrition, less than body requirements, related to poor nutrition before surgery and altered GI system after surgery

PLANNING

The major goals for the patient undergoing gastric surgery may include reduced anxiety, increased knowledge and understanding about the surgical procedure and postoperative course, optimal nutrition and management of the complications that can interfere with nutrition, relief of pain, avoidance of hemorrhage and steatorrhea, and enhanced self-care skills at home.

NURSING INTERVENTIONS

REDUCING ANXIETY

An important part of the preoperative nursing care involves allaying the patient's fears and anxieties about the impending surgery and its implications. The nurse encourages the patient to verbalize fears and concerns and answers the patient's and family's questions. If the patient has an acute obstruction, a perforated bowel, or an active GI hemorrhage, adequate psychological preparation may not be possible. In this event, the nurse caring for the patient after surgery should anticipate the concerns, fears, and questions that are likely to surface and should be available for support and further explanations.

RELIEVING PAIN

After surgery, analgesics may be administered as prescribed to relieve pain and discomfort. It is important to provide adequate pain relief so the patient can perform pulmonary care activities (deep breathing and coughing) and leg exercises, turn from side to side, and ambulate. The nurse assesses the effectiveness of analgesic intervention and consults with other members of the health care team if pain is not controlled adequately. Positioning the patient in the Fowler position promotes comfort and allows emptying of the stomach after gastric surgery.

The nurse maintains functioning of the NG tube to prevent distention and secures the tube to prevent dislocation, which may result in increased pain and tension on the suture line. Normally, the amount of NG drainage after a total gastrectomy is minimal as there is no reservoir where secretions can collect.

PROVIDING TEACHING

The nurse explains routine pre- and postoperative procedures to the patient, which include preoperative medications, NG intubation, IV fluids, abdominal dressings, and the possible need for a feeding tube, pain management, and pulmonary care. These explanations need to be reinforced after surgery, especially if the patient had emergency surgery.

RESUMING ENTERAL INTAKE

The patient's nutritional status is evaluated before surgery. If surgery is performed for gastric cancer, often the patient is malnourished and may require preoperative enteral or, more often, parenteral nutrition. After surgery, parenteral nutrition may be continued to meet caloric needs, to replace fluids lost through drainage and vomiting, and to support the patient metabolically until oral intake is adequate.

After the return of bowel sounds and removal of the NG tube, the nurse may give fluids, followed by food in small portions. Foods are added gradually until the patient is able to eat six small meals a day and drink 120 mL of fluid between meals. The key to increasing the dietary content is to offer food and fluids gradually, as tolerated, and to recognize that each patient's tolerance is different.

RECOGNIZING OBSTACLES TO ADEQUATE NUTRITION

Dysphagia and Gastric Retention. Dysphagia may occur in patients who have had a truncal vagotomy, a surgical procedure that may result in trauma to the lower esophagus. Gastric retention may be evidenced by abdominal distention, nausea, and vomiting. Regurgitation also may occur if the patient has eaten too much or too quickly. It also may indicate that edema along the suture line is preventing fluids and food from moving into the intestinal tract. If gastric retention occurs, it may be necessary to reinstate NPO status and NG suction; pressure must be low in the remaining portion of the stomach to avoid disrupting the sutures.

Bile Reflux. Bile reflux gastritis and esophagitis may occur with the removal of the pylorus, which acts as a barrier to the reflux of duodenal contents. Burning epigastric pain and vomiting of bilious material manifest this condition. Eating or vomiting does not relieve the situation. Agents that bind with bile acid, such as cholestyramine, may be helpful. Antacids and metoclopramide hydrochloride have been used with limited success.

Dumping Syndrome. **Dumping syndrome** is an unpleasant set of vasomotor and GI symptoms that sometimes occur in patients who have had gastric surgery or a form of vagotomy. It is seen in 10% of all patients having gastric surgery (Hui et al., 2021). It may be the mechanical result of surgery in which a small gastric remnant is connected to the jejunum through a large opening. Foods high in carbohydrates and electrolytes must be diluted in the jejunum before absorption can take place, but the passage of food from the stomach remnant into the jejunum is too rapid to allow this to happen. The hypertonic intestinal contents draw extracellular fluid from the circulating blood volume into the jejunum to dilute the high concentration of electrolytes and sugars. The ingestion of fluid at mealtime is another factor that causes the stomach contents to empty rapidly into the jejunum (Hui et al., 2021).

Early symptoms include a sensation of fullness, weakness, faintness, dizziness, palpitations, diaphoresis, cramping pains, and diarrhea. These symptoms resolve once the intestine has been evacuated. Later, there is a rapid elevation of blood glucose, followed by increased insulin secretion. This results in a reactive hypoglycemia, which also is unpleasant for the patient. Vasomotor symptoms that occur 10 to 90 minutes after eating are pallor, perspiration, palpitations, headache, and feelings of warmth, dizziness, and even drowsiness. These symptoms are thought to be partially due to hypovolemia caused by rapid shifts of fluid from the intravascular space into the lumen of the bowel (Hui et al., 2021). Anorexia also may be a result of the dumping syndrome, as the person may be reluctant to eat. There are no symptoms in fasting state.

Steatorrhea (excess fat in feces) also may occur in the patient with gastric surgery. It is partially the result of rapid gastric emptying, which prevents adequate mixing with pancreatic and biliary secretions. In mild cases, reducing the intake of fat and administering an antimotility medication (e.g., loperamide) may control steatorrhea.

Vitamin and Mineral Deficiencies. Other dietary deficiencies that the nurse should be aware of include malabsorption of organic iron, which may require supplementation with oral or parenteral iron, and a low serum level of vitamin B_{12}, which may require supplementation by the intramuscular route. Total gastrectomy results in lack of intrinsic factor, a gastric secretion required for the absorption of vitamin B_{12} from the GI tract. Unless this vitamin is supplied by parenteral injection after gastrectomy, the patient inevitably will suffer vitamin B_{12} deficiency, which eventually leads to a condition identical to pernicious anemia. All manifestations of pernicious anemia, including macrocytic anemia (few, fragile, and larger than normal red blood cells) and combined system disease (neurologic disorders of the central and peripheral nervous systems), may be expected to develop within a period of 5 years or less; they progress in severity thereafter and, in the absence of therapy, are fatal. This complication is avoided by the regular monthly intramuscular injection of vitamin B_{12}. This regimen should be started without delay after gastrectomy. Weight loss is a common long-term problem because the patient experiences early fullness, which suppresses the appetite (Çalapkorur & Küçükkatirci, 2020).

TEACHING DIETARY SELF-MANAGEMENT

Because the patient may experience any of the described conditions affecting nutrition, nursing intervention includes proper dietary instruction (Box 22-3). The nurse also gives

(continued on page 772)

BOX 22-3 **Patient Education**

Dietary Management after Gastric Surgery

- To delay stomach emptying and dumping syndrome, after the meal, the patient should lie down for 20–30 minutes.
- Take antispasmodics as prescribed to aid in delaying the emptying of the stomach.
- Do not drink fluids with meals; instead, drink fluids up to 1 hour before or 1 hour after mealtime.
- Create meals containing more dry items than liquid items.
- Eat fat as tolerated, but keep carbohydrate intake low and avoid concentrated sources of carbohydrates (sugared soda, pastries). Increase or supplement dietary fibers.
- Eat smaller but more frequent meals.
- Take dietary supplements of vitamins and medium-chain triglycerides and injections of vitamin B_{12} and iron as prescribed.

instructions regarding enteral or parenteral supplementation if it is needed.

MONITORING AND MANAGING POTENTIAL COMPLICATIONS

Occasionally, hemorrhage complicates gastric surgery. The patient has the usual signs of rapid blood loss and shock (see Chapter 53) and may vomit considerable amounts of bright red blood. The nurse assesses NG drainage for type and amount; some bloody drainage for the first 12 hours is expected, but excessive bleeding should be reported. The nurse also assesses the abdominal dressing for bleeding. Because this situation is upsetting to the patient and family, the nurse should remain calm. The nurse performs emergency measures, such as NG lavage and administration of blood and blood products, along with vigilant hemodynamic monitoring.

TEACHING PATIENTS SELF-CARE

Patient teaching is based on the assessment of the patient's physical and psychological readiness to participate in self-care. The nurse provides information about nutrition, enteral or parenteral nutrition if required, nutritional supplements, pain management, and the symptoms of dumping syndrome and measures to prevent or minimize these symptoms.

The patient and caregivers benefit from a team approach to discharge planning. The team members include the patient and caregiver along with the nurse, physician, dietitian, and social worker. Written or video instructions about meals, activities, medications, and follow-up care are helpful. After the patient is discharged from the hospital, the home care nurse helps with the transition to home by supervising the administration of any enteral or parenteral feedings, emphasizing information about detection and prevention of untoward effects or complications related to feedings. Information about community support groups and end-of-life care is provided to the patient, family, or significant other when indicated.

EVALUATION

Expected patient outcomes may include:

1. Reports decreased anxiety; expresses fears and concerns about surgery
2. Demonstrates knowledge regarding postoperative course by discussing the surgical procedure and postoperative course
3. Attains optimal nutrition:
   a. Maintains a reasonable weight
   b. Does not have excessive diarrhea
   c. Tolerates six small meals a day
   d. Does not experience dysphagia, gastric retention, bile reflux, dumping syndrome, or vitamin and mineral deficiencies
4. Attains optimal level of comfort
5. Exhibits no complications

DUODENAL TUMORS

Tumors of the duodenum are uncommon and, when present, usually are benign and asymptomatic. They are most often discovered at autopsy. Malignant tumors are more likely to cause specific signs and symptoms leading to diagnosis. Unfortunately, malignant tumors often are not discovered until they have metastasized to distant sites. Benign tumors may place patients at an increased risk for malignancy. The relative rarity of tumors of the duodenum and the nonspecific nature of their manifestations complicate their diagnosis and treatment.

Clinical Manifestations and Assessment

Duodenal tumors often present insidiously with vague, nonspecific symptoms. Most benign tumors are discovered incidentally on an x-ray study, during surgery, or at autopsy. When the patient is symptomatic, benign tumors often present with intermittent pain. The next most common presentation is occult bleeding. Malignant tumors often result in symptoms that lead to their diagnosis, although these symptoms may reflect advanced disease. Most patients have sustained weight loss and are malnourished at diagnosis. Bleeding and pain are common. Perforation of the bowel occurs in approximately 10% of patients (Amini & Lopez, 2021).

The traditional approach to diagnosis is an upper GI x-ray series with small bowel follow-through using oral water-insoluble contrast with frequent and detailed x-rays to follow the contrast through the small bowel. A more sensitive examination is an **enteroclysis**, in which an NG tube is advanced into the small bowel to a position above the area in question; then the area is studied by single-contrast and double-contrast techniques. Abdominal CT is used to determine the extent of disease outside the lumen of the duodenum.

Medical and Nursing Management

Benign tumors of the duodenum include adenomas, lipomas, hemangiomas, and hamartomas (a focal malformation that resembles a neoplasm but, unlike a neoplasm, does not result in compression of adjacent tissue). These tumors may be treated endoscopically by excision/resection or electrocautery if the patient is symptomatic. Routine surveillance may be recommended to assess for malignant transformation.

The most common primary malignant tumor of the duodenum is AC; the second and third portions of the duodenum are most often involved. These tumors may present with bleeding or duodenal obstruction (Floch, 2020). If the tumor is located at the ampulla of Vater, obstructive jaundice is likely. Other rare malignant tumors of the duodenum include carcinoid tumors, lymphoma, and GI stromal tumors. Specialized abdominal surgery may be required to remove these rare tumors. Chemotherapy and RT may also be part of the treatment regimen.

Nursing care of the patient with a duodenal tumor is similar to that of the patient with gastric cancer. Each patient requires specialized care, astute assessment for complications, prompt interventions, and individualized teaching for self-care.

COVID-19 CONSIDERATIONS

One of the more striking memories from the beginning of the severe acute respiratory syndrome *coronavirus 2* (SARS-CoV-2) pandemic was the panic around purchasing toilet paper. As it turns out, this was not a fool's errand. GI symptoms are emerging as one of the more common manifestations of COVID-19.

Clinical Manifestations and Assessment

Various GI symptoms were noted in 3.0% to as high as 79% of patients. Most common symptoms are: anorexia, vomiting, nausea, diarrhea, GI bleeding, and abdominal pain (see Table 22-8). These can often be the heralding symptoms, preceding even fever and respiratory symptoms (Schmulson et al., 2020). Patients with higher severity of disease were found to have a higher instance of diarrhea, nausea, or vomiting (Ma et al., 2020). GI symptoms alone were noted in 3% of patients (Zuo et al., 2020). Worth noting that early studies were with hospitalized patients, who might have been on antibiotics or other treatments that may have exacerbated or caused GI symptoms. The CDC continues to list nausea, vomiting, and diarrhea as main symptoms of disease (CDC, accessed 2021).

TABLE 22-8 Gastrointestinal Symptoms Found in SARS-CoV-2

Symptom	Mean Instance (%)
Anorexia	46.5
Vomiting	44
Nausea	21.3
Diarrhea	12.9
GI bleed	9.6
Abdominal pain	6.0

SARS-CoV-2 can be detected in the stool. This is significant because it suggests it can both exist and replicate in the digestive tract. Fecal calprotectin has been noted to be elevated in patients that did not have inflammatory bowel disease, suggesting inflammation (Schmulson et al., 2020).

Pathophysiology

While new data are emerging almost daily regarding SARS-CoV-2, several concepts are taking hold regarding the GI tract involvement.

The spike glycoprotein of SARS-CoV-2 is thought to leverage the angiotensin-converting enzyme 2 (ACE2) receptors to gain access to cells. This causes replication, proliferation, and suppression of the host's immune response. The initial point of entry is inhaling air droplets into the respiratory tract (Zuo et al., 2020). There are ACE2 receptors distributed in many human organs and ACE2 expression is 100-fold higher in the GI tract. This makes not only the small bowel and colon susceptible, but also oral cavity, tongue, and esophagus (Zuo et al., 2020).

Another explanation for GI involvement is that the SARS-CoV-2 virus might reduce tryptophan absorption via ACE2 receptors. This phenomenon has been seen in mouse studies, but not yet human studies. This theoretically leads into disruption of the gut microbiota and can lead to inflammation (Zuo et al., 2020).

Gut Dysbiosis

Studies have shown that respiratory infections can alter the gut microbiota and SARS-CoV-2 is no different. Gut dysbiota (the microbiome is out of balance) can lead to continued GI symptoms as well as functional gastrointestinal disorders (FGIDs).

Studies have shown disruption of the gut microbiota within COVID-19 patients. The presence of these bacteria correlated with disease severity. Coporobacillus bacterium is known to upregulate colonic expression of ACE2, theoretically creating a more desirable environment for the SARS-CoV-2 virus (Zuo et al., 2020). Some bacteria are being studied as protective against COVID-19 due to their downregulation of ACE2 receptors (Zuo et al., 2020).

Gut inflammation, infection, and dysbiosis are common triggers for long-lasting FGIDs. It was found that alterations in the gut microbiota persisted after SARS-CoV-2 infection had resolved (Zuo et al., 2020). Prolonged virus shedding might be contributing to low-grade inflammation, gut permeability, and bile acid malabsorption (Ma et al., 2020). It is also postulated that psychological factors will also play into post–COVID-19 FGIDs. Post-traumatic stress and other psychological stressors are known to be associated with FGID (Schmulson et al., 2020).

Obesity

Obesity is emerging as a significant risk factor for morbidity and even mortality associated with COVID-19. Complications that have been shown to be increased in patients with obesity are respiratory failure, acute respiratory distress syndrome (ARDS) and bilateral pneumonia. In addition, patients experiencing obesity had more hospitalization days than those with average BMI (Wang et al., 2020). As many Americans gained the "Quarantine 15" during the lockdown, the nurse should discuss weight management and risk for complications of COVID-19 with their patients and offer guidance on resources.

Nursing Management

The management of SARS-CoV-2 is an everchanging field. From a nursing perspective, it is critical to recognize GI symptoms, especially nausea, vomiting, and diarrhea as potential COVID-19 symptoms. GI symptoms have been found to be both heralding symptoms and a barometer for severity of disease. Patients should be treated symptomatically for these issues. The nurse will have a crucial role in educating patients for post–infections FGIDs and psychological stressors associated with the pandemic.

Clinical Judgment Case

A 66-year-old patient comes into the Emergency Room (ER) complaining of chest pain. The pain is described as a "burning sensation, right behind the breastbone." The patient's skin is warm and slightly diaphoretic and vital signs are as follows: 98.7 F, HR 102 and regular, 18 RR with an oxygen saturation of 96% on room air and the blood pressure is 142/92. The patient denies pain in the chest, jaw, back, or arms. Heart Sounds are S1 S2 without murmur, gallops, or rub. Lungs sounds include scattered rhonchi throughout all lung fields, cough is productive of clear mucus. The patient denies shortness of breath, nausea, or vomiting. Abdomen is soft, nondistended and nontender, last BM was this AM, formed brown stool, no evidence of bleeding. There is no peripheral edema, or jugular vein distention, capillary refill is 2 seconds and pedal and posterior tibial pulses are 3+ bil. The patient's history included hypertension (HTN), and smoking history of 10-year pack years. The patient states they are concerned that this may be a "heart attack" since there is a strong family history of cardiac disease. The only medication the patient takes is hydrochlorothiazide, dose not recalled, and it was taken this morning.

Step One: recognize cues where relevant and important information is identified from different sources, such as medical history or vital signs

Answer: The complaints of burning pain behind the sternum, diaphoresis, tachycardia (102), B/P of 142/92, history of HTN, 10-pack-year smoking history, scattered rhonchi, and family history of cardiac disease. The smoking history, scattered rhonchi, and productive cough are also recognized cues.

Step Two: Analyze cues, which is organizing and linking the recognized cues to the patient's clinical presentation.

Answer: You have clustered the symptoms to be associated with a cardiac event or perhaps. Gastroesophageal reflux disease. You link the HTN and family history of cardiac disease with the potential of a cardiac event. You link the symptoms of heart burn, history of smoking and cough with GERD. You link smoking history with scattered rhonchi and productive cough.

Step Three: Prioritize hypotheses, where hypotheses are evaluated and ranked according to priority. This can include urgency, likelihood, risk, difficulty and/or time. In this phase you cluster your findings, to arrive at a list of problems (actual and or potential problems) you believe the patient is experiencing and determine the importance or urgency. What do you think is of greatest concern?

Answer: You prioritize a cardiac event as the greatest risk of injury to the patient than GERD.

Step Four: Generate solutions, which is identifying expected outcomes and using hypotheses to define a set of interventions for the expected outcomes.

Answer: Since a cardiac event is suspected, you recognize the need to place the patient on a cardiac monitor and start an IV in case emergency medications are to be administered. You recognize that up to 25% of patients with an MI are asymptomatic during the acute event, so you alert the ER provider that the patient is complaining of chest pain and anticipate a 12-lead ECG, and blood work consisting of cardiac biomarkers such as troponin will be used to diagnose an MI. You anticipate the administration of nitroglycerin SL. You associate the smoking history with GERD and may continue to ask the patient about alcohol use since that is also a risk factor as well as a history of hiatal hernia (another risk factor).

Step Five: Take action, where the solutions that address the highest priorities are implemented.

Answer: You start the IV, place the patient on a cardiac monitor and move the 12-lead ECG machine to the bedside as the provider comes in to assess the patient. The oxygen saturation is monitored continuously. Nitroglycerin is administered. Cardiac biomarkers are ordered. In case the patient problem is GERD, you ask about symptoms of dysphagia (difficulty swallowing or food getting stuck), odynophagia (pain with swallowing), belching, and epigastric pain (dyspepsia). You repeat the vital signs.

Step Six: Evaluate outcomes, which is comparing observed outcomes against expected outcomes.

Answer: The troponin I level comes back as 0.2 which is normal, the ECG reveals sinus tachycardia with no ST changes. VS repeated are now HR of 92 and regular, RR 16, oxygen saturation of 97% on RA, and BP is now 136/82. An echo was ordered that reveals left ventricular hypertrophy associated with HTN. The nitroglycerin offered no relief from the heartburn. A cardiac event is ruled out and GI providers are called to evaluate the patient for GERD, and allternative causes for symptoms that are not reflux-related. You prioritized well in this case, and you have added to your database of clinical presentations for GERD versus a cardiac event such as a myocardial infarction (MI).

CHAPTER REVIEW

NCLEX-Style Review Questions

1. A 47-year-old patient with epigastric pain is being admitted to the hospital. During the admission assessment and interview, what specific information should the nurse obtain from the patient, who is suspected of having peptic ulcer disease? Select all that apply.
   a. Any allergies to food or medications
   b. Use of nonsteroidal anti-inflammatory drugs (NSAIDs)
   c. Medical history for two previous generations
   d. History of side effects of all medications
   e. History of infection with the gram-negative bacteria *H. pylori*

2. What assessment finding supports a client's diagnosis of gastric ulcer? Select all that apply.
   a. Presence of blood in the client's stool for the past month
   b. Complaints of sharp pain in the abdomen after eating a heavy meal
   c. Periods of pain shortly after eating any food.
   d. Complaints of epigastric burning that moves like a wave
   e. Pain may be relieved by vomiting

3. Which medication should the nurse question before administering it to a patient with peptic ulcer disease? Select all that apply.
   a. E-mycin, an antibiotic
   b. Prilosec, a PPI
   c. Flagyl, an antimicrobial agent
   d. Tylenol, a nonnarcotic analgesic
   e. NSAIDs, nonsteroidal anti-inflammatory

4. The nurse is planning for the discharge of a client with peptic ulcer disease. Which outcome must be included in the plan of care? Select all that apply.
   a. The client's pain is controlled with NSAIDs.
   b. The client understands and maintains lifestyle modifications.
   c. The client takes antacids around the clock.
   d. The client has no episodes of GI bleeding.
   e. The client has smoking cessation plan.

5. Select interventions that you should teach a patient to avoid dumping syndrome that is being discharged after gastric surgery. Select all that apply.

a. Assume high Fowler position for at least 1 hour after meals
b. Do not drink fluids with meals
c. Avoid carbohydrates with meals
d. Restrict intake of fats
e. Eat smaller more frequent meals

REFERENCES AND SELECTED READINGS

References and selected readings associated with this chapter can be found on the website that accompanies the book. Visit **http://thepoint.lww.com/Honan3e** to access the references and other additional resources associated with this chapter.

CHAPTER 23

Nursing Management: Patients With Intestinal and Rectal Disorders

Lindsay R. Grasso

Learning Objectives

After reading this chapter, you will be able to:

1. Describe the health care needs of patients with constipation, diarrhea, or fecal incontinence.
2. Compare the conditions of malabsorption regarding their pathophysiology, clinical manifestations, and management.
3. Describe diverticular disease and the care of patients with diverticulitis.
4. Compare and contrast regional enteritis and ulcerative colitis regarding their pathophysiology and medical, surgical, and nursing management.
5. Identify the care needs of the patient with inflammatory bowel disease.
6. Describe the responsibilities of the nurse in meeting the needs of the patient with an ileostomy.
7. Describe the various types of intestinal obstructions as well as their medical and nursing management.
8. Describe the pathophysiology, assessment, and management regarding cancer of the colon or rectum.
9. Describe anorectal conditions including fissures, fistulas, hemorrhoids, and sexually transmitted anorectal diseases.

There are approximately 60 to 70 million people in the United States diagnosed with some type of disease of the gastrointestinal (GI) tract (Kent, 2021). These diseases account for more than 17.9 million emergency department (ED) visits and 3.8 million hospital admissions annually (Perry et al., 2021). GI conditions cost the health care system a total of $119.6 billion annually (Perry et al., 2021). The types of diseases and disorders that affect the lower GI tract are many and varied.

In all age groups, a fast-paced lifestyle, high levels of stress, irregular eating habits, insufficient intake of fiber and water, and lack of daily exercise contribute to GI disorders. There is a growing understanding of the biopsychosocial implications of GI disease. Nurses can have an impact on these GI disorders by identifying behavior patterns that put patients at risk, by educating the public about prevention and management, and by helping those affected to improve their condition and prevent complications.

DISORDERS RELATED TO FECAL ELIMINATION

CONSTIPATION

Constipation is considered a reduction in bowel frequency or irregularity, less than three bowel movements per week, that are often hard, combined with excessive straining and lower abdominal fullness and often feeling of incomplete evacuation (Ferri, 2022). Variation from normal habits may be considered a problem. Symptoms of constipation are extremely common in adults with a median prevalence of 12% to 19% of adults and 33% of adults 60 and older (Ferri, 2022).

Pearls for Practice

Hemorrhoids and anal fissures can develop resulting from constipation. Hemorrhoids develop because of perianal vascular congestion caused by straining. Anal fissures may result from the passage of the hard stool through the anus, tearing the lining of the anal canal.

Perceived constipation also can be a problem. This subjective problem occurs when a person's bowel elimination pattern is not consistent with what they perceive as normal. Chronic laxative use may contribute to this problem and is a major health concern in the United States.

Pathophysiology

The pathophysiology of constipation is poorly understood, but it is thought to include interference with one of three major functions of the colon: mucosal transport (i.e., mucosal secretions facilitate the movement of colon contents), myoelectric activity (i.e., mixing of the rectal mass and propulsive actions), or the processes of defecation.

The urge to defecate is stimulated normally by rectal distention, which initiates a series of four actions: stimulation of the inhibitory rectoanal reflex, relaxation of the internal sphincter muscle, relaxation of the external sphincter muscle and muscles in the pelvic region, and increased intra-abdominal pressure. Interference with any of these processes can lead to constipation.

If all organic causes are eliminated, idiopathic constipation is diagnosed. When the urge to defecate is ignored, the rectal mucous membrane and musculature become insensitive to the presence of fecal masses, and, consequently, a stronger stimulus is required to produce the necessary peristaltic rush for defecation. The initial effect of fecal retention is irritability of the colon, which at this stage frequently goes into spasm, especially after meals, giving rise to colicky midabdominal or low abdominal pains. After several years of this process, the colon loses muscular tone and becomes essentially unresponsive to normal stimuli. **Atony** or decreased muscle tone occurs with aging. This also leads to constipation because the stool is retained for longer periods.

Risk Factors

Constipation can be caused by certain medications (i.e., tranquilizers, anticholinergics, antidepressants, antihypertensives, bile acid sequestrants, opioids, aluminum-based antacids, iron preparations); rectal or anal disorders (e.g., hemorrhoids, fissures); obstruction (e.g., bowel tumors); metabolic, neurologic, and neuromuscular conditions (e.g., Hirschsprung disease, Parkinson disease, multiple sclerosis); endocrine disorders (e.g., diabetes mellitus, hypothyroidism, pheochromocytoma [rare tumor of adrenal medulla]); lead poisoning; and connective tissue disorders (e.g., scleroderma, systemic lupus erythematosus).

Diseases of the colon, such as irritable bowel syndrome (IBS) and diverticular disease, are commonly associated with constipation. Constipation also can occur with any acute disease process in the abdomen (e.g., appendicitis or cholecystitis) or with any abdominal surgery.

Older adults tend to have decreased food intake, reduced mobility, weak abdominal and pelvic muscles, and multiple chronic illnesses requiring medications that can cause constipation. The astute nurse always will check a patient's medication list for those that may exacerbate constipation.

Low-fiber convenience foods are used widely by people who have lost interest in eating. Dentition is important to consider as people with ill-fitting dentures or poor dentition have increased difficulty chewing and frequently will choose softer, processed foods that are lower in fiber. Some older people reduce their fluid intake if they are not eating regular meals. Depression, weakness, or prolonged bed rest also contributes to constipation by decreasing intestinal motility and anal sphincter tone. Nerve impulses are dulled, and there is a decreased urge to defecate. Prolonged bed rest is also a risk factor in constipation; therefore, nursing care for these patients should include ambulation when possible. Many older people overuse laxatives in an attempt to have a daily bowel movement and become dependent on them, which paradoxically can increase the risk of constipation.

Other causes of constipation may include weakness, immobility, debility, fatigue, and an inability to increase intra-abdominal pressure to facilitate the passage of stools, as may occur in patients with emphysema, for instance. Many people develop constipation because they do not take the time to defecate or they ignore the urge to defecate. In addition, the lack of privacy and interruption of usual bowel regimen are factors associated with constipation in hospitalized patients.

Clinical Manifestations and Assessment

Clinical manifestations of constipation include fewer than three bowel movements per week, abdominal distention, pain and pressure, decreased appetite, headache, fatigue, indigestion, a sensation of incomplete evacuation, straining at stool, and the elimination of small-volume, lumpy, hard, dry stools. Due to the wide range of normal bowel function in people, it is extremely difficult to identify constipation in all patients accurately.

The nurse elicits information about the onset and duration of constipation, current and past elimination patterns, the patient's expectation of normal bowel elimination, and lifestyle information (e.g., exercise and activity level, occupation, food and fluid intake, and stress level) during the health history interview. Medical and surgical history, current medications, and laxative and enema use are important, as is information about the sensation of rectal pressure or fullness, abdominal pain, excessive straining at defecation, and flatulence.

Medical and Nursing Management

Treatment is aimed at the underlying cause of constipation and includes education, bowel habit training, increased fiber and fluid intake, and judicious use of laxatives. Management also may include discontinuing laxative use. Routine

TABLE **23-1 Laxatives: Classification, Agent, Action, and Patient Education**

Classification	Sample Agent	Action	Patient Education
Bulk forming	Psyllium hydrophilic mucilloid	Polysaccharides and cellulose derivatives mix with intestinal fluids, swell, and stimulate peristalsis.	Take with 8-oz water and follow with 8-oz water; do not take dry. Report abdominal distention or unusual amount of flatulence.
Saline agent	Magnesium hydroxide	Nonabsorbable magnesium ions alter stool consistency by drawing water into the intestines by osmosis; peristalsis is stimulated. Action occurs within 2 hours.	The liquid preparation is more effective than the tablet form. Only short-term use is recommended because of toxicity (CNS or neuromuscular depression, electrolyte imbalance). Magnesium laxatives should not be taken by patients with renal insufficiency.
Lubricant	Mineral oil	Nonabsorbable hydrocarbons soften fecal matter by lubricating the intestinal mucosa; the passage of stool is facilitated. Action occurs within 6–8 hours.	Do not take with meals because mineral oils can impair the absorption of fat-soluble vitamins and delay gastric emptying. Swallow carefully, because drops of oil that gain access to the pharynx can produce a lipid pneumonia.
Stimulant	Bisacodyl	Irritates the colon epithelium by stimulating sensory nerve endings and increasing mucosal secretions. Action occurs within 6–8 hours.	Catharsis may cause fluid and electrolyte imbalance, especially in older indivuals. Tablets should be swallowed; not crushed or chewed. Avoid milk or antacids within 1 hour of taking the medication because the enteric coating may dissolve prematurely.
Fecal softener	Dioctyl sodium sulfosuccinate	Hydrates the stool by its surfactant action on the colonic epithelium (increases the wetting efficiency of intestinal water); aqueous and fatty substances are mixed. Does not exert a laxative action.	This can be used safely by patients who should avoid straining (cardiac patients, patients with anorectal disorders).
Osmotic agent	Polyethylene glycol and electrolytes (Colyte)	Cleanses colon rapidly and induces diarrhea	This is a large-volume product. It takes time to consume it safely. It can cause considerable nausea and bloating.

exercise to strengthen abdominal muscles is encouraged. Soluble dietary fiber, such as psyllium, are considered early treatment options for patients, but should be combined with adequate fluid intake (Ferri, 2022). Osmotic agents should be used prior to use of stimulate laxatives.

Daily dietary intake of 6 to 12 teaspoonfuls of unprocessed bran is recommended, especially for the treatment of the older individuals. If laxative use is necessary, one of the following may be prescribed: bulk-forming agents, saline and osmotic agents, lubricants, stimulants, or fecal softeners. The physiologic action and patient education information related to these laxatives are given in Table 23-1. Enemas and rectal suppositories generally are not recommended for treating constipation; they should be reserved for the treatment of impaction. If long-term laxative use is necessary, a bulk-forming agent may be prescribed in combination with an osmotic laxative.

Specific medications may be prescribed to enhance colonic transit by increasing propulsive motor activity. These may include cholinergic agents (e.g., bethanechol), cholinesterase inhibitors (e.g., neostigmine), or prokinetic agents (e.g., metoclopramide).

Patient education and health promotion are important functions of the nurse. Patient education should include establishing a bowel routine, providing dietary information, and reducing patient anxiety. After the health history is obtained, the nurse sets specific goals for teaching. Goals for the patient include restoring or maintaining a regular pattern of elimination by responding to the urge to defecate, ensuring adequate intake of fluids and high-fiber foods, learning methods to avoid constipation, relieving anxiety about bowel elimination patterns, and avoiding complications.

Complications

Complications of constipation include hypertension, fecal impaction, hemorrhoids (dilated portions of anal veins), fissures (tissue folds), and **megacolon** (abnormal enlargement of the colon). Increased arterial pressure can occur with defecation. Straining at stool, can also result in the **Valsalva maneuver** (i.e., forcibly exhaling with the glottis closed), has a striking effect on lowering of the arterial blood pressure. During active straining, the flow of venous blood in the chest is impeded temporarily because of increased intrathoracic pressure. This pressure tends to collapse the large veins in the chest. The atria and the ventricles receive less blood, and, consequently, less blood is ejected by the left ventricle. Cardiac output is decreased, and there is a transient drop in arterial pressure. Thus, bowel regimens to prevent constipation frequently are instituted in patients admitted with cardiac and neurologic problems.

Pearls for Practice

The nurse is aware there are a myriad of causes associated with constipation. However, some red flags that are associated with more significant acute problems include vomiting, GI bleeding, severe pain, persistent hypotension and tachycardia and signs of peritoneal irritation (muscle resistance [guarding], abdominal tenderness, and abdominal rigidity).

Fecal impaction occurs when an accumulated mass of dry feces cannot be expelled. The mass may be palpable on digital examination, may produce pressure on the colonic mucosa that results in ulcer formation, and frequently causes seepage of liquid stools.

Megacolon is caused by a fecal mass that obstructs the passage of colon contents. Symptoms include constipation, liquid fecal incontinence, and abdominal distention. Megacolon can lead to perforation of the bowel.

Pearls for Practice

Care should be taken when performing digital rectal procedures as vagal nerve stimulation may occur, causing a vasovagal response in the patient. In addition, straining to stool may also cause a vasovagal response. Signs and symptoms of a vasovagal response include bradycardia, hypotension, lightheadedness, nausea, feelings of hot or cold, confusion, or loss of consciousness. Treatment should include reducing the risk of injury during the episode, maneuvers to increase blood flow to the brain (recumbent position with lower extremities elevated), and evaluation of any cardiac and neurologic causes of syncope.

DIARRHEA

Diarrhea is defined as an increased frequency of bowel movements of more than three per day, an increased amount of stool (more than 200 g/day), or abnormally liquid stool. It is usually associated with increased urgency, perianal discomfort, or incontinence. Diarrhea lasting less than 2 weeks is considered acute; conversely, diarrhea lasting more than 4 weeks is considered chronic. Acute diarrhea is associated most often with infection and usually is self-limiting; chronic diarrhea persists for a longer period and may return sporadically. Any condition that causes increased intestinal secretions, decreased mucosal absorption, or altered motility can produce diarrhea. IBS, inflammatory bowel disease (IBD), and lactose intolerance are frequently the underlying disease processes that cause diarrhea.

Pathophysiology

Types of diarrhea include secretory, osmotic, and mixed diarrhea. Secretory diarrhea is usually high-volume diarrhea and is caused by increased production and secretion of water and electrolytes by the intestinal mucosa into the intestinal lumen. Osmotic diarrhea occurs when water is pulled into the intestines by the osmotic pressure of unabsorbed particles, slowing the reabsorption of water. Mixed diarrhea is caused by increased **peristalsis** (usually from IBD) and a combination of increased secretion and decreased absorption in the bowel.

Risk Factors

Diarrhea can be caused by certain medications (e.g., thyroid hormone replacement, stool softeners and laxatives, antibiotics, chemotherapy, magnesium-based antacids), certain tube-feeding formulas, metabolic and endocrine disorders (e.g., diabetes, Addison disease, thyrotoxicosis), and viral or bacterial infectious processes (e.g., dysentery, shigellosis, food poisoning). Other disease processes associated with diarrhea include nutritional and malabsorptive disorders (e.g., celiac disease), anal sphincter defect, Zollinger–Ellison syndrome, paralytic ileus, intestinal obstruction, and AIDS.

Clinical Manifestations and Assessment

In addition to the increased frequency and fluid content of stools, the patient usually has abdominal cramps, distention, intestinal rumbling (**borborygmus**), anorexia, and thirst. Painful spasmodic contractions of the anus and ineffective straining (**tenesmus**) may occur with defecation. Other symptoms depend on the cause and severity of the diarrhea but are related to dehydration and imbalances of fluid and electrolytes.

Watery stools are characteristic of disorders of the small bowel, whereas loose, semisolid stools are associated more often with disorders of the large bowel. Large, greasy stools suggest intestinal malabsorption, and the presence of mucus and pus in the stools suggests inflammatory enteritis or colitis. Oil droplets on the toilet water are almost always diagnostic of pancreatic insufficiency. Nocturnal diarrhea may be a manifestation of diabetic neuropathy.

Typically, when the source of the diarrhea is not clear, the following diagnostic tests may be performed: complete blood cell count (CBC); serum chemistries; urinalysis; routine stool examination; and stool examinations for infectious or parasitic organisms, bacterial toxins, blood, fat, and electrolytes. Endoscopy or barium enema may assist in identifying the cause.

Pearls for Practice

Older patients can become dehydrated quickly and develop low potassium levels (i.e., hypokalemia) as a result of diarrhea. The nurse observes for clinical manifestations of muscle weakness, arrhythmias, or decreased peristaltic motility that may lead to paralytic ileus. The older patient taking digitalis (e.g., digoxin) must be aware of how quickly dehydration and hypokalemia can occur with diarrhea. The nurse teaches the patient to recognize the symptoms of hypokalemia because low levels of potassium intensify the action of digitalis, leading to digitalis toxicity.

Medical and Nursing Management

Primary management is directed at controlling symptoms, preventing complications, and eliminating or treating the underlying disease. Medications, such as antibiotics (reserved for cases of bacterial overgrowth) and anti-inflammatory agents, may be used to reduce the severity of the diarrhea and treat the underlying disease. The mainstay of treatment in most cases of diarrhea is oral, or, if severe or symptomatic, intravenous rehydration.

The nurse's role includes assessing and monitoring the characteristics and pattern of diarrhea. A health history should address the patient's medication therapy, medical and surgical history, and dietary patterns and intake. Reports of recent exposure to an acute illness or recent travel to another geographic area are important as treatment can change depending on the patient's illness and travel history. Assessment includes abdominal inspection, auscultation (for hyperactive bowel sounds), and palpation for abdominal tenderness. Vital signs are assessed for fever and evidence of fluid volume deficit (weak pulse, hypotension, narrow pulse pressure). Inspection of the mucous membranes and skin is important to determine hydration status. Stool samples are obtained for testing.

During an episode of acute diarrhea, the nurse encourages bedrest and intake of liquids and foods low in bulk until the acute attack subsides. When the patient is able to tolerate food intake, the nurse recommends a bland diet of semisolid and solid foods. The patient should avoid caffeine, carbonated beverages, and very hot and very cold foods due to stimulation of intestinal motility. It may be necessary to restrict milk products, fat, whole-grain products, fresh fruits, and vegetables for several days. Antidiarrheal medications, such as diphenoxylate or loperamide, may be administered as prescribed to reduce the frequency and amount of stools. IV fluid therapy may be necessary for rapid rehydration in some patients, especially in older patients and in patients with pre-existing GI conditions, such as IBD. It is important to monitor serum electrolyte levels closely as imbalances such as hypokalemia (K^+ less than 3.5 mEq/L) and acute metabolic acidosis due to a direct loss of bicarbonate (HCO_3^- less than 22 mEq/L) can occur. The nurse immediately reports evidence of arrhythmias, muscular weakness, fatigue or flaccid paralysis, and hyporeflexia (associated with a K^+ less than 2.5 mEq/L).

Pearls for Practice

Decreased potassium levels cause cardiac arrhythmias (i.e., atrial and ventricular tachycardia, ventricular fibrillation, premature ventricular contractions) that can lead to death.

The perianal area may become excoriated because diarrheal stool contains digestive enzymes that can irritate the skin. Older individuals have decreased skin turgor and reduced subcutaneous fat layers; therefore, care should be taken to follow a structured perianal skin care routine to reduce irritation and excoriation.

FECAL INCONTINENCE

Fecal incontinence describes the involuntary passage of solid or liquid stool from the rectum. It is estimated that 50% to 70% of residents in extended-care facilities and more than 15% of adults in the community have fecal incontinence (Deb et al., 2020). Factors that influence fecal incontinence include the ability of the rectum to sense and accommodate stool, the amount and consistency of stool, the integrity of the anal sphincters and musculature, and rectal motility. Risk factors for older adults include impaired mobility, comorbidities, dementia, and depression (Deb et al., 2020). It is an embarrassing and socially incapacitating problem that requires a many-tiered approach to treatment and much adaptation on the patient's part.

Pearls for Practice

Management of double incontinence (urine and stool) should include frequent toileting assistance, identifying patients who may most benefit from targeted toileting programs, and treating underlying fecal disorders including chronic constipation.

Pathophysiology

Continence is maintained by tonic contraction of the muscles around the rectum. During defecation, nerves relax the muscles, causing a straightening of the rectoanal angle. Distension of the rectum causes relaxation of the sphincter. Fecal incontinence is a failure of this process and can occur for a variety of reasons.

Risk Factors

Fecal incontinence can result from trauma (e.g., after surgical procedures involving the rectum), neurologic disorders (e.g., stroke, multiple sclerosis, diabetic neuropathy, dementia), inflammation, infection, chemotherapy, radiation treatment, fecal impaction, pelvic floor relaxation, laxative abuse, medications, or advancing age (i.e., weakness or loss of anal or rectal muscle tone).

Clinical Manifestations and Assessment

Patients may have minor soiling, occasional urgency and loss of control, or complete incontinence. Patients also may experience poor control of flatus, diarrhea, or constipation.

The nurse obtains a thorough health history, including information about previous surgical procedures, chronic illnesses, dietary patterns, bowel habits and problems, and current medication regimen. A visual and digital examination of the rectal area is completed, checking for abnormalities (fecal impaction, hemorrhoids, fissures, and fistulas) that may be contributing to the incontinence.

Diagnostic studies are necessary because the treatment of fecal incontinence depends on the cause. A rectal examination and other endoscopic examinations, such as a flexible sigmoidoscopy, are performed to rule out tumors, inflammation, or fissures. X-ray studies, such as barium enema, computed tomography (CT), anorectal manometry, and transit studies, may be helpful in identifying alterations in intestinal mucosa and muscle tone or in detecting other structural or functional problems.

Medical and Nursing Management

Specific management techniques can help the patient achieve a better quality of life. If fecal incontinence is related to diarrhea, the incontinence may disappear when diarrhea is treated successfully. Frequently fecal incontinence is a symptom of a fecal impaction. After the impaction is removed and the rectum is cleansed, normal functioning of the anorectal area can resume. If the fecal incontinence is related to a more permanent condition, other treatments are initiated. Biofeedback therapy can be of assistance if the problem is decreased sensory awareness or sphincter control. Fiber supplement to make stools less liquid is often useful in treating mild incontinence along with an antimotility agent to treat diarrhea (Ferri, 2022). Bowel training programs also can be effective. Surgical procedures include surgical reconstruction, sphincter repair, or fecal diversion.

The nurse initiates a bowel training program that involves setting a schedule to establish bowel regularity. The goal is to help the patient achieve fecal continence. If this is not possible, the goal should be to manage the problem so the person can have predictable, planned elimination. Sometimes, it is necessary to use suppositories to stimulate the anal reflex. After the patient has achieved a regular schedule, the suppository can be discontinued.

Complications

Fecal incontinence may cause problems with perineal skin integrity. Maintaining skin integrity is a priority, especially in the debilitated or older patient. Incontinence briefs, although helpful in containing the fecal material, allow for increased skin contact with the feces and may cause excoriation of the skin. The nurse encourages and teaches meticulous skin hygiene, and, in the hospital setting, interventions, such as turning the patient every 2 hours and applying barrier creams or sprays to protect the skin, may be warranted.

Continence sometimes cannot be achieved, and the nurse assists the patient and family to accept and cope with this chronic situation. The patient can use fecal incontinence devices, which include external collection devices and internal drainage systems. External devices are special, drainable pouches. They are attached to a synthetic adhesive skin barrier specially designed to conform to the buttocks. Internal drainage systems can be used to eliminate fecal skin contact and are useful especially when there is extensive excoriation or skin breakdown. A rectal catheter is inserted into the rectum and connected to a drainage system, and stool is collected in order to preserve skin integrity. Rectal catheters are contraindicated in patients who are postoperative from rectal or prostate surgery, recent myocardial infarction, rectal mucosal disease, bleeding dyscrasia, and impaired immune status. It is important to consider that at present, long-term consequences of indwelling fecal collectors have not been studied yet, although some research suggests that some commercially available catheters may be safe for upward of 30 days. A provider's order is required to place these devices.

IRRITABLE BOWEL SYNDROME

IBS is one of the most common GI conditions. Approximately 1 in 10 people globally are affected by IBS, with rates increasing due to countries adapting a more Western lifestyle and diet (Black & Ford, 2020). Patients can often feel stigmatized by health care professionals upon seeking help for IBS type symptoms, and it is reported that it takes patients an average of 4 years to get properly diagnosed (Black & Ford, 2020). While there is no evidence that those with IBS have an increased risk of mortality, this disorder is shown to reduce overall quality of life (Black & Ford, 2020).

Pathophysiology

IBS results from a functional disorder of intestinal motility. The change in motility may be related to neuroendocrine dysregulation, infection or irritation, or a vascular or metabolic disturbance. The peristaltic waves are affected at specific segments of the intestine and in the intensity with which they propel the fecal matter forward. There is no evidence of inflammation or tissue changes in the intestinal mucosa.

Risk Factors

Although no anatomic or biochemical abnormalities have been found that account for the common symptoms, various

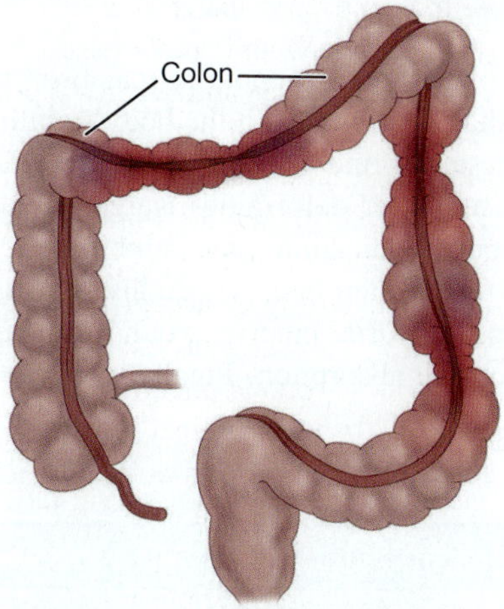

FIGURE 23-1 **In irritable bowel syndrome (IBS), the spastic contractions of the bowel can be seen on x-ray contrast studies.**

factors are associated with the syndrome: heredity, a diet high in fat and sugar or irritating foods, alcohol consumption, history of infective gastroenteritis, smoking, and psychological stress or conditions such as depression and anxiety. In addition, there is a 39% and 29% prevalence in the diagnosis of anxiety or depression, respectively, with IBS (Black & Ford, 2020). IBS is also more commonly diagnosed in females than males (Buttaro et al., 2021).

Clinical Manifestations and Assessment

There is a wide variability in symptom presentation. Symptoms range in intensity and duration from mild and infrequent to severe and continuous. The primary symptom is an alteration in bowel patterns—constipation, diarrhea, or a combination of both. Pain and abdominal distention often accompany changes in bowel pattern. Sometimes the abdominal pain is precipitated by eating, and frequently it is relieved by defecation.

A definite diagnosis of IBS requires tests that confirm the absence of structural or other disorders. Stool studies, contrast x-ray studies, and proctoscopy may be performed to rule out other colon diseases. Barium enema and colonoscopy may reveal spasm, distention, or mucus accumulation in the intestine (Fig. 23-1). Manometry and electromyography (EMG) are used to study intraluminal pressure changes generated by spasticity.

Medical and Nursing Management

The goals of treatment are relieving abdominal pain, controlling the diarrhea or constipation, and reducing stress. Restriction and then gradual reintroduction of foods that are possibly irritating may help determine what types of food are acting as irritants (e.g., beans, caffeinated products, fried foods, alcohol, and spicy foods). A high-fiber diet is prescribed to help control the diarrhea and constipation. Exercise can assist in reducing anxiety and increasing intestinal motility. Patients often find it helpful to participate in a stress reduction or behavior modification program. Hydrophilic colloids (i.e., bulk) and antidiarrheal agents (e.g., loperamide) may be given to control the diarrhea and fecal urgency. Antidepressants can assist in treating underlying anxiety and depression. Anticholinergics (e.g., propantheline) may be taken to decrease smooth muscle spasm, thus decreasing cramping and constipation.

Treatment for IBS includes the use of both pharmacologic and nonpharmacologic management. Current therapies, including laxatives, antidiarrheals, and antispasmodics, are all considered first line use for IBS (Ford et al., 2020). Antidepressants are considered a second line pharmacologic treatment. Nonpharmacologic treatment for IBS includes cognitive behavioral therapy, gut directed hypnotherapy and relaxation therapy. Some research states earlier psychological treatment helps with IBS symptoms, but the research for this treatment options are ongoing (Ford et al., 2020).

The nurse's role is to provide patient and family education. The nurse emphasizes teaching and reinforces good dietary habits. Patients are encouraged to eat at regular times and to chew food slowly and thoroughly. They should understand that although adequate fluid intake is necessary, fluid should not be taken with meals because this results in abdominal distention. Alcohol use and cigarettes should be avoided.

Pearls for Practice

The key to treating IBS in patients is to treat each patient as an individual. Nursing care plans should include interventions that are based on that patient's unique and individual symptoms blending both pharmacologic and psychological-based interventions specific to that particular patient.

MALABSORPTION

Malabsorption is the inability of the digestive system to absorb one or more of the major vitamins (especially A and B_{12}), minerals (i.e., iron and calcium), and nutrients (i.e., carbohydrates, fats, and proteins). Interruptions in the complex digestive process may occur anywhere in the digestive system and cause decreased absorption.

Pathophysiology

The conditions that cause malabsorption can be grouped into the following categories:

- Mucosal (transport) disorders causing generalized malabsorption (e.g., celiac sprue, regional enteritis, radiation enteritis)
- Infectious diseases causing generalized malabsorption (e.g., small bowel bacterial overgrowth, tropical sprue)

- Luminal disorders causing malabsorption (e.g., bile acid deficiency, Zollinger–Ellison syndrome, pancreatic insufficiency)
- Postoperative malabsorption (e.g., after gastric or intestinal resection)
- Disorders that cause malabsorption of specific nutrients (e.g., disaccharidase deficiency leading to lactose intolerance)

Table 23-2 lists the clinical and pathologic aspects of malabsorptive diseases.

Risk Factors

Risk factors predisposing people to malabsorption include any process that interferes with the body's ability to absorb nutrients. These can include pathologic factors, including abdominal diseases or deformities, surgery, radiation therapy, and certain medications that inhibit bacterial growth within the intestine (antibiotics). Bodily fluid losses, from such things as polyuria, emesis, wound drainage, or diarrhea, can decrease absorption. Finally, use of medications,

TABLE **23-2 Characteristics of Diseases of Malabsorption**

Diseases/Disorders	Physiologic Pathology	Clinical Features
Gastric resection with gastrojejunostomy	Decreased pancreatic stimulation because of duodenal bypass; poor mixing of food, bile, pancreatic enzymes; decreased intrinsic factor	Weight loss, moderate steatorrhea (presence of fat within the stool), anemia (combination of iron deficiency, vitamin B_{12} malabsorption, folate deficiency)
Pancreatic insufficiency (chronic pancreatitis, pancreatic carcinoma, pancreatic resection, cystic fibrosis)	Reduced intraluminal pancreatic enzyme activity, with maldigestion of lipids and proteins	History of abdominal pain followed by weight loss; marked steatorrhea, azotorrhea (excess of nitrogenous matter in the feces or urine); also frequent glucose intolerance (70% in pancreatic insufficiency)
Ileal dysfunction (resection or disease)	Loss of ileal absorbing surface leads to reduced bile-salt pool size and reduced vitamin B_{12} absorption; bile in colon inhibits fluid absorption	Diarrhea, weight loss with steatorrhea, especially when more than 100 cm resection, decreased vitamin B_{12} absorption
Stasis syndromes (surgical strictures, blind loops, enteric fistulas, multiple jejunal diverticula, scleroderma)	Overgrowth of intraluminal intestinal bacteria, especially anaerobic organisms, to more than 10^6/mL results in deconjugation of bile salts, leading to decreased effective bile-salt pool size, also bacterial utilization of vitamin B_{12}	Weight loss, steatorrhea; low vitamin B_{12} absorption; may have low D-xylose absorption
Zollinger–Ellison syndrome	Hyperacidity in duodenum inactivates pancreatic enzymes	Ulcer; steatorrhea
Lactose intolerance	Deficiency of intestinal lactase results in high concentration of intraluminal lactose with osmotic diarrhea	Varied degrees of diarrhea and cramps after ingestion of lactose-containing foods; positive lactose intolerance test, decreased intestinal lactase
Celiac disease (gluten enteropathy)	Toxic response to a gluten fraction by surface epithelium results in destruction of absorbing surface	Weight loss, diarrhea, bloating, anemia (low iron, folate), osteomalacia, steatorrhea, azotorrhea, low D-xylose absorption; folate and iron malabsorption
Tropical sprue	Unknown toxic factor results in mucosal inflammation, partial villous atrophy	Weight loss, diarrhea, anemia (low folate, vitamin B_{12}); steatorrhea; low D-xylose absorption, low vitamin B_{12} absorption
Whipple disease	Bacterial invasion of intestinal mucosa	Arthritis, hyperpigmentation, lymphadenopathy, serous effusions, fever, weight loss, steatorrhea, azotorrhea
Certain parasitic diseases (giardiasis, strongyloidiasis, coccidiosis, capillariasis)	Damage to or invasion of surface mucosa	Diarrhea, weight loss; steatorrhea; organism may be seen on jejunal biopsy or recovered in stool
Immunoglobulinopathy	Decreased local intestinal defenses, lymphoid hyperplasia, lymphopenia	Frequent association with *Giardia:* hypogammaglobulinemia or isolated IgA deficiency

such as mineral oil or laxatives, can decrease absorption by increasing peristalsis.

Clinical Manifestations and Assessment

The hallmarks of malabsorption syndrome are diarrhea or frequent, loose, bulky, foul-smelling stools that have increased fat content and often are grayish in color. Patients often have associated abdominal distention, pain, increased flatus, weakness, weight loss, and a decreased sense of well-being. The chief result of malabsorption is malnutrition, manifested by weight loss and other signs of vitamin and mineral deficiency (e.g., easy bruising [vitamin K deficiency], osteoporosis [calcium deficiency], anemia [iron, vitamin B_{12} deficiency]).

Patients with a malabsorption syndrome, if untreated, become weak and emaciated because of starvation and dehydration. Failure to absorb the fat-soluble vitamins A, D, and K causes a corresponding avitaminosis (chronic or long-term vitamin deficiency).

Several diagnostic tests may be prescribed, including stool studies for quantitative and qualitative fat analysis, lactose tolerance tests, D-xylose absorption tests (absorption of sugar), and Schilling tests (B_{12} deficiency). The hydrogen breath test that is used to evaluate carbohydrate absorption is performed if carbohydrate malabsorption is suspected. This test requires the patient to be fasting before they ingest 35 to 50 g of carbohydrate dissolved in water. Exhaled breath is assayed for hydrogen content at baseline and at specific intervals for several hours starting 30 minutes after ingestion. Since hydrogen is not a normal product of human metabolism, any increase in breath hydrogen concentration suggests bacterial fermentation and indicates that unabsorbed carbohydrate has reached an area with high concentrations of intraluminal bacteria, typically the colon (Robles & Priefer, 2020).

Endoscopy with biopsy of the mucosa is the best diagnostic tool. Biopsy of the small intestine is performed to assay enzyme activity or to identify infection or destruction of mucosa. Ultrasound studies, CT scans, and x-ray findings can reveal pancreatic or intestinal tumors that may be the cause. A CBC is used to detect anemia. Pancreatic function tests can assist in the diagnosis of specific disorders.

Medical and Nursing Management

Intervention is aimed at avoiding dietary substances that aggravate malabsorption and at supplementing nutrients that have been lost. Common supplements are water-soluble vitamins (e.g., B_{12}, folic acid), fat-soluble vitamins (e.g., A, D, and K), and minerals (e.g., calcium, iron). Primary disease states may be managed surgically or medically. Dietary therapy is aimed at reducing gluten intake in patients with celiac sprue. Folic acid supplements are prescribed for patients with tropical sprue (see Table 23-2). Sometimes antibiotics (e.g., tetracycline, ampicillin) are needed in the treatment of tropical sprue and bacterial overgrowth syndromes. Antidiarrheal agents may be used to decrease intestinal spasms. Parenteral fluids may be necessary to treat dehydration.

The nurse provides patient and family education regarding diet and the use of nutritional supplements. It is important to monitor patients with diarrhea for fluid and electrolyte imbalances. The nurse conducts ongoing assessments to determine whether the clinical manifestations related to the nutritional deficits have abated. Patient education includes information about the risk of osteoporosis related to malabsorption of calcium (refer to Chapter 40 for information on osteoporosis).

Pearls for Practice: Pathophysiology

Patients who are severely malnourished are at a higher risk of developing refeeding syndrome if fed too rapidly. Excessively high dextrose administration (e.g., peripheral parenteral nutrition [PPN], total parenteral nutrition [TPN]) stimulates insulin release, which rapidly lowers phosphorus, the main characteristic of refeeding syndrome, magnesium, and potassium in the blood (due to intracellular shift and use in carbohydrate metabolic pathways). The hyperinsulinemia also tends to cause sodium and fluid retention. Thiamine also is consumed with high carbohydrate loads. The combination of fluid and sodium retention, decrease in blood electrolyte levels (which can cause arrhythmias), and hypermetabolism due to increased calories can result in heart failure. Measuring daily weights may alert the nurse to signs of fluid retention such as an increase of 0.3 to 0.5 kg/day (Reber et al., 2019). Thus, the complications of refeeding syndrome can include a variety of fluid and electrolyte disturbances, which can include hypoglycemia, tetany (from low calcium and magnesium levels), cardiac arrhythmias, and death. Risk factors for refeeding syndrome include pre-existing malnutrition, electrolyte depletion, or alcoholism, and after prolonged periods of intravenous hydration therapy (e.g., 5% dextrose) without nutrition support for longer than 10 days (Friedli et al., 2020). Consequently, the nurse is suspicious of refeeding syndrome when initiating nutrition in a malnourished patient and is proactive in monitoring serum electrolytes and blood glucose. The adage of start low and go slow applies here and the nutrition is advanced after labs have normalized.

Complications

Complications are related to the underlying disease causing the malabsorption. Depending on the etiology, medical management may include the administration of corticosteroids (for regional enteritis), which may cause a host of adverse effects, such as hypertension, hypokalemia, insomnia, and

TABLE 23-3 **Malabsorption of Nutrients, Water, and Electrolytes**

Nutrient Malabsorbed	Clinical Manifestation
Protein	Wasting, hypoproteinemic edema
Carbohydrate and fat	Diarrhea, abdominal cramps and bloating, weight loss and growth retardation
Fluid	Kidney stones with volume depletion, weight loss, fluid volume deficit (FVD)
Iron	Anemia
Calcium and vitamin D	Bone pain, fractures, tetany
Magnesium	Paresthesias, tetany
Vitamin B_{12} and folate	Anemia, paresthesias, ataxia (vitamin B_{12} only)
Vitamin E	Paresthesias, ataxia, retinopathy
Vitamin A	Night blindness, diarrhea
Vitamin K	Ecchymoses, bruises easily
Selenium	Cardiomyopathy
Malabsorption of bile salts	Increased colonic fluid secretion and watery diarrhea

Adapted from Semrad, C. (2016). Approach to the patient with diarrhea and malabsorption. In L. Goldman & A. I. Schafer (Eds.), *Goldman-Cecil medicine* (25th ed., Table 140-5). Elsevier/Saunders.

euphoria. Antibiotics may reduce vitamin K–producing intestinal flora, resulting in a prolonged prothrombin time (PT) and international normalized ratio (INR) if the patient is concurrently taking warfarin. Refer to Table 23-3 for clinical manifestations of malabsorption.

ACUTE INFLAMMATORY CONDITIONS

APPENDICITIS

The appendix is a small, finger-like appendage about 10 cm (4 in) long that is attached to the cecum just below the ileocecal valve. The appendix fills with food and empties regularly into the cecum. Because it empties inefficiently and its lumen is small, the appendix is prone to obstruction and is particularly vulnerable to infection (i.e., appendicitis).

Appendicitis is the most common reason for emergency abdominal surgery with more than 300,000 visits to the hospital yearly due to appendicitis issues (Jones et al., 2021). The disease is most common in patients between 5 and 45 years of age, an average age of 28, with a slightly higher incidence in males than females (Jones et al., 2021).

Pathophysiology

The appendix becomes inflamed and edematous as a result of becoming kinked or occluded by a fecalith (i.e., hardened mass of stool), tumor, or foreign body. The inflammatory process increases intraluminal pressure, initiating a progressively severe, generalized or periumbilical pain that becomes localized to the right lower quadrant of the abdomen within a few hours. Eventually, the inflamed appendix fills with pus.

Risk Factors

Appendicitis is most prevalent in the young, but it can occur at any age. There is a degree of family predisposition, with increased incidents in male children. Low intake of daily fiber also increases the risk of developing appendicitis (Kornusky & Gilreath-Osoff, 2021).

Clinical Manifestations and Assessment

Vague epigastric or periumbilical pain progresses to right lower quadrant pain and usually is accompanied by a low-grade fever and nausea and, sometimes, vomiting. Loss of appetite is common. In up to 50% of presenting cases, local tenderness is elicited at McBurney point when pressure is applied (Fig. 23-2). Rebound tenderness (production or intensification of pain when pressure is released) may be present. The extent of tenderness and muscle spasm and the existence of constipation or diarrhea depend not so much on the severity of the appendiceal infection as on the location of the appendix. If the appendix curls around behind the cecum, pain and tenderness may be felt in the lumbar region. If its tip is in the pelvis, these signs may be elicited

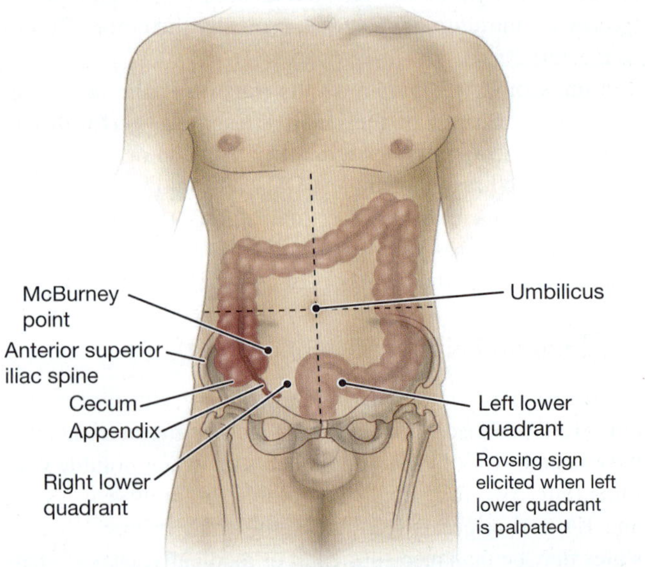

FIGURE 23-2 **When the appendix is inflamed, tenderness can be noted in the right lower quadrant at McBurney point, which is between the umbilicus and the anterior superior iliac spine. Rovsing sign is pain felt in the right lower quadrant after the left lower quadrant has been palpated.**

only on rectal examination. Pain on defecation suggests that the tip of the appendix is resting against the rectum; pain on urination suggests that the tip is near the bladder or impinges on the ureter. Some rigidity of the lower portion of the right rectus muscle may occur. Rovsing sign may be elicited by palpating the left lower quadrant; this paradoxically causes pain to be felt in the right lower quadrant (see Fig. 23-2). If the appendix has ruptured, the pain becomes more diffuse; abdominal distention develops as a result of paralytic ileus, and the patient's condition worsens.

Pearls for Practice

Constipation also can occur with an acute process, such as appendicitis. Laxatives administered in this instance may result in perforation of the inflamed appendix. In general, a laxative or cathartic should never be given when a person has fever, nausea, or pain.

Diagnosis is based on results of a complete physical examination and on laboratory findings and imaging studies. The CBC demonstrates an elevated white blood cell (WBC) count with an elevation of the neutrophils. Abdominal x-ray films, ultrasound studies, and CT scans may reveal a right lower quadrant density or localized distention of the bowel. A diagnostic laparoscopy may be used to rule out acute appendicitis in equivocal cases.

Acute appendicitis is uncommon in the older population. When it does occur, classic signs and symptoms are altered and may vary greatly. Pain may be absent or minimal. Symptoms may be vague, suggesting bowel obstruction or another process. Fever and leukocytosis may not be present. As a result, diagnosis and prompt treatment may be delayed, causing complications and mortality. The patient may have no symptoms until the appendix ruptures. The incidence of perforated appendix is higher in the older population and is associated with a higher mortality rate due to their late presentation and a variety of social factors including lack of transportation, fear of hospitalization, or loss of independence (McGowan, 2020).

Medical and Nursing Management

Typically, immediate surgery is indicated if appendicitis is diagnosed. To correct or prevent fluid and electrolyte imbalance, dehydration, and sepsis, antibiotics and IV fluids are administered until surgery is performed. Appendectomy (i.e., surgical removal of the appendix) is performed as soon as possible to decrease the risk of perforation. It may be performed using general or spinal anesthesia with a low abdominal incision (laparotomy) or by laparoscopy. Both laparotomy and laparoscopy are safe and effective in the treatment of appendicitis with perforation. However, generally recovery after laparoscopic surgery is quicker.

When perforation of the appendix occurs, an **abscess** may form. If this occurs, the patient may be treated initially with antibiotics, and the surgeon may place a drain in the abscess during the operative procedure to facilitate drainage. Subsequent surgical procedures may be performed to ensure complete drainage of the abscess. The postoperative care of the patient with a perforated appendix is more complex and complicated due to the risk of developing sepsis and organ damage.

The nurse prepares the patient for surgery, which includes an IV infusion to replace fluid loss and promote adequate kidney function, and antibiotic therapy to prevent infection. If there is evidence or likelihood of paralytic ileus, a nasogastric tube is inserted. An enema is not administered because it can lead to perforation.

After surgery, the nurse places the patient in a high Fowler position. This position reduces the tension on the incision and abdominal organs, helping to reduce pain. An opioid, usually morphine sulfate, is prescribed to relieve pain. When tolerated, oral fluids are administered. Any patient who was dehydrated before surgery receives IV fluids. Food is provided as desired and tolerated on the day of surgery, once normal bowel sounds are present.

The patient may be discharged on the day of surgery if the temperature is within normal limits, there is no undue discomfort in the operative area, and the appendectomy was uncomplicated. Discharge teaching for the patient and family is imperative. The nurse instructs the patient to make an appointment to have the surgeon remove the sutures between the fifth and seventh days after surgery. Incision care and activity guidelines are discussed; usually normal activity can be resumed within 2 to 4 weeks.

If there is a possibility of **peritonitis**, a drain is left in place at the area of the incision. Patients at risk for this complication may be kept in the hospital for several days and are monitored carefully for signs of intestinal obstruction or secondary hemorrhage. Secondary abscesses may form in the pelvis, under the diaphragm, or in the liver, causing elevation of the temperature, pulse rate, and WBC count.

When the patient is ready for discharge, the nurse teaches the patient and family to care for the incision and perform dressing changes and irrigations as prescribed. A home care nurse may be needed to assist with this care and to monitor the patient for complications and wound healing.

Complications

The major complication of appendicitis is perforation of the appendix, which can lead to peritonitis, abscess formation (collection of purulent material), or portal pylephlebitis, which is septic thrombosis of the portal vein caused by vegetative emboli that arise from septic intestines. Perforation generally occurs 24 hours after the onset of pain if no intervention has occurred. Symptoms include a fever of 37.7°C (100°F) or greater, a toxic appearance, and continued abdominal pain or tenderness. Other complications of appendectomy are listed in Table 23-4.

TABLE 23-4 **Potential Complications and Nursing Interventions after Appendectomy**

Complication	Nursing Interventions
Peritonitis	Observe for abdominal tenderness, fever, vomiting, abdominal rigidity, and tachycardia Employ nasogastric suction Correct dehydration as prescribed Administer antibiotic agents as prescribed
Pelvic abscess	Evaluate for anorexia, chills, fever, and diaphoresis Observe for diarrhea, which may indicate pelvic abscess Prepare patient for rectal examination Prepare patient for surgical drainage procedure
Subphrenic abscess (abscess under the diaphragm)	Assess patient for chills, fever, and diaphoresis. Observe for Hiccups because of diaphragmatic irritation Prepare for x-ray examination Prepare for surgical drainage of abscess
Ileus (paralytic and mechanical)	Assess for bowel sounds Employ nasogastric intubation and suction Replace fluids and electrolytes by intravenous route as prescribed Prepare for surgery if diagnosis of mechanical ileus is established

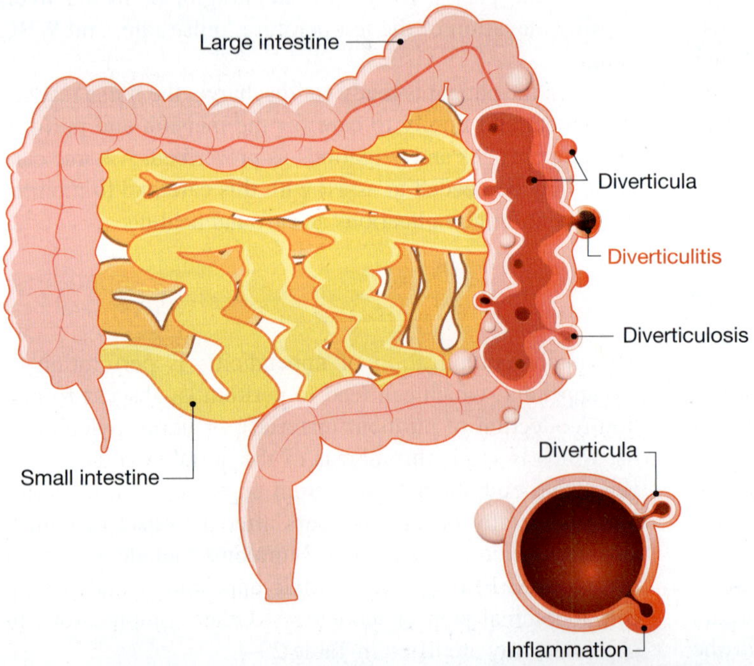

FIGURE 23-3 **Location of diverticula (top), diverticulitis (middle) and diverticulosis (bottom) of the descending colon. (Shutterstock.com ID 1500882671)**

DIVERTICULAR DISEASE

A diverticulum is a sac-like herniation of the lining of the bowel that extends through a defect in the muscle layer. Diverticula may occur anywhere in the small intestine or colon but occur most commonly in the distal sigmoid colon. The incidence of diverticular disease of the colon is 33% to 50% in those over 40 and more than 66% in those over 80 years old (Hunt et al., 2021). The health care cost of diverticular disease is estimated at more than $5.5 billion (Hunt et al., 2021).

Pathophysiology

Diverticula form when the mucosa and submucosal layers of the colon herniate through the muscular wall because of high intraluminal pressure, low volume in the colon (i.e., fiber-deficient contents), and decreased muscle strength in the colon wall (e.g., muscular hypertrophy from hardened fecal masses). Bowel contents can accumulate in the diverticulum and decompose, causing inflammation and infection. The diverticulum also can become obstructed and then inflamed if the obstruction continues. Inflammation and subsequent infection of the diverticulum (i.e., **diverticulitis**) can cause the development of abscesses, which may eventually perforate, leading to peritonitis and erosion of the blood vessels, resulting in bleeding. Diverticulitis may occur as an acute attack or may persist as a continuing, smoldering infection. The symptoms manifested generally result from complications: abscess, fistula formation, obstruction, perforation, peritonitis, and hemorrhage.

Diverticulosis (see Fig. 23-3) exists when multiple diverticula are present without inflammation or symptoms. A low intake of dietary fiber is considered a predisposing factor, but the exact cause has not been identified. Most patients with diverticular disease are asymptomatic, so its exact prevalence is unknown.

Risk Factors

It is estimated that 10% to 25% of people with diverticulosis have diverticulitis at some point in their lives (Strate & Morris, 2020). A congenital predisposition is suspected when the disorder occurs in those younger than 40 years of age.

Clinical Manifestations and Assessment

Chronic constipation often precedes the development of diverticulosis, sometimes by many years. Frequently, no problematic symptoms occur with diverticulosis. Signs and symptoms of diverticulosis are relatively mild and include bowel irregularity with intervals of diarrhea, nausea, anorexia, and abdominal distention. Abdominal pain may radiate to the back, flank, or suprapubic region. With repeated local inflammation of the diverticula, the large bowel may narrow with fibrotic strictures, leading to cramps, narrow stools, and increased constipation or, at times, intestinal obstruction. Weakness, fatigue, and anorexia are common symptoms. With diverticulitis, the patient reports an acute onset of mild to severe pain in the lower left quadrant, accompanied by nausea, vomiting, fever, chills, and leukocytosis (elevated WBC). Rebound tenderness is suggestive of perforation. The condition, if untreated, can lead to septicemia (see Chapter 53).

Typically, diverticulosis is diagnosed by colonoscopy, which permits visualization of the extent of diverticular disease and allows the clinician to biopsy tissue to rule out other diseases as needed. Until recently, barium enema had been the preferred diagnostic test, but now it is used less frequently than colonoscopy. However, if acute diverticulosis is suspected or there are symptoms of peritoneal irritation, a colonoscopy or barium enema is contraindicated because of potential for perforation. CT scan is the diagnostic test of choice if the suspected diagnosis is diverticulitis; it also can reveal one or more abscesses. Abdominal x-rays may demonstrate free air under the diaphragm if a perforation has occurred from the diverticulitis, which causes peritonitis. Laboratory tests that assist in diagnosis include a CBC, revealing an elevated WBC count, and elevated erythrocyte sedimentation rate (ESR).

Gerontologic Considerations

The incidence of diverticular disease increases with age because of degeneration and structural changes in the circular muscle layers of the colon and because of cellular hypertrophy. The symptoms are less pronounced in older individuals than in other adults. Oder indivuals may not have abdominal pain until infection occurs. They may delay reporting symptoms because they fear surgery or are afraid that they may have cancer. Frequently blood in the stool is overlooked, especially in older patients because of a failure to examine the stool or the inability to see changes if vision is impaired.

Pearls for Practice

The nurse understanding that the intestines contain air and fluid under pressure. However, the peritoneal space is free of air! If air is noted (typically under the diaphragm since air will rise to the highest level in the abdomen), then there must be a perforation in an organ containing air. The nurse recognizes that the organ is also spilling its contents into the normally sterile peritoneal space. Examples can include perforation of a gastric or duodenal ulcer, or bowel perforation. This is an emergency and the nurse prepares the patient for surgery.

Medical and Nursing Management

Diverticulitis usually can be treated on an outpatient basis with diet and medication. When symptoms occur, rest, analgesics, and antispasmodics are recommended. Initially, the diet is clear liquid until the inflammation subsides; then a high-fiber, low-fat diet is recommended. This type of diet helps increase stool volume, decrease colonic transit time, and reduce intraluminal pressure. Antibiotics are prescribed for 7 to 10 days. A bulk-forming laxative also is prescribed.

Pearls for Practice

High-fiber foods include items such as fruits, raw vegetables and whole grains help reduce the risk of diverticulitis. In addition, patient teaching can include adding foods such as raspberries and pears as snacks to help increase fiber intake. In the past, it was recommended that people with diverticular disease (diverticulosis or diverticulitis) avoid nuts, corn, popcorn, and seeds for fear that these foods would become lodged in the diverticula and lead to inflammation. However, there is no convincing evidence to support any particular foods that should be favored or avoided (Strate & Morris, 2020).

In acute cases of diverticulitis hospitalization may be required for patients who cannot tolerate PO fluids and food. Measures taken to rest the bowel include withholding oral intake, administering IV fluids and antibiotics, and instituting nasogastric suctioning if vomiting or abdominal distention are present. An opioid is prescribed for pain relief. Historically, morphine was considered to be contraindicated because of a claim that it could increase intraluminal pressure in the colon, thus exacerbating symptoms; however, no research evidence is available to support this claim. Uncomplicated acute diverticulitis can be managed with oral antibiotics for 7 to 10 days in the outpatient setting. Nonsteroidal anti-inflammatory drugs (NSAIDs) are associated with increased risk of perforation and should be avoided.

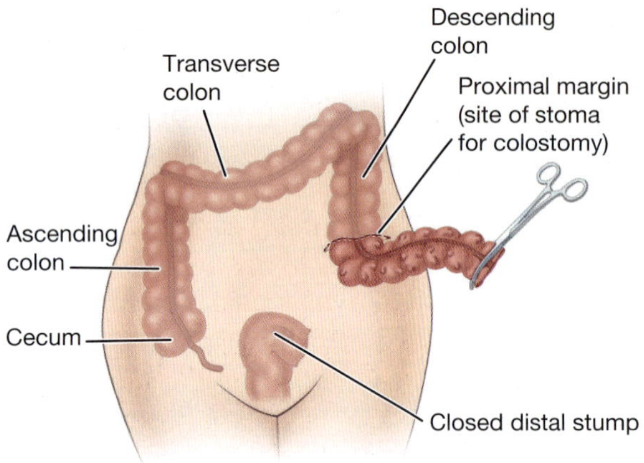

FIGURE 23-4 **The Hartmann procedure for diverticulitis: primary resection for diverticulitis of the colon. The affected segment (*clamp attached*) has been divided at its distal end. In a primary anastomosis, the proximal margin (*dotted line*) is transected and the bowel attached end-to-end. In a two-stage procedure, a colostomy is constructed at the proximal margin with the distal stump oversewn (Hartmann procedure, as shown) or brought to the outer surface as a mucous fistula. The second stage consists of colostomy takedown and anastomosis.**

More often than not, acute diverticulitis will subside with medical management. Immediate surgical intervention is necessary if complications (e.g., perforation, peritonitis, hemorrhage, obstruction) occur. In cases of abscess formation without peritonitis, hemorrhage, or obstruction, CT-guided percutaneous drainage may be performed to drain the abscess, and IV antibiotics are administered. Stabilization of the patient by drainage of the abscess and resolution of the inflammation is complete after approximately 6 weeks; surgery may be recommended to prevent repeated episodes. Typically, two types of surgery are considered either to treat acute complications or to prevent further episodes of inflammation:

- One-stage resection, in which the inflamed area is removed and a primary end-to-end anastomosis is completed
- Multiple-stage procedures for complications such as obstruction or perforation (Fig. 23-4)

The type of surgery performed depends on the extent of complications found during surgery. When possible, the area of diverticulitis is taken out and the remaining bowel is joined end-to-end (i.e., primary resection and end-to-end anastomosis). This is performed through traditional surgical or laparoscopically assisted colectomy. A two-stage resection may be performed in which the diseased colon is removed (as in a one-stage procedure) but no anastomosis is performed; both ends of the bowel are brought out onto the abdomen as stomas. Then this "double-barrel" temporary colostomy is reanastomosed in a later procedure. In a double-barrel colostomy, the proximal stoma serves as an outlet for feces, and the distal stoma leads to the nonfunctioning bowel. The distal opening does not drain feces however will drain mucous and air from the resting bowel. It is also known as a *mucus fistula.* Fecal diversion procedures are discussed later in this chapter.

Complications

Complications of diverticulitis include peritonitis (see below), abscess formation, and bleeding. If an abscess develops, the associated findings are tenderness, a palpable mass, fever, and leukocytosis. An inflamed diverticulum that perforates results in abdominal pain localized over the involved segment, usually the sigmoid; local abscess or peritonitis follows. Abdominal pain, a rigid board-like abdomen, loss of bowel sounds, and signs and symptoms of shock occur with peritonitis. Noninflamed or slightly inflamed diverticula may erode areas adjacent to arterial branches, causing massive rectal bleeding.

PERITONITIS

Peritonitis is inflammation of the peritoneum, the serous membrane lining the abdominal cavity and covering the viscera. Peritonitis is typically a life-threatening emergency that requires prompt surgical intervention and typically involves postoperative critical care monitoring due to the risk of sepsis, organ failure, and subsequent infections.

Pearls for Practice

The development of peritonitis can include a variety of signs and symptoms in patients, including a firm and distended abdomen, rebound tenderness, and guarding by the patient of the abdomen during the examination. These signs and symptoms should cue nurses into suspecting peritonitis in their patients.

Pathophysiology

Peritonitis is caused by leakage of contents from abdominal organs into the abdominal cavity, usually as a result of inflammation, infection, ischemia, trauma, or tumor perforation. Bacterial proliferation occurs. Edema of the tissues ensues, and exudation of fluid develops in a short time. Fluid in the peritoneal cavity becomes turbid (cloudy) with increasing amounts of protein, WBCs, cellular debris, and blood. The immediate response of the intestinal tract is hypermotility, soon followed by paralytic ileus with an accumulation of air and fluid in the bowel.

Risk Factors

Usually, peritonitis is a result of bacterial infection; the organisms come from diseases of the GI tract or, in females, from the internal reproductive organs. Peritonitis also can result from external sources, such as injury or trauma (e.g., gunshot wound, stab wound) or an inflammation that extends from an organ outside the peritoneal area, such as the kidney.

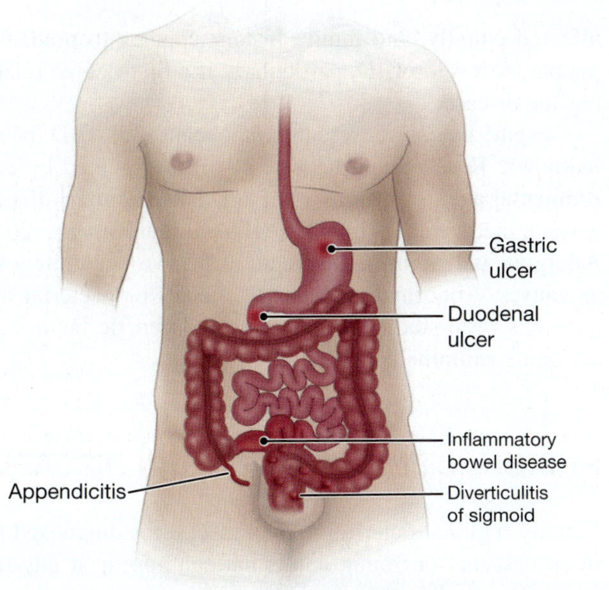

FIGURE 23-5 **Common gastrointestinal causes of peritonitis.**

The most common bacteria implicated, about 75% of peritonitis, are gram-negative organisms (*Escherichia coli, Klebsiella, Proteus*) with gram-positive bacteria (enterococci, streptococci, staphylococci) making up the remainder of cases (Ameer et al., 2021). Inflammation and paralytic ileus are the direct effects of the infection. Other common causes of peritonitis are appendicitis, perforated ulcer, diverticulitis, and bowel perforation (Fig. 23-5). Peritonitis also may be associated with abdominal surgical procedures and peritoneal dialysis.

Clinical Manifestations and Assessment

Symptoms depend on the location and extent of the inflammation. The early clinical manifestations of peritonitis frequently are the symptoms of the disorder causing the condition, aptly nicknamed an "acute abdomen." At first, a diffuse type of pain is felt. The pain tends to become constant, localized, and more intense near the site of the inflammation. Movement usually aggravates it. The affected area of the abdomen becomes extremely tender and distended, and the muscles become rigid. Rebound tenderness and paralytic ileus may be present. Diminished perception of pain in peritonitis can occur in people receiving corticosteroids or analgesics. Patients with diabetes who have symptoms of advanced neuropathy and patients with cirrhosis who have signs of ascites may not experience pain during an acute bacterial episode. Usually, nausea and vomiting occur, and peristalsis is diminished (decreased bowel sounds). A temperature of 100° to 101°F (37.8° to 38.3°C) can be expected, along with an increased pulse rate, tachypnea, dyspnea, and hypotension.

The WBC count is almost always elevated. The hemoglobin and Hct levels may be low if blood loss has occurred. Serum electrolyte studies may reveal altered levels of potassium, sodium, and chloride.

An abdominal x-ray study may show air and fluid levels as well as distended bowel loops. A CT scan of the abdomen may show abscess formation, acute inflammation or infection of one of the major abdominal organs, or a perforation of the small or large bowel. Peritoneal aspiration and culture and sensitivity studies of the aspirated fluid may reveal infection and identify the causative organisms.

Medical and Nursing Management

Fluid, colloid, and electrolyte replacement is the major focus of medical management. The administration of several liters of an isotonic solution is emergently prescribed. Hypovolemia occurs because massive amounts of fluid and electrolytes move from the intestinal lumen into the peritoneal cavity and deplete the fluid in the vascular space.

Analgesics are prescribed for pain. Antiemetics are administered as prescribed for nausea and vomiting. Placement of a nasogastric tube is warranted, and suction is maintained to assist in relieving abdominal distention. Fluid in the abdominal cavity can cause pressure that restricts expansion of the lungs and causes respiratory distress. Oxygen therapy by nasal cannula or mask generally promotes adequate oxygenation, but airway intubation and ventilatory assistance may occasionally be required due to the patient's inability to compensate for the metabolic acidosis that typically occurs with peritonitis.

Antibiotic therapy is initiated early in the treatment of peritonitis. Large doses of a broad-spectrum antibiotic and antifungicide are administered IV until the specific organism causing the infection is identified and appropriate antibiotic therapy can be initiated.

Surgical objectives include removing the infected material and correcting the cause. Surgical treatment is directed toward excision (i.e., appendix), resection with or without anastomosis (i.e., intestine), repair (i.e., perforation), and/or drainage (i.e., abscess). With sepsis accompanying the peritonitis, a fecal diversion may need to be created.

The two most common postoperative complications are wound evisceration and abscess formation. Any suggestion from the patient that an area of the abdomen is tender or painful or "feels as if something just gave way" must be reported. The sudden occurrence of serosanguineous wound drainage strongly suggests wound dehiscence and is a surgical emergency that must be reported promptly to the on-call provider.

Often intensive care is needed. The blood pressure is monitored by arterial line if shock is present. Accurate recording of all intake and output and central venous pressures and/or pulmonary artery pressures assists in calculating fluid replacement. The nurse administers and closely monitors IV fluids response.

In addition, ongoing assessment of pain, GI function, and fluid and electrolyte balance is important. Bladder pressure also is measured routinely to identify abdominal compartment syndrome (refer to Chapter 52, Fig. 52-4). The nurse reports the nature of the pain, its location in the abdomen, and any changes in location. Administering analgesic medication and positioning the patient for comfort are helpful in decreasing pain. The patient is placed on the side with knees flexed; this position decreases tension on the abdominal organs, the head of bed is elevated to prevent pooling of GI contents under the diaphragm.

Signs that indicate that peritonitis is subsiding include a decrease in temperature and pulse rate, softening of the abdomen, return of peristaltic sounds, and passing of flatus and bowel movements. The nurse increases fluid and food intake gradually and reduces parenteral fluids as prescribed. A worsening clinical condition may indicate a complication, and the nurse must prepare the patient for emergency surgery.

Frequently drains are inserted during the surgical procedure, and the nurse must observe and record the character of the drainage postoperatively. Care must be taken when moving and turning the patient to prevent the drains from being dislodged. It is prudent to safety-pin the drains to the patient's gown to limit the chance of accidental dislodgment. Also, it is important for the nurse to prepare the patient and family for discharge by teaching the patient to care for the incision and drains if the patient will be sent home with the drains still in place. Referral for home care or rehabilitation may be indicated for further monitoring and patient and family teaching.

Complications

Frequently, the inflammation is not localized, and the entire abdominal cavity shows evidence of widespread infection. Sepsis is the major cause of death from peritonitis. Shock may result from septicemia or hypovolemia. The inflammatory process may cause intestinal obstruction, primarily from the development of bowel adhesions, and care must be made to monitor the patient's nasogastric tube drainage and input and output closely. The patient is also at high risk of developing pulmonary emboli, and compression stockings, sequential-compression boots, and subcutaneous anticoagulation may be prescribed.

INFLAMMATORY BOWEL DISEASE

IBD refers to two chronic inflammatory GI disorders: regional enteritis (i.e., Crohn disease) and ulcerative colitis (UC). Both disorders have striking similarities but also several differences (Table 23-5); medical and nursing management for both types are similar and discussed jointly.

There are approximately 3 million people in the United States affected by IBD (CDC, 2021). Typically, IBD presents during late childhood or during the second or third decade of life and is attributed to a high morbidity and a decreased quality of life (CDC, 2021). Females and males tend to be affected equally, and family history appears to predispose people to develop IBD, particularly if a first-degree relative has the disease.

Despite extensive research, the cause of IBD is still unknown. Researchers theorize that it is triggered by environmental agents, such as smoking, a Westernized diet and certain medications, like NSAIDs (Buttaro et al., 2021). Allergies and immune disorders also have been suggested as causes. Abnormal response to dietary or bacterial antigens has been studied extensively, and genetic factors also are being examined.

REGIONAL ENTERITIS (CROHN DISEASE)

Usually regional enteritis (Crohn disease) is diagnosed first in adolescents or young adults but can appear at any time in a person's life. The incidence of regional enteritis has risen both nationally and internationally, with rising cases seen in newly industrialized countries in Africa and Asia (Ranasinghe & Hsu, 2022). The most popular theory is that the body's immune system reacts abnormally in people with Crohn disease, mistaking environmental triggers like bacteria, foods, and other substances for dangerous foreign substances, triggering an immune response to protect the body from these environmental factors (Buttaro et al., 2021).

Pathophysiology

Regional enteritis is a subacute and chronic inflammation of the GI tract wall that extends through all layers (i.e., transmural lesion). Although it can occur anywhere in the GI tract, it most commonly occurs in the distal ileum but can be seen in the ascending colon. Regional enteritis is characterized by periods of remission and exacerbation. The disease process begins with edema and thickening of the mucosa. Ulcers begin to appear on the inflamed mucosa. The ulcerations in regional enteritis differ from UC in that they are not continuous or in contact with each other and are separated by normal tissue. Hence, these clusters of ulcers tend to take on a classic "cobblestone" appearance on colonoscopy. Fistulas, fissures, and abscesses form as the inflammation extends down into the peritoneum. **Granulomas** (localized nodular inflammation) occur in 50% of patients. As the disease advances, the bowel wall thickens and becomes fibrotic, and the intestinal lumen narrows. Diseased bowel loops sometimes stick to other loops surrounding those developing adhesions.

Clinical Manifestations and Assessment

Usually, the onset of symptoms is insidious in regional enteritis, with prominent lower right quadrant abdominal pain unrelieved by defecation, fatigue, diarrhea, and weight loss. Scar tissue and the formation of granulomas interfere with the ability of the intestine to transport products of the upper intestinal digestion through the constricted lumen,

TABLE **23-5 Comparison of Regional Enteritis and Ulcerative Colitis**

Factor	Regional Enteritis	Ulcerative Colitis
Course	Prolonged, variable	Exacerbations, remissions
Pathology		
Early	Transmural thickening	Mucosal ulceration
Late	Deep, penetrating granulomas	Minute, mucosal ulcerations
Clinical Manifestations		
Location	Ileum, ascending colon (usually)	Rectum, descending colon
Bleeding	Usually not, but if it occurs, it tends to be mild	Common—severe
Perianal involvement	Common (seen in 30–45% of patients)	Rare—mild
Fistulas	Common	Rare
Rectal involvement	About 20%	Almost 100%
Diarrhea	Less severe	Severe
Diagnostic Study Findings		
Barium series	Regional, discontinuous lesions Narrowing of colon Thickening of bowel wall Mucosal edema Stenosis, fistulas, fissures "String sign" of the terminal ileum, indicating the constriction of a segment of intestine. Ulcerations (the cobblestone appearance)	Diffuse involvement No narrowing of colon No mucosal edema Rare occurrence of stenosis Shortening of colon
Sigmoidoscopy	May be unremarkable unless accompanied by perianal fistulas	Abnormal inflamed mucosa
Colonoscopy	Distinct ulcerations separated by relatively normal mucosa in ascending colon	Friable mucosa with pseudopolyps or ulcers in descending colon
CT scan[a]	May show bowel-wall thickening and fistula formation in regional enteritis (Crohn disease)	Depicts bowel-wall thickening, abscesses, fistulas, and obstructions
Therapeutic Management	Corticosteroids, sulfonamides (sulfasalazine) Antibiotics Parenteral nutrition Partial or complete colectomy with ileostomy or anastomosis Rectum can be preserved in some patients Recurrence common	Corticosteroids, sulfonamides; sulfasalazine useful in preventing recurrence Bulk hydrophilic agents Antibiotics Proctocolectomy, with ileostomy Rectum can be preserved in only a few patients "cured" by colectomy
Systemic Complications	Small bowel obstruction Right-sided hydronephrosis Nephrolithiasis Cholelithiasis Arthritis Retinitis, iritis Erythema nodosum	Toxic megacolon Perforation Hemorrhage Malignant neoplasms Pyelonephritis Nephrolithiasis Cholangiocarcinoma Arthritis Retinitis, iritis Erythema nodosum

[a]Can reveal acute inflammation or infection of one of the major abdominal organs or a perforation of the small or large bowel.

resulting in crampy abdominal pains. Abdominal tenderness and spasm occur. Because eating stimulates intestinal peristalsis, the crampy pain typically occurs after meals. The patient will tend to limit food intake to reduce the crampy pain and, in fact, can reduce the amount and type of food to such a degree that normal nutritional requirements often are not met. As a result, weight loss, malnutrition, and secondary anemia occur.

Ulcers in the membranous lining of the intestine and other inflammatory changes result in a weeping, edematous intestine that continually empties a colonic- and skin-irritating discharge. Disrupted absorption causes chronic diarrhea and associated fluid and electrolyte imbalances (i.e., hypokalemia, hypomagnesemia, hypocalcemia, and low albumin) as well as nutritional deficits. In some patients, the inflamed intestine may perforate, leading to intra-abdominal and anal abscesses. Fever and leukocytosis may occur. Chronic symptoms of regional enteritis may **include steatorrhea** (i.e., excessive fat in the feces).

Abscesses, fistulas, and fissures are common. Manifestations may extend beyond the GI tract and commonly include joint disorders (e.g., arthritis), skin lesions (e.g., erythema nodosum), ocular disorders (e.g., conjunctivitis), and oral ulcers. The clinical course and symptoms can vary; in some patients, periods of remission and exacerbation occur, but in others, the disease follows a fulminating course.

A proctosigmoidoscopy usually is performed initially to determine whether the rectosigmoid area is inflamed. A stool examination also is performed; the result may be positive for occult blood and steatorrhea. Endoscopy, colonoscopy, and intestinal biopsies may be used to confirm the diagnosis. A CT scan may show bowel-wall thickening and fistula formation.

A CBC is performed to assess Hct and hemoglobin levels (usually decreased) as well as the WBC count (may be elevated). The ESR commonly is elevated in relation to the inflammation. Albumin (the long-term marker of nutrition) and protein levels may be decreased, indicating malnutrition.

Pearls for Practice

A low albumin or hypoalbuminemia increases the risk of surgical site infections (SSIs). The reasons for the impaired wound healing include poor tissue healing, decreased collagen synthesis, impaired macrophage activation and leakage of interstitial fluid into the surgical wound, predisposing the patient to SSI (Seidelman & Anderson, 2021). A normal albumin is 3.5 to 5.2 g/dL, levels of 3 to 3.5 g/dL are associated with reduced vaccine response and levels of 2 to 2.5 g/dL are associated with edema (Fischbach, 2022). The nurse is aware that hypoalbuminemia is associated with conditions such as malnutrition, liver disease, sepsis, inflammation, or trauma, and when present is correlated to an increased length of hospital stay and increased mortality.

Complications

Complications of regional enteritis include intestinal obstruction or stricture formation, perianal disease, fluid and electrolyte imbalances, malnutrition from malabsorption, and formation of fistulas and abscesses. The most common type of small bowel fistula caused by regional enteritis is the enterocutaneous fistula (i.e., an abnormal opening between the small bowel and the skin). Abscesses can be the result of an internal fistula that results in fluid accumulation and infection. Patients with regional enteritis are also at increased risk of colon cancer.

Pearls for Practice

A fistula is an abnormal communication between two surfaces. An intestinal fistula can connect from the bowel to the skin as noted previously, or from bowel to bladder (enterovesicular fistula), or recto-vaginal fistula (rectum to vagina). In general, they form secondary to an underlying disease or surgical complication. Crohn disease is a well-known cause of intestinal fistula development since the primary etiology of formation is the loss of the intestinal wall integrity in the area of the underlying disease and chronic inflammation. Treatment is complex as it requires control of the underlying disease, and correction of malnutrition. Since Crohn disease is associated with multiple and recurrent fistula, a surgical fistulotomy is avoided, except for the most superficial fistulae (Madoff & Melton-Meaux, 2020). Options include use of a medical plug to close the fistula, endoscopic fibrin glue injection, placement of a thin surgical cord (seton) into the fistula to help drain any infection (Crohn's & Colitis, n.d.).

ULCERATIVE COLITIS

UC is a recurrent ulcerative and inflammatory disease of the mucosal and submucosal layers of the colon and rectum. The prevalence of UC is highest in those with a family history, Jewish heritage and those that are living in North America and Northern Europe (Ferri, 2022). It affects males and females equally. It is a serious disease, accompanied by systemic complications and a high mortality rate. The risk of colon cancer increases as UC disease progresses, with colorectal cancer risk being 2% after 10 years, 8% after 20 years and 18% by 30 years (De Campos Silva et al., 2020). The worldwide incidence of UC is more common than the incidence of Crohn disease (Ferri, 2022).

Pathophysiology

UC affects the superficial mucosa of the colon and is characterized by multiple ulcerations, diffuse inflammations, and desquamation or shedding of the colonic epithelium.

Bleeding occurs as a result of the ulcerations. The mucosa becomes edematous and inflamed. The lesions are contiguous, occurring one after the other. Abscesses form, and infiltrate can be seen in both the mucosa and submucosa with plasma cells, granulocytes, and lymphocytes (Lynch & Hsu, 2021). The disease process usually begins in the rectum and spreads proximally to involve the entire colon. Eventually, the bowel narrows, shortens, and thickens because of muscular hypertrophy and fat deposits.

Clinical Manifestations and Assessment

The clinical course is usually one of intermittent exacerbations and remissions. The predominant symptoms of UC include bloody diarrhea, passage of mucus, urgency, lower left quadrant abdominal pain, intermittent tenesmus, and fever. Symptoms will differ according to the extent of disease. The bleeding may be mild or severe, and pallor, anemia, and fatigue are the result. The patient may have anorexia, weight loss, vomiting, and dehydration, as well as cramping, the feeling of an urgent need to defecate, and the passage of 10 to 20 liquid stools each day. The disease is classified as mild, severe, or fulminant, depending on the severity of the symptoms. Hypocalcemia and anemia frequently develop. Rebound tenderness may occur in the right lower quadrant. Extraintestinal manifestations include skin lesions (e.g., erythema nodosum), eye lesions (e.g., uveitis), joint abnormalities (e.g., arthritis), and liver disease.

The patient should be assessed for tachycardia, hypotension, tachypnea, fever, and pallor (hypovolemic shock) from rectal bleeding. Bloody diarrhea occurs with most patients with UC and correlates to the severity of the disease and the area of colon involvement, with more distal colonic involvement and rectal involvement resulting in more bloody stools, urgency and rectal bleeding (Kaenkumchorn & Wahbeh, 2020). Treatment is aimed at blood replacement and correction of volume and any clotting abnormalities. Other assessments address level of hydration and nutritional status. The abdomen is examined for bowel sounds, distention, and tenderness. Peripheral edema can occur secondary to hypoalbuminemia. These findings assist in determining the severity of the disease.

The stool can be positive for blood, and laboratory test results reveal low Hct and hemoglobin levels in addition to an elevated WBC count, low albumin levels, and an electrolyte imbalance, including low potassium, magnesium, and calcium levels (Ferri, 2022). Iron-deficiency anemia may be present because of chronic blood loss. Evidence of dehydration is often present during an acute flare up, including elevated creatinine, blood urea nitrogen as well as tachycardia. C-reactive protein (CRP) and ESR, markers of inflammation, will be elevated in severe UC (Kaenkumchorn & Wahben, 2020). The nurse is aware that the patient may also present in metabolic acidosis secondary to loss of base bicarbonate with persistent diarrhea. Abdominal x-ray studies are useful for determining the cause of symptoms. Free air in the peritoneum and bowel dilation or obstruction should be excluded as a source of the presenting symptoms, as peritonitis also can occur.

Colonoscopy should be avoided during acute UC flare due to the risk of perforation. Colonoscopy may reveal friable, inflamed mucosa with exudate and ulcerations. This procedure assists in defining the extent and severity of the disease and helps differentiate between UC and Crohn Disease and to rule out other colorectal diseases like colorectal cancer (Kaenkumchorn & Wahbeh, 2020). With the advent of endoscopy, barium enema studies have been used less often but remain important for certain specific scenarios, such as evaluation of colonic strictures or when certain areas of the colon are difficult to access via colonoscopy (Ud Din et al., 2020), however barium enema *should not* be used in patients with moderate to severe colitis because there is perforation risk when the colon is weakened from inflammation (Buttaro et al., 2021). A barium enema provides information about the presence of distention, obstructions, fistulas, strictures, or tumors (Buttaro et al., 2021). CT scanning can identify abscesses and perirectal involvement, as well as differentiate between diverticulitis and diverticulosis.

Careful examination of the patient's stool for parasites and other microbes is performed to rule out dysentery caused by common intestinal organisms, especially *Entamoeba histolytica* and *Clostridium difficile.*

Complications

Complications of UC include toxic megacolon, perforation, and bleeding as a result of ulceration, vascular engorgement, and highly vascular granulation tissue (Fig. 23-6). In toxic megacolon, the inflammatory process extends into the muscularis, inhibiting its ability to contract and resulting in colonic distention. Symptoms include fever, abdominal pain and distention, vomiting, and fatigue. If the patient with toxic megacolon does not respond within 24 to 72 hours to medical management with nasogastric suction, IV fluids with electrolytes, corticosteroids, and antibiotics, then surgery is required. Then total colectomy is indicated. For many patients, surgery becomes necessary to relieve the effects of the disease and to treat these serious complications; an ileostomy usually is performed. The surgical procedures involved and the care of patients with this type of fecal diversion are discussed later in this chapter. In addition, hypercoagulability is a well-recognized complication of UC, resulting in deep vein thrombosis and pulmonary emboli. The mechanism of increased thrombotic risk is unclear. Standard anticoagulants would be administered. Episcleritis (painless hyperemia of the sclera and conjunctiva without loss of vision) and uveitis (acute or subacute pain in the eye with visual blurring often accompanied by photophobia and headache that can progress to loss of vision) occurs in 2–5% of patients with UC (Malik & Aurelio, 2022). Episcleritis parallels the level of bowel disease and generally responds to anti-inflammatory therapy. In contrast, the occurrence of uveitis increases with the dose and duration of glucocorticoid use. Patients with

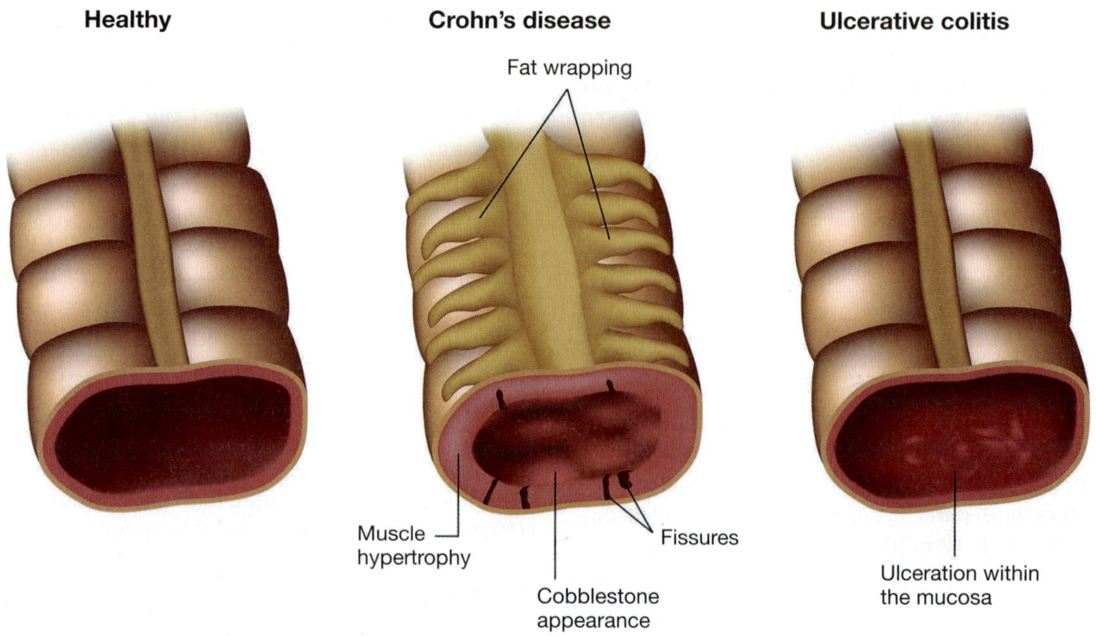

FIGURE 23-6 Irritable bowel disease. A representation of the bowel appearance in Crohn disease and ulcerative colitis when compared to healthy bowel. (Shutterstock.com ID 147789395)

uveitis should receive prompt ophthalmologic examination and treatment with glucocorticoid ocular drops and cycloplegics to prevent progression to blindness. Steroid therapy also can lead to cataracts, thus patients receiving glucocorticoid therapy should receive an annual ophthalmologic examination. It is important that at the time of a new IBD diagnosis, a check-up by an ophthalmologist should be arranged (Castellano et al., 2021).

Patients with IBD also have a significantly increased risk of osteoporotic fractures due to decreased bone mineral density. Corticosteroid therapy also may contribute to the diminished bone density.

Pearls for Practice

The nurse is alert for evidence of improvement including a decrease in abdominal girth and the return of bowel sounds, whereas, the presence of rebound tenderness, increasing abdominal girth, fever and leukocytosis warns the nurse of disease progression.

MEDICAL AND NURSING MANAGEMENT OF INFLAMMATORY BOWEL DISEASE

Medical treatment for regional enteritis and UC is aimed at reducing inflammation, suppressing inappropriate immune responses, providing rest for a diseased bowel so that healing may take place, improving quality of life (Box 23-1), and preventing or minimizing complications. Most patients have long periods of well-being interspersed with short intervals of illness, and management depends on the disease location, severity, and complications.

Oral fluids and a diet that is low residue, high protein, and high calorie with supplemental vitamin therapy and iron replacement are prescribed to meet nutritional needs, reduce inflammation, and control pain and diarrhea. Fluid and electrolyte imbalances from dehydration caused by diarrhea are corrected by IV therapy as necessary if the patient is hospitalized or by oral fluids if the patient is managed at home. Any foods that exacerbate diarrhea are avoided. Milk may contribute to diarrhea in those with lactose intolerance. Smoking is avoided because of increased intestinal motility. Consultation with a dietitian is highly recommended regarding oral diet or enteral feeding; parenteral nutrition has not yielded clinical benefit in this patient population (see Chapter 21).

Aminosalicylate formulations, such as sulfasalazine, often are effective for mild or moderate inflammation and are used to prevent or reduce recurrences in long-term maintenance regimens. Sulfa-free aminosalicylates (e.g., mesalamine) are effective in preventing and treating recurrence of inflammation allowing the patient to maintain remission. Antibiotics (e.g., metronidazole) are used for secondary infections, particularly for purulent complications, such as abscesses, perforation, and peritonitis.

Corticosteroids are used to treat severe and fulminant disease and can be administered orally (e.g., prednisone) in outpatient treatment or parenterally (e.g., hydrocortisone) in hospitalized patients. Topical (i.e., rectal administration) corticosteroids (e.g., hydrocortisone enema, budesonide) also are used widely in the treatment of distal colon disease. When the dosage of corticosteroids is reduced or stopped, the symptoms of disease may return. If corticosteroids are continued, adverse sequelae, such as hypertension, fluid retention, cataracts, hirsutism (i.e., abnormal hair growth), adrenal

BOX 23-1

Nursing Research

Bridging the Gap to Evidence-Based Practice

Effect of Acupuncture in Patients with Irritable Bowel Syndrome: A Randomized Controlled Trial

Does acupuncture help improve IBS symptoms and improve overall quality of life when compared to pharmacologic interventions?

Pei, L., Geng, H., Guo, J., Yang, G., Wang, L., Shen, R., Xia, S., Ding, M., Feng, H., Lu, J., Li, J., Liu, L., Shu, Y., Fang, X., Wu, X., Wang, X., Weng, S., Ju, L., Chen, X., Shen, H., & Sun, J. (2020). Effect of acupuncture in patients with irritable bowel syndrome: A randomized controlled trial. *Mayo Clinic Proceedings 95*(8),1671–1683. https://doi.org/10.1016/j.mayocp.2020.01.042

Purpose

Irritable bowel syndrome is a very common condition in adults that causes abdominal pain and discomfort in patients, leading to overall decreased quality of life. While there are pharmacologic interventions for IBS, these medications are shown to only provide temporary symptom relief. There are nonpharmacologic interventions that have been shown to help improve IBS symptoms, such as acupuncture. Acupuncture has been shown to help IBS symptoms, however, a randomized control trial at multiple centers had not been conducted. Therefore, the purpose of this study was to see if acupuncture, when compared to pharmacologic interventions, resulted in less IBS symptoms and overall, an increase in the participants quality of life.

Design

A multicentred randomized controlled trial was conducted in 7 hospitals. A total of 531 participated with ages ranging from 18 years old to 70 years old. Patients were divided into two groups, those with IBS-Constipation (IBS-C) and IBS-Diarrhea (IBS-D). They were then randomized to the acupuncture group or the medication group, with polyethylene glycol (PEG) 400 for those with IBS-C and pinaverium bromide for those with IBS-D.

The acupuncture group obtained the acupuncture treatment every other day, 3 times a week for a total of 6 weeks with each session lasting 30 minutes. The patients in the IBS-C group received PEG-4000 powder daily for 6 weeks. Participants in the IBS-D group received pinaverium bromide tablets daily for 6 weeks.

Several self-reporting instruments were used throughout the trial to assess patients' quality of life, abdominal pain, bowel habits, and any interference with daily life. It was shown that acupuncture was more effective than both PEG 4000 and pinaverium bromide for IBS treatment, with greater and longer symptom relief, and overall, greater quality of life.

Nursing Implications

This study has shown that acupuncture is an effective, nonpharmacologic intervention to help decrease IBS symptoms and improve quality of life. The nurse plays an important role in educating patients regarding holistic measures to help prevent the symptoms of IBS, including diet modification, adequate hydration, and exercise. It is especially important to consult with pharmacists to confirm that the herbal remedy is safe, as herbals can affect absorption rates, have side effects, etc. The nurse can now educate about acupuncture as a proven intervention, through evidence-based practice, to help reduce symptoms and improve patients' overall quality of life.

suppression, steroid-induced diabetes mellitus (secondary to the hyperglycemia associated with glucocorticoid therapy), poor wound healing, and loss of bone density, may occur.

Immunomodulators (e.g., azathioprine [AZA], 6-mercaptopurine [6-MP], methotrexate, and cyclosporine) and antitumor necrosis factor (anti-TNF) agents have been used to alter the immune response. The exact mechanism of action of these medications in treating IBD is unknown. These medications are useful in maintenance regimens to prevent relapses and decrease the use of steroids. The first-line biologic therapies for UC are both infliximab and vedolizumab and the first-line treatment for CD is infliximab or adalimumab (Chang & Hudesman, 2020). Infliximab is the only anti-TNF with FDA approval for managing fistulization with Crohn disease (Chang & Hudesman, 2020).

When nonsurgical measures fail to relieve the severe symptoms of IBD, surgery may be necessary. While the use of infliximab therapy and other biologic agents have improved disease control and increased remission periods, 60% to 80% of all patients with IBD still require some type of surgery (Lightner, 2020). The most common indications for surgery are medically intractable disease, poor quality of life, or complications from the disease or its treatment. Recurrence of inflammation and disease after surgery in regional enteritis is inevitable.

A common procedure performed for strictures of the small intestines is laparoscope-guided strictureplasty, in which the blocked or narrowed sections of the intestines are widened, leaving the intestines intact. In some cases, a small bowel resection is performed: diseased segments of the small intestines are resected, and the remaining portions of the intestines are anastomosed. Surgical removal of up to 50% of the small bowel usually can be tolerated. In cases of severe regional enteritis of the colon, a total colectomy and ileostomy may be the procedure of choice.

A newer surgical procedure developed for patients with severe regional enteritis is intestinal transplant. Now this technique is available to children and to young and middle-aged adults who have lost intestinal function from disease. Although this procedure is not a cure, eventually it may provide improvement in quality of life for some patients. The associated technical and immunologic problems remain formidable, and the costs and mortality rates remain high.

Approximately 30% of UC patients require surgery and when a proctocolectomy (surgical removal of the colon and rectum) is performed, this surgery can be considered curative (Cohan et al., 2021). A proctocolectomy with ileostomy (i.e., complete excision of colon, rectum, and anus) is recommended when the rectum is severely diseased. If the rectum can be preserved, the procedure of choice is restorative proctocolectomy with ileal pouch anal anastomosis (IPAA). When the colon is surgically removed, the patient is considered "cured" in that extraintestinal manifestations subside and the disease process is otherwise limited to the colon. Indications for surgery include lack of improvement and continued deterioration, profuse bleeding, perforation, continued stricture formation, and cancer. Surgical excision usually improves quality of life.

ILEOSTOMY

Procedures

An **ileostomy**, the surgical creation of an opening into the ileum or small intestine (usually by means of an ileal stoma on the abdominal wall), is commonly performed after a total colectomy (i.e., excision of the entire colon). It allows for drainage of fecal matter (i.e., effluent) from the ileum to the outside of the body. The drainage is typically loose to semiformed and may occur at frequent intervals.

Another procedure involves the creation of a continent ileal reservoir (i.e., **Kock pouch**) by diverting a portion of the distal ileum to the abdominal wall and creating a stoma (Fig. 23-7). This procedure eliminates the need for an external fecal collection bag. Approximately 30 cm of the distal ileum is reconstructed to form a reservoir with a nipple valve that is created by pulling a portion of the terminal ileal loop back into the ileum. GI effluent can accumulate in the pouch for several hours and then be removed by means of a catheter inserted through the nipple valve. In many patients, a total colectomy also is performed with the Kock pouch. Possible indications for a total colectomy with Kock pouch placement (rather than a restorative proctocolectomy with IPAA) include a badly diseased rectum, lack of rectal sphincter

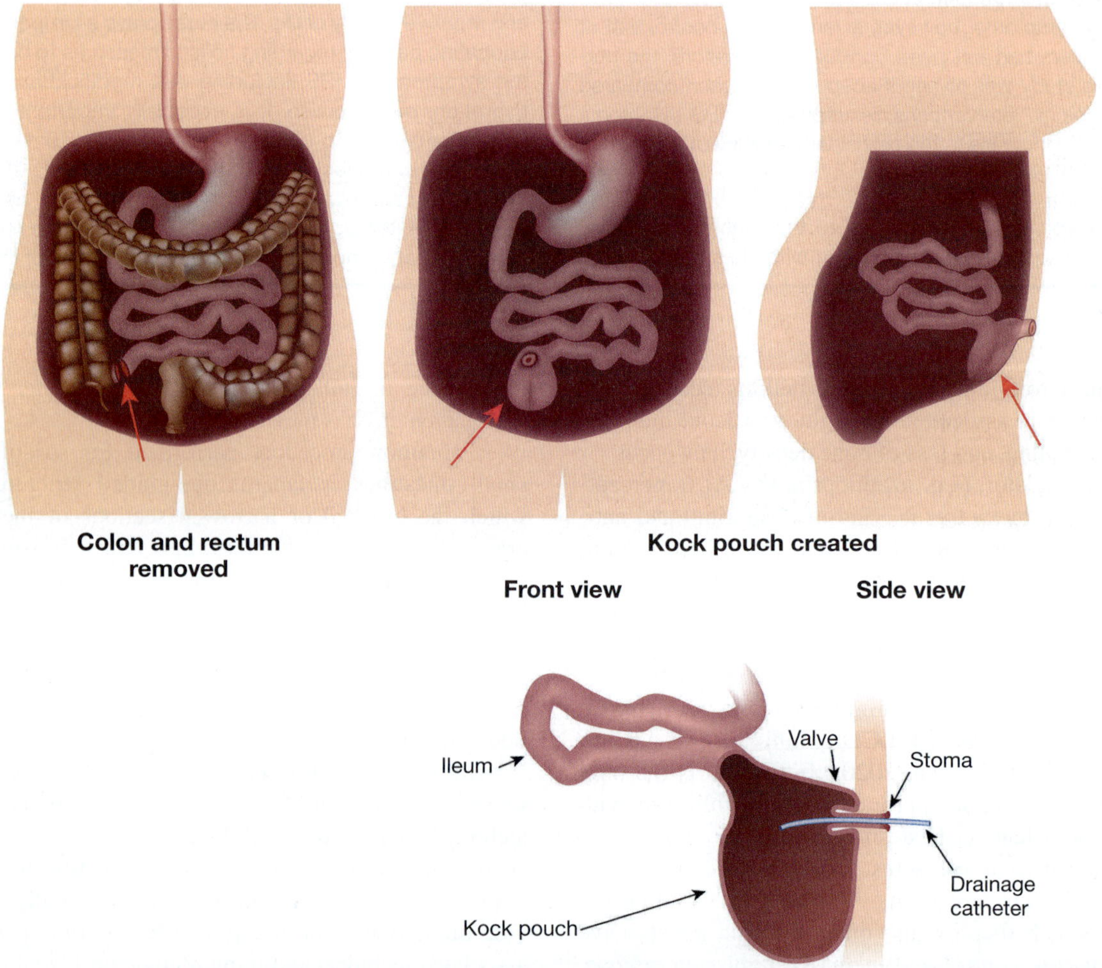

FIGURE 23-7 **Anatomy of a Kock pouch. A Kock pouch is formed by surgically looping part of the distal ileum, stapling the loops together, and opening the inner canals to form a reservoir for the soft, watery stool to be held until catheterized for removal. The nipple valve is formed as shown, by pulling part of the pouch tissue back over the terminal end of the ileum and stapling it closed to reduce the size of the opening and form a canal for the catheter. The length and smaller diameter of the nipple valve prevents waste products from escaping, although some mucus drainage may be expected. (Shutterstock.com ID 147789419 Bottom half of image)**

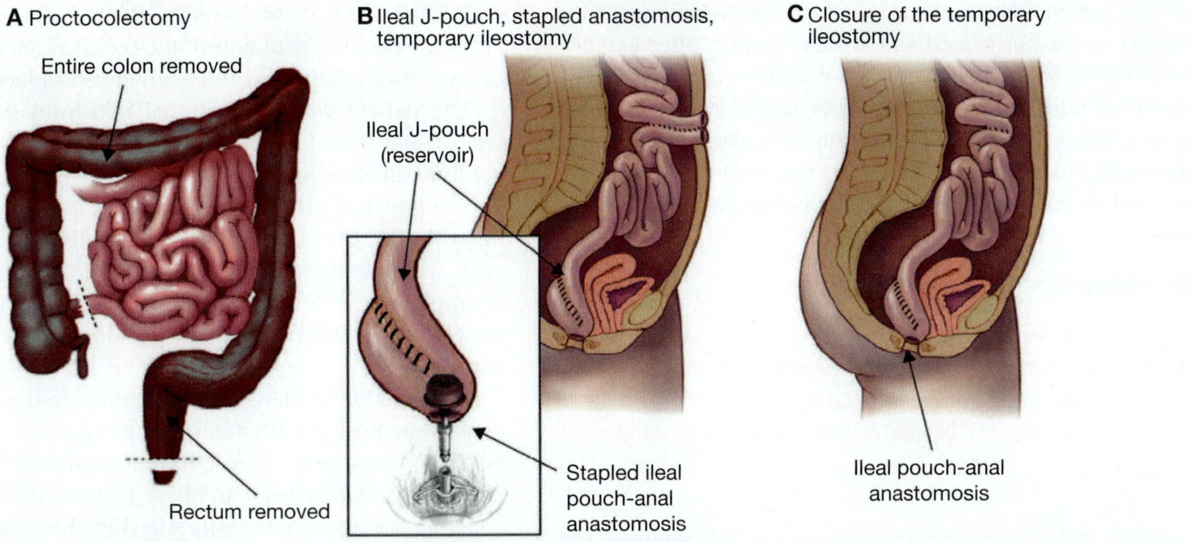

FIGURE 23-8 A. Proctocolectomy. B. Ileal J-pouch, stapled anastomosis, and temporary ileostomy. C. Closure of the temporary ileostomy. The entire surgical procedure is based on four steps: removal of the colon; pelvic dissection and rectum removal sparing the pelvic nerves and the anal sphincter; construction of the ileal pouch, usually with the last 30 to 40 cm of the terminal ileum; and anastomosis of the pouch to the canal anal. (Reprinted with permission from Holzman, R. S., Mancuso, T. J., & Polaner, D. M. [2015]. *A practical approach to pediatric anesthesia* [2nd ed.]. Wolters Kluwer.)

tone, or inability to achieve fecal continence post-IPAA or where IPAA is not a possible option.

There can be many problems associated with Kock pouch's, requiring 30% to 38% of patients to have additional operations to correct these issues (Wu et al., 2020). The major problem with the Kock pouch is malfunction of the nipple valve, with 29.7% of patients experiencing this complication (Wu et al., 2020). The ileocecal nipple valve is used commonly to create a continent, catheterizable channel. However, this nipple valve can slip, leading to bowel obstruction or incontinence (Wu et al., 2020).

A restorative proctocolectomy with IPAA is the surgical procedure of choice in cases in which the rectum can be preserved in that it eliminates the need for a permanent ileostomy. It establishes an ileal reservoir, and anal sphincter control of elimination is retained. The procedure involves connecting a portion of the ileum to the anus (i.e., ileoanal anastomosis) in conjunction with removal of the colon and the rectal mucosa (i.e., total abdominal colectomy and mucosal proctectomy) (Fig. 23-8). A temporary diverting loop ileostomy is constructed at the time of surgery and closed about 3 months later.

With ileoanal anastomosis, the diseased colon and rectum are removed, voluntary defecation is maintained, and anal continence is preserved. The ileal reservoir decreases the number of bowel movements by 50%, from approximately 14 to 20 per day to 7 to 10 per day. Night time elimination is reduced gradually to one bowel movement. Complications of ileoanal anastomosis include irritation of the perianal skin from leakage of fecal contents, stricture formation at the anastomosis site, and small bowel obstruction.

Nursing management of patients with IBD may be medical, surgical, or both. Patients in the community setting or those recently diagnosed may require education about diet and medications as well as referral to support groups. Hospitalized patients with longstanding or severe disease also require careful monitoring, parenteral nutrition, fluid replacement, and possibly emergent surgery. The surgical procedures may involve a fecal diversion with attendant needs for physical care, emotional support, and extensive teaching about management of the ostomy.

Nursing Management for Ileostomy

Some patients with IBD eventually require a permanent fecal diversion with creation of an ileostomy to manage symptoms and to treat or prevent complications. Ileostomy education can be started while the patient is still in the hospital, and with a small amount of planning and care, the patient lives a very normal life. A plan of nursing care for a patient undergoing ostomy surgery is available online at http://thepoint.lww.com/Honan3e.

Providing Preoperative Care

A period of preparation with intensive replacement of fluid, blood, and protein is necessary before surgery is performed. Antibiotics may be prescribed. If the patient has been taking corticosteroids, they will be continued during the surgical phase to prevent steroid-induced adrenal insufficiency. Usually, the patient is provided with frequent, small feedings. All other preoperative measures are similar to those for general abdominal surgery. The abdomen is marked for the proper placement of the stoma by the surgeon or the enterostomal therapist. Care is taken to ensure that the stoma is placed in a convenient location—usually in the right lower quadrant about 2 in below the waist, in an area away from previous scars, bony prominences, skin folds, or fistulas.

The patient must have a thorough understanding of the surgery to be performed and what to expect after surgery. Information about an ileostomy is presented to the patient by means of written materials, models, and discussion. Preoperative teaching includes management of drainage from the stoma, the nature of drainage, and the need for nasogastric intubation, parenteral fluids, and, possibly, perineal packing.

Providing Postoperative Care

Pearls for Practice

A healthy stoma appears pink or red and moist; the nurse alerts the surgeon immediately if the stoma is dusky (dark purple), white, or dark since circulation may be compromised.

General abdominal surgery wound care is required. The nurse observes the stoma for color and size. It should be pink to bright red and shiny. Typically, a temporary plastic bag with an adhesive facing is placed over the ileostomy in the operating room and firmly pressed onto the surrounding skin. The nurse monitors the ileostomy for fecal drainage, which should begin about 72 hours after surgery. The drainage is a continuous liquid from the small intestine because the stoma does not have a controlling sphincter. The contents drain into the plastic bag and thus are kept from coming into contact with the skin. They are collected and measured when the bag becomes full. If a continent ileal reservoir was created, as described for the Kock pouch, continuous drainage is provided by an indwelling reservoir catheter for 2 to 3 weeks after surgery. This allows the suture lines to heal.

As with other patients undergoing abdominal surgery, the nurse encourages those with an ileostomy to engage in early ambulation. It is important to administer prescribed pain medications as required.

Because these patients lose much fluid in the early postoperative period, an accurate record of fluid intake, urinary output, and fecal discharge is necessary to help gauge the fluid needs of the patient. There may be up to 1 L of fluid lost each day, in addition to expected fluid loss through urine, perspiration, respiration, and other sources. With this loss, sodium and potassium are depleted. The nurse monitors laboratory values and administers electrolyte replacements as prescribed. Fluids are administered IV for 4 to 5 days to replace lost fluids.

Nasogastric suction is also a part of immediate postoperative care, with the tube requiring frequent irrigation as prescribed. The purpose of nasogastric suction is to prevent a buildup of gastric contents. After the tube is removed, the nurse offers sips of clear liquids and gradually progresses the diet. It is important to report nausea and abdominal distention immediately because they may indicate intestinal obstruction.

By the end of the first week, rectal packing is removed. Because this procedure may be uncomfortable, the nurse may administer an analgesic an hour before its removal. After the packing is removed, the perineum is irrigated two or three times daily until full healing takes place.

The patient with a traditional ileostomy cannot establish regular bowel habits because the contents of the ileum are fluid and are discharged continuously. The patient must wear a pouch at all times. Stomal size and pouch size vary initially; the stoma should be rechecked 3 weeks after surgery, when the edema has subsided. The final size and type of appliance is selected in 3 months, after the patient's weight has stabilized and the stoma shrinks to a stable shape.

The location and length of the stoma are significant in the management of the ileostomy by the patient. The surgeon positions the stoma as close to the midline as possible and at a location where even an obese patient with a protruding abdomen can care for it easily. Usually, the ileostomy stoma is about 2.5 cm (1 in) long, which makes it convenient for the attachment of an appliance.

Skin excoriation around the stoma can be a persistent problem. Peristomal skin integrity may be compromised by several factors, such as an allergic reaction to the ostomy appliance, skin barrier, or paste; chemical irritation from the effluent; mechanical injury from the removal of the appliance; and infection. If irritation and yeast growth occur, nystatin powder is dusted lightly on the peristomal skin.

Changing an Appliance

A regular schedule for changing the pouch before leakage occurs must be established for those with a traditional ileostomy. The amount of time a person can keep the appliance sealed to the body surface depends on the location of the stoma and on body structure. The usual wearing time is 5 to 7 days. The appliance is emptied every 4 to 6 hours or at the same time the patient empties the bladder. An emptying spout at the bottom of the appliance is closed with a special clip made for this purpose.

Most pouches are disposable and odor-proof. Foods such as spinach and parsley act as deodorizers in the intestinal tract; foods that cause odors include cabbage, onions, and fish. Bismuth subcarbonate tablets, which may be prescribed and taken orally three or four times each day, are effective in reducing odor. Oral diphenoxylate also can be prescribed to diminish intestinal motility, thereby thickening the stool and assisting in odor control.

Changing an ileostomy appliance also allows for examination of the skin around the stoma, and assists in controlling odor if this becomes a problem. The appliance should be changed at any time that the patient complains of burning or itching under the disk or pain in the area of the stoma; routine changes should be performed early in the morning before breakfast or 2 to 4 hours after a meal, when the bowel is least active. See Box 23-2 for guidelines on changing an ostomy appliance.

BOX 23-2

GUIDELINES FOR NURSING CARE

Changing an Ileostomy Appliance

Equipment Needed

- Mild soap
- Clean cloths or towels
- Skin barrier (stoma adhesive, Convatec)
- Cutting guide
- Appliance pouch

Optional Equipment

- Barrier powder
- Antifungal spray or powder
- Barrier washer

Implementation

NURSING ACTION	RATIONALE
1. Promote patient comfort and involvement in the procedure. a. Have the patient assume a relaxed position. b. Provide privacy. c. Explain details of the procedure. d. Expose the ileostomy area; remove the ileostomy belt (if worn).	1. Providing a relaxed atmosphere and adequate explanations help the patient to become an active participant in the procedure.
2. Remove the appliance. a. Have the patient sit on the toilet or on a chair facing the toilet. A patient who prefers to stand should face the toilet. b. The appliance (pouch) can be removed by gently pushing the skin away from the adhesive.	2. These positions facilitate disposal or drainage.
3. Cleanse the skin: a. Wash the skin gently with a soft cloth moistened with tepid water and mild soap; the patient may prefer to bathe before putting on a clean appliance. b. Rinse the soap and dry the skin thoroughly after cleansing.	3. The patient may shower with or without the pouch. a. Micropore or waterproof tape applied to the sides of the faceplate keeps it secure during bathing. b. Moisture or soap residue interferes with appliance adhesion.

Pouching options

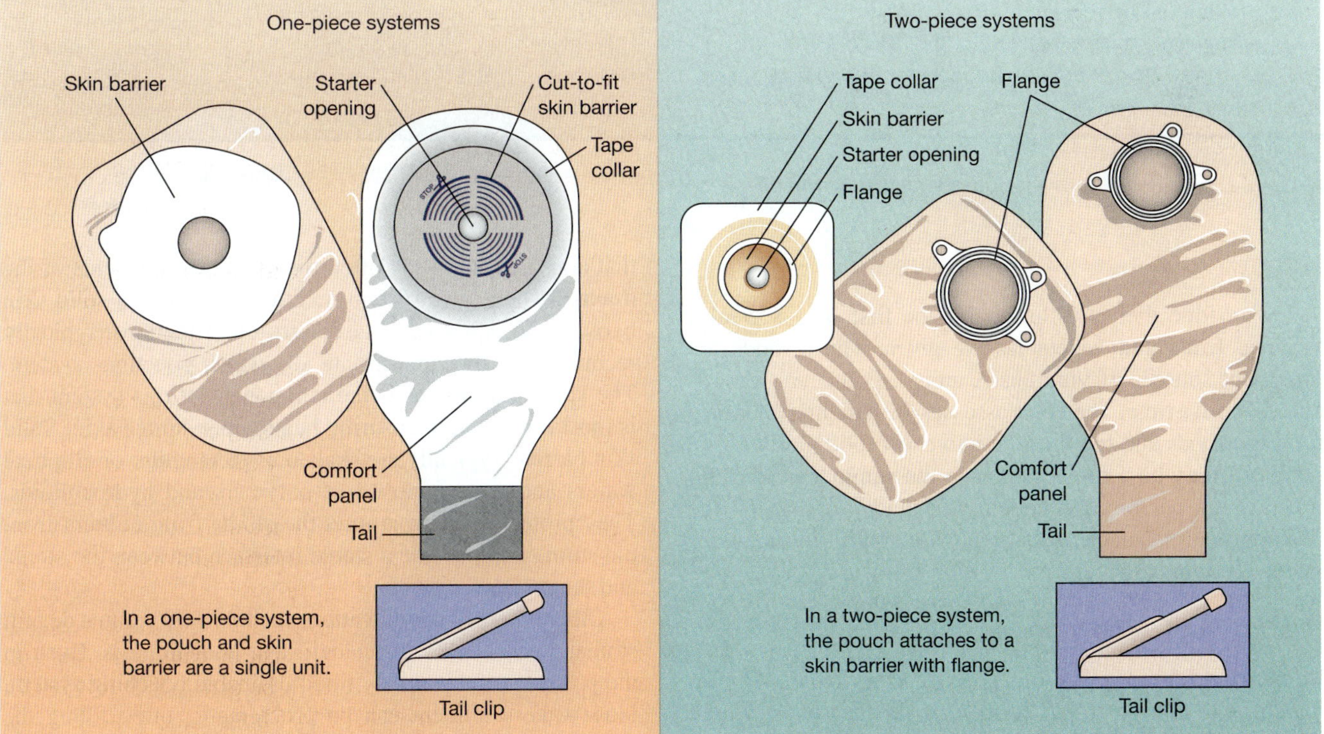

(continued on page 802)

BOX 23-2

GUIDELINES FOR NURSING CARE (*continued*)

Changing an Ileostomy Appliance (*continued*)

NURSING ACTION	RATIONALE
4. Apply appliance: When there is *no* skin irritation: a. An appropriate skin barrier is applied to the peristomal skin before the appliance is applied. b. Remove cover from adherent surface of disk of disposable plastic appliance and apply directly to the skin. c. Press firmly in place for 30 seconds to ensure adherence. When there is skin irritation: a. Cleanse the skin thoroughly but gently; pat dry. Apply barrier powder. b. If more irritation developed, apply Kenalog spray; blot excess moisture with a cotton pledget, and dust lightly with nystatin (Mycostatin) powder. OR Place the sizing guide directly on the skin around the stoma, leaving as little skin as possible around the stoma uncovered. Then, using the guide, cut the appropriate hole in the disk. At times, the stoma site is irregular; if this is the case, the hole should be cut approximating the stoma site as closely as possible. Apply as an alternative a wafer or barrier (Stomahesive, ConvaTec), which is commercially available. The stomal opening should be the same size as the stoma; use a cutting guide (supplied with appliance as indicated). The wafer is applied directly to the skin. Barrier powder can be used to dry irritated skin before barrier application. a. Another alternative is to apply a special barrier washer (e.g., Eakin's Seal). The special barrier adheres well to irritated skin. b. Then the pouch is applied to the treated skin.	4. Many appliances have a built-in skin barrier. The skin should be dried thoroughly before applying the appliance. a. Cleansing removes debris and protects irritated skin under the wafer. b. The corticosteroid preparation (Kenalog) helps decrease inflammation. The antifungal agent (nystatin) treats those types of infections that are common around stomas. A prescription is required for either medication. A skin barrier is a substance that facilitates healing of excoriated skin. It adheres well even to moist, irritated skin. c. A special barrier protects skin from effluent, promotes healing, and helps with adherence. d. This allows skin to heal while the appliance is in place.
5. Check the pouch bottom for closure; use clamp, Velcro closure, or clip provided.	5. Proper closure controls leakage.

Managing Dietary and Fluid Needs

A low-residue diet is followed for the first 6 to 8 weeks. Strained fruits and vegetables are given. These foods are important sources of vitamins A and C. Foods are reintroduced one at a time. The nurse assesses the patient's tolerance for these foods and reminds them to chew food thoroughly.

Fluids may be a problem during the summer when fluid lost through perspiration adds to the fluid loss through the ileostomy. Fluids such as Gatorade are helpful in maintaining electrolyte balance.

Preventing Complications

Monitoring for complications is an ongoing activity for the patient with an ileostomy. Peristomal skin irritation, which results from leakage of effluent, is the most common complication of an ileostomy. A drainable pouching system that does not fit well is often the cause. Components of the drainable pouching system include the pouch, a solid skin barrier, and adhesive. The enterostomal therapist typically recommends the appropriate drainable pouching system. The solid skin barrier is the component of this system that is most important in ensuring healthy peristomal skin. Solid skin barriers typically are shaped as rectangular or elliptical wafers and are composed of polymers and hydrocolloids. They protect the skin around the stoma from effluent from the stoma and provide a stable interface between the stoma and the pouch.

Other common complications include fluid volume deficit, stomal stenosis, urinary calculi, and cholelithiasis. Even in the presence of a properly fitted drainable pouching system, loose watery effluent can be problematic, often filling the pouch (every hour or sooner), which can quickly lead to dehydration and electrolyte losses. Supplemental water, sodium, and potassium are administered to prevent hypovolemia and hypokalemia. Antidiarrheal agents or bile salt sequestrants may be administered to decrease the watery effluent.

Stenosis is caused by circular scar tissue that forms at the stoma site. The scar tissue must be released surgically. Urinary calculi may occur in patients with ileostomies and are attributed, at least partly, to dehydration from decreased fluid intake. Intense lower abdominal pain that radiates to the legs, hematuria, and signs of dehydration indicate that the urine should be strained. Fluid intake is encouraged. Sometimes, small stones are passed during urination; otherwise, treatment is necessary to crush or remove the calculi (see Chapter 27).

Cholelithiasis (i.e., gallstones) occurs more commonly in patients with an ileostomy than in the general population because of changes in the absorption of bile acids that occur postoperatively. Spasm of the gallbladder causes severe upper right abdominal pain that can radiate to the back and right shoulder (see Chapter 24).

MASSES IN THE COLON AND RECTUM

A *polyp* is a mass of tissue that protrudes into the lumen of the bowel. Polyps can occur anywhere in the intestinal tract and rectum. They can be classified as neoplastic (i.e., adenomas and carcinomas) or nonneoplastic (i.e., mucosal and hyperplastic).

NONNEOPLASTIC POLYPS

Although most polyps do not develop into invasive neoplasms, they must be identified and followed closely.

Risk Factors

Nonneoplastic polyps, which are benign epithelial growths, are common in the Western world. They occur more commonly in the large intestine than in the small intestine. Adenomatous (benign) polyps are more common in males. The proportion of these polyps arising in the proximal part of the colon increases with age (after 50 years of age). Prevalence rates vary from 25% to 60%, depending on age. Nonneoplastic polyps occur in 80% of the population, and their frequency increases with age.

Clinical Manifestations and Assessment

Clinical manifestations depend on the size of the polyp and the amount of pressure it exerts on intestinal tissue. The most common symptom is rectal bleeding. Lower abdominal pain also may occur. If the polyp is large enough, symptoms of obstruction occur. The diagnosis is based on history and digital rectal examination, barium enema studies, sigmoidoscopy, or colonoscopy.

Medical and Nursing Management

After a polyp is identified, it should be removed. There are several methods: colonoscopy with the use of special equipment (i.e., biopsy forceps and snares), laparoscopy, or colonoscopic excision with laparoscopic visualization. The latter technique enables immediate detection of potential problems and allows laparoscopic resection and repair of the major complications of perforation and bleeding that may occur with polypectomy. Microscopic examination of the polyp then identifies the type of polyp and indicates what further surgery is required, if any.

COLORECTAL CANCER

Tumors of the colon and rectum are relatively common; the colorectal area (the colon and rectum combined) is now the third most common cause of cancer deaths in both males and females, and when both males and females are combined, colorectal cancer represents the second cause of cancer deaths in the United States (Siegel et al., 2020). Colorectal cancer is the second most common cause of cancer death among males who are 40 to 79 years of age (Siegel et al., 2020). In 2021, approximately 150,000 people have been diagnosed with colorectal cancer, with less than a third of these cases resulting in death (ACS, 2021). Over the last few years, there have been a decrease in the number of older people receiving colorectal cancer diagnoses but an increase in younger people. Overall, the number of people dying from colorectal cancer has decreased over the last two decades, largely due to increased screenings and a decrease in risk factors (Siegel et al., 2020).

Early diagnosis and prompt treatment could save almost three of every four people. If the disease is detected and treated at an early stage, the 5-year survival rate is 91%; however, in the more distal stages of disease, the 5-year survival rate is only approximately 14% (ACS, 2021). Most people are asymptomatic for long periods and seek health care only when they notice a change in bowel habits or rectal bleeding. Prevention and early screening are the keys to detection and reduction of mortality rates.

Pathophysiology

Cancer of the colon and rectum is predominantly adenocarcinoma (i.e., arising from the epithelial lining of the intestine) (ACS, 2020). It may start as a benign polyp but may become malignant, invade and destroy normal tissues, and extend into surrounding structures. Cancer cells may migrate away from the primary tumor and spread to other parts of the body (most often to the liver).

Risk Factors

Colorectal cancer is a disease of Western cultures. The incidence increases with age (the incidence is highest in people over 85 years of age) and is higher in people with a family history of colon cancer and those with IBD or polyps. In males, only the incidence of prostate cancer and lung cancer exceeds that of colorectal cancer. In females, only the incidence of breast and lung cancer exceeds that of colorectal cancer.

Colon cancer in older adults has been closely associated with dietary carcinogens. Diets high in fiber, fresh fruits and vegetables, calcium, vitamin D, and magnesium have been shown to reduce the risk of colorectal cancer (Song et al., 2020). Excess dietary fat, high alcohol consumption, lack of physical activity, and smoking all increase the incidence of colorectal tumors (Siegel et al., 2020).

Clinical Manifestations and Assessment

Symptoms are often insidious. Patients with colorectal cancer usually report fatigue, which is caused primarily by iron-deficiency anemia. In early stages, minor changes in bowel patterns and occasional bleeding may occur. The later symptoms reported most commonly by older individuals are abdominal pain, obstruction, tenesmus, and rectal bleeding.

The symptoms are generally determined by the location of the cancer, the stage of the disease, and the function of the intestinal segment in which it is located. The most common presenting symptom is a change in bowel habits. The passage of blood in the stools is the second most common symptom. Symptoms also may include unexplained anemia, anorexia, weight loss, and fatigue.

The symptoms most commonly associated with right-sided lesions are dull abdominal pain and melena (black, tarry stools). The symptoms most commonly associated with left-sided lesions are those associated with obstruction (abdominal pain and cramping, narrowing stools, constipation, distention), as well as bright red blood in the stool. Symptoms associated with rectal lesions are tenesmus (ineffective, painful straining at stool), rectal pain, the feeling of incomplete evacuation after a bowel movement, alternating constipation and diarrhea, and bloody stool.

Along with an abdominal and rectal examination, the most important diagnostic procedures for cancer of the colon are fecal occult blood testing, barium enema, proctosigmoidoscopy, and colonoscopy (see Chapter 20). The majority of colorectal cancer cases can be identified by colonoscopy with biopsy or cytology smears.

Carcinoembryonic antigen (CEA) studies also may be performed. Although CEA may not be a highly reliable indicator in diagnosing colon cancer because not all lesions secrete CEA, studies show that CEA levels are reliable prognostic predictors. With complete excision of the tumor, the elevated levels of CEA should return to normal within 48 hours. Elevations of CEA at a later date suggest recurrence.

Medical and Nursing Management

The patient with symptoms of intestinal obstruction is treated with IV fluids and nasogastric suction. If there has been significant bleeding, blood component therapy may be required.

Treatment for colorectal cancer depends on the stage of the disease and consists of surgery to remove the tumor, supportive therapy, and adjuvant therapy. Patients who receive some form of adjuvant therapy, which may include chemotherapy, radiation therapy, immunotherapy, or multimodality therapy, typically demonstrate delays in tumor recurrence and increases in survival time.

Radiation therapy is used before, during, and after surgery to shrink the tumor, to achieve better results from surgery, and to reduce the risk of recurrence. For inoperative or unresectable tumors, radiation is used to provide significant relief from symptoms. Intracavitary and implantable devices are used to deliver radiation to the site. The response to adjuvant therapy varies.

Surgery is the primary treatment for most colon and rectal cancers. It may be curative or palliative. Advances in surgical techniques can enable the patient with cancer to have sphincter-saving devices that restore continuity of the GI tract. The type of surgery recommended depends on the location and size of the tumor. Cancers limited to one site can be removed through the colonoscope. Laparoscopic colotomy with polypectomy minimizes the extent of surgery needed in some cases. A laparoscope is used as a guide in making an incision into the colon; then the tumor mass is excised. Use of the neodymium/yttrium-aluminum-garnet (Nd:YAG) laser has proved effective with some lesions as well.

Surgical procedures include the following:

- Segmental resection with anastomosis (i.e., removal of the tumor and portions of the bowel on either side of the growth, as well as the blood vessels and lymphatic nodes) (Fig. 23-9)
- Abdominoperineal resection with permanent sigmoid colostomy (i.e., removal of the tumor and a portion of the sigmoid and all of the rectum and anal sphincter) (Fig. 23-10)
- Temporary colostomy followed by segmental resection and anastomosis and subsequent reanastomosis of the colostomy, allowing initial bowel decompression and bowel preparation before resection
- Permanent colostomy or ileostomy for palliation of unresectable obstructing lesions
- Construction of a coloanal reservoir called a *colonic J pouch*, which is performed in two steps. A temporary loop ileostomy is constructed to divert intestinal flow, and the newly constructed J pouch (made from 6 to 10 cm of colon) is reattached to the anal stump. About 3 months after the initial stage, the ileostomy is reversed and intestinal continuity is restored. The anal sphincter and, therefore, continence are preserved

A colostomy is the surgical creation of an opening (i.e., stoma) into the colon. It can be created as a temporary or permanent fecal diversion. It allows the drainage or evacuation of colon contents to the outside of the body. The

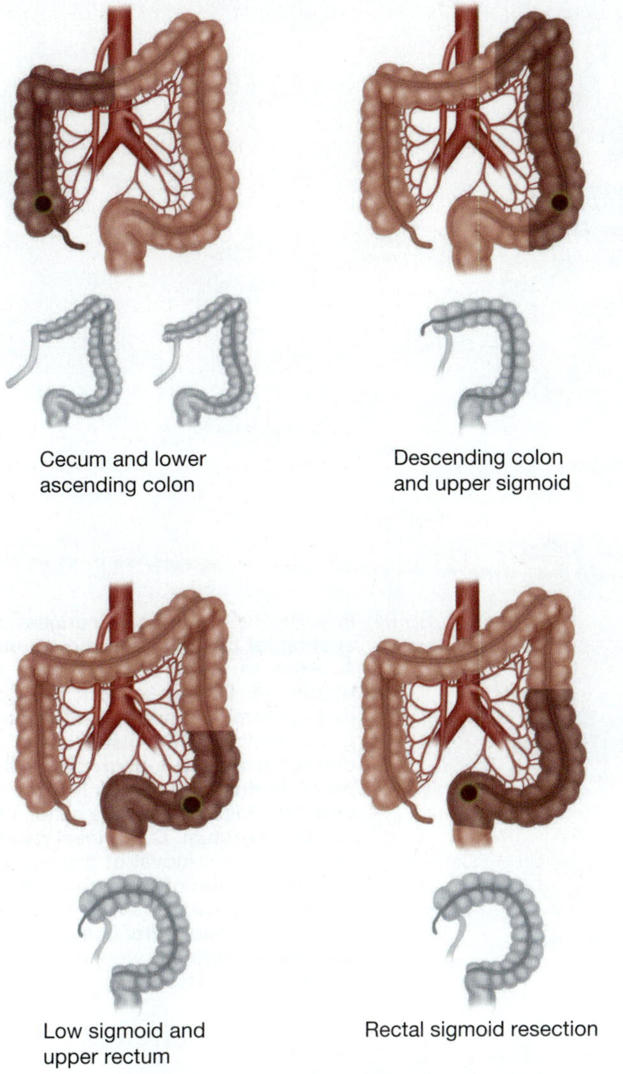

FIGURE 23-9 Examples of areas where cancer can occur, the area that is removed, and how the anastomosis is performed (*small diagrams*).

consistency of the drainage is related to the placement of the colostomy, which is dictated by the location of the tumor and the extent of invasion into surrounding tissues (Fig. 23-11). With improved surgical techniques, colostomies are performed in less than one third of patients with colorectal cancer.

Complications

Tumor growth may cause partial or complete bowel obstruction. Extension of the tumor and ulceration into the surrounding blood vessels result in hemorrhage. Perforation, abscess formation, peritonitis, sepsis, and shock may occur.

Older individuals are at increased risk of complications after surgery and may have difficulty managing colostomy care. Some older patients may have decreased vision, impaired hearing, and difficulty with fine motor coordination. It may be helpful for patients to handle ostomy equipment and simulate cleaning the peristomal skin and irrigating the stoma before surgery. Skin care is a major concern in older patients with a colostomy because of the skin changes that occur with aging—the epithelial and subcutaneous fatty layers become thin, and the skin is irritated easily. To prevent skin breakdown, special attention is paid to skin cleansing and the proper fit of an appliance. Arteriosclerosis causes decreased blood flow to the wound and stoma site. As a result, transport of nutrients is delayed, and healing time may be prolonged. Some patients have delayed elimination after irrigation because of decreased peristalsis and mucus production. Most patients require 6 months before they feel comfortable with their ostomy care.

INTESTINAL OBSTRUCTION

Intestinal obstruction exists when blockage prevents the normal flow of intestinal contents through the intestinal tract. In mechanical obstruction, intraluminal or mural obstructions secondary to pressure on the intestinal wall occur. Examples are intussusception (telescoping of a portion of the intestine within another immediately adjacent portion of intestine), polypoid tumors and neoplasms, stenosis, strictures, adhesions, hernias, and abscesses. Figure 23-12 depicts additional causes of obstruction. In functional obstruction, intestinal musculature cannot propel the contents along the bowel thereby causing a blockage within the intestine. Examples are amyloidosis, muscular dystrophy, endocrine disorders such as diabetes mellitus, or neurologic disorders, such as Parkinson disease. The blockage also can be temporary and the result of the manipulation of the bowel during surgery.

Pearls for Practice

In explaining to patients what adhesions are, the nurse understands that they are bands of scar tissues that develop after previous surgery, radiation, trauma, or infection. The adhesions develop most frequently from previous abdominal surgery (75%) and have the potential to trap the bowel within these bands causing a bowel obstruction.

The obstruction can be partial or complete. Its severity depends on the region of bowel affected, the degree to which the lumen is occluded, and especially the degree to which the vascular supply to the bowel wall is disturbed.

Most bowel obstructions occur in the small intestine. Adhesions are the most common cause of small bowel obstruction, followed by hernias and neoplasms. Other causes include intussusception, **volvulus** (i.e., twisting of the bowel), and paralytic ileus. Most obstructions in the large bowel occur in the sigmoid colon. The most common causes are carcinoma, diverticulitis, inflammatory bowel

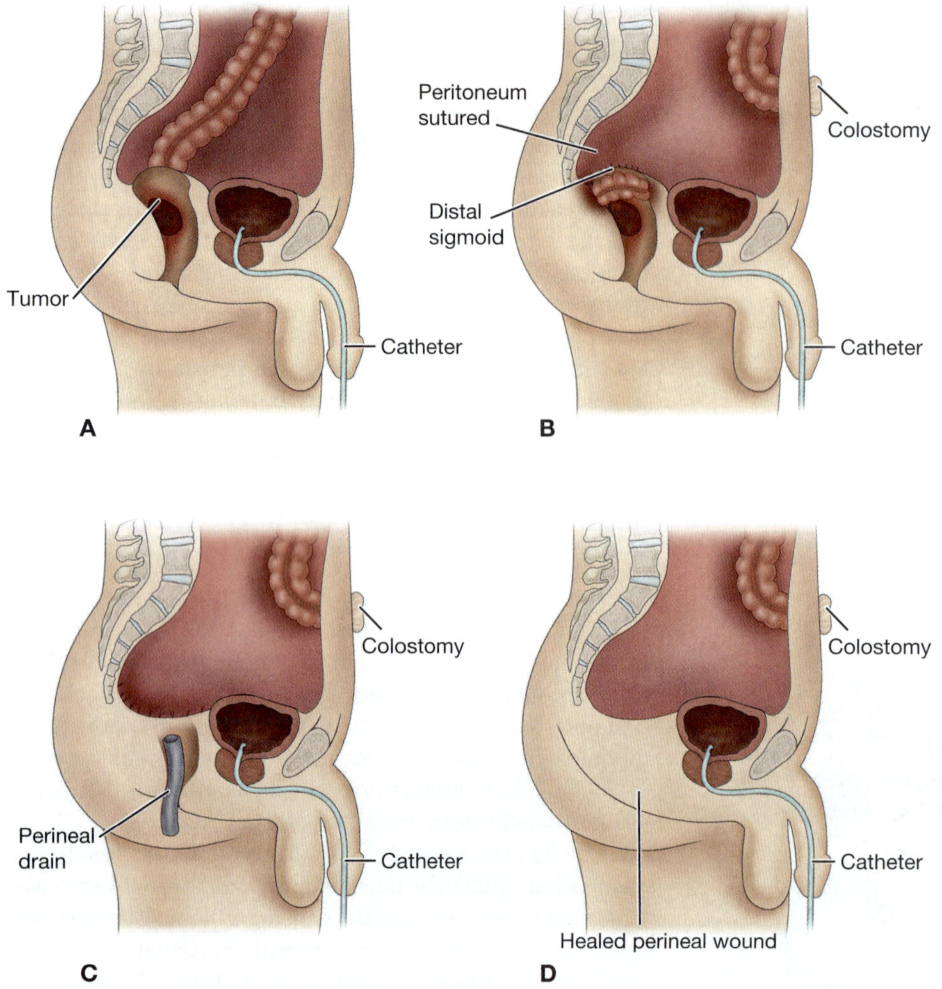

FIGURE 23-10 **Abdominoperineal resection for carcinoma of the rectum. A. Prior to surgery. Note tumor in rectum. B. During surgery, the sigmoid is removed and the colostomy is established. The distal bowel is dissected free to a point below the pelvic peritoneum, which is sutured over the closed end of the distal sigmoid and rectum. C. Perineal resection includes removal of the rectum and free portion of the sigmoid from below. A perineal drain is inserted. D. The final result after healing. Note the healed perineal wound and the permanent colostomy.**

disorders, and benign tumors. Table 23-6 and Figure 23-12 list mechanical causes of obstruction and describe how they occur.

Pearls for Practice

The nurse recognizes that patients with chronically elevated blood sugars (>200 mg/dL) with diabetes (types 1 and 2) are at risk for gastroparesis, which delays gastric emptying and intestinal motility. It is understood that gastric emptying requires the complex coordination of the enteric (intestine) and autonomic nervous systems, smooth muscle cells of the GI tract, and the stomach's specialized pacemaker cells (Aswath et al., 2021). The purported cause is neuropathy affecting the control of gastric and/or intestinal motor function and sensory innervation, along with the use of incretin-based medications which slow stomach emptying. Symptoms include nausea, postprandial fullness, abdominal pain, vomiting of undigested food, reflux. Recommendations may include smaller, more frequent meals, minimizing carbonated beverages, reducing fats, and fiber content (Aswath et al., 2021).

SMALL BOWEL OBSTRUCTION

Pathophysiology

Intestinal contents, fluid, and gas accumulate above the intestinal obstruction. The abdominal distention and retention of fluid reduce the absorption of fluids and stimulate more gastric secretion. Increases in intestinal lumen pressure cause occlusion of capillary blood flow and compromise of venous return and arterial flow. This causes edema, congestion, necrosis, and eventual rupture or perforation of the intestinal wall, with resultant peritonitis.

Reflux vomiting may be caused by abdominal distention. Vomiting results in loss of hydrochloric acid (HCl) and potassium from the stomach, leading to reduction of chlorides and potassium in the blood and to metabolic alkalosis. Dehydration develops from loss of water and sodium. With acute fluid losses, hypovolemic shock may occur.

Clinical Manifestations and Assessment

The initial symptom is usually crampy pain that is wavelike and colicky. The patient may pass blood and mucus but no fecal matter and no flatus. Vomiting occurs. If the obstruction

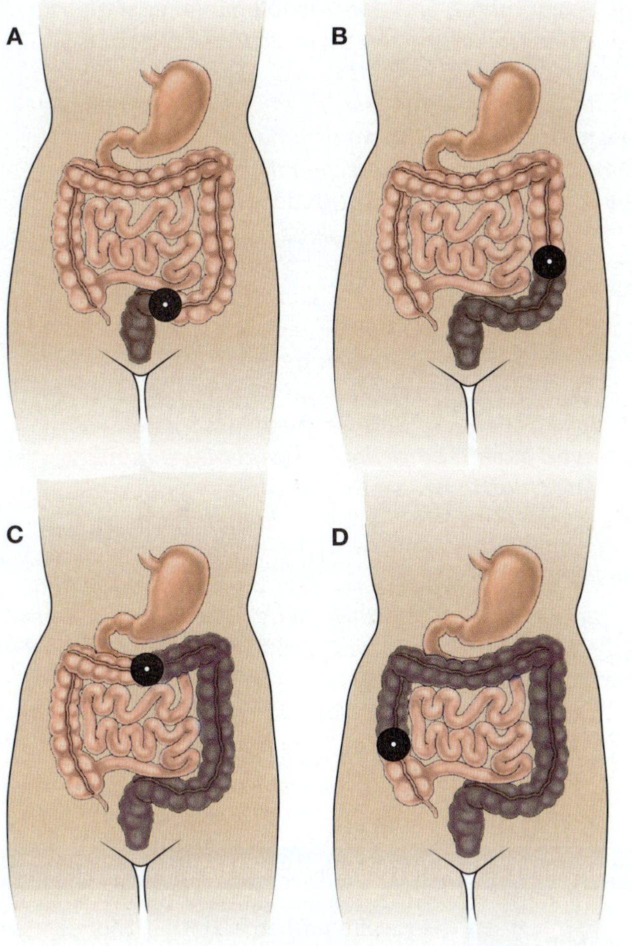

FIGURE 23-11 **Placement of permanent colostomies. The nature of the discharge varies with the site. Shaded areas show sections of bowel removed. With a sigmoid colostomy (A), the feces are solid. With a descending colostomy (B), the feces are semiformed. With a transverse colostomy (C), the feces are unformed. With an ascending colostomy (D), the feces are fluid.**

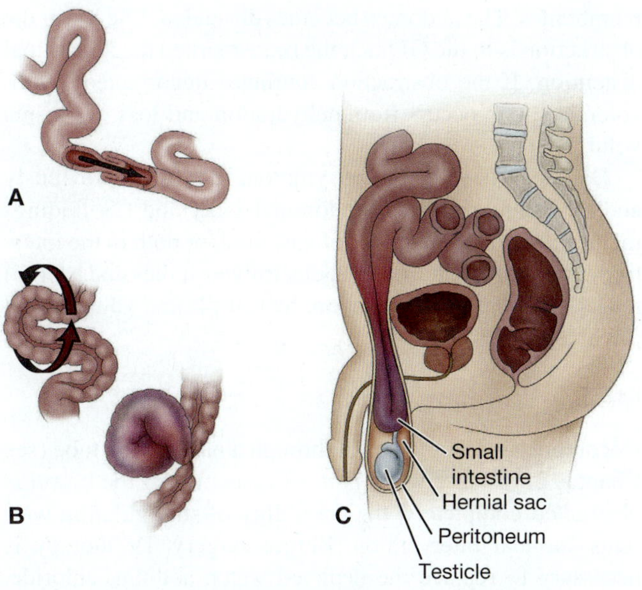

FIGURE 23-12 **Three causes of intestinal obstruction. A. Intussusception invagination or shortening of the colon caused by the movement of one segment of bowel into another. B. Volvulus of the sigmoid colon; the twist is counterclockwise in most cases. Note the edematous bowel. C. Hernia (inguinal). The sac of the hernia is a continuation of the peritoneum of the abdomen. The hernial contents are intestine, omentum, or other abdominal contents that pass through the hernial opening into the hernial sac.**

is complete, the peristaltic waves initially become extremely vigorous and eventually assume a reverse direction, with the intestinal contents propelled toward the mouth instead of toward the rectum. If the obstruction is in the ileum, fecal vomiting takes place. First, the patient vomits the stomach contents, then the bile-stained contents of the duodenum and the jejunum, and finally, with each paroxysm of pain, the darker, fecal-like contents of the ileum. The signs of dehydration become evident: intense thirst, drowsiness, generalized malaise, aching, and a parched tongue and mucous

TABLE 23-6 Mechanical Causes of Intestinal Obstruction

Cause	Course of Events	Result
Adhesions	Loops of intestine become adherent to areas that heal slowly or scar after abdominal surgery.	After surgery, adhesions produce a kinking of an intestinal loop.
Intussusception	One part of the intestine slips into another part located below it (like a telescope shortening).	The intestinal lumen becomes narrowed.
Volvulus	Bowel twists and turns on itself.	Intestinal lumen becomes obstructed. Gas and fluid accumulate in the trapped bowel.
Hernia	Protrusion of intestine through a weakened area in the abdominal muscle or wall.	Intestinal flow may be obstructed completely. Blood flow to the area may be obstructed as well.
Tumor	A tumor that exists within the wall of the intestine extends into the intestinal lumen, or a tumor outside the intestine causes pressure on the wall of the intestine.	Intestinal lumen becomes partially obstructed; if the tumor is not removed, complete obstruction results.

membranes. The abdomen becomes distended. The lower the obstruction is in the GI tract, the more marked the abdominal distention. If the obstruction continues uncorrected, hypovolemic shock occurs from dehydration and loss of plasma volume.

Diagnosis is based on the symptoms described previously and on imaging studies. Abdominal x-ray and CT findings include abnormal quantities of gas, fluid, or both in the intestines. Laboratory studies (i.e., electrolyte studies and a CBC) reveal a picture of dehydration, loss of plasma volume, and possible infection.

Medical and Nursing Management

Decompression of the bowel through a nasogastric tube (see Chapter 21) is successful in most cases. When the bowel is obstructed completely, the possibility of strangulation warrants surgical intervention. Before surgery, IV therapy is necessary to replace the depleted water, sodium, chloride, and potassium.

The surgical treatment of intestinal obstruction depends largely on the cause of the obstruction. In the most common causes of obstruction, such as hernia and adhesions, the surgical procedure involves repairing the hernia or dividing the adhesion to which the intestine is attached. In some instances, the portion of affected bowel may be removed and an anastomosis performed. The complexity of the surgical procedure for intestinal obstruction depends on the duration of the obstruction and the condition of the intestine.

Nursing management of the nonsurgical patient with a small bowel obstruction includes maintaining the function of the nasogastric tube, assessing and measuring the nasogastric output, assessing for fluid and electrolyte imbalance, monitoring nutritional status, and assessing improvement (e.g., return of normal bowel sounds, decreased abdominal distention, subjective improvement in abdominal pain and tenderness, passage of flatus or stool). The nurse reports discrepancies in intake and output, worsening of pain or abdominal distention, and increased nasogastric output. If the patient's condition does not improve, the nurse prepares them for surgery. The exact nature of the surgery depends on the cause of the obstruction. Nursing care of the patient after surgical repair of a small bowel obstruction is similar to that for other abdominal surgeries (see Chapter 22).

Pearls for Practice

The nurse recognizes postoperative ileus, which is slow or absent GI motility, is a common complication of surgical procedures. It is a type of paralytic ileus. Symptoms include hypoactive or absence of bowel sounds, an intolerance of oral intake, nausea, vomiting, abdominal distention, increased abdominal tympany on percussion, and absence of flatus. In general, the etiology is clustered into three categories: neurogenic (e.g., anesthetic medications), inflammatory (e.g., bowel manipulation during surgery), and pharmacologic (e.g., analgesic medications). Although there is debate about the timing of normal resumption of GI function, colonic motility (which is the last to return), is generally restored within 72 hours (Buchanan & Tuma, 2021). Thus, the nurse is concerned if symptoms persist past this window. Data suggest the incidence of prolonged postoperative ileus (>72 hours) after colorectal surgery is between 5% and 30% (Buchanan & Tuma, 2021). Current treatment includes resting the bowel, reduction of oral diet and possibly insertion of a nasogastric tube (NG tube). The nurse assesses opiate administration since it is dose dependent and has been associated with delayed gastric emptying, slowed bowel motility, and decreased peristalsis. The use of nonopiate analgesia is considered. An additional nursing action includes encouraging ambulation very early in the postoperative period for both prevention and treatment of postoperative ileus (Buchanan & Tuma, 2021). There is some evidence that chewing gum acts as a gastric stimulator, encouraging the return of peristalsis and bowel function and prevention of prolonged postoperative ileus however research is ongoing (Devolder, 2019).

Unfolding Patient Stories: S.C. • Part 2

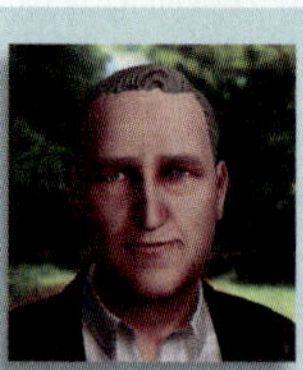

Recall from Chapter 6 S.C., who arrived in the emergency department with severe abdominal pain, is diagnosed with a small bowel obstruction. The patient is NPO and has a nasogastric (NG) tube placed to low intermittent suction. Describe the steps of a focused GI assessment performed by the nurse. How would the nurse explain the rationale for an NG tube and NPO status? What are specific assessments and nursing care responsibilities for an NG tube?

Care for S.C. and other patients in a realistic virtual environment: ***vSim** for Nursing* (thepoint.lww.com/vSimMedicalSurgical). Practice documenting these patients' care in DocuCare (thepoint.lww.com/DocuCareEHR).

LARGE BOWEL OBSTRUCTION

Pathophysiology

As in small bowel obstruction, large bowel obstruction results in an accumulation of intestinal contents, fluid, and gas proximal to the obstruction. Obstruction in the large bowel can lead to severe distention and perforation unless some gas and fluid can flow back through the ileal valve. Large bowel obstruction, even if complete, may be without catastrophic issue if the blood supply to the colon is not disturbed. However, if the blood supply is cut off, intestinal strangulation and necrosis (i.e., tissue death) occur; this condition is life threatening. In the large intestine, dehydration occurs more slowly than in the small intestine because the colon can absorb its fluid contents and can distend to a size considerably beyond its normal full capacity.

Adenocarcinoid tumors account for the majority of large bowel obstructions. Most tumors occur beyond the splenic flexure, making them accessible with a flexible sigmoidoscope, which is able to view the sigmoid and most of the descending colon.

Clinical Manifestations and Assessment

Large bowel obstruction differs clinically from small bowel obstruction in that the symptoms develop and progress relatively slowly. In patients with obstruction in the sigmoid colon or the rectum, constipation may be the only symptom for months. The shape of the stool is altered as it passes the obstruction that is gradually increasing in size. Blood in the stool may result in iron-deficiency anemia. The patient may experience weakness, weight loss, and anorexia. Eventually, the abdomen becomes markedly distended, loops of large bowel become visibly outlined through the abdominal wall, and the patient has crampy lower abdominal pain. Finally, fecal vomiting develops. Symptoms of shock may occur.

Diagnosis is based on symptoms and on imaging studies. Abdominal x-ray and abdominal CT or MRI findings reveal a distended colon and pinpoint the site of the obstruction. Barium studies are contraindicated because of risk of perforation.

Medical and Nursing Management

Restoration of intravascular volume, correction of electrolyte abnormalities, and nasogastric aspiration and decompression are instituted immediately. A colonoscopy may be performed to untwist and decompress the bowel. A cecostomy, in which a surgical opening is made into the cecum, may be performed in patients who are poor surgical risks and urgently need relief from the obstruction. The procedure provides an outlet for releasing gas and a small amount of drainage. A rectal tube may be used to decompress an area that is lower in the bowel. However, the usual treatment is surgical resection to remove the obstructing lesion. A temporary or permanent colostomy may be necessary. An ileoanal anastomosis may be performed if it is necessary to remove the entire large bowel.

The nurse's role is to monitor the patient for symptoms that indicate that the intestinal obstruction is worsening and to provide emotional support and comfort. The nurse administers IV fluids and electrolytes as prescribed. If the patient's condition does not respond to nonsurgical treatment, the nurse prepares the patient for surgery. This preparation includes preoperative teaching as the patient's condition indicates. After surgery, general abdominal wound care and routine postoperative nursing care are provided.

DISEASES OF THE ANORECTUM

Diseases of the anorectum include anal fistulas and fissures, hemorrhoids, sexually transmitted anorectal diseases, and pilonidal cysts. Nursing management of these conditions is discussed in Box 23-3.

ANAL FISTULA

An anal fistula is a tiny, tubular, fibrous tract that extends into the anal canal from an opening located beside the anus (Fig. 23-13A). Fistulas usually result from an infection. They also may develop from trauma, fissures, or regional enteritis. Pus or stool may leak constantly from the cutaneous opening. Other symptoms may be the passage of flatus or feces from the vagina or bladder, depending on the fistula tract. Untreated fistulas may cause systemic infection with related symptoms.

Treatment will depend on the etiology of the fistula. Surgery is recommended because few fistulas heal spontaneously, however new novel therapies are currently under investigation. Commonly, a fistulectomy (i.e., excision of the fistulous tract) is the recommended "gold standard" surgical procedure (Jimenez & Mandava, 2021). The lower bowel is evacuated thoroughly with several prescribed enemas. The fistula is dissected out or laid open by an incision from its rectal opening to its outlet. The wound is packed with gauze and the nurse provides patient and family education regarding dressing changes.

ANAL FISSURE

An anal fissure is a longitudinal tear or ulceration in the lining of the anal canal (see Fig. 23-13B). Fissures generally are caused by the trauma of passing a large, firm stool or from persistent tightening of the anal canal because of stress and anxiety (leading to constipation). Other causes include childbirth, trauma, and overuse of laxatives.

Extremely painful defecation, burning, and bleeding characterize fissures. Bright red blood may be seen on the toilet tissue after a bowel movement.

Most fissures heal if treated by conservative measures, which include dietary modification with addition of fiber supplements, stool softeners and bulk agents, an increase in water intake, sitz baths, and emollient suppositories. A suppository combining an anesthetic with a corticosteroid helps relieve the discomfort. Anal dilation under anesthesia may be required.

If fissures do not respond to conservative treatment, surgery is indicated. Most surgeons consider the procedure of choice to be the lateral internal sphincterotomy with excision of the fissure.

BOX 23-3

Nursing Management of Anorectal Disorders

Relieving Constipation

The nurse encourages intake of at least 2 L of water daily to provide adequate hydration; in addition, the nurse recommends high-fiber foods to promote bulk in the stool and to make it easier to pass fecal matter through the rectum. In patients with pre-existing cardiopulmonary or kidney disease, consultation with the patient's provider regarding fluid intake should occur. Bulk laxatives such as psyllium and stool softeners (e.g., docusate) are administered as prescribed. The patient is advised to set aside a time for bowel movements and to heed the urge to defecate as promptly as possible. It may be helpful to have the patient perform relaxation exercises before defecating to relax the abdominal and perineal muscles, which may be constricted or in spasm. Administering an analgesic before a bowel movement is beneficial.

Reducing Anxiety

Patients facing rectal surgery may be upset and irritable because of discomfort, pain, and embarrassment. The nurse identifies specific psychosocial needs and individualizes the plan of care. The nurse maintains the patient's privacy while providing care and limits visitors, if the patient desires. Soiled dressings are removed from the room promptly to prevent unpleasant odors; room deodorizers may be needed if dressings are foul smelling.

Relieving Pain

During the first 24 hours after rectal surgery, painful spasms of the sphincter and perineal muscles may occur. Control of pain is a prime consideration. The patient is encouraged to assume a comfortable position. Flotation pads under the buttocks when sitting help decrease the pain, as may ice and analgesic ointments. Warm compresses may promote circulation and soothe irritated tissues. Sitz baths taken three or four times each day can relieve soreness and pain by relaxing sphincter spasm. Twenty-four hours after surgery, topical anesthetic agents may be beneficial in relieving local irritation and soreness. Medications may include topical anesthetics (i.e., suppositories), astringents, antiseptics, tranquilizers, and antiemetics. Patients are more compliant and less apprehensive if they are free of pain.

Wet dressings saturated with equal parts of cold water and witch hazel help relieve edema. When wet compresses are being used continuously, petrolatum is applied around the anal area to prevent skin maceration. The patient is instructed to assume a prone position at intervals because this position reduces edema of the tissue.

Promoting Urinary Elimination

Voiding may be a problem after surgery because of a reflex spasm of the sphincter at the outlet of the bladder and a certain amount of muscle guarding from apprehension and pain. The nurse tries all methods to encourage voluntary voiding (i.e., increasing fluid intake, listening to running water, and pouring warm water over the urinary meatus) before resorting to catheterization. After rectal surgery, urinary output is monitored closely.

Monitoring and Managing Complications

The operative site is examined frequently for rectal bleeding. The nurse assesses the patient for systemic indicators of excessive bleeding (i.e., tachycardia, hypotension, restlessness, and thirst). After hemorrhoidectomy, hemorrhage may occur from the veins that were cut. If a tube has been inserted through the sphincter after surgery, blood may be visible on the dressings. If bleeding is obvious, direct pressure is applied to the area, and the surgeon is notified. It is important to avoid using moist heat because it encourages vessel dilation and bleeding.

Promoting Home and Community-Based Care

Teaching Patients Self-Care

Most patients with anorectal conditions are not hospitalized. Those who undergo surgical procedures to correct the condition often are discharged directly from the outpatient surgical center. If they are hospitalized, it is for a short time, usually only 24 hours.

The nurse instructs the patient to keep the perianal area as clean as possible by gently cleansing with warm water and then drying with absorbent cotton wipes. The patient should avoid rubbing the area with toilet tissue. Instructions are provided about how to take a sitz bath and how to test the temperature of the water.

Continuing Care

Sitz baths should follow each bowel movement for 1–2 weeks after surgery. The nurse encourages the patient to respond quickly to the urge to defecate to prevent constipation. The diet is modified to increase fluids and fiber. Moderate exercise is encouraged, and the patient is taught about the prescribed diet, the significance of proper eating habits and exercise, and the laxatives that can be taken safely.

HEMORRHOIDS

Hemorrhoids are dilated portions of veins in the anal canal. They are very common with 40% of the population having hemorrhoids on colonoscopy screenings and 50% of the general population reporting experiencing hemorrhoids at some point in their lifetime (Ferri, 2022). Shearing of the mucosa during defecation results in the sliding of the structures in the wall of the anal canal, including the hemorrhoidal and vascular tissues. Increased pressure in the hemorrhoidal tissue due to pregnancy may initiate hemorrhoids or aggravate existing ones. Hemorrhoids are classified as one of two types: those above the internal sphincter are called *internal hemorrhoids*, and those appearing outside the external sphincter are called *external hemorrhoids* (see Fig. 23-13C).

Hemorrhoids cause itching and pain and are the most common cause of bright red bleeding with defecation. External hemorrhoids are associated with severe pain from the inflammation and edema caused by thrombosis (i.e., clotting of blood within the hemorrhoid). This may lead to ischemia

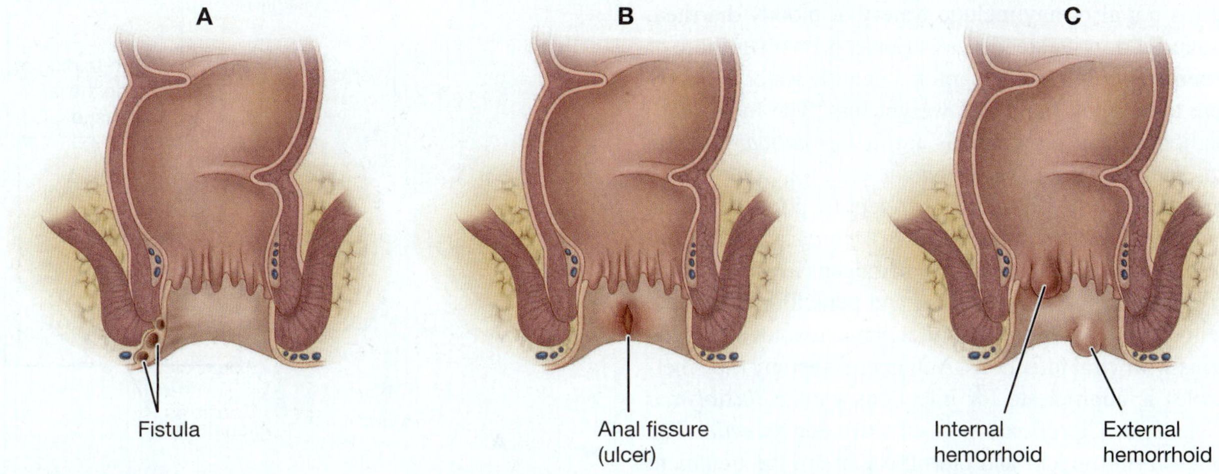

FIGURE 23-13 **Various types of anal lesions. A. Fistula. B. Fissure. C. External and internal hemorrhoids.**

of the area and eventual necrosis. Internal hemorrhoids usually are not painful until they bleed or prolapse when they become enlarged.

Hemorrhoid symptoms and discomfort can be relieved by good personal hygiene and by avoiding excessive straining during defecation. A high-residue diet that contains fruit and bran along with an increased fluid intake may be all the treatment necessary to promote the passage of soft, bulky stools to prevent straining. If this treatment is not successful, the addition of hydrophilic bulk-forming agents such as psyllium may help. Warm compresses, sitz baths, analgesic ointments and suppositories, astringents (e.g., witch hazel), and bed rest allow the engorgement to subside.

Pearls for Practice

In addition to increasing fiber and good personal hygiene, light exercise should be included in patient teaching to help improve peristalsis and improve defecation.

There are several types of nonsurgical treatments for hemorrhoids. Infrared photocoagulation, bipolar diathermy, and laser therapy are used to affix the mucosa to the underlying muscle. Injection of sclerosing agents is also effective for small, bleeding hemorrhoids. These procedures help prevent prolapse.

A conservative surgical treatment of internal hemorrhoids is the rubber-band ligation procedure. The hemorrhoid is visualized through the anoscope, and its proximal portion above the mucocutaneous lines is grasped with an instrument. Then a small rubber band is slipped over the hemorrhoid. Tissue distal to the rubber band becomes necrotic after several days and sloughs off. Fibrosis occurs; the result is that the lower anal mucosa is drawn up and adheres to the underlying muscle. Although this treatment has been satisfactory for some patients, it has proven painful for others and may cause secondary hemorrhage. It also has been known to cause perianal infection.

Cryosurgical hemorrhoidectomy, another method for removing hemorrhoids, involves freezing the hemorrhoid for a sufficient time to cause necrosis. Although it is relatively painless, this procedure is not used widely because the discharge is very foul smelling and wound healing is prolonged. The Nd:YAG laser is useful in excising hemorrhoids, particularly external hemorrhoidal tags. The treatment is quick and relatively painless. Hemorrhage and abscess are rare postoperative complications.

The previously described methods of treating hemorrhoids are not effective for advanced thrombosed veins, which must be treated by more extensive surgery. Hemorrhoidectomy, or surgical excision, can be performed to remove all the redundant tissue involved in the process. During surgery, usually the rectal sphincter is dilated digitally and the hemorrhoids are removed with a clamp and cautery or are ligated and then excised. After the surgical procedures are completed, a small tube may be inserted through the sphincter to permit the escape of flatus and blood; pieces of absorbable gelatin sponge or absorbable hemostatic, noncollagen-based gauze may be placed over the anal wounds.

SEXUALLY TRANSMITTED ANORECTAL DISEASES

Three infectious syndromes that are related to sexually transmitted infections (STIs) have been identified: proctitis, proctocolitis, and enteritis. Proctitis involves the rectum. It is commonly associated with recent anal-receptive intercourse with an infected partner. Symptoms include a mucopurulent discharge or bleeding, pain in the area, and diarrhea. The pathogens most frequently involved are *Neisseria gonorrhoeae, Chlamydia,* herpes simplex virus, and *Treponema pallidum.* Proctocolitis involves the rectum and lowest portion of the descending colon. The most common pathogens causing proctocolitis are *Campylobacter, Shigella, Entamoeba histolytica,* and *Chlamydia trachomatis.* Symptoms are similar to proctitis but also may include watery or bloody diarrhea, cramps, and abdominal tenderness. Enteritis involves more of the descending colon, and symptoms include watery, bloody diarrhea; abdominal pain; and weight loss. The most common pathogens causing enteritis are *E. histolytica, Giardia lamblia, Shigella,* and *Campylobacter.*

Sigmoidoscopy is performed to identify portions of the anorectum involved. Samples are taken with rectal swabs, and cultures are obtained to identify the pathogens involved. Antibiotics (i.e., cefixime, doxycycline, and penicillin G) are the treatment of choice for bacterial infections. Acyclovir is given to patients with viral infections. Antiamebic therapy (i.e., metronidazole) is appropriate for infections with *E. histolytica* and *G. lamblia.* Ciprofloxacin is effective for *Shigella.* The antibiotics erythromycin and ciprofloxacin are the treatment of choice for *Campylobacter* infection.

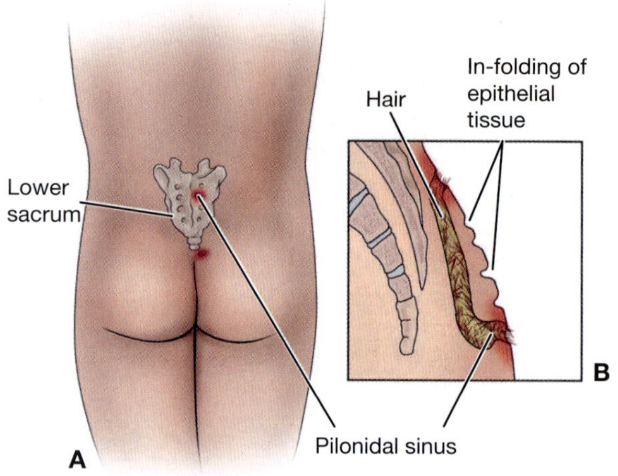

FIGURE 23-14 A. Pilonidal sinus on lower sacrum about 5 cm (2 in) above the anus in the intergluteal cleft. B. Hair particles emerge from the sinus tract, and localized indentations (pits) can appear on the skin near the sinus openings.

PILONIDAL SINUS OR CYST

A pilonidal sinus or cyst is found in the intergluteal cleft on the posterior surface of the lower sacrum (Fig. 23-14). Current theories suggest that it results from local trauma, causing the penetration of hairs into the epithelium and subcutaneous tissue. It also may be formed congenitally by an infolding of epithelial tissue beneath the skin, which may communicate with the skin surface through one or several small sinus openings. Hair frequently is seen protruding from these openings, and this gives the cyst its name, *pilonidal* (i.e., a nest of hair). The cysts rarely cause symptoms until adolescence or early adult life, when infection produces an irritating drainage or an abscess. Perspiration and friction easily irritate this area.

In the early stages of the inflammation, the infection may be controlled by antibiotic therapy, but after an abscess has formed, surgery is indicated. The abscess is incised and drained under local anesthesia. After the acute process resolves, further surgery is performed to excise the cyst and the secondary sinus tracts. The wound is allowed to heal by granulation. Gauze dressings are placed in the wound to keep its edges separated while healing occurs.

Clinical Judgment Case

Your patient is 72 years came into the emergency room complaining of nausea and cramping abdominal pain, particularly in left lower quadrant (LLQ). The patient states the pain was "all over before but now I feel it more on the left." She describes the pain as "cramping, sharp" and graded as 9/10 intensity. The patient began to feel ill 48 hours ago. Last BM of formed stool was yesterday, denies melena or frank blood. The patient's abdomen is firm, tender to touch, hypoactive bowel sounds are noted, no flatus, and the patient is lying on their side with knees toward their chest. Vital signs are T 100.8, HR 112 and regular, RR 28, BP 92/70, O_2 sat is 95% on room air. Lungs are clear to auscultation, S1 S2 without murmur, gallop or rub. Capillary refill 3 seconds, peripheral pulses 3+ bil, no edema, flat neck veins, delayed skin turgor. Patient is anxious and restless and states that "something is terribly wrong, I just know it." Medical history includes, hypertension (HTN), hyperlipidemia, coronary artery disease (CAD), diverticulosis, type 2 diabetes; home medications include hydrochlorothiazide, metformin, a statin, "I can't remember the name," low-dose aspirin, beta blocker, as-needed nitroglycerin, and metamucil daily. Admission lab work reveals a WBC count of 14k, Hgb/Hct 15/50, glucose of 198 mg/dL, sodium 146 mEq/L, K 3.8 mEq/L, Cl 98 mEq/l, and CO_2 20 mEq/L.

Step One: recognize cues where relevant and important information identified from different sources, such as medical history or vital signs

Answer: Nausea and acute sharp, cramping abdominal pain (9/10), now localized to LLQ, hypoactive bowel sounds, no flatus, firm, tender abdomen, guarding by the patient (knee chest position). Temperature of 100.8, tachycardia (112), tachypnea (RR 28), BP 92/70, pulse pressure of 22 mm Hg, capillary refill of 3 seconds, delayed skin turgor, flat neck veins, anxiety, and restlessness. History of CAD, HTN, hyperlipidemia, diverticulosis, and type 2 diabetes. Significant lab work includes

WBC count of 14k, Hgb/Hct 15/50, glucose of 198 mg/dL, sodium 146 mEq/L, and CO_2 20 mEq/L.

Step Two: Analyze cues, which is organizing and linking the recognized cues to the patient's clinical presentation.

Answer: You have clustered the symptoms of nausea and acute cramping abdominal pain (9/10), now localized to LLQ, hypoactive bowel sounds, no flatus, firm, tender abdomen, guarding by the patient (knee chest position), temperature of 100.8, leukocytosis (WBC of 14k), and history of diverticulosis.

You have clustered tachycardia (112), tachypnea (RR 28), BP 92/70, pulse pressure of 22 mm Hg, capillary refill of 3 seconds, delayed skin turgor, flat neck veins, anxiety and restlessness, and CO_2 20 mEq/L.

You have clustered history of DM and glucose of 198 mg/dL with either stress hyperglycemia or uncontrolled DM.

You have clustered the Hct, and sodium, as well as skin turgor, flat neck veins, delayed capillary refill.

Finally, you have clustered history of CAD and hyperlipidemia.

Step Three: Prioritize hypotheses, where hypotheses are evaluated and ranked according to priority. This can include urgency, likelihood, risk, difficulty, and/or time. In this phase you cluster your findings, to arrive at a list of problems (actual and or potential problems) you believe the patient is experiencing and determine the importance or urgency. What do you think is of greatest concern?

Answer: You prioritize the acute abdomen and are concerned that the patient may have perforated the diverticulum (you clustered the abdominal pain, nausea, vomiting, decreased bowel function, fever, and leukocytosis) and has peritonitis. You are concerned that the hypotension, tachycardia, narrow pulse pressure, and delayed capillary refill may be related to shock state (hypovolemic [hemorrhage vs. dehydration] versus septic [if perforation]). You calculate the mean arterial pressure (MAP) and realize that it is 77 mm Hg which maintains perfusion to the organs. You correlate the diastolic pressure and MAP with arteriolar vasoconstriction which you realize rises early in shock and then falls when cardiovascular compensation fails. You are aware that anxiety, along with feelings of doom, are common signs of shock during the early phase of shock. Laboratory evaluation may demonstrate mild organ dysfunction (e.g., increase in baseline creatinine or increase in troponin) or a mild elevation of lactate sometimes precedes hypotension and serves as an early indicator of impaired tissue perfusion. The decreased venous CO_2 (which you know reflects base bicarbonate) is worrisome that lactic acidosis is occurring.

The physical examination finding of flat neck veins, delayed skin turgor, delayed capillary refill, increased sodium and Hct suggest fluid volume deficit. You are aware that with normal fluid balance the Hct is ~ three times the hemoglobin level. When the Hct increases, as well as the sodium a fluid volume deficit is occurring (less water in the blood stream so the percentage of RBCs in blood increases). This is termed hemoconcentration.

The hyperglycemia may be related to the stress of the current situation or uncontrolled DM.

The cardiac history suggests that with fluid repletion, the risk for fluid overload, cardiac event, and heart failure exists.

Step Four: Generate solutions, which is identifying expected outcomes and using hypotheses to define a set of interventions for the expected outcomes.

Answer: The priority is fluid replacement since hypovolemia occurs because massive amounts of fluid and electrolytes move from the intestinal lumen into the peritoneal cavity and deplete the fluid in the vascular space, so IV access is the initial step. You prioritize reassessing vital signs and physical examination findings and given patients cardiac history will want to place cardiac monitoring and pulse oximetry continuously. In addition, diagnostic studies are necessary to reveal the etiology of the acute abdomen. You anticipate an abdominal x-ray to assess for free air and a CT scan of the abdomen may be ordered as it can reveal abscess formation, acute inflammation or infection of one of the major abdominal organs, or a perforation of the small or large bowel. You are aware that placing the patient on their side with knees flexed decreases the tension on the abdominal organs and elevating the head of bed will be done to prevent pooling of GI contents under the diaphragm. You will ensure suction is available as well as O_2 in the room since a nasogastric tube may be placed to prevent vomiting and risk of aspiration. You anticipate the hyperglycemia will be managed with insulin which will increase the risk of hypokalemia (last K^+ level was 3.8), thus you recognize that replacement will be required.

Step Five: Take action, where the solutions that address the highest priorities are implemented.

Answer: You notify the provider of your concerns and start a large-bore IV to prepare for fluid administration and allow simultaneous administration of fluid, medications, and blood component therapy if required. You place the patient on a cardiac monitor and continuous pulse oximetry. The O_2 sat remains at 95% so supplemental oxygen is not needed at this time. An NG tube is inserted by the provider which is draining large amounts of bilious fluid. An IV of lactated Ringer (LR) solution is initiated at 150 mL/hr and a stat abdominal film is ordered. You monitor the vital signs Q 15 minutes and administer broad-spectrum antibiotics as ordered. The x-ray reveals free air and the patient is readied for emergency surgery. An insulin drip is ordered and you prepare the solution by flushing the IV tubing with a volume of 20 mL of the insulin solution to saturate the binding sites before connecting it to the patient, thus ensuring the patient receives the ordered rate of insulin infusion. You realize a target glucose range of 140–180 mg/dL may be recommended. You are aware that K of 4 mEq/L is in each liter of LR but you will continue to monitor the laboratory results. You elevate the head of bed to prevent pooling of GI contents under the diaphragm.

Step Six: Evaluate outcomes, which is comparing observed outcomes against expected outcomes.

Answer: Because of your quick recognition that a perforation may have occurred you alerted the medical and surgical team and early fluid resuscitation and antibiotic initiation certainly improved your patient's outcome. The patient had a temporary ostomy performed and progressed well postoperatively and did not develop abscess formation. Now, teaching begins on how to manage the ostomy; your patient will require emotional support, and you are aware that many patients will require significant time before they feel comfortable with their ostomy care. You are aware that a colonoscopy in 6–8 weeks after surgery will evaluate that the etiology of the peritonitis was diverticulitis versus colorectal cancer. Your patient's ostomy will be reversed, but until then referral for home care may be indicated for further monitoring and patient and family teaching.

CHAPTER REVIEW

NCLEX-Style Review Questions

1. A patient returns to their room following a diagnostic colonoscopy after radiologic evidence of diverticular disease. In Column 1 select the signs and symptoms of concern, in Column 2 identify the possible medical condition the patient may be experiencing (select one) and in Column 3 select the appropriate action to take. Select all that apply.

Select all that apply	Select one	Select all that apply
Temperature of 100.7 F	Colon cancer	Administer enema to relieve constipation
WBC count of 9,000/mm^3	Hemorrhoids	Administer sitz bath
Guarding of the abdomen	Bowel perforation	Prepare the patient for surgery
Free air noted under diaphragm on chest x-ray	Crohn disease	Anticipate IV infusion to replace fluid loss
Abdominal rigidity	Irritable bowel disorder	Monitor vital signs
Normoactive bowel sounds	Constipation	Anticipate antibiotic therapy

2. A patient has a colostomy due to a ruptured diverticulum. On the first postoperative day, the nurse finds no measurable fecal drainage from the client's colostomy stoma. What is the most appropriate nursing intervention? Select all that apply.
a. Call the surgeon and prepare for surgery
b. Obtain an order to irrigate the stoma
c. Place the client on bed rest and notify the provider
d. Continue the current care plan
e. Reassure the patient that functioning is delayed until bowel sounds return

3. A 19-year-old presents with ulcerative colitis. Which of the following signs and symptoms are associated with this disorder? Select all that apply.
a. Bloody diarrhea
b. Positive Murphy sign
c. Abdominal discomfort
d. Ascending colon lesions
e. Psoas sign
f. Stool containing blood and pus.

4. A patient with Crohn disease develops a fever and symptoms of a urinary tract infection. The nurse recognizes that this complication may occur as a result of:
a. Perianal irritation from frequent diarrhea
b. Fistula formation between the bowel and bladder
c. Extraintestinal manifestations of the bowel disease
d. Impaired immunologic response to infectious microorganisms
e. CAUTI with Foley catheter

5. A patient has a bowel perforation from a recent surgery and now has been diagnosed with peritonitis. The patient has hypoactive bowel sounds, a temperature of 100.5°F, and an elevated WBC count. What are the most serious potential complications of peritonitis for which the nurse should monitor? Select all that apply.
a. Nausea
b. Diarrhea
c. Sepsis
d. Abdominal tenderness
e. Hypovolemic shock
f. Leukopenia

REFERENCES AND SELECTED READINGS

References and selected readings associated with this chapter can be found on the website that accompanies the book. Visit **http://thepoint.lww.com/Honan3e** to access the references and other additional resources associated with this chapter.

CHAPTER 24

Nursing Management: Patients With Hepatic and Biliary Disorders

Honore Garrin Kotler • Gregory Eichelzer

Learning Objectives

After reading this chapter, you will be able to:

1. Relate jaundice, portal hypertension, ascites, varices, nutritional deficiencies, and hepatic coma to pathophysiologic alterations of the liver.
2. Describe the medical, surgical, and nursing management of patients with esophageal varices.
3. Compare the various types of hepatitis and their causes, prevention, clinical manifestations, management, prognosis, and home health care needs.
4. Discuss medical and nursing management of patients with liver cancer.
5. Describe the postoperative nursing care of the patient undergoing liver transplantation.
6. Discuss management of cholelithiasis.
7. Differentiate between acute and chronic pancreatitis.
8. Discuss the nursing management of patients with acute pancreatitis.

Liver function is complex, and liver dysfunction affects all body systems. Liver disorders are common and may result from a virus, metabolic disorders, exposure to toxic substances such as alcohol, or tumors. Disorders of the biliary tract and pancreas are also common, including gallbladder stones and pancreatic dysfunction. An understanding of how biliary tract disorders are closely linked with liver disease is necessary to adequately care for patients.

HEPATIC DISORDERS

Understanding and managing liver disorders require expert clinical assessment and management skills. Box 24-1 highlights important considerations for hepatic assessment.

MANIFESTATIONS OF HEPATIC DYSFUNCTION

Jaundice

Yellowing of the skin and sclerae of the eyes are caused by impairment of the liver's ability to metabolize and secrete bilirubin (Fig. 24-1). Jaundice is apparent when the serum bilirubin level exceeds 3 mg/dL. Elevation of serum bilirubin levels can result from acute or chronic liver injury. The differential diagnosis of jaundice can result from the following causes:

- Hepatocellular jaundice caused by viral hepatitis, hepatotoxins (including drugs, and alcohol), metabolic disorders, ischemia, autoimmune hepatitis, or pregnancy
- Obstructive jaundice caused by obstruction of the bile ducts; gallstones; inflammation of bile ducts caused by primary sclerosing cholangitis, biliary strictures, malignancies of the biliary system, pancreatic cancer, liver cancer, or pancreatitis
- Hemolytic jaundice caused by increased production of bilirubin due to hemolysis, hematologic disorders, resorption of a hematoma, or multiple transfusions
- Hereditary hyperbilirubinemia caused by the inherited disorders of bilirubin metabolism, including various syndromes, some of which may require transplantation

PORTAL HYPERTENSION

Portal hypertension is caused by increased resistance to blood flow through the liver and increased blood flow due to vasodilatation in the splanchnic circulation (see Fig. 24-2). The two major complications of portal hypertension are **ascites** and gastroesophageal varices (discussed below) (Garcia-Tso, 2020).

BOX 24-1

Review of Hepatic Assessment

The initial presentation of a patient with liver disease varies greatly and can range from elevated liver enzymes on routine screening with no clinical signs or symptoms of disease to the patient who presents in liver failure with jaundice, hepatic coma, or esophageal bleeding. A comprehensive and complete health history is critical to determine exposure to hepatotoxic substances (including alcohol) or infectious agents causing liver dysfunction and to distinguish between acute and chronic hepatic dysfunction.

Health History Findings

Common Symptoms

- General: Lethargy, weakness, fatigue, fever, jaundice, pruritus (itching)
- Neurologic: Changes in mental acuity, personality changes, sleep disturbances, confusion, and outright coma in advanced chronic liver disease or acute failure
- Cardiopulmonary: Dyspnea resulting from increased fluid retention
- GI: Abdominal pain, increasing abdominal girth, anorexia, nausea, vomiting, hematemesis (vomiting blood), melena (black, tarry stool), hematochezia (stool that contains blood)
- Hematologic/Circulatory: Increased bruising, spontaneous bleeding, dependent and or/pedal edema
- Endocrine: Decreased libido in both males and females

Past Medical History

A prior history of inflammatory bowel disease or ulcerative colitis may lead to the diagnosis of primary sclerosing cholangitis (inflammation of the bile ducts). Chronic liver disease is commonly caused by alcohol and viruses, such as hepatitis B or C. Frequently patients with nonalcoholic fatty liver disease (NAFLD) may have prior medical history of diabetes, hyperlipidemia, and obesity.

Family History

Wilson disease, hemochromatosis, and autoimmune liver disease are genetically based. In α1-antitrypsin deficiency, some people develop cirrhosis rather than emphysema, whereas a family history of inflammatory bowel disease may be associated with primary sclerosing cholangitis (Martin, 2020).

Social History

- *Lifestyle:* Current and prior drug use (i.e., misuse of IV drugs, inhalation of drugs), sexual practices, tattoos, piercings, blood transfusions, needlestick injury, shared razors, toothbrushes
- *Occupational:* Exposure to toxins in workplaces; health care worker exposure to patients in trauma areas, operating rooms, hemodialysis unit or center
- *Travel history:* Recent travel to endemic areas, such as Mexico, Africa, India, or Latin America with ingestion of contaminated food or water, and raw shellfish
- *Alcohol use:* Information regarding current and prior alcohol use should be obtained from both patient and family (i.e., amount of alcohol ingested daily). It is important to recognize that the CDC recommends that adults of legal drinking age can choose not to drink, or to drink in moderation by limiting intake to **2 drinks or less in a day for males or 1 drink or less in a day for females**, on days when alcohol is consumed (CDC, 2022). One alcoholic drink-equivalent totals are: 12 oz of beer (containing an average percentage of 5% alcohol), 5 oz of wine (containing an average percentage of 12% alcohol), or 1.5 fluid ounces of 80-proof distilled spirits (containing an average percentage of around 40% alcohol) (NIH, n.d.). The NIAAA defines heavy alcohol use as consuming more than 4 drinks per day or 14 per week for adult males, and more than 3 drinks per day or 7 per week for adult females. Alcohol consumption reveals a dose-dependent risk increase for liver disease and malignancies, for example consuming 10–19 g/day of alcohol in general or 0–9 g/day as nonwine beverages doubled the risk for advanced liver disease compared to lifetime abstainers (Aberg et al., 2020).
- *Medications:* Review all prescription medications, over-the-counter, herbal supplements or home remedies, and intake of vitamins (especially vitamin A). Medications are frequent culprits in acute hepatic dysfunction and may lead to fulminant hepatic failure (e.g., acetaminophen overdose).

Physical Examination Findings

- *Integumentary and oral:* Jaundice, ecchymosis, spider angiomas and palmar erythema, scleral icterus or yellowing of the sclerae, leukonychia of the nails (white spots on nails), and clubbing of the fingers
- *Oral:* Hepatic fetor, a sweet, mildly fecal breath odor associated with encephalopathy
- *Neurologic:* Impairment of the patient's neurologic or cognitive status (slurred speech, confusion, poor recall, or slowed responses)
- *Musculoskeletal:* Muscle wasting; tremors or asterixis (flapping of the hands when wrists dorsiflexed) with altered mental status indicate hepatic encephalopathy.
- *Abdominal:* Signs of abdominal distention indicating ascites, or prominent dilated veins visible through the skin. Umbilical hernia or ventral hernias also may be observed. The patient with liver disease may also show striae, excoriations, or petechiae of the abdominal skin. Palpation of the liver is important to determine its size, shape, and consistency, and percussion is necessary to assess for ascites. The normal liver has a sharp, smooth edge and is firm, but not hard, with a nonpalpable left lobe. Presence of an enlarged, firm liver and surface irregularity is suspicious for liver disease (Bickley et al., 2021).
- *Other:* Pitting edema of the lower extremities; males may demonstrate gynecomastia and testicular atrophy (while the association of gynecomastia with liver disease is apparent, current data are conflicting and the mechanism remains unclear) (Swerdloff & Ng, 2019).

Diagnostic Evaluation

Diagnostic evaluation includes liver biopsy, liver function tests, and ultrasound (see Chapter 20).

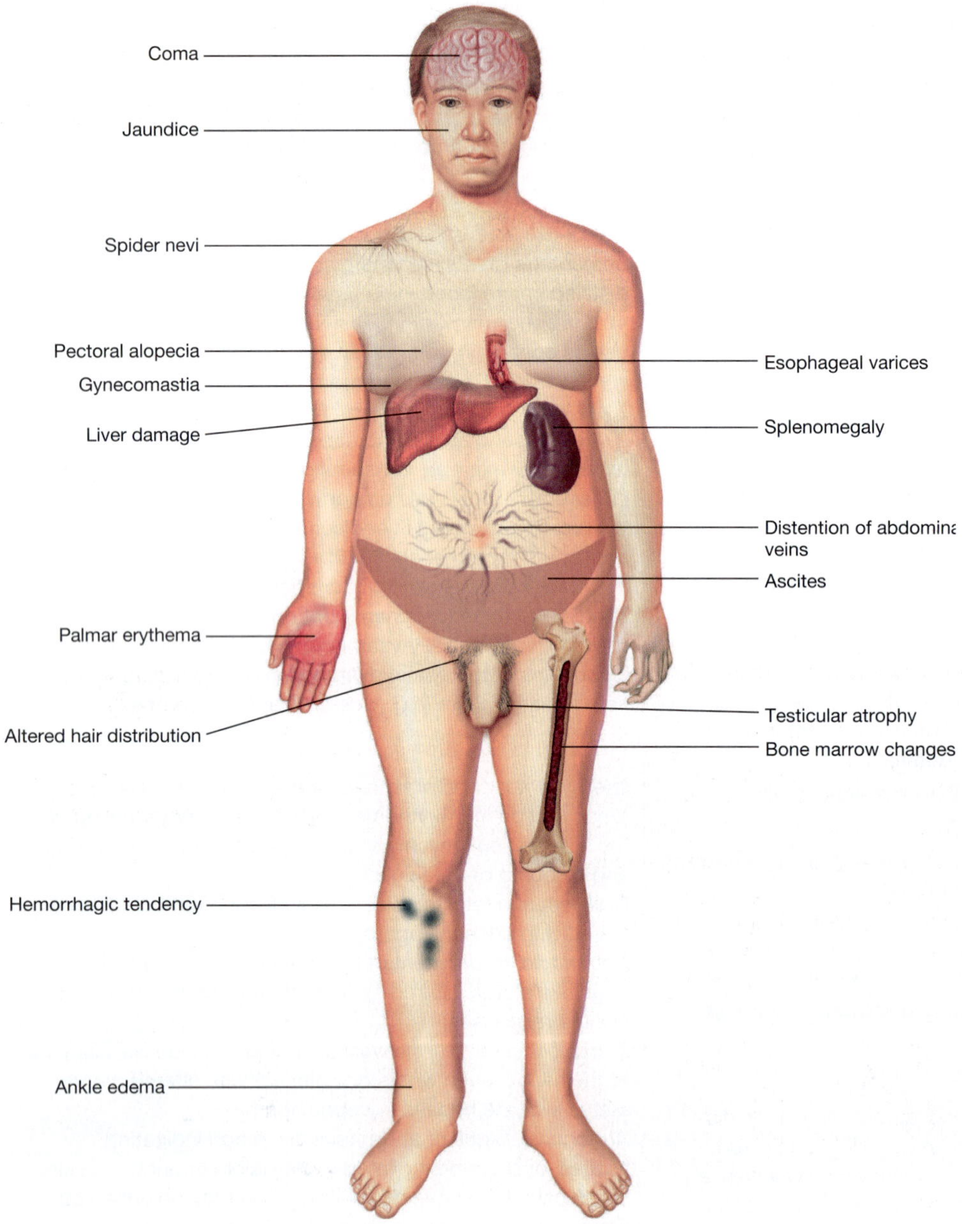

FIGURE 24-1 **Signs of liver failure. (With permission from Lippincott Williams & Wilkins. [2009]. *ACC Atlas of Pathophysiology* [3rd ed., p. 203]. Wolters Kluwer Health.)**

ASCITES

In ascites, fluid accumulates in the peritoneal cavity. Increased blood flow in the veins draining the portal system results in dilation and the development of varicose veins. The cause of ascites in 85% of cases is cirrhosis (Roussel et al., 2023).

Pathophysiology

The mechanisms responsible for the development of ascites are not entirely understood. However, a large body of evidence supports renin-angiotensin-aldosterone system (RAAS) and the sympathetic nervous system as a key mechanism related to ascites caused by cirrhosis (Solà & Gièes, 2021). Portal hypertension and the resulting increase in capillary pressure and obstruction of venous blood flow through the damaged liver are contributing factors. The vasodilation that occurs in the splanchnic circulation is also a suspected causative factor. The failure of the liver to metabolize aldosterone increases sodium and water retention by the kidney. Sodium and water retention, increased intravascular fluid volume, increased lymphatic flow, and decreased synthesis of albumin (hypoalbuminemia) by the damaged liver all contribute to the movement of fluid from the vascular system into the peritoneal space. The process becomes self-perpetuating as loss of fluid into the peritoneal space causes further sodium and water retention by the kidney to maintain the vascular fluid volume. As a result of liver damage, large amounts of albumin-rich fluid, 15 L or more, may accumulate in the peritoneal cavity as ascites (Solà & Gièes, 2021). Figure 24-3 illustrates the pathogenesis of ascites.

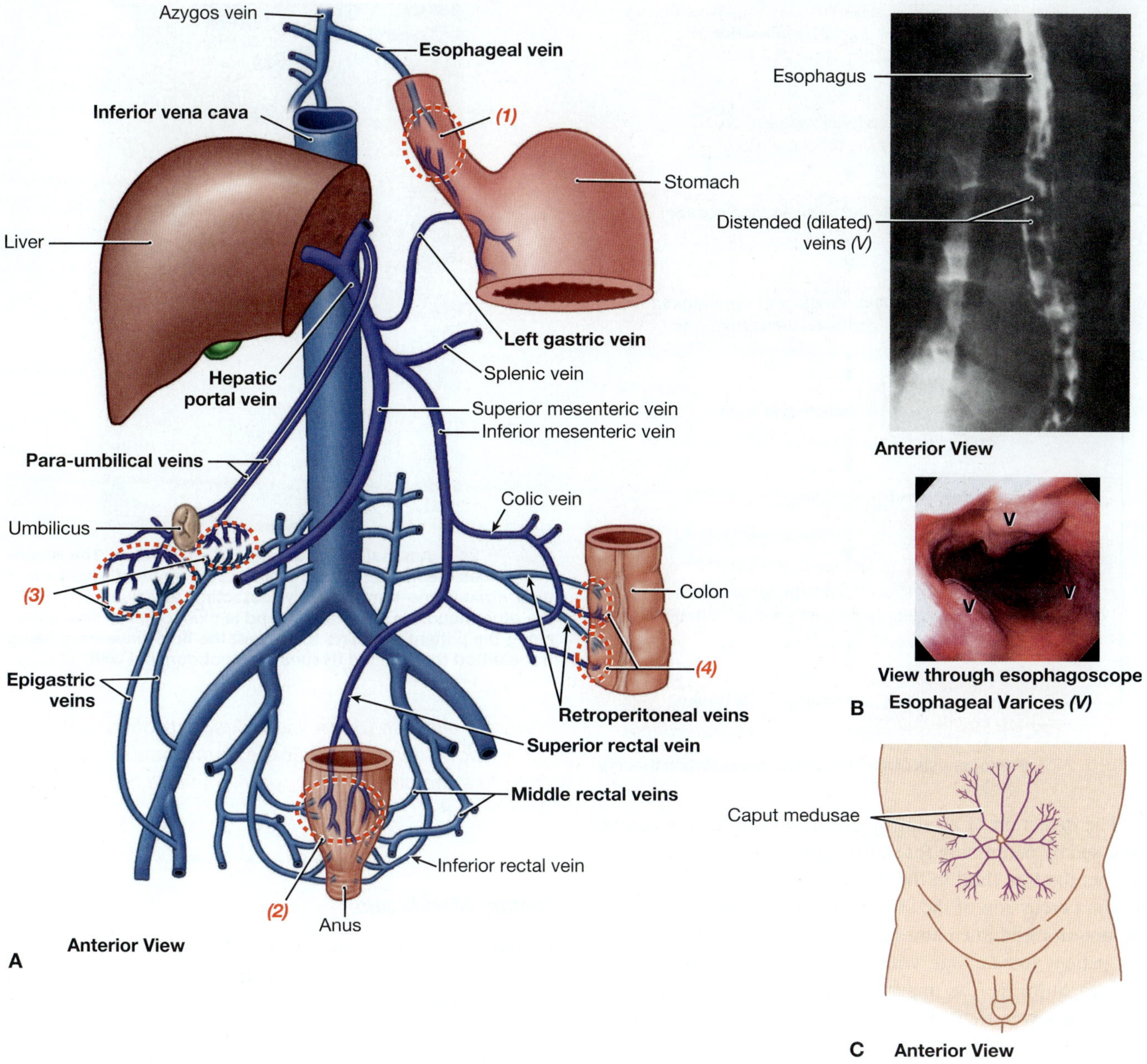

FIGURE 24-2 **A. Portacaval system. In this diagram, portal tributaries (*dark blue*) and systemic tributaries and communicating veins (*light blue*). In portal hypertension (as in hepatic cirrhosis), the portal blood cannot pass freely through the liver, and the portocaval anastomoses become engorged, dilated, or even varicose; as a consequence, these veins may rupture. The sites of the portocaval anastomosis shown are between (1) esophageal veins draining into the azygos vein (systemic) and left gastric vein (portal), which when dilated are esophageal varices; (2) the inferior and middle rectal veins, draining into the inferior vena cava (systemic), and the superior rectal vein continuing as the inferior mesenteric vein (portal) (hemorrhoids result if the vessels are dilated); (3) paraumbilical veins (portal) and small epigastric veins of the anterior abdominal wall (systemic), which when varicose form "caput medusae" (so named because of the resemblance of the radiating veins to the serpents on the head of Medusa, a character in Greek mythology); and (4) twigs of colic veins (portal) anastomosing with systemic retroperitoneal veins. B. Esophageal varices. C. Caput medusae. (Source: Agar, M. R., & Dalley, A. F. [2021]. *Grant's atlas of anatomy* [15th ed.]. LWW. A. Modified from Moore, K. L., Dalley, A. F., & Agur, A. M. R. [2018]. *Clinically oriented anatomy* [8th ed.]. Wolters Kluwer. B. [MRI]. Courtesy of Dr. E. L. Lansdown, University of Toronto, Ontario, Canada. B [photo]. Courtesy of Mission Hospital Regional Center, Mission Viejo, California.)**

Clinical Manifestations and Assessment

Common symptoms of the patient presenting with ascites include increased abdominal girth, weight gain, and swelling of the lower extremities (pedal edema). Dyspnea may be present as the result of abdominal distention or pleural effusions. Abdominal hernias due to increased intra-abdominal pressure may be visible, as well as visible collateral veins and striae (stretch marks). The patient also may experience early satiety, anorexia, and general weakness (Solà & Gièes, 2021).

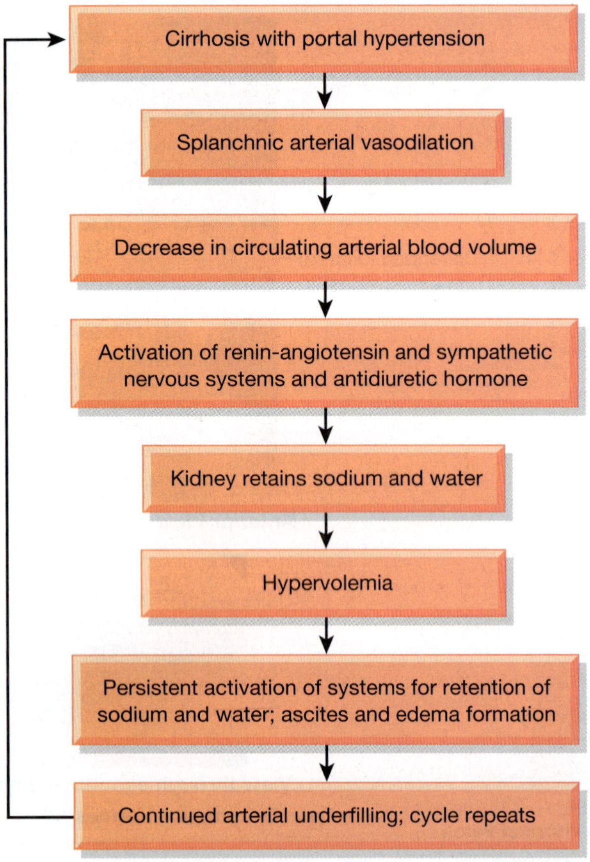

FIGURE 24-3 **Pathogenesis of ascites (arterial vasodilation theory).**

The detection of ascites by physical examination can be assessed by percussion for shifting dullness. With the patient supine, the free fluid in the abdomen will accumulate in the flanks; percussion of the abdomen will reveal tympany over the anterior abdomen and dullness over the flanks. Turning the patient to one side with repeat percussion will reveal shifting dullness (the uppermost area will sound tympanic while the lower area will sound dull to percussion). Assessing for abdominal fluid wave also detects ascites (Fig. 24-4). Bulging flanks also may reveal the presence of ascites. Accurate physical assessment of ascites through examination may be decreased if ascitic fluid is less than 1,500 mL or if the patient is obese (Vintila et al., 2020).

Ultrasonography of the liver and abdomen will definitively confirm the presence of ascites (Vintila et al., 2020). Diagnostic paracentesis (discussed in Chapter 20) is performed routinely on patients presenting with ascites upon hospital admission to detect the presence of spontaneous bacterial peritonitis (SBP). This complication of cirrhosis has a high mortality rate and will be discussed later in the chapter (Adinolfi et al., 2020).

Pearls for Practice

The nurse recognizes that ascites does not necessarily equate with fluid volume excess. In fact, in those patients who develop ascites due to an inability to generate albumin (decreased plasma protein), edema will be significant, however the intravascular space is depleted, the patient is hypovolemic and fluid volume deficit exists (Lough, 2022).

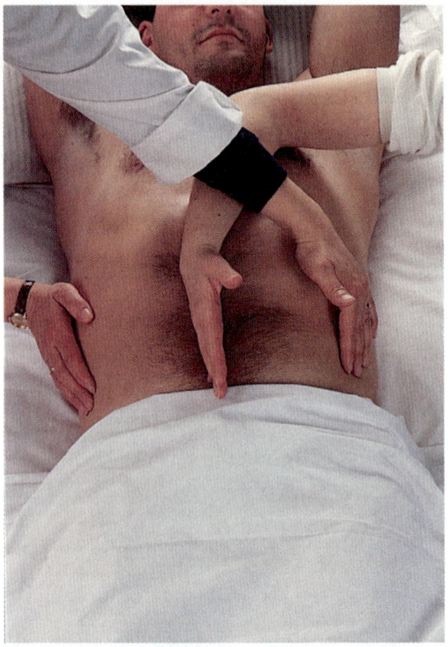

FIGURE 24-4 **Assessing for abdominal fluid wave. The examiner places the hands along the sides of the patient's flanks and then strikes one flank sharply, detecting any fluid wave with the other hand. An assistant's hand is placed (ulnar side down) along the patient's midline to prevent the fluid wave from being transmitted through the tissues of the abdominal wall.**

Medical and Nursing Management

Dietary Modification

Dietary restriction of salt intake is the mainstay of treatment of ascites to achieve a negative sodium balance to reduce fluid retention. The recommended daily sodium intake of patients with ascites should be 2 g or 90 mmol/day (Biggins et al., 2021). To achieve this, a "no salt added" diet is recommended and preprepared foods are avoided. Taking a more aggressive approach to sodium restriction can lead to nutritional deficiencies and hyponatremia (Solà & Gièes, 2021). Patients on sodium-restricted diets should receive nutritional education and guidance on foods that contain high sodium content (i.e., all processed foods, frozen and canned foods not indicated as low sodium) and avoid the use of added salt in meals and food preparation. Ongoing patient education and referral to a licensed nutritionist will facilitate dietary adherence.

Diuretics

The primary role of diuretic therapy is to improve urinary sodium excretion (Aithal et al., 2021). In patients with first episode of ascites, spironolactone is used alone. Combination drug therapy using spironolactone, an aldosterone-blocking agent, and furosemide, a loop diuretic agent, is the most effective regimen to control ascites for subsequent episodes of ascites and for patients who do not respond to spironolactone alone upon first episode. Patients should be monitored for daily weight changes (not to exceed 0.5 kg/day gain or loss in patients without peripheral edema), and up to 1 kg/day in patients with ascites and peripheral edema (Solà & Gièes, 2021). Frequently, failure to achieve weight reduction and decrease in ascites with the use of therapeutic doses of diuretics is due to low salt restriction (Aithal et al., 2021).

Possible complications of diuretic therapy include dehydration, volume depletion, and electrolyte abnormalities, such as hypokalemia or hyperkalemia, hyponatremia, kidney impairment, and hepatic encephalopathy. Gynecomastia is a common side effect caused by spironolactone. If patients with ascites develop dilutional hyponatremia (serum sodium below 134 mmol/L), then diuretics should be discontinued and fluid restriction initiated (Solà & Gièes, 2021).

Paracentesis

Paracentesis is the removal of fluid (ascites) from the peritoneal cavity through a puncture or a small surgical incision through the abdominal wall under sterile conditions. Therapeutic paracentesis provides only temporary removal of fluid; ascites rapidly recurs, necessitating repeated fluid removal. See Chapter 20 for detailed discussion of paracentesis.

Transjugular Intrahepatic Portosystemic Shunt

Transjugular intrahepatic portosystemic shunt (TIPS) is a method of treating ascites in which a cannula is threaded into the portal vein by the transjugular route (Fig. 24-5). To reduce portal hypertension, an expandable stent is inserted to serve as an intrahepatic shunt between the portal circulation and the hepatic vein. This diverts blood flow from a high-pressure vascular bed (portal) to a lower-pressure vascular bed (hepatic veins/inferior vena cava), allowing for the return of blood to the heart and decompressing portal hypertension. It is extremely effective for improving the renal response to diuretic therapy, and preventing recurrence of fluid accumulation (Tripathi, 2020).

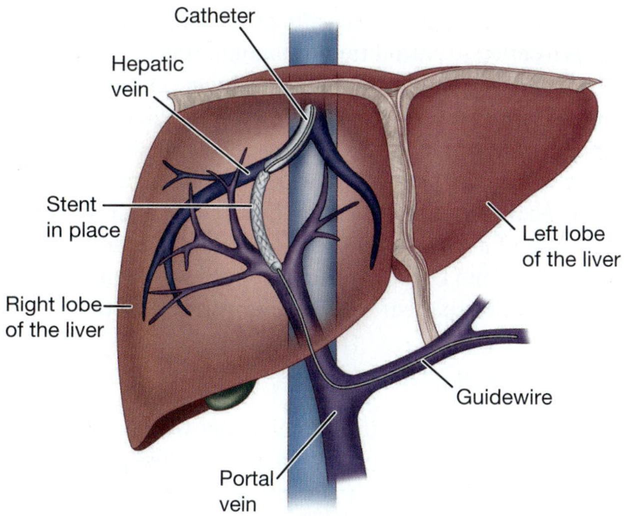

FIGURE 24-5 **Transjugular intrahepatic portosystemic shunt (TIPS). A stent is inserted via catheter to the portal vein to divert blood flow and reduce portal hypertension.**

Although TIPS is an effective treatment for patients with refractory ascites, it does not increase survival benefit and may increase hepatic encephalopathy, which is discussed shortly (Garcia-Tsao, 2020).

Complications

An important complication of ascites is the development of SBP, an infection that may develop in the ascitic fluid, usually from *Escherichia coli*, a gram-negative bacteria. Prompt detection of SBP is required as this complication has a high mortality rate. Diagnostic paracentesis should be performed in all patients with cirrhosis and ascites admitted to the hospital and in any inpatient with cirrhosis showing signs of infection (i.e., fever, chills, abdominal pain) or with abnormalities in liver or kidney function. This procedure removes a small amount of ascitic fluid from the abdomen percutaneously and can be performed at the bedside. The specimen is analyzed for cell count and differential, albumin, total protein, and susceptible organisms (Biggins et al., 2021). The treatment of SBP includes the use of IV antibiotics or oral treatment if tolerated. Long-term prophylaxis with oral antibiotic therapy is recommended to prevent future infection in patients who have had a diagnosis of SBP (Garcia-Tsao, 2020; Solà & Gièes, 2021).

ESOPHAGEAL VARICES

Gastroesophageal varices are present in 40% to 95% of patients with cirrhosis and ~14–20% of those with varices will bleed within 1 to 3 years; varices are the most life-threatening complication in patients with chronic liver disease (Roberts et al., 2021). Bleeding or hemorrhage from esophageal varices is associated with significantly decreased overall lifespan with a mortality rate as high as 20% within the first 6 weeks of initial bleeding episode (Garcia-Tsao, 2020).

Pathophysiology

Esophageal varices are dilated, tortuous veins that usually are found in the submucosa of the lower esophagus but may develop higher in the esophagus or extend into the stomach. Portal hypertension is the primary mechanism by which collateral circulation develops.

Because of increased obstruction of the portal vein, venous blood from the intestinal tract and spleen seeks an outlet through collateral circulation (new pathways for return of blood to the right atrium). The effect is increased pressure, particularly in the vessels in the submucosal layer of the lower esophagus and upper part of the stomach. These collateral vessels are not very elastic; rather, they are tortuous and fragile, and they bleed easily (Suzuki & Sakamoto, 2020). Gastroesophageal bleeding (Fig. 24-6) is due to high

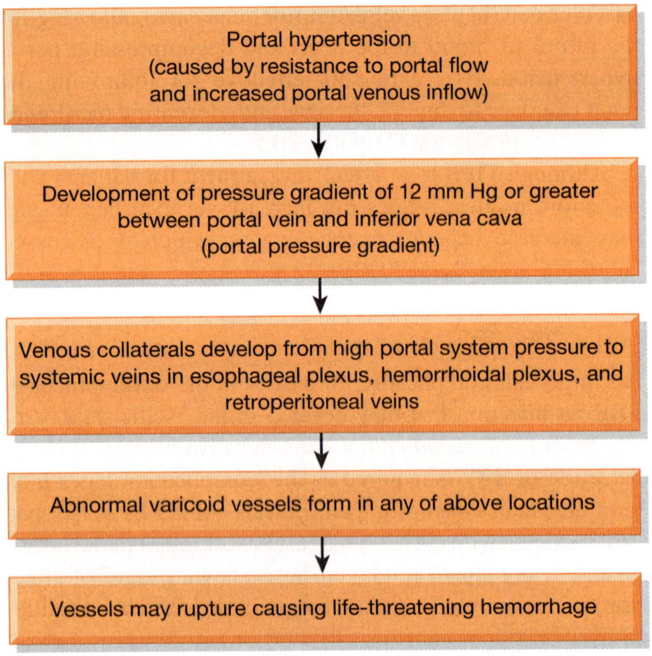

FIGURE 24-6 **Pathogenesis of bleeding esophageal varices.**

portal pressure and increased collateral blood flow, causing dilation and thinning of varices. Any additional increase in pressure or defect in the varices will cause rupture and hemorrhage. Factors that may precipitate hemorrhage are alcohol intake, physical exercise, and any activity that would increase intra-abdominal pressure (e.g., lifting, straining to pass stool, vomiting, coughing) (Garcia-Tsao, 2020).

Bleeding esophageal varices are life-threatening and can result in hemorrhagic shock that produces decreased cerebral, hepatic, and renal perfusion. In turn, there is an increased nitrogen load from bleeding into the GI tract and an increased serum ammonia level, increasing the risk for encephalopathy.

Clinical Manifestations and Assessment

The patient with bleeding esophageal varices may present with hematemesis, melena, or general deterioration in mental or physical status and often has a history of alcohol use disorder. Signs and symptoms of hypovolemic shock include decreasing urine output (<0.5 mL/Kg/hr), oliguria, hypotension, with decreased pulse pressure, flat neck veins, altered mental status (anxiety may be earliest symptom), delayed capillary refill, pallor, cool extremities, tachycardia, and tachypnea. Recall that hypotension typically occurs when 30% of the patient's total blood volume is lost. Endoscopic evaluation (or esophagogastroduodenoscopy [EGD]) is used in the diagnosis and treatment of varices, in both the acute and outpatient settings. Assessment of variceal size, location, and features are used to predict the risk of bleeding. Variceal size is an important factor that determines both pharmacologic and endoscopic therapies to prevent and manage risk of bleeding. In the acute setting, endoscopy should take place within 12 hours after stabilization of the patient (Garcia-Tsao, 2020; Jung et al., 2020).

Medical Management

Acute bleeding from esophageal varices is an emergency that can quickly lead to hemorrhagic shock. The patient is critically ill, requiring aggressive medical care and expert nursing care, and they should be transferred to the intensive care unit (ICU) for close monitoring and management. Assessment and protection of the patient's airway and peripheral venous access is required. Endotracheal intubation may be necessary to prevent aspiration of blood (Garcia-Tsao, 2020; Richardson et al., 2020).

The extent of bleeding is evaluated, and vital signs are monitored continuously if hematemesis (vomiting bright red or brown, "coffee grounds" emesis), hematochezia (bright red stools), and melena (black, tarry, or dark red-colored stool) are present. Signs of potential hypovolemia are noted, such as cold clammy skin, tachycardia, a drop in blood pressure, decreased urine output, restlessness, and weak peripheral pulses. The volume of circulating blood may be estimated and monitored with a central venous catheter or pulmonary artery catheter. Blood pressure is monitored noninvasively or via an arterial catheter. Oxygen is administered to prevent hypoxia and to maintain adequate blood oxygenation, which is evaluated via pulse oximetry or arterial blood gases (ABGs).

Because patients with bleeding esophageal varices have intravascular volume depletion and are subject to electrolyte imbalance, IV fluids with electrolytes and volume expanders are provided to restore fluid volume and replace electrolytes. Transfusion of blood components also may be required to maintain hemodynamic stability and correct coagulopathy with the aim of maintaining a hemoglobin level of 7 to 8 g/dL (Mehta & Fallon, 2021). Caution must be taken with volume resuscitation so that overhydration does not occur because this would raise portal pressure and increase bleeding (Facciorusso, 2020). Usually an indwelling urinary catheter is inserted to permit frequent monitoring of urine output.

Although a variety of pharmacologic, endoscopic, and surgical approaches are used to treat bleeding esophageal varices, none is ideal, and most are associated with considerable risk to the patient. Nonsurgical treatment of bleeding esophageal varices still is preferable because of the high mortality rate of emergency surgery to control bleeding esophageal varices and because of the poor physical condition that is typical of the patient with severe liver dysfunction.

Pharmacologic Therapy

The medical management of the patient with acute variceal hemorrhage includes the use of antibiotic therapy (IV ciprofloxacin, or ceftriaxone in patients with advanced cirrhosis) to prevent infection and improve survival. The most effective specific therapy for the control of active variceal hemorrhage is the combination of a vasoconstrictor with endoscopic therapy or endoscopic variceal ligation or banding which is discussed shortly. Vasoconstrictors include somatostatin or octreotide because they decrease the splanchnic arterial blood and decrease portal pressure with fewer side effects and equal efficacy compared with vasopressin (discussed below). Octreotide has a longer half-life than somatostatin (100 minutes vs. 2 to 3 minutes) and, as a result, has become the agent of choice in managing acute variceal hemorrhage (Gelabert et al., 2019). Octreotide is maintained for 2 to 5 days in conjunction with endoscopic therapy (discussed below). Nonselective beta blockers are used for the prevention of variceal bleeding in patients with cirrhosis and also to reduce episodes of rebleeding after an initial episode (Garcia-Tsao, 2020).

In a patient who is actively bleeding, medications are administered initially because other therapies take longer to take effect. Although vasopressin is no longer considered first-line therapy in the management of active bleeding varices, it may be used to slow variceal hemorrhage because it produces constriction of the splanchnic arterial bed and decreases portal pressure (Boregowda et al., 2019). However, a recent Cochrane review found that vasopressin analogs alone (with supportive therapy) "probably result in increased mortality, compared to endoscopic sclerotherapy" and that "vasopressin analogues alone and band ligation alone probably result in fewer adverse events compared to endoscopic sclerotherapy" (Roberts et al., 2021, p. 2). If prescribed, it is administered by continuous IV infusion. It is important to note that vasopressin also stimulates the contraction of vascular smooth muscle in coronary, GI, pancreatic, skin, and muscular vascular beds. Because of the coronary artery vasoconstriction, it is always use in combination with IV nitroglycerin to prevent the side effects cardiac ischemia, arrhythmias, and hypertension (Gelabert et al., 2019; Gold Standard, 2022). Stable vital signs and the decreasing presence or absence of blood in the gastric aspirate indicate the effectiveness of vasopressin. Monitoring of fluid intake and output and electrolyte levels is necessary because hyponatremia may develop, and vasopressin may have an antidiuretic effect.

Pearls for Practice

If vasopressin is administered in acute esophageal bleed (because of its vasoconstrictive properties in the splanchnic, portal, and intrahepatic vessels), the nurse understands that this medication also causes coronary artery constriction that may dispose patients with coronary artery disease to cardiac ischemia. Thus the nurse observes the patient for evidence of chest pain, electrocardiogram (ECG) changes, and vital sign changes. A high degree of suspicion is maintained as many patients may have silent ischemia. Nitroglycerin is administered concurrently with vasopressin. In addition, the nurse observes for cerebral, bowel and limb ischemia (Pezzotti, 2020).

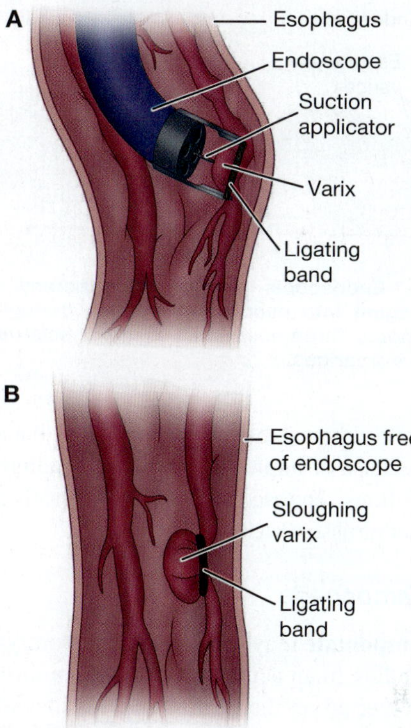

FIGURE 24-7 Esophageal banding. A. A rubber band–like ligature is slipped over an esophageal varix via an endoscope. B. Necrosis results, and the varix eventually sloughs off.

Endoscopic Therapies

Esophageal Banding Therapy (Variceal Band Ligation)

In **variceal banding** (Fig. 24-7), an EGD is performed using a modified endoscope loaded with an elastic rubber band that is passed through an overtube directly onto the varix (singular) or varices (plural) to be banded. It is also called rubber band ligation. After the bleeding varix is suctioned into the tip of the endoscope, the rubber band is slipped over the tissue, causing necrosis, ulceration, and eventual sloughing of the varix. Complications include post-banding bleeding in 2.7% to 7.3% of patients with even less incidence of chest pain and esophageal stricture (Facciorusso, 2020).

Esophageal banding is the most effective therapy to treat acute hemorrhage. Recently this procedure has demonstrated better hemostasis, decreased side effects (ulcer, stricture), a reduced rate of early rebleeding, and a decreased rate of early mortality compared to sclerotherapy (Boregowda et al., 2019). After an acute episode of bleeding, the combination of beta-blocker therapy and routine esophageal banding is the treatment of choice and has been shown to effectively prevent rebleeding and improve survival (Garcia-Tsao, 2020).

Endoscopic Injection Sclerotherapy

In endoscopic injection **sclerotherapy** (EIS), a sclerosing agent is injected through a fiberoptic endoscope into the bleeding esophageal varices to promote thrombosis and eventual sclerosis (Fig. 24-8). This therapy is used only to

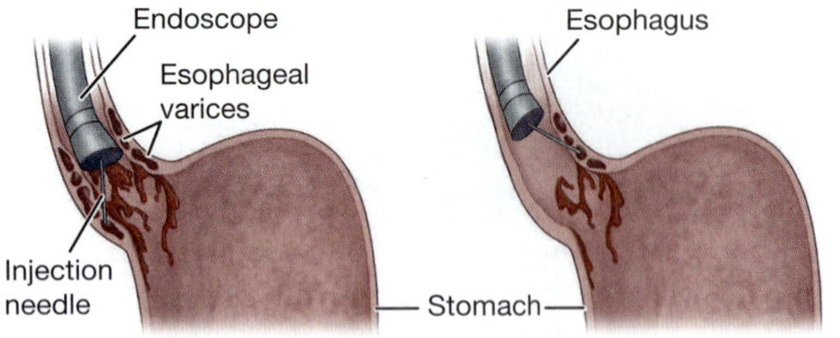

FIGURE 24-8 **Endoscopic injection sclerotherapy. Injection of sclerosing agent into esophageal varices through an endoscope promotes thrombosis and eventual sclerosis, thereby obliterating the varices.**

treat an acute variceal bleed if esophageal banding is not feasible. Because of unproven efficacy and a high incidence of complications, endoscopic variceal sclerotherapy use is limited (Facciorusso, 2020).

Balloon Tamponade

Balloon tamponade may be used as a temporary measure to control bleeding in an active hemorrhage. In this procedure, pressure is exerted on the cardia (upper orifice of the stomach) and against the bleeding varices by a double-balloon tamponade (Sengstaken-Blakemore tube) (Fig. 24-9). The tube has four openings, each with a specific purpose: gastric aspiration, esophageal aspiration, gastric balloon inflation, and esophageal balloon inflation. This method effectively controls bleeding in 80% of patients; however, it is associated with lethal complications, including esophageal rupture, aspiration, and rebleeding, and it carries a high risk of mortality. Its use is restricted to patients with uncontrolled bleeding and as a temporary bridge to other treatments, such as TIPS or endoscopy (Facciorusso, 2020).

Pearls for Practice

The patient being treated with balloon tamponade must remain under close observation in the ICU because of the risk for serious complications. The patient must be monitored closely and continuously. Precautions must be taken to ensure that the patient does not pull on or inadvertently displace the tube.

Transjugular Intrahepatic Portosystemic Shunting

A TIPS procedure is indicated for the treatment of an acute episode of variceal bleeding refractory to pharmacologic or endoscopic therapy. In 10% to 20% of patients for whom urgent band ligation and medications are not successful in eradicating bleeding, a TIPS procedure can control acute variceal hemorrhage effectively by rapidly lowering portal pressure. TIPS is also indicated for those patients who rebleed after pharmacologic or endoscopic prophylaxis has failed. This technique also is used as a bridge to liver transplantation. Most common complications include hepatic encephalopathy, variceal bleeding, and stent malfunction. Contraindications include heart failure, tricuspid valve regurgitation, and pulmonary hypertension (Tripathi et al., 2020).

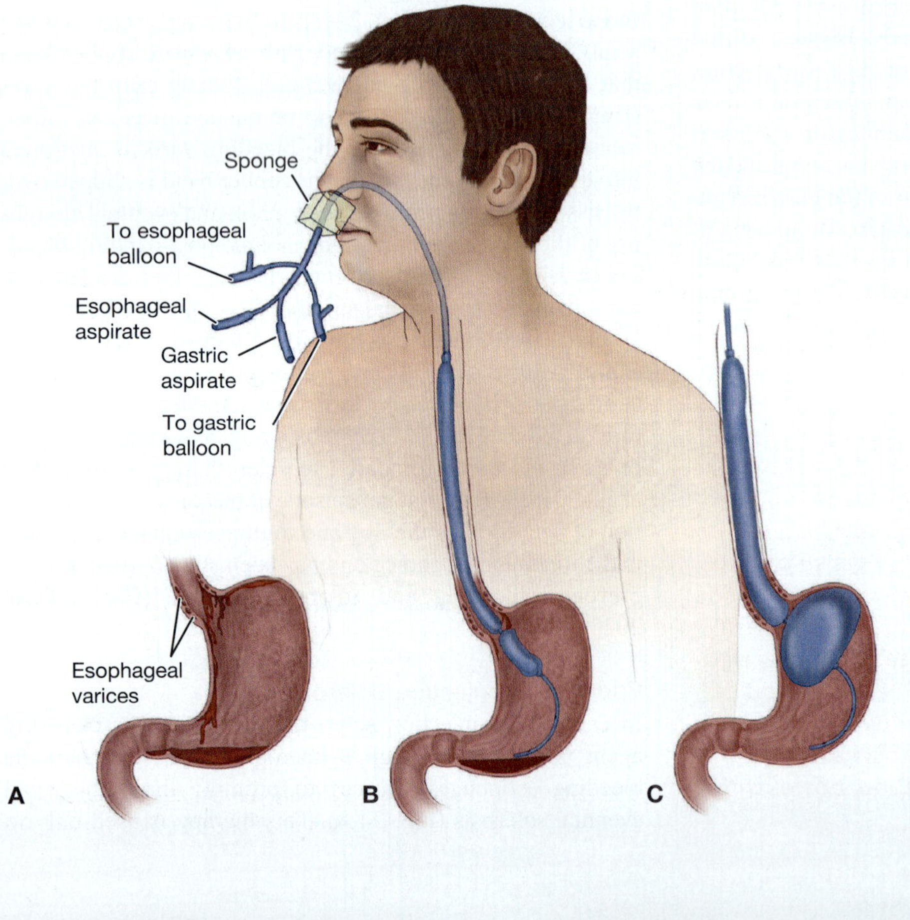

FIGURE 24-9 **Balloon tamponade to treat esophageal varices. A. Dilated, bleeding esophageal veins (varices) of the lower esophagus. B. A four-lumen esophageal tamponade tube with balloons (uninflated) in place. C. Compression of bleeding esophageal varices by inflated esophageal and gastric balloons. The gastric and esophageal outlets permit the nurse to aspirate secretions.**

Nursing Management

After treatment for acute hemorrhage, the patient must be observed for bleeding, perforation of the esophagus, aspiration pneumonia, and esophageal stricture. Antacids, histamine-2 antagonists such as cimetidine, or proton pump inhibitors such as pantoprazole may be administered after the procedure.

After the examination, fluids are not given until the gag reflex returns. Lozenges and gargles may be used to relieve throat discomfort if the patient's physical condition and mental status permit. If the patient is actively bleeding, oral intake will not be permitted, and the patient will be prepared for further diagnostic and therapeutic procedures.

Overall nursing assessment includes monitoring the patient's physical condition and evaluating emotional responses and cognitive status. The nurse monitors and records vital signs and assesses the patient's nutritional and neurologic status. This assessment assists in identifying hepatic encephalopathy, which results from the breakdown of blood in the GI tract and a rising serum ammonia level. Manifestations range from drowsiness to encephalopathy and coma.

If complete rest of the esophagus is indicated because of bleeding, parenteral nutrition is initiated. Gastric suction usually is initiated to keep the stomach as empty as possible and to prevent straining and vomiting. The patient often complains of severe thirst, which may be relieved by frequent oral hygiene and moist sponges to the lips. The nurse closely monitors the blood pressure. Vitamin K therapy and multiple blood transfusions often are indicated because of blood loss and coagulation abnormalities. A quiet environment and calm reassurance may help to relieve the patient's anxiety and reduce agitation.

Bleeding anywhere in the body is anxiety-provoking, resulting in a crisis for the patient and family. If the patient has been a heavy user of alcohol, delirium secondary to alcohol withdrawal can complicate the situation. The nurse provides support and explanations about medical and nursing interventions. Close monitoring of the patient helps in detecting and managing complications. Management modalities and nursing care of the patient with bleeding esophageal varices are summarized in Table 24-1.

Pearls for Practice

When the patient has bleeding esophageal varices, the nurse recognizes that the priority actions will relate to airway maintenance, volume resuscitation, and management of hemodynamics (heart rate, blood pressure). If there is ongoing hematemesis, the nurse anticipates endotracheal intubation to protect the patient's airway. Two large-gauge IV lines are inserted to establish access for fluid administration. Common crystalloid fluids used for fluid resuscitation include 0.9% sodium chloride solution (normal saline) and lactated Ringer (LR) solution and potentially blood products such as packed red blood cells. However, both normal saline and LR carry risks and the choice will depend on the clinical scenario. With LR, the exogenous lactate in LR is converted to bicarbonate by the liver and with liver disease this solution may worsen acidosis, whereas the sodium and chloride load in normal saline may cause hypernatremia and non-anion gap metabolic acidosis from hyperchloremia. In addition, since coagulopathies commonly occur in liver disease, the nurse recognizes that fresh frozen plasma (to maintain a reasonable prothrombin time) and vitamin K may be administered. The administration of platelets is expected if thrombocytopenia exists or the platelet count is below 50,000/mcL (normal, 150,000–400,000/mcL) (Pezzotti, 2020).

Hepatic Encephalopathy and Coma

Hepatic encephalopathy, a life-threatening complication of liver disease, occurs with profound liver failure and may result from the accumulation of ammonia and other toxic metabolites in the blood. Hepatic coma represents the most advanced stage of hepatic encephalopathy.

Pathophysiology

Ammonia is produced in the liver as a by-product of protein and amino acid breakdown. The colon and small intestine are also sites of ammonia production resulting from bacterial action. The liver converts ammonia into urea, which is excreted into the urine. In normal liver function, this process prevents the toxic build-up of ammonia in the blood (Woreta & Mezina, 2020). Damaged liver cells fail to detoxify and convert the ammonia to urea, and the elevated quantity of ammonia enters the bloodstream.

Circumstances that increase serum ammonia levels tend to aggravate or precipitate hepatic encephalopathy. The largest source of ammonia is the enzymatic and bacterial digestion of dietary and blood proteins in the GI tract. Ammonia from these sources increases as a result of GI bleeding (i.e., bleeding esophageal varices, chronic GI bleeding), a high-protein diet, bacterial infection, or uremia. In the presence of alkalosis or hypokalemia, increased amounts of ammonia are absorbed from the GI tract and from the renal tubular fluid. Conversely, serum ammonia is decreased by elimination of protein from the diet, administration of nonabsorbable disaccharides such as lactulose, and by the administration of antibiotic agents such as rifaximin or neomycin sulfate, reducing the amount of ammonia produced and absorbed in the intestine (Garcia-Tsao, 2020). Other factors unrelated to increased serum ammonia levels that can cause hepatic encephalopathy in susceptible patients include excessive diuresis, dehydration, infections, constipation,, and some medications (sedatives, narcotics that depress brain function, and diuretics that cause potassium loss). The increased ammonia concentration in the blood causes brain dysfunction and damage, resulting in hepatic encephalopathy. Table 24-2 presents the stages of hepatic encephalopathy,

TABLE 24-1 **Management Modalities and Nursing Care for the Patient With Bleeding Esophageal Varices**

Treatment Modality[a]	Action	Nursing Priorities
Nonsurgical Modalities		
Pharmacologic Agents		
Propranolol/nadolol	Reduces portal pressure by beta-adrenergic blocking action	*Propranolol* and *nadolol*—decreased pulse pressure, impaired cardiovascular response to hemorrhage.
Somatostatin/octreotide	Reduces portal pressure by selective vasodilation of portal system	Support patient during treatment.
Vasopressin	Reduces portal pressure by constricting splanchnic arteries	Observe response to therapy. Monitor for side effects: *vasopressin*—angina; nitroglycerin is prescribed to prevent or treat angina.
Balloon tamponade	Exerts pressure directly to bleeding sites in esophagus and stomach	Explain procedure to patient briefly to obtain cooperation with insertion and maintenance of esophageal/gastric tamponade tube and reduce patient's fear of the procedure. Monitor closely to prevent inadvertent removal or displacement of tube, subsequent airway obstruction, and aspiration. Provide frequent oral hygiene.
Room-temperature saline lavage	Clears blood and secretions before endoscopy and other procedures	Ensure patency of the nasogastric tube to prevent aspiration. Observe gastric aspirate for blood and cessation of bleeding.
Injection sclerotherapy	Promotes thrombosis and sclerosing of bleeding sites by injection of sclerosing agent into the esophageal varices	Observe for aspiration, perforation of the esophagus, and recurrence of bleeding after treatment.
Variceal banding	Provides thrombosis and mucosal necrosis of bleeding sites by band ligation	Observe for recurrence of bleeding, esophageal perforation.
Surgical Modalities		
Transjugular intrahepatic portosystemic shunt (TIPS)	Reduces portal pressure by creating a shunt within the liver between the portal and systemic venous systems	Observe for rebleeding and signs of infection. Observe for development of portal-systemic encephalopathy (altered mental status, neurologic dysfunction), liver failure, hypertension due to increased volume after surgery, and coagulopathy. Requires intensive, expert nursing care for prolonged period. Follow-up may include ultrasound with Doppler to evaluate for shunt patency.
Surgical ligation of varices	Ties off blood vessels at the site of bleeding	Observe for rebleeding.
Esophageal transection and devascularization	Separates bleeding site from portal system	Observe for rebleeding.

[a]Several modalities may be used concurrently or in sequence.

TABLE **24-2 Stages of Hepatic Encephalopathy and Possible Nursing Diagnoses**[a]

Stage	Clinical Symptoms	Clinical Signs	Electroencephalogram (EEG) Changes	Selected Potential Nursing Diagnoses
1	Normal level of consciousness with periods of lethargy and euphoria; reversal of day–night sleep patterns	Asterixis; impaired writing and ability to draw line figures	Normal EEG	Activity intolerance Self-care deficit Sleep deprivation
2	Increased drowsiness; disorientation; inappropriate behavior; mood swings; agitation	Asterixis; fetor hepaticus	Abnormal EEG with generalized slowing	Impaired social interaction Ineffective role performance Injury risk
3	Stuporous; difficult to rouse; sleeps most of time; marked confusion; incoherent speech	Asterixis; increased deep tendon reflexes; rigidity of extremities	EEG markedly abnormal	Malnutrition risk Impaired mobility Impaired verbal communication
4	Comatose; may not respond to painful stimuli	Absence of asterixis; absence of deep tendon reflexes; flaccidity of extremities	EEG markedly abnormal	Aspiration risk Impaired gas exchange Altered tissue integrity risk Effective sensory perception

[a]Nursing diagnoses are likely to progress so that most nursing diagnoses present at earlier stages will continue during later stages as well. Effective sensory perception (2019). Used with permission from *International Classification for Nursing Practice (ICNP®) Nursing Diagnosis and Outcome Statements.* International Council of Nurses.

common signs and symptoms, and potential nursing diagnoses for each stage (Garcia-Tsao, 2020).

Clinical Manifestations and Assessment

The earliest symptoms of hepatic encephalopathy include minor mental changes and motor disturbances. The patient appears slightly confused and unkempt and has alterations in mood and sleep patterns. The patient tends to sleep during the day and have restlessness and insomnia at night. As hepatic encephalopathy progresses, the patient may become difficult to awaken, eventually resulting in coma (Garcia-Tsao, 2020).

Asterixis (flapping tremor of the hands) may occur (Fig. 24-10). Simple tasks, such as handwriting, become difficult. A handwriting or drawing sample (e.g., star figure), taken daily, may provide graphic evidence of progression or reversal of hepatic encephalopathy; *constructional apraxia* is the inability to reproduce a simple figure (Fig. 24-11). In the early stages of hepatic encephalopathy, the deep tendon reflexes are hyperactive; with worsening of the encephalopathy, these

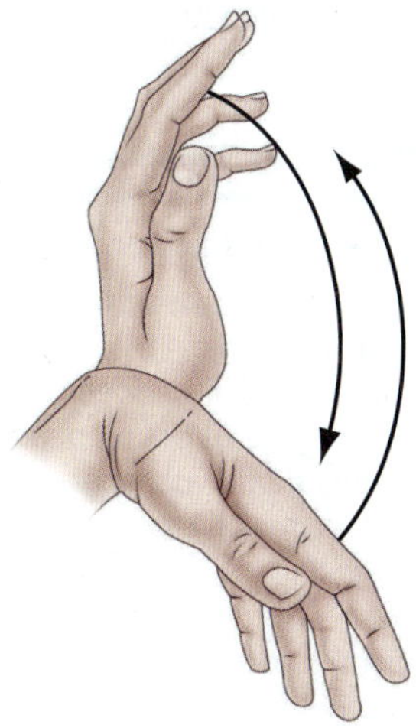

FIGURE 24-10 Asterixis or "liver flap" may occur in hepatic encephalopathy. The patient is asked to hold the arm out with the hand held upward (dorsiflexed). Within a few seconds, the hand falls forward involuntarily and then quickly returns to the dorsiflexed position.

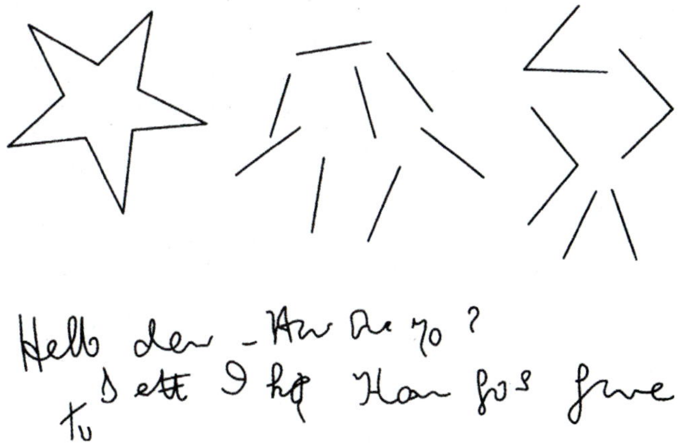

FIGURE 24-11 Effects of constructional apraxia. Deterioration of handwriting and inability to draw a simple star figure occurs with progressive hepatic encephalopathy. (With permission from Sherlock, S., & Dooley, J. [2002]. *Diseases of the liver and biliary system* [11th ed.]. Blackwell Scientific Ltd.)

reflexes disappear and the extremities may become flaccid (Mehta & Fallon, 2021).

The electroencephalogram (EEG) shows generalized slowing, an increase in the amplitude of brain waves, and characteristic triphasic waves (Garcia-Tsao, 2020). Occasionally, **fetor hepaticus**, a sweet, slightly fecal odor to the breath that is presumed to be of intestinal origin, may be noticed. The odor also has been described like freshly mowed grass, acetone, or old wine. Fetor hepaticus is prevalent with extensive collateral portal circulation in chronic liver disease. In a more advanced stage, there are gross disturbances of consciousness and the patient is completely disoriented with respect to time and place (Garcia-Tsao, 2020; Martin, 2020; McGee, 2018; Mehta & Fallon, 2021).

Medical Management

Medical management of hepatic encephalopathy focuses on identifying and correcting the precipitating cause if possible. Common triggering causes include GI bleeding, infection (including SBP, pulmonary, urinary tract infections), hypokalemia and/or metabolic alkalosis, kidney failure, hypovolemia, hypoxia, sedatives or tranquilizers, hypoglycemia and constipation (Ferenci, 2022). Lactulose is administered to reduce serum ammonia levels. It acts by several mechanisms that promote the excretion of ammonia in the stool:

- Ammonia is kept in the ionized state, resulting in a decrease in colon pH, reversing the normal passage of ammonia from the colon to the blood.
- Evacuation of the bowel takes place, which decreases the ammonia absorbed from the colon.
- Fecal flora are changed to organisms that do not produce ammonia from urea.

Two or three soft stools per day are desirable; this indicates that lactulose is performing as intended.

Possible side effects include intestinal bloating and cramps, which usually disappear within a week. To mask the sweet taste, which some patients dislike, lactulose can be diluted with fruit juice. The patient is monitored closely for hypokalemia (due to GI loss of potassium) and dehydration. Other laxatives are not prescribed during lactulose administration because their effects disturb dosage regulation. Lactulose may be administered by nasogastric (NG) tube or retention enema (held for 30 to 60 minutes) for patients who are comatose or for those in whom oral administration is contraindicated or impossible (Clinical Overview, 2021; Mehta & Fallon, 2021).

Pearls for Practice

The patient receiving lactulose is monitored closely for the development of watery diarrheal stools because they indicate a medication overdose.

The addition of antibiotic therapy to alter the intestinal flora and reduce nitrogenous waste from the gut can be used as adjunct therapy to lactulose. Agents such as rifaximin and neomycin have been used; only short-term use (5 to 6 days) of neomycin is recommend due to possible ototoxicity due to eighth cranial nerve toxicity (Clinical Overview, 2021).

Other aspects of management include IV administration of glucose to minimize protein breakdown, administration of vitamins to correct deficiencies, and correction of electrolyte imbalances (especially potassium). Additional principles of management of hepatic encephalopathy include the following (Garcia-Tsao, 2020; Woreta & Mezina, 2020):

- Therapy is directed toward treating or removing the cause.
- Neurologic status is assessed frequently.
- Mental status is monitored by keeping a daily record of handwriting and arithmetic performance.
- Fluid intake and output and body weight are recorded each day.
- Vital signs are measured and recorded every 4 hours.
- Potential sites of infection (peritoneum, lungs, urine) are assessed frequently, and abnormal findings are reported promptly.
- Serum ammonia level is monitored.
- Protein intake is moderately restricted in patients who are comatose or who have encephalopathy that is refractory to lactulose and antibiotic therapy (Box 24-2).
- Reduction in the absorption of ammonia from the GI tract is accomplished using gastric suction, enemas, or oral antibiotics.
- Electrolyte status is monitored and corrected if abnormal.
- Sedatives, tranquilizers, and analgesic medications are discontinued.
- Benzodiazepine antagonists, such as flumazenil, may be administered to improve encephalopathy, whether or not the patient has taken benzodiazepines previously.

Nursing Management

The nurse is responsible for maintaining a safe environment to prevent injury, bleeding, and infection. The nurse

BOX 24-2 Pearls for Practice: Nutrition

Management of Hepatic Encephalopathy

- Prevent the formation and absorption of toxins, principally ammonia, from the intestine.
- Keep daily protein intake between 1.2 and 1.5 g/kg, depending on the degree of decompensation.
- Avoid protein restriction if possible, even in those with encephalopathy. If necessary, implement temporary restriction of 0.5–0.8 g/kg.
- For patients who are truly protein-intolerant, provide additional nitrogen in the form of an amino acid supplement. Use of branched-chain amino acids is still controversial.
- Provide small, frequent meals and an evening snack of complex carbohydrates to avoid protein loading.
- Substitute vegetable protein for animal protein in as high a percentage as possible.

administers the prescribed treatments and monitors the patient for the numerous potential complications. The nurse also communicates with the patient's family to inform them about the patient's status, and supports them by explaining the procedures and treatments that are part of the patient's care. If the patient recovers from hepatic encephalopathy and coma, rehabilitation will likely be prolonged. Therefore, the patient and family will need assistance to understand this severe complication's causes and recognize that it may recur.

Vitamin Deficiency

Decreased production of several clotting factors may be partly due to deficient absorption of vitamin K from the GI tract. This probably is caused by the inability of liver cells to use vitamin K to make prothrombin. Absorption of the other fat-soluble vitamins (vitamins A, D, and E), as well as dietary fats, may also be impaired because of decreased secretion of bile salts into the intestine (Mehta & Fallon, 2021; Squires & Balistreri, 2021).

Another group of problems common to patients with severe chronic liver dysfunction results from inadequate intake of sufficient vitamins. These include the following:

- Vitamin A deficiency, resulting in night blindness and eye and skin changes
- Thiamine deficiency, leading to beriberi, polyneuritis, and Wernicke–Korsakoff psychosis
- Riboflavin deficiency, resulting in characteristic lesions of the skin and mucous membrane
- Vitamin B_6 deficiency, resulting in lesions of the skin and mucous membrane and neurologic changes
- Vitamin C deficiency, resulting in hemorrhagic lesions of scurvy
- Vitamin K deficiency, resulting in hypoprothrombinemia, characterized by spontaneous bleeding and ecchymosis
- Folic acid deficiency, resulting in macrocytic anemia

Because of these avitaminoses (vitamin deficiencies), the diet of patients with chronic liver disease (especially if alcohol-related) is supplemented with vitamins (Hall & Hall, 2021; Pham & McClave, 2021).

Pearls for Practice

Patients with liver disease frequently have abnormal bleeding times. If the prolonged prothrombin time (PT) is due to a vitamin K deficiency, generally, the PT will normalize within 24 to 48 hours after parenteral repletion. However, suppose the etiology of the prolonged PT is due to decreased synthesis of clotting factors (which is reflective of hepatocyte dysfunction). In that case, there may be little or no response to vitamin K (Berk & Korenblat, 2020).

Other Manifestations

Patients with advanced chronic liver disease and cirrhosis will frequently develop other systemic complications, such as altered respiratory or cardiac function, resulting from hepatopulmonary syndrome (HPS) and renal function hepatorenal syndrome (HRS). HPS symptoms include exertional dyspnea, clubbing, and cyanosis; vascular spiders may be observed on physical examination. HPS is related to pulmonary capillary dilatation. Usually one red blood cell fits through the pulmonary capillary, facilitating oxygenation; with pulmonary dilation, many RBCs are passing through the capillary, resulting in a large number of red cells that are not oxygenated. This is equivalent of a right-to-left shunt where the deoxygenated blood from the right side of the heart flows into the left side bypassing the lungs (see Chapter 9). HRS is a type of prerenal kidney injury that occurs in patients with cirrhosis and ascites. It is the result of maximal peripheral vasodilation and maximal activation of hormones that cause the retention of sodium and water and intense vasoconstriction of the renal arteries (Garcia-Tsao, 2020).

Hematologic abnormalities in patients with cirrhosis are common due to a decrease in clotting factors, resulting from vitamin K deficiency, decreased platelets (thrombocytopenia), anemia, and decreased white cells (neutropenia). The patient with cirrhosis will demonstrate easy bruising and bleeding and increased susceptibility to infection (Garcia-Tsao, 2020). Endocrine dysfunction in the regulation of glucose control and altered synthesis of sex hormones by the liver result in gynecomastia, testicular atrophy, and decreased libido and impotence in males. Females may have irregular or absent menstrual cycles and decreased sexual function as well.

VIRAL HEPATITIS

Viral hepatitis is a systemic, viral infection in which necrosis and inflammation of liver cells produce a characteristic cluster of clinical, biochemical, and cellular changes. To date, several types of viral hepatitis have been identified: hepatitis A, B, C, D, and E (Pawlotsky, 2020a) (Table 24-3). Hepatitis G virus was identified in the late 1990s and little is known about it, although it is transmitted sexually and through blood (Buttaro, 2021). It is also possible that HGV infection can be transmitted from the mother to the fetus via the placenta however evidence suggests it does not cause hepatitis in humans and is prevalent as a coinfection in people who have chronic hepatitis B or hepatitis C infections, and it is associated with acute and chronic liver disease (Mehta & Reddivari, 2022). As yet there is no test or treatment for it (Buttaro, 2021). These viruses infect the liver and can result in either acute or chronic liver dysfunction and disease. Initial presentation of viral hepatitis may be asymptomatic or result in fulminant liver failure or chronic liver disease. Patients may have nonspecific symptoms of malaise, GI distress, or present with frank jaundice and elevations of aminotransferases (Pawlotsky, 2020a). Terms associated with viral hepatitis are listed in Box 24-3.

TABLE **24-3 Comparison of Major Forms of Viral Hepatitis**

	Hepatitis A	Hepatitis B	Hepatitis C	Hepatitis D	Hepatitis E
Previous Names	Infectious hepatitis	Serum hepatitis	Non-A, non-B hepatitis		
Epidemiology					
Cause	Hepatitis A virus (HAV)	Hepatitis B virus (HBV)	Hepatitis C virus (HCV)	Hepatitis D virus (HDV)	Hepatitis E virus (HEV)
Mode of transmission	Fecal–oral route; poor sanitation. Person-to-person contact Waterborne; foodborne Transmission possible with oral–anal contact during sex	Parenterally; by intimate contact with carriers or those with acute disease; sexual and oral–oral contact Perinatal transmission from mothers to infants An important occupational hazard for health care personnel	Transfusion of blood and blood products; exposure to contaminated blood through equipment or drug paraphernalia Transmission possible with sex with infected partner; risk increased with STD	Same as HBV HBV surface antigen necessary for replication; pattern similar to that of hepatitis B	Fecal–oral route; person-to-person contact may be possible, although risk appears low
Incubation (days)	14–35 days	60–150 days	14–160 days	21–140 days	14–65 days
Immunity	Average: 30 days Homologous	Average: 70–80 days Homologous	Average: 50 days Second attack may indicate weak immunity or infection with another agent.	Average: 35 days Homologous	Average: 42 days Unknown
Nature of Illness					
Signs and symptoms	May occur with or without symptoms; flulike illness *Preicteric phase:* Headache, malaise, fatigue, anorexia, fever *Icteric phase:* Dark urine, jaundice of sclera and skin, tender liver	May occur without symptoms May develop arthralgias, rash	Similar to HBV; less severe and anicteric	Similar to HBV	Similar to HAV; very severe in pregnant females
Outcome	Usually mild with recovery. Fatality rate: less than 1% No carrier state or increased risk of chronic hepatitis, cirrhosis, or hepatic cancer	May be severe. Fatality rate: 1–10%. Carrier state possible Increased risk of chronic hepatitis, cirrhosis, and hepatic cancer	Frequent occurrence of chronic carrier state and chronic liver disease Increased risk of hepatic cancer	Similar to HBV but greater likelihood of carrier state, chronic active hepatitis, and cirrhosis	Similar to HAV except very severe in pregnant females

BOX 24-3

Hepatitis Terms and Abbreviations

Hepatitis A	
HAV	Hepatitis A virus; etiologic agent of hepatitis A (formerly infectious hepatitis)
IgG anti-HAV IgM anti-HAV	Antibody to hepatitis A virus; appears in serum soon after onset of symptoms; persists indefinitely, indicates lifelong immunity: IgM antibody to HAV; indicates recent infection with HAV; positive up to 6 months after infection
Hepatitis B	
HBV	Hepatitis B virus; etiologic agent of hepatitis B (formerly serum hepatitis)
HBsAG	Hepatitis B surface antigen (Australian antigen); indicates acute or chronic hepatitis B or carrier state; indicates infectious state
Anti-HBs	Antibody to hepatitis B surface antigen; indicates prior exposure and immunity to hepatitis; may indicate passive antibody from HBIG or immune response from hepatitis B vaccine
HBeAg	Hepatitis B e-antigen; present in serum early in course; indicates highly infectious stage of hepatitis B; persistence in serum indicates progression to chronic hepatitis
Anti-HBe	Antibody to hepatitis B e-antigen; suggests low titer of HBV
HBcAg	Hepatitis B core antigen; found in liver cells; not easily detected in serum
Anti-HBc	Antibody to hepatitis B core antigen; most sensitive indicator of hepatitis B; appears late in the acute phase of the disease; indicates infection of HBV at some time in the past
IgM anti-HBc	IgM antibody to HBcAg; present for up to 6 months after HBV infection
Hepatitis C	
HCV	Hepatitis C virus (formerly non-A, non-B virus); may be more than one virus
Hepatitis D	
HDV	Hepatitis D virus (delta agent); etiologic agent to hepatitis D; HBV required for replication
HDAg	Hepatitis delta antigen; detectable in early acute HDV infection
Anti-HDV	Antibody to HDV; indicates past or present infection with HDV
Hepatitis E	
HEV	Hepatitis E virus; etiologic agent of hepatitis E

Hepatitis A Virus

Pathophysiology

The mode of transmission of hepatitis A virus (HAV) occurs through the fecal–oral route, primarily through person-to-person contact and/or ingestion of fecally contaminated food or water. Uncooked food or poor food-handling practices are common methods of transmission of HAV.

HAV replicates in the liver, is excreted in bile, and is shed in the stool. The incubation period is 2 to 4 weeks, with signs and symptoms typically lasting less than 2 months (although in some patients, these can extend up to 6 months). The peak period for transmission of HAV from one person to another occurs in the 2-week period prior to development of jaundice or symptoms, when the concentration of virus in the stool is highest (Sjogren & Cheatham, 2021). Typically, persons infected with HAV spontaneously recover; however, adults over 50 years of age or those with chronic liver disease may progress to fulminant liver failure (Pawlotsky, 2020).

Clinical Manifestations and Assessment

Infection by HAV can present either asymptomatically or with acute symptoms such as fever, malaise, anorexia, nausea, diarrhea, vomiting, abdominal pain, and jaundice. Jaundice presents in over 70% of patients, primarily in adults. Serologic testing is required for accurate diagnosis of hepatitis A infection. A positive anti-HAV (IgM) signifies serum IgM antibodies that are reactive to the HAV and confirms an acute infection.

Anti-HAV (IgG) becomes positive shortly after the onset of infection, will remain positive throughout the person's life, and confers immunity. Total positive anti-HAV and negative anti-HAV (IgM) indicate exposure or vaccination (Pawlotsky, 2020a).

Prevention

Current recommendations to prevent the transmission of HAV are to vaccinate all children routinely, to identify and vaccinate persons at high risk for contracting HAV, and to vaccinate any person who wishes to prevent HAV (Pawlotsky, 2020).

At-risk persons who should be vaccinated include:

- Travelers or visitors to countries with increased incidence of HAV (Mexico, Latin America, Africa, Middle East, Asia, India)
- Men having sex with men
- Intravenous drug use

- Persons with occupational risk (e.g., research with primates or HAV in laboratory settings)
- Persons with chronic liver disease
- Persons with HIV infection
- Persons experiencing homelessness
- Persons who are incarcerated
- Persons living in group setting for those with developmental disabilities
- Adults >40 years

Active immunization for HAV is through vaccination with hepatitis A antigen in two dose schedules and is administered intramuscularly in the deltoid muscle. Passive immunization is achieved through administration of immune globulin–containing hepatitis A antibodies to persons for prophylaxis after exposure to the virus. Its use is indicated for patients with no evidence of immunity (Nelson & Advisory Committee on Immunization Practices [ACIP], 2020).

Box 24-4 discusses community prevention of hepatitis A.

Medical Management

Acute HAV infection in most patients is managed with supportive care. The patient may experience decreased appetite due to alterations in GI function. Dehydration should be prevented; if necessary, IV fluids may be administered. Patients can participate in physical activity as tolerated. Signs and symptoms indicating possible fulminant liver failure, such as altered mental status or severe vomiting, should be identified promptly with referral to a liver transplant center (Sjogren & Cheatham, 2021).

Nursing Management

Management usually occurs in the home unless symptoms are severe. Therefore, the nurse assists the patient and family in coping with the temporary disability and fatigue that are common in hepatitis and instructs them to seek additional health care if the symptoms persist or worsen. The patient and family also need specific guidelines about diet, rest, follow-up blood work, and the importance of avoiding alcohol, as well as sanitation and hygiene measures (particularly hand washing after bowel movements and before eating) to prevent spread of the disease to other family members, environmental sanitation (safe food and water supply, effective sewage disposal), proper food storage, and thorough cooking of foods to recommended temperatures.

BOX 24-4 Community Prevention of Hepatitis A

- Proper community and home sanitation
- Conscientious individual hygiene with emphasis on handwashing
- Safe practices for preparing and dispensing food
- Effective health supervision of schools, dormitories, extended-care facilities, barracks, and camps
- Community health education programs
- Mandatory reporting of viral hepatitis to local health departments
- Vaccination for travelers to developing countries, injection and noninjection drug use, men who have sex with men (MSM), and persons with chronic liver disease
- Vaccination to interrupt community-wide outbreaks
- Travelers to hepatitis A–endemic countries should be advised to eat only properly cooked food, avoid uncooked vegetables and shellfish, and consume only treated or purified water and ice (Averhoff et al., 2020).

HEPATITIS B VIRUS

Hepatitis B virus (HBV) infection is an important global public health problem with as many as 4 billion people worldwide chronically infected. HBV has caused 880,000 deaths due to hepatocellular carcinoma (HCC) and cirrhosis (Suzuki & Sakamoto, 2020).

Pathophysiology

HBV is transmitted primarily through blood (percutaneous and mucosal routes). HBV can be found in blood, saliva, and semen and can be transmitted through mucous membranes and breaks in the skin. HBV is also transferred from carrier mothers to their babies, especially in areas with a high incidence (Pawlotsky, 2020a). HBV is primarily transmitted by perinatal, percutaneous, sexual exposure, and close person-to-person contact via contact with open cuts or sores or by use of shared razors or toothbrushes. HBV-contaminated surfaces also are possible sources of infection as the virus can survive outside of the body for extended periods (Pawlotsky, 2020a).

HBV has a long incubation period. It replicates in the liver and remains in the serum for relatively long periods, allowing transmission of the virus. More than 95% of those who contract HBV infection develop antibodies and recover spontaneously (Pawlotsky, 2020a). The risk of developing chronic HBV infection is significantly higher in persons from endemic countries and when infected from birth (e.g., chronicity rate higher than 95% among patients infected at birth) (Pawlotsky, 2020a). Acute HBV infection can result in fulminant liver failure or progress to chronic infection. Patients with chronic HBV infection eventually may develop cirrhosis, end-stage liver disease, and cancer of the liver (Pawlotsky, 2020a; Terrault et al., 2018).

Risk Factors

Those at risk for development of hepatitis B include individuals born in areas with high rates of HBV infection. Risk factors for HBV infection are summarized in Box 24-5 (Pawlotsky, 2020a).

Clinical Manifestations and Assessment

Signs and symptoms of acute hepatitis B may be insidious and variable. The patient may have anorexia, sleep

BOX 24-5
Risk Factors for Hepatitis B

- Frequent exposure to blood, blood products, or other body fluids
- Being a health care worker: hemodialysis staff, oncology and chemotherapy nurses, personnel at risk for needlesticks, operating room staff, respiratory therapists, surgeons, dentists
- Birth (mother to baby during childbirth)
- Hemodialysis
- Men who have sex with men (MSM) and bisexual activity
- IV/injection drug use
- Close contact with carrier of HBV
- Travel to or residence in area with uncertain sanitary conditions
- Multiple sexual partners
- Recent history of sexually transmitted disease
- Receipt of blood or blood products (e.g., clotting factor concentrate)

disturbances, fevers, dyspepsia, pain in the upper right quadrant, generalized aching, malaise, and weakness. Jaundice may or may not be evident. Skin rashes and arthralgias (pain in the joints) may occur (Thio & Hawkins, 2020). Chronic hepatitis B may remain largely asymptomatic until the development of cirrhosis and signs of hepatic decompensation (Pawlotsky, 2020).

The evaluation of a patient with HBV infection includes a complete history and physical examination, a family history of liver disease, and potential risk factors for disease transmission.

Laboratory testing should include complete blood counts (CBC with platelets), hepatic function panel, and prothrombin time and international normalized ratio (INR). Laboratory tests to detect hepatitis B replication and other viral coinfections (HAV, HCV, HIV) should be included in the assessment (Terrault et al., 2018).

Prevention

The goals of prevention are to interrupt the chain of transmission, to protect people who are at high risk by active immunization through the use of hepatitis B vaccine, and to use passive immunization for unprotected people exposed to HBV (Terrault et al., 2018).

Preventing Transmission

Recommendations to prevent transmission of hepatitis B include vaccination of sexual contacts of individuals with chronic hepatitis B, use of barrier protection during sexual intercourse, avoidance of sharing toothbrushes and razors with others, and covering of open sores or skin lesions. Blood spills should be cleaned with bleach diluted to a 10:1 concentration. Persons with HBV infection should be advised to avoid donation of blood, organs, or sperm.

Active Immunization: Hepatitis B Vaccine

The most effective strategy to prevent hepatitis B infection is through vaccination. Current prevention recommendations include

- All infants and persons aged 0 to 59 years
- Adults aged ≥60 with risk factors for hepatitis B:
  - Persons at risk by sexual exposure (partner positive, multiple sex partners, persons seeking treatment for sexually transmitted infection, men who have sex with men (MSM))
  - Persons at risk for infection by percutaneous or mucosal exposure to blood (injection drug use, positive household contacts, residents and staff members of facilities for persons with developmental disabilities, health care and public safety personnel, patients on dialysis, patients with diabetes)
  - Others: International travelers, persons who are incarcerated, or persons with hepatitis C infection, chronic liver disease, or HIV infection

The hepatitis B vaccine series is administered in three doses intramuscularly: the initial injection, then 1-month, and 6-month intervals for adults (Weng & ACIP, 2022). For those who do not respond to the first series, revaccination is suggested and effective in 80% of individuals (Ledoux, 2022).

Pearls for Practice

The U.S. Food and Drug Administration (FDA) has approved a combined vaccine for both hepatitis A and B (Twinrix) for vaccination of people 18 years of age and older with indications for both hepatitis A and B vaccination. Vaccination consists of three doses on the same schedule as that used for single-antigen hepatitis B vaccine (Weng & ACIP, 2022).

Passive Immunity: Hepatitis B Hyperimmune Globulin

Hepatitis B hyperimmune globulin (HBIG) provides passive immunity to hepatitis B and is indicated for people exposed to HBV who have never had hepatitis B, who have had sexual exposure, infants who have had exposure at birth, and those who have never received hepatitis B vaccine. A second dose of HBIG is given in 1 month for those refusing vaccine, those who have not been vaccinated or vaccine nonresponders (Gold Standard 2019; Thio & Hawkins, 2020). It has demonstrated efficacy in the prevention of HBV infection in high-risk persons (exposure to blood-containing HBV, sexual partners of patients with hepatitis B, and newborn infants of HBsAg-positive mothers) (Gold Standard, 2019).

Medical Management

The goals of treatment for hepatitis B are to prevent replication of active HBV (viral suppression) and reduce the effects of chronic liver inflammation. The ultimate goal of medical management of hepatitis B is to prevent cirrhosis, liver failure, and HCC (Pawlotsky, 2020a). Multiple antiviral therapies are available to treat hepatitis B; of these, pegylated interferon alfa, adefovir, entecavir, telbivudine, lamivudine, and tenofovir are the preferred medications, either as single agents or in combination. Patients with HBV infection should have periodic laboratory testing to assess elevations in liver function and replication of HBV DNA. Patients at high risk for HCC (discussed later in this chapter), including patients with cirrhosis, should receive ultrasound screening every 6 months (Terrault et al., 2018).

Nursing Management

In patients with acute hepatitis B, management of the symptoms of malaise, anorexia, nausea, vomiting, and fever primarily is supportive to maintain nutrition, fluid intake, and adequate rest during recovery. The nurse must be vigilant for signs of progression to fulminant liver failure (discussed later in the chapter); however, alterations in mental status, severe vomiting, and increasing jaundice should initiate referral to a tertiary care center or liver transplant center. In patients with chronic hepatitis B, the nursing role is geared to patient education in the prevention of transmission and avoidance of lifestyle factors that may exacerbate existing liver disease.

HEPATITIS C VIRUS

Hepatitis C virus (HCV) infection is the leading cause of liver disease and is the primary indication for liver transplantation (Pawlotsky, 2020a). With the advent of direct-acting antiviral agents (DAAs), HCV is the only known curable chronic viral infection. Although blood screening prevention measures for those who use injectable drugs have significantly impacted infection rates in industrialized countries, HCV remains endemic throughout the world (Adinolfi et al., 2020; Holmes & Chung, 2021; Pawlotsky, 2020a).

Pathophysiology

HCV is a blood-borne RNA virus and is avidly replicated in the liver. Transmission of hepatitis C occurs primarily through injection of drugs and through transfusion of blood products prior to 1992. Its route is through parenteral contact with blood. Sexual transmission also may occur, with high risk associated with multiple sex partners. Other less common modes of transmission include via hemodialysis, health care worker exposure to needlestick injury or contaminated blood, and tattooing (AASLD/IDSA HCV Guidance Panel, 2018; Pawlotsky, 2020a). Box 24-6 summarizes risk factors for hepatitis C.

BOX 24-6

Risk Factors for Hepatitis C

- Receiving blood products or organ transplant before 1992 or clotting factor concentrates before 1987
- Being a health care or public safety worker (needlestick injuries or mucosal exposure to blood)
- Being a child born to a female infected with hepatitis C virus
- Past/current illicit IV/injection drug use
- Past treatment with chronic hemodialysis
- Multiple sex partners, history of sexually transmitted disease, unprotected sex

Patients infected with this virus spontaneously clear the acute infection in 20% to 50% of cases; the majority of individuals will develop chronic infection, with evidence of hepatitis C RNA viremia (presence of virus in the blood) (Pawlotsky, 2020b). Unlike other hepatitis viruses, the acute stage of hepatitis C often is asymptomatic for decades. Hepatitis C infection with progression to cirrhosis occurs in up to 20% of patients over a period of 20 years or longer if untreated. Factors contributing to the severity of liver disease include increased alcohol use, male gender, older age at infection, HIV or HBV coinfection, and obesity (AASLD/IDSA HCV Guidance Panel, 2018; Pawlotsky, 2020b). Individuals with HCV cirrhosis are at higher risk of developing hepatic decompensation and HCC, and in industrialized countries, hepatitis C remains the most common cause of HCC (Pawlotsky, 2020b).

Pearls for Practice

Nurse should educate patients that if they drink alcohol on a regular basis, they should consume no more than 3,000 mg of acetaminophen a day (Rosenthal & Rosenjack Burchum, 2021), and lower doses may be advised if liver fibrosis or cirrhosis is present.

Clinical Manifestations and Assessment

Most patients with acute or chronic hepatitis C are asymptomatic. Some patients will develop jaundice, nausea, vomiting, and malaise during the acute stage (Pawlotsky, 2020a). Patients with chronic hepatitis C frequently will be diagnosed incidentally during routine laboratory testing or not until cirrhosis develops. Extrahepatic signs of hepatitis C are common, such as skin rashes, joint aches, and purpura (small blood vessels leaking under the skin and causing purple bruising) (Pawlotsky, 2020a).

The diagnosis of HCV infection is confirmed by serology with anti-HCV antibodies present and measurement of viremia through HCV RNA. Genotype testing and liver biopsy will provide information to assist in the management and treatment of hepatitis C as well as to stage the severity of disease. Other tests to assess the extent of liver disease include laboratory tests (i.e., bilirubin, sodium, albumin, aminotransferases, prothrombin time, and INR). Ultrasound or other imaging may be used to assess for cirrhosis or the presence of lesions (AASLD/IDSA HCV Guidance Panel, 2018; Hou et al., 2020; Naggie & Wyles, 2020).

Medical and Nursing Management

Treatment of hepatitis C aims to reduce mortality by preventing the progression of fibrosis and evolution to cirrhosis by reducing HCV RNA levels to nondetectable levels. A nondetectable viral load or HCV RNA 12 weeks after completion of therapy is considered curative. This is called a *sustained viral response (SVR)*. New antiviral therapies with direct acting agents (DAAs), called protease inhibitors, have revolutionized treatment of hepatitis C. Use of these drugs and drug combinations is evolving rapidly, resulting in SVR in genotypes or comorbidities that previously had been difficult to treat. Clinical trial evidence has demonstrated protease inhibitor therapy is well tolerated with less to no symptomatic complaints from patients during treatment course unlike its predecessor, pegylated interferon, given weekly by injection and associated with many side effects (AASLD/IDSA HCV Guidance Panel, 2018; Pawlotsky, 2020b). The specific protease inhibitor or drug combination, dosage, and length of therapy are determined by HCV genotype, history or prior HCV treatment, and presence of cirrhosis and level of decompensation. Patients who previously failed therapy with interferon and/or other types of protease inhibitors and patients with recurrent HCV after liver transplant are eligible to receive alternative regimens in hopes of achieving SVR as well. Patients are monitored with serum laboratory testing, including CBC, metabolic panel, hepatic function panel, and HCV viral load testing at prescribed intervals in conjunction with telephone and monitoring visits to evaluate adherence, tolerance, and compliance (AASLD/IDSA HCV Guidance Panel, 2018; Naggie & Wyles, 2020).

It is important for the nurse to educate the patient with hepatitis C to avoid sharing razors, toothbrushes, nail clippers with sexual partners and family members and discuss the importance of safe sexual practices including barrier contraception as they await SVR (Dienstag, 2020).

HEPATITIS D VIRUS

Hepatitis D virus (delta agent) (HDV) infection occurs in some cases of hepatitis B. Because the virus requires hepatitis B surface antigen for its replication, only individuals with hepatitis B are at risk for hepatitis D. Anti-HDV antibodies (IGg) in patients with chronic hepatitis B confirms the diagnosis (Blum, 2020; Pawlotsky, 2020b).

The symptoms of hepatitis D are similar to those of hepatitis B, however these patients are more likely to develop fulminant hepatitis and to progress to chronic active hepatitis and cirrhosis. Current treatment for hepatitis D is the use of interferon or pegylated interferon alfa for 12 months (Pawlotsky, 2026b).

HEPATITIS E VIRUS

It is believed that hepatitis E virus (HEV) is transmitted by the fecal–oral route, principally through contaminated water in endemic areas with poor sanitation. This form of hepatitis usually is self-limiting, with acute onset and subsequent recovery with no chronicity. HEV is responsible for most cases of fulminant hepatitis in India. Pregnant persons infected with hepatitis E infection have a high mortality rate (between 15% and 25%); this is increased during the last trimester (Aggarwal, 2021; Blum, 2020). Currently, there is no vaccine or specific treatment for HEV; however, research in vaccine development may be promising in the near future.

Prevention of transmission is focused on improvement of sanitation, development of clean water supplies in endemic countries, and safe food-handling practices (Pawlotsky, 2020a).

NONVIRAL HEPATITIS

Liver inflammation and disease can be caused by nonviral etiologies, such as toxins, infections, alcoholic overuse, and autoimmune disorders.

ALCOHOLIC LIVER DISEASE (ALCOHOLIC HEPATITIS)

Excessive ingestion or abuse of alcohol is a common cause of acute hepatitis, and chronic use results in cirrhosis. Alcoholic liver disease (ALD) is a major public health problem and accounts for approximately 44% of deaths related to cirrhosis of the liver. It is estimated that fatty liver results from alcohol in 80% to 90% of heavy drinkers, while 30% to 40% of that population progress toward more problematic forms of liver disease, such as fibrosis, cirrhosis, and HCC (Chalasani, 2020; Szabo & McClain, 2021).

The impact of alcohol ingestion upon the liver is dose-dependent; females will develop advanced liver disease at lower amounts of alcohol than will males. Other cofactors contributing to the development of cirrhosis in ALD is hepatitis C infection, smoking, and obesity. The amount of alcohol consumed to result in significant liver disease is 20 to 40 g of alcohol daily in females and 40 to 80 g of alcohol daily in males over a 10- to 12-year period (Clinical Overview, 2022; Szabo & McClain, 2021). Those with ALD are often drinking about 15 drinks per day (Chalasani, 2020; Szabo & McClain, 2021).

Pathophysiology

Ethanol (alcohol) is metabolized by the liver by alcohol dehydrogenases, cytochrome P450, and catalase. The resultant product, acetaldehyde, is toxic to the liver, resulting in impairment of liver function and cells. Other factors contributing to the pathogenesis of ALD are oxidative stress, hypoxia or oxygen depletion of cells, and mitochondrial injury. Fatty infiltration of liver cells (hepatic steatosis) is a common finding in liver biopsies of patients with ALD (Chalasani, 2020; Vatsalya & Hassan, 2020).

Clinical Manifestations and Assessment

Patients presenting with alcoholic hepatitis are universally jaundiced. The patient may have symptoms of anorexia, nausea, vomiting, and abdominal pain. Fever, muscle wasting, and *stigmata*—such as spider angiomas (Fig. 24-12) or palmar erythema (redness of the palm)—are common findings. The liver may be enlarged, or hard and small. The spleen will be enlarged, and late signs of hepatic decompensation may be evident, such as ascites, pedal edema, and hepatic encephalopathy (Chalasani, 2020).

There is no specific evaluation or test for the diagnosis of ALD; the clinical history and physical presence of liver disease correlated with information regarding alcohol overuse is diagnostic. An AST/ALT ratio of greater than two is a common finding in ALD (Chalasani, 2020; Szabo & McClain, 2021).

A complete history and physical examination is important in the assessment of patients with ALD. Patients should be screened for frequency, amount of alcohol use, type of alcohol, and patterns of alcohol use. Several evidence-based screening instruments for assessment of alcohol dependence exist, such as the CAGE and AUDIT tools to assist clinicians with detection and diagnosis (Szabo & McClain, 2021). Additional information regarding the negative impact of alcohol use upon employment, health (i.e., falls, fractures), or driving status provides more data to assess the extent of alcohol use (Martin, 2020; Szabo & McClain, 2021).

Pearls for Practice

CAGE (Cut down, Annoyed, Guilty, and Eye-opener)

Ask your patients these four questions and use the scoring method described below to determine if substance use disorder exists and needs to be addressed.

CAGE Questions

1. *Have you ever felt you should cut down on your drinking?*
2. *Have people annoyed you by criticizing your drinking?*
3. *Have you ever felt bad or guilty about your drinking?*
4. *Have you ever had a drink first thing in the morning to steady your nerves or to get rid of a hangover (eye-opener)?*

Scoring: Item responses on the CAGE questions are scored 0 for "no" and 1 for "yes" answers, with a higher score being an indication of alcohol problems. A total score of two or greater is considered clinically significant.

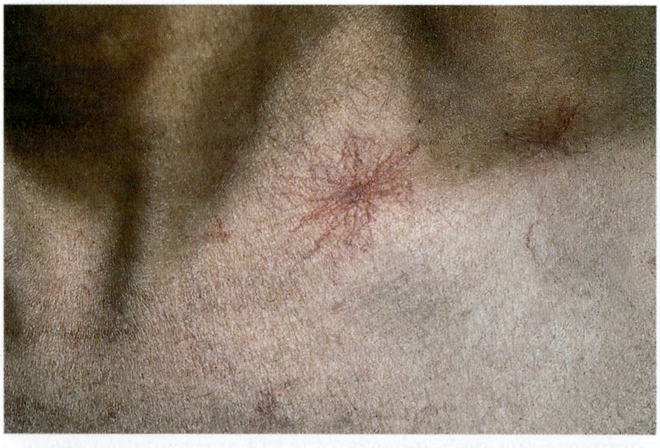

FIGURE 24-12 Spider angioma. This vascular (arterial) spider appears on the skin. Beneath the elevated center and radiating branches, the blood vessels are looped and tortuous.

Medical Management

The mainstay of treatment for ALD is abstinence from alcohol and either oral or enteral nutritional therapy. Patients with ALD frequently are malnourished, with depleted protein stores and vitamin deficiencies; the complex nutritional management of these patients is best suited to clinical nutritionists with expertise in this area. In patients with severe alcoholic hepatitis, prednisolone may be used. Clinical trials have demonstrated improved survival of patients treated for severe alcoholic hepatitis with corticosteroids; however, this remains only for select patients with severe ALD and is contraindicated in the presence of infection, bleeding, or renal impairment. Research on drugs to treat ALD is ongoing and broad (Szabo & McClain, 2021). Box 24-7 reviews dietary management appropriate for patients with hepatitis.

General management includes supportive care with adequate rest, correction of bleeding abnormalities, treatment of infection, and management of fluid overload. Providers trained in alcohol addiction and community resources should be employed once the patient is able to engage in therapy to maintain abstinence.

BOX 24-7 **Pearls for Practice: Nutrition**

Dietary Management of Viral or Drug-Related Hepatitis

- Recommend small, frequent meals.
- Provide intake of 2,000–3,000 kcal/day during acute illness.
- Although early studies indicate that a high-protein, high-calorie diet may be beneficial, advise patient not to force food and to restrict fat intake.
- Carefully monitor fluid balance.
- If anorexia and nausea and vomiting persist, enteral feedings may be necessary.
- Instruct patient to abstain from alcohol during acute illness and for at least 6 months after recovery.
- Advise patient to avoid substances (medications, herbs, illicit drugs, and toxins) that may affect liver function.

NONALCOHOLIC FATTY LIVER DISEASE (NAFLD)

NAFLD is becoming more widely known due to the growing problem with obesity in Western nations and as a component of metabolic syndrome (critical components of metabolic syndrome include hyperglycemia, dyslipidemia, abdominal obesity, and hypertension). The most common cause of transaminase elevation, it is also becoming the most common cause of chronic liver disease (Chalasani, 2020). Nonalcoholic steatohepatitis (NASH) is a more advanced form of NAFLD, that is characterized by macrovesicular steatosis, ballooning degeneration of the hepatocytes, and sinusoidal fibrosis (Chalasani, 2020). Patients diagnosed with NASH experience higher morbidity and mortality and will likely become the main indication for liver transplantation in the United States. Defined as macrovesicular fat accumulation in more than 5% of hepatocytes, NAFLD is likely the cause of most cases of cryptogenic cirrhosis (cirrhosis of uncertain etiology that lacks definitive clinical and histologic criteria), and is associated with better outcomes than alcoholic hepatitis although similar histologically (Torres & Harrison, 2021). A diagnosis of NASH and NAFLD is made in the absence of heavy use of alcohol or alcohol use disorder.

Pathophysiology

Hepatic steatosis results from abnormalities related to regulation of fatty acid metabolism in the liver resulting in steatosis, leaving the hepatocytes susceptible to additional insults from the environment or due to genetic abnormalities (Chalasani, 2020). Other conditions that may cause steatohepatitis include diabetes mellitus, dyslipidemia, obesity, starvation, various medications including cytotoxic and cytostatic drugs, metals, genetic disorders, and surgical procedures within the GI tract (Torres & Harrison, 2021).

Clinical Manifestations and Assessment

Presence of clinical symptoms in NAFLD are rare, however laboratory features of significantly increased ALT and AST may be present. Rarely, patients may experience vague abdominal pain or fatigue (Torres & Harrison, 2021). Routine serum chemistry tests with liver function analysis accompanied by antinuclear antibodies (ANA) should be drawn. Liver imaging studies with ultrasound (US), computed tomography (CT) or magnetic resonance imaging (MRI) will be ordered. Diagnosis of steatosis is easily made with imaging modalities and liver biopsy is rarely ordered solely for this purpose.

Medical Management

Modification of lifestyle with increased exercise and diet modification are prioritized in the treatment of NAFLD. Monitored weight loss according to established guidelines should first be attempted. Some patients may benefit from bariatric weight loss surgery. These patients may also see long-term improvement in liver biopsy findings following surgery, preventing progression of liver fibrosis and cirrhosis.

Medications commonly prescribed for their influence on improving signs of worsening NASH and NAFLD include Vitamin E, statins, and thiazolidinedione insulin sensitizers may be considered. As understanding of this disease process improves and clinical drug trials are underway, new medications currently under investigation may demonstrate significant improvement in efficacy and preventing disease (Chalasani, 2020).

DRUG-INDUCED LIVER DISEASE (DRUG-RELATED HEPATITIS)

Drug-induced hepatotoxicity is very common and can range from mild elevations in aminotransferases to fulminant liver failure due to ingestion or exposure to medications, toxins, or herbal remedies alone or in combination. It is the leading cause of acute liver failure in the United States and developed countries (Teschke & Danan, 2020).

Pathophysiology

Although any medication can affect liver function, use of acetaminophen (found in many over-the-counter medications used to treat fever and pain) has been identified as a leading cause of acute liver failure (Lee, 2020). Other medications commonly associated with liver injury include antibiotics, anticonvulsants, NSAIDs, and antituberculosis agents (Suzuki & Sakamoto, 2020).

Clinical Manifestations and Assessment

Manifestations of sensitivity to a medication may occur on the first day of its use or not until several months later, depending on the medication. Usually the onset is abrupt, with chills, fever, rash, pruritus, arthralgia, anorexia, and nausea. Later, there may be jaundice, dark urine, and an enlarged and tender liver (Lee, 2020; Teschke & Danan, 2020). After the offending medication is withdrawn, symptoms may subside gradually. However, reactions can be severe, or even fatal, even if the medication is stopped. If fever, rash, or pruritus occurs from any medication, its use should be stopped immediately. A thorough history of all medications, over-the-counter medications, and supplements should be obtained from all patients presenting with signs or symptoms of acute or chronic liver disease.

Medical and Nursing Management

The management of drug-induced liver injury includes discontinuation of the suspected medication or medications; evaluation of liver damage, including hospitalization if jaundice or impaired hepatic function is present; and, in cases of fulminant or acute liver failure, referral to a liver transplant center. Antidotes should be delivered if available. N-acetylcysteine is administered routinely in the setting of overdose of acetaminophen by restoring hepatic concentration of glutathione (Chitturi et al., 2021; Lewis, 2021). In acetaminophen overdose glutathione stores are depleted and once they are <30% of normal, irreversible hepatic necrosis occurs; N-acetylcysteine may be protective against liver toxicity if given within 8 hours after acetaminophen ingestion (Agrawal & Khazaeni, 2022).

Although its efficacy is uncertain, a short course of high-dose corticosteroids may be used in patients with severe hypersensitivity (Chitturi et al., 2021).

Pearls for Practice

The liver metabolizes many medications, such as barbiturates, opioids, sedative agents, anesthetics, and amphetamines. Metabolism generally results in inactivation of the medication, although in some cases activation of the medication may occur. One of the important pathways for medication metabolism involves conjugation (binding) of the medication with a variety of compounds to form more soluble substances that may be excreted in the feces or urine, similar to bilirubin excretion. Bioavailability is the fraction of the administered medication that actually reaches the systemic circulation. The bioavailability of an oral medication (absorbed from the GI tract) can be decreased if the medication is metabolized to a great extent by the liver before it reaches the systemic circulation; this is known as first-pass effect. Some medications have such a large first-pass effect that their use is limited essentially to the parenteral route, or oral doses must be substantially larger than parenteral doses to achieve the same effect. If medications are administered that have a high hepatic metabolism, bioavailability increases and hepatic clearance decreases in liver disease. It is important for the nurse to understand the clearance of medications and to observe patients for signs of further deterioration.

FULMINANT HEPATIC FAILURE

Fulminant hepatic failure is the clinical syndrome of sudden and severely impaired liver function in a previously healthy person.

Pathophysiology

Fulminant liver failure is caused by many different etiologies. Viral hepatitis caused by A, B, and E is a common culprit worldwide (O'Grady & Bernal, 2021). Acetaminophen overdose, drug-induced liver injury, viral and autoimmune hepatitis, metabolic disorders such as Wilson disease, poisonous mushroom ingestion, acute hepatic ischemia, obstruction to hepatic blood flow (**Budd–Chiari syndrome**), acute fatty liver of pregnancy, and infiltrating cancer are the most common causes of acute liver failure in the United States (Everson, 2020).

Clinical Manifestations and Assessment

The clinical manifestations of fulminant liver failure are **hepatic encephalopathy**, jaundice, nausea, anorexia, vomiting, and coagulopathy in a patient with no history of prior liver disease (Toma, 2020). The onset is abrupt, and the patient or family may or may not be able to identify the precipitating event.

Medical and Nursing Management

The clinical decision whether a patient will recover from acute liver injury with intense medical management or require liver transplantation typically is made on a case-by-case basis after careful evaluation of the patient. Multiple selection criteria have been developed to determine survival outcome (i.e., risk of death with or without transplant) and assist in the selection of patients appropriate for liver transplant, including time from jaundice to encephalopathy, prothrombin time, and levels of bilirubin, arterial pH, and creatinine (Everson, 2020).

Currently, in the United States, the United Network for Organ Sharing (UNOS) has defined criteria to determine which patients qualify for urgent transplant listing for fulminant liver failure:

- Onset of hepatic encephalopathy within 8 weeks of first symptoms of liver disease
- Absence of pre-existing liver disease
- Transaminases ALT/AST of greater than 3,000
- INR greater than 2.0

Patients may require one of the following interventions:

- Ventilator dependence
- Dialysis or continuous veno-venous hemofiltration (CVVH) or continuous veno-venous hemofiltration with dialysis (CVVD) (refer to Chapter 26)
- Care within an ICU

Patients with fulminant liver failure must have a life expectancy of less than 7 days without liver transplant to qualify for the highest active status for liver allocation, status 1A (United Network of Organ Sharing [UNOS], 2022).

The key to optimized treatment is rapid recognition of acute liver failure and intensive intervention. Supporting the patient in the ICU and assessing the indications for and feasibility of liver transplantation are hallmarks of management in this population. Often fulminant hepatic failure is accompanied by coagulation defects, kidney failure and electrolyte disturbances, cardiovascular abnormalities, infection, hypoglycemia, encephalopathy, and cerebral edema. The use of antidotes for certain conditions may be indicated, such as *N*-acetylcysteine for acetaminophen toxicity (Everson, 2020).

In patients who have fulminant liver failure with stage three (somnolent but can be aroused) or four (coma) encephalopathy, or elevated serum ammonia, there is a high risk for cerebral edema, a life-threatening complication. These patients may require intracranial pressure monitoring, with consideration for concomitant treatment of their coagulopathy. Measures to promote adequate cerebral perfusion include careful fluid balance and hemodynamic assessments, a quiet environment, and diuresis with mannitol, an osmotic diuretic. Use of barbiturate anesthesia or pharmacologic paralysis and sedation is indicated to prevent surges in intracranial pressure related to agitation. Other support measures include monitoring for and treating hypoglycemia, coagulopathy, kidney impairment, and infection. Despite these treatment modalities, the mortality rate remains high. Consequently, liver transplantation (discussed later) has become the treatment of choice for fulminant hepatic failure (Everson, 2020).

CIRRHOSIS

The most common causes of chronic liver disease are viral hepatitis B and C, ALD, nonalcoholic fatty liver disease (NAFLD), primary biliary cholangitis and autoimmune disorders of the liver. Primary biliary cholangitis (previously termed primary biliary cirrhosis) is a chronic, variably progressive disease characterized by autoimmune destruction of intralobular bile ducts leading to portal inflammation, hepatic cell necrosis, fibrosis, cirrhosis and, ultimately, liver failure (Smith & Ibrahim, 2022). Acute forms of liver dysfunction and failure can occur from viral agents, drug hepatotoxicity, toxins, parasites, or metabolic disorders, such as Wilson disease (Garcia-Tsao, 2020). The development of cirrhosis is the final stage of all chronic liver disease and is one of the leading causes of death in the United States (Garcia-Tsao, 2020; Kamath & Shah, 2021).

Pathophysiology

Cirrhosis of the liver occurs when the normal liver tissue is replaced by fibrotic tissue in response to damage to liver cells, resulting in accumulation of extracellular matrix or "scar." The progression from fibrosis to cirrhosis results in the loss of normal structure and function in the liver (Kamath & Shah, 2021). The progression and severity of chronic liver disease can be classified as either compensated or decompensated cirrhosis.

Clinical Manifestations and Assessment

Typically, compensated cirrhosis is asymptomatic. The transition from compensated cirrhosis to decompensated cirrhosis results in the development of jaundice, ascites, bleeding from esophageal varices, and hepatic encephalopathy. Box 24-8 provides guidelines for assessing cirrhosis. The development of any of these complications of hepatic dysfunction signals that the patient has progressed to decompensated cirrhosis. The hallmarks of decompensated cirrhosis are the development of jaundice, ascites (fluid collection in the peritoneum), pedal edema, gastroesophageal varices, and hepatic encephalopathy. Other complications, such as SBP, HRS (kidney dysfunction), and HPS (causes symptoms such as shortness of breath and hypoxemia) may occur as well (Garcia-Tsao, 2020).

BOX 24-8 **Focused Assessment**

Cirrhosis

Be alert for the following signs and symptoms:

Compensated Cirrhosis

- Intermittent mild fever
- Vascular spiders
- Palmar erythema (reddened palms)
- Unexplained epistaxis
- Ankle edema
- Vague morning indigestion
- Flatulent dyspepsia
- Abdominal pain
- Firm, enlarged liver
- Splenomegaly

Decompensated Cirrhosis

- Ascites
- Jaundice
- Weakness
- Muscle wasting
- Weight loss
- Continuous mild fever
- Clubbing of fingers
- Purpura (due to decreased platelet count)
- Spontaneous bruising
- Epistaxis
- Hypotension
- Sparse body hair
- White nails
- Gonadal atrophy

Medical Management

NURSING PROCESS
The Patient With Cirrhosis

ASSESSMENT

Nursing assessment focuses on the onset of symptoms and the history of precipitating factors, particularly long-term alcohol use, as well as dietary intake and changes in the patient's physical and mental status. The patient's past and current patterns of alcohol use (duration and amount) are assessed and documented (CAGE or AUDIT tools may be helpful). It is also important to document any exposure to toxic agents

(continued on page 840)

encountered in the workplace or during recreational activities. The nurse documents and reports exposure to potentially hepatotoxic substances, including medications, IV/injection drug use, inhalants, and general anesthetic agents.

The nurse assesses the patient's mental status during the interview and other interactions with the patient; orientation to person, place, and time is noted. The patient's ability to carry out a job or household activities provides some information about physical and mental status. The patient's relationships with family, friends, and coworkers may give some indication about incapacitation secondary to alcohol use and cirrhosis. Abdominal distention, GI bleeding, bruising, and weight changes are noted.

The nurse assesses nutritional status, which is of major importance in cirrhosis, by obtaining daily weights and monitoring plasma proteins, transferrin, and creatinine levels. A plan of nursing care for a patient with impaired liver function is available online at http://thepoint.lww.com/Honan3e.

DIAGNOSIS

Nursing diagnoses may include the following:

- Activity intolerance related to fatigue, general debility, muscle wasting, and discomfort
- Malnutrition risk, related to chronic gastritis, decreased GI motility, and anorexia
- Altered skin integrity related to compromised immunologic status, edema, and poor nutrition
- Injury and bleeding risk related to altered clotting mechanisms

Potential complications may include the following:

- Bleeding and hemorrhage
- Hepatic encephalopathy
- Fluid volume excess

PLANNING

The goals for the patient may include increased participation in activities, improvement of nutritional status, improvement of skin integrity, decreased potential for injury, improvement of mental status, and absence of complications.

NURSING INTERVENTIONS

PROMOTING REST

The patient with active liver disease requires rest and other supportive measures to permit the liver to re-establish its functional ability. If the patient is hospitalized, weight and fluid intake and output are measured and recorded daily. The nurse adjusts the patient's position in bed for maximal respiratory efficiency, which is especially important if ascites is marked because it interferes with adequate thoracic excursion. Oxygen therapy may be required in liver failure.

Rest reduces the demands on the liver and increases the liver's blood supply. Because the patient is susceptible to the hazards of immobility, efforts to prevent respiratory, circulatory, and vascular disturbances are initiated, such as range-of-motion exercises, turning every 2 hours, and the use of an incentive spirometer (IS) every hour while awake. These measures may help prevent such problems as pneumonia, thrombophlebitis, and pressure ulcers. After nutritional status improves and strength increases, the nurse encourages the patient to increase activity gradually. Activity and mild exercise, as well as rest, are planned.

IMPROVING NUTRITIONAL STATUS

The patient with cirrhosis who has no ascites or edema and exhibits no signs of impending hepatic coma should receive a nutritious, high-protein diet, if tolerated, supplemented by vitamins of the B complex and others as indicated (including vitamins A, C, K, and folic acid). Because proper nutrition is so important, the nurse makes every effort to encourage the patient to eat. Proper nutrition is as important as any medication. Often, small, frequent meals are better tolerated than three large meals because of the abdominal pressure exerted by ascites. Protein supplements also may be indicated.

Patient preferences are considered. Patients with prolonged or severe anorexia and those who are vomiting or eating poorly for any reason may receive nutrients by the enteral or parenteral route.

Patients with fatty stools (**steatorrhea**) should receive water-soluble forms of fat-soluble vitamins—A, D, and E (Aquasol A, D, and E). Folic acid and iron are prescribed to prevent anemia. If the patient shows signs of impending or advancing coma, the amount of protein in the diet is decreased temporarily. In the absence of hepatic encephalopathy, a moderate-protein, high-calorie intake is provided, with protein foods of high biologic value. A diet containing 1.2–1.5 g of protein per kilogram of ideal body weight per day is required unless the patient is malnourished. Protein is restricted if encephalopathy develops. Incorporating vegetable protein to meet protein needs may decrease the risk for encephalopathy. Also sodium restriction is indicated to prevent ascites.

PROVIDING SKIN CARE

Providing careful skin care is important because of subcutaneous edema, the patient's immobility, jaundice, and increased susceptibility to skin breakdown and infection. Frequent changes in position are necessary to prevent pressure ulcers. To prevent trauma to the skin, it is important to avoid irritating soaps and the use of adhesive tape. Lotion may be soothing to irritated skin; the nurse takes measures to minimize scratching by the patient.

REDUCING INJURY RISK

The nurse protects the patient with cirrhosis from falls and other injuries. The side rails should be in place and padded with blankets or other materials in case the patient becomes agitated or restless. To minimize agitation, the nurse orients the patient to time and place and explains all procedures. The nurse instructs the patient to ask for assistance to get out of bed. The nurse carefully evaluates any injury because of the possibility of internal bleeding.

Pearls for Practice

Because of the risk for bleeding from abnormal clotting, the patient should use an electric razor rather than a safety razor. A soft-bristled toothbrush helps minimize bleeding gums, and pressure applied to all venipuncture sites helps minimize bleeding.

MONITORING AND MANAGING POTENTIAL COMPLICATIONS

Bleeding and Hemorrhage. The patient is at increased risk for bleeding and hemorrhage because of decreased production of prothrombin and decreased ability of the diseased liver to synthesize the necessary substances for blood coagulation. Precautionary measures include protecting the patient with padded side rails, applying pressure to injection sites, and avoiding injury from sharp objects. The nurse observes for melena and assesses stools for blood (signs of possible internal bleeding). Vital signs are monitored regularly. Precautions are taken to minimize rupture of esophageal varices by avoiding further increases in portal pressure (see earlier discussion). Dietary modification and appropriate use of stool softeners may help prevent straining during defecation. The nurse closely monitors the patient for GI bleeding and keeps readily available equipment (e.g., balloon tamponade tube), IV fluids, and medications needed to treat hemorrhage from esophageal and gastric varices.

If hemorrhage occurs, the nurse helps the provider initiate measures to halt the bleeding and administers fluid and blood component therapy and medications. The patient with massive hemorrhage from bleeding esophageal or gastric varices is transferred to the ICU and requires emergency surgery or other treatment modalities. The patient and family require explanations about the event and the necessary treatment.

HEPATIC ENCEPHALOPATHY

Hepatic encephalopathy and coma, possible complications of cirrhosis, may manifest as deteriorating mental status and dementia or as physical signs, such as abnormal voluntary and involuntary movements. Hepatic encephalopathy is caused mainly by the accumulation of ammonia in the blood and its effect on cerebral metabolism. Many factors predispose the patient with cirrhosis to hepatic encephalopathy. Therefore, the patient may require extensive diagnostic testing to identify hidden sources of bleeding and increased ammonia production.

Treatment may include the use of lactulose and nonabsorbable intestinal tract antibiotics to decrease ammonia levels, modification of medications to eliminate those that may precipitate or worsen hepatic encephalopathy, and bed rest to minimize energy expenditure.

Monitoring is an essential nursing function to identify early deterioration in mental status. The nurse monitors the patient's mental status closely and reports changes, so that treatment of encephalopathy can be initiated promptly. Because electrolyte disturbances can contribute to encephalopathy, serum electrolyte levels are carefully monitored and corrected if abnormal. Oxygen is administered if oxygen desaturation occurs. The nurse monitors for fever or abdominal pain, which may signal the onset of bacterial peritonitis or other infection (see earlier discussion of hepatic encephalopathy).

Pearls for Practice

Signs and symptoms of bacterial peritonitis include fever, jaundice, abdominal pain, nausea, vomiting, and diarrhea; however, in patients with cirrhosis, a low-grade temperature with or without abdominal pain may be noted (Biggins et al., 2021; Garcia-Tsao, 2020).

Fluid Volume Excess. Patients with advanced chronic liver disease develop cardiovascular abnormalities. These occur due to an increased cardiac output and decreased peripheral vascular resistance, possibly resulting from the release of vasodilators. A hyperdynamic circulatory state develops in patients with cirrhosis, and plasma volume increases. The greater the degree of hepatic decompensation, the more severe the hyperdynamic state. Close assessment of cardiovascular and respiratory status is of key importance for the care of patients with this disorder. Pulmonary compromise, which is always a potential complication of ESLD because of plasma volume excess, makes prevention of pulmonary complications an important role for the nurse. Administering diuretics, implementing fluid restrictions, and enhancing patient positioning can optimize pulmonary function. Fluid retention may be noted in the development of ascites, anasarca, lower extremity swelling, and dyspnea. Monitoring of intake and output, daily weight changes, changes in abdominal girth, and edema formation is part of nursing assessment in the hospital or in the home setting. Patients also are monitored for any changes in kidney function.

PROMOTING HOME AND COMMUNITY-BASED CARE

During the hospital stay, the nurse and other health care providers prepare the patient with cirrhosis for discharge, focusing on dietary instruction. Of greatest importance is the exclusion of alcohol from the diet. The patient may need referral to Alcoholics Anonymous, psychiatric care, or counseling or may benefit from support from a spiritual advisor. Also the patient who is post transplant (discussed shortly) should avoid the consumption of raw meats and shellfish due to the increased risk of foodborne illness in immunosuppressed patients.

Sodium restriction will continue for a considerable time, if not permanently. The patient will require written instructions, teaching, reinforcement, and support from the staff as well as family members.

Successful treatment depends on convincing the patient of the need to adhere completely to the therapeutic plan. The nurse also instructs the patient and family about symptoms of impending encephalopathy, possible bleeding tendencies, and susceptibility to infection.

(*continued on page 842*)

Recovery is neither rapid nor easy; there are frequent setbacks and apparent lack of improvement. Many patients find it difficult to refrain from using alcohol for comfort or escape. The nurse plays a significant role in offering support and encouragement to the patient.

EVALUATION

Expected patient outcomes may include the following:

1. Participates in activities:
   a. Plans activities and exercises to allow alternating periods of rest and activity
   b. Reports increased strength and well-being
   c. Participates in hygiene care
2. Increases nutritional intake:
   a. Demonstrates intake of appropriate nutrients and avoidance of alcohol as reflected by diet log
   b. Gains weight without increased edema and ascites formation
   c. Reports decrease in GI disturbances and anorexia
   d. Identifies foods and fluids that are nutritious and allowed on or restricted from the diet
   e. Adheres to vitamin therapy regimen
   f. Describes the rationale for small, frequent meals
3. Exhibits improved skin integrity:
   a. Has intact skin without evidence of breakdown, infection, or trauma
   b. Demonstrates normal turgor of skin of the extremities and trunk, and decreased edema
   c. Changes position frequently and inspects bony prominences daily
   d. Uses lotions to decrease pruritus
4. Avoids injury:
   a. Is free of ecchymotic areas or hematoma formation
   b. States rationale for side rails and asks for assistance to get out of bed
   c. Uses measures to prevent trauma (e.g., uses electric razor and soft toothbrush, blows nose gently, arranges furniture to prevent bumps and falls, avoids straining during defecation)
5. Is free of complications:
   a. Reports absence of frank bleeding from the GI tract (i.e., absence of melena and hematemesis)
   b. Is oriented to time, place, and person and demonstrates normal attention span
   c. Has a serum ammonia level within normal limits
   d. Identifies early, reportable signs of impaired thought processes

HEPATOCELLULAR CARCINOMA

HCC is the most common hepatic malignancy. It is the third leading cause of cancer death worldwide and the ninth leading cause of cancer death in the United States (Di Bisceglie & Befeler, 2021).

Risk Factors

HCC is strongly linked to cirrhosis and chronic hepatitis B and C infections. ALD, nonalcoholic steatohepatitis (NASH) (inflammation and fat accumulation of the liver), primary biliary cholangitis, and hemochromatosis (excessive retained iron in the body) also are thought to increase risk for HCC. Increasing age and male gender (2–4 ×'s higher compared to females) also increase the likelihood of HCC developing in patients with cirrhosis; American Indian/Alaskan Natives and Hispanics have the highest incidence of HCC in the United Sates (Gilles et al., 2022). HCC may arise in patients without cirrhosis; typically these are individuals with chronic hepatitis B infection (Di Bisceglie & Befeler, 2021; Marrero et al., 2018).

Clinical Manifestations and Assessment

As early diagnosis becomes more common due to improving surveillance monitoring, many patients are diagnosed before symptoms are noticeable. If symptomatic, usually the clinical manifestations of HCC are found in the context of the patient with known cirrhosis: jaundice, ascites, varices, and the stigmata of chronic liver disease are common features. Unintentional weight loss, anorexia, and right upper quadrant pain may be additional presenting signs. In late cases, the patient may present with intra-abdominal bleeding from tumor rupture. In patients deemed high risk, routine screening with abdominal imaging and measurement of alpha fetoprotein levels has improved the detection of liver cancer (Di Bisceglie & Befeler, 2021; Kelley & Venook, 2020; Marrero et al., 2018). Alpha-fetoprotein (AFP) is a plasma protein normally produced by the fetal liver and yolk sac that is dominant in the first trimester of life and diminishes to very low levels by the age of 1 year (Pagana et al., 2023). It is also normally found in very low levels in the adult where normal levels are <40 ng/mL or <40 mcg/L. In nonpregnant persons and males, elevated levels are associated with cancers, particularly liver cancer but increased levels are also found in testicular and ovarian cancer. Levels greater than 200 ng/mL in cirrhotic patients suggest HCC (Adigun et al., 2022).

The diagnosis of liver cancer is based on clinical signs and symptoms, the history and physical examination, and the results of laboratory and imaging studies. Increased serum levels of bilirubin, alkaline phosphatase, GGT, and most importantly, AFP, and AFP variants may be present. Anemia is a common finding, and leukocytosis (increased white blood cells [WBCs]), hypercalcemia, hypoglycemia, and hypocholesterolemia also may be seen on laboratory assessment (Kelley & Venook, 2020).

Confirmation of the diagnosis of HCC is made radiologically with use of computed tomography (CT) scan imaging or magnetic resonance imaging (MRI) to determine the number, size, and location of tumors and if vascular invasion has occurred. In equivocal cases, liver biopsy may be used to obtain tissue samples of the lesion to determine malignancy (Kelley & Venook, 2020; Marrero et al., 2018).

Medical and Nursing Management

Currently there are multiple treatment options for the patient with HCC. Surgical resection is the preferred treatment for patients without cirrhosis and with adequate hepatic reserve; average 5-year survival outcomes after resection nears 70%; however, recurrence rates are as high as 70% at 5 years (Marrero et al., 2018). In patients with HCC and cirrhosis, liver transplantation (discussed in detail below) is the treatment of choice. Liver transplantation is curative for patients with both HCC and ESLD; however, careful patient selection is critical to achieve good outcomes (Di Bisceglie & Befeler, 2021; Marrero et al., 2018).

Other treatments for HCC are percutaneous ethanol injection (PEI) and radiofrequency (RFA) or microwave ablation (MWA), which directly induce tumor necrosis. Transarterial chemoembolization (TACE) is used to block the hepatic blood flow feeding the tumor and is used in combination with chemotherapeutic agents (Di Bisceglie & Befeler, 2021; Kelley & Venook, 2020). Systemic chemotherapy includes sorafenib and other agents; currently multiple clinical trials are underway to study the effectiveness of chemotherapeutic agents to treat HCC (Crissien & Frenette, 2014). Combining sorafenib with immunotherapy agents has become standard of care for treatment in some patients with more advanced HCC with intact liver function (Kelley & Venook, 2020).

LIVER TRANSPLANTATION

Due to recent advances in surgical techniques, immunosuppressant medications, and increased knowledge of immunology, liver transplantation has become the treatment of choice for patients with ESLD and acute liver failure. Because liver transplantation now is recognized as an established therapeutic modality, rather than an experimental procedure to treat these disorders, the number of liver transplantation centers is increasing. Often patients requiring transplantation are referred from distant hospitals to these sites. To prepare the patient and family for liver transplantation, nurses in all settings must understand the processes and procedures of liver transplantation.

The transplantation procedure involves total surgical removal of the diseased liver and replacement with a healthy donor organ in the same anatomic location (**orthotopic liver transplantation** [OLT]). The efficacy of this therapeutic modality is demonstrated by deceased donor survival outcomes greater than 75% at 5 years (Kwong et al., 2022). The important benefit of this option for patients with ESLD or fulminant liver failure is limited by the shortage of cadaveric donor organs. As of 2022, 11,336 patients were on the national UNOS transplant list awaiting liver transplant (HRSA/OPTN, 2022).

Indications and Contraindications

Indications for liver transplantation include:

- Advanced chronic liver disease
- Fulminant hepatic failure
- Metabolic liver diseases
- HCC
- Hepatocellular liver diseases (e.g., viral hepatitis, drug- or alcohol-induced liver disease, Wilson disease)
- Cholestatic diseases (interruption in bile flow seen in primary biliary cholangitis, sclerosing cholangitis, and biliary atresia)

Other less common diseases requiring liver transplantation are polycystic liver disease, vascular disease (Budd–Chiari), and rare metabolic disorders (Everson, 2020).

Medical contraindications for liver transplant include uncontrolled infection, extrahepatic malignancy or advanced hepatobiliary metastatic disease, irreversible brain damage, anatomic difficulties, acute liver failure with increased intracranial pressure or decreased perfusion pressure, and multiorgan failure. Psychosocial contraindications may include active substance use, medical nonadherence, and severe psychiatric instability (Carrion & Martin, 2021). Other factors that may present obstacles to successful transplant are comorbidities, such as advanced cardiac or pulmonary disease, and poor psychosocial support.

Selection and Evaluation for Liver Transplant

The selection and evaluation of a patient for liver transplantation is a multidisciplinary process that requires a complete assessment of the patient, including etiology and stage of liver disease, and evaluation of comorbidities and/or contraindications, psychosocial support status, and any medical or surgical issues. The patient being considered for liver transplantation frequently has many systemic problems that influence preoperative and postoperative care. The medical condition of the patient must be optimized as well as possible to prevent complications and to ensure optimal outcomes. Patients must undergo complete medical, surgical, and psychosocial testing to determine if liver transplant is feasible, and for organ matching (Carrion & Martin, 2021).

Once the patient is evaluated and deemed appropriate for liver transplant by the transplant center, they are placed on the national transplant wait-list administered by the UNOS. The priority for obtaining a cadaveric liver organ is determined by the Model of End Stage Liver Disease (MELD) score, which stratifies the level of illness of those awaiting a liver transplant. The MELD score is derived from a complex formula incorporating sodium levels, bilirubin levels, prothrombin time (reported as INR), and creatinine levels. The MELD score is an indicator of short-term mortality for those with ESLD. Additional priority beyond the patient's physiologic MELD score may be provided for selected diseases that increase the patient's mortality risk, such as HCC, HPS, and metabolic diseases of the liver. The highest priority on the transplant wait-list is provided to patients with acute or fulminant liver failure (HRSA/OPTN, 2022; Marrero et al., 2018).

Surgical Procedure

The transplant operation involves total removal of the diseased liver, or hepatectomy, replacement with the donor organ, vascular anastomoses of the donor liver to the recipient, and biliary reconstruction. This complex surgical procedure is divided in three stages or phases: hepatectomy, anhepatic (no liver) phase, and reperfusion phase.

The first stage involves the total removal of the diseased liver. Vascular clamps are placed on the portal vein and the inferior vena cava above and below the liver, and the native liver is dissected from the recipient. Hemostasis is maintained using sutures and cauterization of bleeding vessels. After preparation of the donor liver, anastomoses of the suprahepatic inferior vena cava, infrahepatic inferior vena cava, and portal vein surgically connect the donor liver to the recipient. Reperfusion of the new donor liver is achieved by removal of vascular clamps and perfusion of portal venous blood. Then hepatic artery anastomosis is performed and, last, biliary reconstruction.

Multiple surgical innovations have been developed to prevent complications, such as bleeding, bile leaks, and reperfusion injury of the new graft, to improve outcomes (Carrion & Martin, 2021).

Liver transplantation is a long surgical procedure, partly because the patient with liver failure often has portal hypertension that requires the ligation of many venous collateral vessels. Blood loss during the surgical procedure may be extensive. If the patient has adhesions from previous abdominal surgery, lysis of adhesions is often necessary. If a shunt procedure was performed previously, it must be surgically reversed to permit adequate portal venous blood supply to the new liver. During the lengthy surgery, it is helpful to provide regular updates to the family about the progress of the operation and the patient's status.

Complications

Immediate postoperative complications may include bleeding, infection, rejection, and delayed graft function. Other complications include biliary leaks and obstruction, hepatic artery thrombosis, and portal vein thrombosis (Everson, 2020).

Primary Graft Nonfunction

Although it continues to decline in incidence, primary graft nonfunction is the most severe complication of liver transplant and occurs in up to 8.5% of deceased donor cases. Ongoing encephalopathy, coagulopathy, jaundice, metabolic acidosis, and hemodynamic instability are clinical indications of primary graft nonfunction (Everson, 2020). Transplant recipients with primary graft nonfunction require immediate retransplantation and receive priority on the transplant wait-list (HRSA/OPTN, 2022).

Bleeding

Bleeding is common in the postoperative period and may result from coagulopathy, portal hypertension, and fibrinolysis (breakdown of fibrin clots) caused by ischemic injury to the donor liver. Hypotension may occur in this phase, secondary to blood loss. Administration of platelets, fresh-frozen plasma, or other blood products may be necessary. Hypertension is more common, although its cause is uncertain. Blood pressure elevation that is significant or sustained is treated.

Infection

Infection is a life-threatening complication after liver transplantation. Pulmonary and fungal infections are common; susceptibility to infection is increased by the immunosuppressive therapy that is needed to prevent rejection (Everson, 2020). Therefore, precautions must be taken to prevent health care–associated infections. The nurse uses strict asepsis when manipulating central venous catheters, arterial lines, and drainage systems for urine, bile, and any body fluids; when obtaining specimens; and when changing dressings. Meticulous hand hygiene and contact precautions are crucial to prevent infection in the recipient of a liver transplant.

Rejection

Rejection is a primary concern. A transplanted liver is perceived by the immune system as a foreign antigen. This triggers an immune response, leading to the activation of T lymphocytes that attack and destroy the transplanted liver. Immunosuppressive agents are used as long-term therapy to prevent this response and rejection of the transplanted liver. These agents inhibit the activation of immunocompetent T lymphocytes to prevent the production of effector T cells. Transplant centers may use two or three immunosuppressants in combination to prevent rejection (Carrion & Martin, 2021). The recipient of the liver transplant requires intensive education in dosing, side effects, and the drug interactions of these medications and will require lifelong immunosuppression.

Although the 1- and 5-year survival rates have increased dramatically with the use of new immunosuppressive therapies, these therapies are not without side effects. Both cyclosporine and tacrolimus have important side effects, such as kidney dysfunction, hypertension, hyperlipidemia, and hyperkalemia. Neurotoxicity may occur with use of tacrolimus, and patients may experience tremors to more severe complications, such as psychosis or seizures. Optimal dosing of immunosuppression must be monitored carefully and individualized to patient condition to prevent rejection and to reduce side effects (Carrion & Martin, 2021).

Despite the success of immunosuppression in reducing the incidence of rejection of transplanted organs, liver transplantation is not routine and may be accompanied by complications related to the lengthy surgical procedure, immunosuppressive therapy, infection, and the technical difficulties encountered in reconstructing the blood vessels and biliary tract.

Nursing Management

The patient considering transplantation, together with the family, must make difficult choices about treatment, use of financial resources, and relocation to another area to be closer to the medical center. They also must cope with the patient's longstanding health problems and any social and family problems associated with behaviors that may have caused the patient's liver failure. As a result, considerable emotional stress occurs while the patient and family consider liver transplantation and wait for an available liver. The nurse must be aware of these issues and attuned to the emotional and psychological status of the patient and family. Referral to a psychiatric liaison nurse, psychologist, psychiatrist, or spiritual advisor may help them cope with the stressors associated with ESLD and liver transplantation.

Preoperative Nursing Interventions

The nurse, surgeon, hepatologist, and other members of the health care team provide the patient and family with full explanations about the procedure, the chances of success, and the risks, including the side effects of long-term immunosuppression. The need for close follow-up and lifelong compliance with the therapeutic regimen, including immunosuppression, is explained to the patient and family.

The nurse coordinator is an integral member of the transplant team and plays an important role in preparing the patient for liver transplantation. The nurse serves as advocate for the patient and family and assumes the important role of liaison between the patient and the other members of the transplant team. The nurse also serves as a resource to other nurses and members of the health care team involved in evaluating and caring for the patient.

Postoperative Nursing Interventions

The patient is maintained in an environment as free from bacteria, viruses, and fungi as possible because immunosuppressive medications reduce the body's natural defenses. In the immediate postoperative period, cardiovascular, pulmonary, renal, neurologic, and metabolic functions are monitored continuously. Mean arterial pressures and pulmonary artery pressures (PAPs) also are monitored. Ventilator support and airway management are priorities. Cardiac output (CO), central venous pressure (CVP), PAPs, pulmonary capillary wedge pressure (PCWP), arterial and mixed venous blood gases, oxygen saturation, oxygen demand and delivery, urine output, heart rate, and blood pressure are used to evaluate the patient's hemodynamic status and intravascular fluid volume (refer to Chapter 54). Liver function tests, electrolyte levels, the coagulation profile, chest x-ray, electrocardiogram, and fluid output (including urine, bile from the T tube, and output from NG and drainage tubes) are monitored closely. Because the liver is responsible for the storage of glycogen and the synthesis of protein and clotting factors, these substances need to be monitored and replaced in the immediate postoperative period. The nurse monitors for signs of excess bleeding in the immediate postoperative period and notifies the provider immediately if bleeding is suspected (hypotension, tachycardia, tachypnea, decreasing CO, melena, increasing abdominal girth, bloody NG drainage, etc.).

There is a high risk for atelectasis and an altered ventilation–perfusion ratio, caused by insult to the diaphragm during the surgical procedure, prolonged anesthesia, immobility, and postoperative pain. Because of this risk, the patient will have an endotracheal tube in place and will require mechanical ventilation during the initial postoperative period. Suctioning is performed as required, and sterile humidification is provided.

As the vital signs and condition stabilize, efforts are made to assist the patient to recover from the trauma of this complex surgery. After removal of the endotracheal tube, the nurse encourages the patient to use an IS to decrease the risk for atelectasis. The patient is then assisted to get out of bed, to ambulate as tolerated, and to participate in self-care to prevent the complications associated with immobility. Close monitoring for signs and symptoms of liver dysfunction and rejection continues throughout the hospital stay. Plans are made for close follow-up after discharge as well. Teaching is initiated during the preoperative period and continues after surgery.

Promoting Home and Community-Based Care

Teaching the patient and family about long-term measures to promote health is crucial for the success of transplantation and represents an important role of the nurse. The patient and family must understand why they need to adhere continuously to the therapeutic regimen, with special emphasis on the methods of administration, rationale, and side effects of the prescribed immunosuppressive agents. The nurse provides written as well as verbal instructions about how and when to take the medications. To avoid running out of medication or skipping a dose, the patient must make sure that an adequate supply of medication is available. Also, instructions are provided about the signs and symptoms that indicate problems necessitating consultation with the transplant team.

The nurse emphasizes the importance of follow-up blood tests and appointments with the transplant team. Trough blood levels (the lowest concentration reached by a medication before the next dose is administered) of immunosuppressive agents are obtained along with other blood tests that assess the function of the liver and kidneys. During the first months, the patient is likely to require blood tests two or three times a week. As the patient's condition stabilizes, blood studies and visits to the transplant team are less frequent. The importance of routine ophthalmologic examinations is emphasized because of the increased incidence of cataracts and glaucoma associated with the long-term corticosteroid therapy used with transplantation. Regular oral hygiene and follow-up dental care, with administration of prophylactic antibiotics before dental examinations and treatments, are recommended because of the immunosuppression. The patient is reminded to avoid the consumption of raw meats and shellfish due to the increased risk of foodborne illness in immunosuppressed patients.

The nurse reminds the patient that preventing rejection and infection leads to a successful transplantation and increases the chances for survival and living a more normal life than before transplantation. Many patients have lived successful and productive lives after receiving a liver transplant.

DISORDERS OF THE GALLBLADDER

Several disorders affect the biliary system and interfere with normal drainage of bile into the duodenum. These disorders include inflammation of the biliary system and carcinoma that obstructs the biliary tree. Gallbladder disease with gallstones is the most common disorder of the biliary system. Most patients with gallstones are asymptomatic; 36 million Americans with gallstones have no pain and are unaware of the presence of stones (Fogel & Sherman, 2020).

CHOLELITHIASIS

Calculi, or gallstones, usually form in the gallbladder from the solid constituents of bile; they vary greatly in size, shape, and composition (Fig. 24-13).

Pathophysiology

There are two major types of gallstones: those composed predominantly of pigment and those composed primarily of cholesterol. Pigment stones form when unconjugated pigments in the bile precipitate to form stones. The risk of developing such stones is increased in patients with cirrhosis, hemolysis, and infections of the biliary tract. Pigment stones cannot be dissolved and must be removed surgically.

Cholesterol stones account for over 70% to 80% of gallbladder disease in the United States. Cholesterol, a normal constituent of bile, is insoluble in water. Its solubility depends on bile acids and lecithin (phospholipids) in bile. In patients who are gallstone prone, there is decreased bile acid synthesis and increased cholesterol synthesis in the liver, resulting in bile supersaturated with cholesterol, which precipitates out of the bile to form stones. The cholesterol-saturated bile predisposes to the formation of gallstones and acts as an irritant that produces inflammatory changes in the gallbladder (Fogel & Sherman, 2020).

Risk Factors

Gallstones are uncommon in children and young adults but become increasingly prevalent after 40 years of age, especially in females (Box 24-9).

Clinical Manifestations and Assessment

Gallstones may be silent, producing no pain and only mild GI symptoms. Such stones may be detected incidentally during surgery or evaluation for unrelated problems.

The patient with gallbladder disease resulting from gallstones may develop two types of symptoms: those due to disease of the gallbladder itself, and those due to obstruction of

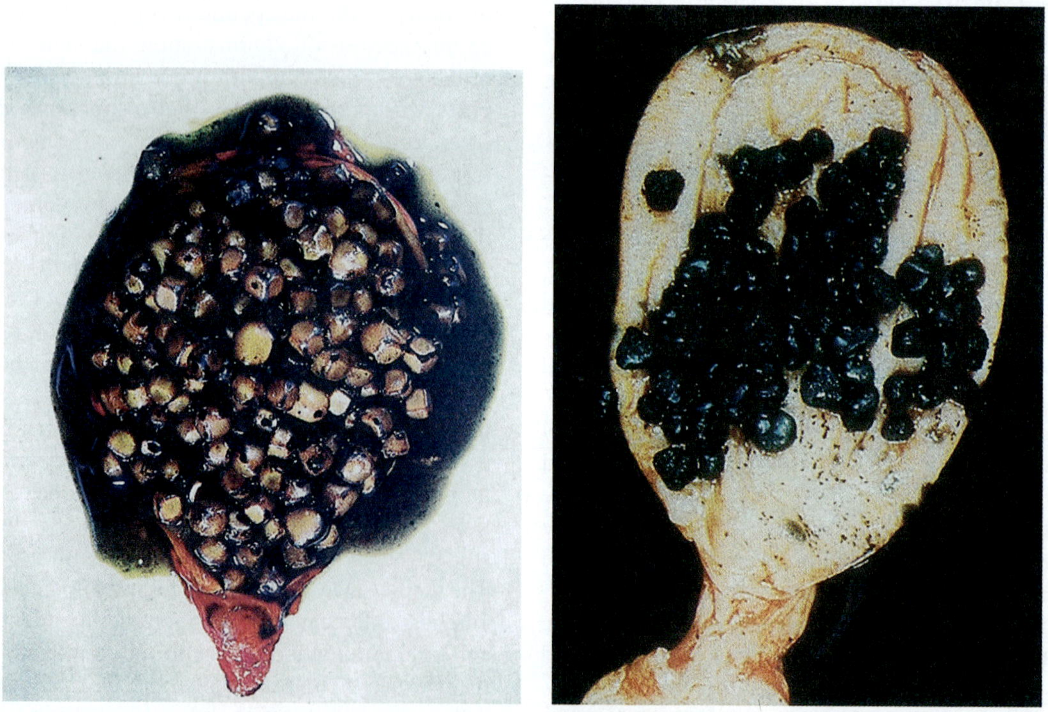

FIGURE 24-13 **Examples of cholesterol gallstones (*left*) made up of a coalescence of multiple small stones and pigment gallstones (*right*) composed of calcium bilirubinate. (From Rubin, R., & Strayer, D. S. [2008]. *Rubin's pathology* [5th ed.]. Lippincott Williams & Wilkins.)**

BOX 24-9

Risk Factors for Cholelithiasis

- Obesity (35% of females with BMI over 32 kg/m^2 have gallstones) (Clinical Overview, 2022b)
- Female gender, especially females who have had multiple pregnancies or who are of Native American or U.S. Southwestern Hispanic ethnicity
- Increasing age (4–10 times higher in older people) (Clinical Overview, 2022b)
- Frequent changes in weight
- Rapid weight loss (leads to rapid development of gallstones and high risk of symptomatic disease)
- Treatment with high-dose estrogen (e.g., in prostate cancer)
- Low-dose estrogen therapy; a small increase in the risk of gallstones
- Ileal resection or disease
- Gastric bypass
- Total parental nutrition
- Diets high in cholesterol, fatty acids, and carbohydrates
- Cystic fibrosis
- Diabetes mellitus
- Cirrhosis
- Family history

the bile passages by a gallstone. The symptoms may be acute or chronic. Epigastric distress, such as fullness, abdominal distention, and vague pain in the right upper quadrant of the abdomen, may occur. This distress may follow a meal rich in fried or fatty foods. Clinical manifestations of gallstones are largely asymptomatic; however, 15% to 20% of patients with gallstones will develop pain and biliary colic with repeated episodes of obstruction. Increased frequency of biliary colic typically will result in cholecystitis. If the gallstone is dislodged and no longer obstructs the cystic duct, the gallbladder drains and the inflammatory process subsides after a relatively short time. If the gallstone continues to obstruct the duct, abscess, necrosis, and perforation with generalized peritonitis may result.

Pearls for Practice

The nurse is alert to the signs and symptoms of peritonitis, including abdominal pain that initially may be vague and generalized but becomes increasingly severe and constant; abdominal distention and tenderness with rebound tenderness; anxiety, paleness, and diaphoresis; anorexia; nausea; vomiting; inability to pass feces and flatus; rigidity of the abdomen; an absence of bowel sounds; cautious movement; and knee–chest position for comfort.

If a gallstone obstructs the cystic duct, the gallbladder becomes distended, inflamed, and, eventually, infected (acute cholecystitis). The patient develops a fever and may have a palpable abdominal mass. The patient may have biliary colic with excruciating upper right abdominal pain that radiates to the back or right shoulder. Usually biliary colic is associated with nausea and vomiting, and it is noticeable several hours after a heavy meal. The patient moves about restlessly, unable to find a comfortable position. The pain will fluctuate, lasting from 30 minutes to up to 6 hours. The patient may experience other symptoms, including nausea, chills, and gastric distress, including belching and bloating.

Such a bout of biliary colic is caused by contraction of the gallbladder, which cannot release bile because of obstruction by the stone. This produces marked tenderness in the right upper quadrant on deep inspiration and prevents full inspiratory excursion when the examiner's fingers are under the liver border, known as *Murphy sign* (Fogel & Sherman, 2020). See management under cholecystitis.

CHOLECYSTITIS

Cholecystitis is acute inflammation of the gallbladder. An empyema of the gallbladder develops if the gallbladder becomes filled with purulent fluid (pus). Repeated episodes of obstruction of the cystic duct by gallstones will cause cholecystitis.

Pathophysiology

Calculous cholecystitis is the cause of more than 80% to 85% of cases of acute cholecystitis (Fogel & Sherman, 2020). In calculous cholecystitis, a gallbladder stone obstructs bile outflow. Bile remaining in the gallbladder initiates a chemical reaction; autolysis and edema occur. The gallbladder becomes inflamed and distended due to increased pressure and vascular compromise, resulting in ischemia and necrosis. The release of inflammatory agents additionally plays a role in the pathophysiology of acute cholecystitis. Secondary infection with bacteria complicates the course of this disorder in up to 50% of patients (Fogel & Sherman, 2020).

Acalculous cholecystitis describes acute gallbladder inflammation in the absence of obstruction by gallstones. It occurs after major surgical procedures, severe trauma, or burns. Other factors associated with this type of cholecystitis include heart failure, diabetes mellitus, cystic artery embolism, immunosuppression, abdominal vasculitis, multiorgan failure, and acute kidney failure. It is speculated that acalculous cholecystitis is caused by further progression of multiple systemic failures, resulting in gallbladder stasis, increased bacterial colonization, and ischemia. Bile stasis (lack of gallbladder contraction) and increased viscosity of the bile are also thought to play a role (Afdhal, 2022; Fogel & Sherman, 2020).

Clinical Manifestations and Assessment

Cholecystitis causes pain, tenderness, and rigidity of the upper right abdomen; usually the pain radiates to the back or right shoulder or scapula. Nausea and vomiting are common.

The patient will have leukocytosis (elevated WBCs), and physical examination may reveal a positive Murphy sign (right subcostal tenderness) (Fogel & Sherman, 2020).

Pearls for Practice

The nurse understands that if there is obstruction of the bile ducts, the bile will not be able to progress to the intestine and clay-colored (gray or white or acholic [without bile]) and steatorrhea (excessive fat in stool due lack of bile acid in the intestine leading to fat malabsorption will be seen) (Bickley et al., 2021). In addition, the bile will be reabsorbed by the blood stream and released by the kidney resulting in dark and foamy urine, and jaundice and icterus will be seen.

Medical Management

The major objectives of medical therapy are to reduce the incidence of acute episodes of gallbladder pain and cholecystitis by supportive and dietary management and, if possible, to remove the cause of cholecystitis by pharmacologic therapy, endoscopic procedures, or surgical intervention. Asymptomatic cholelithiasis can be treated with prophylactic cholecystectomy, especially with findings of large gallstones (greater than 3 cm) due to their malignant potential. Initial management of cholecystitis involves bowel rest (i.e., nothing by mouth [NPO]), management of fluids and electrolyte balance, pain management, and antibiotic coverage (Fogel & Sherman, 2020).

Pharmacologic Therapy

Ursodeoxycholic acid (UDCA) and chenodeoxycholic acid (chenodiol or CDCA) have been used to dissolve small, radiolucent gallstones composed primarily of cholesterol in patients with symptomatic cholecystitis. Because of the high long-term risk of recurrence, laparoscopic cholecystectomy (50% within 5 years), and widespread availability of laparoscopic cholecystectomy, rarely is this method of treatment used today. However, it may be beneficial in prevention of gallstone disease during periods of rapid weight loss (Fogel & Sherman, 2020).

Surgical Management

Laparoscopic or open cholecystectomy is more appropriate for symptomatic patients with acceptable operative risk. Removal of the gallbladder (**cholecystectomy**) through traditional surgical approaches was considered the standard treatment for more than 100 years. There is now widespread use of **laparoscopic cholecystectomy** (removal of the gallbladder through a small incision through the umbilicus). As a result, surgical risks have decreased, along with the length of hospital stay and the long recovery period required after standard surgical cholecystectomy (Fogel & Sherman, 2020).

Laparoscopic Cholecystectomy

Laparoscopic cholecystectomy (Fig. 24-14) has dramatically changed the approach to the management of cholecystitis. It

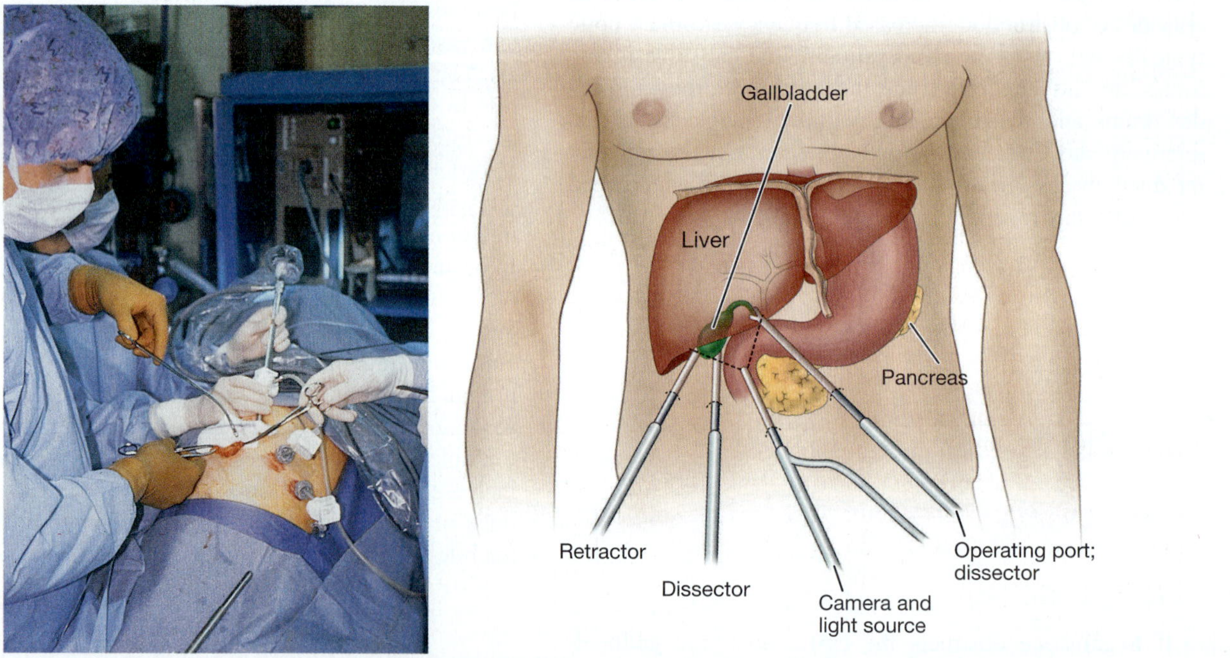

A B

FIGURE 24-14 **In laparoscopic cholecystectomy (A), the surgeon makes four small incisions (less than 12 in each) in the abdomen (B) and inserts a laparoscope with a miniature camera through the umbilical incision. The camera apparatus displays the gallbladder and adjacent tissues on a screen, allowing the surgeon to visualize the sections of the organ for removal.**

has become the new standard for therapy of symptomatic gallstones. Approximately 750,000 patients in the United States require surgery each year for removal of the gallbladder, and greater than 90% of them are candidates for laparoscopic cholecystectomy (Fogel & Sherman, 2020). Contraindications for this surgery include patients with suspected or diagnosed cancer of the gallbladder, third trimester of pregnancy, generalized peritonitis, septic shock, previous surgery that prevents access, and poor pulmonary or cardiac reserve (Neil, 2023).

Before the procedure, the patient is informed that an open abdominal procedure may be necessary, and general anesthesia is administered. Laparoscopic cholecystectomy is performed through a small incision or puncture made through the abdominal wall at the umbilicus. The abdominal cavity is insufflated with carbon dioxide (pneumoperitoneum) to assist in inserting the laparoscope and to aid in visualizing the abdominal structures. The fiberoptic scope is inserted through the small umbilical incision. Several additional punctures or small incisions are made in the abdominal wall to introduce other surgical instruments into the operative field. The surgeon visualizes the biliary system through the laparoscope; a camera attached to the scope permits a view of the intra-abdominal field to be transmitted to a television monitor. After the cystic duct is dissected, the common bile duct can be visualized by ultrasound or cholangiography (imaging of the bile ducts with contrast medium) to evaluate the anatomy and identify stones. The cystic artery is dissected free and clipped. The gallbladder is separated from the hepatic bed and dissected. Then the gallbladder is removed from the abdominal cavity after bile and small stones are aspirated. Stone forceps also can be used to remove or crush larger stones.

Advantages of the laparoscopic procedure are that the patient does not experience the paralytic ileus that occurs with open abdominal surgery and has less postoperative abdominal pain. Early laparoscopic cholecystectomy (within 24 of symptoms) is the preferred intervention for treatment of acute cholecystitis and results in reduced length of stay, fewer surgical complications, and faster recovery for the patient (Fogel & Sherman, 2020).

Pearls for Practice

A common complaint after laparoscopy cholecystectomy surgery is shoulder pain (63%) that involves a multimodal approach to pain that may include opioids, nonsteroidal anti-inflammatory drugs (NSAIDs), corticosteroids, and local anesthetics (Kim et al., 2021). The etiology of the shoulder pain (commonly right sided) is theorized to be associated with diaphragmatic irritations from direct injury, stretching, or retained CO_2 gas in the abdominal cavity (pneumoperitoneum) resulting in phrenic nerve-mediated referred pain to the shoulder. While a variety of intraoperative techniques are suggested to decrease the incidence of shoulder pain (low-pressure pneumoperitoneum, postprocedure saline lavage, and aspiration of pneumoperitoneum) (Barazanchi et al., 2018), some postoperative interventions suggested in recent research include use of lidocaine patch (Kim et al., 2021), use of incentive spirometry since it expands the alveoli and the chest which, in turn, increases the movements of the diaphragm and stimulate it downward reducing the abdominal CO_2 (Saremirad et al., 2021), early mobilization which prevents venous stasis, promote peristalsis, voiding, absorption of insufflated gas, and decreases abdominal distention (Connick, 2019), positioning the patient is an exaggerated lithotomy position (legs are elevated and folded sheets or a pillow placed under the sacrum and lumbar area) has been shown to be a fast and effective method of reducing postoperative shoulder pain after laparoscopic cholecystectomy (Aydemir et al., 2018), and chewing gum since it stimulates intestinal activity in the early postoperative period (Urcanoglu & Yildiz, 2021). Additional studies are needed to elucidate best practices.

Conversion to a traditional abdominal surgical procedure may be necessary if problems are encountered during the laparoscopic procedure; this occurs in 3% of reported surgical cases (Fogel & Sherman, 2020). Careful screening of patients and identification of those at low risk for complications limit the frequency of conversion to an open abdominal procedure. However, with increasing use of laparoscopic procedures, the number of such conversions may increase. The most serious complication after laparoscopic cholecystectomy is a bile duct injury, which may be identified and corrected at the time of the procedure. However, as many as 28% may be missed and >14% present more than a month after the procedure; presenting signs and symptoms include right upper quadrant pain, nausea, vomiting, fever, and jaundice (Parker & Manning, 2021). If suspected a CT of the abdomen and pelvis with contrast, MRI or US may be diagnostic. Bile duct injuries may result in fluid accumulations that typically will require endoscopic stent placement or percutaneous drainage, and some patients will require surgery. Bile peritonitis, a more serious but rare complication, may result in critical illness or death.

Because of the short hospital stay with uncomplicated laparoscopic cholecystectomies, it is important to provide written and verbal instructions about managing postoperative pain and reporting signs and symptoms of intra-abdominal complications, including loss of appetite, vomiting, pain, distention of the abdomen, and temperature elevation. Although recovery from laparoscopic cholecystectomy is rapid, patients are drowsy afterward. The patient must have assistance at home during the first 24 to 48 hours. Box 24-10 details patient self-care after a laparoscopic cholecystectomy.

BOX 24-10 **Patient Education**

Managing Self-Care after Laparoscopic Cholecystectomy

Resuming Activity
- Begin light exercise (walking) immediately.
- Take a shower or bath after 1 or 2 days.
- Wait to drive a car for 3 or 4 days.
- Avoid lifting objects exceeding 5 lb after surgery, usually for 1 week.
- Resume sexual activity when cleared by surgical team.

Caring for the Wound
- Check puncture site daily for signs of infection.
- Wash puncture site with mild soap and water.
- Allow special adhesive strips on the puncture site to fall off. Do not pull them off.

Resuming Eating
- Resume your normal diet.
- If you had fat intolerance before surgery, gradually add fat back into your diet in small increments.

Managing Pain
- You may experience pain or discomfort in your right shoulder from the gas used to inflate your abdominal area during surgery. Use of a heating pad may ease the discomfort (see previous clinical pearl regarding shoulder pain).
- Take analgesics as needed and as prescribed. Report to surgeon if pain is unrelieved even with analgesic use.

Managing Follow-Up Care
- Make an appointment with your surgeon for 7–10 days after discharge.
- Call your surgeon if you experience any signs or symptoms of infection at or around the puncture site: redness, tenderness, swelling, heat, or drainage.
- Call your surgeon if you experience a fever of 37.7°C (100°F) or more for 2 consecutive days.
- Call your surgeon if you develop nausea, vomiting, or abdominal pain.

Cholecystectomy

In cholecystectomy, the gallbladder is removed through an abdominal incision (usually right subcostal) after the cystic duct and artery are ligated. The procedure is performed for acute and chronic cholecystitis. In some patients, a drain is placed close to the gallbladder bed and brought out through a puncture wound if there is a bile leak. A small leak should close spontaneously in a few days, with the drain preventing accumulation of bile. Usually, only a small amount of serosanguineous fluid drains in the initial 24 hours after surgery; afterward, the drain is removed. If a drain or T-Tube is placed, it is positioned in the common bile duct to ensure patency of the duct (see Fig. 24-15). Bile duct injury is a rare but serious complication of cholecystectomy, but it occurs less frequently than with the laparoscopic approach. Patients with multiple comorbidities or with high surgical risk may be treated with the open cholecystectomy (Fogel & Sherman, 2020).

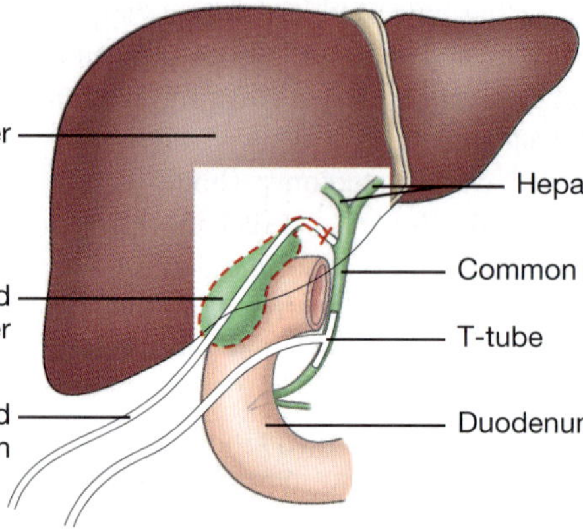

FIGURE 24-15 **Cholecystectomy and T-Tube placement in common bile duct. (Redrawn, with permission, from Macleod, J. (2021). Patients requiring upper gastrointestinal surgery. In I. Peate (Ed.), *Nursing the surgical patient* (pp. 291–312; Figure 16.6). Elsevier Inc.)**

Pearls for Practice

The liver produces averages ~620 mL bile /day and when the T tube is placed, the nurse anticipates approximately 300 to 450 mL in the first 24 hours postoperatively in the T-tube drainage bag (Almaiid & Sugamar, 2022; Macleod, 2021). This amount of drainage will decrease as the edema in the common bile duct subsides (Macleoud, 2021). The nurse suspects T-tube obstruction if the following signs and symptoms are noted: jaundice, pale stools, decreased T-tube drainage, pain, nausea and vomiting (Macleoud, 2021) and the surgeon is notified. Also, the skin surrounding the T-tube should be observed for any redness and excoriation, and protected with a dressing, since bile leakage can irritate the skin and increase patient's discomfort. The T-tube may be clamped before it is removed (based on surgeon preference), and if the patient complains of pain post clamping, the clamp is immediately removed and the surgeon notified. A postoperative cholangiogram is performed to explore the common bile duct for patency of the duct following the cholecystectomy, and in general, the T-Tube is removed 2 weeks postoperatively.

DISORDERS OF THE PANCREAS

Pancreatitis

Pancreatitis (inflammation of the pancreas) is a serious disorder. The most basic classification system used to describe or categorize the various stages and forms of pancreatitis divides the disorder into acute and chronic forms. Acute pancreatitis can be a medical emergency associated with a high risk for life-threatening complications and mortality, whereas chronic pancreatitis may not be detected until significant **exocrine** and endocrine tissue is destroyed. Approximately 80% of patients with acute pancreatitis will recover quickly without developing severe disease (Forsmark, 2020). Common causes for pancreatitis are due to alcohol use disorder or gallstones; however, drugs, trauma, infection, autoimmune disease, or infection also may result in pancreatitis (Forsmark, 2020; Shimizu et al., 2022).

Although the mechanisms causing pancreatic inflammation are unknown, pancreatitis is commonly described as autodigestion of the pancreas. It is believed that the pancreatic duct becomes temporarily obstructed, accompanied by hypersecretion of the exocrine enzymes of the pancreas. These enzymes enter the bile duct, where they are activated and, together with bile, back up (reflux) into the pancreatic duct, causing pancreatitis (Vege, 2020).

ACUTE PANCREATITIS

Acute pancreatitis ranges from a mild, self-limited disorder to a severe, rapidly fatal disease that does not respond to any treatment. Mild acute pancreatitis is characterized by edema and inflammation confined to the pancreas. Minimal organ dysfunction is present and return to normal function usually occurs within 6 months. Although this is considered the milder form of pancreatitis, the patient is acutely ill and at risk for hypovolemic shock, fluid and electrolyte disturbances, and sepsis. A more widespread and complete enzymatic digestion of the gland characterizes severe acute pancreatitis. In this situation, for some unknown reason the normally inactive digestive enzymes are prematurely activated within the pancreas itself, leading to the autodigestion of pancreatic tissue (Close, 2022). Enzymes damage the local blood vessels, and bleeding and thrombosis can occur. The tissue may become necrotic, with damage extending into the retroperitoneal tissues. Local complications consist of pancreatic cysts or abscesses and acute fluid collections in or near the pancreas. Patients who develop systemic complications with organ failure, such as pulmonary insufficiency with hypoxia, shock, kidney failure, and GI bleeding, also are characterized as having severe acute pancreatitis (Forsmark, 2020; Vege, 2020). The severity of acute pancreatitis and its outcomes can be predicted based on clinical and laboratory data (Box 24-11).

Pathophysiology

Self-digestion of the pancreas by its own proteolytic enzymes, principally **trypsin** is a critical initial step, causing acute pancreatitis. Activation of the enzymes can lead to, inflammation, necrosis, erosion, and hemorrhage. This cascade of events also may result in multiorgan failure (Forsmark, 2020).

The two most common causes of acute pancreatitis are gallstone migration and alcoholism, which account for 80% of all cases (Close, 2022). Long-term use of alcohol is commonly associated with acute episodes of pancreatitis, but the patient usually has had undiagnosed chronic pancreatitis before the first episode of acute pancreatitis occurs.

Other, less common causes of pancreatitis include bacterial or viral infection, with pancreatitis occasionally developing as a complication of a virus, such as cytomegalovirus (CMV) and mumps (Forsmark, 2020). Blunt abdominal trauma, peptic ulcer disease, ischemic vascular disease, hyperlipidemia, hypercalcemia, and the use of corticosteroids, thiazide diuretics, oral contraceptives, and other medications also have been associated with an increased incidence of pancreatitis. Acute pancreatitis may develop after surgery on or near the pancreas or after instrumentation of the pancreatic duct. Acute idiopathic pancreatitis accounts for up to 10% of the cases of acute pancreatitis. In addition, there is a small incidence of hereditary pancreatitis (Forsmark, 2020; Vege, 2020).

BOX 24-11

Criteria for Predicting Severity of Pancreatitis[a]

Criteria on Admission to Hospital

- Age over 55 years
- WBC more than 16,000 mm^3
- Serum glucose greater than 200 mg/dL (greater than 11.1 mmol/L)
- Serum LDH greater than 350 IU/L (greater than 350 U/L)
- AST greater than 250 U/mL (120 U/L)

Criteria within 48 Hours of Hospital Admission

- Fall in hematocrit greater than 10% (greater than 0.10)
- BUN increase greater than 5 mg/dL (greater than 1.7 mmol/L)
- Serum calcium less than 8 mg/dL (less than 2.0 mmol/L)
- Base deficit greater than 4 mEq/L (greater than 4 mmol/L)
- Fluid retention or sequestration greater than 6 L
- PO_2 less than 60 mm Hg
- Two or fewer signs, 1% mortality; three or four signs, 15% mortality; five or six signs, 40% mortality; more than six signs, 100% mortality

[a]The more risk factors a patient has, "the greater the severity and likelihood of complications or death."

AST, aspartate aminotransferase; *BUN,* blood urea nitrogen; *LDH,* lactate dehydrogenase; *WBC,* white blood cells.

Clinical Manifestations and Assessment

Severe abdominal pain is the major symptom of pancreatitis that causes the patient to seek medical care. Typically, the pain occurs in the midepigastrium and left upper quadrant abdominal pain (Vege, 2022). Frequently pain is acute in onset, occurring 24 to 48 hours after a very heavy meal or alcohol ingestion, and it may be diffuse and difficult to localize or in 50% of patients may radiate to the back (Vege, 2022). In general, it is more severe after meals and is unrelieved by antacids. Pain may be accompanied by abdominal distention; a poorly defined, palpable abdominal mass; and decreased peristalsis with hypoactive bowel sounds due to an ileus secondary to inflammation. Pain caused by pancreatitis is accompanied frequently by vomiting that fails to relieve the pain or nausea.

The patient appears acutely ill. Abdominal guarding is present and the patient may assume a semifetal position. A rigid or board-like abdomen may develop and is generally an ominous sign; the abdomen may remain soft in the absence of peritonitis. Ecchymosis (bruising) in the flank (Grey–Turner sign) or around the umbilicus (Cullen sign) may indicate severe pancreatitis with retroperitoneal hemorrhage (see Chapter 26, Fig. 26-12). Nausea and vomiting are common in acute pancreatitis. The emesis is usually gastric in origin but also may be bile-stained. Fever, jaundice, mental confusion, and agitation also may occur.

Hypotension is typical and reflects hypovolemia and shock caused by the loss of large amounts of protein-rich fluid into the tissues and peritoneal cavity. In addition to hypotension, the patient may develop tachycardia, cyanosis, and cold, clammy skin. Respiratory distress and peritonitis also are associated with acute pancreatitis (Forsmark, 2020). In addition, the patient may develop a pleural effusion which would present as dullness to percussion on the affected lung.

Pearls for Practice

Although tachycardia (when the patient is at rest) is an early symptom of pathology; it is compensatory response to exercise or stress. The nurse is aware that even in the presence of pathology patients who are on beta-blockers may not present with tachycardia. The nurse remains vigilant with other symptoms such as dyspnea, chest pain, lightheadedness, dizziness, syncope, abnormal heart, and lung sounds.

The diagnosis of acute pancreatitis is based on a history of abdominal pain, the presence of known risk factors, and findings from the physical examination and diagnostics. While serum **amylase** and **lipase** levels are used in making the diagnosis of acute pancreatitis, since they will be elevated three times the upper limit of normal in most cases, the serum lipase is more pancreas-specific than amylase and a more accurate marker for acute pancreatitis (Close, 2022). In addition, the serum lipase rises earlier (within 4 to 8 hours of the onset of symptoms), peaks at 24 hours, and lasts longer (returning to normal within 8 to 14 days), and lipase is also more sensitive when compared with amylase in patients with pancreatitis secondary to alcohol use (Vege, 2022).

A history of gallstones, alcohol use, and viral infection is used to diagnose acute pancreatitis. Usually the WBC count is elevated; hypocalcemia is present in many patients and correlates well with the severity of pancreatitis. Transient hyperglycemia and glucosuria and elevated serum bilirubin levels occur in some patients with acute pancreatitis. Plasma lipids and calcium are additional laboratory tests used to diagnose acute pancreatitis. C-reactive protein (CRP) level which is a marker for inflammation are elevated (normal is <10 mg/L); a level above 150 mg/L at 48 hours is associated with severe pancreatitis (Fischbach et al., 2020; Vege, 2022).

Ultrasound and contrast-enhanced CT or MRI scans are used to identify an increase in the diameter of the pancreas and to detect pancreatic cysts, abscesses, or pseudocysts (discussed shortly). CT or MRI imaging is the modality of choice for the assessment of both acute and chronic pancreatitis (Forsmark, 2020; Shimizu, 2022).

Medical Management

The overall mortality rate of patients with severe acute pancreatitis is high because of shock, anoxia, hypotension, or fluid and electrolyte imbalances. Attacks of acute pancreatitis may result in complete recovery, may recur without permanent damage, or may progress to chronic pancreatitis. The patient who is admitted to the hospital with a diagnosis of pancreatitis is acutely ill and needs expert nursing and medical care (Forsmark, 2020; Shimizu, 2022).

Management of acute pancreatitis is directed toward relieving symptoms and preventing or treating complications. All oral intake is withheld to inhibit stimulation of the pancreas and its secretion of enzymes. The current recommendation is that, whenever possible, the enteral route should be used to meet nutritional needs in patients with pancreatitis. This strategy also has been found to prevent infectious complications and is safe and cost effective in doing so.

The mainstay of therapy for acute pancreatitis is analgesic management of pain, IV fluids to maintain intravascular volume, and elimination of oral intake. Aggressive IV therapy (Ringer's lactate may be preferred for initial fluid resuscitation) will be needed in patients with severe pancreatitis; however, it is important to prevent fluid overload because of the potential development of abdominal compartment syndrome (refer to Chapter 52) (Close, 2022). While prophylactic antibiotics are not recommended, in cases of sepsis, abscess or biliary calculi they are indicated (Close, 2022; Forsmark, 2020). During the acute attack, fluid may collection around the pancreas move into retroperitoneal and peritoneal spaces forming a rounded and circumscribed fluid collection, called a pseudocyst (Forsmark, 2020). Much of this inflammatory fluid will resolve, but if symptomatic fluid aspiration via interventional radiology or endoscopic ultrasound (EUS) may be beneficial. Of note, a pseudocyst is fluid collection that is encapsulated with fibrous tissue. The mark of a true cyst is an epithelial lining, and since this localized collection of fluid does not have one, it is termed *pseudo*cyst. However, after acute necrotizing pancreatitis, areas of pancreatic and peripancreatic necrosis can also develop a surrounding wall and begin to soften and liquefy, thereby becoming "walled-off pancreatic necrosis" (Forsmark, 2020). This takes several weeks to occur, however, the higher the amount of necrosis is correlates with a > risk for adverse outcomes. Treatment will depend the location, however endoscopic drainage may be preferable in patients with high surgical risk (Collins et al., 2023).

Although surgery is often risky because the acutely ill patient is a poor surgical risk, it may be performed to assist in the diagnosis of pancreatitis (diagnostic laparotomy), to establish pancreatic drainage, or to resect or debride a necrotic pancreas (Forsmark, 2020; Shimizu, 2022).

Nursing Management

A plan of nursing care for a patient with acute pancreatitis is available online at http://thepoint.lww.com/Honan3e.

Relieving Pain and Discomfort

Because the pathologic process responsible for pain is autodigestion of the pancreas, the objectives of therapy are to relieve pain and decrease secretion of pancreatic enzymes. The pain of acute pancreatitis is often very severe, necessitating the liberal use of analgesics. The current recommendation for pain management in this population is parenteral narcotics, such as hydromorphone (Forsmark, 2020; Shimizu, 2022). Oral feedings are withheld to decrease the formation and secretion of **secretin**. The patient is maintained on parenteral fluids and electrolytes to restore and maintain fluid balance. NG suction may be used to relieve nausea and vomiting or to treat abdominal distention and paralytic ileus (refer to Chapter 21 for care of NG tube). The nurse provides frequent oral hygiene and care to decrease discomfort from the NG tube and relieve dryness of the mouth.

The acutely ill patient is maintained on bed rest to decrease the metabolic rate and reduce the secretion of pancreatic and gastric enzymes. If the patient experiences increasing severity of pain, the nurse reports this to the provider because the patient may be experiencing hemorrhage of the pancreas or the dose of analgesic may be inadequate.

The patient with acute pancreatitis often has a clouded sensorium because of severe pain, fluid and electrolyte disturbances, and hypoxia. Therefore, the nurse provides frequent and repeated but simple explanations about the need for withholding fluids, maintenance of gastric suction, and bed rest.

Improving Breathing Pattern

The nurse maintains the patient in a semi-Fowler position to decrease pressure on the diaphragm by a distended abdomen and to increase respiratory expansion. Frequent changes of position are necessary to prevent atelectasis and pooling of respiratory secretions. Pulmonary assessment and monitoring of pulse oximetry or ABGs are essential to detect changes in respiratory status so that early treatment can be initiated. The nurse instructs the patient in techniques of deep breathing and in the use of an IS to improve respiratory function, and the nurse encourages and assists the patient to perform these activities every hour. Intubation may be necessary to support ventilation.

Improving Nutritional Status

In the past, the patient with acute pancreatitis has not been permitted food or oral fluid intake. However, recent studies suggest that maintaining NPO and the use of enteral nutrition with nasojejunum tubes, prevents pancreatic enzyme release, maintains gut integrity, enhances immune system functioning, and demonstrates lower complication rates when compared to keeping the patient solely NPO (Pham & McClave, 2021). It is important to assess the patient's nutritional status and to note factors that alter the patient's nutritional requirements (e.g., temperature elevation, surgery, drainage). Laboratory test results and daily weights are useful to monitor the nutritional status.

In addition to administering enteral or parenteral nutrition, the nurse monitors serum glucose levels every 4 to 6 hours. As the acute symptoms subside, the nurse gradually reintroduces oral feedings. Between acute attacks, the patient receives a diet that is high in carbohydrates and low in fats and proteins. The patient should avoid heavy meals and alcoholic beverages.

Improving Skin Integrity

The patient is at risk for skin breakdown because of poor nutritional status, enforced bed rest, and restlessness, which may result in pressure ulcers and breaks in tissue integrity. In addition, the patient who has undergone surgery may have multiple drains or an open surgical incision and is at risk for skin breakdown and infection. The nurse carefully assesses the wound, drainage sites, and skin for signs of infection, inflammation, and breakdown. The nurse carries out wound care as prescribed and takes precautions to protect intact skin from contact with drainage. It is important to turn the patient every 2 hours; use of specialty beds may be indicated to prevent skin breakdown. Often consultation with an **enterostomal therapist** (also referred to as a wound care specialist or wound-ostomy-continence nurse) is helpful in identifying appropriate skin care devices and protocols.

Monitoring and Managing Potential Complications

Fluid and electrolyte disturbances are common complications because of nausea, vomiting, movement of fluid from the vascular compartment to the peritoneal cavity, diaphoresis, fever, and the use of gastric suction. The nurse assesses the patient's fluid and electrolyte status by noting skin turgor and moistness of mucous membranes. The nurse weighs the patient daily and carefully measures fluid intake and output, including urine output, NG secretions, and diarrhea. In addition, it is important to assess for other factors that may affect fluid and electrolyte status, including increased body temperature and wound drainage. Inflammation can lead to significant fluid depletion as well as extravasation of fluid into the retroperitoneal space and abdominal cavity.

The nurse assesses the patient for ascites and measures abdominal girth daily if ascites is suspected.

Fluids are administered intravenously and may be accompanied by infusion of blood or blood products to maintain the blood volume and to prevent or treat hypovolemic shock. It is important to keep emergency medications readily available because of the risk for circulatory collapse and shock. The nurse promptly reports decreased blood pressure and reduced urine output because these signs may indicate hypovolemia and shock or kidney failure. Low serum calcium and magnesium levels may occur and require prompt treatment.

Pearls for Practice

The nurse is aware that early fluid replacement is associated with decreased rates of systemic inflammatory response syndrome (SIRS) and organ failure (refer to Chapter 53) (Close, 2022). Cues that suggest adequate fluid replacement are assessed by improvement in vital signs (mean arterial pressure is >65 mm Hg), urine output (>0.5 to 1 cc/kg/hr) (Vege, 2022).

Pancreatic necrosis is a major cause of morbidity and mortality in patients with acute pancreatitis. The patient who develops necrosis is at risk for hemorrhage, septic shock, and multiple organ failure (refer to Chapter 53). The patient may undergo diagnostic procedures to confirm pancreatic necrosis; surgical debridement or insertion of multiple drains may be performed. The patient with pancreatic necrosis is usually critically ill and requires expert medical and nursing management, including hemodynamic monitoring in the ICU.

In addition to carefully monitoring vital signs and other signs and symptoms, the nurse is responsible for administering prescribed fluids, medications, and blood products; assisting with supportive management, such as use of a ventilator; preventing additional complications; and attending to the patient's physical and psychological care.

Shock and multiple organ failure may occur with acute pancreatitis. Hypovolemic shock may occur as a result of hypovolemia and sequestering of fluid in the peritoneal cavity. Hemorrhagic shock may occur with hemorrhagic pancreatitis. Septic shock may occur with bacterial infection of the pancreas. Cardiac dysfunction may occur as a result of fluid and electrolyte disturbances, acid–base imbalances, and release of toxic substances into the circulation.

The nurse closely monitors the patient for early signs of neurologic, cardiovascular, renal, and respiratory dysfunction. The nurse must be prepared to respond quickly to rapid changes in the patient's status, treatments, and therapies. In addition, it is important to inform the family about the status and progress of the patient and to allow them to spend time with the patient.

Promoting Home and Community-Based Care

The patient who has survived an episode of acute pancreatitis has been acutely ill. A prolonged period is needed to regain strength and return to the previous level of activity. Often the patient is still weak and debilitated for weeks or months after an acute episode of pancreatitis. Because of the severity of the acute illness, the patient may not recall many of the explanations and instructions given during the acute phase. Teaching often needs to be repeated and reinforced. The nurse instructs the patient about the factors implicated in the onset of acute pancreatitis and about the need to avoid high-fat foods, heavy meals, and alcohol. It is important to give the patient and family verbal and written instructions about signs and symptoms of acute pancreatitis and possible complications that should be reported promptly to the provider.

If acute pancreatitis is a result of biliary tract disease, such as gallstones and gallbladder disease, additional explanations are needed about required dietary modifications. If the pancreatitis is a result of alcohol use, the nurse reminds the patient of the importance of eliminating all alcohol.

Often a referral for home care is indicated. This enables the nurse to assess the patient's physical and psychological status and adherence to the therapeutic regimen. The nurse also assesses the home situation and reinforces instructions about fluid and nutrition intake and avoidance of alcohol. The nurse provides specific information about resources and support groups that may be of assistance in avoiding alcohol in the future. Referral to Alcoholics Anonymous or other appropriate support groups is essential.

CHRONIC PANCREATITIS

Chronic pancreatitis is an inflammatory disorder that is characterized by progressive anatomic and functional destruction of the pancreas.

Pathophysiology

As cells are replaced by fibrous tissue with repeated attacks of pancreatitis, pressure within the pancreas increases. The end result is mechanical obstruction of the pancreatic and common bile ducts and the duodenum. In addition, there is atrophy of the epithelium of the ducts, inflammation, and destruction of the secreting cells of the pancreas.

Alcohol consumption in Western societies and malnutrition worldwide, frequently associated with cigarette smoking, are the major causes of chronic pancreatitis. Excessive and prolonged consumption of alcohol accounts for 50% of cases of chronic pancreatitis in the United States, although 25% of cases may be attributed to smoking alone (Forsmark, 2020). Long-term alcohol consumption causes hypersecretion of protein in pancreatic secretions, resulting in protein plugs and calculi within the pancreatic ducts. Alcohol also has a direct toxic effect on the cells of the pancreas. Some research suggests that hypertriglyceridemia, dyslipidemia, and diet also may contribute to the development of chronic pancreatitis. Less common causes of chronic pancreatitis are due to genetic mutations, autoimmune pancreatitis, duct obstruction, and idiopathic pancreatitis. Patients with chronic pancreatitis are at increased risk for the development of pancreatic cancer (Forsmark, 2020).

Clinical Manifestations and Assessment

Chronic pancreatitis is characterized by recurring attacks of severe upper abdominal and back pain, accompanied by vomiting. Often attacks are so painful that opioids, even in large doses, do not provide relief. As the disease progresses, recurring attacks of pain are more severe, more frequent, and of longer duration. Some patients experience continuous severe pain, others have a dull, nagging constant pain, and a small percentage of other patients does not have pain and instead presents with exocrine (steatorrhea, weight loss) or endocrine (diabetes) pancreatic insufficiency (Forsmark, 2020). The risk of opioid dependence is increased in pancreatitis because of the chronic nature and severity of the pain.

Weight loss is a major problem in chronic pancreatitis: more than 75% of patients experience significant weight loss, usually caused by decreased dietary intake secondary to anorexia or fear that eating will precipitate another attack. Malabsorption occurs late in the disease due to decreases in lipase production. As a result, digestion, especially of proteins and fats, is impaired. The stools become frequent, frothy, and foul-smelling because of impaired fat digestion, which results in stools with a high-fat content (referred to as **steatorrhea**). As the disease progresses, calcification of the gland may occur, and calcium stones may form within the ducts. Diabetes mellitus occurs due to loss of pancreatic beta cells.

Various imaging procedures, including MRI, CT scans, and ultrasound, have been useful in the diagnostic evaluation of patients with suspected pancreatic disorders. A CT scan or ultrasound study also is helpful to detect pancreatic cysts or pseudocysts which develop in 10% of patients with chronic pancreatitis (Dholaria et al., 2021). Steatorrhea can be confirmed by laboratory analysis of fecal fat content and determination of exocrine pancreatic insufficiency via the secretin-cholecystokinin test. In most cases, the diagnosis of chronic pancreatitis is based upon clinical findings, history, and imaging modalities such as ERCP, CT, and MRI to detect abnormalities of the pancreas (Forsmark, 2020; Shimizu, 2022).

Pearls for Practice

Endoscopic retrograde cholangiopancreatography (ERCP) provides detail about the anatomy of the pancreas and the pancreatic and biliary ducts, and it is helpful in obtaining tissue for analysis and differentiating pancreatitis from other conditions, such as carcinoma. However, because of its risk, ERCP should be undertaken only when therapy involving the pancreatic duct is appropriate.

Medical Management

Nonsurgical Management

Nonsurgical approaches are focused primarily on complete abstinence of alcohol and tobacco, pain management, nutritional management, and treatment of diabetes mellitus. Pain management is achieved through use of analgesics as first-line therapy and for refractory pain. Pancreatic enzyme replacement is indicated for the patient with malabsorption and steatorrhea. A proton pump inhibitor (omeprazole, lansoprazole) is administered with enzyme therapy to reduce gastric acid inactivation of enzymes. Also supplementation of fat-soluble vitamins is indicated. Improved nutrition and resolution of steatorrhea usually are indicators of clinical improvement in the patient with chronic pancreatitis.

Diabetes mellitus resulting from dysfunction of the pancreatic islet cells is treated with diet, insulin, or oral antidiabetic agents. Use of insulin is the preferred therapy; however, administration should be adjusted carefully to avoid hypoglycemic events (Forsmark, 2020).

Surgical Management

Surgery or interventional therapies are used primarily to address complications of pancreatitis and to relieve abdominal pain and discomfort, restore drainage of pancreatic secretions, and reduce the frequency of acute attacks of pancreatitis. The type of surgery that is performed depends on the anatomic and functional abnormalities of the pancreas, including the location of disease within the pancreas, the presence of diabetes, exocrine insufficiency, biliary stenosis, and pseudocysts of the pancreas.

Pancreaticojejunostomy (also referred to as Roux-en-Y), with a side-to-side anastomosis or joining of the pancreatic duct to the jejunum, allows drainage of the pancreatic secretions into the jejunum. Other surgical procedures may be performed for different degrees and types of underlying disorders. These procedures include revision of the sphincter of the ampulla of Vater, internal drainage of a pancreatic cyst into the stomach, insertion of a stent, and wide resection or removal of the pancreas. A Whipple resection (pancreaticoduodenectomy) can be carried out to relieve the pain of chronic pancreatitis. Endoscopic therapy is used for pancreatic duct stones and strictures. The use of surgical and endoscopic treatment is based upon patient presentation, complications, and the availability of surgical expertise (Forsmark, 2020).

PANCREATIC CANCER

Pancreatic cancer is the fourth leading cause of cancer death in the United States. Cancer may develop in the head, body, or tail of the pancreas; most pancreatic cancers originate in the head of the pancreas. Patients usually do not seek medical attention until late in the disease; most patients have an advanced, unresectable tumor when first detected. In fact, pancreatic carcinoma has a survival rate of only 8% at 5 years. Although pancreatic cancer comprises only 7% of all cancer diagnoses, it is projected to become the second leading cause of cancer death by 2030 (Modi & Shires, 2021).

Risk Factors

Males are affected more than females (1.3:1), and African Americans have a higher prevalence of pancreatic cancer

BOX 24-12

Nursing Research

Bridging the Gap to Evidence-Based Practice

Chung, V., Sun, V., Ruel, N., Smith, T. J., & Ferrell, B. R. (2022). Improving palliative care and quality of life in pancreatic cancer patients. *Journal of Palliative Medicine*, *25*(5), 720–727. https://doi.org/10.1089/jpm.2021.0187.

Purpose

Pancreatic cancer patients often present with complications, which can impact treatment tolerance. Thus, symptom management is a vital component of treatment in addition to traditional chemotherapeutics. Concurrent palliative care with an emphasis on aggressive symptom management may sustain both clinical and patient-centered outcomes during treatment. The purpose of this article is to explore the impact of a concurrent palliative care intervention in patients with pancreatic cancer treated on phase I clinical trials.

Design

This is a secondary analysis of a National Cancer Institute (NCI)-funded randomized trial of an advanced practice nurse–driven palliative care intervention for solid tumor patients treated on phase I clinical trials. Only pancreatic cancer patients were included in the analysis. Patients received two educational sessions around the quality of life (QOL) domains and completed the Functional Assessment of Cancer Therapy-General (FACT-G), patient-reported outcomes version of the common terminology criteria for adverse events (PRO-CTCAE), and the psychological distress thermometer at baseline, 4 and 12 weeks. Mixed model with repeated measures analysis was used to explore outcomes by study arm.

Findings

Of the 479 patients accrued to the study, 42 were diagnosed with pancreatic cancer (26 intervention, 16 usual care). A trend toward improvement in the physical, social, emotional, and functional FACT-G QOL subscales and psychological distress (baseline to 12 weeks) were observed for the intervention arm. Patients reported moderate severity in psychological and physical stress. In this secondary analysis, a nurse-led palliative care intervention may improve the QOL and psychological distress of pancreatic cancer patients. A phase III trial focused on patients with pancreatic cancer is needed to determine the effectiveness of the intervention.

Nursing Implications

Palliative care is an integral part in the management of pancreatic cancer patients. This study has shown a positive impact of a palliative care intervention improving QOL measures across pancreatic cancer patients enrolled in phase I trials. Other recent studies showed that monitoring and fixing symptoms in advanced cancer patients leads to substantially improved survival. In pancreatic cancer patients, the authors hypothesize that early palliative care will impact survival. To answer that question, they have designed a randomized phase III clinical trial of a primary palliative care intervention to improve QOL in metastatic pancreatic cancer patients. With the shortage of palliative care physicians, they designed a scalable approach to provide palliative care to a population in need. With centrally located advanced practice nurses, needs can potentially be identified early to guide interventions by the local teams to positively impact our patients and family caregivers' QOL. Nurses should continue to await result of nurse researchers as they evaluate the efficacy of these interventions.

(Ward, 2022). Use of tobacco, obesity, advanced age, and nonhereditary chronic pancreatitis also are risk factors for pancreatic cancer. Diabetes mellitus is also associated with pancreatic cancer; however, whether it is a risk factor or a manifestation of pancreatic cancer is unclear (Collins et al., 2023). Genetic predisposition also may play a role; up to 10% of patients with this cancer have a first-degree relative diagnosed with pancreatic cancer (Modi & Shires, 2021).

Clinical Manifestations and Assessment

The majority of patients present with pain and/or jaundice, which, along with weight loss, are considered classic signs of pancreatic carcinoma. However, they often do not appear until the disease is far advanced. Other signs include rapid, profound, and progressive weight loss as well as vague upper or midabdominal pain or discomfort that is unrelated to any GI function and is often difficult to describe. Such discomfort radiates as a boring pain in the midback and is unrelated to posture or activity. Often it is progressive and severe, requiring the use of opioids. The formation of ascites is common. An important sign, if it is present, is the onset of symptoms of insulin deficiency: glucosuria, hyperglycemia, and abnormal glucose tolerance. Therefore, diabetes may be an early sign of carcinoma of the pancreas. Meals often aggravate epigastric pain, which usually occurs before the appearance of jaundice and pruritus. Diarrhea and steatorrhea also commonly are present in pancreatic cancer (Modi & Shires, 2021). Unexplained recurring migrating thrombophlebitis, also termed *Trousseau syndrome* which is named after the physician who made the link between cancer and hypercoagulability associated thrombosis may be associated with pancreatic cancer and other types of malignancy primarily gastric and pulmonary (Stoyanov et al., 2019). The thrombophlebitis can involve the upper and lower limbs, thoracic and abdominal wall, and the major blood vessels of the abdomen (Stoyanov et al., 2019). The thrombus can detach resulting in a pulmonary emboli which can be fatal.

CT and MRI imaging are currently the most useful preoperative imaging technique. CT or MRI can accurately image pancreatic masses, show dilatation of pancreatic duct, and indicate if metastases are present in the liver or peritoneum. Endoscopic retrograde pancreatography (ERCP), endoscopic ultrasound (EUS), and magnetic resonance cholangiopancreatography (MRCP) also are used to diagnose pancreatic cancer. Cells obtained during ERCP/EUS are sent to the laboratory for histologic analysis. Although cancer-associated antigen (CA 19-9) serum levels may be elevated, this tumor marker is used primarily to monitor disease progression and treatment efficacy (Modi & Shires, 2021).

Medical Management

Only 10% to 20% of patients with pancreatic cancer benefit from surgical resection; the majority of patients present at a late stage, frequently with metastatic spread to other organs or vascular invasion. In patients with early-stage disease, the Whipple procedure (pancreaticoduodenectomy) is used to remove the pancreatic head, duodenum, part of the jejunum, common bile duct, and gallbladder (Fig. 24-16). Use of adjuvant therapy (i.e., chemotherapy and/or immunotherapy) continues to be controversial and nonstandard in this small group of surgical patients, with ongoing clinical trials to evaluate potential benefits of treatment (Timmer et al., 2021). The chemotherapy agent gemcitabine alone or in combination with other chemotherapeutic agents remains the treatment of choice for most patients with pancreatic cancer. Overall, patients with pancreatic cancer have a high mortality rate and poor survival outcomes even with chemotherapy or surgical treatment. Palliative measures to address symptoms of pancreatic cancer include nutritional support and pain management (Modi & Shires, 2021).

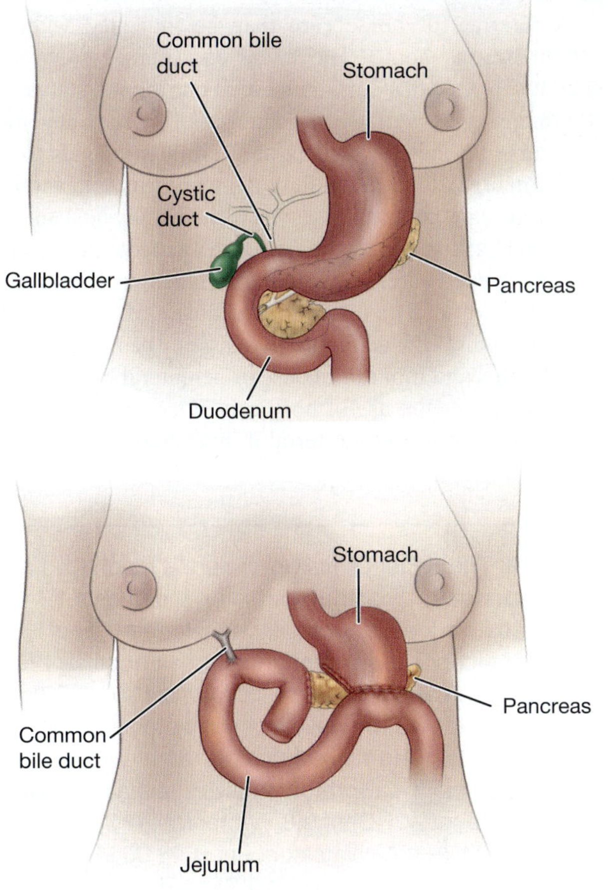

FIGURE 24-16 Pancreatoduodenectomy (Whipple procedure or resection). End result of resection of carcinoma of the head of the pancreas or the ampulla of Vater. The common duct is sutured to the end of the jejunum, and the remaining portion of the pancreas and the end of the stomach are sutured to the side of the jejunum.

Nursing Management

Pain management and attention to nutritional requirements are important nursing measures that improve the level of patient comfort. Refer to Chapter 6 for treatment of cancer pain. Skin care and nursing measures are directed toward relief of pain and discomfort associated with jaundice, anorexia, and profound weight loss. Specialty mattresses are beneficial and protect bony prominences from pressure. Pain associated with pancreatic cancer may be severe and may require liberal use of opioids; patient-controlled analgesia should be considered for the patient with severe, escalating pain.

Because of the poor prognosis and likelihood of short survival, end-of-life preferences are discussed and honored. If appropriate, the nurse refers the patient to hospice care (see Chapter 2 for further discussion).

The postoperative management of patients who have undergone a pancreaticoduodenectomy is similar to the management of patients after extensive GI or biliary surgery. The patient's physical status is often suboptimal, increasing the risk for postoperative complications. Hemorrhage, vascular collapse, and hepatorenal failure remain the major complications of these extensive surgical procedures. The mortality rate associated with these procedures has improved because of advances in nutritional support and improved surgical techniques. An NG tube with suction, NPO status, and nutrition that allows the GI tract to rest while promoting adequate nutrition is anticipated (Fig. 24-17).

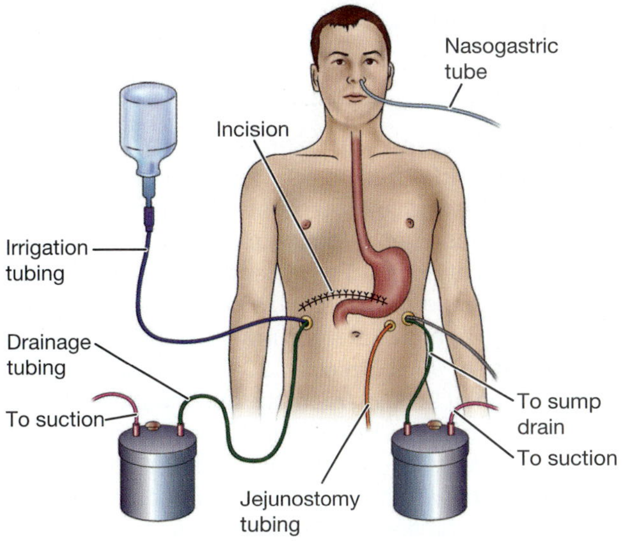

FIGURE 24-17 Multiple sump tubes are used after pancreatic surgery. Triple-lumen tubes consist of ports that provide tubing for irrigation, air venting, and drainage.

Preoperatively and postoperatively, nursing care is directed toward promoting patient comfort, preventing complications, and assisting the patient to return to and maintain as normal and comfortable a life as possible. The nurse closely monitors the patient in the ICU after surgery; in the immediate postoperative period, multiple IV and an arterial line are used for fluid and blood replacement and hemodynamic monitoring, and a mechanical ventilator is used. It is important to note and report changes in vital signs, ABGs and pressures, pulse oximetry, laboratory values, and urine output. The nurse also must consider the patient's compromised nutritional status and risk for bleeding. Depending on the type of surgical procedure performed, malabsorption syndrome and diabetes mellitus are likely; the nurse must address these issues during acute and long-term patient care.

Although the patient's physiologic status is the focus of the health care team in the immediate postoperative period, the patient's psychological and emotional state must be considered, along with that of the family. The patient has undergone a major high-risk surgery and is critically ill; anxiety and depression may affect recovery. The immediate and long-term outcomes of this extensive surgical resection are uncertain, and the patient and family require emotional support and understanding in the critical and stressful preoperative and postoperative periods.

Promoting Home and Community-Based Care

The specific teaching for the patient and family varies with the stage of disease and the treatment choices made by the patient. The patient who has undergone this extensive surgery requires careful and thorough preparation for self-care at home. The nurse instructs the patient and family about the need for modifications in the diet because of malabsorption and hyperglycemia resulting from the surgery. It is important to instruct the patient and family about the continuing need for pancreatic enzyme replacement, a low-fat diet, and vitamin supplementation.

The nurse teaches the patient and family strategies to relieve pain and discomfort, along with strategies to manage drains, if present, and to care for the surgical incision. The patient and family members may require instruction about use of patient-controlled analgesia, enteral/parenteral nutrition, wound care, skin care, and management of drainage. It is important to describe, verbally and in writing, the signs and symptoms of complications and to teach the patient and family about indicators of complications that should be reported promptly.

Discharge of the patient to a long-term care or rehabilitation facility may be warranted after surgery as extensive as a pancreaticoduodenectomy, particularly if the patient's preoperative status was not optimal. Information about the teaching that has been provided is shared with the long-term care staff so that instructions can be clarified and reinforced.

If the patient elects to receive chemotherapy, the nurse focuses teaching on prevention of side effects and complications of the agents used. If surgery is performed to relieve obstruction and establish biliary drainage, teaching addresses management of the drainage system and monitoring for complications. The nurse instructs the family about changes in the patient's status that should be reported to the provider.

A referral for home care may be indicated when the patient returns home. The home care nurse assesses the patient's physical status, fluid and nutritional status, and skin integrity as well as the adequacy of pain management. The nurse teaches the patient and family strategies to prevent skin breakdown and relieve pain, pruritus, and anorexia. The home care nurse assesses the patient's physical and psychological status and the ability of the patient and family to manage needed care. The home care nurse provides needed physical care and monitors the adequacy of pain management. In addition, it is important to assess the patient's nutritional status and monitor the use of parenteral nutrition. The nurse discusses the use of hospice services with the patient and family and makes a referral if indicated.

Clinical Judgment Case

A 58-year-old patient is admitted to your medical unit with GI bleeding (melena), increasing edema of the legs and abdomen, weight gain (5 lb in 3 days) and shortness of breath. The patient's skin is warm and dry, no jaundice, icterus, bruising, or clubbing, pale conjunctiva, and vital signs are as follows: 98.7°F, heart rate of 96 and regular, 20 RR with an oxygen saturation of 98% on room air, and the blood pressure is 108/54 mm Hg. Heart sounds are normal, without gallop or murmur, bibasilar crackles are noted on auscultation, abdomen is distended, nontender, bowel sounds are present in all 4 quadrants, capillary refill is 2 seconds and pedal and posterior tibial pulses are 3+ bil. The patient's history included smoking ½ pack per day (15-pack year history), cirrhosis, esophageal varices, hepatic encephalopathy, and history of alcohol use disorder (has been abstinent for 3 years). Medications at home include lactulose 30 g TID, furosemide 40 mg daily, spironolactone 25 mg daily, folic acid 1 mg daily, thiamine 100 mg daily, and multivitamin daily. Laboratory analysis reveals white blood cell count (WBC) of 9.8, hemoglobin of 5.8 g/dL, hematocrit of 19.2%, platelet count is 98,000/ mm^3, BUN is 38 mg/dL, creatinine is 1.2 mg/dL, and potassium is 3.8 mEq/L. The international normalized ratio (INR) is elevated at 2.1. The ammonia level is 13 mg/dL (within normal limits [WNL]). The patient is to receive two units of packed red blood cells (PRBCs), and is scheduled for endoscopy as soon as transfusion is complete as long as there is no evidence of decompensation.

Step One: Recognize cues where relevant and important information is identified from different sources, such as medical history or vital signs

Answer: Recent GI bleeding (melena), increasing edema of the legs and abdomen, weight gain (5 lb in 3 days), shortness of breath, bibasilar pulmonary crackles, pale conjunctiva. Medical history of smoking ½ pack per day (15-pack year history), cirrhosis, esophageal varices, hepatic encephalopathy, and history of alcohol use disorder (has been abstinent for 3 years). Home medications of lactulose 30 g TID, furosemide 40 mg daily, spironolactone 25 mg daily, folic acid 1 mg daily, thiamine 100 mg daily, and multivitamin daily. Laboratory analysis results of significance are hemoglobin of 5.8 g/dL, hematocrit of 19.2%, platelet count of 98,000/ mm^3, BUN is 38 mg/dL, and INR of 2.1. The patient is to receive 2 units of PRBCs, and once infused will have endoscopy procedure post transfusions.

Step Two: Analyze cues, which is organizing and linking the recognized cues to the patient's clinical presentation.

Answer: You have clustered the symptom of melena and decreased Hgb/Hct, elevated BUN, history of cirrhosis and esophageal varices to be associated with upper GI bleed (etiology unknown at this point however you are aware that melena or black tarry stools occurs from digestion of blood from an upper GI hemorrhage). You cluster the shortness of breath, decreased Hgb/Hct, and pale conjunctiva with anemia. The history of cirrhosis, and portal hypertension, and associated deficient absorption of vitamin K from the GI tract are associated with decreased platelet count (normal count is ~150,000–450,000/mm^3), coagulopathy and an international normalized ratio (INR) that is elevated at 2.1. You have clustered the weight gain, increased edema of extremities and abdomen, decreased hemoglobin with cirrhosis, and portal hypertension. Signs of fluid volume excess include edema, bilateral crackles, shortness of breath, and weight gain. You analyze the vital signs and recognize that there is no tachycardia, tachypnea, and although the blood pressure of 108/54 mm Hg is low, when you calculate the mean arterial pressure (MAP) which is systolic pressure (108 mm Hg), plus the diastolic pressure (54 mm Hg) x's 2/3 (108+ 108 = 216/3 = 72 mm Hg. Since the MAP is >65 mm Hg, you are aware that perfusion to major organs is maintained. However, you are aware that hypovolemic shock can occur and you will be alert to signs and symptoms such as decreasing urine output (<0.5 mL/Kg/hr), oliguria, hypotension, with narrow pulse pressure, decreased MAP, flat neck veins, skin will be cool, altered mental status (anxiety may be earliest symptom), delayed capillary refill, pallor, cool extremities, tachycardia, and tachypnea. You cluster the medical history of cirrhosis, previous history of hepatic encephalopathy, usual dose of lactulose and normal ammonia level with stable management at this point, however you are aware that ammonia increases as a result of GI bleeding (i.e., bleeding esophageal varices, chronic GI bleeding). History of smoking increases risk for pulmonary complications during hospitalization. You cluster the combination drug therapy of spironolactone, an aldosterone-blocking agent, and furosemide, a loop diuretic agent, as the regimen to control ascites. You also cluster the multiple vitamins with avitaminoses (vitamin deficiencies), associated with chronic liver disease (especially if alcohol-related).

Step Three: Prioritize hypotheses, where hypotheses are evaluated and ranked according to priority. This can include urgency, likelihood, risk, difficulty, and/or time. In this phase you cluster your findings, to arrive at a list of problems (actual and/or potential problems) you believe the patient is experiencing and determine the importance or urgency. What do you think is of greatest concern?

Answer: You prioritize current GI hemorrhage and restoring circulating blood volume. Potential problems are hypovolemic shock, risk of aspiration, potential bleeding from thrombocytopenia and coagulopathy, and lack of knowledge regarding the current regimen.

Step Four: Generate solutions, which is identifying expected outcomes and using hypotheses to define a set of interventions for the expected outcomes.

Answer: Expected outcomes are to improve the Hgb/Hct levels by administering 2 units of packed cells without complications, such as acute hemolytic reaction and transfusion-associated circulatory overload (TACO) which can develop if the blood is infused too quickly, hypervolemia occurs. In addition, a risk factor for TACO is hypoalbuminemia which is associated with chronic and advanced hepatic cirrhosis. Transfusion of blood components also may be required to maintain hemodynamic stability and correct coagulopathy with the aim of maintaining a hemoglobin level of 7–8 g/dL. Monitoring the platelet count and coagulation studies is also required since excess bleeding may occur with a platelet count of 50,000–100,000/mm^3. The goal is to maintain hemodynamic stability via IV and blood transfusion with vital signs remaining in the normal range until endoscopy therapy can be initiated with the ultimate aim of absent of frank and occult blood in stools.

Step Five: Take action, where the solutions that address the highest priorities are implemented.

Answer: You start the IV, place the patient on a cardiac monitor and apply the oxygen saturation device. You elevate the head of the bed for patient comfort to semi-Fowler's to promote optimal gas exchange. You bring nasal cannula and flow meter to the bedside in case the saturation decreases (currently 96% on room air). You ask the patient about to previous reactions to transfusions and perform a systematic physical assessment that includes assessing the lungs, oxygen saturation, heart sounds, noting presence of neck vein distention, noting extent and presence of pitting edema, and observe skin for icterus and repeat the vital signs. In the event of a transfusion reaction, a comparison of these findings can help you differentiate between types of reactions and measurement of baseline vital signs is imperative before transfusing any blood product. An IV of normal saline (0.9% NaCl) is infusing and you obtain the first unit of PRBCs from the blood bank after the IV line is started and vital signs are assessed. (Institution policy may limit release to only one unit at a time.) You double-check the labels with another licensed provider to make sure that the ABO group and Rh type agree with the compatibility record. You check to see that the number and type on the donor blood label and on the patient's chart are correct and assess the patient's identification by using two forms of identification (can include the patient's name, date of birth, and medical record number) comparing the blood product label to the patient identification bracelet. Also, you can ask the patient to confirm their name and date of birth. You make sure the PRBC transfusion is initiated within 30 minutes after removal of the PRBCs from the blood bank refrigerator and remain alert for signs and symptoms of an acute hemolytic reaction which is the most dangerous, and potentially life-threatening type of transfusion reaction occurs when the donor blood is incompatible with that of the recipient. Symptoms consist of fever, chills, nausea, vomiting, chest tightness, dyspnea, hypotension, flank pain, hematuria, oliguria, bleeding, and anxiety. For the first 15 minutes, you run the transfusion slowly—no faster than 5 mL/min and observe the patient carefully for adverse effects. If no adverse effects occur during the first 15 minutes, then you increase the flow rate unless the patient is at high risk for circulatory overload. Signs of TACO that you are alert to include increased dyspnea, orthopnea (shortness of breath [SOB] on lying down), tachycardia, sudden anxiety, jugular vein distention, an S3 gallop, increasing crackles (recall the patient already presented with crackles) and an increase in blood pressure can also occur. If the transfusion is continued, pulmonary edema can develop, as manifested by severe dyspnea and coughing up of pink, frothy sputum. For any adverse reaction you are prepared to stop the infusion immediately, notify the health care provider, and follow your agency's transfusion reaction policy. You also track and trend the blood counts and are aware that 1 unit of PRBCs will raise the hemoglobin by 1 g and Hct by 3%, if the patient is not bleeding or hemolyzing. You will also monitor for early signs and symptoms of thrombocytopenia by closely observing the client's skin for petechiae and bruising and alert the provider if noted. The 2 units are infused and the patient is transferred to the GI special procedures unit. In the event of further clinical deterioration, you would alert the nursing supervisor regarding ICU bed availability and are prepared to insert a second large-gauge IV for fluid resuscitation.

Step Six: Evaluate outcomes, which is comparing observed outcomes against expected outcomes.

Answer: The patient remained stable and a bleeding gastric ulcer was found and treated, the patient tolerated the procedure without complications and was subsequently discharged home with the addition of pantoprazole along with their preadmission medication regimen. As a new RN, administering blood for the first time can be intimidating but you reviewed the hospital protocol and remembered that every action has both a benefit and a risk and you reviewed the risks, so you were prepared from the outset with a list of signs and symptoms to observe. This patient's story was certainly complex but you made multiple connections in your learning and each day you will continue to add to your knowledge and skill base. Keep going....

CHAPTER REVIEW

NCLEX-Style Review Questions

1. A patient has advanced cirrhosis and has developed hepatic encephalopathy. The nurse would assess the patient for? Select all that apply.
a. Fetor hepaticus
b. Rhinorrhea
c. Acetone breath
d. Hand tremors
e. Mental status changes

2. A patient with hepatitis A is admitted to a general medical-surgical floor. The nurse knows that this type of hepatitis is spread through which mode of transmission?
a. Injection of drugs
b. Blood
c. Uncooked food
d. Semen
e. Fecally contaminated food or water

3. A patient is being seen in the clinic to rule out pancreatitis. The nurse expects which diagnostic test will be performed to diagnose this disease process? Select all that apply.
a. MR/CT
b. Abdominal ultrasound
c. Lumbar puncture
d. Endoscopy
e. Lipase

4. Which of the following findings would indicate the development of portal hypertension in a client with cirrhosis?
1. Esophageal varices
2. Hemorrhoids
3. Ascites
4. Hyperalbuminemia

a. Only 1 and 4 are correct
b. Only 1, 3, and 4 are correct
c. Only 1 and 3 are correct
d. Only 1, 2, and 3 are correct

5. A 50-year-old patient has a long history of hospital admissions related to alcohol use and consequent liver failure. During this present admission, the patient has been diagnosed with hepatic encephalopathy and prescribed lactulose. During morning report, the nurse learns that the previous nurse withheld the patient's latest dose of lactulose because the patient had two loose bowel movements yesterday. How should the nurse interpret the previous nurse's action?
a. The previous nurse acted correctly because loose bowel movements present a threat to the patient's fluid and electrolyte balance.
b. The previous nurse should have known that two or three soft stools per day are desirable.
c. The previous nurse should have administered the lactulose because it is necessary to remove excess ammonia.
d. The previous nurse should have administered a partial dose of the lactulose in spite of the patient's bowel movements.
e. The previous nurse should have obtained an order for a stool softener to replace the scheduled lactulose.

REFERENCES AND SELECTED READINGS

References and selected readings associated with this chapter can be found on the website that accompanies the book. Visit **http://thepoint.lww.com/Honan3e** to access the references and other additional resources associated with this chapter.

UNIT SEVEN

Problems Related to Urinary Tract Function

A nurse is caring for a patient diagnosed with kidney failure. The patient is currently receiving hemodialysis three times a week and is very anxious about the lifestyle changes that are occurring due to the health problems.

- **What areas of teaching would be important for the nurse to emphasize for this patient?**
- **Explain the various treatment modalities available for this patient population.**
- **Discuss areas of nursing management that would apply to this patient.**

CHAPTER 25

Nursing Assessment: Renal and Urinary Tract Function

Deborah Bain Fahs

Learning Objectives

After reading this chapter, you will be able to:

1. Describe the anatomy and physiology of the renal and urinary systems.
2. Discuss the role of the kidney in regulating fluid and electrolyte balance, acid–base balance, and blood pressure.
3. Identify the assessment parameters used for determining the status of upper and lower urinary tract function.
4. Describe the diagnostic studies used to determine upper and lower urinary tract function.

Proper function of the renal and urinary systems is essential to life. Dysfunction of the kidneys and lower urinary tract is common and may occur at any age and with varying degrees of severity. Assessment of upper and lower urinary tract function is part of every health examination and necessitates an understanding of the anatomy and physiology of the urinary system as well as of the effects of changes in the system on other physiologic functions.

ANATOMY AND PHYSIOLOGY OVERVIEW

The primary function of the renal and urinary systems is to maintain the body's state of homeostasis by carefully regulating fluid and electrolytes, removing wastes, and providing hormones that are involved in red blood cell (RBC) production, bone metabolism, and blood pressure. A thorough understanding of the renal and urinary systems is necessary for assessing people with acute or chronic dysfunction and implementing appropriate nursing care (Gawlick et al., 2020).

Anatomy of the Renal and Urinary Systems

The renal and urinary systems include the kidneys, ureters, bladder, and urethra. Urine is formed by the kidney and flows through the other structures to be eliminated from the body (Gawlick et al., 2020).

Kidneys

The kidneys are a pair of bean-shaped, brownish-red structures located retroperitoneally (behind and outside the peritoneal cavity) on the posterior wall of the abdomen—from the 12th thoracic vertebra to the 3rd lumbar vertebra in the adult (Fig. 25-1A). The average adult kidney weighs approximately 113 to 170 g (about 4.5 oz) and is 10- to 12-cm long, 6-cm wide, and 2.5-cm thick. The right kidney is slightly lower than the left due to the location of the liver (Gawlick et al., 2020; Norris, 2019).

The kidneys are well protected by the ribs and by the muscles of the abdomen and back. Internally, fat deposits surround each kidney, providing protection against jarring. The kidneys and surrounding fat are suspended from the abdominal wall by renal fascia made of connective tissue. The fibrous connective tissue, blood vessels, and lymphatics surrounding each kidney are known as the *renal capsule* (Norris, 2019) (Fig. 25-1B).

An adrenal gland lies on top of each kidney. Each organ is independent in terms of its function, blood supply, and innervation (Gawlick et al., 2020).

The renal parenchyma (organ tissue) is divided into two parts: the cortex and the medulla. The medulla is the inner portion of the kidney. It contains the loop of Henle, the vasa recta, and the collecting ducts of the juxtamedullary nephrons. The collecting ducts from both the juxtamedullary and the cortical nephrons connect to the renal pyramids, which are triangular and are situated with the base facing the concave surface of the kidney and the point (papilla) facing the hilum, or pelvis. Each kidney contains approximately 8 to 18 pyramids which correlates with the number of kidney lobes. The pyramids drain into minor calices, which drain into major calices that open directly into the renal pelvis. The renal pelvis is the beginning of the collecting system and is composed of structures that are designed to collect and transport urine. Once the urine leaves the renal pelvis,

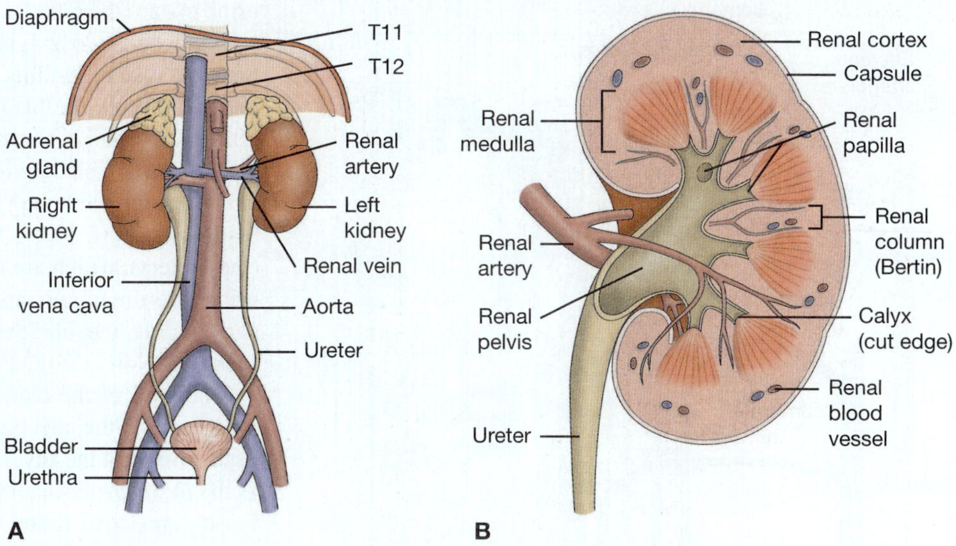

FIGURE 25-1 **A. Kidneys, ureters, and bladder. (The right kidney is usually lower than the left.) B. Internal structure of the kidney. (Grossman, S., & Porth, C. M. [2014].** ***Porth's pathophysiology concepts of altered health states*** **[9th ed.]. Wolters Kluwer/Lippincott Williams & Wilkins.)**

the composition or amount of urine does not change (Norris, 2019). The reddish-brown–colored cortex is located farthest from the center of the kidney and around the outermost edges. It contains the glomeruli, blood vessels and **nephrons** (the functional units of the kidney) (Norris, 2019), which are discussed below.

Blood Supply to the Kidneys

The hilum, or pelvis, is the concave portion of the kidney through which the renal artery enters and the ureters and renal vein exit. The kidneys receive 20% to 25% of the total cardiac output; all of the body's blood circulates through the kidneys approximately 12 times per hour. The renal artery arises from the abdominal aorta and divides into smaller and smaller vessels, eventually forming the afferent arterioles. Each afferent arteriole branches to form a **glomerulus**, which is the capillary bed responsible for glomerular filtration. Blood leaves the glomerulus through the efferent arteriole and flows back to the inferior vena cava through a network of capillaries and veins (Norris, 2019).

Pearls for Practice

The nurse auscultates for renal artery bruits, which indicate turbulent blood flow and are associated with a narrowing of the blood vessel or increased flow. Any patient with hypertension should be evaluated for bruits. Typically, they are noted with renal artery stenosis just above (2 cm) and to the right or left of the umbilicus. A whooshing sound is indicative of a bruit.

Nephrons

Each kidney has 1 million nephrons, which usually allow for adequate kidney function even if the opposite kidney is damaged or becomes nonfunctional. The nephrons are the structures located within the renal parenchyma that are responsible for the initial formation of urine. If the total number of functioning nephrons is less than 20% of normal, renal replacement therapy (RRT) needs to be considered (Gawlick et al., 2020; Muller, 2019).

There are two kinds of nephrons. The cortical nephrons, making up 80% to 85% of the total number, are located in the outermost part of the cortex. The juxtamedullary nephrons, distinguished by long loop of Henle, make up the remaining 15% to 20%, are located deeper in the cortex, and are surrounded by long capillary loops called *vasa recta* that dip into the medulla of the kidney. The length of the tubular component of the nephron is related directly to its ability to concentrate urine (Norris, 2019).

Nephrons are made up of two basic components: a filtering element composed of an enclosed capillary network (the glomerulus) and the attached tubule (Fig. 25-2). The glomerulus is a unique network of capillaries suspended between the afferent and efferent blood vessels, which are enclosed in an epithelial structure called *Bowman capsule*. The glomerular membrane is composed of three filtering layers: the capillary endothelium, the basement membrane, and the epithelium. This membrane normally allows filtration of fluid and small molecules yet limits passage of larger molecules, such as blood cells and albumin. Pressure changes and the permeability of the glomerular membrane of Bowman capsule facilitate the passage of fluids and various substances from the blood vessels, filling the space within Bowman capsule with this filtered solution (Norris, 2019).

The tubular component of the nephron begins in the Bowman capsule. The filtrate created in the Bowman capsule travels first into the proximal tubule, then the loop of Henle, the distal tubule, and either the cortical or medullary collecting ducts. Changes are made continually as the filtrate travels through the tubules until it enters the collecting system and is expelled as urine from the body (see Fig. 25-2) (Norris, 2019).

The structural arrangement of the tubule allows the distal tubule to lie in close proximity to where the afferent and efferent arteriole, respectively, enter and leave the glomerulus.

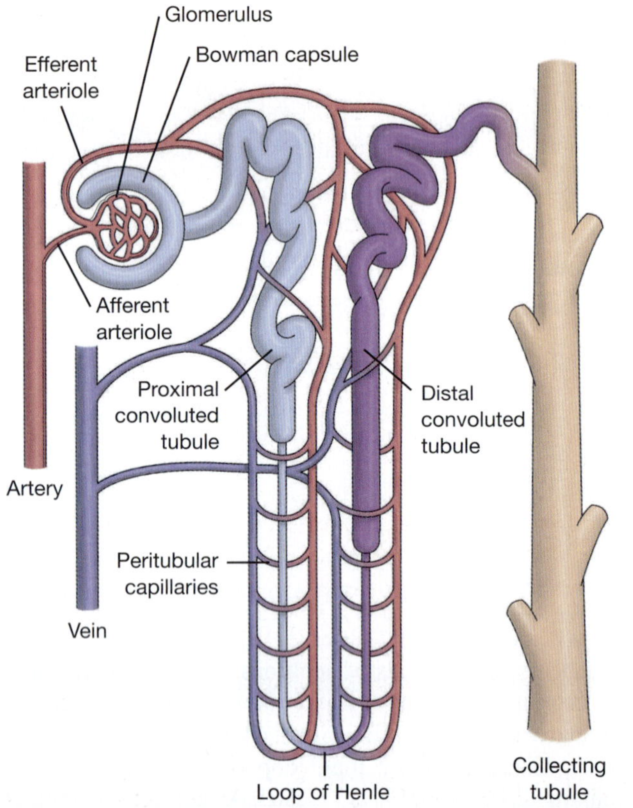

FIGURE 25-2 Representation of a nephron. Each kidney has about 1 million nephrons, which take two forms: cortical and juxtamedullary. Cortical nephrons are located in the cortex of the kidney; juxtamedullary nephrons are adjacent to the medulla.

The distal tubular cells located in this area, known as the *macula densa*, function with the adjacent afferent arteriole and create what is known as the *juxtaglomerular apparatus*. This is the site of renin production. Renin is a hormone involved directly in the control of arterial blood pressure; it is essential for proper functioning of the glomerulus (see later discussion) (Norris, 2019).

Ureters, Bladder, and Urethra

The urine formed in the nephrons flows into the renal pelvis and then into the ureters, which are long fibromuscular tubes that connect each kidney to the bladder. Each ureter is 24- to 30-cm long and 3 mm in diameter (Gawlick et al., 2020; Muller, 2019), originates at the lower portion of the renal pelvis, and terminates in the trigone of the bladder wall (Gawlick et al., 2020).

The lining of the ureters is made up of transitional cell epithelium called *urothelium.* The urothelium maintains bladder and blood impermeability as well as monitors for the presence of foreign substances or bacteria (Grochmal, 2020). The movement of urine from each renal pelvis through the ureter into the bladder is facilitated by peristaltic contraction of the smooth muscles in the ureter wall (Hall & Hall, 2021; Kalidonis & Liatsikos, 2021). These peristatic contractions extend to the renal pelvis and to the ureter which propels urine toward the bladder. Ureteral peristaltic contractions are strengthened by parasympathetic stimulation while the sympathetic system inhibits contractions. Urine flows from the ureters through the bladder detrusor muscles (Hall & Hall, 2021; Kalidonis & Liatsikos, 2021).

The urinary bladder is a muscular, hollow sac located just behind the pubic bone. The functional capacity of the adult bladder is about 300 to 500 mL. The bladder has two inlets (the ureters), which are angled to prevent retrograde flow of urine into the ureters and one outlet (the urethra). The area surrounding the bladder neck is called the *urethrovesical junction* (Norris, 2019).

The wall of the bladder contains four layers. The outermost layer is the adventitia, which is made up of connective tissue. Beneath the adventitia is a smooth muscle layer known as the *detrusor*; beneath the detrusor is a submucosal layer of loose connective tissue that serves as an interface between the detrusor and the innermost layer, a mucosal lining. This inner layer contains specialized transitional cell epithelium, a membrane that is impermeable to water and prevents reabsorption of urine stored in the bladder (Norris, 2019).

When the detrusor muscle contracts, urine is released from the bladder; thus, the detrusor is responsible for **micturition** (voiding). This muscle is continuous with the bladder neck, which forms a portion of the urethral sphincter often referred to as the *internal urethral sphincter.* When the bladder is relaxed, the muscle fibers are closed and functions as the sphincteric mechanism which helps maintain continence. Another muscle involved in continence is the external urinary sphincter at the anterior urethra, the segment most distal from the bladder. During micturition, increased intravesical pressure keeps the ureterovesical junction closed and keeps urine within the ureters. As soon as micturition is completed, intravesical pressure returns to its normal low baseline value, allowing efflux of urine to resume. The only time that the bladder is completely empty is in the last seconds of micturition, before efflux of urine resumes (Norris, 2019).

The urethra arises from the base of the bladder: In the male, it passes through the penis; in the female, it opens just anterior to the vagina. In the male, the prostate gland, which lies just below the bladder neck, surrounds the urethra posteriorly and laterally (Norris, 2019).

Functions of the Upper and Lower Urinary Tracts

Urine Formation

The healthy human body is composed of approximately 60% water. Water balance is regulated by the kidneys and results in the formation of urine. Urine is formed in the nephrons through a complex three-step process: glomerular filtration, **tubular reabsorption**, and **tubular secretion** (Fig. 25-3). The various substances normally filtered by the glomerulus, reabsorbed by the tubules, and excreted in the urine include sodium, chloride, bicarbonate, potassium, urea, creatinine,

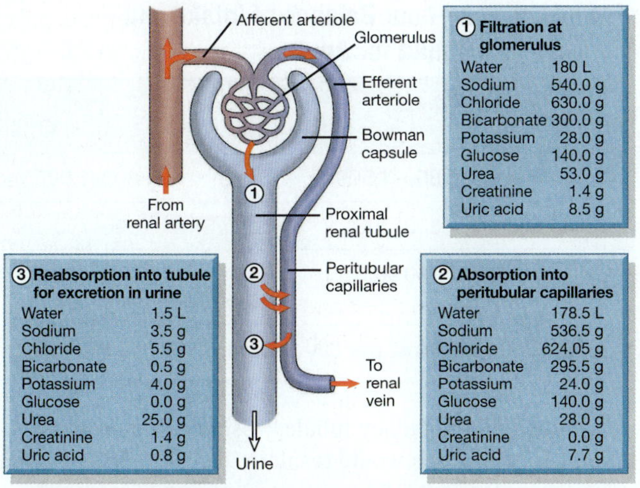

FIGURE 25-3 **Urine is formed in the nephrons in a three-step process: filtration, reabsorption, and excretion. Water, electrolytes, and other substances, such as glucose and creatinine, are filtered by the glomerulus; varying amounts of these substances are reabsorbed in the renal tubule or excreted in the urine. Approximate normal volumes of these substances during the steps of urine formation are shown at the top. Wide variations may occur in these values depending on diet.**

and uric acid. Within the tubule, some of these substances are reabsorbed selectively into the blood to maintain electrolyte and acid–base balance. Others are secreted from the blood into the filtrate as it travels down the tubule (Norris, 2019).

Usually, amino acids and glucose are filtered at the level of the glomerulus and reabsorbed so that neither is excreted in the urine. Normally, glucose does not appear in the urine. However, glycosuria occurs if the amount of glucose in the blood and glomerular filtrate exceeds the amount that the tubules can reabsorb. **Renal glycosuria** occurs in cases of diabetes mellitus (DM) and is the most common clinical expression of a blood glucose level exceeding the kidneys' reabsorption capacity. In general, the serum glucose level is greater than 180 to 200 mg/dL when glycosuria is seen (Norris, 2019).

Protein molecules also are not usually found in the urine; however, low–molecular-weight proteins (globulins and albumin) may be excreted periodically in small amounts. Recall that the glomerulus filters the blood, similar to a strainer. Therefore, when significant **proteinuria** is found, glomerular disease is suspected. Levels of greater than 3.5 g/day are indicative of severe proteinuria and are associated with nephrotic syndrome as well as a variety of glomerular disorders (Haider & Aslam, 2021) (see Chapter 26).

Glomerular Filtration

The normal blood flow through the kidneys is about 1,200 mL/min. As blood flows into the glomerulus from an afferent arteriole, filtration occurs. The filtered fluid enters the renal tubules. Under normal conditions, about 20% of the blood passing through the glomeruli is filtered into the nephron, amounting to about 180 L/day of filtrate. The filtrate normally consists of water, electrolytes, and other small molecules, whereas larger molecules stay in the bloodstream. Efficient filtration depends on adequate blood flow that maintains a consistent pressure through the glomerulus. Many factors can alter this blood flow and pressure, including hypotension, decreased oncotic pressure in the blood, and increased pressure in the renal tubules from an obstruction (Norris, 2019).

Tubular Reabsorption and Tubular Secretion

The second and third steps of urine formation occur in the renal tubules. In tubular reabsorption, a substance moves from the filtrate back into the peritubular capillaries or vasa recta. In tubular secretion, a substance moves from the peritubular capillaries or vasa recta into tubular filtrate. Of the 180 L (45 gallons) of filtrate that the kidneys produce each day, 99% is reabsorbed into the bloodstream, resulting in the formation of 1,000 to 1,500 mL of urine each day. Although most reabsorption occurs in the proximal tubule, reabsorption does occur along the entire tubule. Reabsorption and secretion in the tubule frequently involve passive and active transport. Filtrate becomes concentrated in the distal tubule and collecting ducts under hormonal influence and becomes urine, which then enters the renal pelvis (Norris, 2019).

Osmolarity and Osmolality

Osmolarity and osmolality refer to the ratio of solute (e.g., sodium, chloride, potassium, urea, and glucose) to water in blood or urine. While osmolarity refers to measuring the ratio of the number of solutes (milliosmoles) to water using liters (expressed as mOsm/L), osmolality calculates the ratio of the number of solutes (milliosmoles) to water using weight or kilograms (expressed as mOsm/kg). The terms are confusing and often misused; what is important to remember is that clinicians are attempting to determine the concentration of blood or urine. Because 1 L is roughly equivalent to 1 kg, generally they are similar. The regulation of salt and water is paramount for control of the extracellular volume and both serum and urine osmolarity. Controlling either the amount of water or the amount of solute can change the concentration of blood and urine. Osmolarity and ionic composition are maintained by the body within very narrow limits. Sodium is the most abundant cation in the extracellular space and therefore largely determines the serum osmolarity (increased number of solute atoms or molecules); an increase of 1% to 2% in osmolality will cause a conscious desire to drink and conservation of water by the kidneys (Toffaletti & Rackley, 2022). Serum osmolality is useful in determining a possible cause of seizures and in evaluating ascites, hydration status, acid–base balance, suspected ADH abnormalities as well as suspected poisoning (Fischbach et al., 2022). It is important for nurses to recognize that cognitive impairments can interfere with recognition of cues of thirst and predispose a patient to dehydration.

Pearls for Practice

The terms isotonic, hypotonic, and hypertonic refer to the osmolarity of body fluids (measure of the number of dissolved particles). A serum osmolality test measures the amount of chemicals dissolved in the fluid portion of blood (serum). It could be imagined visually as the total number of molecules floating in the fluid. Normal serum osmolality equals 275 to 295 mOsm/kg of body weight (Fischbach et al., 2022). Different hospital laboratories may use slightly different numbers, such as 280 to 300 mOsm/kg (Lough, 2022). When a hypotonic solution is administered intravenously (IV), the RBCs will swell; conversely, a hypertonic solution will cause the cells to shrink (Norris, 2019). An isotonic solution will not cause a change in the size of the RBCs. Sodium chloride 0.9% (AKA normal saline) is an example of an IV isotonic solution, sodium chloride 0.45% (AKA half saline) is an example of a hypotonic solution, and sodium chloride 3% is an example of a hypertonic solution.

Pearls for Practice

Nurses need to have some understanding of the concentration of an intravenous (IV) solution's osmolarity and its relationship to clinical practice. Isotonic solutions are equal to normal osmolarity (approximately 300 mOsm/L; e.g., lactated Ringer's [275 mOsm/L] and normal saline [308 mOsm/L]); hypotonic solutions have fewer molecules and more water in the solution (less than 275 mOsm/L; e.g., half-normal saline [154 mOsm/L]); and hypertonic solutions have a higher number of molecules and are more concentrated solutions (over 300 mOsm/L; e.g., dextrose 5% in half-normal saline [405 mOsm/L]). Any fluid or medication with an osmolarity greater than 900 mOsm/L, any vesicant, or total parenteral nutrition ***should not*** *be infused through a peripheral catheter; instead a peripherally inserted central catheter (PICC) is recommended by the Infusion Nurses Society (Collins, 2022; Nickel, 2019).*

Regulation of Water Excretion

Regulation of the amount of water excreted is an important function of the kidney. **Antidiuretic hormone (ADH)**, also known as *vasopressin*, plays a key role in the regulation of extracellular fluid by excreting or retaining water. ADH is secreted by the posterior portion of the pituitary gland and acts on the kidney in response to changes in osmolality of the blood; that is, ADH is secreted or suppressed depending on blood concentration or dilution, respectively. An increase in blood osmolality is seen with decreased water intake or increased water loss, stimulating ADH release. Consequently, a small volume of concentrated urine is excreted. ADH increases reabsorption of water and returns the osmolality of the blood to normal. With excess water intake or increased retention of water, as occurs in many disease states such as kidney failure, the blood becomes dilute, resulting in suppression of ADH secretion, causing less water to be reabsorbed by the kidney tubule. Assuming maintenance of kidney function, this would result in increased urine volume (diuresis) (Norris, 2019).

TABLE 25-1 24-hour Balance of Intake and Output for Adults

Water Input	Input Volume (mL)	Output	Output Volume (mL)
Liquid	800–1,500	Urine	800–1,500
Solid	500–700	Lung/Skin	600–700
Oxidative metabolism	150–250	Sweat Stool	0–100 100–200
Total ~ 1,500–2,500 mL per day		**Total ~ 1,500–2,500 mL**	

In general, over 2 L of water is ingested via food and beverages in 24 hours. Of the fluid ingested, the main source of loss is through the urine (800 to 1,500 mL/day) but is highly dependent upon fluid intake; approximately 800 mL is lost through the skin and mucosal airways (called *insensible loss*), and 100 to 200 mL through feces (Norris, 2019; Tkacs et al., 2020). The kidneys require of minimum of 300 to 500 mL of urinary output per day to effectively eliminate waste products and prevent the accumulation of metabolic wastes in the blood (azotemia). Normal urine output is approximately 1.5 L in 24 hours (Norris, 2019) and intake is roughly equivalent to output in a healthy person (see Table 25-1). Fluid imbalance may occur secondary to hemorrhage, dehydration resulting from vomiting or diarrhea or as a result from strenuous exertion during extremely hot weather conditions. Imbalances may also occur from more chronic conditions such as heart failure (HF), liver failure, diabetes insipidus, Addison disease, DM, and chronic lung disease. Normal kidney functioning is essential to maintaining fluid and electrolyte balance. It is important to consider all fluid gained and lost when evaluating total fluid status. Daily weight measurements are a reliable means of determining overall fluid status. One-pound equals approximately 500 mL therefore a weight change of as little as 1 lb might suggest an overall fluid gain or loss of 500 mL (Lough, 2022). Edema may be caused by heart or liver failure (Tkacs et al., 2020). The nurse is aware that edema is not present until 2.5 to 3 L of interstitial fluid has been retained (Kattula et al., 2021), and that pitting edema is associated with ~4.5 kg (10 lb) fluid accumulation (Suneja et al., 2020).

Pearls for Practice

It is important to maintain consistency when assessing daily weight: the nurse uses the same scale, with the patient wearing the same clothes at the same time daily.

Regulation of Electrolyte Excretion

When the kidneys are functioning normally, the volume of electrolytes excreted per day is equal to the amount ingested. For example, the average American daily diet contains 3,400 mg of salt (Centers for Disease Control and Prevention, 2021) and approximately the same amount is excreted in the urine.

Sodium

Normal serum sodium levels are between 135 and 145 mmol/L, making sodium the most plentiful extracellular ion (see Chapter 3). Sodium plays an important role in controlling the fluid and electrolyte balance: where sodium goes, water follows. Sodium is linked inseparably to both blood volume and blood pressure. The kidneys are responsible for regulating electrolyte loss, and approximately 65% to 80% of sodium is reabsorbed by the proximal tubule and 20% to 25% in the loop of Henle (Norris, 2019; Van Leeuwen & Bladh, 2019).

As water from the filtrate follows the reabsorbed sodium, the body's osmotic balance is maintained. If more sodium is excreted than ingested, fluid deficit results; if less sodium is excreted than ingested, fluid retention results. Under normal circumstances, the kidneys are quite efficient at preserving or excreting sodium depending on its loss via the gastrointestinal (GI) tract or skin as well as its gain via diet, medications, or IV therapy (Hall & Hall, 2021; Norris, 2019).

The regulation of sodium volume excreted depends on **aldosterone**, a hormone synthesized and released from the adrenal cortex. With increased aldosterone in the blood, less sodium is excreted in the urine, as aldosterone causes renal reabsorption of sodium. The release of aldosterone from the adrenal cortex is largely under the control of angiotensin II, the most effective physiologic vasoconstrictor known. Angiotensin II levels are controlled by renin, a proteolytic enzyme released from specialized juxtaglomerular cells in the renal afferent arteriole (see Fig. 25-4). Renin secretion is controlled by three distinct but overlapping regulatory systems: (1) renal afferent arteriolar pressure (if it decreases renin secretion increases); (2) cardiopulmonary baroreceptors that are capable of modulating sympathetic nervous system outflow (a fall in blood pressure increases renin secretion by increasing sympathetic tone); and (3) the delivery of NaCl to the macula densa, a group of modified distal tubular cells (a decrease in NaCl delivery to these cells increases renin secretion while an increase in NaCl delivery has the opposite effect). Activation of this system (by dehydration, e.g., shock or hypotension) will increase NaCl reclamation and therefore water retention culminating in an expansion of the intravascular fluid volume. The net result is the maintenance of pressure within the glomerulus to ensure adequate glomerular filtration pressure and renal function (Norris, 2019).

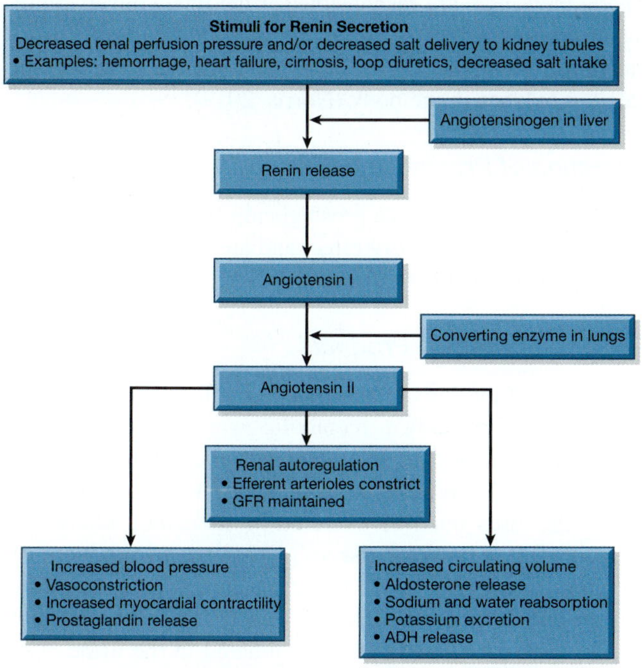

FIGURE 25-4 The renin–angiotensin system. ADH, antidiuretic hormone; GFR, glomerular filtration rate.

Pearls for Practice

The nurse recognizes that a mean arterial pressure (MAP) should be at least 65 mm Hg or higher in order to maintain renal perfusion. A normal MAP is between 70 and 105 mm Hg. A MAP <65 for an extended period can result in end-organ ischemia (deficient supply of blood) and infarction (death of tissues),

Potassium

Potassium is the most abundant intracellular ion; about 98% of the total body potassium is located intracellularly. To maintain a normal serum potassium balance (see Chapter 3), the kidneys are responsible for excreting more than 80% to 90% of the total daily potassium intake during normal activity; 10% to 20% is excreted via the stool. Aldosterone causes the kidneys to excrete potassium, in contrast to its effects on sodium. The acid–base balance, the amount of dietary potassium intake, and the flow rate of the filtrate in the distal tubule also influence the amount of potassium secreted into the urine. Retention of potassium is the most life-threatening effect of kidney failure (McGregor & Jones, 2021).

Pearls for Practice

When the level of potassium is above 6.5 mEq/L, it represents a medical emergency, primarily due to its effect on the heart. Renal perfusion is essential for excretion of potassium; when the MAP decreases to less than 70 mm Hg, urine volumes begin to decrease, resulting in impaired potassium excretion. Therefore, the nurse is alert to minimal urinary output hourly (0.5 to 1.0 mL/kg/hr) and its effect on K^+. The nurse is aware that ECG changes include a progression from peaked T waves to a prolonged PR interval, and then to a widened QRS and heart block; a K^+ level above 7 mEq/L is associated with serious arrhythmias.

Regulation of Acid–Base Balance

The normal serum pH is about 7.35 to 7.45 and must be maintained within this narrow range for optimal physiologic function (Hall & Hall, 2021). The kidney reabsorbs and returns bicarbonate from the urinary filtrate to the body's circulation. It also excretes acid in the urine. Because bicarbonate is a small ion, it is filtered freely at the glomerulus and reabsorbed in the urinary filtrate. To replace any lost bicarbonate, new bicarbonate is generated by the renal tubular cells and then reabsorbed by the tubules and returned to the body (Norris, 2019).

The body's acid production is the result of the breakdown of proteins, which produces acid compounds. The normal daily diet also includes a certain amount of acid materials. Unlike carbon dioxide (CO_2), the phosphoric and sulfuric acids produced are nonvolatile (solid) and cannot be eliminated by the lungs. If these acids were not excreted in the urine, accumulation of these acids in the blood would lower its pH and inhibit cell function. A person with normal kidney function excretes about 70 mEq of acid each day. The kidney is able to excrete some of this acid directly into the urine until the urine pH reaches 4.5, which is 1,000 times more acidic than blood (Norris, 2019). More acid may need to be eliminated from the body than can be secreted directly as free acid in the urine. These excess acids are bound to chemical buffers so that they can be excreted in the urine. Two important chemical buffers are phosphate ions and ammonia (NH_3). Through the buffering process, the kidney can excrete large quantities of acid in a bound form, without further lowering the pH of the urine (Norris, 2019).

Autoregulation of Blood Pressure

Regulation of blood pressure is also a function of the kidney. Specialized vessels of the kidney, called the *vasa recta*, constantly monitor blood pressure as blood begins its passage into the kidney. When the vasa recta detect a decrease in blood pressure, specialized juxtaglomerular cells near the afferent arteriole, distal tubule, and efferent arteriole secrete the hormone renin. Renin does not affect blood pressure directly. It converts a circulating plasma protein named angiotensinogen to angiotensin I, which is converted to angiotensin II and causes the blood pressure to increase by its vasoconstrictor properties and secretion of aldosterone (Norris, 2019). Aldosterone causes renal reabsorption of sodium and water by the distal tubules and collecting ducts; thus volume is returned to systemic circulation. Any etiology that results in poor perfusion or increasing serum osmolality, such as hemorrhage or diarrhea, will cause activation of renin, which leads to activation of angiotensin II and aldosterone secretion. The result is an increase in blood pressure. When the vasa recta recognize the increase in blood pressure, renin secretion stops. Failure of this feedback mechanism is one of the primary causes of hypertension (Norris, 2019).

Renal Clearance

Renal clearance refers to the ability of the kidneys to clear solutes from the plasma. A 24-hour collection of urine is the primary test of renal clearance. Renal clearance depends on several factors: how quickly the substance is filtered across the glomerulus, how much of the substance is reabsorbed along the tubules, and how much of the substance is secreted into the tubules. It is possible to measure the renal clearance of any substance, but the one measure that is particularly useful is the creatinine clearance: as renal function declines, creatinine clearance decreases; that is, the patient's serum creatinine rises (Norris, 2019; Shahbaz & Gupta, 2021).

Creatinine is an endogenous waste product of skeletal muscle that is filtered at the glomerulus, passed through the tubules with minimal change, and excreted in the urine, making creatinine clearance a good measure of the **glomerular filtration rate (GFR)**. To calculate creatinine clearance, a 24-hour urine specimen is collected. Midway through the collection, the serum creatinine level is measured (Norris, 2019; Van Leeuwen & Bladh, 2019). The normal rate of creatinine clearance is approximately 115 to 125 mL/minute (Norris, 2019).

Regulation of Red Blood Cell Production

When the kidneys sense a decrease in the oxygen tension in renal blood flow, they release erythropoietin. Erythropoietin stimulates the bone marrow to produce RBCs, thereby increasing the number of circulating RBCs, raising the O_2 carrying capacity of the blood. Some conditions, such as chronic kidney disease often manifest by anemia, requiring that patients receive exogenous erythropoietin to maintain RBC production (Norris, 2019).

Vitamin D Synthesis

The kidneys also are responsible for the final conversion of inactive vitamin D to its active form, 1,25-dihydroxycholecalciferol. Vitamin D is necessary for maintaining normal calcium balance in the body (Norris, 2019).

Secretion of Prostaglandins

The kidneys also produce prostaglandin E and prostacyclin, which have a vasodilatory effect and are important in maintaining renal blood flow (Steinmetz-Spah et al., 2021).

Excretion of Waste Products

The kidney functions as the body's main excretory organ, eliminating the body's metabolic waste products. The major waste product of protein metabolism is urea, of which about 25 to 30 g are produced and excreted daily. All of this urea must be excreted in the urine; otherwise, it accumulates in body tissues. Other waste products of metabolism that must be excreted are creatinine, phosphates, and sulfates. Uric acid, formed as a waste product of purine metabolism, also is eliminated in the urine. The kidneys serve as the primary mechanism for excreting drug metabolites (Norris, 2019).

Pearls for Practice

The kidneys are responsible for excretion of waste products that account for a daily solute load of approximately 600 mOsm. It is approximated that 500 mL of urine is required daily to excrete that solute load. Without that excretion of 300 to 500 mL, toxins and waste products will rise in the serum or blood value. The term azotemia refers to the buildup of excessive nitrogenous wastes in the blood (refer to Chapter 26 for additional detail).

Urine Storage and Innervation

The bladder is a hollow, distensible, muscular organ whose size, shape, and position vary in relation to the amount of urine it contains (Lanzotti et al., 2021). Both filling and emptying of the bladder are mediated by coordinated sympathetic and parasympathetic nervous system control mechanisms involving the detrusor muscle and the bladder sphincters. Micturition or voiding involves the interplay between voluntary control and the sympathetic and parasympathetic systems. Receptors in the bladder wall relay information to the spinal cord and to the brain. Parasympathetic control originates in S2 to S4 spinal cord segments, are excitatory and causes contraction of the bladder (known as reflex voiding center). Whereas the sympathetic innervation of the bladder is inhibitory and originates from thoracic or T10 to lumbar or L2 spinal cord segments. Since bladder control is located in this region there will be a loss of voluntary bladder control with spinal cord injury in this area, but reflex emptying can still occur. In addition to bladder innervation at the detrusor muscle, there is innervation of the vesical sphincter which is a ringlike muscle that connects the bladder to the urethra and controls the release of urine from the urethra and bladder by relaxing to open or constricting to close. In this region the parasympathetic innervation is inhibitory which causes the sphincter to relax and the bladder pushes urine out of the urethra; when urination is completed, the vesical sphincter constricts (sympathetic response) and urine leakage is prevented. Any damage to the detrusor or sphincter innervation can result in urinary leakage, urinary retention, or overflow incontinence. To summarize, when the bladder is full, there is increased parasympathetic tone and decreased sympathetic activity causes the internal sphincter to relax and the bladder to contract. Finally, there is voluntary control of the external sphincter urethrae, that provides voluntary control of urine flow from the bladder to the urethra; the pudendal nerve (S2–S4) innervates this sphincter. This sphincter can be damaged in childbirth stretching of the ligaments and dysfunction of the pelvic floor muscles, resulting in incontinence (Samet al., 2021).

Bladder compliance is due to the smooth muscle lining of the bladder and collagen deposits within the wall of the bladder, as well as to neuronal mechanisms that inhibit the detrusor muscle from contracting (specifically, adrenergic receptors that mediate relaxation). To maintain adequate kidney filtration rates, bladder pressure during filling must remain lower than 40 to 50 cm H_2O. This low pressure allows the urine to leave the renal pelvis and enter the ureters freely (Norris, 2019). The bladder can hold 400 to 600 mL of urine before a person senses bladder fullness (under normal circumstances), however when the bladder is distended to 150 to 250 mL, sensations are already being transmitted to the spinal cord and then the cerebral cortex. The term functional capacity refers to the volume the bladder typically holds during normal routines before emptying and is best gained through the use of a voiding diary for three days (Griebling, 2021; Wilcox & Rove, 2021). Neurologic changes to the bladder at the level of the supraspinal nerves, the spinal nerves, or the bladder wall itself can cause abnormally high volumes of urine to be stored due to a decreased or absent urge to void (Bickley et al., 2021; Norris, 2019).

At night, the release of vasopressin in response to decreased fluid intake causes a decrease in the production of urine and makes it more concentrated. It allows the bladder to continue filling making them able to sleep for longer periods before needing to void. This process, which is less pronounced in the older population, coupled with decreasing bladder compliance, and decreased vasopressin (ADH) levels, often causes **nocturia** (Boltz, 2020; Norris, 2019; Weiss & Everaert, 2019).

Bladder Emptying

Micturition is activated via the micturition reflex arc within the sympathetic and parasympathetic nervous system, which causes a coordinated sequence of events. Initiation of voiding occurs when the efferent pelvic nerve, which originates at S1–S4, stimulates the bladder to contract, resulting in complete relaxation of the striated urethral sphincter. This is followed by a decrease in urethral pressure, contraction of the detrusor muscle, opening of the vesicle neck and proximal urethra, and flow of urine. This coordinated effort by the parasympathetic system is mediated by muscarinic and, to a lesser extent, cholinergic receptors within the detrusor muscle. The pressure of the bladder must be less than the pressure in the urethra to avoid incontinence. If the intravesical pressure is continually elevated (>40 to 50 cm H_2O), backflow of urine from the bladder to the ureters is likely to occur known as vesicoureteral reflux. The sphincter pressure is maintained at 45 to 65 cm H_2O so that urine is not lost as the bladder fills.

If the spinal pathways from the brain to the urinary system are destroyed (e.g., after a spinal cord injury), reflex contraction of the bladder is maintained, but voluntary control over the process is lost; a loss of sensation in bladder fullness occurs and generally the contractions are insufficient to empty the bladder completely so residual urine (urine left in the bladder after voiding) remains. This places the patient at risk for significant morbidity including UTIs and kidney damage (Mansoor & Rathore, 2019). Normally, residual urine amounts to no more than 50 mL in the middle-aged adult and less than 50 to 100 mL in the older adult (Ballstaedt & Woodbury, 2021).

Pearls for Practice

Any anatomical or functional disorder causing urinary obstruction or stasis places the individual at risk for urinary tract infections (UTIs) (Lainhart et al., 2023). A post-void residual (PVR) of less than 50 mL is considered normal bladder emptying, whereas large and persistent PVRs have also been associated with UTI in those at risk (e.g., DM, kidney diseases, HF, and neurologic diseases [e.g., Parkinson disease, multiple sclerosis, cerebrovascular disease, spinal cord injury, or prolapsed intervertebral disc impinging on the spinal cord]) (Wilcox & Rove, 2021). Of note, there are no officially established volumes that define normal or impaired emptying. The Agency for Healthcare Policy and Research (AHCPR) suggests that a PVR less than 50 cc represents adequate emptying and a PVR greater than 200 cc represents inadequate emptying (Lucioni & Kobashi, 2021).

Gerontologic Considerations

Blood flow to the kidneys decreases with aging, and kidney mass also decreases after 65 years of age, leading to a decrease in the GFR of approximately 10 mL/min per decade, reaching about 50% by age 80 (Griebling, 2021). Creatinine levels do not necessarily demonstrate increased levels in tandem with decreasing GFRs owing to decreasing muscle mass in the older adult. Overall, a decrease in tubular function occurs with age as does the ability to properly maintain or excrete water, sodium, potassium, and other electrolytes however this does not necessarily impair an older individual's ability to maintain a normal fluid and electrolyte balance in an otherwise healthy older adult. The older individual is more susceptible to acute and chronic kidney failure due to the structural and functional changes in the kidney. Upper and lower urinary tract function changes with age (Table 25-2). Symptoms indicative of lower urinary tract dysfunction such as an overactive bladder, urinary frequency, urgency, nocturia, hesitancy, abnormal stream, incomplete bladder emptying and incontinence, increase in severity as one ages, approximately doubling between 40 and 49 years of age and at age 80 years. These age-related symptoms occur in males and females, however overactive bladder appears to occur more prevalently in females.

Pearls for Practice: Aging and Medications

Approximately 26% of all adults over the age of 70 years have some degree of chronic renal impairment, which can have substantial impact on dosing of medications that are cleared by the kidneys (Griebling, 2021). The nurse considers that due to changes in kidney function and polypharmacy, lower doses of medications may be adequate to achieve clinical effects, and "typical" dosages may lead to toxicity or untoward side effects. The nurse observes the older person for adverse drug effects and drug–drug interaction, since they are at increased risk (Greibling, 2021).

Older individuals are more prone to develop hypernatremia and fluid volume deficit because increasing age also is associated with diminished osmotic stimulation of thirst. Thirst is a subjective sensory symptom that is defined as an awareness of the desire to drink. The older population, because of both decreased thirst and/or diminished access to fluids and/or impaired urinary concentrating ability, are at the highest risk of developing hypernatremia (Boltz, 2020) (an increase in the plasma Na^+ concentration >145 mEq/L).

Likewise, many older adults may be placed on diuretics, such as furosemide, to control HF meaning excess sodium may be lost in the urine resulting in hyponatremia. In addition, hypervolemic hyponatremia commonly occurs when patients have excess free water relative to serum sodium levels (e.g., kidney failure, cardiac failure, liver failure) (Boltz, 2020). Therefore, the nurse is alert to sodium levels (hypernatremia or hyponatremia) and is aware of common causes and clinical presentation in order to alert practitioners to reverse this potentially life-threatening condition.

Structural or functional abnormalities that occur with aging also may prevent complete emptying of the bladder. This may be due to decreased bladder wall contractility, secondary to muscle tissue changes such as the decreased ratio of smooth muscle to collagen in the wall of the bladder which may lead to decreased contractile strength (Griebling, 2021) or neurogenic factors, or it may be related to bladder outlet obstruction, such as in BPH. Vaginal and urethral tissues atrophy (become thinner) in aging females due to decreased estrogen levels, resulting in decreased blood supply to the urogenital tissues, with subsequent urethral and vaginal irritation and possible urinary incontinence (Bickley et al., 2021; Norris, 2019).

UTIs increase as individuals age and it is the most common infection among the older adult population. And while UTIs are more common in younger females than in males, the gap narrows as people age. Risk factors include patients residing in convalescent facilities as well as patients with chronic catheterizations and increasing antibiotic resistance. Some older patients present with symptoms of delirium and incontinence, and it is important that the nurse recognize UTIs may lead to urosepsis (septicemia because of a UTI), which has a higher mortality rate in the aged (Griebling, 2021). Symptoms present differently and more subtly than in younger adults and may include increasing confusion, loss of appetite, nausea and vomiting and abdominal pain. In addition, older adults with impaired cognitive functioning may have difficulty communicating symptoms.

Nocturia is common in older adults, resulting in disturbed sleep that impacts daytime fatigue. Because the individual

TABLE **25-2 GERONTOLOGIC CONSIDERATIONS / Age-Related Changes in the Renal System**

Component	Structural and Functional Changes	History and Physical Findings
Kidney	Kidney weight and volume (primarily of the cortex) decline	Progressive decline of kidney reserve (the ability to respond to changes in water or electrolyte imbalances to external stresses) (Boltz, 2020)
Renal blood flow	Blood flow decreases Renal arteries thicken (similar to other vascular changes) Sclerosis of the glomerulus results in atrophy of the afferent and efferent arteriole	Increased risk for kidney failure due to polypharmacy, comorbidities, and decreased kidney function
Nephron	The number of nephrons declines and is associated with decline in GFR The glomerular basement membrane thickens (Papacocea et al., 2021)	Yearly decline in GFR of 1 mL per minute (after age 40) Older individuals are at risk for altered drug excretion and drug–drug interaction
Tubule system	Decrease in the number of tubules and thickening of the tubular basement membrane (Papacocea et al., 2021)	Ability to conserve sodium or excrete hydrogen is decreased, predisposing the older population to fluid and electrolyte and acid–base disturbances. Decline in maximal concentrating capacity, with increased difficulty in excreting a salt load or conserving water in the face of dehydration
Bladder	Reduced bladder tone Residual bladder urine volume increases Decreased bladder capacity In females, decreased estrogen causes changes to the urethral sphincter	Increased sense of urgency In females, increased risk of urinary incontinence Incomplete emptying of bladder, leading to urinary tract infection Increased irritability of bladder with advancing age and may generate less power, which is a problem especially in males with prostatic hypertrophy
Prostate	Enlargement of the prostate	Obstruction to urine flow, leading to frequency, oliguria, anuria
General	Decrease in muscle mass results in decreased production of creatinine Decreased vitamin D synthesis. Vaginal and urethral atrophy	Serum creatinine levels remain constant; creatinine clearance is a better indicator of kidney function Osteomalacia Predisposition of females to urinary tract infections

must awaken at night to void, the risk of falls increases and may results in fractures. Other urologic symptoms such as urinary frequency, urgency, and incontinence may be caused by weakening bladder muscles, decreased bladder capacity, urinary retention, a delayed micturition reflex, and prostate disorders. As individuals age, the density of smooth muscle to connective tissue in the bladder decreases, increasing the likelihood of detrusor fibrosis. Because bladder capacity is reduced, patients may experience a decrease in the force of urinary stream, increased hesitancy, inability to empty the bladder fully, and urinary dribbling; although it may be unclear which symptoms are caused by comorbidities or are a result of aging.

Orthostatic hypotension may occur when the older adult is volume depleted (due to impaired response to thirst and diminished ability of the kidneys to maintain adequate intravascular volume in situations with reduced fluid intake) and the nurse is alert for the signs and symptoms of volume depletion such as decreased urine output (<.5 mL/kg/hr), decreased systolic blood pressure, decreased pulse pressure (normal is 40 mm Hg), orthostatic hypotension (a 20 mm Hg decrease in systolic pressure or a 10 mm Hg decrease in diastolic pressure with position change), rising blood osmolarity, delayed skin turgor, weight loss [refer to Chapter 3]).

Pearls for Practice

Orthostatic hypotension occurs when patient's position changes from supine to upright position because of the redistribution of intravascular volume (between 300 and 800 mL of blood pools in the lower

extremities and splanchnic circulation) due to gravity (Magkas et al., 2019). This transient reduction in venous return to the right heart, causes a decreased stroke volume and cardiac output (up to 40%) which decreases the BP. Therefore, the nurse teaches patients to change positions slowly when moving from a lying or sitting position to a standing position and to use supportive devices, such as handrails and walkers, to prevent falls that could result from dizziness.

Hypertension increases in the geriatric population, contributing to kidney disease and a systematic review and meta-analysis found that hypertension is more likely to result in chronic kidney disease or end stage kidney disease (ESKD) in males rather than in females (Weldegiorgis & Woodward, 2020). It is doubtful, however that this disparity is solely a result of biologic differences but instead, may be explained by the long-term effects and severity of albuminuria, DM, cardiovascular disease, obesity, socioeconomic status, and the possibility that males are not as likely to adhere to their antihypertensive medication regimen, participate in poorer lifestyle habits and embody more pre-existing conditions, placing them at greater risk for hypertension (Weldegiorgis & Woodward, 2020). Polypharmacy is another factor impacting urologic health, resulting in drug-induced urgency, frequency, retention, and urinary incontinence (Baruth et al., 2019). Urinary incontinence is common in adults over 65 years of age and it is estimated that one in three females and 15% to 20% of males suffer from some form of incontinence. In addition, reported prevalence of bladder incontinence is 75.8% for long-term care residents in extended-care facilities (Griebling, 2021). It is important that the nurse is aware that incontinence is a symptom rather than a diagnosis and there may be multiple causes associated with it (Griebling, 2021). Incontinence impacts quality of life causing some individuals to feel socially isolated and depressed and frailty is considered a major risk factor. It is important that the nurse employ a sensitive patient approach in addressing this potentially embarrassing issue. For those individuals with gait disorders who also experience nocturia or nocturnal incontinence, the risk for injurious falls is significant (Griebling, 2021). The nurse should teach bladder-training exercises, such as Kegel maneuvers (refer to Chapter 32, Box 32-9). Medications may also be considered as treatment based upon the type of incontinence such as alpha-adrenergic agonists for stress incontinence or alpha-adrenergic antagonists for overflow incontinence (Tran & Puckett, 2022). Incontinence caused by urinary or vaginal prolapse should be referred to a specialist. UTIs always should be considered as a cause of incontinence along with the use of medications, such as diuretics, antidepressant medications, sedative hypnotics, adrenergic agonists, anticholinergics, and calcium channel blockers. Whether estrogen replacement improves incontinence remains controversial, with some noting that estrogen does not improve urinary incontinence (Koothirezhi & Ranganathan, 2021).

ASSESSMENT

Obtaining a comprehensive health history is the first step in assessing a patient with upper or lower urinary tract dysfunction (Jarvis & Eckhardt, 2020).

Health History

Obtaining a urologic health history requires excellent communication skills because many patients are embarrassed or uncomfortable discussing genitourinary function or symptoms. It is important to use language the patient can understand and to avoid medical jargon while reviewing risk factors, particularly for those patients who are at high risk.

When obtaining the health history specific to the renal and urinary systems, the nurse should inquire about the following:

- The patient's chief concern or reason for seeking health care, the onset of the problem, and its effect on the patient's quality of life (Bickley et al., 2021; Jarvis & Eckhardt, 2020).
- The location, character, and duration of pain, if present, and its relationship to voiding; factors that precipitate pain and those that relieve it (Bickley et al., 2021).
- History of UTIs, including past treatment or hospitalization for UTI (Bickley et al., 2021; Jarvis & Eckhardt, 2020).
- Presence of fever or chills, nausea, vomiting or flank pain (Bono & Reygaert, 2021).
- Previous renal or urinary diagnostic tests (Bickley et al., 2021).
- Use of indwelling urinary catheters, suprapubic tubes, condom catheters, or intermittent catheterization (Bono & Reygaert, 2021).
- Dysuria, frequency, or painful urination which may occur at initiation or termination of voiding (Bickley et al., 2021; Bono & Reygaert; 2021).
- Hesitancy, straining, or pain during or after urination (Bickley et al., 2021; Bono & Reygaert, 2021).
- Urinary incontinence (stress incontinence, urge incontinence, overflow incontinence, or functional incontinence) (Bickley et al., 2021).
- Hematuria (blood in urine) or change in color or volume of urine (Bono & Reygaert, 2021).
- The presence of nocturia and number of episodes nightly (Bickley et al., 2021).
- Sudden onset of severe, unilateral, colicky flank pain that becomes steadier with time, history of renal calculi (kidney stones), passage of stones or gravel in urine (Bickley et al., 2021; Glazer et al., 2021).
- Female patients: Number and type (vaginal or caesarean) of deliveries; use of forceps; vaginal infection, discharge, or irritation; contraceptive practices (Bickley et al., 2021).
- History of polyuria, flank pain, or reduced stream (Bickley et al., 2021).

- Presence or history of genital lesions or sexually transmitted diseases (Bickley et al., 2021).
- Use of tobacco, alcohol, or recreational drugs (Bickley et al., 2021).
- Any prescription and over-the-counter medications (including those prescribed for renal or urinary problems) (Bickley et al., 2021).

Common Complaints

Fatigue, pain, changes in voiding, and GI symptoms are particularly suggestive of urinary tract disease. Dysfunction of the kidney can produce a complex array of symptoms throughout the body.

Fatigue

Gradual kidney dysfunction can be insidious in its presentation, although fatigue and malaise are common symptoms (Lerma et al., 2019). Fatigue, shortness of breath, headaches, dizziness, decreased concentration, and exercise intolerance all result from the condition known as *anemia of chronic kidney disease* and usually develops when over 50% of kidney functioning is lost. While the severity of anemia tends to worsen as kidney disease progresses, the severity of erythropoietin deficiency and subsequent anemia do not always correlate with the severity of kidney failure. Ninety per cent of patients undergoing dialysis will experience anemia of chronic disease and HF, myocardial infarction and death may result from anemia of renal disease. The common diagnostic workup includes CBC with differential, peripheral smear, iron indices which include iron, ferritin, TIBC and transferrin saturation, vitamin B, folate levels, and thyroid function tests. Measuring hemoglobin levels is recommended as this measurement is a better assessment of the oxygen transport ability of the blood (Van Leeuwwen & Bladh, 2019). Erythropoietin-stimulating agents (ESAs) are used to manage anemia in chronic kidney disease and are known to improve survival rate and quality of life as well as to enhance cardiac function and lower hospitalizations and health care costs. When treating anemia with ESAs, the goal hemoglobin is less than 11.5 g/dL as higher levels were associated with worsening outcomes such as increased rates of thrombosis, adverse cerebrovascular and cardiovascular events as well as higher mortality rates. These appear to occur because of ESAs effect on vascular remodeling and vasoconstriction (Shaikh & Aeddula, 2021).

Pain

Usually, genitourinary pain is caused by distention of some portion of the urinary tract because of obstructed urine flow or inflammation and swelling of tissues. Severity of pain is related to the sudden onset rather than the extent of distention (Bickley et al., 2021). It is important for the nurse to elicit the character, duration, location, pattern, and severity of pain in order to formulate the cause. Doubling over, severe, colicky type pain that is intermittent but becomes steadier is generally associated with renal calculi particularly if the patient notices blood in the urine. The patient may also describe pain in the flank or costovertebral angle area which may radiate to the umbilicus. Flank pain is also associated with pyelonephritis (bacterial infection causing inflammation of the kidneys) and the patient may describe symptoms of vomiting, fever, and chills. Burning and painful urination sometimes felt as a dull pressure over the bladder may be indicative of cystitis. Acute overdistention of the bladder can be an excruciating type of pain while chronic overdistention may be painless (Bickley et al., 2021).

Studies have reported that 58% of patients experience pain with chronic kidney disease and 49% describe the pain as moderate to severe in nature whether or not they are undergoing dialysis. Pain in patients with kidney failure stems from their primary disease such as polycystic kidney disease, neuropathy associated with uremia and metabolic bone disease (Davison, 2019).

Table 25-3 lists the various types of genitourinary pain, characteristics of the pain, associated signs and symptoms, and possible causes. Initially a gradual decline in kidney functioning (stages 1 and 2) may be asymptomatic and only noted when the patient presents for routine examination. Individuals presenting with stage 3 or 4 kidney disease are more likely to present with clinical and laboratory signs and symptoms, an elevation in serum creatinine, a decreased GFR, or an abnormal urinalysis which may be the first clue to kidney disease (Benjamin & Lappin, 2021). However, some patients present with hypertension, nausea and vomiting, muscle cramps, pruritis (skin irritation resulting in scratching), weight loss or change in mental status which are signs and symptoms associated with uremia (Zemaitis et al., 2021) leading the nurse to further explore kidney function.

Changes in Voiding

Micturition is normally a painless function that occurs approximately eight times in a 24-hour period. The average person voids approximately 1,500 mL of urine in 24 hours (Norris, 2019), although this amount varies depending on fluid intake, sweating, environmental temperature, vomiting, or diarrhea. Common problems associated with voiding include **frequency**, urgency, dysuria, hesitancy, incontinence, **polyuria** (more than 3 L/day of urine), **oliguria** (less than 400 mL/day), and hematuria (>3 RBCs per high-powered field or a positive dipstick) (Fischbach et al., 2022) (Table 25-4). Pain that may be associated with an overdistended bladder, difficulty starting the stream of urine or decrease in amount of urine or straining to void all may be symptoms of urinary retention (Bickley et al., 2021) and should be evaluated.

Gastrointestinal Symptoms

GI symptoms may occur with urologic conditions because of shared autonomic and sensory innervation and renointestinal reflexes (Tortora & Derrickson, 2020). For example, with kidney stones (nephrolithiasis) in the renal pelvis, ureter, or

TABLE **25-3 Identifying Characteristics of Genitourinary Pain**

Type	Location	Character	Associated Signs and Symptoms	Possible Etiology
Kidney	Costovertebral angle, may extend to umbilicus	Dull constant ache; if sudden distention of capsule, pain is severe, sharp, stabbing, and colicky in nature	Nausea and vomiting, diaphoresis, pallor, signs of shock	Acute obstruction, kidney stone, blood clot, acute pyelonephritis, trauma
Bladder	Suprapubic area	Dull, continuous pain, may be intense with voiding, may be severe if bladder full	Urgency, pain at end of voiding, painful straining	Overdistended bladder, infection, interstitial cystitis; tumor
Ureteral	Costovertebral angle, flank, lower abdominal area, testis, or labium	Severe, sharp, stabbing pain, colicky in nature	Nausea and vomiting, paralytic ileus	Ureteral stone, edema or stricture, blood clot
Prostatic	Perineum and rectum	Vague discomfort, feeling of fullness in perineum, vague back pain	Suprapubic tenderness, obstruction to urine flow; frequency, urgency, dysuria, nocturia	Prostatic cancer, acute or chronic prostatitis
Urethral	Male: along penis to meatus; female: urethra to meatus	Pain variable, most severe during and immediately after voiding	Frequency, urgency, dysuria, nocturia, urethral discharge	Irritation of bladder neck, infection of urethra, trauma, foreign body in lower urinary tract

bladder, patients will complain of intense pain and the location of the pain will vary with the site of the stone. When the problem is at the renal pelvis the patient will complain of flank and upper abdominal pain, whereas ureteral obstruction will produce pain in the upper abdomen, lower abdomen, pelvis, testicles, and perineum. Finally, bladder outlet obstruction will produce pain in the pelvis (Suneja et al., 2020). The most common signs and symptoms are nausea, vomiting, diarrhea, abdominal discomfort, and abdominal distention.

Risk Factors

Various diseases or clinical situations can increase a patient's risk for renal and urinary tract dysfunction. Data collection about previous health problems or diseases provides the health care team with useful information for evaluating the patient's current urinary status. For example, the nurse needs to be aware that multiparous women delivering their children vaginally have a high risk for stress **urinary incontinence**. About 50% to 80% of females will develop at UTI at least once in their lifetime and while in general UTIs occur more often in females than in males, after age 50, the incidence becomes about the same since a number of males suffer from obstructive prostatic hypertrophy predisposing them to UTIs. Risk factors for developing a UTI include recent sexual intercourse, DM, and incontinence. During pregnancy asymptomatic bacteriuria or bacteria in the urine greater than 100,000 colony-forming units per milliliter without associated symptoms, is associated with pyelonephritis, therefore screening is indicated. Any anatomic or functional anomaly resulting in urinary stasis or obstruction may result in a UTI (Quallich & Lajiness, 2020). Other risk factors include catheterizations, estrogen deficiency, urinary retention, use of diaphragms and or spermicides, spinal cord injuries, neurologic disorders such as multiple sclerosis and acquired immunodeficiency disease (McAninch & Lue 2020; Quallich & Lajiness, 2020).

Risk factors for specific disorders and kidney and lower urinary tract dysfunction are summarized in Table 25-5 and discussed in Chapters 26 and 27.

Family History

People with a family history of urinary tract problems are at increased risk for renal disorders, such as autosomal dominant polycystic kidney disease (PCKD), a progressive disorder in which cysts form on the kidneys (and may also involve other organs such as the pancreas, liver, and spleen) causing the organs to be enlarged. PCKD is the most common genetic cause of renal failure, and 4 to 7 million individuals are affected worldwide and by 60 years of age, 50% of patients will require RRT as it is a progressive disorder and symptoms increase with age (Akbar & Bokhari, 2021). Other inherited diseases include hereditary nephritis also called Alport syndrome caused by gene mutations in type 1V collagen manifested by hematuria, proteinuria and resulting progressive renal disease, visual changes, and deafness (Lusco & Fogo, 2021). Urolithiasis has also been found to be familial (Thakore & Liang, 2021).

TABLE **25-4 Problems Associated with Changes in Voiding**

Problem	Definition	Possible Etiology
Frequency	Frequent voiding; more than every 3 hours	Infection, obstruction of lower urinary tract leading to residual urine and overflow, anxiety, diuretics, benign prostatic hyperplasia, urethral stricture, diabetic neuropathy, interstitial cystitis (IC), neurologic conditions
Urgency	Strong desire to void	Infection, chronic prostatitis, urethritis, obstruction of lower urinary tract leading to residual urine and overflow, anxiety, diuretics, benign prostatic hyperplasia, urethral stricture, diabetic neuropathy, IC, neurologic conditions
Dysuria	Painful or difficult voiding	Lower urinary tract infection, inflammation of bladder or urethra, acute prostatitis, stones, foreign bodies, tumors in bladder, IC
Hesitancy and retention	Delay, difficulty in initiating voiding	Benign prostatic hyperplasia, surgical nerve damage, foreign object, compression of urethra, outlet obstruction, neurogenic bladder, organ prolapse (Dougherty & Rawla, 2021)
Nocturia	Wakening from sleep to void more than twice a night	Decreased renal concentrating ability, heart failure, diabetes mellitus, incomplete bladder emptying, excessive fluid intake at bedtime, nephrotic syndrome, cirrhosis with ascites
Incontinence	Involuntary loss of urine	External urinary sphincter injury, obstetric injury, lesions of bladder neck, detrusor dysfunction, infection, neurogenic bladder, medications, neurologic abnormalities
Enuresis	Involuntary voiding during sleep	Delay in functional maturation of central nervous system (bladder control usually achieved by 5 years of age), obstructive disease of lower urinary tract, genetic factors, failure to concentrate urine, urinary tract infection, psychological stress, neurologic conditions
Polyuria	Increased volume of urine voided (generally over 3 L/day)	Diabetes mellitus, diabetes insipidus, use of diuretics, excess fluid intake, lithium toxicity, some forms of kidney disease (hypercalcemic and hypokalemic nephropathy)
Oliguria	Urine output less than 400 mL/day	Acute or chronic kidney failure (see Chapter 26), inadequate fluid intake
Anuria	Urine output less than 50 mL/day	Acute or chronic kidney failure (see Chapter 26), complete obstruction
Hematuria	Red blood cells in the urine	Cancer of genitourinary tract, acute glomerulonephritis, kidney stones, renal tuberculosis, blood dyscrasia, trauma, extreme exercise, rheumatic fever, hemophilia, leukemia, sickle cell trait or disease, polycystic kidney disease, prostatitis
Proteinuria	Abnormal amounts of protein in the urine	Acute and chronic kidney disease, nephrotic syndrome, vigorous exercise, heat stroke, severe heart failure, diabetic nephropathy, multiple myeloma

Social History

It is especially important to obtain a thorough medication history when assessing older patients, for whom the increased occurrence of chronic illness often leads to polypharmacy (concurrent use of multiple medications) (Carr et al., 2021). Aging affects the way the body absorbs, metabolizes, and excretes drugs, placing the older patient at risk for adverse reactions (Maher et al. 2021).

Other key information to obtain includes an assessment of the patient's psychosocial status, level of anxiety, perceived threats to body image, available support systems, and sociocultural patterns. Obtaining this information during the initial and subsequent nursing assessments enables the nurse to uncover special needs, misunderstandings, lack of knowledge, and need for patient teaching (Bickley et al., 2021; Jarvis & Eckhardt, 2020).

Physical Examination

Several body systems can affect upper and lower urinary tract dysfunction, and that dysfunction can affect several end organs; therefore, a head-to-toe assessment is indicated. Areas of emphasis include the abdomen, suprapubic region, genitalia, lower back, and lower extremities.

Palpation of the Kidneys

Because the kidneys are retroperitoneal, they are generally not palpable although a normal right kidney may be palpable

TABLE **25-5 Risk Factors for Selected Renal or Urologic Disorders**

Risk Factor	Possible Renal or Urologic Disorder
Childhood diseases: "strep throat" impetigo, nephrotic syndrome	Chronic kidney failure
Advanced age	Incomplete emptying of bladder, leading to urinary tract infection
Instrumentation of urinary tract, cystoscopy, catheterization	Urinary tract infection, incontinence
Low fluid intake, elevated BMI, DM, gout, acidic urine, UTI, family hx (Nojaba & Guzman, 2021)	Kidney stone formation
Occupational (heavy metal exposure, mining, agricultural, chemical industry) or environmental air exposure including second-hand smoke in children	Kidney disease
Diabetes mellitus	Chronic kidney failure, neurogenic bladder
Hypertension	Renal insufficiency, chronic kidney failure
Multiple sclerosis	Incontinence, neurogenic bladder
Parkinson disease	Incontinence, neurogenic bladder
Systemic lupus erythematosus	Nephritis, chronic kidney failure
Gout, hyperparathyroidism, Crohn disease, ileostomy	Kidney stone formation
Sickle cell anemia, multiple myeloma	Chronic kidney failure
Benign prostatic hyperplasia	Obstruction to urine flow, leading to frequency, oliguria, anuria
Radiation therapy to pelvis	Cystitis, strictures, and fistulas (Matta et al., 2019)
Recent pelvic surgery	Inadvertent trauma to ureters or bladder
Pregnancy	Proteinuria, frequent voiding
Obstetric injury, tumors	Incontinence, fistulas
Spinal cord injury	Neurogenic bladder, urinary tract infection, incontinence

especially in very thin patients with relaxed abdominal muscles; however, a left kidney is not usually palpated. Palpation of the kidneys may detect an enlargement that could prove to be very important. The correct technique for palpation is illustrated in Figure 25-5. Renal dysfunction may produce tenderness over the costovertebral angle, which is the angle formed by the lower border of the 12th rib and the spine (Bickley et al., 2021) (Fig. 25-6).

Inspection, Palpation, Percussion, and Auscultation of the Abdomen

The abdomen (just slightly to the right and left of midline in both upper quadrants) is auscultated to assess for bruits (low-pitched murmurs that indicate renal artery stenosis or an aortic aneurysm) (Fig. 25-7). The abdomen also is assessed for the presence of ascites (accumulation of fluid in the peritoneal cavity), which may occur with dysfunction of the kidney as well as the liver. On inspection, with the patient lying down, a distended abdomen is noted with bulging flanks (sides) due to the weight of fluid accumulation pressing against the flanks. On percussion, dullness is noted on the flank area (where the water is), whereas tympanic sounds are heard on the upper abdomen as the gas-filled intestines rise above the ascites fluid (refer to Chapter 20 for further details and techniques). If the kidneys are tender to palpation, the nurse should percuss the kidneys placing the ball of the hand at the costovertebral angle and striking the hand with the ulnar area of the fist. If the patient experiences pain during this maneuver, pyelonephritis is suspected particularly if the patient is febrile (Bickley et al., 2021).

Percussion of the Bladder

To check for residual urine, the bladder may be percussed after the patient voids. Recall the bladder is in the pelvic cavity and the urinary bladder is not palpable unless it is distended above the symphysis pubis. Percussion of the bladder begins at the midline just below the umbilicus and proceeds downward. The sound changes from tympanic to dull when

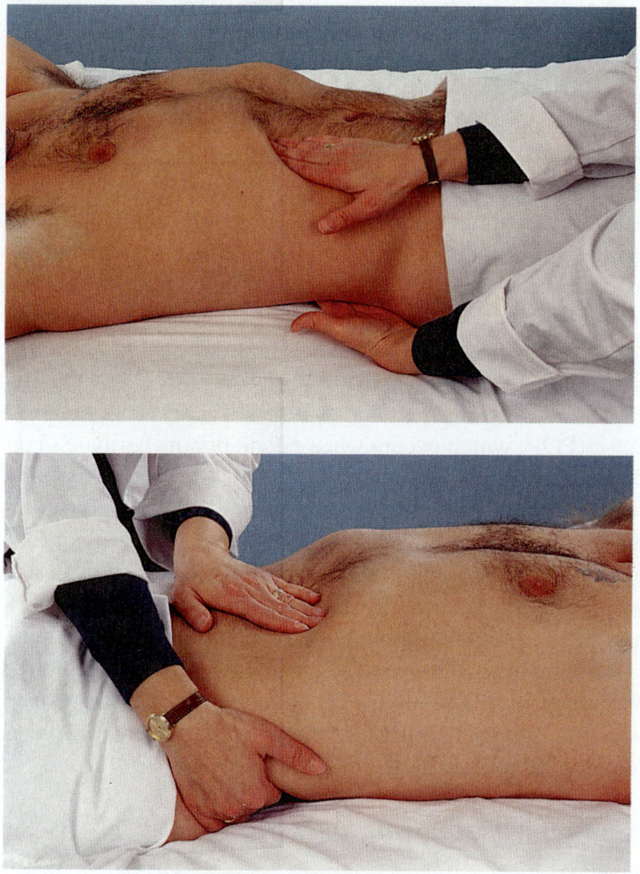

FIGURE 25-5 Technique for palpating the right kidney (*top*). Place one hand under the patient's back with the fingers under the lower rib. Place the palm of the other hand anterior to the kidney with fingers above the umbilicus. Push the hand on top forward as the patient inhales deeply. The left kidney (*bottom*) is palpated similarly by reaching over to the patient's left side and placing the right hand beneath the patient's lower left rib. (From Weber, J. W., & Kelley, J. [2013]. *Health assessment in nursing* [4th ed.]. Lippincott Williams & Wilkins.)

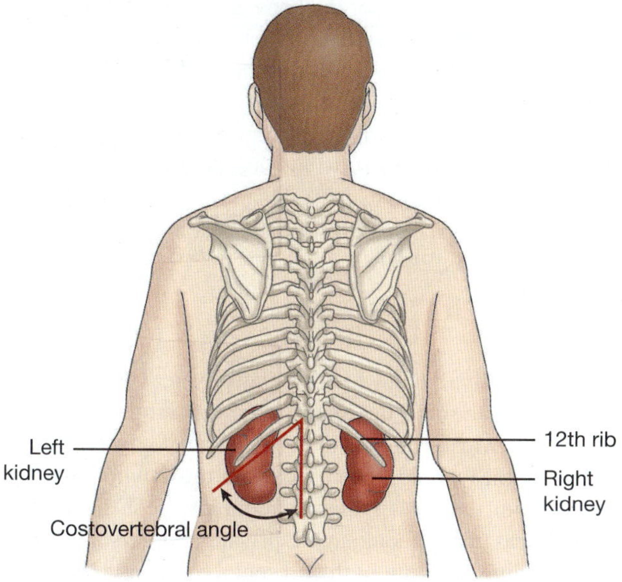

FIGURE 25-6 Location of the costovertebral angle.

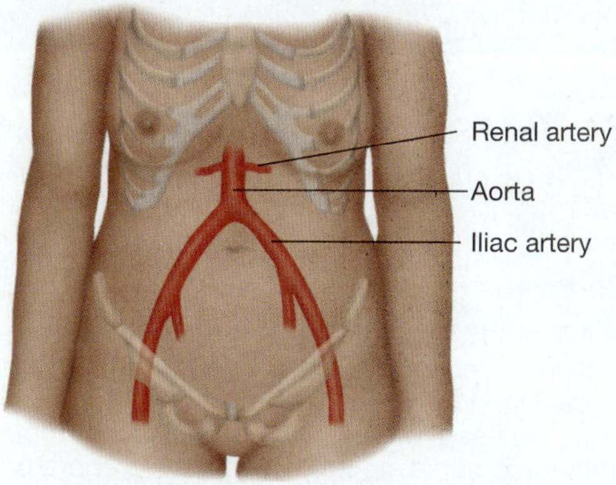

FIGURE 25-7 Arterial bruits with both systolic and diastolic components suggest partial occlusion of the aorta or large arteries. Partial occlusion of a renal artery may cause and explain hypertension. (From Bickley, L. S., & Szilagyi, P. [2003]. *Bates' guide to physical examination and history taking* [8th ed.]. Lippincott Williams & Wilkins.)

percussing over the bladder. If dullness is noted, the bladder volume is typically 400 to 600 mL. The bladder, which can be palpated only if it is moderately distended, feels like a smooth, firm, round mass rising out of the abdomen, usually at midline (Fig. 25-8). Dullness to percussion of the bladder after voiding indicates incomplete bladder emptying. Bladder distention may occur because of a urethral stricture, enlarged prostate, stroke or multiple sclerosis and other neurologic disorders as well as from medications (Bickley et al., 2021). A bladder scan can be performed to assess volume of urine retained after voiding.

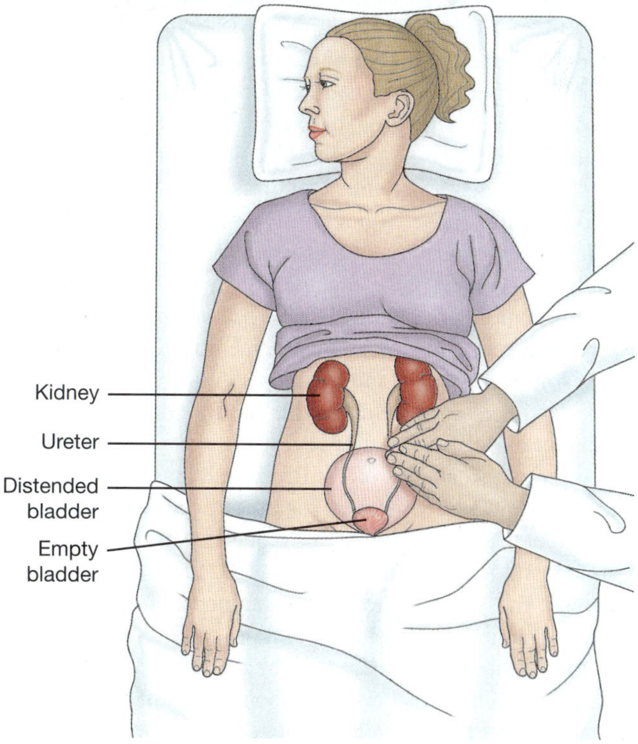

FIGURE 25-8 Palpation of the bladder.

Unfolding Patient Stories: L.B. • Part 2

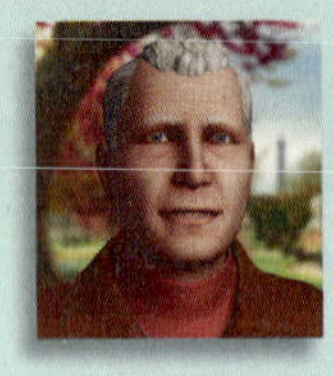

Recall from Chapter 18 **L.B.**, who presented to the emergency department with a hip fracture. What effect can significant blood loss from surgery to repair the fracture have on renal function? What clinical findings would indicate to the nurse that kidney function is impaired? What clinical assessment findings would alert the nurse of potential trauma to the urinary tract resulting from the hip fracture? What diagnostic tests may be used to identify a urinary tract complication that the nurse would consider for preparatory patient education?

Care for L.B. and other patients in a realistic virtual environment: ***vSim** for Nursing* (thepoint.lww.com/vSimMedicalSurgical). Practice documenting these patients' care in DocuCare (thepoint.lww.com/DocuCareEHR).

Palpation of the Prostate and Inguinal Area

In older males, BPH or prostatitis can cause difficulty with urination. The prostate gland is palpated by digital rectal examination (DRE) as part of the yearly physical examination in males 50 years of age and older (see Chapters 31 and 33). The decision to assess the prostate via the prostate-specific antigen (PSA) blood level varies among expert taking into consideration risk versus benefit. The PSA has been noted as a reliable marker for monitoring *recurrence* of prostate cancer, however it does not have the sensitivity or specificity (20% to 40%) needed to be considered an ideal tumor marker (Fischbach et al., 2022). The U.S. Preventive Task Force Services recommends males 55 to 69 years of age make individual informed decisions regarding whether to undergo PSA screening based on in depth discussions with their health care provider. The information provided should include risks, benefits, and limitations of screening at age 50, however those with a family history of prostate cancer diagnosed prior to age 65 (particularly in first-line relatives) or black males, also considered at risk, should receive this information prior to age 50. The American Urologic Association recommends against screening for males aged 40 to 54 at average risk and for those 55 or over considered at risk, the decision should be with careful consideration by the patient and provider after reviewing risk versus benefit. The American Academy of Family Physicians recommends against routine screening and for those aged 55 to 69 who do consider screening, an informed decision should be made as noted previously (Jain & Sapra, 2021). If a PSA is to be drawn, the sample should be obtained before the DRE because manipulation of the prostate can cause the PSA level to increase temporarily (Fischbach et al., 2022). Refer to Chapter 33 for further details on prostate cancer. The inguinal area is examined for enlarged nodes or an inguinal or femoral hernia.

Inspection and Palpation of the Female Genitalia

In females, the vulva, urethral meatus, and vagina are examined; refer to Chapter 32 for additional details regarding the vaginal examination. The urethra orifice is inspected for discharge, polyps, caruncles (a bright, red lesion protruding from the urethra meatus and generally asymptomatic) and fistulas (abnormal connection between two epithelial surfaces). The nurse should inspect for inflammation, irritation, or dilation which may result from urinary tract infections or the insertion of a foreign object. The vagina should be inspected for swelling, discoloration, discharge, masses, fistulas, or fissures (Bickley et al., 2021; Jarvis & Eckardt, 2020). The vagina should be examined for pelvic organ prolapse (POP) which occurs when pelvic organs herniate to or beyond the vaginal wall. In the past, POP was commonly referred to as cystocele, urethrocele, and rectocele, however these terms are no longer used as they fail to provide information related to the structures on the side of the vaginal bulge which is particularly true regarding females who have had pelvic organ surgery in the past. Presenting signs and symptoms may include vaginal bulge and pressure, voiding and defecation and sexual dysfunction. While these may occur in younger females, POP typically presents in older females (Bhadana, 2020).

Assessment for Edema and Body Weight

The patient is assessed for edema and changes in body weight. Edema may be observed, particularly in the face and dependent parts of the body, such as the ankles and sacral areas, and suggests fluid retention. An increase in body weight commonly accompanies edema. A weight gain of 1 kg equals approximately 1,000 mL of fluid (1 lb ≈ 500 mL).

Assessment of Lower Extremities

The deep tendon reflexes of the knee are assessed for quality and symmetry. This is an important part of testing for neurologic causes of bladder dysfunction because the sacral area, which innervates the lower extremities, is the same peripheral nerve area responsible for urinary continence. The gait pattern of the person with bladder dysfunction is also noted, as well as the patient's ability to walk heel to toe. These tests evaluate possible supraspinal causes for urinary incontinence (Bickley et al., 2021; Norris, 2019).

Diagnostic Evaluation

A comprehensive health history and physical examination are used to determine the appropriate laboratory and diagnostic tests. Most patients undergoing urologic testing or imaging studies are apprehensive, even those who have had these tests in the past. Patients frequently feel discomfort and embarrassment about such a private and personal function as voiding. Voiding in the presence of others frequently can cause guarding, a natural reflex that inhibits voiding due to situational anxiety. Because the outcomes of these studies determine the plan of care, the nurse must help the patient relax by providing as much privacy and explanation about the procedure as possible. The following sections review some of the tests that might be used.

Urinalysis and Urine Culture

The urinalysis provides important clinical information about kidney function and helps diagnose other diseases, such as liver and hematopoietic disorders, hydration status and DM. The urine culture determines whether bacteria are present in the urine, as well as their strains and concentration. Urine culture and sensitivity (C&S) also identify the antimicrobial therapy that is best suited for the strains identified, taking into consideration the antibiotics that have the best rate of resolution in that geographic region (Van Leeuwen & Bladh, 2019). Most organisms begin to grow within 24 hours within the laboratory setting, thus a preliminary report can be established, however it takes approximately 48 to 72 hours for organism growth and identification, therefore potential antibiotic therapy should not be initiated until the specimen has been collected. Therapy should be selected based on the most effective, safest, and least expensive medication. Appropriate evaluation of any abnormality can assist in detecting serious underlying diseases. Refer to Table 25-6 for the details regarding urinalysis components and potential significance.

TABLE **25-6 Select Urinalysis Components**

Component	Discussion
Color	Colorless to pale yellow (possible causes: Dilute urine due to diuretics, alcohol consumption, diabetes insipidus, glycosuria, excess fluid intake, renal disease) Yellow to milky white (possible causes: Pyuria, infection, vaginal cream) Bright yellow (possible causes: Multiple vitamin preparations) Deep yellow may be caused by riboflavin. Pink to red (possible causes: Hemoglobin breakdown, red blood cells, gross blood, menses, bladder or prostate surgery, porphyrin, beets, blackberries, rhubarb, medications [phenytoin, rifampin, phenothiazine, cascara, senna products]) Blue, blue green (possible causes: Dyes, methylene blue, *Pseudomonas* species organisms, medications [amitriptyline, triamterene, phenyl salicylate]), green-colored breath mints and oxidized bilirubin. Orange to amber (possible causes: Concentrated urine due to dehydration, fever, bile, excess bilirubin or carotene, rhubarb, medications [phenazopyridium HCl, nitrofurantoin, sulfasalazine, docusate calcium, thiamine]) Brown to black (possible causes: Old red blood cells, urobilinogen, bilirubin, melanin, porphyrin, extremely concentrated urine due to dehydration, medications [cascara, metronidazole, iron preparations, quinine, senna products, methyldopa, nitrofurantoin]; myoglobinuria) Smokey-colored-presence of red blood cells (Van Leeuwen & Bladh, 2021).
Specific gravity	Evaluates ability of kidneys to concentrate solutes in urine and is altered by the presence of blood, protein, and casts in the urine. Disorders or conditions that cause *decreased* urine specific gravity (i.e., dilute urine) include diabetes insipidus, glomerulonephritis, and severe kidney damage, which may cause a fixed specific gravity of 1.010. Glucose, protein, or dyes excreted in the urine *increase* the specific gravity (concentrated urine); therefore, etiologies include diabetes mellitus, patients who recently received high-density radiopaque dyes, and fluid deficit.
Osmolality	Concentrating ability is lost early in kidney disease; these test findings may disclose early defects in kidney function.
Red blood cells (hematuria)	Can develop from an abnormality anywhere along the genitourinary tract and is more common in females than in males. Common causes include acute infection (cystitis, urethritis, or prostatitis), renal calculi, and neoplasm. Other causes include systemic disorders, such as bleeding disorders; malignant lesions; and medications, such as warfarin and heparin.
White blood cells	Should be very few; increased numbers indicate infection or inflammation.
Protein	Occasional loss of up to 150 mg/day of protein in the urine primarily is considered normal and usually does not require further evaluation. Urine concentration, pH, hematuria, and radiocontrast materials all affect the results. Microalbuminuria (excretion of 20–200 mg/dL of protein in the urine) is an early sign of diabetic nephropathy. Common benign causes of transient proteinuria are fever, strenuous exercise, and prolonged standing. Causes of persistent proteinuria include glomerular diseases, malignancies, collagen diseases, diabetes mellitus, pre-eclampsia, UTI, hyperthyroidism, hypertension, heart failure, amyloidosis, multiple myeloma, and use of a wide variety of medications (Van Leeuwen & Bladh, 2019).
Glucose	Should be absent; its presence is suspicious for DM.

TABLE **25-7 Additional Tests of Renal Function**

Test	Description	Normal Range		
Creatinine clearance	Detects and evaluates progression of kidney disease. Test measures volume of blood cleared of endogenous creatinine in 1 minute, which provides an approximation of the glomerular filtration rate. Sensitive indicator of kidney disease used to follow progression of disease.	Measured in mL/min/1.73 m^2		
		Age	Male	Female
		Under 30 years	88–146	81–134
		30–40 years	82–140	75–128
		40–50 years	75–133	69–122
		50–60 years	68–126	64–116
		60–70 years	61–120	58–110
		70–80 years	55–113	52–105
Creatinine level	Measures effectiveness of kidney function. In normal function, the level of creatinine remains fairly constant in the body.	0.6–1.2 mg/dL (50–110 mmol/L)		
Urea nitrogen (blood urea nitrogen [BUN])	Serves as index of kidney function. Urea is a nitrogenous end product of protein metabolism. Test values are affected by protein intake, tissue breakdown, and fluid volume changes.	7–18 mg/dL Patients over 60 years: 8–20 mg/dL		
BUN to creatinine ratio	Evaluates hydration status. An elevated ratio is seen in hypovolemia (may rise to 20:1); a normal ratio with an elevated BUN and an elevated creatinine is seen with intrinsic kidney disease.	About 10:1		

Renal Function Tests

Renal function tests are used to evaluate the severity of kidney disease and to assess the status of the patient's kidney function. These tests also provide information about the effectiveness of the kidney in carrying out its excretory function. Renal function test results may be within normal limits until the GFR is reduced to less than 50% of normal. Renal function can be assessed most accurately if several tests are performed, and their results are analyzed together. Common tests of renal function include serum creatinine which is a waste product of skeletal muscle metabolism and **blood urea nitrogen** which measures urea produced as a waste product of protein breakdown; both of which should be completely eliminated by the kidneys (BUN) levels (Norris, 2019; Van Leeuwen & Bladh, 2019). Table 25-7 describes the purpose and gives the normal range for each test. Other tests for evaluating kidney function that may be helpful include serum electrolyte levels (see Chapter 3). A plan of nursing care for a patient undergoing diagnostic testing of the renal/urologic system is available online at http://thepoint.lww.com/Honan3e.

Pearls for Practice

The nurse understands that a normal BUN/creatinine (Cr) ratio is approximately 10:1. As kidney function declines, both the BUN and the Cr rise, thus although elevated the ratio remains within normal limits. If a BUN is elevated but the creatinine is normal (BUN/Cr greater than 20:1), the nurse must assess for causes excluding renal dysfunction. Reasons may include GI bleeding such as gastric ulcers, duodenal ulcers, and gastric cancer (digestion of RBCs elevates the protein level which is transported to the liver and metabolized to BUN), or dehydration (less water available in the intravascular space) where the BUN may increase in a higher proportion than the creatinine, thus indicators of intravascular depletion include an elevated hematocrit value, and a BUN/Cr ratio of greater than 20:1. In situations where the BUN/Cr ratio is less than 10:1, the nurse considers conditions where there is decreased urea synthesis such as severe liver disease or starvation, syndrome of inappropriate ADH (increased water in the intravascular space), and pregnancy (since the GFR increases 50% in pregnancy, there is a resultant decrease in serum creatinine).

Pearls for Practice: Lifting the Lens: The Use of Race in Medical Tests and Its Contribution to Health Disparities and Structural Racism

Recently, there has been an awareness that the use of race in medical testing such as the estimated glomerular filtration rate or eGFR has resulted in delay in referral and treatment for patients at highest risk for kidney diseases. To clarify, the direct measurement of GFR is time-consuming, costly, and not immune to measurement error (Kuppachi et al., 2021). Thus, in 2009, the Chronic Kidney Disease Epidemiology Collaboration (CKD-EPI) equation was established to standardize traditional serum creatinine–based measures of kidney function (Boulware et al., 2022). You are aware that creatinine is a byproduct of muscle metabolism and that it is produced at a constant rate

if muscle mass is consistent. Therefore, the creatinine is used to give an approximation of the GFR. The eGFR uses the creatinine level and variables such as gender, age and race, specifically Black individuals versus non-Black individuals. The race variable was based upon differences in serum creatinine observed among Black individuals in the study population and assumed to be related to higher muscle mass, and not substantiated by rigorous scientific evidence (Boulware et al., 2021). Fast forward to today, where we recognize race as a social construct and not a biologic one requiring increased scrutiny of medical tests that use race as a variable. The race variable in the eGFR systematically raises the value by 16% for Black individuals compared with all others, resulting in an estimate of better kidney function than actually exists. In fact, in a study of self-reported Black participants with chronic kidney disease, the race coefficient in the eGFR was associated with delayed kidney transplant referral and eligibility (Zelnick et al., 2021). As a result, some institutions have already omitted race as a variable in the calculation of the eGFR, others suggest substituting objective data on body size and composition, such as height or weight (Eneanya et al., 2019), and advocate for ongoing research on evidence-based substitutes for race (Levey et al., 2020). Most recently, CKD-EPI (the same organization that developed the initial measure for the eGFR from serum creatinine level) revised the eGFR without a race coefficient; the adoption of which is recommended by a national task force (Walther et al., 2022). While there is now awareness of the eGFR bias, systems are slow to change and it will behoove nurses to keep a skeptical viewpoint when race is used as a variable in medical tests or devices and advocate for the removal of race as a variable in medical testing.

Imaging Modalities

Several imaging modalities play a vital role in the evaluation of renal and urologic disease.

X-Ray: Kidneys, Ureters, Bladder (KUB)

This x-ray delineates the size, shape, and position of the kidneys and reveals abnormalities, such as calculi in the kidneys or urinary tract, cysts, tumors, ascites, ruptures, gas, intestinal obstruction, intestinal perforation, trauma, bleeding from trauma or kidney displacement by abnormalities in surrounding tissues (Van Leeuwen & Bladh, 2019).

Computed Tomography and Magnetic Resonance Imaging

Computed tomography (CT) scans and magnetic resonance imaging (MRI) are noninvasive techniques that provide excellent cross-sectional views of the kidney and urinary tract. They are used to evaluate genitourinary masses, nephrolithiasis, polycystic kidney disease, hydronephrosis, absence of a kidney, hematoma, pheochromocytoma, abscesses, bleeding or hyperplasia of the adrenal glands, size of kidney following kidney transplant, adrenal tumors, fluid accumulation around the kidneys, metastatic disease, and soft tissue abnormalities (Van Leeuwen & Bladh, 2019). An oral or IV radiopaque contrast agent may be used in CT scanning to enhance visualization, although the use of a CT scan should consider the patient's previous exposures to radiation via imaging studies. In addition, the risks associated with contrast agents should be considered. Contrast-induced nephropathy is associated with a pre-existing renal insufficiency, history of DM, left ventricular dysfunction, anemia, HTN, and reduced intravascular volume (Modi et al., 2021). Pregnancy is generally a contraindication to any procedure involving radiation; therefore, the patient should be questioned about last menstrual period (LMP) (Van Leeuwen & Bladh, 2019). Preprocedural hydration, along with recognition of the lowest dose of contrast as possible for the study, is recommended. If ionated contrast is used and the patient is taking metformin or any medication containing metformin, the medication should be discontinued the day of the procedure and held post procedure for 48 hours, although this may vary depending on the institution (Van Leeuwen & Bladh, 2019). A specialized procedure called CT nephrotomography may be performed to evaluate the kidneys, renal pelvis, and ureters to detect ureteral stones or tumors in the collecting ducts, however significant radiation exposure occurs with this procedure. A CT urogram can be performed to identify the presence of ureteral stones. This procedure has increased over the last 5 years, and the radiation dose in the same period has decreased as a result of technical advances and better scanners (Pietropaolo et al., 2019).

Intravenous Urography

This test shows the kidneys, ureters, and bladder via x-ray imaging as a radiopaque contrast agent that is administered intravenously moves through the upper and then the lower urinary system. It may be used as the initial assessment of many suspected urologic problems, especially lesions in the kidneys and ureters, kidney trauma, hematomas, lacerations in the renal artery, kidney, pelvis, ureters, and bladder and provides an approximate estimate of kidney function (Van Leeuwen & Bladh, 2019).

Retrograde Pyelography

If an IV urography provides inadequate visualization of the collecting systems, a retrograde pyelography may be performed. It involves advancing catheters through the ureters into the renal pelvis by means of cystoscopy, followed by injection of a contrast agent (Van Leeuwen & Bladh, 2019).

Cystography

In cystography, a catheter is inserted into the bladder, and a contrast agent is instilled to outline the bladder wall. This study aids in evaluating vesicoureteral reflux (backflow of urine from the bladder into one or both ureters), recurrent UTIs, hematomas and in assessing for bladder injury (Fischbach et al., 2022).

Voiding Cystourethrography

In a voiding cystourethrography, a urethral catheter is inserted, and a contrast agent is instilled into the bladder. When the bladder is full and the patient feels the urge to void, the catheter is removed, and the patient voids. This study uses fluoroscopy to visualize the lower urinary tract and assesses urine storage in the bladder. It is used as a diagnostic tool to identify vesicoureteral reflux, bladder lacerations or trauma, evaluate for the presence of obstructions or strictures in the urethra and/or ureter, bladder tumors, to evaluate chronic urinary tract infections and detect hematomas. Retrograde urethrography, in which a contrast agent is injected retrograde into the urethra, is always performed before urethral catheterization if urethral trauma is suspected (Van Leeuwen & Bladh, 2019).

Pearls for Practice

The presence of urethral injury should be ruled out prior to Foley catheter placement in patients with blood at the urethra and suspicion of injury to the lower urinary tract. Catheter placement may potentially convert a partial urethral tear to a complete urethral disruption (Gawronski, 2023).

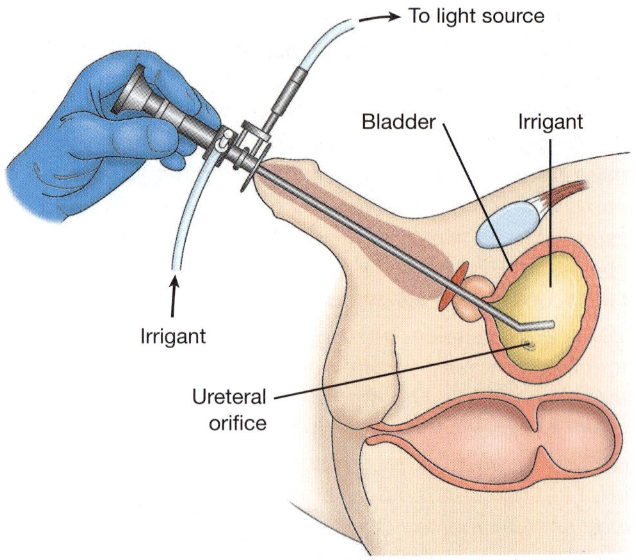

FIGURE 25-9 Cystoscopic examination. A rigid or semirigid cystoscope is introduced into the bladder. The upper cord is an electric line for the light at the distal end of the cystoscope. The lower tubing leads from a reservoir of sterile irrigant that is used to inflate the bladder.

Nuclear Scans

A nuclear scan requires injection of a radioisotope into the circulatory system; then the isotope is monitored as it moves through the blood vessels of the kidneys. The test provides information about kidney perfusion and function. It is used to evaluate acute kidney injury (AKI) and chronic kidney failure, renal masses, and blood flow before and after kidney transplantation (Van Leeuwen & Bladh, 2019).

Renal Angiography

In renal angiography, a catheter is threaded up, generally via the femoral and iliac arteries into the aorta or renal artery. A contrast agent is injected to opacify the renal arterial supply. Angiography is used to evaluate renal blood flow, to differentiate renal cysts from tumors, to evaluate hypertension, and preoperatively, for renal transplantation (Van Leeuwen & Bladh, 2019).

Bladder Ultrasonography

Ultrasonography is a noninvasive procedure that uses sound waves passed into the body through a transducer to detect abnormalities of internal tissues and organs. A bladder ultrasonography is a noninvasive method used to evaluate urinary retention, obstruction, distention, tumors, inflammation, or bleeding. The test requires a full bladder; therefore, fluid intake should be encouraged before the procedure. This test also can be used to determine if a patient is emptying the bladder after urination (Van Leeuwen & Bladh, 2019).

Urologic Endoscopic Procedures

Endourology, or urologic endoscopic procedures, can be performed in one of two ways: using a cystoscope (Fig. 25-9)

TABLE **25-8 Common Urologic Procedures**

Procedure	Description	Purpose
Cystoscopy	Cystoscope is inserted through the urethra into the bladder.	Used to visualize the urethra and bladder directly, as well as the urethral orifices and prostatic urethra. Calculi may be removed from the urethra, bladder, and ureter.
Renal and ureteral brush biopsy	Ureteral catheter is introduced via cystoscope, followed by a biopsy brush that is passed through the catheter.	Suspected lesion is brushed back and forth to obtain cells and surface tissue fragments for histologic analysis.
Kidney biopsy	Small section of renal cortex is obtained either percutaneously (needle biopsy) or by open biopsy through small flank incision.	Helps diagnose and evaluate the extent of kidney disease. Indications for biopsy include unexplained acute kidney failure, persistent proteinuria/hematuria, transplant rejection, glomerulopathies.

inserted into the urethra, or percutaneously, through a small incision and is used to evaluate hematuria, urgency, dysuria, urinary frequency, retention, recurrent UTIs, and the removal of foreign bodies (Albakr et al., 2021; Van Leeuwen & Bladh, 2019) (Table 25-8).

Bladder Scan

A portable ultrasound device provides a 3D image of the bladder and measures bladder volume noninvasively, providing immediate details on the volume of urine retained within the bladder (Van Leeuwen & Bladh, 2019).

CHAPTER REVIEW

NCLEX-Style Review Questions

1. A 72-year-old patient with a history of an enlarged prostate is brought to the emergency room complaining of an inability to void for the past 12 hours. Select all methods when assessing for bladder distention.
  a. Inspect and palpate for a smooth, firm, round mass rising in suprapubic region
  b. Percuss for dullness in the suprapubic region
  c. Palpate for rebound tenderness below the symphysis
  d. Inspect for discharge from the urethral meatus
  e. Using a bladder scan to assess the volume of urine in the bladder

2. A male patient is concerned about changes to his urinary stream. Which of the following are associated with lower urinary tract symptoms? Select all that apply.
  a. Urgency
  b. Flank pain
  c. Frequency
  d. Dribbling
  e. Costovertebral angle (CVA) tenderness

3. Which of the following disorders in the patient history places the patient at risk for urinary tract infection? Select all that apply.
  a. Hypertension
  b. Hypothyroidism
  c. Diabetes mellitus
  d. Hormonal contraceptive use
  e. Increased residual urine

4. The nurse knows that a frequent cause of red blood cells (RBCs) in the patient's urine is which condition? Select all that apply.
  a. INR of 4.0
  b. Hypertension
  c. Bladder cancer
  d. Genitourinary infection
  e. Prostate enlargement

5. A 42-year-old male patient complains of nausea, vomiting, and right flank pain. What is the most likely cause of these symptoms? Select all that apply.
  a. Distention of the bladder
  b. Pyelonephritis
  c. Enlarged prostate
  d. Irritation to the bladder neck
  e. Renal calculi

REFERENCES AND SELECTED READINGS

References and selected readings associated with this chapter can be found on the website that accompanies the book. Visit **http://thepoint.lww.com/Honan3e** to access the references and other additional resources associated with this chapter.

CHAPTER 26

Nursing Management: Patients With Renal Disorders

Andrea Rothman Mann • Linda Honan

Learning Objectives

After reading this chapter, you will be able to:

1. Compare and contrast the pathophysiology, assessment, nursing management, and medical management of the glomerular diseases.
2. Identify causes of acute kidney injury and chronic kidney failure.
3. Summarize the nursing management of the patient with kidney failure.
4. Describe renal replacement therapies.
5. Provide education for the patient undergoing kidney transplantation.
6. Describe assessments for the patient sustaining renal trauma.
7. Evaluate outcomes of care for the patient with kidney disorders.

The renal system is an important regulator of the body's internal environment and is essential for the maintenance of life. The kidneys regulate fluid volume and electrolyte balance; they also play a role in acid–base balance, excrete waste products, regulate blood pressure (BP) and blood osmolarity, contribute to red blood cell (RBC) production and vitamin D metabolism. Kidney dysfunction may be acute or chronic and can affect all body systems. Renal disease is often asymptomatic or presents with nonspecific complaints. Its presentation and severity is determined by the existing renal function and comorbid conditions. This may occur before the glomerular filtration rate (GFR) has reached the stage of kidney failure (Norris & Tuan, 2020). Various factors contribute to kidney dysfunction; Box 26-1 addresses gerontologic considerations. This chapter addresses glomerular dysfunction, acute kidney injury (AKI), chronic kidney disease (CKD), and treatment options, as well as kidney trauma and transplant.

GLOMERULAR DISEASES

Diseases of the glomerulus can generally be classified into one of three major syndromes: nephritic syndrome, nephrotic syndrome, and non-nephrotic proteinuria, with some overlap in the clinical presentations. Nephritic syndrome is characterized by an inflammatory process in which a patient has glomerular hematuria, proteinuria, urinary sediment, renal insufficiency, and often hypertension (HTN) (Fig. 26-1). The "nephritic syndrome" is how patients with acute glomerulonephritis (GN) typically present; it may be caused by an intrinsic renal disease or a systemic disease process. Nephrotic syndrome will be discussed shortly.

Acute Glomerulonephritis

Acute glomerulonephritis is inflammation of the glomerular capillaries encompassing a variety of renal diseases including an untreated infection that damages the glomerulus (primary GN), but may result from systemic diseases such as systemic lupus erythematosus (SLE), which is termed secondary GN (Norris & Tuan, 2020). Acute GN is more common in children, but it can occur at any age.

Pathophysiology

Acute GN comprises a specific set of renal diseases in which an immunologic mechanism triggers inflammation and proliferation of glomerular tissue that can result in damage to the basement membrane, mesangium (thin membrane supporting the capillary loops in renal glomeruli), or capillary endothelium (Norris & Tuan, 2020). The infection, while typically bacterial, may result from viral, fungal, helminthic (parasitic worm), or protozoal infections (Jameson et al., 2020).

Acute poststreptococcal glomerulonephritis (PSGN) may result from impetigo or pharyngitis caused by group A beta-hemolytic streptococci, or staphylococci or viruses and parasites such as malaria (Norris & Tuan, 2020). Chronic illnesses causing glomerular disease can include SLE, Goodpasture

BOX 26-1 **Highlighting Gerontology**

Kidney Dysfunction

Changes in kidney function with normal aging increase the susceptibility of older adults to kidney dysfunction and kidney failure. In addition, the incidence of systemic diseases, such as atherosclerosis, HTN, heart failure, diabetes, and cancer, increases with advancing age, predisposing older adults to kidney disease associated with these disorders. Therefore, acute problems need to be prevented, recognized, and treated quickly to avoid kidney damage. Nurses in all settings should be alert for signs and symptoms of renal dysfunction in older patients.

Because alterations in renal perfusion, glomerular filtration, and renal clearance increase the risk for medication-associated changes in renal function or toxicities, precautions and surveillance are warranted. When older patients undergo diagnostic testing or when new medications (e.g., diuretic agents) are added, precautions must be taken to prevent dehydration, which can compromise marginal renal function and lead to kidney failure.

With aging, the kidney is less able to respond to acute fluid and electrolyte changes. Older patients may develop atypical and nonspecific signs and symptoms of impaired renal function as well as fluid and electrolyte imbalances. Recognition of these problems is hampered further by the misconception that they are normal changes of aging are associated with pre-existing disorders (Eliopoulos, 2022).

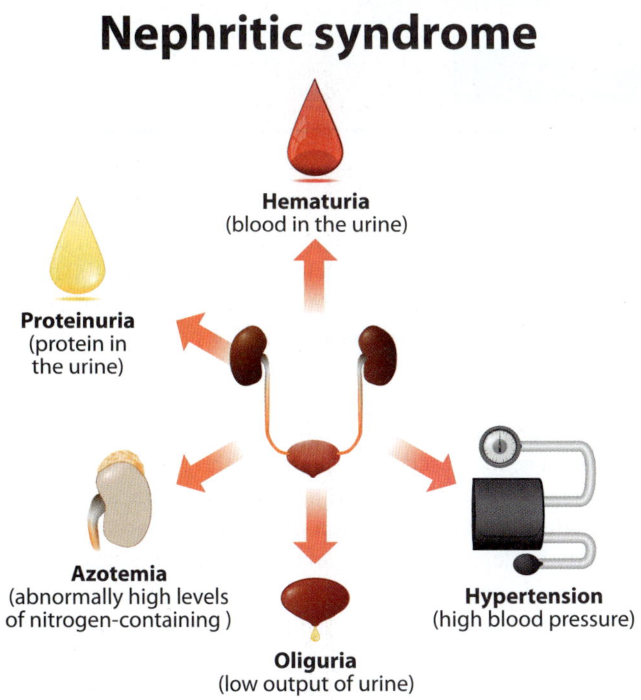

FIGURE 26-1 Nephritic syndrome or acute nephritic syndrome. (Image from Shutterstock.)

syndrome, Berger disease (also known as immunoglobulin A [IgA]) nephropathy and human immunodeficiency virus infection (HIV) (Norris & Tuan, 2020). Acute nephritic syndrome results from glomerular inflammation. In acute GN, the kidneys become large, edematous, and congested. All renal tissues, including the glomeruli, tubules, and blood vessels, are affected to varying degrees. Box 26-2 depicts the pathophysiology of GN.

Acute GN caused by certain strains of group A beta-hemolytic streptococcal infections are referred to as post-streptococcal glomerulonephritis or PSGN. Failure to receive treatment causes an immune-mediated antigen–antibody reaction and inflammation which is noticeable 7 to 12 days after infection, resulting in increased permeability of the glomerular capillary wall. Insoluble immune complexes become trapped in the glomeruli; protein, RBCs, and RBC casts enter the urine (Norris & Tuan, 2020). Sudden onset of hematuria, proteinuria, edema, HTN, and reduced renal function ensues (Norris & Tuan, 2020). RBC degradation causes the smoky or coffee-colored urine, which may be the first sign of the disorder. Often this clinical picture is accompanied by HTN, azotemia (i.e., decreased GFR, rising blood urea nitrogen [BUN], and creatinine). Retention of renal salt and water, causes edema, particularly of the face (periorbital), hand and scrotal regions (Dirkx & Woodell, 2022; Norris & Tuan, 2020).

Treatment focuses on maintaining normal glomerular function. The inflammation typically lasts about 2 weeks, with individuals rarely developing chronic disease. When acute GN is associated with chronic infections, the underlying infections must be treated (Norris & Tuan, 2020).

Pearls for Practice: Azotemia versus Uremia

Azotemia is a term that refers to an increase in the blood urea nitrogen (BUN), and creatinine [Cr]) which results from a severe decrease in kidney function and may be associated with oliguria (less than 400 mL or <0.5 mL/kg/hr), or anuria (less than 100 mL), which is important to quantify when suspecting acute kidney injury (AKI), but is not always associated with it (Jacob et al., 2020; National Institute for Health and Care Excellence [NICE], 2021). Whereas uremia refers to the altered fluid, electrolyte, acid–base balance; impaired body function (HTN, anemia, pruritus, osteodystrophy, etc.) associated with worsening kidney function as in chronic and end-stage kidney disease (ESKD). ESKD is the name formerly used for stage 5 chronic kidney disease or when the patient requires dialysis or transplant for survival.

Risk Factors

Risk factors include a family history of GN; a pre-existing history of known diseases, such as a streptococcal infection of the upper respiratory tract or skin; other infections such as viral diseases, that is, hepatitis, mumps, and varicella zoster may be implicated. In addition, other diseases, such as Goodpasture

BOX 26-2

Focus on Pathophysiology

Acute Glomerulonephritis

Acute glomerulonephritis (AG) is an inflammatory disease of the glomeruli frequently associated with an antigen–antibody response to infection. Group A beta-hemolytic streptococcal infection of the throat is an infectious cause that precedes the onset of glomerulonephritis by 2–3 weeks. AG may also follow impetigo (infection of the skin), visceral abscesses, and acute viral infections (upper respiratory tract infections, mumps, varicella zoster virus, Epstein–Barr virus, hepatitis, and HIV infection). In some patients, antigens outside the body (e.g., medications, foreign serum) initiate the process, resulting in antigen–antibody complexes being deposited in the glomeruli. In other patients, the kidney tissue itself serves as the inciting antigen.

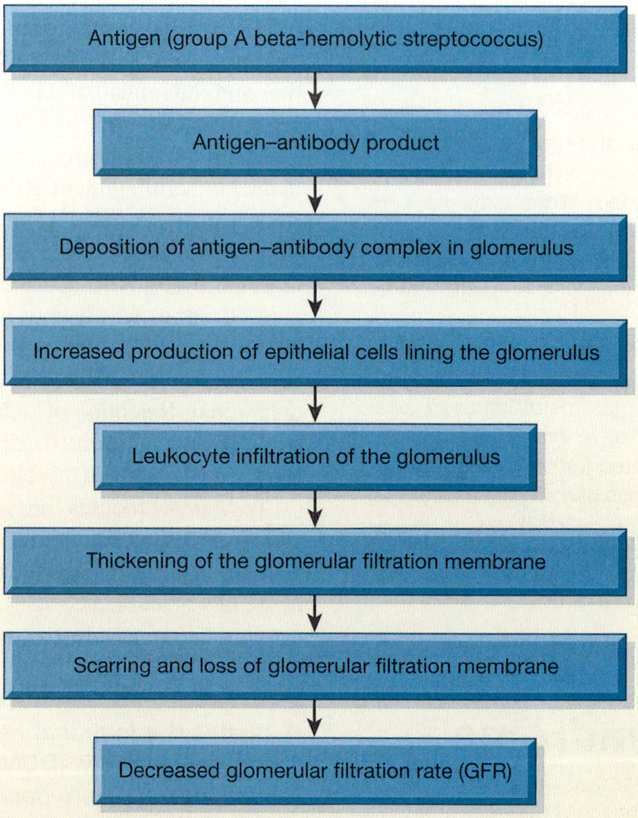

syndrome, Wegener granulomatosis, SLE, subacute bacterial endocarditis, and sepsis have also been identified. While PSGN rarely causes CKD, other disorders such as the autoimmune diseases described above may affect progression.

Clinical Manifestations and Assessment

The primary presenting features of acute GN are a "nephritic picture" of a decreased GFR, hematuria, edema, oliguria, HTN, an active urinary sediment, azotemia (excessive nitrogenous wastes in the blood), and proteinuria (dipstick +2 or >100 mg/dL) (Baumgarten et al., 2022). Hematuria may be microscopic or macroscopic (gross or visible to the eye). The urine is dark and may be described as brown, cola-colored, or coffee colored. RBC and cellular debris called casts are often conclusive for GN and indicate microscopic amount of bleeding associated with glomerular permeability or tubular damage (Landry & Bazari, 2020).

GN may be mild, and the hematuria may be discovered incidentally through a routine microscopic urinalysis, or the disease may be severe, with AKI, oliguria (less than 400 mL), and shortness of breath. Additional assessments to detect underlying causes include assessment for pharyngitis, impetigo, or a heart murmur of endocarditis (Van Leeuwen & Bladh, 2019).

Some degree of edema and HTN is present in most patients. The increased permeability of the glomerular membrane leads to proteinuria and hypoalbuminemia, associated with pitting edema and edema of the hands, face, and feet (initially in dependent areas and areas with low tissue tension) (Van Leeuwen & Bladh, 2019). BUN and serum creatinine levels increase as urine output decreases. In addition, anemia may be present.

In the more severe form of the disease, patients also complain of headache, malaise, and flank pain (pain on sides below ribs and above the pelvis). Older patients may experience circulatory overload with dyspnea, engorged neck veins, cardiomegaly, and pulmonary edema. Atypical symptoms include confusion, somnolence, and seizures, which often are confused with the symptoms of a primary neurologic disorder.

Cultures of throat and skin lesions to rule out Streptococcus species may be obtained. Diagnostic tests include assessing for increasing antistreptolysin O (ASO) titer (a test that checks for a strep infection), which confirms recent infection. Titers begin to increase in 1 to 3 weeks, peak in 3 to 5 weeks, and then return to normal in 6 months. ASO titer is unrelated to severity, duration, or prognosis of disease. In patients with skin infection, anti-DNAase B (ADB) titers are more sensitive than ASO titers for infection with *Streptococcus*. The antinuclear antibody test is useful for patients with acute GN and symptoms of underlying systemic illness, such as SLE and polyarteritis nodosa. Blood culture is indicated in patients with fever, immunosuppression, history of intravenous (IV) drug use, indwelling shunts, or catheters. Other laboratory testing may reveal elevated complement C3 and others as well as increased cryoglobulins (large immune complexes) (Norris & Tuan, 2020).

In most patients, kidney function recovery depends on timely intervention, which, if not done, may lead to a progressive disease (Kazi & Hashmi, 2021). While others, after a period of apparent recovery may insidiously develop chronic GN. The presence of underlying renal disease is associated with the development of **uremia** (discussed later in this chapter).

Medical and Nursing Management

Management consists primarily of symptom management, interventions to preserve kidney function, and prompt treatment of complications. When there is no evidence of malnutrition, dietary protein is restricted when renal insufficiency and nitrogen retention (elevated BUN) develop. Carbohydrates are given liberally to provide energy and reduce the catabolism of protein. Sodium is restricted when the patient has HTN, edema, or heart failure (HF). Treatment will depend on the etiology and severity of acute GN and may include antibiotics, corticosteroids, or cytotoxic agents (Papadakis et al., 2021). Diuretic and antihypertensive medications may be prescribed to control HTN. Plasmapheresis may be used to remove antibodies and mediators of inflammation when antiglomerular basement antibodies are present (Kazi & Hashmi, 2021).

The nurse teaches the patient about fluid restriction for treatment of signs and symptoms of fluid retention (e.g., edema, pulmonary edema, SOB, weight gain). Bed rest is recommended until signs of glomerular inflammation and circulatory congestion subside.

The nurse carefully measures intake and output (I&O), recording and analyzing trends in the data. Fluids are given according to the patient's fluid losses and daily body weight. Insensible fluid loss of approximately 1 L (lungs, stool and skin) is considered when estimating fluid loss. Diuresis usually begins about 1 week after the onset of symptoms, with a decrease in edema and BP. Proteinuria and microscopic hematuria may persist for many months. Recovery from acute GN occurs as inflammation abates, which takes about 2 weeks. Some patients may develop chronic GN characterized by oliguria, shortness of breath, weakness, and periorbital and generalized edema (anasarca). The patient should be instructed to report these symptoms to the health care provider immediately.

Pearls for Practice

The most accurate indicator of fluid loss or gain in an acutely ill patient is weight, as accurate I&O and assessment of insensible losses may be difficult. A weight gain of 1 kg is equal to 1,000 mL of retained fluid (Lough et al., 2022).

Nursing interventions focus on patient education about the disease process, explanations of laboratory and other diagnostic tests, and preparation for safe and effective self-care at home. Patient education is directed toward symptom management and monitoring for complications. The nurse emphasizes fluid and diet restrictions to avoid worsening of edema and HTN. The patient is instructed to notify the primary care provider (PCP) if symptoms of kidney failure occur, including fatigue, nausea, vomiting, diminishing urine output, or at the first sign of any infection. Information for patient education should be given verbally and in writing.

The nurse educates the patient on the importance of follow-up evaluations of BP, urinalysis for protein, and serum BUN and serum creatinine levels to evaluate for disease progression in the patient. A referral for home care may be indicated, giving the nurse an opportunity for assessment and detection of early signs and symptoms of renal insufficiency. If corticosteroids, immunosuppressant agents, or antibiotic medications are prescribed, the nurse uses the opportunity to review the dosage, desired actions, and adverse effects of medications and the precautions to be taken.

Complications

Complications of acute GN include hypertensive encephalopathy, HF, and pulmonary edema. Hypertensive encephalopathy is a medical emergency, characterized by signs of cerebral edema that occur after a severe episode of HTN. Symptoms include headache, nausea, vomiting, followed by neurologic symptoms of restlessness, confusion, seizures, and potentially coma (Potter & Schaefer, 2021). Therapy is directed toward reducing the BP without impairing kidney function. If treated promptly, the symptoms of encephalopathy are usually reversed (Potter & Schaefer, 2021).

Rapidly progressive GN is characterized by a rapid decline in kidney function. Without treatment, kidney failure develops in a matter of weeks or months. Signs and symptoms are similar to those of acute GN (hematuria and proteinuria), but the course of the disease is more severe and rapid. Crescent-shaped cells accumulate in Bowman space (the filter within the glomerulus), disrupting the filtering process. Plasma exchange (plasmapheresis) and treatment with high-dose corticosteroids and cytotoxic agents have been used to reduce the inflammatory response. Dialysis is initiated in acute GN if signs and symptoms of uremia are severe. The prognosis for patients with acute GN is favorable, with most patients recovering.

CHRONIC GLOMERULONEPHRITIS

Pathophysiology

Chronic GN represents the chronic phase of varying nephritis (inflammation of the kidney), which can be related to immunologic, metabolic or hereditary disorders. Diabetes mellitus (DM) and HTN may be a major clinical manifestation. Diabetic nephropathy or glomerulosclerosis is the most common cause of kidney failure treated by renal replacement therapy (RRT) in the United States. As the sclerotic process progresses the nephron is destroyed and renal function declines. Microalbuminuria, defined as urinary albumin excretion of greater than 30 mg in 24 hour, develops (Van Leeuwen & Bladh, 2019). HTN and smoking have been implicated in progression of diabetic nephropathy. Hypertensive glomerular disease causes nephrosclerosis (chronic damage to blood vessels, glomeruli, and tubulointerstitium). The glomeruli and their tubules become inflamed, scarred and/or fibrotic, narrowing arteries and reducing blood flow to the kidneys.

Risk Factors

DM, uncontrolled HTN, hyperlipidemia, chronic tubulointerstitial injury, or hemodynamically mediated glomerular sclerosis place the patient at risk for chronic GN. Secondary glomerular diseases with systemic effects include SLE and Goodpasture syndrome (autoimmune diseases), among others. Renal involvement is seen in 40% to 80% of people with SLE and is more common in females than males (8:1 or 10:1 ratio of females to males) and three- to fourfold more prevalent in African American and American Indian females than in White females (Crow, 2020). The glomerular damage can progress to kidney failure.

Clinical Manifestations and Assessment

The symptoms of chronic GN vary with the underlying disorder and often appear after kidney damage has occurred. Patients, even with severe disease, can be asymptomatic for many years. Their condition may be discovered when HTN is discovered, elevated BUN and serum creatinine levels are detected, or during a routine eye examination when vascular changes or retinal hemorrhages are seen. Many patients report that their feet are slightly edematous at night. Most patients also have general symptoms, such as fatigue, loss of appetite, decreased strength, increasing irritability; headaches, dizziness, and digestive disturbances are common.

As chronic GN progresses, signs and symptoms of kidney failure may develop. The patient appears poorly nourished, with a yellow-gray pigmentation of the skin due to uremia. Periorbital and peripheral (dependent) edema with a normal or severely elevated BP may be noted. Mucous membranes are pale due to anemia. Cardiomegaly, a gallop rhythm (S3), distended neck veins, and other signs and symptoms of HF may be present. Crackles can be heard in the lungs.

Peripheral neuropathy with diminished deep tendon reflexes and neurosensory changes occur late in the disease. The patient becomes confused and demonstrates a limited attention span. An additional late finding includes evidence of pericarditis with or without a pericardial friction rub (see Chapter 15).

A number of laboratory abnormalities occur. Urinalysis reveals a fixed specific gravity of about 1.010, variable proteinuria, and **urinary casts**, which are proteins secreted by damaged kidney tubules. As kidney failure progresses and the GFR falls, the following changes occur:

- Hyperkalemia due to decreased potassium excretion, acidosis, catabolism, and excessive potassium intake from food and medications
- Metabolic acidosis from decreased acid secretion by the kidney and inability to regenerate and reabsorb bicarbonate
- Anemia secondary to decreased erythropoiesis (production of RBCs)
- Hypoalbuminemia with edema secondary to protein loss through the damaged glomerular membrane
- Increased serum phosphorus level due to its decreased renal excretion
- Decreased serum calcium level (calcium and phosphorus exist in an inverse ratio in the body) and decreased vitamin D activation
- Mental status changes due to buildup of nitrogenous wastes
- Impaired nerve conduction due to electrolyte abnormalities and uremia

Kidney biopsy is the gold standard for diagnosis of glomerular disease since it helps to determine the severity of the disease, as well as the underlying cause of the glomerular injury; the GFR indicates the degree of renal function (Kazi & Hashmi, 2021).

Pearls for Practice

Microalbuminuria refers to urinary albumin excretion greater than the normal rate of 30 mg/24 hours and may precede the development of nephropathy by 5 to 7 years (Van Leeuwen & Bladh, 2019). While dipsticks detect albumin excretion, they do not quantify it, therefore, a 24-hour urine collection for protein is performed (Norris & Tuan, 2020).

TABLE 26-1 **Common Fluid and Electrolyte Disturbances in Renal Disorders**

Disturbance	Manifestations	General Management Strategies
Fluid volume excess	Acute weight gain of at least 5%, edema, crackles, shortness of breath, decreased BUN, decreased Hct, distended neck veins	Fluid and sodium restriction, diuretics, dialysis
Sodium deficit (often dilutional)	Nausea, malaise, lethargy, headache, abdominal cramps, apprehension, seizures	Low-sodium diet, fluid restriction, normal saline or hypertonic saline solutions during dialysis
Sodium excess	Dry, sticky mucous membranes; thirst; rough dry tongue; fever; restlessness; weakness; disorientation	Fluids, diuretics, dietary restriction
Potassium excess	Diarrhea, colic, nausea, irritability, muscle weakness, electrocardiogram (ECG) changes (tall, tented T waves is usually the earliest sign on the ECG)	Dietary restriction, diuretics, IV glucose and insulin and sodium bicarbonate, cation exchange resin, calcium gluconate, dialysis
Calcium deficit	Abdominal and muscle cramps, stridor, hyperactive reflexes, tetany, positive Chvostek or Trousseau sign, tingling of fingers and around mouth, ECG changes	Diet, phosphate binders, oral or parenteral calcium salt replacement
Bicarbonate deficit	Headache, confusion, drowsiness, increased respiratory rate and depth, nausea and vomiting, warm flushed skin	Bicarbonate replacement (rare), dialysis
Protein deficit	Chronic weight loss, emotional depression, pallor, fatigue, soft flabby muscles	Diet, dietary supplements, total parenteral nutrition, albumin
Magnesium excess	Facial flushing, nausea and vomiting, sensation of warmth, drowsiness, depressed deep tendon reflexes, muscle weakness, respiratory depression, cardiac arrest	Calcium gluconate, IV normal saline with administration of furosemide, dialysis
Phosphorus excess	Tetany, tingling of fingers and around mouth, muscle spasms, soft tissue calcification	Diet restriction, phosphate binders

The signs and symptoms of common fluid and electrolyte disturbances that can occur in patients with renal disorders and their general management strategies are listed in Table 26-1.

Chest x-rays may show cardiac enlargement and pulmonary edema. The electrocardiogram (ECG) may be normal or may indicate left ventricular hypertrophy (LVH) associated with HTN. Signs of electrolyte disturbances, such as tall, tented T waves associated with hyperkalemia or dysrhythmia may appear (Norris & Tuan, 2020). Computed tomography (CT) and magnetic resonance imaging (MRI) scans reveal a decrease in the size of the renal cortex.

Medical and Nursing Management

Treatment is directed toward underlying condition, reversing the renal impairment and eliminating the underlying cause, where possible. Changes in fluid and electrolyte status and in cardiac and neurologic status are reported promptly to the PCP. Often anxiety levels are extremely high for both the patient and family. Throughout the course of the disease and treatment, the nurse gives emotional support by providing opportunities for the patient and family to verbalize their concerns, have their questions answered, and explore their options for treatment if the kidneys fail.

Instructions to the patient include explanations and scheduling for follow-up evaluations of BP, urinalysis for protein and casts, serum BUN and creatinine levels. If long-term dialysis is needed, the patient and family are taught about the procedure, how to care for the access site, dietary restrictions, and other necessary lifestyle modifications. These topics are discussed later in this chapter.

The nurse in the hospital and community setting educates the patient and reinforces the importance of notifying the health care provider for worsening signs and symptoms of kidney failure, including nausea, vomiting, and diminished urine output. Specific teaching includes explanations about recommended diet and fluid modifications and medications (purpose, desired effects, adverse effects, dosage, and administration schedule). The patient is instructed to inform all health care providers about the diagnosis of GN so that all medical management, including pharmacologic therapy, is based on altered kidney function.

Complications

The major complication of chronic GN is ESKD. GN is the second most common cause of kidney failure worldwide and ranks third most common disease-causing kidney failure in the United States after DM and HTN (Norris & Tuan, 2020).

NEPHROTIC SYNDROME

Nephrotic syndrome is not a specific glomerular disease, rather a cluster of clinical findings reflecting underlying damage to the glomerular capillary membrane. This results in increased permeability and loss of plasma proteins in the urine. Nephrotic syndrome can occur with diseases or medications that affect the kidney. Although frequently considered a disorder of childhood, nephrotic syndrome may occur in adults, often as a secondary disorder (Norris & Tuan, 2020).

Pathophysiology

Nephrotic syndrome results from damage to the glomerular capillary membrane, increasing capillary permeability, which allows protein to leak out into the urine (proteinuria). The patient presents with massive proteinuria, resulting in low serum albumin or hypoalbuminemia. A 24-hour urine sample (or urine protein/creatinine ratio) usually shows more than 3 to 3.5 g of proteinuria (Radhakrishnan & Appel, 2020). The nurse is aware that a serum albumin <2.5 g/dL is associated with edema (Fischbach et al., 2022). Hyperlipidemia and lipiduria occur, along with an increased cholesterol >300 mg/dL. Lipiduria is the presence of free lipid or lipid within tubular cells, within casts, or as free globules, suggesting a glomerular disorder (Tapia & Bashir, 2022). The hyperlipidemia likely occurs secondary to increased hepatic synthesis, which is stimulated by the low serum albumin (Baumgarten et al., 2022). Because of the decreased clearance of low-density lipoproteins (LDLs), hypertriglyceridemia occurs in over 50% of patients (Dirkx & Woodell, 2022). In addition, patients with nephrotic syndrome often have a hypercoagulable state and are therefore prone to develop deep venous thrombosis (DVT), pulmonary embolism (PE), or renal vein thrombosis; likely associated with hepatic overproduction of proteins in response to the low serum albumin. This leads to increased levels of procoagulants (promotion of blood clots), enhanced platelet aggregation, and loss of anticoagulants (such as antithrombin III) in the urine, thus increasing the risk of blood clots (Baumgarten et al., 2022).

Generalized edema, the hallmark of nephrotic syndrome, results from loss of colloidal osmotic pressure (COP) in the blood, causing fluid shifts and fluid accumulation in interstitial tissues. An increase in aldosterone and sympathetic nervous system activity with reduction in natriuretic factors increases the generalized edema. Salt and water retention furthers edema. Dyspnea related to pulmonary edema, pleural effusions and diaphragmatic compromise due to ascites may develop (Norris & Tuan, 2020). As globulins (type of protein), are lost in the urine, the patient becomes vulnerable to infection, particularly to staphylococci and pneumococci. In addition, protein-binding sites are decreased, potentially increasing the amount of free (active) drug available (Norris & Tuan, 2020, p. 880). Figure 26-2 depicts the pathophysiology of nephrotic syndrome.

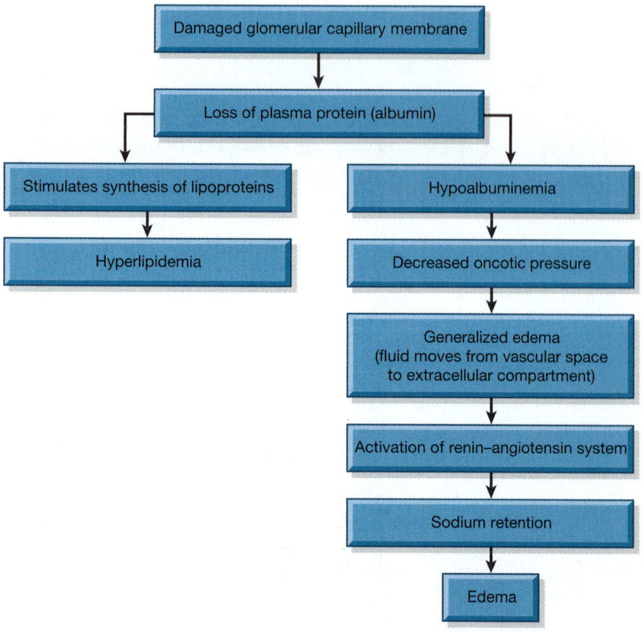

FIGURE 26-2 **Sequence of events in nephrotic syndrome.**

Pearls for Practice: Pathophysiology

Loss of protein causes a decrease in serum colloid osmotic pressure (COP); since there are "less particles to pull (or hold) water in the intravascular space," thus fluid stays in the tissues (edema). Therefore, edema is observable due to the expansion of the interstitial fluid volume; when it is massive and generalized, the excess fluid accumulation is called anasarca. Several clinical conditions such as HF, cirrhosis, and the nephrotic syndrome, as well as local conditions such as venous and lymphatic disease or malignant ascites are associated with the development of edema (Sterns, 2022). Refer to Chapter 11 for details on edema.

Risk Factors

Diabetic nephropathy is the most common cause of nephrotic syndrome, with approximately one third of patients with both type 1 and type 2 DM (who have the disease for 10 years), developing this problem (Sterns 2021, Sharma et al., 2020). Diabetic nephropathy refers to the pathologic structural and functional changes seen in the kidneys of patients with DM resulting from the effects of DM on the kidneys. However, control of blood sugar has been shown to improve albuminuria and halt the rapid decline in kidney function (Maarouf, 2022). Other glomerular diseases may be implicated including SLE, infections (HIV, hepatitis B, hepatitis C) glomerulosclerosis, cancers (leukemias, lymphoma), and nephrotoxicity (Gallo, 2021).

Clinical Manifestations and Assessment

Proteinuria, predominately in the form of albuminuria, where albumin excretion exceeds 3.5 g/day, is the hallmark of nephrotic syndrome (Norris & Tuan, 2020). Hypoalbuminuria with decreased colloid osmotic pressure in the blood is the result. This leads to edema, periorbital edema, scrotal swelling, abdominal distention, weight gain, or anasarca. Fatigue and anorexia may be reported, as well as shortness of breath, pulmonary edema, or HTN. The urine may contain increased white blood cells (WBCs) as well as granular and epithelial casts. The loss of urinary immunoglobulin places the patient at risk for infections. Hyperlipidemia with increased high-density lipoproteins (HDLs) and hypertriglyceridemia places the patient at risk for cardiovascular disease (CVD).

Drug Alert

Decreased serum albumin levels result in decreased protein-binding sites for medications. This allows more free (unbound) medication to circulate, compared to that which is protein bound. Patients with hypoalbuminemia must be observed closely for signs of drug toxicity related to a prolonged half-life (Lehne, 2019, p. 34; Norris & Tuan, 2020). Those medications requiring protein binding, may result in low drug levels (Norris & Tuan, 2020).

A percutaneous needle biopsy of the kidney may be performed for histologic examination of renal tissue to confirm the diagnosis. It involves inserting a needle through the flank to obtain a specimen of cortical and medullary kidney tissue. Before any biopsy is performed the nurse ensures that a complete blood count (CBC), coagulation studies (prothrombin time [PT], partial thromboplastin time [PTT]) and platelet count are evaluated since bleeding and hematoma formation are potential complications. In addition, particular attention is given to the current use of antiplatelet agents, aspirin, nonsteroidal anti-inflammatory drugs (NSAIDs), and anticoagulants, before the procedure.

Medical and Nursing Management

Patients with nephrotic syndrome need education about medication adherence and dietary regimens to promote long-term stability. Reduction in dietary cholesterol and saturated fats helps with lipidemia. Protein intake should be moderate, sufficient to meet protein needs while avoiding excessive intake, which may accelerate renal deterioration and increase urinary protein losses. Salt restriction is essential for managing edema; most patients also require diuretic therapy (Dirkx & Woodell, 2022).

Pearls for Practice

Patients with kidney disease should be evaluated by a renal nutritionist where specific recommendations regarding protein, salt, water, potassium, and phosphorus intake can be made to help prevent disease progression. In general, animal protein intake is reduced to 0.6 to 0.8 g/kg/day, however, significant protein restriction is not advisable in those with cachexia or those with low serum albumin as is seen in nephrotic syndrome (Dirkx & Woodell, 2022).

Due to decreased immunoglobulin, the patient is taught to report any signs of infection promptly, such as a respiratory tract infection, to prevent further glomerular damage. For example, an untreated streptococcal infection may be a risk factor for acute PSGN; pathogens in the bloodstream may lead to sepsis with resulting decreased renal perfusion. Diuretics may be prescribed for the patient with severe edema; however, caution must be used because of the risk of reducing the plasma volume to the point of impaired circulation with subsequent prerenal AKI (discussed later in the chapter). The use of angiotensin-converting enzyme (ACE) inhibitors or angiotensin receptor blocking (ARBs) agents, in combination with diuretics, often reduces the degree of proteinuria (Lehne, 2019). However, since combination therapy of an ACE and ARB increases the risk of AKI and hyperkalemia, the patient must be monitored closely (Dirkx & Woodell, 2022). Statin medications have been shown to improve endothelial function and decrease proteinuria (Lehne, 2019).

Other medications used to treat nephrotic syndrome include immunosuppressant medications and antineoplastic agents with prednisone frequently used as first-line therapy, either daily or on allternative days. Other immunosuppressive drugs, such as cyclophosphamide and mycophenolate mofetil may be used for frequent relapsers, steroid-dependent patients, or steroid-resistant patients (Clinical Overview, 2022). As these medications cause immunosuppression, patients should be taught to protect themselves from infection and to report any infections promptly. In addition, the risk for blood clots is considerable in patients with serum albumin less than 2 g/dL, thus anticoagulation therapy may be necessary if bleeding risk is low (Dirkx & Woodell, 2022).

Complications

Complications of nephrotic syndrome include infection secondary to loss of immunoglobulins, accelerated atherosclerosis secondary to hyperlipidemia, and a hypercoagulable state that may result in thromboembolism (Norris & Tuan, 2020). Body image may be altered due to anasarca and edema, causing a change in appearance.

Non-nephrotic proteinuria

Non-nephrotic proteinuria can be transient, orthostatic (related to sitting/standing or lying down), and persistent (Rovin, 2021). The most common cause of transient proteinuria is fever and heavy exercise, while the etiology of orthostatic proteinuria is unknown and occurs when one loses protein in the urine while in an upright position but not when lying down. In transient and orthostatic proteinuria no treatment is required. Persistent proteinuria occurs in people with underlying kidney disease or other medical conditions such as HTN, DM, or disorders that overproduce protein. Underlying conditions are treated. When persistent low-grade proteinuria is not associated with kidney function or a systemic disease typically no long-term complications are seen, even if untreated (Rovin, 2021). The use an antihypertensive drug, such as an angiotensin-converting enzyme inhibitor (ACEI), may be considered to reduce or eliminate proteinuria. The patient is followed up annually to assess kidney function.

KIDNEY FAILURE

Kidney failure results when the kidneys cannot remove the body's metabolic wastes or perform their regulatory functions. This process may be acute, developing over hours to days, or chronic, developing over months to years. Kidney failure results in azotemia, metabolic derangements, acid–base disturbances, and electrolyte imbalances. Kidney failure is a systemic disease and is a final common pathway of many different kidney and urinary tract diseases.

ACUTE KIDNEY INJURY

Acute kidney injury (AKI), describes a range of acute-onset kidney disorders that can include mild impairment of kidney function progressing to acute kidney failure that requires RRT or dialysis (Lough, 2022). AKI is marked by an abrupt loss of kidney function (sudden increase of serum creatinine of 0.3 mg/dL within 48 hours or 1.5 times baseline serum creatinine over 1 week), decrease in GFR, and abrupt decline in urine output (<0.5 mL/kg/hr for 6 to 12 hours) that can occur over hours or days (Ferri, 2022). AKI occurs in 20% of hospitalized patients and 60% of intensive care unit (ICU) patients. The most common etiologies for AKI are septic shock with positive blood cultures (50%), hypovolemia (34%), drug or medication related (14%), cardiogenic shock (13%), and >40% of hospital-associated AKI is iatrogenic (caused by medical or surgical treatment) (Ferri, 2022; Lough, 2022). The mortality rate in AKI is nearly 25% and approaches 50% to 60% in those that require RRT (Ferri, 2022).

Pearls for Practice

The term acute kidney injury (AKI) has largely replaced the older terminology of acute kidney failure (American Kidney Foundation [AKF]).

Pathophysiology

Although the exact pathogenesis of AKI is not always known, this condition may be reversible if identified and treated before kidney function is impaired permanently. AKI is classified by its etiology, which focuses treatment for the underlying cause.

Classification of Acute Kidney Injury

The major classifications of AKI are prerenal azotemia (problem occurring before the kidneys) caused by hypoperfusion of the kidney; intrarenal (problem occurring within the kidney), in which the renal parenchyma or nephron is damaged; and postrenal (problem occurring after the kidney), in which outflow of urine is obstructed.

Prerenal AKI is caused by reduced blood flow, BP, or perfusion to the kidney with a resulting decrease in the GFR and urine output. A wide variety of factors are associated with a decrease of arterial blood reaching the renal artery (which supplies the kidney) and can include thrombosis (clot), hemorrhage, vasodilation, to low cardiac output states. Therefore, nurses monitor the urinary output hourly and notify the provider when the urine output is <30 mL/hr or <0.5 mL/kg/hr. Common causes of each type of AKI are summarized in Box 26-3.

The nurse monitors the mean arterial pressure (MAP), which is calculated as follows: systolic pressure + (diastolic pressure × 2)/3. A normal MAP is between 70 and 105 mm Hg and the nurse is aware that a MAP of <65 for an extended period can result in end-organ ischemia (deficient supply of blood) and infarction (death of tissues), and that a MAP of >60 mm Hg is necessary to perfuse the coronary arteries; thus, the provider is notified if the MAP is <65 mm Hg. In addition, for patients with a history of HTN and/or renal vascular diseases, higher pressures may be required to maintain renal perfusion. Monitoring and reporting of MAP is a vital nursing action to prevent prerenal AKI.

Pearls for Practice: Pathophysiology

The heart can impact the kidneys and likewise the kidneys can impact the heart. This is the story of cardiorenal syndrome of which there are five types. In type 1, an acute cardiac dysfunction such as cardiogenic shock leads to decreased kidney function. Because of a low cardiac output state, renal vein congestion, or both, the kidney perfusion pressure is affected, and normal compensatory mechanisms are insufficient to maintain blood flow to the kidney. Thus, any acute worsening of cardiac function can lead to renal hypoperfusion. In type 2, it is a chronic cardiac impairment such as HF that leads to the renal impairment; 45% to 65% of patients with HF with reduced ejection fraction (EF) will develop kidney disease (Griffin et al., 2020). In type 3, the acute worsening of kidney function as in AKI causes cardiac decompensation typically related to FVE and metabolic derangements. In type 4, chronic kidney disease leads to heart failure from CKD-associated cardiomyopathy and in type 5, a systemic condition (such as sepsis or DM) causes simultaneous dysfunction of the heart and kidney. Regardless of the type of cardiorenal syndrome, acute or chronic and which came first, it is important to recognize the heart–kidney bond.

BOX 26-3

Causes of Acute Kidney Injury

Prerenal Failure (50–60% of AKI)

- Volume depletion resulting from:
  - Hemorrhage (trauma, surgery, postpartum, GI bleeding)
  - Renal losses (diuretics, osmotic diuresis, diabetes insipidus)
  - GI losses (vomiting, diarrhea, nasogastric suction)
  - Cirrhosis (fluid third-spacing)
  - Skin and mucous membrane losses: burns, hyperthermia, dehydration
  - Excess fluid loss from wounds and drains
- Impaired cardiac efficiency with decreased cardiac output resulting from:
  - Myocardial infarction
  - Heart failure
  - Dysrhythmias
  - Cardiogenic shock
- Vasodilation resulting from:
  - Sepsis
  - Anaphylaxis
  - Antihypertensive medications or other medications that cause vasodilation

Intrarenal Failure (25–40%)

- Prolonged renal ischemia resulting from:
  - Pigment nephropathy (associated with the breakdown of blood cells containing pigments that occlude kidney structures)
  - Myoglobinuria (trauma, crush injuries, burns)
  - Hemoglobinuria (transfusion reaction, hemolytic anemia)
  - Rhabdomyolysis
- Nephrotoxic agents such as:
  - Aminoglycoside antibiotics (gentamicin, tobramycin)
  - Antirejection medications (cyclosporine, tacrolimus)
  - Radiopaque contrast agents
  - Heavy metals (lead, mercury)
  - Solvents and chemicals (ethylene glycol, carbon tetrachloride, arsenic)
  - NSAIDs
  - ACE inhibitors
- Infectious processes such as:
  - Acute pyelonephritis
  - Acute glomerulonephritis

Postrenal Failure (5–10%)

- Urinary tract obstruction, including:
  - Calculi (stones)
  - Tumors
  - Benign prostatic hyperplasia (BPH)
  - Strictures
  - Blood clots

Intrarenal or intrinsic AKI is the result of actual parenchymal damage to the glomeruli or kidney tubules. An ischemic insult is the most common cause of intrarenal AKI where the poor perfusion pathologically affects the internal filtering structure of the kidney. In fact, ischemia of the kidney due to decreased renal perfusion, accounts for more than 50% of cases of intrarenal AKI. It can be considered an advanced stage of prerenal AKI (Lough, 2022). Previously this insult was termed acute tubular necrosis (ATN) owing to the death of tissues associated with poor perfusion, however the newer term of AKI is now used (Lough, 2022). In the early period of renal ischemia, kidney function can be restored completely by improving renal blood flow, typically with IV fluids. If left untreated or when fluid resuscitation is inadequate, AKI will ensue and may become irreversible (Norris & Tuan, 2020).

Other conditions associated with intrarenal AKI include nephrotoxic agents, such as aminoglycosides and radiocontrast dye through direct damage to the nephron. Burns, crush injuries, infections, and severe blood transfusion reactions can lead to rhabdomyolysis (breakdown of skeletal muscles) with **myoglobinuria**. With burns and crush injuries, myoglobin (a protein released from muscle when injury occurs) and hemoglobin are liberated, causing obstruction of renal tubules, renal toxicity, and ischemia (see Box 41-7). Severe transfusion reactions may also cause intrarenal failure; hemoglobin released through hemolysis filters through the glomeruli and becomes concentrated in the kidney tubules to such a degree that precipitation of hemoglobin occurs. Certain medications, especially NSAIDs and ACEIs or ARBs, also may predispose a patient to intrarenal damage. These medications interfere with the normal autoregulatory mechanisms of the kidney and may cause hypoperfusion and eventual ischemia. Infection is also associated with intrarenal AKI as in acute GN and interstitial nephritis (Lough, 2022).

Pearls for Practice

Contrast-induced nephropathy (CIN) is the third most common cause of hospital-acquired AKI, usually occurring within 2 to 3 days, however, can be seen 1 to 3 weeks postexposure. The incidence of CIN-AKI ranges from 6% to 27% and thus the nurse should monitor urinary output and serum creatinine post procedure (Efe et al., 2021). Risk factors for CIN-AKI include pre-existing impaired renal function, diabetes, left ventricular dysfunction, and anemia (Efe et al., 2021; Norris & Tuan, 2020).

Pearls for Practice

Isotonic hydration, such as with normal saline (0.9% NACL), is recommended before, during, and after contrast dye exposure in at-risk individuals. The use of N-acetylcysteine, orally or intravenously and *bicarbonate to prevent CIN have not demonstrated consistent benefit, rather it is suggested that the smallest amount of contrast agent be used, and that repetitive, closely spaced studies are avoided (e.g., <48 hours apart) (Rudnick, 2022).*

Drug Alert

Metformin may cause lactic acidosis, especially those with renal insufficiency, liver disease, or severe infection. Teach patients to report early signs of lactic acidosis, including hyperventilation, somnolence, and myalgia to the health care provider (Lehne, 2019, p. 695).

Pearls for Practice

Low-dose dopamine (0.5 to 3 mcg/kg/min), previously known as renal-dose dopamine, has been commonly administered to increase renal blood flow in an effort to prevent AKI (Sterns, 2022). At higher concentrations (above 5 mcg/kg/min), however dopamine induces renal vasoconstriction which would negatively impact renal perfusion. Although dopamine is effective in increasing urine output in the short-term, it is theorized that tolerance of the dopamine renal receptors occurs in critically ill patients that are most at risk for AKI (Lough, 2020). Low-dose dopamine does not prevent onset of AKI, decrease the need for dialysis, or reduce mortality (Lough, 2020). Thus, the support for routine use of low-dose dopamine for the prevention of AKI remains anecdotal only. That is not to say that therapeutic uses for low-dose dopamine infusions do not exist; it is used frequently in patients with HF in combination with furosemide (Lough, 2022).

Postrenal AKI is the result of a mechanical or functional obstruction resulting in decreased urinary flow and accounts for approximately 5% of AKI cases (Kallenbach, 2022). With an obstruction to urine flow, pressure rises in the kidney tubules and hydronephrosis occurs, compressing normal renal tissue resulting in a decrease in the GFR. Mechanical causes of obstruction are seen with tumors, stones, prostatic hypertrophy, and urethral strictures. While functional causes include diabetic nephropathy, medications such as ganglionic blocking agents that block the autonomic nerve supply to the urinary system, and neurogenic bladder related to spinal cord injury or cerebrovascular accident (Kallenbach, 2022; Norris & Tuan, 2020). Commonly, the postrenal AKI is associated with renal/ureteral calculi, tumors, blood clots, benign prostatic hyperplasia (BPH), or any urethral obstruction (Goyal et al., 2022). Any sudden or complete cessation of urine output with an indwelling catheter should alert the nurse to possible mechanical obstruction. The catheter should be inspected and kinks removed or the catheter irrigated or changed to reestablish urine flow. Renal ultrasonography is the gold standard for diagnosis.

Pearls for Practice

Any abrupt development of anuria should prompt the nurse to verify that the urinary catheter is not occluded (Lough, 2022).

Phases of AKI

There are four clinical phases of AKI: initiation or onset, oliguric, diuretic, and recovery. The onset phase begins with the triggering event and ends when cellular injury and oliguria develop. Common events include significant fluid or blood loss, burns, or diabetes insipidus (Norris & Tuan, 2020, p. 893). A small number of patients develop nonoliguric renal failure, usually associated with nephrotoxic agents; it may also occur with traumatic injury, and the use of halogenated anesthetic agents.

The oliguric period is accompanied by fluid overload and an increase in the serum concentration of wastes, such as urea, creatinine, organic acids, and the electrolytes potassium, phosphorous, and magnesium. The average time period for oliguria is 8 to 14 days, but it may last longer (Norris & Tuan, 2020). Patients should be monitored for fluid volume overload symptoms such as jugular vein distention, crackles, edema, weight gain, and HTN. RRT, such as dialysis, may be needed until kidney function returns.

Pearls for Practice

The nurse is aware that a minimum of 400 mL of fluid or more must be excreted as urine each day to prevent the accumulation of metabolic wastes.

The diuretic phase occurs when the cause of AKI is corrected. This phase is marked by a gradual increase in urine output, which signals that glomerular filtration has started to recover. Urine output may be normal, or the patient may excrete large amounts of dilute urine along with electrolytes. The patient should be observed closely for fluid volume deficit (flat neck veins, delayed skin turgor, weight loss), which may damage the kidney further, as well as for hypokalemia. Abnormal laboratory values plateau and begin to decline.

The recovery period is signaled by the improvement of kidney function and energy level and may take 3 to 6 months. Return to a normal GFR, if it occurs, may take up to 1 year (Kallenbach, 2022). In some instances, residual renal impairment may result (Norris & Tuan, 2020).

Clinical Manifestations and Assessment

Manifestations of AKI include oliguria or anuria with resulting azotemia (increased BUN, and other nitrogenous waste products, and serum creatinine). Acidemia, fluid volume excess, alterations in calcium and phosphorus balance and BP alterations develop rapidly. Erythropoiesis fails with resulting anemia. Almost every system of the body is affected when there is failure of the renal regulatory mechanisms. The patient may appear critically ill and lethargic.

TABLE **26-2 Comparing Clinical Findings among Categories of Acute Kidney Injury**

	Categories		
Characteristics	**Prerenal**	**Intrarenal**	**Postrenal**
Etiology	Hypoperfusion	Parenchymal damage	Obstruction
Blood urea nitrogen value	Increased proportion (greater than 20:1) blood urea nitrogen (BUN) to creatinine	Increased	Increased
Creatinine	Normal or slightly increased	Increased	Increased
Urine output	Decreased	Varies, often decreased	Varies, may be decreased, or sudden anuria
Urine sodium	Typically decreased	Typically increased	Varies
Urinary sediment	Normal, few hyaline casts	Abnormal casts and debris	Usually normal
Urine osmolality	Increased to 500 mOsm	Approximately 350 mOsm, similar to serum	Varies, increased or equal to serum
Urine specific gravity	Increased	Low normal	Varies

Nausea, vomiting, lethargy, headache, muscle twitching, and seizures may occur. Table 26-2 summarizes common clinical findings in all three categories of AKI.

Assessment of the patient with AKI includes evaluation for changes in the urine output, diagnostic tests that evaluate the kidney contour and function, and a variety of laboratory values. See Chapter 25 for information about the normal characteristics of urine, diagnostic findings, and laboratory values in the renal system.

In AKI, oliguria (0.5 mL/kg for >6 hours or less than 400 mL a day) is typically present. Hematuria may be present, and the urine has a low specific gravity (1.010) due to the kidney's inability to concentrate the urine. Differences in urinalysis may be seen depending on whether the AKI is due to prerenal, intrarenal, or postrenal causes. For example, urine in prerenal failure is concentrated, with low sodium, whereas in intrarenal failure due to the nephrons inability to concentrate urine or conserve sodium, casts are seen (evidence of kidney damage). In postrenal failure urine tests will vary depending on the fluid volume status of the patient. Since urine electrolytes are not predictive of outcome in AKI, they are rarely measured (Lough, 2022).

Pearls for Practice

The nurse is aware that the results of urine laboratory tests are valid only in the absence of diuretics.

The BUN level increases steadily at a rate dependent on the degree of protein catabolism, renal perfusion, and fluid or protein intake. Serum creatinine, a more sensitive indicator of kidney function than BUN, increases with glomerular damage and is used to monitor kidney function and disease progression.

Pearls for Practice

The nurse is aware that that BUN is influenced by changes in protein intake, bleeding in the GI tract, cell catabolism, and fluid administration and therefore is unreliable as the sole indicator of kidney injury.

Patients with oliguria (<400 mL/day) and **anuria** (<50 to 100 mL/day) are at high risk for hyperkalemia, a potassium level of more than 5.1 mEq/L (5.1 mmol/L). Hyperkalemia develops as the damaged kidney cannot excrete potassium; protein catabolism and acidosis result in the release of intracellular potassium into the serum, worsening hyperkalemia. The ECG may reveal changes, including tall, tented, or peaked T waves, followed by prolonged PR interval, absent P wave, widened QRS, or bradyarrhythmia. Additional symptoms of hyperkalemia may include weakness, diarrhea, and cardiac arrest. The nurse should be aware of exogenous sources of potassium, such as IV infusions, medications, as well as dietary sources (spinach [green leafy vegetables], potatoes, avocados, pumpkin, spinach, baked potatoes, sweet potatoes, tomatoes, yams, apricots, bananas, nectarines, orange juice, prunes [Kantor, 2019]). Additional contributors to the dietary potassium load include the use of low-sodium products (such as salt substitutes or low-sodium canned soups which have added potassium chloride in place of sodium chloride) (de Waal, 2022).

As metabolic acidosis develops, normal renal buffering mechanisms fail, resulting in hyperventilation. The patient may breathe more rapidly and deeply to "blow off" CO_2 to restore normal serum pH. Hyperventilation as compensation for acidosis may lead to respiratory fatigue or failure, requiring mechanical ventilation.

Serum phosphate levels increase. Calcium levels may decrease in response to decreased absorption of calcium from the intestine as well as a compensatory mechanism for the elevated blood phosphate levels. Anemia is another common laboratory finding in AKI, because of reduced erythropoietin production, reduced RBC lifespan, and blood loss, usually from the GI tract.

Pearls for Practice

Urine output should measure at least 0. 5 mL/kg/hr. Urine output directly reflects GFR in the kidney and, therefore, is a sensitive and early biomarker of AKI (Lough, 2022).

Prevention

Prevention of AKI is essential as mortality rates are as high as 50% or more, especially in patients where multisystem failure is observed (Box 26-4).

The nurse assesses for use of potentially nephrotoxic agents and exposure to environmental toxins. Patients taking nephrotoxic medications, such as aminoglycosides (gentamicin, tobramycin, neomycin), amphotericin B, vancomycin, cyclosporine, certain antineoplastics (Lehne, 2019) or anesthetics, heavy metals such as cisplatin or bismuth, or radiologic contrast agents, should be monitored closely for changes in kidney function. BUN and serum creatinine levels should be obtained at baseline, during treatment, and after therapy is complete, if indicated.

Chronic use of analgesics, particularly NSAIDs, may cause **interstitial nephritis** (inflammation within the renal tissue) and papillary necrosis. Patients with HF or cirrhosis with ascites are at particular risk for NSAID-induced AKI. Increased age, pre-existing kidney disease, and the coadministration of nephrotoxic agents increase the risk for kidney damage.

The nurse identifies those at risk for AKI prior to procedures where contrast media is used (BUN and serum creatinine should be assessed before contrast dye is administered). Patients with GFR <60 mL/min or those with DM should receive preprocedure hydration with isotonic fluids at 3 mL/kg/hr for 1 hour prior to contrast exposure (Rudnick, 2022) and receive as low a dose of contrast as possible for the study. The nurse should withhold metformin, an oral antihyperglycemic medication for patients with non–insulin-dependent diabetes mellitus (NIDDM), prior to procedures requiring IV contrast. Lactic acidosis is a rare side effect of metformin; while not nephrotoxic, the acidosis associated with a complication of kidney failure may worsen when metformin is given and is associated with a 50% mortality rate (Shin, 2021). In general, the medication is withheld for the 48 hours after the vascular procedure and resumed only after renal function has been reassessed.

Biomarkers of kidney injury have been explored for earlier diagnosis of AKI or to separate intrinsic from prerenal causes of AKI, however at the present time the clinical role of biomarkers remains undefined (Udulman, 2022).

BOX 26-4 Health Promotion

Preventing Acute Kidney Injury

- Provide adequate hydration to patients at risk of fluid volume deficit:
  - Perioperative patients
  - Patients on fluid restriction
  - Patients undergoing diagnostic studies with contrast agents (e.g., barium enema, intravenous pyelograms, angiography), especially older patients who may have marginal renal reserve
  - Patients with neoplastic disorders and those receiving chemotherapy
  - Patients with metabolic disorders, such as gout, glycosuria
- Prevent and treat hypotension or shock promptly with fluid and/or blood replacement
- Monitor hourly urine output of patients who are critically ill to promptly detect the onset of oliguria indicating kidney failure. When available, monitor central venous and arterial pressures
- Continually assess renal laboratory values
- Properly identify patients to prevent transfusion reactions, which can precipitate myoglobinuria
- Prevent and treat infections promptly. Infections can lead to sepsis and renal damage
- Intervene promptly with wounds, burns, and other precursors of sepsis
- To prevent infections from ascending in the urinary tract, give meticulous care to patients with indwelling catheters. Remove catheters as soon as possible
- To prevent toxic drug effects, closely monitor dosage, duration of use, and blood levels of all medications metabolized or excreted by the kidneys

Medical and Nursing Management

The kidneys have a remarkable ability to recover from insult. Management includes maintaining fluid and electrolyte balance, avoiding fluid excess, supporting the patient until repair of renal tissue and restoration of function occur.

The underlying cause is identified, treated, and eliminated when possible. If the cause of AKI is related to prerenal factors, then treatment consists of optimizing renal perfusion by repletion of intravascular volume with fluids or treating decreased cardiac output (keeping the MAP above 65 mm Hg). Adequate blood flow to the kidneys in patients with prerenal causes of AKI may be restored by IV fluids or transfusions of blood products. If AKI is caused by hypovolemia secondary to hypoproteinemia, an infusion of albumin may be prescribed. Intrarenal azotemia is treated with supportive therapy, removal of causative agents, and aggressive fluid resuscitation in cases of shock, infection, and rhabdomyolysis. When intrarenal AKI is caused by GN or vasculitis, immunosuppressive therapy is frequently required (Molitoris, 2020). Early dialysis (on a temporary measure) may be required to control rapidly developing complications, such as fluid volume excess (HTN, HF, pericarditis, and pulmonary edema), metabolic acidosis, or hyperkalemia, regardless of BUN or creatinine levels. Also, dialysis may be started prophylactically when BUN reaches 100 mg/dL even if the patient has few or no symptoms (Kallenbach, 2021). However, the best time to start RRT remains controversial (Ronco et al., 2019). While this is expected to be a temporary intervention, a small portion some patients do not recover kidney function and may develop ESKD requiring permanent dialysis (12% to 15% of patients) or kidney transplant (Goyal et al., 2021). Although it is difficult to predict risk for CRF, an older age, higher creatinine level, comorbidities such as HTN, DM, HF, long-term hypotension, ATN, GN, and vasculitic causes of AKI may not fully recover to their baseline renal function (Molitoris, 2020).

Treatment of postrenal failure is aimed at restoring normal outflow of urine by relieving the obstruction. Surgery, such as prostatectomy, percutaneous nephrostomy tubes, stents or indwelling catheters, may be used.

The nurse observes for fluid excess manifested by dyspnea, crackles, tachycardia, HTN, and distended neck veins, as well as generalized edema in the presacral and pretibial areas and any dependent region of the body. The central venous pressure (CVP), when measured, will be elevated (normal CVP is 2 to 8 mm Hg). Fluid and sodium should be restricted in patients with FVE and oliguria or anuria to prevent fluid overload and pulmonary edema. The nurse observes for signs and symptoms of pericarditis (chest pain that increases when lying down or fever and pericardial friction rub) or pericardial effusion (feeling of pressure in the chest, engorged neck veins, distant [muffled] heart sounds, equalizing pressure in heart chambers, pulsus paradoxus), which generally is associated with the need to initiate dialysis. Emergency pericardiocentesis may be required (refer to Chapter 14).

Diuretics, such as furosemide (Lasix), may be prescribed **in the early stages of AKI** to initiate diuresis and maintain renal perfusion when intravascular volume deficits have been corrected, however is of little value once AKI is advanced and established. Careful attention to I&O is required as well as cautious estimates of insensible loss (refer to Chapter 3).

Pearls for Practice

The nurse understands that fluid replacement is essential to prevent progress of AKI secondary to prerenal causes. The aim of fluid administration is to correct the hypovolemia without causing fluid overload and associated complications, including the progression of AKI (Pickkers et al., 2021). However, once the patient presents with fluid volume excess, fluid requirements are calculated on the basis of daily urine volumes and insensible losses. Daily weights and strict intake and output records are essential. Patients with kidney failure are typically restricted to 1 L of fluid per 24 hours if the urine output is 500 mL or less (Lough, 2022).

Hyperkalemia with ECG changes can be treated temporarily with IV insulin, given with glucose to prevent hypoglycemia, to temporarily shift potassium back into the cells. Calcium may be administered to treat the cardiotoxicity that has developed secondary to hyperkalemia since it directly antagonizes the membrane effects of hyperkalemia. It is important to understand that hyperkalemia is the most common metabolic cause of death in patients with AKI (Norris & Tuan, 2020). If these measures are ineffective, RRT is indicated.

Additional measures for hyperkalemia may include administering cation exchange resins (either sodium [sodium polystyrene sulfonate] or calcium [calcium polystyrene sulfonate]) orally, via NG tube, or by retention enema (Lehne, 2019). However, the onset of action is 60 minutes when given rectally and 120 minutes after oral administration (Baxter, 2020). They work by exchanging the cation for potassium across the gastrointestinal wall. For example, sodium polystyrene sulfonate works by exchanging sodium ions for potassium ions in the intestinal tract. Typically, sorbitol is combined with the resin to draw water into the bowel, inducing diarrhea and excretion of potassium contained in the lower gastrointestinal tract. The patient should retain the enema for 30 to 45 minutes. In nonemergency situations, other options to lower serum potassium include aerosolized beta-2 agonists (albuterol) and IV loop diuretics (if the patient is making urine).

High anion-gap acidosis may require sodium bicarbonate therapy—if the arterial pH is less than 7.1 or dialysis. However, hemodialysis may be required because of the sodium in the bicarbonate treatment, increases the risk of fluid volume excess.

In addition, in AKI, the serum phosphorus level rises, and the serum calcium level falls, thus phosphate-binding agents (second and third generations) are given to decrease the absorption of phosphate from the intestinal tract. In the past, aluminum hydroxide gel (short term only) was used short term because of its ability to bind phosphorus effectively in the gastrointestinal tract, however because of the risk of aluminum toxicity it has fallen out of favor. Second-generation dietary phosphorus–binding agents use calcium to bind dietary phosphorus in the gastrointestinal tract which although safer requires monitoring for elevated serum calcium levels and calcium deposits in other areas of the body (Lough, 2022). Third-generation binding medications are non–aluminum-based and non–calcium-based (sevelamer hydrochloride and lanthanum carbonate) have a better safety profile and are frequently prescribed to lower serum phosphorus levels in patients with CKD.

Dialysis may also be used for patients that are intolerant of oral medications or have severe hyperphosphatemia classified as >9 mg/dL (normal ranges vary but in general are 2.5 to 4.5 mg/dL), and symptoms of hypocalcemia (numbness and tingling of the fingers and circumoral region, hyperactive reflexes, and muscle cramps, positive Trousseau or Chvostek sign) (Toffaletti & Rackley, 2022).

Because kidney failure alters the metabolism and action of many drugs, often in ways that are not predictable, medications that are excreted via the kidney require dosage adjustment to prevent toxicity. Commonly used agents requiring adjustment are antibiotics, especially aminoglycosides, digoxin, ACEIs, and magnesium-containing agents.

Pearls for Practice

The nurse is aware that the priority in patients with suspected AKI, is to stop all nephrotoxic medications. In addition, any medications that is cleared or eliminated through the kidneys must have the dose and/or frequency of administration decreased. Pharmacists are consulted and serum medication levels may be monitored.

Nutritional Therapy

Nutritional care for AKI is like that of CKD. AKI causes increased tissue catabolism, impaired glucose use, and synthesis of protein. Azotemia may cause nausea and vomiting. Weight loss may result from negative nitrogen balance. Sufficient calories are given to prevent protein catabolism. Beginning RRT rather than protein restriction should be considered. It RRT is initiated, folate and pyridoxine is supplemented, as they are lost through hemodialysis (Marini & Dries, 2019), and caloric requirements are met with high-carbohydrate meals due to their protein-sparing effect. Dietary restrictions include foods and fluids containing potassium, such as bananas, potatoes, citrus, tomatoes, or melons. Sodium, especially processed food, is avoided. Foods containing phosphorus, including dairy products, chocolate, beans, nuts, legumes, organ meats, and shrimp and dark sodas, are restricted as well. Caffeine also is restricted. The patient may require enteral or parenteral nutrition.

Pearls for Practice

Patients with AKI should receive a diet low in sodium, potassium, phosphorus, which can be liberalized as the patient's renal function improves (Lough, 2022).

Fluid Therapy

Once AKI is established, fluid restriction is indicated to prevent circulatory overload. The fluid requirements are based on 24-hour urine output and insensible losses (perspiration, stool, and water vapor from the lungs—1,000 mL/day) (see Chapter 3). The nurse records daily weights and strict I&O. The nurse suspects fluid retention if the patient develops JVD, SOB, crackles, HTN, edema, or weight gain. Volume overload may be treated with loop diuretics; however if there no response due to progression of AKI, RRT is indicated using hemodialysis or peritoneal dialysis (PD).

In the case of volume depletion as occurs in the diuretic phase of AKI, the nurse anticipates administering fluids (PO or IV) which may require replacing both sensible and insensible loss. As AKI resolves, results of blood chemistry tests are used to determine the amounts of sodium, potassium, and water needed for replacement. The patient is encouraged to resume activities gradually.

Pearls for Practice

If the caloric intake is insufficient to prevent the breakdown of body protein, accumulation of additional nitrogenous waste develops, which may increase uremic symptoms.

Reducing Metabolic Rate

Bed rest may be indicated to reduce exertion and the metabolic rate during the most acute stage of the disorder. Fever and infection, both of which increase the metabolic rate and catabolism, are prevented or treated promptly.

Pearls for Practice

Fever increases insensible water loss by increasing water vapor in the lungs and allowing more water to be lost from the respiratory mucosa (Norris & Tuan, 2020).

Promoting Pulmonary Function

Attention is given to pulmonary function, and the patient is assisted to turn, cough, and deep breathe frequently to prevent atelectasis and respiratory tract infection. Drowsiness and lethargy may prevent the patient from moving and turning without encouragement and assistance. Maintaining a patent airway through oral or endotracheal suction may be necessary.

Preventing Infection

Infection is one of the leading causes of death in patients with AKI related to immune suppression, which predisposes patients to sepsis. Uremia impairs host defenses, particularly leukocyte function, thus strict asepsis is essential with invasive lines and catheters to minimize the risk of infection and subsequent increased metabolism. Any fever, elevated WBC count, erythema (redness) at wound and/or IV catheter sites warrants an assessment and notification of the provider. Of particular concern is the risk of catheter-associated urinary tract infection (CAUTI). Initially, when accurate urine measurements are essential, an indwelling urinary catheter (Foley) may be inserted. The nurse recognizes that an indwelling catheter is a source of infection, thus when the patient is hemodynamically stable, the catheter should be removed as soon as possible. If the patient cannot void urine spontaneously, alternatives to avoid catheter reinsertion include the use of a bladder scanner to estimate quantity of urine in the bladder. Intermittent urinary catheterization (called a *straight catheter*) involves the insertion of a small catheter into the bladder using sterile technique and it is immediately removed after the bladder is emptied. External urine collection options exist for a patient that can void, thus avoiding insertion or reinsertion of a urinary catheter. They include the condom catheter for male patients and an external female collection system that wicks away voided urine via an external tube connected to wall suction for females (Lough, 2022).

Providing Skin Care

The skin may be dry or susceptible to breakdown as a result of edema; therefore, meticulous skin care is important. In addition, excoriation and itching of the skin may result from the deposit of uremic toxins in the patient's tissues. Turning the patient frequently, bathing the patient with cool water, and keeping the patient's skin clean and well moisturized and the fingernails trimmed to avoid excoriation are comforting and prevent skin breakdown.

Pearls for Practice

The nurse recognizes that edematous tissue is fragile and must assess any edematous area for evidence of erythema to prevent skin breakdown.

Providing Support

While AKI is considered potentially reversible, there is variability in the length of time that the patient is ill and the duration of treatment. The patient and family need assistance, explanation, and support during this period. The nurse provides frequent explanations of the purpose and rationale of the treatments, as rising BUN leads to confusion and lethargy. Both the patient and family are included in teaching to allay anxiety and fear. Consistent with the goal of Healthy People 2030, which includes reducing the incidence of kidney disease, and increasing the number of Medicare patients hospitalized with AKI who receive a renal evaluation within 3 months of discharge, the nurse explains the importance of follow-up with a nephrologist (Office of Disease Prevention and Health Promotion [ODPHP], 2021). In addition, the nurse keeps family members informed about the patient's condition, helps them understand the treatments, and provides psychological support. AKI is a serious problem, and the nurse must continue to provide interventions for the underlying disorder (burns, shock, trauma, obstruction of the urinary tract, etc.).

Gerontologic Considerations

The prevalence of kidney dysfunction in Americans older than 65 years of age is 38% (Centers for Disease Control and Prevention [CDC], 2021a). Its prevalence is high in hospitalized populations, especially in ICUs. Despite all the technical and therapeutic advances that have occurred in the last few decades, the overall mortality of AKI patients remains high, reaching 50% in ICU patients. Several conditions predispose a patient to progress with AKI, including age, sepsis, surgeries, and comorbidities, such as HTN, DM, heart disease, neoplasm, and CKD. Several common comorbidities may make older individuals prone to AKI. Among them, the presence of HT, DM, congenital heart disease, and HF standout, according to most studies. Risk factors for progression of AKI to CKD, include age, pre-existing CKD, hypoalbuminemia, and other chronic diseases like arterial hypertension, heart failure, obesity and diabetes mellitus (DM).

The incidence and mortality of AKI is increased in hospitalized older adults due to a decrease in the number of functional nephrons and renal blood flow as well as to atherosclerosis of the renal arteries. The older individual is particularly susceptible to AKI due to limited renal reserve to counteract insults to their kidney function, such as occurs with sepsis and dehydration. Diuretics and chronic NSAID use increase the risk of AKI threefold, as do ACE inhibitors (Norris & Tuan, 2020). The older patient with systemic infection accompanied by vomiting or diarrhea should be kept hydrated, and NSAIDs are avoided, and diuretics, ACEIs or ARBs should be evaluated by the provider. The nurse is reminded to consider that with aging is associated with a decreased clearance of medications and metabolites.

Nurses need to be aware of the risk of AKI in older patients, especially those undergoing diagnostic testing or procedures that can result in dehydration. Suppression of thirst, decreased mobility with lack of access to drinking water, and confusion contribute to the older patient's failure to consume adequate fluids, which may lead to dehydration and further compromise of kidney function (Eliopoulos, 2022). Older individuals are usually scheduled for a large number of tests for which the use of nephrotoxic contrast is necessary. The radiographic contrast, in addition to direct tubular damage, alters renal perfusion and intrarenal hemodynamics. The nurse advocates for spacing of tests if possible.

It is also important to emphasize the correct dosage calculation of medications and the least amount of contrast agents in these patients. Due to the reduction of body mass, overdose of drugs can occur. The nurse carefully monitors fluids and electrolyte balance with a focus on correction of factors such as hypovolemia and hypotension. Regarding the prevention of AKI, the nurse is aware that the optimization of the patient's hemodynamic and volume status (avoidance of anemia, glucose variability; individualized blood pressure management) and avoidance of nephrotoxic insults remain the mainstay of primary prevention (Kashani et al., 2019, p. 9; Krasinski et al., 2020).

Pearls for Practice

Muscle mass and GFR can decrease with age; therefore, even small elevations in creatinine may indicate significant renal impairment in older individuals and should be investigated. Medication dosing should be adjusted as needed. Pharmacy should be consulted as needed.

CHRONIC KIDNEY DISEASE AND END-STAGE KIDNEY DISEASE

"Kidney disease is the silent killer," the eighth leading cause of death in the United States and is a major contributor to global burden of disease (Murabito & Hamark, 2018; Taal, 2020). The association behind the silent nature of CKD is because of the kidney's remarkable ability to sustain its primary function of regulating the extracellular fluid (ECF) volume and composition until late in the course of CKD (Taal, 2020). Kidney failure is a progressive and irreversible deterioration in renal function taking place over months to years. It results in the body's inability to maintain metabolic and fluid and electrolyte balance, resulting in azotemia and subsequent uremia. CKD is the term used with kidney damage or decreased renal function for 3 months or more, with evidence of irreversible nephron loss and scarring. More than 1 in 7 adults in the United States (37 million people) have CKD, and for patients with DM and HTN, that risk is greater (National Institute of Diabetes and Digestive and Kidney Diseases [NIDDK], 2021). For example, nearly one in three people with DM and one in five with HTN have kidney disease.

Currently over 661,000 Americans have kidney failure; 468,00 receive dialysis and 193,000 live with a functioning transplant, while 100,000 are waiting for a kidney transplant. Females are affected more than males; 16% for females compared to 13% for males. According to the National Kidney Foundation (NKF, 2021), one in three people are at risk for kidney disease.

When end-stage kidney failure is reached, RRT with dialysis or kidney transplant is needed to sustain life. The Healthy People initiative is designed to guide national health promotion and disease prevention efforts to improve the health of the nation. Released by the U.S. Department of Health and Human Services (HHS) every decade since 1980, Healthy People identifies science-based objectives with targets to monitor progress and motivate and focus action. Healthy People 2030 has set goals related to kidney failure, including:

- Reduce the proportion of adults with CKD
- Increase the proportion of adults with CKD who know they have it
- Reduce the proportion of adults with CKD who have elevated BP
- Reduce the rate of new cases of ESKD
- Reduce the proportion of adult dialysis patients who rely on catheters for dialysis
- Increase the proportion of people who get a kidney transplant within 3 years of ESKD treatment
- Reduce the proportion of adolescents with CKD
- Increase kidney donation rates
- Reduce the death rate for people on dialysis (ODPHP, n.d.)

The incidence of CKD in people who are 65 years of age and above is 38%, while the incidence of CKD among those 45 to 64 years of age is 6% (CDC, 2021a). CKD is more common in non–Hispanic Black adults (16%) than in non–Hispanic White adults (13%), or non–Hispanic Asian adults (13%). About 14% of Hispanic adults have CKD. Medicare costs for CKD are approximately $84 to $100 billion, and for ESKD are $34 to $36 billion (CDC, 2021a; CDC, 2021b). According to the CDC, 340 people begin treatment with dialysis or transplant each day (CDC, 2021c).

Pearls for Practice: Lifting the Lens: The Impact of Global Warming and Environmental Factors on Our Kidneys

Structural and social determinants of health impact CKD risk, progression, and the onset of complications, including end-stage kidney disease (ESKD) (Weinstein & Kimmel, 2021). And the nurse recognizes that where we live impacts our health. Recent research reveals an increase in CKD, that is not attributable to known causes (DM, HTN, glomerular disease) and has been labeled CKD of unknown origin. To illustrate deaths due to CKD increased by 177% with a death toll being as high as over 20,000 in regions of Central America (Geladari et al., 2021). Scientists are equating the climate impact on kidneys as the canary in the coal mine. Historically, coal miners carried caged canaries in the mines, so that if poisonous gases, such as carbon monoxide leaked, the gases would kill the canary before the miners; thus, it was a warning to get out! The parallel is that our kidneys are becoming injured and scientists are linking the new disease burden to global warming and environmental factors. The nurse needs to consider the impact of global warning on the health of our patients. As world temperatures rise, there is a need to better understand heat stress as a cause of kidney disease, how best to provide adequate hydration, and reduce the negative effects of chronic heat exposure (Johnson et al., 2019). In addition, researchers have found an association between urolithiasis (kidney stones) and heat exposure, related to excessive heat-induced sweating and dehydration, which can lead to increased concentration of calcium and uric acid (Liu et al., 2021). Thus, nurses need to consider the importance of educating patient about hydration when patients develop urolithiasis.

The nurse should consider exposure to heat and heavy labor, exposure to heat waves, and possibly exposure to agrochemicals when assessing risk for kidney disease. Nurses will need to educate patients about preventive measures in extreme heat such as staying hydrated, use of electric fans and/or air conditioning, staying indoors when possible and avoiding outdoor activities where possible, and wearing cool and sun-protective clothing (Liu et al., 2021). Population efforts should include public health efforts to raise awareness, creation of heat warning systems, designing cool spaces for public use, and advancing architecture and urban design to better cope with the temperature rise (Liu et al., 2021).

Pathophysiology

As renal function declines, the end products of protein metabolism, normally excreted in urine, accumulate in the

BOX 26-5

Stages of Chronic Kidney Disease

5 Stages Of Kidney Disease

Stage 1	Stage 2	Stage 3A	Stage 3B	Stage 4	Stage 5
GFR≧90	89≧GFR≧60	59≧GFR≧40	44≧GFR≧30	29≧GFR≧15	GFR<15
Normal or high function	Mildly decreased function	Mild to moderately decreased function		Severely decreased function	Kidney failure

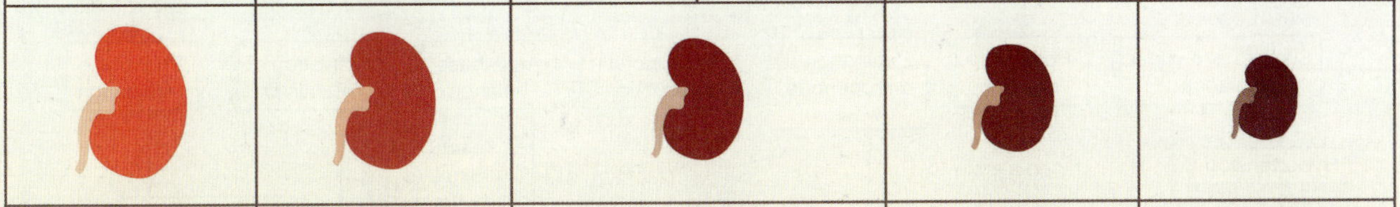

Stages are based on the GFR. The normal GFR is 120–130 mL/min corrected for body size (per 1.73 m^2).

Stage 1: GFR ≥90 mL/min; hematuria, proteinuria, or abnormal renal anatomy

Stage 2 (mild CKD): GFR = 60–89 mL/min; hematuria, proteinuria or abnormal renal anatomy; nephrons highly susceptible to failure

Stage 3a (mildly to moderate CKD): GFR = 45–59 mL/min;

Stage 3b (moderate to severe CKD): GFR = 30–44 mL/min;

Stage 4 (severe CKD): GFR = 15–29 mL/min;

Stage 5 (end-stage CKD): GFR <15 mL/min or kidney failure, treated by dialysis or transplant

From Levin, A., & Stevens, P. E. (2014). Summary of KDIGO 2012 CKD Guideline: Behind the scenes, need for guidance, and a framework for moving forward. *Kidney International, 85*(1), 49–61. https://doi.org/10.1038/ki.2013.444.

blood. As uremia develops, at least two thirds of the nephrons have been destroyed. This differs from azotemia or build up on nitrogenous waste, which may initially develop without symptoms. As the disease progresses, electrolyte and acid–base derangements occur; all body systems are affected. Box 26-5 outlines stages of CKD. Disease progression is based on the amount of renal function present and comorbid conditions, which may appear before the GFR reaches the stage of kidney failure. At the end stage, dialysis and/or renal transplant are needed to prevent coma and death (Norris & Tuan, 2020).

Risk Factors

While the number of new patients with end-stage kidney failure appears to be stabilizing in the United States, the need to reduce both the incidence and prevalence of this devastating complication of kidney disease even further cannot be overemphasized. Undoubtedly the key to success is prevention of both CKD and AKI. Healthy People 2030 identifies five risk factors for kidney failure:

1. DM
2. HTN
3. Proteinuria
4. Family history
5. Increasing age

The CDC identifies the major causes of CKD in order of prevalence as DM, HTN, and GN (2021a). Other causes include **pyelonephritis**, obstruction of the urinary tract, hereditary lesions such as polycystic kidney disease, vascular and autoimmune disorders (such as SLE), infections, medications, or toxic agents. Comorbid conditions that develop during CKD contribute to the high morbidity and mortality among patients with kidney failure (Navaneethan et al., 2020). Environmental and occupational agents that have been implicated in kidney failure include lead, cadmium, mercury, and chromium.

Blood glucose and BP control have been shown to lower the risk of kidney disease. In addition, antihypertensive medications reduce proteinuria, a risk factor for kidney disease (CDC, 2022).

Clinical Manifestations and Assessment

Patients with significant kidney damage may be asymptomatic until 80% of nephrons. CKD is classified as a GFR is <60 mL/min for 3 months or longer, whereas ESKD is a GFR <15 mL/min (Norris & Taun, 2020). Virtually every body system is affected by CKD. Refer to Figure 26-3. Severity of signs and symptoms depends on the degree of renal impairment, other underlying conditions, and the patient's age. Uremia has effects on a variety of organ systems that are detailed below. Some can be managed with dialysis while others cannot.

Systemic Manifestations

- *Neurologic manifestations:* Neurologic changes include lethargy, altered level of consciousness, inability to concentrate, muscle twitching, agitation, confusion, and seizures. Peripheral neuropathy and cramps are present in

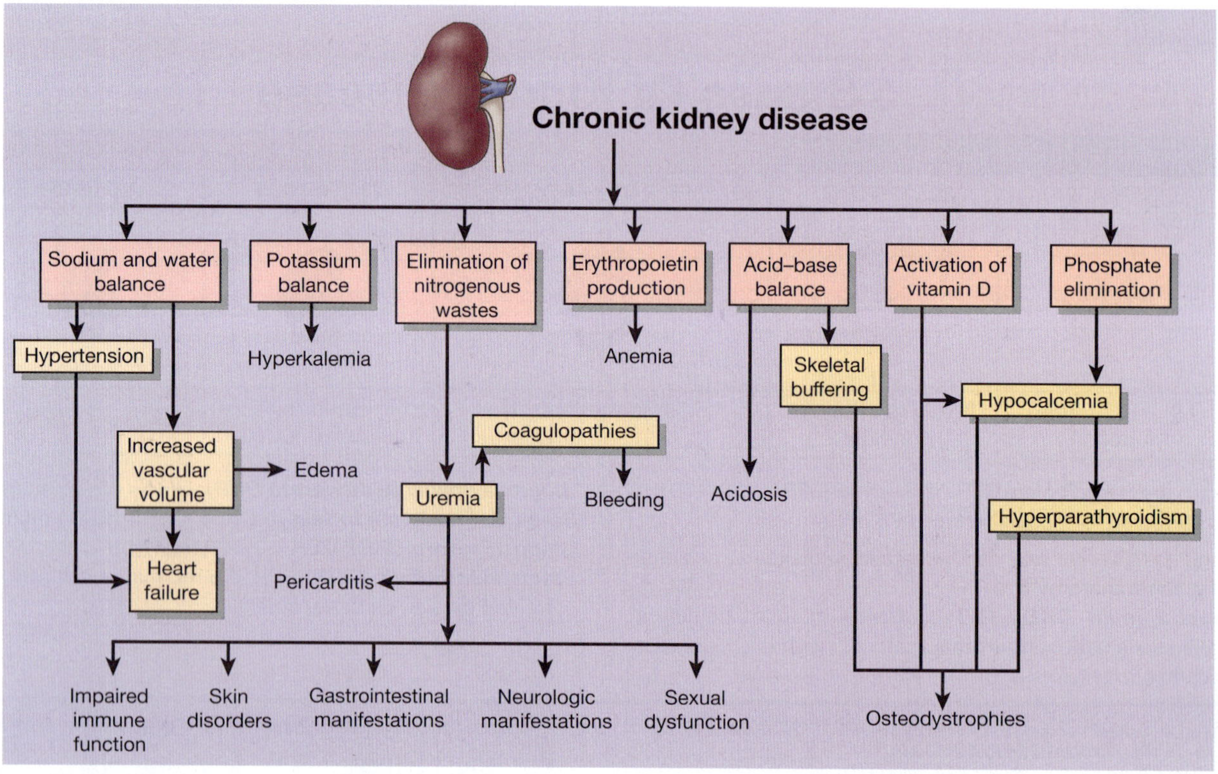

FIGURE 26-3 **Mechanisms and manifestations of chronic kidney disease. (From Norris, T. E. (2019). *Porth's essentials of pathophysiology* (5th ed.). Lippincott Williams & Wilkins; Figure 34-4.)**

some patients. Restless leg syndrome (RLS) and painful or "burning" feet can occur in the early stage of uremic peripheral neuropathy.

- *Cardiovascular manifestations:* HTN, fluid volume excess causes HF and pulmonary edema. Pericarditis (with or without pericardial fluid accumulation) is caused by irritation of the pericardium by uremic toxins and may require dialysis. In addition, the effect of hyperkalemia will be seen in the ECG changes previously discussed on page 897. The nurse is acutely aware that hyperkalemia can result in life-threatening cardiac arrhythmias.
- *GI manifestations:* GI signs and symptoms are common and include anorexia, nausea, vomiting, and hiccups. The patient's breath may have the odor of ammonia or urine (uremic fetor), or the patient may complain of a metallic taste in the mouth.
- *Immunologic manifestations:* Defective granulocytes, B- and T-cell function, and impaired phagocytosis can lead to impaired immune and inflammatory response.
- *Hematology manifestations:* Anemia, secondary to decreased erythropoietin (hormone that stimulates RBC production by the bone marrow) production. Increased bleeding risk because of defective platelet adhesiveness. In general, a normal amount of platelets are seen; however, bleeding time is prolonged.
- *Genitourinary manifestations:* Erectile dysfunction, decreased libido, pain during intercourse (females), and amenorrhea may result.
- *Dermatologic manifestations:* Pruritus is common. Uremic frost, the deposit of urea crystals on the skin, is uncommon today because of early and aggressive treatment of kidney failure with dialysis. The skin may be bronze or waxy yellow or gray, particularly in dark-skinned individuals. The precise mechanisms have not been identified for many of these diverse signs and symptoms.
- *Musculoskeletal manifestations:* Hyperphosphatemia develops due to decrease in renal excretion of phosphate. The calcium levels decrease because of the rise in phosphorus and the inability of the kidney to convert vitamin D to its active form, which facilitates calcium absorption from the gut. Bone and joint problems are associated with disturbances of calcium and phosphate metabolism, resulting in renal osteodystrophy, a clinical entity encompassing several overlapping varieties of bone disease that can cause bone pain or frank fractures (Van Leeuwen & Bladh, 2019).

Box 26-6 summarizes the signs and symptoms seen in kidney failure.

Glomerular Filtration Rate

As glomerular filtration decreases, the serum creatinine and BUN levels increase; the creatinine clearance decreases. Serum creatinine is the more sensitive indicator of kidney function because of its constant production in the body. The BUN is affected not only by kidney disease but also

BOX 26-6

Focused Assessment

Chronic Kidney Disease Progressing to ESKD

The nurse monitors for the following signs and symptoms:

Neurologic
- Weakness and fatigue
- Confusion or behavior changes
- Inability to concentrate
- Disorientation
- Tremors
- Seizures
- Asterixis
- Restless leg syndrome
- Burning of soles of feet

Integumentary
- Gray-bronze skin color
- Dry, flaky skin
- Pruritus
- Ecchymosis or purpura
- Thin, brittle nails
- Coarse, thinning hair

Cardiovascular
- Hypertension
- Pitting edema (feet, hands, sacrum)
- Periorbital edema
- Engorged neck veins
- Pericarditis/pericardial friction rub
- Pericardial effusion or tamponade
- Hyperkalemia
- Hyperlipidemia

Pulmonary
- Crackles
- Thick, tenacious sputum
- Depressed cough reflex
- Pleuritic pain
- Shortness of breath
- Tachypnea
- Kussmaul-type respirations
- Uremic pneumonitis

Gastrointestinal
- Ammonia odor to breath ("uremic fetor")
- Metallic taste
- Mouth ulcerations and bleeding
- Anorexia, nausea, and vomiting
- Hiccups
- Constipation or diarrhea
- Bleeding from GI tract

Hematologic
- Anemia
- Thrombocytopenia

Reproductive
- Erectile dysfunction
- Amenorrhea
- Testicular atrophy
- Infertility
- Decreased libido

Musculoskeletal
- Muscle cramps
- Loss of muscle strength
- Renal osteodystrophy
- Bone pain
- Bone fractures
- Foot drop

by protein intake in the diet, tissue catabolism, fluid intake, parenteral nutrition, and medications such as corticosteroids. Calculation of GFR is discussed in Chapter 25, and the stages of CKD based on GFR can be found in Box 26-5.

Sodium and Water Retention

Some patients retain sodium and water, increasing the risk for edema, HF, and HTN. Dilutional hyponatremia typically occurs. HTN also may result from activation of the renin–angiotensin–aldosterone system and the concomitant increased secretion of aldosterone. Episodes of vomiting and diarrhea may cause sodium and water depletion, which worsens the uremic state (Norris & Tuan, 2020).

Acidosis

In advanced kidney disease, metabolic acidosis occurs because the kidneys are incapable of excreting the acid load (hydrogen ions or H^+) and unable to regenerate and reabsorb base bicarbonate (pH less than 7.35). The kidney tubules are also unable to excrete ammonia (NH_3) which in healthy kidneys neutralizes the daily acid load. There is also decreased excretion of phosphates and other organic acids. The acidosis seems to stabilize as a result of buffering in the bone but may contribute to skeletal disorders (Norris & Tuan, 2020). Symptoms of metabolic acidosis include lethargic, confusion, headache, deep breathing (associated with attempt to "blow off" the respiratory acid to compensate for the acidosis). Refer to Chapter 3 for additional details on metabolic acidosis.

Hyperkalemia

Approximately 90% of potassium excretion is via the kidney. The most common cause of hyperkalemia is reduced renal function, typically the GFR is below 10 mL/min (Norris & Tuan, 2020). The nephron (if capable) adapts to the decrease in GFR by increasing potassium excretion and the GI tract decreases potassium absorption. In general, potassium restriction is unnecessary until the GFR is below 5 to 10 mL/min, at which time the compensatory measures are ineffective and hyperkalemia ensues.

Anemia is caused by inadequate production of erythropoietin by the damaged kidney in addition to chronic blood loss, hemolysis, bone marrow suppression due to retained uremic factors. Erythropoietin, normally produced by the kidneys, stimulates bone marrow to produce RBCs. Anemia is exacerbated further by the shortened lifespan of RBCs due to uremia, nutritional deficiencies, and the patient's tendency to bleed, particularly from the GI tract. Iron deficiency may result from anorexia due to dietary restriction and blood loss during dialysis. The nurse should assess for fatigue, weakness, dizziness, headaches, irritability, shortness of breath and chest pain (Norris & Tuan, 2020).

Calcium and Phosphorus Imbalance

Hyperphosphatemia with resulting hypocalcemia typically develops when the GFR is less than 30 mL/min (Goyal & Jialal, 2022). The decreased serum calcium level causes increased secretion of parathormone from the parathyroid glands, causing calcium to leave the bone. Bone weakness and fractures may result. The active metabolite of vitamin D (1,25-dihydroxycholecalciferol), normally manufactured by the kidney, decreases as kidney failure progresses, impairing calcium absorption and raising PTH levels (Norris & Tuan, 2020). Secondary hyperparathyroidism results. Uremic bone disease or renal osteodystrophy develops from the complex changes in the balance of calcium, phosphate, and parathormone.

Coagulopathies

Platelet production may be normal in patients with CKD, however the platelet function is impaired. Patients with CKD have a 2.3-fold higher risk of hemorrhages, which increases to a 3.5-fold higher bleeding risk in patients when the GFR is <15 mL/min (Baaten et al., 2022). Bleeding may manifest as epistaxis, menorrhagia, GI bleeding, and bruising (Norris & Tuan, 2020). In addition, there is also risk for thrombotic disorders in CKD which may be due to elevated circulating levels of fibrinogen, and coagulation factors thus the nurse observes for both arterial and venous thrombosis, particularly if the patient had nephrotic syndrome. Refer to Figure 26-3.

Medical Management

The goal of management is to maintain nephron function and homeostasis for as long as possible while continuing to treat the underlying disorder(s). Crucial treatment areas include prevention strategies, fluid balance, anemia, pharmacologic therapy, and electrolyte imbalance (Lough, 2022). Lifestyle intervention to address underlying comorbidities and appropriate pharmacologic therapy based on the severity of kidney disease will be provided and modified as kidney function declines (Navaneethan et al., 2020). Special attention to the assessment of the patients BP and management of HTN is essential to prevent or mitigate the significant cardiac complications associated with CKD. Current guidelines from the American College of Cardiology/American Heart Association and the National Kidney Foundation Kidney Disease Outcomes Quality Initiative recommend a goal BP of <130/<80 mm Hg for those with DM and nondiabetic CKD (Reddy, 2022).

The nurse recognizes that referral to a nephrologist is indicated for patients with a GFR <30 mL/min (Reddy, 2022; Winkelman & Duffy, 2021). It is understood that there needs to be discussions about the options and preferences for RRT as kidney disease progresses (discussed in detail later in the chapter).

Prevention Strategies

The nurse is aware of the progressive nature of CKD; thus, the goal is prevention of complications. The aim is to prevent or stave off further deterioration and areas that are important are control of BP, DM, and avoidance of nephrotoxic medications. The clinical pharmacist is consulted as needed. The nurse teaches the patient to avoid NSAIDs in patients with elevated creatinine levels and the use of intravascular contrast dye is avoided (see previous discussion). Smoking has a negative impact on renal function and is nephrotoxic in older adults with HTN, and those with DM (Norris & Tuan, 2020), thus the nurse assists in educating patients on options for smoking cessation.

Pharmacologic Therapy

Complications can be prevented or delayed by treating the underlying cause of the kidney disease. Pharmacologic therapy may include phosphate-binding agents, calcium supplements, antihypertensive and cardiac medications, statins, anticonvulsants, and erythropoietin-stimulating agents (ESAs). Intensive blood glucose control prevents microalbuminuria and the progression of diabetic nephropathy.

Calcium and Phosphorus Binders

Hyperphosphatemia promotes hyperparathyroidism leading to hypercalcemia, a risk for cardiovascular calcification, increased morbidity, and mortality (Burchum & Rosenthal, 2019). Hyperphosphatemia is managed with dietary phosphate restriction, hemodialysis and administering phosphate-binding medications which act in the GI tract to reduce the absorption of phosphate in the intestine. A polymeric phosphate binder, such as sevelamer hydrochloride or more frequently sevelamer carbonate may be used. A side effect of sevelamer hydrochloride is metabolic acidosis, though data do not indicate a better outcome with the carbonate salt (Burchum & Rosenthal, 2019). Lanthanum carbonate is an additional phosphate binder. The goal of hyperphosphatemia treatment should be to reduce serum phosphorus concentrations to ≤5.5 mg/dL (or closer to normal levels) (Fishbane & Nigwekar, 2021). Parathyroid agents, such as cinacalcet, a calcimimetic, may be given for secondary hyperparathyroidism of kidney failure. The medication binds with calcium-sensing receptors in the parathyroid gland, suppressing PTH secretion. When PTH decreases, bone resorption diminishes (Burchum & Rosenthal, 2019), mitigating bone loss.

Pearls for Practice

It is important for nurses to consider the impact of having to take numerous medications daily. For example, patients with kidney disease are frequently treated with phosphate binders which require that they take 1 to 4 binders with each meal or snack (~3 to 5 times per day). This equates to about 11 phosphate-binder pills per day, and the pill burden from this single medication category equivalent to that of nine other therapy types combined (Fishbane & Nigwekar, 2021)! Thus, it is important for nurses to acknowledge the complexity of patient's drug regimen, while assessing their knowledge level about the purpose of the medications and their willingness to adhere to the prescribed regimen. While recognizing the patient's autonomy regarding their health, the nurse understands that the relationship between the patient and nurse can increase the patient's decision-making capacity.

Pearls for Practice

Calcium exists as either bound to albumin or ionized, referring to its free form. Ionized calcium (~45%) is physiologically active whereas bound calcium is inactive. Standard laboratory tests measure the total calcium (ionized and bound). The most common cause of hypocalcemia is low serum albumin, which occurs in patients with nephrotic syndrome and other processes such as starvation or renal cachexia. An ionized calcium level may be ordered or a correction formula for this perceived calcium deficit may be used.

To correct the calcium level, the nurse adds 0.8 g/dL to the total calcium value for every gram of albumin below 4.0 g/dL, using this formula:

$$\text{Corrected calcium} = \text{serum total calcium (mg/dL)} + 0.8 \times (4 - \text{serum albumin [g/dL]})$$

Note: a normal serum calcium level is 8 to 10 mg/dL, which may vary slightly by laboratory; a normal serum albumin is 3.5 to 5.2 g/dL.

Example: Patient has albumin of 2 g/dL (20 g/L), and total serum calcium concentration of 8 mg/dL.

Formula: 8 mg/dL + 0.8 (4 − 2 g/dL)

8 + 0.8(2)

8 + 1.6

9.6 mg/dL = corrected calcium level

Pearls for Practice: Pathophysiology

The parathyroid glands regulate blood calcium and secondary hyperparathyroidism may develop in patients with kidney failure. The parathyroid glands respond to hypocalcemia by increasing the secretion of PTH. PTH works to elevate the blood calcium by stimulating the release of calcium from the bones. Thus, the nurse should assess for bone pain, osteoporosis, and pathologic bone fractures.

Pearls for Practice: Pathophysiology

Under normal circumstances, hypocalcemia results in enhanced calcium uptake by renal collecting tubules. However, in kidney failure, the collecting tubules are unable to reabsorb calcium, and activation of vitamin D also is impaired. With decreased renal synthesis of 1,25-dihydroxyvitamin D (also known as calcitriol, the active form of vitamin D), the intestinal absorption of calcium is decreased. Therefore, kidney diseases place patients at risk for hypocalcemia, secondary hyperparathyroidism, and hyperphosphatemia.

Antihypertensive and Cardiovascular Agents

HTN can be an early manifestation or a consequence of CKD. BP level ≥140/90 mm Hg, is inversely related to the GFR. For example, 92% in patient with a GFR < 30 mL/min have HTN (Thomas, 2019). Aggressive treatment slows the progression of kidney disease. LVH and ischemic heart disease can develop in patients with CKD. HF and pulmonary edema may occur. Lifestyle changes which may include (decreased sodium intake, DASH [dietary approaches to stop hypertension] diet), weight management, physical activity, and moderation in alcohol consumption (see Chapter 12), and pharmacologic management is used along with restriction of sodium and fluids. The patient should be referred to a dietitian for medical nutritional therapy for patients with GFR <50 mL/min and is a Medicare-covered service (Reddy, 2022).

Pharmacologic agents can include thiazide diuretics (preferably chlorthalidone), ACEIs, ARBs, and calcium channel blockers (CCBs) (Thomas, 2019). However, combining ACEs and ARBs can increase the risk of hyperkalemia (Reddy, 2022). Side effects of ACEs and ARBs include cough (>ACEs), angioedema (>ACEs), and hyperkalemia thus, the nurse monitors lab work and teaches patients symptoms of hyperkalemia if they are prescribed (Burcham & Rosenthal, 2019). Diuretics may be used to enhance functional kidney, attempt to recover renal function, or improve fluid balance, in patients with some residual kidney function.

The nurse is aware that CVD is the most common cause of mortality in CKD, even in the early stages. DM, anemia, high LDL cholesterol levels, and vascular calcification are factors that contribute to the incidence of CVD. Statins may reduce cardiovascular risk in stage 2 (GFR = 60 to 89 mL/min) or early stage 3 CKD patients (Mitch, 2020). Studies reveal that treatment with statins contributes to lowering mortality and major cardiovascular events by 20% in people with CKD (Walton, 2022).

Pearls for Practice

Research has shown that ACE (angiotensin-converting enzyme) inhibitors and ARBs (angiotensin II receptor blockers), both medications that treat high blood pressure, can reduce kidney damage in diabetes patients with CKD (ODPHP, 2021).

Anticonvulsants and Neuromuscular Agents

IV diazepam, lorazepam, or phenytoin can be administered to control seizures, which may develop as uremia worsens. The side rails of the bed should be raised and bed in low position to protect the patient. If a seizure occurs, the nurse protects the patient's head, loosens constrictive clothing, and removes patient's eyeglasses. The nursing management of the patient with seizures is discussed in Chapter 45.

About two-thirds of patients receiving dialysis may have RLS manifested by creeping, prickling, and itching sensations at rest; moving the legs allows temporary relief. Avoidance of caffeine, alcohol, and nicotine is recommended since they can exacerbate RLS. Medications such as anticonvulsants, benzodiazepines, dopamine agonists or iron may be prescribed; opioids are used for those not responding to other medications (National Institutes of Health [NIH], 2020).

Erythropoietin

Anemia associated with CKD is treated with recombinant human erythropoietin (rhEPO and erythropoietin-stimulating agents [ESAs]) which include epoetin alfa or darbepoetin alfa (Norris & Tuan, 2020). Initial effects can be seen within 1 to 2 weeks with maximum acceptable hemoglobin of 10 to 11 g/dL in 2 to 3 months. The medication does not prevent progression of renal deterioration (Burcham & Rosenthal, 2019). Iron supplementation is given based on ferritin levels.

Side effects of ESAs include HTN which may require pharmacologic intervention, HF, and thrombotic events including stroke or MI. Dosing should be the lowest needed to gradually raise hemoglobin levels to the lowest level sufficient to reduce the need for RBC transfusion. In most cases the hemoglobin should not exceed 10 to 11 g/dL, which appears sufficient to alleviate the symptoms of anemia (Burcham & Rosenthal, 2019; FDA.gov).

E-poietin is administered intravenously at the end of dialysis or subcutaneously. Adverse effects seen with erythropoietin therapy include headache, arthralgia, nausea, HTN, increased clotting, seizures, and depletion of body iron stores (Burcham & Rosenthal, 2019). The expected outcome for patients receiving e-poietin is higher-energy levels, increased feeling of well-being, better tolerance of dialysis, and improved tolerance of exercise. Blood transfusions may be indicated for patients with chest pain or extreme dyspnea.

Pearls for Practice

Patients with CKD and untreated anemia typically have hemoglobin concentrations in the range of 6 to 8 g/dL. The use of erythropoietin-stimulating agents (ESAs) has been shown to have a significant effect on correcting Hct levels. However, a black-box warning advises clinicians and patients with CKD to "weigh the benefits of ESAs to decrease the need for transfusions against the increased risks for serious, adverse cardiovascular events" associated with ESAs (Burcham & Rosenthal, 2019; FDA, 2017). The adverse cardiovascular events include HTN, increased risk for stroke, and vascular thrombosis. The lowest dose of ESA sufficient to reduce the need for transfusion is recommended and the target Hgb should not exceed 10 to 11 g/dL since Hgb levels >11 g/dL are associated with the adverse events described above.

Iron, in the form of sodium–ferric gluconate complex, iron sucrose, and ferumoxytol may be prescribed to promote an adequate response to erythropoietin in patients with CKD. Oral iron supplements should be stopped prior to use of parenteral iron (Burcham & Rosenthal, 2019).

Nutritional Therapy and Fluid balance

Preventing progression of kidney disease with a cardiac prudent Mediterranean or the DASH diet can reduce HTN, which is responsible for disease progression (de Wall, 2022). These diets are high in fruits, vegetables, and whole grains with adequate amounts of calcium and protein. As kidney failure progresses, the diet, which will be dependent on the stage of kidney disease, and will include restricting fluids, sodium, potassium, phosphorus, and limiting protein intake. A "renal diet" that can be applied to all patients does not exist (Kallenbach, 2021). That is why a registered dietitian is an essential part of the interdisciplinary team and, will make recommendations specific for the patient's treatment plan.

The issue of how much to restrict protein remains controversial. Since protein breaks down to form nitrogenous wastes, a reduction of protein lowers BUN and reduces uremic symptoms (Norris & Tuan, 2020), however adequate amino acids are needed to synthesize proteins and prevent tissue catabolism. Too little protein and malnutrition can cause loss of strength, muscle mass, and weight (Kruzel, 2021). Protein restriction of 0.8 to 10 g/kg/day of ideal body weight can slow the progression of renal disease and improve symptoms of uremia, including nausea and vomiting. The nurse teaches patients, that while popular, high protein diets are contraindicated (de Wall, 2022). At least 50% of the allowed protein must be of high biologic value (HBV), including eggs, meats, and plant-based proteins (Kallenbach, 2021). The nurse is aware that malnutrition and low albumin levels are independent predictors of mortality; therefore, the risk of malnutrition may outweigh any benefit of protein restriction.

Protein restriction can be difficult for patients; the nurse should give positive feedback and express confidence in the patient's ability to adhere to the eating plan. Daily dietary requirements for patients with ESRD will change depending on the type of dialysis chosen (continuous ambulatory peritoneal dialysis [CAPD] vs. hemodialysis). For example, dietary protein is increased slightly to 1.2 g/kg/day during hemodialysis to compensate for loss of protein and amino acids in the dialysate, and 1.3 g/kg/day for PD (Kallenbach,

2021). At the same time, adequate caloric intake and vitamin supplementation must be ensured because a protein-restricted diet does not provide the necessary complement of vitamins, and dialysis results in loss of water-soluble vitamins. Calories are supplied by carbohydrates and fat to prevent wasting resulting in renal cachexia, in severe instances.

The patient must adhere to the prescribed daily fluid allowance which typically combines the previous day's 24-hour urine output and insensible loss (Norris & Tuan, 2020). The nurse teaches the patient different strategies to control intake and thirst, such as sucking on hard candies or mints, chewing gum, rinsing the mouth with refrigerated water, sucking on a lemon wedge, using small glasses instead of large ones, and moisturizing the lips.

Potassium restriction involves limiting citrus fruits and juices, tomatoes, melons, green leafy vegetables, potatoes, and chocolate. In addition, phosphorus is restricted. The patient is taught to control portion size or avoid dairy, peas, beans, nuts (including peanut butter), and cola products. Sodium and MSG are contained in many canned, processed foods (lunch meats), all of which should be avoided (Norris & Tuan, 2020).

Pearls for Practice

Patients with kidney disease must be made aware that some salt substitutes contain potassium chloride and should be avoided.

Dialysis

The patient with increasing symptoms of kidney failure is referred to a dialysis or transplantation center early in the course of progressive disease. Dialysis is initiated when the patient cannot maintain homeostasis with conservative treatment; dialysis is discussed in detail later in the chapter.

Nursing Management

The patient with CKD requires astute nursing care to avoid the complications of reduced kidney function and the stresses and anxieties of dealing with this chronic life-threatening illness.

Nursing care and education are directed toward fluid and electrolyte imbalance, dietary management, and promoting positive feelings by encouraging increased self-efficacy and greater independence. It is extremely important to provide frequent, clear explanations and information to the patient and family concerning kidney failure, treatment options, and potential complications. A plan of nursing care for a patient with kidney failure is available online at http://thepoint.lww.com/Honan3e.

Teaching Patients Self-Care

Encouraging self-management is an essential role of the nurse when caring for patients with kidney failure. Nurses in home care, dialysis centers, hospitals, and outpatient settings all provide ongoing education and reinforcement while monitoring the patient's progress and adherence to the treatment regimen. The nurse provides patient-centered care incorporating the patient's beliefs, values, and concerns in the treatment regimen to improve patient outcomes.

When targeting health education for prevention of CKD, the nurse includes evidence that early detection and treatment of kidney disease may prevent—or at least delay—the progression to ESKD.

The nurse and dietician reinforce the dietary management for patients with kidney disorders as well as fluid restrictions, explaining the correlation between symptoms and nonadherence. The patient can be encouraged to take BP measurements and daily weights at home to illustrate the effect of prescribed antihypertensives and fluid restriction with BP elevations or SOB.

The patient and family should report the following symptoms of worsening kidney function to the health care provider:

- Signs and symptoms of worsening kidney failure, including nausea, vomiting, change in usual urine output, or ammonia/urine odor to the breath
- Signs and symptoms of hyperkalemia, including muscle weakness, diarrhea, abdominal cramps
- If receiving dialysis, signs and symptoms of access problems, such as clotted fistula or graft or signs of infection at the site (discussed shortly)

Continuing Care

The nurse teaches the patient to follow-up with examinations and treatments to prevent and detect progression of kidney disease as well as reinforce care for the primary disorder. The nurse teaches the patient and family about symptoms of worsening condition which should be reported to the health care provider, have treatment options explained, and be offered psychoemotional support. The home care nurse has the opportunity to assess the patient's environment, emotional status, and the coping strategies used by the patient and family to deal with the changes in family roles often associated with chronic illness. The nurse provides ongoing assessment, education, and reinforces adherence to the renal diet and fluid restriction. Reminders about the need for health-promoting activities and health screening, particularly cardiovascular health, are important when caring for the patient with kidney failure.

Gerontologic Considerations

Renal mass gradually decreases by a rate of 10% per decade after the 40th decade, even in the absence of risk factors. The signs and symptoms of renal disease in older individuals may be nonspecific, with HF and HTN or the onset of acute GN as the initial presentation (Norris & Tuan, 2020). Comorbid disorders, such as HF or dementia, can delay diagnosis and complicate treatment.

Older persons are more prone to "white coat hypertension" (refer to Chapter 12); therefore 24-hour monitors should be used to validate a diagnosis of HTN. Systolic HTN also is common in the older population; overtreatment can result in diastolic hypotension or orthostatic hypotension, which may lead to dizziness, falls, and risk for fracture (Eliopoulos, 2022). As discussed earlier ACEIs and ARBs have renal protective effects, yet the use of these medications in older individuals should be undertaken with caution. If the patient's serum creatinine increases or hyperkalemia develops the medication should be reevaluated (Van Leeuwen & Bladh, 2019).

Knowing that CKD is a risk factor for CVD, older adults should receive advice on lifestyle modification and medications, such as antiplatelet and lipid-lowering medications. Available diagnostic criteria and treatment guidelines are not tailored specifically to the older adult. Those at low risk may require medication dosage modifications, BP monitoring, and efforts to avoid medications and procedures that increase the risk of kidney injury. The adage, "start low and go slow" applies to the older patient and refers to starting with low doses and gradually increasing as needed, while watching for orthostatic hypotension and other untoward reactions which may be common in older individuals (Burchum, 2019).

Pearls for Practice

Related to DM, there is uncertainty surrounding the optimal glycemic target in the patient on dialysis although recent epidemiologic data suggest that A1c ranges of 6% to 8%, as well as 7% to 9%, are associated with increased survival rates among diabetic dialysis patients (Alalawi & Bashier, 2021).

Hemodialysis and PD have been used effectively in treating older patients, although neither has proven superior (Norris & Tuan, 2020). While there is no specific age limit for renal transplantation, concomitant disorders, such as coronary artery disease or peripheral vascular disease, have made this option less common for older patient. Treatment for those with CKD should be adapted to suit the patient's comorbidities and life expectancy. When the older adult refuses dialysis or transplantation, conservative management with nutritional therapy, fluid control, and medications may be used. Palliative care, a comprehensive approach that improves quality of life (QOL) for patients and families, has been shown to impact weight gain, fatigue, anxiety and depression, improving the QOL. This differs from hospice care, where survival is not expected to exceed 6 months. The patient is encouraged to explore advanced directives and end-of-life care based on QOL.

Complications

Complications of CKD necessitate a collaborative approach to care and include hyperkalemia, HTN, anemia, metabolic acidosis, hyperphosphatemia, hypocalcemia, bone disease, FVE, HF, pericarditis, pericardial effusion, and pericardial tamponade, hyperparathyroidism, as previously detailed.

RENAL REPLACEMENT THERAPIES

Renal replacement therapy is a term used to encompass life-supporting treatments for kidney failure, including hemodialysis, PD, continuous renal replacement therapies (CRRTs), and renal transplantation. While these treatment modalities are discussed within the context of kidney failure, hemodialysis and PD may be employed to restore homeostasis in patients with AKI as well.

As ESKD approaches, the patient's very survival is threatened. Choosing a treatment option for kidney failure can be overwhelming. Applying best practices and health care navigation for patient with ESKD can improve patient's ability to make informed decisions and increase the numbers of those pursuing transplant. The *My Life, My Dialysis Choice Decision Aid* from the nonprofit Medical Education Institute, Inc. shifts the discussion from *how* to do dialysis to *why* a particular RRT option may be a better fit for the patient's lifestyle (Schatell, 2022). In addition, there is a need to normalize discussions about concerns, fears, preferences, priorities, and future care for those with kidney failure throughout the disease process. For individuals struggling to maintain career and family life and roles while undergoing hemodialysis, there is a need for advanced care planning early in the trajectory of the disease to facilitate development of realistic goals. For the older adult, discussions surrounding QOL should occur (Norris & Tuan, 2020).

DIALYSIS

Dialysis is used to remove fluid and uremic waste products from the body when the kidneys are unable to do so. Methods of therapy include hemodialysis, PD, and CRRT.

Whether kidney disease is acute or chronic, dialysis becomes necessary upon the development of hyperkalemia, fluid overload, or impending pulmonary edema, acidosis, pericarditis, or severe confusion/encephalopathy. It also may be used to remove certain medications or other toxins due to poisoning or medication overdose.

The decision to initiate dialysis is patient centered and reached after thoughtful discussion with the patient, family, providers, and others (social work, spiritual adviser, etc.), as appropriate. Many potentially life-threatening issues are associated with the need for dialysis. The nurse can assist the patient and family by answering their questions, clarifying the information provided, and supporting their decision. Often the lifestyle changes that patients requiring long-term hemodialysis need to make are overwhelming.

Although the costs of dialysis usually are reimbursable, limitations on the patient's ability to work, resulting from illness and dialysis, can impose a great financial burden on the patient and family.

HEMODIALYSIS

Hemodialysis is the most common method of dialysis. Once stable, treatments usually occur three times a week and take about 3 to 5 hours per treatment. The healthy kidney works 24 hours a day; dialysis can only do 10% to 15% of what a normal kidney does (AKF, 2020). The trend in managing CKD is to initiate treatment before the signs and symptoms associated with uremia become severe.

Description

Hemodialysis functions as an artificial kidney, removing toxic nitrogenous substances and excess water from the blood. The patient's blood is diverted to a machine, where toxins are removed, and then the blood is returned to the patient's body. Hemodialysis requires a semipermeable membrane found in the hollow fiber **dialyzer**, or artificial kidney, to replace the function of the impaired kidneys. The dialyzer contains thousands of tiny cellophane tubules through which the blood flows; a **dialysate** solution circulates around the tubules. The exchange of wastes from the blood to the dialysate occurs through the semipermeable membrane by way of **osmosis**, **diffusion**, and **ultrafiltration** (Fig. 26-4). The toxins and wastes in the blood are removed by diffusion, in which particles move from an area of higher concentration in the blood to an area of lower concentration in the dialysate. The dialysate is a solution made up of electrolytes in their ideal extracellular concentrations. The electrolyte level in the patient's blood can be brought under control by adjusting the dialysate. The semipermeable membrane impedes the diffusion of large molecules, such as RBCs and proteins, keeping them in the bloodstream.

Excess water is removed from the blood by osmosis, in which water moves from an area of lower concentration of particulates in the blood (dilute) toward an area of higher concentration of particulates in the dialysate. In ultrafiltration, water moves under high hydrostatic pressure to an area of lower pressure to facilitate water removal, across the dialyzing membrane. That is water moves from the patient to the dialysate.

As hemodialysis uses an extracorporeal circuit where blood circulates outside the body, the blood can clot rapidly.

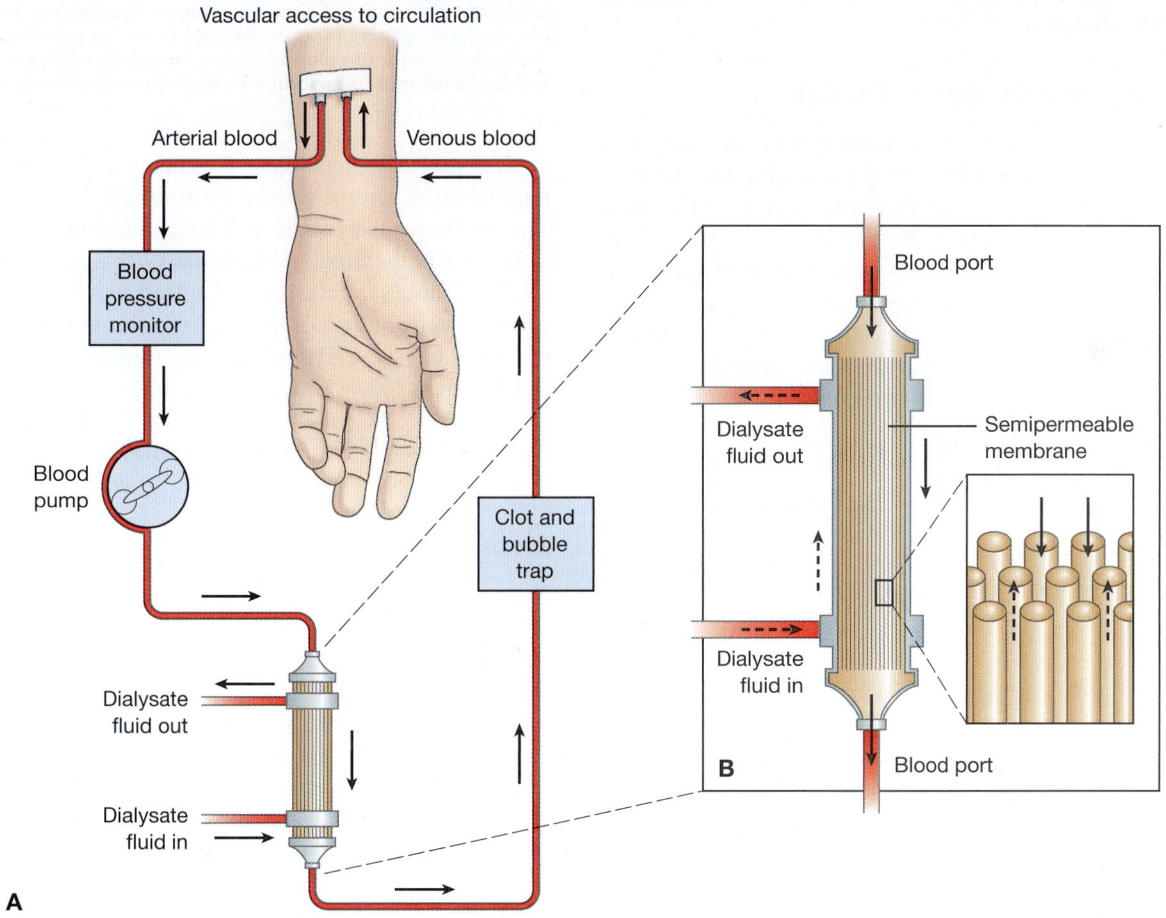

FIGURE 26-4 **Hemodialysis system. A. Blood from an artery is pumped into (B) a dialyzer where it flows through the cellophane tubes, which act as the semipermeable membrane (*inset*). The dialysate, which has the same chemical composition as the blood except for urea and waste products, flows in around the tubules. The waste products in the blood diffuse through the semipermeable membrane into the dialysate.**

Heparin is most commonly used to prevent clotting in the dialysis circuit, although no consensus exists on the optimal method of heparin dosing. When an anticoagulant is dangerous to the patient, such as those with thrombocytopenia, regional anticoagulation can be used. In regional anticoagulation, the anticoagulant is infused continuously into the dialyzer and the antidote is administered as the blood returns to the patient. Heparin-free dialysis has become the method of choice when treating patients with active bleeding and those with an increased risk of bleeding, pericarditis, coagulopathy, or thrombocytopenia (Kallenbach, 2021). For those patients who are allergic to heparin, saline has been used, however, this is controversial, as some studies have suggested that a saline rinses can actually promote clotting (Yuriy, 2022). At the end of the treatment, the dialysate, excess fluid, and waste products are discarded. Most people live 5 to 10 years on dialysis, and many have lived for 20 or more years (AKF, 2020).

Vascular Access

Access to the patient's vascular system must be established to allow blood to be removed, "cleansed," and returned to the patient's vascular system at rapid rates. Several types of access are available.

Temporary Vascular Access Devices

Immediate access to the patient's circulation for emergency hemodialysis is achieved by inserting a double-lumen large-bore catheter into the subclavian, internal jugular, or femoral vein (Kallenbach, 2021) (Fig. 26-5). This method of vascular access involves some risk, such as hematoma, pneumothorax, infection, thrombosis of the subclavian vein, or inadequate flow. For the patient with ESKD, the nurse should emphasize that these are "bridge" catheters and not permanent access; they are used while a method for permanent vascular access is created and heals. Other reasons for use of temporary vascular access devices include a lack of counseling/education/awareness of the disease, emergency need or the nephrologist being unable to predict the timing for need for dialysis, a nonfunctioning fistula created prior to need for dialysis, and a delay in maturation of the fistula (Nakaya, 2021).

Pearls for Practice

Temporary vascular access devices for dialysis (e.g., Quinton catheter or permacath) are typically flushed with heparin at the end of the treatment to maintain patency. The nurse should not use these devices for routine access. In the event of a life-threatening emergency, where no other access is available, the nurse MUST ASPIRATE THE CATHETER PORTS PRIOR to using, to prevent systemic anticoagulation.

The Fistula First Breakthrough Initiative (FFBI) was established in 2005 by the CMS to increase AV fistula use in all appropriate hemodialysis patients and to decrease the placement of central venous catheters (Kallenbach, 2021). The aim is for the patient to have permanent and functioning access at the time that hemodialysis therapy is initiated. Since, a fistula should be placed at least 6 months before it is needed and a graft needs at least 3 to 6 weeks before the start of hemodialysis, early referral and placement is required (Kallenbach, 2021). Due to the continued use of central line dialysis catheters, the original focus of the Fistula First initiative has been transformed to "Fistula First-Catheter Last" Workgroup Coalition (Fatima, 2018; Nakaya et al., 2021).

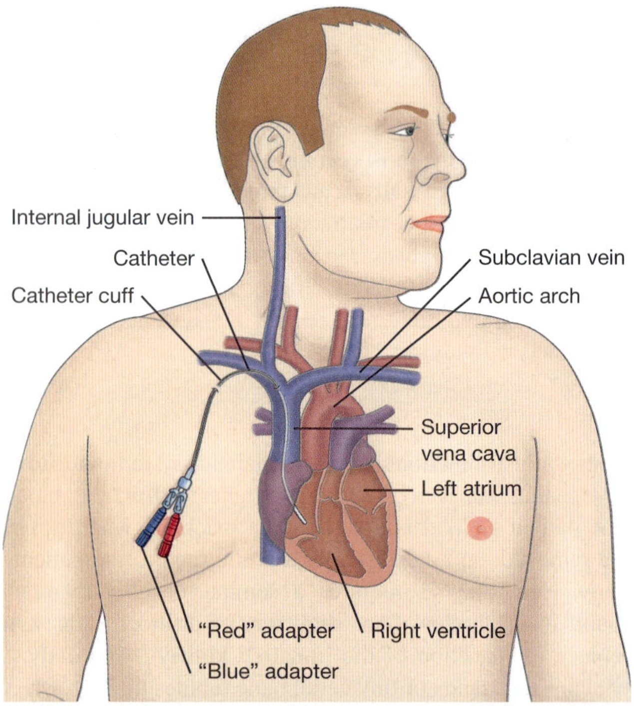

FIGURE 26-5 Double-lumen, cuffed hemodialysis catheter used in acute hemodialysis. The red adapter is attached to a blood line through which blood is pumped from the patient's body to the dialyzer. After the blood passes through the dialyzer (artificial kidney), it returns to the patient's body through the blue adapter.

Arteriovenous Fistula

The gold standard for permanent access is a surgically created **arteriovenous fistula**, usually placed in the forearm (Marsh et al., 2022). The fistula is created by anastomosing (joining) an artery to a vein (Fig. 26-6). This diversion of arterial blood into the vein causes the vein to become enlarged, distended, and prominent, allowing the placement of large-gauge needles for dialysis treatment (Kallenbach, 2021), required for the rapid removal and return of blood. When performing dialysis, two large-bore (15- to 17-gauge) needles are inserted into the fistula; the arterial segment of the fistula is used for flow to the dialyzer and the venous segment for reinfusion of the dialyzed blood. The fistula should be given time to heal and mature (1 to 3 months after surgery); placing the fistula at least 6 months prior to the start

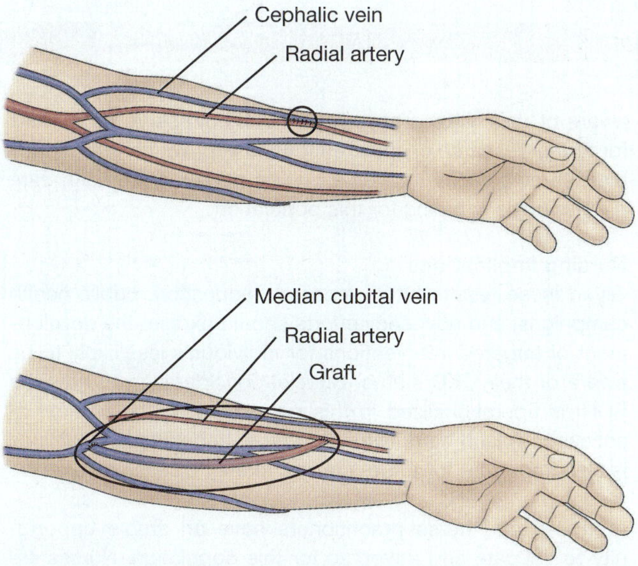

FIGURE 26-6 An internal arteriovenous fistula (top) is created by a side-to-side anastomosis of the artery and vein. A graft (bottom) can also be established between the artery and vein.

of anticipated hemodialysis is preferable. Every attempt is made to use a patient's nondominant arm for the AV fistula and the patient may be encouraged to exercise the arm to promote vessel maturation, such as squeezing a rubber ball, to help the access mature and to increase the size of these vessels (NKF, n.d.b).

Pearls for Practice

A patent fistula or graft has a thrill (vibration or buzz) when palpated gently with the fingers and has a bruit if auscultated with a stethoscope. The extremity should be pink and warm to the touch. No blood pressure measurements, IV infusions, or laboratory phlebotomy procedures are performed on the arm with the fistula or graft.

Arteriovenous Graft

A synthetic **arteriovenous graft** (AV graft) can be of biologic or synthetic material; however, synthetic grafts are used most frequently (Kallenbach, 2021). An AV graft can be created by subcutaneously anastomosing the graft material (e.g., polytetrafluoroethylene or Gortex) between an artery and vein (see Fig. 26-6). Usually, a graft is created in patients who do not have adequate vessels to create an internal AV fistula (Kallenbach, 2021). Infection and thrombosis are the most common complications of arteriovenous grafts. It is best to wait 3 to 6 weeks to access the graft which allows the patient's tissue to grow into the graft, with endothelium similar to the patient's vessels (Kallenbach, 2021).

Preventing complications is essential for patients with grafts and fistulas, however grafts may develop thrombosis, infection, aneurysm and stenosis, more frequently (Morton & Fontaine, 2018; Thrush et al., 2023). In addition, patients should be given information about the appearance of the access and potential changes in body image, which can trigger noncompliance or depression.

Pearls for Practice

The nurse is aware that for grafts and fistulas, firm pressure must be applied to stop any bleeding after needle removal at the end of the hemodialysis treatment (Kallenbach, 2021).

Pearls for Practice

Vascular access failure is the primary cause of morbidity in hemodialysis patients (Steward, 2020). Thus, protection of the dialysis access is a high priority.

Patient Education

The nurse teaches the patient with a fistula or graft to check for a thrill daily. The patient should feel a vibrating or buzzing sensation, over the site and should notify the health care provider or dialysis center if the quality has changed or is absent (Lough, 2022). The nurse assesses for both a thrill and a bruit, a swishing sound heard with the stethoscope, indicating proper function. Further teaching includes avoiding compression of the site; not permitting blood to be drawn, an IV to be inserted, or BP to be taken on the extremity with the dialysis access; not wearing tight clothing or carrying bags or pocketbooks on that side; and not lying on or sleeping on the area. The patient is taught to observe the site daily for redness, swelling, bleeding, drainage, heat, or pain and to report these promptly to the health care provider.

Clotting of the dialysis access increases the risk of life-threatening imbalance of fluids and electrolytes as lack of patency means dialysis cannot be performed. If this occurs, fibrinolysis, surgical thrombectomy, or revision is indicated.

Medical and Nursing Management

During dialysis, the patient, the dialyzer, and the dialysate bath require constant monitoring for complications. The dialysis nurse uses this time for assessing, monitoring, supporting, and educating the patient. The nurse may use this time to discuss the diet for patients with renal disorders or to reinforce fluid restriction, which may cause interdialytic weight gain (Box 26-7). The nurse palpates the fistula or graft for a thrill and auscultates for a bruit (swishing sound), indicating patency of the access.

Pharmacologic Therapy

Just as many medications are excreted wholly or in part by the kidneys, many medications can be removed from the blood during hemodialysis; therefore, dosage adjustments may be needed. Metabolites of drugs that are bound to protein are not removed during dialysis. Removal of other drug metabolites depends on the weight and size of the molecule.

BOX 26-7

Nursing Research

Bridging the Gap to Evidence-Based Practice

Iroegbu, C., Lewis L., & Matura, L. A. (2022). An integrative review: Chronic kidney disease awareness and the social determinants of health inequities. *Journal of Advanced Nursing*, *78*(4), 918–928. https://doi.org/10.1111/jan.15107.

Purpose

Chronic kidney disease is a common and prevalent condition in the United States. However, 90% of individuals with chronic kidney disease are unaware of their diagnosis. To summarize the empirical and theoretical literature to provide a comprehensive understanding of the social determinants of health inequities associated with CKD awareness. Social determinants of health inequities are underlying pathways that shape the health opportunities of individuals based on their social position.

Design

Integrative review (May 2020 through July 2020). Data sources included PubMed, sociologic abstracts, ScienceDirect, CINAHL, and Google Scholar. Quantitative, qualitative, and theoretical articles describing the association of social determinants of health inequities and chronic kidney disease awareness were included. A total of 19 articles were reviewed: two qualitative, one theoretical and 16 quantitative.

Findings

Findings from this review revealed that socioeconomic status, education, race, and gender are consistently associated with patient chronic kidney disease awareness specifically, individuals of higher socioeconomic status and educational attainment, Caucasian race and male gender are more likely to be aware of their CKD. These findings should serve as a basis for further research on interventions to improve chronic kidney disease awareness as well as guide nurses and health care professionals in caring for this population.

Nursing Implications

Given these results future research, education, public health campaigns, and advocacy efforts should explore the development of targeted interventions for individuals less likely to be aware of their CKD status. Special consideration to how the SDHI is operationalized in this population, in the context of access to health care, insurance type, and clinical guidelines is also important for future chronic kidney disease awareness research.

Nurses and nurse practitioners have an ample opportunity to educate and advocate for this population. Nurses are inclined to view the patient holistically, considering all aspects of the patient, not just their diagnosis. This review considers those aspects and proposes that they serve as major contributors to a patient's level of awareness. It is therefore our responsibility, as nurses, to take these findings and apply them as we derive nursing care plans and carry out individualized patient education. In addition, clinical nurses caring for this population should take initiative to advocate for better screening and routine monitoring of this population, particularly those less probably to be aware of their CKD in both inpatient and outpatient clinical settings.

Patients undergoing hemodialysis who require medications, for example, antibiotics, antiarrhythmic medications or cardiac glycosides, are monitored closely to ensure that the blood and tissue levels of these medications are maintained.

The nurse evaluates medications given close to or during dialysis that may promote complications. For example, if an antihypertensive agent is taken prior to dialysis, profound hypotension may result. However, withholding BP medications before dialysis should not be routine practice, but rather determined on a patient-by-patient basis since persistent HTN in seen in some patients during or after treatment (Kanbay et al., 2020; Wang et al., 2019). It is therefore best to confer with the nephrologist before routinely omitting antihypertensive agents prior to dialysis.

Despite recent medical advances, the survival of patients with DM on maintenance dialysis therapy (including hemodialysis and PD [which will be covered shortly]) is lower than that seen in nondiabetics with ESRD (Alalawi & Bashier, 2021). In general, insulin use should be encouraged in dialysis patients particularly those with properties closer to normal human physiology. Some oral agents should either be used cautiously or not at all in dialysis patients, thus demonstrating the complexity of medication administration and need for collaboration between the dialysis nurse, endocrinology, nephrology, and pharmacy. Medications that are taken once daily generally can be delayed until after the dialysis treatment.

Nutritional and Fluid Therapy

Diet is an important factor for patients on hemodialysis because of the effects of uremia. The patient usually requires restriction of sodium, potassium, phosphorous, and fluid. Protein intake is more liberal during hemodialysis but still restricted to about 1.2 ± 0.2 g/kg/day of ideal body weight, with the upper end of the range considered appropriate for protein-malnourished patients (Kallenbach, 2021); protein must be of high biologic quality and consist of the essential amino acids to prevent poor protein use and to maintain a positive nitrogen balance. Examples of foods high in biologic protein content are typically from animal sources and include eggs, meat, milk, cheese, poultry, and fish (Roth, 2019). Usually sodium is restricted to 2,000 mg/day; fluid restrictions include replacing insensible losses plus the 24-hour urine output (Norris & Tuan, 2020; Kallenbach, 2021). The goal for patients on hemodialysis is to keep their interdialytic weight gain under 1.5 kg (recall dialysis is typically performed every 2 to 3 days) (Kallenbach, 2021). In addition, water-soluble vitamins may need to be replaced (Roth, 2019).

Patients may experience social isolation if they feel there are few food choices available for their diet. When dining out, patients may choose food outside of the prescribed diet. Rather than appear impolite, patients will try to prioritize that which is least harmful, such as avoiding foods higher in potassium. Encouragement, empathy, and understanding with an open dialogue about such challenges are recommended. Applying a label of nonadherence to patients may promote feelings of guilt, defensiveness, and anger. Ignoring restrictions can cause life-threatening complications, such as hyperkalemia, HTN, and pulmonary edema. The nurse emphasizes the correlation between dietary indiscretion and the outcome, such as HTN or dyspnea, and promotes self-management of the disease.

Phosphate is limited to 1 g/day. Phosphorus absorption from meat sources is higher than that from plants. Phosphorus added to food, such as phosphoric acid in colas and highly processed foods are well absorbed and contribute to hyperphosphatemia. The word "phosphorus" by itself is not typically included on food labels; education on phosphorus foods is indicated. After hyperphosphatemia is controlled, calcium intake should be approximately 800 mg/day (Saglimbene et al., 2021).

Pearls for Practice

Abrupt weight gain is the most reliable clue of fluid volume excess (Norris & Tuan, 2020). The nurse will hear the term, "dry weight" in clinical practice. It is a term used for patients requiring RRT and refers to the ideal post dialysis weight (after the removal of all or most excess body fluid). Patients who are at dry weight usually have a normal BP whereas if the patient's weight is more than dry weight, the nurse recognizes that this suggests continued fluid volume excess and the patient may be hypertensive. Whereas, if the post dialysis weight is less than dry weight, the patient may be hypovolemic and at risk of hypotension (Kallenbach, 2021).

Providing Psychosocial Care

Often patients requiring long-term hemodialysis are concerned about the unpredictability of the illness and the disruption to their lives. Financial problems, difficulty working, waning sexual desire and impotence, poor-quality sleep, depression from chronic illness, and fear of dying may occur. Younger patients have concerns about marriage, having children, and the burden on their families. Dialysis treatments and restrictions in food and fluid intake often impose challenges to the patient and family. The time required for dialysis and provider visits as well as fatigue and chronic illness can create conflict, frustration, guilt, and depression. The nurse can encourage caregivers and patients to express concerns, anger, or negative feelings; if not expressed, anger may be directed inward and lead to depression, despair, or suicide. If anger is projected outward to other people, it may destroy already-threatened family relationships.

Depression is a common comorbidity in patients receiving dialysis, present in 25% to 68% of patients, that often goes unnoticed or undiagnosed in the CKD patient as the symptoms such as fatigue, lack of appetite, sleeping difficulties, and lack of concentration are misinterpreted as being caused by uremia rather than depression (Cole, 2018; Kallenbach, 2021). Inflammation, uremic toxins, sleep disturbances, pain, fatigue, anorexia, adverse medication effects, dietary constraints, changes in sexual function, role strain, and fear of death may contribute to the development of depression. Depression has been linked to nonadherence to dialysis treatment. Counseling, therapy, and pharmacologic treatment as well as deep slow breathing, music, yoga, acupuncture, and energy therapies may be beneficial (Cole, 2018; Kallenbach, 2021). The sense of loss that the patient experiences cannot be underestimated because every aspect of a "normal life" is disrupted.

Coping strategies include external/family support, emotion management strategies, reliance on faith or spirituality, and self-care practices (Ling et al., 2021). Some patients use denial to deal with the overwhelming array of medical issues. Labels such as "noncompliant" demonstrate a lack of respect for the impact of kidney failure and its treatment on the patient and family. Further, such labels do not encourage positive coping strategies. The term *adherence*, is more neutral and encourages the patient to share difficulties, such as indiscretion in fluid intake, so it can be addressed during dialysis.

Patients and their families should be encouraged to discuss end-of-life options. Studies reveal that between 6% and 49% of patients on hemodialysis have an advanced directive or living will, which leaves the patient's wishes to surrogates (Lupu et al., 2021). The American Nephrology Nurses Association (ANNA) Ethics Committee has developed an end-of-life position statement to foster the nurse's role in these discussions (ANNA, 2020).

Teaching Self-Care

The diagnosis of CKD and the need for dialysis may be overwhelming. Many patients with kidney failure have depressed mentation, a shortened attention span, a decreased level of concentration, and altered perception. Therefore, teaching should occur in brief, 10- to 15-minute sessions, with time added for clarification, repetition, reinforcement, and questions from the patient and family. The nurse needs to convey a nonjudgmental attitude to enable the patient and family to discuss feelings about those treatment options and the material taught.

One study indicated that higher levels of knowledge and greater degree of self-management were associated with significant improvement of function and well-being. Teaching materials at all reading levels are available on the NKF and National Institute of Health (NIH) websites (www.kidney.org, 2021).

Home Hemodialysis

Although most patients who require hemodialysis undergo the procedure in an outpatient setting, home hemodialysis is an option for some. Patients receiving home hemodialysis take less antihypertensive and phosphorus regulating medication, have fewer limits on diet and fluids, have higher-energy levels and improved quality of sleep, and have fewer/shorter hospitalizations. An improved QOL and sense of independent is found in research studies (Ibrahim & Chan, 2019). Home hemodialysis allows the patient to set the schedule, decreases travel and wait times at the dialysis center, and, if done slowly through the night, increases removal of more phosphorus and wastes. Thus, the patient may not require as much dietary restriction or antihypertensive therapy (Flagg, 2018; NIDDK, n.d.).

According to the NIDDK, a patient learns to perform treatments at the dialysis center, working with a dialysis nurse. Most people who do home hemodialysis have a family member, neighbor, or close friend who trains with them at the clinic. The dialysis center supplies the machine and equipment, such as dialysis solution, that will be delivered to the home once or twice a month. The training staff makes sure the patient is confident about performing each task before doing home hemodialysis. Someone from the clinic will be available to answer phone calls 24 hours a day. The health care team never forces a patient to use home hemodialysis because this treatment requires significant changes in the home and family. Home hemodialysis must be the patient's and family's decision. During training, the patient and caregiver learn to:

- Prepare equipment and supplies
- Place the needle in the vascular access
- Monitor the machine, check BP and pulse
- Keep records of the treatments
- Clean the equipment and the room where dialysis is done
- Order supplies

In addition, training includes how to prepare, operate, and disassemble the dialysis machine; maintain and clean the equipment; administer medications (e.g., heparin) into the machine lines; and handle emergency problems, such as hemodialysis dialyzer rupture, electrical or mechanical problems, hypotension, shock, and seizures.

Before home hemodialysis is initiated, resources are assessed in the home environment, household, and community. The home is surveyed to see if electrical outlets, plumbing facilities, and storage space are adequate. The home must have room for the HD machine, supplies, and, in some cases, a water purification machine. Modifications may be needed to enable the patient and caregiver to perform dialysis safely and to deal with emergencies.

Once home dialysis is initiated, the home care nurse visits periodically to evaluate adherence with the recommended techniques, to assess the patient for complications, to reinforce previous teaching, and to provide reassurance. The patient may visit the dialysis center monthly to see the nephrologist, dialysis nurse, and dietitian. Blood tests will be done to evaluate and adjust hemodialysis treatments.

Continuing Care

The health care team's goal in treating patients undergoing hemodialysis is to maximize the patients' vocational potential, functional status, and quality of life. Many patients can resume relatively normal lives, doing the things that are important to them: traveling, exercising, working, or actively participating in family activities. Outcome goals for renal rehabilitation include employment for those able to work, improved physical functioning of all patients, improved understanding about adaptation and options for living well, increased control over the effects of kidney disease and dialysis, and resumption of activities enjoyed before dialysis. Nurses must shift patient care away from the traditional paradigm of management by the health care team to one of self-management.

Gerontologic Considerations

Currently, older adults are commonly accepted for RRT programs if the intervention will increase their quality of life. Outcomes for hemodialysis or PD have not demonstrated one is superior to the other, rather, the mode of therapy should be individualized to the patient's underlying conditions and psychosocial factors. The patient's age should not guide treatment; nor should the patient's age should be the sole factor related to kidney transplant. Guidelines for diagnosis, risk stratification and treatment are similar to those for younger adults (Norris & Tuan, 2020).

Complications

Although hemodialysis can prolong life, it does not alter the natural course of the underlying kidney disease, nor does it completely replace kidney function. The patient is subject to a number of problems and complications. A leading cause of death among patients undergoing maintenance hemodialysis is atherosclerotic CVD. Disturbances of lipid metabolism (hypertriglyceridemia) appear to be accentuated by hemodialysis. Anemia and fatigue contribute to diminished physical and emotional well-being, lack of energy and drive, and apathy. Gastric ulcers and other GI problems result from the physiologic stress of chronic illness, medication, and related problems. Disturbed calcium metabolism leads to renal osteodystrophy that produces bone pain and fractures. Other problems include fluid overload associated with HF, malnutrition, infection, neuropathy, and pruritus.

A majority of people undergoing hemodialysis experience major sleep problems that further complicate their overall health status. Early-morning or late-afternoon dialysis may be a risk factor for developing sleep disturbances. Interventions, such as cooling the dialysate, may prevent temperature elevation, and limiting napping during dialysis may reduce sleep problems in people receiving hemodialysis. Some dialysis centers offer nighttime treatments, three nights a week, while the patient sleeps. These longer treatments mean days are free. There are less dietary changes, fluid allowance is closer to normal and an improved quality of life compared to standard hemodialysis schedules (NIDDK, 2018; NKF, n.d.a).

Other complications during dialysis may include:

- Hypotension and dizziness due to acute reduction in circulating intravascular volume and loss of homeostatic mechanisms.
- Dialysis disequilibrium, is more likely to occur in patients with AKI or those with very high BUN levels. It is thought to be related to cerebral edema (Kallenbach, 2021). Water shifts to the brain after urea removal, resulting in headache, nausea and vomiting, restlessness, decreased level of consciousness, and seizures (Kallenbach, 2021; Moron & Fontaine, 2018).
- Painful muscle cramping as a result of excess fluid removal which decreases intravascular volume and decreases muscle perfusion.
- Exsanguination if blood lines separate or dialysis needles become dislodged.
- Arrhythmias resulting from changes in electrolytes and pH or from removal of antiarrhythmia medications during dialysis.
- Angina from vascular changes (intimal and medial thickening and calcification), and arterial wall stiffening.
- Air embolism, a rare circumstance, but can occur if air enters the vascular system.
- Chest pain, particularly in patients with anemia or arteriosclerotic heart disease.

Pearls for Practice: Pathophysiology

Calciphylaxis (also known as calcific uremic arteriolopathy), is a rare but potentially life-threatening complication that may occur in patients with ESKD on maintenance dialysis. The cause is poorly understood, but contributing factors seem to be hypercalcemia, hyperphosphatemia, and hyperparathyroidism however "many patients have normal values of serum calcium, phosphorus, and parathyroid hormone, making any correlation impossible" (Chiriac et al., 2020, p. 545). Insoluble calcium phosphate crystals develop when the serum phosphorus and calcium rise and the crystals deposit in the soft tissues of the body (lungs, joints, heart valves, cornea, skin). The soft tissue calcifications usually affect the trunk and lower extremities but can also occur in the breast, thigh, abdomen, shoulder, or buttocks. Calciphylaxis generally begins as painful, purplish skin lesions that later form nodules, ulcerate, and ultimately form an eschar with tissue necrosis beneath the lesion (due to diminished blood flow). A high mortality rate occurs when ulcerations develop, with death related to sepsis from infected wounds or skin lesions. Treatment can include hyperbaric therapy, debridement, wound care, antibiotic therapy, lowering the calcium and phosphate levels, and a chelation agent may be used in the dialysis treatment. If the nurse notices these nodules, alerting the providers is important to decrease the morbidity and mortality associated with this complication (Kallenbach, 2021).

ADDITIONAL RENAL REPLACEMENT THERAPIES

Continuous RRT is used with patients at risk for hemodynamic instability such as hypotension, or in those who cannot tolerate the rapid fluid shifts that may occur with hemodialysis (Kallenbach, 2021; Morton & Fontaine, 2018). CRRT (Fig. 26-7) circulates venous blood outside the body through a filter similar to the hemodialysis filter. A pump is used to assist blood flow and the types of CRRT include continuous venovenous hemofiltration (CVVH), continuous venovenous hemofiltration with dialysis (CVVHD), and continuous venovenous hemodiafiltration (CVVHDF). Slow, continuous hemofiltration (SCUF) is performed primarily to remove fluid (Kallenbach, 2021; Morton & Fontaine, 2018). Although the principles of CRRT are the same, the procedures are limited to the critical care setting for the treatment of AKI.

Pearls for Practice

It is important to secure the central venous catheter used for CRRT to prevent dislodgement. The catheter may be sutured and covered with secure dressing (Lough, 2022; Morton & Fontaine, 2018).

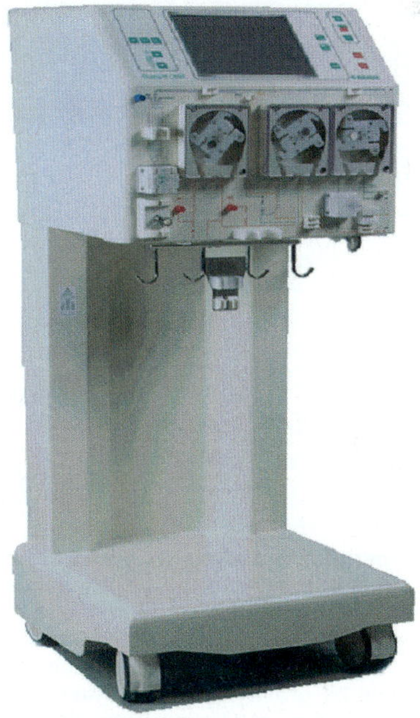

FIGURE 26-7 **Diapact CRRT system.**

PERITONEAL DIALYSIS

The goals of PD are to remove toxic substances and metabolic wastes and to reestablish normal balance of fluids and electrolytes. PD may be performed chronically or for patients who are acutely ill. Patients who are unable or unwilling to undergo hemodialysis or renal transplantation, or who do not have access to the bloodstream, can benefit from PD. In addition, patients who do not tolerate the rapid changes in fluids, electrolytes, and metabolism that occur during hemodialysis experience fewer of these problems with the slower rate of PD.

PD can promote patient independence as it is a self-managed modality. There is increased flexibility in timing of treatments and no travel to a dialysis center, allowing for more personal and family time. PD may preserve residual renal function better than hemodialysis (George, 2019a).

During PD, the thin, serous peritoneal membrane that covers the abdominal organs and lines the abdominal wall serves as the semipermeable or dialyzing membrane. Sterile dialysate fluid is introduced into the peritoneal cavity through a peritoneal or Tenckhoff catheter (Fig. 26-8) with a Dacron cuff to prevent infection. Diffusion across the semipermeable membrane removes urea, creatinine and metabolic end products normally excreted by the kidneys. Excess fluid is removed through osmosis as water moves from an area of lower particle concentration in the patient's blood to an area of higher concentration across a semipermeable membrane into the dialysate. Dialysis solutions are available in concentrations of 1.5%, 2.5%, and 4.25% dextrose. This concentration gradient for fluid removal is created by varying concentrations of glucose; the higher the dextrose concentration, the greater the osmotic gradient which will move more fluid into the abdominal cavity. PD is a slower process than hemodialysis; therefore, it takes longer to reach equilibrium (Lough, 2022; Morton & Fontaine, 2018). At home, patients generally have four peritoneal dialysate exchanges per day or use an automated PD exchange overnight when sleeping (Lough, 2022).

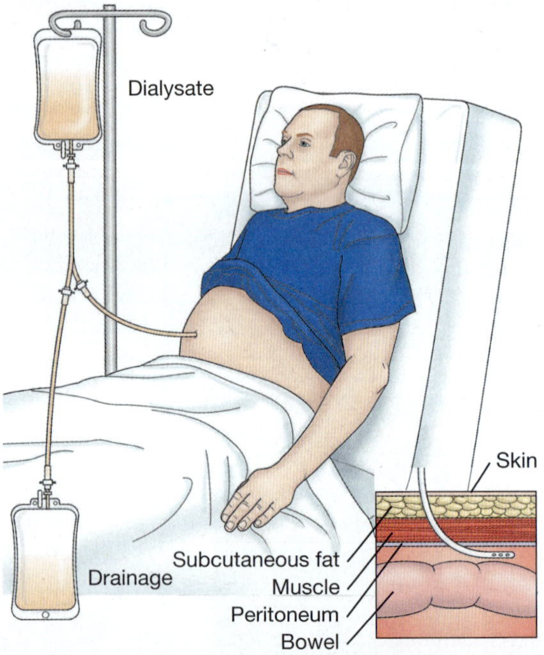

FIGURE 26-8 In peritoneal dialysis (PD) and in acute intermittent PD, dialysate is infused into the peritoneal cavity by gravity, after which the clamp on the infusion line is closed. After a dwell time (when the dialysate is in the peritoneal cavity), the drainage tube is unclamped and the fluid drains from the peritoneal cavity, again by gravity. A new container of dialysate is infused as soon as drainage is complete. The duration of the dwell time depends on the type of PD.

Pearls for Practice

The original postsurgical dressing in kept in place for 5 to 7 days after catheter placement, removing it only in the case of frank bleeding or drainage; trained dialysis personnel should be the first to uncover the original catheter dressing and a mask should always be worn and aseptic technique used while inspecting the exit site (Kallenbach, 2021).

Procedure

Preparing the Patient

Insertion of the peritoneal catheter may be performed at the bedside or in the operating room, depending on acuity of the patient. A broad-spectrum antibiotic may be administered prior to the procedure to prevent postoperative infection. The patient is encouraged to empty the bladder and bowel prior to catheter insertion to reduce the risk of puncturing internal organs. Baseline vital signs, weight, and serum electrolyte levels are recorded. The nurse also assesses the patient's anxiety about the procedure and provides support and instruction.

The catheters used for long-term PD (i.e., Tenckhoff) usually are made of silicone and are radiopaque to permit visualization on x-ray. The catheter has two cuffs, which stabilize the catheter, limit movement, prevent leaks, and provide a barrier against microorganisms. One cuff is placed just distal to the peritoneum, and the other cuff is placed subcutaneously. The subcutaneous tunnel further protects against bacterial infection (Lough, 2022; Morton & Fontaine, 2018) (Fig. 26-9). Unlike the central venous hemodialysis catheter discussed earlier, which can be used immediately after placement, the tissue around the PD catheter requires approximately 2 weeks to form a tight seal to avoid PD fluid leakage. When an "urgent start" is needed (soon after catheter placement), low-volume exchanges with the patient in the supine position to minimize fluid leakage are suggested (Lew, 2021).

Preparing the Equipment

The nurse verifies the physician orders, review the patient's latest laboratory values, inform the patient of the treatment, and gathers necessary supplies. The nurse validates the strength of the prescribed solution (1.5%, 2.5%, or 4.25%), the expiration date of dialysate, the amount of the prescribed solution and checks to ensure the bag is free from leaks and discoloration.

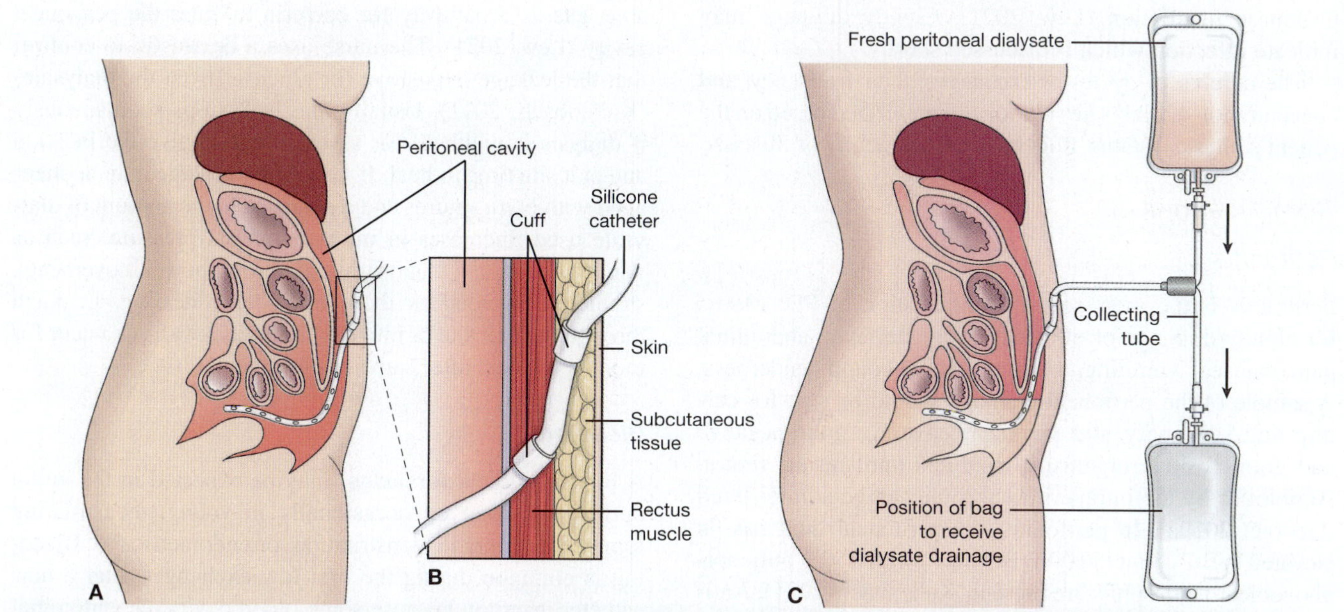

FIGURE 26-9 **Continuous ambulatory peritoneal dialysis. A. The peritoneal catheter is implanted through the abdominal wall. B. Dacron cuffs and a subcutaneous tunnel provide protection against bacterial infection. C. Dialysate flows by gravity through the peritoneal catheter into the peritoneal cavity. After a prescribed period of time, the fluid is drained by gravity, measured and discarded. The new solution is infused into the peritoneal cavity until the next drainage period. Dialysis continues on a 24-hour-a-day basis during which the patient is free to move around and engage in their usual activities.**

Aseptic technique is imperative during PD to prevent peritonitis. The nurse assembles the equipment, including the dialysate and any medications to be added. Heparin may be added to prevent occlusion of the peritoneal catheter, potassium chloride to prevent hypokalemia, and antibiotics to prevent or treat **peritonitis**. The osmotic agent in the dialysate is glucose, which may be absorbed; therefore, regular insulin may be added. Dextrose free, cornstarch-based solutions are available, for example, icodextrin (Kallenbach, 2021).

Pearls for Practice

It is important to remember that peritoneal solutions contain varying concentrations of glucose. Because 30% to 40% of patients receiving PD have diabetes, glucose monitoring is critical.

Before medications are added, the dialysate is warmed to approximate body temperature or the temperature dictated by institutional policy. Warming prevents abdominal discomfort and dilates the vessels of the peritoneum to increase urea clearance. Dry heating using a device for this purpose or per institutional policy is recommended. The dialysate should ***NOT*** be warmed using a microwave because of uneven heating and variations of microwaves; this prevents the danger of burning the peritoneum (Chechamma, 2019b). The nurse primes the PD tubing with the dialysate to prevent air from entering the peritoneal cavity.

Pearls for Practice

The length of time the solution remains in the peritoneal cavity, called the dwell time, and the solution composition affect the outcome. The dwell time affects the amount of fluid removed from the peritoneal capillaries, although a longer dwell time does not remove proportionately more fluid because of osmotic equilibration across the membranes (Lough, 2022).

Performing the Exchange

PD involves a series of exchanges or cycles. An exchange is defined as the infusion, dwell, and drainage of the dialysate. This cycle is repeated throughout the course of the dialysis. The dialysate is infused by gravity into the peritoneal cavity. Typically, 2 L of dialysate inflows over a period of about 5 to 10 minutes. The prescribed dwell, or equilibration time, allows both diffusion and osmosis to occur. At the end of the dwell time, the drainage portion of the exchange begins. The solution drains from the peritoneal cavity by gravity through a closed, sterile system. Usually drainage is completed within 10 to 20 minutes. The effluent or drainage fluid is normally clear, colorless, or straw-colored. Blood-tinged drainage may be seen in the first few exchanges. The nurse documents the strength of dialysate used, total amount returned, clarity and color of the effluent at the end of treatment. Most institutions have PD flowsheets that also include vital signs and patients' response to the treatment. It is important to observe for blood clots and/or fibrin strands that could obstruct the catheter and cause a slowing of the inflow and outflow of dialysate (George, 2019b; Lew, 2021). Management of catheter obstruction may include manual compression of the dialysis tubing and intraperitoneal (IP) heparin infusion, or tissue-type plasminogen activator (t-PA) urokinase instillation (Lew, 2021). Cloudy drainage may indicate infection which is discussed shortly.

The number of cycles or exchanges, their frequency, and concentration of dialysate solution are prescribed based on the patient's physical status, fluid balance, and acuity of illness.

Complications

Peritonitis

Peritonitis is the most serious complication of PD. Assess for cloudy drainage or effluent, low-grade fever, abdominal pain, nausea, vomiting, malaise, and rebound tenderness. A sample of the peritoneal drainage should be sent for culture and sensitivity and treatment covering gram-negative and gram-positive organisms instituted until results return. Antibiotics by the intraperitoneal route can be administered (George, 2019a). In peritonitis, the peritoneal fluid has an elevated WBC count (>100 WBC/mm^3) with >50% polymorphonuclear neutrophils are present (Kallenbach, 2021). Antimicrobial therapy is initiated and adjusted based on culture and sensitivity of the peritoneal fluid. Antimicrobial therapy may be administered intravenously and/or added to the dialysate. Consider special cultures for fungal infections if the patient does not improve in 3 days (George, 2019, p. 233).

Most episodes of peritonitis are due to touch contamination. The nurse should avoid breaking aseptic technique, accidentally disconnecting the PD catheter from the transfer set, or reusing the minicap. To prevent infection, a sign reading "STOP – Procedure in Progress" is placed on the patient's door and the door remains closed during the procedure. Any room fan should be turned off until the procedure is complete and live flowers or plants prohibited due to the potential presence of insects or bacteria (George, 2019b). Masks should be worn during dressing changes to avoid contamination with oral or nasal flora, and the catheter should be handled gently to minimize manipulation which may cause trauma to the exit site and may lead to infection (Kallenbach, 2021). The catheter should be secured to the skin to avoid trauma from accidental tugging. A nonocclusive dressing is recommended because drainage is wicked away from the insertion incision and exit site rather than trapped creating moisture which is associated with exit site infections (Crabtree et al., 2019; Payton & Kennedy, 2021).

Pearls for Practice

To detect rebound tenderness, press one hand firmly into the abdominal wall and quickly withdraw the hand. Rebound tenderness exists when pain occurs upon removal and is associated with inflammation of the peritoneal cavity. Other disorders should be considered as an etiology for a patient's symptoms along with peritonitis.

Leakage

The incidence of dialysate leakage around the catheter site ranges from 0% to 40%, and must be corrected because the area acts as a pathway for bacteria to enter the peritoneal cavity (Lew, 2021). The nurse uses a dextrostix to confirm that the leakage is positive for glucose (from the dialysate) (Kallenbach, 2021). Usually, the leak stops spontaneously if dialysis is withheld for several days to give the incision and exit site time to heal. If necessary, leakage may be managed with extra sutures and a decrease in the amount of dialysate used. Increases in intra-abdominal pressure, such as vomiting, coughing, and straining during bowel movements, should be avoided as these may delay healing. Leakage through the exit site or into the abdominal wall can occur for months or years after catheter placement.

Bleeding

A bloody effluent (drainage) may be expected in the initial outflow or observed occasionally in young, menstruating females (retrograde menstruation, or endometriosis). Bleeding is common during the first few exchanges after a new catheter insertion because some blood enters the abdominal cavity following insertion. During menstruation, the hypertonic fluid pulls blood from the uterus, through the opening in the fallopian tubes, into the peritoneal cavity. Some patients have had bloody effluent from minor trauma. Invariably, bleeding stops in 1 to 2 days and requires no specific intervention. More frequent exchanges during this time may be necessary to prevent blood clots from obstructing the catheter. Gross bleeding at any time indicates a more serious problem and must be investigated immediately.

Incomplete Recovery of Fluid

If the fluid drains slowly or the volume drained is less than the amount inserted, the nurse turns the patient from side to side, elevates the head of the bed, or repositions the patient to facilitate drainage. Complete emptying of the peritoneal cavity during the drain phase is extremely important to ensure the next treatment starts with fresh solution. Mixing new solution with retained fluid in the peritoneum reduces solution potency and results in less effective treatment (George, 2019a).

The nurse should ensure the patient empties the colon through regular bowel movements as the tip of the catheter may come up against the bowel, preventing adequate drainage (George, 2019b). The nurse should not attempt to reposition the catheter.

Another measure to promote drainage includes checking the patency of the catheter by inspecting for kinks, closed clamps, or an air lock. The nurse must ensure that the PD catheter remains secure and that the dressing remains dry.

Pearls for Practice

The most common reason for outflow delay or failure to drain dialysate is constipation, which typically is treated with oral laxatives or an enema. Fluid or diet restrictions as well as the medications, such as phosphate binders,

increase the risk of constipation for patients on PD. After constipation is resolved, the nurse should educate the patient about monitoring their bowel pattern and having an established bowel regimen.

Other Complications

Exit site infections are a potential complication. The site must be cleansed daily and after every shower, for patients managing PD at home. The nurse teaches the patient to assess for redness, swelling, tenderness, hyperthermia, open areas, exudate, crusting, or purulent drainage to initiate timely intervention. Using prophylactic antibiotic ointment is part of successful maintenance of PD (Chechamma, 2019). *Staphylococcus aureus* and *Pseudomonas aeruginosa* are the main bacteria that cause exit site infections. Specific antibiotics for exit site care should match the sensitivity of the organism cultured. Some experts cited improvement with exit site infections by treating *S. aureus* in the nares twice a day for 7 days out of every month, as well as daily antibiotic cream to the exit site for patients with positive nasal cultures (Bridger, 2019). The patient and family need to be educated to avoid creams and lotions around exit site (Lough, 2022).

If patients complain of pain when the dialysate is entering the peritoneum, it may be related to peritoneal catheter migration, rapid infusion of the dialysate, hyperosmolarity of the dialysate (higher glucose solution, ex. 4.25%), or acidity of the dialysate. Interventions include slowing the infusion of the dialysate and may include the addition of $NaHCO_3$ to increase pH of the dialysate; the use of lidocaine (anesthetic) and may include surgical revision or replacement of the catheter (Kallenbach, 2021).

Other complications that may occur with long-term PD include abdominal hernias (incisional, inguinal, diaphragmatic, and umbilical) because of chronically increased intra-abdominal pressures; previous abdominal surgery is also a risk factor for hernia or intestinal obstruction secondary to adhesions.

Approaches to Peritoneal Dialysis

PD can be performed using several different approaches: acute continuous or intermittent PD, CAPD, and continuous cycler PD (CCPD).

Continuous Ambulatory Peritoneal Dialysis

CAPD works on the same principles as other forms of PD; however, there are fewer extreme fluctuations in the patient's laboratory values with CAPD than with intermittent PD or hemodialysis because dialysis is constantly in progress. CAPD is performed at home by the patient or a trained caregiver; the procedure allows the patient reasonable freedom and control of daily activities (Box 26-8).

BOX 26-8

Assessing Suitability for Continuous Ambulatory Peritoneal Dialysis (CAPD)

Although CAPD is not suitable for all patients with kidney failure, it is a viable therapy for those who can perform self-care and exchanges and who can fit therapy into their own routines. Often, patients report having more energy and feeling healthier once they begin CAPD. Nurses can be instrumental in helping patients with kidney failure find the dialysis therapy that best suits their lifestyle. Those considering CAPD need to investigate the advantages and disadvantages along with the indications and contraindications for this form of therapy.

Advantages

- Freedom from a dialysis machine
- Control over daily activities
- Less dietary restrictions, increased fluid intake, higher serum Hct values, improved BP control, venipunctures are avoided, and gains in a sense of well-being

Disadvantages

- Continuous dialysis 24 hours a day, 7 days a week

Indications

- Patient's willingness, motivation, and ability to perform dialysis at home
- Strong family or community support system (essential for success), particularly if the patient is an older adult
- Special problems with long-term hemodialysis, such as dysfunctional or failing vascular access devices, excessive thirst, severe HTN, postdialysis headaches, and severe anemia requiring frequent transfusion
- Interim therapy while awaiting kidney transplantation
- Kidney failure secondary to diabetes because HTN, uremia, and hyperglycemia are easier to manage with CAPD than with hemodialysis

Contraindications

- Adhesions from previous surgery (adhesions reduce clearance of solutes) or systemic inflammatory disease
- Chronic backache and pre-existing disc disease, which could be aggravated by the pressure of dialysis fluid in the abdomen
- Risk of complications, for example, in patients receiving immunosuppressive medications, which impede healing of the catheter site, and in patients with a colostomy, ileostomy, nephrostomy, or ileal conduit because of the risk of peritonitis. The risk for complications is not an absolute contraindication for CAPD therapy but must be taken into consideration
- Diverticulitis, because CAPD has been associated with rupture of the diverticulum
- Severe arthritis or poor hand strength, necessitating assistance in performing the exchange; however, patients who are blind or partially blind and those with other physical limitations can learn to perform CAPD

BOX 26-9

Nursing Management for Peritoneal Dialysis

Caring for the Catheter Site

To reduce the risk of peritonitis in the patient using peritoneal dialysis (PD), use meticulous care to avoid contaminating the catheter, fluid, or tubing and to avoid accidentally disconnecting the catheter from the tubing. Avoid catheter manipulation, and provide meticulous care of the catheter entry site, using a standardized protocol. The patient and other caregivers who are present wear a mask and use strict aseptic technique for preparation of the dialysate and dressing changes.

The nurse takes every opportunity to assess the patient's catheter care technique and offers feedback or corrections to prevent infections. Teach the patient to perform routine catheter site care as recommended, typically daily to three or four times weekly. The patient may perform this care during showering or bathing, using liquid soap. Emphasize that the exit site should not be submerged in (bath) water. During care, both nurse and patient need to ensure that the catheter remains secure, avoiding tension and trauma. The patient may wear a gauze or semi-transparent dressing over the exit site.

Meeting Psychosocial Needs

In addition to the complications of PD previously described, patients who elect continuous ambulatory peritoneal dialysis (CAPD) may experience altered body image because of the abdominal catheter and the bag and tubing. Waist size may increase 1–2 in (or more) with fluid in the abdomen, affecting clothing selection. The patient may feel "fat." Body image may be so altered that patients do not want to look at or care for the catheter for days or weeks. The nurse may arrange for the patient to talk with other patients who have adapted well to CAPD. Although some patients think of the catheter positively, as a life-sustaining device—others feel they are doing exchanges all day long and have no free time, particularly in the beginning. They may experience depression because they feel overwhelmed with the responsibility of self-care.

Patients undergoing CAPD also may experience sexual patterns and/or sexual dysfunction. The patient and partner may be reluctant to engage in sexual activities, in part because psychologically, the catheter is "in the way" of sexual performance. The peritoneal catheter, drainage bag, and about 2 L of dialysate may interfere with the patient's body image as well. Although these problems may resolve with time, some problems may warrant special counseling. Questions by the nurse about concerns related to sexuality and sexual function often provide the patient with a welcome opportunity to discuss these issues and provide a first step toward their resolution.

Teaching Patients Self-Care

Patients are taught to perform PD according to their own learning ability and knowledge level and are given only as much information at one time as they can handle without feeling uncomfortable or becoming overwhelmed.

Because protein loss is higher with PD than with hemodialysis, the patient is instructed to eat a well-balanced diet that is slightly more liberal in protein. It is important to encourage the patient to increase their daily fiber intake to prevent constipation, which can impede inflow and outflow of dialysate. Due to the glucose content of the dialysate, weight gain can occur. Should this occur, patients may be instructed to limit carbohydrate intake to avoid excessive weight gain. Restrictions on potassium, sodium, and fluids are more liberal. Patients commonly lose about 2–3 L of fluid over and above the volume of dialysate infused into the abdomen during a 24-hour period, permitting a more normal fluid intake.

Continuing Care

The nurse validates that strict aseptic technique is being followed. The patient is instructed to not shower for approximately 3–6 weeks, until the PD catheter site is healed and permission is given by the health care provider. Blood chemistry values are followed closely to make certain the therapy is adequate for the patient. The home care nurse assesses the home environment and suggests modifications to accommodate the equipment and facilities needed to carry out CAPD. Additional assessments include monitoring for changes related to kidney disease, complications such as peritonitis, and treatment-related problems such as heart failure, inadequate drainage, and weight gain or loss. The nurse continues to reinforce and clarify teaching about kidney failure and kidney disease while assessing the patient's and family's progress in coping with the procedure.

The patient performs exchanges several times a day, 24 hours a day, 7 days a week, at intervals scheduled throughout the day. The dialysate dwells for the prescribed period of time; 4 to 6 hours is common. The patient is free to ambulate and participate in activities of daily living. At the end of the dwell time, the dialysate is drained from the peritoneal cavity into the empty sterile bag. Box 26-9 provides nursing management for CAPD.

Continuous Cyclic Peritoneal Dialysis

CCPD combines overnight intermittent PD with a prolonged dwell time during the day. The peritoneal catheter is connected to a cycler machine every evening, providing three to five exchanges overnight. Upon arising, the patient infuses 1.5 to 2.5 L of fresh dialysate, then caps off the catheter. This dialysate remains in the abdominal cavity until the tubing is reattached to the cycler at bedtime.

Because there are fewer opportunities for contamination with bag changes and tubing disconnections, CCPD has a lower rate of infection than other forms of PD. It also frees the patient from exchanges during the day, allowing the patient to engage more freely in work and activities of daily living.

KIDNEY TRANSPLANTATION

Kidney transplantation is the optimal treatment for improving survival and quality of life for patients with ESKD. Kidney

BOX 26-10
Kidney Donation

An inadequate number of donor kidneys remain the greatest limitation to treating patients with end-stage kidney disease successfully. For those interested in donating a kidney, the National Kidney Foundation provides written information describing the organ donation program and a card specifying the organs to be donated in the event of death.

The organ donation card is signed by the donor and two witnesses and should be carried by the donor at all times. Procurement of an adequate number of kidneys for potential recipients is still a major problem despite national legislation that requires relatives of deceased patients or patients declared brain-dead to be asked if they would consider organ donation.

In some states in the United States, drivers can indicate their desire to be organ donors on their driver's license, application or renewal.

transplantation involves transplanting a kidney from a living donor or heartbeat-only donor (one who has been pronounced brain dead but whose cardiopulmonary system is maintained artificially) to a recipient who has ESKD (Box 26-10). Traditionally, kidney transplant donors had been blood relatives; however, living donor kidney transplant (LDKT) between spouses, friends, and those on organ registries may be performed with comparable outcomes. Either donor kidney may be transplanted, however the left is preferred as the left renal vein is longer than the right which tends to make anastomosis technically easier to perform (Lam et al., 2020).

Patients choose kidney transplantation for various reasons, including the desire to no longer need dialysis, an improvement in their sense of well-being and the wish to lead a more normal life. In addition, the cost of maintaining a successful transplantation is one third the cost of dialysis treatment. Patients on dialysis have an adjusted all-cause mortality rate that is 6.5 to 7.4 times higher than that of the general population; the rate is 1.1 to 1.6 times higher for transplant patients (www.kidneyfund.org).

Depending on the cause and symptoms of kidney failure, occasionally the removal of the diseased kidneys may be performed (nephrectomy) before transplantation of the donor kidney is placed in the patient's iliac fossa (either side may be used). The renal artery of the donor is anastomosed to the hypogastric, renal, or iliac artery of the recipient. The ureter of the newly transplanted kidney is anastomosed to the ureter of the recipient, and the renal vein is anastomosed to the renal vein of the recipient (Fig. 26-10).

Barriers to Transplant

There are currently over 100,000 patients waiting for a kidney transplant (Kallenbach, 2021). Living donor kidney transplantation is optimal (Thongprayoon, 2020), however the current donor pool utilization does not meet the demand. Some centers are using expanded-criteria donors, such as those over 60 years or with two critical risk factors, to meet this need with positive outcomes. Another alternative approach is to use marginal kidneys not suitable for a single kidney transplant owing to the insufficient nephron mass from older donors, and which otherwise would have been discarded. For example, for adult deceased donor kidneys >60% are ultimately not transplanted. This approach is termed dual kidney transplant, where two marginal kidneys are transplanted. The dual kidney transplant may reduce organ discard and optimize the use of kidneys from marginal deceased donor kidneys (Stratta et al., 2022).

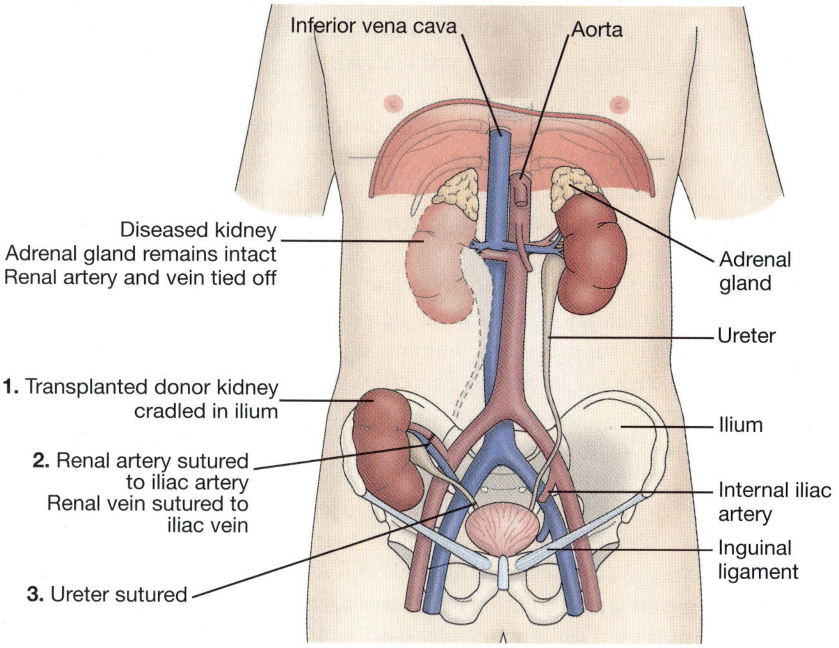

FIGURE 26-10 **Kidney transplantation: (*1*) The diseased kidney may be removed and the renal artery and vein tied off. (*2*) The transplanted kidney is placed in the iliac fossa. (*3*) The renal artery of the donated kidney is sutured to the iliac artery, and the renal vein is sutured to the iliac vein. (*4*) The ureter of the donated kidney is sutured to the bladder or to the patient's ureter.**

The average waiting time to receive a first kidney transplant is 3.6 years (NKF, 2021). In 2020, 22,827 kidney transplants took place with over 5,700 of recipients receiving live donor kidneys (CDC). The average life expectancy for patient's receiving dialysis is 5 years, compared to 8 to 12 years for a deceased donor kidney transplant and 8 to 20 years for a living donor kidney transplant recipient.

Healthy People 2030 calls to increase the proportion of patients with kidney failure who receive a transplant within 3 years. A second goal is to increase kidney donation rates (ODPHP, n.d.). Unfortunately, the donor pool is unable to meet the current demands for those awaiting transplant. See Box 26-10 regarding kidney donation. Researchers are working to develop engineered kidney tissues and organoids (artificially grown mass of cells or tissue that resembles an organ). The laboratory protocols for growing organoids in culture have made impressive strides in producing tissue structures resembling the kidney although kidney development and maturation has not been fully replicated. Work continues using stem cells, scaffolding and chips to create 3D working models (NIDDK, 2020).

Medical and Nursing Management

Preoperative Management

Preoperative management goals include bringing the patient's metabolic state to a level as close to normal as possible, making sure that the patient is free of infection, and preparing the patient for surgery and the postoperative course. Preoperatively, immunosuppressant medication is initiated prior to the transplant to prevent hyperacute, short (acute) and long-term (chronic) rejection of the new kidney.

A complete physical examination is performed to detect and treat any conditions that could cause complications after transplantation. The rules of compatibility that apply to blood transfusion apply to kidney transplant. ABO compatibility, histocompatibility testing are conducted to determine compatibility of the tissues and cells of the donor and recipient. Other diagnostic tests are completed to identify conditions requiring treatment before transplantation. The lower urinary tract is studied to assess bladder neck function and to detect urethral reflux.

The patient must be free of infection and cancers at the time of renal transplantation because medications to prevent transplant rejection suppress the immune response, leaving the patient at risk for infection. Therefore, the patient is evaluated and treated for any infections, including gingival (gum) disease and dental caries.

A psychosocial evaluation is conducted to assess the patient's ability to adjust to the transplant, coping styles, social history, social support available, and financial resources. The nurse assesses for a history of psychiatric illness because psychiatric conditions may be exacerbated by the corticosteroids used for immunosuppression. If a dialysis routine has been established, hemodialysis is performed the day before the scheduled transplantation procedure to optimize the patient's physical status.

The nursing aspects of preoperative care for the patient undergoing renal transplant are similar to those for patients undergoing other types of elective abdominal surgery. Preoperative teaching addresses postoperative pulmonary hygiene, pain management options, dietary restrictions, IV and arterial lines, tubes such as an indwelling catheter and possibly a nasogastric tube, and early ambulation.

Most patients have been on dialysis for months or years before transplantation. Many have waited months to years for a kidney transplant and are anxious about the surgery, possible rejection, and the need to return to dialysis. Helping the patient to deal with these concerns is part of the nurse's role in preoperative management as is teaching the patient about what to expect after surgery. A plan of nursing care for a patient undergoing kidney surgery is available online at http://thepoint.lww.com/Honan3e.

Postoperative Management

The goal of care is to maintain homeostasis until the transplanted kidney is functioning well. The patient whose transplanted kidney functions immediately has a more favorable prognosis than does the patient whose transplanted kidney does not. Nursing care involves the monitoring of surgical wounds, care of drains (if placed), pain management, monitoring the function of the graft, administration of immunosuppressive medication, as well as general postoperative concerns (vital signs, I&O, prevention of atelectasis, infection and venous thromboembolism).

Antirejection Medication

The survival of a transplanted kidney depends on the ability to prevent the body's immune response to the transplanted kidney. To overcome or minimize the body's defense mechanism, immunosuppressive agents, in combination, are administered. There are four classes of medications: corticosteroids, calcineurin inhibitors (CNIs), antiproliferative agents, and mammalian target of rapamycin (mTOR) inhibitors. Corticosteroids are initially part of the immunosuppression regimen. CNIs include cyclosporine or tacrolimus; their mechanism and immunosuppression actions are primarily due to their suppression of T cells. Tacrolimus is similar to cyclosporine, but more potent, allowing the doses used to be much smaller. In most cases, these drugs are used interchangeably rather than in combination (Kallenbach, 2021). Alternative options are considered in pregnancy and lactation due to serious adverse effects of cyclosporine on the fetus or neonate (Burcham & Rosenthal, 2019; Karch, 2020); whereas the risk versus benefit should be considered in pregnancy or with lactation with tacrolimus.

The antiproliferative agent, mycophenolate mofetil, appears to have an improved immunosuppressive effect, including action against B lymphocytes (Karch, 2020), making this medication the only immunosuppressant that may treat chronic rejection (Kallenbach, 2021). It is contraindicated in pregnancy due to teratogenicity and spontaneous abortion. The mTOR inhibitors include sirolimus, which inhibits T-lymphocyte activation and proliferation as well as antibody production, making it unique. Initially this medication is taken in combination with cyclosporine and steroids. Later, cyclosporine can be withdrawn in some patients at a low immunologic risk while the dose of sirolimus is increased. This medication can be used for chronic rejection and is not nephrotoxic (Kallenbach, 2021).

Several monoclonal antibodies have been developed for use in transplantation. This class of medication is either humanized or chimeric antibodies; in other words, the majority of the antibody molecule is from a partial human immunoglobulin, with only a small portion from a murine antibody molecule. This humanization makes it less likely to be recognized as a foreign protein, thus minimizing the first-dose side effects and yielding a prolonged drug half-life. These drugs prevent rejection by interfering with binding of interleukin-2 to lymphocytes (e.g., basiliximab), and are administered intravenously after transplantation (Kallenbach, 2021).

Belatacept, a selective T-cell costimulation blocker, is indicated for prophylaxis of kidney rejection in adult patients that is used in combination with basiliximab, mycophenolate mofetil, and corticosteroids. This agent has been shown to prolong graft survival (Karch, 2020). Given, the burgeoning area of pharmacologic research, the nurse must continue to learn about new treatment options for our patients.

The side effects and risks associated with these medications are numerous and include nephrotoxicity, leukopenia (decreased WBC), iatrogenic Cushing syndrome, adrenal insufficiency, myopathy, sodium and water retention, hyperlipidemia, headache, tremor, and several types of cancers, as well as risk for infection (Burcham & Rosenthal, 2019). In addition, nonimmunologic complications of bone diseases (osteoporosis), cataracts, DM, hyperlipidemia, HTN, and gastrointestinal complications (e.g., ulcers, hyperuricemia, and hyperkalemia) are potential complications (Kallenbach, 2021). Obesity, as well as hirsutism and gingival hyperplasia, may also occur.

While corticosteroids are tapered or discontinued gradually over several weeks to months the nurse reinforces that some form of immunosuppressive therapy is required for the life of the transplanted kidney (Burchum & Rosenthal, 2019).

Drug Alert

Long-term use of corticosteroids is associated with HTN, hyperlipidemia, DM, infection, osteoporosis, avascular necrosis, weight gain, cataracts, and mood changes and may contribute to development or worsening of cardiovascular disease (Burchum & Rosenthal, 2019).

Drug Alert

Echinacea, a complementary and alternative therapy classified as a dietary supplement, is used to treat the common cold and influenza. Because it stimulates immune function its use may interfere with the action of immunosuppressant medications and is to be avoided in transplant patients (Burcham & Rosenthal, 2019).

Drug Alert

Cyclosporine should not be taken with grapefruit juice. A compound in grapefruit juice can raise cyclosporine levels by 50–200%, increasing the risk for toxicity (Burcham & Rosenthal, 2019).

Assessing the Patient for Transplant Rejection

After kidney transplantation, the nurse assesses the patient for signs and symptoms of transplant rejection. A rare event the hyperacute rejection occurs within minutes to hours after transplantation resulting in immediate graft failure. It is rare owing to very sensitive cross-match tests performed before surgery (Williams-Taylor et al., 2022). Although an acute rejection can happen any time after transplant, it usually occurs weeks to months after surgery; the most common occurrence is during the first 3 months after transplant (Naik & Shawar, 2021). Patients who have acute **rejection** may be asymptomatic and evidence of rejection may be a sudden rise of serum creatinine to more than 25% of the baseline value (Naik & Shawar, 2022). However, any new-onset or worsening of proteinuria or HTN should raise the suspicion for rejection. Sometimes a rejecting graft may present with fever, pain, tenderness, or swelling at the graft site, hematuria, dysuria, HTN, fluid retention, and decreased urine output (Naik & Shawar, 2021). Lab work should be evaluated for an increase in serum creatinine, BUN, and a decreased creatinine clearance.

Chronic rejection is the result of repeated episodes of acute rejection resulting in vascular infarction and scarring, progressing for years until it leads to ultimate failure of the transplanted organ (Williams-Taylor et al., 2022). Physical examination findings in chronic rejection are usually nonspecific but may include HTN, peripheral edema and fatigue; the symptoms of fever or graft tenderness are typically absent in chronic rejection (Hassanein & Augustine, 2021). Symptoms which develop over months or years are similar to signs of ESKD (Hassanein & Augustine, 2021). Box 26-11 discusses renal transplant rejection and infection.

Preventing Infection

The nurse monitors the patient closely for infection. Patients are particularly susceptible to impaired wound healing and infection related to immunosuppressant therapy and complications of kidney failure. Infecting organisms may be from the patient's own flora, which pose a threat due to immunosuppression. Fungi, viruses, and protozoan reflect opportunistic

BOX 26-11

Renal Transplant Rejection and Infection

Renal graft rejection and failure may occur immediately (hyperacute), within the first minutes after transplant related to the preformed antibody or ABO incompatibility; rarely seen today owing to very sensitive presurgical cross-match tests. Acute rejection, can happen any time after transplant, usually within days to weeks, and is potentially reversible. It is not uncommon for rejection to occur during the first year after transplantation. Chronic rejection usually develops more than 3 months post-transplant and can either be antibody-mediated or T cell–mediated rejection (Naik & Shawar, 2022). With multiple episodes of acute rejection, the transplanted kidney may steadily lose function after many years (chronic) necessitating a return to dialysis or another transplant.

Detecting Rejection

Ultrasonography may be used to detect enlargement of the kidney; percutaneous renal biopsy (most reliable) and x-ray techniques are used to evaluate transplant rejection. If the body rejects the transplanted kidney, the patient needs to return to dialysis or receive another organ, if eligible. The rejected kidney is not typically removed, depending on the risk for infection if the kidney is left in place.

Risk for Infection

About 75% of recipients of kidney transplant have at least one episode of infection in the first year after transplantation because of immunosuppressant therapy. Immunosuppressants of the past made the transplant recipient more vulnerable to opportunistic infections (candidiasis, cytomegalovirus, *Pneumocystis* pneumonia) and infection with other relatively nonpathogenic viruses, fungi, and protozoa, which can be a major hazard. The antirejection medications, cyclosporine and tacrolimus, have reduced the incidence of opportunistic infections. These medications selectively exert its effect, sparing T cells that protect the patient from life-threatening infections. In addition, combination immunosuppressant therapy and improved clinical care have produced 1-year patient survival rates approaching 100% and graft survival exceeding 90%. Infections, however, remain a major cause of death at all points in time for recipients of kidney transplant.

infections and may include herpes simplex, herpes zoster, CMV, candida, *Pneumocystis carinii*, aspergillus, and cryptococci. Observe for bacterial infections from invasive vascular accesses and urinary catheters, as well as postoperative wound and respiratory infections. Broad-spectrum antibiotics are typically given for 48 hours post-transplant or until invasive lines and drains (if placed) are discontinued (Morton & Fontaine, 2018, p. 939). Even a modest increase in temperature (99° F or 37.2° C) may be significant in this population. Clinical manifestations include shaking, chills, fever, tachycardia, and tachypnea as well as either an increase or a decrease in WBCs (leukocytosis or leukopenia).

Urine cultures are performed frequently because of the high incidence of bacteriuria during early and late stages of transplantation. Any type of wound drainage should be viewed as a potential source of infection because drainage is an excellent culture medium for bacteria. Catheter and drain tips should be cut with sterile scissors, placed in a sterile container, and sent to the laboratory for culture.

The nurse ensures that the patient is protected from exposure to infection through consistent handwashing, good oral care and skin hygiene, frequent assessments of vital signs and complete assessments. Some centers use protective isolation systems with air filtration, gut and skin decontamination and low microbial diets. The nurse advocates for the patient by ensuring hospital staff, visitors, and other patients with active infections protect the patient, especially through scrupulous hand hygiene during all patient contact.

Monitoring Urinary Function

Renal function is related to ischemic injury in the donor kidney either from hypotensive periods in cadaver/heartbeat-only donors or preservation time outside the body over 24 hours. The kidney may begin to function immediately, but may not function optimally for 4 weeks, during which time anuria, oliguria, or polyuria may be present. A baseline radionuclide renal scan can assess renal perfusion 24 hours post-transplant and can be repeated with altered laboratory or clinical changes.

The patient may experience significant changes in fluid and electrolyte status. Therefore, careful monitoring of urine output volume and color should be performed at least every 30 minutes in the PACU, and hourly on the medical surgical unit. If a sudden drop in urinary drainage occurs, suspect clotted, kinked or compressed tubing in the urinary drainage system. The nurse is mindful that the ureter anastomosis to the bladder is fragile, and the bladder must remain decompressed for several days to promote proper healing (Williams-Taylor et al., 2022). If clots occlude the end of the catheter, the nurse follows institutional protocols. For example, some protocols may suggest irrigating the Foley catheter to ensure that clot or tissue has not affected its patency. While others suggest milking the tubing to dislodge a clot rather than gentle irrigation, which may increase the risk for infection (Morton & Fontaine, 2018, p. 926). It may be necessary to change the catheter if the clot cannot be dislodged (Williams-Taylor et al., 2022).

IV fluids are administered on the basis of urine volume and serum electrolyte levels and are prescribed by the provider. In general, the new kidney will be producing large amounts of urine, and fluid replacement, usually maintained in a 1:1 ratio, must be sustained. Hyperkalemia may result from oliguria or anuria, requiring insulin (with glucose) to transport potassium into the cell or oral polystyrene sulfonate to promote GI excretion. Hemodialysis may be necessary postoperatively to maintain homeostasis until the transplanted kidney is functioning well.

Addressing Psychological Concerns

The rejection of a transplanted kidney remains a matter of great concern to the patient, the family, and the health care team. An important nursing function is the assessment of the patient's stress and coping. The nurse uses each visit with the patient to determine if the patient and family are coping effectively and if the patient is adhering to the prescribed medication regimen. If indicated or requested, the nurse refers the patient for counseling.

Psychological disturbances may develop from corticosteroid use. About 60% of patients develop insomnia, anxiety, agitation or irritability; 6% experience delirium, hallucinations, depression, euphoria, mania, and a small percentage may become suicidal. Good mental health does not seem to prevent these side effects (Burcham & Rosenthal, 2019).

Monitoring and Managing Potential Complications

The patient undergoing kidney transplantation is at risk for the postoperative complications that are associated with any surgical procedure. In addition, the patient's physical condition may be compromised because of the complications associated with longstanding kidney failure and its treatment. Therefore, careful assessment for the complications related to kidney failure and corticosteroid use, such as poor wound healing, is an important aspect of nursing care.

GI ulceration and corticosteroid-induced bleeding may occur. Fungal colonization of the GI tract, especially the mouth and urinary bladder, may occur secondary to corticosteroid and antibiotic therapy. Closely monitoring the patient and notifying the provider about the occurrence of these complications are important nursing interventions. In addition, the patient is monitored closely for adverse effects of corticosteroids or signs of adrenal insufficiency when these medications are discontinued.

Pearls for Practice

A two- to threefold higher risk is seen in transplant recipients compared to the general population for certain malignancies such as colon, lung, liver, lymphoma, melanoma, and nonmelanoma skin cancer, therefore patients are encouraged to follow screening guidelines. It should be noted that no single immunosuppressant has been found to increase the risk; rather, the risk increases as the total amount of immunosuppression increases (Kallenbach, 2021).

Teaching Patients Self-Care

The nurse works closely with the patient and family to be sure that they understand the need for continuing immunosuppressive therapy as prescribed. In addition, the patient and family are instructed to assess for and report signs and symptoms of transplant rejection, infection, or significant adverse effects of the immunosuppressive regimen. Have the patient perform a "teach back" to state they should report decreased urine output; weight gain; malaise; fever; respiratory distress; tenderness over the transplanted kidney; anxiety; depression; changes in eating, drinking, or other habits; and changes in BP. The patient is instructed to inform other health care providers (e.g., dentist) about the kidney transplant and the use of immunosuppressive agents. Patients are usually discharged 3 to 5 days after the transplantation procedure (Lam et al., 2020).

Continuing Care

Follow-up care with the transplant team is a lifelong necessity. Individual verbal and written instructions are provided concerning diet, medication, fluids, daily weight, daily measurement of urine, management of I&O, prevention of infection, resumption of activity, and avoidance of contact sports in which the transplanted kidney may be injured. CVD is the major cause of morbidity and mortality after transplantation (Ueki et al., 2021), due in part to the increasing age of patients with transplants.

Malignancy develops more frequently in patients receiving long-term immunosuppressive therapy. Cancer outcomes are generally poor, in this group, especially for those developing melanoma, renal cell carcinoma, and post-transplant lymphoproliferative disease (Al-Adra et al., 2021). Remind the patient of the importance of health-promotion activities, such as wearing sunscreen and health screenings, including regular PAP smears, mammogram, colonoscopy, and breast or testicular self-examination as appropriate. Routine age-appropriate vaccines, and vaccines indicated for immunocompromised patients are generally administered 3 to 6 months following transplantation (Chandraker & Yeung, 2022). Inactivated vaccines are generally considered safe to administer after kidney transplantation; however, any live or live attenuated vaccines are not (Chandraker & Yeung, 2022).

The American Association of Kidney Patients (see Resources) is a nonprofit organization that serves the needs of those with kidney disease. It can provide many helpful suggestions for patients and family members learning to cope with dialysis and transplantation.

RENAL TRAUMA

Genitourinary trauma occurs in approximately 5% of trauma cases, and the kidney is the third most common organ injured with abdominal trauma (Maquillan & Makic, 2020). It is rarely an isolated injury and is associated with blunt injury such as (automobile and motorcycle collisions, falls, athletic injuries, assaults) or penetrating injuries such as those occurring with gunshot wounds, stabbing or impalement (Macquillan & Makic, 2020). Renal trauma is present in up to 24% cases of abdominal trauma (Mann et al., 2019), generally occurring in young males. The nurse should suspect renal injury when the patient presents with blunt abdominal or penetrating flank and back wounds; nearly all patients with renal gunshot wounds have associated injuries of other internal organs (Macquillan & Macik, 2020).

The kidneys are anchored by fascia, surrounded by fat pads and protected by the rib cage and musculature of the back posteriorly and by a cushion of abdominal wall and viscera anteriorly (Macquillan & Makic, 2020). They are highly mobile as they are fixed only at the renal pedicle (stem of renal blood vessels and the ureter). Blunt trauma injury, whether direct or by rapid deceleration may result in kidney injury. This typically occurs during a fall from a height or motor vehicle accident where the individual makes contact with the dashboard, lap belt or steering wheel. Renal artery thrombosis or contusion of the renal parenchyma may result. The most common blunt injury occurs when the kidney is compressed against the lower rib cage and upper lumbar transverse process, stretching the ureter. Pre-existing conditions such as hydronephrosis or cysts create increased susceptibility to injury (Maquillan, 2020).

Blunt renal trauma is classified into one of four groups, as follows:

- *Contusion:* Bruises or hemorrhages under the renal capsule; capsule and collecting system intact
- *Minor laceration:* Superficial disruption of the cortex; renal medulla and collecting system are not involved
- *Major laceration:* Parenchymal disruption extending into cortex and medulla, possibly involving the collecting system
- *Vascular injury:* Tears of renal artery or vein

The most common renal injuries are contusions, lacerations, ruptures, and renal pedicle injuries or small internal lacerations of the kidney (Fig. 26-11). The kidneys receive half of the blood flow from the abdominal aorta; therefore, even a fairly small renal laceration can produce massive blood loss. When gross hematuria or microscopic hematuria occurs, the nurse considers hemorrhage is likely present. The nurse monitors for additional signs of hemorrhage include a decreasing BP, MAP below 65 mm Hg, or tachycardia without a discernible cause, such as pain.

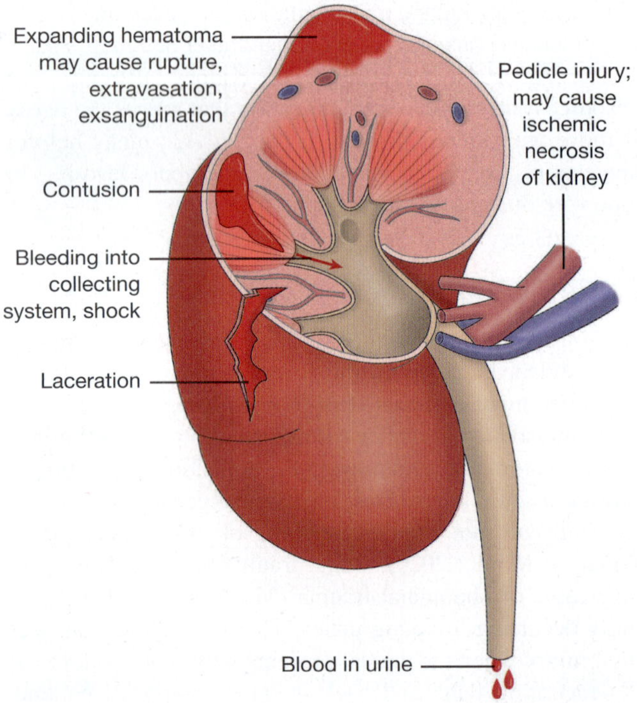

FIGURE 26-11 **Types and pathophysiologic effects of renal injuries: contusions, lacerations, rupture, and pedicle injury.**

Pearls for Practice

The nurse recognizes that a MAP <70 mm Hg places the patient at risk for AKI.

Clinical Manifestations and Assessment

Clinical manifestations of renal injury include pain, renal colic (due to blood clots or fragments obstructing the collecting system), hematuria, mass or swelling in the flank, ecchymosis, and lacerations or wounds of the lateral abdomen and flank. While hematuria is the most common manifestation of renal trauma, there is no relationship between the degree of hematuria and the degree of injury.

The nurse assesses for ecchymosis over the flank (Grey–Turner sign) and periumbilical area (Cullen sign) as well as flank tenderness with palpation and gross hematuria (Fig. 26-12).

Pearls for Practice

Grey–Turner sign and Cullen sign are associated with retroperitoneal bleeds.

Microscopic hematuria may be present; therefore, evaluation of trends in the hemoglobin and Hct is critical. A CT scan of the abdomen may be done to assess penetrating trauma. Free air, injury to the kidney, or a penetrating object is assessed. Any patient with gross hematuria will need to be evaluated, although the nurse should recognize that the amount of hematuria correlates poorly with the magnitude of injury (McQuillan & Makic, 2020).

Medical and Nursing Management

The priorities of care for patients with renal trauma include establishing and maintaining a patent airway, ensure breathing and circulation (Maquillan & Makic, 2020). Additional goals of management are to control hemorrhage and pain, to prevent infection, and to preserve and restore kidney function. The patient is monitored for oliguria and signs of hemorrhagic shock because a pedicle injury or shattered kidney can lead to rapid exsanguination and death. An expanding hematoma may cause rupture of the kidney capsule. A palpable flank or abdominal mass with local tenderness, swelling, and ecchymosis suggests renal hemorrhage. The area of the original mass can be outlined with a marking pen so that the examiner can evaluate the area for change.

Often renal trauma is associated with other injuries to nearby organs; therefore, the patient is assessed for skin

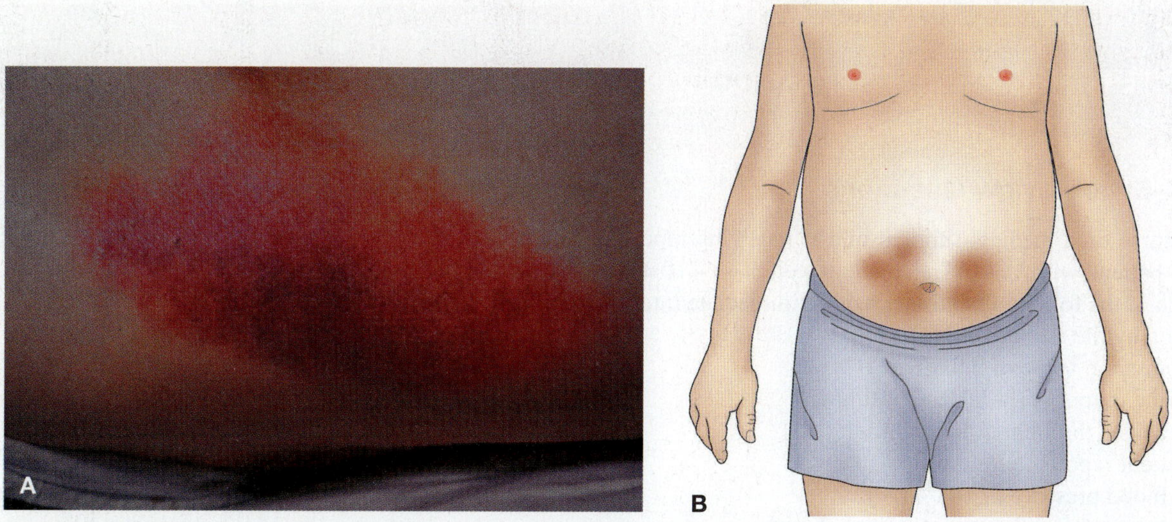

FIGURE 26-12 **Ecchymosis with renal trauma. A. Grey–Turner sign. B. Cullen sign. (A from Berg, D., & Worzala, K. [2006].** ***Atlas of adult physical diagnosis*****. Lippincott Williams & Wilkins.)**

abrasions, lacerations, and entry and exit wounds of the upper abdomen and lower thorax because these may be associated with renal injury. Trauma to the right kidney may be associated with liver injury while trauma to the left kidney may involve injury to the spleen. In rare cases, damage to the adrenal gland may result in adrenal insufficiency and death.

Pearls for Practice

When caring for a trauma patient presenting with blood at the urethral meatus, inability to void, and a perineal hematoma, suspect a urethral injury. DO NOT attempt to insert a urinary catheter until the patient is evaluated by the provider.

Surgical Management

In renal trauma, any sudden change in the patient's condition suggests hemorrhage. For signs of shock, plan to provide aggressive fluid resuscitation. The damaged kidney may have to be removed (nephrectomy) however, angioembolization can be used, even when the patient is hemodynamically unstable (Mann et al., 2019).

Early postoperative complications include rebleeding, formation of a perinephritic abscess, sepsis, urine extravasation, and formation of a fistula. Other complications include formation of stones, infection or abscess, cysts, chronic pyelonephrosis, vascular aneurysms, and loss of kidney function. HTN can be a complication of any renal surgery but usually is a late complication of renal injury.

Instruct the patient who has undergone surgery about incisional care and the importance of adequate fluid intake. Give instructions about changes that should be reported to the provider, such as fever, hematuria, flank pain, or any signs and symptoms of decreasing kidney function. In addition, guidelines for gradually increasing activity, lifting, and driving are provided in accordance with the provider's prescription.

Follow-up nursing care includes BP monitoring and advising the patient to restrict activities for about 1 month after trauma to minimize the incidence of delayed or secondary bleeding. Advise the patient to schedule periodic follow-up assessments of renal function (creatinine clearance, BUN, and serum creatinine). If a nephrectomy was necessary, the patient is advised to wear medical identification.

Gerontologic Considerations

Care for this population is essentially the same; however, older individuals may have chronic disease processes that must be considered. Older adults often have higher mortality following traumatic injury than do younger adults including alterations in the cardiac and respiratory systems that reduce physiologic reserve needed to respond to shock and hypoxia.

CHAPTER REVIEW

NCLEX-Style Review Questions

1. The nurse on a medical surgical unit is receiving report on a patient with AKI. The patient weight is 110 lb. Which of the following findings require immediate intervention by the nurse?
a. Potassium value of 5.0 mEq/L
b. Urine output of 24 mL the past hour
c. Crackles throughout lung fields
d. Patient reports itching skin
e. A blood pressure of 108/44
f. Patient refused fingerstick blood glucose

2. When caring for the patient with end-stage kidney disease (ESKD), the nurse teaches the patient to manage his diet by avoiding which foods? Select all that apply.
a. Green leafy vegetables and citrus
b. Apples and pears
c. Proteins of high biologic value
d. Oat, wheat, and rye-containing products
e. Baked potatoes
f. Low-sodium canned soups

3. During a "teach back" after education on kidney transplant rejection, the nurse recognizes the patient understood the education when the patient states they will monitor for which of these signs and symptoms? Select all that apply.
a. Thrill and bruit over the fistula
b. Weight gain and fever
c. Palpitations and thirst
d. Flank pain and pyuria
e. Swelling of the ankles and around the eyes
f. Loss of appetite and 3 lb weight loss

4. When planning care for the patient with kidney trauma, the nurse notifies the health care provider immediately for which of these findings? Select all that apply.
a. Laboratory reports microscopic hematuria
b. Tachycardia
c. Patient upset and crying over the trauma
d. Scar noted on patient's left flank
e. Blood pressure of 112/40
f. Ecchymosis around the umbilicus

5. The nurse is caring for a patient with nephrotic syndrome. In order to prevent long-term complications, which of these does the nurse include in patient teaching?
a. Observe for dark urine and clay-colored stool.
b. Void every 2 hours on schedule.
c. Signs and symptoms of deep vein thrombosis (DVT) and pulmonary emboli (PE)
d. Minimize the intake of saturated fat.
e. Avoid driving at night.
f. Follow a low sodium diet

REFERENCES AND SELECTED READINGS

References and selected readings associated with this chapter can be found on the website that accompanies the book. Visit **http://thepoint.lww.com/Honan3e** to access the references and other additional resources associated with this chapter.

CHAPTER 27

Nursing Management: Patients With Urinary Disorders

Kassandra August-Marcucio

Learning Objectives

After reading this chapter, you will be able to:

1. Identify factors contributing to upper and lower urinary tract infections (UTIs).
2. Describe nursing care of the patient with a UTI.
3. Differentiate the various adult dysfunctional voiding patterns.
4. Develop a patient education plan for a patient who has mixed (stress and urge) urinary incontinence.
5. Identify potential causes of an obstruction of the urinary tract, and management of the patient with this condition.
6. Develop a teaching plan for the patient undergoing treatment for renal calculi (kidney stones).
7. Discuss the available options for management of urinary cancers.
8. Identify issues relevant to the initial management of trauma to the urinary tract.
9. Identify issues important to patient self-care of urinary diversions.

The urinary system is responsible for providing the route for drainage of urine formed by the kidneys. Nursing requires an understanding of the anatomy, physiology, diagnostic testing, nursing care, and rehabilitation of patients with multiple processes that interfere with the urinary system. This chapter focuses on the nursing management of patients with common urinary conditions.

INFECTIONS OF THE URINARY TRACT

Urinary tract infections (UTIs) are caused by pathogenic microorganisms in the urinary tract (the normal urinary tract should be sterile above the urethra). Lower UTIs include bacterial **cystitis** (inflammation of the bladder), bacterial **prostatitis** (inflammation of the prostate), and bacterial **urethritis** (inflammation of the urethra). Acute or chronic nonbacterial causes of inflammation in any of these areas can be misdiagnosed as bacterial infections. Upper UTIs are much less common and include acute or chronic **pyelonephritis** (inflammation of the kidney and renal pelvis), interstitial nephritis (inflammation of the spaces between the kidney tubules), and renal abscesses (pus-filled cavity of the kidney; Fig. 27-1). Upper and lower UTIs are further classified as uncomplicated or complicated, depending on other patient-related conditions (Box 27-1; e.g., whether the UTI is recurrent, the duration of the infection, and whether the bacteria is community-acquired or hospital-acquired). Uncomplicated UTIs are commonly community-acquired, while complicated UTIs usually occur in people with urologic abnormalities, comorbidities such as diabetes, or recent catheterization.

UTI or acute cystitis is an infection of the bladder which is most commonly caused by coliform bacteria (i.e., *E. coli*) typically ascending from the urethra (Nicolle & Drekonja, 2020). Risk factors for acquiring a UTI are assigned female at birth (AFAB) or female populations, previous UTIs, sexual activity, changes in the bacterial environment of the vagina, pregnancy, advancing age, structural problems within the urinary tract, and poor personal hygiene (Centers for Disease Control and Prevention [CDC], 2021). UTIs are the fifth most common type of health care–associated infection causing close to 63,000 UTIs in acute care hospitals and accounting for more than 9.5% of infections that are reported by acute care hospitals (National Healthcare Safety Network [NHSN], 2022). Instrumentation of the urinary tract remains the most common reason for hospitalized patients' to acquire UTIs.

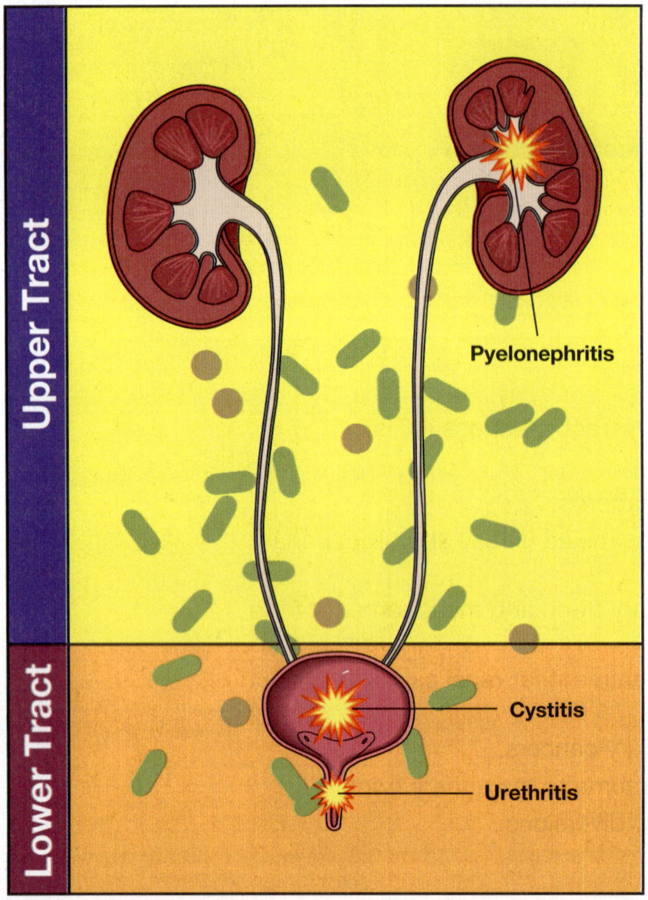

FIGURE 27-1 **Urinary tract infection. (Courtesy of LifeArt, Lippincott, Wolters Kluwer.)**

BOX 27-1

Classifying Urinary Tract Infections

Urinary tract infections (UTIs) are classified by location: the lower urinary tract (which includes the bladder and structures below the bladder) or the upper urinary tract (which includes the kidneys and ureters). They can also be classified as uncomplicated or complicated UTIs.

Lower UTIs

Cystitis, prostatitis, urethritis

Upper UTIs

Acute pyelonephritis, chronic pyelonephritis, renal abscess, interstitial nephritis, perirenal abscess

Uncomplicated Lower or Upper UTIs

Community-acquired infection; common in young AFAB or female patients and not usually recurrent

Complicated Lower or Upper UTIs

Often nosocomial (acquired in the hospital) and related to catheterization; occur in patients with urologic abnormalities, pregnancy, immunosuppression, and diabetes mellitus; obstructions and are often recurrent

LOWER URINARY TRACT INFECTIONS

Pathophysiology

For infection to occur, bacteria must gain access to the bladder, attach to and colonize the epithelium of the urinary tract, evade host defense mechanisms, and initiate inflammation. Many UTIs result from fecal organisms that ascend from the perineum to the urethra and the bladder and then adhere to the mucosal surfaces. Due to the orientation of the urethra, it is uncommon for assigned male at birth (AMAB) or male patients to have UTIs. The short urethra of AFAB people or females and the location of the urethra close to the rectum and proximity to the vagina puts them at higher risk for acquiring UTIs.

Bacterial Invasion of the Urinary Tract

By increasing the normal slow shedding of bladder epithelial cells (resulting in bacteria removal), the bladder can clear even large numbers of bacteria. Glycosaminoglycan (GAG), a hydrophilic protein, normally exerts a nonadherent protective effect against various bacteria by attracting water molecules and forming a water barrier that serves as a defensive layer between the bladder and the urine. GAG may be impaired by certain agents (cyclamate, saccharin, aspartame, and tryptophan metabolites). The normal bacterial flora of the vagina and urethral area also interfere with adherence of *Escherichia coli.*

Reflux

Urethrovesical reflux, which is the reflux of urine from the urethra into the bladder, can be a contributor to development of UTIs (Fig. 27-2). With coughing, sneezing, or straining, the bladder pressure increases, which may force urine from the bladder into the urethra. When the pressure returns to normal, the urine flows back into the bladder, bringing into the bladder bacteria from the anterior portions of the urethra. Urethrovesical reflux is also caused by dysfunction of the bladder neck or urethra. The urethrovesical angle and urethral closure pressure may be altered, combined with vaginal tissue atrophy, increasing the incidence of infection in postmenopausal people.

Ureterovesical or vesicoureteral reflux refers to the backward flow of urine from the bladder into one or both ureters (see Fig. 27-2). The ureters tunnel into the posterior bladder wall, so that the bladder musculature compresses a small portion of the ureter during normal voiding. Vesicoureteral reflux is most common in infants and children as this is likely caused by congenital abnormalities. This condition affects approximately 1% to 3% of children, putting them at risk for development of UTIs (Boston Children's Hospital, 2022).

Uropathogenic Bacteria

Bacteriuria is defined as the presence of bacteria in the urine, which is further classified as symptomatic or asymptomatic (Crader et al., 2022). It is important to differentiate whether

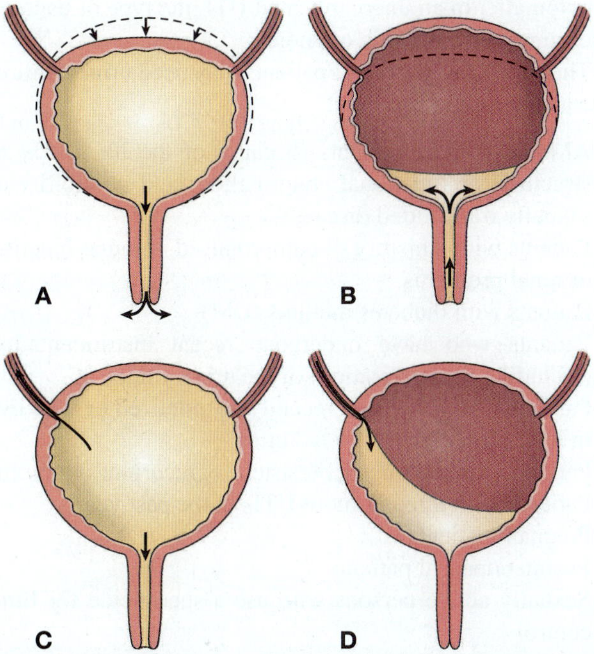

FIGURE 27-2 **Mechanisms of urethrovesical and ureterovesical reflux may cause urinary tract infection. Urethrovesical reflux: With coughing and straining, bladder pressure rises, which may force urine from the bladder into the urethra. (A) When bladder pressure returns to normal, the urine flows back to the bladder (B), which introduces bacteria from the urethra to the bladder. Ureterovesical reflux: With failure of the ureterovesical valve, urine moves up the ureters during voiding (C) and flows into the bladder when voiding stops (D). This prevents complete emptying of the bladder. It also leads to urinary stasis and contamination of the ureters with bacteria-laden urine.**

the sample provided is contaminated. Most commonly, urine samples are contaminated by skin cells due to improper collection of urine. In AFAB or female patients, contamination of the urine sample is more common if the labia are not properly cleaned and are not kept out of the urine stream during sample collection. In AMAB or male patients, contamination of the collected urine sample occurs less frequently; however, uncircumcised patients should be instructed to cleanse the head of the penis and ensure that the foreskin does not touch the urine stream during urine collection. The organisms most frequently responsible for UTIs are those normally found in the lower gastrointestinal (GI) tract such as *E. coli*.

Routes of Infection

Bacteria enter the urinary tract in three well-recognized ways: by the transurethral route (ascending infection), through the bloodstream (hematogenous spread), or by means of a fistula (direct extension). The most common route of infection is transurethral, in which bacteria (often from fecal contamination) colonize the periurethral area and subsequently enter the bladder by means of the urethra. Less common is the formation of fistula of the bowel to the bladder. This should be considered in patients who have recurrent *E. coli* infections, complaint of feelings of passing air with urination, or brown stool-colored urine.

BOX 27-2
Risk Factors for Urinary Tract Infection

- Inability or failure to empty the bladder completely
- Obstructed urinary flow:
  - Congenital abnormalities
  - Urethral strictures
  - Contracture of the bladder neck
  - Bladder tumors
  - Calculi (stones) in the ureters or kidneys
  - Compression of the ureters
  - Neurologic abnormalities
  - Enlarged prostate
- Decreased natural host defenses or immunosuppression
- Instrumentation of the urinary tract (e.g., catheterization, cystoscopic procedures)
- Inflammation or abrasion of the urethral mucosa
- Contributing conditions:
  - Diabetes mellitus (increased urinary glucose levels create an infection-prone environment in the urinary tract)
  - Pregnancy
  - Neurologic disorders
  - Gout
  - Altered states caused by incomplete emptying of the bladder and urinary stasis

Risk Factors

Several mechanisms maintain the sterility of the bladder: the physical barrier of the urethra, urine flow, ureterovesical junction competence, various antibacterial enzymes and antibodies, and antiadherent effects mediated by the mucosal cells of the bladder. Abnormalities or dysfunctions of these mechanisms are contributing risk factors for lower UTIs (Box 27-2).

The American College of Obstetricians and Gynecologists (ACOG) recommends that all pregnant people be screened for asymptomatic bacteriuria. For people at low risk for the development of UTIs during pregnancy, it is unclear of the benefit of treatment of asymptomatic bacteriuria beyond the first trimester (Moore et al., 2018). More solid research on the incidence of premature birth and of the adverse effects of antibiotic treatment during pregnancy for asymptomatic bacteriuria is needed.

Clinical Manifestations and Assessment

Signs and Symptoms

A variety of signs and symptoms are associated with UTI. Those who have asymptomatic bacteriuria do not need antibiotic therapy and should be monitored for signs and symptoms of symptomatic UTI. Signs and symptoms of an uncomplicated lower UTI include **dysuria** (painful or difficult urination), burning with urination, frequency, urgency, **nocturia** (excessive urination at night), and incontinence. Other symptoms can include suprapubic discomfort and gross hematuria (Nicolle & Drekonja, 2020).

Pearls for Practice

Older patients can lack the typical symptoms of UTI and sepsis. Nonspecific symptoms, such as altered mental status, lethargy, anorexia, new incontinence, hyperventilation, and low-grade fever, may be clues to UTI. It is important for the nurse to take into account that these symptoms are present in many disease processes, not just UTI. While UTI should remain in the differential, symptoms should be observed closely, even in the setting of a positive urine culture, to avoid overlooking other acute illnesses.

Pearls for Practice

Asymptomatic bacteriuria, which is the presence of bacteria in the urine that does not demonstrate symptoms of UTI, is the main cause of antibiotic overuse. Inappropriate antimicrobial use drives antimicrobial resistance in the community, as well as in the person being treated (Nicolle et al., 2019). The nurse should carefully question the patient who qualifies for urine collection. In the absence of urinary tract symptoms, the clinical value of checking a random urine sample should be questioned. Urine cultures should be utilized only in populations where symptomatic UTI is suspected.

In patients with complicated UTIs, such as those with indwelling catheters, manifestations can range from asymptomatic bacteriuria to gram-negative sepsis with shock. Complicated UTIs often are due to a broader spectrum of organisms, have a lower response rate to treatment, and tend to recur. The likelihood of patients with long-term catheters having asymptomatic bacteriuria is close to 100% (Nicolle et al., 2019; however, any patient with an indwelling catheter who suddenly develops signs and symptoms of septic shock should be evaluated for **bacteremia** (the presence of bacteria in blood) from a UTI. The kidneys receive approximately 25% of the cardiac output every minute. When a patient has pyelonephritis, the infection is in the kidney parenchyma and can travel from the kidney into the bloodstream, which is termed *bacteremia. Septicemia* is the clinical syndrome associated with the bacteremia that results in vasodilatation, microvascular permeability, and massive inflammatory response that can result in death. Nurses should be aware of signs and symptoms of bacteremia from UTI, including hypothermia or hyperthermia, tachycardia, tachypnea, leukocytosis or leukopenia, and greater than 10% immature (band) forms (bands are immature neutrophils that contain a nucleus, indicating infection). Under normal circumstances only 1% to 3% of neutrophils are band forms. Refer to Chapter 53 for further discussion of sepsis and septic shock.

Diagnostic Tests

The results of the urine culture and the associated sensitivities confirm the diagnosis of UTI in patients who are symptomatic. In an uncomplicated UTI, the type of bacteria determines the antibiotic of choice.

The following groups of patients may need urine cultures when symptoms are present:

- AMAB or male patients (because of the likelihood of structural or functional abnormalities and possibility of sexually transmitted disease)
- Patients with a history of compromised immune function or renal problems
- Patients with diabetes mellitus (DM)
- Patients who have undergone recent instrumentation (including catheterization) of the urinary tract
- Patients who have been recently hospitalized or who live in long-term care (LTC) facilities
- Patients with prolonged, persistent, or recurrent symptoms
- Patients with three or more UTIs in the past year
- Pregnant patients
- Postmenopausal patients
- Sexually active persons who use a spermicide for birth control

A multiple-test dipstick often includes testing for white blood cells (WBCs), known as the *leukocyte esterase test*, and nitrite testing (Griess nitrate reduction test). If the leukocyte esterase test is positive, it is assumed that the patient has pyuria (pus in the urine), since esterase is an enzyme released from WBCs; a UTI is suspected. Treatment should be directed by the results of a urine culture with appropriate sensitivities to prevent antimicrobial resistance.

Pearls for Practice

The nurse is aware that false-positive leukocyte esterase tests can occur if the clean-catch midstream urine collection was not performed correctly or there was contamination from the vagina in the specimen.

Tests for sexually transmitted infections (STIs) should be performed if indicated (see Chapter 34) because acute urethritis caused by sexually transmitted organisms or acute vaginitis infections may be responsible for symptoms similar to those of UTIs. If STI is suspected, it is important to identify the organism in order to treat the patient and their partner within a safe time frame to avoid secondary effects of STI.

Imaging studies are rarely indicated for the evaluation of UTIs, except with suspected anatomic issues or if additional pathology, such as renal lithiasis (stone formation or calculi) or fistula (a false track or abnormal passageway), is suspected. For those with recurrent symptomatic UTIs, imaging may be indicated.

Medical and Nursing Management

Management of UTIs typically involves pharmacologic therapy and patient education. The nurse teaches the patient about medication regimens and infection prevention measures (Box 27-3).

BOX 27-3

Patient Education

Preventing Recurrent Urinary Tract Infections

Hygiene

- After showering, pat the labia dry; avoid douching and excessive cleaning of the vaginal area.
- After each bowel movement, clean the perineum from front to back, away from the urethra and labia toward the rectum reducing concentrations of pathogens near the urethral opening.

Fluid Intake

- Drink liberal amounts of fluids daily to flush out bacteria.
- Limit coffee, tea, soda, juice, alcohol, and other fluids that are urinary tract irritants.

Voiding Habits

- Void every 2–3 hours during the day and completely empty the bladder. This prevents overdistention of the bladder, urinary stasis, and compromised blood supply to the bladder wall. All predispose the patient to UTI.

Therapy

- Take medication *exactly* as prescribed.
- Special timing of administration may be required.
- Notify the primary provider if fever occurs or if signs and symptoms persist.
- Consult the primary provider regularly for follow-up.

Pearls for Practice

Patients who are asymptomatic do not require screening for bacteriuria. It is important to consider that treatment of asymptomatic bacteriuria has not been associated with improved outcomes but is uniformly followed by reinfection with organisms of increasing antimicrobial resistance. Patients who are scheduled for a urologic procedure are the exception. According to the American Urological Association (AUA), single-dose antimicrobial prophylaxis is appropriate for most urologic procedures to prevent surgical site infection and prevent against periprocedural infections, with the secondary goal of reducing antibiotic overuse (AUA, 2019).

Initial Pharmacologic Therapy

Antimicrobial treatment of the patient with symptomatic UTI should be an antibiotic chosen from the resulted sensitivities that will eradicate bacteria from the urinary tract while causing minimal effects on GI and vaginal flora. Disrupting vaginal flora can result in vaginal yeast infections. Yeast vaginitis occurs in as many as 25% of patients treated with antimicrobial agents that affect vaginal flora, causes more symptoms, and is more difficult and thus more costly to treat than the UTI itself. The ideal antimicrobial agent should be affordable, have few adverse effects, have minimal medication interactions, and produce low resistance in the targeted organisms.

Various treatment regimens have been successful in treating uncomplicated lower UTIs in AFAB and female patients: single-dose administration, short-course (3 to 4 days) regimens, or 7- to 10-day regimens. The trend is toward a shortened course of antibiotic therapy for uncomplicated symptomatic UTIs because most cases are cured after 3 to 5 days of treatment (Nicolle et al., 2019). Phenazopyridine, a urinary analgesic, may be prescribed to relieve the discomfort of dysuria and pelvic or perineal pain and urgency associated with the infection (Gold Standard, 2023). Patients should be informed that their urine will turn dark orange with this medication and there is a possibility of experiencing yellowing of the eyes, which is recognized as a side effect. It is important that the nurse encourages and reinforces that completing antibiotics as prescribed is important to prevent antimicrobial resistance.

A fluoroquinolone is a routine choice for short-course therapy of uncomplicated, mild-to-moderate UTIs. There is high patient adherence (95.6%) to the 3-day regimen and a high eradication rate (96.4%) for all pathogens.

Drug Alert

Fluoroquinolones are associated with an increased risk of tendinitis and tendon rupture. This risk is further increased in those over age 60; in kidney, heart, and lung transplant recipients; and with use of concomitant steroid therapy. Providers should advise patients, at the first sign of tendon pain, swelling, or inflammation, to stop taking the fluoroquinolone, to avoid exercise and use of the affected area, and to promptly contact their provider about changing to a nonfluoroquinolone antimicrobial drug (U.S. Food and Drug Administration [FDA], 2017). More recently, the FDA has since added an additional warning that fluroquinolones can increase the risk for abdominal aortic aneurysm (AAA) and should be avoided in older patients and patients who have a history of blood vessel blockages or aneurysms, high blood pressure, and certain genetic conditions such as Marfan syndrome or Ehlers–Danlos syndrome (FDA, 2018). Nurses should be aware of these important risks associated with fluoroquinolones when educating patients about their prescribed antimicrobial therapy.

Nitrofurantoin should not be used in patients with renal insufficiency because it is ineffective at glomerular filtration rates of less than 50 mL/min and may cause peripheral neuropathy.

In a complicated UTI (e.g., pyelonephritis), the general treatment of choice is usually a cephalosporin or an ampicillin/aminoglycoside combination; the choice should be based on culture results. Patients in institutional settings may require 7 to 10 days of medication for the treatment to be effective. Medications such as ampicillin or amoxicillin can be used, but some *E. coli* strains have developed resistance. Longer medication courses are indicated for AMAB or male patients, first-trimester pregnant persons, and AFAB or female patients with pyelonephritis and other types of complicated UTIs. Hospitalization and IV antibiotics may be needed in patients who become acutely ill and are at risk for sepsis.

Long-Term Pharmacologic Therapy

Although the trend in management is brief pharmacologic treatment of UTIs for 3 to 5 days, there is risk for recurrence. Infections that recur within 2 weeks of therapy do so because organisms of the original offending strain remained. Relapses may suggest that the source of bacteriuria may be the upper urinary tract or that initial treatment was inadequate in length or proper antimicrobial choice. For patients who are AMAB or males, recurrent symptomatic UTIs should be evaluated for possible diagnosis of chronic prostatitis. Chronic prostatitis requires further evaluation and treatment beyond basic UTI guidelines.

It is no longer recommended to perform a urine sample to "confirm" treatment success except in pregnancy (Anger et al., 2022). Recurrent UTIs should also be accompanied by the recurrence of the symptoms of UTI such as dysuria, burning with urination, frequency, urgency, and fever. If symptomatic infection recurs after completing antimicrobial therapy, another short course (3 to 4 days) of full-dose antimicrobial therapy can be considered. Choice of antibiotic will be based upon the organism involved, previous UTI strains, and allergic drug history of the patient. Long-term use of antimicrobial agents has not been shown to decrease the risk of reinfection (Nicolle et al., 2019). Development of microbial resistance to prolonged antibiotic administration is a concern, and such treatment should only be implemented by an infectious disease provider after complete evaluation and workup.

If recurrence is caused by persistent bacteria from preceding infections, the cause (e.g., kidney stone, abscess) must be treated. For persons who develop UTI after sexual intercourse, postcoital prophylaxis with low-dose antimicrobials may be prescribed with close follow-up to ensure appropriate and diligent antimicrobial stewardship.

The patient is encouraged to drink liberal amounts of fluids (water is the best choice) to promote renal blood flow and to flush the bacteria from the urinary tract. Current evidence about the effectiveness of daily intake of cranberry juice to prevent UTIs has demonstrated that there is no true benefit but no true harm. Patients who want to pursue cranberry replacement should be aware of other medication interactions, avoid large amounts of the acidic drink to prevent bladder irritation, and avoid sugary versions of cranberry juices. It should not be administered to patients on anticoagulants or antiplatelet drugs because of the potential to affect coagulation or platelet aggregation. Urinary tract irritants (e.g., coffee, tea, citrus, spices, artificial sweeteners, carbonated sodas, alcohol) should be avoided.

The pain associated with UTI is quickly relieved once effective antimicrobial therapy is initiated. Analgesic agents and the application of heat to the perineum help relieve pain and spasm. Effective hydration can also help to relieve the symptoms of burning with urination and suprapubic discomfort.

Gerontologic Considerations

The incidence of symptomatic UTI is known to be higher in the aging population. Several risk factors contribute to the development of UTI, including pelvic prolapse, development of cystocele, rectocele or bladder diverticulum, urinary reflux, urinary incontinence, lack of ability to perform perineal hygiene, vaginal atrophy, and estrogen deficiency or prostate diseases (Alpay et al., 2018). Older patients are more likely to have other comorbidities, which make UTIs harder to treat and identify, such as DM, spinal cord injuries, catheterization (straight catheterization or indwelling catheters), and impaired mobility (Alpay et al., 2018). Asymptomatic bacteriuria should be considered in appropriate patients who have no symptoms and for which the UTI differential does not coincide with disease presentation.

In the older population, structural abnormalities secondary to decreased bladder tone and neurogenic bladder secondary to stroke or autonomic neuropathy of diabetes may prevent the complete emptying of the bladder and may increase the risk for UTI (Scott & Liang, 2021). Older persons often have incomplete emptying of the bladder and urinary stasis. In the absence of estrogen, postmenopausal AFAB or female patients are susceptible to colonization and increased adherence of bacteria to the vagina and urethra. Oral or topical estrogen has been used to restore the glycogen content of vaginal epithelial cells and an acidic pH for some postmenopausal persons with recurrent cystitis.

The antibacterial activity of prostatic secretions that protect AMAB and male people from bacterial colonization of the urethra and bladder decreases with aging. The increase of UTIs in AMAB or male patients as they age is due largely to prostatic hyperplasia, strictures of the urethra, and neuropathic bladder. Catheterization may also contribute to the higher incidence of UTI in this group. The most common cause of recurrent UTIs in older AMAB or male patients is chronic bacterial prostatitis. In institutionalized older patients, such as those in LTC facilities, infecting pathogens are often resistant to many antibiotics and may be chronic, representing asymptomatic bacteriuria.

Diligent hand hygiene, careful perineal care, and frequent toileting may decrease the incidence of UTIs seen in patients in LTC facilities. The organisms responsible for UTIs in people who are institutionalized may differ from those found in patients residing in the community; this may be due to the frequent use of antibiotic agents by patients in LTC facilities. *E. coli* is the most common organism seen in older patients in the community or hospital. However, patients with indwelling catheters are more likely to be infected with *Proteus*, *Klebsiella*, *Pseudomonas*, or *Staphylococcus* species. Patients who have been previously treated with multiple antibiotics may be infected with *Enterococcus* species. Treatment regimens are generally the same as those for younger adults, although age-related changes in the intestinal absorption of medications and decreased renal function and hepatic flow may necessitate alterations in dose.

UPPER URINARY TRACT INFECTIONS

Pyelonephritis is a bacterial infection of the kidney parenchyma and renal pelvis. The most common bacteria strains involved in pyelonephritis are *E. coli*, *Proteus*, *Klebsiella*, *Enterobacter*, and *Pseudomonas* (Wagenlehner, Pilatz & Naber, 2024). Causes involve either the ascending spread of bacteria from the bladder or proliferation of bacteria from systemic sources reaching the kidney via the bloodstream. An incompetent ureterovesical valve or obstruction occurring in the urinary tract increases the susceptibility of pyelonephritis (see Fig. 27-1) because static urine provides a good medium for bacterial growth. Bladder tumors, strictures, benign prostatic hyperplasia (BPH), and urinary stones are some potential causes of obstruction that can lead to infections.

Pyelonephritis may be acute or chronic. Acute pyelonephritis is usually manifested by enlarged kidneys with interstitial infiltrations of inflammatory cells, often associated with acute symptoms of infection. Abscesses may be noted on the renal capsule and at the corticomedullary junction that should resolve with treatment. Atrophy and destruction of tubules and the glomeruli may result if the patient experiences a protracted disease course. When pyelonephritis becomes chronic, the kidneys become scarred, contracted, nonfunctional, and cause chronic kidney disease or failure that can result in the need for therapies such as transplantation or dialysis.

Acute Pyelonephritis

More than 250,000 cases of acute pyelonephritis occur in the United States each year, with 100,000 patients requiring hospitalization. Recurrence of pyelonephritis is significantly less common than with uncomplicated UTIs, with 9% of AFAB or female patients and approximately 6% of AMAB or male patients having a second episode within a year (Medina & Castillo-Pino, 2019).

Clinical Manifestations and Assessment

The patient with acute pyelonephritis is acutely ill with chills, fever, leukocytosis (elevated WBCs), bacteriuria, and pyuria. Low back pain, flank pain (resulting from inflammation and edema of the renal parenchyma), nausea and vomiting, headache, malaise, and painful urination are common findings. Physical examination reveals pain and tenderness in the area of the costovertebral angle (see Chapter 25, Fig. 25-6). In addition, symptoms of lower urinary tract involvement, such as dysuria and frequency, are common but not always present. An ultrasound study or a computed tomography (CT) scan with contrast may be performed to locate any obstruction in the urinary tract. If obstruction is present, then relief of the obstruction is essential to prevent the complications and eventual kidney damage. Urine culture and sensitivity tests are performed to determine the causative organism so that appropriate antimicrobial agents can be prescribed. Blood cultures should also be obtained to determine if the patient has progressed to urosepsis and may need more intensive antibiotic therapy.

Medical and Nursing Management

Patients with acute uncomplicated pyelonephritis are treated on an outpatient basis if they are not exhibiting dehydration, nausea or vomiting, or symptoms of sepsis. A 2-week course of antibiotics is recommended because renal parenchymal disease is more difficult to eradicate than mucosal bladder infections. Antimicrobial treatment will be based upon urine culture and sensitivity results. In the outpatient setting, if the local antibiogram (laboratory results for the sensitivity of an isolated bacterial strain to different antibiotics) demonstrates a local resistance rate for the oral regimen exceeding 10%, then an initial 24-hour intravenous dose of antibiotics may be considered for effective treatment of the microorganism. The patient's renal and liver function should be considered and monitored during certain antibiotic treatments. Pregnant persons may be hospitalized for 2 or 3 days of parenteral antibiotic therapy. Oral antibiotic agents may be prescribed once the patient is afebrile for greater than a 24-hour period and demonstrating clinical improvement. Hydration is essential in all patients with UTIs even when there is adequate kidney function; this helps facilitate "flushing" of the urinary tract and reduces pain and discomfort.

A possible issue in acute pyelonephritis treatment is a chronic or recurring symptomless infection persisting for months or years. After the initial antibiotic regimen, the patient may need antibiotic therapy for up to 6 weeks if evidence of a relapse is seen. Follow-up imaging should be performed within 3 to 4 weeks of completing treatment to ensure resolution of pyelonephritis and to monitor for lasting damage to the kidneys.

Chronic Pyelonephritis

Repeated bouts of acute pyelonephritis may lead to chronic pyelonephritis.

Clinical Manifestations and Assessment

The patient with chronic pyelonephritis usually has no symptoms of infection unless an acute exacerbation occurs.

Noticeable signs and symptoms may include fatigue, headache, poor appetite, polyuria, excessive thirst, and weight loss. Persistent and recurring infection may produce progressive scarring of the kidney resulting in kidney failure (see Chapter 26).

The extent of the disease is assessed by a computerized tomography (CT) or magnetic resonance (MR) urogram, and degree of renal dysfunction via measurements of creatinine clearance, blood urea nitrogen, and creatinine levels. Bacteria, if detected in the urine, are eradicated if possible. Infectious disease consultation should be considered in select populations who experience recurrent or chronic pyelonephritis.

Medical and Nursing Management

The patient may require hospitalization or may be treated as an outpatient. When the patient requires hospitalization, fluid intake and output are carefully measured and recorded. Unless contraindicated, 3 to 4 L of fluids per day is encouraged to dilute the urine, decrease burning on urination, and prevent dehydration. The nurse assesses the patient's temperature per provider or hospital protocol and administers antipyretic and antibiotic agents as prescribed. Symptomatic patients are often more comfortable on bedrest. Patient teaching focuses on prevention of further infection by consuming adequate fluids, emptying the bladder regularly to prevent urinary stasis, and performing recommended perineal hygiene if indicated. The importance of taking antimicrobial medications exactly as prescribed is stressed to prevent multidrug-resistant organisms (MDROs), as is the need for keeping follow-up appointments.

Complications

Complications of chronic pyelonephritis include end-stage kidney disease (ESKD) from progressive loss of nephrons secondary to chronic inflammation and scarring.

ADULT VOIDING DYSFUNCTION

Both neurogenic and nonneurogenic disorders can cause adult voiding dysfunction (Table 27-1). The **micturition** process involves several highly coordinated neurologic responses that mediate bladder function. A functional urinary system allows for appropriate bladder filling and complete bladder emptying (see Chapter 25). If voiding dysfunction goes undetected and untreated, the upper urinary system may be compromised. Chronic incomplete bladder emptying from poor detrusor pressure can result in recurrent bladder infection. Incomplete bladder emptying due to bladder outlet obstruction (such as benign prostatic hyperplasia [BPH]), causing urinary retention, can result in hydronephrosis from the high detrusor pressure that radiates up the ureters to the renal pelvis causing hydronephrosis.

OVERACTIVE BLADDER

It is estimated that more than 33 million Americans have overactive bladder (OAB). OAB is the name for a group of urinary symptoms. OAB is a clinical diagnosis and is not a disease. The most common symptom is a sudden, uncontrolled need or urge to urinate. Other symptoms include the feeling that one needs to pass urine many times during the day and at night (Urology Care Foundation, 2022). Normal frequency is seven voids per day and once at night up until the age of 70 years, where urination can become more frequent based on other comorbidities. OAB can have a significant impact on quality of life. Treatment for OAB is similar to urge incontinence, discussed later in the chapter.

URINARY INCONTINENCE

More than 17 million adults in the United States are estimated to have **urinary incontinence**, with most of them experiencing OAB syndrome, making this disorder more prevalent than diabetes or ulcer disease. Despite widespread media coverage, urinary incontinence remains underdiagnosed and underreported, and it continues to carry stigma. Patients may be too embarrassed to seek help, causing them to ignore or conceal symptoms. Many patients resort to using absorbent pads or other devices without having their condition properly diagnosed and treated. Health care providers must learn to be comfortable asking about private symptoms of incontinence, be alert to subtle cues of urinary incontinence, and stay informed about current management strategies. Cues of urinary incontinence include avoidance of social situations, perineal dermatitis, and depression.

Risk Factors

Urinary incontinence affects people of all ages but is more common among the older population and can decrease an older person's ability to maintain an independent lifestyle. This increases dependence on caregivers and may lead to admittance to LTC facilities. More than half of LTC residents have urinary incontinence. Although urinary incontinence is not a normal consequence of aging, age-related changes in the urinary tract and pelvic floor muscles predispose the older person to incontinence.

Although it is commonly regarded as a condition that occurs in older multiparous AFAB and female persons, it is also seen in young nulliparous AFAB and female persons, especially during vigorous high-impact activity. Age, biologic sex, and number of vaginal deliveries are established risk factors (Box 27-4) that explain, in part, the increased incidence in AFAB and female persons due to pelvic floor muscle dysfunction.

Types of Incontinence

Only with appropriate recognition of the problem, assessment, and referral for diagnostic evaluation can appropriate

TABLE **27-1 Conditions Causing Adult Voiding Dysfunction**

Condition	Voiding Dysfunction	Treatment
Neurogenic Disorders		
Cerebellar ataxia	Incontinence or dyssynergia	Timed voiding; anticholinergics
Cerebrovascular accident	Retention or incontinence	Anticholinergics; beta-3-agonist; bladder retraining
Dementia	Incontinence	Beta-3-agonist; prompted voiding
Diabetes mellitus	Incontinence and/or incomplete bladder emptying	Timed voiding; electromyelogram (EMG)/biofeedback; pelvic floor nerve stimulation; anticholinergics/ antispasmodics; beta-3-agonist; well-controlled blood glucose levels
Multiple sclerosis	Incontinence or incomplete bladder emptying	Timed voiding; EMG/biofeedback to learn pelvic muscle exercises and urge inhibition; pelvic floor nerve stimulation; antispasmodics; beta-3-agonists; intermittent catheterization
Parkinson disease	Incontinence	Anticholinergics/antispasmodics; beta-3-agonists; urinary diversion
Spinal Cord Dysfunction		
Acute injury	Urinary retention	Indwelling catheter; intermittent straight catheterization
Degenerative disease	Incontinence and/or incomplete bladder emptying	EMG/biofeedback; pelvic floor nerve stimulation; anticholinergics; beta-3-agonists; intermittent catheterization
Nonneurogenic Disorders		
"Bashful bladder"	Inability to initiate voiding in public bathrooms	Relaxation therapy; EMG/biofeedback
Overactive bladder	Urgency, frequency, and/or urge incontinence	EMG/biofeedback; pelvic floor nerve stimulation; anticholinergics; beta-3-agonists
Post general surgery	Acute urine retention	Catheterization (indwelling catheter or intermittent)
Post-prostatectomy	Incontinence	*Mild:* biofeedback; pelvic floor nerve stimulation; pelvic floor physical therapy *Moderate/severe:* surgery—artificial sphincter or bladder sling
Stress incontinence	Incontinence with cough, laugh, sneeze, position change	*Mild:* biofeedback; pelvic floor physical therapy; periurethral bulking with collagen *Moderate/severe:* surgery

BOX 27-4 **Risk Factors for Urinary Incontinence**

- Pregnancy: vaginal delivery, episiotomy
- Menopause
- Genitourinary surgery
- Pelvic muscle weakness
- Incompetent urethra due to trauma or sphincter relaxation
- Immobility
- High-impact exercise
- Diabetes mellitus
- Stroke
- Age-related changes in the urinary tract
- Morbid obesity
- Cognitive disturbances: dementia, Parkinson disease
- Medications: diuretics, sedatives, hypnotics, opioids
- Caregiver or toilet unavailable

treatment be outlined and recommended. All patients with incontinence should be considered for evaluation and treatment. Urinary incontinence may be transient or reversible if the underlying cause is successfully treated and the voiding pattern reverts to normal (Box 27-5).

Stress incontinence is the involuntary loss of urine through an intact urethra as a result of sneezing, coughing, or changing position. It can predominantly affect AFAB and female patients who have had vaginal deliveries and is thought to be the result of decreasing ligament and pelvic floor support (pelvic floor dysfunction). In postmenopausal AFAB or female biologic sex patients, decreasing or absent estrogen levels within the urethral walls and bladder base can contribute to stress urinary incontinence. In male biologic sex patients, stress incontinence is often experienced after a radical prostatectomy for prostate cancer because of the loss of

BOX 27-5

Causes of Transient Incontinence: DIAPPERS

Delirium
Infection of urinary tract
Atrophic vaginitis, urethritis
Pharmacologic agents (anticholinergics, sedatives, alcohol, analgesics, diuretics, muscle relaxants, adrenergic agents)
Psychological factors (depression, regression)
Excessive urine production (increased intake, diabetes insipidus, diabetic ketoacidosis)
Restricted activity
Stool impaction

urethral compression that the prostate had supplied before the surgery and disruption of the pelvic floor muscles.

Urge incontinence is the involuntary loss of urine associated with a strong urge to void that cannot be suppressed. The patient is aware of the need to void but is unable to reach a toilet in time. An uninhibited detrusor contraction is the precipitating factor. This can occur in a patient with neurologic dysfunction that impairs inhibition of bladder contraction or in a patient without overt neurologic dysfunction.

Reflex incontinence is the involuntary loss of urine due to hyperreflexia in the absence of normal sensations usually associated with voiding. This commonly occurs in patients with spinal cord injury because they have neither neurologically mediated motor control of the detrusor nor sensory awareness of the need to void (see Chapter 44).

Overflow incontinence is the involuntary loss of urine associated with overdistention of the bladder. Such overdistention results from the bladder's inability to empty normally, despite frequent urine loss. Neurologic abnormalities (e.g., spinal cord lesions), factors that obstruct the outflow of urine (e.g., tumors, strictures, and prostatic hyperplasia), and myogenic abnormalities (problems with bladder contractions) can cause overflow incontinence.

Functional incontinence refers to those instances in which lower urinary tract function is intact but other factors, such as severe cognitive impairment (e.g., Alzheimer dementia), make it difficult for the patient to identify the need to void or physical impairments make it difficult or impossible for the patient to reach the toilet in time for voiding. Often times, these patients can respond well to timed-voiding (bladder is emptied at regular intervals).

Iatrogenic incontinence refers to the involuntary loss of urine due to extrinsic medical factors, predominantly medications. One such example is the use of alpha-adrenergic agents to decrease blood pressure. In some people with an intact urinary system, these agents adversely affect the alpha receptors responsible for bladder neck closing pressure; the bladder neck relaxes to the point of incontinence with a minimal increase in intra-abdominal pressure, mimicking stress incontinence. As soon as the medication is discontinued, the apparent incontinence resolves.

Some patients have several types of urinary incontinence. When the patient presents with evidence of multiple symptoms of overlapping incontinence disorders, this can be classified as mixed urinary incontinence.

Clinical Manifestations and Assessment

Once incontinence is recognized, a thorough history is necessary. This includes a detailed description of the problem and a history of medications, noting those associated with urinary incontinence such as loop diuretics, ACE inhibitors, calcium channel blockers, narcotics, sedatives–hypnotics (including alcohol), anticholinergics, lithium, and NSAIDs (Akoto et al., 2022). The patient's voiding history, a diary of fluid intake and output, and bedside tests (e.g., residual urine, stress maneuvers) may be used to help determine the type of urinary incontinence involved. Urodynamic testing is only indicated in some incontinence patient scenarios. Urinalysis and urine cultures should only be performed if signs and symptoms of infection are evident.

Medical Management

Management depends on the type of urinary incontinence and its causes. Strategies for promoting urinary continence can be found in Box 27-6. Management of urinary incontinence may be behavioral, pharmacologic, or surgical in nature depending on the severity of symptoms and failure of other therapies.

Behavioral Therapy

Behavioral therapies are the first choice to decrease or eliminate urinary incontinence and or symptoms of OAB (Box 27-7). In using these techniques, health care professionals

BOX 27-6

Patient Education

Strategies for Promoting Urinary Continence

- Increase your awareness of the amount and timing of all fluid intake.
- Avoid taking diuretics after 4 PM.
- Limit bladder irritants, such as caffeine, alcohol, and aspartame (NutraSweet).
- Take steps to avoid constipation: Drink adequate fluids, eat a well-balanced diet high in fiber, exercise regularly, and take stool softeners if recommended.
- Void regularly, 5–8 times a day (about every 2–3 hours at first, and increasing duration between voids):
  - First thing in the morning
  - Before each meal
  - Before retiring to bed
  - Once during night if necessary
- Perform all pelvic floor muscle exercises as prescribed, every day.
- Stop smoking (smokers usually cough frequently, which increases incontinence).

BOX 27-7

Behavioral Interventions for Urinary Incontinence

Behavioral strategies are largely carried out, coordinated, and monitored by the nurse. These interventions may or may not be augmented by the use of medications.

Fluid Management

One of the most common approaches is fluid management because adequate daily fluid intake of approximately 50–60 oz (1,500–1,800 mL), taken as small increments between breakfast and the evening meal, helps to reduce urinary urgency related to concentrated urine production, decreases the risk of urinary tract infection, and maintains bowel functioning. (Constipation, resulting from inadequate daily fluid intake, can increase urinary urgency and/or urine retention.) The best fluid is water. Fluids containing caffeine, carbonation, alcohol, or artificial sweetener should be limited because they irritate the bladder wall, thus resulting in urinary urgency. Some patients who have coexisting medical diagnoses, such as heart failure or end-stage kidney disease, need to discuss their daily fluid limit with their primary health care provider.

Weight Management

Obesity is associated with OAB and urinary incontinence; thus, weight control should be considered as a first-line intervention, particularly when the body mass index (BMI) is greater than 30 (National Institute for Health and Care Excellence [NICE], 2019). Studies reveal that weight loss leads to a significant reduction of the stress incontinence (Resnick, 2020).

Standardized Voiding Frequency

After establishing a patient's natural voiding and urinary incontinence tendencies, voiding on a schedule can be very effective in those with and without cognitive impairment, although patients with cognitive impairment may require assistance with this technique from nursing personnel or family members. The object is to purposely empty the bladder before the bladder reaches the critical volume that would cause an urge or stress incontinence episode. This approach involves the following:

- **Timed voiding** involves establishing a set voiding frequency (such as every 2 hours if incontinent episodes tend to occur 2 or more hours after voiding). The person chooses to "void by the clock" at the given interval while awake, rather than wait until a voiding urge occurs.
- **Prompted voiding** is timed voiding that is carried out with assistance from staff or family members when the person has cognitive difficulties that make it difficult to remember to void at set intervals. The caregiver checks the patient to assess if they have remained dry and, if so, assists the patient to use the bathroom while providing positive reinforcement for remaining dry.
- **Habit retraining** is timed voiding at an interval that is more frequent than the person would usually choose. This technique helps to restore the sensation of the need to void in people who are experiencing diminished sensation of bladder filling due to various medical conditions such as a mild cerebrovascular accident (CVA).
- **Bladder retraining** incorporates a timed voiding schedule and urinary urge inhibition exercises to inhibit voiding, or leaking urine, in an attempt to remain dry for a set time. When the first timing interval is easily reached on a consistent basis without urinary urgency or incontinence, a new voiding interval, usually 10–15 minutes beyond the last, is established. Again, the person practices urge inhibition exercises to delay voiding or avoid incontinence until the next preset interval arrives. When an acceptable voiding interval is reached, the patient continues that timed voiding sequence throughout the day.

Pelvic Muscle Exercise

Pelvic muscle exercise (PME) aims to strengthen the voluntary muscles that assist in bladder and bowel continence in all persons. Research shows that written and/or verbal instruction alone is usually inadequate to teach a person how to identify and strengthen the pelvic floor for sufficient bladder and bowel control. Biofeedback-assisted PME uses either electromyography or manometry to help the person identify the pelvic muscles as they attempt to learn which muscle group is involved when performing PME. The biofeedback method also allows assessment of the strength of this muscle area.

PME involves gently tightening the same muscles used to stop flatus or the stream of urine for 5- to 10-second increments, followed by 10-second resting phases. To be effective, these exercises need to be performed 2 or 3 times a day for at least 6 weeks. Depending on the strength of the pelvic musculature when initially evaluated, anywhere from 10 to 30 repetitions of PME are prescribed at each session. Patients of advanced age may need to exercise for an even longer time to strengthen the pelvic floor muscles. Pelvic muscle exercises are helpful for AFAB or female patients with stress, urge, or mixed incontinence and for AMAB or male patients who have undergone prostate surgery.

Vaginal Cone Retention Exercises

Vaginal cone retention exercises are an adjunct to the pelvic muscle (Kegel) exercises. Vaginal cones of varying weight are inserted intravaginally twice a day. The patient tries to retain the cone for 15 minutes by contracting the pelvic muscles.

Transvaginal or Transrectal Electrical Stimulation

Commonly used to treat urinary incontinence, electrical stimulation is known to elicit a passive contraction of the pelvic floor musculature, thus re-educating these muscles to provide enhanced levels of continence. This modality is often used with biofeedback-assisted pelvic muscle exercise training and voiding schedules. At high frequencies, it is effective for stress incontinence. At low frequencies, electrical stimulation can also relieve symptoms of urinary urgency, frequency, and urge incontinence. Intermediate ranges are used for mixed incontinence.

Neuromodulation

Neuromodulation via transvaginal or transrectal nerve stimulation of the pelvic floor inhibits detrusor overactivity and hypersensory bladder signals and strengthens weak sphincter muscles.

help patients avoid potential adverse effects of pharmacologic or surgical interventions. The AUA and the Society of Urodynamics and Female Urology (SUFU) have since put a strong emphasis on behavioral interventions for the treatment of urinary incontinence and OAB to prevent exposure to detrimental side effects of medications, avoid overtreatment, and prevent possible unnecessary surgical interventions (Gormley et al., 2012).

Pharmacologic Therapy

Pharmacologic therapy works best when used as an adjunct to behavioral interventions. Anticholinergic agents inhibit bladder contraction and are considered first-line medications for urge incontinence. Oxybutynin is frequently prescribed as a first-line therapy and has dual actions of relaxing the detrusor muscle and inhibiting bladder contraction. Topical estrogen can be useful for peri- or postmenopausal patients with either stress or urgency incontinence who exhibit vaginal atrophy which can contribute to incontinence (Akoto et al., 2022). Topical vaginal estrogen can be used safely in small pea-sized amounts when applied directly to the vaginal tissues.

Surgical Management

Surgical correction may be indicated in select patients who have not achieved continence using behavioral and pharmacologic therapy. Surgical options vary according to the underlying anatomy and the physiologic problem. Urethral slings are a procedure for the surgical correction of AFAB or female patients with stress urinary incontinence or patients who have undergone radical prostatectomy with mild-to-moderate urinary incontinence. AFAB or female patients with stress incontinence may undergo an anterior vaginal repair, retropubic suspension, or needle suspension to reposition the urethra. Procedures to compress the urethra and increase resistance to urine flow include sling procedures and placement of periurethral bulking agents such as artificial collagen.

Periurethral bulking is a semipermanent procedure in which small amounts of artificial collagen (or other substances) are placed within the walls of the urethra to enhance the closing pressure of the urethra. This procedure takes only 10 to 20 minutes and may be performed under local anesthesia or moderate sedation. A cystoscope is inserted into the urethra, and a small amount of collagen is injected into the urethral wall. The patient is usually discharged home after voiding. More than one collagen bulking session may be necessary if the initial procedure did not halt the stress urinary incontinence. Periurethral bulking with collagen offers an alternative to surgery after failure of behavioral therapies.

An artificial urinary sphincter can be used to close the urethra and promote continence. Two types of artificial sphincters are a periurethral cuff and a cuff inflation pump.

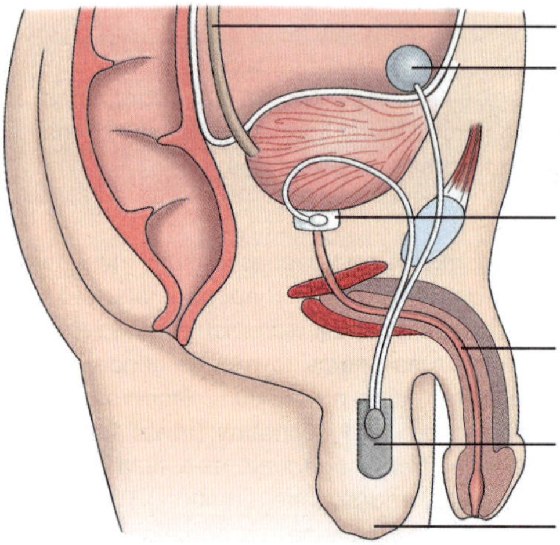

FIGURE 27-3 Male artificial urinary sphincter. The artificial urinary sphincter (AUS) is composed of a circumferential urethral cuff, a pressure-regulating balloon reservoir, and a scrotal pump. An inflatable cuff is inserted surgically around the urethra. The pressure-regulating balloon, which is surgically inserted behind the pelvic bone in a natural open space beside the bladder, uses fluid (typically saline) to open and close the cuff surrounding the urethra. When the patient has to urinate, they will squeeze and release the control pump that is surgically implanted in the scrotal sac. The control pump triggers the system to remove fluid from the cuff. When the cuff is empty of fluid, then the patient can urinate. The cuff will then automatically refill after a few minutes, squeezing the urethra closed.

This therapy is approved for persons who have undergone a radical prostatectomy (Fig. 27-3).

AMAB or male patients with overflow and urge incontinence may undergo a transurethral resection of the prostate (TURP) to relieve symptoms of prostatic enlargement.

Nursing Management

Nursing interventions are directed by the patient's clinical symptoms. For behavioral therapy to be effective, the nurse must provide support and encouragement. Behavioral therapy takes time to improve a patient's level of continence and if the patient is not encouraged to continue they can become discouraged. Patient teaching is important and should be provided verbally and in writing (see Box 27-6).

If pharmacologic treatment is used, it is important to educate patients regarding common side effects of the prescribed medications. Patients who have mixed incontinence (both stress and urge incontinence) should be instructed that anticholinergic and antispasmodic agents can help decrease urinary urgency and frequency and urge incontinence, but they do not decrease the urinary incontinence related to stress incontinence. If surgical correction is considered or undertaken, the procedure, potential surgical complications, and its desired outcomes should be described to the patient and family. Follow-up contact with the patient after all interventions enables the nurse to answer the patient's questions and to provide reinforcement and encouragement.

Gerontologic Considerations

Older persons experience transient episodes of incontinence that tend to be abrupt in onset. When this occurs, the nurse should question the patient, as well as the family if necessary, about the onset of symptoms and any signs or symptoms of a change in other organ systems. Acute UTI, infection elsewhere in the body, constipation, stool impaction, a change in a chronic disease pattern, such as elevated blood glucose levels in patients with diabetes or decreased estrogen levels in menopausal persons, can provoke the onset of urinary incontinence. If the cause is identified, modified, or eliminated early at the onset of incontinence, the incontinence itself may be eliminated. Although the bladder of the older person is more vulnerable to altered detrusor activity (bladder capacity does not change, but sensation and contractility decrease), age alone is not a risk factor for urinary incontinence (Resnick, 2020).

URINARY RETENTION

Urinary retention is the inability to empty the bladder completely during attempts to void. Acute urinary retention in AMAB or male persons is frequently associated with obstruction such as BPH or acute prostatitis. Acute retention occurs infrequently in AFAB or female persons, with the exception of postoperative retention due to anesthesia effects or organ prolapse. Chronic urine retention often leads to overflow incontinence (from the pressure of the retained urine in the bladder). **Residual urine** is urine that remains in the bladder after voiding. In a healthy adult younger than 60 years, complete bladder emptying should occur with each voiding. In adults older than 60 years, 50 to 100 mL of residual urine may remain after each voiding because of the decreased contractility of the detrusor muscle, which is a normal finding and does not necessarily require intervention.

Urinary retention can occur postoperatively in any patient who received spinal or general anesthesia. General anesthesia reduces bladder muscle innervation and suppresses the urge to void, impeding bladder emptying. A number of medications have been implicated in the development of urinary retention and are briefly discussed below. Other etiologies that should be considered in acute urinary retention are trauma, infection (prostatitis, cystitis), and neurologic and psychiatric disorders.

Pathophysiology

Urinary retention may result from diabetes; prostatic enlargement; urethral pathology (infection, urethral strictures, tumor, calculus; trauma (pelvic injuries); pregnancy; or neurologic or myogenic disorders such as stroke, spinal cord injury, multiple sclerosis (MS), Guillain–Barré syndrome, or Parkinson disease.

Some medications cause urinary retention, either by inhibiting bladder contractility or by increasing bladder outlet resistance, namely anticholinergics and sympathomimetic agents. Medications that cause retention by inhibiting bladder contractility include antispasmodic agents (oxybutynin chloride, belladonna, and opioid suppositories) and tricyclic antidepressant medications (imipramine, doxepin). Medications that cause urine retention by increasing bladder outlet resistance include alpha-adrenergic agents (ephedrine sulfate, pseudoephedrine), beta-adrenergic blockers (propranolol), and estrogens.

Sympathomimetics "mimic" the sympathetic nervous system and therefore have the anticipated result of increasing heart rate and contractility, dilating bronchioles and pupils, and—pertinent to this chapter—relaxing the bladder wall and thus closing the sphincter, affecting urinary retention. Anticholinergics work by blocking the parasympathetic nervous system response, which causes contraction of the bladder and relaxation of the sphincter. Thus, since this response is blocked, clinically the effects are similar to the sympathomimetics; hence, both drugs are implicated in urinary retention.

Clinical Manifestations and Assessment

The assessment of a patient for urinary retention is multifaceted because the signs and symptoms may be easily overlooked. The following questions serve as a guide in assessment:

- What was the time of the last urination, and how much urine was voided?
- Is the patient voiding small amounts of urine frequently?
- Is the patient dribbling urine?
- Does the patient complain of pain or discomfort in the lower abdomen? (Discomfort may be relatively mild if the bladder distends slowly or absent.)
- Is the pelvic area rounded and swollen, indicating urine retention and a distended bladder?
- Does percussion of the suprapubic region elicit dullness, possibly indicating urine retention and a distended bladder?
- Are other indicators of urinary retention present, such as restlessness and agitation?
- Does a postvoid bladder ultrasound test reveal residual urine?

The patient may verbalize an awareness of bladder fullness and a sensation of incomplete bladder emptying. Signs and symptoms of UTI (urgency, frequency, nocturia, and dysuria) may be present. Hematuria may be present due to the extent of bladder muscle distention, especially in retention in excess of 1 L of urine. A series of urodynamic studies, described in Chapter 25, may be performed to identify the type of bladder dysfunction and to aid in determining appropriate treatment. The patient may complete a voiding diary to provide a written record of the amount of urine voided and the frequency of voiding. Postvoid residual urine may be assessed either using straight catheterization or an ultrasound bladder scanner and is considered diagnostic of urinary retention if there is more than 200 mL of residual urine.

Medical Management

Management strategies are instituted to prevent overdistention of the bladder and to treat infection or correct underlying etiology for the retention. Immediate management involves decompression of the bladder via catheterization, which is discussed later in this chapter.

Nursing Management

Many problems can be prevented with careful assessment and appropriate nursing interventions. The nurse explains why normal voiding is not occurring and monitors urine output closely. The nurse also provides reassurance about the possible temporary nature of retention and successful management strategies.

In the case of acute urinary retention, decompression with a urethral catheter is commonly required. Nurses need to assess, however, if the patient recently underwent surgery, such as a radical prostatectomy or urethral reconstruction, since catheterization via urethra would be contraindicated. If there are no contraindications to urinary catheterization, the nurse chooses a 14- to 18-French Foley catheter to decompress the bladder. If the patient has a past history of prostatic disease, a *coude* catheter is recommended to facilitate passage through the posterior urethra to accommodate enlargement of the prostatic tissue. A complication associated with emergent catheterization for urinary retention is hypotension (from rapid volume redistribution) and hematuria (from overdistention of the bladder muscle).

Promoting Urinary Elimination

Nursing measures to encourage normal voiding patterns include providing privacy; ensuring an environment and a position conducive to voiding; and assisting the patient with the use of the bathroom or bedside commode, rather than a bedpan, to provide a more natural setting for voiding. The AMAB or male patient may stand beside the bed while using the urinal if this position is more comfortable for urination.

Additional measures include applying warmth to relax the sphincters (e.g., sitz baths, warm compresses to the perineum, showers), offering the patient hot tea, and offering encouragement and reassurance. Simple trigger techniques, such as turning on the water faucet while the patient is trying to void, may also be used. After surgery or childbirth, prescribed analgesics should be administered because pain in the perineal area makes voiding difficult.

When the patient cannot void, catheterization is used to prevent overdistention of the bladder (see later discussion of neurogenic bladder and catheterization). Rarely is a suprapubic tube used for BPH except in instances when the patient continually fails voiding trials and requires long-term management of urinary retention.

Promoting Home Care

Modifications to the home environment can provide simple and effective ways to assist in treating urinary incontinence and retention. For example, the patient may need to remove obstacles, such as throw rugs or other objects, to provide easy, safe access to the bathroom. Other modifications that the nurse may recommend include installing support bars in the bathroom; placing a bedside commode, bedpan, or urinal within easy reach; leaving lights on in the bedroom and bathroom; and wearing clothing that is easy to remove quickly.

Complications

Urine retention can lead to chronic infection and, if left unresolved, predispose the patient to renal calculi (urolithiasis or nephrolithiasis), pyelonephritis, and sepsis. Acute or chronic kidney failure may develop secondary to renal obstruction (refer to Chapter 26). If hydronephrosis has occurred due to large volumes of retained urine, renal insufficiency may develop and progress to kidney failure and bladder areflexia.

NEUROGENIC BLADDER

Neurogenic bladder is a dysfunction that results from a lesion of the nervous system and leads to urinary incontinence. It may be caused by spinal cord injury, spinal tumor, herniated vertebral disk, MS, congenital disorders (spina bifida or myelomeningocele), myogenic disorders, infection, or DM.

Pathophysiology

The two types of neurogenic bladder are spastic (or reflex) bladder and flaccid bladder. Spastic bladder is more common and is caused by any spinal cord lesion above the voiding reflex arc (upper motor neuron lesion). The result is a loss of conscious sensation and cerebral motor control. A spastic bladder empties on reflex, with minimal or no controlling influence to regulate its activity.

Flaccid bladder is caused by a lower motor neuron lesion, commonly resulting from trauma, but increasingly recognized in patients with DM. The bladder continues to fill and becomes greatly distended, and overflow incontinence occurs. The bladder muscle does not contract forcefully at any time. Because sensory loss may accompany a flaccid bladder, the patient feels no discomfort. This can also occur with BPH with obstructive component.

Clinical Manifestations and Assessment

Evaluation for neurogenic bladder involves measurement of fluid intake, urine output, and residual urine volume, urinalysis, and assessment of sensory awareness of bladder fullness and degree of motor control. Comprehensive urodynamic studies may be performed.

Medical Management

The problems resulting from neurogenic bladder disorders vary considerably from patient to patient. Several long-term objectives are appropriate for all types of neurogenic bladders:

- Preventing overdistention of the bladder
- Emptying the bladder regularly and completely
- Maintaining urine sterility with no stone formation or development of UTIs
- Maintaining adequate bladder capacity with no reflux

Specific interventions include continuous or intermittent self-catheterization (ISC), use of an external condom-type catheter, and encouragement of mobility and ambulation. A liberal fluid intake is encouraged to reduce the urinary bacterial count, reduce stasis, decrease the concentration of calcium in the urine, and minimize the precipitation of urinary crystals and subsequent stone formation.

A bladder retraining program may be effective in treating a spastic bladder or urinary retention. Use of a timed voiding schedule may be established. The patient may be taught to "double void": after each voiding, the patient is instructed to remain on the toilet, relax for 1 to 2 minutes, and then attempt to void again in an effort to further empty the bladder.

Pharmacologic Therapy

Alpha blockers were originally developed for hypertension; these drugs block the adrenergic system and help persons with BPH by relaxing smooth muscle tissue found in the prostate and the bladder neck, thereby facilitating urine outflow. The four alpha medications approved by the U.S. Food and Drug Administration (FDA) are terazosin (Hytrin), doxazosin (Cardura), tamsulosin (Flomax), and alfuzosin (Uroxatral).

Surgical Management

In some cases, surgery may be carried out to correct bladder neck contractures, prostatic obstruction, or vesicoureteral reflux, or to perform some type of urinary diversion procedure.

Catheterization

In patients with a urologic disorder or with marginal kidney function, care must be taken to ensure that urinary drainage is adequate and that kidney function is preserved. When urine cannot be eliminated naturally and must be drained artificially, catheters may be inserted directly into the bladder, the ureter, or the renal pelvis. Catheters vary in size, shape, length, material, and configuration. The type of catheter used depends on its purpose, and catheterization is performed to achieve the following:

- Relieve urinary tract obstruction
- Assist with postoperative drainage in urologic and other surgeries
- Provide a means to monitor accurate urine output in critically ill patients
- Promote urinary drainage in patients with neurogenic bladder dysfunction or urine retention
- Prevent urinary leakage in patients with stage III to IV pressure ulcers (see Chapter 51)

A patient should be catheterized only if necessary, because instrumentation can potentially lead to UTI. Catheters impede most of the natural defenses of the lower urinary tract by obstructing the periurethral ducts, irritating the bladder mucosa, and providing an artificial route for organisms to enter the bladder. Organisms may be introduced from the urethra into the bladder during catheterization, or they may migrate along the epithelial surface of the urethra or external surface of the catheter.

Indwelling Catheters

Virtually all health care–associated UTIs are caused by instrumentation of the urinary tract. Catheter-associated urinary tract infection (CAUTI) is associated with increased morbidity, mortality, hospital cost, and length of stay (IHI, 2022). When an indwelling catheter cannot be avoided, a closed drainage system is essential. This drainage system is designed to prevent any disconnections, thereby reducing the risk of contamination. The spout (or drainage port) of any urinary drainage bag can become contaminated when opened to drain the bag. Bacteria enter the urinary drainage bag, multiply rapidly, and then migrate to the drainage tubing, catheter, and bladder. By keeping the drainage bag lower than the patient's bladder and not allowing urine to flow back into the bladder, this risk is minimized.

Triple-lumen indwelling urinary catheters are commonly used after transurethral prostate surgery (TURP) and for patients who are suffering from continuous gross hematuria secondary to cystitis or bladder cancer (see Chapter 33). This system has a triple-lumen indwelling urethral catheter attached to a closed sterile drainage system. With the triple-lumen catheter, urinary drainage occurs through one channel. The retention balloon of the catheter is inflated through the second channel, and the bladder is continuously irrigated with sterile irrigating solution through the third channel.

Pearls for Practice

After a patient undergoes a TURP, they will have a three-way catheter system in place that fulfills several roles: irrigation, tamponade, drainage, and traction. Precise intake and output records must be maintained, especially if total resection time was greater than 90 minutes. These patients are at risk for TUR syndrome, a result of the absorption of irrigation fluid intraoperatively, which can lead to hyponatremia, bradycardia, and confusion.

Accurate intake and output and assessment are essential to avoid the complication of hyponatremia and volume overload associated with instillation of large volumes of irrigating solution during surgery. Solutions used for urinary irrigation are electrolyte-free and thus hypo-osmotic and in general are glycine, sorbitol, and mannitol. During a TURP, the hypotonic solution can be absorbed into the prostatic veins with resultant volume overload and dilutional hyponatremia. The nurse is alert for signs of fluid overload such as dyspnea, decreasing O_2 saturation, jugular vein distention, development of S_3 gallop, hypertension, or hypotension (with the development of heart failure [HF]), and arrhythmias. Early signs of dilutional hyponatremia are mental status changes, headache, nausea and vomiting, muscle twitching, and respiratory distress. The provider is notified of any change in patient condition. The rate of irrigant infusion is aimed at maintaining clear to pink-colored urine. When clots are present, the rate of infusion is increased to prevent clot retention. Since the draining irrigant and urine are both returning to the urinary drainage bag, the nurse must keep an accurate record of amount of irrigant solution instilled and subtract the volume of the irrigant from the total drainage amount in the urinary drainage bag, which is recorded as urine. Thus, if 2 L were instilled over the past 4 hours and the urinary drainage bag contained 2,150 mL, the urine output for the past 4 hours is recorded as 150 mL.

Suprapubic Catheters

Suprapubic catheterization allows bladder drainage by inserting a catheter or tube into the bladder through a suprapubic (above the pubis) incision or puncture (Fig. 27-4). The catheter or suprapubic drainage tube is then threaded into the bladder and secured with sutures or tape, and the area around the catheter is covered with a sterile dressing. The catheter is connected to a sterile closed drainage system, and the tubing is secured to prevent tension on the catheter. This may be a temporary or permanent measure to divert the flow of urine from the urethra when the urethral route is impassable (because of injuries, strictures, prostatic obstruction), after gynecologic or other abdominal surgery when bladder dysfunction is likely to occur, and occasionally after pelvic fractures. Suprapubic bladder drainage may be maintained continuously for several weeks. Suprapubic bladder drainage can also be a permanent necessary modality to divert urine in patients who experience bladder areflexia.

Suprapubic drainage offers certain advantages. Patients can usually void sooner after surgery than is possible with urethral catheters, and they may be more comfortable. The suprapubic catheter allows greater mobility and permits measurement of residual urine without urethral instrumentation. The suprapubic catheter is removed when it is no longer required, and a dressing is placed over the site.

The patient requires liberal amounts of fluid to prevent encrustation around the catheter. Other potential problems include the formation of bladder stones, acute and chronic infections, and problems collecting urine. A **wound care specialist**/enterostomal therapist, also referred to as a wound-ostomy-continence nurse, may be consulted to assist the patient and family in selecting the most suitable urine collection system and to teach them about its use and care.

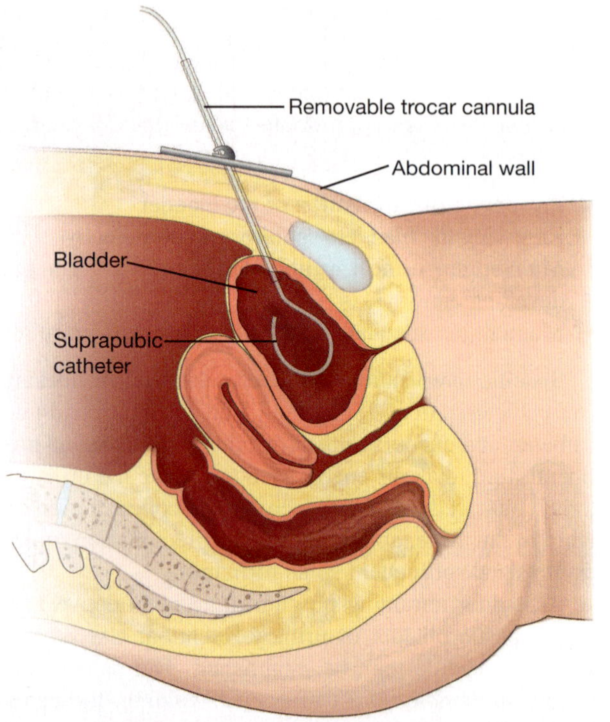

FIGURE 27-4 Suprapubic bladder drainage. A trocar cannula is used to puncture the abdominal and bladder walls. The catheter is threaded through the trocar cannula, which is then removed, leaving the catheter in place. The catheter is secured by tape or sutures to prevent unintentional removal.

Nursing Management during Catheterization

Assessing the Patient and the System

For patients with indwelling catheters, the nurse assesses the drainage system to ensure that it provides adequate urinary drainage. An accurate record of fluid intake and urine output provides essential information about the adequacy of renal function and urinary drainage. The nurse observes the catheter to make sure that it is properly anchored, to prevent pressure on the urethra at the meatus and labia, and to prevent tension and traction on the tubing in both male and female patients. Care is taken to ensure that the catheter position permits leg movement. In AMAB or male patients, the drainage tube (not the catheter) is taped laterally to the thigh to prevent pressure on the urethra at the penoscrotal junction, which can eventually lead to formation of a urethrocutaneous fistula. In AFAB or female patients, the drainage tubing attached to the catheter is taped to the thigh to prevent tension and traction on the bladder and the bladder neck.

Patients are at high risk for UTI from catheterization due to instrumentation of the urethra and need to be monitored carefully. Comorbidities such as advanced age and patients who are debilitated, malnourished, chronically ill, immunosuppressed, or have diabetes should be identified early on and monitored accordingly. The nurse observes these patients for signs and symptoms of UTI that have been discussed previously. The area around the urethral orifice is observed for drainage and excoriation.

Older patients with an indwelling catheter or patients with neurologic conditions (MS, stroke, spinal cord injury) may not exhibit the typical signs and symptoms of infection. Any subtle change in physical condition or mental status must be considered a possible indication of infection and promptly investigated because sepsis may occur before the infection is diagnosed. It is important for the nurse to understand that even if urinary infection is suspected, other differential diagnoses should be investigated per clinical presentation. Figure 27-5 summarizes the sequence of events leading to infection and leakage of urine that often follow long-term use of an indwelling catheter in an older patient.

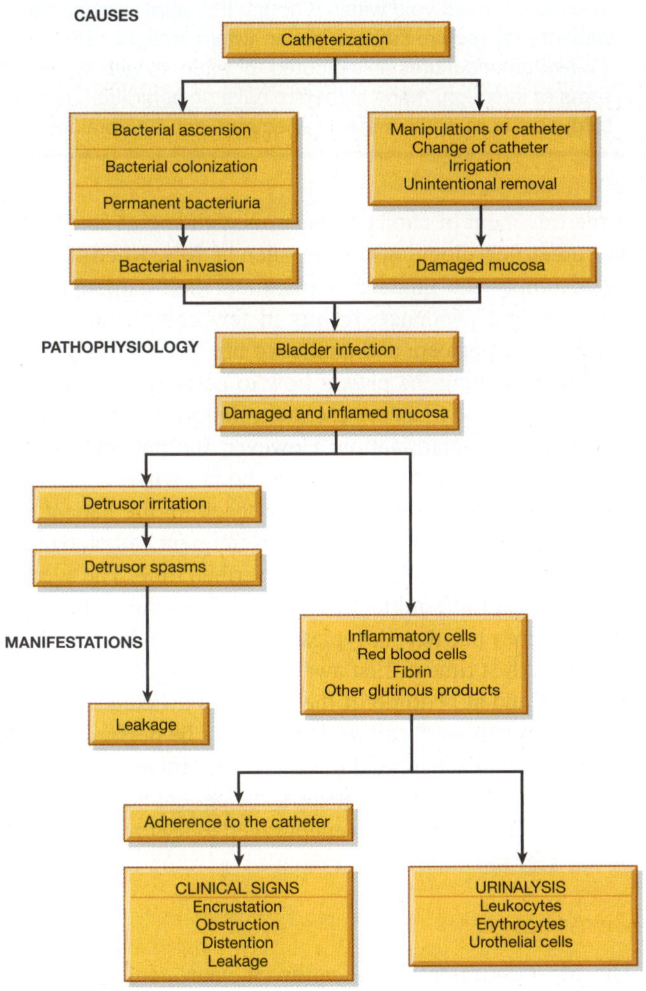

FIGURE 27-5 Pathophysiology and manifestations of bladder infection in long-term catheterized patients.

Preventing Infection

Certain principles of care are essential to prevent infection in patients with a closed urinary drainage system (Box 27-8). The catheter is a foreign body in the urethra and produces a reaction in the urethral mucosa with some urethral discharge.

Bacteriuria is considered inevitable in patients with indwelling catheters (Nicolle et al., 2019). Continual observation for fever, chills, and other signs and symptoms of systemic infection is necessary.

Minimizing Trauma

Trauma to the urethra during catheterization can be minimized by:

- Using an appropriate-sized catheter
- Lubricating the catheter adequately with a water-soluble lubricant during insertion
- Inserting the catheter far enough into the bladder to prevent trauma to the urethral tissues when the retention balloon of the catheter is inflated

Manipulation of the catheter is the most common cause of trauma to the bladder mucosa in the catheterized patient. Infection can occur when urine invades the damaged mucosa. Special care should be taken to ensure that any patient who has altered mental status does not remove the catheter with the retention balloon still inflated because this could cause bleeding and considerable injury to the urethra.

Retraining the Bladder

When an indwelling urinary catheter is in place, the detrusor muscle does not actively contract the bladder wall to stimulate emptying because urine is continuously draining from the bladder. The detrusor may not immediately respond to bladder filling when the catheter is removed, resulting in either urine retention or urinary incontinence. This condition, known as *postcatheterization detrusor instability*, can be managed with bladder retraining (Box 27-9).

Immediately after the indwelling catheter is removed, the patient is placed on a timed voiding schedule, usually every 2 to 3 hours. After voiding, the bladder is scanned using a portable ultrasonic bladder scanner. The provider will set a parameter of a maximum of total volume in the urine that would require straight catheterization for complete bladder emptying. After a few days, as the nerve endings in the bladder wall become aware of bladder filling and emptying, bladder function usually returns to normal. If the person has had an indwelling catheter in place for an extended period, bladder retraining may take longer.

Assisting With Intermittent Self-Catheterization (ISC)

ISC provides periodic drainage of urine from the bladder. By promoting drainage and eliminating excessive residual urine, intermittent catheterization protects the kidneys, reduces the incidence of UTIs, and improves continence. It

BOX 27-8

Preventing Infection in the Catheterized Patient

- Use scrupulous aseptic technique during insertion of the catheter. Use a preassembled, sterile, closed urinary drainage system.
- To prevent contamination of the closed system, *never* disconnect the tubing. The drainage bag must *never* touch the floor. The bag and collecting tubing are changed if contamination occurs, if urine flow becomes obstructed, or if tubing junctions start to leak at the connections.
- If the collection bag *must* be raised above the level of the patient's bladder, pinch the drainage tubing. This prevents backflow of contaminated urine into the patient's bladder from the bag.
- Ensure a free flow of urine to prevent infection. Improper drainage occurs when the tubing is kinked or twisted, allowing pools of urine to collect in the tubing loops.
- To reduce the risk of bacterial proliferation, empty the collection bag at least every 8 hours through the drainage spout—more frequently if there is a large volume of urine.
- Avoid contamination of the drainage spout. A receptacle in which to empty the bag is provided for each patient.
- Never irrigate the catheter routinely. If the patient is prone to obstruction from clots or large amounts of sediment, use a three-way system with continuous irrigation.
- Never disconnect the tubing to obtain urine samples or to ambulate or transport the patient.
- Never leave the catheter in place longer than is necessary.
- Avoid routine catheter changes. The catheter is changed only to correct problems such as leakage, blockage, or encrustations.
- To remove obvious encrustations from the external catheter surface, the area can be washed gently with soap during the daily bath. Using silicone catheters results in significantly less crust formation. A liberal fluid intake, within the limits of the patient's cardiac and renal reserve, and an increased urine output must be ensured to flush the catheter and to dilute urinary substances that might form encrustations.
- Avoid unnecessary handling or manipulation of the catheter by the patient or staff.
- Carry out hand hygiene before and after handling the catheter, tubing, or drainage bag.
- Wash the perineal area with soap and water at least twice a day; avoid a to-and-fro motion of the catheter. Vigorous cleansing of the meatus while the catheter is in place is discouraged because the cleansing action can move the catheter back and forth, increasing the risk of damage. Dry the area well, but avoid applying powder because it may irritate the perineum.
- Monitor the patient's voiding when the catheter is removed. The patient must void within 8 hours; if unable to void, the patient may require catheterization with a straight catheter.
- Collect urine cultures as indicated for patients with symptoms of infection; many catheters have an aspiration (puncture) port from which a sterile specimen can be obtained.

BOX 27-9

Bladder Retraining After Indwelling Catheterization

- Instruct the patient to drink a measured amount of fluid from 8 AM to 10 PM to avoid bladder overdistention. Offer no fluids (except sips) after 10 PM.
- At specific times, ask the patient to void by applying pressure over the bladder; tapping the abdomen; or with spinal cord injuries (SCI), stretching the anal sphincter with a finger to trigger the bladder.
- Immediately after the voiding attempt, assess the postvoid residual (PVR) urine either using straight catheterization or an ultrasound bladder scanner. Residual urine of more than 200–300 mL is considered diagnostic of urinary retention.
- Measure the volumes of urine voided and obtained by catheterization if indicated.
- Palpate the bladder at repeated intervals to assess for distention. If there is suspicion of urinary retention, percuss the bladder (refer to Chapter 25).
- Instruct the patient who has no voiding sensation to be alert for any signs that indicate a full bladder, such as perspiration, cold hands or feet, or feelings of anxiety.
- Lengthen the intervals between catheterizations as the volume of residual urine decreases. Catheterization is usually discontinued when the volume of residual urine is less than 100 mL.

is the treatment of choice in patients with spinal cord injury and other neurologic disorders, such as MS, when the ability to empty the bladder is impaired. Self-catheterization promotes independence, results in few complications, and enhances self-esteem and quality of life.

When teaching the patient how to perform self-catheterization, the nurse must use aseptic technique to minimize the risk of cross-contamination. However, the patient may use a "clean" (nonsterile) technique at home, where the risk of cross-contamination is reduced. In teaching the patient, the nurse emphasizes the importance of frequent catheterization and emptying the bladder at the prescribed time. The average daytime clean intermittent catheterization schedule is three to four times per day. A typical schedule can be structured as at breakfast time or first awakening, at lunch time, at dinner time, and at bedtime. If the patient is awakened at night with an urge to void, catheterization may be performed after an attempt is made to void normally. Intermittently between scheduled catheterization times, if the patient has the urge to urinate then they should be encouraged to try to void on their own. Refer to Box 27-10 for details regarding ISC teaching.

Complications

The most common complication of neurogenic bladder is infection resulting from urinary stasis and indwelling urinary catheter (if the patient has one in place). Long-term

BOX 27-10 **Patient Education**

Intermittent Self-Catheterization[a]

AFAB/Females:
- Assume a sitting position.
- Use a mirror to help locate the urinary meatus until comfortable locating it, and then after that feel for the appropriate location.
- Insert the lubricated catheter 7.5 cm (3 in) into the urethra, in a downward and backward direction until urine begins to flow.
- After removal, discard the catheter.
- Consult the primary provider at regular intervals to assess urinary function and to detect complications.

AMAB/Males:
- Assume a Fowler or sitting position.
- Lubricate the catheter.
- Retract the foreskin of the penis (if uncircumcised) with one hand.
- Grasp the penis and hold it at a right angle to the body. (This maneuver straightens the urethra and makes it easier to insert the catheter.)
- Insert the catheter 15–25 cm (6–10 in) until urine begins to flow.
- After removal, discard the catheter.
- Consult the primary provider at regular intervals to assess urinary function and to detect complications.

[a]If the patient cannot perform intermittent self-catheterization, a family member may be taught to carry out the procedure at regular intervals during the day.

complications include urolithiasis (stones in the urinary tract), vesicoureteral reflux, and hydronephrosis, all of which can lead to destruction of the kidney, resulting in decreased renal function.

UROLITHIASIS AND NEPHROLITHIASIS

Urolithiasis and nephrolithiasis refer to stones (calculi) in the urinary tract and kidney, respectively. Kidney stone disease is a common malady, affecting nearly 1 in 11 people in the United States at some point in a patient's life. There is a high incidence of recurrence of approximately 15% in the first year, with a 50% chance of experiencing another stone within the next 10 years (Blaz, 2021). In addition, the incidence of asymptomatic renal stones has been reported to be approximately 40% (Bishop et al., 2020).

Pathophysiology

Stones are formed in the urinary tract when urinary concentrations of substances such as calcium oxalate, calcium phosphate, and uric acid increase. Referred to as *supersaturation*, this is dependent on the amount of the substance, ionic strength, and pH of the urine (an acid environment promotes calcium excretion). Stones may be found anywhere

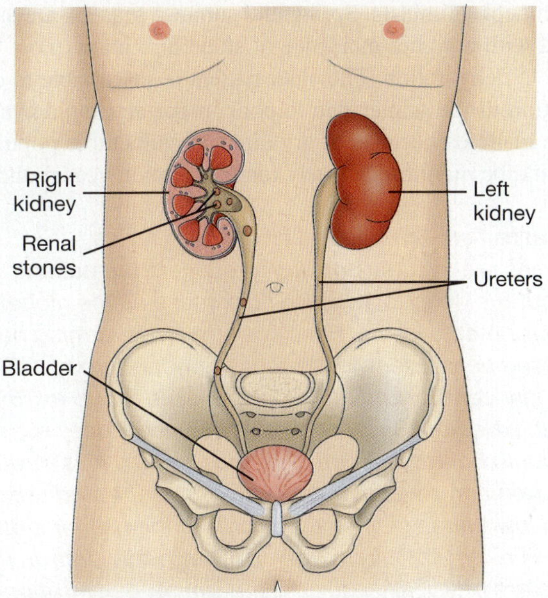

FIGURE 27-6 **Examples of potential sites of calculi formation (urolithiasis) in the urinary tract.**

from the kidney to the bladder (Fig. 27-6) and may vary in size from minute granular deposits, called sand or gravel, to bladder stones as large as an orange.

Stone formation is not clearly understood, and there are a number of theories about their causes and links to systemic conditions such as hypertension, diabetes, gout, metabolic syndrome, primary hyperparathyroidism, and coronary artery disease (CAD; Blaz, 2021). Obesity is associated with insulin resistance and compensatory hyperinsulinemia, which can contribute to stone formation (Blaz, 2021). Theories of stone formation involve either the process of supersaturation of urine with calcium, oxalate, and uric acid, wherein these microscopic crystals form and adhere to the urothelium, creating the formation of stones; or the formation of calcium oxalate stones. More recent theories center on surface molecules that promote or inhibit the formation of crystals (Blaz, 2021). Another theory relates to fluid volume status of the patient (stones tend to occur more often in dehydrated patients). Certain factors favor the formation of stones; however, in many patients, no cause may be found.

Risk Factors

Urinary stones occur predominantly in the fourth to seventh decades of life and affect males/AMAB persons more than females/AFAB persons (11% in males/AMAB persons and 7% in females/AFAB persons, annually), although an increased prevalence is observed across all age groups and in all genders (Blaz, 2021). Anatomic structure of the upper and lower urinary tract may pose a risk as UTIs (struvite calculi) or stasis is associated with stone formation. Metabolic defects such as hyperparathyroidism and hyperuricemia (gout) are also associated with stone formation. Genetic predisposition, such as familial renal tubule acidosis, is strongly associated with nephrolithiasis. Spring and summer seasons are associated with a higher incidence of stone formation, most likely due to dehydration. The older patient is susceptible to dehydration in the winter due to poor intake and rapid evaporation of fluids because of dry air. This vulnerable population should be monitored closely for dehydration year-round.

Pearls for Practice: Lifting the Lens

Nurses are in a key position to educate the patient about the need to increase fluid intake as the global environment warms. Specifically, global warming has caused an increase in the mean temperature of 1.0° C in the last century and is also responsible for up to 75% of heat extremes (Sasai et al., 2021). Since kidney stones occur in hot, dry climates, increasing fluid loss through the skin and respiration results in concentrated urine and low urine volumes that increase the risk for stones (Bushinsky, 2020), rehydration is key particularly in those who are physically active. Quite simply, dehydration increases the risk for nephrolithiasis, and the nurse can teach the need for better hydration, shade, and rest. It is advised that preventive treatment includes teaching the patient to increase oral fluid intake to produce a urine volume greater than 2 L/day, which can reduce recurrent stone formation by about 50% (Bushinsky, 2020).

Clinical Manifestations and Assessment

Signs and symptoms of stones in the urinary system depend on the presence of obstruction, infection, and hydronephrosis. When stones block the flow of urine, obstruction develops, producing an increase in hydrostatic pressure and distending the renal pelvis and proximal ureter. Infection (pyelonephritis and UTI with chills, fever, and dysuria) can be a contributing factor with struvite stones (Bushinsky, 2020). Some stones cause few symptoms while slowly destroying the nephrons of the kidney; others cause excruciating pain and discomfort.

Stones in the renal pelvis may be associated with an intense, deep ache in the costovertebral region (see Chapter 25, Fig. 25-6: location of the costovertebral angle). Hematuria may be present; pyuria may also be noted. Pain originating in the renal area radiates anteriorly and downward toward the bladder and toward the testis. If the pain suddenly becomes acute, with tenderness over the costovertebral area, and nausea and vomiting appear, the patient is having an episode of renal colic. Diarrhea and abdominal discomfort may occur. Stones lodged in the ureter (ureteral obstruction) cause ureteral colic: acute, excruciating, colicky, wavelike pain, radiating down the thigh and to the genitalia. Often, the patient has a desire to void, but little urine is passed, and it usually contains blood (either microscopic or gross) because of the abrasive action of the stone. In general, the patient spontaneously passes stones 0.5 to 1 cm in diameter. Stones larger than 1 cm in diameter usually must be removed or fragmented so that they can be removed or passed spontaneously. Stones lodged in the bladder usually produce symptoms of irritation and may be associated with UTI and hematuria. If the stone obstructs the bladder neck, urinary retention occurs. Stones that are in the bladder should be observed carefully because if they are not expelled and remain in the bladder they can grow significantly in size and require invasive surgical removal.

The diagnosis is confirmed by x-rays of the kidneys, ureters, and bladder (KUB) or by ultrasonography (although ultrasound cannot identify the location of ureteral stones), IV urography, or retrograde pyelography. Blood chemistries and a 24-hour urine test for measurement of calcium, uric acid, creatinine, sodium, pH, and total volume are part of the diagnostic workup. Dietary and medication histories and family history of renal stones are obtained to identify factors predisposing the patient to the formation of stones.

When stones are recovered (stones may be freely passed by the patient or removed during surgical intervention of stones), chemical analysis is carried out to determine their composition. Stone analysis can provide a clear indication of the underlying disorder and steer further treatment steps for the patient (Table 27-2, p. 951).

Medical Management

The goals of management are to eradicate the stone, determine the stone type, prevent nephron destruction, control infection, and relieve any obstruction that may be present. The immediate objective of treatment of renal or ureteral colic is to relieve the pain until its cause can be eliminated. Opioid analgesics are administered; nonsteroidal anti-inflammatory drugs (NSAIDs) also have demonstrated efficacy in treating renal stone pain. In addition, NSAIDs inhibit the synthesis of prostaglandin E, reducing swelling and facilitating passage of the stone. Hot baths or moist heat to the flank areas may also be useful. Fluids are encouraged to increase the hydrostatic pressure behind the stone, assisting it in its downward passage.

Nutritional Therapy

Nutritional therapy plays an important role in preventing renal stones (Bushinsky, 2020). Fluid intake is the mainstay of most medical therapy for renal stones. Unless fluids are contraindicated, patients with renal stones should drink approximately 2 L of water daily or have IV fluids prescribed to keep the urine dilute. A urine output exceeding 2 L a day is advisable. Further nutritional advisement for the patient will be based on the type of stone (calcium oxalate or uric acid) that is diagnosed.

Procedures for Treatment of Stone Disease

If the stone does not pass spontaneously or if complications occur, common interventions include endoscopic or other procedures—for example, ureteroscopy, extracorporeal shock wave lithotripsy (ESWL), or endourologic (percutaneous) stone removal (Fig. 27-7). Refer to discussion of surgical treatment in Table 27-3 on page 953.

Surgical intervention is indicated if the stone does not respond to other forms of treatment, and to correct anatomic

TABLE **27-2 Comparison of Renal Stones**

Stone Type	Causes	Treatment
Calcium (~75% of renal stones)	• Hypercalcemia (high serum calcium) and hypercalciuria (high urine calcium) • Hyperparathyroidism • Renal tubular acidosis • Cancers • Granulomatous diseases (e.g., sarcoidosis, tuberculosis), which may cause increased vitamin D production by the granulomatous tissue • Excessive intake of vitamin D • Excessive intake of milk and alkali • Myeloproliferative diseases (leukemia, polycythemia vera, multiple myeloma), which produce an unusual proliferation of blood cells from the bone marrow • Insufficient fluid intake	• If type II absorptive hypercalciuria (half of all patients with calcium stones), restricted calcium intake • Liberal fluid intake encouraged • Dietary restriction of protein and sodium • Dietary restriction of foods high in oxalates • Medications, such as ammonium chloride, may be used • Thiazide diuretics may be beneficial in reducing calcium loss in the urine and lowering elevated parathormone levels
Uric acid (~5–10% of stones)	• Gout • Myeloproliferative disorders	• Dietary management is key (low-purine diet) • Foods high in purine (shellfish, anchovies, asparagus, mushrooms, and organ meats) are avoided • Sustained alkalization of urine with potassium citrate or sodium bicarbonate results in dissolution of existing stones • Recommended urine output 30 mL/kg/24 hr • Allopurinol may be prescribed to reduce serum uric acid levels and urinary uric acid excretion
Struvite (~15% of stones)	• Form in persistently alkaline, ammonia-rich urine caused by the presence of urease-splitting bacteria such as *Proteus, Pseudomonas, Klebsiella, Staphylococcus,* or *Mycoplasma* species • Predisposing factors for struvite stones include neurogenic bladder, foreign bodies, and recurrent urinary tract infections (UTIs)	• Fluid intake is increased
Cystine (1–2% of all stones)	• Occur exclusively in patients with a rare inherited defect in renal absorption of cystine (an amino acid)	• Low-protein diet • Urine is alkalinized • Fluid intake is increased
All stone types	• Infection, urinary stasis, and periods of immobility, all of which slow renal drainage and alter calcium metabolism • Anatomic derangements such as polycystic kidney disease, horse-shoe kidneys, chronic strictures, and medullary sponge disease; also inflammatory bowel disease and in ileostomy or bowel resection (patients absorb more oxalate)	• Cease taking medications that cause stones reoccurrence including antacids, atazanavir (HIV medication), carbonic anhydrase inhibitors (e.g., acetazolamide, topiramate), triamterene (K^+ sparing diuretic) and felbamate (anticonvulsant; Clinical Overview, 2022). • A sodium intake of 3–4 g/day is recommended. Table salt and high-sodium foods should be reduced because sodium competes with calcium for reabsorption in the kidneys. • Avoid intake of oxalate-containing foods (e.g., spinach, strawberries, rhubarb, tea, peanuts, wheat bran). • Drink two glasses of water at bedtime and an additional glass at each nighttime awakening to prevent urine from becoming too concentrated during the night. • Avoid activities leading to sudden increases in environmental temperatures that may cause excessive sweating and dehydration. • Contact your primary provider at the first sign of a UTI.

abnormalities within the kidney to improve urinary drainage. If the stone is in the kidney, the surgery performed may be a nephrolithotomy (incision into the kidney with removal of the stone) or a nephrectomy, only in circumstances of the kidney being nonfunctional secondary to infection or hydronephrosis. Stones in the kidney pelvis are removed by a pyelolithotomy, those in the ureter by ureterolithotomy, and those in the bladder by cystotomy. If the stone is in the bladder, an

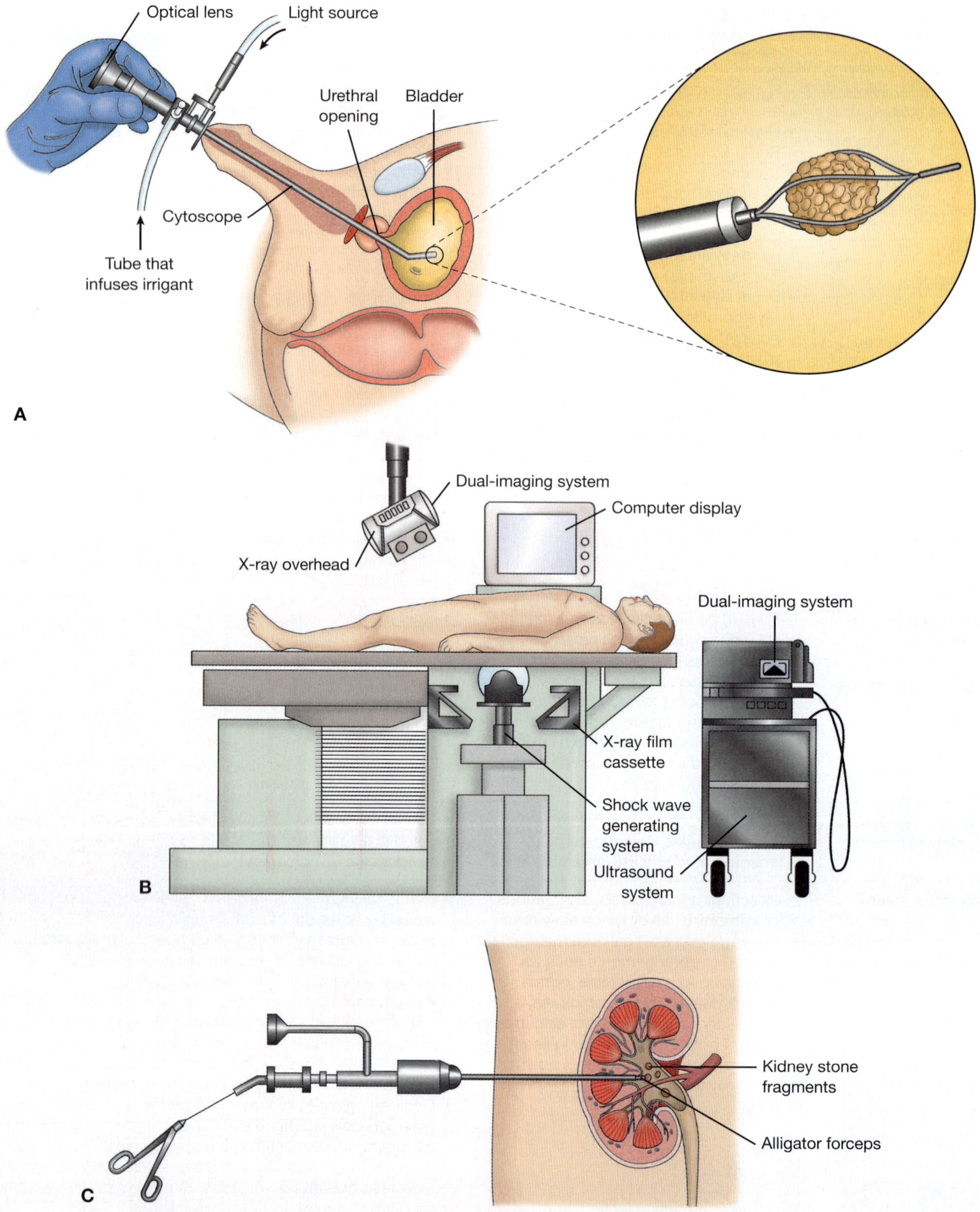

FIGURE 27-7 Methods of treating renal stones. A. During a ureteroscopy, which is used for removing small stones located in the ureter close to the bladder, a ureteroscope is inserted into the ureter to visualize the stone. The stone is then fragmented or captured and removed. B. Extracorporeal shock wave lithotripsy (ESWL) may be used for symptomatic, nonpassable upper urinary tract stones. Electromagnetically generated shock waves are focused over the area of the renal stone. The high-energy dry shock waves pass through the skin and fragment the stone. C. Percutaneous nephrolithotomy is used to treat larger stones. A percutaneous tract is formed and a nephroscope is inserted through it. Then the stone is extracted or pulverized.

TABLE **27-3 Surgical Treatment of Renal Stones**

Procedure	Description	Postprocedure Care
Ureteroscopy (see Fig. 27-7A)	Access to the stone is accomplished by inserting a ureteroscope into the ureter and then, depending on the size of the stone, either basketing or inserting a laser, electrohydraulic lithotripter, or ultrasound device through the ureteroscope to fragment and remove the stones. A stent may be inserted and left in place for 48 hours or more after the procedure to keep the ureter patent.	***For all procedures:*** • Increase fluid intake to assist in the passage of stone fragments. • Monitor for signs and symptoms that indicate complications, such as fever, decreasing urine output, and pain. ***For all procedures except electrohydraulic lithotripsy:*** • Expect hematuria (it is anticipated in all patients), but it should disappear within 4–5 days.
Extracorporeal shock wave lithotripsy (ESWL) (see Fig. 27-7B)	A high-energy amplitude of pressure, or shock wave, is generated by the abrupt release of energy and transmitted through water and soft tissues; this is a noninvasive procedure used to break up stones in the calyx of the kidney. After the stones are fragmented to the size of grains of sand, the remnants of the stones are spontaneously voided. The patient is observed for obstruction and infection resulting from blockage of the urinary tract by stone fragments.	
Endourologic methods (see Fig. 27-7C) percutaneous nephrostomy; percutaneous nephrolithotomy	A nephroscope is introduced through a percutaneous route into the renal parenchyma. Depending on its size, the stone may be extracted with forceps or by a stone retrieval basket.	
Electrohydraulic lithotripsy	An electrical discharge is used to create a hydraulic shock wave to break up the stone. A probe is passed through the cystoscope, and the tip of the lithotripter is placed near the stone. After the stone is extracted, the percutaneous nephrostomy tube is left in place for a time to ensure that the ureter is not obstructed by edema or blood clots.	

instrument may be inserted through the urethra into the bladder, and the stone is crushed in the jaws of this instrument. Such a procedure is called a cystolitholapaxy. Nursing management following kidney surgery is discussed in Chapter 26.

NURSING PROCESS
The Patient With Kidney Stones

ASSESSMENT

The patient with suspected renal stones is assessed for pain and discomfort as well as associated symptoms such as nausea, vomiting, diarrhea, and abdominal distention. The severity and location of pain are determined, along with any radiation of the pain. Nursing assessment also includes observing for signs and symptoms of UTI and obstruction. The urine is inspected for blood and bacteria and is strained for stones or gravel. The history focuses on factors that predispose the patient to urinary tract stones or that may have precipitated the current episode of renal or ureteral colic. The patient's knowledge about renal stones and measures to prevent their occurrence or recurrence is also assessed.

DIAGNOSIS

Appropriate nursing diagnoses of the patient with kidney stones may include:

- Acute pain related to inflammation, obstruction, and abrasion of the urinary tract
- Lack of knowledge regarding prevention of recurrence of renal stones
- Lack of knowledge regarding the role of diet in the treatment of renal stones
- Impaired urinary elimination due to presence of renal stones

Potential complications may include the following:

- Infection and urosepsis (from UTI and pyelonephritis)
- Obstruction of the urinary tract by a stone or edema with subsequent acute kidney failure

(*continued on page 954*)

PLANNING

The major goals for the patient may include relief of pain and discomfort, prevention of recurrence of renal stones, and absence of complications.

NURSING INTERVENTIONS

RELIEVING PAIN

Severe and acute pain is often the presenting symptom of a patient with renal and urinary calculi and requires immediate attention. Opioid analgesic agents (IV or intramuscular) may be prescribed and administered to provide rapid relief along with an IV or PO NSAID. The patient is encouraged and assisted to assume a position of comfort. If activity brings pain relief, the patient is assisted to ambulate. The pain level is monitored closely, especially after administration of pain relief, and an increase in severity, or pain that is not responsive to intervention, is reported promptly so that potential relief can be provided and additional treatment initiated.

MONITORING AND MANAGING POTENTIAL COMPLICATIONS

Increased fluid intake is encouraged to prevent dehydration and increase hydrostatic pressure within the urinary tract to promote passage of the stone. If the patient cannot take adequate fluids orally, IV fluids are prescribed. The total urine output and patterns of voiding are monitored. Ambulation is encouraged as a means of moving the stone through the urinary tract.

All urine is strained because uric acid stones may crumble. Any blood clots passed in the urine should be crushed and the sides of the urinal and bedpan inspected for clinging stones. Because renal stones increase the risk of infection, sepsis, and obstruction of the urinary tract, the patient is instructed to report decreased urine volume and bloody or cloudy urine.

Patients with calculi require frequent nursing observation to detect the spontaneous passage of a stone. The patient is instructed to immediately report any sudden increases in pain intensity because of the possibility of a stone fragment obstructing a ureter. Vital signs, including temperature, are monitored closely to detect early signs of infection. UTIs may be associated with renal stones due to an obstruction from the stone or from the stone itself. All infections should be treated with the appropriate antibiotic agent before efforts are made to dissolve the stone.

Because the risk of recurring renal stones is high, the nurse provides education about the causes of kidney stones and recommendations to prevent their recurrence (see Table 27-2). The patient is encouraged to follow a regimen to avoid further stone formation, including maintaining a high fluid intake because stones form more readily in concentrated urine. A patient who has shown a tendency to form stones should drink enough fluid to excrete greater than 2,000 mL for the rest of their life.

CONTINUING CARE

The patient is monitored closely in follow-up care to ensure that treatment has been effective and that no complications, such as obstruction, infection, renal hematoma, or hypertension, have developed.

The patient's ability to monitor urinary pH and interpret the results is assessed during follow-up visits to the clinic or health care provider's office. Because of the high risk of recurrence, the patient with renal stones needs to understand the signs and symptoms of stone formation, obstruction, and infection, and the importance of reporting these signs promptly. If medications are prescribed for the prevention of stone formation, the actions and importance of the medications are explained. Supporting literature and handouts referencing patient education should be provided to enhance adherence to recommendations.

EVALUATION

Expected patient outcomes may include:

1. Reports relief of pain
2. States increased knowledge of health-seeking behaviors to prevent recurrence:
   a. Consumes increased fluid intake (at least 2 L of fluid per day)
   b. Participates in appropriate physical activity
   c. Consumes diet prescribed to reduce dietary factors predisposing to stone formation
   d. Recognizes symptoms (fever, chills, flank pain, hematuria) to be reported to the provider
   e. Monitors urinary pH as directed
   f. Takes prescribed medication as directed to reduce stone formation
3. Experiences no complications:
   a. Reports no signs or symptoms of infection or urosepsis
   b. Voids 200 to 400 mL per void of clear urine without evidence of hematuria
   c. Experiences absence of dysuria, frequency, and hesitancy
   d. Maintains normal body temperature

GENITOURINARY TRAUMA

Various types of injuries of the flank, back, or upper abdomen may result in trauma to the ureters, bladder, or urethra. Renal injury occurs in 3% of all trauma cases and occurs in up to 10% of abdominal trauma cases (Bacidore, 2020).

Pearls for Practice

If a patient is admitted with pelvic fractures, blunt trauma, with trauma related to a motor vehicle crash, or with penetrating injuries, or has recently had urethral or bladder neck surgery, do not perform a urinary catheterization unless a urology provider has evaluated the patient for urethral tear.

Specific Injuries and Clinical Manifestations

Urethral Trauma

Urethral injuries usually occur with blunt trauma to the lower abdomen or pelvic region. Many patients also have associated pelvic fractures. Classic symptoms include blood at the urinary meatus (present in 80% to 90% of patients with urethral injury); penile, scrotal, or perineal hematoma or swelling; an inability to void; and a distended bladder. The nurse is aware that urinary catheterization is contraindicated if blood is noted at the urinary meatus, until urethral tear has been ruled out by the appropriate urology provider.

Ureteral Trauma

Penetrating trauma and unintentional injury during surgery are the major causes of trauma to the ureters. Gunshot wounds account for 95% of ureteral injuries, which may range from contusions to complete transection. Unintentional injury to the ureter may occur during gynecologic or urologic surgery. There are no specific signs or symptoms of ureteral injury; many traumatic injuries are discovered during exploratory surgery. If the ureteral trauma is not detected and urine leakage continues, fistulas can develop. IV urography detects 90% of ureteral injuries and can be performed on the operating table in patients undergoing emergent surgery. Surgical repair with placement of stents (to divert urine away from an anastomosis) is usually necessary.

Bladder Trauma

Injury to the bladder may occur with pelvic fractures and multiple traumas or from a blow to the lower abdomen when the bladder is full (lap belt or steering wheel injuries). The fuller the bladder is, the greater the risk for bladder injury (Bacidore, 2020). Signs and symptoms to be alert for may include gross hematuria, suprapubic pain and tenderness, difficulty voiding, abdominal distention, guarding, or rebound tenderness (Bacidore, 2020). Blunt trauma may result in contusion, evident as an ecchymosis—a large, discolored bruise resulting from escape of blood into the tissues and involving a segment of the bladder wall—or in rupture of the bladder extraperitoneally, intraperitoneally, or both. Complications from these injuries include hemorrhage, shock, sepsis, and extravasation of blood into the tissues.

Pearls for Practice

The nurse is suspicious for GU trauma in any patient with pelvic fracture; blunt trauma to the lower chest or flank; contusions, hematoma, or tenderness over the flank, lower abdomen, or perineum; genital swelling or discoloration; blood at the urethral meatus; hematuria after Foley catheter placement; or difficulty with micturition (Mondor, 2022).

Medical Management

The goals of management in patients with genitourinary trauma are to control hemorrhage, pain, and infection and to maintain urinary drainage. Genitourinary trauma is frequently associated with renal trauma. Hematocrit and hemoglobin levels are monitored closely; decreasing values may indicate hemorrhage within the genitourinary system. The patient is also monitored for oliguria, signs of hemorrhagic shock, and signs and symptoms of acute peritonitis.

Surgical Management

Surgery is indicated for hemodynamic instability, ongoing bleeding, or urinary extravasation. However, minimally invasive techniques, such as angiographic embolization for hemorrhage and stenting for urinary extravasation, may allow renal salvage. In fact, recent studies indicate that 84% to 95% of renal trauma has been managed nonoperatively (Coppola & Moskovitz, 2019). In the case of urethral trauma, unstable patients who need monitoring of urine output may need a suprapubic catheter or a nephroureterectomy tube (NU tube) inserted. The patient is catheterized after urethrography is performed to minimize the risk of urethral disruption and extensive, long-term complications, such as stricture, incontinence, and impotence. Surgical repair may be performed immediately; however, delayed surgical repair tends to be the favored procedure because it is associated with fewer long-term complications. After surgery, an indwelling urinary catheter may remain in place for 1 month or longer depending on the extent of the injury, repair, and overall status of the patient status post injury.

Nursing Management

The patient with genitourinary trauma should be assessed frequently during the first few days after injury to detect flank and abdominal pain, muscle spasm, and swelling over the flank.

During this time, patients can be instructed about care of the incision and the importance of an adequate fluid intake. In addition, instructions about changes that should be reported to the provider, such as fever, hematuria, flank pain, or any signs and symptoms of decreasing kidney function, are provided. The patient with a ruptured bladder may have gross hematuria for several days after repair. Guidelines for increasing activity gradually, lifting, and driving are also provided in accordance with the provider's orders or directions.

Follow-up nursing care includes monitoring the blood pressure to detect hypotension and advising the patient to restrict activities for about 1 month after trauma to minimize the incidence of delayed or secondary bleeding.

CANCER OF THE BLADDER

Urinary tract cancers include those of the urinary bladder; kidney and renal pelvis; ureters; and other urinary structures, such as the prostate. The American Cancer Society (ACS) reports that in 2022 there will be approximately 81,200 new cases of bladder cancer diagnosed with about 17,100 of those resulting in death (ACS, 2022). Bladder cancer can span the spectrum from non–life-threatening to invasive tumors that demonstrate metastases to other body structures. The three types of bladder cancer are transitional cell carcinoma (TCCa) (95%), squamous cell carcinoma (1% to 2%), adenocarcinoma (1%), and small cell tumors (<1%; Maliski, 2020a). More than 90% of identified urothelial tumors originate in the urinary bladder, while 8% will be found in the renal pelvis; the remaining 2% originate in the ureter or urethra (National Comprehensive Cancer Network [NCCN], 2022).

Risk Factors

Bladder cancer has a high worldwide incidence, and when combined with prostatic cancer, is the most common urologic malignancy, accounting for 90% of all tumors seen. Cancers arising from the prostate, colon, and rectum and from the lower gynecologic tract may metastasize to the bladder. Box 27-11 summarizes risk factors.

Clinical Manifestations and Assessment

Bladder tumors usually arise at the base of the bladder and involve the ureteral orifices and bladder neck. Painless gross hematuria is the most common symptom of bladder cancer. Infection of the urinary tract is a common complication, producing frequency, urgency, and dysuria, and can often delay referral of patients to urology providers for workup. Recent research indicates that a significant barrier to a timely diagnosis of bladder cancer is poor referral rates to a urology provider for workup. Hematuria is often seen in primary care and urgent care settings where patients rely on those providers to determine when referral is appropriate. It is unclear regarding the knowledge gap of providers pertaining to guidelines, as well as complicated patient conditions such as UTIs, kidney stones, or BPH that may prevent the provider from referring patients to urology providers (Gold & Lotan, 2022). Any alteration in voiding or change in the urine may indicate cancer of the bladder. Pelvic or back pain may occur with metastasis.

The diagnostic evaluation includes cystoscopy (the mainstay of diagnosis), excretory urography, CT or MR urogram, ultrasonography, and bimanual examination with the patient anesthetized. Biopsies of the tumor and adjacent mucosa are the definitive diagnostic procedures providing tissue for evaluation. TCCAs and carcinomas in situ shed recognizable cancer cells. Urine cytology should be evaluated for patients who present with gross hematuria or are identified as high-risk microscopic hematuria patients per the AUA guidelines (American Urologic Association [AUA], 2022).

Although the current diagnostic tools such as cytology and CT/MRI have a high detection rate, they are costly. Newer diagnostic tools such as bladder tumor antigens, nuclear matrix proteins, adhesion molecules, cytoskeletal proteins, and growth factors are being studied to support the early detection and diagnosis of bladder cancer. To date, no universal screening test has been promoted.

BOX 27-11 Risk Factors for Bladder Cancer

- Cigarette smoking: risk proportional to number of packs smoked daily and number of years of smoking (associated with 50% of bladder cancers in the United States)
- Exposure to environmental carcinogens: dyes, rubber, leather, ink, paint, metals, and petroleum; consider military specific exposures (e.g., agent orange or contaminated water)
- Recurrent or chronic bacterial infection of the urinary tract
- Bladder stones
- High urinary pH
- High cholesterol intake
- Pelvic radiation therapy
- Cancers arising from the prostate, colon, and rectum
- Diets rich in beef, pork, and animal fat (Rathore, 2023)
- Age, incidence increases with age: higher after the age 60 years, uncommon younger than 40 years median age at diagnosis is 69 years in males/AMAB persons and 71 years in females/AFAB persons (Rathore, 2023)

Medical and Nursing Management

Treatment of bladder cancer depends on the grade of the tumor (the degree of cellular differentiation), the stage of tumor growth (the degree of local invasion and the presence or absence of metastasis), and the multicentricity (having many centers) of the tumor. Refer to Chapter 5 for further details on cancer. The patient's age and physical, mental, and emotional status are considered when discussing treatment modalities. Specific nursing care will be dictated by the treatment plan. The nurse is integral in supporting the patient with information, counseling, and guidance for all modalities of treatment including surgical intervention, intravesical treatment, radiation therapy, or palliative care.

Surgical Management

Transurethral resection of a bladder tumor (TURBT) or fulguration (cauterization) may be performed. These procedures eradicate the tumors through surgical incision or electrical current with the use of instruments inserted through the urethra. After this surgery, intravesical administration of bacille Calmette-Guérin (BCG) or intravesical gemcitabine (anticancer drug that belongs to a class of drugs known as antimetabolites) may be appropriate. BCG is an attenuated live strain of *Mycobacterium bovis*, the causative agent for tuberculosis. Instillation of BCG after TURBT has been shown to significantly decrease the risk of bladder cancer recurrence, followed by an induction and maintenance protocol (NCCN, 2022).

A simple **cystectomy**, radical cystectomy or cystoprostatectomy is performed for invasive or multifocal bladder cancer. Radical cystoprostatectomy in AMAB or male patients involves removal of the bladder, prostate, and seminal vesicles and immediate adjacent perivesical tissues. In AFAB or female patients, radical cystectomy involves removal of the bladder, lower ureter, uterus, fallopian tubes, ovaries, anterior vagina, and urethra. Removal of the bladder requires a urinary diversion procedure. Radical cystectomy remains the primary standard of care for invasive bladder cancer in the United States for patients who are appropriate surgical candidates.

Pharmacologic Therapy

Chemotherapy with a combination of methotrexate, 5-fluorouracil, vinblastine, doxorubicin (Adriamycin), and cisplatin has been effective in producing partial remission of TCCa of the bladder in some patients. Topical chemotherapy (intravesical chemotherapy or instillation of antineoplastic agents into the bladder, resulting in contact of the agent with the bladder wall) is considered when there is a high risk of recurrence, when cancer in situ is present, or when tumor resection has been incomplete, and it delivers a high concentration of medication to the tumor to promote tumor destruction.

BCG is now considered the most effective intravesical agent for recurrent bladder cancer, especially superficial TCCa, because it is an immunotherapeutic agent that enhances the body's immune response to cancer. BCG is particularly effective in the treatment of carcinoma in situ, eradicating it in more than 80% of cases. Once the bladder is full, the patient must retain the intravesical solution for 2 hours before voiding. At the end of the procedure, the patient is encouraged to void and to drink liberal amounts of fluid to flush the medication from the bladder.

Radiation Therapy

Radiation is most commonly used in the adjuvant setting. Patients with locally advanced disease (pT3–4) are known to have high rates of pelvic recurrence and poor overall survival after radical cystectomy and perioperative chemotherapy (NCCN, 2022). Data are limited and further studies are needed to validate if adjuvant radiation may improve these outcomes. A 2019 systematic review that evaluated adjuvant radiation for bladder cancer compared to usual guideline therapy found there was no clear demonstratable benefit of adjuvant radiation therapy following radical cystectomy or cystoprostatectomy; however, there may be some role for the combination of adjuvant radiation with chemotherapy in locally advanced disease (NCCN, 2022). Radiation therapy is not recommended as monotherapy for the treatment of bladder cancer.

URINARY DIVERSIONS

Urinary diversion procedures are performed to divert urine from the bladder to a new exit site, usually through a surgically created opening (stoma) in the skin. These procedures are primarily performed when a bladder tumor necessitates cystectomy. Urinary diversion has also been used in managing pelvic malignancy, birth defects, strictures, trauma to the ureters and urethra, neurogenic bladder, chronic infection causing severe ureteral and renal damage, and intractable **interstitial cystitis**.

Controversy exists about the best method of establishing permanent diversion of the urinary tract. New techniques are frequently introduced in an effort to improve patient outcomes and quality of life. The age of the patient, condition of the bladder, body build, weight, degree of ureteral dilation, status of renal function, and the patient's learning ability and willingness to participate in postoperative care are all taken into consideration when determining the appropriate surgical procedure. Acceptance of a urinary diversion depends to a large degree on the location or position of the stoma, whether the drainage device (pouch or bag) establishes a watertight seal to the skin, the patient's ability to manage the pouch and drainage apparatus, and the patient's ability to mentally and emotionally handle body image changes caused by formation of a stoma.

There are two types of urinary diversion. In a cutaneous urinary diversion, urine drains through an opening created in the abdominal wall and skin (Fig. 27-8, p. 958). In a **continent urinary diversion**, a portion of the intestine is used to create a new reservoir for urine (Fig. 27-9, p. 959).

CUTANEOUS URINARY DIVERSIONS

Ileal Conduit

The **ileal conduit**, or ileal loop, is the oldest and most common of the urinary diversion procedures in use because of the low number of complications and surgeons' familiarity with the procedure. The urine is diverted by implanting the ureters into a 12-cm loop of ileum that is led out through the abdominal wall. This loop of ileum is a simple conduit (passageway) for urine from the ureters to the surface. The resected ends of the remaining intestine are anastomosed (connected) to provide an intact bowel. A loop of the sigmoid colon may also be used. An ileostomy bag is used to collect the urine.

Stents are placed in the ureters to prevent occlusion secondary to postsurgical edema. Bilateral ureteral stents allow urine to drain from the kidney to the stoma and provide a method for accurate measurement of urine output. They may be left in place 10 to 21 days postoperatively. Jackson–Pratt tubes or other types of drains are inserted to prevent the accumulation of fluid in the space created by removal of the bladder.

After surgery, a skin barrier and a transparent, disposable urinary drainage bag are applied around the conduit and connected to drainage. A custom-cut appliance is used until the edema subsides and the stoma shrinks to its final size. The

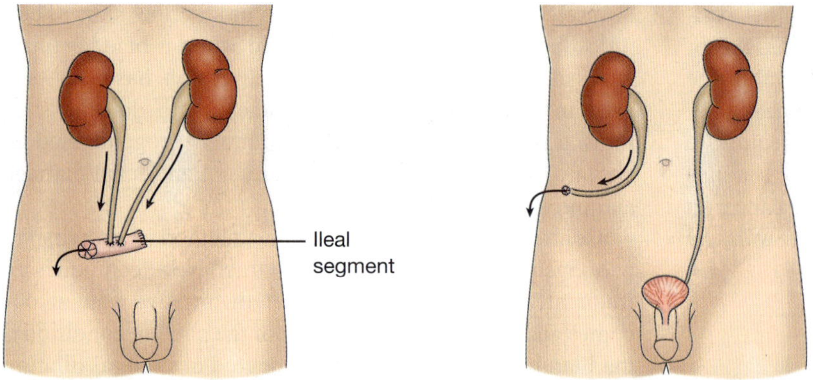

A Conventional ileal conduit.
The surgeon transplants the ureters to an isolated section of the terminal ileum (ileal conduit), bringing one end to the abdominal wall. The ureter may also be transplanted into the transverse sigmoid colon (colon conduit) or proximal jejunum (jejunal conduit).

B Cutaneous ureterostomy.
The surgeon brings the detached ureter through the abdominal wall and attaches it to an opening in the skin.

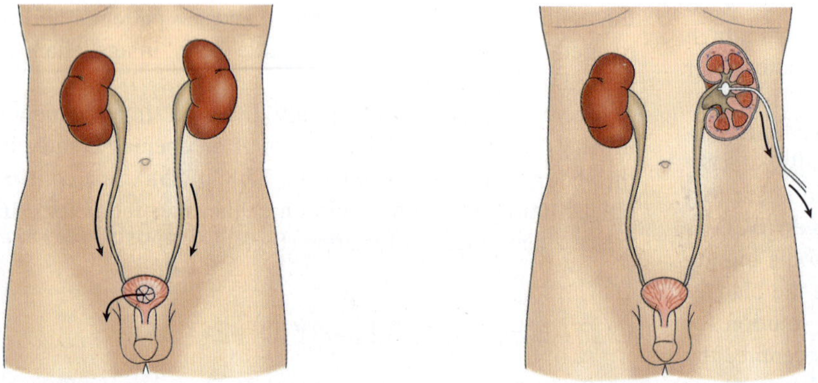

C Vesicostomy.
The surgeon sutures the bladder to the abdominal wall and creates an opening (stoma) through the abdominal and bladder walls for urinary drainage.

D Nephrostomy.
The surgeon inserts a catheter into the renal pelvis via an incision in the flank or by percutaneous catheter placement into the kidney.

FIGURE 27-8 Types of cutaneous diversions include (A) the conventional ileal conduit, (B) cutaneous ureterostomy, (C) vesicostomy, and (D) nephrostomy.

clear bag allows the stoma to be inspected and the patency of the stent and the urine output to be monitored. The ileal bag drains urine (not feces) continuously. The appliance usually remains in place as long as it is watertight; it is changed when necessary to prevent leakage of urine.

Pearls for Practice

The stoma should be pink or red in color. If it appears dusky, the nurse suspects impaired perfusion and alerts the surgeon immediately.

Complications

Complications that may follow placement of an ileal conduit include wound infection or wound dehiscence, urinary leakage, ureteral obstruction, hyperchloremic acidosis, small-bowel obstruction, ileus, and gangrene of the stoma. Delayed complications include ureteral obstruction, contraction or narrowing of the stoma (stenosis), renal deterioration due to chronic reflux, pyelonephritis, incisional hernia, and renal calculi. Approximately 15% of patients with ileal conduits will demonstrate hyperchloremic acidosis (especially in those patients with impaired renal function); it can occur both shortly after the procedure or as a longer-term consequence due to retention of urinary ammonium from the mucosa of the colon and loss of bicarbonate (Tanna et al., 2022).

Stoma Ischemia and Necrosis

The stoma is monitored because ischemia and necrosis of the stoma can result from tension on the mesentery blood vessels, twisting of the bowel segment (conduit) during surgery, or arterial insufficiency. The new stoma must be inspected at least every 4 hours to assess the adequacy of its blood supply. The stoma should be red or pink. If the blood supply to the stoma is compromised, the color changes to purple, brown, or black. These changes are significant for oxygen deprivation to the stoma and can be the first indications of

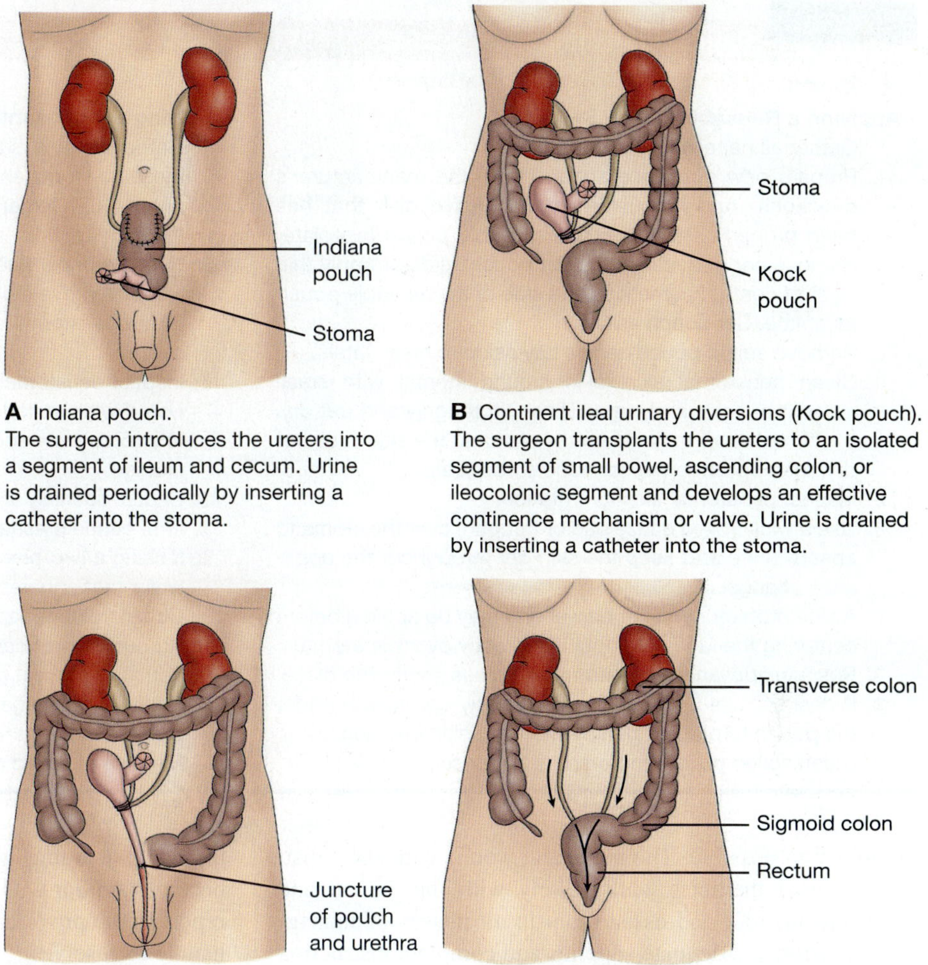

A Indiana pouch.
The surgeon introduces the ureters into a segment of ileum and cecum. Urine is drained periodically by inserting a catheter into the stoma.

B Continent ileal urinary diversions (Kock pouch). The surgeon transplants the ureters to an isolated segment of small bowel, ascending colon, or ileocolonic segment and develops an effective continence mechanism or valve. Urine is drained by inserting a catheter into the stoma.

C
In male patients, the Kock pouch can be modified by attaching one end of the pouch to the urethra, allowing more normal voiding. The female urethra is too short for this modification.

D Ureterosigmoidostomy.
The surgeon introduces the ureters into the sigmoid colon, thereby allowing urine to flow through the colon and out of the rectum.

FIGURE 27-9 Types of continent urinary diversions include (A) the Indiana pouch; (B) and (C) the Kock pouch, also called a continent ileal diversion; and (D) a ureterosigmoidostomy.

impending ischemia of the site. These changes are reported *immediately* to the surgeon. The surgeon or wound care specialist/enterostomal therapist may insert a small, lubricated tube into the stoma and shine a flashlight into the lumen of the tube to assess for superficial ischemia or necrosis. A necrotic stoma requires immediate surgical intervention, but if the ischemia is superficial, the dusky stoma is observed and may slough its outer layer in several days.

Stoma Retraction and Separation

Stoma retraction and separation of the mucocutaneous border can occur as a result of trauma or tension on the internal bowel segment used for creation of the stoma. Mucocutaneous separation can occur if the stoma does not heal as a result of accumulation of urine on the stoma and mucocutaneous border. Using a collection drainage pouch with an antireflux valve is helpful because the valve prevents urine from pooling on the stoma and mucocutaneous border. Meticulous skin care to keep the area around the stoma clean and dry promotes healing. If a separation of the mucocutaneous border occurs, surgery is not usually needed. The separated area is protected by applying karaya powder, stoma adhesive paste, and a properly fitted skin barrier and pouch. By protecting the separation, healing is promoted. If the stoma retracts into the peritoneum, surgical intervention is mandatory.

If surgery is needed to manage these complications, the nurse provides explanations to the patient and family. The need for additional surgery is usually perceived as a setback by the patient and family. Emotional support of the patient and family is provided along with physical preparation for surgery.

Nursing Management

Teaching Patients Self-Care

A major postoperative objective is to assist the patient to achieve the highest level of independence, self-care, and body

BOX 27-12

Patient Education

Using Urinary Diversion Collection Appliances

Applying a Reusable Pouch System

1. Gather all necessary supplies.
2. Prepare new appliance according to the manufacturer's directions: Apply double-faced adhesive disk that has been properly sized to fit the reusable pouch faceplate. Remove paper backing and set pouch aside or apply thin layer of contact cement to one side of the reusable pouch faceplate. Set pouch aside.
3. Remove soiled pouch gently. Lay aside to clean later.
4. Clean peristomal skin (skin around stoma) with small amount of soap and water. Rinse thoroughly and pat dry. If a film of soap remains on the skin and the site does not dry, the appliance will not adhere adequately.
5. Inspect peristomal skin for irritation.
6. Use a wick (rolled gauze pad or tampon) over the stoma to absorb urine and keep the skin dry throughout the appliance change.
7. A skin protector wipe or barrier ring may be applied before centering the faceplate opening directly over the stoma.
8. Position appliance over stoma and press gently into place.
9. If desired, use a pouch cover or apply cornstarch under the pouch to prevent perspiration and skin irritation.
10. Clean soiled pouch and prepare for reuse.

Applying a Disposable Pouch System

1. Gather all necessary supplies.
2. Measure stoma and prepare an opening in the skin barrier about 1/8-in larger than the stoma and the same shape as the stoma.
3. Remove paper backing from skin barrier and set aside.
4. Gently remove old appliance and set aside.
5. Clean peristomal skin with warm water and pat dry thoroughly.
6. Inspect peristomal skin (skin around stoma) for irritation.
7. Use a wick (rolled gauze pad or tampon) over the stoma to absorb urine and keep the skin dry during the appliance change.
8. Center opening of skin barrier over stoma and apply with firm, gentle pressure to attain a watertight seal.
9. If using a two-piece system, snap pouch onto the flanged wafer that adheres to skin.
10. Close drainage tap or spout at bottom of pouch.
11. A pouch cover can be used or cornstarch applied under pouch to prevent perspiration and skin irritation.
12. Apply hypoallergenic tape around the skin barrier in a picture-frame manner.
13. Dispose of soiled appliance.

positivity as possible. The nurse and wound care specialist/enterostomal therapist work closely with the patient and family to instruct and assist them in all phases of managing the ostomy. Adequate supplies and complete instruction are necessary to enable the patient and a family member to develop competence and confidence in their skills. Written and verbal instructions are provided, and the patient is encouraged to contact their provider with follow-up questions. Follow-up telephone calls from the nurse to the patient and family after discharge may provide added support and provide another opportunity to answer their questions. Follow-up visits and reinforcement of correct skin care and appliance management techniques also promote skin integrity. Specific techniques for managing the appliance are described in Box 27-12.

The patient is encouraged to participate in decisions regarding the type of collecting appliance and the time of day to change the appliance. The patient is assisted and encouraged to look at and touch the stoma early to overcome any fears. The nurse should assist the patient and their family in connecting with support groups to further help the patient adapt to the new normal of their life. The patient and family need to know the characteristics of a normal stoma:

- Pink and moist, like the inside of the mouth
- Insensitive to pain because it has no nerve endings
- Vascular and may bleed when cleaned

In addition, if a segment of the GI tract was used to create the urinary diversion, mucus likely will be visible in the urine. By learning what is normal, the patient and family become familiar with what signs and symptoms they should report to the provider or nurse and what problems they can handle themselves.

Information provided to the patient and the extent of involvement in self-care are determined by the patient's physical recovery and ability to accept and acquire the knowledge and skill needed for independence. The patient is given the opportunity to practice and demonstrate the knowledge and skills needed to manage urinary drainage. The nurse should help the patient correct any incorrect application of the device and encourage the patient when proper care is taken of the stoma.

Continuing Care

Follow-up care is essential to determine how the patient has adapted to the body image changes and lifestyle adjustments. Visits from a home care nurse are important to assess the patient's adaptation to the home setting and management of the ostomy. Teaching and reinforcement may assist the patient and family to cope with altered urinary function. It is also necessary to assess for long-term complications that may occur, such as pouch leakage or rupture, stone formation, stenosis of the stoma, deterioration in renal function, or incontinence.

Long-term monitoring for anemia is performed to identify vitamin B deficiency, which may occur when a significant portion of the terminal ileum is removed. This may take several years to develop and can be treated with vitamin B injections.

Cutaneous Ureterostomy

A cutaneous ureterostomy (see Fig. 27-8, p. 958), in which the ureters are directed through the abdominal wall and attached to an opening in the skin, is used for selected patients with ureteral obstruction (e.g., advanced pelvic cancer) because it requires less extensive surgery than other urinary diversion procedures. It is an appropriate procedure for patients who have had previous abdominal irradiation.

A urinary appliance is fitted immediately after surgery. The management of the patient with a cutaneous ureterostomy is similar to the care of the patient with an ileal conduit, although the stomas are usually flush with the skin or normally retracted.

CONTINENT URINARY DIVERSIONS

Continent Ileal Urinary Reservoir (Indiana Pouch)

The most common continent urinary diversion is the Indiana pouch, created for the patient whose bladder is removed or no longer functions. The Indiana pouch uses a segment of the ileum and cecum to form the reservoir for urine (see Fig. 27-9A, p. 959). The ureters are tunneled through the muscular bands of the intestinal pouch and anastomosed. The reservoir is made continent by narrowing the efferent portion of the ileum and sewing the terminal ileum to the subcutaneous tissue, forming a continent stoma flush with the skin. The pouch is sewn to the anterior abdominal wall around a cecostomy tube. Urine collects in the pouch until a catheter is inserted and the urine is drained (Maliski, 2020b).

The pouch must be drained at regular intervals (typically every 4 to 6 hours) by a catheter to prevent absorption of metabolic waste products from the urine, reflux of urine to the ureters, and UTI (Maliski, 2020b). Postoperative nursing care of the patient with a continent ileal urinary pouch is similar to nursing care of the patient with an ileal conduit. These patients usually have additional drainage tubes (cecostomy catheter from the pouch, stoma catheter exiting from the stoma, ureteral stents, Penrose drain, and a urethral catheter). All drainage tubes must be carefully monitored for patency and amount and type of drainage. In the immediate postoperative period, the cecostomy tube is irrigated two or three times daily to remove mucus and prevent blockage.

Other variations of continent urinary reservoirs include the Kock pouch (U-shaped pouch constructed of ileum, with a nipple-like one-way valve; see Fig. 27-9B, C) and the Charleston pouch (uses the ileum and ascending colon as the pouch, with the appendix and colon junction serving as the one-way valve mechanism), although these types of pouches are not commonly performed (Maliski, 2020b).

Ureterosigmoidostomy

Ureterosigmoidostomy, another form of continent urinary diversion, is an implantation of the ureters into the sigmoid colon (see Fig. 27-8D). It is usually performed in patients who have had extensive pelvic irradiation, previous small bowel resection, or coexisting small bowel disease.

After surgery, voiding occurs from the rectum (for life), and an adjustment in lifestyle will be necessary because of urinary frequency. Drainage has a consistency equivalent to watery diarrhea, and the patient has some degree of nocturia. Patients usually need to plan activities around the frequent need to urinate, which in turn may affect the patient's social life. However, this provides the advantage of urinary control without having to wear an external appliance.

CHAPTER REVIEW

NCLEX-Style Review Questions

1. An 80-year-old assigned female at birth (AFAB)/female patient presents to the emergency department because of persistent dysuria, perineal pain, right flank pain, fever, chills, and nausea. The patient reports that they have not felt well for the past 3 days. They also report increasing weakness and fatigue. The triage nurse assesses vital signs and does a quick assessment of the patient. The first table lists the nurse's findings.

Vital Signs	
Temperature	101.2° F
Heart rate	110 beats/minute
Respirations	26 breaths/minute
Blood pressure	96/45 mm Hg
Oxygen saturation	96% on Room Air
Physical Assessment	
Orientation	3/3 oriented to person, place, and time
PERRLA	Present; pupils 3 mm
HEENT	Normal gaze, equal smile, no tongue deviation
Motor	No drift, equal strength ×4 extremities
Sensory	No sensory loss
Language	No aphasia; no dysarthria

Abdomen	Pain with palpation in the right lower quadrant; normal bowel sounds ×4 quadrants; positive CVA tenderness on right
Cardiac	S1S2 without murmur, gallop or rub, flat neck veins
Pulmonary	Normal to auscultation in all lung fields
Vascular	No lower extremity edema

Select all abnormal findings in the data provided

2. The triage nurse gives the report to the ED nurse. Use an X to indicate whether the following nursing actions are Indicated (appropriate or necessary), Contraindicated (could be harmful), or Non-Essential (make no difference or are not necessary) for the patient's care at this time.

Nursing Action	Indicated	Contraindicated	Non-Essential
Establish IV access for administration of fluid/medications as needed			
Administer oxygen via nasal cannula			
Draw a comprehensive metabolic profile (CMP or Chem 7)			
Obtain a urine culture and routine specimen			
Anticipate drawing blood cultures to determine if the patient has progressed to urosepsis			

3. Forty-five minutes later, the laboratory posted the findings listed below. Select the values that are of concern to you and require follow-up.

Laboratory Test Results	Current
Hemoglobin	12.5 g/dL (normal in Female: 12–16 g/dL)
Platelet count	221 mm^3 (normal 150–400,000/mm^3)
White blood cell count	12,000 μL (normal is 5,000–10,000/μL)
Serum potassium	4.9 mEq/L (normal is 3.5–5.2 mEq/L)
Blood urea nitrogen	22 mg/dL (patients over 60 years: 8–20 mg/dL)
Creatinine	2.1 mg/dL (0.6–1.2 mg/dL)
Blood culture	Pending
Urine culture	Pending
Urinalysis	Appearance: Cloudy Color: Amber pH: 6.0 Specific Gravity: 1.020 Nitrites: Positive Ketones: None Bilirubin: None Crystals: None Casts: Rare Glucose: None Leukocytes: 56/HPF RBCs: >189/HPF

4. The patient is transferred to a medical-surgical unit and continues to exhibit decline. Which of the following laboratory test results indicate further decline?

Laboratory Test Results	Current
Hemoglobin	12.5 g/dL
Platelet count	221 mm^3
White blood cell count	14,000 μL
Serum potassium	4.6 mEq/L
Blood urea nitrogen	22 mg/dL
Creatinine	2.6 mg/dL
Blood culture	Negative
Urine culture	*E. coli* >100,000 CFU

5. The medical-surgical unit nurse shares the patient's laboratory findings with the critical care unit (CCU) nurse through face-to-face bedside report. The nurse informs the CCU nurse that the patient is receiving additional IV fluid replacement with normal saline and has started receiving a dose of IV ciprofloxacin. The patient's blood

pressure prior to the transfer to the CCU was 81/40 mm Hg (MAP of 54 mm Hg). Which of the following actions are appropriate for the CCU nurse to perform? Select all that apply.

A. Redraw a creatinine in 6 hours
B. Take vital signs every 15 minutes
C. Anticipate administration of vasopressors
D. Assist with central line insertion
E. Insert an indwelling urinary catheter
F. Perform frequent cardiac assessments
G. Perform frequent skin assessments
H. Insert a nasogastric tube

REFERENCES AND SELECTED READINGS

References and selected readings associated with this chapter can be found on the website that accompanies the book. Visit **http://thepoint.lww.com/Honan3e** to access the references and other additional resources associated with this chapter.

Problems Related to Endocrine Function

A 70-year-old patient with type 1 diabetes is being seen in the endocrinology clinic because of a foot wound that will not heal. The patient states that their blood sugar levels have been ranging from 78 to 350 mg/dL and admits to eating "sweets" at every meal. A culture of the wound was sent to the laboratory.

- **What questions are pertinent to ask the patient regarding the fluctuating blood sugar levels?**
- **What teaching areas would you reinforce regarding wound healing in this patient?**
- **What would help the patient keep an accurate record of blood sugar times and levels?**

CHAPTER 28

Nursing Assessment: Endocrine Function

Gayge J. Maggio

Learning Objectives

After reading this chapter, you will be able to:

1. Identify the major endocrine glands of the body, their anatomic location, and the hormones they secrete.
2. Summarize the major action of the hormones secreted from each of the glands.
3. Describe the negative feedback mechanism and its importance in the regulation of biologic processes.
4. Summarize the role of the hypothalamus and the pituitary in regulation of hormone secretion from the thyroid and the adrenal glands.
5. Name the disorders produced by over- and undersecretion of hormones from the endocrine glands.
6. Describe components of a health history and physical examination of the endocrine system.
7. Identify the diagnostic tests used to assess altered function of the endocrine glands.

Understanding the function of the endocrine glands and the consequences of dysfunction enables the health care professional to anticipate physiologic changes. Symptoms of endocrine disorders usually manifest according to hormone over- or undersecretion. The assessment of the endocrine system is not as straightforward as other systems because it is difficult to inspect and palpate these glands due to their anatomic locations, and patients present with a wide variety of symptoms. The health care professional must understand the function of endocrine hormones and attentively assess a patient's symptoms and diagnostic findings to detect an endocrine disorder.

ANATOMY AND PHYSIOLOGY OVERVIEW

Function and Regulation of Hormones

The **endocrine** system consists of groups of organs involved in regulating metabolism, tissue function, reproduction, growth, and development by synthesizing and releasing specific hormones. **Hormones** are chemical messengers that, when released, have specific "target" tissue, where the hormone binds and impacts cellular functions and reactions (Fig. 28-1). The endocrine system maintains optimal internal functional cell integrity; thus, its influence impacts almost every cell, organ, and function of the body. The endocrine glands include the pituitary, thyroid, parathyroids, adrenals, pancreatic islets, ovaries, and testes (Fig. 28-2). Endocrine glands secrete their hormones either directly into the bloodstream (anterior pituitary) or via nerve tracts (posterior pituitary), which differentiates them from **exocrine** glands, such as sweat glands, which secrete their products through ducts onto epithelial surfaces of the skin, or the salivary glands, which secrete directly into the digestive tract. The endocrine glands are composed of secretory cells arranged in minute clusters known as *acini.* No ducts are present, but the glands have a rich blood supply so the hormones they produce rapidly enter the bloodstream.

The hypothalamus is the link between the nervous system and the endocrine system. The hypothalamus controls the pituitary, which influences the target glands through the action of the secreting hormones. Table 28-1 lists the major hormones, their target tissue, and some of their properties.

In the healthy physiologic state, hormone concentrations in the bloodstream are maintained at a relatively constant level according to need, primarily through negative feedback mechanisms. In a negative feedback loop, when hormone concentration increases, further production of that hormone is inhibited. When hormone concentration decreases,

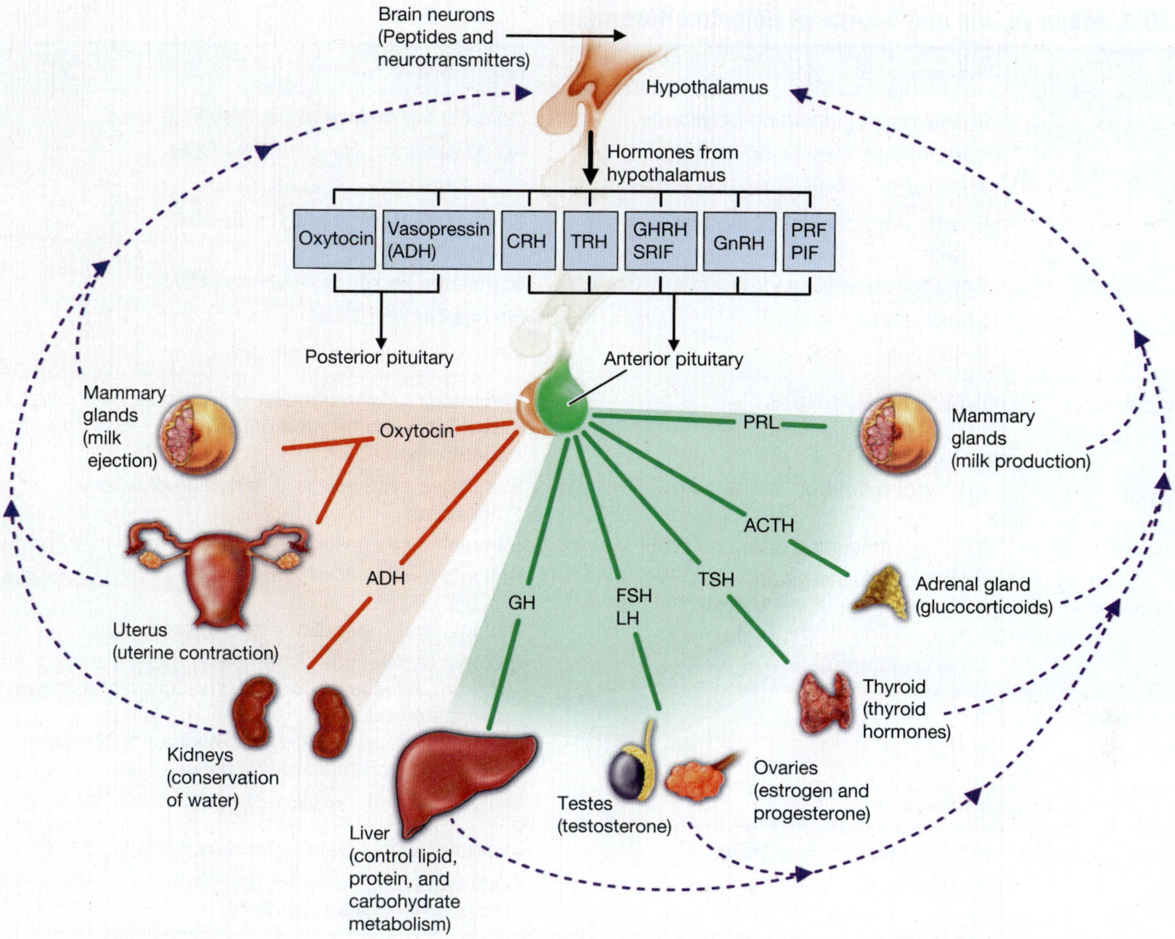

FIGURE 28-1 **Hypothalamic and pituitary hormones and their target organs. The hypothalamus produces hormones that act on the anterior pituitary or are stored in the posterior pituitary. The anterior pituitary produces hormones that act on various body tissues and stimulate production of other hormones. T3, triiodothyronine; T4, thyroxine; TRH, thyrotropin-releasing hormone; TSH, thyroid-stimulating hormone.**

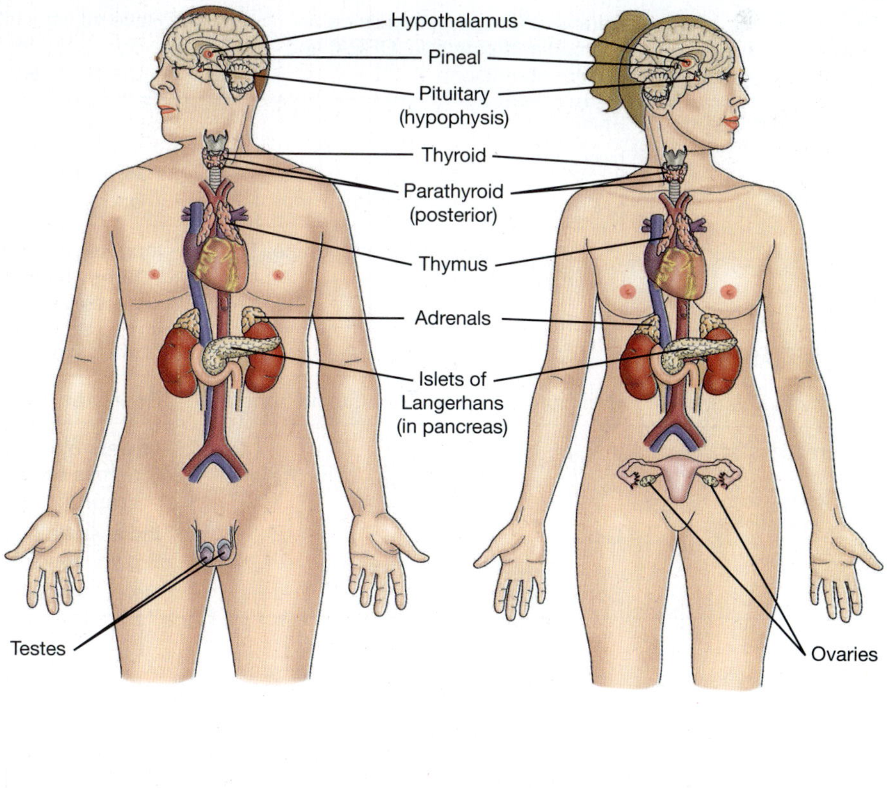

FIGURE 28-2 **Major hormone-secreting glands of the endocrine system.**

TABLE **28-1 Major Action and Source of Selected Hormones**

Source	Hormone	Major Action
Hypothalamus	Releasing and inhibiting hormones	Controls the release of pituitary hormones
	Corticotrophin-releasing hormone (CRH)	ACTH secretion stimulated by CRH
	Thyrotropin-releasing hormone (TRH)	Stimulates the release of TSH
	Growth hormone–releasing hormone (GHRH)	GH secretion stimulated by GHRH
	Gonadotropin-releasing hormone (GnRH)	Stimulates secretion of LH and FSH
	Somatostatin	Inhibits GH and TSH
	Dopamine	Inhibits secretion of prolactin
Anterior pituitary	Growth hormone (GH)	Stimulates growth of bone and muscle, promotes protein synthesis and fat metabolism, decreases carbohydrate metabolism
	Adrenocorticotropic hormone (ACTH)	Stimulates synthesis and secretion of adrenal cortical hormones
	Thyroid-stimulating hormone (TSH)	Stimulates synthesis and secretion of thyroid hormone
	Follicle-stimulating hormone (FSH)	Biologic female: stimulates growth of ovarian follicle, ovulation Biologic male: stimulates sperm production
	Luteinizing hormone (LH)	Biologic female: stimulates development of corpus luteum, release of oocyte, production of estrogen and progesterone Biologic male: stimulates secretion of testosterone, development of interstitial tissue of testes
	Prolactin	Biologic female: prepares breast for breastfeeding
Posterior pituitary	Antidiuretic hormone (ADH)	Increases water reabsorption by kidney
	Oxytocin	Stimulates contraction of pregnant uterus, milk ejection from breasts after childbirth
Adrenal cortex	Mineralocorticosteroids, mainly aldosterone	Increases sodium absorption, potassium loss by kidney
	Glucocorticoids, mainly cortisol	Affects metabolism of all nutrients; regulates blood glucose levels, affects growth, has anti-inflammatory action, and decreases effects of stress
	Adrenal androgens, mainly dehydroepiandrosterone (DHEA) and androstenedione	Have minimal intrinsic androgenic activity; they are converted to testosterone and dihydrotestosterone in the periphery
Adrenal medulla	Epinephrine Norepinephrine	Serve as neurotransmitters for the sympathetic nervous system; the flight or fight response specifically increases heart rate, blood flow to skeletal muscle, and production of glucose
Thyroid (follicular cells)	Thyroid hormones: triiodothyronine (T_3), thyroxine (T_4)	Increase the metabolic rate, increase protein and bone turnover, increase responsiveness to catecholamines, necessary for fetal and infant growth and development
Thyroid C cells	Calcitonin	Lowers blood calcium and phosphate levels
Parathyroid glands	Parathormone (PTH, parathyroid hormone)	Regulates serum calcium
Pancreatic islet cells	Insulin	Lowers blood glucose by facilitating glucose transport across cell membranes of muscle, liver, and adipose tissue
	Glucagon	Increases blood glucose concentration by stimulation of glycogenolysis and glyconeogenesis
	Somatostatin	Delays intestinal absorption of glucose

Source	Hormone	Major Action
Kidney	1,25-Dihydroxyvitamin D	Stimulates calcium absorption from the intestine
	Renin	Activates renin–angiotensin–aldosterone system
	Erythropoietin	Increases red blood cell production
Ovaries	Estrogen	Affects development of biologic female sex organs and secondary sex characteristics
	Progesterone	Influences menstrual cycle, stimulates growth of uterine wall, maintains pregnancy
Testes	Androgens, mainly testosterone	Affect development of biologic male sex organs and secondary sex characteristics, aid in sperm production

Norris, T., & Tuan, R. (2020). *Essentials of pathophysiology* (5th ed.). Wolters Kluwer.

the rate of production of that hormone increases. In addition, hormones are regulated by the central nervous system (CNS)—a sympathetic or parasympathetic response can stimulate or suppress hormone production.

Glands of the Endocrine System

Pituitary Gland

Because the endocrine and nervous systems are so closely associated, they are collectively called the *neuroendocrine system*. The pituitary gland, or hypophysis, is a round structure about 1.27 cm (½ in) in diameter located on the inferior aspect of the brain. Commonly referred to as the *master gland*, the pituitary secretes hormones that control the secretion of additional hormones by other endocrine glands (Fig. 28-3). The pituitary gland is divided into the anterior and posterior lobes.

The pituitary itself is controlled by the hypothalamus, an adjacent area of the brain that is connected to the pituitary by the pituitary stalk. The hypothalamus produces and releases factors that act on cells of the pituitary gland: Growth hormone releasing hormone (GHRH), gonadotropin-releasing hormone (GnRH), thyrotrophic-releasing hormone (TRH), and corticotrophin-releasing hormone (CRH) act on the anterior pituitary, and oxytocin and vasopressin are produced here before traveling to the posterior pituitary.

Anterior Pituitary Gland

The major hormones of the anterior pituitary are follicle-stimulating hormone (FSH), luteinizing hormone (LH), prolactin, **adrenocorticotropic hormone** (ACTH), **thyroid-stimulating hormone** (TSH), and growth hormone (GH) (also referred to as somatotropin). The releasing factors secreted by the hypothalamus, described above, control the secretion of these hormones. These releasing factors reach the anterior pituitary by way of the bloodstream in a special circulation called the *pituitary portal blood system*. Other hormones secreted by the anterior pituitary include melanocyte-stimulating hormone (MSH), which regulates skin pigmentation and beta-lipotropin; the function of lipotropin is poorly understood.

The hormones released by the anterior pituitary enter the general circulation and are transported to their target organs. The main function of FSH, LH, ACTH, and TSH is the release of hormones from other endocrine glands. Prolactin acts directly on the breast to stimulate milk production. Hormones that stimulate other organs and tissues are discussed in conjunction with their target organs later in this chapter.

Growth Hormone

GHRH from the hypothalamus stimulates cells in the anterior lobe of the pituitary to secrete GH, also known as *somatotropin*. GH impacts all tissues, particularly bone and cartilage (Fig. 28-4). It increases the rate of protein synthesis, stimulating growth of all organs except the brain. It increases mobilization of fatty acids and decreases the rate of carbohydrate metabolism. In addition, it increases muscle mass and stimulates the immune system. GH is considered anti-insulin since it limits insulin's ability to uptake glucose in peripheral tissues and enhances glucose synthesis in the liver, resulting in hyperglycemia.

Posterior Pituitary

Important hormones secreted by the posterior lobe of the pituitary (called the *neurohypophysis*) include **vasopressin**, also termed *antidiuretic hormone* or *ADH*, and **oxytocin**. These hormones are synthesized in the hypothalamus and travel from the hypothalamus to the posterior pituitary gland via nerve tracts. Vasopressin (ADH) release will result in reabsorption of water into the bloodstream rather than excretion by the kidneys; its secretion is stimulated by an increase in blood osmolality (concentrated blood) or by a decrease in blood pressure as additional water is needed to return to the bloodstream. Oxytocin secretion is stimulated during pregnancy and at childbirth. It facilitates milk ejection during lactation and increases the force of uterine contractions during labor and delivery.

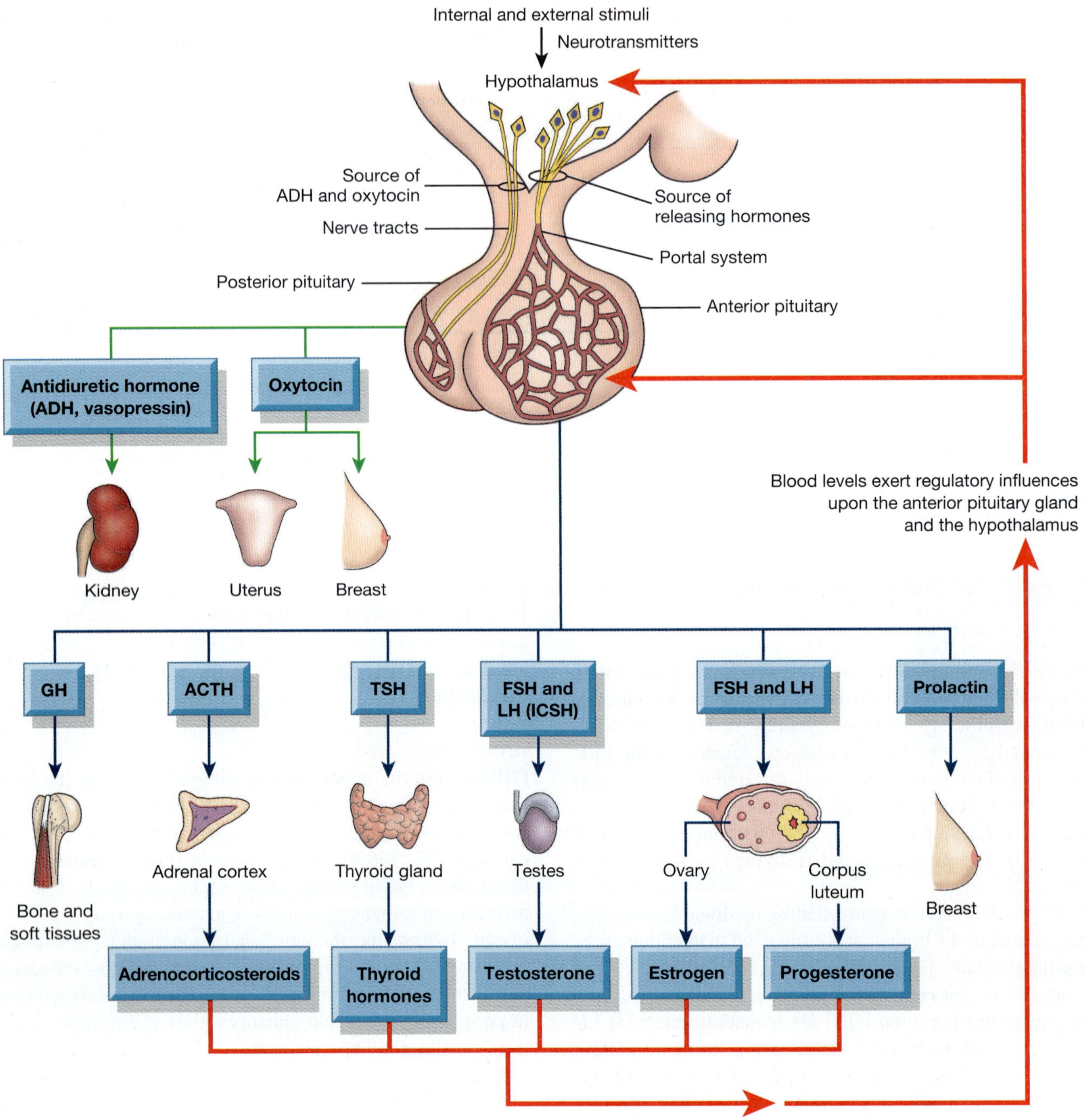

FIGURE 28-3 The pituitary gland, the relationship of the brain to pituitary action, and the hormones secreted by the anterior and posterior pituitary lobes.

Thyroid Gland

TSH (also called *thyrotropin*) acts on the thyroid gland, a butterfly-shaped organ located in the lower neck, anterior to the trachea. It consists of two lateral lobes connected by an isthmus. The gland is about 5 cm long and 3 cm wide and weighs about 30 g. Blood flow to the thyroid is very high (about 5 mL/min per gram of thyroid tissue, approximately five times the blood flow to the liver), reflecting the high metabolic activity of the thyroid gland. The thyroid produces three hormones: thyroxine (T_4), triiodothyronine (T_3), and **calcitonin**. T_4 and T_3 are referred to collectively as *thyroid hormone.* Iodine is essential to the thyroid for synthesis of its hormones.

Thyroid Hormones

The primary function of thyroid hormones is to control cellular metabolic activity. Thyroxine (T_4), a relatively weak hormone, maintains body metabolism in a steady state. Triiodothyronine (T_3) is about five times as potent as T_4 and has a metabolic action that is more rapid. These hormones

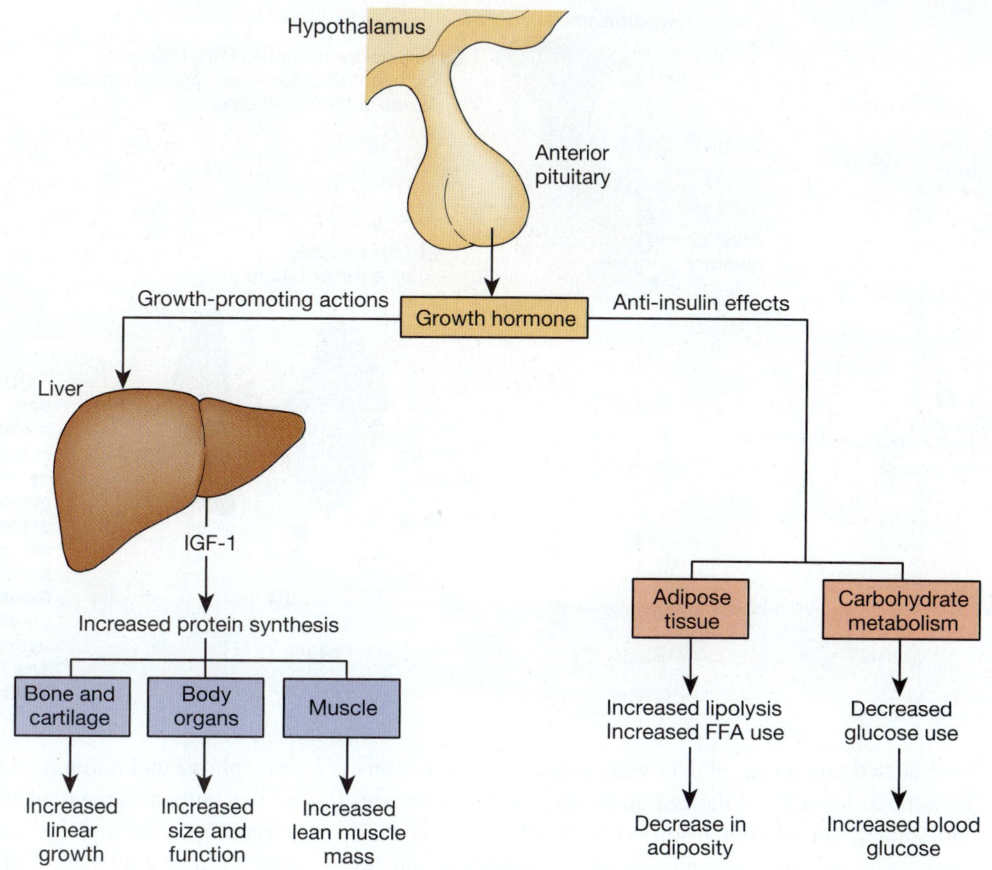

FIGURE 28-4 Feedback mechanism for growth stimulation. Regulation of growth hormone by growth hormone–releasing hormone (GHRH) promotes growth through the action of insulin-like growth factor 1 (IGF-1). Increases in IGF-1 trigger an increase in somatostatin to inhibit growth. Dysregulation can result in gigantism or acromegaly. (Reprinted with permission from Felner, E. I., & Umpierrez, G. E. [2014]. ***Endocrine pathophysiology*****. Lippincott Williams & Wilkins.)**

accelerate all bodily processes that contribute to oxygen consumption and alter the responsiveness of tissues to other hormones. Thyroid hormones influence cell replication, are important in brain development, and are necessary for normal growth. Thyroid hormones influence every major organ system through their widespread effects on cellular metabolism. The secretion of T_3 and T_4 by the thyroid is controlled by TSH from the anterior pituitary gland. TSH controls the rate of release of thyroid hormones. In turn, the level of thyroid hormones in the blood determines the release of TSH. If the concentration of thyroid hormones in the blood decreases, the release of TSH increases, which causes increased output of T_3 and T_4 (this is an example of negative feedback). The term **euthyroid** refers to thyroid hormone production that is within normal limits. Thyrotropin-releasing hormone (TRH) exerts a modulating influence on the release of TSH from the pituitary. Environmental factors, such as a decrease in temperature, may lead to increased secretion of TRH, resulting in elevated secretion of thyroid hormones. Figure 28-5 shows the hypothalamic–pituitary–thyroid axis, which regulates production of thyroid hormones.

Parathyroid Glands

The parathyroid glands (normally four in number) are situated in the neck and embedded in the posterior aspect of the thyroid gland (Fig. 28-6). Parathormone (parathyroid hormone or PTH), the protein hormone produced by the parathyroid glands, regulates metabolism of calcium and phosphorus. Increased secretion of parathormone results in osteoclast growth and bone resorption. When bone resorption is increased, calcium is released from the bone into the blood, thereby increasing the serum or blood calcium level. Some actions of this hormone are increased by the presence of vitamin D. Parathormone also tends to lower the level of phosphorus in the blood. The serum level of ionized calcium regulates the output of parathormone. Increased serum calcium results in decreased parathormone secretion, another example of a negative feedback system (Fig. 28-7).

Calcitonin

Calcitonin is secreted in response to high plasma levels of calcium, and it reduces the plasma level of calcium by increasing its deposition in bone.

Adrenal Glands

There are two adrenal glands, one attached to the upper portion of each kidney. CRH from the hypothalamus stimulates the pituitary gland to secrete ACTH, which in turn stimulates the adrenal cortex to secrete the adrenal hormones (glucocorticoids, mineralocorticoids, and androgens). Increased levels of the adrenal hormones then inhibit the production or secretion of CRH and ACTH. Each adrenal

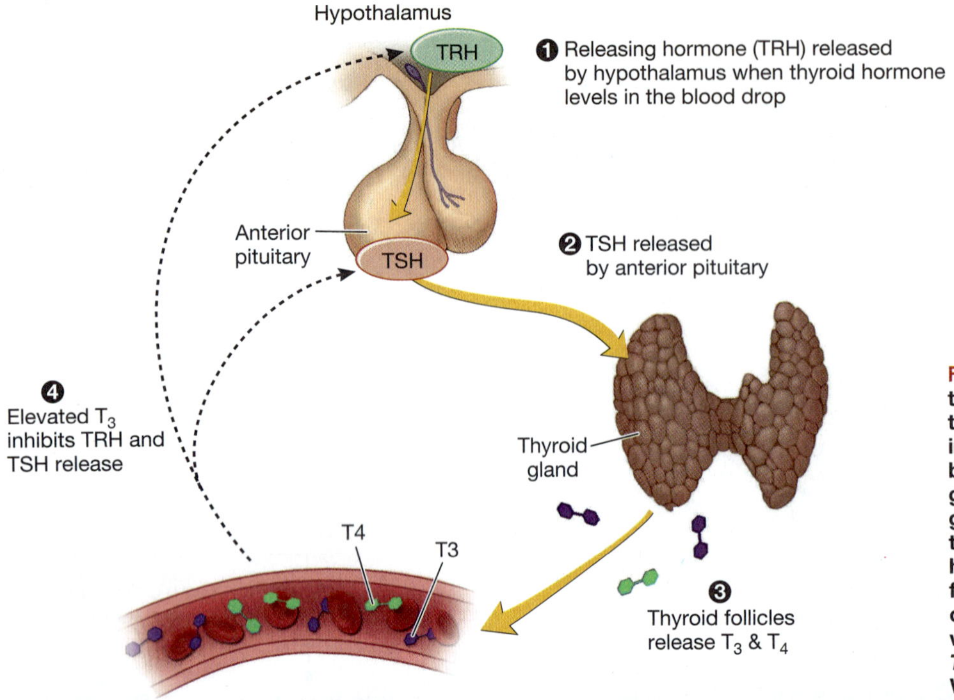

FIGURE 28-5 **Thyroid hormone regulation. (1) TRH is secreted by the hypothalamus when thyroid hormone levels in the blood decline. (2) TSH is released by the anterior lobe of the pituitary gland. (3) In response to TSH, the thyroid gland releases thyroid hormones into the bloodstream. (4) Elevated thyroid hormone levels provide the negative feedback signal to the hypothalamus, causing TRH to be reduced. (Reprinted with permission from Wingerd, B. [2014]. *The human body*. Lippincott Williams & Wilkins.)**

gland is two endocrine glands with independent functions. The adrenal medulla at the center of the gland secretes catecholamines, and the outer portion of the gland, the adrenal cortex, secretes glucocorticoids, mineralocorticoids, and sex hormones (Fig. 28-8). The hypothalamic–pituitary–adrenal axis regulates secretion of hormones from the adrenal glands.

Adrenal Medulla

The adrenal medulla functions as part of the autonomic nervous system. Stimulation of preganglionic sympathetic nerve fibers, which travel directly to the cells of the adrenal medulla, causes release of the catecholamine hormones epinephrine and norepinephrine. About 90% of the secretion of the human adrenal medulla is epinephrine (also called *adrenaline*). The major effect of epinephrine release is to prepare to meet a challenge (the fight-or-flight response). This causes decreased blood flow to tissues that are not needed in emergency situations, such as the gastrointestinal (GI) tract, and increased blood flow to tissues that are important for effective fight or flight, such as cardiac and skeletal muscle. Catecholamines regulate metabolic pathways to promote catabolism of stored fuels to meet caloric needs from endogenous sources, induce the release of free fatty acids, increase the basal metabolic rate, and elevate the level of blood glucose.

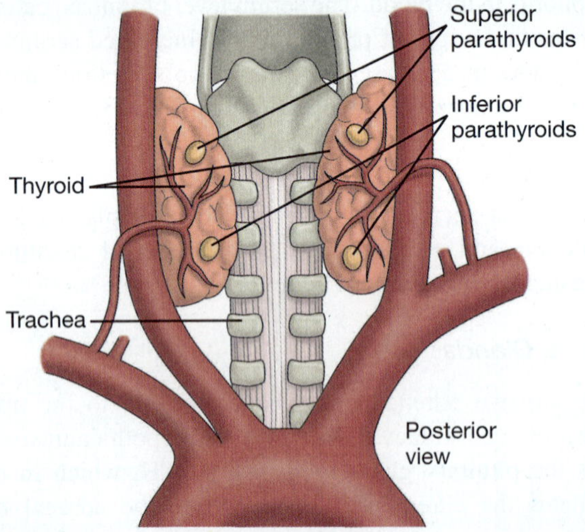

FIGURE 28-6 **The parathyroid glands are located behind the thyroid gland. The parathyroids may be embedded in the thyroid tissue.**

Pearls for Practice: Stress Hyperglycemia

The nurse recognizes the role of cortisol, catecholamines, and proinflammatory cytokines mediated by the hypothalamic–pituitary–adrenal axis (see Chapter 30) and elevation of blood sugar. In clinical practice you will note that acutely ill patients who have no history of diabetes mellitus (DM) may present with high blood sugar, which will be termed stress hyperglycemia. You understand that increased blood sugar provides fuel for the immune system and the brain at time of stress; however, stress hyperglycemia is also associated with adverse outcomes. For example, research reveals increased morbidity and mortality in trauma patients; those undergoing surgical procedures; or patients with infectious diseases (sepsis and pneumonia), cardiovascular diseases, or cerebrovascular diseases who present with stress hyperglycemia

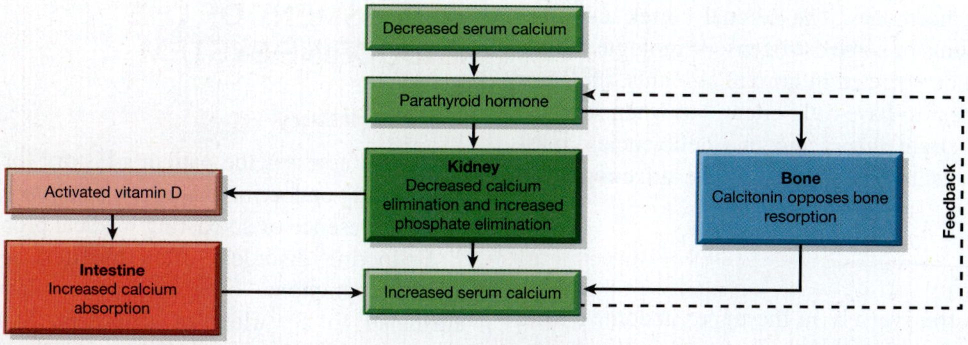

FIGURE 28-7 As extracellular calcium decreases, the parathyroid gland increases secretion of its hormone, P.T.H., which acts on bone tissue to release calcium into the blood. It also acts on the kidneys and intestines to increase the reabsorption of calcium. Calcitonin, which is produced and secreted by the thyroid gland, decreases serum calcium levels by opposing bone resorption. A low calcium level is called hypocalcemia. A high calcium level is called hypercalcemia.

(Pratiwi et al., 2021). Thus, it is not something to ignore. A hemoglobin (Hb) A1c can differentiate undiagnosed DM from stress hyperglycemia since the A1c reflects the glucose over the past 3 months. In general, however, stress hyperglycemia associated with acute disease resolves spontaneously after resolution of the acute illness (Russo et al., 2021).

Adrenal Cortex

A functioning adrenal cortex is necessary for life; adrenocortical secretions make it possible for the body to adapt to stress of all kinds. The adrenal cortex secretes three types of

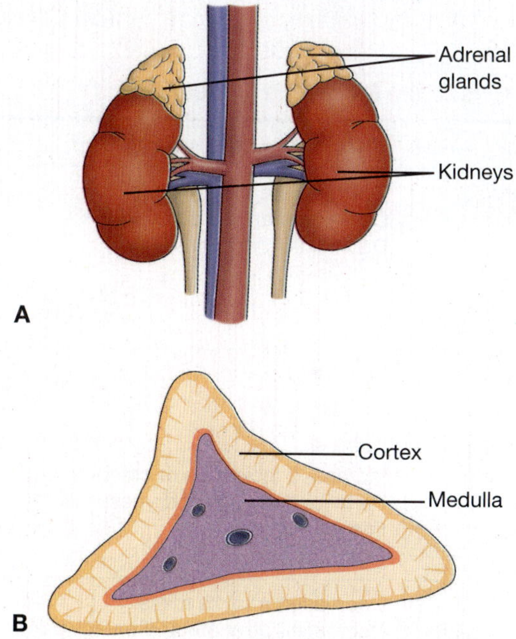

FIGURE 28-8 A. The adrenal glands sit on top of the kidneys. B. Each gland is composed of an outer cortex and an inner medulla. Each area secretes specific hormones. The adrenal medulla secretes catecholamines—epinephrine and norepinephrine; the adrenal cortex secretes glucocorticoids, mineralocorticoids, and sex hormones.

steroid hormones produced by the adrenal cortex: **glucocorticoids**, the prototype of which is hydrocortisone; **mineralocorticoids**, mainly aldosterone (which is important in NA^+/K^+ regulation); and sex hormones, mainly **androgens** (male sex hormones).

Glucocorticoids. The adrenal cortex secretes glucocorticoids in response to the release of ACTH from the anterior lobe of the pituitary gland. Glucocorticoids have major effects on the metabolism of almost all organs because of their influence on glucose metabolism (elevation of blood glucose levels) as well as their ability to inhibit the inflammatory response to tissue injury and suppress allergic manifestations. Without the adrenal cortex, severe stress would cause peripheral circulatory failure, circulatory shock, and prostration. Survival in the absence of a functioning adrenal cortex is possible only with replacement of nutritional components, electrolytes, fluids, and appropriate exogenous adrenocortical hormone.

Mineralocorticoids. Mineralocorticoids exert their major effects on electrolyte metabolism. Aldosterone is the primary mineralocorticoid and is the primary hormone for the long-term regulation of sodium balance. It influences fluid balance through the renin–angiotensin–aldosterone system (RAAS). When sensing decreased perfusion pressure in the body, renin is released from the kidney into the bloodstream. The renin cascade results in an increase in angiotensin II, which stimulates the release of aldosterone and elevates blood pressure by constricting arterioles. Increased aldosterone levels act principally on the renal tubule to cause increased absorption of sodium ions in exchange for excretion of potassium or hydrogen ions. This tends to restore blood pressure to normal and increases renal excretion of potassium. Therefore, the release of aldosterone also can be increased in the presence of hyperkalemia.

Biologic Sex Hormones. ACTH controls the secretion of adrenal androgens, which exert effects similar to those of biologic male sex hormones. The adrenal cortex also may secrete small amounts of some estrogens, or biologic female sex hormones. When secreted in normal amounts, the adrenal androgens appear to have little effect, but when secreted in excess, as in certain inborn enzyme deficiencies, masculinization may result. This is termed the **adrenogenital syndrome**.

Pancreatic Islets

The pancreas lies transversely in the upper abdomen, with the head of the pancreas resting at the curve of the duodenum and the body beneath the stomach. The beta cells of the pancreas secrete insulin, which facilitates glucose transport into body cells, lowering the blood glucose levels when they are above normal. When blood glucose levels are low, alpha cells of the pancreas secrete the hormone glucagon. This promotes gluconeogenesis to raise the blood glucose level. Because its action is opposite to insulin, it may be termed a *counter-regulatory hormone.* The delta cells of the pancreas secrete somatostatin, which reduces the rate at which food is absorbed from the GI tract. See Chapter 29 for more detailed discussion of insulin.

Gerontologic Considerations

As a result of aging, the endocrine glands have decreased ability to secrete hormones, or the target organs lose their ability to respond to the hormones produced by the different glands.

These gerontologic changes are summarized in Table 28-2.

ASSESSMENT OF THE ENDOCRINE SYSTEM

Health History

The nurse assesses the patient's history for the presence of pre-existing endocrine disorders, adherence to medications, and the presence of coexisting medical problems.

Endocrine disorders often manifest with nonspecific, atypical symptoms or common complaints that can be attributed to a variety of disorders. Symptoms include weight gain or loss, constipation or diarrhea, tachycardia or bradycardia, hypotension or hypertension, depression or anxiety, heat or cold intolerance, etc. In addition, endocrine disease may be masked or associated with other comorbidities. For example, the symptoms of an older patient admitted with heart failure (HF) may be attributed to pre-existing cardiac disease without considering thyroid disease. Because the endocrine system impacts nearly all cells and organs, the nurse must have a suspicion of potential endocrine disorders in all hospitalized patients. In addition, it is the clustering of signs and symptoms, correlated with the nurse's knowledge of normal physiologic endocrine function, that will alert the nurse to an underlying endocrine disorder. Clinical presentations of endocrine disorders are discussed below according to specific endocrine glands.

Pituitary Dysfunction

Hormonal imbalances of the pituitary involve FSH, LH, ACTH, GH (somatotropin), TSH, MSH, and prolactin from

TABLE **28-2 GERONTOLOGIC CONSIDERATIONS / Age-Related Changes to the Endocrine System**

Endocrine Gland	Age-Related Changes	History and Physical Findings
Thyroid	Atrophy and fibrosis of the thyroid gland with decreased activity of the thyroid gland, resulting in decreased basal metabolic rate Reduced uptake of radioactive iodine and decreased secretion and release of thyrotropin Increased nodularity of the thyroid	Cold intolerance Decreased appetite Decreased vital signs
Parathyroid gland	Decreased absorption and activation of vitamin D, which can lead to increased loss of bone minerals and decreased bone mass	Increased risk for fractures
Adrenal gland	Decreased adrenal function; adrenocorticotropic hormone (ACTH) secretion decreases with age with resultant decreased estrogen, progesterone, androgen, and glucocorticoids	Increased incidence of osteoporosis Perineal and vaginal dryness Fragile skin tissue
Pituitary gland	The volume of the pituitary decreases Decreased ACTH, thyroid-stimulating hormone (TSH), follicle-stimulating hormone (FSH), luteinizing hormone (LH)	Decreased muscle mass Decreased strength and energy tolerance Thin and dry skin
Pancreas	Decreased secretion of insulin and decreased sensitivity to circulating insulin	Reduced ability to metabolize glucose

Adapted from Eliopoulos, C. (2021). *Gerontological nursing* (10th ed.). Wolters Kluwer.

the anterior pituitary as well as ADH and oxytocin from the posterior pituitary.

During the health history, the nurse asks the patient about history of weakness, lethargy, muscular weakness, changes in sexual function (loss of libido), and secondary sex characteristics, as well as any menstrual disturbances in females. In addition, assessment for galactorrhea (spontaneous, inappropriate flow of milk from male or female breast in the absence of pregnancy or breastfeeding/chestfeeding) is indicated to assess for prolactinomas (a pituitary tumor causing excessive prolactin). The nurse asks about changes in weight, height, enlargement of peripheral body parts, in the texture of the skin or hair; and in urination or body temperature. Owing to the proximity of the pituitary to the optic chiasm, complaints of headaches and visual disturbances are not uncommon and should be evaluated. Neurologic assessment data should consider the patient's level of consciousness, orientation, ability to obey commands, and appropriate response to stimuli. The nurse also inquires about symptoms of hyper/hypotension, heat or cold intolerance, palpitations, tremors, and mood changes.

Growth Hormone Dysfunction

Males and females are affected equally by GH dysfunction. In adults, assess for bony changes, such as increase in the width and thickness of bones—enlarged hands, feet, sinuses, spine, mandible (protruding jaw), and nose. If there is pressure on the optic nerve, changes in vision and headaches may occur. As GH can cause complications with insulin secretion, including glucose intolerance, leading to diabetes, blood sugar should be assessed.

Thyroid Gland Dysfunction

During the health history, the nurse asks the patient about changes in weight and appetite, bowel movements, heart rate and respiration, any marked tremors, nervousness, excitability, apprehension or impaired memory, decreased initiative, and slow thought processes. The nurse also asks about changes in the patient's tolerance to heat and cold as well as excessive sweating or feeling very cold, lethargy or apathy, and changes in hair and skin. The presence of exophthalmos, which is an abnormal protrusion of one or both eyeballs that produces a startled expression, also should be assessed. It is associated with thyroid eye disease, especially Graves diseases (discussed in Chapter 30) (Cioffi & Liebmann, 2020).

Parathyroid Dysfunction

During the health history, the nurse considers that hypofunction of the parathyroids is associated with hypocalcemia. Calcium and phosphorus have an inverse relationship; thus, when serum calcium levels are low (due to parathyroid hyposecretion), phosphate levels rise. If hypofunction is suspected, the nurse assesses for neuromuscular irritability as nerve cells become excited and overstimulate muscle cells in the presence of hypocalcemia. Clinical manifestations include complaints of paresthesias (perioral or extremities) and fasciculations (muscle twitching); therefore, the nurse asks the patient about neuromuscular manifestations. Hypocalcemia has an impact on cardiac function and can prolong the QT interval, causing cardiac arrhythmias, hypotension, and potential cardiac failure. The nurse inquires about complaints of palpitations, shortness of breath, dizziness, and presence of peripheral edema. In addition, since chronic hypocalcemia is associated with cataract formation, the nurse asks about visual changes. The mechanism for the development of cataracts may be related to changes in the surface tension of the lens and instability of aqueous humor, leading to the development of cataracts in the presence of low calcium.

Hyperfunction of the parathyroids may result in hypercalcemia as excessive parathyroid hormone causes the release of calcium from bones (Cheng, 2022). If hyperfunction of the parathyroid is suspected, the nurse understands that symptoms of hypercalcemia may be vague and include complaints in the following systems: GI (anorexia, nausea, vomiting, bowel hypomotility, and constipation), musculoskeletal (muscle weakness, bone pain), neurologic (fatigue, decreased concentration), or renal (polyuria as hypercalcemia decreases the concentrating ability in the distal tubule). Also, the patient may make complaints that are more severe. For example, hyperparathyroidism is associated with an increased incidence of peptic ulcer disease; therefore, the nurse should ask about the presence of melena (dark tarry stools containing decomposing blood). In addition, the patient is asked about cardiac complaints since hypercalcemia is associated with shortened QT interval, bradycardia, and hypertension. Finally, the formation of stones in one or both kidneys may cause symptoms due to renal calculi, such as back or flank pain, nausea, vomiting, and dysuria. Primary hyperparathyroidism is overproduction of PTH by the parathyroids, whereas secondary hyperparathyroidism is associated with increased PTH production in response to low calcium or vitamin D states, most commonly in chronic kidney disease (Cheng, 2022). See Chapter 30 for details.

Adrenal Dysfunction

The nurse asks the patient about symptoms of fluid imbalance (related to aldosterone); symptoms of hyper/hypoglycemia (related to cortisol); and changes in voice, hair, and sexual drive (related to androgens).

To address hypersecretion of the adrenal cortex (known as Cushing disease, covered in Chapter 30), the nurse should inquire about problems with acne or hirsutism (related to hypersecretion of androgens), muscle weakness and paresthesia (hypersecretion of aldosterone), or history of fractures (hypersecretion of cortisol). When considering failure of the adrenal cortex (known as Addison disease, also covered in Chapter 30), the nurse asks about symptoms of weakness, fatigue, poor appetite, and weight loss. If a problem with the adrenal medulla is suspected, the nurse assesses the patient's level of stress (related to catecholamines), such as headache, anxiety, nervousness, complaints of a racing heart, and sweating.

Physical Examination

General Appearance

To assess for endocrine dysfunctions, the nurse notes the appearance of facial features, presence of hair, skin condition, and overall proportion. Excessive adrenocortical hormones may cause facial hair in patients who were assigned female at birth, "moon face" (swollen and round face), "buffalo hump" (accumulation of fatty deposits at the base of the neck), thinning of the skin, obesity of the trunk and thinness of the extremities, purple striae (stretch marks), and slow healing of minor cuts and bruises. Masculinization in patients assigned female at birth and truncal obesity may be seen with adrenal hypersecretion. With hyposecretion of the adrenal cortex, a bronze-pigmented skin color in the creases of the hands or over the metacarpophalangeal (finger) joints, elbows, and knees as well darkening of scars is seen. This increased pigmentation is associated with excessive MSH.

Vital Signs

The nurse performs a thorough cardiac assessment, including vital signs, noting rate and rhythm of the heart and auscultation of heart sounds. Bradycardia is associated with hypothyroidism; tachycardia is associated with hyperthyroidism. Diabetes insipidus, which causes profound polyuria, may cause clinical signs of volume depletion, such as tachycardia and hypotension.

Parathyroid problems may cause calcium derangements, which profoundly impact the cardiac system. Hypocalcemia decreases myocardial contractility, prolongs the QT interval (predisposing patients to ventricular arrhythmias), and is associated with hypotension secondary to reduced cardiac output. Hypercalcemia alters myocardial function; causes rhythm disturbances, such as bradycardia, first-, second-, and third-degree heart blocks, and a shortened QT interval; and is associated with hypertension. When a parathyroid problem is suspected, the nurse should assess for pathologic fractures or symptoms due to renal calculi. Assess for neuromuscular irritability (tetany) related to hypocalcemia (refer to Chapter 30 for assessment cues). Pheochromocytoma, a tumor of the adrenal medulla that causes excess secretion of catecholamines, results in episodic severe hypertension and tachycardia.

Thyroid

The nurse inspects and palpates the thyroid gland routinely in all patients. Inspection begins with identification of landmarks. The nurse inspects the lower neck region between the sternocleidomastoid muscles for swelling or asymmetry. The nurse instructs the patient to extend the neck slightly and swallow. Thyroid tissue rises normally with swallowing. The thyroid is palpated for size, shape, consistency, symmetry, and the presence of tenderness. Each of the lobes is palpated in detail. The nurse may examine the thyroid from an anterior or a posterior position (Fig. 28-9). If palpation discloses an enlarged thyroid gland, check for thrills and auscultate both lobes using the bell of the stethoscope to identify any bruits (Box 28-1).

Eyes and Vision

The nurse assesses central vision and visual fields. Loss of color discrimination, diplopia (double vision), or blindness in a portion of a field of vision may be related to pressure of a pituitary tumor on the optic chiasm (located anterior to the pituitary stalk). See Chapter 48 for information on assessing vision and extraocular movements (EOM). Exophthalmos or *proptosis* is an anterior bulging of the eyeballs associated with hyperthyroidism.

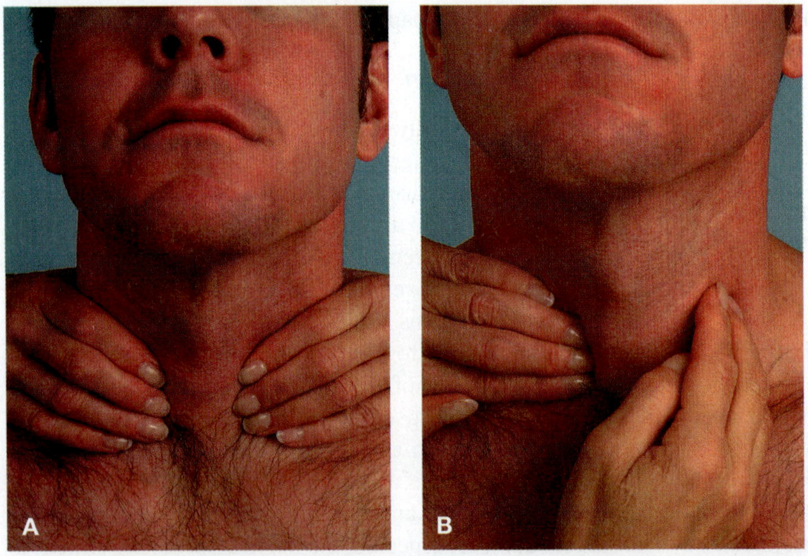

FIGURE 28-9 Palpating the thyroid. A. Posterior approach. B. Anterior approach. (From Rhoads, J. [2006]. *Advanced health assessment and diagnostic reasoning*. Lippincott Williams & Wilkins.)

BOX 28-1

Physical Assessment of an Enlarged Thyroid

In Graves disease, hypertrophy (enlarged cells) and hyperplasia (increased number of cells) of the thyroid may cause the gland to grow to two to three times its normal size. If the thyroid is retrosternal, goiters may not be visible, so it is important to assess for difficulty in swallowing. When the nurse places the hands on the thyroid, they feel increased blood flow to the thyroid (thrills). Often thrills are described as sensation of a purring cat. Auscultation using a stethoscope assesses for a bruit (blowing or whooshing sound), which signifies turbulent blood flow and may be found on one side or on the entire gland.

Diagnostic Evaluation

Diagnostic evaluation is described related to the glands.

Anterior Pituitary Gland Tests

Computed tomography (CT) scan and magnetic resonance imaging (MRI) can be done to identify the presence or extent of tumors. Serum levels of pituitary hormones, along with hormones of target glands, may be indicated to evaluate for increased or decreased activity of each gland. For example, an increased thyrotrophic hormone–releasing factor (TRF), which targets the thyroid, is associated with hyperthyroidism. An increase in ACTH, which targets the adrenal cortex, is found in Cushing disease, whereas a decrease in ACTH will be seen in adrenal insufficiency or Addison disease.

Posterior Pituitary Gland Tests

Plasma levels of ADH can indicate increased or decreased levels. A fluid deprivation test may be indicated for diabetes insipidus. In this test, plasma and urine osmolality are measured, and these levels may be altered in disease. Refer to Chapter 30 for more details on this test.

Urine osmolality is assessed for syndrome of inappropriate secretion of antidiuretic hormone (SIADH). Because patients with SIADH do not excrete dilute urine, the urine osmolality will be increased. Also, serum sodium levels will be recorded as low because of the retention of water. SIADH will be covered in Chapter 30.

Thyroid Gland Tests

Several tests can be performed to test the functioning of the thyroid gland. Serum TSH is the best screening test for thyroid disorders and helps differentiate disorders of the thyroid gland itself from disorders of the pituitary and hypothalamus. High levels of serum TSH will indicate normal function or hypothyroidism, whereas low values indicate hyperthyroidism. This is an example of the negative feedback system. If the thyroid hormones (T_3 and T_4) are not secreted by the thyroid, TSH is increased to help stimulate the thyroid to produce these hormones. If T_3 and T_4 are excreted in large amounts, as occurs in hyperthyroidism, TSH is decreased. TSH is also used to monitor thyroid replacement regimen.

Free T_4 levels measure the level of unbound thyroxine in the blood that is free to enter cells and produce its effects (Ferri, 2022). More than 99% of T_3 and T_4 are bound to proteins. Thus, levels of serum-free T_4 will be increased in hyperthyroidism. T_4 decreases in hypothyroidism. Total levels of T_3 or T_4–T_3 increase in hyperthyroidism.

Antithyroid antibodies will be seen in autoimmune thyroid disease, like Hashimoto thyroiditis and Graves disease. A radioactive iodine uptake test also can be done. This indicates the rate of iodine uptake by thyroid gland. It increases in hyperthyroidism and decreases in hypothyroidism. Needle aspiration biopsy can be done to evaluate thyroid cell structure.

Thyroid imaging can be used in the differential diagnosis of masses. Often increased functioning of nodules, or "hot" nodules, is associated with benign adenomas but not always, whereas "cold" areas refer to decreased functioning (Braimon & Rieke, 2021). Cancer of the thyroid often manifests as a "cold" area.

Parathyroid Tests

Serum calcium and PTH levels, as well as bone density tests, may be ordered.

In primary hyperparathyroidism, the serum PTH and calcium will increase, whereas the serum PTH will decrease with hypercalcemia that is related to an etiology other than the parathyroid hypersecretion. Phosphate levels may be decreased but, in general, are in the lower range of normal. Bone density tests may reveal decreased density owing to the increased osteoclast activity. In secondary hyperparathyroidism due to chronic kidney disease the serum PTH will be elevated; however, the serum calcium is typically low or low-normal due to the inability to synthesize vitamin D (refer to Chapter 26 and see Chapter 30, Box 30-8).

In hypoparathyroidism, the levels of serum calcium will be lower and phosphate levels are elevated.

Adrenal Medulla Tests

Although there is no consensus on the best test for pheochromocytoma (a rare tumor of the adrenal medulla), there will be increased levels of catecholamine and metanephrine (metanephrines are the breakdown product of catecholamines [epinephrine and norepinephrine]) in urine and plasma and elevated serum levels of epinephrine and norepinephrine. The plasma-free metanephrines test may be the first choice for excluding a tumor (Patrick et al., 2022). A 24-hour urine specimen for fractionated metanephrines (metanephrine and normetanephrine) and creatinine is performed when pheochromocytoma is suspected. An additional 24-hour urine for catecholamines (epinephrine, norepinephrine, and dopamine) is obtained if the patient is symptomatic (Cooper & Van Uum, 2022). While pheochromocytoma-secreted catecholamine levels fluctuate, metanephrine is constant, which is the reason this test is preferred (Lough, 2022). Before the metanephrine blood level is drawn, the patient should avoid acetaminophen for 48 hours since it interferes with the testing of metanephrines, and they may be asked to lie down and rest quietly for 15 to 30 minutes before sample collection (Pagana et al., 2021).

Imaging studies to locate the neoplasm may include CT, MRI, ultrasound, and scintigraphy (a two-dimensional picture that is produced through the detection of radiation emitted by a radioactive substance administered into the body).

Adrenal Cortex Tests

In adrenal insufficiency (Addison disease), the adrenal glands produce too little cortisol, lowering serum cortisol and blood glucose. Reduced levels of aldosterone cause decreased serum sodium and increased potassium levels. A patient with primary adrenal insufficiency will present with a low serum cortisol level and a simultaneously high serum ACTH level. A patient with secondary adrenal insufficiency (pituitary disease) will have low serum cortisol and ACTH levels. Refer to Chapter 30 for more details of primary versus secondary adrenal insufficiency.

To assess for adrenal hypersecretion (Cushing syndrome), a variety of tests can evaluate the functioning of the adrenal cortex, such as an overnight dexamethasone suppression test, plasma ACTH, plasma and urinary cortisol, and 24-hour urinary free cortisol level.

CHAPTER REVIEW

NCLEX-Style Review Questions

1. Increased growth hormone is associated with which of the following? Select all that apply.
   a. Hypoglycemia
   b. Increased muscle mass
   c. Increased adipose tissue
   d. Increased protein synthesis
   e. Liver gluconeogenesis

2. When assessing the thyroid gland, the nurse inspects, palpates, and auscultates for which of the following? Select all that apply.
   a. Size
   b. Tenderness
   c. Murmurs
   d. Thrills
   e. Bruits

3. Match each age-related change in the endocrine system to the related history, risk, or physical examination findings.

Column 1	Column 2
a. Decreased thyroid Function	1. Osteoporosis
b. Decreased estrogen, progesterone, androgen	2. Risk of hyperglycemia
c. Decreased sensitivity to circulating insulin	3. Cold intolerance
d. Decreased absorption and activation of vitamin D	4. Perineal and vaginal dryness

4. A 47-year-old patient with a history of kidney disease presents to the primary care provider complaining of bone pain. Routine laboratory studies reveal an increased PTH levels. Which of the following are the potential diagnoses? Select all that apply.
   a. Graves disease
   b. Secondary hyperparthyroidism
   c. Addison disease
   d. Primary hyperparathyroidism
   e. Cushing disease

5. You are evaluating a patient with suspected hyperthyroidism. Select all the expected laboratory findings associated with this disorder.
   a. Decreased TSH
   b. Increased TSH
   c. Increased free T4
   d. Decreased free T4
   e. Increased T3
   f. Decreased T3

REFERENCES AND SELECTED READINGS

References and selected readings associated with this chapter can be found on the website that accompanies the book. Visit **http://thepoint.lww.com/Honan3e** to access the references and other additional resources associated with this chapter.

CHAPTER 29

Nursing Management: Diabetes Mellitus

Kathryn Shugrue Tierney

Learning Objectives

After reading this chapter, you will be able to:

1. Differentiate between type 1 and type 2 diabetes.
2. Describe etiologic factors associated with diabetes.
3. Relate the clinical manifestations of diabetes to the associated pathophysiologic changes.
4. Identify the diagnostic and clinical significance of glucose test results.
5. Explain the dietary modifications recommended for management of people with diabetes.
6. Describe the relationships among diet, exercise, and medication for people with diabetes.
7. Develop a plan for teaching insulin self-management.
8. Identify the role of noninsulin glucose-lowering agents in diabetes therapy.
9. Differentiate between diabetic ketoacidosis and hyperosmolar nonketotic syndrome.
10. Explain management strategies for a person with diabetes to use during "sick days."
11. Describe the major macrovascular and microvascular complications of diabetes.
12. Use the nursing process as a framework for care of hospitalized patients with diabetes.

Diabetes mellitus is a group of metabolic diseases characterized by elevated levels of glucose in the blood (**hyperglycemia**). Diabetes is a chronic illness that requires medical care and patient self-management to prevent or decrease the risk of complications. It affects multiple organ systems and has potentially far-reaching and devastating physical, social, and economic consequences. It is a significant risk factor in the development of heart disease and stroke, and it is the leading cause of nontraumatic amputations, blindness in working-age adults, and end-stage kidney disease (ESKD; Centers for Disease Control and Prevention [CDC], 2020).

The economic cost of diabetes continues to rise because of increasing health care costs and an aging population. Costs related to diabetes are estimated to be $327 billion annually, including direct medical care expenses and indirect costs attributable to disability and premature death (CDC, 2020).

Nursing management of patients with diabetes can involve treatment of a wide variety of physiologic disorders, depending on the patient's health status and whether the patient is newly diagnosed or seeking care for an unrelated health problem. Because all patients with diabetes must master the concepts and skills necessary for long-term management and avoidance of potential complications of diabetes, patient education is necessary for competent self-care and is an ongoing focus of nursing care.

DIABETES MELLITUS

Diabetes affects more than 34.2 million people in the United States, or approximately 10.5% of the population (CDC, 2020). Of this number, 21 million are diagnosed with diabetes, and an estimated 7.3 million are undiagnosed. As many as 88 million people are thought to have **prediabetes**, a condition that indicates increased risk for the development of diabetes (CDC, 2020). The occurrence of both type 1 and type 2 diabetes is increasing in all age groups. Diabetes is especially prevalent among persons over 65 years of age (CDC, 2020).

Classification

The major classifications of diabetes are type 1 diabetes, type 2 diabetes, and gestational diabetes. Other types of diabetes are caused by genetic conditions, surgery, medications, pancreatic disease, and other illnesses (American Diabetes Association [ADA], 2022a).

Table 29-1 summarizes the major classifications of diabetes, current terminology, and major clinical characteristics. This classification system is dynamic in two ways. First, there can be many differences among people within each category. Second, except for people with type 1 diabetes, patients may move from one category to another. For example, a patient with gestational diabetes may, after delivery, move into the type 2 category. Also, metabolic processes typically associated with one diagnosis, such as insulin resistance in type 2 diabetes, may be present in other settings, such as type 1 diabetes. Older terms, such as "insulin-dependent diabetes," "non–insulin-dependent diabetes," "juvenile diabetes," "adult-onset diabetes," and others have been eliminated to reduce confusion.

Pathophysiology

Insulin is a hormone produced by the pancreas that controls blood glucose levels by regulating the production, use, and

TABLE **29-1 Classification of Diabetes Mellitus and Related Glucose Intolerances**

Current Classification	Previous Classifications	Clinical Characteristics and Clinical Implications
Type 1 (5–10% of all diabetes)	Juvenile diabetes Juvenile-onset diabetes Ketosis-prone diabetes Brittle diabetes Insulin-dependent diabetes mellitus (IDDM)	Onset any age, but usually young Etiology includes genetic, immunologic, and environmental factors (e.g., virus) Often have positive islet cell or glutamic acid decarboxylase (GAD) antibodies Little or no endogenous insulin production Dependent on exogenous insulin Acute complication of hyperglycemia due to lack of insulin: diabetic ketoacidosis
Type 2 (90–95% of all diabetes)	Adult-onset diabetes Maturity-onset diabetes Ketosis-resistant diabetes Stable diabetes Non–insulin-dependent diabetes (NIDDM)	Onset any age Risk factors include obesity, heredity, and environmental factors Negative for islet cell and GAD antibodies Decrease in endogenous insulin, or increased with insulin resistance Glucose lowering medications may improve blood glucose levels if hyperglycemia not resolved with dietary modification and exercise May need insulin on a short- or long-term basis to prevent hyperglycemia Ketosis uncommon, except in stress or infection Acute complication of hyperglycemia: hyperglycemic hyperosmolar nonketotic syndrome
Latent autoimmune diabetes of adult (LADA)	Type 1.5 diabetes	Age of onset >30 years Presence of glutamic acid decarboxylase antibodies Insulin independence for at least 6 months after diagnosis (typically not insulin dependent initially and are often misclassified as having type 2 DM)
Diabetes mellitus associated with other conditions or syndromes	Secondary diabetes	Accompanied by conditions known or suspected to cause the disease: pancreatic diseases, hormonal abnormalities, use of medications such as corticosteroids and estrogen-containing preparations Depending on the ability of the pancreas to produce insulin, the patient may require treatment with insulin
Gestational diabetes	Gestational diabetes	Onset during pregnancy, usually in the second or third trimester Due to hormones secreted by the placenta, increased insulin resistance Above-normal risk for perinatal complications, especially macrosomia Changes in diet and exercise, as well as insulin if needed, to maintain blood glucose at target levels Occurs in about 2–5% of all pregnancies Glucose intolerance transitory but may recur: • In subsequent pregnancies • 50–60% will develop overt diabetes (usually type 2) within 10 years (especially if other risk factors present) • Risk factors are the same as for type 2 diabetes, as well as previous history of GDM or previous baby with macrosomia (over 9 lb) All pregnant patients between 24 and 28 weeks of gestation should be screened with oral glucose tolerance test

Current Classification	Previous Classifications	Clinical Characteristics and Clinical Implications
Prediabetes (impaired glucose tolerance)	Borderline diabetes Latent diabetes Chemical diabetes Subclinical diabetes Asymptomatic diabetes	Oral glucose tolerance test value between 140 mg/dL and 199 mg/dL or A1c 5.7–6.4% Should be screened for diabetes yearly
Prediabetes (impaired fasting glucose)		Fasting plasma glucose between 100 mg/dL and 125 mg/dL or A1c 5.7–6.4% Should be screened for diabetes yearly Institute therapeutic lifestyle modifications

storage of glucose. It is secreted by beta cells, in the islets of Langerhans of the pancreas. In patients with diabetes glucose metabolism is disrupted due to a decrease or absence of insulin production, a reduction in insulin efficacy at the level of the receptor (commonly known as "insulin resistance"), or both. Insulin is an anabolic, or storage, hormone. When a person eats a meal, insulin secretion increases and moves glucose from the blood into muscle, liver, and fat cells. Once inside the cells, insulin functions in the following ways:

- Transports and metabolizes glucose for energy
- Stimulates storage of glucose as glycogen in the liver and muscle cells
- Signals liver cells to stop the release of stored glucose
- Enhances storage of dietary fat in adipose tissue
- Accelerates transport of amino acids into cells
- Facilitates the transport of potassium into the cells
- Inhibits the breakdown of stored glucose, protein, and fat (Norris, 2019)

Another hormone involved in glucose regulation is *glucagon*. Glucagon is secreted by the alpha cells of the islets of Langerhans in the pancreas and stimulates the liver to release stored glucose (glycogen), thereby increasing the blood sugar. Insulin and glucagon work together to maintain normal serum glucose levels.

In people with diabetes, hyperglycemia occurs when one or more of the following changes occur: reduction or loss of insulin production, resistance to insulin at the level of the cell, inappropriate secretion of glucagon.

Pearls for Practice

Approximately 50% of the total insulin secreted daily by the pancreas is basal insulin, and the remainder is in response to food intake. Basal insulin is sometimes called background insulin and provides a constant level of insulin action throughout the day, whereas bolus insulin controls blood sugar before meals. Minutes after eating, the serum insulin level rises, peaking in 3 to 5 minutes and returning to baseline within 2 to 3 hours (Norris, 2019. To attain glycemic control, nurses may be required to manage insulin drips or basal bolus insulin regimens.

Type 1 Diabetes

Type 1 diabetes affects approximately 5% to 10% of people with the disease. It is often characterized by an acute onset and most commonly affects children and young adults, although it can occur at any age (ADA, 2022a). Type 1 diabetes is characterized by destruction of the pancreatic beta cells. The diagnosis is further defined as type 1a, or immune-mediated diabetes, which represents 5% to 10% of newly diagnosed diabetes (Domenichini & Ferri, 2022). The etiology of type 1a diabetes is primarily autoimmune. Autoimmune diseases are caused by abnormal immune responses in which antibodies are directed against normal tissues of the body, responding to those tissues as if they were foreign. Immune destruction of the beta cells, caused by autoantibodies against islet cells and insulin, is associated with certain types of human leukocyte antigen (HLA). It is believed that destruction by the immune system of the beta cells is initiated by a combination of genetic, immunologic, and environmental factors, such as viruses or toxins. The risk of developing type 1 diabetes is three to five times higher in people with certain types of HLA. People do not inherit type 1 diabetes itself; rather, they may have a genetic predisposition, or tendency, toward development of the disease.

Regardless of the specific cause, beta-cell destruction results in hyperglycemia due to decreased insulin production and unregulated glucose production by the liver. In addition, glucose derived from food cannot be stored in the liver but instead remains in the blood and contributes to postprandial (after meals) hyperglycemia. If the concentration of glucose in the blood exceeds the renal threshold for glucose, usually 180 to 200 mg/dL, the kidneys cannot reabsorb all of the filtered glucose; glucose then appears in the urine (glycosuria). Glucose is an osmotic agent; water follows it. As the glucose is excreted in the urine, it is accompanied by excessive loss of fluids and electrolytes. This is termed *osmotic diuresis.*

Because insulin normally inhibits glycogenolysis (breakdown of stored glucose) and gluconeogenesis (production of new glucose from amino acids and other substrates), these processes occur unrestrained in people with insulin deficiency and contribute further to hyperglycemia. In addition, fat breakdown occurs, resulting in an increased production of **ketones**, which are organic acids. If excessive amounts of ketones are present in the blood, ketoacidosis develops.

Glucose levels can be measured in several ways, including serum levels, capillary glucose, glycated hemoglobin (A1c), and continuous glucose monitoring (CGM). Serum levels are measured by laboratory testing after a venous blood draw. Capillary glucose is measured using blood from a fingerstick that is placed on a glucose test strip. This type of testing is available to patients at home and is used to determine glucose levels day to day. The hemoglobin A1c is a measure of average glucose levels over a period of approximately 3 months. Because it is an average, it does not give any information regarding patterns of blood sugar or periods of hyper or hypoglycemia, but it is a useful longitudinal measure of glucose control over time. CGMs measure interstitial glucose levels and provide real-time data on glucose levels as well as direction and rate of change. Each of these methods of measuring glucose control has potential risks and benefits as well as situations in which they are not as accurate.

Type 2 Diabetes

Type 2 diabetes affects approximately 90% to 95% of people with the disease. Although type 2 diabetes is commonly associated with older age, its incidence is increasing in younger people (CDC, 2020). Hyperglycemia in type 2 diabetes is most commonly related to insulin resistance and impaired insulin secretion. *Insulin resistance* refers to decreased tissue sensitivity to insulin. Normally, insulin binds to receptors on cell surfaces and initiates a series of reactions involved in glucose metabolism. In type 2 diabetes, these intracellular reactions are diminished, making insulin less effective in stimulating glucose uptake by the cells and at regulating glucose release by the liver (Fig. 29-1). The exact mechanisms that lead to insulin resistance and impaired insulin secretion in type 2 diabetes are unknown, although increasing age, increased weight, and lack of physical exercise as well as genetic factors are thought to play a role (ADA, 2022a).

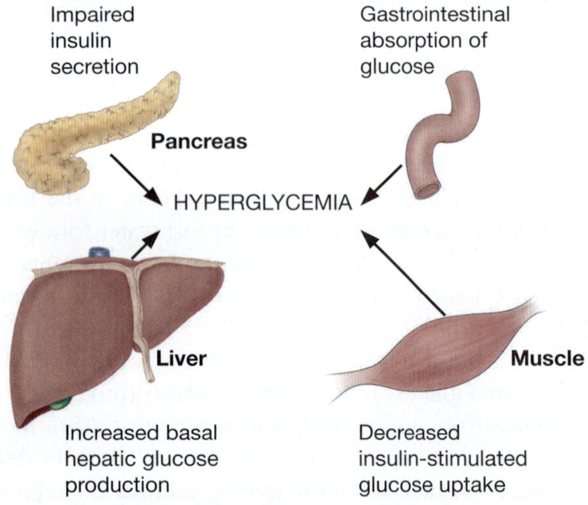

FIGURE 29-1 **Pathogenesis of type 2 diabetes.**

To overcome insulin resistance and prevent the buildup of glucose in the blood, increased amounts of insulin must be secreted to maintain a normal glucose level. However, when the beta cells cannot meet the increased demand for insulin, the glucose level rises, and hyperglycemia develops.

Diabetic ketoacidosis (DKA) does not typically occur in type 2 diabetes mellitus because there is usually enough insulin present to prevent the breakdown of fat and the accompanying production of ketones. However, severe hyperglycemia may lead to *hyperglycemic hyperosmolar nonketotic syndrome* (HHNS), another acute complication of type 2 diabetes discussed later in this chapter.

Because type 2 diabetes is usually associated with slow, progressive glucose intolerance, its onset may go undetected for many years. If the patient experiences symptoms, they are frequently mild and may include fatigue, irritability, increased urination, increased thirst, poor wound healing, frequent infections, or changes in vision.

Many patients with type 2 diabetes are diagnosed as a result of routine laboratory tests or during ophthalmoscopic examinations. One consequence of undetected diabetes is that long-term microvascular (diabetic retinopathy, neuropathy, and nephropathy) and macrovascular complications (peripheral vascular, coronary disease, and stroke) may have developed before the actual diagnosis of diabetes is made (ADA, 2020a).

Latent Autoimmune Diabetes of Adult Onset (LADA)

As the classification implies, LADA is a progressive form of autoimmune diabetes that develops in adults; it may also be termed type 1.5 DM. Clinical features include age of onset >30 years, the presence of glutamic acid decarboxylase antibodies and insulin independence for at least 6 months after diagnosis (Clinical Overview, 2021). As noted, these patients are typically not insulin dependent initially and are often misclassified as having type 2 DM (Domenichini & Ferri, 2022).

Gestational Diabetes

Gestational diabetes mellitus (GDM) is any degree of hyperglycemia with onset occurring during pregnancy and is estimated to affect up to 10% of pregnant people (CDC, 2020b). Hyperglycemia can develop during pregnancy because of the secretion of placental hormones, which causes insulin resistance. It also can develop when the physiologic stress of pregnancy reveals glucose tolerance abnormalities that were not apparent prior to pregnancy. Hyperglycemia during pregnancy increases the risk for congenital anomalies and other complications (ADA, 2022k).

Risk assessment for gestational diabetes should be completed prior to conception or during the first prenatal visit. People at high risk for GDM include those with obesity, personal history of GDM, glycosuria, or a strong family history of diabetes. If the patient is at high risk the blood glucose should be tested as soon as possible in the first trimester and retested between 24 and 28 weeks of gestation, if initial glucose was normal. People at low-to-moderate risk for gestational diabetes should be tested between 24 and 28 weeks of pregnancy (ADA, 2022k).

Initial management of gestational diabetes includes diet and exercise changes as well as blood glucose monitoring. Insulin is indicated if glucose levels are not at goal with these changes alone. Goals for blood glucose levels during pregnancy are 95 mg/dL or less before meals, less than or equal to 140 mg/dL 1 hour after meals, and less than or equal to 120 mg/dL 2 hours after meals (ADA, 2022k).

After delivery of the placenta, blood glucose levels in people with GDM usually return to normal. However, people who have had GDM are at risk for developing type 2 diabetes later in life and should be screened at least every 3 years. A person who has had GDM should be counseled to maintain a healthy body weight and to exercise regularly to reduce the risk for type 2 diabetes.

Risk Factors

Certain ethnic groups are disproportionately affected by diabetes. Age-adjusted population differences demonstrate the highest prevalence among Native American and Alaska Native people (14.7%), followed by Hispanic people (12.5%), and non-Hispanic Black people (11.7%), compared with 9.2% for Asian American people and 7.5% for non-Hispanic White people (CDC, 2020).

Pearls for Practice: Lifting the Lens

In a recent report by the ADA regarding structural and social determinants of health, five domains (socioeconomic status, neighborhood and physical environment, food environment, health care, and social context) were analyzed for their impact on the risk for diabetes and outcomes (Hill-Briggs et al., 2021). Across all five domains, structural or systems-level root inequities were related to worsened diabetes prevalence, diabetes disease control, and diabetes-related deaths (Hill-Briggs et al., 2021; Ogunwole & Golden, 2021). As an example, when a patient is discharged with newly diagnosed DM, it is important to consider structural issues such as availability of green spaces for physical activity, access to affordable and healthy food, ability to pay for the cost of medical treatment, and exposure to environmental chemicals, among others. It is understood that local, state, and federal policy-level interventions are needed to remove the SSDOH as a barrier to health equity, and your voice as an RN is important as we as a profession advocate for the changes needed to achieve health equity for all our patients.

Screening is recommended for all people over the age of 35 because changes in glucose levels do not always cause overt clinical symptoms initially. Screening should be done sooner and more frequently for people with risk factors for developing diabetes. Box 29-1 summarizes risk factors for diabetes mellitus. Given the increase in incidence of type 2 diabetes in children, screening is recommended for at-risk children at any age (ADA, 2022a).

BOX 29-1

Risk Factors for Diabetes Mellitus

- Family history of diabetes (e.g., parents or siblings with diabetes)
- Obesity (i.e., BMI over 25 kg/m^2)
- Ethnicity (e.g., African American, Latino, Native American, Asian American, Pacific Islander)
- Age 45 years or older
- Previously identified impaired glucose tolerance or impaired fasting glucose
- Hypertension (over 140/90 mm Hg or on antihypertensive therapy)
- HDL cholesterol level <35 mg/dL (0.90 mmol/L) and/or triglyceride level over 250 mg/dL (2.82 mmol/L)
- History of gestational diabetes or delivery of babies over 9 lb

Adapted from American Diabetes Association. (2022). Standards of medical care in diabetes. *Diabetes Care*, *45*(S1), S2.

Clinical Manifestations and Assessment

Clinical manifestations depend on the patient's level of hyperglycemia. Classic clinical manifestations of all types of diabetes include the "three Ps": polyuria, polydipsia, and polyphagia. Polyuria (increased urination) and polydipsia (increased thirst) occur as a result of the excess loss of fluid associated with osmotic diuresis. Patients may experience polyphagia (increased appetite) resulting from the catabolic state induced by insulin deficiency and the breakdown of proteins and fats. Other symptoms include dehydration, weight loss, fatigue, weakness, transient vision changes, tingling or numbness in the hands or feet, dry skin, skin lesions, wounds that are slow to heal, and recurrent infections.

Pearls for Practice

Hyperglycemia impairs immune function (decreases white blood cell function), promotes inflammation, increases blood viscosity, favors the growth of yeast organisms, and is associated with changes in the blood vessel walls, resulting in increased risk for infection, microvascular and macrovascular complications, and foot ulcers.

A blood glucose level that is abnormally elevated is the basic criterion for the diagnosis of diabetes. There are three ways to diagnose diabetes: fasting plasma glucose (FPG) levels of 126 mg/dL or higher, a random plasma glucose level exceeding 200 mg/dL in a patient with classic symptoms of hyperglycemia, or an A1c level of 6.5% or higher (ADA, 2022a). It is recommended that in the absence of overt symptoms of hyperglycemia, the tests should be repeated or two of the three tests should be used simultaneously to confirm the diagnosis (ADA, 2022a). Normal fasting glucose for a person without diabetes is 80 to 90 mg/dL with a range of 70 to 120 mg/dL. Prediabetes is diagnosed when the FPG is 100 to 125 mg/dL. The oral glucose tolerance test (OGTT) is no longer recommended for routine clinical use in nonpregnant adults. See Box 29-2 for ADA diagnostic criteria for diabetes mellitus.

In addition to assessment and diagnostic evaluation for diabetes, other important components of care include ongoing specialized assessment of patients with known diabetes and evaluation for complications in patients with newly diagnosed diabetes. Parameters that should be assessed regularly are shown in Box 29-3.

Gerontologic Considerations

The overall prevalence of diabetes is increasing, with the greatest increase occurring in the aging population (CDC, 2020), necessitating assessment in older people. The cause of age-related changes in carbohydrate metabolism is not clear. Possibilities include poor diet, physical inactivity, altered insulin secretion, and insulin resistance.

Elevated levels of blood glucose commonly appear in the fifth decade of life and increase in frequency with advancing age. Almost 30% of people over 65 years of age have diabetes (CDC, 2020). Because people with diabetes are living

BOX 29-2

Criteria for the Diagnosis of Diabetes Mellitus

1. A1c of 6.5% or greater
   Or
2. Symptoms of diabetes plus random plasma glucose concentration equal to or greater than 200 mg/dL (11.1 mmol/L). "Random" is defined as any time of day without regard to time since last meal. The classic symptoms of diabetes include polyuria, polydipsia, and unexplained weight loss.
   Or
3. Fasting plasma glucose greater than or equal to 126 mg/dL (7.0 mmol/L). Fasting is defined as no caloric intake for at least 8 hours.
   Or
4. Two-hour postload glucose equal to or greater than 200 mg/dL (11.1 mmol/L) during an oral glucose tolerance test. The test should be performed as described by the World Health Organization, using a glucose load containing the equivalent of 75 g anhydrous glucose dissolved in water.

In the absence of unequivocal hyperglycemia with acute metabolic decompensation, these criteria should be confirmed by repeat testing on a different day. The fourth measure is not recommended for routine clinical use.

Adapted from American Diabetes Association. (2022a). Classification and Diagnosis of Diabetes: Standards of Medical Care in Diabetes-2022. *Diabetes Care*, *45*(1), S17–S3846.

BOX 29-3

Assessing the Patient With Diabetes

History

- Symptoms related to the diagnosis of diabetes:
  Symptoms of hyperglycemia
  Symptoms of hypoglycemia
  Frequency, timing, severity, and resolution
- Results of blood glucose monitoring
- Status, symptoms, and management of chronic complications of diabetes:
  Eye, kidney, nerve, genitourinary, sexual, and gastrointestinal
- Cardiac, peripheral vascular, foot complications associated with diabetes
- Dietary management plan
- Activity or exercise regimen, including potential barriers to exercising safely
- Pharmacologic treatment, including potential barriers to getting or taking medication
- Use of tobacco, alcohol, and prescribed and over-the-counter medications
- Lifestyle, cultural, psychosocial, and economic factors that may affect diabetes treatment
- Effects of diabetes or its complications on functional status (e.g., mobility, vision)

Physical Examination

- Blood pressure
- Body mass index (height and weight)
- Fundoscopic examination and visual acuity
- Foot examination (lesions, signs of infection, pulses)
- Skin examination (lesions and insulin-injection sites)
- Neurologic examination:
  Vibratory and sensory examination using monofilament
  Deep tendon reflexes
- Oral examination

Laboratory Examination

- A1c (glycated hemoglobin)
- Fasting lipid profile
- Urine microalbumin
- Serum creatinine level
- Urinalysis
- Electrocardiogram

Referrals

- Ophthalmology
- Podiatry
- Dietitian
- Diabetes educator
- Others if indicated

BOX 29-4

Highlighting Gerontology

Age-Related Changes that May Affect Diabetes and Its Management

Sensory Changes
- Decreased vision
- Decreased smell
- Taste changes
- Decreased proprioception
- Diminished thirst

Gastrointestinal Changes
- Dental problems
- Appetite changes
- Delayed gastric emptying
- Decreased bowel motility

Activity/Exercise Pattern Changes
- Potentially more sedentary

Kidney Function Changes
- Decreased function
- Decreased drug clearance

Affective/Cognitive Changes
- Medications/meals omitted or taken erratically

Socioeconomic Factors
- Fad diets
- Loneliness/living alone
- Lack of money/lack of support system

Chronic Diseases
- Hypertension
- Arthritis
- Neoplasms
- Acute/chronic infections

Potential Drug Interactions
- Use of another person's medications
- Consulting multiple health providers for different illnesses
- Unhealthy alcohol use

longer, both type 1 and type 2 diabetes are seen more frequently in the older population.

Older patients with diabetes are likely to have coexisting illnesses, such as hypertension, heart disease, stroke, and other health care problems that complicate diabetes management. Normal physiologic changes of aging may mask the symptoms of diabetes, making diagnosis more difficult. Finally, age-related health problems, such as polypharmacy, depression, cognitive impairment, urinary incontinence, falls, and chronic pain increase the risk for complications of diabetes (ADA, 2022j).

Regardless of the type or duration of diabetes, the goals of diabetes treatment may need to be altered when caring for older patients. The focus is on quality-of-life issues, such as maintaining independent functioning and promoting general well-being. Periods of prolonged hyperglycemia should be avoided, but overall glucose targets may be higher in older patients than in the general population. Box 29-4 presents age-related changes that may affect diabetes and its management.

Medical Management

The therapeutic goal for diabetes management is to achieve normal levels of blood glucose (euglycemia) without hypoglycemia while maintaining a high quality of life. Diabetes management has five components:

- Nutrition
- Exercise
- Monitoring
- Medication
- Education

Patients with type 1 diabetes produce little or no insulin and require exogenous insulin to control levels of blood glucose. The primary treatment of type 2 diabetes is decreasing insulin resistance with lifestyle changes and medication. Exercise is important in improving the effectiveness of insulin for all patients with diabetes. In patients with type 2 diabetes, noninsulin glucose lowering agents may be added if meal planning, diet therapy, and exercise are not successful in controlling blood glucose levels. Multiple noninsulin agents may be needed to reduce glucose to goal levels. Insulin may be added to other therapies, or the patient may be changed to insulin therapy entirely. Some patients require insulin on an ongoing basis; others require insulin on a temporary basis during periods of acute physiologic stress, such as illness or surgery. The types and number of agents used initially depend on the severity of the hyperglycemia at the time of diagnosis.

Pearls for Practice

The stress response results in hyperglycemia because it activates the sympathetic nervous system. The ensuing increase in catecholamines, systemically derived from the adrenal gland or released locally at the level of the liver, increases hepatic glycogenolysis and the release of large quantities of glucose into the bloodstream while inhibiting the release of insulin. Thus, all patients who are under stress are at risk for hyperglycemia.

Diabetes management should be reassessed at regular intervals to account for changes in lifestyle and physical and emotional status as well as because of advances in treatment methods. Treatment plans should be a collaborative effort between the health care team, the patient, and the patient's family. The individual patient must manage an often complex therapeutic regimen and should be at the center of all treatment decisions.

Nutrition

Nutrition is a significant part of diabetes management. Nutrition management can be associated with reversal or significant improvement of hyperglycemia. The most important objectives in the dietary management of diabetes are control of total caloric intake to attain or maintain a reasonable body weight, control of blood glucose levels, and normalization of lipids and blood pressure to prevent heart disease. However, achieving these goals is not always easy. A registered dietician trained in diabetes management should have the primary responsibility for designing and teaching this aspect of the therapeutic plan given that medical nutrition therapy (nutritional therapy) for diabetes is complex. Nurses and other members of the health care team must be knowledgeable about nutrition therapy and supportive of patients who need to implement diet and exercise changes. Nutrition management of diabetes should consider patient's food preferences, lifestyle, usual eating times, and ethnic and cultural circumstances and food availability (ADA, 2022e).

For patients who require insulin to help control blood glucose levels, maintaining as much consistency as possible in the amounts of calories and carbohydrates ingested at each meal can be helpful. In addition, consistency in the approximate time intervals between meals, with the addition of snacks if necessary, can help prevent hypoglycemic reactions and maintain overall control of blood glucose.

For patients whose weight is above target and who have diabetes, weight loss can sometimes improve glucose levels. A 5% decrease in total weight is recommended through diet and exercise changes to help improve blood glucose levels (ADA, 2022e). Some patients with type 2 diabetes who require glucose lowering agents to control blood glucose levels may be able to reduce or eliminate the need for medication through weight loss.

Consistently following a meal plan is one of the most challenging aspects of diabetes management. However, pacing food intake throughout the day and decreasing overall caloric intake places more manageable demands on the pancreas and can lead to weight loss. For obese patients with diabetes who do not take insulin or other agents, consistent meal content or timing is important but not as critical.

Pearls for Practice

It is important to assess the patient's blood sugar BEFORE meals when an insulin correction scale is ordered since the patient's blood sugars will rise after ingesting food.

Meal Planning

Advances in diabetes management and insulin therapy allow greater flexibility in the timing and content of meals. This contrasts with the older concept of maintaining a constant dose of insulin, which required patients to adjust their schedule to the actions and duration of the insulin.

When teaching about meal planning, clinical dietitians use various educational tools, materials, and approaches. Initial education addresses the importance of the relationship of food and insulin, and the provision of an individualized meal plan. In-depth follow-up education then focuses on management skills such as eating at restaurants; reading food labels; and adjusting the meal plan for exercise, illness, and special occasions. The nurse plays an important role in communicating pertinent information to the dietitian and reinforcing the patient's understanding.

For some patients, certain aspects of meal planning may be difficult to learn. This may be related to limitations in the patient's intellectual level or to emotional issues, such as difficulty accepting the diagnosis of diabetes or feelings of deprivation. In any case, it helps to emphasize that nutritional management of diabetes provides a new way of thinking about food, rather than a new way of eating. It is also important to simplify information as much as possible and to provide opportunities for the patient to practice and repeat activities and information.

Caloric Requirements and Distribution. Calorie-controlled diets are planned by first calculating a person's energy needs and caloric requirements based on age, gender, height, and weight. Then an activity element is factored in to provide the actual number of calories required for weight maintenance. To promote a 1- to 2-lb weight loss per week, 500 to 1,000 calories are subtracted from the daily total. The calories are distributed into carbohydrates, proteins, and fats, and a meal plan is developed with consideration of the patient's lifestyle and food preferences. The ADA and the American Dietetic Association recommend that the percentages of carbohydrate, protein, and fat of any diet be tailored specifically to each individual (ADA, 2022b).

Carbohydrates. Carbohydrates are an important source of energy. In general, carbohydrates have the greatest effect on blood glucose levels because they are more quickly digested than other foods and are converted into glucose rapidly.

Sources of carbohydrates include grains, fruits, vegetables, legumes, and milk. The majority of carbohydrate selections in the diet should come from these sources. Foods containing sucrose (sugar) may be included; however, foods high in fat and that lack vitamins, minerals, and fiber, as well as sucrose-containing foods and beverages, should be limited. All carbohydrates should be eaten in moderation to avoid high postprandial (after meal) levels of blood glucose (ADA, 2022b).

Fats. There is no difference in recommendations for people with and without diabetes regarding fat content in the diet. Increased intake of foods containing long-chain omega-3 fatty acids, such as fish, is recommended (ADA, 2022b).

Protein. The amount of protein intake in people with diabetes should be tailored to their specific needs. Because protein appears to have minimal effect on glucose level, foods with significant protein content should be avoided for treatment of hypoglycemia (ADA, 2022b).

Food Classification Systems. To teach diet principles and to help patients with meal planning, several systems have been developed in which foods are organized into groups with common characteristics, such as number of calories, composition of foods, or effect on blood glucose levels. Food intake can be managed several ways, including carbohydrate counting, food lists, and calorie counting.

Carbohydrate Intake. Because carbohydrates are the main nutrients in food that influence blood glucose, monitoring carbohydrate intake by carbohydrate counting or experience-based estimation can be effective ways to achieve control of blood glucose (ADA, 2022b).

Carbohydrate counting provides flexibility in food choices and can be less complicated to understand than other systems. It also allows for more accurate management with medication and exercise, particularly with insulin. Insulin-to-carbohydrate (I:C) ratios are patient specific and can change over time with changes in weight and other health issues. For example, a patient with an I:C ratio of 1:15 would take 1 unit of insulin for every 15 g of carbohydrate consumed. All food sources of carbohydrates should be considered when developing a meal plan using carbohydrate counting. Insulin-to-carbohydrate calculations have the potential to allow for more flexible eating habits and more predictable glucose control. Recommendations for specific percentage of calories from carbohydrates, protein, or fat are individualized rather than based on a "one size fits all" approach (Watts & Yelverton, 2021).

Other Dietary Concerns

Alcohol. Alcohol has the potential to cause significant adverse effects in people with diabetes. Patients with diabetes do not need to give up alcoholic beverages entirely, but they should be aware of the potential adverse effects of alcohol specific to diabetes. Alcohol is absorbed before other nutrients and does not require insulin for absorption. Large amounts can be converted to fats, increasing the risk for DKA (discussed later in the chapter). In general, the same precautions regarding the use of alcohol by people without diabetes should be applied to patients with diabetes. Patient teaching about alcohol intake must emphasize moderation in the amount of alcohol consumed. Moderate intake is considered to be one alcoholic beverage per day for females and two per day for males (ADA, 2022b).

Hypoglycemia is a significant risk with consumption of alcohol, especially for patients who take insulin or secretagogues (an agent that stimulates secretion of another substance; in relation to diabetes, secretagogues stimulate insulin secretion). Alcohol may decrease the normal physiologic reactions in the body that produce glucose (gluconeogenesis). Therefore, if a patient with diabetes consumes alcohol on an empty stomach, there is an increased likelihood of hypoglycemia. In addition, excessive alcohol intake may impair the patient's ability to recognize and treat hypoglycemia or to follow a prescribed meal plan to prevent hypoglycemia. To reduce the risk of hypoglycemia, the patient should be cautioned to consume food with alcohol.

Sweeteners. There are two main types of sweeteners: nutritive and non-nutritive. Nutritive sweeteners contain calories; non-nutritive sweeteners have few or no calories in the amounts normally used. It is unclear whether the use of non-nutritive sweeteners is acceptable for patients with diabetes. Effort should be made to encourage water intake rather than use beverages that are sweetened with any type of sweetener (ADA, 2022b).

Misleading Food Labels. Food manufacturers are required to include the nutrition content of foods on package labels. Reading food labels is an important skill for patients to learn and use when food shopping.

Foods labeled "sugarless" or "sugar-free" may still contain calories equal to those of the equivalent sugar-containing products if they are made with nutritive sweeteners. Therefore, these products may not always be useful and may still cause elevated blood glucose levels if eaten in sufficient quantity.

Foods labeled "dietetic" are not necessarily reduced-calorie foods. They may be lower in sodium or have other special dietary uses. Patients are advised that foods labeled "dietetic" still may contain significant amounts of sugar or fat.

Patients also must be taught to read the labels of "health foods"—especially snacks—because they may contain carbohydrates, such as honey, brown sugar, and corn syrup. In addition, they may contain saturated vegetable fats (e.g., coconut or palm oil), hydrogenated vegetable fats, or animal fats, which may be contraindicated in people with elevated blood lipid levels.

Exercise

Benefits

Exercise is extremely important in diabetes management because of its effects on lowering blood glucose, reducing cardiovascular risk factors, easing stress, and maintaining a sense of well-being. Exercise lowers blood glucose levels by increasing the uptake of glucose by body muscles and by improving insulin utilization. Exercise also alters blood lipid concentrations, increasing levels of high-density lipoproteins (HDLs) and decreasing levels of total cholesterol and triglycerides. This is especially important for people with diabetes because of their increased risk of cardiovascular disease.

Exercise Precautions

Exercise in the setting of insulin deprivation can lead to worsening hyperglycemia and ketosis. Patients should monitor urine ketones prior to exercise and should not begin exercising until urine test results are negative for ketones.

Hyperglycemia in the absence of ketonuria is not a contraindication for exercise.

Exercising facilitates glucose uptake; therefore, patients also should be instructed to take steps to avoid activity-induced hypoglycemia. Patients who require insulin or insulin secretagogues should be taught to check a blood glucose level prior to exercising. If the blood glucose is less than 90 mg/dL (5 mmol/L), carbohydrate may need to be consumed prior to starting the exercise (ADA, 2022b). Insulin doses may need to be altered around the time of exercise to avoid hypoglycemia. The exact change in insulin dose and amount of food needed varies from person to person and should be determined by monitoring blood glucose. Hypoglycemia may also occur many hours after exercise. To avoid postexercise hypoglycemia, especially after strenuous or prolonged exercise, the patient may need to eat a snack at the end of the exercise session and at bedtime as well as monitor the blood glucose level more frequently. Other participants or observers should be aware that the person exercising has diabetes, and they should know how to assist if hypoglycemia occurs.

Regular daily exercise, rather than sporadic exercise, should be encouraged. Exercise recommendations must be altered as necessary for patients with complications of diabetes, such as retinopathy, autonomic neuropathy, sensorimotor neuropathy, and cardiovascular disease (ADA, 2022b). Increased blood pressure associated with exercise may worsen retinopathy and increase the risk of a hemorrhage into the vitreous or retina. Patients with ischemic heart disease risk triggering angina or a myocardial infarction. Avoiding trauma to the lower extremities is especially important in patients with changes in balance and stability related to neuropathy.

In general, a slow, gradual increase in the exercise period is encouraged. For many patients, walking is a safe and beneficial form of exercise that, other than proper shoes, requires no special equipment. People with diabetes should discuss exercise with their health care providers and undergo medical evaluation before starting an exercise program (ADA, 2022b).

Monitoring Glucose Levels and Ketones

Self-Monitoring of Blood Glucose

Home blood glucose monitoring is a cornerstone of diabetes management. **Self-monitoring of blood glucose (SMBG)** levels by patients has altered diabetes care dramatically. Using frequent SMBG and learning how to respond to the results enables people with diabetes to adjust their treatment regimen to obtain optimal control of blood glucose. This allows for detection and prevention of hypoglycemia and hyperglycemia and plays a crucial role in normalizing blood glucose levels, which, in turn, may reduce the risk of long-term complications of diabetes.

SMBG is a key component of treatment for any intensive regimen of insulin therapy and for diabetes management during pregnancy. It is also recommended for patients with unstable diabetes, those with a tendency to develop severe ketosis or hypoglycemia, and for patients who have hypoglycemia unawareness (discussed shortly).

Selecting an SMBG System. Various methods for SMBG are available. Fingerstick monitors involve applying a drop of blood to a special reagent strip and allowing the blood to stay on the strip for the amount of time specified by the manufacturer. Blood glucose meters give a digital readout of the blood glucose value. CGM systems utilize subcutaneous filaments to monitor glucose levels in the subcutaneous fluid. The chosen method for SMBG must match the skill level of the patient. Factors affecting SMBG performance include visual acuity, fine motor coordination, cognitive ability, comfort with technology and willingness to use it, and cost.

Nurses play an important role in providing initial teaching about techniques for SMBG. Equally important is evaluating the techniques of patients who are experienced in self-monitoring. Patients should be discouraged from purchasing SMBG products from stores or catalogs that do not provide direct education. The accuracy of the monitor should be considered when choosing a specific product.

Frequency. For most patients who require intensive insulin, fingerstick monitoring is recommended four to six or more times daily, usually before meals and at bedtime (ADA, 2022d). An alternative option is to use a CGM system. Patients not receiving insulin may be instructed to assess their blood glucose levels at least two or three times a week, including a 2-hour postprandial test. For all patients, testing is recommended whenever hypoglycemia or hyperglycemia is suspected. Patients should increase the frequency of SMBG with changes in medications, activity, or diet and with stress or illness. Keeping a record or logbook of blood glucose levels can be helpful in detecting patterns. SMBG instruction should include parameters for contacting the primary or endocrine provider.

Continuous Glucose Monitoring System

A **continuous glucose monitor (CGM)** uses technology capable of monitoring blood glucose continuously. A sensor capable of measuring glucose in the interstitial fluid is inserted subcutaneously, and the information is transmitted to a receiver or blue-tooth enabled device. The glucose is measured approximately every 5 minutes, providing real-time information regarding glucose level and rate of change in either direction. The currently available commercial CGM systems are either real-time (does not require action from the wearer to retrieve information) and intermittent-scan (requires wearer to scan the device to retrieve the glucose level). Information from the CGM is especially useful for patients using insulin pumps and intensive insulin regimens in that it can warn the patient of hypoglycemia and hyperglycemia, as well as provide information regarding patterns of diabetes control over specific periods of time. Figure 29-2 shows a CGM.

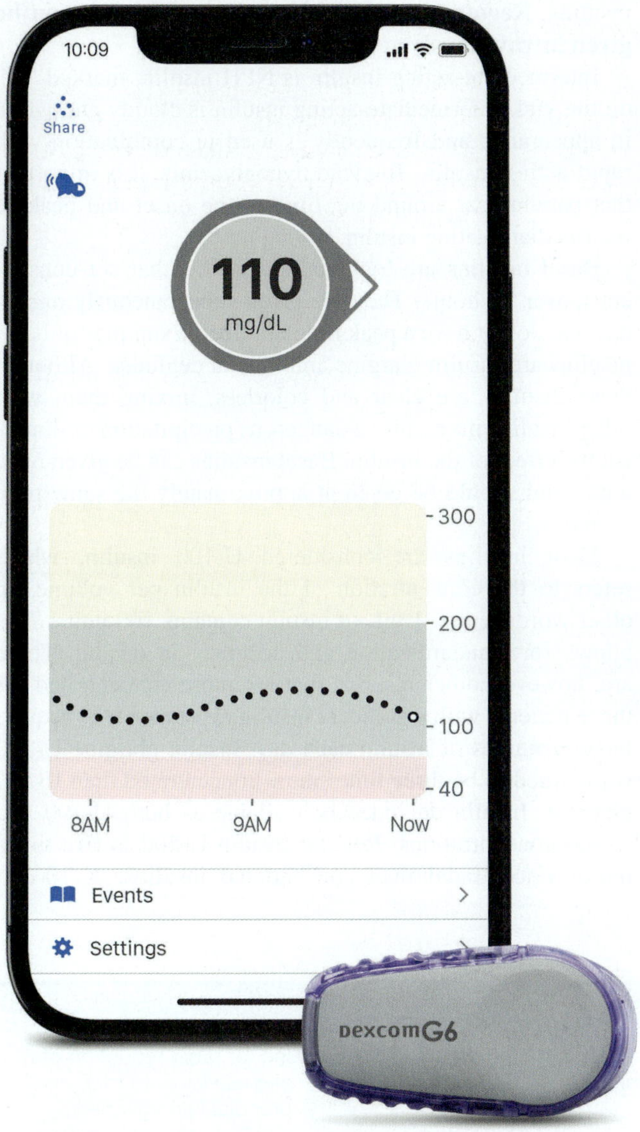

FIGURE 29-2 **The Dexcom G6 Continuous Glucose Monitoring (CGM) System including wearable glucose monitoring device, smart device, and receiver, which sends real-time glucose readings automatically to a compatible smart device, Dexcom receiver, or sensor augmented pump system. Compatible smart devices sold separately. For more information visit www.dexcom.com/g6. (Reproduced with permission from Dexcom.)**

Measuring Glycated Hemoglobin

A1c is a blood test that reflects average blood glucose levels over a period of approximately 3 months (ADA, 2022c). When blood glucose levels are elevated, glucose molecules attach to hemoglobin in red blood cells. The longer the amount of glucose in the blood remains above normal, the more glucose binds to hemoglobin and the higher the glycated hemoglobin level becomes. The glucose remains attached to the hemoglobin for the life of the individual red blood cell, approximately 90 to 120 days. If near-normal blood glucose levels are maintained, with only occasional increases, the overall value will not be significantly elevated. However, if the blood glucose values are consistently elevated, then the A1c will also be elevated. If the patient reports mostly normal results of SMBG but the A1c is elevated there may be errors in the methods used for glucose monitoring, errors in recording results, or frequent elevations in glucose levels at times during the day when the patient is not usually monitoring blood sugar levels. Normal values differ slightly from test to test and from laboratory to laboratory but typically range from 4% to 6%.

It should be noted that the A1c can be affected by changes in red blood cell turnover and that A1c levels do not correlate with SMBG or CGM data in some patients. Also, because the A1c represents average glucose levels, it does not provide any information regarding the variability in a particular patient's blood glucose (ADA, 2022c).

Urine Glucose Testing

Before SMBG was available, urine glucose testing was the only way to monitor diabetes on a daily basis. Its advantages are that it is less expensive than SMBG, noninvasive, and painless. However, urine glucose testing is not recommended because the results do not accurately reflect blood glucose level at the time of the test and because the renal threshold for glucose, 180 to 200 mg/dL, is well above target blood glucose levels. Finally, urine testing for glucose cannot detect or measure hypoglycemia.

Testing for Ketones

Ketones (or ketone bodies) are byproducts of fat breakdown that accumulate in the blood and urine in the absence of insulin. Ketones in the urine signal that the body has started to break down stored fat for energy and the risk of DKA is high. Urine testing is the most common method used for self-testing of ketone bodies by patients. A urine dipstick is used to detect ketonuria or both ketonuria and glucosuria.

Urine ketone testing should be performed whenever patients with type 1 diabetes have glycosuria, have persistently elevated blood glucose levels, or are symptomatic for DKA, as well as during illness and pregnancy.

Pharmacologic Therapy

As previously stated, insulin is secreted by the beta cells of the islets of Langerhans and works to lower the blood glucose level after meals by facilitating the uptake and utilization of glucose by muscle, fat, and liver cells. In the absence of adequate insulin levels or utilization, pharmacologic therapy is essential.

Insulin Therapy

In people with type 1 diabetes, exogenous insulin must be administered daily for life because the body no longer produces adequate insulin. In type 2 diabetes, insulin may be necessary on a long-term basis to control glucose levels if other agents are ineffective. In addition, some patients may require insulin temporarily during illness, infection, pregnancy, surgery, or other stressful events.

Sources of Insulin. In the past, all insulins were obtained from pork and beef pancreas. Currently, recombinant DNA technology is used to create "human" insulin. Human source insulin, which is designed to act more like insulin from the human pancreas, is now standard therapy.

Insulin Preparations. Insulin is available in the following preparations: rapid-acting, short-acting, intermediate-acting, and long-acting. In general, the rapid- and short-acting insulins are expected to cover the increase in glucose levels after meals soon after injection; the intermediate-acting insulins are expected to cover subsequent meals; and the long-acting insulins provide a relatively constant (or basal) level of insulin. Table 29-2 summarizes categories of insulin.

Rapid-acting or "bolus" insulins, such as insulin lispro, insulin aspart, and insulin glulisine, produce a rapid effect that attempts to mimic the normal physiologic response of the pancreas to food intake. These insulins must be timed to the meal because of their rapid onset. The patient should be instructed to eat within 15 minutes of taking the insulin. The short duration of action of these insulins usually requires that patients with type 1 diabetes and some patients with type 2 or gestational diabetes receive additional longer-acting insulin to maintain glucose control.

Short-acting insulin, called regular insulin and marked "R" on the vial, is an unmodified clear solution that usually is administered 20 to 30 minutes before a meal. It can be given either alone or in combination with modified longer-acting insulins. **Regular insulin is the only insulin that can be given intravenously** and is used to treat DKA.

Intermediate-acting insulin is NPH insulin, marked "N" on the vial. Intermediate-acting insulin is cloudy and white in appearance and frequently is used in combination with rapid-acting insulin. To avoid hypoglycemia, it is important that patients eat around the time of the onset and peak of intermediate-acting insulin.

Basal insulins are long-acting insulins that act consistently over 24 hours. They are given subcutaneously once a day and do not have a peak time of effect. Examples of basal insulins are insulin glargine and insulin degludec. Although these insulins are clear and colorless, mixing them with other insulins may cause a dangerous precipitation or diminish the effect of the insulin. Basal insulins can be given once a day and should be given at approximately the same time each day.

Most insulins are considered U-100 insulin, which refers to the concentration of the insulin per volume. In other words, every 1 mL of insulin contains 100 units. This allows for standardization and accuracy in dosing. There are, however, other insulins that are more concentrated for those patients with significant insulin resistance who require larger volumes of insulin each day. Insulin glargine U-300 is modified to be three times more concentrated than U-100 glargine. Insulin degludec is available as both U-100 and U-200 concentrations. Regular insulin U-500 is five times more concentrated than conventional insulins. A 10-unit

TABLE **29-2 Categories of Subcutaneous Insulin**

Time Course	Agent	Onset	Peak	Duration	Indications
Rapid-acting	Lispro (Humalog and Humalog U-200) Aspart (Novolog) Glulisine (Apidra)	15 minutes 15 minutes 15 minutes	1 hour 40–50 minutes 1 hour	3–5 hours 3–5 hours	Used for rapid reduction of glucose level, to treat postprandial hyperglycemia, and/or to prevent nocturnal hypoglycemia Commonly referred to as "meal-time" or "bolus insulin"
Ultra-rapid acting	Lispro-AABC (Lyumjev) Aspart-(Fiasp)	1 minute 2.5 min	57 minutes 40–50 min	Shorter duration of action than regular insulin	
Short-acting	Regular (Humulin-R, Novolin-R)	½–1 hour	2–3 hours	4–6 hours	Usually administered 20–30 minutes before a meal; may be taken alone or in combination with longer-acting insulin
Intermediate-acting	NPH (Humulin N, Novolin N)	2–4 hours	6–8 hours	12–16 hours	Usually taken after food
Long-acting	Glargine (Lantus, Basaglar, Semglee) Glargine U-300 (Toujeo) Detemir (Levemir) Degludec (Tresiba and Tresiba U-200)	2 hours	Continuous (no defined onset or peak)	24 hours 42 hours	Used to approximate endogenous basal insulin secretion

dose change in U-500 is equivalent to a 50-unit dose change in conventional U-100 insulin. Insulin lispro is also available as U-200 insulin.

Afrezza is the only inhaled insulin approved for use in the United States. This insulin is used as a pre-meal dose and is delivered through an inhaler device. Afrezza is a rapid-acting or bolus insulin and is available in 4-, 8- and 12-unit cartridges. Multiple cartridges can be used consecutively for higher insulin requirements. Patients must undergo spirometry testing prior to using inhaled insulin. Afrezza is contraindicated in patients with chronic lung disease, and only patients who do not smoke or who have not smoked for at least 6 months can use the medication.

Insulin Regimens. Insulin regimens vary from one to four or more injections a day. Usually there is a combination of short-acting insulin and longer-acting insulin in order to more closely approximate insulin secretion of a system without diabetes. The normally functioning pancreas continuously secretes small amounts of insulin. In addition, whenever blood glucose increases, such as after ingestion of food, there is a rapid burst of insulin secretion in proportion to the glucose-raising effect of the food. The goal of all but the simplest, one-injection insulin regimens is to mimic this normal pattern of insulin secretion in response to food intake and activity patterns. Table 29-3 illustrates several insulin regimens, including the potential advantages and disadvantages of each.

The more intensive regimens require significant education and close follow-up by the health care team. There is a greater risk of hypoglycemia with the intensive regimens, but often they are more effective at controlling glucose more closely.

Conventional Insulin Therapy. One approach to insulin use is to simplify the regimen as much as possible, with the goal of avoiding acute complications of diabetes (hypoglycemia and symptomatic hyperglycemia). Conventional insulin therapy typically involves one injection per day of long-acting insulin, but other insulins, such as short-acting or mixed insulins, can be used depending on the patient's blood glucose pattern.

Intensive Insulin Therapy. A second approach is to use more frequent insulin injections to achieve levels of blood glucose that are as close to normal as is safe and practical. An intensive insulin therapy regimen involves three to four injections of insulin a day using both long-acting and short-acting insulin or using insulin pump therapy. Although intensive treatment is beneficial in reducing the risk of complications, not all people with diabetes are candidates for this approach to diabetes management.

Pearls for Practice

When administering insulin, it is very important to read the label carefully and to be sure that the correct type of insulin is administered. Take care to avoid mistaking Lantus insulin for Lispro insulin (because both begin with "L") or Lantus for regular insulin because both are clear.

Teaching Patients to Self-Administer Insulin. Insulin injections are self-administered into the subcutaneous tissue. A variety of insulin-specific syringes, insulin pens, and injection-aid devices are available.

Storing Insulin. All insulins, including spare pens and vials not in use, should be refrigerated. Extremes of temperature should be avoided; insulin should not be allowed to freeze and should not be kept in direct sunlight or in high temperatures. The insulin pen or vial in use should be kept at room temperature to reduce local irritation at the injection site. Typically, insulin can be kept at room temperature for 1 month, but the patient should consult the package insert for individual instructions for each type of insulin.

Vials of intermediate-acting insulin also should be inspected for flocculation, which is a frosted, whitish coating inside the bottle. If a frosted, adherent coating is present, some of the insulin is bound and should not be used. Pens or vials of insulin that have been in use for more than the manufacturer's specified time, or those that have passed the expiration date also should be discarded.

Selecting Syringes. Syringes must be matched with the insulin concentration (e.g., U-100). Currently, three sizes of U-100 insulin syringes are available:

- 1-mL syringes that hold 100 units
- 0.5-mL syringes that hold 50 units
- 0.3-mL syringes that hold 30 units

Insulin syringes are disposable and have a 31-gauge needle; varying lengths of the needle are available. The smaller syringes are marked in 1-unit increments and may make it easier for patients with visual deficits and those taking very small doses of insulin to dose more accurately. The 1-mL syringes are marked in 1- and 2-unit increments.

Preparing the Injection: Mixing Insulins. Regular and NPH insulins can be mixed together in the same syringe. Regular insulin must be inspected for clarity and not used unless it is crystal clear. NPH will be cloudy and should be mixed carefully by rolling the vial gently. The regular insulin is drawn into the syringe first, followed by the NPH. Injecting cloudy insulin into a vial of clear insulin contaminates the entire vial of clear insulin and alters its action.

Patients who have difficulty mixing insulins have two options. They may use premixed insulin in a vial or in a prefilled insulin pen. A prefilled insulin pen is shown in Figure 29-3; it is also discussed in detail below. Premixed insulins are available in different ratios of NPH insulin to regular insulin. The ratio of 70/30 (70% NPH and 30% regular insulin in one vial) is most common; this combination is available as Novolin 70/30 (Novo-Nordisk) and Humulin 70/30 (Lilly). Humulin is also available in a 50/50 ratio (Humulin 50/50).

For patients who can inject insulin but who have difficulty drawing up a single or mixed dose, syringes may be prefilled with the help of home care nurses or family and friends.

TABLE **29-3 Insulin Regimens**

Schematic Representation	Description	Advantages	Disadvantages
Normal pancreas 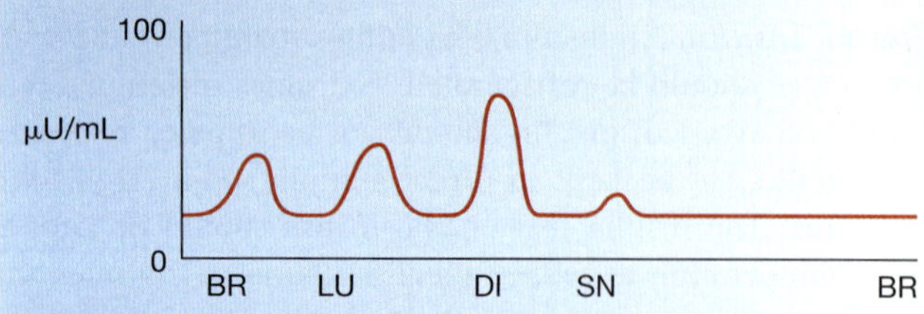	Release of insulin increases when levels of blood glucose rise and continues at a low, steady rate between meals		
One injection per day 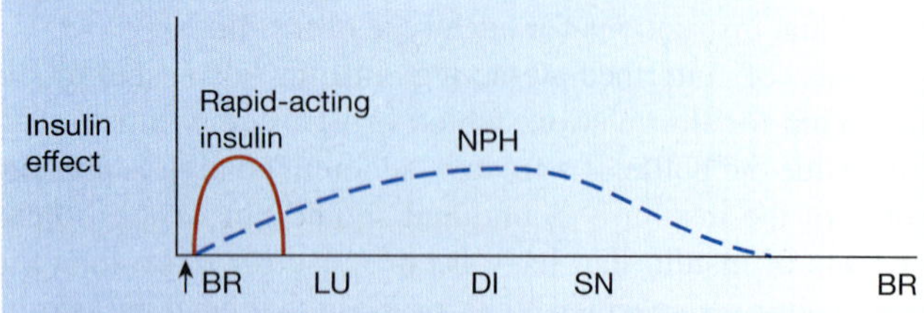	Morning or night: • Long-acting (basal) insulin	Simple regimen	Depending on post-prandial glucose levels, may not be able to sufficiently control fasting numbers without increasing risk for daytime hypoglycemia
Two injections per day-mixed 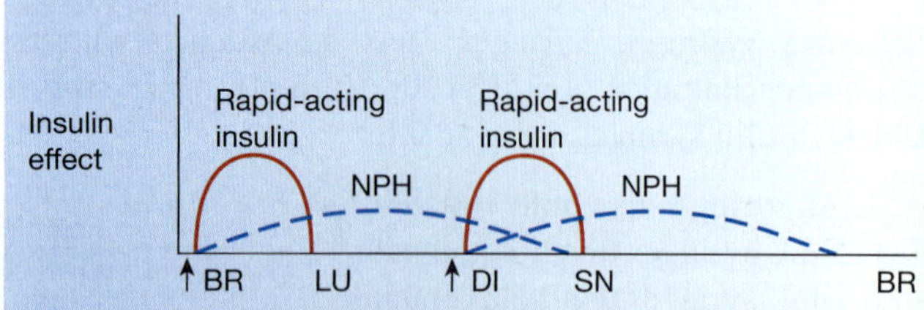	Before breakfast and dinner: • NPH or • NPH with rapid-acting insulin or • Premixed insulin	Simplest regimen that attempts to mimic normal pancreas	Need relatively fixed schedule of meals and exercise Cannot independently adjust NPH or regular insulin if premixed insulin is used
Three or four injections per day 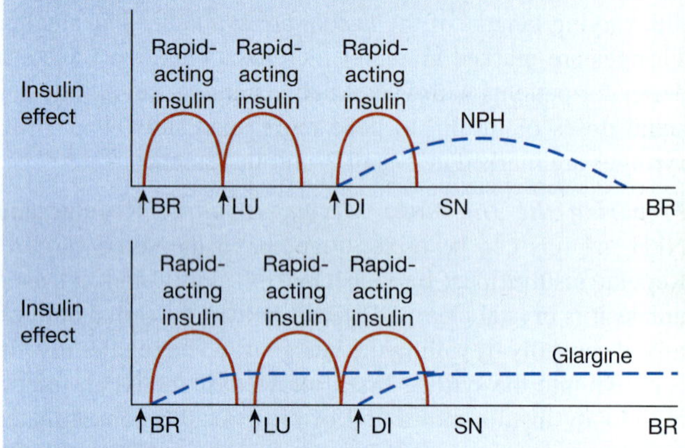	Rapid-acting insulin before each meal with: • basal insulin daily	More closely mimics normal pancreas than two-injection regimen Each premeal dose of bolus insulin is determined independently More flexibility with meals and exercise	Requires more injections than other regimens Requires multiple blood glucose tests on a daily basis Requires intensive education and follow-up
Insulin pump 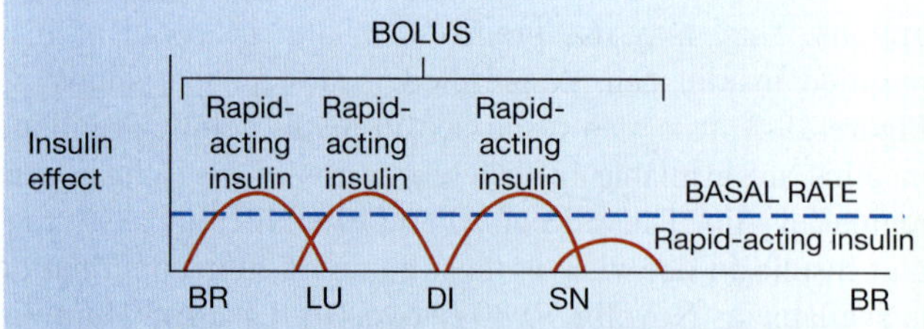	Uses ONLY rapid-acting insulin (lispro, aspart, glulisine) infused at continuous rate called *basal rate* (commonly 0.5–2 units/hr) and premeal *bolus doses* activated by pump wearer	Most closely mimics normal pancreas Decreases unpredictable peaks of intermediate-acting and long-acting insulins Increases flexibility around meals and exercise	Requires intensive training and frequent follow-up Potential for pump or pump site failure Requires multiple blood glucose tests daily or use of CGM Potential increase in expenses (depending on insurance coverage)

Schematic Representation	Description	Advantages	Disadvantages
Sensor augmented insulin pump	Used in conjunction with a continuous glucose monitor; pump is able to adjust insulin delivery to reduce fluctuations in glucose levels, and reduce hyper- and hypoglycemia	As with insulin pumps above Improvement in time with glucose levels at goal, reduction in hypoglycemia	As with insulin pumps above Requires use of continuous glucose monitor to use the internal pump algorithms

BR, breakfast; LU, lunch; DI, dinner; SN, snack. Rapid-acting insulin; lispro, aspart, or glulisine.

A 3-week supply of insulin syringes may be prepared and kept in the refrigerator. Prefilled syringes should be stored with the needle in an upright position to avoid clogging of the needle. Like insulin in vials, prefilled syringes should be rotated gently between the hands to mix and warm the insulin before injection.

Selecting and Rotating the Injection Site. As shown in Figure 29-4, the four main areas for injection are the abdomen, the posterior surface of the upper arms, the anterior surface of the thighs, and the flank area. Insulin is absorbed faster in some areas of the body than in others. The rate of absorption is greatest in the abdomen and decreases progressively in the arm, thigh, and hip, respectively.

Systematic rotation of injection sites within an anatomic area is recommended to prevent localized changes in fatty tissue (lipohypertrophy). Areas of existing lipohypertrophy should be avoided to ensure consistent insulin absorption (ADA, 2022f).

Pearls for Practice

If the patient plans to exercise, insulin should not be injected into the limb that will be exercised because this can cause faster absorption and may result in hypoglycemia.

Insulin Injection. The injection site is cleansed prior to insertion of the needle. To inject insulin, the skin is gently pinched and the needle inserted at a 90-degree angle. For patients with less subcutaneous tissue, a 45-degree angle can be used to avoid inadvertently injecting into muscle. Injection sites should be at least 1 in apart. An injection that is

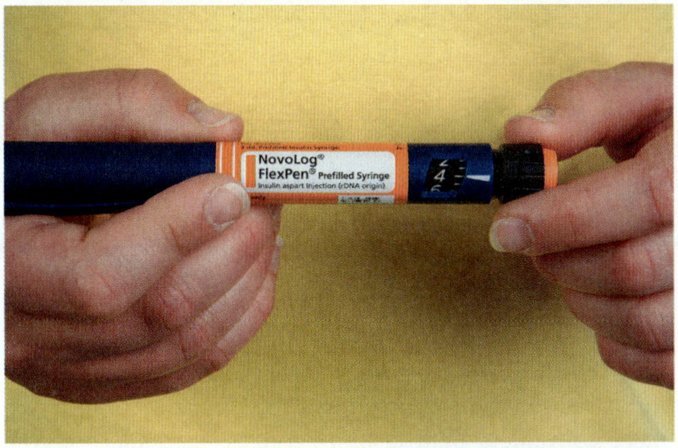

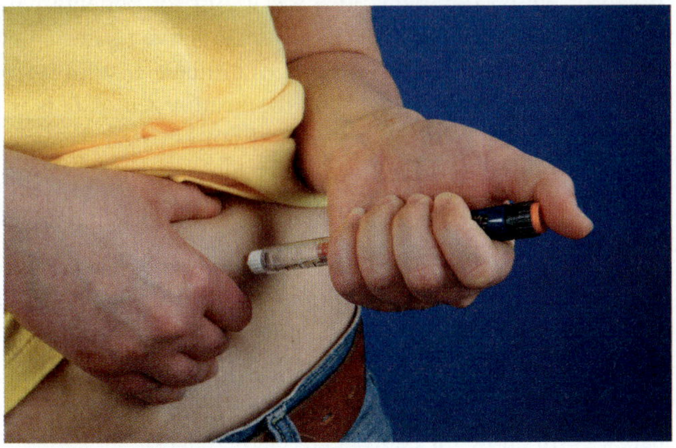

FIGURE 29-3 **Prefilled insulin syringe.**

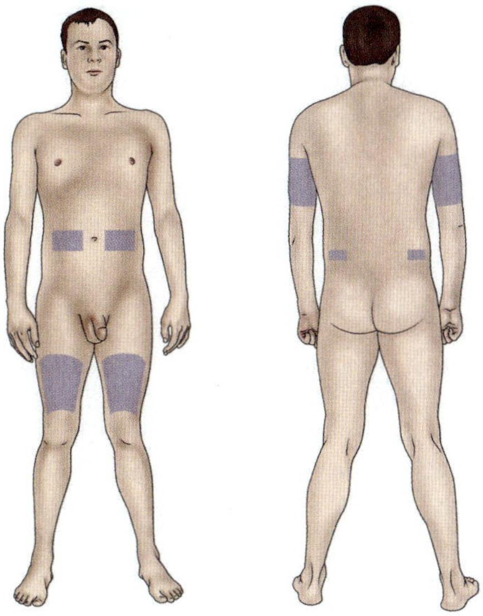

FIGURE 29-4 **Suggested areas for insulin injection.**

BOX 29-5 **Patient Education**

Self-Injection of Insulin

1. With one hand, stabilize the skin by spreading it or pinching up a large area.

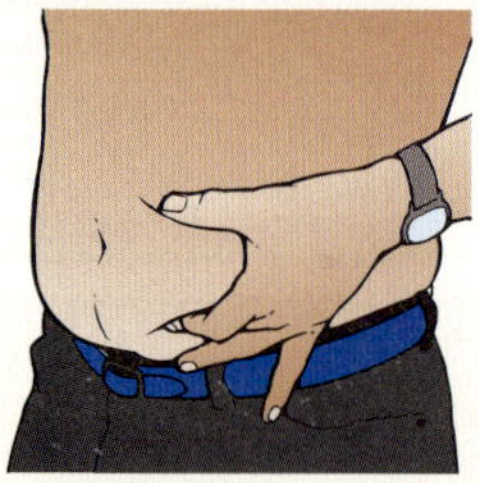

Pinching the skin

2. Pick up the syringe with the other hand and hold it as you would a pencil. Insert the needle straight into the skin.[a]

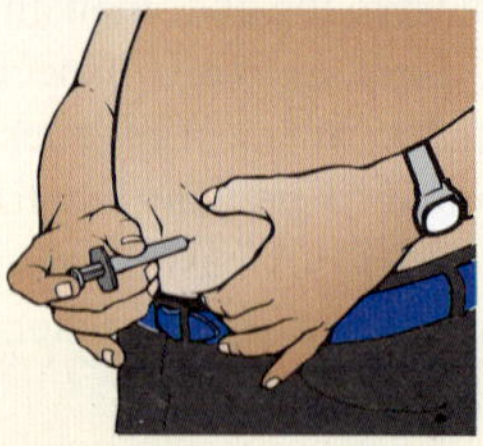

Inserting the needle into the skin

3. To inject the insulin, push in the plunger all the way.

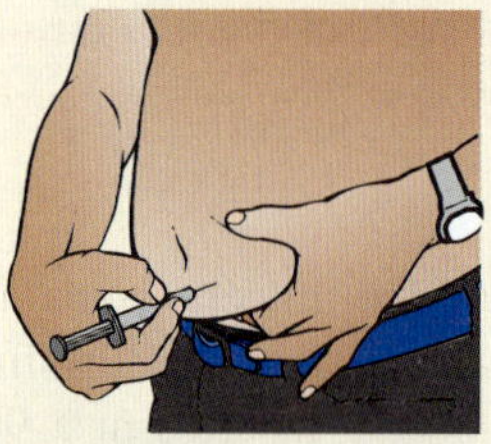

Injecting the insulin

4. Pull the needle straight out of the skin. Press a cotton ball over the injection site for several seconds.

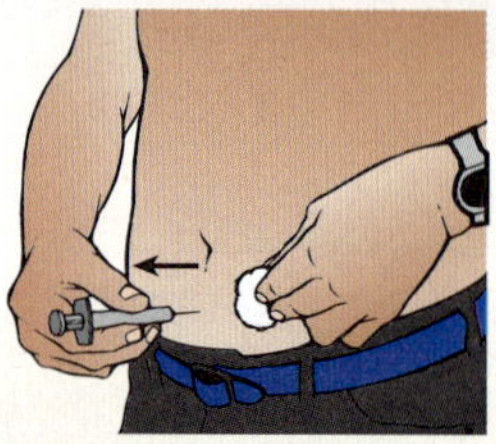

Removing the needle and holding cotton ball over site

5. Use a disposable syringe *only once* and discard it into a hard plastic container (with a tight-fitting top), such as an empty bleach or detergent container. Follow state regulations for disposal of syringes and needles.

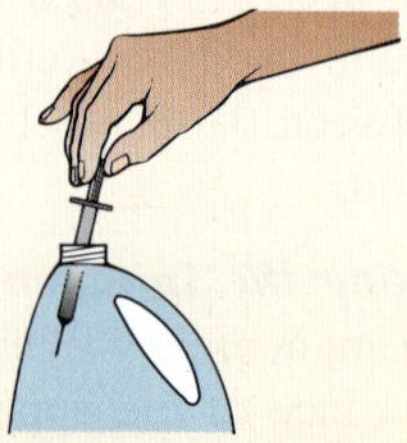

Disposing of syringe

[a]Some patients may be taught to insert the needle at a 45-degree angle.

too deep or too shallow may affect the rate of absorption. Because insulin is injected into subcutaneous tissue, routine aspiration to assess for blood being drawn into the syringe is not necessary. Box 29-5 illustrates patient education for insulin injection. Box 29-6 details how to evaluate the effectiveness of self-injection of insulin education.

Pearls for Practice

*When administering insulin subcutaneously, the injection site should **not** be massaged because massaging can interfere with insulin absorption.*

Insulin Pens. Insulin pens are prefilled devices for insulin delivery that provide more accurate insulin delivery. Each pen typically holds 300 units of insulin. Rather than having to measure the insulin in a syringe, the pen device allows the patient to select the correct number of units by turning a knob on the end of the pen. A one-time-use pen needle is attached to the pen prior to using and can be discarded the same way as insulin syringes. Insulin pens are generally more convenient than insulin syringes, particularly during travel or eating out. They also are useful for patients with impaired manual dexterity, vision, or cognitive function that makes the use of traditional syringes difficult. Insulin injection technique is the same with the insulin pen as it is for insulin syringe. Insulin pens should not be used for more than one person as blood and other biologic material may transfer into the insulin and cause transmission of blood-borne pathogens between patients.

Selecting Insulin Pen Needles. There are a variety of sizes of pen needles available. In general, all brands are interchangeable and can be used on all insulin pens. Sizes range from 4 mm/32-gauge to 12.7 mm/29-gauge. For most patients, the smaller needles will allow for equivalent glucose control but less pain on injection compared to the larger needles (ADA, 2022f).

BOX 29-6

Outcome Criteria for Determining Effectiveness of Self-Injection of Insulin Education

Equipment

Insulin

1. Identifies information on label of insulin vial or pen:
   - Type (e.g., long-acting or short-acting)
   - Species (human, biosynthetic, pork)
   - Concentration (e.g., U-100, U-200, U-300, or U-500)
   - Expiration date
2. Checks appearance of insulin:
   - Clear or milky white
   - Checks for flocculation (clumping, frosted appearance)
3. Identifies where to purchase and store insulin:
   - Indicates approximately how long vial or pen will last (1,000 units per bottle U-100 insulin, 300 units per pen U-100 insulin)
   - Indicates how long opened vials or pens can be used

Syringes

1. Identifies concentration (U-100) marking on syringe; U-100 = 100 units per 1 mL.
2. Identifies size of syringe (e.g., 100-unit, 50-unit, 30-unit). The most common syringe used for insulin administration is a U-100.
3. Describes appropriate disposal of used syringe.

Preparation and Administration of Insulin Injection

1. Draws up correct amount and type of insulin
2. Properly mixes two insulins if necessary
3. Inserts needle and injects insulin
4. Describes site rotation:
   - Demonstrates injection with all anatomic areas to be used
   - Describes pattern for rotation, such as using abdomen only or using certain areas at the same time of day
   - Describes system for remembering site locations, such as horizontal pattern across the abdomen as if drawing a dotted line

Knowledge of Insulin Action

1. Lists prescription:
   - Type and dosage of insulin
   - Timing of insulin injections
2. Describes approximate time course of insulin action:
   - Identifies long- and short-acting insulins by name
   - States approximate time delay until onset of insulin action
   - Identifies need to delay food consumption until 5–15 minutes after injection of rapid-acting insulin (lispro, aspart, glulisine)

Incorporation of Insulin Injections Into Daily Schedule

1. States proper order of premeal diabetes activities:
   - May use mnemonic device such as the word "tie," which helps the patient remember the order of activities ("t" = test [blood glucose], "i" = insulin injection, "e" = eat).
   - Describes daily schedule, such as test, insulin, eat before breakfast and dinner; test and eat before lunch and bedtime.
2. Describes information regarding hypoglycemia:
   - Symptoms: shakiness, sweating, nervousness, hunger, weakness
   - Causes: too much insulin, increased exercise, not enough or delay in food intake
   - Treatment: 15-g concentrated carbohydrate, such as two or three glucose tablets, 1 tube glucose gel, or ½ cup of juice
   - After initial treatment, follow with snack that includes starch and protein, such as cheese and crackers, milk and crackers, half sandwich
3. Describes information regarding prevention of hypoglycemia:
   - Avoids delays in meal timing
   - Eats a meal or snack approximately every 4–5 hours (while awake)
   - Avoid skipped meals
   - Increases food intake before exercise if blood glucose level is less than 100 mg/dL
   - Checks blood glucose regularly
   - Identifies safe modification of insulin doses consistent with management plan
   - Carries a form of fast-acting sugar at all times
   - Wears a medical identification bracelet
   - Teaches family, friends, coworkers about signs and treatment of hypoglycemia
   - Has family, roommates, traveling companions who learn to use injectable glucagon for severe hypoglycemic reactions
4. Maintains regular follow-up for evaluation of diabetes control:
   - Keeps written record of blood glucose, insulin doses, hypoglycemic reactions, variations in diet
   - Sees health care provider regularly (usually two to four times per year)
   - States how to contact health care provider in case of emergency
   - States when to call health care provider to report variations in blood glucose levels

Alternative Methods of Insulin Delivery. Alternative methods of insulin delivery include the use of insulin pumps and jet injectors.

Continuous Subcutaneous Insulin Infusion (CSII): Insulin Pumps. Continuous subcutaneous insulin infusion (CSII), or insulin pump therapy, involves the use of small devices worn externally that more closely mimic the insulin production of a pancreas that is functioning normally. Insulin pumps contain a special syringe, called a reservoir, and are connected to a subcutaneous needle by a thin, narrow-lumen tube with a needle or catheter attached to the end. The patient inserts the needle or catheter into subcutaneous tissue, usually on the abdomen, and secures it with tape or a transparent dressing. The needle or catheter is changed and the reservoir is refilled at least every 2 to 3 days. Figure 29-5 illustrates CSII equipment.

In order to more closely approximate the action of a pancreas that is functioning normally, the insulin pump is

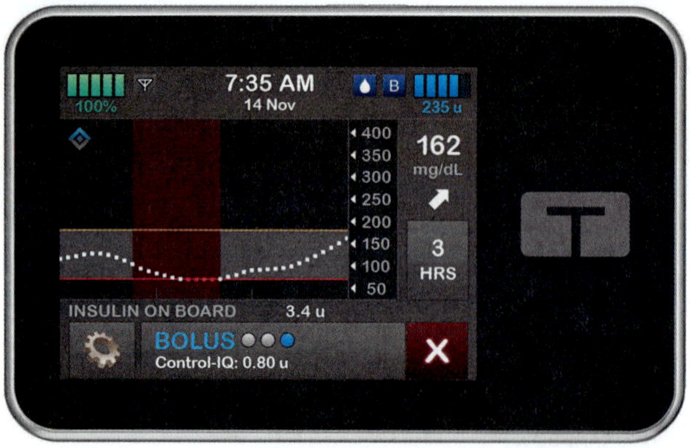

FIGURE 29-5 This is an example of a hybrid closed-loop insulin pump. (Used with permission of Tandem Diabetes Care, Inc.)

programmed to deliver rapid-acting insulin in both a basal and bolus manner. The basal rate is infused continuously over 24 hours, though the rate itself can be tailored to the patient's specific needs at specific times of day. For instance, the basal rate is set at a higher rate overnight if the patient has a history of dawn phenomenon (abnormal early-morning increase in blood sugar—usually between 3 and 8 AM) or abnormal nocturnal rise in blood glucose due to release of hormones. Boluses at meals can be calculated by the pump after the patient inputs the blood glucose at the time of the bolus and the amount of carbohydrate that they intend to consume. Because the pump is infusing rapid-acting insulin, the patient has increased control over delivery of the insulin and, therefore, has more flexibility regarding meal times, food choices, and exercise timing. The pump can easily be disconnected for limited periods for showering, exercise, or sexual activity.

In general, only rapid-acting insulins, such as lispro, aspart, and glulisine, are used in the insulin pump. In rare cases, Humulin R U-500 insulin may be used for patients who have insulin requirements of over 300 units per day.

One disadvantage of insulin pumps is that unexpected disruptions in the flow of insulin from the pump may happen if the tubing or needle becomes occluded, if the supply of insulin runs out, or if the battery is depleted. These occurrences can lead to DKA. Another potential disadvantage is the risk for infection at the sites of needle insertion. Effective patient teaching minimizes these risks. Hypoglycemia also may occur with insulin pump therapy; however, this usually is related to the lowered level of blood glucose achieved by many patients rather than to a specific problem with the pump itself.

Candidates for the insulin pump must be willing to assess their blood glucose level several times daily. In addition, they must be psychologically stable and open about having diabetes because the insulin pump is a visible sign to others and a constant reminder to patients that they have diabetes. Most important, patients using insulin pumps must have extensive education in the use of the pump and in self-management of blood glucose and insulin doses.

The newest insulin pumps combine continuous glucose sensors with insulin infusions and are able to change insulin delivery to help prevent or treat hypo- and hyperglycemia. Currently these systems use only insulin, but research is ongoing for systems that use dual hormone infusions with both insulin and glucagon.

Disposing of Syringes and Needles. Insulin syringes and pens, needles, and lancets should be disposed of according to local regulations. Some areas have special programs for needle disposal to prevent sharps from being discarded in the main waste disposal system. If community disposal programs are unavailable, used sharps should be placed in a puncture-resistant container. The patient should contact local authorities for instructions about proper disposal of filled containers; containers of sharps should never be mixed with containers to be recycled.

Complications of Insulin Therapy. Reactions to insulin therapy and other complications may occur.

Local Allergic Reactions. A local allergic reaction (redness, swelling, tenderness, and induration) may appear at an injection site 1 to 2 hours after insulin administration. These reactions are becoming rare because of the increased use of human insulins.

Systemic Allergic Reactions. Systemic allergic reactions to insulin also are uncommon, affecting 0.1% to 3% of patients treated with insulin (Tian et al., 2021). When they do occur, there is an immediate local skin reaction that gradually spreads into generalized urticaria (hives). Treatment is desensitization with the administration of small doses of a different insulin formulation, usually human insulins, although some studies use desensitization with insulin analogs in gradually increasing amounts (Heinzerling, 2022). Occasionally, these rare reactions are associated with generalized edema or anaphylaxis.

Insulin Lipodystrophy. Lipodystrophy refers to a localized reaction at the insulin injection site, in the form of either lipoatrophy or lipohypertrophy. Lipoatrophy is loss of subcutaneous fat; it appears as slight dimpling or pitting of subcutaneous fat. Lipohypertrophy is the development of a fibrofatty mass; it appears as raised, hardened tissue. Because injection into a damaged site may delay absorption of insulin, use of these areas should be delayed until the lipodystrophy is resolved. The use of human insulin, site rotation, and administration of insulin at room temperature decreases the risk of lipodystrophy.

Resistance to Injected Insulin. Many patients have some degree of insulin resistance at one time or another for various reasons. Clinical insulin resistance has been defined as a daily insulin requirement of 200 units or more. Approaches to increased insulin requirements include using insulin sensitizers or using a more concentrated insulin preparation, such as U-200 or U-500.

Fasting Hyperglycemia. An elevated level of blood glucose upon arising in the morning or after a period of fasting is

TABLE **29-4 Causes of Morning Hyperglycemia**

Characteristic	Treatment
Insulin Waning	
Progressive rise in blood glucose from bedtime to morning	Increase dose of long-acting insulin, or, if using intermediate-acting insulin increase the evening or bedtime dose.
Dawn Phenomenon	
Relatively normal blood glucose until about 3 AM, when the level begins to rise	Change time of injection of evening intermediate-acting insulin from dinnertime to bedtime.
Somogyi Effect	
Normal or elevated blood glucose at bedtime, a decrease at 2–3 AM to hypoglycemic levels, and a subsequent increase caused by the production of counterregulatory hormones	Decrease evening (predinner or bedtime) dose of intermediate-acting insulin, or increase bedtime snack.

caused by an insufficient level of insulin or lack of suppression of glucagon. Particular processes, including dawn phenomenon, the Somogyi effect, or insulin waning, also may be present. The *dawn phenomenon* is characterized by a blood glucose level that is relatively normal until approximately 3 AM, when blood glucose levels begin to rise. This phenomenon is thought to result from nocturnal surges in growth hormone secretions, which create a greater need for insulin in the early morning hours in patients with type 1 diabetes. The dawn phenomenon must be distinguished from *insulin waning* (the progressive increase in blood glucose from bedtime to morning) and from the *Somogyi effect* (nocturnal hypoglycemia followed by rebound hyperglycemia).

It may be difficult to tell from a patient's history which of the above causes is responsible for morning hyperglycemia. To determine the cause, the patient must be awakened once or twice during the night to test blood glucose levels, or a continuous glucose sensor may be used. Testing at bedtime, at 3 AM, and on awakening or reviewing glucose patterns provided by a glucose sensor provides information that can be used to make adjustments in insulin to avoid morning hyperglycemia. Table 29-4 summarizes the differences among insulin waning, the dawn phenomenon, and the Somogyi effect.

Noninsulin Glucose Lowering Agents

Noninsulin glucose lowering agents may be effective for patients with type 2 diabetes who do not reach target levels with diet and exercise alone. These agents include biguanides, dipeptidyl peptidase 4 (DPP-4) inhibitors, glucagon-like peptide 1 (GLP-1) analogs, sodium-glucose transporter 2 (SGLT-2) inhibitors, sulfonylureas, alpha-glucosidase inhibitors, nonsulfonylurea insulin secretagogues (meglitinides and phenylalanine derivatives), and thiazolidinediones (glitazones). Table 29-5 provides a summary of glucose lowering agents with nursing implications.

Patients must understand that glucose lowering medications are prescribed as an addition to, not as a substitute for, diet and exercise. Use of glucose lowering medications may need to be stopped temporarily and insulin prescribed during illness, pregnancy, or hospitalization.

In time, as beta cells continue to decline, noninsulin glucose lowering agents may no longer be adequate in controlling type 2 diabetes. In such cases, the patient is treated with insulin. Approximately half of all patients who initially use noninsulin glucose lowering agents eventually require insulin. Because mechanisms of action vary, use of multiple medications with different actions is common. For some patients with type 2 diabetes, the use of noninsulin agents in combination with insulin is indicated. Mechanisms of action for noninsulin glucose lowering agents are shown in Figure 29-6.

Biguanides. Metformin, the most commonly used biguanide, produces its glucose lowering effects by decreasing hepatic production of glucose and facilitating the action of insulin on peripheral receptor sites. Biguanides have no effect on pancreatic beta cells. Metformin is contraindicated in patients with kidney impairment and in those at risk for acute kidney dysfunction. Metformin-induced lactic acidosis is a serious complication of biguanide therapy in patients with kidney failure. Metformin should not be administered for 2 days before any diagnostic testing that may require use of a contrast agent, and normal kidney function should be confirmed before the medication is restarted after the procedure.

DPP-4 Inhibitors. The DPP-4 inhibitors act by reducing the activity of the DPP-4 enzyme, whose primary action is to degrade glucagon-like peptide 1 (GLP-1). This prolongs the availability of GLP-1, whose actions are to stimulate insulin production, slow gastric emptying, and suppress glucagon secretion.

GLP-1 Receptor Agonists. GLP-1 receptor agonists are a class of medications that work to increase endogenous insulin secretion, delay gastric emptying, promote satiety, and suppress glucagon secretion. GLP-1 medications are injected once daily or once weekly depending on the preparation or can be given daily in tablet form. Whereas most

TABLE **29-5 Glucose Lowering Agents**

Generic (Trade) Name	Action/Indications	Side Effects	Implications
Sulfonylureas			
First- and Second-Generation Sulfonylureas	Stimulate beta cells of the pancreas to secrete insulin; may improve binding between insulin and insulin receptors or increase the number of insulin receptors	Hypoglycemia Mild GI symptoms Weight gain Drug–drug interactions (nonsteroidal anti-inflammatory drugs, warfarin, sulfonamides)	Monitor patient for hypoglycemia Patients at high risk for hypoglycemia: advanced age, renal insufficiency When taken with beta-adrenergic blocking agents, may mask usual warning signs and symptoms of hypoglycemia Instruct patients to avoid use of alcohol Use caution in history of sulfa allergy
Second-Generation Sulfonylureas Glipizide Glyburide Glimepiride	Have more potent effects than first-generation sulfonylureas	Same as above	Same as above
First-Generation Sulfonylureas Chlorpropamide Tolazamide Tolbutamide	Used infrequently in the United States today		
Biguanides			
Metformin and metformin ER	Inhibit production of glucose by the liver Increase body tissues' sensitivity to insulin Decrease hepatic synthesis of cholesterol	Lactic acidosis Hypoglycemia if metformin is used in combination with insulin or other antidiabetic agents Drug–drug interactions GI disturbances, primarily diarrhea Contraindicated in patients with impaired kidney or liver function, respiratory insufficiency, severe infection, or alcohol use disorder	Monitor for lactic acidosis and hypoglycemia Patients taking metformin are at increased risk of acute kidney failure and lactic acidosis with use of iodinated contrast material for diagnostic studies; metformin should be stopped 48 hours prior to and for 48 hours after use of contrast agent or until kidney function is evaluated and normal.
Alpha-Glucosidase Inhibitors			
Acarbose Miglitol	Delay absorption of complex carbohydrates in the intestine and slow entry of glucose into systemic circulation Do not increase insulin secretion Used in type 2 diabetes to control blood glucose levels Can be used alone or in combination with sulfonylureas, metformin, or insulin to improve glucose control	Hypoglycemia (risk increased if used with insulin or other antidiabetic agents) GI side effects (abdominal discomfort or distention, diarrhea, flatulence) Drug–drug interactions	Must be taken with first bite of food to be effective Monitor for GI side effects (diarrhea, abdominal distention) Monitor for blood glucose levels to assess effectiveness of therapy Monitor liver function studies every 3 months for 1 year, then periodically afterward Contraindicated in patients with GI or renal dysfunction or cirrhosis

Generic (Trade) Name	Action/Indications	Side Effects	Implications
Nonsulfonylurea Insulin Secretagogues			
Repaglinide categorized as a meglitinide Neteglide categorized as a D-phenylalanine derivative	Stimulate rapid and short insulin secretion from the pancreas Used in type 2 diabetes to control blood glucose levels by decreasing postprandial increases in blood glucose Can be used alone or in combination with metformin or thiazolidinediones to improve glucose control	Hypoglycemia/weight gain less likely than with sulfonylureas Drug–drug interactions (with ketoconazole, fluconazole, erythromycin, rifampin, isoniazid)	Monitor blood glucose levels to assess effectiveness of therapy Has rapid action and short half-life Monitor patients with impaired liver and/or renal function Has no effect on plasma lipids Is taken before each meal
Thiazolidinediones (or Glitazones)			
Pioglitazone	Sensitize body tissue to insulin; stimulate insulin receptor sites to lower blood glucose and improve action of insulin May be used alone or in combination with sulfonylurea, metformin, or insulin	Weight gain, edema Decrease effectiveness of oral contraceptives Possible liver dysfunction Drug–drug interactions Hyperlipidemia (has variable effect on lipids; pioglitazone may be preferred choice in patients with lipid abnormalities) Impaired platelet function	Monitor for signs of fluid overload Monitor liver function Avoid use in patients with heart failure
DPP-4 Inhibitors			
Sitagliptin Saxagliptin Linagliptin	Blocks enzymatic breakdown of endogenous GLP-1, indirectly promoting release of insulin and reducing secretion of glucagon	Nasopharyngitis Possible acute pancreatitis	Weight neutral, does not cause hypoglycemia
GLP-1 Agonists			
Exenatide and exenatide extended-release Liraglutide Dulaglutide Semaglitide	Stimulates release of insulin; prevents secretion of glucagon; slows gastric emptying; reduces appetite, promotes weight loss	GI side effects, including nausea and decreased appetite	Use with caution in patients with gastroparesis Use caution in patients with history of pancreatitis Contraindicated in patients with a personal or family history of medullary thyroid cancer or MEN-2
SGLT-2 Inhibitors			
Canagliflozin Dapagliflozin Empagliflozin Ertugliflozin	Promotes insulin-independent renal excretion of glucose	Polyuria; mycotic infection; possible normoglycemic DKA	Helpful in controlling blood pressure and promoting weight loss

other noninsulin glucose lowering agents are weight neutral or cause weight gain, GLP-1 receptor agonists promote weight loss. They also are glucose dependent and generally do not cause hypoglycemia unless combined with other medications such as sulfonylureas or insulin. Side effects are typically mild but can include nausea.

SGLT-2 Inhibitors. Sodium glucose co-transporter-2 (SGLT-2) inhibitors are oral medications that work primarily by inhibiting reabsorption of glucose in the proximal renal tubules, which promotes loss of glucose through the urine, thereby reducing blood glucose levels. Weight loss and improved blood pressure also are seen with these medications. Common side effects include increased urinary frequency and genital mycotic infections, and some patients have developed DKA while taking the medication.

Sulfonylureas. The sulfonylureas exert their primary action by stimulating the pancreas directly to secrete insulin. Therefore, a functioning pancreas is necessary for these agents to be

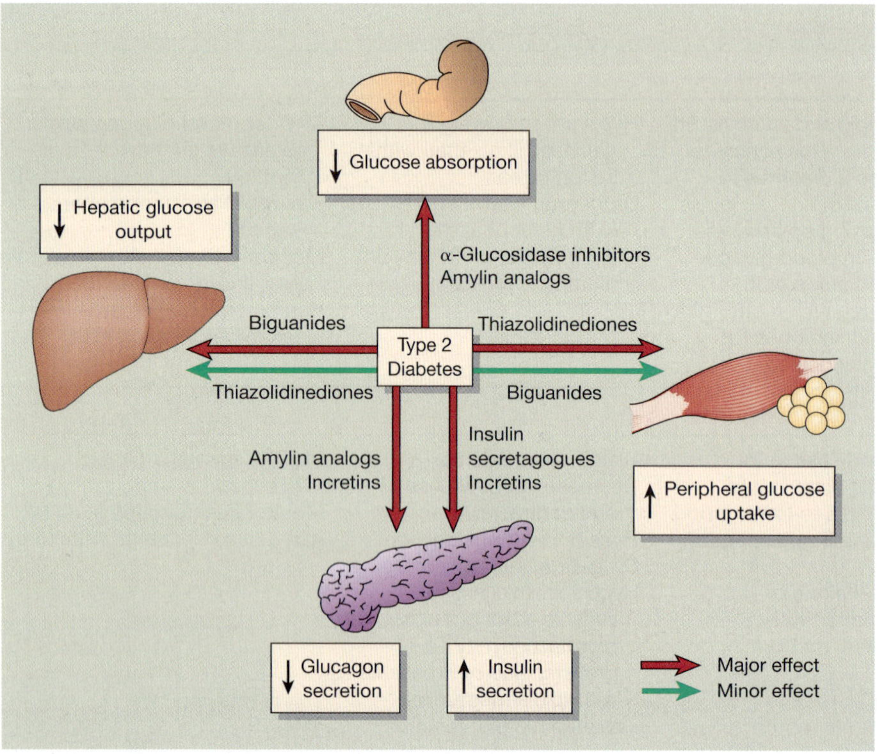

FIGURE 29-6 **Sites of action of oral glucose lowering agents.**

effective, and they are not indicated in patients with type 1 diabetes. Sulfonylureas improve insulin action at the cellular level and also may directly decrease glucose production by the liver.

The most common side effect of sulfonylureas is hypoglycemia. Second-generation sulfonylureas (glipizide, glyburide, glimepiride) have fewer side effects and drug interactions than do first-generation sulfonylureas since they are excreted by both the liver and the kidneys, thus making them safer to use in older individuals. However, if renal or hepatic insufficiency is suspected, patients must be monitored for hypoglycemia. Because the second-generation drugs are a safer option, first-generation sulfonylureas are seldom used today.

Nonsulfonylurea Insulin Secretagogues. Repaglinide and nateglinide act similarly to sulfonylureas but have a different chemical structure. Both lower the blood glucose level by stimulating insulin release from the pancreatic beta cells. These drugs have a very rapid onset and a short duration and *must be taken with meals*; they should not be taken if a meal is skipped.

Alpha-Glucosidase Inhibitors. Acarbose and miglitol are alpha-glucosidase inhibitors. They work by delaying the absorption of glucose in the intestines, which results in a lower level of postprandial blood glucose. Reduction in plasma glucose results in improved diabetes control and lower A1c levels.

The advantage of alpha-glucosidase inhibitors is that they are not systemically absorbed, making them safer to use. Side effects include diarrhea and flatulence. These effects may be minimized by starting at a very low dose and increasing the dose gradually. Because acarbose and miglitol affect food absorption, they must be taken immediately before a meal, making therapeutic adherence a potential problem.

Thiazolidinediones (TZDs). Pioglitazone is an oral glucose lowering medication categorized as a thiazolidinedione (TZD). This class of medication enhances insulin action at receptor sites without increasing insulin secretion from the beta cells of the pancreas. These medications can be used alone or in combination with other glucose lowering agents. These medications may impair liver function and also may increase the risk of myocardial infarction and heart failure. Liver function studies must be performed at baseline and at frequent intervals throughout treatment.

Other Pharmacologic Therapy

Pramlintide is a synthetic analog of human amylin, a hormone that is secreted by the beta cells of the pancreas. It is used as an adjunct in the treatment of type 1 and type 2 diabetes when insulin alone cannot control blood glucose levels. Pramlintide is used with insulin, not in place of insulin.

Transplantation of Pancreatic Cells

Transplantation of the whole pancreas or a segment of the pancreas is performed on a limited population, mostly in patients with diabetes who are receiving kidney transplantation simultaneously. The main issue involves weighing the risks of antirejection medications against the advantages of pancreas transplantation.

Nursing Management

Nursing management of patients with diabetes can involve treatment of a wide variety of physiologic disorders, depending on the patient's health status and whether the patient is newly diagnosed or seeking care for an unrelated health problem. Because all patients with diabetes must master the concepts and skills necessary for long-term management and avoidance of potential complications of diabetes, a solid educational foundation is necessary for competent self-care and is an essential component of nursing care.

Diabetes mellitus is a chronic illness that requires a lifetime of special self-management behaviors. Because diet, physical activity, and physical and emotional stress affect glucose control, patients must learn to balance a multitude of factors. They must learn daily self-care skills to prevent acute fluctuations in blood glucose, and they also must incorporate into their lifestyle many preventive behaviors for avoidance of long-term diabetic complications. Patients must become knowledgeable about nutrition, medication effects and side effects, exercise, disease progression, prevention strategies, blood glucose monitoring techniques, and medication adjustment. In addition, they must learn the skills associated with monitoring and managing diabetes and must incorporate many new activities into daily routines. An understanding of the depth and breadth of knowledge and skills that patients with diabetes must acquire helps nurses provide effective patient education and counseling.

Developing a Diabetes Teaching Plan

Changes in the health care system as a whole have had a major impact on education and training for patients with diabetes. Patients with new-onset type 1 diabetes are hospitalized for much shorter periods or may be managed completely on an outpatient basis. Patients with new-onset type 2 diabetes are rarely hospitalized for initial care. Because many patients with diabetes are admitted to the hospital for reasons other than diabetes or its complications, all nurses play a vital role in identifying patients with diabetes, assessing self-care skills, providing basic education, reinforcing teaching, and referring patients for follow-up care after discharge. Regardless of the setting, all encounters with patients with diabetes are opportunities for support and reinforcement of self-management skills.

All patients with diabetes should be assessed for self-care needs. The ADA recommends that teaching include three levels of care. The first, survival skills, provides the patient with basic knowledge and skills for diabetes management. An outline of survival information includes the following:

1. Simple pathophysiology:
   a. Basic definition of diabetes
   b. Normal blood glucose ranges and target blood glucose levels
   c. Effect of insulin and exercise
   d. Effect of food and stress, including illness and infections
   e. Basic treatment approaches
2. Treatment modalities:
   a. Administration of insulin and oral medications
   b. Meal planning
   c. Monitoring of blood glucose and urine ketones
3. Recognition, treatment, and prevention of acute complications:
   a. Hypoglycemia
   b. Hyperglycemia
4. Practical information:
   a. Where to buy and store insulin, syringes, and supplies for monitoring glucose
   b. When and how to contact the primary provider

When patients have mastered basic skills and information, they are ready for home management, the second level of teaching. This level involves providing the patient with detailed information, beyond basic survival skills, to foster self-reliance and independence for diabetes management at home.

More advanced patient education includes skills and information to improve lifestyle and individualization of diabetes self-management. The degree of advanced diabetes education provided depends on the patient's interest and ability.

Unfolding Patient Stories: S.H. • Part 2

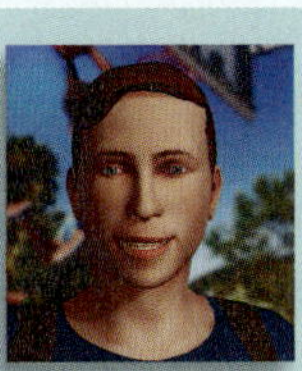

Recall from Chapter 3 **S.H.,** a high school student recently diagnosed with type 1 diabetes. Outline a diabetes education plan for the patient and parents. What are important patient education topics, resources, and methods for the nurse to consider? How would the nurse evaluate whether the patient and family understand the education provided?

Care for S.H. and other patients in a realistic virtual environment: ***vSim** for Nursing* (thepoint.lww.com/vSimMedicalSurgical). Practice documenting these patients' care in DocuCare (thepoint.lww.com/DocuCareEHR).

Assessing Readiness to Learn

The nurse must assess the patient's readiness to learn before initiating diabetes education. When patients are first diagnosed with diabetes, or first told of the need for insulin, they often go through various stages of the grieving process. The amount of time it takes for the patient and family members to accept the realities of living with diabetes varies.

Once the patient's questions have been answered and possible misconceptions are corrected, the nurse focuses attention on concrete survival skills. Because of the immediate need for multiple new skills, teaching is initiated as soon as possible after diagnosis. Nurses whose patients are in the hospital rarely have the luxury of waiting until the patient feels ready to learn; short hospital stays necessitate initiation of survival skill education as early as possible. This gives the patient the opportunity to practice skills with supervision by the nurse before discharge. Follow-up by home health nurses often is necessary for reinforcement of survival skills.

Determining Teaching Methods

Patient teaching must be flexible and planned to meet the needs of the individual patient. Teaching skills and providing information in a logical sequence is not always the most helpful approach for patients. For example, many patients fear self-injection. Before they learn how to prepare insulin, patients should be taught to insert the needle and inject insulin. Once they have actually performed injections, most patients are better prepared to hear and to comprehend other information necessary for insulin administration. Ample opportunity should be provided for patients and families to practice skills under supervision. Refer to Chapter 1 for details on Teaching Techniques and Learning Readiness.

Implementing the Plan

Teaching Experienced Patients

Nurses should continue to assess the skills and self-care behaviors of patients who have had diabetes for many years. Assessment of experienced patients should include direct observation of skills, not just the patient's self-report of self-care behaviors. In addition, these patients must be fully aware of preventive measures related to foot care and eye care as well as management of risk factors.

Teaching Patients Self-Care

Patient teaching and support for diabetes self-management is an important nursing responsibility. Patients who are having difficulty following the diabetes treatment plan must be approached with care and understanding. If problems with glucose control or with the development of preventable complications exist, the nurse should assess the patient to determine possible reasons. Often problems can be corrected simply by providing complete information and ensuring that the patient understands the information. The focus of diabetes education is on patient empowerment, highlighting the knowledge, skills, and attitudes needed to maintain and improve one's health.

If knowledge deficit is not the problem, certain physical or emotional factors may be impairing the patient's ability to perform self-care skills. For example, decreased visual acuity may interfere with the patient's ability to administer insulin accurately, measure the blood glucose level, or inspect the skin and feet. Decreased joint mobility or other disability also may impair a patient's ability to inspect the bottom of the feet. Emotional factors, such as depression or financial barriers, may impair the patient's ability to carry out multiple daily self-care measures. Sometimes family, personal, or work problems are given priority over diabetes management. As noted earlier, the SSDOH have a significant impact on diabetes prevalence, diabetes disease control, and diabetes-related deaths (Hill-Briggs et al., 2021; Ogunwole & Golden, 2021). It is also important to assess the patient for infection or emotional stress, which can lead to elevated blood glucose levels despite adherence to the treatment regimen.

Providing Continuing Care

Continuing care of patients with diabetes is critical in managing and preventing complications. The degree to which patients interact with health care providers to obtain ongoing care depends on many factors. Age, socioeconomic level, existing complications, type of diabetes, and other health problems all may influence the frequency of follow-up visits. Home health nurses are an excellent resource for ongoing diabetes education, wound care, insulin preparation, or assistance with glucose monitoring. Even patients who achieve excellent glucose control and have no complications should see their primary provider at least twice a year for ongoing evaluation. In addition, the nurse should remind the patient about the importance of participating in other health promotion activities, such as immunizations and recommended age-appropriate health screenings. Participation in support groups is encouraged for patients who have had diabetes for many years as well as for those who are newly diagnosed. Those who participate in support groups often have an opportunity to share valuable information and experiences and to learn from others.

ACUTE COMPLICATIONS OF DIABETES

The three major acute complications of diabetes are caused by short-term imbalances in blood glucose levels. They are hypoglycemia, DKA, and HHNS, also called hyperglycemic hyperosmolar syndrome (HHS).

Hypoglycemia

Hypoglycemia (low blood glucose) occurs when the blood glucose falls below normal. Level 1 hypoglycemia is a glucose <70 mg/dL but ≥54 mg/dL and Level 2 hypoglycemia is <54 mg/dL. Level 3 hypoglycemia is any event requiring external assistance because of mental or physical alterations.

Pathophysiology

Hypoglycemia is caused primarily by medication, such as insulin or oral hypoglycemic agents. Common factors that affect the action of those medications include inadequate food intake or increased physical activity. Hypoglycemia may occur at any time of the day or night. Common factors that increase risk of hypoglycemia include exercise, delayed or missed meals, or change in medication dosing.

Clinical Manifestations and Assessment

The clinical manifestations of hypoglycemia are grouped into two categories, based on where they are apparent; they are symptoms of the autonomic nervous system (ANS) and of the central nervous system (CNS).

At the onset of hypoglycemia, the parasympathetic system is activated, causing hunger (Norris, 2019). This is followed by activation of the sympathetic nervous system, resulting in a surge of epinephrine and norepinephrine. This causes symptoms such as diaphoresis, tremor, tachycardia, palpitation, anxiety, and hunger.

In moderate hypoglycemia, the fall in blood glucose level deprives the brain cells of needed fuel for functioning. Signs of impaired function of the CNS may include inability to concentrate, headache, lightheadedness, confusion, memory lapses, numbness of the lips and tongue, slurred speech, impaired coordination, emotional changes, irrational or combative behavior, diplopia (double vision), and drowsiness. Any combination of these symptoms may occur.

In patients with severe cases of hypoglycemia, CNS function is so impaired that the patient needs the assistance of another person for treatment of hypoglycemia. Symptoms may include disoriented behavior, seizures, difficulty arousing from sleep, or loss of consciousness.

Pearls for Practice

The brain relies almost entirely on glucose for energy. Since, the brain cannot synthesize or store more than a few minutes' supply of glucose, symptoms of cerebral function deterioration are noted with hypoglycemia (Norris, 2019).

Symptoms of hypoglycemia may occur suddenly and unexpectedly and vary considerably from person to person. To some degree, this may be related to the actual level to which the blood glucose falls or to the rate at which it falls. For example, patients who usually have a blood glucose level in the hyperglycemic range (e.g., 200 mg/dL or greater) may feel hypoglycemic symptoms when the blood glucose falls rapidly to 120 mg/dL or less. This is commonly referred to as *relative hypoglycemia*. Conversely, patients who frequently have a glucose level in the low range of normal (e.g., 80 to 100 mg/dL) may be asymptomatic until the blood glucose falls to less than 50 mg/dL. Some patients who have had diabetes for many years experience hypoglycemic unawareness. This condition occurs when the normal compensatory response to low blood sugar fails to cause symptoms, thus, the patient is unaware of the problem and may experience profound hypoglycemia without any warning.

Medical and Nursing Management

Giving Carbohydrates

Immediate treatment must be given when hypoglycemia occurs. The usual recommendation is that 15 to 20 g of a fast-acting concentrated source of glucose be taken orally. Sources of glucose for the treatment of hypoglycemia include:

- Three or four commercially prepared glucose tablets
- 4 to 6 oz of fruit juice or regular soda
- 6 to 10 hard candies
- 2 to 3 teaspoons of sugar or honey

Sugar should *not* be added to juice, even if it is labeled as unsweetened juice. Adding table sugar to fruit juice may cause a sharp increase in the blood glucose level, causing prolonged hyperglycemia.

The blood glucose level should be retested in 15 minutes and retreated with another 15 g of carbohydrate if the patient is still hypoglycemic. If the symptoms persist for longer than 15 minutes after initial treatment, the treatment is repeated even if blood glucose testing is not possible. It is important that people with diabetes, especially those receiving insulin or oral hypoglycemic agents, have a source of carbohydrates readily available at all times.

Pearls for Practice

If a patient with hypoglycemia is unresponsive, a glucagon injection or bolus of IV dextrose according to hospital protocol is administered rather than risking aspiration with carbohydrates by mouth.

Initiating Emergency Measures

For adult patients experiencing hypoglycemia who are unconscious or unable to swallow safely, an injection of glucagon 1 mg can be administered either subcutaneously or intramuscularly. **Glucagon** is a hormone produced by the alpha cells of the pancreas that stimulates the liver to convert glycogen to glucose. Because of glycogen's short duration of action, the patient should be given both a concentrated source of carbohydrate followed by a snack once they regain consciousness. This will prevent recurrence of hypoglycemia and help replenish the glucose stored in the liver.

Glucagon is sold by prescription only and should be part of the emergency supplies available to patients with diabetes who require insulin. Family members, friends, and coworkers should be instructed in the use of glucagon, especially for patients who have little or no warning of hypoglycemic episodes. There are now three commercially available preparations of glucagon including an injection kit, a nasal spray, and an auto-injector pen.

Patients who are hospitalized and experience severe hypoglycemia are generally given 25 to 50 mL of 50% dextrose in water ($D_{50}W$) via IV push at a rate of 10 mL/min; actual amounts are dictated by hospital protocol. This intervention is effective in achieving an increase in the blood glucose within minutes.

Diabetic Ketoacidosis

DKA is a life-threatening complication of diabetes caused by an absence or markedly inadequate amount of insulin.

This deficit of insulin results in disorders in the metabolism of carbohydrates, proteins, and fats. The primary clinical features of DKA are hyperglycemia, ketosis, dehydration, electrolyte loss, and metabolic acidosis.

Pathophysiology

Without insulin, the amount of glucose entering the cells is reduced, and production and release of glucose by the liver is increased. Both factors lead to hyperglycemia. In an attempt to rid the body of the excess glucose, the kidneys excrete excess glucose, causing an osmotic diuresis, leading to dehydration and marked loss of electrolytes. The hyperosmolality of the extracellular fluid leads to the stimulation of thirst, resulting in polydipsia and fluid shifting from intracellular to extracellular space. This fluid shifting causes low or normal levels of serum sodium despite water losses with polyuria. This low serum sodium level is referred to as *pseudohyponatremia.*

Pearls for Practice

One of the causes of pseudohyponatremia is related to the significantly elevated glucose level, which raises the serum tonicity; this in turn pulls water out of cells, thus lowering the serum sodium level. A correction formula exists: For every 100 mg/dL increase in serum glucose over 100 mg/dL, the hypertonicity will cause the sodium concentration to fall by approximately 2 mEq/L (Hoorn & Sterns, 2022). The nurse is aware that other correction formulas exist such as adding 1.6 mmol/L to the measured serum sodium level for every 100 mg/dL increase of serum glucose >100 mg/dL (Hehar & Shill, 2022); thus, it is recommended that institutional protocol be followed.

Another effect of insulin deficiency is the breakdown of fat (lipolysis) into free fatty acids and glycerol. The free fatty acids are converted into ketone bodies by the liver. In DKA, the excessive production of ketone bodies leads to the development of metabolic acidosis. A characteristic response to this acidemia is for the respiratory center to blow off its respiratory acid, leading to rapid deep respirations known as **Kussmaul respirations**.

Pearls for Practice

Since ketones are a volatile acid, as they are exhaled, they may manifest as acetone breath that has a fruity odor similar to overripe apples.

Causes of DKA include new onset of type 1 diabetes, insufficient or missed doses of insulin, physical or emotional stress, and illness or infection. Infection is the most common precipitating cause of DKA (30% to 40%) (Lough, 2022). Additional conditions that may precipitate DKA include myocardial infarction, cerebrovascular accident, sepsis, pancreatitis, or use of drugs or medications (e.g., cocaine, glucocorticoids, higher-dose thiazide diuretics, sympathomimetic agents and second-generation "atypical" antipsychotic agents; Hirsch & Emmett, 2022). An insulin deficit may result from an insufficient dosage of insulin prescribed or from insufficient insulin being administered by the patient. Physical and emotional stress increases the level of the counter regulatory ("stress") hormones—glucagon, epinephrine, norepinephrine, and cortisol—all of which cause an increase in blood glucose. Finally, illness and infection are associated with insulin resistance, which puts the patient at risk for hyperglycemia. If insulin is not increased during times of stress, illness, and infection, hyperglycemia may progress to DKA. For some patients with undiagnosed or untreated type 1 diabetes, DKA is the initial manifestation of diabetes (occurrence is 20% to 25% of cases; Hirsch & Emmett, 2022).

Clinical Manifestations and Assessment

Hyperglycemia leads to polyuria, polydipsia, weakness, and malaise. In addition, the patient may experience blurred vision due to osmotic changes on the lens related to hyperglycemia. Clinical manifestations of DKA are depicted in Figure 29-7. Patients with marked intravascular volume depletion may present with orthostatic hypotension; warm, dry skin; decreased skin turgor; flat neck veins; and dry mucous membranes. Volume depletion also may lead to frank hypotension and a weak, rapid pulse.

The ketosis and acidosis of DKA lead to gastrointestinal (GI) symptoms, such as anorexia, nausea, vomiting, and abdominal pain. The patient may have acetone breath (a fruity odor) as well as Kussmaul respirations representing the body's attempt to decrease the acidosis, counteracting the effect of ketone accumulation. Mental status changes in DKA vary widely; the patient may be alert, lethargic, or comatose, usually depending on the severity of the abnormality of plasma osmolality.

Pearls for Practice

The Kussmaul respirations are an increased rate and depth of breathing in an effort to "blow off" or exhale carbonic acid in the form of carbon dioxide (CO_2). This is an attempt to correct for the metabolic acidosis.

Pearls for Practice

Ketone bodies are acids that disturb the acid–base balance of the body when they accumulate in excessive amounts. The resulting DKA may cause signs and symptoms such as abdominal pain; nausea; vomiting; hyperventilation; a fruity breath odor; and, if left untreated, altered level of consciousness, coma, and death. Initiation of insulin treatment, along with fluid and electrolytes as needed, is essential to treat hyperglycemia and DKA and rapidly improves the metabolic abnormalities.

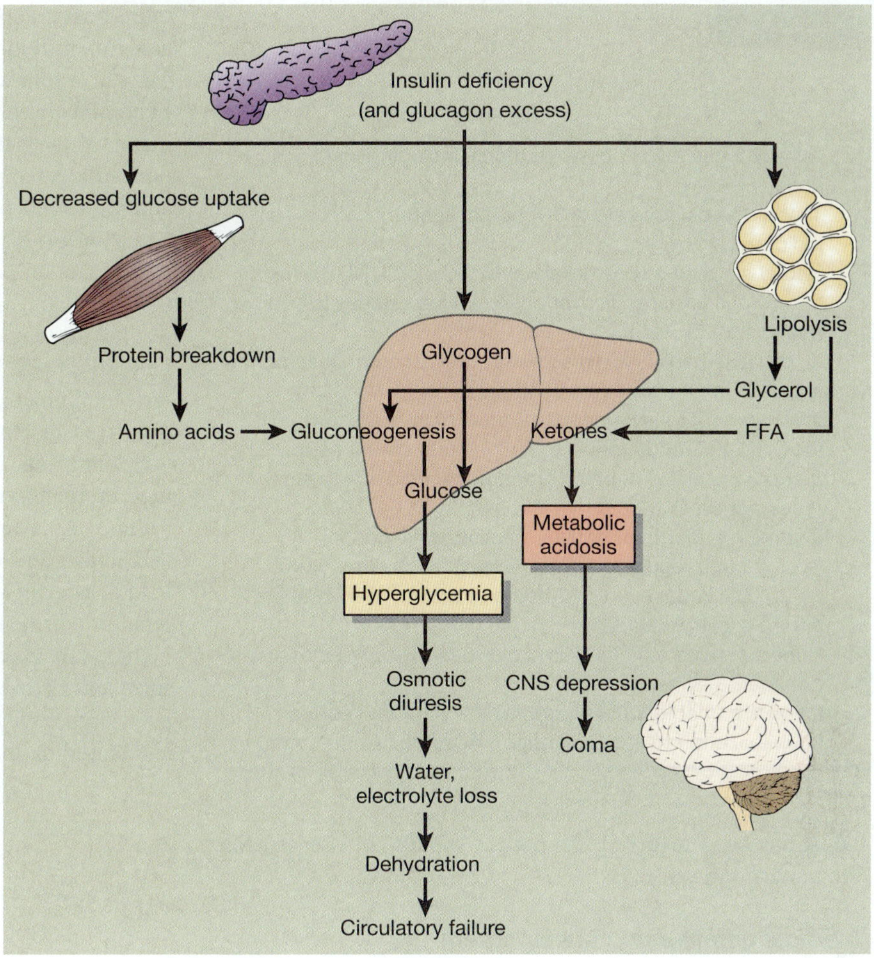

FIGURE 29-7 **Mechanisms of diabetic ketoacidosis (DKA). DKA is associated with very low levels of insulin and extremely high levels of glucagon, catecholamines, and other counterregulatory hormones. Increased levels of glucagon and the catecholamines lead to mobilization of substrates for gluconeogenesis and ketogenesis by the liver. Gluconeogenesis in excess of that needed to supply glucose for the brain and other glucose-dependent tissues produces a rise in blood glucose levels. Mobilization of free fatty acids from triglyceride stores in adipose tissue leads to accelerated production of ketones and ketosis. FFA, free fatty acids; CNS, central nervous system. (From Porth, C. M. [2015].** ***Essentials of pathophysiology*** **[4th ed.]. Lippincott Williams & Wilkins.)**

Diagnostic findings include:

- Blood glucose levels greater than 250 mg/dL
- Low serum pH (<7.3)
- Low serum bicarbonate (<18 mEq/L; Hirsch & Emmett, 2022)
- Accumulation of serum and urine ketones
- Presence of glucose in the urine
- Abnormal levels of serum electrolytes (sodium, potassium, and chloride)

Pearls for Practice: Pathophysiology

Plasma ketones are used by the body as an energy source when glucose is low or unavailable for cellular metabolism. With the breakdown of stored fat (lipolysis), liberated fatty acids are oxidized to ketone bodies, such as acetone (least abundant of all serum ketones), acetoacetate (a ketoacid), and beta-3-hydroxybutyrate (hydroxy acid). Testing urine for ketones evaluates only acetoacetate and acetone but NOT hydroxybutyrate. Elevated plasma beta-3-hydroxybutyrate is associated with high anion gap metabolic acidosis. Bedside testing or point-of-care testing (such as glucose finger sticks) and serum testing for plasma beta-3-hydroxybutyrate are recommended rather than a urine dip test for ketones as a screening for DKA. Urine or blood beta-hydroxybutyrate in DKA is >3 mmol/L (normal is <0.4 to 0.5 mmol/L; Lough, 2022; Pagana et al., 2021). Note, in the absence of hyperglycemia, the presence of high levels of beta-hydroxybutyrate is associated with alcoholic ketoacidosis (Pagana et al., 2021).

Prevention

For prevention of DKA related to illness, patients must be taught "sick day" rules for managing their diabetes when ill. Box 29-7 lists sick day rules. The most important concept to teach patients is not to eliminate insulin doses when nausea and vomiting occur. Instead, the patient should take the usual insulin dose, or previously prescribed "sick day" doses, and then attempt to consume frequent small portions of carbohydrates. Drinking fluids every hour is important to prevent dehydration. Blood glucose and urine ketones must be assessed every 3 to 4 hours.

If the patient cannot take fluids without vomiting, or if elevated glucose or ketone levels persist, the patient must contact their health care provider. After the acute phase of

BOX 29-7 **Patient Education**

Guidelines to Follow During Periods of Illness ("Sick Day Rules")

- Take glucose lowering medications, including insulin, as usual.
- Test blood glucose every 3–4 hours. Test urine ketones if indicated.
- Report elevated glucose levels (over 300 mg/dL [16.6 mmol/L] or as otherwise specified) or positive urine ketones to your health care provider.
- If you take insulin, you may need supplemental doses of rapid-acting insulin every 3–4 hours.
- If you cannot follow your usual meal plan, substitute soft foods (e.g., 3 cups regular gelatin, 1 cup cream soup, 2 cups custard, 3 squares graham crackers) six to eight times per day.
- If vomiting, diarrhea, or fever persists, take liquids (e.g., 2 cups regular cola or orange juice, 2 cups broth, 1 cup Gatorade) every 1–2 hours to prevent dehydration and to provide calories.
- Report nausea, vomiting, and diarrhea to your health care provider.
- If you are unable to retain oral fluids, you may require hospitalization to avoid diabetic ketoacidosis and coma.

DKA has been resolved, the patient should be assessed for the underlying cause.

Medical and Nursing Management

In addition to treating hyperglycemia, management of DKA is directed toward correcting dehydration, electrolyte loss, and acidosis.

Rehydration

In patients who are dehydrated, rehydration is important for maintaining tissue perfusion. In addition, fluid replacement enhances the excretion of excessive glucose by the kidneys. The optimal rate of initial isotonic *saline* infusion (0.9% NACL or normal saline) to replace fluid losses caused by polyuria, hyperventilation, diarrhea, and vomiting and to expand extracellular volume and stabilize cardiovascular status will depend upon the patient's clinical presentation.

For patients who present in shock (severe hypovolemia), many protocols call for administration of 1 L per hour (Hirsch & Emmett, 2022). For hypovolemic patients without shock (unless contraindicated due to underlying heart failure), isotonic *saline* is infused at a rate of 15 to 20 mL/kg lean body weight for the first couple of hours, with a maximum of <50 mL/kg in the first 4 hours), depending on the patient's response (Hirsch & Emmett, 2022). The subsequent IV fluid replacement will depend on the sodium level and level of dehydration; typically it will be either normal saline or half-strength normal saline solution. Moderate-to-high rates of infusion (250 to 500 mL/hr) may continue for several more hours, depending on the patient's vital signs, physical assessment findings, serum electrolytes, and urinary output. The nurse follows the institution's protocol regarding IV rate of administration. Administration of IV fluid that is too rapid increases the risk of cerebral edema and the development of noncardiogenic pulmonary edema (Hirsch & Emmett, 2022), and while the patient clinically may present with hypovolemic shock, it is essential to monitor the patient closely to avoid cerebral edema and respiratory distress while correcting the fluid volume deficit. When the blood glucose level reaches 200 mg/dL or less, change to IV solutions containing glucose (D_5NS, $D_5$1/2NS) to prevent a precipitous decline in the blood glucose level with insulin administration, which is discussed shortly (Hirsch & Emmett, 2022).

Monitoring of fluid volume status involves frequent measurements of vital signs; respiratory, cardiac, and neurologic assessment; and evaluation of serum electrolytes and intake and output. Monitoring for signs of fluid overload is especially important for patients who are older, have renal impairment, or who are at risk for heart failure. Signs include crackles, distended neck veins, edema, weight gain, shortness of breath, orthopnea, paroxysmal nocturnal dyspnea, hypertension, moist mucous membranes, and a full and bounding pulse.

Pearls for Practice

A normal serum chloride is 98 to 106 mEq/L or 98 to 106 mmol/L and the amount of chloride in the normal saline solution is 154 mEq/L which can lead to hyperchloremia. If a large volume of normal saline is used in fluid resuscitation an overload of chloride ions into the blood can occur. The excess chloride forces bicarbonate to move intracellularly, thereby reducing the available base bicarbonate leading to the acidosis (Sharma et al., 2022). Recent research suggests a balanced electrolyte solution such as lactated Ringer's and Plasma-Lyte as an alternative to normal saline in an effort to prevent hyperchloremic metabolic acidosis (Catahay et al., 2022). Future research will evaluate whether protocols will change.

Insulin

Intravenous regular insulin is the insulin used most commonly to treat DKA. Typically, the initial insulin infusion rate is 0.1 to 0.14 U/kg/hr depending on whether a bolus dose of 0.1 unit/kg was administered intravenously (optional) (Masharani & Kroon, 2021). The nurse must convert hourly rates of insulin infusion (frequently prescribed as "units per hour") to IV drip rates. In a 70-kg patient the infusion would be 7 units of insulin per hour. Therefore, if 100 units of regular insulin are mixed in 500 mL of 0.9% NS, then 1 unit of insulin equals 5 mL; therefore, an initial insulin infusion rate of 7 units/hr would equal 35 mL/hr. The insulin solution is infused separately from rehydration solutions to allow for the frequent changes in the rate and concentration of the latter.

The nurse monitors the blood glucose hourly and expects blood glucose to decrease by approximately 50 to 70 mg/dL (2.8 to 3.9 mmol/L) per hour (Hirsch & Emmett, 2022). If the serum glucose does not fall by this amount in the first hour, the nurse assesses the IV site to ensure that the insulin is being delivered and that no IV line filters that may bind insulin have been inserted into the line (Hirsch & Emmett, 2022). After these possibilities are eliminated, the insulin infusion rate is increased according to the institutional protocol until a steady decline of the serum glucose occurs. See Pearls for Practice regarding priming the IV insulin drip shortly. Once the blood glucose level reaches 200 mg/dL or less, prevention of hypoglycemia necessitates changing the IV solution to one containing glucose. The rate of insulin is subsequently decreased according to institutional protocol with a typical target blood glucose of 140 to 180 mg/dL until there is resolution of DKA (Nasrullah et al., 2022). Insulin is infused continuously until subcutaneous administration of insulin can be resumed. Even if blood glucose levels are decreasing and returning to normal, the insulin drip must not be stopped until subcutaneous insulin therapy has been started. Usually, blood glucose levels are corrected before acidosis is corrected. Therefore, IV insulin must be continued until the serum bicarbonate level improves to at least 15 mEq/L and the anion gap is 12 or less (Hirsch & Emmett, 2022).

Pearls for Practice

The intravenous administration of regular insulin is faster than subcutaneous administration. In general, when regular insulin is administered IV, its half-life is about 4 to 5 minutes, and steady state is reached in approximately 20 to 30 minutes (Nyce et al., 2022). Therefore, when monitoring blood glucose levels, the nurse is aware that the IV regular insulin is continuing to exert its action.

Pearls for Practice

To minimize the effect of adsorption of insulin to the IV container or tubing, it is recommended that the nurse "coat the IV line" by flushing the tubing with the insulin solution. A priming volume of 20 mL is sufficient to saturate the binding sites before connecting it to the patient, thus ensuring the patient receives the ordered rate of insulin infusion (Recznik, 2020).

Pearls for Practice

Overly aggressive hydration and rapid correction of hyperglycemia may play a role in the development of cerebral edema. The goal is to decrease the serum glucose level by 50 to 70 mg/dL/hr to prevent this complication. When the serum osmolality is decreased too rapidly, fluid shifts into the CNS, causing the cerebral edema. The nurse is alert for complaints of headache and changes in level of consciousness and cranial nerve function and monitors hourly glucose and IV rates as well as intake and output. The provider is alerted to any of these changes.

Restoring Electrolytes

Potassium is the major electrolyte of concern during treatment of DKA. The initial plasma concentration of potassium may be low because of renal loss due to osmotic diuresis, or normal or high because of the shifting of potassium out of the cell to accompany the movement of hydrogen into the cells because of acidemia. Laboratory measurements are essential to evaluate the patient's serum potassium. If the potassium level is <3.3 mEq/L, the insulin therapy is deferred until potassium replacement is administered (Hirsch & Emmett, 2022). Hourly measures of serum potassium are expected until the serum potassium is above 3.3 mEq/L (Hirsch & Emmett, 2022). When the potassium level is >3.3 mEq/L, the insulin treatment is initiated. Conversely, if the potassium level is >5.3 mEq/L, potassium replacement is withheld until serum levels fall to normal; this prevents the possibility of cardiac arrest from hyperkalemia. The serum level of potassium will decrease with insulin administration as insulin facilitates the movement of potassium intracellularly' therefore, the nurse expects to monitor the serum potassium at least every 2 hours when an insulin drip is in use with the goal of maintaining the serum potassium concentration in the range of 4 to 5 mEq/L (Nyce et al., 2022). In addition, the nurse is aware that rehydration will lead to increased plasma volume and subsequent decreases in the concentration of serum potassium as well as increased urinary excretion of potassium. It is critical that serum potassium levels be monitored carefully since the most life-threatening electrolyte derangement during treatment of DKA is hypokalemia (Nyce et al., 2022).

Pearls for Practice

Potassium levels must be assessed prior to starting insulin therapy in the acute care setting. Insulin facilitates movement of potassium into the cell and therefore can exacerbate hypokalemia. Potassium must be replaced prior to starting insulin. Every 10 mEq of parenteral potassium should increase the serum level by approximately 0.1 mEq/L. Most protocols require the serum potassium level be greater than 3.3 mEq/L prior to starting insulin. Cautious but timely potassium replacement is vital to avoid arrhythmias that may occur with hypokalemia. An ECG should be done on admission, and continuous cardiac monitoring is anticipated until the crisis is resolved. To prevent hyperkalemia, urine output is monitored to ensure adequate kidney function before potassium is administered. If the potassium is higher than 5.3 or the patient is oliguric, potassium replacement is withheld. Frequent laboratory measurements of potassium levels are expected.

Pearls for Practice

Signs and symptoms of hypokalemia generally are not seen until the serum level is less than 3.0 mEq/L. The most profound effects are on cardiac function and may lead to cardiac arrhythmias; predisposition to digitalis toxicity; and electrocardiographic (ECG) changes, such as prolonged PR interval, ST segment depression, the development of a U wave often seen in the lateral precordial leads V4 to V6, and prolongation of the QT interval (Mount, 2022). In addition, patients complain of muscle weakness and fatigue. If the potassium is less than 2.5 mEq/L, muscle weakness, rhabdomyolysis (see Box 41-7), and paralysis of the respiratory muscles can occur (Mount, 2022).

Reversing Acidosis

Accumulation of ketone (acetone) bodies occurs as a result of fat breakdown. The acidosis that occurs in DKA is reversed with insulin, which inhibits further fat breakdown. The use of bicarbonate is generally not required or recommended unless the pH is ≤6.9 and the patient has decreased cardiac contractility, vasodilatation that can impair tissue perfusion, or life-threatening hyperkalemia (Hirsch & Emmett, 2022). In hyperkalemia, bicarbonate administration is used to drive potassium intracellularly, thus lowering the intravascular or serum potassium concentration. Repeat ABGs, and electrolytes, particularly potassium and bicarbonate, are monitored to evaluate response to treatment; bicarbonate is repeated until pH >7.0 (Hirsch & Emmett, 2022).

Hyperglycemic Hyperosmolar Nonketotic Syndrome

HHNS is a serious life-threatening condition characterized by hyperosmolality (usually >320 mOsm/L) and hyperglycemia (at least 600 mg/dL) with or without alterations in level of consciousness (Hehar & Shill, 2022). The plasma osmolality could reach 380 mOsmol/kg, and neurologic symptoms present (including coma) in 25 to 50 percent of cases (Hirsch & Emmett, 2022). Ketosis is minimal or absent. Persistent hyperglycemia causes osmotic diuresis, which results in losses of water and electrolytes. The higher the serum glucose, the more profound the dehydration, and the greater the risk for renal impairment and mental status changes. Table 29-6 compares DKA and HHNS. Other terms include HHS and hyperglycemic hyperosmolar nonketotic coma.

Pathophysiology

HHNS occurs in people who have no known history of diabetes (~20%) or who have type 2 diabetes. HHNS often can be traced to a precipitating event, such as infection (32% to 60%) such as pneumonia, UTI, sepsis, acute or chronic illness (e.g., myocardial infarction, stroke); medications that exacerbate hyperglycemia; or therapeutic procedures, such as surgery, dialysis, inadequate insulin treatment, or nonadherence (21% to 41%; Hirsch & Emmett, 2022). The history may include days to weeks of polyuria and polydipsia. What distinguishes HHNS from DKA is that ketosis and acidosis generally do not occur in HHNS, partly because of

TABLE **29-6 Comparison of Diabetic Ketoacidosis (DKA) and Hyperglycemic Hyperosmolar Nonketotic Syndrome (HHNS)**

Characteristics	DKA	HHNS
Patients most commonly affected	Can occur in type 1 or type 2 diabetes; more common in type 1 diabetes	Can occur in type 1 or type 2 diabetes; more common in type 2 diabetes, especially older patients with type 2 diabetes
Precipitating event	Omission of insulin; physiologic stress (infection, surgery, stroke, MI)	Physiologic stress (infection, surgery, stroke, MI)
Onset	Rapid (less than 24 hours)	Slower (over several days)
Blood glucose levels	Usually over 250 mg/dL (over 13.9 mmol/L); often in the 350–500 mg/dL (19.4 to 27.8 mmol/L) range	Usually over 600 mg/dL (over 33.3 mmol/L); frequently exceeds 1,000 mg/dL (56 mmol/L)
Arterial pH level	Below 7.3	Normal
Serum and urine ketones	Present	Absent
Serum osmolality	300–350 mOsm/L	Greater than 350 mOsm/L
Plasma bicarbonate level	Less than 18 mEq/L	Normal
BUN and creatinine levels	Elevated	Elevated
Mortality rate	Less than 1%	5–20%

MI, myocardial infarction.

differences in insulin levels (those with type 2 diabetes usually continue to secrete some insulin). In DKA, no insulin is present, and this promotes the breakdown of stored glucose, protein, and fat, which leads to the production of ketone bodies and ketoacidosis. In HHNS, the insulin level is too low to prevent hyperglycemia and subsequent osmotic diuresis, but it is high enough to prevent fat breakdown; thus, there is little or no ketoacid accumulation.

Clinical Manifestations and Assessment

The clinical picture of HHNS is one of hypotension, profound dehydration (dry mucous membranes, poor skin turgor, sunken eyes, low jugular venous pressure), tachycardia, and variable neurologic signs (e.g., alteration of sensorium, seizures, hemiparesis). As HHNS tends to occur in older people, many of whom have coexisting comorbidities such as cardiac and renal disease, the mortality rate ranges from 5% to 20%, usually related to an underlying illness, the vulnerability of the older patient, and the severity of HHNS.

Diagnostic assessment reveals very high blood glucose, usually 600 to >1,000 mg/dL, and high serum osmolality that may reach 380 mOsm/kg. Levels of electrolytes and blood urea nitrogen (BUN) are consistent with the clinical picture of profound dehydration. Mental status changes and neurologic deficits are common secondary to cerebral dehydration that results from extreme hyperosmolality. Postural hypotension results from the dehydration.

Medical Management

The overall approach to the treatment of HHNS is similar to that of DKA: replacement of fluids, correction of electrolyte imbalances, and administration of insulin. Because patients with HHNS are typically older, close monitoring of volume and electrolyte status is important for prevention of fluid overload, heart failure, and cardiac dysrhythmias. Fluid treatment is started with 0.9% or 0.45% NS, depending on the patient's sodium level and the severity of volume depletion. Fluid replacement is guided by central venous or hemodynamic pressure monitoring. Potassium is added to IV fluids when urinary output is adequate and is guided by continuous ECG monitoring and frequent laboratory determinations of potassium. As in DKA, the initiation of insulin therapy is delayed if the serum potassium is below 3.3 mEq/L since insulin will worsen the hypokalemia by driving potassium into the cells (Hirsch & Emmett, 2022).

Extremely elevated concentrations of blood glucose decrease as the patient is rehydrated. Insulin plays a less important role in the treatment of HHNS compared to DKA because it is not needed for reversal of acidosis, and, therefore, the patient may have lower insulin requirements. Insulin is administered at a continuous low rate to treat hyperglycemia.

Replacement IV fluids with dextrose are administered after the glucose level has decreased to the range of 250 to 300 mg/dL (Hirsch & Emmett, 2022).

Other therapeutic modalities are determined by the underlying illness and the results of continuing clinical and laboratory evaluation. It may take 3 to 5 days for neurologic symptoms to resolve; treatment of HHNS usually continues well after metabolic abnormalities are resolved. After recovery from HHNS, many patients can control their diabetes with diet alone or with diet and noninsulin glucose lowering medications. Insulin may not be needed once the patient has recovered from the acute hyperglycemic episode. Frequent self-blood glucose monitoring (SBGM) is important in preventing recurrence of HHNS.

Nursing Management

Nursing care of patients with HHNS includes close monitoring of vital signs, fluid status, and laboratory values. In addition, strategies are implemented to maintain safety and prevent injury related to changes in the sensorium secondary to HHNS. Fluid status and urine output are monitored closely because of the high risk of kidney failure secondary to severe dehydration. In addition, the nurse must direct care to the condition that may have precipitated the onset of HHNS, such as MI, infection, illness, or extreme stress (burns, trauma, etc.), inadequate diabetes management. The nurse will also consider iatrogenic treatments, such as TPN/PPN, enteral feedings, or sympathomimetics. Because HHNS tends to occur in older patients, the physiologic changes that occur with aging should be noted. Careful assessment of cardiovascular, pulmonary, and renal function throughout the acute and recovery phases of HHNS is important.

LONG-TERM COMPLICATIONS OF DIABETES

Long-term complications, which are becoming more common as people live longer with diabetes, can affect almost every organ system of the body and are a major cause of death and disability. The general categories of long-term complications of diabetes are macrovascular disease, microvascular disease, and neuropathy.

The specific causes and pathogenesis of each type of complication are not thoroughly understood. However, it appears that increased levels of blood glucose predispose patients with diabetes to microvascular complications and risk factors contributing to macrovascular complications. Hypertension is most likely another contributing factor, especially in both macrovascular and microvascular diseases.

Long-term complications are seen in patients with both type 1 and type 2 diabetes. Because patients with type 2 diabetes can go undiagnosed for many years, evidence of complications may be present at the time of diagnosis.

Macrovascular Complications

Diabetic macrovascular (macroangiopathy) complications result from changes in medium to large blood vessels. Blood vessel walls thicken, sclerose, and become occluded by plaque that adheres to the vessel walls. Eventually, blood flow is blocked. These atherosclerotic changes tend to occur more often and at an earlier age in patients whose glucose control is not at goal. Coronary artery disease, cerebrovascular disease, and peripheral vascular disease are the three main types of macrovascular complications that occur frequently in people with diabetes.

Cardiovascular disease is the major cause of illness and death for people with diabetes (ADA, 2022g). People with diabetes are two to four times more likely to develop cardiovascular disease that those without diabetes (Domenichini & Ferri, 2022). One unique feature of coronary artery disease in patients with diabetes is that typical ischemic symptoms may be absent. Therefore, the patient may not experience the early warning signs of decreased coronary blood flow and may have a "silent" myocardial infarction. This lack of ischemic symptoms may be secondary to autonomic neuropathy. Cardiac disease is discussed in detail in Chapter 13.

Cerebral blood vessels are affected similarly by accelerated atherosclerosis. Occlusive changes or an embolus elsewhere in the vasculature that lodges in a cerebral blood vessel can lead to transient ischemic attacks and strokes. For patients who present with ischemic stroke, approximately 15% to 33% have diabetes (Goldstein, 2020). Recovery from a stroke is likely to be more difficult for patients with elevated blood glucose levels at the time of, and immediately after, a stroke. Because symptoms of cerebrovascular disease may be similar to symptoms of acute diabetic complications (HHNS or hypoglycemia), it is very important to assess the blood glucose level and treat abnormal levels rapidly so that testing and treatment of cerebrovascular disease can be initiated promptly, if indicated.

Atherosclerotic changes in the large blood vessels of the lower extremities are responsible for a two to three times higher incidence of occlusive peripheral arterial disease in people with diabetes. Signs and symptoms of peripheral vascular disease include diminished peripheral pulses and intermittent claudication (pain in the buttock, thigh, or calf during walking). Severe arterial occlusive disease in the lower extremities is largely responsible for the increased incidence of gangrene and subsequent amputation in patients with diabetes. Refer to Chapter 11 for assessment of ankle-brachial index (ABI). Foot ulcers occur in approximately 15% of people with diabetes (annual incidence rate 2%) and are the leading causes of hospital admission; factors associated with ulcerations include peripheral vascular insufficiency, repeated trauma (unrecognized because of sensory loss), and superimposed infection (Domenichini & Ferri, 2022).

Medical and Nursing Management

The focus of management is aggressive modification and reduction of risk factors. Diet and exercise are important in managing diabetes, hypertension, and hyperlipidemia. Smoking cessation is essential. If blood pressure goals are not met within 3 months of lifestyle changes, angiotensin-converting enzyme (ACE) inhibitors or angiotensin receptor blockers (ARBs) are recommended for blood pressure control, if not otherwise contraindicated. Cholesterol lowering medications (e.g., statins) may be added. Aspirin therapy is recommended as a primary prevention strategy in those patients who have a 10-year risk for cardiovascular disease of at least 10% (Domenichini & Ferri, 2022). However, aspirin is not recommended routinely for all patients (ADA, 2022g).

When macrovascular complications do occur, patients may require medication changes or intensification of their regimen to get glucose levels to goal. Target A1c and blood glucose goals are person-dependent and should be modified to avoid hypoglycemia, with higher A1c targets particularly in those patients who are older or have known coronary artery disease.

Microvascular Complications

Diabetic microvascular disease (microangiopathy) is characterized by thickening of the membrane of the capillary basement. The basement membrane surrounds the endothelial cells of the capillary. Increased blood glucose levels react through a series of biochemical responses to thicken the basement membrane to several times its normal thickness. Two areas affected by these changes are the retina and the kidneys.

Diabetic Retinopathy

Diabetic retinopathy accounts for 8% of all causes of legal blindness in the United States. It occurs in patients with both type 1 and type 2 diabetes. After 20 years of a person having diabetes, >90% with type 1 and >60% of those with type 2 diabetes will develop some degree of retinopathy (Clinical Overview, 2022). Glaucoma, cataracts, and other disorders of the eye occur earlier and more frequently in people with diabetes (ADA, 2022i). Table 29-7 summarizes the complications of diabetes that affect vision.

Diabetic retinopathy is caused by changes in the small blood vessels in the retina, the area of the eye that receives images and sends information about the images to the brain. The retina is richly supplied with blood vessels of all kinds: small arteries and veins, arterioles, venules, and capillaries. Figure 29-8 shows the difference between a healthy retina and a retina affected by diabetes.

The risk for retinopathy increases with the length of time a person has had diabetes. Chronic hyperglycemia and hypertension also increase the risk for retinopathy (ADA, 2022i). Changes in the microvasculature include microaneurysms, intraretinal hemorrhage, hard exudates, and focal capillary closure.

Retinopathy has three stages: nonproliferative, preproliferative, and proliferative.

- *Stage I:* Nonproliferative retinopathy is characterized by macular edema and occurs in approximately 10% of

TABLE 29-7 **Ocular Complications of Diabetes**

Eye Disorder	Characteristics
Retinopathy	Deterioration of the small blood vessels that nourish the retina
Nonproliferative (background)	Early-stage, asymptomatic retinopathy. Blood vessels within the retina develop microaneurysms that leak fluid, causing swelling and forming deposits (exudates). In some cases, macular edema causes distorted vision.
Preproliferative	Represents increased destruction of retinal blood vessels
Proliferative	Abnormal growth of new blood vessels on the retina. New vessels rupture, bleeding into the vitreous and blocking light. Ruptured blood vessels in the vitreous form scar tissue, which can pull on and detach the retina.
Cataracts	Opacity of the lens of the eye; cataracts occur at an earlier age in patients with diabetes.
Lens changes	The lens of the eye can swell when blood glucose levels are elevated. For some patients, visual changes related to lens swelling may be the first symptoms of diabetes. It may take up to 2 months of improved blood glucose control before hyperglycemic swelling subsides and vision stabilizes. Therefore, patients are advised not to change eyeglass prescriptions during the 2 months after discovery of hyperglycemia.
Glaucoma	Results from occlusion of the outflow channels by new blood vessels. Glaucoma may occur with slightly higher frequency in people with diabetes.

people with type 1 or type 2 diabetes. It may lead to visual distortion and loss of central vision.

- *Stage II:* Preproliferative retinopathy involves more widespread vascular changes and loss of nerve fibers. Approximately 10% to 50% of patients with preproliferative retinopathy develop proliferative retinopathy in a short time, some within a year.
- *Stage III:* Proliferative retinopathy is characterized by production of new blood vessels and formation of scar tissue. The new vessels are prone to bleeding. Fibrous scar tissue places traction on the retina that may cause hemorrhage or retinal detachment, with subsequent loss of vision.

Clinical Manifestations and Assessment

Retinopathy is typically painless. In nonproliferative and preproliferative retinopathy, blurry vision secondary to macular edema occurs in some patients, although many patients are asymptomatic. Even patients with a significant degree of proliferative retinopathy and some hemorrhaging may not experience major visual changes. Symptoms indicative of hemorrhaging include floaters or cobwebs in the visual field, sudden visual changes including spotty or hazy vision, or complete loss of vision.

Diagnosis of retinopathy is made by direct visualization of the retina through dilated pupils with an ophthalmoscope by an ophthalmologist or optometrist.

Medical Management

The primary focus of the management of retinopathy is prevention through blood glucose control. Other strategies that may slow the progression of diabetic retinopathy include control of hypertension and smoking cessation. Laser photocoagulation in patients with retinopathy is effective at preventing vision loss. Routine screening for diabetic retinopathy allows for earlier access to this important procedure (ADA, 2022i).

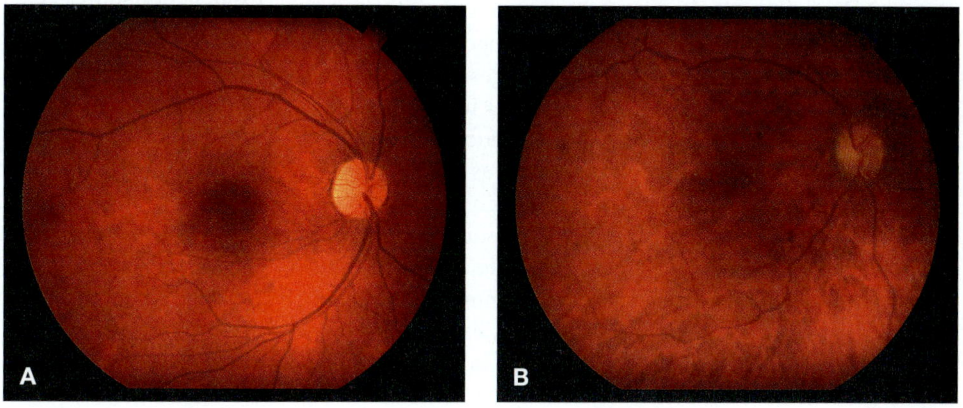

FIGURE 29-8 **Diabetic retinopathy. (A) In a normal eye, the light circular area over which a number of blood vessels converge is the optic disc, where the optic nerve meets the back of the eye. (B) The photograph of a patient with diabetic retinopathy shows hard exudates in circinate ring. (Reproduced, with permission, from Wu, G. [2010].** ***Diabetic retinopathy*****. Wolters Kluwer Health. Figures 1–5 and 2–6.)**

Nursing Management

Nursing management of patients with diabetic retinopathy or other eye disorders focuses on patient education about the importance of prevention through regular ophthalmologic examinations and control of blood glucose. The effectiveness of early diagnosis and prompt treatment is emphasized. If vision loss occurs, nursing care also must address the patient's adjustment to impaired vision and use of adaptive devices for diabetes self-care as well as activities of daily living. Nursing care for patients with low vision or loss of vision is discussed in detail in Chapter 48.

Diabetic Nephropathy

Diabetic nephropathy, or renal disease secondary to microvascular changes in the kidney, is the single leading cause of ESKD (ADA, 2022h). In fact, approximately 40% of patients in a given dialysis center have a diagnosis of diabetes (Domenichini & Ferri, 2022). It is characterized by albuminuria (protein in the urine), hypertension, and progressive renal insufficiency. Some patients eventually require dialysis or kidney transplantation.

Patients with type 1 diabetes frequently show initial signs of renal disease after 10 to 15 years, while patients with type 2 diabetes may develop renal disease within 10 years after diagnosis. However, because many patients with type 2 diabetes have had diabetes for many years before diagnosis, there can be evidence of nephropathy at the time of diagnosis.

Pathophysiology

If blood glucose levels are elevated consistently for a significant period of time, the kidney's filtration mechanism is stressed, allowing blood proteins to leak into the urine. As a result, the pressure in the blood vessels of the kidney increases. It is thought that this elevated pressure serves as the stimulus for the development of nephropathy.

Clinical Manifestations and Assessment

Most of the signs and symptoms of renal dysfunction in patients with diabetes are similar to those seen in patients without diabetes. For patients with diabetes, as kidney failure progresses, the catabolism (breakdown) of both exogenous and endogenous insulin decreases, causing increased risk for hypoglycemic episodes. Insulin needs change as a result of changes in the catabolism of insulin, changes in diet related to the treatment of nephropathy, and changes in insulin clearance that occur with decreased kidney function. Other medications excreted through the kidney, such as sulfonylureas, may also need to be adjusted to avoid hypoglycemia.

Nephropathy is characterized by the presence of albumin in the urine. Routine urine screening can detect even slight elevations in albumin levels. Urine albumin to creatinine ratio of $\geq$30 mg/g is abnormal and signals early nephropathy. People with diabetes should have their urine checked at least annually for the presence of albumin (ADA, 2022h).

Hypertension, whether it is a downstream effect of diabetic nephropathy or a comorbid condition, should be managed aggressively.

Medical Management

In addition to achieving and maintaining near-normal blood glucose levels, management for all patients with diabetes should include careful attention to control of hypertension and promoting smoking cessation to decrease or delay the onset of early albuminuria. Other concerns include prevention or vigorous treatment of urinary tract infections and avoidance of nephrotoxic medications. As kidney function changes, adjustment of medications may be necessary.

For patients who have developed albuminuria, an ACE inhibitor or ARB should be prescribed. These medications lower blood pressure and reduce albuminuria, thereby protecting the kidney. This preventive strategy should be part of the standard of care for all people with diabetes. In chronic or end-stage kidney failure, two types of treatment are available: dialysis (hemodialysis or peritoneal dialysis) and kidney transplantation.

Diabetic Neuropathy

Diabetic neuropathy refers to a group of diseases that affect all types of nerves, including peripheral (sensorimotor) and autonomic nerves. The disorders are clinically diverse and depend on the location of the affected nerve cells. They may be focal or diffuse (ADA, 2022i).

The etiology of neuropathy appears to be related to elevated levels of blood glucose over a period of years. The pathogenesis of neuropathy may be attributed to either vascular or metabolic mechanisms, or both. Thickening of the membrane of the capillary basement and closure of capillaries disrupt blood supply to nerves. Also, demyelinization of nerves, which is thought to be related to hyperglycemia, and accumulation of sorbitol in nerve cells slow nerve conduction.

The two most common types of diabetic neuropathy are sensorimotor polyneuropathy and autonomic neuropathy. Sensorimotor polyneuropathy, also called *peripheral neuropathy*, most commonly affects the distal portions of the nerves, especially the nerves of the lower extremities. Mononeuropathies (e.g., cranial neuropathies affecting the oculomotor nerve) affect a single nerve. Autonomic neuropathies cause a variety of clinical manifestations, depending on the area involved.

Peripheral Neuropathy

Clinical Manifestations and Assessment

Initial symptoms of neuropathy may include paresthesias (numbness or tingling) and aching or burning sensations, especially at night. A decrease in proprioception (awareness of posture and movement of the body and of position and weight of objects in relation to the body) and a decreased sensation of light touch may lead to an unsteady gait. Decreased sensations of pain and temperature place patients with neuropathy at increased risk for injury and undetected foot infections. Joint deformities may result from abnormal weight distribution on joints, resulting from lack of proprioception. Sensation can be assessed using a monofilament device (see Fig. 29-10).

On physical examination, there may be a decrease in deep tendon reflexes and vibratory sensation. For patients who have few or no symptoms of neuropathy, these physical findings may be the only indication of neuropathic changes.

Medical and Nursing Management

Pain, particularly of the lower extremities, is a disturbing symptom for many people with neuropathy due to diabetes. The first step in pain management is to achieve optimal control of blood glucose. Pharmacologic treatment of pain may include analgesics, antidepressants, and antiseizure medications, as well as use of transcutaneous electrical nerve stimulation (TENS).

Autonomic Neuropathies

Neuropathy of the ANS can result in a broad range of dysfunctions affecting many organ systems. Three manifestations of autonomic neuropathy are related to the cardiac, GI, and urogenital systems. Cardiovascular symptoms may range from resting tachycardia, exercise intolerance, and orthostatic hypotension to silent, or painless, myocardial ischemia and infarction.

GI symptoms of early satiety, bloating, nausea, vomiting, and constipation or diarrhea may occur as a result of delayed gastric emptying. Decreased gastric motility may result in poor control of blood glucose caused by delayed absorption of glucose from ingested foods, which leads to increased variability in blood glucose levels and increased risk of hypoglycemia.

Urinary retention, a decreased sensation of bladder fullness, and other urinary symptoms of neurogenic bladder may result from autonomic neuropathy. The patient with a neurogenic bladder is predisposed to development of urinary tract infections because of the inability to empty the bladder completely. This is especially true of patients with poorly controlled diabetes because hyperglycemia impairs resistance to infection.

Sexual dysfunction is a complication of diabetes. Erectile dysfunction occurs with greater frequency in males with diabetes. Some people with autonomic neuropathy have normal erectile function and can experience orgasm but do not ejaculate normally. The effects of autonomic neuropathy on female sexual functioning include reduced vaginal lubrication, decreased libido, and lack of orgasm. Vaginal infection, which is more common in people with diabetes, may be associated with decreased lubrication, itching, and tenderness.

Medical and Nursing Management

Management strategies depend on symptoms and focus on modification and management of risk factors. Early recognition and appropriate management of neuropathy is important. Effective treatment options for symptomatic diabetic neuropathy are available and may relieve symptoms.

For example, treatment of delayed gastric emptying includes a low-fat diet, frequent small meals, and close monitoring of blood glucose. Metoclopramide is now reserved for the most severe cases of gastroparesis, and treatment duration should be limited (ADA, 2022i). Treatment of diabetic diarrhea may include bulk-forming laxatives or antidiarrheal agents. Constipation is treated with a high-fiber diet and adequate hydration; medications, laxatives, and enemas may be necessary if constipation is severe. Treatment of erectile dysfunction may include medication (e.g., phosphodiesterase type-5 inhibitors) and mechanical devices (ADA, 2022i).

Complications of the Feet and Legs

Amputation and foot ulcers, consequences of diabetic neuropathy and/or peripheral artery disease, are common and major causes of death and disability in people with diabetes. Early recognition and management of risk factors can prevent or delay these complications of diabetes (ADA, 2022i).

As shown in Figure 29-9, the typical sequence of events in the development of a diabetic foot ulcer begins with a soft tissue injury of the foot, formation of a fissure between the toes or in an area of dry skin, or formation of a callus. Patients with an insensitive foot do not feel injuries, which may be thermal (e.g., from using heating pads, walking barefoot on hot concrete, testing bath water with the foot), chemical (e.g., burning the foot while using caustic agents on calluses, corns, or bunions), or traumatic (e.g., injuring skin while cutting nails, walking with an undetected foreign object in the shoe, or wearing ill-fitting shoes and socks).

If the patient is not in the habit of thoroughly inspecting both feet on a daily basis, the injury or fissure may go unnoticed until a serious infection has developed. Drainage, swelling, redness of the leg, or gangrene may be the first sign of foot problems that the patient notices. Treatment of

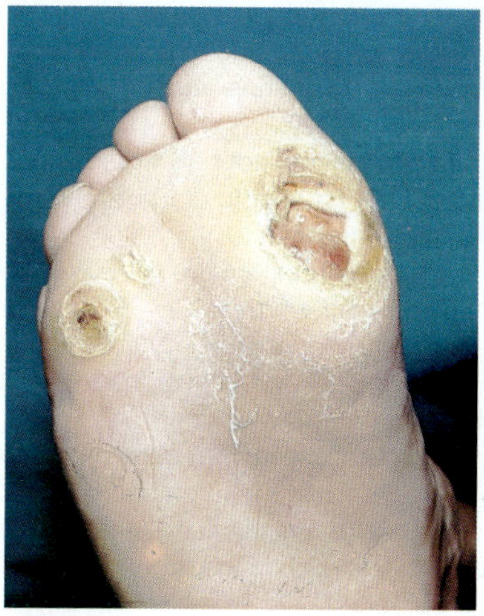

FIGURE 29-9 Neuropathic ulcers occur on pressure points in areas with diminished sensation in diabetic polyneuropathy. The ulcer may go unnoticed if sensation is absent.

foot ulcers typically involves antibiotics and debridement. Controlling glucose levels, which tend to increase when infections occur, is important for promoting wound healing. In addition, smoking cessation should be promoted aggressively. In patients with peripheral vascular disease, foot ulcers may not heal because of the decreased ability of oxygen, nutrients, and antibiotics to reach the injured tissue due to decreased circulation. Amputation may be necessary to prevent the spread of infection.

The risk of amputation and other problems involving the lower extremities is especially high for patients who have had diabetes for more than 10 years, those with poor blood glucose control, and those with peripheral vascular disease and peripheral neuropathy. Foot assessment and foot care instructions are vitally important for patients who are at high risk for foot infections.

Medical and Nursing Management

Teaching patients proper foot care is a nursing intervention that can prevent costly and painful complications that result in disability. Box 29-8 provides foot care tips for patient education. Preventive foot care begins with careful daily assessment of the feet. The feet must be inspected for redness, blisters, fissures, calluses, ulcerations, changes in skin temperature, or development of foot deformities. For patients with visual impairment or decreased joint mobility, use of a mirror or the help of a family member to inspect the bottoms of both feet may be necessary. The interior surfaces of shoes also should be inspected for any rough spots or foreign objects. In addition to daily visual and manual inspection of the feet, the feet should be examined during every health care visit or at least once a year by a health care provider. Patients with diabetes also should undergo neurologic and circulatory evaluation by an experienced examiner. Neurologic examination can be done using a monofilament device, shown in Figure 29-10. Circulation can be assessed by palpating for pulses in the lower extremities or by Doppler ultrasound. Patients with pressure areas, such as calluses, or thick toenails should be treated by a podiatrist.

Blood glucose control is important for preventing infection and diabetic neuropathy. The patient may be referred by the health provider to a wound care center for management of persistent wounds of the feet or legs.

SPECIAL ISSUES IN DIABETES CARE

Patients with Diabetes Who Are Undergoing Surgery

During periods of physiologic stress, such as surgery, blood glucose levels tend to increase because of changes in stress hormones. If hyperglycemia is not controlled during surgery,

BOX 29-8 **Patient Education**

Foot Care Tips

- Take care of your diabetes:
  - Work with your health care team to keep your blood glucose level within a normal range.
- Inspect your feet every day:
  - Look at your bare feet every day for cuts, blisters, red spots, and swelling.
  - Use a mirror to check the bottoms of your feet, or ask a family member for help if you have trouble seeing.
  - Check for changes in temperature.
- Wash your feet every day:
  - Wash your feet in warm, not hot, water.
  - Dry your feet well. Be sure to dry between the toes.
  - Do not soak your feet.
  - Do not check water temperature with your feet; use a thermometer or your elbow.
- Keep the skin soft and smooth:
  - Rub a thin coat of skin lotion over the tops and bottoms of your feet but not between your toes.
  - Have corns and calluses trimmed by a podiatrist.
- Inspect toenails. All people with diabetes should seek a qualified podiatrist for maintenance of feet and nails.
- Wear shoes and socks at all times:
  - Never walk barefoot.
  - Wear comfortable closed-toe shoes that fit well and protect your feet.
  - Stockings should fit well (without folds, wrinkles, or seams), be comfortable, and be changed daily.
  - Feel inside your shoes before putting them on each time to make sure the lining is smooth and there are no objects inside.
  - Wear sandals in public showers.
- Protect your feet from hot and cold:
  - Wear shoes at the beach or on hot pavement.
  - Wear socks at night if your feet get cold.
- Keep the blood flowing to your feet:
  - Put your feet up when sitting.
  - Wiggle your toes and move your ankles up and down for 5 minutes, two or three times a day.
  - Do not cross your legs for long periods of time.
  - Do not smoke.
- Check with your health care provider:
  - Have your health care provider check your bare feet and find out whether you are likely to have serious foot problems. Remember that you may not feel the pain of an injury.
  - Call your health care provider right away if there is a cut, sore, blister, or bruise on your foot that does not begin to heal after 1 day.
  - Follow your health care provider's advice about foot care.
  - Do not self-medicate or use home remedies or over-the-counter agents to treat foot problems.

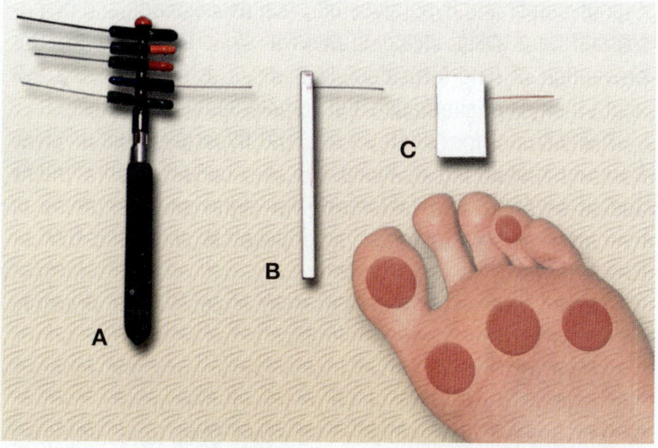

FIGURE 29-10 **The monofilament test is used to assess the sensory threshold in patients with diabetes. The test instrument—a monofilament (A, B, and C are examples of monofilaments)—is gently applied to about five pressure points on the foot (as shown in image on left). The examiner applies the monofilament to the test area to determine whether the patient feels the device. (Adapted with permission from Cameron, B. L. [2002]. Making diabetes management routine. *American Journal of Nursing*, 102[2], 26–32.)**

the resulting osmotic diuresis may lead to excessive loss of fluids and electrolytes. Patients with type 1 diabetes also are at risk of developing ketoacidosis during periods of stress.

Hypoglycemia is a concern in patients with diabetes who are undergoing surgery. This is a concern especially during the preoperative period if surgery is delayed beyond the time when the patient received their injection of long-acting insulin.

There are various approaches to managing glucose levels during the perioperative period. Frequent monitoring of blood glucose is essential throughout the preoperative and postoperative periods, regardless of the method used for glucose control.

During the postoperative period, patients with diabetes also must be monitored closely for cardiovascular complications because of the increased prevalence of atherosclerosis, wound infection, and skin breakdown.

Patients with Diabetes Who Are Hospitalized

At any one time, 10% to 20% of hospitalized general medical-surgical patients have diabetes. This number may increase as older patients make up an increasing proportion of the hospitalized population. Often, diabetes is not the primary medical diagnosis, yet problems with control of diabetes frequently result from changes in the patient's normal routine or from surgery or illness. Some of the main issues pertinent to nursing care of patients with diabetes who are hospitalized are presented below.

Self-Care Issues

All patients admitted to the hospital must relinquish control of some aspects of their daily care to the hospital staff. For patients with diabetes who are actively involved in diabetes self-management, relinquishing control over meal timing, insulin timing, and insulin dosage can be particularly difficult. It is important for the nurse to acknowledge the patient's concerns and involve the patient in the plan of care as much as possible. If the patient disagrees with certain aspects of nursing or medical care related to diabetes, the nurse must communicate this to other members of the health care team and, where appropriate, make changes in the plan to meet the patient's needs.

Hyperglycemia During Hospitalization

Hyperglycemia may occur in patients who are hospitalized as a result of the illness that precipitated the hospitalization. Other factors that may contribute to hyperglycemia during hospitalization include:

- Changes in usual treatment regimen
- Use of medications and IV fluids, such as partial parenteral nutrition (PPN) and total parenteral nutrition (TPN), that increase blood sugar
- Inappropriate withholding of insulin or inappropriate use of "sliding scales," or the progressive increase in **insulin** doses based on predefined blood glucose ranges
- Mismatched timing of meals and insulin

Nursing actions to correct or manage these factors are important for avoiding hyperglycemia.

Hypoglycemia During Hospitalization

Hypoglycemia in hospitalized patients is often the result of too much insulin or delays in eating. Causes of hypoglycemia in hospitalized patients include:

- Overuse of "sliding scale" insulin
- Lack of change in insulin dosage when dietary intake is changed
- Overly aggressive treatment of hyperglycemia
- Delayed meal after insulin administration
- Older adults with diabetes due to alterations in adaptive physiologic responses to low glucose levels. In addition, comorbidities including cognitive and functional decline may impact rapid identification of hypoglycemia (Lowery & Triplett, 2022)
- Heart failure or kidney or liver disease

The nurse must assess the pattern of glucose values and avoid giving doses of insulin that repeatedly lead to hypoglycemia. Successive doses of subcutaneous rapid-acting insulin should be administered no more frequently than every 3 to 4 hours. To avoid hypoglycemic reactions caused by delayed food intake, the nurse should arrange for snacks to be given to the patient if meals are postponed because of procedures, physical therapy, or other activities.

Assisting with Hygiene

Nurses caring for patients with diabetes who are hospitalized must focus attention on oral hygiene and skin care. Because these patients are at increased risk for periodontal disease, it is important for the nurse to assist the patient with daily dental care. The patient also may require assistance in keeping the skin clean and dry, especially in the groin and axillary areas and under the breasts, where chafing and fungal infections tend to occur.

For patients who must remain in bed, nursing care must emphasize the prevention of skin breakdown at pressure points. The heels are particularly susceptible to breakdown because of loss of sensation of pain and pressure associated with sensory neuropathy.

Feet should be cleaned, dried, lubricated with lotion, and inspected frequently. If the patient is in the supine position, pressure on the heels can be alleviated by elevating the lower legs on a pillow, with the heels positioned over the edge of the pillow. When the patient is seated in a chair, the feet should be positioned so that pressure is not placed on the heels. If the patient has an ulcer on one foot, it is important to provide preventive care to the unaffected foot as well as to give special care to the affected foot. As always, every opportunity should be taken to teach the patient about diabetes self-management, including daily oral, skin, and foot care.

Managing Stress

Physiologic stress, such as infections and surgery, contributes to hyperglycemia and may precipitate DKA or HHNS. Emotional stress can have a negative impact on diabetes control as well. An increase in stress hormones leads to an increase in glucose levels, especially if intake of food and insulin remains unchanged. In addition, during periods of emotional stress, people with diabetes may alter their usual pattern of meals, exercise, and medication. This can contribute to hyperglycemia or hypoglycemia.

People with diabetes must be made aware of the potential deterioration in glucose control that can accompany emotional stress. Nursing care must include encouraging the patient to follow the diabetes treatment plan as much as possible during times of stress. In addition, learning strategies for minimizing stress and coping with stress are important aspects of diabetes education.

NURSING PROCESS
The Patient With Diabetes as a Secondary Diagnosis

Patients with diabetes frequently seek medical attention for problems not directly related to control of blood glucose. However, during the course of treatment for the primary medical diagnosis, blood glucose control may worsen. Therefore, it is important for nurses caring for patients with diabetes to focus attention on the diabetes as well as on the primary health issue.

NURSING ASSESSMENT

In addition to nursing assessment for the primary problem, assessment of the patient with diabetes also must focus on hypoglycemia and hyperglycemia, skin assessment, and diabetes self-care skills, including survival skills and measures for prevention of long-term complications. The nurse should ask about the use of alternative and complementary therapies.

Assessment for hypoglycemia and hyperglycemia involves frequent monitoring of blood glucose, usually before meals and at bedtime, and monitoring for signs and symptoms of hypoglycemia or prolonged hyperglycemia, including DKA or HHNS.

Careful assessment of the skin, especially at pressure points and on the lower extremities, is important. The skin is assessed for dryness, cracks, skin breakdown, and redness. The patient is asked about symptoms of neuropathy, such as tingling and pain or numbness of the feet. Deep tendon reflexes are assessed.

The nurse should assess the patient's diabetes self-care skills as soon as possible to determine whether further diabetes teaching is required. The nurse observes the patient preparing and injecting the insulin, monitoring blood glucose, and performing foot care. The patient's knowledge about diet can be assessed with the help of a dietitian through direct questioning and review of the patient's menu choices. The patient is asked about signs and symptoms, treatment, and prevention of hypoglycemia and hyperglycemia. The patient's knowledge of risk factors for microvascular and macrovascular disease, including hypertension, increased lipids, and smoking, is assessed. In addition, the patient is asked the date of the last eye examination, which included dilation of the pupils. Also it is important to assess the patient's use of preventive health measures, such as an annual influenza vaccination, date of the most recent pneumonia and COVID-19 vaccinations, as well as current medication regimen.

NURSING DIAGNOSIS

Appropriate nursing diagnoses may include:

- Imbalanced nutrition related to increase in stress hormones secondary to the primary medical problem and imbalances in insulin, food, and physical activity
- Risk for impaired skin integrity related to immobility and decreased sensation
- Deficient knowledge about diabetes self-care skills related to new diagnosis, lack of basic diabetes education, or lack of continuing in-depth diabetes education
- Potential complications from inadequate control of blood glucose may include:
  - Hyperglycemia, hypoglycemia
  - DKA or HHNS

PLANNING AND GOALS

The major goals for the patient may include improved nutritional status, maintenance of skin integrity, and ability to perform basic diabetes self-care skills as well as preventive care for the avoidance of chronic complications of diabetes and absence of complications.

NURSING INTERVENTIONS

IMPROVING NUTRITIONAL STATUS

The patient's food intake is planned with the primary goal of maintaining target glucose levels and reducing risk for hyper- and hypoglycemia. The dietary plan also must consider the primary health problem in addition to lifestyle, cultural background, activity level, and food preferences. Alterations may be required because of the patient's primary health problem. The patient may be NPO in preparation for diagnostic or surgical procedures. Other common alterations for the patient who is hospitalized include special diets, tube feedings, and parenteral fluids. All of these treatments require special consideration for the patient with diabetes. The patient's nutritional intake is monitored carefully along with blood glucose and daily weight.

MAINTAINING SKIN CARE

The skin is assessed daily for dryness or breaks. The feet are cleaned with warm water and soap. Excessive soaking of the feet is avoided. The feet are dried thoroughly, especially between the toes, and lotion is applied to the entire foot, except between the toes. For patients who are confined to bed, the heels are elevated off the bed with a pillow placed under the lower legs and the heels resting over the edge of the pillow. Dermal ulcers are treated as indicated and prescribed. The nurse promotes optimal control of blood glucose in the patient with skin breakdown.

ADDRESSING KNOWLEDGE DEFICITS

Hospital admission of the patient with diabetes provides an ideal opportunity for the nurse to assess the patient's level of knowledge about diabetes and its management. The nurse uses this opportunity to assess the patient's understanding of diabetes management, including blood glucose monitoring, administration of medications, meal planning, exercise, and strategies to prevent long- and short-term complications of diabetes. The nurse also assesses the adjustment of the patient and family to diabetes and its management and identifies any misconceptions they may have.

MONITORING AND MANAGING POTENTIAL COMPLICATIONS

Inadequate control of blood glucose levels may hinder recovery from the primary health problem. Blood glucose levels are monitored, and insulin is administered as prescribed. It is important for the nurse to ensure that the prescribed insulin dosage is modified as needed to compensate for changes in the patient's schedule or eating pattern. Treatment is given for hypoglycemia or hyperglycemia. Blood glucose records are assessed for patterns of hypoglycemia and hyperglycemia at the same time of day, and findings are reported to the primary care provider. In the patient with prolonged elevations in blood glucose, laboratory values and the patient's physical condition are monitored for signs and symptoms of DKA or HHNS.

Development of acute complications of diabetes secondary to inadequate control of blood glucose levels may be associated with other health care problems because of changes in activity level and diet, and physiologic alterations related to the primary health problem itself. Therefore, the patient must be monitored for hyperglycemia and hypoglycemia, and measures must be implemented for their prevention and early treatment.

PROVIDING CONTINUING CARE

A patient who is hospitalized for another health problem may require referral for home care for that problem or if gaps in knowledge about self-care are found. The home care nurse reinforces the teaching provided during hospitalization and assesses the home care environment to determine its adequacy for self-care and safety.

EVALUATION

Expected patient outcomes may include the following:

1. Achieves optimal control of blood glucose:
   a. Takes steps to avoid significant hypoglycemia and hyperglycemia
   b. Takes steps to resolve rapidly any hypoglycemic episodes
2. Maintains skin integrity:
   a. Maintains intact skin without dryness and cracking
   b. Avoids ulcers caused by pressure and neuropathy
3. Demonstrates/verbalizes diabetes survival skills and preventive care
4. Exhibits understanding of treatment modalities:
   a. Demonstrates correct technique for administering insulin or other glucose lowering medications and assessing blood glucose
   b. Demonstrates appropriate knowledge of diet through proper menu selections and identification of pattern used for selecting foods at home
   c. Verbalizes signs and symptoms, appropriate treatment, and prevention of hypoglycemia and hyperglycemia
5. Demonstrates proper foot care:
   a. Inspects feet, including inspection for cracks or infections between toes
   b. Washes feet with warm water and soap; dries feet thoroughly
   c. Applies lotion to entire foot, except between toes
   d. Identifies strategies that decrease the risk of foot ulcers, including wearing shoes at all times; using hand or elbow, not foot, to test temperature of bath water; avoiding use of heating pad on feet; avoiding constrictive shoes; wearing new shoes for brief periods only; avoiding home remedies for treatment of corns and calluses; having feet examined at every appointment with the health care provider; and consulting a podiatrist for regular nail care if necessary
6. Takes steps to prevent eye disease:
   a. Verbalizes need for yearly or more frequent thorough eye examinations with pupil dilation by an ophthalmologist
   b. Verbalizes that retinopathy usually does not cause change in vision until serious damage to the retina has occurred

(continued on page 1018)

c. States that early laser treatment along with good control of blood glucose and blood pressure may prevent visual loss from retinopathy
d. Identifies hypoglycemia and hyperglycemia as two causes of temporary blurred vision

7. States measures to control risk factors:
   a. Smoking cessation
   b. Limitation of fats and cholesterol
   c. Control of hypertension
   d. Exercise
   e. Regular monitoring of kidney function
8. Reports absence of acute complications:
   a. Maintains blood glucose and urine ketones within normal limits
   b. Experiences no signs or symptoms of hypoglycemia or hyperglycemia
   c. Identifies signs and symptoms of hypoglycemia or hyperglycemia
   d. Reports appearance of symptoms so that treatment can be initiated

Clinical Judgment Case

A 54-year-old patient comes into the emergency room (ER) complaining of weakness, dizziness, and weight loss. The patient's skin is warm and dry with delayed skin turgor and vital signs are as follows: 98.7° F, HR 112 and regular, 28 RR with an oxygen saturation of 96% on room air, and blood pressure 102/52 mm Hg. There is a "fruity" odor to the patient's breath. The patient denies pain in the chest, jaw, back, or arms. Heart sounds are S1 S2 without murmur, gallops, or rub; neck veins are flat. Lungs sounds are clear. The patient denies shortness of breath, nausea or vomiting. Abdomen is soft, nondistended; upon palpation the patient states there is some tenderness at the umbilicus; last BM was yesterday, formed brown stool, no evidence of bleeding. There is no peripheral edema, capillary refill is 4 seconds, and pedal and posterior tibial pulses are 2+ to 3+ bil. The patient's history included diabetes type 1 (40-year history) and hyperlipidemia. The patient states they are concerned that their "diabetes may be out of whack." The only medications the patient takes is a "statin but can't recall the name," and their insulin regimen is "glargine 30 units once daily and insulin lispro approximately 10 units at each meal," adjusted for meal type and glucose at the time of the meal. The patient's A1c is "generally in the range of 6.5–7."

Step One: Recognize cues where relevant; important information is identified from different sources, such as medical history or vital signs.

Answer: History of diabetes for 40 years and hypercholesterolemia. Complaints of weakness, dizziness, and weight loss. Physical examination findings of delayed skin turgor, flat neck veins, abdominal tenderness at the umbilicus, and capillary refill of 4 seconds. Cues of concern related to vital signs: HR of 112 and regular, 28 RR with fruity odor, and blood pressure 102/52.

Step Two: Analyze cues, which is organizing and linking the recognized cues to the patient's clinical presentation.

Answer: You have clustered the symptoms to be associated with a hyperglycemic emergency, and given patient's history of type 1 diabetes you suspect DKA. Signs of fluid volume deficit include hypotension, tachycardia, delayed skin turgor, delayed capillary refill (normal <2 seconds), and flat neck veins. The deep and rapid respiratory rate you link to Kussmaul respirations, which you associate with metabolic acidosis as the body is attempting to "blow off the respiratory acid," which is carbonic acid in the form of CO_2. The characteristic fruity odor is associated with ketosis. You link the age of the patient, history of diabetes, and hypercholesteremia with the potential of a cardiac event. You link the abdominal tenderness at the umbilicus with a potential cause of the hyperglycemia (e.g., appendicitis, pancreatitis) or acidemia or hyponatremia.

Step Three: Prioritize hypotheses, where hypotheses are evaluated and ranked according to priority. This can include urgency, likelihood, risk, difficulty, and/or time. In this phase you cluster your findings to arrive at a list of problems (actual and or potential problems) you believe the patient is experiencing and determine the importance or urgency. What do you think is of greatest concern?

Answer: You prioritize an FVD as the greatest risk of injury to this patient. The blood pressure is 102/52, which correlates to a mean arterial pressure or MAP of 68.7. You are aware that a normal MAP is >70 mm Hg and that if the MAP is <65 mm Hg for an extended period, it can result in end-organ ischemia as you await evaluation by the ER provider.

Step Four: Generate solutions, which is identifying expected outcomes and using hypotheses to define a set of interventions for the expected outcomes.

Answer: Since a hyperglycemic emergency is suspected, you recognize the need for IV fluids, insulin, and monitoring of electrolytes and pH. You perform a point-of-care glucose testing and the glucose is 350.

Step Five: Take action, where the solutions that address the highest priorities are implemented.

Answer: You alert the provider of the high point-of-care glucose reading and start an IV, place the patient on a cardiac monitor, and monitor the oxygen saturation continuously. You repeat the vital signs and reassess the patient's abdominal exam and neurologic status. A 12 lead ECG is performed and there is no evidence of hypokalemia which includes prolonged PR interval, ST segment depression, and the development of a U wave. You are aware that central nervous system (CNS) depression can lead quickly to coma. You assess the patient's neurologic status and note that pupils are equal and reacting to light at 3 mm bil. There is no weakness noted; however, patient is less responsive now. Blood work is drawn stat, which includes troponin level, lipase, CBC, chemistry profile, and ABGs; as you await the results, an IV of normal saline is administered. You are aware that the IV normal saline will help to dilute the hyperglycemia. An insulin drip is ordered but you await the results of the electrolytes because if the potassium is less than 3.3 mEq/L, you cannot start the insulin drip since insulin facilitates movement of potassium intracellular. You also orient the patient to the treatment plan since you are aware that stress increases catecholamines which stimulate glycogenolysis, lipolysis, and gluconeogenesis, allowing more glucose to surge into the bloodstream. You prepare the insulin drip, aware that you must "coat the IV line" by flushing the tubing with the insulin solution with a volume of 20 mL to saturate the binding sites before connecting it to the patient, thus ensuring the patient receives the ordered rate of insulin infusion. The potassium level is 4.2 mEq/L and the insulin drip is started. The pH is 7.3 and the bicarbonate level is 16 mEq/L, so you are aware correction of the metabolic acidosis with base bicarbonate IV is not required at this time. You monitor the electrolytes and glucose hourly, paying close attention to the potassium level since it the most life-threatening electrolyte derangement during treatment of DKA and note that the glucose dropped from 350 mg/dL to 240 mg/dL in the first hour. You are aware that a rapid correction of hyperglycemia may play a role in the development of cerebral edema. The goal is to decrease the serum glucose level by 50 to 70 mg/dL/hr to prevent this complication. You follow institutional protocol and decrease the insulin drip since the last hour's insulin IV continues to exert action.

Step Six: Evaluate outcomes, which is comparing observed outcomes against expected outcomes.

Answer: You continue to evaluate vital signs and physical examination findings since monitoring for signs of fluid overload is important and the patient has now received 2 L of normal saline. You note resolution of the tachycardia (HR is now 92 and regular), capillary refill has improved to <2 seconds, lungs remain clear, and heart sounds are normal. The RR returned to 14 bpm and oxygen saturation was maintained over 95%. The BP has now increased to 120/72 with a MAP of 88 mm Hg, and the IV is changed to ½ normal saline. You have continued to monitor hourly glucose and electrolytes and when the glucose reached 200 mg/dL, the IV was changed to $D_5$1/2 NS, once again to prevent hypoglycemia from the action of IV insulin. The patient's slowness has improved, and they ask you, "What happened? How come my normal insulin dose was not enough to prevent this?" You explain that the providers will now investigate the potential causes of DKA, of which infection is the most common precipitating cause. You are aware that additional conditions that may precipitate DKA include myocardial infarction, cerebrovascular accident, sepsis, or pancreatitis as well as medications. The patient is subsequently admitted to the medical step-down unit, and you are to be commended because of your quick connection of the patient's clinical presentation and immediate assessment with a point-of-care glucometer.
Kudos to you and your astute clinical judgment and thoughtful care. Note on followup, the troponin I level, which is a newer-generation "high-sensitivity" cardiac biomarker, came back as 0.2, which is normal; however, the WBCs were elevated and abdominal pain subsequently migrated to the RLQ and a diagnosis of appendicitis was made.

CHAPTER REVIEW

NCLEX-Style Review Questions

1. Which should be included when teaching a patient newly diagnosed with diabetes about the dietary management of the disease? Select all that apply.
   a. Food intake should be decreased before exercise.
   b. Consistency between food intake and activity is important.
   c. Consistency in the amounts of calories and carbohydrates ingested at each meal is encouraged.
   d. Insulin and other glucose lowering agents decrease the need for dietary management.
   e. Foods high in fat and that lack vitamins, minerals, and fiber should be limited.

2. A patient presents to the clinic complaining of polyuria, polydipsia, and unexplained weight loss that suggest diabetes mellitus. What criteria would support a diagnosis of diabetes mellitus? Select all that apply.
   a. A1c—6.9
   b. Oral glucose tolerance test, 2-hour postload glucose 140 mg/dL
   c. Fasting plasma glucose >110 mg/dL
   d. Fasting plasma glucose >126 mg/dL
   e. Random glucose 220 mg/dL

3. The nurse would expect that insulin may be substituted for other glucose lowering agents in which of the following patients? Select all that apply.
   a. A patient with a history of diabetes hospitalized for an acute infection
   b. A patient whose A1c is at goal
   c. A patient experiencing hypoglycemia
   d. A patient who is newly diagnosed with borderline hyperglycemia
   e. A patient with a history of diabetes hospitalized with a myocardial infarction

4. A patient has just been admitted to the emergency department after being found disoriented at the grocery store. A medical alert bracelet indicates that the patient has type 1 diabetes. A diagnosis of DKA is made. Which of the following clinical signs do you anticipate finding upon assessment? Select all that apply.
   a. Hyperglycemia
   b. Kussmaul respiration
   c. Hypertension
   d. Hypokalemia
   e. Fruity odor of breath

5. Which of the following adverse events are associated with administration of insulin intravenously? Select all that apply.
   a. Hypoglycemia
   b. Hypocalcemia
   c. Hypernatremia
   d. Hypokalemia
   e. Hyperchloremia

REFERENCES AND SELECTED READINGS

References and selected readings associated with this chapter can be found on the website that accompanies the book. Visit **http://thepoint.lww.com/Honan3e** to access the references and other additional resources associated with this chapter.

CHAPTER 30

Nursing Management: Patients With Endocrine Disorders

Elaine Siow

Learning Objectives

After reading this chapter, you will be able to:

1. Identify the disorders associated with each of the endocrine glands.
2. Describe the underlying pathophysiology of each of the endocrine disorders.
3. Identify the risk factors associated with each of the endocrine disorders.
4. Describe the clinical manifestations and assessment of each of the endocrine disorders.
5. Summarize the medical and nursing management of each of the endocrine disorders.

Disorders of the endocrine system are common and have the potential to affect the function of every organ system in the body, such as growth, development, metabolism, and fluid and electrolyte balances. When considering pathology of the endocrine system, it is helpful to consider that disorders commonly reflect either too little hormone (undersecretion), too much hormone (oversecretion), or tumors. Refer to Table 30-1 for a list of disorders associated with hormone oversecretion and undersecretion (each will be presented in this chapter). Endocrine disorders can occur from a primary condition or from a secondary disorder that resulted in altered endocrine function.

PITUITARY DISORDERS

Oversecretion (hypersecretion) is the most common cause of pituitary disorders. It usually involves hypersecretion of adrenocorticotropic hormone (ACTH) that leads to Cushing syndrome or hypersecretion of growth hormone (GH) leading to **acromegaly** or **gigantism**. While oversecretion of the pituitary may affect a singular hormone, such as GH, undersecretion (hyposecretion) usually involves all of the **anterior pituitary hormones** and is termed *panhypopituitarism.* In this condition, the thyroid gland, the adrenal cortex, and the gonads atrophy because of loss of the trophic-stimulating hormones (influencing the activity of a gland). Hypopituitarism can result from destruction of the anterior lobe of the pituitary gland.

Recall that the **posterior lobe of the pituitary gland** secretes antidiuretic hormone (ADH), also known as *vasopressin*; too little ADH results in diabetes insipidus (DI), while too much ADH leads to **syndrome of inappropriate ADH** (SIADH).

PITUITARY TUMORS

Pathophysiology

Pituitary tumors are usually benign, although their location and effects on hormone production by target organs can cause life-threatening effects. Although local symptoms, such as headache and visual changes, may be seen as the tumor causes pressure within the brain, systemic effects are varied depending on the over/undersecretion of particular hormones. Prolactinomas are the most common form of pituitary tumor, causing a hypersecretion of prolactin that may lead to amenorrhea (loss of menstruation), galactorrhea (spontaneous, inappropriate flow of milk from male or female breasts in the absence of pregnancy or breast or chestfeeding.), and infertility in females. In males, these tumors can cause hypogonadism, decreased libido, and impotence.

If the tumor is large and the disorder is not diagnosed early, symptoms such as visual alterations due to pressure on the optic chiasm (Fig. 30-1) and headaches are common findings.

Risk Factors

Multiple endocrine neoplasia, type 1 (MEN1), also known as *Wermer syndrome*, is a rare autosomal dominant hereditary condition that is strongly associated with developing pituitary tumors (Cohen-Cohen et al., 2020).

Clinical Manifestations and Assessment

A normal anterior pituitary gland is formed by multiple cell types, including eosinophilic, basophilic, and chromophobic cells. Eosinophilic tumors that develop early in life can result in gigantism, as the epiphyseal plates have not yet fused. The

TABLE **30-1 Disorders Associated With Hormone Oversecretion and Undersecretion**

Hormone	Disorders Caused by Oversecretion	Disorders Caused by Undersecretion
Adrenocorticotropic hormone (ACTH)	Cushing syndrome	Addison disease
Thyroid-stimulating hormone (TSH)	Hyperthyroidism	Hypothyroidism
Growth hormone	In adults: acromegaly In children: gigantism	In children: congenital GH deficiency
Antidiuretic hormone (ADH; vasopressin)	Syndrome of inappropriate antidiuretic hormone (SIADH) secretion	Diabetes insipidus
Thyroid hormone	Hyperthyroidism	In children and adults: hypothyroidism or myxedema During fetal and neonatal development: congenital hypothyroidism (stunted body growth and mental development)
Parathormone	Hyperparathyroidism	Hypoparathyroidism
Insulin	Hypoglycemia	Diabetes mellitus

excess GH stimulates hepatic secretion of insulinlike growth factor-1 (IGF-1), which causes most of the clinical manifestations of acromegaly (Melmed & Katznelson, 2021). The affected person may be more than 7 ft tall and large in all proportions, but the person may be so weak and lethargic that they can hardly stand. If the disorder begins during adult life, the excessive skeletal growth occurs only in the feet, the hands, and the superciliary ridge (bony ridge located above the eye sockets); facial features (nose, lips, ears, and forehead) become broader and larger, the tongue enlarges, the space between the teeth increases, and the lower jaw grows, resulting in an underbite and extended lower jaw (Melmed & Katznelson, 2020a), which is called *acromegaly.* It is a slowly progressive insidious disorder resulting in a significant delay in diagnosis which is on average is 8 to 10 years

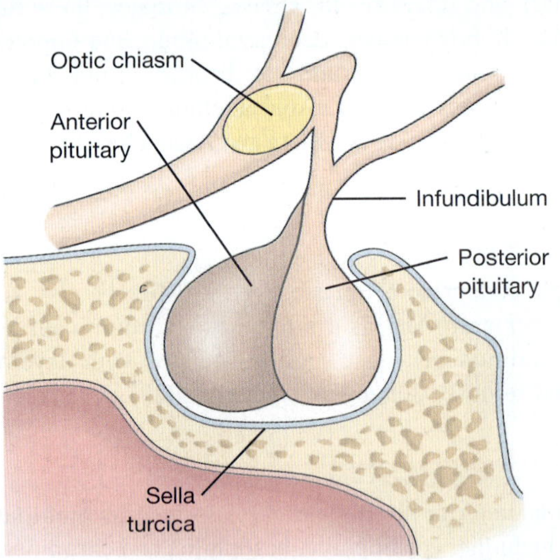

FIGURE 30-1 Relationship of the pituitary gland to the optic chiasm.

(Clinical Overview, 2022). Enlargement also can involve all tissues and organs of the body including the thyroid, heart, liver, lungs, and kidneys (Melmed & Katznelson, 2020a). As an example, because of soft tissue enlargement, carpal tunnel syndrome is noted frequently in patients with acromegaly when carpal tunnel growth compresses on the median nerve. Patients typically suffer from severe headaches and visual disturbances due to tumor compression on the optic nerves (resulting in bitemporal hemianopia) and palsies of the cranial nerves III, IV, and VI (Norris & Tuan, 2020). Assessments of central vision and visual fields may indicate loss of color discrimination, diplopia (double vision), or temporal hemianopia (loss of vision of one half of the visual field). In addition, the nurse asks about changes in shoe, ring, glove, or hat size. These tumors promote protein synthesis, which stimulates the growth of all organs; liver gluconeogenesis, causing hyperglycemia; decalcification of the skeleton; muscular weakness; and endocrine disturbances (refer to Fig. 30-2). Skeletal changes that occur with acromegaly are not reversible, whereas soft tissue changes may be. Cardiovascular disorders are the leading cause of death in acromegaly. Hypertension (HTN) occurs in 50% of patients with acromegaly and it is associated with cardiomyopathy, decreased ejection fraction (EF), valvular disease, arrhythmias, and atherosclerosis (Clinical Advisor, 2022). Diagnosis is based on biochemical measurement of GH and IGF-1 (insulinlike growth factor 1) levels, which are elevated. With treatment, the characteristic soft tissue overgrowth and metabolic abnormalities, such as diabetes mellitus (DM) improve; however, the bony changes generally do not regress and joint symptoms persist (Melmud & Katznelson, 2020b).

Basophilic tumors that give rise to Cushing disease have manifestations that are associated with excessive secretion of ACTH in the pituitary gland. This can lead to masculinization

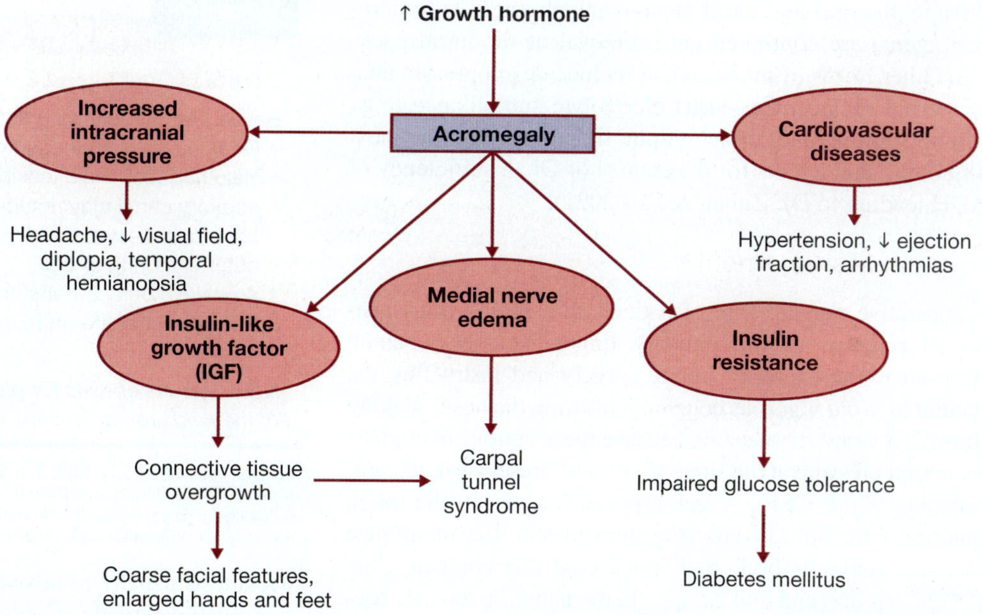

FIGURE 30-2 **Clinical manifestations of acromegaly.**

and amenorrhea in females, truncal obesity, HTN, thin skin, moon face, purple skin striae, and osteoporosis.

Chromophobic tumors represent 90% of pituitary tumors. These tumors usually produce no hormones but destroy the rest of the pituitary gland, causing hypopituitarism. Because the pituitary gland releases GH, thyroid-releasing hormone (TRH), ACTH, luteinizing hormone, follicle-stimulating hormone, and prolactin, signs and symptoms vary depending on the specific hormones that are deficient but may include weight loss; somnolence; fine, scant hair; dry, soft skin; a pasty complexion; short stature; and small bones. Patients also experience headaches, loss of libido, and visual defects progressing to blindness. Other signs and symptoms include polyuria, polyphagia, a lowering of the **basal metabolic rate**, and a subnormal body temperature.

Diagnosis requires a careful history and physical examination, including assessment of visual acuity and visual fields. Computed tomography (CT) and magnetic resonance imaging (MRI) reveal the presence and extent of pituitary tumors. If other information is inconclusive, serum levels of pituitary hormones may be obtained, along with measurements of hormones of target organs (e.g., thyroid and adrenal) to assist in diagnosis.

Medical Management

Hypophysectomy using a transsphenoidal approach is the treatment of choice for patients with a pituitary tumor, as the approach offers direct access to the sella turcica with minimal risk of trauma and hemorrhage. Tumors within the sella turcica and small adenomas of the pituitary can be removed through a transsphenoidal approach: an incision is made beneath the upper lip (sublabial) or via an endonasal approach (via the nares), in which entry is gained successively into the nasal cavity, sphenoidal sinus, and sella turcica with minimal risk of trauma and hemorrhage. Microsurgical techniques used in the transsphenoidal approach provide improved illumination, magnification, and visualization so that nearby vital structures can be avoided. The transsphenoidal approach also avoids the risks of craniotomy, and the postoperative discomfort is similar to that of other transnasal surgical procedures.

Preoperatively, the patient undergoes a series of baseline endocrine tests, such as measurement of serum prolactin, GH, cortisol (excessive corticosteroids for Cushing syndrome), and thyroid hormones (such as triiodothyronine, thyroxine, follicle-stimulating hormone [FSH], and luteinizing hormone [LH]; Zubair & Das, 2021). It is important to measure baseline thyroid and cortisol hormones to determine if supplements are needed prior to surgery (Zubair & Das, 2021). Funduscopic and visual field examination are performed because sometimes the pituitary tumor may create localized pressure on the optic nerve or chiasm. In addition, the nasopharyngeal secretions are cultured to detect a sinus infection, which is a contraindication to using the transsphenoidal approach.

Corticosteroids may be administered before and after surgery because the pituitary is the source of ACTH. In addition, the absence of the pituitary gland can alter the function of many body systems. For instance, cessation of menstruation and infertility can occur after total or near-total ablation of the pituitary gland. Corticosteroid replacement therapy and thyroid hormone replacement is necessary. In addition, prior to surgery, octreotide may be used to shrink the pituitary tumor and inhibit the production or release of GH, improving the patient's clinical condition.

The initial postoperative management focuses on preventing infection and promoting healing because the procedure disrupts the oral and nasal mucous membranes. Antimicrobial agents are continued until removal of the nasal packing. Other forms of management include desmopressin and/or steroid replacement, strict electrolyte surveillance (e.g., serum sodium and urine output monitored for the next 48 hours), and agents for the control of DI (insufficiency of ADH leading to DI; Zubair & Das 2021).

Nursing Management

Preoperative nursing care of patients undergoing transsphenoidal removal of the pituitary tumor includes teaching deep-breathing exercises before surgery and instructing the patient to avoid vigorous coughing, blowing the nose, sucking through a straw, or sneezing because these actions may place increased pressure at the surgical site and cause a leak of cerebrospinal fluid (CSF). A leak represents a tear in the tough outermost meningeal dura (the dura mater), the membrane that surrounds the brain and spinal cord that contains CSF. If CSF can descend and escape via the nares, so too can bacteria ascend into the meninges. Therefore, the nurse assesses for signs of meningeal irritation, such as nuchal rigidity (stiff neck), temperature elevation, and changes in mental status (see Chapter 45). The nurse teaches patients to avoid certain activities, such as bending over or straining during urination or defecation, because they can raise intracranial pressure (ICP).

Postoperative nursing care includes monitoring vital signs, such as hemodynamic, cardiac, and respiratory status. The nurse assesses visual acuity and visual fields at regular intervals because of the close anatomic proximity of the pituitary gland to the optic chiasm. One method is to ask the patient to count the number of fingers held up by the nurse. Evidence of decreasing visual acuity may suggest an expanding hematoma. In addition, the nurse raises the head of the bed to 15 to 30 degrees with the patient's head in the midline position to limit neck vein compression, decrease pressure on the sella turcica, and promote cerebral venous drainage (reducing potential for elevated ICP). Measurement of the patient's serum electrolytes and intake and output guide replacement of fluid and electrolytes and assess for DI. The urine specific gravity is measured after each voiding. The patient's daily weight is monitored to determine fluid status. The nurse recalls that 1 L of fluid equals 1 kg, or approximately 2.2 lb. Usually fluids are given after nausea ceases, after which the patient may be able to progress to a regular diet.

The nurse should check the nasal packing inserted during surgery frequently for blood or CSF drainage (Box 30-1). Often patients are instructed to breathe through their mouth instead of the nose, and oral care should be offered every 4 hours or more frequently as the patient can experience excessive mouth dryness. If a sublabial approach is used, the patient is advised not to brush their teeth until the incision above the teeth has been healed. Measures to help the patient maintain oral care and moist mucous membranes include offering warm saline mouth rinses, using a mist vaporizer, applying lip balm, and using a room humidifier. The nasal packing is usually removed within 48 to 72 hours of insertion postoperatively (Caulley et al., 2020). Following this, the area around the nares may be cleaned with the prescribed nasal solution to remove crusted blood and discharge, and to moisten the mucous membranes. Oral antibiotics are administered as ordered while packing is in place to protect the patient from infection (Caulley et al., 2020).

BOX 30-1 **Focused Assessment**

Cerebrospinal Fluid Leak

Be alert for the following signs and symptoms:

- Copious clear drainage from nose or ear.
- Halo ring test: Fluid leaking from the nose or external auditory canal may result in the double ring sign on absorbent tissue, which is a central circle of blood and an outer clear ring of CSF.
- A positive beta-2-transferrin test (a carbohydrate-free isoform of transferrin found in CSF) indicates that CSF fluid is present.

Note: Results of tests for glucose, chloride, and total protein of the fluid are not specific or conclusive for CSF.

Data from Ramayya A.G., & Sinha S, & Grady M (2019). Neurosurgery. Brunicardi F, & Andersen D.K., & Billiar T.R., & Dunn D.L., & Kao L.S., & Hunter J.G., & Matthews J.B., & Pollock R.E.(Eds.), *Schwartz's Principles of Surgery*, 11e. McGraw Hill. https://accesssurgery.mhmedical.com/content.aspx?bookid=2576&sectionid=216212278

DIABETES INSIPIDUS

DI is characterized by a deficiency of ADH, also known as *vasopressin or AVP*. ADH is produced in the hypothalamus, stored in the posterior pituitary gland, and controls the ability of water to pass through the cells of the collecting ducts. If no ADH is present, then no water can be reabsorbed, and the urine output is massive. DI can occur if (1) the hypothalamus produces insufficient ADH, (2) the posterior pituitary fails to release ADH, or (3) the kidney nephron is resistant (unresponsive) to ADH (Lough, 2022). In general, this disorder is characterized by excessive thirst (polydipsia) and large volumes of dilute urine. It is helpful to remember the three Ds: **D**iabetes insipidus, **D**ecreased ADH, and **D**iuresis. There are three types of DI: neurogenic, nephrogenic, and psychogenic polydipsia.

Pathophysiology

Neurogenic DI is characterized by an acute onset resulting from the destruction of the posterior pituitary gland, resulting in a lack of vasopressin. Nephrogenic DI generally results from drug-related damage to the renal tubules, resulting in the inability of kidney tubules to respond to circulating ADH. Psychogenic DI is caused by excessive water intake.

Risk Factors

DI may develop as a result of head trauma, brain tumor, surgical ablation, or irradiation of the pituitary. It also may occur with infections of the central nervous system (CNS;

e.g., meningitis, encephalitis, or tuberculosis) or with tumors (e.g., metastatic disease and lymphoma of the breast or lung). Another cause of DI is failure of the renal tubules to respond to ADH. This nephrogenic form of DI may be related to hypokalemia, hypercalcemia, or medications that impair the kidneys' ability to reabsorb water. While congenital nephrogenic DI is a rare inherited X-linked recessive AVPR2 genetic mutation, the different forms of mutations by race remains unclear (Kim et al., 2020). In a multicenter retrospective chart review conducted in 16 medical centers in the United States, around 30% of pediatric patients with nephrogenic DI did not have a positive family history or genetic testing conducted (D'Alessandri-Silva et al., 2020). The incidence of acute DI in patients with a severe head injury is high, especially in penetrating injuries. Independent risk factors for DI include a Glasgow Coma Scale (GCS) of 8 or less, and cerebral edema. Psychogenic DI is seen in many psychiatric conditions but is more commonly seen in schizophrenia (Kotagiri & Kutti, 2021). See Chapter 44 for details on GSC (Box 44-6). DI is often associated with increased mortality and poor functional health outcomes in patients with severe traumatic brain injury (Gempeler et al., 2020).

Clinical Manifestations and Assessment

Without the action of ADH on the distal nephron of the kidney, a patient with ADH likely will have an enormous daily output of very dilute urine (3 to 20 L) with nocturia, frequency, and a specific gravity of 1.001 to 1.005. Signs and symptoms of fluid volume deficit that occur as patients are unable to compensate for the massive urinary loss include:

- Weight loss
- Poor skin turgor
- Dry mucous membranes
- Increased heart rate
- Hypotension

Due to intense thirst, the patient tends to drink 2 to 20 L of fluid daily and often prefers cold water. The onset of DI may be abrupt or insidious. The disease cannot be controlled by limiting fluid intake because the high-volume loss of urine continues even without fluid replacement. Fluid restriction can cause the patient to experience an insatiable craving for fluid and to develop hypernatremia and severe dehydration.

To diagnose DI, an accurate 24-hour urine collection is obtained to measure for volume and creatinine. A urine volume of less than 2 L/24 hours (without hypernatremia) rules out DI.

If central DI is suspected, a *vasopressin challenge test* may be used (Box 30-2). Desmopressin (DDAVP; desamino-arginine vasopressin) is administered intranasally, subcutaneously, or intravenously (IV) with subsequent measurement of urine volume, specific gravity, and/or urine osmolality. If DI is secondary to central or neurogenic DI, administration of ADH results in an elevation of urine osmolality by more than 50%. However, if the etiology is nephrogenic, there is a small or no increase in urine osmolality as the kidneys are not responsive to ADH. In addition, levels of serum plasma are obtained to screen for DM (glucose), dehydration and azotemia (urea nitrogen), hypercalcemia (calcium), hypokalemia (potassium), and hyperuricemia (uric acid).

BOX 30-2

Vasopressin Challenge Test

1. Typically vasopressin test is performed in the morning with the patient having fasted.
2. An IV line has to be inserted to facilitate delivery of medications.
3. Blood samples are obtained to measure serum corticotropin (ACTH) and serum cortisol.
4. The vasopressin test involves administration of intramuscular arginine-vasopressin (AVP; 10 pressor units) or intravenous desmopressin (10 mcg).
5. Before administration of vasopressin, blood samples are obtained 15 minutes before, immediately before, and then afterward at the following intervals: 15, 30, 45, 60, 90, and 120 minutes.

Data from Lacroix, A., & Raff, H. (2013). Vasopressin and desmopressin simulation test. *UpToDate*. http://www.uptodate.com/contents/vasopressin-and-desmopressin-stimulation-test.

Other diagnostic procedures include concurrent measurements of plasma levels of ADH and plasma and urine osmolality. Table 30-2 summarizes laboratory findings. A fluid deprivation test may be considered, but it is contraindicated if the patient's serum sodium is elevated. This test involves withholding fluids for 8 to 12 hours or until 3% to 5% of the body weight is lost, and plasma and urine osmolality studies are performed at the beginning and end of the test. DI is likely if the patient continues to excrete large volumes of urine with low specific gravity and osmolality or experiences weight loss, increasing serum osmolality, and elevated levels of serum sodium. During the deprivation test, ADH or vasopressin can be given subcutaneously as described previously. However, the patient's condition needs to be monitored frequently due to the risk of severe dehydration. The test will be terminated if the patient develops tachycardia, excessive weight loss, or hypotension.

Once the diagnosis is confirmed but the cause (e.g., head injury) is unclear, the patient will be assessed further for presence of tumors that may be causing the disorder.

Pearls for Practice: Pathophysiology

ADH is also known as vasopressin or by its chemical name, arginine vasopressin or AVP. When ADH activity is present, small volumes of concentrated urine are excreted; whereas if ADH is absent, large amounts of diluted urine are excreted. Increased ADH is associated with SIADH, while decreased levels are associated with DI (central). Normal levels are below 2.5 pg/mL or below 2.3 pmol/L (Fischbach et al., 2022).

TABLE **30-2 Laboratory Tests for Diabetes Insipidus**

Test	Normal Values	Critical Values	Nursing Implications
Serum osmolality Urine osmolality Urine specific gravity	288–291 mOsm/Kg 700–1,400 mOsm/Kg At least 1.015	Over 295 mOsm/kg Under 200 mOsm/kg 1.001–1.005	Patients will not be given fluid for 4–18 hours. The nurse will measure hourly urine osmolality, urine specific gravity, and patient weight. If patient loses at least 3% of body weight, the nurse will measure serum osmolality.
Plasma sodium	135–145 mEq/L	Over 145 mEq/L	Patient will be monitored for hypernatremia due to hypothalamic lesions, which cause impaired osmotic regulation but intact volume regulation of ADH secretion.
Serum ADH levels	1.3–4.1 pg/mL (values may vary slightly among different laboratories)	Look for low serum ADH levels in diabetes insipidus; e.g., in central diabetes insipidus, look for values below 1.1 pg/mL. High serum ADH levels are seen in nephrogenic diabetes insipidus.	If three successive hourly tests of urine osmolality indicate no change, administer 5 units of vasopressin and measure urine osmolality 1 hour later. Serum ADH is used to determine type of diabetes insipidus; e.g., primary diabetes insipidus ranges from 3 to 7.5 pg/mL, and nephrogenic diabetes insipidus ranges from 12 to 13 pg/mL. The nurse should be aware that serum ADH levels are always interpreted relative to serum osmolality.

Adapted from Williamson, M. A., & Snyder, L. M. (2015). *Wallach's interpretation of diagnostic tests*. Lippincott Williams & Wilkins.

Medical Management

The objectives of medical therapy are to replace ADH (which is usually a long-term therapeutic program), to ensure adequate fluid replacement, and to identify and correct the underlying intracranial pathology.

Desmopressin/DDAVP, a synthetic vasopressin, is used to control fluid balance and prevent dehydration. Desmopressin does not have the vascular effects of natural ADH. Thus, it is particularly valuable due to its longer duration of action and fewer adverse effects compared to other preparations previously used to treat the disease. Desmopressin can be administered orally as tablets or intranasally using a metered-dose nasal inhaler or a calibrated rhinal tube (intranasal). Usually one or two administrations daily (every 12 to 24 hours) are needed to control the symptoms, and the dose is then individualized according to the response. However, sometimes nasal decompression can cause rhinitis or conjunctivitis (Fitzgerald, 2022).

Other medications used to treat patients with DI include intramuscular administration of vasopressin, chlorpropamide, thiazide diuretics (potentiate the action of vasopressin), and/or prostaglandin inhibitors (e.g., ibuprofen, indomethacin, and aspirin). Intramuscular administration of ADH, vasopressin tannate in oil, is used if the intranasal route is not possible. The medication is administered every 24 to 96 hours. The vial of medication should be warmed or shaken vigorously before administration. The injection is administered in the evening so that maximum results are obtained during sleep. Abdominal cramps are a side effect of this medication. Rotation of injection sites is necessary to prevent lipodystrophy. The patient receiving chlorpropamide should be warned of the possibility of hypoglycemic reactions. If the DI is renal in origin, the previously described treatments are ineffective. Thiazide diuretics, mild salt depletion, and prostaglandin inhibitors (ibuprofen, indomethacin, and aspirin) are used to treat the nephrogenic form of DI. While there is no effective treatment for psychogenic DI, antipsychotics with high affinity to dopamine D_2 receptors may lead to a higher risk of polydipsia, and clozapine may be an effective treatment for polydipsia (Kirino et al., 2020). Sometimes the only help for these patients is to prevent water intoxication by limiting fluid intake, including antipsychotic medications, and using behavioral and psychosocial interventions to reduce symptoms of polydipsia (Havens et al., 2022).

Nursing Management

The nursing management of the patient with DI includes maintaining adequate fluid volume, monitoring the patient's weight, administering vasopressin, monitoring vital signs, and monitoring the patient's intake and output. Due to vasoconstrictive properties, vasopressin should be avoided in patients with pre-existing coronary artery disease (CAD) or vascular disease. The patient with possible DI needs support while undergoing studies for a possible cranial lesion. Prior to discharge, the nurse informs the patient and family about follow-up care and emergency measures, provides specific verbal and written instructions, demonstrates how to administer the medications, and observes return demonstrations as appropriate. The nurse should provide instructions on measuring daily weights to determine how much body fluid has been gained or lost. This information will allow the provider to titrate the dosage of vasopressin accordingly to avoid doses that are too high or too low. High doses of vasopressin will lead to fluid retention and weight gain. On the other hand, insufficient or low doses of vasopressin will lead to excess urine production (polyuria) and weight loss. In addition, the nurse should advise the patient to wear a medical identification bracelet and to carry medication and information about this disorder at all times.

SYNDROME OF INAPPROPRIATE ANTIDIURETIC HORMONE (SIADH)

SIADH is a syndrome characterized by excessive secretion of ADH, causing significant retention of water. As a result, the sodium level becomes dilute, and hyponatremia ensues. It is the most frequently cited cause of euvolemic hyponatremia. Almost 14% of hospitalized patients have hyponatremia, and nearly 50% can be attributed to SIADH (Farber & Yee, 2022). Table 30-3 details the characteristics of DI versus SIADH.

Pathophysiology

SIADH is a disorder of impaired water excretion caused by the inability to stop the secretion of ADH. As a result, excessive ADH can be secreted from the posterior pituitary gland directly into the bloodstream or by abnormal synthesis and secretion of vasopressin by tumors. Patients with this disorder cannot excrete diluted urine. They retain water and develop a subsequent sodium deficiency known as **dilutional hyponatremia**. With too much H_2O in the bloodstream, the kidneys cannot excrete dilute urine, and the water moves from the extracellular compartment to the intracellular region, causing brain cells to swell. This has a significant impact on the CNS (brain and spinal cord) because of brain edema and increased ICP. If the sodium level becomes low enough (approximately 115 mEq/L), seizures may occur.

Risk Factors

SIADH is often of nonendocrine origin. The established risk factors and potential causes of SIADH include age 60 years and older, biologic females, lower body weight and lower volume of distribution (which exacerbates the impact of ADH dysregulation and decreased glomerular filtration rate), history of hyponatremia, polypharmacy, and medical comorbidity (Pinkhasov et al., 2021). The syndrome may also occur in patients with malignancies, pulmonary disorders, disorders of the nervous system, and medication use. Carcinomas (lung, GI tract [stomach, duodenum, pancreas], GU tract [ureter, bladder, prostate, endometrium], and lymphoma) that synthesize and release ADH can lead to SIADH. SIADH has occurred in patients with pulmonary disease, such as advanced tuberculosis, severe pneumonia, positive-pressure ventilation, and other disorders of the lungs (Noris & Tuan, 2020). Disorders of the CNS, such as head injury, brain surgery or tumor, vascular (stroke, subdural hematoma, subarachnoid hemorrhage), and infection (brain abscess, meningitis, encephalitis), can produce SIADH by direct stimulation of the pituitary gland. HIV infection associated with the development of SIADH may be related to an underlying pulmonary infection (*Pneumocystis jirovecii* [formerly called *Pneumocystitis carinii*]) or symptomatic infection of the CNS or malignancy (Sterns, 2022a). Medications, such as vincristine, phenothiazines, tricyclic antidepressants (SSRIs, tricyclic, MAOI), thiazide diuretics, anticonvulsants, antidiabetic drugs, and nicotine, can cause SIADH, either by directly stimulating the pituitary gland or by increasing the sensitivity of renal tubules to circulating ADH.

TABLE **30-3 Differentiating Features of DI Versus SIADH**

Value	Diabetes Insipidus	SIADH
ADH	⇓	⇑
Serum sodium (Na)	⇑	⇓
Urine output	⇑ urine output	⇓ urine output
Urine osmolality	⇓ (for what would be expected)	⇑ (for what would be expected)
Specific gravity	⇓ <1.005	⇑ >1.030

Clinical Manifestations and Assessment

The clinical manifestations of SIADH include the following:

- Hyponatremia (serum sodium below 135 mEq/L)
- Decreased serum osmolality (less than 275 mOsm/kg) with inappropriately increased urine osmolality (greater than 100 mOsm/kg—reveals impaired ability of the kidneys to dilute the urine)
- Urine sodium over 40 mEq/L (with normal dietary salt intake; Faber & Yee, 2022; Yasir & Mechanic, 2022)

Pearls for Practice

In SIADH, there is increased renal reabsorption of water, causing serum hyponatremia (sodium <135 mEq/L). The urine is concentrated due to the water reabsorption; thus, the urine sodium may be elevated (greater than 40 mEq/L), matching with the concentrated urine output of SIADH. However, the nurse is aware that the use of diuretics negates the reliability of the urine sodium as well as urine osmolality levels, if obtained. The nurse recognizes that serum hyponatremia with a decreased urine output and urine sodium of ~≥40 mEq/L (certainly a U_{Na^+} >20 mEq/L) in the clinical setting of head trauma, pulmonary disease, etc. are consistent with SIADH (Winter & Harris, 2021).

Obtain a detailed history to rule out other causes of hyponatremia, such as heart failure, adrenal insufficiency, and kidney failure. On assessment, patients usually present with normal vital signs, moist mucous membranes, normal skin turgor, and no edema. The reabsorbed water tends to be intracellular rather than interstitial, and, therefore, patients appear euvolemic (normal volume). Patients with SIADH resulting in severe hyponatremia often exhibit more acute symptoms, such as confusion, lethargy, weakness, myoclonus, asterixis, depressed reflexes, generalized seizures, and coma related to ensuing cerebral edema.

Medical Management

Medical management includes identifying and eliminating the underlying cause. Brain and chest imaging may be obtained to identify a potential etiology, such as CNS or lung pathology. Laboratory testing is performed to rule out other cause of hyponatremia, such as infection (white blood cell [WBC] count) or dysfunction of a number of systems: thyroid (thyroid-stimulating hormone [TSH] level), adrenal (cortisol), cardiac (ECG, echocardiogram, brain natriuretic peptide [BNP]), liver (liver function tests), and kidney (BUN and serum creatinine). Elevated plasma arginine vasopressin (AVP) level is expected. Treatment will depend on the speed of onset of the hyponatremia and the clinical presentation. In asymptomatic patients, fluid restriction is the treatment of choice (less than 800 mL water per day), whereas in acutely symptomatic patients (profound hyponatremia is present with Na below 120 mEq/L), an IV of 3% sodium chloride (hypertonic saline) will be infused slowly via a central line or a peripherally inserted central catheter (PICC), and IV pump. You are aware that a chest x-ray is required to confirm placement of the central or PICC line before use (Kang et al., 2021). Diuretics, such as furosemide (Lasix) IV, will prevent extracellular fluid volume expansion by causing diuresis. Because retained water is excreted slowly through the kidneys, the extracellular fluid volume contracts and the serum sodium concentration gradually increases toward normal. It is important not to correct the sodium level too rapidly; the rate of correction aims to increase the serum sodium 8 mEq/L during the first 24 hours since rapid correction can cause demyelination (osmotic demyelination syndrome [ODS], formerly referred to as central pontine myelinolysis [CPM]) and damage to the CNS (Kheetan et al., 2021; Sterns, 2022b). See Chapter 3 Pearls for Practice on page 72 for details on ODS.

Nursing Management

Nursing management includes close monitoring of fluid intake and output (fluid restriction is a mainstay of therapy in most patients with SIADH, with a suggested goal intake of less than 800 mL/day), daily weight, urine and blood chemistries, and neurologic status. The sodium level will be evaluated at regular intervals—typically every 4 to 6 hours with any active treatment—until the sodium level stabilizes. The nurse assesses for neurologic signs caused by hyponatremia, such as confusion, seizures, and delirium as well as cardiopulmonary status (hypervolemia, including HTN, pulmonary crackles, pleural effusions, tachypnea, decreased O_2 saturation, ascites, JVD, and peripheral edema). If ordered, the nurse carefully monitors hypertonic saline administration because a complication of overaggressive treatment with 3% saline is ODS (Box 30-3). Providing supportive measures and explanations of procedures helps the patient with this disorder.

> BOX 30-3 **Focus on Pathophysiology**
>
> **Osmotic Demyelination Syndrome (ODS) or Central Pontine Myelinolysis (CPM)**
>
> ODS or CPM is a serious complication that develops after aggressive treatment of hyponatremia. The rapid rise in serum sodium with resultant change in serum osmolality causes water to be pulled from the brain cells. The changes in the brain cell volume (shift in water out of brain cells) cause injury to the myelin sheath (myelin sheath protects the nerves). These changes can result in significant neurologic morbidity and mortality. The most common presentation is a decreased level of consciousness.

Pearls for Practice

As appropriate, use seizure precautions to protect the patient from injury and prevent aspiration. Keep oxygen and suctioning equipment at the bedside. See Box 45-2 on page 1444 for details on seizure precautions. In the event of a seizure, lower the head of the bed (remove eyeglasses if applicable) and place the patient on their side to prevent aspiration and protect the airway.

DISORDERS OF THE THYROID GLAND

The thyroid gland lies in the anterior neck, below the larynx and next to and around to the trachea; it controls cellular metabolic activity. As a reminder, the hypothalamus secretes thyrotropin-releasing hormone (TRH) that stimulates the anterior pituitary gland to produce thyroid-stimulating hormone (TSH). The TSH stimulates the thyroid gland to produce and secrete the thyroid hormones: triiodothyronine or T3 (smaller amount ~20%) and thyroxine or T4 (greater amount ~80%; Pirahanchi et al., 2022). T_4 is rapidly transformed into T_3, the more active form of thyroid hormone (Carroll & Schoenl, 2020). Levels of T3 and T4 exert negative feedback on the production of TRH and TSH. That is, the higher the levels of T3 and T4, the less stimulation of TRH and TSH. In contrast, low levels of thyroid hormone (T3 and T4) increase TRH and TSH. Iodine is essential for thyroid hormone production. T3 has three iodine molecules and T4 has four. Refer to Box 30-4 for symptoms of undersecretion (hypothyroidism) and oversecretion (hyperthyroidism).

BOX 30-4 **Focused Assessment**

Hyperthyroidism Versus Hypothyroidism

Be alert for the following signs and symptoms of hyperthyroidism:

- Weight loss
- Warm, moist, flushed skin
- Tremors, emotionally hyperexcitable
- Tachycardia, irregular pulse
- Heat intolerance, hyperthermia
- Increased GI function
- Thinning of hair
- Exophthalmos (visual protrusion of the eye), corneal ulcerations
- Patients may have a staring gaze, a rim of sclera visible between the upper eyelid and the superior margin of the iris during downward gaze (lid lag)
- Systolic murmur, thrill, bruit

Be alert for the following signs and symptoms of hypothyroidism:

- Weight gain
- Dry skin, nonpitting edema
- Fatigue, mental and physical sluggishness
- Bradycardia
- Cold intolerance
- Constipation
- Coarse hair, loss of eyebrows
- Carpal tunnel syndrome
- Pleural and pericardial effusions

HYPOTHYROIDISM

Hypothyroidism results from insufficient levels of thyroid hormone. Thyroid deficiency can affect all body functions, and symptoms range from mild, subclinical forms to myxedema coma, a life-threatening hypothyroidism.

Often patients with hypothyroidism may have *primary* or *thyroidal hypothyroidism*, which refers to dysfunction of the thyroid gland itself. If the cause of the thyroid dysfunction is failure of the pituitary gland, the hypothalamus, or both, then the hypothyroidism is known as *central hypothyroidism.* If the cause is entirely a pituitary disorder, then it may be referred to as *pituitary* or *secondary hypothyroidism.* If the cause is a disorder of the hypothalamus resulting in inadequate secretion of TSH due to decreased stimulation by TRH, then it is referred to as *hypothalamic* or *tertiary hypothyroidism.* If thyroid deficiency is present at birth, then the hypothyroidism is known as *congenital hypothyroidism.* In such instances, the birthing parent also may have thyroid deficiency. In North America, because of iodine supplementation, iodine deficiency is rare; however, a deficiency of iodine can be the cause of hypothyroidism where dietary iodine is insufficient (Carroll & Schoenl, 2020). See Figure 30-3 and Table 30-4.

TABLE **30-4 Varieties of Hypothyroidism and Their Causes**

Name	Cause
Primary or *thyroidal hypothyroidism*	Dysfunction of the thyroid gland itself
Central hypothyroidism	Failure of the pituitary gland, the hypothalamus, or both
Pituitary or secondary hypothyroidism	A pituitary disorder
Hypothalamic or tertiary hypothyroidism	Disorder of the hypothalamus resulting in inadequate secretion of TSH due to decreased stimulation by TRH
Congenital hypothyroidism	Thyroid deficiency present at birth, the birthing parent also may have thyroid deficiency

Pathophysiology

In hypothyroidism, the decreased production of thyroxine (T_4) leads to the stimulation of TSH in the anterior pituitary

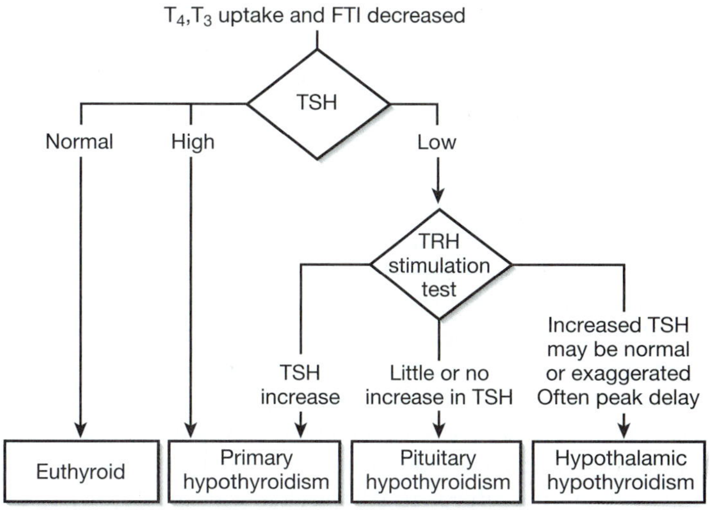

FIGURE 30-3 Algorithm for diagnosis of hypothyroidism. The sensitive thyroid-stimulating hormone (TSH) test is the preferred primary screening test for thyroid disease. Low TSH obviates the need for the thyroid-releasing hormone (TRH) test in most patients. T_4, thyroxine; T_3, triiodothyronine; FTI, free thyroxine index. (From Talreia, D. T., Talreia, R. R., & Talreia, R. S. [2005]. ***Internal medicine peripheral brain*****. Lippincott Williams & Wilkins.)**

gland. Subsequently, TSH stimulates the secretion of triiodothyronine (T_3) to increase production of T_4, leading to hypertrophy of the thyroid gland. Laboratory findings include decreased T_3 and T_4 and an increased TSH.

Pearls for Practice

In clinical practice, you will see TSH and free T4 are monitored to assess for thyroid disease. Why not T3, you may ask? The rationale is that serum T_3 level remains within the general reference range until severe stages of hypothyroidism, and it is the last to be depleted. Therefore, it is unlikely to be helpful in the diagnosis of most cases (Clinical Overview, 2021). Free T4 (vs. bound T4, which is unavailable as it is already bound to proteins) is the reservoir for T3 conversion (the active worker of the thyroid hormones), so T4 levels are critical for proper thyroid function. It is the "free" T4 or T3 or unbound that can enter and affect the body tissues. In addition, the half-life of T4 is 7–10 days compared to hours only for T3; thus, "free" T4 is frequently measured for thyroid function.

Risk Factors

The most common cause of hypothyroidism in adults is autoimmune thyroiditis (**Hashimoto disease**), in which the immune system attacks the thyroid gland. Hypothyroidism can occur in patients with previous hyperthyroidism treated with radioiodine or antithyroid medications or **thyroidectomy**. There is an increased incidence of hypothyroidism in patients who have undergone radiation therapy for head and neck cancer. Therefore, thyroid function tests are recommended for all patients who receive such treatment.

Hypothyroidism has been shown to affect females five times more frequently than males and occurs most often in people between 30 and 60 years of age. Despite females being more likely to suffer from thyroid disease, females were significantly less likely to be screened compared to males (odds ratio: 1.38, 95% CI: 0.74–2.6) (Stoll, 2019). In contrast, findings from the NHANES 2007 to 2012 survey showed that inadequate treatment of hypothyroidism was associated with being biologic male, younger age, Hispanic ethnicity, and lack of health care access (Ettleson et al., 2021). In addition, longstanding mild-to-moderate hypothyroidism often is seen in the older population. The explanation for the higher prevalence of hypothyroidism among older people may be related to alterations in immune function with age. Subclinical disease is common among older females and can be asymptomatic or mistaken for other medical conditions. For instance, subtle symptoms of hypothyroidism, such as fatigue, muscle aches, and mental confusion, may be attributed to the normal aging process by the patient, family, and health care provider. Hence, screening of TSH levels over a 3- to 6-month interval is recommended for nonpregnant adults to confirm or rule out abnormal findings before making a diagnosis or considering any treatment strategies (U.S. Preventive Task Force [USPSTF], 2015). Racial disparities observed in thyroid screening rates reveal that being White was associated with three times greater odds of receiving thyroid screening than underrepresented groups (Stoll, 2019). Gerontologic considerations are discussed in Box 30-5.

Clinical Manifestations and Assessment

Clinical manifestations of hypothyroidism are divided into early and late symptoms and represent slowing of the metabolic process. The early symptoms of hypothyroidism are nonspecific and can range from fatigue to somnolence, loss of libido to amenorrhea, apathy to mental and physical sluggishness, and nonpitting edema to pleural and pericardial effusions. Reports of hair loss, brittle nails, and dry skin are

BOX 30-5 Highlighting Gerontology

Hypothyroidism

The older population often presents with atypical signs and symptoms of hypothyroidism. For instance, the older patient may have few or no symptoms until the dysfunction is severe. Depression, apathy, and decreased mobility are major initial symptoms that may be accompanied by significant weight gain despite a poor appetite. In addition, constipation is common and affects one fourth of older patients with hypothyroidism. In the older patient with mild-to-moderate hypothyroidism, thyroid hormone replacement must be started with low dosages and increased gradually to prevent serious cardiovascular and neurologic side effects. (Remember "start low and go slow.") In general, thyroid replacement begins at one fourth to one half the expected dose and is increased in small increments no less than 4 to 6 weeks apart. Angina may occur with rapid thyroid replacement in the presence of coronary artery disease secondary to the hypothyroid state or pre-existing atherosclerosis. Heart failure and tachyarrhythmias may worsen during the transition from the hypothyroid state to the normal metabolic state. Dementia may become more apparent during early replacement of thyroid hormone in the older patient.

Older patients with severe hypothyroidism and atherosclerosis may become confused and agitated if their metabolic rate is increased too quickly. Marked clinical improvement follows the administration of hormone replacement; such medication must be continued for life. The older patient requires periodic follow-up monitoring of levels of serum TSH. In addition, older people should be reminded that failure to adhere to current therapy may lead to complications. A careful history can identify the need for further teaching about the importance of safe medication administration.

Complications, such as myxedema and myxedema coma, usually occur exclusively in patients older than 50 years of age. The high mortality rate of myxedema coma mandates immediate IV administration of thyroid hormone as well as supportive care and monitoring for cardiac complications, particularly in patients with ischemic heart disease.

common. The patient frequently complains of constipation. Paresthesia (numbness and tingling of the fingers) and nerve entrapment syndrome have been linked with endocrine disorders, such as hypothyroidism, but the etiology is poorly understood. Also, hearing loss may occur.

Late symptoms include slow speech, subdued emotional responses, apathy, absence of sweating, cold intolerance, constipation, thickening of skin (due to accumulation of mucopolysaccharides in subcutaneous tissues), dyspnea, weight gain, thinning of hair, alopecia, and deafness. On assessment, patients usually present with swelling of eyelids, pitting edema, bradycardia, hypotension, and hypothermia. Figure 30-4 illustrates clinical manifestations of hypothyroidism.

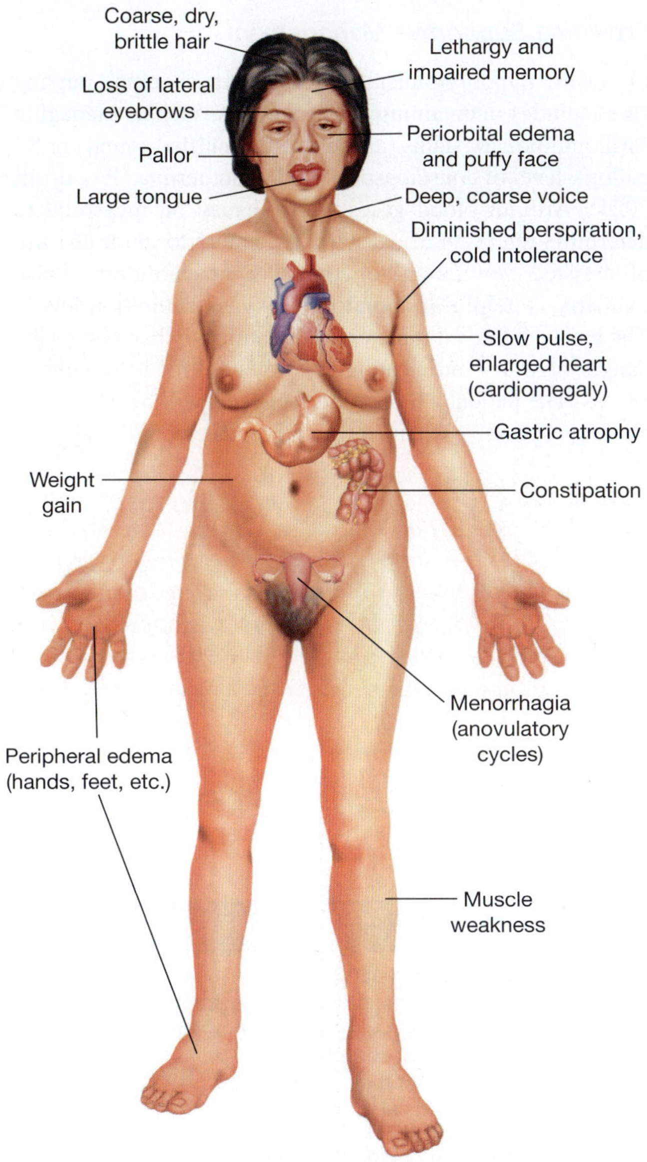

FIGURE 30-4 Dominant clinical features of hypothyroidism. (From Porth, C. M. [2015]. *Essentials of pathophysiology: Concepts of altered health states* [4th ed.]. Lippincott Williams & Wilkins.)

Advanced hypothyroidism may produce personality and cognitive changes that are characteristic of dementia. Respiratory manifestations include pleural effusion, respiratory muscle weakness, inadequate ventilation, and sleep apnea.

Severe hypothyroidism is associated with an elevated level of serum cholesterol, atherosclerosis, CAD, poor left ventricular function, and pericardial effusion. In addition, the patient with severe hypothyroidism often presents with subnormal temperature and pulse rate (bradycardia). The patient usually begins to gain weight even without an increase in food intake, although they may be cachectic. The hair thins and falls out, and the face becomes expressionless and masklike. The patient often complains of being cold, even in a warm environment.

Pearls for Practice

The patient with advanced hypothyroidism is profoundly hypothermic (91° to 95° F) and abnormally sensitive to sedatives, opioids, and anesthetic agents. Therefore, these medications are administered with extreme caution. If these medications are used, closely monitor the patient's vital signs (heart rate, blood pressure, body temperature, and respiration rate).

Myxedema coma describes the most extreme, severe stage of hypothyroidism, in which the patient is hypothermic and unconscious. Increasing lethargy may progress to stupor and then to coma. Myxedema leads to the accumulation of mucopolysaccharides in subcutaneous and other interstitial tissues; this causes nonpitting edema and doughy skin. The fluid accumulation causes a characteristic puffy appearance to the face and eyes (periorbital edema). The patient's tongue can be enlarged, and the voice becomes hoarse and husky. Sometimes myxedematous fluid that collects in the interstitial spaces can lead to mucopolysaccharide deposits in the heart that cause generalized cardiac dilation, bradycardia, and other signs of altered cardiac function (Norris & Tuan, 2020). Myxedema coma may also develop with undiagnosed hypothyroidism and may be precipitated by infection, systemic disease, or the use of sedatives or opioid analgesic agents. The patient's respiratory drive is depressed, resulting in alveolar hypoventilation, progressive carbon dioxide retention, narcosis, and coma. These symptoms, along with cardiovascular collapse and shock, require aggressive and intensive therapy if the patient is to survive. Myxedema coma is a medical emergency; even with early vigorous therapy, mortality rate is high.

Medical Management

Hormone Replacement

The primary objective in the medical management of hypothyroidism is to restore a normal metabolic state by replacing the missing hormone, levothyroxine (thyroxine; T_4).

Synthetic levothyroxine is the preferred preparation for treating hypothyroidism and suppressing nontoxic **goiters** (enlargements of the thyroid gland). The dosage for hormone replacement is based on the concentration of the patient's serum TSH. If replacement therapy is adequate, the symptoms of myxedema disappear and normal metabolic activity is resumed.

Cardiac Management

The patient who has lived with hypothyroidism for a long period of time is likely to have coronary-related diseases, such as atherosclerosis and CAD. Recall that there is elevated serum cholesterol in hypothyroidism, which is largely accounted for by an increase of LDL cholesterol, which is a risk factor for coronary heart disease. As long as metabolism is subnormal and the tissues, including the myocardium, require relatively little oxygen, a reduction in blood supply is tolerated without overt symptoms of CAD. When thyroid hormone is administered, the myocardial oxygen demand increases without increasing the myocardial oxygen supply; therefore, patients should be monitored for cardiac complications, such as chest pain and heart failure. Patients also may be treated for angina or arrhythmias due to the release of catecholamines that may be activated during thyroid replacement therapy. In the event of angina or arrhythmias, the nurse should notify the primary care provider immediately and discontinue administration of the thyroid hormone. The thyroid hormone replacement can be resumed at a later time at a lower prescribed starting dosage under the close observation of the prescribing provider and the nurse.

Nursing Management

A plan of nursing care for a patient with hypothyroidism is available online at http://thepoint.lww.com/Honan3e.

Monitoring Physical Status

The nurse closely monitors the patient's vital signs and cognitive level to detect any deterioration of physical and mental status, signs and symptoms indicating that treatment has resulted in a metabolic rate exceeding the ability of the cardiovascular and pulmonary systems to respond, and continued limitations or pleural and pericardial effusions (complications of myxedema). The normal levels of pericardial fluid are from 30 to 50 mL and pleural fluid of less than 10 to 20 mL (Norris & Tuan, 2020). Table 30-5 discusses pleural and pericardial effusions. Vital signs, thyroid levels, weight, and physical examination findings are recorded to provide baseline assessment before treatment. The nurse monitors the pulse for rate and rhythm and notifies the provider if there is a marked increase in the HR and/or tremors; anxiety; change in appetite, bowel movements, weight, and/or sleep pattern, or physical examination findings when treatment is initiated (Kizior & Hodgson, 2022).

Providing Supportive Management

In severe hypothyroidism and myxedema coma, nursing care includes maintaining vital functions, such as managing cardiopulmonary status (auscultate for muffled sounds or S3 gallop), level of consciousness, and hypothermia (Woodruff, 2021). Arterial blood gases (ABGs) may be measured to determine retention of carbon dioxide and to guide the use of assisted ventilation to combat hypoventilation. Pulse oximetry is helpful in monitoring oxygen saturation levels. The nurse should administer fluids cautiously because of the danger of water intoxication and potential for fluid volume excess. The patient's blood glucose levels will be monitored closely, especially when on thyroid replacement therapy.

Pearls for Practice

Hypoglycemia may be seen with hypothyroidism. The etiology of this finding is associated with a sluggish liver, increasing the patient's susceptibility to low blood sugar. Hyponatremia is present in approximately 50% of patients with myxedema coma, and it is thought to be associated with impairment of free water excretion by the kidneys due to inappropriate excess vasopressin secretion, excess ADH release, or renal impairment (Ross, 2021).

TABLE **30-5 Pericardial and Pleural Effusion**

Effusion	Description	Assessment Findings
Pericardial effusion	When fluid accumulates in the pericardium, the intrapericardial pressure increases around the heart, causing a cardiac tamponade. As a result, the ventricles are unable to fill properly, leading to a low stroke volume.	Beck triad: When pericardial effusion increases significantly enough to impair cardiac function, a cardiac tamponade develops (the three **D's**): • **D**istant heart sounds • **D**istention of the jugular veins • **D**ecreased cardiac output
Pleural effusion	Fluid accumulates in the pleural space, causing symptoms of dyspnea, nonproductive cough, and pleuritic chest pain.	The three **D's** of pleural effusion: • **D**ull to percussion on affected side • **D**ecreased breath sounds on affected side • **D**ecreased respiratory excursion on affected side

Pearls for Practice

If hypoglycemia is evident, concentrated glucose may be prescribed to provide glucose without precipitating fluid overload. Oral antidiabetic agents or insulin may be administered to reduce the effect of hyperglycemia that results from thyroid replacement therapy.

Preventing Medication Interactions

The nurse should take precautions during the course of therapy because of the interaction of thyroid hormones with other medications. Thyroid hormones may increase blood glucose levels, which may necessitate adjustment in the dosage of insulin or oral antidiabetic agents in patients with diabetes. The effects of thyroid hormone may be increased by phenytoin and by tricyclic antidepressant agents. Thyroid hormones also may increase the pharmacologic effects of digitalis glycosides, anticoagulant agents, and indomethacin, necessitating careful observation and assessment by the nurse for side effects. Also bone loss and osteoporosis may occur with thyroid therapy.

Even in small doses, hypnotic and sedative agents may induce profound somnolence, lasting far longer than anticipated. Furthermore, they are likely to cause respiratory depression, which can easily be fatal because of decreased respiratory reserve and alveolar hypoventilation. If their use is necessary, the dose should be one half or one third of that ordinarily prescribed in patients of similar age and weight with normal thyroid function. If these medications must be used, the patient must be monitored closely for signs of impending narcosis (stupor-like condition) or respiratory failure.

Pearls for Practice

To help absorption, levothyroxine should be taken on an empty stomach (30 to 45 minutes before breakfast), if possible, to maximize absorption and reduce insomnia if taken at night (Carroll & Schoenl, 2020). In addition, proton pump inhibitors (PPIs) and elemental supplements such as calcium and ferrous sulfate affect the absorption of levothyroxine, so it is prudent to ask patients to separate administration by several hours (Surks, 2021). Finally, a consistent formulation or brand of levothyroxine is important as there are slight variations in the dose of the generic formulations, which can have a clinical impact in very sensitive hypothyroid patients; if a switch occurs by the pharmacy and the patient is concerned, a TSH level may be obtained 4–6 weeks later to ensure TSH levels remain within therapeutic range (Carroll & Schoenl, 2020).

Encouraging Mobility

Encouraging participation in activities within established tolerance can help prevent complications of immobility. The patient with hypothyroidism experiences decreased energy and moderate-to-severe lethargy. As a result, the risk of complications from immobility increases. The patient's ability to exercise and to participate in activities is further limited by the changes in cardiovascular and pulmonary status that occur secondary to hypothyroidism. The nurse assists the patient with care and hygiene while encouraging the patient to participate within their ability.

Promoting Comfort and Safety

The patient often experiences chilling and extreme intolerance to cold, even if the room feels comfortable or hot to others. The nurse provides extra clothing and blankets and protects the patient from drafts. Heating pads and electric blankets should be avoided because of the risk for peripheral vasodilatation, further loss of body heat, and vascular collapse. In addition, the patient is at risk of experiencing burns from these items without being aware of it because of their delayed responses and decreased mental status associated with hypothyroidism.

Enhancing Coping Mechanisms

The patient with moderate-to-severe hypothyroidism may experience severe emotional reactions to changes in appearance and body image and the frequent delay in diagnosis. The nonspecific, early symptoms may have produced negative reactions by family members and friends, who may have labeled the patient mentally unstable, uncooperative, or unwilling to participate in self-care activities. As hypothyroidism is treated successfully and symptoms subside, the patient may experience depression and guilt as a result of the progression and severity of symptoms that occurred. The nurse informs the patient and family that the symptoms and inability to recognize them are common and are part of the disorder itself. The patient and family may require assistance and counseling to deal with the emotional concerns and reactions that result.

HYPERTHYROIDISM

Hyperthyroidism is the second most prevalent endocrine disorder, after DM.

Pathophysiology

Hyperthyroidism occurs as a result of the overproduction of T_3, T_4, or both from the thyroid gland. Oversecretion of thyroid hormones (hyperthyroidism) is manifested by a greatly increased metabolic rate. Other characteristics of hyperthyroidism result from the increased response to circulating catecholamines (epinephrine and norepinephrine). Refer to Box 30-4. Usually oversecretion of thyroid hormones is associated with an enlarged thyroid gland (goiter).

Graves disease is a common cause of hyperthyroidism. It is an autoimmune disease of the thyroid gland that results in the binding of antibodies to TSH, which causes the overproduction of thyroid hormones T_3 and T_4. Females are eight times more likely to be affected with this disease than males, with an onset usually between 20 and 40 years of age (Fitzgerald, 2015). An approximately 25% prevalence rate of hyperthyroidism has been reported in adults aged 65 years and older (Diab et al., 2019). Hyperthyroidism symptoms may appear after an emotional shock, stress, or an infection, but the exact significance of these relationships is not understood. Other less common causes of hyperthyroidism include thyroiditis (inflammation of the thyroid), overmedication with synthetic thyroid hormone, and thyroid nodules. Symptoms of hyperthyroidism also may occur with the release of excessive amounts of thyroid hormone as a result of inflammation after irradiation of the thyroid or destruction of thyroid tissue by tumor.

Patients with well-developed hyperthyroidism exhibit a typical group of signs and symptoms associated with hypermetabolism similar to those produced by enhanced sympathetic nervous system activity (Norris & Tuan, 2020). The course of the disease may be mild, characterized by remissions and exacerbations, and terminating with spontaneous recovery in a few months or years. When untreated, the disease may progress relentlessly, leading to emaciation, nervousness, delirium, disorientation, and heart failure. The term **thyrotoxicosis** refers to *symptomatic* hyperthyroxinemia. While hyperthyroidism is a type of thyrotoxicosis, they are not the same. Although thyrotoxicosis can be caused by hyperthyroidism, other examples of thyrotoxicosis are associated with inflammation of the thyroid gland or ingestion of thyroid hormone. In these circumstances, there is an increased in either release of stored thyroid hormone or ingestion of exogenous hormone but not accelerated synthesis. Finally, a life-threatening complication of hyperthyroidism, in which profound hypermetabolism involves multiple systems, is called *thyrotoxic crisis* or *thyroid storm.*

Clinical Manifestations and Assessment

Patients with hyperthyroidism often present with symptoms of nervousness. Often these patients are emotionally hyperexcitable, irritable, and apprehensive. They cannot sit quietly. Cardiac complaints may include palpitations. Rapid resting pulse rates typically range between 90 and 160 beats per minute. The systolic blood pressure is elevated; and electrocardiogram (ECG) findings may reveal sinus tachycardia or atrial fibrillation. Patients tolerate heat poorly and perspire unusually freely (hyperhydrosis–excessive sweating). The skin appears flushed and feels warm, soft, and moist. Older individuals may report dry skin and diffuse pruritus. A fine tremor of the hands and tongue may be observed. Patients typically exhibit **exophthalmos** (bulging eyes associated with abnormal fluid accumulation behind the eyes), which produces a startled facial expression. Other manifestations include increased dietary intake, progressive weight loss, abnormal muscular fatigability, weakness (e.g., difficulty climbing stairs and rising from a chair), amenorrhea, decreased fertility, and changes in bowel patterns (increased peristalsis). Also, osteoporosis and fracture are associated with hyperthyroidism because of increased loss of bone minerals.

On physical assessment, the thyroid gland is enlarged, feels soft, and may pulsate; often a thrill can be palpated, and a bruit is heard over the thyroid arteries. These are signs of increased blood flow through the thyroid gland. If the thyroid becomes hypertrophied, compression may be noted on the trachea or esophagus. Assess for respiratory distress, stridor, or dysphagia. Cardiac effects on the ECG may include sinus tachycardia or arrhythmias. In addition, the physical examination may reveal increased pulse pressure and palpitations. These changes may occur due to the increased sensitivity to catecholamines or to changes in neurotransmitter turnover. Myocardial hypertrophy and heart failure may occur if the hyperthyroidism is severe and untreated. Systolic murmurs may be noted. Cardiac decompensation in the form of heart failure is common, especially in the older population; note the presence of dyspnea, crackles, peripheral edema, jugular vein distention, and the S_3 heart sound. See Box 30-6 for additional

BOX 30-6

Highlighting Gerontology

Hyperthyroidism

Hyperthyroidism is less common in the older population than hypothyroidism. Patients older than 60 years of age account for 10–15% of the cases of hyperthyroidism. Clinical manifestations may be as vague as anorexia and weight loss or isolated atrial fibrillation with an absence of ocular signs, making disorders difficult to detect. New or worsening heart failure or angina is more likely to occur in older patients than in younger patients. Patients also may report other cardiovascular symptoms and difficulty climbing stairs or rising from a chair due to muscle weakness.

Spontaneous remission of hyperthyroidism is rare in older people. Assessment of TSH levels are indicated in the older population who have unexplained physical or mental deterioration. In general, the use of radioactive iodine is recommended for treatment of thyrotoxicosis in older people unless an enlarged thyroid gland is pressing on the airway. The hypermetabolic state of thyrotoxicosis must be controlled by antithyroid medications before radioactive iodine is administered because radiation therapy may precipitate thyroid storm by increasing the release of thyroid hormones.

In general, antithyroid medications are not recommended for older patients because of the increased incidence of side effects, such as granulocytopenia, and the need for frequent monitoring. The dosage of other medications used to treat other chronic illnesses in older patients may need to be modified because of the altered rate of metabolism in hyperthyroidism. In addition, antithyroid medications are considered to be less effective in the treatment of toxic nodular goiter, the most common cause of thyrotoxicosis in the older population.

Use of beta-adrenergic blocking agents (e.g., propranolol) may be indicated to decrease the cardiovascular and neurologic signs and symptoms of thyrotoxicosis. These agents must be used cautiously in older people to minimize adverse effects on cardiac function, such as heart failure.

gerontologic considerations. Laboratory findings include a decrease in serum TSH (with primary disease), increased T_3 and T_4, and an increase in radioactive iodine uptake.

Medical Management

Appropriate treatment of hyperthyroidism depends on the underlying cause and often consists of a combination of therapies, including radioactive iodine, antithyroid agents, and surgery. Treatment of hyperthyroidism aims to reduce thyroid hyperactivity, relieve symptoms, and prevent complications. Radioactive iodine (^{131}I) is the preferred choice of treatment for Graves disease; in some cases, antithyroid medications may be needed to make the patient euthyroid in preparation for surgery (Reismann, 2021).

Radioisotope Iodine 131 (^{131}I) Therapy

The goal of radioactive iodine therapy (^{131}I) is to destroy the overactive thyroid cells. Almost all the iodine that enters and is retained in the body becomes concentrated in the thyroid gland. Therefore, the radioactive isotope of iodine becomes concentrated in the thyroid gland, where it destroys thyroid cells without jeopardizing other radiosensitive tissues. Over a period of several weeks, thyroid cells exposed to the radioactive iodine are destroyed, resulting in reduction of the hyperthyroid state and, inevitably, hypothyroidism.

The patient is instructed about what to expect with this tasteless, colorless radioiodine, which may be administered by the radiologist. About 95% of patients are cured by one dose of radioactive iodine. The additional 5% of patients require two doses; rarely is a third dose necessary. Radioactive iodine ablation initially causes an acute release of thyroid hormone from the thyroid gland and may cause an increase of symptoms. The patient is observed for signs of **thyroid storm** (Box 30-7). The use of beta-adrenergic blocking agents, such as propranolol, is helpful in controlling these symptoms. Because a higher rate of treatment failure was reported among patients taking methimazole, it is sometimes discontinued for at least 3 to 4 days before radioisotope therapy and if the therapeutic dose of radioiodine therapy is adjusted upward (Fitzgerald, 2022).

After treatment with radioactive iodine, the patient is monitored closely until a **euthyroid** (normal thyroid) state is reached. Sometimes the symptoms of hyperthyroidism can persist for months to years after radioactive iodine treatment (Fitzgerald, 2022). Close follow-up is required to evaluate thyroid function because the incidence of hypothyroidism after this form of treatment is very high. Around 80%

BOX 30-7

Thyroid Storm (Thyrotoxic Crisis, Thyrotoxicosis)

Thyroid storm (thyrotoxic crisis) is a form of severe hyperthyroidism, usually of abrupt onset. It is fatal if left untreated, but with proper treatment, the mortality rate is reduced substantially. The patient with thyroid storm or crisis is critically ill and requires astute observation and aggressive and supportive nursing care during and after the acute stage of illness.

Clinical Manifestations

Thyroid storm is characterized by:

- High fever (hyperpyrexia) above 38.5° C (101.3° F), as high as 41° C (105.8° F)
- Extreme tachycardia (more than 130 bpm), tachyarrhythmias
- Exaggerated symptoms of hyperthyroidism with disturbances of a major system—e.g., GI (weight loss, diarrhea, abdominal pain), cardiovascular (chest pain, dyspnea, palpitations), and skin (diaphoresis, heat intolerance)
- Altered neurologic or mental state, which frequently appears as marked anxiety, agitation, delirium, psychosis, somnolence, or coma

Usually life-threatening thyroid storm is precipitated by stress, such as injury, infection, thyroid and nonthyroidal surgery, tooth extraction, insulin reaction, diabetic ketoacidosis, pregnancy, digitalis intoxication, abrupt withdrawal of antithyroid medications, extreme emotional stress, or vigorous palpation of the thyroid. These factors can precipitate thyroid storm in a patient whose hyperthyroidism is partially controlled or completely untreated. Current methods of diagnosis and treatment for hyperthyroidism have greatly decreased the incidence of thyroid storm, making it uncommon today.

Management

Immediate objectives are reduction of body temperature and heart rate and prevention of vascular collapse. Measures to accomplish these objectives include:

- A hypothermia mattress or cooling blanket, a cool environment, hydrocortisone, and acetaminophen. Salicylates are not used because they displace thyroid hormone from binding proteins and worsen the hypermetabolism.
- Humidified oxygen is administered to improve tissue oxygenation and meet the high metabolic demands. ABG levels or pulse oximetry may be used to monitor respiratory status.
- IV fluids containing dextrose are administered to replace liver glycogen stores that have been decreased in the hyperthyroid patient.
- PTU or methimazole is administered to impede formation of thyroid hormone and block conversion of T_4 to T_3, the more active form of thyroid hormone.
- Hydrocortisone is prescribed to treat shock or adrenal insufficiency.
- Iodine is administered to decrease output of T_4 from the thyroid gland. For cardiac problems, such as atrial fibrillation, arrhythmias, and heart failure, sympatholytic agents may be administered. Propranolol, combined with digitalis, has been effective in reducing severe cardiac symptoms. Beta-adrenergic blockers are used with caution in patients with severe HF or bronchospasm.
- The nurse monitors for fluid overload in older people and in those with pre-existing cardiovascular disease or kidney failure.

of patients develop hypothyroidism following radioiodine therapy (Reismann, 2021). Thus, patients are informed of this possibility before treatment and require close follow-up during the first year and annually for thyroid function tests. When necessary, small doses of thyroid hormone replacement are prescribed with gradually increasing doses over a period of months (up to about 1 year) until the free T_4 and TSH levels stabilize within normal ranges.

Radioactive iodine has been used to treat toxic adenomas, multinodular goiter, and most varieties of thyrotoxicosis (rarely with permanent success); it is preferred for treating patients beyond the childbearing years who have diffuse toxic goiter. Radioiodine treatment is contraindicated during pregnancy because it crosses the blood-placental barrier and may cause fetal death, fetal hypothyroidism, fetal thyroid ablation, malformation, growth restriction, and intellectual and developmental disabilities later in life (Iijima, 2021). The guidelines by the American Thyroid Association indicated that pregnancy should be postponed for at least 6 to 12 months after treatment due to risks of radiation to the eggs within the ovaries (Alexander et al., 2017).

A major advantage of treatment with radioactive iodine is that it avoids many of the side effects associated with antithyroid medications. However, some patients and their families fear medications that are radioactive. For this reason, patients may elect to take antithyroid medications rather than radioactive iodine.

Antithyroid Drug Therapy

Antithyroid medications are summarized in Table 30-6. The objective of pharmacotherapy is to inhibit one or more stages in thyroid hormone synthesis or hormone release. Antithyroid agents block the utilization of iodine by interfering with the iodination of tyrosine and the coupling of iodotyrosines in the synthesis of thyroid hormones. This prevents the synthesis of thyroid hormone. Most commonly, propylthiouracil (PTU) or methimazole is used until the patient is euthyroid. These medications block the conversion of T_4 to T_3. T_3 is about four times more potent than T_4.

The therapeutic dose is determined on the basis of clinical criteria, including changes in pulse rate, pulse pressure, body weight, size of the goiter, and results of laboratory studies of thyroid function. Antithyroid medications do not interfere with release or activity of thyroid hormones that were formed previously. As a result, it may take several weeks until relief of symptoms occurs. At that time, the maintenance dose is established, and a gradual withdrawal of the medication over the next several months follows.

Toxic complications of antithyroid medications are relatively uncommon. Nevertheless, the importance of periodic follow-up is emphasized because of medication sensitization, such as fever, rash, urticaria, or even agranulocytosis (a marked decrease in the number of granulocytes) and thrombocytopenia (decreased platelets) may develop. With

TABLE **30-6 Pharmacologic Agents Used to Treat Hyperthyroidism**

Agent	Action	Nursing Considerations
Propylthiouracil (PTU)	Blocks synthesis of hormones (conversion of T_4 to T_3)	Monitor cardiac parameters. Observe for conversion to hypothyroidism. Must be given by mouth. Watch for rash, nausea, vomiting, agranulocytosis, lupus syndrome.
Methimazole	Blocks synthesis of thyroid hormone	More toxic than PTU Watch for rash and other symptoms as for PTU.
Sodium iodide	Suppresses release of thyroid hormone	Given 1 hour after PTU or methimazole. Watch for edema, hemorrhage, GI upset.
Potassium iodide	Suppresses release of thyroid hormone	Discontinue for rash. Watch for signs of toxic iodine levels.
Saturated solution of potassium iodide (SSKI)	Suppresses release of thyroid hormone	Mix with juice or milk. Given by straw to prevent staining of teeth.
Dexamethasone	Suppresses release of thyroid hormone	Monitor input and output. Monitor glucose. May cause hypertension, nausea, vomiting, anorexia, infection.
Beta blocker (e.g., propranolol)	Beta-adrenergic blocking agent	Monitor cardiac status. Hold for patients with bradycardia or decreased cardiac output. Use with caution in patients with heart failure.

Adapted from Morton, P. G., & Fontaine, D. K. (2013). *Essentials of critical care nursing: A holistic approach.* Wolters Kluwer Health/Lippincott Williams & Wilkins.

any sign of infection, especially pharyngitis and fever or the occurrence of mouth ulcers, the patient is advised to notify the provider immediately and undergo hematologic studies. Agranulocytosis, the most serious toxic side effect, occurs in approximately 0.5% of patients. Its incidence is higher in patients older than 40 years of age. It usually occurs within the first 3 months but may occur up to 1 year after therapy is started.

Patients taking antithyroid medications are instructed not to use decongestants for nasal stuffiness because these agents are poorly tolerated. PTU is usually the treatment of choice during the first trimester of pregnancy, with a switch to methimazole in the second trimester of pregnancy to decrease the risk of liver failure in the birthing parent (Alexander et al., 2017; Braimon & Rieke, 2021). As thyroid function improves, the dose is tapered as antithyroid medications can cross the placenta to cause fetal hypothyroidism, fetal TSH hypersecretion, and fetal goiter (Fitzgerald, 2022).

Another goal of therapy is to reduce the amount of thyroid tissue, with resulting decreased production of thyroid hormone. Occasionally thyroid hormone is administered with antithyroid medications to put the thyroid gland at rest. In this approach, hypothyroidism from excess antithyroid medication is avoided, as is stimulation of the thyroid gland by TSH. Levothyroxine sodium is the most common thyroid hormone preparation used. It takes approximately 10 days of its administration to achieve full effect. Liothyronine sodium has a more rapid onset, and its action is of short duration.

Adjunctive Therapy

Iodine or iodide compounds, once the only therapy available for patients with hyperthyroidism, are no longer used as the sole method of treatment. Such compounds decrease the release of thyroid hormones from the thyroid gland and reduce the vascularity and size of the thyroid. Compounds such as potassium iodide (KI), commonly known as Lugol Iodine solution, and saturated solution of potassium iodide (SSKI) may be used in combination with antithyroid agents or beta-adrenergic blockers to prepare the patient with hyperthyroidism for surgery. These agents reduce the activity of the thyroid hormone and the vascularity of the thyroid gland, making the surgical procedure safer. They are not intended for long-term treatment of hyperthyroidism since after a varying period of time, the beneficial effects diminish and the condition may return in its initial intensity or become more severe (Gold Standard, 2022a). Solutions of iodine and iodide compounds are more palatable in milk or fruit juice and are administered through a straw to prevent staining of the teeth. These compounds reduce the metabolic rate more rapidly than antithyroid medications, but their action does not last as long. Beta-adrenergic blocking agents are important in controlling the effects of hyperthyroidism on the sympathetic nervous system. For example, propranolol generally is used to control nervousness, tachycardia, tremor, anxiety, and heat intolerance. The patient continues taking propranolol until the free T_4 is within the normal range and the TSH level approaches normal.

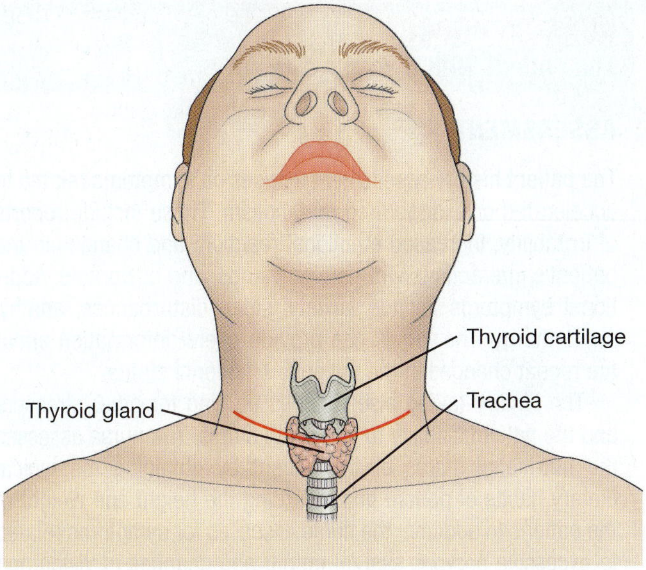

FIGURE 30-5 **Thyroidectomy incision.**

Thyroidectomy

Thyroidectomy, the surgical removal of most of the thyroid gland, was once the primary method of controlling hyperthyroidism (Fig. 30-5). The surgical removal of about five sixths of the thyroid tissue (subtotal thyroidectomy) reliably results in prolonged remission in most patients with exophthalmic goiter. Surgery for the treatment of hyperthyroidism is performed soon after the thyroid function has returned to normal (4 to 6 weeks). Preoperatively, PTU is administered until signs of hyperthyroidism have disappeared. A beta-adrenergic blocking agent (propranolol) may be used to reduce the heart rate and other signs and symptoms of hyperthyroidism; however, this does not create a euthyroid state. Iodine (Lugol Iodine solution or KI) may be prescribed in an effort to reduce blood loss; however, the effectiveness of this treatment is unknown.

Presently, the surgical option is reserved only for special circumstances, such as for patients with nodular goiters with suspicion of malignancy, obstructing goiters despite radioactive iodine and antithyroid therapy, patients who refuse radioactive iodine and cannot be adequately managed with antithyroid medication, pregnant patients inadequately managed with antithyroid medications, recurrent thyroid cysts, goiters, and patients who are allergic to or unable to take antithyroid medications (AORN, 2021; Ferri, 2022a). Surgery for the treatment of hyperthyroidism is performed soon after the thyroid function has returned to normal (4 to 6 weeks). Pre- and postoperative care of patients undergoing thyroidectomy is reviewed shortly.

NURSING PROCESS
The Patient With Hyperthyroidism

ASSESSMENT

The patient history assessment focuses on symptoms related to accelerated or exaggerated metabolism. These include reports of irritability; increased emotional reaction; and changes in the patient's interactions with family, friends, and coworkers. Additional symptoms include anxiety, sleep disturbances, apathy, and lethargy. The family can provide useful information about the recent changes in the patient's emotional status.

The history-taking also includes probing for other stressors and the patient's ability to cope with stress. The nurse assesses the nutritional status of the patient by obtaining the typical dietary habits of patient and recording the height and weight of the patient. In addition, the nurse assesses for symptoms related to excessive nervous system output and changes in vision and appearance of the eyes. Periodically, the nurse should assess and monitor the patient's cardiac status, including heart rate and rhythm, heart sounds, blood pressure, and peripheral pulses.

DIAGNOSIS

Appropriate nursing diagnoses may include:

- Malnutrition risk, related to exaggerated metabolic rate, excessive appetite, and increased gastrointestinal (GI) activity
- Coping impairment related to irritability, hyperexcitability, apprehension, and emotional instability
- Situational low self-esteem related to changes in appearance, excessive appetite, and weight loss
- Altered body temperature related to hypermetabolic status
- Discomfort related to eye changes secondary to hyperthyroidism

Potential complications may include the following:

- Thyrotoxicosis or thyroid storm
- Impaired cardiac output due to alterations in heart rate or rhythm
- Hypothyroidism

PLANNING

The goals for the patient may be improved nutritional status, improved coping ability, improved self-esteem, maintenance of normal body temperature, and absence of complications.

NURSING INTERVENTIONS

IMPROVING NUTRITIONAL STATUS

Hyperthyroidism affects all body systems, including the GI system. The appetite is increased but may be satisfied by several well-balanced meals of small size, up to six meals a day. Foods and fluids are selected to replace fluid lost through diarrhea and diaphoresis and to control the diarrhea that results from increased peristalsis. Rapid movement of food through the GI tract may result in nutritional imbalance and further weight loss. The nurse should monitor fluid and electrolytes to assess for unusual loss due to increased GI motility. To reduce diarrhea, highly seasoned foods and stimulants such as coffee, tea, cola, and alcohol are discouraged. The nurse encourages high-calorie, high-protein foods. A quiet atmosphere during mealtime may aid digestion. The nurse records weight (500 mL = 1 lb), dietary intake, and input/output (I&O) to monitor nutritional status.

ENHANCING COPING MEASURES

The patient with hyperthyroidism needs reassurance that the emotional reactions being experienced are a result of the disorder and that, with effective treatment, those symptoms will be controlled. Because of the negative effect these symptoms have on family and friends, they too need reassurance that the symptoms are expected to disappear with treatment. It is important to use a calm, unhurried approach with the patient and to minimize stressful experiences. For instance, the patient should not be placed in a room with other patients who are very ill or talkative. The nurse introduces relaxing activities, such as listening to soft music or keeps the room quiet. The nurse minimizes noises, such as loud music, conversation, and equipment alarms, as much as possible. If thyroidectomy is planned, the patient needs to know that pharmacologic therapy is necessary to prepare the thyroid gland for surgical treatment. The nurse reminds the patient to take the medications as prescribed. Because of hyperexcitability and shortened attention span, the patient may require repetition of this information and written instructions.

IMPROVING SELF-ESTEEM

The patient with hyperthyroidism is likely to experience changes in appearance, appetite, and weight. These factors, along with the patient's inability to cope well with family and the illness, may result in loss of self-esteem. The nurse must convey an understanding of the patient's concern about these problems and assist the patient in developing effective coping strategies. The patient and family need to know that these changes are a result of the thyroid dysfunction and are, in fact, out of the patient's control.

If changes in appearance are very disturbing to the patient, mirrors may be covered or removed. In addition, the nurse reminds family members and personnel to avoid bringing these changes to the patient's attention. The nurse explains to the patient and family that these physical changes are expected to disappear with effective treatment.

MAINTAINING NORMAL BODY TEMPERATURE

It is important for the patient to maintain a normal body temperature. The patient with hyperthyroidism frequently finds a normal room temperature too warm because of an exaggerated metabolic rate and increased heat production. To ensure a normal body temperature, the nurse maintains the environment at a cool, comfortable temperature and changes bedding and clothing as needed. Instructions to the patient and family emphasize that cool baths and cool or cold fluids may provide relief. However, shivering is to be avoided as it increases metabolic energy expenditure. The nurse explains the reason for the patient's discomfort and the importance of providing a cool environment to the family and staff.

PROVIDING EYE CARE

Relief of symptoms related to excessive output by the nervous system and changes in vision and appearance of the eyes is indicated when necessary. For instance, if the patient experiences eye changes secondary to hyperthyroidism, eye care, and protection may be necessary. The patient may need instructions about instillation of eye drops or ointment prescribed to soothe the eyes and protect the exposed cornea.

MONITORING AND MANAGING POTENTIAL COMPLICATIONS

Thyrotoxicosis or Thyroid Storm. The nurse closely monitors the patient with hyperthyroidism for signs and symptoms that may be indicative of thyroid storm. The nurse assesses cardiac and respiratory functions by obtaining vital signs, monitoring ECG (arrhythmias such as atrial fibrillation and tachyarrhythmia), physical examination including heart (e.g., systolic murmurs; S3 if acute heart failure [HF] develops) and lung sounds (e.g., crackles if pulmonary edema or HF develops), ABGs, and pulse oximetry. Assessment continues after treatment is initiated because of the potential effects of treatment on cardiac function. If applicable (O_2 sat <95%), oxygen is administered to prevent hypoxia, to improve tissue oxygenation, and to meet the high metabolic demands. IV fluids may be necessary to maintain levels of blood glucose and to replace lost fluids. Decrease in body temperature is achieved by use of a cooling blanket and the antipyretic agent acetaminophen. Salicylates (aspirin) are contraindicated because they displace thyroid hormone from its binding protein, increasing the level of free, metabolically active thyroid hormone (Lough, 2022). Antithyroid medications (e.g., PTU or methimazole) may be prescribed to reduce thyroid hormone levels. In addition, propranolol and digitalis may be prescribed to treat cardiac symptoms. If shock develops, treatment strategies must be implemented.

Hypothyroidism. Hypothyroidism is likely to occur with any of the treatments used for hyperthyroidism; periodically monitor the patient for signs and symptoms of hypothyroidism. In addition, as part of the teaching for the patient and family, include instructions on the importance of continuing therapy indefinitely after discharge and a discussion of the consequences of failing to take medication.

EVALUATION

Expected patient outcomes may include the following:

1. Demonstrates improvement in nutritional status:
   a. Reports adequate dietary intake and decreased hunger
   b. Identifies high-calorie, high-protein foods; identifies foods to be avoided
   c. Avoids use of alcohol and other stimulants
   d. Reports decreased episodes of diarrhea
2. Demonstrates effective coping methods in dealing with family, friends, and coworkers:
   a. Explains reasons for irritability and emotional instability
   b. Avoids stressful situations, events, and people
   c. Participates in relaxing, nonstressful activities
3. Achieves increased self-esteem:
   a. Verbalizes feelings about self and illness
   b. Describes feelings of frustration and loss of control
   c. Describes reasons for increased appetite
4. Maintains normal body temperature
5. Experiences relief of symptoms
6. Absence of complications:
   a. Has levels of serum thyroid hormone and TSH within normal limits
   b. Identifies signs and symptoms of thyroid storm and hypothyroidism
   c. Vital signs, ECG, ABGs, and pulse oximetry are within normal limits
   d. States importance of regular follow-up and lifelong maintenance of prescribed therapy

THYROIDITIS

Thyroiditis refers to the inflammation of the thyroid gland that may result in abnormalities in its functioning. The clinical classification of thyroiditis is based on the onset and duration of the disease, resulting from causes that are acute, subacute, or chronic. Thyroiditis can result in the swelling of the thyroid gland, manifesting symptoms in the form of acute and subacute thyroiditis. The chronic form of thyroiditis often presents with painless enlargement of the thyroid gland.

Pathophysiology

Acute thyroiditis is a rare disorder caused by infection of the thyroid gland by bacteria, fungi, mycobacteria, or parasites. The most common cause of acute thyroiditis is *Staphylococcus aureus* and other staphylococci. Subacute thyroiditis occurs after a viral infection, resulting in painful thyroid swelling for 2 to 3 months (Ferri, 2022a). Chronic thyroiditis occurs frequently in females between 30 and 50 years of age. It has been termed as *Hashimoto disease* or *chronic lymphocytic thyroiditis*. The diagnosis is based on the histologic appearance of the inflamed gland. Cell-mediated immunity may play a significant role in the pathogenesis of chronic thyroiditis, and there may be a genetic predisposition to it. If left untreated, the disease runs a slow, progressive course, eventually leading to hypothyroidism.

Clinical Manifestations and Assessment

In acute thyroiditis, often pharyngitis or pharyngeal pain is present. Physical examination may reveal warmth, erythema (redness), and tenderness over the thyroid gland. The condition manifests as a painful swelling in the anterior neck that lasts between 1 and 2 months and then disappears spontaneously without residual effect. It often follows a respiratory infection. The thyroid enlarges symmetrically and may be painful. The overlying skin is often red and warm. Swallowing may be difficult and uncomfortable. Irritability, nervousness, insomnia, weight loss, chills, fever, and manifestations of hyperthyroidism are common. In subacute thyroiditis the enlarged thyroid is exquisitely tender, fever is present, and signs of hyperthyroidism are present initially (as described above); however, signs of hypothyroidism can subsequently develop (Ferri, 2022b). In contrast to acute thyroiditis, the chronic forms are not accompanied by pain, pressure symptoms, or fever, and thyroid activity is normal or low rather than increased. The most common presentation in a patient suspected to have chronic thyroiditis is an enlarged, painless firm mass that is not frequently palpable over the thyroid gland. In addition, patients are likely to present with symptoms of hypothyroidism (Fitzgerald, 2022).

Medical Management

The medical management of acute thyroiditis includes antimicrobial agents and fluid replacement. Surgical incision and drainage may be needed if an abscess is present. In subacute thyroiditis, the treatment aims to control the inflammation. Nonsteroidal anti-inflammatory drugs are commonly used to relieve neck pain. Acetylsalicylic acid (aspirin) is avoided because of displacement of thyroid hormone from its binding sites resulting in increased amount of free circulating hormone. Beta-adrenergic blocking agents (e.g., propranolol) may be used to control symptoms of hyperthyroidism. Antithyroid agents that block the synthesis of T_3 and T_4 are not effective in thyroiditis because the associated thyrotoxicosis results from the release of stored thyroid hormones rather than from their increased synthesis. In more severe cases, oral corticosteroids may be prescribed to reduce swelling and relieve pain. In some cases, temporary hypothyroidism may develop and may necessitate thyroid hormone therapy.

In chronic thyroiditis, the objective of the treatment is to reduce the size of the thyroid gland and prevent hypothyroidism. Thyroid hormone therapy is prescribed to reduce thyroid activity and the production of thyroglobulin. If hypothyroid symptoms are present, thyroid hormone therapy is prescribed. Surgery may be required if pressure symptoms persist.

Nursing Management

The nursing management of patients with thyroiditis includes educating patients about their condition, specifically on pain management and the use of medications. Most patients who present with thyroiditis are given patient education on how to manage the symptoms of the disease and usually do not require in-patient admission.

THYROID TUMOR AND CANCER

Classification of tumors of the thyroid gland includes benign or malignant, presence or absence of associated thyrotoxicosis, and diffuse or irregular quality of the glandular enlargement. A goiter is present if the enlargement is sufficient to cause a visible swelling in the neck. All grades of goiter may occur, from barely visible to those producing disfigurement. The histopathology differs depending on the etiology of goiter. For instance, some are symmetric and diffuse; others are nodular. Often toxic goiters are accompanied by hyperthyroidism. Nontoxic goiters, on the other hand, are associated with a euthyroid state that does not result from an inflammatory or neoplastic cause.

Thyroid cancer is less prevalent than other forms of cancer; only about 1 in 20 thyroid nodules is cancerous. According to the American Cancer Society (2022), an estimated 43,800 new cases of thyroid cancer are diagnosed each year, 31,940 in females and 11,860 in males. About 1,160 females and 1,070 males die annually from this malignancy (American Cancer Society, 2022). The increased risk of thyroid carcinoma has been linked to modifiable risk factors such as exposure to ionizing radiation, inorganic and organic environmental contaminants (e.g., perchlorate, brominated flame retardants, and bisphenols), and abnormal iodine nutritional intake (Tang et al., 2020).

Pathophysiology

The most common type of goiter, a simple or colloid goiter, often is encountered in geographic regions where there is lack of iodine (e.g., the Great Lakes areas of the United States). If too little iodine exists, the level of T_4 will decrease, causing the stimulation of TSH from the anterior pituitary. This stimulation causes the enlargement of the thyroid. Simple goiter also may be caused by an intake of large quantities of goitrogenic substances in patients with unusually susceptible glands. These substances include excessive amounts of iodine or lithium, often used in the treatment of bipolar disorders. Too much iodine can cause enlargement of the thyroid, resulting in the development of excess secretion of thyroid hormone. Keep in mind that many patients receive IV iodine in the hospital as a result of diagnostic studies that require contrast, such as cardiac catheterization and CT scans.

Simple goiter represents a compensatory hypertrophy of the thyroid gland, caused by stimulation by the pituitary gland. Such goiters usually cause no symptoms, except for the swelling in the neck, which may result in tracheal compression when excessive. Many goiters of this type recede after the iodine imbalance is corrected. Supplementary iodine, such as SSKI, is prescribed to suppress the pituitary's thyroid-stimulating activity.

Some thyroid glands are nodular because of areas of hyperplasia (overgrowth). No symptoms may arise unless these nodules increase in size and descend into the thorax, where symptoms of local pressure may manifest. Some nodules become malignant, and some are associated with a hyperthyroid state. The patient with many thyroid nodules eventually may require surgery.

Clinical Manifestations and Assessment

Most patients with simple goiters are asymptomatic and may complain of pressure in the neck. On assessment, the patient may present with a soft, diffusely enlarged nodule over the neck. As the goiter progresses, the patient may experience symptoms, such as difficulty breathing and swallowing (dysphagia). Late symptoms also include hoarseness, cough, dysphonia (difficulty speaking), stridor, or choking sensation due to tracheal compression or vocal cord paralysis, and facial plethora (redness) due to compression of the thoracic inlet (junction between the neck and the chest through which vital structures pass) by the enlarged thyroid (Clinical Overview, 2022). Patients usually present in euthyroid state with normal levels of TSH and T_4.

On the other hand, lesions that are single, hard, and fixed on palpation or associated with cervical lymphadenopathy suggest malignancy. Although thyroid function tests may be helpful in evaluating thyroid nodules and masses, the results are rarely conclusive. Fine-needle biopsy (FNB) of the thyroid gland often is used to establish the diagnosis of thyroid cancer. The purpose of the biopsy is to differentiate cancerous thyroid nodules from noncancerous nodules and to stage the cancer if detected. The procedure is safe and usually requires only a local anesthetic. Another type of aspiration or biopsy uses a large-bore needle rather than the fine needle. This method often is used to detect rapid-growing tumors or when the results of the FNB are inconclusive. Other diagnostic studies include ultrasound, MRI, CT, thyroid scans, radioactive iodine uptake studies, and thyroid suppression tests.

Medical Management

Most patients with small, simple goiters and euthyroid states do not require treatment. Patients with large goiters generally receive exogenous thyroid hormones and iodine to reduce thyroid growth. Surgery is not required unless the goiter continues to grow (1) despite pharmacologic treatment, (2) causing airway difficulties, and (3) leading to suspected malignancy.

Surgical removal, however, is the treatment of choice for thyroid cancers. Total or near-total thyroidectomy is performed if possible. Patients whose thyroid cancer is detected early and who are appropriately treated usually do very well. Patients who have had papillary cancer, the most common (about 80% of all thyroid cancers) and least aggressive tumor, have a 10-year survival rate of 97% (Fitzgerald, 2022). Survival rates associated with follicular thyroid cancer were low (26%) in patients presenting with metastasis at the time of diagnosis compared with patients who developed metastasis during follow-up (Wu et al., 2022). Hence, continuing thyroid hormone therapy and periodic follow-up with diagnostic testing are important to ensure the patient's well-being.

A modified neck dissection or more extensive radical neck dissection is performed if there is lymph node involvement. Efforts are made to spare parathyroid tissue to reduce the risk of postoperative hypocalcemia with resultant tetany. Ablation procedures are carried out with radioactive iodine to eradicate residual thyroid tissue if the tumor is radiosensitive.

Postoperatively, the patient is instructed to take exogenous thyroid hormone to prevent hypothyroidism. If the remaining thyroid tissue is inadequate to produce sufficient thyroid hormone, thyroxine is required permanently. Free T_4, TSH, and levels of serum calcium and phosphorus are monitored to determine whether the thyroid hormone supplementation is adequate and to note whether calcium balance is maintained. Although local and systemic reactions to radiation may occur and may include neutropenia or thrombocytopenia, these complications are rare when radioactive iodine is used. The use of total thyroid surgery in combination with radioactive iodine may be considered on an individual basis rather than "one size fits all" for patients with thyroid cancer (Wang et al., 2020).

Posthospitalization follow-up includes clinical assessment for recurrence of nodules or masses in the neck and signs of hoarseness, dysphagia, or dyspnea. Total-body scans are performed 2 to 4 months after surgery to detect residual thyroid tissue or metastatic disease. Thyroid hormones are stopped for about 6 weeks before the tests. Care must be taken to avoid iodine-containing foods and contrast agents. A repeat scan is performed 1 year after the initial surgery. If measurements are stable, a final scan is obtained in 3 to 5 years.

Nursing Management

Providing Preoperative Teaching

Preoperative patient education is important to gain the patient's confidence and reduce anxiety. The nurse instructs the patient about the importance of eating a diet high in carbohydrates and proteins. A high daily caloric intake is necessary because of the increased metabolic activity and rapid depletion of glycogen reserves. Supplementary vitamins, particularly thiamine and ascorbic acid, may be prescribed. The nurse advises the patient to avoid tea, coffee, cola, and other stimulants. The nurse explains the purpose of preoperative tests and what preoperative preparations to expect. In addition, special efforts are made to ensure a good night's rest before surgery, although many patients are admitted to the hospital on the day of surgery. Preoperative teaching includes demonstrating to the patient how to support the neck with the hands after surgery to prevent stress on the incision. This involves raising the elbows and placing the hands behind the neck to provide support and reduce strain and tension on the neck muscles and the surgical incision.

Assessing the Postoperative Patient

Postoperatively, the nurse periodically assesses the surgical dressings and reinforces them if necessary. The nurse observes the sides and the back of the neck as well as the anterior dressing for bleeding. In addition to monitoring the pulse and blood pressure for any indication of internal bleeding, it is important to be alert for complaints of a sensation of pressure or fullness at the incision site, frequent swallowing, or choking. Such symptoms may indicate subcutaneous hemorrhage and hematoma formation. In addition, the nurse notes vocal changes or hoarseness, as this may indicate injury to the laryngeal nerve or laryngeal edema, which may develop postoperatively. If drains are inserted intraoperatively, the nurse records the color, amount, and consistency of the drainage and maintains function of the device.

Maintaining the Airway

Respiratory difficulties can occur as a result of edema of the glottis, hematoma formation, or injury to the recurrent laryngeal nerve. This complication requires insertion of an airway. It is vital to have a tracheostomy set by the bedside at all times because, in the event of significant edema, placement of an endotracheal tube (ETT) is unlikely because of narrowing of the airway. If the respiratory distress is caused by hematoma, a surgical evacuation is required.

Managing Pain

The nurse assesses the intensity of pain and administers analgesic agents as prescribed. The nurse should anticipate apprehension in the patient and inform the patient that oxygen will assist breathing. When moving and turning the patient, the nurse must carefully support the patient's head and avoid tension on the sutures. The most comfortable patient position is the semi-Fowler position, with the head elevated and supported by pillows.

Administering Hydration Therapy

IV fluids are administered during the immediate postoperative period. Nurses can anticipate that when PO fluids are allowed, patients report little difficulty in swallowing. Serving small amounts of cold fluids and ice is recommended.

Managing Safety

The nurse advises the patient to talk as little as possible to reduce edema to the vocal cords. Items that are needed frequently are kept within easy reach so the patient does not need to turn the head to reach for them. An overbed table provides easy access to items, such as tissues, a water pitcher and glass, and a small emesis basin. It is also convenient to use this table when vapor-mist inhalations are prescribed for the relief of excessive mucus accumulation.

Encouraging Nutrition and Physical Activity

The patient is permitted to get out of bed as soon as possible but must support their neck to reduce strain on the neck muscles. The nurse encourages the patient to eat soft foods. A well-balanced diet high in calories and protein may be prescribed to promote weight gain.

Providing Postoperative Patient Education

Patient teaching emphasizes the importance of taking prescribed medications, discusses postoperative appointment(s), describes suture removal, and provides postoperative recommendations for follow-up. Usually the patient is discharged from the hospital on the day of surgery or soon afterward if the postoperative course is uncomplicated. Also the patient who is undergoing radiation therapy is instructed in how to assess and manage side effects of treatment.

Managing Postthyroidectomy Complications

Hemorrhage, hematoma formation, edema of the glottis, and injury to the recurrent laryngeal nerve are complications discussed above. Hypoparathyroidism occurs in 4% of patients and vocal cord paralysis in 1% (Ferri, 2022b). Recall that parathyroid hormone regulates the level of calcium within the blood. Sometimes the parathyroid glands are removed during thyroid surgery, resulting in altered calcium metabolism. As the blood calcium level falls (hypocalcemia), hyperirritability of the nerves occurs, with spasms of the hands and feet and muscle twitching. This group of symptoms is termed *tetany*. Ensure adequate opening of the airway because laryngospasm, although rare, may occur and obstruct the airway. Usually tetany is treated with IV calcium gluconate. Hypocalcemia is temporary after thyroidectomy unless all parathyroid tissue was removed. See later discussion of hypocalcemia and Figure 30-7.

DISORDERS OF THE PARATHYROID GLANDS

HYPERPARATHYROIDISM

Pathophysiology

Hyperparathyroidism is characterized by having excess parathormone (PTH), leading to a markedly increased level of serum calcium that can present as a potentially life-threatening situation.

Pearls for Practice

Hypercalcemia is a total calcium concentration greater than 10.5 mg/dL; hypocalcemia is a total calcium concentration of less than 8.5 mg/dL.

The actions of PTH are increased by the presence of vitamin D. The serum level of ionized calcium regulates the

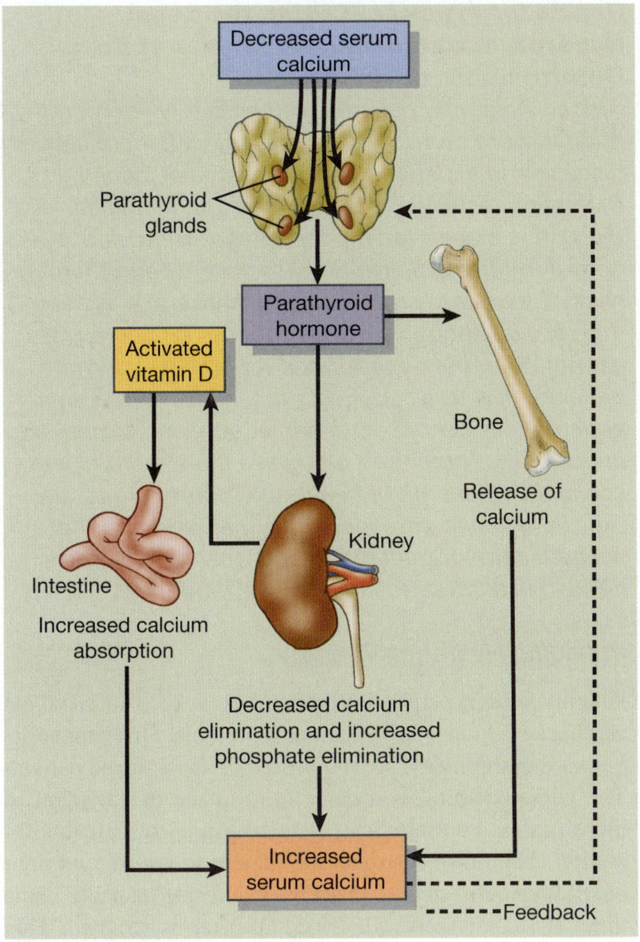

FIGURE 30-6 Regulation of serum calcium concentration by parathyroid hormone. (From Porth, C. M. [2015]. *Essentials of pathophysiology: Concepts of altered health states* [4th ed.]. Lippincott Williams & Wilkins.)

output of parathormone (Fig. 30-6). Increased serum calcium leads to a decreased secretion of parathormone, thus creating a negative feedback system. When the product of serum calcium and serum phosphorus rises, calcium phosphate may precipitate and calcify in various organs of the body, such as the kidneys.

Risk Factors

About 100,000 new cases of hyperparathyroidism are detected each year in the United States. The incidence of this disorder increases 10-fold between 15 and 65 years of age. Primary hyperparathyroidism (tumor or hyperplasia of the parathyroids) occurs three to four times more often in females than in males and is most common in people between 60 and 70 years of age, peaking in the seventh decade (Cheng, 2022). Secondary hyperparathyroidism is seen most often in patients with chronic kidney failure (Box 30-8). Primary hyperparathyroidism has the highest prevalence among African American people (Fieber et al., 2020).

BOX 30-8 **Focus on Pathophysiology**

Kidney Failure and Secondary Hyperparathyroidism

Phosphate excretion becomes impaired when kidney function deteriorates, resulting in an elevated level of serum phosphate. There is an inverse relationship between calcium and phosphorus: as the level of serum phosphate rises, the level of serum calcium falls.

This hypocalcemia stimulates PTH release with resultant increase in calcium release from the bone. In kidney failure, the kidneys' ability to synthesize vitamin D becomes impaired, which leads to decreased intestinal absorption of calcium. Hypocalcemia in this situation will stimulate the release of PTH, leading to hyperparathyroidism. The sustained elevation in parathyroid hormone (PTH) levels can cause high-turnover bone disease and fracture and can contribute to the development of calciphylaxis, where insoluble calcium phosphate crystals deposit in the soft tissues of the body (lungs, joints, heart valves, cornea, skin). See Chapter 26 for additional details on calciphylaxis.

Clinical Manifestations and Assessment

Half of the people diagnosed with hyperparathyroidism are asymptomatic. Most cases were detected by high levels of serum calcium during routine blood tests. Secondary hyperparathyroidism manifests signs and symptoms similar to those of primary hyperparathyroidism.

The patient may experience signs and symptoms resulting from involvement of several body systems; Box 30-9 summarizes symptoms of hypercalcemia. The development of symptoms varies in severity and rapidity of disease progression and reflects both the hypercalcemia and hyperparathyroid components of the disease process (Cheng, 2022). Apathy, fatigue, muscle weakness, nausea, vomiting, and constipation may occur due to the increased concentration of calcium in the blood. The direct effect of calcium on the brain and nervous system can cause psychological manifestations, such as irritability, neurosis, or psychoses. Cardiac responses to elevated serum calcium levels include HTN, increased cardiac contractility, shortened QT interval, ventricular hypertrophy, vascular stiffening, vascular and valvular calcification, and the development of ventricular arrhythmias (Silverberg & Fuleihan, 2021). It is important for the nurse to assess patients

BOX 30-9 **Focused Assessment**

Hypercalcemia

Be alert for the following signs and symptoms:

- **Stones:** Kidney
- **Bones:** Bone pain, osteoporosis, pathologic fractures
- Abdominal **Moans:** Nausea, vomiting, and abdominal pains (hypercalcemia can lead to development of peptic ulcer and acute pancreatitis)
- Psychic **Groans:** Mental irritability, neurosis, confusion

on digitalis as this drug accentuates the cardiac response of hypercalcemia.

The formation of stones in one or both kidneys, related to the increased urinary excretion of calcium and phosphorus, occurs in 55% of patients with primary hyperparathyroidism. Renal damage results from the precipitation of calcium phosphate in the renal pelvis and parenchyma, which causes renal calculi (kidney stones), obstruction, pyelonephritis, and kidney failure.

Musculoskeletal symptoms accompanying hyperparathyroidism—such as skeleton pain and tenderness, especially of the back and joints, pain on weight bearing, pathologic fractures, deformities, and shortening of body stature—may be caused by demineralization of the bones or by bone tumors composed of benign giant cells, resulting from overgrowth of osteoclasts. Oversecretion of PTH causes excessive osteoclast growth, which, in turn, promotes bone resorption. Because there is not enough calcium in the bone, the bones demineralize causing kyphosis, compression fractures, and boney cysts that cause fragile bones, increasing the risk for fracture. Hypercalcemia may stimulate gastric secretions, causing increased incidence of peptic ulcer and abdominal pain. Pancreatitis may develop as a result of stones in the pancreatic ducts.

Primary hyperparathyroidism is diagnosed by persistent elevation of serum calcium levels and an elevated concentration of PTH. **Radioimmunoassay** for PTH is sensitive and differentiates primary hyperparathyroidism from other causes of hypercalcemia in more than 90% of patients with elevated serum calcium levels. An elevated serum calcium level alone is a nonspecific finding because serum levels may be altered by diet, medications, and kidney disease and bone changes. Bone changes on x-ray or bone scans indicate advanced disease. The double-antibody parathyroid hormone test distinguishes between primary hyperparathyroidism and malignancy as a cause of hypercalcemia. Ultrasound, MRI, thallium scan, and FNB evaluate the parathyroid functions and localize parathyroid cysts, adenomas, or hyperplasia.

Medical and Nursing Management

The recommended treatment of primary hyperparathyroidism is the surgical removal of abnormal parathyroid tissue (parathyroidectomy). It is the only definitive treatment for symptomatic primary hyperparathyroidism since it can normalize calcium levels, decrease the risk for kidney stones, improve BMD, decrease fracture risk, and enhance quality-of-life (QOL) measures (Cheng, 2022). In some patients who are without symptoms and have serum calcium concentrations that are only mildly elevated and normal kidney function, surgery may be delayed, and the patient is monitored closely for worsening of hypercalcemia, bone deterioration, renal impairment, or the development of kidney stones. Nursing management involves providing hydration, encouraging mobility, administering nutrition and medications, providing emotional support, and observing for and managing hypercalcemic crisis.

Pearls for Practice: Lifting the Lens: Hyperparathyroidism and Impact of Social Determinants of Health

African American patients with primary hyperparathyroidism were more likely to present with more severe disease and experienced higher rates of incomplete evaluation resulting in delays in treatment (Fieber et al., 2021). It is disheartening, though not surprising, that persistent disparities in disease severity and thoroughness of a workup prior to surgical referral was seen in this study. Although surgical success and cure rates did not differ between African American and White patients, this study suggests that African American patients may benefit from earlier surgical referral. It is important for nurses to recognize the structural and social determinants of health that contribute to the prevalent health care inequities that exist and that we advocate for patients to access the care that is needed in a timely fashion, and without bias.

Providing Hydration Therapy

Patients with hyperparathyroidism are at risk for renal calculi because kidney involvement is possible. Strict intake and output measurements are monitored in hospitalized patients. The nurse encourages a daily fluid intake of 2,000 mL or more (unless contraindicated) to help prevent calculus formation. The nurse instructs the patient to report symptoms of renal calculi, such as sharp back and side pain and hematuria. If kidney stones develop, all urine is strained. Thiazide diuretics are avoided because they decrease the renal excretion of calcium and further elevate levels of serum calcium. Because of the risk for hypercalcemic crisis, the nurse should instruct the patient to avoid dehydration and to seek immediate attention if conditions that commonly produce dehydration (e.g., vomiting and diarrhea) occur.

Encouraging Mobility

The nurse encourages the patient to ambulate using a walker. For those with limited mobility, use a rocking chair because bones that are subjected to normal stress give up less calcium. Bedrest increases calcium excretion and the risk for renal calculi. Oral phosphates lower the serum calcium level in some patients; however, long-term use is not recommended due to the risk of ectopic calcium phosphate deposition into the soft tissues.

Administering Nutrition and Medication

Dietary calcium is dependent on the patient's serum calcium level. In general, 1,000 mg/day of calcium is recommended since a low-calcium diet may lead to further increases in PTH secretion and could aggravate bone disease (Cheng, 2022). However, if the serum calcitriol (active form of vitamin D) concentration is high, calcium intake of <800 mg/day is suggested (Silverberg & Fuleihan, 2021). If the patient has a coexisting peptic ulcer, prescribed antacids and protein feedings are necessary. Measures to prevent constipation (a common occurrence postoperatively) include offering prune juice or stool softeners and increasing physical activity and fluid intake.

Providing Emotional Support

The insidious and chronic onset of hyperparathyroidism together with diverse and vague symptoms may lead to depression and frustration. The family may have considered the patient's illness to be psychosomatic. Increasing awareness of the course of the disorder with patient education may help the patient and family deal with their reactions and feelings.

Managing Hypercalcemic Crisis

Acute hypercalcemic crisis can occur with extreme elevation of serum calcium levels. Serum calcium levels of greater than 15 mg/dL (3.7 mmol/L) result in neurologic, cardiovascular, and renal symptoms that can be life-threatening. Treatment involves rehydration with large volumes of IV fluids (2 to 4 L/day) to keep urine output above 100 mL/hr (normal saline expands volume and inhibits calcium resorption), diuretic agents (to promote renal excretion of excess calcium), and phosphate therapy (to correct hypophosphatemia and decrease serum calcium levels by promoting calcium deposition in bone and reducing the GI absorption of calcium; Cheng, 2022). The patient's fluid status must be monitored due to large volume of IV fluids, particularly in patients with cardiac dysfunction or renal insufficiency to avoid fluid volume excess. Cytotoxic agents (e.g., mithramycin), calcitonin, and dialysis may be used in emergency situations to decrease serum calcium levels quickly. Effective results occur within 24 hours but last only about 1 to 2 weeks. A combination of calcitonin and corticosteroids has been administered in emergencies to reduce the serum calcium level by increasing calcium deposition in bone. Other agents that may be administered to decrease serum calcium levels include bisphosphonates (e.g., etidronate, pamidronate). Refer to Chapter 3 for more details on hypercalcemia.

Careful assessment and care are required to minimize complications and reverse the life-threatening hypercalcemia. It is important to pay particular attention to cardiac function as hypercalcemic crisis can result in death caused by cardiac arrest (Norris & Tuan, 2020). Medications are administered with care, and attention is given to fluid and electrolyte balance. Supportive measures are necessary for the patient and family.

HYPOPARATHYROIDISM

Pathophysiology

Hypoparathyroidism results from hyposecretion of the parathyroid glands, leading to low levels of PTH that eventually result in hypocalcemia and hyperphosphatemia. In the absence of PTH, there is increased blood phosphate (hyperphosphatemia) and a resultant decreased level of blood calcium (hypocalcemia) due to the inverse relationship between serum phosphorus and calcium described in Box 30-8. Without PTH, there is also decreased intestinal absorption of dietary calcium as well as decreased resorption of calcium from bone and through the renal tubules, causing hypocalcemia.

The most common cause of hypoparathyroidism is surgical removal of parathyroid gland tissue during thyroidectomy, parathyroidectomy, or radical neck dissection. These small glands are easily overlooked and can be removed inadvertently during thyroid surgery.

Hypoparathyroidism also may occur in patients who have undergone a subtotal resection or total parathyroidectomy with parathyroid autotransplantation. Other risk factors include genetic predisposition, carcinoma, infection, exposure to heavy metals (e.g., copper, iron), and magnesium depletion (hypomagnesemia: less than 1.2 mg/dL; Fitzgerald, 2022). There appears to be a possible link between cognitive function deficits and lower serum calcium and higher serum phosphate levels in people with hypoparathyroidism that remains to be further examined (Rubin et al., 2022).

Clinical Manifestations and Assessment

Hypocalcemia causes irritability of the neuromuscular system and contributes to the chief symptom of hypoparathyroidism, tetany. Tetany is a general muscle hypertonia, with tremor and spasmodic or uncoordinated contractions occurring with or without efforts to make voluntary movements. Symptoms of latent tetany are numbness, tingling, and cramps in the extremities, and the patient complains of stiffness in the hands and feet. In overt tetany, the signs include bronchospasm, laryngeal spasm, carpopedal spasm (flexion of the elbows and wrists and extension of the carpophalangeal joints and dorsiflexion of the feet), dysphagia, photophobia, cardiac arrhythmias, and seizures. Other symptoms include anxiety, irritability, depression, and even delirium. ECG changes, such as prolonged QT intervals, and hypotension also may occur.

A positive **Trousseau sign** or a positive **Chvostek sign** on physical assessment suggests latent tetany (Fig. 30-7).

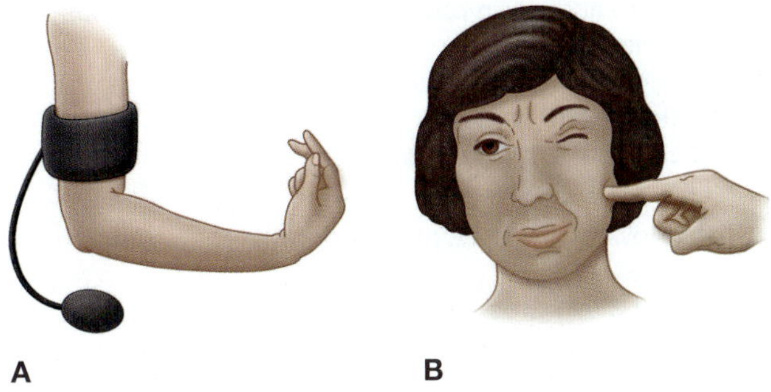

FIGURE 30-7 **Tetany is caused by tonic spasm of the intrinsic hand muscles. Evaluate the patient for Trousseau sign (A) or Chvostek sign (B).**

Trousseau sign is positive when carpopedal spasm is induced by occluding the blood flow to the arm for 3 minutes with a blood pressure cuff. Chvostek sign is positive when a sharp tapping over the facial nerve just in front of the parotid gland and anterior to the ear causes spasm or twitching of the mouth, nose, and eye.

The diagnosis of hypoparathyroidism often is difficult because of the vague symptoms, such as aches and pains. Therefore, laboratory studies are especially helpful. Tetany develops at serum calcium levels of 5 to 6 mg/dL (1.2 to 1.5 mmol/L) or lower. Serum phosphate levels are increased, and x-rays of bone show increased density. Calcification is detected on x-rays of the subcutaneous or paraspinal basal ganglia of the brain.

Medical Management

The goal is to increase the serum calcium level to 8 to 9 mg/dL (2.0 to 2.25 mmol/L) and to eliminate the symptoms of hypoparathyroidism and hypocalcemia. When hypocalcemia and tetany occur after a thyroidectomy, the immediate treatment is administration of IV 10% calcium gluconate. If this does not decrease neuromuscular irritability and seizure activity immediately, sedative agents, such as pentobarbital, may be administered. Parenteral PTH can be administered to treat acute hypoparathyroidism with tetany. The patient receiving PTH is monitored closely for allergic reactions and changes in serum calcium levels.

Treatment for chronic hypoparathyroidism is determined after serum calcium levels are obtained. A diet high in calcium and low in phosphorus is prescribed (Box 30-10). Oral calcium salts, such as calcium gluconate, may be used to supplement the diet. Aluminum hydroxide gel or aluminum carbonate may be used after meals to bind phosphate and promote its excretion through the GI tract. Other variable dosages of a vitamin D preparation—dihydrotachysterol (synthetic vitamin D), ergocalciferol (vitamin D), or cholecalciferol (vitamin D)—are usually required and enhance calcium absorption from the GI tract.

If the patient develops respiratory distress resulting from neuromuscular irritability, the patient may require tracheostomy or mechanical ventilation along with bronchodilating medications.

BOX 30-10 Pearls for Practice: Nutrition Nuggets

Hypoparathyroidism

Patients with hypoparathyroidism are prescribed a diet high in calcium and low in phosphorus. The following foods are recommended:

- Rice milk or nondairy creamer
- Refined white bread
- Green beans, broccoli, cucumbers
- Fish

The following foods are restricted:

- Egg yolks
- Milk and milk products (although high in calcium, these are restricted because they also contain high levels of phosphorus)
- Spinach (contains oxalate that forms insoluble calcium substances)

Nursing Management

Nursing management of the patient with acute hypoparathyroidism includes the care of patients who have undergone thyroidectomy, parathyroidectomy, or radical neck dissection. Care is directed toward detecting early signs of hypocalcemia and anticipating signs of tetany, seizures, and respiratory difficulties. To anticipate emergencies, calcium gluconate should be readily available along with equipment necessary for IV administration. Calcium gluconate is administered slowly in patients who have a current cardiac disorder, such as arrhythmias, and in patients who are currently receiving digitalis.

The patient requires continuous cardiac monitoring and careful assessment because calcium and digitalis increase systolic contraction and also potentiate each other, which can produce potentially fatal arrhythmias.

Patient education about medications and diet therapy is essential. The patient needs to know the reason for high calcium and low phosphate intake and the symptoms of hypocalcemia and hypercalcemia. In addition, the nurse teaches the patient to contact the primary provider if these symptoms occur.

DISORDERS OF THE ADRENAL GLANDS

PHEOCHROMOCYTOMA

Pheochromocytoma is a rare disease, with two to eight new cases per million annually. Around 0.1% of patients with high blood pressure have this tumor that can cause severe hypertensive crisis (Canu et al., 2021).

Pathophysiology

Pheochromocytoma begins with benign growth of a tumor inside the adrenal medulla and usually secretes both epinephrine and norepinephrine (Fitzgerald, 2022). In 90% of patients, the tumor arises in the medulla but can arise in other extra-adrenal chromaffin tissue located in or near the aorta, ovaries, spleen, or other organs. This clinical syndrome is characterized by a massive release of catecholamines that causes severe HTN. The release may be paroxysmal rather than continuous, causing intermittent episodes of headaches, tremor, nervousness, and marked variability in blood pressure (Norris & Tuan, 2020).

Risk Factors

Pheochromocytoma can happen at any age. Around 40% of patients with pheochromocytoma have a genetic mutation that makes them prone to developing the tumor (Fitzgerald, 2022). In most cases, 10% of the tumors are bilateral, and 10% are malignant. Although rare, there has been evidence that germline mutations in multiple endocrine neoplasia type 2 (MEN-2) may predispose a person to having pheochromocytoma in 50% of cases (Amodru et al., 2020). MEN-2 is a rare inherited disease that leads to overactivity and enlargement of the endocrine glands (e.g., overproduction of adrenaline in the adrenal glands). Because of the risk of pheochromocytoma in family members of affected people, the patient's family members should be alerted and examined for pheochromocytoma.

Clinical Manifestations and Assessment

The nature and severity of symptoms of functioning tumors of the adrenal medulla depend on the relative proportions of epinephrine and norepinephrine secretion (Table 30-7). Typical presentation of a patient with pheochromocytoma includes the five **H**'s:

- **H**ypertension (severe)
- **H**eadache
- **H**yperhydrosis (excessive sweating)
- **H**ypermetabolism
- **H**yperglycemia (conversion of liver and muscle glycogen to glucose due to epinephrine secretion)

Other symptoms may include tremor, flushing, and anxiety. Approximately 8% of patients are completely asymptomatic. Paroxysmal symptoms of pheochromocytoma usually develop in the fifth decade of life.

Typically, pheochromocytoma is characterized by acute, unpredictable attacks lasting seconds or several hours. The attacks can be triggered by events, such as use of intravenous contrast dyes or glucagon injection, needle biopsy of the mass, anesthesia, or surgical procedures; exercise; bending; lifting; emotional stress; and drugs (e.g., MAO inhibitors, caffeine, nicotine, decongestions, and amphetamines; Fitzgerald, 2022). Symptoms usually begin abruptly and subside slowly. During these attacks, the patient is extremely anxious, tremulous, and weak. The patient may experience headache, vertigo, blurring of vision, tinnitus, air hunger, and dyspnea. Other symptoms include polyuria, nausea, vomiting, diarrhea, abdominal pain, and a feeling of impending doom. Headache is the most common symptom reported in 90% of symptomatic patients that can range from mild to severe in duration (Young, 2021). Blood pressures exceeding 250/150 mm Hg have been recorded. Such elevations in blood pressure are life-threatening and can cause severe complications, such as cardiac arrhythmias, dissecting aneurysm, stroke, and acute kidney injury. Postural hypotension (decrease in systolic blood pressure, lightheadedness, dizziness on standing) occurs in 70% of patients with untreated pheochromocytoma.

Diagnostic measurements of urine and plasma levels of catecholamine and their metabolites (metanephrine [MN], vanillylmandelic acid [VMA]) are the most direct and conclusive tests for overactivity of the adrenal medulla. CT and MRI studies detect tumors and possible metastases. A negative test result for catecholamines virtually excludes pheochromocytoma; however, increased levels of at least one catecholamine or MN can occur in 10% of patients with essential HTN. In most cases, pheochromocytoma can be diagnosed or confirmed based on a properly collected 24-hour urine sample of free catecholamine, MN, and VMA; levels as high as twice the normal level may be found. The use of combined serum and urine tests increases the diagnostic accuracy of testing. A number of medications and foods, such as coffee and tea (including decaffeinated varieties), bananas, chocolate, vanilla, and aspirin, may alter the results of these tests. Therefore, the patient must be given instructions to avoid such items.

The total concentration of plasma catecholamine (epinephrine and norepinephrine) is measured with the patient supine and at rest for 30 minutes. To prevent elevation of catecholamine levels resulting from the stress of venipuncture, a butterfly needle, scalp vein needle, or venous catheter may be inserted 30 minutes before the blood specimen is obtained. Factors that may elevate catecholamine concentrations must be controlled to obtain valid results; these factors include the dietary items noted earlier, use of tobacco, emotional and physical stress, and use of many prescription and over-the-counter medications (e.g., amphetamines, nose drops or sprays, decongestant agents, bronchodilators).

Medical Management

Although uncommon, other conditions may be associated with this tumor, including cardiac complications, hypotension,

TABLE 30-7 Laboratory Tests for Epinephrine and Norepinephrine

Test	Normal Values	Critical Values	Nursing Implications
Plasma level of epinephrine Plasma level of norepinephrine	100 pg/mL (590 pmol/L) Less than 100–550 pg/mL (590–3,240 pmol/L)	Greater than 400 pg/mL (2,180 pmol/L) diagnostic of pheochromocytoma Greater than 2,000 pg/mL (11,800 pmol/L) diagnostic of pheochromocytoma	The nurse should ensure that the patient is not on epinephrine drugs, such as nose drops and cough mixtures, and norepinephrine drugs, such as Levophed, because these drugs may lead to false increases in levels of plasma epinephrine and norepinephrine. In addition, the patient's blood should be drawn in a nonstressful environment.

shock, and sudden death. Once pheochromocytoma is diagnosed, surgical treatment should not be delayed with the removal of adrenal glands and possible resection of local and distant metastases (Amodru et al., 2020). A laparoscopic removal of the tumor is often the treatment of choice, but open laparotomy is required if tumors are large and invasive in nature (Fitzgerald, 2022).

The patient will be admitted to the intensive care unit for close monitoring (especially ECG) and careful administration of alpha-adrenergic blocking agents (e.g., phentolamine) or smooth muscle relaxants (e.g., sodium nitroprusside) to lower the blood pressure quickly. Phenoxybenzamine, a long-acting alpha blocker, may be used after the blood pressure is stable to prepare the patient for surgery. Calcium-channel blockers, such as nifedipine, usually are well tolerated by patients and have reduced requirements for perioperative fluids. However, calcium-channel blockers should not be used in patients with severe heart failure (Fitzgerald, 2022). Usually calcium-channel blockers are coadministered with alpha-adrenergic blocking agents or used alone. Beta-adrenergic blocking agents, such as propranolol, may be used in patients with cardiac arrhythmias and in those not responsive to alpha blockers. Alpha-adrenergic and beta-adrenergic blocking agents must be used with caution because patients with pheochromocytoma may have increased sensitivity to them. Catecholamine synthesis inhibitors, such as alpha-methyl-*p*-tyrosine, also may be used preoperatively if adrenergic blocking agents do not reduce the effects of catecholamines. Insulin may be required to maintain normal serum glucose levels.

Nursing Management

The nursing management of the patient includes close monitoring of the patient's vital signs (especially heart rate and blood pressure) for several days in the intensive care unit. Most importantly, the nurse monitors the patient closely for excessive rapid decrease in blood pressure that may cause underperfusion to the vital organs (e.g., brain and kidneys). Other management includes monitoring of patient's mental status, acute ECG changes, arterial pressures, fluid and electrolyte balance, and blood glucose levels. Several IV lines are inserted for administration of fluids and medications. Despite large doses of medications used to lower the blood pressure, some patients may continue to be hypertensive. This is due to the effect of poor elasticity of the damaged blood vessels from chronic HTN.

During the phases of care, the nurse informs the patient about the importance of follow-up monitoring to ensure that pheochromocytoma does not recur undetected. For instance, due to the risk for recurrence of HTN, periodic checkups are required, especially in young patients and in those whose families have a history of pheochromocytoma. The patient is scheduled for periodic follow-up appointments to observe for return of normal blood pressure and plasma and urine levels of catecholamines.

ADDISON DISEASE

Addison disease, or primary adrenocortical insufficiency, occurs when adrenal cortex function is inadequate to meet the patient's need for cortical hormones. The three adrenal corticosteroids are glucocorticoids (primarily cortisol, which decreases inflammatory reaction, decreases WBC migration to the inflamed area, increases fat metabolism, and raises serum glucose), mineralocorticoids (primarily aldosterone, which causes sodium reabsorption and, with it, water, along with renal excretion of potassium), and androgens (sex hormones).

Pathophysiology

A primary adrenal insufficiency originates in the adrenal glands themselves and is likely associated with autoimmune or idiopathic atrophy of the adrenal cortex when cell-mediated immune mechanisms result in decreased production of adrenocortical hormones (e.g., cortisol and aldosterone). While primary adrenal insufficiency is an uncommon disorder, autoimmunity is responsible for about 90% of spontaneous cases in industrialized countries (Fitzgerald, 2022). In contrast, secondary adrenal insufficiency can be due to either a lack of anterior pituitary ACTH secretion, or hypothalamic corticotropin-releasing hormone (CRH) dysfunction. This causes a resultant decrease production of cortisol but not aldosterone. ACTH only minimally influences aldosterone secretion, as it is secreted primarily in response to the presence of angiotensin II in the bloodstream.

Risk Factors

The risk factors for Addison disease include surgical removal of both adrenal glands and infection of the adrenal glands. Tuberculosis is the most common cause of Addison disease; other less common causes include carcinoma of adrenal glands, surgical removal of adrenals and bleeding, genetic disposition, and repeated fungal infections requiring use of antifungal medicines known to destroy adrenal gland tissue (National Institute of Diabetes and Digestive and Kidney Disease [NIDDK], 2018). Although autoimmune destruction has replaced tuberculosis as the principal cause of Addison disease, tuberculosis should be considered even though TB treatment has improved over the years. Inadequate secretion of ACTH from the pituitary gland results in secondary adrenal insufficiency because of decreased stimulation of the adrenal cortex. Symptoms of adrenocortical insufficiency also may result from the sudden cessation of exogenous adrenocortical hormonal therapy, which suppresses the body's normal response to stress and interferes with normal feedback mechanisms. Hence, corticosteroids should never be stopped abruptly. Daily administration of corticosteroids has the potential to suppress function of the adrenal cortex. It has been shown that suppression of HPA axis is present in patients receiving high doses of glucocorticoids (>20- to 30-mg hydrocortisone or equivalent) for more than 3 weeks

(Alexandraki et al., 2018). It may also be seen in the setting of chronic high-dose inhaled corticosteroids, due to systemic absorption (Atteih & Ratner, 2021).

Pearls for Practice

HPA axis refers to the interaction of the hypothalamic–pituitary gland–adrenal glands that helps us respond to stress. In short, the hypothalamus sensing a stress releases CRH, which is transported via the blood stream to the pituitary gland (anterior), which then produces ACTH. The released ACTH is transported via the blood stream to the adrenal glands resulting in the production of cortisol from the adrenal cortex to assist us in weathering the stressor. Now consider that when placed on "steroids" (typically because of their anti-inflammatory and pharmacologic effects in a variety of conditions), the hormone is in your system (exogenous); thus, there is no production (endogenous) from the adrenal gland, which means there is suppression of the HPA axis. Now consider if you suddenly stop taking the exogenous steroid that you have been on long term or have an additional stressors (e.g. trauma, infection, or surgery), you are now at risk for adrenal crisis. That is why you will see tapering of corticosteroids based on the duration of therapy. For example, if a patient has been prescribed corticosteroids for less than 2 weeks, the medication can be discontinued abruptly. If, however, the patient has been on corticosteroids for 2 to 4 weeks, then the dose can be expected to be tapered over 1 to 2 weeks to prevent the suppression of the HPA axis. If a patient has been on corticosteroids for >1 month, then there is a slow taper over 1 to 2 months to a physiologic dose (approximately 2.5 mg/m^2/day of prednisolone) with discontinuation after assessment of adrenal function has demonstrated recovery (Gold Standard, 2022b).

Clinical Manifestations and Assessment

Addison disease is characterized by muscle weakness, anorexia, GI symptoms, fatigue, emaciation, skin pigmentation changes (Box 30-11), and hypotension as well as low blood glucose, low serum sodium, and high serum potassium levels. Depression, emotional lability, apathy, and confusion are present in 60% to 80% of patients. With decreased glucocorticoids, mineralocorticoids, and androgens, there is stimulation of the anterior pituitary to increase ACTH. This releases the melanocyte hormone, which results in a bronze-pigmented rash (Fig. 30-8). Hyperpigmentation is more prominent in palmar creases, buccal mucosa, pressure points (elbows, knees, knuckles), perianal mucosa, around areolas of nipples, and scars (Ferri, 2022). Since pigmentation of the palmar creases may be normal in darker-skinned individuals, it is suggested that comparison with other family members for the presence or absence of hyperpigmentation be considered (Nieman, 2020). Figure 30-8 details the clinical manifestations of Addison disease and specifies the relationship of signs and symptoms to specific hormone deficiency.

BOX 30-11 **Focused Assessment**

Skin Changes in Addison Disease

Be alert for the following signs and symptoms:

- Skin pigmentation changes of bronzed or suntanned appearance (seen in primary Addison disease because the persistently low levels of cortisol cause hypersecretion of ACTH from the pituitary gland; increased melanin synthesis is associated with an increase in ACTH; thus, hyperpigmentation occurs)
- Increased pigmentation at skin creases, pressure points (knuckles, elbows, knees), scars, and buccal mucosa

In severe cases, the disturbance of the metabolism of sodium and potassium may be marked by depletion of sodium and water and severe chronic dehydration. **Addisonian crisis** is an acute life-threatening event that develops with disease progression. It may also be referred to as acute adrenal insufficiency or adrenal crisis. Acute hypotension is characterized by cyanosis and the classic signs of circulatory shock: pallor, apprehension, rapid and weak pulse, rapid respirations, and low blood pressure. In addition, the patient may complain of headache, nausea, abdominal pain, and diarrhea and may show signs of confusion and restlessness. Even slight overexertion, exposure to cold, acute infection, or a decrease in salt intake may lead to circulatory collapse, shock, and death if untreated. The stress of surgery or dehydration resulting from preparation for diagnostic tests may precipitate an Addisonian or hypotensive crisis. The nurse anticipates laboratory analysis will reveal hyponatremia and hyperkalemia due to the lack of aldosterone and hypoglycemia related to the lack of glucocorticoids.

Symptoms of secondary adrenal insufficiency are the same as those for primary adrenal insufficiency with a few exceptions, most notably the lack of hyperpigmentation, as ACTH secretion is not increased. In addition, symptoms are due to glucocorticoid rather than mineralocorticoid deficiency. Therefore, signs of hypoglycemia are present, while signs of hyperkalemia are not because of the continued presence of aldosterone.

The diagnosis is confirmed by laboratory test results. Combined measurements of early-morning serum cortisol and plasma ACTH are performed to differentiate patients with primary adrenal insufficiency from those with secondary adrenal insufficiency.

Patients with primary insufficiency have a plasma ACTH level that is greatly increased (over 22.0 pmol/L) and a serum cortisol concentration lower than the normal range (less than 165 nmol/L) or in the low-normal range. Other laboratory findings include decreased levels of blood glucose

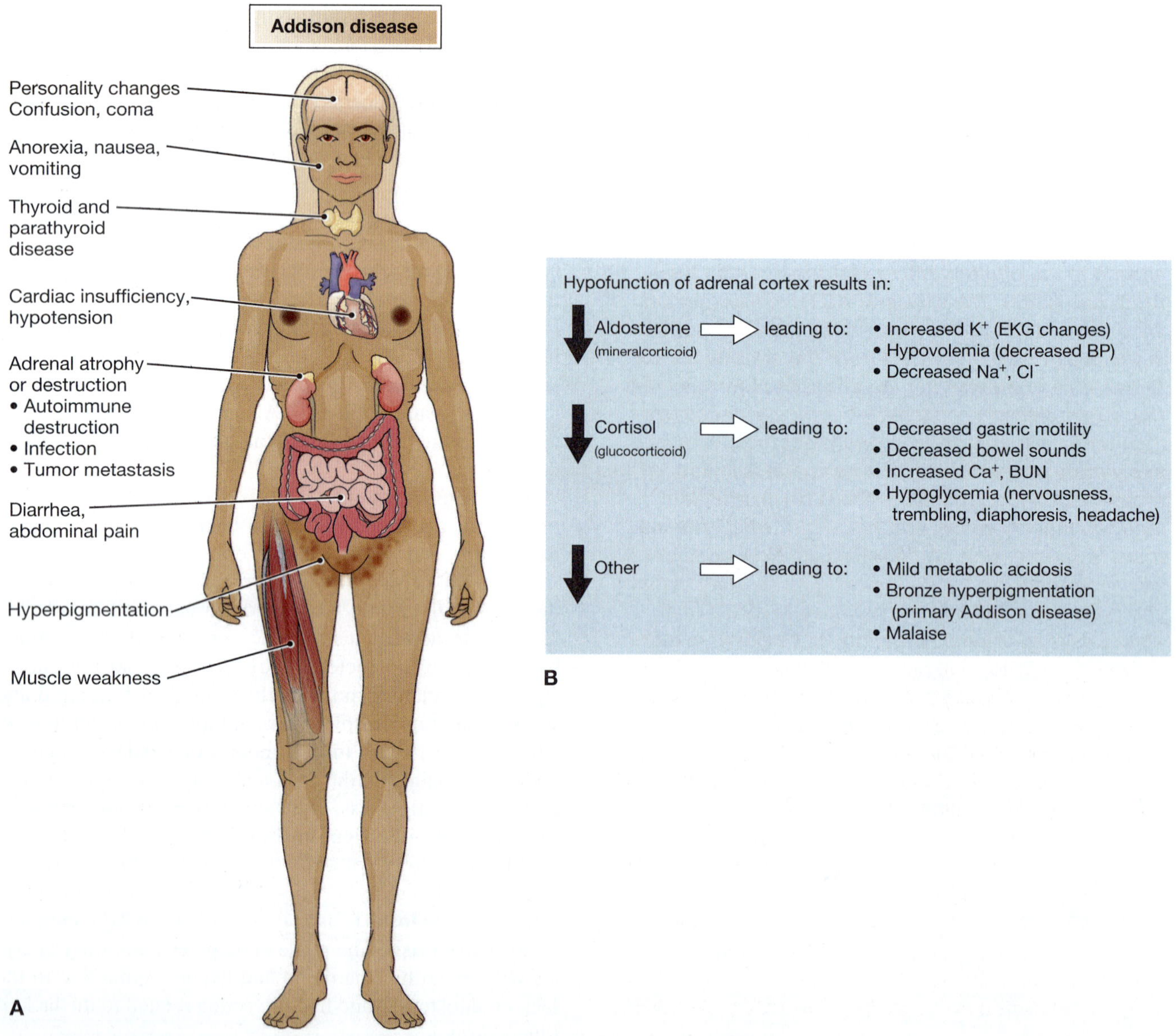

FIGURE 30-8 (A) Clinical manifestations of Addison disease. (From Porth, C. M. [2015]. *Essentials of pathophysiology: Concepts of altered health states* [4th ed.]. Lippincott Williams & Wilkins.) (B) Chart detailing the signs and symptoms of Addison disease and relationship to specific hormone deficiencies. (Reprinted with permission from Diepenbrock, N. H. [2015]. *Quick reference to critical care* [5th ed.]. Lippincott Williams & Wilkins.)

(hypoglycemia) and sodium (hyponatremia), an increased concentration of serum potassium (hyperkalemia), and an increased WBC count (leukocytosis). If the adrenal cortex is destroyed, baseline cortisol values become low, and ACTH administration fails to cause the normal increase in plasma cortisol and urinary 17-hydroxycorticosteroids. Secondary adrenal insufficiency is characterized by low pituitary dysfunction. The adrenal gland is healthy, but it is not being stimulated properly by the pituitary. In this situation, low levels of adrenocortical hormones in the blood or urine and decreased serum cortisol levels are seen. A normal response to repeated doses of exogenous ACTH is seen (adrenal gland is normal), but no response occurs after the administration of metyrapone, which stimulates endogenous ACTH.

Medical Management

Immediate treatment is directed toward combating circulatory shock: restoring blood circulation, administering fluids and corticosteroids, monitoring vital signs, and placing the patient in a recumbent position with the legs elevated. Corticosteroid use is discussed in Box 30-12 and Table 30-8. Hydrocortisone is administered intravenously, followed by 5% dextrose in normal saline. Oral hydrocortisone replacement is resumed once intravenous infusion is discontinued. Vasopressor amines may be required if hypotension persists. Broad-spectrum antibiotics may be administered if infection has precipitated adrenal crisis in a patient with chronic adrenal insufficiency. In addition, the patient is assessed closely to identify other factors, stressors, or illnesses that led to the acute episode.

BOX 30-12

Using Corticosteroids in the Treatment of Adrenal Disease

Synthetic corticosteroids are administered for a variety of clinical conditions, including adrenal insufficiency, suppressing inflammation and autoimmune reactions, controlling allergic reactions, and reducing the rejection process in transplantation. Choices for corticosteroids include prednisone, methylprednisolone, and dexamethasone, which are all synthetic compositions of cortisol (hydrocortisone). The dosage of corticosteroids is determined by the nature and chronicity of the illness as well as the patient's other medical conditions. Side effects include the development of diabetes mellitus, osteoporosis, peptic ulcer, increased protein breakdown resulting in muscle wasting and poor wound healing, and redistribution of body fat. Therefore, the adverse effects of corticosteroids must be weighed against the benefits to the patient's current condition.

Depending on the severity of disease, corticosteroids may be used for a period of time and gradually reduced or tapered as the symptoms subside so as to avoid undesirable effects, such as adrenal suppression.

Once the primary disorder is resolved, corticosteroid dosages are tapered to allow the return of normal adrenal function and to prevent steroid-induced adrenal insufficiency. However, up to 1 year or longer after use of corticosteroids, the patient still may be at risk for adrenal insufficiency in times of stress. If surgery is necessary, the patient is likely to require IV corticosteroids during and after surgery to reduce the risk for acute adrenal crisis. The nurse plays an important role in providing education about the dosage, taper schedule, and side effects of corticosteroids. Table 30-7 provides an overview of the effects of corticosteroid therapy and their nursing implications. In general, it is believed that clinically significant adrenal suppression does not occur with prednisone treatment of 5 mg/day or less (Karlet, 2023).

In keeping with the natural secretion of cortisol, the best time of day for the total corticosteroid dose is in the early morning, between 7 and 8 AM. The half-life of synthetic steroids is approximately 8 hours. Therefore, if a large dose is administered at 8 AM (when the adrenal gland is most active), maximal suppression of the adrenal gland occurs. The adrenal suppressive effect can last for 12–24 hours. If symptoms of the disorder being treated are suppressed, alternate-day therapy may be helpful in reducing pituitary–adrenal suppression in patients requiring prolonged therapy. Since large amounts of glucocorticoids administered exogenously in the blood inhibit the release of ACTH and endogenous glucocorticoids, atrophy of the adrenal cortex can develop with long-term use. If exogenous glucocorticoid administration is discontinued suddenly, adrenal insufficiency can occur due to the inability of the atrophied cortex to respond adequately.

Although the synthetic corticosteroids are safe for some patients because of relative freedom from mineralocorticoid activity, most natural and synthetic corticosteroids produce similar kinds of side effects. Mineralocorticoids have major effects on electrolyte metabolism, acting principally on the renal tubular and GI epithelium to cause increased absorption of sodium ions in exchange for excretion of potassium or hydrogen ions. ACTH only minimally influences aldosterone secretion. It is primarily secreted in response to the presence of angiotensin II in the bloodstream. Angiotensin II is a substance that elevates the blood pressure by constricting arterioles. Its concentration is increased when renin is released from the kidney in response to decreased perfusion pressure. The resultant increased levels of aldosterone promote sodium reabsorption by the kidney and the GI tract, which tends to restore blood pressure to normal. The release of aldosterone also is increased by hyperkalemia.

Nursing Management

Restoring Fluid Status

Along with dietitian referral, the nurse encourages the patient to consume foods and fluids that assist in restoring and maintaining fluid and electrolyte balance and teaches the patient to select foods that are high in sodium during GI disturbances and in very hot weather. The nurse instructs the patient and family to administer hormone replacement as prescribed and to modify the dosage during illness and other stressful situations. Written and verbal instructions are provided about the administration of mineralocorticoid (fludrocortisone) or corticosteroid (prednisone).

Prior to fluid replacement therapy, the nurse monitors the patient for any signs and symptoms of fluid imbalances by monitoring the blood pressure and pulse rate as the patient moves from a lying to a standing position. A decrease in systolic pressure (20 mm Hg or more) indicates fluid volume deficit, as evidenced by the patient's narrowed pulse pressure, delayed capillary filling, and flat neck veins. The nurse monitors the patient for manifestations of hypovolemic shock: hypotension, rapid weak pulse, rapid respiratory rate, pallor, and extreme weakness. Other key considerations include checking for weight loss, measuring intake and output, assessing for muscle weakness and fatigue, and investigating any illness or stress that may have precipitated the acute crisis.

Reducing Stress

Until the patient's condition is stabilized, unnecessary activity and stress that could precipitate another hypotensive episode are avoided. The nurse assesses for signs of infection or the presence of other stressors. Even minor events or stressors may be excessive in patients with adrenal insufficiency. During the acute crisis, the nurse maintains a quiet, nonstressful environment and performs all activities (e.g., bathing, turning) for the patient. Maintaining communication and explaining all procedures to the patient and family can help reduce their anxiety. During stressful procedures or significant illnesses, additional supplementary therapy or higher doses of glucocorticoids are required to prevent an Addisonian crisis.

TABLE **30-8 Side Effects of Corticosteroid Therapy and Implications for Nursing Practice**

Side Effects	Collaborative Interventions
Cardiovascular Effects	
Hypertension Thrombophlebitis Thromboembolism Accelerated atherosclerosis	Monitor for elevated blood pressure. Assess for signs and symptoms of deep venous thrombosis (DVT): redness, warmth, tenderness, and unilateral edema of an extremity. Remind the patient to avoid positions and situations that restrict blood flow (e.g., crossing legs, prolonged sitting in same position, use of knee highs or girdles). Encourage foot and leg exercises when recumbent. Encourage low sodium intake. Encourage limited intake of fat.
Immunologic Effects	
Increased risk of infection and masking of signs of infection	Assess for subtle signs of infection and inflammation. Encourage the patient to avoid exposure to people with upper respiratory infection. Monitor the patient for fungal infections. Encourage handwashing.
Ophthalmologic Changes	
Glaucoma Corneal lesions	Encourage frequent eye examinations. Refer the patient to an ophthalmologist if changes are detected in visual acuity.
Musculoskeletal Effects	
Muscle wasting Poor wound healing Osteoporosis with vertebral compression fractures, pathologic fractures of long bones, aseptic necrosis of head of the femur	Encourage high intake of protein and vitamin C or supplementation of protein and vitamin C, if indicated. Encourage a diet high in calcium and vitamin D or supplementation of calcium and vitamin D, if indicated. Take measures to avoid falls and other trauma. Use caution in moving and turning patient. Encourage postmenopausal patients on corticosteroids to consider bone mineral density testing and treatment, if indicated. Instruct the patient to rise slowly from the bed or chair to avoid falling.
Metabolic Effects	
Alterations in glucose metabolism Steroid withdrawal syndrome	Monitor blood glucose levels at periodic intervals. Instruct the patient about medications, diet, and exercise prescribed to control blood glucose level. Report signs of adrenal insufficiency. Administer corticosteroids and mineralocorticoids as prescribed. Monitor fluid and electrolyte balance. Administer fluids and electrolytes as prescribed. Instruct the patient about the importance of taking corticosteroids as prescribed without stopping therapy abruptly. Encourage the patient to obtain and wear a medical identification bracelet. Advise the patient to notify all health care providers (e.g., dentist) about the need for corticosteroid therapy.
Changes in Appearance	
Moon face Weight gain Acne	Encourage a low-calorie, low-sodium diet. Assure the patient that most changes in appearance are temporary and will disappear if and when corticosteroid therapy is no longer necessary.

Maintaining Self-Care

Because of the need for lifelong replacement of adrenal cortex hormones to prevent Addisonian crises, the patient and family members receive explicit verbal and written instructions about the rationale for replacement therapy and proper dosage. In addition, they learn about how to modify the medication dosage and increase salt intake in times of illness, very hot weather, and other stressful situations. The patient also learns how to modify diet and fluid intake to help maintain fluid and electrolyte balance.

The patient and family are aware about the need for lifelong corticosteroid replacement therapy and are prescribed preloaded, single-injection syringes of corticosteroid for use in emergencies. Instruction must be provided on how and when to inject cortisol in emergencies, as should demonstration of the "teach back" method of injection technique (see Chapter 1). It is important to instruct the patient to inform other health care providers, such as dentists, about the use of corticosteroids, to wear a medical alert bracelet, and to carry information at all times about the need for corticosteroids. The patient and family need to know the signs of excessive or insufficient hormone replacement. The development of edema or weight gain may signify the dose is too high; postural hypotension and weight loss frequently signify the dose is too low.

Monitoring and Managing Addisonian Crisis

Physical and psychological stressors must be avoided since the patient with Addison disease is at risk for an Addisonian crisis, which presents as complete circulatory collapse and shock. Triggers include exposure to cold, overexertion, infection, and emotional distress. The patient with an Addisonian crisis requires immediate treatment with IV administration of fluid, glucose, and electrolytes, especially sodium; replacement of missing steroid hormones; and vasopressors. In addition, the patient must avoid exertion; therefore, the nurse must anticipate the patient's needs and take measures to meet them. Careful monitoring of symptoms, vital signs, weight, and status of fluids and electrolytes is essential to assess the patient's progress and return to a precrisis state. To reduce the risk of future episodes of an Addisonian crisis, efforts are made to identify and reduce the factors that may have led to the crisis.

CUSHING SYNDROME/DISEASE

Pathophysiology

Cushing syndrome, or hypercortisolism, is a disorder characterized by high levels of serum cortisol—too much ACTH is at work in the body. Three important causes of Cushing syndrome are:

- A pituitary tumor that overproduces ACTH, termed Cushing disease
- An adrenal tumor that overproduces ACTH, termed Cushing syndrome
- Long-term glucocorticoid pharmacologic therapy, termed iatrogenic

Pathophysiology

Cushing syndrome is commonly caused by chronic use of synthetic corticosteroid medications and infrequently is due to excessive production of corticosteroid secondary to hyperplasia or tumor of the adrenal cortex. Overproduction of endogenous corticosteroids may be caused by several mechanisms, including a tumor of the pituitary gland that produces ACTH and stimulates the adrenal cortex to increase its hormone secretion despite production of adequate amounts (as noted earlier, technically termed *Cushing disease*). Primary hyperplasia of the adrenal glands in the absence of a pituitary tumor is less common. Another less common cause of Cushing syndrome is the ectopic production of ACTH by malignancies; bronchogenic carcinoma is the most common type of these malignancies. Regardless of the cause, the normal feedback mechanisms that control the function of the adrenal cortex become ineffective, and the usual diurnal pattern of cortisol is lost.

Risk Factors

The chronic use of corticosteroids is a common risk factor of developing Cushing syndrome. Females are three to eight times more likely than males to develop Cushing syndrome, and the age of onset or diagnosis ranged from 25 to 45 years of age (Nieman, 2022a). Although racial disparities do not appear to be significant risk factor in Cushing syndrome, Black patients had a borderline lower remission rates at 3 months postoperatively than did White patients (Ioachimescu et al., 2022). The main factor of remission in White patients was tumor growth in the pituitary gland. Other less common risk factors that may result in Cushing syndrome include primary hyperplasia of the adrenal glands in the absence of a pituitary tumor and ectopic production of ACTH by malignancies.

Clinical Manifestations and Assessment

The signs and symptoms of Cushing syndrome are primarily due to oversecretion of glucocorticoids and androgens (sex hormones), although mineralocorticoid secretion also may play a role. Overproduction of the adrenal cortical hormone leads to an arrest of height, obesity, musculoskeletal changes, and glucose intolerance. Altered fat metabolism results in a classic picture of Cushing syndrome in the adult: central-type obesity, a protruding abdomen, a fatty "buffalo hump" in the neck and supraclavicular areas, and a round "moon-faced" appearance (Fig. 30-9). The skin is thin, fragile, and easily traumatized; ecchymoses (bruises) and purple striae develop (secondary to stretching of the weakened skin). The patient complains of weakness and lassitude. Sleep is disturbed due to altered diurnal secretion of cortisol.

Muscle weakness, wasting, and thin extremities are caused by protein wasting. Excessive catabolism of bone protein can result in osteoporosis. Kyphosis, backache, and compression fractures of the vertebrae may result.

Retention of sodium and water occurs as a result of increased mineralocorticoid activity, producing HTN, hypokalemia, and heart failure. Hyperglycemia or overt diabetes may develop. The patient may report weight gain, increased susceptibility to infection, and slow healing of minor cuts.

In females of all ages, virilization may occur as a result of excess androgens. Virilization is characterized by the appearance of masculine traits and the recession of feminine traits.

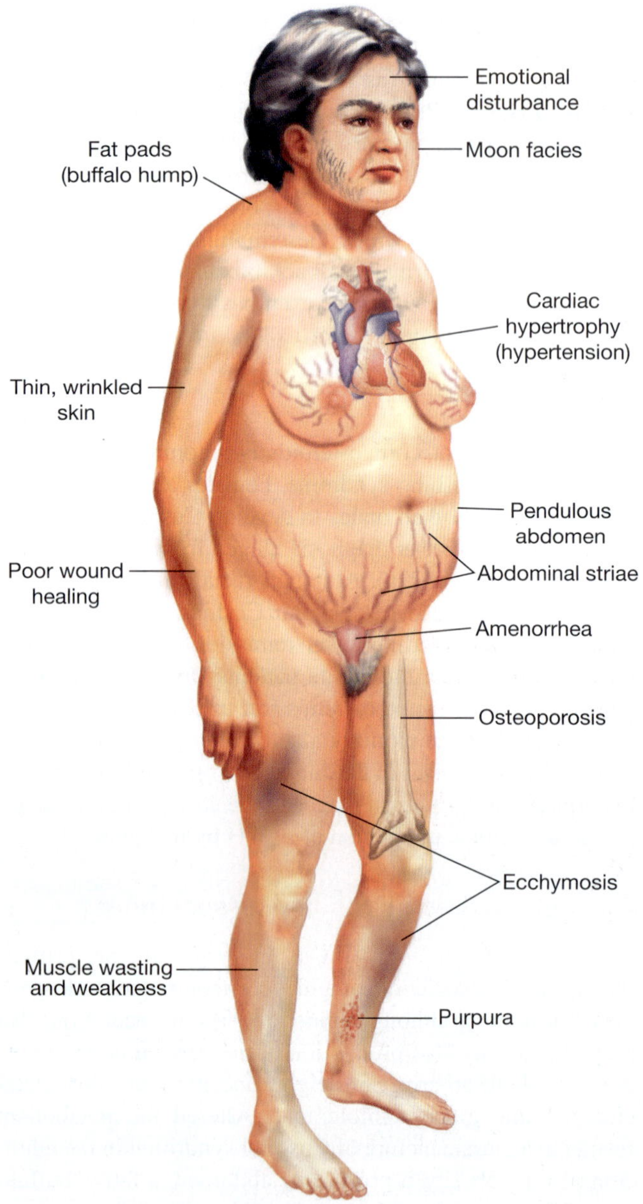

FIGURE 30-9 Major clinical manifestations of Cushing syndrome. (From Porth, C. M. [2015]. *Essentials of pathophysiology: Concepts of altered health states* [4th ed.]. Lippincott Williams & Wilkins.)

There is an excessive growth of hair on the face (hirsutism), the breasts atrophy, menses cease, the clitoris enlarges, and the voice deepens. Libido is lost in males and females.

Changes occur in mood and mental activity, and psychosis may develop. Distress and depression are common and are increased by the severity of the physical changes that occur with this syndrome. If Cushing disease is a consequence of a pituitary tumor, visual disturbances may occur because of pressure of the growing tumor on the optic chiasm.

The initial diagnostic assessment involves:

1. 24-hour urine free cortisol (2 measurements),
2. late night salivary cortisol (2 measurements), and/or
3. dexamethasone suppression test: low-dose 1 mg (Galm & Tritos, 2020).

The diagnosis of Cushing disease is determined when at least two different test results are abnormal (Nieman, 2022). The 1-mg overnight dexamethasone suppression test is widely used and the most sensitive screening for the diagnosis of pituitary and adrenal causes of Cushing disease (Norris & Tuan, 2020). In general, 1 mg of dexamethasone is administered orally at 11:00 PM to 12:00 AM (MIDNIGHT), and a plasma cortisol level is obtained at 8:00 AM the next morning. Suppression of cortisol to less than 5 mg/dL indicates that the hypothalamic–pituitary–adrenal axis is functioning properly. Stress; obesity; depression; and medications, such as antiseizure agents, estrogen (during pregnancy or as oral medications), and rifampin; can falsely elevate cortisol levels. Studies have shown that nighttime salivary cortisol levels show promise in screening effectively for Cushing syndrome. Although not a routine diagnostic test in the United States, salivary cortisol concentrations are shown to be reflective of active free cortisol in plasma. Traditionally, salivary cortisol is collected in the evening or midnight either by providing saliva samples in a plastic tube or by chewing a piece of cotton salivette. Compared with the standard urine-free cortisol levels, midnight salivary cortisol test offers some advantage as an accurate and reliable alternative diagnostic tool for Cushing syndrome (Lin et al., 2019). However, there is some evidence to indicate that having multiple salivary cortisol measurement (6 AM, 8 AM, 12 noon, 6 PM, and 10 PM) may be a better method to evaluate the diurnal rhythm of cortisol in Cushing syndrome (Yoshida et al., 2018). This may be used in patients who are suspected of having cyclic or intermittent Cushing syndrome (Nieman, 2022). Saliva samples can be obtained easily in a nonstressful environment (e.g., at home) and does not require hospitalization. The test is relatively safe and easy to administer, with a sensitivity of 98% and a specificity of 100% (Lin et al., 2019).

Pearls for Practice

Sensitivity refers to the proportion of patients with a disease testing positive for it (i.e., how well a test detects actual disease). In the example above, 98% of patients with Cushing disease test positive; thus, sensitivity refers to TRUE positive. Specificity refers to the proportion of patients without the disease who would test negative (i.e., how well a test detects the absence of disease). In the case above, the test correctly identifies 100% of patients who did not have the disease, or a TRUE negative. They help us evaluate the accuracy and reliability of diagnostic tests.

Indicators of Cushing syndrome include an increase in levels of serum sodium (hypernatremia) and blood glucose (hyperglycemia), a decrease in serum potassium (hypokalemia), a reduction in the number of blood eosinophils, and disappearance of lymphoid tissue. Measurements are obtained of plasma and urinary cortisol levels. Several blood samples may be collected to determine whether the normal diurnal variation in plasma levels is present; frequently this variation is absent in adrenal dysfunction. If several blood samples are required, they must be collected at the times specified, and the time of collection must be noted on the requisition slip.

Radioimmunoassay measurement of plasma ACTH is used together with the high-dose suppression test to distinguish pituitary tumors from ectopic sites of ACTH production. Elevation of ACTH and cortisol indicates pituitary or hypothalamic disease. Low ACTH with high cortisol level indicates adrenal disease. CT, ultrasound, or MRI is performed to localize adrenal tissue and detect tumors of adrenal gland.

Medical Management

Treatment is directed at the pituitary gland if Cushing is caused by pituitary tumors rather than tumors of the adrenal cortex. Successful surgical removal of the tumor by transsphenoidal hypophysectomy is the treatment of choice, and it has early postoperative remission rates in around 90% of patients with microadenomas and 65% of patients with macroadenomas (Tritos & Biller, 2019). In addition, radiation of the pituitary gland has been successful, but it may take several months for control of the symptoms. **Adrenalectomy** is the treatment of choice in patients with primary adrenal hypertrophy or when other therapies have failed. For patients requiring surgery, the peak age of surgery was found to be 10 years later in Black patients compared with White patients; this may be due to a possibility of diagnostic delays in middle-aged Black females and older Black patients (Ioachimescu et al., 2022).

Postoperatively, symptoms of adrenal insufficiency may begin to appear 12 to 48 hours after surgery because of the reduction of high levels of circulating adrenal hormones. Temporary replacement therapy with hydrocortisone may be necessary for several months, until the adrenal glands begin to respond normally to the body's needs. If both adrenal glands have been removed (bilateral adrenalectomy), patients should be educated that a lifetime replacement of adrenal cortex hormones is necessary, and they should be taught how to identify signs of acute Addisonian crisis.

Adrenal enzyme inhibitors, such as metyrapone, aminoglutethimide, mitotane, and ketoconazole, are used to reduce hyperadrenalism if the syndrome is caused by ectopic ACTH secretion by a tumor that cannot be eradicated. Close monitoring is necessary because symptoms of inadequate adrenal function may result due to possible side effects of these medications.

If Cushing syndrome is a result of the administration of corticosteroids, an attempt is made to reduce or taper the medication to the minimum dosage needed to treat the underlying disease process (e.g., autoimmune, allergic disease, or rejection of transplanted organ). Frequently, alternate-day therapy decreases the symptoms of Cushing syndrome and allows recovery of the adrenal glands' responsiveness to ACTH.

Nursing Management

Decreasing Risk of Injury

Establishing a protective environment helps prevent falls, fractures, and other injuries to bones and soft tissues. The patient who is very weak may require assistance in ambulating to avoid falling or bumping into sharp corners of furniture. Foods high in protein, calcium, and vitamin D are recommended to minimize muscle wasting and osteoporosis. Referral to a dietitian may assist the patient in selecting appropriate foods that are also low in sodium and calories.

Decreasing Risk of Infection

The patient should avoid unnecessary exposure to people with infections. The nurse frequently assesses the patient for subtle signs of infection because the anti-inflammatory effects of corticosteroids may mask the common signs of inflammation and infection.

Encouraging Rest and Activity

Weakness, fatigue, and muscle wasting make it difficult for the patient with Cushing syndrome to carry out normal activities; however, the nurse encourages moderate activity to prevent complications of immobility and promote increased self-esteem. Insomnia often contributes to the patient's fatigue. It is important to help the patient plan and space rest periods throughout the day. Efforts are made to promote a relaxing, quiet environment for rest and sleep.

Promoting Skin Integrity

Proper skin care is necessary to avoid traumatizing the patient's fragile skin. The nurse avoids use of adhesive tape because it can irritate and tear the skin when the tape is removed. The nurse frequently assesses the skin and bony prominences and encourages and assists the patient to change positions frequently to prevent skin breakdown.

Improving Body Image

If the cause of Cushing syndrome can be treated successfully, the major physical changes disappear in time. The patient may benefit from discussion of the effect the changes have had on their self-concept and relationships with others. Weight gain and edema may be modified by recommending a low-carbohydrate, low-sodium, and high-protein diet.

Improving Thought Processes

Explanations to the patient and family members about the cause of emotional instability are important in helping them cope with the mood swings, irritability, and depression that may occur. Psychotic behavior may occur in a few patients and should be reported. The nurse encourages the patient and family members to verbalize their feelings and concerns.

Monitoring and Managing Addisonian Crisis

The patient with Cushing syndrome or disease whose symptoms are treated by the withdrawal of corticosteroids, by adrenalectomy, or by removal of a pituitary tumor is at risk for adrenal hypofunction and Addisonian crisis. If high levels of circulating adrenal hormones have suppressed the function of the adrenal cortex, atrophy of the adrenal cortex is likely. If the level of circulating hormones is decreased rapidly because of surgery or abrupt cessation of corticosteroid agents, manifestations of adrenal hypofunction and Addisonian crisis may develop. The nurse monitors the patient closely for hypovolemia (hypotension, rapid weak pulse, rapid respiratory rate, pallor, flat neck veins, and extreme weakness), hyponatremia, and hyperkalemia. Efforts are made to identify factors that may have led to the crisis. The patient may require IV administration of fluid, electrolytes, and corticosteroids before, during, and after treatment or surgery. The nurse assesses the status of fluid and electrolytes by monitoring laboratory values and daily weights. If Addisonian crisis occurs, the patient is treated for circulatory collapse and shock.

Monitoring and Managing Fluid Volume Excess, Hypokalemia, and Hyperglycemia

Retention of sodium and water from mineralocorticoids may result in the development of edema and HTN; therefore, assessment of vital signs and fluid volume excess is warranted (JVD, presence of S3 and/or S4 gallop, crackles on pulmonary exam, pitting edema). In addition, observe for signs and symptoms of hypokalemia (K^+ below 3.5 mEq/L), which can have a profound impact on cardiac and neurologic function. ECG changes associated with hypokalemia include T-wave flattening, ST depression, and the appearance of a U wave. Older patients are at the highest risk for arrhythmias, as are those with heart disease and patients receiving digoxin or antiarrhythmic drugs (Castro & Sharma, 2021). The nurse understands that the magnesium level will also be assessed since repletion of magnesium is required in order to raise the potassium level. When magnesium is depleted, intracellular potassium is liberated to the ECF, which causes an increase in the excretion of potassium by the kidney and hypokalemia ensues (Reddy, 2022). Thus, both potassium and magnesium replacement may be required, even when the serum magnesium level is within the reference range, to ensure maintenance of intracellular potassium level (Clinical Overview, 2021). Blood glucose monitoring should be followed closely because of the increased risk for glucose intolerance and hyperglycemia with Cushing syndrome and hypoglycemia if the patient is now at risk for adrenal hypofunction due to interventions to treat Cushing syndrome.

Teaching Self-Care Measures

Upon discharge, the patient and family should understand that stopping the use of the corticosteroid abruptly and without medical supervision is likely to result in acute adrenal insufficiency as well as reappearance of the underlying symptoms of the chronic disease. The nurse emphasizes the need to ensure an adequate supply of the corticosteroid because running out of the medication or skipping doses can precipitate adrenal insufficiency and Addisonian crisis. The need for dietary modifications is stressed; the nurse reminds the patient and family that it is important to ensure adequate calcium intake without increasing the risks for HTN, hyperglycemia, and weight gain. Recall the catabolic effects of cortisol causes loss of the protein matrix of bone leading to bone disease (Mayer & Jones, 2019). The patient and family may be taught to monitor blood pressure, blood glucose levels, and weight. Wearing a medical alert bracelet and notifying health care providers (e.g., dentist) of the patient's condition are important.

PRIMARY ALDOSTERONISM

Pathophysiology

Primary aldosteronism, also known as *Conn syndrome*, is a condition in which the adrenal cortex produces too much aldosterone because of hyperplasia or tumor. The principal action of aldosterone is to conserve body sodium; thus, excessive aldosterone will result in increased renal reabsorption of sodium and an increase in extracellular fluids and blood pressure. In primary aldosteronism, there is decreased plasma renin activity.

Secondary hyperaldosteronism also can occur from a nonadrenal cause of elevated aldosterone and/or nonsuppressed plasma renin activity, such as renal artery stenosis, renin-secreting tumors, kidney disease, and malignant HTN.

Risk Factors

Excessive production of aldosterone occurs in some patients with functioning tumors of the adrenal gland. Primary aldosteronism is common among males with a peak incidence between 50 and 60 years of age (Fitzgerald, 2022). Other risk factors for primary aldosteronism include unilateral or bilateral adrenal hyperplasia (caused by overactivity of one or both adrenal glands), familial hyperaldosteronism, and aldosterone-producing adrenal adenoma (Fitzgerald, 2022).

Clinical Manifestations and Assessment

Patients with hyperaldosteronism exhibit a profound decline in the serum levels of potassium (hypokalemia) and hydrogen ions (alkalosis, leading to tetany) as demonstrated by an increase in pH and serum bicarbonate concentration. The serum sodium level is normal or typically elevated depending on the amount of water reabsorbed with the sodium or water loss in the urine. HTN is the most prominent sign of aldosteronism. The prevalence of primary aldosteronism among normotensive people, stage 1 and 2 untreated HTN, and resistant HTN was 11%, 38%, and 22%, respectively (Brown et al., 2020).

Hypokalemia leads to muscle weakness, cramping, and fatigue as well as an inability on the part of the kidneys to acidify or concentrate the urine, leading to polyuria. Serum sodium becomes abnormally concentrated, contributing to excessive thirst (polydipsia) and arterial HTN. A secondary increase in blood volume and possible direct effects of aldosterone on nerve receptors, such as the carotid sinus, result in HTN.

Hypokalemic alkalosis may decrease the level of ionized serum calcium and predispose the patient to tetany and paresthesia. Glucose intolerance may occur because hypokalemia interferes with insulin secretion from the pancreas.

In addition to a high or normal serum sodium level and a low serum potassium level, diagnostic studies for primary hyperaldosteronism indicate high serum aldosterone and low serum renin levels. The measurement of the aldosterone excretion rate after salt loading is a useful diagnostic test for hyperaldosteronism. The renin–aldosterone stimulation test and bilateral adrenal venous sampling are useful in differentiating the cause of primary aldosteronism. Antihypertensive medication may be discontinued up to 2 weeks before testing.

Medical Management

Treatment of primary aldosteronism usually involves surgical removal of the adrenal tumor through adrenalectomy. Adrenalectomy is performed through an incision in the flank or the abdomen using laparoscopic techniques. In general, postoperative care resembles that for other abdominal surgeries. The patient is susceptible to fluctuations in adrenocortical hormones and requires administration of corticosteroids, fluids, and other agents to maintain blood pressure and prevent acute complications. If the adrenalectomy is bilateral, lifetime replacement of corticosteroids will be necessary. If one adrenal gland is removed, the replacement therapy may be only temporary because of the suppression of the remaining adrenal gland by high levels of adrenal hormones. A normal level of serum glucose is maintained with insulin, IV fluids, and dietary modifications. Hypokalemia resolves for all patients after surgery, but HTN may persist. Spironolactone (potassium-sparing diuretic) and eplerenone (aldosterone antagonist type of potassium-sparing diuretic) may be prescribed to control HTN and minimize hypokalemia.

Nursing Management

Nursing management during the postoperative period includes frequent assessment of vital signs to detect early signs and symptoms of adrenal insufficiency and crisis or hemorrhage. Explaining all treatments and procedures, providing comfort measures, and providing rest periods can reduce the patient's stress and anxiety level.

Clinical Judgment Case

A patient, J.K., is on your surgical unit after undergoing a lobectomy for small cell carcinoma of the left lung. Today is postoperative day 3 and the chest tube was recently removed by the surgeon. The left chest dressing is dry and intact. You have cared for J.K. for the past 2 days and notice today that the patient is increasingly lethargic. You assess vital signs at 2 PM which are: T 98.2° F, P 88 and regular, 16 RR with pulse oximetry of 96% on room air. B/P is 122/78. Physical examination reveals S1, S2 without murmur, gallop or rub; lungs are decreased breath sounds to mid on the left, crackles of left lower lobe; trach is midline; abdomen is soft, nondistended, nontender; bowel sounds (BS)+ in all 4 Q, + flatus; no BM. Pedal and posterior tibial pulses are 3+ bil, there is no peripheral edema, capillary refill is 2 seconds all extremities. Pupils equal and reacting to light (PEARL) 3 mm bil. Pt is moving all extremities, strength 5/5. Pt is oriented to person and place but not time and is increasing sluggish when you ask questions. Patient's diet was increased from clear liquids to full diet. However, the patient is now complaining of a headache. Morning laboratory data taken at 6 AM are as follows: Na of 125 mEq/L, K^+ of 3.7, Cl of 98, CO_2 25. Complete blood count (CBC) is within normal limits (WNL).

Step One: Recognize cues where relevant; important information is identified from different sources, such as medical history or vital signs.

Answer: From patient history: small cell carcinoma of the left upper lobe, post left lobectomy, post op day 3, chest tube removed, decreased lung sounds to mid on the left, crackles of left lower lobe, increasing lethargy, sluggish responses, oriented times 2 only (person and place), Na of 125 mEq/L at 6 AM. It is now 8 hours since blood draw. Recent complaint of headache.

Step Two: Analyze cues, which is organizing and linking the recognized cues to the patient's clinical presentation.

Answer: You realize that lung cancer is associated with the production of ADH-like hormone and associate the diagnosis with the early morning hyponatremia, the patient appearing euvolemic, the increasing lethargy and sluggishness, and the new complaint of a headache. You are concerned that the sodium has further decreased and the headache may be associated with brain swelling and increasing intracranial pressure (ICP).

You associate the decreased breath sounds and crackles with atelectasis postsurgical intervention. The oxygen saturation is stable; however, you will return to the patient and assess use of incentive spirometry and cough effort. If it is productive, you will note the color, amount, and consistency of the sputum. You are aware that the patient is afebrile and WBC are WNL.

Step Three: Form and prioritize hypotheses, where hypotheses are evaluated and ranked according to priority. This can include urgency, likelihood, risk, difficulty, and/or time. In this phase you cluster your findings to arrive at a list of problems (actual and or potential problems) you believe the patient is experiencing and determine the importance or urgency. What do you think is of greatest concern?

Answer: Your priority is to assess the sodium level again since your concern for SIADH outweighs your concern for atelectasis (stable oxygen saturation on room air). You will notify the surgeon about your concerns of decreasing orientation (2/4), decreasing sensorium, hyponatremia from this AM, and recent complaint of headache. You are aware that appearance of euvolemia is associated with SIADH. You are concerned about atelectasis of the left lung causing the crackles, but as noted above, given the oxygen saturation is WNL on room air and there is no fever, trach is midline (trach deviates toward an atelectasis), and WBC is WNL, the priorities are the increasing ICP and the potential for seizures.

Step Four: Generate solutions, which is identifying expected outcomes and using hypotheses to define a set of interventions for the expected outcomes.

Answer: You anticipate the need for repeat electrolytes, a serum and urine osmolality to evaluate if the hyponatremia has worsened and assessment of urine sodium. You anticipate removing the PO liquids and are aware that if SIADH is confirmed, a central line or peripherally inserted central catheter (PICC) may need to be placed due to the osmolality of 3% NaCl solution, and an IV pump is required. Seizure precautions will be initiated since seizures can occur with hyponatremia. You will remove patient's eyeglasses and ensure suction and oxygen are available at the bedside.

Step Five: Take action, where the solutions that address the highest priorities are implemented.

Answer: You notify the surgeon; a stat electrolyte panel is ordered, as are urine and serum osmolality and urine for sodium. The stat sodium is 119 mEq/L, and the serum osmolality is 265 mOsm/kg, and you recognize that the patient's I&O will be strictly monitored. Fluid restriction is initiated (800 mL per day or 400 mL per 12-hour shift). Since the patient had PO intake this AM you will remove the water pitcher from the bedside. You repeat the vital signs and neuro assessment. You are awaiting a consult from endocrinology and prepare for insertion of a central line or PICC, since the patient is symptomatic. You recognize that an IV of 3% sodium chloride (hypertonic saline) may be ordered. You also alert radiology that a portable chest film will be needed stat to confirm placement of the PICC or central line before it is used. Since 3% NaCl is hyperosmolar (513 mEq of Na and 513 mEq of Cl [1,026 mOsm/L]), it must be administered via a central line and IV pump. You ask the providers about administering furosemide IV to prevent extracellular fluid volume expansion by causing diuresis. You anticipate repeating labs Q4 hours and are aware that the sodium level should not rise more than 8 mEq/L during the first 24 hours to prevent osmotic demyelination syndrome (ODS), formerly referred to as central pontine myelinolysis (CPM). You institute seizure precautions to protect the patient from injury and prevent aspiration. Oxygen and suctioning equipment are already at the bedside. In the event of a seizure, your will lower the head of the bed (you have already removed the patient's eyeglasses). If a seizure occurs, you will place the patient on their side to prevent aspiration and protect the airway.

Step Six: Evaluate outcomes, which is comparing observed outcomes against expected outcomes.

Answer: By 6 PM, the patient's sodium is 121 mEq/L and the patient's headache is improving. Fluid restrictions are maintained. There has been no seizure activity. Endocrinology is now consulting, a PICC line was inserted, chest film confirmed placement, and 3% saline was initiated. The patient's sensorium has improved; they are now oriented to person, time, place, and situation. You continue to monitor the patient and are aware that the patient will require additional treatment. However, you were able to connect the patient's diagnosis, symptomatology, and lab work with SIADH. You were able to give the surgeon a comprehensive but succinct summary of your concerns and anticipated the additional lab work, potential need for central line insertion, and chest film to confirm placement; and you prepared for seizure precautions. Because of your anticipated needs and actions for the patient, care was delivered in a timely manner. Kudos to you, well done.

CHAPTER REVIEW

NCLEX-Style Review Questions

1. Upon evaluation of the patient's laboratory data and clinical signs and symptoms, the nurse suspects that the patient may have pheochromocytoma. Which of the following is directly related with pheochromocytoma? Select all that apply.

a. Severe headache; pain score of 9 out of 10
b. Diaphoresis
c. Blood pressure 80/90 mm Hg
d. Blood sugar of 160 mg/dL
e. Lethargy

2. A patient presented to the unit with an ADH-secreting tumor. Upon diagnostic and physical evaluation, the nurse suspects the patient is experiencing SIADH. Which of the following is a clinical manifestation of SIADH? Select all that apply.

a. Hyponatremia
b. Hypernatremia
c. Increased serum osmolality
d. Reduced serum osmolality
e. Dry mucous membranes
f. Low urine output

3. The nursing management of a patient who underwent a sublabial approach for transsphenoidal removal of a pituitary tumor yesterday includes which of the following actions? Select all that apply.

a. Providing oral care
b. Removing nasal pack to check for bleeding and CSF leak
c. Instructing the patient to avoid blowing the nose or using a straw for PO intake
d. Raising the head of the bed 15 to 30 degrees to promote drainage
e. Brushing teeth with a hard toothbrush to prevent bacterial overgrowth

4. A patient who has been taking high-dose corticosteroid therapy for approximately 2 months to treat a severe inflammatory condition, which has now resolved, asks you why they need to continue taking the corticosteroids. What is your best response? Select all that apply.

a. It is possible for the inflammation to recur when corticosteroid therapy is halted.
b. Corticosteroids are a type of hormone. Once you have been started on a replacement hormone, you must continue the hormone replacement therapy for the rest of your life.
c. The drug suppressed your own adrenal gland secretion of corticosteroids. Slowly decreasing the dose over time allows your adrenal glands to start adequate secretion again.
d. The drug suppressed your immune system while you were taking it. Slowly decreasing the dose over time prevents your immune system from starting up too quickly and initiating allergic reactions.
e. There should be no problem stopping the therapy since you have only been on it for 2 months.

5. A patient is admitted to your emergency room with a history of hyperthyroidism; they recently underwent dental extraction. The patient's vital signs on admission are as follows: T 104.7° F, HR 136, RR 32, O_2 sat is 92% on RA, B/P is 92/42. In Column 1 choose *three* actions to take; in Column 2 select *one* potential condition; and in Column 3 select *three* priority parameters to monitor.

Action to take	Potential condition	Parameters to monitor
Place patient on cardiac monitor	Addison disease	**Electrocardiogram**
Start a peripheral IV	Syndrome of inappropriate antidiuretic hormone (SIADH)	**Pulse oximetry**
Administer aspirin for the fever	**Thyroid storm or thyrotoxicosis**	Orthostatic blood pressure
Insert a Foley catheter	Hyperglycemia hyperosmolar nonketotic syndrome (HHNK)	**B/P monitoring**
Administer oxygen at 2 LPM via nasal cannula		Bowel sounds

REFERENCES AND SELECTED READINGS

References and selected readings associated with this chapter can be found on the website that accompanies the book. Visit **http://thepoint.lww.com/Honan3e** to access the references and other additional resources associated with this chapter.

UNIT NINE

Problems Related to Reproductive Function

A 40-year-old patient has been diagnosed with a low-grade squamous intraepithelial lesion of the cervix following an abnormal Pap test. Today the certified nurse midwife is seeing the patient for a follow-up visit to discuss the next steps. The patient is very worried about the prognosis.

- **Assess the patient's current knowledge of the diagnosis, readiness for information, and their concerns at this time.**
- **Discuss their possible diagnosis of cervical cancer, prognosis, and recommended next steps.**
- **What is the purpose of a colposcopy?**
- **Review postprocedure teaching and expectations.**
- **Discuss medical/surgical management of cervical cancer.**
- **Consider how a trauma-informed lens can be applied to this patient encounter.**

CHAPTER 31

Nursing Assessment: Assigned Female at Birth (AFAB) and Assigned Male at Birth (AMAB) Reproductive Function

Erin M. Morelli • Michelle L. Telfer • Susanne A. Quallich

Learning Objectives

After reading this chapter, you will be able to:

1. Describe the structures and functions of the reproductive system of a person assigned female at birth (AFAB).
2. Discuss the nursing assessment of the reproductive system of a person AFAB.
3. Describe structures and functions of the reproductive system of a person assigned male at birth (AMAB).
4. Discuss the nursing assessment of the reproductive system of a person AMAB.
5. Identify the recommended preventive screenings for the reproductive systems of patients AFAB and AMAB.
6. Understand the diagnostic tests that may be ordered by the provider to complement the assessment of the reproductive system for patients AFAB and AMAB.

ASSIGNED FEMALE AT BIRTH (AFAB) REPRODUCTIVE SYSTEM

This chapter seeks to use inclusive language. While many patients with a uterus and a vagina identify using words such as *woman* and *she, her, hers* and many with a penis use *man* and *he, his, him*, this does not apply to all patients. Therefore, one goal of this chapter is to introduce you, if you are not already familiar with it, to gender-inclusive terminology. It is of the utmost importance to ensure that nurses are mindful of the language patients prefer to use for identifying themselves and the parts of their bodies.

An understanding of the normal anatomy and physiology of the AFAB reproductive system is necessary and important for the nurse. It is integral to recognizing the complex issues that can occur within the reproductive system for those AFAB throughout the lifespan from menarche through menopause. Patients seeking health care for these body systems may be evaluated by a gynecologist, a certified nurse-midwife, or an advanced practice nurse practitioner (APRN).

ANATOMY AND PHYSIOLOGY OVERVIEW

Anatomy of the Assigned Female at Birth (AFAB) Reproductive System

The AFAB reproductive system consists of the external and internal genital structures as well as the mammary glands located on the chest. The hypothalamus and pituitary glands drive the reproductive system through the release and modulation of hormones. Hormones influence the cyclic changes throughout the reproductive life of a person, and the cessation of the changes results in menopause.

External Genitalia

The external genital structures, referred to as the vulva, consist of the mons pubis; labia majora; labia minora; clitoris; and the vestibule of the vagina, which contains the hymen, the urethral and vaginal orifice, and the greater vestibular glands (Bartholins) and the paraurethral glands (Skenes; Fig. 31-1). The mons pubis consists of fatty tissue at the junction of the thighs and torso, while the labia majora are two prominent cutaneous lateral folds of adipose tissue that form the outer border of the vulva. In addition to adipose tissue, they contain the distal ends of the round ligaments and a rich supply of sebaceous, apocrine, and eccrine sweat glands. Both lateral surfaces are covered by pubic hair after puberty, while the insides remain smooth and hairless. The labia minora are highly innervated, thinner, smooth, hairless folds of tissue internal to the labia majora that cover the urethral meatus and vaginal introitus. The upper portions of the labia minora unite anteriorly to form a partial covering or prepuce; the clitoris and posteriorly merge with the labia majora at the posterior fourchette (opening to vaginal vault). The labia minora is composed of thick connective tissue containing elastic fibers and small blood vessels, which forms erectile tissue

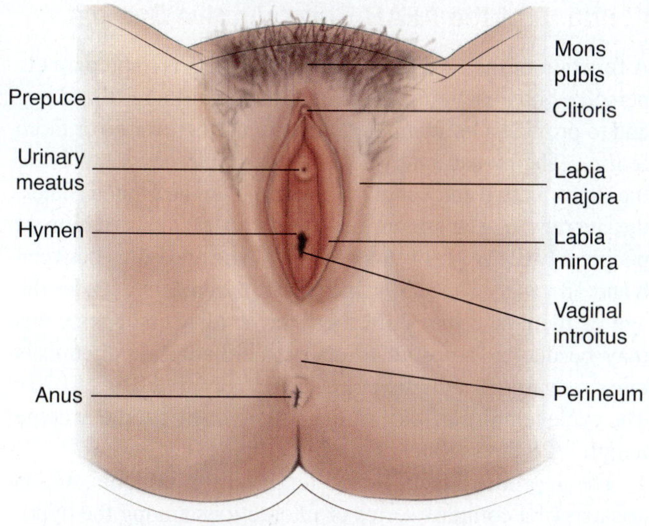

FIGURE 31-1 **External AFAB genitalia.**

similar to the penile corpus spongiosum. Normal variation of the dimensions of the labia minora can be significant and is not cause for concern. The average length ranges from 2 to 10 cm, and width varies from 0.7 to 5 cm, and the labia may be asymmetric. The clitoris, the most critical anatomic structure for AFAB sexual arousal and orgasm, is a complex structure with internal structures of paired crura, root, suspensory ligament, and vestibular bulbs and external structures of body or shaft, glans, and prepuce. It also has an intimate physiologic and anatomic relationship with the distal urethra and vagina, and the term "clitoral urethral complex" has been used to describe this important area. The clitoris is highly innervated, and the glans is made of erectile tissue that can range in length from 1 to 2 cm (Levin, 2018). The urethral meatus lies below and posterior to the clitoris, and the urethra connects to the bladder and can range from 4.8 cm to 5.1 cm in length (Shin et al., 2018). The vaginal introitus lies just posterior to the urethral meatus and is covered posteriorly by a thin membrane, the hymen. The hymen is a nonfunctional structure made of hairless skin that is variable in shape appearing as a ring or semilunar fold that can be disturbed at any point in the person's life by activities from bicycle or horseback riding, insertion of tampons and intercourse. This disruption of the hymenal tissue may be noticed as a brief painful episode followed by some spotting of blood or may not be noticed at all. The periurethral glands are mucus-secreting structures that are set in the wall of the urethra. The greater vestibular glands are bean-sized structures on each side of the vaginal orifice that also secrete mucus. The smooth, hairless area between the vagina and rectum is called the perineum and can vary in length from 2.5 to 5.0 cm; the perineum stretches, especially during childbirth or sexual arousal.

Internal Reproductive Structures

The internal structures of the AFAB reproductive system are the vagina, uterus, ovaries, and salpinges (Fig. 31-2).

The vagina is a dynamic canal that is lined with a mucous membrane that extends from the vulva to the cervix. The vagina serves as a barrier to the uterus being colonized by harmful bacteria. The vagina is colonized by healthy microbiota, including *Lactobacillus acidophilus*, that secrete lactic acid to reduce the chance of growth of pathogenic microorganisms (Chumduri & Turco, 2021). The walls of the vaginal vault are lined with rugae, ribbed or ruffled folds of skin, which stretch and expand during sexual arousal and birth. The upper part of the vagina, the **fornix**, surrounds the **cervix** (the inferior part of the uterus). The fornices are divided into anterior and superior in relation to the cervix. The uterus is a pear-shaped, muscular organ, which can vary in size depending on parity (number of births) and uterine abnormalities (e.g., fibroids). The uterus lies posterior to the bladder and is held in position by several ligaments. The uterus consists of the cervix, which projects into the vagina; the corpus or body of the uterus; and the fundus or uppermost part of the uterus. The uterus is composed of two layers, the myometrium or thick layer of smooth muscle, and the endometrium, the inner mucosal layer (Chumduri & Turco, 2021). The triangular inner portion of the fundus narrows to a small canal in the cervix that has constrictions at each end, referred to as the external os and internal os. The cervix acts as a physical barrier between the internal uterus and the external vaginal canal (Chumduri & Turco, 2021). The cervix is a dynamic tubular structure approximately 4 cm in length in a nongravid (nonpregnant) person; it is made up of collagen matrices that soften and change during the menstrual cycle and labor and birth. The cervix secretes mucus which changes throughout the menstrual cycle and can be used to help track fertility. The upper lateral parts of the uterus are called the cornua. From here, the oviducts, or salpinges (fallopian tubes), extend outward to meet the ovaries.

The **ovaries** lie behind and below the salpinges and are kept in place by the ovarian ligaments, which attach to the uterus. The ovaries have two functions: to act as an endocrine organ secreting estrogen and progesterone and to mature and release eggs (oocytes) for fertilization. They are oval bodies about 3 cm long (Chumduri & Turco, 2021). Ovaries contain

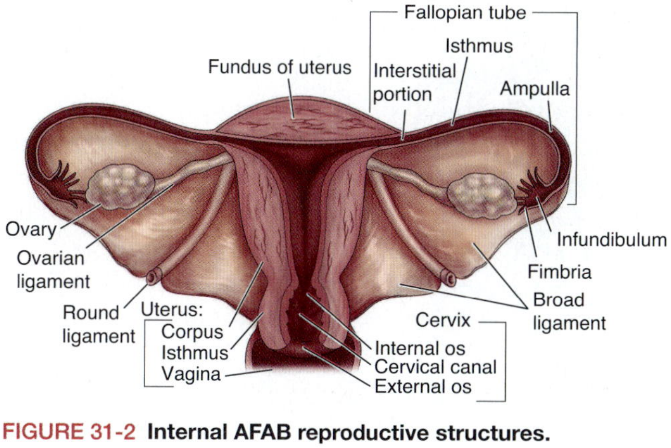

FIGURE 31-2 **Internal AFAB reproductive structures.**

thousands of tiny egg cells or *ova* that are present at the time of birth and decline in number as menarche begins. The ovaries and the salpinges together are referred to as the **adnexa**.

Breasts

The breasts lie over the pectoralis muscle from the sternum to the midaxillary line. Breast tissue is composed of milk glands, milk ducts, fascia, and fatty tissue. Breast tissue extends into the axilla and the axillary process (tail of Spence) and should be included in any breast palpation exam. Suspensory ligaments (Cooper ligaments) support the breast on the chest wall to the clavicle and help maintain the shape of the breast. Secondary breast development occurs during puberty and is known as **thelarche**, or breast budding. During puberty, a rise in estrogen stimulates growth of the adipose and ductal tissues, and progesterone causes lobular growth and alveolar budding. This development usually occurs from 10 to 16 years of age, although the range can vary from 8 to 18 years of age with a wide range of normal (Khaja & DeSilva, 2019). After puberty, the breasts are not considered fully developed as further development occurs during pregnancy and lactation.

Each fully developed breast (Fig. 31-3) is made up of glandular lobules and ducts bound and separated by fibrous tissue and fat. Approximately 15 to 20 lobules are grouped together to form cone-shaped lobes. Fibrous tissue surrounds the lobes and ducts. Fatty tissue fills the spaces between lobes and ducts and gives the breast a soft texture. During lactation, milk is produced in the lobules and is carried through the ducts to the areola. The areolae vary in size and color and contain sebaceous glands known as areolar glands (Montgomery tubercles), which provide lubrication and enlargement during pregnancy and lactation.

Function of the AFAB Reproductive System

A function of the AFAB reproductive system is to prepare the person's body each month for implantation of a fertilized egg and to provide a nourishing environment to grow one or more fetuses. The menstrual cycle is a complex process involving the reproductive and endocrine systems. In the United States, the average age at **menarche** (the start of menstruation in people AFAB) is 11.9 years of age with an age range between 8 and 18 years of age (Martinez, 2020). In recent decades the age of menarche has shifted earlier; evidence suggests this may be due to exposure to endocrine-disrupting chemicals or extraovarian production of estrogen (Smith & Biro, 2020). The cycle length can vary from 21 to 35 days, but the average length is 28 days (Ricci et al., 2021).

The reproductive cycle of females and patients AFAB consists of a complex series of interactions among the hypothalamic–pituitary system, the ovarian system, the endometrial system, and the various hormones secreted by each of those systems.

The Menstrual Cycle

Estrogen and progesterone are two hormones integral to proper functioning of the reproductive system for a patient with ovaries. The ovaries produce several types of **estrogen** as well as progesterone. Estrogen is responsible for development and maintenance of the reproductive organs, secondary sex characteristics of the adult AFAB, breast development, and the monthly uterine changes associated with menstruation. **Progesterone** plays a role in regulating uterine changes during the menstrual cycle; preparing the **endometrium**, via the **corpus luteum,** for implantation of a fertilized ovum; and maintaining pregnancy via the placenta (Ricci et al., 2021).

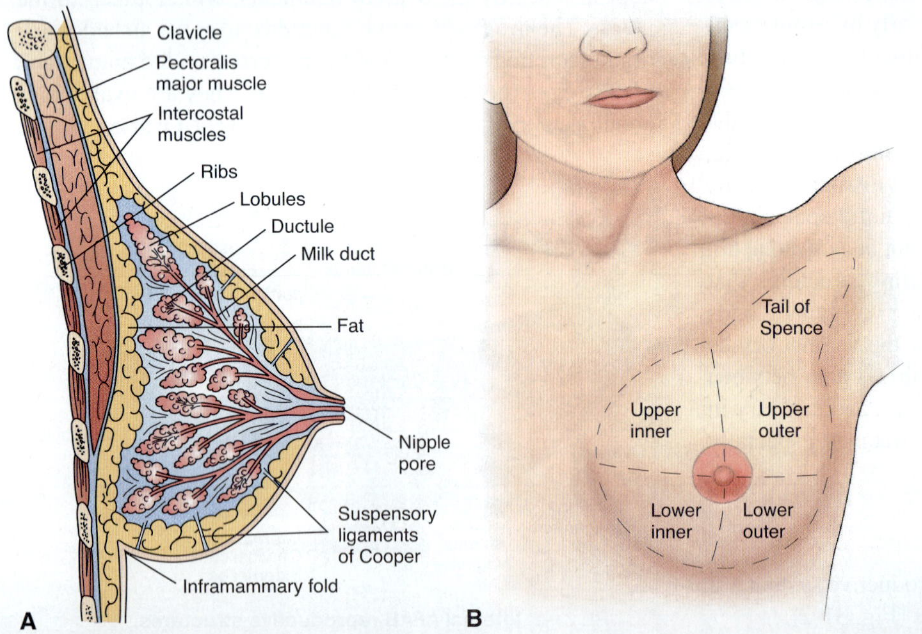

FIGURE 31-3 **A. Anatomy of the breast. B. Areas of breast, including the tail of Spence.**

Together, progesterone and estrogen and many other hormones help prepare the breasts for lactation (Alekseev, 2021). **Androgens** are hormones that are produced by the ovaries and the adrenals in small amounts; they influence early follicular development as well as the libido (Ricci et al., 2021).

In a patient AFAB, the pituitary gland releases the gonadotropic hormones **follicle-stimulating hormone** (FSH) and **luteinizing hormone** (LH). FSH is responsible primarily for stimulating the ovaries to secrete estrogen and triggering follicles in the ovary to mature into eggs, while LH is responsible primarily for stimulating progesterone production as well as encouraging the release of mature eggs. LH surges at the midpoint of the menstrual cycle and is secreted in the urine. Detection of urinary LH is the mechanism that is used in ovulation predictor kits that patients who are trying to conceive utilize. Another way for a patient to detect ovulation is by watching their cervical mucus and looking for mucus that resembles egg white: clear, slippery, and stretchy. Feedback mechanisms help to regulate secretion of FSH and LH. Elevated estrogen levels in the blood inhibit FSH secretion but promote LH secretion. Release of FSH and LH also is influenced by gonadotropin-releasing hormone (GnRH), which is secreted from the hypothalamus. This complex feedback system results in the cyclic changes in the uterine endometrium and ovaries as well as the process of menstruation (Table 31-1).

In the beginning of the menstrual cycle, low estrogen levels signal the hypothalamus to release FSH and begin follicular maturation. Maturing follicles release estrogen, which stimulates the release of LH. This surge of LH encourages **ovulation**, which is the release of the mature egg from the ovary. Ovulation generally occurs mid-way (14 days) through a typical 28-day menstrual cycle. The egg is released into the fallopian tubes, where it awaits fertilization. If fertilization does not occur, hormone levels decrease and the menstrual phase of the cycle begins.

Pearls for Practice

Some people are aware of the release of the egg from the ovary and note it as a cramp or pain on one side of the abdomen. This midcycle pain is called mittelschmerz (Ricci et al., 2021).

Menstruation is the cyclic shedding of the uterine endometrial lining that occurs when an egg is not fertilized. This menstrual flow is discharged through the cervix and into the

TABLE 31-1 Hormonal Influences and Menstrual Cycle

(Times approximate) Phase	Menstrual	Follicular	Ovulation	Luteal	Premenstrual
Day	1 2 3 4 5 6 7 8 9 10 11 12 13 14 15 16 17 18 19 20 21 22 23 24 25 26 27 28 1 2				
Ovary					
	Degenerating corpus luteum; beginning follicular development	Growth and maturation of follicle	Ovulation	Active corpus luteum	Degenerating corpus luteum
Estrogen Production					
	Low	Increasing	High	Decreasing, then a secondary rise	Decreasing
Progesterone Production					
	None	Low	Low	Increasing	Decreasing
FSH Production					
	Increasing	High, then decreasing	Low	Low	Increasing
LH Production					
	Low	Low, then increasing	High	High	Decreasing
Endometrium					
	Degeneration and shedding of superficial layer. Coiled arteries dilate and then constrict again.	Reorganization and proliferation of superficial layer	Continued growth	Active secretion and glandular dilation; highly vascular; edematous	Vasoconstriction of coiled arteries; beginning degeneration

vagina, and it usually lasts an average of 3 to 7 days. The amount of menstrual flow varies but averages 1 oz or a range of approximately 2/3 to 2-2/3 oz in volume per cycle. The beginning of the menstrual flow marks the end of one menstrual cycle and the start of a new one (Ricci et al., 2021).

Perimenopause

Perimenopause is the transition between the reproductive years and menopause. This transition begins with menstrual irregularities and is completed when menses have ceased for 1 year. The mean duration of perimenopause is 4 to 5 years, but symptoms may begin 8 years or more before the final menstrual period. The average age at onset of menstrual irregularity is 47.5 years of age. In addition to menstrual irregularities, there are vasomotor symptoms (VMS) such as hot flashes and night sweats. Psychological symptoms, sleep disturbances, sexual and urogenital dysfunction can occur (Guerin et al., 2022; Troìa et al., 2021). Up to 80% of people AFAB seek care for symptoms from providers during this period, making this an important point of contact for providers (Minkin, 2019). The decline in estrogen affects the vaginal mucosa, resulting in loss of rugae, elasticity, and an increase in pH often leading to itching, dryness, and dyspareunia (pain during sexual intercourse). Ovulatory cycles can be unpredictable and irregular, with surges of hormones leading to unintended pregnancies. Forty-eight percent of all pregnancies in patients in their 40s are unplanned, making this the second most common age cohort for unplanned pregnancies. This statistic shows the need for improved education and counseling of all people anticipating and experiencing perimenopause, especially for contraceptive needs. For many patients, hormonal contraception (with appropriate counseling) not only prevents unexpected pregnancies, but is often the most effective treatment for many of the perimenopausal symptoms (Troia et al., 2020). Each person experiences perimenopause differently and the variation in symptoms, their intensity, frequency, and duration is wide. Perimenopause is an important time to engage patients about strategies for health promotion and disease prevention beyond menopause, including cardiac, colon, lipid, and mental health changes.

Menopause

Menopause marks the end of reproductive capacity and generally occurs between 45 and 52 years of age. Menopause is defined retrospectively by 12 months of amenorrhea and loss of ovarian follicular activity. It is a major transition in a person's life and can be accompanied by a multitude of symptoms and health concerns. With menopause, the ovaries are no longer active, and the reproductive organs become smaller in the absence of estrogen. Menopause is not a pathologic phenomenon but a normal part of aging and maturation. In addition to the effects of reduced estrogen on the reproductive system, neuroendocrinologic, biochemical, and metabolic changes related to aging occur throughout the person's body (Table 31-2). Early menopause may occur if the ovaries are surgically removed or are destroyed by radiation or chemotherapy, or because of an unknown etiology. For many people, menopause may be a liberating time, free from the worries of conception and reproduction. Others may view it more negatively as it connotes aging, and many experience symptoms that interfere with day-to-day life. In addition to the side effects on the physical body, psychosocial changes that many go through at the same time include children leaving or returning home,

TABLE **31-2 Changes in the AFAB Reproductive System During Perimenopause and Menopause**

Structural Change	Functional Change	Symptoms and Physical Findings
Cessation of ovarian function and decreased estrogen production; thinning of urinary and genital tracts; thinning of pubic hair and atrophy of the labia and vagina Metabolic changes	Decreased ovulation Onset of perimenopause and menopause Vasomotor instability and hormonal fluctuations Decreased bone formation, bone loss Decreased vaginal lubrication Increased vaginal pH Slower metabolism, changes in fat distribution and storage	Decreased/lost ability to conceive; increased infertility or unexpected pregnancy Irregular menses with eventual cessation of menses Hot flashes or flushing; night sweats, sleep disturbances; mood swings; fatigue Psychological changes (depression, anxiety) Increased risk for osteoporosis and osteoporotic fractures; loss of height Dyspareunia Increased risk for urinary tract infection Increased incidence of inflammation (atrophic vaginitis) with discharge, itching, and vulvar burning Decreased libido and sexual satisfaction Weight gain
Relaxation of pelvic musculature	Prolapse of uterus, cystocele, rectocele	Dyspareunia, urinary incontinence, constipation and difficulty with bowel elimination, feelings of perineal pressure or protrusion of organs

care of older family members, partner issues, and challenges in the workforce related to aging (Minkin, 2019). By considering a patient's concerns, values, and preferences, nurses have the potential to support and enhance a patient's sense of well-being, not only at menopause but for the rest of their life (Santen et al., 2020). Box 31-1 discusses the management of symptoms and nursing care of patients in perimenopause and menopause.

BOX 31-1

Assessment and Management of Perimenopause and Menopausal Symptoms

The multitude of symptoms a person experiences during perimenopause and through menopause vary widely from person to person in the onset, duration, intensity, and impact on day-to-day function and health. Patients approaching menopause often have many concerns about their health based on family histories including heart disease, osteoporosis, or cancer. Symptoms need to be evaluated carefully as they also may indicate other more serious disorders.

Each patient's experience must be considered on an individual basis, and nurses need to be sensitive to the range of patients' feelings toward this significant change in their lives. Patients' reactions and feelings related to loss of reproductive capacity may vary. Some patients may experience role confusion, whereas others experience a sense of sexual and personal freedom. Each person needs to be as knowledgeable as possible about their options and should be encouraged to discuss their concerns in order to make an informed decision about managing symptoms and maintaining their health.

Vasomotor Symptoms (VMS)

Seventy-five percent of menopausal patients experience VMS persisting on average 4–5 years, but for nearly 25% they will persist as long as 10 years (Santoro et al., 2021). VMS vary in intensity from a barely perceptible warm feeling from time to time to a sensation of extreme warmth accompanied by profuse sweating, sometimes multiple times an hour, causing discomfort, sleep disturbances, and subsequent fatigue. Treatment of these symptoms can include nonprescription therapies; prescription nonhormonal therapy; and hormone therapy (HT), which includes contraceptives during the perimenopausal time.

Nonprescription therapies include simple lifestyle changes to reduce VMS, such as avoiding alcohol and other potential triggers; wearing layered clothing; use of fans and cooling mattresses at night; relaxation techniques, such as slow breathing and yoga; and exercise (Minkin, 2019). While patients widely use herbal products and vitamins, there is little evidence to demonstrate efficacy beyond the placebo effect. Soy, a weak plant estrogen, has been demonstrated to have a modest effect on VMS, though it remains controversial with concerns of stimulating breast tissue. Any patient at increased breast cancer risk should discuss the use of any supplement, especially those with soy, with their oncologist (Minkin, 2019).

Prescription nonhormonal therapies include selective serotonin reuptake inhibitors (SSRIs) and selective norepinephrine reuptake inhibitors (SNRIs), which have been shown to reduce hot flashes even at lower doses than used for depression; however, if a patient is also experiencing depression and anxiety these may be most beneficial at optimal dosing (Minkin, 2019).

Prescription Hormonal Therapy (HT)

Through the perimenopausal period, hormonal contraceptives offer an excellent option for both symptomatic treatments and for prevention of unplanned pregnancy. A recent systematic review found the levonorgestrel-intrauterine device (IUD) with additional estrogen when indicated at the lowest dose for the shortest period to provide the most effective relief of symptoms with the best long-term benefits for those with a uterus. Other combined hormonal contraceptives and progesterone-only methods can be used but may have more bleeding and less efficacy for symptoms (Guerin et al., 2022). Menopausal HT went through a controversial period after the 2002 publication of the Women's Health Initiative, after which there was a dramatic decline in the usage of HT. With further results and context, HT is the most effective intervention for menopausal symptoms including VMS and genitourinary; it also prevents bone loss and fracture (Minkin, 2019).

Estrogens: Transdermal forms of estradiol are the recommended forms; these include patches, gels, sprays, and a vaginal ring. The major contraindications to estrogen are undiagnosed vaginal bleeding, previous breast cancer, coronary heart disease, severe liver disease, and personal history of thromboembolic disease. Transdermal estrogens are not associated with increased thromboembolic events.

Progestogens: Patients with a uterus need to take a progestogen when taking systemic estrogen to reduce the risk of endometrial hyperplasia or cancer. Transdermal patches, oral, vaginal, and IUDs are all acceptable methods of delivery. Side effects can include breast tenderness, mood swings, and bleeding.

Nonestrogen therapies: Paroxetine is the only FDA-approved nonhormonal therapy approved for VMS. Gabapentin has shown benefits compared to a placebo in several studies to reduce VMS (Minkin, 2019; Santoro et al., 2021).

Mood Swings, Headaches, Cognitive Symptoms, Depression and Anxiety

Patients with a history of depression are at increased risk, but 16% of those with no previous history will experience new-onset depression and/or anxiety during menopause. Hormone changes and neurosteroids are believed to play a role in increasing vulnerability to depression during this time (Santoro et al., 2021).

Nonpharmacologic methods to manage these symptoms are similar to those for VMS and include mindfulness, meditation, yoga, physical activity, and cognitive behavioral therapy. Avoidance of alcohol, caffeine, a sedentary lifestyle, and other potential triggers can be helpful.

Pharmacologic therapies include HT as well as SSRIs and SNRIs as discussed above.

(*continued*)

BOX 31-1 **Assessment and Management of Perimenopause and Menopausal Symptoms (*continued*)**

Genitourinary Symptoms

Genitourinary syndrome of menopause (GSM) is a term that includes various symptoms and signs including genital symptoms (atrophy, dryness, burning), sexual symptoms (dyspareunia, impaired function), and urinary symptoms (urgency, incontinence, urinary tract infections; Pertyńska-Marczewska & Pertyński, 2021). Many patients may be reluctant to disclose these symptoms, though they can significantly impact quality of life. It is important for the nurse to ask about these symptoms during routine exams and provide anticipatory education and guidance.

Nonpharmacologic therapies include the use of pH-balanced lubricants and pelvic floor physical therapy. There is one nonhormonal pharmacologic therapy, ospemifene, which stimulates moisture in the vagina and is taken orally daily. Topical dehydroepiandrosterone (DHEA), called prasterone, can also be used for GSM; while not technically HT, its mechanism of action is to stimulate estrogen and androgens in the vaginal cells (Minkin, 2019).

Estrogen HT, discussed above, is the most effective therapy for GSM for the appropriate patient and includes transdermal patch, vaginal rings, creams, and oral sprays (Santoro et al., 2021).

Finding the right approach for each patient will require a careful assessment of symptoms, health history, and the goals and preferences of the patient. Treatment plans should be a shared decision-making process that will evolve over time as symptoms change and ebb. There is no definitive time for stopping HT, and the American Congress of Obstetrics and Gynecologists 2018 Committee Opinion "recommends against routine discontinuation of systemic estrogen at age 65 years" and instead recommends HT should be individualized as with those younger (American College of Obstetricians and Gynecologists [ACOG], 2018; Minkin, 2019).

The decisions patients make related to the use of HT must be individualized and based on each patient's current health, risk factors, family history, and severity of symptoms.

ASSESSMENT

Nurses obtaining health history information and performing physical assessments are in an ideal position to discuss health issues, health promotion, and health-related concerns of the reproductive system. Relevant topics include contraception, mental health, physical activity, nutrition, cardiovascular risks, health screening, sexuality, menopause, safety and violence screening, health risk behaviors, and immunizations. Recommendations for health screening are summarized in Table 31-3. Screening and health history are key to early recognition of ways to optimize health.

Sexuality and sexual function are often discussed with providers in the gynecologic and obstetric care arenas, but all nurses should consider these issues part of a routine health assessment.

Health History

In addition to obtaining a general health history, information related to past health issues and experiences specific to reproductive health are necessary. It is important for the nurse to create a welcoming, inclusive, and nonjudgmental environment.

Pearls for Practice

Nurses should share their pronouns and inquire about the patient's pronouns and preferred name.

In addition to basic information related to medical and surgical history, data should be collected about the following:

- Menstrual history (including menarche, length of cycles, length and amount of flow, bleeding between periods or after intercourse, bleeding after menopause), pain with menses, pain with intercourse, pelvic pain
- Sexual history, including contraceptive use, pregnancy intention, sexual health, sexual practices, sexual orientation, history of sexually transmitted infections (STIs), and current use of STI protection. Risk reduction is the framework of these sexual history questions; rooting the questions around number of partners is often not helpful. Consider focusing more on if there have been any new partners since their last visit and offering STI screening to all patients to allow those who may not feel comfortable answering questions to opt in (Mintz & Moore, 2022)
- History of abnormal Pap tests, date of last Pap test, history of HPV vaccination
- Obstetric history (number of pregnancies, outcomes of pregnancies)
- Exposure to medications (immunosuppressive agents, diethylstilbestrol [DES], others)
- Current medication use (prescriptions, over-the-counter [OTC], vitamins, herbs, supplements)
- Vaginal symptoms: abnormal discharge, odor, or itching
- History of urinary problems: urinary function, including frequency, urgency, and incontinence
- History of bowel problems: constipation, irritable bowel syndrome, Crohn disease
- History of or current fertility treatments or hormone therapy
- History of breast health
- History or current sexual, physical, or emotional abuse
- History of surgery or other procedures on structures within the reproductive tract or breasts (including female genital cutting/circumcision [FGC] and breast augmentation/reduction)
- History of chronic illness or disability that may affect health status, reproductive health, need for health screening, or access to health care

TABLE 31-3 **Summary of Health Screening and Counseling Issues for Patients AFAB[a]**

Component	Screening and Counseling		
	Ages 19–39	**Ages 40–64**	**Ages 65+**
Sexual and reproductive health issues	Pelvic examination if indicated Annual clinical breast examination Contraceptive needs vs. preconception care Sexual health and satisfaction High-risk sexual behaviors	Pelvic examination if indicated Annual clinical breast examination Contraceptive needs vs. preconception care Sexual health and satisfaction High-risk sexual behaviors Menopausal concerns	Pelvic examination if indicated Annual clinical breast examination Sexual health and satisfaction High-risk sexual behaviors Menopausal concerns
Health and risk behaviors	Hygiene Injury prevention Nutrition Exercise patterns Risk for interpersonal violence Use of tobacco, drugs, and alcohol Life stresses Immunizations	Hygiene Bone loss and injury prevention Nutrition Exercise patterns Risk for interpersonal violence Use of tobacco, drugs, and alcohol Life stresses Immunizations	Hygiene Bone loss and injury prevention Nutrition Exercise patterns Risk for interpersonal violence Use of tobacco, drugs, and alcohol Life stresses Immunizations
Screening tests to consider	Pap test Screening for sexually transmitted infections (STIs) as indicated	Pap test Mammography[b] Cholesterol and lipid profile Fasting glucose Colorectal cancer screening Bone mineral density testing Thyroid-stimulating hormone testing Hearing and eye examinations Screening for sexually transmitted infections (STIs) as indicated	Pap test Mammography Cholesterol and lipid profile Fasting glucose Colorectal cancer screening Bone mineral density testing Thyroid-stimulating hormone testing Hearing and eye examinations Screening for sexually transmitted infections (STIs) as indicated

[a]Each individual's risks (family history, personal history) influence the need for specific assessments and their frequency.

[b]Recent recommendations include regular screening with mammography at age 50 and then every 2 years through 74 years of age.

Data from http://www.ahrq.gov/professionals/clinicians-providers/guidelines-recommendations/guide/cpsguide.pdf.

- Psychosocial information (availability of resources and support)
- Family history of breast or reproductive tract disorders

(Bonifacino & Corbelli, 2021)

Sexual History

Incorporation of the sexual health history into the general health history can provide the opportunity to clarify myths and explore areas of concern that the patient may not have felt comfortable discussing in the past.

Pearls for Practice

Nurses should reflect on their comfort and biases prior to beginning to take sexual health histories.

The nurse can begin by explaining the purpose of obtaining a sexual history and reiterating that all that is shared is confidential. It can sometimes be helpful to normalize with the patient that these conversations are a common part of health care. Patients use a variety of terms when describing their anatomy and sexual practices. History-taking includes gathering data about present and past sexual activity, sexual orientation, types of sexual activity the patient engages in, sexual satisfaction, and function/dysfunction. It is also important to discuss intentions around pregnancy. Sexual complications may be related to medication, life changes, disability, or the onset of physical or mental illness. By initiating an assessment about sexual concerns, the nurse can provide a safe environment for discussing sensitive topics as well as validation that these topics are appropriate for discussion (Mintz & Moore, 2022).

Sexually Transmitted Infections

Individual risk for STIs should be assessed during the patient interview. Risk is much higher for patients who are not using barrier methods of protection such as condoms and dental dams consistently and when they have sexual encounters with new partners. Patients should understand that certain STIs (e.g., chlamydia and gonorrhea) can be asymptomatic and if left untreated can result in pelvic inflammatory disease, ectopic pregnancy, and infertility. Risk-reduction discussion and preventive health care should be the framework for these conversations with patients (Brookmeyer et al., 2021; Mintz & Moore, 2022). (For further details, refer to Chapter 34.)

Female Genital Cutting/Circumcision

FGC includes procedures that intentionally alter or cause injury to the vulva, clitoral structures, and vagina, for nonmedical reasons, sometimes including partial or total removal of the external genitalia or narrowing of the vaginal opening. FGC is carried out mostly on young girls at some point between infancy and age 15 in some cultures. There are more than 200 million girls and females alive today who have experienced FGC in the 30 countries in Africa and the Middle East where FGC is concentrated (World Health Organization [WHO], 2022). FGC is carried out mostly by traditional circumcisers, who often play other central roles in communities, such as attending childbirths; however, approximately 26% of all FGC is performed by health care providers, and the trend toward medicalization is increasing (Leye et al., 2019). The causes of FGC include a mix of cultural, religious, and social factors within families and communities. FGC is considered to be a rite of passage and is a culturally acceptable practice as it is believed to promote hygiene, protect virginity and family honor, prevent promiscuity, improve female attractiveness and male sexual pleasure, and enhance fertility (WHO, 2022). There are four types of FGC (Table 31-4).

From a medical perspective, FGC has no health benefits, and it harms patients in many ways. Immediate complications can include severe pain, shock, hemorrhage, tetanus or sepsis, urinary retention, open sores in the genital region, and injury to nearby genital tissue. Long-term consequences can include recurrent infections in the bladder and urinary tract, painful menses, cysts, infertility, an increased risk of childbirth complications and newborn deaths, and the need for later surgeries. Patients who have undergone FGC may not think of themselves as harmed. Nurses who care for these patients must be sensitive, be knowledgeable, maintain cultural humility, and remain nonjudgmental. Respect for others' health beliefs, practices, and behaviors and recognition of the complexity of issues involved are crucial (WHO, 2022).

TABLE **31-4 Types of Female Genital Cutting (FGC)**

Type	Description
Type 1 FGM (Clitoridectomy)	Partial or total removal of the clitoris (a small, sensitive, and erectile part of the female genitals) and, rarely, the prepuce (the fold of skin surrounding the clitoris) as well
Type II FGM (Excision)	Clitoridectomy with partial or total excision of the labia minora, with or without excision of the labia majora
Type III FGM (Infibulation)	Narrowing of the vaginal opening through the creation of a covering seal, formed by cutting and repositioning the inner or outer labia, with or without the removal of the clitoris. Type III is more likely than other types of FGM to result in infertility.
Type IV FGM (Other)	All other harmful procedures to the AFAB genitalia for nonmedical purposes, e.g., pricking, piercing, incising, scraping, and cauterizing the genital area.

Data from World Health Organization. (2022). *Female genital mutilation*. https://www.who.int/news-room/fact-sheets/detail/female-genital-mutilation.

Domestic and Family Violence

Domestic violence is a broad term that includes child abuse, older adult abuse, and abuse of adults. Abuse can be emotional, physical, sexual, or economic, and it involves fear of one partner by another and control by threats; intimidation; neglect; bullying; repressing; defacing; stalking; criticizing; physical, emotional, and/or sexual abuse; and financial exploitation (Annals of Emergency Medicine, 2019; WHO, 2021). The majority of victims are AFAB—"globally, an estimated 27% of females and girls aged 15 years or older have experienced physical or sexual Intimate Partner Violence (IPV)—but high rates of IPV are also experienced by other groups, including sexual and gender minorities, people with disabilities, migrants, and people from marginalised (sic) ethnic or Indigenous groups" (Oram et al., 2022). As many as 10 million people in the United States are affected by domestic and family violence, and the number is expected to rise as the population ages (Houseman & Semien, 2022). Although all patients are at potential risk for abuse, factors that elevate risk include young age, substance and alcohol use disorder, mental health disorders, marital discord, low education, pregnancy, history of abuse as a child, unemployment, new HIV diagnosis, and economic hardships, among others (Houseman & Semien, 2022). The COVID-19 pandemic, which required people to stay in their own homes, increased the risk for domestic and family violence. Although it remains underreported, a 60% increase in emergency calls due to domestic violence was recently reported in Europe (Mahase, 2020). Violence is rarely a one-time occurrence in a relationship; it usually continues and escalates in severity. All patients should be screened for domestic violence but in particular those who are pregnant should be screened over the course of the pregnancy, including at the first prenatal visit, at least once per trimester, and at the postpartum checkup; the estimates of perinatal emotional, physical or sexual abuse affect 28.4%, 13.8%, and 8% of pregnant people during those times, respectively (Stewart et al., 2017; Wong et al., 2022). Given the prevalence of domestic and family violence, the nurse should maintain a high index of suspicion and screen patients using trauma-informed care (TIC) interventions (discussed shortly). Institutional protocols should be followed regarding referral, documentation, and follow-up.

Incest and Childhood Sexual Abuse

As many as 1 in 12 patients have experienced childhood sexual abuse (McNiss et al., 2021). Victims of sexual assault are more likely to suffer from depression or posttraumatic stress disorder, abuse alcohol or drugs, and contemplate suicide. The nurse should plan to offer support and appropriate referrals to psychiatric mental health professionals, community resources, and self-help groups (Kim et al., 2021).

Rape, Sexual Assault, Abuse, and Human Trafficking

In 2019, there were an estimated 463,634 victims of rape and sexual assault in the United States. That means every 68 seconds, a person is sexually assaulted in the United States. Most episodes of sexual assault are not reported. Screening for abuse, rape, violence, and human trafficking should be part of the routine assessment for all health visits because patients often do not report or seek treatment for assault. Often, the assailant is a partner, spouse, or date (ACOG, 2020; Rape, Abuse & Incest National Network [RAINN], 2022). Eighty-seven percent of victims of human trafficking reported that they came into contact with a health care professional who did not recognize that they were being trafficked. Trafficking is a global challenge with more than 40 million people experiencing human trafficking (Peck & Doiron, 2022).

Nurses need to be prepared to look for signs of abuse, violence, and trafficking. While none of these signs guarantee that a patient is experiencing abuse or being trafficked, it should cause the nurse to further assess for safety.

These signs may include:

- a disconnect between the history shared and the clinical picture
- bruises in various stages of healing
- repeated visits after incidents of personal injury—often blamed on clumsiness
- presenting for care with a companion who is overly involved in the visit or refuses to leave the patient alone in the exam room
- patient not making eye contact with the person who brings them to the visit or with health care team members
- a support person who insists on translating
- a support person who holds onto all documents such as identification cards and insurance cards
- answers to questions that seem to be memorized or scripted
- age of the patient that does not match the clinical appearance
- burns, branding, or other physical signs of ownership

Nurses who suspected a patient is a victim of abuse, assault, or trafficking should ask additional questions about the patient's living and working environments such as:

- Can you leave your home and workspaces freely?
- Are you afraid of anyone you see daily in your home or workplace?
- Has anyone threatened you?
- Are you able to spend time with friends and other family members as you wish?
- Has anyone forced you to use drugs or alcohol?

(Costa et al., 2019)

Nurses who identify victims should share resources and engage with the health care team regarding the optimal plan of care for the patient. This may include giving resources to the patient, helping the patient to make a safety plan, or sometimes involving the police or the Department of Children and Families.

For more information on resources:
https://www.thehotline.org
https://humantraffickinghotline.org/

Pearls for Practice

Some nurses receive additional training in forensic nursing and become sexual assault nurse examiners (SANEs). They provide high-quality tailored care for patients in acute settings following sexual assault and violence and collect specimens for use by law enforcement (Shaw & Coates, 2021).

Physical Assessment

The nurse can use the physical assessment time to educate patients on their reproductive health, including normal physiologic processes, like menstruation and menopause, and to assess possible abnormalities. This section focuses on physical assessment, including gynecologic and breast examinations. Many patients have a gynecologic examination as part of their physical. The gynecologic portion is often the last portion of the physical examination as care providers tend to move from less sensitive areas to more sensitive ones. This also gives the patient a chance to become comfortable with the examination and their provider. Recommendations for frequency of breast and pelvic examinations have changed over time. Current guidelines advise that a pelvic exam be performed "when indicated by medical history or symptoms" (ACOG, 2018).

Trauma-Informed Care (TIC)

Approximately half of American patients have experienced at least one traumatic event in their lifetime. It is essential that the nurse takes this into account when interviewing patients for their health history and when providing care. TIC is a concept that includes centering the patient and ensuring that the provision of care does not retraumatize them. It also includes being aware of the frequency of trauma and recognizing when a patient may be a current victim and screening and supporting them appropriately (Guest, 2021). There are six key principles that have been identified by the Substance Abuse and Mental Health Services Administration (SAMHSA): safety; trustworthiness and transparency; peer support; collaboration; empowerment; and gender, historical, and cultural humility and responsiveness (Trauma-Informed Care Implementation Resource Center, 2021). TIC is a broad concept that extends far beyond the reproductive health assessment; however, the focus here will be on how to bring this important lens to each patient encounter.

Nurses will provide care for patients with infections or pregnancies related to sexual assault who require support, understanding, and comprehensive care. Patients who have experienced rape or sexual abuse may be very anxious about pelvic or breast examinations, labor, pelvic or breast irradiation, or any treatment or examination that involves hands-on treatment or requires removal of clothing. This is one area where TIC is absolutely required.

During a trauma-informed health visit, the provider:

- invites the patient to share their goals for the visit;
- obtains consent from the patient before proceeding in each step of the visit;
- explains each part of the visit and clarifies as needed;
- asks permission before touching the patient;
- maintains eye contact with the patient;
- uses draping to cover all body parts not being examined;
- offers modifications, such as self-collection of swabs or self-insertion of speculum;
- invites the patient to get into a position that makes them most comfortable (including not using footrests for pelvic examinations);
- strives to be positioned at the same level of the patient to not assert dominance;
- stops immediately if the patient requests it or enquires about ceasing if the patient appears uncomfortable; and
- includes the patient in decision-making about their plan of care.

(White et al., 2022)

Consent

Informed consent includes a discussion of the risks and benefits of the proposed examination or treatment. Complete consent also discusses the alternatives and the option of no exam and no treatment. With TIC, treatment is not withheld in order to coerce the patient to consent. A certified medical interpreter should be used for staff or providers who do not share the same language as the patient; a provider may also be certified in the patient's language as an interpreter. Consent should not be interrupted or coerced by the support person/people who the patient brings with them to the visit. If a patient does not consent, it should be documented as "patient declined" or "patient decided against" as it is more respectful of patient autonomy than "patient refused" (Tillman, 2020).

Breast Examination

The American Cancer Society (ACS) recommends that females and patients AFAB at average risk for breast cancer undergo a clinical breast examination at least every 3 years while in their 20s and 30s and then annually thereafter (see Chapter 32). In the normal progression of a general physical examination, the breasts would be examined before the genitals as the provider moves from "head to toe." Before the examination, the patient should be asked if they have any known palpable masses and if there is any associated pain, swelling, redness, nipple discharge, or skin changes.

Research has not shown a clear benefit of regular physical breast exams done by either a health provider (clinical breast exams) or by the patient themself (breast self-exams). There is little evidence that these tests help detect breast cancer early when the patient also has screening mammograms. Most often, breast cancer is detected because of symptoms (such as a lump), or a patient discovers the symptom during usual activities such as bathing or dressing. Patients should be familiar with how their breasts normally look and feel and report any changes to a health care provider right away (ACS, 2022). Breast cancers that are found because they are causing symptoms tend to be larger and are more likely to have already spread beyond the breast. In contrast, breast cancers found during screening examinations are more likely to be smaller and still confined to the breast (ACS, 2022).

Inspection

Examination begins with inspection. The patient disrobes to the waist and sits in a comfortable position facing the examiner. The breasts are inspected for size and symmetry. A slight variation in size between the breasts is common and generally normal. Inspect the skin for color, venous pattern, thickening, and edema. Nipple inversion of one or both breasts is common and is significant only when of recent origin. Ulceration or rashes require evaluation. Then the breasts are inspected while the patient raises both arms overhead and again while they place their hands on their waist, pushing their shoulders in. These movements cause contraction of the pectoral muscles and should not alter the breast contour or nipple direction. Dimpling or retraction observed during these position changes suggests an underlying mass. The nurse observes for deep pin-point dimpling of the skin similar to an orange's skin (termed *peau d'orange*), which is associated with carcinoma. The clavicular and axillary regions are visually inspected before palpation (Bickley, 2020).

Erosions. Very small erosions (1 to 2 mm) of the nipple epithelium may be the only manifestation of Paget carcinoma (a rare type of breast cancer that occurs in the ducts adjacent to the nipple and areola and spreads to the skin of the nipple and the areola). It accounts for less than 3% of breast cancers and may be associated with ductal carcinoma in situ (DCIS). It is often not seen on mammograms and is only diagnosed by biopsy (Sisti et al., 2020). Refer to Chapter 32 for additional details.

Nipple Discharge. A more common issue providers may find affecting the nipple is discharge. Nipple discharge in a person who is not lactating may be related to many causes. Any discharge that is spontaneous, persistent, or unilateral is of concern. Clear discharge on expression is usually normal, while green discharge could indicate an infection. Bloody discharge does not always indicate malignancy. Tumors of

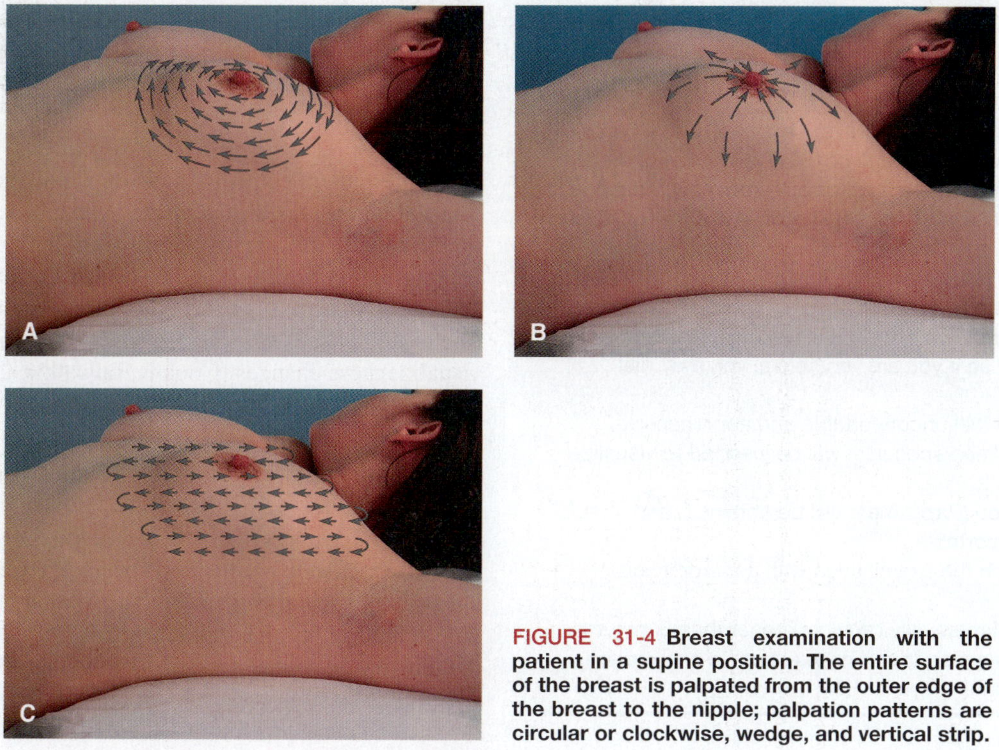

FIGURE 31-4 **Breast examination with the patient in a supine position. The entire surface of the breast is palpated from the outer edge of the breast to the nipple; palpation patterns are circular or clockwise, wedge, and vertical strip.**

the pituitary or thyroid gland or brain, encephalitis (a brain infection), and head injuries also can cause a nipple discharge. Oral contraceptives, pregnancy, hypertension, chlorpromazine-type medications, and frequent breast stimulation may be contributing factors. Among patients who have an abnormal discharge, benign conditions are much more common than breast cancer; in fact, breast cancer is the cause in approximately 5% to 12% of cases (Barsic et al., 2022). However, if a patient AMAB has nipple discharge, the likelihood of malignancy is 23% to 57% and should be evaluated immediately (Gupta et al., 2021).

Discharge from one breast is likely to be caused by a problem with that breast, such as a noncancerous or cancerous breast tumor. Discharge from both breasts is more likely to be caused by a problem outside the breast, such as an imbalance of hormones made by the pituitary or thyroid gland or by medications. If nipple discharge persists for more than one menstrual cycle or seems unusual to the patient, they should seek evaluation. Postmenopausal patients who have nipple discharge should seek evaluation promptly.

Pearls for Practice

Patients should be asked about the presence of nipple discharge during history-taking. If no discharge has been noted by the patient, then the provider should not attempt to elicit discharge during the physical exam (Bickley, 2020).

Palpation

Both breasts are palpated with the patient sitting up (upright) and lying down (supine) with the ipsilateral (same side) arm above or behind their head to flatten tissue as much as possible. The entire surface of the breasts and axillary tails are palpated systematically in progression from superficial tissue to deeper tissue. The finger pads of the examiner, not the fingertips, are generally used. There are several methods of palpation techniques: Concentric circles, rows, "wagon wheel" or vertical strips can all be utilized. However, it is important that the provider chooses a method and is consistent to improve accuracy in dime-sized circles, from the outer limits of the breast toward the nipple in a clockwise direction (Fig. 31-4). If a mass is detected, it is described by its location (e.g., left breast, 2 cm from the nipple at 2 o'clock position). Size, shape, consistency, border delineation, and mobility are included in the description. Different phases of the menstrual cycle cause changes in the breast tissue.

Pelvic Examination

The pelvic portion of the assessment consists of external and internal inspection and palpation of structures and organs. Gynecologic examinations may be uncomfortable or even distressing for some patients. It is important, then, that the nurse employs assessment techniques that help patients feel more comfortable and less vulnerable. It is important to minimize the inherent power differential of patient and health care team members (O'Laughlin et al., 2021). Patient education is essential as appropriate and accurate information can help to minimize the fear and negative feelings that some associate with gynecologic examinations (Box 31-2).

Before the examination begins, the patient should be offered to empty their bladder. The nurse should explain to

BOX 31-2
Patient Education

Pelvic Examination

A pelvic examination includes assessment of the appearance of the vulva, vagina, and cervix and the size and shape of the uterus and ovaries to ensure reproductive health and absence of illness. The nurse should share the following information with the patient in order to help make the examination proceed more smoothly:

- You may have a feeling of fullness or pressure during the examination, but you should not feel pain. It is important to relax because if you are very tense, you may feel discomfort.
- It is normal to feel uncomfortable and apprehensive.
- A narrow, warmed speculum will be inserted to visualize the cervix.
- A Papanicolaou (Pap) smear will be obtained, and should not be uncomfortable.
- You may watch the examination with a mirror if you choose.
- The examination usually takes no longer than 5 minutes.
- Draping will be used to minimize exposure and reduce embarrassment.

the patient that this can aid in the examination as a full bladder can make palpation of pelvic organs challenging for the examiner and increase discomfort to the patient.

The American College of Obstetricians and Gynecologists (ACOG) advises that a chaperone be present for all physical examinations of breast, chest, genital, and rectal areas. The presence of a chaperone is recommended regardless of the sex or gender of the patient or the examiner. Patients can choose to decline a chaperone; however, an examiner can also choose not to examine sensitive areas without a chaperone. Family members, friends of the patient, or students should not be used as chaperones (ACOG, 2020).

Positioning

Although several positions may be used for the pelvic examination, the supine lithotomy position is used most commonly. In this position, the patient lies on the table with their feet in footrests, buttocks at the edge of the table, and thighs abducted. The head of the bed should be raised so that the patient and the examiner can make eye contact during the examination. Supine lithotomy is more comfortable for most patients, and it may also facilitate the bimanual examination. It is increasingly more common not to use the footrests (aka stirrups) and to instead have patients put the soles of their feet together and bend their knees outward for the exam. Seehusen et al. (2006) conducted a well-designed study on how patients felt about exams that did not use stirrups and found that patients felt they had much more control and felt less vulnerable. In the United States, the lithotomy position and stirrups are more common; however, they are not often used in the rest of the world. Some patients may prefer to be positioned on their left side with their right leg bent at a 90-degree angle. This may be used with a patient who prefers this position or who has mobility challenges that make this positioning more suitable (Seehusen et al., 2006).

Inspection

After the patient is positioned, the examiner inspects the external genitalia. Lesions of any type are evaluated. Structural changes include **cystocele** (bulging of bladder into the vagina), **rectocele** (bulging of rectum into the vagina), or **uterine prolapse** (uterus falling out of normal position). The examiner may ask the patient to bear down in order to visualize these changes (Cook & Talwalkar, 2019).

Palpation

Palpation begins with an evaluation of the inguinal lymph nodes. Then, using the fingers of a gloved hand, the examiner gently separates the labia and palpates the lower part of the vagina. If an examination is necessary for a patient who has not had vaginal penetration, the **hymen** may be palpated within the vaginal opening if still present. Remnants of the hymen may be palpated as a rim of incongruous tissue at the introitus. The greater vestibular glands (Bartholin glands) lie between the labia minora and the hymenal ring and should be free of abscess and drainage (Bickley, 2020).

Speculum Examination

The speculum is an instrument used to open the vaginal walls for internal inspection of the vagina and cervix as well as for performance of the Papanicolaou (Pap) smear. Patients should be offered to see and touch the speculum prior to insertion. In addition, letting patients know that they can ask you to slow down, stop, or remove the speculum at any time during the exam is an important part of trauma-informed and patient-centered care. Speculums are either metal or plastic. If metal, warming the speculum prior to insertion can be more comfortable for the patient; this can be done by keeping speculums in a drawer on a heating pad or with warm water. Lubrication of the outer superior and inferior blade of the speculum with a water-soluble lubricant gel decreases the friction and discomfort associated with insertion and opening of the speculum without affecting the quality of the cytology results during the collection of specimens (O'Laughlin et al., 2021).

When the speculum is positioned properly, it is opened slowly to visualize the cervix (Fig. 31-5). The examiner inspects the cervical surface for any lesions or anomalies. The cervix typically is 2 to 3 cm wide and pink in color with a smooth appearance. Discharge from the cervical os may be cultured as needed to rule out infection. If indicated for health maintenance and consent has been obtained by the patient, a Papanicolaou (Pap) smear can be obtained from the cervix (this test is discussed in more detail in the section on diagnostic evaluation) (Bickley, 2020; Ricci et al., 2021).

While withdrawing the speculum, the provider inspects the vagina for lesions and vaginal discharge, which may be

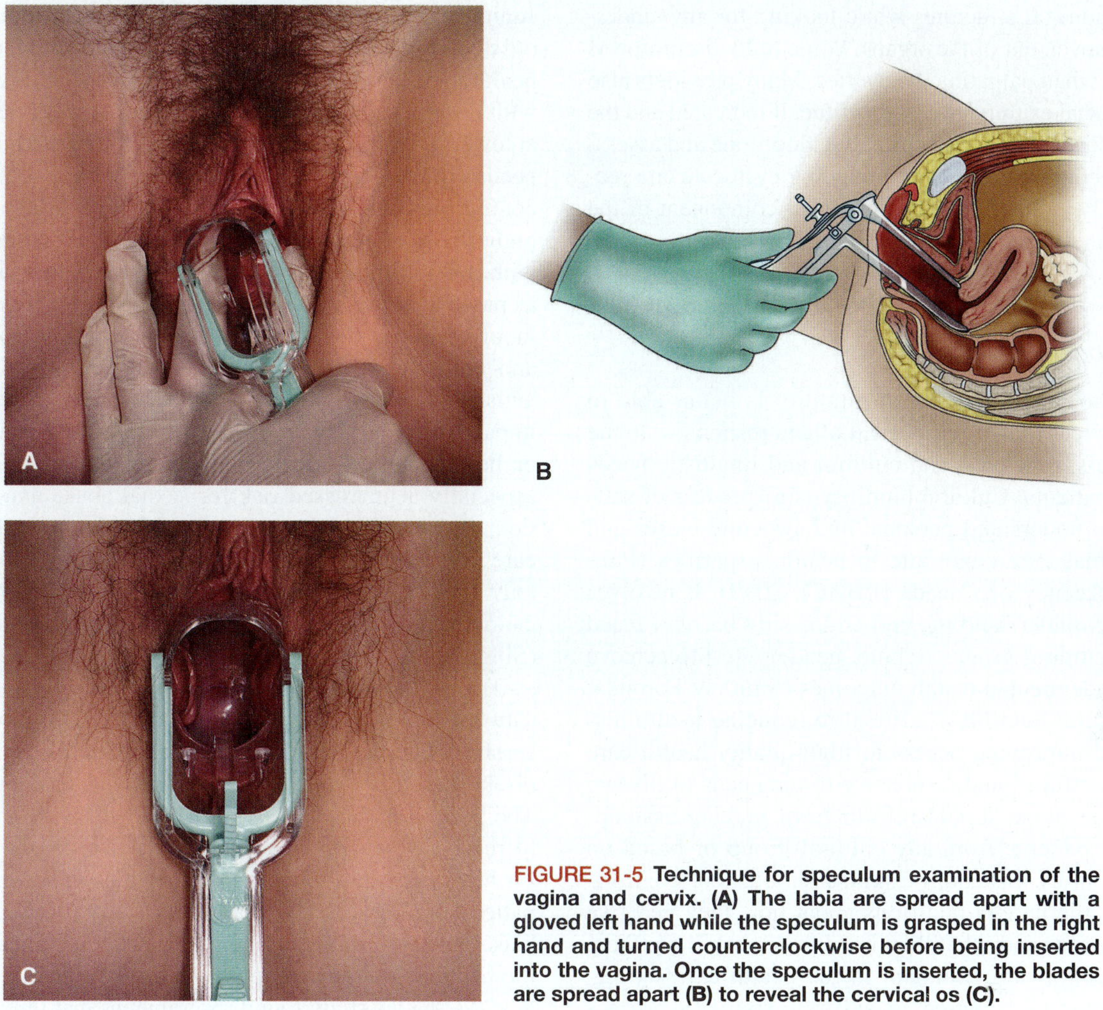

FIGURE 31-5 **Technique for speculum examination of the vagina and cervix. (A) The labia are spread apart with a gloved left hand while the speculum is grasped in the right hand and turned counterclockwise before being inserted into the vagina. Once the speculum is inserted, the blades are spread apart (B) to reveal the cervical os (C).**

normal or may result from vaginitis (Table 31-5). As mentioned during the patient interview section, patients should be offered screening for STIs prior to a pelvic exam. If desired by the patient, cultures for gonococcal, chlamydial, and trichomonas organisms can be collected (Bickley, 2020). In addition, a wet mount can be done to determine if the patient has candidiasis, bacterial vaginosis, or trichomonas.

Bimanual Palpation

After the internal inspection, a bimanual examination of the pelvic organs may be conducted. After receiving consent, the provider slowly inserts two gloved lubricated fingers from one hand into the vagina of the patient while the other hand compresses from the outside to assess the reproductive organs. The provider assesses size and position of the

TABLE **31-5 Vaginal Discharge Characteristics**

Cause of Discharge	Symptoms	Odor	Consistency/Color
Physiologic	None	None	Mucus/white
Candida infection	Itching, irritation	Yeast odor or none	Thin to thick, curd-like/white
Bacterial vaginosis	Odor	Fishy, often noticed after intercourse	Thin/grayish or yellow
Trichomonas infection	Irritation, odor	Malodorous	Copious, often frothy/yellow-green
Atrophic	Vulvar or vaginal dryness	Occasional mild malodor	Usually scant and mucoid/may be blood-tinged

uterus and adnexal structures while looking for any tenderness upon movement of the organs. Some mild discomfort is not unusual when palpating the ovaries. Many providers also perform a rectal examination at this time, if indicated and the patient consents. Assessment of pelvic floor tone and assessment for pelvic organ prolapse including cystocele and rectocele may be done during the bimanual component of the pelvic exam (Aboseif & Liu, 2020).

Special Considerations in Health Assessment

Cultural Considerations

A nurse who practices cultural humility is better able to provide services that are respectful of and responsive to the health beliefs, practices, and cultural and linguistic needs of diverse patients. Cultural humility is a "process of self-reflection to understand personal and systemic biases and privilege" that may contribute to health disparities (Public Health Agency of Canada [PHAC], 2019). It involves recognizing, understanding, and addressing barriers faced by certain cultural groups (ethnic, gender, etc.) to achieve positive academic and health outcomes (Smith & Foronda, 2021). Cultural humility is critical to reducing health disparities and improving access to high-quality health care that is respectful of and responsive to the needs of diverse patients. The nurse should refrain from making assumptions about patients from any cultural group or based on their own biases. Instead, the nurse should feel comfortable asking the patient questions about how they perceive their health care and what they need in order to help them feel comfortable and confident in the health care setting. Cultural humility is based in self-reflexivity: a process for health care professionals to recognize their own bias, privilege and the limits of their own knowledge. It results in health care professionals acknowledging patients' own expertise in their cultural knowledge and being open to learning from their patients. Effective communication and positive relationships are essential to developing collaborative culturally respectful care and shared decision-making that result in a person's greater understanding of their health care plans, satisfaction, and improved health outcomes (Lekas et al., 2020).

Patients with Disabilities

Patients with disabilities may require special care to address their individual needs, but they should always receive the same general health care screenings and assessments as patients without disabilities. However, research has shown patients with disabilities do not receive regular health screenings within recommended guidelines (Centers for Disease Control and Prevention [CDC], 2020). About 61 million adults in the United States live with a disability, with approximately 1 in 4 people who identify as females living with disabilities (CDC, 2020). People with disabilities have increased barriers to accessing and receiving equitable health care. Up to one third of adults 18 to 44 years old do not have a usual health care provider and have unmet health care needs due to cost (CDC, 2020). AFAB people with disabilities are screened for breast and cervical cancer at lower rates than those without disabilities and have unmet needs around contraception, preconception, and pregnancy counseling (CDC, 2020; Sonalkar, 2019). Studies also show higher rates of death related to breast cancer among patients with a disability, even when diagnosed at the same stage as patients without a disability. Disabilities can range from mobility issues due to spinal cord injuries, cerebral palsy, and multiple sclerosis to intellectual disabilities, such as autism and Down syndrome that can have wide ranging impacts from mild to severe, and disabilities related to sight or hearing loss. Patients with intellectual disabilities are especially at increased risk for sexual abuse and exploitation, and careful screening should be carried out. Health care professionals, due to lack of knowledge and training, may avoid discussing sexual health, abuse, or sexual education as they may feel it is not necessary or inappropriate (Singh Shrestha et al., 2021).

The lack of training and knowledge among not just health care providers but also among office staff in how to successfully interact with and care confidently for persons with disabilities leads to grave disparities and inadequate care. The needed additional time for a person with a disability to receive a sensitive and unhurried visit can be a barrier for health care providers and lead to bias in accepting such patients in their offices. One recent study found providers' biases and discriminatory attitudes play a significant role in the health disparities people with disabilities face (Lagu et al., 2022). This study found several areas that impacted care and the challenges of each (Table 31-6; Lagu et al., 2022). The presence of a disability does not justify skipping any parts of the physical assessment that are deemed to be essential for high-quality care, including the pelvic examination. In order to successfully complete a thorough pelvic exam for a person with significant intellectual disabilities, several techniques may need to be employed, including adequate preparation time, emotional support, and the utilization of relaxation and deep breathing exercises to facilitate an exam. With consent, the use of safe, short-acting oral or injectable sedatives prior to a procedure can allow many patients to safely and comfortably complete an assessment (Singh Shrestha et al., 2021; see Box 31-3).

Gerontologic Considerations

By 2030 it is projected that 50% of females and people AFAB will live to 90 years old or beyond and will encounter and live with more physical and medical limitations with aging (Lambrinoudaki et al., 2022). While diagnostic screening measures are appropriate, preventative health issues may have more of a positive impact on quality and longevity of life and therefore may be appropriate for the provider to discuss with older patients. Nurses engaging

TABLE 31-6 Themes of Identified Barriers to Care of People With Disabilities

Barrier	Issues
Physical accommodations	Exam room not big enough to accommodate a wheelchair Scale to weigh people using wheelchairs Motorized tables to help with transfer
Communication accommodations	Patients without needed hearing aids American Sign Language interpreters Writing boards or pictographic boards
Knowledge, experiences, skills	Knowing what durable medical equipment would be most beneficial for patients How to assess and educate patients
Structural barriers	15-minute visits, reimbursement rates that do not account for the extra time required, lack of care coordination Not knowing ahead of time that a person has a disability and how to accommodate it
Attitudes toward people with disabilities	Avoiding ableist language People with disabilities feeling burdensome and demanding Some offices outright denying care for people with disabilities or discharging them from care if deemed too difficult
Knowledge of ADA	Little or no training provided to providers in school ADA is difficult to enforce

Based on Lagu et al. (2022).

with postmenopausal patients should use this time to discuss concerns of their patients and provide education and reassurance of the normal aging processes. There is insufficient data to support routine pelvic exams; they should be performed when patients present with symptoms that need further evaluation but not done routinely for asymptomatic patients (United States Preventive Task Force [USPTF], 2022).

Caring for older patients with gynecologic concerns requires the nurse to be prepared for a wide spectrum of age-related changes. The optimal treatment modality for the older patient should not be based on age alone. Many older patients, regardless of advancing chronologic age, remain in excellent health. Therefore, the patient's health status and treatment preferences must play a role in the shared decision-making process. This should include discussions of preventative health activities that may be just as important, if not more so, to their continued health as diagnostic procedures (Toi et al., 2022).

BOX 31-3 Assessment of People AFAB With Disabilities

Additional Health History

Address questions directly to the patient rather than to people accompanying them. Ask about:

- Self-care limitations resulting from the disability (ability to feed and dress, use of assistive devices, transportation requirements, other assistance needed)
- Sensory limitations (lack of sensation, low vision, hearing impairment)
- Accessibility issues (ability to get to health care provider, transfer to examination table, accessibility of office/clinic, previous experiences with health care providers, health screening practices, understanding of physical examination)
- Cognitive or developmental changes that affect understanding
- Limitations secondary to disability that affect general health issues and reproductive health and health care
- Sexual function and concerns
- Menstrual history and menstrual hygiene practices
- Physical, sexual, or psychological abuse (including abuse by care providers; abuse by neglect or withholding or withdrawing assistive devices or personal health care)
- Presence of secondary disabilities (e.g., those resulting from the patient's primary disability: pressure ulcers, spasticity, osteoporosis, etc.)
- Health concerns related to aging with a disability

Physical Assessment

Provide instructions directly to the patient, rather than to people accompanying them; provide written or audiotaped instructions.

Ask the patient what assistance they need for the physical examination, and provide assistance if needed for the following:

- Undressing and dressing
- Providing a urine specimen
- Standing on scale to be weighed (provide alternative means of obtaining weight if they are unable to stand on scale)
- Moving on and off the examination table
- Assuming, changing, and maintaining positions

Consider the fatigue experienced by the person during a lengthy examination, and allow them time to rest.

Provide assistive devices and other aids/methods needed to allow adequate communication with the patient (interpreters, signers, large-print written materials).

Complete the examination as it would be indicated for any other person; having a disability is *never* justification for omitting parts of the physical examination, including the pelvic examination, if indicated.

Diagnostic Evaluation

Papanicolaou (Pap) Cytologic Test: Screening for Cervical Cancer

Often cervical cancer can be found early, and sometimes even prevented entirely, through HPV vaccination and Pap tests. If detected early, cervical cancer is one of the most successfully treatable cancers. Deaths from cervical cancer are higher in populations around the world where patients do not have access to routine screening for cervical cancer and HPV vaccination and can be seen as a measure of inequity (Vale et al., 2021). In fact, cervical cancer is the major cause of cancer deaths in many patients in developing countries. Usually these patients are diagnosed with late-stage cancers rather than precancers or early cancers (Vale et al., 2021). In high resource countries, however, the death rate from cervical cancer has declined by more than 70%. This is thought to be mainly related to the effectiveness of routine Pap test screening guidelines and HPV vaccination (Bus-Kuwofie et al., 2019).

Pearls for Practice

Pap testing should begin at age 21. Many organizations (ASCCP, ACOG, USPTF, AAFP) have guidelines stating patients should have a Pap test every 3 years until age 29. After age 30, patients should have a Pap test every 5 years with HPV co-testing. The ACS has recommended starting Pap tests and HPV co-testing at age 25. All groups agree that after age 65 or after a hysterectomy, Pap test screening should end, unless the patient has a history of abnormal pap smears in the past 10 years or a history of cervical cancer. Nurses should include asking about abnormal Paps and HPV vaccination during history-taking (ACS, 2020; American Society of Colposcopy and Cervical Pathology [ASCCP], 2019; Shami & Coombs, 2021).

During the Pap test, a sample of cells are lightly scraped or brushed from the external and internal surfaces of the cervix. If the cervix has been removed, the cells will be sampled from the upper part of the vagina, known as the vaginal cuff. This test should not be performed when a patient is heavily menstruating, as blood can interfere with interpretation. Although the Pap test is an excellent screening system, it is not a diagnostic test; both false-positive and false-negative results may occur.

The Bethesda Classification system has been developed to promote consistency in reporting Pap results. Although patients may assume (incorrectly) that an abnormal Pap smear signifies cancer, this is not generally the case. It simply means that it is abnormal. Under the microscope, the appearance of a few cells differs in some way from the classic appearance of healthy, intact cervical cells. The difference could be due to local irritation, a non-HPV infection, a low-risk or high-risk HPV type, or even an error in the preparation of the cell sample. An abnormal Pap result requires prompt notification and follow-up as abnormalities detected in a Pap test may signify cellular changes that may lead to cancer if left untreated (Box 31-4). The nurse should provide simple and clear explanations as well as emotional support designed to meet the needs of the specific patients that may encourage appropriate and timely follow-up. The follow-up may include evaluation with colposcopy, cervical biopsy, or a repeat Pap test in a year. Treatment may include cryotherapy, laser therapy, cone biopsy, or loop electrical excision procedure (LEEP) (Shami & Coombs, 2021) (Box 31-5).

BOX 31-4 **Bethesda Classification System for Pap Smears**

- Negative for intraepithelial lesion or malignancy (NILM): follow routine cervical screening guidelines
- For all other Pap test results, management should follow ASCCP risk-based consensus guidelines: https://www.asccp.org/management-guidelines
- Atypical squamous cells of undetermined significance (ASCUS): mild changes, may resolve spontaneously, needs closer follow-up, most common abnormal pap smear result
- Atypical squamous cells, cannot exclude high-grade squamous intraepithelial lesion (ASC-H): more likely associated with precancer or cancer
- Low-grade squamous intraepithelial lesion (LSIL): mild changes, may resolve spontaneously
- High-grade squamous intraepithelial lesion (HSIL): more likely associated with precancer or cancer
- Atypical glandular cells of undetermined significance (AGUS): more likely associated with precancer or cancer

(Shami & Coombs, 2021; ASCCP, 2019)

Uterine Diagnostics

Certain uterine conditions, such as dysfunctional uterine bleeding, may require diagnostic testing as well. Diagnostic tests performed on uterine and peritoneal tissues include endometrial (aspiration) biopsy, dilation and curettage (D&C), laparoscopy, hysteroscopy, and **endometrial ablation**. For information on these procedures, refer to Table 31-7.

Mammography

Mammography is an x-ray breast-imaging technique performed in a hospital radiology department or independent imaging center that can detect nonpalpable lesions and assist in diagnosing palpable masses. The breast is mechanically compressed from top to bottom (craniocaudal view) and side to side (mediolateral oblique view; Fig. 31-6). Although usually two views of each breast are taken for a screening mammogram, for some patients, such as those with breast implants, with large breasts, or having their first mammogram, additional pictures may be needed. Experience of slight discomfort is due to the maximum compression necessary for proper visualization. Although mammography may detect a breast tumor before it is clinically palpable (i.e., smaller

BOX 31-5

Diagnostic Testing and Management of Abnormal Pap Test Results

Colposcopy

Some abnormal Pap tests are evaluated by colposcopy, while some are closely monitored with repeat Pap test in 1 year. Nurse practitioners, nurse-midwives, and gynecologists require special training in this diagnostic technique.

The colposcope is a portable microscope used to visualize the cervix and obtain samples of abnormal tissue for analysis. The examiner applies acetic acid (similar to vinegar) to the cervix to highlight suspect areas.

A cervical biopsy or endocervical curettage may be performed during colposcopy. Tissue analysis is used to determine whether abnormal changes have occurred. If these biopsy specimens show cervical intraepithelial neoplasia (CIN), the patient may require further intervention (cryotherapy, laser therapy, or a cone biopsy).

Cervical Biopsy

Abnormal colposcopy findings indicating the need for biopsy include leukoplakia (white plaque visible before applying acetic acid), acetowhite tissue (white epithelium after applying acetic acid), punctuation (dilated capillaries occurring in a dotted or stippled pattern), mosaicism (a tile-like pattern), and atypical vascular patterns.

Biopsy involves taking a sample of tissue from the cervix for further analysis.

Cryotherapy and Laser Therapy

Both are outpatient procedures that can be performed in an office setting or same-day procedure setting with sedation. Cryotherapy is the freezing of suspect cervical tissue with nitrous oxide. It is good for small areas of mild to moderate dysplasia. It can be used to treat carcinoma in situ of the cervix (stage 0) but not invasive cancer.

Cryotherapy may result in cramping and occasional feelings of faintness (vasovagal response). A watery discharge is normal for a few weeks after the procedure as the cervix heals. It is not precisely controlled, so abnormal cells may be left behind.

Laser treatment uses a tiny beam of light to vaporize abnormal cervical cells. The laser beam is directed through a colposcope, is more precise than cryosurgery, and has the benefit of targeting only the diseased cervical tissues. Healing is much faster than with freezing. Not all offices have lasers, thus increasing costs to patients if treatment is carried out in the hospital. This, too, can be used to treat carcinoma in situ of the cervix (stage 0) but not invasive cancer.

Cone Biopsy and Loop Electrosurgical Excision Procedure

If endocervical curettage findings indicate abnormal changes or if the lesion extends into the canal, the patient may undergo a cone biopsy. The cone biopsy can be performed surgically or with a procedure called loop electrosurgical excision procedure (LEEP).

LEEP can be performed in the outpatient setting and has a high success rate in removal of abnormal cervical tissue. The provider uses a fine wire loop with electrical energy flowing through it to remove abnormal cervical tissue. Samples are sent to pathology.

Usually cone biopsy is done in an operating room with a laser or conventional surgical instruments (cold-knife cone). A cone- or cylinder-shaped piece of the cervix is removed. Also a diagnostic cone may treat the problem. There should be a shared decision-making approach about whether to proceed with this surgical procedure, including a conversation about plans for future childbearing.

than 1 cm), mammography has limitations. Overall, screening mammograms do not find about one in five instances of breast cancer. They do not work as well in patients with dense breasts since dense breasts can hide a tumor. Dense breasts are more common in younger patients, pregnant patients, and those who are lactating, but a finding of dense breasts is common for many patients. When this is noted on the mammogram report, a bilateral breast ultrasound is recommended for a more complete evaluation with breast imaging.

Digital breast tomosynthesis (DBT) is emerging as a new standard of care in breast screening, especially for persons with dense breast tissue. DBT is a type of digital mammography that takes multiple images which are then assembled to provide highly focused 3-D images of the breast, which improves the sensitivity and specificity of the exam. DBT has been covered by Medicaid since 2015; however, not all commercial insurers cover this test. DBT has been shown to reduce screening recall rates and to have the potential to detect cancers at an earlier stage across all breast densities (Chong et al., 2019; Narayan et al., 2020).

Current screening guidelines of the ACS recommend a mammogram every year beginning at 40 years of age. The ACS also has guidelines for older people and people at increased risk of breast cancer. Professional organization guidelines vary (Table 31-8). Three other diagnostic tests to detect/view breast masses are galactogram (ductogram), ultrasound (US), and magnetic resonance imaging (MRI; Table 31-9).

Other Radiologic Tests for Abnormal Nipple Discharge and Breast Masses

Less than 5% of clinical breast concerns are for nipple discharge, and only 10% to 15% of those will be cancerous, but it can cause significant stress and mental discomfort for those who have it (Kim et al., 2020; Tao et al., 2021). A mammogram is the first line in diagnosing abnormal nipple discharge (Tao et al., 2021). A galactogram, also called a ductogram, uses x-rays and iodine-enhanced mammography to diagnose the cause of abnormal nipple discharge;

TABLE **31-7 Uterine Diagnostic Tests**

Test	Description
Endometrial (aspiration) biopsy	Method of obtaining endometrial tissue by placing a flexible suction tube through the cervix into the uterus. This tissue sample permits diagnosis of cellular changes in the endometrium. Indicated in cases of midlife irregular bleeding, postmenopausal bleeding, and irregular bleeding while taking hormone therapy or tamoxifen.
Dilation and curettage (D&C)	Can be used as a diagnostic or therapeutic tool. Cervical canal is dilated and the endometrium is scraped or suctioned. Can be used to gather endometrial tissue for cytologic examination, to control abnormal uterine bleeding, and as a therapeutic measure for incomplete miscarriage.
Laparoscopy (pelvic peritoneoscopy)	Involves inserting laparoscope into peritoneal cavity through small incision below the umbilicus to allow visualization of the pelvic structures. Used for diagnostic purposes (e.g., in cases of pelvic pain when no cause can be found) as well as for surgical procedures, including tubal ligation, ovarian biopsy, hysterectomy, and adhesion lysis.
Hysteroscopy (transcervical intrauterine endoscopy)	Allows direct visualization of all parts of the uterine cavity by means of a lighted optical instrument. Under a local anesthetic, the hysteroscope is passed into the cervical canal and advanced 1 or 2 cm under direct vision. Uterine-distending fluid is infused through the instrument to dilate the uterine cavity and enhance visibility. Often done at the same time as D&C.
Endometrial ablation (destruction of the uterine lining)	Performed in cases of severe bleeding not responsive to other therapies. Performed under general, regional, or local anesthesia, the uterus is distended with a fluid infusion. Providers use a hysteroscope and resector (cutting loop), roller ball (a barrel-shaped electrode), or laser beam to destroy the lining of the uterus. Hemorrhage, perforation, and burns can occur. Some patients experience pelvic pain as a delayed side effect. This rapid procedure is an alternative to hysterectomy for some patients.
Hysterosalpingography (HSG)	Radiographic study of the uterus and fallopian tubes performed to evaluate infertility or tubal patency and to detect abnormal conditions in the uterine cavity. With the patient in lithotomy position, the cervix is exposed with a speculum. A cannula is inserted into the cervix, and a contrast agent is injected into the uterine cavity and the fallopian tubes. Then x-rays are taken to show the path and the distribution of the contrast agent.
Ultrasonography (ultrasound [US])	Useful adjunct to physical examination for patients with abnormal pelvic findings. Based on transmission of pulsed ultrasonic sound waves via a transducer that is either placed on the abdomen (abdominal scan) or through a vaginal probe (vaginal US). The entire procedure takes usually less than 10 minutes and involves no ionizing radiation. Sometimes saline is infused into the uterus for better imaging of the uterine lining; this is helpful for diagnosis of polyps and fibroids. This procedure is called a sonohysterogram.
Computed tomography (CT)	Demonstrates tumor and any extension into the retroperitoneal lymph nodes and skeletal tissue. In some cases it provides better imaging than US. Does expose the patient to radiation. More costly than US procedures.
Magnetic resonance imaging (MRI)	Produces patterns that are finer and more definitive than other imaging procedures; does not expose patients to radiation. High cost is the major drawback.

this once was the only method for accurately showing mammary ducts (Schulz-Wendtland et al., 2018; Tao et al., 2021). However, recent advances in both the availability of MRIs and the introduction of DBT has made the use of galactograms less common as a solo diagnostic. More recent studies demonstrate higher sensitivity and specificity with combined DBT with galactogram or with second-look ultrasound after galactogram (Kim et al., 2020; Tao et al., 2021). In settings where access to MRIs is limited, the galactogram remains an important, cost-effective procedure for diagnosing nipple discharge.

Ultrasound (US), also known as sonography, uses sound waves to look inside a part of the body. This test is painless and has no radiation exposure. Breast US is used most often to evaluate breast problems that are found during a mammogram or physical examination and to guide a needle biopsy of a suspicious mass. In someone with a breast tumor, US also may be used to assess lymph nodes under the arm. Breast US may be helpful to use along with a mammogram when screening a person with dense breast tissue.

Magnetic resonance imaging (MRI) of the breast is a highly sensitive technology that uses magnets and radio waves instead of x-rays to produce very detailed, cross-sectional pictures. It is a useful diagnostic adjunct to mammography without exposure to radiation. The procedure cannot always distinguish accurately between malignant and benign breast conditions. This is why MRI is not recommended as a screening test for patients at average risk of

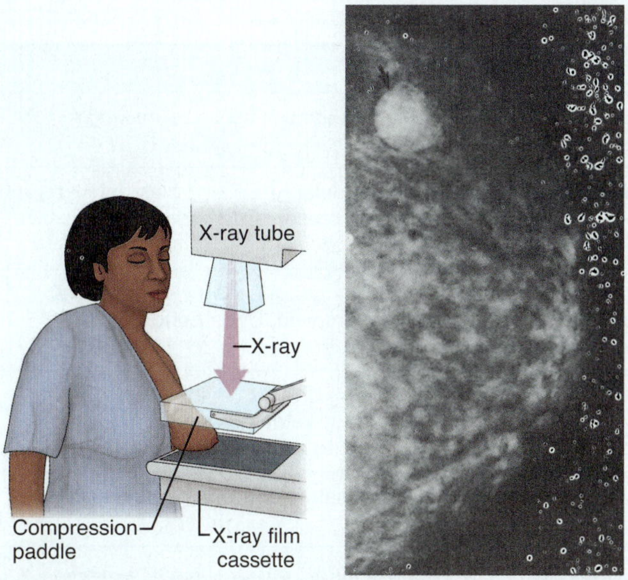

A B

FIGURE 31-6 The mammography procedure (A) relies on x-ray imaging to produce the mammogram (B), which, in this case, reveals a breast lump.

breast cancer, as it would result in unneeded biopsies and other tests in many of these patients.

MRI is most useful when assessing for disease that is either multifocal (more than one tumor in the same quadrant of the breast) or multicentric (more than one tumor in different quadrants of the breast), chest wall involvement, tumor recurrence, or response to chemotherapy.

For patients with breast augmentation, MRI also can identify occult (undetectable) breast cancer and determine the integrity of saline or silicone breast implants.

Disadvantages of MRI include high cost, variations in technique and interpretation, and the potential for patient distress from claustrophobia in the MRI machine.

Breast Tissue Analysis

Diagnostic tests performed on breast tissue are described in Table 31-8.

AMAB REPRODUCTIVE SYSTEM

In AMAB individuals, several organs serve as parts of both the urinary tract and the reproductive system. Disorders in the AMAB reproductive organs may interfere with the functions of one or both systems. As a result, a urologist commonly treats diseases of the AMAB reproductive system.

ANATOMIC AND PHYSIOLOGIC OVERVIEW

The structures in the AMAB reproductive system include the testes; the vas deferens (ductus deferens) and seminal vesicles; the penis; and certain accessory glands, such as the prostate gland and Cowper gland (bulbourethral gland; Fig. 31-7).

The testes are formed in the embryo, within the abdominal cavity, near the kidney. During the last month of fetal life, the testes descend posterior to the peritoneum, pierce the abdominal wall in the groin, and progress along the inguinal canal into the scrotum. In this descent, they are accompanied by blood vessels, lymphatics, nerves, and ducts, all of which support the tissue and make up the spermatic cord. This cord extends from the internal inguinal ring through the

TABLE **31-8 Breast Cancer Screening Guidelines for People AFAB**

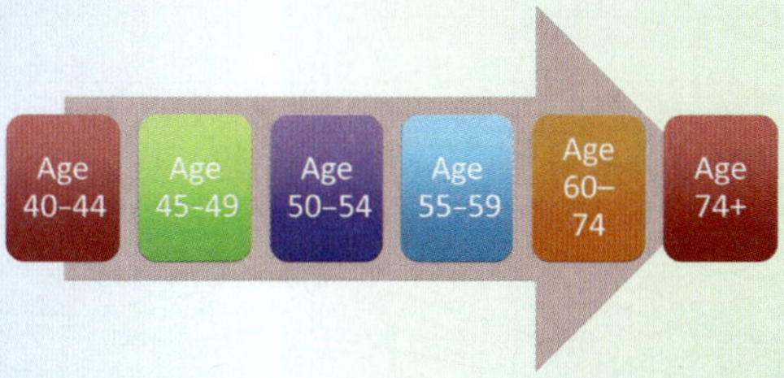

	Age 40–44	Age 45–49	Age 50–54	Age 55–59	Age 60–74	Age 74+
USPSTF	Individual Decision	Individual Decision	Every 2 Y	Every 2 Y	Every 2 Y	Insufficient evidence
ACS	Individual Decision	Every Year	Every Year	Every 1–2 Y	Every 1–2 Y	Continue as long as their overall health is good, life expectancy >10 y
ACR	Every Year	Every Year	Every Year	Every Year	Every Year	Appropriate when life expectancy exceeds 5 to 7 y

Source: Narayan, A. K., Lee, C. I., & Lehman, C. D. (2020). Screening for breast cancer. *Medical Clinics of North America*, *104*(6), 1007–1021. https://doi.org/10.1016/j.mcna.2020.08.003

TABLE **31-9 Procedures for Breast Tissue Analysis**

Procedure	Description
Percutaneous biopsy	Samples palpable and nonpalpable lesions via needle or core biopsy that obtains tissue by making a small puncture in the skin. It is less invasive than a surgical biopsy.
Fine-needle aspiration (FNA)	Small-gauge needle with a syringe is inserted into the mass or area of nodularity. Cellular material obtained during the procedure is spread on a glass slide or placed in a preservative and sent for analysis.
Core needle biopsy	Similar to FNA except that a needle with a larger gauge is used (usually 14 gauge). It allows for a more definitive diagnosis than FNA because actual tissue, not just cells, is removed. Often performed for relatively large tumors that are close to the skin surface.
Stereotactic core biopsy	Performed on nonpalpable lesions detected by mammography. After using digital mammography to determine the exact coordinates of the lesion, a core needle is inserted to retrieve samples of the tissue for pathologic examination. Stereotactic biopsy often allows the patient to avoid a surgical biopsy.
Ultrasound-guided core biopsy	Performed on nonpalpable lesions found by ultrasound; does not use radiation and is faster and less expensive than stereotactic core biopsy.
Excisional biopsy (lumpectomy)	Standard procedure for complete pathologic assessment of a palpable breast mass. The entire mass, plus a margin of surrounding tissue, is removed.
Incisional biopsy	Surgical removal of a portion of a mass when complete excision of the area may not be possible or immediately beneficial to the patient. Incisional biopsy is becoming less common as pathologic information can be obtained from the core needle biopsy.
Wire needle localization	Technique used to precisely locate nonpalpable masses detected on a mammogram, ultrasound, or MRI that require an excisional biopsy. A long, thin wire is inserted through a needle and guided into the area of abnormality using an x-ray or ultrasound. The needle is withdrawn, and the wire is left in place to mark the precise location.

abdominal wall and the inguinal canal to the scrotum. As the testes descend into the scrotum, a tubular extension of peritoneum accompanies them. This tissue is obliterated during fetal development; the only remaining portion is that which covers the testes, the tunica vaginalis.

The testes are encased in the scrotum, which keeps them at a slightly lower temperature than the rest of the body to facilitate spermatogenesis. The **testes** have a dual function: **spermatogenesis** (production of sperm) and secretion of the male sex hormone **testosterone**, which induces and preserves the male sex characteristics. The testes consist of numerous seminiferous tubules in which the spermatozoa form. Collecting tubules transmit the spermatozoa into the epididymis, a hood-like structure lying on the testes and containing winding ducts that lead into the vas deferens. This firm, tubular structure passes upward through the inguinal canal as part

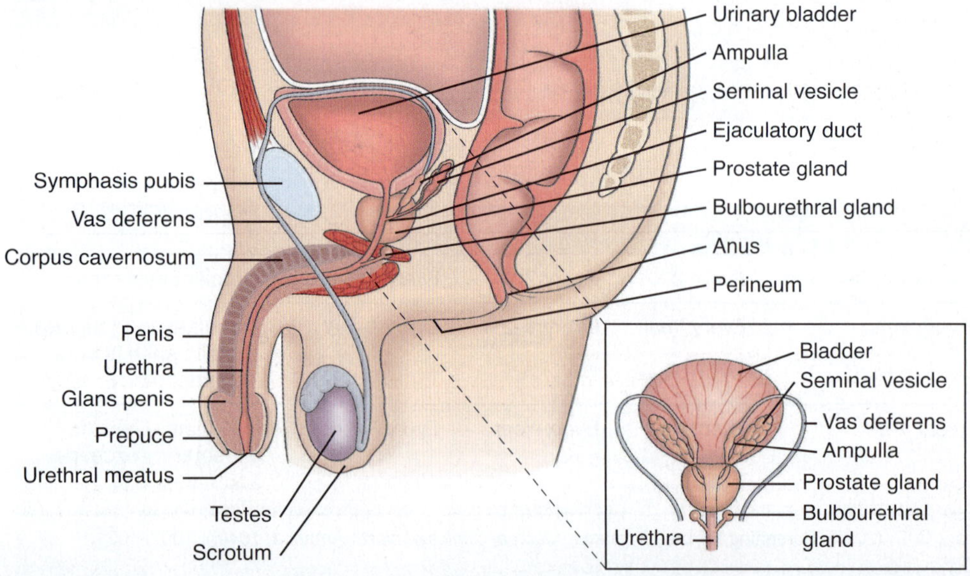

FIGURE 31-7 Structures of the AMAB reproductive system.

of the spermatic cord to enter the abdominal cavity behind the peritoneum. It then extends downward toward the base of the bladder. An outpouching from this structure is the seminal vesicle. The tract is continued as the ejaculatory duct, which passes through the prostate gland to enter the urethra. Secretions from the seminal vesicles join secretions from the prostate and exit the penis during ejaculation.

The **penis** has a dual function: it is the organ for copulation and for urination. Anatomically, it consists of the glans penis, the body, and the root. The glans penis is the soft, rounded portion at the distal end of the penis. The urethra opens at the tip of the glans. The glans is naturally covered or protected by elongated penile skin—the foreskin—which may be retracted to expose the glans. However, many males and people AMAB had the foreskin removed (circumcision) as newborns. The body of the penis is composed of erectile tissues containing numerous blood vessels that become distended, leading to an erection during sexual excitement. The urethra, which passes through the penis, extends from the bladder through the prostate to the distal end of the penis, ending at the meatal opening.

The **prostate gland** lies just below the neck of the bladder. It surrounds the urethra and is traversed by the ejaculatory duct, a continuation of the vas deferens. This gland produces a secretion that is suitable both chemically and physiologically to the needs of the spermatozoa in their passage from the testes. Cowper gland lies below the prostate, within the posterior aspect of the urethra. This gland empties its secretions into the urethra during ejaculation, providing lubrication.

Gerontologic Considerations

As people AMAB age, the prostate gland enlarges, prostate secretion decreases, the scrotum may hang lower, the testes become smaller and less firm, and pubic hair becomes sparser. Changes in gonadal function include a slow decline in plasma testosterone levels and reduced production of progesterone (Table 31-10). Other potential changes include decreased sexual function, slowed sexual responses and longer refractory period, an increased risk for cancer of the genitourinary tract, and possible urinary incontinence or retention.

Male reproductive capability is maintained with advancing age. Although degenerative changes occur in the seminiferous tubules, spermatogenesis continues. However, libido (sexual desire) and potency decrease (Swerdloff & Wang, 2020).

Pearls for Practice

If the patient is concerned about sexual function, the nurse can ask about whether the patient on waking has an early morning erection. If the patient does, this argues against an organic cause (neurologic, vascular, or endocrinologic) and suggests a functional problem. A thorough history focusing on the onset and progression of symptoms, libido, medications, surgery, and psychosocial issues is important in the evaluation. Screening for depression, hypothyroidism, hypogonadism, and diabetes can be considered (Swerdloff & Wang, 2020; Griebing, 2021).

Hypogonadism occurs in up to one fourth of older males and people AMAB. The prevalence increases with comorbidities such as diabetes and obesity, among others. The average decrease in serum total testosterone levels with aging is 1% to 2% per year with prevalence rates of 23% among people in their 70s (Ferri, 2022). This decline is more evident in those older than 60 years of age. In older males and people AMAB, the sexual response slows, attaining an erection takes longer, and full erections may not be attained, although ability to climax is preserved. Sexual function can be affected by several factors, such as:

- Psychological problems
- Comorbidities (vasculogenic [atherosclerotic disease, occlusions to vasculature after pelvic trauma, liver failure])
- Neurogenic factors (spinal cord injury, Parkinson disease, stroke, tumors, trauma)
- Endocrine factors (hypogonadism, hyper- and hypothyroidism)
- Mixed causation (diabetes, uremia)
- Medication (opioids, alcohol, antihypertensive, steroids, antidepressants, cardiac medications [e.g., digoxin], beta blockers, diuretics, and others)

Cancers of the kidney, bladder, prostate, and penis all have increased incidence in people AMAB older than 50 years of age. Digital rectal examination (DRE) and screening tests for hematuria may uncover a higher percentage of malignancies at earlier stages and lead to lower morbidity associated with treatment as well as a lower mortality rate.

Urinary incontinence or retention in the older AMAB adult may have many causes, including medications and age-

TABLE 31-10 GERONTOLOGIC CONSIDERATIONS / Age-Related Changes in the AMAB Reproductive System

Structural Changes	Functional Changes	History and Physical Findings
Decrease in secretion of sex hormones, especially testosterone Decreased muscle strength and sexual energy Shrinkage and loss of firmness of testes; thickening of seminiferous tubules Enlargement of prostate gland	Changes in sexual response: prolonged time to reach full erection, rapid penile detumescence (decreased rigidity) and prolonged refractory period Possible decline in libido Decrease in number of viable sperm	Smaller testes Erectile dysfunction Weakening of prostatic contractions Hyperplasia of prostate gland Signs and symptoms of obstruction of lower urinary tract (urgency, frequency, nocturia)

related conditions, such as neurologic disease or benign prostatic hyperplasia (BPH). Diagnostic tests are performed to exclude reversible causes of urinary incontinence.

ASSESSMENT

Health History

Male sexuality is a complex phenomenon that is strongly influenced by personal, cultural, and social factors. Sexuality and AMAB reproductive function become concerns in the presence of illness (Jensen & Albaugh, 2020). Assessment of AMAB reproductive function begins with an evaluation of urinary function and symptoms. This assessment also includes a focus on sexual function and on manifestations of sexual dysfunction.

The patient is asked about their usual state of health and any recent change in general physical and sexual activity. Any symptoms or changes in function are explored fully and described in detail. These symptoms may include those associated with an obstruction caused by an enlarged prostate gland: increased urinary frequency, decreased force of urine stream, or "double" voiding (the patient needs to urinate two or three times over a period of several minutes to completely empty their bladder). The patient also is assessed for dysuria (painful urination) and hematuria (blood in the urine).

Assessment of sexual function is an essential part of every health history. The extent of the history depends on the patient's presenting symptoms and the presence of factors that may affect sexual function: chronic illnesses (e.g., diabetes, multiple sclerosis, stroke, cardiac disease), use of medications that affect sexual function (e.g., many antihypertensive and anticholesterolemic medications, psychotropic agents), stress, and alcohol use.

Often patients are hesitant to initiate a discussion about sexual issues with their health care providers. By initiating an assessment of sexual concerns, the nurse demonstrates that changes in sexual functioning are valid topics for discussion and provides a safe environment for discussing these sensitive topics.

Physical Assessment

Physical assessment includes examination of the penis and scrotum, the DRE, and assessment of the male breasts.

Penis and Scrotal Examination

The AMAB genitalia are inspected for abnormalities and palpated for masses. The scrotum is palpated carefully for nodules, masses, or inflammation. Examination of the scrotum can reveal such disorders as hydrocele (accumulation of serous fluid in the scrotal sac), varicocele (enlargement of the veins of the spermatic cord), or tumor of the testis. The penis is inspected and palpated for ulcerations, plaques, inflammation, and discharge. The testicular examination provides an excellent opportunity to instruct the patient about techniques for testicular self-examination (TSE) and its importance in early detection of testicular cancer (see Chapter 33). TSE could begin during adolescence, although this practice has been called into question with recommendations that TSE is not emphasized due to potential harms which may include false-positive results, anxiety, and harms from a substantial number of extra medical examinations and diagnostic tests (Clinical Overview, 2021; Einhorn, 2020). That said, early detection and therapeutic intervention can lead to a 90% survival rate (ACS, n.d.). The European Association of Urology (EAU) guidelines recommend advising patients with a familial history of testicular cancer, as well as their family members, to perform regular self-examination of testes (Languna et al., 2021).

Digital Rectal Examination

The DRE is recommended as part of the regular health checkup for every AMAB person older than 50 years of age; it is invaluable in screening for cancer of the prostate gland. The DRE enables the examiner to estimate the size, shape, and consistency of the prostate gland (Fig. 31-8). Tenderness of the prostate gland on palpation and the presence and consistency of any nodules are noted. Although this examination may be awkward for the patient, it is an important screening tool.

Assessment of the Male Breasts

Breast cancer can occur in males and people AMAB. Examination of the male breasts and axillae should be included in a physical examination. The nipple and areola are inspected for masses and nipple discharge.

Gynecomastia is the firm enlargement of glandular tissue beneath and immediately surrounding the areola of the male.

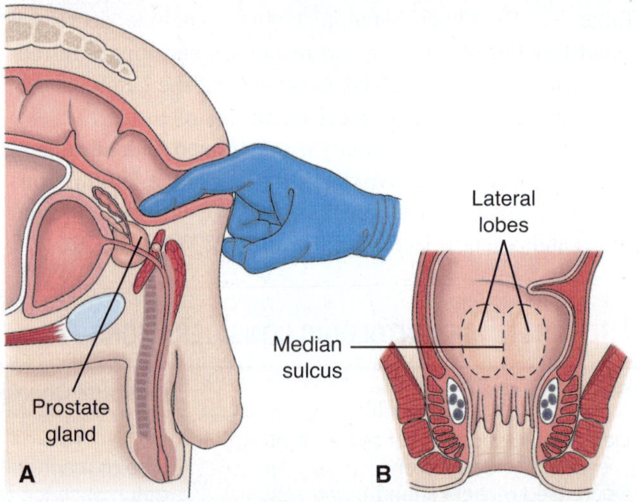

FIGURE 31-8 A. Palpation of the prostate gland during digital rectal examination (DRE) enables the examiner to assess the size, shape, and texture of the gland. B. The prostate is round, with a palpable median sulcus or groove separating the lateral lobes. It should feel rubbery and free of nodules and masses.

This is different from the enlargement of soft, fatty tissue, which is caused by obesity.

Diagnostic Evaluation

Prostate-Specific Antigen Test

The prostate gland produces a substance known as prostate-specific antigen (PSA). It can be measured in a blood specimen, and levels increase with certain pathologies: prostate cancer, BPH, acute urinary retention, and acute prostatitis are the most common examples. In most laboratories, the range of values generally considered normal is 0.2 to 4.0 ng/mL, with levels greater than 4.0 considered elevated, especially depending on age. The use of age-specific reference ranges for populations helps minimize unnecessary biopsies (American Urological Association [AUA], 2018; Trabulsi et al., 2021).

Prostate cancer screening with serum PSA testing has become common practice, although its overall utility has recently come into question (AUA, 2018). The AUA recommends PSA testing beginning at 55 years of age, along with DRE, and then screening at 2- to 4-year intervals, although screening needs to be discussed with each person individually, based on history and risk. Screening should begin at 40 years of age for those at high risk, including those with a family history of prostate cancer (first-degree relative [father, brother, or son] diagnosed with prostate cancer at an early age [under 65 years of age]) and Black males (AUA, 2018). PSA is also useful to monitor patients for recurrence after treatment for cancer of the prostate.

Ultrasonography

Transrectal ultrasound (TRUS) may be offered to patients with abnormalities detected by DRE and those with elevated PSA levels; a lubricated, condom-covered rectal probe transducer is inserted into the rectum, along the anterior wall. Needle biopsies of the prostate are commonly guided by TRUS.

Prostate Fluid or Tissue Analysis

Specimens of prostate fluid or tissue may be obtained for culture if disease or inflammation of the prostate gland is suspected, but this is uncommonly performed.

Tests of AMAB Sexual Function

If the patient cannot engage in sexual intercourse to their satisfaction, a detailed history is obtained. A panel of screening lab work to rule out common contributors to erectile issues will be considered and can include screening for diabetes, cholesterol derangements, and low testosterone. A Rigiscan test may be ordered, or nocturnal penile tumescence tests may be conducted in a sleep laboratory to monitor changes in penile circumference during sleep. The results help identify the cause of erectile dysfunction. Additional tests, including penile Doppler studies or psychological evaluations, also can be part of the diagnostic workup and usually are conducted by a specialized team of health care providers.

CHAPTER REVIEW

NCLEX-Style Review Questions

1. A 19-year-old patient complains of vaginal irritation. They say they were out for an evening a week ago at a club with friends but do not remember leaving the club. The patient states that they have never been sexually active but now fear they may have been assaulted. What are the appropriate steps for the nurse to take? Select all that apply.
   a. Tell the patient you are sure nothing bad happened to them if they left willingly. Their friends would not have let them leave with a dangerous person.
   b. Tell the patient that you believe them, this is not their fault, and you want to help them.
   c. Tell the patient that they probably decided to have sex, they likely now have a sexually transmitted infection (STI), and they need to accept responsibility for their own actions.
   d. Offer emotional support and referral for counseling, but caution that medical treatment at this time is not necessary as it has been too long since the incident.
   e. Offer emotional support and referral for counseling, and explain each part of the visit such as options for pregnancy and sexually transmitted infection testing.
2. Examples of nursing actions that represent trauma-informed care (TIC) include which of the following? Select all that apply.
   a. Obtain consent from the patient before proceeding in each step of the visit.
   b. Explain each part of the visit and clarify as needed.
   c. Explain that the faster you collect the specimens, the more quickly they can move on.
   d. Maintain eye contact with the patient.
   e. Use draping to cover all body parts not being examined.
3. Changes expected in postmenopausal patients AFAB include which of the following? Select all that apply.
   a. Sleep disturbances
   b. Increased risk for osteoporosis
   c. Anemia

d. Hypernatremia
e. Difficulty with bowel elimination

4. A 51-year-old cisgender Black male patient who has been given written information on the PSA test states he has heard conflicting advice about the usefulness of this test and asks why it has been recommended he have this done. Which of the following can independently suggest a screening PSA is warranted? Select all that apply.
a. The patient is Black.
b. The patient's cousin had prostate cancer at age 76.
c. The patient is White.
d. The patient's father had prostate cancer at age 52.
e. The patient's brother was diagnosed with prostate cancer at age 50.
f. The patient's son had testicular cancer at age 18.
g. The patient has parasitic infections of the bladder.

5. A 61-year-old AMAB patient is complaining of erectile dysfunction. The nurse reviews the patient's medical/surgical history. What data in the patient's chart are associated with erectile dysfunction? Select all that apply.
a. Hypertension
b. Hyperlipidemia
c. GERD
d. Asthma
e. Pelvic fracture
f. Diabetes
g. ORIF of the left arm

REFERENCES AND SELECTED READINGS

References and selected readings associated with this chapter can be found on the website that accompanies the book. Visit **http://thepoint.lww.com/Honan3e** to access the references and other additional resources associated with this chapter.

CHAPTER 32

Nursing Management: Patients With Breast and Female Reproductive Disorders

Yolanda Bone • Vanessa Pomarico-Denino • Maura Murphy Abbott

Learning Objectives

After reading this chapter, you will be able to:

1. Describe common benign breast problems.
2. Identify risk factors for breast cancer.
3. Identify screening and diagnostic tests used to detect breast disorders.
4. Describe different treatment modalities for breast cancer.
5. Use the nursing process as a framework for care of the patient undergoing breast cancer treatment.
6. Describe the distinct types of menstrual disorders and their management.
7. Differentiate bacterial vaginosis and candidiasis.
8. Identify factors associated with pelvic organ prolapse.
9. Understand risk factors for gynecologic cancers.
10. Describe differences between the types of hysterectomies.
11. Identify appropriate care for the transgender patient.

The breast and female reproductive organs play a significant role in normal and abnormal physiology as well as in a person's sexuality and body image. Disorders of the breast or reproductive system, whether minor or serious, can cause great anxiety. Some disorders require only limited intervention. Other diagnoses may require significant interventions, some of which may even be life-threatening. All breast disorders necessitate nurses to have knowledge, understanding, and skill in patient education involving all aspects of care, including prevention, etiology, and treatment.

BREAST DISORDERS

Benign Conditions of the Breast

Most benign breast disorders result from normal physiologic processes. They represent a spectrum of conditions that receive clinical attention and may present as imaging abnormalities, palpable lesions, irregularities found on physical examination, or pain. Once a benign diagnosis has been confirmed, treatment typically focuses on symptom management and patient education. Benign epithelial breast lesions are classified in three categories: nonproliferative, proliferative without atypia, and **atypical hyperplasia**. The latter refers to abnormal epithelial proliferative breast lesions that are not qualitatively or quantitatively abnormal enough to be classified as carcinoma in situ but confer a mild to moderate increase in a patient's risk for developing breast cancer and indicate the need for further evaluation, increased screening recommendations, and a discussion of risk-reduction strategies (Myers & Wall, 2022). The nurse should work as an integral member of the interdisciplinary team to ensure a thorough history and physical examination are completed and that all diagnostic and treatment options are made available to the patient. In addition, the nurse is an invaluable resource and provider of patient education. Table 32-1 compares distinct types of benign and malignant breast masses.

Breast Pain

Mastalgia, or breast pain, is one of the most common breast complaints. Cyclic breast pain, the most common type of breast pain, accounts for nearly 75% of all complaints (ElSherif & Valente, 2022). It is usually related to hormonal fluctuations during the **luteal phase** of the menstrual cycle that stimulate the proliferation of normal glandular tissue and subsequently cause pain. Noncyclic pain is far less common, can be constant or intermittent, and does not vary with the menstrual cycle. Patients who experience muscle

TABLE **32-1 Comparison of Various Breast Masses**

The most common breast masses are due to cysts, fibroadenomas, or malignancy. Biopsy is usually needed for confirmation, but the following characteristics are diagnostic clues:

Characteristics	Cysts	Fibroadenomas	Malignancy
	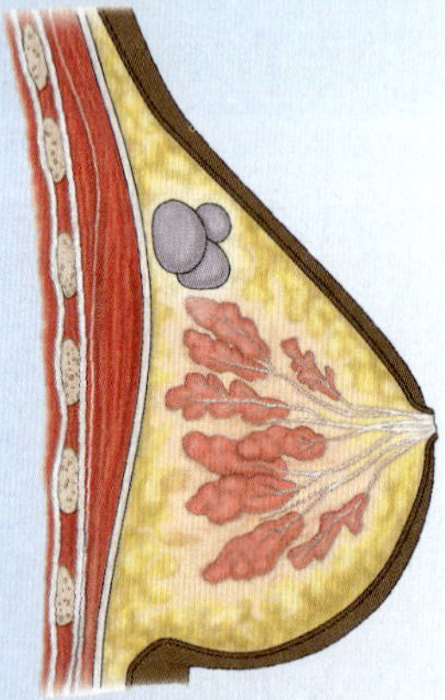	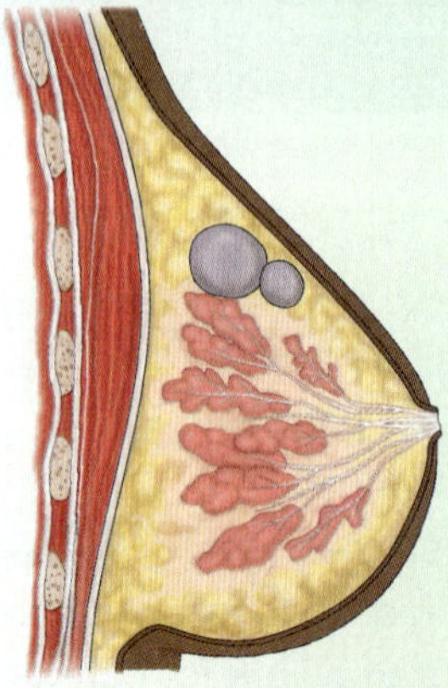	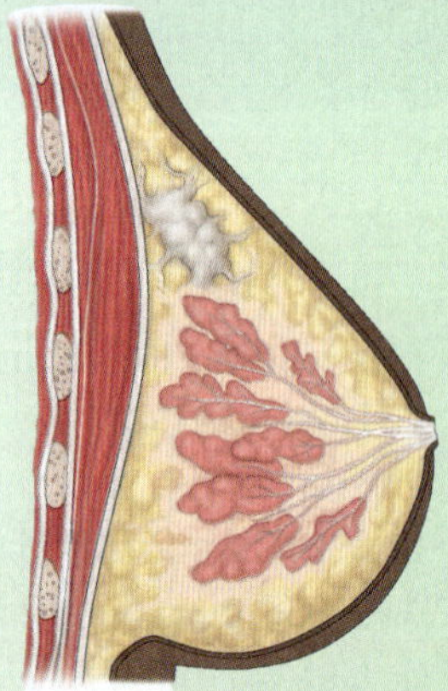
Age	30–55 years of age, regress after menopause except with use of estrogen therapy	Puberty to menopause	At least 30–90+ years of age, most common in postmenopausal years
Number	Single or multiple	Usually single, may be multiple	Usually single
Shape	Round	Round, disk, or lobular	Irregular or stellate
Consistency	Soft to firm, usually elastic	Usually firm	Firm or hard
Mobility	Mobile	Mobile	May be fixed to skin or underlying tissues
Tenderness	Usually tender	Usually nontender	Usually nontender
Retraction signs	Absent	Absent	May be present

strain or trauma to the breast may experience noncyclic pain. Patients should be reassured that breast pain is rarely indicative of cancer. A patient should seek attention from their health care provider for persistent pain. Elimination of methylxanthines, including caffeine, theophylline, and theobromine, may alleviate breast pain. These substances are found in coffee, tea, chocolate, and cola beverages. Lowering dietary fat also may improve cyclic pain, and nonsteroidal anti-inflammatory drugs (NSAIDs) often are initiated. There is some evidence that evening primrose oil, vitamin E, and flaxseed may provide some relief for patients who prefer remedies that are more natural. The attenuated androgen danazol may be implemented for severe, persistent pain and is effective due to its ability to suppress pituitary gonadotropins. However, there are significant side effects to this treatment option, and it is not easily tolerated. Because of this, it is rarely used. Similarly, tamoxifen (a selective estrogen receptor modulator) is an option to treat severe symptoms, but it also carries with it a host of often intolerable side effects (increased risk for endometrial cancer and DVT; common side effects include hot flashes, irregular periods, vaginal discharge, peripheral edema, hypertension, mood changes, pain, depression, skin changes and skin rashes, nausea and vomiting, weakness, arthritis, arthralgia, lymphedema, and pharyngitis); thus, it too is not prescribed often (Dolan & Walsh, 2023; Farrar & Jacobs, 2022). The nurse may recommend that the patient wear a supportive bra both day and night, decrease caffeine intake, and take NSAIDs as needed for breast pain. Oftentimes, this combination of therapies alleviates symptoms significantly (Tahir & Shamsudeen, 2022).

Breast Cysts

Cysts are the most common nonproliferative breast lesions. They are fluid-filled, round or ovoid masses, derived from the terminal duct lobular unit, and develop due to cystic lobular involution (regression of breast lobules). Cysts occur most commonly in females of childbearing age and may be exacerbated during perimenopause when hormonal fluctuations increase. Acute enlargement of cysts, which may occur immediately prior to menses, may cause sudden-onset severe, localized pain. Fibrocystic disease is not a risk factor for the development of breast malignancy; however, atypia (or atypical ductal hyperplasia [ADH]) in fibrocystic disease does have a malignant potential (Kowalski & Okoye, 2022).

Simple Cysts

Simple cysts are benign by definition and do not require intervention. On ultrasound, they are well circumscribed, anechoic (low degree of sound reverberation), and have posterior acoustic enhancement and an absence of solid components. Often aspiration is performed to relieve discomfort, but simple, nonpainful cysts identified incidentally on ultrasound do not require intervention.

Complicated Cysts

Complicated cysts meet most, but not all, criteria for simple cysts on ultrasound examination. They may have internal echoes, fluid or debris components, and an imperceptible wall and may lack posterior acoustic enhancement. They are very rarely malignant but should be aspirated to confirm diagnosis or are followed with repeat imaging.

Complex Cysts

Complex cysts have mixed components that are both cystic and solid in nature with a thick wall and/or internal septa (thin wall or partition) and do require a core biopsy to rule out malignancy. These lesions are more likely than simple or complicated cysts to be cancerous. The risk of malignancy is 23% to 31% for complex cysts (Ortman et al., 2022). The nurse should educate the patient about the diagnostic workup process and provide support to alleviate anxiety.

Fibrocystic Breast Conditions

Often breast pain is attributed to **fibrocystic breast changes** and may be the patient's presenting complaint. Fibrocystic breast changes also can produce a transient breast mass. Both breast discomfort and breast nodularity are common and are often a normal response to hormonal changes during the menstrual cycle, with estrogen primarily being the underlying causative factor. Pathologists also may use the term "fibrocystic" in reference to microscopic findings, such as fibrosis, adenosis, papillomatosis, ductal epithelial hyperplasia, and cysts (Giuliano & Hurvitz, 2022).

Fibroadenomas

Fibroadenomas are proliferative lesions without atypia (cell abnormalities) in which the underlying etiology is the estrogenic effects on breast tissue. They usually present as firm, round, movable, benign tumors that contain glandular and stromal tissue (connective tissue cells). In many cases, multiple fibroadenomas will occur in the same breast or bilaterally. They can occur from puberty to menopause and are most common from the late teens through the early 30s. Fibroadenomas usually do not require treatment. Diagnosis is best confirmed through a "triple test": clinical examination, imaging, and tissue biopsy. Fibroadenomas larger than 2 cm are more likely to persist and commonly are excised. Fibroadenomas also are sometimes excised when they are painful or when the presence of a palpable mass is too anxiety-provoking for the patient to tolerate. Patients with a negative "triple test" (nonsuspicious clinical examination, benign appearance on imaging, and benign pathology results) do not require treatment but should have short-term interval follow-up with clinical examination and age-appropriate imaging (American Cancer Society [ACS], 2022; Sabel, 2023).

Atypical Ductal Hyperplasia

ADH is usually an incidental finding from biopsy of a radiographic abnormality or palpable mass. It is characterized by an abnormal growth of ductal cells in the breast and the presence of atypia (structural abnormality in a cell) without either the cytologic or architectural criteria necessary for a diagnosis of ductal carcinoma in situ (DCIS). The presence of ADH increases the for breast cancer to four to five times that of the general population. Multifocal ADH lesions can present an even higher risk for developing breast cancer (ACS, 2022; Tomlinson-Hansen et al., 2023).

Lobular Carcinoma in Situ

Lobular carcinoma in situ (LCIS) is characterized by an abnormal proliferation of cells within the breast lobules; it is frequently found in the opposite breast (Hayes & Lippman, 2022). LCIS is usually found incidentally from a breast biopsy as it cannot be seen mammographically and may not form a palpable mass. Actually, the term is a bit misleading because this condition is not "carcinoma," or cancer. Historically, LCIS was considered a premalignant condition but is now considered more of a marker of increased risk for invasive breast cancer. The subsequent invasive carcinoma can be either ductal or lobular in origin and can develop in either breast. LCIS increases the of breast cancer about 7 to 11 times when compared with that of the general population (ACS, 2022). Patients with LCIS should be referred to a breast cancer specialist for full discussion of treatment options due to the significantly higher risk for developing breast cancer. These options include increased surveillance, chemoprevention to reduce the risk of developing breast cancer, and consideration for enrollment in breast cancer prevention trials. Patients also may consider bilateral **prophylactic mastectomy** dependent upon the level of risk, family history, and other factors, although it is no more effective in prolonging survival than the less aggressive approach (Hayes & Lippman, 2022; Sabel, 2023).

MALIGNANT CONDITIONS OF THE BREAST

Breast cancer occurs when cells in the breast undergo changes in cellular DNA, do not undergo apoptosis, and grow out of control. Some breast cancers are in situ, which is the earliest stage of cancer and is considered "noninvasive." Breast cancer is the most commonly diagnosed malignancy in female patients, except for nonmelanoma skin cancer. The ACS estimates that 287,850 new cases of invasive breast cancer were diagnosed in the United States in 2022 as well as an additional estimated 51,400 cases of DCIS breast cancer; 43,250 females were expected to die from breast cancer in the United States in 2022. Lung cancer is the only cancer that causes more deaths in females. Although much rarer, males can develop breast cancer. In 2022, it was estimated that 2,710 males were diagnosed with breast cancer, accounting for about 1% of all breast cancer diagnoses. Breast cancer death rates have been decreasing steadily since 1989, for an overall decline of 43% through 2020. The decrease in death rates is believed to be the result of finding breast cancer earlier through screening and increased awareness, as well as better treatments (ACS, 2022). In 2022, there were approximately 3.8 million females living with a history of breast cancer or currently undergoing treatment for the disease (ACS, 2022).

Risk Factors

The two most significant risk factors for developing breast cancer are being female and growing older. Eighty-five percent of females who develop breast cancer have no risk factors other than age and biologic sex. Age is considered the most significant risk factor for the development of breast cancer, rising rapidly until the early 60s, peaking in the 70s, and then declining (Giuliano & Hurvitz, 2023). Whereas most breast cancers are "sporadic," a small percentage (5% to 10%) are due to having an inherited genetic mutation, such as in the ***BRCA1*** or ***BRCA2*** genes. Those who carry these mutations have a lifetime risk of 45% to 85% of developing breast cancer (55% to 85% of people who inherit a harmful BRCA1 variant and 45% to 69% of people who inherit a harmful BRCA2 variant will develop breast cancer by 70 to 80 years of age) (Giuliano & Hurvitz, 2023; NCI, 2020). Box 32-1 lists other risk factors for developing breast cancer.

BOX 32-1 Risk Factors for Breast Cancer

- Being an assigned female at birth (AFAB)
- Increasing age
- Inherited genetic mutation for breast cancer, such as *BRCA1* and/or *BRCA2* or other cancer susceptibility genes
- Family history of breast cancer, particularly with a first-degree relative diagnosed with breast cancer at an early age (under 50 years of age)
- Personal history of breast cancer
- History of benign proliferative breast disease, especially those with atypia
- History of high-dose radiation therapy to the chest, such as patients who have undergone treatment for Hodgkin disease or non-Hodgkin lymphoma
- Hormonal factors:
    - Early menarche (before 12 years of age)
    - Late menopause (after 55 years of age)
    - Nulliparity or no full-term pregnancies
    - Late age at first full-term pregnancy (after 30 years of age)
    - Recent contraceptive use
    - Long-term use of estrogen and progestin (hormone replacement therapy)
- History of ovarian cancer or endometrial cancer
- Obesity, particularly postmenopausal
- Alcohol consumption
- Ashkenazi Jewish ethnicity related to BRCA1/2 mutation carrier risk

Screening and Prevention

While many risk factors like sex and age are not modifiable, other risk factors, such as maintaining a healthy weight or limiting alcohol intake, mitigate the risk of developing breast cancer. As important as prevention is, screening and early detection especially in high-risk patients is equally or perhaps even more important. Early diagnosis generally is associated with better clinical outcomes and overall survival. This is why screening mammograms and prompt attention for any breast abnormality are extremely important.

Males can experience breast cancer, as well, with the risk being 1 in 1,000 males or 1 in every 100 breast cancer diagnoses in the United States (Center for Disease Control and Prevention [CDC], 2022). Since it is so rare in males, they are not offered routine screening, and male breast cancer is not addressed in detail in this chapter. Any breast mass or abnormality should be evaluated in male patients, and male BRCA mutation carriers, due to their increased risk of developing breast cancer, are followed with increased breast cancer surveillance. Upon diagnosis, male breast cancer is treated similarly to breast cancer in females (ACS, 2022; NCCN, 2023).

Protective Factors

People can choose to maximize their overall health by maintaining a normal weight, particularly after menopause, engaging in regular physical activity, and avoiding or limiting alcohol consumption. People who breast or chestfeed for an extended period of time (for a year or longer) may have some added protection. Females at high risk for breast cancer may be candidates for chemoprevention and opt to take selective estrogen receptor modulators (SERMs); medications such as tamoxifen, raloxifene, or aromatase; or inhibitors such as exemestane to reduce their risk (ACS, 2021; NCCN, 2023).

Screening Recommendations

While the ACS does not recommend regular clinical breast exams or breast self-exams as part of a routine breast cancer screening schedule, this does not mean that these exams should never be done. In some situations, particularly for patients at higher-than-average risk, health care providers may still offer clinical breast exams, along with providing counseling about risk and early detection. The risks and benefits of prevention strategies should be discussed in detail, weighing the potential benefits with the risks of the interventions.

Prevention Strategies in the High-Risk Patient

By identifying the population of patients who are at highest risk for breast cancer, prevention and earlier detection are possible. Patients who have risk factors should talk with their health care provider to assess their risk and implement an individualized plan for surveillance and risk reduction. The decision whether or not to undergo genetic testing and the risks and benefits of prevention strategies should be discussed in detail, weighing the potential benefits with the risks of the interventions. Some patients might still be more comfortable doing regular self-exams as a way to keep track of how their breasts look and feel. But it's important to understand that there is very little evidence that doing these exams routinely is helpful for people at average risk of breast cancer (ACS, 2022). People who are at increased risk for breast cancer should talk to their health care provider to establish the optimal age to begin screening as people at high risk often begin clinical breast examinations and breast imaging at younger ages (ACS, 2022; NCCN, 2023).

Long-Term Surveillance

Some people at high risk choose a conservative approach, with more frequent or earlier screening and additional imaging modalities, such as magnetic resonance imaging (MRI). More frequent clinical breast examinations and breast self-awareness are emphasized. The NCCN Clinical Practice Guidelines in Oncology offer patient-specific recommendations for screening in this population (2023).

Chemoprevention

Chemoprevention with a variety of medications has demonstrated significant reduction in breast cancer in people at high risk. The National Surgical Adjuvant Breast and Bowel Project (NSABP) Breast Cancer Prevention Trial showed that treatment with tamoxifen resulted in a 49% decrease in short-term risk for breast cancer in healthy females at increased risk (Vogel, 2001). Raloxifene has also demonstrated effectiveness in risk reduction and has a lower side-effect profile than tamoxifen (although the risk for DVT remains) (Dolan & Walsh, 2023). Both tamoxifen and raloxifene, which are categorized as selective estrogen receptor modulators (SERMs), are FDA approved for chemoprevention. Another medication, exemestane, an aromatase inhibitor, also has demonstrated effectiveness in reducing the risk for breast cancer in healthy people who are high risk. Though its use is recognized by the NCCN and the American Society of Clinical Oncology (ASCO), exemestane is not FDA approved for that use (Dolan & Walsh, 2023). When considering chemoprevention, the risks and benefits should be weighed carefully by the patient and their health care provider.

Prophylactic Mastectomy

Prophylactic bilateral **total mastectomy** is an option for carefully selected patients with significant breast cancer risk and/or extreme anxiety associated with potential diagnosis. This surgery as a method of breast cancer prevention has demonstrated a significant risk reduction in patients who are known to have *BRCA1* or *BRCA2* mutations. The decision to undergo prophylactic mastectomy should be made carefully and with the input of the multidisciplinary team (NCCN, 2023). All breast tissue should be removed, but sentinel node biopsy is not routinely recommended unless breast cancer is detected upon pathologic examination of the tissue (Thompson et al., 2023).

Clinical Manifestations

Breast cancers can occur anywhere in the breast but usually are found in the upper outer quadrant, where the most breast tissue is located. In general, the lesions are nontender, tend to be fixed rather than mobile, and may be harder with irregular borders.

With the increased use of screening mammography, more patients are being diagnosed early and are seeking treatment for earlier-stage disease. These patients often present with no signs or symptoms other than having a mammographic abnormality. However, some patients seek initial treatment after ignoring symptoms. Oftentimes, those patients present with advanced stage disease. Advanced signs may include skin dimpling, nipple retraction, or skin ulceration.

Breast Imaging

Breast imaging includes all of the radiographic imaging modalities used to detect and diagnose breast abnormalities and diseases. Mammography is the most common imaging modality and has improved dramatically over the past several decades. Other common imaging modalities include ultrasound and MRI. Newer types of tests are now being developed for breast imaging. Some of these, such as breast tomosynthesis (3D mammography), are already being used in some centers. Other tests are still being studied, and it will take time to see if they are as good as or better than those used today (ACS, 2022).

Mammography

Mammography is a specific type of radiographic imaging that utilizes low-dose x-ray for examination of the breasts (Iranmakani et al., 2020). Mammography is the best and most universally accepted screening tool available to detect breast cancer at its earliest and most treatable stages, and it is currently the only imaging modality recommended for routine breast cancer screening in the general population.

There are two types of mammograms: screening and diagnostic. Screening mammograms are for routine use at recommended intervals to detect unanticipated breast cancer in asymptomatic females. Screening mammography must be performed on a regular basis in order to reduce breast cancer mortality. Diagnostic mammograms are performed either when a radiographic abnormality is detected on a screening mammogram or when the patient or their caregiver notices a change or a problem in their breast. Also mammography is used to assist in interventional breast procedures, such as stereotactic breast biopsy and needle localization.

Newer, digital mammography techniques provide dramatic improvements in the visualization of lesions for interpreting physicians and greater ease of examination for the patient.

The mammography examination takes only a few minutes and has minimal radiation exposure. During a mammogram, the breast is manually compressed in the mammography unit by a registered mammography technologist in two different views: the craniocaudal view (compression from top to bottom) and the mediolateral oblique view (from side to side). Other views may be obtained when a patient has a palpable or image-detected abnormality requiring more focused or directed examination. The nurse should educate the patient on the importance of regular screening mammography; immediate pursuit of attention upon discovery of any palpable abnormality; and the availability of comfort options, such as disposable foam pads to ease discomfort during compression.

Ultrasound

Ultrasonography (ultrasound) is used as a screening or diagnostic adjunct to mammography. The procedure consists of spreading thin coating of lubricating jelly over the area to be imaged. Then a transducer is placed on the breast. The transducer transmits high-frequency sound waves through the skin toward the area of concern. The sound waves that are reflected back form a two-dimensional image, which is then displayed on a computer screen. No radiation is emitted during the procedure. The technique is used often to determine if a mass is cystic versus solid but cannot rule out malignant lesions definitively. Due to its limited specificity, ultrasound should not be used for routine screening but has recently been advocated as a valuable screening tool in patients who have mammographically dense breasts (ACS, 2022b; Spear & Mendelson, 2021).

Magnetic Resonance Imaging

MRI of the breast produces incredibly detailed cross-sectional images using magnetic fields rather than x-rays. An IV injection of gadolinium, a contrast dye, is given to improve visibility. The patient lies face down and the breast is placed through a depression in the table. A coil is placed around the breast, and the patient is placed inside the MRI machine. The entire procedure takes about 30 to 40 minutes.

MRI is most useful in patients with proven breast cancer, when assessing for multifocal (more than one tumor in the same quadrant of the breast), multicentric (more than one tumor in different quadrants of the breast), or bilateral disease; chest wall involvement; tumor recurrence; or response to chemotherapy (Sumkin et al., 2019). The procedure also can identify occult (undetectable) breast cancer and determine the integrity of saline or silicone breast implants. It is not recommended for routine screening in the general population, but it is recommended for people who have a lifetime risk of greater than 20% to 25% based on predictive models; who have a known or suspected genetic predisposition to breast cancer; or with other elevating risk factors, such as prior radiation exposure. The risks of false-positive and false-negative examination results should be addressed, and MRI screening should be performed after a detailed discussion with the patient (Giuliano & Hurvitz, 2023).

Some disadvantages of MRI include high cost, variations in technique and interpretation, and the potential for patient claustrophobia. Breast MRI is extremely sensitive but has low specificity so the procedure cannot always distinguish malignant and benign breast conditions accurately. MRI is contraindicated in patients with implantable metal devices, such as aneurysm clips, pacemakers, and ports of tissue expanders, because of the magnetic force acting on metallic objects. Removal of all metal from the patient's body and clothing (MRI is a strong magnetic field), including foil-backed medication patches, is necessary prior to MRI to avoid thermal injury (Pagana et al., 2021).

Breast Biopsy

Percutaneous needle biopsy, either by fine-needle aspiration (FNA) or by tissue core biopsy, is the simplest biopsy technique and should always be the first modality considered for breast tissue sampling. This type of biopsy allows for definitive diagnosis with lower morbidity than open surgical biopsy and a lower cost for the procedure. The nurse educates the patient prior to the procedure, answers questions, and offers emotional support. Approximately "60% of lesions clinically thought to be cancer prove on biopsy to be benign, while about 30% of clinically benign lesions are found to be malignant," demonstrating the fallibility of clinical judgment and the need for a biopsy (Giuliano & Hurvitz, 2022).

Fine-Needle Aspiration

Fine-needle aspiration (FNA) is a noninvasive biopsy technique that is generally well tolerated by most patients. A local anesthetic may or may not be used. For palpable masses, a surgeon performs the procedure. A small-gauge needle (25- or 22-gauge) attached to a syringe is inserted into the mass or area of nodularity. Suction is applied to the syringe, and multiple passes are made through the mass. A simple cyst often disappears on aspiration, and the fluid is usually discarded, though it may be sent for pathologic examination. If no fluid is obtained on aspiration, then any cellular material obtained in the hub of the needle is spread on a glass slide or

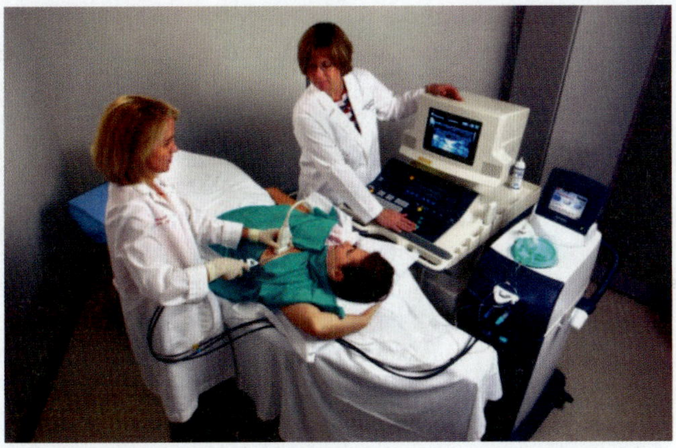

FIGURE 32-1 Ultrasound-guided breast biopsy. (Courtesy of Mammotome.)

placed in a preservative and sent to the laboratory for analysis. For nonpalpable masses, the same procedure can be performed by a radiologist or surgeon using ultrasound guidance.

FNA is less expensive than other diagnostic methods, and usually results are available quickly; however, due to risk of a false-negative result and the inability to distinguish between noninvasive and invasive cancers close clinical correlation is necessary (Giuliano & Hurvitz, 2022).

Ultrasound-Guided Breast Biopsy

Ultrasound-guided breast biopsy is a minimally invasive procedure wherein the physician uses the ultrasound to visualize the lesions and guide the needle for sampling (Fig. 32-1). It is the preferred biopsy modality for all lesions visible by ultrasound. For the procedure, the patient lies supine on a table and the physician inserts a needle to obtain specimens after thoroughly cleaning the skin, injecting subcutaneous analgesia such as lidocaine, and making a small nick in the skin. The needle may or may not have vacuum assistance to help obtain adequate specimens. The biopsy needle is typically 12- to 18-gauge without vacuum assistance and 7- to 12-gauge with vacuum assistance. Several tissue samples are obtained and sent to the laboratory for analysis. A small titanium clip should be placed in the biopsy cavity for documentation of correct sampling site, for future mammogram evaluation, and for locating the site should further treatment be warranted.

Stereotactic Breast Biopsy

Stereotactic core biopsy is another minimally invasive procedure that uses x-ray guidance to obtain breast tissue samples (Fig. 32-2). It is the preferred biopsy modality for microcalcifications and lesions not visible by ultrasound. The patient lies prone on the stereotactic table, and the breast is suspended through an opening and compressed between two x-ray plates. Digital mammography images are obtained, and the exact coordinates of the lesion to be sampled are located with the aid of a computer. After sterilizing the skin, a local anesthetic is injected into the entry site on the breast. A small

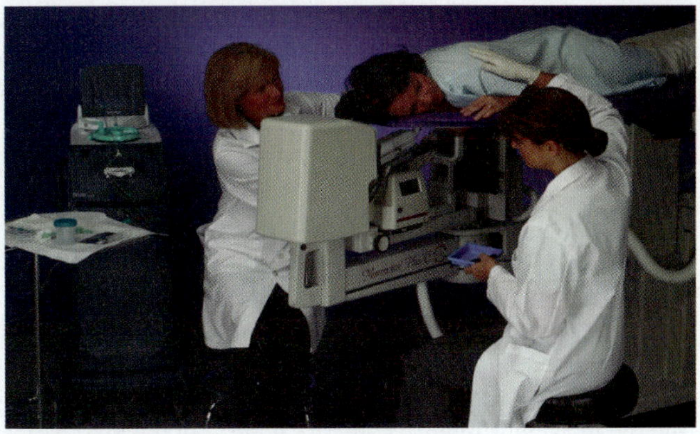

FIGURE 32-2 Stereotactic breast biopsy. (Courtesy of Mammotome.)

nick is made in the skin, a core needle is inserted, and samples of the tissue are taken for pathologic examination. Often, several passes are taken to ensure adequate tissue sampling. Clip placement is necessary for this type of biopsy as well.

Magnetic Resonance Imaging–Guided Breast Biopsy

MRI-guided breast biopsy is logistically similar to **stereotactic biopsy** and is used increasingly for lesions that cannot be visualized under mammography or ultrasound. Special concern is necessary for equipment safety in the magnetic field, and MRI-specific biopsy equipment is used.

Surgical Biopsy

When minimally invasive breast biopsy is not feasible, an excisional or surgical biopsy may be used to remove an entire lesion with minimal tissue loss. This type of biopsy also may be referred to as a *lumpectomy.* Depending on the clinical situation, a frozen-section analysis of the specimen may be performed at the time of the biopsy by the pathologist, who does an immediate intraoperative reading and provides a provisional diagnosis. Surgical biopsy is usually performed using local anesthesia and IV sedation and often follows *wire needle localization*, wherein mammography or ultrasonography are used to locate the lesion and place a guidewire through the skin and into the area of suspicion. Then the surgeon may follow the guidewire down to the lesion for precise removal and minimal tissue loss.

The nurse plays a significant role in surgical breast biopsy. During the preoperative visit, the nurse assesses the patient for specific educational, physical, or psychosocial needs. The nurse should review medical and psychosocial history and facilitate conversation regarding fears, concerns, and questions. Often patients are worried not only about the procedure but also about the potential implications of the pathology results. The nurse should provide a thorough explanation and written materials to reinforce education.

The patient should discontinue any anticoagulant therapy prior to the procedure. The patient may be instructed not to eat or drink for several hours or after midnight the night before the procedure, depending on the type of biopsy planned. Most breast biopsy procedures today are performed with the use of moderate sedation and local anesthesia.

Immediate postoperative assessment includes monitoring the effects of the anesthesia and inspecting the surgical dressing for any signs of bleeding. Once the sedation has worn off, the nurse reviews the care of the biopsy site, pain management, and activity restrictions with the patient. Prior to discharge from the ambulatory surgical center or the office, the patient must be able to tolerate fluids, ambulate, and void. The patient must have someone to drive them home. Usually, the dressing covering the incision is removed after 48 hours, but the Steri-Strips, which are applied directly over the incision, should remain in place for approximately 7 to 10 days. The use of a supportive bra following surgery is encouraged to limit movement of the breast and to reduce discomfort. A follow-up telephone call from the nurse 24 to 48 hours after the procedure can provide the patient with the opportunity to ask any questions and can be a source of great comfort and reassurance.

Most people return to their usual activities the day after the procedure but are encouraged to avoid jarring or high-impact activities for 1 week to promote healing of the biopsy site. Usually discomfort is minimal, and most patients find acetaminophen sufficient for pain relief, although a mild opioid may be prescribed if needed. Follow-up after the biopsy includes a return visit to the surgeon for discussion of the final pathology report and assessment of the healing of the biopsy site.

Staging

There are three primary staging systems for cancer. The most clinically relevant, the American Joint Committee on Cancer (AJCC)'s TNM system classifies tumors using information on the size of the tumor and the extent of spread within the breast (T), involvement in lymph nodes (N), and spread to distant organs (M). Refer to Chapter 5 for more information on staging of cancer. This staging system is used very commonly in clinical settings and assigns a stage of I, II, III, or IV according to the determined T, N, and M classification. Stage I indicates an early-stage breast cancer, and IV indicates the most advanced. The Extent of Disease system used by the National Cancer Institute (NCI)'s Surveillance, Epidemiology, and End Results (SEER) program and the Summary Stage system are other classification systems that are used often in data reporting and state tumor registries (NCI, n.d.). The American Joint Committee on Cancer and the International Union Against Cancer have a joint TNM (tumor, regional lymph nodes, distant metastases) staging system for breast cancer that recently included biologic markers to modify the anatomic staging (Giuliano & Hurvitz, 2022).

Prognosis

The most important prognostic factors for breast cancer patients at diagnosis are stage of disease and grade of disease. Stage refers to the size of the tumor; if the cancer has spread into the lymph nodes; and, if there are metastases, whether they are local or distant. The smaller the tumor size and the less it has spread, the lower the stage and the more favorable the outcomes in comparison to larger tumors with wider spread. Grade refers to how aggressive the cancer cells are. The more aggressive the cancer, the higher the grade leading to a worse prognosis. Another prognostic factor that also helps determine treatment is hormone receptor positivity, as there are treatments that can target hormonal positive tumors such as estrogen and progesterone. Patients who are diagnosed at a more advanced stage have a lower 5-year relative survival rate, as do patients with larger tumor size at diagnosis. The 5-year relative survival rate for localized disease (stages 0–I) is near or equal to 100%, for regional disease (stages II–III) is approximately 86%, and for distant-stage disease (stage IV) it is 29% (ACS, 2022). Overall survival rate for all SEER stages of breast cancer is 90% (ACS, 2022). The most common route of regional spread is to the axillary lymph nodes (Fig. 32-3). Other sites of lymphatic spread include the internal mammary and supraclavicular nodes. Distant metastasis can affect any organ, but the most common sites are bone, lung, liver, pleura, adrenals, skin, and brain. Amplification of certain genes, such as *HER2/neu* (discussed later in this chapter), or excessive amounts of their protein product may represent a poorer prognosis. Box 32-2 lists other prognostic factors.

Types

Ductal Carcinoma in Situ

Ductal carcinoma in situ (DCIS) is characterized by the proliferation of malignant cells inside the milk ducts without invasion into the surrounding tissue. Frequently, DCIS is manifested on a mammogram with the appearance of calcifications, and it is considered stage 0 breast cancer. Treatment options include breast-conserving surgery and radiation therapy with or without tamoxifen, total mastectomy with or without tamoxifen, and breast-conserving surgery without radiation therapy (NCI, 2020).

Infiltrating Ductal Carcinoma

Infiltrating ductal carcinoma (IDC), the most common histologic type of breast cancer, accounts for 80% of all cases. The tumors arise from the duct system and invade the surrounding tissues. They often present as a solid mass in the breast.

Infiltrating Lobular Carcinoma

Infiltrating lobular carcinoma (ILC) accounts for approximately 10% of breast cancers and is the second most common type of breast cancer after IDC. These tumors arise from the lobular epithelium and typically occur as an area of ill-defined thickening in the breast. They are often multicentric and can be bilateral.

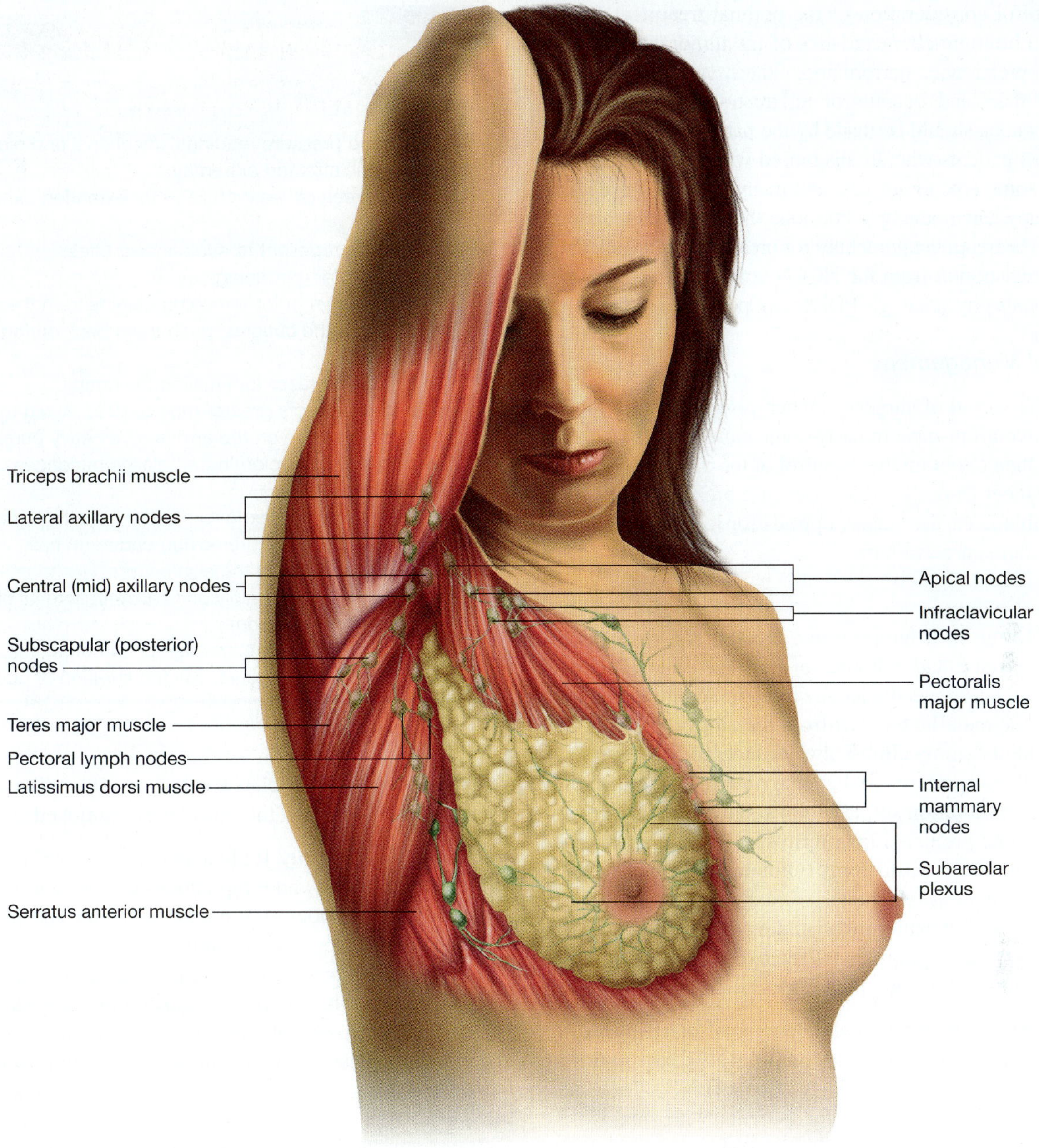

FIGURE 32-3 Lymphatic drainage of the breast. (Reprinted from Lippincott Williams & Wilkins [LWW]. [2016]. Breast and axilla. In L. M. Willis [Ed.], *Health assessment made incredibly visual!* [3rd ed., Chapter 7, p. 346]. Wolters Kluwer.)

BOX 32-2

Factors Affecting Prognosis for Breast Cancer

- Age and menopausal status of the patient
- Stage of disease
- Histologic and nuclear grade of the primary tumor
- Estrogen and progesterone receptor status of the primary tumor
- Proliferative capacity of the tumor
- *HER2/neu* gene amplification

From PDQ® Adult Treatment Editorial Board. *PDQ breast cancer treatment*. National Cancer Institute. Retrieved July 19, 2023, from https://www.cancer.gov/types/breast/hp/breast-treatment-pdq

Medullary Carcinoma of the Breast

Medullary carcinoma is a rare subtype of IDC and accounts for about 5% of breast cancers. It tends to be diagnosed more often in the patient's 40s to early 50s. The tumor is usually a soft, fleshy mass that tends to be low grade, and it is not likely to spread outside of the breast tissue. Because of this, the prognosis is often favorable.

Medical and Nursing Management

A multidisciplinary team approach to treatment for breast cancer allows for an individualized plan of care based upon careful consideration of the optimal treatment for the stage and biologic characteristics of the tumor; the patient's personal preference, performance status, and age; and the potential risks and benefits of all treatment options. Treatment decisions should be made by the patient and their physician. Most patients who are diagnosed with breast cancer will undergo some type of surgery, and many also will have radiation therapy, chemotherapy, hormone therapy, and/or biologic therapy. The treatment guidelines for breast cancer are available via free registration from the NCCN at https://www.nccn.org/professionals/physician_gls/PDF/breast.pdf (NCCN, 2023).

Surgical Management

The primary goal of surgery is when possible to be curative and remove all disease in early-stage cancers and when not possible then to obtain local control of the disease by removing the cancer from the breast. Because breast cancer is now diagnosable at earlier stages, options for less invasive surgical procedures are available.

Procedures

Lumpectomy. In a lumpectomy, the surgeon removes the cancerous tissue and a border of normal tissue. This usually follows a wire needle localization procedure to mark the tumor or the metallic clip left from the biopsy. Patients who undergo lumpectomy almost always undergo 5 to 7 weeks of radiation therapy afterward. Patients who have a lumpectomy or breast conservation surgery followed by radiation therapy have the same predicted long-term survival as patients who choose to undergo mastectomy (Giuliano & Hurvitz, 2022). Appropriate patient selection is critical when planning surgical intervention. A patient who undergoes lumpectomy also may have regional lymph nodes removed to determine if the cancer has spread beyond the breast.

Simple Mastectomy. In a simple or total mastectomy, the entire breast and nipple–areola complex (NAC) are removed, without axillary lymph node dissection (ALND). Total mastectomy may be performed for patients with noninvasive breast cancer or DCIS, which does not have a tendency to spread to the lymph nodes. It also may be performed prophylactically for patients who are at substantial risk for breast cancer. Also, a total mastectomy may be performed in conjunction with **sentinel lymph node** biopsy (SLNB) for patients with invasive breast cancer.

Modified Radical Mastectomy. Modified radical mastectomy is performed to treat invasive breast cancer. The procedure involves removal of the entire breast tissue, including the NAC. In addition, a portion of the axillary lymph nodes are removed (ALND). Box 32-3 discusses hand and arm care after ALND.

If immediate breast reconstruction is desired, the patient is referred to a plastic surgeon prior to the mastectomy so that they have the opportunity to explore all available options. In modified radical mastectomy, the pectoralis major and pectoralis minor muscles are left intact, unlike in radical mastectomy, in which the muscles are removed.

BOX 32-3 Patient Education

Hand and Arm Care after Axillary Lymph Node Dissection (ALND)

- Avoid blood pressure readings, injections, and blood draws in the affected extremity.
- Use sunscreen (at least 15 SPF) for extended exposure to the sun.
- Apply insect repellent to avoid insect bites.
- Wear gloves for gardening.
- Use a cooking mitt for removing objects from the oven.
- Avoid cutting the cuticles; push them back during manicures.
- Use an electric razor for shaving the armpit.
- Avoid lifting objects greater than 5–10 lb. Avoid too much increased pressure on the arm (e.g., a heavy purse).
- Avoid tight jewelry, clothing, or elastic bandages on the affected arm.
- Avoid chemical hair removers under the affected arm, and avoid nicks and cuts if removing underarm hair.
- If a trauma or break in the skin occurs, wash the area with soap and water, and apply an OTC antibacterial ointment (Bacitracin or Neosporin).
- Observe the area and extremity for 24 hours; if redness, swelling, or a fever occurs, call the surgeon or nurse.

Radical Mastectomy. Radical mastectomy includes removal of the entire breast and lymph nodes under the arm as well as removal of the underlying pectoralis major and minor muscles. This technique is currently used very rarely due to the proven effectiveness and significantly decreased morbidity associated with less aggressive procedures, such as modified radical mastectomy, total mastectomy, and lumpectomy.

Newer mastectomy techniques, including skin-sparing and NAC sparing, are gaining popularity as the cosmetic outcome is often favorable compared to traditional mastectomy procedures. However, these techniques are not appropriate for everyone and require a careful evaluation and discussion between the patient and their surgeon.

Breast Conservation Therapy. The goal of **breast conservation treatment**, including lumpectomy, wide excision, partial or segmental mastectomy, and quadrantectomy (one quarter of the breast tissue removed) is to excise the tumor in the breast completely and obtain clear margins while achieving an acceptable cosmetic result. If the procedure is being performed to treat a noninvasive breast cancer, lymph node removal is not necessary. For an invasive breast cancer, lymph node removal is indicated. The lymph nodes are removed through a separate semicircular incision in the axilla. Breast conservation along with radiation therapy in stage I and stage II breast cancers has demonstrated survival rates equal to that of modified radical mastectomy.

Sentinel Lymph Node Biopsy. SLNB is used for pathologic axillary staging for patients with breast cancer. The sentinel lymph nodes are the first nodes in the lymphatic basin to receive drainage from the primary tumor in the breast and are identified by injecting a radioactive tracer, blue dye, or both around the tumor in the breast. The tracer travels via the lymphatic pathways to the sentinel nodes. The surgeon locates the nodes, excises them, and sends them for pathologic analysis. If cancer cells are present in the sentinel nodes, the likelihood of cancer in other lymph nodes is high, so the surgeon performs a complete ALND. If the sentinel lymph nodes are free of cancer, ALND is not necessary. SLNB is considered best practice, and it is the standard of care for staging invasive breast cancer as it is accurate and spares patients considerable morbidity and sequelae associated with complete dissection. Figure 32-3 shows the lymphatic drainage of the breast.

Although SLNB is a less invasive procedure than ALND and results in a shorter recovery period, a patient who has undergone SLNB still may experience complications, such as lymphedema, related to the procedure. The nurse's role is to educate the patient on methods to manage lymphedema, listen to the patient's concerns, provide emotional support, and refer the patient to appropriate specialists when indicated.

Complications for the Surgical Patient

Lymphedema. Lymphedema results from impaired flow of lymph fluid through the draining lymphatic vessels after lymph node dissection. An accumulation of lymph fluid develops in the surrounding and dependent tissues, leading to swelling, fibrosis of the soft tissues, neurologic complications such as pain and paresthesias, and infection. Continuous assessment and early identification of signs and symptoms of lymphedema should be integral in the care of patients undergoing therapy for breast cancer. Risk for lymphedema depends on the type of therapy received and is more common in patients who undergo ALND. Recent research noted that manual lymphatic drainage in the early stages following breast cancer surgery may help prevent progression to clinical lymphedema (Thompson et al., 2021). Referral to a lymphedema specialist is key to management of this complication (Sleigh & Manna, 2022).

Pearls for Practice

To prevent lymphedema or lymphangitis (infection of the lymph vessels), nurses should place a sign above the bed of a patient following mastectomy or node dissection not to perform blood pressures, blood draws, injections, or IV insertions on the side where the operation was performed. Lymphatic drainage is altered due to node dissection, causing the potential for fluid to accumulate in the affected extremity. Tight or restrictive clothing or jewelry is avoided on the same side as the surgical procedure. Complications of infiltration, phlebitis, or trauma can result if the affected extremity is used. Some patients will obtain a medical alert bracelet with this warning.

Hematoma and Seroma Formation. Hematoma, a collection of blood inside the surgical cavity, may occur after either mastectomy or breast conservation and usually develops within the first 12 hours after surgery. The nurse assesses for signs and symptoms of hematoma at the surgical site; this may include swelling, tightness, pain, and bruising of the skin. The surgeon should be notified immediately for gross swelling or increased bloody output from the drain, typically a Jackson-Pratt. While most hematomas are small and resolve without intervention, some must be evacuated surgically. Refer to Box 32-4 for drain care.

A seroma, a collection of serous fluid, may accumulate under the breast incision after mastectomy or breast conservation or in the axilla. Signs and symptoms include swelling, heaviness, discomfort, and a sloshing of fluid. Seromas may develop temporarily after the drain is removed or if the drain is in place and becomes obstructed. Seromas rarely pose a threat, and the surgeon or health care provider may unclog the drain or manually aspirate the fluid with a needle and syringe.

Infection. Infection is a risk after any surgical procedure. This risk may be higher in patients with accompanying conditions, such as diabetes, immune disorders, and advanced age, as well as in those with poor hygiene. Patients are taught to monitor for signs and symptoms of infection, such as redness, warmth around the incision, tenderness, foul-smelling drainage, temperature greater than 100.4°F, and chills and to contact the surgeon or nurse for evaluation should they notice any of these. For more severe infections, treatment consists of oral or IV antibiotics for 1 or 2 weeks.

Nursing management for patients undergoing surgery is discussed in the nursing process section later in this chapter.

Reconstructive Surgery

A variety of reconstructive options is available today for those who desire a correction in the size or the shape of the breast, including reduction **mammoplasty**, augmentation mammoplasty, and mastopexy (discussed shortly). Several options are also available to reconstruct the breast after a mastectomy.

Reconstructive Surgeries for Lumpectomy. Reconstructive surgeries include reduction mammoplasty, augmentation mammoplasty, and mastopexy.

Reduction mammoplasty is most commonly performed on people who have large breasts. It is an outpatient procedure that is performed under general anesthesia. Most commonly, an anchor-shaped incision that circles the areola is made, extending downward and following the natural curve of the inframammary fold. Depending on the size of the breast, the nipple may be moved up to a higher position while still attached to the breast tissue, or it may be separated

BOX 32-4

Surgical Breast Cancer Patient With a Drainage Device

A drain is placed in the surgical wound at the time of surgery to evacuate drainage from the surgical site. The tubing has multiple perforations on the distal end (in the wound site), and the tubing is attached to a device externally that collects the drainage. Suction is maintained by compression of the device. Usually the drain is sutured to the skin. The typical device used for breast surgery is called a *Jackson Pratt* (JP), a bulb-like device (see the figure below).

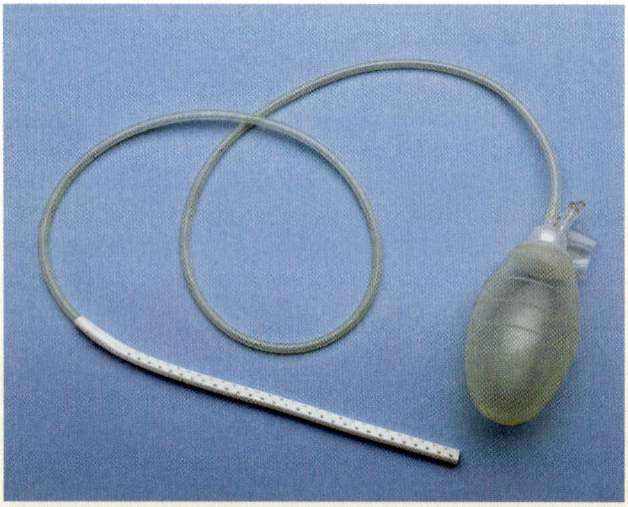

The nurse and patient or caregiver are aware that the device must be compressed to maintain suction at the wound bed. If the device is inflated fully, it must be emptied to maintain the vacuum necessary to facilitate drainage away from the wound bed.

The nurse explains the procedure to the patient and/or caregiver, brings a measuring device such as an ounce medicine cup (if limited drainage is expected) or a graduated cylinder, and explains the importance of hand washing before the procedure (maximum capacity of the JP is approximately 100 mL). Nonsterile gloves are donned.

The JP drainage device is unclipped from the patient's gown, and, using sterile technique, the spout plug is opened on the JP bulb. The device will expand fully since the suction has been released (image above reveals fully expanded JP; no vacuum exists). The nurse is careful not to touch the inside of the spout or plug and teaches this to the patient and/or caregiver. The device is emptied by turning the bulb over and squeezing the bulb so that the contents can escape from the device. The amount and appearance of the drainage is recorded. The JP bulb is NEVER squeezed unless the spout plug is released.

An alcohol wipe can be used to clean the spout and plug. Maintaining sterile technique, the JP is compressed completely flat with one hand, and, while compression is maintained, the plug is reattached with the other hand.

The nurse is aware that the system must be airtight to function. If rapid reinflation is noted after plugging the spout, an air leak should be suspected; the nurse attempts to compress and plug the device again, and if the device remains inflated, the provider should be notified. The nurse secures the device to the patient's gown, below the wound (to facilitate drainage) to prevent pulling on the wound site and/or potential dislodgment. The nurse removes and discards gloves and washes hands thoroughly.

If multiple drains are used, they are labeled numerically (1, 2) or alphabetically (a, b), and drainage per drain is recorded as deemed by institutional policy or surgeon protocol.

Depending on surgeon preference and quality of the drainage, the patient may be instructed on how to "milk clots" through the tubing of the drainage device, which requires gentle compression of the tubing between the thumb and index finger while stabilizing the exit site to prevent dislodgment of the tubing with the nondominant hand. Holding the tube securely above the obstruction is necessary to avoid pulling the tube out of the incision. *Note: This is only done depending on surgeon preference.*

The nurse teaches the patient and/or caregiver which observations of the drain site require contacting the physician or nurse (e.g., sudden change in color of drainage, sudden cessation of drainage, signs or symptoms of an infection) per the surgeon's recommendation.

The nurse reinforces that the drain is typically ready for removal by the surgeon when draining is less than 30 mL for a 24-hour period.

and transplanted to a new location. Drains are placed in the incision and remain for 2 to 5 days.

Augmentation mammoplasty is performed on those who desire larger or fuller breasts. Usually this procedure is performed by placing a silicone or saline breast implant under the pectoralis muscle. The incision line can be placed in the inframammary fold, in the axilla, or around the areola. The procedure is performed as an outpatient procedure under general anesthesia. A drain is not necessary.

Mastopexy is performed when the patient is content with the size of their breasts but wishes to have the shape changed and a lift performed. The procedure is also an outpatient surgery.

Reconstructive Procedures after Mastectomy. Breast reconstruction can provide a significant psychological benefit for patients who are already struggling with the emotional distress of losing a breast. A consultation with a plastic surgeon can help the patient understand procedures for which they are a candidate and the pros and cons of each option. Factors to consider include body size and shape; comorbidities, such as hypertension, diabetes mellitus, or obesity; personal habits, such as smoking; and patient preference. The patient must be informed that although breast reconstruction can provide a good cosmetic result, it will never precisely duplicate the natural breast. Realistic preparation can help the patient avoid unrealistic expectations. Reconstruction is considered an integral component in the surgical treatment of breast cancer and is usually covered by insurance companies.

Many patients elect immediate reconstruction at the time of the mastectomy operation. Delayed reconstruction may

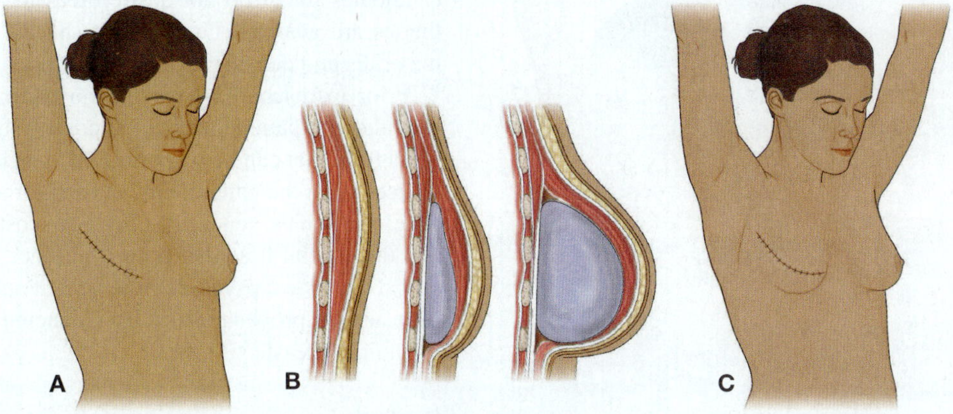

FIGURE 32-4 **Breast reconstruction with tissue expander. A. Mastectomy incision line prior to tissue expansion. B. The expander is placed under the pectoralis muscle and is filled gradually with saline solution through a port to stretch the skin enough to accept a permanent implant. C. The breast mound is restored. Although permanent, scars will fade with time. The nipple and areola are reconstructed later. (Adapted from American Society of Plastic and Reconstructive Surgeons. *Breast reconstruction*. Author.)**

be preferable to patients who are having a difficult time deciding on whether reconstruction is desired at all or if they are unsure as to the type of reconstruction they prefer. In patients with advanced disease, such as in inflammatory breast cancer, treatments should be given without delay so immediate reconstruction is not recommended. Delays in healing after immediate reconstruction may interfere with the initiation of treatment, particularly radiation therapy.

Tissue Expander Followed by Permanent Implant. Breast reconstruction using a tissue expander followed by a permanent implant is commonly used. To accommodate an implant, the skin remaining after a mastectomy and the underlying muscle must be stretched gradually by a process called *tissue expansion.* The surgeon places a balloon-like device through the mastectomy incision underneath the pectoralis muscle. A small amount of saline is injected through a metal port intraoperatively to partially inflate the expander, this is followed by additional saline injections through the port at weekly intervals until the expander is fully inflated. It remains fully expanded for about 6 weeks to allow the skin to loosen. Then the expander is exchanged for a permanent implant.

Advantages are a shorter operating time and a shorter recuperation period than for autologous (using the patient's own tissue) reconstruction. A disadvantage is a tendency for the implant to feel firm and round, with little natural ptosis, or sag. Patients with a small to medium contralateral breast with little ptosis are good candidates for this procedure. Patients who have had prior radiation or who have connective tissue disease are not good candidates because of the decreased elasticity of the skin.

The patient may be instructed not to have an MRI while the tissue expander is in place as often the port contains metal. This is not an issue once the permanent implant is in place. Figure 32-4 shows breast reconstruction with a tissue expander.

Tissue Transfer Procedures. Autologous reconstruction is the use of the patient's own tissue to create a breast mound. A flap of skin, fat, and muscle with its attached blood supply is rotated to the mastectomy site to create a mound that simulates the breast. Donor sites may include the **transverse rectus abdominis myocutaneous (TRAM) flap** (Fig. 32-5), gluteal flap, or the latissimus dorsi flap (Fig. 32-6). The results more closely resemble a real breast because the skin and fat from the donor sites are similar in consistency to a natural breast. These procedures are far more complex and involve longer recuperation than a procedure with a tissue expander. The risk for potential complications, such as infection, bleeding, and flap necrosis, is also greater.

The TRAM flap is the tissue transfer procedure that is performed most commonly. This involves completely detaching the skin, fat, muscle, and blood supply from the body and then

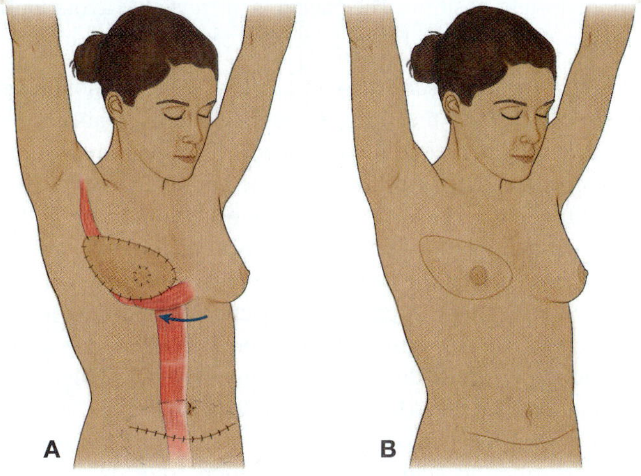

FIGURE 32-5 **Breast reconstruction: transverse rectus abdominis myocutaneous (TRAM) flap. A. A breast mound is created by tunneling abdominal skin, fat, and muscle to the mastectomy site. B. Final location of scars. (Adapted from American Society of Plastic and Reconstructive Surgeons. *Breast reconstruction*. Author.)**

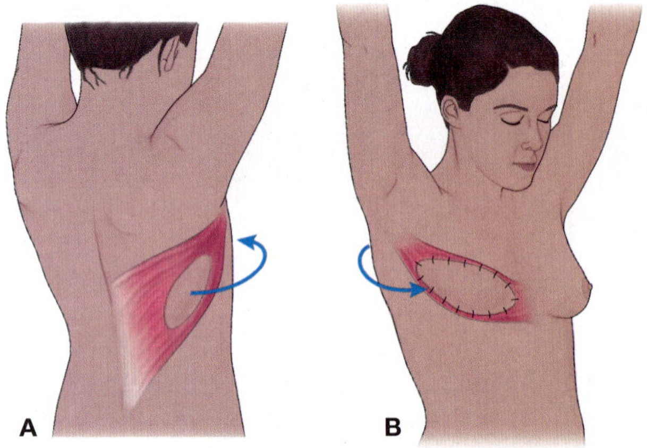

FIGURE 32-6 **Breast reconstruction: latissimus dorsi flap. A. The latissimus muscle with an ellipse of skin is rotated from the back to the mastectomy site. B. Because the flap usually is not bulky enough to provide an adequate breast mound, often an implant is also required. (Adapted from American Society of Plastic and Reconstructive Surgeons. *Breast reconstruction.* Author.)**

transplanting them to the mastectomy site using microvascular surgery. Postoperatively, patients who have undergone TRAM procedures often face a lengthy recovery of 8 to 10 weeks and have incisions both at the mastectomy site and at the donor site in the abdomen. The nurse must assess the newly constructed breast site for changes in color, circulation, and temperature because flap loss is a potential complication. Mottling or an obvious decrease in skin temperature is reported to the surgeon immediately. Breathing and leg exercises are essential because the patient is more limited in their activity and is at greater risk for respiratory complications and deep vein thrombosis (DVT). Measures to help the patient reduce tension on the abdominal incision during the first postoperative week include elevating the head of the bed 45 degrees. Once the patient is able to ambulate, they can protect the surgical incision by splinting it and gradually will achieve a more upright position. The patient is instructed to avoid high-impact activities and lifting to prevent stress on the incision.

Nipple–Areolar Reconstruction. After the breast mound has been created and the site has healed, some patients choose to have nipple–areolar reconstruction. This is a minor surgical procedure performed either in the physician's office or at an outpatient surgical facility. The most common method of creating a nipple is with the use of local flaps of skin and fat from the center of the new breast mound, which are wrapped around each other to create a projecting nipple. The areola is created using a skin graft. The most common donor site is the upper inner thigh because this skin has darker pigmentation than the skin on the reconstructed breast. After the nipple graft has healed, micropigmentation or tattooing can be performed to achieve a more natural color. Usually the surgeon can match the reconstructed NAC with that of the contralateral breast for an acceptable cosmetic result.

Prosthetics. A breast prosthesis, an external form that simulates the breast, is an option for patients who are not candidates for or do not desire breast reconstruction. Prosthetics are available in different shapes, sizes, colors, and materials and can be placed inside a bra.

Prior to discharge from the hospital, the nurse usually provides the patient with a temporary, lightweight, cotton-filled form that can be worn until the surgical incision is well healed. Then the patient can be fitted for a prosthesis. Insurance companies generally cover the cost of the prosthesis and the special bras that hold it in place. A breast prosthesis can provide a psychological benefit and assist the patient in resuming proper posture by balancing the weight of the remaining breast.

Radiation

Patients may undergo radiation therapy to destroy any residual microscopic cancer cells in the breast, chest wall, axilla, internal mammary, or supraclavicular nodes following surgery (NCCN, 2023).

Breast conservation treatment followed by radiation therapy for stage I and II breast cancers results in a survival rate equal to that of a modified radical mastectomy. If radiation therapy, a component of breast conservation treatment, were contraindicated, then a mastectomy would be indicated. Also radiation treatment is recommended after mastectomy in patients whose breast cancer tumors were large (greater than 5 cm) or when the lymph nodes were involved.

Types

Patients may undergo external beam radiation (EBR) therapy or internal radiation, also known as **brachytherapy**.

External Beam Radiation. EBR typically begins about 6 weeks after breast conservation surgery to allow the surgical site to heal. If systemic chemotherapy is indicated, radiation therapy usually begins after its completion. Before radiation begins, the patient undergoes a planning session called a *simulation*, in which the anatomic areas to be treated are mapped out and then identified with small permanent ink markings. EBR delivers high-energy photons from a linear accelerator and usually is administered to the entire breast region. Each treatment lasts only a few minutes and generally is given 5 days a week for 5 to 7 weeks. In patients whose surgery consisted of breast conservation, after completion of radiation to the entire breast, many patients receive a "boost," a dose of radiation to the lumpectomy site where the cancer was removed. If a mastectomy was performed, radiation treatments are targeted at the chest wall. The treatments are not painful.

Accelerated breast irradiation is a newer technique that is gaining favor. It is similar to standard EBR, but it is given at a slightly higher dose over a 3-week period as opposed to 5 to 6 weeks. Breast cancer recurrence rates at 10 years are equal in both groups. Even more accelerated approaches in radiation treatment are being implemented in some settings. These include even larger doses of radiation over a 5-day period as well as intraoperative radiation therapy (IORT), which is single-dose treatment given in the operating room after lumpectomy is performed.

Internal Radiation Therapy. Internal radiation therapy, or brachytherapy, involves inserting a radioactive substance sealed in needles, seeds, catheters, or wires directly into the breast. MammoSite, Savi, Axxent, and Contura are varieties of internal radiation treatment options in which radiation is administered twice a day over a 5-day period.

Some patients receive both internal and external radiation. The type of radiation and the frequency depend on the classification, stage, and location of the tumor (Giuliano & Hurvitz, 2022).

Nursing Management of the Patient Undergoing Radiation Therapy

In general, radiation therapy is well tolerated. Acute side effects consist of mild to moderate erythema, breast edema, and fatigue. Occasionally, skin breakdown may occur in the inframammary fold or near the axilla toward the end of treatment. Frequent trips to the radiation oncology unit for treatment can exacerbate fatigue and may be accompanied by depression. The patient needs to be reassured that the fatigue is normal and not a sign of recurrence. Side effects usually resolve within a few weeks to a few months after treatment is completed. Rare long-term effects of radiation therapy include pneumonitis, rib fracture, breast fibrosis, and lymphedema (if radiation treatment also included the axilla).

Self-care instructions for patients receiving radiation are provided to assist in the maintenance of skin integrity during the treatments and for several weeks after completion. They pertain only to the area being treated and not to the rest of the body. The instructions include the following:

- Use mild soap with minimal rubbing.
- Avoid perfumed soaps or deodorants.
- Use hydrophilic lotions (e.g., Lubriderm, Eucerin, Aquaphor) for dryness.
- Use a nondrying, antipruritic soap (e.g., Aveeno) if pruritus occurs.
- Avoid tight clothes, underwire bras, excessive temperatures, and ultraviolet light.

Follow-up care includes teaching the patient to minimize sun exposure to the treated area, such as using sunblock with an SPF of 15 or above, and reassuring the patient that minor twinges and shooting pain in the breast are normal after radiation treatment.

Systemic Therapy

Systemic treatment uses anticancer, or antineoplastic, drugs that are given intravenously or orally and travel throughout the body in the bloodstream with the goal of destroying cancer cells that have escaped the breast and axillary lymph nodes before they metastasize. Chemotherapy, targeted therapy which includes biologic and hormonal therapy and immunotherapy are types of systemic treatment. **Neoadjuvant therapy** (drug treatment given prior to surgery) allows for assessment of the tumor's response to the chemical agent and is used to shrink a tumor before surgery. When successful tumor shrinkage occurs, breast conservation surgery without the need for mastectomy can be performed. **Adjuvant therapy** is administered after surgery and is used to eradicate any residual cancer cells in the body. The type of systemic therapy used depends on the tumor type/grade, immunohistology, hormonal status, size, lymph node status, angiolymphatic invasion (cancer cells seen in small blood or lymph vessels), and age and performance status of the patient (NCCN, 2023).

For some patients who have metastatic disease, or breast cancer that has traveled beyond the breast and into other organs or parts of the body, surgery may no longer be advisable, and systemic therapy is the primary treatment of choice.

Biologic Therapy

HER2/neu is a growth-promoting protein that is present in about 15% to 30% of breast cancers and results in faster growth and a higher recurrence rate than in tumors that do not overproduce it. Trastuzumab is a monoclonal antibody that targets this protein and reduces the recurrence rate and mortality in patients with both metastatic and early-stage breast cancer. Lapatinib, bevacizumab, and pertuzumab are other biologic therapies that are used to treat advanced breast cancer in appropriate patients (NCCN, 2023).

Endocrine (Hormone) Therapy

Estrogen is a hormone produced in the ovaries that can promote breast cancer growth. Females whose breast cancers have positive hormone receptors may take hormone therapy to block the effects of estrogen on tumor growth. Both premenopausal and postmenopausal patients may take tamoxifen if their tumors test positive for hormone receptors. Tamoxifen works by blocking the effects of estrogen on breast tissue. Tamoxifen is recommended for a 5- to 10-year course of therapy after surgery and has demonstrated significant reduction in the recurrence rate and improved survival. Sequelae of tamoxifen include menopausal symptoms, fatigue, mood swings, and an increased risk of endometrial cancer and blood clots (NCCN, 2023).

Aromatase inhibitors, such as letrozole, anastrozole, and exemestane, are another hormone therapy option for postmenopausal patients. These drugs work by blocking aromatase, an enzyme whose role is to convert the hormone androstenedione to estrogen in the body after menopause, thus decreasing levels of circulating estrogen. Aromatase inhibitors cannot stop the ovaries from making estrogen, so they are not effective in premenopausal patients. They are prescribed for a 5-year course of therapy and may be given alone or following a course of tamoxifen. Aromatase inhibitors have a lower side-effect profile than tamoxifen

TABLE **32-2 Adverse Reactions Associated With Adjuvant Hormonal Therapy Used to Treat Breast Cancer**

Therapeutic Agent	Adverse Reactions/Side Effects
Selective Estrogen Receptor Modulator	
Tamoxifen	Hot flashes, vaginal dryness/discharge/bleeding, irregular menses, nausea, mood disturbances, increased risk for endometrial cancer, increased risk for thromboembolic events (deep vein thrombosis, pulmonary embolism, superficial phlebitis)
Aromatase Inhibitors	
Anastrozole Letrozole Exemestane	Musculoskeletal symptoms (arthritis, arthralgia [joint pain], myalgia [muscle pain]), increased risk of osteoporosis/fractures, nausea/vomiting, hot flashes, fatigue, mood disturbances

but can cause osteoporosis, bone fractures, and musculoskeletal problems (ACS, 2022). Table 32-2 lists potential adverse effects of different hormonal therapies for breast cancer. Box 32-5 addresses side-effect management of hormonal agents.

Chemotherapy

The indication for chemotherapy depends on the size of the tumor, lymph node involvement, the presence or absence of hormone receptors in the tumor, and the amount of HER2/neu present in the breast cancer cells. Combination chemotherapy, or the use of more than one drug, has proven to be more effective than single-drug regimens. The most common drugs recommended for use in breast cancer are cyclophosphamide, docetaxel, doxorubicin, epirubicin, fluorouracil, and paclitaxel. Most chemotherapy regimens are given in 2- to 3-week cycles for a total of 3 to 6 months of therapy (ACS, 2022; NCCN, 2023).

Immunotherapy

Immunotherapy is the use of medicines to boost a person's own immune system to recognize and destroy cancer cells more effectively. Immunotherapy typically works on specific proteins involved in the immune system to enhance the immune response. These drugs have side effects different from those of chemotherapy. Some immunotherapy drugs, for example, monoclonal antibodies, work in more than one way to control cancer cells and may also be considered targeted therapy because they block a specific protein on the cancer cell to keep it from growing. Immunotherapy is used to treat some types of breast cancer, specifically triple negative breast cancer (ACS, 2022). An example of an immunotherapeutic agent is pembrolizumab that targets PD-1 (a protein on immune system T cells that normally helps keep them from attacking other cells in the body). By blocking PD-1, these drugs boost the immune response against breast cancer cells. This can often shrink tumors (ACS, 2022).

BOX 32-5 **Patient Education**

Managing Side Effects of Adjuvant Hormonal Therapy in Breast Cancer

Hot Flashes
- Wear breathable, layered clothing.
- Avoid caffeine and spicy foods.
- Perform breathing exercises (paced respirations).
- Consider medications (vitamin E, antidepressants) or acupuncture.

Vaginal Dryness
- Use vaginal moisturizers for everyday dryness (e.g., Replens, vitamin E suppository).
- Apply vaginal lubrication during intercourse (e.g., Astroglide, K-Y jelly).

Nausea and Vomiting
- Consume a bland diet.
- Try to take medication in the evening.

Musculoskeletal Symptoms
- Take nonsteroidal analgesics as recommended.
- Take warm baths.

Risk of Endometrial Cancer
- Report any irregular bleeding to a gynecologist for evaluation.

Risk for Thromboembolic Events
- Report any redness, swelling, or tenderness in the lower extremities or any unexplained shortness of breath.

Risk for Osteoporosis or Fractures
- Undergo a baseline bone density scan.
- Perform regular weight-bearing exercises.
- Take calcium supplements with vitamin D.
- Take bisphosphonates (e.g., alendronate) or calcitonin as prescribed.

Common side effects associated with immunotherapy are skin rashes, fatigue, diarrhea, endocrine problems, and other immune-mediated systemic effects.

Nursing Management of the Patient Undergoing Chemotherapy

Common physical side effects of chemotherapy for breast cancer vary with the type of treatment given and may include nausea, vomiting, bone marrow suppression, taste changes, alopecia (hair loss), mucositis (painful inflammation and ulcerations of the mucous membranes in the digestive tract), skin changes, and fatigue. A weight gain of more than 10 lb occurs in about half of all patients; the cause is unknown. Premenopausal patients also may experience temporary or permanent **amenorrhea** (absence of menstrual period) leading to sterility. Nurses play a key role in helping patients manage the physical and psychosocial sequelae of chemotherapy. Instructing the patient about the use of antiemetics and reviewing the optimal dosage schedule can help minimize nausea and vomiting. Measures to ease the symptoms of mucositis may include rinsing with normal saline solution, avoiding hot and spicy foods, and using a soft toothbrush. Some patients may require hematopoietic growth factors to minimize the effects of chemotherapy-induced neutropenia and anemia. Granulocyte colony–stimulating factors (G-CSFs) boost the white blood cell count, helping reduce the incidence of neutropenic fever and infection. Erythropoietin growth factor increases the production of red blood cells, thus decreasing the symptoms of anemia. The nurse instructs the patient and family on proper injection technique of hematopoietic growth factors and about symptoms that require follow-up with their provider.

The nurse may assist the patient in finding a wig prior to hair loss to alleviate the stress associated with alopecia. The nurse may provide a list of wig suppliers in the patient's geographic region. Familiarity with creative ways to use scarves and turbans may help minimize the patient's distress. The patient needs reassurance that new hair will grow back when treatment is completed, although the color and texture may be different. The ACS offers a program called "Look Good, Feel Better," which began in 1989 and provides useful tips for applying cosmetics during chemotherapy.

Chemotherapy may negatively affect the patient's self-esteem, sexuality, and sense of well-being. This, combined with the stress of a potentially life-threatening disease, can be overwhelming. Providing support and promoting open communication are important aspects of nursing care. Referring the patient to a dietitian, social worker, psychiatrist, or spiritual advisor can provide additional support. Numerous community support and advocacy groups are available for patients and their families. Complementary therapies, such as guided imagery, meditation, and relaxation exercises, also can be used in conjunction with conventional treatments. Refer to Chapter 5 for details on cancer care.

Pearls for Practice

The nurse recognizes that many patients will experience chemotherapy-induced nausea and vomiting (CINV), which may persist for several days after chemotherapy. For patients at high risk for CINV, antiemetics are given prior to initiation of treatment, and the nurse reviews the discharge medication plan for breakthrough nausea and vomiting. Refer to Chapter 5 for details on CINV.

Treatment for Recurrent or Metastatic Breast Cancer

Breast cancer may recur locally (on the chest wall or in the conserved breast), regionally (in the remaining lymph nodes), or systemically (in distant organs). In metastatic disease, the bone, usually the hips, spine, ribs, or pelvis, is the most common site of spread. Other sites of metastasis include the lungs, liver, pleura, and brain.

The overall prognosis and optimal treatment are determined by a variety of factors, such as the site and extent of recurrence, the time to recurrence from the original diagnosis, history of prior treatments, the patient's performance status, and any existing comorbid conditions. Patients with bone metastases generally have a longer overall survival compared with metastases in visceral organs.

Local recurrence in the absence of systemic disease is treated aggressively with surgery, radiation, and hormonal therapy. Chemotherapy also may be used for tumors that are not hormonally sensitive. Local recurrence may be an indicator that systemic disease will develop in the future, particularly if it occurs within 2 years of the original diagnosis.

Metastatic breast cancer involves control of the disease rather than cure. Treatment includes hormonal therapy, chemotherapy, immunotherapy, and targeted therapy. Surgery or radiation may be indicated in select situations. Premenopausal patients who have hormonally dependent tumors may eliminate the production of estrogen by the ovaries through **oophorectomy** or suppression of estrogen synthesis by luteinizing hormone–releasing hormone (LHRH) agonists, such as leuprolide or goserelin.

Patients with advanced breast cancer are monitored closely for signs of disease progression. Baseline studies are obtained at the time of recurrence. These may include complete blood count; comprehensive metabolic panel; tumor markers; bone scan; CT of the chest, abdomen, and pelvis; and MRI of symptomatic areas. Additional x-rays may be performed to evaluate areas of pain or abnormal areas seen on bone scan. These studies are repeated at regular intervals to assess for effectiveness of treatment and to monitor progression of disease (NCCN, 2023).

Nursing Management of the Patient With Recurrent or Metastatic Breast Cancer

Nurses play a vital role in not only educating patients and managing their symptoms but also in providing emotional support. Many patients find that recurrence of the disease is more distressing than the initial cancer diagnosis. In addition to coping with further treatments, they are faced with a greater uncertainty about their future and long-term survival. The nurse can help the patient identify coping strategies and set priorities to optimize quality of life (QOL). Family members and significant others should be included in the treatment plan and follow-up care. Referrals to support groups, psychiatry, social work, and complementary medicine programs, such as guided imagery, meditation, and yoga, should be made as indicated.

Nurses are also key members of the interdisciplinary team providing palliative care. The highest priorities should include alleviating pain and providing comfort measures. A frank discussion with the patient and family regarding their preferences for end-of-life care should occur before the need arises to ensure a smooth transition without disruption of care. Referrals to hospice and home health care should be initiated as necessary.

Survivorship and Quality of Life

With increased early detection and improved treatment modalities, people with breast cancer have become the largest group of cancer survivors. Sequelae of diagnosis and treatment may affect the patient and their family for an extended period of time. It is important that nurses learn about these long-term effects and intervene appropriately to optimize QOL. The nurse can be pivotal in providing education and support to the patient as they make very difficult and emotional decisions. The patient should be prepared early for the potential long-term complications of the disease and its treatments so that they can make informed decisions, have realistic expectations, and be proactive in obtaining the support that is needed.

Many breast cancer survivors have difficulty with issues pertaining to sexuality and menopausal symptoms. Estrogen withdrawal due to chemotherapy-induced menopause and hormone therapy can cause a variety of symptoms, including hot flashes, vaginal dryness, urinary tract infections (UTIs), weight gain, decreased sex drive, and increased risk for osteoporosis. Some of these symptoms also can lead to fatigue and sleep disturbances. Hormone replacement therapy (HRT) to alleviate menopausal symptoms is contraindicated with breast cancer, so patients need to rely on alternative remedies. Certain chemotherapeutic agents can cause long-term cardiac effects and impaired cognitive functioning, such as difficulty concentrating. Rare long-term effects of radiation can include pneumonitis and rib fractures. Long-term sequelae after breast surgery may include lymphedema (mainly after ALND), pain, and sensory disturbances.

Pearls for Practice

Cardiac function must be assessed in patients undergoing chemotherapy and/or radiation since common cardiac complications in patients with breast cancer involve dysfunction of the cardiovascular system manifested by damage of cardiomyocytes (cardiac muscle cell). Patients can develop asymptomatic left ventricular dysfunction or even heart failure, abnormal valve function, cardiac arrhythmias and conduction disorders, myocarditis, pericarditis, endothelial damage, premature development of atherosclerosis, and thromboembolic complication (Bikiewicz et al., 2021); cardiotoxicity is also associated with some chemotherapy agents (Giuliano & Hurvitz, 2022). The nurse is aware that echocardiography, Holter monitoring, cardiac and pulmonary assessments, and laboratory work, such as brain natriuretic peptide (BNP) and troponin levels, may be monitored.

Long-term psychosocial ramifications may include anxiety, depression, uncertainty about the future, and fear of recurrence. Many of these sequelae can affect the patient's partner and children. In the workplace, the patient may suffer from fear of discrimination, concern over coworkers' reactions, fear of losing benefits, and lack of physical stamina. The nurse should facilitate open conversation with the patient about their fears and concerns and provide referrals to support groups and counseling as needed.

NURSING PROCESS
The Patient Undergoing Surgery for Breast Cancer

ASSESSMENT

The health history is a valuable tool to assess the patient's reaction to the diagnosis and their ability to cope with it. Pertinent questions include the following:

- How is the patient responding to the diagnosis?
- What coping mechanisms does the patient find most helpful?
- What psychological or emotional supports does the patient have and use?
- Is there a partner, family member, or friend available to assist them in making treatment choices?
- What are their educational needs?
- Is the patient experiencing any pain or discomfort?

DIAGNOSIS

Major preoperative nursing diagnoses may include the following:

- Knowledge deficiency about the planned surgical treatments
- Anxiety related to the diagnosis of cancer
- Fear related to specific treatments and body image changes
- Coping impairment (individual or family) related to the diagnosis of breast cancer and related treatment options
- Decisional conflict related to treatment options

Major postoperative nursing diagnoses may include the following:

- Pain and discomfort related to surgical procedure
- Disturbed sensory perception related to nerve irritation in affected arm, breast, or chest wall
- Altered body image perception related to loss or alteration of the breast
- Risk for impaired adjustment related to the diagnosis of cancer and surgical treatment
- Self-care deficit related to partial immobility of upper extremity on operative side
- Risk for sexual dysfunction related to loss of body part, change in self-image, and fear of partner's responses
- Knowledge deficiency:
  - Drain management after breast surgery
  - Arm exercises to regain mobility of affected extremity
  - Hand and arm care after an ALND

Potential complications may include the following:

- Lymphedema
- Hematoma/seroma formation
- Infection

PLANNING

The major goals may include increased knowledge about the disease and its treatment; reduction of preoperative and postoperative fear, anxiety, and emotional stress; improvement of decision-making ability; pain management; improvement in coping abilities; improvement in sexual function; and the absence of complications.

INTERVENTIONS

Both pre- and postoperative nursing care greatly impact the patient's surgical experience.

PREOPERATIVE NURSING INTERVENTIONS

Providing Education and Preparation About Surgical Treatments. Patients with newly diagnosed breast cancer are expected to absorb an abundance of new information during a very emotionally challenging time. The nurse plays a key role in reviewing treatment options by reinforcing information provided to the patient and answering any questions. The nurse fully prepares the patient for what to expect before, during, and after surgery. Patients undergoing breast conservation with ALND, or a total or modified radical mastectomy, generally remain in the hospital overnight (or longer if they have immediate reconstruction). Surgical drains will be inserted in the mastectomy incision and in the axilla if the patient undergoes an ALND. The patient should be informed that they will go home with the drain(s) and that complete instructions about drain care will be provided prior to discharge. In addition, the patient should be informed that often they will have decreased arm and shoulder mobility after an ALND and that they will be shown range-of-motion exercises prior to discharge. Refer to Box 32-6 for exercises after breast surgery. The patient also should be reassured that appropriate analgesia and comfort measures will be provided to alleviate any postoperative discomfort. In addition, the nurse can inform the patient about educational materials that are available on the web by the National Comprehensive Cancer Network for **DCIS breast cancer** (https://www.nccn.org/patientresources/patient-resources/guidelines-for-patients/guidelines-for-patients-details?patientGuidelineId=30), **invasive breast cancer** (https://www.nccn.org/patients/guidelines/content/PDF/breast-invasive-patient.pdf), and **metastatic breast cancer** (https://www.nccn.org/patients/guidelines/content/PDF/stage_iv_breast-patient.pdf). These guidelines are developed by a multidisciplinary panel of breast cancer experts and contain the most recent recommendations for patients. More than 60 guidelines have been created by NCCN and can be accessed at Guidelines for Patients (nccn.org).

Reducing Fear and Anxiety and Improving Coping Ability. The nurse must help the patient cope with the physical as well as the emotional effects of surgery. Many fears may emerge during the preoperative phase. These can include fear of pain, mutilation (after mastectomy), and loss of sexual attractiveness; concern about inability to care for oneself and one's family; concern about taking time off from work; and coping with an uncertain future. Providing the patient with realistic expectations about the healing process and expected recovery can help alleviate fears. Maintaining open communication and assuring the patient that they can contact the nurse at any time with questions or concerns can be a source of comfort. The patient also should be made aware of available resources at the treatment facility as well as in the breast cancer community, such as social workers, psychiatrists, and support groups. Some patients find it helpful and reassuring to talk to a breast cancer survivor who has undergone similar treatments.

Promoting Decision-Making Ability. Choosing the optimal treatment can be very overwhelming for patients. The nurse can be instrumental in ensuring that the patient and family members truly understand their options and can weigh the risks and benefits of each option. The patient may be presented with the option of having breast conservation treatment followed by radiation or a mastectomy. The nurse can explore the issues with the individual patient by asking questions such as the following:

- How would you feel about losing your breast?
- Are you considering breast reconstruction?
- If you choose to retain your breast, would you consider undergoing radiation treatments 5 days a week for 5–6 weeks?

Questions such as these can help the patient focus. Once the patient's decision is made, it is especially important to support it.

POSTOPERATIVE NURSING INTERVENTIONS

Relieving Pain and Discomfort. Many patients tolerate the breast surgery quite well and have minimal pain during the postoperative period. Patients who have had more invasive procedures, such as a modified radical mastectomy with

(continued on page 1106)

BOX 32-6

Patient Education

Exercise after Breast Surgery

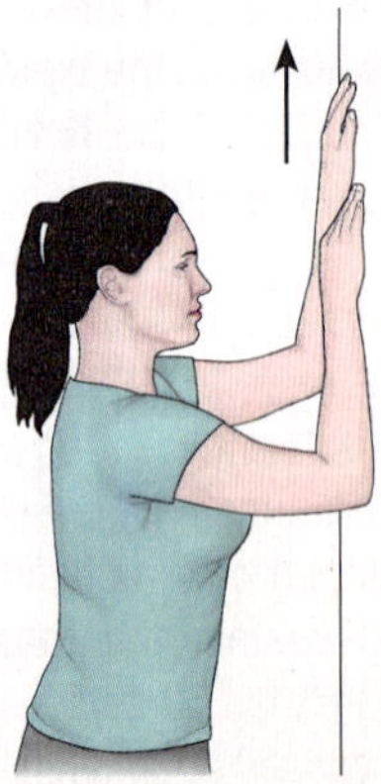

1. *Wall handclimbing*. Stand facing the wall with feet apart and toes as close to the wall as possible. With elbows slightly bent, place the palms of the hand on the wall at shoulder level. Flexing the fingers, work the hands up the wall until arms are fully extended. Then reverse the process, working the hands down to the starting point.

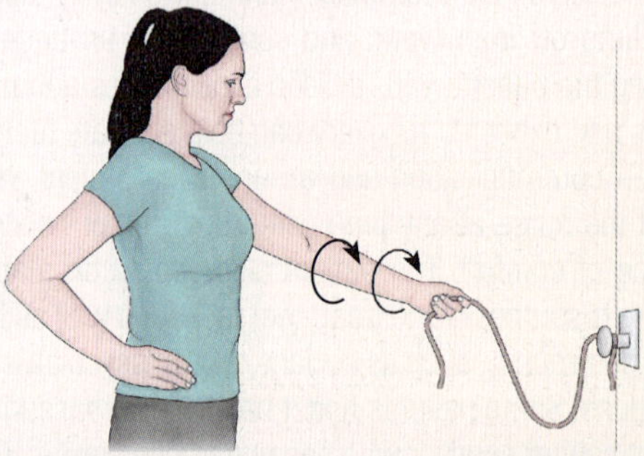

2. *Rope turning*. Tie a light rope to a doorknob. Stand facing the door. Take the free end of the rope in the hand on the side of surgery. Place the other hand on the hip. With the rope-holding arm extended and held away from the body (nearly parallel with the floor), turn the rope, making as wide swings as possible. Begin slowly at first; speed up later.

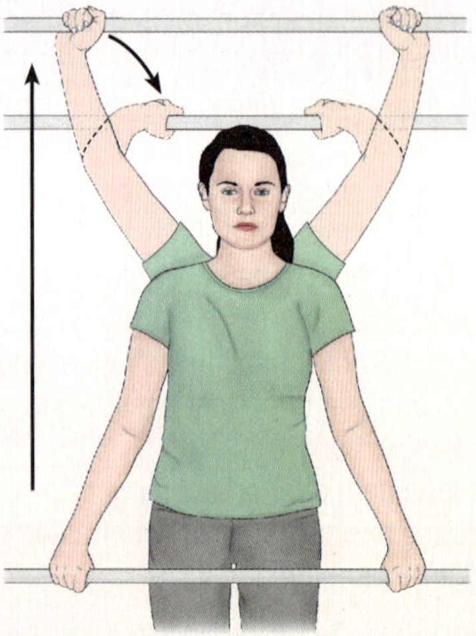

3. *Rod or broomstick lifting*. Grasp a rod with both hands, held about 2 ft apart. Keeping the arms straight, raise the rod over the head. Bend elbows to lower the rod behind the head. Reverse the maneuver, raising the rod above the head, and then return to the starting position.

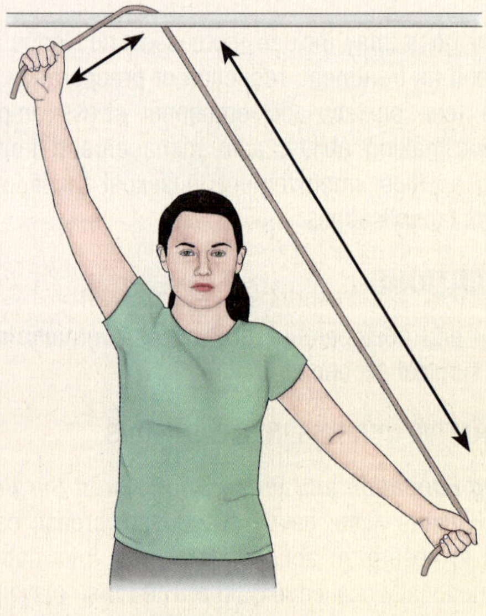

4. *Pulley tugging*. Toss a light rope over a shower curtain rod or doorway curtain rod. Stand as nearly under the rope as possible. Grasp an end in each hand. Extend the arms straight and away from the body. Pull the left arm up by tugging down with the right arm, then the right arm up and the left down in a see-sawing motion.

immediate reconstruction, may have considerably more pain. All patients are discharged home with an analgesic and are encouraged to take it if needed. Sometimes patients complain of a slight increase in pain after the first few days of surgery as they regain sensation around the surgical site and become more active. Patients who report severe pain must be evaluated to rule out any potential complications. Alternative methods of pain management, such as taking warm showers and using distraction methods such as guided imagery, also may be helpful.

Managing Postoperative Sensations. Because nerves in the skin and axilla often are cut or injured during breast surgery, patients

BOX 32-7

Talking With Patients and Partners

For patients in the diagnostic phase: We've talked about your recent breast cancer diagnosis. It's natural for you to be full of feelings, concerns, and fears for yourself and your family. Sometimes it's hard to find someone to speak freely with. Would you like to share what you've been thinking about, feeling, and worrying about recently?

For partners in the diagnostic phase: We've talked about your partner's recent breast cancer diagnosis. It's natural for you to have a lot of feelings, concerns, and fears for your partner, yourself, and your family. Partners often feel that they have to be strong for the patient or for others and that they aren't entitled to express their own concerns. Would you like to share what you've been thinking about, feeling, or worrying about recently?

For patients in the postsurgical phase: Many people who have had breast surgery, especially mastectomy or extensive lumpectomy, are concerned not only with their own loss but also with how their partner will accept it. How have you felt about losing [part of] your breast? How has it changed your body image? Your sense of your sexuality? Your desire for intimacy?

For partners in the postsurgical phase: Many partners of people who have had breast surgery are concerned, as are the patients themselves, about how they'll respond to the loss. How have you felt about your partner's losing [part of] their breast? How has it changed their attractiveness for you? Your sexual feelings toward them? Your desire for intimacy?

For patients in the adjuvant therapy phase: Given the type of therapy (radiation, chemotherapy, hormone therapy) you're going to have, what side effects do you anticipate? What do you know about them? Let's talk about ways to reduce and handle potential side effects.

For partners in the adjuvant therapy phase: Given the type of therapy (radiation, chemotherapy, hormone therapy) your partner is going to have, what side effects do you anticipate? What do you know about them? Let's talk about ways to reduce and handle potential side effects and how it might help you to be familiar with them.

For patients in the ongoing recovery phase: As you plan your return to a full work schedule, what measures—setting priorities, delegating responsibility, managing stress—might help you make the necessary physical and emotional adjustments? What have you learned about balancing work, family, and play in your life?

For partners in the ongoing recovery phase: As your partner plans their return to a full work schedule, what strategies have you thought about using to make your own physical and emotional adjustments so that you don't continue to be overburdened at work and at home?

From Hoskins, C. N., & Haber, J. (2000). Adjusting to breast cancer. *American Journal of Nursing*, *100*(4), 26–32.

experience a variety of sensations, such as tenderness, soreness, numbness, tightness, pulling, and twinges along the chest wall, in the axilla, and along the inside aspect of the upper arm. After mastectomy, some patients experience phantom sensations and report a feeling that the breast and/or nipple are still present. Sensations usually persist for several months and then begin to diminish. Patients should be reassured that this is a normal part of healing and that these sensations are not indicative of a problem.

Promoting Positive Body Image. Patients who have undergone mastectomy often find it very difficult to view the surgical site for the first time. No matter how prepared the patient may think they are, the appearance of an absent breast can be very emotionally distressing. Some patients who have undergone breast conservation treatment may find it difficult to view their surgical incisions, although this is rare. Ideally, the patient sees the incision for the first time when they are with the nurse or another health care provider who is available for support. The nurse first assesses the patient's readiness and provides gentle encouragement and a private setting.

Promoting Positive Adjustment and Coping. Providing ongoing assessment of how the patient is coping with their diagnosis of breast cancer and their surgical treatment is important in determining their overall adjustment. Assisting the patient in identifying and mobilizing their support systems can be beneficial to their well-being. The patient's spouse or partner may need guidance, support, and education as well. The patient and partner may benefit from a wide network of available community resources, including the Reach to Recovery program of the ACS, advocacy groups, or a spiritual advisor. Encouraging the patient to discuss issues and concerns with other patients who have had breast cancer may help them to understand that their feelings are normal and that other people who have had breast cancer can provide invaluable support and understanding.

The patient also may have considerable anxiety about the treatments that will follow surgery and their implications. Providing information about the plan of care and referral to the appropriate members of the health care team also promote coping during recovery. Some patients require additional support to adjust to their diagnosis and the changes that it brings. Box 32-7 lists talking points for patients and partners.

Improving Sexual Function. Once discharged from the hospital, most patients are physically allowed to engage in sexual activity. However, any change in the patient's body image or self-esteem or the response of their partner may increase their anxiety level and affect sexual function. Some partners may have difficulty looking at the incision, whereas others may be completely unaffected. Encouraging the patient to openly discuss how they feel and possible reasons for a decrease in libido, such as fatigue, anxiety, and self-consciousness, may help to clarify issues. Helpful suggestions for the patient may include varying the time of day for sexual activity; such as when the patient is less tired; assuming positions that are more comfortable; and expressing affection using alternative measures such as hugging, kissing, and manual stimulation.

(*continued on page 1108*)

Most patients and their partners adjust with minimal difficulty if they openly discuss their concerns. However, if issues cannot be resolved, a referral may be helpful. The ambulatory care nurse in the outpatient clinic or hospital should inquire whether the patient is having difficulty with sexuality issues because many patients are reluctant or embarrassed to bring it up themselves.

EVALUATION

Expected preoperative patient outcomes may include:

1. Exhibits knowledge about diagnosis and surgical treatment options:
   a. Asks relevant questions about diagnosis and available surgical treatments
   b. States rationale for surgery
   c. Describes advantages and disadvantages of treatment options
2. Verbalizes willingness to deal with anxiety and fears related to the diagnosis and the effects of surgery on self-image and sexual functioning
3. Demonstrates ability to cope with diagnosis and treatment:
   a. Verbalizes feelings appropriately and recognizes normalcy of mood lability
   b. Proceeds with treatment in timely fashion
   c. Discusses impact of diagnosis and treatment on family and work
4. Demonstrates ability to make decisions regarding treatment options in timely fashion

Expected postoperative patient outcomes may include:

1. Reports that pain has decreased and states that pain and discomfort management strategies are effective
2. Identifies postoperative sensations and recognizes that they are a normal part of healing
3. Exhibits clean, dry, and intact surgical incisions without signs of inflammation or infection
4. Lists the signs and symptoms of infection to be reported to the nurse or surgeon
5. Verbalizes feelings regarding change in body image
6. Discusses meaning of the diagnosis, surgical treatment, and fears appropriately
7. Participates actively in self-care activities:
   a. Performs exercises as prescribed
   b. Participates in self-care activities as prescribed
8. Discusses issues of sexuality and resumption of sexual relations
9. Demonstrates knowledge of postdischarge recommendations and restrictions:
   a. Describes follow-up care and activities
   b. Demonstrates appropriate care of incisions and drainage system
   c. Demonstrates arm exercises and describes exercise regimen and activity limitations during postoperative period
   d. Describes care of affected arm and hand and lists indications to contact the surgeon or nurse
10. Experiences no complications:
    a. Identifies signs and symptoms of reportable complications (e.g., redness, heat, pain, edema)
    b. Explains how to contact appropriate health care providers in case of complications

REPRODUCTIVE DISORDERS

MENSTRUAL DISORDERS

Menstrual disorders consist of any irregularity within the menstrual cycle. Previous terminology used to describe deviations in uterine bleeding has included **amenorrhea** (absence of menses), **dysmenorrhea** (painful menses), **menorrhagia** (excessive menstrual bleeding), **metrorrhagia** (excessive and prolonged menstrual bleeding), irregular bleeding patterns, **premenstrual syndrome** (PMS), and **premenstrual dysphoric disorder** (PMDD). Normal menstrual cycles typically occur every 21 to 45 days (ACOG, 2021b).

Any menstrual cycle changes should be discussed with the patient's health care provider, so that appropriate diagnosis, management, and treatment can occur.

AMENORRHEA

Amenorrhea is divided into two types: primary, which is the absence of menses by age 13 without secondary sex characteristics or by age 15 regardless of presence of secondary sex characteristics. Secondary amenorrhea is the absence of regular menstruation for 3 months or irregular menstruation for 6 months in people who have had a regular pattern of menstrual cycles that was previously established (McCance & Huether, 2019).

Pathophysiology

Primary amenorrhea is caused by hypothyroidism, **Turner syndrome**, pituitary disorders, hyperandrogenism, disorders of sexual development, pregnancy, anatomic abnormalities, or in utero exposure to DES (diethylstilbestrol; McCance & Huether, 2019; Titus et al., 2019). Those with Turner syndrome have only one normal "X" chromosome and have absence of breast or pubic hair development. DES was a drug given to pregnant people between 1938 and 1970 to help prevent miscarriages. It was discovered later that the drug affected the reproductive organs of female offspring, causing infertility. These patients will have secondary sex characteristics but incomplete development of reproductive organs, specifically uterine and fallopian tube abnormalities (National Cancer Institute at the National Institutes of Health [NIH], 2021).

When menses do not occur for 6 months or more after a regular pattern of cycles has been established, it is considered **secondary amenorrhea**. Pathologic causes of secondary amenorrhea include eating disorders, pregnancy, excessive weight loss, body mass index (BMI) of less than 22% of average, excessive exercise, endocrine dysfunction such as polycystic ovarian syndrome (PCOS), hypothalamic or pituitary dysfunction, medications, or anatomic deviations such as **cervical stenosis** or **imperforate hymen** (McCance & Heuther, 2019; Obstetrics & Gynecology, 2019)

Exercise-associated amenorrhea, also known as the *female athlete triad*, is a type of amenorrhea that is common among athletes and those with rapid weight loss due to bariatric surgery or starvation dieting. Amenorrhea also may be caused by hormonal contraceptives, such as oral contraception, Depo-Provera, implanted long-term progesterone contraception, or the presence of a progesterone-only intrauterine device (IUD). Patients with eating disorders are at risk for developing menstrual irregularities due to suppression in the hypothalamic–pituitary–ovarian axis (McCance & Heuther, 2019).

Pearls for Practice: Pathophysiology

The female athlete triad is an association between low-energy availability (with or without eating disorders), amenorrhea, and osteoporosis. It is a state of insufficient caloric intake (excessive exercise or reduced energy intake), low estrogen, and elevated cortisol. The elevated cortisol inhibits the release of gonadotropins, which results in suppression of ovulation and decreased estrogen production. The negative impact on bone density occurs because of the decreased estrogen availability and suppression of hormones that stimulate bone growth. As a result, amenorrhea and decreased bone mineral density are seen (American Academy of Orthopedic Surgeons, 2020).

Clinical Manifestations and Assessment

Patients who have an established menstrual cycle pattern will report a history of the absence of menstruation or other symptoms that are associated with the underlying cause of amenorrhea. Those patients 15 years of age who have developed secondary sex characteristics generally will seek medical evaluation if they have not experienced any menstruation, as will 13-year-olds who have not developed any secondary sex characteristics. A detailed menstrual history is critical in determining abnormality in menstrual patterns and should be accompanied by pregnancy and sexual histories, contraception use, medications, exercise patterns, and detailed history on any intentional or unintentional changes in weight.

Once pregnancy has been excluded, appropriate labs should include thyroid-stimulating hormone (TSH) and prolactin levels, follicle-stimulating hormone (FSH), luteinizing hormone (LH, also known as lutropin), dehydroepiandrosterone sulfate (DHEAS), and serum testosterone. If the patient is short in stature, genetic testing for Turner syndrome should be considered (McCance & Huether, 2019). Physical examination of the external and internal genitalia by a health care provider will determine any anatomic deviations that may cause obstruction of the vaginal outlet.

Medical and Nursing Management

A withdrawal bleed occurs with the administration of medroxyprogesterone acetate (MPA) (Provera) 10 mg for 7 to 10 days. Depending upon risk factors, an oral contraceptive pill (OCP) then can be initiated to assist with regulation of the menstrual cycle. Alternatively, the patient can be prescribed progesterone the first week of each month or every 3 months for a withdrawal bleed. It is important to instruct the patient that if a menstrual period has been missed for several months, a heavy flow can be expected after taking MPA, and severe cramping may be experienced as a result. Therapies for painful menstruation are listed below.

Also, a pelvic ultrasound may be ordered to confirm the absence of a uterus or any other structural abnormalities that may be a contributing factor in amenorrhea (ACOG, 2021c).

DYSMENORRHEA

Painful menstruation, or dysmenorrhea, has two classifications: primary and secondary. Primary dysmenorrhea occurs at the onset of menarche and the early following years after establishing a cycle and may become more severe over time (McCance & Huether, 2019). It is considered one of the most common causes of pelvic pain, with rates as high as 90%. Approximately 10% to 15% of adolescent females report severe pain from their menstrual cycles, resulting in lost time from work or school (Shields & Kho, 2021). Secondary dysmenorrhea begins well after the menstrual cycle has been established and is typically caused by organic or structural causes (McCance & Huether, 2019).

Pathophysiology

The classic characterization of primary dysmenorrhea is crampy pain in the abdomen and/or lower back just before the onset of bleeding and persisting for the first few days into the menstrual flow. It is due to an excessive production of **prostaglandins** in the lining of the uterus, which causes contractions of the smooth muscle (Shields & Kho, 2021). The onset of primary dysmenorrhea typically occurs 6 to 24 months after the menstrual cycle has been established (Shields & Kho, 2021).

Secondary dysmenorrhea begins well after the onset of menarche, usually after age 20, but can occur as late as the third or fourth decade of life and is suggestive of an underlying pathology, such as **endometriosis** (most common cause), fibroids (discussed later in this chapter), or a pelvic infection. It may be related to IUDs, congenital anomalies, ovarian cysts, or benign or malignant tumors (McCance & Huether, 2019).

Clinical Manifestations and Assessment

Often primary dysmenorrhea is characterized by sharp, intermittent abdominal pain that is accompanied by

TABLE 32-3 **Comparing Primary and Secondary Dysmenorrhea**

Aspect	Primary Dysmenorrhea	Secondary Dysmenorrhea
Definition	Menstrual pain without organic disease	Menstrual pain associated with an identifiable disease or structural cause
Quality of pain	Sharp, intermittent pain	Recurrent, crampy, suprapubic pain
Timing	Begins with onset of menarche	Symptoms begin earlier in cycle and last longer
Age of onset	Occurs with menarche	Occurs between 30 and 40 years of age
Additional symptoms	Headache, fatigue, backache, dizziness, nausea, diarrhea, and constipation	Change in bowel habits, rectal pressure, painful defecation, dyspareunia

headache, fatigue, backache, nausea, diarrhea, insomnia or constipation. The gastrointestinal (GI) symptoms are caused by prostaglandins triggering uterine vasoconstriction and prolonged contractions or cramping (McCance & Huether, 2019; Sheilds & Kho, 2021). Symptoms for secondary dysmenorrhea begin earlier in the cycle and last longer. There is also a change in bowel habits, rectal pressure, and painful defecation due to the influence of prostaglandins. Table 32-3 compares primary and secondary dysmenorrhea.

Medical Management

Nonsteroidal anti-inflammatories (NSAIDs) and hormonal contraceptives are the mainstay and first-line therapy for treating primary dysmenorrhea due to their antiprostaglandin effect (McCance & Huether, 2019; Shields & Kho, 2021).

Ibuprofen and naproxen are available over the counter (OTC). Other NSAIDs available by prescription include mefenamic acid, prescription-strength ibuprofen and naproxen, and cyclooxygenase (COX)-2 inhibitors. By blocking the production of prostaglandin, pain usually will not occur or will be mild in comparison.

While effective, NSAIDs can have a negative impact on the GI system; therefore, care must be taken to avoid long-term use of these medications. Combined oral contraceptives (COCs) are greatly beneficial in treatment for this condition as the combined hormones inhibit ovulation as well as decrease uterine flow and thereby decrease uterine contractility (Dunphy et al., 2019). COCs are an excellent choice for sexually active patients who desire birth control as well as relief from dysmenorrhea.

Management of secondary dysmenorrhea is aimed at identification of the causative factor through the use of the appropriate diagnostic tests. The same medications listed above also may be used to alleviate pain.

Nursing Management

Nurses can teach patients how to accurately keep a menstrual diary that will assist in tracking patterns of menstrual discomfort and pain (Fig. 32-7). Advising the patient to take an OTC NSAID 1 to 2 days prior to the onset of menses will help to inhibit prostaglandin production and help to decrease the amount of abdominal pain and cramping. Patients who take proton pump inhibitors (PPIs), which are available OTC or by prescription, need to be instructed on the proper administration of these drugs, which will help to protect the lining of the stomach from the effects of the NSAIDs. It is recommended that PPIs be taken on an empty stomach. The patient should eat something 30 to 60 minutes after taking the PPI to allow the medication to start working. Also, taking the NSAID with food will help to minimize stomach upset.

Nonpharmacologic therapy includes supplementation with magnesium, calcium, and fish oil supplement, but further studies are currently underway to accurately define appropriate dosages and outcomes (McGuirk, 2022). Low-level localized heat, such as a heating pad or wrap, for 15 to 20 minutes intermittently can be beneficial in easing uterine contractility. It is important to instruct the patient not to use heat that is too high or for prolonged periods of time due to the risk of burns. In addition, alternative therapies such as acupuncture and herbal remedies have demonstrated some benefit in decreasing uterine contractions in some small studies (Dunphy et al., 2019).

ABNORMAL UTERINE BLEEDING

Any uterine bleeding that deviates from a patient's usual pattern is considered abnormal uterine bleeding (AUB). This includes bleeding between periods, postmenopausal bleeding, postcoital bleeding, bleeding heavier than usual or for greater length of time, or bleeding between menstrual cycles for at least 6 months (McCance & Huether, 2019). Approximately 1.4 million people report AUB annually (Dehn, 2020). The International Federation of Gynecology and Obstetrics (FIGO) developed a classification system that describes deviations in menstrual bleeding in nonpregnant patients. PALM-COEIN, is an acronym that refers to polyps, adenomyosis, leiomyoma, malignancies, coagulopathies, ovulatory dysfunction, iatrogenic, not yet classified. PALM refers to structural etiologies that contribute to the development of AUB, whereas COEIN are nonstructural contributors (Santoro & Clain, 2021). Despite the new classification recommendations, much of the literature still uses the following terms to describe and categorize abnormal bleeding patterns:

Menstrual Cycle Log

Month and Date	Bleeding Y/N	Symptoms	Length of Time	Intensity	Treatment	Impact
1						
2						
3						
4						
5						
6						
7						
8						
9						
10						
11						
12						
13						
14						
15						
16						
17						
18						
19						
20						
21						
22						
23						
24						
25						
26						
27						
28						
29						
30						
31						

KEY:

Symptoms:

NS, no symptoms
N/V, nausea/vomiting
TS, trouble sleeping
S, sensitive to light, sight, or sound
D, disturbances in sight/vision
B, bleeding: heavy, moderate, light
GI, diarrhea or constipation
BE, binge eating
FC, food cravings
I-irritable
FN-feeling nervous
T-tired
C-abdominal cramping or pain
H-headache
M-mood: depressed, anxious

Intensity:

Mild
Moderate
Severe

Treatment:

M-medicine
BR-bed rest
HCP-contacted health care provider

FIGURE 32-7 Menstrual log.

- Any change in a normal menstrual cycle is referred to as *abnormal uterine bleeding* (AUB)
- Bleeding that occurs at regular intervals but is in excessive amounts and/or duration is known as *menorrhagia* or *heavy menstrual bleeding (HB).*
- Excessive bleeding can lead to iron-deficiency anemia due to chronic blood loss and its associated symptoms.
- Unpredictable bleeding patterns, including irregular, prolonged, or heavy bleeding are considered to be *anovulatory bleeding.*

Bleeding that occurs frequently but irregularly is known as *metrorrhagia. Menometrorrhagia* is now the term used to refer to heavy and prolonged menstrual bleeding (HPMB) and is heavy bleeding of prolonged duration occurring at irregular intervals. Any persistent AUB can lead to iron-deficiency anemia if left undiagnosed and untreated. Cycles greater than 35 days are known as **oligomenorrhea**, and cycles occurring in less than 21 days are known as **polymenorrhea**.

Causes

Coagulation disorders, such as thrombocytopenia (low platelet count) or Von Willebrand disease (most common inherited bleeding disorder in humans, refer to Chapter 19), are causes of AUB and should be ruled out as an underlying factor. Females who take unopposed estrogen are likely to develop AUB, as are those with liver diseases that impair fibrinogen synthesis. Certain endocrine disorders, including Cushing syndrome, Addison disease, thyroid disorders, and PCOS;

extreme fluctuations in weight; or excessive exercise can cause irregular uterine bleeding. Pregnancy should always be excluded when AUB is present (Dunphy et al., 2019).

Other causes include pelvic infections caused by sexually transmitted infections (STIs; gonorrhea, *Chlamydia*, trichomonas), weight loss or weight gain, recent systemic infections, endometriosis, trauma, benign tumors, or lesions (Yaşa & Uğurlucan, 2020). Refer to Chapter 34 for details on STIs.

Medical and Nursing Management

Nursing care must include vital signs, including orthostatic blood pressures, pulse rate to evaluate for tachycardia or arrhythmias, and a BMI. Menstrual pad counts assist the health care provider in determining the approximate amount of blood loss through the description of the saturation of sanitary pads or tampons on an hourly basis. Characteristics of the flow, such as the color of blood and presence of clots, are to be noted as well. Physical examination of the genitalia and a Pap smear are performed. It is important that the patient undergo appropriate diagnostic testing to determine underlying pathology of AUB prior to treatment. This may include a pelvic ultrasound and endocrine tests, as described earlier. A CBC with differential, TSH, prothrombin time (PT), and partial prothrombin time (PTT) are indicated in the workup for AUB. Also, an iron panel should be included to determine the presence of iron-deficiency anemia (Yaşa & Uğurlucan, 2020). An endometrial biopsy is considered the first-line diagnostic test to rule out endometrial hyperplasia or malignancy in patients over 35 years of age or in those under 35 years of age who are morbidly obese or who have chronic anovulation or PCOS (Davis & Sparzak, 2021).

Once any pathology has been ruled out, it is appropriate for the patient to be treated with hormonal contraception that will regulate the menstrual cycle, decrease bleeding and cramping associated with heavy bleeding, and decrease any incidence of anemia associated with excessive blood loss. Progestin-releasing IUDs reduce blood flow, as does implanted progesterone (Dunphy et al., 2019).

PREMENSTRUAL SYNDROME AND PREMENSTRUAL DYSPHORIC DISORDER

PMS is the name given to a cluster of behavioral, emotional, and physical symptoms that typically occur the week prior to menstruation and may continue into the first week of the menstrual cycle (McCance & Huether, 2019). Symptoms usually resolve with the onset of menstrual flow but can persist for the first few days of bleeding. PMDD is a more severe form of PMS and is recognized by diagnostic criteria developed by the American Psychiatric Association (APA), ACOG, and the World Health Organization (WHO). Symptoms must be present consistently during the luteal phase (second half of the menstrual cycle) and have a negative impact to some degree on the person's life. The severity of the symptoms experienced by the patient and the impact on daily functioning are what delineates PMDD from PMS (Dunphy et al., 2019).

It is estimated that approximately 75% of females of reproductive age are affected by symptoms related to menstrual cycle changes that interfere with daily lifestyle and relationships (Casper, 2021). There is no known cause of PMS/PMDD, although research indicates these symptoms are most likely due to fluctuating levels of estrogen, progesterone, and serotonin.

Clinical Manifestations and Assessment

More than 100 physical and behavioral symptoms are associated with PMS/PMDD and range from mild to severely disabling (Box 32-8).

Symptoms may be misdiagnosed as menopause, anxiety, bipolar disorder, metabolic disorders (such as diabetes), chronic fatigue syndrome, or rheumatologic diseases. It is important that health care providers take a comprehensive, systematic approach to accurately diagnosing patients with PMS/PMDD so that appropriate therapy may be initiated. Patients may experience some of the symptoms or a constellation of symptoms at any one time during the luteal phase, including breast pain, bloating, ankle swelling, perceived weight gain, food cravings, and functional and cognitive impairments (McCance & Huether, 2019).

BOX 32-8 **Focused Assessment**

Premenstrual Syndrome

Be alert for the following signs and symptoms:

Physical:

- Weight gain
- Abdominal bloating
- Constipation or diarrhea
- Breast tenderness
- Acne
- Headache
- Heart palpitations

Behavioral:

- Irritability
- Depression
- Mood swings
- Increased appetite
- Overwhelming fatigue
- Insomnia
- Crying spells
- Change in libido

Cognitive:

- Decreased concentration
- Paranoia
- Indecision
- Sensitivity to rejection
- Suicidal ideation

Medical Management

Menstrual cycle diaries (see Fig. 32-7) are kept for two to three menstrual cycles (Dunphy et al., 2019). The presence or absence of symptoms is to be noted daily, along with the impact of symptoms on daily activities. Providers are able to view trends of symptoms based on these logs that correlate with the menstrual cycle. Nurses can encourage lifestyle changes that will impact the severity of symptoms. These lifestyle changes include regular exercise, which promotes increased circulation of endorphins released from exercise; avoidance of excessive caffeine (coffee, soda, tea, energy drinks, and chocolate) and sodium-rich foods; decreased alcohol intake; and smoking cessation. Randomized trials of patients taking increased complex carbohydrates during the luteal phase have revealed a decrease in the severity of PMS symptoms due to increased levels of serotonin (Dunphy et al., 2019). Low serum calcium can cause muscle irritability; therefore, it is recommended that the patient ensure a daily intake of 1,200 to 1,600 mg of calcium. Complementary and alternative therapies including botanicals have been used for centuries to help treat symptoms of menstrual irregularities (Salkar et al., 2020).

Use of vitamin B_6 from 50 to 500 mg/day has been met with mixed success. Other nonpharmacologic therapies include oral magnesium, vitamin D, vitamin E supplements, and evening primrose oil (Carlini et al., 2022; Morehead & McInnis, 2021). Results of recent studies of evening primrose oil and the effect on PMS have demonstrated that this provides some improvement of PMS symptoms (Aguilar-Aguilar, 2021).

There are some results on the use of chasteberry for its dopaminergic effects on the emotional and physical symptoms of PMS and PMDD, but the exact mechanism is unknown (Salkar et al., 2020). For patients who do not respond to nonpharmacologic therapy, pharmacologic management is considered. The use of oral contraceptives has proven to be of great benefit for those with physical and emotional symptoms of PMS. Continuous contraception for 3 months' duration or longer often alleviates PMS symptoms (Dunphy et al., 2019; McCance & Huether, 2019).

Selective serotonin reuptake inhibitors (SSRIs) and serotonin-norepinephrine reuptake inhibitors (SNRIs) have shown efficacy in mood stabilization. Pulsed or cyclical dosing of SSRIs also can be used during the 2 weeks prior to and including the week of menstrual flow (Casper, 2021; Dunphy et al., 2019).

Gonadotropin-releasing hormone (GnRH) agonists (leuprorelin or medroxprogesterone) suppress the menstrual cycle, but long-term use can produce consequences of menopause due to the lack of estrogen, which may lead to irreversible osteoporosis. NSAIDs are beneficial for physical symptoms, including headache and dysmenorrhea.

Nursing Management

Nurses must take accurate and detailed health and nutritional histories and screen for symptoms of anxiety and/or depression as well as assess for current or past suicidal and homicidal ideation.

If the nurse recognizes any signs of an inability to manage anger, suicide/homicide ideation, depression, or anxiety, they should encourage the patient to seek evaluation by an appropriate health care provider. Nurses also may help patients with stress reduction and management techniques, adherence to medication, and therapeutic lifestyle changes (such as smoking cessation; regular exercise; and eating a low-fat, low-cholesterol, low-sodium diet). Pain management is similar to that discussed under dysmenorrhea (NSAIDs, PPIs, and heat pad use).

VULVOVAGINAL INFECTIONS

Fungal and bacterial infections in the vagina are common, self-limited gynecologic conditions that occur in people of all ages due to a disruption in the normal pH of the vagina, overgrowth of normal vaginal flora, sexually transmitted infections, or lack of estrogen (McCance & Huether, 2019). The pH of the vagina is 3.5 to 4.5; this provides the normal environment for *Lactobacillus acidophilus* to exist. This is a healthy bacterium that thrives in the vaginal ecosystem and provides protection against infections by inhibiting growth of anaerobes (Dehn et al., 2021).

Lactobacillus metabolizes glycogen to lactic acid in the vagina and maintains normal vaginal pH. Antibiotics, menopause (or estrogen deficiency), oral contraceptives, spermicides, diabetes, douching, frequent intercourse, and smoking are known to decrease or alter the number of healthy lactobacilli (McCance & Huether, 2019). In addition, newer generation medications used to treat type 2 diabetes mellitus such as the SGLT-2 inhibitors and immunosuppressant medications may also contribute to the development of vulvovaginal candidiasis (Dehn et al., 2021).

Without the lactobacillus, there is a proliferation of anaerobic activity, the pH of the vagina is altered, and an overgrowth of bacteria is produced. Table 32-4 summarizes types of vaginal infections and vaginitis. **Bacterial vaginosis** (BV) and **vulvovaginal candidiasis** (VVC) are discussed in detail below.

Nurses play a vital role in helping patients to understand the mode of infection, treatment, and self-care modalities. Although not considered STIs, BV and VVC can coexist with STIs; therefore, appropriate screening for these infections is important. Also, it is important to note that the creams and suppositories used in the treatment of VVC and BV have been known to weaken latex condoms, diaphragms, and cervical caps; therefore, caution should be taken to avoid sexual intercourse during treatment.

BACTERIAL VAGINOSIS

The most common vaginal infection is BV or Gardnerella with an estimated 29% prevalence among females between

TABLE **32-4 Vaginal Infections and Vaginitis**

Infection	Cause	Clinical Manifestations	Management Strategies
Candidiasis	*Candida albicans, glabrata,* or *tropicalis*	Inflammation of vaginal epithelium, producing itching, reddish irritation White, cheese-like discharge clinging to epithelium	Eradicate the fungus by administering an antifungal agent. Frequently used antifungal medications include miconazole, clotrimazole, tioconazole, fluconazole, terconazole, and nystatin. Review other causative factors (e.g., antibiotic therapy, nylon underwear, tight clothing, pregnancy, oral contraceptives). Assess for diabetes and HIV infection in patients with recurrent infections.
Gardnerella-associated bacterial vaginosis	*Gardnerella vaginalis* and vaginal anaerobes	Usually no edema or erythema of vulva or vagina Gray-white to yellow-white discharge clinging to external vulva and vaginal walls	Administer metronidazole with instructions about avoiding alcohol while taking this medication. If infection is recurrent, may treat partner.
Trichomonas vaginalis vaginitis (STD)	*Trichomonas vaginalis*	Inflammation of vaginal epithelium, producing burning and itching Frothy yellow-white or yellow-green vaginal discharge	Relieve inflammation, restore acidity, and reestablish normal bacterial flora; provide oral metronidazole for patient and partner.
Bartholinitis (infection of greater vestibular gland)	*Escherichia coli* *Trichomonas vaginalis* *Staphylococcus* *Streptococcus* *Gonococcus*	Erythema around vestibular gland Swelling and edema Abscessed vestibular gland	Drain the abscess; provide antibiotic therapy; excise gland of patients with chronic bartholinitis; instruct patient to take warm sitz baths.
Cervicitis: acute and chronic	*Chlamydia* *Gonococcus* *Streptococcus* Many pathogenic bacteria	Profuse purulent discharge Backache Urinary frequency and urgency	Determine the cause: Perform cytologic examination of cervical smear and appropriate cultures. Selected oral antibiotic treatment regimens should also be effective against *Neisseria gonorrheae* because of the high frequency of concomitant infection. Eradicate other causes.
Atrophic vaginitis	Lack of estrogen; glycogen deficiency	Discharge and irritation from alkaline pH of vaginal secretions	Provide topical vaginal estrogen therapy; improve nutrition if necessary; relieve dryness through use of moisturizing medications.

the ages of 14 and 49. It is not considered a sexually transmitted infection but its increased prevalence can be associated with sexual activity.

Risk Factors

Risk factors for developing BV include new or multiple sexual partners, douching, an increase in sexual activity, retained foreign body in the vagina (such as a tampon, broken condom, or sex toy), and coexisting STIs (CDC, 2020a). BV also may be present after a menstrual cycle due to the increase in the vaginal pH. If left untreated in patients who are pregnant, BV is a risk factor for premature labor as well as post-abortion endometritis and cuff cellulitis (infection) after hysterectomy.

Clinical Manifestations and Assessment

The majority of people who have BV are asymptomatic (CDC, 2020a). Patients with symptomatic BV will report an increased malodorous vaginal discharge or leukorrhea (a whitish discharge of mucus from the vagina) that is grayish white in color. Amines commonly found in the vagina become unstable when the pH is altered; they release the characteristic "fishy" odor. The odor is generally more noticeable after sexual intercourse, sexual activity, or menses. Unprotected intercourse will produce the malodorous discharge due to the interaction of semen and normal vaginal amines. Sometimes patients will report vaginal itching, dysuria, or pelvic pressure similar to that of a UTI due to the localized irritation of the urinary meatus from the discharge.

A swab of vaginal discharge taken from the vaginal walls and applied to two glass slides is known as a *wet mount.* One slide has saline added; the other slide has potassium hydroxide (KOH) added and then is viewed under a microscope. The presence of characteristic *clue cells* (vaginal epithelial cells that are coated with bacteria) on the saline slide is a hallmark for diagnosing BV. The KOH-prepared slide will release amines and is known as a "whiff test." The presence of a fishy odor on the whiff test suggests BV (Papadakis et al., 2022). Nitrazine paper determines the pH, which will be greater than 4.5 for BV.

Medical and Nursing Management

The preferred medication for treatment of BV is metronidazole 500 mg twice daily for 7 days. If the patient is nonadherent, a single 2-g dose may be administered, although higher cure rates occur with the 7-day dose. The CDC no longer recommends the single-dose therapy due to its low efficacy (CDC, 2020a). Metronidazole gel 0.75% administered in one 5-g applicator vaginally at bedtime for 7 nights is an alternative and is preferred to avoid any GI upset caused by oral medications. If an allergy to metronidazole exists, alternative therapies are oral clindamycin 300 mg twice daily for 7 days; clindamycin 2% cream, one 5-g application vaginally at bedtime for 7 days; or clindamycin ovules 100 mg intravaginally once at bedtime for 3 days. Tinidazole, a newer-generation medication that is chemically related to metronidazole, was approved in 2007 by the U.S. Food and Drug Administration (FDA) for treatment of BV. Improved patient adherence due to once-a-day dosing and shorter duration of therapy is observed (CDC, 2020a).

It is extremely important that the nurse educate the patient on avoidance of all alcohol while taking metronidazole and for 3 days after the last dose due to the disulfiram (Antabuse)-type reaction that is induced; this causes nausea, vomiting, flushing of the skin, chest pain, blurred vision, mental confusion, sweating, breathing difficulty, and anxiety.

VULVOVAGINAL CANDIDIASIS

VVC is caused predominantly by *Candida albicans.* Other nonalbicans species that cause VVC include *C. tropicalis* and *C. glabrata* (Jeanmonod & Jeanmonod, 2021). It is estimated that approximately 25% of all vaginal infections are VVC, but that number is difficult to determine because it is not a reportable condition and because the availability of OTC treatments makes it hard to determine how many people are affected.

Risk Factors

Risk factors include use of broad-spectrum antibiotics (such as penicillins, cephalosporins, and tetracyclines), exogenous hormones, or corticosteroids, as well as pregnancy (Papadakis, 2022). Other risk factors for VVC include uncontrolled diabetes, obesity, and diets high in sugars or artificial sweeteners (Weerasekera et al., 2018). New sexual partners, contaminated sex toys, or an increase in sexual activity also may change the pH of the vagina, making it more susceptible to infection. Males who are uncircumcised and do not practice good hygiene may harbor yeast and pass on the infection to their partners.

Clinical Manifestations and Assessment

The most common complaint is vulvar pruritus. Patients also complain of dysuria related to inflammation of the urinary meatus by means of the vaginal discharge. A urine specimen should be obtained to rule out any other source of infection. **Dyspareunia**, or pain with intercourse, may also be reported.

VVC differs from BV in that the discharge is generally thick, white, and curd-like, much like the appearance of cottage cheese, and is odorless. It is adherent to the vaginal walls on speculum examination. On physical examination, the external genitalia are erythematous, and adherent white discharge may be noted on the vaginal walls and labia. Diagnosis is established based on a wet mount (a swab of the vaginal discharge on a glass slide that has been mixed with KOH). Under microscopic examination, the presence of hyphae is visible, and Nitrazine will reveal a normal pH of 4.0 to 4.5. If there are clue cells or trichomonads present, it is indicative of a coexisting BV or trichomonas infection (CDC, 2021a). A 48-hour culture will diagnose the predominant causative factor definitively.

Medical Management

Many people will self-diagnose and treat based on symptoms with OTC topical preparations containing azole. This practice is not encouraged as patients may be self-treating for an infection that may not be VVC, or the yeast will become resistant to the OTC treatment. It is important to educate patients to seek evaluation by a health care professional who can diagnose and treat any vaginal infection appropriately.

Topical antifungal agents that are used vaginally offer the most rapid relief. Terconazole cream is available in both 3- and 7-day preparations. This medication covers all three species of yeast, whereas the OTC preparations cover only *C. albicans.* Fluconazole is a single-dose oral medication that is effective against *Candida*, but there is a delay in symptom relief of up to 3 days. It is, however, an effective treatment, particularly when treating a patient with coexisting BV who is using a vaginal preparation of metronidazole. Oral fluconazole is a category C drug and should be used with caution during the first trimester of pregnancy. There are some risks of congenital musculoskeletal malformations when oral fluconazole is used repeatedly during the first trimester (Zhu et al., 2020).

Nursing Management

The nurse's role in educating a patient with BV or VVC includes assessing for high-risk behaviors, such as multiple sexual partners and unprotected sexual intercourse. If a patient is having recurrent vaginal infections, it is important for the patient to be evaluated by a health care professional to determine the cause.

Recurrent infections can be caused by nonadherence to medication therapy and poor hygiene. Those with recurrent infections may benefit from suppressive therapy with weekly oral fluconazole for a duration of 6 months (Jeanmonod & Jeanmonod, 2021). Also, it is important to assess any cross-contamination with sexual toys. Teaching patients and their partners about proper hygiene in addition to sterilization of sex toys can decrease recurrent infections.

Pearls for Practice

Normalizing use of devices to aid in sexual function is important as some patients consider there is bias associated with their use. The nurse educates the patient in proper cleaning that includes using a damp, soapy washcloth with antibacterial soap to clean electric toys (without submerging electrical components). They should be stored in a container or pouch (to keep them clean) and in a cool, dry place. Silicone toys may be cleaned in the dishwasher (on top rack); batteries must be removed first. The patient is informed to follow the manufacturer's directions.

If the cause is determined to be from diabetes, the nurse can assist the patient with adherence to dietary guidelines, proper management of blood glucose, and hygienic practices as well as referral to appropriate health care providers for further management.

STRUCTURAL DISORDERS

Physical strain and hormone deficiencies compromise the ability of the pelvic musculature to support pelvic organs. Weakening of this musculature causes pelvic organs to displace downward into the pelvic cavity to varying degrees (Fig. 32-8).

PROLAPSE

The pelvic organs are supported by a complex system of ligaments and muscles that are protected by the bony pelvis. The bony pelvis serves as an attachment site for these ligaments and muscles. The uterus is located deep within the bony pelvis but is freely movable during physical examination. A series of muscles known as the pubococcygeal muscles extend from the pubic bone to the coccyx, encompassing the urethra, vagina, anus, and rectum.

If the muscles and ligaments are weakened, the uterus and bladder prolapse or herniate into the vaginal canal. Patients may or may not be aware of these structural defects until they become symptomatic or are discovered on physical examination. Types of prolapse include:

- *Cystocele:* The herniation of the bladder into the anterior vagina (Fig. 32-8A)
- *Rectocele:* The extrusion of the rectum into the posterior vagina (Fig. 32-8B)
- *Enterocele:* The descent of the small intestine into the vaginal vault (Fig. 32-8C)
- *Uterine prolapse:* Downward descent of the uterus into the vagina (Fig. 32-9)
- *Vault prolapse:* Prolapse of the top of the vagina after a hysterectomy

Incidence of pelvic organ prolapse (POP) increases with age with the majority of patients experiencing POP being over the age of 50 (McCance & Huether, 2019). Patients are more likely to develop prolapse once the muscles and ligaments begin to loosen or relax. Approximately 25% of females in the Unites States are affected by POP (Shaw et al., 2021).

Risk Factors

Increased pressure on the abdomen and pelvic floor from pregnancy or obesity causes the ligaments of the pelvic floor

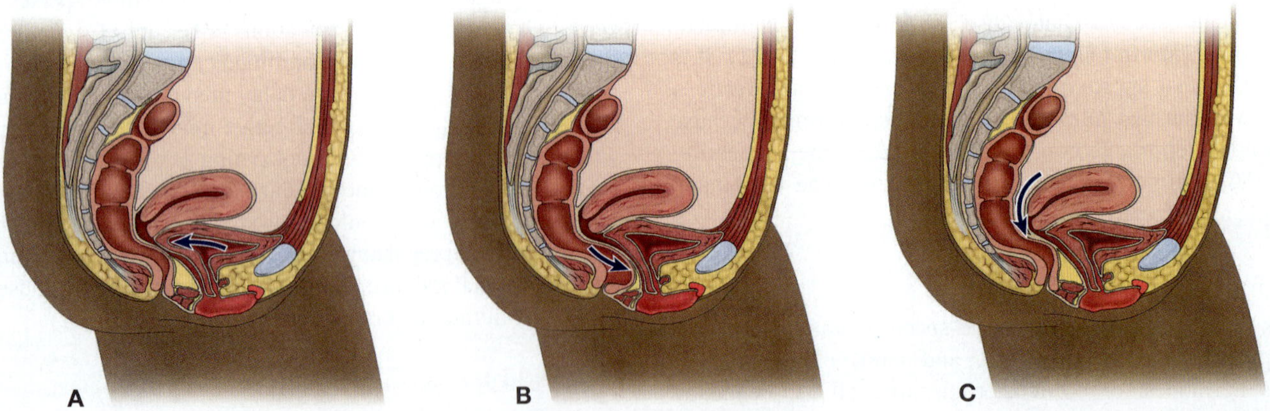

A B C

FIGURE 32-8 Diagrammatic representation of the three most common types of pelvic floor relaxation: (A) cystocele, (B) rectocele, and (C) enterocele. *Arrows* depict sites of maximum protrusion.

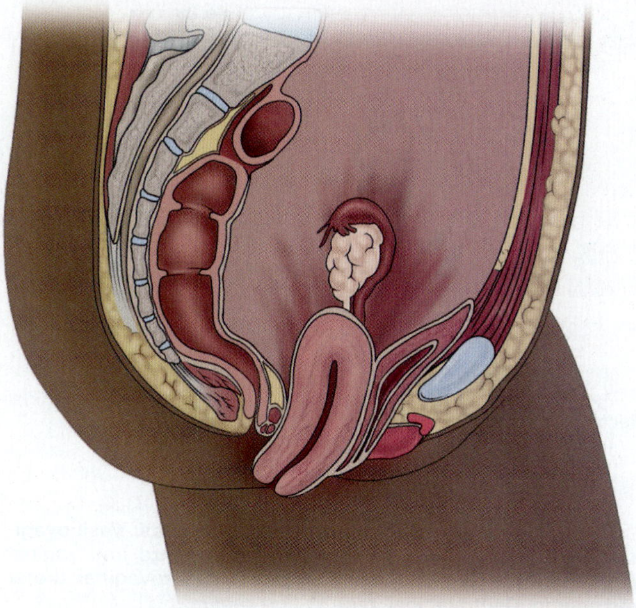

FIGURE 32-9 Complete prolapse of the uterus through the introitus.

to weaken. Direct injury to the levator ani or the stretching of the pudendal nerves during childbirth impairs the elasticity of the pelvic floor muscles. People who have more than one vaginal birth are at higher risk for developing prolapse, with risk increasing with each subsequent vaginal delivery (Papadakis et al., 2022). Estrogen helps with maintaining pelvic structure; therefore, patients who are menopausal are more likely to develop a prolapse due to lack of estrogen. Other predisposing factors for developing POP include connective tissue disease, chronic constipation, prolonged standing, and neurologic disorders (McCance & Huether, 2019; Papadakis et al., 2022). Increasing strength of the pelvic floor can be correlated to the strengthening effect of exercising the core and abdominal muscles; this can prevent pelvic organs from displacement.

Regardless of age, straining from constipation and increased intra-abdominal pressure from coughing are other risk factors for prolapse.

Clinical Manifestations and Assessment

Many patients who have a uterine or bladder prolapse will be asymptomatic, while others may seek evaluation by a health care provider because of a noticeable "bulge" in the vaginal area. Back pain in the absence of trauma may be present. Urinary incontinence is a common complaint with a bladder prolapse accompanied by pelvic pressure. Frequently, patients will complain of a UTI when, in fact, it is the prolapse that is producing the symptoms. Patients also may report difficulty having a bowel movement and often will need to place pressure on their perineal or vaginal areas in order to facilitate a bowel movement. Incomplete rectal evacuation or fecal incontinence may occur as a result of prolapse.

Medical and Nursing Management

Treatment depends upon the severity of the symptoms and degree of prolapse involved. The patient's general state of health and activity is also of concern if considering surgical intervention. Urodynamic testing evaluates bladder function. For mild uterine prolapse, a **pessary** is the first line of treatment. Pessaries are removable devices made of silicone, latex, plastic, or rubber that are inserted into the vagina to provide support. A variety of styles is available, and they are cost-effective while providing immediate relief of symptoms (Shaw et al., 2021; Fig. 32-10).

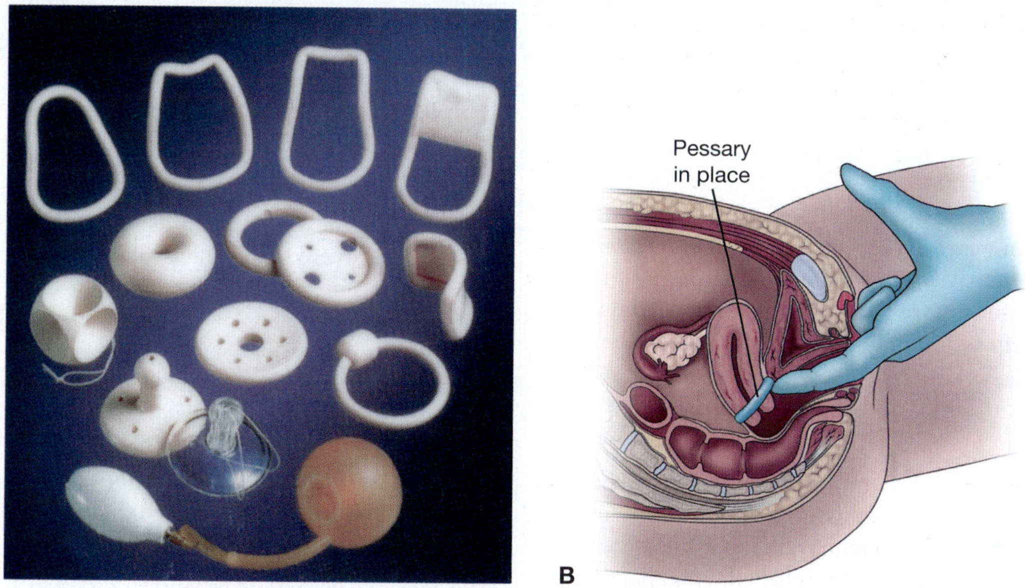

A B

FIGURE 32-10 Examples of pessaries. **A.** Various shapes and sizes of pessaries available. **B.** Insertion of one type of pessary.

BOX 32-9

Patient Education: Performing Kegel (Pelvic Muscle) Exercises

Purposes: To strengthen and maintain the tone of the pubococcygeal muscle, which supports the pelvic organs; to reduce or prevent stress incontinence and uterine prolapse; to enhance sensation during sexual intercourse; and to hasten postpartum healing:

1. Become aware of pelvic muscle function by "drawing in" the perivaginal muscles and anal sphincter as if to control urine or defecation, but not contracting the abdominal, buttock, or inner thigh muscles.
2. Sustain contraction of the muscles for up to 10 seconds, followed by at least 10 seconds of relaxation.
3. Perform these exercises 30–80 times a day.

Pelvic floor rehabilitation or pelvic floor muscle training (PFMT) offers a nonsurgical approach to patients who are motivated to adhere to the exercise schedule. These exercises help to strengthen the pelvic floor muscles so they can better support pelvic organs. **Kegel exercises** are a form of PFMT (Box 32-9). Physical therapists or urogynecologists who are specifically trained in PFMT teach the patient exercises that increase the strength of the pelvic floor muscle. Biofeedback programs feature assisted pelvic floor exercises utilizing a functional electrical stimulator (FES) and are used to help patients contract the appropriate pelvic muscles. Nurses can become trained in PFMT and are able to effectively teach patients about proper use of FES equipment.

Reconstructive pelvic surgery depends upon the impact of the severity of symptoms on the patients' daily living. Sacrospinous fixation, also referred to as an *anterior–posterior repair*, utilizes the surrounding ligaments to tighten and attach lax musculature onto the bony pelvis (Favre-Inhofer et al., 2021). Vaginal hysterectomy is the most common surgical treatment for patients beyond childbearing age who have a uterovaginal prolapse; however, surgical repair with or without hysterectomy should be considered a last resort option (McCance & Hueterh, 2019).

Nurses provide important patient teaching. Educating the patient on weight loss, smoking cessation, and avoiding heavy lifting enables the patient to care for themself. Proper insertion, removal, and cleaning of pessary devices will help the patient to avoid vaginal infections. Nurses can discuss appropriate ways to avoid unnecessary straining and constipation. Anticipatory guidance regarding procedures or surgery will help to alleviate any patient anxiety about the surgical process.

FISTULAS

A fistula is an abnormal, tortuous opening between two internal organs or between an internal hollow organ and the exterior of the body. Fistulas may be simple or complex. Figure 32-11 depicts vaginal fistulas. Rectovaginal fistulas (RVFs) are abnormal openings that occur between the vagina and the rectum, allowing fecal material and flatulence to leak into the vagina, causing fecal incontinence. Anal fistulas generally develop as a result of an anal abscess and may be an indication of a neoplasm (Papadakis et al., 2022). Vesicovaginal fistulas occur between the bladder, vagina, and anus causing urinary and/or fecal incontinence. These conditions occur as a result of congenital anomalies, trauma due to childbirth or surgery, radiation therapy, Crohn disease, diverticular diseases, or neoplasm of the rectum or vagina. Postpartum infections also may result in fistula formation due to third- and fourth-degree perineal tears or tissue breakdown, but these are considered uncommon in developed countries due to the availability of caesarean sections and improved birthing therapies (Reisenauer et al., 2021). This condition causes severe pain and risk for urosepsis due to recurrent UTIs and has social ramifications related to urinary and fecal incontinence.

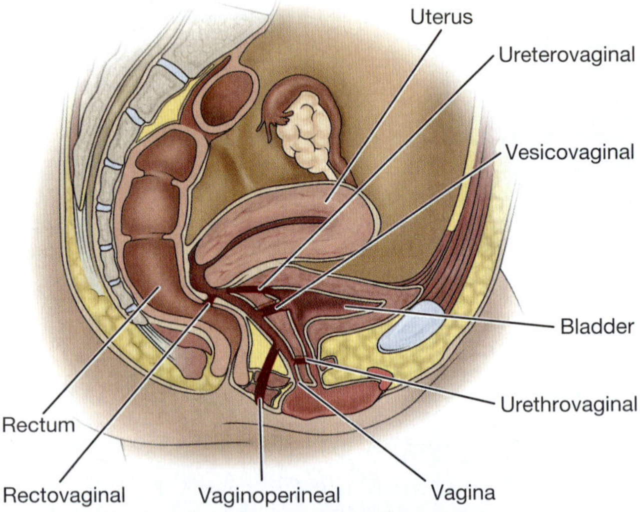

FIGURE 32-11 **Common sites for vaginal fistulas: Vesicovaginal, bladder and vagina. Urethrovaginal, urethra and vagina. Vaginoperineal, vagina and perineal area. Ureterovaginal, ureter and vagina. Rectovaginal, rectum and vagina.**

Clinical Manifestations and Assessment

Depending upon the type of fistula, symptoms will vary. If caused by an obstetric or surgical complication, fistulas may not be apparent for up to 30 days after the initial injury or may be discovered incidentally during the 6-week postpartum follow-up visit. An obstetric-related RVF is the most common form of fistulas (Tuma et al., 2021). Urinary or fecal incontinence are the main reasons why patients will seek evaluation by a health care provider. Fecal discharge through the vagina produces a malodorous discharge and may be mistaken for a vaginal infection. An accurate history of onset, timing, and location, along with symptoms the patient is experiencing, is important to help locate the structural abnormality. Physical assessment of the genital area will help to identify the affected area. The fistula may be palpable on digital rectal examination or vaginal examination. A sigmoidoscopy, colonoscopy, small bowel imaging, cystoscopy, or intravenous pyelography will aid in definitive diagnosis.

Medical and Nursing Management

If the fistula is due to Crohn disease or diverticular disease, treatment is aimed at the causative disease and should be followed by a gastroenterologist.

Surgical repair is the only option if the fistula does not heal spontaneously. There is a high rate of recurrence of fistulas in spite of surgical repair. Nurses play an important role in helping the patient to understand the importance of cleanliness and hygiene and to understand the signs and symptoms of recurrent infection or surgical failure to repair the fistula. Regular sitz baths and changing of perineal pads help prevent infection. It is important for the nurse to inspect the patient's skin for any signs of erythema or breakdown.

It is also imperative that the nurse assess the impact fistulas play on the patient's psychological state. Many patients suffer from physical and social distress as well as sexual dysfunction as a result of urinary and fecal incontinence due to fistulas (Mernoff, 2020). Assessing the patient's support system as well as appropriate referrals to pain management and surgeons familiar with this type of surgery is imperative.

BENIGN DISORDERS

OVARIAN CYSTS

Ovaries produce estrogen, progesterone, and a small amount of testosterone necessary for female reproductive function as well as formation of oocytes or eggs. Follicles are structures within the ovary containing a single ovum or egg. Follicular growth is stimulated by FSH once a month. After ovulation occurs (release of the egg), the graafian follicle that houses the ovum becomes the corpus luteum. This structure undergoes transformation and regresses with the onset of menses. Ovaries are a common site for cysts to form as a result of hormonal influence on the formation of the **graafian follicle** and subsequent corpus luteum. When this series of hormonal transitions does not occur, a cyst may develop (McCance & Huether, 2019). Any graafian follicle that is over 2 cm is considered a cyst. Ovarian cysts are classified as functional or nonfunctional. Statistically, females under age 50 are more likely to have a benign cyst, whereas females over age 50 are more likely to have a cyst that is malignant. These cysts manifest more commonly during the reproductive years with the majority of cysts being benign (Mobeen & Apostol, 2021).

Types

Functional cysts are also known as *simple cysts* due to their appearance on ultrasound. These types of cysts rupture and hemorrhage and occasionally cause pain. The condition is self-limiting. Pain that occurs during ovulation, known as **mittelschmerz**, also produces unilateral ovarian pain and generally is relieved with symptomatic treatment, such as OTC NSAIDs (Brott & Le, 2021; Papadakis et al., 2022). Ovarian follicles that rupture during ovulation release fluid, cause pain, and may be noted on ultrasound as an incidental finding.

Nonfunctional cysts, or endometriomas, are also known as "chocolate cysts" due to their characteristic appearance on ultrasound. The cysts develop as a result of sloughed off endometrial tissue that has formed a cystic mass on the ovary; they are brown in appearance (Mobeen & Apostol, 2021).

Dermoid cysts or benign teratomas are nonfunctional and are comprised of embryonic cells containing hair, teeth, bone, cartilage, and nails (McCance & Huether, 2019). Since the histologic features and clinical behaviors of dermoid cysts or germ-cell tumors have been well established, there has been little new research performed in this area for the past two decades.

Patients with nonfunctional dermoid cysts are diagnosed by pelvic ultrasound after they have had a missed menstrual cycle and have a false-positive pregnancy test. Transvaginal ultrasound is the diagnostic test of choice to differentiate a benign or malignant mass (Mobeen & Apostol, 2021). These cysts have characteristic microscopic fat detected that appears to be echogenic within the mass on ultrasound (CDC, 2020b; Saleh et al., 2021).

Ovaries with multiple cysts due to chronic anovulatory cycles and hyperandrogenism are known as *polycystic ovarian syndrome* (PCOS). PCOS is the most common endocrine disorder that affects approximately 5% to 10% of females of reproductive age (Papadakis et al., 2022). It is a complex disorder of androgen excess, insulin resistance, and an imbalance in the ratios of luteinizing hormone and FSH, causing **anovulation** (lack of ovulation). Androgen excess coupled with disproportionate amounts of LH and FSH and decreased sex hormone–binding globulins (SHBGs) causes the occurrence of anovulatory cycles. This fluctuation in the normal levels of hormones results in insulin resistance due to the influence of hormone production from the pituitary. Patients affected by PCOS are at risk for developing type 2 diabetes, acne, endometrial cancer, hyperlipidemia, obesity, hirsutism, and infertility (CDC, 2020b).

Clinical Manifestations and Assessment

Patients experiencing rupture of functional cysts present with a sudden onset of unilateral lower abdominal pain. Nausea and vomiting may be present. Pain typically increases with movement. A typical presentation of PCOS will include a history of irregular menstrual cycles (can be over 35 days per cycle or fewer than eight menses annually). Characteristics of bleeding include heavy flow with increased abdominal cramping and also may include large clots. The patient may be hirsute on the face and chest or between the breasts and demonstrate mild to severe acne. Male pattern baldness or alopecia may be present. Forty to 80% of people with PCOS have central obesity

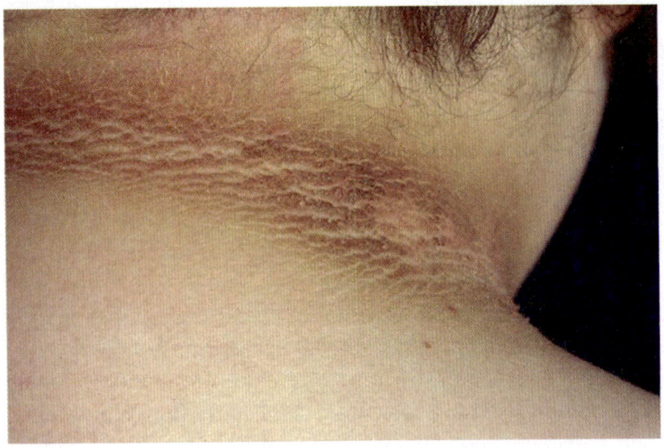

FIGURE 32-12 Acanthosis nigricans. Hyperpigmentation of skin folds, velvety in appearance commonly seen in axilla, groin, and neck. (From *Danforth obstetrics and gynecology*. Lippincott Williams & Wilkins.)

and 50% to 90% will develop type 2 diabetes mellitus (Barber et al., 2019a). **Acanthosis nigricans** is a hyperpigmentation of the skin around the neck (see Fig. 32-12) but also may be noted in the axilla, groin, or the dorsal aspect of hands, and the patient also may have an excessive number of skin tags around the neck, under the arms and breasts, or in the groin (McCance & Huether, 2019). It is commonly associated with insulin resistance. See Figure 32-12. In order to be diagnosed with PCOS, the patient must meet the Rotterdam criteria: (1) amenorrhea or oligomenorrhea, (2) hyperandrogenism (biochemical or clinical signs), and (3) polycystic ovaries on ultrasound (Perla Health, 2021). Pelvic ultrasound utilizing color Doppler will reveal 25 or more follicles with a "string of pearls" appearance varying in size less than 10 mm (Ponnatapura et al., 2019). Patients with unilateral right lower quadrant pain must be evaluated for the potential of appendicitis.

Medical and Nursing Management

Functional cysts are self-limiting and generally respond to the use of OTC NSAIDs, such as ibuprofen or naproxen. Once a diagnosis of ovarian cysts is made, and depending upon the size of the cyst, hormonal contraception is recommended to induce suppression of FSH. This decreases the incidence of formation of ovarian follicles, limits or halts an increase in the size of any established cysts, and halts the future formation of cysts. If pain persists longer than 48 hours, an exploratory laparoscopy may be performed to rule out the presence of ovarian torsion (twisting of the ovary, primarily affecting the right ovary).

Patients with PCOS require extensive blood work and a transvaginal ultrasound to rule out any other causative factors. Labs include FSH, LH, beta-human chorionic gonadotropin (β-hCG), SHBG, free testosterone, prolactin, lipid panel, thyroid studies, and a fasting glucose. A 2-hour glucose tolerance test is useful in determining glucose intolerance. The LH-to-FSH ratio in patients with PCOS is usually greater than 2:1 or 3:1, but a normal ratio is not a diagnosis of exclusion (Saadia, 2020).

It is important that blood work not be performed while the patient is taking oral contraceptives as this will alter the accuracy of results and delay diagnosis.

Treatment of PCOS is aimed at the primary concerns (acne, infertility, obesity). Due to the incidence of insulin resistance with PCOS, patients should follow a regular program of exercise and eat a low-fat diet. If, in spite of therapeutic lifestyle changes, the patient is unable to lose weight or ovulate, metformin is initiated to assist with decreasing insulin resistance and to allow for spontaneous ovulation. Metformin is an insulin-sensitizing agent that lowers testosterone levels and induces ovulation once hormone levels are balanced. The most common side effect of this medication is transient nausea and diarrhea. Slowly increasing the dosage of metformin and dosing at mealtime will help alleviate these side effects and increase patient compliance. Weight loss decreases insulin resistance, which improves PCOS (Dileep et al., 2021). The method of birth control used (either oral contraceptive, patch, or vaginal rings) while on metformin should be discussed with the patient because treatment can restore fertility. Patients with PCOS should be evaluated by a reproductive endocrinologist.

COCs help patients with PCOS regulate menstrual cycles and decrease blood flow with menses and the cramping associated with heavy menses. In addition, COCs improve SHBG production, which helps bind-free testosterone. This improves acne, hirsutism, and alopecia. People who do not have regular menstrual cycles are at risk for endometrial cancer due to the prolonged exposure of estrogen and overgrowth of the endometrial lining and, therefore, may need to have an endometrial biopsy if there has not been menses in 1 year.

Spironolactone is a blood pressure medication that has antiandrogenic effects that is beneficial to those who experience hirsutism (Papadakis et al., 2022). Because this is a potassium-sparing diuretic, patients with PCOS should have their electrolytes monitored periodically, particularly the potassium level. COCs that contain *drospirenone*, a newer-generation progesterone has the same antiandrogenic effects as spironolactone. Patients with PCOS may also benefit from an insulin-sensitizing agent such as metformin (McCance & Huether, 2019).

Nurses can assist patients with weight loss and exercise guidelines as well as with adherence to medications. It is important to help patients understand the implications of this disease on QOL and infertility. Nurses play a key role in supporting patients with this disease and recognizing if patients need referral to a dietician or for psychological support.

UTERINE FIBROIDS

Leiomyomas or myomas are common, benign growths of the uterus (Fig. 32-13). It is estimated that 20% to 80% of females will develop leiomyomas by age 50 (U.S. Department of

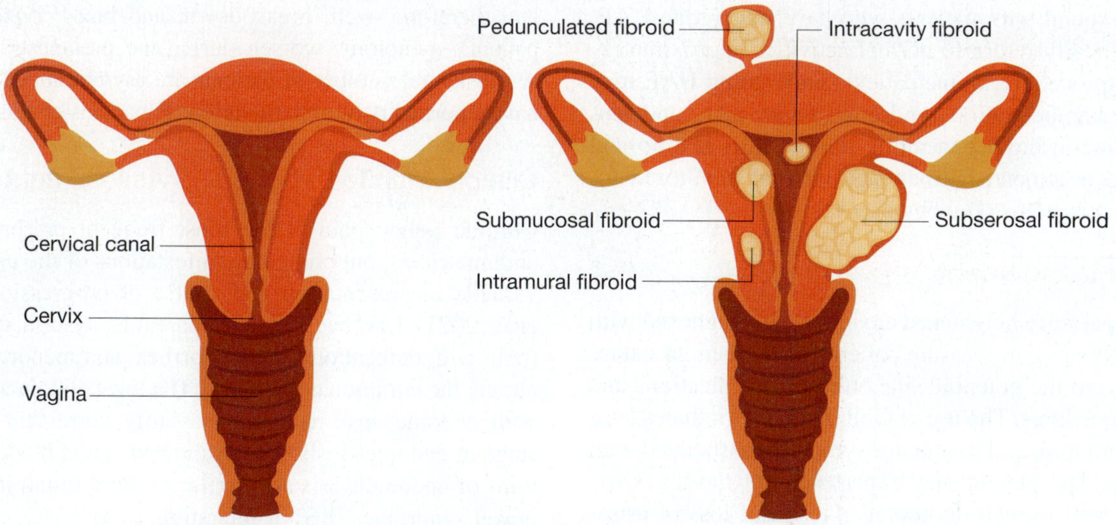

FIGURE 32-13 **Uterine fibroids (myomas). (From Shutterstock; ID 1712984434.)**

Health and Human Services [USDHHS], Office on Women's Health, 2019a). Risk factors include early menarche, use of oral contraception before the age of 16, and/or being overweight (McCance & Huether, 2019). The high prevalence of uterine fibroids is the cause of high disease burden at the cost of approximately $34.4 billion in the United States annually (Giuliani et al., 2020). Approximately 50% of cases will require surgical intervention. Symptoms largely depend on the size and number of fibroids. The incidence of fibroids increases with age. Box 32-10 describes the types of uterine fibroids.

Clinical Manifestations and Assessment

The majority of patients with fibroids are asymptomatic until the fibroid has enlarged and is impeding on other organs. Fibroids cause significant symptoms, including heavy menstrual bleeding, dyspareunia, disabling pelvic pain, rectal pressure, and infertility (Dunphy et al., 2019; Papadakis et al., 2022). Diagnosis is made with pelvic ultrasound, which confirms the presence, size, and location of fibroids. Fibroids may be palpated initially on bimanual pelvic examination. Often the uterus is enlarged as a result of the growth.

It is important to rule out pregnancy with a patient who is experiencing these signs and symptoms. There is a risk for miscarriage as the fibroid distorts the uterus impacting on fetal growth. Fibroids may grow rapidly in early pregnancy (Papadakis et al., 2022).

BOX 32-10

Types of Uterine Fibroids

- *Subserosal fibroids* grow on the outer edge of the uterus underneath the outer covering called the serosa and grow toward the pelvic cavity.
- *Intramural fibroids* grow within the wall of the uterine muscle (myometrium) and are the most common type.
- *Submucosal fibroids* grow inside the uterus immediately below the inner uterine surface and into the uterine cavity.
- *Pedunculated fibroids* arise from inside or outside the surface of the uterine muscle and project outward.

Medical Management

There are several treatments for fibroids. Medical management is indicated for patients who are considered surgical risks or who decline surgical intervention (Dunphy et al., 2019). GnRH agonists, such as Lupron, are used to decrease the size of the fibroid by effectively suppressing the hormonal production that feeds the fibroid. Hysterectomy is another treatment (see discussion later in the chapter). For patients who have fibroids and want to preserve their fertility, a **myomectomy** is performed. This is a surgical procedure that removes the fibroid but leaves the uterus intact. Myomectomies can be performed laparoscopically, hysteroscopically (inspection of the uterine cavity by laparoscopy), or via robotic-assisted laparoscopy.

Alternatives to invasive surgeries include uterine artery embolization (UAE) using minimally invasive plastic or gelatin particles that are injected into the uterine arteries to occlude blood flow to the fibroid (McCance & Huether, 2019). This type of procedure is used only on patients who have completed childbearing. Magnetic resonance–guided high-frequency focused ultrasound energy (MRgFUS) uses high-intensity ultrasound with increased temperature to destroy fibroid cells without damaging collateral tissue (Giuliani et al., 2020). In general, this type of procedure is confined to premenopausal patients with symptomatic fibroids. The advantage to this procedure is that patients generally can return to normal activities the day after treatment. Cryoablation, or radiofrequency of individual fibroids, is now FDA approved and is proven safe and effective in reducing the size of fibroids. Cryoablation also has been found to provide a reduction in severity of symptoms 12 months after the procedure without concerns of postembolization syndrome commonly found with patients who have undergone UAE. Patients typically return to normal activities approximately 5 days postprocedure. Some patients undergoing UAE may develop postembolization syndrome: fever, pain, and leukocytosis due to the degenerating fibroid. This is a normal response to treatment, but patients must be monitored for worsening symptoms (Dunphy et al., 2019).

Nursing Management

Patients experience heightened anxiety when diagnosed with a fibroid. Nurses can reassure patients of the benign nature of fibroids and the potential side effects of medications and surgical procedures. The use of GnRH agonists induces temporary menopause and vasomotor symptoms associated with menopause. The patient may experience hot flashes, sleep disruption, and vaginal dryness as a result of loss of estrogen. These symptoms are reversible once the medication has been discontinued. Due to the high level of bleeding associated with any myomectomy or surgical procedure, all aspirin and aspirin-containing products should be discontinued 3 to 4 weeks before the procedure is performed. Aggressive pain management is advised due to the increased amount of cramping from the infarction of the fibroid. Instructing patients on patient-controlled analgesia (PCA) pumps (refer to Chapter 6) and regular administration of NSAIDs and antiemetics will ensure adequate pain control. Patients are coping not only with the physical loss but also the psychological loss of fertility if the patient is not undergoing fertility-sparing surgery, so nurses need to address those concerns and offer referrals to therapists if needed.

ENDOMETRIOSIS

Endometriosis is a progressive, benign gynecologic disorder affecting females in their childbearing years and causing chronic inflammation and formation of adhesions. It does not continue after menopause. Approximately 6% to 10% of females suffer from endometriosis, with as high as 80% of these people reporting chronic pelvic pain; it is the third most common reason for a hysterectomy (McCance & Huether, 2019). This disease may be disabling and chronic. It impacts the woman's sexual relations as well as their physical, social, and psychological well-being.

Pathophysiology

Endometriosis is the presence of endometrial-like tissue that proliferates outside of the uterine cavity, causing persistent pelvic pain and scarring that leads to infertility. The pathophysiology of this disease is largely unknown, but many theories exist (McCance & Huether, 2019). It is thought to be caused by the retrograde flow during menses of endometrial tissue through the fallopian tubes and into the peritoneal cavity, where this tissue seeds, forming adhesions in the pelvic, bladder, and bowel areas. The peritoneal endometrial tissues are influenced by the hormonal changes of the menstrual cycle and therefore swell, break down, and bleed; typically, the patient's symptoms worsen during the premenstrual phase. A substantial number of patients are asymptomatic and may have a normal pelvic examination (Papadakis et al., 2022).

Clinical Manifestations and Assessment

Chronic pelvic pain is the most frequent presentation of endometriosis, but clinical manifestations of the disease are variable in presentation and course of progression (Christ et al., 2021). Low back pain, dyspareunia, dysuria, **dyschezia** (pain with defecation), dysmenorrhea, and menorrhagia are among the common complaints. The level of pain associated with endometriosis is not necessarily correlated with the stage of endometriosis. The cyclic bowel and bladder symptoms of endometriosis are similar to those found in irritable bowel syndrome (IBS) or interstitial cystitis (IC), making it difficult to differentiate the disorders.

A detailed health history regarding the patient's symptoms in relation to their menstrual cycle will help the health care provider establish a pattern. Any tenderness of the fallopian tubes, ovaries, or uterus on bimanual examination is an indication for further evaluation. The most common finding is tenderness with palpation of the posterior vaginal fornix, but a definitive diagnosis cannot be established without further diagnostic testing. Transvaginal ultrasound visualizes the uterine cavity and endometrium for any adhesions. This examination is unable to visualize smaller lesions; therefore, misdiagnosis may be made. Currently, direct visualization of the adhesions through surgical intervention remains the preferred method for definitive diagnosis. Lysis of adhesions may improve fertility through laparoscopic ablation of the endometrial implants (Dunphy et al., 2019).

Medical and Nursing Management

The first line of treatment for endometriosis consists of the use of NSAIDs for pain, progestins, or combined hormonal contraceptives to treat the condition. The combined hormones in COCs suppress ovulation and growth of endometrial implants, thereby decreasing inflammation and pain. GnRH agonists (such as Leuprorelin), androgenic agents, depot MPA, and levonorgestrel IUD are considered second-line therapy for 3 months (Tsamantioti & Mahdy, 2021). Any of these medications suppresses ovulation and endometrial growth and reduces or eliminates menses, thus alleviating the chance of retrograde flow into the pelvic cavity. Use of continuous contraception provides prolonged suppression of ovulation, inhibiting growth of endometrial tissue. There are no differences in the outcomes of the use of COCs over GnRH, although patients given GnRH agonists have higher incidence of complaints of hot flashes, vaginal dryness, and other vasomotor symptoms associated with menopause. These symptoms are reversible once GnRH therapy has been discontinued.

Surgical intervention is considered the last line of therapy especially if it follows a minimum of 3- to 9-month use of hormonal therapies such as OCPs, GnRH analogs that suppress ovulation, androgenic agents, a testosterone derivative, and MPA 9 (Dunphy et al., 2019; Papadakis et al., 2022). Exploratory laparoscopy with lysis of adhesions is considered the gold standard and temporarily decreases the pain and bleeding associated with endometriosis. Total abdominal hysterectomy (TAH) remains the definitive therapy for patients who have completed their childbearing and is effective for patients who suffer from debilitating pain (Papadakis et al., 2022).

Complementary and alternative therapies are useful in patients who suffer from endometriosis and should be a part of the plan of care. Due to the issues surrounding loss of fertility with this disease, stress management should be included. Yoga may help with stress reduction and also increases core and abdominal strength, which will help patients who undergo surgical intervention to have an easier recovery. Specifically trained physical therapists can help alleviate and manage the symptoms associated with chronic pelvic pain.

Educating the patient affected by endometriosis and their family and support network will help them to understand the significant impact of this disease on their physical and psychological health. Many patients have sought the opinions of multiple medical providers regarding the treatment of endometriosis, and many have had a negative experience or may be in denial of the ramifications of the disease; therefore, establishing trust between the patient and the health care provider is crucial. A collaborative effort among all members of the health care team, including the nurse, health care provider, pharmacist, pain management specialist, and social worker, must exist to help improve the patient's outcome.

MALIGNANT CONDITIONS

CANCER OF THE CERVIX

Cervical cancer is the third most common reproductive cancer in the world (Papadakis et al., 2022). Rates for cervical cancer, however, have been decreasing since 1975 largely due to increased access to cervical cancer screening as well as HPV vaccination (CDC, 2021; McCance & Huether, 2019). According to the ACS, approximately 14,000 new cases of cervical cancer diagnoses are projected for the year 2021 (ACS, 2021b).

The most common type of cervical cancer is squamous cell carcinoma (SCC), accounting for approximately 80% of all cervical cancer cases, but the incidence of SCC is decreasing while the incidence of cervical adenocarcinoma is on the rise (Papadakis et al., 2022). Scientists researching triggers to changes in the cervical tissue that led to cancer have implicated human papilloma virus (HPV) as the most common causative factor in development of cervical cancer (CDC, 2021b). Cervical cancer has a slow progression from certain strains of oncogenic HPV to invasive cervical cancer and may take years to progress. HPV has over 100 strains, some of which have oncogenic potential and are known to cause cervical abnormalities. Patients are asymptomatic unless they have external genital warts, or **condyloma**. In general, infection with HPV during a female's younger years is cleared spontaneously or is suppressed to undetectable levels. The HPV vaccine was developed in 2006, and the quadrivalent vaccine covers four of the oncogenic strains (6, 11, 16, 18) while the bivalent vaccine covers two of the oncogenic strains. This is a primary prevention measure to reduce cervical cancer cases and deaths, and while vaccinations rates are rising, the literature demonstrates that the vaccine continues to be underused (MMWR, 2021).

Screening and Prevention

The Pap smear is a screening tool used to detect any abnormalities of the cervix (Table 32-5). In recent years, liquid-based cytology has been developed to improve specimen adequacy, making it superior to traditional glass slide specimens.

Cytologic screening tests are the most effective preventative measure for screening and diagnosing invasive cervical cancer.

TABLE 32-5 **American Congress of Obstetricians and Gynecologists (ACOG) Cervical Cytology Screening Guidelines**

Patient Population	Frequency
<21 years of age	No screening
21–29 years of age	Every 3 years
30–65 years of age	Every 3 years with HPV cotesting every 5 years
65 years of age and older	Discontinue if no abnormal Pap tests for 10 years and no previous history of moderate–severe dysplasia or cancer
Patients having had a hysterectomy for noncancerous reasons	Discontinue after hysterectomy *unless* patient has had a supracervical hysterectomy, then above guidelines apply
Patients with high-risk factors: HIV, diethylstilbestrol (DES) exposure, or cervical intraepithelial neoplasm (CIN) 2 or 3	Every 6 months or as directed by health care provider

Data from ACOG. (2020). *Updated cervical cancer screening guidelines*. https://www.acog.org/clinical/clinical-guidance/practice-advisory/articles/2021/04/updated-cervical-cancer-screening-guidelines

BOX 32-11 **Risk Factors for Cervical Cancer**

- Early age of first coitus
- Multiple sexual partners
- High parity (high number of births)
- STIs
- Cigarette smoking
- Exposure to human papillomavirus (HPV)
- Immunocompromised state (e.g., having HIV, or taking immunosuppressant drugs for an autoimmune condition)
- Using oral contraceptive pills (OCPs) for a prolonged period of time
- Having a mother who took DES between 1940 and 1971 (a hormone to prevent miscarriage)

DES, diethylstilbestrol.

Risk Factors

Risk factors for cervical cancer include multiple sexual partners, use of oral contraceptives, smoking, infection with HIV, and CIN of pap tests (CDC, 2021b; Papadakis et al., 2022). Lesbian women are at higher risk for HPV and cervical cancer due to misinformation as well as insufficient knowledge and screening. Lesbians are underrepresented in current research due to privacy concerns, lack of inquiries on the part of the health care provider regarding sexual orientation, and fear of repercussions (Lee et al., 2020; USDHHS, 2019b). Box 32-11 lists other risk factors for cervical cancer.

Clinical Manifestations and Assessment

Routine screening for cervical cancer increases a person's chances of being diagnosed at an earlier stage. Advanced disease will manifest itself with irregular vaginal bleeding as well as pelvic pain and pressure. Malodorous vaginal discharge occurs as a result of tumor necrosis. Dyspareunia and rectal pressure also are common as the tumor increases in size and extent, invading surrounding tissue and causing other symptoms to develop. The standard of care for an abnormal Pap test is to follow-up with a **colposcopy** and directed biopsy. Colposcopy is a high-powered magnification of the cervix, which has had an acetic acid solution applied to it to help differentiate the cervical cells. Biopsies are taken in areas of visible abnormal vascular patterns.

The squamocolumnar junction of the cervix is rich with squamous cells; this is known as the transformational zone. Cellular abnormalities develop over time, leading to the development of squamous cell dysplasia or cervical intraepithelial neoplasia (CIN) (McCance & Huether, 2019). There are no overt signs or symptoms of CIN, and it is strictly diagnosed via liquid cytology, which provides superior sensitivity to detection of cancer cells. Low-grade lesions correlate with CIN 1, which is mild dysplasia that generally resolves spontaneously without treatment and is monitored through serial cytology to determine any progression to a higher-grade lesion. High-grade lesions are consistent with CIN 2 and CIN 3 and are considered precancerous lesions (Khieu & Butler, 2021). High-grade lesions (severe dysplasia) are more likely to progress to cervical cancer if not treated. Biopsy confirms whether or not the lesion is SCC or adenocarcinoma. Cervical cancer screening should begin at 21 years of age, regardless of sexual debut. Between 21 and 29 years of age, females should have cervical cytology screening without HPV testing every 3 years. All females over 30 years of age should have cervical cytology screening and cotesting for HPV every 3 to 5 years, unless an abnormality is detected. If an abnormal cytology is detected, then appropriate follow-up should occur based on current algorithm guidelines for abnormal cytology. All patients 65 years of age and older who have had normal cervical cytology without prior history of CIN should no longer undergo cervical cytology due to the low incidence of disease in this age group (American Society for Colposcopy and Cervical Pathology [ASCCP], 2020).

Delayed diagnosis of cervical cancer will result in a more advanced disease state.

Staging is the next step, once the diagnosis for invasive cervical cancer has been made. Staging is performed on a scale of 0 to IVB. Stage 0 is known as carcinoma in situ (CIS). Stage IVB is consistent with distant metastasis when the disease has spread to the remainder of the reproductive organs, bladder, rectum, liver, and/or lungs. Treatment is dependent upon type of carcinoma and extent of disease. As the tumor size increases, so does the risk of treatment failure. Pelvic ultrasound is an easy and noninvasive way to evaluate any cervical pathology due to its ability to visualize the size and location of a cervical mass. A chest x-ray and abdominal/pelvic imaging, such as CT scan or MRI, are performed to rule out metastasis to other areas of the body.

Medical Management

Abnormal Pap smears that reveal high- or low-grade squamous intraepithelial lesions (HGSILs or LGSILs) are followed up with a colposcopy and cervical biopsy. Once diagnosis has been established, a cervical *conization* or cone biopsy is performed. Cold knife conization and loop electrosurgical excision procedure (LEEP) are other procedures that may be performed to treat HGSIL or LGSIL, which are precursors to cervical cancer. These types of procedures remove cone-shaped wedges high in the cervical canal with enough surrounding tissue to ensure clear margins. This is accomplished using a surgical scalpel, laser, or electrocautery. Prognosis is excellent for patients treated with these types of procedures. Cervical conization alone is adequate for patients who want to preserve childbearing ability (Cooper et al., 2021). Invasive cervical cancer is rare under the age of 20 years, but there has been a documented increased risk for premature births among people who have had excisional cervical procedures for dysplasia prior to conception.

Patients diagnosed with a stage of IB or IIA undergo a radical hysterectomy: removal of the uterus and upper one third of the vagina, including the cervix, but sparing the ovaries. Bilateral pelvic lymph node sampling is also done. Pelvic radiation and chemotherapy may follow depending upon the size and extent of the tumor. Stage IB carries an increased risk of recurrence. Neoadjuvant (administered before surgery) chemotherapy has demonstrated success in decreasing tumor size and increasing survival when used prior to a radical hysterectomy. Patients diagnosed with locally advanced cervical cancer have a higher rate of recurrence than those patients diagnosed with early-stage disease. The survival rate for a patient diagnosed with stage IB is approximately 92% (Cancer.net, 2021).

In clinical trials, HPV vaccinations has a near 100% efficacy in preventing CIN 2, CIN 3 and adenocarcinoma in situ, and 99% efficacy preventing genital warts (CDC, 2020c). There are currently two HPV vaccines available: bivalent, which prevents types 16 and 18, and quadrivalent, which prevents types 6, 11, 16, and 18. Routine vaccination should be administered as follows:

- For both males and females at 11 or 12 years of age but can begin at the age of 9 years
- For both females and males through 26 years of age who have not been vaccinated previously or who have not completed the 3-dose series (CDC, 2020d)

In addition, adults between the ages of 27 and 45 who have not received the recommended HPV vaccinations can discuss whether or not they would benefit from getting the HPV series. It is unclear why but persons in this age range who may have been exposed to HPV previously do not mount the same immune response as those who are younger (CDC, 2020d).

The HPV vaccines are a series of three vaccines administered at 2 and 6 months after the initial injection. It is important to receive the entire series of three vaccinations. It is recommended that patients remain in the office for at least 15 minutes after administration of the vaccine to ensure there is no reaction.

For females over age 26 years, the best way to prevent cervical cancer is to get routine cervical cancer screening, as recommended.

Nursing Management

Nurses working in a variety of settings have the opportunity to educate patients on cervical cancer screenings. Availability of access to care is prevalent with federally funded cervical cancer screening programs through public health departments, hospital-based primary care centers, and community health care clinics. Educating parents and young people about HPV vaccination is important when considering that vaccination is so efficacious. Clinical trials of the vaccine demonstrated a 93% efficacy in prevention of cervical precancers of types 16 and 18 in females who were exposed to HPV. There is a reported 98% antibody response in all studies of the bivalent vaccine 1 month after completion of the series (CDC, 2020c).

If a patient has undergone any cervical biopsy procedures, it is important to provide instruction on the importance of pelvic rest (such as abstinence and no vaginal penetration) as well as observing for and reporting to their provider any fever, increased bleeding, pelvic pain, or malodorous vaginal discharge. Ensure that the patient has the phone number of their health care provider or local hospital in the event that any of these symptoms occur after their procedure.

CANCER OF THE UTERUS

Cancer of the endometrium or uterus is the most common gynecologic malignancy in resource-abundant countries, and occurs in approximately 3% of all females, peaking between the ages of 60 and 70 (Plaxe & Mundt, 2022). The 5-year survival rate is 69% with localized or regional disease (Cancer.org, 2021). Usually it is diagnosed early, and better outcomes are reported with surgical intervention. It is rarely diagnosed in people under 50 years of age and is generally attributed to chronic anovulation and/or obesity (Plaxe & Mundt, 2022). Cervical cytology may show atypical endometrial cells, but these are considered poor predictors of pathology. Abnormal uterine bleeding (AUB) is the presenting sign in 90% of all endometrial cases (Papadakis et al., 2022). Endocervical and endometrial sampling is considered the gold standard for diagnosis of this type of cancer (Dunphy et al., 2019; Papadakis et al., 2022).

Most endometrial cancers are considered endometrioid. Less common are the nonendometrioid lesions, including serous, clear cell, and carcinosarcomas. Nonendometrioid cancers are more aggressive, with an increased mortality rate.

Unopposed estrogen causes endometrial hyperplasia, or an overgrowth of the uterine lining. Simple hyperplasia often spontaneously regresses, but complex hyperplasia and atypical hyperplasia are more likely to progress to cancer (Doherty et al., 2020). The prognosis for type 1 endometrial cancer is good as opposed to type 2, which carries a higher mortality rate. Fertility-sparing progestin therapy is recommended for those who wish to preserve fertility and presumably have type 1 endometrial adenocarcinoma (Casdio et al., 2020). Oral MPA is the most commonly used progestin in this population and should be used for 12 weeks prior to evaluating response to treatment.

Risk Factors

Risk factors are discussed in Box 32-12. Nurses should encourage those with hereditary nonpolyposis colorectal cancer (HNPCC) (Box 32-13) or who are high risk for it to begin annual screening with endometrial biopsies and transvaginal ultrasound beginning at 25 years of age. Some patients may reduce their risk of endometrial cancer through the use of OCPs levonorgestrel IUD, or cyclic progestin therapy (Papadakis et al., 2022).

BOX 32-12

Risk Factors for Endometrial Cancer

- Use of estrogen after menopause
- Early onset of menarche (under 12 years of age) or late menopause (over 50 years of age)
- Nulliparous (never given birth)
- Polycystic ovarian syndrome (PCOS)
- Use of tamoxifen
- Obesity, especially if BMI at age 18 was high
- Diabetes
- Prior pelvic radiation
- Personal or family history of breast, colon, or ovarian cancer; or endometrial hyperplasia

Clinical Manifestations and Assessment

Abnormal vaginal bleeding is the most common early symptom of endometrial cancer; 80% of patients will present with abnormal vaginal bleeding as their chief complaint. Postmenopausal patients also may present with complaints of vaginal bleeding well after menses has ceased. Any unexplained vaginal bleeding or an irregularity in menstrual cycle should be evaluated by a health care provider.

Traditionally diagnosis has been made based on the tissue pathology from a dilation and curettage (D&C); however, endometrial biopsy is the preferred method since it is a simple procedure performed in the health care provider's office and does not involve anesthesia. If the biopsy is inconclusive or suggests endometrial cancer, a D&C is the gold standard. Hysteroscopic-directed biopsy is another alternative that is performed with the insertion of a scope through the cervix and directly into the uterus, allowing for complete visualization of the endometrium. A transvaginal ultrasound may be performed in addition to taking measurements of the endometrial thickness. Greater than 11 mm is a predictor of abnormal pathology; in postmenopausal patients, greater than 5 mm is considered pathologic (Tofiloska et al., 2019).

BOX 32-13

Hereditary Nonpolyposis Colorectal Cancer (HNPCC) Syndrome or Lynch Syndrome

Hereditary nonpolyposis colorectal cancer (HNPCC) syndrome increases a person's risk of developing ovarian, colon, endometrial, renal, bladder, brain, and stomach cancer.

It is an inherited cancer susceptibility syndrome occurring in approximately 5% of all cancers.

A person is at higher risk for HNPCC if they have three or more first-degree relatives with colon or endometrial cancer, with at least two of them having been diagnosed with colon cancer at age 50 or younger.

Genetic testing for HNPCC is available and recommended to those at risk.

Pearls for Practice

D&C is a brief surgical procedure that can be performed in a medical office or outpatient surgical center in which the cervix is dilated and a special instrument called a curette, or a suction curettage (also called vacuum aspiration for evacuations for terminations or abortions), is used to scrape the uterine lining. An anesthetic is administered (spinal, general, or local anesthetizing of the cervix) and a sample of the uterine contents may be sent for analysis.

Medical Management

Once the diagnosis has been established, and depending upon the stage and extent of cancer, treatment varies. Hyperplasia is generally treated with levonorgestrel IUD or oral progestin therapy. Megestrol acetate 40 mg BID to QID for 3 months is an alternative with a repeat biopsy in 3 months (Dunphy et al., 2019). Invasive disease necessitates surgical intervention including hysteroscopy D&C, but the standard treatment is a TAH with bilateral salpingo-oophorectomy (BSO; removal of fallopian tubes and ovaries). Lymph node biopsy is performed if there are clinically suspicious nodes and is done on patients who have a tumor >2 cm, type II endometrial cancer, or myometrial invasion of more than 50% as this increases the risk of metastasis (Dunphy et al., 2019). Type of hysterectomy has little bearing on outcome, although some believe that an open hysterectomy is optimal in visualizing the peritoneum over a laparoscopic-assisted vaginal hysterectomy, in which the peritoneum is not as well visualized; however, this has not been proven in the literature. Choice of type of hysterectomy varies and is dependent upon a variety of factors. Studies on minimally invasive surgeries have demonstrated lower rates of peri- and postoperative complications (Chen & Berek, 2021). Surgical staging is the most precise method to determine metastasis to surrounding tissues and organs; it involves abdominal and pelvic washings and periaortic lymph node evaluation.

Stage I is curable by surgery alone as it is considered low risk and the disease is confined to the uterus. High-risk stage I and some stage II cancers will require postoperative adjuvant radiation therapy or vaginal brachytherapy as the disease has lymph node involvement, is outside of the uterus, or contains high-risk cell types (papillary or clear cell). Radiation affects the ability of cells to proliferate and decreases growth of cancer cells. Vaginal brachytherapy is used to decrease vaginal recurrence in patients with intermediate risk endometrial cancer (Plaxe & Mundt, 2021). Vaginal brachytherapy consists of the placement of a device containing sealed radioactive material into the vagina postoperatively for 3 to 4 days; it is then removed. This method is preferred over EBR due to its lessened side effects. It delivers low- or high-dose radiation directly into the tumor. Brachytherapy decreases the incidence of regional recurrence and offers less toxicity than EBR (Zhang et al., 2020). The patient is on strict bed rest for the entire duration of therapy. Patients are kept on a diet of clear liquid or low-residue foods to avoid stool formation. Stool softeners and medications to decrease peristalsis are administered. Patients are isolated from other patients, and a camera mounted on the wall of the room allows monitoring of the patient while minimizing caregivers' exposure to radiation. Lead absorbs more radiation than any other material; therefore, a portable lead shield is placed at the bedside behind which all caregivers stand to administer medications, change IV bags, or deliver food trays. Nurses wear film badges or dosimeters to measure the amount of radiation exposure. Refer to Chapter 5 for details on brachytherapy.

Patients with diseases in high-risk stages II and III will receive both radiation and chemotherapy. There are limited data on the efficacy of the role of adjuvant chemotherapy alone or with concurrent radiation.

Nursing Management

Educating patients who have high-risk factors and discussing strategies to reduce risk factors is considered primary prevention. Decreasing obesity and controlling diabetes are two ways to decrease the risk of the development of endometrial cancer.

Nurses can stress the importance of evaluation for any abnormal vaginal bleeding. Use of oral contraceptives as a younger adult also provides some protection against developing endometrial cancer.

Nurses caring for patients receiving brachytherapy must take precautions against occupational exposure to radioactive material. **Time**, **distance**, and **shielding** make up the rules for protecting against unnecessary exposure. A long-handled forceps and lead container are kept in the patient's room after the radioactive material has been placed into the patient. It is imperative that staff never pick up the radioactive source with their bare hands if it becomes displaced from the patient's vagina. The institution's radiation safety team should be notified in the event this occurs. Also, patients should be made aware of the side effects of radiation therapy, including radiation enteritis, nausea, loss of appetite, bladder irritation, early menopause, vaginal dryness, and loss of interest in sexual intercourse (Athanasiou et al., 2020). See Chapter 5 for more details on radiation therapy.

CANCER OF THE OVARY

Ovarian cancer is referred to as a cancer that "whispers" because its clinical manifestations are not apparent until the tumor has invaded surrounding structures and is causing symptoms. It is the leading cause of death from cancers of the reproductive tract. The majority of patients diagnosed (50% to 70%) with ovarian cancer are usually diagnosed at stage 3 with advanced disease (ACS, 2021b; Ovarian Cancer Research Alliance [OCRA], 2021; Komatsu et al., 2021). It carries a high fatality rate due to the aggressiveness of the malignancy. Five-year survivorship rate is foreseeable if the cancer is diagnosed at an early stage, but only 15% of patients with ovarian cancer are diagnosed at that stage and have a 90% 5-year survival rate (OCRA, 2021). More than half of patients diagnosed are over 65 years of age, and 5% to 10% have genetic links (Dunphy et al., 2019). See Box 32-14 for additional risk factors. Use of oral contraceptives has been proven to decrease risk of developing ovarian cancer by 50% with long-term protection benefits. Hormonal contraception causes reversible anovulation, thus decreasing the cumulative cycles of the ovary over a person's lifetime. The longer the duration of use of OCPs, the greater the decrease in the risk of ovarian cancer; every 5 years of use of oral contraceptives equates to a risk reduction of approximately 20% (Huber et al., 2020; Joy, 2019).

BOX 32-14 Risk Factors for Cancer of the Ovary

- Age over 40 or postmenopausal
- Nulliparous
- Personal history of breast, colon, or endometrial cancer
- Personal history of hereditary nonpolyposis colorectal cancer or Lynch syndrome
- Obesity (BMI over 30)
- Use of fertility drugs
- Long-term use of hormone replacement therapy (HRT)
- Genetic predisposition; positive family history of ovarian cancer

Cancers of the ovary occur in the epithelial cells lining the ovary. There are several different types of ovarian tumors: those that are germ cell tumors, originating from cells that produce eggs from the ovary; surface cell tumors; and sex cord stromal tumors. Malignant ovarian cells shed from the ovary implant onto the surfaces of the peritoneal cavity. Then these cancerous cells undergo transformation into ovarian surface epithelium (McCance & Huether, 2019). There are two hereditary syndromes that are affiliated with ovarian cancer presenting at younger ages. These are hereditary breast-ovarian cancer (HBOC) syndrome and Lynch syndrome (also called hereditary nonpolyposis colorectal cancer syndrome; Joy, 2019). Although poorly understood, some newer theories point to endometriosis as the predisposing factor for development of ovarian cancer due to damage from inclusion cysts on the ovary or exposure to mullerian factors (specific sensitive tumor marker for ovaries) during menstruation (Bulun et al., 2019).

Clinical Manifestations and Assessment

Symptoms of ovarian cancer are subtle and start with persistent bloating, early satiety, or a change in bowel or bladder habits. Typically, patients will complain of weight gain confined to their abdominal area. Due to the close proximity of the ovaries to the intestines, patients will complain of GI symptoms; as a result, this cancer carries a high rate of misdiagnosis, with patients commonly receiving treatment for a variety of disorders, including IBS, gastroesophageal reflux (GERD), menopause, or UTIs. Ascites (fluid accumulation in the peritoneal cavity) is considered a late-stage symptom, and prognosis is poor (Dunphy et al., 2019; Papadakis et al., 2022).

No reliable screening tools are available for this disease. Treatment is hindered by late diagnosis, when the disease has already invaded peritoneal tissues and surrounding structures.

Bimanual examinations diagnose approximately one third of ovarian masses. Pelvic ultrasounds and blood tests for CA 125, a tumor marker, are the first diagnostics performed when ruling out an ovarian mass. If either of these tests is suggestive of a tumor, an abdominal and pelvic CT scan is performed. Patients are always referred to an oncologic gynecologist for management of this disease.

Medical Management

Surgical staging identifies tumor histologic grade and volume, which allows for the identification of treatment options and determines the prognosis based on tumor type (Table 32-6). During surgery, the suspicious tissue that is removed and sent to the laboratory for immediate analysis is known as a *frozen section.* If positive, the surgeon then performs extensive cytoreduction surgery or **debulking** to obtain clean tissue margins. This includes a TAH with BSO, removal of the omentum, peritoneal washings, and partial colectomy if there is any colon involvement (Dunphy et al., 2019; Papadakis et al., 2022).

Stage IA or IB tumors are considered low risk and favorable to treatment, if well- or moderately well-differentiated tumors are confined to the ovary. Absence of tumor on the external surfaces, absence of ascites, and negative peritoneal washings are also favorable signs. Stage IA or IB with poorly differentiated tumors, tumors notable on the external surface of the ovary, ruptured tumor capsule, and positive peritoneal washings all are considered high risk and unfavorable. Advanced stages III and IV require combination chemotherapy after surgical staging has been performed to determine tumor sensitivity to a particular chemotherapeutic agent.

TABLE **32-6 Stages of Ovarian Cancer**

Stage	Description
Stage I	Tumor confined to ovary
Stage II	Involves one or both ovaries and extends into pelvis
Stage III	Involves one or both ovaries, as well as peritoneal metastasis and/or lymph node involvement
Stage IV	Distant metastasis beyond peritoneal cavity, including the liver

Chemotherapy treats residual tumor and helps to control any metastatic disease. Advance tumors receive chemotherapy first to decrease the size of the tumor; then the patient undergoes surgical debulking to remove as much tumor as possible. Carboplatin combined with paclitaxel is currently the standard first-line therapy in the management of ovarian cancer, typically yielding a response rate of approximately 65% and a median progression-free survival (PFS) ranging from 16 to 21 months (Paoletti et al., 2020). Patients whose tumors are resistant to platinum receive single-agent therapy. A blood test for CA 125 is a sensitive indicator of disease relapse. A newer therapy that is currently being used for an alternative first-line therapy for ovarian cancer is a class of medications known as poly-adenosine-diphosphate-ribose-polymerase (PARP) inhibitors (olaparib, niraparib, veliparib; Previs, 2021).

Nursing Management

Education and support begin preoperatively and continue through discharge. Care must be individualized based on the patient's psychological and physical status, stage of illness, and treatment plan. Patients will need anticipatory guidance regarding postoperative infections, pain management, and potential side effects from chemotherapeutic agents. Postoperatively, patients will need to be monitored for signs and symptoms of infection, ileus, DVT, pulmonary embolus (PE), and bleeding. Encouraging the patient in the regular use of incentive spirometry, as well as regular ambulation, will help to decrease the development of DVT and atelectasis.

Emotional support is extremely important as the patient recovers from surgery and has to cope with a diagnosis of cancer. Side effects from chemotherapy should be discussed with the patient and their support system. Hair loss, nutrition, neuropathies, and nausea and vomiting as well as self-image alterations should be addressed regularly with the patient during their preoperative assessment and should be ongoing during their treatment. Refer to Chapter 5 for details on cancer care.

CANCER OF THE VULVA

Vulvar cancer is rare and represents just 4% to 5% of all cancers of the female reproductive tract (PDQ, 2021; Mazzotta et al., 2021). Its incidence has been increasing slowly since 1973, however, and research now reveals that condyloma or squamous dysplasia precedes the development of vulvar cancer. HPV infections account for 40% to 50% of vaginal and vulvar cancers (Preti et al., 2020). There is increased evidence of young females with HPV being diagnosed with vulvar intraepithelial neoplasia (VIN), but the disease has a high cure rate after surgical resection and radiotherapy. People diagnosed with vulvar cancer are usually between 65 and 70 years of age (Papadakis et al., 2022). Approximately 86% of patients will be diagnosed with localized disease (Cancer.net, 2021).

The majority (90%) of cases of vulvar cancer are SCC (VSCC), and approximately 40% to 60% of subtypes are largely due to high-risk strains of HPV, most commonly HPV 16 subtype (Mazzotta et al., 2021). VIN is more complex, is deeply invasive, and is considered the precancerous condition of HPV types 16, 18, 31, and 33. Patients who have been treated for condyloma, HPV, or abnormal cervical cytology, and those who smoke cigarettes or have an increased number of sexual partners, have increased risk of developing cancer of the vulva. It is more common for younger females to be diagnosed with HPV-related VSCC, while older people have a propensity for developing vulvar high-grade squamous intraepithelial lesions (VHSIL; Preti et al., 2020). The 5-year survival rate for localized disease is approximately 86%, but that percentage drops to approximately 51% for those with disease that has spread to the lymph nodes (Cancer.net, 2021).

Clinical Manifestations and Assessment

Longstanding external labial itching or burning of the external genitalia are early signs often self-treated by patients with OTC cortisone or anti-itch creams. Only about half of patients will present with dyspareunia, vulvar edema, or pain. Later-stage manifestations include ulcerated lesions that are indicative of cancer. Older patients are more likely to have advanced disease at the time of diagnosis (Preti et al., 2020). Lesions occur in the vulvar area but may extend into the perianal and rectal areas, and lesions occur most commonly in areas that do not have hair. A Keyes punch biopsy or tissue biopsy is the gold standard for diagnosing vulvar cancer.

Medical Management

As with all cancerous lesions, early diagnosis of vulvar cancer is paramount. Vulvar biopsy can be performed in the office if short-term medical therapies have been proven unsuccessful or if there is a high index of suspicion for cancer. Vulvar colposcopy may be performed, but laser ablation or a wide excision of the affected area or a vulvectomy (removal of the vulva) with lymph node sampling for clear margins is dependent upon the size, depth, and focality of lesions. As a result, preservation of the clitoral area may or may not occur (Helm, 2021). For those patients who prefer to avoid surgery, the use of chemoradiation has demonstrated more favorable outcomes than with radiation alone (Mazzotta et al., 2021). An alternative to surgery for early-stage lesions is the use of imiquimod, which is a topical immune-response modifier with antiviral and antitumor properties typically used for the treatment of external genital warts. Depending upon the extent of the vulvectomy, use of chemotherapy, biologics, and radiation treatments also may be indicated. If there is evidence of disease spread to adjacent organs or regional lymph nodes, lymphadenectomy (excision of one or more lymph nodes) will be performed. There is a statistically significant correlation between extent of reconstructive surgery and disease outcomes, with local reconstructive surgery demonstrating a better prognosis with significant reduction in relapse rate.

Nursing Management

Patients are at higher risk for infection depending upon the size and extent of the surgical site. Monitoring patients postoperatively for wound infections, fever, discharge, and pain is a priority. Avoidance of cross-contamination of body fluids (such as urine or feces) will help to decrease infection. Foley care and assessment of skin are important in identifying any potential site of entry for infection.

Pearls for Practice

Catheter-associated urinary tract infection (CAUTI) is one of the most common causes of hospital-acquired infection (HAI); therefore, the nurse plays a key role in detection and prevention of UTIs. The following interventions are recommended:

- *Insert catheters only for appropriate indications, and remove them as soon as possible.*
- *Ensure that only professionally trained persons insert and maintain catheters; insert catheters using sterile technique and sterile equipment. Catheter size should be individualized to the needs of the patient, use as small a catheter as possible to minimize urethral trauma.*
- *Maintain a closed drainage system. Empty the collecting bag regularly using a separate collecting container for each patient. Avoid touching the draining spigot to the collecting container.*
- *Maintain unobstructed urine flow (keep the collecting bag* ***below*** *the level of the bladder at all times; do not place the bag on the floor; keep the catheter and collecting tube free from kinking). Properly secure indwelling catheters after insertion to prevent movement and urethral traction.*
- *Maintain hand hygiene and follow standard (or appropriate isolation) precautions. Routine hygiene (e.g., cleansing of the meatal surface during daily bathing or showering) is appropriate.*
- *If a urine specimen is needed, collect a small sample by aspirating urine from the needleless sampling port with a sterile syringe/cannula adaptor after cleansing the port (CDC, 2017).*

Postoperative requirements for prolonged bed rest underscore the importance of assessing the patient for the development of DVT and PE, to avoid tension on the surgical site and promote healing. Frequent position changes and the use of compression stockings and intermittent pneumatic compression boots, along with regular use of incentive spirometry, will aid in avoiding the formation of DVTs and PEs.

Patients who have undergone a vulvectomy may suffer from distorted body image as a result of surgical resection; however, there are gaps in the literature that supports this theory. Decreased sensation, vaginal dryness, and dyspareunia all affect a person's ability to enjoy sexual relations. There is also a risk of pelvic floor dysfunction due to the severing of the delicate nerve supply in the vulvar area. Discussion with the surgeon regarding the extent of surgery will help the nurse to answer any questions the patient may have postoperatively. Frequently reported concerns of patients with gynecologic cancer are the fear of recurrence and difficulty with changes in their sexual health (Götze et al., 2019). Partner involvement and a social work or mental health referral are beneficial to help patients and their partners understand what to expect after discharge from the hospital.

HYSTERECTOMY

Surgical removal of the female reproductive organs is performed for a variety of reasons: dysfunctional uterine bleeding, benign or malignant masses, POP, pelvic pain, endometriosis, or trauma. Hysterectomies are the most common nonobstetric major surgery performed in the United States. Approximately 1:3 females will undergo a hysterectomy by the age of 60 years (CDC, 2020e). The majority of hysterectomies are performed for benign uterine disorders that impact the QOL for patients suffering from uterine disease or menstrual disorder.

Minimally invasive surgical techniques are now preferred due to reduced blood loss, decreased postoperative complications, and quicker recovery time; however, supracervical hysterectomies may serve to preserve risk of bladder prolapse but run the risk of spotting and a rare incidence of future cervical malignancy (Beyan et al., 2020; Spuentrup et al., 2021). Hysterectomies consist of surgical removal of the uterus and fallopian tubes; however, conservation of the ovaries and cervix may be considered depending upon the patient's age and reason for surgery. Bilateral oophorectomy is associated with a decreased risk of breast and ovarian cancer. Fifty percent of people who undergo hysterectomy between 40 and 44 years of age will have both ovaries removed at the time of surgery. That percentage increases to 78% for people between 45 and 64 years of age. Surgical removal of the ovaries results in immediate cessation of production of both estrogen and androgen, causing surgical menopause. Subtotal hysterectomy or sparing of the cervix has no proven benefits (Giugale et al., 2021). It is important for patients to know if they have not had their cervix removed; people with an intact cervix will need to continue to undergo annual Pap smear screening for cervical cancer.

Types

Deciding on whether a TAH versus a total vaginal hysterectomy (TVH) should be performed is largely dependent upon a patient's BMI and other comorbid conditions. TVH allows for less blood loss, quicker recovery, shorter hospital stay, fewer infections, and less pain than the abdominal approach, which requires incisions through the abdominal musculature. TVH and laparoscopic-assisted vaginal hysterectomy (LAVH) can be done in a 1-day surgery center, whereas TAH and radical hysterectomies require a longer hospital stay. The use of laparoscopic and hysteroscopic (inspection of the uterine cavity by endoscopy) approaches are other alternatives to be considered and are dependent upon the surgeon's skill and experience with the equipment; robotic-assisted surgery is another approach. Vaginal hysterectomies are associated with better outcomes and less complications for obese patients (ACOG, 2019). Radical hysterectomies, performed for malignant conditions, consist of the complete removal of all the reproductive organs, including the surrounding tissue margins, the upper one third of the vagina, and pelvic lymph node sampling. The number of hysterectomies performed overall is lower now due to the development and use of endometrial ablation, progestin IUDs, and UAE.

Nursing Management

All patients with hysterectomies are surgical patients and therefore must be cared for like any other surgical patient. Attention to pain management; postoperative complications, such as DVT, PE, wound infections, and UTIs; and return of bowel function are the primary concerns for nurses. The nurse assesses the patient's lung sounds and encourages regular use of incentive spirometry. The nurse also monitors for return of bowel functions, as an ileus (absence of peristalsis; usually accompanied by abdominal pain, distention, and occasionally nausea and vomiting; and typically occuring following abdominal surgery) may occur due to manipulation of the bowel during surgery and the effects of anesthesia and analgesia on peristalsis.

Encouraging patients to walk with assistance as soon as the effects from general anesthesia have resolved helps with circulation and prevents formation of blood clots. Many patients undergoing hysterectomy also are dealing with the loss of fertility and, possibly, a cancer diagnosis. The nurse allows the patient to verbalize their concerns and feelings and makes referrals to mental health providers if needed.

Discharge planning should include pelvic rest for 4 to 6 weeks and teaching the patient wound care and signs and symptoms of infection. Patients are allowed to shower and should be encouraged to resume regular activity gradually per the surgeon's recommendation. Patients who have had a TAH generally are not permitted to drive for 4 to 6 weeks. They should avoid any heavy lifting, pushing, or pulling (such as vacuum cleaning) until their surgeon clears them to resume those activities. It is normal for people who have had hysterectomies to have some vaginal discharge. Patients who have undergone TAH normally will have some vaginal bleeding for up to 1 week postoperatively; patients who have undergone TVH and LAVH may have some vaginal discharge consisting of blood and mucus for several weeks postoperatively. Any foul-smelling vaginal discharge, unusual pain, or fever should be reported to the surgeon immediately. If there is evidence of unilateral swelling of the lower extremities, shortness of breath, or any discharge or redness around their incision sites, the patient should contact their health care provider.

Unfolding Patient Stories: Doris Bowman • Part 2

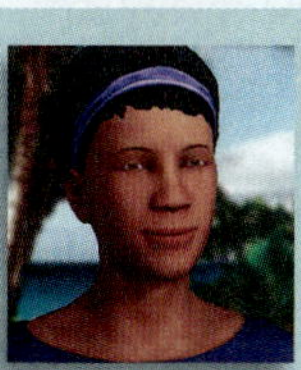

Recall from Chapter 5 **D.B.**, who is undergoing a TAH with BSO. What are potential postoperative complications that the nurse should consider? What assessments and interventions are done by the nurse to monitor for early detection or to prevent these complications? Describe the discharge education provided by the nurse on self-care monitoring required of the patient at home and what should be reported to the health care provider.

Care for D.B. and other patients in a realistic virtual environment: ***vSim** for Nursing* (thepoint.lww.com/vSimMedicalSurgical). Practice documenting these patients' care in DocuCare (thepoint.lww.com/DocuCareEHR).

HEALTH CARE FOR TRANSGENDER PEOPLE

Health Care Disparities

There is an increasing awareness of **transgender** patients and their lack of access to health care. It is paramount that nurses and health care providers educate themselves in the care of this underserved and marginalized population. This patient population is largely uninsured, experiences social stigmatization, and is at higher risk for PCOS, HIV exposure, interpersonal violence, and suicide. Transgender people are persons whose gender identity differs from their birth sex or whose gender expression is different from what is typically considered to be societal norms. *Gender dysphoria* is a term used to describe the physical and emotional discomfort in one's assigned birth sex (Ferri, 2022; IOM, 2011). If left untreated or if a person was unable to express or live as the gender with which they identify, that could lead to increased depression and, often, suicide. There are a disproportionate number of transgender people, especially teens and young adults, who become homeless due to familial isolation, loss of income, and inability to secure employment or housing. They may be placed inappropriately in emergency shelters and become victims of violence.

Previous surveys performed by the National Center for Transgender Equality and the National Gay and Lesbian Task Force revealed that 50% of the respondents reported having to teach their health care provider about transgender care (National Center for Transgender Equality, 2021). Forty-one percent of transgender people reported suicide attempts versus the national average of 1.6%; this population also reported HIV rates that are four times that of the national average. The results also include that a staggering 24% have been discriminated against by a health care provider, and 19% were denied care from a health care provider completely. All patients deserve the same respect regardless of gender identity, preference, or expression. Refer to Box 32-15 for a glossary of gender terminology.

When a person is transgender, they often live socially as a member of the sex with which they identify, through clothing and perhaps a name change. This is known as "transition." Some will choose to take hormones, such as testosterone or estrogen, for the desired physical

BOX 32-15 Glossary of Gender Terminology

Term	Definition
Agender	Describes someone who does not claim any gender, for whom gender is not a significant identity marker.
Cisgender	Describes a person whose gender aligns with the gender associated with their assigned sex at birth.
Gender-expansive	A wider range and greater flexibility of gender identity and/or expression than the binarism of male/female. May indicate a state of individual exploration of gender expression and/or gender identity.
Genderfluid	Describes a person whose gender identity is "fluid" or in flux.
Genderqueer	Describes a fluidity of identity that lies outside both the gender binary and, often, the typical or binary-inflected categories of sexual orientation.
Nonbinary	A nonbinary person does not identify exclusively as "man" or "woman," but, as the term suggests, may identify as a combination of the two, something in between, or something totally outside the gender binary. Can be used as a broad category encompassing gender identities such as agender, bigender, genderqueer, or genderfluid.
Transgender	Describes someone whose gender identity differs from the gender identity commonly aligned with their assigned sex at birth. This may include male-to-female transgender people; female-to-male transgender people; or those whose gender is nonbinary, fluid, or otherwise exists outside the male/female binary.

From Human Rights Campaign. Glossary of terms. (n.d.). https://www.hrc.org/resources/glossary-of-terms; National LGBT Health Education Center. (2020). *LGBTQIA+ glossary of terms for health care teams*. Boston: Fenway Institute. https://www.lgbtqiahealtheducation.org/wp-content/uploads/2020/10/Glossary-2020.08.30.pdf characteristics of the gender with which they identify. Many insurance companies deny coverage of hormone therapy for these patients. Others may have gender-affirming surgery, such as chest reconstruction (this is not to be referred to as a mastectomy as it is an entirely different surgical approach than that of a breast cancer surgery), breast implants, orchiectomy, vaginoplasty, or phalloplasty while others may never have surgery at all. Some transgender persons may or may not choose to take hormones. Many patients who are in transition may have difficulty securing health care insurance, and some insurances may initially deny coverage for any procedures related to patients' transitions, mental health therapy, facial-feminization, or gender-affirming surgery. However, federal law prohibits any discrimination by insurance companies in covering gender-confirming procedures (National Center for Transgender Equality, 2021). In addition, health insurance plans cannot have a categorical exclusion of specific transition-related procedures. Many patients who are unemployed, uninsured or underinsured may choose to purchase hormones via the internet or from unreliable sources. If patients become hospitalized, they may be anxious that they will not receive their hormones. Frequently they are discriminated against by members of the health care profession due to lack of knowledge, training, or personal bias on the part of the provider. The patient's level of anxiety may be escalated, and the provider may perceive them as a "difficult" patient. A person who has had to turn to sex work to survive or who has been discriminated against repeatedly throughout life may turn to negative behaviors in times of crisis. Older transgender persons are increasingly at risk for death from treatable chronic diseases or cancer due to their fear of stigmatization and previous discrimination or lack of health insurance. End-of-life issues and health care directives become a worrisome issue for older transgender persons due to the absence of a legal marriage and subsequent legal inability to allow partners to make health care decisions (Chidiac et al., 2021). Many states that do not recognize same-sex marriage also do not allow partners to make health care decisions so it falls onto the next of kin. This becomes a legal debate especially in the context of end-of-life care particularly if the patient does not have a living will or if the patient lives in a state that does not recognize domestic partnerships or same-sex marriages.

Fear and anxiety often will dissipate once a relationship of trust with care providers has been formed. It is difficult to find culturally competent and compassionate providers who have experience with transgender patients. The goal of Healthy People 2030 is to "improve the health, safety, and well-being of lesbian, gay, bisexual, and transgender people" (Healthy People 2030, 2021).

Nursing Management

It is important for nurses to be culturally diverse at all levels of practice. Nurses need to understand the specific needs of transgender patients and demonstrate acceptance with increased sensitivity and remain nonjudgmental while delivering care. It is equally important for nurses to educate other members of the health care team who may not have experience with this population to avoid any compromise in patient care due to bias or ignorance. Any bias or ignorance should not be tolerated by any member of the health care team. Refer to Box 32-16 for summary of best practices for transgender and gender diverse care.

Due to the historically poor treatment of the transgender population by the health care profession, many will seek care only in an emergency and when routine health conditions have exacerbated into a serious condition. It is vital that nurses treat the patient, not the gender, and accept and encourage involvement of the patient's partner, significant other, and any other person who is considered family by that patient. Nurses also must be familiar with individual institution policies regarding nonblood relatives as next-of-kin for patients.

Nurses are in a unique position to establish a trusting relationship with patients. It is important to use gender-neutral terms and to ask the patient for their preferred name and pronouns. Other important interventions for this patient population include:

- Assessing the patient for high-risk behaviors, including IV drug use, prostitution, or use of hormones obtained via the internet, on the street, or from the patient's friends.
- Offering to help transgender patients with their breast binder (if they wear one) after a shower, or assisting with padded bras and undergarments.
- Offering support and reassurance for those undergoing invasive examinations, such as a breast or pelvic

BOX 32-16 Best Practices for Transgender and Gender Diverse Care

- **Introduce** yourself to *all* patients using your name and pronouns, and invite patients to share these with you as well.
- **Document** your patient's name, gender, and the pronouns they use anywhere you can in the electronic health record.
- **Confirm** whether family members to whom your patient is not "out" may be calling about them, and make sure you know how you will protect their privacy.
- **Communicate** your patient's name and pronouns to the health care team and advocate for your patient by correcting others if needed.
- **Acknowledge** mistakes you make with your patient's name and pronouns briefly, correct yourself, and quickly move on.

Nye, C. M., & Anderson, A. (2021). Transgender and gender diverse nursing care. *AJN, American Journal of Nursing, 121*(10), 53–57. https://doi.org/10.1097/01.NAJ.0000794272.25624.e5; National LGBT Health Education Center. (2020). *Affirmative services for transgender and gender-diverse people: best practices for frontline health care staff.* Boston: Fenway Institute. https://www.lgbtqiahealtheducation.org/wp-content/uploads/2020/03/TFIE-40_Best-Practices-for-Frontline-Health-Care-Staff-Publication_web_final.pdf examination, as transgender patients may have emotional conflict between their actual body and what they perceive their body to be.

Hysterectomies are routine gynecologic procedures performed for specific medical and surgical needs, as previously discussed in this chapter. Hysterectomies are considered gender-affirming surgeries for transgender men. These surgeries are considered "medically necessary transition-related care" for those who suffer from gender dysphoria as a result of having female reproductive organs and regular menstrual cycles. In order to be considered a surgical candidate for a hysterectomy, the patient will need to undergo a gynecologic examination. It is important to note that a vast majority of transgender patients undergoing this surgery are either nulliparous or have never had vaginal penetration. If the patient has been using testosterone, a significant amount of vaginal atrophy will occur. Any transgender patient who has not had a hysterectomy or has had a supracervical hysterectomy will need to continue with routine cervical screening. ACOG (2021) recommends routine age-appropriate preventative screenings, including prostate and breast examinations, regardless of gender identity.

Any transgender patient who has any type of gender-affirming surgery should be treated like any other postoperative patient with the same risk factors.

CHAPTER REVIEW

NCLEX-Style Review Questions

1. Which of the following procedures are avoided (if possible) on patients who had a mastectomy with lymph node dissection performed for breast cancer? Select all that apply.
   a. IV insertion should be performed on the opposite side of the surgical procedure
   b. Blood pressure can be taken on the same side as the surgical procedure.
   c. Blood draws can occur on the same side as the surgical procedure.
   d. Injections should be administered on the opposite side of the surgical procedure.
   e. Tight or restrictive clothing or jewelry should be avoided on the same side as the surgical procedure.

2. A patient suspects that they may have **premenstrual dysphoric disorder** (PMDD). The nurse should ask the patient about which symptoms? Select all that apply.
   a. Symptoms that occur during the luteal phase of the menstrual cycle
   b. Symptoms that occur during the follicular phase of the menstrual cycle
   c. Symptoms that worsen during menopause
   d. Symptoms that persist throughout the entire menstrual cycle
   e. Symptoms including weight gain, abdominal bloating, and acne
   f. Symptoms of depression, mood swings, and overwhelming fatigue

3. Which patient would be at highest risk for subsequent development of lymphedema? Select all that apply.
   a. A 75-year-old with a single focus of biopsy-proven localized ductal carcinoma in situ
   b. A 65-year-old with a known benign cyst
   c. A 50-year-old with a biopsy-confirmed fibroadenoma
   d. A 62-year-old with biopsy-proven invasive ductal carcinoma with palpable axillary lymph nodes and positive node fine-needle aspiration
   e. A 68-year-old who is postmodified radical mastectomy with axillary node dissection and a portion of the axillary lymph nodes removed (ALND)

4. Your patient is complaining of urinary incontinence and sensation of increased pressure of the pelvic floor. The patient is 51 years of age, gravida 4, para 4 (gravida means pregnancies and para means live births), is 5 ft 2 in, and weighs 132 lb (BMI of 24.1, which is typical weight). The patient denies problems with constipation. Vital signs are 97.6 degrees, HR 88 and regular, RR 16, B/P 138/84, and O_2 sat on room air is 96%. The patient works as a barista, was recently diagnosed with hypertension, and recently started on antihypertensive medications. Select from the options below the risk factors or symptoms suggestive of bladder prolapse.
   a. Age of 51 years
   b. Gravida 4, para 4
   c. BMI 24.1
   d. Denies constipation
   e. Works as a barista
   f. History of hypertension

5. For the patient in item 4, after diagnosis of a urinary prolapse, which of the following interventions, do you anticipate teaching them as management? Select all that apply.

a. Pessary usage
b. Weight loss
c. Pelvic floor muscle training
d. Avoiding constipation
e. Kegel exercises

REFERENCES AND SELECTED READINGS

References and selected readings associated with this chapter can be found on the website that accompanies the book. Visit **http://thepoint.lww.com/Honan3e** to access the references and other additional resources associated with this chapter.

CHAPTER 33

Nursing Management: Care of the Assigned Male at Birth (AMAB) Patients With Reproductive Disorders

Kassandra August-Marcucio

Learning Objectives

After reading this chapter, you will be able to:

1. Discuss the causes and management of assigned male at birth (AMAB) sexual dysfunction.
2. Compare the treatments for prostate cancer, including advantages and disadvantages.
3. Use the nursing process as a framework for care of the patient undergoing prostatectomy.
4. Describe the various conditions affecting the testes, including pathophysiology, clinical manifestations, and management.
5. Describe the various conditions affecting the penis, including pathophysiology, clinical manifestations, and management.

Disorders of the assigned male at birth (AMAB) patient's reproductive system involve the genitalia and, in some instances, sexuality. Discussion and diagnosis of these conditions can include feelings of anxiety and embarrassment and can invoke past traumatic events; thus, evaluation must include an empathetic nursing approach that incorporates trauma-focused care. The effects of trauma, chronic illness, and physical disability of sexual function can be profound. A patient's willingness to discuss these issues is influenced directly by culture, religion, social community, and overall comfort with one's sexuality.

DISORDERS OF AMAB SEXUAL FUNCTION

ERECTILE DYSFUNCTION

Erectile dysfunction (ED) is the inability to achieve or maintain an erection sufficient for satisfactory sexual activity. Satisfactory sexual activity can include penetration (both anal and vaginal), oral sexual encounters, foreplay, and masturbation. Up to 30 million AMAB persons in the United States and 150 million worldwide are estimated to be affected by ED (AUA, 2018).

Pathophysiology

The physiology of erection and ejaculation is complex and involves sympathetic and parasympathetic components. Achieving an erection involves the release of nitric oxide into the corpus cavernosum during sexual stimulation; this releases cyclic guanosine monophosphate (cGMP) and causes relaxation of the smooth muscles. This allows flow of blood into the corpus cavernosum. Both neurologic and vascular functions are necessary for an erection. Once blood flows into the corpora, the dorsal vein must remain compressed to result in erection.

ED has both psychogenic and organic causes. Psychogenic causes include anxiety, fatigue, depression, pressure to perform sexually, and past sexually traumatic events. Organic causes include occlusive vascular disease, endocrine disease (diabetes, hypogonadism, hyperthyroidism, and hypothyroidism), cirrhosis, chronic kidney failure, postsurgical causes (retroperitoneal or major abdominal surgery), neurologic disorders (neuropathies, parkinsonism, spinal cord injury, and multiple sclerosis), trauma to the pelvic or genital area, alcohol, medications (Box 33-1), and substance use disorder.

Clinical Manifestations and Assessment

The diagnosis of ED requires a sexual and medical history; an analysis of presenting symptoms; a physical examination, including a neurologic examination; a detailed assessment of the usage of any medications, alcohol, and drugs; and per the most recent AUA guidelines, laboratory studies such as follicle-stimulating hormone (FSH), luteinizing hormone (LH), testosterone (both free testosterone and standard) prolactin, estradiol, and sex-binding globin (SBG) (Burnett et al., 2018). Psychological evaluation for relationship issues and past sexual trauma should be considered in select patients.

BOX 33-1

Classes of Medications Associated With Erectile Dysfunction

- Antiadrenergics and antihypertensives
- Anticholinergics and phenothiazines
- Antiseizure agents
- Antifungals
- Antiandrogen medications (prostate cancer treatment)
- Antipsychotics
- Antispasmodics
- Anxiolytics, sedative–hypnotics, tranquilizers
- Beta blockers
- Calcium-channel blockers
- Carbonic anhydrase inhibitors
- H_2 antagonists
- Thiazide diuretics
- Tricyclic antidepressants

Because ED can occur secondary to a variety of disorders and pharmacologic agents, nurses are encouraged to ask patients questions about erectile function. Numerous tools are available to help nurses introduce the topic of sexual health with their patients, including the sexual health inventory for males (SHIM) or the erection hardness scale (EHS; Burnett et al., 2018). The patient may report decreased frequency of erections, inability to achieve a firm erection, or rapid detumescence (subsidence of erection). Figure 33-1 describes the evaluation and treatment of ED.

Medical Management

Treatment can be medical, surgical, or both, depending on the cause (Table 33-1). Nonsurgical therapy includes treating associated conditions, such as diabetes, and adjusting antihypertensive agents, SSRIs, or other medications as appropriate. Endocrine therapy may reverse the condition if related to such conditions such as hypo/hyperthyroidism; hypogonadism should not be treated specifically for monotherapy of ED. Patients with ED from psychogenic causes should be referred to a sex therapist or other qualified provider to discuss underlying psychological issues affecting their ability to engage in sexual intercourse. Patients with ED secondary to organic causes may be candidates for penile implants.

Pharmacologic Therapy

Phosphodiesterase-5 (PDE-5) inhibitors are oral medications that are used to treat ED. Sildenafil citrate, the first of these agents, was introduced in the 1990s in the United States. Other PDE-5 inhibitors are vardenafil HCl, avanafil, and tadalafil. PDE-5 is an enzyme that destroys cGMP, the nucleotide that causes the cavernosal relaxation necessary for erection to occur. By inhibiting PDE-5, cGMP can accumulate, thus facilitating relaxation of corporeal smooth muscle in response to sexual stimulation. When PDE-5 inhibitors are taken about 30 to 45 minutes before sexual activity, they

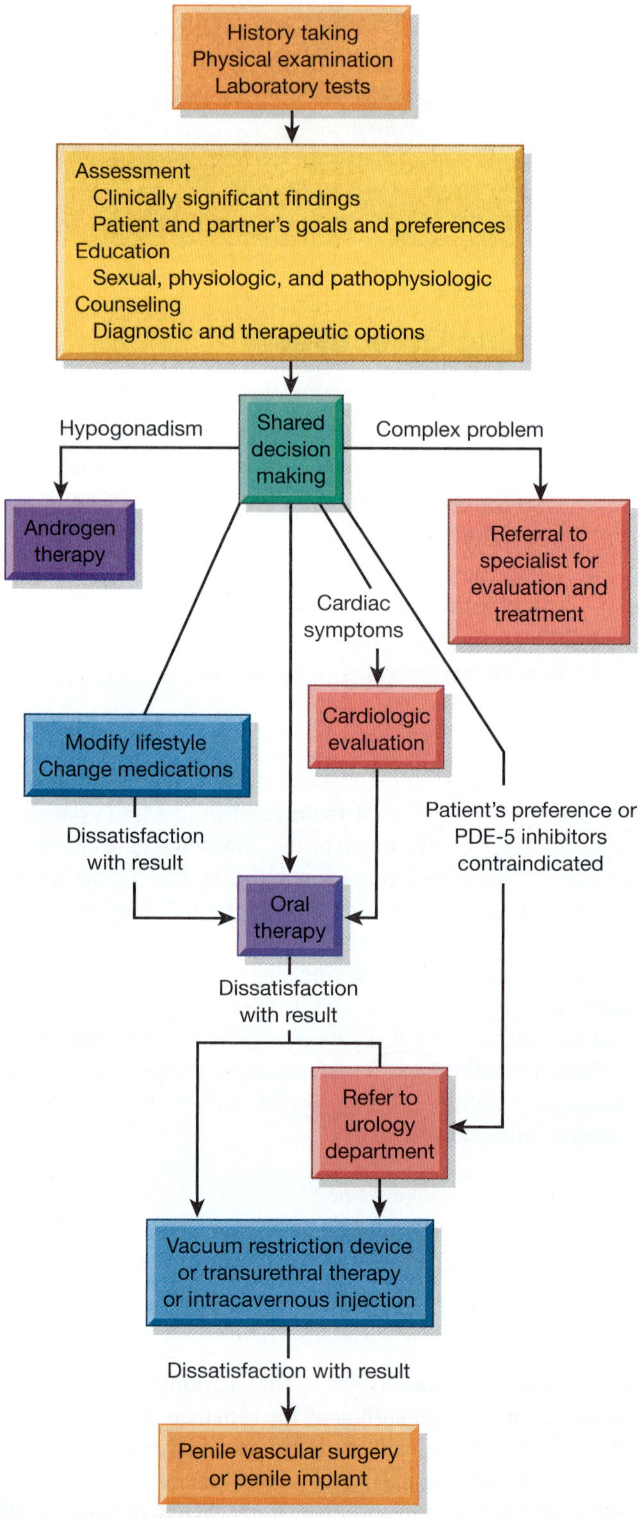

FIGURE 33-1 **Evaluation and treatment of males with erectile dysfunction. (From Lue, T. F. [2000]. Erectile dysfunction. *New England Journal of Medicine*, *342*[24], 1807. © 2000 Massachusetts Medical Society. All rights reserved. Used with permission.)**

TABLE **33-1 Treatments for Erectile Dysfunction**

Method	Description	Advantages and Disadvantages	Duration
Pharmacologic therapy • Oral medication (sildenafil citrate; vardenafil HCl; avanafil; tadalafil) 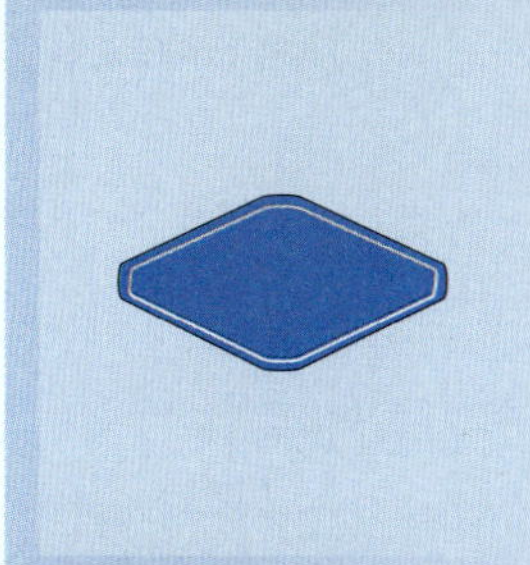 Oral medication	Smooth muscle relaxant causing blood to flow into penis	Can cause headache and sinus stuffiness Contraindicated for patients taking nitrate medications Used with caution in patients with retinopathy or poor exercise tolerance Renal dosing may be required for patients with kidney failure Some formulations require medications be taken on an empty stomach to be effective	Taken orally 30–60 minutes prior to intercourse Stimulation required to achieve erection
• Injection (alprostadil, alprostadil, papaverine, and phentolamine) 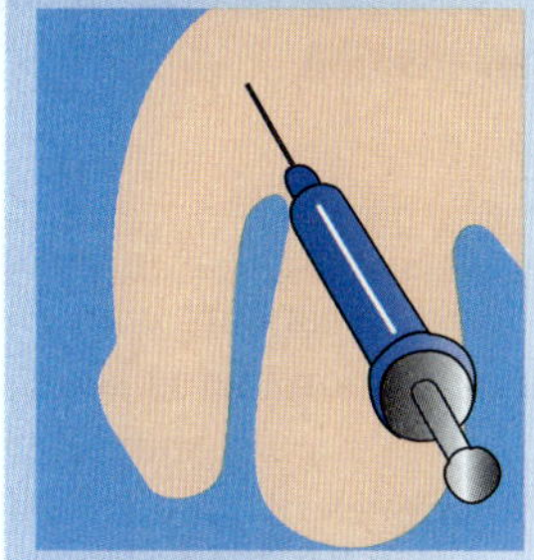 Penile injection	Smooth muscle relaxant increasing blood to flow into penis	Firm erections are achievable in more than 50% of cases Pain at injection site; plaque formation, risk of priapism Risk for Peyronie disease with consistent plaque formation over time Potential for Priapism	Injection 5–20 minutes before intercourse Erection can last up to 1 hour
• Urethral suppository (alprostadil) 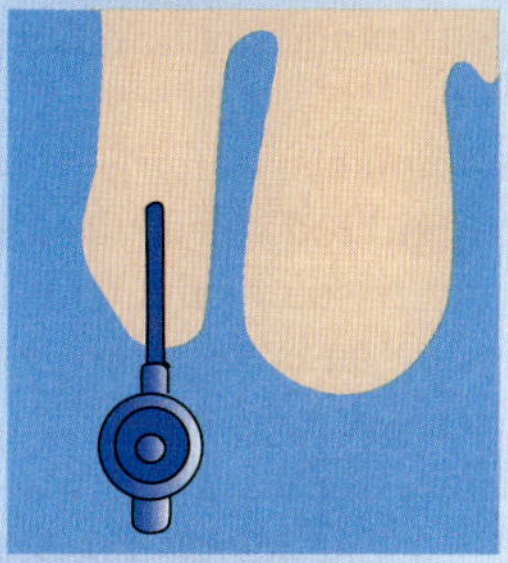 Penile suppository	Smooth muscle relaxant increasing blood flow into penis	May be used twice a day Not recommended with partners who are pregnant or trying to become pregnant as it can dilate the cervix and cause miscarriage Potential for priapism Dysuria or irritation of the urethra from insertion	Inserted 20–30 minutes before intercourse Erection can last up to 1 hour.
Penile implants • Semirigid rod • Inflatable 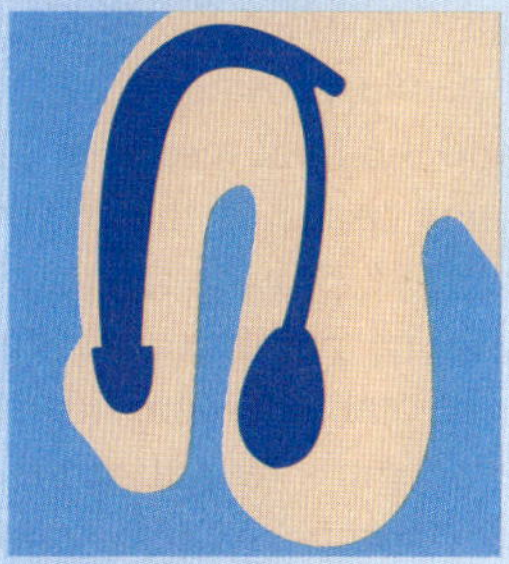 Penile implant	Surgically implanted into corpus cavernosum	Reliable Requires surgery Healing takes up to 3–6 weeks Semirigid rod results in permanent semierection If patient elects to remove penile implant they will have no erections	Indefinite—must be deflated manually (inflatable device) Inflatable prosthesis: Saline returns from penile receptacle to reservoir

(continued)

TABLE 33-1 **Treatments for Erectile Dysfunction (*continued*)**

Method	Description	Advantages and Disadvantages	Duration
Negative-pressure (vacuum) devices 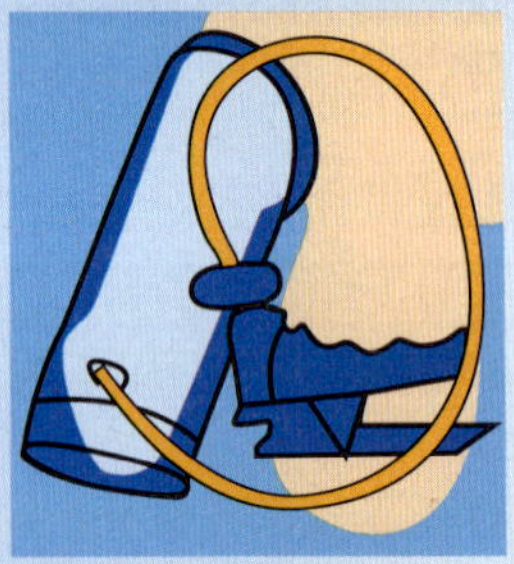 Penile vacuum pump	Induction of erection with vacuum; maintained with constriction band around base of penis	Few side effects Patients may find it cumbersome to use Vasocongestion of penis can cause pain or numbness If no lubricant is used, pain and irritation to the external skin of the penis	To prevent penile injury, constriction band must not be left in place for longer than 1 hour

may be effective in producing, *with stimulation*, an erection that can last 60 to 120 minutes. It is important to counsel patients that these medications are dependent on stimulation for erection to occur. Patients who are prescribed PDE-5 inhibitors should not take organic nitrates (e.g., nitroglycerin for chest pain) because together these drugs can cause severe hypotension. Side effects of PDE-5 inhibitors that patients should be aware of include flushing; headache; sweating; heartburn; dizziness or lightheadedness; and prolonged erection lasting greater than 4 hours, which is called **priapism**. It is important that a patient seek emergent or urgent care for an erection that lasts for 4 hours or more. Neglecting to treat this condition can cause permanent damage to the penis. With sildenafil citrate use, a blue visual haze in the peripheral vision due to the inhibition of the PDE-5 pathway can occur. Table 33-2 summarizes the dosing and nursing implications of these medications.

Another pharmacologic measure that can be considered is an injectable vasoactive agent. Alprostadil and combination of alprostadil, papaverine, and phentolamine are local vasodilators that can be injected into the corpora cavernosa of the penis. These medications cause vasodilation of the surrounding blood vessels and channels blood flow from the iliac arteries and the pelvis to the penis to create an erection. Repeated injections into the penis can cause the development of fibrotic plaques. Over time, fibrotic plaques can cause scarring to occur within the corpora, which will manifest as curvature to the penis, or a disease process called Peyronie disease. Other potential side effects that the patient should be aware of are pressure or pain at the injection site or bleeding after injection.

Alprostadil is a local vasodilator for treatment of erectile dysfunction that can also come in a gel pellet and applicator. This may be an alternative option for patients who are not interested or who are fearful of penile injections. The patient places the applicator into the urethra of the penis and expels the gel pellet from the applicator. Once the pellet is in the urethra, the patient is instructed to massage the penis to encourage the gel pellet to dissolve. Once the alprostadil is absorbed into the surrounding tissues, dilation of local blood vessels will result in blood flow to the penis, causing an erection.

Penile Implants

Penile implants are a surgical option for patients who are suffering from refractory erectile dysfunction that is largely nonresponsive to medication therapy. Patients should be encouraged to trial all medication therapies, if they are eligible, prior to selecting surgical intervention with penile implant. It is important to remember that penile implants are a highly elective procedure and patients should undergo thorough evaluation to ensure their risk of death during surgery is low. High surgical risk patients should not be referred for penile implant.

There are two types of penile implants: semirigid rod (malleable) and inflatable. The semirigid rod is a device that has two rods that replace the spongy tissue of the corpora cavernosa, enabling the patient to have an erection without the use of medications. Semirigid rods are a good choice for patients who have physical limitations, for example, weakness of a hand or arm after cerebrovascular accident (CVA), as they would not need the dexterity to compress the bulb as in an inflatable device. Patients who choose semirigid rod placement should be informed that they will always have an erection, but the device is flexible enough to be discreet.

The inflatable prosthesis generally includes three pieces. The three pieces of the inflatable penile prosthesis include the inflatable cylinders, the pump, and the fluid reservoir. The inflatable cylinders replace the spongy tissue of the corpora cavernosa in the penis and, when inflated, provide the patient with an erection for sexual activity. The pump for inflating the device is implanted within the scrotal sac alongside the testicles, usually on the side of the patient's dominant hand. The inflatable cylinders are inflated by compressing the pump

TABLE **33-2 Pharmacologic Treatment of Erectile Dysfunction**

	Sildenafil Citrate	Vardenafil HCl	Avanavil	Tadalafil
Recommended dose	Dosage range is 25–100 mg, based on individual response. Take only once in 24 hours.	Dosage range is 5–20 mg, based on individual response. Take only once in 24 hours.	Dosage range is 50– 200 mg, based on individual response. Take only once in 24 hours.	Dosage range is 5–20 mg, based on individual response. Take only once in 24 hours. For patients with decreased liver or kidney function, the maximum dose is 10 mg every 48 hours.
When to take	Take the medication 30–60 minutes before sexual activity. *There must be sexual stimulation to produce an erection.*	Take the medication 1 hour before sexual activity. The peak action occurs in 30–120 minutes. *There must be sexual stimulation to produce an erection.*	Take the medication at least 15 minutes before sexual activity. The peak action occurs in 30–120 minutes. *There must be sexual stimulation to produce an erection.*	Take the medication before sexual activity. Effect peaks at 2–6 hours; effect may last up to 36 hours. *There must be sexual stimulation to produce an erection.*
Side effects	Side effects include headache, flushing, indigestion, nasal congestion, and blue vision.	Side effects include headache, flushing, runny nose, indigestion, and sinusitis.	Side effects include headache, flushing, runny nose, and back pain.	Tadalafil may cause back pain and muscle aches. The patient should tell the provider if they experience any of these side effects.
Note	Patients must be counseled to seek medical attention for an erection lasting longer than 4 hours. Patients must be counseled to seek medical attention in the event of sudden loss of vision in one or both eyes. Taking more than one of these mediations is not advised; combinations have not been evaluated formally for efficacy or safety. If combination therapy is necessary, this should be monitored by a qualified urology provider. These medications can potentiate the effects of nitrates, alpha blockers, antihypertensives, and alcohol.			
Contraindications	Do not take if you are taking nitrate medications, such as nitroglycerin or isosorbide mononitrate. Do not take if you have high uncontrolled blood pressure or coronary artery disease or have had a heart attack in the last 6 months without having an in-depth discussion with your cardiology provider. Do not take if you have been diagnosed with a cardiac arrhythmia or kidney or liver dysfunction—discuss with your provider to ensure proper dosing.			
Drug interactions	These medications can interact with other medications that you may be taking. Provide your provider with a complete list of all prescribed medications as well as over-the-counter medications, including herbal supplements, that you are using.			

between the fingers through the scrotal wall. The fluid maintained in the reservoir, which is implanted behind the retropubic space, is then pumped through the contained system to the inflatable cylinders within the penis. A three-piece penile prosthetic implant can be beneficial to patients who desire a more natural appearing flaccid penis when the device is not in use.

Counseling for Device Placement

Factors to consider in choosing a prosthesis include the expectations of the patient and their partner. Involving the partner in discussions regarding penile prosthesis ensures that proper expectations are set and that the procedure is understood by both parties. Risks of surgical intervention should be discussed with the patient, including postoperative swelling, pain, and risk for incisional infection, device infection, or device rejection. The risks and benefits of pursuing an elective procedure should be discussed with the patient and the general health of the patient confirmed prior to surgical intervention. Erosion of the prosthetic device through one or both corpora cavernosa cavities (see Chapter 31, Fig. 31-7), or through the urethra, is a long-term risk of intra-penile prosthetic devices. It is important that the penile implant is evaluated for erosion at well visits. Signs and symptoms of penile prosthetic device erosion may include burning with urination, decreased urinary stream, perineal pain, or visualization of the device through the penile tissue. The most common cause for prosthetic erosion is an ill-fitting implant; therefore, encouraging the patient to find a certified and experienced urologic surgeon is important before proceeding with penile implantation.

Vacuum Erection Devices

Negative-pressure (vacuum) devices also may be used to induce an erection. A plastic cylinder is placed over the flaccid penis, and negative pressure is applied. When an erection is attained, a constriction band is placed around the base of the penis to maintain the erection. The patient should be instructed to lubricate the penis with a water-based lubricant prior to use to avoid injury or discomfort to the penis.

Nursing Management

Personal satisfaction and the ability to satisfy a partner sexually are common concerns of patients. Persons with illnesses and disabilities may need the assistance of a sex therapist to find, implement, and integrate their sexual beliefs and behaviors into a healthy and satisfying lifestyle. The nurse should assess the patient's needs and make appropriate resources available, including information regarding referral to a specialized sex therapist, such as the American Association of Sexuality Educators, Counselors and Therapists (www.aasect.org).

DISORDERS OF EJACULATION

The spectrum of disorders of ejaculation responses ranges from occasional ejaculation through intercourse or self-stimulation to complete inability to ejaculate under any circumstances. Premature ejaculation (PE) is the occurrence of ejaculation before or shortly after penetration, without a sense of control, with the patient experiencing distress related to this (Shindel et al., 2022). When considering the instance of self-reported PE, few have an ejaculation latency time (the time between penetration and ejaculation) of less than 2 minutes, making the actual prevalence of clinical PE less than 5% (Shindel et al., 2022). Treatment modalities include behavioral therapy to delay ejaculation or partner involved therapy. Medical therapy of PE includes utilizing SSRIs, select tricyclic antidepressants (TCAs), topical local anesthetics, tramadol, PDE-5s, and alpha-adrenergic blockers. Topical anesthetics can also be considered, such as lidocaine, prilocaine, or benzocaine, to decrease the sensitivity of the glans of the penis. The use of TCA and SSRIs prolong ejaculation by manipulating the serotonin system and 5-HT receptors that are involved in the ejaculatory process (Shindel et al., 2022).

Neurologic disorders (e.g., spinal cord injury, multiple sclerosis, neuropathy secondary to diabetes), surgery (prostatectomy), and medications are the most common causes of inhibited ejaculation. Chemical, vibratory, and electrical methods of stimulation have been used with some success.

CONDITIONS OF THE PROSTATE

PROSTATITIS

Prostatitis is an inflammation of the prostate gland that is caused by infectious agents; it is most often caused by bacteria ascending via the urethra or from intraprostatic reflux.

Pathophysiology

Escherichia coli is the most common organism identified in prostatitis in greater than 50% of cases, followed by *Pseudomonas aeruginosa*. It is important to note that prostatitis can be caused by sexually transmitted diseases such as *Chlamydia trachomatis*, *Neisseria gonorrhoeae*, and *Trichomonas vaginalis*. Structurally, bacteria are introduced into the urethra and ascend the urethral tract, causing AMAB patients to develop prostatitis. Another way that bacteria can be introduced into the urethral tract is by instrumentation, such as cystoscopy or catheterization, or via fine needle biopsy of the prostate.

Clinical Manifestations and Assessment

Diagnosis of prostatitis should begin with careful history taking of the patient. First, the patient should be questioned regarding recent unprotected sexual activity. This conversation should be approached carefully as patients can be reluctant to divulge personal sexual encounters. It is important to notify and assure the patient that the patient–provider relationship and interview is confidential. If prostatitis is related to a sexually transmitted disease, then immediate treatment would be warranted and may affect what type of antibiotic therapy is initiated.

Symptoms of prostatitis may include perineal discomfort, dysuria (painful or difficult urination), urgency, frequency, and pain with or after ejaculation. **Prostatodynia** (pain in the prostate) is manifested by pain on voiding or perineal pain without evidence of inflammation or bacterial growth in the prostate fluid.

Acute bacterial prostatitis may present with sudden fever and chills and pain in the perineum, rectum, or low back. Urinary symptoms, such as dysuria, frequency, urgency, and **nocturia** (awakening at night to urinate), may occur. Chronic bacterial prostatitis is a major cause of relapsing urinary tract infection (UTI). Symptoms are usually mild, consisting of frequency; dysuria; and, occasionally, urethral discharge. Complications of prostatitis include swelling of the prostate gland, urinary retention, epididymitis, bacteremia, and pyelonephritis (discussed in Chapter 26).

Digital rectal examination (DRE) can be helpful in the diagnosis of prostatitis. A DRE is usually not recommended if the patient is suffering from acute prostatitis. It is important that the provider does not perform the DRE vigorously in a patient who is being evaluated for prostatitis as this may cause the patient increased pain and may increase the risk of bacteremia. On physical examination with DRE, the prostate may feel tender, enlarged, or boggy (soft and spongy).

Urine studies should be collected prior to DRE. Common findings on urinalysis can demonstrate elevated red blood cells or elevated white blood cells; depending on what bacteria may be present, nitrates may be evident on urine studies. If prostatitis is suspected, culture should be sent prior to initiating antibiotic therapy to ensure appropriate antibiotic therapy is being utilized to avoid multidrug resistant organism formation. Although it is important to evaluate the urine for bacteria, up to 35% of urinary studies in patients presenting with prostatitis symptoms will not grow an identifiable organism (Coker & Dierfeldt, 2016). If there is urethral discharge, it should be collected and sent for analysis.

A complete blood count (CBC) may be ordered to rule out blood infection related to prostatitis. In severe cases, a blood culture may be performed when septicemia is suspected. A **prostate-specific antigen** (PSA) test may or may not be obtained since in many patients the acute inflammatory process causes temporary elevation and may not be a good indicator of success of treatment. The PSA may remain elevated for months following the infection before returning to baseline.

In settings of chronic prostatitis, prostatic massage with urine collection before and after may be indicated to identify bacteria. Prostatic massage should never be performed on a patient suspected of acute prostatitis due to the risk of septicemia.

Medical Management

The goal of therapy for acute bacterial prostatitis is to avoid the complications of abscess formation and septicemia. A broad-spectrum antibiotic, frequently a fluoroquinolone, is administered for 14 to 30 days. A longer course of antibiotics is favored to have ideal penetration into the prostatic tissue. More recent research shows that certain fluoroquinolones, such as ciprofloxacin, have severe side effects that should be considered. These include potential rupture of abdominal aneurysm, ligament injuries, and temporal mandibular joint necrosis. Comfort is promoted with analgesic agents, antispasmodic medications, bladder sedatives (to relieve bladder irritability), sitz baths (to relieve pain and spasm), and stool softeners (to prevent pain from straining to defecate).

Chronic bacterial prostatitis can be difficult to treat because most antibiotics diffuse poorly from the plasma into the prostatic fluid and longer courses of antibiotics may be required. The risks and benefits of longer treatment with antibiotics versus conservative management should be evaluated. Treatment may include alpha-adrenergic blockers to promote relaxation of the bladder and prostate.

The treatment of nonbacterial prostatitis is directed toward relief of symptoms. This would include conservative management with rest, sitz baths, avoiding physical activity that would impact the perineum, and NSAIDs as tolerated and directed per the provider's instruction. Antibiotics should be avoided to avoid multidrug-resistant organisms.

Nursing Management

A person experiencing symptoms of acute prostatitis may be hospitalized for IV antibiotic therapy. Nursing management includes administration of prescribed antibiotics and provision of comfort measures, including prescribed analgesic agents and sitz baths. In addition, the patient is cautioned to avoid activities that result in repetitive perineal trauma, such as cycling, horseback riding, motorcycling, and vigorous sexual activity.

The patient with chronic prostatitis is treated on an outpatient basis and is instructed about the importance of continuing antibiotic therapy until all prescribed doses are completed. The nurse will assist the patient with hot sitz baths for 10- to 20-minute intervals, this may be done several times daily for comfort. Other supportive nursing interventions are providing fluids for hydration, administering prescribed antipyretics and analgesics, and instructing the patient to avoid sitting for long periods to minimize discomfort. In rare instances, prostatitis can cause urinary obstruction that can require urinary catheterization, either intermittently or indwelling.

BENIGN PROSTATIC HYPERPLASIA

Benign prostatic hyperplasia (BPH) is prevalent in persons with a prostate as they increase in age. Per the American Urological Association (AUA) guidelines, BPH is a histologic diagnosis that results in the proliferation of glandular epithelial tissue, smooth muscle, and the connective tissue in the prostatic transitional zone. The risk of BPH increases with age and presents in over 70% of older AMAB patients. BPH can cause several bothersome obstructive urinary tract symptoms that can affect a patient's quality of life (Lerner, 2021).

Pathophysiology

The enlargement of the prostate is caused by hyperplasia of the lateral lobes of the prostate that obstruct the vesical neck or prostatic urethra, causing obstructive urinary symptoms. Obstructive symptoms include feelings of incomplete emptying, poor urinary stream, urgency, frequency, trouble initiating a urine stream, intermittency of urination, and urinary retention. Over time, retention can cause a gradual dilation of the ureters (hydroureter) and kidneys (hydronephrosis). The patient suffering from urinary retention may be at higher risk for UTI or bacteriuria resulting from urinary stasis. Retained urine serves as an ideal medium for infective organism growth.

Clinical Manifestations and Assessment

There is no agreed-upon definition of BPH because the etiology of enlarged prostate is unknown. Assessment of BPH begins with obtaining a complete review of symptoms of the urinary system. The obstructive and irritating symptoms associated with BPH include increased frequency of urination, nocturia, urgency, hesitancy in starting urination, abdominal straining with urination, decrease in the volume, poor urinary stream, interruption of the urinary stream, dribbling, a sensation of incomplete emptying, possible acute urinary retention, and history of recurrent UTIs. BPH can have a progressive natural history that can be more profound in persons who have a larger prostate gland and/or a higher PSA (AUA, 2021).

DRE may reveal a large, rubbery, and nontender prostate gland, although the size of the prostate correlates poorly with symptom report. A post-void residual (PVR) can help determine whether the provider should be concerned regarding urinary retention. Initially, medical management should be the pathway of choice for treatment of BPH, followed by reassessment of symptoms and possible discussion of surgical interventions, which is discussed later in this chapter.

Diagnostic studies are only indicated in cases of refractory urinary retention or compromised renal function, or they may be ordered preoperatively. Urodynamic studies are used when it is unclear if symptoms are solely being caused by BPH or by overactive bladder symptoms.

Medical Management

The AUA outlines the best practice statements for the treatment of BPH. Initial treatment of BPH that does not present with acute urinary retention is medical management with follow-up to determine treatment effectiveness. If medical therapies are unsuccessful, then surgical interventions can be discussed with the patient if appropriate.

Acute urinary retention related to BPH always requires emergency intervention, often with catheterization, either with an indwelling catheter or intermittent catheterization. The ordinary catheter may be too soft and pliable to advance through the urethra into the bladder. A Coude catheter (45-degree, semirigid curved tip) is recommended to facilitate passage through the prostatic urethra. If a catheter cannot be placed, typically a urologic team can place a catheter using a camera and wire-guidance. Rarely, an incision is made into the bladder and a suprapubic tube is placed to provide drainage. Further details are discussed in Chapter 27 under urinary retention.

Pharmacologic Therapy

Pharmacologic treatment for BPH includes use of alpha-adrenergic blockers and 5-alpha-reductase inhibitors. Alpha-adrenergic blockers relax the smooth muscle of the bladder neck and prostate, improve urine flow, and relieve BPH symptoms. Side effects include lightheadedness, dizziness, and retrograde ejaculation, and they can interfere with PDE-5s used for erectile dysfunction. Medications called 5-alpha-reductase inhibitors interfere with the conversion of testosterone to dihydrotestosterone (DHT), which is associated with prostate growth. Decreased levels of DHT lead to decreased activity of glandular cells and prostate size. Recent studies suggest that the use of 5-alpha-reductase inhibitors in persons with prostates less than 30 to 40 g does not demonstrate any significant improvement in BPH symptoms. Persons with larger prostate glands and lower urinary flow rates appear to benefit the most from treatment with 5-alpha-reductace inhibitors (Lerner, 2021). Side effects may include gynecomastia, ED, low-volume ejaculate, and flushing.

Saw palmetto is an herbal product some patients find helpful in addressing symptoms associated with BPH. In theory, it functions by interfering with the conversion of testosterone to DHT. The lack of standardization of herbal products should be a source of concern for health care providers, and the nurse should warn patients that formulations may be different with each purchase.

Surgical Interventions

Surgical interventions for BPH range from minimally invasive to invasive procedures. Treatment options include UroLift®, Rezum®, Green Light Laser, transurethral incision of the prostate (TUIP), transurethral resection of the prostate (TURP), and Holmium laser enucleation of the prostate (HOLEP). Surgical approach of choice depends on the size of the gland, the severity of obstruction, the age of the patient, comorbidities, and the overall function of the bladder (see Box 33-3). Treatment of BPH with surgical intervention aims to eliminate the obstructive prostate tissue to open the prostatic urethra to allow passage of urine out of the bladder.

Conservative Management

In "watchful waiting," another option chosen by many, patients are monitored periodically for severity of symptoms. If the patient is stable with their symptoms and their kidney function is within normal limits, they can be monitored for their BPH conservatively. In select patients, it may be acceptable to allow for higher PVR levels if monitored appropriately (see Chapter 25 for details on PVR). A shared decision-making discussion that includes the option to "do nothing" should always be had with the patient, their family members, or other legal health care decision makers; in this discussion, the risks and benefits of possible options are weighed and detailed.

CANCER OF THE PROSTATE

Prostate cancer is the most common cancer in AMAB populations other than nonmelanoma skin cancer. In 2021, it was estimated that 248,530 new cases of prostate cancer would be diagnosed, accounting for almost 26% of new cancer cases in the AMAB population (National Comprehensive Cancer Network [NCCN], 2022). Despite significant improvement in treatment and identifying prostate cancer, 10.7% of AMAB cancer deaths in 2021 were related to prostate cancer (NCCN, 2022). When considering all stages of prostate cancer, the 5-year relative survival rate for prostate cancer is approximately 98% (NCCN, 2022).

Risk Factors

Prostate cancer risk factors include age, family history of prostate cancer, ovarian or BRCA 1 breast cancer familial genetic mutations, abnormal DRE, and PSA at the time of diagnosis. There is evidence to suggest that smoking history and exposures may be related to prostate cancer diagnosis.

There has been a long-held belief that Black populations carried the highest incidence of prostate cancer; however, more recent research indicates that racism, lack of intersectionality and poor sampling, has led to a falsely higher incidence of prostate cancer in Black populations. Cultural differences in viewing health care, distrust of the medical system from years of generational trauma, and lack of understanding of race as a social construct, have contributed to incorrect assumptions that certain populations have higher incidence of prostate cancer, when in fact, the incidence is similar when adjusted for social factors and accounting for largely saturated White study sampling (Schenk et al., 2022).

Prostate cancer in persons younger than 40 is very rare; however, the risk of having prostate cancer increases substantially over the age of 50 years (ACS, 2022). It is well established that family history is a significant risk factor for prostate cancer. In genetic studies, prostate cancer has been linked to other hereditary cancers such as breast and ovarian cancer and Lynch syndrome, due to germline mutations (NCCN, 2022). Approximately 11% of prostate cancer patients who have an additional primary cancer will be found to carry at least one germline mutation (NCCN, 2022). During the family history review, it is important that the nurse have the patient identify any family members who may have had prostate cancer, breast cancer, ovarian cancer, or Lynch syndrome.

Clinical Manifestations and Assessment

It is rare that patients presenting with prostate cancer will exhibit symptoms due to the current use of preventative screening protocols. If the neoplasm is large enough to encroach on the bladder neck, signs and symptoms of urinary obstruction occur (difficulty and frequency of urination, urinary retention, and decreased size and force of the urinary stream). Hematuria may result if the cancer invades the urethra or bladder, or both.

In advance stages of prostate cancer, it can metastasize to the bone and lymph nodes. Symptoms related to metastases include backache, hip pain, perineal and rectal discomfort, anemia, weight loss, weakness, nausea, and oliguria (less than 400 mL/day). These symptoms may be the first indications of prostate cancer, although due to current early screening guidelines by several organizations, it is uncommon for AMAB people to present at this advanced stage.

The AUA (Carter et al., 2013) recommendation states that "the highest-quality evidence for benefit (lower prostate cancer mortality) was found in persons ages 55 to 69 screened at 2- to 4-year intervals," and the organization "does not recommend routine screening in persons between ages 40 and 54 years at average risk." It is important that there is a shared decision-making conversation regarding the risks of screening. There is significant risk of overtreatment and overdiagnosis of prostate cancer tumors that will not need treatment. The NCCN recognizes the risks related to identifying low-risk prostate cancer tumors; however, maximizing the ability to identify high-grade aggressive prostate cancer tumors continues to evolve.

There has been controversy over the use of PSA screening over the last several years. In 2012, the United States Preventative Services Task Force (USPSTF) changed their recommendation for PSA screening to a grade D recommendation. A grade D recommendation suggests discouraging the use of this service (USPSTF, 2018). In 2017, the USPSTF reversed their decision and upgraded PSA screening to a grade C recommendation. A grade C recommendation states that there no determination made either for or against the service. The review of the guidelines and current practices found fair evidence to improve health outcomes, but the balance between risks and benefits were too close to justify a general recommendation (USPSTF, 2018). The reversal of this decision is based on evidence that in the period between the downgrade of the recommendation to the reversal there was a demonstratable increase in prostate cancer diagnoses (Catalona, 2018).

In direct contrast, the American Cancer Society (ACS, 2015) does not support routine PSA screening but recommends that "asymptomatic persons who have at least a 10-year life expectancy should have an opportunity to make an informed decision with their health care provider about screening for prostate cancer after receiving information about the uncertainties, risks, and potential benefits associated with screening." These tests are recommended for patients (40 to 45 years of age) if they are at high risk for prostate cancer; namely, persons who have a first-degree relative (father, brother, or son) diagnosed with prostate cancer at an early age (under 65 years of age; ACS, 2015b).

The level of PSA in the blood is proportional to the total prostatic mass and does not necessarily indicate malignancy. However, there are limitations in the relationship between serum PSA and prostate cancer volume. Each patient identified to have an elevated PSA should have a complete assessment when considering if the finding of an elevated PSA requires referral to a urology provider to discuss further management.

If prostate cancer is detected early, the likelihood of cure is high. This is limited by the methods used to identify prostate cancer from abnormal findings on DRE and serum PSA elevations. Both of those tools have significant issues related to sensitivity and specificity, adding to the continued lack of consensus regarding "best screening" tools. DRE has experienced the most debate regarding its usefulness in detecting prostate cancer. Several meta-analyses, including one by Okpua et al. (2021) demonstrate the inconsistencies that may occur when utilizing DRE as a risk assessment tool. The authors note "that [the] examiners' skill, patients' positioning during DRE, anal tone and the nature, including the length of the examiners' index fingers, are factors behind the variation seen across different DRE results" (Okpua et al., 2021, p. 8). Routine repeated rectal palpation of the gland (preferably by the same examiner) may assist in early cancer detection as a nodule within the substance of the gland, which may prompt a workup for prostate cancer.

Needle biopsies of the prostate are guided by transrectal ultrasound (TRUS); this may be indicated for patients who have elevated PSA levels, abnormal DRE findings, and associated risk factors. Prostate cancer is a pathologic diagnosis and is reported on a Gleason score. In 2014, the International Society of Urological Pathology Consensus Conference on Gleason Grading of Prostatic Carcinoma developed a grade group scoring system that would allow for universal consensus regarding pathology results. Despite this new grading system being simpler and more accurately reflecting prostate cancer biology, it is recommended by the World Health Organization (WHO) that the grade group system be used in conjunction with Gleason grading (Gordetsky & Epstein, 2016).

New modalities for prostate biopsy incorporate magnetic resonance imaging (MRI) to take multiparametric images of the prostate to identify concerning lesions. MRI-fusion biopsies, or Artemis, a 3D semirobotic prostate fusion biopsy system, have been demonstrated in studies over the last 5 years to be useful in risk identification for intermediate- and high-risk prostate cancers (Nordstrom et al., 2021). Potential risks and benefits of the procedure are the same as standard biopsy, and studies suggest that there is no change in infection risk (Borghesi et al., 2017). Identified lesions on an MRI of the prostate are rated using the Prostate Imaging Reporting and Data System (PIRADS) scale that was developed by the American College of Radiology (ACR). The most recent version of the PIRADS v.2 discusses the grading score on a scale of 1 to 5. A PIRADS lesion score of 1 has a low likelihood of clinically significant prostate cancer, while a PIRADS 5 lesion score has a high likelihood of clinically significant prostate cancer (ACR, 2019). While MRI-fusion biopsy is now present in many prostate cancer detection guidelines, the technology may not be readily available in many hospitals and radiology centers; thus, standard prostate biopsy remains a feasible option for initial detection of prostate cancer (NCCN, 2022).

With the identification of intermediate- or high-risk prostate cancer, other testing to identify spread of disease is recommended by the NCCN based on risk stratification. Further testing to establish the extent of disease includes bone scan, computed tomography (CT) scan, or prostate-specific membrane antigen (PSMA) scan. Depending on the patient's Gleason (or grade group), metastatic workup may be warranted. Prostate cancer often first metastasizes to the bone or the pelvic lymph nodes. Bone scan can be useful in identifying concerning osseous (bone)metastases; however, a patient's previous history of broken bones or degenerative bone diseases should be noted when interpreting results. CT of the abdomen and pelvis with contrast is useful in identifying possible metastases in the pelvis. PSMA scan, which has now received FDA approval, can be used in place of bone scan and CT of the abdomen and pelvis and has demonstrated that it is substantially more likely to detect metastatic tumors in patients with prostate cancer recurrence than traditional imaging workup (NCI, 2020).

Medical and Nursing Management

Treatment is based on initial risk stratification tools to identify initial workups; this is dependent on a thorough evaluation of the patient's 10-year life expectancy. If the patient's life expectancy is not likely to be equal to or greater than 10 years and they have low-risk prostate cancer, an in-depth shared decision-making conversation should be had regarding the risks and benefits of treatment. If the patient's health demonstrates a less than 10-year life expectancy, it is questionable whether they will benefit from treatment in their lifetime.

If the patient's life expectancy is expected to be 10 years or greater, their prostate cancer risk is determined to be intermediate or high, comorbidities are managed and those comorbidities are not expected to impact life expectancy, then a shared decision-making conversation should be had with the patient regarding potential treatment options.

Surgical Management

Radical prostatectomy is the complete surgical removal of the prostate; seminal vesicles; and often the surrounding fat, nerves, lymph nodes, and blood vessels. It is considered one of the standard first-line treatment options for prostate cancer; however, radiation therapy techniques have improved substantially over the last 10 years, making it a feasible option for patients with equal benefit. Significant side effects of radical prostatectomy are erectile dysfunction, urinary incontinence, and penile shortening; all of these can impact the patient's quality of life. It is important for health care providers to have in-depth conversations reviewing these potential life-changing side effects prior to surgical intervention. Robotically assisted laparoscopic prostatectomy (RALP) offers advantages of low morbidity and more rapid discharge postprocedure (see below for discussion).

Radiation Therapy

Radiation therapy can be a feasible option for initial treatment at all stages of prostate cancer. The decision to proceed with radiation therapy should be made with an informative shared decision-making conversation with the patient's urology team. Two major forms of radiation therapy are used to treat cancer of the prostate: teletherapy (external) and brachytherapy (internal). Refer to Chapter 5 for details on radiation therapy.

Teletherapy (external-beam radiation therapy or EBRT) involves 6 to 8 weeks of daily (5 days/week) radiation treatments. A radiation oncologist will determine the set dose for treatment. New technologies map and restrict the dose of radiation exposure to adjacent structures, such as the bladder and the rectum. It is thought to be accurate within 1 to 3 mm, with some newer technology that can hold or stop radiation treatment until the prostate is in the field, thus accommodating for patient movement, breathing, or stool in the bowel.

Brachytherapy involves the implantation of interstitial radioactive seeds under anesthesia, via the perineum, into the prostate. Eighty to 100 seeds are placed directly into the prostate, and the patient returns home after the procedure. Exposure of others to radiation is minimal, but the patient should avoid close contact with pregnant persons and infants for 2 to 3 months. Brachytherapy is not commonly used, as it is typically only used to treat low-grade prostate cancers. The majority of patients who would qualify for brachytherapy also qualify for active surveillance under more recent guidelines; this prevents overtreatment of prostate cancer.

Side effects of teletherapy and brachytherapy include inflammation of the rectum, bowel, and bladder due to their proximity to the prostate and the radiation doses, also known as irradiation cystitis (bladder inflammation) or proctitis (inflammation of the anus and rectum). While the erectile dysfunction experienced by patients after RALP is most often immediate, patients are likely to suffer a decline in erectile function with time after radiation therapy. Table 33-3 discusses nursing interventions to minimize side effects. Combination therapy (radiation therapy followed by hormonal therapy) may improve overall survival in some risk stratification categories.

TABLE 33-3 Management of Radiation-Induced Symptoms

Symptom	Intervention
Cystitis	Maintain hydration Encourage patient to take prescribed medications (bladder antispasmodics, alpha blockers, analgesics) Avoid known bladder irritants (see Chapter 27)
Diarrhea	Provide low-residue diet Maintain hydration Administer antidiarrheals as indicated Give dietary bulking agents as indicated
Erectile dysfunction	Assess for level of distress and suggest sexual therapist as appropriate Provide education regarding appropriate medication Instruct patient to take medications as prescribed
Proctitis (inflammation of the rectum)	Offer sitz baths Recommend water-based lubricants Maintain hydration to avoid constipation Adjust diet to avoid constipation

Hormonal Therapy

Hormonal therapy for advanced prostate cancer suppresses androgenic stimuli to the prostate by decreasing the level of circulating plasma testosterone or interrupting the conversion to or binding of DHT. This significantly decreases the level of testosterone, slowing the progression of prostate cancer. The effect of hormonal therapies is to achieve castration chemically. A patient could opt for surgical castration (**orchiectomy**) to achieve a similar effect; however, in the setting of modern medical therapies that can induce chemical castration, this is not often chosen or preferred by patients.

Effective hormonal alternatives to orchiectomy include the nonsteroidal antiandrogens (bicalutamide, enzalutamide, nilutamide), luteinizing hormone-releasing hormone (LHRH, i.e., leuprolide and goserlin), and antiandrogen agents. LHRH suppresses testicular androgen, while antiandrogens cause suppression of adrenal androgen. LHRH agonists are used for the following: (1) in the adjuvant and neoadjuvant setting (e.g., before use of hormonal suppressive agents) in combination with radiation therapy, and (2) in the treatment of prostate cancer recurrence indicated by an elevation in the PSA or evident metastases on imaging. Hormonal symptoms, including hot flashes, emotional liability, breast tenderness, and fatigue, all similar to menopausal symptoms, may be experienced by patients receiving hormonal therapy for the treatment of prostate cancer. Patients should be effectively counseled regarding the possible side effects of hormonal therapy, especially the increased risk of stress fracture or bone fracture. Supplementation with vitamin D and calcium should be considered for all patients receiving hormonal therapy for the treatment of prostate cancer.

Second-Line Medical Treatment

The management of hormone-refractory cancer of the prostate should be managed by an experienced genitourinary oncologist. Many FDA-approved second-line therapies are available to patients, including clinical trials with immunotherapy. Abiraterone has demonstrated promise in improving overall survival in patients with castrate-resistant prostate cancer as reported in the STAMPEDE trial (James et al., 2017). The CHAARTED trial demonstrated that there was significant improvement in overall survival with the use of docetaxel (Puente, 2017). The patient should immediately be referred to a capable oncologist if castrate-resistant prostate cancer is detected or if metastatic disease is found on imaging.

Other Therapies

Ablation Therapies of the prostate are used to ablate prostate cancer in qualifying patients who prefer to not pursue surgery and in those with recurrent prostate cancer. Some of the procedures that are categorized as ablation therapies include high-intensity focused ultrasound (HIFU), cryoablation, irreversible electroporation (IRE), transurethral ultrasound ablation (TULSA), Tookad, and focal laser ablation. In recent noninferiority trials, for patients with low-to-intermediate grade prostate cancer there are data to suggest that ablation therapies when compared with prostatectomy have similar cancer treatment outcomes at 7 years with potentially fewer side effects (Nyk et al., 2022). Transperineal probes are inserted into the prostate under ultrasound guidance to freeze the tissue directly. Few centers have surgeons who are certified to perform cryotherapy. The patient should be sure to research and find the best provider for them with experience in cryotherapy/surgery. It is important to note that cryotherapy has not yet demonstrated whether it is comparative to radical prostatectomy, EBRT, or Active Surveillance protocols in long-term survival outcomes for low-to-intermediate grade prostate cancer (Marra et al., 2021).

For patients with advanced prostate cancer, palliative measures, such as pain management, complementary and alternative medicine (CAM), and androgen deprivation, can be options. Although cure is unlikely with advanced prostate cancer, many patients survive for a long period of time with several treatments that can delay the progression of prostate cancer.

Bone lesions resulting from metastasis of prostate cancer can be very painful. Opioid and nonopioid medications are used to control the pain. External-beam radiation therapy can be delivered to certain skeletal lesions to relieve pain, while radiopharmaceuticals can be injected intravenously to treat multiple sites of bone metastasis.

More than one third of patients with a diagnosis of prostate cancer elect to use some form of CAM. Because of lack of research on many forms of CAM, patients often have to rely on anecdotal information or information gained via the internet to make decisions about its use.

Complications

Each treatment for prostate cancer has some incidence of sexual dysfunction. With nerve-sparing radical prostatectomy, the likelihood of recovering the ability to have erections is better for patients who are younger and in whom both neurovascular bundles (the erectile nerves and blood vessels called neurovascular bundles run along the surface of each side of the prostate) are spared. Hormonal therapy also affects the central nervous system mechanisms that mediate sexual desire and arousability. PDE-5 inhibitors may be effective for treatment of ED in younger patients after radical retropubic prostatectomy, especially if the neurovascular bundles were preserved. They may improve erectile function in patients with partial or moderate ED after radiation therapy for localized prostate cancer. Other pharmacologic interventions for erectile dysfunction were discussed previously.

PROSTATE SURGERY

Simple prostatectomy or robot-assisted laparoscopic prostatectomy (RALP) may be indicated for the patient with BPH or prostate cancer. Prostate surgery should be performed before acute urinary retention develops and damages the upper urinary tract and collecting system or before cancer progresses.

Procedures

Several approaches can be used to remove the hypertrophied portion of the prostate gland: TURP, UroLift®, Rezum®, green light laser, TUIP, HOLEP, and prostatectomy (Table 33-4). Hyperplastic tissue is removed, leaving behind the capsule of the prostate.

NURSING PROCESS
Patient Undergoing Prostatectomy

ASSESSMENT

The nurse assesses how the underlying disorder (BPH or prostate cancer) has affected the patient's lifestyle. The nurse asks about family history of cancer, heart or kidney disease, diabetes, previous abdominal procedures, and other potentially life-limiting comorbidities. In addition, the nurse observes for weight loss, pallor, ability to get in and out of bed without assistance, and ability to perform activities of daily living (ADL). This information helps determine how soon the patient will be able to return to normal activities after prostatectomy; typical recovery time ranges from 6 to 8 weeks.

DIAGNOSIS

Based on the assessment data, the patient's major nursing diagnoses may include the following:

- Preoperative nursing diagnoses:
  - Anxiety related to surgery and its outcome
  - Knowledge deficit related to disease process
  - Acute pain related to surgical intervention
  - Deficient knowledge about factors related to the disorder and the treatment protocol
- Postoperative nursing diagnoses:
  - Acute pain related to the surgical incision, catheter placement, and bladder spasms
  - Deficient knowledge about postoperative care and management
- Based on the assessment data, the potential complications may include the following:
  - Hemorrhage and shock
  - Infection
  - Deep vein thrombosis (DVT)
  - Catheter obstruction
  - Urine leak at the site of anastomosis
  - Sexual dysfunction

(*continued on page 1149*)

TABLE 33-4 **Surgical Approaches for Treatment of Prostate Disorders**

Surgical Approach	Images	Advantages	Disadvantages	Nursing Implications
Transurethral resection of the prostate (TURP) is carried out through endoscopy: the surgical instrument is introduced via the urethra to the prostate, which can then be viewed directly. The gland is removed in small chips with an electrical cutting loop. This procedure may be used for glands of varying size. The procedure is ideal for patients who have small glands and poor surgical risks.	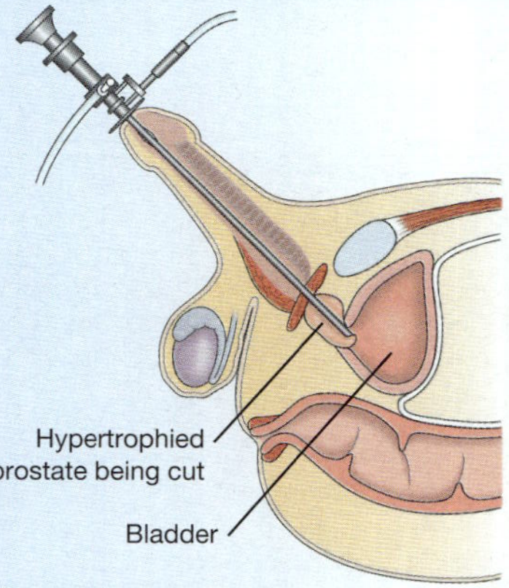	Avoids abdominal incision Safer for patients with surgical risk as it prevents major abdominal surgery Lower morbidity rate Causes less pain	Recurrent obstruction, urethral trauma, and stricture may develop. Delayed bleeding may occur. Recurrent bleeding may occur. Retrograde ejaculation due to removal of prostatic tissue at the bladder neck, which causes the seminal fluid to flow backward into the bladder	Monitor for TUR syndrome. Monitor for hemorrhage. Observe for symptoms of urethral stricture (dysuria, straining, weak urinary stream).
Suprapubic approach Suprapubic prostatectomy is one method of removing the gland through an abdominal incision. An incision is made into the bladder, and the prostate gland is removed from above.	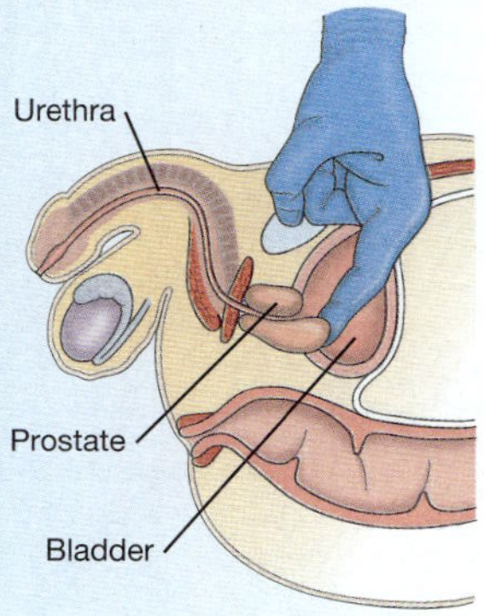	Technically simple (shorter surgical time than robotic approach) Offers wide area of exploration Permits exploration for cancerous lymph nodes Allows more complete removal of obstructing gland Permits treatment of associated bladder lesions	Requires surgical approach through the bladder Difficult to control hemorrhage Urine may leak around the suprapubic tube. Recovery may be prolonged and uncomfortable.	Monitor for indications of hemorrhage and shock. Provide meticulous aseptic care to the area around suprapubic tube. Monitor for signs and symptoms of urinary tract infection. Provide wound care to prevent surgical site infection.
Perineal approach Perineal prostatectomy involves removal of the gland through an incision in the perineum.	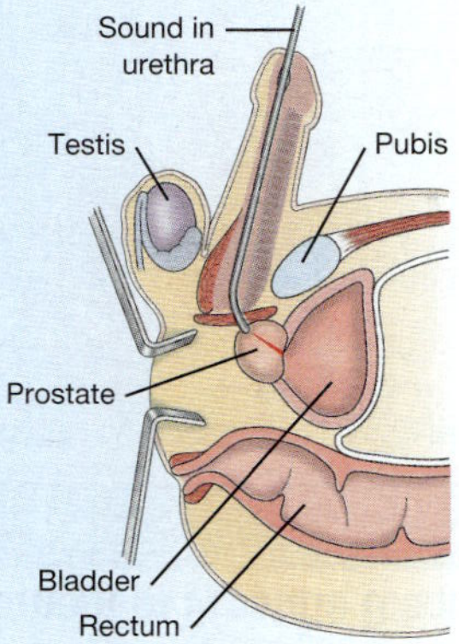	Offers direct anatomic approach Permits gravity drainage of catheter Particularly effective for radical cancer therapy Allows hemostasis under direct vision Low mortality rate Low incidence of shock	Higher postoperative incidence of impotence and urinary incontinence Possible damage to rectum and external sphincter Restricted operative field Possible development of a long-term fistula	Avoid using rectal tubes or thermometers and enemas after perineal surgery. Use drainage pads to absorb excess urinary drainage. Possible urinary leakage around the wound after the catheter is removed Monitor for signs and symptoms of urinary tract infection.

(continued)

TABLE **33-4 Surgical Approaches for Treatment of Prostate Disorders (*continued*)**

Surgical Approach	Images	Advantages	Disadvantages	Nursing Implications
Retropubic approach Retropubic prostatectomy is more common than the suprapubic approach. A low abdominal incision is made, and the prostate gland can be reached between the pubic arch and the bladder without entering the bladder.	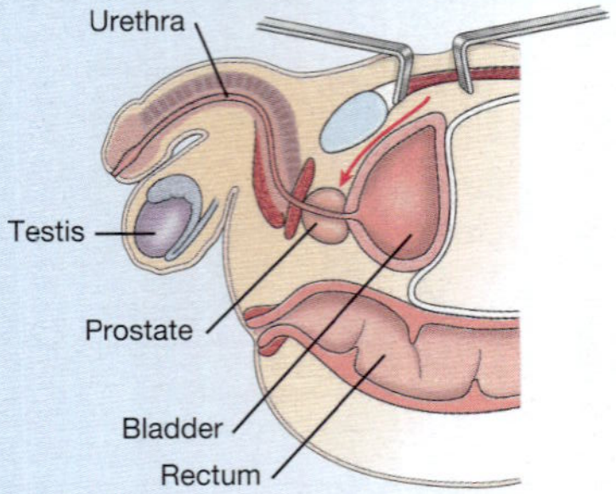	Avoids incision into the bladder Permits surgeon to see and control bleeding Shorter recovery period Less damage to the bladder sphincter	Cannot treat associated bladder disease Increased incidence of hemorrhage from prostatic venous plexus	Monitor for hemorrhage. Anticipate urinary leakage for several days after removing the catheter.
Transurethral incision of the prostate (TUIP) is indicated when the prostate gland is small (30 g or less), and it is an effective treatment for many cases of BPH. An instrument is passed through the urethra. Incisions are made in the prostate and prostate capsule to reduce the prostate's pressure on the urethra and to reduce urethral constriction.	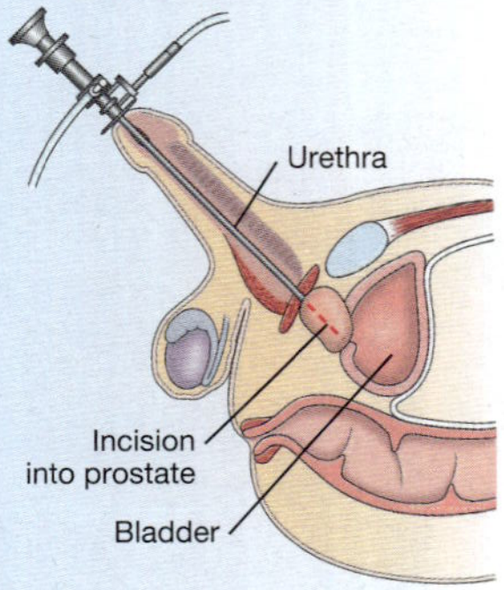	Results comparable to TURP Low incidence of erectile dysfunction and retrograde ejaculation No contracture of the bladder neck Outpatient procedure Low complication rate	Recurrent obstruction and urethral trauma Delayed bleeding	Monitor for hemorrhage.
Robotic prostatectomy (Da Vinci prostatectomy) Laparoscopic prostatectomy provides better visualization of the surgical site and surrounding areas.	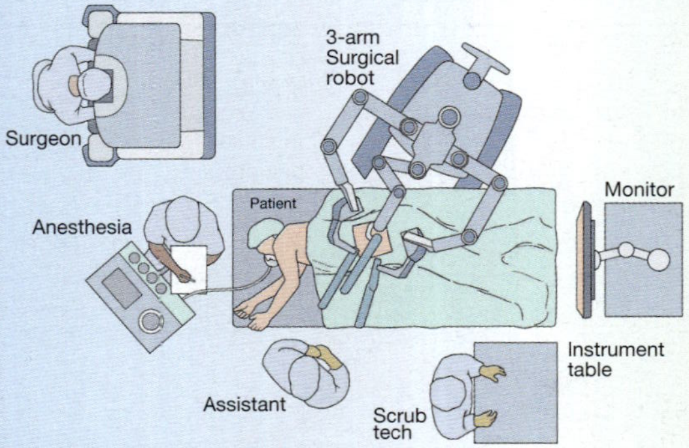	Minimally invasive technique Improved patient satisfaction and quality of life Short convalescence More rapid return to normal activity Short indwelling catheter duration (approx. 1 week) Decreased blood loss Improved magnification of operative field	Technically demanding skill set for surgeon Lack of tactile sensation available with open prostatectomy Inability to palpably assess for induration and palpable nodules Inability to delineate the proximity of involvement of the neurovascular bundles due to lack of palpation	Observe for symptoms of urethral stricture (dysuria, straining, weak urinary stream). Monitor for hemorrhage and shock. Provide meticulous aseptic care to the surgical incision site. Avoid using rectal tubes or thermometers and enemas after perineal surgery. Use drainage pads to absorb excess urinary drainage. Anticipate urinary incontinence after the catheter is removed.

Postoperative complications depend on the type of prostatectomy performed and may include hemorrhage, clot formation, catheter obstruction, urinary incontinence, and sexual dysfunction.
All prostatectomies carry a risk of impotence because of potential damage to the pudendal nerves; despite new nerve-sparing procedures, patients should be informed of this risk. The anatomic changes in the posterior urethra lead to retrograde ejaculation or the absence of ejaculate. Due to the removal of the prostate, the patient will experience noticeable penile shortening. For the patient with resulting ED that does not resolve, options are available to produce erections sufficient for sexual intercourse: prosthetic penile implants, vacuum devices, and pharmacologic interventions.

PLANNING

The major preoperative goals for the patient may include reduced anxiety and learning about their prostate disorder and the perioperative experience. The major postoperative goals may include maintenance of fluid volume balance, relief of pain and discomfort, ability to perform self-care activities, maintenance of the indwelling catheter, and prevention of complications.

PREOPERATIVE NURSING INTERVENTIONS

REDUCING ANXIETY

The nurse must establish communication with the patient to assess their understanding of the diagnosis and of the planned surgical procedure. The nurse clarifies the nature of the surgery and expected postoperative outcomes, familiarizes the patient with the preoperative and postoperative routines, and initiates measures to reduce anxiety. Because the patient may be sensitive and embarrassed discussing problems related to the genitalia and sexuality, the nurse provides privacy and establishes a trusting and professional relationship. The patient is encouraged to verbalize their feelings and concerns.

RELIEVING DISCOMFORT

During hospitalization of the postoperative prostatectomy patient, the nurse monitors the patient's voiding patterns, watches for bladder distention, and assists with maintenance of the indwelling catheter. The catheter helps to decompress the bladder. If the patient cannot tolerate a urinary catheter, they are prepared for a cystostomy (surgical creation of an opening into the bladder, usually with a catheter [e.g., suprapubic tube, see Chapter 27]).

PROVIDING INSTRUCTION

Before surgery, the nurse reviews with the patient the anatomy of the affected structures and their function in relation to the urinary and reproductive systems, using diagrams and other teaching aids if indicated. This instruction often takes place during the preadmission testing visit or in the urologist's office. The nurse explains what will take place as the patient is prepared for surgery (depending on the type of prostatectomy planned). The nurse also describes the type of incision, which varies with the surgery chosen, and informs the patient about the likely type of urinary drainage system and the recovery room procedure. It is important that the patient be given appropriate information to ensure informed consent prior to the procedure.

PREPARING THE PATIENT

If the patient is scheduled for a prostatectomy, the preoperative preparation described in Chapter 4 is provided.

POSTOPERATIVE NURSING INTERVENTIONS

MAINTAINING FLUID BALANCE

During the postoperative period, the patient is at risk for imbalanced fluid volume due to irrigation of the surgical site during and after surgery. With irrigation of the urinary catheter to prevent its obstruction by blood clots, fluid may be absorbed through the open surgical site and retained, increasing the risk of excessive fluid retention, fluid imbalance, and water intoxication. The patient is observed for signs of fluid volume excess, such as jugular vein distention (JVD), the development of an S_3 gallop, and pulmonary crackles. The urine output and the amount of fluid used for irrigation must be monitored closely to determine whether irrigation fluid is being retained and to ensure adequate urine output. An intake and output record, including the amount of fluid used for irrigation, must be maintained closely. The patient is monitored for electrolyte imbalances (e.g., hyponatremia), increasing blood pressure, confusion, and respiratory distress. Refer to Box 33-2 for details on dilutional hyponatremia after a transurethral prostatectomy (TURP). In addition, since the prostate is a vascular organ, hemorrhage is an immediate danger postoperatively; thus, the nurse monitors the patient for hypotension, tachycardia, tachypnea, gross hematuria, restlessness, pallor, delayed capillary refill and decreasing levels of hemoglobin and hematocrit. If deterioration of the patient's condition occurs, the surgeon is notified immediately. The nurse anticipates fluid resuscitation with IV fluids and blood products.

Pearls for Practice

In assessing urinary output, the nurse anticipates output at a minimum 0.5 mL/kg/hr; thus, if the patient weighs 70 kg, 35 mL of urine is expected hourly. To calculate the actual urine output, the nurse must consider all irrigating fluids instilled against the total drainage of the urine collection bag. If large amounts of irrigating solutions are required postoperatively, the nurse empties the collection bag frequently to prevent overfilling and back pressure within the bladder. Meticulous recording of the urinary output is required.

RELIEVING PAIN

If pain is present, the cause and location are determined, and the severity of pain and discomfort is assessed using a pain scale. The pain may be incisional, referred to the flank area, or caused by bladder spasms. Patients experiencing bladder spasms typically describe the pain as severe cramping and spasmodic in the suprapubic region. They may note a feeling of pressure or fullness in the bladder, and the nurse may encounter leakage from the urethra around the catheter rather than through the catheter.

Pearls for Practice

Bladder spasms are associated with irritation to the detrusor muscle, causing spasm of the muscle. If spasms are present, the nurse ensures that the urinary drainage system is patent since obstruction is associated with spasms. In addition, the nurse administers antispasmodic medication as prescribed.

(continued on page 1150)

BOX 33-2

Transurethral Resection Syndrome (Symptomatic Dilutional Hyponatremia)

Transurethral resection (TUR) syndrome is a rare (less than 2%) but potentially serious complication of transurethral prostatectomy (TURP). Risk factors are related to size of the gland (larger >45 g) and length of surgical time (>90 minutes) (Helo et al., 2021). Signs and symptoms are caused by neurologic, cardiovascular, and electrolyte imbalances associated with absorption of the solution used to irrigate the surgical site during the surgical procedure. Hyponatremia, hypo-osmolality, and hypervolemia are dominant findings. Symptoms usually are detected by assessing the patient's neurologic status and evaluating the serum sodium level; if the serum sodium is less than 120 mEq/L, a significant dilution exists that may lead to coma or seizure (Helo et al., 2021). The dilutional hyponatremia leads to cerebral edema; thus, neurologic symptoms are observed. Of note, the use of isotonic, iso-osmolar irrigating solution and newer surgical techniques have decreased the risk of hyponatremia significantly (Helo et al., 2021). If the irrigating solution used was normal saline, then hyponatremia will not occur; however, volume overload may be seen with symptoms of dyspnea, hyper- or hypotension, hyperchloremia, and full, bounding pulse. If there is poor left ventricular function, pulmonary edema may develop. Given the age of many persons undergoing TURP and possible comorbidities of cardiac disease, type of surgical technique, and irrigating solution used, the nurse is aware that fluctuating intravascular volume and myocardial compromise may result in hypotension.

Signs and Symptoms of TUR Syndrome

- Lethargy and confusion
- Hypertension
- Tachycardia
- Nausea and vomiting
- Visual disturbances, such as decreased visual acuity, blurred vision, and blindness (self-limited) if glycine is used as an irrigant, as it is a neurotransmitter for the retina (Emmett et al., 2022)
- Headache
- Muscle spasms
- Seizures

Interventions

- If the patient presents with the aforementioned signs and symptoms, the intraoperative irrigating solution of glycine, sorbitol/mannitol, or water is discontinued and replaced with normal saline.
  - Monitor the amount of irrigation solution absorbed intraoperatively; 1,000 mL has been suggested to temporarily halt the procedure and 2,000 mL to terminate the procedure (Emmett et al., 2022).
  - Monitor the serum electrolytes.
- If saline was used for irrigation, the risk for hyponatremia is low but heart failure can develop. Administer diuretics as prescribed to facilitate excretion of absorbed fluid.
- Monitor intake and output.
- Monitor the patient's vital signs and level of consciousness
- Differentiate the lethargy and confusion of TUR syndrome from postoperative disorientation and hyponatremia.
- Maintain the patient's safety during times of confusion.
- Assess lung and heart sounds for indications of pulmonary edema, heart failure, or both.

The nurse monitors the drainage tubing and irrigates the system as prescribed to relieve any obstruction that may cause discomfort. Usually, if clots impede urinary drainage, the catheter is irrigated with 50–60 mL of irrigating fluid at a time. It is important to make sure that the same amount is recovered in the drainage receptacle. Securing the catheter drainage tubing to the patient's leg or lower abdomen can help decrease tension on the catheter and prevent bladder irritation.

After the patient is ambulatory, they are encouraged to walk but not to sit for prolonged periods because this increases intra-abdominal pressure and the possibility of discomfort and bleeding.

MONITORING AND MANAGING POTENTIAL COMPLICATIONS

After prostatectomy, the patient is monitored for major complications, such as hemorrhage, infection, DVT, catheter obstruction, and sexual dysfunction.

Hemorrhage. The immediate dangers after a prostate surgery are bleeding and hemorrhagic shock. This risk is increased with BPH because a hyperplastic prostate gland is very vascular. Bleeding may result in the formation of clots, which then obstruct urine flow. The drainage normally begins as reddish-pink and then clears to a light pink within 24 hours after surgery. Bright red bleeding with increased viscosity and numerous clots usually indicates arterial bleeding and requires surgical intervention. Venous bleeding, which is dark red in color, may be controlled by the provider via "overinflating" the urinary catheter balloon and applying traction to the catheter so that the balloon holding the urinary catheter in place applies pressure to the prostatic fossa. If after 20 minutes the bleeding is not controlled, surgical exploration may be considered. Since bleeding is increased when the patient is in the sitting position, which increases bladder and venous pressure, the patient is encouraged to rest in bed with the head of the bed slightly elevated.

Nursing management includes assistance in implementing strategies to stop the bleeding and to prevent or reverse hemorrhagic shock. If hemorrhagic shock occurs, treatments described in Chapter 53 are initiated.

Nursing interventions include closely monitoring vital signs; administering medications, IV fluids, and blood component therapy as prescribed; maintaining an accurate record of intake and output; and carefully monitoring drainage to ensure adequate urine flow (avoiding kinks in the catheter) and patency of the drainage system.

Infection. After prostatectomy, the surgeon usually changes the dressing on the first postoperative day. Careful aseptic technique is used because the potential for infection is great. Rectal thermometers, rectal tubes, and enemas are avoided because of the risk of injury and bleeding in the prostatic fossa. Sitz baths are used to promote healing.

UTIs and epididymitis (infection of the epididymis, discussed later in the chapter) are possible complications after prostatectomy, and the patient is assessed for their occurrence. Because the risk for infection continues after discharge from the hospital, the patient and caregivers need to be instructed to monitor for signs and symptoms of infection (fever, chills, sweating, myalgia [muscle pain], dysuria, urinary frequency, and urgency).

Deep Vein Thrombosis. Because patients undergoing prostatectomy have a high incidence of DVT and pulmonary embolism, the provider may prescribe prophylactic anticoagulation. The nurse assesses the patient frequently after surgery for manifestations of DVT and applies elastic compression stockings and sequential compression devices as needed. Nursing and medical management of DVT and pulmonary embolism are described in Chapters 9 and 17, respectively.

Obstructed Catheter. After any procedure involving the prostate in which a catheter is placed, the catheter must drain well. An obstructed catheter produces distention of the prostatic capsule and resultant hemorrhage. A diuretic may be prescribed to promote urination and initiate postoperative diuresis, thereby helping to keep the catheter patent. The nurse observes the lower abdomen for increasing distention to ensure that the catheter has not become blocked. On percussion of a patient with a blocked catheter, increased dullness will be noted in the suprapubic region. A bladder scan can be performed to assess volume of urine retained in the bladder.

The drainage bag, dressings, and incisional site are examined for bleeding. The color of the urine is noted and documented; a change in color from red to pink to amber indicates reduced bleeding. Blood pressure, pulse, and respirations are monitored and compared with baseline preoperative vital signs to detect hypotension. The nurse also observes for cues such as restlessness, diaphoresis, pallor, hypotension, tachypnea, an increasing pulse rate, and capillary refill >3 seconds and alerts the provider.

Drainage of the bladder may be accomplished by gravity through a closed sterile drainage system. A three-way drainage system is useful in irrigating the bladder and preventing clot formation (Fig. 33-2); one port is for balloon inflation, another port is used for irrigation inflow to the bladder, and the third port is for outflow of irrigation fluid and urine output into the urinary drainage bag. Continuous bladder irrigation (CBI) may be used after a TURP to maintain the drainage of the urinary catheter; remove blood clots from the bladder that are the result of the procedure and cleanse the surgical area to promote healing as well as to prevent potentially obstructing clots. The amount of fluid recovered in the drainage bag must equal the amount of fluid infused, plus the patient's urinary output. Overdistention of the bladder is avoided because it can induce secondary hemorrhage by stretching the coagulated blood vessels

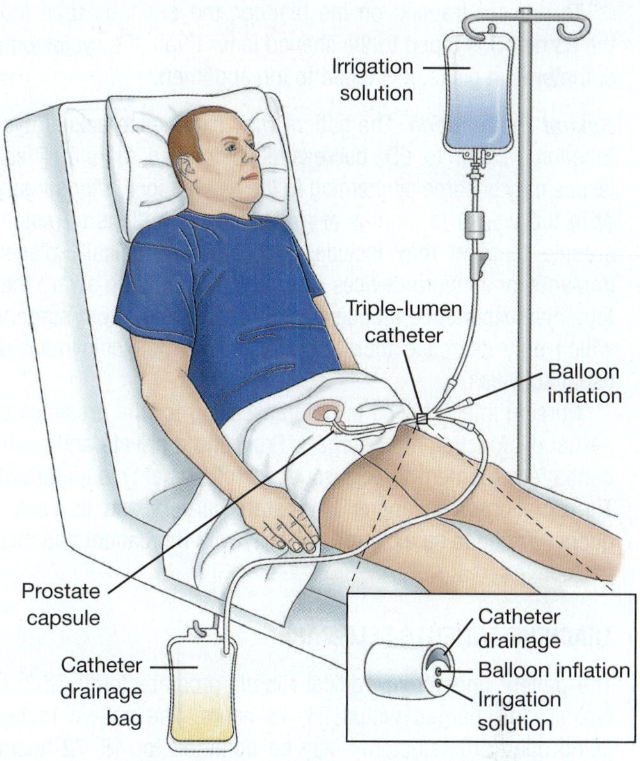

FIGURE 33-2 **A three-way system for bladder irrigation.**

in the prostatic capsule. The nurse monitors the inflow of the irrigation fluid and the outflow via the catheter drainage port and maintains meticulous measurement of I&O. The infusion of the continuous bladder irrigation fluid is maintained at a rate to keep the urine drainage light pink without clots. It is not a "set rate" of infusion but rather is dependent on the color of the urinary output and presence or absence of clots. For example, if the drainage becomes red with clots, the flow rate of the irrigation is increased rapidly until the drainage color becomes pink to clear, at which time the rate is decreased.

Pearls for Practice: Calculating the Urine Output With CBI

The nurse understands that when CBI is used, the urinary drainage bag will contain a combination of the irrigating solution infused into the bladder and the patient's urine output. To calculate the actual urinary output, the urinary drainage bag is emptied and measured and compared to the amount of irrigation fluid that was infused. For example, if 2,000 mL of irrigation solution was infused and the urinary drainage bag emptied 2,400 mL, the urinary output for this patient was 400 mL. The nurse notifies the surgeon when urinary output falls below the expected minimum, which is 0.5 mL/kg per hour. In addition, the nurse notifies the surgeon if the amount of outflow drainage in the urinary drainage bag is less than what was infused as this may suggest bladder rupture at the suture line.

(continued on page 1152)

To prevent traction on the bladder, the drainage tube (not the catheter) is taped to the shaved inner thigh. If a cystostomy catheter is in place, it is taped to the abdomen.

Sexual Dysfunction. The patient may experience sexual dysfunction related to ED, decreased libido, and fatigue. These issues may become concerning to the patient soon after surgery or in the weeks to months of rehabilitation. Options to restore erectile function may include medications, surgically placed implants, or vacuum devices. The patient should be aware that they may experience fatigue during rehabilitation from surgery, which may decrease their libido and alter their enjoyment of usual activities.

Nursing interventions include assessing for the presence of sexual dysfunction after surgery. Providing a private and confidential environment to discuss issues of sexuality is important. The emotional challenges of prostate surgery and its consequences need to be explored carefully with the patient and their partner.

TEACHING PATIENTS SELF-CARE

The patient undergoing radical robotic prostatectomy (RRP) is typically discharged within 24–48 hours. The patient undergoing open prostatectomy may be admitted for 48–72 hours. The patient and caregivers require instructions about how to manage the urinary drainage system, how to assess for complications, and how to promote recovery. Verbal and written instructions should be provided, and the patient and family need to know about signs and symptoms that should be reported to the provider (e.g., blood in urine, decreased urine output, fever, change in wound drainage, calf tenderness; Box 33-3).

BOX 33-3 Patient Education

Self-Care after a Prostatectomy

- Perform Kegel exercises after the catheter is removed as they may help with regaining urinary control:
  - Tense the perineal muscles by pressing the buttocks together; hold this position; relax. This exercise can be performed 10–20 times each hour while sitting or standing.
  - Try to interrupt the urinary stream after starting to void; wait a few seconds and then continue to void.
- While the prostatic fossa heals (6 to 8 weeks), avoid activities that produce Valsalva effects (straining, heavy lifting) as this may increase venous pressure and produce hematuria.
- Avoid long motor trips and strenuous exercise, which increase the tendency to bleed.
- Note that spicy foods, alcohol, and coffee may cause bladder discomfort.
- Maintain fluid intake to avoid dehydration, which increases the tendency for a blood clot to form and obstruct the flow of urine.
- Report to the urologist signs of complications, such as bleeding, passage of blood clots, a decrease in the urinary stream, urinary retention, or symptoms of UTI.

After the catheter is removed (usually when the urine appears clear), urine may leak out around the wound for several days. Some urinary incontinence may occur after catheter removal, and the patient is informed that this is likely to subside over time. The patient should be counseled that they can have full incontinence for 2–3 months after prostatectomy, and the nurse should ensure availability of incontinence supplies for the patient.

CONTINUING CARE

Referral for home care may be indicated if the patient is older or has other health problems, if the patient and family cannot provide care in the home, or if the patient lives alone without available supports. The home care nurse assesses the patient's physical status and provides catheter and wound care. The home care nurse encourages the patient to ambulate and to carry out perineal exercises as prescribed. Perineal exercises should only be performed after the indwelling catheter is removed. If the prostatectomy was performed to treat prostate cancer, the patient and family also are instructed about the importance of follow-up and monitoring with the urologist.

EVALUATION

Expected postoperative patient outcomes may include the following:

1. Reports relief of discomfort
2. Exhibits fluid and electrolyte balance:
   a. Irrigation fluid and urinary output are within parameters determined by surgeon
   b. Experiences no signs or symptoms of fluid retention
3. Participates in self-care measures:
   a. Increases activity and ambulation daily
   b. Produces urine output within normal ranges and consistent with intake
   c. Performs perineal exercises and interrupts urinary stream to promote bladder control
   d. Avoids straining and lifting heavy objects
4. Is free of complications:
   a. Maintains vital signs within normal limits
   b. Exhibits wound healing without signs of inflammation or hemorrhage
   c. Maintains acceptable level of urinary elimination
   d. Maintains optimal drainage of catheter and other drainage tubes
   e. Reports understanding of changes in sexual function

CONDITIONS AFFECTING THE TESTES AND ADJACENT STRUCTURES

ORCHITIS AND EPIDIDYMITIS

Orchitis is an inflammation of the testes, with or without infection. **Epididymitis** is an inflammation of the epididymis, with or without infection. Bacterial causes of epididymitis and orchitis usually descend from an infected prostate (prostatitis) or urinary tract. Recommended treatments include rest, elevation of the scrotum, ice packs to reduce scrotal edema, antibiotics, analgesic agents, and anti-inflammatory medications.

Pathophysiology

In AMAB patients younger than 35 years of age, the major cause of epididymitis or orchitis is *Chlamydia trachomatis.* The infection passes upward through the urethra and the ejaculatory duct and then along the vas deferens to the epididymis, and it can migrate to the testis as well.

Clinical Manifestations and Assessment

The patient may complain of unilateral pain and soreness in the inguinal canal along the course of the vas deferens and may develop pain and swelling in the scrotum and the groin. The epididymis becomes swollen and extremely painful. Bacteriuria may be evident, but not in all cases. With acute orchitis or epididymitis the patient may present with chills, fever, nausea, urinary frequency, urgency, or dysuria. Laboratory assessment includes urinalysis and gram stain of urethral drainage if there is suspicion of sexually transmitted infection (STI). If epididymitis is untreated, it can progress to involve the testis.

Medical Management

Treatment with scrotal support, ice, and antibiotic therapy are anticipated on an outpatient basis. If the epididymitis is caused by a chlamydial infection, the patient *and their sexual partner* must be treated with antibiotics. If no improvement occurs within 2 weeks, an extended course of antibiotics should be considered (15 to 30 days of antibiotics). An epididymectomy (excision of the epididymis from the testis) may be performed as a last resort for patients who have recurrent, incapacitating episodes of epididymitis or for those with chronic, painful conditions; however, this is rare.

Nursing Management

The scrotum is elevated with a scrotal bridge or folded towel to prevent traction on the spermatic cord, to promote venous drainage, and to relieve pain. A folded hand towel is secured under one thigh, allowing the penis and scrotum to be elevated on the midsection of the towel, and then the edge of the towel is secured under opposite thigh. Anti-inflammatory agents are administered as prescribed until the acute inflammation subsides. Analgesic medications can be administered as needed for pain relief, such as ibuprofen and acetaminophen as first-line agents. Antibiotics should be administered as prescribed, and the patient is encouraged to complete the entire course. Intermittent cold compresses to the scrotum may help ease the pain. Later, local heat or sitz baths may help resolve the inflammation.

The nurse should provide education to the patient to avoid straining, lifting, and sexual activity until the infection is resolved. The patient should continue taking analgesic agents and antibiotics as prescribed and using ice packs if necessary to relieve discomfort. The patient should be educated that it may take 2 to 3 months for the epididymis to return to normal and for scrotal swelling to subside.

TESTICULAR CANCER

Testicular cancer is the most common cancer in AMAB patients between 15 and 40 years of age, with an average age at diagnosis of 33 years of age; however, it can occur in AMAB patients of any age. It is a highly treatable and usually curable form of cancer, with a cure rate of greater than 90% for all stages of the disease. The ACS expected that in 2022, there would be 9,910 new cases of testicular cancer diagnosed in the United States and approximately 460 deaths (ACS, 2022). Testicular cancer is a rare carcinoma accounting for only 1% of AMAB cancers (NCCN, 2022).

Classification of Testicular Tumors

The testicles contain several types of cells, each of which may develop into one or more types of cancer. The type of cancer determines the appropriate treatment and affects the prognosis. Testicular cancers are classified as germinal, having their origins within the germ cells of the gonads (testes), or nongerminal (stromal).

Pure Seminoma Testicular Tumors

Testicular germ cell tumors are the most common type of testicular tumors and comprise 95% of malignant tumors of the testicle (NCCN, 2022). Germ cell tumors originate from the cells in the gonads (testes).

Non-Seminomatous Testicular Tumors

Testicular cancer also may develop in the supportive and hormone-producing tissues, or stroma, of the testicles. The two main types of stromal tumors are Leydig cell tumors and Sertoli cell tumors.

Risk Factors

Risk factors for testicular cancer include undescended testicles (**cryptorchidism**); a family history of testicular cancer; and cancer of one testicle, which increases the risk in the other testicle.

Clinical Manifestations and Assessment

The symptoms of testicular cancer often present as a painless or painful testicular nodule, mass, enlargement, or induration (hardening; NCCN, 2022). In the case of metastatic disease from testicular cancer, the patient may present with enlarged lymph nodes of the lower neck or upper chest (supraclavicular), a retroperitoneal mass, gynecomastia,

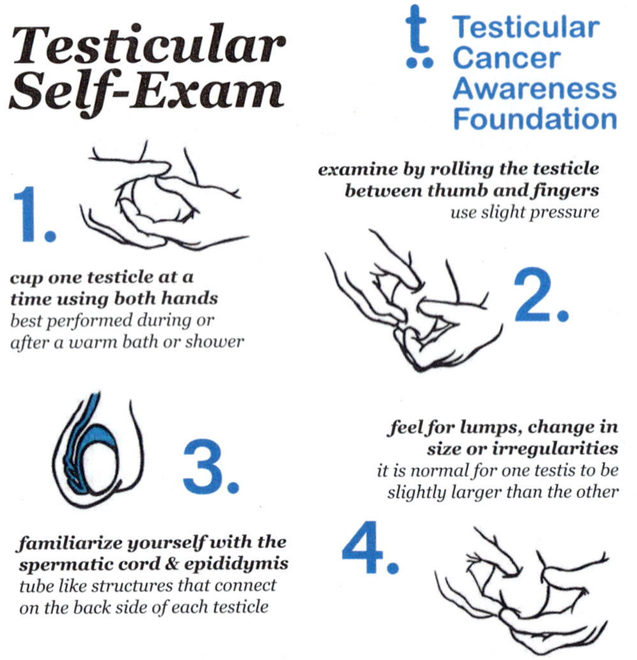

FIGURE 33-3 Monthly testicular self-exams. (Reproduced with permission from the Testicular Cancer Awareness Foundation. https://www.testicularcancerawarenessfoundation.org/self-exam)

venous thrombosis, or pulmonary embolism (NCCN, 2022). Enlargement of the testis without pain is a significant diagnostic finding. Monthly testicular self-examinations is a Grade B recommendation by the USPSTF as of 2018 (Fadich et al., 2018). A Grade B recommendation notes that the service should be offered to eligible patients as it is supported by fair evidence that the service improves important health outcomes and concludes that the benefits outweigh harms. Nurses should provide education to patients between the ages of 15 and 40 on how to effectively perform a monthly self-examination of the testicles (see Fig. 33-3). They should review with the patient the abnormal findings that would require further evaluation by a provider.

Serum tumor markers human chorionic gonadotropin (hCG) and alpha-fetoprotein (AFP) are critical in determining prognosis and determining treatment outcomes (NCCN, 2022). Lactate dehydrogenase (LDH) levels are elevated in 50% of the patients diagnosed with testicular cancer; however, is not as specific a marker as beta-hCG and AFP (NCCN, 2022). Scrotal ultrasound is a critical tool in the workup of a testicular mass. Ultrasound will help to determine the presence, location, and size of the testicular mass. Testicular tumors on ultrasound appear as heterogeneous (tissue that appears to look different from one area to the next), hypoechoic (tissue that is more dense than usual), and vascular (NCCN, 2022). A CT of the abdomen and pelvis may be performed to determine the extent of the disease in the retroperitoneum and pelvis. A chest x-ray should be performed to assess for possible lung metastasis. PET scans should not be used for staging in testicular cancer. Tissue diagnosis is performed at the time of orchiectomy. Transcrotal biopsies of the testes are not recommended for initial diagnosis of testicular cancer because violating the scrotum increases the risk of local or atypical regional recurrence and can complicate treatment (NCCN, 2022).

Pearls for Practice: Why CT Scan With Testicular Cancer?

The testes descend during gestation from within the abdomen to the inguinal region, and lymph drainage from the testes occurs via the para-aortic lymph nodes. They carry their blood supply as they descend. Cancers can spread to the lymph nodes near the origin of the arteries and veins which arise from the aorta and the inferior vena cava (just inferior to the kidneys). The lymph nodes may appear enlarged on CT scan. Thus, if metastatic disease is suspected a CT scan of the abdomen is performed to evaluate for retroperitoneal lymph node disease. Metastatic retroperitoneal disease may present as back pain.

Medical Management

Testicular cancer staging is based on the extent of disease and assessment of postorchiectomy serum marker levels. For patients with seminomas (all stages combined), the cure rate exceeds 90% and for patients with low-stage seminomas (NCI, 2022). The goals of management are to eradicate the disease and achieve a cure. Treatment selection is based on the cell type and the anatomic extent of the disease. During orchiectomy, the testis is removed through an inguinal incision with a high ligation of the spermatic cord. A retroperitoneal lymph node dissection (RPLND) may be performed during or after orchiectomy if there is evidence of lymph node metastasis. Although libido and climax are usually unimpaired after RPLND, the patient may develop ejaculatory dysfunction.

It is important to discuss sperm banking with patients diagnosed with testicular cancer. Undergoing therapeutic treatment for testicular cancer may negatively affect future fertility of patients. Ideally, if sperm banking is desired, this should be completed prior to the treatment of testicular cancer. This discussion is most important for patients who are of reproductive age or patients who desire to preserve their fertility for future conception (NCCN, 2022).

Treatment of pure seminoma testicular cancers is largely dictated by stage of disease and can be complex. Treatments may include orchiectomy, lymph node dissection, chemotherapy (adjuvant or salvage), and in some cases radiation therapy. Patients diagnosed with testicular cancer should have an in-depth shared decision-making conversation with a qualified genitourinary oncologist regarding treatment options and implications on quality of life.

High-grade, metastatic, or recurrent testicular cancer requires higher levels of care by a qualified genitourinary oncologist and medical oncologist team. Overall survival rates of these populations decrease significantly when compared to Stage I/II disease states. For example, the prognosis of patients with brain metastases from testicular cancer is poor, with greater than 50% of patients dying within 1 year of diagnosis (NCCN, 2022).

Nursing Management

Nursing management includes assessment of the patient's physical and psychological status and monitoring of the patient for response to and possible effects of surgery, chemotherapy, and radiation therapy (see Chapter 5). Operative care is described in Chapter 4. Because the patient may have difficulty coping with their condition, issues related to body image and sexuality are addressed. The patient needs to know that radiation therapy will not necessarily prevent them from conceiving children, and unilateral excision of a testis will not necessarily decrease virility.

Banking Sperm

Cryopreserving semen in a sperm bank is an option for persons who are about to undergo a procedure or treatment (e.g., radiation therapy to the pelvis, chemotherapy, RPLND, prostatectomy) that may affect their fertility. All patients undergoing cancer treatment should be offered the opportunity for sperm cryopreservation. This requires visits to a fertility clinic, where the sperm is produced by masturbation and collected in a sterile container for storage.

HYDROCELE

A **hydrocele** is a collection of peritoneal fluid between the parietal and visceral layers of the tunica vaginalis, which directly surrounds the testis and the spermatic cord (Eyre, 2021a). Most hydroceles are idiopathic in nature. Other causes for hydrocele can be inflammation or acute injury to the testicle. Transillumination is a bedside technique that can be used to differentiate a hydrocele from a hernia. Because hydroceles are a collection of fluid, the hydrocele will glow red, whereas the dense tissue of a hernia will not illuminate. For definitive diagnosis, a scrotal ultrasound should be performed.

Therapy is not required unless the hydrocele becomes tense or if the scrotal mass becomes large, uncomfortable, or embarrassing. In the surgical treatment of hydrocele, called a hydrocelectomy, an incision is made through the wall of the scrotum down to the distended tunica vaginalis. The sac is resected and is sutured together to collapse the wall. Postoperatively, the patient should be encouraged to keep the incisional site clean, wear supportive underwear, avoid strenuous activity, ice the scrotum, and rest. Complications of the hydrocelectomy procedure can be infection of the incision site, swelling of the scrotum, pelvic pain disorder, or recurrence of the hydrocele.

VARICOCELE

A **varicocele** is an abnormal dilation of the veins of the pampiniform venous plexus in the scrotum (the network of veins from the testis and the epididymis that constitute part of the spermatic cord) and is present in 15% to 20% of AMAB people (Fig. 33-4). Varicoceles usually occur in the veins on the upper portion of the left testicle in adults because of the angle in which the left spermatic cord inserts into the left renal vein, while the right spermatic cord enters the inferior vena cava. Varicoceles can be associated with infertility in some AMAB persons; however, patients should be reassured that studies indicate that 75% of patients will be fertile and 80% have normal sperm parameters (Eyre, 2021a). Few symptoms may be produced by the enlarged spermatic vein, and no treatment is required unless fertility is a concern or there is pain. Options to repair varicocele are surgery, microsurgical repair, or percutaneous venous embolization. Traditional surgical repair consists of ligating the gonadal vein branches so retrograde blood flow no longer reaches the plexus of veins within the scrotum (Eyre, 2021b). This can also be performed microsurgically, which may contribute to lower recurrence rates. Percutaneous venous embolization can be utilized in some patients; however, there is evidence of a high recurrence of varicoceles. Complications are minimal. Postoperatively, an ice pack may be applied to the scrotum for the first few hours after surgery to relieve edema. Then the patient wears a scrotal supporter.

CONDITIONS AFFECTING THE PENIS

PHIMOSIS AND PARAPHIMOSIS

Phimosis is a condition in which the foreskin is constricted so that it cannot be retracted over the glans. It can occur congenitally or from inflammation and edema. If the preputial area is not cleaned, normal secretions accumulate (smegma), causing inflammation (balanitis), which can lead to adhesions and fibrosis. It is seen more commonly in adult patients with poorly controlled diabetes and obesity. In older people, it can be related to penile adhesions causing the inability to pull back the foreskin. Penile carcinoma may develop and go undetected in the patient suffering from phimosis. Phimosis is corrected by circumcision or dorsal slit.

Paraphimosis is a condition in which the foreskin is retracted behind the glans and, because of narrowness and subsequent edema, cannot be returned to its usual position covering the glans. It is a true urologic emergency, and patients should be directed to the nearest emergency department for treatment. Initial treatment of paraphimosis involves firmly compressing the glans to reduce its size and then pushing the glans back while simultaneously moving the prepuce forward. If the provider is unable to compress the paraphimosis, the patient will require emergent circumcision. Paraphimosis is commonly caused when health care providers do not replace the foreskin over the glans after performing catheterization or peri-care or bathing the patient.

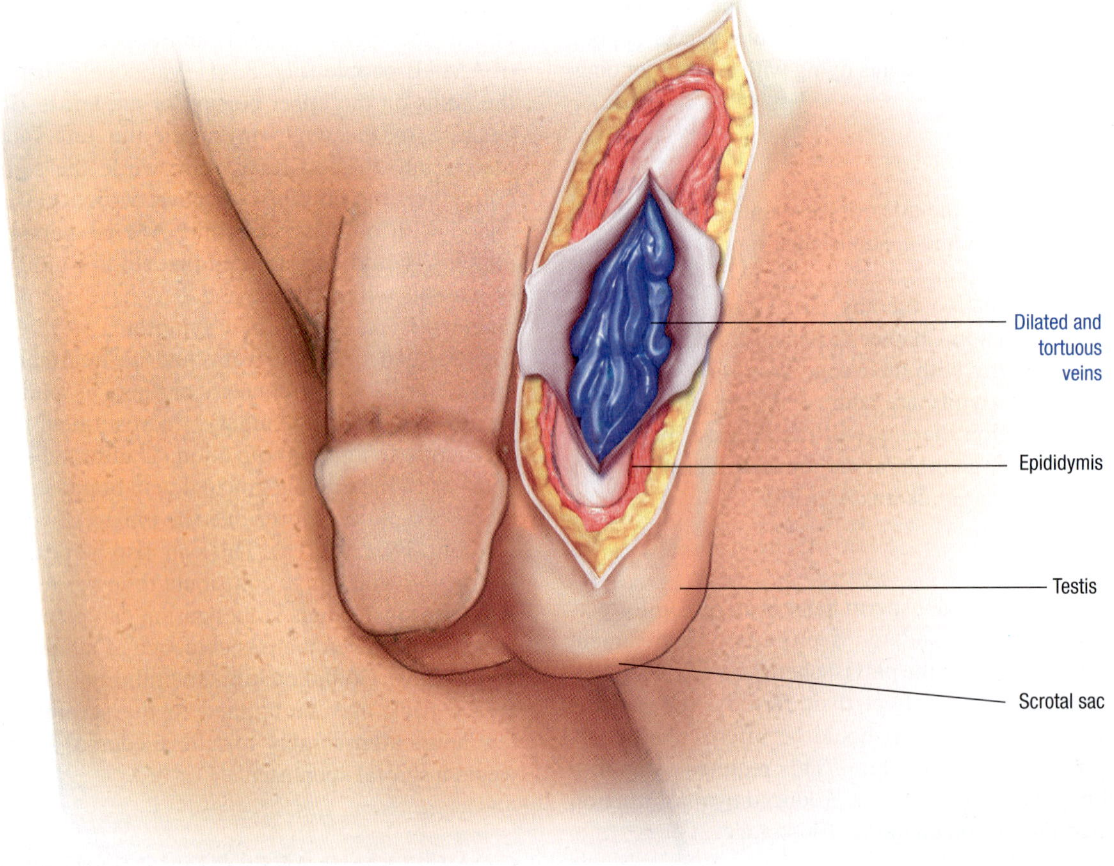

FIGURE 33-4 **Varicocele.**

Pearls for Practice

To catheterize an uncircumcised AMAB person, the nurse retracts the foreskin and uses soap and water to clean away the smegma (whitish sebaceous secretion that collects between the glans penis and foreskin) before beginning the sterile procedure. The glans and foreskin are rinsed thoroughly. The nurse follows institutional protocols for biologic male catheterization. Immediately after catheterization, the foreskin is returned to its normal position to prevent an accumulation of fluid within the glans, which may cause ***paraphimosis*** *(the inability to retract the foreskin to its natural position because of venous and lymphatic congestion caused by constriction by the foreskin). The provider should be notified immediately if the nurse is unable to retract the foreskin.*

PRIAPISM

Priapism is a persistent erection that causes the penis to become large, hard, and painful. It results from either neural or vascular causes, including sickle cell thrombosis, leukemic cell infiltration, and tumor invasion of the penis or its vessels. It may occur with use of medications that affect the central nervous system, antihypertensive agents, antidepressant medications, PDE-5 inhibitors, and substances injected into the penis to treat ED.

Priapism is a true urologic emergency. The goal of therapy is to improve venous drainage of the corpora cavernosa to prevent ischemia, fibrosis, and impotence. The corpora may be irrigated with an anticoagulant, which allows stagnant blood to be aspirated. Shunting procedures to divert the blood from the turgid corpora cavernosa to the venous system or into the corpus spongiosum–glans penis compartment may be attempted.

Clinical Judgment Case

An 82-year-old patient is admitted to your surgical unit after undergoing a transurethral resection of the prostate (TURP). Vital signs were stable in the PACU, and you have received an oral report on the patient's status. On transfer to your unit, you note that the patient's skin is warm and dry and vital signs are as follows: 98.7° F, HR 92 and regular, RR of 26 with an oxygen saturation of 93% on room air, and blood pressure of 142/92 mm Hg. Heart sounds are S1, S2 without murmur, gallops, or rub. Lung sounds include fine crackles at the bases bilaterally; cough is nonproductive. The patient is complaining of some shortness of breath but denies chest pain, nausea, or vomiting. Abdomen is soft, nondistended, and nontender. There is no peripheral edema, capillary refill is 2 seconds, and pedal and posterior tibial pulses are 3+ bil. The patient is alert; is oriented to person, time, place, and situation; and denies headache. Pupils are equal and reacting to light, 3 mm bil. No weakness noted. There is a continuous bladder irrigation (CBI) catheter in place, and normal saline is the irrigation that is infusing. You note that the urinary drainage is dark red with some clots in the urinary drainage tubing and drainage bag. The patient has a history of coronary artery disease (CAD) and denies COPD, or diabetes.

Step One: Recognize cues where relevant and important information is identified from different sources, such as medical history or vital signs.

Answer: The complaints of shortness of breath, RR of 26, oxygen saturation of 93% on room air, bibasilar crackles, hypotension, and the clots and dark red drainage in urinary drainage tubing and drainage bag are of concern, as is your patient's history of CAD.

Step Two: Analyze cues, which is organizing and linking the recognized cues to the patient's clinical presentation.

Answer: You have clustered the symptoms of SOB, tachypnea (RR 26), hypertension (142/92), bibasilar crackles, decreased oxygen saturation (93%) with potential for a cardiac event due to the stress of surgery, age of the patient, and cardiac history of heart failure (left-sided) associated with the irrigation of normal saline intraoperatively and postoperatively resulting in volume overload. You will review the intraoperative notes to confirm that saline was used as the irrigant during the surgery, versus a hypotonic solution. You will also assess the intraoperative notes to evaluate the amount of irrigation solution administered during surgery. You are aware that the use of a hypotonic solution for irrigation is associated with hyponatremia, which will present with neurologic changes (patient's neuro status was within normal limits when you received the patient from the PACU). You recognize that red urinary drainage with clots is related to bleeding at the surgical site and respond by increasing the rate of the irrigating solution rapidly until the drainage color becomes pink to clear, at which time the rate is decreased.

Step Three: Prioritize hypotheses, where hypotheses are evaluated and ranked according to priority. This can include urgency, likelihood, risk, difficulty, and/or time. In this phase you cluster your findings to arrive at a list of problems (actual and or potential problems) you believe the patient is experiencing and determine importance or urgency. What do you think is of greatest concern?

Answer: You prioritize notifying the surgeon regarding vital sign changes, decreased oxygen saturation, and physical examination findings (crackles) and concern for FVE versus a cardiac event. However, recognizing that it is critical to remove the blood clots because of the procedure, you will increase the rate of irrigant flow to prevent potentially obstructing clots.

Step Four: Generate solutions, which is identifying expected outcomes and using hypotheses to define a set of interventions for the expected outcomes.

Answer: You will notify the provider and reassess the patient's heart and lung sounds, vital signs, and oxygen saturation. You will administer low-flow oxygen (2 L nasal cannula) per standing order and anticipate possible need for an ECG and cardiac biomarkers, BNP to evaluate for heart failure, and electrolytes to evaluate the sodium level. You will increase the rate of irrigant flow to prevent potentially obstructing clots until the drainage clears. You will continue to monitor for neurologic changes from both possible hyponatremia from CBI and from hypoxemia.

Step Five: Take action, where the solutions that address the highest priorities are implemented.

Answer: You place a call to the provider, and while awaiting the call you increase the rate of irrigation; the urine pinks and clears, so you decrease the rate again as you reassess vital signs and heart and lung sounds. You administer low-flow oxygen (2 L via nasal cannula), elevate the head of bed for patient comfort, and place the patient on continuous pulse oximetry reading. You repeat the vital signs, and the oxygen saturation is now 97% on 2 L, and the RR is now 20. The BP remains elevated at 144/94; the pulse is full and bounding at a regular rate of 94. The crackles at both bases continue; however, they have not increased, and there is no S3 (associated with HF) or S4 (associated with MI or hypertension). You place the patient on a cardiac monitor while you await the provider's call. They respond and agree that a 12 lead ECG should be performed and that stat serum electrolytes, BNP, and cardiac biomarkers should be obtained. A portable chest film is also ordered. You maintain strict I&O record and continue to evaluate the patient's vital signs and physical examination findings.

Step Six: Evaluate outcomes, which is comparing observed outcomes against expected outcomes.

Answer: The stat blood work reveals a troponin I of less 0.2 ng/mL, and you are aware that a normal level is less than 0.5 ng/mL. The 12 lead ECG is unremarkable; however, the brain natriuretic peptide (BNP) is 380 pg/mL. You know that a normal BNP is less than 100 pg/mL and an elevated BNP is a good marker for HF. The higher the level of BNP, the more severe the HF. The stat electrolytes reveal sodium of 140 mEq/L, and other electrolytes are within normal limits. The chest film reveals mild heart failure, and the provider orders stat diuretics intravenously to facilitate excretion of absorbed fluid.

Because of your astute clinical observations, you alerted the provider immediately to your concerns of cardiac compromise given this patient's history of CAD, age, TURP, and irrigating solution used (normal saline), and treatment was initiated to treat the pulmonary edema that developed. Your patient required potassium replacement after the diuretic was administered; however, your patient had an uneventful postoperative course and was discharged home on postop day 3. Job well done for your clinical judgment and decision-making!

CHAPTER REVIEW

NCLEX-Style Review Questions

1. A 45-year-old patient complains of swelling in the scrotum. The nurse assesses the patient for which conditions? Select all that apply.
   a. Prostatitis
   b. Hydronephrosis
   c. Hydrocele
   d. Acute orchitis
   e. Cystitis

2. A patient is received on your medical-surgical unit after undergoing a TURP procedure from the PACU. Continuous bladder irrigation with normal saline is infusing, and the urinary drainage has turned from pink to dark red with some small clots. Which actions are your priorities? Select all that apply.
   a. Increase the rate of the CBI solution
   b. Ensure there are no kinks in the drainage tubing
   c. Decrease the rate of the CBI solution
   d. Monitor I and O
   e. Set the irrigation solution on IV pump at 100 mL/hr

3. Which of the following symptoms suggest that the patient is experiencing transurethral resection (TUR) syndrome after undergoing a transurethral prostatectomy (TURP) where a hypotonic irrigating solution was used intraoperatively? Select all that apply.
   a. Confusion
   b. Constipation
   c. Hyponatremia
   d. Seizures
   e. Skin rash

4. An 80-year-old patient is being treated presumptively for acute prostatitis. The nurse is asked why the course of antibiotics is so long and if it is related to their age. Select the nurse's best responses.
   a. The infection is resistant to most antibiotics.
   b. Most antibiotics diffuse poorly from the plasma into the prostatic fluid.
   c. Most of the antibiotic is excreted in the urine, requiring a longer course.
   d. The liver is preventing the antibiotic from working effectively.
   e. Age is unrelated to medical regimen; all patients need a prolonged antibiotic course.

5. A 58-year-old patient has had a prostatectomy. The nurse is preparing them for discharge. What information is important for the nurse to incorporate in the teaching plan? Select all that apply.

a. Try to interrupt the stream after starting to void.
b. Increased activity is permitted.
c. Limit fluid intake to prevent hypervolemia.
d. Spicy foods, alcohol, and coffee may cause bladder discomfort.
e. You should expect immediate return of erectile function.

REFERENCES AND SELECTED READINGS

References and selected readings associated with this chapter can be found on the website that accompanies the book. Visit **http://thepoint.lww.com/Honan3e** to access the references and other additional resources associated with this chapter.

CHAPTER 34

Nursing Management: Patients With Sexually Transmitted Infections

Christa Palancia Esposito

Learning Objectives

After reading this chapter, you will be able to:

1. Differentiate among colonization, infection, and disease.
2. Compare the various types of sexually transmitted infections (STIs) and the signs, symptoms, and treatments of each.
3. Use the nursing process as a framework for care of patients with an STI.
4. Develop a teaching plan for the patient with an STI.

A sexually transmitted infection (STI), also known as a sexually transmitted disease (STD), is an infection acquired through sexual contact with an infected person. STIs are the most common infectious diseases in the United States and are epidemic in most parts of the world. To understand the pathophysiology of STIs, it is important to understand the infectious process.

THE INFECTIOUS PROCESS

An infectious disease is any disease caused by the growth of pathogenic microbes in the body. It may or may not be communicable (i.e., contagious). The nurse plays an important role in infection control and prevention. Educating patients can decrease their risk of becoming infected or decrease the sequelae of infection.

The Chain of Infection

A complete chain of events is necessary for infection to occur. The necessary elements for infection to occur are described in Box 34-1.

Colonization, Infection, and Infectious Disease

Relatively few anatomic sites are sterile (brain, blood, bone, heart, vascular system). Bacteria found throughout the body usually provide beneficial **normal flora** to compete with potential pathogens, to facilitate digestion, or to work in other ways symbiotically with the host.

Colonization

The term *colonization* is used to describe microorganisms present without host interference or interaction. Organisms reported in microbiology test results often reflect colonization rather than infection. *Colony count* represents a visual count of microbes present in a sample. In general, providers use a colony count of greater than 100,000/mL or 10^5 bacteria/mL to represent an infection. However, astute providers also will consider other local and systemic signs of infection at lower colony counts, such as fever, leukocytosis (elevated white blood cells [WBCs]), erythema (redness), purulent exudate, inflammation, warmth, and the like.

Infection

Infection indicates a host interaction with an organism. A patient colonized with *Staphylococcus aureus* may have staphylococci on the skin without any skin interruption or irritation. However, if the patient had an incision, *S. aureus* could enter the wound, be seen as foreign, and result in an immune system reaction of local inflammation and migration of WBCs to the site. Infection may be suggested based on clinical evidence of erythema, heat, and pain as well as laboratory evidence of WBCs on the wound specimen smear.

Infectious Disease

It is important to recognize the difference between infection and infectious disease. While infection merely indicates interaction between the host and the organism, **infectious disease** is the state in which the infected host displays a decline in wellness due to the infection. When the host

BOX 34-1

Chain of Infection

The chain of infection requires the following elements:

- A causative organism
- A reservoir of available organisms
- A portal or mode of exit from the reservoir
- A mode or route of transmission from reservoir to host
- A susceptible host
- A mode of entry to host

Causative Organism

The types of microorganisms that cause infections are bacteria, rickettsiae (gram-negative bacteria carried by ticks, fleas, and lice), viruses, protozoa, fungi, and helminths (parasitic worms).

Reservoir

Reservoir is the term used for any person, plant, animal, substance, or location that provides nourishment for microorganisms and enables their further dispersal.

Mode of Exit

The organism must have a mode of exit from a reservoir. An infected host must shed organisms to another host or to the environment before transmission can occur. Organisms exit through the respiratory tract, the gastrointestinal tract, the genitourinary tract, the skin, or the blood.

Route of Transmission

A route of transmission is necessary and specific to each pathogen in order to connect the infectious source with its new host. Organisms may be transmitted through sexual contact, skin-to-skin contact, percutaneous injection, or through infectious particles carried in the air. A person who carries or transmits an organism but does not have apparent signs and symptoms of infection is called a *carrier.*

Susceptible Host

For infection to occur, the host must be susceptible (not possessing immunity to a particular pathogen). Previous infection or vaccine administration may render the host immune (not susceptible) to further infection with an agent. Although exposure to potentially infectious microorganisms occurs essentially on a constant basis, our elaborate immune systems generally prevent infection from occurring. A person who is immunosuppressed has much greater susceptibility to infection than does a healthy person.

Portal of Entry

A portal of entry is needed for the organism to gain access to the host. For example, airborne *Mycobacterium tuberculosis* does not cause disease when it settles on the skin of an exposed host; the only entry route for *M. tuberculosis* is through the respiratory tract.

interacts immunologically with an organism but remains symptom free, the definition of infectious disease has not been met. The microbiology laboratory report is the primary source of bacterial infection identification and should be viewed as a tool to be used along with clinical indicators to determine whether a patient is colonized, infected, or diseased. Microbiology reports from clinical specimens usually show three components: the smear and stain, the culture and organism identification, and the antimicrobial susceptibility (i.e., sensitivity). As a marker for the likelihood of infection, the smear and stain (referred to as *gram stain*) generally provide the most helpful information because they describe the mix of cells present at the anatomic site at the time of specimen collection and are a guide to the choice of antibiotic pending the culture results. The gram stain will classify organisms as either gram positive or gram positive. The culture will detail the exact organism(s), while the sensitivity will specify antimicrobials most likely to be effective against the organism(s).

SEXUALLY TRANSMITTED INFECTIONS

STIs are acquired through sexual contact with an infected person. Table 34-1 identifies infections that can be classified as STIs and their routes of transmission. Portals of entry of STI-causing microorganisms and sites of infection include the skin and mucosal linings of the urethra, cervix, vagina, rectum, and oropharynx.

Education about prevention of STIs includes information about risk factors and behaviors that can lead to infection. Refer to Box 34-2 for risk factors associated with STIs. The placement of a condom or protective barrier (i.e., dental dam) before any sexual contact is imperative to help prevent the acquisition or transmission of an STI. Refer to Box 34-3 for the application of a male condom and Figure 34-1 for the application of a female condom.

TABLE 34-1 **Conditions Classified as Sexually Transmitted Diseases (STDs) and Their Routes of Transmission**

Disease	Route(s) of Transmission
Chlamydia	Sexual
Gonorrhea	Sexual
Herpes simplex	Sexual, percutaneous, perinatal
Human papillomavirus (HPV)	Sexual, percutaneous
Syphilis	Sexual, perinatal
Trichomoniasis	Sexual

BOX 34-2

Risk Factors for Sexually Transmitted Infections and Diseases

- Having unprotected sex
- Having multiple partners
- Being under 26 years of age
- Starting sex at an early age
- Using alcohol or illegal drugs
- Using IV drugs
- Having a history of STI
- Participating in prostitution
- Using oral contraceptives as only form of contraception
- Poverty
- Social segregation
- Unemployment
- Cultural norms

Pearls for Practice

Infection with one STI suggests the possibility of infection with other diseases as well. After one STI is identified, diagnostic evaluation for others should be performed.

SYPHILIS

Pathophysiology

Syphilis is an acute and chronic infectious disease caused by the spirochete *Treponema pallidum.* It is acquired primarily through sexual contact although rarely may be congenital in origin; that is, it can be passed from birthing parent to child during pregnancy or childbirth.

Risk Factors

Risk factors include having unprotected sex and being infected with other STIs. Although the rate of syphilis is increasing since 2000 across all demographics, the majority of cases occur in men who have sex with men (MSM) (Centers for Disease Control and Prevention [CDC], 2018; Ghanem et al., 2020).

Clinical Manifestations and Assessment

In the untreated person, the course of syphilis can be divided into three stages: primary, secondary, and tertiary. These stages reflect the time from infection and the clinical manifestations observed in that period and are the basis for treatment decisions.

Primary syphilis occurs 2 to 3 weeks after initial inoculation with the organism. A painless lesion at the site of infection is called a *chancre* (Fig. 34-2). Untreated, these lesions usually resolve spontaneously within about 2 months.

Secondary syphilis occurs when the hematogenous spread (distributed or spread by way of the bloodstream) of organisms from the original chancre leads to generalized infection.

BOX 34-3

Patient Education

Use of Male Condoms

1. Put on a new condom before any kind of sex.
2. Hold the condom by the tip to squeeze out the air.

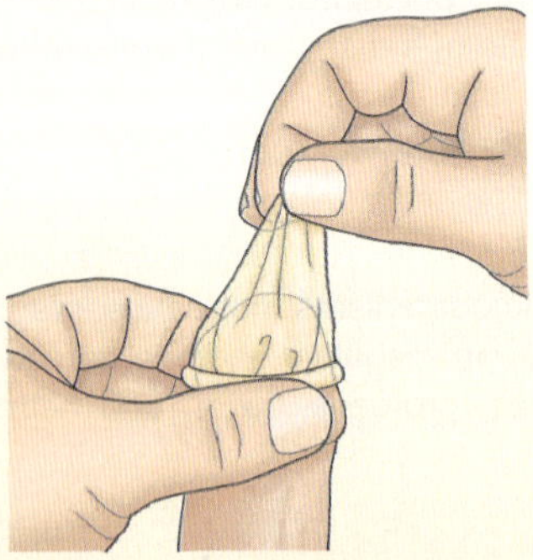

3. Unroll the condom all the way over the erect penis.

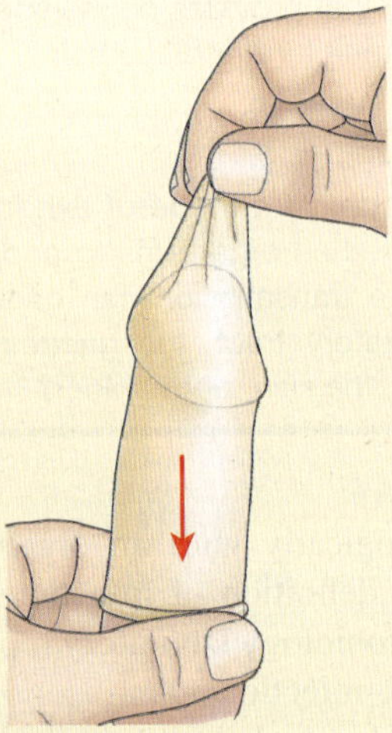

4. Have sex.
5. Hold the condom so it cannot come off the penis.
6. Pull out.
7. Use a new condom if you want to have sex again or if you want to have sex in a different place (e.g., in the anus and then in the vagina).

Keep condoms cool and dry. Never use skin lotions, baby oil, petroleum jelly, or cold cream with condoms. The oil in these products will cause the condom to break. Products made with water (such as K-Y jelly or glycerin) are safer to use.

The rash of secondary syphilis occurs about 2 to 8 weeks after the chancre and involves the trunk and the extremities, including the palms of the hands and the soles of the feet. Transmission of the organism can occur through contact with these lesions. Generalized signs of infection may include lymphadenopathy (abnormal enlargement of lymph nodes), arthritis, meningitis (inflammation of the pia mater, arachnoid, and subarachnoid space), hair loss, fever, malaise, and weight loss. After the secondary stage, there is a period of **latency (delay)**, when the infected person has no signs or

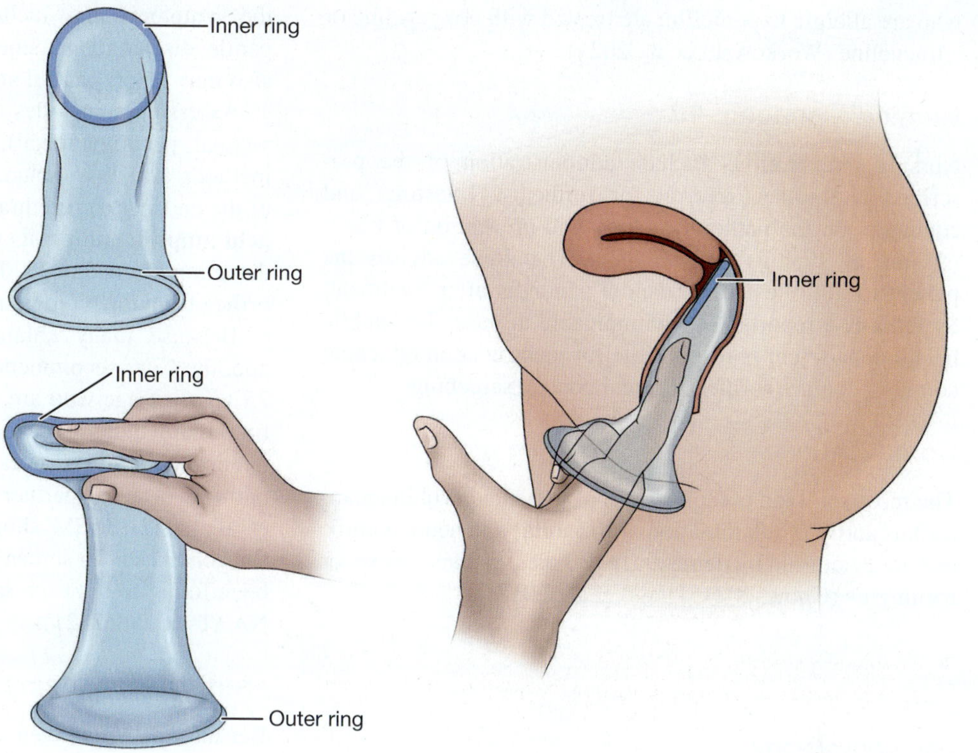

FIGURE 34-1 **Female condom. To insert the female condom, hold the inner ring between the thumb and middle finger. Put the index finger on the pouch between the thumb and other fingers and squeeze the ring. Slide the condom into the vagina as far as it will go. The inner ring keeps the condom in place.**

symptoms of syphilis. Latency can be interrupted by a recurrence of secondary syphilis.

Tertiary syphilis is the final stage in the natural progression of the disease. It is estimated that between 20% and 40% of those infected do not exhibit signs and symptoms in this final stage. Tertiary syphilis has become uncommon in the era of antibiotics and presents as a slowly progressive inflammatory disease with the potential to affect multiple organs (O'Byrne & MacPherson, 2019).

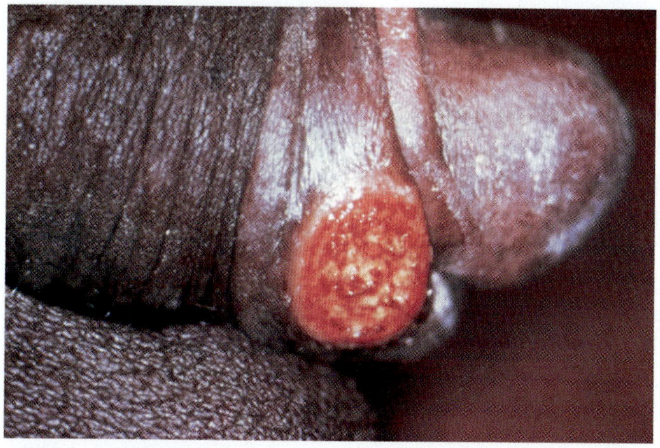

FIGURE 34-2 **The first stage of a syphilis infection is the appearance of a chancre, a round, usually solitary, painless sore that appears on the glans penis or the shaft of the penis, or it may lie within the urethra. If left untreated, it will heal; however, secondary syphilis will develop. (From Goodheart, H. [2003].** ***Goodheart's photoguide of common skin disorders*****. Lippincott Williams & Wilkins.)**

The conclusive diagnosis of syphilis can be made by direct identification of the spirochete obtained from the chancre lesions of primary syphilis. Serologic tests used in the diagnosis of secondary and tertiary syphilis require clinical correlation in interpretation. The serologic tests are summarized as follows:

- Nontreponemal or reagin tests, such as the Venereal Disease Research Laboratory (VDRL) or the rapid plasma reagin circle card test (RPR-CT), generally are used for screening and diagnosis. After adequate therapy, the test result is expected to decrease quantitatively until it is read as negative, usually about 2 years after therapy is completed.
- Treponemal tests, such as the fluorescent treponemal antibody absorption test (FTA-ABS) and the microhemagglutination assay test (MHA-TP), are used to verify that the screening test did not represent a false-positive result. Positive results usually are positive for life and therefore are not appropriate to determine therapeutic effectiveness.

Medical Management

Administration of antibiotics is the treatment for all stages of syphilis. A single dose of penicillin G benzathine intramuscular injection is the medication of choice for early syphilis or early latent syphilis of less than 1 year's duration. Patients with late latent or latent syphilis of unknown duration should receive three injections at 1-week intervals. Usually, patients who are allergic to penicillin are treated with doxycycline or tetracycline (Workowski et al., 2021).

Nursing Management

Nursing interventions include administration of the prescribed antibiotics, referral for further STI testing, and education on the pathophysiology and prevention of transmission of syphilis and all STIs. The nurse advises the patient to get retested at 6 and 12 months after treatment. Syphilis is a reportable communicable disease. The public health department is responsible for identification of sexual contacts, contact notification, and contact screening.

Complications

The most common complications of untreated syphilis manifest as aortitis (inflammation of the aorta) and neurosyphilis and are evidenced by dementia, psychosis, paresis, stroke, or meningitis (Chow, 2021; Drago et al., 2018).

CHLAMYDIA TRACHOMATIS AND NEISSERIA GONORRHOEAE

Pathophysiology

Chlamydia trachomatis and *Neisseria gonorrhoeae* are the most commonly reported bacterial STIs. Coinfection with *Chlamydia* often occurs in patients infected with *N. gonorrhoeae. Chlamydia* and *N. gonorrhoeae* are transmitted during sexual relations or may be transmitted from birthing parent to child during vaginal birth.

Risk Factors

Any sexually active person can be infected with *Chlamydia* or *N. gonorrhoeae*, and the risk increases with the number of sexual partners. The group with the greatest risk for *Chlamydia* infection is young people who were assigned female at birth (AFAB) who are 24 years of age and younger; risk may be associated with a cervix that has not matured fully (Workowski et al., 2021). The risk for *N. gonorrhoeae* also includes sexually active young people AFAB as well as MSM.

Clinical Manifestations and Assessment

Both *Chlamydia* and *N. gonorrhoeae* infections frequently do not cause symptoms in AFAB and thus are often referred to as "silent" in regard to clinical presentation. When symptoms are present, the most frequent finding is mucopurulent cervicitis with exudates in the endocervical canal. Females with gonorrhea also can present with symptoms of urinary tract infection (UTI) or vaginitis.

Although males are more likely than females to have symptoms when infected, infection with *N. gonorrhoeae* and/or *Chlamydia* also can be asymptomatic. When symptoms are present in assigned male at birth (AMAB) patients, the symptoms may include burning during urination and penile discharge. Patients with *N. gonorrhoeae* infection also may report painful swollen testicles.

Assessment includes noting fever, discharge (urethral, vaginal, penis, or rectal), and signs of arthritis. Diagnostic methods available include urine testing or swab specimens of the endocervix, urethra, anal canal, and pharynx. **Nucleic acid amplification tests (NAAT)** are most sensitive for the detection of chlamydia. The gram stain best identifies gonorrhea from the biologic male urethra.

Because many chlamydial infections are asymptomatic, the CDC recommends all AFAB patients younger than 25 years of age who are sexually active be tested routinely for chlamydial infection (CDC, 2021), as should AFAB patients older than 25 years if they have new or multiple sex partners or a sex partner with a diagnosed STI (Fischbach et al., 2022). MSM should be screened at least annually for gonorrhea. To screen anyone, self-collected swabs have been found to have the same accuracy as provider-obtained NAATs (CDC, 2021).

Medical Management

Because patients often are infected with both gonorrhea and chlamydia simultaneously, the CDC recommends dual therapy if chlamydia has not been ruled out by NAAT. The CDC-recommended treatment for chlamydia is doxycycline, alternatively azithromycin or levofloxacin. For gonorrhoea, a single dose of intramuscular ceftriaxone is recommended; the dose is weight dependent. Patients weighing greater than 150 kg (about 330 lb) receive twice the dose.

Nursing Management

Gonorrhea and chlamydia are reportable communicable diseases. The target group for preventive patient teaching about gonorrhea and chlamydia is the adolescent and young adult population. Along with reinforcing the importance of abstinence, when appropriate, education should address postponing the age of initial sexual exposure, limiting the number of sexual partners, and use of condoms or barrier protection. Moreover, patient counseling includes abstinence for 1 week after treatment in addition to the completion of the partner's treatment. Test of cure is not recommended unless medication adherence is in question; however, the retesting of AFAB patients 3 months' posttreatment is recommended due to the possibility of reinfection. Education for males includes that they must inform their AFAB partners of infection, and they must provide literature on STIs and the risk of **pelvic inflammatory disease** (PID) to them (discussed later in this chapter).

Complications

In AFAB patients, PID, **ectopic pregnancy**, endometritis, and infertility are possible complications of either *N. gonorrhoeae* or *Chlamydia* infection. Figure 34-3 demonstrates how microorganisms spread in pelvic infection.

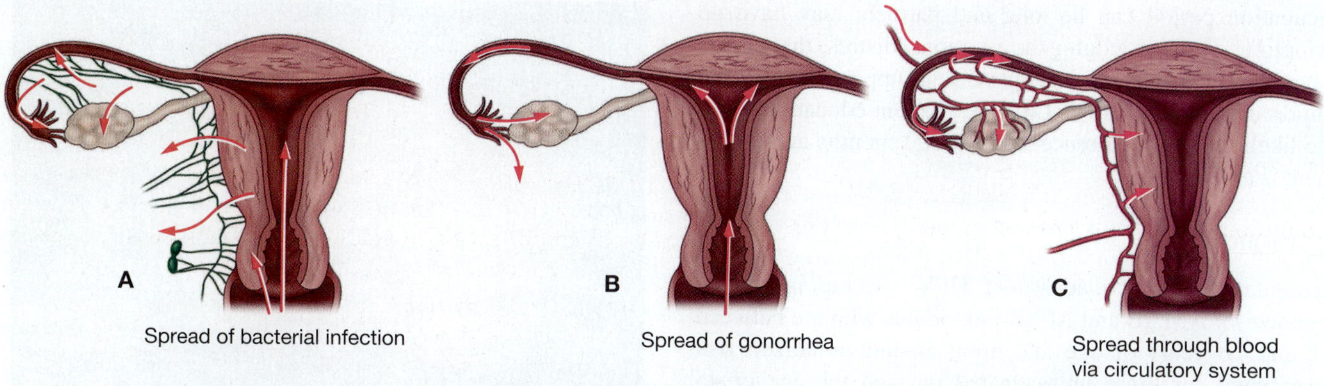

FIGURE 34-3 Pathway by which microorganisms spread in pelvic infections. (A) Bacterial infection spreads up the vagina, into the uterus, and through the lymphatics. (B) Gonorrhea spreads up the vagina, into the uterus, and then to the tubes and ovaries. (C) Bacterial infection can reach the reproductive organs through the bloodstream (hematogenous spread).

In AMAB individuals, epididymitis, a painful disease that may lead to infertility, may result from infection with either bacterium. In people of any gender, *N. gonorrhoeae* may cause arthritis or bloodstream infection.

HUMAN PAPILLOMAVIRUS

Human papillomavirus (HPV) infection is the most common viral STI among young, sexually active people. Millions of Americans are infected with HPV; many are unaware they carry the virus. Most sexually active people acquire genital HPV infection at some point in their lives (Workowski et al., 2021).

Pathophysiology

The virus affects the skin and mucous membranes through sexual contact (i.e., naked rubbing and vaginal/anal intercourse). At least 40 HPV types can infect the genitalia and perineum, including the skin of the penis, vulva, and anus as well as the linings of the vagina, cervix, and rectum. Certain types of HPV can cause the cells of the cervix to become abnormal, contributing to approximately 92% of cervical cancer cases (Senkomago et al., 2019; refer to Chapter 32 for additional details). Other strains of HPV cause genital warts. The virus can be present in the body for a long period of time before detection or symptoms occur (CDC, 2021). Psychologically, the diagnosis of HPV on a Papanicolaou (Pap) test can be upsetting to patients. This is particularly stressful and difficult to understand for some patients after testing negative for years. Explaining the latency of viruses can facilitate understanding. Often HPV is self-limiting due to an effective immune system response; however, smoking has been associated with increased morbidity. Persistent HPV can lead to cervical cancer, but with proper management and patient adherence morbidity and mortality are easily minimized. Therefore, best practice Pap follow-up is patient specific. Newer guidelines assist providers on making the determination whether to Pap test yearly or up to every 3 to 5 years depending on risk factors, history, and age.

Risk Factors

Risk factors include being sexually active, having multiple sex partners, and having sex with a partner who has or has had multiple partners.

Clinical Manifestations and Assessment

More than 150 strains of HPV exist, and infection can be latent (asymptomatic and detected only by DNA hybridization tests for HPV), subclinical (visualized only after application of acetic acid followed by inspection under magnification), or clinical (visible warts).

The most common strains of HPV, 6 and 11, usually cause **condylomata** (genital warts) on the genitalia and can be found in the mouth. Often these lesions are visible, flesh-colored, flat, verrucous, or papillary.

Some HPV strains (16, 18, 31, 33, and 45) affect the cervix, resulting in abnormal Pap tests, and are strongly associated with cervical cancer (CDC, 2021). Thus, the Pap test is the detection vehicle identifying HPV DNA. **Colposcopy**-derived biopsies diagnose any cellular changes or dysplasia (changes in cervical cells).

Medical and Nursing Management

Treatment of external genital warts includes topical application of trichloroacetic acid, podophyllin, and chemotherapeutic agents as well as injections of interferon administered by a health care provider. Topical agents that can be applied by patients to external lesions include podofilox and imiquimod. Electrocautery and laser therapy are alternative therapies that may be indicated for patients with a large number or area of genital warts (Workowski et al., 2021).

AFAB patients with HPV should have an annual Pap test because of the potential of HPV to cause dysplasia. Use of condoms can reduce the likelihood of transmission, but transmission also can occur during skin-to-skin contact in areas not covered by a barrier such as condoms or dental dams.

In many cases, patients are angry about having warts or HPV and do not know who infected them because the incubation period can be long and partners may have no symptoms. Acknowledging the emotional distress that occurs when an STI is diagnosed and providing support and facts are important nursing actions. Likewise, patient education about the likelihood of recurrence in the first 3 months after treatment is encouraged.

Complications

Preventatively, the quadrivalent HPV vaccine is recommended for AMAB and AFAB individuals who are between 11 and 26 years of age and upon an individualized risk assessment for those unvaccinated through the age of 45 (Meites et al., 2019). Immunization will not replace other strategies important in the prevention of HPV or the need for cervical cancer screening. Loss of the uterus and death from invasive cancer should be avoidable with proper care and follow-up.

HERPES VIRUS TYPE 2 INFECTION (HERPES GENITALIS, HERPES SIMPLEX VIRUS)

Herpes genitalis is a recurrent, lifelong viral infection that causes herpetic lesions (blisters) on the vulva, vagina, and cervix in AFAB patients and the penis in AMAB patients. There are two types of herpes simplex virus (HSV): HSV-1 and HSV-2, which are clinically indistinguishable.

Pathophysiology

HSV-1 is known as the oral type and can be transmitted to the genitalia by oral sex or self-inoculation (i.e., touching a cold sore and then touching the genital area). HSV-2 is always transmitted sexually. Usually the initial infection is very painful and lasts about 1 week, but it also can be asymptomatic. Most HSV infections occur via asymptomatic transmission when neither the carrier nor the recipient manifests lesions (Workowski et al., 2021).

Recurrences are more common with HSV-2 than HSV-1, are less painful, and usually produce minor itching and burning. Some patients have few or no recurrences, whereas others have frequent bouts. Often recurrences are associated with stress, sunburn, dental work, or inadequate rest or nutrition—all situations that may tax the immune system. When viral replication diminishes, the virus ascends the peripheral sensory nerves and remains inactive in the nerve ganglia. Similar to HPV, HSV can lay dormant without symptoms.

Risk Factors

Risk factors include contact with an infected person's mouth, oropharynx, mucosal surface, vagina, or cervix.

Clinical Manifestations and Assessment

Itching and pain accompany the process as the infected area becomes red and edematous. Primary infection may begin with macules (small flat spots on skin) and papules (small circumscribed elevations) and progress to vesicles (small, serous-filled elevated spots) and ulcers. The vesicular state often appears as a blister, which later coalesces, ulcerates, and encrusts (Fig. 34-4). Influenza-like symptoms may occur 3 or 4 days after the lesions appear. Often inguinal lymphadenopathy (enlarged lymph nodes in the groin), minor temperature elevation, malaise, headache, myalgia (aching muscles), and dysuria (pain on urination) are noted. Pain is evident during the first week and then decreases. The lesions subside in about 2 weeks unless secondary infection occurs.

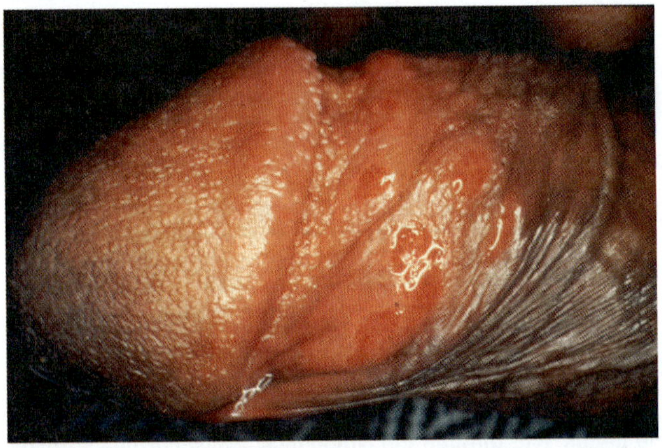

FIGURE 34-4 Herpes simplex may manifest as a painful open ulcer or cluster of superficial vesicles (fluid-filled) with an erythematous base. (From Goodheart, H. [2003]. *Goodheart's photoguide of common skin disorders*. Lippincott Williams & Wilkins.)

The gold standard for HSV diagnosis is an NAAT culture of the lesion. Type-specific serologic enzyme immunoassays (EIAs) can diagnose HSV; low index values of less than 3.0 should have confirmatory testing by Western blot (Workowski et al., 2021). For many, the diagnosis of HSV comes with emotional distress and sigma necessitating emotional support and reassurance.

Medical Management

There is currently no cure for HSV infection; treatment is aimed at relieving the symptoms. Antiviral dosing varies, depending on primary, recurrent, or suppressive management. Management goals include preventing the spread of infection, making patients comfortable, decreasing potential health risks, and initiating a counseling and education program. The antiviral agents acyclovir, valacyclovir, and famciclovir are recommended to suppress the viral load and decrease recurrence and shedding (Workowski et al., 2021).

Nursing Management

Patient education is paramount in preventing the transmission of HSV. Counseling regarding suppressive therapy should be offered to patients who have frequent recurrences (six or more recurrences per year) and has been shown to decrease the risk of recurrence by 75% (Dinulos, 2021). The nurse informs patients of their potential to transmit the virus without symptoms or lesions. In addition, patients have a moral and potentially legal obligation to disclose their diagnosis to sexual partners. Moreover, the use of barrier methods to prevent the transmission is imperative. Often, emotional support is needed for the patient who is diagnosed with HSV since herpes can be present without symptoms for years (Workowski et al., 2021).

Concept Mastery Alert

HSV can be transmitted whether lesions are present or not. A patient's consistent use of condoms with sexual activity is a measure to reduce the risk of transmission and recurrences.

Complications

Rarely, complications may arise from extragenital spread of HSV, such as to the buttocks, upper thighs, or even the eyes as a result of touching lesions and then touching other areas. Patients should be advised to wash their hands after contact with lesions. Other potential problems are aseptic meningitis, neonatal transmission, and severe emotional stress related to the diagnosis.

FEMALE REPRODUCTIVE INFECTIONS ASSOCIATED WITH SEXUAL ACTIVITY

PELVIC INFLAMMATORY DISEASE

PID is an inflammatory condition of the pelvic cavity that may begin with cervicitis (inflammation of the uterine cervix) and may involve the uterus (endometritis), fallopian tubes (salpingitis), ovaries (oophoritis), pelvic peritoneum, or pelvic vascular system. Infection may be acute, subacute, recurrent, or chronic and localized or widespread, and infection usually is caused by bacteria but may be attributed to a virus, fungus, or parasite. Gonorrheal and chlamydial organisms are the most likely causes.

Pathophysiology

PID arises from a polymicrobial infection that ascends upward from the vagina and into the uterus, fallopian tubes, and peritoneal cavity. In bacterial infections that occur after childbirth or abortion, pathogens are disseminated directly through the tissues that support the uterus by way of the lymphatics and blood vessels.

In gonorrheal infections, the gonococci pass through the cervical canal and into the uterus, where the environment, especially during menstruation, allows them to multiply rapidly and spread to the fallopian tubes and into the pelvis (see Fig. 34-3B). Usually the infection is bilateral.

Pelvic infection is caused most commonly by sexual transmission but also can occur with invasive procedures, such as endometrial biopsy, surgical abortion, hysteroscopy, or insertion of an intrauterine device (IUD). Bacterial vaginosis (BV), a vaginal infection, may predispose AFAB people to pelvic infection.

Figures 34-3 and 34-5 illustrate the path that organisms can travel from the vagina to the sterile peritoneum, resulting in peritonitis (inflammation of the peritoneum).

Risk Factors

Risk factors for PID include early age at first intercourse, multiple sexual partners, frequent intercourse, intercourse without condoms, intercourse with a partner with an STI, and a history of STIs or previous pelvic infection (CDC, 2021).

Clinical Manifestations and Assessment

Symptoms of pelvic infection usually begin with vaginal discharge, **dyspareunia** (painful sexual intercourse), lower abdominal pelvic pain, and tenderness that occurs after menses. Pain may increase with voiding or with defecation. The minimal criteria for diagnosis and treatment include one or more of the following:

- Uterine tenderness
- Adnexal tenderness (adnexa are the "appendages" of the uterus, namely the ovaries, fallopian tubes, and ligaments that hold the uterus in place)
- Cervical motion tenderness

Other symptoms include fever, general malaise, anorexia, nausea, headache, and possibly vomiting (CDC, 2021).

Medical Management

AFAB patients with mild infections may be treated as outpatients with ceftriaxone IM and doxycycline with metronidazole, but hospitalization may be necessary if a patient is nonresponsive to medication, if a surgical emergency (e.g., appendicitis) or abscess formation is suspected, or if the patient is pregnant and salpingitis (inflammation of the fallopian tubes) is suspected (CDC, 2021). Intensive therapy includes bed rest, IV fluids, and IV antibiotic therapy. If the patient has abdominal distention or **ileus** (temporary arrest of intestinal peristalsis), nasogastric intubation and suction are initiated. Careful monitoring of vital signs and symptoms assists in evaluating the status of the infection. Treatment of sexual partners is necessary to prevent reinfection.

Nursing Management

A hospitalized patient is maintained on bed rest and usually is placed in the semi-Fowler position to facilitate dependent drainage. The nurse administers analgesic agents as prescribed for pain relief. Heat applied safely to the abdomen also may provide some pain relief and comfort. On an outpatient basis, confirming patient follow-up 3 days after treatment is imperative to assess symptom abatement.

Patient teaching consists of explaining how pelvic infections occur, how they can be controlled and avoided, and

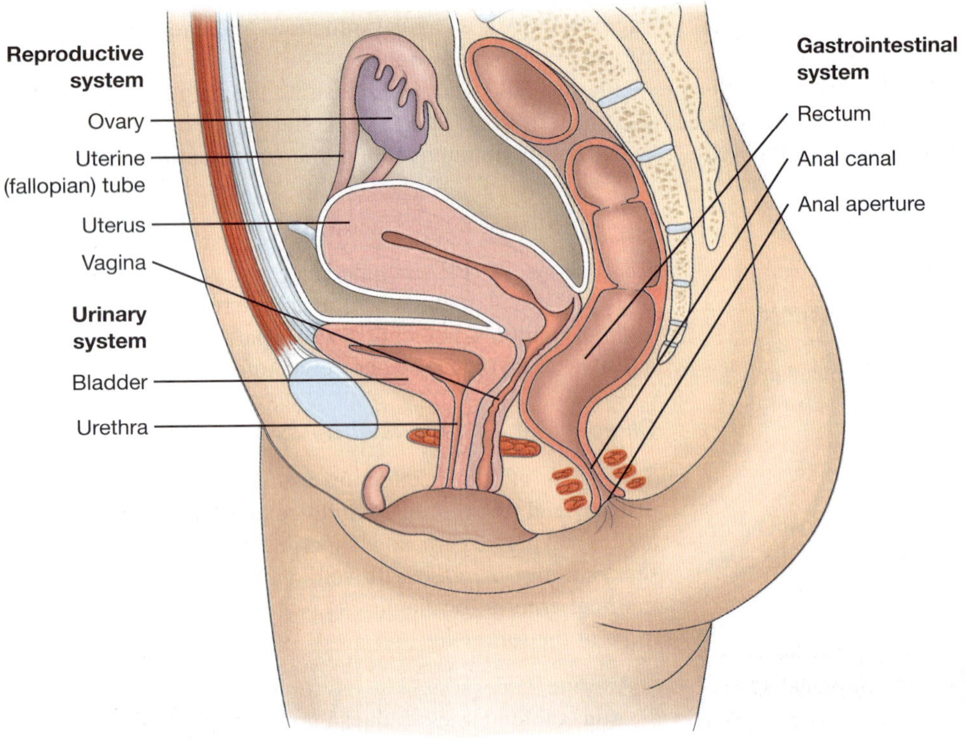

FIGURE 34-5 Assigned female at birth anatomy. Note the relationship of the reproductive organs to the pelvic peritoneum.

their signs and symptoms. All patients who have had PID need to be informed of the signs and symptoms of ectopic pregnancy (pain, abnormal bleeding, delayed menses, faintness, dizziness, and shoulder pain) because they are prone to this complication.

Complications

PID can result in tubo-ovarian abscess, recurrent disease, pelvic or generalized peritonitis, strictures, fallopian tube obstruction, ectopic pregnancy, and infertility. Adhesions are common and often result in chronic pelvic pain. Other complications include bacteremia with septic shock and thrombophlebitis with possible embolization.

BACTERIAL VAGINOSIS (BV)

The vagina is protected against infection by its normally low pH (3.5 to 4.5), which is maintained in part by *Lactobacillus acidophilus*, the dominant bacteria in a healthy vaginal ecosystem. These bacteria suppress the growth of anaerobes (occurring in the absence of free oxygen) and produce lactic acid, maintaining normal pH. Factors that may initiate or predispose a patient to infections include contact with an infected partner and wearing tight, nonabsorbent, and heat- and moisture-retaining clothing. BV and trichomoniasis are two vulvovaginal infections that are sexually associated.

Pathophysiology

BV is caused by an alteration in the vaginal microbiome, an overgrowth of anaerobic bacteria, including *Gardnerella vaginalis,* and an absence of **lactobacilli**. It is characterized by a fish-like odor that is particularly noticeable after sexual intercourse or during menstruation as a result of an increase in vaginal pH. Usually it is accompanied by a heavier-than-normal discharge.

Risk Factors

Douching, multiple sex partners of any gender, tobacco use, and sexual activity in general are risk factors for BV (Clinical Overview, 2022; Kenyon et al., 2018).

Clinical Manifestations and Assessment

Although more prevalent with menses, BV can occur throughout the menstrual cycle and can be asymptomatic. Discharge is thin, milk-like, and gray to yellowish white and smoothly coats the vaginal walls. The fish-like odor can be detected before or after adding a drop of potassium hydroxide to a glass slide with a sample of vaginal discharge. Under the microscope, vaginal cells are coated with bacteria and are described as *clue cells.* Usually the pH of the discharge is greater than 4.7 because of the amines that are released from the bacterial overgrowth. Lactobacilli, which serve as a natural host defense, are usually absent. Vaginal NAAT cultures with gram stains are also diagnostic.

Medical Management

Metronidazole administered orally twice a day for 1 week is as efficacious as a vaginal gel preparation. Clindamycin vaginal cream or ovules (oval suppositories) are also effective.

BV is not considered an STI exclusively but is associated with sexual activity. Treatment of patients' partners is not proven to be effective, but use of condoms may be helpful.

Nursing Management

Some patients complain of an unpleasant but transient metallic taste when taking metronidazole.

Clindamycin creams are oil-based and will decrease the efficacy of latex condoms. The nurse teaches proper perineal hygiene for prevention (Workowski et al., 2021).

Complications

BV is not considered a serious condition; however, it has been associated with acquisition of other STIs, premature labor, endometritis, and PID (Workowski et al., 2021).

TRICHOMONIASIS

Pathophysiology

Trichomonas vaginalis (aka "trich") is a flagellated protozoan that causes a common sexually transmitted vaginitis. It may be transmitted by an asymptomatic carrier who harbors the organism in the urogenital tract.

Clinical Manifestations and Assessment

Clinical manifestations include a vaginal discharge that is thin (sometimes frothy), yellow to yellow-green, malodorous, and very irritating. An accompanying vulvitis may result, with vulvovaginal burning and itching. Trich often causes urethritis in AMAB people. Diagnosis is made most accurately with NAAT, detecting more infections than wet mount microscopic analysis or vaginal culture (Workowski et al., 2021). Inspection with a speculum often reveals vaginal and cervical erythema (redness) with multiple small petechiae ("strawberry spots"). Testing of a trichomonal discharge demonstrates a pH greater than 4.5.

Medical and Nursing Management

For AFAB patients, the recommended treatment for trichomoniasis is metronidazole 500 mg orally twice daily for 7 days, alternatively, tinidazole 2 g once. AMAB patients receive a one-time loading dose of metronidazole 2 g. Retesting is recommended 3 months after treatment due to the high rate of reinfection (Workowski et al., 2021).

Nursing education on abstaining from sexual activity until both partners are treated is imperative.

MALE REPRODUCTIVE INFECTIONS ASSOCIATED WITH SEXUAL ACTIVITY

Several infections affect the AMAB genitourinary tract, including prostatitis (see Chapter 33), epididymitis, and orchitis, often caused by STIs.

Epididymitis usually descends from an infected prostate or urinary tract. The infection passes upward through the urethra, ejaculatory duct, and vas deferens to the epididymis and commonly develops from STIs, such as gonorrhea and chlamydia. In younger AMAB people, the major cause of epididymitis are *C. trachomatis* and *N. gonorrhoeae* (McGowan, 2021).

Orchitis is an inflammation of the testes (testicular congestion) that can be caused by a number of factors: bacterial, viral, spirochetal, parasitic, traumatic, chemical, or unknown. Bacterial causes usually spread from an associated epididymitis in AMAB people who are sexually active. Causative organisms include *N. gonorrhoeae, C. trachomatis, Escherichia coli, Klebsiella, Pseudomonas aeruginosa, Staphylococcus* species, and *Streptococcus* species. In addition, a more common cause of isolated orchitis is mumps. When postpubertal AMAB people contract mumps, about one in five develop some form of orchitis 4 to 7 days after the jaw and neck swell, and the testes may show some atrophy. Therefore mumps vaccination is recommended for postpubertal AMAB people who have not had mumps or previous mumps vaccination in childhood. Further details related to epididymitis and orchitis may be found in Chapter 33.

NURSING PROCESS
The Patient With a Sexually Transmitted Infection

ASSESSMENT

During the physical examination, the examiner looks for rashes, lesions, drainage, discharge, or swelling. Inguinal nodes are palpated to elicit tenderness and to assess swelling (Fig. 34-6). AFAB patients are examined for abdominal or uterine tenderness.

(*continued on page 1170*)

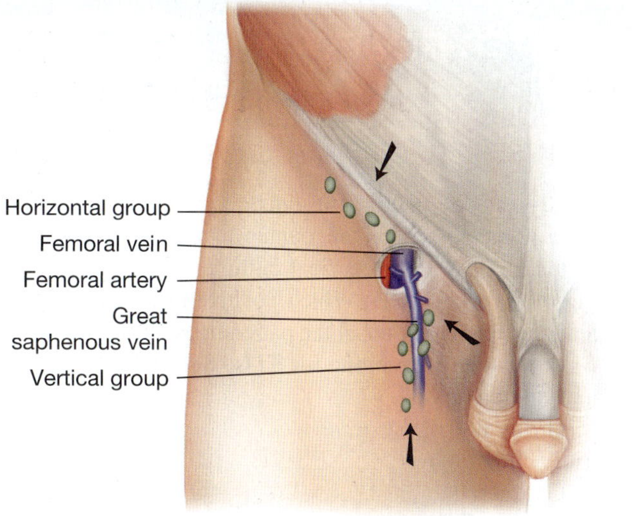

FIGURE 34-6 **Superficial inguinal lymph nodes. (Courtesy of Bickley, L. [2013].** ***Bates' pocket guide to physical examination and history taking*****. Lippincott Wolters Kluwer.)**

DIAGNOSIS

Appropriate nursing diagnoses of the patient with an STI may include:

- Deficient knowledge about the disease and risk for spread of infection and reinfection
- Anxiety related to anticipated stigmatization and to prognosis and complications
- Ineffective health maintenance related to high-risk sexual behaviors
- Risk for infection transmission related to lack of measures for STI prevention
- Risk of infection transmission from birthing parent to child during delivery

PLANNING AND GOALS

Major goals are increased patient understanding of the natural history and treatment of the infection, reduced anxiety, increased adherence to therapeutic and preventive goals, and absence of complications.

NURSING INTERVENTIONS

INCREASING KNOWLEDGE AND PREVENTING SPREAD OF DISEASE

Often, education about STIs and prevention of the spread to others are accomplished simultaneously. Explanation includes covering the causative organism, the usual course of the infection (including the interval of potential communicability to others), and possible complications. The nurse stresses the importance of following therapy as prescribed and the need to report any side effects or progression of symptoms. The nurse emphasizes that the same behaviors that led to infection with one STI increase the risk for any other STI. Methods used to contact sexual partners should be discussed. The patient should understand that until the partner has been treated, continued sexual exposure to the same person may lead to reinfection. The nurse discusses the relative value of condoms in reducing the risk for infection with STIs.

REDUCING ANXIETY

When appropriate, the nurse encourages the patient to discuss anxieties and fear associated with the diagnosis, treatment, or prognosis. Patients may need help in planning discussion with partners. If the patient is especially apprehensive about this aspect, referral to a social worker or other specialist may be appropriate.

INCREASING COMPLIANCE

In group settings or in a one-to-one setting, open discussion about STI information facilitates patient teaching. Discomfort can be reduced by factual explanation of causes, consequences, treatments, and prevention. Patients can obtain more information by accessing the CDC website (see References and Selected Readings at the end of the chapter).

EVALUATION

Expected patient outcomes may include the following:

1. Understands infection and treatment:
   a. Verbalizes understanding of infectious process
   b. Demonstrates adherence to medications, barriers, and behaviors
2. Absence of complications, such as ectopic pregnancy, infertility, neurosyphilis, gonococcal meningitis/arthritis, and prostatitism

CHAPTER REVIEW

NCLEX-Style Review Questions

1. A 22-year-old patient presents requesting STI testing after a recent sexual encounter ended with a broken condom. They have cervical cultures but declined having blood work done. Which positive test results would lead the nurse to counsel the patient to seek further blood work related to screening for STIs? Select all that apply.

a. Candida yeast
b. Group B *Streptococcus*
c. Trichomoniasis
d. Gardnerella
e. Chlamydia trachomatis

2. A 16-year-old patient presents with recurrent painful vulvar lesions. The nurse obtains subsequent test results from the patient's pelvic evaluation and confirms the identification of HSV-2. What counseling is most appropriate for this patient? Select all that apply.

a. HSV-2 is self-limiting and will go away again on its own; no medication needed.
b. HSV-2 can be transmitted and acquired without obvious symptoms or sores.
c. A blood test can determine if this is a new infection or subsequent outbreak.
d. Stress caused the sores; exercise and stress management will prevent them.
e. HSV-2 is always transmitted sexually.

3. A 29-year-old patient presents with pelvic pain, fever, and irregular bleeding. Lungs are clear, BS + in all 4 quadrants, Hct of 45%. The patient has been trying to get pregnant and fears they are is having a miscarriage. Upon examination, the patient yells when their uterus is palpated bimanually and almost jumps off the table with cervical motion tenderness. The pregnancy test is negative. In Column 1, select all the symptoms that are concerning; in Column 2, select the one likely cause of the patient's issues; and in Column 3, select what nursing interventions are most appropriate for this patient.

Select All that Apply	Select One	Select All that Apply
Pelvic pain	Bowel perforation	Reassure the patient that they are not pregnant.
Cervical tenderness	Appendicitis	Refer patient to a fertility specialist.
Hct 45%	Pelvic inflammatory disease	Administer the antibiotics as prescribed.
BS in all 4 quadrants	Ectopic pregnancy	Apply heat safely to the abdomen to provide some pain relief and comfort.
Fever		Place the patient in the semi-Fowler position.

4. A 26-year-old patient recently had a colposcopy that detected cervical dysplasia and HPV types 16 and 18, necessitating the removal of part of their cervix. The patient returns for their postoperative follow-up appointment and says, "I'm glad the cancer thing is over and I don't have to come back again for a long time." Which nursing response is most appropriate? Select all that apply.

a. "You are fortunate the cancer was caught early and you healed fast."
b. "You still need to return for frequent Pap tests to monitor your cervix."
c. "Good for you, not smoking helps keep the HPV away for good."
d. "There will be a problem getting pregnant now after your surgery."
e. "You should use condoms or dental dams regularly for safer sex"

5. A 24-year-old patient complains about an ulcer on the shaft of their penis as well as fever and enlarged nodes in the inguinal region. The patient is diagnosed with syphilis and discharged after receiving one dose of penicillin IM. Which comments made by the patient would alert the nurse of the need to review the management plan with this patient? Select all that apply.

a. "I am aware that all my sexual partners will need to be treated."
b. "I know that my blood work (VDRL or RPR titer) may take 12 months to become negative."
c. "This disease cannot be cured, and I will likely develop complications."
d. "I am aware that I must wear a condom every time I have sex."
e. "If my pregnant partner also tests positive for syphilis, they will not be able to transmit it to the baby."

REFERENCES AND SELECTED READINGS

References and selected readings associated with this chapter can be found on the website that accompanies the book. Visit **http://thepoint.lww.com/Honan3e** to access the references and other additional resources associated with this chapter.

UNIT TEN

Problems Related to Immunologic Function

A 65-year-old patient with a history of diabetes and hyperlipidemia has tested positive with a home rapid antigen test for COVID-19. The patient is complaining of cough, fever, and fatigue that began 2 days ago, and is not immunized against COVID-19 but would like to discuss treatment for this illness. The medication list includes metformin, atorvastatin, and fluoxetine.

- **What medications would the nurse expect the health care provider to order for this patient?**
- **How do the patient's past medical history and current medications affect COVID-19 treatment options?**
- **What are important components of nursing management for this patient?**

CHAPTER 35

Nursing Assessment: Immune Function

Mary E. Bartlett

Learning Objectives

After reading this chapter, you will be able to:

1. Discuss the body's general immune response.
2. Discuss the stages of the immune response.
3. Differentiate humoral and cellular immune responses.
4. Complete an assessment on the function of the immune system.

The most basic abilities of the human body to protect itself from disease and illness derive from the various components of the immune system. The term ***immunity*** refers to the body's specific protective response to an invading foreign agent or organism. The immune system functions as the body's defense mechanism against invasion and allows a rapid response to foreign substances in a specific manner. Responses occur at the genetic and cellular levels.

Immune function is affected by a variety of factors, such as central nervous system integrity; emotional status; medications; and the stress of illness, trauma, or surgery. Dysfunctions involving the immune system occur across the lifespan. When the functions of the immune system are diminished or disturbed, autoimmune and other disorders may develop. Disorders of the immune system may stem from excesses or deficiencies of immunocompetent cells, alterations in the function of these cells, immunologic attack on self-antigens, or inappropriate or exaggerated responses to specific antigens (Table 35-1).

ANATOMY AND PHYSIOLOGY OVERVIEW

One of the most effective defense mechanisms is the body's capacity to equip itself rapidly with weapons (antibodies) individually designed to meet each new invader (antigens). Antibodies react with antigens by:

- Coating antigens' surfaces
- Neutralizing the antigens if they are toxins
- Precipitating the antigens out of solution if they are dissolved

Although this system is normally protective, in some cases, the body produces inappropriate or exaggerated responses to specific antigens, and the result is an allergic or hypersensitivity reaction. Another example of an inappropriately robust immune reaction occurs with the cytokine storm of COVID-19. Before looking at immunity and immune response more closely, it is helpful to understand the basic components of the immune system.

Anatomy of the Immune System

The immune system is composed of an integrated collection of various cell types, each with a designated functional role in defending against infection and invasion by other organisms. Supporting this system are molecules that are responsible for the interactions, modulations, and regulation of the system. These molecules and cells participate in specific interactions with immunogenic **epitopes** or antigenic determinants, which are substances that, when introduced into the body, stimulate the production of an antibody. These epitopes are present on foreign materials and initiate a series of actions in a host, including the inflammatory response, the lysis of microbial agents, and the disposal of foreign toxins. The major components of the immune system include the bone marrow; the white blood cells (WBCs); the lymphoid tissues (including the thymus gland, the spleen, the lymph nodes, and the tonsils and adenoids); and similar tissues in the gastrointestinal (GI), respiratory, and reproductive systems (Fig. 35-1).

Stem cells (undifferentiated cells) in the bone marrow generate lymphocytes (a type of WBC; Fig. 35-2). There are two types of lymphocytes: **B lymphocytes (B cells)**, which mature in the bone marrow and enter the circulation as precursors to antibody-secreting cells or memory cells, and **T lymphocytes (T cells)**, which move from the bone marrow to the thymus, where they mature into several kinds of cells with different helper functions (Fig. 35-3).

TABLE **35-1 Immune System Disorders**

Disorder	Description
Autoimmunity	Normal protective immune response paradoxically turns against or attacks the body, leading to tissue damage
Hypersensitivity	Body produces inappropriate or exaggerated responses to specific antigens
Gammopathies	Immunoglobulins are overproduced
Immune Deficiencies	
Primary	Deficiency results from improper development of immune cells or tissues; usually congenital or inherited
Secondary	Deficiency results from some interference with an already developed immune system; usually acquired later in life

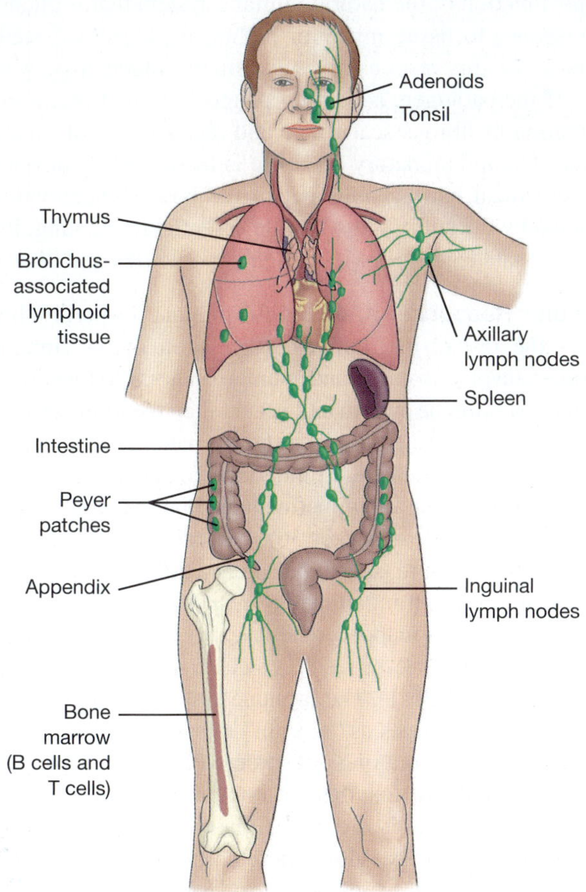

FIGURE 35-1 **Central and peripheral lymphoid organs and tissues. (From Grossman, S., Porth, C. M., Conelius, J., Gerard, S. O., Moriber, N., O'Shea, E. R., & Wheeler, K. [2014].** ***Porth's pathophysiology: Concepts of altered health states*****. Wolters Kluwer Health/Lippincott Williams & Wilkins.)**

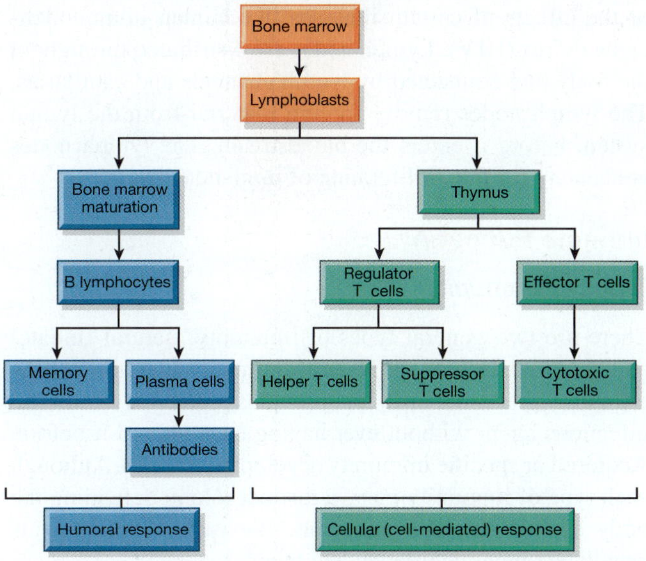

FIGURE 35-2 **Development of cells of the immune system.**

The thymus is a double-lobed organ found in the upper mediastinum. The spleen is located in the left upper quadrant of the abdomen. It is composed of red pulp (where old and injured red blood cells [RBCs] are destroyed) and white pulp (which contains concentrations of lymphocytes), and it acts like a filter. While it is possible to live without a spleen, its loss affects future health care decisions about immunization

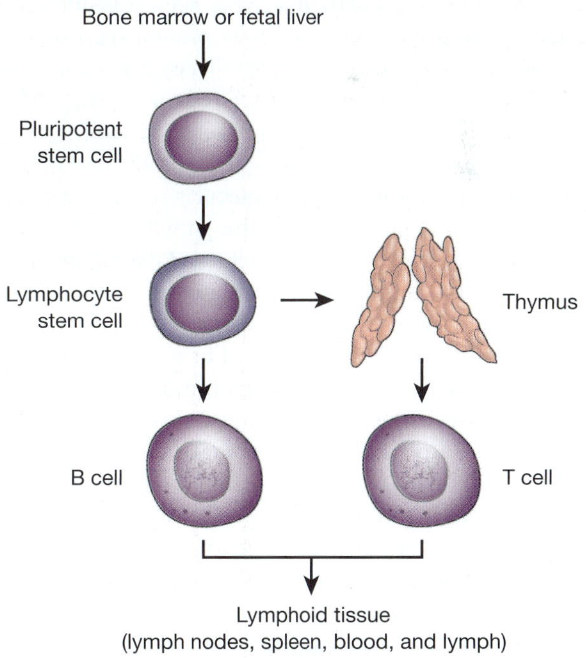

FIGURE 35-3 **Lymphocytes originate from stem cells in the bone marrow. B lymphocytes mature in the bone marrow before entering the bloodstream, whereas T lymphocytes mature in the thymus, where they also differentiate into cells with various functions. (From Grossman, S., Porth, C. M., Conelius, J., Gerard, S. O., Moriber, N., O'Shea, E. R., & Wheeler, K. [2014].** ***Porth's pathophysiology: Concepts of altered health states*****. Wolters Kluwer Health/Lippincott Williams & Wilkins.)**

or the effects of certain illnesses like human immunodeficiency virus (HIV). Lymph nodes are distributed throughout the body and connected by lymph channels and capillaries. The lymph nodes remove foreign material from the lymph system before it enters the bloodstream. The lymph nodes are centers for the proliferation of immune cells.

Immune Function

Types of Immunity

There are two general types of immunity: natural (innate) and acquired (adaptive). Natural immunity is a nonspecific immunity present at birth that provides protection against an infectious agent without ever having encountered it before. Acquired or specific immunity develops after birth. Although each type of immunity plays a distinct role in defending the body against harmful pathogens, the various components usually act in an interdependent manner.

Natural Immunity

Natural immunity provides a nonspecific response to any foreign pathogen, regardless of the pathogen's composition. Because of its lack of specificity, natural immunity maintains a broad spectrum of defense against and resistance to infection. The basis of this defense mechanism is the ability to distinguish between "self" and "nonself." Recent research in transplantation medicine demonstrates that this is a very simplistic differentiation. **Natural killer** (NK) cells also recognize "missing self" cells that have been transformed or infected by pathogens and no longer present the usual cell membrane markers (Delves, 2021). Thus, NK cells represent both innate and acquired immune characteristics (Mujal et al., 2021). Natural (innate) immunity coordinates the initial response to pathogens through the production of cytokines, which are hormone-like molecules released by cells; they have a profound impact on the growth, development, and activation of immune system cells and the inflammatory response. Natural immunity also responds to pathogens via other effector molecules, which either activate cells for control of the pathogen (by elimination) or promote the development of the acquired immune response. The cells involved in this response include macrophages, dendritic cells, and NK cells. These cells directly recognize and respond to a wide variety of pathogens long before the development of antigen-specific acquired immunity. The early events in this immune response are critical in determining the nature of the adaptive immune response. Innate immune mechanisms can be divided into two stages: immediate (generally occurring within 4 hours) and delayed (occurring between 4 and 96 hours after exposure).

The development of immunity occurs via physical and chemical barriers, inflammatory response, and immune response.

Physical and Chemical Barriers. Activation of the natural immunity response is enhanced by processes inherent in physical and chemical barriers. The processes prevent or delay the entry into the body of various pathogens before infection can develop. Physical surface barriers include intact skin, mucous membranes, and cilia of the respiratory tract, which prevent pathogens from gaining access to the body. The cilia of the respiratory tract, along with coughing and sneezing responses, filter and clear pathogens from the upper respiratory tract before they can invade the body further. Chemical barriers, such as mucus, acidic gastric secretions, enzymes in tears and saliva, and substances in sebaceous and sweat secretions, act in a nonspecific way to destroy invading bacteria and fungi. In addition, the actions of digestive enzymes, acidic conditions, and the secretion of defensins (small peptides that quickly kill gram-negative and gram-positive microorganisms by disrupting the microbial membrane) destroy pathogens present in food or swallowed mucus (Norris & Tuan, 2020). Viruses are countered by other means, such as **interferon** (IFN). IFN, one type of biologic response modifier, is a nonspecific viricidal protein that is naturally produced by the body and is capable of activating other components of the immune system.

Inflammatory Response. The inflammatory response is a major function of the natural immune system that is elicited in response to tissue injury or pathogens. Chemical mediators assist this response by minimizing blood loss, walling off the pathogen, activating phagocytes, and promoting formation of fibrous scar tissue and regeneration of injured tissue. The inflammatory response is facilitated by physical and chemical barriers inherent in the body. Inflammation, denoted by the suffix "-itis," while essential for healing, in a chronic state leads to a wide range of pathology and illness.

Immune Response. A successful immune response eliminates the responsible antigen. Regulation of the immune response involves balance and counterbalance. Dysfunction of the natural immune system can occur when the immune components are inactivated or when they remain active long after their effects are beneficial. Immunodeficiencies are characterized by inactivation or impairment of immune components (described further in Chapter 36). Disorders with an inflammatory component (e.g., asthma, allergy, arthritis) are characterized by persistent inflammatory responses. In some cases, the body produces inappropriate or exaggerated responses to specific antigens, and the result is an allergic or hypersensitivity reaction (Box 35-1). The immune system's recognition of the body's own tissues as "foreign" rather than as self is the basis for many autoimmune disorders (refer to Chapters 37 and 38). Despite the fact that the immune response is critical to the prevention of disease, it must be well controlled to curtail immunopathology. Most microbial infections, including COVID-19, induce an inflammatory response mediated by T cells and cytokines, which, in excess, can cause tissue damage. Because COVID-19 infects respiratory tissue, inflammatory responses such as edema leads to pneumonia and acute respiratory distress syndrome (ARDS). As the storm builds,

BOX 35-1 Focus on Pathophysiology

Allergic Reaction

An allergic reaction is a manifestation of tissue injury resulting from interaction between an antigen and an antibody. Allergy is an inappropriate and often harmful response of the immune system to substances that are normally harmless. In this case, the inappropriate substance is termed an *allergen*.

Mast cells located in tissues throughout the body can be activated by a variety of stimuli, causing immediate allergic inflammation. The binding of the antigen and antibodies on the mast cells causes the release of mediators that affect blood vessel, smooth muscle, and glandular secretions. The powerful chemical mediators released from the mast cells cause a sequence of physiologic events, resulting in symptoms of immediate hypersensitivity. There are two types of chemical mediators: primary and secondary. Primary mediators are preformed and are found in mast cells or basophils. Secondary mediators are inactive precursors that are formed or released in response to primary mediators (e.g., leukotrienes, bradykinin, and serotonin).

When in contact with an allergen, the body produces large amounts of IgE, thus causing a hypersensitivity or allergic response (see figure on next page). IgE-producing cells are located in the respiratory and intestinal mucosa. Two or more IgE molecules bind together to an allergen and trigger mast cells or basophils to release chemical mediators, such as histamine and leukotrienes. Maximal intensity of histamine release is reached within about 15 minutes after antigen contact. Effects of histamine release include erythema; localized edema in the form of wheals; pruritus; contraction of bronchial smooth muscle, resulting in wheezing and bronchospasm; widespread vasodilation, capillary permeability, and potentially catastrophic vascular collapse; and increased secretion of gastric and mucosal cells, resulting in diarrhea. Histamine action results from stimulation of histamine-1 (H_1) and histamine-2 (H_2) receptors found on different types of lymphocytes, particularly T-lymphocyte suppressor cells and basophils. H_1 receptors are found predominantly on bronchiolar and vascular smooth muscle cells; H_2 receptors are found on gastric parietal cells.

Certain medications are categorized by their action at these receptors. Diphenhydramine is an example of an antihistamine, a medication that displays an affinity for H_1 receptors. Cimetidine and ranitidine target H_2 receptors to inhibit gastric secretions in cases of peptic ulcer disease.

Leukotrienes, another chemical mediator released by mucosal mast cells, cause smooth muscle contraction, bronchial constriction, mucus secretion in the airways, and the typical wheal-and-flare reaction of the skin. Compared with histamine, leukotrienes are 100 to 1,000 times more potent in causing bronchospasm. Many manifestations of inflammation can be attributed in part to leukotrienes. Medications categorized as leukotriene antagonists or modifiers block the synthesis or action of leukotrienes and prevent the signs and symptoms associated with asthma.

Hypersensitivity

A hypersensitivity reaction is an abnormal, heightened reaction to any type of stimulus. Usually it does not occur with the first exposure to an allergen, but it is a reflection of excessive or atypical immune responses. To promote understanding of the immunopathogenesis of disease, hypersensitivity reactions have been classified into four specific types of reactions: anaphylactic (type 1) hypersensitivity, cytotoxic (type II) hypersensitivity, immune complex (type III) hypersensitivity, and delayed-type (type IV) hypersensitivity. Most allergies are identified as either type I or type IV hypersensitivity reactions.

Anaphylactic (Type I) Hypersensitivity

The most severe form of hypersensitivity reaction or immune-mediated reaction is **anaphylaxis**. An unanticipated severe allergic reaction that is often explosive in onset, anaphylaxis is characterized by edema in many tissues, including the larynx, and often is accompanied by hypotension, bronchospasm, and cardiovascular collapse in severe cases. Mast cells in any organ system may be involved; however, the primary foci are the cardiovascular, skin, respiratory, and gastrointestinal systems (sites where mast cells are abundant; Graham, 2022). Type I or anaphylactic hypersensitivity is an immediate reaction beginning within minutes of exposure to an antigen. This reaction is mediated by IgE antibodies and typically occurs on re-exposure to a specific antigen. If chemical mediators continue to be released, a delayed reaction may occur up to 24 hours after allergen exposure. Refer to Chapter 37 for more details on anaphylaxis.

Cytotoxic (Type II) Hypersensitivity

Type II, or cytotoxic, hypersensitivity occurs when the system mistakenly identifies a normal constituent of the body as foreign. This reaction may be the result of a cross-reacting antibody, possibly leading to damage to cells and tissues. Several disorders are associated with type II hypersensitivity reactions, including myasthenia gravis, in which the body mistakenly generates antibodies against normal nerve ending receptors; or Goodpasture syndrome, in which antibodies are generated against lung and renal tissue, producing lung damage and kidney failure; or they may be associated with drug-induced immune hemolytic anemia, Rh-hemolytic disease of the newborn, and incompatibility reactions in blood transfusions.

Immune Complex (Type III) Hypersensitivity

Type III, or immune complex, hypersensitivity involves immune complexes that are formed when antigens bind to antibodies. These complexes are cleared from the circulation by phagocytic action. If these type III complexes are deposited in tissues or vascular endothelium, two factors contribute to injury: the increased amount of circulating complexes and the presence of vasoactive amines. As a result, there is an increase in vascular permeability and tissue injury. The joints and kidneys are particularly susceptible to this type of injury. Type III hypersensitivity is associated with systemic lupus erythematosus, rheumatoid arthritis, certain types of nephritis, and some types of bacterial endocarditis.

(*continued*)

BOX 35-1

Focus on Pathophysiology (*continued*)

Delayed-Type (Type IV) Hypersensitivity

Type IV, or delayed-type hypersensitivity, also known as cellular hypersensitivity, occurs 24–72 hours after exposure to an allergen. It is mediated by sensitized T cells and macrophages. An example of this reaction is the effect of an intradermal injection of tuberculin antigen or purified protein derivative (PPD). Sensitized T cells react with the antigen at or near the injection site. Lymphokines are released and attract, activate, and retain macrophages at the site. These macrophages then release lysozymes, causing tissue damage. Edema and fibrin are responsible for the positive tuberculin reaction.

Another example of a type IV hypersensitivity reaction is contact dermatitis resulting from exposure to allergens, such as cosmetics, adhesive tape, topical agents (e.g., povidone-iodine), medication additives, and plant toxins. The most common immune-mediated reaction to local anesthetics is a type IV hypersensitivity reaction. The primary exposure results in sensitization. Re-exposure causes a hypersensitivity reaction with resultant symptoms, such as pruritus, erythema, and raised lesions.

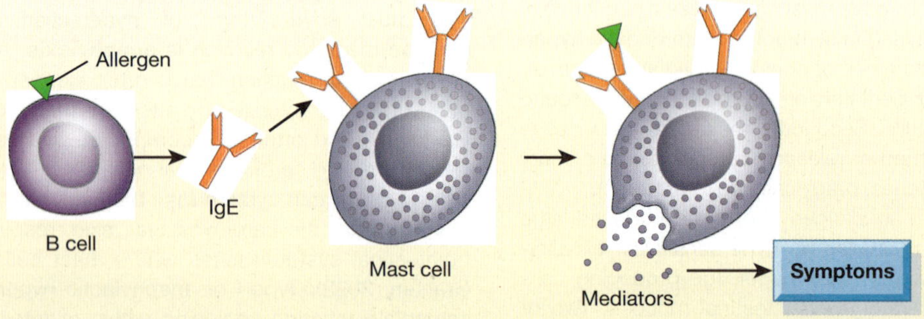

Allergen triggers the B cell to make IgE antibody, which attaches to the mast cell. When that allergen reappears; it binds to the IgE and triggers the mast cell to release its chemicals. (Courtesy of the U.S. Department of Health and Human Services, National Institutes of Health.)

cytokine release affects other organs including the brain, heart, blood vessels, kidneys, and liver with further effects of inflammation. During the first waves of COVID-19, patients died of multi-organ failure brought on by the over-activation of cytokines, the cytokine storm, and other immune system elements (Montazersahe et al., 2022). Figure 35-4 details the clinical picture of cytokine storm. Regulatory mechanisms must be in place to suppress or halt the immune response in order to minimize tissue damage. This is achieved mainly by the transformation of growth factors that inhibit macrophage activation. In some cases, T-cell activation is so overwhelming that these mechanisms fail, and pathology results. With COVID-19, research into "long COVID" focuses on patients with persistent symptoms from a prior COVID-19 infection. Knowledge of this basic pathophysiology of the cytokine storm enables understanding of the global effect on patients' acute and chronic disease trajectories (Peluso, 2022). Since the initial infection by COVID-19 affects the brain and blood vessels, symptoms of long COVID-19 such as brain "fog," fatigue, and postural orthostatic tachycardic syndrome (POTS) make pathophysiologic sense.

Pearls for Practice

Postural orthostatic tachycardic syndrome is an unusually significant increase in heart rate (≥30 bpm) that occurs when a person changes position such as lying to standing position within 10 minutes in the absence of orthostatic hypotension (Zhao & Tran, 2022).

One of the most actively researched areas of immunology involves the inflammatory response and its contribution to chronic conditions, such as diabetes, autoimmune disease, and cancer. Previously, when cells underwent apoptosis (programmed cell death) or phagocytosis (the engulfing of microorganisms or other cells and foreign particles by phagocytes), the death of cells was thought to be a null response that did not contribute to further actions by the immune system. Research into the role of damage-associated molecular pattern molecules (DAMPs) changes this belief and contributes to the evidence that inflammation may be the most important factor of any disease process. DAMPs, also known as alarmins, consist of a wide variety of proteins and other byproducts of cell damage that trigger cascading events in the inflammatory response. Recent research demonstrates a relationship between the presence of DAMPs and the severity of infection with COVID-19 (Parthasarathy et al., 2022). One of the reasons that people who are obese are more likely to have complications due to COVID-19 infection relates to adipose tissue as an endocrine organ. The higher the body mass index, the more likely a person will have a hyperacute immune response to infection triggering the cytokine storm. The growing body of research about COVID-19, the immune response, and the role of inflammation contributes to better understanding of chronic illness and its prevention (Pahwa, 2021). Weight loss continues to provide the most effective means to prevent and treat chronic illnesses.

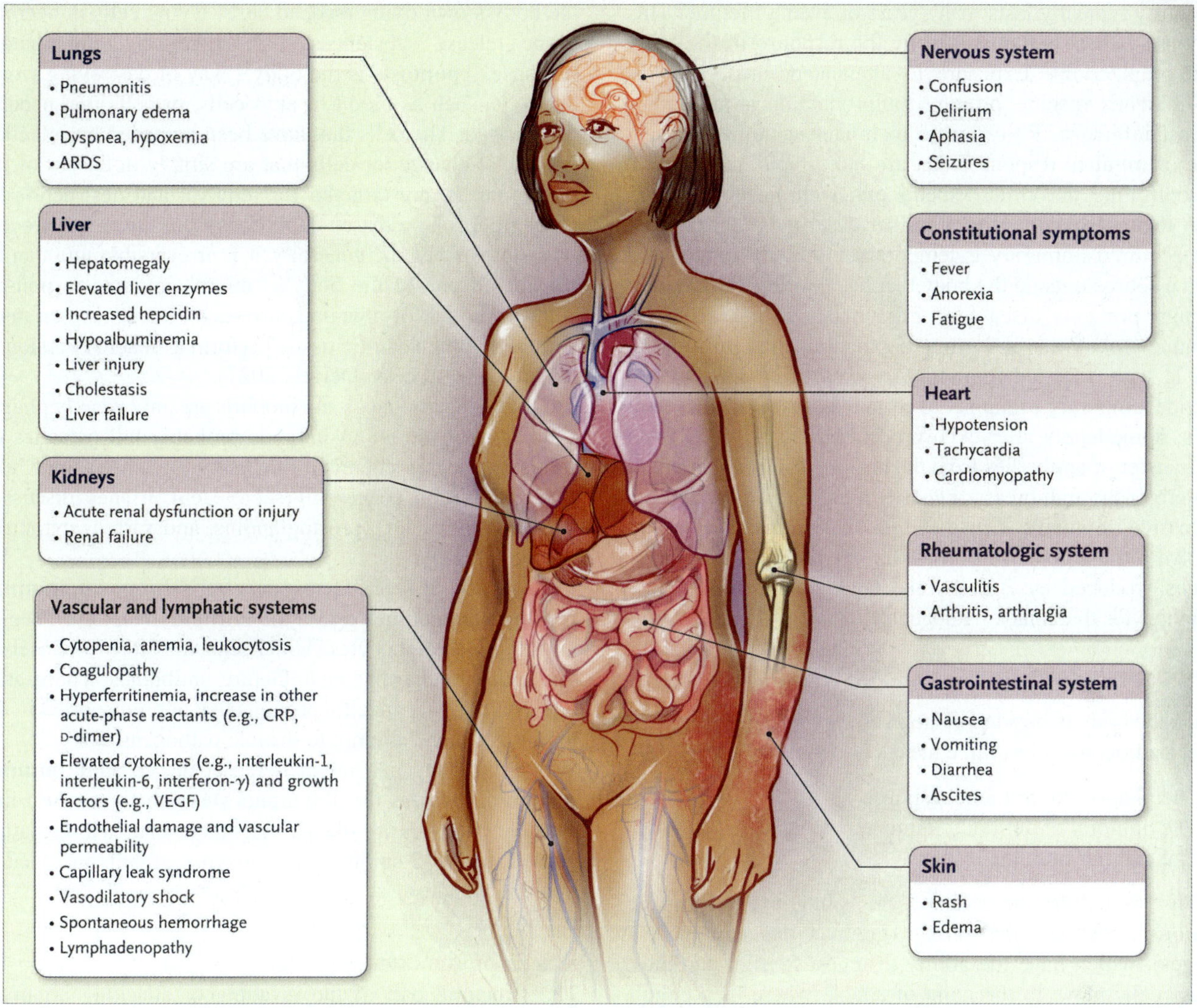

FIGURE 35-4 Clinical picture of cytokine storm, which is an umbrella term encompassing several disorders of immune dysregulation characterized by constitutional symptoms, systemic inflammation, and multiorgan dysfunction that can lead to multiorgan failure if inadequately treated. (Reproduced with permission from Fajgenbaum, D. C., & June, C. H. [2020]. Cytokine storm. *The New England Journal of Medicine*, *383*[23], 2255–2273; Figure 1. https://doi.org/10.1056/NEJMra2026131)

Acquired Immunity

Acquired immunity—immunologic responses acquired during life but not present at birth—usually develops as a result of exposure to an antigen through immunization (vaccination) or by contracting a disease, both of which generate a protective immune response. Weeks or months after initial exposure to the disease or vaccine, the body produces an immune response that is sufficient to defend against the disease on re-exposure. In contrast to the rapid but nonspecific innate immune response, this form of immunity relies on the recognition of specific foreign antigens. The two components of the immune response are strongly interrelated. Events occurring early in infection dictate the direction of the adaptive response and activate the acquired immune effector mechanisms, which have direct feedback on the cells of the innate (natural) system. The acquired immune response is broadly divided into two mechanisms: the cell-mediated response, involving T-cell activation, and effector mechanisms, involving B-cell maturation and the production of antibodies. With the combination of innate and acquired immune responses, the body is capable of protecting itself immediately as well as against future challenges to its integrity. Current practice and thought supports our changing approach to the COVID pandemic; enough people have either been immunized, sick with COVID, or both that lifting of many isolation restrictions is possible. The change from a pandemic that demanded work and school from home, social distancing, and personal protective equipment (PPE) to the new strategy that encourages people to learn to understand and minimize their own personal risks of contracting COVID are a function of the capabilities of innate and acquired immune responses.

The two types of acquired immunity are known as active and passive. In active acquired immunity, the immunologic defenses are developed by the person's own body. This immunity typically lasts many years or even a lifetime. This response is best demonstrated by the response of the body to immunizations. Exposure to attenuated virus, such as the influenza vaccine, prompts the production of antibodies against influenza. Re-exposure to influenza initiates a cascade of immune responses that are more rapid and capable of controlling the virus. Patients either eliminate the virus from their system or have a milder case of influenza. Passive acquired immunity is temporary immunity transmitted from a source outside the body that has developed immunity through previous disease or immunization. For example, immune globulin or antiserum, obtained from the plasma of people with acquired immunity, is used in emergencies to provide temporary immunity to certain diseases, such as hepatitis, immediately after exposure. Immunity resulting from the transfer of antibodies from the birthing parent to an infant in utero or through breast or chestfeeding is another example of passive immunity. Active and passive acquired immunity involve immunologic responses that are both humoral (antibodies produced by B cells) and cellular (cell-mediated T lymphocytes that attack pathogens).

Response to Invasion

When the body is invaded or attacked by bacteria, viruses, or other pathogens, it has three means of defense:

- The phagocytic immune response
- The humoral or antibody immune response
- The cellular immune response

The first line of defense, the **phagocytic immune response**, involves the WBCs (granulocytes and macrophages), which have the ability to ingest foreign particles. These cells move to the point of attack, where they engulf and destroy the invading agents. Phagocytes also remove the body's own dying or dead cells. Dying cells in necrotic tissue release substances that trigger an inflammatory response. **Apoptosis** is the body's way of destroying worn-out cells, such as blood or skin cells, or cells that need to be renewed. The cells that have been damaged by infection or genetic change, or cells that are simply in excess of the body's needs, are targeted for removal and destruction by a subgroup of proteases called *caspase*. Once the process of apoptosis begins, generally it is irreversible and can be considered one of the body's "micro" immune responses. Nurses who perform wound care such as occurs when manually debriding necrotic tissue perform a "macro" version of this immune process (Delves, 2021).

Unlike macrophages, eosinophils are only weakly phagocytic. On activation, eosinophils probably kill parasites by releasing specific chemical mediators into the extracellular fluid. In addition, eosinophils secrete leukotrienes (discussed later in the chapter), prostaglandins, and various cytokines (Delves, 2021).

A second protective response, the **humoral immune response** (sometimes called the **antibody** response), begins with the B lymphocytes, which can transform themselves into plasma cells that manufacture antibodies. These antibodies are highly specific proteins that are transported in the bloodstream and attempt to disable pathogens.

The third mechanism of defense, the **cellular immune response**, involves the T lymphocytes, which can turn into special cytotoxic (or killer) T cells that can attack the pathogens. Table 35-2 summarizes the types of cells involved in immune response.

Basics of Immune Response

The structural part of the invading or attacking organism that is responsible for stimulating antibody production is

TABLE 35-2 Lymphocytes Involved in Immune Responses

Type of Immune Response	Cell Type	Function
Humoral	B lymphocyte	Produces antibodies or immunoglobulins (IgA, IgD, IgE, IgG, IgM)
Cellular	T lymphocyte	
	Helper T	Attacks foreign pathogens (antigens) directly Initiates and augments inflammatory response
	Helper T_1	Increases activated cytotoxic T cells
	Helper T_2	Increases B-cell antibody production
	Suppressor T	Suppresses the immune response
	Memory T	Remembers contact with an antigen and on subsequent exposures mounts an immune response
	Cytotoxic T (killer T)	Lyses cells infected with virus; plays a role in graft rejection
Nonspecific	Non-T, non–B lymphocyte (L lymphocytes)	Amplify T-cell proliferation
	Null cell	Destroys antigens already coated with antibody
	Natural killer (NK) cell (granular lymphocyte)	Defends against microorganisms and some types of malignant cells; produces cytokines

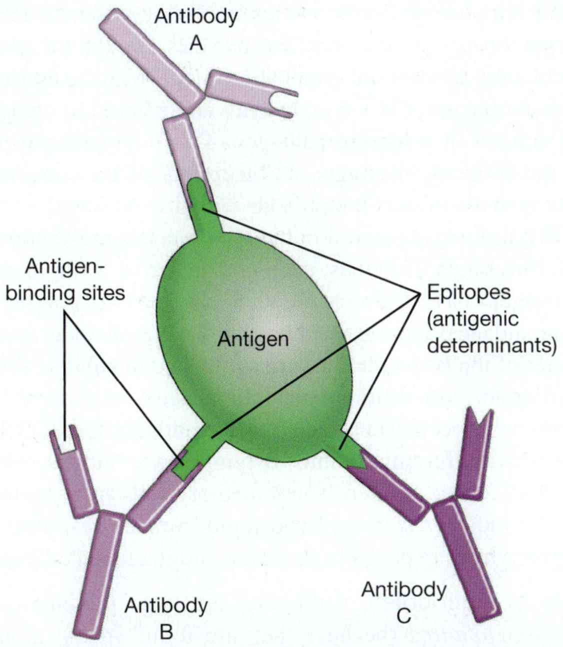

FIGURE 35-5 Complement-mediated immune responses. (Grossman, S., Porth, C. M., Conelius, J., Gerard, S. O., Moriber, N., O'Shea, E. R., & Wheeler, K. [2014]. *Porth's pathophysiology: Concepts of altered health states*. Wolters Kluwer Health/ Lippincott Williams & Wilkins.)

called an **antigen** (or an immunogen). An antigen can be a small patch of proteins on the outer surface of a microorganism. Some antigens are naturally immunogenic or able to stimulate an immune response directly. Most antigens must be coupled with other molecules to stimulate the immune response. A single bacterium or large molecule, such as a diphtheria or tetanus toxin, may have several antigens, or markers, on its surface, thus inducing the body to produce a number of different antibodies. Once produced, an antibody is released into the bloodstream and carried to the attacking organism. There, it combines with the antigen, binding with it like an interlocking piece of a jigsaw puzzle (Fig. 35-5). Currently, there are more than 200 commercial antigen tests to detect COVID-19. Most of these test for nucleocapsid proteins such as the spike protein found on the virus's surface. Many tests check for the N gene and are 100% specific. The downside of this level of specificity with COVID-19 means a single base pair mutation of the N gene by a new variant could increase the rate of false-negative tests (Centers for Disease Control and Prevention [CDC], 2022).

There are four well-defined stages in an immune response: recognition, proliferation, response, and effector.

Recognition Stage. Recognition of antigens as foreign, or nonself, by the immune system is the initiating event in any immune response. The body accomplishes recognition using lymph nodes and lymphocytes for surveillance. Lymph nodes continuously discharge lymphocytes into the bloodstream. These lymphocytes patrol the tissues and vessels that drain the areas served by that node.

Circulating lymphocytes recognize antigens on foreign surfaces through complex rearrangements of genes that produce T-cell antigen receptors (TCRs) during cell differentiation and maturation in the thymus. T cells present in primary lymphoid tissue that have not been presented with an antigen are called *naïve*, as they are capable of responding to a vast array of antigens (Delves, 2021). Macrophages play an important role in helping the circulating lymphocytes process the antigens. Both macrophages and neutrophils have receptors for antibodies and *complement* (a system of proteins found in normal blood plasma that combines with antibodies to destroy pathogens, to be discussed later in this chapter); as a result, they coat microorganisms with antibodies, complement, or both, enhancing phagocytosis. Then the engulfed microorganisms are subjected to a wide range of toxic intracellular molecules. When foreign materials enter the body, circulating lymphocytes come into physical contact with the surfaces of these materials. Upon contact with the foreign material, naïve lymphocytes, with the help of macrophages, either remove the antigen from the surface or obtain an imprint of its structure, initiating the process of acquired immunity and antigen recognition in preparation for subsequent re-exposure to the antigen (Delves, 2021).

Proliferation Stage. The circulating lymphocyte containing the antigenic message returns to the nearest lymph node. Once in the node, the sensitized lymphocyte stimulates some of the resident dormant T and B lymphocytes to enlarge, divide, and proliferate. T lymphocytes differentiate into cytotoxic (or killer) T cells, whereas B lymphocytes produce and release antibodies. Enlargement of the lymph nodes in the neck in conjunction with a sore throat is one example of the inflammatory response during immune activation.

Response Stage. In the response stage, the differentiated lymphocytes function in either a humoral or a cellular capacity. The production of antibodies by the B lymphocytes in response to a specific antigen begins the humoral response. *Humoral* refers to the fact that the antibodies are released into the bloodstream and, therefore, reside in the plasma (fluid fraction of the blood).

With the initial cellular response, the returning sensitized lymphocytes migrate to areas of the lymph node other than those areas containing lymphocytes programmed to become plasma cells. Here, they stimulate the residing lymphocytes to become cells that will attack microbes directly, rather than through the action of antibodies. These transformed lymphocytes are known as *cytotoxic (killer) T cells*. The T stands for *thymus*, signifying that, during embryologic development of the immune system, these T lymphocytes spent time in the thymus of the developing fetus. Viral rather than bacterial antigens induce a cellular response. This response is manifested by the increasing number of T lymphocytes (lymphocytosis) seen on the complete blood counts (CBC) of people with viral illnesses, such as infectious mononucleosis (cellular immunity is discussed in further detail later in this chapter).

BOX 35-2

Examples of Humoral and Cellular Immune Responses

Humoral Responses (B Cells)

- Bacterial phagocytosis and lysis
- Anaphylaxis
- Allergic hay fever and asthma
- Immune complex disease
- Bacterial and some viral infections

Cellular Responses (T Cells)

- Transplant rejection
- Delayed hypersensitivity (tuberculin reaction)
- Graft-versus-host disease
- Tumor surveillance or destruction
- Intracellular infections
- Viral, fungal, and parasitic infections

It is important for the nurse to understand that the social determinants of health impact health outcomes for our patients. With rates of STDs increasing, emphasis on sexual behaviors alone is insufficient. A concerted effort at eradicating the barriers to health will require an interprofessional approach of policy makers, health care providers, and researchers (Tapp & Hudson, 2020).

Most immune responses to antigens involve both humoral and cellular responses, although one usually predominates. For example, during transplant rejection, the cellular response predominates, whereas in cases of bacterial pneumonias and sepsis, the humoral response plays the dominant protective role (Box 35-2).

Effector Stage. In the effector stage, either the antibody of the humoral response or the cytotoxic (killer) T cell of the cellular response reaches and connects with the antigen on the surface of the foreign pathogen. The connection initiates a series of events that, in most instances, results in the total destruction of the invading microbes or the complete neutralization of the toxin. The events involve interplay of antibodies (humoral immunity), complement, and action by the cytotoxic T cells (cellular immunity). Figure 35-6 summarizes the stages of the immune response.

Humoral Immune Response

The humoral response is characterized by the production of antibodies by B lymphocytes in response to a specific antigen. Although the B lymphocyte is ultimately responsible for the production of antibodies, both the macrophages of natural immunity and the special T-cell lymphocytes of cellular immunity are involved in recognizing the foreign substance and in producing antibodies.

Antigen Recognition. B lymphocytes recognize and respond to invading antigens in more than one way. The B lymphocytes appear to respond to some antigens by triggering antibody formation directly; however, in response to other antigens, they need the assistance of T cells to trigger antibody formation. The T lymphocytes are part of a surveillance system that is dispersed throughout the body and recycles through the general circulation, tissues, and lymphatic system. With the assistance of macrophages, the T lymphocytes are believed to recognize the antigen of a foreign pathogen. The T lymphocyte picks up the antigenic message, or "blueprint," of the antigen and returns to the nearest lymph node with that message.

B lymphocytes stored in the lymph nodes are subdivided into thousands of clones, each responsive to a single group of antigens having almost identical characteristics. When the antigenic message is carried back to the lymph node, specific clones of the B lymphocyte are stimulated to enlarge, divide, proliferate, and differentiate into plasma cells capable of producing specific antibodies to the antigen. Other B lymphocytes differentiate into B-lymphocyte clones with a memory for the antigen. These memory cells are responsible for the more exaggerated and rapid immune response in a person who is exposed to the same antigen repeatedly.

Role of Antibodies. Antibodies are large proteins called *immunoglobulins* (because they are found in the globulin fraction of the plasma proteins). All immunoglobulins are glycoproteins and contain a certain amount of carbohydrate. Each antibody molecule consists of two subunits, each of which contains a light and a heavy peptide chain. Each subunit has a portion, referred to as the fragment antigen binding (Fab) fragment, that serves as a binding site for a specific antigen. The Fab fragment (antibody-binding site) binds to the antigenic determinant, similar to a lock-and-key mechanism. The Fab fragment provides the "lock" portion that is highly specific for an antigen. An additional portion, known as the Fc fragment, which contains the c-terminal and does not contain antigen-binding sites, allows the antibody molecule to take part in the complement system (Delves, 2021).

Antibodies defend against foreign pathogens in several ways, and the type of defense employed depends on the structure and composition of both the antigen and the immunoglobulin. The antibody molecule has at least two combining sites, or Fab fragments. One antibody can act as a cross-link between two antigens, causing them to bind or clump together. This clumping effect, referred to as **agglutination**, helps clear the body of the pathogen by facilitating phagocytosis. Agglutination is used in several laboratory tests, such as those for syphilis, to recognize and enumerate the presence of antibody–antigen complexes, indicative of infection. Some antibodies assist in removal of offending organisms through **opsonization**. In this process, the antigen–antibody molecule is coated with a sticky substance that also facilitates phagocytosis. The immune system, like social media, creates hashtags such as #virus or #bacteria as a label for pathogens to search and eliminate them from the body.

Antibodies also promote the release of vasoactive substances, such as histamine and slow-reacting substance, two of the chemical mediators of the inflammatory response. Antibodies do not function in isolation; rather, they mobilize other components of the immune system to defend against

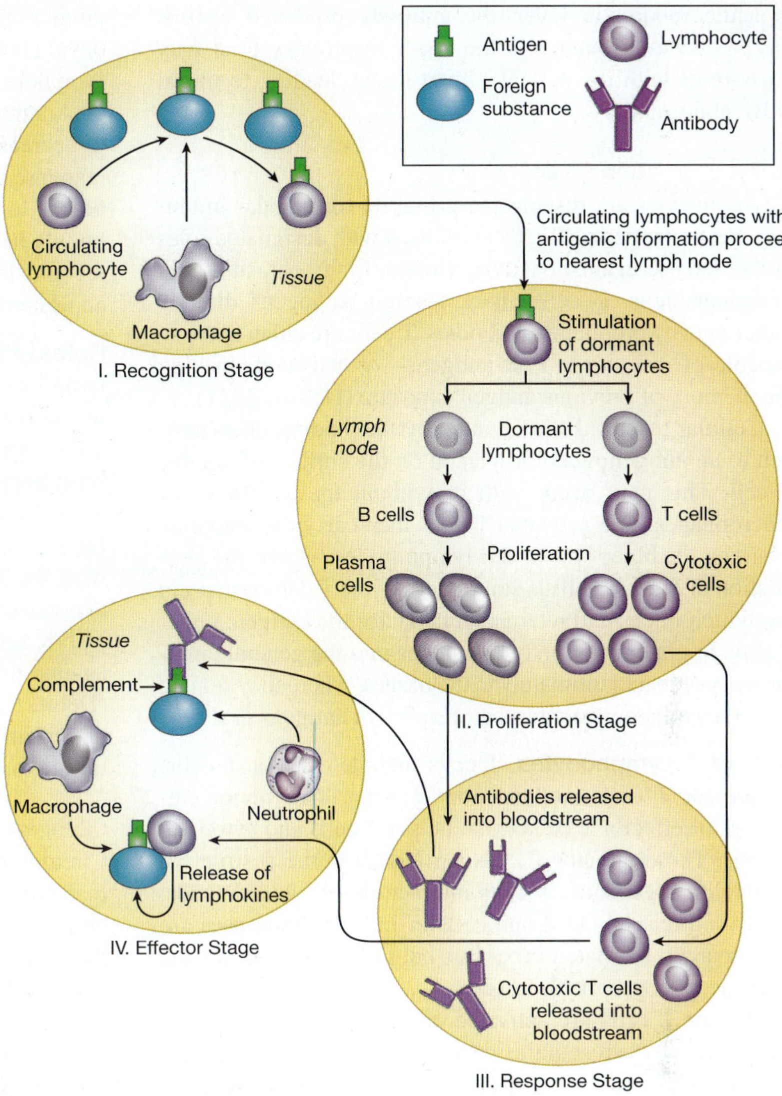

FIGURE 35-6 Stages of the immune response. (I) In the *recognition stage,* antigens are recognized by circulating lymphocytes and macrophages. (II) In the *proliferation stage,* the dormant lymphocytes proliferate and differentiate into cytotoxic (killer) T or B cells responsible for formation and release of antibodies. (III) In the *response stage,* the cytotoxic T cells and the B cells perform cellular and humoral functions, respectively. (IV) In the *effector stage,* antigens are destroyed or neutralized through the action of antibodies, complement, macrophages, and cytotoxic T cells.

the pathogen. The typical role of antibodies is to focus components of the natural immune system on the pathogen. This includes activation of both the complement system and phagocytosis (Delves, 2021).

The body can produce five different types of immunoglobulins (Ig). Each of the five types, or classes, is identified by a specific letter of the alphabet derived from the name of the heavy chain present on the immunoglobulin: IgA for alpha (α), IgD for delta (δ), IgE for epsilon (ε), IgG for gamma (γ), and IgM for mu (μ). Classification is based on the chemical structure and biologic role of the individual immunoglobulin.

Antigen–Antibody Binding. The portion of the antigen involved in binding with the antibody is referred to as the **antigenic determinant**. The most efficient immunologic responses occur when the antibody and antigen fit like a lock and key (Fig. 35-7). Poor fit can occur with an antibody that was produced in response to a different antigen. This phenomenon is known as *cross-reactivity*. For example,

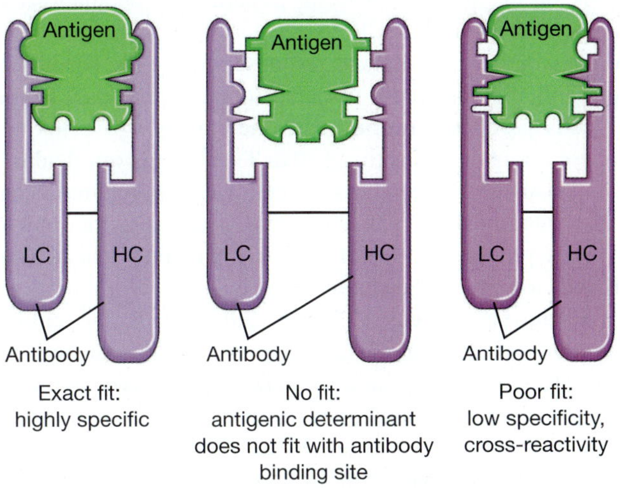

FIGURE 35-7 Antigen–antibody binding. (*Left*) A highly specific antigen–antibody complex. (*Middle*) No match and, therefore, no immune response. (*Right*) Poor fit or match with low specificity; antibody reacts to antigen with similar characteristics, producing cross-reactivity.

in acute rheumatic fever, the antibody produced against *Streptococcus pyogenes* in the upper respiratory tract may cross-react with the patient's heart tissue, leading to mitral valve abnormalities.

Cellular Immune Response

T lymphocytes are responsible primarily for cellular immunity. Several types of T cells exist, each with designated roles in the defense against bacteria, viruses, fungi, parasites, and malignant cells. T cells attack foreign pathogens directly rather than by producing antibodies. T cells are either naïve—capable of reacting to new antigens—or activated—having the memory of previous antigen exposure (Delves, 2021).

Cellular reactions are initiated by the binding of an antigen to an antigen receptor located on the surface of a naïve T cell. This may occur with or without the assistance of macrophages. The activated T cells then carry the antigenic message, or blueprint, to the lymph nodes, where the production of other T cells is stimulated. Some T cells remain in the lymph nodes and retain a memory for the antigen. Other T cells migrate from the lymph nodes into the general circulatory system and ultimately to the tissues, where they remain until they either encounter their respective antigens or die.

Role of T Lymphocytes. T cells include effector T cells, suppressor T cells, and memory T cells. Two major categories of effector T cells exist: helper T cells and cytotoxic T cells. These effector T cells participate in the destruction of foreign organisms. T cells interact closely with B cells, indicating that humoral and cellular immune responses are not separate, unrelated processes but rather branches of the immune response that interact.

Helper T cells are activated on recognition of antigens and stimulate the rest of the immune system. When activated, helper T cells secrete **cytokines**, which attract and activate B cells, cytotoxic T cells, NK cells, macrophages, and other cells of the immune system. Separate subpopulations of helper T cells produce different types of cytokines and determine whether the immune response will be the production of antibodies or a cell-mediated immune response. Helper T cells produce **lymphokines**, one category of cytokines. These lymphokines activate other T cells (e.g., interleukin-2 [IL-2]), natural and cytotoxic T cells (e.g., IFN-gamma), and other inflammatory cells (e.g., tumor necrosis factor). Helper T cells produce IL-4 and IL-5, lymphokines that activate B cells to grow and differentiate.

Cytotoxic T cells (killer T cells) attack the antigen directly by altering the cell membrane and causing cell lysis (disintegration) and by releasing cytolytic enzymes and cytokines. Lymphokines can recruit, activate, and regulate other lymphocytes and WBCs. These cells then assist in destroying the pathogen. Delayed-type hypersensitivity is an example of an immune reaction that protects the body from antigens through the production and release of lymphokines (see later discussion). While some types of hypersensitivity reactions are instantaneous due to the presence of circulating antibodies, a delayed reaction occurs over hours, days, or weeks depending on the rate of the production of lymphokines.

Another type of cell, the **suppressor T cell**, has the ability to decrease B cell production, thereby keeping the immune response at a level that is compatible with health (e.g., sufficient to fight infection adequately without attacking the body's healthy tissues). **Memory cells** are responsible for recognizing antigens from previous exposure and mounting an immune response.

Roles of Null Lymphocytes and Natural Killer Cells. Null lymphocytes and NK cells are other lymphocytes that assist in combating organisms. These cells are distinct from B and T cells and lack the usual characteristics of those cells. **Null lymphocytes**, a subpopulation of lymphocytes, destroy antigens already coated with antibody. These cells have special Fc receptor sites on their surface that allow them to connect with the Fc end of antibodies; this is known as *antibody-dependent, cell-mediated cytotoxicity*.

NK cells, another subpopulation of lymphocytes, defend against microorganisms and some types of malignant cells (Delves, 2021). NK cells are capable of directly killing pathogens and producing cytokines. The helper T cells contribute to the differentiation of null and NK cells.

Complement System

Circulating plasma proteins, known as **complement**, are made in the liver and other sites and activated when an antibody connects with its antigen. There are more than 35 of these plasma or membrane proteins, and they are an important additional component of the immune system (Delves, 2021). Destruction of an invading or attacking organism or toxin is not achieved merely by the binding of the antibody and antigens; destruction also requires activation of complement, the arrival of killer T cells, or the attraction of macrophages. Complement has three major physiologic functions: defending the body against bacterial infection, bridging natural and acquired immunity, and disposing of immune complexes and the byproducts associated with inflammation.

The proteins that comprise complement interact sequentially with one another in a cascading or "falling domino" effect. The complement cascade is important to modifying the effector arm of the immune system. Activation of complement allows for the occurrence of important events, such as removal of infectious agents and initiation of the inflammatory response. These events involve active parts of the pathway that enhance chemotaxis of macrophages and granulocytes, alter blood vessel permeability, change blood vessel diameters, cause cells to lyse, alter blood clotting, and cause other points of modification. In a patient, these events manifest as erythema due to blood vessel changes and edema as substances are transported to the site of infection. These macrophages and granulocytes continue the body's defense by devouring the antibody-coated microbes and by releasing antibacterial products.

Role of Interferons

IFNs are cytokines. They have antiviral and antitumor properties. In addition to responding to viral infection, IFNs are produced by T lymphocytes, B lymphocytes, and macrophages in response to antigens. They modify the immune response by suppressing antibody production and cellular immunity. They also facilitate the cytolytic (cell destruction) role of lymphocytes, macrophages, and NK cells. Research continues on the pathways that IFNs use to transmit signals from cell membranes to the nucleus. IFNs are undergoing extensive testing to evaluate their effectiveness in treating tumors and chronic infections such as AIDS (Schroeder, 2020; Tompa et al., 2021).

Pearls for Practice

The nurse recognizes that the immune system has the potential to recognize cancer or tumor-associated antigens as foreign or dangerous; as a result, immune therapies are currently being investigated as a tool to bolster the immune response in cancer. An example is the use of alpha interferon produced by recombinant DNA techniques to bind with target cancer cell membrane to augment cytotoxic intracellular events (Schroeder, 2020).

Advances in Immunology

Genetic Engineering

One of the more remarkable evolving technologies is **genetic engineering**, which uses recombinant DNA technology. Genetic engineering is used in everything from the production of insulin and human growth hormone to the production of experimental mice. One type of genetic engineering permits scientists to combine genes from one type of organism with genes of a second organism. This type of technology allows cells and microorganisms to manufacture proteins, monokines, and lymphokines that can alter and enhance immune system function. This type of technology also produces genetically modified organisms (GMOs) that have been the source of much controversy in the food industry. The second use of recombinant DNA technology involves gene therapy (Fogel & Gerschwind, 2022). If a particular gene is abnormal or missing, experimental recombinant DNA technology may be capable of restoring normal gene function. For example, a recombinant gene is inserted onto a virus particle. When the virus particle splices its genes, the virus automatically inserts the missing gene and theoretically corrects the genetic anomaly. Extensive research into recombinant DNA technology and gene therapy is ongoing; cautious optimism exists that "in the future effective, durable, and safe therapies will provide benefit to patients—not only those with single-gene disorders but those with complex acquired diseases as well" (Anguela et al., 2019, p. 273).

Stem Cells

Stem cells are potentially immortal cells that are capable of self-renewal and differentiation; they continually replenish the body's entire supply of both RBCs and WBCs. Some stem cells, described as *totipotent cells*, have tremendous capacity to self-renew and differentiate. Embryonic stem cells, described as *pluripotent*, give rise to numerous cell types that are able to form tissues (Delves, 2021). Research and clinical trials have shown that stem cells can restore an immune system that has been destroyed. Stem cell transplantation therapy has been developed for numerous types of conditions, such as severe combined immunodeficiency (SCID), acute myeloid leukemia, periodontal disease, and other types of cancer (Shalapour et al., 2020). Clinical trials using stem cells as therapy are underway in patients with a variety of disorders having an autoimmune component, including systemic lupus erythematosus (SLE), rheumatoid arthritis, scleroderma, multiple sclerosis, and heart disease, specifically in the repair of endothelial cells (Ebrahimi et al., 2021).

Gerontologic Considerations

People at the extremes of the lifespan are more likely than middle-aged adults to develop problems related to the functioning of the immune system (Table 35-3). The greatest impact of aging on the immune system is on cell-mediated immunity; age has a lesser but substantial impact on humoral immunity. The frequency and severity of infections are increased in older people, possibly due to a decreased ability to respond adequately to pathogens. Both the production and the function of T and B lymphocytes may be impaired. Responses to antigen stimulation may be altered, with increasing proportions of lymphocytes becoming unresponsive with age. An example of this is the recent development of a vaccine for older patients against herpes zoster and postherpetic neuralgia caused by the varicella virus. The antigen present in this vaccine has 14 times the amount of live attenuated virus present in the varicella vaccine for children (Gabutti et al., 2019). The impact of aging on the immune system can best be summarized as *immunosenescence*, a condition thought to be a result of involution of the thymus (Nguyen et al., 2019). In addition, comorbidities often causes a reduced local innate immunity such as in chronic obstructive pulmonary disease (COPD), where impaired mucociliary clearance, alveolar macrophage dysfunction, and suppressed cough mechanism increase the risk for pulmonary infections in older patients (High, 2020). Other innate immune components that decline with age include physical barriers such as skin integrity, and gastric acid secretion.

ASSESSMENT OF THE IMMUNE SYSTEM

Assessment of the immune system involves nearly every organ system of the body.

TABLE 35-3 **GERONTOLOGIC CONSIDERATIONS / Age-Related Changes in Immunologic Function**

Body System	Structural and Functional Changes	History and Physical Findings
Immune	Impaired function of B and T lymphocytes Failure of lymphocytes to recognize mutant or abnormal cells Decreased antibody production Failure of immune system to differentiate "self" from "non-self" Suppressed phagocytic immune response	Suppressed responses to pathogenic organisms with increased risk for infection Increased incidence of cancers Anergy (lack of response to antigens applied to the skin [PPD, allergens]) Increased incidence of autoimmune diseases Absence of typical signs and symptoms of infection and inflammation Dissemination of organisms usually destroyed or suppressed by phagocytes (e.g., reactivation or spread of tuberculosis)
Gastrointestinal	Decreased gastric secretions and motility Decreased phagocytosis by the liver's Kupffer cells Altered nutritional intake with inadequate protein intake	Proliferation of intestinal organisms, resulting in gastroenteritis and diarrhea Increased incidence and severity of hepatitis B; increased incidence of liver abscesses Suppressed immune response
Urinary	Decreased kidney function and changes in lower urinary tract function (enlargement of prostate gland, neurogenic bladder) Altered flora in the genitourinary tract	Urinary stasis and increased incidence of UTIs
Pulmonary	Impaired ciliary action due to exposure to smoke and environmental toxins	Impaired clearance of pulmonary secretions; increased incidence of respiratory infections
Integumentary	Thinning of skin with less elasticity; loss of adipose tissue	Increased risk of skin injury, breakdown, and infection
Circulatory	Impaired microcirculation	Stasis and pressure ulcers
Neurologic function	Decreased sensation and slowing of reflexes	Increased risk of injury, skin ulcers, abrasions, and burns

Health History

Common Complaints

Accurately assessing a patient's immune system can include consideration of nonspecific signs and symptoms, such as fatigue, impaired wound healing, recurrent infections, weight loss, or lymphadenopathy (Fig. 35-8). The signs and symptoms may be more specific, such as a butterfly (malar) rash in SLE; joint deformities in rheumatoid arthritis; thrush in HIV; or erythema, hoarseness, and dyspnea with anaphylactic reaction.

Past History

The nurse asks the patient about childhood and adult immunizations and childhood diseases. Known past or present exposure to tuberculosis is assessed, and the dates and results of any tuberculin tests (PPD or tine test) and chest x-rays are obtained. The nurse elicits information related to any recent exposure to any infections and the exposure dates. Take note of illness with COVID-19 and possible long-term effects. It is important for the nurse to assess whether the patient has been exposed to any sexually transmitted infections (STIs) or bloodborne pathogens, such as hepatitis A, B, or C viruses and HIV virus. A history of STIs, such as gonorrhea, syphilis, HPV infection, and chlamydia, can alert the nurse that the patient may have been exposed to HIV infection or to

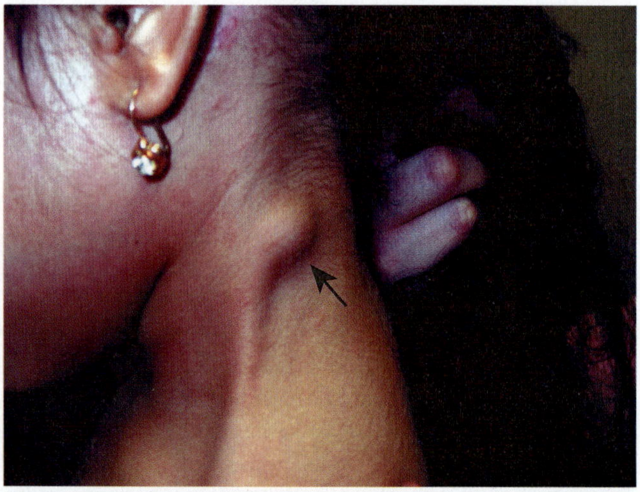

FIGURE 35-8 **Lymphadenopathy. An enlarged cervical lymph node. (Courtesy of J. S. Gehrig, *Patient assessment tutorials* [3rd ed.]. Lippincott, Wolters, Kluwer.)**

hepatitis. The CDC recommends universal HIV testing of all patients over the age of 13, with risk assessment determining the need for repeat testing. The nurse obtains a history of past and present infections and the dates and types of treatments along with a history of any multiple persistent infections, fevers of unknown origin, lesions or sores, or any type of drainage.

Allergy

The nurse asks the patient about any allergies, including types of allergens (e.g., pollens, dust, plants, cosmetics, food, medications, vaccines, latex), the symptoms experienced, and seasonal variations in occurrence or severity in the symptoms. A history of testing and treatments, including prescribed and over-the-counter medications that the patient has taken or is currently taking for these allergies and the effectiveness of the treatments, is obtained. Ensure comprehensive documentation that includes supplements, probiotic use, and complementary and homeopathic remedies. Read back the list you have compiled and ask: "Other than food and water, is there anything else you put in or on your body that is not on this list?" All medication and food allergies are listed on an allergy alert sticker and placed on the front of the patient's health record if paper and in the electronic health record. Continued assessment for potential allergic reactions in the patient is vital.

Autoimmune Disorders

Autoimmune disorders affect people of all genders, ages, ethnicities, and social classes. The nurse asks the patient about any autoimmune disorders, such as lupus erythematosus, rheumatoid arthritis, or psoriasis. The patient is asked to describe the onset, severity, remissions and exacerbations, functional limitations, treatments they have received or are currently receiving, and the effectiveness of the treatments. Although most specific autoimmune disorders are rare, together they affect approximately 5% of the U.S. population. The occurrence of different autoimmune diseases within a family strongly suggests a genetic predisposition to more than one autoimmune disease (Delves, 2021).

Neoplastic Disease

If there is a history of cancer in the family, the nurse takes note of the type of cancer, age at onset, and relationship (maternal or paternal) of the patient to the affected family member(s). Dates and results of any cancer screening tests for the patient are obtained. A history of cancer in the patient is also obtained, along with the type of cancer, date of diagnosis, and treatment modalities used. Immunosuppression contributes to the development of cancers; however, cancer itself is immunosuppressive. Hematologic cancers, such as leukemia and lymphoma, are associated with altered production and function of WBCs and lymphocytes (Delves, 2021).

The nurse records data about all treatments that the patient has received or is currently receiving, such as radiation or chemotherapy, in the health history. Radiation destroys lymphocytes and decreases the ability to mount an effective immune response. The size and extent of the irradiated area determine the extent of immunosuppression. Whole-body irradiation may leave the patient totally immunosuppressed. Chemotherapy also affects bone marrow function, destroying cells that contribute to an effective immune response and resulting in immunosuppression. Should the cancer recur, previous chemotherapy regimens affect the choice of subsequent treatments. Encourage your patient to maintain comprehensive records of these treatments.

Chronic Illness and Surgery

The nurse notes any history of chronic illness, such as diabetes mellitus, kidney disease, COPD, or fibromyalgia. The onset and severity of illness, as well as treatment that the patient is receiving for the illness, are obtained. Chronic illness may contribute to immune system impairments in various ways. Kidney failure is associated with a deficiency in circulating lymphocytes. In addition, immune defenses may be altered by acidosis and uremic toxins. In diabetes, hyperglycemia impairs immune function (decreases the function of WBCs), promotes inflammation, favors the growth of yeast organisms, and is associated with changes in the walls of the blood vessels, resulting in increased risk for infection as well as both microvascular and macrovascular dysfunctions. Recurrent respiratory tract infections are associated with COPD as a result of altered inspiratory and expiratory function and ineffective airway clearance.

Special Problems

Conditions such as burns and other forms of injury and infection may contribute to altered immune system function. Major burns cause impaired skin integrity and compromise the body's first line of defense. Loss of large amounts of serum occurs with burn injuries and depletes the body of essential proteins, including immunoglobulins. The physiologic and psychological stressors associated with surgery or injury stimulate cortisol release from the adrenal cortex; increased serum cortisol also contributes to suppression of normal immune responses.

Social History

Poor nutritional status, poor sleep habits, smoking, excessive consumption of alcohol, illicit drug use, STIs, and occupational or residential exposure to environmental radiation and pollutants have been associated with impaired immune function. The nurse needs to assess all these factors in a detailed patient history. Many electronic health records contain flowsheets that assist in documentation of social determinants of health.

Nutrition

The importance of optimal nutrition in enhancing immunity is gaining greater recognition. Inadequate intake of vitamins that are essential for synthesis of both DNA and protein may lead to protein–calorie deficiency and, subsequently, to impaired immune function. Vitamins also help in the regulation of cell proliferation and maturation of immune cells. Excess or deficiency of trace elements (i.e., copper, iron, manganese, selenium, or zinc) in the diet generally suppresses immune function.

Fatty acids are the building blocks that make up the structural components of cell membranes. Lipids are precursors of vitamins A, D, E, and K, as well as cholesterol. Both excess and deficiency of fatty acids have been found to suppress immune function.

Depletion of protein reserves results in atrophy of lymphoid tissues, depression of antibody response, reduction in the number of circulating T cells, and impaired phagocytic function. As a result, susceptibility to infection is greatly increased. During periods of infection or serious illness, nutritional requirements may be altered further, potentially contributing to depletion of stores of protein, fatty acid, vitamin, and trace elements and causing even greater risk of impaired immune response and sepsis. Patients whose nutritional status is compromised have a delayed postoperative recovery and often experience more severe infections and delayed wound healing. The nurse must assess the patient's nutritional status and caloric intake. The nurse is responsible for assuming a proactive role in ensuring the best possible nutritional intake for all patients as a vital step in preventing untoward treatment outcomes.

Medications and Blood Transfusions

The nurse obtains a list of past and present medications that the patient has used or is using. In large doses, antibiotics, corticosteroids, cytotoxic agents, salicylates, nonsteroidal anti-inflammatory drugs (NSAIDs), and anesthetics can cause immune suppression (Table 35-4). The overuse of antibiotics, their effect on the intestinal microbiome, and the use of fecal transplants to restore a depleted microbiome are areas that the nurse may explore with the patient during an assessment of the immune system.

The nurse obtains a history of blood transfusions because previous exposure to foreign antigens through transfusion may be associated with the current abnormal immune function. In addition, although the risk of HIV transmission through blood transfusion is extremely low in patients who received a transfusion after 1985 (the year that testing of blood for HIV was initiated in the United States), a small risk remains. The nurse also assesses for signs or symptoms of hepatitis in patients who have received blood products.

Travel and Occupation

Patients who are immunocompromised should be asked about travel history and occupational history to determine exposure to specific pathogens. For example, patients from the Southwest United States are more likely to be infected with certain types of fungi that are more prevalent in the desert.

Psychoneuroimmunologic Factors

The patient assessment also addresses psychoneuroimmunologic factors. The bidirectional pathway between the brain and immune system is referred to as *psychoneuroimmunology*, a field that has been the focus of research and discussion over the last several decades (Bower et al., 2022). It is thought that the immune response is regulated and modulated in part by neuroendocrine influences. Lymphocytes and macrophages have receptors that are capable of responding to neurotransmitters and endocrine hormones. Lymphocytes can produce and secrete adrenocorticotropic hormone and endorphin-like compounds. Cells in the brain, especially in the hypothalamus, can recognize prostaglandins, IFNs, and interleukins, as well as histamine and serotonin, which are released during the inflammatory process. Like all other biologic systems functioning to promote homeostasis, the immune system is integrated with other psychophysiological processes and is subject to regulation and modulation by the brain.

Conversely, the immune processes can affect neural and endocrine function, including behavior. Growing evidence indicates that a measurable immune system response can be influenced positively by biobehavioral strategies, such as relaxation and imagery techniques, biofeedback, humor, hypnosis, and conditioning. Therefore, the assessment should address the patient's general psychological status and the patient's use of and response to these strategies.

Physical Assessment

Immune dysfunction may have manifestations in various body systems (Box 35-3). In addition to the assessment components described below, the nurse assesses the patient's respiratory, cardiovascular, genitourinary, and neurosensory status for signs and symptoms indicative of immune dysfunction.

Assessment of the Skin

The nurse assesses the skin and mucous membranes for color, lesions, dermatitis, purpura (subcutaneous bleeding), urticaria (hives), inflammation (angioedema [Fig. 35-9]), or any discharge. Purpura may indicate life-threatening infections like meningitis; urticaria indicates an acute or chronic response to allergens, pathogens, or autoimmune disorders.

Assessment of Eyes, Ears, Nose, and Throat

The nurse assesses for redness of the conjunctivae; periorbital tissues may be swollen and darkened with allergic disorders. The nares may show pale and edematous nasal mucous membranes and swollen turbinates. Assess secretions (typically clear) of the nasal passages or in the posterior pharynx. Thick secretions (yellow or green) may suggest infection. Percussion over the maxillary or frontal sinuses may elicit tenderness in acute sinusitis.

TABLE **35-4 Selected Medications and Effects on the Immune System**

Drug Classification (and Examples)	Effects on the Immune System
Antibiotics (in large doses)	**Bone marrow suppression**
ceftriaxone	Eosinophilia, hemolytic anemia, hypoprothrombinemia, neutropenia, thrombocytopenia
cefuroxime sodium	Eosinophilia, hemolytic anemia, hypoprothrombinemia, neutropenia, thrombocytopenia
chloramphenicol	Leukopenia, aplastic anemia
dactinomycin	Agranulocytosis, neutropenia
fluoroquinolones	Hemolytic anemia, methemoglobinemia, eosinophilia, leukopenia, pancytopenia
gentamicin sulfate	Agranulocytosis, granulocytopenia
macrolides	Neutropenia, leukopenia
penicillins	Agranulocytosis
streptomycin	Leukopenia, neutropenia, pancytopenia
vancomycin	Transient leukopenia
Antithyroid drugs	
propylthiouracil (PTU)	Agranulocytosis, leukopenia
Nonsteroidal anti-inflammatory drugs (NSAIDs; in large doses)	**Inhibit prostaglandin synthesis or release**
aspirin	Agranulocytosis
COX-2 inhibitors	Anemia, allergy, no other major adverse effects to the immune system
ibuprofen	Leukopenia, neutropenia
indomethacin	Agranulocytosis, leukopenia
phenylbutazone	Pancytopenia, agranulocytosis, aplastic anemia
Adrenal corticosteroids	**Immunosuppression**
prednisone	Suppression or prevention of cell-mediated immune reactions reducing leukocyte, monocyte, and eosinophil levels Decreased immunoglobulin binding to cell surface receptors inhibiting interleukin synthesis
Antineoplastic agents (cytotoxic agents)	**Immunosuppression**
alkylating agents	Leukopenia, bone marrow suppression
cyclophosphamide	Leukopenia, neutropenia
mechlorethamine HCl	Agranulocytosis, neutropenia
cyclosporine	Leukopenia, inhibition of T-lymphocyte function
Antimetabolites	**Immunosuppression**
fluorouracil (pyrimidine antagonist)	Leukopenia, eosinophilia
methotrexate (folic acid antagonist)	Leukopenia, aplastic bone marrow
mercaptopurine (6-MP) (purine antagonist)	Leukopenia, pancytopenia

BOX 35-3 **Focused Assessment**

Immune Dysfunction

Be alert for the following signs and symptoms:

Respiratory System
- Changes in respiratory rate
- Cough (dry or productive)
- Abnormal lung sounds (wheezing, crackles, rhonchi, stridor)
- Rhinitis
- Hyperventilation
- Bronchospasm
- Hypoxemia

Cardiovascular System
- Hypotension
- Tachycardia
- Arrhythmia
- Vasculitis
- Anemia

Gastrointestinal System
- Hepatosplenomegaly
- Colitis
- Vomiting
- Diarrhea

Genitourinary System
- Frequency and burning on urination
- Hematuria
- Discharge

Musculoskeletal System
- Joint mobility
- Edema
- Pain

Skin
- Rashes
- Pruritus
- Lesions
- Dermatitis
- Hematomas or purpura
- Edema, angioedema, or urticaria
- Inflammation
- Flushing
- Discharge

Neurosensory System
- Cognitive dysfunction
- Hearing loss
- Visual changes
- Headaches and migraines
- Ataxia
- Tetany

Assessment of the Lungs

The nurse inspects the patient for work of breathing, respiratory rate, use of accessory muscles, presence of retractions or bulging at intercostal space and/or supra- and infraclavicular area, and clubbing; the nurse auscultates the lungs for adventitious sounds. Patients with acute asthma may display tachypnea and auditory wheezes, dyspnea, retractions, and use of accessory muscles of respiration. Patients with *Pneumocystis jirovecii* pneumonia (PJP) or Pneumocystis pneumonia (PCP) or COVID-19 infections may have increased work of breathing after minor exertions such as climbing stairs. Assess with an ambulatory oxygen saturation measurement.

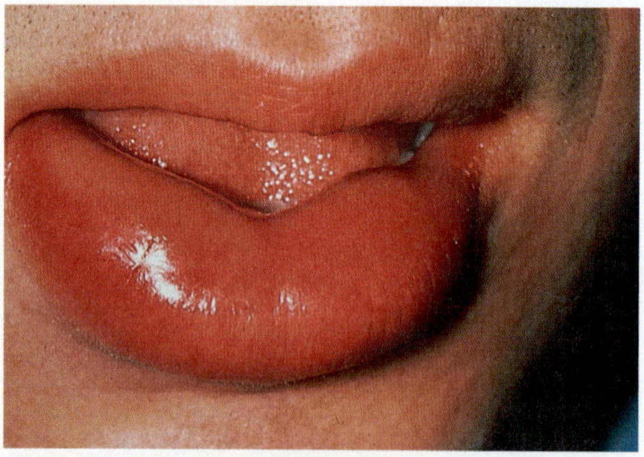

FIGURE 35-9 Angioedema is a diffuse, nonpitting, tense swelling of the dermis and subcutaneous tissue that can develop rapidly. Although usually allergic in nature and sometimes associated with hives, angioedema does not itch. (From Neville, B., Damm, D. D., & White, D. K. [1991]. *Color atlas of clinical oral pathology*. Lea & Febiger. Used with permission.)

Assessment for Signs of Infection

The nurse notes any signs of infection (erythema, warmth, tenderness, drainage). The patient's temperature is recorded, and the patient is observed for chills and sweating. Fever often accompanies infection; however, older patients or patients who are immunocompromised may not exhibit high fevers.

Assessment of the Lymph Nodes

The lymph nodes and thyroid are palpated for enlargement. If palpable nodes are detected, their location, size, consistency, and reports of tenderness on palpation are noted. Lymphadenopathy indicates activation of the immune system against pathogens. Generalized lymphadenopathy, which is manifested by swollen lymph nodes in multiple sites, is often one of the first signs of infection with HIV.

Assessment of the Joints

Joints are assessed for tenderness, swelling, increased warmth, and limited range of motion. These findings indicate inflammation and infiltration by leukocytes, including macrophages and cytokines.

Diagnostic Evaluation

The nurse needs to be aware that patients undergoing evaluation for possible immune system disorders experience not only physical pain and discomfort with certain types of diagnostic procedures but also many psychological reactions. For example, patients may fear test results that demonstrate decreased immune function because the diminished immune system can make them more prone to certain infections, cancers, and other disorders. It is the nurse's role to counsel, educate, and support patients throughout the diagnostic process. Further, many patients may be extremely anxious about the results of diagnostic tests and the possible implications of those results for their employment, insurance, and personal relationships. This is an ideal time for the nurse to provide counseling and education, should these interventions be warranted.

Immune Competence Testing

A series of blood and skin tests and a bone marrow biopsy may be performed to evaluate the patient's immune competence. Specific laboratory and diagnostic tests are discussed in greater detail along with individual disease processes in subsequent chapters in this unit. Selected laboratory and diagnostic tests used to evaluate immune competence are summarized in Box 35-4.

Allergy Testing

Diagnostic evaluation of the patient with allergic disorders commonly includes blood tests, smears of body secretions (nasal, conjunctival, or sputum secretions), skin tests (intradermal injections of solutions at several sites that may provoke an allergic response), and the radioallergosorbent test (RAST). Many health organizations recommend that RAST be phased out in favor of more sensitive tests such as fluorescence enzyme-labeled assays.

Results of laboratory blood studies provide supportive data for various diagnostic possibilities; however, they are not the major criteria for the diagnosis of allergic disease.

BOX 35-4

Selected Tests for Evaluating Immunologic Status

Various laboratory tests may be performed to assess activity or dysfunction of the immune system. The studies assess leukocytes and lymphocytes, humoral immunity, cellular immunity, phagocytic cell function, complement activity, hypersensitivity reactions, specific antigen–antibodies, or HIV infection.

Leukocyte and Lymphocyte Tests

- White blood cell count and differential
- Bone marrow biopsy

Humoral (Antibody-Mediated) Immunity Tests

- B-cell quantification with monoclonal antibody
- In vivo immunoglobulin synthesis with T-cell subsets
- Specific antibody response
- Total serum globulins and individual immunoglobulins (by electrophoresis, immunoelectrophoresis, single radial immunodiffusion, nephelometry, isohemagglutinin techniques)

Cellular (Cell-Mediated) Immunity Tests

- Total lymphocyte count
- T-cell and T-cell subset quantification with monoclonal antibody
- Delayed hypersensitivity skin test
- Cytokine production
- Lymphocyte response to mitogens, antigens, and allogenic cells
- Helper and suppressor T-cell functions

Phagocytic Cell Function Tests

- Nitroblue tetrazolium reductase assay

Complement Component Tests

- Total serum hemolytic complement
- Individual complement component titrations
- Radial immunodiffusion
- Electroimmunoassay
- Radioimmunoassay
- Immunonephelometric assay
- Immunoelectrophoresis

Hypersensitivity Tests

- Scratch test
- Patch test
- Intradermal test
- Radioallergosorbent test (RAST)
- Immunofluorescence

Specific Antigen–Antibody Tests

- Radioimmunoassay
- Immunofluorescence
- Agglutination
- Complement fixation test

HIV Infection Tests

- Enzyme-linked immunosorbent assay (ELISA)
- P24 antigen test
- Western blot, replaced by the fourth-generation antigen/antibody tests
- CD4 and CD8 cell counts
- Polymerase chain reaction (PCR)

Pearls for Practice

With allergic condition, the WBC count is usually normal, except with infection. Eosinophils, which are granular leukocytes, normally make up 1% to 3% of the total number of WBCs. A level between 5% and 15% is nonspecific but suggests an allergic reaction. Moderate eosinophilia is defined as 15% to 40% eosinophils and is found in patients with allergic disorders; in patients with malignancy, immunodeficiencies, parasitic infections, or congenital heart disease; and in patients receiving peritoneal dialysis. Severe eosinophilia is defined as 50% to 90% eosinophils and is found in patients with idiopathic hypereosinophilic syndrome. In addition, look at the absolute count for eosinophils and neutrophils. If the total count of WBCs is low, the percentages of these components may be falsely elevated.

Skin Tests

If a skin test is indicated, there is a reasonable suspicion that a specific allergen is producing symptoms in an allergic patient. However, several precautionary steps must be observed before skin testing with allergens is performed:

- Testing is not performed during periods of bronchospasm.
- Epicutaneous tests (scratch or prick tests) are performed before other testing methods in an effort to minimize the risk of systemic reaction.
- Emergency equipment must be readily available to treat anaphylaxis. See Box 35-5.

Pearls for Practice

In the event of an anaphylactic reaction resulting from the administration of a medication, blood, or blood product, the infusion should be immediately discontinued, and the nurse should immediately notify the provider and rapid response team (if available). The nurse will continually assess the patient's respiratory status (RR, lung sounds, pattern of breathing, oxygen saturation); monitor their hemodynamic status, which will include pulse rate, rhythm (via ECG), and blood pressure; and ensure IV access is available. In addition, interventions include administering epinephrine (administered by intramuscular injection into the anterolateral thigh), facilitating ventilation (positioning the patient to assist with breathing and instructing the patient to breathe slowly and deeply, oxygen administration), administering volume replacement

BOX 35-5

Nursing Research

Bridging the Gap to Evidence-Based Practice

Noh, Y., & Lee, I. A mixed-methods approach-based study of anaphylaxis awareness and educational needs among nursing students. *International Journal of Environmental Research and Public Health*, *18*(17), 9280. https://doi.org/10.3390/ijerph18179280.

In this mixed-methods study, the authors identified anaphylaxis awareness among nursing students through a survey and the needs for anaphylaxis education through focus group interviews (FGIs).

Purpose

There has been a sixfold increase in the incidence of anaphylaxis worldwide over the past 3 decades with a recurrence rate of one in three. The purpose of this study was to evaluate nursing students, "anaphylaxis awareness," which refers to the degree of understanding of the causes, symptoms, and treatment of anaphylaxis.

Design

Anaphylaxis awareness was surveyed from 10 June–30 July 2018 using a structured questionnaire with 221 junior or senior nursing students. To assess the needs for anaphylaxis education, 14 senior nursing students were interviewed using focus group interviews (FGI) from 10 to 22 June 2018. Quantitative data were analyzed descriptively using SPSS, and qualitative data were assessed using thematic analysis.

Findings

Nursing students' awareness of anaphylaxis was identified by correct answers to items concerning symptoms (33.0%), causes (64.6%), and treatments (55.8%), with an overall average of 51.5%. The thematic analysis identified four themes reflecting students' educational needs: the need for anaphylaxis education, various education **methods**, field training-based study of educational content, and repeated education. Nursing students' anaphylaxis awareness is low.

Nursing Implications

Since anaphylaxis is a systemic allergic reaction that can lead to death owing to rapidly developing diverse symptoms in several organs over a short period, when symptoms appear, proper and quick emergency treatment is essential. This study revealed a need for anaphylaxis education to be planned (and repeated) in the nursing curriculum. For example, when asked about the epinephrine injection site, only 46.6% chose correctly (i.e., thigh), and when asked about whether antihistamines and steroids are good substitutes for epinephrine, only 24.0% answered correctly. The students suggested that current education does not keep up with the growing increase in prevalence of anaphylaxis. While 89.2% of the students received lectures on anaphylaxis, none were trained in practice. Incorporating the authors, suggestions in future education programs may promote students' confidence in treating anaphylaxis.

(rapidly administering IV prescribed fluids), providing comfort and emotional support, and maintaining surveillance for and preventing (when possible) recurrent reactions and complications (Graham, 2022).

Methods of **skin testing** include prick skin tests, scratch tests, and intradermal skin testing. After negative prick or scratch tests, intradermal skin testing is performed with allergens that are suggested by the patient's history to be problematic. The back is the most suitable area of the body for skin testing because it permits the performance of many tests. The multitest applicator is a commercially available device with multiple test heads that allows simultaneous administration of antigens by multiple punctures at different sites. A negative response on a skin test cannot be interpreted as absence of sensitivity to an allergen. Such a response may occur with insufficient sensitivity of the test or with use of an inappropriate allergen in testing. Therefore, it is essential to observe the patient undergoing skin testing for an allergic reaction, even if the previous response was negative.

The results of skin tests complement the data obtained from the history. They indicate which of several antigens are most likely to provoke symptoms and provide some clue to the intensity of the patient's sensitization. Also the dosage of the antigen (allergen) injected is important. Most patients are hypersensitive to more than one allergen. Under testing conditions, they may not react (although they usually do) to the specific allergens that induce their attacks.

Familiarity with and consistent use of a grading system with skin tests are essential. The grading system used should be identified on a skin test sheet for later interpretation. A positive reaction, evidenced by the appearance of an urticarial wheal (round, reddened skin elevation; Fig. 35-10), localized **erythema** (diffuse redness) in the area of inoculation or contact, or pseudopodia (irregular projection at the end of a wheal) with associated erythema is considered indicative of sensitivity to the corresponding antigen.

False-negative results may occur because of improper technique, outdated allergen solutions, or prior use of medications that suppress skin reactivity. Corticosteroids and antihistamines, including over-the-counter allergy medications, suppress skin test reactivity and usually are withheld for 48 to 96 hours before testing, depending on the duration of their activity. False-positive results may occur because of improper preparation or administration of allergen solutions.

Interpretation of positive or negative skin tests must be based on the history, physical examination, and other laboratory test results. The following guidelines are used for the interpretation of skin test results:

- Skin tests are more reliable for diagnosing atopic sensitivity in patients with allergic rhinoconjunctivitis (nasal congestion, runny nose, postnasal drip, sneezing, red eyes [conjunctivitis], and itching of the nose or eyes) than in patients with asthma.

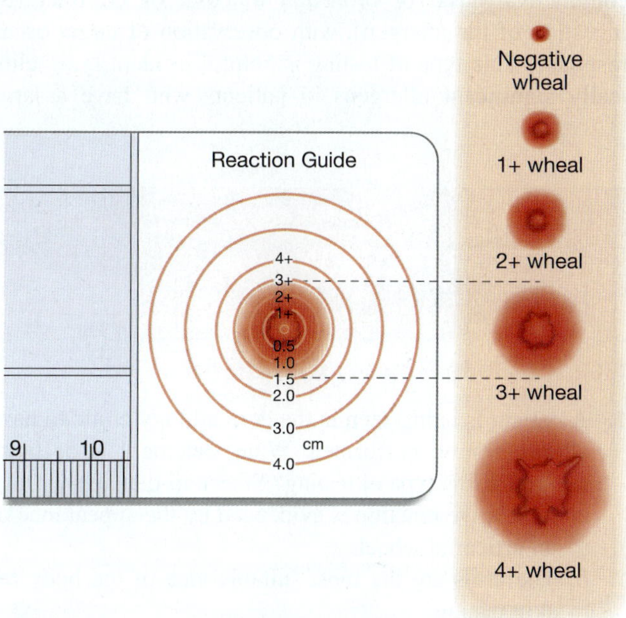

FIGURE 35-10 **Interpretation of reactions: Negative = wheal soft with minimal erythema. 1+ = wheal present (5 to 8 mm) with associated erythema. 2+ = wheal (7 to 10 mm) with associated erythema. 3+ = wheal (9 to 15 mm) with slight pseudopodia possible with associated erythema. 4+ = wheal (12 mm+) with pseudopodia and diffuse erythema.**

- Positive skin tests correlate highly with food allergy.
- The use of skin tests to diagnose immediate hypersensitivity to medications is limited because usually metabolites of medications, not the medications themselves, are responsible for causing hypersensitivity.

In cases of doubt about the validity of the skin tests, a radioallergosorbent testing (RAST) or a provocative challenge test may be performed.

Radioallergosorbent Testing

RAST is a radioimmunoassay that measures allergen-specific IgE in the patient's blood. In addition to detecting an allergen, RAST indicates the quantity of allergen necessary to evoke an allergic reaction. Values are reported on a scale from 0 to 5. Values of 2 or greater are considered significant. The major advantages of RAST over other tests include decreased risk of systemic reaction, stability of antigens, and lack of dependence on skin reactivity modified by medications. The major disadvantages include limited allergen selection and reduced sensitivity compared with intradermal skin tests, lack of immediate results, and higher cost. RAST is being replaced by the more sensitive fluorescence enzyme-labeled assays such as ImmunoCAP, a quantitative test for IgE proteins.

Provocative Testing

Provocative testing involves the direct administration of the suspected allergen to the sensitive tissue, such as the conjunctiva, nasal or bronchial mucosa, or GI tract (by ingestion of the allergen), with observation of target organ response. This type of testing is helpful in identifying clinically significant allergens in patients who have a large number of positive tests. Major disadvantages of this type of testing are the limitation of one antigen per session and the risk of producing severe symptoms, particularly bronchospasm, in patients with asthma.

CHAPTER REVIEW

NCLEX-Style Review Questions

1. A patient is being seen in the dermatology clinic to have allergy testing performed. What statement is accurate regarding this type of testing? Select all that apply.
   a. A positive reaction is evidenced by the appearance of an urticarial wheal.
   b. The arms are the most suitable area of the body for skin testing.
   c. A negative response can be interpreted as an absence of sensitivity to an allergen.
   d. There is no risk of a false-negative result.
   e. Allergy testing is not performed during periods of bronchospasm.

2. Age-related changes associated with immunologic function in the older adult include which of the following? Select all that apply.
   a. Suppressed responses to pathogenic organisms with increased risk for infection
   b. Increased incidence of cancers
   c. Possible presence of anergy in response to antigens applied to the skin [PPD, allergens]
   d. Decreased incidence of autoimmune diseases
   e. Presence of exaggerated signs and symptoms of infection and inflammation

3. In an allergic reaction, the nurse recognizes that histamine release causes which of the following effects? Select all that apply.
   a. Erythema (redness)
   b. Localized edema in the form of wheals
   c. Dilation of bronchial smooth muscle
   d. Constriction of blood vessels
   e. Decreased gastric acid secretion

4. In the event of an anaphylactic reaction to an IV medication, what are appropriate nursing interventions? Select all that apply.
   a. Stop the IV medication.
   b. Monitor the patient's vital signs, including O_2 sat.
   c. Administer epinephrine subcutaneously.
   d. Decrease the rate of the IV medication.
   e. Ensure IV access.

5. A patient is exhibiting anaphylaxis after eating shellfish. What type of reaction is the patient experiencing?
   a. Type I
   b. Type II
   c. Type III
   d. Type IV
   e. Type V

REFERENCES AND SELECTED READINGS

References and selected readings associated with this chapter can be found on the website that accompanies the book. Visit **http://thepoint.lww.com/Honan3e** to access the references and other additional resources associated with this chapter.

CHAPTER 36

Nursing Management: Patients With Immunodeficiency, HIV Infection, and AIDS

Mary E. Bartlett

Learning Objectives

After reading this chapter, you will be able to:

1. Describe the basic aspects of primary immunodeficiency.
2. Describe the essential aspects of secondary immunodeficiency.
3. Summarize the epidemiology of HIV infection and AIDS.
4. Explain the gerontologic considerations of HIV/AIDS in the United States.
5. Describe the pathophysiology, modes of transmission, and prevention of HIV infection.
6. Explain postexposure prophylaxis for health care workers.
7. Explain pre-exposure prophylaxis for patients at high risk.
8. Summarize the clinical manifestations, assessment, and treatment of patients of HIV infection.
9. Use the nursing process as a framework for care of the patient with AIDS.

Nurses have been at the forefront of caring for patients with human immunodeficiency virus (HIV) even before the cause and infectious nature of the virus was known. Today, nurses work as clinicians, researchers, patient advocates, and educators. For many of those nurses who worked the frontlines of the HIV epidemic, COVID-19 brought a sense of déjà vu. Certification for registered nurses and advanced practice nurses is offered through the HIV/AIDS Nursing Certification Board (HANCB). Certification is highly valued and provides formal recognition of HIV/AIDS nursing knowledge. Through the concerted effort of policy makers, researchers, and providers developing best practices and strategies, nurses are in a unique position to meet the challenges of HIV care. Because the field of HIV nursing and medicine changes rapidly, readers should refer to the most recent guidelines and recommendations at www.iasusa.org.

Immunodeficiency, or the inability for the body's natural defenses to protect itself from outside pathogens, presents in one of its most complicated forms in patients with the infection that causes **acquired immunodeficiency syndrome (AIDS).**

PRIMARY AND SECONDARY IMMUNODEFICIENCIES

Immunodeficiencies are classified as either primary or secondary and are further classified by the affected components of the immune system. Primary immunodeficiency diseases are genetic in origin and manifest most commonly in infancy and childhood as abnormally recurrent infections. About 80% of patients with primary immunodeficiency are less than 20 years of age. Many primary immunodeficiencies may occur alone or as part of a syndrome. More than 400 have been described that affect different components of the immune system, affecting more than 500,00 people (NIAID, 2021). Transmission of these inborn errors is predominantly X-linked; therefore, more than 70% of affected patients are male. Primary immunodeficiencies, classified by the main component of the immune system that is dysregulated, affect B lymphocytes (or IgG), T lymphocytes, natural killer (NK) cells, phagocytic cells, or complement proteins. Primary immunodeficiencies are divided into five broad categories based on the part of the immune system that is affected:

- Antibody deficiencies—an antibody is also known as an immunoglobulin, which is a protein used by the immune system to identify and neutralize foreign objects, such as pathogenic bacteria and viruses.
- Combined immunodeficiencies—a genetic condition of the immune system resulting in defects in the immune system.
- Phagocytic cell deficiencies—neutrophils and monocytes are phagocytic white blood cells (they circulate and migrate through tissues to ingest and destroy both microbes and cellular debris).

4. Immune dysregulation—a dysregulated immune disorder occurs when the body can't control or restrain an immune response.
5. Complement deficiencies—complements are a complex system of more than 30 proteins that act in concert to help eliminate infectious microorganisms; if deficiencies exist there is a reduced level of specific proteins or complements involved in proper immune functioning.

More than 50% of primary immunodeficiency is caused by errors in B lymphocytes, causing decreases in production of immunoglobulin and antibodies. The most common B-cell disorder is combined variable immunodeficiency (CVID). The usual presentation is recurrent and frequent (>4 yearly) sinus and chest infections in children or adults (ASCIA, 2021).

In contrast, secondary immunodeficiencies affect the normal immune system of the patient, resulting in increased susceptibility to infection and certain types of cancer. Extrinsic and intrinsic factors, such as nonimmune systemic disorders like HIV infection, immunosuppressive therapy, prolonged illness or hospitalization, and aging, trigger secondary immunodeficiency. These factors cause impaired immune response through loss or destruction of lymphocytes, such as CD4 cell depletion, or decreased production of lymphocytes, as in the effects of irradiation on bone marrow lymphocyte production (Justiz Vaillant & Qurie, 2022). Patients with immunosuppression from secondary immunodeficiencies are referred to as *immunocompromised hosts.* The most common secondary immunodeficiency is AIDS and worldwide it is the effects of malnutrition. Obesity is also linked to suppression of the immune system (Alwarawrah et al., 2018) and may explain the disproportionate mortality and morbidity of COVID-19 among people in racial and ethnic minority groups (Centers for Disease Control and Prevention [CDC], 2022).

HUMAN IMMUNODEFICIENCY VIRUS AND ACQUIRED IMMUNODEFICIENCY SYNDROME

The CDC estimates that more than 1.2 million people are living with HIV/AIDS in the United States. The CDC estimates that there were >29,000 new infections in 2020 with a decline by one third in new diagnoses since 2014. Overall, in the United States, the rate of new infections has declined by two thirds from the height of the epidemic in the 1980s and 1990s. In the past several years, the reduction in the rate of new infections among young men who have sex with men (MSM) reflects increasing success of the use of antiretroviral medications to treat and prevent HIV. Preliminary numbers for January to September of 2021 demonstrate no decline in new infections in spite of COVID-19 isolation guidelines. Worldwide, there were 1.5 million new cases of HIV in 2020, a reduction of 25% from 2014. At the end of 2020, UNAIDS/WHO estimated that 37.7 million people are living with HIV/AIDS in the world, and 73% of those people have access to highly active antiretroviral (ARV) treatment (HAART). While many advances have been made in the treatment and long-term survival of people living with HIV/AIDS, new infections continue. Worldwide, 16% of people infected with HIV are unaware of their diagnosis; these patients are the ones responsible for transmitting most new infections. The recommendation by the CDC is for universal testing for all people between 13 and 65 years of age to lead to early diagnosis and treatment of people infected with HIV and to slow the rate of new infections in the United States (CDC, 2022).

Epidemiology

Over the past 40 years since the first CDC report of five gay men in Los Angeles with a rare pneumonia (PEPFAR, n.d.), 75 million people have been infected worldwide with more than 32 million deaths. Most theories about the origin and spread of AIDS point to a mutated simian immunodeficiency virus (SIV) that crossed species to humans, similar to the changes seen with bird and swine influenza viruses today (McDow, 2018). The earliest blood sample with confirmed HIV infection dates to 1959 in Kinshasa, the Democratic Republic of Congo.

An analysis of people with a diagnosis of HIV infection by race/ethnicity and risk factor underscores the disproportionate impact of HIV among communities of color and MSM of all races. In the United States, new infection rates by race/ethnicity are 42.1 per 100,000 for African Americans and 21.7 for Hispanic and Latino people. Although African Americans make up only 13% of the population of the 34 states surveyed, their rate of HIV infection is 60% higher than that of White people. The rate of new infections in males is five times higher than in females. By transmission category, MSM continue to account for the largest number of diagnoses overall at 69% of newly diagnosed cases and 81% of males with a new HIV diagnosis (CDC, 2019). Transgender people account for 2% of new HIV diagnoses, with 93% among people who identify as male to female (MTF).

Worldwide, AIDS killed more than 680,000 people in 2020, and 75% of those deaths occured in sub-Saharan Africa (WHO, 2021). Between 2000 and 2020, new HIV infections decreased by 49%, and 15.3 million people are alive because of treatment with ARV medications. In sub-Saharan Africa, where millions of children were orphaned by HIV, significant reductions have been achieved by access to inexpensive generic medications.

New research finds that many patients live longer due to the use of ARV agents but are increasingly susceptible to age-associated non-AIDS diseases. The mechanism suspected is a chronic inflammatory process caused by HIV or the long-term use of ARV medications. In resource-rich countries, such as the United States, the epidemic has changed to one in which patients who are motivated can achieve long term, if not lifelong, suppression of the virus with safe and tolerable medications. Patients who access and adhere to therapy rarely suffer AIDS-related complications. More likely, these patients will have many non–AIDS-defining cancers, cardiovascular disease, kidney disease, osteopenia/osteoporosis, liver failure, frailty, and neurologic decline. These normal age-related processes occur sooner and more severely in patients infected with HIV (National Institute on Aging [NIA], 2021; Merrick et al., 2020).

Gerontologic Considerations

Of the 29,000 patients newly diagnosed with HIV infections in 2020, about 3,000 were over the age of 55 years. Ninety-one percent of these patients were linked to care within 1 month of diagnosis (CDC, 2021). HIV infection in middle-aged and older populations may be underreported and underdiagnosed because some health care professionals erroneously believe that older adults are not at risk for HIV infection. In addition, HIV-related dementia in the older adult may mimic Alzheimer disease and may be misdiagnosed.

In fact, several factors put older adults at risk for HIV infection:

- Older adults recently widowed or divorced are dating again and may not be aware of the risks of HIV infection.
- Many older adults are sexually active but do not use condoms, viewing them only as a means of unneeded birth control.
- Older adults may be IV/injection substance users.
- Older adults may have received HIV-infected blood through transfusions before 1985.
- Normal age-related changes include a reduction in immune system function, which puts the older adult at greater risk for infections, cancers, and autoimmune disorders. Many older adults also experience the loss of loved ones, resulting in depression and bereavement, factors that are associated with depressed immune function.

Physical and mental stress of long-term caregiving and the number of comorbidities are significant predictors of the adequacy of social support in older adults with HIV.

Transmission

HIV is a bloodborne, sexually transmissible virus. **HIV-1** is transmitted in body fluids containing HIV or infected $CD4^+$ T lymphocytes. These fluids include blood, seminal fluid, vaginal secretions, amniotic fluid, and human milk. Mother-to-child transmission of HIV-1 may occur in utero or through breast or chestfeeding, but most perinatal infections are thought to occur after exposure during delivery (CDC, 2023; Abbas et al., 2021). Inflammation and breaks in the skin or mucosa result in the increased probability of exposure to HIV. HIV is not transmitted through casual contact. Because HIV is harbored within lymphocytes, a type of white blood cell (WBC), any exposure to infected blood results in a significant risk of infection. The amount of virus and infected cells in the body fluid, as well as other host factors, is associated with the risk of new infection after exposure to that fluid.

Transfusion of blood and blood products can transmit HIV to recipients. However, the risk associated with transfusions has been virtually eliminated because of voluntary self-deferral, completion of a detailed health history, extensive testing, heat treatment of clotting factor concentrates, and more effective methods of virus inactivation. Donated blood is tested for antibodies to HIV-1, **HIV-2**, and p24 antigen (an early marker for HIV infection); in addition, since 1999, nucleic acid amplification testing (NAAT) has been performed (Justiz et al., 2022). However, blood donated during the window period after infection is highly infectious even if it tests negative for HIV antibodies. The window period is the period between initial infection with HIV and development of a positive antibody test for HIV. Development of a positive HIV antibody test generally occurs within 2 to 4 weeks, but incubation periods as long as 10 months have been observed (Sax, 2022).

Until an effective vaccine is developed, preventing HIV by eliminating or reducing risky behaviors is essential (Box 36-1). Primary prevention efforts through effective educational programs are vital for control and prevention. As noted earlier, HIV is not transmitted by casual contact.

Prevention and Education

Nearly 20 years ago, in an effort to reduce further the incidence of HIV infection, the CDC announced an initiative advancing HIV prevention (AHP). This initiative includes four strategies: making HIV testing a routine part of medical care, implementing new models for diagnosing HIV infections outside medical settings, preventing new infections by working with HIV-infected people and their partners, and further decreasing perinatal transmission of HIV. More recently, additional strategies include: prevent new HIV infections, improve health outcomes for persons living with HIV, reduce HIV-related disparities and health inequities, and continually improve effectiveness and efficiency of operations (CDC, 2022b). Today, the CDC website provides customized information about HIV and AIDS, risk of getting or transmitting HIV, and ways to mitigate individual risks (CDC, n.d.).

BOX 36-1

Risk Behaviors Associated With HIV Infection and AIDS

- Sharing injection drug use equipment (aka "works")
- Having sexual relations with infected individuals (both male and female, cis- or transgender)
- Receiving HIV-infected blood or blood products (especially before blood screening was instituted in 1985)
- Being born to a birthing parent with HIV infection not taking ART medication

Initiation of effective educational programs educates the public regarding safer sexual practices and decreases the risk of transmitting HIV-1 infection to sexual partners (Box 36-2). Other than abstinence, consistent and correct use of condoms is the only method proven to decrease the risk for sexual transmission of HIV infection (see Chapter 34, Box 34-3, Fig. 34-1). Latex condoms should be used during vaginal or anal intercourse. Nonlatex condoms made of natural materials, such as lambskin, are available for people with latex allergy but will not protect against HIV infection. Condoms made from polyurethane provide protection against STDs and HIV comparable to that of latex condoms (CDC, 2022a). A condom should be used for oral contact with the penis, and a dental dam (a piece of latex used by dentists to isolate a tooth for treatment) should be used for oral contact with the vagina or rectum.

The use of a microbicide, nonoxynol-9 (N-9), was widely advocated to reduce the risk of HIV infection until a clinical trial conducted in almost 1,000 female commercial sex workers in African countries revealed that those who used N-9 intravaginally along with condoms were 50% more likely to be infected with HIV than those who did not use the N-9 gel. Based on these results, it is now recommended that intravaginal application of N-9 not be used as a means of HIV prevention. Further research throughout the world continues to investigate the use of other microbicides, especially since the female sex partner controls its use. The challenge lies in developing a microbicide that is antiviral yet not irritating to the genital mucosa.

Other topics important in preventive education include avoiding sexual practices that might cut or tear the lining of the rectum, penis, or vagina, and avoiding sexual contact with multiple partners or people who are known to be HIV-positive or IV/injection drug users. In addition, people who are HIV positive or who use injection drugs should be instructed not to donate blood or share drug equipment with others.

Clinical evidence demonstrates that durable undetectable viral load translates into no risk of transmission of HIV. This is based on years of cohort studies of serodiscordant couples in which the HIV-positive partner maintains an undetectable viral load, nonadherence to condom use, and no infection of the HIV-negative partner. Durably undetectable viral load is defined as at least 6 months of undetectable viral load after starting medications (CDC, 2022).

Increasingly, needle exchange programs are available so that IV/injection drug users can obtain sterile drug equipment at no cost. Extensive research has demonstrated that needle exchange programs do not promote increased drug use; however, they have been found to decrease the incidence of blood-borne infections in people who use IV/injection drugs (CDC, 2022). In the absence of needle exchange programs, IV/injection substance users should be instructed on methods to clean their syringes and advised to avoid sharing cotton and other drug use equipment. Substance users interested in treatment programs should be referred to those programs.

Pre-exposure prophylaxis (PrEP), when taken consistently, has been shown in several clinical trials to reduce the rate of sexual transmission of HIV up to 99% and transmission via injection substance use by at least 74% (CDC, 2021). A combination pill of tenofovir and emtricitabine is taken daily to prevent HIV infection among people whose behavior may increase their risk of exposure through sex or injection drug use. This regimen has shown efficacy and safety for people at substantial risk of acquiring HIV infection. However, people on PrEP must commit to medication adherence and regular follow-up with their health care provider (CDC, 2021). To increase adherence rates, a new depot formulation of PrEP is available as an intermuscular injection every 2 months.

BOX 36-2 Health Promotion

Safer Sexual Behaviors

- Encourage patients to be tested for HIV.
- Encourage HIV-positive patients to take ARV medication to sustain an undetectable viral load for 6 months.
- Encourage HIV-negative patients to take PrEP.
- Advise patients to abstain from sharing sexual fluids.
- Advise patients to reduce the number of sexual partners to one.
- Encourage patients to use latex condoms always. If the patient is allergic to latex, polyurethane condoms should be used.
- Advise patients to avoid using cervical caps or diaphragms without using a condom as well.
- Recommend patients always use dental dams for oral–genital or anal stimulation.
- Advise patients to use water-based lubricants to decrease condom breakage.
- Advise patients to avoid anal intercourse because this practice may injure tissues.
- Advise patients to avoid manual–anal intercourse.
- Encourage patients not to ingest urine or semen.
- Educate patients about nonpenetrative sexual activities, such as body massage, social kissing (dry), mutual masturbation, fantasy, and sex films.
- Advise patients to avoid sharing needles, razors, toothbrushes, sex toys, or blood-contaminated articles.
- Encourage patients who are HIV positive to inform previous, present, and prospective sexual and drug-using partners of their HIV-positive status. If the patient is concerned for their safety, advise the patient that many states have anonymous partner notification programs through the public health department to notify people who have been exposed to HIV.
- Advise HIV-positive patients to avoid donating blood, plasma, body organs, or sperm.

Pearls for Practice

Due to the rapidly changing and evolving guidelines for HIV care, it is essential to access reliable internet resources. On December 20, 2021, the FDA approved

the first long-acting extended-release suspension for HIV prevention. Cabotegravir is administered as an IM injection every 2 months as PrEP for adolescent and adult high-risk patients to reduce sexual transmission of HIV (FDA, 2021). Currently, just 25% of the more than 1 million people eligible for PrEP are consistently taking it. With the introduction of a long-acting, well-tolerated injectable, expectations are that more people will begin and adhere to its use.

Related Reproductive Education

Because HIV infection in females often occurs during the childbearing years, family planning issues need to be addressed. Attempts to achieve pregnancy by couples in which only one partner has HIV, referred to as serodiscordant, exposes the unaffected partner to the virus. An undetectable viral load (defined as two plasma viral loads measured 3 months apart), will prevent sexual transmission of HIV to the uninfected partner and, for pregnant people with HIV, minimize the risk of transmission to the infant (Bhatt & Douglas, 2020). In addition, if the HIV-negative partner is female, timing condom-less intercourse to the time of ovulation and taking PrEP will further reduce the risk of sexual transmission of HIV (HIV.gov, 2022). These advances in HIV prevention expand the pregnancy possibilities for people of the full spectrum of sexual and gender identities living with HIV (Pralat et al., 2021). Birthing parents who are HIV positive with a detectable viral load should be instructed not to breast or chestfeed their infants because HIV is transmitted through human milk. Transmission through breast or chestfeeding can be reduced to 1% to 2% with an undetectable maternal viral load. This is a reasonable approach in sub-Saharan countries where many children die from unsanitary water sources and formula is unavailable (Blanche, 2020). Due to effective ARV medications and universal testing of pregnant persons and newborns in the United States, mother-to-child transmission rates have dropped dramatically. The use of medications coupled with avoiding breast or chestfeeding has allowed the risk of transmission of HIV from birthing parent to child to drop from 25% to less than 1% in the Western world (Blanche, 2020). If ARV treatment is begun before pregnancy to a sustained, undetectable level and maintained throughout pregnancy and birth, the transmission rate from birthing parent to child is zero. The complete elimination of pediatric HIV/AIDS has become attainable (Blanche, 2020). The few failures that occur in maternal–child transmission occur with HIV-negative people who become infected after their first trimester screening. Therefore, HIV testing in the second and third trimesters as well as condom use and PrEP are essential to prevent new infections.

Certain contraceptive methods may pose additional health risks for females. The message must be that contraception and prevention of HIV or other sexually transmitted infections (STIs) are two separate considerations. Estrogen and progesterone may increase a female's risk for HIV infection through changes in the cervical mucosa. In addition, females infected with HIV who use estrogen oral contraceptives have shown increased shedding of HIV in vaginal and cervical secretions, putting their partner at increased risk for HIV transmission in serodiscordant couples. Research continues to find a method that reduces risks of HIV infection and pregnancy that is effective and discreet (Achilles et al., 2021). The female condom (see Chapter 34, Fig. 34-1) is as effective in preventing pregnancy as other barrier methods, such as the diaphragm and the male condom. Unlike the diaphragm, the female condom also is effective in preventing the transmission of HIV infection and STIs. The female condom has the distinction of being the first barrier method that can be controlled by the female partner.

Postexposure Prophylaxis

Standard Precautions

In 1996, the CDC and its Hospital Infection Control Practices Advisory Committee (HICPAC) developed guidelines to reduce the risk for exposure of health care workers to HIV through the development of standard precautions. Standard precautions incorporate the major features of universal precautions (designed to reduce the risk of transmission of bloodborne pathogens) and body substance isolation (designed to reduce the risk of transmission of pathogens from moist body substances); these standards are applied to all patients in health care facilities regardless of their diagnosis or presumed infectious status (Box 36-3). Standard precautions apply to blood; all body fluids, secretions, and excretions (except sweat), regardless of whether they contain visible blood; nonintact skin; and mucous membranes (CDC, 2021). The primary purpose of standard precautions is to prevent the transmission of nosocomial infection. The first tier, referred to as standard precautions, reduces the risk for exposure from all recognized or unrecognized sources of infections in hospitals. New elements, such as respiratory hygiene/cough etiquette, safe injection practices, and the use of masks during catheter placement, effectively address those specific issues centered on patient protection. Many elements of standard precautions have been updated to address the increasing use of personal protective equipment (PPE) for health care workers during the COVID-19 pandemic.

Large-scale studies of exposed health care workers continue to be conducted by the CDC and other groups. In November 2000, the Needle-Stick Safety and Prevention Act became law, mandating that health care facilities use devices to protect against sharps injuries. A plan of nursing care for a patient with an infectious disease is available online at http://thepoint.lww.com/Honan3e.

Postexposure Prophylaxis for Health Care Providers

Postexposure prophylaxis in response to the exposure of health care personnel to blood or other body fluids reduces the risk for HIV infection. According to the CDC, there

BOX 36-3

Standard Precautions

The following guidelines prevent the transmission of infection during patient care for all patients, regardless of known or unknown infectious status. Barrier protection should be used at all times to prevent contamination of the skin and mucous membrane with blood, body fluids containing visible blood, other body fluids (cerebrospinal, synovial, pleural, peritoneal, pericardial, amniotic fluids, and semen and vaginal secretions). Barrier protection should be used with *all* tissues. The type of barrier protection used should be appropriate for the type of procedure being performed and the type of exposure anticipated. Examples of barrier protection include disposable laboratory coats, gloves, and eye and face protection. Private rooms and rooms specially equipped with ventilation systems should be used as indicated.

- **Protective body clothing**, such as disposable laboratory coats, should be worn whenever there is potential for splashing of blood or body fluids:
  - Wear a clean, nonsterile gown to protect the skin and prevent soiling of clothing during procedures and patient care activities that are likely to generate splashes or sprays of blood, body fluids, secretions, or excretions.
  - Remove a soiled gown promptly, avoiding contact with clean clothes, and wash hands/perform hand hygiene to prevent the transfer of microorganisms to other patients or environments.
- **Gloves** are to be worn when there is a potential for hand or skin contact with blood, other potentially infectious material, or items and surfaces contaminated with these materials.
  - Clean, nonsterile gloves can be used to protect the nurse's hands.
  - Change gloves after contact with materials that may contain a high concentration of microorganisms, even when working with the same patient.
  - Remove the gloves promptly after use, and wash hands immediately before touching noncontaminated items and environmental surfaces and before going to another patient.
- **Face protection** (face shield, mask, and eye protection) should be worn during procedures that are likely to generate droplets of blood or body fluid to prevent exposure to mucous membranes of the mouth, nose, and eyes.
  - Masks are used for three primary purposes in health care settings:
    1. On health care personnel to protect them from contact with infectious material from patients, e.g., respiratory secretions and sprays of blood or body fluids, consistent with Standard Precautions and Droplet Precautions
    2. On health care personnel when engaged in procedures requiring sterile technique to protect patients from exposure to infectious agents carried in a health care worker's mouth or nose
    3. On coughing patients to limit potential dissemination of infectious respiratory secretions from the patient to others

    Masks should not be confused with particulate respirators that are used to prevent inhalation of small particles that may contain infectious agents transmitted via the airborne route.
- Environmental control includes the following:
  - Ensure that the hospital has adequate procedures for the routine care, cleaning, and disinfection of environmental surfaces, beds, bed rails, bedside equipment, and other surfaces that are touched frequently.
  - Ensure that procedures are being followed.
  - Advocate for the purchase and correct use of the safest equipment.
- Patient care equipment:
  - Used patient care equipment that is soiled with blood, body fluids, secretions, or excretions should be handled in a manner that prevents exposure of the skin and mucous membrane, contamination of clothing, and transfer of microorganisms to other patients and the environment.
  - Ensure that reusable equipment is not used for the care of another patient until it has been cleaned and reprocessed appropriately.
  - Ensure that single-use items are discarded properly.
  - Use mouthpieces, resuscitation bags, or other ventilation devices as an alternative to mouth-to-mouth resuscitation methods.
  - Used linen that is soiled with blood, body fluids, secretions, or excretions should be handled, transported, and processed in a manner that prevents exposure of the skin and mucous membranes, contamination of clothing, and transfer of microorganisms to other patients and environments.
- **Wash hands** thoroughly and immediately if contaminated with blood, body fluids containing visible blood, or other body fluids to which universal precautions apply:
  - Use soap and water or an antimicrobial agent or waterless antiseptic agent.
  - Wash the hands during procedures for the same patient to prevent cross-contamination of different body sites.
  - Wash the hands and other skin surfaces immediately after gloves are removed.
- **Avoid accidental injuries** that can be caused by needles, scalpel blades, laboratory instruments, and so on when performing procedures, cleaning instruments, handling sharp instruments, disposing of used needles or pipettes, and similar activities. Used needles, disposable syringes, scalpel blades, pipettes, and other sharp items are to be placed in puncture-resistant containers marked with a biohazard symbol for disposal:
  - Use "needleless" systems correctly whenever possible.
  - Never recap used needles or otherwise manipulate them by using both hands or use any technique that involves directing the point of the needle toward any part of the body.
  - Use either a one-handed scoop technique or a mechanical device designed for holding the needle sheath.
  - Do not remove used needles from disposable syringes by hand, and do not bend, break, or otherwise manipulate used needles by hand.
  - Place used disposable syringes and needles, scalpel blades, and other sharp items in appropriate puncture-resistant containers as close as practical to the area in which the items were used.
  - Place reusable syringes and needles in a puncture-resistant container for transport to the reprocessing area.

Adapted from Siegel, J. D., Rhinehart, E., Jackson, M., Chiarello, L., & Health care Infection Control Practices Advisory Committee. (2022). 2007 Guideline for isolation precautions: Preventing transmission of infectious agents in health care settings. https://www.cdc.gov/infectioncontrol/guidelines/isolation/index.html

have been only 58 confirmed cases of HIV transmission through occupational exposure, only 1 of which was after 1999 (CDC, 2021). The CDC recommends that all health care providers who have sustained a significant exposure to HIV be counseled and offered anti-HIV postexposure prophylaxis, if appropriate (Box 36-4). More providers are prescribing postexposure prophylaxis for patients exposed to HIV because of high-risk sexual behavior or possible contact through injected substance use. The rationale and process for prescribing postexposure prophylaxis is the same whether the exposure was accidental, such as a needlestick or sexual assault; injection substance use; or another high-risk behavior. Postexposure prophylaxis should not be considered an acceptable method of preventing HIV infection, but is used for reducing risk after a possible transmission. For patients at increased risk for acquiring HIV infection, the nurse should encourage PrEP.

The medications recommended for postexposure prophylaxis are those used to treat established HIV infection. Prophylaxis should be started immediately after exposure; therapy started more than 72 hours after exposure is thought to offer no benefit due to rapid increases in viral load upon initial infection.

The recommended course of therapy involves taking the prescribed medications for 4 weeks. Those who choose post-exposure prophylaxis must be prepared for the side effects of the medications and must be adherent to treatment or risk sero-conversion and possible viral resistance. Cost should not be a concern; the average wholesale price of a medication regimen for 28 days is less than $1,000 but is available for free from most emergency rooms, from Planned Parenthood, and through programs sponsored by pharmaceutical companies (CDC, 2021). Most health care employers and agencies provide access to treatment and medication through Occupational Health Services.

BOX 36-4

Postexposure Prophylaxis for Health Care Providers

If you sustain a puncture injury, such as a needle stick, take the following actions immediately:

- Wash the area thoroughly with soap and water.
- Alert your supervisor/nursing faculty and initiate the injury-reporting system used in the setting.
- Identify the source patient, who may need to be tested for HIV, hepatitis B, and hepatitis C. State laws will determine whether written informed consent must be obtained from the source patient before their testing. Rapid testing should be used, if possible, if the HIV status of the source patient is unknown because results can be available within 20 minutes.
- Report as quickly as possible to employee health services, the emergency department, or other designated treatment facility. This visit should be documented in your confidential medical record.
- Give consent for baseline testing for HIV, hepatitis B, and hepatitis C. Confidential HIV testing can be performed up to 72 hours after the exposure but should be performed as soon as you can give informed consent for baseline testing.
- Get postexposure prophylaxis for HIV in accordance with CDC guidelines. If possible, start the prophylaxis medications within 2 hours after exposure. Postexposure prophylaxis must be initiated within 72 hours of exposure to be effective. Make sure that you are being monitored for symptoms of toxicity. Practice safer sex until follow-up testing is complete. Continue the HIV medications for 4 weeks.
- Follow up with postexposure testing at 1 month, 3 months, and 6 months.
- Document the exposure in detail for your own records, as well as for your employer.

Pathophysiology

Because HIV infection is an infectious disease, it is important to understand how HIV integrates itself into a person's immune system and how immunity plays a role in the course of infection. This knowledge is also essential for understanding medication therapy and vaccine development.

Viruses are intracellular parasites. HIV belongs to a group of viruses known as **retroviruses**. These viruses carry their genetic material in the form of ribonucleic acid (RNA) rather than deoxyribonucleic acid (DNA). As shown in Figure 36-1, HIV consists of a viral core containing the viral RNA, surrounded by an envelope consisting of protruding glycoproteins (gp). For HIV to enter the targeted cell, the membrane of the viral envelope must be fused with the plasma membrane of the cell, a process mediated by the envelope glycoproteins of HIV and other coreceptors (National Institutes of Health [NIH], 2021; Norris & Tuan, 2020).

All viruses target specific cells. Lymphocytes (a type of WBC) consist of three major populations: T cells, B cells, and NK cells. Mature T cells are phenotypically (characteristics of the cells) composed of two major subpopulations, defined by cell surface reciprocal expression of CD4 or CD8. Approximately two thirds of peripheral blood T cells are $CD4^+$, and approximately one third are $CD8^+$. Most people have about 700 to 1,500 $CD4^+$ cells/mm^3, but a count as low as 500 cells/mm^3 can be considered "normal." HIV targets cells with the CD4 glycoprotein expressed on the surface of T lymphocytes, **monocytes**, dendritic cells, and brain microglia. Monocytes and macrophages serve as long-lived reservoirs of HIV. Most primary clinical isolates of HIV use the chemokine coreceptor **CCR5** for cell entry. HIV must attach to both the CD4 and the CCR5 coreceptor binding sites in order to infect $CD4^+$ cells.

A mutation of CCR5 that is common among Caucasians but no other ethnic groups has been identified. About 1% of Caucasians lack functional CCR5 and are highly protected against HIV infection even if exposed (although protection is not absolute); about 18% are not markedly protected against infection but, if infected, demonstrate significantly slower

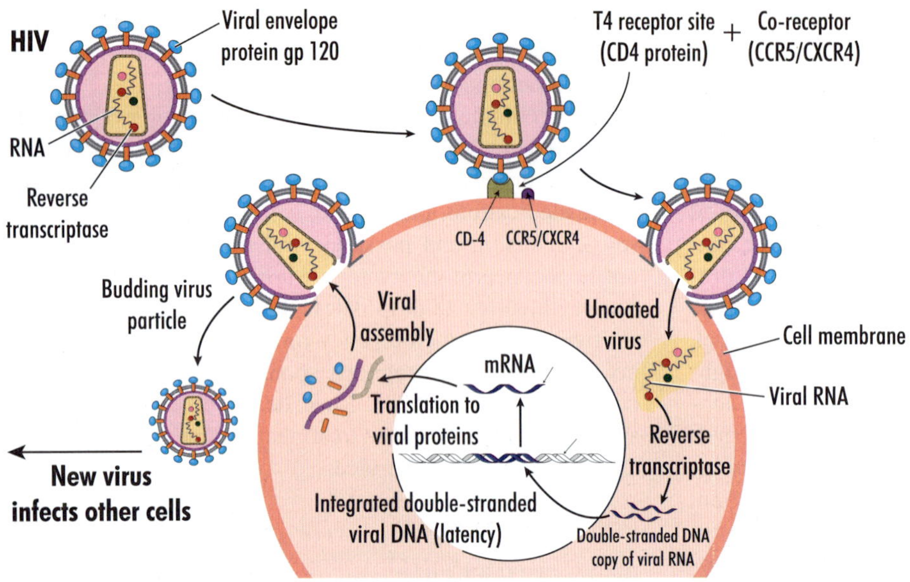

FIGURE 36-1 **HIV virus. (From shutterstock.com. ID: 198678155.)**

rates of disease progression (Tebas et al., 2014). Reports of a male treated in Berlin, Germany, who received a stem cell transplant for treatment of acute myeloid leukemia from a donor with the Delta 32 mutation at the CCR5-binding site shows promise for further research for HIV treatment. After total intentional destruction of the patient's bone marrow, a procedure with a 30% mortality rate, this patient had no detectable virus 20 months after transplant and discontinuation of ARV therapy (Symons et al., 2014).

The HIV life cycle is complex (see Fig. 36-1) and consists of the following:

- The HIV gp120 and gp41 attach to the uninfected $CD4^{+}$ lymphocyte at the CD4 receptor and one of two coreceptors, fusing with the cell membrane.
- The viral core contents are emptied into the host cell, a process known as *uncoating*.
- HIV enzyme **reverse transcriptase** converts the viral genetic material from RNA into double-stranded DNA.
- Double-stranded DNA is spliced into the cellular DNA by the action of integrase, another HIV enzyme.
- During transcription, the integrated DNA or **provirus** makes new viral proteins and viral RNA. Provirus may remain inactive for months to years within the $CD4^{+}$ cell and other components of the immune system.
- HIV protease cleaves the new proteins (polyproteins).
- The new proteins join the viral RNA into new viral particles.
- New viral particles bud from the cell and start the process all over.

In resting (nondividing) cells, HIV can apparently survive in a latent state as an integrated provirus that produces few or no viral particles. These resting $CD4^{+}$ T cells as well as monocytes and macrophages can be stimulated to produce new particles if something reactivates them. Activation of the infected cell may be achieved by antigens; mitogens; certain cytokines (tumor necrosis factor-α [TNF] or interleukin-1 [IL-1]); or virus gene products of such viruses as **cytomegalovirus** (CMV), Epstein–Barr virus, herpes simplex virus, and hepatitis viruses. Consequently, whenever the infected T cell is activated, HIV replication and budding occur, which often destroys the host cell. Then newly formed HIV is released into the blood plasma and infects other $CD4^{+}$ cells (see Fig. 36-1). If inadequately suppressed, HIV mutates at a relatively constant rate, enabling it to blunt or completely suppress the effects of HIV medications.

Assessment and Diagnosis

Diagnostic tests are summarized in Table 36-1.

TABLE 36-1 **Selected Laboratory Tests for Diagnosing and Tracking HIV and Assessing Immune Status**

Test	Findings in HIV Infection
Enzyme immunoassay (EIA)	Antibodies are detected, resulting in positive results. May have false-negative results within the window period.
Antigen/antibody	Detects HIV antibodies and p24 antigen; detects early acute infection.
Viral load	Quantifies HIV RNA in the plasma. Monitors efficacy of ART through virologic suppression. Goal is for load to be undetectable.
CD4/CD8 ratio	These are markers found on lymphocytes. HIV kills $CD4^{+}$ cells, which results in a significantly impaired immune system. Used in decision to initiate ART and use of prophylactic medications.

HIV Antibody Tests

Before an HIV antibody test is performed, the meaning of the test and possible test results are explained, and informed consent for the test is obtained from the patient. The CDC recommends universal testing of all patients 13 to 75 years of age through opt-out testing. However, some states still require written informed consent and face-to-face results counseling. Consult state laws about specific requirements related to testing for HIV. When the result of the HIV antibody test is received, it is carefully explained to the patient in private (Box 36-5). All test results are kept confidential. Education and counseling about the test result and about preventing transmission are essential. The patient's psychological response to a seropositive test result may include feelings of panic, depression, and hopelessness. The social and interpersonal consequences of a positive test result can be devastating. The patient may lose their sexual partner because of disclosure. The patient may experience discrimination in employment and housing, as well as social ostracism. For these reasons and others, a patient who tests positive may need ongoing counseling, as well as referrals for social, financial, medical, and psychological support services.

Patients whose test results are seronegative may develop a false sense of security, possibly resulting in continued high-risk behaviors or feelings that they are immune to the virus. These patients may need ongoing counseling to help modify high-risk behaviors and to encourage returns for repeated testing. Other patients may experience anxiety regarding the uncertainty of their status.

BOX 36-5

HIV Test Results: Implications for Patients

Interpretation of Positive Test Results

- Antibodies to HIV are present in the blood (the patient has been infected with the virus, and the body has produced antibodies).
- HIV is active in the body, and the patient can transmit the virus to others.
- Despite HIV infection, the patient does not necessarily have AIDS.
- The patient is not immune to HIV (the antibodies do not indicate immunity).

Interpretation of Negative Test Results

- Antibodies to HIV are not present in the blood at this time, which can mean that the patient has not been infected with HIV or, if infected, the body has not yet produced antibodies (the patient may be in the window period—usually 4 weeks to 6 months).
- The patient should continue taking precautions. The test result does not mean that the patient is immune to the virus, nor does it mean the patient is not infected; it just means that the body may not have produced antibodies yet. Recommend repeat testing if at high risk for HIV.

During initial infection with HIV, the immune system responds by producing antibodies against the virus, usually within 4 to 12 weeks after infection. In 1985, the U.S. Food and Drug Administration (FDA) licensed the first HIV-1 antibody assay that used approximately 5 to 7 mL of blood. The **enzyme immunoassay (EIA)** test, formerly referred to as the enzyme-linked immunosorbent assay (ELISA) test, identifies antibodies directed specifically against HIV. As of 2014, the CDC recommends testing with the newer fourth-generation test for HIV-1 and HIV-2 antibodies and HIV-1 p24 antigen using an immunoassay process. The p24 antigen is detectable as early as 14 days after exposure (Huynh & Kahwaji, 2022). If an HIV infection is suspected (before 14 days), an **HIV** RNA test can detect an infection that may be present before the p24 antigen is detected (Huynh & Kahwaji, 2022).

Home-based testing for HIV antibodies using a small amount of blood was first proposed in 1985 but was not approved by the FDA until 1995. Although home testing kits are commercially available using oral swabs, they raise concerns because of the lack of counseling and the possibility of inaccurate results, including both false-positive and false-negative results.

Viral Load Tests

Target amplification methods quantify HIV RNA or DNA levels in the plasma and have replaced p24 antigen capture assays. Target amplification methods include reverse transcriptase–**polymerase chain reaction** (RT-PCR) and nucleic acid sequence–based amplification (NASBA). A widely used **viral load test** measures plasma HIV RNA levels. Currently, these tests track viral load and response to treatment of HIV infection. RT-PCR is also used to detect HIV in high-risk seronegative people before antibodies are measurable, to confirm a positive EIA result, and to screen neonates. Viral load is a better predictor of the risk for HIV disease progression than the $CD4^+$ count. The lower the viral load, the longer the time to AIDS diagnosis and the longer the survival time. Increased presence of the virus causes lymphoid dysfunction and other inflammatory responses that affect long-term survival (CDC, 2021).

Stages of HIV Disease

The stage of HIV disease is based on clinical history, physical examination, laboratory evidence of immune dysfunction, signs and symptoms, opportunistic infections, and malignancies. The CDC standard case definition of AIDS categorizes HIV infection and AIDS in adults and adolescents based on clinical conditions associated with HIV infection and $CD4^+$ T-cell counts. The classification system groups clinical conditions into one of three categories, denoted A, B, and C. Each category represents clinical progression of HIV infection in the patient, from asymptomatic (category A) to "full blown" AIDS (category C). Although a patient's health and immune status may improve, the CDC classification of the patient's illness does not change. Universal testing coupled with early diagnosis and treatment attempts to intervene in the natural progression of HIV to maintain as functional an immune system as possible.

Primary Infection (Acute HIV Infection, Acute Retroviral Syndrome)

The period from infection with HIV to the development of antibodies to HIV is known as **primary infection**. This period is characterized by intense viral replication and widespread dissemination of HIV throughout the body. During primary infection, a window period occurs, during which a person with HIV infection tests negative on the HIV antibody blood test. Although antibodies to the HIV envelope glycoproteins typically can be detected in the sera of HIV-infected individuals by 2 to 3 weeks after infection, most of these antibodies lack the ability to inhibit virus infection. By the time neutralizing antibodies can be detected, HIV-1 is firmly established in the host. During this period, there are high levels of viral replication and destruction of $CD4^+$ T cells, resulting in high levels of HIV in the blood and a dramatic drop in $CD4^+$ T-cell counts from the normal range of 500 to 1,500 cells/mm^3 of blood. Detectable levels of virus can occur as early as 72 hours after exposure; this provides the rationale for immediate initiation of prophylaxis.

About 3 weeks into this acute phase, the person may display symptoms similar to mononucleosis, such as fever, enlarged lymph nodes, rash, muscle aches, and headaches. These symptoms resolve within another 1 to 3 weeks as the immune system begins to recuperate. That is, the $CD4^+$ T-cell population responds in ways that cause other immune cells, such as $CD8^+$ lymphocytes, to increase their killing of infected, virus-producing cells. The body produces antibody molecules in an effort to contain the virus; they bind to free HIV particles (outside cells) and assist in their removal. This balance between the amount of HIV in the body and the immune response is referred to as the **viral set point**; it results in a steady state of infection that can last for years.

Primary HIV infection, the time during which the viral burden set point is achieved, includes the acute symptomatic and early infection phases. During this initial stage, viral replication is associated with dissemination in lymphoid tissue (lymph nodes, spleen, tonsils and adenoids, and the thymus) and a distinct immunologic response. The final level of the viral set point is inversely correlated with disease prognosis; that is, the higher the viral set point, the poorer the prognosis. The primary infection stage is part of CDC category A.

HIV Asymptomatic (CDC Category A: More Than 500 $CD4^+$ T Lymphocytes/mm^3)

When a viral set point is reached, a chronic, clinically asymptomatic state begins. Despite its best efforts, the immune system rarely, if ever, fully eliminates the virus. By about 6 months, the rate of viral replication reaches a lower but relatively steady state that is reflected in the maintenance of viral levels at a set point. This set point varies greatly from patient to patient and dictates the subsequent rate of disease progression; on average, 8 to 10 years pass before a major HIV-related complication develops. In this prolonged, chronic stage, patients feel well and have few if any symptoms. Apparent good health continues because $CD4^+$ T-cell levels remain high enough to preserve defensive responses to other pathogens.

HIV Symptomatic (CDC Category B: 200 to 499 $CD4^+$ T Lymphocytes/mm^3)

Over time, the number of $CD4^+$ T cells gradually falls. Category B consists of symptomatic conditions in HIV-infected patients that are not included in the conditions listed in category C. These conditions also must meet one of the following criteria: (1) the condition is due to HIV infection or a defect in cellular immunity, or (2) the condition is considered to have a clinical course or to require management that is complicated by HIV infection.

AIDS (CDC Category C: Fewer Than 200 $CD4^+$ T Lymphocytes/mm^3)

When the $CD4^+$ T-cell level drops below 200 cells/mm^3 of blood, the person has AIDS. As levels decrease to fewer than 100 cells/mm^3, the immune system is significantly impaired. Once a patient has had a category C condition, they maintain a permanent diagnosis of AIDS even if the immune system recuperates. This classification has implications for entitlements (e.g., disability benefits, housing, and food stamps) because these programs are often linked to an AIDS diagnosis. Although the revised classification system of the CDC emphasizes $CD4^+$ T-cell counts, it allows for the count of $CD4^+$ T-cells to be expressed as a percentage of $CD4^+$ T cells compared with total lymphocytes. The $CD4^+$ percentage is less subject to variation on repeated measurements than is the absolute $CD4^+$ T-cell count. A $CD4^+$ percentage of less than 14% of the total lymphocytes is consistent with an AIDS diagnosis. The percentage, as compared with the absolute number of $CD4^+$ T cells, becomes particularly important when the patient has a heightened immune response to infections in addition to HIV.

Clinical Manifestations

During the first stage of HIV infection, the patient may be asymptomatic or may exhibit various signs and symptoms. The patient's health history should alert the health care provider about the need for HIV screening based on the patient's sexual practices, IV/injection drug use, and receipt of blood transfusions. Patients who are in later stages of HIV infection may have a variety of symptoms related to their immunosuppressed state. HIV often causes **opportunistic infections (OIs)**. With widespread availability and improved effectiveness of ARVs, clinical occurrence of OIs has plummeted. Unfortunately, there still are parts of the world with limited availability of ARVs. For nurses who travel to work in these areas, OIs and other common manifestations are discussed below.

Respiratory Manifestations

Dyspnea (labored breathing), cough, chest pain, and fever are associated with various OIs, such as those caused by *Pneumocystis jirovecii, Mycobacterium avium-intracellulare,* CMV, and *Legionella* species.

Pneumocystic Pneumonia

The most common infection in people with AIDS is *Pneumocystic* pneumonia (PCP). The current guidelines on treatment of OIs (Sax et al., 2023) refer to the causative organism as *P. jirovecii* instead of *P. carinii,* although the infection is still abbreviated as PCP. PCP was one of the first OIs described in association with AIDS, and it is the most common OI resulting in the diagnosis of AIDS. Without prophylactic therapy, 80% of all people infected with HIV will develop PCP.

The clinical presentation of PCP in patients with HIV infection is generally less acute than in people who are immunosuppressed because of other conditions. The time between the onset of symptoms and the actual documentation of disease may be weeks to months. Patients with AIDS initially develop nonspecific signs and symptoms, such as nonproductive cough, fever, chills, dyspnea, and occasionally chest pain. PCP may be present despite the absence of crackles. Arterial oxygen concentrations in patients who are breathing room air may be mildly decreased, indicating minimal hypoxemia. Pulse oximetry after exercise, such as walking up and down a flight of stairs, is a simple, noninvasive test for outpatient use.

If left untreated, PCP eventually progresses and causes significant pulmonary impairment and respiratory failure. Some patients have a dramatic onset and a fulminating course involving severe hypoxemia, cyanosis, tachypnea, and altered mental status. Respiratory failure can develop within 2 to 3 days after the initial appearance of symptoms.

PCP can be diagnosed definitively by identifying the organism in lung tissue or bronchial secretions. This is accomplished by such procedures as sputum induction, bronchial-alveolar lavage, and transbronchial biopsy (by fiberoptic bronchoscope).

Tuberculosis

Mycobacterium tuberculosis tends to occur with IV/injection drug use and others with a pre-existing high prevalence of tuberculosis (TB) infection (refer to Chapter 9). TB that occurs late in HIV infection is characterized by the absence of a delayed type of hypersensitivity response mediated by T lymphocytes to the tuberculin skin test. This is known as **anergy**, and it occurs because the compromised immune system can no longer respond to the TB antigen. For this reason, TB testing is essential upon initial diagnosis of HIV, with appropriate treatment for patients demonstrating latent TB infection. Nurses administer the Mantoux test to determine infection with TB (refer to Chapter 9 for details). In the later stages of HIV infection, TB may be associated with dissemination to extrapulmonary sites (miliary TB), such as the central nervous system (CNS), bone, pericardium, stomach, peritoneum, and scrotum. Multidrug-resistant strains of the bacillus have emerged and often are associated with a lack of adherence to regimens for antituberculosis medication.

Immune reconstitution syndrome (also known as *paradoxical reactions*) seems to occur more often among patients with TB. Patients can experience high fevers, worsening lymphadenopathy, or transient to severe worsening of pulmonary infiltrates and expanding CNS lesions. Reduction of HIV-1 RNA levels and marked increases in $CD4^+$ T-lymphocyte counts have been associated with the occurrence of paradoxical reactions in patients with TB disease or *Mycobacterium avium* complex (MAC). A common mycobacterium, MAC may cause infection in immunosuppressed patients. While affecting the lungs primarily, it can have extrapulmonary impact on the lymph nodes, bones, skin, and other tissues. However, a MAC infection cannot be passed from one person to another. Although the majority of reactions occur within the first 3 months after initiation of ART, it can also occur in those whose CD4 T lymphocyte (CD4) cell counts <50 cells/mm^3 (French & Meintjes, 2020; HIV.gov, 2022).

Gastrointestinal Manifestations

The gastrointestinal (GI) manifestations of AIDS include loss of appetite, nausea, vomiting, oral and esophageal candidiasis, and chronic diarrhea. Diarrhea is a problem in 50% to 90% of all AIDS patients. GI symptoms may be related to the direct effect of HIV on the cells lining the intestines. Some of the enteric pathogens that occur most frequently, identified by stool cultures or intestinal biopsy, are *Cryptosporidium muris, Salmonella* species, *Isospora belli, Giardia lamblia,* CMV, *Clostridium difficile,* and *M. avium-intracellulare.* In patients with AIDS, the effects of diarrhea can be devastating in terms of profound weight loss (more than 10% of body weight), fluid and electrolyte imbalances, perianal skin excoriation, weakness, and inability to perform the usual activities of daily living.

Candidiasis

Candidiasis or *thrush,* a fungal infection, occurs in almost all patients with AIDS and AIDS-related conditions. It commonly precedes other life-threatening infections and is characterized by adherent creamy-white patches in the oral cavity (Fig. 36-2). When left untreated, oral candidiasis progresses to involve the esophagus and stomach. Associated signs and symptoms include difficult, painful swallowing, and retrosternal pain. Some patients also develop ulcerating oral lesions and are particularly susceptible to dissemination of candidiasis to other body systems.

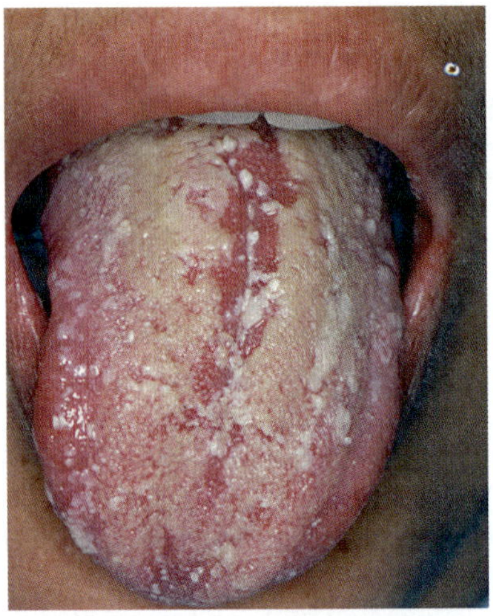

FIGURE 36-2 **Oral candidiasis. (From Goodheart, H. P. [2015]. *Goodheart's photoguide of common skin disorders* [4th ed.]. Lippincott Williams & Wilkins.)**

Wasting Syndrome

Wasting syndrome is part of the category C case definition for AIDS. Diagnostic criteria include profound involuntary weight loss exceeding 10% of baseline body weight and either chronic diarrhea for more than 30 days or chronic weakness and documented intermittent or constant fever in the absence of any concurrent illness that could explain these findings. This protein–energy malnutrition is multifactorial. In some AIDS-associated illnesses, patients experience a hypermetabolic state in which excessive calories are burned and lean body mass is lost. This state is similar to that seen in sepsis or trauma and can lead to organ failure. The distinction between cachexia (wasting) and malnutrition, or between cachexia and simple weight loss, is important because the metabolic derangement seen in wasting syndrome may not be modified by nutritional support alone.

Progressive tissue wasting may occur with only modest GI involvement and without diarrhea. TNF and IL-1 are cytokines that play important roles in AIDS-related wasting syndrome and the inflammatory processes that complicate its course. Both act directly on the hypothalamus to cause anorexia. Cytokine-induced fever accelerates the body's metabolism by 14% for every 1°F increase in temperature. TNF causes inefficient use of lipids by reducing enzymes that are needed for fat metabolism, whereas IL-1 triggers the release of amino acids from muscle tissue. It is believed that infections and sepsis lead to transient increases in TNF, IL-1, and other cell mediators above the chronically elevated levels that often are seen with AIDS (refer to Chapter 53 for discussion of sepsis). These transient increases in TNF and IL-1 trigger muscle wasting. People with AIDS generally experience increased protein metabolism in relation to fat metabolism, which results in significant decreases in lean body mass due to muscle and protein breakdown. Hypertriglyceridemia, seen in people with AIDS and attributed to chronically elevated cytokine levels, can persist for months without tissue wasting and loss of lean body mass. It is also caused by **protease inhibitors** (PIs) and increases the risk for pancreatitis.

Oncologic Manifestations

Patients with AIDS have a higher than usual incidence of cancer, possibly related to HIV stimulation of developing cancer cells or to the immune deficiency that allows cancer-causing substances, such as viruses, to transform susceptible cells into malignant cells. Kaposi sarcoma (KS), certain types of B-cell lymphomas, and invasive cervical carcinoma are included in the CDC classification of AIDS-related malignancies. Carcinomas of the skin, stomach, pancreas, rectum, and bladder also occur more frequently in people with AIDS.

Kaposi Sarcoma

KS, the most common HIV-related malignancy, is a disease that involves the endothelial layer of blood and lymphatic vessels. Since the introduction of ARVs, there has been a significant decrease in the incidence of KS. It is associated with transmission of human herpes virus 8 (HHV-8). Acquired KS occurs in patients who are treated with immunosuppressive agents and commonly in patients who have undergone organ transplantation. In such patients, KS usually resolves once the dose of the immunosuppressive medication is decreased or discontinued. In people with AIDS, epidemic KS is seen most often among gay and bisexual males. Although the histopathology of all forms of KS is virtually identical, the clinical manifestations differ: AIDS-related KS exhibits a more variable and aggressive course, ranging from localized cutaneous lesions to disseminated disease involving multiple organ systems. Cutaneous signs may be the first manifestation of HIV, appearing in more than 90% of HIV-infected patients as the immune functions deteriorate. These skin signs correlate to low $CD4^+$ counts, usually less than 50. Cutaneous lesions can appear anywhere on the body and are brownish pink to deep purple. They may be flat or raised and surrounded by ecchymoses (hemorrhagic patches) and edema (Fig. 36-3). Rapid development of lesions involving large areas of skin is associated with extensive disfigurement. The location and size of some lesions can lead to venous stasis, lymphedema, and pain. Ulcerative lesions disrupt skin integrity and increase discomfort and susceptibility to infection. The most common sites of visceral involvement are the lymph nodes, GI tract, and lungs. Involvement of internal organs may eventually lead to organ failure, hemorrhage, infection, and death.

Proper identification of these lesions is difficult with darkly pigmented skin; biopsy confirms the diagnosis. Prognosis depends on the extent of the tumor, the presence of other symptoms of HIV infection, and the $CD4^+$ count. Death may result from tumor progression.

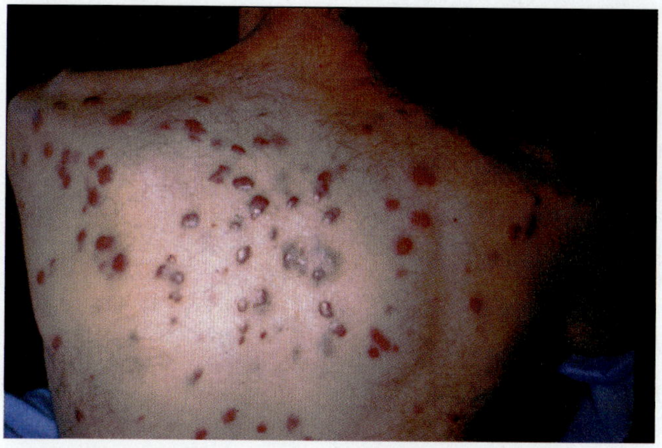

FIGURE 36-3 **Lesions of AIDS-related Kaposi sarcoma. Whereas some patients may have lesions that remain flat, others experience extensively disseminated, raised lesions with edema.**

B-Cell Lymphomas

B-cell lymphomas are the second most common malignancy occurring in people with AIDS. Lymphomas associated with AIDS usually differ from those occurring in the general population. Patients with AIDS are typically much younger than the usual population affected by non-Hodgkin lymphoma. In addition, AIDS-related lymphomas tend to develop outside the lymph nodes, most commonly in the brain, bone marrow, and GI tract. These types of lymphomas are characteristically of a higher grade, indicating aggressive growth and resistance to treatment.

The course of AIDS-related lymphomas includes multiple sites of organ involvement and complications related to OIs. Although aggressive combination chemotherapy is frequently successful in the treatment of non-Hodgkin lymphoma in the patient who is HIV negative, treatment is less successful in people with AIDS because of severe hematologic toxicity and complications of OIs.

Neurologic Manifestations

An estimated 80% of all patients with AIDS experience some form of neurologic involvement during the course of HIV infection. Many neuropathologic disorders are underreported because patients may have neurologic involvement without overt signs or symptoms. Neurologic complications involve central, peripheral, and autonomic functions. HIV-associated neurocognitive disorders (HAND) can affect memory, attention, language, and executive functioning. Neurologic dysfunction results from direct effects of HIV on nervous system tissue, OIs, primary or metastatic neoplasms, cerebrovascular changes, metabolic encephalopathies, or complications secondary to therapy. Immune system response to HIV infection in the CNS includes inflammation, atrophy, demyelination, degeneration, and necrosis.

HIV Encephalopathy

HIV encephalopathy or HIV-associated dementia (HAD) was formerly referred to as *AIDS dementia complex.* The clinical syndrome is characterized by a progressive decline in cognitive, behavioral, and motor functions. Substantial evidence exists showing that HIV encephalopathy is a direct result of HIV infection in brain macrophages and microglia. HIV infection is thought to trigger the release of lymphokines and other inflammatory factors that result in cellular dysfunction or interference with neurotransmitter function rather than cellular damage.

Signs and symptoms may be subtle and difficult to distinguish from fatigue, depression, or the adverse effects of treatment for infections and malignancies. Early manifestations include memory deficits, headache, difficulty concentrating, progressive confusion, psychomotor slowing, apathy, and ataxia. Later stages include global cognitive impairments, delay in verbal responses, a vacant stare, spastic paraparesis (a slight weakness or paralysis of both lower extremities), hyperreflexia, psychosis, hallucinations, tremor, incontinence, seizures, mutism, and death.

Confirming the diagnosis of HIV encephalopathy can be difficult. Extensive neurologic evaluation includes a computed tomography (CT) scan, which may indicate diffuse cerebral atrophy and ventricular enlargement. Other tests that may detect abnormalities include magnetic resonance imaging (MRI), analysis of CSF through lumbar puncture, and brain biopsy.

Cytomegalovirus

Retinitis is the most common clinical manifestation of CMV. Before the use of ARVs, 30% of patients experienced CMV retinitis with a high incidence of blindness. The incidence of CMV retinitis has been reduced by 80% with these medications.

Peripheral retinitis might be asymptomatic or present with floaters, scotomata (a loss of vision within the visual field), or reduced visual acuity. CMV retinitis has characteristic fluffy yellow-white retinal lesions with or without intraretinal hemorrhage visualized on funduscopic examination. Blood vessels near the lesions might appear to be sheathed. Patients with $CD4^+$ counts of less than 50 should be examined by an ophthalmologist on a yearly basis (Sax et al., 2023).

Other Neurologic Disorders

Other common infections involving the nervous system include *Toxoplasma gondii, M. tuberculosis*, and syphilis. Additional neurologic manifestations include both central and peripheral neuropathies. Vascular myelopathy is a degenerative disorder that affects the lateral and posterior columns of the spinal cord, resulting in progressive spastic paraparesis, ataxia (inability to coordinate body movements), and incontinence. HIV-related peripheral neuropathy is thought to be a demyelinating disorder. It is associated with pain and numbness in the extremities, weakness, diminished deep tendon reflexes, orthostatic hypotension, and impotence. Peripheral neuropathy is a common adverse effect of many HIV medications.

Depressive Manifestations

The prevalence of depression among people with HIV infection is two to three times the rate of the general population (Perazzo et al., 2020). The causes of depression are multifactorial and may include a history of pre-existing mental illness, neuropsychiatric disturbances, and psychosocial factors. Depression also occurs in people with HIV infection in response to the physical symptoms, including pain and weight loss, as well as isolation. People with HIV/AIDS who are depressed may experience irrational guilt and shame, loss of self-esteem, feelings of helplessness and worthlessness, and suicidal ideation.

Integumentary Manifestations

Cutaneous manifestations are associated with HIV infection and the accompanying OIs and malignancies. KS (described earlier) and OIs, such as herpes zoster and herpes simplex, are associated with painful vesicles that disrupt skin integrity. Molluscum contagiosum is a viral infection characterized by multiple grouped lesions. Seborrheic dermatitis is associated with an indurated, diffuse, scaly rash involving the scalp and face (see Chapter 51). Patients with AIDS also may exhibit a generalized eosinophilic folliculitis associated with dry, flaking skin or atopic dermatitis, such as eczema or psoriasis. Up to 60% of patients treated with trimethoprim-sulfamethoxazole (TMP-SMZ) develop a drug-related rash that is pruritic with pinkish-red macules and papules. Regardless of the origin of these rashes, patients experience discomfort and are at increased risk for additional infection from disrupted skin integrity. See Chapter 50 for how to assess and describe rashes.

Pearls for Practice

The viral exanthem associated with acute retroviral syndrome during initial infection with AIDS is one of the few rashes accurately described as maculopapular (flat, erythematous rash on the skin that is covered with small confluent [merging] bumps).

Gynecologic Manifestations

Persistent, recurrent vaginal candidiasis or bacterial vaginosis may be the first sign of HIV infection in female patients. Past or present genital ulcer disease is a risk factor for the transmission of HIV infection. Females with HIV infection are more susceptible to and have increased rates of incidence and recurrence of genital ulcer disease and venereal warts. Ulcerative STIs, such as chancroid, syphilis, and herpes, are more severe in females with HIV infection. Human papillomavirus (HPV) causes venereal warts and is a risk factor for cervical intraepithelial neoplasia, a cellular change that is frequently a precursor to cervical cancer. Females with HIV are 10 times more likely to develop cervical intraepithelial neoplasia than are those not infected with HIV. HIV-seropositive females with cervical carcinoma present at a more advanced stage of disease and have more persistent and recurrent disease and a shorter interval to recurrence and death than females without HIV infection.

A significant percentage of patients who require hospitalization for pelvic inflammatory disease (PID) have HIV infection. Female patients with HIV are at increased risk for PID, and the associated inflammation may potentiate the transmission of HIV infection (see Chapter 34 for information related to PID). Moreover, people with HIV infection appear to have a higher incidence of menstrual abnormalities, including amenorrhea or bleeding between periods, than do people without HIV infection.

Immunologic Manifestations

Immune reconstitution inflammatory syndromes (IRIS) have been described for mycobacterial infections, including disease caused by MAC and *M. tuberculosis*, PCP, toxoplasmosis, hepatitis B and hepatitis C, CMV infection, varicella-zoster virus infection, cryptococcal infection, and progressive multifocal leukoencephalopathy. Immune reconstitution syndromes are characterized by fever and worsening of the clinical manifestations of the OI, or the appearance of new manifestations developing during the first 3 months after the initiation of ART. It is important to determine the absence or reappearance of the underlying OI, new drug toxicity, or a new OI; any or all of these can occur in the patient as the immune system recovers. Treatment is directed toward appropriate antimicrobial therapy for the provoking infection; terminating ART is only considered when treatment options have failed and life-threatening disease exists (French & Meintjes, 2020). If the syndrome represents an immune restoration response, corticosteroids may be used to alleviate the inflammatory reaction, nonsteroidal anti-inflammatory agents (NSAIDs) are reserved for patients with severe inflammation, particularly when it is life threatening, or significant symptoms (French & Meintjes, 2020). The nurse should be alert to signs of immune reconstitution syndrome and advise the patient to seek health care if they are feeling sicker with no clear explanation.

Medical and Nursing Management

Treatment Regimen

Protocols for treatment of HIV disease change frequently. The U.S. DHHS periodically convenes a team of HIV specialists from across the country to evaluate the latest evidence and make recommendations that are widely disseminated (DHHS, 2022). In general, ARV medications should be offered to all people, regardless of CD4 cell count to reduce the morbidity and mortality of HIV infection (DHHS, 2022). In addition, ARV therapy (ART) is recommended to prevent HIV transmission. Even with these overriding recommendations from the DHHS, treatment decisions are individualized based on several factors, including $CD4^+$ T-cell count, HIV RNA (viral load), severe symptoms of HIV disease or AIDS, and willingness of the patient to adhere to a lifelong treatment regimen. In addition, the nurse assesses patient comorbidities and possible interactions with current medications and ensures pretreatment HIV genotypic resistance testing. New HIV medications are easier to take, have fewer adverse reactions, and are effective and potent. Monitoring the DHHS website for updates to the recommendations is essential before caring for patients with HIV/AIDS (DHHS, 2021). Research into broadly neutralizing anti-HIV antibodies (bNAbs) demonstrates the future possibility of a few infusions in the early stages of infection that may eliminate daily ART (Science Daily, 2022).

ART may be complex, have major side effects, pose difficulties regarding adherence, and carry serious potential consequences; these include viral resistance resulting from nonadherence to the medication regimen or suboptimal levels of ARV agents. Adherence to ART facilitates long-term success of initial regimens that are easily tolerated and convenient. Poor adherence allows the development of resistance to ART necessitating the use of less tolerable and more complicated regimens. Patient education about adherence continues to be an essential intervention by nurses. The increasing number of ARV agents (Table 36-2) and the rapid evolution of new

TABLE **36-2 Commonly Used Antiretroviral Agents**[a]

Generic Name (Abbreviation)	Food Effect	Adverse Events
Nucleoside Reverse Transcriptase Inhibitors (NRTIs)		
emtricitabine emtricitabine and tenofovir	Can be taken without regard to meals	Minimal toxicity; lactic acidosis with hepatic steatosis (rare but potentially life-threatening toxicity with use of NRTIs); combined with tenofovir as part of the PrEP regimen
tenofovir disoproxil fumarate tenofovir alafenamide	Can be taken without regard to meals	Asthenia (loss of strength and energy), headache, diarrhea, nausea, vomiting, and flatulence; renal insufficiency; lactic acidosis with hepatic steatosis (rare but potentially life-threatening toxicity with use of NRTIs)
Non-Nucleoside Reverse Transcriptase Inhibitors (NNRTIs)		
efavirenz	High-fat/high-caloric meals increase peak plasma concentrations of capsules by 39% and tablets by 79%; take on an empty stomach	Rash (rare cases of Stevens–Johnson syndrome have been reported); central nervous system symptoms (dizziness, somnolence, insomnia, abnormal dreams, confusion, abnormal thinking, impaired concentration, amnesia, agitation, depersonalization, hallucinations, and euphoria); increased transaminase levels (ALT/AST or liver enzymes); false-positive cannabinoid test; teratogenic
Protease Inhibitors (PIs)		
atazanavir dolutegravir/lamivudine	Administration with food increases bioavailability Should be taken with food; avoid taking with antacids	Indirect hyperbilirubinemia; prolonged PR interval—some patients experienced asymptomatic first-degree AV block; use with caution in patients with underlying conduction defects or on concomitant medications that can cause PR prolongation; hyperglycemia; fat maldistribution; possible increased bleeding episodes in patients with hemophilia
Fusion Inhibitors		
enfuvirtide	Injected subcutaneously	Local injection site reactions—almost 100% of patients (pain, erythema, induration, nodules and cysts, pruritus, ecchymosis); increased rate of bacterial pneumonia; hypersensitivity reaction—symptoms may include rash, fever, nausea, vomiting, chills, rigors, hypotension, or elevated serum liver enzymes
CCR5 Antagonists		
maraviroc	No food effect; take with or without food	Abdominal pain; cough; dizziness; musculoskeletal symptoms; pyrexia; rash; upper respiratory infections; hepatotoxicity; orthostatic hypotension
Integrase Inhibitors		
raltegravir	Take with or without food	Nausea, headache; diarrhea; pyrexia; CPK elevation

[a]Regimens should be individualized based on the advantages and disadvantages of each combination, such as pill burden, dosing frequency, toxicities, drug–drug interaction potential, comorbid conditions, and level of plasma HIV-RNA. Complete listing of medications, adverse effects, and patient education available at https://aidsinfo.nih.gov/contentfiles/lvguidelines/adultandadolescentgl.pdf.
The nurse is advised to refer to pharmacologic resources for additional information.

information have introduced extraordinary complexity into the treatment of HIV infection in the patient with a resistant virus. The goals of treatment include maximal and sustained suppression of viral load, restoration or preservation of immunologic function, improved quality of life, and reduction of HIV-related morbidity and mortality. Treatment as prevention is a reality given the Undetectable = Untransmissible findings. The DHHS guidelines recommend viral load testing at the time of diagnosis of HIV disease and every 3 to 4 months thereafter; $CD4^+$ cell counts should be measured at diagnosis and usually every 3 to 6 months thereafter (DHHS, 2021). The overall goals to reduce morbidity and mortality during viral suppression should focus on reducing the risks associated with chronic illness. Nursing interventions aimed at smoking cessation; exercise; diet; and adherence to treatment for comorbidities like diabetes, hypertension, and hyperlipidemia are effective in maximizing health and longevity for all patients, not just those with HIV (HIV.gov treatment guidelines, 2021).

Medications

More than 30 approved ARV agents, belonging to seven classes, are available for the design of combination regimens. Effective regimens contain at least three virologically active medications from at least two classes called triple therapy. The seven classes currently approved by the FDA are as follows:

- Nucleoside/nucleotide reverse transcriptase inhibitors (NRTIs)
- Non-nucleoside reverse transcriptase inhibitors (NNRTIs)
- PIs
- Integrase strand transfer inhibitors (INSTIs)
- CCR5 antagonist
- Fusion inhibitor
- Post-attachment inhibitors (the newest class; see Table 38-2 [NIH, 2021]).

Each of these medications attacks HIV at different stages of viral replication in the $CD4^+$ lymphocyte.

As new medications are developed and research is completed, the number and types of recommended drug combinations continue to change (DHHS, 2021). In addition, some pharmaceutical companies have combined two to three agents into one tablet or capsule (such as Dovato, which is a combination of dolutegravir/lamivudine) so that a patient may be taking one tablet or capsule that contains two different medications. With a decrease in the number of tablets or capsules that the patient must take ("pill burden"), the patient is more likely to adhere to prescribed regimens and achieve sustained viral suppression. Efforts are underway to develop additional combinations of ARV medications. The first single tablet for once-a-day use was made available in 2006; Atripla combined efavirenz (Sustiva), emtricitabine (Emtriva), and tenofovir disoproxil fumarate (Viread). Today, there are eleven of these well-tolerated combination pills available (NIH FDA, 2021). Simplifying treatment regimens and decreasing the number of medications that must be taken each day increase patients' adherence to therapy (DHHS, 2021).

Adherence

It is difficult to predict which patients will adhere to medication regimens. Adherence rates of 95% minimize the risks of developing a resistant virus. Patients should understand that the first regimen prescribed has the best chance for long-term treatment success with minimal impact on daily functioning and prevention of resistance. Individualized plans of care that take into consideration housing and social support issues, in addition to health indicators, are essential. Adherence to the ART plan involves very complex behavior that can change over the duration of the medication regimen. Self-reported adherence measures can distinguish clinically meaningful patterns of medication-taking behaviors; therefore, nurses should ask patients if they are taking their medications as prescribed. Factors associated with nonadherence include active substance use, depression, lack of social support, and treatment fatigue. Gender, race, pregnancy, and history of past substance use have not been associated with nonadherence (DHHS, 2021). Box 36-6 summarizes various strategies that health care providers can use to encourage adherence to the treatment regimen. Every health care encounter should be used as an opportunity to briefly review the treatment regimen and identify any new issues.

Patients who elect to interrupt therapy should be counseled that the HIV viral load will increase, usually to pretreatment levels, resulting in an increased risk for transmission to others during risky behaviors, such as unsafe sex

BOX 36-6

Patient Education: Adhering to the Medication Therapy for HIV

With the advent of one daily pill for treatment for most patients, adherence is significantly simplified. To help ensure adherence with more complicated therapy regimens, you need to be able to:

- Correctly identify each medication, preferably by name
- State the action of each medication
- State the correct times that medication is to be taken
- Identify special guidelines to follow when taking medications (e.g., with meals, on an empty stomach, medications that are not to be taken together)
- Demonstrate methods of tracking and storage of the medication regimen and use reminders such as beepers and/or pillboxes
- Identify specific laboratory tests, such as viral load, that are necessary to monitor the effectiveness of the medication regimen
- List expected side effects of each medication
- Identify side effects to report to health care providers
- Explain the importance of and necessity for adherence
- Demonstrate correct administration of intramuscular, subcutaneous, or IV medications
- Demonstrate correct use and safe disposal of needles, syringes, and other IV equipment
- Discuss episodes of nonadherence to the medication regimen

and sharing needles. Because of drug toxicities, drug resistance, quality-of-life issues, and the high cost of medications, some patients may choose to take a "drug holiday" or structured treatment interruption. Through an open, honest partnership between the health care provider and the patient, these options can be explored and their effectiveness maximized. Structured intermittent therapy, characterized by alternating short periods on and off medication, appears to be ineffective and may increase mortality.

Evaluation of Therapy

Viral load tests evaluate the results of therapy (DHHS, 2021). Viral load levels should be measured immediately before initiation of ART and again after 2 to 8 weeks. In most patients, adherence to a regimen of potent ARV agents should result in a significant decrease in the viral load by 2 to 8 weeks. The viral load should continue to decline over the following weeks, and, in most individuals, it will drop below detectable levels (currently defined as less than 50 RNA copies/mL) by 16 to 20 weeks. The rate of viral load decline toward undetectable levels is affected by the baseline T-cell count, the initial viral load, the potency of the medication, adherence to the medication regimen, prior exposure to ARV agents, and the presence of any OIs. The confirmed absence of a viral load response in an adherent patient should prompt the health care team to re-evaluate the regimen and check for resistant mutations through HIV genotype testing. The $CD4^+$ count should increase by 100 to 150 cells/mm^3 per year, with an accelerated response in the first 3 months (DHHS, 2021).

Side Effects

Many of the ARV agents that prolong life may simultaneously cause lipodystrophy syndrome and place the person at risk for early-onset hypercholesterolemia, heart disease, and diabetes. Fat redistribution syndrome, which consists of lipoatrophy (Fig. 36-4), lipohypertrophy, or both in localized areas, is also known as *lipodystrophy syndrome.* This syndrome is one of the most frequent systemic side effects associated with the use of ARV medications, especially PIs, with estimates ranging from 10% to more than 80% of patients (Glesby, 2022). Many people who have lipodystrophy experience an increase in fat loss in the legs, arms, face, or a build-up of fat around the abdomen and at the base of the neck, or both. Patients also may experience an increase in breast size. All of these adverse effects can have a profound impact on a patient's psychological well-being due to the increased stress of stigmatization.

Facial wasting, characterized as a sinking of the cheeks, eyes, and temples caused by the loss of fat tissue under the skin, may be treated by injectable fillers such as poly-L-lactic acid.

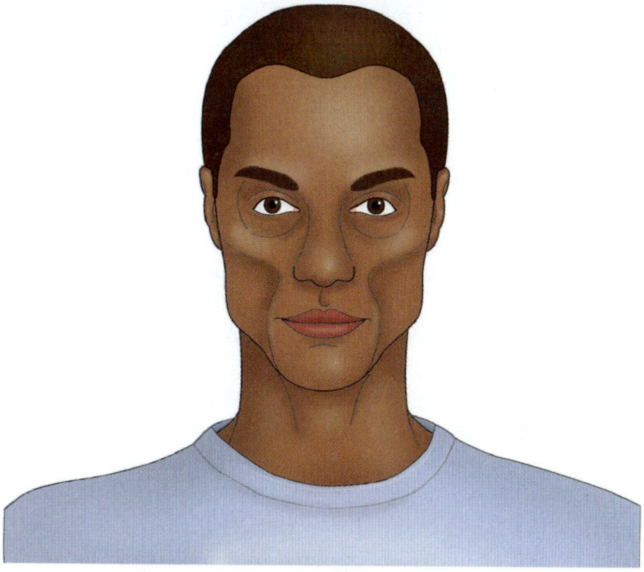

FIGURE 36-4 Facial lipoatrophy.

Drug Resistance

Drug resistance can be broadly defined as the ability of pathogens to withstand the effects of medications that are intended to be toxic to them. Resistance develops because of spontaneous genetic mutation of the pathogens or in response to exposure to the medication. Factors associated with the development of drug resistance include serial monotherapy (taking one medication at a time), common during early clinical trials, inadequate suppression of virus replication with suboptimal treatment regimens, difficulty with adherence to complex and toxic regimens, and initiation of therapy late in the course of HIV infection. HIV-1 may find refuge beyond physiologic protective adaptations, such as behind the blood–brain barrier, where diminished drug concentrations in the CNS might induce the development of drug-resistant mutants. HIV-1 persists in lymphoid tissue even in people who appear to have responded well to antiviral therapy; this is another factor that is limiting discovery of a cure or vaccine for HIV.

Resistance testing has a number of limitations and is more helpful in the elimination of ARV agents rather than in deciding which ones should be used. Deciding whether a medication regimen is effective or ineffective is a complex phenomenon. Some patients demonstrate inconsistent results on virologic, immunologic, and clinical parameters. In general, virologic failure occurs first, followed by immunologic failure, and finally by clinical progression. These events may be separated by months to years (DHHS, 2021). Genotypic testing allows detection of amino acid mutations that are either proved or suspected to be associated with phenotypic resistance. Phenotypic testing predicts the susceptibility of resistant virus to inhibition by a particular drug (DHHS, 2021).

In addition to resistance testing, several factors must be considered in choosing medications for a new regimen once the prior one has failed. These factors include the patient's treatment history, viral load, and medication tolerance; the likelihood of the patient's adherence to the medication regimen; and concomitant medical conditions or medications.

Resistance testing is of greatest value when it is performed before drugs are discontinued or immediately afterward (within 4 weeks). Most HIV providers perform genotype testing during the initial diagnosis stage as some patients with HIV are infected with a resistant virus. Drug resistance testing is not advised for patients with a viral load of less than 1,000 copies/mL because amplification of the virus is unreliable (DHHS, 2021).

Vaccines

Vaccine research for HIV has two potential areas of application: prevention of new infections and therapy for people already infected with HIV (therapeutic vaccine). Since HIV-1 was discovered, researchers have been working to develop a vaccine. A vaccine is a substance that triggers the production of antibodies to destroy the offending organism. Creation of an HIV vaccine is feasible, but researchers have had difficulty finding an adequate animal model in which to test new vaccines. Because HIV can attack the human immune system as either a cell-free or cell-associated virus, a vaccine against HIV must be capable of producing both antibodies and cytotoxic lymphocytes.

Treatment of Opportunistic Infections

Pneumocystis jirovecii pneumonia (formerly called *Pneumocystis carinii* pneumonia or PCP)

In the past several years, many advances have been made in the treatment of *Pneumocystis jirovecii* pneumonia. TMP-SMZ (a sulfa-containing regimen), is the treatment of choice for PCP in patients with AIDS and in immunocompromised patients without HIV infection; it is available in both IV and oral preparations. TMP-SMZ is an antibacterial agent used to treat various organisms causing infection. People with HIV infection who have a T-cell count of less than 200 cells/mm^3 should receive chemoprophylaxis against PCP with TMP-SMZ. PCP prophylaxis can be safely discontinued in patients who are responding to highly active ART (HAART) with a sustained increase in T lymphocytes. TMP-SMZ also confers cross-protection against toxoplasmosis and some common respiratory bacterial infections. Patients with AIDS who are treated with TMP-SMZ experience a high incidence of adverse effects, such as fever, rashes, leukopenia (decreased WBC count), thrombocytopenia (decreased platelet count), and kidney dysfunction. Treatment for PCP should continue until the patient's CD4 is sustained at levels >200 cells/mm^3.

Pentamidine, an antiprotozoal medication, is used as an alternative agent for combating PCP. Avoid intramuscular administration because of the potential for painful formation of a sterile abscess. In addition, IV pentamidine can cause severe hypotension if it is administered too rapidly. Other adverse effects include impaired glucose metabolism leading to the development of diabetes mellitus from damage to the pancreas, kidney damage, liver dysfunction, and neutropenia. Initially, the success of aerosolized pentamidine led to its use as a treatment for mild-to-moderate PCP. However, it has proved to be less effective and more costly than TMP-SMZ, and early relapses are common. Because of these limitations, aerosolized pentamidine should not be used (DHHS, 2021).

Mycobacterium Avium Complex

Chemoprophylaxis against disseminated MAC is indicated for people infected with HIV whose T-cell count is lower than 50 cells/mm^3. Treatment for MAC infections involves use of either clarithromycin or azithromycin. Secondary prophylaxis for disseminated MAC may be discontinued in patients who have sustained increases in CD4 counts (at least 100 cells/mm^3) in response to HAART, have completed 12 months of MAC therapy, and have no signs or symptoms attributable to MAC. Primary prophylaxis for disseminated MAC may be discontinued in patients who have responded to HAART with CD4 counts of 100 cells/mm^3 or higher for at least 3 months and may be reintroduced if counts decrease to 50 to 100 cells/mm^3 (DHHS, 2021).

Cytomegalovirus Retinitis

Retinitis caused by CMV is a leading cause of blindness in patients with AIDS. Prophylaxis with oral ganciclovir may be considered for people infected with HIV who have CD4$^+$ T-cell counts of less than 50 cells/mm^3. Two antiviral agents, ganciclovir and foscarnet, offer effective treatment but not a cure for CMV retinitis. Because ganciclovir and foscarnet do not kill the virus but instead control its growth, they must be taken for life. Relapse rates associated with the two agents are similar. Discontinuation of the medication is associated with the relapse of retinitis within 1 month.

A common adverse reaction to ganciclovir is severe neutropenia, which limits the concomitant use of zidovudine. Intravitreal injections of ganciclovir have been effective for patients who cannot tolerate systemic ganciclovir because of severe neutropenia, infection at the venous access site, or the need to take zidovudine. Zidovudine may be given with foscarnet. Common adverse reactions to foscarnet are nephrotoxicity, including acute kidney failure; and electrolyte imbalances, including hypocalcemia, hyperphosphatemia, and hypomagnesemia, which can be life-threatening. Other common adverse effects include seizures, GI disturbances, anemia, phlebitis at the infusion site, and low back pain. Possible bone marrow suppression (producing a decrease in WBC and platelet counts), oral candidiasis, and liver and kidney impairments require close patient monitoring.

Other Infections

Oral acyclovir, famciclovir, or valacyclovir may be used to treat infections caused by herpes simplex or herpes zoster. Patients coinfected with HSV and HIV are more likely to transmit and infect others if not treated for herpes. Esophageal or oral candidiasis is treated topically with clotrimazole (Mycelex) oral troches or nystatin suspension. Chronic refractory candidiasis (thrush) or esophageal involvement is treated with ketoconazole or fluconazole.

Antidiarrheal Therapy

Although many forms of diarrhea respond to treatment, it is not unusual for this condition to recur and become a chronic problem for the patient with HIV. Therapy with octreotide acetate, a synthetic analog of somatostatin, has been shown to be effective in managing chronic severe diarrhea. High concentrations of somatostatin receptors have been found in the GI tract and in other tissues. Somatostatin inhibits many physiologic functions, including GI motility and intestinal secretion of water and electrolytes.

Chemotherapy

Kaposi Sarcoma

Usually, management of KS is difficult because of the variability of symptoms and the organ systems involved. KS is rarely life-threatening except when there is pulmonary or GI involvement. The treatment goals are to reduce symptoms by decreasing the size of the skin lesions, to reduce discomfort associated with edema and ulcerations, and to control symptoms associated with mucosal or visceral involvement. No one treatment has been shown to increase survival. Localized treatment includes surgical excision of the lesions or application of liquid nitrogen to local skin lesions, and injections of intraoral lesions with dilute vinblastine. Injection of intraoral lesions has been associated with local pain and skin irritation. Radiation therapy is effective as a palliative measure to relieve localized pain due to tumor mass (especially in the legs) and for KS lesions that are in sites such as the oral mucosa, conjunctiva, face, and soles of the feet.

Interferon is known for its antiviral and antitumor effects. Patients with cutaneous KS treated with **alpha-interferon** have experienced tumor regression and improved immune system function. Positive responses have been observed in 30% to 50% of patients, with the best responses seen in those with limited disease and no OIs. Alpha-interferon is administered by the IV, intramuscular, or subcutaneous route. Patients may self-administer interferon at home or receive interferon in an outpatient setting. Rituximab infusions are monoclonal antibodies effective in the treatment of KS and non-Hodgkin lymphoma but may cause a fatal infusion reaction and are administered in the inpatient setting so that the patient can be observed during administration.

Lymphoma

Successful treatment of AIDS-related lymphomas has been limited because of the rapid progression of these malignancies. Combination chemotherapy and radiation therapy regimens may produce an initial response, but it is usually short-lived. Because standard regimens for non-AIDS lymphomas have been ineffective, many providers suggest that AIDS-related lymphomas should be studied as a separate group in clinical trials.

Antidepressant Therapy

Treatment for depression in people with HIV infection involves psychotherapy integrated with pharmacotherapy. If depressive symptoms are severe and of sufficient duration, treatment with antidepressants may be initiated. Antidepressants, such as imipramine, desipramine, and fluoxetine, may be used because these medications also alleviate the fatigue and lethargy associated with depression. A psychostimulant, such as methylphenidate, may be used in low doses in patients with neuropsychiatric impairment. Electroconvulsive therapy may be an option for patients with severe depression who have not responded to pharmacologic interventions.

Nutrition Therapy

Malnutrition increases the risk for infection and may increase the incidence of OIs. Nutrition therapy should be integrated into the overall management plan and should be tailored to meet the nutritional needs of the patient, whether by oral diet, enteral tube feedings, or parenteral nutritional support, if needed. As with all patients, a healthy diet is essential for the patient with HIV infection. For all patients with AIDS who experience unexplained weight loss, calorie counts should be obtained to evaluate nutritional status and initiate appropriate therapy. The goal is to maintain the ideal weight and, when necessary, to increase weight.

Appetite stimulants have been used successfully in patients with AIDS-related anorexia. Megestrol acetate, a synthetic oral progesterone preparation used to treat breast cancer, promotes significant weight gain and inhibits cytokine IL-1 synthesis. In patients with HIV infection, it increases body weight primarily by increasing body fat stores. Dronabinol, which is a synthetic tetrahydrocannabinol (THC), the active ingredient in marijuana, has been used to relieve nausea and vomiting associated with cancer chemotherapy. Many states now allow the use of medical marijuana for patients who are HIV positive.

Oral supplements may be used to improve diets that are deficient in calories and protein. Ideally, oral supplements should be lactose-free as many people with HIV infection are lactose intolerant. Parenteral nutrition is the final option because of its prohibitive cost and associated risks, including risk of infections.

Complementary and Alternative Medicine (CAM)

Traditional Western or allopathic medicine focuses on the treatment of disease. These treatments or interventions are taught in medical and nursing schools and are used by health care providers in the care of patients. Complementary and alternative medicine (CAM) is often viewed as consisting of unconventional and unorthodox treatments or interventions. These modalities and therapies stress the need to treat the whole person, recognizing the interaction of the body, mind, and spirit. People with HIV infection report substantial use of CAM for symptom management. The use of CAM in patients with HIV infection and AIDS often results because of disillusionment with standard medical treatment, which to date has provided no cure. Combined with standard medical therapies, CAM may improve the patient's overall well-being. However, there can be adverse drug–drug interactions between certain CAM therapies (e.g., St. John wort) and some ARV medications (DHHS, 2021).

CAM can be divided into four categories:

- Spiritual or psychological therapies, which may include humor, hypnosis, faith healing, guided imagery, and positive affirmations.
- Nutritional therapies, which may include vegetarian or macrobiotic diets or supplements of vitamin C or beta-carotene. Also Chinese herbs are used, in addition to compound Q (a Chinese cucumber extract) and *Momordica charantia* (bitter melon).
- Drug and biologic therapies, including medications and other substances not approved by the FDA. Examples are *N*-acetylcysteine, pentoxifylline, and 1-chloro-2, 4-dinitrobenzene.
- Treatment with physical forces and devices, which may include acupuncture, acupressure, massage therapy, reflexology, therapeutic touch, and yoga.

Although there is insufficient research on the effects of CAM, a growing body of literature reports benefits for modalities involving nutrition, exercise, psychosocial treatment, and traditional Chinese medicine.

Many patients who use these therapies do not report use of CAM to their health care providers. To obtain a complete health history, the nurse should ask about the patient's use of alternative therapies, including all over-the-counter drugs, nutritional supplements, and vitamins. Patients may need to be encouraged to report their use of CAM to their primary health care provider. Problems may arise, for example, when patients are using CAM while participating in clinical drug trials; alternative therapies can have significant adverse side effects, making it difficult to assess the effects of the medications in the clinical trial. The nurse needs to become familiar with the potential adverse side effects of these therapies. The nurse who suspects that CAM is causing a side effect needs to discuss this with the patient, the alternative therapy provider, and the primary health care provider. It is important for the nurse to view CAM with an open mind and to try to understand the importance of this treatment to the patient. This approach will improve communication with the patient and reduce conflict.

NURSING PROCESS
The Patient With AIDS

The nursing care of patients with AIDS is challenging because of the potential for any organ system to be the target of infections or cancer. In addition, this disease is complicated by many emotional, social, and ethical issues.

ASSESSMENT

Nursing assessment includes identification of potential risk factors, including a history of high-risk sexual practices or IV/injection drug use. The nurse assesses the patient's physical and psychological status and should explore all factors affecting the immune system and its function.

NUTRITIONAL STATUS

The nurse assesses nutritional status by obtaining a dietary history and identifying factors that may interfere with oral intake, such as anorexia, nausea, vomiting, oral pain, or difficulty swallowing. In addition, the nurse evaluates the patient's ability to purchase and prepare food. Weight history (e.g., changes over time); anthropometric measurements; and levels of blood urea nitrogen (BUN), serum protein, albumin, and transferrin provide objective measurements of nutritional status.

Pearls for Practice

Transferrin, which is synthesized in the liver, is a transport protein that regulates iron absorption by transporting it from the intestines to the bloodstream; therefore, it may be monitored to evaluate iron saturation of the blood. Low levels of transferrin impair hemoglobin production, resulting in anemia. Transferrin levels also decrease with liver disease and poor protein intake; thus, this laboratory test may be ordered to assess liver function and nutritional status. High levels of transferrin are associated with immune function and the ability to deal with infection. Normal transferrin levels for adults are 215 to 365 mg/dL or 2.15 to 3.65 g/L for males and 250 to 380 mg/dL or 2.5 to 3.8 g/L for females. Decreased transferrin levels are seen in microcytic (small red blood cells) anemia, protein calorie malnutrition, chronic infection, acute liver disease, hypoproteinemia, and nephrotic disease (protein loss in urine) (Pagana et al., 2021).

SKIN INTEGRITY

The nurse inspects the skin and mucous membranes daily for evidence of breakdown, ulceration, or infection. Monitoring the oral cavity for redness, ulcerations, and the presence of creamy-white adherent patches detects candidiasis. Assessment of the perianal area for excoriation and infection in patients with profuse diarrhea is important. Cultures of wounds may be indicated and performed by the nurse to identify infectious organisms, especially methicillin-resistant *Staphylococcus aureus* (MRSA).

RESPIRATORY STATUS

The nurse assesses respiratory status by monitoring the patient for cough, sputum production (i.e., amount and color), dyspnea on exertion, orthopnea, tachypnea, and chest pain. Auscultation detects the quality of breath sounds. Other measures of pulmonary function include chest x-ray results, arterial blood gas values, pulse oximetry, and pulmonary function tests.

NEUROLOGIC STATUS

The nurse determines neurologic status by assessing level of consciousness; orientation to person, place, and time; and memory lapses. Assessment of mental status as early as possible during initial care provides a baseline. The nurse assesses the patient for sensory deficits (visual changes, headache, or numbness and tingling in the extremities), motor involvement (altered gait, paresis [slight or partial paralysis], or paralysis), and seizure activity.

FLUID AND ELECTROLYTE BALANCE

Fluid and electrolyte status is determined by examining the skin and mucous membranes for turgor and dryness. Dehydration may be indicated by increased thirst, decreased urine output, postural hypotension, weak and rapid pulse, and urine specific gravity of 1.025 or more. Electrolyte imbalances, such as decreased serum sodium, potassium, calcium, magnesium, and chloride, typically result from profuse diarrhea. The nurse assesses the patient for signs and symptoms of electrolyte deficits, including decreased mental status, muscle twitching, muscle cramps, irregular pulse, nausea, vomiting, and shallow respirations.

KNOWLEDGE LEVEL

The nurse evaluates the patient's level of knowledge about the disease and the modes of disease transmission. In addition, the nurse assesses the patient's family's and friends' level of knowledge. The patient's psychological reaction to the diagnosis of HIV infection or AIDS is important to explore. Reactions vary among patients and may include denial, anger, fear, shame, withdrawal from social interactions, and depression. The nurse should identify the patient's resources for support.

DIAGNOSIS

The list of potential nursing diagnoses is extensive because of the complex nature of this disease. However, based on assessment data, major nursing diagnoses for the patient may include the following:

- Impaired skin integrity related to cutaneous manifestations of HIV infection, excoriation, and diarrhea
- Diarrhea related to enteric pathogens, HIV infection, or ARV medications
- Risk for infection related to immunodeficiency
- Activity intolerance related to weakness, fatigue, malnutrition, impaired fluid and electrolyte balance, and hypoxia associated with pulmonary infections
- Disturbed thought processes related to shortened attention span, impaired memory, confusion, and disorientation associated with HIV-related cognitive decline
- Ineffective airway clearance related to PCP, increased bronchial secretions, and decreased ability to cough related to weakness and fatigue
- Pain related to impaired perianal skin integrity secondary to diarrhea, KS, and peripheral neuropathy
- Imbalanced nutrition, less than body requirements, related to decreased oral intake
- Social isolation related to stigma of the disease, withdrawal of support systems, isolation procedures, and fear of infecting others
- Anticipatory grieving related to changes in lifestyle and roles and unfavorable prognosis
- Deficient knowledge related to HIV infection, means of preventing HIV transmission, and self-care

Based on the assessment data, possible complications may include the following:

- OIs
- Impaired breathing or respiratory failure
- Wasting syndrome and fluid and electrolyte imbalance
- Adverse reaction to medications

PLANNING

Goals for the patient may include achievement and maintenance of skin integrity, resumption of usual bowel patterns, absence of infection, improved activity tolerance, improved thought processes, improved airway clearance, increased comfort, improved nutritional status, increased socialization, expression of grief, increased knowledge regarding disease prevention and self-care, and absence of complications.

NURSING INTERVENTIONS

PROMOTING SKIN INTEGRITY

The nurse routinely assesses the skin and oral mucosa for changes in appearance, location and size of lesions, and evidence of infection and breakdown. The nurse assists immobile patients to change position every 1 to 2 hours. Devices such as alternating-pressure mattresses and low–air-loss beds are used to prevent skin breakdown. Patients should avoid scratching; use nonabrasive, nondrying soaps; and apply nonperfumed skin moisturizers to dry skin surfaces. Regular oral care is also encouraged.

The nurse applies medicated lotions, ointments, and dressings to affected skin surfaces as prescribed. Adhesive tape is avoided. Protect the patient's skin from friction and rubbing by keeping bed linens free of wrinkles and avoiding tight or restrictive clothing. The nurse advises patients with foot lesions to wear cotton socks and shoes that do not cause the feet to perspire. Antipruritic, antibiotic, and analgesic agents are administered as prescribed.

The nurse assesses the perianal region frequently for impairment of skin integrity and infection. The patient should keep the area as clean as possible. The perianal area should be cleaned after each bowel movement with nonabrasive soap and water

(continued on page 1216)

to prevent further excoriation and breakdown of the skin. If the area is very painful, soft cloths or cotton sponges may be less irritating than washcloths. In addition, sitz baths or gentle irrigation may facilitate cleaning and promote comfort. It is important to dry the area thoroughly after cleaning. Topical lotions or ointments may be prescribed to promote healing. If infection is suspected, wounds should be cultured to initiate the appropriate antimicrobial treatment. The nurse assists debilitated patients in maintaining hygienic practices.

PROMOTING USUAL BOWEL PATTERNS

The nurse assesses bowel patterns for diarrhea. The nurse monitors the frequency and consistency of stools and the patient's reports of abdominal pain or cramping associated with bowel movements. Factors that exacerbate frequent diarrhea should be avoided. The nurse measures the quantity and volume of liquid stools to document fluid volume losses and obtains stool cultures to identify pathogenic organisms.

The nurse counsels the patient about ways to decrease diarrhea. Recommendations may include restricting oral intake to rest the bowel during periods of acute inflammation associated with severe enteric infections. As the patient's dietary intake is increased, the patient avoids foods that act as bowel irritants, such as raw fruits and vegetables, popcorn, carbonated beverages, and spicy foods. Small, frequent meals help to prevent abdominal distention. The nurse administers prescribed medications, such as anticholinergics, antispasmodics, or opioids, which decrease diarrhea by decreasing intestinal spasms and motility. Administering antidiarrheal agents on a regular schedule may be more beneficial than administering them on an as-needed basis. Also, antibiotics and antifungal agents may be prescribed to combat pathogens identified by stool cultures. The nurse also assesses the self-care strategies being used by the patient to control diarrhea, including the use of probiotics.

PREVENTING INFECTION

The nurse instructs the patient and caregivers to monitor for signs and symptoms of infection: fever; chills; night sweats; cough with or without sputum production; shortness of breath; difficulty breathing; oral pain or difficulty swallowing; creamy-white patches in the oral cavity; unexplained weight loss; swollen lymph nodes; nausea; vomiting; persistent diarrhea; frequency, urgency, or pain on urination; headache; visual changes or memory lapses; redness, swelling, or drainage from skin wounds; and vesicular lesions on the face, lips, or perianal area. The nurse monitors laboratory test results that indicate infection, such as the WBC count and differential. Culture specimens of wound drainage, skin lesions, urine, stool, sputum, and blood as well as a culture from the patient's mouth are obtained to identify pathogenic organisms and the most appropriate antimicrobial therapy. The nurse instructs the patient to avoid others with active infections, such as upper respiratory infections.

IMPROVING ACTIVITY TOLERANCE

The nurse assesses activity tolerance by monitoring the patient's ability to ambulate and perform activities of daily living. Patients may be unable to maintain their usual levels of activity because of weakness, fatigue, shortness of breath, dizziness, and neurologic involvement. Assistance in planning daily routines that maintain a balance between activity and rest may be necessary. In addition, patients benefit from instructions about energy conservation techniques, such as sitting while washing or while preparing meals. Personal items that are used frequently should be kept within the patient's reach. Measures such as relaxation and guided imagery may be beneficial because they decrease anxiety, which contributes to weakness and fatigue.

Collaboration with other members of the health care team may uncover other factors associated with increasing fatigue and strategies to address them. Physical therapists participate in the plan of care of patients with AIDS at long-term care facilities to increase endurance and tolerance for activities of daily learning. If fatigue is related to anemia, administering epoetin alfa (Epogen) as prescribed may relieve fatigue and increase activity tolerance.

MAINTAINING THOUGHT PROCESSES

The nurse assesses the patient for alterations in mental status that may be related to neurologic involvement, metabolic abnormalities, infection, side effects of treatment, and coping mechanisms. Manifestations of neurologic impairment may be difficult to distinguish from psychological reactions to HIV infection, such as anger and depression.

If the patient experiences altered mental or cognitive status, the nurse instructs family members to speak to the patient in simple, clear language and give the patient sufficient time to respond to questions. Family members orient the patient to the daily routine by talking about what is taking place during daily activities. They are encouraged to provide the patient with a regular daily schedule for medication administration, grooming, mealtimes, bedtimes, and awakening times. Posting the schedule in a prominent area (e.g., on the refrigerator), providing nightlights for the bedroom and bathroom, and planning safe leisure activities allow the patient to maintain a regular routine in a safe manner. The nurse encourages activities that the patient previously enjoyed. These should be easy to accomplish and fairly short in duration. Around-the-clock supervision may be necessary, and strategies can be implemented to prevent the patient from engaging in potentially dangerous activities, such as driving or using the stove. The nurse uses strategies for improving or maintaining functional abilities and for providing a safe environment for patients with HIV-related cognitive decline.

IMPROVING AIRWAY CLEARANCE

At least daily, the nurse assesses respiratory status, including rate, rhythm, use of accessory muscles, breath sounds, mental status, and skin color. Any cough and the quantity and characteristics of sputum are documented. The nurse obtains sputum specimens for infectious organism analysis as indicated. Pulmonary therapy (coughing, deep breathing, postural drainage, percussion, and vibration) as often as every 2 hours may be required to prevent stasis of secretions and promote airway clearance. Because of weakness and fatigue, many patients require assistance in attaining a position (such as a semi-Fowler position) that facilitates breathing and airway clearance. The nurse evaluates fluid volume status so that adequate hydration can be maintained. Daily intake is 3 L of fluid unless contraindicated because of renal or cardiac disease. Humidified oxygen may be prescribed, and nasopharyngeal or tracheal suctioning, intubation, and mechanical ventilation may be necessary to maintain adequate ventilation.

RELIEVING PAIN AND DISCOMFORT

The nurse assesses the patient for the quality and severity of pain associated with impaired perianal skin integrity, the lesions of KS, and peripheral neuropathy. In addition, the nurse explores the effects of pain on elimination, nutrition, sleep, affect, and communication, along with exacerbating and relieving factors. Cleaning the perianal area as previously described can promote comfort. Topical anesthetics or ointments may be prescribed. The nurse increases patient comfort while sitting with the use of soft cushions or foam pads. If necessary, systemic analgesic agents also may be prescribed. Frequently, pain from KS is described as a sharp, throbbing pressure and heaviness if lymphedema is present. Pain management may include use of NSAIDs and opioids, plus nonpharmacologic approaches, such as relaxation techniques. When NSAIDs are administered to patients who are receiving zidovudine, the nurse is aware that hepatic and hematologic status is evaluated.

The patient with pain related to peripheral neuropathy frequently describes it as burning, numbness, and "pins and needles." Pain management approaches may include opioids, tricyclic antidepressants, and elastic compression stockings to equalize pressure. Tricyclic antidepressants potentiate the actions of opioids and can be used to relieve pain without increasing the dose of the opioid. Ongoing assessment by the nurse of the use and potential abuse of opioids is part of the collaborative model of pain management.

IMPROVING NUTRITIONAL STATUS

The nurse assesses nutritional status by monitoring weight; dietary intake and output; and levels of serum albumin, BUN, protein, and transferrin. The patient is assessed for factors that interfere with oral intake, such as anorexia, candidal infection, nausea, pain, weakness, fatigue, and lactose intolerance. Based on the results of assessment, the nurse implements specific measures to facilitate oral intake. A dietitian helps to determine the patient's nutritional requirements.

Control of nausea and vomiting with antiemetic medications administered on a regular basis may increase the patient's dietary intake. Inadequate food intake resulting from pain caused by oral lesions or a sore throat may be managed by administering prescribed opioids and viscous lidocaine. In addition, the nurse encourages the patient to eat foods that are easy to swallow and to avoid rough, spicy, or sticky food items and foods that are excessively hot or cold. The patient should perform oral hygiene before and after meals; in the debilitated patient with AIDS, the nurse will assist in these activities. If fatigue and weakness interfere with intake, the nurse encourages the patient to rest before meals. If the patient is hospitalized, meals should be scheduled so that they do not occur immediately after painful or unpleasant procedures. The nurse advises the patient with diarrhea and abdominal cramping to avoid foods that stimulate intestinal motility and abdominal distention, such as fiber-rich foods or lactose, if the patient is intolerant to lactose. The nurse instructs the patient about ways to enhance the nutritional value of meals. Supplements, such as puddings, powders, milkshakes, and Advera (a nutritional product specifically designed for people with HIV infection or AIDS) also may be useful. Patients who cannot maintain their nutritional status through oral intake may require enteral feedings or parenteral nutrition.

DECREASING THE SENSE OF ISOLATION

People with AIDS are at risk for double stigmatization. Judgments about disease acquisition and lifestyle choices isolate many patients who are HIV positive. Many people with AIDS are young adults at a developmental stage that is usually associated with establishing intimate relationships, personal goals, and career goals, as well as having and raising children. Their focus changes as they are faced with a disease that threatens their quality of life with no cure. In addition, they may be forced to reveal hidden lifestyles or behaviors to family, friends, coworkers, and health care providers. As a result, people with HIV infection may be overwhelmed with emotions such as anxiety, guilt, shame, and fear. They also may be faced with multiple losses, such as loss of financial security, normal roles and functions, self-esteem, privacy, ability to control bodily functions, ability to interact meaningfully with the environment, and sexual functioning, as well as rejection by sexual partners, family, and friends. Some patients may harbor feelings of guilt because of their lifestyle or because they may have infected others in current or previous relationships. Other patients may feel anger toward sexual partners who transmitted the virus to them. Infection control measures used in the hospital or at home may further contribute to the patient's emotional isolation. Any or all of these stressors may cause the patient with AIDS to withdraw both physically and emotionally from social contact.

Nurses are in a key position to provide an atmosphere of acceptance and understanding for people with AIDS and their families and partners. The nurse assesses the patient's usual level of social interaction as early as possible to provide a baseline for monitoring changes in behaviors that suggest social isolation (e.g., decreased interaction with staff or family, hostility, noncompliance). Patients are encouraged to express feelings of isolation and loneliness with the assurance that these feelings are not unique or abnormal.

(*continued on page 1218*)

Providing information about how to protect themselves and others may help patients avoid social isolation. The nurse reassures patients, family, and friends that AIDS is not spread through casual contact. Patient care conferences that address the psychosocial issues associated with AIDS may help sensitize the health care team to patients' needs.

COPING WITH GRIEF

The nurse helps the patient verbalize feelings and explore and identify resources for support. In addition, the nurse works with the patient to establish mechanisms for coping, especially when the patient is grieving anticipated losses. The patient is encouraged to maintain contact with family, friends, and coworkers and to use local or national AIDS support groups and hotlines. If possible, losses are identified and addressed. The nurse encourages the patient to continue usual activities whenever possible. Consultations with mental health counselors are useful for many patients.

MONITORING AND MANAGING POTENTIAL COMPLICATIONS

Opportunistic Infections. Patients who are immunosuppressed are at risk for OIs. Therefore, anti-infective agents may be prescribed and laboratory tests obtained to monitor their effect. The nurse should report signs and symptoms of OIs, including fever, malaise, difficulty breathing, nausea or vomiting, diarrhea, difficulty swallowing, and any occurrences of swelling or discharge.

Respiratory Failure. Impaired breathing is a major complication that increases the patient's discomfort and anxiety and may lead to respiratory and cardiac failure. The nurse monitors respiratory rate and pattern and auscultates the lungs for abnormal breath sounds. The patient should report shortness of breath and increasing difficulty in carrying out usual activities. The nurse monitors pulse rate and rhythm, blood pressure, and oxygen saturation. Suctioning, if indicated, and oxygen therapy ensure an adequate airway and prevent hypoxia. Using universal precautions, a face shield, mask, and goggles should be worn in the event of secretion spray with suctioning. Mechanical ventilation may be necessary for the patient who cannot maintain adequate ventilation because of pulmonary infection, fluid and electrolyte imbalance, or respiratory muscle weakness. Arterial blood gas values will be obtained to guide ventilator management. Instruct intubated patients in methods to allow communication with the nurse and others. The patient receiving mechanical ventilation should be assessed regarding coping with the stress associated with intubation and ventilator assistance. The possible need for mechanical ventilation in the future should be discussed early in the course of the disease, when the patient is able to make known their preferences about treatment. The use of mechanical ventilation should be consistent with the patient's decisions about end-of-life treatment.

Cachexia and Wasting. Wasting syndrome and fluid and electrolyte disturbances, including dehydration, are common complications of HIV infection and AIDS. The nurse evaluates the patient's nutritional and electrolyte status by monitoring weight gains or losses, skin turgor, ferritin (blood cell protein that contains iron) levels, hemoglobin, hematocrit, and electrolyte levels. Fluid and electrolyte status is monitored on an ongoing basis; fluid intake and output and urine specific gravity may be monitored daily if the patient is hospitalized with complications. The nurse assesses the skin for dryness and adequate turgor. Vital signs are monitored for decreased systolic blood pressure or increased pulse rate on sitting or standing. The nurse documents and reports to the provider signs and symptoms of electrolyte disturbances, such as muscle cramping, weakness, irregular pulse, decreased mental status, nausea, and vomiting. The nurse also monitors serum electrolyte values and reports abnormalities.

The nurse helps the patient select foods that will replenish electrolytes, such as oranges and bananas (potassium) and cheese and soups (sodium). Fluid intake is 3 L or more per day, unless contraindicated, to replace fluid lost with diarrhea, and measures to control diarrhea are initiated. If fluid and electrolyte imbalances persist, the nurse administers IV fluids and electrolytes as prescribed. The nurse also monitors effects of parenteral therapy.

Side Effects of Medications. Adverse reactions are of concern in patients who receive many medications to treat HIV infection or its complications. Many medications can cause severe toxic effects. The nurse provides information about the purpose of the medications, their correct administration, side effects, and strategies to manage or prevent side effects. Patients and their caregivers need to know which signs and symptoms of side effects should be reported immediately to their primary health care provider (see Table 36-2).

In addition to medications used to treat HIV infection, other medications that may be required include opioids, tricyclic antidepressants, and NSAIDs for pain relief; medications for treatment of OIs; antihistamines (diphenhydramine) for relief of pruritus; acetaminophen or aspirin for management of fever; and antiemetic agents for control of nausea and vomiting. Concurrent use of these medications can cause many drug interactions, resulting in hepatic and hematologic abnormalities. Therefore, careful monitoring of laboratory test results is essential.

During each contact with the patient, it is important for the nurse to ask not only about side effects but also about how well the patient is adhering to the medication regimen.

TEACHING PATIENTS SELF-CARE

The nurse instructs patients, families, and friends about the routes of transmission of HIV. As discussed earlier, the nurse discusses precautions the patient can use to avoid transmitting HIV sexually or through exposure to blood and other bodily fluids. Patients and their families or caregivers must receive instructions about how to prevent disease transmission, including handwashing techniques and methods for safely handling and disposing of items soiled with body fluids. Clear guidelines about avoiding and controlling infection, maintaining regular health care appointments; managing symptoms; and getting adequate nutrition, rest, and exercise are necessary. Emphasize the importance of personal and environmental hygiene. The nurse teaches caregivers the guidelines (standard precautions) described in Box 36-3. Patients and caregivers should clean kitchen and bathroom surfaces regularly with disinfectants to prevent growth of fungi and bacteria. Patients with pets should have another person clean the areas soiled by animals, such as birdcages and litter boxes. If this is not possible, patients should use gloves and should wash their hands after they clean the area. Patients should avoid exposure to others who are sick or who have recently received live vaccines. The nurse emphasizes the importance of avoiding smoking, excessive alcohol, and over-the-counter and street drugs. Instruct patients who are HIV positive or who inject substances not to donate blood. IV/injection drug users who are unwilling to stop using should avoid sharing drug equipment with others.

The nurse teaches caregivers how to administer medications, including IV preparations, in the home. Often the medication regimens used for patients with HIV infection and AIDS are complex and expensive. If the patient requires enteral or parenteral nutrition, provide instruction to the patient and family about how to administer nutritional therapies at home. Home care nurses provide ongoing teaching and support for the patient and family.

PROVIDING CONTINUING CARE

Many people with AIDS remain in their community and continue their usual daily activities, whereas others can no longer work or maintain their independence. Families or caregivers may need assistance in providing supportive care. Many community-based organizations provide a variety of services for people living with HIV infection and AIDS; nurses can help identify these services.

Nurses may refer patients to community programs that offer a range of services for patients, friends, and families, including help with housekeeping, hygiene, and meals; transportation and shopping; individual and group therapy; support for caregivers; telephone networks for the homebound; and legal and financial assistance. These services are typically provided by both professionals and nonprofessional volunteers. A social worker can identify sources of financial support, if needed.

Home care and hospice nurses are called on to provide physical and emotional support to patients and families as patients with AIDS enter the terminal stages of disease. This support takes on special meaning when people with AIDS lose friends and when family members fear the disease or feel anger concerning the patient's lifestyle. The nurse encourages the patient and family to discuss end-of-life decisions and to ensure that care is consistent with those decisions, all comfort measures are employed, and the patient is treated with dignity at all times. Refer to Chapter 2 for details on end-of-life care.

EVALUATION

Expected patient outcomes may include:

1. Maintains skin integrity
2. Resumes usual bowel habits
3. Experiences no OIs
4. Maintains adequate level of activity tolerance
5. Maintains usual level of thought processes
6. Maintains effective airway clearance
7. Experiences increased sense of comfort and less pain
8. Maintains adequate nutritional status
9. Experiences decreased sense of social isolation
10. Progresses through grieving process
11. Reports increased understanding of AIDS and participates in self-care activities
12. Remains free of complications

A plan of nursing care for a patient with AIDS is available online at http://thepoint.lww.com/Honan3e.

Emotional and Ethical Concerns

Nurses in all settings provide care for patients with HIV infection. In doing so, they encounter not only the physical challenges of this epidemic but also emotional and ethical concerns. The concerns raised by health care professionals involve issues such as fear of infection, responsibility for giving care, values clarification, confidentiality, developmental stages of patients and caregivers, and poor prognostic outcomes.

Health care providers may have fear and anxiety about disease transmission despite education concerning infection control and the low incidence of transmission to health care providers. Nurses are encouraged to examine their personal beliefs and to use the process of values clarification to approach controversial issues. The American Nurses Association's Code of Ethics for Nurses also can be used to help resolve ethical dilemmas that might affect the quality of care given to patients with HIV infection and AIDS (refer to Chapter 1, Box 1-1).

Nurses are responsible for protecting the patient's right to privacy by safeguarding confidential information. Inadvertent disclosure of confidential patient information may result in personal, financial, and emotional hardships for the patient. The controversy surrounding confidentiality concerns the circumstances in which information may be disclosed to others. Many patients avoid necessary health care appointments due to confidentiality concerns. Health care team members need accurate patient information to conduct assessment, planning, implementation, and evaluation of patient care. Failure to disclose HIV status could compromise the quality of patient care. Sexual partners of patients who are HIV-infected should know about the potential for infection and the need to engage in safer sex practices as well as the possible need for testing and health care. State health departments offer confidential partner notification services. In situations in which a patient cannot or will not inform others, "duty to warn" regulations vary by state. Nurses are advised to discuss concerns about confidentiality with nurse administrators and to consult professional nursing organizations, such as the Association of Nurses in AIDS Care (ANAC), and legal experts in their state to identify the most appropriate course of action.

AIDS has had a high mortality rate, but advances in ARV and multidrug therapy have demonstrated promise in controlling disease progression. It is not known whether current treatment regimens will remain effective because viral drug resistance has developed with many medications. However, most experts agree that educated, adherent patients can expect to survive for decades, living a life that is relatively complication-free. In spite of these advances, many young and middle-aged adults will experience serious illness and may die during the usual course of the disease process. Unlike cancer or other diseases, AIDS is associated with controversies challenging our legal and political systems as well as religious and personal beliefs. Contributing to this stress are personal fears of contagion or disapproval of the patient's lifestyle and behaviors. Nurses who feel stressed and overburdened may experience physical and mental distress in the form of fatigue, headache, changes in appetite and sleep patterns, helplessness, irritability, apathy, negativity, and anger.

Many strategies have been used by nurses to cope with the stress associated with caring for patients with AIDS. Education and provision of up-to-date information help to alleviate apprehension and prepare nurses to deliver safe, high-quality patient care. Interdisciplinary meetings allow participants to support one another and provide comprehensive patient care. Staff support groups give nurses an opportunity to solve problems and explore values and feelings about caring for patients with AIDS and their families; the groups also provide a forum for grieving. Other sources of support include nursing administrators, peers, and spiritual advisors.

CHAPTER REVIEW

NCLEX-Style Review Questions

1. A patient with a $CD4^+$ count of 100 cells/mm^3 and not taking any antiretroviral medications is admitted to the hospital after a motor vehicle crash. In addition, the patient has a productive cough, fever, lymphadenopathy, and a history of night sweats. The patient's **purified protein derivative** (PPD) test is negative. What is the nurse's best action? Select all that apply.

a. Use standard precautions alone because the patient does not have tuberculosis.
b. Use airborne precautions alone because the patient has not started appropriate therapy for HIV.
c. Use standard precautions and airborne precautions because the patient has tuberculosis.
d. Use standard and airborne precautions until the infectious disease providers verify the patient does not have tuberculosis, and then continue using standard precautions.
e. Transfer patient to a negative-pressure room.

2. Which finding in the patient with HIV who started ARV treatment 3 months ago indicates that the treatment is effective? Select all that apply.

a. Increased CD4 cells
b. Decreased CD4 cells
c. Decreased viral load
d. Increased CD8 cells
e. Decreased HIV antibody levels

3. A 44-year-old patient with a longstanding diagnosis of AIDS has been admitted to the hospital with an absolute neutrophil count (ANC) of 185/mm^3, an Hct of 40%, a platelet count of 150,000 mm^3. When planning the patient's care, what action should the nurse prioritize? Select all that apply.

a. Placing the patient on neutropenic precautions
b. Obtaining the patient's blood type and cross-matching in anticipation of transfusion
c. Providing the patient with supplementary oxygen by simple face mask
d. Padding hard surfaces on the patient's bed and observing for petechiae
e. Stressing the importance of frequent handwashing, avoiding crowds, and using an electric razor to avoid potential injury

4. Kaposi sarcoma, once a common manifestation of AIDS before ART was available, is seldom seen. A patient with AIDS wants to know how Kaposi sarcoma presents. What is the nurse's best response? Select all that apply.

a. Thick, white exudate in the mouth
b. A purple-red lesion on the body
c. Weight loss
d. An increase in respiratory secretions
e. Lesion may be flat or raised

5. A patient with a new diagnosis of HIV has a CD4 count of 700. The client is asymptomatic. What is the expected course of action? Select all that apply.

a. Since the patient is asymptomatic, they can negotiate a time to start therapy

b. Expect that the patient will be asked to recheck the laboratory results in 1 month. If the count remains the same, then treatment may commence

c. Expect that medication therapy will start now and you will need to teach about the importance of adherence

d. Anticipate that medication therapy will not begin until the patient becomes symptomatic

e. Educate the patient on ways to mitigate transmission risk

REFERENCES AND SELECTED READINGS

References and selected readings associated with this chapter can be found on the website that accompanies the book. Visit **http://thepoint.lww.com/Honan3e** to access the references and other additional resources associated with this chapter.

CHAPTER 37

Nursing Management: Patients With Allergic Disorders

Nicole C. Colline

Learning Objectives

After reading this chapter, you will be able to:

1. Describe the management of patients with allergic disorders.
2. Describe measures to prevent and manage anaphylaxis.
3. Discuss the different allergic disorders according to type.

Autoimmune reactions occur when self-antigens are recognized by the body's normal defense mechanisms as foreign. With the presence of these "foreign" antigens, B cells become hyperactive, and increased amounts of immunoglobulin E (IgE) are produced, thus causing a hypersensitivity or allergic response. **Hypersensitivity** is an amplified or inappropriate response to an antigen on second exposure (see Pathophysiology), leading to inflammation or illness resulting in destruction of healthy tissue and/or somatic symptoms. The cause may result from genetic, hormonal, and environmental factors; many times, the etiology is unclear. The reaction time varies and can be within minutes to hours of exposure or may be delayed for days to weeks. Refer to Chapter 35 for details of types of allergic classifications (Table 35-1). Symptoms will vary depending on the classification and may range from a local reaction to the life-threatening systemic response of anaphylaxis.

Health care personnel play a vital role in the recognition and management of individuals suffering with allergic responses. It is important for nurses to recognize signs and symptoms of allergic reactions, understand the risk factors associated with reaction, and become familiar with treatment and management.

There are two types of IgE-mediated allergic reactions: atopic (local) and nonatopic disorders. Although the underlying immunologic reactions of the two types of disorders are the same, the predisposing factors and manifestations are different. The atopic disorders are characterized by a hereditary predisposition and production of a local reaction to IgE antibodies causing allergic responses in the nose, eyes, skin, and lungs (e.g., allergic rhinitis, asthma, angioedema, and atopic dermatitis/eczema; Delves, 2020). Nonatopic disorders have symptoms similar to atopic variants but lack increased serum IgE levels and/or antigen-specific IgE.

Allergic or hypersensitivity reactions are further classified into "types": Types I, II, III, and IV. Type I, II, and III reactions occur within 24 hours of exposure to an allergen. They are called "immediate" hypersensitivity reactions. Type I reactions include bronchial asthma, allergic rhinitis, food allergies, and anaphylaxis. Type II reactions include immune thrombocytopenia, autoimmune hemolytic anemia and neutropenia. Type III reactions include lupus and serum sickness. Type IV reactions are called "delayed hypersensitivity" reactions as they commonly occur 48 to 72 hours after exposure to the allergen. Examples include contact dermatitis, tuberculosis, and fungal infections (Allarakha & Jacob, 2022; Albright, Larkin & Chong, 2023).

Unfolding Patient Stories: J.H. • Part 2

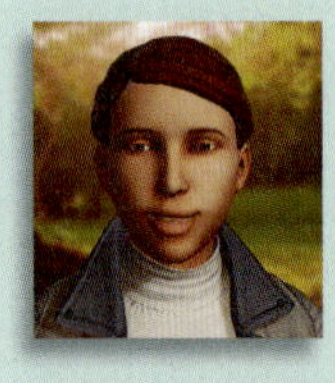

Recall from Chapter 10 that J.H. came to the clinic with continued symptoms of asthma. The nurse confirmed the patient was following the asthma action plan; however, J.H. now returns to the clinic with worsening symptoms. What assessment findings would indicate to the nurse that this patient is having a hypersensitivity reaction to an allergen(s)? What questions can assist the nurse in identifying the causative agent(s)? What interventions should be implemented when allergen(s) are identified?

Care for J.H. and other patients in a realistic virtual environment: ***vSim** for Nursing* (thepoint.lww.com/vSimMedicalSurgical). Practice documenting these patients' care in DocuCare (thepoint.lww.com/DocuCareEHR).

ANAPHYLAXIS

Anaphylaxis is defined as a severe systemic hypersensitivity reaction that is rapid in onset and can cause various reactions including death. Anaphylaxis is a clinical response to an immediate (type I hypersensitivity) immunologic reaction

BOX 37-1 **Focus on Pathophysiology**

Anaphylaxis

The chain of events for anaphylaxis:

1. Response to antigen. Immunoglobulin (Ig) E recognizes and binds to the antigen.
2. Release of chemical mediators. Activated IgE on basophils promotes release of mediators (histamine, serotonin, and leukotrienes).
3. Intensified response. Mast cells are stimulated and release more histamine and other inflammatory mediators.
4. Respiratory distress. In the lungs, histamine causes bronchial constriction, endothelial cell destruction, and fluid leakage into the alveoli.
5. Deterioration. Meanwhile, mediators increase vascular permeability, causing fluid to leak from the vessels. The face and tongue can become severely swollen. Blood vessels dilate throughout the body, resulting in hypotension and shock.
6. Failure of compensatory mechanisms. Endothelial cell damage causes basophils and mast cells to release heparin and mediator-neutralizing substances. Anaphylaxis is now irreversible.

Adapted from Lippincott. (2017). *Pathophysiology: An incredibly visual! pocket guide.* Lippincott Williams & Wilkins.

between a specific **antigen** and an **antibody**. The reaction results from a rapid release of IgE-mediated chemicals, which can induce a severe, life-threatening reaction. Anaphylaxis involves multiple organs and body systems, is rapid in onset, and is potentially fatal. The most common causes of anaphylactic reactions include food, medications, and insect venom (Motosue et al., 2022).

Pathophysiology

Anaphylaxis occurs when the body's immune system produces specific IgE antibodies toward a substance that is normally nontoxic (e.g., food such as a peanut; Box 37-1). When the person first ingests the peanut, for example, there are no physical reactions manifested. Instead, antibodies are produced for that specific substance, and then those antibodies are stored in the immune system for future re-exposure. If the substance is ingested again, the body releases excess amounts of the protein **histamine**. Large amounts of histamine released into the body may cause flushing, urticaria (hives), angioedema, hypotension, and bronchoconstriction (Fig. 37-1). These rapid systemic changes (occurring most commonly in the dermatologic, respiratory, cardiovascular, and gastrointestinal [GI] tracts) characteristically produce clinical manifestations within seconds or minutes after antigen exposure. In severe cases, these symptoms may cause shock. If no medical intervention is sought, death may ensue (LoVerde et al., 2018).

Box 37-2 lists substances that most commonly cause anaphylaxis.

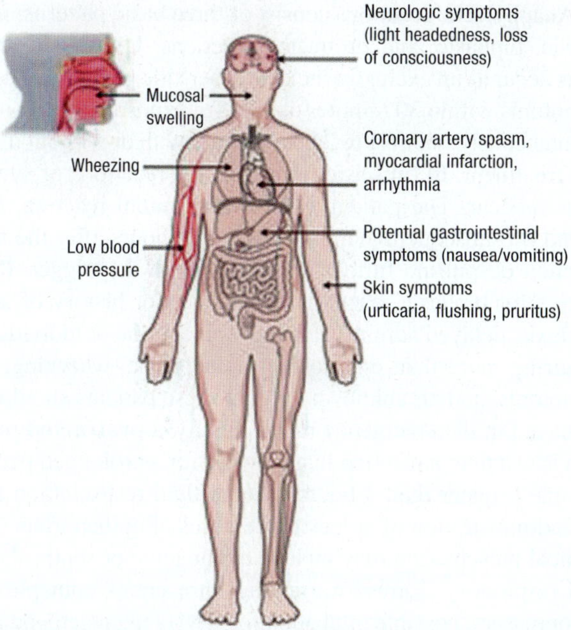

FIGURE 37-1 Anaphylaxis: Systemic symptoms. (Miller, M. D., Chhabra, A. B., Konin, J., & Mistry, D. [2013]. *Sports medicine conditions: Return to play: recognition, treatment, planning.* Lippincott Williams & Wilkins.)

Clinical Manifestations and Assessment

The severity of previous anaphylactic reactions does not determine the severity of subsequent reactions, which could be the same, more severe, or less severe. The severity depends on the degree of **allergy** and the dose of **allergen**.

BOX 37-2 **Common Causes of Anaphylaxis**

Foods

Peanuts, tree nuts (e.g., walnuts, pecans, cashews, almonds), shellfish (e.g., shrimp, lobster, crab), fish, cow milk, eggs, soy, wheat

Medications

Antibiotics (especially penicillin, cephalosporins, and sulfonamides), along with aspirin and other NSAIDs, allopurinol, radiocontrast agents, anesthetic agents (lidocaine, procaine), vaccines, hormones (insulin, vasopressin, adrenocorticotropic hormone [ACTH]), and newer biologic modifiers such as omalizumab, infliximab, and cetuximab

Other Pharmaceutical/Biologic Agents

Animal serums (tetanus antitoxin, snake venom antitoxin, rabies antitoxin), antigens used in skin testing, transfusion products, methylmethacrylate (bone cement)

Insect Stings

Honeybees, wasps, hornets, yellow jackets, ants (including fire ants), snakes, jellyfish

Latex

Medical and nonmedical products containing latex

Anaphylactic reactions consist of three basic patterns: uniphasic, biphasic, and protracted reactions. **Uniphasic** reactions occur as an exclusive incident where the patient develops symptoms within 30 minutes of allergen exposure that resolve spontaneously within 1 to 2 hours, either with or without medical treatment. In **biphasic** responses, the reactions or symptoms reoccur. The patient will have an initial reaction, followed by subsequent symptoms up to 72 hours after the first reaction despite no further interaction with the trigger. Risk factors for biphasic reactions include a prior history of anaphylaxis, delayed administration of epinephrine or individuals requiring more than one dose of epinephrine, wheezing, GI symptoms, and an unknown trigger. These patients should be managed in the emergency room. Finally, a **protracted** reaction is just that: a reaction that may last for a prolonged period of time (greater than 4 hours) despite fluid resuscitation and postadministration of at least three doses of epinephrine. The clinical presentation may include cardiogenic or septic shock and respiratory distress warranting intravenous epinephrine, vasopressors, possible intubation for airway management, and a stay in the intensive care unit (Gorham, 2022).

Mild systemic reactions consist mainly of cutaneous symptoms (e.g., generalized erythema/flushing, pruritus). Nasal congestion, periorbital swelling, generalized erythema, pruritus (itching) and urticaria, sneezing, and tearing of the eyes also can be expected. *Moderate* systemic reactions may include flushing, warmth, tingling of the extremities, anxiety (feeling of impending doom), nausea, vomiting, and diarrhea in addition to any of the milder symptoms. Both mild and moderate reactions begin within 2 hours of exposure. More *serious* reactions include confusion, syncope, bronchospasm and edema of the airways or larynx with dyspnea, cough, and wheezing. Moderate symptoms can progress rapidly to severe symptoms such as bronchospasm, laryngeal edema, cyanosis, and circulatory and respiratory failure if not promptly treated. Stridor, drooling, and tongue or facial edema are ominous signs, suggestive of impending airway obstruction, and it is urgent that the airway is maintained by either intubation or if needed emergency needle cricothyrotomy or cricothyrotomy (McHugh & Repanshek, 2022). Cardiac arrest and coma may follow (Mikhall et al., 2021).

Monitoring the patient with anaphylaxis includes continual assessment of the patient's respiratory rate and pattern, oxygen saturation, assessing for breathing difficulties or abnormal lung sounds, checking for changes to mentation, ECG/telemetry monitoring, and assessing for hemodynamic stability (pulse rate and rhythm, blood pressure, mean arterial pressure [MAP]). Two large-bore IVs are inserted to prepare for fluid administration and medications because significant intravascular volume can be lost due to increased capillary permeability (McHugh & Repanshek, 2022). If patients are hypotensive, they should be placed in the supine position with lower extremities slightly elevated to increase cerebral and cardiac perfusion and pregnant individuals in the semirecumbant position on their left side to avoid compression of the inferior vena cava by the gravid uterus and prevent circulatory collapse (Clinical Overview, 2022; Navalpakam et al., 2022; Schwartz, 2020). Proper positioning can prevent cardiac arrest and death. If the patient's respiratory status is compromised, they may need to remain in the upright position (Navalpakam et al., 2022). Supplemental oxygen is administered if hypoxemia occurs, and preparation should be made for potential endotracheal intubation as warranted. Table 37-1 summarizes the clinical manifestations of various pathophysiologic changes.

Prevention

Any patient who has experienced an anaphylactic reaction in the past is at greater risk of experiencing one in the future

TABLE 37-1 Clinical Manifestations of Anaphylaxis

Change	Signs and Symptoms
Activation of IgE and subsequent release of chemical mediators	Feeling of impending doom or fright
Histamine release	Sweating; sneezing; shortness of breath; nasal pruritus, urticaria, and angioedema (swelling of the deep dermis or subcutaneous or submucosal tissues); nasal mucosal edema; profuse watery rhinorrhea; itching; nasal congestion
Increased vascular permeability, subsequent decrease in peripheral resistance and leakage of plasma fluids	Hypotension, decreased MAP, shock, and possible cardiac arrhythmias
Increased capillary permeability and mast cell degranulation	Edema of upper respiratory tract, resulting in hypopharyngeal and laryngeal obstruction
Bronchiole smooth muscle contraction and increased mucus production	Hoarseness, shortness of breath, stridor, wheezing, hypoxemia, and use of accessory muscles
Smooth muscle contraction of intestines and bladder	Severe stomach cramps, nausea, diarrhea; urinary urgency and incontinence

(Gorham, 2022). Long-term management of anaphylaxis is necessary to decrease morbidity and mortality. This includes prevention of reoccurrence. For those with a history of or predisposition to anaphylaxis, strict avoidance of potential allergens is essential. Furthermore, prevention includes thorough education to both the patient and caregiver(s) on identifying and eliminating the causative agent, followed by the use of emergency medication and seeking immediate medical treatment. Annual follow-up with an allergist and/or immunologist will aid in individualized care.

When avoidance is impossible (e.g., patients at risk for anaphylaxis from insect stings should avoid areas populated by insects and should use appropriate clothing, insect repellent, and caution to avoid further stings) or one has previously experienced an idiopathic or exercise-induced anaphylactic reaction, an emergency kit that contains epinephrine should be carried at all times. The EpiPen (epinephrine injection) from Viatris Pharmaceuticals is a commercially available first-aid device that delivers premeasured doses of 0.3 mg (EpiPen) or 0.15 mg (EpiPen Jr) of epinephrine (Fig. 37-2). The autoinjection system requires no preparation, and the self-administration technique is uncomplicated. The patient must be given an opportunity to demonstrate the correct technique for use; an EpiPen training device can be used for teaching correct technique. Verbal and written information about the emergency kit, as well as strategies to avoid exposure to threatening allergens, also must be provided. Failure to administer epinephrine promptly and properly has proven to be fatal in severe anaphylactic reactions.

Patients with known anaphylaxis to any substance should be provided with two epinephrine autoinjectors. After being taught how to use the autoinjector, patients should "teach back" the administration technique to the nurse or medical provider. They should be instructed to call 911 and go to the emergency department for medical care if they need to use the EpiPen.

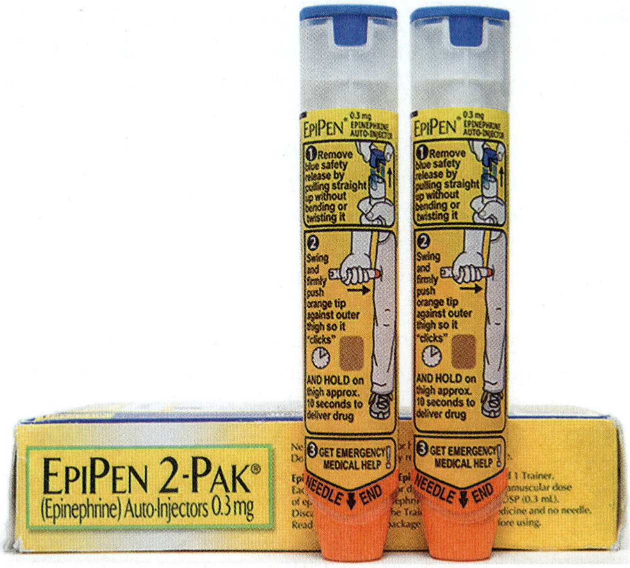

FIGURE 37-2 **The EpiPen. Autoinjectors are commercially available first-aid devices that administer premeasured doses of epinephrine. An EpiPen training device is available for patients to practice correct self-injection technique. (Courtesy of Amy Kerkemeyer/Shutterstock.)**

Screening for allergies before a medication is prescribed or first administered is an important preventive measure. A careful history of any sensitivity to suspected antigens must be obtained before administering any medication, particularly in parenteral form, because this route is associated with the most severe anaphylaxis. Nurses caring for patients in any setting (hospital, home, outpatient diagnostic testing sites, long-term care facilities) must assess patients' risks for anaphylactic reactions. Patients are asked about previous exposure to contrast agents used for diagnostic tests and any allergic reactions as well as reactions to any medications, foods, insect stings, and latex.

People who are predisposed to anaphylaxis should wear some form of identification, such as a medical alert bracelet, or carry a wallet card that names allergies to medications, food, and other substances. They should also work with their medical provider on developing an anaphylaxis action plan in case of repeat exposure to an allergen or reoccurrence of an anaphylactic reaction.

Long-term preventative measures include proper management of a patient's chronic condition(s), such as asthma, cardiovascular disease, etc., followed by detailed education regarding treating an acute anaphylactic reaction. All patients are to be informed that anaphylaxis can be deadly and that immediate treatment can be the difference between life and death.

Medical Management

Delays in diagnosing and treating anaphylaxis have significant effects on patient morbidity and mortality. The diagnosis of anaphylaxis is predominantly based on objective findings during clinical examination. Serum IgE, plasma tryptase (a protease of human mast cells that has been implicated as a pathologic mediator of numerous allergic and inflammatory conditions), and urinary histamine levels are commonly elevated, but false-negative results are possible and they are therefore not considered among the criteria to diagnose an anaphylactic reaction (LoVerde et al., 2018).

Anaphylaxis continues to be underdiagnosed, largely in part from patient under-reporting: not describing all their symptoms and undermining their expressed symptoms. Similarly, medical providers are not well versed in the complexity of anaphylaxis in part due to the lack of a gold standard for diagnosis and absent point-of-care testing (Motosue et al., 2022). As the prevalence of anaphylaxis is rising, proper diagnosis and medical management is imperative to save lives.

Management should be focused on the early use of epinephrine and assessing and maintaining airway function and circulation (Navalpakam et al., 2022). Acute management depends on the severity of the reaction. Initially, respiratory and cardiovascular functions are evaluated. If the patient is in cardiac arrest, cardiopulmonary resuscitation is instituted. Oxygen is provided in high concentrations during cardiopulmonary resuscitation or if the patient is cyanotic, dyspneic, or wheezing. At first response, epinephrine, in a 1:1,000 dilution, is administered intramuscularly into the anterolateral thigh. This injection may be repeated once or twice in 5- to 15-minute intervals if symptoms persist or are worsening. If under the care of medical professionals, intramuscular epinephrine administration may be followed by a continuous IV infusion if needed. If the adult patient is hypotensive, 1 to 2 L or 20 mL/kg of isotonic fluid is administered (McHugh & Repanshek, 2022). Epinephrine is the first-line treatment of anaphylaxis as it is the only medication that may halt cardiac or respiratory arrest and subsequent fatality, which can occur within 5 to 30 minutes of allergen exposure (Curry, 2021; LoVerde et al., 2018; Shaker et al., 2020, Tanno et al., 2019).

Most adverse events associated with administration of epinephrine ("adrenaline") occur when the dose is excessive or given intravenously. More common symptoms include headache, tachycardia, tremor, and pallor. Though rare, severe adverse reactions to epinephrine include pulmonary edema, ventricular arrhythmias, myocardial infarction, malignant hypertension, and intracranial hemorrhage. Patients at risk for adverse effects include older patients and those with hypertension, arteriopathies (diseases of the arteries), or known ischemic heart disease. In those with cardiovascular disease, risks and benefits should be weighed prior to the administration of epinephrine, but as the heart is a potential target for effects from anaphylaxis, the use of epinephrine is usually warranted (Navalpakam et al., 2022; McLendon & Sternard, 2022; Tanno et al., 2019).

Drug Alert

To avoid mishaps in dosing, premeasured fixed doses are available in many emergency departments for both adult and pediatric EpiPens, which provide the standard adult or pediatric dose (EpiPen, 0.3-mg epinephrine for adults; EpiPen Jr, 0.15-mg epinephrine for infants and children weighing 15–24 kg, 0.1 mg for infant/child weighing 7.5–14 kg; Clinical Overview, 2022).

Antihistamines and corticosteroids also may be administered to prevent recurrences of the reaction and to treat urticaria and angioedema, although they are not the first-line treatment. Their use should not delay the administration of epinephrine as waiting can result in a patient fatality. Antihistamines take up to 80 minutes to suppress histamine levels by 50% and only treat milder symptoms, such as pruritus. Steroids generally work very slowly once administered and play a role in decreasing systemic inflammation. IV fluids (e.g., normal saline solution), volume expanders, and vasopressor agents are administered to maintain blood pressure and normal hemodynamic status (LoVerde et al., 2018; McHugh & Repanshek, 2022).

In patients with episodes of bronchospasm or a history of bronchial asthma or chronic obstructive pulmonary disease, aminophylline and corticosteroids may be administered to improve airway patency and function. If hypotension is unresponsive to isotonic crystalloid fluid and vasopressors, glucagon may be administered intravenously for its acute inotropic and chronotropic effects. Glucagon may be administered in those patients not responding to epinephrine along with additional vasopressors. Glucagon stimulates the enzyme adenylate cyclase, and its activation results in the intracellular accumulation of the second messenger cyclic adenosine monophosphate (cAMP). Increased levels of cAMP improve the suppressive actions that epinephrine exerts on the biochemical events responsible for the anaphylactic response. Its administration may result in nausea, vomiting, hypoglycemia, and hyperglycemia in patients with diabetes (LoVerde et al., 2018).

Patients who have experienced anaphylactic reactions and received epinephrine should be transported to the local emergency department for observation and monitoring because of the risk for a "rebound" (or reoccurrence) reaction usually within 4- to 10 hours after the initial allergic reaction. Patients with severe reactions are monitored closely for 12 to 24 hours in a facility that can provide emergency care, if needed.

Nursing Management

If a patient is experiencing an acute allergic response, the nurse's initial action is to assess the patient for signs and symptoms of anaphylaxis. The nurse assesses the airway, breathing pattern, and other vital signs. The patient is observed for signs of increasing edema and respiratory distress. Prompt notification of the provider (or calling 911 if in the community) and preparation for initiation of emergency measures (intubation, administration of emergency medications, insertion of IV lines, fluid administration, oxygen administration) are important to reduce the severity of the reaction and to restore cardiovascular function. The nurse documents the interventions used, timeline of events including times of medication administration, the patient's vital signs, and response to treatment. Large volumes of IV fluid may be required to restore intravascular volume, and the nurse monitors for signs of over resuscitation (JVD, crackles on pulmonary exam, edema, S3 heart sound).

Pearls for Practice

In the event of an acute allergic reaction, the nurse recognizes that ET intubation may be difficult or impossible because it can result in increased laryngeal edema, bleeding, and further narrowing of the glottic opening. Fiberoptic ET intubation, needle cricothyrotomy (followed by transtracheal ventilation), or cricothyrotomy may be necessary (LoVerde et al., 2018).

Pearls for Practice

The nurse is aware that high-risk medications associated with anaphylaxis include chemotherapy agents (carboplatin, docetaxel, oxaliplatin, paclitaxel, liposomal doxorubicin, and cetuximab) and monoclonal antibiotics (blinatumomab, rituximab, trastuzumab, and cetuximab). The nurse observes the patient for changes: dermatologic (angioedema, flushing, urticaria), pulmonary (shortness of breath, wheezing, stridor), cardiac (tachycardia, hypotension, decreasing MAP, chest pain), gastrointestinal (nausea, vomiting, cramping), and neurologic (headache, dizziness, blurred vision). If any of these symptoms occur, the infusion is immediately stopped, a rapid response is called, and the medical provider is notified.

The patient who has recovered from anaphylaxis needs an explanation of what occurred as well as instruction about avoiding future exposure to antigens and how to administer emergency medications to treat anaphylaxis. All patients who have experienced an anaphylactic reaction should receive a prescription for preloaded syringes of epinephrine; they should carry two syringes at all times. The nurse instructs the patient and family in their use and has the patient and family demonstrate correct administration of the medication (Box 37-3).

Stinging insects are a common cause of anaphylactic reactions. People who are allergic to insect venom may require venom immunotherapy (VIT), which is used as a control measure and not a cure. Immunotherapy administered after an insect sting is very effective in reducing the risk of anaphylaxis from future stings (Adams et al., 2022).

Similarly, those with anaphylaxis to many foods and medications (e.g., insulin-allergic patients with diabetes) can have desensitization therapy while under the care of an allergist if use or consumption of the allergen is necessary. Desensitization is very high risk and complex: it is based on controlled anaphylaxis with a gradual release of mediators. Under the supervision of a skilled medical provider or allergist, patients introduce small amounts of the allergen to their immune system multiple times over a 6- to 12-month time frame. With each office visit, the amount of allergen ingested increases. The goal is to consume the medication or food at normal intervals and not experience an allergic reaction (Madrigal-Burglaeta, 2022). Patients who undergo desensitization are cautioned that there should be no lapses in therapy because this may lead to the reappearance of the allergic reaction when the use of the medication is resumed. During desensitization, it is imperative to have emergency equipment available in case of an anaphylactic reaction. See further discussion of immunotherapy later in this chapter.

BOX 37-3 Patient Education

Self-Administration of Epinephrine

1. After removing the EpiPen autoinjector from its carrying tube, grasp the unit with the orange tip (injecting end) pointing downward. Form a fist around the unit with the orange tip down; with your other hand, remove the blue safety release cap.
2. Hold the orange tip near the outer thigh. Swing and **jab firmly** into the outer thigh until a click is heard with the device perpendicular (90-degree angle) to the thigh.
3. Hold the device firmly against the thigh for approximately 3 seconds.
4. Remove the unit from the thigh, and massage the injection area for 10 seconds. Call 911, and seek immediate medical attention. Carefully place the used EpiPen, needle-end first, into the device storage tube without bending the needle. Screw on the storage tube completely, and take it with you to the hospital emergency room.
5. Medication should be stored at temperature between 68° and 77°F and should be protected from light.

Note: The EpiPen and EpiPen Jr Auto-Injector may come packaged with an EpiPen Trainer and separate Trainer Instructions for Use. **The EpiPen Trainer has a gray color. The gray EpiPen Trainer contains no medicine and no needle.**

ALLERGIC RHINITIS

Allergic **rhinitis** (AR [hay fever]) is the most common form of chronic upper airway inflammation, characterized by rhinorrhea, sneezing, nasal congestion, and nasal itching. It is most commonly seen in the spring/summer months. Its incidence is on the rise, affecting 40% of the U.S. population, especially those who are genetically predisposed, and affecting individuals with a diagnosis of asthma four to six times more than those without asthma (Correia & Baroody, 2019).

Allergic rhinitis (AR) is a type I hypersensitivity reaction that has become a global health problem causing extensive burden and disability worldwide. It is one of the more common reasons for visits to primary practitioners, and it contributes to school and work absences, lack of work productivity, and decreased outdoor involvement. The etiology of this disease is poorly understood, but genetic and environmental factors influence its prevalence (Bousquet et al., 2020; Correia & Baroody, 2019; Meng et al., 2019; Trikojat et al., 2017).

There are two main types of AR: seasonal and perennial. Seasonal rhinitis affects those who are sensitive to the circulating pollens of certain plants that are present in the air during a particular season. Perennial rhinitis is year-round; individuals are sensitive to the pollens in the air during almost every month of the year. Rhinitis is considered to be the allergic form if the symptoms are caused by an allergen-specific IgE-mediated immunologic response. However, a sizable proportion of patients with rhinitis have mixed rhinitis, or coexisting allergic and nonallergic rhinitis (NAR). NAR carries similar symptoms to allergic rhinitis, though it is not provoked by a specific allergen and is most common in autumn/winter months (Avdeeva et al., 2022).

The proportion of patients with the allergic form of rhinitis is greatest among children yet is on the rise among adults. It often occurs with other conditions, such as allergic conjunctivitis, sinusitis, and asthma. AR is more prevalent in high-income countries, but severity of symptoms is higher in low- and middle-income countries. If symptoms are severe, AR may interfere with sleep, leisure, and school or work activities. If left untreated, many complications may result, such as allergic asthma; chronic nasal obstruction; chronic otitis media with hearing loss; anosmia (absence of the sense of smell); and, in children, orofacial dental deformities. Early diagnosis and adequate treatment are essential to relieve current symptoms and reduce comorbidities later in life (Bousquet et al., 2020).

Because AR is induced by airborne pollens or molds, it is activated by the following seasonal occurrences:

- Early spring: Tree pollen (oak, elm, poplar), mold spores
- Early summer: Rose pollen (rose fever), grass pollen (timothy, red-top)
- Early fall: Weed pollen (ragweed), mold spores

Each year, attacks begin and end at about the same time. Airborne mold spores require warm, damp weather. Although there is no rigid seasonal pattern, these spores appear in early spring, are rampant during the summer, and then taper off and disappear by the first frost.

Clinical Manifestations and Assessment

Typical signs and symptoms of allergic rhinitis include sneezing and nasal congestion; clear, watery nasal discharge; itchy eyes and nose; and lacrimation (Bousquet et al., 2020). Drainage of nasal mucus into the pharynx, called "postnasal drip," results in multiple attempts to clear the throat and a dry cough, hoarseness, or scratchy throat. Headache, pain over the paranasal sinuses, and epistaxis can accompany AR. The symptoms of this chronic condition depend on environmental exposure and intrinsic host responsiveness. AR can affect quality of life by also producing fatigue, loss of sleep, poor concentration, and interference with physical activities. Of great concern is the risk of developing persistent asthma and other comorbid conditions (chronic otitis media and sinusitis, obstructive sleep apnea, airway inflammation, etc.) if AR is not controlled (Correia & Baroody, 2019; Trikojat et al., 2017).

Studies have shown that individuals suffering with AR are 1.7 times more likely to experience depression and anxiety during inflammation phases and have reduced academic performance and work productivity, impaired sexual performance, and lower quality of life scores (deShazo & Kemp, 2022; Trikojat et al., 2017). Nasal congestion leading to mouth breathing, postnasal drip, and intense coughing can lead to interrupted sleep patterns resulting in daytime fatigue. This fatigue may result in reduced work performance, decreased socialization, and feelings of inadequacy. Symptoms of sadness and worry can follow.

Diagnosis of AR is based on history, physical examination, and diagnostics. A thorough history of symptomology is imperative to properly diagnose AR. Intermittent AR comes and goes, and symptoms last for greater than 1 hour per day when faced with an allergen. Persistent AR occurs for more than 4 days for 4 weeks at a time and is further classified as mild, moderate, or severe depending on if symptoms interfere with activities of daily life or sleep (Bousquet et al., 2020). On objective examination, a patient suffering with allergic rhinitis may appear fatigued (the patient may complain of not feeling well rested after a full night's sleep) and may also present with any of the following conditions:

- Allergic "shiners" (gray-black discoloration below lower eye lids that some refer to as "raccoon eyes")
- Puffy eyes
- Clear or cloudy fluid surrounding the tympanic membranes
- Nasal congestion or rhinorrhea
- Marked erythema of palpebral conjunctivae associated with increased tearing
- Enlarged nasal turbinates that are a pale bluish color and boggy in texture
- Enlarged anterior cervical lymph nodes
- Cobblestoned appearance on the posterior pharynx (due to chronic postnasal drip and nasal congestion)
- Sinus tenderness on palpation (Bousquet et al., 2020)

Diagnostic tests include nasal smears, peripheral blood counts, total serum IgE, epicutaneous and intradermal testing, radioallergosorbent test (RAST), food elimination and challenge, and nasal provocation tests. Results indicative of allergy as the cause of rhinitis include increased levels of IgE and eosinophil and positive reactions on allergen testing. False-positive and false-negative responses to these tests, particularly skin testing and provocation tests, may occur, yet they still are considered a highly effective means of identifying agents that are causative of allergic responses (Ansotegui et al., 2020).

It is imperative that patients with AR are diagnosed properly and their treatment is individualized according to the severity of their disease. Patients must then be able to verbalize understanding of their diagnosis, proper treatment modalities, and when to seek follow-up care.

Medical Management

The goal of therapy is to provide relief from symptoms and encourage adherence to therapeutic regimens. Therapy may include one or all of the following interventions: avoidance therapy; pharmacotherapy; immunotherapy; homeopathic modalities; and, in cases resistive to other treatments, surgery. Verbal instructions must be reinforced by written information. Knowledge of general concepts regarding assessment and therapy in allergic diseases is important so that the patient can learn to manage certain conditions as well as prevent severe reactions and illnesses.

Avoidance Therapy

In avoidance therapy, every attempt is made to remove the allergens that act as precipitating factors. Often, simple measures and environmental controls are effective in decreasing symptoms. Examples include using air cleaners/purifiers, humidifiers, and dehumidifiers; keeping windows closed during periods of high pollen counts and windy conditions; using air conditioning as much as possible in the warmer months; sleeping with windows closed; removing dust-catching furnishings (carpets, stuffed animals, feather bedding, window coverings); removing pets from the home or bedroom; removing cockroaches by professional extermination followed by regular cleaning of the infested area(s); using pillow and mattress covers that are impermeable to dust mites; washing bedding materials biweekly in hot water (55°C); and maintaining a smoke-free environment (Correia & Baroody, 2019).

Because multiple allergens are often implicated, multiple measures to avoid exposure to allergens are often necessary. High-efficiency particulate air (HEPA) purifiers and vacuum cleaner filters also may be used to reduce allergens in the environment, though they are ineffective if used as the only means to decrease the allergen exposure. The patient is instructed to reduce exposure to people with upper respiratory tract infections. If an upper respiratory infection occurs, the patient is encouraged to take deep breaths and to cough frequently to ensure adequate gas exchange and to prevent atelectasis. The patient is instructed to seek medical attention because the presence of allergy symptoms along with an upper respiratory tract infection may compromise adequate lung function (Correia & Baroody, 2019).

Research has shown that multiple avoidance strategies tailored to a person's risk factors can reduce the severity of symptoms, the number of work or school days missed because of symptoms, and the number of unscheduled health care visits for treatment. In many cases, it is impossible to avoid exposure to all environmental allergens, so pharmacologic therapy or immunotherapy is needed.

Pharmacologic Therapy

Although allergen avoidance is clearly the safest and most effective means of treating symptoms associated with AR, some individuals may require pharmacologic therapy to further suppress the effects of histamine on the body. The ultimate goal of pharmacologic therapy is to target the specific symptom(s) and treat them with the most appropriate medication.

Antihistamines

Antihistamines, now classified as H_1-receptor antagonists (or H_1 blockers), are used in the management of *mild* allergic disorders. H_1 blockers bind selectively to H_1 receptors, preventing the actions of histamines at these sites. They do not prevent the release of histamine but rather protect the surrounding tissue from the effects of the histamine release.

Oral antihistamines, which are readily absorbed, are most effective when given at the first occurrence of symptoms because they prevent the development of new symptoms. The effectiveness of these medications is limited to certain patients with hay fever, vasomotor rhinitis, urticaria (hives), and mild asthma.

Antihistamines are further classified into first- and second-generation drugs. First-generation antihistamines include diphenhydramine and are lipophilic with anticholinergic side effects. Second-generation antihistamines (e.g., loratadine, fexofenadine, and cetirizine) are less lipophilic, have a longer half-life, and possess fewer sedating effects as they do not as readily cross the blood–brain barrier. For this reason, second-generation antihistamines are preferred for treating ocular symptoms, sneezing, and itching in both children and young adults. Oral antihistamines are minimally effective in treating nasal congestion; therefore, intranasal remedies are widely used for treating AR (Correia & Baroody, 2019). Most antihistamines and intranasal preparations are available over-the-counter in local pharmacies. Refer to Table 37-2 for details.

Pearls for Practice

It is important for patients to understand that medications for allergy control should be used only when the allergy is apparent. This is usually on a seasonal or intermittent basis. Continued use of medications when not required can cause an increased tolerance to the medication, with the result that the medication will not be effective when needed.

Adrenergic Agents/Decongestants

Adrenergic agents, vasoconstrictors of mucosal vessels, are used topically (nasal and ophthalmic formulations) in addition to the oral route. These medications help relieve severity of symptoms by narrowing blood vessels in the nasal passageways, therefore decreasing nasal congestion; however, these medications will not treat the underlying cause of nasal congestion, sinus pressure, etc.

The most commonly used oral adrenergic agent is pseudoephedrine hydrochloride. Although considered safe if used as directed, pseudoephedrine hydrochloride has been known to cause in some patients mild shakiness, heart palpitations, and anxiety shortly after ingestion. Pseudoephedrine is to be used cautiously or avoided in patients with underlying cardiac conditions, anxiety disorders, patients who are or plan on becoming pregnant, patients with asthma, and those who use herbal supplements on a regular basis. Potential side effects include hypertension, arrhythmias, palpitations, central nervous system stimulation, irritability, tremor, insomnia, and tachyphylaxis (acceleration of hemodynamic status). Due to

TABLE **37-2 Selected H_1-Antihistamines**

H_1-Antihistamine	Contraindications	Major Side Effects	Nursing Implications and Patient Teaching
First-Generation H_1-Antihistamines (Sedating)			
Diphenhydramine	Allergy to any antihistamines Generally not recommended in last 2 weeks of pregnancy Use with caution if breast or chestfeeding Use cautiously with closed-angle glaucoma, asthma, stenosing peptic ulcer, benign prostatic hypertrophy or bladder neck obstruction, older patients	Drowsiness, confusion, dizziness, dry mouth, nausea, vomiting, urinary retention, insomnia, nervousness, tremors, blurred vision, and gastrointestinal disturbance	Administer with food if gastrointestinal upset occurs. Caution patients to avoid alcohol, driving, or engaging in any hazardous activities due to sedative effects of this medication. Suggest sucking on sugarless lozenges or ice chips for relief of dry mouth. Assess for urinary retention; monitor urinary output.
Chlorpheniramine	Allergy to any antihistamines Not recommended in last 2 weeks of pregnancy Use with caution during breast or chestfeeding Use cautiously with closed-angle glaucoma, asthma, stenosing peptic ulcer, BPH or bladder neck obstruction, older patients	Drowsiness, sedation, and dizziness, although less than other sedating agents; confusion, dry mouth, nausea, vomiting, urinary retention, epigastric distress, thickening of bronchial secretions	Caution patients to avoid alcohol, driving, or engaging in any hazardous activities until CNS response to medication is stabilized. Suggest sucking on sugarless lozenges or ice chips for relief of dry mouth. Recommend the use of a humidifier.
Hydroxyzine	Allergy to hydroxyzine or cetirizine, pregnancy, lactation; contraindicated in patients with a known history of QT prolongation and in first trimester of pregnancy Use cautiously with closed-angle glaucoma, BPH, moderate-to-severe renal impairment, and older adults	Drowsiness; dry mouth; involuntary motor activity, including tremor and seizures	Caution patients to avoid alcohol, driving, or engaging in any hazardous activities until CNS response to medication is stabilized. Suggest sucking on sugarless lozenges or ice chips for relief of dry mouth. Instruct patients to report tremors.
Second-Generation H_1-Antihistamines (Nonsedating)			
Cetirizine	Allergy to any antihistamines; used cautiously in those with renal failure or renal impairment There is no adequate information regarding the effects of cetirizine on the breast or chestfed infant or the effects on milk production Self-medication with cetirizine (nonprescription or OTC formulations) during pregnancy is not recommended	Dry nasal mucosa, thickening of bronchial secretions	Can be taken without regard to meals. Instruct patients to use caution if driving or performing tasks that require alertness. Ethanol ingestion should be avoided, and coadministration with other CNS depressants should be approached with caution. Recommend the use of a humidifier.
Desloratadine	Allergy to loratadine Lactation Use cautiously with kidney or liver impairment or with pregnancy	Somnolence, nervousness, dizziness, fatigue, dry mouth; may result in thickened bronchial secretions in the respiratory tract, thereby aggravating asthma or an asthmatic attack.	Can be taken without regard to meals. Suggest sucking on sugarless lozenges or ice chips for relief of dry mouth. Recommend the use of a humidifier.

H_1-Antihistamine	Contraindications	Major Side Effects	Nursing Implications and Patient Teaching
Loratadine	Allergy to any antihistamines; use with caution in patients with asthma; use cautiously in those with renal failure, renal impairment, or liver disease; those breast or chestfeeding are advised to consult a health care professional prior to using loratadine	Headache, nervousness, dizziness, depression, edema, increased appetite; result in thickened bronchial secretions in the respiratory tract, thereby aggravating an acute asthmatic attack	Instruct patients to avoid alcohol and to use caution if driving or performing tasks that require alertness. Suggest sucking on sugarless lozenges or ice chips for relief of dry mouth. Recommend the use of a humidifier.
Fexofenadine	Allergy to any antihistamines Pregnancy Lactation Use with caution with liver or kidney impairment and in older patients	Fatigue, drowsiness, GI upset	Should not be administered within 2 hours of ingestion of antacids; avoid taking with apple, grapefruit, or orange juice. Instruct patients to use caution if driving or performing tasks that require alertness. Recommend the use of a humidifier.
Levocetirizine	Allergy to any antihistamines; dosage should be selected with caution in older patients (start at low dosage range) because of the greater frequency of decreased liver, kidney, and/or cardiac function and of concomitant disease and drug therapy; not recommended for patients who are breast or chestfeeding Self-medication with cetirizine (OTC formulations) during pregnancy is not recommended Contraindicated in children 6 months–11 years of age with renal impairment. Contraindicated for use in patients with end-stage renal disease/renal failure (CrCl less than 10 mL/min) and those undergoing dialysis. Levocetirizine is also contraindicated for use in pediatric patients less than 12 years of age with any amount of renal impairment.	Somnolence, nasopharyngitis, fatigue, dry mouth, and pharyngitis	Avoid concomitant use with alcohol or other CNS depressants; take once daily in the evening; may take with or without food

its side effect profile, pseudoephedrine should be avoided in children (Correia & Baroody, 2019).

Adrenergic nasal decongestants are applied topically to the nasal mucosa for the relief of nasal congestion. They activate the alpha-adrenergic receptor sites on the smooth muscle of the nasal mucosal blood vessels, reducing local blood flow, fluid exudation, and mucosal edema.

Topical ophthalmic drops (e.g., olopatadine) are used for symptomatic relief of eye irritations caused by allergies. Common ocular complaints warranting use of ophthalmic drops include tearing, scleral and/or conjunctival erythema, and itching.

Topical decongestants such as catecholamines (phenylephrine) or imidazoline derivatives (xylometazoline or oxymetazoline) work extremely well on nasal congestion, the primary symptom of AR, but have bothersome effects if overused. When overused or used for a prolonged period, discontinuation of the medication can cause rhinitis medicamentosa, or rebound nasal congestion. This effect is not seen with oral decongestants, though the systemic route does not have such a positive impact on nasal congestion compared to their topical counterpart (Correia & Baroody, 2019).

Mast Cell Stabilizers

Mast cell stabilizers are used prophylactically (before exposure to allergens) to prevent the onset of symptoms and to treat symptoms once they occur. They are also used therapeutically in chronic AR. Intranasal cromolyn sodium is a spray that acts by stabilizing the mast cell membrane, thus reducing the release of histamine and other mediators of the allergic response (Rosenthal & Burchum, 2021). This spray is as effective as an antihistamine but less effective than intranasal corticosteroids in the treatment of seasonal AR. The patient must be informed that the beneficial effects of the medication may take a week or so to manifest.

Corticosteroids

Intranasal **corticosteroids** (INCS) are regarded as some of the most efficacious treatments for AR and are considered first-line treatment for those with moderate-to-severe symptoms. Their anti-inflammatory properties reduce nasal congestion, sneezing, itching, and rhinorrhea in people of all ages, thus improving sleep and overall quality of life. In addition, ICNS are more effective in controlling ocular symptoms caused by AR than oral antihistamines. INCS have proven to be more effective than other medications (e.g., oral antihistamines, leukotriene receptor agonists) in controlling nasal and sinus symptoms associated with AR. Examples of these medications include beclomethasone, budesonide, dexamethasone, flunisolide, fluticasone, and triamcinolone. Studies have proven that INCS are the most effective *maintenance* therapy for chronic allergic rhinitis, regardless of the patient's age, sex, race, or gender. These findings are based on their ability to prevent progression to more severe disease, along with their ability to decrease the likelihood of the evolution of a sleep-related breathing disorder or asthma (Bousquet et al., 2020; Correia & Baroody, 2019).

INCS are administered by metered-spray devices. If the nasal passages are blocked, a topical decongestant may be used to clear the passages before the administration of the INCS. Patients must be aware that full benefit may not be achieved for several days to 2 weeks. Adverse effects of INCS are mild and include drying of the nasal mucosa, potentially causing **epistaxis** (bloody nose) which is resolved with discontinuing the medication for a few days. They can also have an aftertaste, cause blood-tinged secretions, have a bothersome "smell," and cause burning and itching sensations in the nose and throat ("throat rundown"). INCS have been approved by the FDA for use in children and have shown neither detrimental effects on growth effects in children nor the development of ocular disease (e.g., glaucoma; Bousquet et al., 2020; Correia & Baroody, 2019).

Leukotriene Modifiers

The only leukotriene modifier (LM; "antileukotriene") approved for use in AR in the United States is montelukast. LMs are not first-line treatment for AR but are beneficial to those with ocular and nasal symptoms who also concomitantly suffer with asthmatic lung disease. Their side effect profile is minimal, though changes in behavior and mental health have been documented. It is common to see antihistamines used in conjunction with LMs as combination therapy for patients with AR and asthma or poorly controlled AR (Cooreia & Baroody, 2019; Shen et al., 2018).

Immunotherapy

Allergen desensitization (allergen immunotherapy, hyposensitization) is primarily used to treat IgE-mediated diseases by repeated exposure to allergen extracts. When allergy symptoms remain poorly controlled with avoidance measures and pharmacotherapy, immunotherapy may be warranted. Immunotherapy involves the administration of gradually increasing quantities of specific allergens to the patient until a dose is reached that is effective in reducing disease severity from natural exposure (Bousquet et al., 2020). Immunotherapy is treatment in the form of vaccine therapy (better known as "allergy shots" or subcutaneous immunotherapy [SCIT]), sublingual administration (sublingual immunotherapy [SLIT]), and intralymphatic immunotherapy (ILIT). Although severe systemic reactions occur in fewer than 1% of patients receiving immunotherapy, the risk for systemic and potentially fatal anaphylaxis does exist. It tends to occur most frequently at the induction or "up-dosing" phase.

Goals of immunotherapy include reducing the level of circulating IgE, increasing the level of blocking antibody IgG, and reducing the sensitivity of mediator cells. Subcutaneous treatments can be curative, whereas sublingual ones are preventive. Immunotherapy has been most effective for ragweed pollen; however, treatment also has been effective for grass, tree pollen, cat dander, and house dust mite allergens. Indications and contraindications for immunotherapy are presented in Box 37-4.

Unlike antiallergy medication, allergen immunotherapy has the potential to alter the allergic disease course after 3 to 5 years of therapy. Because it may prevent progression or development of asthma or multiple or additional allergies, it is also considered to be a potential preventive measure. The patient must understand what to expect and the importance of continuing therapy for several years before immunotherapy is accomplished.

Pearls for Practice

Immunotherapy should not be initiated during pregnancy; for patients who have been receiving immunotherapy before pregnancy, the dosage should not be increased during pregnancy provided the patient is tolerating and benefiting from the injections.

Subcutaneous immunotherapy treatment consists of injecting the patient with extracts of the known allergen(s) causing bothersome symptoms. Injections begin with very small amounts that are increased gradually, usually at weekly intervals, until a maximum tolerated dose is attained. Maintenance booster injections are administered at 2- to 4-week intervals, frequently for a minimum of 3 years. Positive effects of SCIT are noted around week 12 of injections and will continue to increase over the subsequent 1 to 2 years. Long-term benefit seems to be related to the cumulative dose of vaccine given over time, lasting at least 2 years after therapy has stopped (Correia & Baroody, 2019).

BOX 37-4

Allergen immunotherapy: Indications and Contraindications

Indications

- Allergic rhinitis, conjunctivitis, or allergic asthma
- History of a systemic reaction to *Hymenoptera* (large order of insects, including sawflies, wasps, bees, and ants) and specific IgE antibodies to *Hymenoptera* venom
- Food allergies
- Desire to avoid the long-term use, potential adverse effects, or costs of medications
- Lack of control of symptoms by avoidance measures or use of medications

Contraindications

- Use of beta-blocker or angiotensin-converting inhibitor therapy, which may mask early signs of anaphylaxis
- Presence of significant pulmonary or cardiac disease or organ failure, autoimmune diseases and malignancies
- Pregnancy before the start of AIT
- Inability of the patient to recognize or report signs and symptoms of a systemic reaction
- Nonadherence of the patient to other therapeutic regimens and low probability that patient will adhere to immunization schedule (often weekly for an indefinite period)
- Inability to monitor the patient for at least 30 minutes after administration of immunotherapy
- Absence of equipment or adequate personnel to respond to allergic reaction if one occurs

Subcutaneous immunotherapy should always be administered by a skilled medical provider, and patients should expect to wait in the office for 30 minutes after their injection to monitor for adverse reactions. Common adverse reactions include itching and redness at the site of injection. Those with poorly controlled asthma and pregnant individuals should avoid SCIT due to the rare risk of anaphylaxis (Bousquet et al., 2020; Correia & Baroody, 2019; Terada & Kawata, 2022).

Sublingual immunotherapy involves daily ingestion of liquid or tablet extracts of the allergen (most commonly ragweed, various grasses, and dust mites) approximately 8 weeks before the onset of the targeted pollen season. The efficacy of SLIT is similar to SCIT, and adherence to therapy is high due to ease of use. The first dose is always administered under the direct observation of a skilled provider. Subsequent doses can be self-administered at home. Benefits of SLIT include self-administration at home, no pain during administration, improvement in comorbid conditions (e.g., asthma, conjunctivitis), and reduced risk of anaphylaxis. Adverse effects include potential bad taste, oral mucosal irritation, nasal congestion, and risk of nonadherence. For the maximum benefit to be achieved, SLIT must be taken daily for 3 years during allergy season; this should grant at least 2 years of symptom resolution (Bousquet et al., 2020; Terada & Kawata, 2022). Candidates for SLIT therapy are chosen carefully after analyzing the risk/benefit ratio.

Rarely utilized, SLIT has been beneficial for those with allergies to cat dander and pollen. With SLIT, antigens are administered into the lymph nodes and are then directly delivered to the antigen-presenting cells. This presentation activates T and B cells, which allows for antibody production and cell recognition. After three allergen extraction injections, tolerance to the allergen has likely been achieved (Terada & Kawata, 2022). The benefits of SLIT include less time required for treatment to achieve clinical effectiveness.

Concept Mastery Alert

Allergy control by immunotherapy usually requires treatment for at least 3 years.

Pearls for Practice

Because the injection of an allergen may induce systemic reactions, such injections are administered only in a setting (e.g., physician's office, clinic) where epinephrine is immediately available.

Therapeutic failure is evident when a patient does not experience a decrease of symptoms within 12 to 24 months, fails to develop increased tolerance to known allergens, and cannot decrease the use of medications to reduce symptoms. Potential causes of treatment failure include misdiagnosis of allergies, inadequate doses of allergen, newly developed allergies, and inadequate environmental controls.

Homeopathic Modalities

Anecdotally, the health benefits of traditional Chinese medicine (TCM), which include herbal therapies and acupuncture, have been reported for years. Clinical trials have highlighted the use of acupuncture on those suffering with AR and asthma. Researchers found a significant reduction in nasal congestion, which consequently improved quality of life when the patient underwent acupuncture treatments (Meng et al., 2019). Furthermore, a meta-analysis evaluated the effects herbal concoctions used in TCM had on allergy symptoms. Though serum IgE levels did not decrease, upper airway itchiness and nasal symptoms decreased when compared to controls (Chan & Ng, 2020). Case studies regarding incorporating TCM into pharmacologic medicine are ongoing and promising. Supplements, such as Sulphur and Allium cepa, have had positive effects on symptom relief in individuals struggling with AR (Gandhi et al., 2021). Further studies are needed to expand the data on use of TCM in allergic diseases, but those that have been completed are reassuring.

Surgery

If avoidance techniques, pharmacotherapy, immunotherapy, and the use of homeopathic remedies have been unsuccessful in managing AR symptoms, patients may be referred for surgical evaluation and intervention. The primary symptom relieved with surgery is nasal obstruction, which thus improves the quality of life of the patient. Patients should understand that surgery is a last resort; it may be recommended after all other treatments have failed, and its primary indication is for symptom relief. Follow-up with an otolaryngologist is part of the surgical treatment plan.

CONTACT DERMATITIS

Contact dermatitis, a type IV delayed hypersensitivity reaction, is an acute or chronic skin inflammation that results from direct skin contact with chemicals or allergens.

Types

There are five basic types: allergic, photoallergic, irritant, photoirritant (phototoxic), and protein (Table 37-3). The most common form of CD is irritant dermatitis, accounting for 80% of cases (Scheinman et al., 2021). Symptoms arise after excessive exposure to or additive effects of irritants (e.g., soap and water, cosmetics, dust, foods, degreasing agents, detergents, plants, solvents). Skin sensitivity may develop after brief or prolonged periods of exposure, and the clinical picture may appear hours or weeks after the sensitized skin has been exposed. Risk factors for developing CD include underlying inflammatory skin disease(s) (e.g., stasis dermatitis), genetic predisposition, and lighter skin tone.

Clinical Manifestations and Assessment

Symptoms include itching, burning, **erythema**, skin lesions (vesicles), and edema, followed by weeping, crusting, and, finally, drying and peeling of the skin. In severe responses, hemorrhagic bullae may develop. Repeated reactions may be accompanied by thickening of the skin and pigment changes, a clinical finding termed "lichenification." Secondary invasion by bacteria, most commonly *Staphylococcus aureus*, may develop in skin that is abraded by rubbing or scratching. Usually, there are no systemic symptoms unless the eruption is widespread. See Figure 37-3.

The location of the skin eruption and the history of the exposure aid in determining the condition (see Table 37-3). However, in cases of obscure irritants or an unobservant patient, the diagnosis can be extremely difficult, often involving many trial-and-error procedures before the cause is determined. Patch tests on the skin with suspected offending agents may clarify the diagnosis. Management is discussed in Table 37-3.

ATOPIC DERMATITIS

Atopic dermatitis is a type I immediate hypersensitivity disorder characterized by symmetric distribution of inflammatory, pruritic lesions the severity of which fluctuates. It is further identified by periods of relapse, most commonly seen with seasonal and environmental changes. Although most commonly seen in children, the chronicity of symptoms is experienced well into adulthood. The greatest risk factors for developing atopic dermatitis include personal or family histories of allergic rhinitis or asthma, immune systems producing an abundance of immunoglobulin of IgE antibodies, low socioeconomic status, young age at onset, and non–White ethnicity (Langan et al., 2020). Other terms used to describe this skin disorder include *atopic eczema, atopic dermatitis/eczema,* and *atopic dermatitis/eczema syndrome* (AEDS).

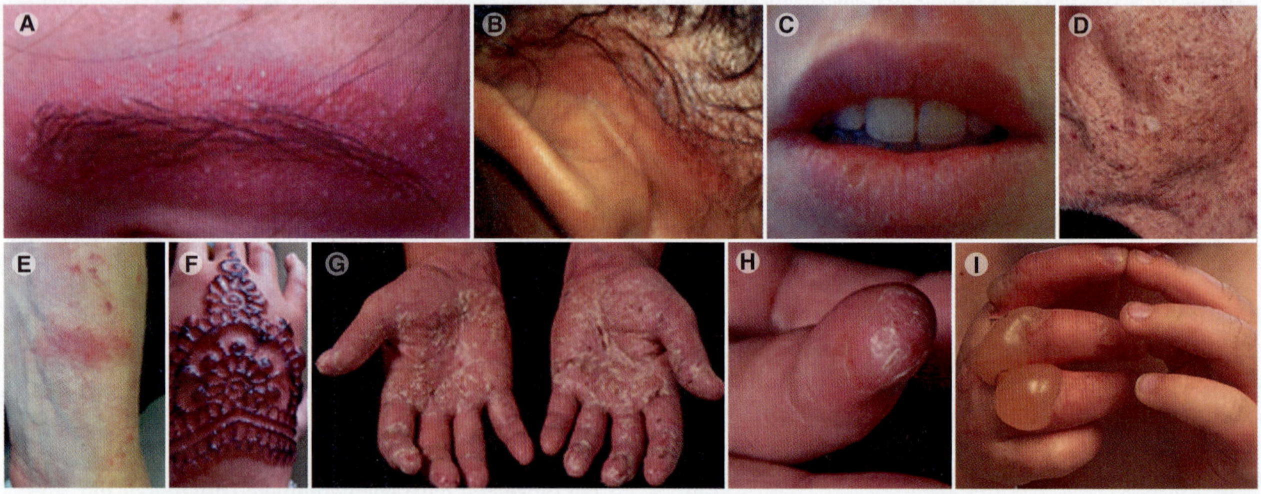

FIGURE 37-3 Typical CD reactions to various chemicals. Reaction caused by allergic contact dermatitis (CD) to hair dye products used on eyebrows (part a) and scalp (part b), fragrances in a lipstick (part c), shaving foam (part d), chromium found in a leather wristwatch strap (part e), *p*-phenylenediamine used in a semipermanent tattoo on the hand (part f), rubber chemicals in gloves (part g), and glues used in dental care (part h), photoirritant CD reaction to citrus juice (part i). (Reproduced, with permission, from Scheinman, P. L., Vocanson, M., Thyssen, J. P., Johansen, J. D., Nixon, R. L., Dear, K., Botto, N. C., Morot, J., & Goldminz, A. M. [2021]. Contact dermatitis. *Nature Reviews Disease Primers*, *7*[1], 38. Figure 4.)

TABLE 37-3 Types, Testing, and Treatment of Contact Dermatitis

Type	Etiology	Clinical Presentation	Diagnostic Testing	Treatment
Allergic	Results from contact of skin and allergenic substance. Allergic contact dermatitis develops within 12–48 hours of an antigen exposure and persists for 3 or 4 weeks.	Inflammation—the intensity depends on the degree of sensitivity and the concentration of the antigen. Inflammation may correspond exactly to the shape of the offending substance (e.g., the area under a watchband, ring, or elastic waistband, or if offending irritant is a plant [e.g., poison ivy] linear lesions will be seen)	Patch testing (contraindicated in acute, widespread dermatitis, nor it is useful in irritant contact dermatitis)	Avoidance of offending material Burow solution (aluminium acetate in water), a drying agent[a] for weeping skin lesions; or oatmeal baths or cool water compress Dinulos, J. (2021) Systemic corticosteroids (prednisone) for 7–10 days Topical corticosteroids for mild cases Oral antihistamines to relieve pruritus
Irritant	Results from contact with a substance that chemically or physically damages the skin on a nonimmunologic basis. Occurs after first exposure to irritant or repeated exposures to milder irritants over an extended time. Nickel is the most common contact allergen in industrialized countries globally (found in jewelry, belts, snaps, and eyeglasses).	Inflammation—the intensity is related to the concentration of the irritant and the length of exposure. Mild irritants cause dryness, fissuring, and erythema; a mild eczematous reaction may occur with continuous exposure. Continuous exposure to moisture in areas such as the hand, the diaper area, or the skin around a colostomy may eventually cause eczematous inflammation. Strong chemicals may produce an immediate reaction.	Clinical picture Appropriate negative patch tests	Identification and removal of source of irritation Application of hydrophilic cream or petrolatum to soothe and protect Topical corticosteroids and compresses for weeping lesions Antibiotics for infection and oral antihistamines for pruritus
Photoirritant (phototoxic)	Resembles the irritant type but requires sun and a chemical in combination to damage the epidermis; can occur minutes to hours after exposure.	Similar to irritant dermatitis; resembles exaggerated sunburn or blisters	Photopatch test	Same as for allergic and irritant dermatitis
Photoallergic	Resembles allergic dermatitis but requires light exposure in addition to allergen contact to produce immunologic reactivity; occurs 24–72 hours after exposure to sun-exposed skin; may spread to unexposed areas.	Similar to allergic dermatitis	Photopatch test	Same as for allergic and irritant dermatitis
Protein	Commonly found in individuals who handle food in the workplace.	Inflammatory perionyxis (paronychial inflammation) and immediate erythema with pruritus; skin lesions, with a chronic and recurring course, are analogous with the clinical picture in allergic contact dermatitis and irritant contact dermatitis; usually appear on the skin of hands, wrists and forearms, more rarely they concern only the fingertips.	Prick tests with the suspected protein-containing material are essential, as patch tests have in most cases negative results.	Strict avoidance of handling and touching the offending proteins products, for example, by wearing gloves; topical treatment with corticosteroids.

[a]Contact Dermatitis and Patch Testing.

Dinulos, J. (2021). Contact dermatitis and patch testing. In J. Dinulos (Ed.), *Habif's clinical dermatology* (7th ed., pp. 125–148). Elsevier Inc.

Clinical Manifestations and Assessment

Most patients with atopic dermatitis have significant elevations of serum IgE and peripheral eosinophilia. Pruritus and hyperirritability of the skin (most commonly seen in flexural folds) are the most consistent features of atopic dermatitis and are related to large amounts of histamine in the skin (Fig. 37-4). Excessive dryness of the skin with resultant itching is related to changes in lipid content, sebaceous gland activity, and sweating. In response to stroking of the skin, immediate redness appears on the skin and is followed in 15 to 30 seconds by pallor, which persists for 1 to 3 minutes. Years of chronically irritated skin resulting in excessive itching can cause **lichenification**, or a leathery hardened appearance of the affected area. Lesions develop secondary to the trauma of scratching and appear in areas of increased sweating and hypervascularity.

It is important to note that atopic dermatitis is often the first step in a process that leads to asthma, allergic rhinitis, and rhinoconjunctivitis (inflammatory disorder of allergic etiology affecting the mucous membrane of the nasal cavity and the conjunctiva of the eye), otherwise known as the "atopic march." It is the result of interactions among susceptibility genes, the environment, defective function of the skin barrier, and immunologic responses. Goals of care should be focused on prevention of recurrences; maximizing quality of life, which includes preserving emotional, physical, and social well-being; and providing cost-effective treatments to decrease the economic burden this disease may cause.

Medical Management

Treatment of patients with atopic dermatitis must be individualized. Guidelines for treatment include decreasing itching and scratching by wearing cotton fabrics; washing with a mild detergent; humidifying dry heat in winter; maintaining room temperature at 20°C to 22.2°C (68°F to 72°F); using antihistamines, such as diphenhydramine (Benadryl); and avoiding animals, dust, sprays, and perfumes. Keeping the skin moisturized with daily baths to hydrate the skin and the use of topical skin emollients is encouraged and remains the main treatment for atopic dermatitis. Topical anti-inflammatory therapies, such as corticosteroids, are used to treat diffuse inflammation, and any secondary infection is treated with antibiotics to eliminate *S. aureus* when indicated. Use of immunosuppressive agents, such as cyclosporine, tacrolimus, and pimecrolimus, may be effective in inhibiting T cells and mast cells involved in atopic dermatitis, but their efficacy is reduced compared to topical corticosteroids.

If atopic dermatitis cannot be controlled with topical agents, phototherapy may be considered. With phototherapy, ultraviolet light is applied to the affected area three to five times over a 2- to 3-month time frame. Risks include photodamage, skin carcinoma, and melanoma induction (theorized to activate the carcinogenic process when ultraviolet [UV] radiation is absorbed by melanin in melanocytes). Systemic treatments are also available if topical agents and phototherapy fail (or if phototherapy is not desired). Such therapies include immunotherapy (e.g., ciclosporin, methotrexate) and oral steroids (e.g., prednisone). Systemic treatments should be used for the shortest duration possible, as long-term safety profiles of these medications are not well understood.

Nursing Management

Patients who experience atopic dermatitis and their families require assistance and support from the nurse to cope with the disorder. Often the symptoms are disturbing to the patient and disruptive to the family. The appearance of the skin may affect the patient's self-esteem and their willingness to interact with others. Researchers have proven that atopic dermatitis has significant effects on levels of anxiety and depression; therefore, proper screening should be in place at every follow-up visit (Silverberg et al., 2019).

Instructions and counseling about strategies to incorporate preventive measures and treatments into the lifestyle of the family may be helpful. Education points include counseling the patient and family on various triggers of atopic dermatitis (e.g., workplace allergens, winter months, heat or exercise [sweating], emotional stress, hormonal fluxes, consumption of alcohol, the common cold, skin irritants [perfumes], and microorganisms [bacteria, fungi, viruses, and yeast]) that may lead to an exacerbation. The patient and family need to be aware of signs of secondary infection and of the need to seek treatment if infection occurs. The nurse also teaches the patient and family about the side effects of medications used in treatment.

DERMATITIS MEDICAMENTOSA (DRUG RASH)

Dermatitis medicamentosa, a type I hypersensitivity disorder, is the term applied to skin rashes associated with certain medications. Although people react differently to each medication, certain medications tend to induce eruptions of similar types. Rashes are among the most common adverse reactions to medications, and up to 2% are severe and life threatening.

Clinical Manifestations and Assessment

In general, drug rashes appear suddenly, have a particularly vivid color, manifest with characteristics that are more intense than the somewhat similar eruptions of infectious origin, and, with the exception of bromide and the iodide rashes, disappear rapidly after the medication is withdrawn. In individuals with lighter skin tones, the skin becomes erythematous. In more pigmented skin tones, drug rashes may appear as a hyperpigmented or darker, violaceous shade

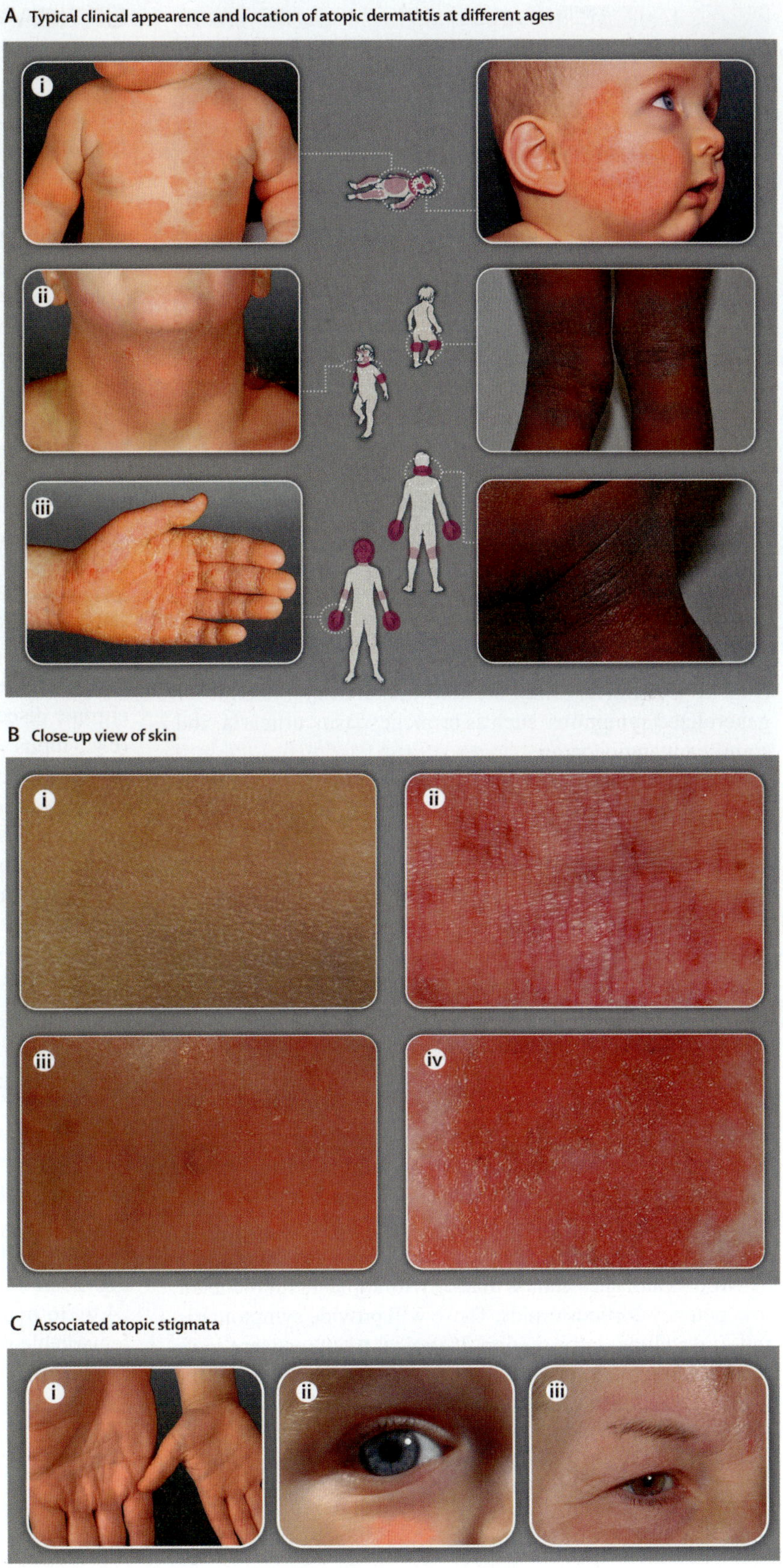

FIGURE 37-4 The typical clinical appearance and locations of atopic dermatitis are shown at different ages (A). In infants (Ai), eczema lesions are often more acute than in adults and are mainly located on the face and the extensor surfaces of the limbs. The trunk might be affected, but the diaper area is typically spared. From ages 1 to 2 years and onward (Aii), polymorphous manifestations with different types of skin lesions are seen, particularly in flexural folds. In adolescents and adults (Aiii), lichenified and excoriated plaques are often found, particularly at flexures, wrists, ankles, and eyelids; in the head-and-neck type, the upper trunk, shoulders, and scalp are involved. Adults might have only chronic hand eczema, or they might present with prurigolike lesions. Close-up views of the skin (B) show nonlesional (Bi), acute (Bii), subacute (Biii), and chronic (Biv) lesions of atopic dermatitis. Atopic stigmata (C), such as palmar and plantar hyperlinearity (mostly seen in patients with FLG mutations or ichthyosis vulgaris [Ci]), Dennie–Morgan infraorbital folds (Cii), and Hertoghe sign (thinning of the lateral part of eyebrow [Ciii]) are more common in patients with atopic dermatitis than in the general population and can help establish the diagnosis. The images on the right in Aii and Aiii have been reproduced from *Harper's Textbook of Pediatric Dermatology*, fourth edition, by permission of John Wiley & Sons. All other images are the author's own.

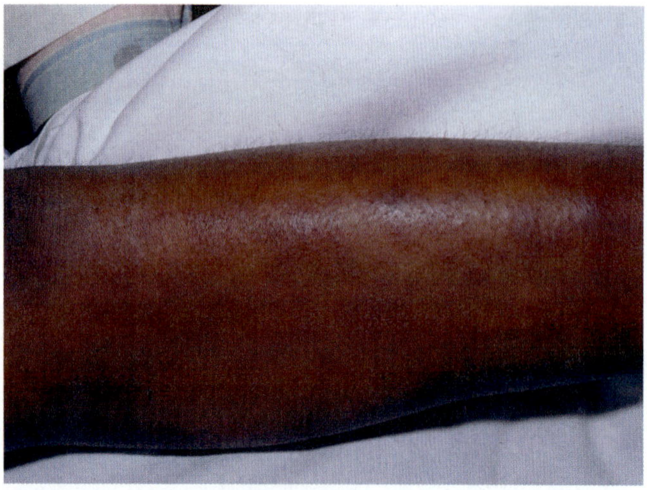

FIGURE 37-5 **DRESS with phenytoin-induced eosinophilia, hepatomegaly, splenomegaly, and lymphadenopathy. (Reproduced with permission from Lugo-Somolinos, A., McKinley-Grant, L., Goldsmith, L. A., Papier, A., Adigun, C. G., Culton, D., Davey, M., Diamantis, S., Fredeking, A., Lee, I. [2011].** ***VisualDx: Essential Dermatology in Pigmented Skin.*** **Lippincott Williams & Wilkins.)**

(Fig. 37-5). Rashes may be accompanied by systemic or generalized symptoms, such as bronchospasm, urticaria, and significant angioedema.

Medical and Nursing Management

Upon discovery of a medication-related drug rash, the causative agent must be discontinued immediately and treatment initiated for any symptoms the patient is experiencing. Once stable, the patient is warned that they have a hypersensitivity to a particular medication and is advised not to take it again. Patients should carry with them at all times information identifying the hypersensitivity and subsequent reaction experienced.

Skin eruptions or simple drug reactions related to medication therapy may suggest more serious hypersensitivities. Frequent assessment and prompt reporting of the appearance of any eruption is important so that early treatment can be initiated. Some cutaneous drug reactions can further develop into more serious reactions that involve other organs. These are known as **complex drug reactions**.

Mild skin rashes can be treated with topical emollients or low-potency corticosteroids. These will provide symptomatic relief of itching and irritation. If topical treatments are ineffective for symptom control, antihistamines can be used for a short duration. Discontinuation of the offending medication will usually relieve symptoms; oral treatments are rarely needed.

Pearls for Practice

Caution should be given with antihistamine use in the older and pediatric populations due to risk of central nervous system effects (e.g., delirium) and generalized fatigue.

URTICARIA AND ANGIONEUROTIC EDEMA

Urticaria (hives) is a type I hypersensitive allergic reaction of the skin characterized by the sudden appearance of pinkish, edematous elevations (commonly called "**wheals**") with central pallor that vary in size and shape. Urticaria commonly itches and can even burn (Fig. 37-6). They may involve any part of the body, including the mucous membranes (especially those of the mouth), the larynx (occasionally with serious respiratory complications), and the GI tract. Urticaria typically last for 30 minutes to 24 hours and can be associated with angioneurotic edema (angioedema). Urticaria have many causes, the most common being food products, medications, infections, genetic causes, insect stings, environmental factors (e.g., temperature changes), and underlying medical diseases (Guo & Saltoun, 2019).

Each hive remains for a few minutes to several hours before disappearing. For hours or days, clusters of these lesions may come, go, and return episodically. If this sequence continues for longer than 6 weeks, the condition is called **chronic urticaria**. Chronic urticaria affects up to 1% of the population and typically coexists with other chronic disease states, most commonly autoimmune disease (e.g., lupus, rheumatoid arthritis, thyroid disease). Though its prevalence is on the rise, chronic urticaria is difficult to diagnose, and treatments are sparse as the understanding of the disease is limited.

Angioneurotic edema involves the deeper layers of the skin, resulting in more diffuse swelling rather than the discrete lesions characteristic of hives. The skin will swell, be either slightly erythematous or skin-colored, and be painful to touch. The skin does not pit on pressure, as ordinary edema does. The regions most often involved are the lips, eyelids, cheeks, hands, feet, genitalia, and tongue; the mucous membranes of the larynx, the bronchi, and the GI canal also may be affected, particularly in the hereditary type. Swellings may appear suddenly, in a few seconds or minutes, or slowly, in 1 or 2 hours. In the latter case, often their appearance is preceded by itching or burning sensations. Seldom does more than a single swelling appear at one time, although one may develop while another is disappearing. Infrequently, swelling recurs in the same region. Individual lesions usually last 24 to 36 hours. On rare occasions, swelling may recur with remarkable regularity at intervals of 3 to 4 weeks.

FOOD ALLERGY

Pathophysiology

Adverse food reactions are classified as immune mediated (food allergy, celiac disease; rapid onset; clinical symptoms within minutes of food ingestion) or nonimmune mediated (food intolerance). IgE-mediated food allergy, a type I

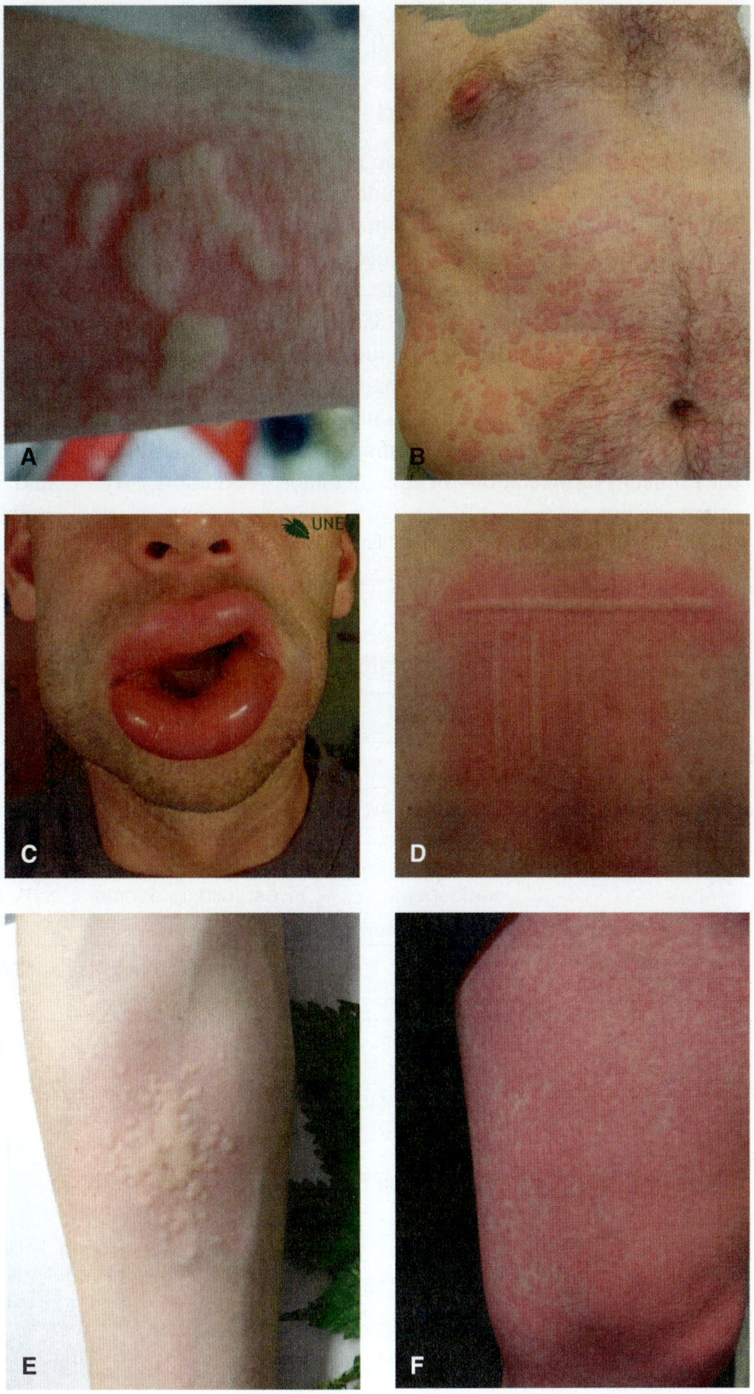

FIGURE 37-6 **Wheals and angioedema in urticaria. (A) Wheals at an early stage of development in a patient with chronic spontaneous urticaria. (B) Wheals of several hours duration in a patient with chronic spontaneous urticaria. (C) Angioedema in a patient with chronic spontaneous urticaria. (D) Wheals induced by scratching of the skin in a patient with symptomatic dermographism. (E) Wheals induced by skin contact with a stinging nettle (contact urticaria). (F) Wheals with pronounced erythema in a patient with cholinergic urticaria. (Reprinted with permission from Maurer, M., Zuberbier, T., Metz, M. [2022]. The classification, pathogenesis, diagnostic workup, and management of urticaria: An update. *Handbook of Experimental Pharmacology*, *268*, 117–133. Figure 1. https://doi.org/10.1007/164_2021_506.)**

hypersensitivity reaction, is an abnormal immune response to food proteins or derivatives that cause physical illness or harm. Its prevalence is on the rise, affecting 8% of children and 4% of adults (Krajewski & Krajewski, 2022). People who have a genetic predisposition combined with exposure to allergens early in life through the GI or respiratory tract or nasal mucosa tend to be at higher risk of developing an IgE-mediated food allergy. Clinical presentations will vary, though a timely diagnosis is imperative as many adverse reactions can become life threatening.

Almost any food can cause allergic symptoms, some even resulting in anaphylaxis. The most common offenders are seafood (lobster, shrimp, crab, clams, fish), legumes (peanuts, peas, beans, licorice), seeds (sesame, cottonseed, caraway, mustard, flaxseed, sunflower seeds), tree nuts, berries, egg white, buckwheat, milk, and chocolate. Peanut and tree nut (e.g., cashew, walnut) allergies are responsible for severe food allergy reactions in children and may result in anaphylactic death. Anaphylactic mortality in adults tends to be related to nuts, seafood, and insect stings, whereas in pediatrics the culprit tends to be food related, commonly milk and nut products (Turner et al., 2017).

Clinical Manifestations and Assessment

The clinical symptoms are classic allergic symptoms (urticaria, sneezing, rhinorrhea, conjunctival irritation, and dermatitis), lower respiratory symptoms (wheezing, cough, laryngeal edema, angioedema), and GI symptoms (itching; swelling of lips, tongue, and palate; abdominal pain; nausea; cramps; vomiting; and diarrhea). Cardiovascular symptoms may be present as well. These include syncope, palpitations, feeling of faintness, and chest pain. Swelling, respiratory, and cardiovascular symptoms should be treated as an emergency as they are indications of anaphylaxis. See Table 37-4 for clinical manifestations of IgE-mediated food allergy by organ system.

A careful diagnostic workup is required in any patient with a suspected food hypersensitivity. Included are a detailed allergy history, a physical examination, and pertinent diagnostic tests. Skin testing is used to identify the source of symptoms and is useful in identifying specific foods as causative agents.

Medical Management

Therapy for food hypersensitivity includes elimination of the food responsible for the hypersensitivity. Pharmacologic therapy is necessary for patients who cannot avoid exposure to offending foods and for patients with multiple food sensitivities not responsive to avoidance measures. Medication therapy involves the use of H_1 blockers, antihistamines, adrenergic agents, corticosteroids, and cromolyn sodium.

An essential aspect of management is teaching patients and family members to recognize symptoms associated with an anaphylactic reaction, when and how to administer life-saving medication (epinephrine), and when to call for emergency help. Those with a previous history of

TABLE **37-4 Clinical Manifestations of IgE-Mediated Food Allergy by Organ System**

Organ Systems	Symptoms	Mild	Moderate	Severe
Skin	Rash	Faint erythema	Erythema	Generalized marked erythema (more than 50% of the body surface area)
	Urticaria/angioedema	Fewer than 3 areas of hives; mild lip edema	More than 3 areas of hives; significant lip or face edema	Generalized involvement of swelling face/lips/eyelids
	Pruritus	Occasional scratching	Scratching continuously	Continuous scratching; excoriations
Upper airway	Sneezing/itching	Occasional sniffing	Intermittent rubbing of nose or eyes; frequent sniffing	Continuous rubbing of nose or eyes; periocular swelling; persistent rhinorrhea
Lower airway	Wheezing	Expiratory wheezing	Inspiratory and expiratory wheezing	Use of accessory muscles; audible wheezing; increased work of breathing
	Laryngeal manifestation	Episodes of throat clearing or cough; persistent throat tightness	Hoarseness, frequent cough	Stridor
Gastrointestinal tract	Subjective symptoms	Nausea or mild abdominal pain	Moderate abdominal pain with normal activity	Notably distressed due to GI symptoms with decreased activity
	Objective symptoms	1 episode of emesis or diarrhea	More than 1 but fewer than 3 episodes emesis or diarrhea	More than 3 episodes of emesis or diarrhea
Cardiovascular/neurological		Subjective weakness, dizziness; tachycardia	Drop in blood pressure; significant change in mental status (anxiety, confusion)	Severe cardiovascular collapse; unconsciousness
Other			Loss of bladder control	Pelvic pain

Reproduced with permission from Anvari, S., Miller, J., Yeh, C. -Y., & Davis, C. M. (2018). Ig-E mediated food allergy. *Clinical Reviews in Allergy & Immunology*, *57*, 244–260. https://doi.org/10.1007/s12016-018-8710-3

anaphylactic reaction to any food substance should have an individualized anaphylaxis action plan created with the assistance of their primary provider.

Many food allergies disappear with time, particularly in children. About one third of proven allergies disappear in 1 to 2 years if the patient carefully avoids the offending food; however, allergies to peanuts, shellfish, fish, and tree nuts have been reported to persist throughout adulthood in 20% of people. Some patients may follow with an allergist who will provide an oral food challenge in hopes of obtaining an official diagnosis. Many patients then go on to participate in oral immunotherapy (OIT) in which, under the close observation of a medical provider, a small amount of allergen is consumed. Over time, with an increasing amount of allergen at each visit, the patient's immune system becomes desensitized. This process can be very dangerous and is also very time consuming as it is usually performed over a month's time frame. If successful, OIT can drastically improve someone's quality of life (Anvari et al., 2018).

Nursing Management

In addition to participating in management of the allergic reaction, the nurse focuses on preventing future exposure of the patient to the food allergen. If a severe allergic or anaphylactic reaction to food allergens has occurred, the nurse must instruct the patient and family about strategies to prevent its recurrence. The patient is instructed about the importance of carefully assessing foods prepared by others for obvious as well as hidden sources of food allergens, and of avoiding locations and facilities where those allergens are likely to be present. This includes careful reading of food labels and monitoring the preparation of food by others to be sure that exposure to even minute amounts of allergenic foods is avoided. One of the dangers of food allergens is that they may be hidden in other foods and not apparent to people who are susceptible to the allergen. For example, often peanuts and peanut butter are used in salad dressings and Asian, African, and Mexican cooking and may result in severe allergic reactions, including anaphylaxis. Previous contamination of equipment with allergens (e.g., peanuts) during preparation of another food product (e.g., chocolate cake) is enough to produce anaphylaxis in people with severe allergy.

The patient and family must be knowledgeable about early signs and symptoms of allergic reactions and must be proficient in emergency administration of epinephrine if a reaction occurs. The nurse should advise the patient to wear a medical alert bracelet or to carry identification and emergency equipment at all times. The nurse can assist the patient in updating the anaphylaxis action plan in conjunction with the medical provider at each follow-up visit. They can assist in referrals to allergists when an oral food challenge is desired. Patients' food allergies should be noted on their medical records because there may be risk of allergic reactions not only to food but also to some medications containing similar substances.

SERUM SICKNESS

Pathophysiology

Serum sickness is an immune-complex type III hypersensitivity reaction and occurs in 30% of all medication adverse reactions. In type III hypersensitivity reactions, the immune system becomes dysregulated and antibodies and antigens combine and form complexes which destroy cells and cause tissue damage. If these type III complexes are deposited in tissues or vascular endothelium, there is an increase in vascular permeability and tissue injury, resulting in a vasculitis (inflammation of blood vessels).

Traditionally, serum sickness has resulted from the administration of therapeutic antisera of animal sources for the treatment or prevention of infectious diseases, such as tetanus, pneumonia, rabies, diphtheria, and botulism, as well as the bites of venomous snakes and black widow spiders. With the advent of human antitetanus serum and antibiotics, classic serum sickness is much less common now; however, various medications (primarily penicillin) may cause a serum-sickness–like reaction (SSLR) similar to that caused by foreign sera. Serum-sickness–like reaction caused by medications occurs due to repeated or overuse of the agent. The medications most commonly associated with SSLR include antidepressants, antiarrhythmics, antihypertensives, antiepileptics, antineoplastics, and antimicrobials (beta-lactam antibiotics: penicillin, sulfonamides, cephalosporins, and macrolides) (McNamara et al., 2020).

Clinical Manifestations and Assessment

Symptoms are caused by a reaction and immunologic attack on the serum or medication. Antibodies appear to be of the IgE and IgM classes. Early manifestations, beginning 6 to 10 days after administration of the medication, include an inflammatory reaction at the site of injection of the medication, followed by regional and generalized lymphadenopathy, arthritis, abdominal pain, edema, and fever. Symptoms may appear as late as 3 weeks afterward. There is usually a skin rash, which may be urticarial or purpuric. Joints are frequently tender and swollen. Vasculitis may occur in any organ but is observed most commonly in the kidney, resulting in proteinuria and hematuria. An elevated sedimentation rate and leukocytosis may also occur.

Medical and Nursing Management

The primary goal in serum sickness therapy is to treat the clinical syndrome symptomatically. This hypersensitivity reaction lasts for several days to a few weeks if untreated, but the patient responds promptly and completely with immediate discontinuation of the culprit medication followed by use of nonsteroid anti-inflammatory drugs (NSAIDs), antihistamines, or corticosteroids (McNamara et al., 2020; Yorulmaz et al., 2017). Resolution of symptoms is usually seen in 1 to 2 weeks. Aggressive therapy, including ventilator support, may be necessary if peripheral neuritis and Guillain–Barré syndrome occur. If symptoms are severe enough to warrant ventilator support or if hemodynamic instability ensues, the patient is admitted to an intensive care unit. See Chapter 45 for nursing management of Guillain–Barré syndrome.

LATEX ALLERGY

Latex allergy, the allergic reaction to natural rubber proteins, has been implicated in rhinitis, conjunctivitis, contact dermatitis, urticaria, asthma, and anaphylaxis. Currently, up to 6% of Americans are affected by a latex allergy, many of whom experience life-threatening symptoms. Over the past 80 years, the number of individuals affected with this allergy has dropped drastically due to the processing of nonlatex materials and nonpowdered latex gloves used in occupational settings. Despite numbers and studies confirming this, the severity of illness associated with a latex allergy remains a nursing priority.

Risk Factors

Latex is the most common cause of occupational urticaria (Parisi et al., 2021). Populations at risk include health care workers, patients with atopic allergies or multiple surgeries, people working in factories that manufacture latex products, patients with spina bifida or spinal cord injuries, individuals with increased need for surgical procedures, and people with congenital abnormalities of the genitourinary tract. Due to more frequent contact with latex-containing products, medical personnel, restaurant employees, emergency personnel, construction workers, condom wearers, florists, hairdressers, and others, are at higher risk of developing a sensitivity or allergy to latex. See identified and potential risk factors in Table 37-5.

Anaphylaxis to latex-containing products typically occurs during medical procedures: surgery, dental exams, catheter insertions, medical device placement, gynecological procedures. Some researchers hypothesize this is due to the reaction between latex and water-soluble antigens found in body tissue(s). Its diagnosis is difficult as patients are not always able to express their concerns and physical ailments, especially under anesthesia, but cardiovascular collapse and bronchospasm lead to an eventual diagnosis.

When latex proteins become airborne, people may unknowingly breathe them in and develop systemic reactions. They may experience shortness of breath, abdominal pain, swollen oral mucosa/lips, upper respiratory symptoms, palpitations, or dizziness. If untreated, these symptoms can lead to shock and death. It is important to note that cross-reactions have been reported in people who are allergic to certain food products, such as kiwis, bananas, papaya, peaches, pears, nectarines, pineapples, mangos, passion fruit, avocados, celery, and chestnuts (Nguyen et al., 2022).

Pathophysiology

Routes of exposure to latex products can be cutaneous, percutaneous, mucosal, parenteral, or aerosol. Allergic reactions are more likely with exposure via the mucous membrane or from the parenteral route but also can occur with cutaneous contact or inhalation. The most frequent source of exposure is cutaneous, which usually involves the wearing of natural latex gloves. The powder used to facilitate putting on latex gloves can become a carrier of latex proteins from the gloves; when the gloves are put on or removed, the particles become airborne and can be inhaled or settle on the skin, mucous membranes, or clothing. Mucosal exposure can occur from the use of latex condoms, catheters, airways, and baby bottle nipples. Parenteral exposure can occur from IV lines or hemodialysis equipment. In addition to latex-derived medical devices, many household items also contain latex. Examples of medical and household items containing latex are found in Table 37-6.

TABLE 37-5 Identified and Potential Risk Groups Patients for Natural Rubber Latex (NRL) Sensitization and Allergy

Occupations and Other Situations With Frequent Contact With Latex	Medical Conditions With an Increased Predisposition for Latex Sensitization
• Physicians and other health care professionals • Food handlers/restaurant workers • Domestic workers • Hairdressers • Rubber industry workers • Security personnel, police officers, and firefighters • Condom users • Construction workers • Painters • Funeral home workers • Florists	• Spina bifida • Urogenital abnormalities • Anorectal malformations • Tracheoesophageal fistula • Multiple congenital anomalies • Ventriculoperitoneal shunt • Cerebral palsy • Quadriplegia • Preterm infants • Atopic individuals (hereditary predisposition to developing allergic reactions)

Reproduced with permission from Parisi, C. A. S., Kelly, K. J., Ignacio, J. A., Gonzalez-Díaz, S. N., Bilò, M. B., Cardona, V., Park, H-S., Braschi, M. C., Macias-Weinmann, A., Piga, M. A., Acuña-Ortega, N., Sánchez Borges, M., & Yañez, A. (2021). Update on latex allergy: New insights into an old problem. *World Allergy Organization Journal*, *14*(100569), 1–15. Table 1. http://doi.org/10.1016/j.waojou.2021.100569

TABLE 37-6 **Selected Products Containing Natural Rubber Latex**

Hospital Environment
Ace bandage (brown)
Adhesive bandages, Band-Aid dressing, Telfa
Anesthesia equipment
Blood pressure cuff, tubing, and bladder
Catheters
Catheter leg bag straps
Crutch axillary pads and hand grips, tips
ECG pads
Elastic compression stockings
Gloves
IV catheters
IV rubber injection ports
Levin tubes
Medication vials
Penrose drains
Prepackaged enema kits
Pulse oximeters
Resuscitation bags
Stethoscope tubing
Single-use syringes (Monoject, B & D)
Suction tubing
Tapes
Thermometer probes
Tourniquets
Thera-Bands
Home Environment
Balloons
Diapers, incontinence pads
Condoms, diaphragms
Feminine hygiene pad
Wheelchair cushions
Latex dishwashing gloves
Pacifiers/baby bottle nipples/teething rings

Clinical Manifestations and Assessment

Several different types of reactions to latex are possible: irritant contact dermatitis, allergic dermatitis, and latex allergy. Table 37-7 lists the causes, symptoms, and management of each.

The diagnosis of latex allergy is based on the history and diagnostic test results. Sensitization is detected by skin testing, RAST, or enzyme-linked immunosorbent assay (ELISA). Skin tests should be performed only by providers who have expertise in their administration and interpretation and who have the necessary equipment available to treat local or systemic allergic reactions to the reagent.

Medical Management

See Table 37-5 for medical management.

Nursing Management

The nurse can assume a pivotal role in the management of latex allergies in both patients and staff. All patients should be asked about latex allergy, although special attention should be given to those at particularly high risk (e.g., patients with spina bifida, patients who have undergone multiple surgical procedures). Every time an invasive procedure must be performed, the nurse should consider the possibility of latex allergies. Nurses working in operating rooms, intensive care units, short-term procedure units, and emergency departments need to pay particular attention to latex allergy. Medical facilities should strive to be "latex-safe" environments and eliminate as many sources of potential allergens as possible. Any medical equipment or device that contains latex should be labeled.

Although the type I reaction is the most significant of the reactions to latex, care must be taken in the presence of irritant contact dermatitis and delayed hypersensitivity reaction to avoid further exposure of the person to latex. Patients with latex allergy are advised to notify their health care providers and to wear a medical information bracelet. Patients must become knowledgeable about what products contain latex and what products are safe, nonlatex alternatives. Also, they must become knowledgeable about signs and symptoms of latex allergy as well as emergency treatment and self-injection of epinephrine in case of allergic reaction.

Pearls for Practice

Chronic exposure to latex and a history of skin atopy increases the risk of sensitization for health care providers. If a patient is exposed to latex through frequent medical procedures utilizing latex products (e.g., repeated urinary catheterization), they, too, should be considered at increased risk for developing a latex allergy.

Nurses can be instrumental in establishing and participating in multidisciplinary committees to address latex allergy and to promote a latex-free environment. Latex allergy protocols and education of staff about latex allergy and precautions are important strategies to ensure assessment and prompt treatment of affected people.

TABLE **37-7 Types of Reactions to Latex**

Type of Reaction	Cause	Signs/Symptoms	Treatment
Irritant contact dermatitis	Damage to skin because of irritation and loss of epidermoid skin layer; not an allergic reaction. Can be caused by excessive use of soaps and cleansers, multiple hand-washings, inadequate hand drying, mechanical irritation (e.g., sweating, rubbing inside powdered gloves), exposure to chemicals added during the manufacturing of gloves, and alkaline pH of powdered gloves. Reaction may occur with first exposure, is usually benign, and is not life-threatening.	Acute: redness, edema, burning, discomfort, itching Chronic: dry, thickened, cracked skin	Referral for diagnostic testing Avoidance of exposure to irritant Thorough washing and drying of hands Use of powder-free gloves with more frequent changes of gloves Changing glove types Use of water- or silicone-based moisturizing creams, lotions, or topical barrier agents Avoidance of oil- or petroleum-based skin agents with latex products because they cause breakdown of the latex product
Allergic contact dermatitis	Delayed hypersensitivity (type IV) reaction. Usually affects only area in contact with latex; cause of reaction is T cell–mediated sensitization to additives of latex. Reaction is not life-threatening and is far more common than a type I reaction. Slow onset; occurs 24–48 hours after exposure, and is localized. Resolves within 3–4 days after exposure. More severe reactions may occur with subsequent exposures.	Localized pruritus, swelling, and blisters.	Referral for diagnosis (patch tests) and treatment Thorough washing and drying of hands Use of water- or silicone-based moisturizing creams, lotions, or topical barrier agents Avoidance of oil- or petroleum-based products unless they are latex-compatible Avoidance of identified causative agent because continued exposure to latex products in the presence of breaks in skin may contribute to latex protein sensitization
Latex allergy	Type I IgE-mediated immediate hypersensitivity to plant proteins in natural rubber latex. In sensitized people, anti-latex IgE antibody stimulates mast cell proliferation and basophil histamine release. Exposure can be through contact with the skin, mucous membranes, or internal tissues, or through inhalation of traces of powder from latex gloves. Severe reactions usually occur shortly after parenteral or mucous membrane exposure. People with any type I reaction to latex are at high risk of anaphylaxis.	Local: swelling, redness, edema, itching Mild systemic: rhinitis, flushing, conjunctivitis Severe systemic: urticaria, laryngeal edema, bronchospasm, asthma, severe vasodilation angioedema, anaphylaxis, cardiovascular collapse, and death All above reactions can occur within minutes after exposure	Immediate treatment of reaction with epinephrine, fluids, vasopressors, corticosteroids, and airway and ventilator support, with close monitoring for recurrence for next 12–14 hours Prompt referral for diagnostic evaluation Treatment and diagnostic evaluation in latex-free environment Strict avoidance of allergy testing and management Assessment of all patients for symptoms of latex allergy Teaching of patients and family members about the disorder and about the importance of preventing future reactions by avoiding latex Encouraging wearing of a medical alert bracelet that identifies latex allergy for emergency situations Warning labels can be attached to car windows to alert police and paramedics about the driver's or passenger's latex allergy in case of a motor vehicle crash Carrying an EpiPen at all times and being prepared and able to use it

Clinical Judgment Case

A 42-year-old patient comes into the emergency room (ER) after a bee sting (~30 minutes ago) with a known history of insect allergy. The patient is complaining of severe "scratching of the throat," slight swelling of the lips (angioedema), and shortness of breath; there are urticaria (hives) and wheals noted on the extremities, chest, and abdomen. Vital signs are as follows: 98.7°F, HR 122 and regular, 28 RR with an oxygen saturation of 88% on room air, blood pressure 98/42 mm Hg. Heart sounds are S1 S2 without gallop or murmur; the point of maximum impulse (PMI) is nondisplaced (5th intercostal space [ICS], midclavicular line). Inspiratory and expiratory wheezing is found in all lung fields; no stridor is noted. The patient is complaining of abdominal cramping; abdomen is soft, nondistended; bowel sounds are present in all 4 quadrants; denies nausea and vomiting. Skin is warm and flushed, capillary refill is 3 seconds, and pedal and posterior tibial pulses are 1+ bil. The patient's only medical history is allergy to insect sting and a previous acute anaphylactic reaction at age 12. The patient self-administered an EpiPen over an hour ago in anterior lateral thigh through clothes and is worried that the expiration date has long since passed. The EpiPen was left in the field, but the patient believes it is at least 5 years old. The patient is anxious and becoming increasingly restless.

Step One: Recognize cues where relevant and important information is identified from different sources, such as medical history or vital signs.

Answer: History of insect allergy and anaphylactic reaction to bee sting. Unknown but assumed expired EpiPen since they usually expire 18 months from the manufacture date. Complaints of shortness of breath and abdominal cramping, increasing restlessness and anxiety, "scratching of the throat." Physical examination findings of shortness of breath; flushed warm skin; slight swelling of the lips; urticaria; wheals noted on the extremities, chest, and abdomen, inspiratory and expiratory wheezing throughout all lung fields; no stridor; delayed capillary refill; and 1+ pedal and posterior tibial pulses. Cues of concern related to vital signs: HR of 122 and regular, 28 RR, O_2 sat of 88%, and blood pressure 98/42.

Step Two: Analyze cues, which is organizing and linking the recognized cues to the patient's clinical presentation.

Answer: You have clustered the patient's symptoms to be associated with anaphylactic shock. You associate the tachycardia with the body's attempt to increase the CO in the setting of shock. The blood pressure of 98/42 mm Hg is hypotensive, and you calculate the mean arterial pressure (MAP), which is systolic pressure (98 mm Hg) plus the diastolic pressure (42 mm Hg) x's 2/3 (98 + 84 = 182/3 = 61 mm Hg). Since the MAP reflects perfusion to major organs, you are aware that a MAP below 65 mm Hg for an extended period can cause end-organ ischemia, and infarction can occur. A MAP >60 mm Hg is needed to perfuse the coronary arteries, risking cardiovascular collapse. If the MAP drops <60 mm Hg, blood will not be able to perfuse cerebral tissues as well; there will be a loss of consciousness, and neuronal death will quickly ensue. The oxygen saturation of 88%, inspiratory and expiratory wheezing, anxiety, tachypnea, and restlessness are associated with signs of airway obstruction and hypoxemia. You cluster the persistence of the signs and symptoms of anaphylaxis after EpiPen injection with expiration of the medication or worsening anaphylactic reaction.

Step Three: Prioritize hypotheses, where hypotheses are evaluated and ranked according to priority. This can include urgency, likelihood, risk, difficulty, and/or time. In this phase you cluster your findings to arrive at a list of problems (actual and or potential problems) you believe the patient is experiencing and determine the importance or urgency. What do you think is of greatest concern?

Answer: The potential hypotheses include (1) anaphylactic shock since the patient is presenting with tachycardia, tachypnea, and hypotension (you recall that the mast cell release of vasoactive substances can cause profound vasodilatation resulting in erythema, decreased venous return to the heart [up to 35% of the intravascular volume can be lost into the interstitial space within 10 minutes], decreased cardiac output and distributive shock); (2) urgent need to support the airway; (3) urgent need to restore vascular tone; and (4) patient's lack of knowledge regarding management for allergic reactions. In the moment, you prioritize anaphylactic shock, which includes management of airway constriction and hypotension, as the greatest risk of injury to this patient.

Step Four: Generate solutions, which is identifying expected outcomes and using hypotheses to define a set of interventions for the expected outcomes.

Answer: Since anaphylactic shock is suspected, you follow the ABC priority for care (**A**irway, **B**reathing, **C**irculation) since respiratory or cardiac arrest and death can occur within minutes. You will want to establish and protect the airway and administer oxygen to improve the oxygen saturation which on admission was 88% on room air. Since the hypoxemia is related to airway constriction, the immediate action is also to administer epinephrine, which will relax bronchial smooth muscle and improve vascular tone and permeability, thereby counteracting bronchospasm, hypotension, and tissue edema and prepare for intubation if needed. You will monitor the oxygen saturation continuously and vital signs every 15 minutes at a minimum. You recognize that while elevation of the head of bed (HOB) may improve the hypoxemia, the B/P may decline further because of blood redistribution with gravity. The patient is already significantly hypotensive with a MAP of 61mm Hg; therefore, the patient is placed in the supine position with lower extremities slightly elevated to increase cerebral and cardiac perfusion. You will have the "crash cart" brought to the patient's bedside. You recognize the hypotension is due to the capillary permeability and that rapid fluid replacement IV is required.

Step Five: Take action, where the solutions that address the highest priorities are implemented.

Answer: Since the goals are to establish and protect the airway, to restore intravascular volume, to reverse the sequence of events leading to inadequate tissue perfusion, and to correct the underlying cause of the fluid loss as quickly as possible, you start two large-gauge IV lines to establish access for fluid administration, place the patient on a cardiac monitor, monitor the oxygen saturation continuously, and administer oxygen via high-flow nasal cannula as prescribed. You anticipate fluid resuscitation in anaphylactic shock will be 0.9% sodium chloride solution (normal saline) solution while waiting for the epinephrine to take effect. You will administer prescribed 0.3–0.5 mg intramuscular epinephrine (1:1,000 concentration) in the anterior lateral thigh and prepare to repeat the dose (every 5–30 minutes as prescribed; IV administration may be required. You are aware that the earlier the epinephrine is administered, the better the outcome. You also prepare and administer diphenhydramine IV as prescribed to improve cutaneous erythema and pruritus. You page respiratory therapy to administer stat albuterol treatment to control the bronchospasm (wheezing). You continue to monitor lung sounds, assessing for stridor, and are aware that drooling and tongue or facial edema are ominous signs, suggestive of impending airway obstruction. You know it is urgent that the airway is maintained by either intubation or, if needed, emergency needle cricothyrotomy or cricothyrotomy (the crash cart is at the bedside). If the patient's oxygen saturation does not improve, you are aware that the patient will need to be intubated and transferred to a critical care unit.

Step Six: Evaluate outcomes, which is comparing observed outcomes against expected outcomes.

Answer: The patient responded to IM injections of epinephrine (required two doses) and IV administration of diphenhydramine, as well as nebulized albuterol treatments. Currently, the patient is maintained on 40% fraction of inspired oxygen (FIO_2), with a saturation of 96%. The patient also received 2 L of normal saline, and their BP is currently 110/50 with a MAP of 70 mm Hg. The patient is now aware that having one anaphylactic event as a child is associated with a much greater risk of having another in their lifetime. The patient will be monitored in the ER because of the risk for a "rebound" (or reoccurrence) reaction, usually within 4–10 hours after the initial allergic reaction. Since this patient had a severe reaction, you can anticipate that the patient will be monitored closely for 12–24 hours. Before discharge, the patient will be provided with two prescribed epinephrine autoinjectors, given training on proper use, and instructed if there is a return of symptoms following ER discharge they should use their injector in the lateral thigh and then return to the ER. Although this was a stressful situation, you kept your composure and followed the priorities of ABC. Because of your quick, adept nursing care and marshaling of other health care professionals, this patient's story had a successful conclusion. Now, it is time to teach and review your patient's understanding of the anaphylaxis plan and the need to follow up with an allergy specialist.

CHAPTER REVIEW

NCLEX-Style Review Questions

1. During a clinical post-conference, the nursing instructor is discussing factors related to the risk of anaphylaxis. Which statements properly describe allergic and anaphylactic reactions? Select all that apply.
   a. The severity increases with the age of the patient.
   b. The severity of previous reactions determines the severity of subsequent reactions.
   c. The severity depends on the dose of the allergen.
   d. The severity of previous reactions does not determine the severity of subsequent reactions.
   e. The severity depends on the degree of allergy.

2. Which reaction would be consistent with a mild reaction to an allergen? Select all that apply.
   a. Bronchospasm
   b. Sneezing
   c. Wheezing
   d. Tearing of the eyes
   e. Syncope

3. You are caring for a patient receiving first chemotherapy which is *carboplatin*. In Column 1 select cues that are of concern, in Column 2 select the potential etiology, and in Column 3 select appropriate actions.

Cues	Potential Etiology	Appropriate Actions
Angioedema	Hypovolemic shock	Stop IV infusion of carboplatin
Increasing MAP	Septicemia	Encourage PO intake of clear liquids
Stridor	Anaphylaxis	If hypotensive, place supine with legs elevated
O_2 saturation of 96% on room air	Cardiogenic shock	Notify provider
Abdominal cramping	Neurogenic shock	Monitor oxygen saturation

4. A patient is being seen in the dermatology clinic for urticaria. The nurse would expect which medication to be prescribed for the patient? Select all that apply.
   a. Pseudoephedrine
   b. Diphenhydramine
   c. Dexamethasone
   d. Cromolyn sodium
   e. Loratadine

5. Which of the following are at risk of developing a latex allergy? Select all that apply.
   a. Health care workers
   b. Patients with spina bifida or spinal cord injuries
   c. Patients on hemodialysis
   d. Patients requiring first surgery
   e. Patient requiring urinary catheterization (first time)

REFERENCES AND SELECTED READINGS

References and selected readings associated with this chapter can be found on the website that accompanies the book. Visit **http://thepoint.lww.com/Honan3e** to access the references and other additional resources associated with this chapter.

CHAPTER 38

Nursing Management: Patients With Rheumatic Disorders

Linda Alessie Podolak

Learning Objectives

After reading this chapter, you will be able to:

1. Explain the pathophysiology of rheumatic diseases and disorders.
2. Describe the assessment and diagnostic findings seen in patients with a suspected diagnosis of rheumatic disease or disorder.
3. Describe the systemic effects of a connective tissue disease.
4. Discuss the pharmacologic, medical, and nursing management associated with rheumatic disorders.
5. Apply the nursing process as a framework for the care of the patient with a rheumatic disorder.
6. Identify appropriate nursing interventions based on nursing diagnoses that commonly occur with rheumatic disorders.

Rheumatic disorders affect the joints, bones, muscles, and connective tissues. These conditions can be minor illnesses, or they can be life threatening. Systemic effects caused by rheumatic disorders or diseases result in obvious limitations in mobility and activities of daily living (ADL) as well as more subtle manifestations, such as pain, fatigue, insomnia, and altered body image perception. Organ failure and death may be an end result for some rheumatic disorders. The rheumatic condition may be the patient's primary health problem or a secondary diagnosis. Thorough understanding of rheumatic conditions and their effects on a patient's function and well-being is key to developing an interprofessional plan of care.

OVERVIEW

Commonly called arthritis (inflammation of a joint) and thought of as one condition, the rheumatic diseases are actually more than 100 different types of disorders that primarily affect joints, bones, skeletal muscles, and connective tissues. They collectively affect an estimated 58.5 million (23.7%) U.S. adults aged ≥18 years (Centers for Disease Control and Prevention [CDC], 2021; Theis et al., 2021). Some disorders are more likely to occur at a particular time of life or to affect people of one sex more than the other (see Box 38-1). The symptom that most commonly causes a person to seek medical attention is pain. Other common symptoms include joint swelling, limited movement, stiffness, weakness, and fatigue. The onset of these conditions may be acute or insidious, with a course possibly marked by periods of remission (a period when disease symptoms are reduced or absent) and exacerbation (a period when symptoms occur or increase).

Assessment includes a complete health history followed by a complete physical examination combined with a functional assessment. Inspection of the patient's general appearance occurs during initial contact. Gait, posture, and general musculoskeletal size and structure are observed. Gross deformities and abnormalities in movement are noted. Also, the symmetry, size, and contour of other connective tissues, such as the skin and adipose tissue, are noted and recorded. The functional assessment is a combination of history (what the patient reports that they can and cannot do) and examination (observation of activities is made: the patient demonstrates what they can and cannot do, such as dressing and getting in and out of a chair). Observation also includes the adaptations and adjustments the patient may have made (sometimes without awareness); for example, with shoulder or elbow involvement, the person may bend over to reach a fork, rather than raising the fork to the mouth.

The history and physical assessment data are supplemented by supportive or confirming diagnostic test findings. Common serum laboratory tests used for patients with rheumatic disorders are described in Table 38-1. Radiologic investigations facilitate early diagnosis, guide treatment,

BOX 38-1 **Highlighting Gerontology**

Although people of all ages may be affected, rheumatic disease is commonly thought of by the patient, family, and society as an inevitable consequence of aging. Many older people expect and accept the immobility and self-care problems related to the rheumatic disorders and do not seek help, thinking that nothing can be done. Ageist attitudes exist that assume older people are frail and a burden to society. An incorrect assumption that changes induced by disease are age-related leads to therapeutic neglect of potentially treatable conditions. Careful diagnosis and appropriate treatment are crucial and can improve the quality of life for older people. An adequate support system for the older population is also a critical factor in the ability to follow an interdisciplinary plan of care that includes exercise, nutrition, general health maintenance, pharmacotherapy, and nonpharmacologic management. Biologically, aging results from the impact of molecular and cellular changes over time, leading to a functional decline. However, the rheumatic disorders do have some special implications for the older adult.

Age alone causes changes in serologic studies (e.g., ESR, ANA, CRP), making interpretation of laboratory values more difficult. Decreased vision and altered balance, often present in older people, may be problematic if rheumatic disease in the lower extremities affects locomotion. Also, the combination of decreased hearing and visual acuity, memory loss, and depression can contribute to failure to follow the treatment regimen in older patients.

Pharmacologic treatment of rheumatic disease in older patients is more difficult. Aging brings many physical and metabolic changes that may increase the older patient's sensitivity to both the therapeutic and toxic effects of some drugs, making overtreatment or inappropriate treatment possible. If therapeutic medications influence the senses (hearing, cognition), this effect is intensified in the older population. The cumulative effect of these medications is accentuated because of the physiologic changes of aging. For example, decreased kidney function in older adults alters the metabolism of certain medications, such as NSAIDs. In addition, older patients are more prone to side effects associated with the use of multiple-drug therapy for various disorders (Burchum & Rosenthal, 2022; Chalise, 2019; Marill, 2022; Stein, 2022; World Health Organization [WHO], 2021).

and, ultimately, impact prognosis. Scans, computed tomography (CT), and magnetic resonance imaging (MRI) are not the most cost-effective methods for detection of early disease and are not performed routinely at the time of diagnosis. In some instances, many tests are used to monitor the course of the disease. For example, contrast radiography and MRI play a role in diagnosing advancing systems affected in scleroderma; the erythrocyte sedimentation rate (ESR) reflects inflammatory activity and, indirectly, the progression or remission of disease. Ultimately, the health care provider determines which tests are necessary based on the symptoms, stage of disease, cost, and likely benefit of the test.

Pearls for Practice

The ESR is a measure of the rate of sedimentation of red blood cells (RBCs) in an anticoagulated whole blood sample over a specified period of time; it is commonly referred to as a "sed" rate. Often, increased "sed" rates are associated with inflammatory states. Normally, the distance an RBC falls in 1 hour is less than 15 mm/hr for males and slightly higher in females. The speed with which the RBC moves is related to the clumping of RBCs. The more clumping, the heavier and higher the speed that an RBC falls. Inflammatory states produce proteins that encourage this clumping; thus, high ESR levels are associated with inflammation. The ESR does not diagnose a problem, but it is used to monitor status of a disease and response to therapy (Van Leeuwen & Bladh, 2021).

Treatment can be simple, aimed at localized relief, or it can be complex, directed toward relief of systemic effects. The chronic nature of most of these disorders mandates that the patient understand the disease, have the information necessary to make good self-management decisions, be referred to appropriate community agencies (such as the Arthritis Foundation) for support, and be presented with a therapeutic program that is compatible with their lifestyle. The concept of treat-to-target (T2T) is now recognized as a treatment paradigm and an international initiative for many of the rheumatic disorders. T2T includes any management strategy in which therapy is altered based on the goal of achieving a prespecified target (March & Richards, 2019). The goals and strategies of management of basic rheumatic diseases are outlined in Table 38-2. The T2T trend in management is toward a more aggressive pharmacologic approach earlier in the disease presentation.

Pharmacologic management of rheumatic disorders is used to manage symptoms, control pain and inflammation, and—in some diseases, such as rheumatoid arthritis (RA)—modify the disease course. However, disease typically advances steadily and, as a result, pharmacologic therapy is chronic; thus, success requires motivation and cooperation by the patient. Selection of medication is based on the patient's needs, the stage of disease, and the risk of side effects (March & Richards, 2019).

Antiarthritic drugs fall into three major groups: nonsteroidal anti-inflammatory drugs (NSAIDs) including salicylates (e.g., aspirin), disease-modifying antirheumatic drugs (DMARDs), and glucocorticoids (adrenal corticosteroids). These groups differ with reference to time course of effects, toxicity, and ability to slow disease progression. Table 38-3 reviews the medications commonly used in rheumatic disorders, particularly RA.

Nonpharmacologic treatment measures include the use of heat or cold, weight reduction, joint rest and avoidance of joint overuse, orthotic devices (e.g., splints, braces) to support inflamed joints, and an exercise regimen. Occupational and

TABLE **38-1 Common Serum Laboratory Tests for Rheumatic Diseases**

Test	Normal Value	Implications
Serology		
Erythrocyte Sedimentation Rate (ESR)		
Measures the rate at which red blood cells (RBCs) settle out of unclotted blood in 1 hour	Westergren method *Males,* 0–15 mm/hr, over 50 years of age: 0–20 mm/hr *Females,* 0–20 mm/hr, over 50 years of age: 0–30 mm/hr	Usually, increase is seen in inflammatory connective tissue diseases (e.g., RA, SLE, scleroderma), gout, can be seen in older adults. An increase indicates rising inflammation; the higher the ESR, the greater the inflammatory activity
Uric Acid		
Measures level of uric acid in serum	*Males,* 3.4–7 mg/dL (202–416 µmol/L) *Females,* 2.4–6 mg/dL (143–357 µmol/L) *Biologic Crystallization Point,* at least 6.8 mg/dL (408 µmol/L)	Increase is seen with gout, where there is an overproduction of uric acids that occurs when there is excessive cell breakdown and catabolism of nucleonic acids
Serum Immunology		
Antinuclear Antibody (ANA)		
Measures antibodies that react with a variety of nuclear antigens Usually the first step; if antibodies are present, further testing determines specific circulating antibodies to extractable nuclear antigens (anti-dsDNA, anti-RNP, anti–Ro-SSA).	Screen: negative by ELISA and IFA methods, repeat use Hep-2 cell line If positive by IFA, specimen is titered. Titer: less than 1:160 Low titers are present in older and some healthy adults	Positive test is associated with systemic rheumatic disease, such as mixed connective tissue disease, SLE, RA, scleroderma, CREST syndrome, can be seen in older adults The higher the titer, the greater the inflammation Some negative ANA findings have been found to have positive anti-Ro (SSA)
Anticentromere Antibody Test		
A specific autoantibody, detected by using Hep-2 cells in various stages of cell division, centromere region of the cell chromosomes will stain if positive	Screen: negative by ELISA and IFA methods If positive by IFA, specimen is titered.	Positive test is associated with the CREST syndrome in scleroderma Present in 90% of those with CREST
Anticyclic Citrullinated Peptide (Anti-CCP)		
Disease-specific autoantibody, highly specific diagnostic and prognostic markers for RA Detects patients with early RA at baseline (after 3–6 months of symptoms) Second-generation test: CCP2 assay, even higher sensitivity	Negative	Positive in RA Predictive of erosive disease Sensitivity of anti-CCP comparable to rheumatoid factor (RF) but has higher specificity (90–95%) Differentiates other entities that can resemble RA and, at times, be RF positive
Anti–double-stranded DNA (anti-dsDNA)		
Specific autoantibody to extractable nuclear antigens; differentiates native (i.e., double-stranded) DNA antibodies from other nonnative antibodies; 95% specific for SLE, making it a valuable disease marker	Negative: less than 25 IU by ELISA	DNA–anti-dsDNA immune complexes play a role in SLE pathogenesis, found in 70% of SLE patients Positive: 31–200 IU; strongly positive: over 200 IU Anti-dsDNA concentrations may decrease with successful therapy, may increase with exacerbation of SLE
Autoantibodies, Others		
Specific autoantibodies to extractable nuclear antigens (*anti-RNA, anti-Sm, anti-scl-70*); may reflect disease-specific immune mechanisms but are not pathogenetic by themselves	Negative: less than 20 U/mL by ELISA	Positive: greater than 26 U/mL *Anti-RNA:* mixed connective tissue disease (MCTD), 35–40% of SLE patients *Anti-Sm* (Smith): SLE, MCTD *Anti-scl-70:* Scleroderma

Test	Normal Value	Implications
Complement Levels—C3, C4		
Complement component levels: done if a reduction/consumption of complement component concentration is suspected C3 constitutes 70% of the total protein in the complement system (antigen–antibody complexes)	C3: 75–175 mg/dL (or 0.75–1.75 g/L) C4: 14–40 mg/dL (or 140–400 mg/L)	Decrease may be seen in active SLE, immune complex disease (i.e., RA) Decrease indicates autoimmune activity
C-Reactive Protein Test (CRP)		
Measures the presence of abnormal glycoprotein in response to inflammatory cytokines	Less than 1 mg/dL (less than 10 mg/L)	A positive reading indicates active inflammation Often is positive for RA and SLE More sensitive than ESR test
Immunoglobulin Electrophoresis		
Measures the values of immunoglobulins	IgG: 700–1,500 mg/dL (7.0–15.0 g/L) IgM: 60–300 mg/dL (600–3,000 mg/L)	Increased levels of IgG occur in RA, autoimmune disorders (i.e., SLE) Increased levels of IgM occur in RA, SLE
Rheumatoid Factor (RF)		
Measures RFs, antibodies directed against the Fe fragment of IgG Determines the presence of abnormal antibodies seen in connective tissue disease	0–20 U/mL Negative titer	Positive titer greater than 1:80 Present in 80% of those with RA; positive RF also may suggest SLE, MCTD Low titers can be seen in OA The higher the titer (number at right of colon), the greater the inflammation

physical therapy can help the patient adopt self-management strategies. Other nonpharmacologic modalities, such as massage, yoga, pulsed electromagnetic fields, transcutaneous electrical nerve stimulation (TENS), and music therapy, have been used in the treatment of arthritis (Cuccurullo et al., 2021; Heiberg et al., 2019; Hinman et al., 2019; Misra et al., 2021). In addition, iontophoresis can be used to deliver medication through the skin using direct electrical current. A combination of methods may be required because different methods often work better at different times.

Common choices of complementary and alternative medicine (CAM) used by patients with rheumatologic disorders include dietary supplements, herbal therapies, mind/body and spiritual practices, manual/manipulative therapies, biostimulation, vagus nerve stimulation, and topical ointments (Berman et al., 2019; Misra et al., 2021). It is essential that health care providers remain informed on appropriate indications for use, risks, and limitations of such therapies or practices.

For rheumatology patients hospitalized for COVID-19 and requiring high-flow oxygen, noninvasive ventilation,

TABLE **38-2 Goals and Strategies for Rheumatic Diseases**

Major Goals	Management Strategy
Suppress inflammation and the autoimmune response	Optimize pharmacologic therapy (anti-inflammatory and disease-modifying agents)
Control pain	Protect joints; ease pain with splints/orthoses, thermal modalities, relaxation techniques
Maintain or improve joint mobility	Implement exercise programs for joint motion and muscle strengthening and overall health
Maintain or improve functional status	Make use of adaptive devices and techniques
Increase patient's knowledge of disease process	Provide and reinforce patient teaching
Promote self-management by patient adherence to the therapeutic regimen	Promote social support and encouragement of change-based interventions compatible with therapeutic regimen and lifestyle

TABLE **38-3** **Medications Used in Rheumatic Diseases**

Medication	Action, Use, and Indication	Nursing Considerations
Nonsteroidal Anti-Inflammatory Drugs (NSAIDs)		
Salicylates		
Acetylated Aspirin *Nonacetylated* Choline salicylate, salsalate, sodium salicylate	*Action:* anti-inflammatory, analgesic, antipyretic Acetylated salicylates are platelet aggregation inhibitors Anti-inflammatory doses will produce blood salicylate levels of 20–30 mg/dL	Administer with meals to prevent gastric irritation Assess for tinnitus, gastric intolerance, gastrointestinal (GI) bleeding, and purpuric tendencies Monitor for possible confusion in older adults
Nonsalicylates		
First-Generation Diclofenac, diflunisal, etodolac, flurbiprofen, ibuprofen, indomethacin, ketoprofen, meclofenamate, meloxicam, nabumetone, naproxen, oxaprozin, piroxicam, sulindac, tolmetin sodium	*Action:* anti-inflammatory, analgesic, antipyretic, inhibition of platelet aggregation, inhibition of prostaglandin synthesis Anti-inflammatory effect occurs 2–4 weeks after initiation NSAIDs are first-line therapy in several rheumatic diseases All NSAIDs are useful for short-term treatment of acute gout attack	Administer NSAIDs with food Monitor for GI, CNS, cardiovascular, renal, hematologic, and dermatologic adverse effects All prescription-strength NSAIDs carry a boxed warning regarding risk for thrombotic events, GI ulceration, and bleeding Avoid salicylates; use acetaminophen for additional analgesia Need to be used regularly for maximal effect Watch for possible confusion in older adults
Second-Generation COX-2 Inhibitors Celecoxib	*Action*: Selective prostaglandin inhibition; inhibit only cyclooxygenase (COX)-2 enzymes, which are produced during inflammation; and spare COX-1 enzymes, which can be protective to the stomach	Monitoring the same as for other NSAIDs Increased risk of cardiovascular events, including myocardial infarction and stroke Appropriate for older adults and patients who are at high risk for gastric ulcers
Related Agent Acetaminophen	*Action*: Inhibits the synthesis of prostaglandins; antipyretic, analgesic, no anti-inflammatory properties	Chronic excessive use of more than 3 g/day may lead to hepatotoxicity or renal or cardiac damage Concurrent use of NSAIDs increases the risk of adverse renal effects
Disease-Modifying Antirheumatic Drugs (DMARDs)		
Nonbiologic DMARDs—Conventional (Traditional) Drugs		
Immunosuppressives Methotrexate	*Action:* Immune suppression; inhibits folic acid reductase, leading to inhibition of DNA synthesis and other cellular effects Acts faster than other DMARDs Methotrexate is gold standard for RA treatment; also useful in SLE, SSc Therapeutic effects may develop in 3–6 weeks	Assess for bone marrow suppression, GI ulcerations, pneumonitis, liver disease, skin rashes, bladder toxicity, increased infections. Common adverse effects include nausea, hair loss, and stomatitis Monitor CBC, platelets, liver enzymes, creatinine every 2–4 weeks Caution with NSAID use Folic acid supplementation recommended Advise patient of contraceptive measures because of teratogenicity
Antimalarials Hydroxychloroquine, chloroquine	*Action:* Anti-inflammatory, inhibits lysosomal enzymes Slow-acting, onset may take 3–6 months Useful in RA and SLE	Administer concurrently with NSAIDs Assess for visual changes, GI upset, skin rash, headaches, photosensitivity, bleaching of hair Retinopathy may occur; emphasize ophthalmologic examinations (every 6–12 months)

Medication	Action, Use, and Indication	Nursing Considerations
Sulfonamides sulfasalazine	*Action:* Anti-inflammatory, reduces lymphocyte response, inhibits angiogenesis Useful in RA, seronegative spondyloarthropathies	Periodically monitor CBC and platelet counts Do not use in patients with allergy to sulfa medications or salicylates Emphasize adequate fluid intake Assess for GI upset, skin rash, headache, liver abnormalities, anemia
Pyrimidine Synthesis Inhibitor Leflunomide	*Action:* Has antiproliferative and anti-inflammatory effects, powerful immunosuppressant Used in moderate-to-severe RA; SLE May be used alone or in combination with other DMARDs (except methotrexate) About as effective as methotrexate but more adverse effects	Assess for diarrhea, respiratory infection, alopecia, skin rash, mouth sores, nausea Monitor liver function tests, risk of severe hepatic impairment Risk for serious infections Contraindicated in patients who are pregnant and breast or chestfeeding
Nonbiologic DMARDs—Minor Drugs Used Infrequently		
Cyclosporine	*Action:* Immune suppression by inhibiting T lymphocytes Used for severe, progressive RA, unresponsive to other DMARDs Used in combination with methotrexate Used in SLE	Assess slow dose titration upward until response noted or toxicity occurs Assess for toxic effects: bleeding gums, fluid retention, hair growth, tremors Monitor blood pressure and creatinine every 2 weeks until stable
Gold-Containing Compounds Aurothioglucose, gold sodium thiomalate, auranofin	*Action:* Inhibits T- and B-cell activity, suppresses synovitis during active stage of rheumatoid disease Slow-acting, onset may take 3–6 months IM preparations are given weekly for about 6 months and then every 2–4 weeks	FDA black-box warning regarding gold toxicity manifested by serious blood dyscrasias, stomatitis, profuse diarrhea, proteinuria, hematuria, and rash Monitor CBC and urinalysis with every other injection
Penicillamine	*Action:* Anti-inflammatory, inhibits T-cell function, impairs antigen presentation Slow-acting, therapeutic effects take 3–6 months Restricted to severe cases RA and systemic sclerosis unresponsive to other treatment	Associated with serious toxicity—bone marrow suppression Assess for GI irritation, decreased taste, skin rash or itching, bone marrow suppression, proteinuria with CBC; monitor urinalysis every 2–4 weeks
Minor Immunosuppressants Azathioprine, cyclophosphamide	*Action:* Immune suppression, affects DNA synthesis and other cellular effects Have teratogenic potential; azathioprine and cyclophosphamide reserved for more aggressive or unresponsive disease Used in RA; SLE	Assess for bone marrow suppression, GI ulcerations, skin rashes, alopecia, bladder toxicity, increased infections Monitor CBC, liver enzymes, creatinine every 2–4 weeks Advise patient of contraceptive measures because of teratogenicity
Biologic DMARDs—Immunomodulators		
Tumor Necrosis Factor (TNF) Inhibitors Adalimumab, etanercept, infliximab, golimumab, certolizumab pegol	*Action:* Biologic response modifier that binds to TNF, a cytokine involved in inflammatory and immune responses Used in moderate-to-severe RA unresponsive to methotrexate Can be used alone or with methotrexate or other DMARDs Humira is administered every 1–2 weeks, and Enbrel is administered twice a week Simponi is the first treatment that is administered once a month	Patient should be tested for tuberculosis before beginning this medication Teach patient subcutaneous self-injection of adalimumab or etanercept Infliximab is administered by IV over 2 hours or more Medication must be refrigerated Monitor for injection site reactions Educate patient about increased risk for serious infection and to withhold medication if fever occurs Contraindicated in HF class III/IV, and at risk for new onset of heart failure

(*continued*)

TABLE **38-3 Medications Used in Rheumatic Diseases (*continued*)**

Medication	Action, Use, and Indication	Nursing Considerations
T-Cell Activation Inhibitors Abatacept	*Action:* selectively modulates T-cell activation, altering immune response (costimulatory blocker) Alternative treatment of moderate-to-severe RA when conventional DMARDs and TNF inhibitors are inadequate	Contains maltose, may falsely elevate blood glucose High risk for serious infections (TB, zoster) Do not give live vaccines
B-Cell Depleting Agents Rituximab	*Action:* monoclonal antibody directed at the CD20 antigen expressed on mature B and pre-B cells B-cell depletion therapy: a course of two IV infusions, 2 weeks apart with a repeat treatment interval of 6–12 months Used in RA; SLE	Premedicate with acetaminophen and diphenhydramine to decrease infusion reactions; glucocorticoid can be used Severe mucocutaneous reactions can occur 1–3 weeks after infusion Use caution in patients with cardiac and pulmonary diseases
Interleukin (IL)-1 Receptor Antagonist Anakinra	*Action:* Human IL-1 receptor antagonist; blocks IL-1 receptors, decreasing inflammatory and immunologic responses Used in moderate-to-severe RA unresponsive to one or more conventional DMARDs, e.g., methotrexate Can be used alone or with methotrexate or DMARDs but not with TNF inhibitors Can be used in gout	Teach patient subcutaneous self-injection and to monitor for site reactions Medication must be refrigerated at 36–46°F (2–8°C) and warmed to room temperature for 30 minutes prior to injection Educate patient about increased risk for infection and to withhold medication if fever occurs
Interleukin (IL)-6 Receptor Antagonist Tocilizumab, sarilumab	*Action*: Human IL-6 receptor antagonist; blocks IL-6 receptors, decreasing inflammatory and immunologic responses Used in moderate-to-severe RA unresponsive to other DMARDs Can be used alone or with methotrexate but not with TNF inhibitors or other DMARDs that increase the risk for infection Tocilizumab used in severe COVID-19 patients	Fully diluted tocilizumab solutions should be refrigerated at 36–46°F (2–8°C) and warmed to room temperature for 30 minutes prior to infusion Risk for serious infections and other serious adverse effects, e.g., liver injury, GI perforation, neutropenia, and thrombocytopenia; monitor transaminase, neutrophil and platelet levels every 4–8 weeks during treatment Can reduce blood levels of other drugs, e.g., oral contraceptives, statins
Targeted DMARDs		
Janus Kinase (JAK) Inhibitor Tofacitinib citrate, baricitinib, upadacitinib	*Action*: JAK inhibitor works deep inside the cell (intracellular) to disrupt activities occurring in signaling pathways that play a role in the inflammatory and immune responses associated with RA Used in moderate-to-severe RA patients who can't take methotrexate or unresponsive to it Baricitinib used in severe COVID-19 patients	All oral agents Should not be given if lymphocyte count, neutrophil count, or red blood cell count is too low or liver tests are too high FDA safety alert warns of increased risk of blood clots, heart problems, and cancer High risk for serious infections (TB, zoster) Do not give live vaccines
Glucocorticoids		
Adrenal Corticosteroids Prednisone, hydrocortisone sodium succinate, methylprednisolone sodium succinate, methylprednisolone acetate, intra-articular injection	*Action:* Anti-inflammatory; may also delay disease progression Used for shortest duration and at lowest dose possible to minimize serious toxicity (e.g., osteoporosis, gastric ulceration, adrenal suppression) Useful for unremitting RA, SLE Fast-acting; onset in days Intra-articular injections useful for joints unresponsive to NSAIDs	Assess for toxicity: cataracts, GI irritation, hyperglycemia, hypertension, fractures, avascular necrosis, hirsutism, psychosis If NSAIDs and glucocorticoids are prescribed together, risk for adverse GI effects may increase fourfold, recommended to discontinue NSAID therapy Joints most amenable to injections include ankles, knees, hips, shoulders, and hands Repeated injections can cause joint damage

CBC, complete blood count; CNS, central nervous system; RA, rheumatoid arthritis; SLE, systemic lupus erythematosus; WBCs, white blood cells.
Data from Borham, L., & Hafiz, W. (2021). Pharmacotherapy in systemic rheumatic diseases. In H. Almoallim & M. Cheikh (Eds.), *Skills in rheumatology*. Springer. https://doi.org/10.1007/978-981-15-8323-0_4; Burchum, J., & Rosenthal, L. (2022). *Lehne's pharmacology for nursing care* (11th ed.). Elsevier; Ward, I. M., & Knott, A. (2018). Practical pearls about current rheumatic medications. *Primary Care: Clinic Office of Practice*, *45*, 193–212. https://doi.org/10.1016/i.pop.2018.02.003.

intermittent ventilation (IMV) or extracorporeal membrane oxygenation (ECMO), the National Institutes of Health (NIH) recommends four immunomodulators as potential therapies. The two preferred are baricitinib and tocilizumab, while tofacitinib and sarilumab are listed in the NIH guidelines as alternatives. Baricitinib and tofacitinib are janus kinase (JAK) inhibitors, which have anticytokine effects (in RA there is an overproduction of cytokines which play a role in inflammation, and JAK inhibitors impede this process and is discussed in more detail shortly). Baricitinib also has potential antiviral effects, interfering with the ability of a virus to enter and infect susceptible cells and has shown to reduce mortality among patients with COVID-19. Tocilizumab and sarilumab are interleukin-6 (IL-6) antagonists that reduce inflammation and cytokine storm associated with increased morbidity and mortality from COVID-19 (Santangelo & Ramey, 2022).

Nurses need to understand the classification of rheumatic diseases. Yazdany and Manno (2022e) emphasize two clinical clues in the examination of the patient as useful in classifying and diagnosing arthritis: the joint pattern and the presence or absence of extra-articular manifestations (e.g., fatigue). One basic system is to classify disease as either monoarticular (affecting a single joint) or polyarticular (affecting multiple joints) and then to further classify it as either inflammatory (e.g., RA) or degenerative, noninflammatory (e.g., osteoarthritis [OA]). This chapter groups the conditions into those affecting the joints, bones, and muscles and those affecting the connective tissues.

BOX 38-2

Focus on Pathophysiology

Rheumatic Disorders

Each **synovial** joint has a given range of motion, and the synovial fluid within a joint has three primary functions: lubrication, nutrient distribution, and shock absorption. Inflammation is manifested in the joints as **synovitis**. Rheumatic disorders always involve damage to the articular cartilages. Because articular cartilages involve some degree of inflammation and degeneration, the rheumatic disorders can be classified as either inflammatory (e.g., RA) or degenerative, noninflammatory (e.g., OA).

In the inflammatory rheumatic disorder classification, the primary process starts with inflammation due to an altered immune function. The inflammatory reaction includes swelling, pain, and loss of function (see Chapter 35 for the inflammatory and immunologic processes). Degeneration then occurs as a secondary process, spreading to the articular surfaces. The cause of degeneration of the articular cartilage is poorly understood but believed to be metabolically active and, therefore, is more accurately called *degradation.*

On the other hand, in the degenerative (noninflammatory) rheumatic disorder classification, inflammation occurs as a secondary process. The resultant secondary synovitis is usually milder, is more likely to be seen in advanced disease, and represents a reactive process. The synovitis is thought to result mainly from degeneration due to mechanical irritation of two bone surfaces. As the articular cartilage becomes damaged, the matrix (noncellular component of tissue) begins to break down; the exposed cartilage changes from a slick, smooth gliding surface to a rough fibrous network of collagen fibers. Later this network may be converted to bone, locking the articulating elements into position. Fixation of a joint, called **ankylosis**, eliminates the friction but at the drastic cost of immobility.

CONDITIONS AFFECTING THE JOINTS, BONES, AND MUSCLES

Despite the diversity of rheumatic disorders, the joint is the area most commonly affected and involves some degree of inflammation and damage to the articular cartilages, which may occur simultaneously. Understanding normal anatomy and physiology of **articulations**, or joints, is the key to understanding the pathophysiology of the rheumatic disorders (Box 38-2).

Osteoarthritis

Osteoarthritis, also known as degenerative joint disease, is a chronic, noninflammatory (even though synovial inflammation plays a pivotal role in the pathogenesis of OA), progressive disorder that causes cartilage deterioration in synovial joints and vertebrae. It particularly affects the weight-bearing joints, knees and hips, and joints of the distal interphalangeal (DIP) and proximal interphalangeal (PIP) joints of the fingers (Gelber, 2021; Sen & Hurley, 2022; Yazdany & Manno, 2022b). OA is the most common and most frequently disabling of the joint disorders; evidence has emerged that OA is a serious disease with increasing impact worldwide (Allen et al., 2022; Kloppenburg & Berenbaum, 2020; Kraus & Vincent, 2020). OA is overdiagnosed and trivialized and frequently over- or undertreated. The functional impact of OA on quality of life, especially for older patients, is often ignored.

OA has been classified as both primary (idiopathic), with no prior event or disease related to the OA, and secondary, resulting from previous joint injury or inflammatory disease. The distinction between primary and secondary OA is not always clear, but often the clinical presentation and symptoms are similar.

Risk Factors

Risk factors for OA are summarized in Box 38-3. Age is the risk factor most strongly correlated with OA, while obesity is now well recognized as an important contributing factor (Allen et al., 2022; Hunter & Bierma-Zeinstra, 2019).

OA generally affects adults 40 years of age and above (American College of Rheumatology [ACR], 2021; Yazdany & Manno, 2022b). Prevalence of arthritis in the United States

BOX 38-3 **Risk Factors for Osteoarthritis (OA)**

- Aging
- Obesity (mechanical loading from a higher body mass index is associated with an increased risk of knee OA; the link between OA and adipose-derived leptin is now recognized as a metabolically active contributor to inflammatory cascades)
- Genetic predisposition
- Joint location (joint-specific, age-related articular cartilage changes, varying joint responsiveness to cytokines)
- Malalignment of joints (can lead to rapid development of OA; congenital and developmental disorders, e.g., poorly reduced intra-articular fractures, developmental dysplasia of the hip)
- Trauma (also can lead to rapid development of OA; overuse or abuse of joints, as occurs in high-impact sports; previous joint damage; and excessive loading or forces, such as that seen in shoulders and elbows of pneumatic drill operators and baseball pitchers and in knees of basketball players).
- Sex (females are twice as likely to develop OA than males; differences in incidence after 50 years of age may be the result of postmenopausal estrogen deficiency; articular chondrocytes possess functional estrogen receptors)

Adapted from Di Cesare, P. E., Haudenschild, D. R., Abramson, S. B., & Samuels, J. (2021). Pathogenesis of osteoarthritis. In G. S. Firestein, R. C. Budd, S. E. Gabriel, G. A. Koretzky, I. B. McInnes & J. R. O'Dell. (Eds.), *Firestein & Kelley's textbook of rheumatology* (11th ed., pp. 1770–1788). Elsevier.

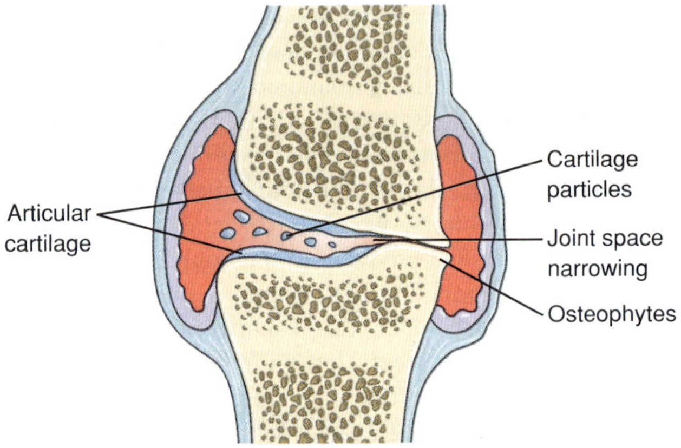

FIGURE 38-1 Osteoarthritic degenerative joint changes: hypertrophy of bone margins resulting in characteristic osteophytes (bone spurs) and narrowing of joint space.

for adults 25 years of age and older having clinical OA of some joint was estimated at nearly 30.8 million (Abramoff & Caldera, 2020; Kraus & Vincent, 2020). Because of the aging of Western populations and because of the increased prevalence of obesity, a major risk factor, the occurrence of OA is on the rise. Radiologic OA is more prevalent than symptomatic OA. OA of the hand, hip, and knee become more frequent with age, and more females are affected than males after 50 years of age (CDC, 2020b; Gelber, 2021).

In addition, the genetic risk of OA is associated with a range of biologic mechanisms. What is promising is that ethnic groups, who have been underrepresented, are now starting to be included in research, giving a more equitable picture of the genetic architecture of OA at a more global population level (Aubourg et al., 2021).

Furthermore, having OA may increase the risk for cardiovascular disease (CVD). Research shows people with OA are almost three times more likely to develop CVD or heart failure than those without OA. The Arthritis Foundation (2022) recommends educating patients to maintain a healthy weight; stay active and exercise; limit pain reliever use; and monitor blood sugar, blood pressure, and cholesterol levels.

Pathophysiology

OA may be thought of as the result of many factors that, when combined, predispose the patient to the disease. In OA, changes in articular cartilage occur first; eventually, changes to secondary soft tissue may occur. OA is characterized by erosion of the articular cartilage combined with hypertrophy of bone at the joint margins, resulting in formation of new bone known as **osteophytes** or bone spurs (Fig. 38-1) and subchondral (the bony plate that supports the articular cartilage) sclerosis. In addition, OA is characterized by a range of biochemical and morphologic alterations of the synovial membrane and joint capsule. In general, a combination of cartilage degradation, bone stiffening, and reactive inflammation of the synovium occurs (Di Cesare et al., 2021; Grandi & Bhutani, 2020; Kraus & Vincent, 2020). Understanding of OA has been expanded greatly beyond what previously was thought of as simply a passive, degenerative "wear and tear" disorder related to aging to an active, dynamic disease affecting the whole joint.

Clinical Manifestations and Assessment

The general clinical manifestations of OA are pain, stiffness, and functional disability (Allen et al., 2021; Nelson, 2021; Sen & Hurley, 2022). Pain in one or more joints typically is worsened by activities and is alleviated by rest. Although osteoarthritic pain is unusual during the night or at rest, there are exceptions, including in patients with mild OA using joints for several hours, in patients with advanced OA with destructive arthropathy, and in patients with an acute inflammatory flare-up of OA. Stiffness may be defined as a sensation of a gelling or tightening of the involved joint that usually occurs after inactivity, such as in the morning or when rising after sitting for a prolonged period. Morning stiffness usually resolves after less than 10 minutes (no more than 30 minutes' duration), in contrast to prolonged stiffness seen in inflammatory disorders. Functional impairment is reflected in limited range of motion (ROM) and patient report of limited ability to perform day-to-day activities.

The diagnosis of OA is complicated by many contributing factors. The ACR has established clinical classification criteria for OA of specific joints to promote consistency in the diagnosis of OA. Typically, OA is diagnosed by an overall clinical impression based on the patient's age and history, location of joint abnormalities, and radiographic findings. Limited passive movement can be the first and only physical sign of symptomatic OA. During joint examination, crepitus, a continuous grating sensation, may be felt or heard as the joint goes through ROM. Physical assessment of the musculoskeletal system reveals joint enlargement, resulting from **joint effusion** or bony swelling or both. This is most easily detected in the patient's knees by the evidence of patellar tap or by the elicitation of a fluid thrill (wave test). Joint deformities reflect advanced disease with joint destruction, which then contributes to misalignment, joint instability (causing a sensation in the knees of "giving way" or "locking"), and limb shortening. Fingers also can be misaligned in the presence of Heberden (enlargements of DIP joints) or Bouchard nodes (enlargements of PIP joints; Fig. 38-2).

Radiographic assessment has long been considered the gold standard to diagnose OA and to establish severity of joint damage; to monitor disease activity, progression, and response to therapy; and to search for complications of the disorder or the treatment. Standard x-rays of affected joints show osteophytes, the most characteristic feature of OA, and, in more advanced disease, joint space narrowing and sclerosis. One method of classifying the severity of OA (with or without symptoms) is on a plain radiograph using the Kellgren–Lawrence (KL) grading scale. This overall joint scoring system, used extensively in research for more than five decades, grades OA in five levels from 0 (no osteophytes or joint space narrowing) to 4 (large osteophytes, severe joint space narrowing with subchondral sclerosis); generally, a grade of 2 is considered diagnostic of OA (Abramoff & Caldera, 2020; Nelson, 2021). MRI can be used to assess the quantity and function of cartilage, synovium, and bone. Arthroscopy is a more appropriate gold standard in the evaluation of OA, allowing direct visualization of cartilage surface integrity. Routine laboratory testing is rarely required and is primarily used to rule out other conditions, such as metabolic or inflammatory arthropathies. A positive C-reactive protein (CRP) and rheumatoid factors (RFs) can be found in low-grade inflammation in OA. Synovial fluid analysis can be done to differentiate OA from RA. According to the World Health Organization (WHO), biomarkers are an important aspect for clinical diagnosis and treatment for arthritis in general and OA research for drug development. Therefore, molecular biomarkers are currently being explored for clinical utility, such as urinary C-telopeptide fragments of type II collagen (u-CTXII). However, the lack of clinically validated biomarkers, in particular early OA biomarkers, hinders therapeutic advancements necessary to develop disease-modifying drugs (Hosnijeh et al., 2019).

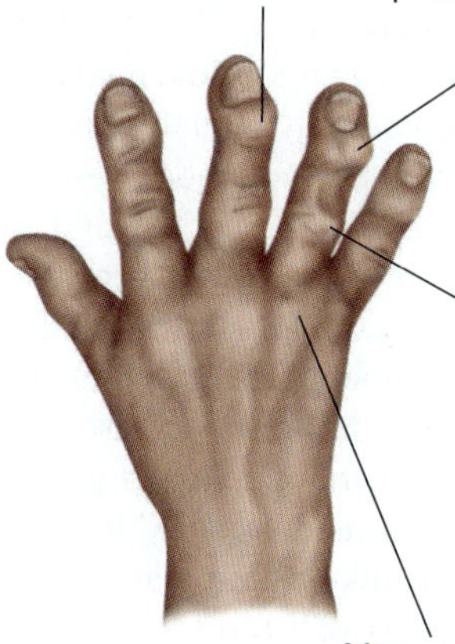

FIGURE 38-2 Heberden and Bouchard nodes. (From Bickley, L. S. [2009]. *Bates' guide to physical examination and history taking* [10th ed.]. Lippincott Williams & Wilkins.)

Medical and Nursing Management

No treatment halts the degenerative process of OA; as a result, management focuses on:

- educating patients about OA,
- reducing pain and inflammation,
- optimizing and maintaining physical function, and
- attempting to prevent or slow the progression of structural damage (Hunter & Bierma-Zeinstra, 2019).

Nonpharmacologic treatment measures mentioned earlier in the chapter are the core for OA management and should be maintained throughout the patient's course of the disease. Interventions mainly center around rest, joint protection, and heat application with some use of cold. CAM therapies for symptom management have become an increasingly popular avenue of treatment, particularly movement therapies (Bannuru et al., 2019; Brown, 2020; Kraus & Vincent, 2020; Misra et al., 2021; National Institute of Arthritis and Musculoskeletal and Skin [NIAMS], 2019). According to the 2019 ACR and Arthritis Foundation guidelines (Kolasinski et al., 2020; Pearson, 2020), strong recommendations were made for exercise; weight loss; self-efficacy and self-management programs; tai chi and canes; and orthoses; which are braces and other devices to correct alignment or provide support. The ACR recommends that the use of TENS and traditional Chinese acupuncture be reserved for patients who are candidates for total joint reconstructive surgery but are either unwilling to undergo the surgery or have medical contraindications to these procedures. In addition, a national public health intervention of preventing injuries, such as from falls, can help avoid OA later in life and can benefit from muscle strengthening and balance training (CDC, 2020b; Osteoarthritis Action Alliance, CDC, & Arthritis Foundation, 2020). Regarding nutritional supplements (e.g., glucosamine, often in combination with chondroitin), more research is needed because study findings on glucosamine are inconsistent as to the effectiveness of pain management in OA.

Pharmacologic therapy is used in conjunction with nonpharmacologic measures. It is important to obtain a complete blood count, chemistry panel including glucose and creatinine, and liver function tests before initiation of pharmacologic therapy for OA due to an increased risk for adverse events. In OA, the initial analgesic therapy has traditionally been acetaminophen (Tylenol), known as paracetamol (Panadol) in Europe and much of the world, with doses up to 1,000 mg four times daily (Shagroni et al., 2021). Recently a network meta-analysis showed that acetaminophen had a nearly null effect on pain symptoms and thus is no longer considered appropriate as a single agent for managing OA pain. However, for regular users of acetaminophen, total daily dose of 3 g and under is considered the maximal safe dose. Study results suggest that high doses (over 3,000 mg) place patients at risk for upper gastrointestinal (GI) complications and hepatic toxicity (Bannuru et al., 2019; Heimgartner, 2021; Misra et al., 2021; Primorac et al., 2021). To promote excretion of the drug, adequate water intake of at least 2,000 mL/day is encouraged.

Pearls for Practice

Nurses need to educate patients who are taking acetaminophen to avoid the concomitant use of alcohol and over-the-counter (OTC) products that contain acetaminophen, such as cold preparations and combination opioid analgesics such as Tylenol #3 (acetaminophen and codeine). Use of these substances simultaneously with acetaminophen can lead to the possibility of hepatic toxicity (Arthritis Foundation [AF], 2021; Heimgartner, 2021).

The ACR/AF OA guidelines recommend NSAIDs as the first line of therapy, preferably with topical use before oral for knee OA. If the patient is at risk for or experiences GI complications with an NSAID, supplemental treatment with a protective agent, such as misoprostol, or with the addition of a proton pump inhibitor (PPI), may be indicated. As an alternative to traditional NSAIDs, treatment with the cyclooxygenase (COX)-2 inhibitors celecoxib or etoricoxib may be considered in selected patients. The use of COX-2 inhibitors in the management of RA will be discussed later.

Other medications that may be considered are the opioids and topical analgesics, such as capsaicin and methyl salicylate. Another therapeutic approach is the intra-articular injection of hyaluronic acid, referred to as *viscosupplementation*. Viscosupplementation is used in patients with OA and is thought to act as a short-term lubricant and provide a biomechanical benefit as well as an analgesic effect by buffering synovial nerve endings directly; it also may have some anti-inflammatory effects, and it may stimulate synovial lining cells to produce hyaluronic acid, which acts like a lubricant and shock absorber in the joints.

However, modifying OA structural progression and symptomatic consequences has become a focus of drug development as well as epigenome-based therapeutics (the information encoded in the DNA sequence is modifiable in some way to regulate the levels of activity of specific genes). There are many compounds with potential disease-modifying effects in late stages of development that show promise (Grandi & Bhutani, 2020; Hunter & Bierma-Zeinstra, 2019).

For persistent, moderate-to-severe OA and erosive RA, reconstructive surgery and corticosteroids are used often. Reconstructive surgery is indicated when pain cannot be relieved by conservative measures and the threat of loss of independence is eminent. Surgical procedures include synovectomy (excision of the synovial membrane), arthrodesis (surgical fusion of the joint), tenorrhaphy (suturing of a tendon), and osteotomy (to alter the distribution of weight within the joint). The procedure used most is **arthroplasty**, surgical repair of the joint done through small incisions. If joint damage cannot be repaired, a joint replacement is needed. Surgery is not performed during disease flare-ups.

Tidal irrigation (lavage) and joint debridement of the knee involve the introduction of a large volume of saline into the joint through cannulas and then removal of debris with this fluid. In some cases, this procedure provides pain relief for up to 6 months. A new treatment for OA of the knee is autologous chondrocytes implantation (ACI), a procedure to repair injuries. It involves collecting cells that form cartilage from the patient's own joints, growing the cells in a laboratory, and then injecting the cultured cells into the patient's joint (Gerjo & van Osch, 2022). Approved by FDA in 2016, it is designed to grow new cartilage and improve symptoms.

Gout

Gout is now the most common inflammatory arthritis in the United States. Gout is a disease of both metabolism and inflammation. Its pathogenesis requires the intersection of two distinct processes; a metabolic disorder marked by the deposition of monosodium urate crystals within joints and other tissues and an inflammatory response to the crystals formed (Dehlin et al., 2020; Keenan et al., 2021). Gout is a heterogeneous group of conditions related to a genetic defect of purine metabolism that results in hyperuricemia (excessive uric acid, a purine end product). The prevalence of gout is reported to be less than 1% to 6.8%, and it appears to be on the rise. It occurs more commonly in males than in females, and the incidence of gout is less common in Asian and Hispanic individuals than in African-American and White individuals (Dalbeth, 2021, p. 1844). The general incidence increases with age, body mass index, and increasing levels of serum uric acid (urate) (Dalbeth, 2021; Dehlin et al., 2020). While hyperuricemia may indicate an increased risk of gout, the association between hyperuricemia and gout is unclear. Typically, the higher the uric acid level and longer the length of the elevation, the more likely that gout will occur, and tophi (deposits of uric acid) will form. On the other hand, some patients with hyperuricemia do not develop gout, and other patients with repeated gout attacks have normal or low levels of serum uric acid. Therefore, the exact level of uric acid that is considered pathologic is not yet known.

Pearls for Practice

The normal uric acid level is 3.4 to 7 mg/dL for males and 2.4 to 6 mg/dL for females. However, it is recommended that since a saturation point of 6.8 mg/dL is associated with urate crystals precipitation, levels should be lower. In hospitalized patients, an elevated uric acid level is a significant risk factor for acute kidney injury (AKI). The least common cause of the elevation is gout; thus, nurses monitor I&O and BUN and creatinine and report any deviation from the patient's baseline (Fischbach et al., 2022).

Primary gout is characterized by hyperuricemia caused by an overproduction of uric acid, a decreased urate excretion in the kidney, or a combination of the two mechanisms. However, less than 5% of patients with gout are hyperuricemia because of urate overproduction (Yokose & Choi, 2021). Often primary gout is caused by an inherited disorder in purine metabolism, with a 50% incidence (Choi, 2019; Keenan et al., 2021). Secondary gout is related to a wide number of diseases or drugs that decrease the kidney's ability to excrete uric acid, increase the production of uric acid, or a combination of both. Conditions associated with secondary gout include diabetic ketoacidosis, severe dieting or starvation, metabolic syndrome, and chronic kidney disease. Disorders such as multiple myeloma and leukemia result in increased production of uric acid because of a greater cell turnover and an increase in cell breakdown. Altered renal tubular function, either as a major action or as an unintended side effect of certain pharmacologic agents (e.g., diuretics such as thiazides and furosemide), low-dose salicylates, or ethanol, can contribute to uric acid underexcretion. An excessive intake of foods that are high in purines (shellfish, organ meats) may result in symptoms of gout in susceptible persons.

Pathophysiology

Hyperuricemia denotes an elevated level of uric acid (urate) in the blood, and in recent years it has been recognized that the reference ranges are quite wide. The laboratory reference ranges of hyperuricemia often are reported based on population norms, and values vary depending on the population being evaluated. To define individuals with hyperuricemia, current evidence-based reviews recommend that it is more clinically relevant to use the biologic value of 6.8 mg/dL or 408 μmol/L, a level of serum uric acid above the saturation point for crystal formation (Keenan et al., 2021; Yazdany & Manno, 2022a; Yokose & Choi, 2021). Asymptomatic hyperuricemia is a laboratory finding, not a disease, but it can lead to gout pathogenesis. Attacks of gout appear to be related to sudden increases or decreases of serum uric acid levels. When the uric acid precipitates and then deposits within a joint as urate crystals, an inflammatory response occurs, and an attack of gout begins. With repeated attacks, accumulations of sodium urate crystals, called **tophi**, are deposited in peripheral areas of the body, such as the great toe, the hands, and the ear (lower temperature areas). Renal urate lithiasis (kidney stones), with chronic renal disease secondary to urate deposition, may develop.

Clinical Manifestations and Assessment

Manifestations of the gout syndrome include acute gouty arthritis (recurrent attacks of severe articular and periarticular inflammation), tophi (crystalline deposits accumulating in articular tissue, osseous tissue, soft tissue, and cartilage), gouty nephropathy (renal impairment), and uric acid urinary calculi. Four phases (or stages) of gout can be identified: asymptomatic hyperuricemia, acute gouty arthritis, intercritical or interval gout, and chronic tophaceous gout (acute and intercritical gout together are sometimes noted as one phase). Phase 1, asymptomatic hyperuricemia, is when the serum urate level is high, but gout manifested by arthritis or nephrolithiasis has not yet occurred. People can remain asymptomatic throughout their lifetimes. The subsequent development of gout is directly related to the duration and magnitude of the hyperuricemia. Therefore, the commitment to lifelong pharmacologic treatment of hyperuricemia is deferred until there is an initial attack of gout (phase 2).

Acute arthritis is the most common early clinical manifestation of gouty arthritis. The patient experiences excruciating pain and inflammation in one or more small joints. The metatarsophalangeal (MTP) joint of the big toe is the joint affected most commonly (up to 90% of patients) and is referred to as **podagra** (Dalbeth, 2021; Schlesinger, 2019; Yazdany & Manno, 2022a). The tarsal area, ankle, or knee also may be affected. Less commonly, the wrists, fingers, and elbows may be affected. Trauma, alcohol ingestion, dieting, medications, surgical stress, or illness may trigger the acute attack (Fig. 38-3). The abrupt onset often occurs

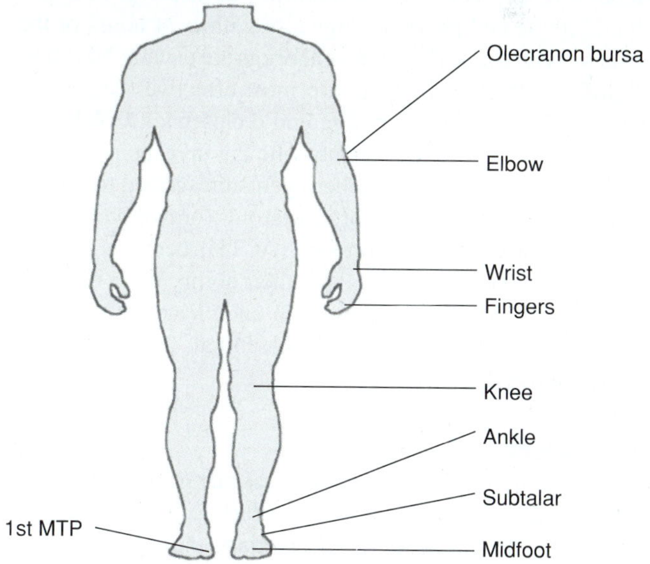

FIGURE 38-3 **Gout: common sites of involvement. MTP (metatarsophalangeal) or gout of the knee. (From Stoller, J. K., Nielsen, C., Buccola, J., & Brateanu, A. [2014]. *The Cleveland clinic foundation intensive review of internal medicine* [6th ed.]. Wolters Kluwer Health.)**

at night, awakening the patient with severe pain, redness, swelling, and warmth of the affected joint. Early attacks tend to subside spontaneously over 3 to 10 days even without treatment. The attack is followed by a symptom-free period (the intercritical stage or phase 3) until the next attack, which may not come for months or years. However, with time, attacks tend to occur more frequently, involve more joints, last longer, and lead to long-term sequelae (phase 4).

In general, tophi are associated with more frequent and severe inflammatory episodes. Higher serum concentrations of uric acid also are associated with more extensive tophus formation. Tophi most commonly occur in the synovium, olecranon bursa, subchondral bone, infrapatellar and Achilles' tendons, and subcutaneous tissue on the extensor surface of the forearms and overlying joints. Also, they have been found in the aortic walls, heart valves, nasal and ear cartilage, eyelids, cornea, and sclerae. Joint enlargement may cause a loss of joint motion. Uric acid deposits may cause kidney stones and kidney damage.

Imaging methods, such as ultrasound and dual energy CT scan, can assist with gout diagnosis. A definitive diagnosis of gouty arthritis is established by polarized light microscopy of the synovial fluid of the involved joint (Dalbeth, 2021; Yokose & Choi, 2021). Uric acid crystals are seen within the polymorphonuclear leukocytes in the fluid. Although the gold standard for diagnosis is correct identification of crystals, clinical impressions are most frequently used.

Medical Management

Treatment of gout is managed in two major phases: management of acute gouty inflammation and long-term management to prevent flare ups and to control hyperuricemia. According to recent ACR guidelines, an acute gout attack should be treated pharmacologically within 24 hours of the onset of symptoms. First-line oral drugs are usually NSAIDs. NSAIDs with short half-life are most effective (e.g., indomethacin, naproxen, ibuprofen, and diclofenac). Colchicine is currently reserved for patients who are unresponsive to or intolerant of safer agents. Other agents prescribed to relieve an acute attack of gout are corticosteroids (oral or parenteral) or adrenocorticotropic hormones (ACTH) because of their anti-inflammatory properties and their ability to be used for short periods of time, so long-term complications can generally be avoided (Burchum & Rosenthal, 2022; Dalbeth, 2021; Yokose & Choi, 2021).

Drug Alert

Selection of NSAIDs, colchicine, or corticosteroids is influenced by the patient's comorbid conditions (e.g., renal, cardiac, hepatic, or GI disease). Aging itself is an important risk factor. For instance, age-related decline in kidney function and the use of diuretics in older individuals are common risk factors for NSAID-induced renal injury.

Low-dose colchicine has been used for prophylaxis after resolution of attacks, but it does not prevent accumulation of tophi and urate in joints. Usually management of hyperuricemia, tophi, joint destruction, and kidney disorders is initiated after the acute inflammatory process has subsided. Three classes of agents may be used to lower the serum uric acid: xanthine oxidase inhibitors (allopurinol or febuxostat), uricosuric agents, and uricase (pegloticase). Allopurinol, a xanthine oxidase inhibitor, is considered the drug of choice for preventing the precipitation of an attack and tophi formation and for promoting the regression of existing tophi. Febuxostat is a nonpurine xanthine oxidase inhibitor that mimics the action of allopurinol and is an effective alternative for patients who experience severe reactions to allopurinol. Uricosuric agents, such as probenecid, correct hyperuricemia and stimulate renal urate excretion. Sulfinpyrazone is very similar to probenecid, but it is more potent and has been discontinued in the United States due to hepatic safety issues. Urolithiasis can occur as a side effect of uricosurics, and all patients should maintain a high fluid intake (2 L/day). Drugs that metabolize uric acid, such as rasburicase and pegloticase, are called *uricolytic agents*. Rasburicase is approved to decrease uric acid levels associated with malignancy and not for management of gout. The use of pegloticase, a new uricase, is reserved for refractory tophaceous gout. However, pegloticase carries an FDA black-box warning, advising to administer the drug only in health care settings and by health care professionals prepared to manage anaphylactic and other serious infusion reactions (Burchum & Rosenthal, 2022; Dalbeth et al., 2021; Shagroni et al., 2021; Terkeltaub, 2019; Yazdany & Manno, 2022a; Yokose & Choi, 2021).

When reduction of the serum urate level is indicated, uricosuric agents are the medications of choice. The recommended target goal of therapy is a serum uric acid level of less than 6 mg/dL, a level below the saturation point of 6.8 mg/dL at which urate crystals precipitate from solution (Fitzgerald et al., 2020; Shagroni et al., 2021; Yazdany & Manno, 2022a; Yokose & Choi, 2021). Current practice trends have shown that reducing and maintaining the serum uric acid levels result in crystal dissolution from joints, a reduction in gout attacks (flares), and the prevention or reduction in tophaceous deposits. If the patient has, or is at risk for, renal insufficiency or renal calculi (kidney stones), allopurinol is also effective at a lowered adjusted dose. New therapies for acute gout targeting interleukin-1 β blockage are currently under investigation and show promise for successful gout treatment. Canakinumab was approved by the FDA in 2011 and has been shown to extend the time to the next attack and reduce the frequency of subsequent attacks. Although not FDA approved, anakinra may be prescribed by health care providers for very severe attacks of gout (Dalbeth, 2021; Terkeltaub, 2019; Yokose & Choi, 2021). Corticosteroids may be used in patients who have no response to other therapy. If the patient experiences several acute episodes or there is evidence of tophi formation, prophylactic treatment is considered. Specific treatment is

TABLE **38-4 Medications Used to Treat Gout**

Medication	Actions and Use	Nursing Implications
Colchicine	Lowers the deposition of uric acid and interferes with leukocyte infiltration, thus reducing inflammation; does not alter serum or urine levels of uric acid; used in acute and chronic management	Second-line choice for treating gout flare; NSAIDs are recommended as first line *Acute management:* Administer colchicine when attack begins; dosage increased until pain is relieved or diarrhea develops Do not take with grapefruit juice
Probenecid	Uricosuric agent; inhibits renal reabsorption of urates and increases the urinary excretion of uric acid; prevents tophi formation	Recommended to take with food to lessen GI effects Risk of uric acid deposition in kidney; patient should ingest large volumes of fluids
Allopurinol, febuxostat	Inhibits xanthine oxidase; interrupts the breakdown of purines before uric acid is formed; inhibits xanthine oxidase because it blocks uric acid formation	Monitor for GI reactions (nausea, vomiting, diarrhea, and abdominal pain) and neurologic effects (drowsiness, headache, metallic taste) Serious adverse effects include bone marrow depression and hepatotoxicity
Pegloticase	Recombinant form of uric acid oxidase; pegloticase is an enzyme that converts uric acid to allantoin, a water-soluble compound that is readily excreted by the kidney	Monitor for infusion reactions, such as urticaria, dyspnea, chest discomfort, erythema, and pruritus Premedicate with an antihistamine and glucocorticoid Reactions usually occur within 2 hours after infusion

based on the serum uric acid level, 24-hour urinary uric acid excretion, and renal function. Table 38-4 lists the common medications used in treating gout.

Nursing Management

Pain management is the primary concern during the acute phase of an attack. The joint should be rested and elevated, and application of ice, not heat, may help with reducing discomfort. Keeping the bedclothes away from the affected joint using a "bed cage" if available can be of benefit. The management of the intercritical and chronic phases of gout involves teaching self-care measures to decrease the risk of attacks (e.g., avoidance of aspirin [because doses below 2 to 3 g/day impair renal excretion of uric acid retention and higher doses are associated with high renal excretion of uric acids], trauma, stress, alcohol, smoking) and to avoid long-term complications (e.g., importance of medication compliance). During the intercritical period, the patient feels well and may abandon preventive behaviors, which may result in an acute attack. Health care providers recommend that patients restrict consumption of foods high in purines, especially organ meats and shellfish; others believe that limiting protein foods such as red meats, lamb and pork or avoiding trigger foods are sufficient. Patients should be taught to limit alcohol intake; avoid fad starvation diets; and avoid sugary drinks and food that are high in fructose such as fructose corn syrup, sweetened soda, and processed foods. As fructose breaks down in the body, purines are released. The breakdown of purines produces uric acid, the substance that forms painful crystals in the joints and causes gout. Uric acid levels rise within minutes after drinking high fructose drinks. It is important that patients drink plenty of fluids, at least 2,000 mL daily, to avoid dehydration and lessen renal involvement and the development of urinary stones (Dalbeth, 2021; Fitzgerald et al., 2020; Yazdany & Manno, 2022a). Maintenance of normal body weight should be encouraged. Dietary vitamin C supplementation has been shown to reduce the risk of gout. Also, dietary restriction of sodium, fat, and cholesterol can lead to a reduction in gout symptoms and decrease effects associated with coexisting metabolic syndrome. Although research is limited, first acute gout attacks may commonly precede the diagnosis of metabolic abnormalities and associated diseases. Gout studies have shown to be associated with poorer physical health-related quality of life (HRQOL). Both gout-specific features (attack frequency and intensity, intercritical pain, and number of joints involved) and comorbid disease were associated with poor HRQOL in all domains. Therefore, success of lifelong treatment is dependent on the patient's commitment to treatment. Nurses need to explain lifestyle changes and drug management to the patient as they play a vital role in increasing treatment adherence and, therefore, considerable improvements in patient-centered outcomes. When compared with usual general practice care, studies have shown that nurse-led care was associated with higher adherence to medications and greater improvements in gout flares, tophi, physical function, and patient-reported gout impact (Dalbeth, 2021; Dalbeth et al., 2021).

Fibromyalgia

Fibromyalgia (FM) is a chronic syndrome characterized by widespread nonarticular musculoskeletal pain or multiple tender points lasting more than 3 months and other general symptoms, such as fatigue and sleep disturbances (NIAMS, 2021; Siracusa et al., 2021). The pain in FM is not due to tissue damage or inflammation; this makes it fundamentally different from other rheumatic disorders and many other pain conditions. The pathogenesis of FM is not well known, and the diagnosis is made clinically at present. To date, no objective tests or biomarkers demonstrate sufficient diagnostic accuracy. According to the 1990 ACR criteria, which specify 11 or more tender points, FM affects females more frequently than males (10:1 ratio). However, according to alternative ACR criteria for FM, females are only 2 times more likely than males to experience chronic widespread pain (CWP) (Clauw, 2019). The newer criteria established in 2010 do not require performing a tender point count, and they are recommended for clinical diagnosis versus the 1990 criteria intended for research. A hallmark of FM is that individuals display diffuse hyperalgesia (increased pain to normally painful stimuli) and/or allodynia (pain to normally nonpainful stimuli). This suggests that these individuals have a fundamental problem with central dysfunction (pain processing mechanisms) that results in central pain sensitization. These findings of centralization of pain have been corroborated by advanced neuroimaging techniques and appear to be due, in part, to imbalances in levels of neurotransmitters that affect pain and sensory transmission (Clauw, 2019; Crofford, 2021; Siracusa et al., 2021). The overall prevalence rate remains at 2% to 4% worldwide (ACR, 2021).

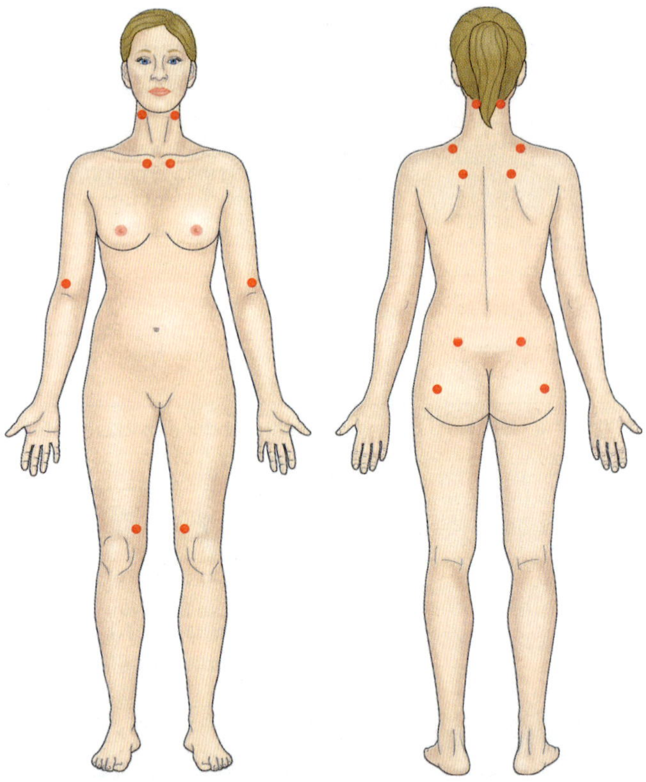

FIGURE 38-4 **Fibromyalgia tender points.**

Clinical Manifestations and Assessment

The core features of CWP and tenderness are almost invariably accompanied by a wide range of symptoms, the most common of which are sleep disturbances, fatigue, morning stiffness, muscle weakness, paresthesias, cognitive dysfunction ("fibro fog"), chronic headaches, mood disturbances, and irritable bowel syndrome (ACR, 2021; CDC, 2020c; Clauw, 2019; Crofford, 2019; Siracusa et al., 2021; Yazdany & Manno, 2022c). CWP is pain that typically is both above and below the waist on both sides of the body and involves the axial skeleton (neck, back, or chest). The patient complains of a widespread burning pain and often is unable to discriminate if pain occurs in the muscles, joints, or soft tissues. Physical examination typically reveals point tenderness at 11 or more of 18 identified sites characteristically described in ACR 1990 criteria (Fig. 38-4).

Medical Management

It is recommended to use symptom-based pharmacology therapy together with nonpharmacologic therapies. Paying attention to the specific symptoms reported by the patient is important. Patient education, exercise, and cognitive therapy, along with medication, are frequently used. The current standard of care for FM is to use a stepped care model where multiple therapies are layered atop one another to achieve meaningful improvement. It is suggested that health care professionals can do their best with combinations of nonpharmacologic and pharmacologic therapies using a joint decision-making approach that accounts for patient preferences and broadens the focus to more than pain (Mascarenhas et al., 2021; Silveira et al., 2021; Yazdany & Manno, 2022c). Refer to recent research in Box 38-5.

The pharmacotherapy of FM is mechanism-based; many have been tested to a greater or lesser extent. NSAIDs may be used to treat the diffuse muscle aching and stiffness. Tramadol is the only opiate shown to provide some relief. Many drugs have been used off-label to treat FM. Pregabalin, an analgesic, anxiolytic, and anticonvulsant ($\alpha_{2\text{-}\delta}$ receptor ligand agent) was the first to receive FDA approval for FM use. Psychotropic agents have been used to reduce pain centrally, even in the absence of depression; these include serotonin noradrenaline reuptake inhibitors or SNRIs (duloxetine, milnacipran), least selective serotonin reuptake inhibitors or SSRIs (fluoxetine, paroxetine), dopaminergic agents (pramipexole), and antidepressants, particularly tricyclics (Clauw, 2019; Crofford, 2021; Hagler et al., 2020a; Yazdany & Manno, 2022c). The two SNRIs, duloxetine and milnacipran, were shown to be effective and are approved by the FDA for symptom relief in FM. Also, tricyclic antidepressants in low doses can be used to improve or restore normal sleep patterns. Other drugs acting on the central nervous system also have been used or are under investigation (e.g., gabapentin was found to be effective and similar to pregabalin; cannabinoid use suggests modest efficacy). Individualized programs of exercise are used to decrease muscle weakness and discomfort and to improve the general deconditioning that occurs in affected patients. Meditative movements such as tai chi and yoga have been reported to be safe and effective for overall symptoms and physical functioning. In addition, neurostimulation therapies such as peripheral nerve stimulation (PNS), occipital nerve stimulation (ONS), etc., have found to be helpful, as has cognitive behavioral therapy (e.g., cognitive restructuring, behavioral training, mindfulness-based stress reduction, operant behavioral therapy). However, other nonpharmacologic therapies (e.g., massage, biofeedback, hydrotherapy, acupuncture) have been tested and found to have insufficient evidence to recommend their use for FM (Crofford, 2021).

Nursing Management

Typically, patients with FM have endured their symptoms for a long period of time. They may feel as if their symptoms have not been taken seriously. Nurses need to undertake a holistic assessment to identify the influence of any factors on the pain experienced and management strategies. The assessment should include the following:

- Beliefs and thoughts about the cause of the condition. Talking about how the pain started can lead to shared insight and provide direction for management strategies.
- Level of functional activity. FM has been associated with lower levels of health-related quality of life and more work productivity loss (CDC, 2020c).
- Mood status. The nurse should help the patient identify existing psychological stressors that are having an adverse effect on the pain experienced.
- Sleep patterns. If pain is interfering with the quality of sleep, the patient will often awaken unrefreshed and experience difficulties with cognitive functioning, including concentration, sentence formation, and memory recall.
- Patient's role. The nurse should assess if the patient is experiencing emotional or physical difficulties in the workplace or the family setting (Rose et al., 2020).

Nurses need to pay special attention to supporting these patients and providing encouragement as they begin their program of therapy. The goal of FM treatment is to improve the physical and mental health of patients and their quality of life. Interventions or strategies should be developed to promote better functioning. Greater education, lower-intensity fatigue, and using aerobic or strength training exercises were predictors of physical functioning (Winser et al., 2020). Other studies suggest that a large proportion of FM patients use complementary and alternative medicine (e.g., tai chi, yoga, meditation), and found these treatments offer beneficial effects to these patients such as higher quality of life and self-reported lower pain levels (Cheng et al., 2019; Prabhakar et al., 2019; Pfalzgraf et al., 2020). Nurses need to work with patients to increase independence, avoiding complications of deconditioning, work disability, and the inability to fulfill social roles. In addition, self-reported or perceived fatigue is associated with the incidence of falls or risk of falling among older adults (Pana et al., 2021); this supports the belief that stretching, aerobic exercise, and strength training should be in every patient's exercise plan.

Pearls for Practice

Nurses should focus on patient safety. Nurses caring for people with FM should assess for potential risk factors of falling and offer plans for individualized fall-prevention strategies. One of the Joint Commission (JC) 2022 National Patient Safety Goals for the Nursing Care Center Program aims at reducing the risk of falls. The JC recommends a patient evaluation include fall history; review of medications and alcohol consumption; gait and balance screening; assessment of walking aids, assistive technologies, and protective devices; and environmental assessments.

Motivational interviewing (MI) is a patient-centered approach that nurses can use to promote behavioral changes (see the Nursing Process section later in the chapter). Meta-analysis of studies using MI delivered in brief consultations showed efficacy in medical settings for a wide range of behavioral issues, such as exercise, self-management of pain, and medication adherence (Jamil et al., 2021; Kinnett-Hopkins et al., 2022; Pas & Bradshaw, 2021). MI can be helpful when the patient is considering making a change. Thirty years of evidence has shown the efficacy of MI across a variety of conditions (Lianov, 2020). Other management approaches include patient support groups and the use of meditation, prayer, and other spiritual practices. Reflective listening to patients' descriptions of their concerns and symptoms is essential to helping patients make the changes that are necessary to improve their quality of life (Vowell, 2020b).

DIFFUSE CONNECTIVE TISSUE DISEASES

Rheumatic disorders with diffuse inflammation and degeneration in the connective tissues are referred to as *connective tissue diseases*. These disorders share similar clinical features and may affect some of the same organs. The characteristic clinical course is one of exacerbations and remissions. Although the diffuse connective tissue diseases have unknown causes, they are thought to be the result of immunologic abnormalities in which the immune system loses its ability to tell the difference between foreign invaders and the body's normal cells. The common connective tissue diseases RA, systemic lupus erythematosus (SLE), and scleroderma are presented in detail.

Rheumatoid Arthritis

RA is the most common inflammatory arthritic disorder and serves as a prototype for the study of many inflammatory and immune-mediated diseases. RA affects 1% of the general population worldwide, with a female-to-male ratio of 3:1. RA can begin at any age, but the peak is in the fourth or fifth decade for females and the sixth to eighth decades for males (DiBaise & Kohn, 2021; Veale et al., 2021; Yazdany & Manno, 2022d). The gold standard for the classification of RA was the 1987 American College of Rheumatology (ACR) criteria. This was designed for application in clinical research studies only and not for clinical diagnosis. A definition that is uniform, incorporates clinical characteristics, and has a high sensitivity and specificity for classifying patients with RA was needed. Thus, the 2010 RA classification criteria were developed collaboratively by the ACR and the European League Against Rheumatism (EULAR). It is currently the standard for RA disease classification, which includes presence of preclinical phase serum autoantibodies, and provides a framework for accurate diagnosis of early RA (Brasington & Miner, 2019; Deane, 2019; Liao, 2019).

Pathophysiology

A variety of predetermined genes (e.g., human leukocyte antigens [HLA]), random events, and environmental (e.g., pathogens, smoking) factors contribute to RA susceptibility and pathogenesis. In RA, numerous cell types are involved, including macrophages, T cells, B cells, fibroblasts, chondrocytes (cells found in cartilage connective tissue that maintain tissue homeostasis), and dendritic cells (a special type of immune cell that boosts antigen-presenting white blood cells found in bone marrow or lymph-derived leukocytes [they are not nerve cells; the term relates to their shape, "tree-like"]). The autoimmune reaction primarily occurs in the synovial tissue. Adaptive and innate immune responses in the synovium have been implicated in the pathogenesis of RA. RF antibodies against immunoglobulin G (IgG) develop in the synovium to form immune complexes. The activation of the complement system and release of lysosomal enzymes from leukocytes leads to inflammation. It is unknown why the body produces an antibody (RF) against its own antibody (IgG) and, in consequence, transforms IgG to an antigen or foreign protein that must be destroyed. Phagocytosis produces enzymes (proinflammatory cytokines such as interleukin [IL]-1, interleukin-6 [IL-6], and tumor necrosis factor [TNF]) within the joint. These cytokines are the primary factors that drive the inflammatory response in RA. The enzymes (especially cytokines) break down collagen, causing edema; proliferation of the synovial membrane; and, ultimately, formation of **pannus** (Fig. 38-5). Pannus, formation of vascular granulation tissue, is a characteristic of RA that differentiates it from other forms of inflammatory arthritis. Pannus has a destructive effect on the adjacent

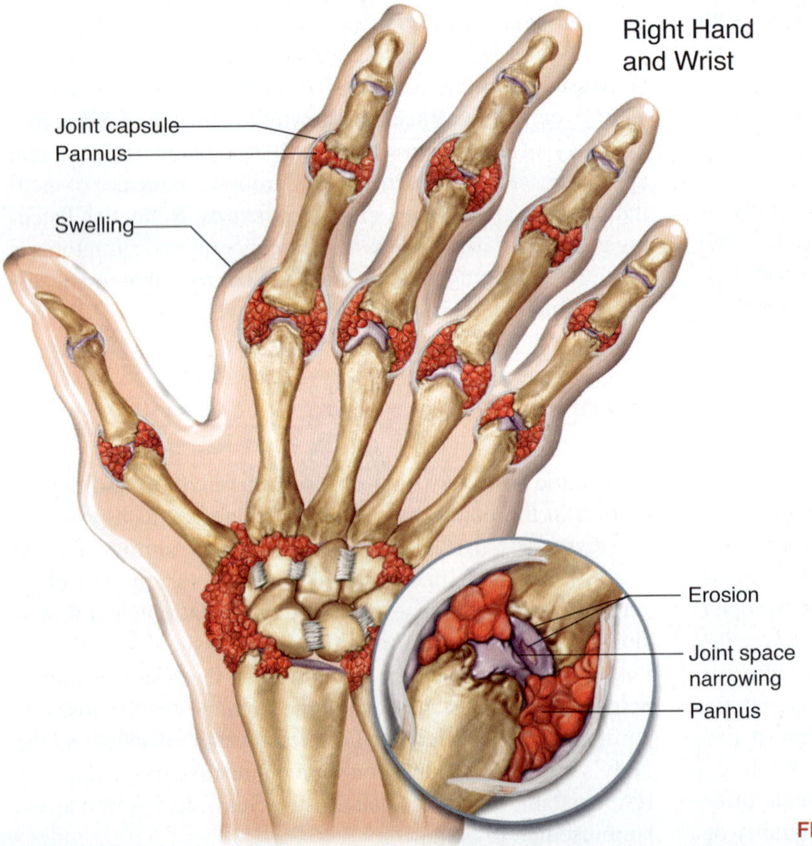

FIGURE 38-5 **Joints affected by rheumatoid arthritis.**

cartilage and bone. If the response is not suppressed, the disease progresses and the consequences are loss of articular surfaces and joint motion. Muscle fibers also undergo degenerative changes. Tendon and ligament elasticity and contractile power are lost.

Clinical Manifestations and Assessment

Clinical manifestations of RA vary, usually reflecting the stage and severity of the disease. Physical signs of RA are associated with the pathophysiology of the disease. The manifestations of RA can be categorized as early or late disease and as articular (joint) or extra-articular. Joint pain, swelling, warmth, erythema (redness), and lack of function are classic symptoms. Palpation of the joints reveals spongy or boggy tissue. Often, fluid can be aspirated from the inflamed joint. The hallmark of RA is synovial proliferation and tenderness in multiple joints, particularly in the small joints of the hands, wrists, and feet. As the disease progresses, the knees, shoulders, hips, elbows, ankles, cervical spine, and temporomandibular joints are affected. In addition to joint pain and swelling, a cardinal sign of inflammatory arthritis that can appear even before pain is morning stiffness lasting for more than an hour (Brasington & Miner, 2019; England & Mikuls, 2021).

Deformities of the hands and feet are common in RA (Fig. 38-6). Often the PIP and metacarpophalangeal (MCP) joints of the hands are involved initially. The deformity may be caused by misalignment resulting from swelling, progressive joint destruction, or the subluxation (partial dislocation) that occurs when one bone slips over another and eliminates the joint space.

RA is a systemic disease with multiple extra-articular features. Most common are fever, weight loss, fatigue, anemia, lymph node enlargement, and Raynaud phenomenon (cold- and stress-induced vasospasm causing episodes of digital blanching or cyanosis). Extra-articular disease manifestations occur in about 40% of patients at some time in the course of the disease (Myasoedova et al., 2019). Rheumatoid nodules may be noted in patients with more advanced RA in about 20% of patients (Brasington & Miner, 2019). These nodules are usually nontender and movable in the subcutaneous tissue. They usually appear over bony prominences, most often on extensor surfaces or pressure points, such as the elbow; are varied in size; and can disappear spontaneously. Nodules occur only in people positive for RF. The nodules often are associated with rapidly progressive and destructive disease. Other extra-articular features include arteritis (inflammation of the walls of arteries), neuropathy, scleritis (inflammation of the sclera), pericarditis, splenomegaly, and Sjögren syndrome (dry eyes and dry mucous membranes).

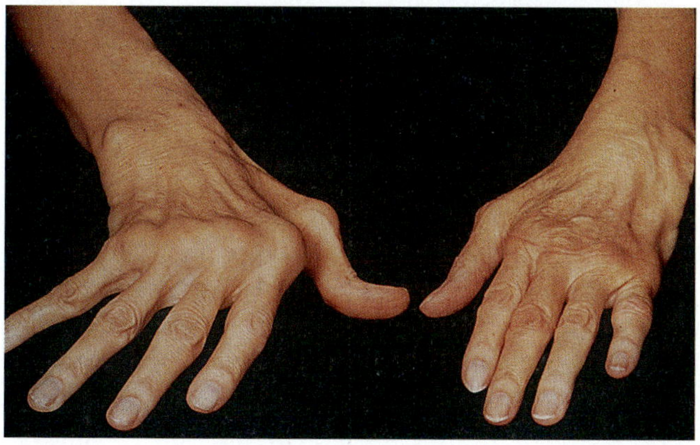

FIGURE 38-6 Deformity to the hands caused by rheumatoid arthritis.

A clinical examination of all synovial joints should be undertaken for evidence of tenderness, swelling, and range of movement. Evidence for synovitis should be seen by a rheumatologist, ideally within 6 weeks after the onset of symptoms, to facilitate early diagnosis and clinical management and to achieve optimal outcomes for patients (Brasington & Miner, 2019; DiBaise & Kohn, 2021; England & Mikuls, 2021). Presence of deformities, such as hyperextension of PIP joints (swan neck), flexion of PIP joints (Boutonniere), and ulnar deviation, in which fingers point toward the ulna, may be noted on examination. The patient is also assessed for extra-articular changes, such as weight loss, sensory changes, lymph node enlargement, and fatigue (Mills, 2021).

Pearls for Practice

Patients commonly have the inability to "wring out a washcloth," need to hold a cup with both hands, and may complain of the sensation of having a "stone in my shoe."

According to the ACR/EULAR 2010 RA classification criteria, in addition to active synovitis in at least one joint that cannot be better explained by another diagnosis, additional criteria added include positivity for antibodies to citrullinated proteins (ACPAs or anti-CCP) and abnormal levels of inflammatory markers, such as ESR and CRP levels. RF is present in up to 70% to 80% of patients with RA, but its presence alone is not diagnostic of RA. Anticyclic citrullinated peptide (anti-CCP) is a marker that has similar sensitivity but potentially greater specificity to RF (Abdulkhaliq & Alotaibi, 2021; Brasington & Miner; 2019; Deane, 2019; DiBaise & Kohn, 2021; Feist & Burmester, 2019; Gravallese & Monach, 2019; Liao, 2019). Some laboratories are currently doing a second generation of the test, called the CCP2 assay. The RBC count and complement C3 and C4 levels are decreased. Complements may be decreased as they are "used up" in some antigen-antibody reactions. Results of antinuclear antibody (ANA), the screening test for autoantibodies (antibodies that form against self), also may be positive. **Arthrocentesis** shows abnormal synovial fluid that is cloudy, milky, or dark yellow and contains numerous inflammatory components, such as leukocytes and complement. The enzyme MMP-3 is increased in the synovial fluid of the patient with RA, and it may be a marker of progressive joint damage. Synovial biopsy can detect inflammatory cells associated with RA. Radiologic studies are not specifically diagnostic in the early stages of RA; however, they do show characteristic bony erosions and narrowed joint spaces occurring later in the disease and help in monitoring the progression of disease and effectiveness of treatment.

Medical and Nursing Management

Drugs remain the cornerstone of RA treatment. Joint inflammation is the main driver of joint damage and is the most important cause of functional disability in the early stages of disease; thus, changes in the therapeutic landscape in RA are seen. Today, treatment is more aggressive. The treatment paradigm changed to adopt a "patient-centered" and "treat-to-target" approach aiming at disease remission. Current guidelines recommend starting a course of DMARDs early, within 3 months of RA diagnosis to delay joint degeneration. DMARDs work in diverse ways by modifying the immune system's inflammatory response. It has been found that management of RA early, in the first 12 weeks of symptoms (referred to as a therapeutic "window of opportunity"), might prevent persistent disease (Buch & Nam, 2019; Burchum & Rosenthal, 2022). NSAIDs provide fast relief of symptoms but do not prevent joint damage or slow disease progression. Because the effects of DMARDs take weeks or months to develop, whereas the effects of NSAIDs are immediate, an NSAID is given until the DMARD has had time to act.

The use of traditional NSAIDs (salicylates and nonsalicylates) inhibits the production of prostaglandins and provides anti-inflammatory effects as well as analgesia. Effectiveness, side effects, cost, and dosing schedules are considered in the selection of an NSAID. The incidence of adverse reactions (e.g., gastric irritation, kidney damage, changes in liver function) to the NSAIDs increases with age and long-term use. A second-generation NSAID, the COX-2 inhibitor, has been shown to inhibit inflammatory processes, but it does not inhibit the protective prostaglandin synthesis in the GI tract. Therefore, patients who are at increased risk for GI complications, especially GI bleeding, have been managed effectively with COX-2 inhibitors.

Drug Alert

COX-2 inhibitors such as celecoxib and etoricoxib must be used with caution because of the associated risk of cardiovascular (CV) disease including cardiovascular thromboembolism, myocardial infarction, or stroke. It is recommended the lowest effective dose for the shortest possible duration is used since the increased CV risk is consistently observed at higher doses.

The DMARDs can be subdivided into three categories: conventional (traditional nonbiologic) DMARDs, biologic DMARDs, and targeted DMARDs. The conventional nonbiologic agent, methotrexate, is one of the first-choice DMARDs and has become the drug of choice due to its potency and time of action (faster than all other DMARDs). Therapeutic effects or improvement may develop in 3 to 6 weeks, compared to other DMARDs, which can take 3 to 4 months to work (Burchum & Rosenthal, 2022). A black-box warning exists for unexpected, severe, and sometimes fatal myelosuppression; aplastic anemia (see Chapter 19); and GI toxicity reported with methotrexate (usually high dose) in combination with some NSAIDs. In addition, methotrexate is teratogenic (capable of causing birth defects); therefore, a pregnancy test should be performed if a decision is made to begin treatment in a patient who can become pregnant. Finally, methotrexate does not cause direct renal toxicity; however, since it is primarily excreted via the kidneys, if a patient has impaired renal function (beyond CKD stage 3) they require dose adjustment (Jayatilleke, 2021).

Pearls for Practice

Nurses should alert patients that taking extra doses of methotrexate is dangerous. The drug is administered weekly or twice a week. Nurses need to encourage feedback to ensure that the patient understands the weekly dosing schedule and that the medication should not be used "as needed" for symptom control. (Institute for Safe Medication Practices [ISMP]; www.ismp.org)

Another preferred conventional nonbiologic DMARD, hydroxychloroquine, a drug with antimalarial actions, can be initiated early and used with mild symptoms, but as a rule it is used in combination with methotrexate. By itself, hydroxychloroquine does not slow disease progression; however, early use can improve long-term outcomes.

Leflunomide, a nonbiologic small-molecule DMARD, is a relatively new and powerful immunosuppressant used for patients with RA. Compared with methotrexate, leflunomide is about equally as effective but more dangerous because of the incidence of liver failure; it is reserved for second-line use. Other minor nonbiologic DMARDs, cyclosporine, gold salts, penicillamine, and azathioprine, have been available for many years. These have been used frequently in the past, but their use today is limited. The drugs are generally reserved for patients with severe, progressive RA disease whose RA has not responded to safer DMARDs.

Biologic agents (also referred as *immunomodulators*) are expensive, whereas the conventional nonbiologic small-molecule DMARDs cost much less and are easier to manufacture.

Biologic drugs can be categorized based on their mechanism of action; they target specific components of the inflammatory process. They can be used to treat patients with moderate-to-severe disease that has not responded to DMARDs or in combination therapy with an established DMARD, such as methotrexate. Some biologic agents or modifiers interfere with the action of TNF: etanercept, infliximab, and adalimumab. Most recently, golimumab and certolizumab pegol have been approved for use in RA. The immunosuppressant actions of TNF inhibitors can increase the patient's risk of serious infections, including bacterial sepsis, invasive fungal infection, and tuberculosis. As a result, prior to initiation of TNF inhibitors, patients should be tested for tuberculosis. A different biologic agent, anakinra, interferes with IL-1, which modulates immune and inflammatory responses and thus has efficacy with rheumatic disorders. Like the TNF inhibitors, anakinra poses a risk of serious infections; therefore, anakinra should not be used in combination with TNF inhibitors.

Pearls for Practice

Do not give live vaccines to patients on a biologic agent. Nurses need to monitor for signs of infection (e.g., fever, cough, flu-like symptoms, open sores on body). Also, nurses should monitor for heart failure in patients on etanercept or infliximab.

The emerging agents show that a new era in treatment has begun, newly targeting B lymphocyte cells, T-cell activation, and IL-6. These constitute new principles for interference with the disease process (Burchum & Rosenthal, 2022; Choquette et al., 2021; MacDougall & Bathon, 2019; Radu & Bungau, 2021). Tofacitinib, also a type of DMARD, is the first oral medication in a new class of treatments called Janus kinase (JAK) inhibitors and is FDA approved for moderate-to-severe RA in which methotrexate did not work well. As most biologics fight inflammation from outside the cell, the JAK inhibitor works deep inside the cell to disrupt activities occurring in signaling pathways. These JAK pathways are believed to be involved in the production of cytokines and in the inflammation of RA (Angelini et al., 2020; Choquette et al., 2021; Fragoulis et al., 2019; Singh & Singh, 2020).

The third major group of antiarthritic drugs is the glucocorticoids (adrenal corticosteroids). These are powerful anti-inflammatory drugs used in RA especially during exacerbations ("flare ups") of the disease or when needing a "bridging" medication while waiting for the slower DMARDs (e.g., methotrexate) to begin taking effect. Oral glucocorticoids, such as prednisone and prednisolone, are indicated for patients with generalized symptoms. Long-term therapy can cause serious toxicity (e.g., osteoporosis, gastric ulceration, adrenal suppression, diabetes), so glucocorticoids should be limited to patients with RA that has not responded adequately to all other treatment options. Intra-articular injections, commonly used in severe RA, may be employed if only one or two joints are affected. Antibiotics, the tetracycline derivatives minocycline and doxycycline, are given to improve symptoms (morning stiffness, joint pain and tenderness) and enhance ADL in patients with RA. These antibiotics have been found to decrease the action of enzymes on cartilage degradation. Usage is seen in patients who have not responded to DMARDs.

The *Prosorba Column*, a blood filtration device used in apheresis, has been approved by the FDA for use in treating patients with more severe and longstanding RA who have had no response to or are intolerant of DMARDs. The device, a protein A immunoadsorption column, is used in 12-weekly 2-hour apheresis treatments to bind IgG (i.e., circulating immune complex). As the patient's blood passes through the column, RF is removed.

Drug Alert

If the patient is on an angiotensin-converting enzyme (ACE) inhibitor, it should be discontinued prior to treatment using Prosorba Column, as the risk of serious hypotension exists with this treatment.

Through all stages of RA, depression and sleep deprivation may require the short-term use of low-dose antidepressant medications, such as amitriptyline, paroxetine, or sertraline, to reestablish an adequate sleep pattern and to manage chronic pain. Patient education should be considered as an effective nonpharmacologic intervention in improving clinical outcomes and psychological status in patients with RA. A self-management program that focuses on joint protection and physical activities has shown improvement in physical functioning, self-efficacy, and self-management behaviors (Shao et al., 2021; Wu et al., 2022). Furthermore, adults with RA are at high risk of falls and fall-related injuries. Strategies to prevent falls should be implemented (Meyer et al., 2021; Mikos et al., 2020; Muhammad et al., 2021; Stanmore et al., 2021; Wiegmann et al., 2022).

Systemic Lupus Erythematosus

SLE is a chronic inflammatory multisystem autoimmune disease with variable presentations, courses, and prognoses characterized by remissions and exacerbations. National incidence data are difficult to obtain because SLE onset is difficult to determine along with other factors such as lack of a singular diagnostic test, racial/ethnic disparities in SLE susceptibility and mortality, and differing case definitions. The Lupus Foundation of America estimates that 1.5 million Americans have one of the four forms of lupus. The CDC funded five population-based registries to study U.S. populations diagnosed with SLE or discoid lupus. A meta-analysis from the CDC found the pooled prevalence of SLE from 4 state-specific registries was 72.8 per 100,000 person-years. Also, an overall prevalence of approximately 200,000 people in the United States meet the ACR 1997 revised classification criteria for SLE. The number of cases was generated by applying sex/race-stratified estimates to the 2018 U.S. Census population (Dall'Era & Wofsy, 2021; Izmirly et al., 2021; Liebowitz, 2021). Occurrence peaks up to 10 to 15 times more frequently in females than in males (predominantly during the childbearing years), and Black individuals and Hispanic individuals are affected more frequently than are White individuals. The American Indian/Alaska Native population had the highest race-specific SLE estimates, among both females and males (Izmirly et al., 2021).

Pathophysiology

SLE is a result of disturbed immune regulation that causes an exaggerated production of autoantibodies and antigens. The immune abnormalities that characterize SLE occur in five phases: susceptibility (genes and environmental factors), abnormal innate and adaptive immune responses, autoantibodies immune complexes, inflammation, and damage. Interactions of predisposing factors (genes, female sex, and environment) result in abnormal immune responses, specifically in B cells and T cells. These responses produce pathogenic autoantibodies and immune complexes that activate complement, form in tissue, and cause inflammation. Inflammation stimulates antigens, which, in turn, stimulate additional antibodies. The cycle repeats and, over time, leads to irreversible organ damage. Some individuals do not progress through all phases (Gupta & Kaplan, 2019).

Drug Alert

Certain medications, such as hydralazine, procainamide, isoniazid, chlorpromazine, and some antiseizure medications, can trigger an exaggerated immune response and cause a chemical- or drug-induced SLE.

Clinical Manifestations and Assessment

The onset of SLE may be insidious or acute. For this reason, SLE may remain undiagnosed for many years. The most common presenting manifestations are constitutional symptoms (fever, fatigue, and/or weight loss), cutaneous manifestations, and articular manifestations (arthritis and/or arthralgia). Each of these manifestations appears to be present in at least 50% of patients with lupus at the time of diagnosis (Dall'Era, 2021; Dall'Era & Wofsy, 2021; Yazdany & Manno, 2022f). SLE is an autoimmune systemic disease that can affect any body system. Clinical manifestations can resemble RA and may be mistaken for it, especially early in the course of the disease. Unlike RA, the arthritis is nonerosive and not seen on x-ray.

Several different types of skin manifestations are prevalent in 80% to 90% of patients with SLE. Photosensitivity rashes are most common; however, the most characteristic skin manifestation is an acute cutaneous lesion consisting of a butterfly-shaped rash across the bridge of the nose and cheeks (Dall'Era, 2021; Dall'Era & Wofsy, 2021; Hagler et al., 2020c; Wallace & Weisman, 2019; Fig. 38-7). This malar rash manifests as an erythematous, flat or raised lesion; is pruritic (itchy) or painful; and can be transient and heal without scarring. In some cases of discoid lupus erythematosus (DLE), only skin involvement occurs. Discoid (coinlike) lesions are scarring and ring-shaped lesions that may result in erythematous, scaling plaques, and alopecia (hair loss). In some patients with SLE, the initial skin involvement is the precursor to more systemic involvement. The lesions often worsen during exacerbations (flares) of the systemic disease and possibly are provoked by sunlight or artificial ultraviolet B light.

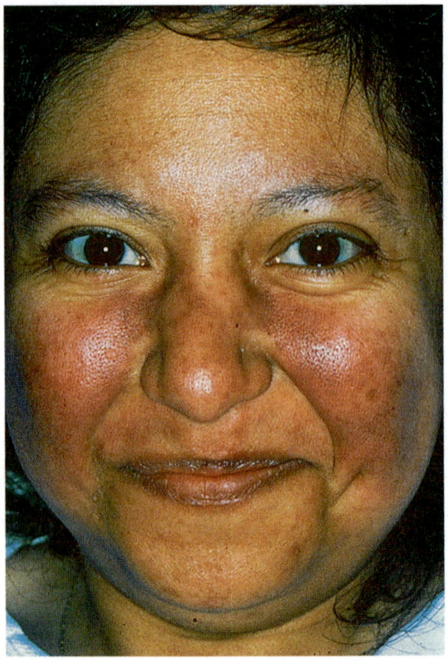

FIGURE 38-7 The characteristic butterfly rash of systemic lupus erythematosus.

Pearls for Practice

The nurse should teach patients to avoid sunlight or ultraviolet (UV) exposure and to protect themselves with clothing and sunscreen with at least a sun protection factor (SPF) of 30.

Central nervous system involvement is widespread, encompassing the entire range of neurologic disease (60% prevalence). The varied and frequent neuropsychiatric presentations of SLE are now widely recognized. In general, these are demonstrated by subtle changes in behavior patterns or cognitive ability. Headaches, psychiatric disorders (mood disorder, depression, and psychosis), cognitive dysfunction, and seizures are the most frequent manifestations, although only psychosis and seizures are included in the ACR criteria for SLE (Hagler et al., 2020c; Wallace & Weisman, 2019).

Pericarditis (inflammation or infiltration of the pericardium) and pleuritis (inflammation of the pleura) are the most common cardiopulmonary disorders (refer to Chapters 9 and 15). Females who have SLE are also at risk for early atherosclerosis. Kidney involvement is one of the more serious manifestations and is associated with increased morbidity and mortality. Serum creatinine levels and urinalysis are used in screening, and early detection allows for prompt treatment so that kidney damage can be prevented. Kidney involvement may lead to hypertension, which also requires careful monitoring and management.

Diagnosis of SLE is based on a complete history, physical examination, and diagnostic tests. SLE has an extreme range of clinical manifestations without classic presentation. Diagnosis is made difficult by the variable manifestations of the disease and relies on the overall clinical picture with the correlation of diagnostic laboratory and imaging studies, possibly including skin biopsy.

The presence of at least four of the criteria established by the ACR is required to make the diagnosis of SLE. Cutaneous manifestations comprise 4 of the 11 diagnostic ACR criteria (malar rash, discoid rash, photosensitivity, and oral ulcers). When performing an assessment, it is critical to inspect skin for erythematous rashes. The nurse asks the patient about the existence of photosensitivity, fatigue, oral ulcers, or pain in joints. In addition, systemic involvement may encompass several organ systems; therefore, the nurse must review laboratory values or findings that might suggest that the effects of inflammation are targeting organs (e.g., ESR, complete blood count—anemia or thrombocytopenia, creatinine, hematuria).

No single laboratory test confirms SLE. Laboratory features include both hematologic abnormalities (e.g., hemolytic anemia, leukopenia, thrombocytopenia) and immunologic findings indicative of autoimmunity. Most patients with SLE (more than 98%) demonstrate elevated serum levels of antinuclear antibodies (ANA), which is another ACR criterion for SLE diagnosis (see Table 38-1). A small percent of patients will test negative for ANA. More recently, enzyme-linked immunosorbent assays (ELISA) containing a mixture of nuclear antigens are being used to detect ANA; these have lower sensitivity for the detection of ANA than the Hep-2 technique. A negative ANA by ELISA should be repeated on a Hep-2 cell line to increase the sensitivity of the test (Dall'Era, 2021). Other diagnostic immunologic tests that support SLE diagnosis in the presence of clinical manifestations are CRP, anti–double-stranded DNA (anti-ds DNA; 95% specificity for SLE but lack sensitivity), anti-RNA, anti-La (SSB), anti-Sm (Smith; 99% specificity for SLE but lack sensitivity) or antiphospholipid antibodies, and high-titer IgG antibodies. The double-stranded DNA test, C3, and C4 indicate whether there is a genetic component that is common in patients with SLE (Dall'Era & Wofsy, 2021; Feist & Burmester, 2019; Feldman & Costenbader, 2019; Yazdany & Manno, 2022f).

Pearls for Practice: Sensitivity Versus Specificity

Sensitivity of a laboratory test reveals how often a test is positive in those who actually have a particular disease (e.g., 100% sensitivity correctly identifies every person who has a disease), whereas specificity of a laboratory test reveals how often the test is negative in patients who do not have the disease (e.g., 100% specificity correctly identifies every person who does not have the disease).

Medical and Nursing Management

SLE can be life threatening; however, advances in its treatment have led to improved survival and reduced morbidity. Treatment of SLE includes management of acute and chronic disease. The goals of treatment include preventing progressive loss of organ function, reducing the likelihood of acute disease, minimizing disease-related disabilities, and preventing complications from therapy. Management of SLE involves regular monitoring to assess disease activity and therapeutic effectiveness.

The mainstay of SLE treatment is based on pain management and nonspecific immunosuppression. Therapy includes NSAIDs; DMARDs (including antimalarials) alone or in combination with glucocorticoids (a class of corticosteroids); and, in severe SLE cases, immunosuppressive agents (azathioprine, mycophenolate mofetil, methotrexate). Hydroxychloroquine has a central role for long-term treatment. A number of medications have recently been made available. In 2011, the biologic belimumab became the first FDA-approved drug for treatment of mild-to-moderate SLE, and anifrolumab, a monoclonal antibody, was approved in July 2021 for the treatment of SLE (Liebowitz, 2021; Yazdany & Manno, 2022f).

Corticosteroids are the single most important medication available for SLE. These drugs are used topically for cutaneous manifestations, in low oral doses for minor disease activity, and in high doses for major disease activity. IV administration of corticosteroids is an alternative to traditional high-dose oral use (Fanouriakis et al., 2021; Khosroshahi & Lim, 2021). Important risk factors associated with the use of corticosteroids are osteoporosis and fractures (refer to Table 30-8 for side effects of corticosteroid therapy). Corticosteroid toxicity is a major problem, and tapering of the dosage is a primary concern. Treatment of moderate-to-severe SLE consists of a period of intensive immunosuppressive therapy (induction therapy) followed by a longer period of less intensive maintenance therapy. The main objective of the induction therapy is to stop injury, recover function, and induce remission by managing immunologic activity. The combination of high-dose glucocorticoids with pulses of intravenous cyclophosphamide (CYC), a cytotoxic agent, remains the standard of care for severe SLE with major organ involvement. B-cell–depleting therapies, such as the monoclonal antibodies rituximab and epratuzumab (humanized anti-CD22 antibody), are reserved for patients who have serious forms of SLE that have not responded to conservative therapies.

Nurses also need to be sensitive to the psychological reactions of the patient with SLE. Patient education and emotional support are especially important. The disease or its treatment may produce dramatic changes in appearance and considerable distress for the patient. The changes and unpredictable course of SLE necessitate expert assessment skills and nursing care.

Scleroderma

Scleroderma ("hard skin") is a relatively rare disease that is poorly understood; the cause is unknown. Potential triggers include genetic factors and exposure to certain environmental and occupational agents (e.g., silica dust, heavy metals, polyvinyl chloride) and drugs (e.g., bleomycin, cocaine, fenfluramine appetite suppressants), infection, and human cytomegalovirus (CMV) and other viruses (Varga, 2021; Wigley & Boin, 2021). Scleroderma is classified into localized and systemic (systemic sclerosis), with subclassifications within each. Two forms of systemic sclerosis are recognized: limited (80% of patients) and diffuse (20%) (Yazdany & Manno, 2022g). Incidence estimates 20 people per million per year (Barnes & Mayes, 2019; Mandal & Boin, 2021). Similar to other connective tissue diseases, scleroderma is more frequent in females than males (2–3:1). Also, African Americans and Native Americans tend to have a more severe disease course and worse outcomes compared Caucasians.

Pathophysiology

Like other diffuse connective tissue diseases, scleroderma has a variable course, featuring remissions and exacerbations. Systemic scleroderma (SSc) is a progressive, chronic, devastating, and debilitating disease with a prognosis not as optimistic as that of SLE. Pathogenesis integrates three cardinal features: vascular injury and damage, activation of innate and adaptive arms of the immune system autoimmunity, and generalized interstitial and vascular fibrosis.

The clinical manifestations and disease activity can be highly variable. It is a result of a dynamic biologic process unique to scleroderma, exhibiting levels of activity that vary with time and that can shift in nature at different stages. During the initial phase of the disease, signs of classic inflammatory events are often present and visible in the skin and soft tissues. SSc commonly begins with skin involvement. Mononuclear cells cluster on the skin and stimulate lymphokines to stimulate procollagen. Insoluble collagen is formed and accumulates excessively in the tissues. Initially, the inflammatory response causes edema formation, with a resulting skin appearance that is taut, smooth, and shiny. Skin tightening is the most readily recognizable feature of scleroderma. The skin then undergoes fibrotic changes, leading to loss of elasticity and movement. Eventually, the tissue degenerates and becomes nonfunctional. This chain of events, from inflammation to degeneration, also occurs in blood vessels; synovium; skeletal muscles; and internal organ(s) of the heart, lungs, GI tract, and kidneys (Hagler et al., 2020b; Lafyatis & Varga, 2019; Mandal & Boin, 2021; Wigley & Boin, 2021).

Clinical Manifestations and Assessment

Scleroderma starts insidiously with Raynaud phenomenon and swelling in the hands. The hallmark of scleroderma is when the skin and the subcutaneous tissues become increasingly hard and rigid and cannot be pinched up from the underlying structures (fibrosis). Wrinkles and lines are obliterated. The skin is dry because sweat secretion over the involved region is suppressed. The extremities stiffen and lose mobility. The condition spreads slowly; for years, these changes may remain localized in the hands and the feet. The face appears masklike, immobile, and expressionless, and the mouth becomes rigid.

The changes within the body, although not visible directly, are vastly more important than the visible changes. The left ventricle of the heart is involved, resulting in heart failure. The esophagus hardens, interfering with swallowing. The lungs become scarred, impeding respiration. Digestive disturbances occur because of hardening (sclerosing) of the intestinal mucosa. Progressive kidney failure may occur.

The patient may manifest a subset of limited cutaneous SSc symptoms referred to as the CREST syndrome (Box 38-4). Previously, this acronym was used as a synonym for the subtype limited scleroderma; however, this term has fallen out of favor because many patients do not have all five of these manifestations. Furthermore, patients with subtype diffuse scleroderma can have all of these features as well; therefore, the "CREST" is no longer considered to only denote subtype limited scleroderma.

Assessment focuses on the hallmark sclerotic changes (thickening) in the skin, contractures in the fingers, and color changes or ulcerations in the fingertips due to poor circulation (Bukiri & Volkmann, 2022; Denton & Ong, 2019; Wigley & Boin, 2021). Assessment of systemic involvement requires a review of systems with special attention to GI, pulmonary, renal, and cardiac symptoms. Limitations in mobility and self-care activities should be assessed along with the impact the disease has had (or will have) on body image.

There is no one conclusive test to diagnose scleroderma, and testing depends on the possibility or extent of organ involvement. A skin biopsy is performed to identify cellular changes specific to scleroderma. Pulmonary studies show ventilation–perfusion abnormalities. Echocardiography evaluates left ventricular function and pulmonary arterial pressure and identifies pericardial effusion (often present with cardiac involvement). Esophageal studies demonstrate reflux esophagitis (early discriminator) and dysmotility in most patients with scleroderma. Autoantibody testing,

BOX 38-4 **Focused Assessment**

Cutaneous Symptoms of Scleroderma

Be alert for the CREST symptoms:

- **C**alcinosis (calcium deposits in the tissues)
- **R**aynaud phenomenon (spasm of blood vessels in response to cold or stress)
- **E**sophageal dysfunction (acid reflux and decrease in mobility of esophagus)
- **S**clerodactyly (thickening and tightening of skin on fingers and hands)
- **T**elangiectasia (capillary dilation that forms vascular red marks on surface of skin)

particularly ANA, is the most useful laboratory test, with a positive result common in more than 95% of patients with scleroderma and antisclerodermal antibody (anti-scl) 70 (Khanna, 2019; Wigley & Boin, 2021; Yazdany & Manno, 2022g). In the presence of CREST syndrome, 90% have a positive anticentromere antibody test. Other autoantibodies demonstrate an association between scleroderma and a specific clinical pattern, such as anti-topoisomerase I antibodies and lung fibrosis or anti-RNA polymerase I/III and scleroderma renal crisis.

Medical and Nursing Management

Management of scleroderma depends on the patient's clinical manifestations and is based on disease comorbidities (Hagler et al., 2020b; Steen, 2019; Yazdany & Manno, 2022g). In scleroderma, treatment includes management of both acute and chronic disease. Acute conditions require interventions directed at controlling increased disease activity or exacerbations that can involve any organ system. Management of the more chronic condition involves periodic monitoring and recognition of meaningful clinical changes requiring adjustments in therapy. Because this is a life-altering disease that has no cure, all patients should receive counseling, during which realistic individual goals may be determined. As in the other rheumatic disorders, support measures include strategies to decrease pain, limit disability, maintain moderate exercise, and prevent joint contractures. No specific medication regimen has proved effective in modifying the disease process in scleroderma, but, along with antiarthritic drugs, various medications are used to treat organ system involvement. Calcium-channel blockers may provide improvement in symptoms of Raynaud phenomenon. ACE inhibitors appear to have improved survival of renal scleroderma crisis, and now there are many therapeutic agents approved for use in pulmonary hypertension (Steen, 2019; Yazdany & Manno, 2022g; Zanatta et al., 2020).

In addition to the common problems of rheumatic disorders, nurses need to identify other patient difficulties or needs related to scleroderma and plan accordingly. For instance, patients with scleroderma have problems associated with impaired skin integrity and imbalanced nutrition that is less than what the body requires. The patient with advanced disease also may have impaired gas exchange, decreased cardiac output, impaired swallowing, and constipation. There has been increased attention on psychosocial issues in SSc, but currently there are no evidence-based interventions (Spiritovic, 2019).

Providing meticulous skin care and preventing the effects of Raynaud phenomenon are major nursing challenges. Nurses teach patients to avoid the cold and to protect fingers with mittens. In addition, warm socks and properly fitting shoes are helpful in preventing foot ulcers. Careful, frequent inspection for early ulcers is important, and smoking cessation is critical.

NURSING PROCESS
The Patient With a Rheumatic Disorder

ASSESSMENT

The health history and physical and psychological assessments focus on current and past symptoms, such as fatigue, weakness, pain, stiffness, fever, or anorexia and the effects of these symptoms on the patient's lifestyle and self-image. Also the patient's social support systems are assessed as well as their ability to participate in daily activities, adhere to the treatment regimen, and manage self-care (Box 38-5). Additional areas assessed include the patient's understanding, motivation, knowledge, coping abilities, past experiences, preconceptions, and fears. The impact of the rheumatic disorder on the patient must be assessed to understand the patient's problems so that a plan of care specific to their issues can be developed. The nurse assesses the impact of the condition by asking, "Are there things that you cannot do now that you could do a year ago?" "What is it about your condition that you find most frustrating?" "What do you most enjoy doing?" "What things do you find difficult that you would like to be able to do?" and "How do you manage to get around the tasks that are difficult?" Find out the patient's frustrations and concerns. Learn how the patient copes with the limitations and the amount of support they have at home and at work (Woolf, 2019). The nurse's assessment and patient's responses to these questions may lead to identifying issues and concerns that can be addressed by nursing interventions, and, through collaboration with other interprofessional members, expected patient outcomes can be achieved (Cuccurullo et al., 2021; Hinman et al., 2019; Iversen, 2019; McCabe et al., 2019; Ward & Reuben, 2022).

DIAGNOSIS

Nursing diagnoses for patients with rheumatic disorders may include but are not limited to the following:

- Acute and chronic pain related to inflammation and/or progression of joint deterioration, tissue damage, fatigue, lowered tolerance level, or ineffective pain/comfort measures
- Fatigue related to inflammatory process and increased disease activity, pain, inadequate sleep/rest, impaired physical and psychosocial functioning (including emotional stress/depression), and inadequate nutrition
- Insomnia related to pain, anxiety/stress, depression, and medications
- Impaired physical mobility related to musculoskeletal impairment, decreased ROM, muscle weakness, pain on movement, limited endurance, or lack of or improper use of ambulatory devices
- Self-care deficits related to limitations secondary to progression of disease, pain, fatigue, contractures, or loss of motion
- Ineffective health management related to complexity of chronic health problem and medication adherence, decisional

(continued on page 1272)

BOX 38-5

Nursing Research

Bridging the Gap to Evidence-Based Practice

What Is the Evidence of the Effects of an Online Nursing Consultation in People with Fibromyalgia?

Garcia-Perea, E., Pedraz-Marcos, A., Martinez-Rodriguez, S. H., Otones-Reyes, P., & Palmer-Santos, A. M. (2021). Effectiveness of a fibromyalgia online nursing consultation in the quality of life: A randomized controlled trial. *Pain Management Nursing*, *23*(4), P478–485. https://doi.org/10.1016/j.pmn.2021.09.001

Purpose

Fibromyalgia (FM) is a complex rheumatic disorder with an identity of its own that affects the physical and mental health of those who suffer it. FM is a disorder of centrally amplified and maintained musculoskeletal pain with objective evidence of altered pain processing in the spinal cord and brain. Although pain is the defining symptom of FM, fatigue, unrefreshing sleep, cognitive complaints, and mood disturbances such as depression and anxiety also have significant impact on health-related quality of life. Nurses have a pivotal role in helping patients move forward after getting a diagnosis of FM. Information and communication technologies (ICT) are a potential alternative and complementary aid in the management of diverse chronic pathologies, particularly demonstrated during the period of maximum impact of the COVID-19 pandemic. The purpose of this study is to evaluate the effectiveness of an online nursing consultation through the internet platform Red Sinapsis (RS) in improving the perceived quality of patients with FM.

Design

The study was a parallel trial design, on a simple randomization scheme with 1:1 ratio, to evaluate the effectiveness on quality of life of using ICT in online nursing consultations at 3 months and 6 months. The study was conducted at a pain management clinic in Madrid, Spain, that deals with cases referred by other professionals for intense or unresponsive pain, from February 2015 to February 2016. The study population consisted of patients diagnosed with FM per the criteria of the American College of Rheumatology who met the following conditions for inclusion: (1) aged >18 years; (2) Spanish speakers; and (3) access to a computer to participate in the study. Those participants suffering severe cognitive or mental disorder preventing following instructions were excluded. Patients with post-traumatic stress disorder (PTSD) and mood disorders were not excluded. Assumption was that clinically relevant improvement in health-related quality of life (HRQoL) by 20% of the intervention group (IG) versus the control group (CG) with an alpha value of 0.005 and a power of 80% would require 33 patients in each study arm, 66 in total. This sample was overestimated by 15% to cover losses in the follow-up program. Patients were selected consecutively as they came for consultation at the center, then randomization was applied using a program to generate pseudo-random numbers. From the 80 randomized patients, 40 were assigned to the CG and 40 to the IG. The intervention variable was the online nursing consultation on the IT platform Red Sinapsis. This online tool provides patients with information on their illness, access to their clinical history, and a messaging system for communicating with the nursing or medical staff at any time. The patients assigned to the IG were given access to this tool throughout the duration of the study. The CG received usual care. They attended two face-to-face consultations with the principal researcher, at which time patients' knowledge of their condition, its treatment, and the repercussions on their family environment was explored, at 6 months and 12 months into the study. The results variables were the perceived state of health and emotional state regarding anxiety and depression of all the subjects in the study, measured through the following questionnaires: Fibromyalgia Impact Questionnaire (FIQ) and 36-item Short-Form Health Survey. These variables were measured over a span of 1 year, at the first consultation, at 6 months, and at 12 months.

Findings

The IG showed a 65% improvement in the perception of their state of health at 12 months into the study, compared with an improvement of 5.6% in the CG ($P < .001$). The IG also achieved better results for emotional status with more than 2 points in the anxiety variable (from 7.64 to 5.36) that remained constant in the CG. The depression variable showed constant improvement over the 12 months of the study in the IC, changing from an average of 7.72 (standard deviation [SD] = 2.05) to 5.33 (SD = 1.65), while in the CG a slight deterioration was observed. In both cases, the difference in mood evolution was significant ($P < .001$).

Nursing Implications

Online nursing follow-up for people with fibromyalgia conducted over an IT platform (Red Sinapsis) enhanced patients' perceived quality of life related to their welfare and emotional state. This study has shown that people affected by FM may benefit from the use of ITC through a follow-up program provided by nursing professionals who are able to offer assistance and coaching focused on the disorder in a simple and accessible manner. Complementarily to face-to-face consultations, patients could benefit from the advantages that online platforms can offer for maintaining healthy lifestyle habits, controlling the evolution of their pain, learning about their disorder, and becoming more committed to their treatment.

conflicts, economic difficulties, and deficient knowledge regarding disease management

- Altered body image perception related to physical (e.g., joint abnormalities) and psychological (e.g., depression) changes, loss of body function, and dependency imposed by chronic illness
- Coping impairment related to actual or perceived lifestyle or role changes, chronicity of disease, poor prognosis, and sense of powerlessness
- Injury risk related to adverse effects of medications, high risk of falls, and potential complications

PLANNING

The major goals for the patient may include relief of pain and discomfort, relief of fatigue, promotion of nutrition and restorative sleep, increased mobility and exercise, maintenance of self-care, motivation, adherence to therapeutic regimen, improved body image, effective coping, absence of complications, and promotion of home care.

NURSING INTERVENTIONS

Pain management and optimal functional ability, including the promotion of a healthy, positive life course adaptation, are major goals of nursing intervention. Patient teaching is an essential nursing intervention in the care of the patient with a rheumatic disorder. Education is the key to successfully enabling the patient to maintain as much independence as possible, to take medications accurately and safely, and to use adaptive devices correctly. Patient teaching focuses on the disorder itself, the possible changes related to the disorder, and the therapeutic regimen prescribed to treat it. Additional teaching is centered on the potential side effects of medications, strategies to maintain independence and function, and patient safety.

RELIEVING PAIN AND DISCOMFORT

Pain has quite different effects on different patients. The response to pain and the degree to which it disrupts the patient's life give a more meaningful indication of severity. Does the pain affect their sleep? How has pain affected their mood? What specific functions or activities does it limit? Understanding the problems it causes can guide how best to manage the patient's pain.

The nurse teaches patients to differentiate between joint pain and stiffness. Medications are used on a short-term basis to relieve acute pain. Because the pain may be persistent, non-opioid analgesics, such as NSAIDs, are often used. After administering medications, the nurse needs to reassess pain levels and response to treatment. With persistent pain, assessment findings should be compared with baseline measurements; evaluations of additional measures include exploring coping skills and strategies that have worked in the past.

The nurse teaches the patient about self-administration of pharmacologic agents and the need for safety in doing so. The patient needs to understand the importance of taking medications, such as NSAIDs and DMARDs, exactly as prescribed to achieve maximum benefits. These benefits include relief of pain and anti-inflammatory action as the disease is brought under control. Because disease control and pain relief are delayed, the patient may mistakenly believe the medication is ineffective or may think of the medication as merely "pain pills," taking them only sporadically and failing to achieve control over the disease activity. Alternatively, the patient may not understand the need to continue the medication for its anti-inflammatory actions once pain control has been achieved.

Heat applications are also helpful in relieving pain, stiffness, and muscle spasm. Superficial heat may be applied in the form of warm tub baths or showers and warm, moist compresses. Paraffin baths (dips), which offer concentrated heat, are helpful to patients with wrist and small-joint involvement. Therapeutic exercises can be carried out more comfortably and effectively after heat has been applied. However, in some patients, heat actually may increase pain, muscle spasm, and synovial fluid volume. If the inflammatory process is acute, cold applications in the form of moist packs or an ice bag may be tried. Both heat and cold are analgesic to nerve pain receptors and can relax muscle spasms (Cuccurullo et al., 2021; Hinman et al., 2021). The nurse teaches safe use of heat and cold application, in 15- to 20-minute intervals, usually three to four times a day. The nurse checks the temperature of warm soaks and covers cold packs with a towel, particularly for patients with impaired sensation. Further study of the effectiveness of these modalities is needed.

The nurse encourages measures to protect affected joints. There is no clear indication that the use of orthotic devices, such as braces, splints, collars, and shoe modifications, provides pain relief. However, there is preliminary evidence to support the use of extra-depth shoes, with or without semi-rigid insoles, to relieve pain on walking and weight bearing (Cuccurullo et al., 2021). Patients should be taught to avoid stooping, bending, or overreaching and to rest 5 to 10 minutes when trying to complete a task. The nurse educates the patient regarding other strategies for decreasing pain, such as relaxation techniques, imagery, meditation, and distraction.

DECREASING FATIGUE

Fatigue is a common problem for patients with rheumatic disorders (Tournadre et al., 2019; Woolf, 2019; Zielinski et al., 2019). Fatigue related to rheumatic disorders can be both acute (brief and relieved by rest or sleep) and chronic. Chronic fatigue related to the disease process is persistent, cumulative, and not eliminated by rest, but it is influenced by biologic, psychological, social, and personal factors. The nurse discusses related causes of fatigue with patients. Disease-related factors that may influence the amount and severity of fatigue include persistent pain, sleep disturbance, impaired physical activity, and disease duration. Pain increases fatigue because additional physical and emotional energy is required to deal with it. Pain also may cause the patient to expend more energy to do tasks in a way that causes less pain. A plan of nursing care for a patient with a rheumatic disorder is available online at http://thepoint.lww.com/Honan3e.

PROMOTING NUTRITION

Dietary intake of high-quality food has declined in most Western cultures. Americans are eating an increased amount of processed animal products and foods (high in trans fatty acids and omega-6 free fatty acids), food additives, preservatives, and high–glycemic-index foods (Stamp & Cleland, 2021). These factors directly or indirectly stimulate inflammation by increasing levels of arachidonic acid, a key component of many inflammatory mediators. Evidence has suggested incorporating an anti-inflammatory diet to improve serologic and symptomatic markers of inflammation. Fish oil supplements and omega-3 or omega-6 fatty acids can be added to the diet.

An anti-inflammatory diet is a predominantly plant-based diet, avoiding excess and high-glycemic-load calories. There is a strong

(continued on page 1274)

emphasis on avoidance of foods that may potentially exacerbate the inflammatory response (e.g., trans fats, refined sugars, high saturated fats, alcohol, and caffeine in excess). The majority of the diet should be derived from four areas: whole-grain products, fresh fruits and vegetables, legumes, and seeds and nuts. These sources provide several anti-inflammatory components, such as fiber, isoflavones (e.g., soybeans and soy products), carotenoids, and omega-3 free fatty acids (e.g., flaxseed). Patients can be told to keep a journal to assist in monitoring ongoing diet and symptom changes and not to expect immediate results, allowing at least 12 weeks before reevaluating for any benefits. Consultation with a dietitian is highly recommended for understanding the overall diet and suggestions for meal planning.

Pearls for Practice

Some medications (e.g., oral corticosteroids) used in the treatment of rheumatic diseases stimulate the appetite and, when combined with decreased activity, may lead to weight gain. Therefore, patients may need to be counseled about eating a healthy calorie-restricted diet.

PROMOTING RESTORATIVE SLEEP

Restful sleep is important in helping the patient to cope with pain, minimize physical fatigue, and deal with the changes necessitated by a chronic disease. In patients with acute disease, sleep time is frequently reduced and fragmented by prolonged awakenings. Also stiffness, depression, and medications may compromise the quality of sleep and increase daytime fatigue. A sleep-inducing routine, medication, and comfort measures may help improve the quality of sleep. The nurse encourages patients to take a warm bath or shower before bedtime to relax muscles; showering first thing in the morning may be beneficial to reduce morning stiffness.

Teaching sleep hygiene strategies may be helpful in promoting restorative sleep. These strategies include establishing a set time to sleep and wake up, creating a quiet sleep environment with a comfortable room temperature, avoiding factors that interfere with sleep (e.g., use of alcohol and caffeine), maintaining proper positioning of joints, using relaxation exercises, and getting out of bed and engaging in another activity (e.g., reading) if unable to fall asleep within 20 to 30 minutes (Yeager, 2019).

INCREASING MOBILITY

Maintaining some degree of joint mobilization and load on the joints is essential to the preservation of articular cartilage integrity. If the patient is overweight, a weight reduction program is a critical element in relieving stress on painful joints. Proper body positioning is essential to minimize stress on inflamed joints and prevent deformities that limit mobility. All joints should be supported in a position of optimal function. When in bed, the patient should lie flat on a firm mattress, with feet positioned against a footboard and with only one pillow under the head because of the risk of dorsal kyphosis. A pillow should not be placed under the knees, because this promotes flexion contracture. It is best for the patient to lie prone several times daily to prevent hip flexion contracture.

Care must be taken so that splinting for comfort does not restrict mobility later. Regularly removing the splint and exercising the joint through an ROM should be done to prevent joint "freezing." Splint modification may be needed when changes occur in joint structure.

In addition, assistive devices may be necessary for mobility. They should be fitted properly, and the patient should be instructed in their correct and safe use. A cane long enough to allow for only a slight bend of the elbow should be held in the hand opposite the affected side. Forearm-trough style crutches (platform crutches) may be needed to protect the upper extremities if the disease also involves the hands and wrists. This is especially important for the patient undergoing rehabilitation after reconstructive surgery on a joint in the lower extremity. Assistive devices can mean the difference between dependence and independence in mobility. However, keep in mind also that use of assistive devices may alter the patient's body image, which can become a barrier to adherence to the treatment regimen.

ENCOURAGING EXERCISE

The ACR has identified exercise as a fundamental part in the management of rheumatic disorders. Active and active/self-assisted ROM exercises are encouraged because they prevent joint stiffness and increase mobility (Hinman et al., 2019). Active/self-assisted exercises involve the use of overhead pulleys or wand exercises (shoulder exercises using a wand, stick, or cane). Measures to reinforce proper body posture and increase mobility include walking erect and using chairs with straight backs. When seated, the patient should rest the feet flat on the floor and the shoulders and hips against the back of the chair.

A formal program with occupational and physical therapy should be prescribed to educate the patient about principles of joint protection, pacing activities, work simplification, ROM, and muscle-strengthening exercises. An individualized exercise program is crucial to movement. Exercises appropriate for promoting mobility in patients with rheumatic disorders are summarized in Table 38-5. Appropriate programs of moderate pressure massage therapy and exercise, including tai chi and balance training, have been shown to decrease pain, improve function, and improve quality of life (Berman et al., 2019; Iversen, 2019; McCabe et al., 2019; Rodriquez, 2020). The major challenge for the patient and the health care provider is the need to adjust all aspects of treatment according to the activity of the disease. Especially for the patient with an active diffuse connective tissue disease, such as RA or SLE, activity levels may vary from day to day and even within a single day.

FACILITATING SELF-CARE

Self-care includes practices that patients undertake to promote their own health and well-being despite having a chronic illness. Self-care practices must be taught and reinforced so the patient

TABLE **38-5 Exercises to Promote Mobility**

Type of Exercise	Purpose	Recommended Performance	Precautions
Stretching (Flexibility)	Maintain or increase muscle flexibility	Stretch to the point of feeling tightness; 5–10 minutes daily	Hold position 5–15 seconds; build toward 20–30 seconds holds
Range of motion (Flexibility)	Maintain flexibility and joint motion	Active or active/self-assisted at least daily	Reduce number of repetitions when inflammation is present
Isometric resistance (Strengthening)	Improve muscle tone, static endurance, and strength; prepare for dynamic and weight-bearing exercises	Perform at 40–60% of maximal voluntary contraction (MVC) daily; 6–10 repetitions of each range	Monitor blood pressure; isometric exercises may increase blood pressure and decrease blood flow to muscles
Isotonic resistance (Strengthening)	Maintain or increase dynamic strength and endurance; increase muscle power; enhance synovial blood flow; promote strength of bone and cartilage	Start with repetitions against gravity and add progressive resistance; perform 2–3 days per week	May increase biomechanical stress on joints that are unstable or misaligned
Aerobic exercise (cardiorespiratory conditioning)	Improve cardiovascular fitness and endurance	Perform 3–5 days/week for 30 min/day of moderate-intensity exercise; 150 minutes/week	Progress slowly as activity tolerance and fitness improve; can speak normally—no SOB
Aquatic exercise	Water supports or resists movement; warm water may provide muscle relaxation and ease of movement	Provides buoyant medium for performance of dynamic or aerobic exercise	Recommended water temperature (88–93°F); deep water to minimize joint compression; nonslip footwear for safety

Adapted from Hinman, R. S., Nicolson, P. J., & Bennell, K. L. (2019). Principles of rehabilitation: Physical and occupational therapy. In M. C. Hochberg, E. M. Gravallese, A. J. Silman, J. S. Smolen, M. E. Weinblatt, & M. H. Weisman (Eds.), *Rheumatology* (7th ed., pp. 426–433). Elsevier.

does not develop self-care deficits. The nurse needs to keep in mind that a patient's deformity does not necessarily equate with the severity of limitations or disability. For example, swollen (edematous) hands may be quite limiting.

The nurse should assist the patient in identifying any self-care deficit and those factors that interfere with the ability to perform self-care activities. The nurse in a hospital or extended-care facility can help preserve the patient's independence by making available adaptive equipment for eating, toileting, bathing, and dressing. In the home, the nurse can encourage use of these devices. Also, the nurse should reemphasize the importance of relief for pain, stiffness, and fatigue and its impact on increasing the patient's ability to perform self-care.

PROMOTING MOTIVATION AND ENHANCING HEALTH MANAGEMENT

Motivating patients to make behavioral changes is an important nursing intervention. MI, proved effective in treating addictions, has been adapted for managing chronic illnesses. MI is a skillful clinical style for eliciting from patients their own good motivations for making behavior changes in the interest of their health through exploring and resolving ambivalence (Tooley & Kolahi, 2022; Vowell, 2022a). MI is an evidence-based counseling approach that can be used by nurses to help patients adhere to health regimens and can be applied in very brief, 10- to 15-minute patient encounters (Haque & D'Souza, 2019). A key to understanding MI is knowing the phenomenon of ambivalence (Vowell, 2022a). Patients may feel ambivalent about change. Conflicting motivations are normal and common, to simultaneously want and not want. "I want to exercise, but it hurts," "I mean to take my medicine, but I keep forgetting." Nurses need to recognize the telltale sign of ambivalence is the "but" in the middle of their narrative. The nurse's task is to elicit "change talk" rather than resistance from the patient. Resistance is the patient's way of trying to resolve the discomfort created by ambivalence. Resistance is best handled by restating, using a "but" statement. For example, "You say you want to exercise, but it hurts. What things can you do to help ease the pain with activity?" The nurse refrains from persuading and confronting but guides the patient toward an acceptable resolution that triggers change. Patient motivation and readiness to change are dynamic states that can be greatly influenced by interactions between nurse and patient. By guiding the patient on what are seen as obstacles (the "buts"), nurses can play a vital role in motivating the patient toward change. The first MI-related textbook was published by Miller and Rollnick in 1991 introducing fundamental concepts; in 2013 they developed a new four-process model of MI and guiding principles (Box 38-6).

(*continued on page 1276*)

BOX 38-6
Four Guiding Principles of Motivational Interviewing (Acronym RULE)

R: Reflect Resistance

When the nurse suggests change and the patient is resisting and arguing against it, the nurse should "roll with the patient's resistance" (i.e., the nurse acknowledges that resistance to change is expected). The patient is the primary source of arguments and solutions. The nurse should reflect resistance nonjudgmentally.

U: Understand

The nurse expresses empathy and communicates acceptance of the patient's experience, including the patient's ambivalence about change. Be interested in the patient's own concerns, values, and motivations.

L: Listen

By listening to what patients say, the nurse can tell how likely they are to change. Listen for verbs in patient narrative indicating change talk, statements in relation to desire, ability, reasons, need, commitment, and taking action.

E: Empower

Nurses assist patients to explore how they can make a difference in their own health, emphasizing the patient's ability to choose and carry out a plan for change. Outcomes are best when patients take an active role in their own health care.

Data from Haque, S. F., & D'Souza, A. (2019). Motivational interviewing: The RULES, PACE, and OARS. Current Psychiatry, 18(1), 27–28; Miller, W. R., & Rollnick, S. (2013). *Motivational interviewing: Helping people change* (3rd ed.). The Guilford Press.

As part of standard nursing practice, patient education is the cornerstone to effective health management. Nurses should use therapeutic skills, such as reflective listening and asking open questions, prior to informing (Vowell, 2022b). Ask the patient what they already know about the topic before preceding—use the "ask–provide–ask–formula" or "teach back" (see Chapter 1).

Educational topics should include information about the nature and treatment of the disease, pain management strategies, correct posture and body mechanics, correct use of assistive devices, principles of joint protection, energy conservation and pacing techniques, balanced nutrition, weight and stress management, and an individualized exercise program. In the spirit of motivation and enhancement, it is crucial to form a partnership (collaboration) between nurse and patient; the nurse needs to listen and elicit information from the patient, understand the patient's own perspectives (evocation), and recognize that the patient can and does make choices about the course of their life (autonomy). In the end, the patient should express confidence in their ability to make treatment decisions and to carry out a health regimen.

IMPROVING BODY IMAGE AND COPING

All aspects of the patient's life, including work role, social life, sexual function, financial status, and perception of self may be altered because of the impact and unpredictability of the course of a rheumatoid disorder. Body image changes can lead to social isolation and depression. Hence, the nurse and the family need to understand and be sensitive to the patient's emotional reactions to the disease and provide support and assistance when appropriate.

The nurse should encourage the patient and family to verbalize feelings, perceptions, and fears related to the disease. In addition, the nurse facilitates communication and aids the patient and family in identifying areas in which they have some control over disease symptoms and treatment. By taking action and involving others, the patient develops or draws on coping skills and possibly community support. The role of the nurse aims at addressing these psychological challenges to optimize the physical and psychological status of each patient (Crow, 2021; de Wit, 2019). The nurse also assists the patient to identify past coping mechanisms as well as use of effective coping strategies, which are key to positive outcomes.

MONITORING AND MANAGING POTENTIAL COMPLICATIONS

Medications used for treating rheumatic disorders have the potential for serious and adverse effects. Therefore, an important aspect of care is avoiding medication-induced complications. The provider bases the prescribed medication regimen on clinical findings and medical history and then monitors for side effects with periodic clinical assessments and laboratory testing. The nurse plays a major role in working with the primary provider and pharmacist to help the patient recognize and deal with medication side effects. If side effects occur, the medication may need to be stopped or the dose reduced. The patient may experience an increase in symptoms while the complication is being resolved or a new medication is being initiated. In such cases, the nurse's counseling regarding symptom management may relieve potential anxiety and distress.

PROMOTING HOME CARE

Depending on the severity of the disorder and the patient's resources and supports, referral for home care may or may not be warranted. The patient who is older or frail, has a rheumatic disorder that limits function significantly, and lives alone may need a referral for home care. A dietary consultation may be indicated to ensure that the patient is knowledgeable about dietary recommendations given the increased risk of cardiovascular disease. The patient and family should be informed about support services such as Meals on Wheels and local chapters of the Arthritis Foundation.

During home visits, the nurse has the opportunity to assess the home environment and its adequacy for patient safety and management of the disorder. Adherence to the treatment program can be monitored more easily in the home setting, where physical and social barriers to adherence are more readily identified. For example, a patient with diabetes who requires insulin may be unable to fill the syringe accurately or be unable to administer the insulin because of impaired joint mobility. Often, appropriate adaptive equipment needed for increased independence is identified more readily when the nurse sees how the patient functions in the home. Any barriers to adherence are identified, and appropriate referrals are made. Referrals to physical and occupational therapists may be made as problems are identified and limitations increase.

Furthermore, with each home visit the nurse assesses the patient's physical and psychological status, adequacy of symptom management, and adherence to the management plan. Previous teaching is reinforced, with emphasis on potential side effects of medications and changes in physical status that indicate disease progression and the need to contact the health care provider for reevaluation. Because of the increased risk of involvement of multiple organ systems, the importance of follow-up appointments is emphasized to the patient and family.

EVALUATION

Expected patient outcomes may include the following:

1. Experiences relief of pain or improved comfort level:
   a. Identifies factors that cause or increase pain
   b. Identifies realistic goals for pain relief
   c. Uses pain management strategies safely and effectively
   d. Reports decreased pain and increased comfort level
2. Experiences reduction in level of fatigue:
   a. Identifies factors that contribute to fatigue
   b. Verbalizes the relationship of fatigue to disease activity
   c. Schedules periodic rest periods, and identifies and uses other measures to prevent or modify fatigue
   d. Reports decreased level of fatigue
   e. Practices energy conservation strategies
   f. Discusses the relationship of the inflammatory process to fatigue and nutrition
3. Improves sleep patterns:
   a. Reports fewer nighttime awakenings
   b. Adheres to sleep-inducing routine
   c. Reports feeling rested on awakening
4. Increases or maintains level of mobility:
   a. Identifies factors that impede mobility
   b. Demonstrates normal or acceptable body alignment and posture
   c. Uses assistive devices appropriately and safely
   d. Participates in activities and exercises that promote or maintain mobility
5. Maintains self-care activities:
   a. Participates in self-care activities within capabilities
   b. Uses adaptive equipment and alternative methods to increase participation in self-care activities
   c. Maintains self-care at highest possible level
6. Enhances motivation and health management:
   a. Self-initiates goal-directed behavior
   b. Expresses belief in ability to perform activities
   c. Develops contract for health management with mutually agreeable goals for treatment
   d. Performs self-care and health-related activities consistent with ability
   e. Balances treatment, exercise, work, leisure, rest, and nutrition
7. Experiences improved body image and coping:
   a. Verbalizes concerns about the impact of rheumatic disease on appearance and function
   b. Sets and achieves meaningful goals
   c. States acceptance of self-worth
   d. Adapts to body image changes caused by disease
   e. Identifies and uses effective coping strategies
8. Experiences absence of complications:
   a. Takes medications as prescribed
   b. States potential side effects of medications and names reportable side effects
   c. Verbalizes understanding of rationale for monitoring
   d. Adheres to recommendations for monitoring
   e. Identifies strategies to reduce risks of side effects and potential risks for falling

Clinical Judgment Case

A 22-year-old patient was admitted for the first time to the hospital for shortness of breath (SOB). The patient was recently diagnosed with systemic lupus erythematosus (SLE). Symptoms related to SLE that the patient presents with include oral painless ulcers, tenderness, and swelling of joints in wrist and knees and fatigue. The SOB began suddenly this morning. Currently, skin is dry, there is delayed skin turgor, no malar rash, jugular veins are flat, and vital signs are as follows: 98.7°F, HR is 102 and regular, RR 26 and shallow, with an oxygen saturation of 91% on room air and blood pressure of 152/86 mm Hg. The patient is complaining of pain in the left chest; however, they deny jaw, back, or arm pain. When asked what makes the pain worse, the patient replies, "breathing and moving, and it feels worse when I lay down;" "it's like there's a 'catch' stopping me from breathing;" also "my left shoulder hurts." Heart sounds are S1 and S2, without gallop or murmur; the point of maximum impulse (PMI) is nondisplaced. A friction rub of left lung heard and decreased breath sounds of left lung fields are noted on pulmonary exam, no wheezes. There is no clubbing of digits or cyanosis. Denies cough. Abdomen is soft, nondistended, nontender, last BM was yesterday, formed brown stool, denies melena. Capillary refill is 2 seconds and pedal and posterior tibial pulses are 3+ bil. The patient's history also includes asthma and current medications are prednisone 7.5 mg daily (corticosteroid), hydroxychloroquine 200 mg daily (disease-modifying anti-rheumatic drug [DMARD]), and nonsteroidal anti-inflammatory drugs (NSAIDs) prn for joint pain. The patient has albuterol for asthma PRN but has not used it in over a year.

Step One: Recognize cues where relevant and important information is identified from different sources, such as medical history or vital sign.

Answer: Sudden onset SOB, recent diagnosis of SLE, asthma history. Cues related to SLE that are important are oral painless ulcers, tenderness and swelling of joints in wrist and knees, and fatigue. Physical examination findings of importance are dry skin; delayed skin turgor; flat jugular veins; left-sided chest pain that "catches" and is aggravated by breathing, moving, and lying flat; left shoulder pain; a friction rub on the left; and decreased breath sounds at left lung fields. Vital signs concerns include tachycardia at HR of 102, tachypnea at RR of 26 and shallow, oxygen saturation of 91% on room air, and hypertension with a blood pressure of 152/86 mm Hg.

Step Two: Analyze cues, which is organizing and linking the recognized cues to the patient's clinical presentation.

Answer: You have clustered the sudden onset SOB, chest pain that is aggravated by lying down and breathing, decreased O_2 sat, tachycardia, tachypnea, friction rub, and decreased breath sounds of left lung with the potential of pleural effusion or pleuritis (inflammation of the pleura—which can occur with or without an effusion). The left shoulder pain may be referred pain versus joint pain of SLE since other joints (wrist and knees) are also tender and edematous. You are also concerned about the history of asthma given the decreased breath sounds and decreased O_2 saturation. The tachycardia may be related to the hypoxia or fluid-volume deficit. Specifically, signs of fluid-volume deficit include dry skin, flat neck veins, delayed skin turgor, tachycardia, and tachypnea. The hypertension may be related to systemic corticosteroids, which increase sodium reabsorption and therefore water, but also may be associated with kidney involvement; despite this patient's age, you are aware that SLE accelerates atherosclerosis. The joint tenderness, fatigue, and oral lesions are symptoms of SLE, and you are aware that the symptoms are primarily clustered to a flare-up of this chronic condition. You are also concerned that the sudden change in the patient's status is anxiety producing and aim to provide comfort and emotional support and begin to build a trusting relationship.

Step Three: Prioritize hypotheses, where hypotheses are evaluated and ranked according to priority. This can include urgency, likelihood, risk, difficulty, and/or time. In this phase you cluster your findings to arrive at a list of problems (actual and/or potential problems) you believe the patient is experiencing and determine the importance or urgency. What do you think is of greatest concern?

Answer: You prioritize the decreased oxygen saturation, tachypnea, and SOB as priority and aim to improve the patient's comfort and low oxygen saturation. Next will be providing comfort and emotional support, given this is the patient's first hospital admission. You are also concerned about symptoms of fluid-volume deficit. Another important actual problem relates to the patient's hypertension, which you will continue to monitor as the providers identify the etiology and determine if treatment is needed. Finally, you will maintain surveillance of the multiple systems affected (renal, cardiac, pulmonary, skin) by this presumed flare-up of SLE.

Step Four: Generate solutions, which is identifying expected outcomes and using hypotheses to define a set of interventions for the expected outcomes.

Answer: You want to promote ventilation and oxygenation, and interventions that you can employ include elevating the head of the bed for comfort and applying supplemental low-flow oxygen to improve the oxygen saturation. You expect that a chest x-ray will be ordered and a consult with rheumatology will be called in to evaluate this patient; this is necessary to treat the underlying cause of the sudden change in the patient's condition. You will also want to limit the patient's expenditure of oxygen and monitor urinary output since you are concerned that the hypertension may be related to renal involvement in the flare-up. You anticipate laboratory analysis will be ordered that includes a urinalysis (check for hematuria, proteinuria); complete blood count; and chemistry profile, including electrolytes, BUN, and creatinine to evaluate kidney function. You also expect an order for ECG to rule out cardiac versus pulmonary involvement and assess for arrhythmias, which you are aware are associated with hypoxia. You also understand that an IV is necessary for fluid administration and emergency medication administration (if needed). You will monitor the oxygen saturation continuously and reassess vital signs and pulmonary examination.

Step Five: Take action, where the solutions that address the highest priorities are implemented.

Answer: You bring the pulse oximetry into the room and supplemental oxygen is initiated at 2 L to increase oxygen delivery and improve tissue perfusion. You elevate the HOB 30–45 degrees and suggest the patient lay on the left side (affected side) since that may relieve pain due to limitation of expansion. You also realize that repositioning (at least every 2 hours) will optimize the patient's ventilatory pattern and *ventilation/perfusion* matching. To limit the patient's expenditure of oxygen you will bring a bedpan or commode to the bedside; this is also important because, given concerns over kidney involvement that occurs with SLE, monitoring of intake and output is also important. You also will continue to monitor the patient's RR, accessory muscle use, oxygenation status, vital signs, and pulmonary exam. You are aware that blood work will be obtained along with chest x-ray, ECG, and perhaps other procedures to determine the exact cause of the SOB, so it will be important to allow resting between all the diagnostic studies. You will explain all procedures to the patient as you are aware that anxiety can increase the SOB. In addition, you will explain all activities and the purpose and effects of tests or therapies.

Step Six: Evaluate outcomes, which is comparing observed outcomes against expected outcomes.

Answer: The chest x-ray revealed a pleural effusion, which required an ultrasound-guided thoracentesis with specimens sent to the lab for analysis. VS repeated are now HR of 90 and regular, RR 18, oxygen saturation of 97% on 2 L, and BP is now 122/68 mm Hg. The rheumatology providers are at the bedside, and they are discussing next steps. You are right by the patient's side supporting them through this crisis, repeating information as needed and defining medical terms if required.

You have learned that despite an age of 22, this chronic inflammatory disease can affect many systems and that multiple specialties are needed to manage and monitor the patient's progress. In this case, dermatology (lesions), cardiology/nephrology (HTN), rheumatology (SLE), and pulmonology (pleural effusion) are involved in this patient's care. This case also reminded you that the basics of nursing care cannot be underestimated. In positioning of this patient, monitoring and optimizing oxygenation and ventilation, providing comfort and emotional support, maintaining surveillance for complications, and educating the patient, you have witnessed the breadth and importance of nursing care.

CHAPTER REVIEW

NCLEX-Style Review Questions

1. When assessing a patient, the nurse knows that which clinical manifestations are shared by rheumatoid arthritis and OA? Select all that apply.
   a. Decreased C4 level
   b. Symmetric knee involvement
   c. Tophi
   d. Joint swelling
   e. Pain

2. The nursing diagnosis identified for a patient with OA is acute pain. Which action(s) by the patient warrants intervention by the visiting nurse? Select all that apply.
   a. Acetaminophen taken PO of more than 4,000 mg/day
   b. Capsaicin applied topically as needed 3 to 4 times a day
   c. Cold application to localized area for 40 minutes 4 to 5 times a day
   d. Paraffin dips providing concentrated heat applied to the wrist before bedtime
   e. Warm moist compresses to the right upper quadrant (RUQ) for acute pain

3. A patient with SLE is admitted to the hospital for evaluation and management of acute joint inflammation. Which information obtained in the admission laboratory testing results is of concern to the nurse? Select all that apply.
   a. Elevated blood urea nitrogen (BUN)
   b. Increased C-reactive protein
   c. Positive ANA
   d. Positive RF
   e. Elevated creatinine

4. Which statement indicates the patient requires further teaching regarding the nutritional management of gout? Select all that apply.
   a. "I need to limit my alcohol intake such as grain liquors."
   b. "I need to follow a high-protein diet."
   c. "I need to eliminate fructose drinks like sweetened soda."
   d. "I need to avoid fad starvation diets."
   e. "I need to limit my fluid intake to 1,500 mL per day."

5. Which of the following cues should alert you to the complication of pericarditis in a patient admitted with SLE? Select all that apply.
   a. Sharp chest pain that may improve by sitting up and leaning forward
   b. Cardiac gallop marked by distinct S3 and S4 heart sounds
   c. Flat neck veins observed when patient is lying at a 30-degree angle
   d. Pericardial friction rub producing a grating, to-and-fro sound
   e. Carotid artery bruit auscultated during breath-holding

REFERENCES AND SELECTED READINGS

References and selected readings associated with this chapter can be found on the website that accompanies the book. Visit **http://thepoint.lww.com/Honan3e** to access the references and other additional resources associated with this chapter.

UNIT ELEVEN

Problems Related to Musculoskeletal Function

A 26-year-old patient is being seen in the orthopedic clinic for complaints of low back pain radiating down the left leg. The back pain started after lifting a steel beam at work. The patient is employed as a construction worker.

- **Discuss evaluative data that would be important to gather on this patient.**
- **Describe diagnostic procedures that would lead to a definitive diagnosis.**
- **Discuss medical and nursing management for this patient.**

CHAPTER 39

Nursing Assessment: Musculoskeletal Function

Linda Honan

Learning Objectives

After reading this chapter, you will be able to:

1. Describe the basic structure and function of the musculoskeletal system.
2. Discuss the relationship of the health history to the assessment of musculoskeletal health.
3. Describe the significance of physical assessment findings to the diagnosis of musculoskeletal dysfunction.
4. Specify the diagnostic tests used for assessment of musculoskeletal function.

The musculoskeletal system includes the bones, joints, muscles, tendons, ligaments, and bursae of the body. The functions of these components are highly integrated; therefore, disease in or injury to one component adversely affects the others. For instance, an infection in a joint (septic arthritis) causes degeneration of the articular surfaces of the bones within the joint and local muscle atrophy.

Diseases and injuries that involve the musculoskeletal system are commonly implicated in disability and death. In fact, trauma is the fifth leading cause of death in persons >65 years of age, and falls are responsible for 70% of accidental deaths in persons ≥75 years of age (Ferri, 2022, p. 611). Over 3 million visits to the emergency department (ED) for injurious falls occur annually, which accounts for 10.5% of all ED visits among older individuals (CDC, 2019; Uiterwyk et al., 2022). In addition, 29.6% of these visits required hospital admission (Uiterwyk et al., 2022), and such falls a leading cause of traumatic brain injury and fractures in older adults (Stark et al., 2021). The nurse is aware that musculoskeletal diseases and injuries can significantly affect overall productivity, independence, and quality of life (QOL) in people of all ages. Regardless of your nursing practice area, you will encounter patients with disruption in musculoskeletal function.

ANATOMY AND PHYSIOLOGY OVERVIEW

The health and proper functioning of the musculoskeletal system is interdependent with that of the other body systems. The musculoskeletal system has important functions, including providing protection for vital organs (e.g., brain, heart, liver, kidneys, lungs, spleen) and providing a sturdy framework to support body structures. It also makes mobility possible. Joints hold the bones together and allow the body to move. The muscles attached to the skeleton contract, moving the bones and producing heat that helps maintain body temperature. Movement facilitates the return of deoxygenated blood to the right side of the heart by compressing the venous vasculature. In addition, the musculoskeletal system serves as a reservoir for immature blood cells and essential minerals, including calcium, phosphorus, magnesium, and fluoride. More than 98% of total body calcium is present in the bones (Rosenthal & Rosenjack Burchum, 2021). In addition, the red bone marrow located within bone cavities produces red blood cells (RBCs), white blood cells (WBCs), and platelets through a process referred to as **hematopoiesis**.

Structure and Function of the Skeletal System

The shape and construction of a specific bone are determined by its function and the forces exerted on it.

Bone Types and Tissue

Bones are constructed of two types of bone tissue: **cancellous** (trabecular) or **cortical** (compact). Cancellous bone, or spongy bone, is found in the interior of bones and forms a lattice-like pattern. Red (responsible for blood-cell production) or yellow bone marrow (primarily fat) fills the lattice network. Cortical, or compact, bone forms the outer shell of a bone. It has a densely packed, calcified intercellular matrix, making the cortical bone more rigid than cancellous bone (Norris, 2019). Varying amounts of both cancellous and cortical bone are found throughout the body in differing proportions depending on the function of the bone.

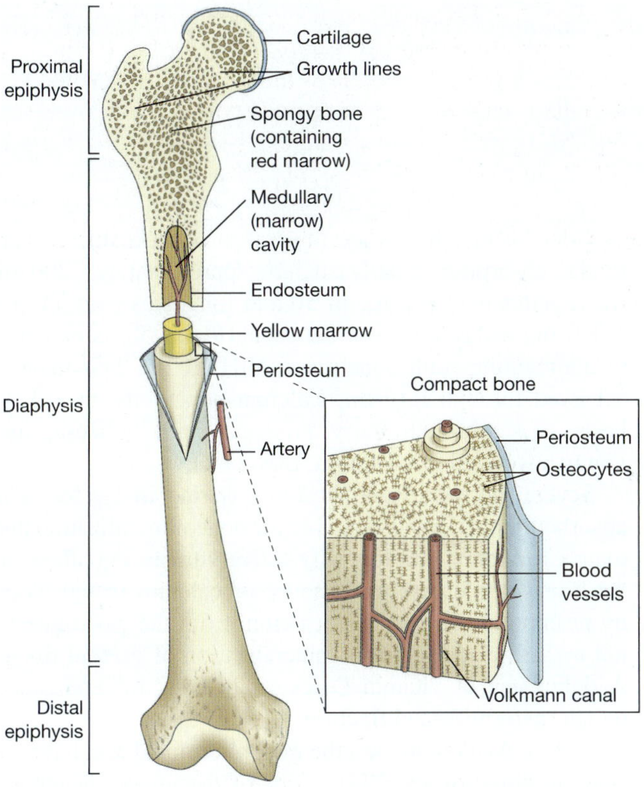

FIGURE 39-1 **Structure of a long bone; composition of compact bone.**

There are 206 bones in the human body, divided into four categories:

- Long bones (e.g., femur)
- Short bones (e.g., metacarpals)
- Flat bones (e.g., sternum)
- Irregular bones (e.g., vertebrae)

Long bones are shaped like rods or shafts with rounded ends (Fig. 39-1). The shaft, known as the **diaphysis**, is primarily cortical bone. The ends of the long bones, called **epiphyses**, are primarily cancellous bone. The epiphyseal plate separates the epiphyses from the diaphysis, and this plate is the center for longitudinal growth in children; thus, it can be a critical indicator of potential growth problems if fractured in children. The epiphyseal plate or growth plate is calcified in adults (once skeletal maturity is reached). The ends of long bones are covered at the joints by articular **cartilage**, which is tough, elastic, avascular (without blood vessels) tissue. Long bones are designed for weight-bearing and movement. Short bones consist of cancellous bone covered by a layer of compact bone. Flat bones are important sites of hematopoiesis and frequently provide protection for vital organs. They are made of cancellous bone layered between compact bone. Irregular bones, for example the vertebrae, have unique shapes related to their function.

Bone is composed of four basic cell types—**osteoprogenitor cells**, **osteoblasts**, **osteocytes**, and **osteoclasts**. Osteoprogenitor cells are stem cells located in the bone marrow that are the precursors to the more specialized bone cells (osteoblasts and osteoclasts) (Norris, 2019). Osteoblasts function in bone formation by secreting bone matrix. The term *blast* refers to immature or precursor cell; osteoblasts are foundational for bone formation (Norris, 2019). Bone matrix consists of collagen and other proteins that provide a framework in which inorganic mineral salts are deposited. These minerals are composed primarily of calcium and phosphorus. Osteoblasts also secrete the enzyme alkaline phosphatase, which is thought to raise calcium and phosphate levels for precipitation to occur (Norris, 2020, p. 1179). Collagen fibers provide bone's tensile strength (the ability to resist pulling and stretching forces), while the mineral content of bone enables it to resist compression forces that occur during weight-bearing and movement (Scanga & Curci, 2020, p. 619).

Osteoclasts are involved in dissolving and resorbing bone. The fourth type of bone cell, the osteocyte is involved in bone maintenance by communicating signals that attract, activate, or repress osteoclasts and osteoblasts (Bergwitz & Wysolmerski, 2022). The osteocyte determines where new bone formation is needed and/or where osteoclastic bone resorption is required, which is essential for proper bone remodeling.

The microscopic functioning unit of mature cortical bone is the **osteon** or Haversian system. Within the osteon, the Haversian canal contains blood vessels and occasionally axons (part of nerve cells) for the osteon (Standring, 2021). Covering the bone is a dense, fibrous membrane known as the **periosteum** that contains the osteoprogenitor cells needed for bone growth and development (Norris, 2019). This membranous structure nourishes bone and facilitates its growth. The periosteum contains blood vessels and also provides for the attachment of tendons, which connect muscles to bones, and ligaments, which connect bones to bones. The **endosteum** is a thin, vascular membrane that lines the inner surface of the bone marrow cavity of long bones and the spaces in cancellous bone.

Bone marrow is vascular tissue located in the medullary (shaft) cavity of long bones and in flat bones. Red bone marrow, located mainly in the sternum, ilium, vertebrae, and ribs in adults, is responsible for producing RBCs, WBCs, and platelets. In adults, the long bone is filled with fatty, yellow marrow.

Bone tissue is well vascularized. Cancellous bone receives a rich blood supply through metaphyseal and epiphyseal vessels. Periosteal vessels carry blood to compact bone through minute openings called *Volkmann canals.* In addition, nutrient arteries penetrate the periosteum and enter the medullary cavity through foramina (small openings). Nutrient arteries supply blood to the marrow and bone. The venous system may accompany arteries or may exit independently.

Pearls for Practice: Laboratory: Alkaline Phosphatase

The nurse is aware that in cases of bone injury or fractures, the serum alkaline phosphatase can increase secondary to the activity of osteoblasts (Norris, 2019).

Bone Formation

Osteogenesis (bone formation) begins long before birth. **Ossification** is the process by which the bone matrix (collagen fibers and other proteins) is formed and hard mineral crystals composed of calcium and phosphorus are bound to the collagen fibers. The mineral components of the bone give it its characteristic strength, whereas the collagen gives bone its resilience.

Bone Maintenance

Bone is a dynamic tissue in a constant state of turnover. During childhood, bones grow and form by a process called *modeling*. By early adulthood (i.e., late 20s to early 30s), **remodeling** is the primary process that occurs. Remodeling maintains bone structure and function through simultaneous **resorption** (removal/destruction of tissue) and osteogenesis (bone formation). The balance between bone resorption and formation is influenced by physical activity; dietary intake of certain nutrients, especially calcium; and several hormones, including calcitriol (i.e., active vitamin D), parathyroid hormone (PTH), calcitonin, thyroid hormone, cortisol, growth hormone, and the sex hormones estrogen and testosterone. Physical activity, particularly weight-bearing activity, stimulates bone formation and remodeling. Bones subjected to continued weight-bearing tend to be thick and strong. Conversely, people who are unable to engage in regular weight-bearing activities, such as those on prolonged bed rest or those with disabilities, have increased bone resorption from calcium loss, and their bones become osteopenic and weak. These weakened bones may fracture easily.

Pearls for Practice: Pathophysiology

Bone remodeling is a lifelong process that involves removal and replacement of bone tissue. It is an interplay between osteoblast (building up bone) and osteoclast (breaking down bone or bone resorption) activity. Similar to the maintenance of a building, some workers are actively removing old windows or walls (osteoclasts), while other workers are putting in new windows or walls (osteoblasts). Both processes are occurring concurrently and are regulated by calcium-controlling hormones, such as vitamin D and parathyroid hormone (see Chapter 28). Other influences include sex steroids, growth factors, and cytokines. With age, there is a slowing of the bone builders while the workers that break down bone continue their pace. Thus, it is understood that in postmenopausal females and older males, an imbalance develops between the bone resorption activity of osteoclasts and the building up activity of osteoblasts, leading to decreased bone density and a predisposition to osteoporosis (Scanga & Curci, 2020).

Pearls for Practice

Maximum bone growth is completed by the early fourth decade when bone is the most robust. After age 40, the resorption of bone exceeds bone formation, which increases the risk of osteoporosis-related fractures (Wilson et al., 2021).

Good dietary habits are integral to bone health. In particular, absorption of daily calcium, approximately 1,200 mg for females over the age of 50 and for males over 71 and 1,000 mg a day for those between 19 and 50, is essential to maintaining adult bone mass (NIH, 2021). This may be achieved through ingesting calcium-rich foods on a daily basis (e.g., through dairy products [milk, cheese, and yogurt], fortified cereals, tofu; Box 39-1).

Several hormones are vital in ensuring that calcium is absorbed properly and available for bone mineralization and matrix formation. Biologically active vitamin D (calcitriol) functions to increase the amount of calcium in the blood by promoting absorption of calcium from the gastrointestinal tract. It also facilitates mineralization of osteoid tissue. A deficiency of vitamin D results in bone mineralization deficit, deformity, and fracture.

PTH and calcitonin are the major hormonal regulators of calcium homeostasis. PTH is one of the important regulators of the concentration of calcium and phosphate in the blood. PTH promotes movement of calcium and phosphorus from the bone into the extracellular fluid. In response to low calcium levels in the blood, levels of PTH increase, promoting the mobilization of calcium from the bone, conservation of calcium by the kidney, enhanced intestinal absorption of calcium, and reduction of phosphate levels. Conversely, calcitonin, which is also called thyrocalcitonin, is secreted by the thyroid gland and lowers blood calcium levels. Calcitonin is excreted in response to elevated blood calcium levels. It inhibits bone resorption (the breakdown of bone), reduces the renal reabsorption of calcium and phosphate, and increases the deposit of calcium in bone (Norris, 2019).

Both thyroid hormone and cortisol have multiple systemic effects with specific effects on bones. Excessive production of thyroid hormone in adults (e.g., Graves disease) can result in increased bone resorption over new bone formation, leading to net bone loss. Increased levels of cortisol have these

BOX 39-1 **Pearls for Practice: Nutrition**

Bone Health

Calcium is important for bone health. Sources of calcium include:

- Milk, yogurt, and cheese
- Rhubarb, cooked collard greens, Chinese cabbage, kale, and broccoli
- Sardines, oysters, clams, and canned salmon with bones
- Tofu
- Calcium-fortified fruit juices, fruit drinks, and cereals

same effects. Patients receiving long-term synthetic cortisol or corticosteroids (e.g., prednisone) are at increased risk for steroid-induced osteopenia and fractures.

Growth hormone has direct and indirect effects on skeletal growth and remodeling. It indirectly stimulates the liver and, to a lesser degree, the bones to produce insulin-like growth factor-1 (IGF-I), which accelerates linear bone growth in children. Growth hormone also directly stimulates skeletal growth in children and adolescents. It is believed that the low levels of both growth hormone and IGF-I that occur with aging may be partly responsible for decreased bone formation and resultant osteopenia.

The sex hormones testosterone and estrogen have important effects on bone remodeling. Estrogen stimulates osteoblasts and inhibits osteoclasts; therefore, bone formation is enhanced and resorption is inhibited. Low levels of estrogen or increased levels of corticosteroids cause disruption in normal osteoclast and osteoblast homeostasis. Testosterone has both direct and indirect effects on bone growth and formation. Testosterone directly causes skeletal growth in adolescence and has continued effects on skeletal muscle growth throughout the lifespan. Increased muscle mass results in greater weight-bearing stress on bones, resulting in increased bone formation. In addition, testosterone converts to estrogen in adipose tissue, providing an additional source of bone-preserving estrogen for older males. This conversion is important for preservation of healthy bone metabolism during aging that likely reduces fractures (Hammes & Levin, 2019).

Blood supply to the bone also affects bone formation. With diminished blood supply or hyperemia (congestion), osteogenesis and bone density decrease. Bone necrosis occurs when the bone is deprived of blood.

Bone Healing

Although the exact process of fracture healing is open to debate, stages of bone healing are identified below (Norris, 2019). When a bone is fractured, the bone regenerates itself.

1. *Hematoma formation—Day 1–5:* When there is a fracture, the torn blood vessels in the periosteum, adjacent muscles, and soft tissue bleed into the injured tissue, forming a hematoma. This hematoma facilitates the formation of fibrin, which will become the framework upon which new bone will grow. Macrophages (large phagocytic WBCs) invade the fracture site and remove damaged, necrotic tissue (recall that any time there is a disruption of blood flow there is ischemia and potentially infarction or tissue death). Inflammatory cells migrate to the injured area, releasing growth factors that stimulate osteoclast and osteoblast activity. Inflammation, swelling, and pain are present.
2. *Inflammatory phase--Day 5–11:* New capillaries infiltrate the hematoma, and fibroblasts (cells that produce collagen, the major protein of bone) from the periosteum, endosteum, and bone marrow produce a bridge between the fractured bones. This bridge made of tissue not yet ossified—termed a soft tissue **callus**—establishes a connection between the bone fragment and will, in time, become bone. Under the influence of signaling molecules, cell proliferation and differentiation occur. Simultaneously, a layer of woven bone is laid down by the osteoprogenitor cells (Sheen & Garla, 2021).
3. *Reparative phase--Day 11–28:* Chondrocytes (cartilage cells) in the cartilage callus form matrix vesicles, which regulate calcification of the cartilage. Enzymes within these matrix vesicles prepare the cartilage for calcium release and deposit. The calcified cartilage, referred to as *bony callus*, is invaded by blood vessels and becomes resorbed by chondroblasts and osteoclasts. It is replaced by woven bone similar to that of the growth plate. Minerals continue to be deposited until the bone is firmly reunited. With major adult long bone fractures, ossification (the making of bone) takes 3 to 4 months.
4. *Remodeling--6 weeks onward:* The final stage of fracture repair consists of remodeling the new bone into its former structural arrangement. Remodeling may take months to years, depending on the extent of bone modification needed, the function of the bone, and the functional stresses on the bone.

Serial x-rays are used to monitor the progress of bone healing. The rate of fracture healing is influenced by the type of bone fractured, the adequacy of blood supply, the surface contact of the fragments, and the age and general health of the person. Adequate immobilization is essential until there is x-ray evidence of bone formation with ossification.

When fractures are treated with open fixation techniques, the bony fragments can be placed in direct contact. Primary bone healing occurs through cortical bone (Haversian) remodeling. Little or no cartilaginous callus develops. Immature bone develops from the endosteum. There is an intensive regeneration of new osteons, which develop in the fracture line by a process similar to normal bone maintenance. Fracture strength is obtained when the new osteons have become established.

Structure and Function of the Articular System

The junction of two or more bones is called a **joint** (articulation). There are two basic kinds of joints: solid or synarthroses, and synovial or diarthrodial (movable and contain a cavity; Norris, 2019). Synarthrosis joints can be fibrous or cartilaginous. The skull sutures are an example of fibrous joints that are immovable. Cartilaginous joints can be subdivided into synchondroses and symphyses. Synchondrosis joints are where bones are joined by hyaline cartilage, such as the epiphyseal or growth plates, while symphyses joints are where two separate bones connect via cartilage, such as the pubic symphysis or intervertebral disks (Norris, 2019).

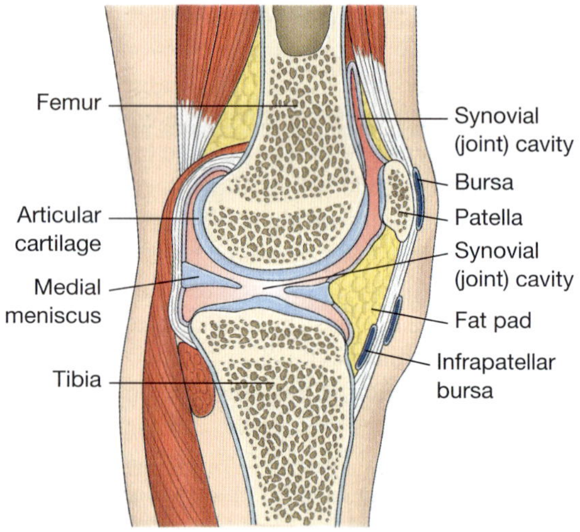

FIGURE 39-2 **Hinge joint of the knee.**

Synovial or diarthrodial joints are classified as freely movable joints; however, movement ranges from minimal (e.g., sacroiliac joint), to simple hinge movement (e.g., elbow and knee), to ball and socket or spheroidal (e.g., the hip and the shoulder; Fig. 39-2). Additional joints are classified as saddle joints, such as the base of the thumb; *pivot* joints such as the radius and the ulna that permit rotation for activities as turning a doorknob; and *gliding* joints that allow for limited movement in all directions, such as the joints of the carpal bones in the wrist. The diarthrosis joints are frequently affected by rheumatic disorders (Norris, 2019).

The ends of the articulating bones of a typical movable joint are covered with smooth hyaline cartilage. A tough, fibrous sheath called the **joint capsule** surrounds the articulating bones. The capsule is lined with a membrane, the **synovium**, which secretes the lubricating and shock-absorbing synovial fluid into the joint capsule. Therefore, bone surfaces do not directly touch each other. In some synovial joints (e.g., the knee), fibrocartilage disks (e.g., medial meniscus) are located between the articular cartilage surfaces. These disks provide shock absorption. Normal synovial fluid is clear or pale yellow, does not clot, and contains fewer than 100 cells/mm^3 (Norris, 2019).

Ligaments (fibrous connective tissue bands) bind the articulating bones together. Ligaments and muscle tendons, which pass over the joint, provide joint stability. In some joints, intracapsular ligaments (e.g., the cruciate ligaments of the knee) are found within the capsule and add stability to the joint.

A **bursa** is a thin-walled sac lined with synovial fluid that facilitates the movement of tendons and muscles over bony prominences. Bursae are found at the elbow, shoulder, knee, and some other joints.

Structure and Function of the Skeletal Muscle System

Muscles are attached by tendons (cords of fibrous connective tissue) or aponeuroses (broad, flat sheets of connective tissue) that attach muscles to bones, connective tissue, other muscles, soft tissue, or skin. The muscles of the body are composed of parallel groups of muscle cells (fasciculi) encased in fibrous tissue called **fascia** (or epimysium). The more fasciculi contained in a muscle, the more precise the movements. Muscles vary in shape and size according to the activities for which they are responsible. Skeletal (striated) muscles are involved in body movement, posture, and heat-production functions.

Muscle Tone

The contraction of muscle fibers can result in either isotonic or isometric contraction of the muscle. In **isometric contraction**, the length of the muscles remains constant but the force generated by the muscles is increased; an example of this is pushing against an immovable wall. **Isotonic contraction**, on the other hand, is characterized by shortening of the muscle with no increase in tension within the muscle; an example of this is flexing the forearm. In normal activities, many muscle movements are a combination of isometric and isotonic contraction.

Relaxed muscles demonstrate a state of readiness to respond to contraction stimuli. This state of readiness, known as muscle **tone (tonus)**, is produced by the maintenance of some of the muscle fibers in a contracted state. Muscle spindles, which are sense organs in the muscles, monitor muscle tone. Muscle tone is minimal during sleep and is increased when the person is anxious. A muscle that is limp and without tone is described as **flaccid**; a muscle with greater-than-normal tone is described as **spastic**. In conditions characterized by destruction of lower motor neurons (e.g., polio), denervated muscle becomes **atonic** (soft and flabby) and atrophies.

Muscle Actions

Muscles accomplish movement by contraction. Through the coordination of muscle groups, the body is able to perform a wide variety of movements (Fig. 39-3). The prime mover is the muscle that causes a particular motion. The muscles assisting the prime mover are known as *synergists*. The muscles causing movement opposite to that of the prime mover or synergists are known as *antagonists*. An antagonist must relax to allow the prime mover to contract, producing motion. For example, when contraction of the biceps causes flexion of the elbow joint, the biceps are the prime movers, and the triceps are the antagonists. A person with muscle **paralysis** (a loss of movement, possibly from nerve damage) may be able to retrain functioning muscles within the synergistic group to produce the needed movement. Muscles of the synergistic group then become the prime movers.

Exercise, Disuse, and Repair

Muscles need to be exercised to maintain function and strength. When a muscle repeatedly develops maximum or

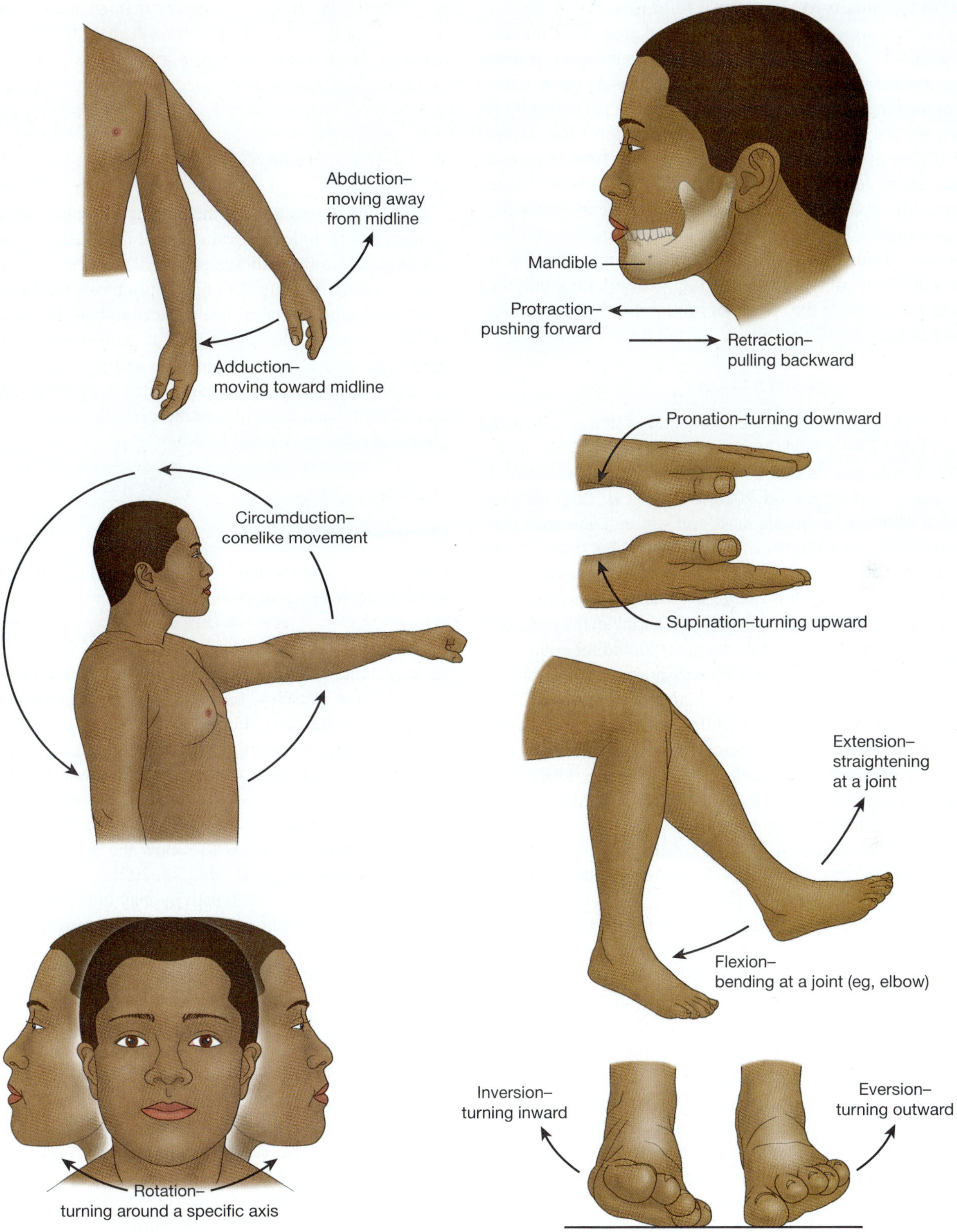

FIGURE 39-3 **Body movements produced by muscle contraction.**

close to maximum tension over a long time, as in regular exercise with weights, the cross-sectional area of the muscle increases. This enlargement, known as **hypertrophy**, results from an increase in the size of individual muscle fibers without an increase in their number. Hypertrophy persists only if the exercise is continued. The opposite phenomenon occurs with disuse of muscle over a long period of time. Age and disuse cause loss of muscular function as fibrotic tissue replaces the contractile muscle tissue. The decrease in the size of a muscle is called **atrophy**. Bed rest and immobility cause loss of muscle mass and strength. When immobility is the result of a treatment modality (e.g., casting, traction), the patient can decrease the effects of immobility by performing isometric exercise of the muscles of the immobilized part.

Gerontologic Considerations

Multiple changes in the musculoskeletal system occur with aging (Table 39-1). Peak bone mass is reached by the early fourth decade and then bone density decreases at a rate of 0.5% annually (Fingerhood, 2020; Wilson et al., 2021). There is also a decrease in muscle mass and strength and an actual loss in the size and number of muscle fibers due to myofibril atrophy with fibrous tissue replacement. The decreased contractile muscle force with increased weakness predisposes to muscle fatigue and poor exercise tolerance (Fingerhood, 2021). Numerous metabolic changes, including reduction of estrogen, testosterone and growth hormone and related decreased physical activity, contribute to **osteoporosis**. The osteoblast activity is reduced while osteoclast activity continues, resulting in a deterioration of bone architecture and strength particularly in cancellous or trabecular bone, such as the vertebral body (Fingerhood, 2021). In older people, the articular cartilage degenerates in weight-bearing areas and heals less readily. Ultimately, ligaments become weak, and this contributes to the development of **osteoarthritis** (degenerative joint disease). Decrease in muscle mass and range of motion (ROM) can cause functional impairment in older individuals. Diminished neuron stimulation and nutritional deficiencies also contribute to loss of muscle strength. In addition, past musculoskeletal problems for which the patient has compensated may become new problems with age-related changes. For example, people who have had polio and who have been able to function normally by using synergistic muscle groups may discover increasing incapacity because of a reduced compensatory ability. However, many of the effects of aging can be slowed with physical activity, particularly strength training, and adequate intake of energy and protein (Fingerhood, 2021).

Pearls for Practice

Nurses are aware that the incidence of falls increase with age and annually one third of those over 65 years of age will fall. Fractures are the likely outcome of falls, particularly in those patients with a history of osteoporosis. Predictors of future fractures are those patients with a history of previous fractures; thus nurses should inquire about history of falls and sequela when interviewing patients (Wilson et al., 2021).

ASSESSMENT

The nursing assessment of the patient with musculoskeletal dysfunction includes an evaluation of the effects of the musculoskeletal problem on the patient. The nurse is concerned with assisting patients who have musculoskeletal problems to maintain their general health, accomplish their activities of daily living, and manage their treatment programs. The nurse encourages optimal nutrition and teaches the patient strategies to minimize problems related to mobility. Through an individualized plan of nursing care, the nurse helps the patient achieve maximum health.

Health History

Common Complaints

Common musculoskeletal complaints include pain or tenderness and altered sensations.

Pain

Most patients with diseases and traumatic conditions or disorders of the muscles, bones, and joints experience pain. Bone pain is characteristically described as a dull, deep nagging pain that is "boring" in nature and can be localized, whereas muscular pain is described as soreness or aching and is referred to as "muscle cramps." Fracture pain is sharp and piercing, whereas nerve pain is described as sharp, burning, or shooting and tends to follow the distribution of the affected nerves (Magee & Manske, 2021).

Pain that increases with activity may indicate joint sprain or muscle strain, whereas steadily increasing pain points to the progression of an infectious process (osteomyelitis), degenerative changes, a malignant tumor, or neurovascular complications. Radiating pain occurs in conditions in which pressure is exerted on a nerve root. Pain is variable, and its assessment and nursing management must be individualized. It is important that the patient's pain and discomfort be managed successfully (see Chapter 6). The nurse notes body positioning and the influence of appliances, such as casts, traction, and surgical pins, when considering the patient's pain. Effective pain management is associated with decreased length of stay (LOS), improved functioning, decreased readmissions, and earlier recovery (Torani & Byrd, 2020).

Altered Sensations

Frequently, sensory disturbances are associated with musculoskeletal problems. The patient may describe **paresthesias**, which are burning, tingling sensations, or numbness.

TABLE 39-1 **GERONTOLOGIC CONSIDERATIONS / Age-Related Changes of the Musculoskeletal System**

Musculoskeletal System	Structural Changes	Functional Changes	History and Physical Findings
Bones	Gradual, progressive loss of bone mass Vertebrae collapse; decreased osteoblastic activity (reduced production of new bone)	Bones fragile and prone to fracture: vertebrae, hip, wrist	Loss of height Posture changes Kyphosis Loss of flexibility Flexion of hips and knees Back pain Osteoporosis Fracture
Muscles	Increase in collagen and resultant fibrosis Decreased size (atrophy) and number of muscle fibers; wasting Tendons less elastic	Loss of strength and flexibility Weakness Fatigue Stumbling Falls	Loss of strength Diminished agility Decreased endurance Prolonged response time (diminished reaction time) Diminished tone Wide based gait History of falls
Joints	Cartilage shows progressive deterioration Thinning of intervertebral discs Decreased viscosity of synovial fluid	Stiffness, reduced flexibility, and pain interfere with activities of daily living	Diminished range of motion Stiffness Loss of height
Ligaments	Lax ligaments (less than normal strength; weakness)	Postural joint abnormality Weakness	Joint pain on motion; resolves with rest Crepitus Joint swelling/enlargement Osteoarthritis (degenerative joint disease)

Box 39-2 provides assessment questions related to altered sensation. These sensations may be caused by pressure on nerves or by circulatory impairment. Soft tissue swelling or direct trauma can impair function.

Past, Family, and Social History

When taking the history, the nurse assesses for past history pertinent to the musculoskeletal system (e.g., a history of fractures or musculoskeletal diseases, such as rheumatoid arthritis). The nurse notes any history of family members who have had limitations that prevented performing functional activities. The nurse inquires about the use of any assistive devices such as canes, walkers, crutches, and/or wheelchairs and also assesses the patient's activity level. For example, does the patient do weight-bearing exercises on a regular basis? Is the patient involved in high-risk activities

BOX 39-2
Assessing Altered Sensation

Questions that the nurse should ask regarding altered sensations include the following:

- Is the patient experiencing any abnormal sensations or numbness?
- If the abnormal sensation or feeling of numbness involves an extremity, how does this feeling compare to sensation in the unaffected extremity?
- When did the condition begin? Is it getting worse?
- Does the patient also have pain? (If the patient has pain, then the assessment for pain should include questions related to sensation, numbness, onset, duration, location, characteristics, aggravating factors, alleviating factors, etc. Refer to Chapter 6 for aspects of pain assessment.)
- If the affected part is an extremity, the nurse compares the overall appearance in relation to the unaffected extremity, noting size, shape, and symmetry.
- Can the patient move the affected part?
- What is the color of the part distal to the affected area? Is it pale? Dusky? Mottled? Cyanotic? Has the color changed?
- Does rapid capillary refill occur? (The nurse can gently squeeze a nail until it blanches, and then release the pressure. The amount of time for the color under the nail to return to normal is noted. Color normally returns within 2 seconds. The return of color is evidence of capillary refill.
- Note the temperature of the limb. Is it different from the unaffected extremity?
- Is a pulse palpable distal to the affected area? If the affected area is an extremity, how does the pulse compare to that felt in the unaffected extremity?
- Is edema present? If so, is it pitting?
- Is any constrictive device (ring, watch, etc.) or clothing causing nerve or vascular compression?

and sports that may put them at risk for injury? This may evolve into an opportunity for safety education, such as wearing a helmet when bicycle riding.

Physical Assessment

An examination of the musculoskeletal system ranges from a basic assessment of functional capabilities to sophisticated physical examination maneuvers that facilitate diagnosis of specific bone, muscle, and joint disorders. The extent of assessment depends on the patient's physical complaints, health history, and physical clues that warrant further exploration. The nursing assessment is primarily a functional evaluation, focusing on the patient's ability to perform activities of daily living.

Techniques of inspection and palpation are used to evaluate the patient's posture, gait, bone integrity, joint function, and muscle strength and size. In addition, assessing the skin and neurovascular status is an important part of a complete musculoskeletal assessment. When specific symptoms or physical findings of musculoskeletal dysfunction are apparent, the nurse carefully documents the examination findings and shares the information with the provider, who may decide that a more extensive examination and a diagnostic workup are necessary.

Special precautions must be taken when assessing a patient with a musculoskeletal injury (Box 39-3).

Posture

The normal curvature of the spine is convex through the thoracic portion and concave through the cervical and lumbar portions. Common deformities of the spine include **kyphosis**, an increased forward curvature of the thoracic spine, frequently seen in older patients with osteoporosis and in some patients with neuromuscular diseases. **Lordosis**, an exaggerated curvature of the lumbar spine, is seen during pregnancy related to adjustment of posture in response to changes in the center of gravity. **Scoliosis** is a lateral curving deviation of the spine (Fig. 39-4). The two main types are adolescent idiopathic (without an identifiable cause) scoliosis and adult

BOX 39-3

The Patient With Musculoskeletal Injury

Special precautions must be taken when assessing a patient who has sustained trauma. If there is injury to an extremity, it is important to assess for soft tissue trauma, deformity, and neurovascular status. If the patient might have a cervical spine injury and is wearing a cervical collar, the collar must not be removed until the absence of spinal cord injury is confirmed by appropriate imaging studies. When the x-ray confirms no fracture and the collar is removed, the cervical spine area is assessed gently for swelling, tenderness, deformity, and skin integrity. With pelvic trauma, injuries may occur to abdominal organs. The patient is assessed for abdominal pain, tenderness, hematomas, distention, and the presence or absence of femoral pulses. If blood is present at the urinary meatus, the nurse should suspect bladder and urethral injury, and the patient should not be catheterized. Instead, such findings should be reported immediately to the emergency department provider or the surgeon.

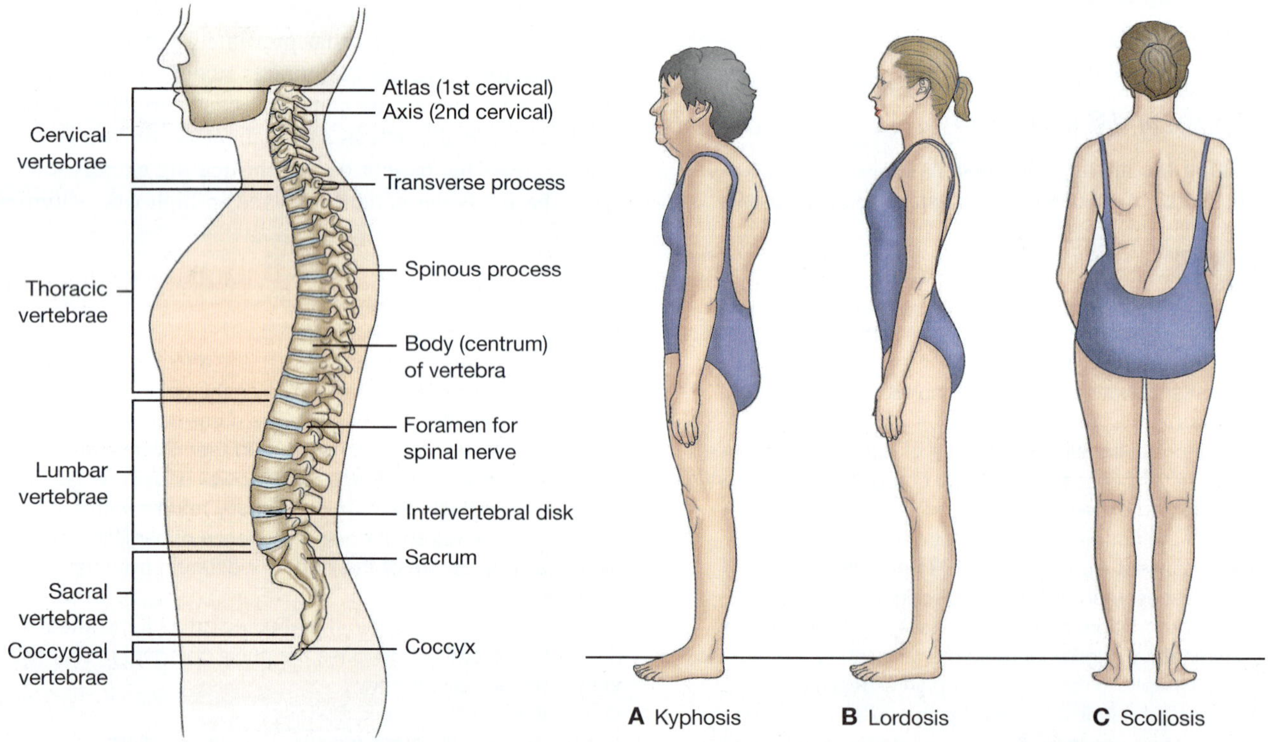

FIGURE 39-4 **A normal spine and three abnormalities. A. Kyphosis: an increased convexity or roundness of the spine's thoracic curve. B. Lordosis: swayback; exaggeration of the curve of the lumbar spine. C. Scoliosis: a lateral curvature of the spine.**

degenerative scoliosis; these are distinguished by age of onset (Szilagyi, 2021).

Gait

Gait is assessed by having the patient walk away from the examiner for a short distance. The nurse observes the patient's gait for smoothness and rhythm. Any unsteadiness or irregular movements are considered abnormal. Limited joint motion may affect gait. In addition, a variety of neurologic conditions are associated with abnormal gaits, such as a spastic hemiparesis gait, in which patients may drag their toes, circle their leg stiffly outward and forward, or lean their trunk to the contralateral side to clear the affected leg during walking (stroke); steppage gait, in which patients either drag the feet or lift them high, with knees flexed, and bring them down with a slap onto the floor, appearing to be walking upstairs (lower motor neuron disease); and shuffling gait, in which steps are short and shuffling with involuntary hastening (Parkinson disease; Bickley et al., 2021).

Bone Integrity

The bony skeleton is assessed for deformities, alignment, and symmetry. During the examination, body parts are compared from side to side. Shortened extremities, amputations, and body parts that are not in anatomic alignment are noted. Fracture findings may include abnormal angulation of long bones, motion at points other than joints, and crepitus (a grating sound) at the point of abnormal motion. Movement of fracture fragments must be minimized to avoid additional injury.

Joint Function

Evaluate joints by noting symmetry to the other extremity—is the change to the joint limited to one side of the body or both? Note any deformity or malalignment of joints or bones (Bickley et al., 2021). The tissues surrounding joints are examined for nodule formation, color changes, skin integrity, temperature, and injury. ROM is evaluated both actively (the joint is moved by the muscles surrounding the joint without assistance from the nurse) and passively (the joint is moved by the examiner). The nurse needs to be familiar with the normal ROM of major joints. Limited ROM may be the result of skeletal deformity, joint pathology, or **contracture** (shortening of surrounding joint structures) of the surrounding muscles, tendons, and joint capsule. With contractures, there is a loss of full movement resulting from a fixed resistance caused either by tonic spasm of muscle (reversible) or by fibrosis of joint structures (permanent). In older patients, limitations of ROM associated with osteoarthritis may reduce their ability to perform activities of daily living.

If joint motion is compromised or the joint is painful, the joint is examined for **effusion** (excessive fluid within the capsule), swelling, and increased temperature that may reflect active inflammation. An effusion is suspected if the joint is swollen and the normal bony landmarks are obscured. The most common site for joint effusion is the knee. If inflammation or fluid is suspected in a joint, consultation with a provider is indicated.

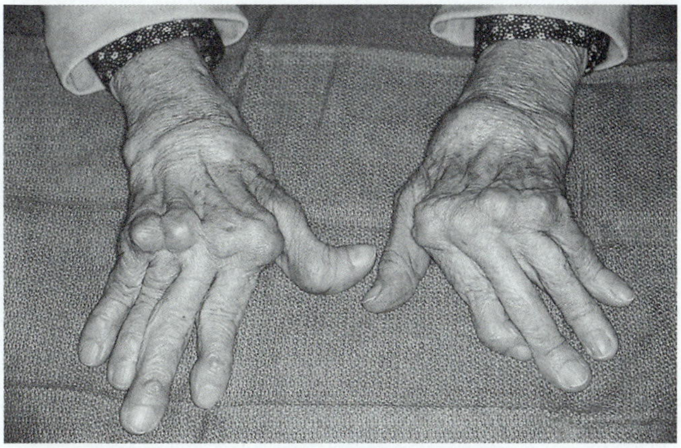

FIGURE 39-5 A patient with rheumatoid arthritis with involvement of the metacarpophalangeal joints. Note the severe ulnar drift of the fingers. (From Koopman, W. J., & Moreland, L. W. [2005]. *Arthritis and allied conditions: A textbook of rheumatology* [15th ed., Figure 45-6]. Lippincott Williams & Wilkins.)

Joint deformity may be caused by contracture, dislocation (complete separation of joint surfaces), subluxation (partial separation of articular surfaces), or disruption of structures surrounding the joint. Weakness or disruption of joint-supporting structures may result in a weak joint that requires an external supporting appliance (e.g., brace).

Palpation of the joint while it is moved passively provides information about the integrity of the joint. Normally, the joint moves smoothly. A snap or crack may indicate that a ligament is slipping over a bony prominence. Slightly roughened surfaces, as in arthritic conditions, result in **crepitus** (grating, crackling sound, or sensation) as the irregular joint surfaces move across one another.

Nodule formation is associated with rheumatoid arthritis (Fig. 39-5), gout, and osteoarthritis. While the subcutaneous nodules of rheumatoid arthritis are soft and occur within and along tendons, the nodules of gout are hard and lie within and immediately adjacent to the joint capsule itself. Osteoarthritic nodules are hard and painless and represent bony overgrowth that has resulted from destruction of the cartilaginous surface of bone within the joint capsule. They are seen frequently in older adults (refer to Chapter 38 for additional details).

Muscle Strength and Size

The muscular system is assessed by noting muscular strength and coordination, the size of individual muscles, and the patient's ability to change position. Weakness of a group of muscles might indicate a variety of conditions. By palpating the muscle while passively moving the relaxed extremity, the nurse can determine the muscle tone. The nurse assesses muscle strength by having the patient perform certain

TABLE 39-2 **Muscle Strength**

Grade	Strength	Physical Findings
0	None	No contraction
1	Trace	Palpable contraction only
2	Poor	Moves joint without gravity
3	Fair	Moves joint against gravity
4	Good	Moves against gravity and resistance
5	Normal	Normal strength

Reproduced from Staheli, L. T. (2016). *Fundamentals of pediatric orthopedics* (5th ed.). Wolters Kluwer Health.

maneuvers with and without added resistance (Table 39-2). For example, when the biceps are tested, the patient is asked to extend the arm fully and then to flex it against resistance applied by the nurse. A simple handshake may provide an indication of grasp strength.

The nurse may elicit muscle **clonus** (rhythmic contractions of a muscle) in the ankle or wrist by sudden, forceful, sustained dorsiflexion of the foot or extension of the wrist. **Fasciculation** (involuntary twitching of muscle fiber groups) may be observed (Fig. 39-6).

The nurse measures the girth of an extremity to monitor increased size due to exercise, edema, or bleeding into the muscle. Girth may decrease due to muscle atrophy. The unaffected extremity is measured and used as the reference standard for the affected extremity. Measurements are taken at the maximum circumference of the extremity. It is important that the measurements be taken at the same location on the extremity and with the extremity in the same position, with the muscle at rest. Distance from a specific anatomic landmark (e.g., 10 cm below the tibial tuberosity for measurement of the calf muscle) should be indicated in the patient's record so that subsequent measurements can be made at the same point. For ease of serial assessment, the nurse may indicate the point of measurement by marking the skin. Unilateral calf swelling that is more than 3 cm larger than the opposite limb is a clinical variable associated with deep vein thrombosis (DVT; Bickley et al., 2021).

Skin

In addition to assessing the musculoskeletal system, the nurse inspects the skin for edema, temperature, and color. Palpation of the skin can reveal whether any areas are warmer, suggesting increased perfusion or inflammation, whereas cooler skin suggests decreased perfusion or the presence of edema. Cuts, bruises, and evidence of decreased circulation or inflammation can influence nursing management of musculoskeletal conditions.

Neurovascular Status

Neurovascular status is important for the nurse to perform frequent neurovascular assessments of patients with musculoskeletal disorders (especially of those with fractures) because of the risk for tissue and nerve damage. The nurse uses the 6 Ps as a cue for neurovascular assessment: **P**ain, **P**allor, **P**oikilothermia (referring to cold temperature), **P**ulses (includes capillary refill), **P**aresthesia, and **P**aralysis. Table 39-3 summarizes peripheral vascular assessment. One complication that the

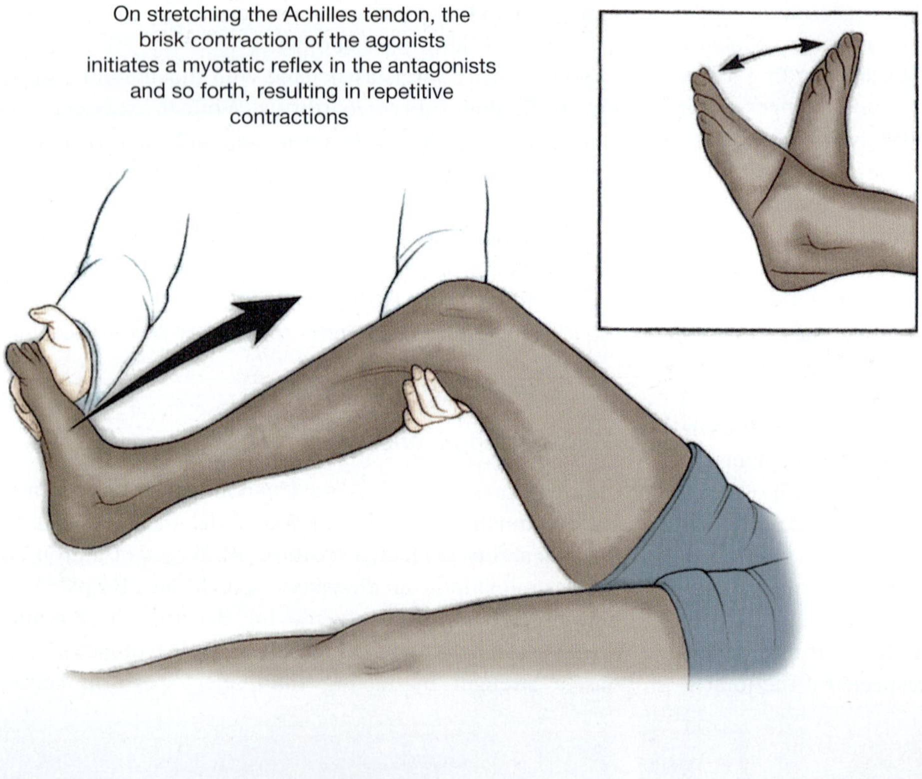

FIGURE 39-6 **Clonus. (From Young, P. A., Young, P. H., & Tolbert, D. L. [2015]. *Basic clinical neuroscience* [3rd ed., Figure 6-8]. Wolters Kluwer.)**

TABLE 39-3 Assessing for Peripheral Nerve Function

Assessment of peripheral nerve function has two key elements: evaluation of sensation and evaluation of motion. The nurse may perform one or all of the following during a musculoskeletal assessment.

Nerve	Test of Sensation	Test of Movement
Peroneal nerve	Stimulate the skin midway between the great and second toe. 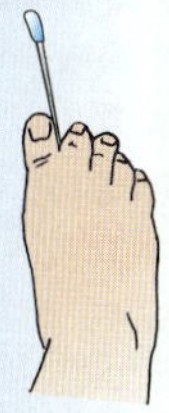	Ask the patient to dorsiflex the foot and extend the toes. 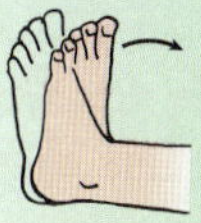
Tibial nerve	Stimulate the medial and lateral surface of the sole. 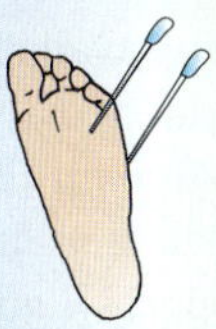	Ask the patient to plantar flex toes and foot. 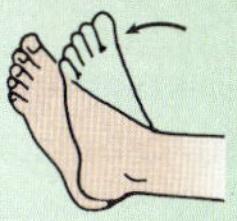
Radial nerve	Stimulate the skin midway between the thumb and index finger. 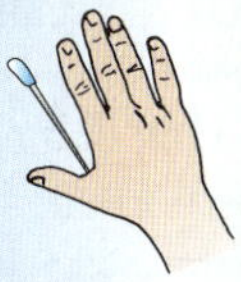	Ask the patient to extend the wrist; if too painful, ask them to extend the thumb. 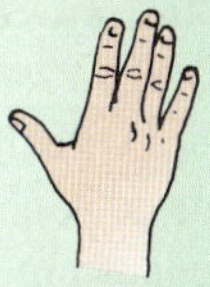
Ulnar nerve	Stimulate the distal fat pad of the small finger. 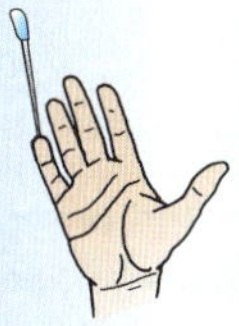	Ask the patient to spread all their fingers. 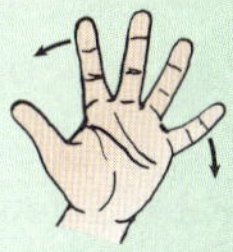
Median nerve	Stimulate the top or distal surface of the index finger. 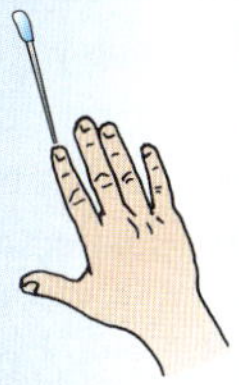	Ask the patient to touch the thumb to the little finger. Have the patient make an OK sign by touching the tip of the thumb to the tip of the index finger. 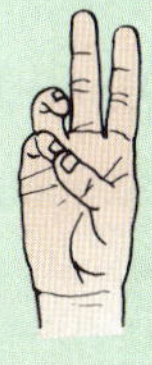

BOX 39-4 Indicators of Peripheral Neurovascular Dysfunction

Circulation

- *Color:* Pale, cyanotic, or mottled
- *Temperature:* Cool
- *Capillary refill:* More than 2 seconds
- Pulses: Grade pulses 0–4+ (refer to Chapter 11)

Motion

- Weakness
- Paralysis

Sensation

- Paresthesia (tingling or pricking ["pins and needles"])
- Unrelenting pain
- Pain on passive stretch
- Absence of feeling

nurse needs to be alert for when assessing the patient is *compartment syndrome*, which is described in detail later in this unit. This major neurovascular problem is caused by pressure within a muscle compartment that increases to such an extent that microcirculation diminishes, leading to nerve and muscle anoxia and necrosis. Function can be lost permanently if the anoxic situation continues for longer than 6 hours (Orman & Evans, 2022). Assessment of neurovascular status is frequently referred to as assessment of CSM (circulation, sensation, and movement). Symptoms of neurovascular dysfunction are discussed in Box 39-4.

Diagnostic Evaluation

During the period of assessment, the patient requires support and nursing care, including physical and psychological preparation for examinations and tests. Patient education before the tests (what is to be done; why it is being done; what the patient can expect to experience, including tactile, visual, and auditory sensations; and what patient participation is expected) reduces anxiety and enables the patient to be an active participant in care. The resulting medical diagnosis and prescribed treatment regimen affect the nursing management of the patient.

Imaging Procedures

X-Ray Studies

X-ray studies are important in evaluating patients with musculoskeletal disorders since they are readily available and inexpensive. Bone x-rays determine bone density, texture, erosion, and changes in bone relationships. X-ray study of the cortex of the bone reveals any widening, narrowing, or signs of irregularity. Joint x-rays reveal fluid, irregularity, spur formation, narrowing, and changes in the joint structure. Multiple views are needed for full assessment of the structure being examined. Serial x-rays may be indicated to determine if healing of a fractured bone is progressing normally or to determine if a bone affected by disease is stable, deteriorating, or responding to prescribed therapy. After being positioned for the study, the patient must remain still while the x-rays are taken.

Computed Tomography

A computed tomography (CT) scan shows in detail a specific plane of involved bone and can reveal tumors of the soft tissue or injuries to the ligaments or tendons. It is used to identify the location and extent of fractures in areas that are difficult to evaluate (e.g., acetabulum). CT studies, which may be performed with or without the use of contrast agents, can last up to 1 hour. If an intravenous (IV) contrast agent is used, the patient must be assessed before the CT scan for a contrast agent allergy. The contrast is iodine based. Refer to Chapter 42 for additional details regarding CT scans.

Magnetic Resonance Imaging

Magnetic resonance imaging (MRI) is a noninvasive imaging technique that uses magnetic fields, radiowaves, and computers to demonstrate abnormalities (e.g., tumors or narrowing of tissue pathways through bone) of soft tissues, such as muscle, tendon, cartilage, nerve, and fat. It is based on the activity of hydrogen atoms when placed in a magnetic field. Because an electromagnet is used, patients with any metal implants, clips, or pacemakers are not candidates for MRI. Refer to Chapter 42 for additional details regarding MRIs.

Pearls for Practice

Jewelry, hair clips, hearing aids, credit cards with magnetic strips, and other metal-containing objects must be removed from the patient before the MRI is performed; otherwise, they can become dangerous projectile objects or cause burns. Credit cards with magnetic strips may be erased, and nonremovable cochlear devices can become inoperable. Also, transdermal patches that have a thin layer of aluminized backing must be removed before MRI because they can cause burns. The provider should be notified before the patches are removed.

Arthrography

Arthrography can identify acute or chronic tears or injuries of the joint capsule or cartilage, ligament, and tendon. It provides excellent visualization of the shoulder, elbow, knee, ankle, hip, and wrist. A radiopaque contrast agent is injected into the joint cavity, often using fluoroscopic guidance, to outline soft tissue structures and the contour of the joint. The joint is put through its ROM to distribute the contrast agent. During the fluoroscopic portion of the examination, "real-time" tracking of contrast as it passes into and fills the joint can highlight abnormalities such as abnormal contrast leakage out of the joint (Ferri, 2019). However, this imaging modality has now been largely replaced by cross-sectional imaging techniques and is only performed as part of CT (CT arthrography) using direct injection of iodine contrast within the joint cavity, or MR arthrography using a dilute gadolinium solution for imaging (De Smet et al., 2021). It is contraindicated in patients with a skin infection at the site of injection (Ferri, 2019).

After an arthrogram, a compression elastic bandage may be applied and the joint rested; the nurse provides comfort measures (mild analgesia, ice) as appropriate.

Pearls for Practice

If contrast agents will be used for CT scan, MRI, or arthrography, the nurse carefully assesses the patient for previous contrast agent allergy. The nurse assesses risk of pregnancy before decisions are made regarding the use of contrast materials.

Bone Densitometry (Dual-Energy X-Ray Absorption [DEXA] Scan)

Bone densitometry is a readily available, noninvasive test used to estimate bone mineral density (BMD), which is responsible for 70% of bone strength (Bickley et al., 2021). BMD of the wrist, femoral neck, and lumbar spine are used to estimate the extent of osteoporosis and to guide treatment decisions, with the femoral neck considered the best predictor of hip fracture. It is recommended for those older than 65 years of age (postmenopausal) and for other people younger than 65 years at increased risk for osteoporosis-related fractures (Ferri, 2019). DEXA scan results are reported as a T and a Z score. The T score shows the amount of bone compared with that of a young adult of the same sex with peak bone mass. A score above 1 is normal, –1 to –2.5 indicates osteopenia (thin bones), and below –2.5 indicates osteoporosis (porous bones; Pagana et al., 2021). The Z score reflects the amount of bone compared with an age-matched group. See Chapter 40 for a further discussion of osteoporosis risks.

Concept Mastery Alert

BMD is used in diagnosing osteoporosis. Bone scans are used to detect metastatic and primary bone tumors, osteomyelitis, certain fractures, and aseptic necrosis, but not osteoporosis.

Bone Scan

A bone scan is a nuclear medicine test performed primarily to detect metastatic and primary bone tumors, since lesions are seen 6 to 12 months before they appear on x-rays (Fischbach et al., 2021). However, this test also is useful to evaluate unexplained bone pain, suspected infections, stress fractures, and aseptic necrosis. A bone-seeking radioactive tracer is injected IV and the scan is performed 2 to 3 hours after the IV injection. The waiting time allows for the tracer to concentrate in bone. The patient will be asked to drink water while waiting. Radioactive uptake is related to osteoblastic activity and blood flow; thus, bone formation is monitored. A "hot" bone scan is seen in any disorder that results in increased bone formation (Skinner, 2021). Increased activity is seen in primary skeletal disease (osteosarcoma), metastatic bone disease, inflammatory skeletal disease (osteomyelitis), and certain types of fractures. The term "cold spots" refers to areas where the tracers have not accumulated. The procedure takes approximately 1 hour and the patient must lie still during the scan. Before the patient undergoes an imaging study, the nurse assesses for conditions that may require special consideration during the study or that may be contraindications to the study (e.g., pregnancy and/or the inability to tolerate required positioning due to age, debility, or disability). The nurse is aware that medications containing barium and bismuth (Pepto-Bismol and Kaopectate) can interfere with the study and notifies the provider if needed. The patient is asked to void before the procedure since a full bladder masks the pelvic bones (Fischbach et al., 2021). The nurse reassures the patient that the radioactive tracer is excreted readily and no radiation precautions need to be taken. Increased by mouth (PO) fluids aid in the excretion of the radioactive substance, which is usually excreted from the body within 6 to 24 hours (Pagana et al., 2021).

Arthroscopy

Arthroscopy is a procedure that allows direct visualization of a joint to diagnose joint disorders. Treatment of tears, defects, and disease processes may be performed through the arthroscope. The procedure is performed in the operating room under sterile conditions; injection of a local anesthetic into the joint or general anesthesia is used. A large-bore needle is inserted, and the joint is distended with saline. The arthroscope is introduced, allowing for visualization of the joint structures, synovium, and articular surfaces. After the procedure, the puncture wound is closed with adhesive strips or sutures and covered with a sterile dressing. Complications are rare but may include infection, hemarthrosis (bleeding into the joint cavity), neurovascular compromise, thrombophlebitis, stiffness, effusion, adhesions, and delayed wound healing.

The joint is wrapped with a compression dressing to control swelling. In addition, ice may be applied to control edema and discomfort. Frequently, the joint is kept extended and elevated to reduce swelling. It is important to monitor neurovascular status (refer to Box 39-4). The nurse administers prescribed analgesics to control discomfort. The nurse explains when the patient can resume activity and what weight-bearing limits to follow, as prescribed by the orthopedic surgeon. The nurse also explains to the patient and family the symptoms (e.g., swelling, numbness, cool skin) to observe in order to determine whether complications are occurring and the importance of notifying the surgeon of these observations. The nurse's verbal instructions are reinforced with written instructions before discharge. Finally, the nurse explains the surgeon's prescription for analgesic medication.

Other Studies

Arthrocentesis

Arthrocentesis (joint aspiration) is carried out to obtain synovial fluid for purposes of examination or to relieve pain due to effusion. Examination of synovial fluid is helpful in the diagnosis of septic arthritis and other inflammatory arthropathies (any joint disease) and reveals the presence of hemarthrosis (bleeding into the joint space), which suggests trauma or a bleeding disorder. Normally, synovial fluid is clear, pale, straw-colored, and scant in volume. Using aseptic technique, the provider inserts a needle into the joint and aspirates fluid. Anti-inflammatory medications, such as cortisone, may be injected into the joint. A sterile dressing is applied after aspiration. There is a small risk of infection after this procedure. If the patient has a prosthetic joint, an orthopedic specialist should be consulted prior to this procedure; other relative contraindications include cellulitis/inflammation in the area where the needle would be inserted and coagulopathy since bleeding (hemarthrosis) is a potential complication (Purcell et al., 2019).

Nerve Conduction Studies and Needle Electromyography

Nerve conduction studies (NCSs) and electromyography (EMG) provide information about the electrical potential of muscles and the peripheral nerves leading to them. NCSs involve placing electrodes on the skin over the nerve that is being evaluated and stimulating the nerve with electrical impulses. This noninvasive test measures the speed and strength of the electrical impulse in a nerve. An example of when NCS may be ordered is carpal tunnel syndrome. Often the NCS is performed in conjunction with an EMG in which needle electrodes are inserted into selected muscles, and responses to electrical stimuli are recorded on an oscilloscope. The test is performed to evaluate the electrical potential generated by muscle cells when they are activated. The procedure helps to determine any abnormality of function and to differentiate muscle and nerve problems (Leung, 2019). As an example, an EMG may be ordered to evaluate for myasthenia gravis. The patient is forewarned that both procedures are uncomfortable and that in EMGs hematomas may form at needle insertion sites. The application of pressure to the needle site is expected to control potential bleeding. If the patient is on aspirin or anticoagulants, the health care provider is notified before the procedure (Fischbach et al., 2021).

Biopsy

Biopsy may be performed to determine the structure and composition of bone marrow, bone, muscle, or synovium to help diagnose specific diseases. The nurse prepares the patient by providing teaching about the procedure and assuring the patient that analgesic agents will be provided. The

TABLE **39-4 Blood Chemistry Studies Related to Musculoskeletal Conditions**

Blood Chemistry	Musculoskeletal Conditions
Altered serum calcium levels	Osteomalacia, parathyroid dysfunction, Paget disease, metastatic bone tumors, or prolonged immobilization
Serum phosphorus inversely related to calcium levels	Diminished in osteomalacia associated with malabsorption syndrome
Elevated acid phosphatase	Paget disease and metastatic cancer
Elevated alkaline phosphatase	Early fracture healing and diseases with increased osteoblastic activity (e.g., metastatic bone tumors)
Elevated creatine kinase and aspartate	Muscle damage
Elevated erythrocyte sedimentation rate (ESR) or C-reactive protein (CRP)	Inflammation, infection, autoimmune disorders, neoplasia, pregnancy, renal insufficiency, or rheumatologic disorder
Elevated uric acid	Gout, nephrolithiasis
Elevated myoglobin	Muscle trauma
Serum osteocalcin (bone GLA protein)	Indicates rate of bone turnover
Calcitonin levels	Bone metabolism
Parathormone	Bone metabolism
Vitamin D levels	Bone metabolism
Increased urine calcium levels	Bone destruction (e.g., parathyroid dysfunction, metastatic bone tumors, multiple myeloma)

nurse monitors the biopsy site for edema, bleeding, and infection (fever, erythema, swelling, drainage, and tenderness at the site) and asks the patient about their perception of pain. Ice is applied as prescribed to control bleeding and edema. In addition, analgesics are administered as prescribed for comfort.

Laboratory Studies

Examination of the patient's blood and urine can provide information about a primary musculoskeletal problem (e.g., Paget disease), a developing complication (e.g., infection), the baseline for instituting therapy (e.g., anticoagulant therapy), or the response to therapy. The complete blood count includes the hemoglobin level (which is frequently lower after bleeding associated with trauma and surgery) and the WBC count (which is elevated with any inflammatory condition, including acute infections, trauma, acute hemorrhage, and tissue necrosis). Before surgery, coagulation studies are performed to detect bleeding tendencies (because bone is very vascular tissue).

Blood chemistry studies provide data about a wide variety of musculoskeletal conditions; see Table 39-4.

CHAPTER REVIEW

NCLEX-Style Review Questions

1. A cast was applied to a patient's fractured leg 4 hours ago. Which finding is associated with neurovascular compromise? Select all that apply.

a. Capillary refill of 5 seconds
b. Ability to move the toes
c. Full sensation
d. Toes cool to touch
e. Paleness of toes

2. A 45-year-old patient just received DEXA scan results, and the T score was –1.2. Based upon this information, the nurse understands the patient has _____ (select 1 from Column 1), and would benefit from ________ (select 2 from Column 2).

Column 1	Column 2
a. Normal DEXA results	a. Lifestyle strategies
b. Osteoporosis	b. Bisphosphonates therapy
c. Osteopenia	c. Dietary teaching
	d. Hormone therapy

3. Your patient is scheduled for an MRI with contrast. What are appropriate nursing actions? Select all that apply.
  a. Assess for shellfish allergy
  b. Remove transdermal patch
  c. Assess renal function
  d. Remove hearing aids
  e. Alert the patient that they will hear a rhythmic knocking sound during the procedure

4. A patient has sustained multiple injuries in a motor vehicle crash. A cervical collar was applied by EMTs in the field. While in the ER the patient complains that the collar is restricting their breathing. Which of the following are appropriate actions? Select all that apply.
  a. Reassess patient's vital signs
  b. Reassess patient's pulse O_2 saturation
  c. Remove the patient's clothes
  d. Explain to the patient the collar must stay in place until it is determined the cervical spine is clear of injuries or fracture
  e. Administer sedation

5. A patient is scheduled for a bone scan to assess for bone metastasis. What are the nursing responsibilities in preparing this patient? Select all that apply.
  a. The patient is NPO for a bone scan.
  b. The test requires drinking a contrast dye.
  c. The test takes approximately 1 hour.
  d. Barium and bismuth interfere with the scan.
  e. The radiation is lower than with a CT scan.
  f. Radiation safety principles of time, distance, and shielding are required.

REFERENCES AND SELECTED READINGS

References and selected readings associated with this chapter can be found on the website that accompanies the book. Visit **http://thepoint.lww.com/Honan3e** to access the references and other additional resources associated with this chapter.

CHAPTER 40

Nursing Management: Patients With Musculoskeletal Disorders

Stephanie A. Barrett • Cynthia Bautista

Learning Objectives

After reading this chapter, you will be able to:

1. Describe the rehabilitation and health education needs of the patient with low back pain.
2. Describe common conditions and nursing care of the upper and lower extremities.
3. Explain the pathophysiology, pathogenesis, prevention, and management of osteoporosis.
4. Describe management of the patient with Paget disease.
5. Use the nursing process as a framework for care of the patient with osteomyelitis.
6. Describe medical and nursing management as well as potential complications to be encountered in the patient with a bone tumor.

Musculoskeletal disorders carry a heavy economic and health burden. The economic impact of musculoskeletal diseases is multifactorial including lost work days, changes in employment, increased prices for medications and services, new methods of treatments and drugs, and medical care organization costs (Yelin, & Cisternas, 2020). Adding to this burden are the personal, functional, and psychological limitations imposed on the patient. Musculoskeletal disorders are increased in patients with insufficient physical activity. Negative outcomes associated with a sedentary lifestyle include heart disease, diabetes, and depression. Increasing physical activity, which can vary according to the patient's functional level, can improve cardiovascular and respiratory status, reduce the severity of existing health problems, and reduce the impact of physical decline and falls. Nurses must be aware of the clinical manifestations and management of these disorders.

ACUTE LOW BACK PAIN

Low back pain, one of the most common reasons for a visit to a provider, is primarily caused by one of many musculoskeletal problems, including acute lumbosacral strain, unstable lumbosacral ligaments and weak muscles, osteoarthritis of the spine, spinal stenosis, intervertebral disk problems, and unequal leg length.

Older patients may experience back pain associated with osteoporotic vertebral fractures or bone metastasis. Other causes include kidney disorders, pelvic problems, retroperitoneal tumors, and abdominal aortic aneurysms.

In addition, obesity, stress, and, occasionally, depression may contribute to low back pain. Low back pain is so common, more than 80% of people will experience it within their lifetime (Jameson et al., 2020a).

Pathophysiology

The spinal column can be considered an elastic rod constructed of rigid units (vertebrae) and flexible units (intervertebral disks) held together by complex facet joints, multiple ligaments, and paravertebral muscles. Its unique construction allows for flexibility while providing maximum protection for the spinal cord. The abdominal and thoracic muscles help to stabilize the spine and are important in lifting activities, working together to minimize stress on the spinal units. Disuse weakens these supporting muscular structures. Obesity, postural problems such as slouching and poor body mechanics, structural problems such as scoliosis, and overstretching of the spinal supports may result in back pain.

The intervertebral disks change in character as a person ages. A young person's disks are mainly fibrocartilage with a gelatinous matrix. As a person ages, the fibrocartilage becomes dense and irregularly shaped. Disk degeneration is a common cause of back pain. The lower lumbar disks, L4 to L5 and L5 to S1, are subject to the greatest mechanical stress and the greatest degenerative changes. Disk protrusion (herniated nucleus pulposus) or facet joint changes can cause pressure on nerve roots as they leave the spinal canal; this results in pain that radiates along the nerve.

Clinical Manifestations and Assessment

The initial evaluation of acute low back pain (lasting less than 3 months) includes a focused history and physical examination, including general observation of the patient, back examination, and neurologic testing (reflexes, sensory impairment, straight-leg raising, muscle strength, and assessment of muscle atrophy). Signs and symptoms relate to the corresponding dermatome (see Fig. 42-13) or myotome (the group of muscles served by motor neurons of a spinal cord segment). Pressure on the nerve roots or spinal cord will cause symptoms such as abnormal or painful sensations (paresthesias or dysesthesias), loss of sensation, weakness, and autonomic dysfunction (most commonly bladder or bowel incontinence) (Bartleson & Barbano, 2020). Pain may be felt directly along the spine itself or may be referred (e.g., aortic aneurysm may present with back pain), or the patient may report pain radiating down the leg, which is known as **radiculopathy** or **sciatica** (pain from irritation of the sciatic nerve, classically felt from the low back to behind the thigh and radiating down below the knee). The presence of this symptom suggests nerve root involvement. The patient's gait, spinal mobility, reflexes, leg length, leg motor strength, and sensory perception may be affected. Careful examination of both sides will allow the nurse to note subtle differences. Back pain due to musculoskeletal disorders usually is aggravated by activity, whereas pain due to other conditions is not.

Physical examination may disclose paravertebral muscle spasm (greatly increased muscle tone of the back postural muscles) with a loss of the normal lumbar curve and possible spinal deformity. The findings suggest either nonspecific back symptoms or potentially serious problems, such as sciatica, spine fracture, cancer, infection, or a rapidly progressing neurologic deficit. If the initial examination does not suggest a serious condition, no additional testing is performed during the first 4 weeks of symptoms.

The diagnostic procedures described in Box 40-1 may be indicated for the patient with potentially serious or prolonged low back pain. The nurse prepares the patient for these studies, provides the necessary support during the testing period, and monitors the patient for any adverse responses to the procedures.

BOX 40-1

Diagnostic Procedures for Low Back Pain

X-ray of the spine: May demonstrate a fracture, dislocation, infection, osteoarthritis, or scoliosis

Bone scan and blood studies: May disclose infections, tumors, and abnormalities in bone marrow

Computed tomography (CT): Useful in identifying underlying problems, such as obscure soft tissue lesions adjacent to the vertebral column and problems of vertebral disks

Magnetic resonance imaging (MRI): Permits visualization of the nature and location of spinal pathology

Electromyogram (EMG) and Nerve Conduction Studies (NCS): Used to evaluate disorders of the spinal nerve root (radiculopathies)

Medical and Nursing Management

Management focuses on relief of pain and discomfort, activity modification, use of back-conserving techniques of body mechanics, and weight reduction. Most back pain is self-limited and resolves within 4 weeks with analgesics, rest, stress reduction, and relaxation.

Relieving Pain

Given the opioid epidemic with resultant opioid-related overdoses and deaths, nonprescription analgesics are suggested for pain control, such as nonsteroidal anti-inflammatory drugs (NSAIDs). At times, a patient may require the addition of muscle relaxants. If medication is prescribed, the nurse assesses the patient's response to each medication. As the acute pain subsides, medication dosages are reduced as prescribed. Often heat or cold therapy is used and frequently provides temporary relief of symptoms; superficial heat has demonstrated moderate evidence of benefit; however, further study of the effectiveness of heat or cold modalities is needed (Jameson et al., 2020a; Kim et al., 2019). In the absence of symptoms of disease (radiculopathy of the roots of spinal nerves), spinal manipulation performed by a chiropractor or an osteopath may be helpful. Acupuncture, massage, biofeedback, tai chi, and yoga are other modalities the patient may find to be therapeutic. There is no rigorous evidence that these modalities are beneficial; however, there is anecdotal evidence that many patients benefit from alternative modalities (Clinical Overview, 2020). Each patient's plan of care should be individualized, and the nurse will evaluate and note the patient's response to various pain management modalities.

To relieve pain, the nurse encourages the patient to remain active, consider ergonomic equipment such as sit/stand workstation to reduce stress on the back muscles and to change position frequently. The patient is taught to control and modify the perceived pain through behavioral therapies that reduce muscular and psychological tension. Diverting the patient's attention from the pain to another activity (e.g., reading, conversation, watching television) may be helpful in some instances. Guided imagery, in which the relaxed patient learns to focus on a pleasant event, may be used along with other pain-relief strategies.

Improving Physical Mobility

Physical mobility is monitored through continuing assessments. The nurse assesses how the patient moves and stands. Bedrest is discouraged in acute low back pain since it increases pain and prolongs recovery when compared with ambulatory patients (Knight et al., 2021). As the back pain subsides, self-care activities are resumed with minimal strain on the injured structures. Position changes should be made slowly and carried out with assistance as required. The patient should avoid twisting and jarring motions. The nurse encourages the patient to remain active and advises the patient to avoid sitting, standing, or walking for long periods. The patient may find that sitting in a chair with arm rests to support some of the body weight and a soft support at the small of the back provides comfort.

With severe pain, the nurse instructs the patient to limit activities for 1 to 2 days (Bartleson & Barbano, 2020). Extended periods of inactivity are not effective and result in deconditioning. An international campaign (the Victorian WorkCover Authority in Australia), called "Back Pain: Don't Take It Lying Down," is an example of stressing the importance of continued mobility in patients with back pain. Lumbar flexion is increased by elevating the head and thorax 30 degrees using pillows or a foam wedge as well as another pillow to allow the patient to flex the knees slightly. Alternatively, the patient can assume a lateral position with knees and hips flexed (curled position) with a pillow between the knees and legs and a pillow supporting the head. A prone position should be avoided because it accentuates lordosis (inward curvature of the spine). The nurse instructs the patient to get out of bed by rolling to one side and placing the legs down while pushing the torso up, keeping the back straight.

As the patient achieves comfort, activities are resumed gradually, and an exercise program is initiated. Initially, low-stress aerobic exercises, such as short walks or swimming, are suggested. After 2 weeks, conditioning exercises for the abdominal and trunk muscles are started. The physical therapist designs an exercise program for the individual patient to reduce lordosis, increase flexibility, and reduce strain on the back. The nurse encourages the patient to adhere to the prescribed exercise program. Erratic exercising is ineffective. Some patients may find it difficult to adhere to a program of prescribed exercises for a long period. These patients are encouraged to improve their posture, use good body mechanics on a regular basis, and engage in regular exercise activities (e.g., walking, swimming) to maintain a healthy back. Activities should not cause excessive lumbar strain, twisting, or discomfort; for example, activities such as horseback riding, basketball, and weight-lifting should be avoided. If there is no improvement within 1 month, additional assessments for physiologic abnormalities are performed. Management is based on findings.

Using Proper Body Mechanics

Good body mechanics and posture are essential to avoid recurrence of back pain. The patient must be taught how to stand, sit, lie, and lift properly. Providing the patient with a list of suggestions helps in making these long-term changes (Box 40-2). If the patient wears high heels, the nurse

BOX 40-2 **Health Promotion**

Activities to Promote a Healthy Back

Standing

Advise the patient to adhere to the following guidelines:

- Avoid prolonged standing and walking.
- When standing for any length of time, rest one foot on a small stool or box to relieve lumbar lordosis.
- Avoid forward flexion work positions.
- Avoid high heels.

Sitting

Discuss the following strategies with the patient:

- Avoid sitting for prolonged periods.
- Sit in a straight-back chair with back well supported and arm rests to support some of the body weight; use a footstool to position knees higher than hips if necessary.
- Eradicate the hollow of the back by sitting with the buttocks "tucked under."
- Maintain back support; use a soft support at the small of the back.
- Avoid knee and hip extension. When driving a car, have the seat pushed forward as far as possible for comfort.
- Guard against extension strains—reaching, pushing, or sitting with legs straight out.
- Alternate periods of sitting with walking.

Lying

Encourage the patient to do the following:

- Rest at intervals; fatigue contributes to spasm of the back muscles.
- Place a firm bed board under the mattress.
- Avoid sleeping in a prone position.
- When lying on the side, place a pillow under the head and one between the legs, with the legs flexed at the hips and knees.
- When supine, use a pillow under the knees to decrease lordosis.

Lifting

Emphasize the importance of the following strategies:

- When lifting, keep the back straight and hold the load as close to the body as possible.
- Lift with the large leg muscles, not the back muscles.
- Use trunk muscles to stabilize the spine.
- Squat while keeping the back straight when it is necessary to pick up something off the floor.
- Avoid twisting the trunk of the body, lifting above waist level, and reaching up for any length of time.

Exercising

Daily exercise is important in the prevention of back problems.

- Walk daily, and gradually increase the distance and pace of walking.
- Perform prescribed back exercises twice daily, increasing exercise gradually.
- Avoid jumping and jarring activities.

encourages changing to low heels with good arch support. The patient who is required to stand for long periods should shift weight frequently and should rest one foot on a low stool, which decreases lumbar lordosis. Patients who stand in place for a long period of time (e.g., cashiers) should stand on a foot cushion made of foam or rubber. The proper posture can be verified by looking in a mirror to see whether the chest is up, the abdomen is tucked in, and the shoulders are down and relaxed (Fig. 40-1). The patient should avoid locking the knees when standing and bending forward for long periods.

When the patient is sitting, the knees and hips should be flexed, and the knees should be level with the hips or higher to minimize lordosis. The feet should be flat on the floor. The back needs to be supported, so the patient should avoid sitting on stools or chairs that do not provide firm back support.

The nurse instructs the patient in the safe and correct way to lift objects—using the strong quadriceps muscles of the thighs, with minimal use of weak back muscles. With feet placed hip-width apart to provide a wide base of support, the patient should bend the knees, tighten the abdominal muscles, and lift the object close to the body with a smooth motion, avoiding twisting and jarring motions (Fig. 40-2). It takes about 6 months for a person to readjust postural habits. Practicing these protective and defensive postures, positions, and body mechanics results in natural strengthening of the back and diminishes the chance that back pain will recur.

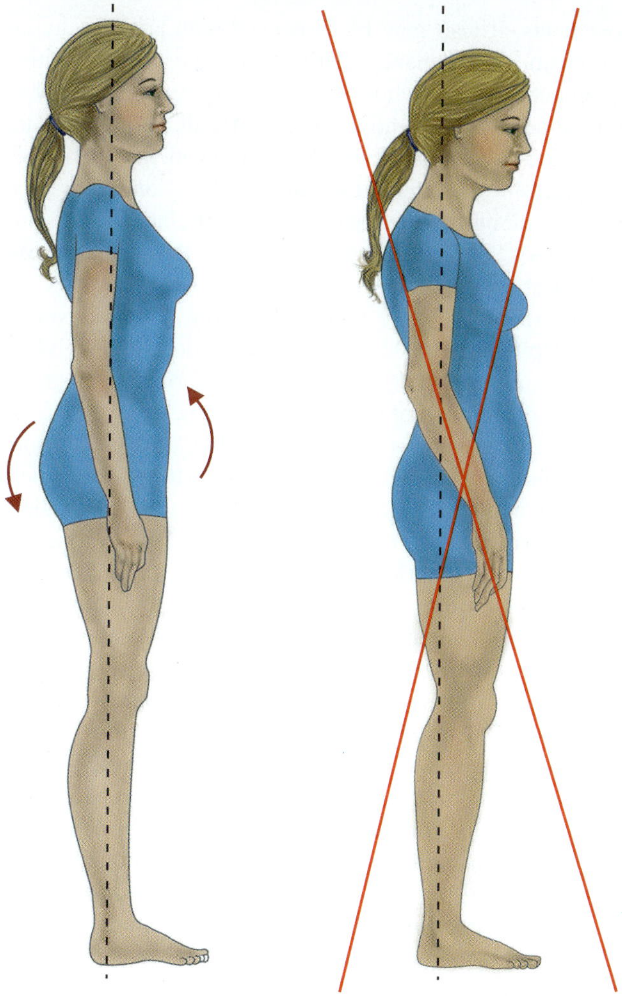

FIGURE 40-1 **Proper and improper standing postures. (*Left*) Abdominal muscles contracted, giving a feeling of upward pull, and gluteal muscles contracted, giving a downward pull. (*Right*) Slouch position, showing abdominal muscles relaxed and body out of proper alignment.**

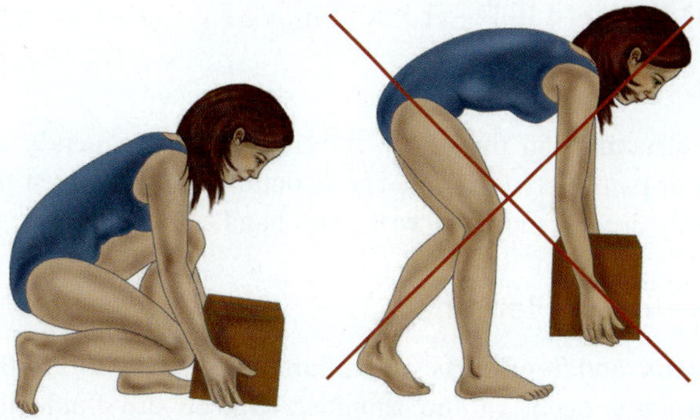

FIGURE 40-2 **Proper and improper lifting techniques. (*Left*) Correct position for lifting. This person is using the long and strong muscles of the arms and legs and holding the object so that the line of gravity falls within the base of support. (*Right*) Incorrect position for lifting because pull is exerted on the back muscles and leaning causes the line of gravity to fall outside the base.**

Pearls for Practice

Nurses, by virtue of their daily work, are a group at high risk for acute back injuries (e.g., through transferring patients, repositioning patients in bed, lifting a patient in bed, making an occupied bed). The national problem with obesity (33.6 % of the U.S. population is classified as obese [Chooi et al., 2019]), compounds this risk. Use of "lift teams" or lift devices should be available to nursing staff and accompanied by ergonomic instruction on body mechanics principles as described above. Risk of musculoskeletal injuries associated with direct patient care can cause as many as 20% of nurses to leave their direct patient care positions (Healthcare—Safe Patient Handling | Occupational Safety and Health Administration [osha.gov]). The nurse would do well to practice and use the postures described above.

Modifying Nutrition for Weight Reduction

Obesity contributes to back strain by stressing the relatively weak muscles of the back and abdomen. Exercises are less effective and more difficult to perform when the patient is overweight. Weight reduction through diet modification may prevent recurrence of back pain. Weight reduction is based on a sound nutritional plan that includes a change in eating habits to maintain desirable weight. Monitoring weight reduction, noting achievement, and providing encouragement and positive reinforcement facilitate adherence. Frequently, back problems resolve as optimal weight is achieved.

COMMON UPPER EXTREMITY PROBLEMS

The structures in the upper extremities are frequently the sites of painful syndromes. The structures affected most frequently are the shoulder, wrist, and hand.

Bursitis and Tendinitis

Bursitis and **tendinitis** are inflammatory conditions that commonly occur in the shoulder. Bursae are fluid-filled sacs that prevent friction between joint structures during joint activity. When inflamed, they are painful. Tendonitis is inflammation of a tendon. Tendons, which connect muscles to bone, are enclosed in sheaths. At points of friction, the sheath is double layered. The space between the two sheaths is filled with fluid similar to synovial fluid. Overuse of the tendon can result in inflammation and degeneration of the tendon (Norris, 2019). Conservative treatment includes rest of the extremity, ultrasound to the joint, and NSAIDs to control the inflammation and pain. Intermittent application of ice (for 20 minutes at a time) may be beneficial for superficially inflamed bursa, while application of heat may be helpful for deep forms of bursitis. The patient is educated not to fall asleep with a heating pad on to avoid thermal burns. Heat, if used, is applied for 20-minute periods (Todd, 2021). Corticosteroid injections may be considered. Stretching and strengthening exercises should be initiated after the acute phase. Further imaging or arthroscopic intervention may be considered if pain and weakness persist.

Impingement Syndrome

Impingement syndrome, or rotator cuff tendinitis, is caused by repeated overhead activity of the shoulder. When the arm is raised overhead, there is decreased space between the humeral head and acromion. The patient may experience dull achy pain, limited movement, and muscle spasm. Complaints such as difficulty in dressing oneself and night pain because of difficulty in positioning the shoulders may be noted. The process may progress to rotator cuff disease (see Chapter 41). Conservative treatment includes rest; application of heat, cold, and ultrasound; NSAIDs; joint injections; and physical therapy (Box 40-3 discusses patient education). Arthroscopic debridement (a minimally invasive surgical procedure that permits evacuation of joint debris) is used for persistent pain. Gentle joint motion is begun after surgery.

BOX 40-3 **Patient Education**

Measures to Promote Shoulder Healing of Impingement Syndrome

- Rest the joint in a position that minimizes stress on the joint structures to prevent further damage and the development of adhesions.
- Support the affected arm on pillows while sleeping to keep from turning onto the shoulder.
- For the first 24–48 hours of the acute phase, apply cold to reduce swelling and discomfort; then, according to the treatment plan, apply heat intermittently to promote circulation and healing.
- Gradually resume motion and use of the joint. Assistance with dressing and other ADLs may be needed.
- Avoid working and lifting above shoulder level or pushing an object against a "locked" shoulder.
- Perform the prescribed daily ROM and strengthening exercises.

Carpal Tunnel Syndrome

Carpal tunnel syndrome (CTS) is an entrapment neuropathy that occurs when the median nerve at the wrist is compressed by a thickened flexor tendon sheath, skeletal encroachment, edema, or a soft tissue mass. Although the exact etiology of increased carpal tunnel pressure is unknown, the syndrome is commonly associated with repetitive hand and wrist movements. It also may be associated with arthritis, hypothyroidism, or pregnancy. Patients who perform repetitive movements or those whose hands are exposed repeatedly to cold temperatures, vibrations, or extreme direct pressure are at a greater risk for developing CTS. The patient experiences pain, paresthesia (numbness and tingling), and, possibly, weakness along the median nerve (thumb, index, and middle fingers). See Table 39-3 for assessing the medial nerve. Phalen test or Tinel sign may be used to help identify CTS (Fig. 40-3). Night pain is common, often waking the patient from sleep (Kothari, 2021). Nerve conduction studies (NCS) and electromyography (EMG) may be performed to diagnose CTS (see description of tests in Chapter 39).

Treatment of CTS is based on the cause of the condition. Symptoms may be relieved by wrist splints to prevent hyperextension and prolonged flexion of the wrist, avoidance of repetitive flexion of the wrist (e.g., making ergonomic changes at work to reduce wrist strain), use of NSAIDs, and carpal canal cortisone injections. Specific yoga postures, relaxation, and acupuncture may be nontraditional alternatives to relieve carpal tunnel symptoms. In pregnancy, symptoms usually resolve spontaneously weeks after delivery (Dwivedi & Dasilva, 2021).

If conservative treatment fails, surgical management options are traditional open nerve release or endoscopic laser surgery. Both of these procedures are performed under local anesthesia and involve making small incisions into the affected wrist and cutting the carpal ligament so that the carpal tunnel is widened. Smaller incisions are made with the endoscopic laser procedure, and there is less scar formation and a shorter recovery time than with the open method. Following either of these procedures, the patient wears a hand splint and limits hand use during healing. The patient may need assistance with personal care and activities of daily living (ADLs). Full recovery of motor and sensory function

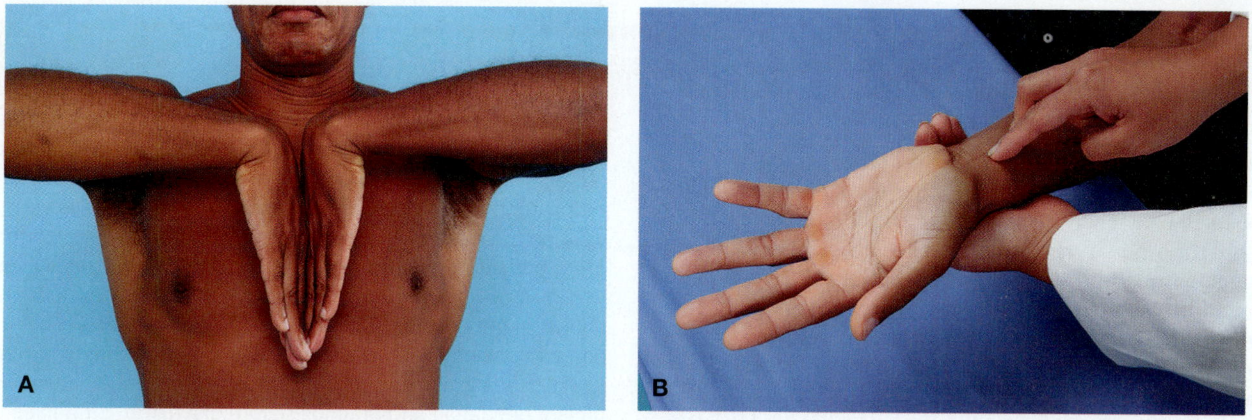

FIGURE 40-3 **There are two ways to assess for carpal tunnel syndrome: Phalen test and Tinel sign. A. To perform Phalen test, have the patient hold the position shown for 60 seconds. B. To elicit Tinel sign in a patient, percuss lightly over the median nerve, located on the inner aspect of the wrist. If the patient reports tingling, numbness, and pain, the test for Phalen and Tinel sign is considered positive. (From Weber, J. W., & Kelley, J. [2021].** ***Health assessment in nursing*** **[7th ed.; Fig. 24-21]. Wolters Kluwer Health, Lippincott Williams & Wilkins.)**

may take several weeks or months after either type of nerve release surgery.

Ganglion

A ganglion, a collection of gelatinous material near the tendon sheaths and joints, appears as a round, firm, compressible, cystic swelling, usually on the dorsum of the wrist (60% to 70%). They may be caused by injury or repetitive activity. The ganglion may or may not be locally tender. The pain may be described as aching and can be aggravated by extreme flexion or extension. Ganglion cysts may occur in any age group, but they are found most commonly in people between 20 and 40 years of age (De Keyser, 2021). Asymptomatic ganglions are monitored, since approximately 50% will resolve without treatment. Other treatments may include aspiration, corticosteroid injection, or surgical excision. After treatment, a compression dressing and immobilization splint are used.

Dupuytren Disease

Dupuytren disease results in a slowly progressive **contracture** of the palmar fascia, called Dupuytren contracture, which causes flexion of the fourth and fifth fingers and, frequently, the middle finger (Fig. 40-4). This renders the fingers more or less useless. It is caused by an inherited autosomal dominant trait and occurs most frequently in males who are older than 50 years of age and who are of northern European descent. While strongly inheritable, it is also associated with drug therapy for epilepsy, diabetes, and alcohol use disorder (Karbowiak et al., 2021). It starts as a nodule of the palmar fascia. The nodule may not change, or it may progress so that the fibrous thickening extends to involve the skin in the distal palm and produces a contracture of the fingers. The patient may experience dull aching discomfort, morning numbness, cramping, and stiffness in the affected fingers. The patient often seeks care because contracture of the fingers alters the function of the hand. This condition starts in one hand, but eventually both hands can be affected. With contracture development, patients are referred to a hand specialist. Nonsurgical options of treatment include percutaneous needle fasciotomy (fascia is cut to relieve tension or pressure) and injection of collagenase into the palmer cord. The collagenase breaks down the fibrous thickening, and the patient returns to the surgeon for manipulation of the finger, resulting in increased function. Surgical options include palmar and digital fasciectomies. Finger and hand exercises are begun as prescribed on postoperative day 1 or 2.

Box 40-4 discusses nursing interventions for patients undergoing surgery for upper extremity problems.

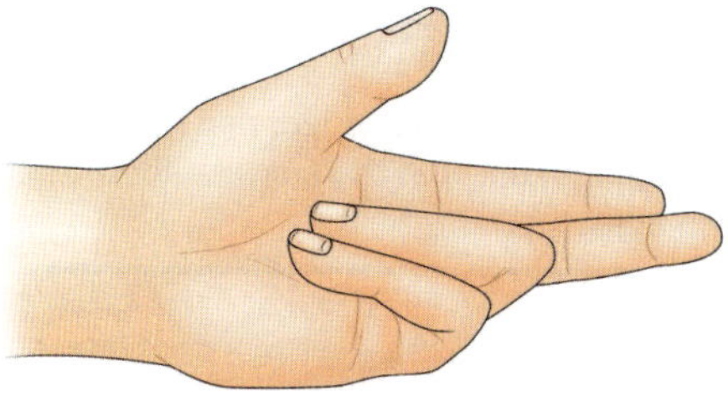

FIGURE 40-4 **Dupuytren contracture, a flexion deformity caused by an inherited trait, is a slowly progressive contracture of the palmar fascia, which severely impairs the function of the fourth, fifth, and, sometimes, the middle finger.**

COMMON FOOT PROBLEMS

Disorders of the foot are commonly caused by poorly fitting shoes, which distort normal anatomy while inducing deformity and pain.

Several systemic diseases affect the feet. Patients with diabetes are prone to develop corns and peripheral neuropathies with diminished sensation, leading to ulcers at pressure

BOX 40-4

Nursing Interventions for the Patient Undergoing Surgery to Treat Upper and Lower Extremity Conditions

Promoting Tissue Perfusion

Neurovascular assessment of the exposed digits every 1–2 hours for the first 24 hours after surgery is essential to monitor the function of the nerves and the perfusion of the tissues. The nurse compares the affected extremity with the unaffected one and the postoperative status with the documented preoperative status. Perfusion is assessed by temperature, color, capillary refill, and grading of peripheral pulses. The nurse asks the patient to describe the sensations in the affected extremity and to demonstrate mobility of the involved area. With tendon repairs and nerve, vascular, or skin grafts, motor function is tested as necessary. Dressings provide support but are not constrictive. If the patient is discharged within several hours after the surgery, the nurse teaches the patient and family how to assess for edema and neurovascular status (circulation, sensation, motion). Compromised neurovascular function can increase the patient's pain.

Relieving Pain

Pain experienced by patients who undergo hand and foot surgery is related to inflammation and edema. Formation of a hematoma may contribute to the discomfort. To control the edema, the extremity should be elevated on several pillows when the patient is sitting or lying. When higher elevation is prescribed for an upper extremity, an elevating sling may be attached to an IV pole or to an overhead frame. If the patient is ambulatory, the affected arm is elevated in a conventional sling with the hand at heart level.

Ice packs applied intermittently to the surgical area during the first 24–48 hours may be prescribed to control edema and provide some pain relief. Dependent positioning of an extremity is uncomfortable, but simply elevating the extremity often relieves the discomfort. Oral analgesics may be used to control the pain. The nurse instructs the patient and family about appropriate use of these medications.

Activity

During the first few days after surgery, the patient may need assistance with ADLs, particularly following surgery of an upper extremity when one hand is bandaged and independent self-care is impaired. The patient may need to arrange for assistance with feeding, bathing and hygiene, dressing, grooming, and toileting. Within a few days, the patient develops skills in one-handed ADLs and is usually able to function with minimal assistance and use of assistive devices. The nurse encourages use of the involved hand, unless contraindicated, within the limits of discomfort. As rehabilitation progresses, the patient resumes use of the injured hand. Physical or occupational therapy–directed exercises may be prescribed. The nurse emphasizes adherence to the therapeutic regimen.

After lower extremity surgery, the patient will have a bulky dressing on the foot, protected by a light cast or a special protective boot. Limits for weight-bearing on the foot will be prescribed by the surgeon. Some patients are allowed to walk on the heel and progress to weight-bearing as tolerated; other patients are restricted to non–weight-bearing activities. Assistive devices (e.g., crutches, walker) may be needed. The choice of the devices depends on the patient's general condition and balance and on the weight-bearing prescription. Safe use of the assistive devices must be ensured through adequate patient education and practice before discharge. Strategies to move around the house safely while using assistive devices are discussed with the patient. As healing progresses, the patient gradually resumes ambulation within prescribed limits. The nurse emphasizes adherence to the therapeutic regimen.

Preventing Infection

Any surgery carries a risk of infection. In addition, percutaneous pins may be used to hold bones in position, and these pins serve as potential sites for infection. Care must be taken to protect the surgical wound from dirt and moisture. When bathing, the patient can secure a plastic bag over the dressing to prevent it from getting wet. Patient instructions concerning aseptic wound care and pin care may be necessary. Refer to Chapter 41 for pin care.

The nurse teaches the patient to monitor for temperature changes and infection. Drainage on the dressing, a foul odor, or increased pain and swelling could indicate infection. The nurse instructs the patient to report any of these findings to the provider promptly. If prophylactic antibiotics are prescribed, the nurse provides instruction about their correct use.

Promoting Home and Community-Based Care

The nurse plans patient teaching for home care, focusing on neurovascular status, pain management, mobility, and wound care.

The nurse instructs the patient to report the following signs and symptoms, which indicate impaired circulation:

- Change in sensation
- Inability to move toes or fingers
- Digits or extremity cool to touch
- Color changes

The nurse also provides instructions for wound care, including:

- Keep the dressing or cast clean and dry
- Report signs of wound infection (e.g., pain, drainage, fever) immediately
- Follow the prescribed antibiotic regimen
- Keep your appointment with the surgeon for the initial dressing change

points of the foot. Patients with peripheral vascular disease and arteriosclerosis can develop ulcers as a result of ischemia. Complaints of burning and itching feet can be seen, resulting in scratching and skin breakdown. Foot deformities may occur with rheumatoid arthritis. Dermatologic problems commonly affect the feet in the form of fungal infections and plantar warts.

The discomforts of foot strain are treated with rest, elevation, physiotherapy, and orthotic devices. The patient must inspect the foot and skin under pads and orthotic devices daily for pressure and skin breakdown. If a "window" is cut into shoes to relieve pressure over a bony deformity, the skin must be monitored daily for breakdown from pressure exerted at the window area. Active foot exercises promote circulation and help strengthen the feet. Walking in properly fitting shoes is considered the ideal exercise.

Plantar Fasciitis

Plantar fasciitis is an inflammation of the foot-supporting fascia. Often, patients experience severe heel pain with the first steps in the morning. The pain is localized to the anterior medial aspect of the heel and diminishes with gentle stretching of the foot and Achilles tendon. Management includes stretching exercises, wearing shoes with support, orthotic devices (e.g., heel cups, arch supports), weight loss for obese patients, and NSAIDs. In approximately 80% of patients, symptoms of plantar fasciitis will resolve in 12 months (Trojian & Tucker, 2019). Unresolved plantar fasciitis may progress to fascial tears at the heel and eventual development of heel spurs.

Hallux Valgus

Hallux valgus (HV; commonly called a bunion) is a deformity in which the great toe deviates laterally (Fig. 40-5A). Associated with this is a marked prominence of the medial aspect of the first metatarsophalangeal joint. There is also osseous enlargement (exostosis) of the medial side of the first metatarsal head, over which a bursa may form (secondary to pressure and inflammation). Acute bursitis symptoms include a reddened area, edema, and tenderness.

Although the precise etiology of HV deformity is unknown, factors contributing to bunion formation may include heredity, ill-fitting shoes, a loss of arch height, and gradual lengthening and widening of the foot associated with aging. Frequently osteoarthritis is associated with HV. Treatment depends on the patient's age, the degree of deformity, and the severity of symptoms. If a bunion deformity is uncomplicated, wearing a shoe that conforms to the shape of the foot or that is molded to the foot to prevent pressure on the protruding portions may be the only treatment needed. A low heel, wider toebox, or focused stretching of the shoe upper is recommended (Ferrari, 2021).

Corticosteroid injections may be considered to control acute inflammation. Surgical removal of the bunion

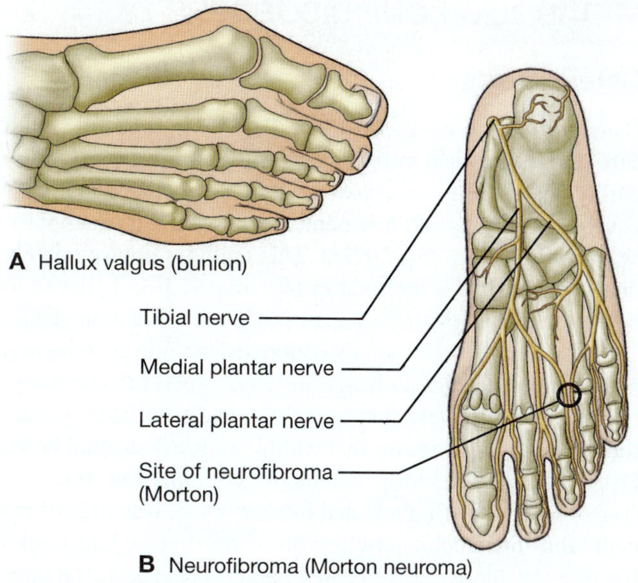

FIGURE 40-5 Common foot deformities.

(exostosis) and osteotomies to realign the toe may be required to improve function and appearance. Complications related to bunionectomy include limited range of motion (ROM), paresthesias, tendon injury, and recurrence of deformity.

Postoperatively, the patient may have intense throbbing pain at the operative site, requiring analgesic medication. The foot is elevated to the level of the heart to decrease edema and pain. The neurovascular status of the toes is assessed by noting temperature, color, sensation, movement, and capillary refill of the affected toes. The duration of immobility and initiation of ambulation depend on the procedure used. Toe flexion and extension exercises are initiated to facilitate walking. Shoes that fit the shape and size of the foot are recommended.

Morton Neuroma

Morton neuroma (plantar digital neuroma, neurofibroma) is a thickening of the tissues around the third (lateral) branch of the medial plantar nerve (see Fig. 40-5B). The third digital nerve, which is located in the third intermetatarsal (web) space, is most commonly involved. Microscopically, digital artery changes cause an ischemia of the nerve.

The result is a throbbing, burning pain in the foot that is usually relieved when the patient rests. Conservative treatment consists of inserting innersoles and metatarsal pads designed to spread the metatarsal heads and balance the foot posture. Local injections of hydrocortisone and a local anesthetic may provide relief. If these fail, surgical excision of the neuroma is necessary. Pain relief and loss of sensation are immediate and permanent.

See Box 40-4 for interventions for patients undergoing surgery for foot problems.

METABOLIC BONE DISORDERS

Osteoporosis

Osteoporosis is a costly disorder, not only in terms of health care dollars but also in terms of human suffering, pain, disability, and death. Approximately 54 million Americans have osteoporosis and low bone mass (National Osteoporosis Foundation [NOF], 2021a). This includes approximately one in two females and one in four males. It is believed to be the underlying cause of 2 million fractures a year (NOF, 2021). Characteristics of osteoporosis include a reduction of bone density and a change in bone structure. The bones become progressively porous, brittle, and fragile; they fracture easily under stresses that would not break normal bone. Osteoporosis frequently results in compression fractures (Fig. 40-6) of the thoracic and lumbar spine, fractures of the neck and intertrochanteric region of the femur, and Colles fractures of the wrist (refer to Chapter 41). These fractures may be the first clinical manifestation of osteoporosis. Fracture risk increases with increasing age and is greatest in White females.

Pathophysiology

It is thought that 60% to 80% of a person's peak bone mass is genetically determined. Bone mineral density (BMD) in adults is determined by the magnitude of bone acquisition during adolescence and young adulthood coupled with the rate of bone loss that ensues thereafter (Norris, 2019). Typically, peak bone mass is achieved by the early fourth decade, but after this age, rates of bone loss of 0.5% per year are seen; the rate of bone resorption (the lysis or breakdown of bone) is greater than the rate of bone formation, resulting in a reduced total bone mass (Fingerhood, 2021; Wilson et al., 2021). As individuals age, mismatches in bone remodeling, due to reduced formation, increased resorption, or a combination of both, result in greater rates of bone loss (Weber, 2020).

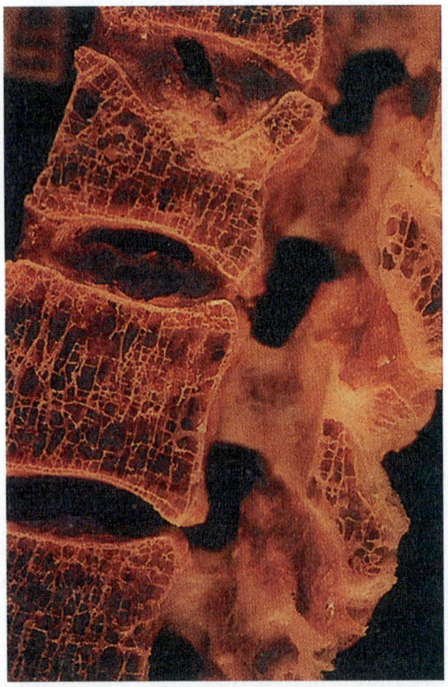

FIGURE 40-6 Progressive osteoporotic bone loss and compression fractures. (From Rubin, E., Gorstein, F., Schwarting, R., Rubin, R., Schwarting, R., & Strayer, D., Eds. (2004). *Rubin's Pathology: Clinicopathologic Foundations of Medicine* [4th ed.]. Lippincott Williams & Wilkins.)

Pearls for Practice

Nurses are aware that bone density issues in later years are correlated to bone acquisition in younger years. It is important that nurses stress the need for bone health for children and young adults. Early identification of at-risk teenagers and young adults, increased calcium intake, participation in regular weight-bearing exercise, and modification of lifestyle (e.g., reduced use of caffeine, cigarettes, carbonated soft drinks, and alcohol) are interventions that decrease the risk of osteoporosis, fractures, and associated disability later in life.

Primary osteoporosis is the loss of bone mass due to aging and decreased gonadal function, not to any other chronic illness (Ferri, 2022, p. 1109). Type 1 osteoporosis is related to the withdrawal of estrogens at menopause or with oophorectomy which causes accelerated bone resorption that continues during the postmenopausal years. Females develop osteoporosis more frequently and more extensively than males because of lower peak bone mass and the effect of estrogen loss during menopause. Fractures of the spine, hip, and wrist are associated with type 1, whereas type 2 osteoporosis occurs after age 70 (in both males and females) due to the imbalance between bone building and bone resorption (described earlier). Fractures of the spine, long bones, and hip are associated with type 2 (Ford & Heinle, 2022).

Secondary osteoporosis is associated with chronic conditions such as nutritional deficiencies and with medications. Coexisting medical conditions, such as gastric bypass, malabsorption syndromes, lactose intolerance, alcohol use disorder, kidney failure, liver failure, Cushing syndrome, hyperthyroidism, and hyperparathyroidism, contribute to bone loss and the development of osteoporosis. Medications, including corticosteroids, antiseizure medications, heparin, tetracycline, aluminum-containing antacids, and thyroid supplements, affect the body's use and metabolism of calcium. The degree of osteoporosis is related to the duration of medication therapy. When the therapy is discontinued or the metabolic problem is corrected, the progression of osteoporosis is halted, but restoration of lost bone mass usually does not occur. Specific disease states (e.g., celiac disease, hypogonadism) and medications (e.g., corticosteroids, antiseizure medications) that place patients at risk need to be identified and therapies instituted to reverse the development of osteoporosis. Calcium metabolism is illustrated in Figure 40-7.

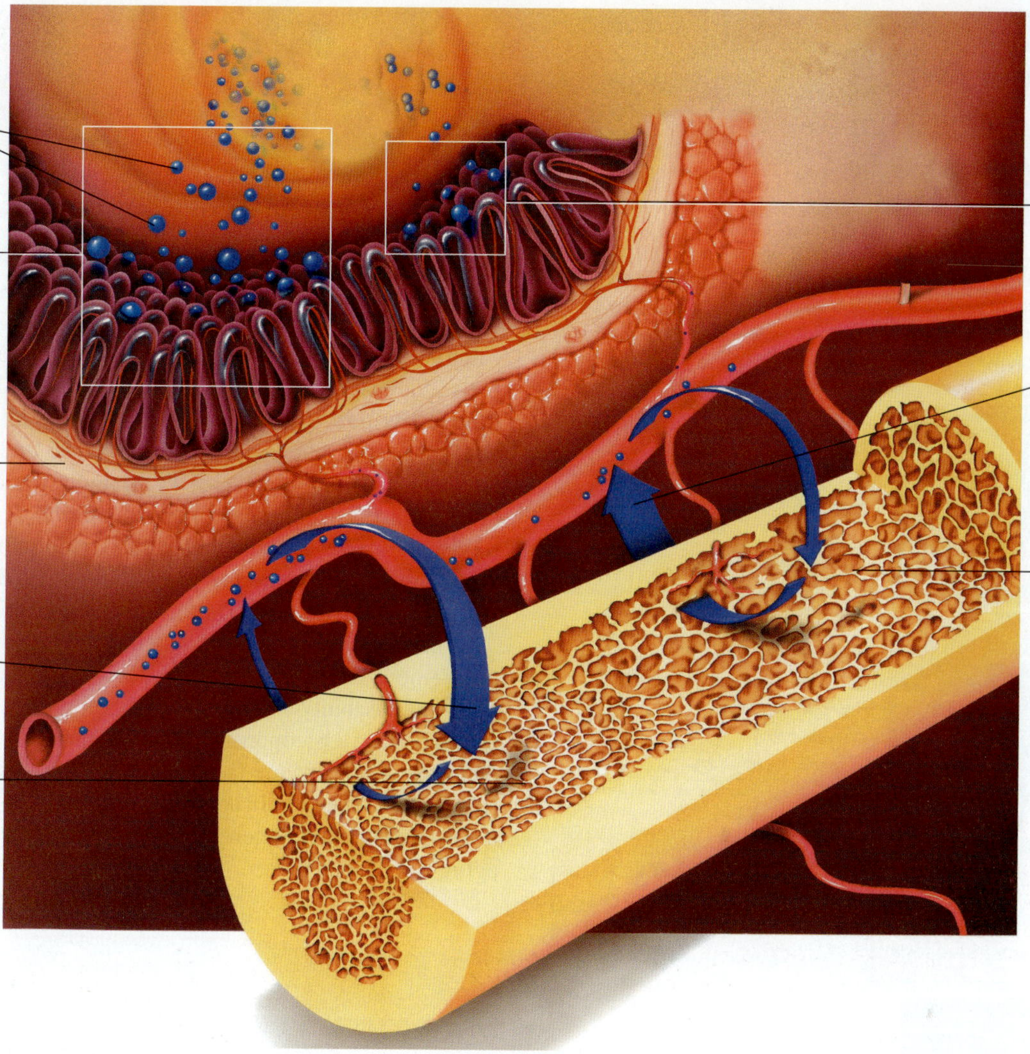

FIGURE 40-7 Calcium metabolism in osteoporosis. Normally, blood absorbs calcium from the digestive system and deposits it into bone. In osteoporosis, blood levels of calcium are reduced. To maintain blood calcium levels, reabsorption of calcium from the bones is increased.

Risk Factors

Females who are small-framed, with low body weight (<58 kg), are at the greatest risk for osteoporosis (Ford & Heinle, 2022). Males have a greater peak bone mass and do not experience sudden estrogen reduction. As a result, osteoporosis occurs in males at a lower rate and at an older age (about one decade later) (Weber, 2020). It is believed that testosterone and estrogen are important in achieving and maintaining bone mass in males.

Nutritional factors contribute to the development of osteoporosis. A diet that includes adequate calories and nutrients needed to maintain bone, calcium, and vitamin D must be consumed. Vitamin D is necessary for calcium absorption and for normal bone mineralization. Dietary calcium and vitamin D must be adequate to maintain bone remodeling and body functions. While there is some controversy, it appears that vitamin D deficiency is more prevalent than previously thought (Weber, 2020) as more than 75% of individuals in the United States are either vitamin D deficient or insufficient (Weber, 2020).

Bone formation is enhanced by the stress of weight and muscle activity. Resistance and impact exercises are most beneficial in developing and maintaining bone mass. Immobility contributes to the development of osteoporosis. Additional clinical risk factors for osteoporotic fractures are previous fragility fracture (s), a family history of hip fracture, and a history of falls (Ford & Heinle, 2022). Refer to Figure 40-8 for a summary of risk factors for osteoporosis.

Pearls for Practice: Lifting the Lens

There is ongoing debate about the risk of fracture and osteoporosis across all ethnic groups beyond Chinese and White individuals (see Fig. 40-8). In addition, "the beneficial role of dairy products in bone health has been more extensively established in Chinese and Caucasian girls and females, but these results could

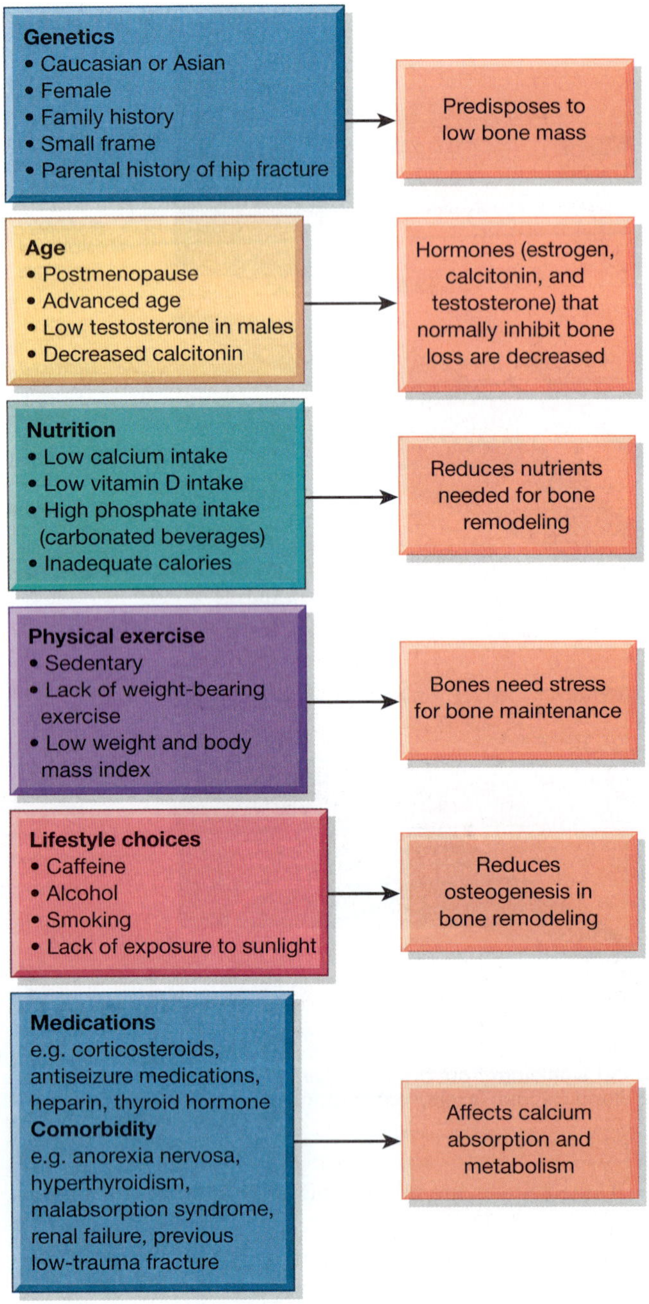

FIGURE 40-8 **Risk factors for osteoporosis and the effects of these factors on bone.**

not be replicated for other populations (Muñoz-Garach et al., 2020, p. 3)." In addition, the fracture risk algorithm (FRAX) systematically underestimates the risk in non-White populations by using a correction factor based on studies conducted 30–40 years ago resulting in lower calculated fracture risk among people of color (Reid, 2021). Thus, the nurse should recognize that there is a need for additional research regarding the impact of osteoporosis across racial and ethnic minorities, for thoughtful analysis regarding clinical algorithms whose use of race may perpetuate inequities in clinical care, and for supporting the need for research on the influence of bone health-promoting diets in specific ethnic groups. In sum, ***do not*** *assume that any of your patients are not at risk for this common disorder because of race or ethnicity.*

Gerontologic Considerations

The prevalence of osteoporosis increases with age; although this disorder is not gender specific, there is an increased incidence in females. Furthermore, older people absorb dietary calcium less efficiently and excrete it more readily through their kidneys; therefore, postmenopausal females and older individuals need to ensure daily calcium intake as well as vitamin D. For females older than age 50 and males older than age 70, a daily intake of 1,200 mg/day and 800 IU/day of vitamin D is suggested and consumption of calcium-rich foods and beverages is preferred. Calcium intake above 2,500 mg/day is avoided to prevent potential risk of kidney stones and constipation (Das & Choudhuri, 2021).

With the aging of the population, the incidence of fractures (more than 9 million osteoporotic fractures per year), pain, and disability associated with osteoporosis is increasing (International Osteoporosis Foundation, 2021). Most residents of long-term care facilities have a low BMD and are at risk for bone fracture. In addition, restricted sun exposure and a reduced capacity to generate previtamin D in the skin with aging is a consideration.

Pearls for Practice

Nurses are aware that corticosteroids are the most frequent cause of medication-related osteoporosis. Often patients with arthritis are prescribed long-term steroids. The combination of the medication and the disease process itself places patients at increased risk for fractures.

Clinical Manifestations and Assessment

Osteoporosis may be undetectable on routine x-rays until there has been 25% to 40% demineralization, resulting in radiolucency of the bones. Frequently, postmenopausal females lose height from vertebral collapse. The gradual collapse of a vertebra may be asymptomatic (one third in height loss per year per decade over 50 years of age); it is observed as progressive kyphosis or "dowager's hump" (Fig. 40-9). Multiple compression fractures of the vertebrae result in skeletal deformity. The postural changes result in relaxation of the abdominal muscles and a protruding abdomen. Also the deformity may produce pulmonary insufficiency. Many patients complain of fatigue.

Osteoporosis is diagnosed by dual-energy x-ray absorptiometry (DEXA), which provides information about BMD at the spine and hip. DEXA of the forearm, hip, or spine are the gold standard in screening for osteoporosis and predicting the risk of hip and nonvertebral fracture. Current

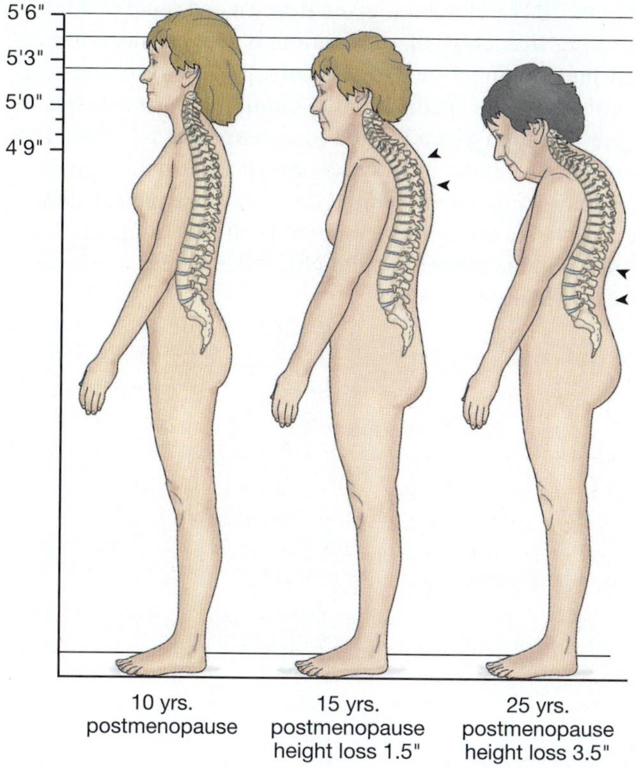

FIGURE 40-9 Typical loss of height associated with osteoporosis and aging.

evidence-based guidelines recommend the use of BMD (spine and hip) as the first-line screening test for osteoporosis (The International Society for Densitometry, 2021) for all postmenopausal females and males over 50 years of age. The DEXA scan data are analyzed and reported as T scores (the number of standard deviations [SDs] above or below the average BMD value for a healthy adult at 30 years of age). A normal BMD is less than 1 SD below the young adult mean value. According to Burt et al. (2019), BMD is known to correlate with bone strength and is considered an important component in predicting future fracture risk. It is critical to rule out other conditions associated with low BMD. There is also a fracture risk algorithm (FRAX) developed by the World Health Organization (WHO) to evaluate specific risk factors to assess the 10-year absolute fracture risk for all osteoporotic fractures. The WHO defines osteoporosis as being present when the T score is at least 2.5 SD below the young adult mean value on BMD scan (NOF, 2021b). In all transgender and gender nonconforming individuals aged 50 years or older, regardless of hormone status, a T score of <–2.5 or less should be used to diagnose osteoporosis (The International Society for Densitometry, 2021). Low bone mass (osteopenia) is diagnosed when the BMD T score is between 1 and 2.5 SD below the young adult mean value. Fracture risk increases progressively as the SD of the T score falls below the mean value.

BMD studies are useful in identifying low bone mass and osteoporotic bone and in assessing response to therapy. Bone loss and osteoporosis can be reduced through early screening (using both assessment of risk factors and BMD scans), promotion of adequate dietary intake of calcium and vitamin D, encouragement of lifestyle changes, and early institution of preventive medications, resulting in a reduced incidence of fracture.

Other possible medical diagnoses that contribute to bone loss (e.g., multiple myeloma, osteomalacia, hyperparathyroidism, malignancy, celiac disease, hypogonadism in males) can be excluded through the use of x-ray studies or laboratory studies, such as serum calcium, serum phosphate, vitamin D 25OH, bone-specific alkaline phosphatase, urine calcium excretion, testosterone and estrogen studies, Hct, and erythrocyte sedimentation rate (ESR). In the future, quantitative ultrasound may be used to predict fracture risk because of its decreased costs and lack of exposure to radiation; however, additional research is needed to establish its utility in diagnosis and management of osteoporosis (Ford & Heinle, 2022).

Medical and Nursing Management

All people should continue to obtain sufficient calcium, vitamin D (Box 40-5), sunshine, and weight-bearing exercise to slow the progression of osteoporosis.

BOX 40-5

Pearls for Practice: Nutrition

Calcium and Vitamin D

A diet rich in calcium and vitamin D throughout life, with an increased calcium intake during adolescence, young adulthood, and the middle years, protects against skeletal demineralization. Such a diet includes three glasses of skim or whole vitamin D–enriched milk (a cup of milk or calcium-fortified orange juice contains about 300 mg of calcium) or other foods high in calcium (e.g., cheese and other dairy products, steamed broccoli, canned salmon with bones) daily.

The RAI level for adults 19–50 years of age is 1,000 mg/day, and the RAI level for adults 51 years of age and older is 1,200 mg/day.

The Bone Health and Osteoporosis Foundation (formerly the National Osteoporosis Foundation) (2021) recommends an intake of 800–1,000 international units (IU) of vitamin D per day for adults 50 years of age and older. Inadequate intake of calcium or vitamin D over a period of years results in decreased bone mass and the development of osteoporosis.

To ensure adequate calcium intake, a calcium supplement with vitamin D may be prescribed and taken with meals or with a beverage high in vitamin C to promote absorption. The recommended daily dose should be split and not taken as a single dose. Common side effects of calcium supplements are abdominal distention and constipation. Because GI symptoms and abdominal distention are frequent side effects of calcium supplements, the nurse instructs the patient to take the calcium supplements with meals. Also, it is important to teach the patient to drink adequate fluids to reduce the risk of renal calculi.

Pharmacologic Therapy

Medications commonly prescribed to treat osteoporosis are classified based on their mechanism of action: anticatabolic (i.e., antiresorptive or against bone breakdown) and anabolic (i.e., bone building). Anticatabolic medications, or antiresorptives, inhibit osteoclast activity, resulting in reductions in skeletal turnover and bone loss. Oral bisphosphonates, such as alendronate and risedronate, reduce spine and hip fractures associated with osteoporosis through inhibition of osteoclast activity, reducing bone resorption and turnover. Adequate calcium and vitamin D intake is needed for maximum effect. Side effects of bisphosphonates include gastrointestinal (GI) symptoms (e.g., dyspepsia, nausea, flatulence, diarrhea, constipation), and some patients may develop esophageal ulcers, esophagitis, gastric ulcers, or osteonecrosis of the jaw related to bisphosphonate use. Patients must take these medications on an empty stomach with a full glass of water upon arising in the morning, and they must sit upright for 30 to 60 minutes after the administration. Other bisphosphonates are administered intravenously; however, oral bisphosphonates are generally the initial therapy owing to their efficacy, favorable cost, and the availability of long-term safety data (Rosen & Drezner, 2021).

At natural or surgical menopause, hormone therapy with estrogen and progesterone had been the mainstay of therapy to slow bone loss and reduce the occurrence of fractures. Estrogen replacement decreases bone resorption and increases bone mass, reducing the incidence of osteoporotic fractures. However, studies have demonstrated greater risks, including strokes, venous thromboemboli, and breast cancer, than the benefits of osteoporosis preventive treatment could justify. Although hormone therapy is approved to conserve bone mass and prevent osteoporosis-related fractures, the lowest effective dose for the shortest amount of time is recommended (NOF, 2021c).

Denosumab, is a human monoclonal antibody that inhibits osteoclast formation and prevents resorption for treatment of postmenopausal osteoporosis. It may be used for patients at high risk for fractures who cannot tolerate other therapy (Ford & Heinle, 2022), since it has been shown to decrease the risk for spine, hip, and nonvertebral fracture in females and males (Weber, 2020). It is administered subcutaneously and should not be used in patients who have had a myocardial infarction or stroke in the past year (Ford & Heinle, 2021).

Another class of medications are anabolic or "bone-building" drugs such as teriparatide (Forteo), or abaloparatide (Tymlos), a recombinant human parathyroid hormone. This class stimulates osteoblasts to build bone matrix and facilitates overall calcium absorption. The medication is administered subcutaneously into the thigh or abdominal wall once daily for the treatment of osteoporosis in postmenopausal females and males at risk for fracture. In research studies bone mass density improved and a reduction in fracture rates were similar with abaloparatide and teriparatide (Rosen, 2021). However, given the cost and route of administration, this class of medication is not considered as a first-line treatment for osteoporosis. It is not recommended that this class of medication be continued for more than a 2-year duration given limited long-term research data. The nurse is also aware that symptoms of orthostatic hypotension may occur with the initial dose; thus, the patient should be in either a sitting or recumbent position during administration and the nurse should monitor the patient's pulse and blood pressure.

Pearls for Practice

Postural (orthostatic) hypotension is a significant decrease in BP with a change in body position from supine to sitting/standing or from sitting to standing. It may be accompanied by dizziness, lightheadedness, or syncope. An increase in heart rate of 15 bpm with either a 20 mm Hg decrease in systolic pressure or a 10 mm Hg decrease in diastolic pressure within 3 minutes are abnormal findings (Bickley et al., 2021). The patient will remain in the recumbent position and the provider notified if the patient is symptomatic.

Preventing Injury

Physical activity is essential to strengthen muscles, improve balance, prevent disuse atrophy, and slow progressive bone demineralization. Regular weight-bearing exercise promotes bone formation. It is recommended that patients perform 20 to 30 minutes of aerobic exercise (e.g., walking), 3 days or more a week. Weight training stimulates an increase in BMD. In addition, exercise improves balance, reducing the incidence of falls and fractures. Tai chi and yoga may be helpful to improve balance, increase muscle tone, and reduce fall risk in those over 65 years (Clinical Overview, 2021). Isometric exercises can strengthen trunk muscles. The nurse encourages walking, good body mechanics, and good posture. Daily weight-bearing activity, preferably outdoors in the sunshine to enhance the body's ability to produce vitamin D, is encouraged. Sudden bending, jarring, and strenuous lifting are avoided.

Fracture Management

Fractures of the hip are managed surgically by joint replacement or by closed or open reduction with internal fixation (e.g., hip pinning). Surgery, early ambulation, intensive physical therapy, and adequate nutrition result in decreased morbidity and improved outcomes. In addition, patients need to be evaluated for osteoporosis and treated, if indicated. Refer to Chapter 41 for details on nursing management of patients with a fracture.

One of the more common fractures associated with osteoporosis is vertebral compression fracture. It can affect approximately 25% of postmenopausal females and 750,000 individuals annually (American Associate of Neurosurgeons

BOX 40-6

Highlighting Gerontology

Fall Prevention

Older adults fall frequently as a result of environmental hazards, neuromuscular disorders, diminished senses, cardiovascular responses, and responses to medications. The patient and family need to be included in planning for care and preventive management regimens. For example, the home environment should be assessed for safety and elimination of potential hazards (e.g., scatter rugs, cluttered rooms and stairwells, toys on the floor, pets underfoot). Then a safe environment can be created (e.g., well-lighted staircases with secure hand rails, grab bars in the bathroom, properly fitting footwear).

[AANS], 2021). Compression fractures can lead to significant deformity and pain, causing disability and decreased quality of life (QOL). Typically osteoporotic compression fractures of the vertebra are managed conservatively with analgesics, external braces, and physical therapy. However, patients with ongoing severe pain may choose vertebral body augmentation, such as kyphoplasty or percutaneous vertebroplasty. Percutaneous vertebroplasty/kyphoplasty includes injection of polymethylmethacrylate bone cement into the fractured vertebra, followed by inflation of a pressurized balloon to restore the shape of the affected vertebra. This procedure can provide rapid relief of acute pain and improve QOL. Patients who have not responded to first-line approaches to the treatment of vertebral compression fracture can be considered for the procedure. It is contraindicated in the presence of infection, old fractures, uncorrected coagulopathies, and allergic sensitivity to any of the required components.

Box 40-6 discusses fall prevention. Box 40-7 discusses the impact of nurse practitioners on osteoporosis management.

Paget Disease

Paget disease (osteitis deformans) is a disorder of localized rapid bone turnover, most commonly affecting the skull, femur, tibia, pelvic bones, humerus, scapula, and vertebrae. The disease occurs in about 3% of the population older than 50 years of age and up to 10% in those more than 90 years of age (Tucci, 2022). The incidence is slightly greater in males than in females and increases with aging (Tucci, 2022). A family history has been noted, with siblings often developing the disease. The cause of Paget disease is not known.

Pathophysiology

In Paget disease, there is a primary proliferation of osteoclasts, which produces bone resorption. This is followed by a compensatory increase in osteoblastic activity that replaces the bone. As this chaotic bone turnover continues, a classic mosaic (disorganized) pattern of bone develops. Because the diseased bone is of poor quality, highly vascularized, and structurally weak, pathologic fractures occur. Structural bowing of the legs causes malalignment of the joints of the hip, knee, and ankle, which contributes to the development of arthritis and back and joint pain.

Clinical Manifestations and Assessment

Paget disease is insidious; most patients never experience symptoms but have skeletal deformity. A few patients have symptomatic deformity, and up to 40% of patients who come to medical attention present with bone pain (Tucci, 2022). The condition is identified most frequently on x-ray studies performed during a routine physical examination or during a workup for another problem. Sclerotic changes, skeletal deformities (e.g., bowing of the femur and tibia, enlargement of the skull, deformity of pelvic bones), and cortical thickening of the long bones occur.

BOX 40-7

Nursing Research

Bridging the Gap to Evidence-Based Practice

Collins, L., Cata, D. M., & Conley, N. S. (2020). A comparison study- oral patient-controlled analgesia (PCA) versus traditional delivery of pain medication following orthopaedic procedures. *Orthopaedic Nursing*, *39*(5), 324–332.

Purpose

The purpose of this timing study was to examine if the use of the oral PCA device would reduce the nursing time to accomplish the delivery of PRN oral pain medication compared to the manual administration by nursing staff.

Design

This study took place on an inpatient orthopedic surgical unit. It was a descriptive comparative timing study that compared the nursing time to accomplish the manual administration of a single dose of oral PRN pain medication with the nursing time utilizing the PCA device.

Findings

The mean nursing time to provide manual administration of a single dose of PRN pain medication was 12.7 minutes. The mean time to provide a single dose of pain medication using the oral PCA device was 2.06 minutes. The reduction in nursing time from 12.7 to 2.06 minutes per single dose delivered is 10.7 minutes or an 84% reduction in the nursing time necessary to deliver pain medication.

Nursing Implications

Nurses working on inpatient orthopedic units spend a significant portion of their time addressing the pain needs of their patients. Utilizing an oral PCA device for the delivery of single-dose PRN pain medication can help nurses provide care in an increasingly demanding work environment. The additional time that is made available for the nurse allows for greater nursing presence at the bedside.

In most patients, skeletal deformity involves the skull or long bones. The skull may thicken, and the patient may report that a hat no longer fits. In some cases, the cranium, but not the face, is enlarged. This gives the patient's face a small, triangular appearance. Most patients with skull involvement have impaired hearing from cranial nerve compression and dysfunction. Other cranial nerves also may be compressed.

The femurs and tibiae tend to bow, producing a waddling gait. The spine is bent forward and is rigid; the chin rests on the chest. The thorax is compressed and immobile on respiration. The trunk is flexed on the legs to maintain balance, and the arms are bent outward and forward and appear long in relation to the shortened trunk. Nerve entrapment may be seen.

Pain, tenderness, and warmth over the bones may be noted. The pain is mild to moderate, deep, and aching; it increases with weight-bearing if the lower extremities are involved. Pain and discomfort may precede skeletal deformities of Paget disease by years and often are wrongly attributed by the patient to old age or arthritis.

The temperature of the skin overlying the affected bone increases because of increased bone vascularity. The nurse is aware that due to the vascularity of pagetic bone, excessive bleeding during orthopedic surgery is a concern (Charles, 2021a).

Increased osteoblastic activity is reflected by elevated serum alkaline phosphatase (sAP), and the bone-specific alkaline phosphatase (bAP), is frequently elevated (Charles, 2021a). Conditions that affect bone growth or cause increased activity of bone cells affect serum ALP and excretion of urinary N telopeptide (a measure of bone turnover). Higher values suggest more active disease. In most patients with Paget disease normal levels of blood calcium and phosphorus are seen.

Concept Mastery Alert

Elevated serum alkaline phosphatase (SAP) levels, but a normal serum calcium level, are indicative of Paget disease.

X-rays confirm the diagnosis of Paget disease. Local areas of demineralization and bone overgrowth produce characteristic mosaic patterns and irregularities. Bone scans demonstrate the extent of the disease. Bone scintigraphy is the most sensitive test to detail the extent and site of pagetic lesions. Bone biopsy may aid in the differential diagnosis.

Medical and Nursing Management

Several medications reduce bone turnover, reverse the course of the disease, relieve pain, and improve mobility. Pain usually responds to NSAIDs. Gait problems from bowing of the legs are managed with walking aids, shoe lifts, and physical therapy. Weight is controlled to reduce stress on weakened bones and malaligned joints. A diet adequate in calcium and vitamin D is important, as is periodic monitoring to prevent hypocalcemia and secondary hyperparathyroidism during therapy (Norris, 2019).

Bisphosphonates are used to treat Paget disease as they help to suppress further pain and spread of the disease. The preferred option is a one-time dose of zoledronic acid (5 mg IV), which has been associated with controlling symptoms for up to 5 to 6 years and some for as long as 10 years (Charles, 2021b; Tucci, 2022). They produce rapid reduction in bone turnover and relief of pain. They also reduce bone-specific alkaline phosphatase and urinary N telopeptide levels. If the patient wishes to avoid IV medication, oral bisphosphonates (alendronate or risedronate) can be used. As noted earlier, food inhibits absorption of these medications; therefore, patients ingest the medications on an empty stomach (refer to previous discussion of bisphosphonates in this chapter). In the rare patient intolerant of both parenteral and oral bisphosphonates, calcitonin, a polypeptide hormone, may be used as it slows bone resorption by decreasing the number and availability of osteoclasts. Calcitonin therapy facilitates remodeling of abnormal bone into normal lamellar bone, relieves bone pain, and helps alleviate neurologic and biochemical signs and symptoms. Calcitonin is administered subcutaneously or by nasal inhalation. Side effects include flushing of the face and nausea. The effect of calcitonin therapy is evident in 3 to 6 months through reduction of bone loss and pain.

Fractures, arthritis, and hearing loss are complications of Paget disease. Fractures are managed according to location. Healing occurs if fracture reduction, immobilization, and stability are adequate. Severe degenerative arthritis may require total joint replacement. Loss of hearing, which is associated when Paget disease affects the skull, is managed with hearing aids and communication techniques used with people who are hearing-impaired (e.g., speech reading, body language).

Gerontologic Considerations

Because Paget disease tends to affect older people, careful assessment of a patient's pain and discomfort is necessary. It is estimated that up to 10% in those aged >90 years has this disease (Ferri, 2022). Patient teaching helps the patient understand the treatment regimen, the need for a diet with adequate calcium and vitamin D, and how to compensate for altered musculoskeletal functioning. The home environment is assessed for safety to prevent falls and to reduce the risk of fracture. Strategies for coping with a chronic health problem and its effect on QOL need to be developed.

MUSCULOSKELETAL INFECTIONS

Osteomyelitis

Osteomyelitis is an infection of the bone; it can be acute or chronic and is usually bacterial in nature. The bone becomes infected in one of three ways:

- Extension of soft tissue infection (e.g., infected pressure or vascular ulcer, incisional infection)

- Direct bone contamination from bone surgery (e.g., surgical fixation), open fracture, or traumatic injury (e.g., gunshot wound)
- Hematogenous (blood-borne) spread from other sites of infection (e.g., urinary tract infection, intravascular catheterization sites, skin and soft tissues and the endocardium are the most commons sites [Jameson et al., 2020b]).

The risk for osteomyelitis increases with age and includes patients with impaired immune systems, trauma and open fractures; those persons who inject drugs; those with chronic illnesses (e.g., diabetes, neuropathy, and arterial insufficiency) or orthopedic hardware; and those receiving long-term corticosteroid therapy or immunosuppressive agents.

Pearls for Practice

The nurse is aware that all orthopedic surgeries carry the risk of osteomyelitis. Consider that with surgery, the protective barrier of the skin is disrupted, allowing bacteria from the skin to enter the wound and invade bone tissue (Hofstee et al., 2020). Therefore the nurse maintains a high degree of suspicion and observes for symptoms such as pain, swelling, purulent drainage, wound breakdown, erythema, increased local temperature, dull pain, malaise, and sometimes fever and chills. The surgeon is notified of the nurse's concerns.

Acute osteomyelitis may present gradually with the onset appearing over a few days, but it usually manifests within 2 weeks, whereas chronic osteomyelitis manifests more slowly (Momodu et al., 2021). The nurse is aware that postoperative surgical wound infections can occur within 30 days after surgery. They are classified as incisional (superficial, located above the deep fascia layer) or deep (involving tissue beneath the deep fascia). If an implant has been used, deep postoperative infections may occur within a year. Deep sepsis after arthroplasty (surgical procedure that replaces damaged joints) may be classified as follows:

- *Stage 1, acute fulminating:* Occurring during the first 3 months after orthopedic surgery; frequently associated with hematoma, drainage, or superficial infection
- *Stage 2, delayed onset:* Occurring between 4 and 24 months after surgery
- *Stage 3, late onset:* Occurring 2 or more years after surgery, usually as a result of hematogenous spread

Bone infections are more difficult to eradicate than are soft tissue infections because the infected bone is mostly avascular (without blood vessels) and not accessible to the body's natural immune response. Also, there is decreased penetration by antibiotics.

Pathophysiology

Bone infections are commonly caused by *Staphylococcus aureus* (~40–50% of cases) *and Streptococcus.* Other pathogenic organisms that frequently are found in osteomyelitis include MRSA: methicillin-resistant *S. aureus, Pseudomonas aeruginosa, Escherichia coli, Neisseria gonorrhoeae, Haemophilus influenzae, Fungi, and Salmonella* (Norris, 2019). There is increasing incidence of infections that are penicillin resistant, nosocomial, gram negative, and anaerobic.

The initial response to infection is inflammation, increased vascularity, and edema. After 2 or 3 days, thrombosis of the blood vessels occurs in the area, resulting in ischemia with bone necrosis. The infection extends into the medullary cavity and under the periosteum and may spread into adjacent soft tissues and joints. Unless the infective process is treated promptly, a bone abscess forms. The resulting abscess cavity contains dead bone tissue (the **sequestrum**), which does not easily liquefy and drain. Therefore, the cavity cannot collapse and heal as it does with abscesses in soft tissue. New bone growth (the **involucrum**) forms and surrounds the sequestrum (Fig. 40-10). Although healing appears to take place, a chronically infected sequestrum remains and produces recurring abscesses throughout the patient's life. This is referred to as chronic osteomyelitis.

Clinical Manifestations and Assessment

The hallmark of osteomyelitis is localized pain over the infected bones. When the infection is blood-borne, the onset is usually sudden, occurring often with the clinical and laboratory manifestations of sepsis (e.g., chills, high fever, rapid pulse, and general malaise). The systemic symptoms, such as fever, may overshadow the local signs at first. As the infection extends through the cortex of the bone, it involves the periosteum and the soft tissues. The infected area becomes painful, swollen, and extremely tender. The patient may describe a constant, pulsating pain that intensifies with movement as a result of the pressure of the collecting pus. When osteomyelitis occurs from spread of adjacent infection or from direct contamination, there may be symptoms of sepsis. The area is swollen, warm, painful, and tender to touch.

In acute osteomyelitis, x-ray findings demonstrate soft tissue swelling, areas of irregular decalcification, bone necrosis, periosteal elevation, and new bone formation. However, these radiographic changes associated with osteomyelitis are delayed for approximately 14 days. Radioisotope bone scans, particularly the isotope-labeled white blood cell (WBC) scan, and magnetic resonance imaging (MRI) help with early definitive diagnosis. Of all the diagnostic imaging options, the MRI has the highest combined sensitivity and specificity for detecting osteomyelitis (within 3 to 5 days of disease onset) (Momodu et al., 2021). Blood studies reveal leukocytosis (elevated WBCs) and an elevated ESR and C-reactive protein in hematogenous and acute osteomyelitis, but those counts may be normal in chronic contiguous osteomyelitis. Wound and blood culture studies are performed to identify the offending organisms so appropriate antibiotic therapy can be instituted.

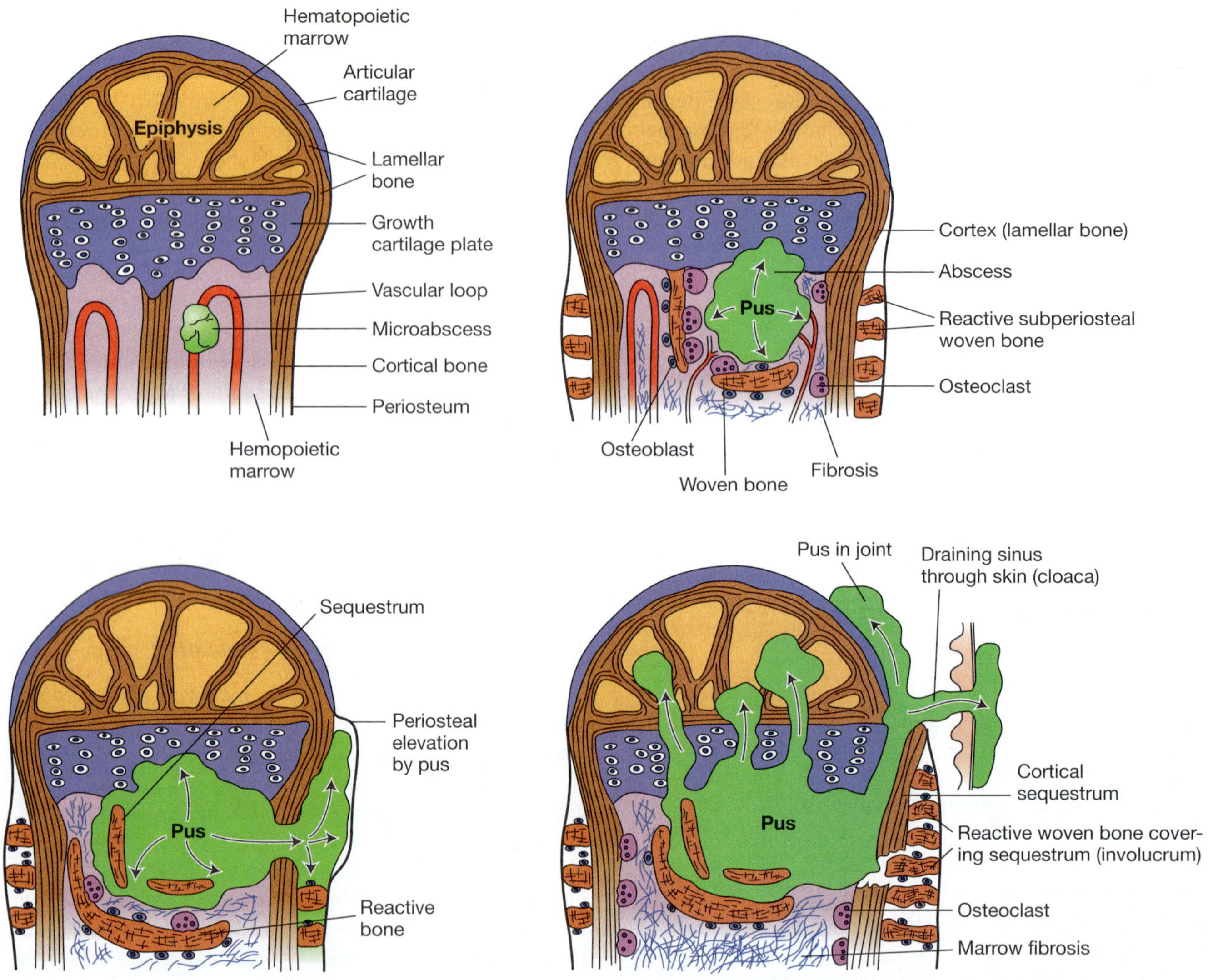

FIGURE 40-10 Stages of osteomyelitis.

With chronic osteomyelitis, large, irregular cavities, raised periosteum, sequestra, or dense bone formations are seen on x-ray. Bone scans may be performed to identify areas of infection. Usually, the ESR and the WBC count are normal. Anemia, associated with chronic infection, may be evident. The abscess is cultured to determine the infective organism and appropriate antibiotic therapy. While both acute and chronic osteomyelitis are associated with infections of the bone, they are differentiated by the presence of dead bone in the latter.

Prevention

Prevention of osteomyelitis is the goal. Elective orthopedic surgery should be postponed if the patient has a current infection [e.g., urinary tract infection, pharyngitis (sore throat)] or a recent history of infection. During orthopedic surgery, careful attention is paid to the surgical environment and to techniques to decrease direct bone contamination. Prophylactic antibiotics, administered to achieve adequate tissue levels at the time of surgery and for 24 hours after surgery, are helpful. Urinary catheters and drains are removed as soon as possible to decrease the incidence of hematogenous spread of infection.

Treatment of focal infections diminishes hematogenous spread. Aseptic postoperative wound care reduces the incidence of superficial infections and osteomyelitis. Prompt management of soft tissue infections reduces extension of infection to the bone. When patients who have had joint replacement surgery undergo dental procedures or other invasive procedures (e.g., cystoscopy), prophylactic antibiotics are recommended frequently. In order to decrease the incidence of osteomyelitis of the foot in patients with diabetes, therapy should be aimed at controlling the blood sugar, decreasing the incidence of peripheral vascular disease.

Medical Management

The initial goal of therapy is to control and halt the infective process. Antibiotic therapy depends on the results of blood and wound cultures. Frequently, the infection is caused by more than one pathogen. General supportive measures (e.g., hydration, a balanced diet, correction of anemia) should be instituted. If necessary, the area affected with osteomyelitis is immobilized to decrease discomfort and to prevent pathologic fracture of the weakened bone.

Pharmacologic Therapy

As soon as the culture specimens are obtained, IV antibiotic therapy begins. The aim is to control the infection before the blood supply to the area diminishes as a result of thrombosis. Around-the-clock dosing is necessary to achieve a sustained high therapeutic blood level of the antibiotic. After results of the culture and sensitivity studies are known, an antibiotic to which the causative organism is sensitive is prescribed. IV antibiotic therapy usually continues for 6 weeks for acute osteomyelitis; chronic osteomyelitis may require a longer course of medication (Fort, 2022). After the infection appears to be controlled, the antibiotic may be administered orally for up to 3 months. To enhance absorption of the orally administered medication, antibiotics should not be administered with food.

Surgical Management

If the infection is chronic, surgical debridement may be indicated. The infected bone is surgically exposed, the purulent and necrotic material is removed, and the area is irrigated with sterile saline solution. Antibiotic-impregnated beads may be placed in the wound for direct application of antibiotics for 2 to 4 weeks. IV antibiotic therapy is continued.

In chronic osteomyelitis, antibiotics are adjunctive therapy to surgical debridement. A sequestrectomy (removal of enough involucrum to enable the surgeon to remove the sequestrum) is performed. In many cases, sufficient bone is removed to convert a deep cavity into a shallow saucer (saucerization). All dead, infected bone and cartilage must be removed (to the extent possible) before permanent healing can occur. This is, followed by culture-directed IV antibiotic therapy.

The wound is either closed tightly to obliterate the dead space or packed and closed later by granulation or possibly by grafting. The debrided cavity may be packed with cancellous bone graft to stimulate healing. With a large defect, the cavity may be filled with a vascularized bone transfer or muscle flap (in which a muscle is moved from an adjacent area with blood supply intact). These microsurgery techniques enhance the blood supply. The improved blood supply facilitates bone healing and eradication of the infection. These surgical procedures may be staged over time to ensure healing. A wound-assisted vacuum device may help with closure of the wound. Because surgical debridement weakens the bone, internal fixation or external supportive devices may be needed to stabilize or support the bone to prevent pathologic fracture.

NURSING PROCESS
The Patient With Osteomyelitis

ASSESSMENT

The patient reports an acute onset of signs and symptoms (e.g., localized pain, edema, erythema, abrupt fever with acute osteomyelitis, and persistent low-grade temperature with chronic osteomyelitis); also the patient may describe recurrent drainage of an infected sinus tract with associated pain, edema, and low-grade fever. The nurse assesses the patient for risk factors (e.g., older age, diabetes, long-term corticosteroid therapy, PVD) and for a history of previous injury, infection, or orthopedic surgery. The patient avoids pressure on the area and guards movement. In acute hematogenous osteomyelitis, the patient exhibits generalized weakness due to the systemic reaction to the infection.

Physical examination reveals an inflamed, markedly edematous, warm area that is tender. Purulent drainage may be noted. The patient has an elevated temperature with acute osteomyelitis; with chronic osteomyelitis, the temperature elevation may be low grade, occurring in the afternoon or evening.

Pearls for Practice

The nurse recognizes there is a normal oral temperature in 99% of the population with ranges from 36.0°C (96.8°F) to 37.7°C (99.8°F) with a circadian variation of 1°C or more between the morning nadir and the evening peak (Leggett, 2020).

NURSING DIAGNOSES

Appropriate nursing diagnoses may include:

- Acute pain related to inflammation and edema
- Impaired physical mobility related to pain, use of immobilization devices, and weight-bearing limitations
- Risk for extension of infection: bone abscess formation
- Knowledge deficiency related to the treatment regimen

PLANNING

The patient's goals may include relief of pain, improved physical mobility within therapeutic limitations, control and eradication of infection, and knowledge of the treatment regimen.

NURSING INTERVENTIONS

RELIEVING PAIN

The affected part may be immobilized with a splint to decrease pain and muscle spasm. The nurse monitors the neurovascular status of the affected extremity. Frequently the wounds are very painful, and the extremity must be handled with great care and gentleness. Elevation reduces swelling and associated discomfort. Pain is controlled with prescribed analgesics and other pain-reducing techniques.

(*continued on page 1316*)

IMPROVING PHYSICAL MOBILITY

Treatment regimens may consist of activity restriction. The bone is weakened by the infective process and must be protected by immobilization devices and by avoidance of stress on the bone. The patient must understand the rationale for the activity restrictions. The nurse encourages full participation in ADLs within the physical limitations to promote general well-being.

CONTROLLING THE INFECTIVE PROCESS

The nurse monitors the patient's response to antibiotic therapy and observes the IV access site for evidence of phlebitis, infection, or infiltration. With long-term, intensive antibiotic therapy, the nurse monitors the patient for signs of superinfection (e.g., oral or vaginal candidiasis, loose or foul-smelling stools).

If surgery is necessary, the nurse takes measures to ensure adequate circulation to the affected area (wound suction to prevent fluid accumulation, elevation of the area to promote venous drainage, avoidance of pressure on the grafted area), to maintain needed immobility, and to ensure the patient's adherence to weight-bearing restrictions. The nurse changes dressings using aseptic technique to promote healing and to prevent cross-contamination.

The nurse continues to monitor the general health and nutrition of the patient. A diet high in protein and vitamin C promotes a positive nitrogen balance and healing. The nurse encourages adequate hydration as well.

TEACHING PATIENTS SELF-CARE

The patient and family are taught about the importance of strictly adhering to the therapeutic regimen of antibiotics and preventing falls or other injuries that could result in bone fracture. They need to learn to maintain and manage the IV access and IV administration equipment in the home. Teaching includes medication name, dosage, frequency, administration rate, safe storage and handling, adverse reactions, and necessary laboratory monitoring. In addition, aseptic dressing and warm compress techniques are taught.

The nurse carefully monitors the patient for the development of additional sites that are painful or for sudden increases in body temperature. The nurse instructs the patient and family to observe for and report elevated temperature, drainage, odor, signs of increased inflammation, adverse reactions, and signs of superinfection.

If warranted, the nurse completes a home assessment to determine the patient's and family's and caregiver's abilities regarding continuation of the therapeutic regimen. If the patient's support system is questionable, or if the patient lives alone, a home care nurse may be needed to assist with IV administration of the antibiotics. The nurse monitors the patient for response to the treatment, signs and symptoms of superinfections, and adverse drug reactions. The nurse stresses the importance of follow-up health care appointments and recommends age-appropriate health screening.

EVALUATION

Expected patient outcomes may include:

1. Experiences pain relief:
   a. Reports decreased pain
   b. Experiences no tenderness at site of previous infection
   c. Experiences no discomfort with movement
2. Increases physical mobility:
   a. Participates in self-care activities
   b. Maintains full function of unimpaired extremities
   c. Demonstrates safe use of immobilizing and assistive devices
   d. Modifies environment to promote safety and to avoid falls
3. Shows absence of infection:
   a. Takes antibiotic as prescribed
   b. Reports normal temperature
   c. Exhibits no edema
   d. Reports absence of drainage
   e. Laboratory results indicate normal WBC count and ESR
   f. Wound cultures are negative
4. Adheres to therapeutic plan:
   a. Takes medications as prescribed
   b. Protects weakened bones
   c. Demonstrates proper wound care
   d. Reports signs and symptoms of complications promptly
   e. Consumes a diet high in protein and vitamin C
   f. Keeps follow-up health care appointments
   g. Reports increased strength
   h. Reports no elevation of temperature or recurrence of pain, edema, or other symptoms at the site

Septic (Infectious) Arthritis

Septic arthritis refers to infection of a joint by a microorganism. It is an important medical emergency with high morbidity and mortality; inappropriate or delayed treatment can lead to joint damage and a mortality rate of about 10% to 15% (Abram et al., 2020).

Pathophysiology

Joints can become infected through spread of infection from other parts of the body (hematogenous spread) or directly through trauma or surgical instrumentation. Previous trauma to joints, joint replacement, coexisting arthritis, diabetes mellitus, rheumatoid arthritis, osteoarthritis, alcohol use disorder, cutaneous ulcers, and diminished host resistance contribute to the development of an infected joint. Those who use IV drugs or who have intravenous catheters in place to treat other medical conditions are at particular risk for unusual bacterial infection. Patients taking glucocorticosteroids, other immunosuppressive agents, and biologic response modifiers to manage autoimmune diseases, such as rheumatoid arthritis and inflammatory bowel disease, are also at risk. *S. aureus* causes most adult joint infections, followed by *Streptococci*, accounting for 90% of cases of septic arthritis (Matteson

& Osmon, 2020). Prompt recognition and treatment of an infected joint are important because accumulating purulent material results in chondrolysis (destruction of hyaline cartilage), which can cause destruction of the surface of the bones.

Clinical Manifestations and Assessment

The patient with acute septic arthritis usually presents with a warm, painful, swollen joint with decreased ROM. The knee is involved in more than 50% of cases (Matteson & Osmon, 2020). Systemic chills, fever, and leukocytosis are present. Older patients and patients taking corticosteroids or immunosuppressive medications may not exhibit typical clinical manifestations of infection and may not have a marked febrile response. Therefore, they require ongoing assessment to detect infection as early as possible in the infective process. An assessment for the source and cause of infection is performed. Blood cultures, ESR, C-reactive protein, and complete blood count are evaluated. Diagnostic studies include aspiration, examination, and culture of the synovial fluid. Evaluation of the synovial fluid can be critical when choosing the appropriate antibiotic and treatment plan for the patient. Computed tomography (CT) and MRI may reveal inflammation and damage to the joint and may be helpful in assessing osteomyelitis. Radioisotope scanning may be useful in localizing the infective process.

Medical and Nursing Management

Prompt treatment is essential and may save a joint prosthesis for patients who have one. Broad-spectrum IV antibiotics are started promptly and then changed to organism-specific antibiotics after culture results are available. The IV antibiotics are continued until symptoms disappear. The synovial fluid is monitored for sterility and decrease in WBCs.

In addition to prescribing antibiotics, the provider may aspirate the joint with a needle to remove excessive joint fluid, exudate, and debris. This promotes comfort and decreases joint destruction caused by the action of proteolytic enzymes in the purulent fluid. Occasionally, arthrotomy (incision into a joint) or arthroscopy is used to drain the joint and remove dead tissue.

The inflamed joint is supported and immobilized in a functional position by a splint that increases the patient's comfort. Analgesics may be prescribed to relieve pain. The patient's nutrition and fluid status is monitored. Progressive ROM exercises are prescribed after the infection subsides.

If septic joints are treated promptly, recovery of normal function is expected. The patient is assessed periodically for recurrence. If the articular cartilage was damaged during the inflammatory reaction, joint fibrosis and diminished function may result.

The nurse describes the septic arthritis process to the patient and teaches the patient how to relieve pain using pharmacologic and nonpharmacologic interventions. The nurse also explains the importance of supporting the affected joint, adhering to the prescribed antibiotic regimen, and observing weight-bearing and activity restrictions. In addition, the nurse demonstrates and encourages the patient to practice safe use of ambulatory aids and assistive devices.

The nurse teaches the patient strategies to promote healing through aseptic dressing changes and proper wound care. Then the patient is encouraged to perform ROM exercises after the infection subsides.

BONE TUMORS

Neoplasms of the musculoskeletal system are of various types, including osteogenic (bone), chondrogenic (cartilage), fibrogenic (fibrous), muscle (rhabdomyogenic), and marrow (reticulum) cell tumors as well as nerve, vascular, and fatty cell tumors (lipoma). They may be primary tumors or metastatic tumors from primary cancers elsewhere in the body (e.g., breast, lung, prostate, kidney). Metastatic bone tumors are more common than primary bone tumors.

Benign Bone Tumors

Benign tumors of the bone and soft tissue are more common than malignant primary bone tumors. Benign bone tumors generally are slow growing, well circumscribed, and encapsulated; present few symptoms; and are not a cause of death.

Benign primary neoplasms of the musculoskeletal system include osteochondroma, enchondroma, bone cyst (e.g., aneurysmal bone cyst), osteoid osteoma, rhabdomyoma, and fibroma. Some benign tumors, such as giant cell tumors, have the potential to become malignant.

Osteochondroma is the most common benign bone tumor. It usually occurs as a large projection of bone at the end of the long bones (at the knee or shoulder). It develops during growth and then becomes a static bony mass. In fewer than 1% of patients, the cartilage cap of the osteochondroma may undergo malignant transformation after trauma, and a chondrosarcoma or osteosarcoma may develop.

Enchondroma is a common tumor of the hyaline cartilage that develops in the hand, femur, tibia, or humerus. Usually, the only symptom is a mild ache. Pathologic fractures may occur.

Bone cysts are lesions that expand within the bone. Aneurysmal (widening) bone cysts are seen in young adults, who present with a painful, palpable mass of the long bones, vertebrae, or flat bone. Unicameral (single cavity) bone cysts occur in children and cause mild discomfort and possible pathologic fractures of the upper humerus and femur, which may heal spontaneously. Approximately two thirds of patients with single-cavity bone cysts present with fractures, commonly of the ilium and calcaneus in adults (Subramanian et al., 2021).

Osteoid osteoma is a painful tumor that occurs in children and young adults. The neoplastic tissue is surrounded by reactive bone formation that can be identified by x-ray. The pain typically occurs at night and is relieved with NSAIDs (Dookie &Joseph, 2021).

Giant cell tumors (osteoclastomas) are benign for long periods but may invade local tissue and cause destruction. They occur in young adults and are soft and hemorrhagic. Eventually, giant cell tumors may undergo malignant transformation and metastasize.

Malignant Bone Tumors

Primary malignant musculoskeletal tumors are relatively rare and arise from connective and supportive tissue cells (sarcomas) or bone marrow elements (multiple myeloma; see Chapter 19). Malignant primary musculoskeletal tumors include osteosarcoma, chondrosarcoma, and Ewing sarcoma. Soft tissue sarcomas include liposarcoma, fibrosarcoma of soft tissue, and rhabdomyosarcoma. These arise in fat cells, fibrous connective tissue, or soft tissue, respectively. Bone tumor metastasis to the lungs is common.

Osteogenic sarcoma (osteosarcoma) is the primary malignant bone tumor that is most common and most often fatal. Prognosis depends on whether the tumor has metastasized to the lungs at the time the patient seeks health care. Osteogenic sarcoma appears most frequently in males between 10 and 25 years of age (in bones that grow rapidly; approximately 75% of cases), in older people with Paget disease, and as a result of radiation exposure (after age 50, peaking at 70 years of age) (Arora & Shaikh, 2021). Clinical manifestations include pain, edema, limited joint or limb motion, pain on weight-bearing, and weight loss (which is considered an ominous finding). The bony mass may be palpable, tender, and fixed, with an increase in skin temperature over the mass and erythema. The primary lesion may involve any bone, but the most common sites are the distal femur, the proximal tibia, and the proximal humerus. Treatment consists of neoadjuvant (started before second method of treatment) chemotherapy, followed by surgery and chemotherapy. This regimen has resulted in an increase in limb salvage rates from 53% in the 1980s to greater than 90% today (Arora & Shaikh, 2021).

Malignant tumors of the hyaline cartilage are called chondrosarcomas. These tumors are the second most common primary malignant bone tumor, accounting for 20% of all primary malignant bone tumors (Limaiem et al., 2021). They are large, bulky, slow-growing tumors that affect adults. Symptoms include localized swelling and pain. The usual tumor sites include the pelvis, femur, humerus, spine, scapula, and tibia. Metastasis to the lungs occurs in fewer than half of patients. When these tumors are well differentiated, large bloc excision or amputation of the affected extremity results in increased survival rates. These tumors may recur. Refer to a pediatric text for details of the Ewing family of tumors.

Metastatic Bone Disease

Metastatic bone disease (secondary bone tumor) is more common than any primary bone tumor. It is the third most common site of metastatic disease after lung and liver, owing to the rich arterial supply of the bone (Jayarangaiah et al., 2021). Tumors arising from tissues elsewhere in the body may invade the bone and produce localized bone destruction (lytic lesions) or bone overgrowth (blastic lesions). The most common primary sites of tumors that metastasize to bone are the kidney, prostate, lung, breast, ovary, and thyroid. Metastatic tumors most frequently attack the skull, spine, pelvis, femur, and humerus, and they often involve more than one bone (polyostotic).

Pathophysiology

A tumor in the bone causes the normal bone tissue to react by osteolytic response (bone destruction) or osteoblastic response (bone formation). Primary tumors cause bone destruction, which weakens the bone, resulting in bone fractures. Adjacent normal bone responds to the tumor by altering its normal pattern of remodeling. The bone's surface changes and the contours enlarge in the tumor area.

Malignant bone tumors invade and destroy adjacent bone tissue. Benign bone tumors, in contrast, have a symmetric, controlled growth pattern and place pressure on adjacent bone tissue. Malignant invading bone tumors weaken the structure of the bone until it can no longer withstand the stress of ordinary use; pathologic fracture commonly results.

Clinical Manifestations and Assessment

Patients with primary malignant and benign bone tumors present with night pain (described frequently as deep and boring), swelling, and, occasionally, pathologic fracture of the involved bone (Jayarangaiah et al., 2021; Jones, 2020). Patients with metastatic bone tumors may have a wide range of associated clinical manifestations. They may be symptom free or have varying degrees of disability, and, at times, obvious bone growth. Unintentional weight loss, malaise, and fever may be present. The tumor may be diagnosed only after pathologic fracture has occurred.

With spinal metastasis, spinal cord compression may occur (refer to Chapter 43). The vertebra is the most common site affected (Jayarangaiah et al., 2021). It can progress rapidly or slowly. Neurologic deficits (e.g., progressive pain, weakness, gait abnormality, paresthesia, paraplegia, urinary retention, loss of bowel or bladder control) must be identified early and treated with decompressive laminectomy to prevent permanent spinal cord injury.

The differential diagnosis is based on the history, physical examination, and diagnostic studies, including CT, bone scans, myelography, arteriography, MRI, biopsy, and biochemical assays of the blood and urine. Frequently, serum ALP levels are elevated with osteogenic sarcoma. With metastatic carcinoma of the prostate, serum acid phosphatase levels are elevated. Hypercalcemia is present with bone metastases from breast, lung, or kidney cancer. Symptoms of hypercalcemia include muscle weakness, fatigue, anorexia,

TABLE **40-1 Hypercalcemia of Malignancy**

Levels of Hypercalcemia	Serum Calcium Level	Assessment
Mild	>10.3; <12 mg/dL	Symptoms may be present
Moderate	>12 mg/dL	Critical laboratory value
Severe	>14 mg/dL	Emergency measures required

Adapted from Mayo Clinic Laboratories. Test ID: CA: calcium, total, serum. https://www.mayocliniclabs.com/test-catalog/Clinical+and+Interpretive/601514. Updated September 17, 2020.

nausea, vomiting, polyuria, cardiac arrhythmias, seizures, and coma. Hypercalcemia must be identified and treated promptly. The nurse is aware that over 50% of patients die within 30 days of receiving a diagnosis of hypercalcemia of malignancy (Green, 2020). Refer to Table 40-1 for classification of hypercalcemia of malignancy. A surgical biopsy is performed for histologic identification. Extreme care is taken during the biopsy to prevent seeding and resultant recurrence after excision of the tumor.

Chest x-rays are performed to determine the presence of lung metastasis. Surgical staging of musculoskeletal tumors is based on tumor grade and site (intracompartmental or extracompartmental) as well as on metastasis. Staging is used for planning treatment.

During the diagnostic period, the nurse explains the diagnostic tests and provides psychological and emotional support to the patient and family. The nurse assesses coping behaviors and encourages use of support systems.

Medical Management

Primary Bone Tumors

The goal of treatment of a primary bone tumor is to destroy or remove the tumor. This may be accomplished by surgical excision (ranging from local excision to amputation and disarticulation), radiation therapy if the tumor is radiosensitive, and chemotherapy (preoperative [neoadjuvant], intraoperative, postoperative, and adjunctive for possible micrometastases). Preoperative imaging studies determine the extent of tumor penetration and impact on adjacent structures. Survival and QOL are important considerations in procedures that attempt to save the involved extremity.

Typically patients are managed with initial neoadjuvant chemotherapy, delayed resection of the primary tumor, and then further postoperative chemotherapy (Jones, 2020). The SAP level, which often is elevated in patients with osteosarcoma, can be used to monitor disease status. Limb-sparing (salvage) procedures are used to remove the tumor and adjacent tissue. A customized prosthesis, total joint arthroplasty, or bone tissue from the patient (autograft) or from a cadaver donor (allograft) replaces the resected tissue. Soft tissue and blood vessels may need grafting because of the extent of the excision. Complications may include infection, loosening or dislocation of the prosthesis, allograft nonunion, fracture, devitalization of the skin and soft tissues, joint fibrosis, and recurrence of the tumor. Function and rehabilitation after limb salvage depend on positive encouragement and reducing the risk of complications.

Surgical removal of the tumor may require amputation of the affected extremity with the amputation extending well above the tumor to achieve local control of the primary lesion (refer to Chapter 41). Because of the danger of metastasis with malignant bone tumors, combined chemotherapy is started before and continued after surgery in an effort to eradicate micrometastatic lesions. The goal of combined chemotherapy is greater therapeutic effect at a lower toxicity rate with reduced resistance to the medications. There is an improved long-term survival rate when a localized osteosarcoma is removed and chemotherapy is initiated. Soft tissue sarcomas are treated with radiation, limb-sparing excision, and adjuvant chemotherapy.

Secondary Bone Tumors

The treatment of metastatic bone cancer is palliative. The therapeutic goal is to relieve the patient's pain and discomfort while promoting QOL.

If metastatic disease weakens the bone, structural support and stabilization are needed to prevent pathologic fracture. At times, large bones with metastatic lesions are strengthened by prophylactic internal fixation. Internal fixation of pathologic fractures, arthroplasty, or methylmethacrylate (bone cement) reconstruction minimizes associated disability and pain. Patients with metastatic disease are at higher risk than other patients for postoperative pulmonary congestion, hypoxemia, deep vein thrombosis, and hemorrhage.

Hypercalcemia results from breakdown of bone. It needs to be recognized promptly. A normal serum calcium is 8.6 to 10 mg/dL for ages 18 to 59 and 8.8 to 10.2 for those ≥60 years (Mayo Clinic, 2020). Treatment includes hydration with IV administration of normal saline solution often with furosemide diuresis; mobilization; and medications such as bisphosphonates, pamidronate, and calcitonin (refer to Chapter 5 for further details on hypercalcemia). Because inactivity leads to loss of bone mass and increased calcium in the blood, the nurse assists the patient to increase activity and ambulation.

Frequently, hematopoiesis is disrupted by tumor invasion of the bone marrow or by treatment (chemotherapy or radiation). Blood component therapy restores hematologic factors. Pain can result from multiple factors, including the osseous metastasis, surgery, chemotherapy or radiation side effects, and arthritis. Pain must be assessed accurately and managed with adequate and appropriate opioid, nonopioid, and nonpharmaceutical interventions. In the absence of fracture, external beam radiation may be used for painful metastatic sites. Systemic chemotherapy or endocrine therapy also may be considered for palliation. Patients with multiple bony metastases may achieve pain control with systemically administered "bone-seeking" isotopes (e.g., strontium-89).

Nursing Management

The nursing care of a patient who has undergone excision of a bone tumor is similar in many respects to that of other patients who have had skeletal surgery. Vital signs are monitored; blood loss is assessed; and observations are made to assess for the development of complications, such as deep vein thrombosis, pulmonary emboli, infection, contracture, and disuse atrophy. The affected part is elevated to reduce edema, and the neurovascular status of the extremity is assessed.

Providing Patient Education

Patient and family teaching about the disease process and diagnostic and management regimens is essential. Explanation of diagnostic tests, treatments (e.g., wound care), and expected results (e.g., decreased ROM, numbness, change of body contours) helps the patient deal with the procedures and changes. Cooperation and adherence to the therapeutic regimen are enhanced through understanding. The nurse can most effectively reinforce and clarify information given by the provider by being present during these discussions.

Relieving Pain

Accurate pain assessment is the foundation for pain management. Pharmacologic and nonpharmacologic pain management techniques are used to relieve pain and increase the patient's comfort level. The nurse works with the patient in designing the most effective pain management regimen, thereby increasing the patient's control over the pain. Prescribed IV or epidural analgesics are used during the early postoperative period. Later, oral or transdermal opioid or nonopioid analgesics are indicated to alleviate pain. In addition to external radiation, systemic radioisotopes may be used to control pain. See Chapter 6 for further discussion of pain management.

Preventing Pathologic Fracture

Bone tumors weaken the bone to a point at which normal activities or even position changes can result in fracture. During nursing care, the affected extremities must be supported and handled gently. External supports (e.g., splints) may be used for additional protection. At times, the patient may elect to have surgery (e.g., open reduction with internal fixation, joint replacement) in an attempt to prevent pathologic fracture. Prescribed weight-bearing restrictions must be followed. The nurse and physical therapist teach the patient how to use assistive devices safely and how to strengthen unaffected extremities.

Promoting Coping Skills

The nurse encourages the patient and family to verbalize their fears, concerns, and feelings. They need to be supported as they deal with the impact of the malignant bone tumor. Feelings of shock, despair, and grief are expected. Referral to a psychiatric advanced practice nurse, psychologist, counselor, or spiritual advisor may be indicated for specific psychological help and emotional support.

Promoting Self-Care

Independence versus dependence is an issue for the patient who has a malignancy. Lifestyle is changed dramatically, at least temporarily. It is important to support the family in working through the adjustments that must be made. The nurse assists the patient in dealing with changes in body image due to surgery and possible amputation. It is helpful to provide realistic reassurance about the future and resumption of role-related activities and to encourage self-care and socialization. The patient participates in planning daily activities. The nurse encourages the patient to be as independent as possible. Involvement of the patient and family throughout treatment encourages confidence, restoration of self-concept, and a sense of being in control of one's life.

Monitoring and Managing Potential Complications

Delayed Wound Healing

Wound healing may be delayed because of tissue trauma from surgery, previous radiation therapy, inadequate nutrition, or infection. The nurse assesses the patient's nutritional status by monitoring weight, percentage of weight loss, and evaluating the serum albumin or prealbumin level. An unintentional weight loss of 10% of usual body weight in 3 months is a risk factor for malnutrition.

Pearls for Practice

The nurse monitors and reports laboratory markers related to nutritional status. Serum prealbumin has a shorter half-life (2 days) than albumin (21 days) and is not influenced by fluid balance, making it an excellent marker for malnutrition. A normal prealbumin level is 19 to 38 mg/dL with values of 0 to 5, 5 to 10, and 10 to 15 mg/dL reflecting a severe, moderate, and mild protein depletion, respectively (Pagana et al., 2021). Interventions that promote homeostasis and wound healing should be initiated as soon as possible. In addition, the nurse considers that the patient's requirements for calories, protein, vitamins, and minerals will be expected to increase in times of stress.

The nurse minimizes pressure on the wound site to promote circulation to the tissues. Repositioning the patient at frequent intervals reduces the incidence of skin breakdown and pressure ulcers. Special therapeutic beds may be needed to prevent skin breakdown and to promote wound healing after extensive surgical reconstruction and skin grafting.

Inadequate Nutrition

Because loss of appetite, nausea, and vomiting are frequent side effects of chemotherapy and radiation therapy, it is necessary to provide adequate nutrition for healing and health promotion. Antiemetics, relaxation techniques, and acupuncture reduce the adverse GI effects of chemotherapy. Stomatitis is controlled with anesthetic or antifungal mouthwash (see Chapter 5). Adequate hydration is essential. Nutritional supplements and enteral or parenteral nutrition may be prescribed to achieve adequate nutrition.

Osteomyelitis and Wound Infections

Prophylactic antibiotics and strict aseptic dressing techniques are used to diminish the occurrence of osteomyelitis and wound infections. During healing, other infections (e.g., upper respiratory infections) need to be prevented so that hematogenous spread does not result in osteomyelitis. If the patient is receiving chemotherapy, it is important to monitor the WBC count and to instruct the patient to avoid contact with people who have colds or other infections.

Hypercalcemia

Hypercalcemia is a dangerous complication of bone cancer. The symptoms must be recognized and treatment initiated promptly. Symptoms include muscular weakness, incoordination, anorexia, nausea and vomiting, constipation, electrocardiographic changes (e.g., shortened QT interval and ST segment, bradycardia, heart blocks), and altered mental states (e.g., confusion, lethargy, psychotic behavior). See Table 40-1 and Chapter 5, Table 5-6 for a discussion of hypercalcemia and its management.

CHAPTER REVIEW

NCLEX-Style Review Questions

1. Which assessment finding may indicate to the nurse an acute peripheral neurovascular dysfunction for the patient recovering from surgery of the foot? Select all that apply.
   a. Pale skin
   b. Atrophy of the limb
   c. Capillary refill of 4 seconds
   d. Absence of feeling
   e. Thickened toenails
   f. Loss of toe hairs
   g. Cool skin

2. A patient is diagnosed with osteoporosis. Which statements should the nurse include when teaching the patient about the disease? Select all that apply.
   a. Osteoporosis is common after menopause.
   b. Osteoporosis is a degenerative disease characterized by an increase in bone density.
   c. Osteoporosis can increase the risk for fractures.
   d. The recommended daily calcium dose should be taken as a single dose, and the patient should be instructed not to lie down for 30 minutes.
   e. Weight-bearing exercise should be avoided.
   f. The patient's T score is at least 2.5 SD below the young adult mean value on the BMD scan.

3. What places the patient at risk for impaired wound healing after surgery for a primary bone cancer? Select all that apply.
   a. Radiation therapy
   b. Prealbumin level is 28 mg/dL
   c. Weight loss of 18% over the previous 3 months
   d. Anorexia
   e. Hct of 45%

4. A 25-year-old patient experienced an open fracture of the right fibula with major soft tissue damage of the lower leg in a motor vehicle accident. Surgical reduction and fixation of the fibula were performed with debridement of nonviable tissue and drain placement in the damaged soft tissue. For which complication is this patient at risk (select one from Column 1) and for what clinical cues would you observe related to your selection (select all that apply in Column 2)?

Column 1	Column 2
a. Osteoporosis	a. Weight loss
b. Osteomyelitis	b. Purulent drainage
c. Osteosarcoma	c. Erythema
d. Compartment syndrome	d. Progressive kyphosis
	e. Paresthesia
	f. Increased local temperature
	g. Elevated ESR
	h. Normal C-reactive protein

5. A patient is admitted to your hospital unit with a diagnosis of metastatic bone disease secondary to primary lung cancer metastasis. Select in Column 1 the lab work that requires your immediate attention (choose 1 item) and select in Column 2 the symptoms associated with the abnormal blood work (select all that apply).

Column 1

a. Potassium of 3.5 mEq/L
b. WBC of 9.8 per cubic millimeter (cmm)
c. Calcium of 12 mg/dL
d. Hct of 45%

Column 2

a. Constipation
b. Peaked T waves
c. Shortened QT interval
d. Cyanosis
e. Confusion
f. Muscle weakness
g. U waves

REFERENCES AND SELECTED READINGS

References and selected readings associated with this chapter can be found on the website that accompanies the book. Visit **http://thepoint.lww.com/Honan3e** to access the references and other additional resources associated with this chapter.

CHAPTER 41

Nursing Management: Patients With Musculoskeletal Trauma

Linda Honan

Learning Objectives

After reading this chapter, you will be able to:

1. Differentiate among contusions, strains, sprains, and dislocations.
2. Specify the clinical manifestations of a fracture and the emergency management of the patient with a fracture.
3. Describe the principles and methods of fracture reduction, fracture immobilization, and management of open fractures.
4. Describe the prevention and management of complications of fractures.
5. Discuss nursing management of the patient with a cast.
6. Discuss nursing management of the patient undergoing joint replacement or amputation.

Injury to any part of the musculoskeletal system necessitates evaluation of the damaged area, along with assessment of the structures and organs that underlie the fracture. For example, if a bone is broken, the adjacent muscles cannot function, blood vessels and nerves may be injured with resultant neurovascular complications, and the organs that lie beneath the fracture may have damage secondary to the trauma.

Treatment of injury to the musculoskeletal system involves providing support to the injured part until healing is complete. Frequently, management includes the use of internal and/or external devices, such as bandages, splints, casts, skin or skeletal traction, artificial joint replacement, pins, or a combination of these. Pharmacologic treatment often includes anti-inflammatory agents, muscle relaxants, and analgesics. They may help diminish edema and relax muscles at risk for spasm that can cause further injury to inflamed muscles or to fractured bones. Pain relief is an important factor to facilitate healing.

Patient education is essential for optimal outcomes. Nursing care is planned to maximize the effectiveness of treatment modalities, prevent potential complications associated with interventions, and observe for the development of untoward signs and symptoms as soon as possible. After the immediate and painful effects of the injury have passed, treatment efforts are focused on preventing fibrosis and atrophy or degeneration of the injured muscles and joint structures, respectively.

COMMON MUSCULOSKELETAL INJURIES

Contusions, Strains, and Sprains

Pathophysiology

A **contusion** is an injury to soft tissue produced by blunt force, such as a blow, kick, or fall, that results in bleeding into soft tissues (ecchymosis, or bruising); it can involve the skin and the subcutaneous tissues as well as underlying muscle (Zolkoske & Fehr, 2023). A *hematoma* (collection of blood within tissues) develops when the bleeding is sufficient to form an appreciable solid swelling. A muscle **strain**, or a "pulled muscle," is an injury to a musculotendinous unit caused by overuse, overstretching, or excessive stress. It can occur anywhere within the muscle, but it commonly occurs at the distal muscle–tendon junction (Nelson & Gunalda, 2019). Recall that a tendon connects muscle to bone, whereas a ligament connects bone to bone. A **sprain** is a ligamentous injury often caused by a trauma or a wrenching or twisting motion. The injury can range from a mild stretching of the ligament to a complete tear. While a history and physical examination are important, diagnostic studies of the affected extremity may be ordered to determine diagnosis.

Risk Factors

The main risk factor for contusions, strains, or sprains is participation in sports and physical fitness activities. Strains and sprains occur after intense activity or are associated with overuse, repetitive injuries, or trauma, whereas contusions can occur in any soft tissue that suffers blunt trauma. Ankles, knees, and wrists are vulnerable to sprains, while strains frequently occur in the neck, lower back, and hamstring muscle (back of the thigh). Previous injuries are a risk factor for reinjury.

Clinical Manifestations and Assessment

An important question for nurses to ask when assessing for musculoskeletal injury is, "What were you doing at the time of the injury?" For example, many ankle sprains occur because of inversion injury (turning ankle in while walking), while muscle strains occur because of a "pulled muscle" while exercising. The nurse assesses the threes "S's," size, shape, and symmetry, of the involved area in comparison to the opposite region. It is important to note presence of **edema** (swelling), ecchymosis (bruising), tenderness, abnormal joint motion, and pain. Contusions, strains, and sprains can present with similar symptoms of pain, edema, and discoloration from the broken blood vessels. The patient may guard or protect the affected area, and they may have difficulty moving the affected area; increased warmth may be noted at the injury site.

With contusions, the nurse notes ecchymosis and edema of the injured area. The patient may complain initially of dull pain at the site that increases as edema develops and of subsequent stiffness of the area, usually by the next day.

Muscle strains are graded along a continuum based on symptoms and loss of function. A first-degree strain reflects tearing of few muscle fibers and is accompanied by minor edema, tenderness (usually noticed after the activity is over), and mild muscle spasm, without a noticeable loss of function. A second-degree strain involves a tearing of more muscle fibers and is manifested by edema, tenderness, muscle spasm, ecchymosis, and a notable loss of load-bearing strength of the involved extremity. A third-degree strain involves complete disruption of at least one musculotendinous unit that involves separation of muscle from muscle, muscle from tendon, or tendon from bone. Patients present with significant pain, muscle spasm, ecchymosis, a large hematoma, edema, and loss of function. An x-ray should be obtained to rule out bone injury because an avulsion fracture (in which a bone fragment is pulled away from the bone by a tendon) may be associated with a third-degree strain.

Like strains, sprains (ligamentous injuries) are graded to reflect the degree of injury. A mild sprain, termed first-degree sprain (a tear of only a few fibers), may cause minor edema, tenderness, and mild muscle spasm, without a noticeable loss of function. Patients can bear weight with minimal pain. A second-degree sprain is an incomplete tear of the ligament (bone-to-bone); as blood vessels rupture, ecchymosis and edema are expected and there is functional disability; however, there is generally no abnormal motion noted of the joint (Nelson & Gunalda, 2019). The degree of disability and pain increases during the first 2 to 3 hours after the injury because of the associated swelling and bleeding. There is restricted motion of the affected limb, and weight bearing is painful. A third-degree sprain involves complete ligament tear with resultant complaints of significant pain, muscle spasm, ecchymosis, edema, loss of function, and abnormal joint motion. Patients are unable to bear weight on the affected limb. Tenderness at the distal tibia (inner ankle) or fibula (outer ankle) is associated with an inversion or eversion injury and may indicate a fracture.

BOX 41-1 PRICE

*The acronym **PRICE**—**P**rotection, **R**est, **I**ce, **C**ompression, **E**levation—is helpful for remembering treatment interventions for musculoskeletal injuries.*

Protection of the injured area minimizes bleeding from the site of the injury. Rest prevents additional injury and promotes healing. Intermittent application of moist, crushed wetted ice in a plastic bag, or dry cold packs for 20–30 minutes after the injury, produces vasoconstriction, which decreases bleeding, edema, and discomfort, and is suggested for the first 3–7 days after injury. Ensure care to avoid skin and tissue damage from excessive cold. An elastic compression bandage controls bleeding, reduces edema, and provides support for the injured tissues. Elevation controls the swelling.

Medical and Nursing Management

Treatment of contusions, strains, and sprains consists of resting and elevating the affected part, applying cold, and using a compression bandage (Box 41-1). Immobilization of the affected extremity until definite diagnosis is determined may be appropriate to minimize the risk of hemorrhage (Nelson & Gunalda, 2019). It is important to monitor the **neurovascular status** of the injured extremity; this is termed **CSM:** **C**irculation, by way of pulses, color, temperature, and capillary refill; **S**ensation, by noting awareness of light touch; and **M**ovement, by range of motion (ROM) of the most distal digits. The nurse compares the injured limb to the uninjured limb.

Although conclusive evidence regarding the use of cryotherapy (cold) is lacking regarding its effect on inflammation, studies demonstrate its utility for pain relief when applied following soft tissue injury, and to reduce soreness when applied after damaging exercise (Kwiecien & McHugh, 2021). While specific guidelines that detail the duration and frequency of ice application are lacking, many resources suggest cold application for 15 to 20 minutes repeated within intervals of between 30 and 60 minutes since this type of protocol results in a decrease in 3°C to 7°C of intramuscular temperature and in a 50% reduction of intramuscular blood flow (SantAnna, 2022). Interestingly, a recent study discovered that the use of crushed wetted ice in a plastic bag resulted in more effective analgesia when compared to the application of agitated chemical cold pack to the injury site for 20 minutes (Leroux et al., 2021). The application of ice is suggested for the first 3 to 7 days after injury (Nelson & Gunalda, 2019). After a brief immobilization period (usually <1 week), intermittent heat application (for 15 to 30 minutes, four times a day) is suggested to relieve muscle spasm and promote vasodilation, absorption, and repair. Depending on the severity of injury, progressive passive and active exercises may begin (usually within 1 week). Severe sprains and strains may require 1 to 3 weeks of immobilization before exercises are initiated. Excessive exercise early during treatment delays recovery and may result in reinjury. Strains and sprains take weeks or months to heal because ligaments and tendons are relatively avascular. Splinting may be used to prevent reinjury.

JOINT DISLOCATIONS

Pathophysiology

With **dislocation** of a joint, the articular surfaces of the bones forming the joint are no longer in anatomic alignment. The bones are literally "out of joint." Dislocations may be congenital, or present at birth; spontaneous or pathologic; or traumatic, resulting from injury in which the joint is disrupted by force. A **subluxation** is a partial dislocation of the joint. Traumatic dislocations are orthopedic emergencies because the associated joint structures, blood supply, and nerves are distorted and severely stressed.

Pearls for Practice

If the dislocation is not treated promptly, avascular necrosis (AVN) or osteonecrosis, which is tissue death due to anoxia and diminished blood supply, and nerve palsy may occur. The risk of osteonecrosis increases with increasing time to reduction of the dislocation and may complicate 1% to 22% of posterior hip dislocations (Weinlein, 2021). Tenderness at the site, limited ROM, the affected limb being shortened, pain, and asymmetry of limbs is observed. The limb is immobilized, and the provider notified.

Clinical Manifestations and Assessment

Signs and symptoms of a traumatic dislocation include acute pain, change in contour of the joint, change in the length of the extremity (shortening of the affected limb), loss of normal mobility, and change in the axis of the dislocated bones. X-rays confirm the diagnosis and reveal any associated fracture.

Pearls for Practice

Most hip dislocations are posterior, and the nurse observes the injured limb is shortened, internally rotated, and adducted (toward the noninjured limb). In the event of an anterior dislocation, which occurs rarely (<10%), the injured limb is shortened and externally rotated (Weinlein, 2021). The majority of hip dislocations are the result of motor vehicle accidents.

Medical and Nursing Management

The affected joint needs to be immobilized while the patient is transported to the hospital. An x-ray of the pelvis (in the event of a hip dislocation) is performed before any attempt at reduction to rule out fractures since femoral head fractures occur in 5% to 15% of hip dislocations (Weinlein, 2021). Once fracture is ruled out, the dislocation is reduced promptly (i.e., displaced parts are brought into normal position) to preserve joint function. Analgesia, muscle relaxants, and possibly anesthesia are used to facilitate closed reduction (e.g., noninvasive or nonsurgical reduction). The joint is immobilized by bandages, splints, casts, or traction and is maintained in a stable position. Neurovascular status is monitored (temperature, capillary refill, pulses, color, mobility, sensation). Repeat plain films and a CT scan of the pelvis should be obtained after closed reduction to confirm correct alignment of the limb. After reduction, if the joint is stable, then weight bearing is allowed as tolerated on crutches, with progression as pain allows. Patients with posterior hip dislocations are instructed in posterior hip precautions (see Box 41-14) for at least 6 weeks. Patients are followed closely for the first 2 years because if the complication of osteonecrosis occurs, it will do so within this time frame (Weinlein, 2021).

SPECIFIC MUSCULOSKELETAL INJURIES

Common specific musculoskeletal injuries include **rotator cuff** tears, epicondylitis, and injury to the ligaments of the knee. Table 41-1 summarizes key findings and treatment for these common injuries.

FRACTURES

A **fracture** is a break in the continuity of bone caused by a direct blow, crushing force, sudden twisting motion, or extreme muscle contraction. When the bone is broken, adjacent structures also are affected, resulting in soft tissue edema and hemorrhage into the muscles and joints, with potential joint dislocations, ruptured tendons, severed nerves, and damaged blood vessels. Because body organs may be injured by the force that caused the fracture or by fracture fragments, it is important for nurses to have knowledge of the organs that lie beneath the fracture. For example, the nurse is alert for liver injuries with fractures to right ribs 6 through 12 and splenic injuries with fractures to left ribs 9 through 11. In addition to the magnitude of the force on the bone, the nurse needs to consider the strength of the bone, which is related directly to its density. Thus, a lower force may create a fracture because of bone weakness (e.g., osteoporosis or bone cysts).

Types of Fractures

Fractures are defined according to the bone involved (e.g., humerus, femur, tibia) and can be categorized in several

TABLE **41-1 Specific Musculoskeletal Injuries**

Injury	Description	Key Assessment Findings	Treatment
Rotator cuff tears	Tear results from an acute injury or from chronic joint stresses; it occurs when there is damage to one or more of the four muscles and their tendons in the shoulder.	• Acromioclavicular joint pain; in many cases, the patient with a rotator cuff tear experiences night pain and cannot sleep on the involved side • Limited ROM; the patient cannot perform over-the-head activities or activities as simple as putting on a coat • Muscle weakness • Many tears are asymptomatic	• Rest and modalities such as hot packs, ultrasound, or cold applications, with specific ROM exercises as soon as tolerated • Nonsteroidal anti-inflammatory drugs (NSAIDs), but most frequent treatment is steroid injection into the shoulder joint • Arthroscopic debridement (removal of devitalized tissue) • Arthroscopic, mini-open, or open acromioplasty with tendon repair
Epicondylitis (tennis elbow)	Chronic, painful condition that is caused by excessive, repetitive extension and flexion and/or pronation and supination activities of the forearm. These excessive, repetitious activities result in inflammation (**tendinitis**) and minor tears in the tendons at the origin of the muscles on the medial or lateral epicondyles.	• Pain that usually radiates down the extensor (dorsal) surface of the forearm and generally is relieved with rest and avoidance of the aggravating activity • Weakened grasp • May coexist with nerve compression neuropathy (commonly carpal tunnel syndrome)	• Application of ice for pain after the activity • NSAIDs for pain • In some instances, immobilization of the arm in a molded splint or cast is necessary • Local injection of a corticosteroid generally is reserved for patients with severe pain who do not respond to NSAIDs and immobilization because of its degenerative effects on tendons • After pain subsides, rehabilitation exercises that stretch and strengthen the area (including gentle and gradual increased stretching of the tendons) • Occasionally, surgery to release strictures or to debride the joint

Knee injury	Injury to the anterior cruciate ligament (ACL) or the posterior cruciate ligament (PCL), which stabilize forward and backward motion of the femur and tibia, occurs when the foot is firmly planted and the knee is hyperextended and the person twists the torso and femur. Injury to the lateral or medial collateral ligaments of the knee, which provide stability lateral and medial to the knee, occurs when the foot is firmly planted and the knee is struck either medially or laterally.	• Acute onset of pain
		• Point tenderness (e.g., tenderness at the site of injury)
		• Joint instability and inability to walk without assistance
		• Hemarthrosis (bleeding into the joint) may develop, contributing to the pain
			• Treatment will depend on the severity of the injury, but may include:
			  • PRICE
			  • Evaluation of the joint for fracture
			  • Aspiration of joint fluid to relieve pressure
			  • Limited weight bearing
			  • Use of protective elastic bandaging or brace
			  • Surgery, typically performed as ambulatory arthroscopic surgery, in which the surgeon uses an arthroscope to visualize and repair the damage

ways, including the direction of the fracture. A *complete fracture* involves a break across the entire cross-section of the bone, which frequently is displaced (removed from its normal position). An *incomplete fracture* (e.g., greenstick fracture) involves a break through only part of the cross-section of the bone. An *oblique fracture* runs across the bone at a diagonal angle of 45 to 60 degrees. A *comminuted* fracture is one that produces several bone fragments, while an *impacted* fracture is one whose ends are driven into each other. A *closed fracture* (simple fracture) is one that does not cause a break in the skin. An *open fracture* (compound or complex fracture) is one in which the wound to the skin or mucous membrane extends to the fractured bone. Some fractures have specific names, for example, a fracture of the distal radius (wrist) is termed a *Colles fracture. Stress fractures* occur with repeated bone trauma from athletic activities, most frequently involving the tibia and metatarsals. *Compression fractures* are caused by compression of vertebrae and are associated frequently with osteoporosis. Figure 41-1 depicts types of fractures.

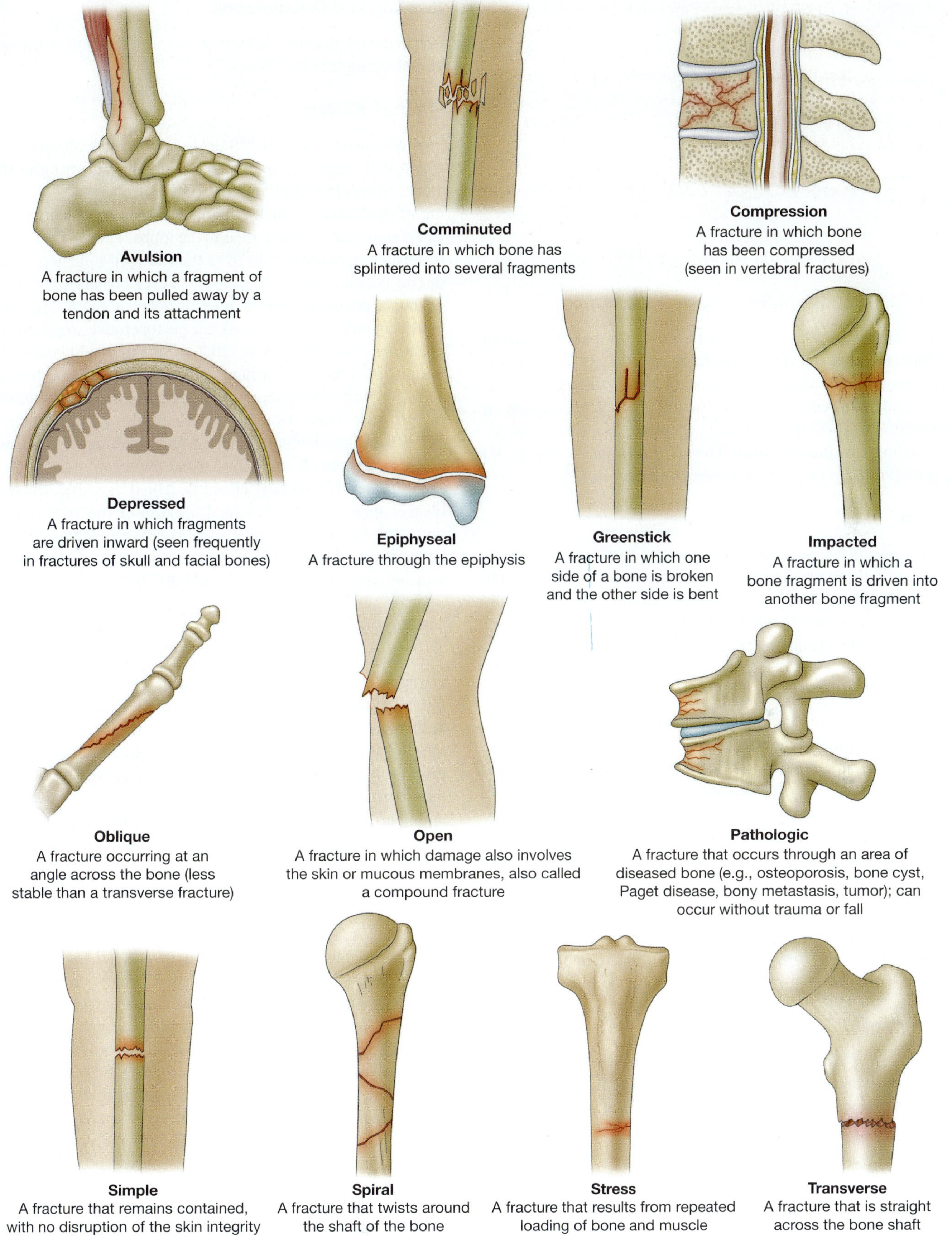

FIGURE 41-1 Specific types of fractures.

Pearls for Practice

On x-rays, long bone fractures will be categorized as proximal (closest to or toward the center of the body), middle, or distal (the portion of the bone that is farthest away). An intra-articular fracture extends into the joint space, whereas fractures not involving the joint are termed extra-articular. In children, fractures are described in relation to the growth plate (physis); thus, if a fracture is seen between the joint and the growth plate, it will be termed an epiphyseal fracture. A diaphysis fracture refers to the shaft of the bone; a metaphysis fracture is between the epiphysis and the diaphysis.

Clinical Manifestations and Assessment

The diagnosis of a fracture is based on the patient's symptoms, the physical signs, and the x-ray findings. Usually, the patient reports having sustained an injury to the area. The clinical manifestations of a fracture include pain, loss of function, deformity, shortening, **crepitus** (described shortly), swelling, and discoloration. These clinical manifestations do not all need to be present in every fracture.

Pain

The pain is immediate, continuous, and increases in severity until the bone fragments are immobilized. The muscle spasms that accompany a fracture begin shortly after the injury and result in increasing pain intensity and further bony fragmentation or malalignment.

Loss of Function

After a fracture, the extremity cannot function properly because normal function of the muscles depends on the integrity of the bones to which they are attached. Pain contributes to the loss of function. In addition, abnormal movement (false motion) may be present.

Deformity

Displacement, angulation, or rotation of the fragments in a fracture or soft tissue swelling causes a visible or palpable deformity. Movement may be noted at the fracture site, whereas under normal circumstances, movement of bones occurs only at the joint.

Shortening

In fractures of long bones, there is actual shortening of the extremity because of the contraction of the muscles that are attached distal (furthest away) and proximal (nearest) to the site of the fracture.

Crepitus

Palpation of the extremity reveals a grating sensation, called crepitus, caused by the rubbing of the bone fragments against each other.

Swelling and Discoloration

Localized edema and ecchymosis occur as a result of trauma and bleeding into the tissues.

Fracture Blisters

Fracture blisters are tense blisters or bullae (large blister) associated with high-energy injuries commonly occurring in the ankle, elbow, foot, and/or knee. These sites have less anchoring of epidermal–dermal junction and little subcutaneous fat cushioning than do other areas in the limbs. They are the result of separation of the dermis from the stratified squamous layer due to edema (Bove et al., 2021). Fever blisters occur 6 to 72 hours postinjury and if present delay definitive fracture treatment and increase the risk for postoperative wound complications (Tosounidis et al., 2020). Nurses should be alert to the potential for compartment syndrome (discussed shortly) since fracture blisters represent underlying increased interstitial pressure. Other factors associated with the development of fever blisters include hypertension, smoking, alcohol use disorder, peripheral vascular disease, lymphatic obstruction, and diabetes (Tosounidis et al., 2020). If possible, fracture blisters should not be disrupted because of risk of infection with skin flora. An ointment such as silver sulfadiazine may be applied to the blister to promote re-epithelialization and to prevent infection (Tosounidis et al., 2020).

Managing Fractures

Immediately after injury, whenever a fracture is suspected, it is important to immobilize the body part before the patient is moved. If an injured patient must be moved before extremity **splints** can be applied, support the limb distal and proximal to the fracture site to prevent rotation as well as angular motion. It is important to recognize that movement of fracture fragments can cause additional pain, soft tissue damage, and neurovascular damage. Splinting a fracture can include bandaging the legs together, with the unaffected extremity serving as a splint for the injured one. In an upper extremity injury, the arm can be bandaged to the chest, a forearm placed in a **sling**, or a finger can be taped to the adjacent digit. Taping, splinting, or bandaging too tightly may cause impaired distal perfusion and thus is avoided. Immobilization is applied to the joints above and below the fracture. Neurovascular status distal to the injury is assessed before and after splinting to determine the adequacy of peripheral tissue perfusion and nerve function. An assessment of the patient also includes observing for the six warning "Ps" associated with acute disruption of arterial flow: **p**ain, **poi**kilothermia (cold limb), **p**allor (paleness), **p**aresthesia (can occur as numbness, "pins and needles," burning, itching, and/or tingling), **p**ulselessness (weak pulses or delayed capillary refill; normal is less than 2 seconds) and **p**aralysis.

If cervical and thoracolumbar spinal injuries are suspected, immobilization of the spine via cervical collar or spinal backboard as well as the avoidance of movement is

BOX 41-2

Type of Closed Bone Fracture and Estimated Blood Loss (EBL)

Closed Bone Fracture	Estimated Blood Loss (EBL)
Femur	500 mL–3 L
Tibia	500–1,000 mL
Radius or Ulna	150–250 mL
Humerus	250 mL
Pelvis	4–6 L

Adapted from Walsh, C., (2020). Musculoskeletal injuries. In K. McQuillan (Ed.), *Trauma Nursing: From Resuscitation Through Rehabilitation*. (5th ed., Chapter 23, pp. 599–638). Elsevier Inc.

essential. The neck is always maintained in the neutral position (Hickey, 2019). If moving is necessary, log rolling with the appropriate number of staff is used. Refer to Chapter 44 for further details regarding spinal fractures.

With an open fracture, the wound is covered with a sterile dressing to prevent contamination of deeper tissues. No attempt is made to reduce the fracture, even if bone fragments are protruding through the wound. The patient is transferred to the hospital for treatment. Tetanus prophylaxis will be administered in the emergency room (ER) if the last known booster was over 5 years ago (Havers et al., 2020).

An immediate priority is maintaining hemodynamic stability. Hypovolemic shock, resulting from hemorrhage (both visible and nonvisible blood loss) and from loss of intravascular volume into the interstitial space, may occur in fractures of the extremities, thorax, pelvis, or spine. Because the bone is very vascular, large quantities of blood may be lost as a result of trauma, especially in fractures of the femur and pelvis. Refer to Box 41-2. An open fracture results in greater blood loss and increased risk of infection. The nurse is aware that bleeding is a common problem with fractures. The older population may be at increased risk if vasoconstriction is insufficient to maintain blood pressure. When an acute loss of >15% of blood volume occurs, a state of inadequate blood volume exists. This has a direct impact on perfusion; as the blood volume decreases, cardiac output falls, and multiple organ failure can occur. Hypovolemic shock occurs when there is a reduction in intravascular volume by 15% to 30%, which represents a loss of 750 to 1,500 mL of blood. Box 41-3 provides focused assessment guidelines for hypovolemic shock. Treatment of shock consists of stabilizing the fracture to prevent further hemorrhage, restoring blood volume and circulation, relieving the patient's pain, providing adequate splinting, and protecting the patient from further injury and other complications.

BOX 41-3

Focused Assessment

Hypovolemic Shock

Be alert for the following signs and symptoms:

- Thirst
- Anxiety, restlessness, altered sensorium
- Elevated heart rate, tachycardia
- Weak pulse (thready)
- Hypotension
- Decreased Mean Arterial Pressure (MAP) below 65 mm Hg
- Cool, clammy skin
- Decreased urine output (<0.5 mL/kg/hr)
- Decreased pulse pressure (difference between the systolic and diastolic pressure)
- Rapid, shallow respirations
- Delayed capillary refill

Surgical Management

Many patients with unstable fractures undergo surgery to correct the condition. Frequent surgical procedures include **open reduction with internal fixation (ORIF)** and closed reduction with internal fixation (the fracture is reduced prior to making a surgical incision for "internal fixation" of the fracture) for fractures; amputation for severe extremity conditions (e.g., massive trauma); **bone graft** for joint stabilization, defect filling, or stimulation of bone healing; and **tendon transfer** for improving motion.

Ongoing Management

Nursing goals include improving function by restoring motion and stability and by relieving pain and disability. The principles of fracture treatment include reduction, immobilization, and regaining of normal function and strength through rehabilitation.

Reduction

Reduction of a fracture ("setting" the bone) refers to restoration of the fracture fragments to anatomic alignment and rotation. Either closed reduction or **open reduction** may be used to reduce a fracture. Before **fracture reduction** and immobilization, the nurse prepares the patient for the procedure, assures permission for the procedure is obtained, and administers an analgesic as prescribed. The nurse gently handles the injured extremity to avoid additional damage.

Closed Reduction. In most instances, closed reduction is accomplished through manipulation and manual traction. The extremity is held in the desired position while the provider applies a cast, splint, or other device. Reduction under anesthesia with percutaneous pinning may be used. The immobilizing device maintains the reduction and stabilizes the extremity for bone healing. X-rays are obtained to verify that the bone fragments are aligned correctly.

Traction (skin or skeletal) may be used to effect fracture reduction and immobilization. Traction is discussed later in the chapter.

Open Reduction. With an open fracture, surgical intervention is needed to align the bone fragments. **Internal fixation** devices (metallic pins, wires, screws, plates, nails, or

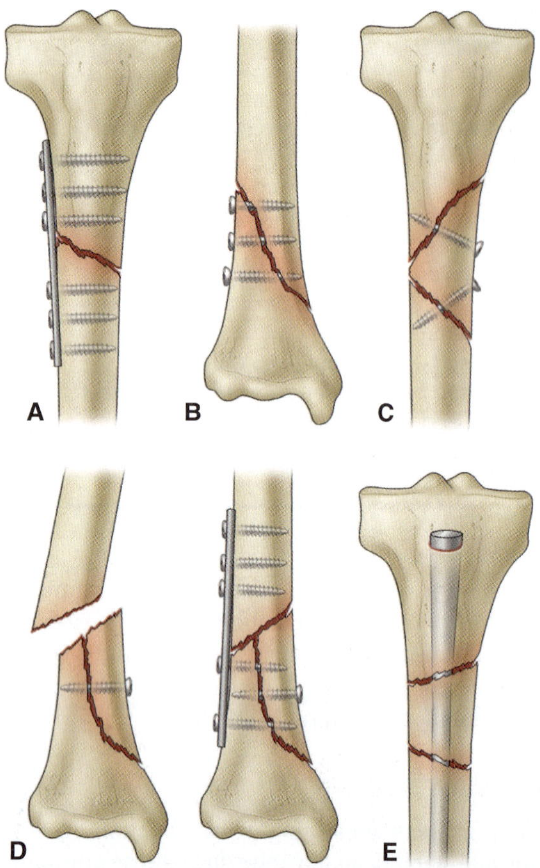

FIGURE 41-2 **Techniques of internal fixation. A. Plate and six screws for a transverse or short oblique fracture. B. Screws for a long oblique or spiral fracture. C. Screws for a long butterfly fragment. D. Plate and six screws for a short butterfly fragment. E. Medullary nail for a segmental fracture.**

rods), which are made of stainless steel, titanium, or cobalt alloys and are nonmagnetic and electrolytically inert, are used to hold the bone fragments in position until bone healing occurs (Fig. 41-2). Internal fixation devices ensure firm immobilization, close approximation, and fixation of the bony fragments. Because they decrease the space between fragments and movement at the fracture site healing seems to take place faster (Phillips & Hornacky, 2021a). They are not designed to support the body's weight, and they can bend, loosen, or break if stressed. The estimated strength of the bone, the stability of the fracture, reduction and fixation, and the amount of bone healing are important considerations in determining weight-bearing limits. Although the incision may appear healed, the underlying bone requires more time to repair and regain normal strength. Some orthopedic procedures require weight-bearing restrictions. The orthopedic surgeon will prescribe the weight-bearing limits and the use of protective devices (orthoses), if necessary, after surgery. Typically, the patient starts non–weight-bearing exercises and progresses to ambulation early, which decreases joint stiffness and muscle atrophy and prevents a long period of rehabilitation (Phillips & Hornacky, 2021a).

Management of an Open Fracture

For patients with open fractures, prompt, thorough wound irrigation with sterile isotonic saline solution and low pressure and **debridement** are necessary to remove foreign bodies, obvious debris, and bacteria (Howe, 2022). Often this is performed in the operating room. Once the wound is cleaned, the fracture is carefully reduced and stabilized by internal and/or external fixation. Ideally, surgery is performed within 8 hours (Phillips & Hornacky, 2021a). All open fractures are considered contaminated and carry risks for osteomyelitis (bone infection), tetanus, and gas gangrene. Approximately 25% of those with open fractures develop osteomyelitis (discussed shortly) (Schmitt, 2022). For this reason, systemic antibiotics are generally prescribed and administered as soon as possible (preferably within 6 hours) after open trauma to reduce the risk of soft tissue infection or osteomyelitis (Phillips & Hornacky, 2021b; Schmitt, 2022). The nurse is mindful that fixation of fractures carries a risk of infection. The objectives of management are to prevent infection of the wound, soft tissue, and bone, and to promote healing of soft tissue and bone. Options include sterile dressing changes to allow drainage of wound and edema from heavily contaminated injuries; the use of a wound vacuum–assisted closure (VAC) device also known as negative pressure wound therapy (NPWT); or re-exploration of the wound with debridement as necessary to remove infected and devitalized (dead) tissue and increase vascularity in the region. After it has been determined that infection is not present, the wound is closed by grafting of autogenous (patient's own tissue) skin, or a flap, or healing by secondary intention (a full-thickness wound heals from the base upward, by laying down new tissue). However, when the wound is closed during the first surgery, reduced rates for infections and nonunion are seen (Rupp et al., 2020). The nurse instructs the patient or family to monitor temperature at regular intervals and report signs of infection to their provider (Box 41-4). Infections must be treated promptly.

Pearls for Practice

While open fractures carry the risk of infection, a greater probability for shock exists with open fractures because of the potential for significant blood loss; thus, the nurse observes for signs and symptoms of hypovolemia (see Box 41-3) (Phillips & Hornacky, 2021b).

BOX 41-4 Focused Assessment

Infection with an Open Fracture: All Open Fractures Are Considered Contaminated

Be alert for signs and symptoms of infection:
- Elevated temperature
- Tachycardia
- Tachypnea
- Redness, warmth, pain or tenderness, swelling, purulent drainage at wound site
- Leukocytosis (elevated WBCs)

Pearls for Practice

Do not rely on fever as a marker for infection in older individuals. Consider change in the level of consciousness an indication.

Immobilization

After the fracture has been reduced, the bone fragments must be immobilized, or held in correct position and alignment, until union occurs. Internal fixation, as described above, or external fixation via bandages, casts, and splints are methods used to immobilize fractures. Casts are discussed later in the chapter.

Unfolding Patient Stories: M.H. • Part 1

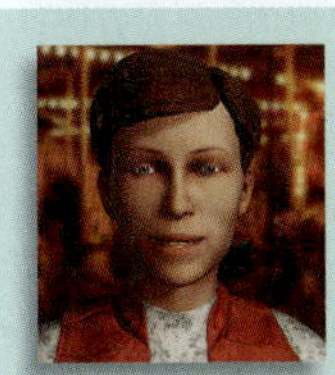

M.H, a 45-year-old, was brought to the emergency department after a fall down icy stairs. The patient is complaining of severe left lower leg pain and is wearing long pants and boots. What are priority assessments and interventions that the nurse should implement for a suspected lower leg fracture? (M.H.'s story continues in Chapter 42).

Care for M.H. and other patients in a realistic virtual environment: ***vSim** for Nursing* (thepoint.lww.com/vSimMedicalSurgical). Practice documenting these patients' care in DocuCare (thepoint.lww.com/DocuCareEHR).

Nursing Management

The major goals for the patient with a fracture include knowledge of the treatment regimen, relief of pain, improved physical mobility, achievement of maximum level of self-care, healing of any trauma-associated lacerations and abrasions, maintenance of adequate neurovascular function, and absence of complications.

Teaching Related to Treatment Regimen

Anticipatory guidance is provided to the patient and significant others by explaining the sights, sounds, and sensations (e.g., heat from the hardening reaction of the plaster) associated with application of the internal or external device chosen to treat the fracture. Specific treatment modalities are discussed later in the chapter. Regardless of the treatment modality chosen for the fracture, patient teaching includes self-care, medication information, monitoring for potential complications, and the need for continuing health care supervision. Fracture healing and restoration of full strength and mobility may take many months.

Relieving Pain

The nurse must carefully evaluate pain associated with musculoskeletal conditions, asking the patient to indicate the exact site, character, and intensity of the pain to help determine its cause. Pain associated with the underlying condition (e.g., fracture) is frequently controlled by immobilization. Pain due to edema that is associated with trauma, surgery, or bleeding into the tissues frequently can be controlled by elevation and, if prescribed, intermittent application of cryotherapy. Ice bags (one third to one half full) or cold application devices are placed on each side of the cast or fixator, if prescribed, making sure not to indent the cast or put undue pressure on external pins. Analgesics are administered as prescribed.

Pain also may be indicative of complications. Unrelenting pain that is unresponsive to usual treatment measures (narcotics, elevation, cold) is associated with compartment syndrome. Severe pain over a bony prominence may warn of an impending pressure ulcer. Discomfort due to pressure on the skin may be relieved by elevation that controls edema or by positioning that alters pressure. However, the affected limb must be elevated no higher than heart level to ensure adequate arterial perfusion. If the fracture is casted, it may be necessary to modify the cast or to apply a new cast.

Pearls for Practice

The nurse must never ignore complaints of pain from the patient in a cast because of the possibility of problems such as impaired tissue perfusion or pressure ulcer formation.

Improving Mobility

Every joint and digit that is not immobilized should be exercised and moved through its ROM to maintain function. The nurse encourages the patient to assist in the repositioning, if not contraindicated, by use of the **trapeze** or bed rail. If a patient has a spica cast (a cast that stabilizes the hips and thighs, also known as a body cast), a stabilizing **abduction** bar may be incorporated into the cast to maintain the legs in an abducted position. This bar should never be used as a turning device. If internal fixation is required to stabilize the fracture, the provider determines weight-bearing activity.

Because deep vein thrombosis (DVT) is a significant risk for the immobilized patient, the nurse encourages the patient to do active flexion–extension foot and ankle exercises and isometric contraction of the calf muscles (calf-pumping exercises) every hour while awake to decrease venous stasis in the unaffected limb. In addition, sequential compression devices (SCDs), such as venous compression (Venodyne) boots, and anticoagulant therapy may be prescribed to help prevent thrombus formation. The nurse encourages the patient to move digits and joints distal to the injury hourly when awake to prevent problems related to inactivity.

Pearls for Practice

The nurse follows hospital protocol regarding the application of an SCD. Contraindications to use of an SCD may include lower extremity cellulitis, gangrene, severe arteriosclerosis, ischemic vascular disease, massive leg edema, suspected DVT, postoperative

incision below the knee, recent skin graft, recent lower extremity fracture, open wound trauma or amputation, and/or absent pedal pulse (LeCuyer et al., 2021). In the event that no contraindications exist, the SCD is applied bilaterally, whereas if a contraindication is present in one leg, the SCD is applied to the unaffected leg only (LeCuyer et al., 2021).

Maintaining Adequate Neurovascular Function

The immobilized extremity's neurovascular status is assessed at least every hour initially, always comparing the affected extremity to the noninjured one. The nurse assesses for the "six P's," as described previously. Edema is a natural response of the tissue to trauma. If the edema is significant, pressure can rise within the area, compromising circulation as well as nerve and motor function. Early recognition of diminished circulation and nerve function, therefore, is essential to prevent loss of function. The affected extremity is adjusted so that it is no higher than heart level to control edema but not impede arterial perfusion. The surgeon is notified at once if signs of compromised neurovascular status are present. The nurse assesses the sensory and motor function of major nerves in the area of injury. Diminished circulation and nerve function must be treated promptly by release of constricting bandages. Refer to Box 41-5 for assessment of peripheral nerves of the upper extremities.

Normal findings of the fractured limb include minimal edema and discomfort, warmth to touch, capillary refill less than 2 seconds, normal sensations, and ability to move fingers or toes. Numbness, tingling, and burning may be caused by nerve injury from pressure at the fracture site. The nurse instructs the patient to report any changes in sensation or movement immediately so that they can be evaluated promptly.

Maintaining and Restoring Function

It is important to teach exercises to maintain the health of unaffected muscles and to increase the strength of muscles needed for transferring and for using assistive devices (e.g., crutches, walker, special utensils). The nurse and physical therapist teach patients how to use assistive devices safely. Isometric and muscle-setting exercises (discussed later in the chapter) are encouraged to minimize disuse atrophy and to promote circulation. Participation in activities of daily living (ADLs) is encouraged to promote independent functioning and self-esteem. Gradual resumption of activities is promoted within the therapeutic prescription. With internal fixation, the surgeon determines the amount of movement and weight-bearing stress the extremity can withstand and prescribes the level of activity. Plans are made to help the patient modify their home environment as needed and to secure personal assistance if necessary.

Monitoring and Managing Potential Complications

Fat Embolism Syndrome

Emboli are clots that travel. In pelvic or long-bone fractures, in trauma patients, or in orthopedic surgeries, the fat globules released when the bone was fractured may occlude the small blood vessels that supply the lungs, brain, kidneys, and other organs (Fig. 41-3).

It is thought that at the time of fracture, fat emboli are released from the bone marrow or adipose tissue at the

BOX 41-5 **GUIDELINES FOR NURSING CARE**

Assessing the Radial, Medial, and Ulnar Nerves

Implementation

NURSING ACTION	RATIONALE
1. To assess the radial nerve, ask the patient to extend the thumb against resistance. If you suspect radial nerve damage, check the sensation at the web space between the thumb and index finger by asking the patient to describe the sensation to light touch.	1. Inability to extend finger or lack of sensation suggests radial nerve abnormality.
2. To test for median nerve integrity, ask the patient to make the "OK" sign using the thumb and forefinger to make a ring. Check the strength of the "O" by trying to open it with your fingers. Assess sensation on the distal surface of the index finger.	2. Weakness indicates a median nerve abnormality.
3. To assess the ulnar nerve, ask the patient to spread their fingers as widely as possible. Also check sensation to the little finger and the ulnar half of the ring finger by asking the patient to describe the sensation as you touch the area described.	3. Difficulty spreading fingers or lack of sensation suggests ulnar neuropathy.

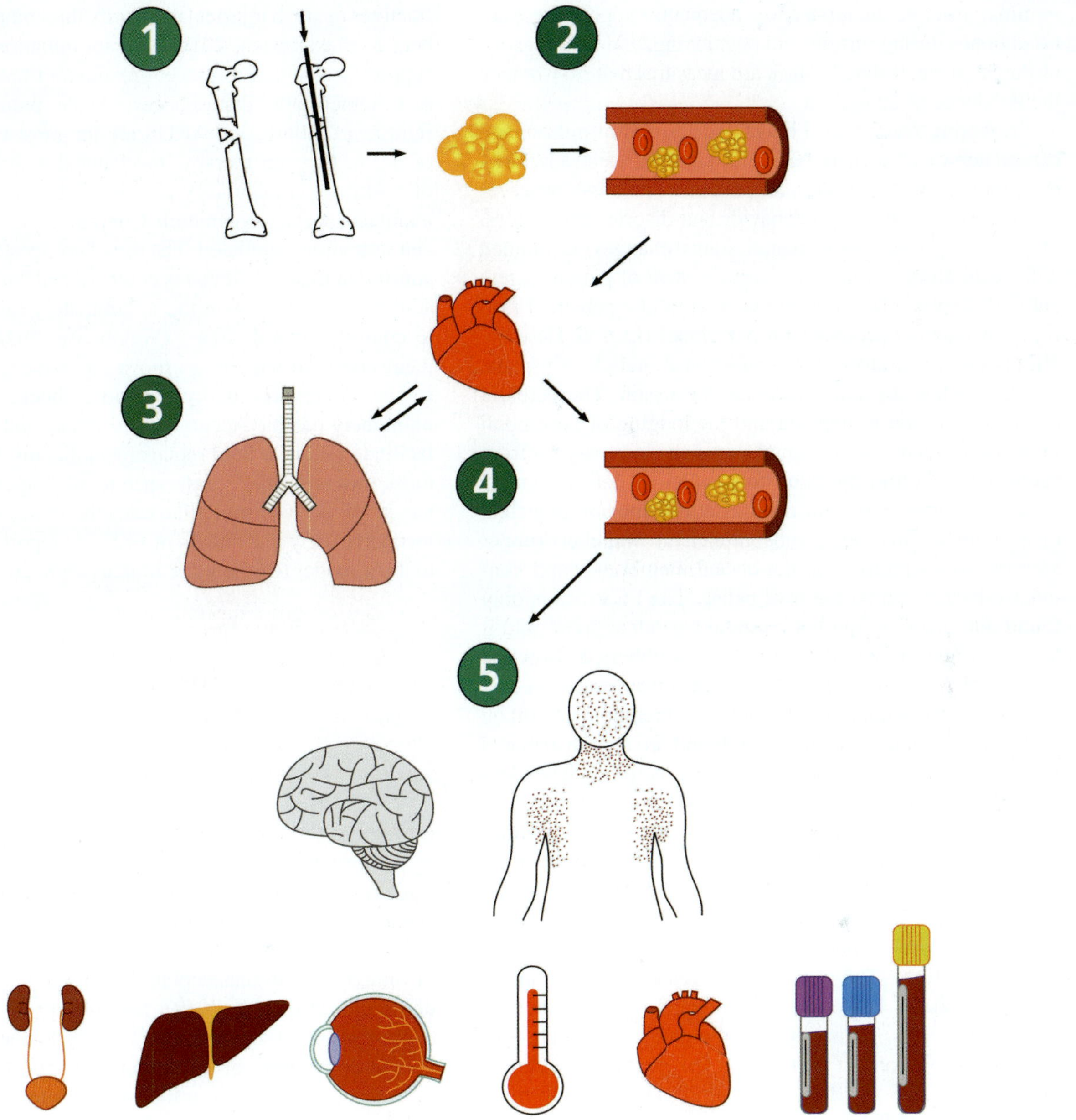

FIGURE 41-3 **Typical clinical progression of fat embolism syndrome. (*1*) Long bone fracture or intramedullary instrumentation causes (*2*) bone marrow fat to enter the venous circulation. (*3*) Fat embolizes to the pulmonary capillary bed causing alveolar damage and dysfunction. (*4*) Fat may enter the systemic circulation via a patent foreman ovale, arteriovenous shunts, the pulmonary capillary bed, or all three. (*5*) Fat subsequently embolizes and damages other organs including neurologic, dermatologic, renal, hepatic, ophthalmic, cardiovascular, and hematologic systems. (Reproduced with permission from Luff, D., & Hewson D. W. [2021]. Fat embolism syndrome. *BJA Education*, *21*[9], 322–328. https://doi.org/10.1016/j.bjae.2021.04.003)**

fracture site into the venous system through torn veins (Norris & Tuan, 2020, p. 1202). The emboli appear to have minimal physiologic effects and most patients display no signs or symptoms; however, a rare potentially fatal result of fat emboli is fat embolism syndrome (FES) that results in end-organ damage. The pathophysiology of FES remains unclear. The onset of symptoms of FES is rapid, usually within 24 to 72 hours of injury, with a median time of 48.5 hours after long bone injury (95% related to fractures of the lower extremities, and it is more common in closed fractures) (Cerepani, 2020; Luff & Hewson, 2021; Rothberg & Makarewich, 2019). However, FES has been observed as soon as 12 hours after injury (Rothberg & Makarewich, 2019). Risk factors for FES include blunt force trauma, fracture of long bones (femur, tibial) or pelvic bones, multiple fractures, crush injuries, or orthopedic surgery (intramedullary nail fixation, fixation of multiple fractures, and total hip arthroplasty [THA]). FES occurs most frequently in young male adults (average age 31 years) (Rothberg & Makarewich, 2019). Immediate immobilization of fractures (including early surgical fixation), minimal fracture manipulation, adequate support for fractured bones during turning and positioning, and maintenance of fluid and electrolyte balance are measures that may reduce the incidence of fat emboli.

Presenting features of FES include a triad of pulmonary, central nervous system (CNS), and skin manifestations; however, they are not present in all patients. The nurse observes for fever and a change in behavior and disorientation (59% of patients present with mental status changes) combined with respiratory compromise (nearly 96% of patients present with hypoxia [$PaO_2 < 60$ mm Hg]) and a petechial rash (33% of patients present with petechiae) (Luff & Hewson, 2021). The respiratory distress response includes dyspnea, crackles, wheezes, and substernal chest pain. The cerebral disturbances (due to hypoxia and the lodging of fat emboli in the brain) manifest in mental status changes varying from headache and mild agitation to confusion, delirium, seizures, and coma. The skin manifestations include petechial rash to the axillary, neck, subconjunctival, and chest (upper anterior torso) regions; in the buccal membranes and conjunctival sacs; and on the hard palate. The FES rash is only found anteriorly on the body in nondependent areas, and it has never been reported on the back (Rothberg & Makarewich, 2019). It is proposed that the rash pattern occurs because when supine, the fat droplets (which float like oil on water) accumulate in the aortic arch and are then distributed through the carotid and subclavian vessels to nondependent areas (Rothberg & Makarewich, 2019).

Occlusion of many small vessels causes the pulmonary pressure to rise. Edema and hemorrhages in the alveoli impair oxygen transport, leading to hypoxia. Arterial blood gas values reveal hypoxemia, with early respiratory alkalosis (hyperventilation) and later respiratory acidosis (hypoventilation). The chest x-ray reveals a typical "snowstorm" infiltrate; however, this finding is associated with other pathologies. Thus, a CT of the chest and, in particular, high-resolution CT (HRCT) is the modality of choice to assess for FES (Luff & Hewson, 2021). Magnetic resonance imaging (MRI) is the radiologic modality of choice to diagnose cerebral fat embolism. Without prompt, definitive treatment, acute pulmonary edema, acute respiratory failure, acute respiratory distress syndrome (ARDS), and right heart failure may develop. Approximately 44% of patients with FES require mechanical ventilation (Luff & Hewson, 2021).

The patient develops a fever greater than >38°C (>100.4°F). Fat globules may be found in the urine, blood, sputum, and bronchoalveolar lavage samples; however, this is a nonspecific finding in the setting of multitrauma and sepsis. There are no laboratory tests specific to FES; however, anemia, thrombocytopenia, and elevated inflammatory markers (**erythrocyte** sedimentation rate [ESR], C-reactive protein [CRP], and inflammatory cytokines) are commonly seen (Rothberg & Makarewich, 2019).

The nurse monitors high-risk patients (adults between 20 and 40 years of age with long-bone, pelvic, or multiple fractures or crush injuries) to identify this complication (Rothberg & Makarewich, 2019). Prompt initiation of respiratory support is essential to prevent respiratory failure and to correct homeostatic disturbances. Acute pulmonary edema, right heart failure, and ARDS are the most common causes of death. Oxygen therapy, mechanical ventilation, and use of positive end-expiratory pressure (PEEP) may be used to maintain arterial oxygenation. Continuous monitoring of oxygen saturation is initiated. The use of corticosteroids (for their anti-inflammatory effects) is controversial but if used may be administered IV to treat the inflammatory lung reaction and to control cerebral edema (Weinhouse, 2022). Vasopressor medications to support cardiovascular function are administered IV to prevent hypotension, shock, and interstitial pulmonary edema. Accurate fluid intake and output records facilitate adequate fluid replacement therapy. In addition, the nurse provides calm reassurance to allay apprehension. FES has a 5% to 20% mortality rate; therefore, the nurse must recognize early indications of FES and report them promptly to the provider (Rothberg & Makarewich, 2019).

Pearls for Practice

Subtle personality changes, restlessness, irritability, or confusion in a patient who has sustained a fracture are indications for immediate reassessment of the patient (vitals, O_2 saturation, physical examination, and laboratory data).

Delayed Union, Malunion, and Nonunion

When prolonged healing (3 to 12 months) for union of the fracture is noted, it is termed **delayed union**. The fracture eventually does heal. In **malunion**, there is flawed union of fractured bone, that is the bone heals in the standard amount of time, but in an unacceptable position with residual bony deformity (Hill et al., 2019). **Nonunion** results from failure of the ends of a fractured bone to unite in normal alignment. Patient complaints of persistent discomfort and abnormal movement or instability at the fracture site indicate potential delayed union, malunion, or nonunion.

Delayed union may be due to inadequate blood supply, inadequate bone-to-bone contact infection, or incorrect immobilization of the fracture. It may be associated with a fracture that involved a significant loss of bone, a hematoma at the fracture site, or comorbidity (e.g., diabetes mellitus, autoimmune disease). Malunion is associated with inadequate reduction of the fracture, misalignment of the fracture at the time of immobilization, or infection at the fracture site, and it presents as a deformity at the site visually or on x-ray; this generally requires surgical intervention. In nonunion, fibrocartilage or fibrous tissue exists between the bone fragments; no bone salts have been deposited. Nonunion is associated with infection, inadequate circulation, malignancy, and noncompliance with activity restrictions. Behaviors associated with both malunion and nonunion include cigarette smoking, excessive alcohol intake, and poor nutrition. Nonunion most commonly occurs with open tibia fractures, scaphoid fractures, fractures of the fifth metatarsal or the hamate (carpal bone in the wrist), talus (lower part of the ankle joint) and, in older people, at the neck of the femur because of their tenuous blood supply. Factors contributing to both nonunion and malunion include interposition of tissue between the bone ends, manipulation that disrupts callus formation, excessive space between bone fragments (bone gap), limited bone contact, bone or soft tissue loss, and impaired blood supply resulting in AVN. Medications that may affect fracture healing include chemotherapy, glucocorticoids, antibiotics (e.g., fluoroquinolones have adverse effects upon cartilage regrowth and bone healing), NSAIDs and older nonselective anti-cyclooxygenase (COX)-2 agents (animal studies suggest decreased healing; however, human studies are inconsistent) (Howe, 2022). Medical conditions that may affect fracture healing include diabetes, obesity, alcohol use disorder, and metabolic bone disease (Shapiro et al., 2022). Finally, a false joint (pseudarthrosis) often develops at the site of the fracture.

Pearls for Practice

Nurses encourage patients with bone fractures to quit smoking since nicotine inhibits vascular ingrowth and early revascularization of bone and diminishes osteoblast activity. In addition, poor nutrition is a risk factor for impaired fracture healing since metabolic requirements increase during fracture healing. Prealbumin and albumin are used conventionally as indicators of nutritional level and a normal albumin is 4.0 to 5.5 g/dL and prealbumin is 19 to 38 mg/dL (Fischbach et al., 2022; Nivati et al., 2021).

Nonunion is treated with internal fixation, bone grafting, electrical bone stimulation (thought to stimulate osteoblasts or bone formation), or a combination of these therapies. Internal fixation stabilizes the bone fragments and ensures bone contact. A bone graft may be an **autograft** (tissue, frequently from the iliac crest, harvested from the patient for their own use) or an **allograft** (tissue harvested from a donor for a recipient). The bone graft fills the bone gap, provides a lattice structure for invasion by bone cells, and actively promotes bone growth.

After grafting, immobilization and non–weight-bearing exercises are required while the bone graft becomes incorporated, and the fracture or defect heals. Depending on the type of bone grafted, healing may take from 6 to 12 months or longer. Bone grafting problems include wound or graft infection, prolonged wound drainage, fracture of the graft, persistent pain, sensory loss, and nonunion (Schmidt, 2021).

Venous Thromboemboli

Venous thromboemboli, including DVT and pulmonary emboli (PE), are associated with reduced skeletal muscle contractions and bed rest. Patients with fractures of the lower extremities and pelvis are at high risk for venous thromboemboli. PEs may cause death several days to weeks after injury.

Depending on the size and location of the emboli, symptoms vary. A large PE can cause an increase in pulmonary arterial resistance, which can lead to right heart failure and hypoxemia (Stacy, 2022). Massive emboli can present as shock and loss of consciousness. The most frequent signs are sudden-onset shortness of breath (dyspnea), restlessness, increased respiratory rate, tachycardia, chest pain, cough, and low-grade fever. Pleuritic pain that increases with inspiration is seen with pulmonary infarct. Moderate hypoxemia occurs, without retention of CO_2, and a cough that is productive of blood-tinged sputum may be seen. It is important that a high degree of suspicion is maintained for PE since patients may have mild or nonspecific symptoms. Refer to Chapters 9 and 17 for details on DVT and PE.

Pearls for Practice

A significant risk factor for DVT is bed rest. The longer the duration of bedrest, the higher the possibility that deep vein thrombosis will develop (Cao et al., 2021). The nurse assesses for signs and symptoms of DVT, which include unilateral limb edema (unrelieved by elevation), warmth, erythema, tenderness/pain, and/or "fullness" of the lower extremities which commonly occurs at least 2 to 5 days after immobilization or surgery (Cannon, 2021).

Disseminated Intravascular Coagulation

Disseminated intravascular coagulation (DIC) is a systemic disorder that results in widespread hemorrhage and microthrombosis with ischemia. Its causes are diverse and can include massive tissue trauma. Early manifestations of DIC include unexpected bleeding after surgery and bleeding from the mucous membranes, venipuncture sites, and gastrointestinal and urinary tracts. The treatment of DIC is discussed in Chapter 19.

Avascular Necrosis of Bone

AVN or osteonecrosis occurs when the bone loses its blood supply and dies. The cause of AVN is not well understood but is associated with trauma and subsequent impairment of blood supply; it is also associated with glucocorticoid treatment, connective tissue disease, sickle cell disease, embolization, alcohol use, smoking, and HIV (Jameson et al., 2020). It may occur after a fracture with disruption of the blood supply (especially of the femoral head). It is also seen with dislocations, bone transplantation, and radiotherapy (called osteoradionecrosis) and chemotherapy (Matthews et al., 2022). The patient develops tenderness of the affected area and experiences limited movement; a click or crepitus may be noted when a joint is put through ROM (Clinical Overview, 2021a). X-rays may reveal loss of mineralized matrix and structural collapse; MRI is the modality of choice. Referral to an orthopedic surgeon is important for surgical treatment of early-stage osteonecrosis because patients diagnosed with precollapse osteonecrosis are likely to progress to collapse within 3 years (Clinical Overview, 2021a). Treatment generally consists of attempts to revitalize the bone with bone grafts, prosthetic replacement, or **arthrodesis** (joint fusion).

Reaction to Internal Fixation Devices

Internal fixation devices may be removed after bony union has taken place. However, in most patients, the device is not removed unless it produces symptoms. The devices are made of nonmagnetic and electrolytically inert metals such as stainless steel, cobalt, and titanium alloys or polymers such as silicone and polyethylene (Phillips & Hornacky, 2021b). Grounds for removal include pain, negative body sensation, device failure, neurologic symptoms, decreased function, infection, or fear of future complications in active individuals (Prediger et al., 2020). In a recent review, more than 90% of internal fixations were removed within 24 months after the initial surgery; however, no clear timing for removal was noted since it is dependent on the time point for bone healing (Prediger et al., 2020). If the device is removed, the bone needs to be protected from refracture related to osteoporosis, altered bone structure, and trauma. Bone remodeling reestablishes the bone's structural strength.

Reaction to External Fixation Devices

Because the screws or pins are inserted externally (Fig. 41-4), infection is a complication for which nurses must be vigilant. Rates of pin tract infections range between 9% and 100% in the literature when looking at external fixation (regardless of site) (Shields et al., 2022). Signs of infection include erythema, purulent drainage, warmth, leukocytosis (elevated white blood cell count), fever, and loosening pins (pins should be immobile in the bone). It is important to note that in a recent review of international protocols of pin-site care where practice varied, no one standard was associated with a 0% infection rate (Shields et al., 2022). Variations in pin care include use of soap and water, iodine cleaning, saline, chlorhexidine, hydrogen peroxide, sulphadiazine, xeroform dressing, plain dressing, combination of hydrogen peroxide with sulphadiazine and xeroform dressings, crust removal or retention, and differences in cleaning routine (e.g., twice daily, daily, or weekly pin care). The study revealed that weekly pin care is as effective as daily care, that low-energy pin-insertion techniques and hydroxyapatite (HA)-coated pins are superior, and that the use of sulphadiazine appears to demonstrate the most promise (Shields et al., 2022). That said, currently no consensus exists about which protocol should be applied universally. The mainstay of prevention and/or reduction of the incidence of pin-site infections is surgical technique during pin insertion and implementation of one of the existing protocols of pin-site care. Thus, pin care is performed according to hospital and provider protocol.

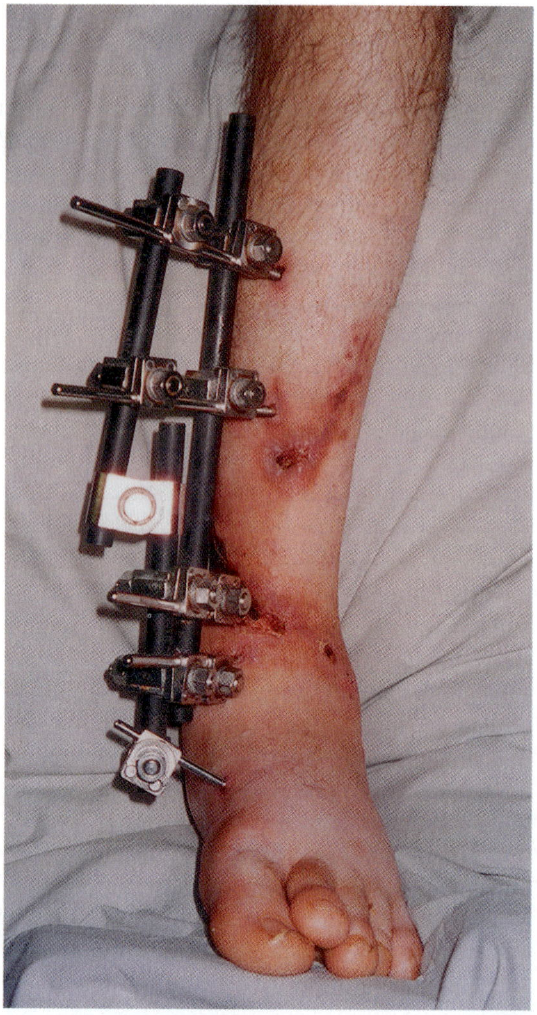

FIGURE 41-4 External fixation device. Pins are inserted into bone. The fracture is reduced and aligned and then stabilized by attaching the pins to a rigid portable frame. The device facilitates treatment of soft tissue damaged in complex fractures.

Complex Regional Pain Syndrome

Complex regional pain syndrome (CRPS), formerly called *reflex sympathetic dystrophy, RSD or CRPS type 1, and causalgia or CRPS type 2 (if associated with nerve injury)* is a painful sympathetic nervous system problem characterized by constant and intense limb pain associated with vasomotor and neurosensory abnormalities, skin changes, and demineralization of bone (Luther, 2023). It is a rare complication that occurs anywhere from 0.05% to 0.2% in older studies and 3% to 7% in more recent studies (Lloyd et al., 2021). The pathogenesis is poorly understood but when it does occur, it is seen most often in postmenopausal females in the sixth decade whose injury was a fracture (16% to 46%), strain or sprain (10% to 29%), postsurgery (3% to 24%), and contusion or crush injury (8% to 18%) (Dinakar, 2022; Luther, 2023).

Clinical manifestations of CRPS typically occur 4 to 6 weeks after direct injury (fracture or surgery) and symptoms include severe pain (described as burning, searing, stabbing, tingling, numbness, or an electric shock that worsens with movement, contact, temperature variation, and stress), swelling, hyperesthesia, limited ROM, discoloration, vasomotor skin changes (e.g., fluctuating warm, red, dry and cold, sweaty, cyanotic), and abnormal nail, skin, and hair changes. *Livedo reticularis* is common in CRPS; *Livedo* describes the red, nonblanchable (i.e., does not turn white when pressed) network pattern (reticulated) in the skin. About 60% of patients may report excessive sweating in the affected limbs (Dinakar, 2022). Temperature asymmetry between the affected and unaffected sides may exceed 1°C (Dinakar, 2022). The cardinal feature of CRPS, excruciating pain and edema of the affected limb, frequently is present; initially it may be very mild; however, it may be so severe that a Doppler test is needed to rule out the possibility of a DVT (Dinakar, 2022). This syndrome is frequently chronic, with extension of symptoms to adjacent areas of the body. Disuse muscle atrophy and bone deossification (osteoporosis) occur with persistence of CRPS. Patients may exhibit ineffective individual coping related to the chronic pain. No single treatment has been found to be universally effective; early detection and an interdisciplinary approach to treatment appear to be key in treating CRPS (Kessler et al., 2020). Recommendations include early (within 6 months of symptom onset) referral for physical and occupational therapy, a short course of oral corticosteroids, bisphosphonates, and transdermal lidocaine patches (Lloyd et al., 2021). Physiotherapy techniques may include the use of mirror therapy, transcutaneous electrical nerve stimulation (TENS), acupuncture, and electroacupuncture (Luther, 2023). Since CRPS is also associated with anxiety and depression, additional therapies may include cognitive-behavioral therapy, relaxation techniques, coping skills, and biofeedback (Cooney & Parikh, 2021). Referral to a pain management specialist is recommended for those with persistent CRPS to discuss additional treatment options which may include ketamine (Ketalar) infusions, intrathecal drug pumps, regional nerve blocks, peripheral nerve stimulators, and sympathetic ganglion blocks (Lloyd et al., 2021).

Prevention may include early mobilization after injury and 500 to 1,500 mg of vitamin C given daily for 50 days (Clinical Overview, 2021b; Giustra et al., 2021; Packham & Holly, 2021). The nurse needs to help the patient cope with CRPS manifestations and explore multiple ways to control pain (see Chapter 6).

Pearls for Practice

Since patients with CRPS feel severe and long-lasting pain in response to light touch, the nurse avoids using the involved extremity for blood pressure measurements and venipunctures.

Heterotopic Ossification

Heterotopic ossification (myositis ossificans) is the abnormal formation of bone in extra-skeletal soft tissue where bone does not usually exist, in response to blunt trauma, fracture, or total joint replacement. It is also commonly seen in patients with traumatic brain injury, spinal cord injury, cerebrovascular accident, burns, traumatic amputations, and joint replacements (Sun et al., 2022). Heterotopic ossification occurs 3 to 12 weeks after inciting injury but can take up to 6 months to present; risk factors include spasticity, older age, pressure ulcer, the presence of DVT, having a tracheostomy, long bone fractures, prior injury to the same area, edema, immobility, long-term coma, and severity of the injury (Sun et al., 2022). Signs and symptoms include pain, decreased ROM, and stiffness of joints. Edema, effusion, erythema, warmth, and tenderness in the tissue or joint may be present (Sun et al., 2022). Early mobilization may prevent its occurrence. NSAIDs (e.g., ibuprofen) to decrease inflammation or bone formation and prophylactic low-dose radiation therapy (a single dose of 700 to 800 g administered up to 24 hours preoperatively or within 72 hours postoperatively) have been shown to help prevent heterotopic ossification after THA. In addition, etidronate (a bisphosphonate) has been approved for prevention of it in spinal cord injuries and complication of THA (Sun et al., 2022). Usually, the bone lesion resorbs over time, but the abnormal bone eventually may need to be excised if symptoms persist. Exercises to maintain joint ROM are considered the foundation of prevention.

Fractures of Specific Sites

Injuries to the skeletal structure may vary from a simple linear fracture to a severe crushing injury. The type and location of the fracture and the extent of damage to surrounding structures determine the therapeutic management. Maximum functional recovery is the goal of management.

Clavicle

Fracture of the clavicle (collar bone) is a common injury that results from a fall or a direct blow to the shoulder. These injuries frequently are associated with equestrian sports and cycling, when a rider is thrown forward and lands on the unprotected shoulder. Head or cervical spine injuries may accompany these fractures. They are also seen in older patients after a low-impact fall. Those with clavicular fractures are typically males between the ages of 15 and 30 years, with a second peak incidence occurring in females older than 80 years (Stelter et al., 2020). When the clavicle is fractured, the patient assumes a protective position, slumping the shoulders and immobilizing the arm to prevent shoulder movements. A deformity of the clavicle may be observed, with obvious local tenderness. The treatment goal is to align the shoulder in its normal position by means of closed reduction and immobilization or, if displaced, an ORIF.

Depending on the site of the clavicular fracture, most minimally displaced or nondisplaced fractures can be treated nonsurgically with a sling or a figure-eight bandage (also called a *clavicular strap* or *broad arm sling*) to pull the shoulders back, reducing and immobilizing the fracture (Fig. 41-5), and 2 to 6 weeks of immobilization, as well as avoidance of

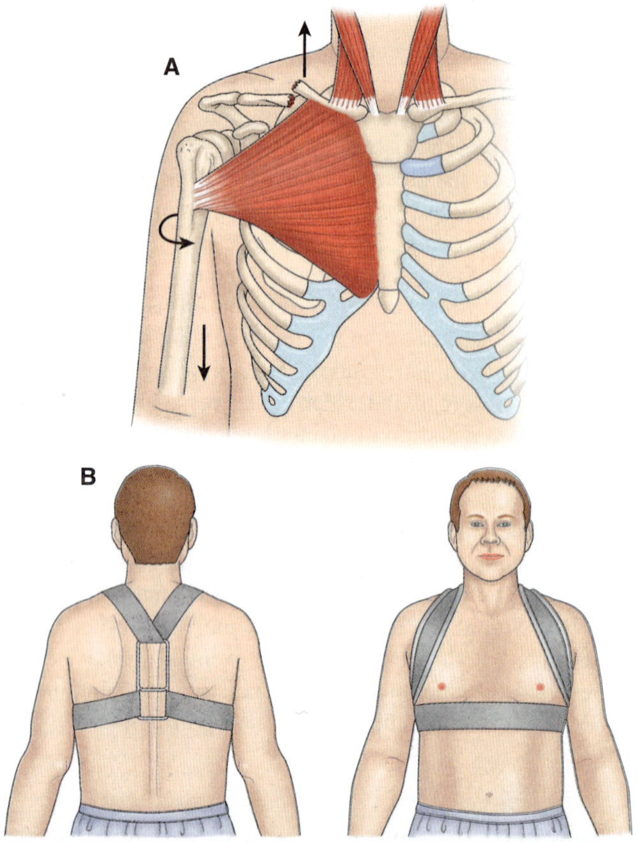

FIGURE 41-5 Fracture of the clavicle. A. Anteroposterior view shows typical displacement in midclavicular fracture. B. Immobilization is accomplished with a clavicular strap.

heavy lifting and contact sports for 4 to 6 months (Yeh & Lee, 2022). In some patients depending on patient comfort, no sling or bandage is required. Each treatment has advantages and disadvantages. When a clavicular strap is used, the axillae are well padded to prevent skin breakdown or a compression injury to the brachial plexus and the axillary artery. If the clavicle is displaced significantly or if there is significant comminution or excessive shortening (more than 2 cm), referral to an orthopedic surgeon is warranted. When internal fixation is indicated, surgery may be performed with either a plate and screws or an intramedullary device.

The nurse monitors the skin integrity and circulation and nerve function of both arms. An arm sling may be used to support the arm and to relieve pain. A sling may cause the elbow to stiffen, so the patient is encouraged to perform gentle elbow ROM exercises to maintain normal function and prevent stiffness. The nurse cautions the patient not to elevate the arm above the shoulder level until the ends of the bone have united (about a minimum of 2 months for solid union [possibly a month longer in adults]). Contact sports should be avoided for 8 to 10 weeks, but the nurse encourages the patient to exercise the elbow, wrist, and fingers as soon as possible. Complications of clavicular fractures include trauma to the nerves of the brachial plexus, injury to the subclavian vein or artery from a bony fragment, and malunion (faulty union of fractured bone) or nonunion (failure of the ends of a fractured bone to unite in normal alignment). Nonunion occurs more frequently with distal clavicular fractures managed nonsurgically.

Pearls for Practice

The nurse recognizes that the apex of the lungs rises 1 to 2 in above the inner 1/3 of the clavicles and in the event of clavicular fractures assesses for pneumothorax (sudden onset of shortness of breath, crepitus, tachypnea, decreased or absent lung sounds, asymmetric lung expansion, hyperresonance on percussion). Instruct the patient to report any shortness of breath immediately (Kalb & Fowler, 2020).

Humeral Shaft

Fractures of the shaft of the humerus may injure the nerves and brachial blood vessels in the affected arm; therefore, neurovascular assessment is essential to identify when immediate attention is required. Table 41-2 provides guidelines for neurovascular evaluation. A wrist drop (the hand hangs flaccidly in a position of flexion when the patient attempts to bring the arm to a horizontal position) is indicative of radial nerve injury (DeCastro & Keefe, 2022). Approximately 3% of all fractures are of the humeral shaft; most can be treated nonoperatively (Perez, 2021). An ORIF of a fracture of the humerus is necessary if the patient has nerve palsy, blood vessel damage, comminuted fracture, humeral shortening >3 cm, or pathologic fracture. There are two distinct populations who are at greater risk for humeral shaft fractures: young adults injured in high-energy motor vehicle accidents, falls from height, or gunshots; and older adults who fall from a standing height.

If the fracture is uncomplicated, well-padded splints, overwrapped with an elastic bandage, are used to immobilize the upper arm initially and to support the arm in 90 degrees of flexion at the elbow. The weight of the hanging arm and splints reduces the fracture. In about 7 to 10 days the splint or hanging arm cast may be converted to a prefabricated functional brace (Perez, 2021). Functional bracing consists of a contoured thermoplastic sleeve that wraps around the midshaft of the humerus and provides circumferential compression, with interlocking fabric (Velcro) closures which immobilize the reduced fracture (Fig. 41-6). As swelling decreases, the sleeve is tightened, and uniform pressure and bone stability is maintained. Functional bracing allows active use of muscles, motion in the shoulder and elbow, and good approximation of fracture fragments. In fact, it is considered the "gold standard" for nonoperative treatment because of its ease of application, adjustability, allowance of shoulder and elbow motion, relatively low cost, and reproducible results (Perez, 2021). The patient may move the elbow in the brace, which is important as this joint is notorious for becoming stiff with possible permanent

TABLE **41-2 Neurovascular Assessment and Expected Findings**

Assessment Component	Technique	Normal Findings
Skin color	Evaluate the injured area in relation to the noninjured area.	No change is noted compared to other parts of the body.
Skin temperature	Palpate using the dorsum of the hand as it is more sensitive to temperature.	No change is noted compared to other parts of the body.
Pulses	Assess proximal and distal pulses. Grade as 0, absent; 1+, weaker than normal; 2+, normal; or 3+, full and bounding.	No change is noted compared to other extremity.
Capillary refill	Depress the nail bed and note return of color.	Capillary refill is less than 2 seconds.
Sensation	With their eyes closed, evaluate the patient's ability to feel light touch of the affected extremity (e.g., assess on the first web space of foot [between great toe and second toe] for the peroneal nerve, or base of thumb [radial nerve], or little finger [ulnar nerve]). Assess presence of numbness or tingling.	No sensory deficit is noted.
Mobility	Observe the ROM in joints or digits distal to the injury.	Full movement of digits is noted.
	Note edema and tenseness of the injured area.	Minimal edema and ecchymosis are noted.
	Mark and measure circumference if concerned.	In a nontraumatized limb, a difference of 1 cm at the ankles and 2 cm at mid-calf is expected.

limitation of motion (Kalb & Fowler, 2020). The use of a sling is discouraged with functional splinting to avoid rotation deformities. After, the first week, pendulum shoulder exercises may be prescribed to provide active movement of the shoulder, thereby preventing adhesions of the shoulder joint capsule. The brace is worn until the patient is pain free and there is radiographic evidence of union. Complications of bracing include skin breakdown and malunion; since skin maceration is a concern, the nurse teaches the importance of daily hygiene (Perez, 2021). If an ORIF was required for the humeral fracture, immediate mobilization of the elbow joint and active-assisted shoulder mobilization should be possible. Isometric exercises may be prescribed to prevent muscle atrophy. Complications that are seen with humeral

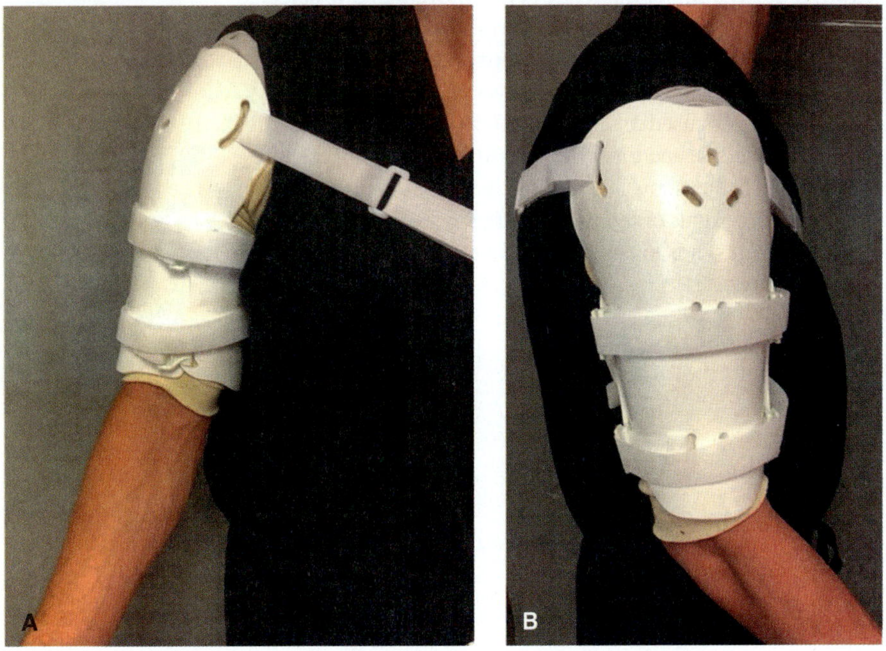

FIGURE 41-6 **Anterior (A) and lateral (B) views of a humeral brace. (From D. S. Horwitz, & D. Suk, [2021].** ***Hoppenfeld's treatment and rehabilitation of fractures*** **[2nd ed., Fig. 13.5]. Wolters Kluwer Health.)**

shaft fractures include delayed union and nonunion (failure of the ends of a fractured bone to unite).

Elbow

Fractures of the elbow result from motor vehicle crashes, falls on the elbow (in the extended or flexed position), or a direct blow. Symptoms include elbow pain and swelling. Radial head fractures are the most common fractures involving the elbow; however, the distal humerus or proximal ulna is also commonly involved. Nondisplaced or minimally displaced fractures can be treated nonoperatively; however, a displaced fracture may require operative treatment. Typically, the arm is placed in a molded posterior plaster splint at 90 degrees; at days 3 to 7, the splint is removed, and the arm is supported in a sling (Perez, 2021). Active and active-assisted exercises are begun to limit the development of stiffness and contracture that can lead to significant functional disability. The sling is discontinued at 3 weeks and exercises are gradually increased as tolerated; however, forceful manipulation of the elbow is never permitted (Perez, 2021).

Elbow fractures may result in injury to the median, radial, or ulnar nerves. The patient is evaluated for paresthesia and signs of compromised circulation in the forearm and hand. The most serious complication is *Volkmann contracture* (an acute compartment syndrome [ACS]), which results from antecubital swelling, hemorrhage, and effusion into the muscles or arterial insufficiency or ischemia of the muscles (Fig. 41-7). It is a claw-like deformity of the hand (Thompson, 2021). Contracture of the fingers and wrist occurs as the result of obstructed arterial blood flow to the forearm and hand. The patient is unable to extend the fingers, describes abnormal sensation (e.g., unrelenting pain, pain on passive stretch), and exhibits signs of diminished circulation to the hand. Although the incidence of Volkmann contracture is low, its devastating complications are preventable if detected early. This serious complication warrants nursing vigilance to minimize limb loss. The nurse needs to monitor the patient regularly for compromised neurovascular status. Refer to Box 41-5 for focused assessment guidelines for evaluation of the radial, medial, and ulnar nerve in upper extremity fractures. Severe pain at the elbow and increasing tenseness of the forearm are worrisome signs of increasing intracompartmental pressure. Compartment syndrome is discussed on pages 1350–1352.

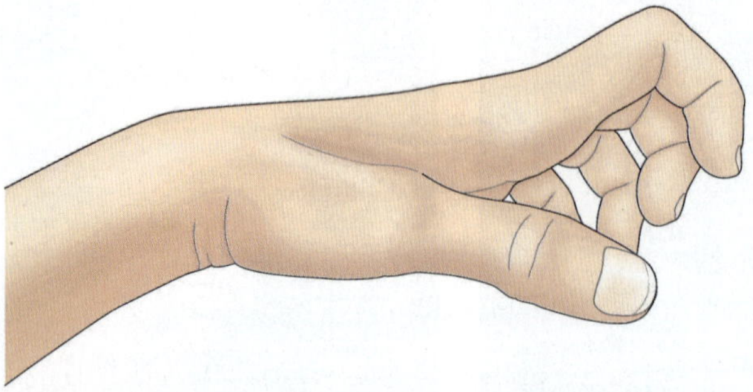

FIGURE 41-7 Volkmann contracture.

Pearls for Practice

Increasing pain that is out of proportion to the injury and worsens with passive stretching of the involved muscles is an early indication that a compartment syndrome is developing (Thompson, 2021). The nurse may note that the forearm is tender and tense with swelling, and sensitivity of the patient's fingertips may be diminished. If found, the nurse notifies the provider. Absence of a radial pulse is a late finding.

Hand

Trauma to the hand often requires extensive reconstructive surgery. The objective of treatment is always to regain maximum function of the hand. Hand fractures account for ~17% of all fractures in adults, with 59% of hand fractures occurring in the phalanges, 33% in the metacarpals, and 8% in the carpal bones (Jemec & Burr, 2022). Scaphoid fractures (bone on the thumb side of the wrist) are the most common carpal bone fractures, far exceeding all other carpal bone injuries; such a fracture typically occurs after falling onto an outstretched hand. The risk of nonunion can be high if the fracture is displaced (Hayat & Varacallo, 2022). There is also a risk for AVN since blood flow to the scaphoid bone is tenuous and typically retrograde. Refer to Figure 41-8 for carpel bones details. Patient complaints include radial-sided wrist pain, tenderness in the anatomic snuff box, bruising, and edema (swelling at the base of the thumb). Treatment (if nondisplaced) may include a long arm or short arm cast with or without immobilization of the thumb; at present there is not enough evidence to suggest whether one option is better than the other (Hayat & Varacallo, 2022). For a nondisplaced fracture of the phalanx (finger bone), the finger is splinted or "buddy taped" to an adjacent finger for stabilization versus

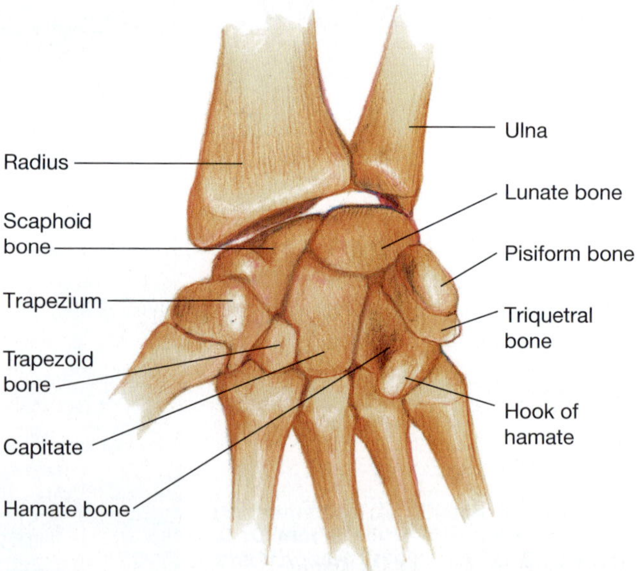

FIGURE 41-8 Palmar view of carpal bones. (Courtesy of Anatomical Chart Company.)

casting for a short period of immobilization, and then progressive ROM and rehabilitation (McDaniel & Rehman, 2022). Displaced fractures and open fractures may require ORIF, using wires or pins.

Arm

The most frequently broken arm bone is the radius, and the site most commonly affected is the distal radius. Termed a Colles fracture (the broken fragment of the radius tilts upward), the distal radius fracture usually is the result of a **f**all **o**n **o**ut**s**tretched **h**and injury (referred to by the acronym "FOOSH injury"). This fracture is frequently seen in older females with osteoporotic bones and weak soft tissues that do not dissipate the energy of the fall or in younger people involved in high impact trauma (e.g., falls, sports injuries). The patient presents with a deformed wrist, radial deviation, pain, swelling, weakness, limited finger ROM, and numbness.

Treatment usually consists of closed reduction and immobilization with a short arm cast if the fracture is nondisplaced or minimally displaced. The extremity may be treated initially in a temporary sugar tong (long U-shaped) splint for 5 to 7 days until swelling subsides and then casted in a short arm cast. For fractures with extensive comminution (bone is broken into a number of pieces) or impaction, ORIF, arthroscopic percutaneous pinning, or external fixation is used to achieve and maintain reduction and to allow for early functional rehabilitation. The wrist and forearm are elevated for 48 hours after reduction to control swelling, and active motion of the fingers and shoulder begins promptly. The nurse monitors for signs of neurovascular compromise, comparing findings on the affected limb to the other limb.

Pearls for Practice

When the fracture is splinted or casted, the nurse educates the patient that severe pain, discoloration of fingers or nail beds, edema, numbness/tingling of the fingers, or decreased finger ROM should be reported to the provider immediately (Summers & Fowles, 2022).

Tibia and Fibula

The most common fractures below the knee are tibia and fibula fractures, and these tend to result from a direct blow, falls with the foot in a flexed position, or a violent twisting motion. The patient presents with pain, deformity, obvious hematoma, and considerable edema. Frequently, these fractures are open and involve severe soft tissue damage because there is little subcutaneous tissue in the area.

The peroneal nerve is assessed for damage that may result in foot drop (inability to lift the foot), by checking for sensation of the web between the great and second toes, and for increased sensitivity of the dorsal surfaces of the foot (top). If nerve function is impaired, the patient cannot dorsiflex the great toe and has diminished sensation in the first web space (between first metatarsal and hallux [big toe]). As with all fractures, the patient is observed for signs of neurovascular complications. The development of ACS (see discussion later in this chapter) requires prompt recognition and resolution to prevent permanent functional deficit. Other complications include delayed union, infection, impaired wound edge healing due to limited soft tissue, and loosening of the internal fixation hardware (if ORIF is performed to repair fracture).

Most closed tibial fractures are treated with closed reduction and initial immobilization in a long leg walking cast, a patellar tendon–bearing cast, hinged knee brace, or walking boot (depending on where the fracture is located). Reduction must be relatively accurate in relation to angulation and rotation. Comminuted fractures may be treated with skeletal traction, internal fixation with intramedullary nails or plates and screws, or external fixation. External support may be used with internal fixation.

Pelvis

Numerous classification systems have been used to describe pelvic fractures in relation to pelvic anatomy, stability, and mechanism of injury. Some fractures of the pelvis do not disrupt the pelvic ring and are termed stable pelvic fractures; others do and are termed unstable (nonintact pelvic ring). The severity of pelvic fractures varies.

Stable Pelvic Fractures

Stable fractures of the pelvis (Fig. 41-9) heal rapidly because the pelvic bones are mostly cancellous bone, which has a rich blood supply. The fractures are treated with a few days of bed rest and symptom management until the pain and discomfort are controlled. However, if a fractured sacrum involves the S2–S5 sacral nerve root then bowel or bladder incontinence and sexual dysfunction could result (Davis et al., 2022).

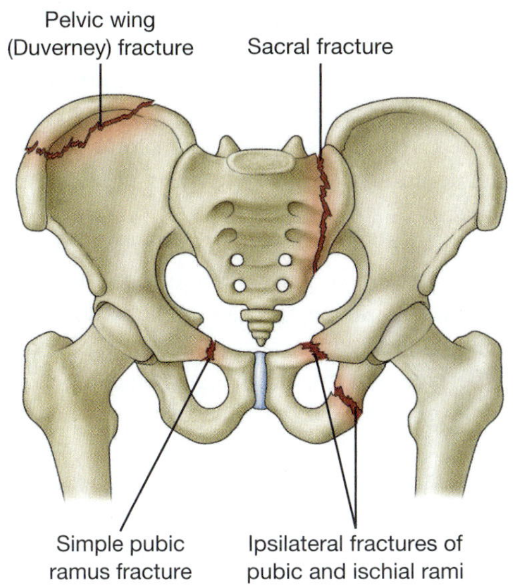

FIGURE 41-9 **Stable pelvic fractures.**

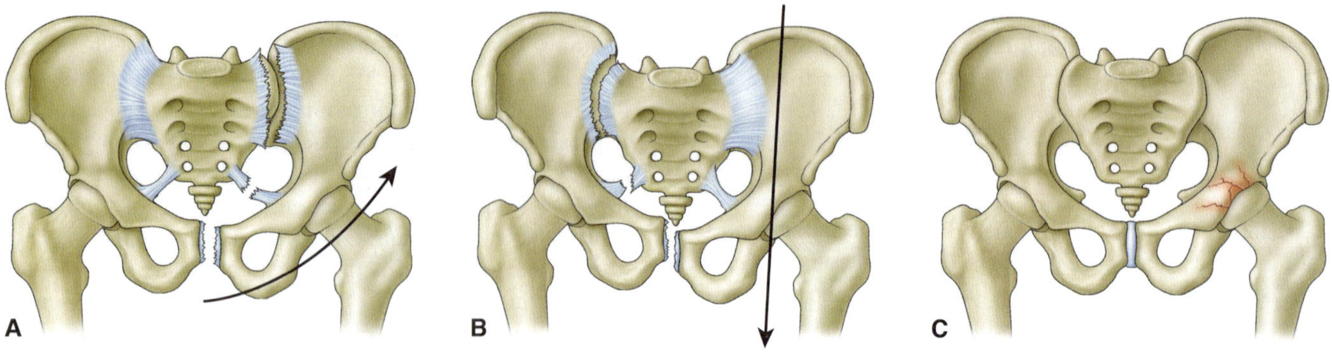

FIGURE 41-10 **Unstable pelvic fracture. A. Rotationally unstable fracture. The symphysis pubis is separated and the anterior sacroiliac, sacrotuberous, and sacrospinous ligaments are disrupted. B. Vertically unstable fracture. The hemipelvis is displaced anteriorly and posteriorly through the symphysis pubis, and the sacroiliac joint ligament is disrupted. C. Undisplaced fracture of the acetabulum.**

Unstable Pelvic Fractures

Unstable fractures of the pelvis may result in rotational instability (e.g., the "open book" type, in which a separation occurs at the symphysis pubis with sacral ligament disruption), vertical instability (e.g., the vertical shear type, with superior–inferior displacement), or a combination of both (Fig. 41-10).

Managing Pelvic Fractures

Falls, motor vehicle crashes, and crush injuries can cause pelvic fractures. The mortality rate in pelvic ring fractures is 19% but is likely higher in older patients and in those presenting with hemodynamic instability; for example mortality rates between 32% to 50% are seen in those that present in hemorrhagic shock when admitted to the hospital (Clinical Overview, 2021c; DeBose et al., 2021). Management of severe, life-threatening pelvic fractures is coordinated with the trauma team. Intra-abdominal bleeding is present in up to 40% of cases, but there also may be thoracic, retroperitoneal, and cranial injuries which have priority over treatment of fractures (Davis et al., 2022). There is a high mortality rate associated with pelvic fractures related to hemorrhage, pulmonary complications, fat emboli, thromboembolic complications, and infection.

Signs and symptoms of pelvic fracture include ecchymosis; tenderness over the symphysis pubis, anterior iliac spines, iliac crest, sacrum, or coccyx; local edema; numbness or tingling of the pubis, genitals, and proximal thighs; and inability to bear weight without discomfort and pain that is exacerbated by movement. Desault sign, which is a superficial hematoma noted above the inguinal ligament or in the scrotum/perineum or thigh, is suggestive of a pelvic fracture (Clinical Overview, 2021c). Neurovascular assessment of the lower extremities is performed to detect injury to pelvic blood vessels and nerves. Figure 41-11 details the pelvic bones. The peripheral pulses of both lower extremities are palpated; absence of a pulse may indicate a tear in the iliac artery or one of its branches. An inability to void may indicate a disrupted urethra (Clinical Overview, 2021c).

Immediate treatment in the emergency department of a patient with an unstable pelvic fracture includes stabilizing the pelvic bones and tamponading or compressing bleeding vessels. A simple method of stabilizing the pelvis is the tying of a sheet circumferentially around the hips at the level of the greater trochanters or the use of a pelvic prefabricated binder (Mondor, 2022). This is often done in the field, and this temporary measure applies pressure, closes the "open-book" pubic symphysis (anteroposterior compression injury to the pelvis), and assists in controlling bleeding.

Hemorrhage and shock are two of the more serious consequences that may occur. The nurse recognizes that with pelvic fractures injuries can occur not only to major vessels and nerves but also to major visceral organs, such as the intestines, bladder, and urethra (Dickson, 2023). Bleeding arises from the cancellous surfaces of the fracture fragments, from laceration of veins and arteries by bone fragments, and possibly from a torn iliac artery. Focused assessment with sonography in trauma (FAST) examination can be used to identify intra-abdominal injuries quickly. Diagnostic peritoneal lavage has largely been replaced with the use of FAST

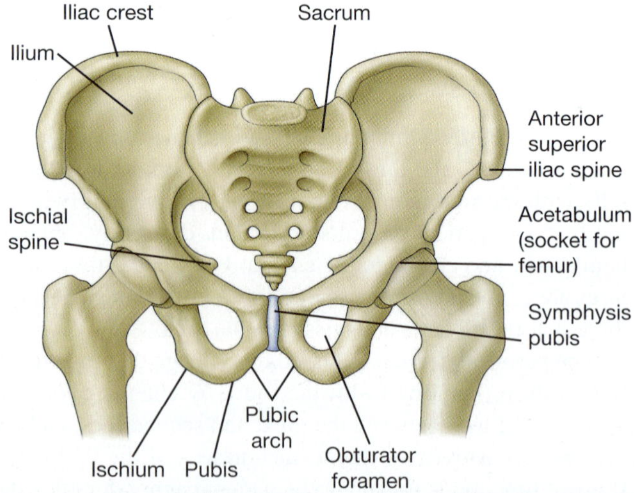

FIGURE 41-11 **Pelvic bones.**

and abdominal CT scanning to detect intra-abdominal hemorrhage and intrapelvis injuries. CT is the gold standard for evaluating pelvic trauma (100% sensitive and specific for pelvic fractures) (Clinical Overview, 2021c). Retrograde cystourethrogram can be performed to diagnose genitourinary injuries; if such injuries are suspected, it should be performed before inserting a Foley catheter.

Pearls for Practice

The risk of hemorrhagic shock from intrapelvic bleeding or associated abdominal injury is high with pelvic fractures; thus, the patient is handled gently to minimize further bleeding and shock. Manual compression of the pelvis should be avoided, and before moving the patient the nurse should know whether the pelvic fracture is classified as stable, which implies that turning or moving the patient will not cause further displacement of the pelvis, or unstable, in which case additional displacement of the pelvis can occur with turning or moving (Mondor, 2022). The use of log rolling patients with pelvic fractures has been questioned by authors who suggest that there is a risk of hemodynamic instability since movement of the pelvis may lead to clot disruption and further blood loss resulting in hypovolemic shock (Rodriques, 2017). The National Institute of Health and Care Excellence (2017) recommends not log rolling patients with suspected pelvic fractures before pelvic imaging if there is hemodynamic instability and an occult (hidden) penetrating injury is suspected. When log rolling is required, it is critical to assess for any evidence of hemodynamic instability (increasing pulse, RR, decreasing BP and MAP).

Injuries to the bladder, urethra, rectum, intestines, other abdominal organs, and pelvic vessels and nerves are associated with pelvic fracture. To assess for urinary tract injury, the patient's urine is examined for blood (hematuria) or blood at the introitus, or if the patient is a male, observed for scrotal hematoma. A urinary drainage catheter should not be inserted until the status of the urethra is known. Ecchymosis of the anterior abdominal wall, flank, or sacral or gluteal region is suggestive of significant internal bleeding. Diffuse and intense abdominal pain, hyperactive or absent bowel sounds, and abdominal rigidity and hyper-resonance or dullness to percussion suggest injury to the intestines or abdominal bleeding. The nurse is aware that the loss of dullness over the liver (normally percusses a dull sound) indicates the presence of free air and that dullness over regions normally tympanic may indicate the presence of blood or fluid.

If major vessels are lacerated, the bleeding may be stopped through emergent embolization using interventional radiology techniques prior to surgery. Patients with pelvic fractures can lose up to 6 L of blood and therefore are at risk for exsanguination. The nurse follows the Advances Trauma Life support (ATLS) guidelines, using the sequential C-ABCD (**C**atastrophic hemorrhage control, **A**irway, **B**reathing, **C**irculation, and **D**isability) to detect and manage potentially life-threatening injuries (see Chapters 53 [hemorrhagic shock] and 55). An emergency laparotomy may be required with pelvic fractures for abdominal injuries. For patients with ongoing hemorrhage and pelvic instability, the use of pelvic external fixation may be used since it provides stability to the pelvic ring. Once the patient is hemodynamically stable, treatment generally involves an ORIF repair. These measures promote hemostasis, hemodynamic stability, comfort, and early mobilization. Long-term complications of pelvic fractures include malunion, nonunion, residual gait disturbances, and back pain from ligament injury.

Acetabular Fractures

Acetabular fractures primarily occur in young adults as a result of high-velocity trauma (Hoge & Chauvin, 2022). Drivers and passengers sitting in the right front seat in motor vehicle crashes may forcibly propel their knees into the dashboard, injuring the knee–thigh–hip complex; the force exerted through the head of the femur extends into the acetabulum. The acetabulum (see Fig. 41-11) is particularly vulnerable to fracture with these types of injuries as well as falls from heights, and extreme sporting events. The initiation of mandatory seat belts has significantly decreased the incidence of acetabular fracture. Treatment depends on the pattern of fracture. Stable, nondisplaced fractures may be managed with traction and protective (toe-touch) weight bearing so that the affected foot is only placed on the floor for balance. Displaced and unstable acetabular fractures are treated with open reduction, percutaneous fixation, joint debridement, and internal fixation or arthroplasty (replacement of all or part of the joint surfaces). Internal fixation permits early non–weight-bearing ambulation and ROM exercise. Percutaneous fixation is useful in patients who are sicker or where extensive approaches are not suitable (Hoge & Chauvin, 2022). Complications seen with acetabular fractures include nerve palsy, AVN, heterotopic ossification, DVT, infection, and posttraumatic arthritis.

Femoral Shaft

Considerable force is required to break the shaft of the femur in adults since it is the longest and strongest bone in the body. Most femoral fractures are seen in young adults who have been involved in a motor vehicle crash, who have fallen from a high place, or who have received a gunshot wound. Older females with osteoporosis are also at risk for femur shaft fractures after ground-level falls (Denisiuk & Afsari, 2022). Frequently, these patients have associated multiple injuries and significant soft tissue damage.

The nurse assesses for the presence and location of the pain, edema, bruising, deformity, and instability. The patient presents with an enlarged, deformed, painful thigh and cannot move the hip or the knee. The fracture may be transverse, oblique, spiral, or comminuted. Frequently, the patient develops shock because the thigh alone can hold around 1,500 mL of blood, and losses to 3 L may be seen (Denisiuk & Afsari, 2022; Walsh, 2020). An expanding diameter of the thigh suggests continued bleeding. If the fracture is open, prompt administration of antibiotics and tetanus is imperative to reduce the risk of infection (Denisiuk & Afsari, 2022).

The fracture is immobilized so that additional soft tissue damage does not occur. In general, skeletal traction or splinting is used to immobilize fracture fragments until the patient is physiologically stable and ready for ORIF procedures.

Internal fixation usually is carried out within a few days after injury. Intramedullary locking nail devices are used for midshaft (diaphyseal) fractures. Depending on the supracondylar fracture pattern, intramedullary nailing or screw plate fixation may be used. Internal fixation permits early mobilization. A thigh cuff orthosis may be used for external support. To preserve muscle strength, the patient is instructed to perform active exercises of the upper and lower extremities on a regular basis. Active muscle movement enhances healing by increasing blood supply and electrical potentials at the fracture site. Prescribed weight-bearing limits are based on the type of fracture. Physical therapy includes ROM and strengthening exercises, safe use of ambulatory aids, and gait training. Functional ambulation stimulates fracture healing. Healing time is 4 to 6 months.

A common complication after fracture of the femoral shaft is restriction of knee motion. Active and passive knee exercises begin as soon as possible, depending on the management approach and the stability of the fracture and knee ligaments. Fat emboli syndrome is prevalent in the polytraumatized patient with femoral shaft fractures (see previous discussion) (Denisiuk & Afsari, 2022).

Femur

The terms hip fracture and neck of femur fracture are synonymous (Emmerson et al., 2022). Fracture of the proximal femur is termed a *hip fracture* and is classified as either intracapsular or extracapsular. Intracapsular fractures include femoral head and femoral neck fractures, while extracapsular fractures includes trochanteric, intertrochanteric, and subtrochanteric fractures (Fig. 41-12). Fractures of the neck of the femur may damage the vascular system that supplies blood to the head and the neck of the femur, and the bone may become ischemic. For this reason, AVN is common in patients with femoral neck fractures. Older people are particularly vulnerable to intertrochanteric fractures and generally have a much worse prognosis than do younger patients. It is important for the nurse to be aware that the mortality rate after hip fracture surgical repair is 2% to 4%, the mortality rate within 1 year in older patients is 20% to 30%, and that 58% of patients require long-term care in a nursing facility after this fracture, which results in loss of independence and

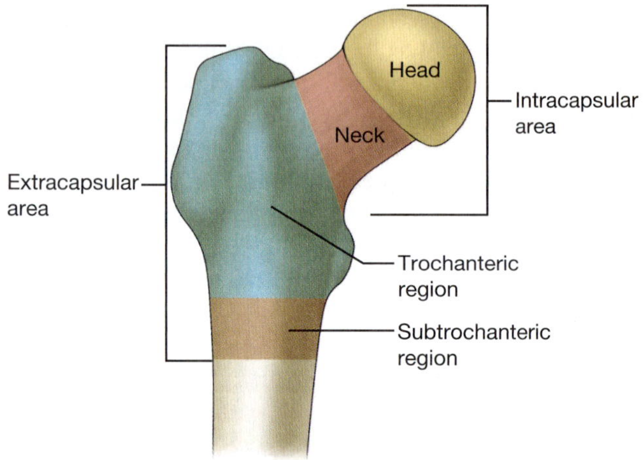

FIGURE 41-12 **Regions of the proximal femur.**

a significant economic burden on health care systems (Dove, 2023).

Clinical Manifestations and Assessment

With displaced fractures of the femoral neck, the leg is shortened, abducted, and rotated (Cerepani, 2020). The patient complains of pain in the hip and groin or knee. Nondisplaced fractures (e.g., stress fractures) will not be shortened or rotated, but the patient will complain of pain. With most fractures of the femoral neck, the patient cannot move the leg without a significant increase in pain. Impacted intracapsular femoral neck fractures cause moderate discomfort (even with movement), may allow the patient to bear weight, and may not demonstrate obvious shortening or rotational changes. With extracapsular femoral fractures of the trochanteric or subtrochanteric regions, the extremity is significantly shortened, externally rotated to a greater degree than in intracapsular fractures, exhibits muscle spasm that resists positioning of the extremity in a neutral position, and has an associated large hematoma or area of ecchymosis. The diagnosis of fractured hip is confirmed with an x-ray.

Gerontologic Considerations

Older people (particularly females) who have brittle bones from osteoporosis and who tend to fall frequently have a high incidence of hip fracture. Weak quadriceps muscles, general frailty due to age, and comorbidities that produce decreased cerebral arterial perfusion (transient ischemic attacks, anemia, emboli, cardiovascular disease, and medication effects) contribute to the incidence of falls. Comorbidities contribute to complications and increased length of stay for older hip fracture patients (Erickson, 2020).

Often, a fractured hip is a catastrophic event that has a negative impact on the patient's lifestyle and quality of life. Over 90% of hip fractures occur in people >65 years of age, with a mean age of 80 years (Dove, 2023). Because of the risk of DVT and PE with hip surgery, regional anesthesia is recommended since it reduces the risk for proximal DVT following total hip replacement. Without prophylaxis, the risk for DVT after hip surgery and knee reconstruction ranges from 45% to 70%, and clinically significant pulmonary embolism occurs in 20% of patients undergoing hip surgery (Schafer, 2020). In addition, the most frequent complication associated with hip fracture in elderly patients is postoperative delirium as a result of the stress of the trauma, unfamiliar surroundings, sleep deprivation, and medications. An incidence rate of 5.15% to 48.37% of postoperative delirium following hip fracture repair in older patients was seen in a recent research study (Kong et al., 2022). Preoperative predictors of postoperative delirium, which is defined as "disturbance of consciousness…with reduced ability to focus, sustain, or shift attention," include a history of delirium, estimated blood loss ≥ 400 mL, duration of surgery ≥ 120 minutes, preoperative albumin ≤ 40 g/L (<4 g/dL) and TSH ≤ 2 mU/L (since thyroid hormone is essential for maintaining the normal CNS functioning and is closely associated with mentation) (Kong et al., 2022; Robertson & Robertson, 2006, p. 2060).

Pearls for Practice

When a patient presents with a change in the level of consciousness, the nurse recalls the mnemonic DOG: Drugs are reviewed to evaluate whether a medication could be associated with the altered sensorium, Oxygen saturation level is assessed for hypoxemia via pulse oximeter, and a Glucose level is obtained via a finger stick to evaluate for hypoglycemia/hyperglycemia since all are associated with altered LOC.

To prevent complications, the nurse must assess the older patient for chronic pre-existing conditions as described above, including polypharmacy. Dehydration and poor nutrition may be present, contributing to hemoconcentration, and this predisposes the patient to the development of venous thromboemboli. Therefore, monitoring intake and output in older individuals and assessing for DVT are particularly important.

Muscle weakness and wasting, which may have initially contributed to the fall and fracture, will be further compromised by bed rest and immobility. The nurse encourages the patient to move all joints except the involved hip and knee. Strengthening of the arms and shoulders will facilitate walking with assistive devices. The nurse educates the older patient in fall reduction lifestyle changes (see Box 41-6). A plan of nursing care for an older patient with a fractured hip is available online at http://thepoint.lww.com/Honan3e.

BOX 41-6 Fall Reduction

Limiting alcohol consumption
Having vision assessed annually
Increasing physical activity as able
Considering balance training (tai chi is effective to reduce falls in people at low or moderate risk of falling) (Blain et al., 2020)
Walking if able, making sure to walk on a flat open surface
Choosing suitable walking shoes; wearing nonskid shoes, avoiding high heels or walking around the house in socks or slippers.
Maintaining healthy body weight
Increasing calcium and vitamin D via diet and/or supplements, if recommended by a provider
Quitting smoking
Using an assistive device, such as a walker, cane, etc., if needed
Clearing clutter in living spaces (removing obstacles such as newspapers, books, and electrical cords)
Picking up or securing scatter rugs or mats to avoid tripping
Having well-lit rooms and hallways
Keeping pets away from pathways
Using handrails when climbing stairs (may require installation of handrails and lighting)
Installing grab bars in the room or bathroom (next to and inside the tub, and next to the toilet)
Adjusting the bed height
Using hip protectors to prevent fall-related injuries
Using digital technology (including wearables) to detect, prevent, or manage falls
For additional resources see:

- Centers for Disease Control and Prevention, STEADI: www.cdc.gov
- Community-Based Fall Prevention Programs: www.cdc.gov
- National Institute on Aging: www.nia.nih.gov

Adapted from Erickson, K. L. B. (2020). Innovations in care of the elderly hip fracture patient; a nightmare no more. *Nursing Clinics of North America*, *55*(2), 149–161.

Medical Management

If surgery cannot be performed immediately, the fracture is immobilized so that additional soft tissue damage does not occur. Temporarily, traction can either be applied as skin or skeletal (pins or wires inserted into bones) traction. Each carries risks. Skin traction can put undue pressure on skin for prolonged periods of time and is limited in the amount of weight that can be applied (5 to 7 lb [2.3 to 3.2 kg] or less). Recent research revealed no significant difference with the application of skin traction versus no traction in pain relief, in reduction of the fracture displacement, or in healing rate, nor does it reduce the risk of pressure ulcers. As a result, it has limited use (Biz et al., 2019; Hill et al., 2019; Sammut et al., 2021). Higher weights risk damage to the skin and neurovascular status of the involved extremity.

Skeletal traction is used more frequently to immobilize fracture fragments until the patient is physiologically stable and ready for surgical treatment. However, skeletal traction can increase the risk of infection since sterile pin(s) are drilled or wires are placed into the bone. The weight for skeletal traction is determined by body size and the extent of the injury. With either choice, continued neurovascular monitoring and assessment of the skin is needed.

In addition, there are several types of traction. *Straight* or *running traction* applies the pulling force in a straight line with the body part resting on the bed. Buck's extension traction is an example of skin traction that is straight traction. It may be used for patients with fractures of the hip as a temporary measure to reduce muscle spasm and immobilize the extremity, but this must be balanced against the risk of complications such as pressure ulcers, discomfort, blisters, compartment syndrome, increased limitation of mobility, and thromboembolism (Hill et al., 2019; Sammut et al., 2021). Another type of traction is *balanced suspension traction* (see Fig. 41-15 on page 1356), in which the affected extremity "floats" or is suspended in the traction apparatus by the balanced weights. The line of traction on the extremity remains fairly constant despite patient movement as long as the pull remains constant.

Pearls for Practice

The nurse must never remove weights from skeletal traction unless an emergency situation occurs. Removal of the weights completely defeats their purpose and may result in injury to the patient.

The goal of surgical treatment of hip fractures is to obtain a satisfactory fixation so that the patient can be mobilized quickly and avoid secondary medical complications. Surgical intervention is carried out as soon as possible after injury; within 24 hours is associated with lower complication rates and lower 30-day mortality (Dove, 2023).

Surgical treatment consists of one of the following:

- Open or closed reduction of the fracture and internal fixation; a thigh cuff orthosis may be used for external support.
- Replacement of the femoral head with a prosthesis (**hemiarthroplasty**). This is usually reserved for fractures that cannot be satisfactorily reduced or securely nailed, for frail patients, or to avoid complications of nonunion and AVN of the head of the femur. It is similar to a total hip replacement but only replaces the ball portion of the hip joint, not the socket (which is replaced in total hip replacement [discussed later in the chapter]). THA may be performed in healthy, active patients (Dove, 2023).
- Closed reduction with percutaneous stabilization for an intracapsular fracture.

Nursing Management

The immediate postoperative care for a patient with a hip fracture is similar to that for other patients undergoing major surgery.

Encouraging Activity. The patient is encouraged to exercise as much as possible by means of the overbed trapeze. This device helps strengthen the arms and shoulders in preparation for protected ambulation (e.g., toe touch, partial weight bearing). A common complication after fracture of the femoral shaft is restriction of knee motion. In general, active and passive knee exercises begin as soon as possible, depending on the management approach and the stability of the fracture and knee ligaments. To preserve muscle strength, the patient is instructed to exercise the noninjured hip and the lower leg, foot, and toes on a regular basis. The surgeon prescribes the degree of weight bearing and the rate at which the patient can progress to full weight bearing. On the day of surgery or first postoperative day, generally, the patient transfers to a chair with assistance and begins assisted ambulation. The amount of weight bearing that can be permitted depends on the stability of the fracture reduction. In general, hip flexion and internal rotation restrictions apply *only* if the patient has had a hemiarthroplasty (replacement of the ball of the hip) or THA (replacement of both the femoral and acetabular components with an artificial prosthesis). Physical therapists work with the patient on ROM and strengthening exercises, safe use of ambulatory aids, and gait training. Functional ambulation stimulates fracture healing. The patient can anticipate discharge to home or to a rehabilitation facility with the use of an ambulatory aid. Some modifications in the home may be needed, such as installation of elevated toilet seats and grab bars (see Box 41-6).

Monitoring and Managing Potential Complications. Attention is given to pain management as well as prevention of secondary medical problems, such as hemorrhagic shock, atelectasis, pneumonia, DVT, heart failure, constipation, pressure ulcer development, bladder control problems, pain, AVN, and nonunion. Age, comorbidities, and immobility increase the risk for developing postoperative complications. Early mobilization of the patient is important so that independent functioning can be restored. Older people with hip fractures are particularly prone to complications that may require more vigorous treatment than the fracture. Frequently, the patient develops shock because blood loss into the tissues is common with these fractures. In addition, blood loss can be extensive during THA; blood can be salvaged through a cell saver for autotransfusion (Phillips & Hornacky, 2021b). Achievement of homeostasis after injury and after surgery is accomplished through careful monitoring of vital signs, wound drainage from dressings and external drains (drains are typically removed 24 to 48 hours after surgery), laboratory results, and physical assessment findings, as well as through collaborative management, including adjustment of therapeutic interventions as indicated. Refer back to Box 41-3 for signs and symptoms of hypovolemic shock.

Pearls for Practice

The use of drains in orthopedic surgery is the subject of debate since there is inconsistent data regarding the benefits of drain application. While drains remove accumulated blood to prevent hematomas and therefore decrease the risk of compartment syndrome, they also risk retrograde migration of bacteria from the skin around the wound and may increase the need for blood transfusions. Thus, many surgeons have reconsidered the need for drainage following total hip arthroplasty. However, if a drain is not used, a hematoma is a good culture medium for bacterial

growth and may hinder rehabilitation because of joint swelling. If drains are used, the nurse uses aseptic technique when measuring the drain output and understands they are removed as quickly as possible (24 to 48 hours).

Neurovascular complications may occur from direct injury to nerves and blood vessels or from increased tissue pressure. Assessment includes checking the neurovascular status of the extremity, especially circulatory perfusion of the lower leg and foot (popliteal, posterior tibial, and pedal pulses; toe capillary refill time; color; temperature; sensation and movement). A Doppler ultrasound device may be needed to assess blood flow. With hip fracture, bleeding into the tissues is expected. Excessive swelling may be observed and may further impair the neurovascular status. Patients may complain of increased pain at the site, and swelling may be noted in the thigh and buttock due to hematoma formation. Ice may be applied to decrease the swelling. The nurse marks the extent of drainage on the dressing by circling the extent and noting initials, date, and time. If excessive, the nurse should notify the provider.

DVT is a common postoperative complication contributing to significant morbidity and mortality in patients undergoing hip fracture surgery. To prevent DVT, the nurse encourages intake of fluids, and ankle and foot exercises. The nurse assesses the patient's legs for signs of DVT, which may include unilateral calf edema, tenderness, warmth, redness, a palpable cord, and Brancroft or Moses sign (pain with calf compression against the tibia) (Orient, 2019). Objective evidence is found in fewer than 50% of patients with these classic signs of DVT; therefore, the nurse maintains a high degree of suspicion for this complication (Patel, 2019). The symptoms are related to inflammatory processes; therefore, the nurse also assesses for low-grade fever, malaise, and elevated white blood cell (WBC) count and sedimentation rate (Norris & Tuan, 2020). The nurse administers the anticoagulant and mechanically based prophylaxis (e.g., sequential compression devices and prophylactic anticoagulant therapy) as prescribed.

Pulmonary complications, which commonly include atelectasis and pneumonia, are a threat to older patients undergoing hip surgery. Deep-breathing exercises, a change of position at least every 2 hours, and the use of an incentive spirometer hourly help prevent respiratory complications. The nurse assesses breath sounds at least every 4 hours to detect adventitious or diminished sounds. Oxygen saturation should be assessed; supplemental oxygen may be ordered to keep the level above 95%. Pain must be treated with analgesic agents; otherwise, the patient may not be able to readily cough, deep breathe, or engage in prescribed activities. Out-of-bed (OOB) activities will be beneficial for lung function as well as muscle strength.

Heart failure is a frequent cause of mortality in older patients with hip fracture. The cumulative effect of trauma, major surgery, and concurrent medical history place the patient at risk for heart failure. The nurse is alert for signs and symptoms associated with left-sided heart failure, including shortness of breath, cough, dyspnea on exertion (DOE), crackles, orthopnea, and paroxysmal nocturnal dyspnea. Right ventricular failure presents with peripheral edema (may be pitting), jugular vein distention, and abdominal distention. Edema will be in dependent areas, so the nurse assesses the sacral area and extremities. Bendopnea (shortness of breath within 30 seconds of bending over at the waist [due to fluid or pressure changes in the abdomen]) is also seen in heart failure. Accurate recording of intake and output (noting decreased urinary output), auscultation of heart (noting presence of S_3) and lung sounds (crackles), and monitoring O_2 saturation and vital signs (noting decreasing blood pressure, tachycardia, and tachypnea) are important nursing responsibilities. The nurse consults with the surgeon if signs and symptoms of excess fluid volume persist or worsen. The nurse expects fluid restriction and administers diuretics as ordered.

Skin breakdown is often seen in older patients with hip fracture. Postoperative dressings should be flexible (to allow early mobilization of the patient), balance permeability and absorbency, manage exudate, protect the wound, and allow gentle removal from aging or fragile skin, to reduce the rates of postoperative blistering (Pickles et al., 2022). Although the literature reveals modern dressings have better outcomes for blistering and patient satisfaction, there is a lack of evidence regarding the superiority of one dressing over any other (Rothfusz et al., 2021). However, for blister prevention, the use of paraffin-tulle gauze rather than a nonadherent primary dressing and the use of secondary compressive spica wraps rather than either perforated cloth or silk tape is suggested (Rothfusz et al., 2021). The nurse ensures that the patient is changing position at least every 2 hours. Proper skin care, especially on the heels, back, sacrum, and shoulders, as well as turning and frequent repositioning and supporting the legs with pillows and lifting the heels off the mattress all help to relieve pressure. Special mattress may provide protection by distributing pressure evenly.

Reduced GI motility, immobility, and the effects of anesthesia may result in constipation. Accurate assessment of intake and output, assessing bowel sounds, and noting distention of the abdomen are important nursing interventions, as prevention of constipation is the goal. A diet high in fiber and fluids may help stimulate gastric motility and since ambulation improves GI peristalsis, the nurse assists the patient in OOB activities and ambulation as prescribed. If constipation develops, therapeutic measures may include stool softeners, laxatives, suppositories, and enemas. To improve the patient's appetite, the nurse identifies and includes the patient's food preferences, as appropriate, within the prescribed therapeutic diet.

Loss of bladder control (incontinence or retention) may occur. In general, the routine use of an indwelling catheter is avoided because of the high risk for urinary tract infection (UTI). If a catheter is inserted at the time of surgery, it usually is removed on the morning of the first postoperative day. Because urinary retention is common after surgery, the nurse must assess the patient's voiding patterns and amounts, noting bladder distention and voiding of small amounts of urine (less than 100 mL) frequently. To ensure proper urinary tract function, the nurse monitors intake, via IV route and/or by mouth if allowed, and output. If no pre-existing cardiac disease (e.g., heart failure, coronary artery disease) exists, then liberal intake of fluids is encouraged. The patient is informed to notify the nurse if complaints of bladder fullness or inability to void are noted. A bladder scan can be performed by the nurse to evaluate postvoid residual, which should be less than 200 mL.

Infection is suspected if the patient complains of persistent, moderate discomfort in the hip, experiences chills or malaise, and has an elevated WBC count and ESR. The nurse observes the surgical incision for erythema, warmth, and tenderness and notes color, amount, and consistency of wound drainage. In older adults, symptoms of infection may be nonspecific (e.g., patients may be afebrile without complaints); an important marker is a decline in the patient's functional status and/or the presence of confusion. The closed-wound drainage system (if used) is observed for color and amount of drainage and functioning of the drainage device. Risk factors for reportable complications, wound complications, and readmission after total joint arthroscopy include dyslipidemia, hypertension, abnormal fasting glucose, and visceral obesity according to the Centers for Medicare & Medicaid Services (Li & Glassman, 2018).

Delayed complications of hip fractures include malunion, delayed union or nonunion, AVN of the femoral head (particularly with femoral neck fractures), and fixation device problems (e.g., protrusion of the fixation device through the acetabulum, loosening of hardware) (discussed earlier in this chapter). Healing time is 4 to 6 months.

Promoting Health. Osteoporosis screening of patients who have experienced hip fracture is important for prevention of future fractures (Box 41-7). Specific patient education is needed regarding dietary requirements, lifestyle changes, and weight-bearing exercise to promote bone health. Prevention of falls is also important and may be achieved through exercises to improve muscle tone, flexibility, and balance and through the elimination of environmental hazards such as throw rugs. Other environmental considerations are reviewed in Box 41-6.

BOX 41-7

Risk Factors for Osteoporosis

- Age
- Female >65 regardless of risk factors
- Ethnicity (White, Asian)
- Small bone structure
- Postmenopausal
- Sedentary lifestyle
- Chronic obstructive pulmonary disease
- Smoking
- Steroid use
- Family history
- Calcium deficiency
- Poor nutrition (lifelong low calcium intake, decreased protein intake)
- Excessive alcohol intake
- Excessive caffeine intake
- Malignancy
- Hyperthyroidism
- Hyperparathyroidism
- Rheumatoid arthritis
- Diabetes mellitus
- Cushing disease
- Gastrectomy
- Inflammatory bowel disease
- Malabsorption
- Multiple myeloma

TREATMENT MODALITIES

Cast

A **cast** is a rigid external immobilizing device whose purpose to immobilize and hold the fracture in proper alignment while minimizing the functional impairment of the limb (Sabeh et al., 2020). It is applied for a variety of medical-surgical disorders including fractures and deformities. Many injuries that were previously treated with casts may now be treated with other immobilization devices (e.g., immobilizers). In general, casts permit patient mobility while restricting movement of a body part. The cast provides adequate stability to the injured area and does not restrict circulation and nerve supply. In addition, it must be smooth and free of ridges to prevent pressure on underlying tissue.

Casting Materials

Casts may be made of plaster or nonplaster materials. Hybrid casts composed of plaster followed by another layer of fiberglass are an additional option that combines advantages of both materials (Sabeh et al., 2020). Refer to Box 41-8 for cast application.

Fiberglass

Nonplaster casts are generally referred to as fiberglass casts. These water-activated polyurethane materials are lightweight strong, water resistant, durable, more radiolucent, and porous, providing more ventilation than plaster casts. They are made of nonabsorbent fabric impregnated with lukewarm water-activated hardeners that bond and reach full rigid strength in minutes. After the cast is applied, the patient should remain immobile with the limb placed on a plastic-coated pillow for at least 20 minutes to avoid pressure and indentations and to allow the cast to set. A fiberglass cast dries in about an hour. The material does not soften when

BOX 41-8

GUIDELINES FOR NURSING CARE

Assisting with Cast Application

Equipment

Tubular stockinette, casting material as specified by the provider (plaster rolls/plaster splints); sink equipped with plaster trap or bucket of water, gloves, padding, sponge or felt padding (if necessary)

Implementation

NURSING ACTIONS	RATIONALE
1. Support extremity or body part to be casted.	1. Minimizes movement; maintains reduction and alignment; increases comfort.
2. Position and maintain body part to be casted in the position indicated by the provider during the casting procedure.	2. Facilitates casting; reduces incidence of complications (e.g., malunion, nonunion, contracture).
3. Drape the patient.	3. Avoids undue exposure; protects other body parts from contact with casting materials.
4. Wash and dry the body part to be casted.	4. Reduces incidence of skin breakdown.
5. Place knitted material (e.g., stockinette) over the body part to be casted. Stockinette should be 1 in longer than the final cast length both proximally and distally (Karim, 2020). • Apply the material in a smooth and nonconstrictive manner.	5. Protects skin from casting materials. Protects the skin from pressure; this extra material is needed to fold the stockinette before applying the last layer of cast material to ensure adequate padding (fiberglass has sharp edges and therefore a well-padded margin using stockinette flipped proximally and distally creates smooth, padded edge); protects skin from abrasion.
6. Wrap soft, nonwoven roll padding smoothly and evenly around the body part. Use additional padding around bony prominences to protect superficial nerves (e.g., head of fibula, olecranon process). A minimum of two layers is needed to ensure adequate padding (Karim, 2020).	6. Protects the skin from pressure of the cast. Protects the skin at bony prominences. Protects superficial nerves.
7. Apply plaster or nonplaster casting material evenly on body part. • Choose bandage of appropriate width. • Overlap preceding turn by half the width of the bandage. • Use continuous motion, maintaining constant contact with the body part. • Use additional casting material (splints) at joints and at points of anticipated cast stress.	7. Creates a smooth, solid, well-contoured cast. Facilitates smooth application. Creates a smooth, solid, immobilizing cast. Shapes the cast properly for adequate support. Strengthens the cast.
8. "Finish" cast: • Smooth the edges. • Trim and reshape with a cast knife or cutter.	8. Protects skin from abrasion. Allows full range of motion of adjacent joints.
9. Remove particles of casting materials from the skin.	9. Prevents particles from loosening and sliding underneath the cast.
10. Support the cast during hardening. • Handle hardening casts with the palms of your hands. • Support the cast on a firm, smooth surface. • Do not rest the cast on hard surfaces or on sharp edges. • Avoid pressure on the cast.	10. Casting materials begin to harden in minutes; maximum hardness of nonplaster cast occurs in minutes; maximum hardness of plaster cast occurs with drying (24–72 hours, depending on environment and thickness of cast). Avoids denting of cast and development of pressure areas.
11. Promote drying of cast. • Leave cast uncovered and exposed to air. • Turn patient every 2 hours, supporting the major joints. • Fans may be used to increase air flow and speed drying.	11. Facilitates drying.
12. Confirm that the fracture is appropriately reduced with biplanar radiographs once the cast has been applied.	12. X-rays are obtained to verify that the bone fragments are aligned correctly.
13. Document the distal neurovascular status before and after fracture reduction and cast application.	13. Determines the adequacy of peripheral tissue perfusion and nerve function.

wet, which allows for hydrotherapy when appropriate. When wet, casts can be air dried in the sun (if weather permits) or with a hair dryer on a cool setting; thorough drying is important to prevent skin breakdown.

Plaster

Traditional casts are made of rolls of plaster bandage that are wet in cool water and applied smoothly to the body. A crystallizing reaction occurs, and heat is given off (an exothermic reaction). The heat given off during this reaction can be uncomfortable, and the patient needs to be informed about the sensation of increasing warmth that generally dissipates after 15 minutes. In addition, the nurse explains that the cast needs to be exposed to air (i.e., uncovered) to allow maximum dissipation of the heat and facilitate drying. Depending on the type of plaster selected it may take 4 to 18 minutes for the plaster to set, and it can take 24 hours or more to dry thoroughly (Phillips & Hornacky, 2021a). Because the plaster cast remains wet and somewhat soft, the cast needs to remain uncovered until it is completely dry. A wet plaster cast appears dull and gray, sounds dull on percussion, feels damp, and smells musty. A dry plaster cast is white and shiny, resonant to percussion, firm, and odorless. Duration of immobilization in a cast will depend on the fracture pattern and age of the patient and is usually 4 to 8 weeks (Sabeh et al., 2020). Evidence of clinical or radiographic union is necessary before discontinuing a cast.

Pearls for Practice

The nurse ensures that all jewelry is removed from the injured limb that is to be casted since edema is expected in fractures.

Nursing Management

Monitoring and Managing Potential Complications

Compartment Syndrome

Compartment syndrome is caused by a significant injury that creates increased pressure within the fascia, which is the thick tissue connected to bones that separates groups of muscles from each other in the arms and legs. The separations are called compartments (Hussey, 2022a). There are three types of compartment syndromes: ACS, chronic compartment syndrome, and crush compartment syndrome. *ACS* involves a sudden and severe decrease in blood flow to the tissues distal to an area of injury that results in ischemic necrosis if prompt, decisive intervention does not occur. It is a potentially limb-threatening complication that occurs when increased pressure occurs within a limited space (e.g., cast, muscle compartment) that compresses the blood vessels and nerves within the area. The pressure within the confined space becomes so high that there is massive compromise to circulation and nerve transmission in the affected extremity. Permanent damage develops within a few hours if action is not taken. Typically, ACS will develop within 48 to 72 hours of injury (Holderread et al., 2023).

Chronic compartment syndrome is characterized by pain, aching, and tightness in a muscle or muscle group that has been subjected to inordinate stress or exercise and may be accompanied by edema. In this instance, muscle volume increases by as much as 20% within a short time, resulting in stretching of the fascia and inflammation. It usually affects young adult high-level athletes (e.g., marathon runners). Symptoms usually resolve within an hour of stopping the activity (Hussey, 2022a). *Crush compartment syndrome* is caused by massive external compression or crushing of a compartment; for instance, this may occur when a car jack fails, and a car falls on a mechanic. This type of massive injury results in systemic effects that include rhabdomyolysis (Box 41-9), which causes acute kidney injury and may eventually lead to multiple organ dysfunction syndrome (MODS), further discussed in Chapter 53.

A specific type of compartment syndrome in the arm is Volkmann contracture (discussed previously). It is frequently associated with supracondylar fractures of the humerus (refer to Fig. 41-7). The following discussion focuses on ACS.

Fascia is tough connective tissue that surrounds muscle groups, organs, nerves, blood vessels, bones, and internal structures. It does not expand readily. Therefore, if a compartment begins to swell, the pressure in the area rises, leading to venous obstruction, compromising circulation and nerve and motor function to the point at which the limb may need to be amputated (Fig. 41-13).

Risk factors for this complication include trauma from accidents, surgery, or crushing injuries, in which massive edema and bleeding is expected. Casts and tight bandages are also associated with this complication as the external devices increase the pressure within the injured area. In addition, it may be caused by any condition that increases the risk of bleeding or edema in a confined space, such as in patients with soft tissue injury, without fractures, who are on anticoagulants or have bleeding dyscrasias (e.g., prolonged malposition, burns, electrocutions, snake venom, stressful athletic activity, contusions, and infiltrations from intravenous [IV] sites). One third of all compartment syndrome cases occur in the absence of bony injury (Agius & Cole, 2021). Long bone fractures (one third of all cases are tibial diaphyseal fractures) and multitrauma patients are implicated in ACS; however, it can occur in other parts, such as the hand, foot, thigh, gluteal region, and abdomen (Hussey, 2022a). Further details on ACS of the abdomen are in Chapter 52.

It is essential to detect this complication early since irreversible nerve damage begins within 1 hour. Muscle necrosis, and other irreversible changes occur within 4 to 6 hours of ischemia (Holderread et al., 2023; Hussey, 2022a). There is loss of light touch sensation in the distribution of the nerve in the compartment (e.g., first web space for lower extremity may be an early finding, see Table 41-2); however, this may be difficult to assess because of altered mentation of patients (unresponsive, uncooperative patient [e.g., ETOH (ethyl alcohol and alcohol), overdose], or those with peripheral nerve deficits). Clinical

BOX 41-9

Focus on Pathophysiology

Rhabdomyolysis

A wide variety of etiologies are associated with rhabdomyolysis, including seizures, drug reactions (e.g., statins), extreme exercise, soft tissue infections, burns, malignant hyperthermia, extended lithotomy position and lateral decubitus positions, use of pneumatic antishock garments or tourniquet ischemia, compartment syndrome, toxins (alcohol, cocaine, heroin, amphetamines, ecstasy, phencyclidine, snakebite), and electrical and crush injuries. With trauma injuries, the nurse is alert for rhabdomyolysis, in which the crushing injury causes the breakdown of skeletal muscle, resulting in the release of muscle cell contents, including myoglobin (a protein released from muscle when injury occurs), creatine phosphokinase (CPK), phosphate, enzymes, and potassium, into the systemic circulation. Clinical symptoms of rhabdomyolysis can be nonspecific: fever, malaise, nausea and vomiting, and tachycardia; more overt symptoms include muscle pain and aches (e.g., myalgia), weakness and swelling of the involved muscle, dark "tea-colored" urine (e.g., myoglobinuria), electrolyte abnormalities (e.g., hyperkalemia, hypophosphatemia, hypocalcemia), metabolic acidosis, elevated serum creatine kinase (CK), and myoglobinuria (Makic, 2019, p. 1282). Myoglobin, which gives skeletal muscle its color, is released from the damaged muscle and filtered by the kidney, resulting in brown- or tea-colored urine. Myoglobinuria does not occur in the absence of rhabdomyolysis; therefore, when present, it is the best marker and diagnostic cornerstone of rhabdomyolysis. However, it may not always be detected (Clinical Overview, 2021d). Urine dipstick for blood may be positive because of the cross-reaction with myoglobin; however, microscopic examination of urine may reveal no red blood cells. The myoglobin is a large molecule that gets lodged in the glomerulus, threatening kidney function due to renal tubular obstruction and direct toxic effects and resulting in acute kidney injury (AKI). In fact, it is the most common complication of rhabdomyolysis, occurring in up to 67% of all cases, regardless of cause (O'Connor & Deuster, 2020; Stanley et al., 2022). The CPK typically begins to rise within 2–12 hours after the injury, peaks within 1–5 days, and declines after 3–5 days in the absence of muscle injury. In general, the CPK is in excess of five times the normal serum level. Anion gap metabolic acidosis may be present due to the release of organic acids from damaged muscle (O'Connor & Deuster, 2020). Goals of management are to prevent acute kidney injury by countering the effects of myoglobin with the use of early and aggressive fluid resuscitation (reduces the accumulation of toxic intracellular contents); up to 30 mL/kg with isotonic saline is typically prescribed and titrated until the serum CPK reaches normal levels (Makic, 2019). The fluid resuscitation goals aim to achieve a urinary output of 2 mL/kg/hr. Bicarbonate administration may be used in specific situations such as when patients have severe rhabdomyolysis with CPK levels above 5,000 units/L or clinical evidence of severe muscle injury such as crush injury (urine that is alkalized lessens myoglobin toxicity). In addition, management of hyperkalemia with insulin/dextrose is expected. The nurse assesses urine output hourly, monitors vital signs, maintains strict intake and output, and assesses for fluid volume deficit (secondary to the trauma) versus fluid volume excess (secondary to overhydration). The ECG is monitored since hyperkalemia is associated with peaked T waves, bradycardia, and arrhythmias (Makic, 2019). The nurse monitors for compartment syndrome in all patients admitted with this diagnosis; it is a well-described late complication as well as a potential cause of rhabdomyolysis (O'Connor & Deuster, 2020).

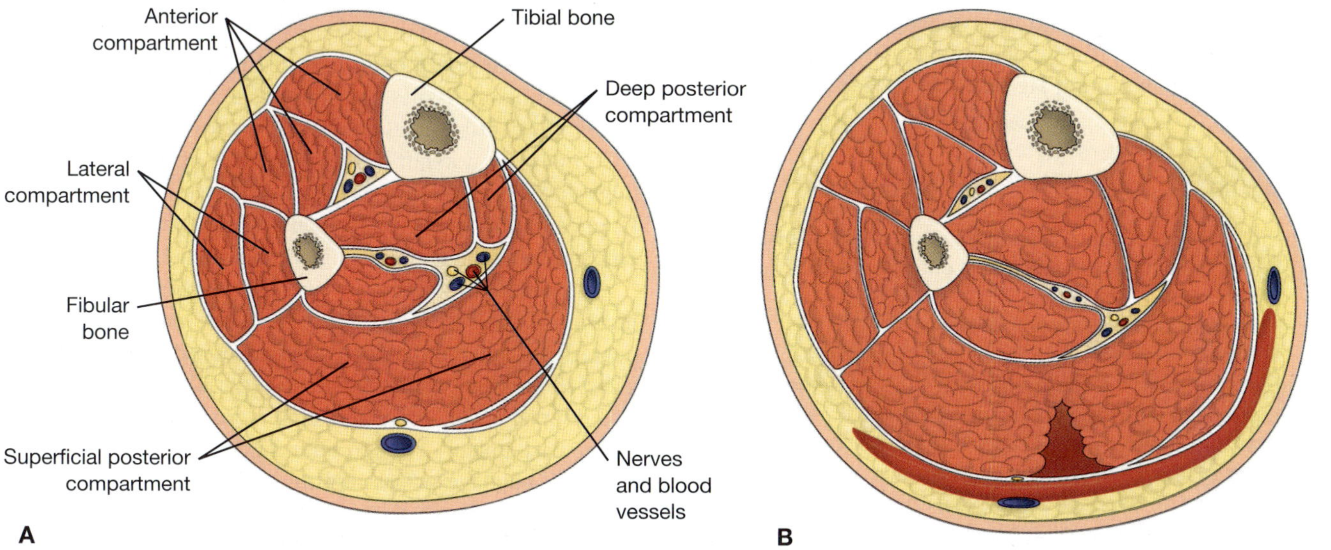

FIGURE 41-13 **A. Cross-section of normal lower leg with muscle compartments. B. Cross-section of lower leg with compartment syndrome. Swelling of muscles causes compression of nerves and blood vessels.**

manifestations include paleness of limb, cool skin temperature, delayed capillary refill, weak pulsations, paresthesia (tingling/burning sensation in the involved muscle), decreased sensation and mobility, tight and full muscle, and pain (progressive—not relieved by position changes, ice, or analgesia, or pain that is disproportional to the injury). A hallmark sign is pain that occurs or intensifies with passive ROM. Ominous ***late*** signs are pallor and loss of pulses. The nurse should measure and monitor the circumference of the affected area (abdomen, limb, etc.) to assess for edema, loosen bandages or castings that are too tight, and if concerned about neurovascular impairment, notify the provider immediately.

Pearls for Practice

It is important to note that late signs of compartment syndrome are pulselessness and pallor. The presence of a pulse does not rule out compartment syndrome. Rather, the nurse recognizes that pain that occurs or intensifies with passive ROM and is disproportional to the injury may be the earliest sign of ACS (Holderread et al., 2023).

If the complication is secondary to a tight bandage or cast, the nurse anticipates that the bandage will be loosened or removed and the cast bivalved (cut in half longitudinally) to release the constriction. While the surgeon is bivalving the cast, the nurse assists in maintaining limb alignment (Box 41-10). The affected limb must be elevated no higher than heart level to ensure arterial perfusion. Intracompartmental pressure monitoring may be required to diagnose compartment syndrome. A variety of commercial systems are available for the provider to measure intracompartmental pressure. A newer technique of monitoring pressures is called near-infrared spectroscopy. This is a noninvasive system that provides continuous monitoring of tissue oxygenation of the affected area (Hussey, 2022a). It uses absorption of light in near-infrared spectrum that corresponds to oxygenated and deoxygenated hemoglobin. The intracompartmental pressure of a normal muscle compartment at rest is less than 10 mm Hg (Hussey, 2022a). A high tissue pressure indicates compartment syndrome. Debate exists on the intracompartmental pressure that mandates fasciotomy, but pressures exceeding 30 mm Hg suggest the need to consider a fasciotomy (Hussey, 2022a). Another reliable method of assessment for ACS is *perfusion pressure* or ΔP of the limb, which is calculated as:

$$\Delta P = \text{diastolic blood pressure} - \text{intracompartmental pressure}$$

A perfusion pressure of less than 30 mm Hg is considered a criterion for fasciotomy (Agius & Cole, 2021).

If pressure is not relieved by removing the bandage or cast, and circulation is not restored, a **fasciotomy** may be necessary to relieve the pressure within the muscle compartment. A fasciotomy is a surgical procedure in which the skin, subcutaneous tissue, and affected compartment's fascia are opened, allowing the pressure to be relieved; the muscle is able to expand and circulation restored. Patients who develop this complication unrelated to a cast or dressing undergo this sterile procedure. The fasciotomy area may be surgically repaired, or wound VAC or graft tissue may be used when the swelling subsides. Complications that may occur after fasciotomy include AVN and infection.

The nurse closely monitors the patient's response to conservative and surgical management of compartment syndrome. Limb assessment of circulation, sensation, and mobility continues as ordered, and the nurse promptly reports changes to the provider.

BOX 41-10 Procedure for Bivalving a Cast

The following procedure is followed when a cast is bivalved.

1. With a cast cutter, a longitudinal cut is made to divide the cast in half.
2. The under padding is cut with scissors.
3. The cast is spread apart with cast spreaders to relieve pressure and to inspect and treat the skin without interrupting the reduction and alignment of the bone.
4. After the pressure is relieved, the anterior and posterior parts of the cast are secured together with an elastic compression bandage to maintain immobilization.
5. To control swelling and promote circulation, the extremity is elevated (but no higher than heart level) to minimize the effect of gravity on perfusion of the tissues.

Pearls for Practice

If ACS is suspected, the injured extremity should not be elevated above the right atrium to decrease edema, as this action will increase the intracompartmental pressure and reduce blood flow to the extremity (Hussey, 2022a). Instead, the extremity should be maintained at heart level (Hussey, 2022a).

Pressure Ulcers

Pressure ulcers are breakdowns in the skin caused by prolonged pressure on a body part. Casts or bandages can put pressure on soft tissues, causing tissue anoxia and pressure ulcers. Susceptible sites in the lower extremity include the heel, malleoli, dorsum of the foot, head of the fibula, tibial tuberosity, and anterior surface of the patella (Fig. 41-14). Upper extremity sites are located at the medial and or lateral epicondyle of the humerus, olecranon, and ulnar styloid.

The pathophysiology of and risk factors for pressure ulcers are discussed in Chapter 51. The nurse has a high degree of suspicion that a pressure ulcer is developing under a cast or dressing when the patient reports pain and tightness in a defined casted area. The area is inspected for drainage on the cast and any emitted odor. In addition, the nurse palpates the bandage or cast noting increasing warmth, which suggests underlying tissue erythema. Even if discomfort does not occur, there may be extensive loss of tissue with skin breakdown and tissue necrosis; therefore, any suspicious findings are reported to the provider.

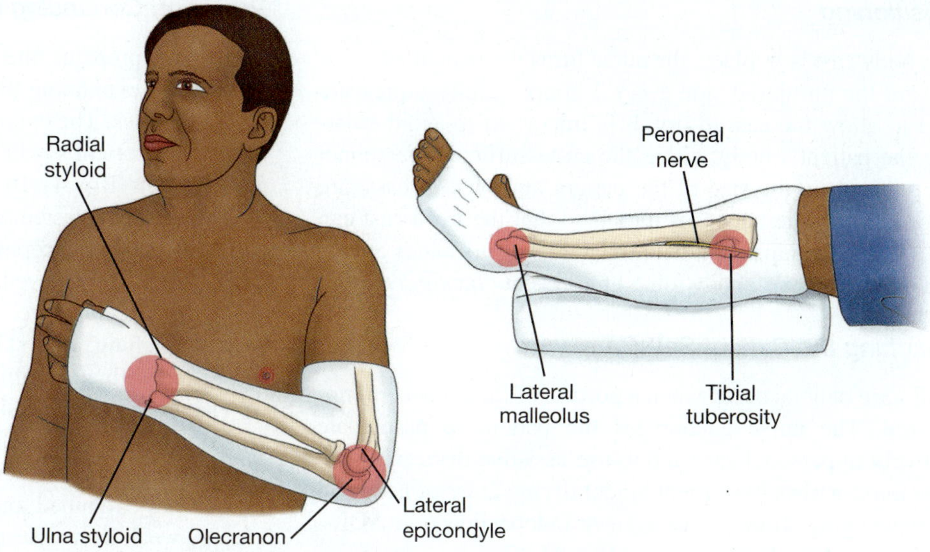

FIGURE 41-14 **Pressure areas in common types of casts.** ***Left,*** **long arm cast.** ***Right,*** **short leg cast.**

The cast may be bivalved or an opening (window) cut in the cast in order to assess for pressure ulcer development. A window allows inspection of the affected area and possibly treatment. The portion of the cast is replaced and held in place by an elastic compression dressing or tape. The nurse assesses for "window edema"—that is, swelling of the underlying tissue through the window, which creates pressure areas around the window margins. Patients who have histories of impaired sensation due to neuropathy or neurologic injury are at high risk for ulcer development; thus, removable braces may be used for management of fractures with frequent skin assessments.

Disuse Syndrome

When a muscle is left inactive, it loses its strength and size. A patient loses 5% muscle strength for every day spent in bed (Meehn et al., 2019). Disuse syndrome is muscular deconditioning and atrophy resulting from inactivity or immobilization; often referred to by the adage, "use it before you lose it." Depending on the status of the patient and length of time since the initial trauma, strengthening exercises may be ordered. The nurse recognizes that approximately 50% of patients who fractured their hip will recover their prefracture function while the remainder experience ongoing limitations in mobility, ADLs, and quality of life (Meehn et al., 2019). The nurse will teach the patient to tense or contract muscles (isometric muscle contraction) without moving the underlying bone. The internal or external devices stabilize the underlying bone. Isometric activity, such as teaching a patient in an arm cast to "make a fist," helps reduce muscle atrophy and maintain muscle strength. Muscle-setting exercises (e.g., quadriceps-setting and gluteal-setting exercises) are important in maintaining muscles essential for walking (Box 41-11). Isometric exercises should be performed hourly while the patient is awake. The physical therapist can assist in developing an exercise regimen for the patient.

Providing Initial Patient Teaching

The nurse teaches the patient and family that the casted extremity must be uncovered until it is completely dry and supported on pillows to the level of the heart to control swelling; ice packs should be applied as prescribed over the fracture site for 1 or 2 days. The patient is taught to elevate the casted arm or leg when seated to promote venous return and control swelling, unless ACS is suspected, where the extremity is at the level of the heart. The patient needs to understand that the body part will be immobilized after casting.

BOX 41-11 Muscle-Setting Exercises

Isometric contractions of the muscle maintain muscle mass and strength and prevent atrophy.

Quadriceps-Setting Exercise

- Position the patient supine with the leg extended.
- Instruct the patient to push their knee back onto the mattress by contracting the anterior thigh muscles.
- Encourage the patient to hold the position for 5–10 seconds.
- Let the patient relax.
- Have the patient repeat the exercise 10 times each hour when awake.

Gluteal-Setting Exercise

- Position the patient supine with legs extended, if possible.
- Instruct the patient to contract the muscles of the buttocks.
- Encourage the patient to hold the contraction for 5–10 seconds.
- Let the patient relax.
- Have the patient repeat the exercise 10 times each hour when awake.

Positioning

If a body cast is in place, the nurse turns the patient as a unit toward the uninjured side every 2 hours to relieve pressure and to allow the cast to dry. It is important to avoid twisting the patient's body within the cast. Sufficient personnel (depending on the size of the patient and type of cast) are needed when the patient is turned so that the fresh cast can be adequately supported with the palms of the hands at vulnerable points (i.e., body joints) to prevent cracking.

Teaching the Patient Self-Care

Self-care deficits occur when a portion of the body is immobilized. The nurse encourages the patient to participate actively in personal care and to use assistive devices safely. The nurse assists the patient in identifying areas of need and in developing strategies to achieve independence in ADLs. Patient teaching is discussed in Box 41-12.

BOX 41-12 **Patient Education**

Cast Care

- Move about as normally as possible, but avoid excessive use of the injured extremity, and avoid walking on wet, slippery floors or sidewalks.
- If the cast is on an upper extremity, a sling may be used when you ambulate. To prevent pressure on the cervical spinal nerves, the sling should distribute the supported weight over a large area and not on the back of the neck. Remove the arm from the sling and elevate it frequently.
- Perform prescribed exercises regularly and, as prescribed.
- Elevate the casted extremity to heart level frequently to prevent swelling. For example: when lying down, elevate the arm so that each joint is positioned higher than the preceding proximal joint (e.g., elbow higher than the shoulder, hand higher than the elbow).
- Do not attempt to scratch the skin under the cast. This may cause a break in the skin and result in the formation of a skin ulcer. Cool air from a hair dryer may alleviate an itch. Do not insert objects, such as coat hangers, inside the cast to scratch itching skin. If itching persists, contact your provider.
- Cushion rough edges of the cast with tape.
- Keep the cast dry, but do not cover it with plastic or rubber because this causes condensation, which dampens the cast and skin. Moisture softens a plaster cast (a wet fiberglass cast must be dried thoroughly with a hair dryer on a cool setting to avoid skin burns).
- Report any of the following to the provider: persistent pain; swelling that does not respond to elevation; changes in sensation; decreased ability to move exposed fingers or toes; changes in capillary refill, skin color, and temperature.
- Note odors around the cast, stained areas, warm spots, and pressure areas. Report them to the provider.
- Report a broken cast to the provider; do not attempt to fix it yourself.

Providing Continuing Care

The nurse prepares the patient for cast removal or cast changes by explaining that the cast is cut with a cast cutter, which vibrates. The cutter does not penetrate deeply enough to hurt the patient's skin. The cast padding is cut with scissors. Refer to Box 41-13.

The formerly casted body part is weak from disuse, stiff, and may appear atrophied. Therefore, support is needed when the cast is removed. The skin, which is usually dry and scaly from accumulated dead skin, is vulnerable to injury from scratching. The skin needs to be washed gently and lubricated with an emollient lotion.

The nurse and physical therapist teach the patient to resume activities gradually within the prescribed therapeutic regimen. Exercises prescribed to help the patient regain joint motion are explained and demonstrated. Because the muscles are weak from disuse, the body part that has been casted cannot withstand normal stresses immediately. In addition, the nurse teaches the patient with noticeable swelling of the affected extremity after cast removal to continue to elevate the extremity to control swelling until normal muscle tone and use are reestablished.

SKIN TRACTION

Skin traction may be used to control muscle spasms and to immobilize an area before surgery. Skin traction is accomplished by using a weight to pull on traction tape or on a foam boot attached to the skin. The amount of weight applied must not exceed the tolerance of the skin. Adhesive tape and weights greater than 7 lb are avoided as they may cause avulsion of the superficial skin layers. Contraindications to skin traction include patients with varicose veins, neurovascular disorders, fragile skin, and diabetes (Biz et al., 2019).

Buck's Extension Traction

Buck's extension traction (unilateral or bilateral) is skin traction to the lower leg. The pull is exerted in one plane when partial or temporary immobilization is desired. In general, this form of traction is used to immobilize fractures of the proximal femur before surgical fixation or when only a light traction weight is necessary.

Before the traction is applied, the nurse inspects the skin for abrasions and circulatory disturbances. The skin and circulation must be in healthy condition to tolerate the traction. The extremity should be clean and dry before the foam boot or traction tape is applied.

To apply Buck's traction, one nurse elevates and supports the extremity under the patient's heel and knee while another nurse places the foam boot under the leg, with the patient's heel in the heel of the boot. Next, the nurse secures Velcro straps around the leg. Traction tape overwrapped

BOX 41-13

GUIDELINES FOR NURSING CARE

Removing a Cast

Equipment

Cast scissors, cast saw, and cast spreader (if necessary); eye protection, Ace wraps, splints as indicated, adhesive tape (optional)

Implementation

NURSING ACTIONS	RATIONALE
1. Inform the patient about the procedure.	1. Facilitates cooperation and reduces fear about the procedure.
2. Reassure the patient that the electric saw or cast cutter will not cut the skin. (Explain that the blade oscillates to cut the cast and vibrations will be felt.)	2. Reduces anxiety.
3. Wear eye protection (patient and operator of the cast cutter).	3. Protects eyes from flying cast particles.
4. Bivalve the cast using a series of alternating pressures and linear movements of the blade along the line to be cut.	4. Cuts cast in halves; avoids burning sensation from prolonged contact of oscillating blade with padding.
5. Cut the padding with scissors.	5. Releases all of the casting materials.
6. Support the body part as it is removed from the cast.	6. Reduces stresses on body part that has been immobilized.
7. Gently wash and dry the area that has been immobilized.[a] Apply emollient lotion.	7. Removes dead skin that has accumulated during immobilization; keeps skin supple.
8. Teach the patient to avoid rubbing and scratching skin.	8. Prevents skin breakdown.
9. Collaborate with the physical therapist to teach the patient to resume active use of the affected body part gradually within the guidelines of the prescribed therapeutic regimen.	9. Protects weakened body part from excessive stress; progressive exercises reduce stiffness and restore muscle strength and function.
10. Teach the patient to control swelling by elevating the extremity or using an elastic bandage if prescribed.	10. Facilitates circulation (i.e., venous return) and controls fluid pooling.

[a]If a new cast is to be applied, follow guidelines for application of a cast and associated nursing care.

with elastic bandage in a spiral fashion may be used instead of the boot. Excessive pressure is avoided over the malleolus and proximal fibula during application to prevent pressure ulcers and nerve damage. The nurse then passes the rope affixed to the spreader or footplate over a pulley fastened to the end of the bed and attaches the weight—usually 5 lb—to the rope.

Pearls for Practice

The nurse must check nonadhesive traction frequently because it tends to slip when the traction weight is applied. Assessment of pressure on the fibula is essential because of the risk of nerve impingement; the peroneal nerve passes around the neck of the fibula just below the knee. Assess for inability to dorsiflex the foot and toes, a foot drop, or sensation in the web between the great toe and second toe.

Skin breakdown, the development of blisters, nerve pressure, and circulatory impairment are complications that may develop as a result of skin traction. Skin breakdown results from irritation caused by contact of the skin with the tape or foam and shearing forces. Older adults are at greater risk for this complication because of their sensitive, fragile skin.

Pearls for Practice

The nurse must promptly investigate every report of discomfort expressed by the patient in traction.

Circulatory impairment is manifested by cold skin temperature, decreased peripheral pulses, slow capillary refill time, and bluish skin. DVT, a serious circulatory impairment, may be manifested by unilateral calf tenderness, warmth, redness, and swelling (see Chapter 17).

SKELETAL TRACTION

The goals of skeletal traction are to maintain alignment of the injured limb and counteract the shortening of the injured limb from muscle spasm before definitive treatment can occur. Skeletal traction is applied directly to the bone. This method of traction is used occasionally to treat fractures of the femur, the tibia, and the cervical spine. The traction is applied directly to the bone by use of a metal pin or wire (e.g., Steinmann or Denham pin or Kirschner wire [K-wire]), which is inserted through the bone distal to the fracture, avoiding nerves, blood vessels, muscles, tendons, and joints. Tongs applied to the head are fixed to the skull to apply traction that immobilizes cervical fractures.

After local anesthesia and skin preparation by the surgeon, using surgical asepsis, a small skin incision is made, and sterile pin(s) are drilled or wire is placed through the bone. The patient feels pressure during this procedure and possibly some pain when the periosteum is penetrated.

After insertion, the pin or wire is attached to the traction bow or caliper. The ends of the pin or wire are covered with corks or tape to prevent injury to the patient or caregivers. The weights are attached to the pin or wire bow by a rope-and-pulley system that exerts the appropriate amount and direction of pull for effective traction. Skeletal traction frequently uses 7 to 11 kg (15 to 24 lb) to overcome muscle tension, restoring the femoral length and reducing muscle spasm (Hill et al., 2019). The nurse is aware that the weights applied initially must overcome the spasms of the affected muscles that pull on the fractured bones and shorten the limb. The nurse routinely checks the patient's neurovascular status, including skin color, pulse, capillary refill, temperature, mobility, and sensation. Changes from baseline or normal value are reported to the surgeon.

Often, skeletal traction is balanced traction, which supports the affected extremity, allows for some patient movement, and facilitates patient independence and nursing care while maintaining effective traction. The Thomas splint with a Pearson attachment (Fig. 41-15) is frequently used with skeletal traction for fractures of the femur. Because upward traction is required, an overbed frame is used.

When skeletal traction is discontinued, the extremity is gently supported while the weights are removed. The pin is cut close to the skin and removed by the physician. Then internal fixation, casts, or splints are used to immobilize and support the healing bone.

External fixators are often used to maintain position of unstable fractures when the use of a cast is prohibited, or the patient's condition is unstable and precludes a surgical procedure to stabilize the fracture. They can also be used to manage open fractures with soft tissue damage or severe comminuted (crushed or splintered) fractures while permitting active treatment of damaged soft tissues. Complicated fractures of the humerus, forearm, femur, tibia, and pelvis are often managed with external skeletal fixators. The fracture is reduced, aligned, and immobilized by a series of pins or screws inserted directly into the bone above and below the fracture and secured with the use of a metal frame. Pin position is maintained through attachment to a portable frame. The fixator facilitates patient comfort, early mobility, and active exercise of adjacent uninvolved joints; thus, complications due to disuse and immobility are minimized.

Pearls for Practice

The nurse never adjusts the clamps on the external fixator frame. It is the surgeon's responsibility to do so.

Nursing Management

Maintaining Effective Traction

When skeletal traction is used, the nurse checks the traction apparatus at least once per shift to see that the ropes are in the wheel grooves of the pulleys, the ropes are not frayed, the weights hang freely, the skeletal pins are secure, the correct weight is in place, and the knots in the rope are tied securely. The nurse also evaluates the patient's position because slipping down in bed results in ineffective traction.

Maintaining Positioning

The nurse must maintain alignment of the patient's body in traction as prescribed to promote an effective line of pull. The nurse positions the patient's foot to avoid footdrop (plantar flexion), inward rotation (inversion), and outward rotation (eversion). The patient's foot may be supported in a neutral position by orthopedic devices (e.g., foot supports).

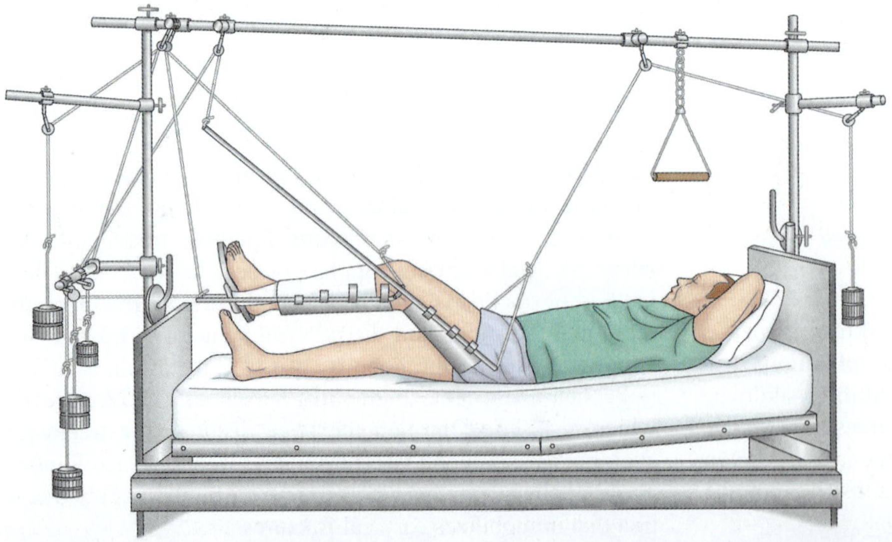

FIGURE 41-15 Balanced suspension skeletal traction with Thomas leg splint. The patient can move vertically as long as the resultant line of pull is maintained.

Preventing Skin Breakdown

The patient's elbows frequently become sore, and nerve injury may occur if the patient repositions by pushing on the elbows. In addition, patients frequently push on the heel of the unaffected leg and elbows when they raise themselves in bed. Therefore, the nurse should protect the elbows and heels and inspect them for pressure ulcers. A trapeze should be suspended above the patient, to encourage movement without using the elbows or heels. Areas that are particularly vulnerable to pressure caused by a traction apparatus applied to the lower extremity include the ischial tuberosity, popliteal space, Achilles tendon, and heel. If the patient is not permitted to turn on one side or the other, the nurse must make a special effort to provide back care and to keep the bed dry and free of crumbs and wrinkles. The patient can assist by holding the overhead trapeze and raising the hips off the bed. If the patient cannot do this, the nurse can push down on the mattress with one hand to relieve pressure on the back and bony prominences and to provide for some shifting of weight. A pressure-relieving air-filled or high-density foam mattress overlay may reduce the risk of pressure ulcers.

For change of bed linens (top to bottom rather than side to side), the patient raises the torso while nurses on both sides of the bed roll down and replace the upper mattress sheet. Then, as the patient raises the buttocks off the mattress, the nurses slide the sheets under the buttocks. Finally, the nurses replace the lower section of the bed linens while the patient rests on the back. Sheets and blankets are placed over the patient in such a way that the traction is not disrupted.

Providing Pin-Site Care

The wound at the pin insertion site requires attention. The goal is to avoid infection and development of **osteomyelitis** (Box 41-14). Osteomyelitis is an acute or chronic inflammation of the bone caused by infection. There is wide variability on pin care, and research on outcomes is scarce; thus, further studies are warranted. There are several possible cleansing solutions identified in the literature, including soap and water, normal saline, chlorhexidine, povidone-iodine solution, and half strength hydrogen peroxide. Several possible dressing protocols include daily cleansing, weekly cleansing, removal or retention of crust, use of a dressing or no dressing, and type of dressing material used. Therefore, the nurse follows their facility's specific policy and procedure pertaining to skeletal pin care (Campbell & Watt, 2020; Shields et al., 2022). General rules include:

- Pins located in areas with considerable soft tissue should be considered at greatest risk for infection.
- Strict handwashing should always take place before and after skeletal pin-site care.
- Patients and families should be taught pin care before discharge. They should be required to demonstrate the prescribed care and provided with written instructions that include signs and symptoms of infection.

BOX 41-14 **Focus on Pathophysiology**

Osteomyelitis

Osteomyelitis is an infection in the bone caused by a variety of microorganisms, most commonly *Staphylococcus aureus*, that are introduced during injury, from the bloodstream, through direct inoculation (chronic infection of skin/soft tissue), or during surgery. Once in the bone, the microorganisms proliferate and spread within the bone shaft, causing an inflammatory response that further destroys the bone. Wound cultures identify the organism and antibiotic sensitivity. Risk factors include diabetes, prosthetic joints, and older age. Difficult to treat, osteomyelitis requires IV therapy, in general, for 6 weeks. Osteomyelitis may be classified as acute (an infection lasting less than 4 weeks that typically develops within 2 weeks of infection) or chronic (more than 4 weeks). Dull pain over the affected bone is the dominant finding in osteomyelitis. Palpation of the involved bone usually elicits tenderness over the infected area. In acute osteomyelitis, increased warmth, erythema, and swelling at the affected segment are typically present, whereas in chronic osteomyelitis, symptoms are often nonspecific. However, pain, swelling, and erythema at the infection site may be seen. The nurse considers osteomyelitis in a chronic poorly healing wound (especially in patients with diabetes) and assesses for the presence of a sinus tract from intact skin. The C-reactive protein level is typically elevated (rising within hours of infection) and typically returns to baseline within 1 week after adequate treatment (therefore this test may be useful to monitor response to therapy) (Clinical Overview, 2022). The erythrocyte sedimentation rate or ESR is also commonly elevated, and elevated WBC levels may be seen in acute infections (but is not reliable). The WBC count may be normal in chronic osteomyelitis.

The nurse must inspect the pin sites daily for reaction (i.e., normal changes that occur at the pin site after insertion) and infection. Signs of reaction may include redness, warmth, and serous or slightly sanguinous drainage at the site. These signs are expected to subside after 72 hours. Signs of infection may mirror those of reaction but also include the presence of edema, purulent drainage, erythema, excessive warmth, tenderness, pin loosening, and odor. In addition, the nurse monitors the patient for fever. Minor infections may be readily treated with antibiotics, whereas infections that result in systemic manifestations may additionally warrant pin removal until the infection resolves. When pins are mechanically stable (after 48 to 72 hours), weekly pin site care may be recommended. Crusting may occur at the pin site, and uncertainties currently exist about whether scabs around the pin sites should be removed. Additional research is needed to determine best practice to prevent infection with external fixators. The nurse follows institutional protocol and teaches the patient and family to perform pin-site care prior to discharge from the hospital. Written follow-up instructions that include the signs and symptoms of infection should be provided.

JOINT REPLACEMENT SURGERY

Joint surgery is one of the most frequently performed orthopedic surgeries. Joint disease, disability, or deformity may necessitate surgical intervention to relieve pain, improve stability, and improve function. Conditions contributing to joint degeneration include osteoarthritis (degenerative joint disease), rheumatoid arthritis, trauma, and congenital deformity. As noted previously, some fractures (e.g., femoral neck fracture) may cause disruption of the blood supply and subsequent AVN, and a **joint replacement** may be elected over an ORIF. Joints frequently replaced include the shoulder, hip, knee (Fig. 41-16), and finger joints. Less frequently, more complex joints (elbow, wrist, or ankle) are replaced.

Timing of these procedures is important to ensure maximum function. Surgery should be performed before surrounding muscles become contracted and atrophied and serious structural abnormalities occur. The surgeon carefully evaluates the patient so that the most appropriate procedure is performed.

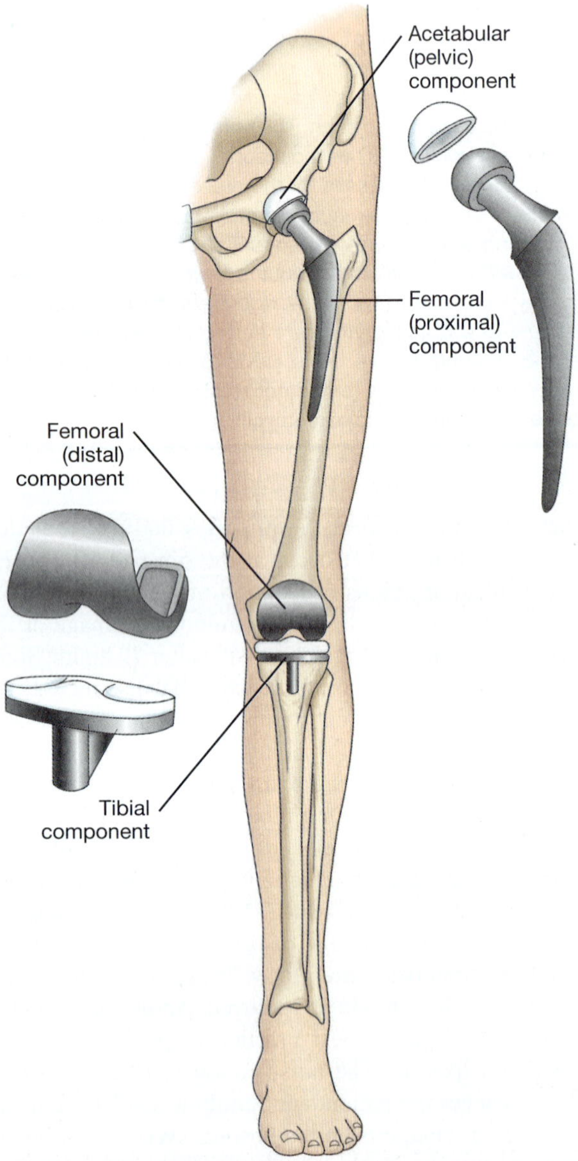

FIGURE 41-16 Examples of hip and knee replacement.

Surgical procedures include excision of damaged and diseased tissue, repair of damaged structures (e.g., ruptured tendon), **arthroplasty** (replacement of all or part of the joint surfaces), and **arthrodesis** (immobilizing fusion of a joint).

Most joint replacements consist of metal, ceramic, or polyethylene components. Selection is typically based on the patient's age and activity level as well as the surgeon's preference. Cementless fixation of the femoral and acetabular component has become the standard procedure in the United States. Accurate fitting and the presence of healthy bone with adequate blood supply are important in the use of cementless components. The healing process in a noncemented prosthesis requires the same amount of time as a long bone cortical fracture, about 3 months (Dickson, 2023). Joint implants may be cemented with a bone-bonding agent; since cemented components typically allow early weight bearing they may be ideal for patient whose activities do not place great demand on the joint but who would benefit from early mobility such as older patients with osteoporosis and poor-quality bone since they may lack the compressive strength to support weight-bearing forces (Phillips & Hornacky, 2021a). Much progress has been made in reducing the prosthesis failure rate through improved techniques, improved materials, and use of bone grafts. The anterior, anterolateral, posterior, or minimally invasive THA approach are used for THA (see next section). The anterior approach avoids disruption of the posterior soft tissues and was thought to have lower dislocation rates; however, in recent research, although the direct anterior approach resulted in less atrophy of the hip musculature compared with a direct lateral or posterior approach, evidence does not reveal outcome differences at 1 year between the surgical approaches (O'Connor & Switzer, 2022; Varacallo et al., 2022; Vasarhelvi et al., 2020). Implant survival rates are 90% to 95% successful at 15 years; however, longevity will vary depending on patient factors, such as weight and activity (Mackenzie & Su, 2020, p. 1785).

With joint replacement, excellent pain relief is obtained in most patients. Return of motion and function depends on preoperative soft tissue condition, soft tissue reactions, and general muscle strength. Early failure of joint replacement is associated with excessive activity and preoperative joint and bone pathology.

Because these are elective procedures, some patients donate their own blood during the weeks preceding their surgery (autologous donation). This blood is used to replace that lost during surgery. Autologous blood transfusions eliminate many of the risks of transfusion therapy. Regarding recommendations related to blood transfusions for patients undergoing a total hip replacement, a threshold hemoglobin no higher than 8 g/dL is appropriate in asymptomatic postoperative hip fracture patients (O'Connor & Switzer, 2022).

TOTAL HIP REPLACEMENT

THA, or surgical replacement of the hip joint with an artificial prosthesis, is indicated for osteoarthritis, acetabular dysplasia, rheumatoid arthritis, AVN, posttraumatic injury, and other causes.

Pearls for Practice

Aspirin and NSAIDs should be discontinued at least 1 week prior to surgery because of the risk of perioperative bleeding.

Preoperative Management

Assessment of the patient and preoperative management are aimed at having the patient in optimal health at the time of surgery. Preoperatively, it is important to evaluate cardiovascular, respiratory, kidney, and liver functions. In addition, the nurse considers many factors, such as age over 60 years, obesity, preoperative leg edema, a history of any venous thromboemboli, varicose veins, cancer, prolonged immobility, estrogen, and a wide variety of hematologic conditions, as they are indicators of risk for postoperative DVT and PE, the most common causes of postoperative mortality in those undergoing total hip replacement, and every effort is made to prevent them.

Preoperatively, it is important also to assess the neurovascular status of the extremity undergoing joint replacement. Postoperative assessment data are compared with preoperative assessment data to identify changes and deficits. For example, a sensory deficit postoperatively is of concern unless it was also noted preoperatively, as nerve palsy can occur as a result of surgery. A plan of nursing care for a patient with a total hip replacement is available online at http://thepoint.lww.com/Honan3e.

Providing Patient Education

Maintenance of the femoral head component in the acetabular cup is essential. The nurse teaches the patient about positioning the leg in **abduction**, which helps prevent dislocation of the prosthesis. The patient is aware that an abduction splint, a wedge pillow, or pillows will be placed between the knees to keep the hip in abduction if a posterior approach is used. For an anterior approach or anterolateral approach, the patient is instructed to avoid hip extension as well as external rotation beyond neutral. With an anterior THA approach, the hip muscles are left intact, generally leading to a more stable hip, lower complication rates (e.g., reduced blood loss), earlier restoration of gait, and decreased postoperative restrictions. The nurse should consult with the surgeon regarding the need for specific postoperative hip restrictions. The patient should be out of bed and moving relatively early; in some instances, the evening of the surgery, but no later than postoperative day 1 (Perkins, 2021). General dislocation precautions include no hip flexion past 90 degrees, avoiding hip adduction and internal or external rotation, and no lying in prone position. In general, hip precautions including raised toilet seats should be employed, as they will minimize hip joint flexion in the postoperative period.

Pearls for Practice

For total hip replacement surgery (posterior approach) the legs should be slightly abducted. Prevent hip flexion beyond 90 degrees, hip adduction, and internal rotation to avoid dislocation of the hip after joint replacement surgery. For an anterior approach, motions that externally rotate the limb as well as hyperextension and flexion of the hip combined with external rotation are avoided.

Preventing Infection

Preoperative assessment of the patient for infections (including skin, urinary tract, and pulmonary infection) is necessary because of the risk for postoperative infection. Any infection 2 to 4 weeks before planned surgery may result in postponement of surgery. Preoperative skin preparation frequently begins 1 or 2 days before the surgery. Prophylactic antibiotics are given immediately preoperatively (while the time varies, administration of antibiotics within 60 minutes of the initial incision and prior to tourniquet inflation has demonstrated efficacy in preventing surgical site infection [SSI]) and continued for 24 to 48 hours postoperatively (Crader & Varacallo, 2022; Dickson, 2023).

Intraoperative Management

Blood is conserved during surgery to minimize loss via a pneumatic tourniquet that produces a "bloodless field." Intraoperative blood salvage with reinfusion may be used when a large volume of blood loss is anticipated, and this has shown to substantially reduce the need for allogeneic transfusions (transfusion of blood collected from someone other than the patient). It involves centrifuging, washing, and filtering the collected blood. Red cells are retained while platelets, plasma, and contaminants are removed; the processed red cells are then re-suspended in a saline solution, which can be transfused back into the patient (Godfrey, 2020). The washed blood can be kept for 6 hours at room temperature (Phillips & Hornacky, 2021a). In addition, the use of perioperative antifibrinolytics such as tranexamic acid (TXA) may block the activation of plasminogen to plasmin and therefore decrease bleeding and blood loss resulting from the trauma of surgery (Qi et al., 2019).

Airborne bacteria that contaminate the wound at the time of surgery cause most deep infections. Therefore, as with any surgery, there is strict adherence to aseptic principles, and the operating area is controlled and made as bacteria-free as possible.

Culture of the joint during surgery, before intraoperative antibiotic therapy is begun, may be important in identifying and treating subsequent infections. If osteomyelitis develops, it is difficult to treat. Persistent infection at the site of the prosthesis usually requires removal of the implant and joint revision, which is a complex procedure. Also, it is not always possible to achieve a functional joint when the reconstruction procedure has to be repeated.

Postoperative Management

Repositioning the Patient and Preventing Dislocation

Depending on the surgical approach, the nurse may turn the patient onto the affected or unaffected extremity as prescribed by the surgeon.

To avoid dislocation, the patient will have either a triangular abduction wedge placed between the legs or pillows placed between the knees prior to positioning, to keep the affected leg in an abducted position and prevent internal rotation. The pillows between the legs are used when in a supine or side-lying position and when turning. The patient's hip is never flexed more than 90 degrees. To prevent hip flexion, the nurse does not elevate the head of the bed more than 60 degrees. Limited flexion is maintained during transfers and when sitting. When the patient is initially assisted out of bed, an abduction splint or pillows are kept between the legs. The nurse encourages the patient to keep the affected hip in extension, instructing the patient to pivot on the unaffected leg with assistance by the nurse, who protects the affected hip from **adduction** (together), flexion, internal or external rotation, and excessive weight bearing.

When the patient is turned onto their side, proper alignment and supported abduction are maintained with pillows or abduction wedge. The nurse ensures that the straps of the abduction wedge are secured before turning the patient onto their unaffected side and that straps do not cause undue pressure on the peroneal nerve or surrounding skin. If the patient needs to use a bedpan, a fracture bedpan is used; the nurse instructs the patient to flex the unaffected hip and use the trapeze to lift the pelvis onto the pan. The patient is also reminded not to flex the affected hip. In addition, the patient is aware that crossing of legs is prohibited. Elevated toilet seats and chairs are suggested, as well as "reaching devices" that will limit hip flexion to less than 90 degrees. Occupational therapists can provide the patient with devices to assist with dressing below the waist.

High-seat (orthopedic) chairs and semireclining wheelchairs may also be used to minimize hip joint flexion. When sitting, the patient's hips should be higher than the knees. The patient's affected leg should not be elevated when sitting. The patient may flex the knee. A cradle boot may be used to prevent leg rotation and to support the heel off the bed, preventing development of a pressure ulcer. In general, the nurse instructs the patient not to sleep on the operative side without consulting the surgeon. Hip precautions should be enforced for 4 or more months after surgery.

Dislocation may occur with positioning that exceeds the limits of the prosthesis. The nurse must recognize dislocation of the prosthesis. Indicators are as follows:

- Increased pain at the surgical site, swelling, and immobilization
- Acute groin pain in the affected hip or increased discomfort
- Shortening of the leg
- Abnormal external or internal rotation
- Restricted ability or inability to move the leg
- Reported "popping" sensation in the hip

Although dislocation after a total hip replacement is decreasing due to surgical approaches, if a prosthesis becomes dislocated, the nurse (or the patient, if at home) immediately notifies the surgeon because the hip must be reduced and stabilized promptly so that the leg does not sustain circulatory and nerve damage. Dislocation is the second most common complication following total hip replacement, following aseptic loosening, affecting up to 11% of patients following initial surgery (Lu et al., 2019). Half of dislocations occur from unexpected movements, such as fall or twist, when hip precautions are less likely to be helpful (Machin et al., 2022). Closed treatment for a first-time dislocation is usually successful in two thirds of cases, after which the hip may be stabilized with Buck's traction or a **brace** to prevent recurrent dislocation. For patients with recurrent dislocations, surgery will normally be required. As the muscles and joint capsule heal, the chance of dislocation diminishes. Stresses to the new hip joint should be avoided for the first 3 to 6 months.

Pearls for Practice

In a recent national study (England) of >229,000 patients who underwent total hip surgery, there was no evidence of an increase in early dislocation or 30-day readmission rates after stopping traditional postoperative hip precautions (Machin et al., 2022). Length of stay in the hospital decreased from 4 to 3 days, and no significant trend in the emergency readmissions within 30 days were seen. Thus, there is a trend to reduce or stop hip precautions. Nurses should follow institutional guidelines and continue to evaluate research findings.

Promoting Ambulation

Patients with total hip replacement begin ambulation with a physical therapist, generally within a day after surgery. The nurse and the physical therapist assist the patient in achieving the goal of independent ambulation. At first, the patient may be able to stand for only a brief period because of orthostatic hypotension.

Pearls for Practice

Orthostatic hypotension is an abnormal drop in blood pressure on change of position from lying to standing. Approximately 500 to 700 mL of blood momentarily

shifts to the lower body when changing position to standing from supine, resulting in decreased venous return and arterial pressure. Complaints of dizziness may be noted. A drop of systolic pressure of 20 mm Hg, a drop in diastolic pressure of 10 mm Hg or more, or an increase in heart rate of 15 bpm within 3 minutes is diagnostic of orthostatic hypotension. It may be related to hypovolemia, dehydration, drug-induced hypotension, or prolonged bed rest. Patients should be encouraged to rise slowly and move their legs prior to rising to facilitate venous return from the extremities.

Specific weight-bearing limits on the prosthesis are determined by the surgeon and are based on the patient's condition, the procedure, and the fixation method. Usually, patients with cemented prostheses can proceed to weight bearing as tolerated. If the patient has a press-fit, cementless, ingrowth prosthesis, weight bearing immediately after surgery may be limited to minimize micromotion of the prosthesis in the bone. As the patient is able to tolerate more activity, the nurse encourages transferring to a chair several times a day for short periods and walking for progressively greater distances. Refer to Box 41-15 for patient education to prevent hip dislocation.

Monitoring for Complications

Complications that may occur include dislocation of the hip prosthesis, excessive wound drainage, thromboembolism, infection, and heel pressure ulcer. Other complications for which the nurse must monitor include those associated with immobility, heterotopic ossification, AVN, and loosening of the prosthesis.

Monitoring Wound Drainage

If extensive blood loss is anticipated after total joint replacement surgery, an autotransfusion drainage system (in which

BOX 41-15

Patient Education

Avoiding Hip Dislocation after Replacement Surgery

Until the hip prosthesis stabilizes after hip replacement surgery, it may be necessary to follow instructions for proper positioning so that the prosthesis remains in place. Dislocation of the hip is a serious complication of surgery that causes pain and loss of function and necessitates reduction under anesthesia to correct the dislocation. Desirable positions include abduction, neutral rotation, and flexion of less than 90 degrees. When you are seated, the knees should be lower than the hip.

Methods for avoiding displacement for posterior hip procedures include the following:

- Keep the knees apart at all times.
- Put two pillows between the legs when sleeping.
- Never cross the legs when seated.
- Avoid bending forward when seated in a chair to pick up an object on the floor.
- Avoid internal rotation of the hip.
- Avoid sitting in a low chair or toilet seat to avoid flexing the hip more than 90 degrees.
- Use a high-seated chair and a raised toilet seat; consider handrails by the toilet.
- Limit sitting to 30 minutes at a time—to minimize hip flexion and the risk of prosthetic dislocation and to prevent hip stiffness and flexion contracture.
- Do not flex the hip to put on clothing such as pants, stockings, socks, or shoes. Consider occupational therapy devices for dressing and reaching.
- Encourage quadriceps setting and ROM exercises, as directed.
- Positions to avoid after total hip replacement are illustrated below.

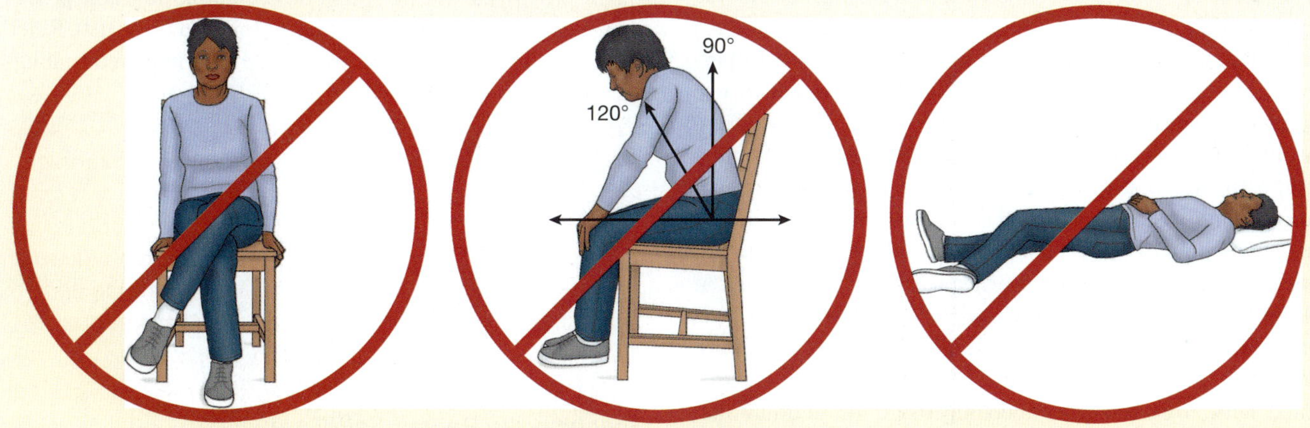

Affected leg should not cross the center of the body

Hip should not bend more than 90 degrees

Affected leg should not turn inward

Nettina, S. M. (2014). *Lippincott manual of nursing practice*, 11 edition. Wolters Kluwer Health.

the drained blood is filtered and reinfused into the patient during the immediate postoperative period) may be used to decrease the need for blood transfusions. Because of the risk of contamination, the blood should be administered within 6 hours of initiation of collection. The nurse should follow institutional protocol.

Fluid and blood accumulating at the surgical site may be drained with a portable suction device (PSD). Traditionally, a PSD was used to prevent accumulation of fluid, which could contribute to discomfort and provide a site for infection. However, recent research reveals that with use of a PSD, patients had improved soft tissue healing and a lower rate of early wound-related complications; however, late infections were not prevented with the use of a PSD (Keeney et al., 2019). In general, the routine use of surgical drains is not recommended for hip and knee replacement (Wainwright et al., 2020); if used they are typically removed by 48 hours after surgery.

Preventing Deep Vein Thrombosis

The risk of venous thromboembolism in total hip and total knee repair is approximately 0.6% to 1.5% (Santana et al., 2020). Without prophylaxis, the incidence of documented DVT in the patient with total joint arthroplasty is reported in the range of 20% to 60% (Wainwright et al., 2020; Yu et al., 2021). The risk of DVT can be reduced with short intraoperative time, epidural anesthesia, intraoperative heparin administration, pneumatic devices, foot flexion-extension exercises, and early ambulation. Since bed rest ≥3 days postoperatively is a risk factor for DVT, the nurse must institute preventive measures such as early ambulation and monitor the patient closely for the development of DVT and PE (Yu et al., 2021). The nurse understands that walking helps propel blood back to the right side of the heart and prevents venous stasis that may lead to development of venous thrombi (Haynes & Henry, 2022). Signs of DVT include unilateral limb pain, swelling, warmth, erythema of the affected limb, and tenderness. Measures to promote circulation and decrease venous stasis are priorities for the patient undergoing hip reconstruction. The nurse encourages the patient to consume adequate amounts of fluids, to perform ankle and foot exercises hourly while awake, to use sequential compression devices as prescribed, and to transfer out of bed and ambulate with assistance beginning on the first postoperative day. There is no consensus on appropriate anticoagulation status post-THA; however, low–molecular-weight heparin (e.g., enoxaparin, dalteparin) or sometimes unfractionated heparin or aspirin (for a minimum of 10 to 14 days and up to 35 days) is prescribed as prophylaxis for DVT after hip replacement surgery (Ortel et al., 2020; Santana et al., 2020). If warfarin is administered (it is associated with slightly higher bleeding risk), the international normalized ratio (INR) should be maintained between 2.0 and 3.0 (Ingason et al., 2022). Prophylactic regimens with anticoagulants decrease the risk of DVT anywhere from 10% to 80%, but given the incidence of breakthrough DVT, the nurse must remain vigilant in assessing for this common complication (Badireddy & Mudipalli, 2022).

Preventing Infection

Infection, a serious complication of total hip replacement, may necessitate removal of the implant. The incidence of periprosthetic joint infection is 1% to 2% (Ahmed et al., 2019). Patients who are experiencing obesity (BMI >35 kg/m^2) or are undernourished and patients who have diabetes, chronic pulmonary disease, dementia, liver disease, heart failure, connective tissue disorders or rheumatoid arthritis, or concurrent infections (e.g., UTI, dental abscess), are at high risk for infection. Prolonged surgical time and prolonged wound drainage >10 days are additional risk factors for joint infections; antibiotics given at the appropriate time, reducing traffic in the operating room, chlorhexidine prep, and betadine wash reduce the rate of periprosthetic joint infection (Ahmed et al., 2019).

Because total joint infections are so disastrous, all efforts are made to prevent them. Potential sources of infection are avoided. Typically, prophylactic antibiotics are prescribed within 60 minutes of the initial incision and prior to tourniquet inflation and continued for 24 to 48 hours postoperatively. If indwelling urinary catheters or PSDs are used, they are removed as soon as possible to avoid infection. Prophylactic antibiotics are prescribed if the patient needs any future surgical or invasive procedures, such as tooth extraction or cystoscopic examination.

Acute infections may occur within 3 months after surgery and are associated with progressive superficial infections or hematomas. Delayed surgical infections may appear 3 to 24 months after surgery and may cause return of discomfort in the hip. Late infections occur more than 2 years after surgery; they are attributed to the spread of infection through the bloodstream from another site in the body. A positive culture result is the gold standard in diagnosing prosthetic joint infection (Ahmed et al., 2019). If an infection occurs, antibiotics are prescribed. Severe infections may require surgical debridement, prolonged use of antibiotics, multiple revision procedures, or removal of the prosthesis (Ahmed et al., 2019). Refer to Box 41-16 for risk factors associated with impaired healing.

Pearls for Practice

When assessing the surgical site, the nurse observes for redness, warmth, swelling, pain, drainage, and loss of function and notifies the provider with any concerns. The clinical observation of the patient and the wound is "more powerful than laboratory investigations and is the most reliable way to identify wound infection" (Copanitsanou & Santy-Tomlinson, 2021, p. 2).

Teaching the Patient Self-Care

Before the patient prepares to leave the acute care setting, the nurse provides thorough teaching to promote continuity of the therapeutic regimen and active participation in the

BOX 41-16

Risk Factors for Delayed Healing

The nurse is aware that patients who present with the following factors are at risk for delayed healing of fractures:

- Extensive local trauma
- Malnutrition
- Bone loss
- Inadequate immobilization
- Space or tissue between bone fragments
- Infection
- Local malignancy
- Metabolic bone disease (e.g., Paget disease)
- Irradiated bone (radiation necrosis)
- Avascular necrosis (AVN)
- Intra-articular fracture (synovial fluid contains fibrolysins, which lyse the initial clot and restrict clot formation)
- Age (older people heal more slowly)
- Use of corticosteroids (inhibit the repair rate)
- Smoking
- Diabetes
- Vascular disease

rehabilitation process. The nurse advises the patient of the importance of the daily exercise program in maintaining the functional motion of the hip joint and strengthening the abductor muscles of the hip and reminds the patient that it will take time to strengthen and retrain the muscles.

Assistive devices (crutches, walker, or cane) are used for a time. After sufficient muscle tone has developed to permit a normal gait without discomfort, these devices are not necessary. In general, by 3 months, the patient can resume routine ADLs. Frequent walks, swimming, and use of a high rocking chair are excellent for hip exercises. Sexual intercourse can be resumed based upon surgeon recommendation (typically 4 to 6 weeks postoperatively).

Assistance in putting on shoes and socks may be needed. The patient should avoid low chairs and maintain restrictions per surgeon's preference. At the present time, weight-bearing restrictions after THA are not standardized and are typically determined by the surgeon's preference. Precautions that minimize hip flexion and risks of prosthetic dislocation, hip stiffness, and flexion **contracture** are reviewed with the patient and significant others. Other activities to avoid typically include tub baths, jogging, lifting heavy loads, and excessive bending and twisting (e.g., shoveling snow, forceful turning).

Pearls for Practice

The risk of dislocation after THA decreases as time passes without a dislocation. If dislocation occurs, typically it is seen early in the postoperative period and frequently is due to either patient-associated or surgical factors. The patient-associated factors that have been implicated include previous surgery, lumbar spine fusion surgery, body mass index (BMI) of 30 kg/m^2 or higher, and/or neurologic impairment (Lu et al., 2019).

TOTAL KNEE REPLACEMENT

Total knee replacement surgery is considered for patients who have severe pain and functional disabilities related to destruction of joint surfaces by arthritis (osteoarthritis, AVN, rheumatoid arthritis, posttraumatic arthritis) or bleeding into the joint (e.g., hemarthrosis), such as may result from hemophilia. The prostheses consist of tibial and patellar components made of high-density polyethylene that articulate with the polished metallic surface of the femoral component (Phillips & Hornacky, 2021a). It is designed to provide the patient with a functional, painless, stable joint. Some surgeons may prefer the patient to make an autologous (from the patient) blood donation before surgery since allogenic (different donor) blood transfusions are associated with an increased risk of prosthetic joint infection when compared with autologous blood transfusion (Perkins, 2020).

Postoperative Management

Postoperatively, the knee is dressed in a compression bandage. Ice may be applied to control edema and bleeding. The nurse assesses the neurovascular status of the leg. It is important to encourage active flexion of the foot every hour when the patient is awake. Efforts are directed at preventing complications (thromboembolism, peroneal nerve palsy, infection, limited ROM). If bleeding is observed on the dressing, the area should be circled, dated, and timed so it can be closely monitored for an increasing amount; the surgeon may complete the first dressing change (Perkins, 2020). If extensive bleeding is anticipated, an autotransfusion drainage system may be used during the immediate postoperative period (see previous discussion). The color, type, and amount of drainage are documented, and any excessive drainage or change in characteristics of the drainage is promptly reported to the surgeon.

The use of a CPM device, a motorized device that continuously moves the knee joint passively through a set degree of ROM, is dependent on the surgeon's preference. Recent research on the use of this device has not demonstrated its efficacy, so it is falling out of favor. If the CPM device is used, the patient's knee must be aligned with the hinge joint of the CPM device to maximize comfort and prevent complications; sheepskin or padding is used to protect skin that is exposed to the CPM device (Rex, 2018). ROM movement usually begins on postoperative day 1 at full extension (0 degrees) and 30 degrees of flexion and generally is advanced 10 degrees per day until discharge.

The nurse assists the patient to get out of bed on the evening of or the day after surgery. The knee may be protected with a knee immobilizer (splint or brace) and is elevated when the patient sits in a chair. Physical therapy teaches the patient how to get in and out of a chair and the use of stairs. The patient should avoid crossing the legs, and kneeling is not recommended following the surgery (Abozead et al., 2022). When the patient is in bed, a pillow should be placed under the operative leg to decrease edema, but never directly under the knee to avoid joint contracture (Farrington, 2021; Perkins 2020). The surgeon prescribes weight-bearing limits. Progressive ambulation, using assistive devices and within the prescribed weight-bearing limits, begins on the day after surgery. The physical therapist supervises exercises for strength and ROM, and progression of rehabilitation will be based upon patient tolerance. Therapy is continued on an outpatient basis.

The overall complication rate of total knee replacement is low (e.g., the incidence of knee joint infection is less than 2%). Potential complications are similar to those for total hip replacement, e.g., DVT and infection (discussed previously) (Farrington, 2021). As with THA, there is no uniform consensus regarding type and duration of anticoagulation therapy after total knee arthroplasty (TKA). Anticoagulants and pneumatic compression devices are often utilized. Patients usually can achieve a pain-free, functional joint and participate more fully in life activities than before the surgery. The expected duration of a TKA is 10 to 15 years or longer (Perkins 2020).

AMPUTATION

Amputation is the removal of a body part, usually an extremity. Amputation of a lower extremity is often necessary because of progressive peripheral vascular disease (often a sequela of diabetes mellitus), fulminating gas gangrene, trauma (crushing injuries, burns, frostbite, electrical burns), congenital deformities, chronic osteomyelitis, or malignant tumor. Of the 185,000 amputations that occur in the United States each year, 82% occur due to vascular disease (Hussey, 2022b; Shahsavari et al., 2020). Amputation of the opposite limb is necessary within 5 years in 30% to 50% of patients who have an amputation due to vascular disease (Ford, 2021). Amputation of an upper extremity occurs less frequently than amputation of a lower extremity and is most often necessary because of either traumatic injury (68.8%), industrial accident (90%–92% of cases), or a malignant tumor (Shahsavari et al., 2020).

Levels of Amputation

Amputation is performed at the most distal point that will heal successfully. The site of amputation is determined by two factors: circulation in the body part and functional usefulness (i.e., meets the requirements for the use of a prosthesis).

The objective of surgery is to conserve as much extremity length as needed to preserve function and possibly to achieve a good prosthetic fit. Amputation should be viewed as an opportunity to reestablish or enhance a patient's functional level and facilitate a return to near-normal movement (Ford, 2021). Preservation of knee and elbow joints is desired. Most amputations involving extremities can be eventually fitted with a prosthesis.

The amputation of toes and portions of the foot causes minor changes in gait and balance. A Syme amputation (modified ankle **disarticulation** amputation) is the most common ankle procedure where the amputation is performed above the ankle joint, and the skin of the heel is used for the flap; it is performed frequently for extensive foot trauma since it produces a painless, durable extremity end that can withstand full weight bearing. Below-knee amputation (BKA) is preferred to above-knee amputation (AKA) because of the importance of the knee joint and the energy requirements for walking. Knee disarticulations are most successful with young, active patients who can develop precise control of the prosthesis. When AKAs are performed, all possible length is preserved, muscles are stabilized and shaped, and hip contractures are prevented for maximum ambulatory potential. Most people who have a hip disarticulation amputation must rely on a wheelchair for mobility.

Complications

Complications that may occur with amputation include hemorrhage, infection, skin breakdown, phantom limb pain, and joint contracture. Because major blood vessels have been severed, massive bleeding may occur. Infection is a risk with all surgical procedures. The risk of infection increases with contaminated wounds after traumatic amputation. Skin irritation caused by the prosthesis may result in skin breakdown. **Phantom limb pain** is caused by the severing of peripheral nerves and involves both the peripheral nervous system and the CNS. Joint contracture is caused by positioning and a protective flexion withdrawal pattern associated with pain and muscle imbalance.

Medical and Nursing Management

There is no consensus in the literature regarding dressing choice and wound care for patients with amputations; therefore, dressings vary according to surgeon preference and may include a closed rigid cast dressing, a removable rigid dressing, or a soft dressing. A closed rigid cast dressing is frequently used to provide uniform compression, control edema, support soft tissues, control pain, prevent joint contractures, and protect the limb from external trauma. Care is taken not to constrict circulation.

For the patient with a lower extremity amputation, the plaster cast may be equipped to attach a temporary prosthetic extension (pylon) and an artificial foot. This rigid dressing technique is used as a means of creating a socket for immediate postoperative prosthetic fitting. The length of the prosthesis is tailored to the individual patient. Weight bearing is limited initially, with bilateral upper extremity support from parallel bars, a walker, or crutches. The cast is changed in about 5 to 7 days; if wound healing is satisfactory, a new rigid dressing or prosthetic cast is applied (Ford, 2021). Elevated body temperature, severe pain, or a loose-fitting cast may necessitate earlier replacement.

A removable rigid dressing may be placed over a soft dressing to control edema, prevent joint flexion contracture, and protect the residual limb (stump) from unintentional trauma during transfer activities. This rigid dressing is removed several days after surgery for wound inspection and is then replaced to control edema. The dressing facilitates residual limb shaping. Within 3 to 4 weeks, the rigid dressing can be changed to a removable temporary prosthesis if there are no skin complications. The patient is shown the proper use of elastic wrapping or a stump shrinker to control edema and help contour the residual limb when not wearing the prosthesis (Ford, 2021).

Commonly a soft dressing (nonadherent dressing on the incision, sterile gauze 4 × 4, rolled gauze holding the prior two in place), with or without compression may be used if there is significant wound drainage, and frequent inspection of the residual limb is desired (Kwasniewski & Mitchel, 2022). An immobilizing splint may be incorporated in the dressing. Stump (wound) hematomas are controlled with wound drainage devices to minimize infection. If drains are used, they are usually removed at 48 hours (Toy, 2021). The wound is assessed for signs and symptoms of infection (erythema, warmth, unexplained increase in pain, purulent drainage, dehiscence of the wound, poor wound healing, and fever); estimates are that infections occur in 17% to 40% of major lower limb amputations (Kwasniewski & Mitchel, 2022). The nurse also assesses for systemic indicators of infection (e.g., elevated temperature, leukocytosis [elevated WBCs] with an increase of at least 10% bands on the differential) and promptly reports indications of infection to the surgeon. Comorbidities, such as diabetes, malnutrition, malignancy, peripheral arterial disease, and smoking are increased risk factors for infection. Wound dehiscence is when the surgical wound edges separate completely; this occurs in approximately 16% of amputations and is associated with underlying infection; hematoma; and comorbidities such as diabetes, smoking, malnutrition, and obesity (Kwaniewski & Mitchel, 2022). Treatment may include a wound vacuum-assisted closure or VAC.

Pearls for Practice

If the cast or elastic dressing inadvertently comes off, the nurse must immediately wrap the residual limb with an elastic compression bandage. If this is not done, excessive edema will develop in a short time, resulting in a delay in rehabilitation. The nurse notifies the surgeon if a cast dressing comes off so that another cast can be applied promptly.

Pearls for Practice

*It is essential to maintain nearby joints in extension to prevent the formation of contractures (joint deformities that develop from persistent shortening of muscles/tendons). Educate the patient **not** to put a pillow under the joint because a flexion contracture of the hip may result.*

Promoting Rehabilitation

Patients who require amputation because of severe trauma are usually, but not always, young and healthy, heal rapidly, and are physically able to participate in a vigorous rehabilitation program. Because the amputation is the result of an injury, the patient needs psychological support in accepting the sudden change in body image and in dealing with the stresses of hospitalization, long-term rehabilitation, and modification of lifestyle. Patients who undergo amputation need support as they grieve the loss, and they need time to work through their feelings about their permanent loss and change in body image. Depression can occur in 20.6% to 63% of patients after amputation (Molina & Faulk, 2022).

The multidisciplinary rehabilitation team (patient, nurse, clinical nurse specialist, physician, social worker, physical therapist, occupational therapist, psychologist, prosthetist, vocational rehabilitation worker) helps the patient achieve the highest possible level of function and participation in life activities. Prosthetic clinics and amputee support groups facilitate this rehabilitation process. Vocational counseling and job retraining may be necessary to help patients return to work.

Psychological issues may be influenced by the type of support the patient receives from the rehabilitation team and by how quickly ADLs and use of the prosthesis are learned. Knowing the full options and capabilities available with the various prosthetic devices can give the patient a sense of control over the resulting disability.

Minimizing Altered Sensory Perceptions

A person who has had an amputation may experience phantom limb pain soon after surgery (70% to 80%), whereas the incidence at 6 months ranges from 60% to 90% (Kwaniewski & Mitchel, 2022). The pain is often described as sharp and electric or burning pain of the amputated limb, and highly fluctuant (Dinakar, 2022). The incidence is increased in those patients who had chronic pain before the amputation, in which case the pain is described as similar to the pain felt in the limb before surgery (Dinakar, 2022).The pathogenesis of the phantom limb phenomenon is unknown. When a patient describes phantom pains or sensations, the nurse acknowledges these feelings and helps the patient modify these perceptions. A multimodal approach that combines both pharmacologic and nonpharmacologic interventions should be considered for treatment. TENS, massage, mirror therapy, use of myoelectric prosthesis, biofeedback, ultrasound, acupuncture, hypnosis, hot and cold modalities, or local anesthetics may provide some relief for patients. In addition, beta blockers may relieve dull, burning discomfort; antiseizure medications control stabbing and cramping pain; and tricyclic antidepressants are used to modify pain signals and improve mood and coping ability. Newer treatment modalities include virtual and augmented reality in an attempt to extinguish maladaptive memory traces of the amputated limb and extinguish the pain (Hanyu-Deutmeyer et al., 2022).

Pearls for Practice

Phantom limb pain may be related, elicited, or exacerbated by physical factors (e.g., changes in weather or pressure on the residual limb) and psychological factors (e.g., emotional stress). Phantom pain commonly occurs after an arm or leg amputation but may also occur after the surgical removal of the breast, rectum, penis, testicle, eye, tongue, or teeth (Dinakar, 2022).

Helping the Patient to Achieve Physical Mobility

Proper positioning prevents the development of hip or knee joint contracture in the patient with a lower extremity amputation. Exercises that preserve essential ROM for hip extension and knee extension also should be part of the therapy program. Abduction, external rotation, and flexion of the lower extremity are avoided. Depending on the surgeon's preference, the residual limb may be placed in an extended position or elevated for a brief period after surgery. Prolonged elevation (after initial 24 hours postoperative) is not recommended, as flexion contractions are to be avoided.

A physical therapist will develop exercises if indicated for muscle strengthening and to prevent abduction and flexion contractures. The nurse encourages the patient to turn from side to side and to assume a prone position, if possible, to stretch the flexor muscles and to prevent flexion contracture of the hip. The nurse discourages sitting for prolonged periods to prevent flexion contracture. The legs should remain close together to prevent an abduction deformity. The nurse encourages the patient to use assistive devices (e.g., reachers) to more readily perform self-care activities and to identify what home modifications should be made to perform these activities in the home environment.

Postoperative ROM exercises are started early because contracture deformities develop rapidly. ROM exercises include hip and knee exercises for BKAs and hip exercises for AKAs. It is important that the patient understand the importance of exercising the residual limb. In general, patients are kept non–weight bearing on the involved extremity until the wounds are healed (Grimm & Potter, 2021).

The upper extremities, trunk, and abdominal muscles are exercised and strengthened. The extensor muscles in the arm and the depressor muscles in the shoulder play an important part in crutch walking. The major problems that can delay prosthetic fitting during this period are (1) flexion deformities, (2) nonshrinkage of the residual limb, and (3) abduction deformities of the hip. In general, fabrication of the temporary prosthesis begins 3 to 4 weeks after amputation. The average time to prosthetic fitting varies widely, however preference is to fit most traumatic, oncologic, and congenital amputations between 4 and 6 weeks postoperatively (longer time is expected for patients with vascular disease) (Grimm & Potter, 2021).

Excessive pressure from the prosthesis can cause skin irritation, pain, skin breakdown, and infection. The nurse observes the operative site for erythema and pain. The patient is taught to wash the stump with care using mild soap, change the stump sock regularly, and clean the prosthesis socket regularly with mild soap and water (Magee & Manske, 2021). In addition, the patient and family are taught to inspect the skin of the entire residual limb carefully, using a mirror if necessary to visualize difficult-to-see areas, particularly areas over bony prominences that may be vulnerable to high pressure within the socket (Gravano & Lusardi, 2020).

Clinical Judgment Case

A 72-year-old patient comes into the emergency room (ER) after a motor vehicle collision (MVC). The cervical spine was stabilized in the field and a c-collar is in place. The patient is complaining of severe left-sided hip and groin pain that increases with movement. The patient's skin is cool, there is ecchymosis and slight edema at the symphysis pubis, a hematoma on the left thigh, and the left lower extremity is not shortened or rotated. Vital signs are as follows: 98.7°F, HR 118 and regular, 24 RR with an oxygen saturation of 93% on room air and the blood pressure is 100/44 mm Hg. Heart sounds are S1 S2 without gallop or murmur; the point of maximum impulse (PMI) is nondisplaced (5th intercostal space [ICS], midclavicular line). Lungs are clear. The patient denies nausea or vomiting. Abdomen is soft, nondistended, tender at the symphysis pubis, last BM was yesterday, formed brown stool, no evidence of bleeding. Capillary refill is 3 seconds and pedal and posterior tibial pulses are 1+ bil; there is delayed skin turgor. The patient's history included hyperlipidemia and hypertension, which are treated with hydrochlorothiazide and atorvastatin. The patient is anxious and becoming restless.

Step One: Recognize cues where relevant and important information is identified from different sources, such as medical history or vital signs.

Answer: History of hyperlipidemia and hypertension. Complaints of restlessness and anxiety, severe pain of the hip and groin, a hematoma of the left thigh, inability to move without increasing pain. Physical examination findings of diminished peripheral pulses, delayed capillary refill, cool skin, ecchymosis, and edema at the symphysis pubis. No rotation or shortening of the left lower extremity (LLE). Cues of concern related to vital signs: HR of 118 and regular,
24 RR, O_2 sat of 93% and blood pressure is 100/44 mm Hg. c-collar in place.

Step Two: Analyze cues, which is organizing and linking the recognized cues to the patient's clinical presentation.

Answer: You have clustered the patient's symptoms to be associated with potential pelvic fracture. Specifically, the MVC, the hematoma of the left thigh (Desault sign), ecchymosis and edema at the symphysis pubis, severe pain, and an inability to bear weight. You recognize that there is a risk of hemorrhagic shock from intrapelvic bleeding or associated abdominal injury with pelvic fractures. You associate the tachycardia with the body's attempt to increase the cardiac output (CO). The blood pressure of 100/44 is hypotensive and you calculate the mean arterial pressure (MAP), which is systolic pressure (100 mm Hg) plus the diastolic pressure (44 mm Hg) × 2/3 (100 + 88 = 188/3 = 63 mm Hg). Since the MAP reflects perfusion to major organs, you are aware that a MAP below 65 mm Hg for an extended period can cause end-organ ischemia, and infarction can occur. You are concerned that the pelvic fracture has caused significant blood loss that has decreased the CO and led to hypovolemic shock. You noted that the painful limb is neither shortened or rotated, which would be the case in a hip fracture or hip dislocation.

Step Three: Prioritize hypotheses, where hypotheses are evaluated and ranked according to priority. This can include urgency, likelihood, risk, difficulty and/or time. In this phase you cluster your findings to arrive at a list of problems (actual and or potential problems) you believe the patient is experiencing and determine the importance or urgency. What do you think is of greatest concern?

Answer: The potential hypothesis includes (1) hypovolemic shock (since the patient is presenting with tachycardia and hypotension, you recognize that at least a 30% loss of the patient's total blood volume has occurred), (2) suspected pelvic fracture, (3) potential intrapelvic bleeding or associated abdominal injury, and (4) hemodynamic instability with movement. In the moment, you prioritize hypovolemic shock as the greatest risk of injury to this patient.

Step Four: Generate solutions, which is identifying expected outcomes and using hypotheses to define a set of interventions for the expected outcomes.

Answer: Since hypovolemic shock is suspected (pelvic fractures can lose up to 6 L of blood and therefore patients are at risk for exsanguination), you recognize the need to place the patient on a cardiac monitor and start two large-gauge IVs for emergency fluid replacement. You follow the Advances Trauma Life support (ATLS) guidelines, using the sequential C-ABCD (**C**atastrophic hemorrhage control, **A**irway, **B**reathing, **C**irculation, and **D**isability) to detect and manage potentially life-threatening injuries. You will want to administer oxygen to improve the oxygen saturation, which on admission was 93% on room air. You will monitor the oxygen saturation continuously and vital signs every 15 minutes at a minimum. You recognize that while elevation of the head of bed (HOB) may improve the hypoxemia, the BP may decline further because of blood redistribution with gravity and the patient is significantly hypotensive with a MAP of 63 mm Hg. You expect Focused Assessment with Sonography in Trauma (FAST) examination and/or abdominal CT scan to identify intra-abdominal injuries quickly. Laboratory testing that will evaluate baseline complete blood count (CBC), and to type and cross-match the blood in anticipation of blood transfusions (blood products may need to be administered, particularly if the cause of the hypovolemic shock is hemorrhage), coagulation studies, lactate level, and chemistry will be obtained.

Step Five: Take action, where the solutions that address the highest priorities are implemented.

Answer: Since the goals are (1) to restore intravascular volume, (2) to reverse the sequence of events leading to inadequate tissue perfusion, and (3) to correct the underlying cause of the fluid loss as quickly as possible, you start two large-gauge IV lines to establish access for fluid administration, place the patient on a cardiac monitor, and monitor the oxygen saturation continuously and administer oxygen at 2 L via nasal cannula. You anticipate fluid resuscitation in hypovolemic shock will be either 0.9% sodium chloride solution (normal saline) or lactated Ringer (LR) solution while waiting for blood products to transfuse. You are aware that despite the significant hypotension, you cannot elevate the patient's legs slightly to improve venous return to the heart, since it is contraindicated in trauma of the hip and pelvis. You recognize that immediate stabilization of the pelvic bones and tamponading or compressing bleeding vessels is needed and that a simple method of stabilizing the pelvis is the tying of a sheet circumferentially around the hips at the level of the greater trochanters. You are aware that in order to apply the sheet, you will need to log roll the patient, which may lead to clot disruption and further blood loss. But since stabilization is also required, it is critical to assess for any evidence of hemodynamic instability (increasing pulse, RR, decreasing BP and MAP) while applying the pelvic "binder." In addition, you are aware that until the cervical spine is clear, the patient must be log rolled with the c-collar in place. A Foley catheter is to be inserted; however, you spoke to the provider about waiting until the diagnostic studies are complete since injuries to the bladder and urethra (as well as abdominal organs and pelvic vessels and nerves) are associated with pelvic fracture. If blood at the introitus or, if the patient has a penis, scrotal hematoma is seen, a urinary drainage catheter should not be inserted until the status of the urethra is known.

Step Six: Evaluate outcomes, which is comparing observed outcomes against expected outcomes.

Answer: The FAST study and CT scan revealed a pelvic ring fracture and iliac vessel injury, and the patient was immediately transferred to interventional radiology for emergent embolization of the iliac vessel. An external fixator was used to stabilize the pelvic fracture. Once the patient was hemodynamically stable, an open reduction and internal fixation (ORIF) of the pelvis was performed. The cervical spine was cleared and the c-collar removed. The patient subsequently recovered from this trauma and was discharged home. It is because of your quick thinking and recognition of the need to individualize care that you astutely did not elevate the lower extremities when the patient presented in shock. You followed ATLS C-ABCD guidelines, you recognized the need to attempt to stabilize the pelvic fracture with a sheet, and you remembered the need to evaluate the status of the urethra before simply following routine standards of care of inserting a Foley. Because of your quick thinking, you helped stabilize this patient. Kudos to you.

CHAPTER REVIEW

NCLEX-Style Review Questions

1. In the immediate postoperative period, select the measures that would best prevent a DVT? Select all that apply.
   a. Active flexion–extension foot and ankle exercises
   b. Early ambulation
   c. Measuring intake and output
   d. Lowering the legs below the level of the heart
   e. Use of sequential compression devices (SCD)

2. A 22-year-old patient is admitted to the emergency department with a crush injury to both lower legs. The patient was pinned under a car for 3 hours and on admission vital signs are stable; patient is alert and oriented and complaining of extreme pain in both legs. Popliteal pulses are strong; pedal and posterior tibial pulses are weak. The ankle and feet appear dusky; the skin is tense, but the skin envelope is not broken. X-rays show no broken bones. Based upon these data, what interventions are most appropriate? Select all that apply.
   a. Notify the provider and anticipate that a stat $\dot{V}/\dot{Q}$ scan will be performed to rule out fat emboli.
   b. Prepare to set up skin traction to decrease the pressure on the calf muscle.
   c. Notify the provider and anticipate that the provider will measure the pressure in the compartment and possibly perform a fasciotomy if elevated pressure is noted.
   d. Prepare IV antibiotics to decrease the risk of osteomyelitis.
   e. Evaluate whether the pain occurs or intensifies with passive ROM and is disproportional to the injury.

3. During assessment of a patient admitted to the emergency room after a motor vehicle collision, the patient becomes semiconscious and continues moaning with pain. Select the symptoms associated with hypovolemic shock.
   a. Tachycardia
   b. Bradypnea
   c. MAP < 65 mm Hg
   d. Urine output < 0.5 mL/kg/hr
   e. Hypotension

4. A 73-year-old patient is placed in skeletal traction prior to surgery for an ORIF of fractured femur. The patient develops chest pain, tachypnea, and tachycardia the second day in traction. What additional symptom would indicate the patient's symptoms are related to a fat emboli syndrome rather than a pulmonary thromboembolic event? Select all that apply.
   a. Hypoxia
   b. Peripheral edema
   c. Petechiae of the anterior chest wall
   d. Warm, reddened areas in the leg
   e. Delirium

5. A 23-year-old patient experienced an open fracture of the left tibia with major soft tissue damage of the lower leg in a bicycle accident. Surgical reduction and fixation of the tibia were performed with debridement of nonviable tissue and drain placement in the damaged soft tissue. Which finding by the nurse would most likely indicate the development of osteomyelitis? Select all that apply.

a. Peripheral pulses 3 +/ 4 + bilaterally
b. Elevated C-reactive protein
c. Numbness in the left leg and toes
d. Muscle spasms around the affected bone
e. Swelling and erythema at the infection site

REFERENCES AND SELECTED READINGS

References and selected readings associated with this chapter can be found on the website that accompanies the book. Visit **http://thepoint.lww.com/Honan3e** to access the references and other additional resources associated with this chapter.

UNIT TWELVE

Problems Related to Neurologic Function

A 65-year-old patient presents to the emergency department by ambulance. The paramedics state that the patient's roommate witnessed the patient's sudden onset of confusion, weakness of the right arm and leg, and difficulty speaking (inability to get the right words out). The symptoms occurred 2 hours prior to arrival at the hospital. The patient has a history of smoking, hypertension, atrial fibrillation, and prior transient ischemic attacks (TIAs). An initial noncontrast head computed tomography (CT) was negative for intracerebral hemorrhage. An acute ischemic stroke in the left hemisphere is suspected.

- **Discuss emergency management of a stroke when a patient presents with suspected stroke symptoms.**
- **What subtype of ischemic stroke is the patient most likely experiencing?**
- **Discuss nursing considerations for the patient receiving tPA.**
- **Describe three of the eight standardized performance measures that are considered for a patient with an ischemic stroke.**

CHAPTER 42

Nursing Assessment: Neurologic Function

Donna M. Avanecean

Learning Objectives

After reading this chapter, you will be able to:

1. Describe the structures and functions of the central and peripheral nervous systems.
2. Differentiate pathologic changes that affect motor control and those that affect sensory pathways.
3. Compare the functioning of the sympathetic and parasympathetic nervous systems.
4. Describe changes in neurologic function associated with aging and their impact on neurologic assessment findings.
5. Describe the significance of physical assessment to the diagnosis of neurologic dysfunction.
6. Describe diagnostic tests used for assessment of suspected neurologic disorders and the related nursing implications.

Nurses in many practice settings encounter patients with altered neurologic function. Disorders of the nervous system can occur at any time during the lifespan and can vary from mild, self-limiting symptoms to devastating, life-threatening disorders. Nurses must be skilled in the assessment of the neurologic system, whether the assessment is generalized or focused on specific areas of function. In either case, assessment requires knowledge of the anatomy and physiology of the nervous system and an understanding of the array of tests and procedures used to diagnose neurologic disorders. Knowledge about the nursing implications and interventions related to assessment and diagnostic testing is also essential.

ANATOMY AND PHYSIOLOGY OVERVIEW

The function of the nervous system is control of all motor, sensory, autonomic, cognitive, and behavioral activities. The nervous system consists of two major divisions: the central nervous system (CNS), including the brain and spinal cord; and the peripheral nervous system (PNS), which includes cranial and spinal nerves that lie outside the brain and spinal cord. The PNS can be further divided into the somatic, or voluntary nervous system, and the autonomic, or involuntary nervous system.

Anatomy of the Nervous System

Cells and Neurotransmitters of the Nervous System

Cells of the brain link the motor and sensory pathways, monitor the body's processes, respond to the internal and external environment, maintain homeostasis, and direct all psychological, biologic, and physical activity through complex chemical and electrical messages. The basic functional unit of the brain is the neuron (Fig. 42-1). It is composed of a cell body, a dendrite, and an axon. The **dendrite** is a branch-type structure with synapses (a gap between two neurons, in which impulses jump from one neuron to another) for receiving electrochemical messages. The **axon** is a long projection that carries impulses away from the cell body. Nerve cell bodies occurring in clusters are called *ganglia* or *nuclei.* A cluster of cell bodies with the same function is called a *center* (e.g., the respiratory center).

Neurotransmitters communicate messages from one neuron to another or from a neuron to a specific target tissue and are responsible for all types of brain activity. Each neurotransmitter has an affinity for specific receptors in the postsynaptic bulb. When released, neurotransmitters cross the synaptic cleft and bind to receptors in the postsynaptic cell membrane. The action of a neurotransmitter is to potentiate, terminate, or modulate a specific action, and it can either excite or inhibit the activity of the target cell. Usually,

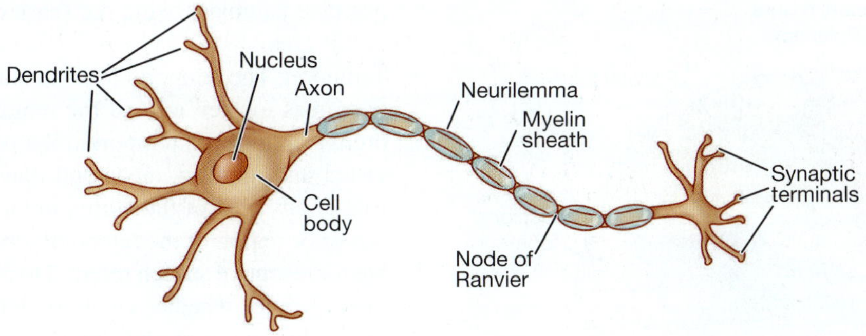

FIGURE 42-1 **Neuron.**

multiple neurotransmitters are at work in the neural synapse. Imbalances or deficiencies of a particular neurotransmitter may cause neurologic dysfunction. Major neurotransmitters are described in Table 42-1.

The Central Nervous System

The Brain

The brain is divided into three major areas: the cerebrum, the brainstem, and the cerebellum. The cerebrum is composed of two hemispheres, the thalamus, the hypothalamus, and the basal ganglia. In addition, connections for the olfactory (cranial nerve I) and optic (cranial nerve II) nerves are found in the cerebrum. The brainstem includes the midbrain, pons, medulla, and connections for cranial nerves III through XII. The cerebellum is located under the cerebrum and behind the brainstem (Fig. 42-2).

Cerebrum. The cerebrum consists of two hemispheres that are incompletely separated by the great longitudinal fissure. This sulcus (a depression or groove) separates the cerebrum into the right and left hemispheres. The two hemispheres are joined at the lower portion of the fissure by the corpus callosum. The outside surface of the hemispheres has many folded layers or convolutions called *gyri,* which increase the surface area of the brain. The external or outer portion of the cerebrum (the cerebral cortex) is made up of gray matter, approximately 2 to 5 mm in depth. White matter makes up the innermost layer and is composed of nerve fibers and neuroglia (support tissue) that form tracts or pathways connecting various parts of the brain. The cerebral hemispheres are divided into pairs of frontal, parietal, temporal, and occipital lobes. The four lobes are as follows (see Fig. 42-2):

- Frontal: The frontal lobe is the largest lobe in the front of the skull. The major functions are concentration, abstract thought, information storage or memory, and motor function. The motor strip, which lies in the frontal lobe, anterior to the central sulcus, is responsible for muscle movement. Refer to Figure 42-3 for specific locations

TABLE **42-1 Major Neurotransmitters**

Neurotransmitter	Source	Action	Example of Dysfunction
Acetylcholine (major transmitter of the parasympathetic nervous system)	Many areas of the brain; autonomic nervous system	Usually excitatory; parasympathetic effects sometimes inhibitory (stimulation of heart by vagal nerve)	↓ Leads to myasthenia gravis
Serotonin	Brainstem, hypothalamus, dorsal horn of the spinal cord	Inhibitory, helps control mood and sleep, inhibits pain pathways	↓ Leads to depression
Dopamine	Substantia nigra and basal ganglia	Usually inhibits, affects behavior (attention, emotions) and fine movement	↓ Leads to Parkinson disease
Norepinephrine (major transmitter of the sympathetic nervous system)	Brainstem, hypothalamus, postganglionic neurons of the sympathetic nervous system	Usually excitatory; affects mood and overall activity	Seen rarely
Gamma-aminobutyric acid (GABA)	Spinal cord, cerebellum, basal ganglia, some cortical areas	Inhibitory	↓ Leads to seizures
Enkephalin, endorphin	Nerve terminals in the spine, brainstem, thalamus and hypothalamus, pituitary gland	Excitatory; pleasurable sensation, inhibits pain transmission	Poor pain control

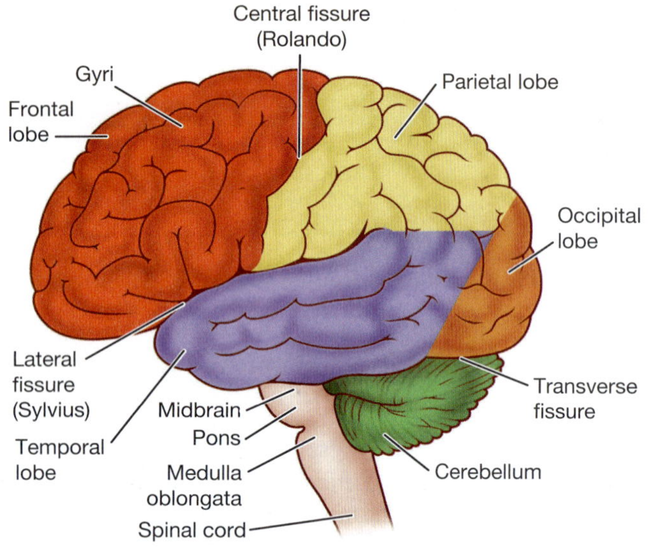

FIGURE 42-2 **View of the external surface of the brain showing lobes, cerebellum, and brainstem.**

of control of motor movement. It also contains Broca's area (left frontal lobe region in most people), critical for motor control of speech. The frontal lobe is responsible in large part for a person's affect, judgment, personality, emotions, attitudes, and inhibitions, and it contributes to the formation of thought processes.

- Parietal: The parietal lobe is the primary sensory cortex, which is located posterior to the motor strip, and is organized topographically similar to the motor strip. This lobe analyzes sensory information such as pressure, vibration, pain, and temperature, and relays the interpretation of this information to the thalamus from the sensory cortex. It is also essential to a person's awareness of their body in space, as well as orientation in space and spatial relations. For example, stereognosis, or the ability to perceive an object using the sense of touch, is processed in this area.
- Temporal: The temporal lobes contain the auditory receptive areas located around the temple regions. The interpretive area of the temporal lobe provides integration of visual and auditory areas and plays the most dominant role of any area of the cortex in thinking. Located in the posterior region of the temporal lobe is the area responsible for receptive speech referred to as *Wernicke's area.* For most people, whether right- or left-handed, Wernicke's area is located in the left lobe. Long-term memory recall is also associated with this lobe.
- Occipital: The occipital lobe located in the posterior portion of the cerebral hemispheres is known as the primary visual cortex. The occipital lobe also assists in some visual reflexes and allows for some involuntary eye movements.

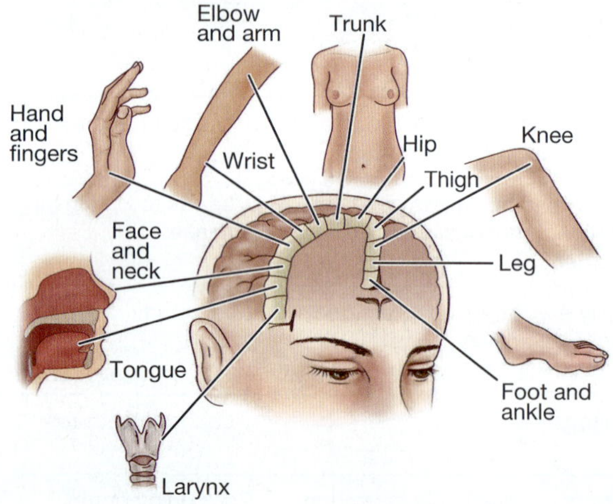

FIGURE 42-3 **Diagrammatic representation of the cerebrum showing locations for control of motor movement of various parts of the body.**

The corpus callosum (Fig. 42-4) is a thick collection of nerve fibers that connects the two hemispheres of the brain and transmits the information from one side of the brain to the other. Right-handed people and some left-handed people have cerebral dominance on the left side of the brain for verbal, linguistic, arithmetical, calculating, and analytic functions. The nondominant hemisphere is responsible for geometric, spatial, visual, pattern, and musical functions.

The basal ganglia are masses of nuclei located deep in the white matter of the cerebral hemispheres and are responsible for control of fine motor movements. The thalamus lies on either side of the third ventricle and acts primarily as a relay station for all sensations except smell. All memory also passes through this section of the brain.

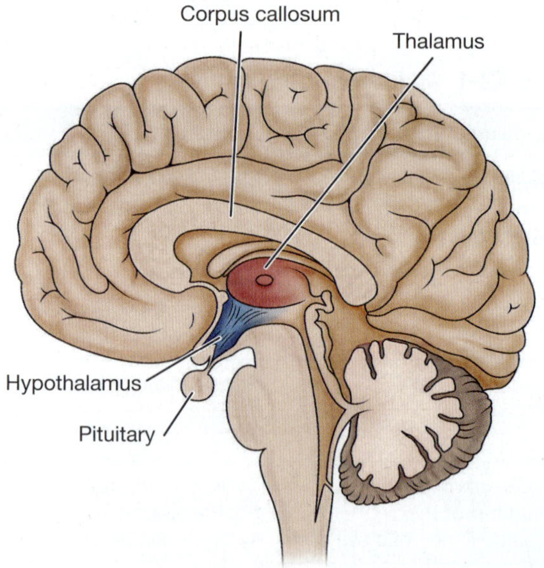

FIGURE 42-4 **Medial view of the brain. The brain is divided into the right and left hemispheres, and the two halves are connected by the corpus callosum. This bundle of nerve tissue contains over 200 million axons (nerve fibers that carry electrical impulses from neurons' cell bodies) by rough estimate. This neural tissue facilitates communication between the two sides of the brain (Healthline, 2015).**

The hypothalamus (see Fig. 42-4) is anterior and inferior to the thalamus and lies next to the third ventricle. It includes the optic chiasm (where the two optic tracts cross) and the mammillary bodies (involved in olfactory reflexes and emotional response to odors). The infundibulum of the hypothalamus connects to the posterior pituitary gland. The hypothalamus, important in the endocrine system, regulates the pituitary secretion of hormones influencing metabolism, reproduction, stress response, and urine production. It works with the pituitary to maintain fluid balance (refer to Chapter 28 for further details). In addition, the hypothalamus, the site of the hunger center, is involved in appetite control. It contains centers that regulate the sleep–wake cycle, blood pressure, aggressive and sexual behavior, and emotional responses (e.g., blushing, rage, depression, panic, and fear). The hypothalamus also controls and regulates the autonomic nervous system and maintains temperature regulation by promoting vasoconstriction or vasodilatation.

The pituitary gland is located in the sella turcica at the base of the brain. In adults, the pituitary is a common site of brain tumors, which are frequently detected by signs and symptoms traced to the pituitary, such as hormonal imbalance or visual disturbances due to pressure on the optic chiasm (see Chapter 30).

Nerve fibers from the cortex converge in each hemisphere and exit in a tight bundle of nerve fibers known as the *internal capsule.* After entering the pons and medulla, each bundle crosses to the corresponding bundle from the opposite side. Although the various cells in the cerebral cortex are quite similar in appearance, their functions vary widely, depending on location.

Brainstem. The brainstem is responsible for automatic functions such as heart rate, breathing, and swallowing. It consists of the **midbrain, pons**, and **medulla oblongata** and contains motor and sensory pathways (see Fig. 42-2). The midbrain connects the pons and cerebellum with the cerebral hemispheres and serves as the center for auditory and visual reflexes. Cranial nerves III and IV originate in the midbrain. The pons is situated in front of the cerebellum, between the midbrain and the medulla, and acts as a bridge between the cerebrum, the cerebellum, and the medulla. Cranial nerves V through VIII originate in the pons and connect the brain to the pons. Portions of the pons also control the heart rate, respiration, and blood pressure.

The medulla oblongata contains motor fibers from the brain to the spinal cord and sensory fibers from the spinal cord to the brain. Most of these fibers cross, or *decussate*, at this level. Cranial nerves IX through XII originate in the medulla and connect the brain to the medulla. The medulla and pons are essential for respiratory function.

Cerebellum. The cerebellum is separated from the cerebral hemispheres by a fold of dura mater, the *tentorium cerebelli.* The cerebellum is largely responsible for coordination of all movement. It also controls fine movement, balance, **position (postural) sense** or proprioception (awareness of where each part of the body is), and integration of sensory input.

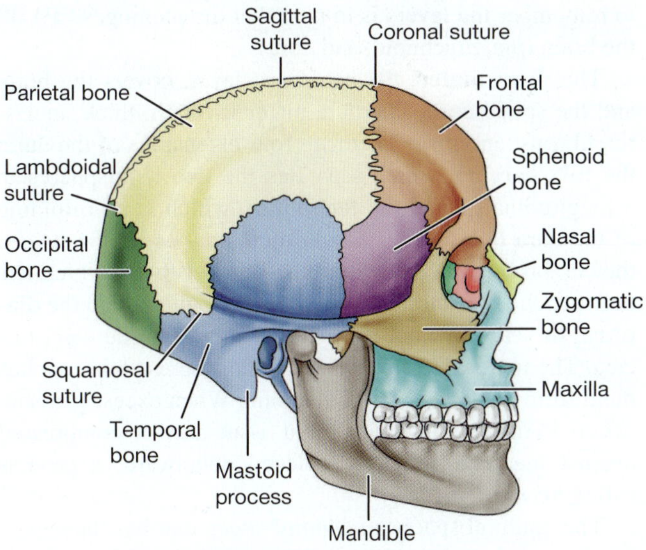

FIGURE 42-5 **Bones and sutures of the skull.**

Structures Protecting the Brain

Skull. The brain is contained in a rigid skull, protecting it from injury. The major bones of the skull are the frontal, temporal, parietal, and occipital bones (Fig. 42-5). These bones join at suture lines.

Meninges. The meninges (fibrous connective tissues) cover the brain and spinal cord, and provide protection, support, and nourishment. The three layers of the meninges are the **dura, arachnoid, and pia mater** (Fig. 42-6). An easy way

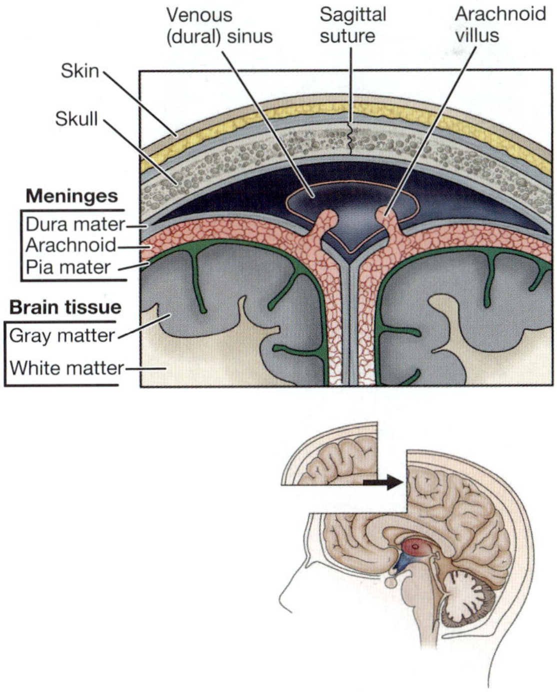

FIGURE 42-6 **Meninges and related structures.**

to remember the layers is to note that the meninges **"PAD"** the brain (*p*ia, *a*rachnoid, and *d*ura).

The **dura mater**, the outermost layer, covers the brain and the spinal cord. The dura mater is tough, thick, inelastic, fibrous, and gray. There are four extensions of the dura: the **falx cerebri**, which separates the two hemispheres in a longitudinal plane; the **tentorium**, which is an infolding of the dura that forms a tough, membranous shelf between the cerebrum and cerebellum; the **falx cerebelli**, which lies between the two lateral lobes of the cerebellum; and the **diaphragm sellae**, which provides a "roof" for the sella turcica. The tentorium supports the hemispheres and separates them from the lower part of the brain. When excess pressure occurs in the cranial cavity, brain tissue may be compressed against the tentorium or displaced downward, a process called ***herniation***.

The epidural space, a *potential space* that has the capacity to expand slightly, lies outside the outermost layer of the dura. In the spinal canal, the dura forms a tubular sheath around the spinal cord. This narrow space between the dura mater and the periosteum (lining of the bones) is where local anesthetic can be injected for pain relief.

The **arachnoid**, the middle membrane, is an extremely thin, delicate membrane resembling a spider web (hence the name arachnoid). It appears white because it has no blood supply. This membrane has unique finger-like projections, **arachnoid villi**, which absorb cerebrospinal fluid (CSF). In a normal adult, approximately 500 mL of CSF is produced each day; all but 125 to 150 mL is absorbed by the villi (Hickey, 2019). When blood enters the system (from trauma or hemorrhagic stroke), the villi become obstructed, and hydrocephalus (increased size of ventricles) may result. The subarachnoid space is between the arachnoid and pia layers and contains CSF.

The pia mater, the innermost membrane, is a thin, transparent layer that hugs the brain closely and extends into every fold of the brain's surface. It is highly vascular.

Cerebrospinal Fluid

CSF, a clear and colorless fluid, is produced in the lateral ventricles by the choroid plexus and is circulated around the brain and spinal cord through the ventricular system. There are four ventricles. The two lateral ventricles, normally containing 25 mL of CSF each, open into the third ventricle at the interventricular foramen or the foramen of Monro. The third and fourth ventricles connect via the aqueduct of Sylvius. The fourth ventricle supplies CSF to the subarachnoid space and down the spinal cord on the dorsal surface. CSF is returned to the brain and then circulated, where it is absorbed by the arachnoid villi.

The composition of CSF is similar to other extracellular fluids (such as blood plasma), but the concentrations of the various constituents differ. The laboratory report of CSF analysis usually contains information on color, specific gravity, protein count, white blood cell (WBC) count, glucose, and other electrolyte levels. Normal CSF contains a minimal number of WBCs and no red blood cells (RBCs). The intracranial pressure (ICP) within the skull results from a combination of

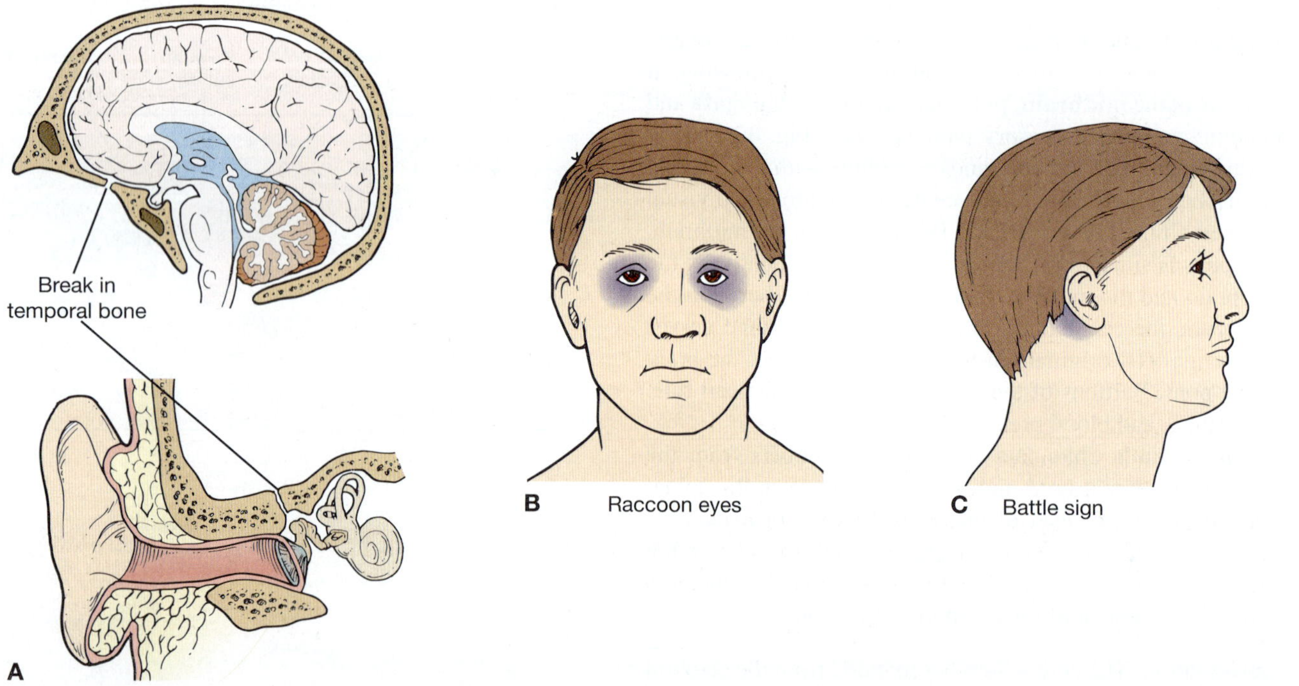

FIGURE 42-7 **A.** Basilar skull fracture in the temporal bone can cause cerebrospinal fluid (CSF) to leak from the nose or ear. **B.** Periorbital ecchymosis, called raccoon eyes. **C.** Battle sign over the mastoid process. (From Rosdahl, C. B., & Kowalski, M. [2021]. *Textbook of basic nursing* [12th ed., Fig. 78-7]. Wolters Kluwer.)

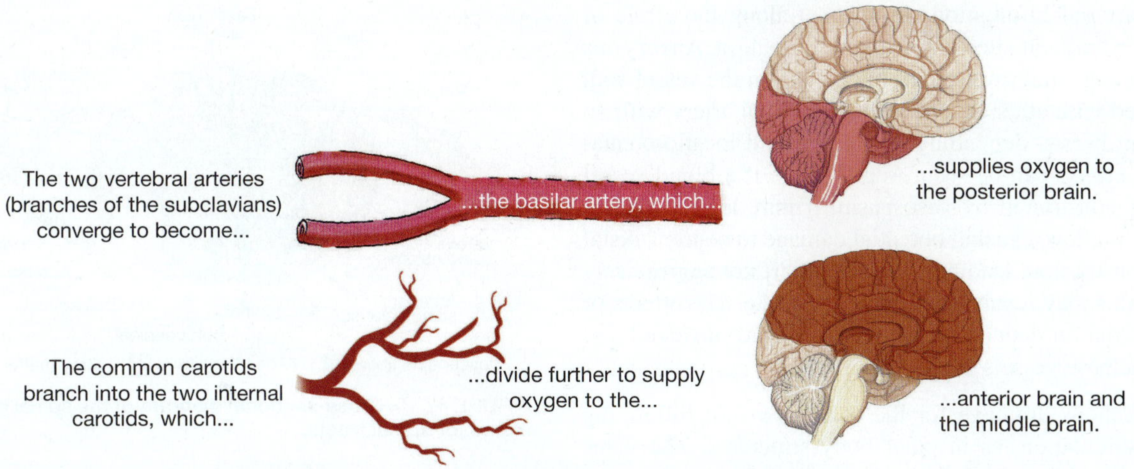

FIGURE 42-8 **Arterial circulation to the brain. (From Dyer, J. G. (2014).** ***Anatomy and physiology made incredibly visual!*** **(2nd ed., p. 62). Lippincott Williams & Wilkins.)**

brain tissue, blood flow, and CSF. Normal CSF pressure is approximately 5 to 15 mm Hg (Hickey, 2019), whereas pressures greater than 20 mm Hg indicate increased ICP.

Pearls for Practice

In the event of a skull fracture, the nurse should be alert for signs of CSF leakage. Suspect rhinorrhea (leakage of CSF via nares) with fractures involving the cribriform plates of the anterior cranial fossa, whereas otorrhea (leakage of CSF via ear) is suspected with fractures involving the basilar skull. Depending on the site of the fracture, the patient may present with ***raccoon eyes*** *(bruising around the eyes) or* ***Battle sign*** *(ecchymosis of the mastoid process of the temporal bone). Leakage of CSF places the patient at risk for meningitis. If a CSF leak is suspected, the nurse should be aware that nothing is allowed into the patient's nose or ears (suction or nasogastric catheters, dressings, tissues, etc.). For example, an orogastric tube (mouth to stomach) would be used rather than a nasogastric tube (nose to stomach). See Figure 42-7.*

Cerebral Circulation

The cerebral circulation receives approximately 15% of the cardiac output, or 750 mL per minute. The brain does not store nutrients, has a high metabolic demand, and requires high blood flow. The brain's blood pathway is unique because it flows against gravity; its arteries fill from below, and the veins drain from above. The brain has poor collateral blood flow, which results in irreversible tissue damage when blood flow is occluded for even short time periods.

Arteries. Two internal carotid arteries and two vertebral arteries and their extensive system of branches provide blood supply to the brain (Fig. 42-8). The internal carotids arise from the bifurcation of the common carotid and supply much of the anterior circulation. The vertebral arteries branch from the subclavian arteries, flow back and upward on either side of the cervical vertebrae, and enter the cranium through the foramen magnum. The vertebral arteries join to become the basilar artery at the brainstem; then the basilar artery divides to form the two branches of the posterior cerebral arteries. The vertebrobasilar arteries supply most of the posterior circulation of the brain.

The circle of Willis is formed from the branches of the anterior circulation and posterior circulation connected by one anterior communicating artery and two posterior communicating arteries (Fig. 42-9). The arteries of the circle of Willis can provide collateral circulation if one or more of the four vessels supplying it becomes occluded.

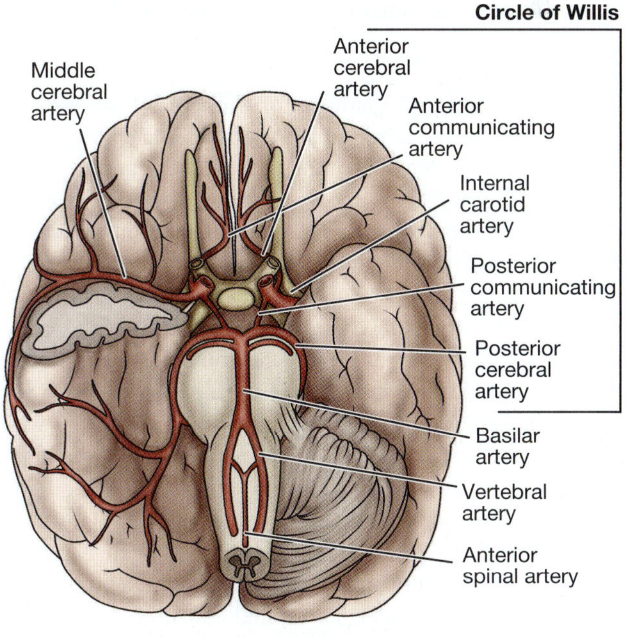

FIGURE 42-9 **Arterial blood supply of the brain, including the circle of Willis, as viewed from the ventral surface.**

The arterial bifurcations (branches) along the circle of Willis are frequent sites of aneurysm formation. Aneurysms may be congenital or result from changes in the vessel wall associated with atherosclerotic disease. If an artery with an aneurysm bursts, depending on its size and location, catastrophic effects can be seen. Additionally, if a blood vessel becomes constricted by vasospasm, it may lead to diminished blood flow, causing potential damage to neurons distal to the constriction, leading to cell death. If not aggressively treated, this may result in an ischemic stroke. The effects of the constriction depend on which vessels are involved and the areas these vessels supply.

Veins. Venous drainage for the brain does not follow the arterial circulation, as in other body structures. The veins reach the brain's surface, join larger veins, then cross the subarachnoid space and empty into the **dural sinuses**, which are the vascular channels lying within the dura mater (see Fig. 42-6). The network of sinuses empties into the internal jugular vein, returning blood to the heart. Cerebral veins and sinuses are unique because, unlike other veins, they do not have valves to prevent blood from flowing backward and depend on both gravity and blood pressure.

Blood–Brain Barrier

The CNS and its neurons are inaccessible to many substances that circulate in the blood plasma (e.g., dyes, medications, and antibiotics) because of the blood–brain barrier. This barrier is formed by the tight junction of the endothelial cells in the brain's capillaries. All substances entering the CSF must filter through the capillary endothelial cells and astrocytes (Hickey, 2019). The blood–brain barrier has a protective function but can be altered by trauma, cerebral edema, and cerebral hypoxemia; this has implications in the treatment and selection of medication for CNS disorders.

Spinal Cord

The spinal cord and medulla form a continuous structure extending from the cerebral hemispheres and serving as the connection between the brain and the periphery. Approximately 45 cm (18 in) long and about the thickness of a finger, it extends from the foramen magnum at the base of the skull to the lower border of the first lumbar vertebra, where it tapers to a fibrous band called the *conus medullaris.* Continuing below the second lumbar space are the nerve roots that extend beyond the conus, which are called the *cauda equina* because they resemble a horse's tail. Similar to the brain, the spinal cord consists of gray and white matter. Gray matter in the brain is external and white matter is internal; in the spinal cord, gray matter is in the center and is surrounded on all sides by white matter (Fig. 42-10). The spinal cord is an H-shaped structure with nerve cell bodies (gray matter) surrounded by ascending and descending tracts (white matter). The spinal cord is encased by the meninges as in the brain including the pia mater, arachnoid, and dura mater.

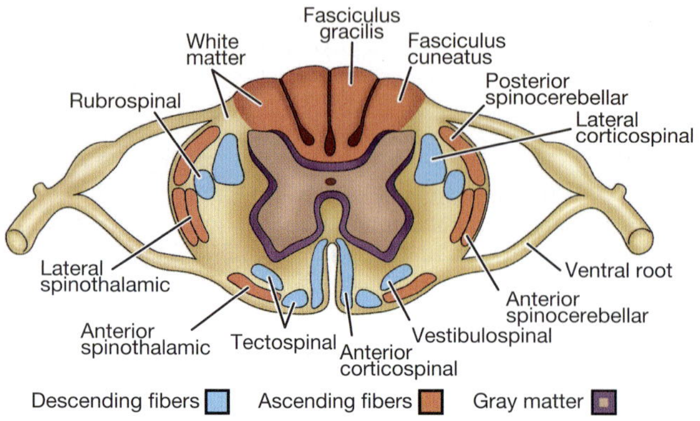

FIGURE 42-10 **Cross-sectional diagram of the spinal cord showing major spinal tracts.**

Pearls for Practice

The nurse understands that the spinal cord extends to L1; therefore, if a lumbar puncture (spinal tap) is to be performed, the site for insertion of the needle will be below L1. Typically the needle is placed in the interspace between L3 and L4 or between L4 and L5, which is a safe distance from the distal spinal cord. The bony landmark for the L4 spinous process is located at the intersection of the line between the top of the iliac crests and the midline of the lumbar spine.

Sensory and Motor Pathways: The Spinal Tracts. The white matter of the cord is composed of **myelinated** and **unmyelinated** nerve fibers. The fast-conducting **myelinated fibers** form bundles that also contain **glial cells**. Fiber bundles with a common function are called ***tracts***.

There are six **ascending** tracts (see Fig. 42-10). Two conduct sensation, principally the perception of touch, pressure, vibration, position, and passive motion from the same side of the body. Before reaching the cerebral cortex, these fibers cross to the opposite side in the medulla. The two spinocerebellar tracts conduct sensory impulses from muscle spindles, providing necessary input for coordinated muscle contraction. They ascend essentially uncrossed and terminate in the cerebellum. The last two spinothalamic tracts are responsible for conduction of pain, temperature, proprioception, fine touch, and vibratory sense from the upper body to the brain. They ascend, cross to the opposite side of the brain, and terminate in the thalamus.

There are eight **descending** tracts. The two corticospinal tracts conduct motor impulses to the anterior horn cells from the opposite side of the brain and control voluntary muscle activity. The three vestibulospinal tracts descend uncrossed and are involved in some autonomic functions (sweating, pupil dilation, and circulation) and involuntary muscle control. The corticobulbar tract conducts impulses responsible for voluntary head and facial muscle movement and crosses at the level of the brainstem. The rubrospinal and reticulospinal tracts conduct impulses involved with involuntary muscle movement.

Vertebral Column. The bones of the vertebral column surround and protect the spinal cord and normally consist of seven **cervical**, twelve **thoracic**, and five **lumbar** vertebrae, as well as the **sacrum** (a fused mass of five vertebrae), and terminate in the **coccyx**. Nerve roots exit from the vertebral column through the intervertebral foramina (openings). The vertebrae are separated by disks, except for the first and second cervical, the sacral, and the coccygeal vertebrae. The vertebral body, arch, pedicles, and laminae all encase and protect the spinal cord.

The Peripheral Nervous System

The PNS includes the **cranial nerves**, the **spinal nerves**, and the **autonomic nervous system**.

Cranial Nerves

Twelve pairs of cranial nerves emerge from the lower surface of the brain and pass through the foramina in the skull (Fig. 42-11). Three are entirely sensory (I, II, VIII), five are motor (III, IV, VI, XI, and XII), and four are mixed (V, VII, IX, and X) because they have both sensory and motor functions. Most cranial nerves innervate the head, neck, and special sense structures. Table 42-2 lists the names and primary functions of the cranial nerves.

Pearls for Practice

Anisocoria is the term for unequal pupils. A difference of 1 mm or less between pupils occurs in approximately 20% of the population. This is termed physiologic anisocoria. However, if the nurse discovers a new pupil asymmetry, this finding must be reported immediately and the patient must be reassessed for other neurologic changes as any change in pupillary reaction can indicate neurologic deterioration (Ryan, 2019).

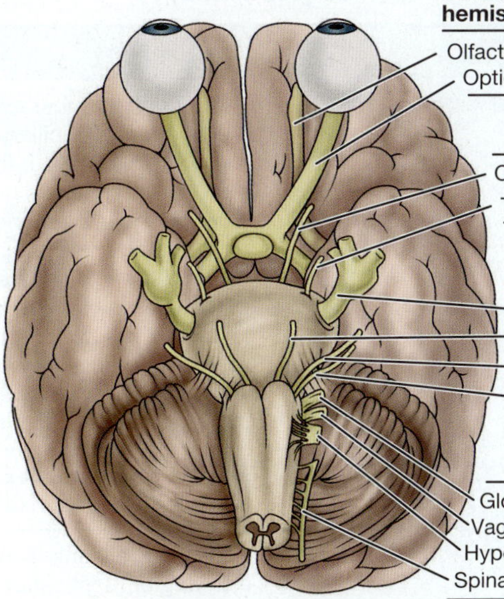

FIGURE 42-11 Diagram of the base of the brain showing entrance or exit of the cranial nerves. The right column shows the anatomic location of the connection of each cranial nerve to the central nervous system.

Spinal Nerves

The spinal cord is composed of 31 **pairs of spinal nerves**: eight cervical, twelve thoracic, five lumbar, five sacral, and one coccygeal. Each spinal nerve has a **ventral** and a **dorsal** root (Fig. 42-12).

The dorsal roots are sensory and transmit sensory impulses from specific areas of the body known as ***dermatomes*** (Fig. 42-13) to the dorsal ganglia. The sensory fiber may be **somatic**, carrying information about pain, temperature, touch, and position sense (proprioception) from

TABLE **42-2 Cranial Nerves**

Cranial Nerve (CN)	Type	Assessment	Dysfunction
I (Olfactory)	Sensory	With eyes closed, the patient should be asked to identify two familiar odors (e.g., coffee, tobacco). Each nostril is tested separately. Avoid using strong odors, such as ammonia, as the trigeminal nerve may be stimulated. Testing of this CN is usually deferred.	Inability to identify odor, termed anosmia
II (Optic)	Sensory	Assess visual acuity using a portable eye chart or, if not available, grossly assess vision by having the patient read a card or newspaper from big print to small. Assess visual fields by testing peripheral vision: stand directly in front of the patient. Ask the patient to close one eye and focus on your nose as you assess the patient's ability to see your fingers that are positioned in four visual fields (upper right and left and lower right and left). In combination with CN III, assess the pupils (the light emitted into the pupil begins the process by which constriction is seen; constriction is the function of CN III).	Decreased visual acuity Decreased visual fields

(continued)

TABLE **42-2 Cranial Nerves (*continued*)**

Cranial Nerve (CN)	Type	Assessment	Dysfunction
III (Oculomotor)	Motor	CN III controls most extraocular eye movement (EOM), eyelid elevation, and pupillary constriction. To assess EOM, ask the patient to follow your finger through the six cardinal positions (use the letter H as a guide to assess the ability of the eye to move to the left superior, left lateral, left inferior, right superior, right lateral, and right inferior). CN III is responsible for all movements except lateral movement (CN VI) and movement of the eye downward and inward (CN IV). While the patient is looking at the six positions, have them hold the position briefly while you assess for nystagmus (rotary oscillation of the eye). Test for pupillary reflexes (constriction of the pupil to light),and inspect the eyelids for ptosis (drooping of the eyelid).	Inability to move the eyes in the visual field described Ptosis of affected eye Nonreactive or dilated pupil
IV (Trochlear)	Motor	This is assessed with EOM as described above. CN IV moves the eye down and in (as if looking toward the nose).	Inability to look down and in
V (Trigeminal)	Mixed	Assess facial sensation, corneal reflex (sensory aspect), and chewing or mastication. Have the patient close the eyes. Touch cotton to the patient's forehead, cheeks, and jaw. Test sensitivity to superficial pain in these same three areas by using the sharp and dull ends of a broken tongue blade. Alternate between the sharp point and the dull end. Patient reports "sharp" or "dull" with each movement. If responses are incorrect, test for temperature sensation. Test tubes of cold and hot water are used alternately. To assess chewing, ask the patient to clench the jaw while you palpate the temporal and masseter muscles. Corneal reflex may be assessed by having the patient look up and away while you brush the cornea with a wisp of cotton; both eyes should blink (Note: use of contact lens decreases this response). Similar to the pupillary reaction (CN II and III), corneal reflexes are a combination CN V and VII.	Absence of corneal reflex Diminished sensation to forehead, maxillary, and mandibular regions Weakness of muscles responsible for chewing
VI (Abducens)	Motor	Abducens moves the eye laterally (side to side or horizontally) and is assessed with EOMs.	Inability to look laterally, double vision
VII (Facial)	Mixed	Assess for symmetry of facial movement. Ask the patient to smile, raise the eyebrows, keep eyes and lips closed while you try to open them, and puff out the cheeks. Taste is also a function of this CN, although testing is often deferred. The motor response of closing the eye in response to stimuli is assessed with corneal reflex (combination of CN V and VII).	Facial paralysis Facial asymmetry, droop of mouth Absent nasolabial fold Decreased ability to taste
VIII (Acoustic)	Sensory	Assess hearing by rubbing your fingers, placing a ticking watch, or whispering near each ear. Equilibrium can be assessed with the Romberg test and is usually deferred.	Decreased hearing in affected ear
IX (Glossopharyngeal)	Mixed	This CN's function is primarily innervation of the pharynx and tongue, pharyngeal muscles, and swallowing. Ask the patient to open the mouth and say "Ah." Note symmetric elevation of the upper palate and uvula in the midline position. Assessing for the gag reflex tests this nerve and CN X, as they travel together. To test gag reflex, use a cotton swab or tongue blade to touch the patient's posterior pharynx; note gag response.	Dysphagia Absence of gag reflex
X (Vagus)	Mixed	This CN is assessed by swallowing and gag reflex as noted above. In addition, the quality of the patient's voice is noted.	Hoarse or nasal quality to voice Slurred speech
XI (Spinal accessory)	Motor	Have the patient shrug the shoulders and turn their head from side to side; assess the sternocleidomastoid and trapezius muscles for symmetry.	Inability to shrug shoulders
XII (Hypoglossal)	Motor	Inspect the patient's tongue for atrophy at rest. To assess movement of the tongue, have the patient stick out the tongue and move it internally from cheek to cheek.	Tongue weakness

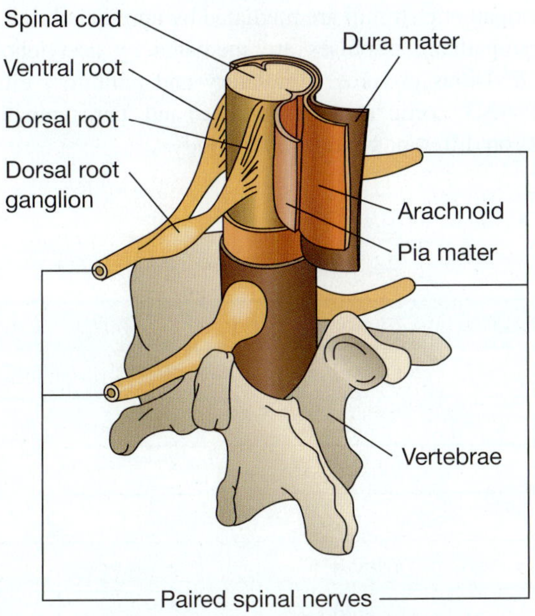

FIGURE 42-12 **Spinal cord and meninges. (From Norris, T. L., & Lalchandani, R. [2018].** ***Porth's pathophysiology*** **[10th ed., Fig. 13.13]. Lippincott Williams & Wilkins.)**

the tendons, joints, and body surfaces; or **visceral**, carrying information from the internal organs.

The ventral roots are motor and transmit impulses from the spinal cord to the body, and these fibers are also either somatic or visceral. The visceral fibers include autonomic fibers that control the cardiac muscles and glandular secretions.

Autonomic Nervous System

The **autonomic nervous system** regulates activities of internal organs, such as the heart, lungs, blood vessels, digestive organs, and glands. Maintenance and restoration of internal homeostasis is largely the responsibility of the autonomic nervous system. There are two major divisions: the **sympathetic nervous system,** with predominantly excitatory responses, most notably the "fight-or-flight" response, and the **parasympathetic nervous system**, which controls mostly visceral functions, known as "rest-and-digest."

The autonomic nervous system is regulated by centers in the spinal cord, brainstem, and hypothalamus. Its regulatory effects are exerted not on individual cells but on large expanses of tissue and on entire organs. The responses elicited do not occur instantaneously but after a lag period.

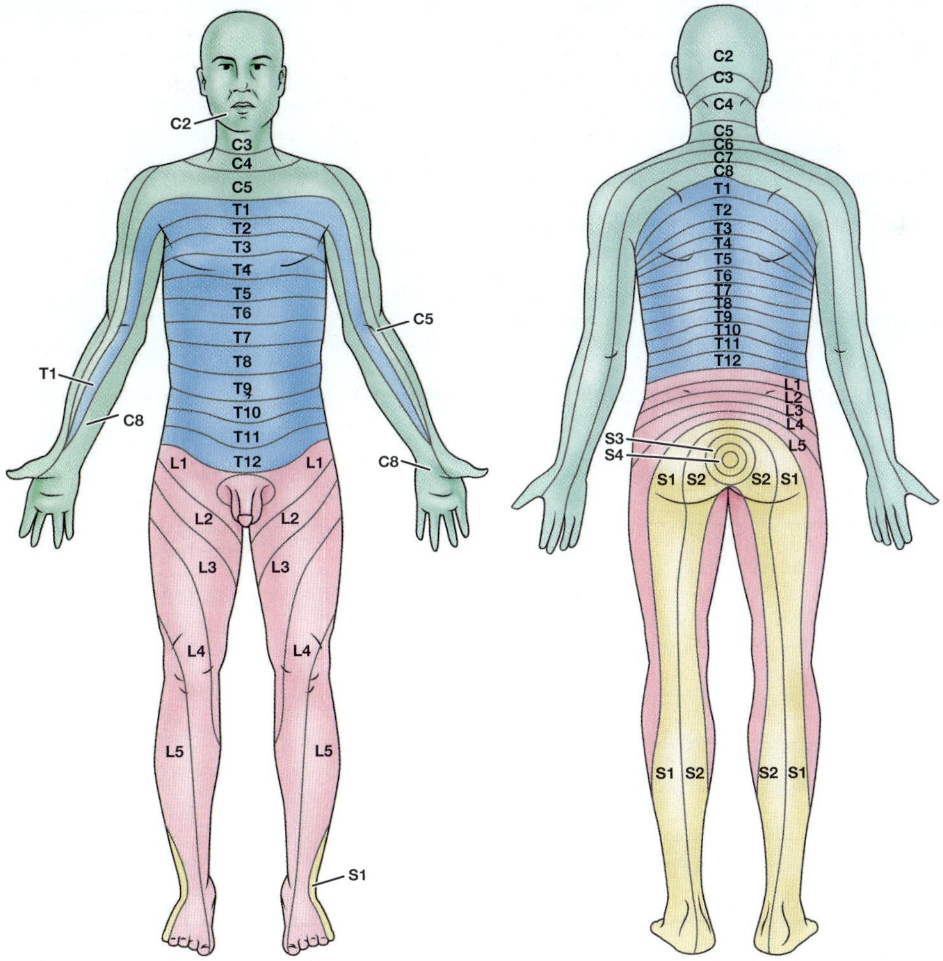

FIGURE 42-13 **Dermatome distribution.**

These responses are sustained far longer than other neurogenic responses to ensure maximal functional efficiency on the part of receptor organs, such as blood vessels. The autonomic nervous system transmits its impulses by way of nerve pathways, enhanced by chemical mediators.

Sympathetic stimuli are mediated by norepinephrine, and parasympathetic impulses are mediated by acetylcholine. Both divisions produce stimulatory and inhibitory effects. Table 42-3 compares sympathetic and parasympathetic effects on different systems of the body.

TABLE **42-3 Autonomic Effects of the Nervous System**

Structure or Activity	Parasympathetic Effects	Sympathetic Effects
Pupil of the Eye	Constricted	Dilated
Circulatory System		
Rate and force of heartbeat	Decreased	Increased
Blood Vessels		
In heart muscle	Constricted	Dilated
In skeletal muscle	[a]	Dilated
In abdominal viscera and the skin	[a]	Constricted
Blood pressure	Decreased	Increased
Respiratory System		
Bronchioles	Constricted	Dilated
Rate of breathing	Decreased	Increased
Digestive System		
Peristaltic movements of digestive tube	Increased	Decreased
Muscular sphincters of digestive tube	Relaxed	Contracted
Secretion of salivary glands	Thin, watery saliva	Thick, viscid saliva
Secretions of stomach, intestine, and pancreas	Increased	[a]
Conversion of liver glycogen to glucose	[a]	Increased
Genitourinary System		
Urinary bladder Muscle walls	Contracted	Relaxed
Sphincters	Relaxed	Contracted
Muscles of the uterus	Relaxed; variable	Contracted under some conditions; varies with menstrual cycle and pregnancy
Blood vessels of external genitalia	Dilated	[a]
Integumentary System		
Secretion of sweat	[a]	Increased
Pilomotor muscles	[a]	Contracted (gooseflesh)
Adrenal Medulla	[a]	Secretion of epinephrine and norepinephrine

[a]No direct effect.

From Hickey, J., & Strayer, A. L. (2019). *Clinical practice of neurological and neurosurgical nursing* (8th ed.). Lippincott Williams & Wilkins.

Motor and Sensory Functions of the Nervous System

Motor System Function

The motor cortex, a vertical band within each cerebral hemisphere, controls the voluntary movements of the body. The exact locations within the brain at which the voluntary movements of the muscles of the face, thumb, hand, arm, trunk, and leg originate are known (see Fig. 42-3). Stimulation of these cells results in muscle contraction. En route to the pons, the motor fibers converge into a tight bundle known as the ***internal capsule***. A comparatively small injury to the capsule results in paralysis in more muscles than does a much larger injury to the cortex itself.

Within the medulla, the motor axons from the cortex form the **corticospinal** or **pyramidal tracts**. Here, most of the fibers cross (or decussate) to the opposite side. The remaining fibers enter the spinal cord on the same side as the direct pyramidal tract. All of the motor fibers of the spinal nerves represent extensions of the anterior horn cells, with each of these fibers communicating with only one particular muscle fiber. The motor system is complex, and motor function depends on the integrity of the corticospinal tracts, the extrapyramidal system, and cerebellar function.

Upper and Lower Motor Neurons

The voluntary motor system consists of two groups of neurons: **upper motor neurons** and **lower motor neurons**. Upper motor neurons originate in the cerebral cortex, the cerebellum, and the brainstem, where they cross over and descend throughout the corticospinal tract. Their fibers make up the descending motor pathways, are located entirely within the CNS, and modulate the activity of the lower motor neurons. Lower motor neurons are located either in the anterior horn of the spinal cord gray matter or within cranial nerve nuclei in the brainstem. Axons of lower motor neurons in both sites extend through peripheral nerves and terminate in skeletal muscle at the myoneural junction. Lower motor neurons are located in both the CNS and the PNS. The clinical features of lesions of upper and lower motor neurons are discussed in Table 42-4.

TABLE 42-4 Comparison of Lesions of the Upper Motor Neurons and Lower Motor Neurons

Upper Motor Neuron Lesions	Lower Motor Neuron Lesions
Loss of voluntary control	Loss of voluntary control
Increased muscle tone	Decreased muscle tone
Muscle spasticity	Flaccid muscle paralysis
No muscle atrophy	Muscle atrophy
Hyperactive and abnormal	Absent or decreased reflexes

Coordination of Movement

The smoothness, accuracy, and strength that characterize muscular movements are attributable to the influence of the cerebellum and the basal ganglia.

The cerebellum (see Fig. 42-2) is responsible for the coordination, balance, and timing of all muscular movements. Through the action of the cerebellum, the contractions of opposing muscle groups are adjusted in relation to each other to maximal mechanical advantage.

The basal ganglia play an important role in planning and coordinating motor movements and posture. Complex neural connections link the basal ganglia with the cerebral cortex. The major effect of these structures is to inhibit unwanted muscular activity; disorders of the basal ganglia result in exaggerated, uncontrolled movements.

Impaired cerebellar function, which may occur as a result of an intracranial injury, cerebrovascular event, or some type of an expanding mass, results in loss of muscle tone, weakness, and fatigue. Cerebellar signs such as ataxia, which is an inability to coordinate voluntary muscular movements and incoordination, or CSF obstruction and compression of the brainstem may be seen. Signs of increased ICP, including vomiting, headache, and changes in vital signs and level of consciousness (LOC), are especially common when CSF flow is obstructed.

Destruction or dysfunction of the basal ganglia leads not to paralysis but to muscle rigidity, with disturbances of posture and movement. The patient tends to have involuntary movements. These may take the form of coarse tremors, most often in the upper extremities, particularly in the distal portions; athetosis (movement of a slow, squirming, writhing, twisting type); or chorea (spasmodic, purposeless, irregular, uncoordinated motions of the trunk and the extremities, and facial grimacing). Disorders due to lesions of the basal ganglia include Parkinson disease, Huntington disease, and spasmodic torticollis (a painful condition where neck muscles contract involuntarily, causing the head to twist or turn to one side).

Sensory System Function

Integrating Sensory Impulses

The thalamus, a major receiving and transmitting center for the afferent sensory nerves, is a large structure connected to the midbrain (see Fig. 42-4). The thalamus integrates all sensory impulses except olfaction. It plays a role in the conscious awareness of pain and the recognition of variation in temperature and touch. The thalamus is responsible for the sense of movement and position and the ability to recognize the size, shape, and quality of objects.

Receiving Sensory Impulses

Afferent impulses travel from their points of origin to their destinations in the cerebral cortex via the ascending pathways directly, or they may cross at the level of the spinal cord or in the medulla, depending on the type of sensation that is registered. Sensory information may be integrated at the level of the spinal cord or may be relayed to the brain. Knowledge of these pathways is important for neurologic assessment and for understanding symptoms and their relationship to various lesions.

Sensory Losses

Destruction of a sensory nerve results in total loss of sensation in its area of distribution. **Transection** of the spinal cord yields complete anesthesia (a lack of feeling or sensation) below the level of injury. Selective destruction or degeneration of the posterior columns of the spinal cord is responsible for a loss of position and vibratory sense in segments distal to the lesion, without loss of touch, pain, or temperature perception. A lesion, such as a cyst, in the center of the spinal cord causes dissociation of sensation—loss of pain at the level of the lesion. This occurs because the fibers carrying pain and temperature cross within the cord immediately on entering; thus, any lesion that divides the cord longitudinally divides these fibers. Damage to the anterior spinal cord would result in loss of motor function, as well as pain and temperature with preservation of vibratory, position, and touch.

Lesions affecting the posterior spinal nerve roots may cause impairment of tactile sensation, including intermittent severe pain that is referred to the area of distribution. Tingling of the fingers and toes can be a prominent symptom of spinal cord disease, presumably due to degenerative changes in the sensory fibers that extend to the thalamus (i.e., belonging to the spinothalamic tract).

Gerontologic Considerations

During the normal aging process, the nervous system undergoes many changes, and it is extremely vulnerable to general systemic illness. Changes throughout the nervous system that occur with age vary in degree. Nerve fibers that connect directly to muscles show little decline in function with age, as do simple neurologic functions that involve a number of connections in the spinal cord. Disease in older patients often makes it difficult to distinguish normal from abnormal changes. It is important for clinicians not to attribute abnormality or dysfunction to aging without appropriate investigation. Pain in the absence of disease, for example, is not a normal part of aging and should be assessed, diagnosed, and treated. Table 42-5 summarizes structural changes.

Structural Changes

A number of alterations occur with increasing age. Brain weight decreases, as does the number of synapses. A loss of neurons occurs in select regions of the brain. Cerebral blood flow and metabolism are reduced. Temperature regulation becomes less efficient. In the PNS, myelin is lost, resulting in a decrease in conduction velocity in some nerves. There is an overall reduction in muscle bulk and the electrical activity within muscles. Taste buds atrophy, and nerve cell fibers in the olfactory bulb degenerate. Nerve cells in the vestibular system of the inner ear, cerebellum, and proprioceptive pathways also degenerate. Deep tendon reflexes can be decreased or, in some cases, absent. Hypothalamic function is modified such that stage IV sleep is reduced. There is an overall slowing of autonomic nervous system responses. Pupillary responses are reduced or may not appear at all in the presence of cataracts.

Motor Alterations

Changes in motor function often result in a flexed posture, shuffling gait, and rigidity of movement. These changes create difficulties for an older person in maintaining or recovering balance. Strength and agility are diminished, and reaction time and movement time are decreased. Repetitive

TABLE **42-5 GERONTOLOGIC CONSIDERATIONS / Age-Related Changes in the Neurologic System**

Structural changes	Brain weight decreases Loss of neurons in the brain Reduced cerebral blood flow Decreased myelin, resulting in decreased nerve conduction in some nerves Decrease in muscle bulk Slowing in deep tendon reflexes Overall slowing of the autonomic and sympathetic nervous system Temperature regulation becomes less efficient Reduced pupillary response
Sensory changes	Atrophy of taste buds Degeneration of olfactory bulb Degeneration of nerve cells in vestibular system of inner ear, cerebellum, and proprioceptive pathways Decreased neural transmission leading to difficulty in discriminating important sounds from background noise; hearing loss becomes more common Stage IV sleep is decreased; sleep apnea becomes more common Presence of cataracts Dulling of tactile sensation

movements and mild tremors may be noted during an examination and may be of concern to the person. Observation of gait may reveal a wide-based gait with balance difficulties.

Sensory Alterations

Sensory isolation due to visual and hearing loss can cause confusion, anxiety, disorientation, misinterpretation of the environment, and feelings of inadequacy. Sensory alterations may require modification of the home environment, such as large-print reading materials or sound enhancement for the telephone, as well as extra orientation to new surroundings. Simple explanations of routines, the location of the bathroom, and how to operate the call bell or light are just a few examples of information an older individual may need when hospitalized.

Temperature Regulation and Pain Perception

Other manifestations of neurologic changes are related to temperature regulation and pain. The older patient may feel cold more readily than heat and may require extra covering when in bed; a room temperature somewhat higher than usual may be desirable. Reaction to painful stimuli may be decreased with age. Because pain is an important warning signal, caution must be used when hot or cold packs are used. The older patient may be burned or suffer frostbite before being aware of any discomfort. Reports of pain, such as abdominal discomfort or chest pain, may be more serious than the patient's perception might indicate and thus require careful evaluation. Two pain syndromes that are common in the neurologic system in older adults are diabetic neuropathies and postherpetic neuropathies (refer to Chapters 29 and 51 for further information).

Taste and Smell Alterations

The acuity of the taste buds decreases with age; along with an altered olfactory sense, this may cause a decreased appetite and subsequent weight loss. Extra seasoning often increases food intake as long as it does not cause gastric irritation. A decreased sense of smell due to atrophy of olfactory organs may present a safety hazard because older people living alone may be unable to detect household gas leaks or fires. Smoke and carbon monoxide detectors, important for all, are critical for older individuals.

Tactile and Visual Alterations

Another neurologic alteration in the older patient is the dulling of tactile sensation. There may be difficulty in identifying objects by touch, and because fewer tactile cues are received from the bottom of the feet, the person may become confused about body position and location.

These factors, combined with sensitivity to glare, decreased peripheral vision, and a constricted visual field, may result in disorientation, especially at night when there is little or no light in the room. Because an older person takes longer to recover visual sensitivity when moving from a light to dark area, night-lights and a safe and familiar arrangement of furniture are essential.

Mental Status

Mental status is evaluated when obtaining the history. Areas of judgment, intelligence, memory, affect, mood, orientation, speech, and grooming are assessed. Family members who bring the patient to the attention of the health care provider may have noticed changes in the patient's mental status. Drug toxicity should always be suspected as a causative factor when the patient has a change in mental status. **Delirium** (mental confusion, usually with delusions and hallucinations) is seen in older patients who have underlying CNS damage or are experiencing an acute condition, such as infection, adverse medication reaction, or dehydration. Many older patients admitted to the hospital have delirium, and the cause is often reversible and treatable (e.g., drug toxicity, vitamin B deficiency, thyroid disease). Depression may produce impairment of attention and memory. In older patients, delirium, which is an acute change in mental status attributable to a treatable medical problem, must be differentiated from dementia, which is a chronic and irreversible deterioration of cognitive status.

Nursing Implications

Nursing care for patients with age-related changes to the nervous system and for patients with a long-term neurologic disability who are aging should include the previously described modifications. In addition, the consequences of any neurologic deficit and its impact on overall function, such as activities of daily living, use of assistive devices, and individual coping, should be assessed and considered in planning patient care.

Patient teaching is also affected because the nurse must understand the altered responses and the changing needs of the older patient before beginning to teach. When caring for the older patient, the nurse adapts activities, such as preoperative teaching; diet therapy; and instruction about new medications, their timing, and doses; to the patient's needs and capabilities. The nurse considers the presence of decline in fine motor movement and failing vision. When using visual materials for teaching or menu selection, adequate lighting without glare, contrasting colors, and large print are used to offset visual difficulties caused by rigidity and opacity of the lens in the eye and slower pupillary reaction.

Even with hearing loss, the older patient often hears adequately if the speaker uses a low-pitched, clear voice; shouting only makes it harder for the patient to understand the speaker. Providing auditory and visual cues aids understanding; if the patient has a significant hearing or visual loss, assistive devices, a signer, or a translator may be needed.

Teaching at an unrushed pace and using reinforcement enhances learning and retention. Material should be short, concise, and concrete. Vocabulary is matched to the patient's ability, and terms are clearly defined. An older patient requires adequate time to receive and respond to stimuli, learn, and react. These measures allow comprehension, memory, and formation of association and concepts.

ASSESSMENT

Health History

The history-taking portion of the neurologic assessment is critical and, in many cases of neurologic disease, leads to an accurate diagnosis. The initial interview provides an excellent opportunity to systematically explore the patient's current condition and related events while simultaneously observing overall appearance, mental status, posture, movement, and affect. Depending on the patient's condition, the nurse may need to rely on yes-or-no answers to questions, a review of the medical record, input from the family, or a combination of these.

Common Concerns

An important aspect of the neurologic assessment is the history of the present illness. Neurologic disease may be acute or progressive, characterized by symptom-free periods as well as fluctuations in symptoms. Therefore, the nurse asks about the onset, character, severity, location, duration, and frequency of symptoms and signs; associated complaints; precipitating, aggravating, and relieving factors; progression, remission, and exacerbation; and the presence or absence of similar symptoms among family members.

The clinical manifestations of neurologic disease are as varied as the disease processes themselves. Symptoms may be subtle or intense, fluctuating or permanent, inconvenient or devastating. An introduction to some of the more common symptoms associated with neurologic disease is given in this chapter. Detailed discussions regarding how specific symptoms relate to a particular disorder are covered in later chapters in this unit.

Pain

Pain is considered an unpleasant sensory perception and emotional experience associated with actual or potential tissue damage or described in terms of such damage. Therefore, pain is viewed as multidimensional and entirely subjective. Pain can be acute or chronic. In general, acute pain lasts for a relatively short period of time and remits as the pathology resolves. In neurologic disease, acute pain is often associated with spinal disk disease, trigeminal neuralgia, or other neuropathic pathology (e.g., postherpetic neuralgia or painful neuropathies). In contrast, chronic or persistent pain extends for long periods of time and may represent a low level of pathology. This type of pain can occur with many degenerative and chronic neurologic conditions (e.g., cerebral palsy).

Headache and Migraine

Headache, or cephalalgia, is one of the most common of all human physical complaints. Headache is a symptom rather than a disease entity; it may indicate organic disease (neurologic or other disease), a stress response, vasodilation (migraine), skeletal muscle tension (tension headache), or a combination of factors. A **primary headache** is one for which no organic cause can be identified. These types of headache include migraine, tension-type, and cluster headaches. **Migraine headache** is characterized by periodic and recurrent attacks of severe headaches lasting from 4 to 72 hours in adults. The cause of migraine has not been clearly demonstrated, but it is primarily a vascular disturbance that occurs more commonly in females and has a strong familial tendency (Pescador-Ruschel & De Jesus, 2021). The typical time of onset is at puberty, and the highest prevalence in adults occurs between 25 and 55 years of age. Migraine headaches may occur with or without an aura (a sensation that precedes the headache); however, most patients do not exhibit auras. Migraine with aura affects 5% of the adult population, and 90% of auras are visual.

A **secondary headache** is a symptom associated with an organic cause, such as a brain tumor or an aneurysm. Although most headaches do not indicate serious disease, persistent headaches require further investigation. Serious disorders related to headache include brain tumors, subarachnoid hemorrhage, stroke, severe hypertension, meningitis, and head injuries.

Temporal arteritis is a cause of headache in the older population, reaching its greatest incidence in those older than 70 years of age. Inflammation of the cranial arteries is characterized by a severe headache localized in the region of the temporal arteries. The inflammation may be generalized (in which case temporal arteritis is part of a vascular disease) or focal (in which case only the cranial arteries are involved) and may be associated with visual loss.

Seizures

Seizures are the result of abnormal paroxysmal discharges in the cerebral cortex, which then manifest as an alteration in sensation, behavior, movement, perception, or consciousness. The alteration may be short, such as a blank stare that lasts only a second, or of longer duration, such as a tonic–clonic seizure that can last several minutes. The type of seizure activity is a direct result of the area of the brain affected. Seizures can occur as isolated events, such as when induced by a high fever, alcohol or drug withdrawal, or hypoglycemia. A seizure may also be the first obvious sign of a brain lesion.

Dizziness and Vertigo

Dizziness is an abnormal sensation of imbalance or movement. It is fairly common in the older people and one of the more common complaints encountered by health professionals. Dizziness can occur as a result of a variety of medical conditions that include viral syndromes, hypotension, cardiac arrhythmia, hypoglycemia, middle ear infections, and others. One difficulty confronting health care providers when assessing dizziness is the vague and varied terms patients use to describe the sensation.

About 50% of all patients with dizziness have **vertigo**, which is defined as an illusion of movement, usually rotation. Vertigo is usually a manifestation of vestibular dysfunction. It can be so severe as to result in spatial disorientation, light-headedness, loss of equilibrium (staggering), and nausea and vomiting.

Visual Disturbances

Visual defects that cause people to seek health care can range from the decreased visual acuity associated with aging to sudden blindness caused by acute glaucoma. Normal vision depends on functioning visual pathways through the retina and optic chiasm and the radiations into the visual cortex in the occipital lobes. Lesions of the eye itself (e.g., cataract), lesions along the pathway (e.g., tumor), or lesions in the visual cortex (from stroke) interfere with normal visual acuity. Abnormalities of eye movement can also compromise vision by causing **diplopia** or double vision.

Weakness

Weakness, specifically muscle weakness, is a common manifestation of neurologic disease. Weakness frequently coexists with other symptoms of disease and can affect a variety of muscles, causing a wide range of disabilities. Weakness can be sudden and permanent, as in stroke; or progressive, as in many neuromuscular diseases, such as amyotrophic lateral sclerosis (ALS). Any muscle group can be affected.

Abnormal Sensation

Numbness, abnormal sensation, or loss of sensation is a neurologic manifestation of both central and peripheral nerve disease. Altered sensation can affect small or large areas of the body. It is frequently associated with weakness or pain and is potentially disabling. Both numbness and weakness can significantly affect balance and coordination.

History

A review of the medical history, including a system-by-system evaluation, is part of the health history. The nurse should be aware of any history of trauma or falls that may have involved the head or spinal cord.

Family History

The nurse may also use the interview to inquire about any family history of genetic diseases, such as Huntington disease, dystonia, and epilepsy.

Social History

The nurse questions the patient regarding the use of alcohol, medications (including over-the-counter medications and supplements), and illicit drugs, and assesses for signs and symptoms of withdrawal. Additionally, the nurse is aware that certain agents, such as sedatives, analgesics, or neuromuscular blocking agents, may interfere with an accurate neurologic assessment.

The nurse assesses the impact that any neurologic impairment has on the patient's lifestyle. Issues to consider include the limitations imposed on the patient by any deficit and the patient's role in society, including family and community roles. The plan of care that the nurse develops needs to address and support adaptation to the neurologic deficit and continued function to the extent possible within the patient's support system.

There is an increasing awareness that the social and structural determinants of health should be considered when assessing patients. When considering a patient's risk for disease, the nurse needs to consider social variables such as educational level, annual household income, insurance status, geographical region, and social support as well as structural variables such as public health and transportation infrastructure, food delivery systems, and cultural norms, among others (Maalouf et al., 2021; Murray, 2021).

Lifting the Lens

The nurse is aware that as the number of social determinants of health affecting a patient increases, so too does that person's incidence of stroke. For example, in those 75 or younger, stroke risk was more than 2.5 times higher for people with three or more social determinants of health than in those with no social determinants of health (Reshetnyak et al., 2020).

Physical Assessment

The neurologic examination is a systematic process that includes a variety of clinical tests, observations, and assessments designed to evaluate the neurologic status of a complex system. Although the neurologic examination is often limited to a simple screening, the examiner must be able to conduct a thorough neurologic assessment when the patient's history or other physical findings warrant it. An example of a simple screening tool for patients with head injury is the Glasgow Coma Scale (GCS; refer to Box 44-6 in Chapter 44). A GCS score is based on three patient responses: eye opening, motor response, and verbal response. The patient receives a score for their best response in each of these areas, and the three scores are added together. The total score will range from 3 to 15; the higher the number, the better. A score of 8 or lower usually indicates coma.

The brain and spinal cord cannot be examined as directly as other systems of the body. Thus, much of the neurologic examination is an indirect evaluation that assesses the function of the specific body part or parts controlled or innervated by the nervous system. A neurologic assessment is divided into five components: cerebral function, cranial nerves, motor system, sensory system, and reflexes. As in other parts of the physical assessment, the neurologic examination follows a logical sequence and progresses from higher levels of cortical function, such as abstract thinking, to lower levels of function, such as the determination of the integrity of peripheral nerves.

Assessing Cerebral Function

Cerebral abnormalities may cause disturbances in mental status, intellectual functioning, and thought content, and in patterns of emotional behavior. There may also be alterations in perception and motor and language abilities, as well as in lifestyle.

Interpretation and documentation of neurologic abnormalities, particularly mental status abnormalities, should be specific and nonjudgmental. Lengthy descriptions and the use of terms such as ***inappropriate*** or ***demented*** are avoided. Terms such as these often mean different things to different people and, therefore, are not useful when describing behavior. The examiner records and reports specific observations regarding LOC, orientation, emotional state, or thought content, all of which permit comparison by others over time. Analysis and the conclusions that may be drawn from these findings usually depend on the examiner's knowledge of neuroanatomy, neurophysiology, and neuropathology.

Level of Consciousness

The first cue to a change in the neurologic function of a patient may be a change in the LOC, which is evaluated clinically as the patient's ability to respond appropriately to stimuli. It involves both wakefulness and cognition. The nurse compares current findings to previous patient baseline and notifies providers when any deterioration is noted. Rather than use broad terms like *stuporous* or *obtunded,* it is beneficial to describe the behavior in detail.

Pearls for Practice

The major source of energy for the brain is glucose. Neurons of the brain are incapable of creating or storing glucose. Therefore, the brain is dependent on blood flow for brain glucose. When blood glucose drops because of insulin administration, patients exhibit signs of decreased mentation, progressing to unconsciousness. If a patient has a history of diabetes or is receiving insulin treatment for other causes, the nurse should perform a glucose fingerstick to assess blood glucose level when a change in the LOC is noted.

Mental Status

An assessment of mental status begins by observing the patient's appearance and behavior, noting dress, grooming, and personal hygiene. Posture, gestures, movements, facial expressions, speech, and motor activity often provide important information about the patient.

Assessing orientation to time, place, and person assists in evaluating mental status. Does the patient know what day it is, what year it is, and where they are? Is the patient aware of who the examiner is and of their purpose for being in the room?

Assessment of mental status also includes both long- and short-term memory, and the ability to concentrate and attend to tasks asked of them as well. A more detailed mental status assessment may also include assessment of an individual's ability to calculate as well as perform abstract reasoning, such as "What would you do if you spotted a fire in your kitchen?"

TABLE 42-6 Types of Agnosia and Corresponding Sites of Lesions

Type of Agnosia	Affected Cerebral Area
Visual	Occipital lobe
Auditory	Temporal lobe (lateral and superior portions)
Tactile	Parietal lobe
Body parts and relationships	Parietal lobe (posteroinferior regions)

Perception

The examiner may now consider more specific areas of higher cortical function. **Agnosia** is the inability to interpret or recognize objects seen through the special senses. The patient may see a pencil but not know what it is called or what to do with it. The patient may even be able to describe it but not interpret its function. The patient may experience auditory or tactile agnosia as well as visual agnosia. Each of the dysfunctions implicates a different part of the cortex (Table 42-6).

Screening for visual and tactile agnosia provides insight into the patient's cortical interpretation ability. The patient is shown a familiar object and asked to identify it by name. Placing a familiar object (e.g., key, coin) in the patient's hand and having them identify it with both eyes closed is an easy way to assess tactile interpretation.

Motor Ability

Nurses assess cortical motor integration by asking the patient to perform a skilled act (comb hair, brush teeth). Successful performance requires the ability to understand the activity desired and normal motor strength. Failure signals cerebral dysfunction.

Language Ability

A person with normal neurologic function can understand and communicate in spoken and written language. Does the patient answer questions appropriately? Can they read

TABLE **42-7 Types of Aphasia and Region of Brain Involved**

Type of Aphasia	Brain Area Involved
Auditory-receptive	Temporal lobe
Visual-receptive	Parietal-occipital area
Expressive speaking	Inferior posterior frontal areas
Expressive writing	Posterior frontal area

a sentence from a newspaper and explain its meaning? Can the patient write their name or copy a simple figure that the examiner has drawn? A deficiency in language function is called *aphasia.* Different types of aphasia result from injury to different parts of the brain (Table 42-7).

Unfolding Patient Stories: M.H. • Part 2

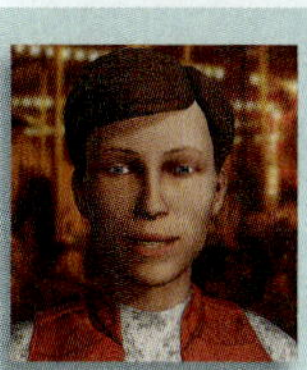

Recall from Chapter 41 the patient who came to the hospital after falling on icy stairs and sustaining a left mid-shaft tibia-fibula fracture requiring surgery. The patient also hit their head and was unresponsive for a short time after the fall. Describe the neurologic assessment performed by the nurse. Why should the nurse report this information promptly to the health care team?

Care for this patient in a realistic virtual environment: ***vSim** for Nursing* (thepoint.lww.com/vSimMedicalSurgical). Practice documenting this patient's care in DocuCare (thepoint.lww.com/DocuCareEHR).

Assessing the Cranial Nerves

Refer back to Table 42-2 on page 1379 for assessment of the cranial nerves. Opposite sides of the face and neck are compared throughout the examination. The assessment of multiple cranial nerves may be combined, such as eye movement (CN III, IV, VI) and **dysphagia**, or difficulty swallowing (CN IX, X, XII).

Examining the Motor System

A thorough examination of the motor system includes an assessment of muscle size, tone, and strength as well as coordination and balance. The muscles are inspected, and palpated if necessary, for their size and symmetry. Any evidence of atrophy or involuntary movements (tremors, tics) is noted. Muscle **tone** (the tension present in a muscle at rest) is evaluated by palpating various muscle groups at rest and during passive movement. Resistance to these movements is assessed and documented. Abnormalities in tone include **spasticity** (increased muscle tone), **rigidity** (resistance to passive stretch), and flaccidity.

Strength

Assessing the patient's ability to flex or extend the extremities against resistance tests muscle strength. The function of an individual muscle or group of muscles is evaluated by placing the muscle at a disadvantage. The evaluation of muscle strength compares the sides of the body to each other.

Clinicians use a five-point scale to rate muscle strength:

- 5 indicates full power of contraction against gravity and resistance or normal muscle strength;
- 4 indicates fair but not full strength against gravity and a moderate amount of resistance or slight weakness;
- 3 indicates just sufficient strength to overcome the force of gravity or moderate weakness;
- 2 indicates the ability to move but not to overcome the force of gravity or severe weakness;
- 1 indicates minimal contractile power (weak muscle contraction can be palpated but no movement is noted) or very severe weakness; and
- 0 indicates no movement.

Distal and proximal strength in both upper and lower extremities is recorded.

Pearls for Practice

There are occasional situations in which weakness of the upper extremities may be so subtle that the nurse is unsure if weakness is present. In these situations, the pronator drift can help assess for weakness. The patient holds their arms out in front of themself with palms facing the ceiling. The patient is asked to hold the position and close their eyes for approximately 20 seconds. If pronation (turning of the palm or the arm inward) or a downward drift of an arm is noted, the limb is weak. A positive pronator drift is associated with upper motor neurons in the brain and spinal cord that control voluntary movement.

Balance and Coordination

Cerebellar influence on the motor system is reflected in balance control and coordination. Coordination in the upper and lower extremities is tested by having the patient perform rapid, alternating movements and point-to-point testing. Speed, symmetry, and degree of difficulty are noted.

Point-to-point testing for coordination of the upper extremities is accomplished by having the patient touch the examiner's extended finger and then their own nose. This is repeated with each arm several times. Coordination in the lower extremities is tested by having the patient run the heel down the anterior surface of the tibia of the other leg. Each leg is tested in turn. **Ataxia** is defined as an inability to coordinate voluntary muscle action, particularly of the muscle groups used in activities such as walking or reaching for objects. The presence of ataxia or tremors (rhythmic, involuntary movements) during these movements suggests cerebellar disease.

The **Romberg test** is a screening test for balance. The patient stands with feet together and arms at the sides, first with eyes open and then with both eyes closed for 20 to 30 seconds. The examiner stands close to reassure the patient of support if they begin to fall. Slight swaying is normal, but a loss of balance is abnormal and is considered a positive Romberg test.

Examining the Reflexes

The motor reflexes are involuntary contractions of muscles or muscle groups in response to abrupt stretching near the site of the muscle's insertion. Common reflexes that may be tested include the deep tendon reflexes (biceps, brachioradialis, triceps, patellar, and ankle reflexes; Fig. 42-14) and

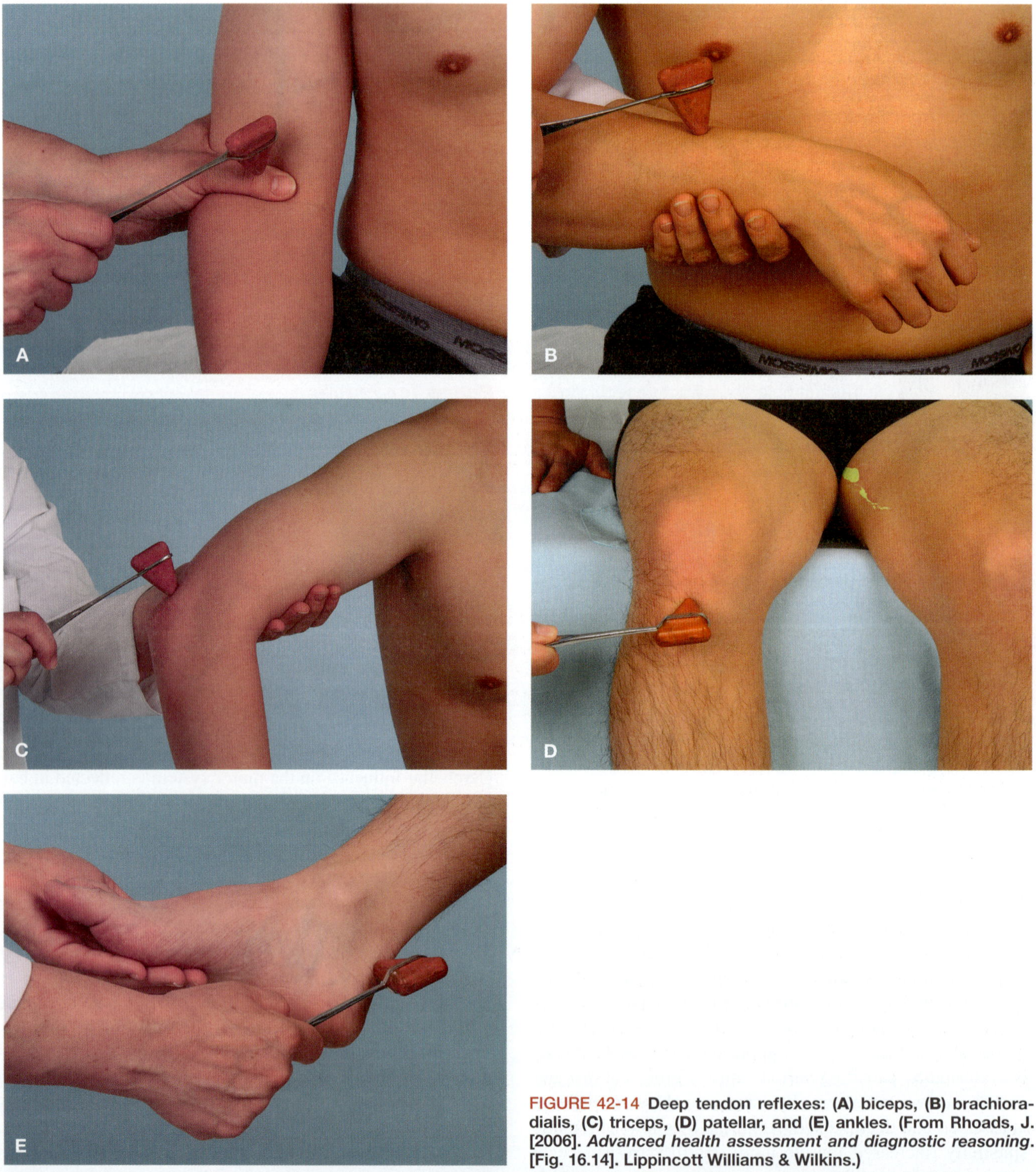

FIGURE 42-14 **Deep tendon reflexes: (A) biceps, (B) brachioradialis, (C) triceps, (D) patellar, and (E) ankles. (From Rhoads, J. [2006].** ***Advanced health assessment and diagnostic reasoning.*** **[Fig. 16.14]. Lippincott Williams & Wilkins.)**

superficial or cutaneous reflexes (abdominal reflexes and plantar or Babinski reflex).

Deep Tendon Reflexes

The tendon is struck directly with a reflex hammer, or indirectly by striking the examiner's digit with the hammer, which is placed firmly against the patient's tendon. Testing these reflexes enables the examiner to assess involuntary reflex arcs that depend on the presence of afferent stretch receptors, spinal synapses, efferent motor fibers, and a variety of modifying influences from higher levels.

Grading. The absence of reflexes is significant, although ankle jerks (Achilles reflex) may be normally absent in older people. Deep tendon reflex responses are often graded on a scale of 0 to 4+. Box 42-1 depicts how to document reflexes using this scale. As stated previously, scale ratings are highly subjective. Findings can be recorded as a fraction, indicating the scale range (e.g., 2/4). Some examiners prefer to use the terms *present*, *absent*, and *diminished* when describing reflexes.

Clonus. When reflexes are very hyperactive, a phenomenon called *clonus* may be elicited. If the foot is abruptly dorsiflexed, it may continue to "beat" two or three times before it settles into a position of rest. Occasionally, with CNS disease, this activity persists, and the foot does not come to rest while the tendon is being stretched but continues the repetitive activity. The unsustained clonus associated with normal but hyperactive reflexes is not considered pathologic. Sustained clonus always indicates the presence of CNS disease and requires further evaluation.

Superficial Reflexes

The major superficial reflexes include corneal, gag or swallowing, upper/lower abdominal, cremasteric (males only), plantar, and perianal. These reflexes are graded differently than the motor reflexes and are noted to be present (+) or absent (−). Of these, only the corneal, gag, and plantar reflexes are commonly tested.

The corneal reflex is tested carefully using a clean wisp of cotton and lightly touching the outer corner of each eye on the sclera. The reflex is present if the action elicits a blink. Conditions such as a stroke or coma might result in loss of this reflex, either unilaterally or bilaterally. Loss of this reflex indicates the need for eye protection and possible lubrication to prevent corneal damage.

The gag reflex is elicited by gently touching the back of the pharynx with a cotton-tipped applicator; first on one side of the uvula and then the other. Positive response is an equal elevation of the uvula and "gag" with stimulation. Absent response on one or both sides can be seen following a stroke and requires careful evaluation and treatment of the resultant swallowing dysfunction to prevent aspiration of food and fluids.

BOX 42-1

Documenting Reflexes

Deep tendon reflexes are graded on a scale of 0 to 4.

0	No response
1+	Diminished (hypoactive)
2+	Normal
3+	Increased (may be interpreted as normal)
4+	Hyperactive (hyperreflexia)

The deep tendon responses and plantar reflexes are commonly recorded on stick figures. The arrow points downward if the plantar response is normal and upward if the response is abnormal.

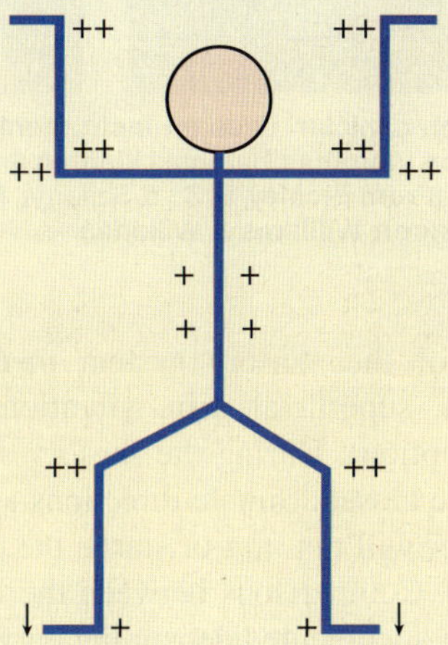

The plantar reflex, also known as the **Babinski reflex**, is elicited by stroking the lateral side of the foot with a tongue blade or the handle of a reflex hammer. In a person with an intact CNS, if the lateral aspect of the sole of the foot is stroked, the toes contract and draw together. However, in a person who has CNS disease of the motor system, the toes fan out. This is normal in newborns; but in adults, a positive Babinski sign indicates brain dysfunction (see Fig. 42-15).

Sensory Examination

The sensory system is even more complex than the motor system because sensory modalities are carried in different tracts located in different portions of the spinal cord. The sensory examination is largely subjective and requires the cooperation of the patient. The examiner should be familiar with dermatomes that represent the distribution of the peripheral nerves that arise from the spinal cord (see Fig. 42-13). Exceptions to this include major destructive lesions of the brain; loss of sensation, which may affect an entire side of the body; and the neuropathies associated with alcoholism, which occur in a glove-and-stocking distribution (i.e., over the entire hand or foot, in areas traditionally covered by a glove or sock).

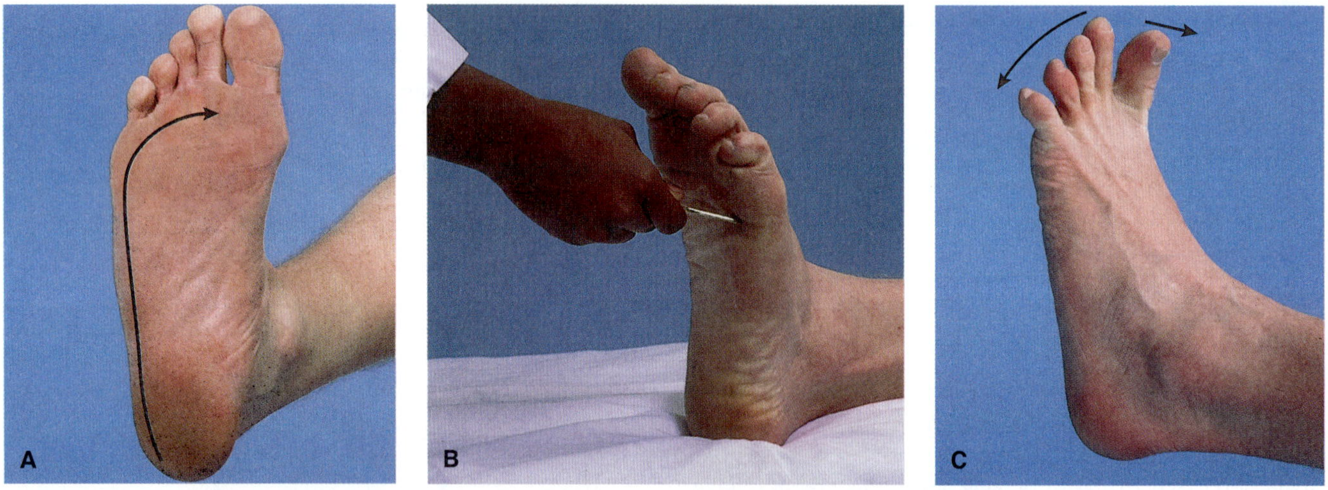

FIGURE 42-15 The clinician uses an instrument to stroke the sole of the patient's foot, beginning at the heel and curving upward, causing toe flexion (negative Babinski sign) (A and B). Toes that fan outward (positive Babinski sign) may indicate injury to the brain or spinal nerves (C). (From Bickley, L. S., & Szilagyi, P. [2003]. *Bates' guide to physical examination and history taking* [8th ed., Unfig. 16-67, 68, and 69]. Lippincott Williams & Wilkins.)

Assessment of the sensory system involves tests for tactile sensation, superficial pain, vibration, and position sense (proprioception). During the sensory assessment, the patient's eyes are closed. Simple directions and reassurance that the examiner will not hurt or startle the patient encourage cooperation. Comparisons between the left- and right-side findings are documented depending on which modality is found to have a deficit.

Diagnostic Evaluation

Computed Tomography Scanning

Computed tomography (CT) scanning makes use of a narrow x-ray beam to scan the body part in successive layers. The images provide cross-sectional views of the brain, with distinguishing differences in tissue densities of the skull, cortex, subcortical structures, and ventricles. The image is displayed on a monitor and is photographed and stored digitally.

Lesions in the brain are seen as variations in tissue density differing from the surrounding normal brain tissue. Abnormalities of tissue indicate possible tumor masses, brain infarction, displacement of the ventricles, and cortical atrophy. An emergency CT scan is performed in a patient with suspected brain bleed (e.g., subarachnoid hemorrhage) since blood within the basal cisterns is generally evident within the first 24 hours, whereas conventional magnetic resonance imaging (MRI) generally is less sensitive than CT scans for detecting blood (Ferri, 2019).

Procedure

CT scanning is usually performed first without contrast material and then with intravenous (IV) contrast enhancement. The patient lies on an adjustable table with the head held in a fixed position while the scanning system rotates around the head or spine and produces cross-sectional images. The patient must lie perfectly still without talking or moving because motion distorts the image.

CT scanning is noninvasive and painless and has a high degree of sensitivity for detecting lesions. With advances in CT scanning, the number of disorders and injuries that can be diagnosed is increasing.

Nursing Interventions

Essential nursing interventions include preparation for the procedure and patient monitoring. Preparation includes teaching the patient about the need to lie quietly throughout the procedure. A review of relaxation techniques may be helpful for patients with claustrophobia. Sedation can be used if agitation, restlessness, or confusion will interfere with a successful study. Ongoing patient monitoring during sedation is necessary.

If an IV contrast agent is used, the patient must be assessed before the CT scan for a contrast agent allergy. The contrast agent is iodine based; however, since early to mid-2000s, a less allergenic, nonionic/low osmolar agent has been used. Previously, it was believed that a shellfish allergy was a risk factor for an allergic reaction to iodine-based dye; however, the shellfish allergen is not a component of IV contrast (Ruff et al., 2021; Wuff et al., 2021).

An IV line for injection of the contrast agent is required prior to the study. Patients who receive an IV or inhalation contrast agent are monitored during and after the procedure for allergic reactions; kidney function; and other side effects, including flushing, nausea, and vomiting. Preprocedure hydration, along with the lowest possible dose of contrast agent for the study, is recommended, since contrast-induced nephropathy (CIN) is a cause of acute kidney injury (AKI). The incidence of CIN-AKI ranges from 6% to 27%; thus, the nurse should monitor urinary output and serum creatinine post procedure (Efe et al., 2021). Risk factors for CIN-AKI include preexisting impaired renal function, diabetes, left ventricular dysfunction, and anemia.

Positron Emission Tomography

Positron emission tomography (PET) is a computer-based nuclear imaging technique that produces images of actual organ functioning.

Procedure

The patient either inhales a radioactive gas or is injected with a radioactive substance that emits positively charged particles. When these positrons combine with negatively charged electrons (normally found in the body's cells), the resultant gamma rays can be detected by a scanning device that produces a series of two-dimensional views at various levels of the brain. This information is integrated by a computer and gives a composite picture of the brain at work.

PET permits the measurement of blood flow, tissue composition, and brain metabolism and thus indirectly evaluates brain function. The brain is one of the most metabolically active organs, consuming 80% of the glucose the body uses. PET measures this activity in specific areas of the brain and can detect changes in glucose use.

In addition, PET is useful in showing metabolic changes in the brain (Alzheimer disease), locating lesions (brain tumor, epileptogenic lesions), identifying blood flow and oxygen metabolism in patients with strokes, evaluating new therapies for brain tumors, and revealing biochemical abnormalities associated with mental illness. The isotopes used have a very short half-life and are expensive to produce, requiring specialized equipment for production.

Nursing Interventions

Key nursing interventions include patient preparation, which involves explaining the test and teaching the patient about inhalation techniques and the sensations (e.g., dizziness, light-headedness, and headache) that may occur. The IV injection of the radioactive substance produces similar side effects. Relaxation exercises may reduce anxiety during the test.

Single-Photon Emission Computed Tomography

Procedure

Single-photon emission computed tomography (SPECT) is a three-dimensional imaging technique that uses radionuclides and instruments to detect single photons. It is a perfusion study that captures a moment of cerebral blood flow at the time of injection of a radionuclide. Gamma photons are emitted from a radiopharmaceutical agent administered to the patient and are detected by a rotating gamma camera or cameras; the image is sent to a minicomputer. This approach allows areas behind overlying structures or background to be viewed, greatly increasing the contrast between normal and abnormal tissues. It is relatively inexpensive, and the duration is similar to that of a CT scan.

SPECT is useful in detecting the extent and location of abnormally perfused areas of the brain, thus allowing detection, localization, and sizing of stroke (before it is visible by CT scan); localization of seizure foci in epilepsy; detection of tumor progression; and evaluation of perfusion before and after neurosurgical procedures. Pregnancy and breastfeeding are contraindications to SPECT.

Nursing Interventions

The nursing interventions for SPECT primarily include patient preparation and patient monitoring. Teaching about what to expect before the test can allay anxiety and ensure patient cooperation during the test. Premenopausal patients are advised to practice effective contraception before and for several days after testing, and the patient who is breastfeeding is instructed to stop nursing for the time period recommended by the nuclear medicine department.

The nurse may need to accompany and monitor the patient during transport to the nuclear medicine department for the scan. Patients are monitored during and after the procedure for allergic reactions to the radiopharmaceutical agent.

Magnetic Resonance Imaging

Procedure

MRI uses a powerful magnetic field to obtain images of different areas of the body. This diagnostic test involves altering hydrogen ions in the body. Placing the patient into a powerful magnetic field causes the hydrogen nuclei (protons) within the body to align like small magnets in a magnetic field. In combination with radiofrequency pulses, the protons emit signals, which are converted to images. An MRI scan can be performed with or without a contrast agent and can identify a cerebral abnormality earlier and more clearly than other diagnostic tests. It can provide information about the chemical changes within cells, allowing the clinician to monitor a tumor's response to treatment. The use of MRI allows visualization of the cerebral vasculature without the administration of an arterial contrast agent, but the clarity of the images is enhanced when a contrast agent is used. MRI does not involve ionizing radiation; and if contrast is required, the agent is gadolinium-based. Noniodinated IV contrast agents are generally considered safe (Ferri, 2019). However, if contrast is used, kidney function must be assessed. At present, MRI is most valuable in the diagnosis of nonacute conditions because the test may take up to an hour to complete.

Nursing Interventions

Patient preparation should include teaching relaxation techniques and informing the patient that they will be able to talk to the staff by means of a microphone located inside the scanner. Many MRI suites provide headphones so that patients can listen to the music of their choice during the procedure.

Before the patient enters the room where the MRI is to be performed, all metal objects and credit cards (the magnetic field can erase them) are removed. This includes medication patches that have a metal backing; these can cause burns if not removed. No metal objects may be brought into the room where the MRI is located; this includes oxygen tanks, traditional ventilators, or even stethoscopes. The magnetic field generated by the unit is so strong that any metal-containing items will be strongly attracted and literally can be pulled away with such force that they fly like projectiles toward the magnet. There is a risk of severe injury and death; furthermore, damage to a very expensive piece of equipment may occur. A patient history is obtained to determine the presence of any metal objects (e.g., aneurysm clips, orthopedic hardware, pacemakers, artificial heart valves). These objects could malfunction, be dislodged, or heat up as they absorb energy. Cochlear implants will be inactivated by MRI; therefore, other imaging procedures are considered.

The patient lies on a flat platform that is moved into a tube housing the magnet; thus, an MRI requires a cooperative patient. The scanning process is painless, but the patient hears loud thumping of the magnetic coils as the magnetic field is being pulsed. Because the MRI scanner is a narrow tube, patients may experience claustrophobia; sedation may be prescribed in these circumstances. Newer versions of MRI machines (open MRI) are less claustrophobic than the earlier devices and are available in some locations. However, the images produced on these machines are not optimal, and traditional devices are preferable for accurate diagnosis.

Pearls for Practice

For patient safety, the nurse must make sure no patient care equipment (e.g., portable oxygen tank) that contains metal or metal parts enters the room where the MRI is located. Oxygen tanks made of aluminum are MRI compatible. The patient must be assessed for the presence of medication patches with foil backing (such as nicotine) that may cause a burn. For a list of medical devices and compatibility with MRI, please refer to the website http://www.mrisafety.com/List.html.

Cerebral Angiography

Procedure

Cerebral angiography is an x-ray study of the cerebral circulation with a contrast agent injected into a selected artery. Cerebral angiography is a valuable tool to investigate vascular disease, aneurysms, and arteriovenous malformations and to define their anatomy. It is still considered the gold standard for diagnosing these conditions.

Most cerebral angiograms are performed by threading a catheter through the femoral artery in the groin and up to the desired vessel. After the groin is shaved and prepared, a local anesthetic is administered to prevent pain at the insertion site and to reduce arterial spasm. A catheter is introduced into the femoral artery, flushed with heparinized saline, and filled with contrast agent. Fluoroscopy is used to guide the catheter to the appropriate vessels. During injection of the contrast agent, images are made of the arterial and venous phases of circulation through the brain.

Nursing Interventions

The patient is NPO for 4 to 6 hours before the test. Before going to the x-ray department, the patient is instructed to void. The locations of the appropriate peripheral pulses are marked with a felt-tip pen. The patient is instructed to remain immobile during the angiogram process and is told to expect a brief feeling of warmth in the face; behind the eyes; or in the jaw, teeth, tongue, and lips, and a metallic taste when the contrast agent is injected.

Nursing care after cerebral angiography includes observation for signs and symptoms of altered cerebral blood flow. In some instances, patients may experience major or minor arterial blockage due to embolism, thrombosis, or hemorrhage, producing a neurologic deficit. Signs of such an occurrence include alterations in the level of responsiveness and consciousness, weakness on one side of the body, motor or sensory deficits, and speech disturbances. Therefore, it is necessary to observe the patient frequently for these signs and to report them immediately if they occur. In addition, the nurse monitors intake and output, looking for renal complications from the dye.

The most common complication post procedure is a groin hematoma (Biller et al., 2022); therefore, the injection site is observed for hematoma formation (a localized collection of blood), and an ice bag may be applied intermittently to the puncture site to relieve swelling and discomfort. Because a hematoma at the puncture site or embolization to a distant artery affects the peripheral pulses, these pulses are monitored frequently. The color and temperature of the involved extremity are assessed to detect possible embolism (the limb would be cool and pale if arterial perfusion is impaired).

Pearls for Practice

The nurse should be aware that with patients undergoing vascular diagnostic studies (angiography or venography) who present with AKI or chronic kidney failure (refer to Chapter 26) and are also prescribed metformin (an oral antihyperglycemic medication for patients with noninsulin-dependent diabetes mellitus), metformin may be withheld due to the rare development of lactic acidosis. Lactic acidosis in this scenario has a 50% mortality rate (Shin, 2021). In general, the medication is withheld for 48 hours after the vascular procedure and resumed only after renal function has been reassessed.

Myelography

Procedure

A myelogram is an x-ray of the spinal subarachnoid space taken after the injection of a contrast agent through a lumbar puncture (LP). It outlines the spinal subarachnoid space and shows any distortion of the spinal cord or spinal dural sac caused by tumors, cysts, herniated vertebral disks, or other lesions. Water-based agents have replaced oil-based agents, and their use has reduced side effects and complications; these agents disperse upward through the CSF. Myelography is performed less frequently today because of the sensitivity of CT and MRI scanning. It is still used occasionally to provide information about the spinal cord and nerve roots and is useful if that patient cannot have an MRI (Rocos, 2020).

Nursing Interventions

Because many patients have misconceptions about myelography, the nurse clarifies the explanation given by the provider and answers questions. The patient is informed about what to expect during the procedure and should be aware that changes in position may be made during the procedure. The meal that normally would be eaten before the procedure is omitted. A sedative may be prescribed to help the patient cope with this rather lengthy test. Patient preparation for LP is discussed later in this chapter.

After myelography, the patient lies in bed with the head of the bed elevated 30 to 45 degrees. The patient is advised to remain in bed in the recommended position for 3 hours or as prescribed by the provider. The patient is encouraged to drink liberal amounts of fluid for rehydration and replacement of CSF. The blood pressure, pulse, respiratory rate, and temperature are monitored, as well as the patient's ability to void. Untoward signs include headache, fever, stiff neck, **photophobia** (sensitivity to light), seizures, and signs of chemical or bacterial meningitis. Headaches occur in approximately 10% to 25% of patients (Ferri, 2019).

Noninvasive Carotid Flow Studies

Procedure

Noninvasive carotid flow studies use ultrasound imagery and Doppler measurements of arterial blood flow to evaluate carotid and deep orbital circulation. The graph produced indicates blood velocity. Increased blood velocity can indicate stenosis or partial obstruction. These tests are often obtained before arteriography, which carries a higher risk of stroke or death. Carotid Doppler, carotid ultrasonography, oculoplethysmography, and ophthalmodynamometry are four common noninvasive vascular techniques that permit evaluation of arterial blood flow and detection of arterial stenosis, occlusion, and plaques. These vascular studies allow noninvasive imaging of extracranial and intracranial circulation.

Nursing Interventions

When a carotid flow study is scheduled, the procedure is described to the patient. The patient is informed that this is a noninvasive test, that a hand-held transducer will be placed over the neck or orbits of the eyes, and that some type of water-soluble jelly is used on the transducer.

Electroencephalography

Procedure

An electroencephalogram (EEG) represents a record of the electrical activity generated in the brain. It is obtained through electrodes applied on the scalp or through microelectrodes placed within the brain tissue. It provides a physiologic assessment of cerebral activity.

The EEG is a useful test for diagnosing and evaluating seizure disorders, coma, or organic brain syndrome. Tumors, brain abscesses, blood clots, and infection may cause abnormal patterns in electrical activity. The EEG is also used in making a determination of brain death.

For a baseline recording, the patient lies quietly with both eyes closed. The patient may be asked to hyperventilate for 3 to 4 minutes and then look at a bright, flashing light for photic stimulation. These activation procedures are performed to evoke abnormal electrical discharges, such as seizure potentials. A sleep EEG may be recorded after sedation because some abnormal brain waves are seen only when the patient is asleep.

Nursing Interventions

To increase the chances of recording seizure activity, it is sometimes recommended that the patient be deprived of sleep on the night before the EEG. Antiseizure agents, tranquilizers, stimulants, and depressants should be withheld 24 to 48 hours before an EEG because these medications can alter the EEG wave patterns or mask the abnormal wave patterns of seizure disorders (England & Plueuger, 2019).

The patient is informed that the standard EEG takes 45 to 60 minutes (12 hours for a sleep EEG). The patient is assured that the procedure does not cause an electric shock and that the EEG is a diagnostic test, not a form of treatment. An EEG requires patient cooperation and ability to lie quietly during the test. Sedation is not advisable because it may lower the seizure threshold in patients with a seizure disorder and it alters brain wave activity in all patients. The nurse needs to check with the physician regarding the administration of antiseizure medication prior to testing.

Routine EEGs use for electrode contact a water-soluble lubricant, which at the conclusion of the study can be wiped off and removed by shampooing. Electrode contact for sleep EEGs involves the use of collodion glue, which requires acetone for removal.

Electromyography

Procedure

An electromyogram (EMG) is obtained by inserting needle electrodes into the skeletal muscles to measure changes in the electrical potential of the muscles and the nerves leading to them. The electrical potentials are shown on an oscilloscope and amplified so that both the sound and appearance of the waves can be analyzed and compared simultaneously.

An EMG is useful in determining the presence of neuromuscular disorders and myopathies. It helps distinguish weakness due to neuropathy (functional or pathologic changes in the PNS) from weakness resulting from other causes.

Nursing Interventions

The procedure is explained, and the patient is warned to expect a sensation similar to that of an intramuscular injection as the needle is inserted into the muscle. The muscles examined may ache for a short time after the procedure.

Lumbar Puncture and Examination of Cerebrospinal Fluid

Procedure

An LP (also referred to as a spinal tap) is an aseptic procedure carried out by inserting a needle into the lumbar subarachnoid space to withdraw CSF. The test may be performed to obtain CSF for examination, to measure and reduce CSF pressure, to assess for infection, and to determine the presence or absence of blood in the CSF. Antibiotics may be administered intrathecally (into the spinal canal) in certain cases of infection or contrast injected for diagnostic purposes.

The needle is usually inserted into the subarachnoid space between the third and fourth or fourth and fifth lumbar vertebrae. Because the spinal cord divides into a sheaf of nerves at the first lumbar vertebra, insertion of the needle below the level of the third lumbar vertebra prevents puncture of the spinal cord.

A successful LP requires that the patient be relaxed; an anxious patient is tense, and this may increase the pressure reading. CSF pressure with the patient in a lateral recumbent position is normally 70 to 200 mm H_2O. This value is position dependent and will change with a horizontal or sitting position (Fischbach & Dunning, 2021). Pressures of more than 200 mm H_2O are considered abnormal.

An LP may be risky in the presence of an intracranial mass lesion because ICP is decreased by the removal of CSF, and the brain may herniate downward through the tentorium and the foramen magnum. To avoid this complication, a CT scan must be done prior to the procedure for patients with a suspected intracranial mass. Additionally, LPs are avoided in patients on antiplatelet therapy or anticoagulants. See Box 42-2 for nursing guidelines for assisting with an LP.

Cerebrospinal Fluid Analysis

The CSF should be clear and colorless. Pink, blood-tinged, or grossly bloody CSF may indicate a subarachnoid hemorrhage. Cloudiness of CSF may be due to increased WBCs or increased protein from microorganisms, whereas xanthochromia (yellow, orange, or brown color) of CNS is usually due to RBC breakdown (Hickey, 2019). Sometimes, with a difficult LP, the CSF initially is bloody because of local trauma but then becomes clearer. Usually, specimens are obtained for cell count, culture, and glucose and protein testing. The specimens should be sent to the laboratory immediately because changes will take place and alter the result if the specimens are allowed to stand.

Post–Lumbar Puncture Headache

A post–lumbar puncture headache, ranging from mild to severe, may occur a few hours to several days after the procedure. This is the most common complication, occurring in 15% to 30% of patients. It is a throbbing bifrontal or occipital headache, dull and deep in character. It is particularly severe on sitting or standing but lessens or disappears when the patient lies down.

The headache is caused by CSF leakage at the puncture site. The fluid continues to escape into the tissues by way of the needle track from the spinal canal. It is then absorbed promptly by the lymphatic system. As a result of this leak, the supply of CSF in the cranium is depleted to a point at which it is insufficient to maintain proper mechanical stabilization of the brain. This leakage of CSF allows settling of the brain when the patient assumes an upright position, producing tension and stretching the venous sinuses and pain-sensitive structures. Both traction and pain are lessened and the leakage is reduced when the patient lies down for 4 to 8 hours (Fischbach, Fischbach & Stout, 2021).

Post–lumbar puncture headache may be avoided if a small-gauge needle is used. The postpuncture headache is usually managed by bed rest, analgesic agents, and hydration. The nurse should follow hospital standards while best practices are being developed. Occasionally, if the headache persists, an epidural blood patch may be used. Blood is withdrawn from the antecubital vein and injected into the epidural space, usually at the site of the previous spinal puncture. The rationale is that the blood acts as a gelatinous plug to seal the hole in the dura, preventing further loss of CSF. The success rate of a single epidural blood patch is estimated between 70% and 98% (Garza et al., 2022).

Other Complications of Lumbar Puncture

Herniation of the intracranial contents, spinal epidural abscess, spinal epidural hematoma, and meningitis are rare but serious complications of LP. Other complications include temporary voiding problems, slight elevation of temperature, backache or spasms, and stiffness of the neck.

BOX 42-2

ASSISTING WITH A LUMBAR PUNCTURE

A needle is inserted into the subarachnoid space through the third and fourth or fourth and fifth lumbar interface to withdraw spinal fluid.

PREPROCEDURE

1. Determine whether written consent for the procedure has been obtained.
2. Explain the procedure to the patient and describe sensations that are likely during the procedure (i.e., a sensation of cold as the site is cleansed with solution, a needle prick when local anesthetic is injected).
3. Determine whether the patient has any questions or misconceptions about the procedure; reassure the patient that the needle will not enter the spinal cord or cause paralysis.
4. Instruct the patient to void before the procedure.

PROCEDURE

1. The patient is positioned on one side (knee to chest position) at the edge of the bed or examining table with back toward the provider; the legs are flexed as much as possible to increase the space between the spinous processes of the vertebrae, for easier entry into the subarachnoid space.
2. A small pillow may be placed under the patient's head to maintain the spine in a horizontal position; a pillow may be placed between the legs to prevent the upper leg from rolling forward.
3. The nurse assists the patient to maintain the position to avoid sudden movement, which can produce a traumatic (bloody) tap.
4. The patient is encouraged to relax and is instructed to breathe normally because hyperventilation may lower an elevated pressure.
5. The nurse describes the procedure step by step to the patient as it proceeds.
6. Using an aseptic technique, the provider cleanses the puncture site with an antiseptic solution and drapes the site.
7. The provider injects local anesthetic to numb the puncture site and then inserts a spinal needle into the subarachnoid space through the third and fourth or fourth and fifth lumbar interspace.
8. A specimen of CSF is removed and usually collected in three test tubes, labeled in order of collection. A pressure reading may be obtained. The needle is withdrawn.

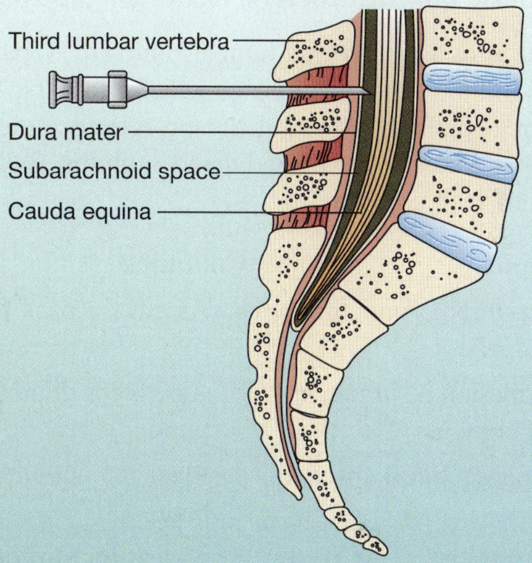

9. The provider applies a small dressing to the puncture site.
10. The tubes of CSF are sent to the laboratory immediately.

POSTPROCEDURE

Typically, patients are instructed to rest in bed for a few hours after an LP, and fluids are encouraged; however, research reveals no definite differences in the effects of bed rest or hydration of patients. Therefore, the nurse should refer to institutional procedures for postprocedure care.

1. Monitor the patient for complications of LP; notify the provider if complications occur:
   a. Common complications: post–lumbar puncture headache, voiding difficulties, slight elevation of temperature, backache or spasms, stiffness of neck. Typical management of postprocedure headache includes maintaining a supine posture, hydration, and analgesia and/or antiemetics prn; however, the nurse follows institutional procedures until best practices are delineated.
   b. Rare complications: herniation of intracranial contents, spinal epidural abscess, spinal epidural hematoma, meningitis

CHAPTER REVIEW

NCLEX-Style Review Questions

1. A patient is undergoing a cerebral angiography to rule out an aneurysm. When preparing the patient for the procedure, what would the nurse include in the instructions? Select all that apply.

a. Expect a metallic taste when the contrast agent is injected.
b. You will need a full bladder prior to the procedure.
c. General sedation will be given prior to procedure.
d. Assess and document peripheral pulses preprocedure.
e. Evaluate if the patient is on metformin preprocedure.

2. A nurse is assisting with a lumbar puncture. What is the most common complication for which the nurse should monitor a patient following the procedure (column 1) and what intervention is indicated (column 2)? Select one from each column.

Column 1	**Column 2**
a. Post–lumbar puncture headache	a. Assess for back pain.
b. Herniation of intracranial contents	b. Assess for dilated pupils.
c. Spinal epidural abscess	c. Place the patient on bedrest.
d. Meningitis	d. Assess for stiff neck.

3. A patient is scheduled for an EEG tomorrow. Which information should the nurse provide to the patient prior to the procedure? (Select all that apply.)

a. Antiseizure medications will be withheld prior to procedure.
b. Sedation will be given during the procedure.
c. There is a slight chance of electric shock.
d. Maintain a sleep-deprived state the night before the procedure.
e. The procedure will be completed in 20 to 30 minutes.
f. Patient cooperation is required, as is the ability to lie quietly during the test.

4. A patient was an unrestrained driver involved in a motor vehicle collision. On arrival, multiple facial lacerations are noted and serosanguinous drainage is noted from both nares bilaterally. A nurse anticipates that the serosanguinous drainage may indicate ______ (select from column 1). Two actions that will be taken are ______ (select two from column 2).

Column 1	**Column 2**
a. Rhinorrhea	a. Nasal packing will be placed in each nare.
b. Otorrhea	b. If required, an orogastric tube should be inserted.
c. Battle sign	c. Monitor for signs and symptoms of meningitis.
d. Raccoon eyes	d. Nasotracheal suctioning is permitted.

5. A nurse is testing the extraocular movements (EOM) of a patient. Which cranial nerves are assessed when evaluating EOMs? (Select all that apply.)

a. Abducens
b. Oculomotor
c. Optic
d. Trochlear

REFERENCES AND SELECTED READINGS

References and selected readings associated with this chapter can be found on the website that accompanies the book. Visit **http://thepoint.lww.com/Honan3e** to access the references and other additional resources associated with this chapter.

CHAPTER 43

Nursing Management: Patients With Oncologic Disorders of the Brain and Spinal Cord

Jill Keller

Learning Objectives

After reading this chapter, you will be able to:

1. Describe the different types of brain and spinal cord tumors, including classification, clinical manifestations, diagnosis, and medical and nursing management.
2. Differentiate primary and metastatic brain tumors.
3. Describe the symptoms and effects of increased intracranial pressure.
4. Describe the symptoms and effects of spinal cord compression.

Tumors affecting the brain and spinal cord can have irreversible side effects. Detecting the first signs of deficits is important to an understanding of the brain and spinal cord anatomy as well as of the cranial nerves. Early intervention can lead to quick diagnosis and possible improved outcomes. Nurses are key when assessing in adults neurologic dysfunctions that may be overlooked in a routine examination.

PRIMARY BRAIN TUMORS

Primary brain tumors are localized intracranial lesions that begin in the brain and occupy space within the skull. The tumor is an abnormal growth of cells that forms a mass, but it also can grow diffusely. The three main areas of the brain include the cerebrum, cerebellum, and brain stem. The effects of neoplasms (tumors or lesions) on the central nervous system (CNS) are proportionate to the location of the brain affected. Signs and symptoms, including seizure activity and focal neurologic signs, are caused by, compression, increased cranial pressure (ICP), or infiltration of tissue, or all of these. Tumors may be benign or malignant. Benign tumors are usually slow growing but can occur in a vital area, where they can grow large enough to cause serious effects. Malignant tumors are rapidly growing in nature, can spread into surrounding tissue, and are considered life-threatening. Primary brain tumors may spread to the spine but rarely spread to other areas of the body.

Oncologic (cancer) disorders of the brain include several types of neoplasms, each with its own biology, prognosis, and treatment options. Because of the unique anatomy and physiology of the CNS, this collection of neoplasms is challenging to diagnose and treat.

Types of Brain Tumors

There are many different types of brain tumors (see Figure 43-1). There are more than 125 different types and subtypes of brain tumors classified by the World Health Organization (WHO) (Box 43-1). They are classified into several groups: those originating within brain tissue (e.g., glioblastoma), those arising from the coverings of the brain (e.g., meningioma), those developing in or on the cranial nerves (e.g., schwannoma), and metastatic lesions originating from cancer elsewhere in the body. Tumors of the pituitary and pineal glands and of cerebral blood vessels are also considered types of brain tumors. Relevant clinical considerations when developing a plan of treatment includes the location, size, histologic character of the tumor and if the tumor can be surgically removed. In addition, researchers have identified genetic mutation of the tumor cell, which helps to identify possible response to treatments. For the sake of this chapter, we will focus on the most common malignant brain tumors according to the National Cancer Institute (NCI, 2021).

Glioblastoma and Anaplastic Astrocytoma

Gliomas are a type of intracerebral brain neoplasm that arise in glial cells. Gliomas are divided into many categories. Glioblastoma (GBM) is a common and aggressive malignant brain tumor. They may arise "de novo," meaning that the tumor begins as a grade 4 with no low-grade precursor. This is unlike secondary glioblastomas that can progress from low grade astrocytic tumors (American Brain Tumor Association [ABTA], n.d.a). Anaplastic astrocytomas also arise from glial cells. They are considered grade 3 or a high-grade tumor. In most all cases, a tissue biopsy, which can be obtained at the time of surgical removal, is needed to confirm the diagnosis. The grade of the tumor is based on cellular

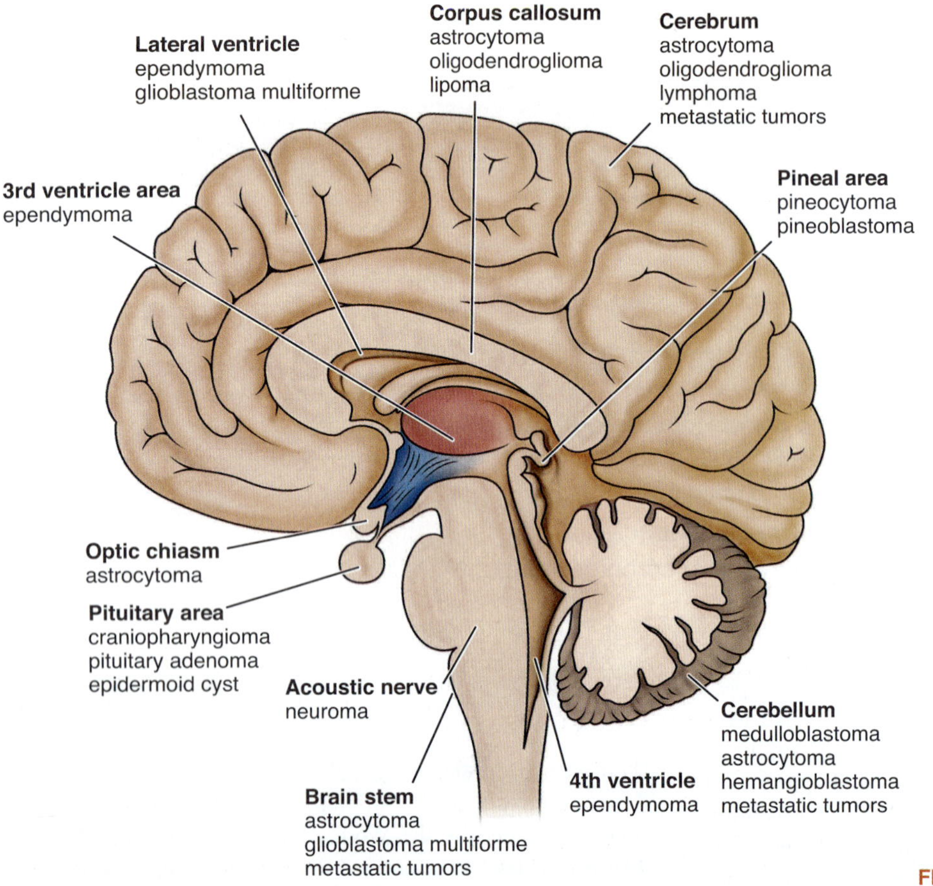

FIGURE 43-1 **Common brain tumor sites.**

density, cell mitosis, and appearance. Usually, these tumors form in the cerebrum and spread by infiltrating the surrounding neural connective tissue. Treatment for this type of tumor may include surgery, radiation therapy, and/or chemotherapy.

BOX 43-1 **World Health Organization Classification of Adult Primary CNS Tumors**

WHO grade I—lesions with low proliferation potential, frequency discrete nature, possible cure following surgery alone.

WHO grade II—lesions that generally infiltrate and with a low mitotic rate but recur more frequently than grade I tumors after local therapy. Some may progress to higher grade malignancy.

WHO grade III—includes lesions with histologic evidence of malignancy, including atypia (not normal) nuclear and increased mitotic rate. They have anaplastic histology (little resemblance to normal cells) and infiltrative capacity. Usually treated with aggressive adjuvant therapy.

WHO grade IV—lesions are mitotically active, necrosis prone, usually associated with rapid pre and postoperative progression and fatal outcomes.

Adapted with permission from National Cancer Institute (NCI). (2021). *Adult central nervous system tumors treatment—Health Professional Version.* https://www.cancer.gov/types/brain/hp/adult-brain-treatment-pdq.

Total surgical resection is difficult due to the "finger-like tentacles" the tumor produces. The goal of surgery is to remove as much tumor as possible without causing any neurologic damage. There are several molecular studies now done on brain tumors. Mutations for GBMs have either IDH-wild-type or IDH-mutant. Unfortunately, the IDH-wild type is more common, more aggressive, and has a poorer prognosis (ABTA, n.d.a). Fewer than 25% of patients survive 2 years, and fewer than 10% will make it to 5 years (Bruce, 2021).

Meningiomas

Meningiomas represent 36.1% of all primary brain tumors and are the most common brain tumor found in adults. Most are characterized as a benign, encapsulated, slow-growing tumor that occurs in people over the age of 60 and found twice as often in females (ABTA, n.d.a). These tumors grow on the membrane covering of the brain, the meninges. Grade 1 meningiomas are the most common type and can be cured by surgery. Due to the slow-growing nature of this tumor, it is not uncommon that people die unaware they have a meningioma. Grade II and III are less common and grow quickly. They can spread to the brain and spinal cord. These tumors have a worse prognosis and usually cannot be completely resected. Manifestations depend on the area involved and are the result of compression rather than invasion of brain tissue. In some cases, this type of tumor can run in families that have the neurofibromatosis type 2 (NF 2) that can increase their risk for developing a brain tumor (National Cancer Institute [NCI], 2021).

Pituitary Tumors

Pituitary tumors (adenoma) represent approximately 10% of all brain tumors (ABTA, n.d.a). They are slow growing in nature. Many of these tumors are benign but, in rare cases, may be malignant. Pituitary tumors are classified as nonfunctioning and functioning. Nonfunctioning or nonsecreting tumors do not produce hormones. Functioning or secreting tumors can produce one or more hormones, normally by the anterior pituitary. Increase may be seen in prolactin hormone, growth hormone, adrenocorticotropic hormone (ACTH), or thyroid-stimulating hormone (TSH). Of the pituitary tumors that cause health issues, females are more affected than males (Dai et al., 2021). Endocrine disorders resulting from these tumors are discussed in Chapter 30.

Magnetic resonance imaging (MRI) is used to visualize the mass. Pressure from a pituitary adenoma may be exerted on the optic nerves, optic chiasm, optic tracts, hypothalamus, or third ventricle. Headache is a common symptom, there can also be visual dysfunction, hypothalamic disorders (diabetes insipidus, sleep disturbances, and changes in appetite), and increased intracranial pressure (ICP). Treatment is dependent on the type of tumor. Transsphenoidal surgery is first-line therapy for growth hormone–secreting tumors and some nonfunctioning tumors. Additional medical treatments include correction of hormone levels.

Schwannoma

Schwannomas are slow growing in nature and are composed of Schwann cells. Of all the cases, 90% are solitary. Those patients found with multiple tumors could be associated with NF 2, schwannomatosis, and Carney complex. The most common schwannoma is the vestibular schwannoma; these are benign (Sheikh & De Jesus, 2021). Schwannomas can be in other areas of the body besides the head and spinal cord since they develop from schwann cells in the peripheral nervous system or nerve root. Symptoms depend on the location of the tumor. The patient can experience loss of hearing, tinnitus, episodes of vertigo, and staggering gait. As the tumor becomes larger, painful sensations of the face may occur on the same side as a result of the tumor causing facial numbness (paresthesia) and pain. MRI is the preferred scan to identify these types of tumors. Benign lesions, if asymptomatic, are often closely observed over time. Surgery is carefully considered, as it can result in permanent nerve damage. Additional options for treatment include stereotactic radiosurgery.

Primary CNS Lymphoma

Primary CNS lymphoma (PCNSL) is a type of non-Hodgkin lymphoma that is aggressive, affecting the brain, eyes, spine and cerebral spinal fluid (CSF). Diagnosis is made through lumbar puncture for CSF analysis or brain biopsy. Patients with suspected PCNSL should avoid steroids until the diagnosis is made, as they can affect biopsy results. Many patients can have nonspecific changes in behavior that make the diagnosis difficult and often delayed. Additional symptoms include weakness of the extremities and bowel and bladder incontinence. In some patients the peripheral nerves can become affected. For those patients with involvement of the eyes, reports of blurred and/or a decrease in vision may be noted. MRI is used to identify lesions. Chemotherapy is the first line of therapy in treatment of PCNSL. Radiation has been linked to increased neurologic side effects. If left untreated, overall prognosis is 1.5 months (Green & Hogg, 2021). B-cell lymphomas have a more favorable prognosis.

Oligodendroglioma

Oligodendroglioma is a type of infiltrating glioma intracranial tumor most commonly seen in the frontal lobe. Low-grade II tumors are noted to be slow growing and are noted to have a good response to treatment. Grade III tumors are more likely to be malignant and have less favorable outcomes. Symptoms of headache and seizures are common. MRI is a useful tool; MRI with spectroscopy and perfusion may assist with grading. Surgical resection is dependent on location of the tumor and the risk factors associated with surgery. Debulking can be done to relieve symptoms when complete resection is not possible. There has been concern that low grade debulked tumors can transition to high-grade tumors. Repeat resection may be an option. Radiation has been shown to decrease symptoms and prolong time to progression. Chemotherapy with radiation after surgery has been found to prolong survival. Low-grade II tumors have a survival of 10 to 12 years. High-grade tumors have median survival of 3.5 years (Tork & Atkinson, 2021).

Low-Grade Astrocytoma

Grade I or low-grade astrocytomas can be classified as Pilocytic astrocytoma and are usually found in the cerebellum. If they can be surgically resected, they will require no further treatment, Pleomorphic xantoastrocytomas are frequently found in the temporal lobe and are usually cured with surgical removal. Subpendymal giant cell astrocytoma (SEGA) is most often seen in younger patients SEGA grows inside the ventricles; again, surgical resection normally leads to a cure.

Medulloblastomas

Medulloblastoma are fast-growing high-grade tumors always located in the cerebellum. The most common symptoms include behavioral changes, changes in appetite, headache, nausea, and vomiting due to increased ICP. Seen more in the pediatric population (ABTA, 2022), treatment includes surgical removal with possible radiation and chemotherapy.

Cerebral Metastases

Metastatic disease is the ability for a malignant cell to travel through the circulation and reestablish itself in a second site. Metastatic brain tumors account for more than half of all brain tumors in adults. Primary sites of cancer that commonly metastasize to the brain include the lung (the most common) follow by melanoma, renal cell, breast, and colorectal (Loeffler, 2021). An increase in brain metastases may be related to earlier detection by MRI, and patients with all forms of cancer are living longer because of improved therapies. Diagnosis of brain metastases depends on the patient's primary cancer. In some cases, a biopsy may be needed to confirm the diagnosis. Treatment is based on the underlying primary diagnosis. Surgery and/or radiation are often primary treatments.

Risk Factors

The incidence of brain tumors appears to have increased in the past few decades. Epidemiologic data suggest that this is due to more aggressive and more accurate diagnosis rather than to an actual rise in incidence. Better access to care and an increase in the aging population may contribute to the increase in rates. An estimated 88,970 new cases of primary brain (nonmalignant and malignant) and CNS tumors will be diagnosed in 2022. Of those tumors, 25,930 will be primary malignant brain tumors. The incidence rate for primary brain and CNS tumors is higher in males than females (Central Brain Tumor Registry of the United States [CBTRUS], 2021).

The cause of most primary brain tumors is unknown. The only known risk factors are exposure to ionizing radiation and cancer-causing chemicals. Additional possible risk factors that require further investigation include nonionizing radiation, consumption of nitrates, cigarette smoking, cell phone use, alcohol intake, exposure to pesticides (among agriculture workers), and exposure to residential power lines (Michaud & Batchelor, 2020).

There has been some suggestion that particular genetic risk factors are associated with certain types of brain tumors. For example, neurofibromatosis type 1 (NF1), also known as von Recklinghausen disease, is a genetic disorder linked to brain and spinal cord tumors. People with this disorder are at higher risk for schwannomas, meningiomas, types of gliomas, and neurofibromas (benign tumor). NF2 is less common and is related to acoustic neuromas. People with a condition called tuberous sclerosis are at risk for low-grade astrocytomas and other benign tumors on the body. Li-Fraumeni syndrome increases the risk for developing gliomas, and Von Hippel-Lindau disease may cause tumors in the blood vessels of the brain and spinal cord as well as, other areas of the body. Other inherited conditions include Gorlin syndrome, Turcot syndrome, and Cowden syndrome (American Cancer Society [ACS], 2020). However, the cause of most brain tumors remains elusive.

BOX 43-2 Primary Brain Tumors in Adults

- Anaplastic astrocytomas and glioblastomas
- Meningiomas and other mesenchymal tumors
- Pituitary tumors
- Schwannomas
- CNS lymphomas
- Oligodendrogliomas
- Ependymomas
- Low-grade astrocytomas
- Medulloblastomas

Adapted with permission from National Cancer Institute (NCI). (2021). *Adult Central Nervous System Tumors Treatment—Health Professional Version.* https://www.cancer.gov/types/brain/hp/adult-brain-treatment-pdq.

Clinical Manifestations

Brain tumors can produce focal (localized) or generalized neurologic symptoms. Symptoms reflect brain invasion, compression by the mass on adjacent structures, or increased ICP. The patient can experience seizures, nausea and vomiting, cognitive impairment, and visual disturbances. In addition, specific signs and symptoms result from tumors that interfere with functions in specific brain regions. These focal symptoms may also include weakness, sensory loss, aphasia, visual dysfunction, and other manifestations related to specific neurologic dysfunction because of localized involvement. Box 43-2 indicates common tumor sites in the brain.

Increased Intracranial Pressure

Symptoms of increased ICP, which is discussed in Chapter 44, result from compression of the brain by the enlarging tumor or edema. Vasogenic (cerebral) edema plays a major role in symptoms related to an increase in mass. Edema can exceed the mass itself, creating increased pressure and disrupting blood flow or CSF. Symptoms often include headache, nausea with or without vomiting, blurred vision, and balance issues. Personality changes and a variety of focal deficits, including motor, sensory, and cranial nerve dysfunction, are common. The nurse remains alert for changes in the patient's level of consciousness (LOC) and notifies the primary care provider of any alterations in mental status. Late signs associated with rising ICP related to the vital signs include hypertension with a widening pulse pressure (the difference between systolic and diastolic pressure), bradycardia, and respiratory depression. This is termed the Cushing triad.

Headache

Headache, although not always present, is most common in the early morning and improves during the day. It is made worse by coughing, straining, or sudden movement. Headache is thought to be caused by the tumor's invading, compressing, or distorting the pain-sensitive structures or by edema that accompanies the tumor (ABTA, n.d.a). Thus, headaches are related to intracerebral edema and increasing

ICP. Over-the-counter medication usually provides little to no relief. Headaches are usually described as deep or expanding or as dull but unrelenting.

Pearls for Practice: Pathophysiology Headache and the Brain

The nurse is aware that headaches in the morning are suggestive of a tumor. When the patient complains of a headache, the nurse assesses the patient's temperature. The nurse knows that fever with headache is associated with an infectious process, such as meningitis or encephalitis, whereas headache without fever may be associated with a tumor or intracerebral bleeding.

Personality Changes

The location, pressure, and degree of infiltration of the tumor and edema, if present, influence the changes in personality and mental status. Changes may be subtle with the patient sleeping more and experiencing loss of interest in activities and difficulty with memory. It is not uncommon for the short-term memory to be affected with long-term memory retained.

Fatigue

Fatigue is a symptom experienced by patients with both malignant and nonmalignant brain tumors. Etiology of fatigue can be multifactorial. The tumor itself, surgery, medications, chemotherapy, and radiation may all contribute to increased fatigue. Patients may complain of a constant feeling of exhaustion, weakness, and lack of energy. It is also important to identify underlying conditions such as stress, anxiety, and depression, which may play a role in fatigue (ABTA, n.d.b).

Vomiting

Vomiting, seldom related to food intake, is usually the result of irritation of the vagal centers in the medulla. Forceful vomiting is described as *projectile vomiting*.

Visual Disturbances

Papilledema is associated with visual disturbances, such as decreased visual acuity, diplopia (double vision), and visual field deficits.

New Onset of Seizures

Seizures are a common symptom among brain tumor patients due to abnormal electrical activity in the brain. They may present upon initial diagnosis or during the course of the disease process. Approximately 33% of those with a brain tumor present with a seizure as their first symptom (Alther et al., 2020). The type and frequency of seizure vary, related to tumor size, site, and type. Simple partial seizures, complex partial seizures, and generalized tonic–clonic seizures are those more commonly seen. Seizures are discussed in Chapter 45.

Localized Symptoms

Common focal, or localized, symptoms include muscle weakness, sensory loss, aphasia (inability to comprehend or formulate language), and visual changes (Wong & Wu, 2021). When specific regions of the brain are affected, there are additional local signs and symptoms, such as motor abnormalities, changes in hearing, alterations in cognition, and language disturbances. The progression of the signs and symptoms is important because it indicates tumor growth and expansion. For example, if a tumor is present in the cerebellar area, the nurse might expect to see changes in balance and coordination. Figure 43-2 reviews specific cerebral structures and function.

Assessment and Diagnostic Findings

The history of the illness and the manner and time frame in which the symptoms evolved are key components in the diagnosis of a brain tumor. A neurologic examination can be helpful in indicating the areas of the CNS that are involved.

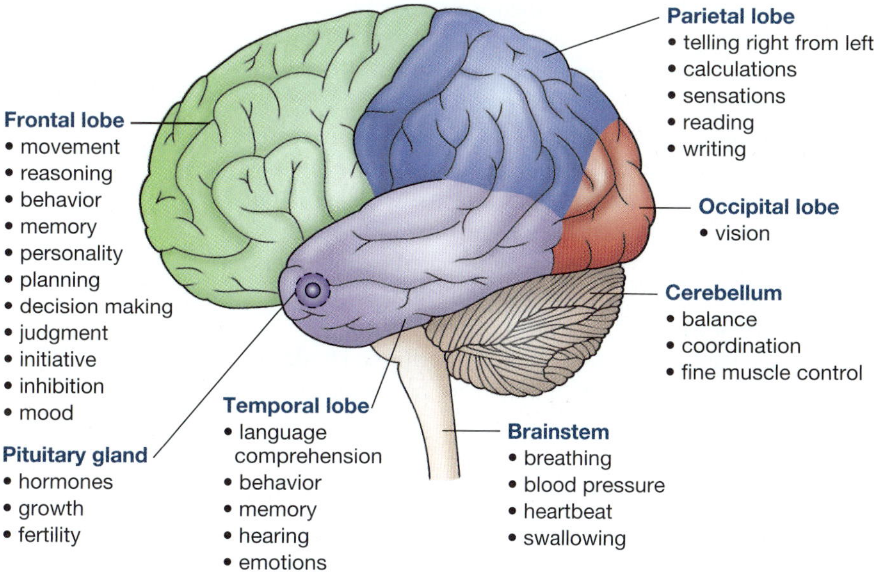

FIGURE 43-2 Brain structures and their function. (Adapted from *The essential guide to brain tumors*. National Brain Tumor Society [2010], page 9. http://www.braintumor.org/patients-family-friends/about-brain-tumors/publications/essentialguide.pdf)

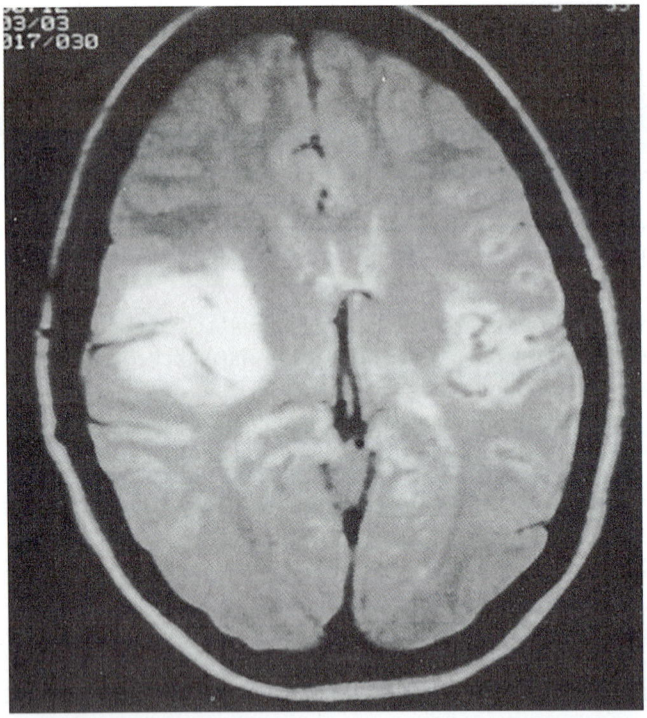

FIGURE 43-3 Low-grade glioma. Magnetic resonance imaging of the brain shows an abnormal density in the right temporal lobe. (Courtesy of the Hospital of the University of Pennsylvania, Nuclear Medicine Section, Philadelphia, PA.)

To assist in identifying the precise location of the lesion, a battery of tests may need to be performed.

MRI is the gold standard for detecting brain tumors (National Comprehensive Cancer Network [NCCN], 2021). Intravenous contrast with gadolinium helps to create a clear image of the brain (Fig. 43-3). Computed tomography (CT), enhanced by a contrast agent, can give specific information concerning the number, size, and density of the lesions or any evidence of bleeding. CT can also provide information about the ventricular system, which is responsible for producing, transporting, and excreting CSF. CT may need to be used for patients who are unable to undergo an MRI due to hardware such as a pacemaker or certain types of implants.

Positron emission tomography (PET), which measures the brain's activity rather than simply its structure, is useful in differentiating a tumor from scar tissue or radiation necrosis. Computer-assisted stereotactic (three-dimensional) biopsy is being used to diagnose deep-seated brain tumors. Cerebral angiography provides visualization of cerebral blood vessels and can localize most cerebral tumors.

Cytologic studies of the CSF may be performed to detect malignant cells because CNS tumors can shed cells into the CSF.

Medical Management of Primary Brain Tumors

A variety of medical treatment modalities, including surgery; chemotherapy; and external-beam radiation therapy, radiosurgery, or radiotherapy can be used alone or in combination with surgical resection. Depending on the type, location, and extent of the tumor, medical treatments may be done for symptom management purposes rather than to cure the patient of the brain tumor. This type of medical management is referred to as palliative care and will help improve the patient's quality of life when a cure is not possible.

Surgical Management

Surgical intervention provides the best outcome for most brain tumor types. The objective of surgical management is removal of part of or the entire tumor without increasing the neurologic deficit and to establish a tissue diagnosis. The surgical approach depends on the type of tumor, its location, and its accessibility. Options include stereotactic biopsy, open biopsy, craniotomy with debulking, and subtotal or complete resection. MRI-guided laser interstitial thermal therapy (LITT) may be considered for patients who are unable to undergo surgery (NCCN, 2021). LITT is a minimally invasive procedure that involves implanting a laser catheter that uses the heat generated by a laser light (65 degrees) to destroy brain lesions by coagulation leading to lesion necrosis under real-time MRI monitoring (NIH, 2022).

Lifting the Lens: Structural and Social Determinants of Health (SDOH) and Neurosurgical Outcomes

In a recent comprehensive literature review to evaluate the influence of SDOH on neurosurgical outcomes, the authors suggest that the effect of gender and race on outcomes is largely mitigated when equal access to care is attained, and socioeconomic factors and comorbidities are controlled for (Glauser et al., 2021). They noted that lower household income significantly decreases survival over time and that socioeconomic status impacts postoperative mortality. As noted in Chapter 1, it is important to recognize that the political economy of health care in the United States impacts one's own health in addition to the health of their patients. The political determinants of health are the systematic processes such as distribution of resources that exacerbate health inequities by directly and indirectly influencing SSDOH, and this study demonstrates that economics are an important driver of postoperative outcomes (Dawes, 2020; Glauser et al., 2021). It is important for all nurses to acknowledge the political determinants of health by exercising their voice concerning the systemic factors that require actionable change in order to impact patients' outcomes. As noted by Florence Nightingale, "I think that feelings waste themselves in words; they ought to be distilled into actions, and into actions which bring results" (AACN, 2019).

Radiation Therapy

Radiation therapy, the cornerstone of treatment for many brain tumors, decreases the incidence of recurrence of incompletely resected tumors. External-beam radiation therapy may be used alone or in combination with surgical resection. Stereotactic radiosurgery may be performed to deep, inaccessible tumors, often in a single session. Precise localization of the tumor is accomplished by the stereotactic approach with precise positioning of the patient.

Pharmacologic Therapy and Chemotherapy

Chemotherapy may be given intravenously, orally, or intrathecally (injected directly into the subarachnoid space). The oral chemotherapy agent temozolomide is often part of the systemic therapy because of its ability to pass through the blood–brain barrier (NCCN, 2021). Chemotherapy that is given by intrathecal injection bypasses the blood–brain barrier. Other chemotherapy agents are usually given as salvage therapy after initial treatments fail. Targeted therapies work differently than chemotherapy and affect the way a cell functions. Bevacizumab may be used to treat some brain and spinal cord tumors. Testing the tumor for biomarkers may make the patient eligible for other inhibitor drugs. For some patients who fail treatment or are resistant to standard therapy, clinical trials may be an alternative option. Corticosteroids are used during treatment to reduce cerebral edema and to reduce the side effects of treatment such as nausea and vomiting. They are also helpful in relieving headache and improving alterations in the LOC. Anticonvulsant agents are used to treat seizures if they occur. Special consideration is given when managing seizures, related to a potential serious interaction between seizure medications and antineoplastic agents. Newer agents are now available with fewer drug interactions and no monitoring of drug levels. Patients with brain tumors are at a higher risk for the development of deep vein thrombosis (DVT) and pulmonary embolism (PE). Careful consideration is taken when prescribing anticoagulant therapy due to the risk of CNS hemorrhage.

Pearls for Practice: Pathophysiology
Salvage Therapy, What Does It Mean?
Salvage therapy is a term that is used to describe treatments that are instituted once the standard treatment is no longer working. It is also known as "rescue" therapy and may include medications, experimental drugs still undergoing clinical trials, radiation, or surgery.

Pain is managed by means of a stepped progression regarding the dosing, delivery method, and type of analgesic agents needed for relief. Headache is often a common complaint of pain in this population of patients. Small doses of morphine are administered at prescribed intervals (refer to Chapter 6).

Medical Management of Metastatic Brain Cancer

The treatment of metastatic brain cancer is palliative and involves eliminating or reducing serious symptoms, thereby improving the quality of life for both patient and family. The therapeutic approach includes radiation therapy, surgery (usually for a single intracranial metastasis), and chemotherapy. Radiosurgery can be considered if a limited number of lesions are present. Survival rates vary, depending on the type and extent of the tumor at the time of diagnosis. The overall prognosis is poor in most cases.

Nursing Management

The effects of increased ICP caused by the tumor mass are reviewed in Chapter 44. The nurse performs neurologic checks, monitors vital signs, maintains a neurologic flow chart, spaces nursing interventions to prevent a rapid increase in ICP, and reorients the patient when necessary to person, time, place, and situation. Patients with changes in cognition caused by their lesions require frequent reorientation and the use of orienting devices (e.g., personal possessions, photographs, lists, and a clock). Supervision of and assistance with self-care, ongoing monitoring, and interventions for prevention of injury may be required. Patients who have seizures are carefully monitored and protected from injury.

The nursing process for patients undergoing neurosurgery is discussed in Chapter 44. The patient with a brain tumor may be at increased risk for aspiration due to cranial nerve dysfunction. If the patient is at risk for aspiration, they should be placed in a side-lying position with HOB elevated 10 to 30 degrees. The nurse must ensure that suction equipment is at the bedside. Preoperatively, the gag reflex and ability to swallow are evaluated by gently touching each side of the posterior pharyngeal wall with a cotton swab or suction catheter and noting the strength of the gag. The nurse expects to observe a simultaneous elevation of the uvula and "gag" with stimulation of the posterior pharynx. Function should be reassessed postoperatively because changes can occur due to alterations in cranial nerves IX (glossopharyngeal) and X (vagus) or the pons or medulla. If the gag reflex is impaired, the health care provider is notified, and food and fluid are withheld until evaluation of swallowing is determined. Box 43-3 explores pain management experience of patients after craniotomy for removal of a brain tumor.

SPINAL CORD TUMORS

Primary spinal tumors are rare, as most spinal tumors will be related to metastatic disease. Tumors within the spine are classified according to their anatomic relation to the spinal cord. Intramedullary tumors arise from within the spinal cord. Intradural–extramedullary tumors are within or under

BOX 43-3

Nursing Research

Bridging the Gap to Evidence-Based Practice

Pain Management Experience Among Hospitalized Postcraniotomy Brain Tumor Patients

Winton, R. E. F., Draucker, C. B., & Von Ah, D. (2021). Pain management experiences among hospitalized postcraniotomy brain tumor patients. *Cancer Nurs. 44*(3), E170–E180. https://dx.doi.org/10.1097/NCC.0000000000000851.

Purpose

The purpose of this study was to assess the level of pain experienced by patients who have undergone a craniotomy for removal of a brain tumor. Pain is often related to scalp, soft tissues or if the dura (the covering the brain) is affected during surgery. Surgery on the subtemporal and suboccipital areas have been found to have a higher rate of pain. Research revealed that little is known about the patient's perspective of pain management postcraniotomy.

Design

The study used qualitative descriptive (QD) methods described by Sandelowski. The method allows patients to share their experiences through interviews. The reports were collected according to the Consolidated Criteria for Reporting Qualitative Research (COREQ). Using semistructured interviews with patients on a 23-bed neurologic step-down unit in an urban teaching hospital in the Midwest United States, researchers focused on how patients experienced postcraniotomy pain and how it was managed. Narratives were analyzed with standard content analytic procedures.

Data were collected from 2/2016 through 12/2016 from patients who had undergone a craniotomy for excision or removal of a primary brain tumor within 2 weeks. Questions assessed how the patient described their pain since surgery, how they dealt with their pain, and how their clinicians managed their pain. Pain intensity ratings and Glasgow Coma scale ratings were obtained daily.

Findings

Twenty-six patients were enrolled in the study. The average age was 58.5 with more female than male participants. The most common tumors were found to be glioma, glioblastoma, oligodendroma, and meningioma. The average length of the interview was 21 minutes. The patients were placed in three different groups. Twelve patients were placed in group 1. Their pain was described as nonsalient or routine. They reported simply getting pills, conferring with staff, waiting pain out and/or having no pain at all. Group 2 consisted of seven patients who described their pain management as definitely getting pain pills and staying on top of the pain. Group 3 had complex pain management issues. Eight patients were in group 3. Five patients reported their pain pattern as not staying on top of it. One patient reported their pain as excruciating. Lastly, three patients reported that everything was done to help them. However, they also experienced other symptoms such as nausea and low heart rate that complicated their pain management.

Overall, pain experiences varied among patients, with some stating that their pain was "no big deal" and manageable. However, there were patients who reported their pain as intense and used words such as "excruciating" or "unbearable."

Nursing Implications

This study will help nurses identify that patients who undergo craniotomies for primary brain tumors may experience different levels of pain. Understanding the location of the surgical site may help identify patients at risk for higher levels of pain. Nurses need to be aware that each patient who undergoes a craniotomy is at risk for pain, and verbal assessment may be helpful in its management.

the spinal dura but not on the actual spinal cord. Extradural tumors are located outside the dura and often involve the vertebral bodies (Welch et al., 2021). These tumors may be either primary or metastatic in nature. Spinal tumors causing cord compression are considered a neurologic emergency.

Metastatic Spinal Cord Tumors

Cancer can spread to the spinal cord. The three most common cancers that metastasize to the spinal cord are breast, lung, and prostate; however, this may also occur with renal, gastrointestinal, and thyroid cancer (Ziu & Mesfin, 2021). Cancer can invade the bone, causing vertebral metastases. The most frequent symptom is dull aching pain in the spine at night. It is estimated that 40% of patients with cancer will develop metastatic spinal disease (Pritts, 2020).

Spinal Cord Compression

Spinal cord compression (SCC) occurs because of tumor extension into the epidural space. The cord can be compressed at any area of the spine, resulting in permanent paralysis if not treated. Patients with myeloma or lymphoma, as well as those with breast, prostate, and lung cancer are at an increased risk for developing SCC (Laufer et al., 2021). Metastatic SCC is seen in 3% to 5% of cancer patients, often affecting the thoracic spine (Beach, 2021).

SCC is considered a medical emergency and requires immediate treatment to prevent permanent neurologic damage. The treatment goal is to relieve cord compression with the use of IV steroids such as dexamethasone (Decadron) to reduce edema. In addition, chemotherapy, radiation, or surgery to debulk the tumor is expected to preserve neurologic function. Early intervention helps to prevent further complications and preserve neurologic function.

Assessment and Diagnostic Findings

Initial symptoms may present as radicular pain (pain that radiates along the dermatome [sensory distribution] of a nerve), weakness, and sensory changes. The nurse is alert for early complaints of back pain, which occurs in the region of the tumor, sometimes described as a "band" or girdle of pain (Oatley & Dunleavey, 2019). Back pain is the most common (95%) and often the first symptom, preceding other symptoms by as much as 2 months (Given, 2021). The pain typically increases when the patient is in the prone position and is worsened by movement, coughing, or sneezing (Pritts, 2020). Symmetric extremity weakness may also be present. Ataxia (diminished balance or coordination) with back pain (secondary to loss of proprioception in legs) should always be a concern for SCC (Patel & Kuris, 2022). Motor weakness and sensory deficits, if left untreated, can progress to paralysis. Neurologic examination and diagnostic studies are used to make the diagnosis. Neurologic examination includes assessment of pain, loss of reflexes above the tumor level, progressive loss of sensation or motor function, and the presence of weakness and paralysis. These changes in neurologic function are related to the mass exerting pressure and compression of the nerve roots or spinal cord. Late symptoms include sphincter dysfunction of bladder and bowel (urinary incontinence or retention; fecal incontinence or constipation). The nurse notifies the provider immediately when any changes or deterioration are noted, since neurologic damage may be reversible if treatment is started within 24 to 48 hours of onset of symptoms (Oatley & Dunleavey, 2019). MRI is the most commonly used diagnostic tool in detecting epidural SCC and metastases. For further details on SCC see Table 5-6.

Medical Management

Treatment of spinal cord tumors depends on the type and location of the tumor, the presenting symptoms, and physical status of the patient. Surgical intervention, if appropriate, is the primary treatment for most tumors. Other treatment modalities include partial removal of the tumor with decompression of the spinal cord. For metastatic lesions of the spine, radiation therapy can be used to decrease the size of the tumor. Chemotherapy for malignant spinal cord neoplasms provides limited benefit except for tumors that are chemosensitive. Dexamethasone is used temporarily to reduce edema and improve neurologic function until other treatments can take effect.

Tumor removal is desirable but not always possible. The goal is to remove as much tumor as possible while sparing uninvolved portions of the spinal cord to avoid neurologic damage. Microsurgical techniques have improved the prognosis for patients with intramedullary tumors. Prognosis is related to the degree of neurologic impairment at the time of surgery, the speed with which symptoms occurred, and the origin of the tumor. Patients with extensive neurologic deficits before surgery usually do not make significant functional recovery, even after successful tumor removal.

Palliative care may be an option for the medical management of some patients. Focus is on improving quality of life, relief from symptoms, pain control, and management of psychosocial and spiritual issues. Patients may receive palliative care at the time of diagnosis and receive treatments such as radiation. Other integrative (complementary/alternative) therapies consist of music, massage, Reiki, and guided imagery.

Nursing Management

Providing Preoperative Care

The objectives of preoperative care include recognition of neurologic changes through ongoing assessments, pain control, and the management of altered activities of daily living (ADLs). The nurse assesses for weakness, muscle wasting, spasticity, sensory changes, bowel and bladder dysfunction, and potential respiratory problems, especially if a cervical tumor is present. Preoperative blood work (e.g., CBC, comprehensive metabolic panel [CMP]) and coagulation studies are obtained for baseline values and to assess for anemia, infection, coagulation deficiencies, or penias (a lack or deficiency in RBC, WBC, or platelets) due to bone marrow invasions. Postoperative pain management strategies are discussed with the patient before surgery.

Assessing the Patient Postoperatively

The patient is monitored for deterioration in neurologic status. A sudden onset of neurologic deficit is an ominous sign and may be due to vertebral collapse associated with spinal cord infarction. Frequent neurologic checks are carried out, with emphasis on movement, strength, and sensation of the upper and lower extremities. Staining of the dressing may indicate leakage of CSF from the surgical site, which may lead to serious infection or to an inflammatory reaction in the surrounding tissues that can cause severe pain in the postoperative period (refer to Chapter 42 for evaluation of CSF leakage).

Approximately 15% of patients with SCC develop a DVT due to blood stasis from paralysis of muscles and hypercoagulopathy (Oatley & Dunleavey, 2019). Since patients are at risk for DVT, the nurse assesses for unilateral limb edema (differences in leg circumference bilaterally from thigh to ankle); increase in the leg's surface temperature, particularly on the calf or ankle; and areas of tenderness or superficial thrombosis. The nurse ensures prophylaxis, which may consist of physical interventions, such as elastic compression stockings, intermittent pneumatic compression devices, body positioning, and exercise. For further details on DVT, see Chapter 17. Postoperatively, DVT prophylaxis may be held initially to prevent development of epidural hematoma after surgery. The optimal timing for initiation of pharmacologic prophylaxis is controversial, and no strict guidelines are currently in place (Patel & Kuris, 2022).

Managing Pain

The prescribed medication should be administered in adequate amounts and at appropriate intervals to relieve pain and prevent its recurrence. Early symptoms of spinal cord tumors include stiffness and pain that continues to worsen. Back pain at night is one of the hallmark signs of spinal metastasis.

The bed is usually kept flat initially. The nurse turns the patient as a unit, keeping shoulders and hips aligned and the back straight. The side-lying position is usually the most comfortable because this position imposes the least pressure on the surgical site. Placement of a pillow between the knees of the patient in a side-lying position helps to prevent extreme knee flexion.

Promoting Home and Community-Based Care

In preparation for discharge, the patient is assessed for the ability to function independently in the home and for the availability of resources such as family members to assist in care giving. Safety is a key component when arranging for home care. Patients with residual sensory involvement are cautioned about the dangers of extremes in temperature. They should be alerted to the dangers of heating devices (e.g., hot water bottles, heating pads, space heaters). The patient is taught to check skin integrity daily. Patients with impaired motor function related to motor weakness or paralysis may require training in ADLs and safe use of assistive devices, such as a cane, walker, or wheelchair.

The patient and family members are instructed about pain management strategies, bowel and bladder management, and assessment for signs and symptoms of neurologic dysfunction, which should be reported promptly.

Clinical Judgment Case

A patient (MW), who is 72 years old, is admitted to your oncology unit. The patient has a history of breast cancer, treated years ago with surgery, chemotherapy, and radiation. MW's chief complaint (CC) is back pain that is described as a "band" across the lower ribs. The pain is described as "tingling" and is rated as 4/10 but increases to 9/10 when they sneeze. Vital signs are as follows: 98.7, HR is 92 and irregular, RR of 18, oxygen saturation of 97% on room air (RA), and B/P is 119/72. Skin is warm and dry. Pupils are equal and reacting to light (PEARL) 3 mm bil. Upper and lower extremity strength is 5/5 bil., pedal and posterior tibial pulses are 3+ bil, capillary refill is <2 seconds. Lung sounds are clear to auscultation, S1S2 without murmurs, gallops, or rub. Abdomen is firm, slightly distended, nontender, bowel sounds are positive (BS+), flatus +, last bowel movement (BM) was four days ago (formed brown). Voided early this morning before admission, has not voided (HNV) since admission (3 hours ago). The patient is on a regular diet, and routine admission orders are in process. Admitting blood work obtained; IID (intermittent infusion device) inserted in left antecub; patient is oriented to the unit, bed, and call bell, which is within patient's reach.

Step One: Recognize cues where relevant and important information is identified from different sources, such as medical history or vital signs.

Answer: History of breast cancer, CC of back pain described as "tingling", 4/10 intensity but increases to 9/10 with sneezing, irregular HR of 92, firm abdomen, no BM in 4 days, has not voided.

Step Two: Analyze cues, which is organizing and linking the recognized cues to the patient's clinical presentation.

Answer: You link the back pain (4/10 that increases to 9/10 with sneezing) and description of "bandlike pain," and radiculopathy ("tingling pain") as potential of spinal cord compression (SCC). You recognize that may mean metastatic disease, as it is seen in 3% to 5% of cancer patients, often those with breast, lung, and prostate cancer, and frequently affects the thoracic spine. You worry that the lack of BM in 4 days and the fact MW HNV may be a late symptom of sphincter dysfunction of bladder and bowel (urinary incontinence or retention; fecal incontinence or constipation). However, since patient has full motor strength, you also reason they may be constipated and HNV since they have had limited PO intake today and may be dehydrated. You recognize that you will go back and assess mucous membranes and skin turgor to help you interpret the reason MW HNV. You are concerned about the irregular heart rate and are worried MW has developed an arrhythmia. Your suspicion is atrial fibrillation since its incidence and prevalence increase with age, especially over 65 years. You review old charts and see the last reading was normal sinus rhythm and there is no history of cardiac arrhythmia.

Step Three: Prioritize hypotheses, where hypotheses are evaluated and ranked according to priority. This can include urgency, likelihood, risk, difficulty, and/or time. In this phase you cluster your findings to arrive at a list of problems (actual and or potential problems) you believe the patient is experiencing and determine the importance or urgency. What do you think is of greatest concern?

Answer: Although you are concerned about the possibility of SCC, constipation, and fluid volume deficit, the priority is to evaluate the patient for atrial fibrillation, since this arrhythmia multiplies mortality from any cause by two and is associated with risk of stroke approximately five times higher than that of the general population.

Step Four: Generate solutions, which is identifying expected outcomes and using hypotheses to define a set of interventions for the expected outcomes.

Answer: You are aware that SCC is an emergency and that motor weakness and sensory deficits if left untreated can progress to paralysis. However, at this time, MW's strength is 5/5. You will repeat the neurologic assessment before change of shift but also ask the patient to call you if the pain worsens or any additional symptoms present. You are aware that the provider would be notified of any changes immediately since neurologic damage may be reversible if treatment is started within 24 to 48 hours of onset of symptoms.

You are making a list of concerns about which you will speak with the PCP, such as the constipation and the fact the patient HNV. You have assessed MW's mucous membranes, which are dry, and skin turgor is delayed. You ask the patient their preferred drink and ensure that it is at the bedside with a full water pitcher. You ask the patient to keep track of the number of glasses they drink. You will continue to monitor intake and output (I&O) and send routine urine to the lab to evaluate the specific gravity. Your unit has portable telemetry units; you realize an admission ECG was not ordered and will notify the provider and also inform them about your concern for fluid volume deficit. You anticipate the IID order will be changed to IV solution. Your priority is assessing the cardiac rhythm since the risk of emboli increases with this arrhythmia. In addition, if this is indeed SCC, then metastasis has occurred, which again increases the risk of hypercoagulopathy.

Step Five: Take action, where the solutions that address the highest priorities are implemented.

Answer: You connect the patient to the portable telemetry unit, which transmits the ECG to a central monitor on the unit. You notify the provider that the rhythm is atrial fibrillation. A 12 lead ECG is also performed. You ask about anticoagulant therapy since the combination of potential metastatic cancer and a fib significantly increases the patient's risk for emboli. You ask about starting an IV since MW has had limited PO intake and discuss with the provider the constipation.

Step Six: Evaluate outcomes, which is comparing observed outcomes against expected outcomes.

Answer: The anticoagulants are ordered; you will continue to monitor I&O. The urine specific gravity was 1.034 and IV of D5 ½ normal saline was ordered. Vital signs have remained stable and there has been no change in the patient's neurological assessment. Cardiology has been called to evaluate MW, and the patient is monitored via telemetry. You have added to your database of prioritizing when multiple problems are present. Great job!

CHAPTER REVIEW

NCLEX-Style Review Questions

1. A patient admitted to the emergency room has a history of a spinal tumor. Which of the following signs and symptoms should alert the nurse to the possibility of SCC? Select all that apply.
   a. Seizures
   b. Headache
   c. Back pain
   d. Diplopia
   e. Radicular pain

2. A patient is admitted for concern of a possible brain tumor. What is the most concerning symptom you would expect them to report? Select all that apply.
   a. Urinary incontinence
   b. Headache upon awakening
   c. Spasticity of the lower extremities
   d. Hyperactive bowel sounds
   e. Seizures

3. Which of the following are **late** signs of rising ICP? Select all that apply.
   a. Papilledema
   b. Change in the LOC
   c. Vomiting
   d. Hypertension
   e. Bradycardia

4. A nurse is caring for a patient who is 4 hours postsurgery for a spinal cord tumor. Neurologic checks should include which of the following? Select all that apply.
   a. Movement of upper and lower extremities
   b. Monitoring sensation
   c. Bowel function
   d. Strength assessment
   e. Liver span

5. A patient has just been admitted to the hospital with a diagnosis of brain tumor. The patient makes a comment that drinking alcohol has caused the brain tumor. The nurse understands that which of the following is a cause of brain tumor? Select all that apply.

a. Smoking
b. Ionizing radiation
c. Diet high in fat
d. Exposure to the sun
e. Exposure to cancer causing chemicals

REFERENCES AND SELECTED READINGS

References and selected readings associated with this chapter can be found on the website that accompanies the book. Visit **http://thepoint.lww.com/Honan3e** to access the references and other additional resources associated with this chapter.

CHAPTER 44

Nursing Management: Patients With Neurologic Trauma

Cynthia Bautista

Learning Objectives

After reading this chapter, you will be able to:

1. Differentiate patients with head injuries according to mechanism of injury, clinical signs and symptoms, diagnostic testing, and treatment options.
2. Describe the multiple needs of the patient with altered level of consciousness.
3. Identify the early and late clinical manifestations of increased intracranial pressure (ICP).
4. Describe the management of the patient with increased ICP.
5. Identify the population at risk for spinal cord injury (SCI).
6. Identify common complications and management of complications in patients with SCIs.
7. Use the nursing process as a framework for care of patients with SCIs.

Trauma involving the central nervous system (CNS) often can be life threatening. Even when not life threatening, brain and spinal cord injuries (SCIs) can result in major physical and psychological dysfunction and can alter the patient's life completely. Neurologic trauma affects the patient, the family, the health care system, and society as a whole because of its major sequelae and the costs of acute and long-term care of patients with trauma to the brain and spinal cord.

Ongoing assessment of the patient's neurologic function and health needs, identification of problems, mutual goal setting, development and implementation of care plans (including teaching, counseling, and coordinating activities), and evaluation of the outcomes of care are nursing actions integral to the recovery of the patient with neurologic trauma. The nurse also collaborates with other members of the health care team to provide essential care, offer a variety of solutions to problems, help the patient and family gain control of their lives, and explore the educational and supportive resources available in the community. The goals are to achieve as high a level of function as possible and to enhance the quality of life for the patient with neurologic trauma and their family.

HEAD INJURIES

Head injury is a broad classification that includes injury to the scalp, skull, or brain. It is the most common cause of death from trauma in the United States. Approximately 2.8 million new cases of head injury occur every year (McNair, 2020). Of these, 2.8 million are treated and released by the emergency room, 100,000 have permanent disabilities, and 50,000 people die (Olson, 2018). Traumatic brain injury (TBI) is the most serious form of head injury. The most common causes of TBI are falls (48%), motor vehicle crashes (14%), being struck by objects (15%), and assaults (10%) (Bautista, 2022; CDC, 2022). Males are at highest risk for TBI (National Data and Statistical Center, 2022). The very young (children under 5 years of age) and older adults (over 75 years of age) are also at increased risk. An estimated 5.3 million Americans today are living with a disability as a result of a TBI (Wilkins, 2019). Despite advances in care, 60% of patients with severe TBI have unfavorable outcomes (Ruet et al., 2019). Patients with TBI often have long-lasting chronic comorbidities, including back pain, depression, hypertension, anxiety, fractures, high blood cholesterol, sleep disorders, panic attacks, osteoarthritis, and diabetes (Hammond et al., 2019). The best approach to head injury is an emphasis on prevention (Box 44-1).

Pathophysiology

Research has shown that not all brain damage occurs at the moment of impact. Damage to the brain from traumatic injury takes two forms: primary injury and secondary injury. Primary injury is the initial damage to the brain that results from the traumatic event. This may include contusions, lacerations, and torn blood vessels due to impact, acceleration/deceleration, or penetration by a foreign object (Norris, 2019). Secondary injury evolves over the ensuing hours and days after the initial injury and can be due to cerebral edema,

BOX 44-1
Health Promotion

Preventing Head and Spinal Cord Injuries

- Advise drivers to obey traffic laws and to avoid speeding.
- Advise patients not to drive when under the influence of drugs or alcohol.
- Advise all drivers and passengers to wear seat belts and shoulder harnesses.
- Caution passengers against riding in the back of pickup trucks.
- Advise motorcyclists, scooter riders, bicyclists, skate-boarders, and roller-bladers to wear helmets.
- Promote educational programs that are directed toward prevention of violence and suicide in the community.
- Provide water safety instruction.
- Teach patients steps that can be taken to prevent falls, particularly in the older population.
- Advise athletes to use protective devices. Recommend that coaches be educated in proper coaching techniques.
- Advise owners of firearms to keep them locked in a secure area where children cannot access them.
- Advise drivers to pay attention to the road and not be a distracted driver; advise against looking away from the road to eat, read, or text while driving.

BOX 44-2
Focus on Pathophysiology

Traumatic Brain Injury

When the brain is injured, there is no room for swelling within the rigid cranial vault. Any bleeding or swelling causes an increase in the amount of intracranial contents, which, in turn, increases intracranial pressure (ICP). The increased pressure causes vasoconstriction and a decrease in blood flow to the brain. This causes hypoxia and ischemia of brain tissue. If ICP continues to rise, eventually the brain will herniate, causing brain death.

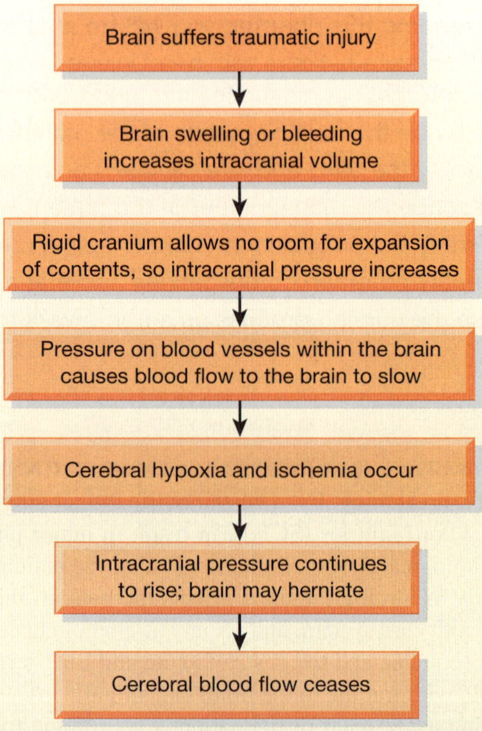

ischemia, seizures, infection, hyperthermia, hypovolemia, and hypoxia (Desai & Jain, 2018).

An injured brain is different from other injured body areas because of its unique characteristics. It resides within the skull, which is a rigid, closed compartment (McNair, 2020). Unlike other areas of the body, the confines of the skull do not allow for the expansion of cranial contents. Any bleeding or swelling within the skull increases the volume of contents and therefore can cause increased **intracranial pressure** (ICP). If the increased pressure is high enough, it can cause **herniation** of the brain through or against the rigid structures of the skull. This causes restriction of blood flow to the brain, with resultant ischemia, infarction, irreversible brain damage, and eventually **brain death** (Box 44-2).

Skull Fractures

A skull fracture is a break in the continuity of the skull caused by forceful trauma. It may occur with or without damage to the brain. Skull fractures can be classified as simple, comminuted, depressed, or basilar. A simple (linear) fracture is a break in the continuity of the bone. A comminuted skull fracture refers to a splintered fracture line. When bone fragments are embedded into brain tissue, the fracture is depressed. A fracture of the base of the skull is called a basilar or basal skull fracture (Norris, 2019). A fracture may be open, indicating a scalp laceration or tear in the dura, (protective covering directly on top of the brain) or closed, in which case the dura is intact.

Clinical Manifestations

The symptoms, apart from those of the local injury, depend on the severity and the distribution of the underlying brain injury. Persistent, localized pain suggests that a fracture is present. Fractures of the cranial vault may or may not produce swelling in the region of the fracture.

Fractures of the base of the skull tend to traverse the paranasal sinus of the frontal bone or the middle ear located in the temporal bone. Therefore, they frequently produce hemorrhage from the nose, pharynx, or ears, and blood may appear under the conjunctiva. An area of ecchymosis (bruising) that may be seen over the mastoid (Battle sign), develops 12 to 24 hours after injury (McNair, 2020). Basilar skull fractures are suspected when cerebrospinal fluid (CSF) escapes from the ears (CSF otorrhea) and the nose (CSF rhinorrhea). A halo sign (a blood stain surrounded by a yellowish stain) may be seen on bed linens or on the head dressing and is highly suggestive of a CSF leak. Patients may also complain of postnasal drip or salty or sweet taste (Holleran, 2023). Drainage of CSF is a serious problem because meningeal infection, abscess formation, and osteomyelitis can occur if organisms gain access to the cranial contents via the nose, ear, or sinus through a tear in the dura.

Assessment and Diagnostic Findings

Radiologic examination confirms the presence and extent of a skull fracture (Norris, 2019). A rapid physical examination and evaluation of neurologic status detects obvious brain injuries, and a computed tomography (CT) scan uses high-speed x-ray scanning to detect less apparent abnormalities.

Magnetic resonance imaging (MRI) is used to evaluate patients with head injury when a more accurate picture of the anatomic nature of the injury is warranted and when the patient is stable enough to undergo this longer diagnostic procedure. See Chapter 42 for further discussion of CT and MRI.

Medical and Nursing Management

Nondepressed skull fractures generally do not require surgical treatment; however, close observation of the patient is essential. Nursing personnel may observe the patient in the hospital, but if no underlying brain injury is present, the patient may be allowed to return home. If the patient is discharged home, specific instructions must be given to the family. Box 44-3 details discharge instructions.

Depressed skull fractures usually require surgery, particularly if contaminated or deformed fractures are present. Large defects can be repaired immediately with bone or artificial grafts; if significant cerebral edema is present, repair of the defect may be delayed for 3 to 6 months. Penetrating wounds require surgical debridement to remove foreign bodies and devitalized brain tissue (devoid of oxygen supply) and to control hemorrhage. IV antibiotic treatment is instituted immediately, particularly with a dural laceration, and blood products are administered if indicated.

As stated previously, fractures of the base of the skull are serious because they are usually open (involving the paranasal sinuses or the middle or external ear). CSF leakage is present in 12% to 30% of patients with skull base fractures (Sivanandapanicker et al., 2019). Clear fluid that is draining from the nose or ears should be collected and tested for glucose. If the drainage is CSF, glucose values of 30 mg/dL or greater are seen (Stacy, 2022a). Suspicion of a CSF leak should be reported immediately to the provider.

The patient who is conscious is cautioned not to blow their nose if there is a CSF leak, as this can worsen the leak. The head is elevated 30 degrees to reduce ICP and promote spontaneous closure of the leak (McNair, 2020). Early detection of a CSF leak may help avoid complications, including meningitis or pneumocephalus (air within the cranial vault). The patient with a basal skull fracture should not have the nose suctioned. If a nasogastric tube is required for patient management, it should be inserted orally. Tears of the dura are commonly seen in basal skull fractures. A suction catheter or nasogastric tube is a potential source of infection and may lead to the development of meningitis. Early CSF rhinorrhea (resolving within 3 to 5 days) usually does not require surgery. Late-onset (7 or more days after the initial injury) and persistent CSF rhinorrhea usually requires surgical intervention to prevent development of meningitis. The majority of CSF leaks tend to resolve spontaneously (Liao et al., 2022).

Pearls for Practice

Any patient with extensive facial fractures or suspected basilar skull fracture may also have a fracture of the cribriform plate (portion of the ethmoid bone that separates the roof of the nose from the cranial cavity). Attempted intubation with a nasogastric tube or nasotracheal tube or suctioning is prohibited to avoid intracranial penetration of the brain with the tube or catheter.

BOX 44-3 Patient and Family Education

Teaching Guidelines Following Concussion

Once the patient is discharged home, they should be closely observed for the next 24 hours and awakened every 2 hours. The patient and family are instructed to observe for the following signs and symptoms and to notify the provider (or bring the patient to the emergency department) if they occur:

- Difficulty in awakening
- Difficulty speaking
- Confusion
- Seizures
- Severe headache
- Vomiting
- Weakness on one side of the body

The patient should also avoid playing contact sports, driving, drinking alcohol, and using heavy machinery until cleared by a health care provider.

BRAIN INJURY

The most important consideration in any head injury is whether or not the brain is injured. Even seemingly minor injury can cause significant brain damage secondary to obstructed blood flow and decreased tissue perfusion. The brain cannot store oxygen or glucose to any significant degree. Because neurons need an uninterrupted blood supply to obtain these nutrients, irreversible brain damage and cell death occur if the blood supply is interrupted for even a few minutes. Clinical manifestations of **brain injury** (injury to the brain that is severe enough to interfere with normal functioning) are listed in Box 44-4. Closed (blunt) brain injury occurs when the head accelerates and then rapidly decelerates or collides with another object (e.g., a wall, the dashboard of a car) and brain tissue is damaged but there is no opening through the skull and dura. Open brain injury occurs when an object penetrates the skull, enters the brain,

BOX 44-4
Focused Assessment

Traumatic Brain Injury

Be on alert for the following signs and symptoms:
- Altered level of consciousness (LOC)
- Confusion
- Pupillary abnormalities (changes in shape, size, and response to light)
- Sudden onset of neurologic deficits
- Changes in vital signs (altered respiratory pattern, widened pulse pressure, bradycardia, tachycardia, hypothermia, or hyperthermia)
- Vision and hearing impairment
- Sensory dysfunction
- Headache
- Seizures

and damages the soft brain tissue in its path (penetrating injury), or when blunt trauma to the head is so severe that it opens the scalp, skull, and dura to expose the brain.

Types of Brain Injury

Concussion

A **concussion** (also referred to as a mild TBI) involves an alteration in mental status that results from trauma and may or may not involve loss of consciousness. This typically lasts no longer than 24 hours and may include symptoms such as headache, nausea, dizziness, auditory disturbances, fatigue, disinhibition, emotional lability, amnesia, and blurry vision (Polinder et al., 2018).

Treatment involves observing the patient for symptoms, including headache, dizziness, lethargy, irritability, anxiety, photophobia, phonophobia (fear of sound or of speaking aloud), difficulty concentrating, and memory difficulties. The constellation of these symptoms beyond the usual recovery period is referred to as *postconcussion syndrome* (Biagianti et al., 2020). Giving the patient information, explanations, and encouragement may reduce some of the problems associated with postconcussion syndrome. The patient is advised to resume normal activities once symptom free at rest (Permenter & Fernández, 2021). Once the patient is discharged home, they should be closely observed for the next 24 hours and awakened every 2 hours in order to detect any changes in mental status. Box 44-3 provides complete instructions to be given to the patient and the family. Neuroimaging (CT and MRI) is generally not indicated in concussion.

Contusion

A **cerebral contusion** is a more severe injury than concussion, involving bruising of the brain, with possible surface hemorrhage. The patient is unconscious for more than a few seconds or minutes. Clinical signs and symptoms depend on the size of the contusion and the amount of associated swelling of the brain (cerebral edema). The patient may lie motionless, with a faint pulse; shallow respirations; and cool, pale skin. The patient may be aroused with effort but soon slips back into unconsciousness. Blood pressure and temperature are subnormal, and the clinical picture is somewhat similar to that of shock. The patient may recover consciousness but pass into a stage of cerebral irritability. In this stage, the patient is conscious and easily disturbed by any form of stimulation, such as noises, light, and voices; they may become hyperactive at times.

Pearls for Practice

When the patient begins to emerge from unconsciousness, every measure that is available and appropriate for calming and quieting the patient should be used. Any form of restraint is likely to be countered with resistance, leading to self-injury or to a dangerous increase in ICP. Therefore, physical restraints should be avoided, if possible.

Gradually, the pulse, respirations, temperature, and other body functions return to normal, but full recovery can be delayed for months. Residual headache and vertigo are common, and impaired mental function or seizures may occur as a result of irreparable cerebral damage.

Diffuse Axonal Injury

Diffuse axonal injury involves widespread damage to axons in the cerebral hemispheres, corpus callosum, and brainstem. It can be seen with mild, moderate, or severe head trauma. The patient experiences immediate coma, global cerebral edema, decorticate and decerebrate rigidity, or *posturing* (Fig. 44-1). **Decorticate** posturing involves abnormal flexion of the upper extremities and extension of the lower extremities and indicates damage to the upper midbrain; **decerebrate** posturing involves extreme extension of the upper and lower extremities and indicates severe damage to the brain at the lower midbrain and upper pons (McNair, 2020). Diagnosis of diffuse axonal injury is made by clinical signs in conjunction with a CT or MRI scan. These tests are usually normal; a definitive diagnosis can be made only at autopsy. Recovery depends on the severity of the axonal injury.

Intracranial Hemorrhage (Intracranial Hematoma)

Hematomas (collections of blood) that develop within the cranial vault are the most serious type of brain injury (McNair, 2020). A hematoma may be epidural (above the dura), subdural (below the dura), or intracerebral (within the brain) (Fig. 44-2). Major symptoms are frequently delayed until the hematoma is large enough to cause distortion of the brain and increased ICP.

Epidural Hematoma (Extradural Hematoma or Hemorrhage)

After a head injury, blood may collect in the epidural (extradural) space between the skull and the dura. This can result

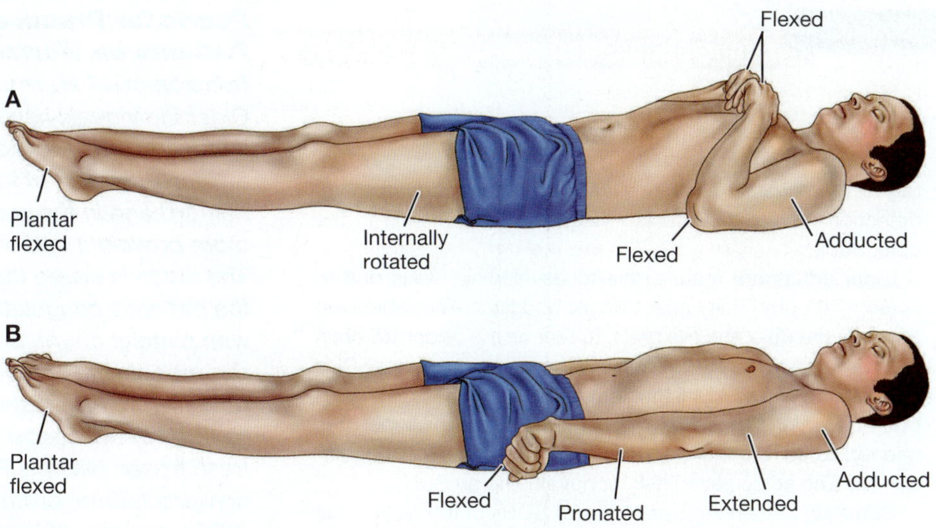

FIGURE 44-1 Abnormal posture response to stimuli. A. Decorticate posturing, involving adduction and flexion of the upper extremities, internal rotation of the lower extremities, and plantar flexion of the feet. B. Decerebrate posturing, involving extension and outward rotation of upper extremities and plantar flexion of the feet.

from a skull fracture that causes a rupture or laceration of the middle meningeal artery, the artery that runs between the dura and the skull, inferior to a thin portion of temporal bone. Hemorrhages from this artery causes a rapid increase in pressure on the brain.

Symptoms are caused by the expanding hematoma. Usually, a momentary loss of consciousness occurs at the time of injury, followed by an interval of apparent recovery (lucid interval). Although the lucid interval is considered a classic characteristic of an epidural hematoma, no lucid interval has been reported in many patients with this lesion (McNair, 2020); therefore, it should not be considered a critical defining criterion. During the lucid interval, compensation for the expanding hematoma takes place by rapid absorption of CSF and decreased intravascular volume, both of which help maintain a normal ICP. When these mechanisms can no longer compensate, even a small increase in the volume of the hematoma produces a marked elevation in ICP. Then, often suddenly, signs of compression appear (usually deterioration of consciousness and signs of focal neurologic deficits, such as dilation and fixation of a pupil or paralysis of an extremity), and the patient's condition deteriorates rapidly.

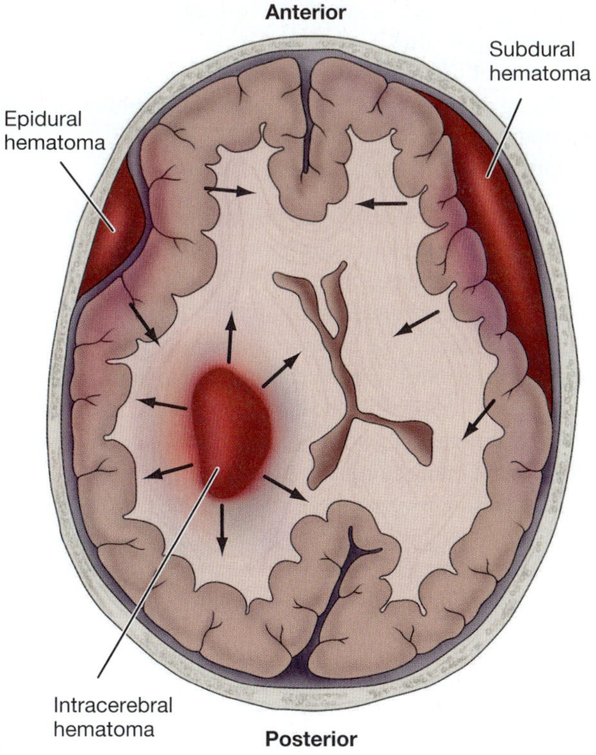

FIGURE 44-2 Location of epidural, subdural, and intracerebral hematomas.

An epidural hematoma is considered an extreme emergency; marked neurologic deficit and respiratory arrest can occur within minutes. Treatment consists of making openings through the skull (burr holes) to decrease ICP emergently, remove the clot, and control the bleeding. A craniotomy (surgical procedure that removes of part of the skull to gain access to the brain) may be required to remove the clot and control the bleeding. A drain may be inserted after creation of burr holes or a craniotomy to prevent reaccumulation of blood.

Subdural Hematoma

A subdural hematoma (SDH) is a collection of blood between the dura and the brain, a space normally occupied by a thin cushion of CSF (see Fig. 44-2). The most common cause of SDH is trauma, but it can also occur as a result of coagulopathies (bleeding disorders) or rupture of an aneurysm. Older adults are at increased risk for subdural hemorrhage secondary to whole brain atrophy, which causes traction on fragile bridging veins and also allows more free space for bleeding (McNair, 2020). Box 44-5 is a discussion of older individuals and SDHs. SDHs can be acute, subacute, or chronic, depending on when the bleed occurred.

Acute and Subacute Subdural Hematoma. Acute SDHs are associated with major head injury involving contusion or laceration. Clinical symptoms develop over 24 to 48 hours. Signs and symptoms include changes in the level

BOX 44-5

Highlighting Gerontology

Subdural Hematomas

Subdural hematomas (SDHs) are more common in older adults, occurring most often in patients in their 60s and 70s. SDHs represent a reversible cause of dementia, so their detection is vital to accurate diagnosis of dementia in the older adult.

Older adults are more prone to developing SDHs due to cerebral atrophy. This causes fragile bridging veins, which run between the dura and the brain, to tear as the atrophied brain pulls away from the dura. Trauma is the leading cause of SDHs and will often be so trivial that the older adult does not remember it occurring. Those with alcohol use disorder (sometimes referred to as "alcoholism") and patients taking anticoagulation are also at increased risk for developing an SDH.

Common presenting symptoms of SDHs in the older adult are gait disturbance, headache, aphasia (inability to speak), altered mental status, and hemiparesis (weakness on one side of the body). The initial presentation of an SDH is often very subtle, with the patient becoming confused and easily agitated. Diagnosis is made by obtaining a CT scan. Treatment typically consists of surgical evacuation of the hematoma.

When caring for the older adult, it is important to consider the risk for development of an SDH. SDHs represent a common cause of reversible dementia that is easily overlooked due to the subtlety of presenting signs and symptoms.

of consciousness (LOC), changes in the reactivity of the pupils, and hemiparesis (weakness on one side of the body). There may be minor or even no symptoms, with small collections of blood. Coma, increasing blood pressure, decreasing heart rate, and slowing respiratory rate are all signs of a rapidly expanding mass requiring immediate intervention (see later discussion of Cushing response).

Subacute SDHs are the result of less severe contusions and head trauma. Clinical manifestations usually appear between 48 hours and 2 weeks after the injury. Signs and symptoms are similar to those of an acute SDH.

If the patient can be transported rapidly to the hospital, an immediate surgery may be performed to open the dura, allowing the subdural clot to be evacuated. Successful outcome also depends on the control of ICP and careful monitoring of respiratory function. The mortality rate for patients with acute or subacute SDH is high because of associated brain damage (McNair, 2020).

Chronic Subdural Hematoma. Chronic SDHs can develop from seemingly minor head injuries and are seen most frequently in older individuals. The time between injury and onset of symptoms can be lengthy (i.e., 3 weeks to many months), so the actual injury may be forgotten.

The treatment of a chronic SDH typically consists of surgical evacuation of the clot if the patient is symptomatic and the bleed is at least 1 cm in size. Smaller bleeds are monitored until the body has fully reabsorbed the blood (McNair, 2020).

Pearls for Practice: Pathophysiology Patients on Warfarin, Aging, and Intracranial Hemorrhage

Older individuals have decreased brain volume, an increased tendency to be on anticoagulants, and an increased risk of falls, which makes intracranial hemorrhage in the warfarin-anticoagulated patient more prevalent and often more difficult to manage. The nurse is aware that laboratory analysis to evaluate the patient's coagulation status will include CBC with platelet count, prothrombin time (PT), partial thromboplastin time (PTT), and international normalized ratio (INR). Immediate interventions may include reversal of anticoagulation (if present) with intravenous fresh frozen plasma (FFP), vitamin K (phytonadione), cryoprecipitate, prothrombin precipitate complex (PCC), and possibly recombinant human factor VIIa (factor VIIa) (Cowell, 2022) to reverse the effects. Approximately 30 minutes following reversal, the nurse expects to recheck the PT/INR (Hull & Garcia, 2022).

Intracerebral Hemorrhage and Hematoma

Intracerebral hemorrhage (ICH) is bleeding into the parenchyma of the brain. It is commonly seen in head injuries when force is exerted to the head over a small area (e.g., bullet wounds and stab injuries). These hemorrhages within the brain may also result from:

- Systemic hypertension, which causes degeneration and rupture of a vessel
- Rupture of a saccular aneurysm (dilatation of vessel wall)
- Vascular anomalies
- Intracranial tumors
- Bleeding disorders, such as leukemia, hemophilia, aplastic anemia, and thrombocytopenia
- Complications of anticoagulant therapy

The onset may be insidious, beginning with the development of neurologic deficits followed by headache. Management includes supportive care; control of ICP; and careful administration of fluids, electrolytes, and antihypertensive medications. Surgical intervention by craniotomy permits removal of the blood clot and control of hemorrhage but may not be possible because of the inaccessible location of the bleeding or the lack of a clearly circumscribed area of blood that can be removed. Decompressive craniectomies that are performed up to 24 hours after the initial injury have been shown to improve outcomes. These procedures are performed to allow for swelling of the brain, which decreases ICP. Early decompressive craniectomy reduces the mortality rate (Fatima et al., 2019).

Management of Brain Injuries

Assessment and diagnosis of the extent of injury are accomplished by the initial physical and neurologic examinations. CT and MRI are the primary neuroimaging diagnostic tools of choice and are useful in evaluating the brain structure.

Cervical spine injuries occur in 1.7% to 8% of patients with TBI. Patients at highest risk for cervical spine injury are those involved in motorcycle crashes and those with lower scores on the Glasgow Coma Scale (GCS) (score of 8 or less) (Dash & Chavali, 2018). The patient is transported from the scene of the injury on a board with the head and neck maintained in alignment with the axis of the body. A hard cervical collar should be applied and maintained until cervical spine x-rays have been obtained and the absence of cervical SCIs is documented.

All therapy is directed toward preserving brain homeostasis and preventing secondary brain injury. Common causes of secondary injury include cerebral edema, hypotension, and respiratory depression. Treatments to prevent secondary injury include stabilization of cardiovascular and respiratory function to maintain adequate cerebral perfusion, control of hemorrhage and hypovolemia, and optimal blood gas values.

Pearls for Practice

Any patient with a head injury is presumed to have a cervical spine injury until such injury is ruled out; therefore, immobilization of the spine via cervical collar and spinal backboard and the avoidance of movement is essential.

ALTERED LEVEL OF CONSCIOUSNESS AND INCREASED INTRACRANIAL PRESSURE

An **altered level of consciousness** (LOC) is apparent in the patient who is not oriented, does not follow commands, or needs persistent stimuli to achieve a state of alertness. LOC is gauged on a continuum, with a normal state of alertness and full cognition (consciousness) on one end and coma on the other end. **Coma** is a clinical state of unarousable unresponsiveness in which there are no purposeful responses to internal or external stimuli, although nonpurposeful responses to painful stimuli and brainstem reflexes may be present (Hickey & Elkamand, 2020). The duration of coma is usually limited to 2 to 4 weeks. *Persistent vegetative state* is a condition in which the unresponsive patient resumes sleep–wake cycles after coma but is devoid of cognitive or affective mental function. The LOC is the most important indicator of the patient's condition.

The volume of the rigid cranial vault is approximately 1,700 mL, containing brain tissue (1,400 mL, or 80%), intravascular blood (150 mL, or 10%), and CSF (150 mL, or 10%). CSF production occurs at a rate of approximately 20 mL/hr, or 500 mL/day (Stacy, 2022b). The volume and pressure of these three components are usually in a state of equilibrium, and together they produce the ICP. An alteration in LOC may be the result of increased ICP. Increased ICP is explained by the Monro-Kellie hypothesis. The **Monro-Kellie hypothesis** states that because of the limited space for expansion within the skull, an increase in any one of the components causes a change in the volume of the others. Because brain tissue has limited space to expand, compensation typically is accomplished by increasing absorption or diminishing production of CSF or decreasing cerebral blood volume. Without such changes, ICP will begin to rise. ICP is usually measured in the lateral ventricles, with normal pressure being 5 to 15 mm Hg. Treatment of increased ICP is generally initiated at a pressure of 20 mm Hg (Hickey & Baumann, 2020).

Pathophysiology

Altered LOC is not a disorder itself; rather, it is the result of multiple pathophysiologic phenomena. The cause may be neurologic (head injury, stroke), toxicologic (drug overdose, alcohol intoxication), or metabolic (liver or kidney failure, diabetic ketoacidosis). Increased ICP affects many patients with acute neurologic conditions. This is because pathologic conditions alter the relationship between intracranial volume and ICP. Elevated ICP is most associated with head injury, although it may also be seen in other neurologic conditions, including brain tumors and subarachnoid hemorrhages. Increased ICP from any cause decreases cerebral perfusion; stimulates further swelling (edema); and may shift brain tissue through openings in the rigid dura, resulting in herniation (Fig. 44-3). The herniated brain tissue exerts pressure on the brain area into which it has shifted, which interferes with the blood supply in that area. Cessation of cerebral blood flow results in cerebral ischemia, infarction, and brain death. Herniation is often a dire, and frequently fatal, event (Hickey & Baumann, 2020).

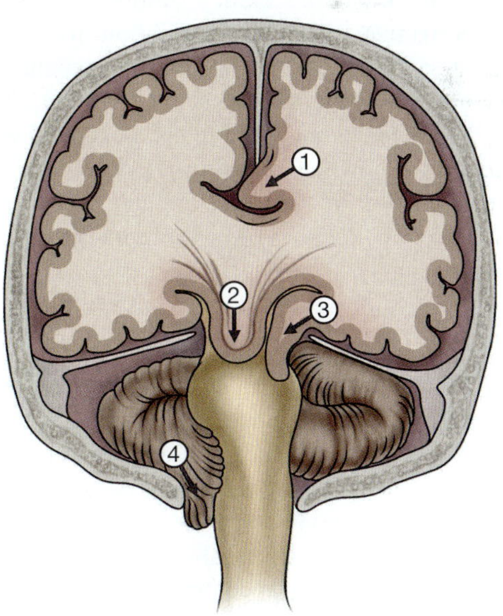

FIGURE 44-3 **Brain with intracranial shifts from supratentorial lesions. (1) Herniation of the cingulate gyrus under the falx cerebri. (2) Central transtentorial herniation. (3) Uncal herniation of the temporal lobe into the tentorial notch. (4) Infratentorial herniation of the cerebral tonsils. (Adapted from Porth, C. M., & Matfin, G. [2013].** ***Pathophysiology: Concepts of altered health states*** **[9th ed.]. Lippincott Williams & Wilkins.)**

Increased ICP may significantly reduce cerebral blood flow, resulting in ischemia and cell death. In the early stages of cerebral ischemia, the vasomotor centers are stimulated, and the systemic pressure rises to maintain cerebral blood flow. This is typically accompanied by a slow, bounding pulse and respiratory irregularities. These changes in blood pressure, pulse, and respiration are important clinically because they suggest increased ICP.

Cerebral edema is defined as an abnormal accumulation of water or fluid in the intracellular space, extracellular space, or both, and is associated with an increase in the volume of brain tissue. Edema can occur in any part of the brain. As brain tissue swells within the rigid skull, several mechanisms attempt to compensate for the increasing ICP. These compensatory mechanisms include autoregulation and decreased production and flow of CSF. **Autoregulation** refers to the brain's ability to change the diameter of its blood vessels automatically to maintain a constant cerebral blood flow during alterations in systemic blood pressure. This mechanism may be impaired in patients who are experiencing a pathologic and sustained increase in ICP.

A clinical phenomenon known as the **Cushing response** (or Cushing reflex) is seen when cerebral blood flow decreases significantly. When ischemic, the vasomotor center triggers an increase in arterial pressure to overcome the increased ICP. A sympathetically mediated response causes an increase in the systolic blood pressure, with a widening of the pulse pressure and cardiac slowing. It is a late sign requiring immediate intervention; however, perfusion may be recoverable if the Cushing response is treated rapidly.

At a certain point, the brain's ability to autoregulate becomes ineffective, and decompensation (ischemia and infarction) begins. When this occurs, the patient exhibits significant changes in mental status and vital signs. The bradycardia, hypertension, and bradypnea associated with this deterioration are known as **Cushing triad**, a grave sign. At this point, herniation of the brainstem and occlusion of the cerebral blood flow occur if therapeutic intervention is not initiated immediately.

Clinical Manifestations

Alterations in LOC occur along a continuum, and the clinical manifestations depend on where the patient is along this continuum. As the patient's state of alertness and consciousness decreases, changes will ultimately occur in the pupillary response, eye opening response, verbal response, and motor response. However, initial alterations in LOC may be reflected by subtle behavioral changes, such as restlessness or increased anxiety. The pupils, normally round and briskly reactive to light, become sluggish (response is slower); as the patient becomes comatose, the pupils become fixed (no response to light). The patient in a coma does not open the eyes, respond verbally, or move the extremities in response to a request to do so.

Pearls for Practice: Pathophysiology
Unequal Pupils

The nurse is aware that most people have equal pupils between 2 and 5 mm bilaterally and that a 1 mm difference between pupils occurs in 16% to 17% of the population; this is termed anisocoria (Burke, 2022). If there is a change or inequality in pupil size, especially in patients without anisocoria, the provider is alerted, as this is a significant finding.

It is important to be familiar with the patient's baseline status as many early signs of increased ICP are subtle; they include sudden onset of restlessness (without apparent cause), confusion, and increasing drowsiness. As ICP increases, the patient becomes stuporous, reacting only to loud or painful stimuli. At this stage, serious impairment of brain circulation is likely taking place, and immediate intervention is required. As neurologic function deteriorates further, the patient becomes comatose and exhibits decorticate or decerebrate posturing or flaccidity (see Fig. 44-1). If the coma is profound, with the patient exhibiting fixed and dilated pupils and impaired or absent respiration, death is usually inevitable.

Assessment and Diagnostic Findings

The patient with an altered LOC is at risk for alterations in every body system. A complete assessment is performed, with particular attention to the neurologic system. Focused neurologic assessments are vital in ensuring early recognition of deterioration (Bell et al., 2021). Such assessment includes an evaluation of mental status, cranial nerve function, cerebellar function (balance and coordination), reflexes, and motor and sensory function.

LOC, a sensitive indicator of neurologic function, can be assessed based on the criteria in the GCS, which include eye opening (E), verbal response (V), and motor response (M). The patient's responses are rated on a scale from 3 to 15. Box 44-6 provides the complete scoring of the GCS. The severity of TBI can be classified based on the score on the GCS. A score of 13 to 15 is classified as mild TBI, 9 to 12 is moderate TBI, and 3 to 8 is severe TBI (Capizzi et al., 2020, McNair, 2020). A score of 3 indicates severe impairment of neurologic function, deep coma, brain death, or pharmacologic inhibition of the neurologic response; a score of 8 or less typically indicates an unconscious patient; a score of 15 indicates a fully alert and oriented patient.

The patient's orientation is assessed by asking the patient to identify their full name; where they are; the day, month, or season; and what happened to them (person, time, place, and situation). Other questions such as "Who is the president?" may be helpful in determining the patient's processing of information in the environment. Verbal response cannot be evaluated if the patient is intubated or has a tracheostomy; this should be clearly documented.

Alertness is measured by the patient's ability to open the eyes spontaneously or in response to a vocal or noxious

BOX 44-6

Focused Assessment

Glasgow Coma Scale

The Glasgow Coma Scale (GCS) is a tool for assessing a patient's response to stimuli. Scores range from 3 (deep coma) to 15 (normal).

Eye opening response	Spontaneous	4
	To voice	3
	To pain	2
	None	1
Best verbal response	Oriented	5
	Confused	4
	Inappropriate words	3
	Incomprehensible sounds	2
	None	1
Best motor response	Obeys command	6
	Localizes pain	5
	Withdraws	4
	Flexion	3
	Extension	2
	None	1
Total		3 to 15

stimulus (pressure or pain). Patients with severe neurologic dysfunction cannot do this. The nurse assesses for periorbital edema (swelling around the eyes) or trauma, which may prevent the patient from opening the eyes, and documents any such condition that interferes with eye opening.

Motor response includes spontaneous, purposeful movement (e.g., the awake patient can move all four extremities with equal strength on command), movement only in response to painful stimuli, or abnormal posturing. If the patient is not responding to commands, the motor response is tested by applying a painful stimulus, using the least amount of pressure to elicit a possible response. Suggestions include using central pressure such as a sternal rub or squeezing the muscle masses and tendons. Central stimulation produces an overall body response, compared to peripheral stimulation via nail bed pressure, which can elicit a reflex response, which is not a true indicator of motor activity (Hickey, 2020). If the patient attempts to push away or withdraw, the response is recorded as purposeful or appropriate ("patient withdraws from painful stimuli"). This response is considered purposeful if the patient can cross the midline from one side of the body to the other in response to painful stimuli. An inappropriate or nonpurposeful response is random and aimless. Movement of only one side is suggestive of hemiparesis, while withdrawal suggests purposeful behavior. The motor response cannot be elicited if pharmacologic paralyzing agents have been administered to the patient. These must be suspended and time must elapse for the effects to wear off before attempting to elicit a motor response.

In addition to LOC, the nurse monitors parameters such as respiratory status, pupillary response, and vital signs on an ongoing basis. Table 44-1 summarizes the assessment and the clinical significance of the findings. Body functions (circulation, respiration, elimination, fluid and electrolyte balance) are examined in a systematic and ongoing manner.

If the patient is comatose and has localized signs, such as abnormal pupillary and motor responses, it is assumed that neurologic disease is present until proven otherwise. If the patient is comatose but pupillary light reflexes are preserved, a toxic or metabolic disorder is suspected. Common laboratory testing and diagnostic procedures performed on patients with decreased LOC and increased ICP are listed in Table 44-2.

Medical and Nursing Management

The first priority of treatment for the patient with altered LOC is to obtain and maintain a patent airway. The patient may be orally or nasally intubated (unless basilar skull fracture or facial trauma is suspected), or a tracheostomy may be performed. Until the ability of the patient to breathe on their own is determined, a mechanical ventilator is used to maintain adequate oxygenation and ventilation. The circulatory status (blood pressure, heart rate) is monitored to ensure adequate perfusion to the body and brain. An IV catheter is inserted to provide access for IV fluids and medications.

Increased ICP is a true emergency and must be treated promptly. Invasive monitoring of ICP is an important component of management. Immediate management to relieve increased ICP requires decreasing cerebral edema, lowering the volume of CSF, and decreasing cerebral blood volume while maintaining cerebral perfusion. These goals are accomplished by administering osmotic diuretics, restricting fluids, draining CSF, controlling fever, maintaining systemic blood pressure and oxygenation, and reducing cellular metabolic demands. Corticosteroids are not recommended in cases of increased ICP resulting from TBI (McNair, 2020). In patients with severe TBI, there was a significant reduction in mortality when clinicians closely followed the guidelines from the Brain Trauma Foundation for control of both ICP and cerebral perfusion pressure (CPP) (Dash & Chavali, 2018).

Monitoring Intracranial Pressure

Nursing management focuses on detecting early signs of increasing ICP because medical interventions are usually ineffective once later signs develop. Frequent neurologic assessments and documentation and analysis of trends will reveal the subtle changes that may indicate increasing ICP.

Detecting Early Indications of Increasing Intracranial Pressure

The nurse assesses for and immediately reports any of the following early signs or symptoms of increasing ICP:

- Change in the LOC, disorientation, restlessness, increased respiratory effort, purposeless movements, and mental confusion: These are early clinical indications of

TABLE **44-1 Nursing Assessment of the Unconscious Patient**

Examination	Clinical Assessment	Clinical Significance
Level of responsiveness or consciousness	Eye opening, verbal and motor responses pupils (size, equality, reaction to light)	Obeying commands is a favorable response and demonstrates a return to consciousness
Pattern of respiration	Respiratory pattern	Disturbances of respiratory center of brain may result in various respiratory patterns
	Cheyne–Stokes respiration	Suggests lesions deep in both hemispheres; area of basal ganglia and upper brainstem
	Hyperventilation	Suggests onset of metabolic problem or brainstem damage
	Ataxic respiration with irregularity in depth/rate	Ominous sign of damage to medullary center
Eyes		
Pupils (size, equality, reaction to light)	Equal, normally reactive pupils Equal or unequal diameter Progressive dilation Fixed dilated pupils	Suggests that coma is toxic or metabolic in origin Helps determine location of lesion Indicates increasing intracranial pressure Indicates injury at level of midbrain
Eye movements	Normally, eyes should move from side to side	Functional and structural integrity of brainstem is assessed by inspection of extraocular movements; usually absent in deep coma
Corneal reflex	When cornea is touched with a wisp of clean cotton, blink response is normal	Tests cranial nerves V and VII; helps determine location of lesion if unilateral; absent in deep coma
Facial symmetry	Asymmetry (sagging, decrease in wrinkles)	Sign of paralysis
Swallowing reflex	Drooling versus spontaneous swallowing	Absent in coma Paralysis of cranial nerves IX, X, and XII
Neck	Stiff neck Absence of spontaneous neck movement	Subarachnoid hemorrhage, meningitis Fracture or dislocation of cervical spine
Response of extremity to noxious stimuli	Firm pressure on a joint of the upper and lower extremity Observe spontaneous movements	Asymmetric response in paralysis Absent in deep coma
Deep tendon reflexes	Tap patellar and biceps tendons	Brisk response may have localizing value Asymmetric response in paralysis No response in deep coma
Pathologic reflexes	Firm pressure with blunt object on sole of foot, moving along lateral margin and crossing to the ball of foot	Flexion of the toes, especially the great toe, is normal except in newborn Dorsiflexion of toes (especially great toe) indicates contralateral pathology of corticospinal tract (Babinski reflex) Helps determine location of lesion in brain
Abnormal posture	Observation for posturing (spontaneous or in response to noxious stimuli) Abnormal flexion (flexion and internal rotation of forearms and hands) Abnormal extension (extension and external rotation)	Deep extensive brain lesion Abnormal flexion indicates damage to the upper midbrain Abnormal extension indicates deeper (brain stem) and more severe dysfunction than does abnormal flexion; implies brain pathology; poor prognostic sign

TABLE 44-2 **Laboratory and Diagnostic Tests for Patients with Traumatic Brain Injury**

Test	Normal Values	Critical Values	Nursing Implications
Complete blood count	WBC: 4.5–10.5 (×1,000/mm^3) WBC for Black adults: 3.2–10.0 (×1,000/mm^3) Hct: females: 36–48%; males: 42–52%	WBC: >30 (×1,000/mm^3) Or <2.0 (×1,000/mm^3) Hct: <20%; >60%	Assess for any signs or symptoms of infection with increased WBC; assess for any signs or symptoms of occult bleeding with decreased Hct.
Glucose	140–180 mg/dL	>180 mg/dL	Hyperglycemia may worsen outcomes; administer insulin if glucose is elevated.
Serum osmolality	275–295 mOsm/Kg	<240 or ≥321 mOsm/L	Osmolality should not exceed 321 mOsm/L to prevent kidney failure in patients receiving mannitol.
Serum sodium	136–145 mEq/L	<125 mEq/L or >152 mEq/L	Hyponatremia may indicate cerebral salt wasting or SIADH. Hypernatremia may indicate diabetes insipidus or be due to mannitol therapy.
Urine specific gravity	1.005–1.030 (usually between 1.010 and 1.025)	<1.005 (dilute) or >1.025 (concentrated)	Low specific gravity can mean diabetes insipidus, while a high level may mean SIADH.
Chest radiograph	Negative for pneumonia or infiltrate	Presence of pneumonia or infiltrate	Ventilated patients are prone to aspiration and development of pneumonias.
Head CT without contrast	Negative for acute hemorrhage	Positive for epidural, subdural, or intracerebral hemorrhage	Observe for any signs or symptoms of intracranial bleeding.
Serum potassium	3.5–5.2 mEq/L	<2.5 mEq/L	Hypokalemia may be a consequence of mannitol therapy.
Magnesium	1.8–2.6 mg/dL	<1.2 mg/dL	Hypomagnesemia may lower the seizure threshold and cause secondary brain injury; low levels should be corrected.

WBC, white blood cell count; Hct, hematocrit; SIADH, syndrome of inappropriate antidiuretic hormone.

Adapted from Fischbach, F., Fischbach, M., & Stout, K. (2021). *Nurses' quick reference to common laboratory and diagnostic tests* (11th ed.). Wolters Kluwer.

increasing ICP because the brain cells responsible for cognition are extremely sensitive to decreased oxygenation.

- Pupillary changes and impaired extraocular movements: These occur as the increasing pressure displaces the brain against the oculomotor and optic nerves (cranial nerves II, III, IV, and VI), which arise from the midbrain and brainstem (see Chapter 42).
- Weakness in one extremity or on one side of the body: This occurs as increasing ICP compresses the pyramidal tracts, which control motor function.
- Headache that is constant, increasing in intensity, and aggravated by movement or straining: This occurs as increasing ICP causes pressure and stretching of venous and arterial vessels in the base of the brain.

Pearls for Practice

The earliest sign of increasing ICP is a change in LOC. Any changes in LOC should be reported immediately.

Detecting Later Indications of Increasing Intracranial Pressure

As ICP increases, the patient's condition worsens, and the following signs and symptoms may be observed:

- LOC continues to deteriorate until the patient is comatose.
- Respiratory rate decreases or becomes erratic, blood pressure and temperature increase. The pulse pressure widens (difference between the systolic and diastolic pressure; normal is 40 mm Hg), and the pulse fluctuates rapidly, varying from bradycardia to tachycardia.
- Altered respiratory patterns develop, including Cheyne–Stokes breathing (rhythmic waxing and waning of rate and depth of respirations alternating with brief periods of apnea) and ataxic breathing (irregular breathing with a random sequence of deep and shallow breaths).
- Projectile vomiting may occur with increased pressure on the reflex center in the medulla.

- Hemiplegia or decorticate or decerebrate posturing may develop as pressure on the brainstem increases; bilateral flaccidity occurs before death.
- Loss of brainstem reflexes, including pupillary, corneal, gag, and swallowing reflexes, occur; this is an ominous sign of impending death.

Because clinical assessment is not always a reliable guide in recognizing increased ICP, especially in comatose patients, monitoring of ICP is an essential part of management (Hickey & Baumann, 2020). ICP is monitored closely for continuous elevation or significant increase over baseline. The trend of ICP measurements over time is an important indication of the patient's underlying status. Vital signs are assessed when an increase in ICP is noted.

ICP can be monitored with the use of an intraventricular catheter (ventriculostomy) or a subarachnoid bolt or screw (Fig. 44-4). When a **ventriculostomy** is used for monitoring ICP, a fine-bore catheter is inserted into a lateral ventricle, preferably in the nondominant hemisphere of the brain (Hickey & Baumann, 2020). The catheter is connected by a fluid-filled system to a transducer, which records the pressure in the form of an electrical impulse. In addition to obtaining continuous ICP recordings, the ventricular catheter allows CSF to drain, particularly during acute increases in pressure. The ventriculostomy can also be used to drain blood from the ventricle. Continuous drainage of CSF under pressure control is an effective method of treating intracranial hypertension. Complications associated with its use include hemorrhage, infection, meningitis, ventricular collapse, misplacement, occlusion of the catheter by brain tissue or blood, and problems with the monitoring system (Hulou et al., 2022). CSF drainage is frequently performed because the removal of CSF with a ventriculostomy drain can dramatically reduce ICP and restore cerebral perfusion. Caution should be used

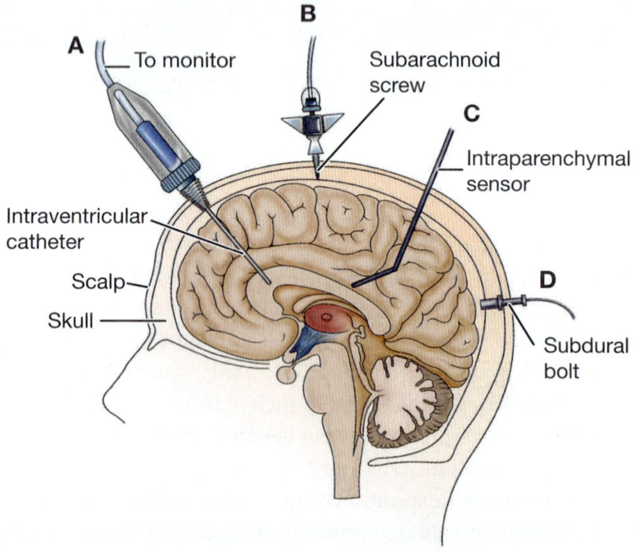

FIGURE 44-4 Intracranial pressure monitoring. A device may be placed in (A) the ventricle, (B) the subarachnoid space, (C) the intraparenchymal space, or (D) the subdural space.

in draining CSF, however, because excessive drainage may result in collapse of the ventricles and herniation.

The **subarachnoid bolt** or **screw** is a hollow device that is inserted through the skull and dura mater into the cranial subarachnoid space (Bautista, 2022). It has the advantage of not requiring a ventricular puncture. The subarachnoid bolt is attached to a pressure transducer, and the output is recorded on an oscilloscope. This technique also has the advantage of avoiding complications from brain shift and small ventricle size. One disadvantage to using a subarachnoid bolt is the inability to obtain CSF for analysis or drainage purposes. Complications include infection and blockage of the bolt by clot or brain tissue, which leads to a loss of pressure tracing and a decrease in accuracy at high ICP readings.

While ICP monitoring is only performed in an ICU setting, CSF drainage may be carried out in the operating room, emergency room, or intensive care unit. A ventriculostomy without the ICP monitoring catheter is known as an *external ventricular drain* (EVD). Box 44-7 provides guidelines on nursing care of the EVD.

Monitoring and Managing Complications

Potential complications for the patient with altered LOC include respiratory failure, pneumonia, pressure ulcers, and aspiration. Respiratory failure may develop shortly after the patient becomes unconscious. If the patient cannot maintain effective respirations, insertion of an airway and mechanical ventilation are initiated to provide adequate ventilation and to protect the airway. Pneumonia is common in patients receiving mechanical ventilation and in those who cannot maintain and clear the airway. The patient with altered LOC is subject to all the complications associated with immobility, such as pressure ulcers, venous stasis, musculoskeletal deterioration, and disturbed gastrointestinal functioning. Aspiration of gastric contents or feedings may occur, precipitating the development of aspiration pneumonia or airway occlusion. For gastric tube feedings, the head of bed (HOB) is elevated to at least 30 degrees and the tube feeding held if the head down position is needed. Refer to Chapter 21 for additional details on gastric tube feedings.

Pearls for Practice: Pathophysiology Aspiration Risk

The nurse is aware that the act of swallowing requires functioning of CN V, VII, IX, X, XI, and XII (Blissitt, 2023). Although symptoms of aspiration can include productive coughing, the nurse recognizes that when there is a weak or absent cough reflex, silent aspiration can occur. The nurse is alert for symptoms of dyspnea, diffuse wheezing, decreasing oxygen saturation, increased respiratory rate and heart rate, and fever (Alipanah-Lechner, 2023).

Endocrine abnormalities, including diabetes insipidus and syndrome of inappropriate antidiuretic hormone (SIADH),

BOX 44-7

GUIDELINES FOR NURSING CARE

Caring for an External Ventricular Drain (EVD)

Nurses in a variety of acute care settings may receive patients who have an external ventricular drain (EVD) in place to drain off excess CSF. The nurse is responsible for maintaining the EVD while monitoring for any signs or symptoms of infection or CSF leak.

Equipment

- Carpenter's level
- Sterile gloves
- Sterile 4 × 4 gauze pad
- Transparent dressing large enough to cover the gauze (e.g., Tegaderm)

Implementation

NURSING ACTION	RATIONALE
1. Position the head of the bed at 30 degrees with the patient's head and neck in the midline position, taking care to avoid neck flexion.	1. Positioning the head of the bed at 30 degrees helps promote venous return, which will assist in keeping ICP within normal limits. Keeping the head and neck in the midline position while avoiding flexion will help prevent any increases in ICP.
2. Using the carpenter's level, set the collection bag even with the external auditory meatus (EAM) of the ear at the level that has been ordered by the physician (measured in centimeters either above or below the EAM).	2. The EAM is level with the foramen of Monro. A level below the EAM will increase drainage of CSF, while a level above the EAM will decrease drainage of CSF.
3. Documentation should include the position of the collection bag, the amount of CSF drainage, and the color and quality of the CSF (clear, cloudy, bloody, etc.).	3. Proper documentation of where the collection bag is placed and the amount of drainage is important for the neurosurgeons to evaluate when to make adjustments to the level and when the EVD is no longer needed. Any change in quality of the CSF may indicate infection or bleeding into the ventricles; such change should be reported immediately.
4. If the patient needs to be turned, the head of the bed needs to be adjusted, or when the patient needs to be moved out of bed, the drainage system should be turned off until it can be returned to the ordered position. Once the patient is back in bed and the system has been re-leveled, the drainage system may be opened again.	4. If the drainage system is not turned off and the patient's head is moved, CSF may be forcefully pulled out of the ventricles, potentially causing herniation of the brain.
5. The EVD should always be handled with sterile technique when changing the dressing covering the insertion site. The dressing consists of a sterile 4 × 4 gauze pad that is folded in order to fully cover the insertion site and then covered with a transparent dressing. The insertion site should be monitored for any signs or symptoms of infection and should be kept clean and dry. If the dressing becomes damp, it should be changed and the provider should be notified.	5. The EVD is a closed, sterile system. Risk for infection is high, and all precautions should be taken to prevent any infection from entering the brain. The gauze needs to be covered with a clear dressing so that the gauze may be readily inspected for the presence of dampness and blood. If the dressing becomes damp with fluid, the fluid is presumed to be CSF. Presence of a damp dressing may indicate a CSF leak.

EAM, external auditory meatus; EVD, external ventricular drain; ICP, intracranial pressure; CSF, cerebrospinal fluid.

are common complications of TBI. Diabetes insipidus is the result of decreased secretion of antidiuretic hormone (ADH). The patient has excessive urine output, decreased urine osmolality, and serum hyperosmolality (>295 mOsm/kg). Therapy consists of administration of fluids, electrolyte replacement, and vasopressin (desmopressin, DDAVP) therapy. SIADH is the result of increased secretion of ADH. The patient becomes volume-overloaded, urine output diminishes, serum sodium concentration becomes dilute (sodium is less than 135 mEq/L), and serum osmolality decreases (less than 275 mOsm/kg). With too much H_2O in the bloodstream, the kidneys cannot excrete dilute urine, and the water moves from the extracellular compartment to the intracellular region, causing brain cells to swell. This has significant impact on the CNS (brain and spinal cord) because of brain edema and increased ICP. Treatment of SIADH includes fluid restriction (typically less than 800 mL/day with no free water), which is usually sufficient to correct the hyponatremia. Severe cases call for judicious administration of a 3% hypertonic saline solution. If hypertonic saline is administered, usually it is necessary to administer furosemide (Lasix) simultaneously to reduce intravascular volume via diuresis. Hyponatremia presents commonly with a change in mental status ranging from mild confusion to coma; seizures are associated with low sodium levels (less than 115 mEq/L). The more quickly this problem has developed, the more profound the signs and symptoms. Aggressive management may be required to correct hyponatremia as delaying treatment may result in irreversible brain damage. However, overcorrection of the sodium level predisposes the patient to central pontine myelinolysis, a disorder in which the white matter of the pons loses myelin (the protective sheath surrounding nerves); this results in tetraplegia with pseudobulbar palsy (lower cranial nerve deficits) (Danyalian & Heller, 2022). To prevent this complication, the nurse monitors results of sodium levels (initially, these may be ordered hourly) and the patient's response to hypertonic saline treatment. As a general guideline, the plasma sodium concentration should probably be raised by no more than 8 mEq during the first 24 hours. For more details on DI and SIADH refer to Chapter 30.

Because the unconscious patient's protective reflexes are impaired, the quality of nursing care provided may literally mean the difference between life and death. The nurse must assume responsibility for the patient until the basic reflexes (coughing, blinking, and swallowing) return and the patient becomes conscious and oriented. Therefore, the major nursing goal is to compensate for the absence of these protective reflexes.

Potential complications include cerebral edema, high fever, alterations in blood pressure and oxygenation, increased metabolic demand, and seizures. The nurse must maintain oral hygiene, monitor for the presence of pressure ulcers, avoid any complications associated with the eyes (eye care is discussed later in this chapter), monitor urinary output and bowel function, and assess nutritional status. The nurse must always remember to be the patient's advocate, as an unconscious patient cannot advocate for themself.

Decreasing Cerebral Edema: Osmotic Diuretics, Fluid Restriction, and Hypothermia

Cerebral edema is one of the more prominent causes of secondary brain injury and is a principal cause of death after a TBI; thus, it is an important target for intervention (Sawant-Pokam et al., 2020). Osmotic diuretics, such as mannitol, may be administered to dehydrate the brain tissue and reduce cerebral edema. Osmotic diuretics work by creating a gradient that draws water across intact membranes, thereby reducing the volume of the swollen brain. Secondarily, they reduce blood viscosity and hematocrit and enhance cerebral blood flow (DeNett & Feltner, 2021). If the patient is receiving osmotic diuretics, serum osmolality should be determined to assess hydration status.

Drug Alert

Mannitol becomes ineffective when the serum osmolality exceeds 320 mOsm.

Pearls for Practice

The serum osmolality is calculated with the following formula:

2 × sodium + glucose/18 + blood urea nitrogen (BUN)/2.8

If a patient's serum sodium is 140 mEq/L, blood sugar is 80 mg/dL, and BUN is 10 mg/dL; then the calculated serum osmolality is

280 (sodium) + 4.4 (glucose) + 3.5 (BUN), for a calculated serum osmolality of 288 mOsm/kg.

Hypertonic saline is another medication that works to reduce cerebral edema. While mannitol is considered the gold standard in reducing increased ICP, hypertonic saline is gaining popularity as an effective osmotic diuretic. Optimal concentration, dosing, timing, and duration of hypertonic saline have yet to be determined (DeNett et al., 2021). The nurse follows institutional policies for hypertonic saline administration.

Another method for decreasing cerebral edema is fluid restriction. Limiting overall fluid intake leads to dehydration and hemoconcentration, which draws fluid across the osmotic gradient and decreases cerebral edema. Fluid needs are met initially by administering the required IV fluids.

Drug Alert

Hypotonic fluids (e.g., 0.45% NaCl, D5W) should be avoided in patients with TBI as those fluids can cause an increase in cerebral edema.

Researchers have long hypothesized that lowering body temperature decreases cerebral edema by reducing the oxygen and metabolic requirements of the brain, thus protecting the brain from continued ischemia. The cerebral metabolic rate increases by 7% per 1°C of increase in body temperature; thus, the higher the temperature, the greater the oxygen consumption, and blood flow must increase to meet tissue demands (Stacy, 2022a). If body metabolism can be reduced by lowering the body temperature, the collateral circulation in the brain may be able to provide adequate blood supply to the brain. The effect of hypothermia on ICP requires more study; thus far, induced hypothermia has not consistently been shown to be beneficial for patients with brain injury. Current literature suggests it is beneficial but only when initiated within 24 hours (Chen et al., 2019). Inducing and maintaining hypothermia is a major clinical treatment that requires resources and reference manuals for the nurse to provide safe administration. Studies that will provide insight into how small variations in temperature can modulate brain injury are needed, until then the nurse should follow institutional guidelines (Scarboro & McQuillan, 2021).

Controlling Fever

High fever in the unconscious patient may be caused by infection of the respiratory or urinary tract, drug reactions, or damage to the hypothalamic temperature-regulating center. Approximately one fifth to one half of fevers are never explained, despite extensive workup. Because of damage to the temperature center in the brain or severe intracranial infection, unconscious patients often develop very high temperatures. Such temperature elevations must be controlled because the increased metabolic demands of the brain can exceed cerebral circulation and oxygenation, resulting in secondary brain injury (McNair, 2020). Studies have shown that monitoring temperature may be warranted with targeted temperature management for reducing potential long-term consequences (Truettner et al., 2018). Persistent hyperthermia with no identified clinical source of infection indicates brainstem damage and a poor prognosis.

Strategies for reducing fever include:

- Removing all bedding over the patient (with the possible exception of a light sheet or small drape)
- Administering acetaminophen as prescribed
- Giving cool sponge baths and allowing a fan to blow over the patient to increase surface cooling
- Using a hypothermia blanket

Frequent temperature monitoring is indicated to assess the patient's response to the therapy and to prevent an excessive decrease in temperature and shivering, which increases heat production and cerebral oxygen consumption.

Pearls for Practice

If an automatic hyperthermia/hypothermia blanket is used for patient care, the nurse understands that the unit directly and continually monitors the patient's temperature by means of a thermistor probe (e.g., rectal, skin) and alternates heating and cooling cycles as necessary to achieve and maintain the desired body temperature. The nurse inserts the thermistor probe into the patient's rectum or axilla and tapes it in place to prevent accidental dislodgment. If the rectal probe (or axillary) is dislodged, it will no longer be measuring the patient temperature and instead will measure the room temperature. The probe should be checked at frequent intervals to ensure correct placement.

Maintaining Blood Pressure, Oxygenation, and Hyperventilation

Patients with TBI may sustain a secondary insult if they become hypotensive or hypoxic. Due to ethical reasons, no randomized controlled trials have been done to study the effects of hypotension and hypoxia. However, a growing body of evidence shows deleterious effects if the patient experiences either of these conditions. It is recommended that systolic blood pressure be maintained at ≥100 mm Hg for patients 50 to 69 years old or ≥110 mm Hg for patients 15 to 49 or >70 years old and oxygen saturation be maintained at greater than 90% (Carney et al., 2017; McNair, 2020).

Hyperventilation, which results in vasoconstriction, was previously used in patients with increased ICP. Research has demonstrated that hyperventilation may not be as beneficial as once thought (Carney et al., 2017). The reduction in partial pressure of carbon dioxide ($PaCO_2$) may result in hypoxia, ischemia, and an increase in cerebral lactate levels (Hickey & Baumann, 2020). Hyperventilation is an option for patients with ICP who are unresponsive to conventional therapies, but it should be used cautiously and should be avoided for the first 24 hours following the initial injury (Carney et al., 2017).

Pearls for Practice: Pathophysiology

Carbon dioxide (CO_2) is a potent vasodilator or vasoconstrictor. A normal PCO_2 is 35 to 45 mm Hg. As the patient hypoventilates, the PCO_2 rises (hypercarbia also known as hypercapnia), which causes vasodilation. Likewise, as the patient hyperventilates, the PCO_2 decreases (hypocarbia), which causes vasoconstriction. It seems reasonable that hyperventilation would cause vasoconstriction and therefore decrease cerebral blood flow with a resulting decrease in ICP. However, on review, when the PCO_2 was lowered to 25 mm Hg, ischemia of the brain and increased mortality was seen. The current trend is to maintain PCo_2 levels on the lower side of normal (35 mm Hg±2) by monitoring arterial blood gas measurements and altering ventilator settings as needed (Stacy, 2022a). In general, normocarbia is preferred.

Reducing Metabolic Demands

Cellular metabolic demands may be reduced through the administration of high doses of barbiturates if the patient is unresponsive to conventional treatment. The mechanism by which barbiturates decrease ICP and protect the brain is through inhibition of free radicals, alterations in vascular tone, and suppression of metabolism (McNair, 2020). Use of high-dose barbiturates should be reserved for patients with refractory increased ICP who do not respond to other medical or surgical treatments. Barbiturates should not be used as prophylaxis to prevent increased ICP (Carney et al., 2017).

Another method of reducing cellular metabolic demand and improving oxygenation is the administration of pharmacologic paralyzing agents, such as pancuronium, vecuronium, and cisatracurium. The patient who receives these agents cannot move; this decreases the metabolic demands and results in a decrease in cerebral oxygen demand. Because the patient cannot respond or report pain, sedation and analgesia must be provided because the paralyzing agents do not provide either.

Patients receiving high doses of barbiturates or pharmacologic paralyzing agents require continuous cardiac monitoring, endotracheal intubation, mechanical ventilation, ICP monitoring, and arterial pressure monitoring.

The ability to perform serial neurologic assessments is lost with the use of barbiturates or paralyzing agents. Therefore, other monitoring tools are needed to assess the patient's status and response to therapy. Important parameters that must be assessed include ICP, blood pressure, heart

BOX 44-8

Risk Factors for Developing Posttraumatic Seizures (PTS)

- Depressed skull fracture
- Penetrating head wound
- Epidural, subdural, or intracerebral hemorrhage
- GCS score below 10
- Cortical contusion
- Seizure within 24 hours of injury

rate, respiratory rate, and response to ventilator therapy (e.g., "bucking" or "fighting" the ventilator). Refer to Chapters 9 and 54 for ventilator considerations. Potential complications include hypotension due to decreased sympathetic tone and myocardial depression (Hickey & Baumann, 2020).

Seizure Prophylaxis

Patients with severe TBI are at risk for developing seizures. Seizures that develop after head injury are known as posttraumatic seizures (PTS) and are classified according to when they occur. If they occur within 7 days of injury, they are known as early PTS; if they occur more than 7 days after the injury, they are known as late PTS (Sun et al., 2021). Box 44-8 lists risk factors for developing PTS. There is evidence to support the use of prophylactic anticonvulsants only for early PTS. It is not recommended that patients be started on seizure prophylaxis more than 1 week after the injury if they have not had any seizures. If the patient develops late PTS, the seizures should be managed in the same way as new-onset seizures (Fordington & Manford, 2020). See Chapter 45 for further discussion on management of seizures.

Preventing DVT

The risk for DVT is high in people with brain injury, and the nurse is alert for cues of DVT, which include unilateral limb edema, low-grade fever, warmth, localized erythema, and limb pain. If DVT is suspected in the lower extremities, the nurse measures the calf circumference (measured 10 cm below tibial tuberosity); if it is 3 cm greater on the affected limb, DVT is suggested. However, the nurse is aware that clinical manifestations are not always present or obvious. Prophylaxis of DVT includes sequential (intermittent) pneumatic compression devices and compression stockings as well as consideration of anticoagulation when the risk of bleeding has decreased and the benefit outweighs the increased risk of intracranial hemorrhage expansion. See additional discussion of DVT related to SCIs in Chapter 17.

Providing Mouth Care

To provide care, the mouth is inspected for dryness, inflammation, and crusting. The unconscious patient requires conscientious oral care because there is a risk of parotitis (inflammation of the salivary glands) if the mouth is not kept scrupulously clean (refer to Chapter 21). The mouth is cleansed and rinsed carefully to remove secretions and crusts and to keep the mucous membranes moist. A thin coating of petrolatum on the lips prevents drying, cracking, and encrustations. If the patient has an endotracheal tube, the tube should be moved to the opposite side of the mouth daily to prevent ulceration of the mouth and lips.

Pearls for Practice

Oral care in patients at risk for increased ICP has been shown to be safe. However, this should be done with caution in patients who already have elevated ICP as oral interventions may cause modest increases in ICP. The nurse is aware that nursing activities such as suctioning, tight tracheostomy tube ties, patient coughing, Valsalva maneuver (bearing down activity such as straining during a bowel movement), and cumulative nursing actions performed in a row are associated with increases in ICP (Stacy, 2022a).

Maintaining Skin and Joint Integrity

Preventing skin breakdown requires continuing nursing assessment and intervention. Special attention is given to unconscious patients because they cannot respond to external stimuli. Assessment includes a regular schedule of turning to avoid pressure, which can cause breakdown and necrosis of the skin. Turning also provides kinesthetic (sensation of movement), proprioceptive (awareness of position), and vestibular (equilibrium) stimulation. After turning, the patient is carefully repositioned to prevent ischemic necrosis over pressure areas.

Preserving Corneal Integrity

Unconscious patients may have their eyes open and have inadequate or absent corneal reflexes. The cornea may become irritated, dried out, or scratched, leading to ulceration. The eyes may be cleansed with cotton balls or gauze moistened with sterile water from inner to outer canthus to remove debris and discharge, using each piece of gauze or cotton ball only once (Edwards & Williams, 2019). In addition, methylcellulose (artificial tears) lubricating drops may be instilled every 1 to 2 hours. Recent research reveals that the use of artificial tears and a polyethylene film that is applied extending beyond the orbits and eyebrows creates a moisture chamber around the cornea and assists in keeping the eyes moist and in the closed position (Ahmadinejad et al., 2020; Nikseresht et al., 2019). It should be noted that in the later study the highest risk of ocular surface disorders of the eye was observed in patients that had their eyelid taped.

In addition, periorbital edema often occurs after cranial surgery. Cold compresses may be prescribed, and care must be exerted to avoid contact with the cornea. Eye patches should be used cautiously because of the potential for corneal abrasion from contact with the patch.

Managing Nutritional Needs

If the patient does not recover quickly and sufficiently enough to take adequate fluids and calories by mouth, a nasogastric

BOX 44-9

Pearls for Practice: Nutrition

Nutritional Support Following Traumatic Brain Injury

- Patients with traumatic brain injury (TBI) have increased metabolic expenditure so they have high caloric needs.
- Full nutritional support should be begun no later than 72 hours after the injury to achieve full caloric replacement by postinjury day 7.
- Protein should comprise 15% of total calories.
- When feedings are initiated, glucose levels should be closely monitored as hyperglycemia is associated with worse outcomes.
- Consultation with a dietician is recommended to provide optimal nutritional support.

tube or gastrostomy tube is inserted for the administration of enteral feedings. A nutritionist should be involved in the care of the unconscious patient to determine the patient's caloric needs and make recommendations for the amount and type of tube feeding that is appropriate. Daily intake and output should be recorded, as should daily weights to ensure the patient has adequate caloric intake (McNair, 2020). Box 44-9 gives nutritional considerations of the patient with decreased LOC and increased ICP.

Preventing Urinary Retention

The patient with an altered LOC is often incontinent or has urinary retention. The bladder is palpated or scanned at intervals to determine whether urinary retention is present. If the patient is not voiding, an indwelling urinary catheter may be inserted and connected to a closed drainage system during the acute phase of illness to monitor urinary output. Because catheters are a major factor in causing urinary tract infection (UTI), the patient is observed for fever, leukocytosis (increased WBCs), and cloudy urine. The urinary catheter is usually removed if the patient has a stable cardiovascular system and if no diuresis, sepsis, or voiding dysfunction existed before the onset of coma. An intermittent catheterization program may be initiated to ensure complete emptying of the bladder at intervals, if indicated.

Promoting Bowel Function

The abdomen is assessed for distention by listening for bowel sounds and measuring the girth of the abdomen with a tape measure. There is a risk for diarrhea from infection, antibiotics, hyperosmolar fluids, and enteral feedings.

Immobility and lack of dietary fiber can cause constipation. The nurse monitors the number and consistency of bowel movements and assesses for signs of fecal impaction. The provider should be alerted if the patient has not had a bowel movement within 3 to 4 days. Stool softeners may be prescribed and can be administered with tube feedings. To facilitate bowel emptying, a glycerin suppository may be indicated. Laxatives can also be added to the regimen in order to prevent constipation (McNair, 2020).

Pearls for Practice

The nurse is aware that straining during bowel movement increases intra-abdominal and/or intrathoracic pressure, which impedes venous return and increases ICP. Therefore a bowel program is initiated to prevent constipation.

Protecting the Patient

Care should be taken to prevent injury from invasive lines and equipment, and other potential sources of injury should be identified. These include restraints, tight dressings, environmental irritants, damp bedding or dressings, and tubes and drains.

Protection also includes protecting the patient's dignity during altered LOC. Simple measures, such as providing privacy and speaking to the patient during nursing care activities, preserve the patient's dignity. Not speaking negatively about the patient's condition or prognosis is also important because patients in a light coma may be able to hear. The patient who is comatose has an increased need for advocacy and requires the nurse to have strong clinical judgment and sharp assessment skills (Mulkey, 2021).

New Therapies

Despite many years of extensive research, no new therapies have been shown to improve outcomes after TBI. Research into this area continues to be important as TBI is a major cause of death and disability in the United States (McCrea et al., 2021). There are no FDA-approved pharmacologic agents that provide improved outcomes following TBI. New therapies need to target multiple stages along the cascade of secondary brain injury (Dekmak et al., 2018).

Intracranial Surgery

Decompressive craniectomy is a surgical procedure that can be used to help relieve increased ICP. A decompressive craniectomy involves removal of a bone flap from the skull to allow expansion of the brain. The bone flap is then implanted into the abdomen, so the bone remains viable. Once cerebral edema has decreased, the bone flap is replaced back on the skull. Use of a craniectomy continues to be controversial as studies have shown no improvement in clinical outcome (Hickey & Baumann, 2020). The nurse positions the head so there is no compression of the unprotected brain, and a protective helmet may be indicated when the patient is out of bed (Holleran, 2023).

BRAIN DEATH

When a patient has sustained a severe neurologic injury incompatible with life, the diagnosis of brain death should be considered. Often, it is the nurse who will first notice signs of decompensation and will begin the process of determining if the patient meets criteria for brain death. Designation of brain death often involves an interprofessional team, which will play a vital role in working with families during the evaluation (Starr et al., 2021).

Brain death was formally defined by the Ad Hoc Committee at Harvard Medical School in 1968 as an "irreversible coma." In 1981, the President's Commission for the Study of Ethical Problems in Medicine and Biomedical and Behavioral Research published *Guidelines for the Determination of Death.* These guidelines clarified that patients who are considered brain dead must have confirmation of cessation of all brain function resulting from an irreversible cause. Reversible conditions, such as shock, hypothermia, and drug intoxication, must be excluded prior to diagnosis. This study served as the basis for the Uniform Death and Determination Act (UDDA), which is now recognized by all 50 states. The UDDA states that death will be determined with accepted medical standards and that death will indicate irreversible loss of all brain function.

Determination of brain death can be done with a clinical examination that demonstrates (1) no evidence of arousal to maximal external stimulation; (2) pupils are fixed in and nonreactive to light; (3) absent corneal, oculocephalic, and oculovestibular reflexes; (4) no facial movement to noxious stimulation; (5) no gag reflex; (6) no cough reflex to deep tracheal suctioning; (7) no motor response to noxious stimulation of the limbs; and (8) no spontaneous respirations with apnea test (Greer et al., 2020).

The nurse may assist in the clinical examination for determination of brain death and in the process of organ procurement. Often, there will be a meeting among the attending physician, nurse, social worker, and representative of the organ procurement organization to inform the family of the organ donation process. The family will often look to the nurse for answers about organ donation and an explanation of questions related to the determination of brain death (Milliken & Uveges, 2020).

SPINAL CORD INJURY

Spinal cord injury (SCI) is a major health problem. An estimated 333,000 people in the United States live each day with a disability from SCIs, and an estimated 18,000 new injuries occur each year (National Spinal Cord Injury Statistical Center [NSCISC], 2022). Males account for 78% of SCIs in a reported national database (NSCISC, 2022). Young people between 16 and 30 years of age account for more than half of the new SCIs each year. The most common cause of SCIs is motor vehicle crashes, which account for 38% of SCIs. Violence-related injuries account for 15% of SCIs, with falls causing 31%, and sports-related injuries causing 8% of SCIs (NSCISC, 2022). The frequency of associated injuries and medical complications in SCIs is high. The frequency with which these risk factors are associated with SCIs serves to emphasize the importance of primary prevention. The same interventions suggested earlier in this chapter for head injury prevention serve to decrease the incidence of SCIs as well (see Box 44-1, p. 1412).

Pathophysiology

Damage to the spinal cord ranges from transient concussion (from which the patient fully recovers) to contusion, laceration, and compression of the cord substance (either alone or in combination), to complete **transection** (severing) of the cord (which renders the patient paralyzed below the level of the injury).

SCIs, like head injuries, can be separated into two categories: primary injuries and secondary injuries (Norris, 2019). Primary injuries are the result of the initial insult or trauma and are usually permanent. Secondary injuries are usually the result of a contusion or tear injury, in which the nerve fibers begin to swell and disintegrate. A secondary chain of events produces ischemia, hypoxia, edema, and hemorrhagic lesions, which in turn result in destruction of myelin and axons (Strayer, 2020). These secondary reactions, believed to be the principal causes of spinal cord degeneration at the level of injury, are now thought to be reversible during the first 4 to 6 hours after injury. Therefore, if the cord has not suffered irreparable damage, some method of early treatment is needed to prevent partial damage from developing into total and permanent damage (Strayer, 2020) (see later discussion).

The vertebrae most frequently involved in SCIs are the fifth, sixth, and seventh cervical (neck) vertebrae (C5–C7), the twelfth thoracic vertebra (T12), and the first lumbar vertebra (L1). These vertebrae are most susceptible because there is a greater range of mobility in the vertebral column in these areas (Norris, 2019).

Clinical Manifestations

Manifestations of SCIs depend on the type and level of injury (Box 44-10). **Incomplete spinal cord lesions** (the sensory or motor fibers, or both, are preserved below the lesion) are classified according to the area of spinal cord damage: central, lateral, anterior, or peripheral. The American Spinal Injury Association (ASIA) provides another standard classification of SCIs according to the degree of sensory and motor function present after injury (Box 44-11). *Neurologic level* refers to the lowest level at which sensory and motor functions are normal. A motor complete SCI (ASIA Grades A and B) involves no motor function below the neurologic level. ASIA Grade A involves no sensory or motor function all the way down to the sacral segments, S4 and S5. ASIA Grade B involves preserved sensory but not motor function below the neurologic level and includes preservation of the sacral segments S4 and S5. A motor incomplete SCI (ASIA Grades C and D) involves preservation of motor function below the neurologic level.

BOX 44-10

Effects of Spinal Cord Injuries (SCIs)

Central Cord Syndrome

- Characteristics: Motor deficits (in the upper extremities compared to the lower extremities; sensory loss varies but is more pronounced in the upper extremities); bowel/bladder dysfunction is variable, or function may be completely preserved.
- Cause: Injury or edema of the central cord, usually of the cervical area. May be caused by hyperextension injuries.

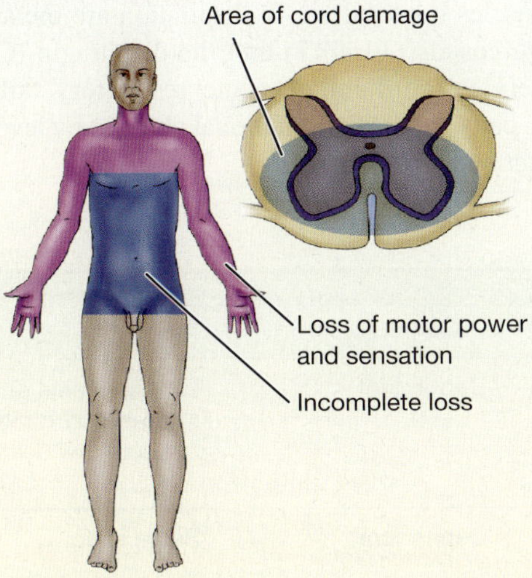

Central Cord Syndrome

Anterior Cord Syndrome

- Characteristics: Loss of pain, temperature, and motor function are noted below the level of the lesion; light touch, position, and vibration sensations remain intact.
- Cause: The syndrome may be caused by acute disk herniation or hyperflexion injuries associated with fracture-dislocation of vertebra. It also may occur as a result of injury to the anterior spinal artery, which supplies the anterior two thirds of the spinal cord.

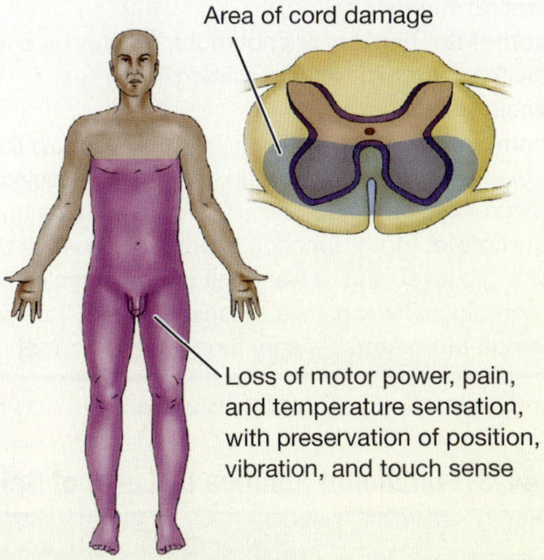

Anterior Cord Syndrome

Brown-Séquard Syndrome (Lateral Cord Syndrome)

- Characteristics: Ipsilateral paralysis or paresis is noted, together with ipsilateral loss of touch, pressure, and vibration and contralateral loss of pain and temperature.
- Cause: The lesion is caused by a transverse hemisection of the cord (half of the cord is transected from north to south), usually as a result of a knife or missile injury, fracture-dislocation of a unilateral articular process, or possibly an acute ruptured disk.

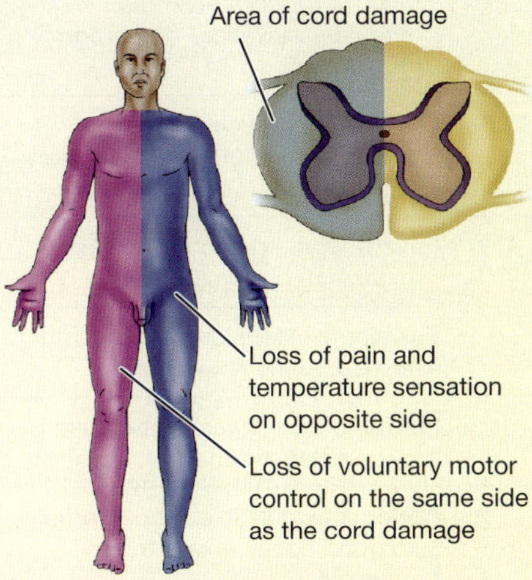

Brown-Séquard Syndrome

Adapted from Strayer, A. L. (2020). Spine and spinal cord injuries. In J. Hickey & A. L. Strayer (Eds.), *The clinical practice of neurological and neurosurgical nursing* (8th ed., Chapter 15). Wolters Kluwer.

ASIA Grade C involves preserved motor function below the neurologic level with at least half of the key muscles having a grade of less than 3 (see Chapter 42 for discussion of grading muscle strength). ASIA Grade D involves preserved motor function below the neurologic level with at least half of the key muscles having a grade of 3 or greater.

A **complete spinal cord lesion** (total loss of sensation and voluntary muscle control below the lesion) can result in **paraplegia** (paralysis of the lower body) or **tetraplegia** (formerly **quadriplegia**—paralysis of all four extremities). Complete SCIs also include loss of all spinal reflexes below the level of the lesion, loss of the ability to perspire

BOX 44-11

ASIA Impairment Scale

A = Complete: No motor or sensory function is preserved in the sacral segments S4–S5.

B = Incomplete: Sensory but not motor function is preserved below the neurologic level, including in the sacral segments S4–S5.

C = Incomplete: Motor function is preserved below the neurologic level, and more than half of key muscles below the neurologic level have a muscle grade of less than 3.

D = Incomplete: Motor function is preserved below the neurologic level, and at least half of key muscles below the neurologic level have a muscle grade of 3 or greater.

E = Normal: Motor and sensory function are normal.

Used with permission of American Spinal Injury Association.

below the level of the lesion, dysfunction of the bowel and bladder, and absence of visceral and somatic sensations below the level of the lesion (Strayer, 2020).

If conscious, the patient usually complains of acute pain in the back or neck, which may radiate along the involved nerve. However, absence of pain does not rule out spinal injury, and a careful assessment of the spine should be conducted if the mechanism of injury has involved significant force (i.e., concomitant head injury).

Respiratory dysfunction is related to the level of injury. The muscles contributing to respiration are the abdominals and intercostals (T1–T11) and the diaphragm (C3–C5). In high cervical cord injury, acute respiratory failure is the leading cause of death. Functional abilities by level of injury are described in Table 44-3.

TABLE **44-3 Functional Abilities by Level of Spinal Cord Injury**

Injury Level	Segmental Sensorimotor Function	Dressing, Eating	Elimination	Mobility[a]
C1	Little or no sensation or control of head and neck; no diaphragm control; requires continuous ventilation	Dependent	Dependent	Limited. Voice or sip-n-puff controlled electric wheelchair
C2–C3	Head and neck sensation; some neck control; independent of mechanical ventilation for short periods	Dependent	Dependent	Same as for C1
C4	Good head and neck sensation and motor control; some shoulder elevation; diaphragm movement	Dependent, may be able to eat with adaptive sling	Dependent	Limited to voice, mouth, head, chin, or shoulder-controlled electric wheelchair
C5	Full head and neck control; shoulder strength; elbow flexion	Independent with assistance	Maximal assistance	Electric or modified manual wheelchair, needs transfer assistance
C6	Fully innervated shoulder; wrist extension or dorsiflexion	Independent or with minimal assistance	Independent or with minimal assistance	Independent in transfers and wheelchair
C7–C8	Full elbow extension; wrist plantar flexion; some finger control	Independent	Independent	Independent; manual wheelchair
T1–T5	Full hand and finger control; use of intercostal and thoracic muscles	Independent	Independent	Independent; manual wheelchair
T6–T10	Abdominal muscle control, partial to good balance with trunk muscles	Independent	Independent	Independent; manual wheelchair
T11–L5	Hip flexors, hip abductors (L1–L3); knee extension (L2–L4); knee flexion and ankle dorsiflexion (L4–L5)	Independent	Independent	Short distance to full ambulation with assistance
S1–S5	Full leg, foot, and ankle control; innervation of perineal muscles for bowel, bladder, and sexual function (S2–S4)	Independent	Normal to impaired bowel and bladder function	Ambulate independently with or without assistance

[a]Assistance refers to adaptive equipment, setup, or physical assistance.

Data from Norris, T. (2018). *Pathophysiology: Concepts of altered health states* (10th ed.). Lippincott Williams & Wilkins.

Pearls for Practice

Ascending edema of the spinal cord in the acute phase of the injury may cause respiratory difficulty that requires immediate intervention. Therefore, the patient's respiratory status must be monitored frequently.

Assessment and Diagnostic Findings

A detailed neurologic examination is performed. Diagnostic x-rays (lateral cervical spine x-rays) and CT are usually performed initially. An MRI may be ordered as further workup if a ligamentous injury is suspected because significant spinal cord damage may exist even in the absence of bony injury. An assessment is made for other injuries because spinal trauma often is accompanied by concomitant injuries, commonly to the head and chest. Continuous cardiac monitoring may be indicated if an SCI is suspected because bradycardia and asystole are common in patients with acute SCIs.

Emergency Management

The immediate management at the scene of the injury is critical because improper handling of the patient can cause further damage and loss of neurologic function. Any patient who is involved in a motor vehicle crash, a diving or contact sports injury, a fall, or any direct trauma to the head and neck should be considered to have an SCI until such an injury has been ruled out. Initial care should include rapid assessment, immobilization, extrication, stabilization or control of life-threatening injuries, and transportation to the most appropriate medical facility (Eli et al., 2021).

At the scene of the injury, the patient should be immobilized on a spinal (back) board, with head and neck in a neutral position, to prevent an incomplete injury from becoming complete. One member of the team must assume control of the patient's head to prevent flexion, rotation, or extension; this is done by placing the hands on both sides of the patient's head at about ear level to limit movement and maintain alignment while a spinal board or cervical immobilizing device is applied. If possible, at least four people should slide the patient carefully onto a board for transfer to the hospital. Any twisting movement may irreversibly damage the spinal cord by causing a bony fragment of the vertebra to cut into, crush, or sever the cord completely (Strayer, 2020). Spine immobilization is necessary to allow for safe transportation from the field to the hospital (Wang et al., 2021).

The standard of care is that the patient is referred to a regional spinal injury or trauma center because of the multidisciplinary personnel and support services required to counteract the destructive changes that occur in the first 24 hours after injury. During treatment in the emergency and x-ray departments, the patient is kept on the transfer board. The patient must always be maintained in an extended position. No part of the body should be twisted or turned, nor should the patient be allowed to sit up. Once the extent of the injury has been determined, the patient may be placed on a rotating bed or in a cervical collar. Later, if SCIs and bone instability have been ruled out, the patient may be moved to a conventional bed or the collar may be removed without harm. If a rotating bed is needed but not available, the patient should be placed in a hard cervical collar and on a firm mattress.

Medical and Nursing Management

The goals of management are to prevent further SCIs and to observe for symptoms of progressive neurologic deficits. Many changes in the treatment of SCIs have occurred during the past 20 years. Treatments such as hypothermia, corticosteroids, and naloxone were investigated and used during the 1980s; of these, high-dose corticosteroids had shown the most promise, but their use has become controversial. In the National Acute Spinal Cord Injury Studies (NASCIS) done in 1990 and 1997, the administration of high-dose corticosteroids, specifically methylprednisolone (Solu-Medrol), was found to improve motor and sensory outcomes at 6 weeks, 6 months, and 1 year if given within 8 hours after injury (Wang et al., 2021). Currently, there is no Level I or II evidence to support the benefits of methylprednisolone; and there is Level I, II, and III evidence that use of high-dose steroids is associated with harmful side effects, up to and including death.

Biologic agents are currently being investigated for the acute and chronic phases of SCIs. Cell-based therapies, including stem cells, have theoretical benefits; while trials so far have not consistently shown efficacy, they do seem to be relatively safe (Muthu et al., 2021).

Nonsurgical Management

Treatment of SCIs attempts to achieve decompression, stabilization, and realignment of the spinal cord while preserving or improving neurologic function (Strayer, 2020). Cervical fractures are reduced, and the cervical spine is aligned with some form of skeletal traction, such as skeletal tongs or with use of the halo device. Cervical traction is used much less frequently due to early surgical stabilization.

A halo device may be used initially with traction or may be applied after removal of the tongs. It consists of a stainless-steel halo ring that is fixed to the skull by four pins. The ring is attached to a removable **halo vest**, a device that suspends the weight of the unit circumferentially around the chest. A metal frame connects the ring to the chest. Halo devices provide immobilization of the cervical spine while allowing early ambulation (Fig. 44-5). Refer to Chapter 41 for nursing responsibilities related to pin care.

Thoracic and lumbar injuries are usually treated with surgical intervention followed by immobilization with a fitted brace. Traction is not indicated either before or after surgery, due to the relative stability of the spine in these regions.

Surgical Management

Surgery is indicated in any of the following instances:

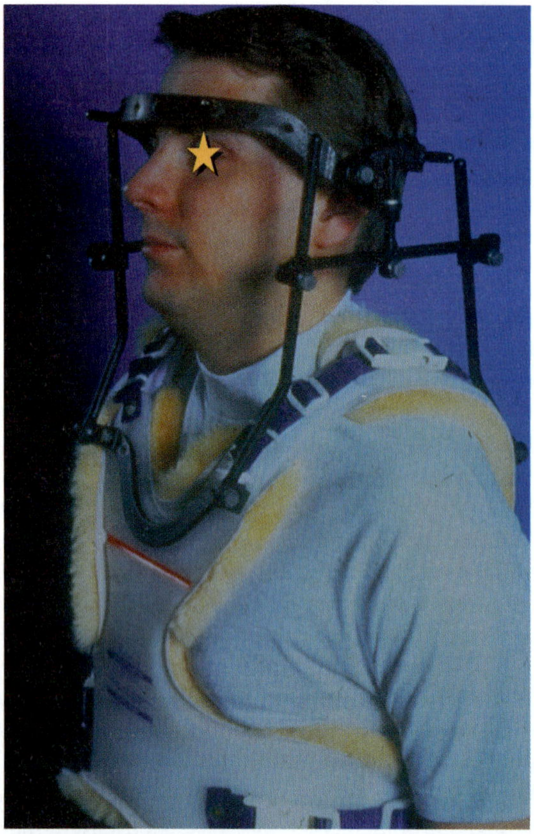

FIGURE 44-5 **Halo vest.**

- Compression of the cord
- Fragmented or unstable vertebral body
- Penetrating wound to the spinal cord
- Bone fragments in the spinal canal
- Deterioration of the patient's neurologic status

Surgery is performed to decompress the spinal cord, reduce the spinal fracture or dislocation, or to stabilize the spinal column. Laminectomy is the most common surgical procedure used to decompress or stabilize the spinal column. A **laminectomy** involves excision of the lamina (a portion of the posterior arch) and spinous processes of a vertebra. Various techniques (e.g., fusion or fixation) are used to create a stable spinal column (Strayer, 2020).

Monitoring and Managing Acute Complications of Spinal Cord Injury

Spinal and Neurogenic Shock

The spinal shock associated with SCIs reflects a sudden depression of reflex activity in the spinal cord (areflexia) below the level of injury. The muscles innervated by the part of the spinal cord segment below the level of the lesion are without sensation and are paralyzed and flaccid. In particular, the reflexes that initiate bladder and bowel function are affected. Bowel distention and paralytic ileus can be caused by depression of the reflexes and are treated with intestinal decompression by insertion of a nasogastric tube (Strayer, 2020).

Neurogenic shock develops due to the loss of autonomic nervous system function below the level of the lesion (Strayer, 2020). The vital organs are affected, causing the blood pressure and heart rate to decrease. This loss of sympathetic innervation causes a variety of other clinical manifestations, including a decrease in cardiac output, venous pooling in the extremities, and peripheral vasodilation, resulting in mild hypotension, bradycardia, and warm skin. In addition, the patient does not perspire on the paralyzed portions of the body because sympathetic activity is blocked; therefore, close observation is required for early detection of an abrupt onset of fever. Further details on neurogenic shock may be found in Chapter 53.

Deep Vein Thrombosis

Thrombophlebitis, inflammation of a vein related to deep vein thrombosis (DVT), is a relatively common potential complication of immobility and is common in patients with SCIs due to the injury itself, hypercoagulability, and/or blood stasis (Piran & Schulman, 2019). DVT occurs in a high percentage of patients with SCIs, placing them at risk for pulmonary embolism (PE), which is the third most common cause of death in patients with SCIs (Piran & Schulman, 2019). The patient must be assessed for symptoms of both DVT and PE. A low-grade fever may be the first sign of DVT as pain and tenderness are not applicable to a patient with SCI. Manifestations of PE include pleuritic chest pain, anxiety, and shortness of breath, and PE occurs in 8% to 14% of all SCI patients (Khanna et al., 2022).

Thigh and calf measurements should be made daily at consistent sites. The patient is evaluated for the presence of DVT if the circumference of one extremity increases significantly. Diagnostic studies used to detect DVT and PE include Doppler ultrasound, radiocontrast venography, ventilation/perfusion lung scans (Strayer, 2020), a computed tomographic pulmonary angiography (CTPA) (Solaru et al., 2021), or spiral CT.

Anticoagulation therapy to prevent DVT and PE is initiated once head injury and other systemic injuries have been ruled out and there is low risk for bleeding. There is a trend to support the use of enoxaparin rather than different types of low–molecular-weight heparin or between low–molecular-weight heparin and unfractionated heparin (Khanna et al., 2022). This may be followed by long-term oral anticoagulation with a vitamin K antagonist (i.e., warfarin) or subcutaneous fractionated heparin injections (Piran & Schulman, 2019). Anticoagulant therapy should be continued for 3 to 6 months after injury (Khanna et al., 2022). The risk of bleeding is substantial during the acute phase as SCI patients are exposed to invasive interventions, falls, infections, and urogenital complications (Eichinger et al., 2018).

Nonpharmacologic measures, including elastic compression stockings or pneumatic compression devices, as well as range-of-motion exercises, are important preventive measures that work to reduce venous pooling and promote venous return. Compression devices should be used for 2 weeks following injury. In some cases, permanent indwelling filters may be placed in the vena cava to prevent emboli (dislodged clots) from migrating to the lungs and causing PE in patients who have developed clots despite receiving anticoagulation (Sabharwal et al., 2019).

Orthostatic Hypotension

For the first 2 weeks following SCIs, blood pressure tends to be unstable and quite low. It gradually returns to preinjury levels, but periodic episodes of severe orthostatic hypotension frequently interfere with efforts to mobilize the patient. Orthostatic hypotension is defined as a reduction in systolic blood pressure of at least 20 mm Hg or diastolic pressure of at least 10 mm Hg, regardless of the patient's symptoms (Wecht, 2022). Patients with SCIs are prone to orthostatic hypotension during position changes due to a loss of reflex vasoconstriction and pooling of blood in the lower extremities and abdominal viscera. Orthostatic hypotension is a particularly common problem for patients with lesions above T7 and those with tetraplegia (Strayer, 2020).

Several techniques can be used to reduce the frequency of hypotensive episodes. Close monitoring of vital signs before and during position changes is essential. Vasopressor medication can be used to treat the profound vasodilation. Elastic compression stockings should be applied to improve venous return from the lower extremities. Abdominal binders may also be used to encourage venous return and provide diaphragmatic support when the patient is upright. Activity should be planned in advance, and adequate time should be allowed for a slow progression of position changes from recumbent to sitting and upright.

Autonomic Dysreflexia

Autonomic dysreflexia, also known as autonomic hyperreflexia, sympathetic storming (excessive and uncontrolled sympathetic output), or autonomic dysfunction syndrome (ADS), is an acute emergency that occurs as a result of exaggerated autonomic responses to stimuli that are harmless in normal people. It usually occurs in SCIs after spinal shock has resolved in patients with cord lesions above T6; however, cases have been reported in patients with SCIs as low as T8–T12. Autonomic dysreflexia may present soon after the initial injury but more commonly becomes symptomatic several months after the SCI (Dobkin, 2022). This syndrome is characterized by a severe, pounding headache with paroxysmal markedly elevated hypertension, profuse diaphoresis (most often of the forehead), nausea, nasal congestion, and bradycardia, pale skin is often observed below the lesion (Strayer, 2020). The sudden increase in blood pressure may cause a rupture of one or more cerebral blood vessels or lead to increased ICP (Krassioukov et al., 2020). Prevention is key.

Several stimuli may trigger this reflex: distended bladder (the most common cause); distention or contraction of the visceral organs, especially the bowel (from constipation, impaction); or stimulation of the skin (tactile, pain, thermal stimuli, pressure ulcer). Because this is an emergency situation, the objectives are to remove the triggering stimulus and to avoid the potentially serious complications.

The following measures are carried out:

- The head of the bed is raised, and the patient is placed immediately in a sitting position to lower blood pressure.
- Rapid assessment is performed to identify and alleviate the cause; inspect for areas of constriction (including clothing).
- The bladder is emptied immediately via a urinary catheter. If an indwelling catheter is not patent, it is irrigated or replaced with another catheter.
- PRN fast-acting short-duration antihypertensive agent (e.g., nifedipine, nitrates, captopril) is administered typically if systolic BP is > 150 mm Hg (Khanna et al., 2022).
- Once BP is within acceptable range (generally <150 mm Hg), the rectum is examined for a fecal mass. If one is present, a topical anesthetic such as lidocaine may be inserted 10 to 15 minutes before the mass is removed because visceral distention or contraction can worsen autonomic dysreflexia. The nurse observes for symptoms of flushing, sweating, nasal congestion, and headache while bowel disimpaction is performed; the procedure is halted if symptoms appear, and blood pressure is reassessed.
- The skin is examined for any areas of pressure, irritation, or broken skin.
- Any other stimulus that could be the triggering event, such as an object next to the skin or a draft of cold air, must be removed.
- The medical record is tagged with a clearly visible note about the risk for autonomic dysreflexia.
- The patient is instructed about prevention and management measures.
- Any patient with a lesion above the T6 segment is informed that such an episode is possible and may occur even years after the initial injury.

NURSING PROCESS
The Patient With Acute Spinal Cord Injury

ASSESSMENT

The breathing pattern is observed, the strength of the cough is assessed, and the lungs are auscultated because paralysis of abdominal and respiratory muscles diminishes coughing and makes clearing of bronchial and pharyngeal secretions difficult.

The patient is monitored closely for any changes in motor or sensory function and for symptoms of progressive neurologic damage. In the early stages of SCIs, determining whether the cord has been severed may be very difficult because signs and symptoms of cord edema are indistinguishable from those of cord transection. Edema of the spinal cord may occur with any severe cord injury and may further compromise spinal cord function.

(*continued on page 1434*)

Motor and sensory functions are assessed through careful neurologic examination. These findings are usually recorded on a flow sheet so that changes in the baseline neurologic status can be monitored closely and accurately. The ASIA classification is commonly used to describe level of function for SCI patients. Box 44-10 gives examples of the effects of altered spinal cord function. At the minimum:

- Motor ability is tested by asking the patient to spread the fingers, squeeze the examiner's hand, and move the toes or turn the feet.
- Sensation is evaluated by gently pinching the skin or touching it lightly with an object such as a tongue blade, starting at shoulder level and working down both sides of the extremities. The patient should have both eyes closed so that the examination reveals true findings, not what the patient hopes to feel. The patient is asked where the sensation is felt.
- Any decrease in neurologic function is reported immediately.

The patient is also assessed for spinal shock, urinary retention, overdistention of the bladder, and paralytic ileus.

DIAGNOSIS

NURSING DIAGNOSES

Based on the assessment data, the patient's major nursing diagnoses may include the following:

- Ineffective breathing patterns related to weakness or paralysis of abdominal and intercostal muscles and inability to clear secretions
- Ineffective airway clearance related to weakness of intercostal muscles
- Impaired bed and physical mobility related to motor and sensory impairments
- Disturbed sensory perception related to motor and sensory impairment
- Risk for altered skin integrity related to immobility and sensory loss
- Urinary retention related to inability to void spontaneously
- Constipation related to presence of atonic bowel as a result of autonomic disruption
- Acute pain and discomfort related to treatment and prolonged immobility

COLLABORATIVE PROBLEMS/POTENTIAL COMPLICATIONS

Potential complications that may develop in patients with SCIs include:

- DVT/PE (thrombophlebitis)
- Orthostatic hypotension
- Autonomic dysreflexia

PLANNING AND GOALS

The goals for the patient may include improved breathing pattern and airway clearance, improved mobility, improved sensory and perceptual awareness, maintenance of skin integrity, relief of urinary retention, improved bowel function, promotion of comfort, and absence of complications.

NURSING INTERVENTIONS

PROMOTING ADEQUATE BREATHING AND AIRWAY CLEARANCE

Oxygen is administered to maintain a normal saturation level because hypoxemia can create or worsen a neurologic deficit of the spinal cord. If endotracheal intubation is necessary, extreme care is taken to avoid flexing or extending the patient's neck, which can result in extension of a cervical injury.

Possible impending respiratory failure is detected by observing the patient, noting rate and depth of respirations, assessing lung sounds, noting accessory muscle use, monitoring oxygen saturation through pulse oximetry, and monitoring arterial blood gas values. Early and vigorous attention to clearing bronchial and pharyngeal secretions can prevent retention of secretions and atelectasis. Suctioning may be indicated, but caution must be used because this procedure can stimulate the vagus nerve, producing bradycardia, which can result in cardiac arrest.

If the patient cannot cough effectively because of decreased inspiratory volume and inability to generate sufficient expiratory pressure, chest physical therapy and assisted coughing may be indicated.

IMPROVING MOBILITY

Proper body alignment is maintained at all times. The patient is repositioned frequently and is assisted out of bed as soon as the spinal column is stabilized. The feet are prone to footdrop; therefore, various types of splints are used to prevent it. When used, the splints are removed and reapplied every 2 hours. Trochanter rolls, applied from the crest of the ileum to the midthigh of both legs, help prevent external rotation of the hip joints.

Patients with lesions above the midthoracic level have loss of sympathetic control of peripheral vasoconstrictor activity, leading to hypotension. These patients may poorly tolerate changes in position and require monitoring of blood pressure when positions are changed. Usually, the patient is turned every 2 hours by log rolling. Log rolling ensures proper spinal alignment during turning of the patient. The patient should not be turned unless the spine is stable and the provider has indicated that it is safe to do so.

Contractures develop rapidly with immobility and muscle paralysis. A joint that is immobilized too long becomes fixed as a result of contractures of the tendon and joint capsule. Atrophy of the extremities results from disuse. Contractures and other complications may be prevented by range-of-motion exercises that help preserve joint motion and stimulate circulation. Passive range-of-motion exercises should be implemented as soon as possible after injury.

PROMOTING ADAPTATION TO SENSORY AND PERCEPTUAL ALTERATIONS

The nurse assists the patient to compensate for sensory and perceptual alterations that occur with SCIs. The intact senses above the level of the injury are stimulated through touch, aromas, flavorful food and beverages, conversation, and music. Additional strategies include the following:

- Providing prism glasses to enable the patient to see from the supine position
- Encouraging use of hearing aids, if indicated, to enable the patient to hear conversations and environmental sounds
- Providing emotional support to the patient
- Teaching the patient strategies to compensate for or cope with these deficits

MAINTAINING SKIN INTEGRITY

Because patients with SCIs are immobilized and have loss of sensation below the level of the lesion, they have the highest prevalence of pressure ulcers in the United States. Around 30% to 40% of patients with SCIs will develop pressure ulcers (Shiferaw et al., 2020). Patients with higher-level SCIs are more likely to develop pressure ulcers than patients with lower-level SCIs (Shiferaw et al., 2020). The most common sites for pressure ulcers are over the ischial tuberosity, the greater trochanter, the sacrum, the gluteal region, and the occiput (back of the head). Patients who wear cervical collars for prolonged periods may develop breakdown from the pressure of the collar under the chin, on the shoulders, and at the occiput. The nurse follows institutional policy regarding collar care, which typically may require changing of pads every 24 hours and inspecting and cleaning the skin every shift. In patients with SCIs, pressure-relieving cushions (e.g., Roho wheelchair cushions) and bed support surfaces are used to lessen the risk of developing pressure ulcer. The nurse is aware that doughnut-shaped devices are NOT to be used because of the reduced blood flow associated with them.

The patient is repositioned every 2 hours, and careful inspection of the skin is made every time the patient is turned. The skin over pressure points is assessed for redness or breakdown. The patient's skin should be kept clean by washing with a mild soap, rinsing well, and blotting dry. Pressure-sensitive areas should be kept well lubricated and soft with hand cream or lotion.

MAINTAINING URINARY ELIMINATION

Immediately after SCIs, the urinary bladder may become atonic and is unable to contract by reflex activity. Urinary retention typically results. Because the patient has no sensation of bladder distention, overstretching of the bladder and detrusor muscle may occur, delaying the return of bladder function.

Intermittent catheterization is carried out to avoid overdistention of the bladder and UTI, typically on a schedule of every 4 to 6 hours (Mondor, 2022). If this is not feasible, an indwelling catheter is inserted temporarily. At an early stage, family members are shown how to carry out intermittent catheterization and are encouraged to participate in this facet of care because they will be involved in long-term follow-up and must be able to recognize complications so that treatment can be instituted.

The patient is taught to record fluid intake, voiding pattern, characteristics of urine, and any unusual sensations that may occur. The management of a neurogenic bladder (bladder dysfunction that results from a disorder or dysfunction of the nervous system) is discussed in detail in Chapter 27.

IMPROVING BOWEL FUNCTION

Immediately after SCIs, a paralytic ileus may develop due to neurogenic paralysis of the bowel; therefore, a nasogastric tube is often required to relieve distention and to prevent vomiting and aspiration.

Bowel activity usually returns within the first week following the injury. As soon as bowel sounds are heard on auscultation, the patient is given a high-calorie, high-protein, high-fiber diet, with the amount of food gradually increased. The nurse administers prescribed stool softeners to counteract the effects of immobility and analgesic agents. A bowel regimen is instituted as early as possible. The types of bowel dysfunction most seen in patients with SCIs are bloating, abdominal distention, incontinence, and constipation. Of these, constipation is the most common and is reported as high as 80% of patients (Qi et al., 2018).

PROVIDING COMFORT MEASURES

A patient who has had pins or tongs placed for cervical stabilization may have a headache or discomfort for several days after the pins are inserted. Patients initially may be bothered by the rather startling appearance of these devices, but usually they readily adapt to them because the devices provide comfort for the unstable neck. The patient may complain of being caged in and of noise created by any object encountering the steel frame of a halo device, but they can be reassured that adaptation to this will occur.

The areas around the four pin sites of a halo device are cleaned daily and observed for redness, drainage, and pain. The pins are observed for loosening, which may contribute to infection. If one of the pins becomes detached, the head is stabilized in a neutral position by one person, while another notifies the neurosurgeon. A torque screwdriver should be readily available in case the screws on the frame need tightening.

The skin under the halo vest is inspected for excessive perspiration, redness, and skin blistering, especially on the bony prominences. The vest is opened at the sides to allow the torso to be washed. The liner of the vest should not become wet because dampness causes skin excoriation. The liner should be changed periodically to promote hygiene and good skin care. If the patient is to be discharged with the vest, detailed instructions must be given to the family, with time allowed for them to demonstrate the necessary skills of halo vest care.

PROMOTING HOME AND COMMUNITY-BASED CARE

Teaching Patient Self-Care. In most cases, patients with SCIs (e.g., patients with tetraplegia or paraplegia) need long-term

(*continued on page 1436*)

BOX 44-12

Nursing Research

Bridging the Gap to Evidence-Based Practice

Hencklein, L. C., da Silva, R. L. F., Campos, D. G., Spagnol, G. S., Silva, J. L. G., de Oliveira Sanfelice, C. F., & de Souza Oliveira-Kumakura, A. R. (2021). Effectiveness of clinical simulation and peer-assisted learning to teaching about the sexuality of people with spinal cord injury. *Journal of Neuroscience Nursing*, *53*(5), 208–214.

Purpose

This study evaluates the effects of an educational intervention (high-fidelity simulation) on nursing students' knowledge acquisition about the sexuality of individuals with SCIs and on the students' self-confidence and satisfaction with the experience.

Design

Quasi-experimental, pre-post-test design was conducted with 54 senior-level nursing students. The intervention was the application of knowledge about sexuality of SCIs by senior-level nursing student on two high-fidelity clinical simulation scenarios. Demographics, knowledge about sexuality of people with SCIs, self-confidence, and satisfaction with the experience data were collected.

Findings

The effect of the simulation on knowledge ranged from the mean of 1.26 in the pre-test to 3.10 in the post-test, which is an increase of 1.84. The means in the scores for satisfaction (4.7) and self-confidence (4.0) were considered excellent.

Nursing Implications

Clinical simulation can promote significant learning for students on topics that are often neglected because of a lack of understanding how to proceed with a complex issue. For nurses working with the sexuality of patients with SCIs, it is important to understand the complexity of the subject. They must consider the limitations, fears, taboos, and uncertainties that the person may be facing after the injury. Simulation can provide great satisfaction and self-confidence in learning a difficult or uncomfortable patient care issue.

rehabilitation. The process begins during hospitalization, as acute symptoms begin to subside or come under better control and the overall deficits and long-term effects of the injury become clear. The goals begin to shift from merely surviving the injury to learning strategies necessary to cope with the alterations that the injury imposes on activities of daily living (ADLs). The emphasis shifts from ensuring that the patient is stable and free of complications to specific assessment and planning designed to meet the patient's rehabilitation needs. Patient teaching may initially focus on the injury and its effects on mobility; dressing; and bowel, bladder, and sexual function. As the patient and family acknowledge the consequences of the injury and the resulting disability, the focus of teaching broadens to address issues necessary for carrying out ADLs and taking charge of their lives. Teaching begins in the acute phase and continues throughout rehabilitation. Interventions are aimed at self-management skills needed to prevent secondary complications; the use of mobile health has made mobile apps a feasible method of delivering these interventions (Mortenson et al., 2019).

Caring for the patient with SCI at home may at first seem a daunting task to the family. They will require dedicated nursing support to gradually assume full care of the patient. Although maintaining function and preventing complications will remain important, goals regarding self-care and preparation for discharge will assist in a smooth transition to rehabilitation and eventually to the community.

Continuing Care. The ultimate goal of the rehabilitation process is independence. The nurse becomes a support to both the patient and the family, assisting them to assume responsibility for increasing aspects of patient care and management. Care for the patient with SCI involves members of all the health care disciplines, which may include nursing, medicine, rehabilitation, respiratory therapy, physical and occupational therapy, case management, and social services. The nurse often serves as coordinator of the management team and as a liaison with rehabilitation centers and home care agencies (Strayer, 2020). The patient and family often require assistance in dealing with the psychological impact of the injury and its consequences; referral to a psychiatric clinical nurse specialist or other mental health care professional is often helpful. Box 44-12 discusses the higher incidence in depression with SCIs and recognition of the importance of assessment of the patient's psychological state early in the rehabilitative process, as early intervention improves long-term patient satisfaction (Strayer, 2020).

As more patients survive acute SCIs, they face the changes associated with aging with a disability. Therefore, teaching in the home and community focuses on health promotion and addresses the need to minimize risk factors that increase the risk of mortality. For the aging SCI patient, there are consequences on functioning and health conditions that impact physical, psychological, and social well-being; nurses need to promote well-being, health, and quality of life (Pili et al., 2018). Home care nurses and others who have contact with patients with SCIs are in a position to teach patients about healthy lifestyles, remind them of the need for health screenings, and make referrals as appropriate. Assisting patients to identify accessible health care providers, clinical facilities, and imaging centers may increase the likelihood that they will participate in health screening.

EVALUATION

EXPECTED PATIENT OUTCOMES

Expected patient outcomes may include the following:

1. Demonstrates improvement in gas exchange and clearance of secretions, as evidenced by normal breath sounds on auscultation:
   a. Breathes easily without shortness of breath
   b. Performs hourly deep-breathing exercises, coughs effectively, and clears pulmonary secretions

   c. Is free of respiratory infection (i.e., has normal temperature, respiratory rate, and pulse; normal breath sounds; absence of purulent sputum)
2. Moves within limits of the dysfunction and demonstrates completion of exercises within functional limitations
3. Demonstrates adaptation to sensory and perceptual alterations:
   a. Uses assistive devices (e.g., prism glasses, hearing aids, computers) as indicated
   b. Describes sensory and perceptual alterations as a consequence of injury
4. Demonstrates optimal skin integrity:
   a. Exhibits normal skin turgor; skin is free of reddened areas or breakdown
   b. Participates in skin care and monitoring procedures within functional limitations
5. Regains control of urinary bladder function:
   a. Exhibits no signs of UTI (e.g., has normal temperature; voids clear, dilute urine)
   b. Has adequate fluid intake
   c. Participates in bladder training program within functional limitations
6. Regains control of bowel function:
   a. Reports regular pattern of bowel movement
   b. Consumes adequate dietary fiber and oral fluids
   c. Participates in bowel training program within functional limitations
7. Reports absence of pain and discomfort
8. Is free of complications:
   a. Demonstrates no signs of DVT or PE
   b. Exhibits no manifestations of PE (e.g., no chest pain or shortness of breath; arterial blood gas values are within normal limits)
   c. Maintains blood pressure within normal limits
   d. Reports no lightheadedness with position changes
   e. Exhibits no manifestations of autonomic dysreflexia (i.e., absence of headache, diaphoresis, nasal congestion, or bradycardia)

Clinical Judgment Case

A 78-year-old patient comes into the Emergency Room (ER). They were found unresponsive at the public library. Efforts to wake the patient were unsuccessful and an ambulance was called. The librarian recalls speaking to the patient earlier and noted the patient was alert, pleasant, and asking for resources. The time last known well was 1 hour ago. The patient's skin is warm and dry with adequate skin turgor and vital signs are as follows: 98.7°F, heart rate 108 and irregular, 18 RR with an oxygen saturation of 96% on room air and the blood pressure is 122/62. Heart sounds are S1 S2 without murmur, gallops, or rub; there is no jugular vein distention (JVD). Lung sounds are clear. Abdomen is soft, nondistended, and nontender. There is no peripheral edema or jugular vein distention, capillary refill is 2 seconds, and pedal and posterior tibial pulses are 3+ bil. Neurologic assessment includes GCS of 7 (not opening eyes [1], localizes pain to painful stimuli [5], and no verbal response [1]), PERL 3 mm bil. and gaze is midline, no nystagmus, no corneal reflex, but gag reflex and cough reflex is present, no head trauma noted or bruising on physical exam, neck is supple (no nuchal rigidity noted). There has been no seizure activity. There is no drainage via the ears (otorrhea) or nose (rhinorrhea). The patient's wallet is examined and license retrieved so that medical records can be accessed, a medical alert bracelet notes atrial fibrillation, and a card in patient's wallet notes an INR of 2.5 last month. Besides warfarin (alternating dosages of 5 mg and 2.5 mg), the patient is prescribed Synthroid 125 mcg daily and a multivitamin. You alert the providers of the history of atrial fibrillation and warfarin anticoagulation.

Step One: Recognize cues where relevant and important information is identified from different sources, such as medical history or vital signs.

Answer: History of atrial fibrillation and hypothyroidism. Sudden loss of consciousness 1 hour ago, comatose, GCS of 7. Irregular pulse, tachycardia, absence of corneal reflex.

Step Two: Analyze cues, which is organizing and linking the recognized cues to the patient's clinical presentation.

Answer: You have clustered the symptom of an irregular pulse and associate it with history of atrial fibrillation. You link the sudden loss of consciousness and coma with GCS of 7 and absence of corneal reflex with a potential structural, metabolic, medication or infectious process. You are aware a GCS of 7 is associated with a severe TBI. Although the patient has no obvious trauma, is afebrile and has no nuchal rigidity, you realize an emergency workup is necessary to begin to identify reversible causes. You are concerned that the change in LOC may be related to the possibility of intracranial hemorrhage since the patient is on warfarin. You see no evidence of Cushing triad (hypertension, bradycardia, and bradypnea), which you know is associated with ICP. You are also curious about the patient's adherence to taking the thyroid medication and about the thyroid function tests

(TSH and free T4) since profound hypothyroidism or myxedema coma presents with an unconscious patient. However, edema is also present, as is hypothermia, in myxedema coma, and the patient does not have either.

Step Three: Prioritize hypotheses, where hypotheses are evaluated and ranked according to priority. This can include urgency, likelihood, risk, difficulty, and/or time. In this phase you cluster your findings to arrive at a list of problems (actual and or potential problems) you believe the patient is experiencing and determine the importance or urgency. What do you think is of greatest concern?

Answer: You prioritize the need to monitor oxygen saturation continuously and reassess the patient's neuro status, place the patient on a cardiac monitor to evaluate their rhythm, start an intravenous line if medications must be administered urgently, and reassess vital signs. You are acutely aware that stat blood work, which includes CBC, bleeding studies (particularly the PT and INR) given the warfarin use, chemistry studies, and thyroid function must be obtained, and that an emergent head computed tomography (CT) scan is needed. You are concerned about the lack of corneal reflex and are aware that corneal abrasions can occur, but the priority is to get the patient monitored and evaluated by the providers and to obtain lab work and transfer the patient for stat CT scan.

Step Four: Generate solutions, which is identifying expected outcomes and using hypotheses to define a set of interventions for the expected outcomes.

Answer: You recognize that comatose patients will have a decreased ability to maintain their airway; therefore, continuous monitoring of the O_2 saturation is needed. If the patient's condition is due to an elevated INR, you are aware that reversal of the anticoagulant is needed and may include intravenous fresh frozen plasma (FFP), vitamin K (phytonadione), among others. You are also aware if this is the cause you will have to apply pressure for 10 minutes or more to bleeding line or venipuncture sites. You anticipate that an intracranial bleed may require surgical evacuation.

If the patient condition is due to an embolic event due to atrial fibrillation (and inadequate anticoagulation), you anticipate the use of TPA since the last known well time was 90 minutes ago. You are aware that time is brain tissue, so the CT scan is a priority.

If the patient's condition is due to an infectious process, then you expect the WBC to be elevated or leukocytosis (elevated WBCs). If this is present, you anticipate a lumbar puncture may be performed.

If the coma is related to hypoglycemia, which is one of the more common reversible causes of coma, you anticipate dextrose administration.

Step Five: Take action, where the solutions that address the highest priorities are implemented.

Answer: The oxygen saturation is monitored continuously and remains >97% on room air. You elevate the head of the bed 30 degrees and maintain the neck in midline position to decrease the risk of increasing ICP. You start the IV, place the patient on a cardiac monitor, and move the 12 lead ECG machine to the bedside as the provider comes in to assess the patient. You do point of care glucose testing—the glucose is 110 mg/dL—and you inform the provider. You repeat the vital signs and reassess the patient's GCS and pupils. Once blood work is obtained, you transfer the patient to radiology for the stat CT scan.

Step Six: Evaluate outcomes, which is comparing observed outcomes against expected outcomes.

Answer: The CT scan reveals a subdural hematoma (SDH), the INR is 2.5, the TSH and free T4 are within normal limits. The ECG reveals atrial fibrillation with no ST changes. VS repeated are now HR of 92 and irregular, RR 16, oxygen saturation of 97% on RA, and BP is now 136/82. The neurosurgeon prepares the patient for emergency evacuation of the SDH. As you prepare the patient for surgery, a family member rushes to the bedside and tells you that 2 weeks ago a light fixture fell on the patient's head; the family member wonders if this could be related. You recognize that as one ages, there is whole brain atrophy which causes traction on fragile bridging veins and also allows more free space for bleeding; that is why the patient is at increased risk for subdural hemorrhage. You prioritized well in this case, and you considered a myriad of possible causes of the patient's condition and recognized that sometimes the actual cause is not on your extensive list—but it is now. Congratulations, you have added to your database of clinical presentations for coma. In addition, the patient tolerated the surgery well, fully recovered, and was back at the library 1 month later.

CHAPTER REVIEW

NCLEX-Style Review Questions

1. The nurse assesses the LOC of a patient who suffered a head injury and determines that the patient's GCS score is 15. Which of the following responses did the nurse assess to determine the GCS score? Select all that apply.
   a. Spontaneous eye opening
   b. Tachycardia, hypotension, bradycardia
   c. Ability to follow commands
   d. Unequal pupil size
   e. Orientation to person, place, and time

2. When caring for a patient with a ventriculostomy, the nurse notices that the intracranial pressure (ICP) is 30 mm Hg. The nurse assesses the patient and the ICP monitor. After opening the drain, which of the following immediate interventions should occur? Select all that apply.
   a. Hypoventilate the patient to increase the PCO_2
   b. Lower the head of the bed to Trendelenburg position
   c. Close the stopcock on the ventriculostomy to prevent drainage of cerebrospinal fluid (CSF)
   d. Elevate the head of the bed to 30 degrees
   e. Ensure the head and neck are in alignment

3. The victim of a motor vehicle crash has been admitted with massive trauma, including traumatic brain injury. Emergency treatment of increased intracranial pressure (ICP) has failed to resolve the problem, and monitoring reveals the ominous presence of Cushing triad. What assessment findings would be consistent with this clinical phenomenon? Select all that apply.
   a. RR 7 breaths per minute
   b. HR 116 beats per minute
   c. B/P 198/100
   d. RR 33 breaths per minute
   e. HR 42 beats per minute
   f. B/P 90/60 mm Hg

4. A Post Anesthesia Care Unit (PACU) nurse is receiving a patient who is postcraniotomy procedure. The patient is mechanically ventilated, and a ventriculostomy drain is in place. The nurse notes the ICP is 40 mm Hg., and the arterial blood gases (ABGs) are as follows: pH 7.3, PCO_2 56 mm Hg, and PaO_2 97 mm Hg. The PACU nurse notifies the anesthesiologist and anticipates which of the following interventions? Select all that apply.
   a. Increasing the respiratory rate or tidal volume
   b. Keeping the head and neck in the midline position while avoiding flexion
   c. Increasing the FiO_2
   d. Assessing that the ventriculostomy drain is open to allow CSF to drain
   e. Elevating the head of bed (HOB) 30 degrees to reduce ICP
   f. Increasing the IV rate

5. Which interventions should the nurse's plan of care include to help prevent autonomic dysreflexia in a patient with SCI? Select all that apply.
   a. Check for fecal impactions.
   b. Monitor blood pressure for hypotension.
   c. Check the urinary drainage system for any obstruction.
   d. Monitor serum electrolytes.
   e. Inspect for areas of constriction (including clothing).

REFERENCES AND SELECTED READINGS

References and selected readings associated with this chapter can be found on the website that accompanies the book. Visit **http://thepoint.lww.com/Honan3e** to access the references and other additional resources associated with this chapter.

CHAPTER 45

Nursing Management: Patients With Neurologic Disorders

Cynthia Bautista

Learning Objectives

After reading this chapter, you will be able to:

1. Identify the various types and causes of seizures.
2. Use the nursing process to develop a plan of care for the patient experiencing seizures.
3. Differentiate the infectious disorders of the nervous system according to causes, manifestations, medical care, and nursing management.
4. Describe the pathophysiology, clinical manifestations, and medical and nursing management of multiple sclerosis, myasthenia gravis, and Guillain–Barré syndrome.
5. Describe neuromuscular disorders and their manifestations and indicated nursing interventions.
6. Use the nursing process as a framework for care of patients with degenerative neurologic disorders.

SEIZURE DISORDERS

SEIZURES, EPILEPSY, AND STATUS EPILEPTICUS

Seizures are a single event of abnormal discharges resulting in an abrupt and temporary altered state of brain function creating a sudden surge of abnormal electrical discharges from chemical changes in brain cells (England & Plueger, 2020). A part or all of the brain may be involved. The term *ictal* refers to an actual seizure or *ictal event.*

Epilepsy is a disease that meets any of the following conditions: (1) at least two unprovoked seizures occurring more than 24 hours apart; (2) one unprovoked seizure and probability of further seizures; (3) diagnosis of an epilepsy syndrome (Katyayan & Diaz-Medina, 2021). Epileptic syndromes are classified by specific patterns of clinical features, including age at onset, family history, and seizure type.

Status epilepticus is continuous seizure activity for more than 5 minutes or two or more sequential seizures without full recovery of consciousness between seizures (England & Plueger, 2020). Seizures that last longer than 5 to 10 minutes are less likely to stop without intervention. Status epilepticus is a neurologic emergency and can be life threatening.

Pearls for Practice

Not all seizures imply epilepsy. Although seizures are the cardinal symptom of epilepsy, seizures also occur as a manifestation of an underlying treatable problem, such as hyponatremia or high fever. Once the cause is identified and treated, the seizures cease. Epilepsy is a disease and refers to recurrent, unpredictable, and unprovoked seizures.

Pathophysiology of Seizures

Messages from the body are carried by the neurons (nerve cells) of the brain by means of discharges of electrochemical energy that sweep along them. These impulses occur in bursts whenever a nerve cell has a task to perform. Sometimes, these cells or groups of cells continue firing after a task is finished. During the period of unwanted discharges, parts of the body controlled by the errant cells may perform erratically. Seizures require three conditions: (1) excitable neurons; (2) increase in excitatory glutaminergic activity (relates to the action of glutamate or to neural or metabolic pathways in which it functions as a transmitter) through recurrent connections to spread the discharge; and (3) reduction in activity of normal inhibitory GABA projection (GABA is an amino acid that is the major inhibitory neurotransmitter in the vertebrate gray matter) (England & Plueger, 2020). When there is an imbalance between inhibition and excitation within the central nervous system (CNS), seizures occur.

Pearls for Practice

Anyone can have a seizure. Although we all have a unique threshold for seizures, an imbalance in that threshold can provoke a seizure. In fact, 10% of Americans will have a seizure in their lifetime. It is a

BOX 45-1

Classification of Seizures

Focal Seizures (seizure activity starts in one area of the brain)

- *Focal*–retains awareness: There is no impairment of consciousness, similar to simple partial seizures; the person may have movement of body parts and may experience an aura.
- *Focal*–altered awareness: There is impairment of consciousness, similar to complex partial seizures; this can spread to both hemispheres of brain.

Partial Seizures

These seizures begin in a part of one hemisphere, generally in the temporal or frontal lobe. The two types of partial seizures, called simple and complex, are based on whether a person remains fully conscious during a seizure.

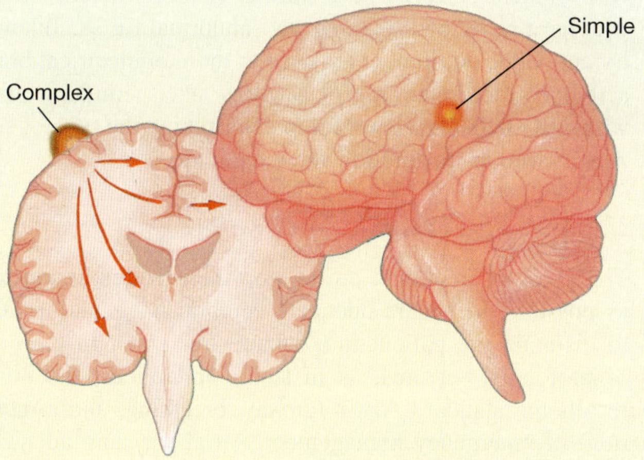

Unknown Seizures (insufficient evidence to classify as focal, generalized, or both)

Generalized Seizures (seizure activity involves both hemispheres of the brain)

Generalized Seizures

These seizures affect both hemispheres of the brain at the same time. Abnormal activity is not focused in one specific area, and there generally is no aura at the start.

- *Tonic–clonic seizures:* Generalized seizures that affect the entire brain; they begin with rigidity (tonic phase), followed by repetitive clonic activity of all extremities, characterized by stiffening or jerking of the body.
- *Tonic seizures:* Seizures characterized by muscle stiffening, dilation of the pupils, and altered respiratory patterns; the body becomes stiff, and the person may fall backward. The seizure usually lasts less than 1 minute, and recovery is rapid.
- *Clonic seizures:* Characterized by jerking movements that involve muscles on both sides of the body
- *Absence seizures:* Short episodes of staring and loss of awareness
- *Atonic seizures:* Sudden loss of muscle tone, resulting in a fall or a "drop" to the ground, with rapid recovery
- *Myoclonic seizure:* Characterized by jerking (myoclonic) movements of a muscle or muscle group, without loss of consciousness

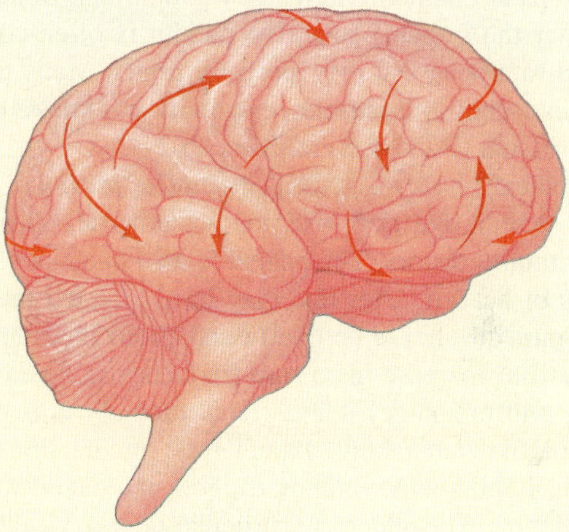

matter of imbalance in excitatory activity in the CNS or a reduction in inhibitory activity.

The international classification of seizures differentiates two main types: focal or partial seizures, which begin in one part of the brain, and generalized seizures, which involve electrical discharges in the whole brain (see Box 45-1). However, it is understood that not all seizures or syndromes fit neatly into these classifications, and patients may have more than one type of seizure.

The specific causes of seizures are varied and can be categorized as idiopathic (genetic, developmental defects) and acquired. Causes of acquired seizures include:

- Cerebrovascular disease
- Hypoxemia of any cause, including vascular insufficiency
- Fever (childhood)
- Head injury
- Hypertension
- CNS infections
- Metabolic and toxic conditions (e.g., kidney failure, hyponatremia, hypocalcemia, hypoglycemia, pesticides)
- Brain tumor
- Drug and alcohol withdrawal; drug toxicity
- Allergies
- Alzheimer disease (see discussion later in this chapter on page 1469)

Clinical Manifestations and Assessment

The initial pattern of the seizure indicates the region of the brain in which the seizure originates (see Box 45-1). In focal seizures in which the patient retains awareness, only a finger or hand may shake, or the mouth may jerk uncontrollably. The person may talk unintelligibly, may be dizzy, and may experience unusual or unpleasant sights, sounds, odors, or tastes but does not experience loss of consciousness.

In focal seizures with altered awareness, the person either remains motionless or moves automatically but inappropriately for time and place, or they may experience excessive emotions of fear, anger, elation, or irritability. Whatever the manifestations, the person does not remember the episode when it is over.

Generalized seizures involve both hemispheres of the brain, causing both sides of the body to react. Intense rigidity of the entire body may occur, followed by alternating muscle relaxation and contraction (generalized tonic–clonic contraction). The simultaneous contractions of the diaphragm and chest muscles may produce a characteristic epileptic cry. The patient may chew the tongue or bite the inner cheek, and the patient may be incontinent of urine and feces. After 1 or 2 minutes, the convulsive movements begin to subside; the patient relaxes and lies in deep coma, breathing noisily. The respirations at this point are chiefly abdominal. In the postictal (after the seizure) state, the patient is often confused and hard to arouse and may sleep for hours. Many patients report headache, sore muscles, extremity weakness, fatigue, and depression (Bazil & Svinivasan, 2021).

A medical history is taken, including previous seizure history, alcohol and drug use, medication use, allergy status, and family history. The patient is also questioned about illnesses or head injuries that may have affected the brain. Female patients should be questioned about their last menstrual period (increase in seizure frequency is noted during menses) and pregnancy status (fetal anomaly is two times higher in females taking antiepileptic medications). The patient is asked about common triggers associated with seizures, which can be olfactory (particular odors), visual (flashing lights), or auditory (certain types of music) in nature, or related to fatigue, sleep deprivation, hypoglycemia, emotional stress, electrical shock, febrile illness, alcohol consumption, certain drugs, drinking too much water, constipation, and hyperventilation (England & Plueger, 2020).

Epilepsy patients who identify as lesbian, gay, bisexual, transgender, queer (LGBTQ+) are concerned with provider-based stigma. It is recommended that nurses receive mandatory LGBTQ+ specific health care education. All LGBTQ+ epilepsy patients should receive the best possible health care (Matsuzaka et al., 2021).

In addition to physical and neurologic evaluations, diagnostic examinations include biochemical, hematologic, and serologic studies. Common diagnostic procedures used include computed tomography (CT) scan, perfusion CT (PCT), magnetic resonance imaging (MRI), magnetic resonance spectroscopy (MRS), and electroencephalogram (EEG). Additional procedures may include single-photon emission computed tomography (SPECT) and positron emission tomography (PET). The EEG, MRI, and PET are essential technologies in verifying brain function through the evaluation of electrical and metabolic activity (Dubendorf, 2022). The SPECT is useful for identifying the epileptogenic zone so that the area in the brain giving rise to seizures can be removed surgically.

The EEG furnishes diagnostic evidence for a substantial proportion of patients with epilepsy and assists in classifying the type of seizure (Dubendorf, 2022). Abnormalities in the EEG usually continue between seizures or, if not apparent, may be elicited by hyperventilation or during sleep. Microelectrodes (depth electrodes) can be inserted deep in the brain to probe the action of single brain cells. Some people with clinical seizures have normal EEGs, whereas others who have never had seizures have abnormal EEGs. Telemetry and video equipment are used to monitor electrical brain activity. Video recording of seizures taken simultaneously with EEG telemetry is useful in determining the type of seizure as well as its duration and magnitude.

Medical and Nursing Management

The goals of treatment are to stop the seizures as quickly as possible, to ensure adequate cerebral oxygenation, and to maintain the patient in a seizure-free state. In the case of prolonged seizures, as in status epilepticus, the nurse recalls the standard ABCs (airway, breathing, and circulation) of emergency management. An airway and adequate oxygenation are established if the patient shows signs of airway obstruction. Oxygen is administered as ordered via nasal cannula, or intubation may be required, and oxygen is administered via the artificial airway and monitored by pulse oximetry. Suctioning of the airway may also be required. An IV line is established, and IV lorazepam, diazepam, or midazolam is administered slowly in an attempt to halt seizures immediately. The IV line is closely monitored because it may become dislodged during seizures. Antiepileptic drugs (AEDs) (levetiracetam, phenytoin, phenobarbital) are administered later to maintain a seizure-free state. In general, a single drug is used to control the seizures. Termed *monotherapy*, the selected drug is determined by the type of seizure, and the dose is increased until symptoms resolve; maximal dose is required; or signs of drug toxicity emerge, at which time alternative therapeutic agents are considered.

Pearls for Practice

Phenytoin, if ordered intravenously, must be administered slowly because of its effect on the myocardium and the potential for arrhythmia development. In addition, it is irritating to the vein; thus, the nurse observes for the development of phlebitis. The rate of administration is no faster than 50 mg/min in normal saline solution since the

drug precipitates in D_5W. If the pre-existing solution contained dextrose, the nurse flushes the IV line with normal saline before administering the medication. Many AEDs are highly bound to plasma protein, and the nurse is aware that only the unbound, or "free," serum concentration is available for use by the body. Patients on high-protein tube feedings (see Chapter 21) may require higher dosages to maintain therapeutic blood levels, while those with hypoalbuminemia because of malnutrition, burns, or liver or kidney disease may require alternative dosing to prevent phenytoin toxicity. The therapeutic range for phenytoin is 10 to 20 mg/L (Madan, 2020).

Blood samples are obtained to monitor serum electrolytes, glucose, blood cell count, and toxicology/drug screen; levels of drugs, such as phenobarbital or phenytoin, may be monitored if the patient has been treated with the medication. If the serum concentration of the AED is below therapeutic level, it suggests that the patient was not taking the medication, the dosage was too low, or factors such as pharmacokinetics of the medication may be involved. EEG monitoring may be useful in determining the nature of the seizure activity. Vital signs and neurologic signs are monitored on a continuing basis. An IV infusion of dextrose is administered if the seizure is caused by hypoglycemia. If initial treatment is unsuccessful, general anesthesia with a short-acting barbiturate may be used. Cardiac involvement or respiratory depression may be life-threatening. The potential for postictal cerebral edema also exists. This varies in clinical presentation and may include deterioration in neurologic signs, ranging from drowsiness to coma, as well as nausea, vomiting, sluggish pupillary response, cardiac arrhythmias, and altered respiratory patterns. The nurse initiates ongoing assessment and monitoring of respiratory and cardiac function because of the risk for delayed depression of respiration and blood pressure secondary to administration of AEDs and sedatives to halt the seizures. Nursing assessment also includes monitoring and documenting the seizure activity and the patient's responsiveness.

A person who has received long-term antiepileptic therapy has a significant risk for fractures resulting from bone disease (osteoporosis, osteomalacia, and hyperparathyroidism), a side effect of therapy. Therefore, during seizures, the patient is protected from injury with the use of seizure precautions, which include placing the bed in a low position, raising the bedside rails, and not letting the patient get up and ambulate without someone's assistance. The patient's room should have suction and oxygen available at the bedside if needed (England & Plueger, 2020). No effort should be made to restrain seizure activity. The patient having a seizure can inadvertently injure nearby people, so nurses should protect themselves. Other nursing interventions for the person having a seizure are presented in Box 45-2.

Severe psychological distress among people with epilepsy was reported during the initial period of the coronavirus disease 2019 (COVID-19) pandemic. There was also an overall increase in seizures with difficulty in accessing medical care for people with epilepsy. The utilization of telemedicine by health care providers was found to be helpful. Ongoing support and care for people with epilepsy is needed to address any unmet health care needs during a pandemic (Cross et al., 2021).

During a Seizure

A major responsibility of the nurse is to observe and record the sequence of signs. Before and during a seizure, the patient is assessed and the following items are documented:

- The circumstances before the seizure (visual, auditory, or olfactory stimuli; tactile stimuli; emotional or psychological disturbances; sleep; hyperventilation)
- The occurrence of an aura (a premonitory or warning sensation that can be visual, auditory, gustatory [taste], visceral, or olfactory) that is experienced at the beginning of a seizure and remembered (England & Plueger, 2020)
- The first thing the patient exhibits in the seizure—in what part of the body the movement or stiffness begins, conjugate gaze position (term that denotes both eyes working in unison), and the position of the head at the beginning of the seizure. This information gives clues to the location of the seizure's origin in the brain. (In recording, it is important to state whether the beginning of the seizure was observed).
- The type of movements in the part of the body involved
- The areas of the body involved (turn back bedding to inspect the patient)
- The size of both pupils and whether the patient's eyes are open
- Whether the patient's eyes or head are/is turned to one side (eyes look away from the side of the seizure)
- The presence or absence of automatisms (involuntary motor activity, such as lip smacking or repeated swallowing)
- Incontinence of urine or stool
- Duration of each phase of the seizure
- Unconsciousness, if present, and its duration
- Any obvious paralysis or weakness of the patient's arms or legs after the seizure
- Inability to speak after the seizure
- Movements at the end of the seizure
- Whether or not the patient sleeps afterward
- Cognitive status (confused or not confused) after the seizure

In addition to providing data about the seizure, nursing care is directed at preventing injury and supporting the patient both physically and psychologically. Steps to prevent or minimize injury are presented in Box 45-2.

After a Seizure

After a patient has a seizure, the nurse's role is to document the events leading to and occurring during and after

BOX 45-2

GUIDELINES FOR NURSING CARE

Nursing Care During a Seizure

- Provide privacy and protect the patient from curious onlookers. The patient who has an *aura* [warning of an impending seizure] may have time to seek a safe, private place.
- Ease the patient to the floor, if possible.
- Protect the head with a pad to prevent injury (from striking a hard surface).
- Loosen constrictive clothing, remove eyeglasses.
- Push aside any furniture that may injure the patient during the seizure.
- If the patient is in bed, remove extra pillows and raise the side rails.
- *Do not attempt to pry open the patient's jaws if they are clenched in a spasm or to insert anything.* Broken teeth and injury to the lips and tongue may result from such an action.
- Do not attempt to restrain the patient during the seizure because muscular contractions are strong and restraint can produce injury.
- If possible, place the patient on one side to facilitate drainage of saliva and mucus. If suction is available, use it if necessary to clear secretions.

Nursing Care After the Seizure

- Keep the patient on one side to prevent aspiration. Make sure the airway is patent.
- There is usually a period of confusion after a tonic–clonic seizure.
- A short apneic period may occur during or immediately after a generalized seizure.
- The patient, on awakening, should be reoriented to the environment.
- If the patient becomes agitated after a seizure (postictal), use calm persuasion.

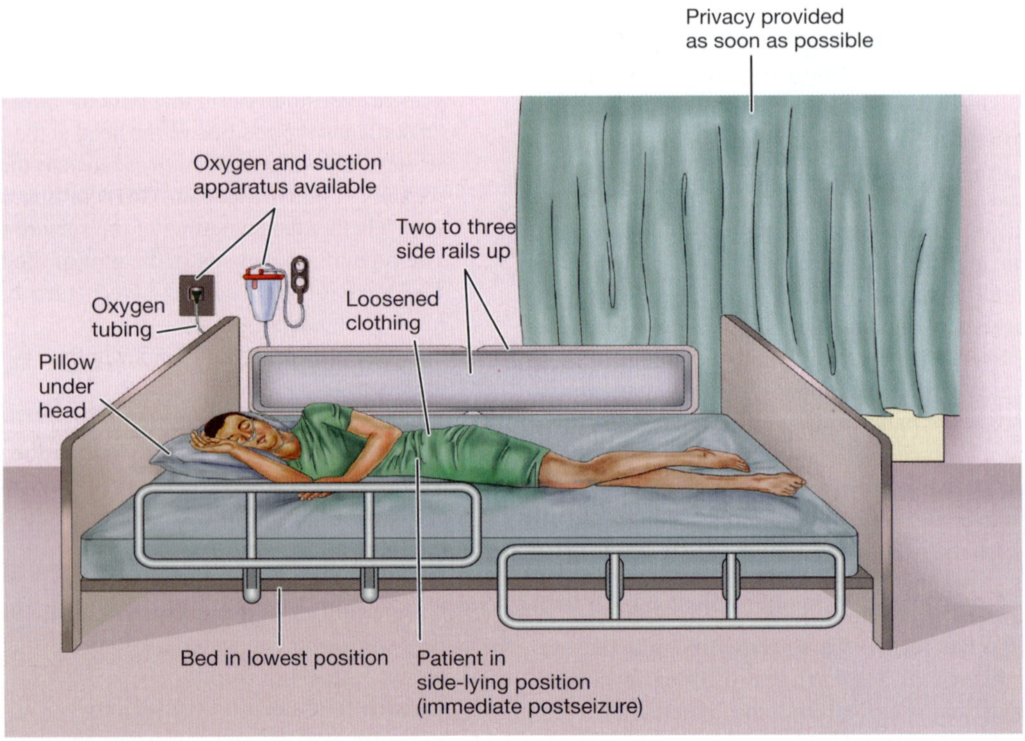

the seizure and to prevent complications (e.g., aspiration, injury). The patient is at risk for hypoxia, vomiting, and pulmonary aspiration. To prevent complications, the patient is placed in the side-lying position to facilitate drainage of oral secretions, and suctioning is performed, if needed, to maintain a patent airway and prevent aspiration (see Box 45-2). Seizure precautions are maintained, including having available functioning suction equipment with a suction catheter. The bed is placed in a low position with two to three side rails up, if necessary, to prevent injury to the patient. The patient may be drowsy and may wish to sleep after the seizure; they may not remember events leading up to the seizure and for a short time thereafter.

Pharmacologic Therapy

Although many medications are available to control seizures, the nurse stresses that the treatment is not curative.

The objective is to achieve seizure control with minimal side effects. Medications are selected on the basis of the patient's type of seizure and the effectiveness and safety of the medications. If properly prescribed and taken, medications control seizures in 70% to 80% of patients with seizures (Lowenstein, 2020). Approximately 35% of patients with epilepsy are resistant to AEDs (England & Plueger, 2020). In these situations, surgery may reduce seizure frequency or provide complete seizure control.

Treatment usually starts with a single medication. The starting dose and the rate at which the dosage is increased depend on the occurrence of side effects. The medication levels in the blood are monitored because the rate of drug absorption varies among patients. Changing to another medication may be necessary if seizure control is not achieved or if toxicity makes it impossible to increase the dosage. The medication may need to be adjusted because of concurrent illness, weight changes, or increase in stress. Stopping these medications without the provider's knowledge can cause seizures to occur with greater frequency or can precipitate the development of status epilepticus (England & Plueger, 2020).

Side effects of AEDs may be divided into three groups: (1) idiosyncratic or allergic disorders, which manifest primarily as skin reactions; (2) acute toxicity, which may occur when the medication is initially prescribed; and (3) chronic toxicity, which occurs late in the course of therapy.

The manifestations of drug toxicity are variable, and any organ system may be involved. Gingival hyperplasia (swollen and tender gums) can be associated with long-term use of phenytoin, for example (Gunturu, 2020). Periodic physical and dental examinations and laboratory tests are performed for patients receiving medications that are known to have hematopoietic, genitourinary, or hepatic effects. Table 45-1 lists the medications in current use.

TABLE **45-1** **Major Antiseizure Medications**

Medication	Dose-Related Side Effects	Toxic Effects
Carbamazepine	Dizziness, drowsiness, unsteadiness, nausea and vomiting, diplopia, mild leukopenia	Severe skin rash, blood dyscrasias, hepatitis
Clonazepam	Drowsiness, behavior changes, headache, hirsutism, alopecia, palpitations	Hepatotoxicity, thrombocytopenia, bone marrow failure, ataxia
Ethosuximide	Nausea and vomiting, headache, gastric distress	Skin rash, blood dyscrasias, hepatitis, systemic lupus erythematosus (SLE)
Gabapentin	Dizziness, drowsiness, somnolence, fatigue, ataxia, weight gain, nausea	Leukopenia, hepatotoxicity
Lamotrigine	Drowsiness, tremor, nausea, ataxia, dizziness, headache, weight gain	Severe rash (Stevens–Johnson syndrome)
Levetiracetam	Somnolence, dizziness, fatigue	Unknown
Oxcarbazepine	Dizziness, somnolence, double vision, fatigue, nausea, vomiting, loss of coordination, abnormal vision, abdominal pain, tremor, abnormal gait	Hepatotoxicity
Phenobarbital	Sedation, irritability, diplopia, ataxia	Skin rash, anemia
Phenytoin	Visual problems, hirsutism, gingival hyperplasia, arrhythmias, dysarthria, nystagmus	Severe skin reaction, peripheral neuropathy, ataxia, drowsiness, blood dyscrasias
Primidone	Lethargy, irritability, diplopia, ataxia, impotence	Skin rash
Tiagabine	Dizziness, fatigue, nervousness, tremor, difficulty concentrating, dysarthria, weak or buckling knees, abdominal pain	Unknown
Topiramate	Fatigue, somnolence, confusion, ataxia, anorexia, depression, weight loss	Nephrolithiasis
Valproate	Nausea and vomiting, weight gain, hair loss, tremor, menstrual irregularities	Hepatotoxicity, skin rash, blood dyscrasias, nephritis
Zonisamide	Somnolence, dizziness, anorexia, headache, nausea, agitation, rash	Leukopenia, hepatotoxicity

Surgical Management

Surgery is indicated for patients whose epilepsy results from intracranial tumors, abscesses, cysts, or vascular anomalies. Some patients have intractable seizure disorders that do not respond to medication. A focal (localized or limited) atrophic process (affecting cells in certain areas of the brain resulting in a loss of function in that area) may occur secondary to trauma, inflammation, stroke, or anoxia. If the seizures originate in a reasonably well-circumscribed area of the brain that can be excised without producing significant neurologic deficits, the removal of the area (termed a *lobectomy*) generating the seizures may produce long-term control and improvement (Lowenstein, 2020).

Epilepsy surgery has been aided by several advances, including microsurgical techniques, EEGs with depth electrodes, improved illumination and hemostasis, and the introduction of neuroleptanalgesic agents (droperidol and fentanyl). These techniques, combined with use of local anesthetic agents, enable the neurosurgeon to perform surgery on an alert and cooperative patient. Using special testing devices, electrocortical mapping, and the patient's responses to stimulation, the boundaries of the epileptogenic focus (the abnormal area of the brain) are determined. The abnormal epileptogenic focus is then excised (lobectomy) (England & Plueger, 2020). Resection surgery significantly reduces the incidence of seizures in patients with refractory epilepsy; however, more research is needed to determine the effect of surgery on quality of life, anxiety, and depression, as all are issues for these patients.

As an adjunct to medication in adolescents and adults with focal seizures, a vagal nerve stimulator may be implanted under the clavicle. The device is connected to the vagus nerve in the cervical area, where it delivers electrical signals to the brain to control and reduce seizure activity (England & Plueger, 2020). An external programming system is used by the physician to change stimulator settings. The patient can turn the stimulator on and off with a magnet. This can be performed as an outpatient surgical procedure.

Gerontologic Considerations

Older people (65 years of age and older) have a high incidence of new-onset epilepsy (England & Plueger, 2020). Cerebrovascular disease is the leading cause of seizures in older individuals, but head trauma, dementia, infection, alcoholism, and aging are also associated risk factors (Elder, 2020). Treatment depends on the underlying cause. Because many older people have chronic health problems, they may be taking other medications that can interact with medications prescribed for seizure control. In addition, the absorption, distribution, metabolism, and excretion of medications are altered in older individuals as a result of age-related changes in kidney and liver function. Therefore, older patients must be monitored closely for adverse and toxic effects of AEDs and for osteoporosis. The cost of AEDs can lead to poor adherence to the prescribed regimen in older patients on fixed incomes.

NURSING PROCESS
The Patient With Epilepsy and Seizures

ASSESSMENT

The nurse elicits information about the patient's seizure history. The patient is asked about the factors or events that may precipitate the seizures. Alcohol and substance use intake is documented. The nurse determines whether the patient has an aura before an epileptic seizure, which may indicate the origin of the seizure (e.g., seeing a flashing light may indicate that the seizure originated in the occipital lobe). Observation and assessment during and after a seizure assist in identifying the type of seizure and its management.

The effects of epilepsy on the patient's lifestyle are assessed. What limitations are imposed by the seizure disorder? Does the patient have a recreational program? Social contacts? Is the patient working, and is it a positive or a stressful experience? What coping mechanisms are used?

DIAGNOSIS

NURSING DIAGNOSES

Based on the assessment data, the patient's major nursing diagnoses may include the following:

- Risk for injury related to seizure activity
- Fear related to the possibility of seizures
- Ineffective individual coping related to stresses imposed by epilepsy
- Deficient knowledge related to epilepsy and its control

COLLABORATIVE PROBLEMS/POTENTIAL COMPLICATIONS

The major potential complications for patients with epilepsy are status epilepticus and medication side effects (toxicity).

PLANNING AND GOALS

Goals for the patient may include prevention of injury, control of seizures, achievement of a satisfactory psychosocial adjustment, acquisition of knowledge and understanding about the condition, and absence of complications.

NURSING INTERVENTIONS

PREVENTING INJURY

Injury prevention for the patient with seizures is a priority. If the type of seizure the patient is having places them at risk for injury, the patient should be lowered gently to the floor (if not in bed), and any potentially harmful items nearby (e.g., furniture, eyeglasses) should be removed. The patient should never be restrained or forced into a position, nor should anyone attempt to insert anything into the patient's mouth once a seizure has begun, as protecting the airway is a priority. Place a pillow under the patient's head to cushion it. Patients for whom seizure precautions are instituted should have the bed in the lowest position and side rails raised when in bed.

Pearls for Practice

Since 50% of deaths associated with epilepsy are accidental (drowning, trauma, burns, choking), the nurse reviews safety issues with the patient, such as never swimming alone, taking showers rather than baths, and avoiding activities that could cause harm if the patient were to have a seizure.

REDUCING FEAR OF SEIZURES

Fear that a seizure may occur unexpectedly can be reduced by the patient's adherence to the prescribed treatment regimen. Cooperation of the patient and family and their trust in the prescribed regimen are essential for control of seizures. The nurse emphasizes that the prescribed AED must be taken on a continuing basis and that drug dependence or addiction does not occur. Periodic monitoring is necessary to ensure the adequacy of the treatment regimen, to prevent side effects, and to monitor for drug resistance.

In an effort to control seizures, factors that may precipitate them are identified, such as emotional disturbances, new environmental stressors, onset of menstruation in female patients, hypoglycemia, or fever. Online programs, such as SeizureTracker.com and "My Seizure Event Diary," are available for patients to document their seizure activity. The patient is encouraged to follow a regular and moderate routine in lifestyle, diet (avoiding excessive stimulants), exercise, and rest (sleep deprivation may lower the seizure threshold). Moderate activity is therapeutic, but excessive exercise should be avoided. An additional dietary intervention, referred to as the *ketogenic diet,* has been suggested for control of seizures in some patients. This diet is high fat and protein and low carbohydrate. Effects of this diet are seen quickly. Because of the high-fat component of this diet and limited replacement of essential nutrients, compliance with this diet is difficult (Zarnowska, 2020).

Photic stimulation (bright flickering lights, television viewing) may precipitate seizures; wearing dark glasses or covering one eye may be preventive. Tension states (anxiety, frustration) induce seizures in some patients. Classes in stress management may be of value. Because seizures are known to occur with alcohol intake, alcoholic beverages should be avoided.

IMPROVING COPING MECHANISMS

The social, psychological, and behavioral problems that frequently accompany epilepsy can be more of a disability than the actual seizures. Epilepsy may be accompanied by feelings of stigmatization, alienation, depression, and uncertainty. The patient must cope with the constant fear of a seizure and the psychological consequences. Adults face potential issues such as the burden of finding employment, restrictions on the ability to drive, concerns about relationships and childbearing, insurance problems, and legal barriers. Alcohol use disorder may complicate matters. Family reactions may vary from outright rejection of the person with epilepsy to overprotection. As a result, many people with epilepsy are at risk for psychological and behavioral problems.

Pearls for Practice

Patients with epilepsy have a depression incidence that is nearly five times higher than that of the general population as well as a higher suicide rate (England & Plueger, 2020). Thus, all patients with epilepsy should be screened for depression.

Counseling assists the patient and family to understand the condition and the limitations it imposes. Social and recreational opportunities are necessary for good mental health. Nurses can improve the quality of life for patients with epilepsy by teaching them and their families about symptoms and their management.

PROVIDING PATIENT AND FAMILY EDUCATION

Perhaps the most valuable facets of care contributed by the nurse to the person with epilepsy are education and efforts to modify the attitudes of the patient and family toward the disorder. The person who experiences seizures may consider every seizure a potential source of humiliation and shame. This may result in anxiety, depression, hostility, and secrecy on the part of the patient and family. Ongoing education and encouragement should be given to patients to enable them to overcome these reactions. The patient with epilepsy should carry an emergency medical identification card or wear a medical information bracelet. The patient and family need to be educated about medications as well as care during a seizure.

MONITORING AND MANAGING POTENTIAL COMPLICATIONS

Status epilepticus, the major complication, was described previously. Another complication is the toxicity of AEDs. The patient and family are instructed about side effects and are given specific guidelines to assess and report signs and symptoms that indicate medication toxicity. Many AEDs require careful monitoring for therapeutic levels. The patient should plan to have serum drug levels assessed at regular intervals. Many known drug interactions occur with AEDs. A complete pharmacologic profile should be reviewed with the patient to avoid interactions that either potentiate or inhibit the effectiveness of the medications.

EVALUATION

EXPECTED PATIENT OUTCOMES

Expected patient outcomes may include the following:

1. Sustains no injury during seizure activity:
   a. Complies with treatment regimen and identifies the hazards of stopping the medication
   b. Patient and family can identify appropriate care during seizure.
2. Indicates a decrease in fear

(*continued on page 1448*)

3. Displays effective individual coping
4. Exhibits knowledge and understanding of epilepsy:
   a. Identifies the side effects of AEDs
   b. Avoids factors or situations that may precipitate seizures (e.g., flickering lights, hyperventilation, alcohol)
   c. Follows a healthy lifestyle by getting adequate sleep and eating meals at regular times to avoid hypoglycemia
5. Absence of complications

INFECTIOUS NEUROLOGIC DISORDERS

Meningitis

Meningitis is an inflammation of the meninges, which are the protective membranes covering the brain and spinal cord. Bacterial or viral infections are the primary causes of meningitis, but it also can be caused by a fungus or parasite. Because of this inflammation close to the brain and spinal cord, meningitis can be life threatening.

Bacterial Meningitis

Bacterial meningitis is caused by bacteria; commonly, *Streptococcus pneumoniae* and *Neisseria meningitidis* (meningococcus) are infecting organisms. *Haemophilus influenzae* was once a common cause of meningitis in children, but because of vaccination, infection with this organism is now rare in the United States. However, it is still a concern for those not immunized for *H. influenzae.* Outbreaks of *N. meningitidis* infection are most likely to occur in dense community groups, such as college campuses and military installations. Although infections occur year-round, incidence of outbreaks is reduced in the summer (VanDemark, 2020). Factors that increase the risk for bacterial meningitis include tobacco use and viral upper respiratory infection because they increase the amount of droplet production. Otitis media and mastoiditis increase the risk for bacterial meningitis because the bacteria can cross the epithelial membrane and enter the subarachnoid space. Patients who are immunosuppressed are at risk for the development of bacterial meningitis (organ transplant, diabetes, cancer, asplenia [spleen removed], chronic steroid therapy, HIV infection, malnutrition, etc.), as well as patients who are very young (less than 2 months of age) and the older population. A study by Sunwoo et al. (2021) found that patients admitted with acute bacterial meningitis in the intensive care unit with low Glasgow Coma Scale scores, old age, and neurologic complications were at high risk for unfavorable outcomes.

Pathophysiology

The brain is protected by the skull, meninges, and the blood–brain barrier. Any violation to these defenses by a pathogen can result in meningitis. Meningeal infections generally originate in one of two ways: through the bloodstream as a consequence of other infections of the heart, lung, or viscera; or by direct spread, such as might occur after a traumatic injury to the facial bones, infection in the skull or spine, sinusitis, otitis, brain abscess, or secondary to invasive procedures, such as lumbar puncture or ventricular shunting procedures.

Pearls for Practice

Given the risk of bacterial meningitis in patients with traumatic injuries, prophylactic antibiotics are administered to patients who present with cerebrospinal fluid (CSF) escaping from the ears (CSF otorrhea) and the nose (CSF rhinorrhea) as is seen in basal skull fractures, dural tears, and compound skull fractures.

Once the causative organism enters the bloodstream, it crosses the blood–brain barrier and proliferates in the CSF. The host immune response disrupts the cellular integrity of the microorganism and the breakdown products (cell wall fragments and lipopolysaccharides [LPS]), which enhances the inflammatory response in the involved meninges. Part of this response is the recruitment of neutrophils to the inflammatory site, resulting in thickening (an increase in viscosity) of the CSF. Because the cranial vault contains little room for expansion, the inflammation may cause increased intracranial pressure (ICP). CSF circulates through the subarachnoid space, where inflammatory cellular materials from the affected meningeal tissue enter and accumulate. The thickened CSF can interfere with CSF absorption, resulting in hydrocephalus. CSF studies demonstrate decreased glucose, increased protein levels, and increased white blood cell count (Fiske & Bloch, 2019).

The prognosis for bacterial meningitis depends on the causative organism, the severity of the infection and illness, and the timeliness of treatment. Acute fulminant presentation may include adrenal damage, circulatory collapse, and widespread hemorrhages (Waterhouse–Friderichsen syndrome). This syndrome is the result of endothelial damage and vascular necrosis caused by the bacteria. Complications include visual impairment, deafness, seizures, paralysis, hydrocephalus, and septic shock.

Clinical Manifestations and Assessment

Headache and fever are frequently the initial symptoms. Fever tends to remain high throughout the course of the illness. An altered level of consciousness (LOC) is frequently seen; however, one third of patients present with normal mentation (Fiske & Bloch, 2019). Meningeal irritation results in a number of other well-recognized signs common to all types of meningitis:

- *Nuchal rigidity (stiff neck):* This is an early sign seen in 30% to 70% of patients (Fiske & Bloch, 2019). Any attempts at flexion of the head are difficult because of

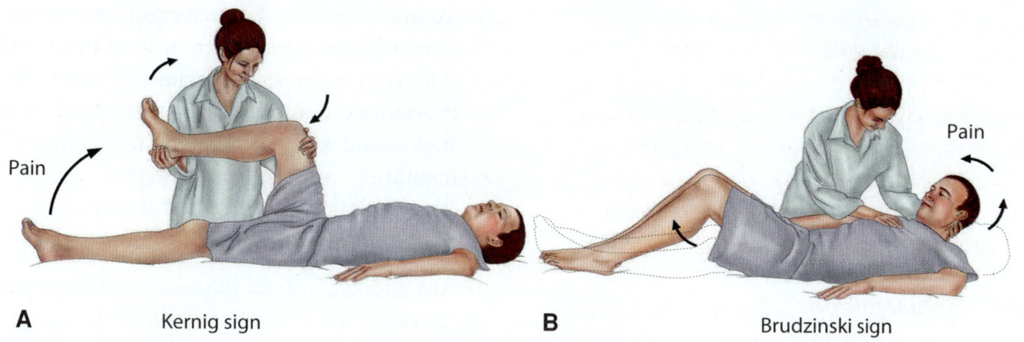

FIGURE 45-1 Testing for meningeal irritation. A. Kernig sign. B. Brudzinski sign.

spasms in the muscles of the neck. With the patient in supine position, the head is gently flexed forward and assessed for rigidity.

- *Positive Kernig sign:* When the patient is lying supine with the hip flexed to a 90-degree angle, resistance to passive extension of the knee is a positive Kernig sign (Fig. 45-1A). This pain is caused by inflammation of the meninges and spinal roots.
- *Positive Brudzinski sign:* When the patient's neck is flexed (after ruling out cervical trauma or injury), flexion of the knees and hips is produced; when the lower extremity of one side is passively flexed, a similar movement is seen in the opposite extremity (see Fig. 45-1B). This sign is caused by exudate that is irritating the root of the lumbar region (VanDemark, 2020).
- *Photophobia (extreme sensitivity to light):* This finding is common, although the cause is unclear.

Pearls for Practice

The classic triad of symptoms of bacterial meningitis is stiff neck/nuchal rigidity, altered LOC, and fever, although all these symptoms are not found routinely. However, 95% of patients with bacterial meningitis suffer from two of the following four symptoms: headache, fever, stiff neck/nuchal rigidity, and altered LOC.

A rash can be a striking feature of *N. meningitidis* infection, occurring in about half of patients with this type of meningitis. Skin lesions develop, ranging from a petechial rash with purpuric lesions to large areas of ecchymosis.

Disorientation and memory impairment are common early in the course of the illness. The changes depend on the severity of the infection and on individual response to the physiologic processes. As the illness progresses, lethargy, unresponsiveness, and coma may develop. Within the first week, seizures occur in 40% to 50% of patients with bacterial meningitis (VanDemark, 2020).

ICP increases secondary to the accumulation of purulent exudate and cerebral edema. The initial signs of increased ICP include decreased LOC and focal motor deficits. Vomiting is a frequent finding associated with rising ICP. If ICP is not controlled, the uncus of the temporal lobe may herniate through the tentorium, causing pressure on the brainstem. Brainstem herniation is a life-threatening event that causes cranial nerve dysfunction and depresses the centers of vital functions, such as the medulla. Refer to Chapter 44 to review vital sign changes termed *Cushing response*. An acute fulminant infection can occur in patients with meningococcal meningitis, producing signs of overwhelming septicemia: an abrupt onset of high fever, extensive purpuric lesions (over the face and extremities), shock, and signs of disseminated intravascular coagulopathy (DIC). Refer to Chapter 19 for details of DIC. Some patients develop hyponatremia or syndrome of inappropriate antidiuretic hormone (SIADH, refer to Chapter 30). Death may occur within a few hours after onset of the infection.

Pearls for Practice

The nurse recognizes that with fever, tachycardia (increased heart rate) and tachypnea (increased respiratory rate [RR]) are expected. If bradycardia and decreased RR are seen, the nurse should consider ICP as an etiology for the decreased HR and RR.

If the clinical presentation suggests meningitis, diagnostic testing is conducted to identify the causative organism. Bacterial culture and Gram staining of CSF and blood are the "gold standard" for definitive diagnosis. These cultures should be obtained immediately when there is a suspicion of bacterial meningitis (Fischbach et al., 2021). CT scanning is useful for detection of abscesses and lesions that may have provided a route for the bacteria.

Medical and Nursing Management

Successful outcomes depend on the early administration of antibiotics that cross the blood–brain barrier into the subarachnoid space in sufficient concentration to halt the multiplication of bacteria. Penicillin antibiotics (e.g., ampicillin, piperacillin) or one of the cephalosporins (e.g., ceftriaxone sodium, cefotaxime sodium) may be used. Vancomycin hydrochloride alone or in combination with rifampin may be used if resistant strains of bacteria are identified. High doses of the appropriate antibiotic are administered IV.

Pearls for Practice

The nurse understands the difference between empiric antimicrobial therapy versus culture-documented therapy. Empiric therapy refers to selection of an antibiotic based upon the "most likely" suspected organism, while considering variables such as the patient's age, predisposing conditions, geographical region, etc. Empiric therapy is initiated immediately after collecting the culture specimens. Premature initiation of antimicrobial therapy before cultures are obtained can suppress bacterial growth and impede the diagnosis. While culture-documented therapy will detail this patient's organism and specific sensitivities and/or resistance to certain antibiotics, there is a lapse of 24 to 72 hours before culture results are returned.

The use of dexamethasone as an adjunct therapy in the treatment of acute bacterial meningitis and in pneumococcal meningitis, if administered before the first dose of antibiotic, has been considered. However, recent results of a meta-analysis did not demonstrate significant reduction in death or neurologic disability in patients with steroid use (Rayanakorn et al., 2020).

Dehydration and shock are treated with fluid volume expanders. Seizures, which may occur early in the course of the disease, are controlled with phenytoin. Some providers may prophylactically use anticonvulsants and histamine-2-receptor antagonists or proton pump inhibitors (PPIs) to prevent GI bleeding. Increased ICP is treated as necessary (see Chapter 44).

The patient with bacterial meningitis is critically ill; therefore, many of the nursing interventions are collaborative with the health care provider, respiratory therapist, and other members of the health care team. The patient's safety and well-being depend on sound nursing judgment.

Neurologic status and vital signs are continually assessed. Pulse oximetry and arterial blood gas (ABG) values are used to quickly identify the need for respiratory support if increasing ICP compromises the patient's LOC. Insertion of a cuffed endotracheal tube (or tracheotomy) and mechanical ventilation may be necessary to maintain adequate tissue oxygenation.

Blood pressure should be monitored to assess for incipient shock, which precedes cardiac or respiratory failure. Rapid IV fluid replacement may be prescribed, but care is taken to prevent fluid overload. Fever also increases the workload of the heart and cerebral metabolism. ICP will increase in response to increased cerebral metabolic demands. Therefore, measures are taken to reduce body temperature as quickly as possible.

Other important components of nursing care include the following measures:

- Protecting the patient from injury secondary to seizure activity or altered LOC.
- Monitoring daily body weight; serum electrolytes; and urine volume, specific gravity, and osmolality, especially if SIADH is suspected (refer to Chapter 30).
- Preventing complications associated with immobility, such as pressure ulcers and pneumonia.
- Instituting infection control precautions until 24 hours after initiation of antibiotic therapy (oral and nasal discharge is considered infectious).

Any sudden, critical illness can be devastating to the family. Because the patient's condition is often critical and the prognosis guarded, the family needs to be informed about the patient's condition. Periodic family visits are essential to facilitate coping of the patient and family. An important aspect of the nurse's role is to support the family and assist them in identifying others who can be supportive of them during the crisis.

Pearls for Practice

Since bacterial meningitis is a contagious disease, isolation precautions must be instituted and will depend on the organism and patient status.

Viral Meningitis

Pathophysiology

Viral meningitis, also known as acute aseptic meningitis or acute benign lymphocytic meningitis, is more common than bacterial meningitis. The most common causes are enteroviruses (coxsackievirus, poliovirus, and echovirus). Patients with HIV can present with acute aseptic meningitis. In most cases no specific organism is identified. Children are most often affected, but all age groups can be affected.

Clinical Manifestations and Assessment

Viral meningitis usually starts with a headache, low-grade fever, stiff neck, photophobia, malaise, and symptoms of an upper respiratory viral illness, similar to bacterial meningitis. However, altered mental status and seizure activity are not associated with this disorder. Assess patient for a recent systemic viral infection. Patient may receive a CT scan to look for increased ICP. A lumbar puncture should be performed, and the CSF will be clear; results will show increased protein and WBC count as well as normal glucose level but will be free of any bacterial organism.

Medical and Nursing Management

Viral meningitis is managed based on the patient's symptoms and supportive nursing care. Patients may need to be hospitalized because of their discomfort and severe vomiting. Supportive care can include bed rest with head of bed (HOB) elevated 30 degrees and the patient's head in neutral alignment (improves venous drainage), a dark quiet environment, fever management, monitoring fluid intake, and pain management. Recovery should occur within 10 days.

ENCEPHALITIS

Encephalitis is an acute inflammatory process of the brain tissue (cerebral cortex) secondary to viruses, bacteria, fungi, or parasites. Viruses are the most common cause of encephalitis in the United States, and herpes simplex virus (HSV) is the most common of these. There are two types of HSV: HSV-1 and HSV-2 (VanDemark, 2020). HSV-1 typically affects children and adults. HSV-2 most commonly affects neonates whose birthing parent was infected during pregnancy (Cole, 2020).

Herpes Simplex Encephalitis

Pathophysiology

HSV-1 causes encephalitis by following a retrograde intraneuronal path to the brain. The olfactory and trigeminal nerves are the paths most commonly involved. A latent virus in brain tissue may reactivate and result in encephalitis. The invading organism causes cerebral edema and petechial hemorrhages of the brain and can directly invade the brain, damaging neurons (VanDemark, 2020).

Clinical Manifestations and Assessment

Initial symptoms include fever, headache, stiff neck, and confusion. Focal neurologic symptoms reflect the areas of cerebral inflammation and necrosis and include behavioral changes, focal seizures, dysphasia, hemiparesis, and altered LOC. Patients may also have auditory and visual hallucinations (VanDemark, 2020).

Neuroimaging studies, EEG, and CSF examination are used to diagnose HSV encephalitis. The EEG demonstrates periodic high-voltage spikes originating in the temporal lobe, and MRI may reveal temporal lobe edema. Lumbar puncture often reveals a high opening pressure and low-glucose and high-protein levels in CSF samples. Viral cultures are almost always negative. The polymerase chain reaction (PCR) is the standard test for early diagnosis of HSV-1 encephalitis. The validity of PCR is very high between the third and tenth days after symptom onset.

Medical and Nursing Management

Acyclovir, an antiviral agent, is the medication of choice in the treatment of HSV. Studies have indicated that early administration of acyclovir improves the prognosis associated with HSV-1 encephalitis and reduces a mortality rate of 60% to 70% down to 30% if treatment is initiated before the onset of coma (VanDemark, 2020). To prevent relapse, treatment should continue for up to 3 weeks. Slow IV administration over at least 1 hour, along with adequate hydration, may prevent crystallization of the medication in the renal tubules, which would be reflected by a rising serum creatinine and blood urea nitrogen (BUN). Assessment of neurologic function is key to monitoring the progression of disease. Comfort measures to reduce headache include dimming the lights, limiting noise, and administering analgesic agents. Opioid analgesic medications may mask neurologic symptoms; therefore, they are used cautiously. Focal seizures and altered LOC require care directed at injury prevention and safety. Nursing care addressing patient and family anxieties is ongoing throughout the illness. Monitoring of blood chemistry test results and hourly urinary output will alert the nurse to the presence of renal complications related to acyclovir therapy.

Arboviral Encephalitis

Arthropod vectors transmit several types of viruses that cause encephalitis. The primary vector in North America is the mosquito. In cases of West Nile virus, humans are the secondary host; birds are the primary host (refer to Fig. 45-2). Arbovirus infection (transmitted by arthropod vectors) occurs in specific geographic areas during the summer or early fall when the vectors are most active. West Nile virus, the most common type of arboviral encephalitis, was first observed in New York City in 1999 (Mukerjl et al., 2021). Older people are primarily affected (Mukerjl et al., 2021). The St. Louis arbovirus is seen in the western United States, and older people are affected more frequently.

Pathophysiology

Viral replication occurs at the site of the mosquito bite. The host immune response attempts to control viral replication. If the immune response is inadequate, viremia will ensue. The virus gains access to the CNS via the cerebral capillaries, resulting in encephalitis. It spreads from neuron to neuron, predominantly affecting the cortical gray matter, the brainstem, and the thalamus. Meningeal exudates compound the clinical presentation by irritating the meninges and increasing ICP.

Clinical Manifestations and Assessment

Arboviral encephalitis begins with early flu-like symptoms, but specific neurologic manifestations depend on the viral type. After a brief febrile prodrome, neurologic symptoms will reflect the area of the brain that is involved. For example, if meninges are involved, patients can present with nuchal rigidity and headache. A unique clinical feature of St. Louis encephalitis is the development of SIADH with hyponatremia in 25% to 33% of affected patients (Mukerjl et al., 2021). (SIADH is detailed in Chapter 30.) Signs and symptoms specific to West Nile encephalitis include a maculopapular or morbilliform rash (erythematous [red] rash resembling that of measles consisting of macules and papules [or maculopapular]) on the neck, trunk, arms, and legs, and flaccid paralysis. Both West Nile and St. Louis encephalitis can result in parkinsonian-like movements, reflecting inflammation of the basal ganglia.

Neuroimaging and CSF evaluation are useful in the diagnosis of arboviral encephalitis. MRI demonstrates inflammation of the basal ganglia in cases of St. Louis encephalitis

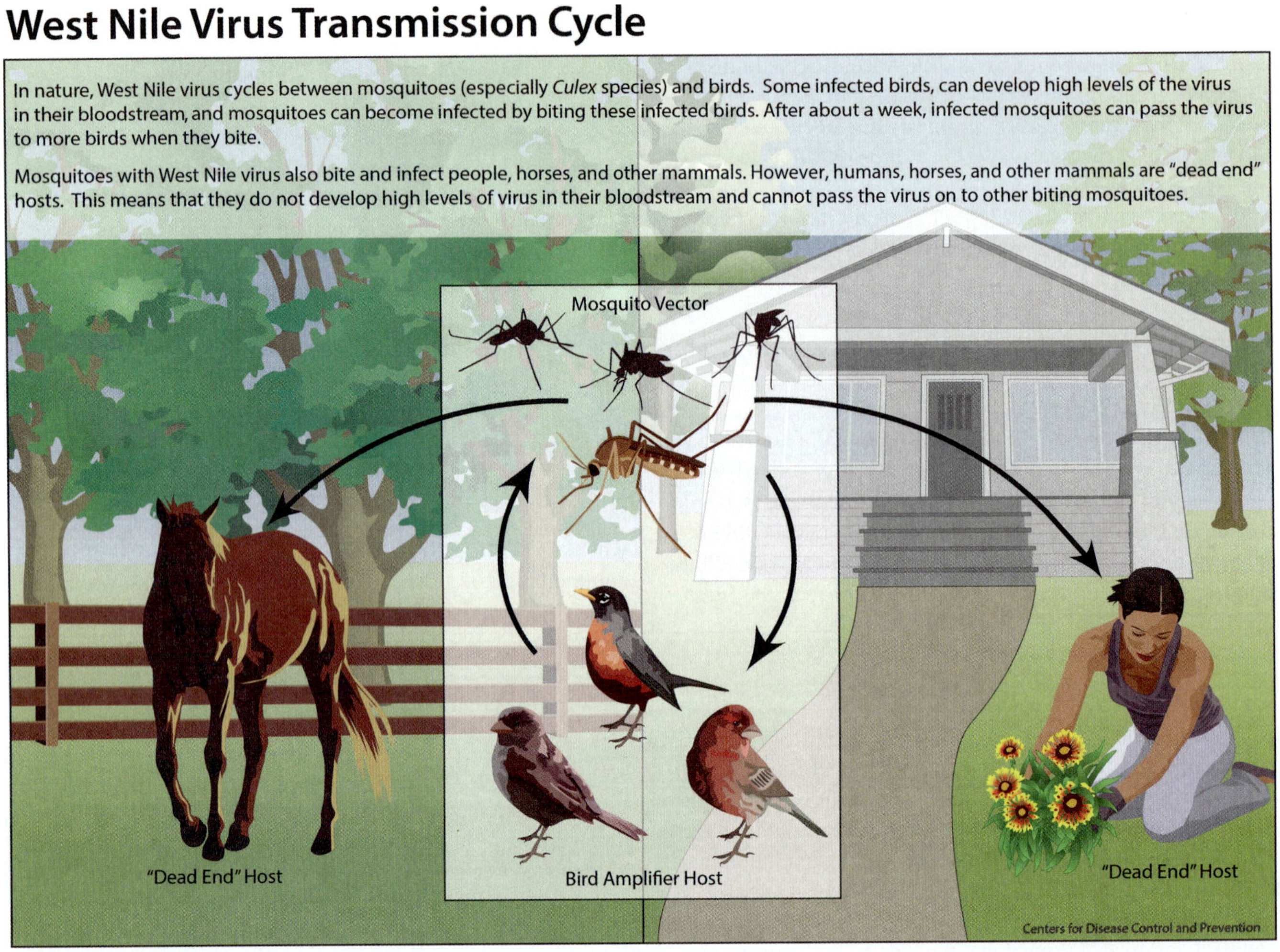

FIGURE 45-2 West Nile transmission cycle. (Used with permission from the Centers for Disease Control and Prevention. [2021]. West Nile virus: Transmission. https://www.cdc.gov/westnile/transmission/index.html)

and inflammation in the periventricular area in cases of West Nile encephalitis. Immunoglobulin M antibodies to West Nile virus are observed in serum and CSF (Beckham et al., 2022). Serum cultures are not useful because the viremia is brief.

Medical and Nursing Management

No specific medication for arboviral encephalitis exists. Medical management is aimed at controlling the seizures and the increased ICP and supporting respiratory function. If the patient is very ill, hospitalization may be required. The nurse carefully assesses neurologic status and identifies improvement or deterioration in the patient's condition. Injury prevention is key in light of the potential for falls and seizures. Arboviral encephalitis may result in death or lifelong residual health issues, such as neurologic deficits and seizures. The family will need support and teaching to cope with these outcomes.

Public education addressing the prevention of arboviral encephalitis is a key nursing role. Clothing that provides coverage and applying Environmental Protection Agency (EPA)–approved insect repellents containing permethrin or another EPA-registered repellent to clothes will give extra protection. This should be used in high-risk areas to decrease mosquito and tick bites. Avoidance of outdoor activities and control of the mosquito vector are important for control of the disease. Screens should be in good repair in the home, and standing water, such as in birdbaths, should be removed or avoided. Blood donation centers screen all blood for West Nile virus. Cases of West Nile virus are reported to the Centers for Disease Control and Prevention (CDC). People must be warned not to handle a dead bird if found and to call the local health department for instructions on reporting and disposing of the body.

BELL PALSY

Bell palsy (facial paralysis) is caused by unilateral inflammation of the seventh cranial nerve, which results in weakness or paralysis of the facial muscles on the ipsilateral, or same side, of the affected facial nerve (Fig. 45-3).

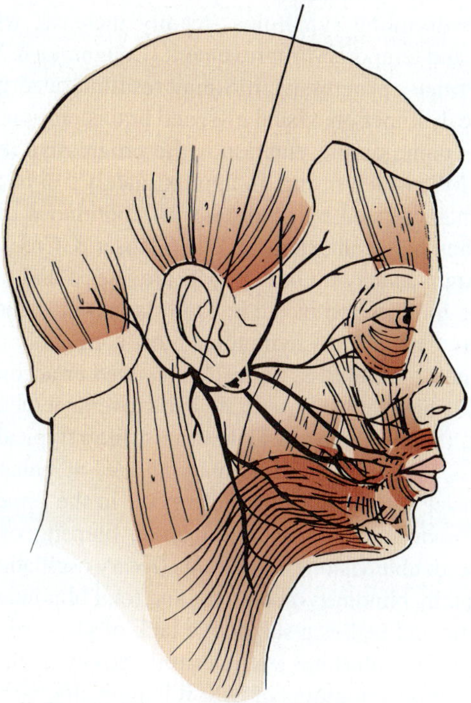

FIGURE 45-3 **Distribution of the facial nerve.**

Pathophysiology

Although the cause is unknown, theories about causes include vascular ischemia, viral disease (herpes simplex, herpes zoster), Lyme disease, autoimmune disease, or a combination of all of these factors. Bell palsy may be a type of pressure paralysis. The inflamed, edematous nerve becomes compressed to the point of damage, or its blood supply is occluded, producing ischemic necrosis of the nerve.

Clinical Manifestations and Assessment

The face is distorted from paralysis of the facial muscles; there are increased lacrimation (tearing) and painful sensations in the face, behind the ear, and in the eye of the affected side. The ear pain may precede the paralysis by 24 to 48 hours. The patient may experience speech difficulties and may be unable to eat on the affected side because of weakness or paralysis of the facial muscles. A disturbance of taste is a common finding. When asking the patient to show their teeth and smile, weakness of the involved nerve will be noted, there will be an absence of wrinkling on the forehead; the affected side will appear mask-like.

Medical and Nursing Management

Corticosteroid therapy (prednisone) may be prescribed to reduce inflammation and edema; this reduces vascular compression and permits restoration of blood circulation to the nerve. Early administration of corticosteroid therapy appears to diminish the severity of the disease, relieve the pain, and prevent or minimize denervation (Pugh, 2022).

Facial pain is controlled with analgesic agents. Heat may be applied to the involved side of the face to promote comfort and blood flow through the muscles. Electrical stimulation may be applied to the face to prevent muscle atrophy.

While the paralysis lasts, nursing care involves protection of the eye from injury. Frequently, the eye does not close completely and the blink reflex is diminished, so the eye is vulnerable to injury from dust and foreign particles. Corneal irritation, corneal abrasion, and ulceration may occur. Distortion of the lower lid alters the proper drainage of tears. To prevent injury, the eye may be covered with a protective shield at night. The eye patch may abrade the cornea, however, because there is some difficulty in keeping the partially paralyzed eyelids closed. Eye ointment may be applied at bedtime to promote adherence of the eyelids to prevent injury during sleep. Artificial tears are typically instilled to maintain eye lubrication. The patient can be taught to close the paralyzed eyelid manually before going to sleep. Wraparound sunglasses or goggles may be worn during the day to decrease normal evaporation from the eye.

NEURODEGENERATIVE AND NEUROMUSCULAR DISORDERS

MULTIPLE SCLEROSIS

Multiple sclerosis (MS), the leading cause of nontraumatic disability in young adults, is an immune-mediated, progressive demyelinating disease of the CNS. *Demyelination* refers to the destruction of myelin, the fatty and proteinaceous material that surrounds certain nerve fibers in the brain and spinal cord; it results in impaired transmission of nerve impulses (Fig. 45-4). MS may occur at any age but typically manifests in young adults between the ages of 20 and 40 years; it affects females more frequently than males and rarely affects those over 60 years (Longbrake & Wesley, 2021).

The etiology of MS is unknown and may result from complex interactions between environmental factors and genetically susceptible individuals that trigger an abnormal immune response that damages the myelin sheath, oligodendrocytes, axons, and neurons (Longbrake & Wesley, 2021). Evidence for a genetic predisposition is seen in an increased risk for White people of northern European ancestry and a decreased risk in others (e.g., Native Americans) (Longbrake & Wesley, 2021). Researchers found that some environmental exposure (i.e., biomarker of Epstein–Barr virus, infectious mononucleosis, smoking) may play a role in the development of MS (Waubant et al., 2019).

Pathophysiology

Sensitized T cells typically cross the blood–brain barrier; their function is to check the CNS for antigens and then

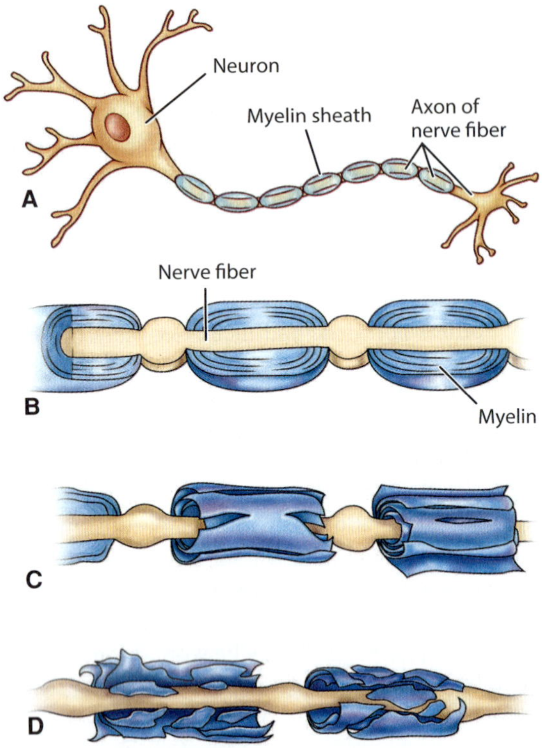

FIGURE 45-4 The process of demyelination. (A) and (B) depict a normal nerve cell and axon with myelin. (C) and (D) show the slow disintegration of myelin, resulting in a disruption in axon function.

leave. B cells and monocytes are also activated; B cells secrete antibodies against myelin. In MS, the sensitized T cells remain in the CNS and promote the infiltration of other agents that damage the immune system. The immune system attack leads to inflammation that damages myelin (which normally insulates the axon and speeds the conduction of impulses along the axon) and the oligodendroglial cells that produce myelin in the CNS.

Demyelination interrupts the flow of nerve impulses and results in a variety of manifestations, depending on the nerves affected. Plaques appear on demyelinated axons, further interrupting the transmission of impulses. Demyelinated axons are scattered irregularly throughout the CNS. The areas most frequently affected are the optic nerves, chiasm, and tracts; the cerebrum; the brainstem and cerebellum; and the spinal cord. Eventually, the axons themselves begin to degenerate, resulting in permanent and irreversible damage (Longbrake & Wesley, 2021).

Clinical Manifestations and Assessment

The course of MS may assume many different patterns (Fig. 45-5). Between 85% and 90% of patients with MS have a relapsing-remitting (RR) course. With each relapse, recovery is usually complete; however, residual deficits may occur and accumulate over time, contributing to functional decline. Approximately 40% of those with the RR course of MS progress to a secondary progressive course, in which disease progression occurs with or without relapses. About 10% to 15% of patients have a primary progressive course, in which disabling symptoms steadily increase, with rare plateaus and temporary improvement (Longbrake & Wesley, 2021). Primary progressive MS may result in quadriparesis, cognitive dysfunction, visual loss, and brainstem syndromes. The least common presentation is the progressive relapsing form of MS, which occurs in approximately 5% of patients and is characterized by relapses with continuous disabling progression between exacerbations (Hauser & Cree, 2021).

The signs and symptoms of MS are varied and multiple, reflecting the location of the lesion (plaque) or combination of lesions. The primary symptoms most commonly reported are unilateral visual loss, typically preceded or accompanied by orbital pain that increases with eye movement (acute optic neuritis), fatigue, depression, weakness, limb (typically legs) numbness, difficulty in coordination, loss of balance, and pain. Visual disturbances due to lesions in the optic nerves or their connections may also include blurring of vision, **diplopia** (double vision), nystagmus (rotary oscillation of the eyes), patchy blindness (scotoma), and total blindness.

Fatigue, defined as a subjective lack of physical or mental energy that interferes with desired activity, is one of the more common symptoms of MS; it is typically worse in the

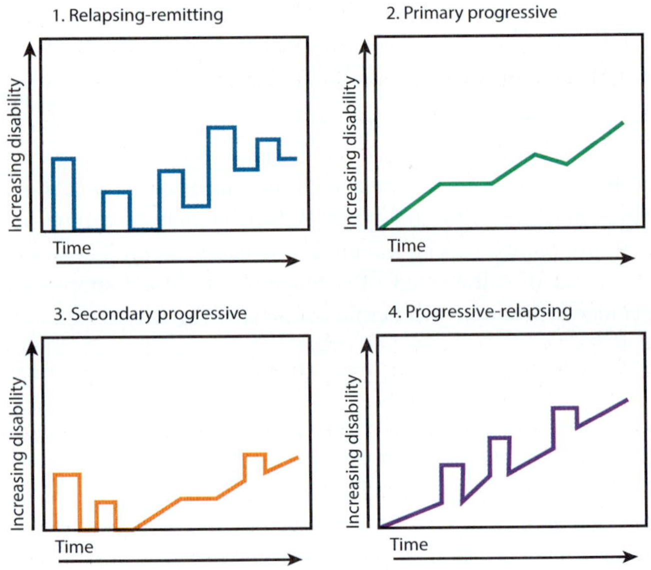

FIGURE 45-5 Types and courses of multiple sclerosis (MS). 1. Relapsing-remitting (RR) MS is characterized by clearly acute attacks with full recovery or with sequelae and residual deficit upon recovery. Periods between disease relapses are characterized by lack of disease progression. 2. Primary progressive (PP) MS is characterized by disease showing progression of disability from onset, without plateaus and temporary minor improvements. 3. Secondary progress (SP) MS begins with an initial RR course, followed by progression of variable rate, which may also include occasional relapses and minor remissions. 4. Progressive-relapsing (PR) MS shows progression from onset but with clear acute relapses with or without recovery. (From Lublin, F. D., & Reingold, S. C. [1996]. Defining the clinical course of multiple sclerosis: Results of an international survey. *Neurology*, *46*[64], 907–911. Used with permission from Lippincott Williams & Wilkins.)

afternoon hours. Depression, heat, anemia, deconditioning, and medication may contribute to fatigue. The etiology of MS-related fatigue is poorly understood; there appears to be no association between fatigue and disease course (Longbrake & Wesley, 2021).

Like fatigue, pain is a symptom that can contribute to social isolation. Approximately 70% of patients with MS report pain at some point (Longbrake & Wesley, 2021). Lesions on the sensory pathways cause pain. Lhermitte sign is described as an electrical sensation that is felt down the arms, back, or lower trunk when the patient flexes the neck. It is theorized this acute pain sensation is related to sclerotic plaques on the dorsal nerve roots (Pagnotta, 2020). Many people with MS need daily analgesics. In some cases, pain is managed with opioids, antiseizure medication, or antidepressants. Rarely, surgery may be needed to interrupt pain pathways.

Additional sensory manifestations include paresthesias (abnormal skin sensations, such as tingling, itching, or burning), dysesthesias (unpleasant, abnormal sense of touch), and loss of proprioception (ability to sense the position, location, orientation, and movement of the body and its parts). An objective sensory loss (position, vibration, shape, texture) is noted in 50% of patients with MS (Pagnotta, 2020). Among perimenopausal people, those with MS are more likely to have pain related to osteoporosis. In addition to estrogen loss, immobility and corticosteroid therapy play a role in the development of osteoporosis among females with MS. Bone mineral density (BMD) testing is recommended for this high-risk group (refer to Chapter 39). Diagnosis and treatment of osteoporosis are discussed in Chapter 40.

Spasticity (muscle hypertonicity) of the extremities (usually the legs) and loss of the abdominal reflexes result from involvement of the main motor pathways (pyramidal tracts) of the spinal cord. The spasticity often occurs with painful spasms, which interfere with mobility, sleep, and activities of daily living (ADLs). Gait abnormalities are common and are usually a result of ataxia, weakness, or spasticity. Disruption of the sensory axons may produce sensory dysfunction (paresthesias, pain). Cognitive and psychosocial problems may reflect frontal or parietal lobe involvement. Some degree of cognitive impairment (e.g., memory loss, decreased concentration) occurs in about 65% of patients, but severe cognitive changes with dementia (progressive organic mental disorder) are rare.

Involvement of the cerebellum or basal ganglia can produce **ataxia** (impaired coordination of movements) and tremor. Loss of the control connections between the cortex and the basal ganglia may occur and cause emotional lability and euphoria. Bladder, bowel, and sexual dysfunctions are common. Bladder dysfunction (urinary urgency, frequency, nocturia, and urge incontinence) affects approximately 75% of patients, and in approximately 15% of these, symptoms can be severe enough to socially isolate the patient (Longbrake & Wesley, 2021).

Secondary complications of MS include urinary tract infections, constipation, pressure ulcers, contracture deformities, dependent pedal edema, pneumonia, reactive depression, and decreased bone density. Emotional, social, marital, economic, and vocational problems may also be a consequence of the disease.

Exacerbations and remissions are characteristic of MS. During exacerbations, new symptoms appear and existing ones worsen; during remissions, symptoms decrease or disappear. Fifteen years after onset, only 20% of patients have no functional limitation (Hauser & Cree, 2021). Precipitation of symptoms may occur with the following events: periods of emotional and physical stress; cold or humid, hot weather; hot baths; overheating; fever; fatigue; and pregnancy (Pagnotta, 2020). There is no single test for the diagnosis of MS. Diagnosis is established based upon clinical examination, results from MRI ("bright spots" of demyelinated lesions or plaques are easily seen in white matter) and evoked potential studies (EPS), and examination of CSF. Approximately 95% of MS patients' MRI studies reveal abnormalities. Electrophoresis of CSF identifies the presence of oligoclonal banding. EPS can help define the extent of the disease process and monitor changes.

Medical and Nursing Management

No cure exists for MS. The goals of treatment are to treat acute exacerbations, delay the progression of the disease, and manage chronic symptoms. Many patients with MS have a stable disease course and require only intermittent treatment, whereas others experience steady progression of their disease. Symptoms requiring intervention include spasticity, fatigue, bladder dysfunction, and ataxia. Management strategies target the various motor and sensory symptoms and effects of immobility that can occur. Smoking cessation is encouraged since it may increase the progression of disability (National Institute for Health and Care Excellence [NIHCE], 2019).

Disease-Modifying Therapies

The disease-modifying medications reduce the frequency of relapse, the duration of relapse, and the number and size of plaques observed on MRI. All of the medications require injection.

Interferon beta-1a and interferon beta-1b are administered subcutaneously (SQ), and another preparation of interferon beta-1a is administered intramuscularly (IM) once a week. Side effects of all the interferon beta medications include flu-like symptoms, which may be minimized by administration at bedtime and can be managed with acetaminophen and ibuprofen; these side effects may resolve after a few months. Additional side effects include injection site reaction (seen more frequently with IM preparations), thrombocytopenia, anemia, leukopenia, potential liver damage, fetal abnormalities, and depression. For optimal control of disability, disease-modifying medications should be started early in the course of the disease.

Pearls for Practice

MS does not affect fertility or carrying a pregnancy to term. Interestingly, patients with MS typically do not have relapses during pregnancy; however, there is a relapse incidence of 20% to 40% in the first 3 months after delivery. The relapse does not impact the risk of long-term disability. Research efforts on the effects of hormones and circulating protein on MS may shed light on the course of MS.

Glatiramer acetate reduces the rate of relapse in the RR course of MS. It decreases the number of plaques noted on MRI and increases the time between relapses. It is administered SQ daily and acts by increasing the antigen-specific suppressor T cells. Side effects and injection site reactions are rare. It is an option for those with an RR course; however, it may take 6 months for evidence of an immune response to appear.

Another therapy is the use of natalizumab, a humanized monoclonal antibody that blocks leukocyte migration into the CNS. It is administered intravenously (IV) and is usually well tolerated, with complaints of mild headaches and flushing during IV administration (Tafti et al., 2022). Ocrelizumab is another IV monoclonal antibody that may be used to treat primary progressive MS and relapsing forms of MS in adults.

IV methylprednisolone, the key agent in treating acute relapse in the RR course, shortens the duration of relapse. It exerts anti-inflammatory effects by acting on T cells and cytokines. One gram is administered IV daily for 3 to 5 days, with or without an oral taper of prednisone (Longbrake & Wesley, 2021). Side effects include mood swings, weight gain, and electrolyte imbalances.

Symptom Management

Medications are also prescribed for management of specific symptoms. Baclofen, a gamma-aminobutyric acid (GABA) agonist, is the medication of choice for treating spasticity. It can be administered orally or by intrathecal injection. Benzodiazepines, tizanidine, and dantrolene may also be used to treat spasticity. Patients with disabling spasms and contractures may require nerve blocks or surgical intervention. Fatigue that interferes with ADLs may be treated with amantadine, pemoline, or fluoxetine. Ataxia is a chronic problem most resistant to treatment. Medications used to treat ataxia include beta-adrenergic blockers, antiseizure agents, and benzodiazepines.

Bladder and bowel problems are often among the more difficult ones for patients, and a variety of medications (anticholinergics, alpha-adrenergic blockers, antispasmodic agents) may be prescribed. Nonpharmacologic strategies also assist in establishing effective bowel and bladder elimination (discussed shortly).

Urinary tract infection is often superimposed on the underlying neurologic dysfunction. Ascorbic acid (vitamin C) may be prescribed to acidify the urine, making bacterial growth less likely. Antibiotics are prescribed when appropriate.

Antidepressants may be prescribed since 25% to 50% of patients with MS are depressed, and the suicide rate is significantly higher than in the general population (Pagnotta, 2020).

An individualized program of physical therapy, rehabilitation, and education is combined with emotional support. An educational plan of care is developed to enable the person with MS to deal with the physiologic, social, and psychological problems that accompany chronic disease.

Promoting Physical Mobility

Relaxation and coordination exercises promote muscle efficiency. Progressive resistive exercises are used to strengthen weak muscles because diminishing muscle strength is often significant in MS.

Exercises. Walking improves the gait and particularly helps with the problem of the loss of the sense of position of the legs and feet. If certain muscle groups are irreversibly affected, other muscles can be trained to compensate. Instruction in the use of assistive devices may be needed to ensure their safe and correct use. Weighted canes, walkers, or limb bracelets may be of value.

Minimizing Spasticity and Contractures. Muscle spasticity is common and, in its later stages, is characterized by severe adductor spasm of the hips, with flexor spasm of the hips and knees. Without relief, fibrous contractures of these joints will occur. Warm packs may be beneficial, but hot baths should be avoided because of risk for burn injury secondary to sensory loss and increasing symptoms that may occur with elevation of the body temperature.

Daily exercises for muscle stretching are prescribed to minimize joint contractures. Special attention is given to the hamstrings, gastrocnemius muscles, hip adductors, biceps, and wrist and finger flexors. Muscle spasticity is common and interferes with normal function. A stretch–hold–relax routine is helpful for relaxing and treating muscle spasticity. Swimming and stationary bicycling are useful, and progressive weight bearing can relieve spasticity in the legs. The patient should not be hurried in any of these activities because this often increases spasticity.

Activity and Rest. The patient is encouraged to work and exercise to a point just short of fatigue. Very strenuous physical exercise is not advisable because it raises the body temperature and may aggravate symptoms. The patient is advised to take frequent short rest periods, preferably lying down. Extreme fatigue may contribute to the exacerbation of symptoms.

Minimizing Effects of Immobility. Because of the decrease in physical activity that often occurs with MS, complications associated with immobility, including pressure ulcers, muscle weakness, and accumulation of bronchial secretions, need to be considered and steps taken to prevent them. Measures to prevent such complications include assessing and maintaining skin integrity and having the patient perform coughing and deep-breathing exercises.

Preventing Injury

If motor dysfunction causes coordination problems and clumsiness, or if ataxia is apparent, the patient is at risk for falling. To overcome this disability, the patient is taught to walk with feet apart to widen the base of support and to increase walking stability. If the loss of sense of position occurs, the patient is taught to watch the feet while walking. Gait training may require assistive devices (walker, cane, braces, crutches, parallel bars) and instruction about their use by a physical therapist. If the gait remains inefficient, a wheelchair or motorized scooter may be the solution. The occupational therapist is a valuable resource in suggesting and securing aids to promote independence. The patient is trained in transfer and ADLs.

Because sensory loss may occur in addition to motor loss, pressure ulcers are a continuing threat to skin integrity. The need to use a wheelchair continuously increases the risk. See Chapter 51 for a discussion of the prevention and treatment of pressure ulcers.

Enhancing Bladder and Bowel Control

In general, bladder symptoms fall into the following categories: (1) inability to store urine (hyperreflexic, uninhibited); (2) inability to empty the bladder (hyporeflexic, hypotonic); and (3) a mixture of both types. The patient with urinary frequency, urgency, or incontinence requires special support. The sensation of the need to void must be heeded immediately so the bedpan or urinal should be readily available. A voiding time schedule is set up (every 1.5 to 2 hours initially, with gradual lengthening of the interval). The patient is instructed to drink a measured amount of fluid every 2 hours and then attempt to void 30 minutes after drinking. Use of a timer or wristwatch with an alarm may be helpful for the patient who does not have enough sensation to signal the need to empty the bladder. The nurse encourages the patient to take the prescribed medications to treat bladder spasticity because this allows greater independence. Intermittent self-catheterization has been successful in maintaining bladder control in patients with MS. If a female patient has permanent urinary incontinence, urinary diversion procedures may be considered. The male patient may wear a condom appliance for urine collection.

Bowel problems include constipation, fecal impaction, and incontinence. Adequate fluids, dietary fiber, and a bowel-training program are frequently effective in solving these problems.

Enhancing Communication and Managing Swallowing Difficulties

If the cranial nerves that control the mechanisms of speech and swallowing are affected, dysarthrias (defects of articulation) marked by slurring, low volume of speech, and difficulties in phonation may occur. **Dysphagia** (difficulty swallowing) may also occur. A speech therapist evaluates speech and swallowing and instructs the patient, family, and health team members about strategies to compensate for speech and swallowing problems. The nurse reinforces this instruction and encourages the patient and family to adhere to the plan. Impaired swallowing increases the patient's risk for aspiration; therefore, strategies are needed to reduce that risk. Such strategies include having a suction apparatus available, performing careful feeding, and ensuring proper positioning for eating. Refer to Chapters 8 and 9 for information related to aspiration.

Improving Sensory and Cognitive Function

Measures may be taken if visual defects or changes in cognitive status occur.

Vision. The cranial nerves affecting vision may be affected by MS. An eye patch or a covered eyeglass lens may be used to block the visual impulses of one eye if the patient has diplopia (double vision). Prism glasses may be helpful for patients who are confined to bed and have difficulty reading in the supine position. People who are unable to read regular-print materials are eligible for the free "talking book" services of the Library of Congress or may obtain large-print or audio books from local libraries.

Cognition and Emotional Responses. Cognitive impairment and emotional lability occur early in MS in some patients and may impose numerous stresses on the patient and family. Some patients with MS are forgetful and easily distracted.

Patients adapt to illness in a variety of ways, including denial, depression, withdrawal, and hostility. Emotional support assists patients and their families to adapt to the changes and uncertainties associated with MS and to cope with the disruption in their lives. The patient is assisted to set meaningful and realistic goals, to remain as active as possible, and to keep up social interests and activities. Hobbies may help the patient's morale and provide satisfying interests if the disease progresses to the stage at which formerly enjoyed activities can no longer be pursued.

The family should be made aware of the nature and degree of cognitive impairment. The environment is kept structured, and lists and other memory aids are used to help the patient with cognitive changes to maintain a daily routine. The occupational therapist can be helpful in formulating a structured daily routine.

Strengthening Coping Mechanisms. The diagnosis of MS is always distressing to the patient and family. They need to know that no two patients with MS have identical symptoms or courses of illness. Although some patients do experience significant disability early, others have a near-normal lifespan with minimal disability. Some families, however, face overwhelming frustrations and problems. MS affects people who are often in a productive stage of life and concerned about career and family responsibilities. Family conflict, disintegration, separation, and divorce are not uncommon. Often, very young family members assume the responsibility of caring for a parent with MS. Nursing interventions in this area include alleviating stress and making appropriate referrals for counseling and support to minimize the adverse effects of dealing with chronic illness.

The nurse, mindful of these complex problems, initiates home care and coordinates a network of services, including social services, speech therapy, physical therapy, and homemaker services. To strengthen the patient's coping skills, as much information as possible is provided. Patients need an updated list of available assistive devices, services, and resources.

Coping through problem solving involves helping the patient define the problem and develop alternatives for its management. Careful planning and maintaining flexibility and a hopeful attitude are useful for psychological and physical adaptation.

Improving Home Management

MS can affect every facet of daily living. Certain abilities are often impossible to regain after they are lost. Physical function may vary from day to day. Modifications that allow independence in home management should be implemented (e.g., assistive eating devices, raised toilet seat, bathing aids, telephone modifications, long-handled comb, tongs, modified clothing). Exposure to heat increases fatigue and muscle weakness, so air conditioning is recommended in at least one room. Exposure to extreme cold may increase spasticity.

Promoting Sexual Functioning

Patients with MS and their partners face problems that interfere with sexual activity, both as a direct consequence of nerve damage and also from psychological reactions to the disease. Easy fatigability, conflicts arising from dependency and depression, emotional lability, and loss of self-esteem compound the problem. Erectile and ejaculatory disorders in male patients and orgasmic dysfunction and adductor spasms of the thigh muscles in female patients can make sexual intercourse difficult or impossible. Bladder and bowel incontinence and urinary tract infections add to the difficulties.

An experienced sexual counselor helps bring into focus the patient's or partner's sexual resources and suggests relevant information and supportive therapy. Sharing and communicating feelings, planning for sexual activity (to minimize the effects of fatigue), and exploring alternative methods of sexual expression may open up a wide range of sexual enjoyment and experiences.

MYASTHENIA GRAVIS

Myasthenia gravis (MG), an autoimmune disorder affecting the neuromuscular junction, is characterized by fatigability and degrees of muscle weakness of the voluntary muscles. According to the Myasthenia Gravis Foundation of America, the prevalence of MG in the United States is estimated to be approximately 20 per 100,000 people. MG occurs in people of all genders at older ages; however before 40 years of age, the disease is three times more common in females (Ulane, 2021). The average age of onset among female patients is 28 years of age, whereas the average age of onset among male patients is 42 years of age. (Cortés-Vicente et al., 2020).

Pathophysiology

Normally, a chemical impulse precipitates the release of acetylcholine from vesicles on the nerve terminal at the neuromuscular junction. The acetylcholine attaches to receptor sites on the motor endplate and stimulates muscle contraction. Continuous binding of acetylcholine to the receptor site is required for muscular contraction to be sustained.

In MG, there is a reduction in the number of acetylcholine receptor sites because antibodies directed at the acetylcholine receptor sites impair transmission of impulses across the neuromuscular junction. Therefore, fewer receptors are available for stimulation, resulting in voluntary muscle weakness that escalates with continued activity (Fig. 45-6). Abnormalities of the thymus (located behind the sternum) are found in most patients with MG (Pugh, 2022).

Clinical Manifestations and Assessment

The initial manifestation of MG usually involves the ocular muscles. Diplopia (double vision) and ptosis (drooping of the eyelids) are common. However, the majority of patients also experience weakness of the muscles of the face and throat (bulbar symptoms) and generalized weakness. Weakness of the facial muscles results in a bland facial expression. Laryngeal involvement produces **dysphonia** (voice impairment) and increases the patient's risk for choking and aspiration. Generalized weakness affects all the extremities and the intercostal muscles, resulting in decreasing vital capacity and respiratory failure. MG is purely a motor disorder with no effect on sensation or coordination.

The hallmark of MG is fluctuating muscle weakness, which intensifies with activity such as exercise, and improves with rest (Koopman, 2020).

An acetylcholinesterase test is used to diagnose MG. The acetylcholinesterase inhibitor stops the breakdown of acetylcholine, thereby increasing availability at the neuromuscular junction. The drug used is edrophonium chloride because it has a rapid onset of 30 seconds and a short duration of 5 minutes (Koopman, 2020). Immediate improvement in muscle strength after administration of this agent represents a positive test and usually confirms the diagnosis.

An ice-pack test can help differentiate MG from other causes of ptosis. An ice pack is applied over the patient's closed eyes for 2 minutes. Improvement of the ptosis that is sustained for several minutes is considered a positive ice-pack test and is suggestive of MG. The rationale behind this test

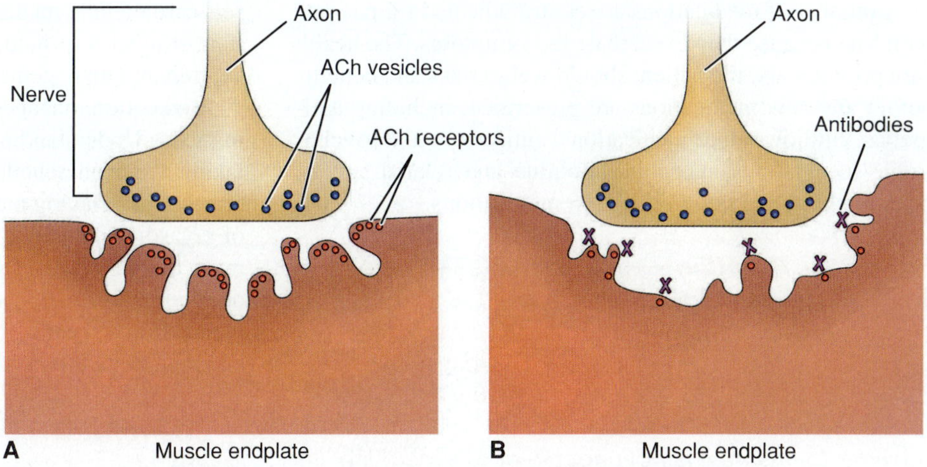

FIGURE 45-6 **Myasthenia gravis (MG). A. Normal acetylcholine (ACh) receptor site. B. ACh receptor site in MG.**

is that by cooling the tissues, which include skeletal muscle fibers, the activity of the acetylcholinesterases is inhibited. This test has the advantage of being noninvasive and inexpensive; however, not all patients with MG present with ptosis.

The presence of acetylcholine receptor antibodies is identified in serum. Repetitive nerve stimulation demonstrates a decrease in successive action potentials. The thymus gland may be enlarged in MG, and a CT scan of the mediastinum is performed to detect thymoma or hyperplasia of the thymus.

Medical and Nursing Management

Management of MG is directed at improving function and reducing and removing circulating antibodies. Therapeutic modalities include administration of anticholinesterase medications and immunosuppressive therapy, plasmapheresis, intravenous immunoglobulin, and thymectomy.

Pharmacologic Therapy

Pyridostigmine bromide, an anticholinesterase medication, is the first line of therapy. It provides symptomatic relief by inhibiting the breakdown of acetylcholine and increasing the relative concentration of available acetylcholine at the neuromuscular junction. The dosage is gradually increased to a daily maximum and is administered in divided doses (usually four times a day). The most common adverse effects are gastrointestinal discomfort, increased bronchial and oral secretions, and muscle fasciculations and cramps (Koopman, 2020). Pyridostigmine tends to have fewer side effects than other anticholinesterase medications (Box 45-3).

If pyridostigmine bromide does not improve muscle strength and control fatigue, the next agents used are immunosuppressant agents. The goal of immunosuppressive therapy is to reduce production of the antibody. Corticosteroids suppress the patient's immune response, decreasing the amount of antibody production; this correlates with clinical improvement. An initial dose of prednisone is given daily; as symptoms improve, the medication is tapered and a maintenance alternative-day dosing schedule may be considered. Since long-term steroids carry substantial risks for a variety of dose-dependent side effects (diabetes, osteoporosis, hypertension), this treatment is usually reserved for patients with ocular symptoms. As the corticosteroid dosage is gradually increased, the anticholinesterase dosage is lowered. Cytotoxic medications are used to treat MG if there is inadequate response to steroids. Azathioprine, an immunosuppressive drug, inhibits T lymphocytes and reduces acetylcholine receptor antibody levels. Therapeutic effects may not be evident for 3 to 12 months. Leukopenia and hepatotoxicity are serious adverse effects, so monthly evaluation of liver enzymes and white blood cell count is necessary.

Pearls for Practice

Prophylactic treatment for osteoporosis and careful follow-up for other side effects is mandatory in all patients managed with long-term prednisone.

BOX 45-3 **Potential Adverse Effects of Anticholinesterase Medications**

Central Nervous System
Irritability
Anxiety
Insomnia
Headache
Dysarthria
Syncope
Seizures
Coma
Diaphoresis

Respiratory
Bronchial relaxation
Increased bronchial
Secretions

Cardiovascular
Tachycardia
Hypotension

Gastrointestinal
Abdominal cramps
Nausea
Vomiting
Diarrhea
Anorexia
Increased salivation

Skeletal Muscles
Fasciculations
Spasms
Weakness

Genitourinary
Frequency
Urgency

Integumentary
Rash
Flushing

A number of medications are contraindicated for patients with MG because they exacerbate the symptoms. The health care provider and the patient should weigh risks and benefits before any new medications are prescribed, including antibiotics, cardiovascular medications, antiseizure and psychotropic medications, morphine, quinine and related agents, beta blockers, and nonprescription medications.

Pearls for Practice

The patient's dentist should be advised of the diagnosis of MG, and procaine should be avoided. Since neuromuscular blocking agents may have a very prolonged effect in patients with MG, any anesthetic medication should be evaluated by the primary care provider to ensure it is not capable of exaggerating myasthenic weakness (Cortez et al., 2020).

Plasmapheresis/Intravenous Immunoglobulin

Plasmapheresis (plasma exchange) is a technique used to treat exacerbations of MG. The patient's plasma and plasma components are removed through a centrally placed large-bore double-lumen catheter. The blood cells and antibody-containing plasma are separated, after which the cells and a plasma substitute are reinfused. Plasma exchange produces a temporary reduction in the level of circulating antibodies. The typical course of plasmapheresis consists of daily or alternative-day treatment, and the number of treatments is determined by the patient's response. IV immunoglobulin (IVIG) treatment involves the administration of pooled human gamma globulin, which usually produces a relatively quick and short-term relief of MG weakness. Although IVIG is easier than plasmapheresis to administer, the response to plasmapheresis is more rapid. No treatments cure MG because they do not stop the production of the acetylcholine receptor antibodies.

Surgical Management

Thymectomy (surgical removal of the thymus gland) can produce antigen-specific immunosuppression and result in clinical improvement. The procedure results in either partial or complete remission. The entire gland must be removed for optimal clinical outcomes; therefore, surgeons prefer the trans-sternal surgical approach. After surgery, the patient is monitored in an intensive care unit, with special attention to respiratory function. The patient is weaned from mechanical ventilation after thorough respiratory assessment. Thymectomy leads to improvement in almost all patients, but it may take months before the patient sees any benefit from the procedure.

Nursing Management

Because MG is a chronic disease and most patients are seen on an outpatient basis, much of the nursing care focuses on patient and family teaching. Educational topics for outpatient self-care include medication management, energy conservation, strategies to help with ocular manifestations, and prevention and management of complications.

Medication management is a crucial component of ongoing care. Understanding the actions of the medications and taking them on schedule is emphasized, as are the consequences of delaying medication and the signs and symptoms of myasthenic and cholinergic crises. The patient can determine the best times for daily dosing by keeping a diary to determine fluctuation of symptoms and to learn when the medication is wearing off. The medication schedule can then be manipulated to maximize strength throughout the day.

Pearls for Practice

Maintenance of stable blood levels of anticholinesterase medications is imperative to stabilize muscle strength. Therefore, the anticholinesterase medications must be administered on time. Any delay in administration of medications may exacerbate muscle weakness and make it impossible for the patient to take medications orally.

To minimize the risk of aspiration, mealtimes should coincide with the peak effects of anticholinesterase medication. In addition, rest before meals is encouraged to reduce muscle fatigue. The patient is advised to sit upright during meals, with the neck slightly flexed to facilitate swallowing. Soft foods in gravy or sauces can be swallowed more easily; if choking occurs frequently, the nurse can suggest puréed food with a pudding-like consistency. Suction should be available at home, with the patient and family instructed in its use. Supplemental feedings may be necessary in some patients to ensure adequate nutrition.

Impaired vision results from ptosis of one or both eyelids, decreased eye movement, or double vision. To prevent corneal damage when the eyelids do not close completely, many providers may instruct the patient to tape or patch the eyes closed for short intervals and to regularly instill artificial tears. If taping is done, it is important to ensure the lid covers the eye to prevent corneal abrasion from the tape or patch. In a recent study of patients who were comatose in an ICU, the use of saline eye drops, artificial eye drops, and polyethylene eye covers were compared, and the polyethylene eye covers significantly reduced the incidence and severity of ocular diseases over eye drop instillation (Khatiban et al., 2021). Although research data are limited as of this edition, nurses need to be alert to subsequent evidence of best practice for eye care. Patients who wear eyeglasses can have "crutches" attached to help lift the eyelids. Patching of one eye can help with double vision.

The patient is reminded of the importance of maintaining health promotion practices and of following health care screening recommendations. Factors that exacerbate symptoms and potentially cause crisis should be noted and avoided: emotional stress, infections (particularly respiratory infections), vigorous physical activity, some medications, and high environmental temperature.

The patient is also taught strategies to conserve energy. To do this, the nurse helps the patient identify the optimal times for rest throughout the day. If the patient lives in a two-story home, the nurse can suggest that frequently used items (e.g., hygiene products, cleaning products, snacks) be kept on each floor to minimize travel between floors. The patient is encouraged to apply for a handicapped license plate to minimize walking from parking spaces and to schedule activities to coincide with peak energy and strength levels. Patients are encouraged to wear a medical alert bracelet identifying them as having MG. The Myasthenia Gravis Foundation of America provides support groups, services, and educational materials for patients, families, and health care providers (www.myasthenia.org).

Complications

Cholinergic Crisis

A cholinergic crisis, which is essentially a problem of overmedication, results in severe generalized muscle weakness, respiratory impairment, and excessive pulmonary secretions that may result in respiratory failure. Weak respiratory muscles do not support inhalation. An inadequate cough and an impaired gag reflex, caused by bulbar weakness, result in poor airway clearance and risk of aspiration. Bulbar weakness specifically involves the muscles of the jaw, face, palate, pharynx, larynx, tongue, glossopharyngeal nerve (IX), vagus nerve (X), and hypoglossal nerve (XII). A downward trend of two respiratory function tests, the negative inspiratory force and vital capacity, is the first clinical sign of respiratory compromise.

Pearls for Practice

The phrase bulbar weakness refers to weakness and fatigue in the neck and jaw, and it is named for the nerves that originate from the bulblike part of the brainstem, the medulla. The nurse anticipates the patient will have difficulty talking, chewing, swallowing, and holding the head erect. Patients should be assessed for their ability to communicate, to tolerate oral intake, and to determine their aspiration risk. A marked decrease in oxygen saturation (as measured by pulse oximetry), tachypnea (increased respiration rate), and coughing to a lesser extent after oral intake suggest aspiration. Weakness of the respiratory musculature can lessen the ability to cough.

Endotracheal intubation and mechanical ventilation may be needed. Cholinesterase inhibitors are stopped when respiratory failure occurs and gradually restarted after the patient demonstrates improvement. Nutritional support may be needed if the patient is intubated for a long period.

Myasthenic Crisis

Myasthenic crisis is a sudden, temporary exacerbation of symptoms of MG. A common precipitating event for myasthenic crisis is an infection. Respiratory distress and varying degrees of dysphagia (difficulty swallowing), dysarthria (difficulty speaking), eyelid ptosis, diplopia, and prominent muscle weakness are symptoms of myasthenic crisis. In addition, in 13% to 20% of patients, myasthenic crisis is the first manifestation of MG (Nikpour, 2020).

Providing ventilatory assistance takes precedence in the immediate management of the patient with myasthenic crisis. Ongoing assessment for respiratory failure is essential. The nurse assesses the respiratory rate and depth, breath sounds, and oxygen saturation and monitors pulmonary function parameters (vital capacity and negative inspiratory force) to detect pulmonary problems before respiratory dysfunction progresses. ABG analysis is performed as needed. Endotracheal intubation and mechanical ventilation may be needed.

Pearls for Practice: Pathophysiology Vital Capacity and Negative Inspiratory Force (NIF)

Vital capacity is the maximal volume of air that can be expired following maximum inspiration and is between 3 and 5 L in a typical adult (Sharoon & Sharma, 2021). Serial measurements of NIF provide the best measure of deteriorating respiratory function in MG (Guptill & Sanders, 2022). It is a relatively easy bedside test and if the NIF is dropping or nears −20 cm water, respiratory support needs to be available. More is discussed shortly on NIF.

If the abdominal, intercostal, and pharyngeal muscles are severely weak, the patient cannot cough, take deep breaths, or clear secretions. Chest physiotherapy, including postural drainage to mobilize secretions and suctioning to remove secretions, may have to be performed frequently. (Postural drainage should not be performed for 30 minutes after feeding because of risk of vomiting and aspiration.)

Several strategies and supportive measures should be performed during this crisis, including monitoring of laboratory work, input and output, and daily weight, along with vigilant pulmonary assessments. If the patient cannot swallow, nasogastric tube feedings may be prescribed. Sedatives and tranquilizers are avoided because they aggravate hypoxia and hypercapnia (excessive carbon dioxide in blood) and can cause respiratory and cardiac depression.

GUILLAIN–BARRÉ SYNDROME

Guillain–Barré syndrome (GBS) is an autoimmune attack on the peripheral nerve myelin. The result is acute, rapid, segmental demyelination of peripheral nerves and some cranial nerves, producing ascending weakness with **dyskinesia** (inability to execute voluntary movements), hyporeflexia, and **paresthesias** (numbness). An antecedent event (most often a viral infection) precipitates clinical presentation. *Campylobacter jejuni*, cytomegalovirus, Epstein–Barr virus, *Mycoplasma pneumoniae, H. influenzae*, and HIV are the most common infectious agents associated with the development of GBS. In a few instances, the patient reports receiving a vaccination prior to the onset of GBS (Guanci et al., 2020).

In North America, approximately 1 to 2 cases of GBS occur for every 100,000 people each year. GBS affects people of all ages and races and females slightly more than males. Given the relationship of GBS to colds and flu-like illnesses, it is expected that GBS would occur more frequently in the fall and winter when these infections are more likely (Guanci et al., 2020).

Pathophysiology

Myelin is a complex substance that covers nerves, providing insulation and speeding the conduction of impulses from the cell body to the dendrites. The cell that produces myelin in the peripheral nervous system is the Schwann cell. In GBS, the Schwann cell is spared, allowing for remyelination in the recovery phase of the disease.

GBS is the result of a cell-mediated and humoral immune attack on peripheral nerve myelin proteins that causes inflammatory demyelination. The immune system cannot distinguish between the two proteins and attacks and destroys peripheral nerve myelin. The exact location of the immune attack within the peripheral nervous system is the ganglioside GM1b. With the autoimmune attack, there is an influx of macrophages and other immune-mediated agents that attack myelin, cause inflammation and destruction, and leave the axon unable to support nerve conduction (Fig. 45-7).

Clinical Manifestations and Assessment

GBS typically begins with muscle weakness and diminished reflexes of the lower extremities. Hyporeflexia and weakness may progress to tetraplegia (paralysis of all four limbs). Demyelination of the nerves that innervate the diaphragm and intercostal muscles results in neuromuscular respiratory failure. Sensory symptoms include paresthesias of the hands and feet and pain related to the demyelination of sensory fibers.

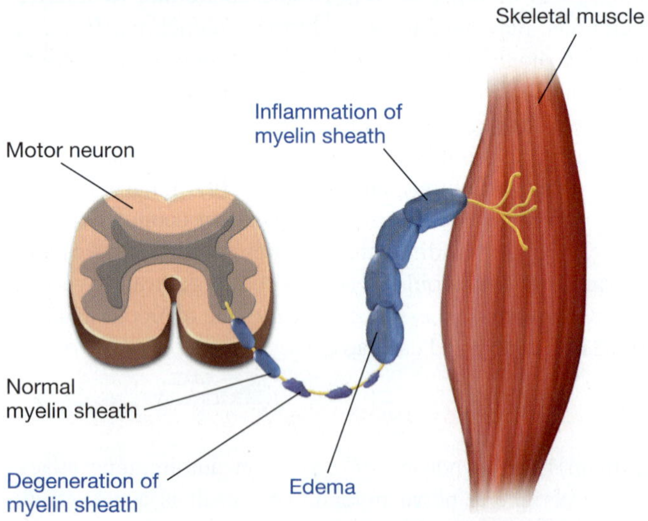

FIGURE 45-7 Peripheral nerve demyelination. (Used with permission from ACC atlas of pathophysiology. [2001]. Lippincott Williams & Wilkins.)

The antecedent event usually occurs 2 weeks before symptoms begin. Weakness usually begins in the legs and progresses upward. Maximum weakness, the *plateau,* varies in length but usually includes neuromuscular respiratory failure and bulbar weakness. The duration of the symptoms is variable; complete functional recovery may take up to 2 years (Guanci et al., 2020). Any residual symptoms are permanent and reflect axonal damage from demyelination.

Cranial nerve demyelination can result in a variety of clinical manifestations. Optic nerve demyelination may result in blindness. Bulbar muscle weakness related to demyelination of the glossopharyngeal and vagus nerves results in the inability to swallow or clear secretions. Vagus nerve demyelination results in autonomic dysfunction, manifested by instability of the cardiovascular system. The presentation is variable and may include tachycardia, bradycardia, hypertension, or orthostatic hypotension. The symptoms of autonomic dysfunction occur and resolve rapidly. GBS does not affect cognitive function or LOC.

Although the classic clinical features include areflexia and ascending weakness, variation in presentation occurs. There may be a sensory presentation with progressive sensory symptoms; an atypical axonal destruction; or the Miller–Fisher variant, which includes paralysis of the ocular muscles, ataxia, and areflexia (Guanci et al., 2020).

The patient presents with symmetric weakness, diminished reflexes, and upward progression of motor weakness. Changes in vital capacity and negative inspiratory force are assessed to identify impending neuromuscular respiratory failure. Serum laboratory tests are not useful in the diagnosis. However, elevated protein levels are detected in CSF evaluation, without an increase in other cells. EPSs demonstrate a progressive loss of nerve conduction velocity.

Medical and Nursing Management

Because of the possibility of rapid progression and neuromuscular respiratory failure, GBS is a medical emergency requiring management in an intensive care unit. After baseline values are identified, assessment of changes in muscle strength and respiratory function alert the provider to the physical and respiratory needs of the patient. Respiratory therapy or mechanical ventilation may be necessary to support pulmonary function and adequate oxygenation. Some clinicians recommend elective intubation before the onset of extreme respiratory muscle fatigue. Mechanical ventilation may be required for an extended period. The patient is weaned from mechanical ventilation after the respiratory muscles can again support spontaneous respiration and maintain adequate tissue oxygenation.

Other interventions are aimed at preventing the complications of immobility. These may include the use of anticoagulant agents and thigh-high elastic compression stockings or sequential compression boots to prevent thrombosis and pulmonary emboli (PE).

Plasmapheresis and IVIG are used to directly affect the peripheral nerve myelin antibody level. Both therapies decrease circulating antibody levels and reduce the amount of time the patient is immobilized and dependent on mechanical ventilation. The cardiovascular risks posed by autonomic dysfunction require continuous electrocardiographic (ECG) monitoring. Tachycardia and hypertension are treated with short-acting medications, such as alpha-adrenergic blocking agents. The use of short-acting agents is important because autonomic dysfunction is very labile. Hypotension is managed by increasing the amount of IV fluid administered.

Maintaining Respiratory Function

Respiratory function can be maximized with incentive spirometry and chest physiotherapy. Monitoring for changes in vital capacity and negative inspiratory force are key to early intervention for neuromuscular respiratory failure. Mechanical ventilation is required if the vital capacity falls, making spontaneous breathing impossible and tissue oxygenation inadequate.

Pearls for Practice: Pathophysiology Maximal Inspiratory Pressures (MIP) or Negative Inspiratory Force (NIF) Among Other Names…

To evaluate respiratory muscle strength, maximal inspiratory pressures (MIP) are obtained using a handheld or electronic device that can be attached to an endotracheal tube (if needed), or the patient can place the device around their lips with a nose clip placed on the nares. The patient is instructed to breathe through the device. The patient must be cooperative to assess MIP or NIF. Other names for measuring NIF are negative inspiratory effort, peak inspiratory pressure (PIP), and peak inspiratory force (Stacy, 2022). The patient exhales the residual volume and then inhales with maximal force; thus, this test assesses whether a patient has enough inspiratory muscle strength to take in an adequate breath. A normal MIP/NIF is usually >–60 cm H_2O; when there is a rapidly decreasing vital capacity or a VC <1,000 mL, a negative inspiratory force <–20 cm H_2O, a PaO_2 <70, or the patient is having significant difficulty clearing secretions or is aspirating, mechanical ventilation may be needed (Sharp, 2022). This simple bedside test also can be used to monitor deterioration or improvement of the strength of the diaphragm and other inspiratory muscles. Respiratory therapy personnel perform this test. A major limitation is that measurement is difficult in those that are severely ill, under sedation, or neurologically impaired.

Parameters for determining the appropriate time to begin mechanical ventilation include a vital capacity of less than 15 mL/kg, among the aforementioned values. At a level of <15 mL/kg, patients have limited respiratory reserve and the need for continued ventilator support (Krawczyk & Heuer, 2022). The potential need for mechanical ventilation should be discussed with the patient and family on admission, to provide time for psychological preparation and decision making. Intubation and mechanical ventilation will result in less anxiety if initiated on a nonemergency basis to a well-informed patient. The patient may require mechanical ventilation for a long period.

Bulbar weakness that impairs the ability to swallow and clear secretions is another factor in the development of respiratory failure in the patient with GBS. Suctioning may be needed to maintain a clear airway.

The nurse assesses the blood pressure and heart rate frequently to identify autonomic dysfunction so that interventions can be initiated quickly if needed. Medications are administered for clinically significant symptoms.

Enhancing Physical Mobility

Nursing interventions to enhance physical mobility and prevent the complications of immobility are key to the function and survival of these patients. The paralyzed extremities are supported in functional positions, and passive range-of-motion (ROM) exercises are performed at least twice daily. Deep venous thrombosis (DVT) and PE are threats to the patient who is paralyzed. Nursing interventions are aimed at preventing DVT. ROM exercises, position changes, anticoagulation, the use of thigh-high elastic compression stockings or sequential compression boots, and adequate hydration decrease the risk for DVT.

Padding may be placed over bony prominences, such as the elbows and heels, to reduce the risk for pressure ulcers. The need for consistent position changes every 2 hours cannot be overemphasized. The nurse evaluates laboratory test results that may indicate malnutrition or dehydration, both of which increase the risk for pressure ulcers. The nurse collaborates with the provider and dietitian to develop a plan to meet the patient's nutritional and hydration needs.

Providing Adequate Nutrition

Paralytic ileus may result from insufficient parasympathetic activity. In this event, the nurse administers IV fluids and parenteral nutrition as prescribed and monitors for the return of bowel sounds and bowel function. If the patient cannot swallow due to **bulbar paralysis** (immobility of muscles), a nasogastric tube or gastrostomy tube may be placed to administer nutrients. The nurse carefully assesses the return of the gag reflex and bowel sounds before resuming oral nutrition.

Improving Communication

Because of paralysis, the patient cannot talk, laugh, or cry and therefore has no method for communicating needs or expressing emotion. Establishing some form of communication with picture cards or an eye blink system provides a means of communication. Collaboration with the speech therapist may be helpful in developing a communication mechanism that is most effective for a specific patient.

Decreasing Fear and Anxiety

The patient and family are faced with a sudden, potentially life-threatening disease, and anxiety and fear are constant themes for them. The impact of disease on the family depends on the patient's role within the family. Referral to a support group may provide information and support to the patient and family.

The family may feel helpless in caring for the patient. Mechanical ventilation and monitoring devices may frighten and intimidate them. Family members often want to participate in physical care; with instruction and support by the nurse, they should be allowed to do so.

In addition to fear, the patient may experience isolation, loneliness, and lack of control. Nursing interventions that increase the patient's sense of control include providing information about the condition, emphasizing a positive appraisal of coping resources, and teaching relaxation exercises and distraction techniques. The positive attitude and atmosphere of the multidisciplinary team are important to promote a sense of well-being.

Diversional activities are encouraged to decrease loneliness and isolation. Encouraging visitors, engaging visitors or volunteers to read to the patient, listening to music or books on tape, and watching television are ways to alleviate the patient's sense of isolation.

Complications

Thorough assessment of respiratory function at regular and frequent intervals is essential because respiratory insufficiency and subsequent failure due to weakness or paralysis of the intercostal muscles and diaphragm may develop quickly. In addition to the respiratory rate and the quality of respirations, serial vital capacity or NIF are monitored at regular intervals so that respiratory insufficiency can be anticipated. In addition, the effectiveness of gas exchange is assessed by monitoring the oxygen saturation and potentially the carbon dioxide levels. Decreasing vital capacity associated with weakness of the muscles used in swallowing, which causes difficulty in both coughing and swallowing, indicates impending respiratory failure. Signs and symptoms include breathlessness while speaking; shallow and irregular breathing; use of accessory muscles; tachycardia; and changes in respiratory pattern, decreasing oxygen saturation and hypercapnia ($PaCO_2 > 45$ mm Hg). However, if the patient has pre-existing COPD, then $PaCO_2$ will routinely be over 45 mm Hg, and/or a pH <7.35 will require the nurse to alert the provider of potential respiratory failure.

Parameters for determining the onset of respiratory failure are established on admission, allowing intubation and the initiation of mechanical ventilation on a nonemergent basis. This also allows the patient to be prepared for the procedure in a controlled manner, which reduces anxiety and complications.

Other complications include cardiac arrhythmias, which necessitate ECG monitoring; transient hypertension; orthostatic hypotension; DVT; PE; urinary retention; and other threats to any patient who is immobilized and paralyzed. These require monitoring and attention to prevent them, and prompt treatment if indicated.

PARKINSON DISEASE

Parkinson disease (PD) is a slowly progressing neurologic movement disorder that eventually leads to disability. The degenerative or idiopathic form is the most common; there is also a secondary form with a known or suspected cause. Although the cause of most cases is unknown, causative factors include genetics, atherosclerosis, excessive accumulation of oxygen-free radicals, viral infections, head trauma, chronic use of antipsychotic medications, and some environmental exposures. Parkinsonian symptoms usually first appear in the fifth decade of life, with diagnosis typically in the sixth or seventh decade of life; however, rare cases have been diagnosed as early as 30 years of age and often suggest a hereditary form of parkinsonism (Jankovic, 2022). It is the second most common **neurodegenerative** disease. PD affects males more frequently than females.

The prevalence and prognosis of COVID-19 patients with PD are comparable to those without PD. Individuals with PD showed multiple patterns of vulnerability, being advanced in age and having chronic conditions and related polypharmacy burden. Significant predictors for contracting COVID-19 in PD patients included a history of diabetes and immunocompromised conditions. There was a decline in motor functions and stress-induced psychiatric problems for those PD patients who contracted COVID-19. PD patients who contracted COVID-19 also had a relatively high mortality and hospital admission rates (El-Qushayri et al., 2021).

Pathophysiology

PD is associated with decreased levels of dopamine resulting from destruction of pigmented neuronal cells in the substantia nigra in the basal ganglia region of the brain. Fibers or neuronal pathways project from the substantia nigra to the corpus striatum, where neurotransmitters are key to the control of complex body movements. Through the neurotransmitters acetylcholine (excitatory) and dopamine (inhibitory), striatal neurons relay messages to the higher motor centers that control and refine motor movements. The loss of dopamine stores in this area of the brain results in more excitatory neurotransmitters than inhibitory neurotransmitters, leading to an imbalance that affects voluntary movement. Clinical symptoms do not appear until 60% of the pigmented neurons are lost and the striatal dopamine level is decreased by 80%.

Cellular degeneration impairs the extrapyramidal tracts that control semiautomatic functions and coordinated movements; motor cells of the motor cortex and the pyramidal tracts are not affected.

Clinical Manifestations and Assessment

PD has a gradual onset, and symptoms progress slowly over a chronic, prolonged course. The cardinal signs are T-R-A-P: **T**remor, **R**igidity of muscles, **A**kinesia/Bradykinesia (without or decreased body movement), and **P**ostural disturbances (gait and balance disorders).

Tremor

The most common reason why individuals seek medical evaluation is the presence of a resting tremor. Resting tremor characteristically disappears with purposeful movement but is evident when the extremities are motionless. The tremor may manifest as a rhythmic, slow-turning motion (pronation–supination) of the forearm and the hand and a motion of the thumb against the fingers as if rolling a pill between the fingers. Tremor is present while the patient is at rest; it increases when the patient is walking, concentrating, or feeling anxious.

Rigidity

Resistance to passive limb movement characterizes muscle rigidity. Cogwheel rigidity is characterized by jerky rhythmic tone on passive muscle stretching (Mastrianni & Harris, 2020). Involuntary stiffness of the passive extremity increases when another extremity is engaged in voluntary active movement. Early in the disease, the patient may complain of shoulder pain due to rigidity.

Akinesia/Bradykinesia

Akinesia means a lack of movement, and *bradykinesia* means a slowness of initiation and execution of movement. Patients may take longer to complete activities and have difficulty initiating movement, such as rising from a sitting position or turning in bed.

Postural Disturbances

A loss of postural reflexes occurs, and the patient stands with the head bent forward and walks with a propulsive gait. The posture is caused by the forward flexion of the neck, hips, knees, and elbows. The patient may walk faster and faster, trying to move the feet forward under the body's center of gravity (shuffling gait). Difficulty in pivoting that causes loss of balance (either forward or backward) places the patient at risk for falls.

Other Manifestations

The effect of PD on the basal ganglia often produces autonomic symptoms that include excessive and uncontrolled sweating, paroxysmal flushing, orthostatic hypotension, gastric and urinary retention, constipation, and sexual dysfunction. Cognitive and psychiatric changes are often interrelated and may be predictive of one another. Depression is common; whether it is a reaction to the disorder or is related to a biochemical abnormality is uncertain. Cognitive changes may appear in the form of judgment, reasoning, decision making, and memory deficits, although intellect is not usually affected. A number of psychiatric manifestations (personality changes, psychosis, dementia, and acute confusion) are common in older patients with PD.

Patients with PD experience sleep disturbances. This may be related to depression, dementia, or medications. Auditory and visual hallucinations have also been reported in PD and may be associated with depression, dementia, lack of sleep, or adverse effects of medications.

Hypokinesia (abnormally diminished movement) is also common and may appear after the tremor. The *freezing phenomenon* refers to a transient inability to perform active movement and is thought to be an extreme form of bradykinesia. In addition, the patient tends to shuffle and exhibits a decreased arm swing. As dexterity declines, **micrographia** (small handwriting) develops. The face becomes increasingly mask-like and expressionless, and the frequency of blinking decreases. Dysphonia (soft, low-pitched, and less audible speech) may occur due to weakness of the muscles responsible for speech and paralysis of the soft palate, resulting in a nasal-sounding speech. In many cases, the patient develops dysphagia, begins to drool, and is at risk for choking and aspiration.

Complications associated with PD are common and are typically related to disorders of movement. As the disease progresses, patients are at risk for respiratory and urinary tract infection, skin breakdown, and injury from falls. The adverse effects of medications used to treat the symptoms are associated with numerous complications, such as dyskinesia (impairment of voluntary movements resulting in fragmented or jerky motions) and orthostatic hypotension.

Early diagnosis can be difficult because patients rarely are able to pinpoint when the symptoms started. Often, a family member notices a change, such as stooped posture, a stiff arm; a slight limp; tremor; or slow, small handwriting. The medical history, presenting symptoms, neurologic examination, and response to pharmacologic management are carefully evaluated when making the diagnosis. Currently, the disease is diagnosed clinically from the patient's history and the presence of two of the four cardinal manifestations: tremor, rigidity, akinesia/bradykinesia, and postural disturbances (Fig. 45-8).

Medical and Nursing Management

Treatment is directed at controlling symptoms and maintaining functional independence. Care is individualized for each patient based on presenting symptoms and social, occupational, and emotional needs. Pharmacologic management is the mainstay of treatment, although advances in research

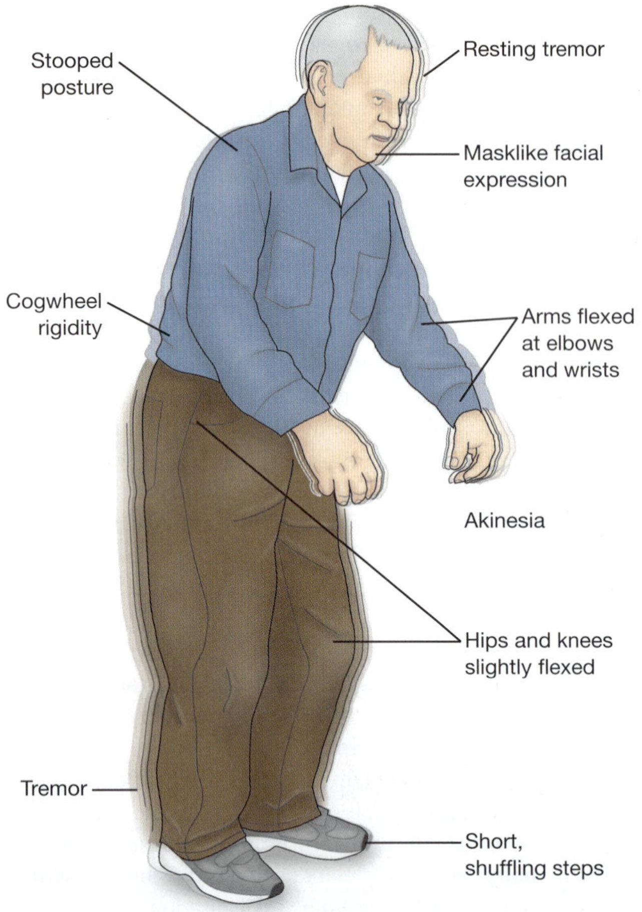

FIGURE 45-8 The clinical features of Parkinson disease: TRAP (Tremor, Rigidity, Akinesia/Bradykinesia, and Postural disturbances). (Adapted from Timby, B. [2010]. *Introductory medical-surgical nursing* [10th ed., p. 535]. Lippincott Williams & Wilkins.)

have led to increased surgical options. Patients are usually cared for at home and are admitted to the hospital only for complications or to initiate new treatments.

Antiparkinsonian Medications

Levodopa is the most effective agent and the mainstay of treatment. Levodopa is converted to dopamine in the basal ganglia, producing symptom relief. The beneficial effects of levodopa are most pronounced in the first few years of treatment. Benefits begin to wane and adverse effects become more severe over time. Confusion, hallucinations, depression, and sleep alterations are associated with prolonged use. Levodopa is usually administered in combination with carbidopa, an amino acid decarboxylase inhibitor, which helps to maximize the beneficial effects of levodopa.

Within 5 to 10 years, most patients develop a response to the medication characterized by **dyskinesia** (abnormal involuntary movements), including facial grimacing, rhythmic jerking movements of the hands, head bobbing, chewing and smacking movements, and involuntary movements of the trunk and extremities. The patient may experience an on–off syndrome, in which sudden periods of near-immobility ("off" effect) are followed by a sudden return of effectiveness of the medication ("on" effect). Refer to Table 45-2 for additional medical therapies.

Drug Alert

MAO-B inhibitors may offer some neuroprotective benefits that could postpone the need for levodopa. Since MAO-B is an enzyme that breaks down dopamine, a medication that helps to block the breakdown of dopamine in the brain makes more dopamine available and reduces some of the motor symptoms of PD. When used together with other medications, MAO-B inhibitors may reduce "off" effect and extend "on" effect as described previously. The patient must be educated to avoid an interaction with products containing tyramine (red wine, aged cheese) since sudden and severe hypertension can occur.

Deep Brain Stimulation

Deep brain stimulation is the delivery of high-frequency electrical stimulation to a select targeted area in the brain (Fig. 45-9).

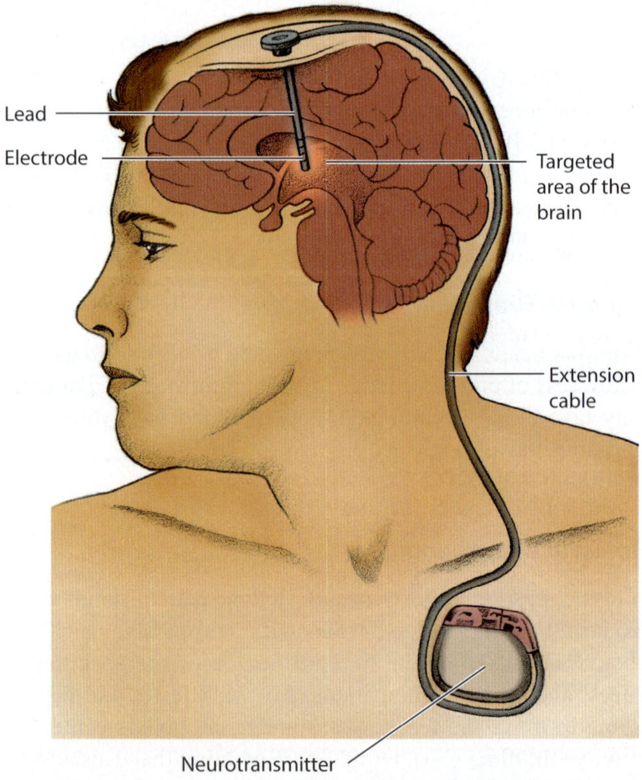

FIGURE 45-9 Deep brain stimulation. The deep brain stimulation system consists of the stimulating lead (which is implanted to the desired target), the extension cable (which is tunneled under the scalp and soft tissues of the neck to the anterior chest wall), and the pulse generator (which is the programmable source of the electrical impulses). This illustration shows the placement of the stimulator in the patient's body. (Used with permission from Lippincott's Nursing Advisor by Lippincott Williams & Wilkins.)

TABLE 45-2 **Antiparkinsonian Medications**

Anticholinergic Therapy Trihexyphenidyl hydrochloride Benztropine mesylate	Used for controlling tremor by counteracting the action of the neurotransmitter acetylcholine; often poorly tolerated in older patients. Intraocular pressure must be closely monitored; these medications are contraindicated in patients with narrow-angle glaucoma. Patients with benign prostate hyperplasia (BPH) are monitored for signs of urinary retention.
Antiviral Therapy Amantadine hydrochloride	Used for symptoms related to akinesia, as well as tremor. A low incidence of side effects is seen but can include psychiatric disturbances (mood changes, confusion, depression, hallucinations), lower extremity edema, orthostatic hypotension, congestive heart failure, nausea, epigastric distress, urinary retention, headache, and visual impairment.
Dopamine Agonists Bromocriptine mesylate Pergolide Ropinirole hydrochloride Pramipexole	Useful in postponing the initiation of carbidopa or levodopa therapy or added to the medication regimen after carbidopa or levodopa loses effectiveness. Adverse reactions to these medications include nausea, vomiting, diarrhea, lightheadedness, hypotension, impotence, and psychiatric effects. Pergolide and pramipexole do not have the potentially serious adverse effects of pergolide and bromocriptine mesylate.
Monoamine Oxidase Inhibitors (MAOIs) Selegiline Rasagiline Zydis selegiline HCl	Used in combination with a dopamine agonist to delay the use of carbidopa or levodopa therapy. Adverse effects are similar to those of levodopa.
Catechol-O-methyltransferase (COMT) inhibitors Entacapone tolcapone	When given in combination with carbidopa or levodopa, they can increase the duration of action. COMT inhibitors block an enzyme that metabolizes levodopa, making more levodopa available for conversion to dopamine in the brain.
Antidepressants	
Tricyclic antidepressants	Used to treat depression; dosing is lower in patients with Parkinson disease, typically one third to one half of the usual dosage.
Amitriptyline hydrochloride	Used for anticholinergic and antidepressant effects.
Serotonin reuptake inhibitors (SRIs) Fluoxetine hydrochloride	Effective for treating depression but may aggravate symptoms of Parkinson disease.
Atypical antidepressants Bupropion hydrochloride	Effective for treating depression but may aggravate symptoms of Parkinson disease.

A CT scan or MRI determines the target area. Unilateral and/or bilateral deep brain stimulation of the subthalamic nucleus or globus pallidus (the site where most of the degenerative changes of PD occurs) improves the symptoms of PD, and early use (when motor complications are developing) results in significant benefit compared to traditional medical treatment (Okun & Lang, 2020). In deep brain stimulation, one or more electrodes is placed in specific areas of the brain and connected to a pulse generator that is implanted in a subcutaneous subclavicular or abdominal pouch. The battery-powered pulse generator sends high-frequency electrical impulses through a wire placed under the skin to a lead anchored to the skull. The electrode blocks nerve pathways in the brain that cause tremors. Deep brain stimulation usually results in patients being at their best for longer periods of the day than they were with medication alone.

Improving Mobility

A progressive program of daily exercise will increase muscle strength, improve coordination and dexterity, reduce muscular rigidity, and prevent contractures that occur when muscles are not used. Walking, riding a stationary bicycle, swimming, and gardening are all exercises that help maintain joint mobility. Stretching (stretch–hold–relax) and ROM exercises promote joint flexibility. Postural exercises are important to counter the tendency of the head and neck to be drawn forward and down. A physical therapist may be helpful in developing an individualized exercise program and can provide instruction to the patient and caregiver on exercising safely. Faithful adherence to an exercise and walking program helps to delay the progress of the disease. Warm baths and massage, in addition to passive and active exercises, help relax muscles and relieve painful muscle spasms that accompany rigidity.

Balance may be adversely affected because of the rigidity of the arms (arm swinging is necessary in normal walking). Special walking techniques must be learned to offset the shuffling gait and the tendency to lean forward. The patient is taught to concentrate on walking erect, to watch the horizon, and to use a wide-based gait (i.e., walking with the feet separated). A conscious effort must be made to swing the arms, raise the feet while walking, and use a heel–toe placement of the feet with long strides. The patient is advised to practice walking to marching music or to the sound of a ticking metronome because this provides sensory reinforcement. Breathing exercises while walking help to move the rib cage and to aerate parts of the lungs. Frequent rest periods aid in preventing frustration and fatigue.

Enhancing Self-Care Activities

Environmental modifications are necessary to compensate for functional disabilities (removing scatter rugs, installing bathroom handrails, ensuring good lighting, etc.). Patients may have severe mobility problems that make normal activities impossible. Adaptive or assistive devices may be useful. At home, a hospital bed with bedside rails, an overbed frame with a trapeze, or a rope tied to the foot of the bed can provide assistance in pulling up without help. An occupational therapist can evaluate the patient's needs in the home, make recommendations regarding adaptive devices, and teach the patient and caregiver how to improvise.

Improving Bowel Elimination

The patient may have severe problems with constipation. Among the factors causing constipation are weakness of the muscles used in defecation, lack of exercise, inadequate fluid intake, and decreased autonomic nervous system activity. The medications used for the treatment of the disease also inhibit normal intestinal secretions. A regular bowel routine may be established by encouraging the patient to set a specific time of day to sit on the toilet without distractions, consciously increase fluid intake, and eat foods with moderate fiber content. Laxatives should be avoided. A raised toilet seat is useful because the patient has difficulty in moving from a standing to a sitting position.

Improving Nutrition

Patients may have difficulty maintaining their weight. Eating becomes a very slow process, requiring concentration due to a dry mouth from medications and difficulty chewing and swallowing. These patients are at risk for aspiration because of impaired swallowing and the accumulation of saliva. They may be unaware that they are aspirating; subsequently, bronchopneumonia may develop.

Monitoring weight on a weekly basis indicates whether caloric intake is adequate. Supplemental feedings increase caloric intake. As the disease progresses, a nasogastric tube or percutaneous endoscopic gastroscopy may be necessary to maintain adequate nutrition. A dietitian can be consulted regarding nutritional needs.

An electric warming tray keeps food hot and allows the patient to rest during the prolonged time that it may take to eat. Special utensils also assist at mealtime. A plate that is stabilized, a nonspill cup, and eating utensils with built-up handles are useful self-help devices. The occupational therapist can assist in identifying appropriate adaptive devices.

Enhancing Swallowing

Swallowing difficulties are common in PD and may be associated with poor head control, tongue tremor, hesitancy in initiating swallowing, difficulty in shaping food into a bolus, and disturbances in pharyngeal motility. To offset these problems, the patient should sit in an upright position during mealtime. A semisolid diet with thick liquids is easier to swallow than solids; thin liquids should be avoided. Thinking through the swallowing sequence is helpful. The patient is taught to place the food on the tongue, close the lips and teeth, lift the tongue up and then back, and swallow. The patient is encouraged to chew first on one side of the mouth and then on the other. To control the buildup of saliva, the patient is reminded to hold the head upright and make a conscious effort to swallow.

Improving Communication

Speech disorders are present in most patients with PD. Their low-pitched, monotonous, soft speech requires that they make a conscious effort to speak slowly, with deliberate attention to what they are saying. The patient is reminded to face the listener, exaggerate the pronunciation of words, speak in short sentences, and take a few deep breaths before speaking. A speech therapist may be helpful in designing speech improvement exercises and assisting the family and health care personnel to develop and use a method of communication that meets the patient's needs. A small electronic amplifier is helpful if the patient has difficulty being heard.

Supporting Coping Abilities

Support can be given by encouraging the patient and pointing out that activities will be maintained through active participation. A combination of physiotherapy, psychotherapy, medication therapy, and support group participation may help reduce the depression that often occurs.

Patients often feel embarrassed, apathetic, inadequate, bored, and lonely. These feelings may be due, in part, to physical slowness and the great effort that even small tasks require. The patient is assisted and encouraged to set achievable goals (e.g., improvement of mobility).

Because PD can lead to withdrawal and depression, patients must be active participants in their therapeutic program, including social and recreational events. A planned program of activity throughout the day prevents too much daytime sleeping as well as disinterest and apathy.

Every effort should be made to encourage patients to carry out the tasks involved in meeting their own daily needs and to remain independent. Doing things for the patient merely to save time undermines the basic goal of improving coping abilities and promoting a positive self-concept.

ALZHEIMER DISEASE

Alzheimer disease (AD) is the most common type of dementia. This disease is a progressive, irreversible, degenerative neurologic disease that begins insidiously and is characterized by gradual losses of cognitive function and disturbances in behavior and affect. Although AD can occur in people as young as 40 years of age, it is uncommon before 65 years of age. AD can be classified into two types: familial, or early-onset AD, and sporadic, or late-onset AD. Familial AD is rare, accounting for only 5% to 10% of all cases, and is frequently associated with genetic mutations (four susceptible genes have been identified). It occurs in middle-aged adults. If family members have at least one other relative with AD, then there is a familial component, which nonspecifically includes both environmental triggers and genetic determinants. Sporadic AD generally occurs in people older than 65 years of age, and it has no obvious pattern of inheritance.

Pathophysiology

Specific neuropathologic and biochemical changes are found in patients with AD. These include neurofibrillary tangles (tangled masses of nonfunctioning neurons) and senile or neuritic plaques (deposits of amyloid protein, part of a larger protein called amyloid precursor protein [APP]) in the brain. The neuronal damage occurs primarily in the cerebral cortex and results in brain atrophy. Similar changes are found in the normal brain tissue of older adults, but to a lesser extent. Cells that use the neurotransmitter acetylcholine are those principally affected by AD. Biochemically, the enzyme active in producing acetylcholine, which is specifically involved in memory processing, is decreased.

Clinical Manifestations and Assessment

In the early stages of AD, forgetfulness and subtle memory loss occur. Patients may experience small difficulties in work or social activities but have adequate cognitive function to hide the loss and function independently. Depression may occur. With further progression of AD, the deficits can no longer be concealed. Forgetfulness is manifested in many daily actions; patients may lose their ability to recognize familiar faces, places, and objects, and they may become lost in a familiar environment. They may repeat the same stories because they forget that they have already told them. Trying to reason with people with AD and using reality **orientation** only increases their anxiety without increasing function. Conversation becomes difficult, and word-finding difficulties occur. The ability to formulate concepts and think abstractly disappears; for example, a patient can interpret a proverb only in concrete terms. Patients are often unable to recognize the consequences of their actions and, therefore, will exhibit impulsive behavior. For example, on a hot day, a patient may decide to wade in the city fountain fully clothed. Patients have difficulty with everyday activities, such as operating simple appliances and handling money.

Personality changes are also usually evident. Patients may become depressed, suspicious, paranoid, hostile, and even combative. Progression of the disease intensifies the symptoms: speaking skills deteriorate to nonsense syllables, agitation and physical activity increase, and patients may wander at night. Eventually, assistance is needed for most ADLs, including eating and toileting, because dysphagia and incontinence develop. The late stages, in which patients are usually immobile and require total care, may last months or years. Occasionally, patients may recognize family members or caregivers. Death occurs as a result of complications, such as pneumonia, malnutrition, or dehydration.

A definitive diagnosis of AD is made based on meeting the clinical criteria and histologic evidence based on examination of brain tissue obtained from biopsy or autopsy. The most important goal is to rule out other causes of dementia or reversible causes of confusion, such as other types of dementia, depression, delirium, alcohol or drug use, or inappropriate drug dosage or drug toxicity. Refer to Table 45-3 for a summary of differences between AD and delirium.

The health history–including medical history, family history, social and cultural history, and medication history–and the physical examination, including functional and mental health status, are essential to the diagnosis of probable AD. Diagnostic tests, including complete blood count, chemistry profile, and vitamin B_{12} and thyroid hormone levels, as well as screening with EEG, CT, MRI, and examination of the CSF may all refute or support a diagnosis of probable AD.

Depression can closely mimic early-stage AD and coexists in many patients. A depression scale is helpful in screening for underlying depression. Tests of cognitive function, such as the Mini-Mental Status Examination and the clock-drawing test, are useful for screening. CT scans and MRIs of the brain are useful for excluding hematoma, brain tumor, stroke, normal-pressure hydrocephalus, and atrophy but are not reliable in making a definitive diagnosis of AD. Infections, physiologic disturbances such as hypothyroidism, PD, and vitamin B_{12} deficiency can cause cognitive impairment that may be misdiagnosed as AD. Biochemical abnormalities can be excluded through examination of the blood and CSF, but the findings are not sufficiently specific to make the diagnosis. AD is a diagnosis of exclusion, and a diagnosis of probable AD is made when the medical history, physical examination, and laboratory tests have excluded all known causes of other dementias.

Medical and Nursing Management

The primary goal in the medical management of AD is to manage the cognitive and behavioral symptoms. There is

TABLE **45-3 Summary of Differences Between Alzheimer Disease and Delirium**

	Alzheimer Disease (AD)	Delirium
Etiology	Familial (genetic [chromosomes 1, 14, 21]) Sporadic	Drug toxicity and interactions; acute disease; trauma; chronic disease exacerbation Fluid and electrolyte disorder
Risk factors	Advanced age; genetics (apoE4 gene)	Preexisting cognitive impairment
Occurrence	50–60% of dementias	20% of hospitalized older people
Onset	Slow, progressive	Rapid, acute onset A harbinger of acute medical illness (e.g., pneumonia, urinary tract infection, myocardial infarction, pain)
Age of onset (years)	Early onset AD: 30–65 years of age Late onset AD: 65+ years of age Most common: 85+ years of age	Any age but predominantly in older people (over 65 years of age) (Rohatgi et al., 2021).
Sex	Males and females equally	Males and females equally
Course	Chronic, irreversible; progressive, regular, downhill	Acute
Duration	2–20 years	Lasts 1 day to 1 month
Symptom progress	Onset insidious. *Early:* Mild and subtle *Middle and late:* Intensified Progression to death (infection or malnutrition)	Symptoms are fully reversible with adequate treatment; can progress to chronicity or death if underlying condition is ignored.
Mood	Early depression (30%)	Variable
Speech/language	Speech remains intact until late in disease *Early:* Mild anomia (cannot name objects); deficits progress until speech lacks meaning; echoes and repeats words and sounds; mutism	Fluctuating; often cannot concentrate long enough to speak
Physical signs	*Early:* No motor deficits *Middle:* Apraxia (70%) (cannot perform purposeful movement) *Late:* Dysarthria (impaired speech) *End stage:* Loss of all voluntary activity; positive neurologic signs	Signs and symptoms of underlying disease
Orientation	Becomes lost in familiar places (topographic disorientation) Has difficulty drawing three-dimensional objects (visual and spatial disorientation) Disorientation to time, place, and person with disease progression	May fluctuate between lucidity and complete disorientation to time, place, and person
Memory	Loss is an early sign of AD; loss of recent memory is soon followed by progressive decline in remote memory as well	Impaired recent and remote memory; may fluctuate between lucidity and confusion
Personality	Apathy, indifference, irritability *Early:* Social behavior intact; hides cognitive deficits *Late:* Disengages from activity and relationships; suspicious; paranoid delusions caused by memory loss; aggressive; catastrophic reactions	Fluctuating; cannot focus attention to converse; alarmed by symptoms (when lucid); hallucinations; paranoid
Functional status, activities of daily living	Poor judgment in everyday activities; has progressive decline in ability to handle money, use telephone, function in home and workplace	Impaired

	Alzheimer Disease (AD)	Delirium
Attention span	Distractable; short attention span	Highly impaired; cannot maintain or shift attention
Psychomotor activity	Wandering, hyperactivity, pacing, restlessness, agitation	Variable; alternatives between high agitation, hyperactivity, restlessness, and lethargy
Sleep–wake cycle	Often impaired; wandering and agitation at nighttime	Takes brief naps throughout day and night

no cure and no way to slow the progression of the disease. Cholinesterase inhibitors, such as donepezil hydrochloride, rivastigmine tartrate, and galantamine hydrobromide, enhance acetylcholine uptake in the brain, thus maintaining memory skills for a period of time. The drug memantine is an N-methyl-D-aspartate receptor antagonist that is thought to interfere with glutaminergic overstimulation. Cognitive ability improves within 6 to 12 months of therapy, but cessation of the medications results in cognitive decline commensurate with disease progression.

Behavioral problems, such as agitation and psychosis, can be managed by behavioral and psychosocial therapies. Providing an environment that is controlled and stable can help with behavior problems. Pharmacologic treatment for psychosis in patients with AD can be complicated; there is a black box warning by the FDA that both conventional and atypical antipsychotics can increase the risk of death (Ballard et al., 2020). Assessment and diagnosis of depression should occur during the initial evaluation. Associated depression can be treated with antidepressants.

Nursing interventions for AD are aimed at promoting patient function and independence for as long as possible. Other important goals include promoting the patient's physical safety, promoting independence in self-care activities, reducing anxiety and agitation, improving communication, providing for socialization and intimacy, promoting adequate nutrition, promoting balanced activity and rest, and supporting and educating family caregivers.

Supporting Cognitive Function

Because dementia of any type is degenerative and progressive, patients display a decline in cognitive function over time. In the early phase of AD, minimal cueing and guidance may be all that are needed for the patient to function fairly independently for a number of years. However, as the patient's cognitive ability declines, family members must provide more and more assistance and supervision. A calm, predictable environment helps people with AD interpret their surroundings and activities. Environmental stimuli are limited, and a regular routine is established. A quiet, pleasant manner of speaking, clear and simple explanations, and use of memory aids and cues help minimize confusion and disorientation and give patients a sense of security. Prominently displayed clocks and calendars may enhance orientation to time. Color-coding the doorway may help patients who have difficulty locating their room. Active participation may help patients maintain cognitive, functional, and social interaction abilities for a longer period.

Promoting Physical Safety

A safe home environment allows the patient to move about as freely as possible and relieves the family of constant worry about safety. To prevent falls and other injuries, all obvious hazards are removed, and hand rails are installed. A hazard-free environment allows the patient maximum independence and a sense of autonomy. Adequate lighting, especially in halls, stairs, and bathrooms, is necessary. Night lights are helpful, particularly if the patient has increased confusion at night (**sundowning**). Driving is prohibited, and smoking is allowed only with supervision. The patient may have a short attention span and be forgetful. Wandering behavior can often be reduced by gentle persuasion or distraction. Restraints should be avoided because they increase agitation. Doors leading from the house must be secured. Outside the home, all activities must be supervised to protect the patient, and the patient should wear an identification bracelet or neck chain in case they become separated from the caregiver.

Promoting Independence in Self-Care Activities

Pathophysiologic changes in the brain make it difficult for people with AD to maintain physical independence. Patients should be assisted to remain functionally independent for as long as possible. One way to do this is to simplify daily activities by organizing them into short, achievable steps so that the patient experiences a sense of accomplishment. Frequently, occupational therapists can suggest ways to simplify tasks or recommend adaptive equipment. Direct patient supervision is sometimes necessary, but maintaining personal dignity and autonomy is important for people with AD, who should be encouraged to make choices when appropriate and to participate in self-care activities as much as possible.

Reducing Anxiety and Agitation

Despite profound cognitive losses, patients are sometimes aware of their diminishing abilities. Patients need constant emotional support that reinforces a positive self-image. When losses of skills occur, goals are adjusted to fit the patient's declining ability.

The environment should be kept familiar and noise-free. Excitement and confusion can be upsetting and may precipitate a combative, agitated state known as a *catastrophic reaction* (overreaction to excessive stimulation). The patient may respond by screaming, crying, or becoming abusive (physically or verbally); this may be the person's only way of expressing an inability to cope with the environment. When this occurs, it is important to remain calm and unhurried. Forcing the patient to proceed with the activity only increases the agitation. It is better to postpone the activity until later, even to another day. Frequently, the patient quickly forgets what triggered the reaction. Measures such as moving to a familiar environment, listening to music, stroking, rocking, or distraction may quiet the patient. Structuring activity is also helpful. Becoming familiar with a particular patient's predicted responses to certain stressors helps caregivers avoid similar situations.

Many older people with AD who have progressed to the late stages of the disease typically reside in nursing homes and are predominantly cared for by nurses' aides. Dementia education for caregivers is essential to minimize patient agitation and can be effectively taught by advanced practice nurses.

Improving Communication

To promote the patient's interpretation of messages, the nurse should remain unhurried and reduce noises and distractions. Use of clear, easy-to-understand sentences to convey messages is essential because patients frequently forget the meaning of words or have difficulty organizing and expressing thoughts. In the earlier stages of AD, lists and simple written instructions that serve as reminders may be helpful. In later stages, the patient may be able to point to an object or use nonverbal language to communicate. Tactile stimuli, such as hugs or hand pats, are usually interpreted as signs of affection, concern, and security.

Providing for Socialization and Intimacy Needs

Because socialization with friends can be comforting, visits, letters, and phone calls are encouraged. Visits should be brief and nonstressful; limiting visitors to one or two at a time helps reduce overstimulation. Recreation is important, and people with AD are encouraged to enjoy simple activities. Realistic goals for activities that provide satisfaction are appropriate. Hobbies and activities, such as walking, exercising, and socializing, can improve the quality of life. The nonjudgmental friendliness of a pet may provide stimulation, comfort, and contentment. Care of plants or of a pet can also be satisfying and an outlet for energy.

AD does not eliminate the need for intimacy. Patients and their spouses may continue to enjoy sexual activity. Spouses should be encouraged to talk about any sexual concerns, and sexual counseling may be necessary. Simple expressions of love, such as touching and holding, are often meaningful.

Promoting Adequate Nutrition

Mealtime can be a pleasant social occasion or a time of upset and distress, and it should be kept simple and calm, without confrontations. Patients prefer familiar foods that look appetizing and taste good. To avoid any "playing" with food, one dish is offered at a time. Food is cut into small pieces to prevent choking. Liquids may be easier to swallow if they are converted to gelatin. Hot food and beverages are served warm, and the temperature of the foods should be checked to prevent burns.

When lack of coordination interferes with self-feeding, adaptive equipment is helpful. Some patients may do well eating with a spoon or with their fingers. If this is the case, an apron or a smock, rather than a bib, is used to protect clothing. As deficits progress, it may be necessary to feed the patient. Forgetfulness, disinterest, dental problems, lack of coordination, overstimulation, and choking may all serve as barriers to good nutrition and hydration.

Promoting Balanced Activity and Rest

Many patients with AD exhibit sleep disturbances, wandering, and behaviors that may be considered inappropriate. These behaviors are most likely to occur when there are unmet underlying physical or psychological needs. Caregivers must identify the needs of patients who are exhibiting these behaviors because further health decline may occur if the source of the problem is not corrected. Adequate sleep and physical exercise are essential. If sleep is interrupted or the patient cannot fall asleep, music, warm milk, or a back rub may help the patient to relax. During the day, patients should be encouraged to participate in exercise because a regular pattern of activity and rest enhances nighttime sleep. Long periods of daytime sleeping are discouraged.

Caregiver Burden

The emotional burden on the families of patients with AD is enormous. The physical health of the patient is often very stable, and the mental degeneration is gradual. Family members are faced with numerous difficult decisions (e.g., when the patient should stop driving, when to assume responsibility for the patient's financial affairs). Aggression and hostility exhibited by the patient are often misunderstood by families or caregivers, who feel unappreciated, frustrated, and angry. Feelings of guilt, nervousness, and worry contribute to caregiver fatigue, depression, and family dysfunction.

In some cases, caregivers themselves can become so fatigued as a result of the stress of caregiving that self-neglect or neglect or abuse of the patient can occur. This has been documented in home situations as well as in institutions. Respite care is a commonly provided service in which caregivers can get away from the home for short periods while someone else tends to the needs of the patient.

Amyotrophic Lateral Sclerosis

Amyotrophic lateral sclerosis (ALS) is a degenerative disease characterized by the loss of both upper and lower motor neurons. As motor neuron cells die, the muscle fibers that they supply undergo atrophic changes. Causes of ALS include multiple genetic and environmental factors (Springer, 2020). It is estimated that 90% of cases of ALS occur sporadically, but 5% to 10% are familial, usually with an autosomal dominant mode of inheritance (Shaw, 2019).

Clinical Manifestations and Assessment

Clinical manifestations depend on the location of the affected motor neurons because specific neurons activate specific muscle fibers. The chief symptoms are fatigue and limb weakness. There is a gradual onset of asymmetric, progressive weakness. Upper extremity onset causes reduced dexterity, and lower extremity symptoms may be tripping, falling, and changes in gait (Springer, 2020). Spasticity usually is present, and the deep tendon stretch reflexes become brisk and overactive. Usually, the function of the anal and bladder sphincters remains intact because the spinal nerves that control muscles of the rectum and urinary bladder are not affected.

In about 25% of patients, weakness starts in the muscles supplied by the cranial nerves, and difficulty in talking, swallowing, and, ultimately, breathing occurs. When the patient ingests liquids, soft palate and upper esophageal weakness cause the liquid to be regurgitated through the nose. Weakness of the posterior tongue and palate impairs the ability to laugh, cough, or even blow the nose. If bulbar muscles are impaired, speaking and swallowing are progressively difficult, and aspiration becomes a risk. The voice assumes a nasal sound, and articulation becomes so disrupted that speech is unintelligible. Some emotional lability may be present, but intellectual function is not impaired. Eventually, respiratory function is compromised.

The prognosis generally is based on the area of CNS involvement and the speed with which the disease progresses. Death usually occurs as a result of infection, respiratory failure, or aspiration.

ALS is diagnosed on the basis of the signs and symptoms because no clinical or laboratory tests are specific for this disease. An electromyogram (EMG) will demonstrate fibrillations, which are signs of denervation, muscle wasting, and atrophy (Shaw, 2019). An MRI scan may show high signal intensity in the corticospinal tracts; this differentiates ALS from a multifocal motor neuropathy.

Medical and Nursing Management

No specific therapy exists for ALS. The main focus of management is on interventions to maintain or improve function, well-being, and quality of life.

Most patients with ALS are managed at home and in the community, with hospitalization for acute problems. The most common reasons for hospitalization are dehydration and malnutrition, pneumonia, and respiratory failure; recognizing these problems at an early stage in the illness allows for the development of preventive strategies.

Riluzole, a glutamate antagonist, is the only drug approved by the FDA. A dose of 100 mg/day (50 mg BID) provides a modest improvement in the survival rate (additional 3 months of survival) (Shaw, 2019). The action of riluzole is not clear, but its pharmacologic properties suggest that it may have a neuroprotective effect in the early stages of ALS. Liver function tests should be monitored at baseline and monthly.

Symptomatic treatment and rehabilitative measures are employed to support the patient. Baclofen, dantrolene sodium, or diazepam may be useful for patients troubled by spasticity, which causes pain and interferes with self-care.

A patient experiencing problems with aspiration and swallowing may require enteral feeding. The American Academy of Neurology practice guidelines suggest the placement of a percutaneous endoscopic gastrostomy tube before the forced vital capacity drops below 50% of the predicted value.

Pearls for Practice

The nurse observes for paradoxical movement of the abdominal wall during inspiration, SOB, and orthopnea, which may be associated with diaphragmatic weakness. Complaints of interrupted sleep, morning headaches, anorexia, and daytime somnolence may reflect nocturnal retention of carbon dioxide.

Respiratory management is guided by the results of vital capacity and negative inspiratory force parameters that are measured at regular intervals. The use of noninvasive positive-pressure ventilation (NPPV) is started as indicated by these measurements (discussed in Chapters 8 and 54). NPPV can be provided in the form of continuous positive airway pressure (CPAP) and bilevel NPPV using face or nasal masks. As the disease progresses, the NPPV will become inadequate, and, if the decision is made to have life prolonged with advanced technology, the patient can proceed to tracheotomy and invasive ventilation (Shaw, 2019).

Decisions about life-support measures are made by the patient and family and should be based on a thorough understanding of the disease, the prognosis, and the implications of initiating such therapy. Patients are encouraged to complete an advance directive or "living will" to preserve their autonomy in decision making.

Degenerative Disk Disease

Low back pain is a significant public health disorder in the United States, although its prevalence is difficult to quantify. Acute low back pain lasts less than 3 months, whereas chronic or degenerative disease has a duration of 3 months or longer (see Chapter 40 for low back pain). It is estimated that disk disease, such as protrusion, accounts for only 5% of all low back problems, whereas degenerative changes are commonly associated with low back pain.

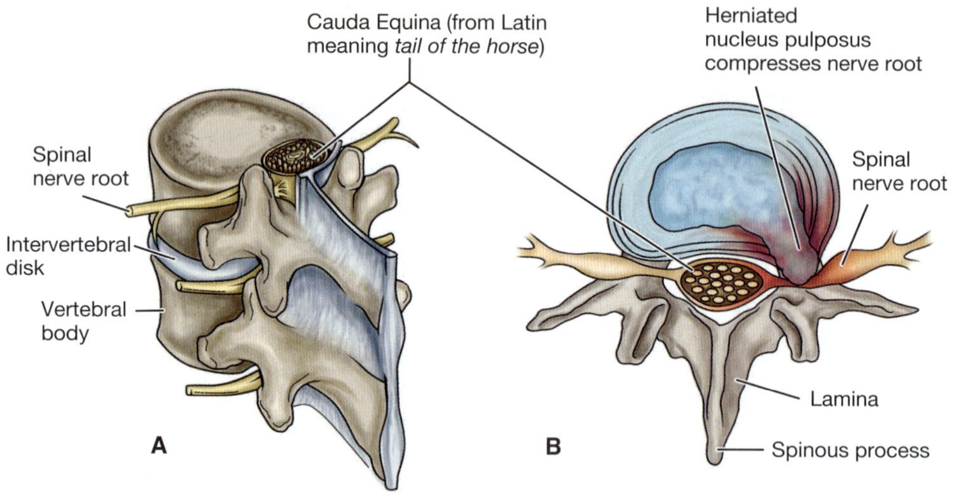

FIGURE 45-10 **A. Normal lumbar spine vertebrae, invertebral disks, and spinal nerve root. B. Ruptured vertebral disk.**

Pathophysiology

The intervertebral disk is a cartilaginous plate that forms a cushion between the vertebral bodies (see Fig. 45-10A). This tough, fibrous material is incorporated in a capsule. A ball-like cushion in the center of the disk is called the *nucleus pulposus.* In herniation of the intervertebral disk (ruptured disk), the nucleus of the disk protrudes into the annulus (the fibrous ring around the disk), with subsequent nerve compression. Protrusion or rupture of the nucleus pulposus usually is preceded by degenerative changes that occur with aging. Loss of protein polysaccharides in the disk decreases the water content of the nucleus pulposus. The development of radiating cracks in the annulus weakens resistance to nucleus herniation. After trauma (falls and repeated minor stresses such as lifting incorrectly), the cartilage may be injured.

For most patients, the immediate symptoms of trauma are short-lived, and those resulting from injury to the disk do not appear for months or years. Then, with degeneration in the disk, the capsule pushes back into the spinal canal, or it may rupture and allow the nucleus pulposus to be pushed back against the dural sac or against a spinal nerve as it emerges from the spinal column (see Fig. 45-10B). This sequence produces pain due to **radiculopathy** (pressure in the area of distribution of the involved nerve endings). Continued pressure may produce degenerative changes in the involved nerve, such as changes in sensation and deep tendon reflexes

Clinical Manifestations and Assessment

Common clinical manifestations are pain, motor and sensory deficits, and alterations of reflexes. A neurologic examination is carried out to determine whether motor, sensory, or reflex impairment from root compression is present and to provide a baseline for future assessment.

MRI has become the diagnostic tool of choice for localizing even small disk protrusions, particularly for lumbar spine disease. If the clinical symptoms are not consistent with the pathology seen on MRI, then CT scanning and myelography are performed. EMG may be used to localize the specific spinal nerve roots involved.

Medical and Nursing Management

Most cases may improve with conservative treatment consisting of 1 to 2 days of bed rest, analgesics, nonsteroidal anti-inflammatory drugs (NSAIDs), progressive exercise, and patient education (Strayer, 2020).

Surgery is usually indicated if the degenerative disk is causing compression on the spinal cord or if the patient has radiculopathy that fails conservative treatment. The most common procedure is a decompression laminectomy, which is the removal of the laminar portion of the vertebrae to gain access to the spinal cord.

INTERVERTEBRAL DISK HERNIATION

CERVICAL SPINE

The cervical spine is subjected to stresses that result from disk degeneration (due to aging, occupational stresses) and **spondylosis** (degenerative changes occurring in a disk and adjacent vertebral bodies with bulging and, occasionally, herniation). Cervical disk degeneration may lead to lesions that can cause damage to the spinal cord and its roots.

Clinical Manifestations and Assessment

A cervical disk herniation usually occurs at the C5–C6 and C6–C7 interspaces. Pain and stiffness may occur in the neck, the top of the shoulders, and the region of the scapulae. Sometimes patients interpret these signs as symptoms of heart trouble or bursitis. Pain may also occur in the upper extremities and head, accompanied by **paresthesia** (tingling or a "pins and needles" sensation) and numbness of the upper extremities. Cervical MRI usually confirms the diagnosis.

Medical and Nursing Management

The goals of treatment are to rest and immobilize the cervical spine to give the soft tissues time to heal and to reduce inflammation in the supporting tissues and the affected nerve roots in the cervical spine. Bed rest (usually 1 to 2 days) is important because it eliminates the stress of gravity and relieves the cervical spine of the need to support the head. It also reduces inflammation and edema in soft tissues around the disk, relieving pressure on the nerve roots. Proper positioning on a firm mattress may bring dramatic relief from pain.

The cervical spine may be rested and immobilized by a cervical collar. A collar allows maximal opening of the intervertebral foramina and holds the head in a neutral or slightly flexed position. The patient may have to wear the collar 24 hours a day during the acute phase. The skin under the collar is inspected for irritation. After the patient is free of pain, cervical isometric exercises are begun to strengthen the neck muscles.

Analgesic agents (e.g., NSAIDs, acetaminophen) are often necessary to manage pain. Narcotics (e.g., hydrocodone/acetaminophen) are reserved for severe pain. Sedatives may be administered to control the anxiety that is often associated with cervical disk disease. Muscle relaxants (cyclobenzaprine, methocarbamol, metaxalone) are administered to interrupt muscle spasm and to promote comfort. NSAIDs (aspirin, ibuprofen, naproxen) or corticosteroids are prescribed to treat the inflammation that usually occurs in the affected nerve roots and supporting tissues. Occasionally, a corticosteroid is injected into the epidural space for relief of radicular (spinal nerve root) pain. Hot, moist compresses (for 10 to 20 minutes) applied to the back of the neck several times daily increase blood flow to the muscles and help relax the patient and reduce muscle spasm.

Surgical excision of the herniated disk may be necessary if there is a significant neurologic deficit, progression of the deficit, evidence of cord compression, or pain that either worsens or fails to improve. A cervical discectomy, with or without fusion, may be performed to alleviate symptoms. An anterior surgical approach may be used through a transverse incision to remove disk material that has herniated into the spinal canal and foramina, or a posterior approach may be used at the appropriate level of the cervical spine. Potential complications with the anterior approach include carotid or vertebral artery injury, recurrent laryngeal nerve dysfunction, esophageal perforation, and airway obstruction. Complications of the posterior approach include damage to the nerve root or the spinal cord due to retraction or contusion of either of these structures, resulting in weakness of muscles supplied by the nerve root or cord.

Microsurgery, such as endoscopic microdiscectomy, may be performed in selected patients through a small incision and using magnification techniques. The patient who undergoes microsurgery usually has less tissue trauma and pain and consequently a shorter hospital stay than after conventional surgical approaches.

Pearls for Practice

Although NSAIDs are often prescribed for cervical disk herniation, when surgery involving bone fusion is considered, NSAIDs are often discontinued because they can interfere with bone healing. The nurse should collaborate with the health care provider to instruct the patient to avoid these drugs prior to and after surgery.

LUMBAR SPINE

The most common site of lumbar disk herniation occurs at the L4–L5 or L5–S1 levels (Strayer, 2020). A herniated lumbar disk causes low back pain accompanied by varying degrees of motor and sensory impairment.

Clinical Manifestations and Assessment

The patient complains of low back pain with muscle spasms, followed by radiation of the pain into one hip and down into the leg (sciatica). Pain is aggravated by actions that increase intraspinal fluid pressure, such as bending, lifting, or straining (as in sneezing or coughing), and usually is relieved by bed rest. Usually there is some type of postural deformity because pain causes an alteration of the normal spinal mechanics. If the patient lies on the back and attempts to raise a leg in a straight position, pain radiates into the leg; this maneuver, called the *straight leg–raising test*, stretches the sciatic nerve. Additional signs include muscle weakness, alterations in tendon reflexes, and sensory loss.

The diagnosis of lumbar disk disease is based on the history and physical findings and the use of imaging techniques, such as MRI, CT, and myelography. Although MRI has largely replaced myelography (fluoroscopy and an injection of contrast material to evaluate the spinal cord, nerve roots and spinal lining), myelography still may be used occasionally to provide information about the spinal cord and nerve roots.

Medical and Nursing Management

The objectives of treatment are to relieve pain, slow disease progression, and increase the patient's functional ability. Bed rest for patients with severe pain in the lumbar region is limited to a short course (2 days or less), followed by resumption of light activity (Strayer, 2020).

Strategies for increasing the patient's functional ability include weight reduction, physical therapy, and biofeedback. Mobilization by walking short distances is recommended. When symptoms subside, stretching, strengthening, and exercise programs should be initiated.

Because muscle spasm is prominent during the acute phase, muscle relaxants are used. NSAIDs and systemic corticosteroids may be administered to counter the inflammation that usually occurs in the supporting tissues and the affected nerve roots. Moist heat and massage help to relax muscles.

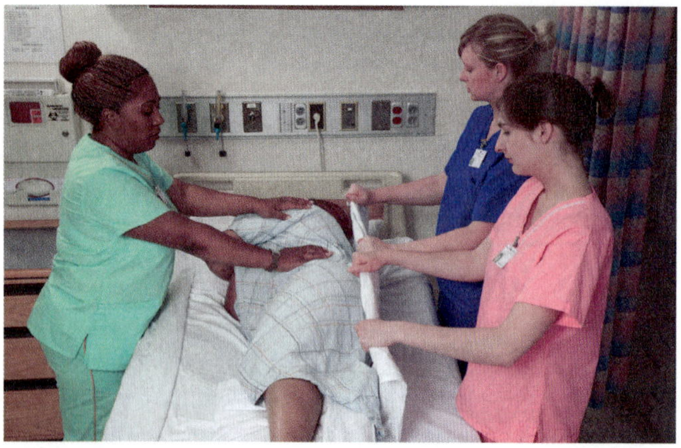

FIGURE 45-11 **Before the patient undergoes spinal surgery, the logrolling technique that will be used for turning the patient should be demonstrated. The patient's arms will be crossed and the spine aligned. To avoid twisting the spine, the patient's head, shoulders, knees, and hips are turned at the same time that the patient rolls over like a log. When in a side-lying position, the patient's back, buttocks, and legs are supported with pillows.**

Most patients fear surgery on any part of the spine and therefore need explanations about the surgery and reassurance that it will not weaken the back. When data are being collected for the health history, any reports of pain, paresthesia, or muscle spasm are recorded to provide a baseline for comparison after surgery. Preoperative assessment also includes an evaluation of movement of the extremities, as well as bladder and bowel function. To facilitate the postoperative turning procedure, the patient is taught to turn as a unit (called *logrolling*) as part of the preoperative preparation (Fig. 45-11). Before surgery, the patient is also encouraged to take deep breaths, cough, and perform muscle-setting exercises to maintain muscle tone.

In the lumbar region, surgical treatment includes lumbar disk excision through a posterolateral laminotomy and the techniques of microdiscectomy and percutaneous discectomy. In microdiscectomy, an operating microscope is used to visualize the offending disk and compressed nerve roots; it permits a small incision (2.5 cm [1 in]) and minimal blood loss and takes about 30 minutes of operating time. In general, the hospital stay is short, and the patient makes a rapid recovery. Percutaneous discectomy is an alternative treatment for herniated intervertebral disks of the lumbar spine. One approach in current use is through a 2.5-cm (1-in) incision just above the iliac crest. A tube, trocar, or cannula is inserted under x-ray guidance through the retroperitoneal space to the involved disk space. Special instruments are used to remove the disk. The operating time is about 15 minutes. Blood loss and postoperative pain are minimal, and usually the patient is discharged within 2 days after surgery. The disadvantage of this procedure is the possibility of damage to structures in the surgical pathway.

Complications that could occur after surgery include herniation relapse, arachnoiditis (inflammation of the arachnoid), neuritis (inflammation of a nerve), or failed disk syndrome (generalized term to describe continued **pain after surgery**). Herniation relapse may occur at the same level or elsewhere so the patient may become a candidate for another disk procedure. Arachnoiditis may occur after surgery (and after myelography [if used]); it involves an insidious onset of diffuse, frequently burning pain in the lower back, radiating into the buttocks. Disk excision can leave adhesions and scarring around the spinal nerves and dura, which then produce inflammatory changes that create chronic neuritis and neurofibrosis. Disk surgery may relieve pressure on the spinal nerves, but it does not reverse the effects of neural injury and scarring and the pain that results.

Because postoperative neurologic deficits may occur from nerve root injury, the motor strength and sensation of the lower extremities are evaluated at specified intervals, along with the color and temperature of the legs and sensation of the toes. Assessing the patient after surgery, the nurse checks vital signs frequently, and the wound is inspected for hemorrhage because vascular injury is a complication of disk surgery. It is important to assess for urinary retention, another sign of neurologic deterioration.

In discectomy with fusion, the patient has an additional surgical incision if bone fragments were taken from the iliac crest or fibula to serve as wedges in the spine. The recovery period is longer than for those patients who underwent discectomy without spinal fusion because bony union must take place.

To position the patient, a pillow is placed under the head, and the knee rest is elevated slightly to relax the back muscles. When the patient is lying on one side, however, extreme knee flexion must be avoided. The patient is encouraged to move from side to side to relieve pressure and is reassured that no injury will result from moving. When the patient is ready to turn, the bed is placed in a flat position and a pillow is placed between the patient's legs. The patient turns as a unit (logrolls) without twisting the back. To get out of bed, the patient lies on one side while pushing up to a sitting position. At the same time, the nurse or family member eases the patient's legs over the side of the bed. Coming to a sitting or standing posture is accomplished in one long, smooth motion. Most patients walk to the bathroom on the same day as the surgery. Sitting is discouraged except for defecation.

Clinical Judgment Case

A patient, K.J., is on your orthopedic unit after a motorcycle collision (without helmet) resulting in multiple injuries including three rib fractures (left 9, 10, and 11), right femur fracture, and a concussion. CT scan on admission was negative for cranial fractures or bleed. Today is hospital day 3 and post op day 2 after an open reduction and internal fixation (ORIF) repair of the right femur fracture. You have cared for K.J. for the past 2 days and notice today that the patient is complaining of a headache and some neck pain. You assess vital signs at 8 am which are: T 98.2 °F, P 88 and regular, 24 RR with pulse oximetry of 94% on room air. BP is 138/82. Physical examination reveals S1S2 without murmur, gallop, or rub; lungs show decreased breath sounds to mid on the left, crackles of left lower lobe; trach is deviating slightly to the left; abdomen is soft, nondistended, nontender; bowel sounds (BS)+ in all 4 Q, + flatus; no bowel movement. Tolerating regular diet well, no nausea or vomiting. Pedal and posterior tibial pulses are 3+ bil; there is some RLE peripheral edema, nonpitting; capillary refill is 2 seconds all extremities. Skin is warm and dry with multiple abrasions noted on lower extremities and left temporal area. Pupils equal and reacting to light (PEARL) 3 mm bil. Pt has 5/5 strength in both upper extremities and left lower extremity (unable to assess full strength of right lower extremity [RLE]). Pt is oriented to person, place, time, and situation. Although the neuro status is unchanged, there is a slowness in K.J.'s responses today as compared to yesterday. Morning laboratory data taken at 6 am are as follows: Na of 140 mEq/L, K+ of 3.7 mEq/L, Cl of 98 mEq/L, CO2 25 mEq/L; glucose of 95 mg/dL. Complete blood count (CBC) is pending.

Step One: Recognize cues where relevant and important information is identified from different sources, such as medical history or vital signs.

Answer: Multiple injuries including three rib fractures (left 9, 10, and 11), right femur fracture, and concussion. Negative CT scan, open reduction and internal fixation (ORIF) repair of the right femur fracture. Complaints of a headache and neck pain, sluggish verbal responses, normal pupils, and full strength of ¾ extremities. Respiratory rate of 24 with pulse oximetry of 94% on room air. B/P is 138/82. Decreased breath sounds to mid on the left, crackles of left lower lobe, trach deviated to left, LLE peripheral edema, multiple abrasions noted on lower extremities and left temporal area. Complete blood count (CBC) is pending. Normal electrolytes and glucose.

Step Two: Analyze cues, which is organizing and linking the recognized cues to the patient's clinical presentation.

Answer: You link left rib fractures 9–11 with potential complication of splenic injury and are awaiting the CBC; however, there is no evidence of hypovolemia as there is no tachycardia or hypotension, capillary refill is normal, and skin is warm and dry.

You also link the left rib fractures with decreased left-sided breath sounds, crackles, tachypnea, tracheal deviation, and decreased oxygen saturation on room air with potential atelectasis.

You link the headache, neck pain, and sluggish verbal responses with the concussion and abrasion of left temporal area; although the CT scan was negative on admission, you are concerned about potential rising intracranial pressure (ICP) and seizures. There are no complaints of nausea or vomiting.

Step Three: Form and prioritize hypotheses, where hypotheses are evaluated and ranked according to priority. This can include urgency, likelihood, risk, difficulty, and/or time. In this phase you cluster your findings to arrive at a list of problems (actual and or potential problems) you believe the patient is experiencing and determine the importance or urgency. What do you think is of greatest concern?

Answer: You rank as your highest priority the concern for rising ICP, headache, neck pain, known head trauma (concussion), and the potential for seizures. Your next concern is the potential atelectasis of the left lung related to multiple fractures, increased respiratory rate, tracheal deviation, and decreasing O_2 sat. Although the patient has no symptoms of hypovolemia, you are aware of the risk of splenic lacerations and are awaiting the CBC to assess trending with yesterday's labs.

Step Four: Generate solutions, which is identifying expected outcomes and using hypotheses to define a set of interventions for the expected outcomes.

Answer: Since your priority is the patient's neurological status, you will ensure oxygen and suction are in the room. You will notify the providers of the new complaint of headache and neck pain, sluggish sensorium, and your concern about potential for ICP and seizures. You will also inform them of the lung sound changes, tachypnea, tracheal deviation, decreasing oxygen saturation, the pending CBC (you are assessing for leukocytosis or elevated WBC) and the need for low flow oxygen. You will also note trending of the H/H related to left 9, 10, 11th rib fractures and continue to monitor vital signs.

Step Five: Take action, where the solutions that address the highest priorities are implemented.

Answer: You continue to monitor neuro signs and prepare in case of seizures, which will involve pushing aside furniture that may injure the patient during a seizure, loosening constrictive clothing and padding and raising the side rails. If the patient wears glasses you may remove them if seizures are anticipated. You notified the provider, and a repeat CT scan is ordered stat. The patient is placed on nasal cannula at 2 L, and a repeat chest film is ordered. You will place the patient on their side in case of seizures to prevent aspiration and protect the airway.

Step Six: Evaluate outcomes, which is comparing observed outcomes against expected outcomes.

Answer: The CT scan reveals a small traumatic intracerebral hemorrhage, and the patient is transferred to the neuro step-down area. The CBC came back within normal limits, and the chest x-ray did reveal atelectasis of the left lower lobe. As soon as the patient stabilizes you will teach the patient about the use of incentive spirometry. The patient remained seizure free, but you are prepared for this potential complication and ensured all needed equipment was at the bedside. You alerted the team to your concerns, and you learned that sometimes complications occur after the first 24 hours and you always need to be alert to subtle changes. You did great!

CHAPTER REVIEW

NCLEX-Style Review Questions

1. A patient with a known history of myasthenia gravis is admitted to your unit with concerns over cholinergic crisis. Which of the following symptoms suggests deterioration in the patient's condition? Select all that apply.
   a. Excessive pulmonary secretions
   b. Negative Inspiratory Force (NIF) of –60 mm Hg
   c. Oxygen saturation of 96%
   d. Impaired gag reflex
   e. Poor airway clearance

2. Which of the following symptoms might a nurse expect a patient with MS to report? Select all that apply.
   a. Diarrhea
   b. Loss of balance
   c. Skin infections
   d. Visual disturbances
   e. Limb numbness

3. Which of the following parameters in a patient admitted with Guillain–Barré syndrome suggests the need for mechanical intervention? Select all that apply.
   a. PaO_2 of 55 mm Hg
   b. Difficulty clearing secretions
   c. Adequate gag reflex
   d. Oxygen saturation of 95%
   e. Use of accessory muscles

4. The patient is admitted with new-onset seizures. Your priorities for nursing care during a seizure include which of the following? Select all that apply.
   a. Protect the airway by turning the patient on the side
   b. Elevate the HOB 30 degrees with the patient's head in neutral alignment
   c. Remove eyeglasses, loosen constrictive clothing
   d. Administer antiseizure medications PO
   e. Administer antiseizure medications IV

5. The nurse knows that the signs and symptoms of meningeal irritation include which of the following? Select all that apply.
   a. Nuchal rigidity and headache
   b. Kernig and Brudzinski signs
   c. Aphasia and motor weakness
   d. Photophobia
   e. Ptosis

REFERENCES AND SELECTED READINGS

References and selected readings associated with this chapter can be found on the website that accompanies the book. Visit **http://thepoint.lww.com/Honan3e** to access the references and other additional resources associated with this chapter.

CHAPTER 46

Nursing Management: Patients With Cerebrovascular Disorders

Karin V. Nyström • Jennifer Picagli • Dawn Wicker

Learning Objectives

After reading this chapter you will be able to:

1. Describe the incidence and epidemiology of stroke.
2. Identify mechanisms that affect cerebral blood flow.
3. Describe the pathophysiology of ischemic and hemorrhagic stroke and transient ischemic attack.
4. Identify risk factors and manifestations of stroke syndromes.
5. Describe collaborative care and drug and mechanical intervention therapies for patients presenting with an acute stroke.
6. Describe the acute care, rehabilitation, drug, and nutritional considerations for patients recovering from stroke.

Cerebrovascular disorder is an umbrella term that refers to abnormalities of the central nervous system (CNS) affecting normal blood supply to the brain and/or spinal cord. There are many vascular abnormalities affecting cerebral blood flow, but the most common cerebrovascular disorder is stroke. The nurse should be well prepared to recognize stroke symptoms, to prompt urgent actions for treatment/management, to care for patients admitted to an acute care facility with a stroke, and to identify the common comorbidities that accompany stroke syndromes. Nurses are also well situated to coordinate secondary prevention strategies as part of stroke education and to assist with transitioning patients back into the community. Nurses work with stroke patients in settings including emergency departments, neurology and hospitalist services, rehabilitation facilities, home care, and outpatient offices. In some cases, the stroke is a precipitating event, bringing a patient into the health care system after a long absence or nonengagement. As such, nurses must be able to develop a plan of care for a stroke patient's recovery that considers both neurologic deficits and potential complications associated with those deficits during both acute recovery and rehabilitation. In addition, the plan should include important stroke prevention strategies, such as pharmacotherapies and lifestyle changes, applicable to patients who have had a stroke as well as for other patient populations at risk for a cerebrovascular event.

STROKE

Even before Hippocrates coined the term "apoplexy" (meaning "struck down with violence" in Attic Greek) to describe the typical stroke syndrome, Babylonian tablets from the second millennium before common era (BCE) described therapies and prognosis "if a man is suffering from facial paralysis and half of his body is paralyzed" (Reynolds & Wilson, 2014; Schutta, 2021). Only in the 20th century did clinicians begin to understand the pathophysiology of ischemic and hemorrhagic stroke and sort the etiologies of these related but idiosyncratic cerebrovascular disorders. While the presentation of stroke is often dramatic, the etiologies of stroke are primarily related to underlying chronic disease states. Rapid recognition and an organized, multidisciplinary approach to patients in the acute stroke phase is associated with decrease in disability and death. Stroke, however, remains the leading cause of adult disability in the United States (American Heart Association [AHA], 2022).

Incidence

According to the Centers for Disease Control and Prevention (CDC) stroke is currently the fifth leading cause of death in the United States, behind heart disease, cancer, chronic respiratory diseases, and accidents (2019); in persons over 65 years of age and Hispanic, Black, and Asian American and Pacific Islander (AAPI) populations, stroke ranks either third or fourth. Approximately 800,000 people experience a stroke each year in the United States; 600,000 of these are first events, and approximately 200,000 are recurrent strokes. Although there has been a slight decrease in incidence since the 1980s, over 7 million adult Americans report having had a stroke, with a prevalence of just over 3% with wide local variability (Tsao et al., 2022). Stroke is the leading cause of serious, long-term adult disability in the United States. It is estimated that approximately 90% of stroke survivors are left with some residual neurologic deficit. The financial impact of stroke is profound, with estimated direct and indirect costs totaling $103.5 billion (Striliciuc et al., 2021). Although strokes can affect people of all ages, older males are more likely to have strokes and older females more frequently tend to die from their stroke. Approximately 10% of strokes happen to adults between 18 and 50 years old. The impact of hypertension and stroke is three times greater for Black individuals than for White individuals (Levine et al., 2020); however, tight BP control (<130 mm Hg) was associated with a 42% lower incidence of stroke compared with standard BP control (130 to 139 mm Hg) (Tsao et al., 2022). Economic and social disparities increase risk of stroke; in the United States, complex sociohistorical conditions have created a higher prevalence "stroke belt" in the south-eastern states (Palacio et al., 2020; AHA, 2022). See Figure 46-1.

Despite the numerous national campaign efforts to increase stroke awareness over the past three decades, several studies have shown that a majority of people cannot name many of the typical stroke symptoms, confuse stroke symptoms with heart attack symptoms, or do not consider calling emergency services for these symptoms (Duncan et al., 2021; Levine et al., 2020). In addition, when considering the disparities in race related to the incidence of stroke, although research studies reveal that interventions can be effective at increasing awareness of stroke symptoms in Black and Hispanic populations, it is important to recognize that relatively few interventions designed to increase stroke knowledge are targeting non-English speaking populations (Levine et al., 2020). Delays in recognizing stroke symptoms and in activating the Emergency Medical System limit treatment options and lead to worsening long-term recovery outcomes. A variety of local, regional, and national programs have been developed to systematize recognition, triage, and treatment, including Stroke Center certification by the Joint Commission (TJC), the AHA/American Stroke Association "Stroke Chain of Survival," and local prehospital approaches based on specific needs and resources (Fassbender et al., 2020). The Stroke Chain of Survival was fashioned after the Heart Chain of Survival for cardiac care. It consists of a prompt prehospital and acute care approach to the evaluation of patients with suspected acute stroke symptoms. Also known as the "7 D's", these components highlight key areas in the recognition of a patient suspected to be having a stroke to reinforce the efficient method for a rapid series of steps in evaluation and management (see Box 46-1). Strokes continue to be one of the most common neurologic emergencies, and both community hospitals and large tertiary referral medical centers admit a high volume of patients with a stroke-related neurologic diagnosis or patients at risk for stroke. Hospitals today are charged with implementing systems of care to treat stroke patients

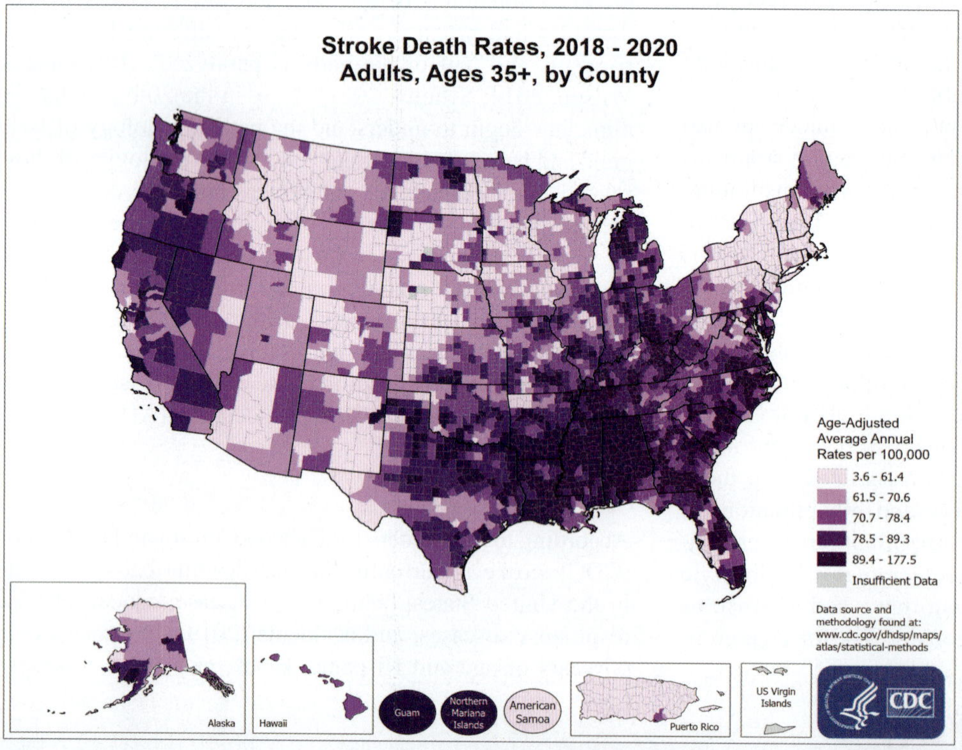

FIGURE 46-1 **Geographic Patterns: Stroke Death Rates for 2018 through 2020 for Adults Aged 35 Years and Older by County. The map shows that concentrations of counties with the highest stroke death rates—meaning the top quintile—are located primarily in the Southeast, with heavy concentrations of high-rate counties in Alabama, Mississippi, Louisiana, Georgia, Kentucky, Tennessee, South Carolina, Arkansas, Guam, and the Northern Mariana Islands. Pockets of high-rate counties are also found in Alaska, Missouri, Oklahoma, Texas, West Virginia, Ohio, Michigan, Indiana, Maryland, North Carolina, and Florida. (Reproduced from the Centers for Disease Control and Prevention, National Center for Chronic Disease Prevention and Health Promotion, Division for Heart Disease and Stroke Prevention. [2022]. Stroke Death Rates, Total Population 35+. https://www.cdc.gov/dhdsp/maps/national_maps/stroke_all.htm)**

BOX 46-1

Stroke Chain of Survival: The 7 D's

1. ***Detection* of the onset of signs and symptoms of acute stroke.** Early recognition of the hallmark signs and symptoms of acute stroke is critical to improved patient outcomes.
2. ***Dispatch* of Emergency Medical Services (EMS) by telephoning 911.** This communication activates EMS systems and ensures prompt EMS response.
3. ***Delivery* of the patient to a medical facility.** The patient should be transported to a stroke hospital or other facility capable of providing acute stroke care, and advanced prehospital notification should be given to the selected medical facility.
4. ***Door* of the emergency department (ED).** Immediately upon arrival, the patient should undergo general and neurologic assessment in the ED.
5. ***Data* collection,** including computer tomography (CT) scan and serial neurologic examinations, along with reviews of the patient's file for potential fibrinolytics (tPA) exclusions.
6. ***Decision* regarding stroke treatment.** If the patient remains a candidate for tissue plasminogen activator (tPA) therapy, review risks and benefits with the patient and family.
7. ***Drug* administration** as appropriate and postadministration monitoring.

in the acute phase of their illness and to direct patients and their families to the appropriate rehabilitative program to optimize recovery and functional outcome (Adeoye et al., 2019).

Pearls for Practice: Lifting the Lens

When considering that mortality rates related to stroke are higher in Black Americans, American Indians, Alaska Natives, Native Hawaiians, and other Pacific Islanders, compared with White Americans, the nurse recognizes that public health interventions and racial equity in care is required to eliminate disparities in health care as all patients should have equal opportunity for health. Interventions must include reducing stroke risk factors (hypertension [prevention/management], diabetes [prevention/management]), increasing awareness of stroke symptoms, and improving social and structural determinants of health such as access to care to promote racial equity in decreasing stroke death rates that exist currently (Levine et al., 2020).

Certified Stroke Centers

In 2003, TJC launched a disease-specific care certification program for medical facilities committed to using evidence-based clinical practice guidelines for best stroke care. TJC's Primary Stroke Center certification program was first developed in collaboration with the American Stroke Association and was based on the 2000 Brain Attack Coalition's "Recommendations for the Establishment of Primary Stroke Centers." In 2011, an update to the recommendation for the establishment of Advanced Primary Stroke Centers as an approach to acute stroke care was published to improve the medical care of stroke patients and included criteria such as an acute stroke team, a dedicated stroke unit, written care protocols, supporting laboratory and imaging services, and mandatory continuing education related to strokes (Alberts et al., 2011). These recommendations followed the 1996 U.S. Food and Drug Administration (FDA) approval of intravenous tissue plasminogen activator (tPA) for the treatment of acute ischemic stroke (NINDS & Stroke rtPA Stroke Study Work Group, 1995). In the past 30 years, intravenous thrombolytic therapy has shown to improve outcomes in patients with acute ischemic stroke if treated within 3 to 4.5 hours from stroke onset and when additional eligibility criteria (discussed later in the chapter) are met. Certified stroke centers are mandated to collect data on a series of specific practice components, including selected performance and outcome measures to monitor and improve the quality of stroke care. These measures apply to patients hospitalized with either an ischemic or hemorrhagic stroke. Currently, 13 stroke performance activities are supported by TJC. Although not inclusive of all important aspects of acute stroke care, initial data from these metrics support the efforts to improve quality of care and to predict functional outcome (Nouh et al., 2022). Table 46-1 outlines the specific stroke performance measures and applicable stroke types.

In the last decade, stroke certification options have expanded to include Acute Stroke Ready Hospitals (for smaller, mostly rural facilities equipped to stabilize and treat acute stroke patients prior to transferring to a higher level of care), Advanced Thrombectomy-capable Stroke Centers (for facilities that meet Advanced Primary Stroke Center criteria and have the capability to perform thrombectomy procedures), and Advanced Comprehensive Stroke Centers (for facilities capable of managing multiple complex stroke patients across the stroke disease trajectory). Today, there are nearly 1,500 hospitals certified as Primary Stroke Centers and over 300 hospitals certified as Comprehensive Stroke Centers (Boggs et al., 2022). Nursing staff working at an advanced certified stroke center will be familiar with evidence-based stroke protocols and will have specific education requirements to maintain their stroke expertise.

Pathophysiology

Stroke is a heterogeneous syndrome characterized by the onset of one or more focal neurologic deficits (corresponding to the affected area of the brain) caused by reduced cerebral blood flow that leads to brain cell death and functional disability. Stroke is now further defined based on both clinical and radiologic features. With advances in computed tomography (CT) and magnetic resonance (MR) imaging, a

TABLE **46-1 Stroke Performance Measures**

Stroke Performance Measures	Stroke Type
NIH Stroke Scale • An initial NIH Stroke Scale score for severity is performed prior to any acute recanalization therapy or within 12 hours of emergency department arrival.	Ischemic stroke
Deep venous thrombosis (DVT) prophylaxis: • Nonambulatory patients should start receiving DVT prophylaxis by the end of day 2	Ischemic stroke Hemorrhagic stroke
Discharged on antithrombotic therapy: • Patients prescribed antithrombotic therapy at discharge	Ischemic stroke
Discharged on anticoagulation for patients in atrial fibrillation: • Patients with atrial fibrillation discharged on anticoagulation	Ischemic stroke
Thrombolytic therapy administered: • Patients with acute ischemic stroke who arrive at the hospital within 120 minutes of time last known well (LKW) and for whom IV tissue plasminogen activator (tPA) was initiated at this hospital within 180 minutes of LKW	Ischemic stroke
Antithrombotic medication by the end of hospital day 2: • Patients received antithrombotic therapy by the end of hospital day 2	Ischemic stroke
Discharged on cholesterol-reducing medication: • Patients with low-density lipoproteins (LDL) above 100 or LDL not measured or on cholesterol-reducer before admission are discharged on cholesterol-reducing drugs	Ischemic stroke
Stroke education: • Patients and caregivers were given education or educational materials prior to discharge to address personal risk factors, stroke warning signs, activation of emergency medical services, need for follow-up after discharge, and medications prescribed	Ischemic stroke Hemorrhagic stroke
Assessed for rehabilitation: • Patients were assessed for rehabilitation	Ischemic stroke Hemorrhagic stroke

stroke can also be defined via radiologic evidence of brain tissue injury, within a shorter time period, and even without clinically evident deficits. The two major stroke types that cause an interruption in cerebral blood flow are an occluded artery that deprives blood flow to part of the brain supplied by that blood vessel (called an *ischemic stroke*, Fig. 46-2), or a ruptured artery resulting in bleeding in or around the brain (called a *hemorrhagic stroke*, Fig. 46-3). Hemorrhagic strokes are further subdivided based on the specific intracranial space that is filled with blood: an intraparenchymal hemorrhage (blood within the brain tissue), and a subarachnoid hemorrhage (SAH) (blood occupying the subarachnoid space). Ischemic strokes account for about 85% of all stroke syndromes. Hemorrhagic strokes account for the remaining 15% (Table 46-2). Regardless of stroke type or mechanism, the concept that **"time is brain"** has become the mainstay for directing a rapid clinical diagnosis and acute treatment options if patients present within a specific time window from the onset of symptoms.

Although patients suffering from an ischemic or hemorrhagic stroke may present with similar neurologic deficits, an initial brain image (i.e., noncontrast head CT) will identify the presence of a hemorrhage shortly after onset; any area of ischemia due to an occluded artery will be typically visible on imaging after 4 to 6 hours from symptom onset. Therefore the rapid diagnosis of an acute ischemic stroke is considered a clinical diagnosis and is based on the patient's presenting symptoms and clinical examination. Treatment options and management will vary depending on stroke type.

Ischemic Stroke

Normally, the brain receives approximately 15% of the total cardiac output. Normal cerebral blood flow is calculated to be 50 to 55 mL of blood per 100 g of brain tissue per minute. For patients who experience an ischemic stroke, disruption of blood flow in or to the brain due to an obstruction of a blood vessel initiates a complex series of circulatory and metabolic events referred to as the *ischemic cascade*. The ischemic cascade begins when cerebral blood flow decreases to less than 25 mL/100 g/min, or about half normal. As neurons are no longer able to maintain aerobic respiration with decreased blood flow, they switch to anaerobic metabolism, which creates a change in cell processes and outputs. These less efficient processes create electrolyte and pH variation which destabilize the cell walls, causing neurons to die (Fig. 46-4). Dead cells closest to the site of the occlusion make up the *core infarct*. The surrounding area of

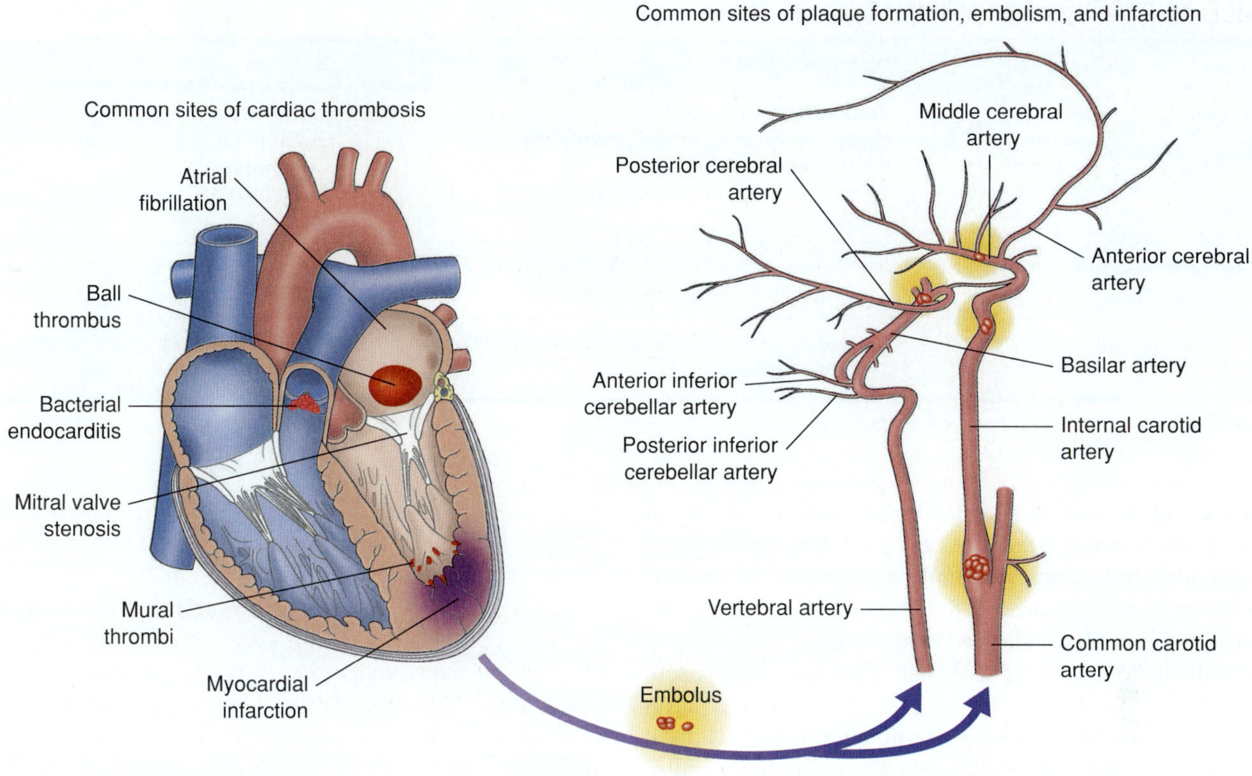

FIGURE 46-2 Ischemic stroke.

affected brain tissue in which blood flow has been reduced is referred to as the *ischemic penumbra*. These cells make up tissue which may be salvageable with rapid treatment to improve local blood flow. In selected patients, the penumbra, or stunned brain tissue, is deemed salvageable with early treatment, such as with thrombolysis (*administration of intravenous thrombolytics*) or with clot retrieval (*using a catheter-based intra-arterial approach to extract the clot*); see Figure 46-5. Specific inclusion and exclusion criteria for the use of these treatment options assist the clinicians in identifying patients who would have the best outcomes after acute stroke.

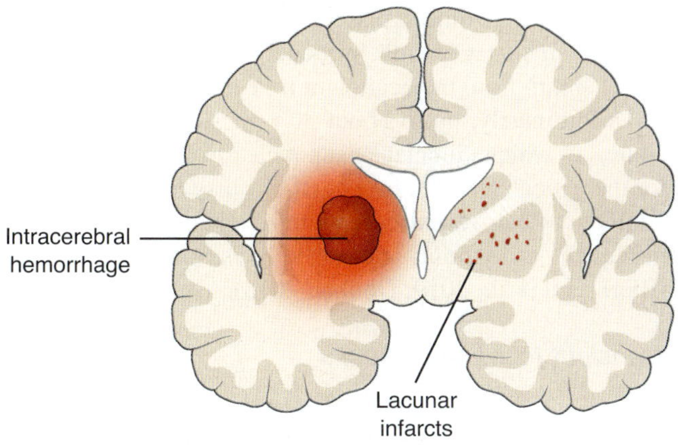

FIGURE 46-3 Common sites of cerebral hemorrhage.

Ischemic strokes are further divided into five subtypes according to a mechanism-based classification system (Adams et al., 1993; Kamel, 2020): large-artery thrombotic strokes (representing 20% of ischemic strokes); small, penetrating artery thrombotic strokes (25%); cardio embolic strokes (20%); cryptogenic strokes (strokes that cannot be attributable to any specific cause) (30%); and "other" (5%). Each stroke subtype has a characteristic pathophysiologic course, but these types have overlapping clinical features. This subtyping directs both therapeutic interventions and long-term prognosis. While the mechanism of the stroke and underlying pathophysiology leading to the stroke vary, the clinical manifestation of the stroke for the patient will depend more strongly on the location of injured brain tissue, rather than the cause.

Large-artery thrombotic strokes are caused by atherosclerotic plaques in the large blood vessels of the brain and/or carotid. Thrombus formation and occlusion occurring at the site of the atherosclerosis can halt blood flow at the site of formation or via embolization, that is, breaking up of the plaque, further "downstream."

Small, penetrating artery thrombotic strokes are also common, occurring in the smaller vessels of the brain, including the brainstem and cerebellum, as well as in deeper brain structures such as the thalamus. In these, the smaller blood vessels have endured damage over time, leading to thrombosis and occlusion. Processes such as longstanding hypertension, hyperlipidemia, diabetes, and some forms of

TABLE **46-2 Comparison of Major Types of Stroke**

Facet	Ischemic	Hemorrhagic
Causes	Large-artery thrombosis Small, penetrating artery thrombosis Cardiogenic embolic Cryptogenic (no known cause) Other	Intracerebral hemorrhage Subarachnoid hemorrhage Cerebral aneurysm Arteriovenous malformation
Main presenting symptoms	Numbness or weakness of the face, arm, or leg, especially on one side of the body	"Exploding headache" Decreased level of consciousness
Additional symptoms	Slurred speech, or difficulty with word finding or comprehension	Nausea/vomiting; visual changes; seizures

Many of these symptoms occur with either stroke type.

autoimmune disease or infection, create injury and inflammation which damage these vessels over time. Small artery thrombotic strokes are frequently referred to as *lacunar strokes or lacunes* because of the small cavities that are created after the death of infarcted brain tissue.

Cardioembolic strokes originate from the heart itself. Emboli, or clots, formed in the heart travel via the carotids and can become lodged in any number of vessels distal to the aortic arch, causing ischemia and infarction. Cardiac arrhythmias, such as atrial fibrillation, are the most common reason for cardiac emboli to form, but disease of the heart valve, including infection, or larger clots in the left ventricle, can also lead to cardioembolic strokes.

Pearls for Practice

Atrial fibrillation is the most common type of cardiac arrhythmia, and it is associated with embolic stroke because of the development of thrombi in the atria due to the turbulent blood flow (the rhythm is irregular) (Nesheiwat et al., 2022). It is critical that the nurse can interpret this rhythm on ECG. Keys for which to observe include an irregular R to R wave and no discernible P wave; instead rapid oscillations or fibrillation wavelets that vary in size, shape, and frequency are seen (particularly visible in the inferior ECG leads II, III, and AVF) (Lough et al., 2022).

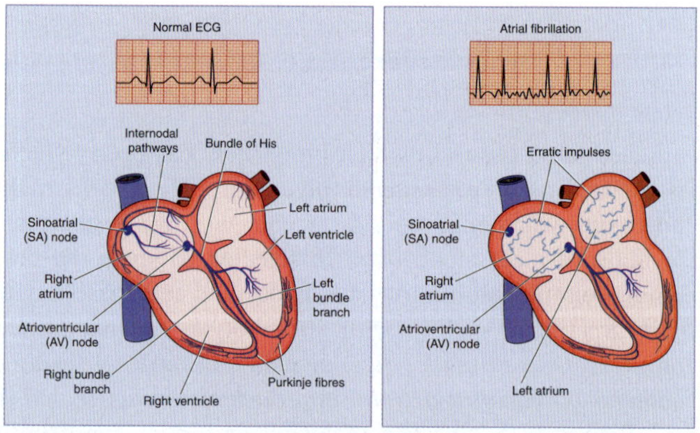

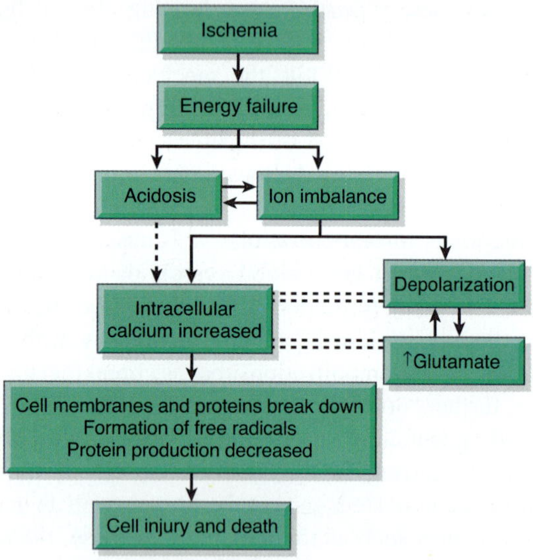

FIGURE 46-4 **Processes contributing to ischemic brain cell injury. Courtesy of the National Stroke Association, Englewood, Colorado.**

The least common identified category of stroke consists of those attributed to less common processes known to cause brain injury, such as hypercoagulable states from autoimmune disease or cancer, platelet and/or endothelial dysregulation from acute illness, dissection of the carotid or vertebral arteries, air or fat emboli introduced from injury, or blood vessel spasm from medication or unregulated drug use.

Unfortunately, up to about 30% of strokes are "cryptogenic," in which clinicians cannot clearly determine a cause for the patient's stroke. Investigations may not reveal a clear etiology or can reveal competing etiologies, for example, infrequent arrhythmia and severely narrowed vasculature (Bjerkreim et al., 2019; Donkor, 2018).

Transient Ischemic Attacks

A transient ischemic attack, or TIA (sometimes incorrectly referred to as a "mini-stroke"), has traditionally been defined as a brief episode of neurologic dysfunction resulting from

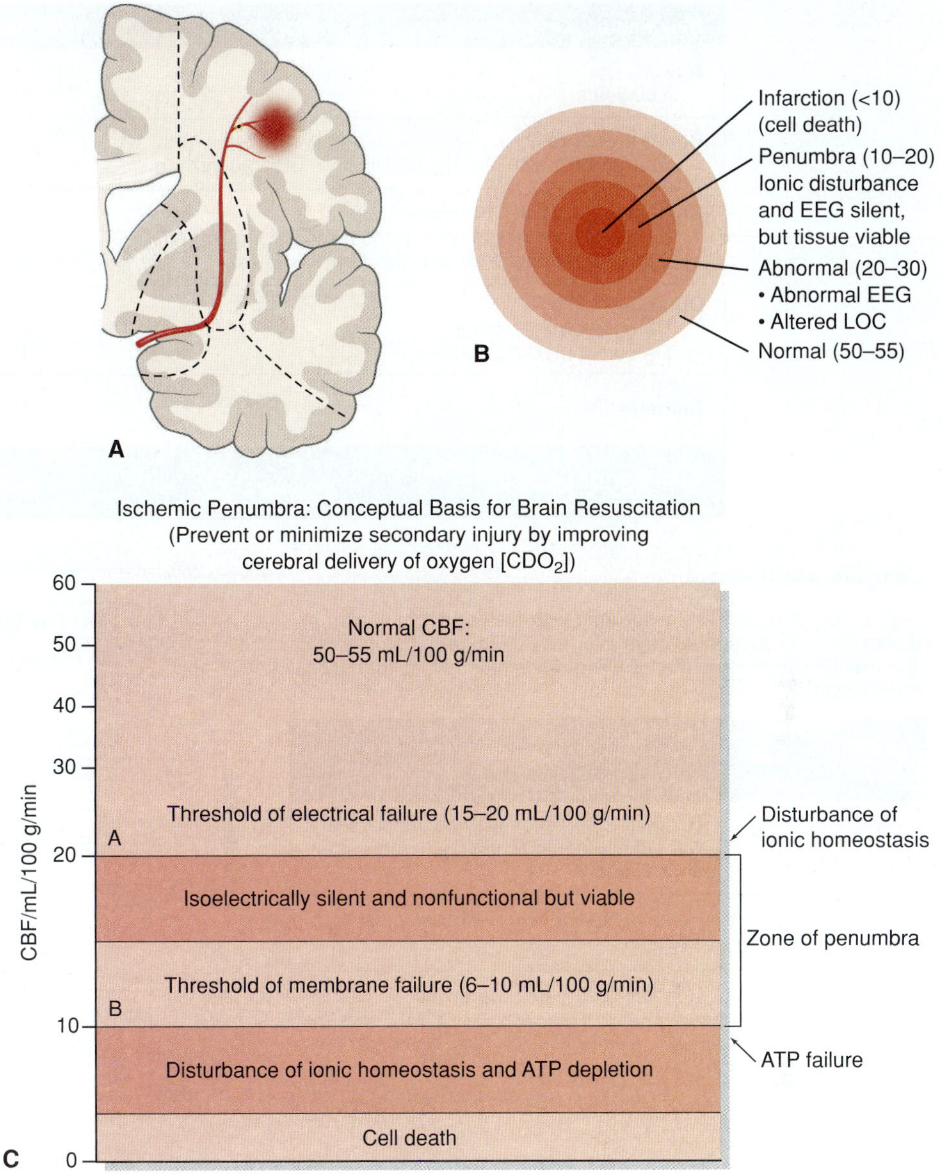

FIGURE 46-5 Cerebral blood supply during ischemic events. A. See distribution of middle cerebral artery and occlusion of a branch. Note area of infarction and surrounding penumbra with viable but nonfunctional cells. These cells will become either infarcted or recover, depending on treatment. B. Ischemic penumbra: normal cerebral blood flow (CBF) = 50 to 55 mL/100 g/min. Variations in CBF are noted. Penumbra is the critical area that may be salvageable with appropriate treatment, or cell death will occur if adequate CBF is not restored. C. Ischemic penumbra: conceptual basis for brain resuscitation. ATP, adenosine triphosphate; EEG, electroencephalogram; LOC, level of consciousness. (Adapted from Hickey J. [2014]. *The clinical practice of neurological and neurosurgical nursing* (7th ed.). Lippincott Williams & Wilkins.)

focal cerebral ischemia not associated with permanent cerebral infarction. A TIA involves the same pathophysiologic mechanism outlined in the ischemic cascade, but symptoms are transient (persisting less than 24 hours) and without evidence of cerebral tissue infarction on follow-up brain imaging studies. TIAs have often been referred to as a warning stroke since the causative process is likely to recur (causing cerebral infarction) if no interventions are undertaken. Unfortunately, many are unrecognized and unreported due to the transient nature of their impairments (Tsao et al., 2022). With the advent of better brain imaging techniques, and recognizing that TIAs typically resolve within 60 minutes, a new definition for a TIA was adopted. It has now been operationally defined as a brief episode of neurologic dysfunction caused by focal brain or retinal ischemia, with clinical symptoms typically lasting less than 1 hour, and without evidence of acute infarction. The corollary is that persistent clinical signs or characteristic imaging abnormalities change the definition to include ischemic infarction. For the purposes of this chapter, ischemic stroke and TIA are considered one disease process that mandates the same evaluative detail in determining cause, implementing a care plan, and supporting secondary stroke prevention measures (Mendelson & Prabhakaran, 2021). A TIA can happen in any blood vessel of the head and neck; if it occurs in a blood vessel of the eye, it is known as *amaurosis fugax or* transient visual loss, where a person has transient monocular visual loss (Tadi et al., 2022). A focal, completed stroke in the eye should be seen by a trained provider with direct visualization of the retina and is unlikely to appear in imaging of the brain.

Patients diagnosed with TIA are at a higher risk for a subsequent stroke (Bjerkreim, 2019; Tsao et al., 2022). Scoring systems have been devised to grade stroke risk for patients with TIA events. As outlined in Figure 46-6, older patients

Risk Factor	Points	Score
Age ≥ 60 years	1	
Blood pressure Systolic BP ≥ 140 mm Hg *OR* Diastolic BP ≥ 90 mm Hg	1	
Clinical features of TIA *(choose one)* Unilateral weakness with or without speech impairment *OR* Speech impairment without unilateral weakness	2 1	
Duration TIA duration ≥ 60 minutes TIA duration 10–59 minutes	2 1	
Diabetes	1	
Total ABCD² score	**0–7**	

Using the ABCD² Score

Higher ABCD² scores are associated with greater risk of stroke during the 2, 7, 30, and 90 days after a TIA (Figure). The authors of the ABCD² score made the following recommendations for hospital observation[1]:

ABCD² Score	2-day Stroke Risk (%)	Comment
0–3	1.0	Hospital observation may be unnecessary without another indication (e.g., new atrial fibrillation)
4–5	4.1	Hospital observation justified in most situations
6–7	8.1	Hospital observation worthwhile

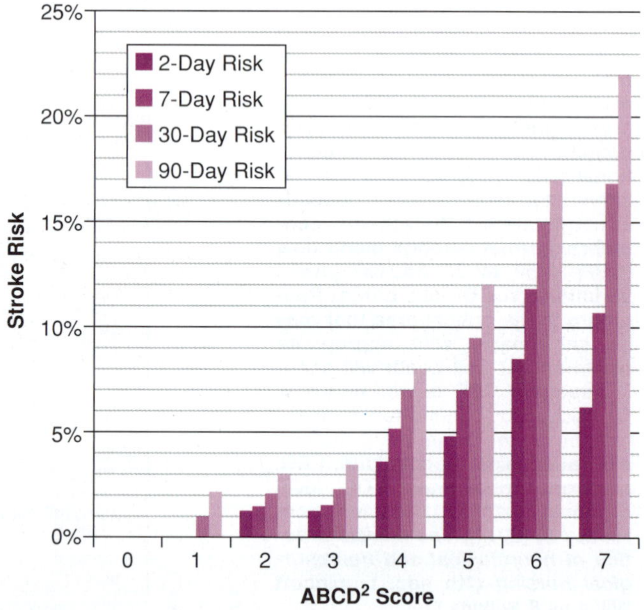

FIGURE 46-6 **Transient ischemic attack (TIA): Prognosis and key management considerations. MR, magnetic resonance; TIA, transient ischemic attack. (Used with permission from Johnston, S. C., Rothwell, P. M., Huynh-Huynh, M. N., Giles, M. F., Elkins, J. S., & Sidney, S. [2007]. Validation and refinement of scores to predict very early stroke risk after transient ischemic attack. *Lancet*, *369*, 283–292; Johnston, S. C., Nguyen-Huynh, M. N., Schwarz, M. E., Fuller, K., Williams, C. E., Josephson, S. A., Hankey, G. J., Hart, R. G., Levine, S. R., Biller, J., Brown, R. D. Jr, Sacco, R. L., Kappelle, L. J., Koudstaal, P. J., Bogousslavsky, J., Caplan, L. R., van Gijn, J., Algra, A., Rothwell, P. M. ... Albers, G. W. [2006]. National Stroke Association guidelines for the management of transient ischemic attacks. *Annals of Neurology*, *60*, 301–313.)**

with elevated blood pressure and multiple symptoms, lasting for a longer duration, were more likely to have a completed stroke in the next 2 to 9 days. Calculating stroke risk based on TIA symptoms helps the provider to determine whether the patient should be admitted for further monitoring or can follow-up for care as an outpatient.

Hemorrhagic Strokes

Hemorrhagic strokes refer to bleeding into the brain tissue (parenchyma), the ventricles, or the subarachnoid space. Although less common than ischemic strokes, they have a higher mortality rate (Stacy, 2022). Normal brain metabolism is disrupted when blood outside the vasculature forms a mass that compresses adjacent brain tissue, causing increased intracranial pressure (ICP), secondary hemorrhage, and/or further ischemia. The rapidity of these changes can be profound. Large volumes and particular locations of bleeding can create *herniation* of the brain tissues, physically moving brain across structures of the skull or even outside the cranium. Blood in or near the ventricles can block outflow of cerebral spinal fluid, leading to acute hydrocephalus, leading to a physical and chemical cascade of injury. Finally, level of consciousness (LOC) can change rapidly, leading to coma and death (Broderick et al., 2021).

Pearls for Practice

Level of consciousness (LOC) includes awareness (the qualitative function of wakefulness) and what arousal or stimulus is necessary for that awareness (walking in room, calling name, touching, stimulation). Assessment of awareness includes the patient's orientation to person, place, time, and situation and requires the patient to accurately answer various questions (Burke, 2022). It is evaluated and documented while noting trends.

Hemorrhagic stroke can be divided into intracerebral hemorrhage (ICH) and SAH. See Figure 46-7. ICH occurs when there is bleeding into any of the spaces within the cranium, including subarachnoid, epidural, and subdural spaces. Bleeding into the subdural and epidural spaces is primarily associated with trauma, after which hypertension is the leading cause in persons over 60 years old. A more diverse etiology can be found in younger patients (Heit et al., 2017). SAHs primarily also occur due to trauma, but of nontraumatic hemorrhage, 80% occur due to bleeding intracranial aneurysms (Long et al., 2017; Stacy, 2022). Congenital or later development of abnormalities in the blood vessels themselves can also increase risk.

Common blood vessel abnormalities include arteriovenous malformations (AVMs) or aneurysms. An intracranial (cerebral) aneurysm is a dilation of the wall of a cerebral artery. These vessel abnormalities may be due to atherosclerosis, congenital defect of the vessel wall, hypertensive vascular disease, head trauma, or advancing age. All of these can create weakness in blood vessel walls, leading to aneurysm and potential later rupture; in some cases, the vessel wall becomes weak without aneurysm formation and is prone to spontaneous rupture. The cerebral arteries most commonly affected by an aneurysm are the internal cerebral artery (ICA), sections of the middle cerebral artery (MCA) and vessels near or at bifurcations around the circle of Willis, especially the anterior communicating artery (ACoA or AComm), posterior communicating artery (PCoA or PComm), or junctions and bifurcations of the MCA (Stojanovic et al., 2019).

A "mycotic aneurysm" is a similar weakening of a blood vessel formed in the setting of infection. This more commonly occurs in the smaller unnamed and distal arteries, and mycotic aneurysms of the brain are often associated with endocarditis or other infections (Yuan & Wang, 2017).

Arteriovenous malformations, or AVMs, are tangles of arteries and veins in the brain lacking a transitional capillary bed; these form during embryonic development. The absence of a capillary bed leads to regionally high blood pressures between arterial and venous flow. Dilation of both arteries and veins can occur, and higher pressure in these weakened, dilated vessels can lead to rupture. AVM is a common cause of hemorrhagic stroke in younger patients (Heit et al., 2017; Hickey & Strayer, 2020). In addition, an association is found with use of sympathomimetic drugs like

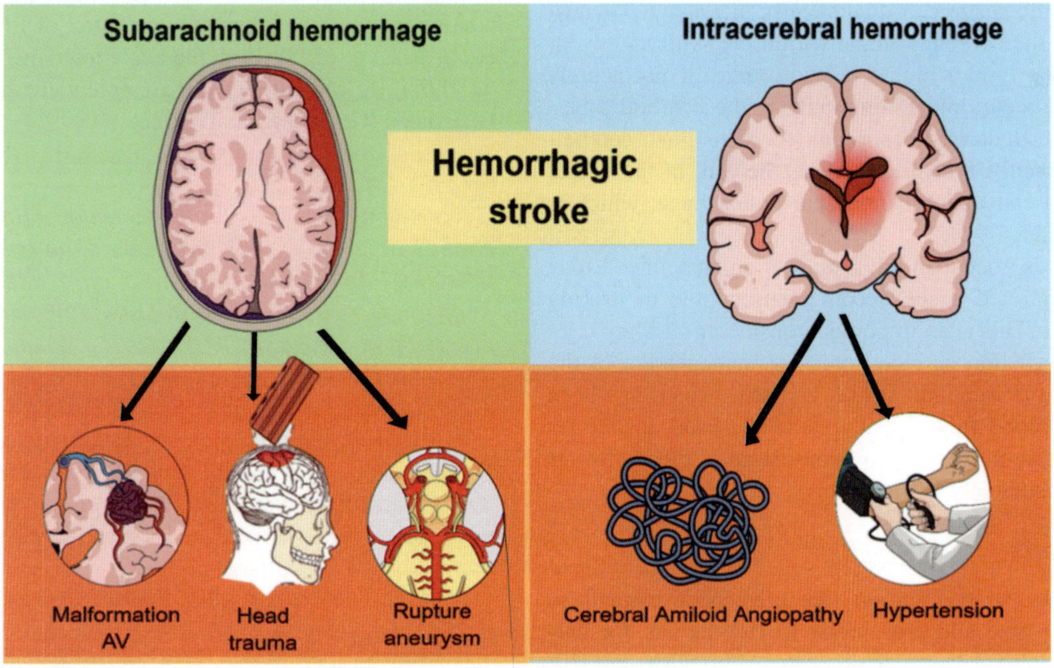

FIGURE 46-7 **The most common types of hemorrhagic stroke. (Reproduced from Gil-Garcia, C. A., Flores-Alvarez, E., Cebrian-Garcia, R., Mendoza-Lopez, A. C., Gonzalez-Hermosillo, L. M., Garcia-Blanco, M. D., & Roldan-Valadez, E. [2022]. Essential topics about the imaging diagnosis and treatment of hemorrhagic stroke: A comprehensive review of the 2022 AHA guidelines. *Current Problems in Cardiology*, *47*[11], 101328. Figure 1.)**

cocaine, heroin, amphetamine, and ephedrine and ICH in young patients (Gil-Garcia et al., 2022).

Less common causes of vessel disruption may be found in patients with vascular disease or vasculopathies. One increasingly recognized cause of hemorrhage is a condition known as "cerebral amyloid angiopathy" or CAA. Fragile amyloid protein deposits will have accumulated in the brain vessels' arterial walls over many years. These vessel walls are much more prone to breakdown, are associated with "microhemorrhage" on MRI, and predispose patients to larger cerebral hemorrhage. MRI evidence of hemorrhages in the cerebral lobes, often numerous and bilateral, may suggest this diagnosis when combined with patient history and clinical presentation; the gold standard remains tissue biopsy, which is rarely pursued. Dementia is associated clinically and there is some familial association (Hostettler et al., 2019). Other rare causes of hemorrhage result from systemic vasculopathy, tumor, or stimulant use or overuse (Hickey & Strayer, 2020). There is an increased risk of ICH linked to a greater number of births (multiparous patients have a significantly higher risk of developing ICH compared to nulliparous or uniparous); increased risk is also seen in longer working hours, more strenuous workdays, and manual work as well as sleeping for extended periods (8 hours or more) (Gil-Garcia et al., 2022).

Primary ICH, from a spontaneous rupture of small arteries or arterioles, accounts for approximately 80% of hemorrhagic strokes and is caused chiefly by uncontrolled hypertension. Blood can accumulate outside the vessels and into the intracranial space over minutes to hours. Symptom presentation can vary from mild deficits to acute loss of consciousness. Because the brain is enclosed in a rigid structure, hemorrhage can dramatically increase ICP, causing shifts in the content volume within the skull and eventual herniation (and a higher mortality rate) if not acutely treated. ICH occurs most commonly in the cerebral lobes, basal ganglia, thalamus, brainstem (the pons), and cerebellum. Occasionally, bleeding ruptures the wall of the lateral ventricle and causes intraventricular hemorrhage, which is frequently fatal.

ICH can also occur in the setting of an ischemic stroke, when the infarcted tissue becomes susceptible to leaking blood vessels. This is an important consideration when considering reperfusion or blood pressure management of the patient with the ischemic stroke, as tissue which has been deprived of blood flow for an extended period appears to be more fragile and prone to hemorrhage if blood flow is strongly and suddenly restored.

Risk Factors

The conditions or risk factors that predispose patients to stroke are diverse and are similar to risk factors for cardiac and peripheral vascular diseases. Although some risk factors are applicable to a specific stroke type, most can apply to both ischemic and hemorrhagic strokes. Identifying patient-specific stroke risk factors is part of the patient and family education process during primary stroke prevention and during stroke recovery. The incidence for Asian and African Americans is particularly high as compared with White Americans and is largely influenced by modifiable risk factor prevalence and control in these groups (Hickey & Strayer, 2020). See Figure 46-8.

Modifiable Risk Factors

Modifiable risk factors are those that can be altered through lifestyle changes and medical treatment. Common modifiable stroke risk factors include hypertension, tobacco use or exposure, diabetes, dyslipidemia, atrial fibrillation, diet, obesity, heavy alcohol use, sleep apnea, and lack of exercise (Gil-Garcia et al., 2020). Analysis by the Global Burden of Diseases and Injuries Collaborators suggests that over 85% of the risk of stroke can be attributed to modifiable risk factors, with almost half related to behavior (Tsao et al., 2022). Hypertension is the most important risk factor for both ischemic and hemorrhagic stroke, and, despite the numerous treatment options, it remains underrecognized and undertreated in most communities. Current best practice recommends an outpatient goal of <130/80 mm Hg in patients with prior stroke, and <120/80 in the general population. (Kleindorfer et al., 2021). In the acute stroke phase, blood pressure is generally liberalized to allow for improved cerebral blood flow, but the general practice in the stroke recovery phase is to lower the systolic BP (SBP) to a target range of 130 to 140 mm Hg in mild to moderate acute ICH in those presenting with systolic blood pressure between 150 mm Hg and 220 mm Hg (Greenberg et al., 2022). Treatment is initiated as soon as possible with careful titration of BP-lowering therapy "to ensure continuous smooth and sustained control of BP" (Greenberg et al., 2022, p. e298). Both the acute lowering of the SBP to <130 mm Hg and elevated BP are potentially harmful and to be avoided (Greenberg et al., 2022).

Pearls for Practice

Control of systemic hypertension is essential, but caution must be exercised because the mean arterial pressure (MAP) must be maintained at a level sufficient to produce adequate cerebral blood flow in the presence of elevated ICP (Burke, 2022). In addition, the nurse monitors the pulse pressure (difference between the systolic and diastolic pressure [normal is 40 mm Hg]), because widening may occur in the late stages of intracranial hypertension. If increased ICP is suspected, the head of bed is elevated to 30 degrees and the head is positioned in neutral position to minimize venous outflow resistance and improve cerebral spinal fluid displacement from the intracranial to the spinal compartment (Sharma et al., 2022).

Diabetes independently increases stroke risk and contributes to the increased prevalence of hypertension and dyslipidemia through microvascular changes throughout the body.

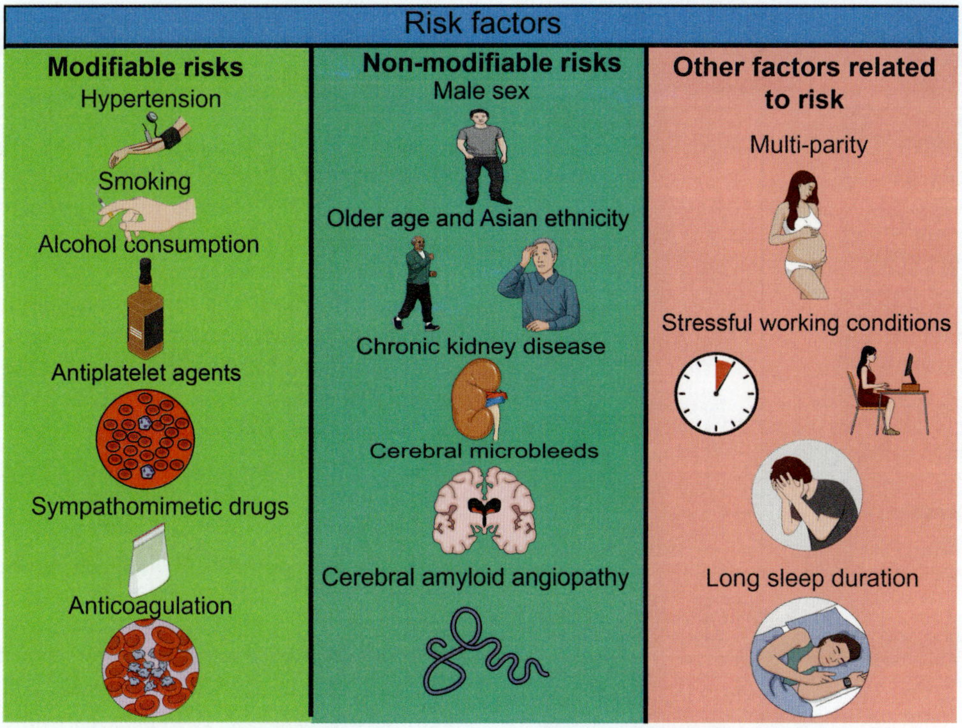

FIGURE 46-8 **Risk factors are classified as (A) modifiable risk, (B) nonmodifiable risk, and (C) other factors related to risk. It is essential to identify an acute treatment for hemorrhagic strokes. (Reproduced from Gil-Garcia, C. A., Flores-Alvarez, E., Cebrian-Garcia, R., Mendoza-Lopez, A. C., Gonzalez-Hermosillo, L. M., Garcia-Blanco, M. D., & Roldan-Valadez, E. [2022]. Essential topics about the imaging diagnosis and treatment of hemorrhagic stroke: A comprehensive review of the 2022 AHA guidelines. *Current Problems in Cardiology*, *47*[11],101328. Figure 3.)**

Glycemic control alone has not been shown to reduce stroke risk, but in combination with blood pressure and lipid management, patients with diabetes can lower their overall risk (van Sloten et al., 2020).

Atrial fibrillation is the most frequently diagnosed arrhythmia in the United States. If left untreated, it puts patients at higher risk for ischemic stroke. Approximately 15% to 20% of ischemic strokes can be attributed to atrial fibrillation. Screening for atrial fibrillation in patients over 40 years of age has been recommended since anticoagulation and rate/rhythm control can reduce stroke risk by up to 68% (AHA/ACC/HRS, 2019).

Obstructive sleep apnea (OSA) is an independent risk factor for stroke, and the mechanism of cause is yet to be elucidated. It has been proposed that intermittent hypoxemia, due to the pauses or decreased quality of breathing in sleep, may cause surges in blood pressure with release of vasoconstrictive peptides such as endothelin; additionally, increased levels of inflammatory biomarkers are seen in sleep-disordered breathing. Patients with OSA have greater functional impairment and higher mortality rates than patients without OSA during an acute stroke. Continuous positive airway pressure (CPAP) treatment is associated with decreased mortality and better functional recovery after stroke (Ifergane et al., 2016).

Smoking and second-hand smoke are prevalent among all age groups and pose an increased stroke risk among females who smoke and who are on oral contraceptives. Smokeless tobacco use is also associated with increased risk. Both ischemic and, more strongly, hemorrhagic stroke are associated with smoking. Cessation programs, including both counseling and nicotine replacement, are recommended by the CDC, although further study is needed to determine optimal approaches (Tsao et al., 2022).

Healthy weight management and exercise are multifactorial and require lifestyle changes that can be more difficult to implement. They are closely linked to hypertension, dyslipidemia, glycemic control and insulin resistance, and sleep apnea. Assisting patients in this is a long-term project among all providers and the individual patient (Kleindorfer et al., 2021). As with tobacco and alcohol cessation, reinforcement of efforts from multiple persons along the health care spectrum is associated with better adherence (Hamdy et al., 2018). See Figure 46-9.

Nonmodifiable Risk Factors

Nonmodifiable risk factors for stroke include age, strong family history of stroke, and race/ethnicity. While these cannot be changed, they should be addressed by the medical team in conjunction with recurrent stroke risk and patient education.

Factors such as age and genetic risk can guide other interventions, including lifestyle modification and particular

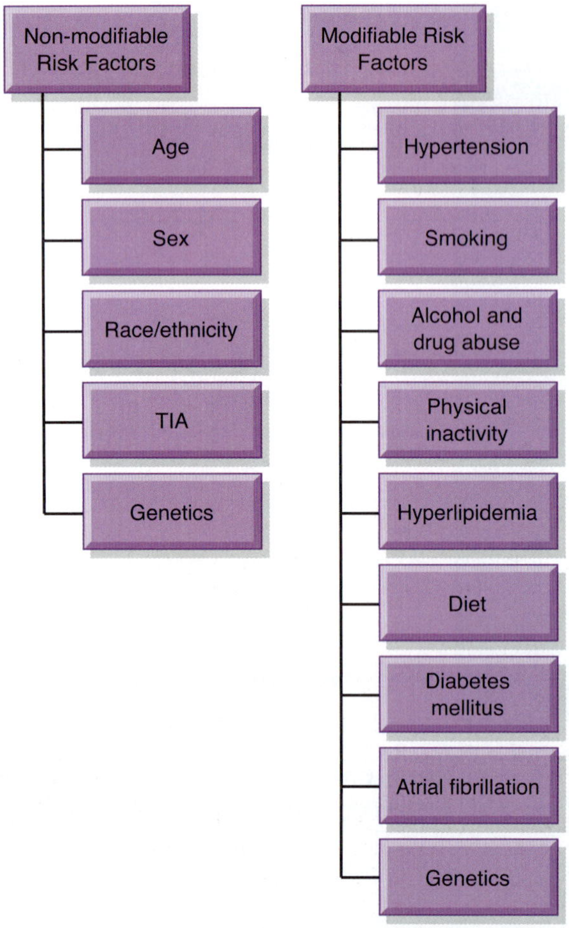

FIGURE 46-9 Risk factors associated with stroke. (Reproduced, with permission from Kuriakose, D., & Xiao, Z. [2020]. Pathophysiology and treatment of stroke: Present status and future perspectives. *International Journal of Molecular Sciences, 21*[20], 7609. Figure 2.)

approaches addressing modifiable risk factors. They may also point toward less common areas of investigation, especially in cryptogenic stroke.

Older age is a risk factor for stroke, and for both ischemic and hemorrhagic strokes the risk doubles every 10 years after 55 years of age. Males tend to have a higher risk for stroke and a higher age-specific stroke incidence rate, but more females tend to die from stroke (Tsao et al., 2022). A holistic approach to aging well and healthily can both reduce the modifiable risk factors and increase wellness to enhance recovery if injury or illness occurs.

Race and ethnicity impact stroke risk among specific populations. Black and Hispanic individuals have a higher incidence of both ischemic and hemorrhagic stroke, and contributing factors may be the higher incidence of diabetes, hypertension, and renal disease in these groups, as well as socioeconomic factors and access to health care. Education and outreach also show greater effect on patient lifestyle modification and medication adherence when taking sociocultural variation into account. In the United States, for example, research has shown differences in response to antihypertensive medications and community outreach among Black Americans (Sulaica et al., 2020). Some populations, such as people with Finnish and East Asian heritage, have increased risks of vascular malformation, such as increased aneurysm formation or Moyamoya disease (Detmer et al., 2019). Finally, while genetic testing is normally of very little benefit for addressing stroke risk, young patients with strong family history of stroke or other nonprovoked thrombotic states may benefit from targeted genetic screening to suggest monitoring or more intensive early therapies for other comorbidities (Zhang et al., 2018).

The relationship between acute ischemic stroke and the corona-19 virus is not entirely clear, but there appears to be an association between traditional stroke risk factors and the compromised immune system (exposed to the virus), which manifests as an inflammatory response, thrombosis, and ischemic injury. Several studies examined the incidence, comorbidities, and outcomes in this patient population and found that while the incidence did not increase appreciably, patients with Covid-19 tended to be younger, with more than one vascular risk factor and a higher in-hospital mortality rate (Mbonde et al., 2022; Nannoni et al., 2020). The long-term effects of Covid-19 in patients with concomitant stroke are unknown.

Clinical Manifestations and Assessment

Common Symptoms

Stroke syndromes produce a wide variety of neurologic deficits, depending on the location in the brain that is affected, the specific cerebral blood vessels that are obstructed, the size and area of underperfused brain tissue, and the amount of collateral (secondary or accessory) blood flow to the affected area. The AHA/ASA advises the public to be aware of the symptoms of stroke and to call 911 immediately. The most common symptoms of stroke include:

- Sudden numbness or weakness of the face, arm, or leg, especially on one side of the body
- Sudden trouble speaking or understanding speech
- Sudden visual disturbances
- Difficulty walking, dizziness, or loss of balance or coordination
- Sudden, severe headache

There are additional, less commonly recognized stroke symptoms that also put patients at risk for disabling and devastating outcomes. These include sudden, unexplained fall; onset of nausea and vomiting; and acute changes in mentation, such as confusion or disorientation. These symptoms have been associated more commonly with strokes that occur in the posterior circulation leading to infarctions in the cerebellum (Arch et al., 2016; Shake et al., 2018).

The provider should be able to correlate commonly presenting neurologic deficits with the location(s) in the brain affected by ischemia or hemorrhage. Box 46-2 compares

BOX 46-2

Focused Assessment

Left and Right Hemispheric Strokes

Be alert for the following signs and symptoms:

Left hemispheric stroke:

- Paralysis or weakness on right side of body
- Right visual field deficit
- Aphasia (expressive, receptive, or global)
- Altered intellectual ability
- Slow, cautious behavior

Right hemispheric stroke:

- Paralysis or weakness on left side of body
- Left visual field deficit
- Spatial-perceptual deficits
- Increased distractibility
- Impulsive behavior and poor judgment
- Lack of awareness of deficits

the symptoms and behaviors seen in patients with right hemispheric strokes with those seen in patients with left hemispheric strokes. Acute neurologic deficits are not stroke-type specific. In general, patients with a hemorrhagic or ischemic stroke can present with similar neurologic deficits, thus making expedited brain imaging an important aspect of the stroke workup.

Posterior circulation strokes and hemorrhagic strokes may present with somewhat different symptoms. A stroke affecting the cerebellum or brainstem may cause severe change in responsiveness or mentation, nausea and vomiting (usually with imbalance or vision change), sudden collapse, or seizure. For patients with cerebral hemorrhages, the most common presenting symptom is a severe headache; there may be vomiting, seizure, neck pain, and LOC change, which may be sudden or insidious. Patients can also have slow hemorrhages that lead to clot formation or an ischemic event which leads to subsequent hemorrhage (Sparaco et al., 2019).

It is important to remember that the presenting signs can determine the location but not the type of stroke. Urgent imaging to determine presence or absence of hemorrhage will guide the time-sensitive next steps in triage and treatment (Greenberg et al., 2022).

Motor

Unilateral motor loss of function is the most common motor deficit in acute stroke, as well as one of the more recognized signs. Injury to upper motor neurons in the cerebrum will lead to dysfunction contralateral to the lesion due to *decussation* (crossing) of most motor tracts at the level of the medullary pyramids in the medulla oblongata. Motor loss can range from complete plegia or paresis on one side to mild weakness of a single isolated muscle group, depending on size and location of the lesion. Input from physical and occupational therapists is essential to recovery of function.

Communication

Language and communication deficits due to stroke are common findings. A majority of persons, both right- and left-handed, rely on the left hemisphere for most language functions. There are several known foci of communication and language in the brain, such as Wernicke and Broca areas, but language deficit can occur with injuries in other regions as well. Speech and language therapists are a vital part of diagnosis and treatment for these impairments. Types of language and communication dysfunction include:

Dysarthria, or "slurred speech": This is caused by injury to the many muscles, tendons, and nerves which allow for enunciation. Dysarthria may be accompanied by swallowing difficulty.

Aphasia, sometimes *dysphasia*: Any degree of language impairment related to the production or comprehension of words. Aphasias can be divided into several types; *expressive aphasia* is impairment with producing usable, correct, and understandable speech, and *receptive aphasia* denotes impairment comprehending language. Spoken, written, and/or signed language may be affected to the same or different degrees. The types may also be "mixed" or "global," indicating both receiving and expressing language have been impaired.

Apraxia is the inability to volitionally do an action; in the context of speech, either to go through the actions to produce speech at all or to organize the sounds and syllables together logically (Klein & Mancinelli, 2021).

Vision

Visual disturbances and vision loss due to stroke can be caused by injury to the visual cortex, nerves, or sensory pathways affecting eye movement, or to vasculature of the eye itself. Common findings include visual field loss; complete, usually unilateral visual loss; diplopia; or, less commonly, perceptual variation or distortion.

Dysphagia

The act of swallowing is a complex process. Strokes may affect any number of nerves or muscles causing some degree of dysphagia. Over half of the cranial nerves and dozens of paired muscles are involved in the process of chewing, moving a food bolus within and beyond the oral cavity, and protecting the trachea. Hemiplegic patients with diaphragmatic dysfunction are also at risk (Wilmskoetter et al., 2020.)

Sensory

Sensory changes after stroke can be independent of, or related to, motor impairment. The degree can be profound or minor and even improve over time. Significant sensory loss increases a patient's risk for injury as they may be unable to recognize an injury, similar to patients with other neuropathies. Paresthesias, or nerve pain, can be devastating to a patient and difficult to treat compared to other forms of pain. This is often described as "pins and needles" or "the feeling of ants (hormiguas)." Sensory neglect occurs when a patient is able to perceive touch or other stimuli, but only when attention is brought to it.

Cognitive and Psychological

Depending on the region affected by the stroke, various cognitive and psychological changes may occur. In addition, the psychological stressors associated with a new major diagnosis and (potential) disability should not be underestimated. Poststroke depression is likely underrecognized but can be addressed with pharmacologic and nonpharmacologic modalities. Strokes in the frontal lobe can cause personality changes and difficulty with executive function. Strokes in other regions may affect short- or long-term memory, ability to calculate, spatial orientation, motivation, or other skills necessary for activities of daily life and social belonging. Allies in this field include physical therapy (PT), occupational therapy (OT), speech-language pathology (SLP), psychology and psychiatry, and peer support groups. Nursing screens for depression or other mood disorders can identify these early and should be part of stroke patient assessments.

Acute Stroke Assessment

Given evidence that shorter time to treatment leads to better outcome for patients recovering from stroke, and the rise of treatment options since the 1990s, it is now a standard of care to have local protocols for acute stroke assessment and triage (Adeoye et al., 2019). These are typically implemented in prehospital medical settings, particularly EMS agencies, and in hospitals. A patient having an acute stroke will usually be a "Level 2 emergency" under the ESI system (see Chapter 55), which means the patient needs immediate assessment. A stroke which leads to unresponsiveness or airway failure leading to immediate or field intubation can also be categorized under ESI Level 1 for the most acute needs.

Nurses in the prehospital setting or at triage in an emergency department should be familiar with the prehospital screening and assessments that are done by members of the EMS team so that they can relay this information to the stroke team prior to arrival and anticipate needed resources (Jauch, 2019). Acute stroke care can be divided into two phases: the hyperacute phase—the first 24 hours of care (Ashcraft et al., 2021) and the acute phase—acute care during hospitalization (Rodgers et al., 2021).

Ideally, patients with stroke symptoms should arrive by EMS with a prenotification to the Emergency Department. Nurses in triage should be in contact with EMS and planning for arrival. Triage of the "walk in" patient requires assessment of the patient's immediate needs at the time of presentation with attention paid to the patient's chief complaint and any obvious signs of stroke. Several algorithms have been developed for the initial workup of a patient presenting with acute stroke symptoms as a template to expedite the diagnostic workup (Fig. 46-10). In general, the triage nurses should confirm the presenting symptoms and the last time the patient was known to be well or otherwise free of the new symptom.

The symptom timeline is extremely important given the time sensitivity of therapeutic options for ischemic stroke. Usually, the time the patient was last known to be at baseline ("last known well") becomes the default time of onset. Some facilities are using emerging imaging technologies or protocols to determine if patients who wake up from sleep with new symptoms may be eligible for therapies.

Certain other information that would help with a risk/benefit calculation for either thrombolytic or mechanical intervention is also important to gather early: medication use, specifically of anticoagulant medications; recent surgeries; and basic labs and vital signs, specifically blood pressure. Information from this assessment can trigger a "stroke code" protocol, alerting a provider or team; in some cases, these can be preactivated if EMS has sufficient information (Ashcraft et al., 2021). Figure 46-11 depicts a typical acute stroke protocol.

Diagnostic Evaluation

The diagnosis of an acute stroke is made by history, a precise neurologic examination, and rapid neuroimaging. Patients with symptoms suggestive of TIA, even if resolved prior to arrival to hospital, should still undergo urgent basic imaging as the course of some strokes may be irregular, or "stuttering," versus having a linear progression. An initial noncontrast head CT scan is performed to assess for the presence of intraparenchymal blood. Ischemia will not be readily visible on initial CT scan when it is performed within the first few hours after symptom onset; however, evidence of bleeding (hemorrhage) will almost always be visible. Providers will also consider the location of the hematoma, the size and presence of blood in the ventricular system, and evidence of increased ICP. Additional diagnostic testing is done to determine if the hemorrhage is due to a ruptured intracranial aneurysm or AVM.

The negative CT head effectively "rules out" hemorrhage, permitting the consideration of thrombolytic therapy in patients with clinical stroke symptoms. Both CT and MRI are acceptable initial studies; however, in most institutions, CT scans are much faster to acquire and put the patient on a more rapid treatment pathway.

If hemorrhage is found, clinicians will consider size, location, presence of blood in the ventricles, and evidence of ICP changes or mass effect of blood on the tissue. Management may be surgical or ICU-based nonsurgical with drains and hyperosmolar therapy. Smaller hemorrhages can be closely monitored without invasive treatment. Further angiography, either computed tomography angiography (CTA) or by interventional radiology procedure, may be done if there is high suspicion of ruptured aneurysm or other vascular malformation or injury which must be surgically repaired.

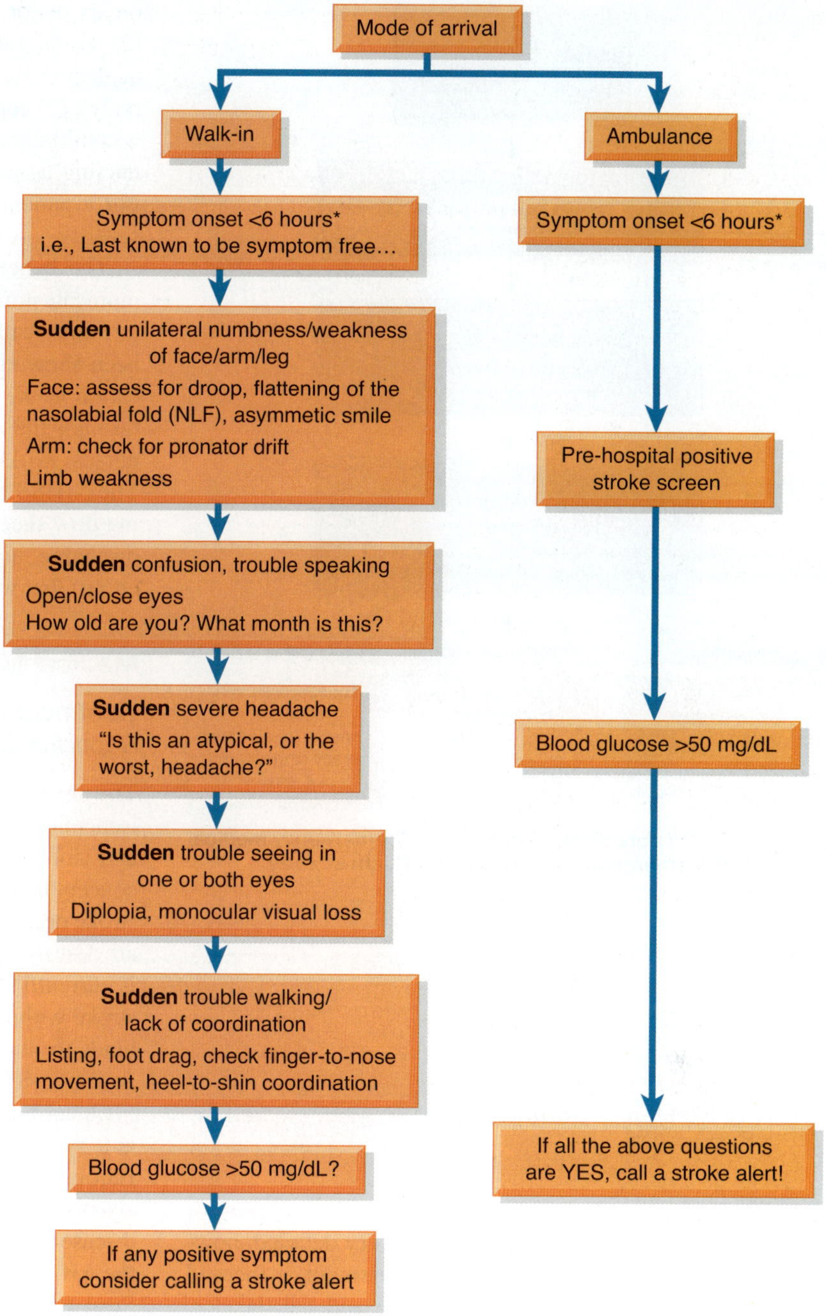

FIGURE 46-10 Triage stroke screen. *While intravenous tPA treatment is administered to eligible patients within 3 to 4.5 hours of symptom onset, patients are frequently evaluated within 6 to 12 hours of symptom onset to determine eligibility for neurointerventional treatment procedures.

It is a common practice at most institutions to also acquire intracranial and extracranial vessel imaging (CTA, magnetic resonance angiography [MRA]) to look for evidence of a significant vessel stenosis, in situ clot, or dissection of a vessel wall that could explain the patient's presenting symptoms and direct treatment options for the patient with acute stroke. If available and appropriate, perfusion imaging can also visualize areas "at risk" for infarction. This imaging helps estimate blockage and delay in blood flow; patients with slow but present blood flow may benefit more from thrombectomy versus patients who have already completely lost flow to affected areas.

Routine blood chemistries, coagulation studies (platelets, prothrombin time/international normalized ratio [INR], activated partial thromboplastin time, blood cell counts, cardiac rhythm status [ECG]), oxygen saturation, and IV access are also obtained as part of the initial evaluation. Key laboratory results (such as the platelet count, glucose, and coagulation profile) will direct decision making regarding treatment options, such as thrombolysis. Table 46-3 details a variety of diagnostic tests or procedures that are commonly recommended. Additional lab studies may be ordered based on patient history, such as medication levels or for specific metabolic concerns.

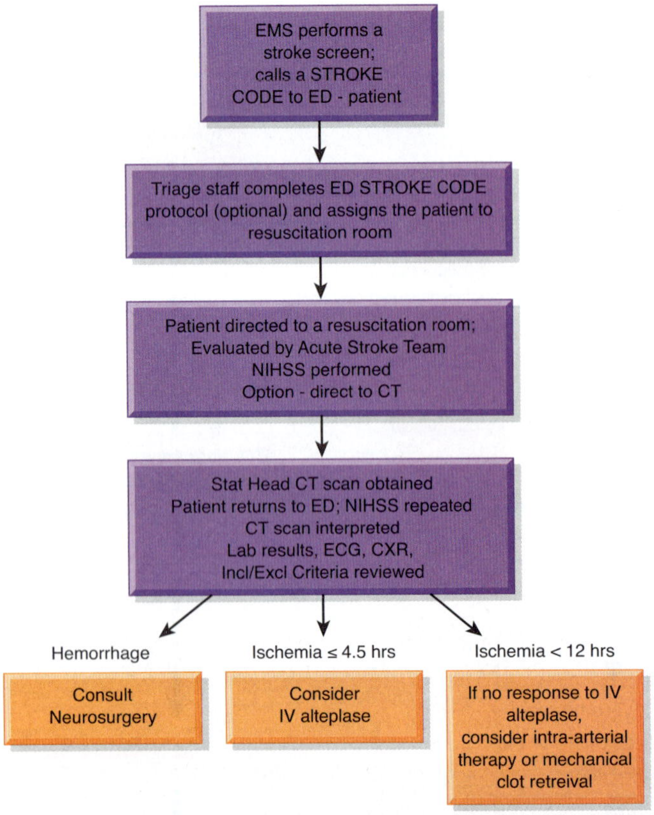

FIGURE 46-11 Acute Stroke Protocol. EMS, emergency medical services; ED, emergency department; CXR, chest x-ray.

Pearls for Practice

The nurse is aware that ICP increases with hypoxemia or hypercapnia (high CO_2) (Sharma et al., 2022). Hypoventilation is common in patients with altered LOC, which will cause the CO_2 to rise (hypercapnia) (Burke, 2022). For O_2 saturation below 94%, oxygen is administered via nasal cannula at 2 to 3 L/min.

The Clinical Examination

The neurologic examination is typically very detailed, however for the purpose of acute stroke assessment, a focused and standardized exam is more suitable and can be performed by providers in different specialties with reliability. This recommended practice has the benefits of identifying common stroke syndromes, and the normalization allows for fluid interteam communication about the patient. Prehospital EMS teams may use a variety of screening tools which can assist with triage, such as the Cincinnati Pre-Hospital Stroke Screen or the Los Angeles Pre-Hospital Stroke Screen score. The National Institutes of Health Stroke Scale (NIHSS) is the most widely accepted assessment tool to quantify stroke severity and to assess patient outcome after stroke treatment (Table 46-4). The NIHSS is a 15-item and 42-point assessment scale, with 3 to 5 options for each item. A score of 0 indicates no current neurologic deficit; scores above 20 generally indicate devastating stroke. The NIHSS focuses on six major areas of the neurologic examination: (1) LOC, (2) visual function, (3) motor function, (4) sensation and neglect (failure to pay attention to stimuli on one side of the body), (5) cerebellar function, and (6) language. The NIHSS was initially used by stroke teams but has become a standard nursing assessment in the ED and hospital wards to monitor a patient's neurologic deficits and to document stroke severity.

The benefits of the NIHSS include the ability to communicate findings via a standardized assessment tool and to numerically quantify progress over time, and they have been shown to correlate with longer-term outcome. Certification in the use of this assessment tool is available online through the ASA training center and is often required for nurses working in Emergency or Neuroscience divisions. The NIHSS has become a standard assessment tool on nursing flow sheets for periodic assessments, during handoffs, at discharge, and when there is a neurologic change (or worsening) that warrants an urgent evaluation.

Medical Management

Treatment for Acute Ischemic Stroke: Reperfusion Therapies

The initial expedited diagnostic workup and treatment of ischemic stroke are driven by time-dependent pharmacologic and clot retrieval device treatment options. This follows the concept that "time is brain," that says for every minute that a stroke occurs and is not treated, nearly two million brain cells are destroyed. Thrombolysis with recombinant tPA (alteplase) is currently the only FDA-approved drug for acute ischemic stroke within a 3-hour window of symptom onset. Alteplase binds to fibrin and converts plasminogen to plasmin, which is responsible for clot breakdown. In the United States, the FDA currently approves recombinant tPA (alteplase), which is a synthetic version of an enzyme made by the body. In Europe and East Asia another similar agent, tenecteplase, is also used; it is currently used in the United States for cardiac disease and "off label" for stroke; for this, it is accepted by the AHA as an alternative agent in selected cases (NINDS & Stroke rtPA Stroke Study Work Group, 1995; Powers et al., 2019). In general, thrombolytics are given intravenously; some occlusions are amenable to intra-arterial administration and are performed by neurointerventionalists, usually as part of a mechanical thrombectomy procedure.

Primary side effects of thrombolytic agents include major bleeding, including in the brain, GI tract, or other parts of the body; or anaphylaxis. Time since stroke onset appears to correlate with the risk of hemorrhage. Initially, the use of tPA was limited to 0 to 3 hours after stroke onset; this was liberalized to 4.5 hours in selected populations after the 2008 European Cooperative Acute Stroke Study (ECASS 3); younger patients, those with fewer comorbidities, and a less severe stroke show benefit from this "extended tPA window" (Hacke et al., 2008). The most recent AHA/ASA guidelines

TABLE **46-3 Diagnostic Procedures for Transient Ischemic Attacks (TIAs) and Stroke**

Diagnostic Procedure	Information Provided
Computed tomography (CT) scan without contrast	Important diagnostic test to quickly assess for the presence of blood (hemorrhage), which will preclude treatment with antithrombotics
CT scan with contrast	Useful to rule out lesions that may mimic ischemia, especially when symptoms are related to hemispheric deficits; hypodense areas on CT scan suggest infarction
Magnetic resonance imaging (MRI)	Offers soft tissue contrast discrimination with superior demarcation of mass lesion from surrounding structures, including areas of ischemia and infarction; good visualization of vascular structures; useful for diagnosis of stroke in first 72 hours; a diffusion-weighted MRI can show ischemia in first few hours
Magnetic resonance angiography (MRA)	Less available and higher cost; noninvasive imaging of the carotid, vertebral, basilar, and major intracranial and extracranial arteries to determine occlusion; useful for clot visualization
Carotid ultrasonography	Noninvasive imaging; widely used for initial diagnosis in patients with carotid territory symptoms for whom carotid endarterectomy (CEA) is considered
Transcranial Doppler (TCD)	Noninvasive monitoring of blood flow velocities of the major cerebral and carotid arteries to assess degree of stenoses; may be included as part of the stroke workup
Cerebral angiography	Ordered for patients to precisely define the percentage of occlusion and in patients with unusual presentation with aneurysm, vasculitis, and high-grade stenosis
Transthoracic echocardiography (TTE)	Helpful to identify cardioembolic sources; TTE is particularly helpful for diagnosing left ventricular thrombi, left atrial myxomas, and thrombi that protrude into the atrial cavity; they are less reliable for small tumors, laminated thrombi, and thrombi limited to the left or right atrium
Transesophageal echocardiography (TEE)	Benefit of TEE is in greater sensitivity for source of cardioembolic (except ventricular disease); TEE provides better visualization of cardiac structures, especially those at greater depth from chest wall and lesions of the atria (atrial appendage thrombi associated with atrial fibrillation), interatrial septum defects (patent foramen ovale, atrial septal defects), mitral valvular vegetation, and atherosclerotic disease of ascending aortic arch
Electrocardiogram (ECG); 12 lead is recommended initially	12 lead ECG recommended immediately because of the high incidence of heart disease in patients with stroke; ECG also useful when cardiogenic embolic stroke or concurrent coronary artery disease is suspected and to evaluate for atrial fibrillation
Ambulatory ECG monitoring	Reserved for patients who have suspicious palpitations, arrhythmias, or enlarged left atrium
Prothrombotic states	Protein C, protein S, antithrombin III, thrombin time, hemoglobin, electrophoresis, anticardiolipin antibody, lupus anticoagulant, and syphilis serology

Adapted from 2019 Guidelines for the early management of adults with ischemic stroke. *Stroke, 50*(12), e344–e418.

(Powers et al., 2019) note limited consideration for use of tPA in strokes of unclear onset time, based on advanced imaging, so long as the patient could be imaged and treated within 4.5 hours of identification of symptoms.

Pearls for Practice

The nurse monitors the patient's neurologic status for signs and symptoms of deterioration and increased ICP that may be related to intracerebral hemorrhage or increasing cerebral edema. Be alert for subtle signs such as drowsiness, to more significant findings such as visual changes (blurred vision, diplopia [double vision], photophobia [sensitivity to light], sluggish pupillary response, severe headache, nausea, vomiting, and seizures). The key parameter that you are alert to is "change"…. Any change in your assessment should be promptly reported (after considering other variables such as medications or other medical conditions that could affect the findings) since early identification of neurologic deterioration is critical to preventing secondary brain injury (Burke, 2022). In addition, the nurse is in a key position to prevent, monitor, and correct hypo- and hypertension, hyperglycemia, or hyperthermia to minimize infarct progression (Sharma & Smith, 2022). Nursing interventions are also enacted to reduce frequent complications, such as aspiration (see Chapter 21), venous thromboembolism (see Chapter 17), and pressure ulcers (see Chapter 51).

Stroke centers generally outline their approach to treatment according to the most current ASA/AHA guidelines.

TABLE **46-4 Summary of National Institutes of Health Stroke Scale (NIHSS)**

Category	Description	Score
1a. Level of consciousness (LOC)	Alert Arousable by minor stimulation Obtunded, strong stimulation to attend Unresponsive, or reflex responses only	0 1 2 3
1b. LOC questions (month, age)	Answers both correctly Answers one correctly Both incorrect	0 1 2
1c. LOC, commands (open, close eyes; make fist, let go)	Obeys both correctly Obeys one correctly Both incorrect	0 1 2
2. Best gaze (eyes open—patient follows examiner's finger or face)	Normal Partial gaze palsy Forced deviation	0 1 2
3. Visual (introduce visual stimulus/threat to patient's visual field quadrants)	No visual loss Partial hemianopsia Complete hemianopsia Bilateral hemianopsia	0 1 2 3
4. Facial palsy (show teeth, raise eyebrows and squeeze eyes shut)	Normal Minor loss Partial loss Complete loss	0 1 2 3
5a. Motor; arm—left (elevate extremity to 90 degrees for 10 seconds and score drift/movement)	No drift Drift but maintains in air Unable to maintain in air No effort against gravity No movement Amputation, joint fusion (explain)	0 1 2 3 4 N/A
5b. Motor; arm—right (elevate extremity to 90 degrees for 10 seconds and score drift/movement)	No drift Drift but maintains in air Unable to maintain in air No effort against gravity No movement Amputation, joint fusion (explain)	0 1 2 3 4 N/A
6a. Motor; leg—left (elevate extremity to 30 degrees for 5 seconds and score drift/movement)	No drift Drift but maintains in air Unable to maintain in air No effort against gravity No movement Amputation, joint fusion (explain)	0 1 2 3 4 N/A
6b. Motor; leg—right (elevate extremity to 30 degrees for 5 seconds and score drift/movement)	No drift Drift but maintains in air Unable to maintain in air No effort against gravity No movement Amputation, joint fusion (explain)	0 1 2 3 4 N/A
7. Limb ataxia (finger-to-nose and heel-to-shin testing)	Absent Present in one limb Present in two limbs	0 1 2
8. Sensory (pin prick to face, arm, trunk, and leg—compare side to side)	Normal Mild to moderate loss Severe to total loss	0 1 2

Category	Description	Score
9. Best language (name items, describe a picture and read sentences)	No aphasia Mild to moderate aphasia Severe aphasia Mute	0 1 2 3
10. Dysarthria (evaluate speech clarity by having patient repeat words)	Normal Mild to moderate dysarthria Severe dysarthria, mostly unintelligible or worse Intubated or other physical barrier	0 1 2 N/A
11. Extinction and inattention (use information from prior testing to score)	No abnormality Visual, tactile, auditory, or other extinction to bilateral simultaneous stimulation Profound hemi-attention or extinction to more than one modality	0 1 2
Total score		

Adapted from the version available at the National Institute of Neurological Disorders and Stroke, National Institutes of Health, Bethesda, MD. http://www.ninds.nih.gov/doctors/NIH_Stroke_Scale.pdf. It is recommended that the full scale with all instructions be used.

Once hemorrhage has been ruled out and the clinical diagnosis of ischemic stroke is made, the acute stroke team must review the eligibility criteria for thrombolytic administration. For a complete list of inclusion and exclusion criteria for IV thrombolysis, see Figure 46-10 and Box 46-3. Many programs consider absolute and relative exclusions based on practice changes, so the nurse must be aware of their institution's guidelines. For example, in many hospitals, the tPA window may be <4.5 hours rather than the 3-hour window noted in the enclosed guidelines.

Nurses are often responsible for administering IV thrombolytics. Both alteplase and tenecteplase are weight based. Alteplase is split into a bolus and an infusion, at 0.9 mg/kg, with a maximum dose of 90 mg. Ten percent of the calculated dose is initially administered as an IV bolus over 1 minute, with the remaining 90% given subsequently via infusion over an hour. Tenecteplase is given only as a single IV bolus at 0.25 mg/kg over 5 seconds (Xiong et al., 2022).

Endovascular revascularization, or mechanical thrombectomy, can be performed in cases where a patient has a large-vessel occlusion; the stroke has not "completed," that is, tissue at risk has not yet infarcted; and the clot is in a blood vessel reachable by catheter-based approaches. Thrombectomy-Capable and Comprehensive Stroke Centers are those with the technology and interventionalists capable of performing these delicate procedures. ICU level of nursing care and monitoring is required after intervention. Major postoperative complications include blood pressure instability, stroke or transient neurologic deficits, cranial nerve injury (facial, vagal), wound hematoma, suture line rupture, TIAs, and hyperperfusion syndromes (characterized by headaches, neurologic deficits, and seizures not caused by cerebral ischemia; commonly associated with an increase in blood pressure) (Lin & Liu, 2020). It is not uncommon for patients to experience blood pressure instability that lasts for approximately 12 to 24 hours postoperatively (Livesay & Hickey, 2020). Once blood flow has been restored, maintenance of a stable systolic pressure of approximately 150 mm Hg is essential. The sudden restoration of high blood flow can lead to ICH, whereas hypotensive episodes can result in ischemic stroke or TIAs (Livesay & Hickey, 2020). Thus, the nurse is vigilant in monitoring vital signs and neurologic status post procedure.

In the most acute phase of suspected stroke, whether or not immediate intervention is performed, ongoing assessments and precise documentation of the patient is paramount. Nursing assessments will include, but may not be limited to: neurologic assessment, usually with the NIHSS, and monitoring of vital signs and pupil changes (change or inequality in pupil size is a significant neurologic sign that should be reported immediately). Patients receiving tPA should additionally be monitored for unexpected bleeding as well as for angioedema (oral/lingual swelling) and anaphylaxis (allergic reaction) to the medication. Angioedema is more likely to occur within the first 2 hours, but precautions should be maintained for identifying signs and symptoms 3 to 24 hours after administration (Maqueda & Perme, 2022). Refer to Chapter 37 for details on angioedema and allergic reaction. Patients who receive thrombectomy require additional monitoring at the access puncture site and potentially for postanesthesia care. A detailed overview of postthrombectomy care is given by the AHA in 2018 (Jadhav et al., 2018; Rodgers et al., 2021).

Results from the 1995 NINDS trial demonstrated a significant improvement in functional outcome at 3 months poststroke in those patients who received tPA within 3 hours after symptom onset (NINDS & Stroke rtPA Stroke Study Work Group, 1995). Results from the 2008 ECASS 3 demonstrated clinically significant improvement in functional outcome in selected patients who received treatment up to

BOX 46-3

Inclusion and Exclusion Characteristics of Patients with Ischemic Stroke Who Could Be Treated With Intravenous Recombinant Tissue-Type Plasminogen Activator (IV r-tPA), or Alteplase

Inclusion Criteria	Exclusion Criteria
1. Symptom onset of <3 hours before beginning treatment 2. Clinical diagnosis of ischemic stroke with measurable deficit 3. Age >18 years	1. Stroke or serious cerebral trauma within previous 3 months 2. Symptoms suggest SAH 3. Arterial puncture at noncompressible site in previous 7 days 4. History of previous intracranial hemorrhage 5. Intracranial neoplasm, AVM, or aneurysm 6. Recent intracranial or intraspinal surgery 7. Elevated blood pressure (SBP >185 or DBP >110 mm Hg) 8. Active internal bleeding 9. Acute bleeding diathesis, including but not limited to platelet count <100,000/mm^3, heparin received within 48 hours resulting in abnormally elevated aPTT above the upper limit of normal, current use of anticoagulant with INR >1.7 or PT >15 seconds, current use of direct thrombin inhibitors or direct factor Xa inhibitors with elevated sensitive laboratory tests (e.g., aPTT, INR, platelet count, ECT, TT, or appropriate factor Xa activity assays) 10. Blood glucose concentration <50 mg/dL 11. CT demonstrates multilobar infarction (hypodensity >1/3 cerebral hemisphere). Relative Exclusion Criteria: Recent experience suggests that under some circumstances, with careful consideration and weighing the risk to benefit, patients may receive fibrinolytic therapy despite ≥1 relative contraindication. Consider risk to benefit of intravenous rtPA administration carefully if any of these relative contraindications is present: 1. Only minor or rapidly improving stroke symptoms (clearing spontaneously) 2. Pregnancy 3. Seizure at onset with postictal residual neurologic impairments 4. Major surgery or serious trauma within previous 14 days 5. Recent GI or GU tract hemorrhage (within previous 21 days) 6. Recent acute myocardial infarction (within previous 3 months)

aPTT, activated partial thromboplastin time; AVM, arteriovenous malformation; CT, computed tomography; ECT, ecarin clotting time; INR, international normalized ratio; PT, partial thromboplastin time; rtPA, recombinant tissue-type plasminogen activator; SAH, subarachnoid hemorrhage; TT, thrombin time.

Source: From Demaerschalk, B. M., Kleindorfer, D. O., Adeoye, O. M., Demchuk, A. M., Fugate, J. E., Grotta, J. C., & Smith, E. E. (2015). Scientific rational for the inclusion and exclusion criteria for intravenous alteplase in acute ischemic stroke. A statement for health care professionals from the American Heart Association/American Stroke Association. *Stroke*, *47*(2), 581–641.

4.5 hours after symptom onset (Hacke et al., 2008; Livesay & Hickey, 2020). Specifically, patients who are under 80 years of age, who have no history of stroke or diabetes, who are not on anticoagulation therapy, and who do not have a severe stroke score of 25 or more are deemed significantly likely to benefit from thrombolysis using this extended time window. This change in practice has afforded more patients the option for treatment and a better functional outcome after stroke. Stroke centers generally outline their approach to treatment according to the most current ASA guidelines. Once a hemorrhage has been ruled out and the clinical diagnosis of ischemic stroke is made, the acute stroke team must review the eligibility criteria for alteplase administration.

Nurses are often responsible for administering thrombolytic medication, and some facilities expect nurses to mix and prepare the medication for administration. It is a weight-based medication; for alteplase, it is dosed at 0.9 mg/kg, with a maximum dose of 90 mg. Ten percent of the calculated dose is administered as an IV bolus over 1 minute. The remaining dose (90%) is administered over 1 hour via an infusion pump. Since bleeding is the most common side effect of alteplase, occurring in 3.0% to 6.4% of all patients treated with tPA, the patient is closely monitored for any suspected bleeding (at IV insertion sites, gums, urine/stools, and intracranially by assessing changes in LOC) (Maqueda & Perme, 2022). Timing of hemorrhagic events after thrombolysis have been noted within the first 5 to 10 hours (50%), and 80% of events occur in the first 12 hours (Chang et al., 2018; Maqueda & Perme, 2022; Powers et al., 2019).

During the hyperacute phase of a suspected acute stroke, ongoing assessments and meticulous documentation of the patient's neurologic and hemodynamic status are essential, regardless of stroke type and whether or not the patient was a candidate for IV treatment.

Acute Stroke Recovery Care

Table 46-5 summarizes the nursing care for thrombolysis and nonthrombolysis treatments for patients with acute ischemic stroke. Poststroke management addresses blood pressure parameters, oxygenation, body temperature, and hyperglycemia. In addition, there are directives for neurologic assessments, deep vein thrombosis (DVT) prophylaxis, body temperature and oxygen status, cardiac monitoring, and screening for impaired swallowing prior to oral intake.

Secondary Stroke Prevention

Patients who have experienced an initial stroke are at increased risk for a second event. This risk is dependent on the etiology of the first stroke and the steps taken to prevent a recurrent stroke. Once the likely etiology of an ischemic stroke is determined, effective secondary stroke prevention will include the selection of the appropriate antithrombotic medication. The use of antithrombotic agents is a primary focus for secondary stroke prevention.

TABLE 46-5 Schedule of Neurologic Assessment and Vital Signs and Other Acute Care Assessments in Thrombolysis-Treated and Nonthrombolysis-Treated Patients

Thrombolysis-Treated Patients	Nonthrombolysis-Treated Patients
Neurologic assessment and vital signs (except temperature) every 15 minutes during alteplase infusion, then every 30 minutes for 6 hours, and then every 60 minutes for 16 hours (total of 24 hours). Note: Frequency of blood pressure (BP) assessments may need to be increased if systolic BP stays greater than 180 mm Hg or diastolic BP stays greater than 105 mm Hg during the first 24 hours. Temperature every 4 hours or as required. Treat temperatures > 99.6°F with acetaminophen as ordered.	In intensive care unit (ICU), every hour with neurologic checks or more frequently if necessary. In a non-ICU setting, depending on patient's condition and neurologic assessments; at a minimum check neurologic assessment and vital signs every 4 hours.
After 24 hours, call provider if systolic BP greater than 185 or less than 110 mm Hg; diastolic BP greater than 105 or less than 60 mm Hg; pulse less than 50 or greater than 110 per minute; respirations 24 per minute; temperature over 99.6°F; or for worsening of stroke symptoms or other decline in neurologic status.	Call provider for further treatment based on provider and institutional preferences/guidelines: Systolic BP above 220 or below 110 mm Hg; diastolic BP above 120 or below 60 mm Hg; pulse below 50 or above 110 per minute; temperature above 99.6°F; respirations 24 per minute; or for worsening of stroke symptoms or other decline in neurologic status.
For O_2 saturation below 94%, give O_2 by cannula at 2–3 L/min	For O_2 saturation below 94%, give O_2 by cannula at 2–3 L/min
Monitor for major and minor bleeding complications	N/A
Continuous cardiac monitoring up to 72 hours or more	Continuous cardiac monitoring for 24–48 hours
Measure intake and output	Measure intake and output
Activity—as ordered by the provider	Activity—as ordered by the provider
IV fluids normal saline (NS) at 75–100 mL/hr	IV fluids NS at 75–100 mL/hr
No heparin, warfarin, aspirin, clopidogrel, or aspirin/extended-release dipyridamole for 24 hours, then start antithrombotic as ordered	Antithrombotics should be ordered before the end of hospital day #2
Brain CT or MRI after rtPA therapy	Repeat brain CT scan or MRI may be ordered 24–48 hours after stroke or as needed

Data from Ashcraft, S., Wilson, S. E., Nyström, K. V., Dusenbury, W., Wira, C. R., & Burrus, T. M.; American Heart Association Council on Cardiovascular and Stroke Nursing and the Stroke Council. (2021). Care of the patient with acute ischemic stroke (prehospital and acute phase of care): an update to the 2009 comprehensive nursing care scientific statement: a scientific statement from the American Heart Association. *Stroke, 52*(5), e164–e178.

For patients whose stroke is thought to be cardiogenic embolic (from atrial fibrillation), warfarin or one of the newer anticoagulants is the most effective treatment to reduce stroke risk. For all other ischemic stroke types, antiplatelet treatment is recommended and can use one of several medications, including aspirin (at doses of 81 to 325 mg), clopidogrel (75 mg daily), and low-dose aspirin in combination with extended-release dipyridamole (50/200 mg). In addition, based on the results of several studies, the use of statins for secondary (and primary) stroke prevention is recommended. A lipid profile is reviewed, and the current goal is for the low-density lipoprotein (LDL) to be less than 70 mg/dL. In general, patients are prescribed a high-dose statin (such as atorvastatin) to achieve the goal LDL. Statins also have shown to have an anti-inflammatory effect, which provides further secondary stroke prevention in the first few months after the event.

Acute Hemorrhagic Stroke

Acute hemorrhagic stroke is initially managed differently than ischemic stroke, although the symptoms at presentation and in deficit may be similar. A higher proportion of hemorrhagic strokes affect LOC, requiring more attention to stabilization needs, for example, maintaining airway breathing and circulation. The major immediate complication of hemorrhage is expansion of bleeding or edema; this in turn leads to what is called "mass effect," or the simple effect of increased, unchecked pressure on the structures of the brain. Increased ICP can lead to acute hydrocephalus as ventricles are blocked, physical injury to brain tissue causes secondary infarct, and ultimately herniation of the brain occurs through the foramen or traumatic openings in the skull (refer to Chapter 44). The presence of blood in the cerebral tissue also acts as an irritant and can lead to seizure.

The immediate goal of treatment is to decrease ICP. High frequency, detailed nursing assessment, and identification and implementation of rapid, appropriate interventions can help decrease the morbidity of these patients. The highest risk of neurodegeneration is in the first 12 to 24 hours after hemorrhage.

Assessment is often initially made with the Glasgow Coma Scale (GCS) as well as the NIHSS. A GCS score, which ranges from 3 for a nonresponsive patient, to 15 for the normally mentating person, is a quick summary of responsiveness. A GCS of 8 or less indicates rapid deterioration of the ability to respond to stimulus; patients with this amount of impairment are often immediately intubated for airway protection. Deterioration must be reported to the health care team. Other assessments include monitoring for changes in standard vital signs or specialized measurements, such as probes for ICP. A too-rapid change in any measurement often portends worse outcome.

The GCS is part of the intracerebral hemorrhage score (ICH), a clinical grading score which considers the GCS, hemorrhage volume, specifics of location of the hemorrhage, and the patient's age to estimate mortality. A higher score is derived from hemorrhages greater than 30 mL, originating in the cerebellum or brainstem, infiltrating the ventricles, substantially affecting LOC, and/or occurring in persons aged 80 or older. These have been shown to increase the risk of mortality (Greenberg et al., 2022).

In patients with SAH specifically, the Hunt and Hess Score is used (Fig. 46-13) to grade patients with SAH to predict surgical mortality. This considers LOC, focal deficit, and headache quality; it can fluctuate during admission. Higher scores portend worse prognoses.

Monitoring of peripheral oxygenation is expected with a pulse oximeter. Nurses will be directed to elevate the head of bed to 30 degrees, monitor sedation if instituted, and prepare for one or more of the following treatment options: anticoagulation reversal if patient is on an anticoagulant; hyperventilation (hypocapnia [low CO_2]) to temporarily cause vascular constriction, resulting in reduced blood flow in vessels not involved with the injury; placement of a ventricular catheter for CSF drainage; or administration of mannitol—all to reduce elevated ICP. Because hyperthermia (temperature above 37.5°C [99.5 F]) is associated with a poorer prognosis following acute stroke, the nurse monitors the patient's temperature and is prepared to initiate measures to prevent and control fever collaboratively with the health care team. In addition, because aspiration is a significant risk, patients should be maintained NPO until they are screened for dysphagia (Hickey & Strayer, 2020).

Providers will report an ICH score early in the assessment of a patient with an intracranial hemorrhage to determine prognosis. The scale in Figure 46-12 reviews specific patient-related characteristics to devise a score that is associated with risk for mortality within the first 30 days after hemorrhage. Components of the ICH score include the GCS score, hemorrhage volume, the presence of infratentorial hemorrhage, location of the hemorrhage, and patient age. The higher scores (5 and 6) predict a 100% mortality and, as such, will assist with decisions related to goals of care.

Concept Mastery Alert

For nonthrombolysis-treated patients, antithrombotics should be administered before the end of day #2.

Surgical evacuation of intracranial bleeding is also considered in selected cases that require immediate intervention and when neurosurgical services are available. Depending on the location and volume of the intracerebral bleed, the degree of neurologic deterioration, and the presence of hydrocephalus and ventricular obstruction, patients may undergo a craniotomy and evacuation of the hematoma. Antihypertensive medications and antiepileptic medications are also mainstays of acute therapy to control bleeding and potential seizures. Blood pressure goals are ordered based on individual patient profiles. Current clinical trials are underway to determine target blood pressure ranges in ischemic stroke; however, generally treatment is avoided unless

GCS	
3–4	2 pts
5–12	1 pt
13–15	0 pts
ICH volume	
≥ 30 cm^3	1 pt
< 30 cm^3	0 pts
IVH	
Yes	1 pt
No	0 pts
Location	
Infratentorial	1 pt
Supratentorial	0 pts
Age	
≥ 80 yrs	1 pt
< 80 yrs	0 pts

ICH score	Mortality
0	No mortality
1	13%
2	26%
3	72%
4	97%
5	100%
6	100%

FIGURE 46-12 **Determination of the intracerebral hemorrhage (ICH) score and risk of mortality. GCS, Glasgow Coma Scale; ICH, intracerebral hemorrhage; IVH, intraventricular hemorrhage. (Hemphill, J. C., Bonovich, D. C., Besmertis, L., Manley, G. T., & Johnston, S. C. [2001]. The ICH score: A simple reliable grading scale for intracerebral hemorrhage. *Stroke*, *32*, 891–897.)**

Hunt-Hess Scale

- **Grade 1:**
  Mild headache, normal mental status, no cranial nerve or motor findings – (GCS score 15, no motor deficits)
- **Grade 2:**
  Severe headache, normal mental status, may have cranial nerve deficit – (GCS score 13–14, no motor deficits)
- **Grade 3:**
  Somnolent, confused, may have cranial nerve or mild motor deficit – (GCS score 13–14, with motor deficits
- **Grade 4:**
  Stupor, moderate to severe motor deficit, may have intermittent reflex posturing – (GCS score 7–12, with or without motor deficits)
- **Grade 5:**
  Coma, reflex posturing or flaccid – (GCS score, 3–6, with or without motor deficits)

FIGURE 46-13 **HUNT-HESS scores. (Data from Hunt, W. E., & Hess, R. M. (1968). Surgical risk as related to time of intervention in the repair of intracranial aneurysms. *Journal of Neurosurgery*, *28*(1), 14–20.)**

the systolic BP is greater than 220 mm Hg or diastolic BP is greater than 120 mm Hg. Pain, fever, and hyperglycemia are addressed in the first 24 hours to reduce further cerebral injury (Hickey & Strayer, 2020).

For patients with a known ruptured aneurysm and subsequent SAH, the 2015 AHA guidelines for SAH describe both surgical clipping and endovascular coiling as beneficial options to reduce the risk of rebleeding. Surgical clipping involves a craniotomy and placement of a clip at the neck of the artery to close the rupture site. Coiling is an endovascular procedure using a catheter that is accessed from the femoral artery and directed through the vasculature to the location of the aneurysm. Multiple coils are then dispensed through the catheter and packed into the dome of the aneurysm to promote clotting and close the aneurysm. The choice of aneurysm treatment depends on the overall health of the patient, the nature and location of the aneurysm, and the available resources at the hospital. Providers also use an assessment scoring tool called the Hunt-Hess Score (Fig. 46-13) to grade patients with SAH to predict surgical mortality. Based on headache quality, focal deficit, and LOC, the patient with a higher score will portend a poor prognosis. Because this score depends on evolving and sometimes fluctuating symptoms, this score can change from what was recorded during the patient's initial admission.

Stroke care in the acute phase is typically designated as the time during which the patient has been admitted to the hospital. The hospital stay can vary from a few days to many weeks, depending on the nature and severity of the stroke and on the deficits and complications associated with recovery. In addition to monitoring for potential complications associated with stroke such as deconditioning, aspiration, infection, bowel and bladder dysfunction, and inability to perform self-care, care plans should include an early initiation of rehabilitation to improve functional outcome.

Stroke Rehabilitation

The potential for recovery after stroke begins in the early phases of hospitalization, often in the ICU, extending beyond the hospital along the different parts of the continuum. There is a plethora of evidence that suggests rehabilitation, particularly early and aggressive rehab, plays a key role for improving functional outcomes and quality of life. Rehabilitation services, PT, OT, and SLP, typically commence when the patient is in the ICU. The goal for stroke rehab in the hospital setting is early mobilization and discharge planning to the next level of care with multiple postacute discharge options. Rehabilitation services work with nursing in coordinating these efforts.

The diagram below depicts the postacute care disposition options along the continuum (see Fig. 46-14). Each stage is working toward maximizing functional recovery, although each stage has benefits and drawbacks.

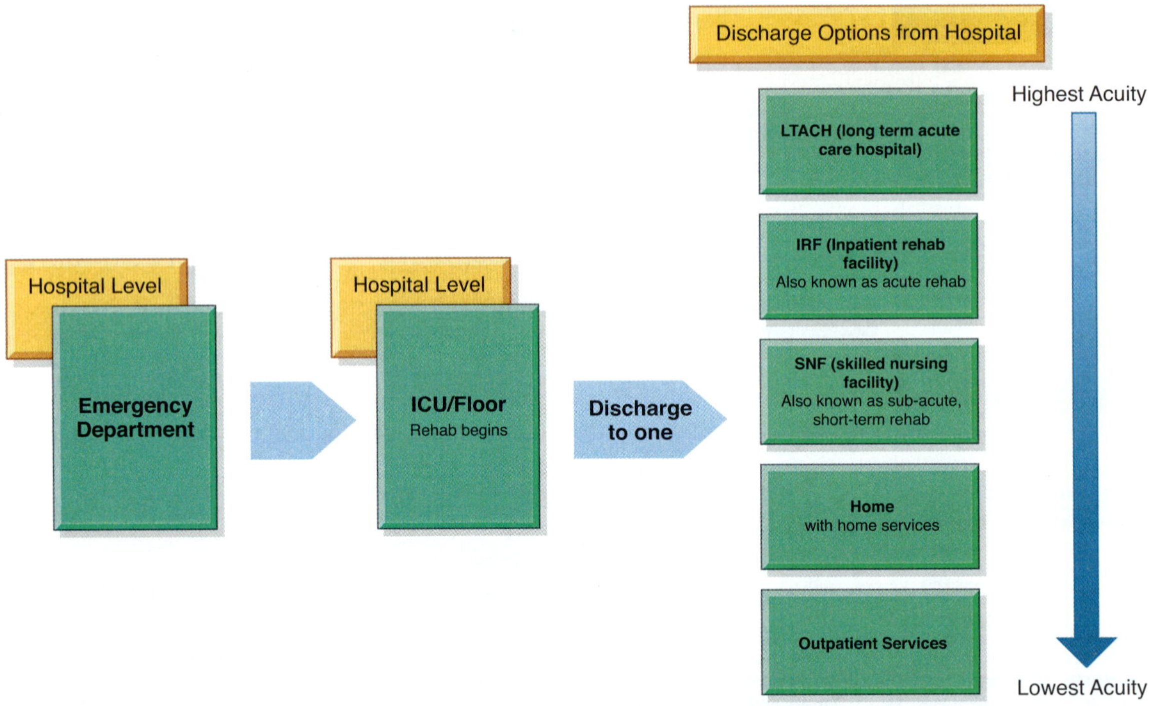

FIGURE 46-14 **Stroke care trajectory from acute care to discharge options.**

Inpatient Rehab facility (IRF), also known as acute rehab, is the most intense option with 3 hours of daily therapy with physical medicine and rehabilitation (physiatry) involvement. In addition, many of the nurses are certified rehabilitation nurses. The goal is to return patients home from this level and continue services in the home and community environment. Long-term acute care hospitals (LTACHs) provide an extension of medical care with daily physician monitoring while beginning rehabilitation. Due to the medical needs, often the rehab is less than the 3 hours. Skilled nursing facilities (SNF), also known as subacute rehab or short-term rehab, offer less intense rehab with 1.5 to 2 hours of therapy. All three of these choices commence in a facility with an inpatient level of care.

After deemed safe and appropriate to return home, patients will transition to home where there will be an extension of rehab services, but not as frequently as the inpatient facilities. Families will be trained and equipment will be provided as necessary. At this stage of their recovery, patients are ready to begin to practice functional tasks in their home environment. There will be continuation of stroke rehab as either home rehab services or outpatient rehab services.

When deciding between home service and outpatient services, one needs to look at the whole picture and consider what would benefit the patient the most. Home care services require patients to be homebound except for religious services or medical appointments. The frequency and length of the visit are limited. In addition, there is limited equipment a therapist can utilize in the home environment. However, if a patient can get to outpatient services there is a myriad of equipment available to utilize in their recovery, and the sessions are longer in duration.

Nursing care is an integral part at each step along the continuum in supporting these patients and preventing potential secondary complications such as aspiration, skin breakdown, falls, incontinence, and depression.

Factors that Affect Discharge Option

There are multiple factors that will impact the discharge plan from the hospital to the next level of care. Facilities all have specific requirements that the patient must meet in order to qualify. Factors that are considered but not limited to are: duration of therapy the patient can tolerate; severity of the stroke; need for all three disciplines of PT, OT, and SLP; nursing care needs; baseline function; level of family support when discharged; insurance barriers; length of stay in the hospital; age; and other active medical issues. The severity of neurologic impairment and level of disability after a stroke are strong predictors for disposition after stroke.

How Discharge Options Affect Stroke Recovery and Outcome Measures

The goal is to maximize functional mobility and limit disability while promoting ability. Advocating for early aggressive rehab at IRF (acute rehab) facilities, if criteria are met, is strongly associated with a more favorable outcome versus going to an SNF.

There are several stroke scales that are utilized as a predictor of disability and outcomes. The NIHSS is a scale used to assess the impairments and neurologic function of the stroke patient. The NIHSS is determined to be a good predictor of outcomes when discharging from a hospital. Most stroke patients with a score of 6 or greater are discharged to an IRF. A second scale often used in the delivery of stroke care is the Modified Rankin Scale (mRS). The mRS is a provider-reported measure of global disability that has been widely applied for evaluating recovery from stroke and as a primary endpoint in randomized clinical trials of emerging acute stroke treatments.

Different Models of Care Utilized in Stroke Rehab

There has been an evolution of team models, particularly with the stroke population, over the last few decades. Facilities vary in which team model they utilize. Understanding the different models and the role of each discipline is important in optimizing the best stroke rehabilitation and outcomes for the patient. Nursing intervention and participation in the different team approaches enhances the recovery, so the approaches are important to understand at each level. The evolution has been from single discipline to multidisciplinary team, to interdisciplinary team and now more facilities are functioning as a transdisciplinary team, which is a team composed of members of several different professions cooperating across disciplines to improve patient care through practice or research. Transdisciplinary teams are now viewed as the gold standard because they provide more integrated service delivery and are a patient centered focus, since in this model all disciplines, including nursing, are responsible for every clinical concern. There is cross communication and cross treatment among all disciplines. The approach fosters awareness of each other's role and lessens the variability of care. Example: When nursing is with the patient, they will carry out what PT has recommended such as transfers with facilitation of the involved side, or speech cues for the aphasic patient. Figure 46-15 provides a visualization of how a transdisciplinary team works. It depicts how there are no boundaries and each discipline wears each other's hats when with the patient. The patient and family are the center of care.

The major goals for the patient (and family) should include all efforts to return the patient to their premorbid functioning. Depending on the location of the initial brain injury, patients are assessed for rehabilitative needs to improve mobility, communication, cognition, coordination, balance, and pain relief (from contractures). Potential complications such as aspiration, incontinence, skin breakdown, falls, depression, and disruption of family dynamics are targets for prevention.

Prevention

In a healthy population, risk factors are identified and addressed in a primordial and primary prevention program. *Primordial prevention* refers to strategies designed to decrease the development of disease risk factors (e.g., efforts

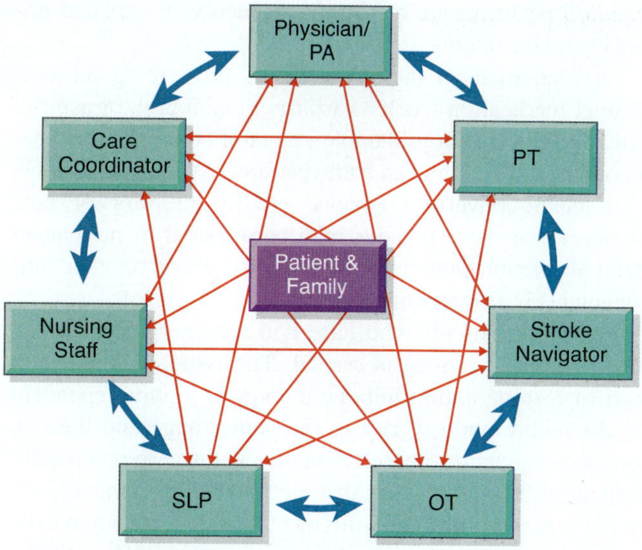

FIGURE 46-15 **Model of transdisciplinary team where the patient and family are at the center of care.**

to decrease the development of obesity, to increase exercise, and to provide a well-balanced diet). Primordial prevention encompasses the entire population and is not limited to individuals with recognized risk factors for stroke or other cardiovascular diseases. The aim is to prevent the development of disease or injury through a focus on social and environmental conditions (Adeoya et al., 2019; Kisling & Das, 2022). The recent focus on addressing the structural and social determinants of health is part of primordial prevention, as we aim to improve the health of the nation (Hayman & Coke, 2020). *Primary prevention* refers to the treatment of established disease risk factors for those healthy patients or populations who have not yet had an event but are susceptible. The 2014 Guidelines for the Primary Prevention of Stroke provide a comprehensive overview of established and emerging modifiable and nonmodifiable stroke risk factors (Meschia et al., 2014). Examples include adhering to a healthy lifestyle (not smoking, following a diet low in sodium and rich in fruits and vegetables, a minimum of 30 minutes of moderate or vigorous physical activity daily, maintaining a body mass index below 25 kg/m^2, consuming no more than one alcoholic drink per day for females and one or two for males). These measures are associated with an 80% lower risk of a first stroke when compared to people who do not follow these measures (Goldstein, 2020).

For patients who have had a stroke, risk factor modification is a critical part of the secondary prevention plan. Stroke education for patients and their families addresses the possible causes of stroke, identifies potential stroke risk factors, reinforces adherence with medications, and discusses pertinent lifestyle changes to reduce stroke risk. The 2014 guidelines for the prevention of subsequent stroke after stroke or TIA highlight the following key risk factors: hypertension, diabetes, dyslipidemia, smoking, alcohol consumption, obesity, and sedentary activity. Patient education has become a standard performance measure for practice at certified primary stroke centers.

Optimal medical therapy includes prescribing an antiplatelet medication (such as aspirin, clopidogrel, or aspirin/extended-release dipyridamole), a statin (such as atorvastatin or simvastatin), and an antihypertensive (thiazide diuretic, angiotensin-converting enzyme [ACE] inhibitor or beta blocker). For those patients with paroxysmal or permanent atrial fibrillation, anticoagulation (with warfarin or other anticoagulant) is also recommended.

For those patients who have had a hemorrhagic stroke, blood pressure control is critical. The issue of whether to start or resume antithrombotic therapy is highly dependent on the nature and severity of the hemorrhage and the risk for a subsequent thrombotic event (as in the case of a patient with atrial fibrillation or with a mechanical heart valve).

For patients with symptoms of TIA or stroke thought to be caused by significant carotid artery stenosis (70% to 99%), a carotid endarterectomy (CEA) may be recommended. A CEA is the removal of an atherosclerotic plaque or thrombus from the ICA to prevent recurrent stroke. Carotid angioplasty and stenting is an alternative (less invasive) procedure performed in selected patients when surgery poses a higher risk and the endovascular approach poses a low perioperative complication risk. These procedures are generally recommended once the patient is hemodynamically stable, usually within the first 2 weeks following their event.

In preparation for discharge, teaching patients and families about what to expect within a home or rehabilitation facility will be a focus for nursing, the rehabilitation staff, and the discharge planner. Resources in the community, such as support groups, regional and national heart and stroke associations, and hospital-based social work support should also be part of the discharge materials.

NURSING PROCESS
The Patient With a Stroke

ASSESSMENT

A nursing flow sheet is maintained for the documentation of a complete neurologic assessment.

A systems approach to examining and documenting findings should include a mental status evaluation (orientation, affect, perception, memory, attention span, speech, and language), motor control, swallowing ability, hydration status, fluid output, skin integrity, and activity level. The ongoing nursing assessment continues to focus on alterations in cognition and functional impairment and directs the appropriate nursing diagnoses.

DIAGNOSIS

Appropriate nursing diagnoses may include:

- Altered hemodynamics related to cardiac arrhythmias, hyper-/hypotension, fluid/electrolyte imbalances
- Impaired physical mobility related to hemiparesis, sensory loss, loss of balance or coordination, or visual field deficit
- Impaired verbal communication related to dysarthria, aphasia, altered cognition
- Impaired swallowing/risk for aspiration related to inability to protect airway or altered LOC
- Risk for infection related to smoking history, invasive lines, Foley catheter, nasogastric (NG) tube
- Risk for ineffective peripheral tissue perfusion related to risk for DVT/immobility
- High risk for injury related to visual field, motor, or perception deficits
- Knowledge deficit related to lack of awareness of stroke risk factors, secondary stroke prevention medications, potential lifestyle changes, physical and occupational therapies

PLANNING

Although rehabilitation begins on the day of admission, the process is intensified during convalescence and requires a coordinated team effort. It is helpful for the team to know the patient's baseline function, medical history, mental and emotional state, behavioral characteristics, and ADLs. In addition, providers should be knowledgeable about the relative importance of predictors of stroke outcome (age, comorbidities such as diabetes, and presenting NIHSS score) in order to provide stroke survivors and their families with a realistic recovery trajectory. For example, the NIHSS score is used commonly to communicate the severity of symptoms associated with stroke and is often conducted on admission, at 24 hours, and at discharge; other institutions will collect the NIHSS score every shift and use the score to communicate patient status (Hickey & Strayer, 2020). Refer to Table 46-4 for the NIHSS scale.

A commonly used assessment scale for measuring disability as it relates to the patient's dependence with daily activities after stroke is the modified Rankin scale. A 0–6 scale is used to describe the trajectory from "zero" or "no symptoms—able to perform all usual activities" to "five" or "severe disability—bedridden and requiring constant 24-hour care." A score of "six" refers to death. This tool has been adopted by providers, rehabilitation specialists, and researchers to determine prestroke capabilities as well as short- and long-term poststroke degree of disability. See Figure 46-16.

The major goals for the patient (and family) may include improved mobility, avoidance of shoulder pain, achievement of self-care, relief of sensory and perceptual deprivation, prevention of aspiration, continence of bowel and bladder, improved thought processes, optimization of communication, maintaining skin integrity, restored family functioning, improved sexual function, and absence of complications.

NURSING INTERVENTIONS

Nursing care has a significant impact on the patient's recovery. Often, many body systems are impaired as a result of the stroke, and conscientious care and timely interventions can prevent

Modified Rankin Scale (MRS)	
0	No symptoms
1	No significant disability, despite symptoms; able to perform all usual duties and activities
2	Slight disability; unable to perform all previous activities but able to look after own affairs without assistance
3	Moderate disability; requires some help, but able to walk without assistance
4	Moderately severe disability; unable to walk without assistance and unable to attend to own bodily needs without assistance
5	Severe disability; bedridden, incontinent, and requires constant nursing care and attention
6	Death

FIGURE 46-16 Modified Rankin scale. (Rankin, J. [1957]. Cerebral vascular accidents in patients over the age of 60. *Scottish Medical Journal*, *2*, 200–215; Bonita, R., & Beaglehole, R. [1988]. Modification of Rankin Scale: Recovery of motor function after stroke. *Stroke*, *19*[12], 1497–1500.)

debilitating complications. During and after the acute phase, nursing interventions include a comprehensive approach to physical care and fostering recovery by listening to the patient and asking questions to elicit the meaning of the stroke experience.

IMPROVING MOBILITY AND PREVENTING JOINT DEFORMITIES

When control of the voluntary muscles is lost, the strong flexor muscles exert control over the extensors. The arm tends to adduct (adductor muscles are stronger than abductors) and to rotate internally. The elbow and the wrist tend to flex, the affected leg tends to rotate externally at the hip joint and flex at the knee, and the foot at the ankle joint supinates and tends toward plantar flexion.

Correct positioning is important to prevent contractures; measures are used to relieve pressure, assist in maintaining good body alignment, and prevent compressive neuropathies, especially of the ulnar and peroneal nerves. Because flexor muscles are stronger than extensor muscles, a posterior splint applied at night to the affected extremity may prevent flexion and maintain correct positioning during sleep. If splints are in place, the nurse assesses the skin for evidence of impaired circulation, sensation, and/or mobility, as well as any evidence of altered skin integrity.

Pearls for Practice

In the acute phase, the goal is to optimize cerebral perfusion so the provider may prescribe the head of bed flat (supine) for 24 hours because of vascular instability (Livesay & Hickey, 2020). The supine position is generally reserved for conscious patients without evidence of dysphagia since they are at low risk for aspiration and can control secretions. The unconscious patient or a patient at risk for aspiration may be positioned in side-lying position with the head of the bed elevated 10 to 30 degrees to facilitate the drainage of secretions from the mouth (Hickey & Strayer, 2020). Results of the HEADPOST study showed no significant difference in outcomes in disability between supine patients for 24 hours and patients with head of bed at 30 degrees for 24 hours (Anderson et al., 2017). Practices for patient positioning are institution-specific and are outlined in stroke recovery care protocols. In general, most practices include an HOB order of 30 degrees, but this will be based on stability of hemodynamics and ICP.

Preventing Shoulder Adduction. To prevent adduction of the affected shoulder while the patient is in bed, a pillow is placed in the axilla when there is limited external rotation; this keeps the arm away from the chest. A pillow is placed under the arm, and the arm is placed in a neutral (slightly flexed) position, with distal joints positioned higher than the more proximal joints (i.e., the elbow is positioned higher than the shoulder and the wrist higher than the elbow). This helps to prevent edema and the resultant joint fibrosis that will limit range of motion (ROM) if the patient regains control of the arm.

Positioning the Hand and Fingers. The fingers are positioned so that they are barely flexed. The hand is placed in slight supination (palm faces upward), which is its most functional position. If the upper extremity is flaccid, a splint can be used to support the wrist and hand in a functional position. Every effort is made to prevent hand edema.

Spasticity, particularly in the hand, can be a disabling complication after stroke. Researchers have reported that repeated intramuscular injections of botulinum toxin A into wrist and finger muscles significantly reduced upper limb spasticity after stroke and improved upper limb motor function for a period of 3 months; however, the evidence on whether botulinum toxin A injections are useful for improving upper limb capacity is lacking (Bavikatte et al., 2021).

Mirror therapy has also demonstrated improvement in motor functions and ADLs that persisted after 6 months. In this therapy, the patient watches a mirror as movements with the unaffected hand are performed, leaving the impression that the affected hand is moving. This therapy is purported to induce neuroplasticity changes in the primary motor cortex that support recovery (Radajewska, 2017; Gandhi et al., 2020).

Establishing an Exercise Program. The affected extremities are exercised passively and put through a full ROM four or five times a day to maintain joint mobility, regain motor control, prevent contractures in the paralyzed extremity, prevent further

(continued on page 1506)

deterioration of the neuromuscular system, and enhance circulation. Repetition of an activity forms new pathways in the CNS and therefore encourages new patterns of motion. At first, the extremities are usually flaccid. If tightness occurs in any area, the ROM exercises should be performed more frequently. Regularity in exercise is most important. Improvement in muscle strength and maintenance of ROM can be achieved only through daily exercise.

The patient is encouraged and reminded to exercise the unaffected side at intervals throughout the day. It is helpful to develop a written schedule to remind the patient of the exercise activities. The nurse supervises and supports the patient during these activities. The patient can be taught to put the unaffected leg under the affected one to assist in moving it when turning and exercising. Flexibility, strengthening, coordination, endurance, and balancing exercises prepare the patient for ambulation. Quadriceps muscle setting and gluteal setting exercises are started early to improve the muscle strength needed for walking; these are performed at least five times daily for 10 minutes at a time.

Preparing for Ambulation. The time to first mobilization after acute stroke should be patient-specific. Although it is generally encouraged to prevent complication such as DVT, skin breakdown, or respiratory illness, a recent clinical trial found outcomes were worse in patients who were mobilized within 24 hours of their stroke event (Livesay & Hickey, 2020). Typically a rehabilitation team is consulted and the patient is assisted out of bed with a provider trained to monitor the patient's consciousness as well as truncal strength and balance. The patient is first taught to maintain balance while sitting and then to learn to balance while standing. If the patient has difficulty in achieving standing balance, a tilt table, which slowly brings the patient to an upright position, can be used. If orthostatic hypotension is a problem, the nurse can gradually elevate the head of the bed and assess blood pressure, pulse, skin color, and any complaints of dizziness or lightheadedness. If hypotension, tachycardia, paleness, diaphoresis, dizziness, or lightheadedness is noted, the head of the bed may be lowered until the symptoms resolve.

The patient is usually ready to walk as soon as standing balance is achieved. Parallel bars are useful in these first efforts. A chair or wheelchair should be readily available in case the patient suddenly becomes fatigued or feels dizzy. As noted earlier, mobilization timing remains controversial and until further studies elucidate the impact of early mobilization on outcomes, the nurse should follow their institutional guidelines (Langhorne et al., 2018; Livesay & Hickey, 2020).

The training periods for ambulation should be short and frequent. As the patient gains strength and confidence, an adjustable cane can be used for support. In general, a three- or four-pronged cane provides a stable support in the early phases of rehabilitation.

PREVENTING SHOULDER PAIN

As many as 70% of stroke patients suffer pain in the shoulder that prevents them from regaining full ROM, and 88% will have some level of upper extremity dysfunction (Winstein, 2016). In fact, in a recent study, 35% of stroke patients reported shoulder pain during the first 3 days following admission, highlighting the importance of preventive strategies (Nadler et al., 2020). Shoulder function is essential in achieving balance and performing transfers and self-care activities. Three problems can occur: painful shoulder; subluxation (partial dislocation) of the shoulder; and poststroke shoulder–hand syndrome (PSSHS) which features hemiplegic shoulder pain, hyperalgesia (abnormally heightened sensitivity to pain [often "burning"]), joint swelling, and limitations when moving. Its prevalence varies from 12% to 49%, and its incidence is about 70% (Wang et al., 2020). PSSHS (painful shoulder and generalized swelling of the hand) can cause a frozen shoulder and, ultimately, atrophy of subcutaneous tissues. When a shoulder becomes stiff, it is usually painful. Refer to Chapter 6 for pain management strategies.

A flaccid shoulder joint may be overstretched by the use of excessive force in turning the patient or from overstrenuous arm and shoulder movement. To prevent shoulder pain, the nurse should never lift the patient by the flaccid shoulder or pull on the affected arm or shoulder. If the arm is paralyzed, subluxation at the shoulder can occur as a result of overstretching of the joint capsule and musculature by the force of gravity when the patient sits or stands in the early stages after a stroke. This results in severe pain.

Many shoulder problems can be prevented by proper patient movement and positioning. The flaccid arm is positioned on a table or with pillows while the patient is seated. Some providers advocate the use of a properly worn sling when the patient first becomes ambulatory to prevent the paralyzed upper extremity from dangling without support. ROM exercises are important in preventing painful shoulder. Overly strenuous arm movements are avoided. The patient is instructed to interlace the fingers, place the palms together, and push the clasped hands slowly forward to bring the scapulae forward; then to raise both their hands above the head. This is repeated throughout the day. The patient is instructed to flex the affected wrist at intervals and move all the joints of the affected fingers. They are encouraged to touch, stroke, rub, and look at both hands. Pushing the heel of the hand firmly down on a surface is useful. Elevation of the arm and hand is also important in preventing dependent edema of the hand. When dressing, the sequence of weaker arm, then head, followed by stronger arm is followed (Winstein, 2016). Patients with continuing pain after attempted movement and positioning may require the addition of analgesia to their treatment program.

Medications are helpful in the management of poststroke pain. Opioids are generally prescribed for acute pain but may be considered for patients with chronic pain. If prescribed, the nurse assesses for side effects, tolerance, dependency, and drug use disorder. Adjuvant drugs, such as antidepressants, anticonvulsants, and anxiolytics, may also be considered. Tricyclic antidepressants are often prescribed for neuropathic pain, while anticonvulsants are used for their ability to stabilize neuronal membranes. Gabapentin is becoming a first-line drug for neuropathic pain (Hickey & Strayer, 2020). The antiseizure medication lamotrigine has been found to be effective for poststroke pain. Topical analgesics, such as lidocaine cream or patch, may also be considered.

ENHANCING SELF-CARE

As soon as the patient can sit up, personal hygiene activities are encouraged. The patient is helped to set realistic goals; if feasible, a new task is added daily. The first step is to carry out all self-care activities on the unaffected side. Such activities as combing the hair, brushing the teeth, shaving with an electric razor, bathing, and eating can be carried out with one hand and are suitable for self-care. Although the patient may feel awkward at first, the various motor skills can be learned by repetition, and the unaffected side will become stronger with use. The nurse must be sure that the patient does not neglect the affected side. Assistive devices will help make up for some of the patient's deficits. For example, a small towel is easier to control while drying after bathing, and boxed paper tissues are easier to use than a roll of toilet tissue.

Return of functional ability is important to the patient recovering after a stroke. An early baseline assessment of functional ability with an instrument such as the Functional Independence Measure (FIM) is important in team planning and goal setting for the patient. The FIM is a widely used instrument in stroke rehabilitation and provides valuable information about motor, social, and cognitive function (Livesay & Hickey, 2020). The patient's morale will improve if ambulatory activities are carried out in street clothes. The family is instructed to bring in clothing that is preferably a size larger than that normally worn. Clothing fitted with front or side fasteners or Velcro closures is the most suitable. The patient has better balance if most of the dressing activities are carried out while seated.

Perceptual problems may make it difficult for the patient to dress without assistance because of an inability to match the clothing to the body parts. To assist the patient, the nurse can take steps to keep the environment organized and uncluttered because the patient with a perceptual problem is easily distracted. The patient has to make many compensatory movements when dressing; these can produce fatigue and painful twisting of the intercostal muscles. Support and encouragement are provided to prevent the patient from becoming overly fatigued and discouraged. Even with intensive training, not all patients can achieve independence in dressing.

MANAGING SENSORY-PERCEPTUAL DIFFICULTIES

Patients with a decreased field of vision should be approached on the side where visual perception is intact. All visual stimuli (e.g., clock, calendar, television) should be placed on this side. The patient can be taught to turn the head in the direction of the defective visual field to compensate for this loss. The nurse should make eye contact with the patient and draw their attention to the affected side by encouraging the patient to move the head. The nurse may also want to stand at a position that encourages the patient to move or turn to visualize who is in the room. Increasing the natural or artificial lighting in the room and providing eyeglasses are important aids to increasing vision.

The patient with homonymous hemianopsia (loss of half of the visual field) turns away from the affected side of the body and tends to neglect that side and the space on that side; this is called *amorphosynthesis*. In such instances, the patient cannot see food on half of the tray, and only half of the room is visible. It is important for the nurse to constantly remind the patient of the other side of the body; to maintain alignment of the extremities; and, if possible, to place the extremities where the patient can see them.

ASSISTING WITH NUTRITION

Stroke can result in swallowing problems (dysphagia). Patients must be observed for paroxysms of coughing, food dribbling out of or pooling in one side of the mouth, food retained for long periods in the mouth, or nasal regurgitation when swallowing liquids. Mental status changes are the earliest signs of aspiration pneumonia in older patients (Clinical Overview, 2022); thus, the nurse keeps a high degree of suspicion of aspiration in all patients with dysphagia. Swallowing difficulties place the patient at risk for aspiration, pneumonia, dehydration, and malnutrition. A speech therapist will evaluate the patient's gag reflexes and ability to swallow. A validated, nurse-directed dysphagia screening assessment has been recommended as part of poststroke care to identify a patient's swallowing difficulty. A speech therapist may be consulted for patients who fail an initial screen and require a more formal evaluation. Even if swallowing function is partially impaired, it may return in some patients over time, or the patient may be taught alternative swallowing techniques, advised to take smaller boluses of food and place food on the unaffected side of their mouth, and taught about types of foods that are easier to swallow. The patient may be started on a thick liquid or puréed diet because these foods are easier to swallow than thin liquids. Having the patient sit upright, preferably out of bed in a chair, and instructing them to tuck their chin toward the chest as they swallow will help prevent aspiration. The diet may be advanced as the patient becomes more proficient at swallowing. If the patient cannot resume oral intake, a gastrointestinal feeding tube will be placed for ongoing tube feedings.

Enteral tubes can be either nasogastric (placed in the stomach) or nasoenteric (placed in the duodenum) to reduce the risk of aspiration. For long-term feedings, a gastrostomy tube is preferred. Refer to Chapter 21 for details on enteral feeding. Nursing responsibilities in feeding include elevating the head of the bed at least 30 degrees to prevent aspiration, checking the position of the tube before feeding, and assessing residuals.

ATTAINING BOWEL AND BLADDER CONTROL

After a stroke, the patient may have transient urinary incontinence due to confusion, inability to communicate needs, and inability to use the urinal or bedpan because of impaired motor and postural control. Occasionally, after a stroke, the bladder becomes atonic, with impaired sensation in response to bladder filling. Sometimes control of the external urinary sphincter is lost

(*continued on page 1508*)

or diminished. During this period, intermittent catheterization with sterile technique is carried out. After muscle tone increases and deep tendon reflexes return, bladder tone increases and spasticity of the bladder may develop. Because the patient's sense of awareness is clouded, persistent urinary incontinence or urinary retention may be symptomatic of bilateral brain damage. The voiding pattern is analyzed, and the urinal or bedpan is offered on a pattern or schedule. The upright posture and standing position are helpful for male patients during this aspect of rehabilitation.

Patients may have problems with bowel control, particularly constipation. Unless contraindicated, a high-fiber diet and adequate fluid intake (2–3 L/day) should be provided, and a regular time (usually after breakfast) should be established for toileting.

IMPROVING THOUGHT PROCESSES

After a stroke, patients may experience changes in cognition and behavior and may exhibit periods of emotional lability. These changes are usually associated with injury to the right hemisphere. Often they are transient; with aggressive rehabilitation, patients can recover.

Screening for these problems is typically incorporated into the initial rehabilitation assessment and then repeated after discharge. Often a neuropsychologist will be consulted to perform formal neuropsychological testing to make recommendations for the appropriate follow-up treatment. A treatment program for addressing any identified deficit is established in collaboration with the patient's neurologist and primary care provider.

The role of the nurse is supportive. The nurse reviews the results of neuropsychological testing; observes the patient's performance and progress; gives positive feedback; and, most importantly, conveys an attitude of confidence and hope. Interventions capitalize on the patient's strengths and remaining abilities while attempting to improve performance of affected functions. Other interventions are similar to those for improving cognitive functioning after a head injury.

IMPROVING COMMUNICATION

Aphasia, which impairs the patient's ability to express themself and to understand what is being said, may become apparent in various ways. The cortical area that is responsible for integrating the myriad pathways required for the comprehension and formulation of language is called the *Broca area.* It is located in a convolution adjoining the middle cerebral artery. This area is responsible for control of the combinations of muscular movements needed to speak each word. Patients who are paralyzed on the right side (due to damage or injury to the left side of the brain) cannot speak, whereas those paralyzed on the left side are less likely to have speech disturbances. The speech therapist assesses the communication needs of the stroke patient, describes the precise deficit, and suggests the best overall method of communication. Most language intervention strategies can be tailored for the individual patient. The patient is expected to take an active part in establishing goals.

Nursing interventions include strategies to make the atmosphere conducive to communication. This includes being sensitive to the patient's reactions and needs and responding to them in an appropriate manner. A consistent schedule, routines, and repetition help the patient to function despite significant deficits. A written copy of the daily schedule, a folder of personal information (birth date, address, names of relatives), checklists, and an audio-taped list help improve the patient's memory and concentration. The patient may also benefit from a communication board, which has pictures of common needs and phrases. When talking with the patient, it is important for the nurse to gain the patient's attention, speak slowly, and keep the language of instruction consistent. One instruction is given at a time, and time is allowed for the patient to process what has been said. The use of gestures may enhance comprehension. In working with the patient with aphasia, the nurse must remember to talk to the patient during care activities. This provides social contact for the patient.

MAINTAINING SKIN INTEGRITY

The patient who has had a stroke may be at risk for skin and tissue breakdown because of altered sensation and inability to respond to pressure and discomfort by turning and moving. Preventing skin and tissue breakdown requires frequent assessment of the skin, with emphasis on bony areas and dependent parts of the body. During the acute phase, a specialty bed (e.g., low-air-loss bed) may be used until the patient can move independently or assist in moving.

A regular turning schedule (at least every 2 hours) must be adhered to even if pressure-relieving devices are used to prevent tissue and skin breakdown. When the patient is positioned or turned, care must be used to minimize shear and friction forces that may tear the skin and expose the patent to additional sources of infection. The patient's skin must be kept clean and dry; gentle massage of healthy (nonreddened) skin and adequate nutrition are other factors that help to maintain normal skin and tissue integrity.

IMPROVING FAMILY COPING

Family members play an important role in the patient's recovery. Family members are encouraged to participate in counseling and to use support systems that will help with the emotional and physical stress of caring for the patient. Involving others in the patient's care and teaching stress management techniques and methods for maintaining personal health also facilitate family coping.

The family may have difficulty accepting the patient's disability and may be unrealistic in their expectations. They are given information about the expected outcomes and are counseled to avoid doing activities for the patient that they can do. They are assured that their love and interest are part of the patient's therapy.

The family needs to be informed that the rehabilitation of the hemiplegic patient requires many months and that progress may be slow. The gains made by the patient in the hospital or rehabilitation unit must be maintained. All caregivers should approach the patient with a supportive and optimistic attitude, focusing on the patient's remaining abilities. The rehabilitation team, the medical and nursing team, the patient, and the family must all be involved in developing attainable goals for the patient at home.

Most relatives of patients with stroke handle the physical changes better than the emotional aspects of care. The family should be prepared to expect occasional episodes of emotional lability. The patient may laugh or cry easily and may be irritable and demanding or depressed and confused. The nurse can explain to the family that the patient's laughter does not necessarily connote happiness, nor does crying reflect sadness, and that emotional lability usually improves with time.

HELPING THE PATIENT COPE WITH SEXUAL DYSFUNCTION

Sexual functioning can be altered by stroke. Sexual dysfunction after stroke is multifactorial. There may be medical reasons for the dysfunction (neurologic and cognitive deficits, previous diseases, medications) as well as various psychosocial factors. A stroke can potentially be such a catastrophic illness that the patient experiences loss of self-esteem and value as a sexual being. These psychosocial factors play an important role in determining sexual drive, activity, and satisfaction after a stroke.

Nurses in the rehabilitation setting play a crucial role in beginning a dialogue between the patient and their partner about sexuality after a stroke. In-depth assessments to determine sexual history before and after the stroke should be followed by appropriate interventions. Interventions for the patient and partner focus on providing relevant information, education, reassurance, adjustment of medications, counseling regarding coping skills, suggestions for alternative sexual positions, and a means of sexual expression and satisfaction.

PROVIDING PATIENT EDUCATION AND PREPARING THE PATIENT FOR THE HOME

Patient and family education is a fundamental component of rehabilitation. The nurse provides teaching about stroke, its causes and prevention, and the rehabilitation process. In both acute care and rehabilitation facilities, the focus is on teaching the patient to resume as much self-care as possible. This may entail using assistive devices or modifying the home environment to help the patient live with a disability. Family members are also encouraged to take part in being assessed for their role as caregivers and their readiness to accept the additional responsibilities associated with a family member with both physical and cognitive disabilities.

An occupational therapist may be helpful in assessing the home environment and recommending modifications to help the patient become more independent. For example, a shower is more convenient than a tub for the patient with hemiplegia because most patients do not gain sufficient strength to get up and down from a tub. Sitting on a stool of medium height with rubber suction tips allows the patient to wash with greater ease. A long-handled bath brush with a soap container is helpful to the patient who has only one functional hand. If a shower is not available, a stool may be placed in the tub and a portable shower hose attached to the faucet. Handrails may be attached alongside the bathtub and the toilet. Other assistive devices include special utensils for eating, grooming, dressing, and writing.

A program of physical therapy can be beneficial in the home environment. One technique that was shown to result in a reduction in motor impairment concentrates on enhanced exercise of the affected limb. Another technique that showed positive outcomes uses sensorimotor training of the upper limb and the wrist.

Depression occurs in 40% to 50% of patients, and patients and families need to be prepared for its potential (Livesay & Hickey, 2020). Counseling and antidepressant therapy may help if depression dominates the patient's life. As progress is made in the rehabilitation program, some problems will diminish. The family can help by continuing to support the patient and by giving positive reinforcement for the progress that is being made.

Community-based stroke support groups may allow the patient and family to learn from others with similar problems and to share their experiences. Support groups take the form of in-person meetings as well as web-based support programs. The patient is encouraged to continue hobbies and recreational and leisure interests and to maintain contact with friends to prevent social isolation. Patients should be supported to keep active, adhere to the exercise program, and remain as self-sufficient as possible.

The nurse should recognize the potential effects of caregiving on the family. Not all families have the adaptive coping skills and adequate psychological functioning necessary for the long-term care of another person. The patient's spouse may be older, with their own health concerns; in some instances, the patient may have been the provider of care to the spouse. Even healthy caregivers may find it difficult to maintain a schedule that includes being available around the clock.

Depressed caregivers are more likely to resort to physical or emotional abuse of the patient and are more likely to place the patient in a nursing home. Respite care (planned short-term care to relieve the family from having to provide continuous 24-hour care) may be available from an adult day care center. Some hospitals also offer weekend respite care that can provide caregivers with needed time for themselves. The nurse encourages the family to arrange for such services and provides information to assist them.

The nurse involved in home and continuing care also needs to remind the patient and family of the need for continuing health promotion and screening practices. Patients who have not been involved in these practices in the past are educated about their importance and are referred to appropriate health care providers, if indicated.

(*continued on page 1510*)

EVALUATION

Expected patient outcomes may include the following:

1. Demonstrates intact neurologic status and normal vital signs and respiratory patterns:
   a. Normal mental status examination, intact cognitive process
   b. Normal speech patterns and language function
   c. Normal/equal strength, movement, and sensation of all four extremities
2. Understands diagnostic procedures and treatment plan:
   a. Review of current and new medications
   b. Proposed physical and occupational therapies
   c. Achieves self-care; uses adaptive equipment
3. Arranges for follow-up appointments with stroke neurologist or primary care provider

Clinical Judgment Case

A 59-year-old patient with known hypertension, hyperlipidemia, hypothyroidism, and a 20 pack-year smoking history (1 pack per day [PPD] for 20 years) presents to the emergency room (ER) by EMS after developing sudden-onset slurred speech and right-sided weakness that had started 30 minutes prior to arrival. The patient's family member witnessed the onset of their symptoms. The family member noticed that the patient had difficulty holding a water glass with their right arm and that their speech sounded slurred. The family member immediately called 911; EMS arrived at their home and did a stroke screening assessment and brought the patient to the emergency department. The patient's family member was encouraged to come to the hospital to provide any additional information to the medical team. The ED medical team confirmed that the patient's last known well (LKW) was 11:30 am. Their first National Institutes of Health Stroke Scale (NIHSS) number on arrival was 11. The patient's skin is warm and dry with delayed skin turgor, and vital signs are as follows: 98.7°F, HR 112 and irregular, 28 RR with an oxygen saturation of 96% on room air, blood pressure 203/96. The patient denies pain in the chest, jaw, back, or arms. Heart sounds are irregular but S1 S2 without murmur, gallops, or rub; neck veins are flat. Scattered rhonchi are noted in lung fields, nonproductive cough. The patient denies shortness of breath, nausea, or vomiting. Abdomen is soft, nondistended, nontender; bowel sounds are present; last BM was yesterday, formed brown stool. There is no peripheral edema, capillary refill is 2 seconds, and pedal and posterior tibial pulses are 3+ bil. Pupils are 3 mm bil and reactive to light, + pronator drift of right arm and weakness of right lower extremity (RLE), 5/5 strength of left upper extremity (LUE) and left lower extremity (LLE). Speech is slightly garbled, and patient is oriented to person, time, place, and situation. There is slight facial weakness. You immediately assess the blood glucose, which is 115. You start an IV and obtain blood work (blood chemistries, coagulation studies [platelets, prothrombin time/international normalized ratio [INR], activated partial thromboplastin time, blood cell counts]) and troponin level, and an ECG is to be performed. You place the patient on the cardiac monitor and pulse oximeter to monitor oxygen saturation and alert the "stroke team." A stat noncontrast CT scan is ordered, and the patient is taken to the scanner for a head CT within 10 minutes of arrival. Patient's medication history includes metformin, "a statin," and levothyroxine (doses are unknown, and name of statin cannot be recalled).

Step One: Recognize cues where relevant and important information is identified from different sources, such as medical history or vital signs.

Answer: History of hypertension, hypothyroidism, and hyperlipidemia. Twenty pack-year smoking history. Complaints of sudden-onset slurred speech and right-sided weakness that started 30 minutes prior to arrival. NIHSS of 11 on arrival. Physical examination findings of delayed skin turgor, flat neck veins, + right pronator drift right arm, weakness of RLE, garbled speech, facial weakness, and scattered rhonchi. Cues of concern related to vital signs: HR of 112 and irregular rate, 28 RR, blood pressure 203/96. Baseline neurologic assessment shows pupils are 3 mm bil reacting to light, oriented times 4, 5/5 strength of LUE and LLE. Blood glucose of 115.

Step Two: Analyze cues, which is organizing and linking the recognized cues to the patient's clinical presentation.

Answer: You have clustered the complaints of sudden onset (30 minutes ago) weakness of RUE and RLE, sudden trouble speaking, + pronator drift of right arm, slightly garbled speech, facial weakness, and hypertension to be associated with a TIA versus embolic stroke versus hemorrhagic stroke. Risk factors for stroke include increased age, hypertension, hyperlipidemia, smoking, and hypothyroidism. You recall that hypothyroidism is associated with elevated serum cholesterol, which is largely accounted for by an increase of

LDL-cholesterol, which is a risk factor for cardiovascular disease. Signs of potential fluid volume deficit include delayed skin turgor, tachycardia, and flat neck veins. You cluster the hyperglycemia with stress reaction with catecholamine release. You cluster the irregular heart rate with the most common arrhythmia-atrial fibrillation, which you know is associated with embolic stroke because of the development of thrombi in the atria due to the turbulent blood flow. You cluster the 20 pack-year smoking history with scattered rhonchi and nonproductive cough. You also consider that the BP of 203/96 is associated with hypertensive emergency (an acute complication of HTN), defined as a severe increase in BP (commonly above 180/120 mm Hg) associated with potentially life-threatening target organ damage such as myocardial infarction (MI), ischemic stroke, hemorrhagic stroke, or pulmonary edema. You are also aware that if an embolic stroke is diagnosed, the BP will have to be treated pre-tPA since an elevated blood pressure (SBP >185 or DBP >110 mm Hg) is one of the exclusion criteria. You await the lab results to evaluate for MI (troponin level and 12 lead ECG results) and await patient return from CT scan.

Step Three: Prioritize hypotheses, where hypotheses are evaluated and ranked according to priority. This can include urgency, likelihood, risk, difficulty, and/or time. In this phase you cluster your findings to arrive at a list of problems (actual and or potential problems) you believe the patient is experiencing and determine the importance or urgency. What do you think is of greatest concern?

Answer: You prioritize a potential stroke as the greatest risk of injury to this patient since "time is brain" because for every minute that a stroke occurs and is not treated, nearly two million brain cells are destroyed. You also are concerned about altered hemodynamics related to atrial fibrillation and hypertension and are concerned about end-organ damage. You are also concerned about potential fluid volume deficit, potential risk for pulmonary complications (given smoking history), and the patient's knowledge base regarding their medical and medication history.

Step Four: Generate solutions, which is identifying expected outcomes and using hypotheses to define a set of interventions for the expected outcomes.

Answer: Since a stroke is suspected, you will continue to use the NIHSS assessment tool to quantify the stroke severity, which requires assessing (1) LOC, (2) visual function, (3) motor function, (4) sensation and neglect (failure to pay attention to stimuli on one side of the body), (5) cerebellar function, and (6) language. Additionally because the use of tPA is time limited (3 to 4.5 hours depending on institutional guidelines), speed is essential in determining the type of stroke (ischemic vs. hemorrhagic) and potential contraindications to tPA. Obtaining a CT scan to determine type of stroke is a top priority. In addition, since atrial fibrillation causes erratic atrial contraction which promotes formation of thrombi within the atria, increasing the risk for an embolic event such as stroke (e.g., patients with AFib have a four to fivefold increase in the risk for stroke and a twofold increase in mortality), management will likely includes measures to control the ventricular rate and to achieve rhythm conversion to sinus rhythm if possible.

Step Five: Take action, where the solutions that address the highest priorities are implemented.

Answer: You repeat the vital signs, monitor the cardiac rhythm and oxygen saturation, and reassess the patient's neurologic and cardiac status. In particular you reassess the blood pressure since you know that an elevated blood pressure (SBP >185 or DBP >110 mm Hg) is a contraindication to tPA. Since the patient's blood pressure was above this limit, a dose of labetalol 10 mg IV was administered per provider order; you reassess the BP, which has now decreased to 179/89. The patient's NIHSS score is unchanged. A 12 lead ECG is performed; there are an irregular R to R wave and no discernible P wave; instead, rapid oscillations or fibrillation wavelets that vary in size, shape, and frequency are seen (particularly visible in the inferior ECG leads II, III, and AVF), which you associate with atrial fibrillation. You talk to the patient about the treatment plan since you are aware that stress increases catecholamines, which stimulate glycogenolysis, lipolysis, and gluconeogenesis, causing hyperglycemia, which is associated with fluid volume deficit. You weigh the patient, as you are aware that tPA if deemed appropriate is a weight-based medication; you note on the electronic record the patient's weight of 70 kg. You elevate the head of the bed 30 degrees and keep the patient's head and neck in neutral position to facilitate venous drainage and to minimize aspiration. An IV of normal saline is started so access is available. You monitor the patient's respiratory status and note that the oxygen saturation remains 96% on room air, so no supplemental oxygen is required at this time. You are aware that hypertension is often present in early stroke phase as a compensatory response and that in most cases, blood pressure is not lowered. The glucose is 115 mg, and you continue to monitor both the glucose and the patient's temperature since hyperthermia (temperature above 37.5°C [99.5°F]) is associated with a poorer prognosis following acute stroke. You are prepared to initiate measures to prevent and control fever collaboratively with the health care team, and you await CT scan results.

Step Six: Evaluate outcomes, which is comparing observed outcomes against expected outcomes.

Answer: CT showed no evidence of hemorrhage, large ischemic stroke, or tumor/mass lesion. A CTA (CT angiogram) showed an occlusion of the left middle cerebral artery. After discussion with the neurologists and patient's family, the provider decided to administer tPA as the patient was within the time window for this treatment and did not have any contraindications to tPA. The pharmacist mixed tPA, and it was administered 36 minutes after arrival. Since alteplase is dosed at 0.9 mg/kg and the patient weighs 70 kg, you verify the dose to be administered is 63 mg. You administer 10% of the calculated dose (63 mg); 6.3 mg is administered as an IV bolus over 1 minute, and the remaining dose is administered over 1 hour via an infusion pump. You monitor the patient for bleeding and are aware that this complication usually occurs within the first 5 to 10 hours (50%) of tPA administration but can occur within 12 hours. Your patient tolerated tPA without complications, and on repeat NIHSS assessment, the patient's neurologic exam improved and NIHSS is now 2 (dysarthria and RUE drift). The patient was a candidate (and also in the time window) for thrombectomy, so they were taken to the interventional radiology suite for the procedure and then to the ICU for recovery. The patient was later transferred to a medical unit for control of the atrial fibrillation. As a novice nurse, the urgency of the situation ("time is brain") certainly adds to the stress of the situation, but you were organized and thorough and can leave work today with a happy story of how a medication can alter the patient's trajectory positively. We hope your positive days in nursing continue.

CHAPTER REVIEW

NCLEX-Style Review Questions

1. A patient being cared for on the neurologic unit has a diagnosis of acute ischemic stroke. It has affected the left hemisphere of the patient's brain. The nurse would expect to assess which deficit in this patient? Select all that apply.
a. Left side of body weakness
b. Aphasia
c. Left field visual deficit
d. Lack of awareness of deficits
e. Right side of body weakness

2. What would the nurse expect to document in a patient diagnosed with a right hemispheric stroke?
a. Aphasia
b. Slow, cautious behavior
c. Left visual field deficit
d. Impulsive behavior
e. Left side of body weakness

3. A patient has been brought to the emergency department (ED) by their distraught spouse who believes that their partner had a stroke. A rapid assessment by the care team confirms that the spouse's suspicions are likely accurate, and the patient is screened for the possible administration of recombinant tissue plasminogen activator (rtPA). Which of the following factors would **contraindicate** the use of tPA? Select all that apply.
a. The brain imaging shows evidence of a lobar hemorrhage.
b. The patient is older than 18 years of age.
c. The patient's platelet count is 79,000/mm^3.
d. The patient has a history of hypertension and type 1 diabetes.
e. The patient had intraspinal surgery 5 days ago.

4. A community health nurse is conducting a workshop for unlicensed care providers who work in a chain of long-term care facilities. The nurse is teaching the participants about the signs and symptoms of stroke. What signs and symptoms should the nurse identify? Select all that apply.
a. Epistaxis
b. Sudden onset of confusion
c. Sudden numbness on one side of the body
d. Visual changes
e. Sudden ear pain

5. Which ECG strip is associated with an embolic stroke?

a.

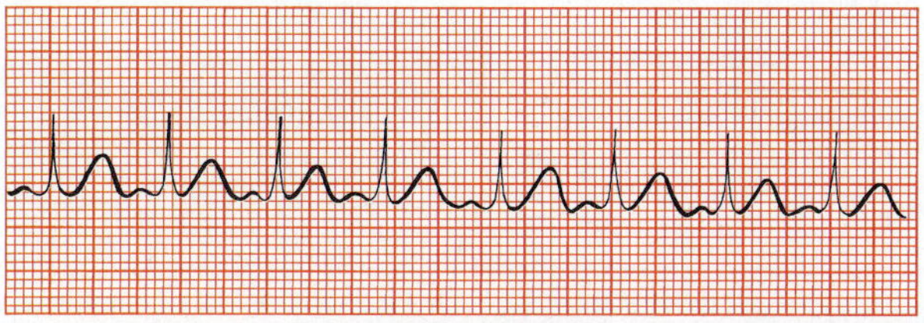

b.

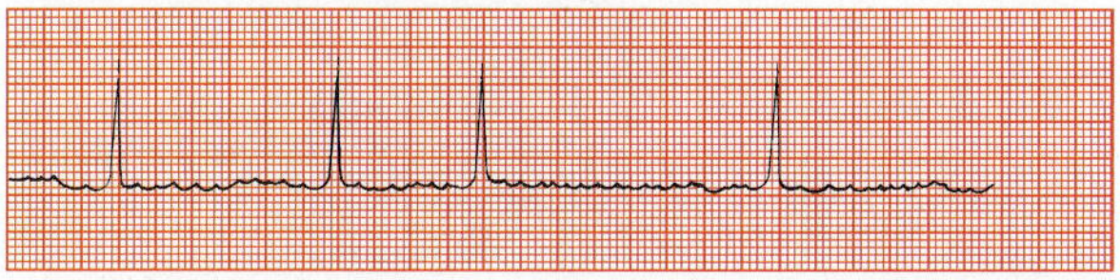

c.

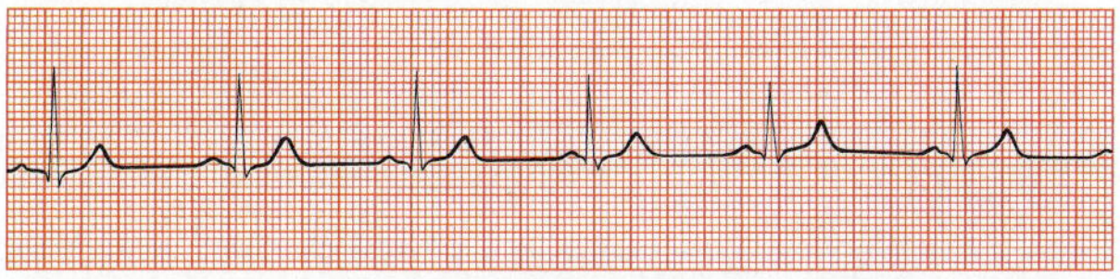

d.

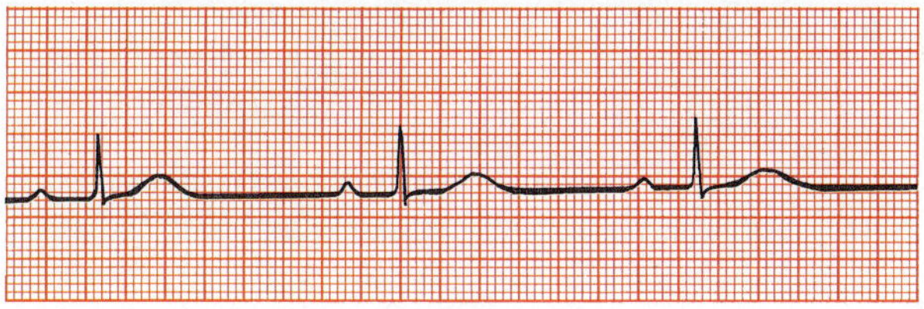

e.

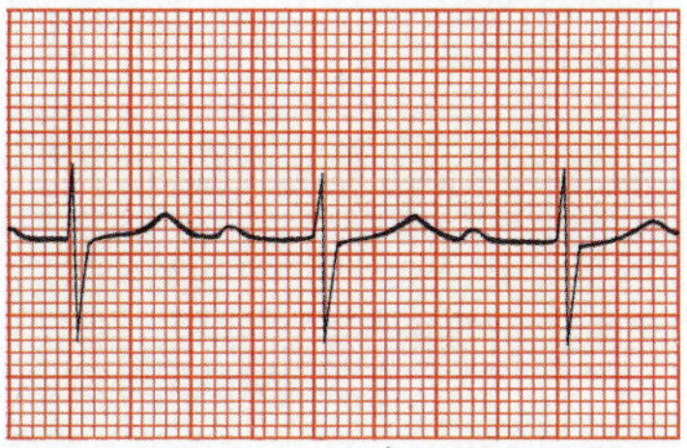

REFERENCES AND SELECTED READINGS

References and selected readings associated with this chapter can be found on the website that accompanies the book. Visit **http://thepoint.lww.com/Honan3e** to access the references and other additional resources associated with this chapter.

UNIT THIRTEEN

Problems Related to Sensorineural Function

A patient with hearing loss in both ears due to trauma is being seen in the hearing clinic. The health care provider is giving the patient information about a cochlear implant.

- **What are the criteria that have to be met to receive a cochlear implant?**
- **What does the surgical procedure involve?**
- **What does the rehabilitation period entail?**

CHAPTER 47

Nursing Assessment: Sensorineural Function

Linda S. Dune

Learning Objectives

After reading this chapter, you will be able to:

1. Identify eye structures and describe their functions.
2. Describe assessment components for the eye.
3. Identify diagnostic tests for assessment of vision and evaluation of visual disabilities.
4. Identify ear structures and describe their functions.
5. Describe assessment components for the ear.
6. Describe methods used to assess hearing and diagnose hearing and balance disorders.

THE EYE

The eye is a sensitive, highly specialized sense organ subject to various disorders, many of which lead to impaired vision. Impaired vision may affect a person's independence in self-care, ability to interact with society and the environment, work and lifestyle choices, sense of self-esteem, safety, and overall quality of life.

Although most people with eye disorders are treated in an ambulatory care setting, many patients receiving health care have an eye disease as a comorbid condition. In addition to understanding the prevention, treatment, and consequences of eye disorders, nurses in all settings assess visual acuity in those at risk, refer patients to eye care specialists as appropriate, implement measures to prevent further visual loss, and help patients adapt to impaired vision.

ANATOMY AND PHYSIOLOGY OVERVIEW

Unlike most organs of the body, the eye is available for external examination, and its anatomy is more easily assessed than many other body parts (Fig. 47-1). The eyeball, or globe, sits in a protective bony structure known as the *orbit.* The optic nerve and the ophthalmic artery enter the orbit at its apex through the optic foramen. The extraocular muscles move the eyeball through all fields of gaze. The four rectus muscles and two oblique muscles (Fig. 47-2) are innervated by cranial nerves (CN) III, IV, and VI. Normally, the movements of the two eyes are coordinated, and the brain perceives a single image.

External Eye

The eyelids, composed of thin, elastic skin that covers striated and smooth muscles, protect the anterior portion of the eye. The eyelids contain multiple glands, including sebaceous, sweat, and accessory lacrimal glands, and they are lined with conjunctival material. The upper lid normally covers the uppermost portion of the iris and is innervated by the oculomotor nerve (CN III). The lid margins contain meibomian glands, which produce an oil-like substance as a constituent of tears that helps to prevent dry eyes in the inferior and superior puncta and the eyelashes. The triangular spaces formed by the junction of the eyelids are known as the *inner* or *medial canthus* and the *outer* or *lateral canthus.*

Tears are vital to eye health. They protect the cornea and sclera with lubrication, nutritional support, moisture, and protection from microbes. Tears also contain immunoglobulins that contribute to the increase in tearing during allergic responses. A healthy tear is composed of three layers: lipoid, aqueous, and mucoid. If there is a defect in the composition of any of these layers, the integrity of the cornea may be compromised. Tears are secreted in response to reflex or emotional stimuli. With every blink of the eyes, the lids wash the cornea and conjunctiva with tears.

Pearls for Practice

In the absence of the patient's corneal reflex, the nurse must protect the patient's affected eye from injury by lubricating it with artificial tears to prevent drying.

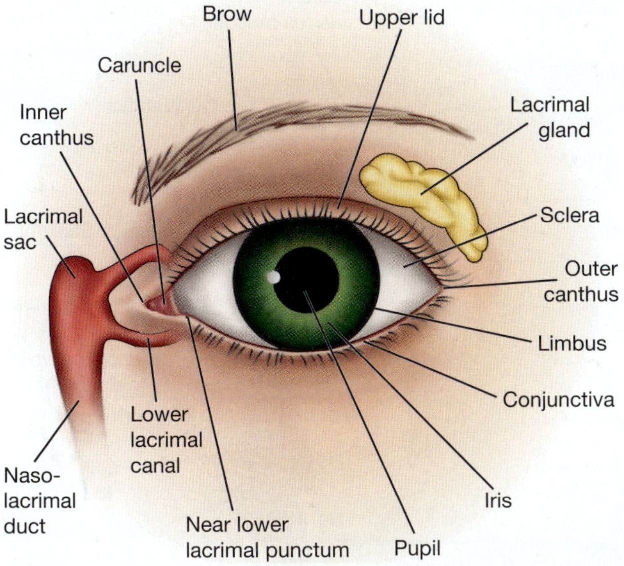

FIGURE 47-1 **External structures of the eye and position of the lacrimal structures.**

Pearls for Practice

The lacrimal apparatus is located in the eyelid and inner canthus and is essential for tear formation and drainage needed to lubricate the eyes. The lacrimal apparatus within the inner canthus contains a tiny fold of mucous membrane that can be blocked by debris when providing eye care (Bickley et al., 2021). When cleaning the eyes, in order to remove crusting or drainage, the nurse moves from the inner to outer canthus. Use only one cotton ball or pledget (small compress) for each eye to remove debris and prevent it from entering the lacrimal duct.

Internal Eye

The conjunctiva, a mucous membrane, provides a barrier to the external environment and nourishes the eye. The goblet

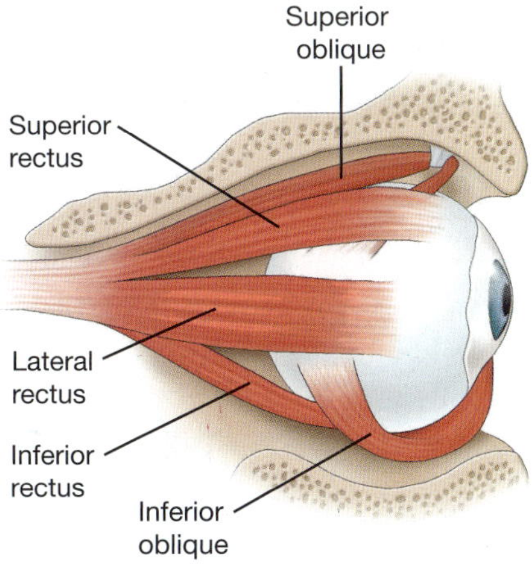

FIGURE 47-2 **The extraocular muscles responsible for eye movement. The medial rectus muscle (not shown) is responsible for opposing the movement of the lateral rectus muscle.**

cells of the conjunctiva secrete lubricating mucus. The bulbar conjunctiva covers the sclera, whereas the palpebral conjunctiva lines the inner surface of the upper and lower eyelids. The junction of the two portions is known as the *fornix*.

The sclera, commonly known as the white of the eye, is a dense, fibrous structure that helps maintain the shape of the eyeball and protects the intraocular contents from trauma (Fig. 47-3). The sclera may have a slightly bluish tinge in young children, a dull white color in adults, a slightly yellowish color in older adults, or a brown color in people with increased melanin; all are variations of normal. Externally, it is overlaid with conjunctiva, which is a thin, transparent mucous membrane that contains fine blood vessels. The conjunctiva meets the cornea at the **limbus** on the outermost edge of the iris.

Pearls for Practice: Lifting the Lens

When increased melanin is observed in the sclera, the term previously used to describe this finding was "muddy sclera." This term was associated with normal findings in Black individuals; however, this variation is also present in Asian or White patients with darker skin tones (Folberg, 2021). A recent article by Folberg (2021) asks us to consider medical language and how it perpetuates harmful bias. The author reminds the reader that it is melanin, not mud, that accounts for the brown color of the sclera. The writer recommends the phrase, "skin tone associated pigmentation" as a more accurate and equitably appropriate term. Understanding historical trauma helps us understand how language can perpetuate social injustice, including with medical terminology; together, we can correct language that is harmful.

The cornea (Fig. 47-4) is a transparent, avascular, domelike structure that covers the iris, pupil, and anterior chamber. It is the most anterior portion of the eyeball and is the main refracting surface of the eye. The epithelial cells of the cornea are capable of rapid replication and are completely replaced every 7 days. Behind the cornea lies the **anterior chamber**, filled with a continually replenished supply of clear aqueous humor that nourishes the cornea. The aqueous humor is produced by the ciliary body, and its production is dependent on a normal intraocular pressure (IOP) of 10 to 21 mm Hg.

The uvea consists of the iris, the ciliary body, and the choroid. The iris, or colored part of the eye, is a highly vascularized, pigmented collection of fibers surrounding the pupil. The pupil is a space that dilates and constricts in response to light. Normal pupils are round and constrict symmetrically when exposed to bright, direct light or for accommodation to objects that are near. Dilation and constriction are controlled by the sphincter and dilator pupillae muscles. The dilator muscles are controlled by the sympathetic nervous system, whereas the sphincter muscles are controlled by the parasympathetic nervous system.

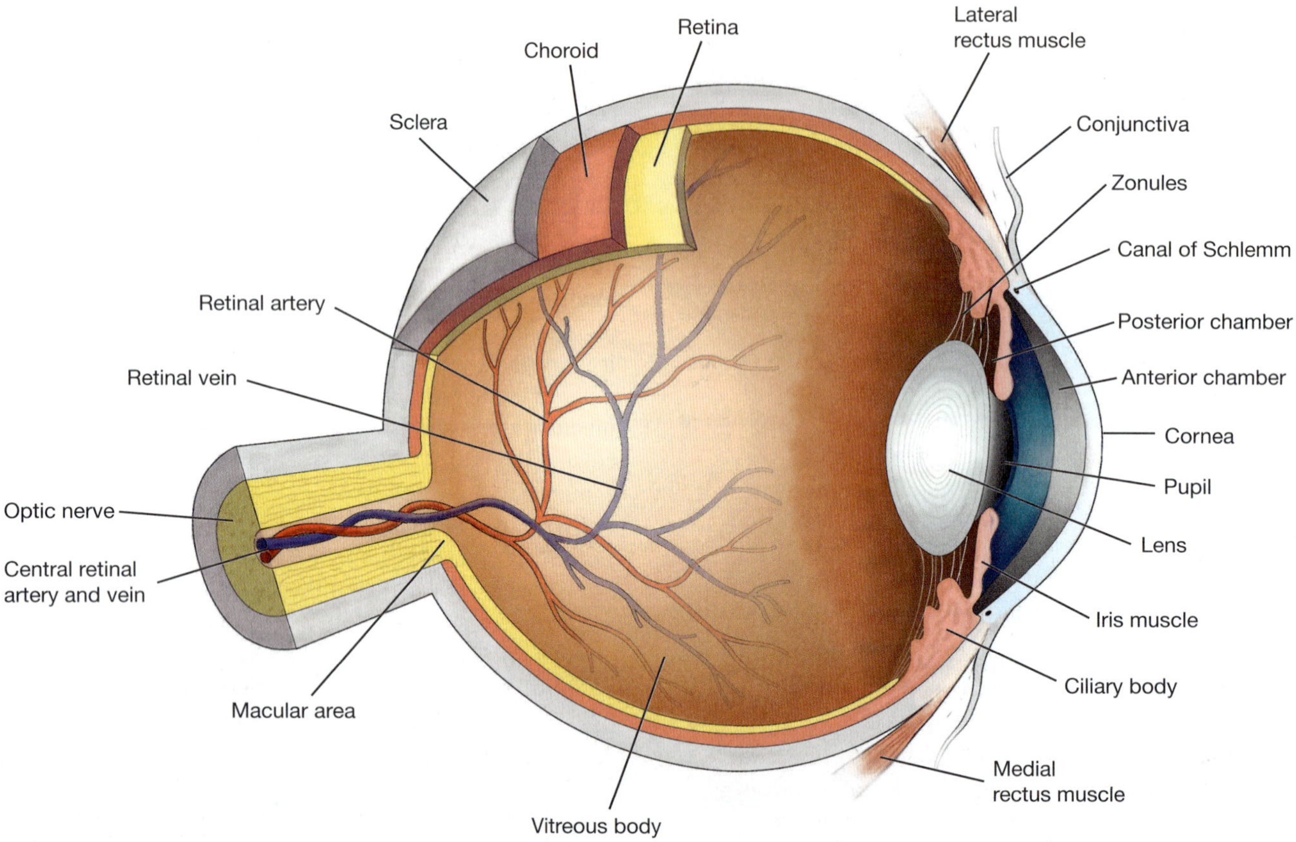

FIGURE 47-3 **Three-dimensional cross-section of the eye.**

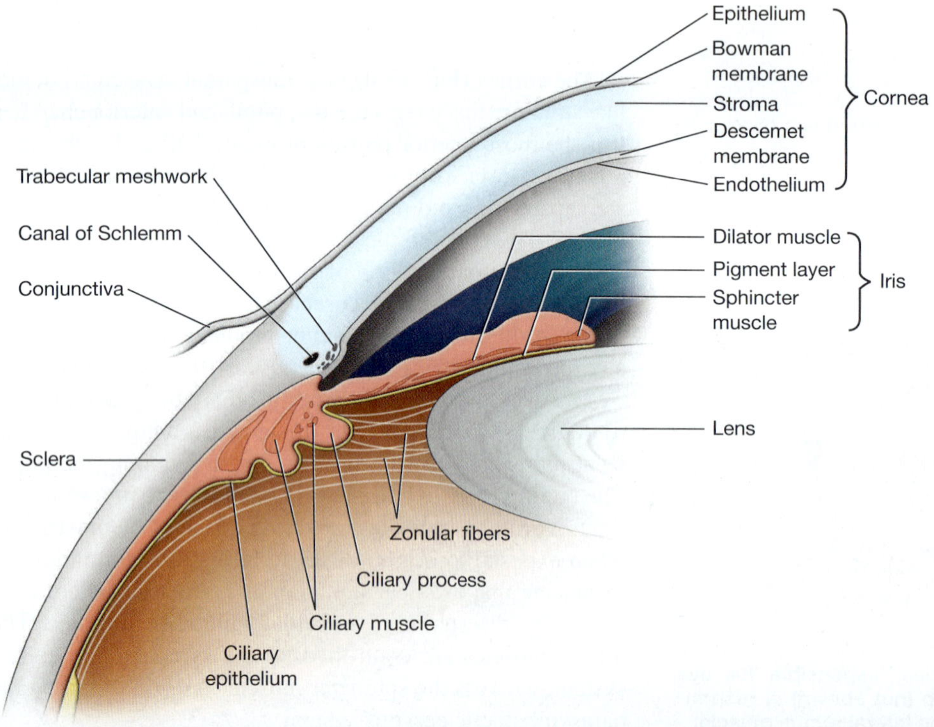

FIGURE 47-4 **Internal structures of the eye. (Redrawn from American Society of Ophthalmic Registered Nurses. [2008].** ***Core curriculum for ophthalmic nursing*****. Kendall/Hall Publishing.)**

Directly behind the pupil and iris lies the lens, a colorless and almost completely transparent biconvex structure. It is avascular and has no nerve or pain fibers. The lens enables focusing for near vision and refocusing for distance vision. The ability to focus and refocus is called **accommodation**. The lens is suspended behind the iris by zonules (string-like fibers) and is connected to the ciliary body. The ciliary body controls accommodation through the zonular fibers and the ciliary muscles (see Fig. 47-4). The aqueous humor is anterior to the lens; posterior to the lens is the vitreous humor. The **posterior chamber** is a small space between the vitreous humor and the iris. The ciliary body in the posterior chamber produces aqueous fluid. This aqueous fluid flows from the posterior chamber into the anterior chamber, from which it drains through the trabecular meshwork into the canal of Schlemm.

The ocular fundus is the largest chamber of the eye and contains the **vitreous humor**, a clear, gelatinous substance composed mostly of water and encapsulated by a hyaloid membrane. The vitreous humor occupies about two thirds of the eye's volume and helps maintain the shape of the eye. It is in continuous contact with the retina and is attached to the retina by scattered collagenous filaments. The choroid lies between the retina and the sclera. It is avascular tissue, supplying blood to the portion of the sensory retina closest to it.

The innermost surface of the fundus is the retina. The retina is composed of 10 microscopic layers and has the consistency of wet tissue paper. It is neural tissue, an extension of the optic nerve. Viewed through the pupil, the landmarks of the retina are the optic disc, the retinal vessels, and the macula. The point of entrance of the optic nerve into the retina is the optic disc. The optic disc is pink; it is oval or circular and has sharp margins. In the disc, a physiologic depression or cup is present centrally, with the retinal blood vessels emanating from it. The retinal tissues arise from the optic disc and line the inner surface of the vitreous chamber. The retinal vessels also enter the eye through the optic nerve, branching out through the retina and forming superior and inferior branches. The macula is the area of the retina responsible for central vision. The rest of the retina is responsible for peripheral vision. In the center of the macula is the most sensitive area, the fovea, which is avascular and surrounded by the superior and inferior vascular arcades (arches of blood vessels). Two important layers of the retina are the retinal pigment epithelium (RPE) and the sensory retina. A single layer of cells constitutes the RPE, and these cells have numerous functions, including the absorption of light. The sensory retina contains the photoreceptor cells: **rods** and **cones**. These are long, narrow cells shaped like rods or cones. The rods are mainly responsible for night vision or vision in low light, whereas the cones provide the best vision for bright light, color vision, and fine detail. Cones are distributed throughout the retina, with their greatest concentration in the fovea. Rods are absent in the fovea (Norris, 2019).

Vision

Visual acuity depends on a healthy, functioning eyeball and an intact visual pathway (Fig. 47-5). This pathway includes the retina, optic nerve, optic chiasm, optic tracks, lateral

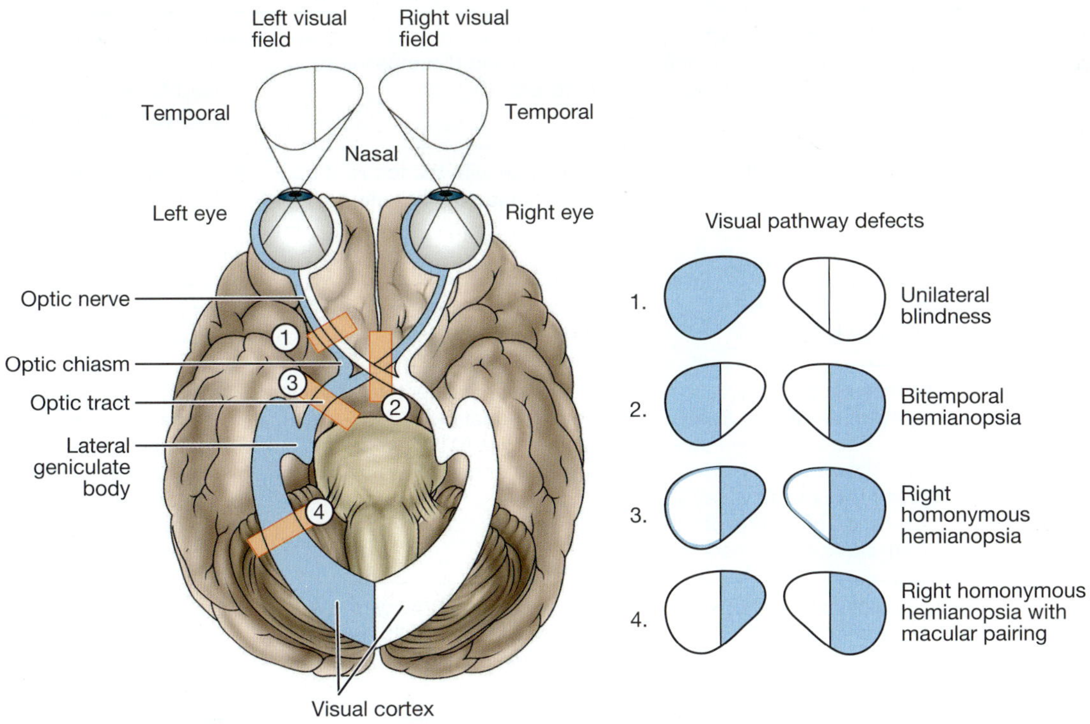

FIGURE 47-5 **The visual pathway. (Redrawn from Fuller, J., & Schaller-Ayers, J. [2000].** ***Health assessment: A nursing approach*** **[3rd ed.]. Lippincott Williams & Wilkins.)**

geniculate bodies, optic radiations, and the visual cortex area of the brain. The pathway is an extension of the central nervous system (CNS). The funduscopic examination allows the only direct visualization of arteries, veins, and the CNS.

The optic nerve is also known as the second cranial nerve (CN II). Its purpose is to transmit impulses from the retina to the occipital lobe of the brain. The optic nerve head, or optic disc, is the physiologic blind spot in each eye. The optic nerve leaves the eye and then meets the optic nerve from the other eye at the **optic chiasm**. The chiasm is the anatomic point at which the nasal fibers from the nasal retina of each eye cross to the opposite side of the brain. The nerve fibers from the temporal retina of each eye remain uncrossed. Fibers from the right half of each eye, which would be the left visual field, carry impulses to the right occipital lobe. Fibers from the left half of each eye, or the right visual field, carry impulses to the left occipital lobe. Beyond the chiasm, these fibers are known as the *optic tract.* The optic tract continues on to the lateral geniculate body, which leads to the optic radiations and then to the cortex of the occipital lobe of the brain.

Gerontologic Considerations

The eye undergoes many changes as the body ages. All cells formed throughout life are retained by the lens, which makes the cell structure of the lens susceptible to the degenerative effects of aging. The lens continues to grow throughout life, laying down fibers in concentric rings. As the body ages, the gel-like characteristics of the vitreous humor are gradually lost, and various cells and fibers cast shadows that the patient perceives as "floaters." The vitreous humor shrinks and shifts with age. Other age-related changes are summarized in Table 47-1.

TABLE **47-1** **GERONTOLOGIC CONSIDERATIONS / Age-Related Changes in the Eye**

Component	Structural Change	Functional Change	History and Physical Findings
Dry eye	Dysfunction of meibomian glands Inflammatory changes to tear proteins	Discomfort and pain with possible vision changes	Patient complains of vision changes, itching, burning, scratching sensation proportional to increased computer screen time
Eyelids and lacrimal structures	Loss of skin elasticity and orbital fat, decreased muscle tone; wrinkles develop	Lid margins turn in, causing lashes to irritate cornea and conjunctiva (entropion); or lid margins may turn out, resulting in increased corneal exposure (ectropion)	Patient reports burning, foreign-body sensation, increased tearing (epiphora); injection, inflammation, and ulceration may occur
Refractive changes; presbyopia	Loss of accommodative power in the lens with age	Reading materials must be held at increasing distance in order to focus	Patient reports difficulty in reading at the usual reading distance; need for increased light; reading glasses or bifocals needed
Cataract	Opacities in the normally crystalline lens	Interference with the focus of a sharp image on the retina	Patient reports increased glare, decreased vision, changes in color values (blue and yellow especially affected)
Posterior vitreous detachment	Liquefaction and shrinkage of vitreous body	May lead to retinal tears and detachment	Patient reports light flashes, cobwebs, floaters
Age-related macular degeneration (AMD)	Drusen (yellowish aging spots in the retina) appear and coalesce in the macula. Abnormal choroidal blood vessels may lead to formation of fibrotic disciform scars in the macula.	Central vision is affected; onset is more gradual in dry AMD, more rapid in wet AMD; distortion and loss of central vision may occur	Patient reports reading vision is affected; words may be missing letters, faded areas appear on the page, straight lines may appear wavy; drusen, pigmentary changes in retina; abnormal submacular choroidal vessels
Low vision	Vision difficulties even with corrective lenses	Vision less than 20/40 with corrective lenses with the best correction possible	Patient reports progressive vision loss in near and far vision with light sensitivity and difficulty seeing at night

Data from Chader, G. J., & Taylor, A. (2013). Preface: The aging eye: Normal changes, age-related diseases, and sight-saving approaches. *Investigative Ophthalmology and Visual Science*, *54*(14), ORSF1–ORSF4.

ASSESSMENT

Health History

The nurse, through careful questioning, elicits the necessary information that can lead to the diagnosis of an ophthalmic condition.

Common Complaints

Common symptoms include changes in vision, pain or discomfort, and discharge. For each of the symptoms, the nurse asks:

- Are both eyes affected?
- Is this a recurrence of a previous condition?
- How has the patient self-treated?
- How is the patient affected by the symptom(s)?
- What makes the symptoms improve or worsen?
- What is the duration of the problem?

Changes in Vision

The nurse asks about changes in vision, including diminished visual acuity and blurred, distorted, or double vision. Changes in vision can be associated with problems such as myopia (distant objects appear blurred or nearsightedness), hyperopia (farsightedness), presbyopia (diminished ability to focus on near objects with age, a form of farsightedness), cataracts (opacity of the lens), glaucoma (abnormally high IOP that can damage the optic nerve), aging, diabetes, hypertension, cranial tumors, head trauma, or increased intracranial pressure (ICP).

Pain or Discomfort

The nurse inquires about the type of pain (sharp or dull) and whether it is worse when blinking. Pain while blinking might be present in superficial trauma events, such as corneal abrasions, corneal lacerations, or presence of a foreign body. Discomfort may include itching or a foreign-body sensation. This sensation of the presence of a foreign body is often present in diseases associated with conjunctival irritation. Conjunctival irritation may be found in conditions such as dry eye, bacterial or viral infections (pink eye), and irritation and allergic reactions (Bickley et al., 2021).

Discharge

It is important to note the color, consistency, and odor of any discharge. Eye discharge commonly results from inflammation or infection of the conjunctiva. Manifestations of other non-eye disorders may include eye discharge, such as erythema multiforme major (Stevens–Johnson syndrome), herpes zoster, and psoriasis vulgaris (refer to Chapter 51).

Past History

The nurse asks if the concern is a recurrence of a previous condition and notes the presence of any systemic diseases and medications used in their treatment. Medications for medical disorders cause many eye disorders as side effects. For example, if long-term steroids are administered for arthritis, cataracts may develop. The nurse also inquires about concurrent ophthalmic conditions and any history of ophthalmic surgery.

Family History

The nurse asks whether any family members have had the same symptoms or condition, such as glaucoma, refraction disorders, and allergies.

Social History

In ophthalmology, the well-being of the patient physically, emotionally, financially, socially, and spiritually can be at risk when vision is threatened. The patient may equate a decrease in visual acuity with a loss of independence. The loss of a driver's license may force a patient to relocate or give up or change their career.

Major goals should include the preservation of vision and the prevention of further visual loss in patients who have already experienced some degree of loss. Lines of communication must be kept open so that the patient is comfortable exploring all treatment options to promote rehabilitation.

Physical Assessment

Visual Acuity Assessment

Following the health history, the patient's visual acuity is assessed. Most people are familiar with the standard Snellen chart. It is composed of a series of progressively smaller rows of letters and is used to test distance vision. The patient is positioned at the prescribed distance, usually 20 ft, from the chart and is asked to read the smallest line visible. The patient should wear distance correction (eyeglasses or contact lenses) if required, and each eye should be tested separately. A card should be provided to cover one eye to prevent the patient from trying to view the chart between the fingers. The fraction 20/20 is considered the standard of healthy vision. The numerator denotes the distance between the patient and the chart, whereas the denominator quantifies the distance at which a healthy eye can read the line of letters. A person whose vision is 20/200 can read print from 20 ft away that a person with 20/20 vision can read at 200 ft (Bickley et al., 2021). Most people can see the letters on the line designated as 20/20 from a distance of 20 ft.

If the patient cannot read the 20/20 line, they are given a pinhole occluder and asked to read again using the eye in question. The patient should be encouraged to read every letter possible. Specific visual acuities are then recorded for each eye. If the patient reads all five letters from the 20/20 line with the right eye and three letters of the 20/15 line with the left eye, the examiner records right eye 20/20, left eye 20/15-2. (Note: Medical abbreviations in the past used

"OD" and "OS" to represent right and left eyes, respectively; however, those abbreviations are no longer recommended because misinterpretation has resulted in harmful medication errors).

If the patient cannot read the largest letter on the chart (the 20/200 line), the patient should be moved toward the chart or the chart moved toward the patient until the patient can identify the largest letter on the chart. If the patient can recognize only the letter E on the top line at a distance of 10 ft, the visual acuity would be recorded as 10/200. If the patient cannot see the letter E at any distance, the examiner should determine if the patient can count fingers. The examiner holds up a random number of fingers and asks the patient to count the number they see. If the patient correctly identifies the number of fingers at 3 ft, the examiner would record "counts fingers/3 ft."

If the patient cannot count fingers, the examiner raises one hand up and down or moves it side to side and asks in which direction the hand is moving. This level of vision is known as hand motion. A patient who can perceive only light is described as having light perception. The vision of a patient who cannot perceive light is described as no light perception.

Near vision testing is performed to identify the need for reading glasses. **Presbyopia** is the term used for impaired near vision and is often found in middle-aged and older persons. A specially designed handheld card is held 14 in away from the patient's eyes, and the patient is asked to read the chart. People with presbyopia are commonly able to read the chart when it is held farther away.

External Eye Examination

After the visual acuity has been recorded, an external eye examination is performed. While standing directly in front of the patient, the nurse notes the position of the eyelids and alignment of the eyes. Commonly, the upper 2 mm of the iris are covered by the upper lid. The patient is examined for **ptosis** (drooping eyelid) and for lid retraction (too much of the eye exposed). Sometimes, the upper or lower lid turns out, referred to as *ectropion*, affecting closure. In addition, the eyelid may invert; this is termed *entropion* and causes irritation of the eye. The lid margins and lashes should have no edema, erythema, or lesions. The examiner looks for scaling or crusting, and the sclera is inspected. A normal sclera is opaque and white (except as noted earlier). Lesions on the conjunctiva, discharge, tearing, and blinking are noted.

The pupils are inspected for size, shape, and symmetry. A normal pupil is black in color, round in shape, and symmetric. Pupil size ranges between 2 and 8 mm depending on extremes of light. In room lighting, usual pupil size is 3 to 5 mm. The room should be darkened so that the pupils can be examined. The nurse checks pupillary response with a penlight to determine if the pupils are equally reactive and regular. The patient is asked to stare at a target; each eye is covered and uncovered quickly while the examiner looks for any shift in gaze. Pupillary inequality of less than 1 mm despite an equal response to light is termed anisocoria. It may be detected in 20% to 30% of healthy people (American Association for Pediatric Ophthalmology and Strabismus [AAPOS], 2021). Anisocoria can be a benign variant (usually less than 1 mm difference between pupils) or a manifestation of disease, termed *pathologic anisocoria* (at least 1 mm difference) (AAPOS, 2021). An artificial eye will have anisocoria. Other notable irregularities may be the result of trauma, previous surgery, or disease.

The pupillary response to light is determined by shining a bright light obliquely into each pupil. Pupils are assessed for *direct reaction*, in which the pupil tested with light constricts, and for *consensual reaction*, in which the pupil of the opposite eye also constricts. The nurse is aware that the pupil of a blind eye will not constrict; however, if a direct light is reflected on the healthy eye, a consensual light reaction may be noted in the impaired eye. There will be no reaction with a prosthetic eye.

The examiner also observes for **nystagmus** (i.e., oscillating movement of the eyeball). The extraocular movements (EOMs) of the eyes are tested by having the patient follow the examiner's finger, a pencil, or a hand light through the six cardinal directions (i.e., up, down, right, left, and both diagonals) of gaze, a wide H pattern. Normal EOMs should produce conjugate movements (simultaneous movement of both eyes) in each direction. This is especially important when screening patients for ocular trauma or for neurologic disorders.

Diagnostic Evaluation

Direct Ophthalmoscopy

A direct ophthalmoscope is a handheld instrument enabling magnification of the cornea, lens, and retina. The patient is normally given mydriatic drops to dilate the pupils and assist in the examination of vision. Contraindications to the use of mydriatic drops include head injury or narrow-angle glaucoma. The patient is given a target at which to gaze. The examiner holds the ophthalmoscope in the right hand and uses the right eye to examine the patient's right eye. The examiner switches to the left hand and left eye when examining the patient's left eye. During this examination, the room should be darkened, and the examiner should be about 15 in away from the patient and 15 degrees lateral to the patient's line of vision. The patient should be relaxed and able to keep both eyes open and steady.

The examiner shines the light on the patient's pupil to examine the fundus (Fig. 47-6). The fundus of the eye is the interior structure opposite the lens that includes the retina, optic disc, macula, fovea, and posterior pole. A normal orange glow is observed as light is applied to the pupil, known as the **red reflex**. Absence of the red reflex may indicate lens opacity, which is consistent with a cataract, detached retina, or retinoblastoma in children. When the fundus is examined,

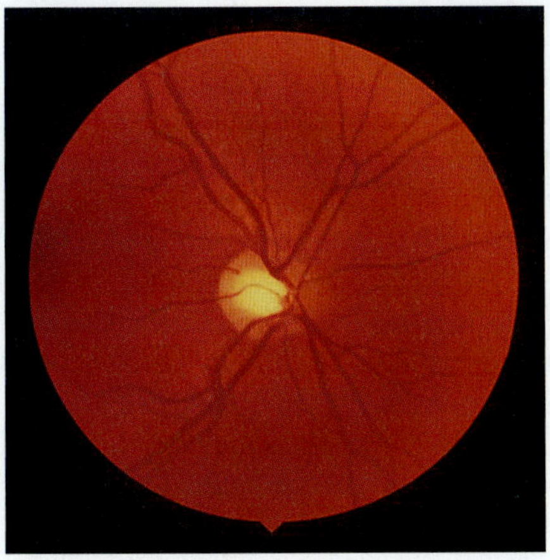

FIGURE 47-6 **Normal fundus.**

the vasculature comes into focus first. The examiner focuses on a large vessel and then follows it as it becomes larger in diameter, leading to the optic disc. The central depression in the disc is known as the *cup*. The normal cup is about one third the size of the disc. The size of the physiologic optic cup should be estimated and the disc margins described as sharp or blurred. The periphery of the retina is examined by having the patient shift their gaze. The last area of the fundus to be examined is the macula, because this area is the most sensitive to light.

The healthy fundus should be free of any lesions. The examiner looks for intraretinal hemorrhages, which may appear as red smudges; if the patient has hypertension, it may look somewhat flame-shaped. A yellow lipid may be present in the retina of patients with hypercholesterolemia or diabetes. The examiner looks for microaneurysms, which look like little red dots, and nevi. *Drusen* (small, hyaline, globular growths), commonly found in macular degeneration, appear as yellowish areas with indistinct edges. The examiner should sketch the fundus and document any abnormalities.

Amsler Grid

The Amsler grid is a test often used for patients with macular problems, such as macular degeneration. It consists of a geometric grid of identical squares with a central fixation point. The grid should be viewed by the patient wearing normal reading glasses. Each eye is tested separately. The patient is instructed to stare at the central fixation spot on the grid and report any distortion in the squares of the grid itself. Patients with macular problems typically note that some of the squares may look wavy, blurred, or distorted. Patients with age-related macular degeneration are commonly given these Amsler grids to take home. The patient is encouraged to check them frequently, as often as daily, to detect any early signs of distortion that may indicate the development of a neovascular choroidal membrane, an advanced stage of macular degeneration characterized by the growth of abnormal choroidal vessels.

Tonometry

Tonometry measures IOP by determining the amount of force or pressure necessary to indent or flatten (applanate) a small anterior area of the globe of the eye. High readings indicate high pressure; low readings indicate low pressure. The procedure is noninvasive and usually painless. A topical anesthetic eye drop is instilled into the lower conjunctival sac, and the tonometer is then used to measure the IOP. Air-puff tonometry may also be done but was found to have minor differences in very high or low pressures as compared to the direct contact method (Luebke, 2019).

Two of the most commonly used tonometers are the applanation tonometer and the Tono-Pen. The applanation tonometer is generally used by the more skilled examiner. A drop of fluorescein dye and an anesthetic drop are instilled in the eye. The applanation tip is pressed against the cornea and the examiner, looking through the slit lamp, obtains the IOP reading. The Tono-Pen is a portable, battery-operated, handheld tonometer that is commonly used in many clinical settings. A disposable cover is placed over the tip of the instrument, and it is held against the anesthetized cornea for a few seconds. The tension reading is displayed in a liquid crystal display window.

Perimetry Testing

Perimetry testing evaluates the field of vision. A *visual field* is the area or extent of physical space visible to an eye in a given position. It has a three-dimensional contour representing areas of relative retinal sensitivity; visual acuity is sharpest at the top of the field and declines progressively toward the periphery. It is most helpful in detecting central **scotomas** (blind areas in the visual field) in macular degeneration and the peripheral field defects in glaucoma and retinitis pigmentosa.

The two methods of perimetric testing are manual and automated perimetry. Manual perimetry involves the use of moving (kinetic) or stationary (static) stimuli or targets. An example of kinetic manual perimetry is the tangent screen. A tangent screen is a wall-mounted black felt material that has a series of concentric circles bisected by straight lines emanating from the center. It tests the central 30 degrees of the visual field. Automated perimetry uses stationary targets, which are more difficult to detect than moving targets. In this test, a computer projects light randomly in different areas of a hollow dome while the patient looks through a telescopic opening and depresses a button whenever the light stimulus is detected. Automated perimetry is more accurate than manual perimetry.

Slit-Lamp Examination

The slit lamp is a binocular microscope mounted on a table. This instrument enables the user to examine the eye with magnification of 10 to 40 times the actual image. The illumination can be varied from a broad to a narrow beam of light for different parts of the eye. For example, by varying the width and intensity of the light, the anterior chamber can be examined for signs of inflammation. Cataracts may be evaluated by changing the angle of the light. When a handheld lens, such as a three-mirror lens, is used with the slit lamp, the angle of the anterior chamber may be examined, as may the ocular fundus.

Color Vision Testing

The ability to differentiate colors has a dramatic effect on the activities of daily living. For example, the inability to differentiate between red and green can compromise traffic safety. Some careers (e.g., commercial art, color photography, airline pilot, electrician) may be closed to people with significant problems differentiating color. Color discrimination allows visualization of a broad spectrum of color. The photoreceptor cells responsible for color vision are the cones, and the greatest area of color sensitivity is in the macula, the area of densest cone concentration. A defect or deficiency in the cones (red, blue, or green) will result in abnormal color vision. There are three basic types of color blindness: red–green, which is the most common deficiency; blue; and total color blindness, also known as *achromatopsia.*

A screening test, such as the polychromatic plates, can be used to establish whether a person's color vision is within normal range. Color vision deficits can be inherited. For example, red–green color deficiencies are inherited in an X-linked manner, affecting approximately 8% of males and 0.5% of females. Acquired color vision losses may be caused by chronic illness (e.g., diabetes, macular degeneration, glaucoma), medications (e.g., digitalis), trauma, exposure to industrial toxins, or aging (e.g., cataracts). A simple test, such as asking a patient if the red top on a bottle of eye drops appears redder to one eye than the other, can be an effective tool. A difference in the perception of the intensity of the color red between the two eyes can be a symptom of a neurologic problem and may provide information about the location of the lesion.

Ultrasonography

Lesions in the globe or the orbit may not be directly visible and are evaluated by ultrasonography. Ultrasonography is a valuable diagnostic technique, especially when the view of the retina is obscured by opaque media, such as cataract or hemorrhage. Ultrasonography can be used to identify orbital tumors, retinal detachment, and changes in tissue composition.

Special techniques can also be used to calculate the power for an intraocular lens implant and to obtain more anatomic information, showing cross-sectional images. Vitreous hemorrhage, retinal detachment, and tumors can be evaluated with minimal discomfort for the patient. Three-dimensional images can be created, and the entire ultrasound examination can be recorded for later use.

Fluorescein Angiography

Fluorescein angiography evaluates clinically significant macular edema, documents macular capillary nonperfusion, and identifies retinal and choroidal neovascularization (growth of abnormal new blood vessels) in age-related macular degeneration. It is an invasive procedure in which fluorescein dye is injected, usually into an antecubital vein. Within 10 to 15 seconds, this dye can be seen coursing through the retinal vessels. Over a 10-minute period, serial black-and-white photographs are taken of the retinal vasculature. The dye may impart a gold tone to the skin of some patients, and urine may turn deep yellow or orange. This discoloration usually disappears in 24 hours.

Pearls for Practice

When the nurse administers eye medications, pressure is applied to the inner canthus while placing the medication on the conjunctival sac to prevent systemic absorption.

THE EAR

The ear is a sensory organ with dual functions—hearing and balance. The sense of hearing is essential for normal development and maintenance of speech, as well as for the ability to communicate with others. Balance, or equilibrium, is essential for maintaining body movement, position, and coordination.

ANATOMY AND PHYSIOLOGY OVERVIEW

External Ear

The **external ear** includes the auricle (**pinna**) and the **external auditory canal** (Fig. 47-7). The external ear is separated from the middle ear by a disc-like structure called the **tympanic membrane** (eardrum). The auricle, attached to the side of the head by skin, is composed mainly of cartilage, except for the fat and subcutaneous tissue in the earlobe. The auricle collects the sound waves and directs vibrations into the external auditory canal.

The external auditory canal is approximately 2.5 cm long. The external auditory canal ends at the tympanic membrane. The skin of the canal contains hair, sebaceous glands, and ceruminous glands, which secrete a waxlike substance called **cerumen** (earwax). Earwax may be honey colored, darkening with a sticky consistency, and range to drier and whitish to gray in color in people of East Asian and Native North American descent (Bickley et al., 2021). The ear's self-cleaning mechanism moves old skin cells and cerumen to the outer part of the ear.

Middle Ear

The **middle ear**, an air-filled cavity, includes the tympanic membrane laterally and the otic capsule medially. The

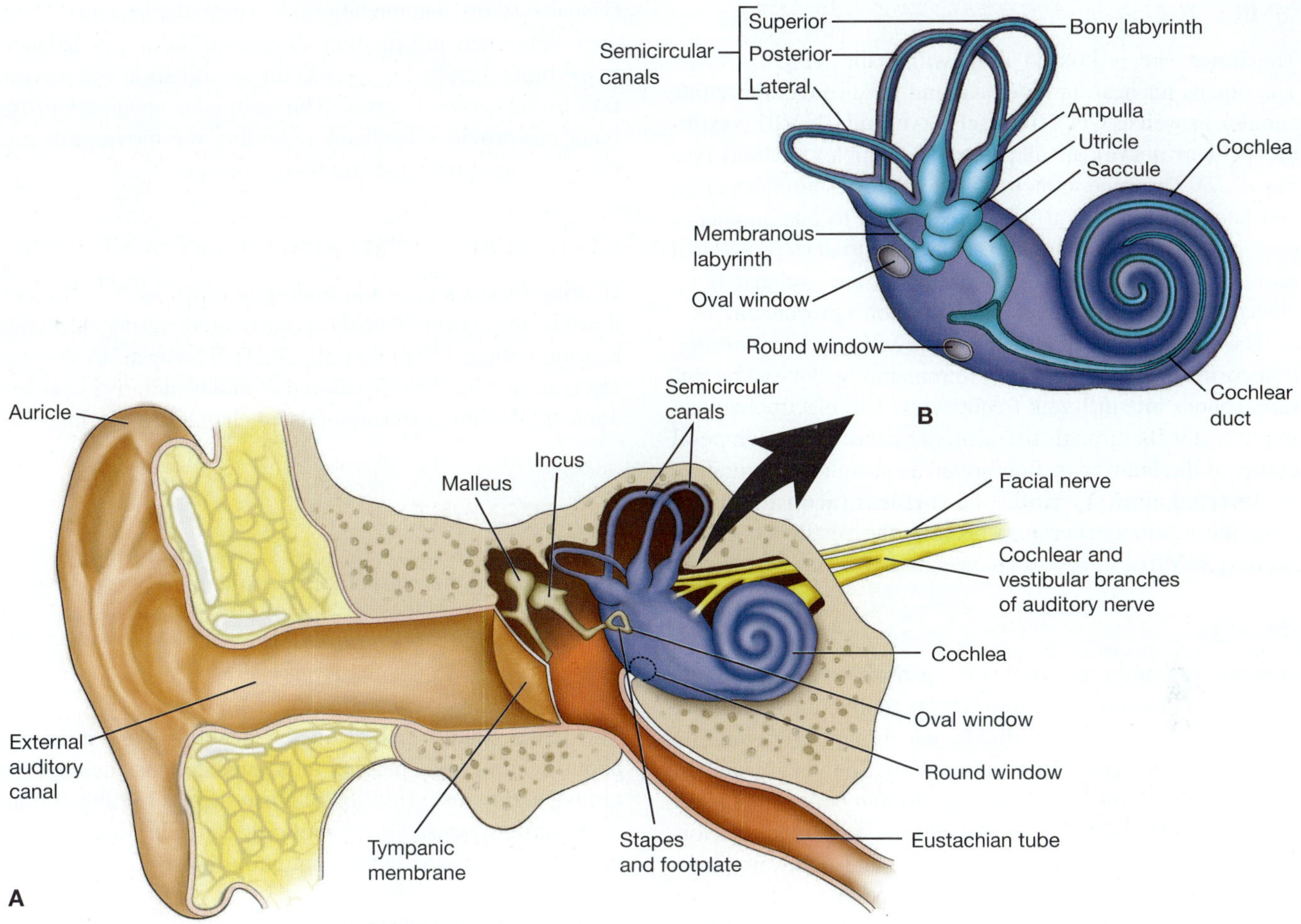

FIGURE 47-7 **A. Anatomy of the ear. B. The inner ear.**

middle ear is connected by the **eustachian tube** to the nasopharynx and is continuous with air-filled cells in the adjacent mastoid portion of the **temporal bone**. Normally, the eustachian tube is closed, but it opens when the person performs a Valsalva maneuver, yawns, or swallows. It drains normal and abnormal secretions of the middle ear and equalizes pressure in the middle ear with that of the atmosphere.

The tympanic membrane (eardrum), about 1 cm in diameter and very thin, is normally pearly gray and translucent. The tympanic membrane protects the middle ear and conducts sound vibrations from the external canal to the **ossicles**. Figure 47-8 illustrates the distinguishing landmarks of the tympanic membrane.

The middle ear contains the three smallest bones (the ossicles) of the body: the **malleus**, the **incus**, and the **stapes**. The ossicles, which are held in place by joints, muscles, and ligaments, assist in the transmission of sound. Two small fenestrae (oval and round windows), located in the medial wall of the middle ear, separate the middle ear from the inner ear. The footplate of the stapes sits in the **oval window**, secured by a fibrous annulus (ring-shaped structure). The footplate transmits sound to the inner ear. The **round window**, covered by a thin membrane, provides an exit for sound vibrations (see Fig. 47-7).

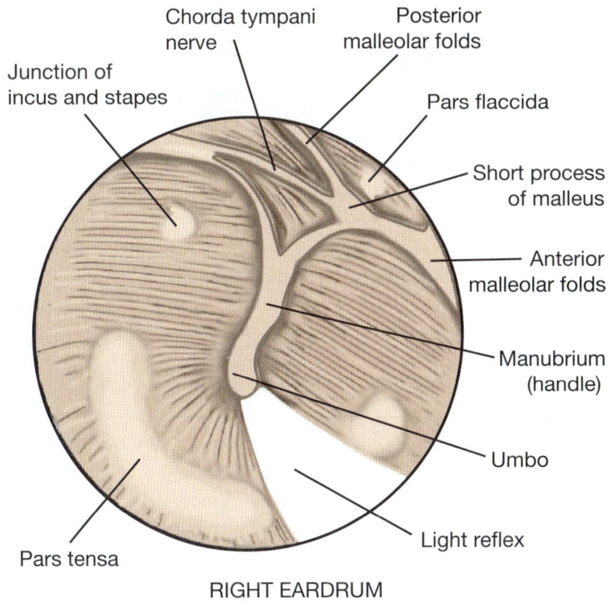

FIGURE 47-8 **The tympanic membrane.**

Inner Ear

The **inner ear** is housed deep within the temporal bone. The organs for hearing (**cochlea**) and balance (**semicircular canals**), as well as CN VII (facial nerve) and CN VIII (**vestibulocochlear nerve**), are all part of this complex anatomy (see Fig. 47-7). The three semicircular canals—posterior, superior, and lateral, which lie at 90-degree angles to one another—contain sensory receptor organs, arranged to detect rotational movement. These receptor end organs are stimulated by changes in the rate or direction of a person's movement.

The **organ of Corti**, also called the *end organ for hearing,* transforms mechanical energy into neural activity and separates sounds into different frequencies. This electrochemical impulse travels through the **acoustic** nerve to the temporal cortex of the brain to be interpreted as meaningful sound. In the **internal auditory canal**, the **cochlear (acoustic) nerve** joins the vestibular nerve to become the vestibulocochlear nerve (CN VIII).

Hearing

Hearing is conducted over two pathways: air and bone (Fig. 47-9). Sounds transmitted by air conduction travel over the air-filled external and middle ear through the vibration of the tympanic membrane and ossicles. Sounds transmitted by bone conduction travel directly through bone to the inner ear, bypassing the tympanic membrane and ossicles. Normally, air conduction is the more efficient pathway. However, a defect in the tympanic membrane or interruption of the ossicular chain disrupts normal air conduction, which results in a **conductive hearing loss**.

Balance and Equilibrium

Body balance is maintained by the cooperation of the muscles and joints of the body (proprioceptive system), the eyes (visual system), and the labyrinth (vestibular system). These areas send their information about equilibrium, or balance, to the brain (cerebellar system) for coordination and perception in the cerebral cortex. The vestibular apparatus of the inner ear provides feedback regarding the movements and the position of the head and body in space.

Gerontologic Considerations

Hearing loss is a common finding in older adults, with two thirds of those over 70 years of age demonstrating detectable hearing deficits (Powell et al., 2021). The term *presbycusis* refers to hearing loss associated with degenerative changes. Table 47-2 summarizes age-related changes in hearing.

ASSESSMENT

Assessment of the ear includes a health history and physical assessment.

Health History

The nurse should include in the health history questions about hearing loss, hearing aids, medications, itching, ear drainage, tinnitus (sensation of noise such as ringing or roaring), vertigo (sensation of motion), ear pain, and environmental exposure to loud or continuous noises.

Common Complaints

The nurse needs to explore common ear complaints, such as changes in hearing acuity, earache, drainage, and tinnitus. Approximately 5% of the world's population suffers from disabling hearing loss (Ferri, 2022). A common complaint of ear pain is associated with a variety of disorders, including

TABLE **47-2 GERONTOLOGIC CONSIDERATIONS / Age-Related Changes in the Ear**

Component	Structural Change	Functional Change	History and Physical Findings
Atrophy of the external ears	Pinna loses flexibility	Thinning and drying of ear canal	Pinna longer and thinner with dry cerumen in the external ear canal
Hardening of cerumen	Dryer, thicker cerumen	Earwax accumulates	Visible earwax and conductive hearing impairment
Thickening of the eardrum	Stiffness of eardrum	Impaired transmission of sound	Mild hearing impairment
Change in vestibulospinal reflex	Loss of vestibular afferents and neurons	Progressive imbalance and increased falls	Balance and gait tests provoke symptoms of dizziness and postural instability
Degeneration of organ of Corti (presbycusis)	Loss of cochlear pathway neurons, atrophy of vascular cochlear tissue	Loss of ability to discriminate words or comprehend conversations	Decreased ability to hear high frequencies or to interpret consonant sounds

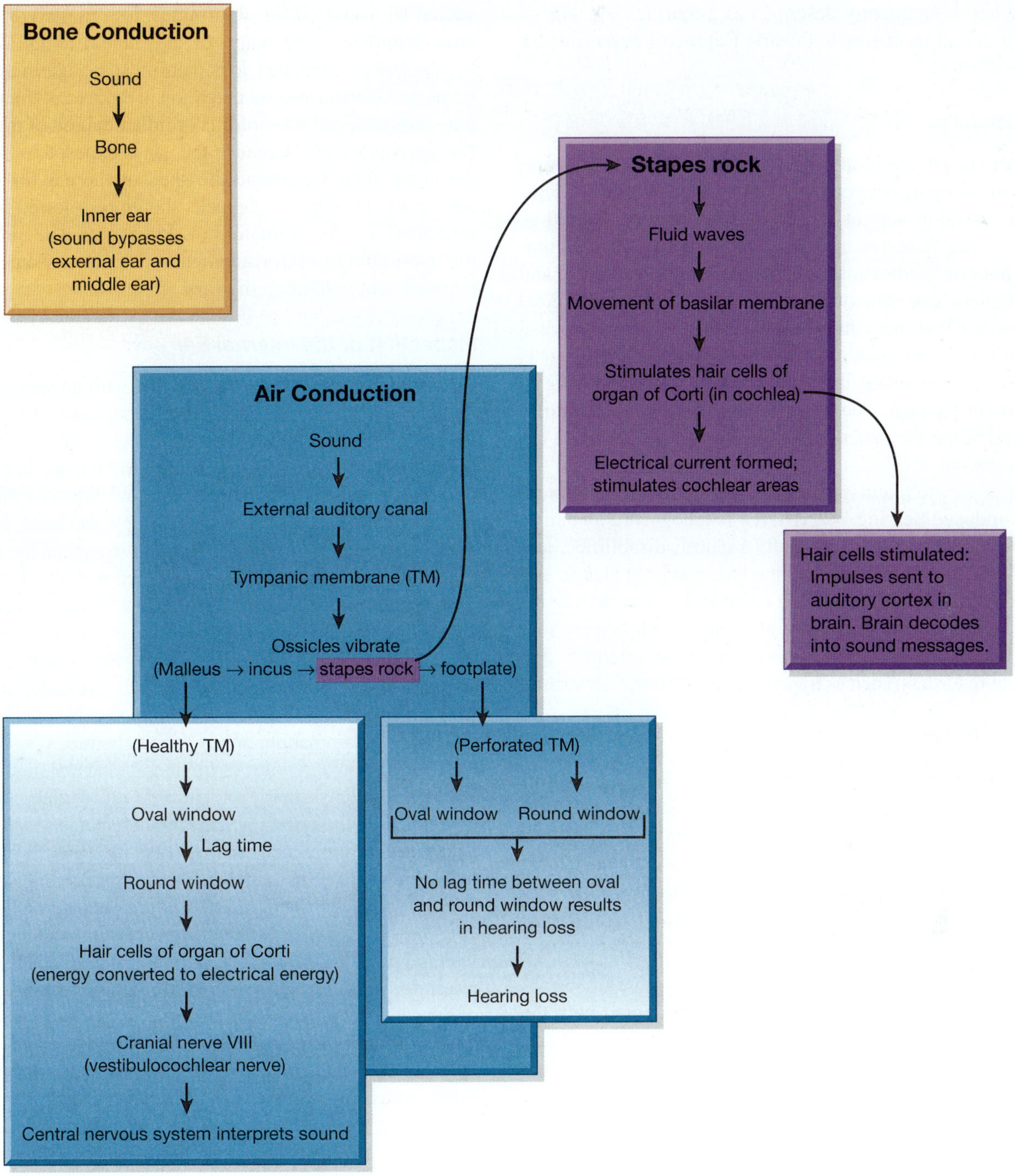

FIGURE 47-9 Bone conduction compared to air conduction.

cerumen impaction, acute external otitis, acute mastoiditis, acute otitis media, and foreign bodies. Impaction of cerumen can cause otalgia (a sensation of fullness or pain in the ear) with or without a hearing loss. If, on manipulation of the auricle, the patient complains of pain, the nurse suspects the etiology of the pain is acute external otitis. Tenderness on palpation in the area of the mastoid may indicate acute mastoiditis or inflammation of the posterior auricular node. Acute otitis media, an acute infection of the middle ear, can occur at any age, though it is seen most commonly in children. Symptoms vary with the severity of the infection. In adults, complaints of pain are usually unilateral, and the pain is relieved after spontaneous perforation or therapeutic incision of the tympanic membrane.

Tinnitus is another common symptom of an underlying disorder of the ear that is associated with hearing impairment and loss, ototoxic substances (see Chapter 49), and a variety of hearing disorders (otosclerosis, Ménière disease, acoustic neuroma) and systemic disorders (thyroid disease, neurologic disorders). Tinnitus may range from mild to severe and is frequently described as a roaring, buzzing, or hissing sound in one or both ears. Refer to Chapter 49 for further details.

Past History

A history of infections affecting the ear may indicate hearing loss caused by diseases of the tympanic membranes. Medications can alter auditory function, so each agent should be evaluated for potential effects on ear disorders. Some common ototoxic medications include antibiotics, diuretics, and nonsteroidal anti-inflammatory agents (NSAIDs). Surgical approaches that may have been performed to improve a patient's auditory function must be explored. If used, it is necessary to evaluate the patient's experience with hearing aids in the past. The effectiveness of previous therapies will determine the patient's options for and decisions on ear interventions.

Exposure to loud noises should also be explored. Noise-induced hearing loss (NIHL) is recognized as one of the most common occupationally induced disabilities, and noise exposure is regulated by the Occupational Health and Safety Administration (OSHA) (Alexander Arts & Adams, 2021). Other related conditions associated with hearing loss include head trauma; brain tumors; multiple sclerosis; and vascular disorders, such as hypertension and arteriosclerosis.

Family History

Many cases of hearing loss are inherited; hereditary disorders of the ear include Hallgren disease, Alport syndrome, Refsum disease, Stickler syndrome, Pendred syndrome, Usher syndrome, Ehlers–Danlos syndrome, and Treacher Collins disease. Some of these disorders are associated with other organ disorders, such as kidney disease.

Social History

The presence of social problems must be explored with the patient who has hearing loss. A patient with decreased hearing may withdraw from situations in which communication skills are needed. They may become depressed and unable to continue in their chosen profession. Explore the patient's ability to work and engage in social interactions. Data regarding the age at onset and severity of hearing loss will help the nurse understand the personal impact of hearing loss.

Physical Assessment

Physical assessment includes inspection and palpation of the external ear, inspection of the internal ear, and hearing evaluation.

Inspection and Palpation of the External Ear

Inspection of the external ear is a simple procedure but is often overlooked. The external ear is examined by inspection and direct palpation; the auricle and surrounding tissues should be inspected for deformities, lesions, and discharge; size; symmetry; and angle of attachment to the head. If manipulation of the auricle is painful, acute external otitis is suspected. Tenderness on palpation in the area of the mastoid may indicate acute mastoiditis or inflammation of the posterior auricular node. Because the ear is exposed to sunlight, the nurse should examine the shell of the ear for lesions. Any lesion lasting over 2 weeks should be referred to a skin care specialist for evaluation of skin cancer. The nurse uses the opportunity to inform patients to apply sunscreen to all exposed skin, including the ears.

Inspection of the Internal Ear

The tympanic membrane is inspected with an otoscope and indirect palpation with a pneumatic otoscope. To examine the external auditory canal and tympanic membrane, the otoscope should be held in the examiner's right hand, in a pencil-hold position, with the examiner's hand braced against the patient's face (Fig. 47-10). Using the opposite hand, the auricle is grasped and gently pulled back to straighten the canal in the adult. If the canal is not straightened with this technique, the tympanic membrane is more difficult to visualize because the canal obstructs the view. The speculum is slowly inserted into the ear canal, with the examiner's eye held close to the magnifying lens of the otoscope to visualize the canal and tympanic membrane. The external auditory canal is examined for discharge, inflammation, or any foreign bodies.

The position and color of the membrane and any unusual markings or deviations from normal are documented (see Fig. 47-8). If the tympanic membrane cannot be visualized because of cerumen, the cerumen may be removed by gently irrigating the external canal with warm water (unless contraindicated). If adherent cerumen is present, a small amount of mineral oil or over-the-counter cerumen softener may be instilled within the ear canal, and the patient is instructed to return for subsequent removal of the cerumen and inspection of the ear. The nurse is aware that ear irrigation is one of the more common causes of iatrogenic injuries treated by otolaryngologists (McHenry, 2020); if performed incorrectly, infection and tympanic membrane perforation can occur. In practice, the final evaluation and irrigation is done by an otolaryngologist; nurse practitioners; or eye, ear, nose, and throat (EENT) provider.

Evaluation of Gross Auditory Acuity

A general estimate of hearing can be made by assessing the patient's ability to hear a whispered phrase or a ticking watch, testing one ear at a time. The Weber and Rinne tests may be used to distinguish conductive loss from sensorineural loss when hearing is impaired.

Whisper Test

To exclude one ear from the testing, the examiner covers the untested ear with the palm of the hand. Then the examiner

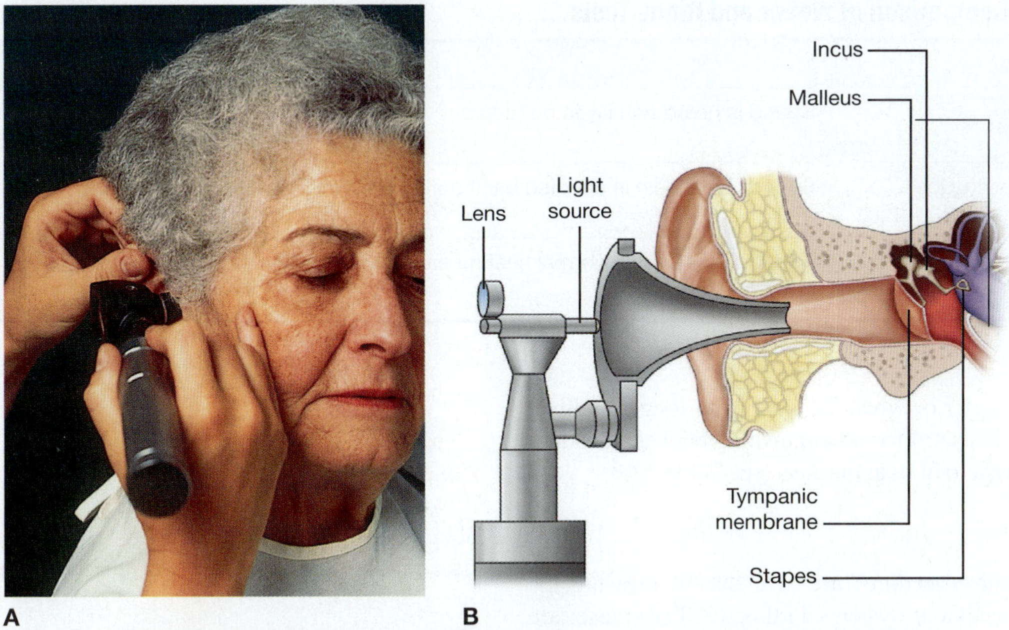

FIGURE 47-10 **Proper technique for examining the ear. A. Hold the otoscope in the right or left hand, in a "pencil-hold" position. B. Steady the hand against the patient's head to avoid inserting the otoscope too far into the external canal.**

whispers softly from a distance of 1 or 2 ft from the unoccluded ear and out of the patient's sight. The patient with normal hearing acuity can correctly repeat what was whispered.

Weber Test

The Weber test uses bone conduction to test lateralization of sound. A tuning fork (ideally, 512 Hz), set in motion, is placed on the patient's head or forehead (Fig. 47-11). The exam is considered normal if the person hears the sound equally in both ears or describes the sound as centered in the middle of the head. The Weber test is useful for detecting unilateral hearing loss (Table 47-3). However, studies reveal that up to 40% of people with normal hearing also lateralize the Weber test, so it should be interpreted only in patients with hearing loss (McGee, 2022).

Rinne Test

In the Rinne test, the examiner shifts the stem of a vibrating tuning fork between two positions: against the mastoid bone (for bone conduction) and, when the sound is no longer audible, 2 in from the opening of the ear canal (for air conduction). As the position changes, the patient is asked to indicate

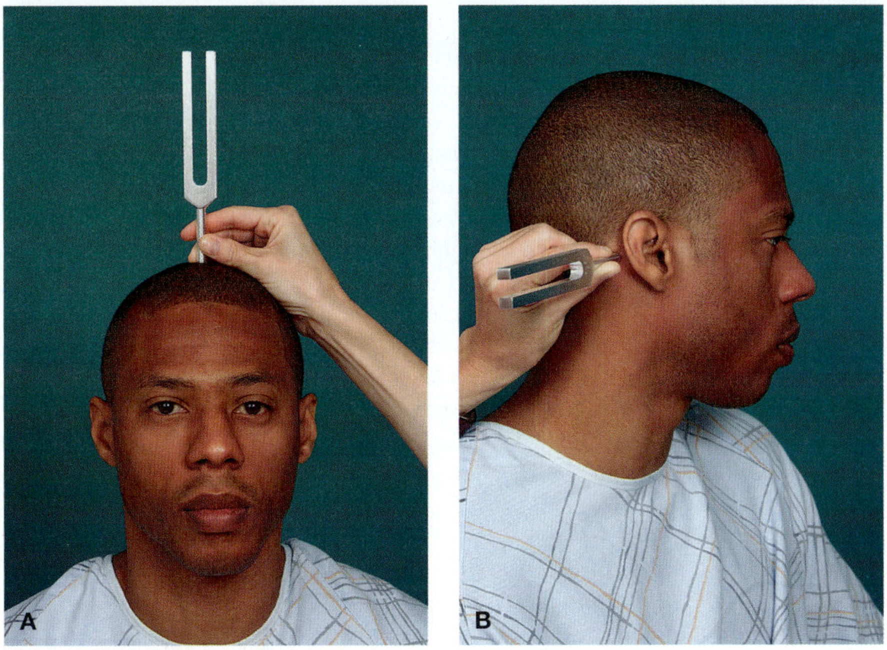

FIGURE 47-11 **A. The Weber test assesses bone conduction of sound. B. The Rinne test assesses both air and bone conduction of sound.**

TABLE **47-3 Comparison of Weber and Rinne Tests**

Hearing Status	Weber	Rinne
Normal hearing	Sound is heard equally in both ears	Air conduction is audible longer than bone conduction
Conductive hearing loss	Sound heard best in affected ear (hearing loss)	Sound heard as long or longer in affected ear (hearing loss)
Sensorineural hearing loss	Sound heard best in normal hearing ear	Air conduction is audible longer than bone conduction in affected ear

which tone is louder or when the tone is no longer audible. The Rinne test is useful for distinguishing between conductive and **sensorineural hearing loss** (see Table 47-3).

Diagnostic Evaluation

Many diagnostic procedures are available to measure the auditory and vestibular systems indirectly. These tests are usually performed by an audiologist whose clinical competence is certified by the American Speech-Language-Hearing Association.

Audiometry

In detecting **hearing loss**, audiometry is the single most important diagnostic instrument. Audiometric testing is of two kinds: *pure-tone audiometry*, in which the sound stimulus consists of a pure or musical tone (the louder the tone before the patient perceives it, the greater the hearing loss), and *speech audiometry*, in which the spoken word is used to determine the ability to hear and discriminate sounds and words. Responses are plotted on a graph known as an *audiogram*, which differentiates conductive from sensorineural hearing loss.

When evaluating hearing, three characteristics are important: frequency, pitch, and intensity. *Frequency* refers to the number of sound waves emanating from a source per second, measured as cycles per second, or Hertz (Hz). The normal human ear perceives sounds ranging in frequency from 20 to 20,000 Hz. *Pitch* is the term used to describe frequency; a tone with 100 Hz is considered of low pitch, and a tone of 10,000 Hz is considered of high pitch. The unit for measuring loudness (*intensity* of sound) is the decibel (dB), the pressure exerted by sound. Hearing loss is measured in decibels, a logarithmic function of intensity that is not easily converted into a percentage. The critical level of loudness is approximately 30 dB. The shuffling of papers in quiet surroundings is about 15 dB. Table 47-4 classifies hearing loss based on decibel level.

Pearls for Practice

Environmental noise has an impact on our patients, ourselves, and visitors, and many efforts are in place for noise reduction. Literature reveals that noise affects the well-being of patients, delaying recovery, disturbing sleep, reducing professional productivity, increasing the occurrence of medical errors, and increasing the incidence of rehospitalization (de Lima et al., 2021; Miranda-Ackerman et al., 2020). Efforts to mitigate noise in hospitals may include changes to architectural design, use of sound absorbing material, alarm management, and traffic studies. In a recent study, the global noise level was 62.66 ± 1.23 dB in the general intensive care unit, but a noise level below 30 to 45 dB is required to facilitate a good sleep environment (Miranda-Ackerman et al., 2020; Tan et al., 2019). Interventions such as the use of ear plugs for patients, white noise to mask background noise, and limiting the volume of alarms of medical devices to 40 dB or lower should be considered (Tan et al., 2019).

Tympanogram

A tympanogram or impedance audiometry is used to evaluate the tympanic membrane and status of the middle ear. This test measures middle ear muscle reflex to sound stimulation (movement of the tympanic membrane) and the compliance of the tympanic membrane by changing the air pressure in the sealed ear canal. Compliance is impaired with middle ear disease, such as fluid accumulation in the middle ear or rupture of the tympanic membrane.

TABLE **47-4 Severity of Hearing Loss**

Loss in Decibels	Interpretation
0–15	Normal hearing
>15–25	Slight hearing loss
>25–40	Mild hearing loss
>40–55	Moderate hearing loss
>55–70	Moderate to severe hearing loss
>70–90	Severe hearing loss
>90	Profound hearing loss

Auditory Brainstem Response

The auditory brainstem response is a detectable electrical potential from CN VIII and the ascending auditory pathways of the brainstem in response to sound stimulation. Electrodes are placed on the patient's forehead. Acoustic stimuli (e.g., clicks) are made in the ear. The resulting electrophysiologic measurements can determine at which decibel level a patient hears and whether there are any impairments along the nerve pathways (e.g., tumor on CN VIII).

Electronystagmography

Electronystagmography is the measurement and graphic recording of the changes in electrical potentials created by eye movements during spontaneous, positional, or calorically evoked nystagmus. It is also used to assess the oculomotor and vestibular systems and their corresponding interaction. It helps diagnose conditions such as Ménière disease and tumors of the internal auditory canal or posterior fossa. Vestibular suppressants, such as sedatives, tranquilizers, antihistamines, and alcohol, are withheld for 24 hours before testing. Prior to the test, the procedure is explained to the patient.

Platform Posturography

Platform posturography is used to investigate postural control capabilities, such as **vertigo**. It can be used to evaluate if a person's vertigo is becoming worse or to evaluate the person's response to treatment. The integration of visual, vestibular, and proprioceptive cues (i.e., sensory integration) with motor response output and coordination of the lower limbs is tested. The patient stands on a platform surrounded by a screen, and different conditions, such as a moving platform with a moving screen or a stationary platform with a moving screen, are presented. The responses from the patient on six different conditions are measured and indicate which of the anatomic systems may be impaired. Preparation for the testing is the same as for electronystagmography.

Sinusoidal Harmonic Acceleration

Sinusoidal harmonic acceleration, or a rotary chair, is used to assess the vestibulo-ocular system by analyzing compensatory eye movements in response to the clockwise and counterclockwise rotation of the chair. Although such testing cannot identify the side of the lesion in unilateral disease, it helps identify disease (e.g., Ménière disease, tumors of the auditory canal) and evaluate the course of recovery. The same patient preparation is required as for electronystagmography.

Middle Ear Endoscopy

With endoscopes of very small diameters and acute angles, the ear can be examined by an endoscopist specializing in otolaryngology. Middle ear endoscopy is performed safely and effectively as an office procedure to evaluate suspected perilymphatic fistula, new-onset conductive hearing loss, the anatomy of the round window before transtympanic treatment of Ménière disease, and the tympanic cavity before ear surgery to treat chronic middle ear and mastoid infections.

The tympanic membrane is anesthetized topically for about 10 minutes before the procedure. Then, the external auditory canal is irrigated with sterile normal saline solution. With the aid of a microscope, a tympanotomy is created with a laser beam or a **myringotomy** knife so that the endoscope can be inserted into the middle ear cavity. Video and photo documentation can be accomplished through the scope.

CHAPTER REVIEW

NCLEX-Style Review Questions

1. You are asked to assess the visual acuity of a patient using the Snellen chart. Which actions are included in the procedure? Select all that apply.
   a. Position the patient 40 ft from the chart.
   b. Test both eyes first, then each separately.
   c. Position the patient 20 ft from the chart.
   d. The patient should wear distance correction (eyeglasses or contact lenses) during testing.
   e. Test each eye separately.
   f. Distance correction (contact lenses or eyeglasses) should be removed during testing.
   g. Record the smallest line visible to the patient.

2. A patient who complains of visual changes is being evaluated for glaucoma. In preparing the patient, how will you educate the patient about the name of the test, the preparation, and what a normal intraocular pressure (IOP) would be? Select all that apply.
   a. 2 to 7 mm Hg IOP
   b. Tonometry
   c. 10 to 21 mm Hg IOP
   d. Amsler grid
   e. The procedure is noninvasive and usually painless
   f. Fluorescein angiography
   g. A topical anesthetic eye drop is instilled into the inner canthus

3. In preparing a patient for cataract surgery, the nurse anticipates administering prescribed eye drops. What medication is anticipated, and how does the nurse instill the eyedrops? Select all that apply.
   a. The eye drops will be administered in the lower conjunctival sac.
   b. A miotic agent will be administered.
   c. A mydriatic medication will be administered.
   d. Pressure is applied to the inner canthus to prevent systemic absorption.
   e. Pumping of the puncta at the inner canthus encourages systemic absorption.
   f. A thiazide diuretic will be administered.
   g. The eye drop is instilled into the inner canthus.

4. The nurse is asked to assess the patient's pupillary response. Which actions are appropriate? Select all that apply.
   a. Darken the room.
   b. Recognize the usual pupil size is 3 to 5 mm.
   c. Shine the bright light directly on each pupil.
   d. Recognize the usual pupil size is 6 to 10 mm.
   e. Shine a bright light obliquely into each pupil.
   f. Pupils are assessed for direct reaction, in which the pupil tested directly with light constricts.
   g. Pupils are assessed for consensual reaction, in which the pupil tested directly with light constricts.

5. In evaluating a patient who is 87 years of age, which age-related changes of the ear are expected? Select all that apply.
   a. Accumulation of earwax
   b. Impaired transmission of sound
   c. Hypertrophy of cochlear tissue
   d. Increased neuron generation
   e. Shortened pinna
   f. Thinning of the ear canal
   g. Thickening of the eardrum

REFERENCES AND SELECTED READINGS

References and selected readings associated with this chapter can be found on the website that accompanies the book. Visit **http://thepoint.lww.com/Honan3e** to access the references and other additional resources associated with this chapter.

CHAPTER 48

Nursing Management: Patients With Eye and Vision Disorders

Carolynn Spera Bruno

Learning Objectives

After reading this chapter, you will be able to:

1. Define low vision and blindness, and differentiate functional and visual impairment.
2. List and describe assessment and management strategies for low vision.
3. Demonstrate orientation and mobility techniques for patients with low vision in a hospital setting.
4. Discuss assessment and management of glaucoma.
5. Discuss assessment and management of cataracts.
6. Discuss assessment and management of retinal disorders.
7. Discuss assessment and management of eye trauma.
8. Discuss assessment and management of infectious and inflammatory eye disorders.
9. Demonstrate the instillation of eye drops and ointment.
10. Discuss the postoperative management and discharge instructions of patients undergoing ocular surgery.

Patients admitted to medical-surgical units may have acute conditions affecting the eye or comorbidities associated with visual impairment. Many of the leading causes of visual impairment are associated with aging (e.g., cataracts, glaucoma, macular degeneration), and two thirds of the population with impaired vision are older than 65 years of age. Younger people are also at risk for eye disorders, particularly traumatic injuries. Understanding the prevention, treatment, and consequences of eye disorders, nurses in all settings assess visual acuity in those at risk (e.g., older patients those with diabetes or AIDS), refer patients to eye care specialists as appropriate, implement measures to prevent further visual loss, and help patients adapt to impaired vision.

IMPAIRED VISION

More than one million Americans are legally blind, and 12 million over the age of 40 years are visually impaired (Centers for Disease Control and Prevention [CDC], 2020). Chief causes of visual impairment or blindness include diabetic retinopathy and age-related eye diseases (e.g., cataracts, macular degeneration, and glaucoma). The World Health Organization (WHO) stated in their World Report of Vision that 80% of all causes of visual impairment can be prevented. The Vision 2020 Global Initiative is an expansive initiative of the International Agency for the Prevention of Blindness (IAPB), which seeks to eliminate causative factors of blindness in the world through providing technical support and advocacy (IAPB, 2022). Given that the population rates within the older demographic are increasing dramatically, along with the recognition that many eye disorders often are undiagnosed, it is essential for nurses to screen for visual impairment and provide education and appropriate resources to their patients.

Refractive Errors, Low Vision, and Blindness

In refractive errors, vision is impaired because a shortened or elongated eyeball prevents light rays from focusing sharply on the retina. Blurred vision from refractive error can be corrected with eyeglasses or contact lenses. The appropriate eyeglass or contact lens is determined by **refraction**. Ophthalmic refraction consists of placing various types of lenses in front of the patient's eyes to determine which lens best improves the patient's vision.

The depth of the eyeball is important in determining refractive error. Patients for whom the visual image focuses precisely on the macula and who do not need eyeglasses or contact lenses are said to have **emmetropia** (normal vision). People who have **myopia** are said to be nearsighted. They have deeper eyeballs; thus, the distant visual image focuses in front of, or short of, the retina. People who are myopic experience blurred distance vision. When people have a shorter depth to their eyes, the visual image focuses beyond the retina; the eyes are shallower and are called *hyperopic*. People with **hyperopia** are farsighted. These patients experience near vision blurriness, whereas their distance vision is excellent.

Another important cause of refractive error is **astigmatism**, an irregularity in the curve of the cornea. Because astigmatism causes a distortion of the visual image, acuity of both distance and near vision can be decreased. Hard or soft toric contact lenses may be used to correct astigmatic errors, in place of eyeglasses.

Ophthalmology has entered the era of customized vision correction, in its desire to achieve "super-normal vision." A new method of measuring refractive error is called *wavefront technology*. The most promising application for this technology is wavefront-guided refractive surgery.

Low vision is a general term describing visual impairment that requires patients to use devices and strategies in addition to corrective lenses to perform visual tasks. Low vision is defined as a best corrected visual acuity (BCVA) of 20/70 to 20/200.

Pearls for Practice: Computer Strain

Many individuals complain of eye strain with increased screen time associated with computer use. The use of blue-blocking glasses has been marketed as a tool to reduce eye strain. However, in a recent double-masked control study blue-blocking lenses did not alter signs or symptoms of eye strain. Thus, to date, there is a paucity of high-quality evidence to support its recommendation. The authors concluded potential factors associated with eye strain that include binocular vision anomalies, screen time over 4 hours, reduced blink rate, reflections and glare, and poor ergonomics are likely contributors to eye strain (Singh et al., 2021).

Blindness is defined as a BCVA that can range from 20/400 to no light perception (NLP). The clinical definition of absolute blindness is the absence of light perception. Legal blindness is a condition of impaired vision in which a person has a BCVA that does not exceed 20/200 in the better eye or whose widest visual field diameter is 20 degrees or less. This definition neither equates with functional ability nor classifies the degrees of visual impairment. Legal blindness ranges from an inability to perceive light to having some vision remaining. A person who meets the criteria for legal blindness may be eligible for government financial assistance, such as social security disability benefits. Nurses may make social service referral for follow-up.

Impaired vision is often accompanied by difficulty in performing functional activities. People with visual acuity of 20/80 to 20/100 and a visual field restriction of 60 degrees to greater than 20 degrees can read at a nearly normal level with optical aids. Their visual orientation is near normal but requires increased scanning of the environment (i.e., systematic use of head and eye movements). Patients with a visual acuity range of 20/200 to 20/400 and a visual field restriction of 20 degrees to greater than 10 degrees can read slowly with optical aids. In this setting, visual orientation is slow, necessitating constant scanning of the environment. People in this category may have the ability to negotiate their environment without auxiliary aids. This ability is termed "travel vision." People with hand motion vision or no vision may benefit from the use of mobility devices (e.g., cane, guide dog) and should be encouraged to learn Braille and to use computer aids.

The most common causes of blindness and visual impairment among adults 40 years of age or older are diabetic retinopathy (refer to Chapter 29), macular degeneration, glaucoma, and cataracts (discussed later in this chapter) (Baloh & Jen, 2022). Macular degeneration is more prevalent among European Americans, whereas glaucoma is more prevalent among African Americans. Age-related changes in the eye are discussed in Chapter 47.

Clinical Manifestations and Assessment

The assessment of low vision includes a thorough history and the examination of distance and near visual acuity, visual field, contrast sensitivity, glare, color perception, and refraction (see Chapter 47). Specially designed, low-vision visual acuity charts are used to evaluate patients.

During history taking, the underlying cause, course, and duration of the patient's visual impairment are identified. Patients with retinitis pigmentosa, for example, have a genetic abnormality. Patients with diabetic macular edema typically experience fluctuating visual acuity. Deterioration of the central portion of the retina causes macular degeneration and central acuity problems. Risk factors of age-related macular degeneration (AMD) include being 50+ years of age, smoking, and family history, and there is a higher incidence among Caucasians than African Americans or Hispanics/Latinos (National Eye Institute [NEI], 2019). Patients with macular degeneration may experience scotomas (partial or complete visual field cuts surrounded by intact visual fields). Central acuity problems cause difficulty in performing activities that require seeing fine details, such as reading. People with peripheral field defects have more difficulties with mobility. The patient's customary activities of daily living (ADLs), medication regimen, habits (e.g., smoking), acceptance of the physical limitations brought about by the visual impairment, and realistic expectations of low-vision aids must be identified and included in the plan of care, including provision of guidelines for safety and referrals to social services.

TABLE **48-1 Activities Affected by Visual Impairment with Suggestions for Low-Vision Aids**

Activity	Optical Aids	Nonoptical Aids
Shopping	Hand magnifier	Lighting, color cues
Fixing a snack	Spectacle magnifier	Color cues, consistent storage plan
Eating out	Hand magnifier	Flashlight, portable lamp
Identifying money	Spectacle, spectacle-mounted or hand magnifier	Arrange paper money in wallet compartments or fold banknotes of different denominations differently
Reading print	Spectacle, spectacle-mounted, dome, hand, or stand magnifier Closed-circuit television	Lighting, high-contrast print, large print, reading slit stand magnifier, electronic books
Writing	Hand magnifier	Lighting, bold-tip pen, black ink
Using a telephone	Telescope hand magnifier	Large print dial or touch tone buttons, hand-printed directory
Crossing streets	Telescope	Cane, ask directions
Finding taxis and bus signs	Telescope	Ask for assistance
Reading medication labels	Hand magnifier	Color codes, large print
Reading stove dials	Hand magnifier	Color codes, raised dots
Adjusting the thermostat	Hand magnifier	Enlarged print model
Using a computer	Spectacle or spectacle-mounted magnifier	High-contrast color, large-print program
Reading signs	Telescope Portable electronic magnifier	Move closer
Watching sporting event	Telescope	Sit in front rows

Adapted from Riordan-Eva, P., & Cunningham, E. (Eds.). (2018). *Vaughan & Asbury's general ophthalmology* (19th ed., table on page 997). McGraw-Hill Companies.

Contrast-sensitivity testing measures visual acuity in different degrees of contrast. The initial test may take the form of simply turning on the lights while testing the distance acuity. If the patient can read better with the lights on, the patient can benefit from magnification. Glare testing enables the examiner to obtain a more realistic evaluation of the patient's ability to function in their environment. Glare can reduce a person's ability to see, especially if they have cataracts. Devices that test glare are calibrated to imitate certain objects that create glare, such as a car's headlights at night.

Medical Management

Managing patients with low vision involves magnification and image enhancement through the use of low-vision aids and strategies, and referrals to social services and community agencies serving those with visual impairment. Since macular degeneration is irreversible, goals are to optimize the patient's remaining vision, whether central or peripheral, and assist the patient to perform customary activities. Low-vision aids include optical and nonoptical devices (Table 48-1). The optical devices include convex lens aids, such as magnifiers and spectacles; telescopic devices; antireflective lenses that diminish glare; and electronic reading systems, such as closed-circuit television and computers with large print. Continuing advances in computer software provide very useful products for patients with low vision. Scanners and the appropriate software enable the user to scan printed material and have it read by computer voice or to enlarge the print for reading. Magnifiers can be handheld or attached to a stand with or without illumination. Telescopic devices can be spectacle telescopes or clip-on or handheld loupes.

The internet continues to expand, and a telephone system has been developed that allows access to the internet and e-mail using voice commands (Box 48-1).

Referrals to community agencies may be necessary for patients with low vision who live alone and cannot self-administer their medications. Community agencies, such as the Lighthouse National Center for Vision and Aging, offer services to patients with low vision that include training in independent living skills, the provision of occupational and recreational activities, and a wide variety of assistive devices for vision enhancement and orientation and mobility.

BOX 48-1
Web Access for the Visually Impaired

People with impaired vision need not be left behind in the computer age. Various technologies are available. A list of general equipment needs follows:

- *Computer:* Software specifically developed for people with visual impairment
- *Internet service provider* (e.g., AOL, Netscape, EarthLink, Xfinity)
- *Screen-reader program:* Converts text on the computer screen to synthesized speech (e.g., JAWS for Windows, Windows Eyes, Slimware Window Bridge, ProTalk 32, Hal Screen Reader, WinVision, outSPOKEN for Windows)
- *Browser program to navigate the World Wide Web* (e.g., Microsoft Internet Explorer, IBM Home Page Reader)

Nursing Management

Coping with blindness involves three types of adaptation: emotional, physical, and social. The emotional adjustment to blindness or severe visual impairment determines the success of the physical and social adjustments of the patient. Successful emotional adjustment means acceptance of blindness or severe visual impairment.

Promoting Coping Efforts

Effective coping may not occur until the patient recognizes the permanence of the blindness. Clinging to false hopes of regaining vision hampers effective adaptation to blindness. A patient who is newly blind and their family members (especially those who live with the patient) undergo the various steps of grieving: denial, anger, loss bargaining, depression, and resolution and acceptance (Kübler-Ross, 1969). The ability to accept the changes that come with visual loss and willingness to adapt to those changes influence the successful rehabilitation of the patient who is blind. Additional aspects to consider are value changes, independence–dependence conflicts, coping with stigma, and learning to function in social settings without visual cues and landmarks.

Promoting Spatial Orientation and Mobility

A person who is blind or severely visually impaired requires strategies for adapting to the environment. ADLs, such as walking to a chair from a bed, require spatial concepts. A patient whose visual impairment results from a chronic progressive eye disorder, such as glaucoma, has better cognitive mapping skills than does the patient who becomes blind suddenly. Patients with progressive eye disorders develop the use of spatial and topographic concepts early and gradually; hence, remembering a room layout is easier for them. Patients who become blind suddenly have more difficulty in adjusting, and emotional and behavioral issues of coping with blindness may hinder their learning. These patients require intensive emotional and physical support.

In the hospital, the bedside table and the call button must always be within reach. The parts of the call button are explained, and the patient is taught to touch and press the buttons or dials until the activity is mastered. The patient must be familiarized with the location of the telephone, water pitcher, and other objects on the bedside table. The food tray's composition is likened to the face of a clock; for example, the main plate may be described as being at 12 o'clock or the coffee cup at 3 o'clock. All articles and furniture must remain in the same positions throughout the patient's hospitalization. Introduction of hospital personnel should be made upon entering and departure from the patient's room.

The nurse should be aware of the importance of techniques in providing physical assistance, encouraging independence, and ensuring safety. Specific guidelines for interacting with the patient with vision loss are presented in Box 48-2. The readiness of the patient and their family to learn must be assessed before initiating orientation and mobility training.

Promoting Home and Community-Based Care

The nurse, social worker, family, and others collaborate to assess the patient's home condition and support system. If available, a low-vision specialist or occupational therapist should be consulted, particularly for patients for whom identifying and administering medications pose problems. Contact information for some private and nonprofit services is included in the Internet Resources for this chapter available at http://thepoint.lww.com/Honan3e.

Other interventions that are appropriate for some people with low vision or blindness include Braille and guide dogs. Guide dogs are specially bred and trained to assist people who have visual impairment. The guide dog is a constant companion to the person who is blind (also referred to as the animal's handler) and is allowed on airplanes and in restaurants, stores, hotels, and other public places. A guide dog in a harness is a working dog and should not be approached without permission of the handler. With the assistance of

Unfolding Patient Stories: V.W. • Part 2

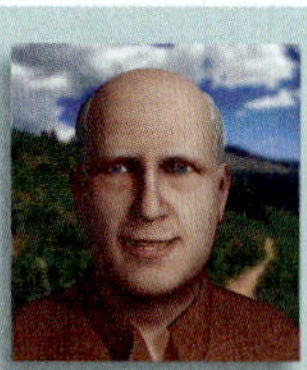

Recall from Chapter 4 V.W., who came to the emergency department with severe abdominal pain and underwent a hemicolectomy for a bowel perforation. During postoperative care the nurse determines that the patient has poor vision. What measures can the nurse take to maintain a safe environment for a patient with visual impairment? How will the discovery of impaired vision impact the nursing plan of care, discharge planning, and delivery of patient education?

Care for V.W. and other patients in a realistic virtual environment: ***vSim** for Nursing* (thepoint.lww.com/vSimMedicalSurgical). Practice documenting these patients' care in DocuCare (thepoint.lww.com/DocuCareEHR).

BOX 48-2
Guidelines for Interacting With People Who Are Blind or Have Low Vision

- Remember that the only difference between you and people who are blind or have low vision is that they are not able to see through their eyes what you are able to see through yours.
- Do not be uncomfortable when in the company of a person who is blind or has low vision. Talk with the person as you would talk with any other individual, honestly and without pity; do not be concerned about using words like "see" and "look." There is no need to raise your voice unless the person asks you to do so.
- Identify yourself as you approach the person and before you make physical contact. Tell the person your name and your role. If another person approaches, introduce them. When you leave the room, be sure to tell the person that you are leaving and if anyone else remains in the room.
- It is appropriate to touch the person's hand or arm lightly to indicate that you are about to speak.
- When talking, face the person and speak directly to them using a normal tone of voice.
- Be specific when communicating direction. Mention a specific distance or use clock cues when possible (e.g., walk left about 2 yards; walk about 20 ft to the right; the telephone is at 2 o'clock). Avoid using phrases such as "over there."
- When you offer to assist someone, allow the person to hold onto your arm just above the elbow and to walk a half-step behind you.
- When offering the person a seat, place the person's hand on the back or the arm of the seat.
- When you are about to go up or down a flight of stairs, tell the person, and place their hand on the banister.
- Make sure that the environment is free of obstacles; close doors and cabinets so they are not in the path.
- Offer to read written information, such as a menu.
- If you serve food to the person, use clock cues to specify where everything is on the plate.
- When the person who is blind or who has low vision is a patient in a health care facility:
  - Make sure all objects the person will need are close at hand.
  - Identify the location of objects that the person may need (e.g., "The call light is near your right hand"; "The telephone is on the table on the left side of your bed.")
  - Remove obstacles that may be in the person's pathway and could cause a fall.
  - Place all assistive devices the person uses close at hand; let the person feel the devices so that they know their location.
- Do not distract the service animal unless the owner has given permission.
- Ask the person, "How can I help you?" At some times, the person needs help, but at other times help may not be needed.

This material is adapted from and based in part on *Achieving Physical and Communication Accessibility,* a publication of the National Center for Access Unlimited; *Community Access Facts,* an Adaptive Environments Center publication; and *The Ten Commandments of Interacting with People with Mental Health Disabilities,* a publication of The Ability Center of Greater Toledo.

the guide dog, the person who is visually impaired can be extremely mobile and accomplish normal activities both within and outside of the home and workplace. There are numerous guide dog organizations, including Fidelco Guide Dog Foundation and Guide Dogs for the Blind, through which potential puppy raisers or handlers can access excellent information and support.

GLAUCOMA

Glaucoma is a group of ocular conditions characterized by optic nerve damage. The optic nerve damage is related to the intraocular pressure (IOP) caused by congestion of aqueous humor in the eye. Ranges of pressures have been considered "normal," but they may be associated with visual loss in some patients. While the average IOP is generally at or below 21 mm Hg, exceptions to this normal value exist. Genetic disposition and central corneal thickness have been implicated in causing ocular hypertension (OHT), a major precursor to glaucoma (Yanoff & Cameron, 2020). Glaucoma is one of the leading causes of irreversible blindness in the world and is the leading cause of blindness among adults in the United States. There is no cure for glaucoma; research is aimed at identifying risk factors and preventing vision loss and blindness.

Pathophysiology

Aqueous humor flows between the iris and the lens, nourishing the cornea and lens. Most (90%) of the fluid then flows out of the anterior chamber, draining through the spongy trabecular meshwork into the canal of Schlemm and the episcleral veins (Fig. 48-1). About 10% of the aqueous fluid exits through the ciliary body into the suprachoroidal space and then drains into the venous circulation of the ciliary body, choroid, and sclera. Unimpeded outflow of aqueous fluid depends on an intact drainage system and an open angle (about 45 degrees) between the iris and the cornea. A narrower angle places the iris closer to the trabecular meshwork, diminishing the angle. The amount of aqueous humor produced tends to decrease with age, in systemic diseases such as diabetes, and in ocular inflammatory conditions.

IOP is determined by the rate of aqueous fluid production, the resistance encountered by the aqueous humor as it flows out of the passages, and the venous pressure of the episcleral veins that drain into the anterior ciliary vein. When aqueous fluid production and drainage are in balance, the IOP is between 10 and 21 mm Hg. When aqueous fluid is inhibited from flowing out, pressure builds up within the eye. Fluctuations in IOP occur with time of day, exertion, diet, and medications. IOP tends to increase with blinking, tight lid

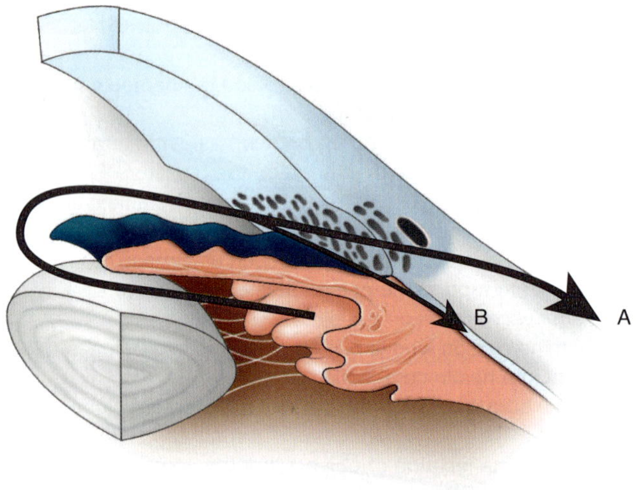

FIGURE 48-1 **Normal outflow of aqueous humor. A. Trabecular meshwork. B. Uveoscleral route. (From Kanski, J. J. [2011].** ***Clinical ophthalmology*****. Butterworth-Heinemann Ltd.)**

squeezing, and upward gazing. Systemic conditions, such as hypertension, and intraocular conditions, such as uveitis and retinal detachment, have been associated with elevated IOP.

There are two accepted theories regarding how increased IOP damages the optic nerve in glaucoma. The direct mechanical theory suggests that high IOP damages the retinal layer as it passes through the optic nerve head. The indirect ischemic theory suggests that high IOP compresses the microcirculation in the optic nerve head, resulting in cell injury and death. Some glaucomas appear as exclusively mechanical, and some are exclusively ischemic types. Typically, most cases are a combination of both. Regardless of the cause of damage, glaucomatous changes typically evolve through clearly discernible stages (Box 48-3).

Classification of Glaucoma

There are several types of glaucoma. Although glaucoma classification is changing as knowledge increases, current clinical forms of glaucoma are identified as open-angle glaucoma, angle-closure glaucoma (also called pupillary block), congenital glaucoma, and glaucoma associated with other conditions, such as developmental anomalies or corticosteroid use. Glaucoma can be primary or secondary, depending on whether associated factors contribute to the rise in IOP. The two common clinical forms of glaucoma encountered in adults are open-angle and angle-closure glaucoma. These are differentiated by mechanisms that cause impaired aqueous outflow. Table 48-2 summarizes the characteristics of the different types of open-angle and angle-closure glaucoma.

Risk Factors

It is estimated that more than three million Americans have glaucoma (Bright Focus Foundation, 2021). Glaucoma is more prevalent among people older than 40 years of age, and the incidence increases with age. It is also more prevalent among males than females and in African American and Asian populations. Inflammatory processes, such as uveitis, known as uveitic glaucoma (UG) are characterized by increased IOP above 21 mm Hg and can lead to optic nerve damage and visual changes (Kesav et al., 2020).

There are multiple mechanisms of IOP, which pose significant challenge when treating UG. Glaucoma associated with uveitis results in cellular debris and protein leakage out of the blood vessels into clear, aqueous fluid, blocking drainage. Initially the angle between the iris and cornea may be open. As IOP rises, the iris can bow forward, sticking to the lens, cornea, or sclera, which closes the angle of the anterior chamber. Collaborative management often requires an ophthalmologist specializing in glaucoma in addition to a rheumatologist (Box 48-4).

BOX 48-3

Progression of Glaucoma

1. **Initiating events**
   Precipitating factors include illness, emotional stress, congenital narrow angles, long-term use of corticosteroids, and use of mydriatics (i.e., medications causing pupillary dilation).
   ↓
2. **Structural alterations in the aqueous outflow system**
   Tissue and cellular changes caused by factors that affect aqueous humor dynamics lead to structural alterations.
   ↓
3. **Functional alterations**
   Conditions such as increased IOP or impaired blood flow create functional changes.
   ↓
4. **Optic nerve damage**
   Atrophy of the optic nerve is characterized by loss of nerve fibers and blood supply. This fourth stage inevitably progresses to the fifth stage.
   ↓
5. **Visual loss**
   Progressive loss of vision is characterized by visual field defects.

Clinical Manifestations and Assessment

Glaucoma is often called the "silent thief of sight" because most patients are unaware that they have the disease until they have experienced visual changes and vision loss. The patient may not seek health care until they experience blurred vision or "halos" around lights, difficulty focusing, difficulty adjusting eyes in low lighting, loss of peripheral vision, aching or discomfort around the eyes, and headache.

The purpose of a glaucoma workup is to establish the diagnostic category, assess the optic nerve damage, and formulate a treatment plan. The patient's ocular and medical history must be detailed to investigate the history of predisposing factors. Diagnostic examination to detect and manage glaucoma includes the following tests: tonometry to measure the IOP; ophthalmoscopy to inspect the optic nerve;

TABLE **48-2 Glaucoma Types, Clinical Manifestations, and Treatment**

Types of Glaucoma	Clinical Manifestations	Treatment
Open-Angle Glaucoma		
Usually bilateral, but one eye may be affected more severely than the other. In all three types of open-angle glaucoma, the anterior chamber angle is open and appears normal.		
Chronic open-angle glaucoma (COAG)	Optic nerve damage, visual field defects, IOP >21 mm Hg	Decrease IOP 20–50%. Additional topical and oral agents added as necessary.
	May have fluctuating IOPs. Usually no symptoms but possible ocular pain, headache, and halos	If medical treatment is unsuccessful, laser trabeculoplasty (LT) can decrease IOP by 20%. Glaucoma filtering surgery if continued optic nerve damage despite medication therapy and LT.
Normal tension glaucoma	IOP ≤21 mm Hg; optic nerve damage, visual field defects	Treatment similar to COAG; however, the best management for normal tension glaucoma is yet to be established. Goal is to lower the IOP by at least 30%.
Ocular hypertension	Elevated IOP Possible ocular pain or headache	Decrease IOP by at least 20%
Angle-Closure (Pupillary Block) Glaucoma		
Obstruction in aqueous humor outflow due to the complete or partial closure of the angle from the forward shift of the peripheral iris to the trabecula. The obstruction results in an increased IOP.		
Acute angle-closure glaucoma (AACG)	Rapidly progressive visual impairment, periocular pain, conjunctival hyperemia, and congestion Pain may be associated with nausea, vomiting, bradycardia, and profuse sweating. Reduced central visual acuity, severely elevated IOP, corneal edema Pupil is vertically oval, fixed in a semi-dilated position, and unreactive to light and accommodation	Ocular emergency, requiring administration of hyperosmotics, acetazolamide, and topical ocular hypotensive agents, such as pilocarpine and beta blockers. Possible laser incision in the iris (iridotomy) to release blocked aqueous fluid and reduce IOP Other eye is also treated with pilocarpine eye drops and/or surgical management to avoid a similar spontaneous attack.
Subacute angle-closure glaucoma	Transient blurring of vision, halos around lights; temporal headaches and/or ocular pain; pupil may be semi-dilated	Prophylactic peripheral laser iridotomy Can lead to acute or chronic angle-closure glaucoma if untreated
Chronic angle-closure glaucoma	Progression of glaucomatous cupping and significant visual field loss; IOP may be normal or elevated; ocular pain and headache	Management is similar to that for COAG: includes laser iridotomy and medications.
Other Types of Glaucoma		
Uveitic glaucoma	IOP ≥21 mm Hg; optic nerve damage, visual field defects	Decrease IOP; medical treatment or surgery may be necessary

BOX 48-4

Risk Factors for Glaucoma

- Family history of glaucoma
- Race (African, Caribbean, Hispanic) (Saeedi et al., 2019)
- Older age (over 60 years of age)
- Diabetes mellitus
- Cardiovascular disease
- Migraine syndromes
- Nearsightedness (myopia)
- Eye trauma
- Prolonged use of topical or systemic corticosteroids

gonioscopy to examine the filtration angle of the anterior chamber; perimetry to assess the visual fields; and pachymetry to measure the thickness of the cornea, which influences IOP readings.

The changes in the optic nerve related to glaucoma are pallor and cupping of the optic nerve disc. The pallor of the optic nerve is caused by a lack of blood supply that results from cellular destruction. Cupping is characterized by exaggerated bending of the blood vessels as they cross the optic disc, resulting in an enlarged optic cup that appears more basin-like compared with a normal cup. The progression of

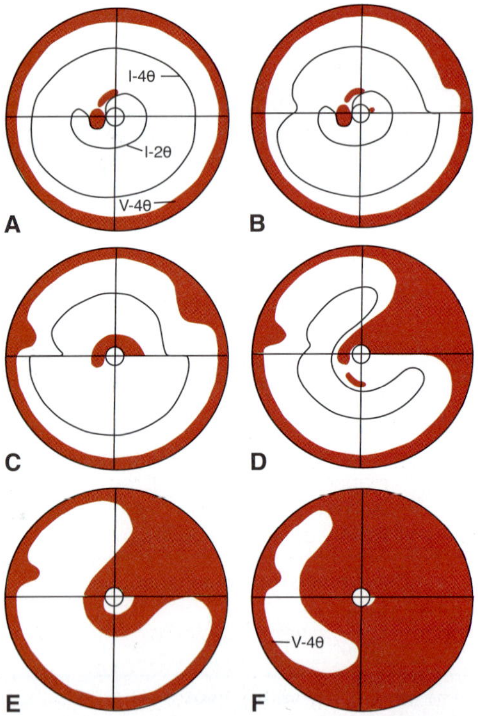

FIGURE 48-2 **Progression of glaucomatous visual field defects. A central scotoma at 10 to 20 degrees of fixation near the blind spot is the initial significant finding (A, B). As the glaucoma progresses, the scotomas enlarge and deepen, resulting in peripheral vision loss. C. Defect within 5 degrees of fixation point nasally. D. Peripheral involvement enlarges. E. Ringlike scotoma. F. Eventually, vision is lost. The resulting "island of vision" becomes the characteristic visual field appearance of glaucoma and correlates with the "tunnel vision," in which peripheral vision is lost. (From Kanski, J. J. [2011].** ***Clinical ophthalmology*****. Butterworth-Heinemann Ltd.)**

cupping in glaucoma is caused by the gradual loss of retinal nerve fibers accompanied by the loss of blood supply, resulting in increased pallor of the optic disc.

As the damage to the optic nerve increases, visual perception in the area is lost. The localized areas of visual loss (i.e., **scotomas**) represent loss of retinal sensitivity and are measured and mapped by perimetry. In patients with glaucoma, there is a distinct pattern that differs from other ocular diseases and is useful in establishing its diagnosis. Figure 48-2 shows the progression of visual field defects caused by glaucoma.

Medical Management

The aim of all glaucoma treatment is prevention of damage to the optic nerve. Lifelong therapy is almost always necessary because glaucoma cannot be cured. Treatment focuses on pharmacologic therapy, laser procedures, surgery, or a combination of these approaches, all of which have potential complications and side effects. The object is to achieve the greatest benefit at the least risk, cost, and inconvenience to the patient. Although treatment cannot reverse damage to the optic nerve, further damage can be controlled. The goal is to maintain an IOP within a range unlikely to cause further damage.

The initial target for IOP among patients with elevated IOP and those with low-tension glaucoma with progressive visual field loss is typically set at 30% lower than the current pressure. The patient is monitored for changes in the appearance of the optic nerve. If there is evidence of progressive damage, the target IOP is lowered again until the optic nerve shows stability.

Medical management of glaucoma relies on systemic and topical ocular medications that lower IOP. Periodic follow-up examinations are essential to monitor IOP, the appearance of the optic nerve, the visual fields, and side effects of medications. Therapy takes into account the patient's health and stage of glaucoma. Comfort, affordability, convenience, lifestyle, and personality are factors to consider in the patient's adherence to the medical regimen.

The patient is usually started on the lowest dose of topical medication and then advanced to increased concentrations until the desired IOP level is reached and maintained. Because of their efficacy, minimal dosing (can be used once each day), and low cost, beta blockers are the preferred initial topical medications. Beta blockers decrease the production of aqueous humor with resultant decrease in IOP. One eye is treated first, with the other eye used as a control in determining the efficacy of the medication; once efficacy has been established, treatment of the other eye is started. If the IOP is elevated in both eyes, both are treated. When results are not satisfactory, a new medication is substituted. The main markers of the efficacy of the medication in glaucoma control are lowering of the IOP to the target pressure, appearance of the optic nerve head, and less deterioration of the visual field.

Surgical management for glaucoma includes several procedures. In laser trabeculoplasty, burns are applied to the inner surface of the trabecular meshwork to open the intratrabecular spaces and widen the canal of Schlemm, thereby promoting outflow of aqueous humor and decreasing IOP. Laser iridotomy, used for pupillary block glaucoma, is an opening made in the iris to eliminate the pupillary block. Laser iridotomy is contraindicated in patients with corneal edema, which interferes with laser targeting and strength.

Filtering procedures for chronic glaucoma are used to create an opening or fistula in the trabecular meshwork to drain aqueous humor from the anterior chamber to the subconjunctival space into a bleb (blister-like fluid collection), thereby bypassing the usual drainage structures. This allows the aqueous humor to flow and exit by different routes (i.e., absorption by the conjunctival vessels or mixing with tears). Trabeculectomy is the standard filtering technique used to remove part of the trabecular meshwork. Complications include hemorrhage, an extremely low (hypotony) or elevated IOP, uveitis, cataracts, bleb failure, bleb leak, and endophthalmitis (refers to bacterial or fungal infection involving the vitreous and/or aqueous humors). Unlike other surgical procedures, the filtering procedure's goal in glaucoma treatment is to achieve incomplete healing of the surgical wound.

Nursing Management

Teaching Patients Self-Care

The medical and surgical management of patients with glaucoma slows the progression of glaucoma but does not cure it. The lifelong therapeutic regimen mandates patient education. The nature of the disease and the importance of strict adherence to the medication regimen must be included in a teaching plan to help ensure compliance. A thorough patient interview is essential to determine systemic conditions, current systemic and ocular medications, family history, and problems with adherence to glaucoma medications. The effects of glaucoma-control medications on vision must also be explained.

Nurses in all settings encounter patients with glaucoma. Even patients with longstanding disease and those with glaucoma as a secondary diagnosis should be assessed for knowledge level and adherence to the therapeutic regimen. Box 48-5 contains points to review with patients with glaucoma.

Pearls for Practice: Miotics, Sympathomimetics, and Beta Blockers

The nurse is aware that miotics decrease the size of the pupil and increase aqueous outflow, which lowers the IOP. Although sympathomimetics reduce the rate of production of aqueous fluid and facilitate its outflow, decreasing IOP, these agents may be contraindicated in some types of glaucoma because they dilate the pupil (Richards & Edwards, 2020). Both medications can result in altered focus; therefore, patients need to be cautious in navigating their surroundings. The mechanism of action of beta blockers includes a blockade of sympathetic nerve endings in the ciliary epithelium, causing a fall in aqueous humor production. Beta blockers may be absorbed systemically and should not be used in patients with asthma, bradycardia, or heart block.

BOX 48-5 **Patient Education**

Managing Glaucoma

- Know your IOP measurement and the desired range.
- Be informed about the extent of your vision loss and optic nerve damage.
- Keep a record of your eye pressure measurements and visual field test results to monitor your own progress.
- Review all your medications (including over-the-counter and herbal medications) with your ophthalmologist, and mention any side effects each time you visit.
- Ask about potential side effects and drug interactions of your eye medications.
- Ask whether generic or less costly forms of your eye medications are available.
- Review the dosing schedule with your ophthalmologist and inform them if you have trouble following the schedule.
- Participate in the decision-making process. Let your provider know what dosing schedule works for you and other preferences regarding your eye care.
- Have the nurse observe you instilling eye medication to determine whether you are administering it properly.
- Be aware that glaucoma medications can cause adverse effects if used inappropriately. Eye drops are to be administered as prescribed, not when eyes feel irritated.
- Ask your ophthalmologist to send a report to your provider after each appointment.
- Keep all follow-up appointments.

Continuing Care

For the patient with severe glaucoma and impaired function, referral to services that assist the patient in performing ADLs may be needed. The loss of peripheral vision can impact mobility, and patients may benefit from low vision and rehabilitation services. Patients who meet the criteria for legal blindness should be offered referrals to agencies that can assist them in obtaining federal assistance.

Reassurance and emotional support are important aspects of care. A lifelong disease involving possible loss of sight has psychological, physical, social, and vocational ramifications. The family must be integrated into the plan of care, and because the disease has a familial tendency, family members should be encouraged to undergo examinations at least once every 2 years to detect glaucoma early.

CATARACTS

A cataract is a lens opacity or cloudiness (Fig. 48-3). Cataracts rank behind only arthritis and heart disease as a leading cause of disability in older adults. In fact, cataracts are the most common cause of treatable blindness. It is estimated that more than 20.5 million Americans have some degree of visual impairment because of cataracts, and that number is

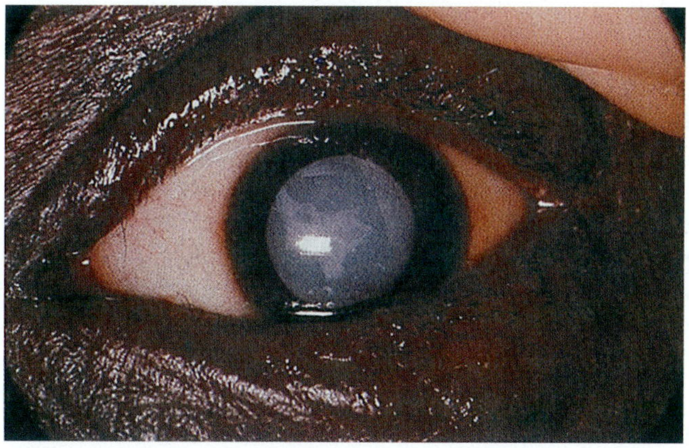

FIGURE 48-3 **A cataract is a cloudy or opaque lens. On visual inspection, the lens appears gray or milky. (From Rubin, E., & Strayer, D. S. [Eds.]. [2014].** ***Rubin's pathology*** **[7th ed.]. Lippincott Williams & Wilkins.)**

BOX 48-6

Risk Factors for Cataract Formation

Aging:

- Loss of lens transparency
- Clumping or aggregation of lens protein (which leads to light scattering)
- Accumulation of a yellow-brown pigment due to the breakdown of lens protein
- Decreased oxygen uptake
- Increase in sodium and calcium
- Decrease in levels of vitamin C, protein, and glutathione (an antioxidant)

Associated ocular conditions:

- Retinitis pigmentosa
- Myopia
- Retinal detachment and retinal surgery
- Infection (e.g., herpes zoster, uveitis)

Toxic factors:

- Corticosteroids, especially at high doses and in long-term use
- Alkaline chemical eye burns, poisoning
- Cigarette smoking
- Calcium, copper, iron, gold, silver, and mercury, which tend to deposit in the pupillary area of the lens

Nutritional factors:

- Reduced levels of antioxidants
- Poor nutrition
- Obesity

Physical factors:

- Dehydration associated with chronic diarrhea, use of purgatives in anorexia nervosa, and use of hyperbaric oxygenation
- Blunt trauma, perforation of the lens with a sharp object or foreign body, electric shock
- Ultraviolet radiation in sunlight and x-ray

Systemic diseases and syndromes:

- Diabetes mellitus
- Down syndrome
- Disorders related to lipid metabolism
- Kidney disorders
- Musculoskeletal disorders

expected to continue to rise (Ansari & Banta, 2021). There is some stage of cataract development present in >50% of persons 65 to 74 years of age and in 65% of those >75 years old (Hoffman, 2022). Cataract surgery is the most common surgical procedure performed in the United States.

Pathophysiology

Cataracts can develop in one or both eyes at any age for a variety of causes (Box 48-6). Visual impairment normally progresses at the same rate in both eyes over many years or in a matter of months. The three most common types of age-related cataracts are defined by their location in the lens: nuclear, cortical, and posterior subcapsular. The extent of visual impairment depends on their size, density, and location in the lens. More than one type can be present in one eye.

A nuclear cataract is caused by central opacity in the lens and has a substantial genetic component. It is associated with myopia (i.e., nearsightedness), which worsens when the cataract progresses. If dense, the cataract severely blurs vision. Periodic changes in prescription eyeglasses help manage this condition.

A cortical cataract involves the anterior, posterior, or equatorial cortex of the lens. A cataract in the equator or periphery of the cortex does not interfere with the passage of light through the center of the lens and has little effect on vision. Cortical cataracts progress at a highly variable rate. Vision is worse in very bright light.

Posterior subcapsular cataracts occur in front of the posterior capsule. This type typically develops in younger people and, in some cases, is associated with prolonged corticosteroid use, diabetes, or ocular trauma. Near vision is diminished, and the eye is increasingly sensitive to glare from bright light (e.g., sunlight, headlights).

Clinical Manifestations and Assessment

Painless, blurry vision is characteristic of cataracts (see Fig. 48-4). The person perceives that surroundings are dimmer, as if their glasses need cleaning. Light scattering is common, and the person experiences reduced contrast sensitivity, sensitivity to glare, and reduced visual acuity. Other effects include myopic shift, astigmatism, monocular **diplopia** (double vision), color shift (the aging lens becomes progressively more absorbent at the blue end of the spectrum), brunescens (color values shift to yellow-brown), and reduced light transmission.

Decreased visual acuity is directly proportionate to cataract density. The Snellen visual acuity test, ophthalmoscopy, and slit-lamp biomicroscopic examination are used to establish the degree of cataract formation. The degree of lens opacity does not always correlate with the patient's

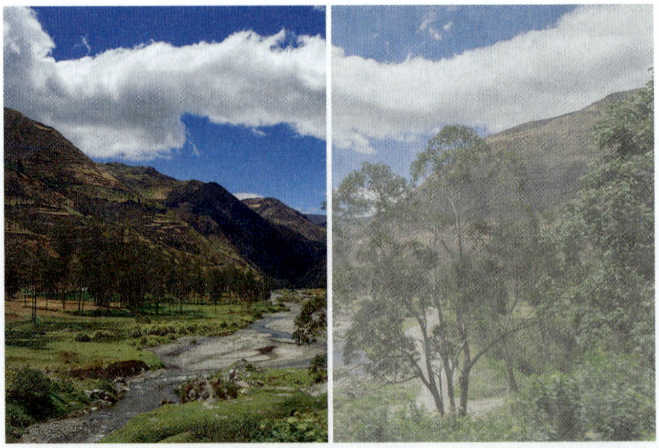

FIGURE 48-4 **Normal view against view of patient suffering from cataract. (Source: Shutterstock.)**

functional status. Some patients can perform normal activities despite clinically significant cataracts. Others with less lens opacification have a disproportionate decrease in visual acuity; hence, visual acuity is one measure of visual impairment and needs to be considered along with other visual screening techniques and assessments.

Medical Management

Nonsurgical Management

Nonsurgical (medications, eyedrops, eyeglasses) treatment has not been found as curative for people with cataracts, nor does it prevent age-related cataracts. Cigarette smoking; long-term use of corticosteroids, especially at high doses; sunlight and ionizing radiation; diabetes; obesity; and eye injuries can increase the risk for cataracts. In the early stages of cataract development, glasses, contact lenses, strong bifocals, or magnifying lenses may improve vision.

Surgical Management

Surgical management of cataracts is considered when reduced vision interferes with normal activities. In deciding when cataract surgery is to be performed, the patient's functional and visual status should be a primary consideration. Surgery is performed on an outpatient basis and usually takes less than 1 hour. Although complications from cataract surgery are uncommon, they can have significant effects on vision. Restoration of visual function through a safe and minimally invasive procedure is the surgical goal.

When both eyes have cataracts, one eye is treated first, with at least several weeks, preferably months, separating the two procedures. Because cataract surgery is performed to improve visual functioning, the delay for the other eye gives time for the patient and the surgeon to evaluate whether the results from the first surgery are adequate to preclude the need for a second operation.

Intracapsular Cataract Extraction

In intracapsular cataract extraction, the entire lens (i.e., nucleus, cortex, and capsule) is removed and fine sutures are used to close the incision. From the late 1800s until the 1970s, it was the technique of choice for cataract extraction. It is infrequently performed today but is still indicated when there is a need to remove the entire lens, such as with a subluxated cataract (i.e., partially or completely dislocated lens).

Extracapsular Cataract Extraction

The extracapsular cataract extraction technique involves smaller incisional wounds (less trauma to the eye) and maintains the posterior capsule of the lens, thus reducing postoperative complications, particularly aphakic (absence of the lens) retinal detachment and cystoid macular edema. A portion of the anterior capsule is removed, allowing extraction of the lens nucleus and cortex. The posterior capsule and zonular support are left intact. An intact zonular–capsular diaphragm provides the needed safe anchor for the posterior chamber intraocular lens (IOL). After the pupil has been dilated and the surgeon has made a small incision on the upper edge of the cornea, a viscoelastic substance (clear gel) is injected into the space between the cornea and the lens. This prevents the space from collapsing and facilitates insertion of the IOL.

Phacoemulsification

This method of extracapsular surgery uses an ultrasonic device that liquefies the nucleus and cortex, which are then suctioned out through a tube. The posterior capsule is left intact. Because the incision is even smaller than the standard extracapsular cataract extraction, the wound heals more rapidly, and there is early stabilization of refractive error and less astigmatism. Hardware and software advances in ultrasonic technology—including modern phaco needles that are used to cut and aspirate the cataract—permit safe and efficient removal of nearly all cataracts through a clear cornea incision. With increasing frequency, self-sealing (sutureless) clear corneal incisions (temporal part of the cornea) are performed with phacoemulsification, minimizing postoperative astigmatism and thus decreasing bleeding and subconjunctival hemorrhage and speeding recovery of visual acuity.

Lens Replacement

After removal of the crystalline lens, the patient is considered to have aphakia (i.e., to not have a lens). The lens, which focuses light on the retina, must be replaced for the patient to see clearly. There are three lens replacement options: aphakic eyeglasses, contact lenses, and IOL implants.

Aphakic glasses, although effective, are rarely used. Objects are magnified by 25%, making them appear closer than they actually are. This magnification creates distortion. Peripheral vision is also limited, and binocular vision (i.e., ability of both eyes to focus on one object and fuse the two images into one) is impossible if the other eye is phakic (normal).

Contact lenses provide patients with almost normal vision, but because contact lenses need to be removed occasionally, the patient also needs a pair of aphakic glasses. Contact lenses are not advised for patients who have difficulty inserting, removing, and cleaning them. Frequent handling and improper disinfection increase the risk for infection.

Insertion of a prosthetic IOL during cataract surgery is the usual approach to lens replacement. After cataract extraction, or phacoemulsification, the surgeon implants an IOL. Extracapsular cataract extraction and posterior chamber IOL are associated with a relatively low incidence of complications (e.g., **hyphema** [bleeding into the anterior chamber of the eye], macular edema, secondary glaucoma, damage to the corneal endothelium). IOL implantation is contraindicated in patients with recurrent uveitis, proliferative diabetic retinopathy, neovascular glaucoma, or rubeosis iridis (condition of new abnormal blood vessels on the surface of the iris).

The most common IOL is the single-focus lens. Eyeglasses are still needed for distant or close vision because the single-focus lens, unlike the natural lens of the eye, cannot alter its shape to bring objects at different distances into focus. Multifocal IOL reduces the need for eyeglasses since the implanted lens accommodate to intermediate and far vision; however, patients can experience reduced nighttime vision, halos, and glare. In the future, older patients may benefit from a combined surgical approach using customized IOL and refractive surgery for customized vision correction.

Toxic Anterior Segment Syndrome

Also known as toxic endothelial cell destruction or sterile endophthalmitis, toxic anterior segment syndrome (TASS) is a noninfectious inflammation caused by a toxic agent that acutely presents 12 to 48 hours following surgery. This disorder is a complication of anterior chamber surgery and is characterized by widespread inflammation including corneal edema, flare, disseminated breakdown of the blood–aqueous barrier, and fibrin formation (Shouchane-Blum et al., 2021).

TASS is characterized by corneal edema less than 24 hours after surgery and an accumulation of white cells in the anterior chamber of the eye. Like the classic endophthalmitis, the symptoms include pain and reduction in visual acuity. In the absence of microorganism growth, improvement has occurred with topical steroid treatment alone.

Nursing Management

The patient with cataracts should receive the usual preoperative care for ambulatory surgical patients undergoing eye surgery.

Providing Preoperative Care

It has been common practice to withhold any anticoagulant therapy (e.g., aspirin, warfarin) to reduce the risk for retrobulbar hemorrhage (after retrobulbar injection) for 5 to 7 days before surgery. Dilating drops are administered every 10 minutes for four doses at least 1 hour before surgery. Additional dilating drops may be administered in the operating room (immediately before surgery) if the affected eye is not fully dilated. Antibiotic, corticosteroid, and anti-inflammatory drops may be administered prophylactically to prevent postoperative infection and inflammation.

Providing Postoperative Care

After recovery from anesthesia, the patient receives verbal and written instructions about how to protect the eye, administer medications, recognize signs of complications, and obtain emergency care. Box 48-7 identifies activities to be avoided. The nurse also explains that there should be minimal discomfort after surgery and instructs the patient to take a mild analgesic agent, such as acetaminophen, as needed. Antibiotic, anti-inflammatory, and corticosteroid eye drops or ointments are prescribed postoperatively.

BOX 48-7 Patient Education

Intraocular Lens Implant

- Wear glasses or metal eye shield at all times following surgery, as instructed by the provider.
- Always wash hands before touching or cleaning the postoperative eye.
- Clean the postoperative eye with a clean tissue; wipe the closed eye with a single gesture from the inner canthus outward.
- Bathe or shower; shampoo hair cautiously or seek assistance.
- Avoid lying on the side of the affected eye the night after surgery.
- Keep activity light (e.g., walking, reading, watching television). Resume the following activities only as directed by the surgeon: driving, sexual activity, unusually strenuous activity.
- Remember not to lift, push, or pull objects heavier than 15 lb.
- Avoid bending or stooping for an extended period.
- Be careful when climbing or descending stairs.
- Know when to contact the surgeon.[a]

[a]Contact the surgeon immediately if any of the following problems occur before the next appointment: (1) vision changes; (2) continuous flashing lights appear to the affected eye; (3) redness, swelling, or pain increase in the eye; (4) the amount or type of eye drainage changes; (5) the eye is injured in any way; (6) significant pain is not relieved by acetaminophen.

Teaching Patients Self-Care

To prevent accidental rubbing or poking of the eye, the patient wears a protective eye patch for 24 hours after surgery, followed by eyeglasses worn during the day and a metal shield worn at night for 1 to 4 weeks. The nurse instructs the patient and family in applying and caring for the eye shield. Sunglasses should be worn while outdoors during the day because the eye is sensitive to light.

Slight morning discharge, some redness, and a scratchy feeling may be expected for a few days. A clean, damp washcloth may be used to remove slight morning eye discharge, moving from inner to outer canthus. Because cataract surgery increases the risk for retinal detachment, the patient must know to notify the surgeon if new floaters (dots) in vision, flashing lights, a decrease in vision, pain, or an increase in redness occurs.

Continuing Care

The eye patch is removed after the first follow-up appointment. The patient may experience blurring of vision for several days to weeks. Sutures, if used, are left in the eye but alter the curvature of the cornea, resulting in temporary blurring and some astigmatism. Vision gradually improves as the eye heals. Patients with IOL implants have functional vision on the first day after surgery. Vision is stabilized when the eye is completely healed, usually within 6 to 12 weeks, when final corrective prescription is completed. Visual correction is needed for any remaining nearsightedness or farsightedness (even in patients with IOL implants).

RETINAL DISORDERS

Although the retina is composed of multiple microscopic layers, the two innermost layers, the sensory retina and the retinal pigment epithelium (RPE), are the most susceptible to common retinal disorders. As the film in a camera captures an image, the retina, the neural tissue of the eye, performs the same function. The rods and cones, the photoreceptor cells, are found in the sensory layer of the retina. Beneath the sensory layer lies the RPE, the pigmented layer. When the rods and cones are stimulated by light, an electrical impulse is generated, and the image is transmitted to the brain.

RETINAL DETACHMENT

Retinal detachment refers to the separation of the RPE from the sensory layer. The four types of retinal detachment are rhegmatogenous, traction, a combination of rhegmatogenous and traction, and exudative. Rhegmatogenous detachment is the most common form. In this condition, a hole or tear develops in the sensory retina, allowing some of the liquid vitreous to seep through the sensory retina and detach it from the RPE (Fig. 48-5). People at risk for this type of detachment include those with high myopia (near sighted) or aphakia (absence of lens) after cataract surgery. Trauma may also play a role in rhegmatogenous retinal detachment. Between 5% and 10% of all rhegmatogenous retinal detachments are associated with proliferative retinopathy, a retinopathy associated with diabetic neovascularization (see Chapter 29).

Tension, or a pulling force, is responsible for traction retinal detachment. An ophthalmologist must ascertain all of the areas of retinal break and identify and release the scars or bands of fibrous material providing traction on the retina. In general, patients with this condition have developed fibrous scar tissue from conditions such as diabetic retinopathy, vitreous hemorrhage, or the retinopathy of prematurity. The hemorrhages and fibrous proliferation associated with these conditions exert a pulling force on the delicate retina.

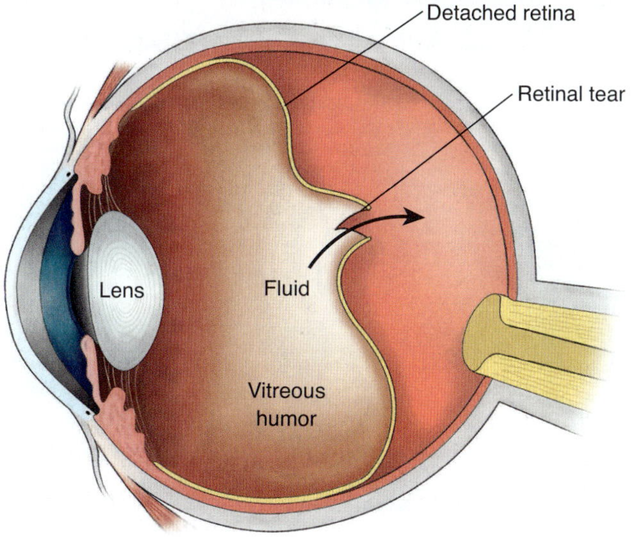

FIGURE 48-5 **Rhegmatogenous detachment, the most common form of retinal detachment.**

Patients can have both rhegmatogenous and traction retinal detachment. Exudative retinal detachments are the result of the production of a serous fluid under the retina from the choroid. Conditions such as uveitis and macular degeneration may cause the production of this serous fluid.

Clinical Manifestations and Assessment

Patients may report the sensation of a shade or curtain coming across the vision of one eye, cobwebs, bright flashing lights, or the sudden onset of a great number of floaters. Patients do not complain of pain.

After visual acuity is determined, the patient must have a dilated **fundus** examination using an indirect ophthalmoscope as well as slit-lamp biomicroscopy. Stereo fundus photography and fluorescein angiography are commonly used during the evaluation.

Increasingly, optical coherence tomography and ultrasound are used for the complete retinal assessment, especially if the view is obscured by a dense cataract or vitreal hemorrhage. All retinal breaks, all fibrous bands that may be causing traction on the retina, and all degenerative changes must be identified.

Medical Management

In rhegmatogenous detachment, an attempt is made to surgically reattach the sensory retina to the RPE. In traction detachment, the source of traction must be removed and the sensory retina reattached. New surgical techniques and advances in instrumentation have led to an increased rate of success of surgical reattachment and better visual outcomes. The most commonly used surgical interventions are the scleral buckle, the pars plana vitrectomy, and pneumatic retinopexy. The scleral buckle is a procedure in which a piece of silicone plastic or sponge is sewn onto the sclera at the site of the retinal tear. The buckle holds the retina against the sclera until scarring seals the tear (Fig. 48-6).

Nursing Management

For the most part, nursing interventions consist of educating the patient and providing supportive care.

Promoting Comfort

Following surgery, patients will require assistance with meals and walking. While some procedures require a hospital stay, many scleral buckling procedures are performed on an outpatient basis. The nurse should advise patients to avoid heavy

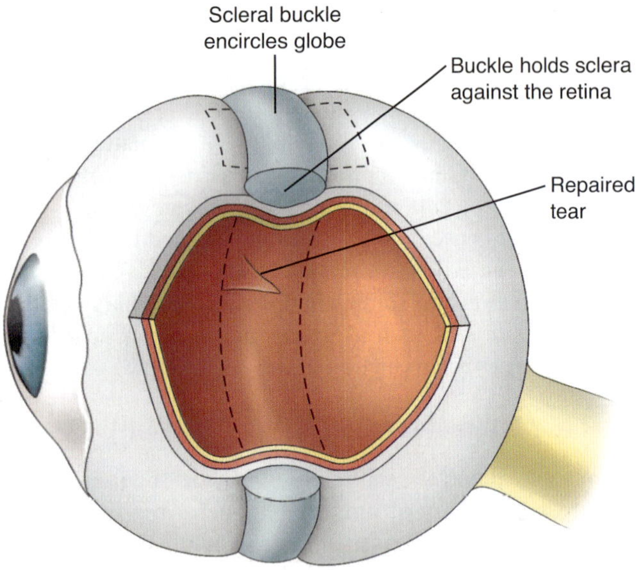

FIGURE 48-6 **Scleral buckle.**

lifting or strenuous activity that could increase IOP. Reading may be restricted until the surgeon gives permission. Patients wear sunglasses during the day and an eye patch at night. Patients often report pain, erythema, and a scratchy sensation after surgery. Ice packs may be applied to counter any edema associated with the conjunctiva. If a vitrectomy was performed with scleral buckling, patients are required to sleep with their head elevated. Air travel must be avoided until the gas bubble, injected during surgery into the vitreous cavity to position the retina, is absorbed. Driving may be restricted until vision stabilizes. Reevaluation of vision and the need for corrective lenses is performed 6 to 8 weeks postoperatively.

Teaching About Complications

Postoperative complications may include increased IOP, endophthalmitis (inflammation of the internal layer of the eye), development of other retinal detachments, development of cataracts, and loss of turgor of the eye. Patients must be taught the signs and symptoms of complications, particularly of increasing IOP and postoperative infection, such as eye pain, sudden change in vision, fever, lid swelling, or conjunctival and/or corneal injection (redness). Excessive pain, swelling, and bleeding must be reported immediately to the surgeon.

MACULAR DEGENERATION

Macular degeneration is the leading cause of severe, irreversible vision loss, particularly in people older than 60 years of age, worldwide affecting 30 to 50 million individuals (Roh & Kim, 2019; Ruia & Kaufman, 2021). Commonly called AMD, it is characterized by tiny, yellowish spots called drusen (Fig. 48-7) beneath the retina. Most people older than 60 years of age have at least a few small drusen. There is a wide range of visual loss in patients with macular degeneration,

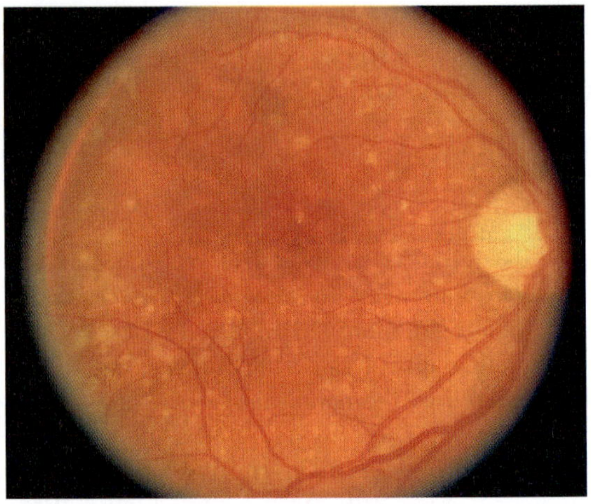

FIGURE 48-7 **Retina showing drusen and age-related macular degeneration (AMD).**

but most patients do not experience total blindness. Central vision is generally the most affected, with most patients retaining peripheral vision (Fig. 48-8). There are two types of AMD, commonly known as the dry type and wet type.

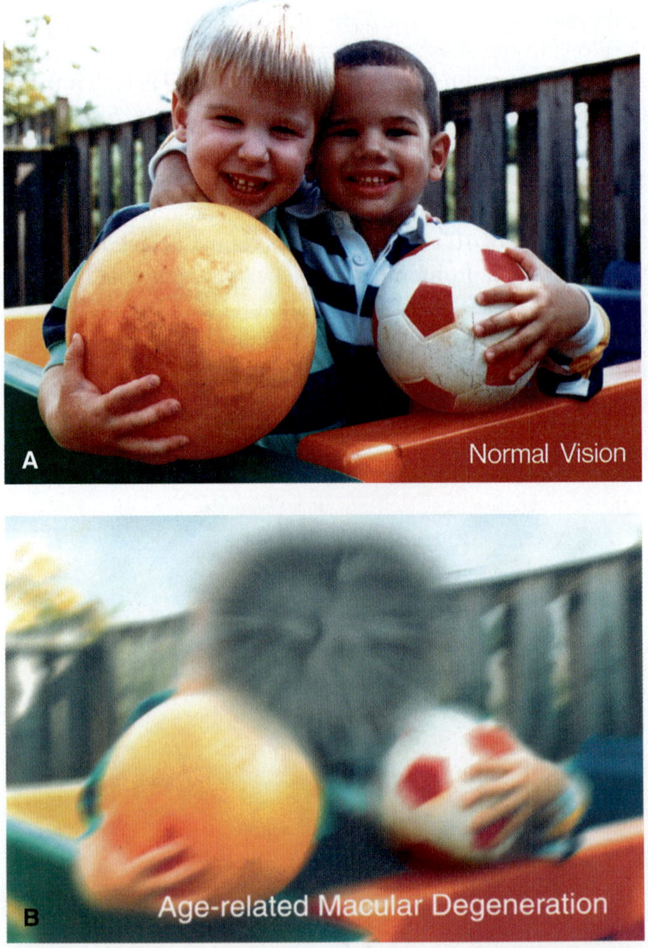

FIGURE 48-8 **A. Normal vision. B. Visual loss associated with macular degeneration. (Photos courtesy of the National Eye Institute/National Institutes of Health.)**

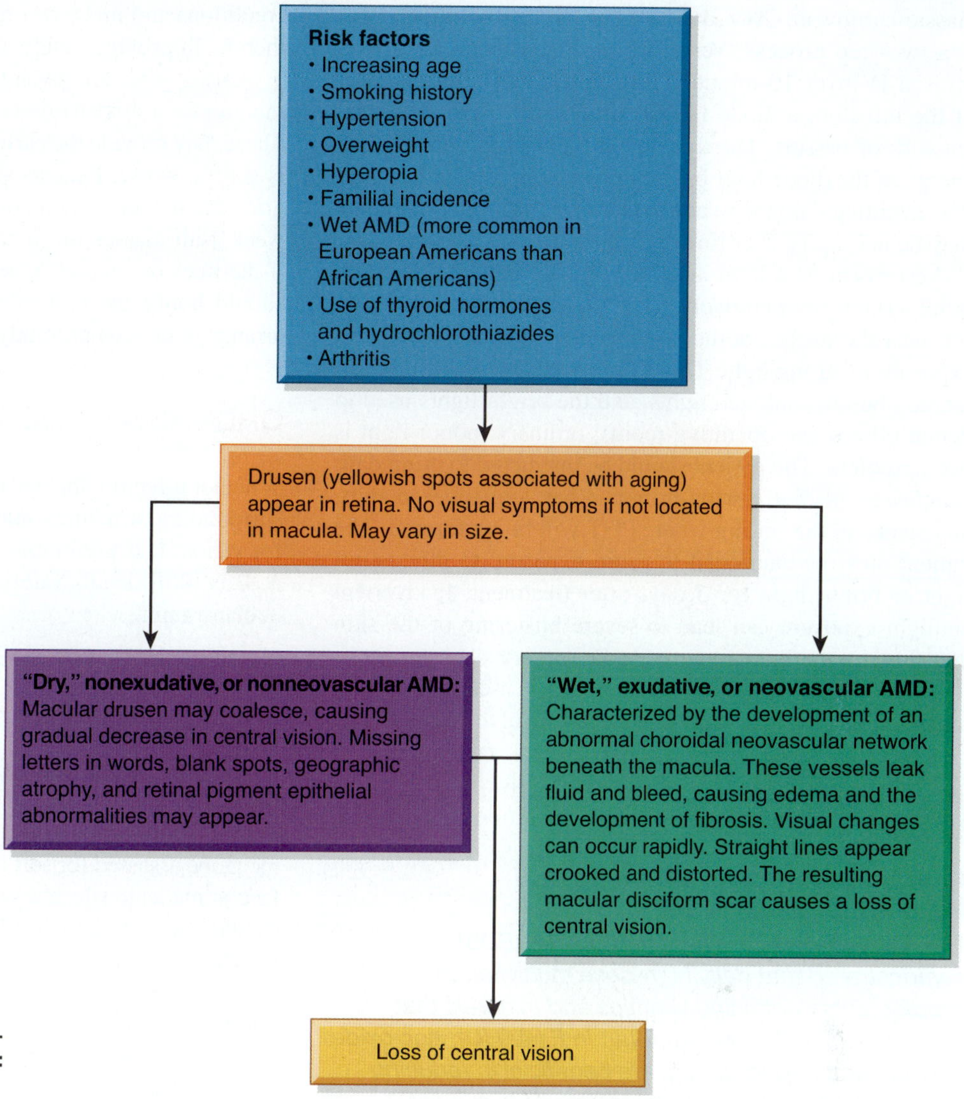

FIGURE 48-9 Progression of age-related macular degeneration (AMD): pathways to vision loss.

Pathophysiology

Approximately 90% of people with AMD have the dry or nonexudative type, which has an insidious onset and leads to a mild to moderate loss of vision, although peripheral vision is preserved. In dry AMD, the outer layers of the retina slowly break down (Fig. 48-9). With this breakdown comes the appearance of drusen. When the drusen occur outside of the macular area, patients generally have no symptoms. When the drusen occur within the macula, however, there is a gradual blurring of vision that patients may notice when they try to read. There is no known treatment that can cure this type of AMD.

Wet or exudative AMD is characterized by **choroidal neovascularization** (CNV), new growth of blood vessels beneath the retina, which if untreated causes severe vision loss in 70% to 90% of AMD cases (Hobbs & Pierce, 2022). Wet AMD may have an abrupt onset. The affected vessels can leak fluid and blood, elevating the retina. Patients report that straight lines appear crooked and distorted, or that letters in words appear broken. Some patients can be treated with the argon laser to stop the leakage from these vessels. However, this treatment is not ideal because vision may be affected by the laser treatment, and abnormal vessels often grow back after treatment.

Medical Management

Vision loss from CNV lesions in AMD is a growing problem. With the growth of these new vessels from the choriocapillary layer, fibrous tissue develops that can, over months, destroy central vision. Laser treatment has been used to close these abnormal vessels, but the very process of photocoagulation carries with it some level of retinal destruction, albeit less than the natural scarring that would occur in the untreated eye.

Photodynamic therapy (PDT) has been developed in an attempt to ameliorate the CNV while causing minimal damage to the retina. Studies have shown that PDT can reduce the risk of visual loss for certain groups of patients who have classic subfoveal CNV due to macular degeneration. PDT is a two-step process. Verteporfin, a photosensitive dye, is infused IV over 10 minutes. Fifteen minutes after the start of the infusion, a diode laser is used to treat the abnormal network of vessels. The dye within the vessels takes up the energy of the diode laser but the surrounding retina does not, thus avoiding damage to adjacent areas. Multiple treatments may be necessary over time.

Verteporfin is a light-activated dye, so patient education is important preoperatively. The dye within the blood vessels near the surface of the skin could become activated with exposure to strong light. This would include bright sunlight, tanning booths, halogen lights, and the bright lights used in dental offices and operating rooms; ordinary indoor light is not a problem. The patient should be instructed to bring dark sunglasses, gloves, a wide-brimmed hat, long-sleeved shirt, and slacks to the setting where PDT will be performed. The patient must be cautioned to avoid exposure to direct sunlight or bright light for 5 days after treatment. Inadvertent sunlight exposure can lead to severe blistering of the skin and sunburn that may require plastic surgery.

Other treatment options are commonly used in the management of advanced wet AMD; they involve intravitreous injection of vascular endothelial growth factor (VEGF) and inhibitor-like medications. Bleeding risk in intravitreal injections is minimal such that anticoagulation is continued.

Pearls for Practice: Vitamins and Macular Degeneration

The Age-Related Eye Disease Study (AREDS) demonstrated that daily high-dose multivitamin supplements containing vitamins and minerals that include vitamin C (500 mg), vitamin E (400 IU), zinc oxide (80 mg), and copper (2 mg) are beneficial in reducing the risk of vision loss in patients with high-risk AMD, and a follow-up study of the AREDS2 demonstrated the beneficial effect of lutein (10 mg) and zeaxanthin (2 mg) (AREDS, 2001; AREDS, 2014; Elessign et al., 2021). In a recent study evaluating the measured quantities of above noted vitamins, the measured quantities of vitamin C, vitamin E, zinc, and copper were slightly higher than labeled but not to an amount that would cause any systemic toxicity if taken at the recommended dosages (Flessig et al., 2021). In addition, it has been found that the B vitamins plus lutein, astaxanthin, zeaxanthin, and meso-zeaxanthin all contribute to slowing the progress of the dry form of macular degeneration (Litwack, 2022).

Nursing Management

Nursing management is primarily educational. Most patients benefit from the use of bright lighting and magnification devices and from referral to a low-vision center. Some low-vision centers send representatives to the patient's home or place of employment to evaluate the living and working conditions and make recommendations to improve lighting, thereby improving vision and promoting safety.

Amsler grids are given to patients to use in their home to monitor for a sudden onset or distortion of vision (Fig. 48-10). These may provide the earliest sign that macular degeneration is getting worse. Patients should be encouraged to use these grids and to look at them, one eye at a time, several times each week with glasses on. If there is a change in the grid (e.g., if the lines or squares appear distorted or faded), the patient should notify the ophthalmologist immediately and should arrange to be seen promptly.

ORBITAL AND OCULAR TRAUMA

Whether affecting the eye or the orbit, trauma to the eye and surrounding structures may have devastating consequences for vision. It is preferable to prevent injury rather than treat it. Box 48-8 details safety measures to prevent orbital and ocular trauma.

Types of Trauma

Orbital Trauma

Injury to the orbit is usually associated with a head injury; hence, the patient's general medical condition must first be stabilized before conducting an ocular examination. Only then is the globe assessed for soft tissue injury. During inspection, the face is meticulously assessed for underlying fractures, which should always be suspected in cases of blunt trauma. To establish the extent of ocular injury, visual acuity is assessed as soon as possible, even if it is only a rough estimate. Soft tissue orbital injuries often result in damage to the optic nerve. Major ocular injuries, indicated by a soft globe, prolapsing tissue, ruptured globe, and hemorrhage, require immediate surgical attention.

Soft Tissue Injury and Hemorrhage

The signs and symptoms of soft tissue injury from blunt or penetrating trauma include tenderness, ecchymosis, lid swelling, **proptosis** (i.e., downward displacement of the eyeball), and hemorrhage. Closed injuries lead to contusions with subconjunctival hemorrhage, commonly known as a *black eye.* Blood accumulates in the tissues of the conjunctiva. Hemorrhage may be caused by a soft tissue injury to the eyelid or by an underlying fracture.

Management of soft tissue hemorrhage that does not threaten vision is usually conservative and consists of thorough inspection, cleansing, and repair of wounds. Cold compresses are used in the early phase, followed by warm compresses. Hematomas that appear as swollen, fluctuating areas may be surgically drained or aspirated; if they are causing significant orbital pressure, they may be surgically evacuated.

Penetrating injuries or a severe blow to the head can result in severe optic nerve damage. Visual loss can be sudden or delayed and progressive. Immediate loss of vision after an ocular injury is usually irreversible. Delayed visual loss

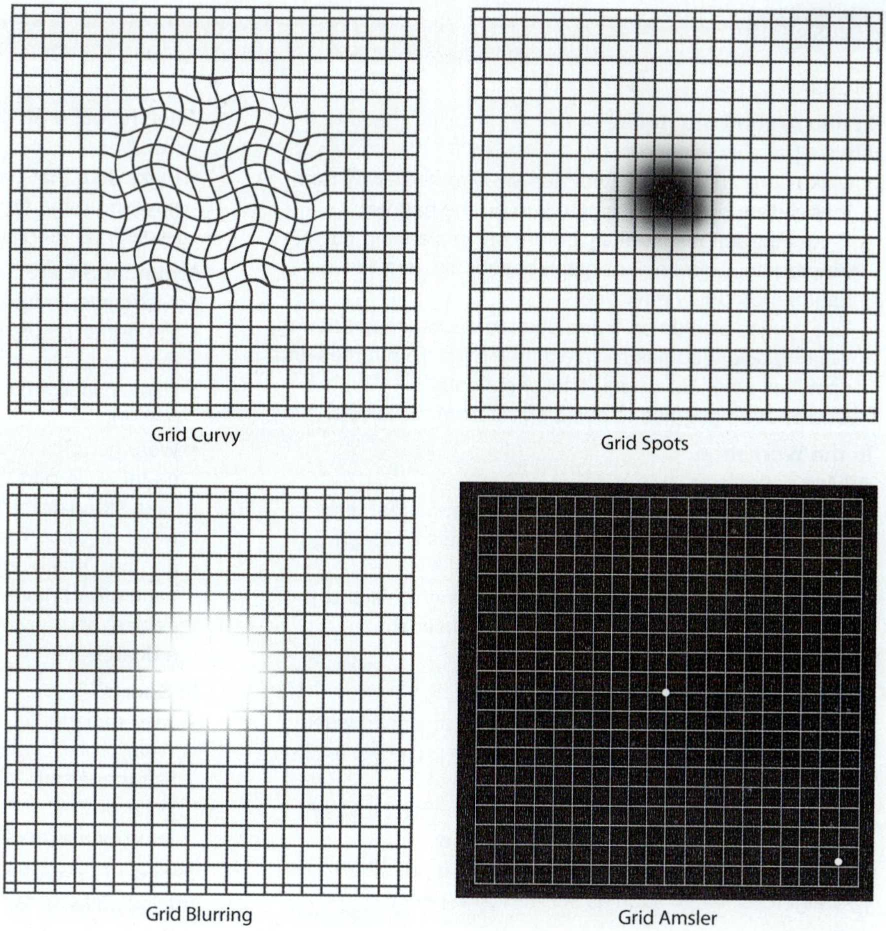

FIGURE 48-10 **Eye examination with an Amsler grid. (Image from Shutterstock.)**

has a better prognosis. Corticosteroid therapy is indicated to reduce optic nerve swelling. Surgery, such as optic nerve decompression, may be performed.

Orbital Fractures

Orbital fractures are detected by facial x-rays. Depending on the orbital structures involved, orbital fractures can be classified as blowout, zygomatic or tripod, maxillary, midfacial, orbital apex, or orbital roof fractures. Blowout fractures result from compression of soft tissue and the sudden increase in orbital pressure when the force is transmitted to the orbital floor, the area of least resistance.

The inferior rectus and inferior oblique muscles, with their fat and fascial attachments, or the nerve that courses along the inferior oblique muscle may become entrapped, and the globe may be displaced inward (i.e., enophthalmos). Computed tomography (CT) can identify the muscle and its auxiliary structures that are entrapped. These fractures are usually caused by blunt small objects, such as a fist, knee, elbow, or tennis or golf ball.

Orbital roof fractures are dangerous because of potential complications to the brain. Surgical management of these fractures requires a neurosurgeon and an ophthalmologist. The most common indications for surgical intervention are displacement of bone fragments disfiguring the normal facial contours, interference with normal binocular vision caused by extraocular muscle entrapment, interference with mastication in zygomatic fracture, and obstruction of the nasolacrimal duct. Surgery is usually nonemergent, and a period of 10 to 14 days gives the ophthalmologist time to assess ocular function, especially the extraocular muscles and the nasolacrimal duct. Emergency surgical repair is usually not performed unless the globe is displaced to the maxillary sinus. Surgical repair is primarily directed at freeing the entrapped ocular structures and restoring the integrity of the orbital floor.

Foreign Bodies

Foreign bodies that enter the orbit are usually tolerated, except for copper, iron, and vegetable materials, such as those from plants or trees, which may cause purulent infection. X-rays and CT scans are used to identify the foreign body. A careful history is important, especially if the foreign body has been in the orbit for a period of time and the incident forgotten. It is important to identify metallic foreign bodies because they prohibit the use of magnetic resonance imaging (MRI) as a diagnostic tool.

After the extent of the orbital damage is assessed, the decision to use conservative treatment or surgical removal is made. In general, orbital foreign bodies are removed if they are superficial and anterior in location; have sharp edges that

BOX 48-8 **Health Promotion**

Preventing Eye Injuries

In and Around the House

Advise patients to:

- Make sure that all spray nozzles are directed away from themselves before pressing down on the handle.
- Read instructions carefully before using cleaning fluids, detergents, ammonia, or harsh chemicals, and to wash hands thoroughly after use.
- Use grease shields on frying pans to decrease spattering.
- Wear special goggles to shield their eyes from fumes and splashes when using powerful chemicals.
- Use opaque goggles to avoid burns from sunlamps.

In the Workshop

Advise patients to:

- Protect their eyes from flying fragments, fumes, dust particles, sparks, and splashed chemicals by wearing safety glasses.
- Read instructions thoroughly before using tools and chemicals, and follow precautions for their use.

Around Children

Advise patients to:

- Pay attention to age and maturity level of a child when selecting toys and games, and to avoid projectile toys, such as darts and pellet guns.
- Supervise children when they are playing with toys or games that can be potentially dangerous.
- Teach children the correct way to handle potentially dangerous items, such as scissors and pencils.

In the Garden

Advise patients to:

- Avoid letting anyone stand at the side of or in front of a moving lawn mower.
- Pick up rocks and stones before going over them with the lawn mower (stones can be hurled out of the rotary blades and rebound off curbs or walls, causing severe injury to the eye).
- Make sure that pesticide spray can nozzles are directed away from the face.
- Avoid low-hanging branches.

Around the Car

Advise patients to:

- Put out all smoking materials and matches before opening the hood of the car.
- Use a flashlight, not a match or lighter, to look at the battery at night.
- Wear goggles when grinding metal or striking metal against metal while performing auto body repair.
- Take standard safety precautions when using jumper cables (wear goggles; make sure the cars are not touching one another; make sure the jumper cable clamps never touch each other; never lean over the battery when attaching cables; and never attach a cable to the negative terminal of a dead battery).

In Sports

Advise patients to:

- Wear protective safety glasses, especially for sports such as racquetball, squash, tennis, baseball, and basketball.
- Wear protective caps, helmets, or face protectors when appropriate, especially for sports such as ice hockey.

Around Fireworks

Advise patients to:

- Wear eye glasses or safety goggles.
- Avoid using explosive fireworks.
- Never allow children to ignite fireworks or stand near others when lighting fireworks.
- Douse firework duds in water instead of attempting to relight them.

may affect adjacent orbital structures; or are composed of copper, iron, or vegetable material. Surgical intervention is directed at preventing further ocular injury and maintaining the integrity of the affected areas. Cultures are usually obtained, and the patient is placed on prophylactic IV antibiotics that are later changed to oral antibiotics.

Ocular Trauma

Ocular trauma is the leading cause of blindness among children and young adults, especially male trauma victims. The most common circumstances of ocular trauma are occupational injuries (e.g., construction industry), sports (e.g., baseball, basketball, racquet sports, boxing), weapons (e.g., air guns, BB guns), assault, motor vehicle crashes (e.g., broken windshields), and explosions (e.g., blast fragments).

There are two types of ocular trauma in which the first response is critical: chemical burn and foreign object in the eye. With a chemical burn, the eye should be immediately irrigated with tap water or normal saline. With a foreign body, no attempt should be made to remove the foreign object. The object should be protected from jarring or movement to prevent further ocular damage. No pressure or patch should be applied to the affected eye. All traumatic eye injuries should be protected using a metal shield, if available, or a stiff paper cup until medical treatment can be obtained (Fig. 48-11).

Clinical Manifestations and Assessment

The nurse obtains a thorough history, particularly assessing the patient's ocular history, such as preinjury vision in the affected eye or past ocular surgery. Details related to the injury that help in the diagnosis and assessment of need for further tests include the nature of the ocular injury (i.e., blunt or penetrating trauma); the type of activity that caused the injury to determine the nature of the force striking the eye; and whether onset of vision loss was sudden, slow, or progressive. For chemical eye burns, the chemical agent must be identified and tested for pH if the agent is available. The nurse examines the corneal surface for foreign bodies,

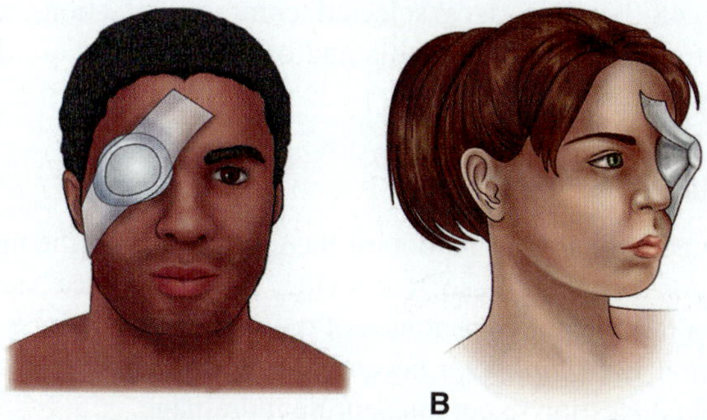

FIGURE 48-11 **Two kinds of eye patches. A. Aluminum shield. B. Stiff paper cup shield (creative substitute when aluminum shield is unavailable).**

wounds, and abrasions and then examines the other external structures of the eye. Pupillary size, shape, and light reaction of the pupil of the affected eye are compared with the other eye. The nurse assesses ocular motility (ability of the eyes to move synchronously up, down, right, and left).

Medical Management

Splash Injuries

Splash injuries are irrigated with normal saline solution before further evaluation occurs. In cases of a ruptured globe, cycloplegic agents (agents that paralyze the ciliary muscle) or topical antibiotics must be deferred because of potential toxicity to exposed intraocular tissues. Further manipulation of the eye must be avoided until the patient is under general anesthesia. Parenteral, broad-spectrum antibiotics are initiated. Tetanus antitoxin is administered, if indicated, as are analgesics. Tetanus prophylaxis is recommended for full-thickness ocular and skin wounds.

Foreign Bodies and Corneal Abrasions

After removal of a foreign body from the surface of the eye, an antibiotic ointment is applied and the eye is patched. The eye is examined daily for evidence of infection until the wound is completely healed.

Contact lens wear is a common cause of corneal abrasion. The patient experiences severe pain and **photophobia** (ocular pain on exposure to light). Corneal epithelial defects are treated with antibiotic ointment and a pressure patch to immobilize the eyelids. Topical anesthetic eye drops must not be given to the patient to take home for repeated use after corneal injury because their effects mask further damage, delay healing, and can lead to permanent corneal scarring. Corticosteroids are avoided while the epithelial defect exists.

Penetrating Injuries and Contusions of the Eyeball

Sharp penetrating injury or blunt contusion force can rupture the eyeball. When the eye wall, cornea, and sclera rupture, rapid decompression or herniation of the orbital contents into adjacent sinuses can occur. In general, blunt traumatic injuries (with an increased incidence of retinal detachment, intraocular tissue avulsion, and herniation) have a worse prognosis than penetrating injuries. Most penetrating injuries result in marked loss of vision with the following signs: hemorrhagic **chemosis** (edema of the conjunctiva), conjunctival laceration, shallow anterior chamber with or without an eccentrically placed pupil, hyphema (hemorrhage within the anterior chamber), or vitreous hemorrhage.

Hyphema is caused by contusion forces that tear the vessels of the iris and damage the anterior chamber angle. Preventing rebleeding and prolonged increased IOP are the goals of treatment for hyphema. In severe cases, the patient is hospitalized with moderate activity restriction. An eye shield is applied. Topical corticosteroids are prescribed to reduce inflammation. An antifibrinolytic agent, aminocaproic acid, stabilizes clot formation at the site of hemorrhage. Aspirin is contraindicated.

A ruptured globe and severe injuries with intraocular hemorrhage require surgical intervention. Vitrectomy, surgical removal of vitreous fluid and stabilization of the retina, is performed for traumatic retinal detachments. Primary **enucleation** (complete removal of the eyeball and part of the optic nerve) is considered only if the globe is irreparable and has NLP. It is a general rule that enucleation is performed within 2 weeks of the initial injury (in an eye that has no useful vision after sustaining penetrating injury) to prevent the risk of **sympathetic ophthalmia** (an inflammation created in the uninjured eye by the affected eye that can result in blindness of the uninjured eye).

Intraocular Foreign Bodies

A patient who complains of blurred vision and discomfort should be questioned carefully about recent injuries and exposures. Patients may be injured in a number of different situations and experience an intraocular foreign body (IOFB). Precipitating circumstances can include working in construction; striking metal against metal; being involved in a motor vehicle crash with facial injury; a gunshot wound; grinding-wheel work; and an explosion.

IOFB is diagnosed and localized by slit-lamp biomicroscopy and indirect ophthalmoscopy, as well as CT or ultrasonography. **MRI is contraindicated because most foreign bodies are metallic and magnetic.** It is important to determine the composition, size, and location of the IOFB and affected eye structures. Every effort should be made to identify the type of IOFB and whether it is magnetic. It is important to identify metallic foreign bodies because they prohibit the use of MRI as a diagnostic tool.

The incidence of endophthalmitis is also high. If the cornea is perforated, tetanus prophylaxis and IV antibiotics are administered.

Ocular Burns

Alkali, acid, and other chemically active organic substances, such as Mace and tear gas, cause chemical burns. Alkali burns (e.g., lye, ammonia) result in the most severe injury because they penetrate the ocular tissues rapidly and continue to cause damage long after the initial injury is sustained. They also cause an immediate rise in IOP. Acids (e.g., toilet bowl cleaners, bleach, car battery fluid, refrigerant) generally cause less damage because the precipitated necrotic tissue proteins form a barrier to further penetration and damage. Chemical burns may appear as superficial punctate keratopathy (i.e., spotty damage to the cornea), subconjunctival hemorrhage, or complete marbleizing of the cornea.

In treating chemical burns, every minute counts. Immediate tap-water irrigation should be started on site before transport of the patient to an emergency department. In the emergency department, only a brief history and examination are performed, then the corneal surfaces and conjunctival fornices are immediately and copiously irrigated with normal saline or any neutral solution. A local anesthetic is instilled, and a lid speculum is applied to overcome blepharospasm (i.e., spasms of the eyelid muscles that result in closure of the lids). Particulate matter must be removed from the fornices using moistened cotton-tipped applicators and minimal pressure on the globe. Irrigation continues until the conjunctival pH normalizes (between 7.3 and 7.6). The pH of the corneal surface is checked by placing a pH paper strip in the fornix. Antibiotics are instilled, and the eye is patched.

The goal of intermediate treatment is to prevent tissue ulceration and promote re-epithelialization. Intense lubrication using nonpreserved (i.e., without preservatives to avoid allergic reactions) artificial tears is essential. Re-epithelialization is promoted with patching or therapeutic soft lenses. The patient is usually monitored daily for several days. Prognosis depends on the type of injury and adequacy of the irrigation immediately after exposure. Long-term treatment consists of two phases: restoration of the ocular surface through grafting procedures and surgical restoration of corneal integrity and optical clarity.

Thermal injury is caused by exposure to a hot object (e.g., curling iron, tobacco, ash), whereas photochemical injury results from ultraviolet irradiation or infrared exposure (e.g., exposure to the reflections from snow, sun gazing, viewing an eclipse of the sun without an adequate filter). These injuries can cause corneal epithelial defect, corneal opacity, conjunctival chemosis (edema) and **injection** (congestion of blood vessels), and burns of the eyelids and periocular region. Antibiotics and a pressure patch for 24 hours constitute the treatment of mild injuries. Scarring of the eyelids may require oculoplastic surgery, whereas corneal scarring may require corneal surgery.

INFECTIOUS AND INFLAMMATORY CONDITIONS

Inflammation and infections of eye structures are common. Eye infection is a leading cause of blindness worldwide. Table 48-3 summarizes selected common infections and their treatment. Conjunctivitis and orbital cellulitis are discussed below.

CONJUNCTIVITIS

Conjunctivitis (inflammation of the conjunctiva) is the most common ocular disease worldwide. Its appearance varies from a mildly pink appearance of the conjunctiva (hence the common term *pink eye*) because of subconjunctival blood vessel congestion to copious purulent drainage.

Clinical Manifestations and Assessment

Conjunctivitis may be unilateral or bilateral, but the infection usually starts in one eye and then spreads to the other eye by hand contact.

Clinical features important to evaluate are the type of discharge (watery, mucoid, purulent, or mucopurulent), presence or absence of lymphadenopathy (enlargement of the preauricular and submandibular lymph nodes where the eyelids drain), important symptoms such as a foreign-body sensation, irritation, a scratching or burning sensation, a sensation of fullness around the eyes, crusting of the eyelids, itching, visual blurring, and photophobia (Tu, 2015; Hoffman, 2022). The main symptoms are redness, discharge, and discomfort (Rutter, 2021).

Common organisms isolated are *Streptococcus pneumoniae, Haemophilus influenzae*, and *Staphylococcus aureus*. Two sexually transmitted agents associated with conjunctivitis are *Chlamydia trachomatis* and *Neisseria gonorrhoeae*. Diagnosis is based on the distinctive characteristics of ocular signs, acute or chronic presentation, and identification of any precipitating events. Positive results of swab smear preparations and cultures confirm the diagnosis.

Types of Conjunctivitis

Conjunctivitis is classified according to its cause. The major causes are microbial infection, allergy, and irritating toxic stimuli. Conjunctivitis can be caused by a wide spectrum of organisms, including bacteria (e.g., *Chlamydia*), viruses, fungi, and parasites. Conjunctivitis can also result from an existing ocular infection or can be a manifestation of a systemic disease.

Microbial Conjunctivitis

Bacterial Conjunctivitis

Bacterial conjunctivitis can be acute or chronic. The acute type can develop into a chronic condition. Signs and symptoms can vary from mild to severe. Chronic bacterial conjunctivitis is usually seen in patients with lacrimal duct obstruction, chronic dacryocystitis (infection of the nasolacrimal sac), and chronic blepharitis (eyelid inflammation). The most common causative microorganisms are *S. pneumoniae, H. influenzae*, and *S. aureus*.

TABLE 48-3 **Common Infections and Inflammatory Disorders of Eye Structures**

Disorder	Description	Management
Hordeolum (stye)	Acute suppurative infection of the glands of the eyelids caused by *Staphylococcus aureus.* The lid is red and edematous, with a small collection of pus in the form of an abscess. There is considerable discomfort.	Warm compresses are applied directly to the affected lid area three to four times a day for 10–15 minutes. If the condition is not improved after 48 hours, incision and drainage may be indicated. Application of topical antibiotics may be prescribed thereafter.
Chalazion	Sterile inflammatory process involving chronic granulomatous inflammation of the meibomian glands; can appear as a single granuloma or multiple granulomas in the upper or lower eyelids.	Warm compresses applied three to four times a day for 10–15 minutes may resolve the inflammation in the early stages. Most often, however, surgical excision is indicated. Corticosteroid injection to the chalazion lesion may be used for smaller lesions.
Blepharitis	Chronic bilateral inflammation of the eyelid margins. There are two types: staphylococcal and seborrheic. Staphylococcal blepharitis is usually ulcerative and is more serious due to the involvement of the base of hair follicles. Permanent scarring can result.	The seborrheic type is chronic and is usually resistant to treatment, but the milder cases may respond to lid hygiene. Staphylococcal blepharitis requires topical antibiotic treatment. Instructions on lid hygiene (to keep the lid margins clean and free of exudates) are given to the patient.
Bacterial keratitis	Infection of the cornea by *S. aureus, Streptococcus pneumoniae,* and *Pseudomonas aeruginosa*.	Fortified (high-concentration) antibiotic eyedrops are administered every 60 minutes around the clock for the first 24–48 hours. When a positive response to treatment is demonstrated, antibiotics may be tapered down to every 2–3 hours for 2 weeks. Systemic antibiotics may be administered to fortify topical antibiotics. Cycloplegics are administered to reduce pain caused by ciliary spasm. Corticosteroid therapy and subconjunctival injections of antibiotics are controversial.
Herpes simplex keratitis	Leading cause of corneal blindness in the United States. Symptoms are severe pain, tearing, and photophobia. The dendritic ulcer has a branching, linear pattern with feathery edges and terminal bulbs at its ends. Herpes simplex keratitis can lead to recurrent stromal keratitis and persist to 12 months, with residual corneal scarring.	Many lesions heal without treatment and residual effects. The treatment goal is to minimize the damaging effect of the inflammatory response and eliminate viral replication within the cornea. Penetrating keratoplasty is indicated for corneal scarring and must be performed when the herpetic disease has been inactive for many months.

Bacterial conjunctivitis manifests with an acute onset of redness, burning, and discharge. There is conjunctival irritation, and injection in the fornices. The exudates are variable but are usually present on waking in the morning. The eyes may be difficult to open because of adhesions caused by the exudate. Purulent discharge occurs in severe acute bacterial infections, whereas mucopurulent discharge appears in mild cases. In gonococcal conjunctivitis, the symptoms are more acute and may present with profuse and purulent exudate, lymphadenopathy, and pseudomembranes.

Chlamydial conjunctivitis includes **trachoma** (a bilateral chronic follicular conjunctivitis of childhood that leads to blindness during adulthood if left untreated) and inclusion conjunctivitis. Trachoma is prevalent in areas with hot, dry, and dusty climates and in areas with poor living conditions. It is spread by direct contact or fomites, and the vectors can be insects such as flies and gnats. Symptoms include red, inflamed eyes, tearing, photophobia, ocular pain, purulent exudates, preauricular lymphadenopathy (anterior to the auricle of the ear), and lid edema. At the middle stage of the disease, an acute inflammation occurs, after which trichiasis (turning inward of hair follicles) and entropion begin to develop, causing corneal erosion and ulceration. The late stage of the disease is characterized by scarred conjunctiva, subepithelial keratitis (inflammation of the cornea), abnormal vascularization of the cornea (pannus), and residual scars from the follicles. Severe corneal ulceration can lead to perforation and blindness.

Inclusion conjunctivitis affects sexually active people who have genital chlamydial infection. Transmission is by oral–genital sex or hand-to-eye transmission. Indirect transmission can occur in inadequately chlorinated swimming pools. The eye lesions usually appear a week after exposure and may be associated with a nonspecific urethritis or cervicitis.

Viral Conjunctivitis

Viral conjunctivitis can be acute and chronic. The discharge is watery, and follicles are prominent. Severe cases include

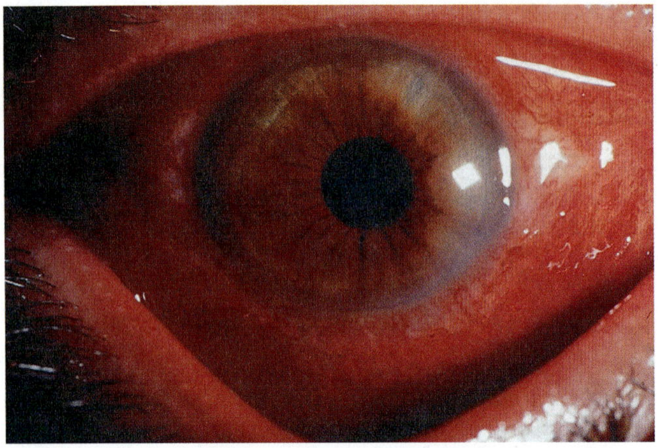

FIGURE 48-12 **Conjunctival hyperemia in viral conjunctivitis.**

pseudomembranes. Pseudomembranes appear as tissue that covers the conjunctiva or sclera but are actually composed of mucus, fibrin, bacteria, or immune system cells. The common causative organisms are adenovirus and herpes simplex virus. Conjunctivitis caused by adenovirus is highly contagious. The condition is usually preceded by symptoms of upper respiratory infection. Corneal involvement causes extreme photophobia. Symptoms include extreme tearing, redness, and foreign-body sensation that can involve one or both eyes. There is lid edema, ptosis, and conjunctival **hyperemia** (dilation of the conjunctival blood vessels) (Fig. 48-12). These signs and symptoms vary from mild to severe and may last for 2 weeks. Viral conjunctivitis, although self-limited, tends to last longer than bacterial conjunctivitis.

Pearls for Practice

The clinical term for hyperemia of the conjunctiva is known as "injected."

Epidemic keratoconjunctivitis (EKC) is a highly contagious viral conjunctivitis that is easily transmitted from one person to another among household members, school children, and health care workers. The outbreak of epidemics is seasonal, especially during the summer, when people use swimming pools. EKC is most often accompanied by preauricular lymphadenopathy and occasionally periorbital pain. EKC can lead to keratopathy (corneal disease).

Allergic Conjunctivitis

Immunologic or allergic conjunctivitis is a hypersensitivity reaction that occurs as part of allergic rhinitis (hay fever), or it can be an independent allergic reaction. Patients often present with a history of atopy (tendency to produce an exaggerated immunoglobulin E [IgE] immune response to otherwise harmless substances in the environment), a genetic predisposition toward hypersensitivity reactions. Atopic conditions include allergies (e.g., food and seasonal), asthma, and atopic dermatitis (e.g., eczema). Allergic conjunctivitis is characterized by extreme pruritus, epiphora (i.e., excessive secretion of tears), injection, and usually severe photophobia. A string-like mucoid discharge is usually associated with rubbing the eyes because of severe pruritus. Vernal conjunctivitis is also known as *seasonal conjunctivitis* because it appears mostly during warm weather.

Toxic Conjunctivitis

Chemical conjunctivitis can be the result of medications; chlorine from swimming pools; exposure to toxic fumes among industrial workers; or exposure to other irritants, such as smoke, hair sprays, acids, and alkalis.

Medical and Nursing Management

The management of conjunctivitis depends on the type (Table 48-4). Most types of mild and viral conjunctivitis are self-limiting, benign conditions that may not require treatment. Box 48-9 includes patient teaching information about viral conjunctivitis. For more severe cases, topical antibiotics, eye drops, or ointments are prescribed. Patients with gonococcal conjunctivitis require urgent antibiotic therapy. If left untreated, this ocular disease can lead to corneal perforation and blindness. The systemic complications can include meningitis and generalized septicemia.

ORBITAL CELLULITIS

Orbital cellulitis is inflammation of the tissues surrounding the eye.

Pathophysiology

Orbital cellulitis may result from bacterial, fungal, or viral inflammatory conditions of contiguous structures, such as the face, oropharynx, dental structures, or intracranial structures. It can also result from foreign bodies and from a pre-existing ocular infection or from generalized septicemia. Infection of the sinuses is the most frequent cause. Infection originating in the sinuses can spread easily to the orbit through the thin bony walls and foramina or by means of the interconnecting venous system of the orbit and sinuses. The most common causative organisms are staphylococci and streptococci in adults and *H. influenzae* in children.

Clinical Manifestations and Assessment

The symptoms include pain, lid swelling, conjunctival edema, **proptosis**, and decreased ocular motility. With such edema, optic nerve compression can occur and IOP may increase.

The severe intraorbital tension caused by abscess formation and the impairment of optic nerve function in orbital cellulitis can result in permanent visual loss. Because of the orbit's proximity to the brain, orbital cellulitis can lead to life-threatening complications, such as intracranial abscess and cavernous sinus thrombosis.

TABLE **48-4 Management of Conjunctivitis**

Conjunctivitis	Management
Bacterial Conjunctivitis	• Acute bacterial conjunctivitis is almost always self-limiting, lasting 2 weeks if left untreated. If treated with antibiotics, it may last a few days, except for gonococcal conjunctivitis. Gonococcal conjunctivitis ceases within hours of topical antibiotic therapy, which may be discontinued 24 hours after treatment. • For trachoma, usually broad-spectrum antibiotics are administered topically and systemically. Surgical management includes the correction of trichiasis (eyelashes growing inward toward the conjunctiva and cornea) to prevent conjunctival scarring. • Adult inclusion conjunctivitis requires 1 week of antibiotics. Prevention of reinfection is important, and affected individuals and their sexual partners must seek treatment for sexually transmitted disease, if indicated.
Viral Conjunctivitis	• Viral conjunctivitis is not responsive to any treatment. Cold compresses may alleviate some symptoms. It is extremely important to remember that viral conjunctivitis, especially epidemic keratoconjunctivitis, is highly contagious. Patient instructions should include an emphasis on hand hygiene and avoiding sharing of hand towels, face cloths, pillowcases, other linens, personal items and eye drops. Tissues should be directly discarded into a covered trash can. Replace all eye cosmetics, if applicable. • All forms of tonometry must be avoided unless medically indicated. All multidose medications must be discarded at the end of each day or when contaminated. Infected employees and others must not be allowed to work or attend school until symptoms have resolved, which can take 3–7 days.
Allergic Conjunctivitis	• Patients with allergic conjunctivitis, especially recurrent vernal or seasonal conjunctivitis, are usually given corticosteroids in ophthalmic preparations. Depending on the severity of the disease, they may be given oral preparations. Use of vasoconstrictors, such as topical epinephrine solution, cold compresses, ice packs, and cool ventilation, usually provides comfort by decreasing swelling.
Toxic Conjunctivitis	• For conjunctivitis caused by chemical irritants, the eye must be irrigated immediately and profusely with saline or sterile water.

Medical and Nursing Management

Immediate administration of high-dose, broad-spectrum, systemic antibiotics is indicated. Cultures and Gram-stained smears are obtained. Monitoring changes in visual acuity, degree of proptosis, central nervous system function (e.g., nausea, vomiting, fever, cognitive changes), displacement of the globe, extraocular movements, pupillary signs, and the fundus is extremely important. Consultation with an

BOX 48-9 **Patient Education**

Instructions for Patients with Viral Conjunctivitis

Viral conjunctivitis is a highly contagious eye infection. It can easily spread from one person to another. The symptoms can be alarming, but they are not serious. The following information will help you understand this eye condition and how to take care of yourself and/or your family member at home.

- Your eyes will look red and will have watery discharge, and your lids will be swollen for about a week.
- You will experience eye pain, a sandy sensation in your eye, and sensitivity to light.
- Symptoms will resolve after about 1 week.
- You may use light, cold compresses over your eyes for about 10 minutes four to five times a day to soothe the pain.
- You may use artificial tears for the sandy sensation in your eye, and mild pain medications, such as acetaminophen.
- You need to stay at home. Children must not play outside. You may return to work or school after 7 days, when the redness and discharge have cleared. You may obtain a doctor's note to return to work or school.
- Do not share towels, linens, makeup, or toys.
- Wash your hands thoroughly and frequently, using soap and water, including before and after you apply artificial tears or cold compresses.
- Use a new tissue every time you wipe the discharge from each eye. You may dampen the tissue with clean water to clean the outside of the eye.
- You may wash your face and take a shower as you normally do.
- Discard all of your makeup articles. You must not apply makeup until the disease is over.
- You may wear dark glasses if bright lights bother you.
- If the discharge from your eye turns yellowish and puslike, or you experience changes in your vision, you need to return to the health care provider for an examination.

otolaryngologist is necessary, especially when sinusitis is suspected. In the event of abscess formation or progressive loss of vision, surgical drainage of the abscess or sinus is performed. Sinusotomy and antibiotic irrigation are also performed.

TREATMENT MODALITIES FOR EYE INJURIES AND DISORDERS

Common treatments discussed in this section include surgery and pharmacologic treatment.

SURGICAL PROCEDURES

Orbital Surgeries

Orbital surgeries may be performed to repair fractures, remove a foreign body, or remove benign or malignant growths. The eyeball is lined with muscle, connective, and adipose tissues and is housed in the bony orbit, which is about 4 cm high, wide, and deep. It is shaped roughly like a four-sided pyramid, surrounded on three sides by the sinuses: ethmoid (medially), frontal (superiorly), and maxillary (inferiorly). Surgical procedures involving the orbit and lids affect facial appearance (cosmesis). The goals are to recover and preserve visual function and to maintain the anatomic relationship of the ocular structures to achieve cosmesis. During the repair of orbital fractures, the orbital bones are realigned to follow the anatomic positions of facial structures.

Orbital surgical procedures involve working around delicate structures of the eye, such as the optic nerve, retinal blood vessels, and ocular muscles. Complications of orbital surgical procedures may include blindness as a result of damage to the optic nerve and its blood supply. Sudden pain and loss of vision may indicate intraorbital hemorrhage or compression of the optic nerve. Ptosis and diplopia may result from trauma to the extraocular muscles during the surgical procedure, but these conditions typically resolve after a few weeks.

Prophylaxis with IV antibiotics is the usual postoperative regimen after orbital surgery, especially with repair of orbital fractures and removal of an intraorbital foreign body. IV corticosteroids are used if there is a concern about optic nerve swelling. Topical ocular antibiotics are typically instilled, and antibiotic ointments are applied externally to the skin suture sites.

For the first 24 to 48 hours postoperatively, ice compresses are applied over the periocular area to decrease periorbital swelling, facial swelling, and hematoma. The head of the patient's bed should be elevated to a comfortable position (30 to 45 degrees).

Discharge teaching should include medication instructions for oral antibiotics, instillation of ophthalmic medications, and application of ocular compresses.

Enucleation

Enucleation is the removal of the entire eye and part of the optic nerve. It may be performed for the following conditions:

- Severe injury resulting in prolapse of uveal tissue (iris, ciliary body, and choroid), or loss of light projection (the ability to identify the direction of the light source) or perception
- An irritated, blind, painful, deformed, or disfigured eye, usually caused by glaucoma, retinal detachment, or chronic inflammation
- An eye without useful vision that is producing or has produced sympathetic ophthalmia (inflammation of the eye or conjunctiva) in the other eye
- Intraocular tumors that are untreatable by other means

The procedure for enucleation involves the separation and cutting of each of the ocular muscles, dissection of the Tenon capsule (fibrous membrane covering the sclera), and cutting of the optic nerve from the eyeball. The insertion of an orbital implant typically follows, and the conjunctiva is closed. A large pressure dressing is applied over the area. Box 48-10 discusses ocular prostheses.

Evisceration

Evisceration involves the surgical removal of the intraocular contents through an incision or opening in the cornea or sclera. Evisceration may be performed to treat severe ocular trauma with ruptured globe, severe ocular inflammation, or severe ocular infection. The optic nerve, sclera, extraocular muscles, and sometimes the cornea are left intact. The main advantage of evisceration over enucleation is that the final cosmetic result and motility after fitting the ocular prosthesis are enhanced. This procedure would be more acceptable to a patient whose body image is severely threatened. The main disadvantage is the high risk of sympathetic ophthalmia (a rare bilateral panuveitis [inflammation of all layers of the uvea of the eye] that occurs following open globe injury).

Exenteration

Exenteration is the removal of the eyelids, the eye, and various amounts of orbital contents. It is indicated in malignancies in the orbit that are life-threatening or when more conservative modalities of treatment have failed or are inappropriate. An example is squamous cell carcinoma of the paranasal sinuses, skin, and conjunctiva with deep orbital involvement. In its most extensive form, exenteration may include the removal of all orbital tissues and resection of the orbital bones.

PHARMACOLOGIC TREATMENT

The main objective of ocular medication delivery is to maximize the amount of medication that reaches the ocular site of action in sufficient concentration to produce a beneficial

BOX 48-10

Ocular Prostheses

Orbital implants and conformers (ocular prostheses usually made of silicone rubber) maintain the shape of the eye after enucleation or evisceration to prevent a contracted, sunken appearance. The temporary conformer is placed over the conjunctival closure after the implantation of an orbital implant. A conformer is placed after the enucleation or evisceration procedure to protect the suture line, maintain the fornices, prevent contracture of the socket in preparation for the ocular prosthesis, and promote the integrity of the eyelids.

All ocular prosthetics have limitations in their motility. There are two designs of eye prostheses (see figure below). The anophthalmic ocular prostheses are used in the absence of the globe. Scleral shells look just like the anophthalmic prosthesis but are thinner and fit over a globe with intact corneal sensation. An eye prosthesis usually lasts about 6 years, depending on the quality of fit, comfort, and cosmetic appearance. When the anophthalmic socket is completely healed, conformers are replaced with prosthetic eyes.

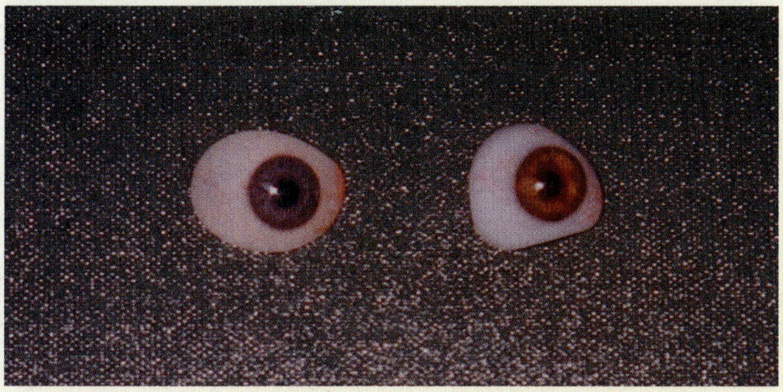

Eye prostheses. (*Left*) Anophthalmic ocular prosthesis. (*Right*) Scleral shell.

An ocularist is a specially trained and skilled professional who makes prosthetic eyes. After the ophthalmologist is satisfied that the anophthalmic socket is completely healed and is ready for prosthetic fitting, the patient is referred to an ocularist. The healing period is usually 6 to 8 weeks. It is advisable for the patient to have a consultation with the ocularist before the fitting. Obtaining accurate information and verbalizing concerns can lessen anxiety about wearing an ocular prosthesis.

Medical Management

Removal of an eye has physical, social, and psychological ramifications for any person. The significance of loss of the eye and vision must be addressed in the plan of care. The patient's preparation should include information about the surgical procedure and placement of orbital implants and conformers and the availability of ocular prosthetics to enhance cosmetic appearance. In some cases, patients may choose to see an ocularist before the surgery to discuss ocular prosthetics.

Nursing Management

Teaching About Postsurgical Care

Patients who undergo eye removal need to know that they will usually have a large ocular pressure dressing, which is typically removed after a week, and that an ophthalmic topical antibiotic ointment is applied in the socket three times daily. When surgical eye removal is immediate and unexpected, as in the case of ocular trauma, the nurse's role in providing emotional support is crucial.

After the removal of an eye, there is a loss of depth perception. Patients must be advised to take extra caution in their ambulation and movement to avoid miscalculations that may result in injury. It may take some time to adjust to monocular vision. Patients using conformers must be advised that the prosthetic may accidentally fall out of the socket. If this happens, the conformer must be washed, wiped dry, and placed back in the socket.

Teaching Patients Self-Care

Patients need to be taught how to insert, remove, and care for the prosthetic eye. Proper hand hygiene must be observed before inserting and removing an ocular prosthesis. A suction cup may be used if there are problems with manual dexterity. Precautions, such as draping a towel over the sink and closing the sink drain, must be taken to avoid loss of the prosthesis. When instructing patients or family members, a return demonstration is important to assess the level of understanding and ability to perform the procedure.

Before insertion, the inner punctal or outer lateral aspects and the superior and inferior aspects of the prosthesis must be identified by locating the identifying marks, such as a reddish color in the inner punctal area. For people with low vision, other forms of identifying markers, such as dots or notches, are used. The upper lid is raised high enough to create a space. The patient slides the prosthesis up, underneath, and behind the upper eyelid. Meanwhile, the patient pulls the lower eyelid down to help put the prosthesis in place and to have its inferior edge fall back gradually to the lower eyelid. The lower eyelid is checked for correct positioning.

To remove the prosthesis, the patient cups one hand on the cheek to catch the prosthesis, places the forefinger of the free hand against the midportion of the lower eyelid, and gazes upward. Gazing upward brings the inferior edge of the prosthesis nearer the inferior eyelid margin. With the finger pushing inward, downward, and laterally against the lower eyelid, the prosthesis slides out, and the patient's cupped hand acts as the receptacle.

Continuing Care

An eye prosthesis can be worn and left in place for several months. Hygiene and comfort are usually maintained with daily irrigation of the prosthesis in place with normal saline solution, hard contact lens solution, or artificial tears. In the case of dry eye symptoms, the use of ophthalmic ointment lubricants or oil-based drops, such as vitamin E and mineral oil, can be helpful. Removing crusting and mucous discharge that accumulate overnight is performed with the prosthesis in place. Malposition may occur when wiping or rubbing the prosthesis in the socket. The prosthesis can be repositioned with the use of clean fingers. Proper wiping of the prosthesis should be a gentle temporal-to-nasal motion to avoid malpositions.

therapeutic effect. This is determined by the dynamics of ocular pharmacokinetics: absorption, distribution, metabolism, and excretion.

Concepts in Ocular Medication Administration

Topical administration of ocular medications results in only a 1% to 7% absorption rate by the ocular tissues. Ocular absorption involves the entry of a medication into the aqueous humor through the different routes of ocular medication administration. The rate and extent of aqueous humor absorption are determined by the characteristics of the medication and the anatomy and physiology of the eye. Natural barriers of absorption that diminish the efficacy of ocular medications include the following:

- *Limited size of the conjunctival sac.* The conjunctival sac can hold only 50 μL, and any excess is wasted. The volume of one eye drop from commercial topical ocular solutions typically ranges from 20 to 35 μL.
- *Corneal membrane barriers.* The epithelial, stromal, and endothelial layers are barriers to absorption.
- *Blood–ocular barriers.* Blood–ocular barriers prevent high ocular tissue concentration of most ophthalmic medications because they separate the bloodstream from the ocular tissues and keep foreign substances from entering the eye, thereby limiting a medication's efficacy.
- *Tearing, blinking, and drainage.* Increased tear production and drainage due to ocular irritation or an ocular condition may dilute or wash out an instilled eye drop; blinking expels an instilled eye drop from the conjunctival sac.

Distribution of an ocular medication into the various ocular tissues varies by tissue type; the various tissues (e.g., conjunctiva, cornea, lens, iris, ciliary body, choroids) absorb medications to varying degrees. Medications penetrate the corneal epithelium by diffusion by passing through the cells (intracellular) or by passing between the cells (intercellular). Water-soluble (hydrophilic) medications diffuse through the intracellular route, and fat-soluble (lipophilic) medications diffuse through the intercellular route. Topical administration usually does not reach the retina in significant concentrations. Because the space between the ciliary process and the lens is small, medication diffusion in the vitreous is slow. When high concentrations of medication in the vitreous are required, intraocular injection is often chosen to bypass the natural ocular anatomic and physiologic barriers.

Aqueous solutions are most commonly used for the eye. They are the least expensive medications and interfere least with vision. However, corneal contact time is brief because tears dilute the medication. Ophthalmic ointments have extended retention time in the conjunctival sac and provide a higher concentration than eye drops. The major disadvantage of ointments is the blurred vision that results after application. In general, eyelids and eyelid margins are best treated with ointments. Contact lenses and collagen shields soaked in antibiotics are alternative delivery methods for treating corneal infections.

Of all these delivery methods, the topical route of administration—instilled eye drops and applied ointments—remains the most common. Topical instillation, which is the least invasive method, permits self-administration of medication and produces fewer side effects.

Preservatives are commonly used in ocular medications. Benzalkonium chloride, for example, prevents the growth of organisms and enhances the corneal permeability of most medications; however, some patients are allergic to this preservative. This may be suspected even if the patient had never before experienced an allergic reaction to systemic use of the medication in question. Eye drops without preservatives can be prepared by pharmacists.

Commonly Used Ocular Medications

Common ocular medications include topical anesthetic, mydriatic, and cycloplegic agents that reduce IOP; anti-infective medications; corticosteroids; nonsteroidal anti-inflammatory drugs (NSAIDs); antiallergy medications; eye irrigants; and lubricants.

Topical Anesthetics

One or two drops of proparacaine hydrochloride and tetracaine hydrochloride are instilled before diagnostic procedures such as tonometry. Topical anesthetics are also used for severe eye pain, to allow the patient to open their eyes for examination or treatment. The nurse must instruct the patient not to rub their eyes while anesthetized because this may result in corneal damage.

Patients with corneal abrasions and erosions experience severe pain and are often tempted to overuse topical anesthetic eye drops. Overuse of these drops results in softening of the cornea. Prolonged use of anesthetic drops can delay wound healing and can lead to permanent corneal opacification and scarring, resulting in visual loss.

Mydriatics and Cycloplegics

Mydriasis, or pupil dilation, is the main objective of the administration of mydriatic and cycloplegic agents (Table 48-5). These two types of medications function differently and are used in combination to achieve the maximal dilation that is needed during surgery and fundus examinations to give the ophthalmologist a better view of the internal eye structures. **Mydriatics** potentiate alpha-adrenergic sympathetic effects that result in the relaxation of the ciliary muscle leading to dilatation of the pupil. The patient may have difficulty reading. The patient is advised to wear sunglasses (most eye clinics provide protective sunglasses). The ability to drive is dependent on the person's age, vision, and comfort level.

TABLE **48-5 Mydriatics and Miotics**

Medication	Forms	Indication/Dosage	Action	Duration	Nursing Considerations
Phenylephrine (Dilate)	Solution (0.12%, 2.5%, 10%)	Instill 1 drop per dose; may repeat in 1 hour for: Mydriasis posterior synechiae and minor eye irritation	Dilates pupil by contracting dilator muscle. Peaks within 10–60 minutes	3–7 hours	Monitor for systemic effects of hypertension if 10% solution is administered.
Atropine	Ointment (1%) Solution (0.5%–2%)	Instill 1–2 drops for acute iritis, uveitis, or cycloplegic refraction, three to four times daily	Dilates pupil by anticholinergic action. Peaks within 30 minutes–3 hours	7–10 days	Have antidote available, physostigmine salicylate (IM or IV). Watch patient for signs and symptoms of glaucoma.
Scopolamine hydrobromide	Solution (0.25%)	Instill 1–2 drops for acute iritis, uveitis, or cycloplegic refraction, once to four times daily	Same action as atropine Peaks within 15–45 minutes	3–7 days	Observe patient closely for disorientation or delirium. May be given to patients sensitive to atropine.
Pilocarpine hydrochloride	Gel (4%) Solution (0.25%–1%)	Apply one ribbon of gel into lower conjunctival sac once daily at bedtime. Instill 1–2 drops of solution for open-angle glaucoma, acute angle-closure glaucoma, or mydriasis caused by mydriatic or cycloplegic drugs	Cholinergic effect of pupil constriction (miosis) and deepening of anterior chamber. Peaks within 30–85 minutes	4–8 hours	Monitor vital signs. Monitor drug administration carefully. If taken by mouth, contact poison control center or take patient to ED immediately.

Pearls for Practice

Mydriatic and cycloplegic agents affect the central nervous system. Their effects are most prominent in children and older patients; these patients must be assessed closely for symptoms, such as increased blood pressure, tachycardia, dizziness, ataxia, confusion, disorientation, incoherent speech, and hallucination. These medications are contraindicated in patients with narrow angles or shallow anterior chambers and in patients taking monoamine oxidase inhibitors or tricyclic antidepressants.

Antiglaucoma Medications

Therapeutic medications for glaucoma are used to lower IOP by decreasing aqueous production or increasing aqueous outflow. Because glaucoma calls for lifetime therapy, the patient must be instructed regarding both the ocular and systemic side effects of the medications.

Most antiglaucoma medications affect the **accommodation** of the lens and limit light entry through a constricted pupil. Visual acuity and the ability to focus may be affected. Factors to consider in selecting glaucoma medications are efficacy, systemic and ocular side effects, convenience, and cost.

Anti-Infective Medications

Anti-infective medications include antibiotic, antifungal, and antiviral agents. Most are available as drops, ointments, or subconjunctival or intravitreal injections. Antibiotics include penicillin, cephalosporins, aminoglycosides, and fluoroquinolones. The main antifungal agent is amphotericin B. Side effects of amphotericin are serious and include severe pain, conjunctival necrosis, iritis, and retinal toxicity. Antiviral medications include acyclovir and ganciclovir. Patients receiving ocular agents are subject to the same side effects and adverse reactions as those receiving anti-infective oral or parenteral medications.

Corticosteroids and Nonsteroidal Anti-Inflammatory Drugs

The topical preparations of corticosteroids are commonly used in inflammatory conditions of the eyelids, conjunctiva,

BOX 48-11

GUIDELINES FOR NURSING CARE

Instilling Eye Medications

Equipment

- Medication(s) as ordered
- Cotton balls or gauze
- Optional: Eye dressing

Implementation

ACTION	RATIONALE
1. Ensure adequate lighting.	1. Adequate lighting ensures the procedure will be carried out using appropriate technique.
2. Perform hand hygiene.	2. Hand hygiene and aseptic technique is important to decrease the risk of contamination of supplies and the spread of further infection.
3. Don clean gloves and, if necessary or required, gently clean any crusts or drainage from the eyelid margins, wiping from the inner to the outer canthus and using a fresh gauze pad or cotton ball moistened with warm water for each stroke.	3. Cleaning the eyes promotes patient comfort and promotes absorption of medications. In addition, debris is removed from the nasolacrimal duct.
4. Prepare medication. Read the label of the eye medication to make sure it is the correct medication. Shake suspensions or "milky" solutions to obtain the desired medication level. Verify which eye is to be treated.	4. Proper checking of medication and which eye is to be treated is an essential right. Mixing of medication in suspension is required.
5. Assume proper position for instillation of eye medications.	5. Positioning of the patient's head in a supine position or, if sitting, hyperextended in a "sniffing position" allows for proper instillation of ophthalmic medication, particularly drops.
6. Do not touch the tip of the medication container to any part of the eye or face. Hold the lower lid down; do not press on the eyeball. Apply gentle pressure to the cheek bone to anchor the finger holding the lid.	6. Maintaining aseptic technique avoids contamination of materials, such as the medication container. Using the cheek bone as a fulcrum to steady the arm allows for improved medication delivery.
7. Apply medication. Instill eye drops before applying ointments. *For eye drops:* Eye drops should be instilled at a distance of approximately 1 in from the eye. Before instilling the eyedrops, instruct the patient to look up and away. The lower lid is gently pulled down to instill the drops in the conjunctival sac. Immediately after instilling eye drops, apply gentle pressure on the inner canthus (punctal occlusion) near the bridge of the nose for 3–5 minutes. Using a clean tissue, gently pat the skin to absorb excess eyedrops that run onto the patient's cheeks. *For eye ointment:* Apply a ½-in ribbon of ointment to the lower conjunctival sac. Immediately after ointment instillation, ask the patient to roll their eyes behind closed lids.	7. Medication is administered into the conjunctival sac, rather than on the eyeball, which can cause discomfort. Gentle pressure on the inner canthus (punctal occlusion) is done to decrease the risk of systemic absorption of the medication. Rolling the eye helps to distribute the medication over the surface of the eyeball.
8. Wait 5 minutes before instilling another eye medication.	8. Allow for absorption of one medication to occur prior to applying another one.
9. Perform hand hygiene.	9. Hand hygiene prevents further contamination post instillation.

cornea, anterior chamber, lens, and uvea. Because these topical eye drops are suspensions, the patient is instructed to shake the bottle several times to promote mixture of the medication and maximize its therapeutic effect. The most common ocular side effects of long-term topical corticosteroid administration are glaucoma, cataracts, susceptibility to infection, impaired wound healing, mydriasis, ptosis, and high IOP. To avoid the side effects of corticosteroids, NSAIDs are used as an alternative in controlling inflammatory eye conditions and postoperatively to reduce inflammation.

Antiallergy Medications

Ocular hypersensitivity reactions are extremely common and result primarily from responses to environmental allergens. Most allergens are airborne or carried to the eye by the hand or by other means, although allergic reactions may also be drug-induced. Corticosteroids are commonly used as anti-inflammatory and immunosuppressive agents to control ocular hypersensitivity reactions.

Ocular Irrigants and Lubricants

Irrigating solutions are used to cleanse the external lids to maintain lid hygiene, to irrigate the external corneal surface to regain normal pH (e.g., in chemical burns), to irrigate the corneal surface to eliminate debris, or to inflate the globe intraoperatively. These solutions have various compositions (sodium, potassium, magnesium, calcium, bicarbonate, glucose, and glutathione) that are safe to use with an intact corneal surface; however, the corneal surface should not be irrigated in cases of threatened corneal perforation. Sterile irrigating solutions, such as Dacriose, for lid hygiene are available. For patients with severe corneal ulcer, specific orders must be obtained regarding whether it is safe to irrigate the corneal surface or just to cleanse the external lids. Although it is good practice to promote hygiene, prevention of complications must be the primary concern.

Lubricants, such as artificial tears, help alleviate corneal irritation, such as dry eye syndrome. Artificial tears are topical preparations of methyl or hydroxypropyl cellulose that are prepared as eye drop solutions, ointments, or ocular inserts (inserted at the lower conjunctival cul-de-sac once each day).

Nursing Management

The objectives in administering ocular medications are to ensure proper administration to maximize the therapeutic effects and to ensure the safety of the patient by monitoring for systemic and local side effects. Absorption of eye drops by the nasolacrimal duct is undesirable because of the potential systemic side effects of ocular medications. To diminish systemic absorption and minimize the side effects, it is important to occlude the puncta (Box 48-11).

Before the administration of ocular medications, the nurse warns the patient that blurred vision, stinging, and a burning sensation are symptoms that ordinarily occur after instillation and are temporary. Risk for interactions of the ocular medication with other ocular and systemic medications must be emphasized; therefore, a careful patient interview regarding the medications being taken must be obtained.

Emphasis must be placed on hand hygiene techniques before and after medication instillation. The tip of the eye drop bottle or the ointment tube must never touch any part of the patient's eye. The medication must be recapped immediately after each use. The patient or the caregiver at home should be asked to demonstrate actual eye drop or ointment instillation and punctal occlusion.

CHAPTER REVIEW

NCLEX-Style Review Questions

1. When the nurse is gathering a history from a patient newly diagnosed with glaucoma, the patient reports the following statement to the nurse. Which statement would be consistent with the patient's diagnosis? Select all that apply.
   a. "I began seeing halos around lights and had dim vision."
   b. "I had a difficult time matching my blue socks."
   c. "My eyes began to tear and itch."
   d. "I could see the street signs better than my hand."
   e. " I feel like I have tunnel vision, like I can't see on the sides"

2. Which statement by the patient diagnosed with viral conjunctivitis indicates that more teaching is necessary? Select all that apply.
   a. "I will wash my hands frequently."
   b. "I will use a washcloth to clean both my eyes, starting with the infected eye and moving to the uninfected eye."
   c. "I will avoid contact with other people until my symptoms are gone."
   d. "I will discard any leftover eye medication when the infection is gone."
   e. "I can return to work today because I started the treatment."

3. The nurse is caring for a baseball player who reports getting hit in the head with a baseball 1 hour prior to admission in the ED. What assessment requires immediate reporting? Select all that apply.
   a. Eye pain
   b. Flashing lights in the visual field
   c. Headache, pain intensity rated as 2/10
   d. Shade across the vision of one eye
   e. Superficial head abrasion

4. The patient with significant visual impairment requires assistance with ADLs. The nurse provides support when serving food by performing which action? Select all that apply.
   a. Leaving the tray on the patient's bedside table
   b. Serving hot food as quickly as possible
   c. Describing the food on the tray in terms of the face of a clock
   d. Ensuring that the food is warm and not hot
   e. Ensuring all food is soft

5. A patient is seen in emergency room with a intraocular foreign body (IOFB) from an explosion causing a blast injury to the eye and requiring emergency surgery. Postoperatively, which of the following interventions are expected? Select all that apply.
   a. Administer IV antibiotics as required
   b. Apply warm compresses to the periocular area
   c. Maintain the bed flat with sandbags at the sides of the head to prevent turning
   d. Ensure that the tetanus prophylaxis was administered (if appropriate)
   e. Allow the patient to proceed to radiology for MRI of the spine

REFERENCES AND SELECTED READINGS

References and selected readings associated with this chapter can be found on the website that accompanies the book. Visit **http://thepoint.lww.com/Honan3e** to access the references and other additional resources associated with this chapter.

CHAPTER 49

Nursing Management: Patients With Hearing and Balance Disorders

Carolynn Spera Bruno

Learning Objectives

After reading this chapter, you will be able to:

1. List the manifestations that may be exhibited by a person with a hearing disorder.
2. Identify ways to communicate effectively with a person with a hearing disorder.
3. Differentiate problems of the external ear from those of the middle ear and inner ear.
4. Compare the various types of surgical procedures used for managing middle ear disorders and appropriate nursing care.
5. Describe the different types of inner ear disorders, including the clinical manifestations, diagnosis, and management.

The delicate structure and function of the ear make early detection and accurate diagnosis of disorders necessary for preservation of normal hearing and balance. Medical surgical nurses will care for patients with hearing loss for a wide variety of reasons. This chapter addresses the assessment and management of hearing and balance disorders common to the adult population.

HEARING LOSS

According to the World Health Organization (WHO), it is estimated that 430 million people require hearing rehabilitation to correct disabling hearing loss; of these, 34 million are children (WHO, 2021). By 2050, it is projected that 2.5 billion people will have hearing loss and 700 million will require rehabilitation (WHO, 2021). *Healthy People 2030* launched a work group to address hearing and other sensory or communication disorders with objectives to improve screening, early detection, and treatment.

Pathophysiology

Hearing loss may be the result of a conduction problem, a sensorineural loss, a mix of both, or a psychogenic issue. Conductive hearing loss usually results from an external ear disorder, such as impacted cerumen (earwax), or a middle ear disorder, such as **otitis media** or otosclerosis (the formation of new bone around the base of the stapes [bone of the middle ear], resulting in progressive hearing loss [discussed later in this chapter]). In such instances, the efficient transmission of sound by air to the inner ear is interrupted. A sensorineural loss involves damage to the cochlea or vestibulocochlear nerve. Patients with mixed hearing loss have conductive loss and sensorineural loss, resulting from dysfunction of air and bone conduction. A functional (or psychogenic) hearing loss is nonorganic and unrelated to detectable structural changes in the hearing mechanisms; it is usually a manifestation of an emotional disturbance.

Many environmental factors have an adverse effect on the auditory system and gradually result in permanent **sensorineural hearing loss**. The most common is noise (unwanted and unavoidable sound), which has been identified as one of today's environmental hazards. The volume of noise that surrounds us daily has increased into a potentially dangerous source of physical and psychological damage.

Risk Factors

About 5% of the world population suffers from disabling hearing loss, with prevalence increasing across age groups (WHO, 2021). Box 49-1 summarizes risk factors.

The National Center for Health Statistics (2021) reports that 13% of adults aged 18 years and older have difficulty with hearing despite the use of hearing aids. Hearing loss is increased among males across all age groups (NCHS, 2021). Hearing difficulties are higher in those of advanced age, 65 years and above, and are associated with cognitive and functional decline (NCHS, 2021).

Among adults, high-frequency hearing loss due to exposure to loud sounds or noise at work or in leisure activities is prevalent. *Noise-induced hearing loss* (NIHL) refers to hearing

BOX 49-1

Risk Factors for Hearing Loss

- Family history of sensorineural impairment
- Congenital malformations of the cranial structure (ear)
- Low birth weight (less than 1,500 g)
- Use of ototoxic medications (e.g., gentamicin, loop diuretics)
- Recurrent ear infections
- Bacterial meningitis
- Chronic exposure to loud noises
- Chronic exposure to loud volume using headphones or earbuds
- Perforation of the tympanic membrane

loss that follows a long period of exposure to loud noise (e.g., heavy machinery, engines, artillery). Occupations such as carpentry, plumbing, and coal mining have the highest risk of noise-induced hearing loss. Recreational activities, such as listening to loud sounds through earbuds or headphones or exposure to loud concerts, as well as exposure to leaf blowers or lawnmowers, can place people at risk for NIHL.

Acoustic trauma refers to hearing loss caused by a single exposure to an extremely intense noise, such as an explosion. Usually, noise-induced hearing loss occurs at a high frequency (about 4,000 Hz). However, with continued noise exposure, the hearing loss can become more severe and include adjacent frequencies. The minimum noise level known to cause NIHL, regardless of duration, is about 85 to 90 dB.

Noise exposure is inherent in many jobs (e.g., mechanic, printer, pilot, musician) and hobbies, such as woodworking and hunting. The Occupational Safety and Health Administration (OSHA) requires that workers wear ear protection to prevent noise-induced hearing loss when exposed to noise above the legal limits. Ear protection against noise is the most effective preventive measure available. There are no medications that protect against NIHL; hearing loss is permanent because the hair cells in the organ of Corti are destroyed.

Clinical Manifestations and Assessment

Early manifestations of deafness and loss may include **tinnitus** (ringing sound in the ear in the absence of an external source), increasing inability to hear when in a group, and a need to turn up the volume of the television. Hearing loss or difficulty hearing also trigger changes in attitude, ability to communicate, awareness of surroundings, and even ability to protect oneself, affecting a person's quality of life. In a classroom, a student who is hard of hearing may appear uninterested and inattentive and may have failing grades. A person at home may feel isolated because of an inability to hear the clock chime, the refrigerator hum, the birds sing, or the traffic pass. A pedestrian who is hard of hearing may attempt to cross the street and fail to hear an approaching car. People with impaired hearing may miss parts of a conversation. Many people are unaware of their gradual hearing loss. Often, it is not the person with the hearing loss but the people with whom they are communicating who recognize the loss first (Box 49-2).

For various reasons, some people with hearing loss refuse to seek medical attention or wear a hearing aid. Others feel self-conscious wearing a hearing aid. Insightful people generally ask those with whom they are trying to communicate to let them know whether difficulties in communication exist. These attitudes and behaviors should be considered when counseling patients who need hearing assistance. The decision to wear a hearing aid is a personal one that is affected by these attitudes and behaviors.

BOX 49-2

Focused Assessment

Hearing Loss

Be alert for the following signs and symptoms:

- *Speech deterioration:* The person who slurs words or drops word endings, or who produces flat-sounding speech, may not be hearing correctly. The ears guide the voice, both in loudness and in pronunciation.
- *Fatigue:* If a person tires easily when listening to conversation or to a speech, this fatigue may be the result of straining to hear. Under these circumstances, the person may become irritable very easily.
- *Indifference:* It is easy for the person who cannot hear what others say to become depressed and disinterested in life in general.
- *Social withdrawal:* Not being able to hear what is going on may cause a person with hearing loss to withdraw from situations that might prove embarrassing.
- *Insecurity:* Lack of self-confidence and fear of mistakes create a feeling of insecurity in many people who are hard of hearing. No one likes to say the wrong thing or do anything that might appear foolish.
- *Indecision and procrastination:* Loss of self-confidence makes it increasingly difficult for a person experiencing hearing loss to make decisions.
- *Suspiciousness:* The person who is hard of hearing, often hears only part of what is being said and may suspect that others are talking about them or that portions of the conversation are deliberately spoken softly so that they will not hear them.
- *False pride:* The person with hearing loss may want to conceal the hearing loss and thus may pretend they are able to hear correctly.
- *Loneliness and unhappiness:* Although many people wish for quiet now and then, *enforced* silence can be boring and even somewhat frightening. People with hearing loss often feel isolated.
- *Tendency to dominate the conversation:* Some people with hearing loss tend to dominate the conversation, believing that as long as it is centered on them and they can control it, they are not as likely to make a mistake and become embarrassed.

Gerontologic Considerations

With aging, changes occur in the ear that may eventually lead to hearing deficits. Although few changes occur in the external ear, cerumen tends to become harder and drier, posing a greater chance of impaction. In the middle ear, the tympanic membrane may atrophy or become sclerotic. In the inner ear, cells at the base of the cochlea degenerate. A familial predisposition to sensorineural hearing loss is also seen, manifested by inability to hear high-frequency sounds, followed in time by the loss of middle and lower frequencies. The term **presbycusis** is used to describe this progressive hearing loss.

In addition to age-related changes, other factors can affect hearing in older adults, such as lifelong exposure to loud noises (e.g., jets, guns, heavy machinery, circular saws). Certain medications, such as aminoglycosides and aspirin, have ototoxic effects when kidney changes (e.g., in the older person) result in delayed medication excretion and increased levels of the medications in the blood. Although the use of quinine for treatment of leg cramps has been banned by the FDA, it was for a time widely used and is found in lower quantities in tonic water. Quinine can cause ringing in the ears or hearing loss. Psychogenic factors and other disease processes (e.g., diabetes mellitus [DM]) also may be partially responsible for sensorineural hearing loss.

When hearing loss occurs, proper evaluation and treatment are warranted. *Healthy People 2030* identified nine objectives for addressing sensory and communication disorders related to hearing loss, including screening and treatment associated with the use of hearing protection devices. *Healthy People 2030* provides specific target measures for addressing hearing disorder objectives. Resources are available in workplaces and in schools. The Individuals with Disabilities Education Act (IDEA) was developed to ensure that children and adults, including older adults, receive the same opportunities in the educational system as those without hearing impairment.

Care of older patients includes recognizing emotional reactions related to hearing loss, such as suspicion of others because of an inability to hear adequately; frustration and anger, with repeated statements such as, "I didn't hear what you said"; and feelings of insecurity because of the inability to hear the telephone or alarms. The Americans with Disabilities Act (ADA) of 1990 required that all emergency services are accessible to people who have text message telephones (TTYs). In addition, in 1998, the Department of Justice mandated that all 911 centers in the United States be accessible to people with Text Telephone (TTYs).

Medical Management

Implanted Hearing Devices

Three types of implanted hearing devices are commercially available: semi-implantable hearing device, fully implantable device, the cochlear implant, and the bone conduction device. Cochlear implants are for patients with little or no hearing and are discussed below. Bone conduction devices, which transmit sound through the skull to the inner ear, are used in patients with a conductive hearing loss if a hearing aid is contraindicated (e.g., those with chronic infection). The device is implanted postauricularly under the skin into the skull, and an external device—worn above the ear, not in the canal—transmits the sound through the skin. Currently there are two types of implantable hearing aid devices, semi-implantable and fully implantable. Semi-implantable devices consist of a magnetic component that is implanted in the auditory ossicle, a receiver, and a sound processor. Fully implantable middle ear devices consist of a sensor and sound processor along with a driver that is connected to the auditory ossicle.

The bone-anchored hearing aid (BAHA) may be fully or partially implantable. It is surgically implanted behind the ear in the mastoid area. The middle ear implantation (MEI) is implanted in the middle ear cavity and designed to move the bones directly rather than only amplifying sound. The BAHA is used for conductive or mixed hearing loss or unilateral sensorineural hearing loss, while the MEI is used for moderate to severe sensorineural hearing loss.

Cochlear Implant

A cochlear implant is an auditory prosthesis used for people with profound bilateral sensorineural hearing loss who do not benefit from conventional hearing aids. The hearing loss may be congenital or acquired. An implant does not restore normal hearing; rather, it amplifies sound so the person detects medium to loud environmental sounds and conversation. The implant provides stimulation directly to the auditory nerve, bypassing the nonfunctioning hair cells of the inner ear. The microphone and signal processor, worn outside the body, transmit electrical stimuli to the implanted electrodes. The electrical signals stimulate the auditory nerve fibers and then the brain, where they are interpreted.

Candidates for a cochlear implant, who are usually at least 1 year of age, are selected after careful screening by otologic history, physical examination, audiologic testing, x-rays, and psychological testing. Children who receive cochlear implants prior to 18 months of age, followed by speech therapy, achieve the greatest hearing, appreciation of sound and music, and development of speech as compared to older children who receive the implants (NIDCD, 2021). Criteria for choosing adults who may benefit from a cochlear implant include the following:

- Profound sensorineural hearing loss in both ears
- Inability to hear and recognize speech well with hearing aids
- No medical contraindication to a cochlear implant or general anesthesia
- Indications that being able to hear would enhance the patient's life (some candidates who are Deaf do not view themselves as having a disability that needs to be cured)

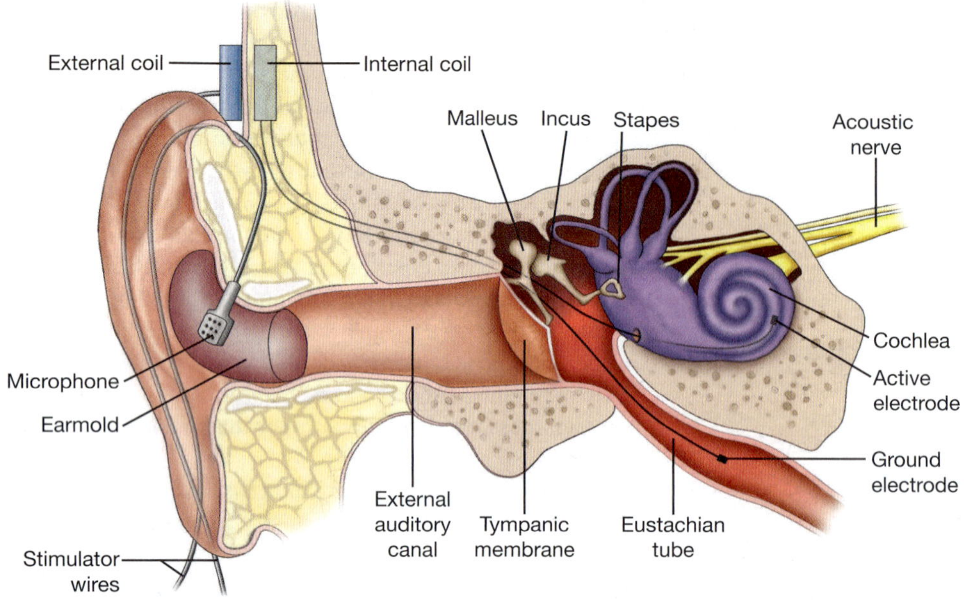

FIGURE 49-1 The cochlear implant. The internal coil has a stranded electrode lead. The electrode is inserted through the round window into the scala tympani of the cochlea. The external coil (the transmitter) is held in alignment with the internal coil (the receiver) by a magnet. The microphone receives the sound. The stimulator wire receives the signal after it has been filtered, adjusted, and modified so that the sound is at a comfortable level for the patient. Sound is passed by the external transmitter to the inner coil receiver by magnetic conduction and then is carried by the electrode to the cochlea.

Concept Mastery Alert

Conductive hearing loss is not an indication for cochlear implants. People with profound bilateral sensorineural hearing loss who do not benefit from conventional hearing aids do qualify as candidates for cochlear implants.

The surgery involves implanting a small receiver in the temporal bone through a postauricular incision and placing electrodes into the inner ear (Fig. 49-1). The microphone and transmitter are worn on an external unit. The patient undergoes extensive cochlear rehabilitation with the multidisciplinary team, which includes an audiologist and speech pathologist. Several months may be needed to learn to interpret the sounds heard. Children and adults who lost their hearing before they learned to speak take much longer to acquire speech. There are wide variations of success with cochlear implants, and there is also controversy about their use, especially among people in the Deaf community. Patients who have had a cochlear implant are cautioned that magnetic resonance imaging (MRI) will inactivate the implant; MRI is to be used only when there is no other diagnostic option.

Aural Rehabilitation

If hearing loss is permanent or cannot be treated by medical or surgical means, or if the patient elects not to undergo surgery, aural rehabilitation may be beneficial. The purpose of aural rehabilitation is to maximize the communication skills of the person who is Deaf. Aural rehabilitation includes auditory training, speech reading, speech training, and the use of hearing aids and hearing guide dogs.

Auditory training emphasizes listening skills so the person who is hearing impaired concentrates on the speaker. Speech reading (formerly known as *lip reading*) can help fill the gaps left by missed or misheard words. The goals of speech training are to conserve, develop, and prevent deterioration of current communication skills.

It is important to identify the type of hearing impairment a person has so that rehabilitative efforts can be directed at their particular need. Surgical correction may be all that is necessary to treat and improve a conductive hearing loss by eliminating its cause. With advances in hearing aid technology, amplification for patients with sensorineural hearing loss is more helpful than ever.

Hearing Aids

A hearing aid is a device through which speech and environmental sounds are received by a microphone, converted to electrical signals, amplified, and reconverted to acoustic signals. Many aids available for sensorineural hearing loss depress the low frequencies, or tones, and enhance hearing for the high frequencies. The evolution in technology has led to the availability of many smaller and more effective hearing aids. The vast majority of all hearing aids sold today are behind-the-ear, in-the-ear, or in-the-canal types (Table 49-1).

A hearing aid should be fitted according to the patient's needs (e.g., type of hearing loss, manual dexterity, and preferences) by a certified audiologist licensed to dispense hearing aids. Many states have consumer protection laws that allow the hearing aid to be returned after a trial use if the patient is not completely satisfied.

A hearing aid makes sounds louder, but it does not improve a patient's ability to discriminate words or understand speech. People who have low discrimination scores (i.e., 20%) on audiograms may derive little benefit from a hearing aid. Hearing aids amplify all sounds, including background noise, which may be disturbing to the wearer. Box 49-3 identifies additional problems associated with hearing aid use. Computerized hearing aids with digital noise

TABLE **49-1 Hearing Aids**

Site (and Range of Hearing Loss)	Advantages	Disadvantages
Body, usually on the trunk (mild–profound)	Separation of receiver and microphone prevents acoustic feedback, allowing high amplification. Generally used in a school setting.	Bulky; requires long wire, which may be cosmetically displeasing; some loss of high-frequency response.
Behind the ear (mild–profound)	Economical; powerful, with no long wires; easily used by children—adapts easily as the child grows, with only the ear mold needing replacement.	Large size, is visible.
In the ear (mild–moderately severe)	The in-the-ear (ITE) is custom molded fitting within the outer ear or partially filling the lower outer ear. One-piece custom fit to contour of ear; no tubes or cords; miniature microphone is located in the ear, which is a more natural placement; more cosmetically appealing due to easy concealment.	Smaller size limits output; patients who have arthritis or cannot perform tasks requiring good manual dexterity may have difficulty with the small size of the aid and/or its battery; can require more repair than the behind-the-ear aid.
In the canal (mild–moderately severe)	In-the-canal (ITC) are custom molded to fit partially in the ear canal and are less visible; completely-in-canal (CIC) or the mini CIC is molded to fit inside the ear canal and is the smallest and least visible type, so more cosmetically pleasing.	Smaller aids require good manual dexterity. CICs are prone to earwax building up and dampening the speaker. Small batteries have a short life and are difficult to handle. There is no volume control.

reduction are available to screen out undesirable background noise and allows amplification at certain programmed frequencies rather than at all frequencies. Adjunctive support to hearing aids include Bluetooth compatibility enabled hearing aids that wirelessly connect to mobile phones and other devices, smartphone applications, and assistive listening devices. Occasionally, depending on the type of hearing loss, binaural aids (i.e., one for each ear) may be indicated. Box 49-4 provides tips for hearing aid care.

Hearing Guide Dogs

Specially trained service dogs are available to assist the person with hearing loss. People who live alone are eligible to apply for a dog trained by, for example, International Hearing Dog, Inc. The dog reacts to the sound of a telephone, a doorbell, an alarm clock, a baby's cry, a knock at the door, a smoke alarm, or an intruder. The dog alerts its handler by physical contact; the dog then runs to the source of the noise. In public, the dog positions itself between the person

BOX 49-3

Hearing Aid Problems

Improper Aid Selection

Consumers often find they cannot adjust to the hearing aid, but there are many hearing aids on the market from which to choose. One consideration is sound amplification. The amplifier is a transformer that increases the amplitude of the electrical signal sent to the receiver. The receiver takes the sound and transmits it to the ear. A mismatch between receiver and amplifier increases sound distortion and may become intolerable to patients. The open mold provides a full shell or half shell instrument. Aids need to transmit sound well, fit comfortably, and be aesthetically pleasing.

Inadequate Amplification

- Dead batteries
- Cerumen in ear
- Cerumen or other material in mold
- Wires or tubing disconnected from aid
- Aid turned off or volume too low
- Improper mold
- Improper aid for degree of loss

Pain from Mold

- Improperly fitted mold
- Ear skin or cartilage infection
- Middle ear infection
- Ear tumor
- Unrelated conditions of the *temporomandibular* joint, throat, or larynx

Whistling Noise

- Loose ear mold
- Improperly made
- Improperly worn
- Worn out

BOX 49-4 **Patient Education**

Tips for Hearing Aid Care

Cleaning

- Behind the ear (BTE) hearing aids may be washed infrequently using soap and water. Ensure that the device is dried thoroughly after cleaning.
- It is recommended to use a soft cotton cloth to clean and remove dried cerumen for most hearing aid devices, such as in-the-ear hearing aids (ITE).
- Many hearing aid manufacturers advertise online information including cleaning directions.
- Clean the cannula with a small pipe cleaner-like device.
- Prevent complications by proper care of the ear device and keeping the ear canal clean and dry.

Malfunctioning

Inadequate amplification, a whistling noise, or pain from the mold can occur when a hearing aid is not functioning properly.

- Check for malfunctions:
  - Is the switch on properly?
  - Are the batteries charged and positioned correctly?
- If the hearing aid is still not working properly, notify the hearing aid dealer.
- If the unit requires extended time for repair, the dealer may lend you a hearing aid until the repair can be accomplished.

Recognizing Complications

Common medical complications include external otitis media and pressure ulcers in the external auditory canal.

- Be alert for signs and symptoms of these infections, including painful ear, especially when the external ear is touched; canal swelling; redness; difficulty hearing; pain radiating to the jaw area; and fever.
- If any of these symptoms are present, notify your health care provider for evaluation. You may need medication to treat infection, pain, or both.

with hearing impairment and any potential hazard that the person cannot hear, such as an oncoming vehicle or a loud, hostile person. In most states, a certified hearing guide dog is legally permitted access to public transportation, public eating places, and stores, including food markets.

Nursing Management

Communicating Effectively

Nurses who understand the different types of hearing loss are more successful in adopting a communication style to fit the needs and preferences of every patient. Trying to speak in a loud voice to a person who cannot hear high-frequency sounds only makes understanding more difficult. However, strategies such as talking into the less-impaired ear and using gestures and facial expressions can help (Box 49-5).

A major issue for many people who are Deaf or hearing-impaired is that they have other health problems that often do not receive attention, in large part because of communication barriers with their health care practitioners and the physical environment. The American Disabilities Act and Section 504 of the 1973 Rehabilitation Act mandates that people with disabilities have access to health care facilities and programs, thereby reducing disparity among individuals who are sensory and physically impaired. To meet the health care needs of patients who are hearing-impaired, practitioners are legally obligated to make accommodations for a patient's inability to hear. Providing interpreters for people who can communicate through sign language is essential in many situations so that the practitioner can effectively communicate with the patient.

During health care and screening procedures, the health care practitioner must be aware that patients who are Deaf or hearing-impaired have certain limitations and must document these in the electronic health record. They are unable to read lips, see a signer, or read written materials in the dark rooms required during some diagnostic tests. The same situation exists if the practitioner is wearing a mask or is not in the direct line of vision. Nurses and other health care practitioners must work with patients who are Deaf or hearing-impaired and their families to identify practical and effective means of communication and to ensure accommodations are made. Refer to agency protocols for assistance when communicating with individuals who are hearing-impaired during a health care visit.

Maintaining a Quiet Environment

Loud, persistent noise has been found to cause constriction of peripheral blood vessels, increased blood pressure and heart rate (because of increased secretion of adrenalin), and increased gastrointestinal activity, as well as to disturb patterns of sleep. Although research is needed to address the overall effects of noise on the human body, a quiet environment is generally more conducive to peace of mind (Box 49-6). A person who is ill typically feels more at ease when noise is kept to a minimum. The WHO sets noise guidelines for hospitals since noise negatively affects patient outcomes and staff performance (Berglund et al., 1999). Infrastructure designs, such as noiseless call bell systems and sound-masking floors and walls, represent attempts to decrease noise in hospitals.

CONDITIONS OF THE EXTERNAL EAR

CERUMEN IMPACTION

Cerumen normally accumulates in the external canal in various amounts and colors. Although wax does not usually need to be removed, impaction occasionally occurs.

BOX 49-5

Communicating with People Who are Deaf

For the person who is Deaf whose speech is difficult to understand:

- Consider how the person prefers to communicate with others. Do not assume that writing, gestures, or other means are the best or preferred technique.
- Consider if the person uses sign language. Interpreters are available in person or by video from the American Sign Language Inc., Interpreting Service (ASLI). These specialists provide the best means of communication and provide accurate, professional services.
- Devote full attention to what the person is saying. Look and listen—do not try to attend to another task while listening.
- Engage the speaker in conversation when it is possible for you to anticipate the replies. This enables you to become accustomed to any peculiarities in speech patterns.
- Try to determine the essential context of what is being said; you can often fill in the details from context.
- Do not try to appear as if you understand if you do not.
- If you cannot understand at all or have serious doubt about your ability to understand what is being said, have the person write the message rather than risk misunderstanding. Having the person repeat the message in speech after you know its content also aids you in becoming accustomed to the person's pattern of speech.
- Written communication is an excellent resource. Written material should be written at a third-grade level so that the majority of people can understand it.

For the person who is hearing-impaired who speech reads:

- If you need to get the patient's attention, wave your hand in front of their visual field.
- When speaking, always face the person and smile.
- Make sure your face is as clearly visible as possible. Locate yourself so that your face is well lighted; avoid being silhouetted against strong light. Do not obscure the person's view of your mouth in any way; avoid talking with any object held in your mouth.
- Be sure that the patient knows the topic or subject before going ahead with what you plan to say. This enables the person to use contextual clues in speech reading.
- Speak slowly and distinctly, pausing more frequently than you would normally.
- If you question whether some important direction or instruction has been understood, check to be certain that the patient has the full meaning of your message.
- If for any reason your mouth must be covered (as with a mask), and you must direct or instruct the patient, write the message.

BOX 49-6

Nursing Research

Bridging the Gap to Evidence-Based Practice

Jun, J., Kapella, M. C., & Hershberger, P. E. (2021). Non-pharmacological sleep interventions for adult patients in intensive care units: A systematic review. *Intensive Critical Care Nursing*, *67*, 103124. https://doi.org/10.1016/j.iccn.2021.103124

Purpose

The purpose is to synthesize and evaluate current nonpharmacologic sleep interventions for critically ill adult patients in intensive care units and provide recommendations for future studies of nonpharmacologic means of improving this population's sleep quality.

Design

A systematic review was conducted following PRISMA guidelines. Seven databases (CINAHL, PsycINFO, Embase, Medline, Cochrane Library, Web of Science, and Scopus) and three keywords (sleep, intervention, and intensive care unit) were employed. All possible combinations of the keywords and similar words were considered. Included studies were primary studies, involved adult intensive care unit patients, focused on nonpharmacologic sleep interventions, measured subjective and/or objective sleep quality, and were published in English between January 2010 and September 2020. The 20 included studies examined different types of nonpharmacologic sleep interventions involving use of earplugs, an eye mask, white noise, music, aromatherapy, massage, acupressure, light intensity, a sleep hygiene protocol, quiet time, and minimization of nursing care. Of 18 studies employing an experimental design, most reported that nonpharmacologic interventions improved sleep quality. All these interventions involved environmental factors or complementary relaxation strategies.

Findings

Nonpharmacologic sleep interventions can have a positive influence on sleep quality in critically ill patients, but more research is needed to determine their effectiveness. For example, white noise for auditory masking helped to improve sleep quality by decreasing the effects of ambient noise and inducing relaxation. One hour of white noise at 40–50 dB for 3 nights significantly improved sleep quality in the intervention group ($P = .008$), resulting in a significant difference in mean sleep quality compared with the control group ($P < .001$).

Nursing Implications

Critical illness and the unfamiliar ICU environment induce sleep disturbances in patients. Thus, to improve patients' sleep quality, routine nursing care activities should include assessing and enhancing modifiable components of the ICU environment. The most frequently used interventions were aromatherapy as a single intervention and combined earplugs and eye mask as a bundled intervention. Intensive care unit nurses should carefully evaluate the influence of all modifiable environmental factors that may affect patients' sleep quality. Greater attention should be paid to smell/odor (e.g., chemical agent, diarrhea, and vomit odors) and inappropriate room temperature (i.e., too hot or too cold) since they were disruptive factors affecting sleep quality not addressed by the interventions reported.

Clinical Manifestations and Assessment

Impaction causes **otalgia**, a sensation of fullness or pain in the ear, with or without a hearing loss. Accumulation of cerumen as a cause of hearing loss is especially significant in the older population. Attempts to clear the external auditory canal with cotton-tipped applicators, matches, hairpins, and other implements are dangerous because trauma to the skin, infection, and damage to the tympanic membrane can occur.

Medical and Nursing Management

Cerumen can be removed by irrigation, suction, or instrumentation. Unless the patient has a perforated eardrum or an inflamed external ear (i.e., **otitis externa**), gentle irrigation with tap water usually helps remove impacted cerumen, particularly if it is not tightly packed into the external auditory canal. For successful removal, the water stream must flow behind the obstructing cerumen to move it first laterally and then out of the canal. To prevent injury, the lowest effective pressure should be used. However, if the eardrum behind the impaction is perforated, water can enter the middle ear, producing acute pain, vertigo, and infection. If irrigation is unsuccessful, a trained health care provider can perform direct visual, mechanical removal on a cooperative patient.

Instilling a few drops of warmed water, saline, glycerin, or mineral oil into the ear canal for 30 minutes can soften cerumen before its removal. Cerumenolytic agents, such as peroxide in glyceryl (Debrox), are available; however, these compounds may cause an allergic dermatitis reaction. There is no high-quality evidence suggesting that one cerumenolytic is more effective than another. Water and saline are equally as effective as cerumenolytics, additionally no differences are seen in efficacy between oil-based and water-based treatments (Percy, 2021). Using any softening solution two or three times a day for several days is generally sufficient. If the cerumen cannot be dislodged by these methods, instruments such as an ear curette, aural suction, and a binocular microscope for magnification can be used by a provider with specialized training.

FOREIGN BODIES

Children may insert objects into their ear canal. Occasionally, beads or parts to toys are found in the external ear canal. Some objects are inserted intentionally into the ear by adults who may have been trying to clean the external canal or relieve itching. Insects may also enter the ear canal. In either case, the effects may range from no symptoms to profound pain and decreased hearing.

Removing a foreign body from the external auditory canal can be quite challenging and in unskilled hands may be dangerous. The object may be pushed completely into the bony portion of the canal, lacerating the skin and perforating the tympanic membrane. The three standard methods for skilled practitioners to remove foreign bodies are the same as those for removing cerumen: irrigation, suction, and instrumentation. The contraindications for irrigation are also the same. Foreign vegetable bodies and insects tend to swell; thus, irrigation is contraindicated. Usually, an insect can be dislodged by instilling mineral oil, which will suffocate the insect and allow it to be removed using alligator forceps or a loop-wired instrument. A referral to a specialist in Ears, Eyes, Nose Throat may be indicated. In some circumstances, the foreign body may have to be extracted in the operating room with the patient under general anesthesia.

CONDITIONS OF THE MIDDLE EAR

TYMPANIC MEMBRANE PERFORATION

Perforation of the tympanic membrane is usually caused by infection or trauma. Sources of trauma include skull fracture, explosive injury, or a severe blow to the ear. Less frequently, perforation is caused by foreign objects (e.g., cotton-tipped applicators, bobby pins, keys) that have been pushed too far into the external auditory canal. In addition to tympanic membrane perforation, injury to the ossicles and even the inner ear may result; thus, attempts by patients to clear the external auditory canal should be discouraged. During infection, the tympanic membrane can rupture if the pressure in the middle ear exceeds the atmospheric pressure in the external auditory canal.

Clinical Manifestations and Assessment

Symptoms of tympanic membrane perforation include whistling sounds upon sneezing and blowing the nose, reduced hearing, purulent drainage from ear(s), and/or otalgia.

Medical and Nursing Management

Although most tympanic membrane perforations heal spontaneously within weeks after rupture, some may take several months to heal. Some perforations persist because scar tissue grows over the edges of the perforation, preventing extension of the epithelial cells across the margins and healing. In the case of a head injury or temporal bone fracture, a patient is observed for evidence of cerebrospinal fluid: **otorrhea** or **rhinorrhea**, a clear, watery drainage from the ear or nose, respectively. If present, the nurse is aware that this represents an abnormal communication between the subarachnoid space and the tympanomastoid space, with a risk of a central nervous system (CNS) infection (refer to Chapter 44). While healing, the ear must be protected from water.

Perforations that do not heal on their own may require surgery. The decision to perform a **tympanoplasty** (surgical repair of the tympanic membrane) is usually based on the need to prevent potential infection from water entering the ear or the desire to improve the patient's hearing. Performed on an outpatient basis, tympanoplasty may involve a variety of surgical techniques. In all techniques, tissue (commonly from the temporalis fascia) is placed across the perforation to allow healing. Surgery is usually successful in closing the perforation

BOX 49-7

Patient Education

Self-Care after Middle Ear or Mastoid Surgery

Postoperative instructions for patients who have had middle ear and mastoid surgery may vary among otolaryngologists. General teaching guidelines for the patient may include:

- Take antibiotics and other medications as prescribed.
- Blow the nose gently, one side at a time, for 1 week after surgery.
- Sneeze and cough with the mouth open for a few weeks after surgery.
- Avoid heavy lifting (over 10 lb), straining, and bending over for a few weeks after surgery.
- Popping and crackling sensations in the operative ear are normal for approximately 3–5 weeks after surgery.
- Temporary hearing loss is normal in the operative ear due to fluid, blood, or packing in the ear.
- Report excessive or purulent ear drainage to the surgeon. Some slightly bloody or serosanguineous drainage from the ear is normal after surgery.
- Change the cotton ball in the ear as needed.
- Avoid getting water in the operative ear for 2 weeks after surgery. You may shampoo the hair 2–3 days postoperatively if the ear is protected from water by saturating a cotton ball with petroleum jelly (or some other water-insoluble substance) and loosely placing it in the ear. If the postauricular suture line becomes wet, pat (do not rub) the area and cover it with a thin layer of antibiotic ointment.

permanently and improving hearing. Postoperative instructions after middle ear surgery are found in Box 49-7.

OTOSCLEROSIS

Otosclerosis involves the stapes and is thought to result from the formation of new, abnormal spongy bone, especially around the oval window, with resulting fixation of the stapes. The efficient transmission of sound is prevented because the stapes cannot vibrate and carry the sound as conducted from the malleus and incus to the inner ear. Otosclerosis is more common in females and is frequently hereditary, and pregnancy may worsen it.

Clinical Manifestations and Assessment

Otosclerosis may involve one or both ears and manifests as a progressive conductive or mixed hearing loss. The patient may or may not complain of tinnitus. Otoscopic examination usually reveals a normal tympanic membrane. Bone conduction is better than air conduction on Rinne testing. The audiogram confirms conductive hearing loss or mixed loss, especially in the low frequencies.

Medical and Nursing Management

There is no known nonsurgical treatment for otosclerosis. Some providers prescribe sodium fluoride to slow the progression of the otosclerosis; however, its efficacy is still debated (Zafar et al., 2021). Amplification with a hearing aid also may help.

One of two surgical procedures may be performed, the stapedectomy or the stapedotomy. A stapedectomy involves removing the stapes superstructure and part of the footplate and inserting a tissue graft and a suitable prosthesis (Fig. 49-2). The surgeon drills a small hole into the footplate to hold a prosthesis. The prosthesis bridges the gap between the incus and the inner ear, providing better sound conduction. Stapes surgery is very successful; approximately 95% of patients experience resolution of conductive hearing loss. Balance disturbance or true vertigo, which rarely occurs in other middle ear surgical procedures, may occur during the postoperative period for several days. For a few patients, hearing aids may be needed after surgical treatment.

MIDDLE EAR MASSES

Other than **cholesteatoma** (middle ear or mastoid tumor), masses in the middle ear are rare. A glomus jugulare tumor is one that arises from the jugular vein and appears as a red blemish on or behind the tympanic membrane upon examination with an otoscope. Glomus jugulare tumors are rarely malignant; however, due to their location, treatment may be necessary to relieve symptoms. The treatment for glomus tumors is surgical excision, except in poor surgical candidates, in whom radiation therapy is used.

A facial nerve neuroma is a tumor on cranial nerve VII (the facial nerve). These types of tumors are usually not visible on otoscopic examination but are suspected when a patient presents with a facial nerve paresis. X-ray evaluation is used to identify the site of the tumor along the facial nerve. The treatment is surgical removal.

CONDITIONS OF THE INNER EAR

Almost 8 million American adults are affected by a chronic problem with balance, and an additional 2.4 million are affected by dizziness alone. Balance or vestibular problems are reported in approximately 9% of the adult population over 65 years of age. In the United States, there are 3 million older adults who are treated for falls in emergency departments each year (Moreland, Kakara, & Henry, 2020). Disorders of balance are a major cause of falls in the older population. Body balance is maintained by the cooperation of the muscles and joints of the body (proprioceptive system), the eyes (visual system), and the labyrinth (vestibular system). These areas send their information about equilibrium, or balance, to the brain (cerebellar system) for coordination and perception in the cerebral cortex. Since the brain obtains its blood supply from the cardiovascular system, arteriosclerosis can also cause a disturbance in balance. Likewise, impaired vision can have an impact on equilibrium. The vestibular apparatus of the inner ear provides feedback regarding the movements and the position of the head and body in space.

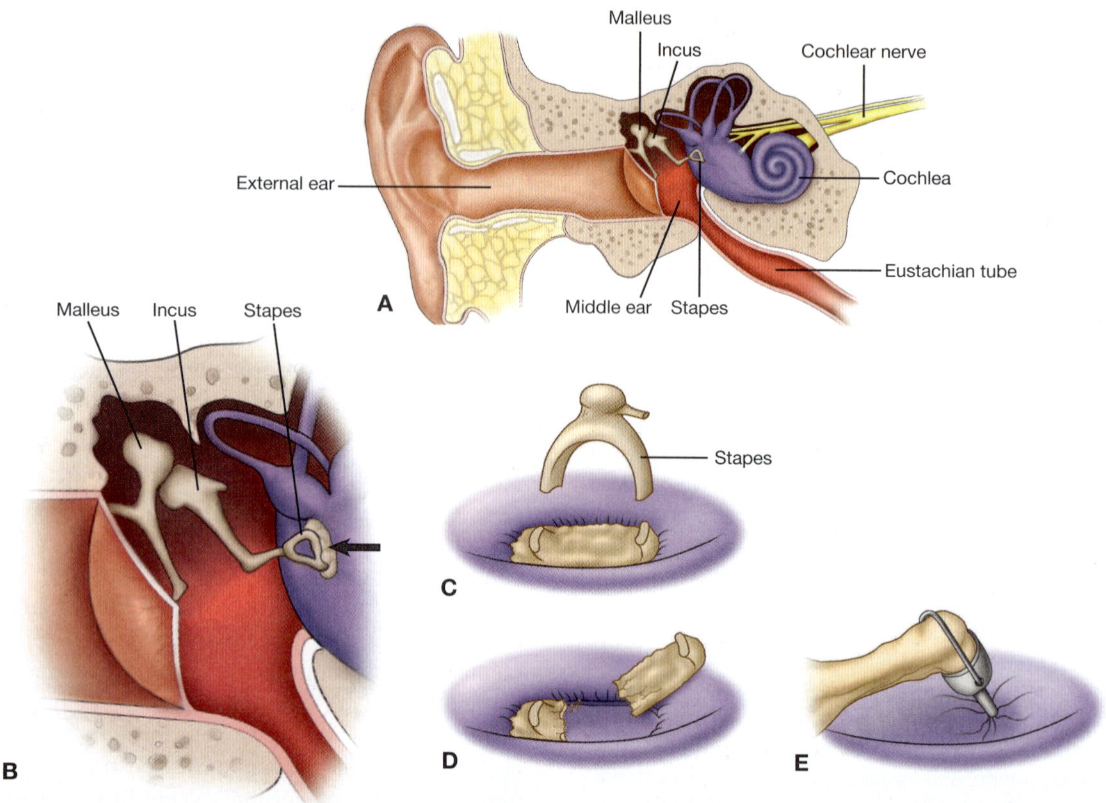

FIGURE 49-2 **Stapedectomy for otosclerosis. A. Normal anatomy. B.** ***Arrow*** **points to sclerotic process at the foot of the stapes. C. Stapes broken away surgically from its diseased base. The hole in the footplate provides an area where an instrument can grasp the plate. D. The footplate is removed from its base. Some otosclerotic tissue may remain, and tissue is placed over it. E. Robinson stainless-steel prosthesis in position.**

Patients and health care providers frequently use the term *dizziness* to describe any altered sensation of orientation in space. **Vertigo** is defined as the misperception or illusion of motion of the person or the surroundings. Most people with vertigo describe a spinning sensation or say they feel as though objects are moving around them. *Ataxia* is a failure of muscular coordination and may be present in patients with vestibular disease. Syncope, fainting, and loss of consciousness are not forms of vertigo and usually indicate disease in the cardiovascular system.

Nystagmus is an involuntary rhythmic movement of the eyes, and slight oscillation may be a normal variant. However, when nystagmus is pathologic, it is an ocular disorder associated with vestibular dysfunction. Nystagmus can be horizontal, vertical, or rotary and can be caused by a disorder in the central or peripheral nervous system.

MOTION SICKNESS

Motion sickness is a disturbance of equilibrium caused by constant motion. For example, it can occur aboard a ship, while riding on a merry-go-round or swing, or in the back seat of a car.

Clinical Manifestations and Assessment

Motion sickness manifests itself with diaphoresis, pallor, nausea, and vomiting caused by vestibular overstimulation. These manifestations may persist for several hours after the stimulation stops.

Medical and Nursing Management

Over-the-counter antihistamines, such as dimenhydrinate or meclizine hydrochloride, may provide some relief of nausea and vomiting by blocking the conduction of the vestibular pathway of the inner ear. Anticholinergic medications, such as scopolamine patches, may also be effective because they antagonize the histamine response. These must be replaced every few days. Common side effects, such as dry mouth and drowsiness, may occur. Potentially hazardous activities, such as driving a car or operating heavy machinery, should be avoided.

MÉNIÈRE DISEASE

Ménière disease is a disorder of the inner ear that causes vertigo, tinnitus, a feeling of fullness or pressure in the ear, and fluctuating hearing loss that significantly impacts a patient's quality of life (Koenen & Andaloro, 2021).

Pathophysiology

Ménière disease is believed to be the result of fluctuating pressure within the inner ear or the mixing of inner ear fluids. The membranous labyrinth of the inner ear contains a fluid called *endolymph*. The membranes can become dilated because of malabsorption of the fluid in the endolymphatic sac or a blockage in the drainage of fluid in the endolymphatic duct within the labyrinth. This dilation is termed **endolymphatic hydrops** or a ballooning of the membranous labyrinth, which results in increased pressure in the system or rupture of the inner ear membrane producing symptoms of Ménière disease.

Risk Factors

According to the National Institute on Deafness and Other Communication Disorders (NIDCD), Ménière disease has a prevalence of approximately 200 cases/100,000 persons in the United States (less than 0.2% of the population) (Hain, 2021). More common in adults, it has an average age of onset in the 40s, with symptoms usually beginning between 20 and 60 years of age. Ménière disease appears to be equally common in all genders and occurs bilaterally in about 20% of patients. About 50% of the patients who have Ménière disease have a positive family history of the disease. Patients who present at greater risk also include those with a recent viral illness or upper respiratory infection, allergy sufferers, smokers, those with stress or fatigue, alcohol users, and those who take aspirin.

Clinical Manifestations and Assessment

Symptoms of Ménière disease include fluctuating, progressive sensorineural hearing loss; tinnitus or a roaring sound; a feeling of pressure or fullness in the ear; and episodic, incapacitating vertigo, often accompanied by nausea and vomiting. These symptoms range in severity from a minor nuisance to extreme disability, especially if the attacks of vertigo are severe. At the onset of the disease, perhaps only one or two of the symptoms are manifested.

Some clinicians believe that there are two subsets of the disease, known as atypical Ménière disease: cochlear and vestibular. Cochlear Ménière disease is recognized as a fluctuating, progressive sensorineural hearing loss associated with tinnitus and aural pressure in the absence of vestibular symptoms or findings. Vestibular Ménière disease is characterized as the occurrence of episodic vertigo associated with aural pressure but no cochlear symptoms. Patients may experience either cochlear or vestibular disease symptoms; however, eventually all of these symptoms develop.

Vertigo is usually the most troublesome complaint related to Ménière disease. A careful history is taken to determine the frequency, duration, severity, and character of the patient's vertigo attacks. Vertigo may last minutes to hours, possibly accompanied by nausea or vomiting. Diaphoresis and a persistent feeling of imbalance or disequilibrium may awaken patients at night. Some patients report that these feelings last for days. However, they usually feel well between attacks. Hearing loss may fluctuate, with tinnitus and aural pressure waxing and waning with changes in hearing. These feelings may occur during or before attacks, or they may be constant. Long periods of remission may occur.

Physical examination findings are usually normal, with the exception of those of cranial nerve VIII. Sounds from a tuning fork (Weber test) may lateralize to the unaffected ear. Using a Rinne test, the normal finding of air conduction remaining greater than bone conduction usually is found. An audiogram typically reveals a sensorineural hearing loss in the affected ear. This can be in the form of a "Pike's Peak" pattern, which looks like a hill or mountain. A sensorineural loss in the low frequencies occurs as the disease progresses. The electronystagmogram may be normal or may show reduced vestibular response. Imaging using magnetic resonance may also prove useful in diagnosis of CNS lesions.

Medical Management

Most patients with Ménière disease can be successfully treated with diet and medication. Many patients can control their symptoms by adhering to a low-sodium (2,000 mg/day) diet with no caffeine, alcohol, or smoking. Box 49-8 describes dietary guidelines that may be useful in Ménière disease. The amount of sodium is one of many factors that regulate the balance of fluid within the body. Sodium and fluid retention disrupts the delicate balance between endolymph and perilymph in the inner ear. Medications to control allergies or improve blood circulation of the inner ear prove helpful. Eliminating tobacco use and stress reduction can also decrease the severity of symptoms. Psychological evaluation may be indicated, as comorbidity of vertigo and anxiety is well established in the literature. A plan of nursing care for a patient with vertigo is available online at http://thepoint.lww.com/Honan3e.

BOX 49-8 **Pearls for Practice: Nutrition**

Dietary Guidelines for Patients with Ménière Disease

Advise patients to:

- Limit foods high in salt or sugar. Be aware of foods with hidden salts and sugars.
- Eat meals and snacks at regular intervals to stay hydrated. Missing meals or snacks may alter the fluid level in the inner ear.
- Eat fresh fruits, vegetables, and whole grains. Limit the amount of canned, frozen, or processed foods with high sodium content.
- Drink plenty of fluids daily. Water, milk, and low-sugar fruit juices are recommended. Limit intake of coffee, tea, and soft drinks. Avoid caffeine because of its diuretic effect.
- Limit alcohol intake. Alcohol may change the volume and concentration of the inner ear fluid and may worsen symptoms.
- Avoid monosodium glutamate (MSG), which may increase symptoms.
- Avoid aspirin and aspirin-containing medications. Aspirin may increase tinnitus and dizziness.

Pharmacologic Therapy

Pharmacologic therapy for Ménière disease consists of antihistamines, such as meclizine, which suppress the vestibular system. Benzodiazepines, such as diazepam, may be used in acute instances to help control vertigo. Antiemetics, such as promethazine suppositories, help control the nausea, vomiting, and vertigo because of their antihistamine effect. Betahistine hydrochloride and diuretic therapy may reduce the severity of symptoms by lowering the pressure in the endolymphatic system. Intake of foods containing potassium (e.g., bananas, cantaloupe, oranges) is necessary if the patient takes a diuretic that causes potassium loss. There is no scientific basis for the use of vasodilators, such as nicotinic acid, papaverine hydrochloride, and methantheline bromide, to alleviate the symptoms, but they are often used in conjunction with other therapies. Corticosteroids are useful in reducing edema of the labyrinth and inflammation in order to improve healing of the inner ear structures.

Surgical Management

Although most patients respond well to conservative therapy, some continue to have disabling attacks of vertigo. If these attacks reduce their quality of life, patients may elect to undergo chemical treatment or surgery for relief. Vestibular rehabilitation can assist to restore function in patients with permanent disorder. Surgical procedures such as labyrinthectomy, which leads to a complete hearing loss in the affected side; vestibular neurectomy; or endolymphatic sac decompression may be considered.

Endolymphatic Sac Decompression

Endolymphatic sac decompression, or shunting, theoretically equalizes the pressure in the endolymphatic space. A shunt or drain is inserted in the endolymphatic sac through a postauricular incision. Many otolaryngologists favor this procedure as a first-line surgical approach to treat the vertigo of Ménière disease because it is relatively simple and safe and can be performed on an outpatient basis.

Middle and Inner Ear Perfusion

Ototoxic medications, such as streptomycin or gentamicin, can be administered to patients by infusion into the middle and inner ear. These medications are used to destroy vestibular function and decrease vertigo. The success rate for eliminating vertigo is about 85%, but the risk of significant hearing loss is high. After the procedure, many patients have a period of imbalance that lasts several weeks.

Intraotologic Catheters

In an attempt to deliver medication directly to the inner ear, catheters are being developed to provide a conduit from the outer ear to the inner ear. The route of the catheter is from the external ear canal through or around the tympanic membrane and to the round window niche or membrane. Medicinal fluids can be placed against the round window for a direct route to the inner ear fluids.

Potential uses of these catheters include treatment for sudden hearing loss and various disorders causing intractable vertigo. Future applications may include tinnitus and slowly progressing sensorineural hearing loss. Intratympanic injections of ototoxic medications for round window membrane diffusion can be used to decrease vestibular function. Established surgical techniques can be used for the patient with vertigo who has not responded to medical or physical therapeutic modalities.

Vestibular Nerve Sectioning

Vestibular nerve sectioning provides the greatest success rate (98%) in eliminating the attacks of vertigo. It can be performed by a translabyrinthine approach (i.e., through the hearing mechanism) or in a manner that can conserve hearing (i.e., suboccipital or middle cranial fossa), depending on the degree of hearing loss. Most patients with incapacitating Ménière disease have little or no effective hearing. Cutting the nerve prevents the brain from receiving input from the semicircular canals. This procedure requires a brief overnight hospital stay.

TINNITUS

Tinnitus is a symptom of an underlying disorder of the ear that is associated with hearing loss. This condition affects approximately 10% of the U.S. population between 40 and 70 years of age. The severity of tinnitus may range from mild to severe. Patients describe tinnitus as a roaring, buzzing, or hissing sound in one or both ears. Numerous factors may contribute to the development of tinnitus, including several ototoxic substances (Box 49-9). Underlying disorders that contribute to tinnitus may include thyroid disease, hyperlipidemia, vitamin B_{12} deficiency, psychological disorders

BOX 49-9 Selected Ototoxic Substances

- *Diuretics:* Ethacrynic acid, furosemide, acetazolamide
- *Chemotherapeutic agents:* Cisplatin, nitrogen mustard
- *Antimalarial agents:* Quinine, mefloquine, chloroquine
- *Anti-inflammatory agents:* Salicylates (aspirin), indomethacin
- *Chemicals:* Alcohol, arsenic
- *Aminoglycoside antibiotics:* Amikacin, gentamicin, kanamycin, netilmicin, neomycin, streptomycin, tobramycin
- *Other antibiotics:* Erythromycin, minocycline, polymyxin B, vancomycin
- *ACE inhibitors:* Enalapril, moexipril, ramipril
- *Acetic acids:* Diclofenac, indomethacin, ketorolac
- *Alpha blockers:* Doxazosin
- *Antiarrhythmics:* Flecainide, propafenone, quinidine, tocainide
- *Calcium-channel blockers:* diltiazem, nifedipine, nisoldipine
- *H_1-blockers:* Cetirizine, fexofenadine
- *Metals:* Gold, mercury, lead

(e.g., depression, anxiety), fibromyalgia, otologic disorders (Ménière disease, acoustic neuroma), and neurologic disorders (head injury, multiple sclerosis).

A physical examination should be performed to determine the cause of tinnitus. Diagnostic testing determines if hearing loss is present. An audiograph speech discrimination test or a tympanogram may be used to help determine the cause. Some forms of tinnitus are irreversible; therefore, patients may need teaching and counseling about ways of adjusting to their treatment and dealing with tinnitus in the future.

BENIGN PAROXYSMAL POSITIONAL VERTIGO

Benign paroxysmal positional vertigo (BPPV) is a brief period of incapacitating vertigo that occurs when the position of the patient's head is changed with respect to gravity, typically by placing the head back with the affected ear turned down. The onset is sudden and followed by a predisposition for positional vertigo, usually for hours to weeks but occasionally for months or years. Other symptoms may include lightheadedness, blurred vision, and nausea and vomiting.

Pathophysiology

BPPV is thought to be due to the disruption of debris in the labyrinth, termed **otoconia** (small crystal particles of calcium carbonate that detach and float in the endolymph and cause symptomatology). This is frequently stimulated by head trauma, infection (particularly of the respiratory tract), or other events. Precipitating factors include sneezing or coughing, or the vertigo may be induced by any change in head positioning. Bed rest is recommended for patients with acute symptoms.

Clinical Manifestations and Assessment

Diagnosis of BBPV is performed after an ear examination, audiogram, and test of nerve responses and use of the Dix–Hallpike test, also called the Nylen–Barany test. The test involves making the patient undergo a rapid change from an erect seated position to a supine position with the head hanging over the edge of the examination table to the left, right, or center. Dizziness and peripheral vertigo will be elicited with the affected ear pointing downward. The eyes are examined for a brief period for nystagmus present while the head is maintained in a provoking position, which also commonly accompanies vertigo. Nystagmus and vertigo may be present for less than 30 seconds during maneuvers.

Medical and Nursing Management

Repositioning techniques can be used to treat vertigo, such as the Epley maneuver. The maneuver is designed to reposition the canalith and involves quick movements of the head. The noninvasive procedure is performed by placing the patient in a sitting position and turning the head to a 45-degree angle on the affected side and 30 to 45 degrees backward. Then the patient is quickly moved to the supine position. The procedure is repeated, tilting the head to the opposite side. The patient must not lie flat for 48 to 72 hours after repositioning to prevent the particles from reentering the posterior canal. The procedure is safe, inexpensive, and easy to perform.

Patients with acute vertigo are treated with medications that target vertigo and its related symptoms of nausea, vomiting, and anxiety. Vestibular suppressants that are commonly used originate from classes of anticholinergics (scopolamine), antihistamines (meclizine, dimenhydrinate), and benzodiazepines. Meclizine is often the drug of choice, with patients treated for a 1- to 2-week course of therapy. Antiemetic medications, such as phenothiazines, are used to treat nausea. Meclizine has both vestibular suppressant and antiemetic effects.

Vestibular rehabilitation can be used in the management of vestibular disorders. This strategy promotes active use of the vestibular system through an interdisciplinary team approach, including medical and nursing care, stress management, biofeedback, vocational rehabilitation, and physical therapy. A physical therapist prescribes balance exercises that help the brain compensate for the impairment to the balance system.

OTOTOXICITY

A variety of medications may have adverse effects on the cochlea, vestibular apparatus, or cranial nerve VIII (vestibulocochlear, also known as acoustic or auditory nerve). All but a few, such as aspirin and quinine, cause irreversible hearing loss. At high doses, aspirin toxicity can produce bilateral tinnitus. IV medications, especially the aminoglycosides, are the most common cause of ototoxicity, and they destroy the hair cells in the organ of Corti (see Box 49-9).

To prevent loss of hearing or balance, patients receiving potentially ototoxic medications should be counseled about the side effects of these medications. These medications should be used with caution in patients who are at high risk for complications, such as children, older individuals, pregnant patients, patients with kidney or liver problems, and patients with current hearing disorders. Blood levels of the medications should be monitored, and patients receiving long-term IV antibiotics should be monitored with an audiogram twice each week during therapy.

Pearls for Practice

Many intravenous medications require careful monitoring of the highest (peak) and lowest (trough) concentration of the drug in the patient's blood to ensure that the dosage is within the therapeutic range and to prevent toxicity. The trough is drawn just before a drug is scheduled to be given, whereas the peak is drawn after the drug is administered (typically 30 minutes).

ACOUSTIC NEUROMA

Acoustic neuromas develop in 1 of every 10,000 people per year. These neuromas account for 5% to 10% of all intracranial tumors and seem to occur with equal frequency in males and females of any age, although most occur during middle age.

Pathophysiology

Acoustic neuromas are slow-growing, benign tumors of cranial nerve VIII, usually arising from the Schwann cells of the vestibular portion of the nerve. Most acoustic tumors arise within the internal auditory canal and extend into the cerebellopontine angle to press on the brainstem, possibly destroying the vestibular nerve.

Clinical Manifestations and Assessment

The most common assessment findings of patients with acoustic neuromas are unilateral tinnitus and hearing loss with or without vertigo or balance disturbance. If the tumor is large, the trigeminal nerve may be involved, resulting in facial paresthesia, hypesthesia (sensitivity to touch), and discomfort. Facial paresis and disturbance in taste result from facial nerve involvement, which occurs less commonly. It is important to identify asymmetry in audiovestibular test results so that further workup can be performed to rule out an acoustic neuroma. MRI with a paramagnetic contrast agent (i.e., gadolinium) is the imaging study of choice. If the patient is claustrophobic or cannot undergo an MRI for other reasons, or if the scan is unavailable, a computed tomography (CT) scan with contrast dye is performed; however, MRI is more sensitive than CT in delineating a small tumor.

Medical and Nursing Management

Surgical removal of acoustic tumors is the treatment of choice because these tumors do not respond well to radiation or chemotherapy. Because treatment of acoustic tumors crosses several specialties, the interdisciplinary treatment approach involves a neurologist and a neurosurgeon. The objective of the surgery is to remove the tumor while preserving facial nerve function. Most acoustic tumors have damaged the cochlear portion of cranial nerve VIII, and hearing is impaired. In these patients, the surgery is performed using a translabyrinthine approach, and the hearing mechanism is destroyed. If hearing is still good before surgery, a suboccipital or middle cranial fossa approach to removing the tumor may be used. This procedure exposes the lateral third of the internal auditory canal and preserves hearing.

Complications of surgery include facial nerve paralysis, cerebrospinal fluid leakage, meningitis, and cerebral edema. Death from acoustic neuroma surgery is rare. Recurrence is not common after surgery, but tinnitus may worsen in some patients (Greene & Al-Dhahir, 2021).

CHAPTER REVIEW

NCLEX-Style Review Questions

1. A 56-year-old patient who is hard of hearing is scheduled for a colonoscopy. Which nursing action is most appropriate in performing patient education prior to the procedure? Select all that apply.
   a. Face the patient directly, smile, and speak slowly.
   b. Continue to administer medications while educating the patient.
   c. Nod to make up for awkward silence, even if you don't know what is being said.
   d. Use only gestures to communicate the highlights of content to be covered.
   e. If you are wearing a mask, and you need to instruct the patient, write the message.

2. The nurse caring for the patient with Ménière disease restricts the following foods in the dietary plan. Select all that apply.
   a. Coffee
   b. Wine
   c. Baked potato
   d. Canned soup
   e. Milk

3. During preoperative teaching, the 25-year-old patient receiving cochlear implants states, "I will be able to fully regain my hearing with the implants." What is the nurse's best response to the patient?
   a. "The implants will assist you to detect medium to loud environmental sound and conversation rather than restoring normal hearing."
   b. "The implant will assist you to restore normal hearing fully."
   c. "The implants will be immediately effective."
   d. "The implant will require minimal rehabilitation in order for you to recognize sounds."
   e. "If an MRI is needed, the new implants allow them to be performed"

4. How might a patient with tinnitus describe to the nurse how they hear sounds? Select all that apply.
   a. Sputtering
   b. Muffled

c. Loud
d. Buzzing
e. Whooshing sound

5. Which of the following factors are associated with ototoxicity? Select all that apply.
a. Co-administration of multiple antibiotics including aminoglycosides, such as gentamycin
b. Elevated serum drug levels
c. Administering IV medications slowly and at a low dose
d. Use of antineoplastic medications particularly those using platinum, such as cisplatin
e. Combining known ototoxic pharmacologic agents

REFERENCES AND SELECTED READINGS

References and selected readings associated with this chapter can be found on the website that accompanies the book. Visit **http://thepoint.lww.com/Honan3e** to access the references and other additional resources associated with this chapter.

UNIT FOURTEEN

Problems Related to Integumentary Function

A 22-year-old college student has come to the burn center via helicopter after a house fire, with full-thickness (third-degree) burn of arms, hands, chest, and abdomen that will need autografting.

- **Describe the nursing management of this patient in the emergent phase of burn injury.**
- **Discuss graft site care and donor site care following an autograft.**
- **What are the long-term complications for this patient?**

CHAPTER 50

Nursing Assessment: Integumentary Function

Captain Patina S. Walton-Battle

Learning Objectives

After reading this chapter, you will be able to:

1. Identify the structures and functions of the skin.
2. Differentiate the composition and function of each skin layer: epidermis, dermis, and subcutaneous tissue.
3. Describe the normal aging process of the skin and skin changes common in older patients.
4. List appropriate questions that help elicit information during an assessment of the skin.
5. Describe the components of physical assessment that are most useful when examining the skin, hair, and nails.
6. Identify and describe primary and secondary skin lesions and their pattern and distribution.
7. Discuss common skin tests and procedures used in diagnosing skin and related disorders.

The skin is the largest organ in the body and makes up approximately 12% of body weight. The skin's structure serves as the body's initial barrier against pathogens, UV light, chemicals, and mechanical injury. It also regulates body temperature, maintains normal fluid and electrolyte balance, detects sensation, and protects from infection and the environment (Yousef et al., 2022). Nurses care for patients with burns, skin infections, surgical wounds, chronic wounds, and secondary skin abnormalities associated with systemic disease; this chapter provides the knowledge necessary to assess, diagnose, and manage skin abnormalities and describes when to seek referrals to the primary care provider or specialist.

ANATOMIC AND PHYSIOLOGIC OVERVIEW

The integumentary system is composed of multiple subunits that work simultaneously. The system includes the epidermis, dermis, hypodermis, associated sweat and sebaceous glands, hair, and nails (Kim & Dao, 2022).

Anatomy of the Skin

The skin is composed of three layers: epidermis (outermost layer), dermis (inner layer), and hypodermis (innermost layer) (Fig. 50-1). Five distinct layers compose the epidermis; from innermost to outermost they are the stratum basale, stratum spinosum, stratum granulosum, stratum lucidum, and stratum corneum (Yousef et al., 2022). Each layer becomes more differentiated (i.e., mature and with more specific functions) as it rises from the basal stratum germinativum layer to the outermost stratum corneum layer. The stratum lucidum is found only on the skin of the palms and soles (Yousef et al., 2022). The basement membrane zone lies at the interface between the epidermis and the dermis and strongly attaches these layers to each other. It also serves as a support for the avascular epidermis (Sullivan & Myers, 2022). The dermis, which is the thickest layer of skin, is composed principally of collagen, a fibrous protein synthesized primarily by fibroblast cells, which are important in remodeling and repairing skin. This layer is split up into two regions, the papillary dermis and reticular dermis. This connective tissue layer contains nerve endings, sensory receptors, capillaries, and elastic fibers.

Epidermis

The epidermis consists of continuously dividing cells covered on the surface by dead cells that were originally deeper in the dermis but were pushed upward by the newly developing, more differentiated cells underneath. This external layer is almost completely replaced every 3 to 4 weeks. The dead cells contain large amounts of **keratin**, an insoluble, fibrous protein that forms the outer barrier of the skin and has the

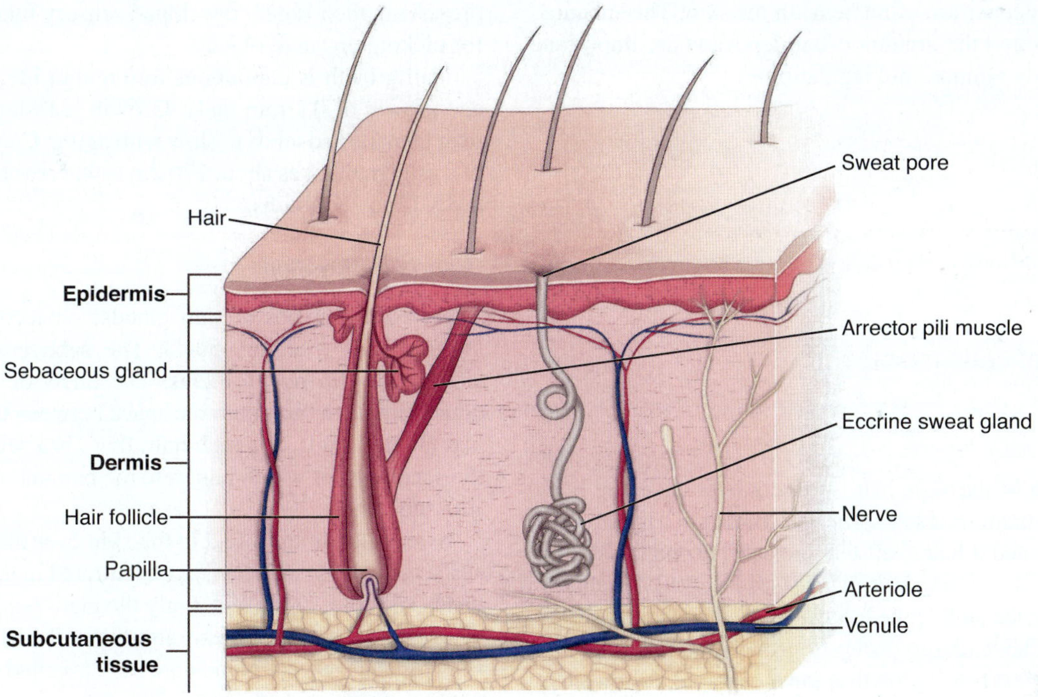

FIGURE 50-1 **Anatomic structures of the skin.**

capacity to repel pathogens and prevent excessive fluid loss from the body. Keratin is the principal hardening ingredient of the hair and nails.

Melanocytes are the special cells of the epidermis that are primarily involved in producing the pigment **melanin**, which colors the skin and hair. Most of the skin of dark-skinned people and the darker areas of the skin on light-skinned people (e.g., the areola) contain larger amounts of this pigment. Albinism is associated with a lack of melanin and is discussed later in the chapter. Production of melanin is controlled by a hormone secreted from the hypothalamus of the brain called *melanocyte-stimulating hormone.* Melanin provides natural protection against the harmful effects of ultraviolet light; however, it does not provide complete protection from the sun's damaging rays.

Two other types of cells are common to the epidermis: Merkel and Langerhans cells. **Merkel cells** are receptors that transmit stimuli to the axon through a chemical synapse and therefore are associated with the sense of touch. **Langerhans cells** are accessory cells of the afferent immune system that play a role in cutaneous (skin) immune system reactions. These cells process invading antigens and transport the antigens to the lymph system to activate the T lymphocytes.

The junction of the epidermis (basement membrane zone, BMZ) and dermis is an area of many undulations and furrows called **rete ridges**. This junction anchors the epidermis to the dermis and permits the free exchange of essential nutrients between the two layers. If the BMZ (dermal–epidermal junction) is damaged, it must reconstruct to successfully achieve skin integrity (Aleemardani et al., 2021).

Dermis

The dermis makes up the largest portion of the skin, providing strength and structure. It is composed of two layers: papillary and reticular. The papillary dermis lies directly beneath the epidermis and is composed primarily of fibroblast cells capable of producing one form of collagen, a component of connective tissue. The reticular layer lies beneath the papillary layer and also produces collagen and elastic bundles. The dermis is also made up of blood and lymph vessels, nerves, sweat and sebaceous glands, and hair roots. The dermis is often referred to as the "true skin." It is especially thick on the palms and soles, while thin over the eyelids and scrotum; thus, it is not surprising that in conditions of fluid volume excess, patients develop edema in thin skinned areas, resulting in periorbital and scrotal edema. An infection of the dermis that spreads rapidly within the skin and subcutaneous structures is termed *cellulitis.* It is usually caused by *Staphylococci* or *Streptococci* and presents with redness, warmth, swelling, and tenderness, usually of the limbs.

Hypodermis

The subcutaneous tissue, or hypodermis, is the innermost layer of the skin. It is primarily adipose tissue, which provides a cushion between the skin layers, muscles, and bones. It promotes skin mobility, molds body contours, and insulates the body. Fat is deposited and distributed according to the person's sex and in part accounts for the difference in body shape between males and females. Overeating results in increased deposition of fat beneath the skin. The subcutaneous tissues and the amount of fat deposited are important factors in body temperature regulation.

Pearls for Practice

An area of skin indurated (hardened) from collagen deposits in the cutaneous and subcutaneous tissue as a result of chronic inflammation is termed sclerosis. Examples include keloid formation, stasis dermatitis, and scleroderma.

Anatomy of Hair, Nails, and Glands of the Skin

Hair

An outgrowth of the skin, hair is present over the entire body except for the palms and soles. The hair consists of a root formed in the dermis and a hair shaft that projects beyond the skin. It grows in a cavity called a *hair follicle* (see Fig. 50-1). Proliferation of cells in the bulb of the hair causes the hair to form.

Hair follicles undergo cycles of growth and rest. The rate of growth varies; beard growth is the most rapid, followed by hair on the scalp, axillae, thighs, and eyebrows. The growth or **anagen phase** may last up to 6 years for scalp hair, whereas the telogen or resting phase lasts approximately 4 months. During telogen, hair is shed from the body. The hair follicle recycles into the growing phase spontaneously, or it can be induced by plucking out hairs. Growing and resting hairs can be found side by side on all parts of the body. About 90% of the 100,000 hair follicles on a normal scalp are in the growing phase at any one time, and 50 to 100 scalp hairs are shed each day. In conditions in which inflammation causes damage to the root of the hair, regrowth is possible. However, if inflammation causes damage to the hair follicle, stem cells are destroyed and the hair does not grow.

Hair in different parts of the body serves different functions. The hairs of the eyes (i.e., eyebrows and lashes), nose, and ears filter out dust, microbes, and airborne debris. Hair color is supplied by various amounts of melanin within the hair shaft. Gray or white hair reflects the loss of pigment. Hair quantity and distribution can be affected by endocrine conditions. For example, Cushing syndrome causes **hirsutism** (excessive hair growth), especially in females; hypothyroidism (i.e., underactive thyroid) causes coarse hair; while hyperthyroidism (i.e., overactive thyroid) is associated with fine hair. In many cases, chemotherapy and radiation therapy cause hair thinning or weakening of the hair shaft, resulting in partial or complete **alopecia** (hair loss) from the scalp and other parts of the body.

Nails

On the dorsal surface of the fingers and toes, a hard, transparent plate of keratin, called the *nail*, overlies the skin. The nail grows from its root, which lies under a thin fold of skin called the *cuticle*. The nail protects the fingers and toes by preserving their highly developed sensory functions, such as for picking up small objects.

Nail growth is continuous throughout life, with an average growth of 0.1 mm daily. Growth is faster in fingernails than toenails and tends to slow with aging. Complete renewal of a fingernail takes about 170 days, whereas toenail renewal takes 12 to 18 months.

Glands of the Skin

There are two types of skin glands: sebaceous glands and sweat glands (see Fig. 50-1). The **sebaceous glands** are associated with hair follicles. The ducts of the sebaceous glands empty **sebum** onto the space between the hair follicle and the hair shaft. For each hair, there is a sebaceous gland, the secretions of which lubricate the hair and render the skin soft and pliable.

Sweat glands are found in the skin over most of the body surface, but they are heavily concentrated in the palms of the hands and soles of the feet. Only the glans penis, the margins of the lips, the external ear, and the nail bed are devoid of sweat glands. Sweat glands are subclassified into two categories: eccrine and apocrine.

The eccrine sweat glands are found in all areas of the skin. Their ducts open directly onto the skin surface. The thin, watery secretion called *sweat* is produced in the basal, coiled portion of the eccrine gland and is released into its narrow duct.

The apocrine sweat glands are larger than eccrine sweat glands and are located in the axillae, anal region, scrotum, and labia majora. Their ducts generally open onto hair follicles. The apocrine glands become active at puberty. In females, they enlarge and recede with each menstrual cycle. Apocrine glands produce a milky sweat that is sometimes broken down by bacteria to produce the characteristic underarm odor.

Functions of the Skin

Protection

Skin acts as a primary protective barrier against external agents such as heat, light, infection, and injury. Also, it regulates the temperature of the body and the exchange of fluids. Skin contains a vast network of nerves, glands, and vessels that enable sensing of heat, touch, pressure, and pain, and is also a crucial interface that regulates body temperature and stores water and lipids to maintain a healthy metabolism (Pissarenko & Meyers, 2020). The thickened skin of the palms and soles protects against the effects of the constant trauma that can occur in these areas.

The stratum corneum, the outer layer of the epidermis, provides the most effective barrier to epidermal water loss to maintain a homeostatic environment and penetration of environmental factors, such as chemicals, microbes, and insect bites. Various lipids are synthesized in the stratum corneum and are the basis for the barrier function of this layer. These are long-chain lipids that are better suited than phospholipids for water resistance. The presence of these lipids in the stratum corneum creates a relatively impermeable barrier for water egress and for the entry of toxins, microbes, and other substances that come in contact with the surface of the skin.

Some substances do penetrate the skin but meet resistance in trying to move through the channels between the cell layers of the stratum corneum. Microbes and fungi, which are part of the body's normal flora, cannot penetrate unless there is a break in the skin barrier.

Sensation

The receptor endings of nerves in the skin allow the body to constantly monitor the conditions of the immediate environment. The primary functions of the receptors in the skin are to sense temperature, pain, light touch, and pressure (or heavy touch). Different nerve endings respond to each of the different stimuli. Although the nerve endings are distributed over the entire body, they are more concentrated in some areas than in others. For example, the fingertips are more densely innervated than the skin on the back.

Fluid Balance

The stratum corneum, the outermost layer of the epidermis, has the capacity to absorb water, thereby preventing an excessive loss of water and electrolytes from the internal body and retaining moisture in the subcutaneous tissues. When skin is damaged, as occurs with a severe burn, large quantities of fluids and electrolytes may be lost rapidly, possibly leading to circulatory collapse, shock, and death.

The skin is not completely impermeable to water. Small amounts of water continuously evaporate from the skin's surface. This evaporation, called *insensible perspiration*, amounts to approximately 600 mL daily in a normal adult. Insensible water loss varies with the body and ambient temperature. In a person with a fever, the fluid loss increases. If the fever is above 38°C (100.4°F), insensible loss increases by 10% per every degree rise (Kamat, 2019). In addition, insensible loss occurs during surgery. For example, it is estimated that in open abdominal surgery, there is a loss of 1 mL/kg/hr fluid occurs when the abdomen is open (Kamat, 2019).

Thermoregulation

The body continuously produces heat as a result of the metabolism of food, which produces energy. This heat is dissipated primarily through the skin.

Evaporation from the skin aids heat loss by conduction. Heat is conducted through the skin into water molecules on its surface, causing the water to evaporate. The water on the skin surface may be from insensible perspiration, sweat, or the environment.

Under normal conditions, metabolic heat production is balanced by heat loss, and the internal temperature of the body is maintained constant at approximately 37°C (98.6°F). The rate of heat loss depends primarily on the surface temperature of the skin, which is a function of the blood flow to the skin. Increased blood flow to the skin results in more heat delivered to the skin and a greater rate of heat loss from the body. In contrast, decreased skin blood flow decreases the skin temperature and helps conserve heat for the body. When the temperature of the body begins to fall, as occurs on a cold day, the blood vessels of the skin constrict, thereby reducing heat loss from the body.

Sweating is another process by which the body can regulate the rate of heat loss. Sweating does not occur until the core body temperature exceeds 37°C (98.6°F), regardless of skin temperature. In extremely hot environments, the rate of sweat production may be as high as 1 L/hr. Under some circumstances (e.g., emotional stress), sweating may occur as a reflex and may be unrelated to the need to lose heat from the body.

Vitamin Synthesis

Skin exposed to ultraviolet light can convert substances necessary for synthesizing vitamin D (cholecalciferol). Vitamin D is essential for the normal absorption of calcium and phosphorous, which are required for healthy bones (Biga et al., 2019). Vitamin D is essential for preventing osteoporosis and rickets, a condition that causes bone deformities and results from a deficiency of vitamin D, calcium, and phosphorus (Box 50-1). Also, normal skin contains high concentrations of vitamin C, which supports important and well-known functions, stimulating collagen synthesis and assisting in antioxidant protection against UV-induced photodamage (Gold Standard, 2022; Pullar et al., 2017).

Immune Response Function

Recent research has confirmed a definite action of **Langerhans cells** (specialized cells in the skin) in the recognition, uptake, processing, and presentation of antigens to sensitized T lymphocytes (James et al., 2020). These specialized cells are of the monocyte-macrophage lineage (cells that are responsible for defending against diverse pathogens) and originate in bone marrow. They are important in the induction of delayed-type sensitivity as well as humoral immunity (refer to Chapter 35). Langerhans cells, along with others, play a pivotal role in the pathogenesis of atopic dermatitis and other allergic diseases (Boguniewicz & Leung, 2020).

COVID-19

Coronavirus disease-19 (COVID-19) is an ongoing global pandemic caused by the "severe acute respiratory syndrome coronavirus 2" (SARS-CoV-2), which was isolated for the first time in Wuhan (China) in December 2019. COVID-19-associated cutaneous manifestations are classified into six main clinical patterns: (1) urticarial rash, (2) confluent (a rash pattern where separate rashes of the same kind, merge together, appearing as one rash) erythematous/

BOX 50-1

Nursing Research

Bridging the Gap to Evidence-Based Practice

An, S., Kim, K., Moon, S., Ko, K. -P., Kim, I., Lee, J. E., & Park, S. K. (2021). Indoor tanning and the risk of overall and early-onset melanoma and non-melanoma skin cancer: Systematic review and meta-analysis. *Cancers*, *13*(23), 5940. https://doi.org/10.3390/cancers13235940

Purpose

The authors investigated the association between indoor tanning and early-onset melanoma and nonmelanoma skin cancer (NMSC). A systematic review of the literature published until July 2021 was performed using PubMed, EMBASE, and MEDLINE. In this study, a total of 54 studies were examined in regard to the association between indoor tanning device use and overall and early-onset skin cancer. The study found that indoor tanning is associated with increased risk for early-onset melanoma and NMSC and has a dose–response relationship with first exposure at an early age and the frequency of exposure. Therefore, this study emphasizes the importance of avoiding indoor tanning risk in younger adults.

Findings

The findings provide evidence that supports policies regulating the excessive use of tanning devices, especially in the vulnerable younger population, to reduce the additional risk of skin cancer.

Nursing Implications

This study supports the evidence for prevention policies regulating modifiable behaviors to reduce the risk between indoor tanning and melanoma risk and suggests that some guidelines or regulations on the use of tanning devices in younger adults should be actively formulated. Nurses can play a pivotal role in educational efforts.

maculopapular/morbilliform (fine, discrete maculopapules) rash, (3) papulovesicular exanthem (skin rash), (2) chilblain (painful inflammation of small blood vessels in the skin)-like acral (refers to extremities) pattern, (5) livedo (reddish, purplish) reticularis (weblike)/racemosa (irregular)-like pattern, and (6) purpuric "vasculitic" (inflamed blood vessels in the skin) pattern. Although COVID-19-associated skin manifestations have been increasingly reported, their pathophysiologic mechanisms are continuously being extensively explored (Genovese et al., 2021).

Pearls for Practice

Localized opening of the normally tight endothelial junctions leads to interstitial edema in the deep layers of the skin and subcutaneous tissue of the face, tongue, hands, face, and genitalia. Occasionally, the tongue or pharynx can be involved. It may be related to allergy or idiopathic in nature. Histamine that is contained in mast cells is released with a variety or immunologic, nonimmunologic, physical, and/or chemical stimuli. The released histamine causes hyperpermeability of the microvessels, which allows fluid to leak out into affected areas and causes the characteristic appearance. Nurses observe for the tense swelling of the lips that develops rapidly. Angioedema is frequently associated with an allergic reaction and may present with hives. If shortness of breath is also noted, the medical provider must be contacted immediately as severe swelling of the airway and tongue can be life threatening.

Gerontologic Considerations

The skin undergoes many physiologic changes associated with normal aging. A lifetime of excessive sun exposure, systemic diseases, and poor nutrition can increase the range of skin problems and the rapidity with which they appear. In addition, certain medications (e.g., antihistamines, antibiotics, diuretics) are photosensitizing and increase the damage that results from sun exposure. The outcome is an increasing vulnerability to injury and to certain diseases. Skin problems are common among older people. Refer to Table 50-1 for skin changes in older individuals.

Many skin changes and lesions are part of normal aging. Recognizing these lesions enables the examiner to assist the patient to feel less anxious about changes in skin. Box 50-2 summarizes some changes that are expected to appear as the skin ages. These are normal and require no special attention unless the skin becomes infected or irritated.

ASSESSMENT

Some conditions may subject the patient to a protracted illness, leading to feelings of depression, frustration, self-consciousness, poor self-image, and rejection. Itching and skin irritations, which are features of many skin diseases, may be a constant annoyance. These discomforts may result in loss of sleep, anxiety, and depression, all of which reinforce the general distress and fatigue that frequently accompany skin disorders.

For patients suffering such physical and psychological discomforts, the nurse needs to provide understanding, explanations of the problem, appropriate instructions related to treatment, nursing support, and encouragement. It is imperative to overcome any aversion that may be felt when caring for patients with unattractive skin disorders. The nurse should show no sign of hesitancy when approaching patients with skin disorders. Such hesitancy only reinforces the psychological trauma of the disorder.

Because patients with skin conditions may be viewed negatively by others, these patients may become distraught and avoid interaction with people. Skin conditions can lead to disfigurement, isolation, job loss, and economic hardship.

TABLE **50-1** **GERONTOLOGIC CONSIDERATIONS/Age-Related Changes of the Skin**

Structural Changes	Associated Physical Findings
Thinning at the junction of the dermis and epidermis results in fewer anchoring sites between the two skin layers, which means that even minor injury or stress to the epidermis can cause it to shear away from the dermis	Increased vulnerability of aged skin to trauma
The epidermis and dermis thin and flatten	Wrinkles, sags, and overlapping skin folds
Loss of the subcutaneous tissue substances of elastin, collagen, and fat	Decreased protection and cushioning of underlying tissues and organs, decreased muscle tone, and loss of the insulating properties of fat
Cellular replacement slows as a result of aging, and there is thinning of the dermal layers	Skin becomes fragile and transparent
The blood supply to the skin also changes with age. Vessels, especially the capillary loops, decrease in number and size	Vascular changes are associated with delayed wound healing
Sweat and sebaceous glands decrease in number and functional capacity	Dry and scaly skin
Reduced hormonal levels of androgens	Associated with declining sebaceous gland function
Hair growth gradually diminishes, especially over the lower legs and dorsum of the feet. Thinning is common in the scalp, axilla, and pubic areas	Decreased hair growth, hair loss
Photoaging (damage from excessive sun exposure)	Profound wrinkling; increased loss of elasticity; mottled, pigmented areas; cutaneous atrophy; and benign or malignant lesions

Health History

During the health history interview, the nurse asks about any family and personal history of skin allergies; allergic reactions to food, medications, and chemicals; previous skin problems; and skin cancer. The names of cosmetics, soaps, shampoos, and other personal hygiene products are obtained if there have been any recent skin problems noticed with the use of these products. The health history contains specific information about the onset, signs and symptoms, location, and duration of any pain, itching, rash, or other discomfort experienced by the patient. The nurse inquires about tattoos because they involve the injection of ink into the dermis of the skin and are associated with an increased risk for blood-borne disease, skin infections, and allergic reactions. Box 50-3 lists selected questions useful in obtaining appropriate information.

BOX 50-2 **Benign Changes in Skin for Older Adults**

- Cherry angiomas (bright red "moles")
- Diminished hair, especially on scalp and pubic area
- Dyschromias (color variations):
  - Solar lentigo (liver spots)
  - Melasma (dark discoloration of the skin)
  - Lentigines (freckles)
- Neurodermatitis (itchy spots)
- Seborrheic keratoses (crusty brown "stuck-on" patches)
- Spider angiomas (network of dilated capillaries radiating from a central arteriole)
- Telangiectasias (red marks on skin caused by stretching of the superficial blood vessels)
- Wrinkles (a small fold, ridge, or crease in the skin)
- Xerosis (dryness)
- Xanthelasma (yellowish waxy deposits on upper and lower eyelids)
- Ichthyosis (fish scale appearance of the skin)
- Senile purpura (purple or red bruises that have an irregular shape)

Unfolding Patient Stories: VB • Part 2

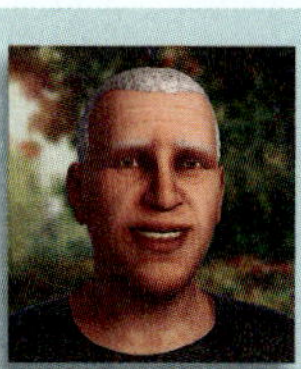

Recall from Chapter 1 that V.B. has chronic obstructive pulmonary disease (COPD) and spends most of the day in a recliner chair smoking and has a poor nutritional intake due to shortness of breath. V.B. is admitted to the hospital with COPD exacerbation. What are the factors related to the diagnosis? What background information can influence skin breakdown? Describe the skin assessment performed by the nurse.

Care for V.B. and other patients in a realistic virtual environment: ***vSim** for Nursing* (thepoint.lww.com/vSimMedicalSurgical). Practice documenting these patients' care in DocuCare (thepoint.lww.com/DocuCareEHR).

BOX 50-3

Health History Related to Skin Disorders

Patient history relevant to skin disorders may be obtained by asking the following questions:

- When did you first notice this skin problem? (Also investigate duration and intensity)
- Has it occurred previously?
- Are there any other symptoms?
- What site was first affected?
- What did the rash or lesion look like when it first appeared?
- Where and how fast did it spread?
- Do you have any itching, burning, tingling, or crawling sensations?
- Is there any loss of sensation?
- Is the problem worse at a particular time or season?
- How do you think it started?
- Do you have a history of hay fever, asthma, hives, eczema, or allergies?
- Who in your family has skin problems or rashes?
- Did the eruptions appear after certain foods were eaten? Which foods?
- When the problem occurred, had you recently consumed alcohol?
- What relation do you think there may be between a specific event and the outbreak of the rash or lesion?
- What medications are you taking?
- What topical medication (ointment, cream, salve) have you put on the lesion (including over-the-counter medications)?
- What skin products or cosmetics do you use?
- What is your occupation?
- What in your immediate environment (plants, animals, chemicals, infections) might be precipitating this disorder? Is there anything new, or are there any changes in the environment?
- Does anything touching your skin cause a rash?
- How has this affected you (or your life)?
- Is there anything else you wish to talk about in regard to this disorder?

Physical Assessment

Assessment of the skin involves the entire skin area, including the mucous membranes, scalp, hair, and nails. The skin is a reflection of a person's overall health, and alterations commonly correspond to disease in other organ systems. Inspection and palpation are techniques commonly used in examining the skin. The room must be well lighted and warm. A penlight may be used to highlight lesions. The patient completely disrobes and is adequately draped. Gloves are worn during skin examination if a rash or lesions are to be palpated.

The general appearance of the skin is assessed by observing color, temperature, moisture or dryness, skin texture (rough or smooth), lesions, vascularity, mobility, and the condition of the hair and nails. Skin turgor, possible edema, and elasticity are assessed by palpation.

Assessing Color

Skin color varies from person to person and ranges from ivory to deep brown to almost pure black. The skin of exposed portions of the body, especially in sunny, warm climates, tends to be more pigmented than the rest of the body.

Almost every process that occurs on the skin causes some color change. For example, **hypopigmentation** may be caused by a fungal infection, eczema, or **vitiligo** (loss of skin color in patches); **hyperpigmentation** can occur after sun injury, as a result of aging, or with disease processes such as Addison because of stimulation of melanocyte-stimulating hormone (refer to Chapter 30). The vasodilation that occurs with fever, sunburn, and inflammation produces a pink or reddish hue to the skin. Pallor is an absence of or a decrease in normal skin color and vascularity and is best observed in the conjunctivae or around the mouth. Assessing for pallor in the palms and soles of patients with dark skin may be helpful (Bickley et al., 2021).

In people with dark skin, melanin is produced at a faster rate and in larger quantities than in people with light skin. Healthy dark skin has a reddish base or undertone. The buccal mucosa, tongue, lips, and nails normally are pink. Dark pigment responds with discoloration after injury or inflammation, and patients with dark skin more often experience postinflammatory hyperpigmentation than do those with lighter skin. The hyperpigmentation eventually fades but may require months to a year to do so. Table 50-2 provides an overview of color changes in people who are light-skinned and dark-skinned.

Concept Mastery Alert

Pallor can best be determined by examining conjunctivae or around the mouth. Nail beds are not necessarily a reliable area when assessing for pallor.

In general, people with dark skin suffer the same skin conditions as those with light skin. They are less likely to have skin cancer but more likely to have keloid or scar formation and disorders resulting from occlusion or blockage of hair follicles.

Lifting the Lens: Our Textbooks and Your Preparation

In a review of four medical textbooks on dermatology, there was significant over-representation of images on lighter-skinned patients as compared to people of color (Reilley-Luther et al., 2020). This impacts students' ability to recognize dermatologic disorders and their preparation for practice with

TABLE **50-2 Color Changes in Light and Dark Skin**

Etiology	Light Skin	Dark Skin
Pallor		
Anemia: Decreased hematocrit Shock: Decreased perfusion, vasoconstriction	Generalized pallor	Brown skin appears yellow-brown, dull; black skin appears ashen gray, dull. (Observe areas with least pigmentation: conjunctivae, mucous membranes)
Local arterial insufficiency	Marked localized pallor (lower extremities, especially when elevated)	Ashen gray, dull; cool to palpation
Albinism: Total absence of pigment melanin	Whitish pink	Tan, cream, white
Vitiligo: A condition characterized by destruction of the melanocytes in circumscribed areas of the skin (may be localized or widespread)	Patchy, milky white spots, often symmetric bilaterally	Same
Cyanosis		
Increased amount of unoxygenated hemoglobin	Dusky blue	Dark but dull, lifeless; only severe cyanosis is apparent in skin. (Observe conjunctivae, oral mucosa, nail beds)
Central: Chronic heart and lung diseases cause arterial desaturation	Bluish discoloration of skin, mucous membranes, and nail beds	
Peripheral: Exposure to cold, anxiety	Nail beds dusky	
Erythema		
Hyperemia: Increased blood flow through engorged arterial vessels, as in inflammation, fever, alcohol intake, blushing	Red, bright pink	Purplish tinge, but difficult to see because epidermal melanin may alter disease presentation by masking erythema. (Palpate for increased warmth with inflammation, taut skin, and hardening of deep tissues)
Polycythemia: Increased red blood cells, capillary stasis	Ruddy blue in face, oral mucosa, conjunctivae, hands, and feet	Well concealed by pigment. (Observe for redness in lips)
Carbon monoxide poisoning	Bright, cherry red in face and upper torso	Cherry red nail beds, lips, and oral mucosa
Stasis dermatitis (venous stasis): Poor venous return in the lower extremities causing hemosiderin staining and cracking of the skin (skin breakdown) that causes stasis ulcers or venous ulcers	Brown or rusty discoloration of the skin resulting from a buildup of hemosiderin (iron-containing pigment derived from the breakdown of hemoglobin) in the interstitial fluid	May be more difficult to detect signs of venous insufficiency such as hemosiderin staining (reddish, brown color) in melanin-rich skin
Venous disease	Edema, hyperpigmentation surrounding the skin (reddish or brown due to hemosiderin), warmth at feet with palpable pulses (exception if no coexisting arterial disease)	Edema, hyperpigmentation surrounding the skin (reddish or brown due to hemosiderin), warmth at feet with palpable pulses (exception if no coexisting arterial disease)

(*continued*)

TABLE **50-2 Color Changes in Light and Dark Skin (*continued*)**

Etiology	Light Skin	Dark Skin
Jaundice		
Increased serum bilirubin concentration (>2.5–3 mg/dL) due to liver dysfunction or hemolysis, as after severe burns or some infections	Yellow first in sclerae, hard palate, and mucous membranes; then over skin	Check sclerae for yellow near limbus; do not mistake normal yellowish fatty deposits in the periphery under eyelids for jaundice. (Jaundice is best noted at junction of hard and soft palate, on palms)
Carotenemia: Increased level of serum carotene from ingestion of large amounts of carotene-rich foods	Yellow-orange tinge in forehead, palms and soles, and nasolabial folds, but no yellowing in sclerae or mucous membranes	Yellow-orange tinge in palms and soles
Uremia: Kidney failure causes retained urochrome pigments in the blood	Orange-green or gray overlying pallor of anemia; may also have ecchymoses and purpura	Easily masked. (Rely on laboratory and clinical findings)
Brown-Tan		
Addison disease: Cortisol deficiency stimulates increased melanin production	Bronzed appearance, an "external tan"; most apparent around nipples, perineum, genitalia, and pressure points (inner thighs, buttocks, elbows, axillae)	Easily masked. (Rely on laboratory and clinical findings)
Café-au-lait spots: Caused by increased melanin pigment in basal cell layer	Tan to light brown, irregularly shaped, oval patch with well-defined borders	Often not visible in a person with very dark skin

diverse populations. Students and practitioners need examples to learn, and current resources are inadequate to serve patients. One solution is Project Improving Medicine's Power to Address Care and Treatment (IMPACT), which is a global effort to reduce disparities in medicine and highlight the tools used to bridge gaps of knowledge and improve care. One of their aims is to create images and information at the point of care to reduce biases in medicine by bridging knowledge gaps. Refer to https://www.visualdx.com/projectimpact for current resources. In addition, the society is "committed to the education of health care providers and the general public on dermatologic health issues related to skin of color," and their website includes a resource library (https://skinofcolorsociety.org/skin-of-color-dermatology-textbooks/nd).

Erythema

Erythema is redness of the skin caused by the congestion of capillaries. In dark-skinned persons, erythema is difficult to perceive (James et al., 2020). To determine possible inflammation, the skin is palpated for increased warmth and for smoothness (i.e., edema) or hardness (i.e., intracellular infiltration).

Cyanosis

Cyanosis is the bluish discoloration that results from a lack of oxygen in the blood. It appears with shock or with respiratory or circulatory compromise. In people with light skin, cyanosis manifests as a bluish hue to the lips, fingertips, and nail beds (Fig. 50-2). In people who are dark-skinned, the skin may appear blue and dull or assume a gray hue. The term *central cyanosis* refers to desaturation of oxygen in the blood; this is reflected in the mucous membranes and skin, whereas *peripheral cyanosis* implies increased oxygen extraction from the blood because of sluggish blood flow, or vasoconstriction related to exposure to cold environments, which is reflected in the extremities. The nurse assesses the patient for additional indications of decreased tissue perfusion, including cold, clammy skin; a rapid, thready pulse; and rapid, shallow respirations. The conjunctivae of the eyelids are examined for pallor and **petechiae**.

Pearls for Practice

Cyanosis is a late sign and symptom of hypoxemia, as 5 g of hemoglobin (normal level is 15 g/dL)

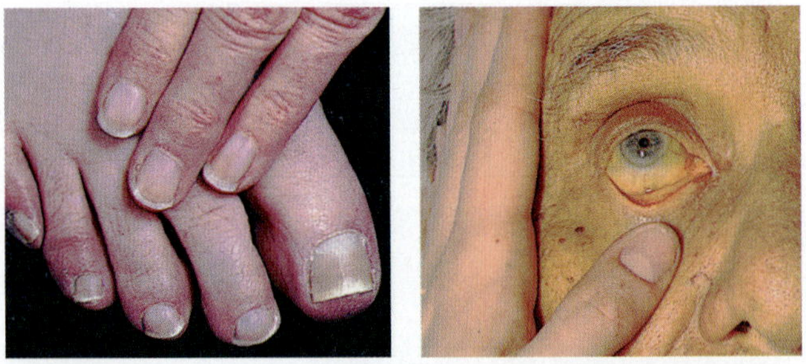

FIGURE 50-2 **Examples of skin color changes: the bluish tint of cyanosis (*left*) and the yellow hue of jaundice (*right*).**

are desaturated before cyanosis is evident. In cases of carbon monoxide poisoning, the level of carboxyhemoglobin does not affect color; therefore, the patient may be profoundly hypoxemic without evidence of cyanosis.

Jaundice

Jaundice, a yellowing of the skin, is directly related to elevations in serum bilirubin and is often first observed in the sclerae and mucous membranes (see Fig. 50-2). The term *icterus* is used to describe yellowing of the sclerae (white of the eyes).

Striae

The nurse assesses for striae (stretch marks), which occur when the elastic fibers in the reticular dermis rupture. Striae are seen in conditions of weight gain, such as pregnancy and obesity, in muscle building, with prolonged use of oral or topical corticosteroids, or in Cushing syndrome (increased adrenal cortical activity) (see Chapter 30).

Assessing Rash

In instances of pruritus (i.e., itching), the patient is asked to indicate which areas of the body are involved. The skin is then stretched gently to decrease the reddish tone and make the rash more visible. Pointing a penlight laterally across the skin may highlight the rash, making it easier to observe. The differences in skin texture are then assessed by running the tips of the fingers lightly over the skin. The borders of the rash may be palpable. The patient's mouth and ears are included in the examination (sometimes rubeola, or measles, causes a red cast to appear on the ears). The patient's temperature is assessed, and the lymph nodes are palpated.

Assessing Skin Lesions

Skin lesions are the most prominent characteristics of dermatologic conditions. They vary in size, shape, and cause and are classified according to their appearance and origin. Skin lesions can be described as primary or secondary. Primary lesions are the initial lesions and are characteristic of the disease itself. Secondary lesions result from external causes, such as scratching, trauma, infections, or changes caused by wound healing. Depending on the stage of development, skin lesions are further categorized according to type and appearance (Table 50-3). The degree of pigmentation of the patient's skin may affect the appearance of a lesion. In patients with darker skin, lesions may be black, maroon, purple, or gray instead of the tan or red seen in patients with light skin.

TABLE **50-3 Primary and Secondary Skin Lesions**

Lesion	Description	Examples
Primary Lesions		
Macule, patch 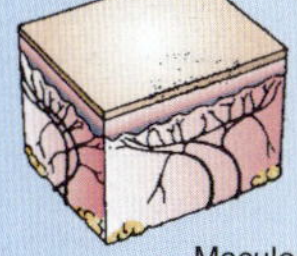 Macule 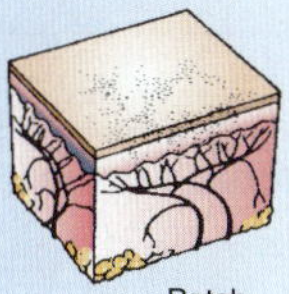 Patch	Flat, nonpalpable skin color change (color may be brown, white, tan, purple, red) • *Macule:* less than 1 cm, circumscribed border • *Patch:* greater than 1 cm, may have irregular border	Freckles, flat moles, petechia, rubella, vitiligo, port wine stains, ecchymosis
Papule, plaque 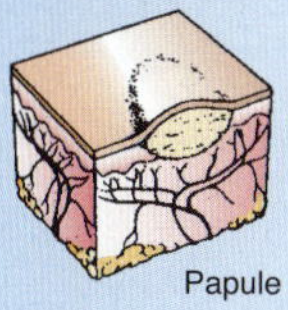 Papule 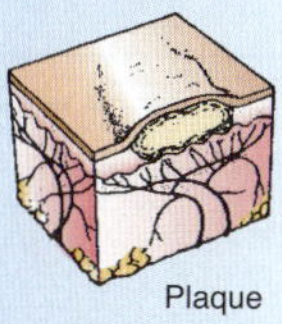 Plaque	Elevated, palpable, solid mass with a circumscribed border Plaque may be coalesced papules with flat top • *Papule:* less than 0.5 cm • *Plaque:* greater than 0.5 cm	*Papules:* Elevated nevi, warts, lichen planus *Plaques:* Psoriasis, actinic keratosis
Nodule, tumor 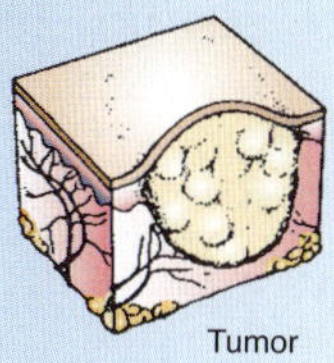 Tumor	Elevated, palpable, solid mass that extends deeper into the dermis than a papule • *Nodule:* 0.5–2 cm; circumscribed • *Tumor:* greater than 1–2 cm; tumors do not always have sharp borders	*Nodules:* Lipoma, squamous cell carcinoma, poorly absorbed injection, dermatofibroma *Tumors:* Larger lipoma, carcinoma

(*continued*)

TABLE **50-3 Primary and Secondary Skin Lesions (*continued*)**

Lesion	Description	Examples
Vesicle, bulla 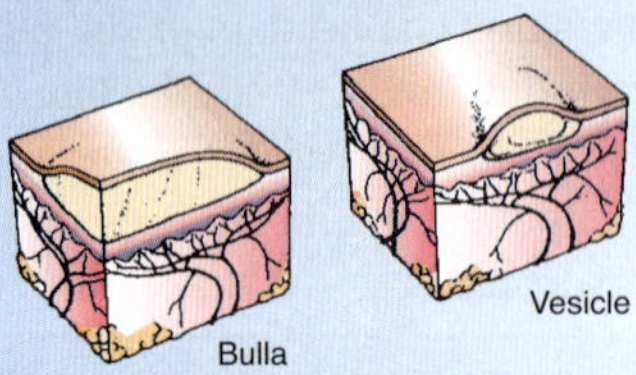 Bulla Vesicle	Circumscribed, elevated, palpable mass containing serous fluid • *Vesicle:* less than 0.5 cm • *Bulla:* greater than 0.5 cm	*Vesicles:* Herpes simplex/zoster, chickenpox, poison ivy, second-degree burn (blister) *Bulla:* Pemphigus, contact dermatitis, large burn blisters, poison ivy, bullous impetigo
Wheal 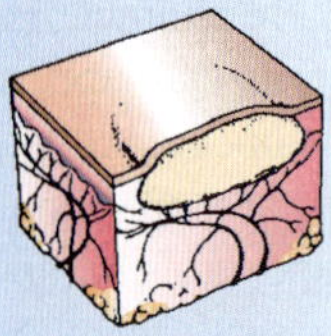 Wheal	Elevated mass with transient borders; often irregular; size and color vary Caused by movement of serous fluid into the dermis; does not contain free fluid in a cavity (as, e.g., a vesicle does)	Urticaria (hives), insect bites
Pustule 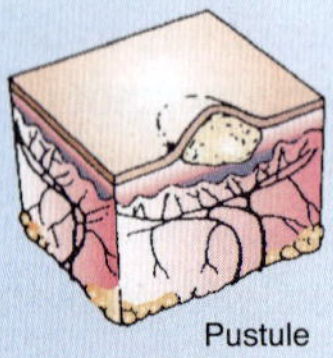 Pustule	Pus-filled vesicle or bulla	Acne, impetigo, furuncles, carbuncles
Cyst 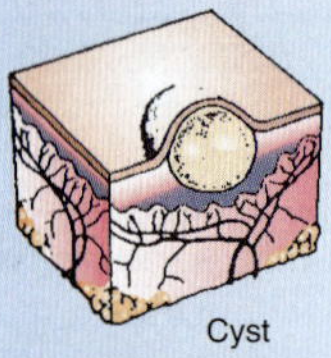 Cyst	Encapsulated fluid-filled or semisolid mass in the subcutaneous tissue or dermis	Sebaceous cyst, epidermoid cysts
Secondary Lesions		
Erosion 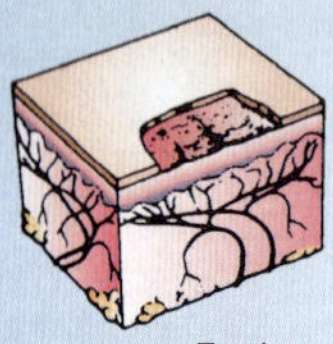 Erosion	Loss of superficial epidermis that does not extend to dermis; depressed, moist area	Ruptured vesicles, scratch marks
Ulcer 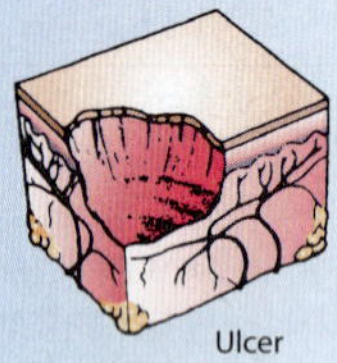 Ulcer	Skin loss or damage at or extending past the epidermis. May include necrotic tissue development, bleeding, or scarring	Stasis ulcer of venous insufficiency, pressure ulcer

Lesion	Description	Examples
Fissure 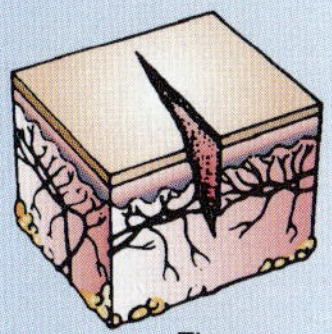 Fissure	Linear crack in the skin that may extend to dermis	Chapped lips or hands, athlete foot
Scales 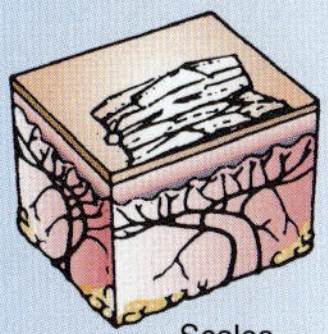 Scales	Flakes secondary to desquamated, dead epithelium that may adhere to skin surface; color varies (silvery, white); texture varies (thick, fine)	Dandruff, psoriasis, dry skin, pityriasis rosea
Crust 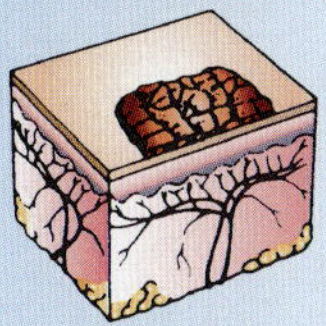 Crust	Dried residue of serum, blood, or pus on skin surface Large, adherent crust is a scab	Residue left after vesicle rupture: impetigo, herpes, eczema
Scar (cicatrix) 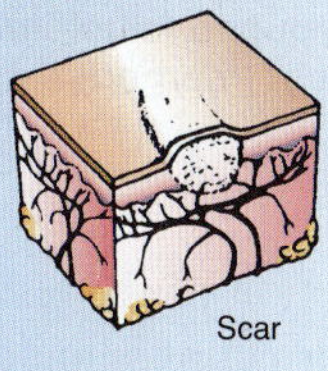 Scar	Skin mark left after healing of a wound or lesion; represents replacement by connective tissue of the injured tissue • *Young scars:* red or purple • *Mature scars:* white or glistening	Healed wound or surgical incision
Keloid 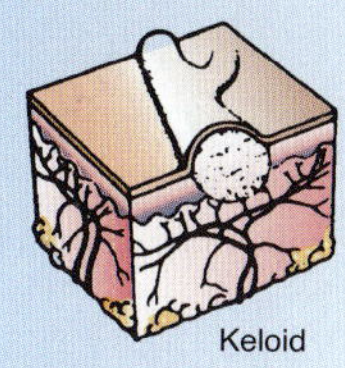 Keloid	Hypertrophied scar tissue secondary to excessive collagen formation during healing; elevated, irregular, red In Black skin fibroblasts are found to be numerous, large, and multinucleated, explaining the manifestation of keloids (Cherry et al., 2021; Iwuala & Taylor, 2022).	Keloid of ear piercing or surgical incision
Atrophy 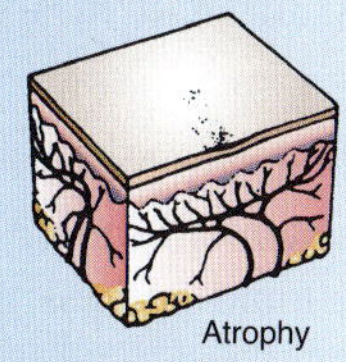 Atrophy	Thin, dry, transparent appearance of epidermis; loss of surface markings; secondary to loss of collagen and elastin; underlying vessels may be visible	Aged skin, arterial insufficiency
Lichenification 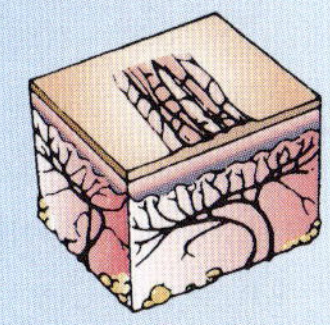 Lichenification	Thickening and roughening of the skin or accentuated skin markings that may be secondary to repeated rubbing, irritation, scratching	Contact dermatitis

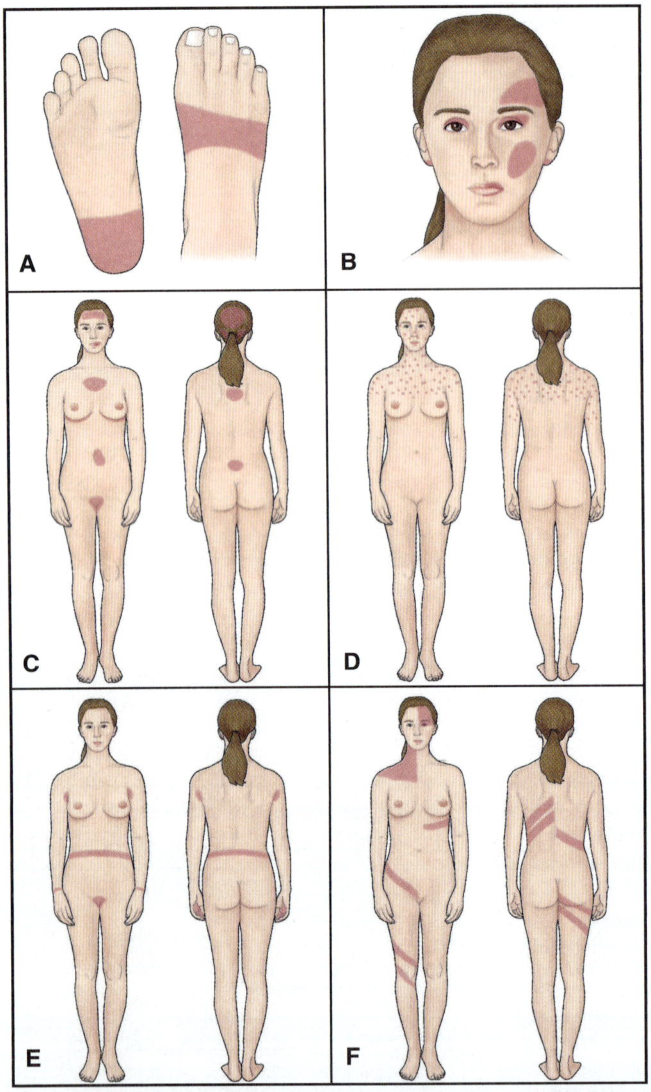

FIGURE 50-3 **Anatomic distribution of common skin disorders. A. Contact dermatitis (shoes). B. Contact dermatitis (cosmetics, perfumes, earrings). C. Seborrheic dermatitis. D. Acne. E. Scabies. F. Herpes zoster (shingles).**

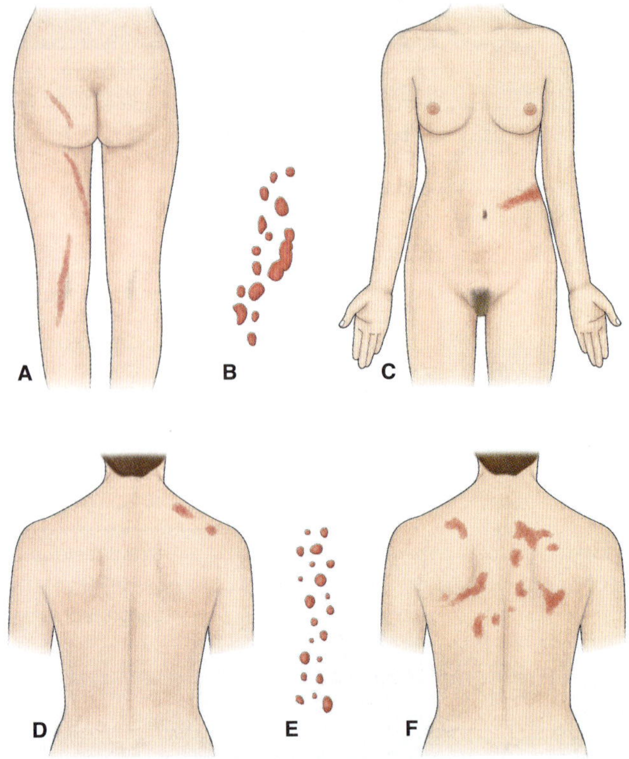

FIGURE 50-4 **Skin lesion configurations. A. Linear (in a line). B. Annular and arciform (circular or arcing). C. Zosteriform (linear along a nerve route). D. Grouped (clustered). E. Discrete (separate and distinct). F. Confluent (merged).**

A preliminary assessment of the eruption or lesion helps identify the type of **dermatosis** (skin disease) and indicates whether the lesion is primary or secondary. At the same time, the anatomic distribution of the eruption should be observed because certain diseases affect certain sites of the body and are distributed in characteristic patterns and shapes (Figs. 50-3 and 50-4). To determine the extent of the regional distribution, the left and right sides of the body should be compared while the color and shape of the lesions are assessed. After observation, the lesions are palpated to determine their texture, shape, and border and to see if they are soft and filled with fluid or hard and fixed to the surrounding tissue.

A disposable metric ruler is used to measure the size of the lesions so that any further extension can be compared with this baseline measurement. Skin lesions are described clearly and in detail on the patient's health record, using precise terminology.

Characteristics of Lesions

After the characteristic distribution of the lesions has been determined, the following information should be obtained and described clearly and in detail:

- Color of the lesion
- Any redness, heat, pain, or swelling
- Size and location of the involved area
- Pattern of eruption (e.g., macular, papular, scaling, oozing, discrete, confluent)
- Distribution of the lesion (e.g., bilateral, symmetric, linear, circular)
- Evolving (e.g., lesion looks different in size, shape, or color)

If acute open wounds or lesions are found on inspection of the skin, a comprehensive assessment should be made and documented. This assessment should address the following issues:

- *Wound bed:* Inspect for necrotic, slough (yellow, white or grey dead tissue), granulation (new reddish connective tissue that forms on the surface of a wound when the wound is healing, often described as "cobblestone-like" in appearance) or epithelial tissue, exudate, color, and odor.
- *Wound edges and margins:* Observe for undermining (i.e., extension of the wound under the surface skin) or epibole (rolled edges) and evaluate for condition.

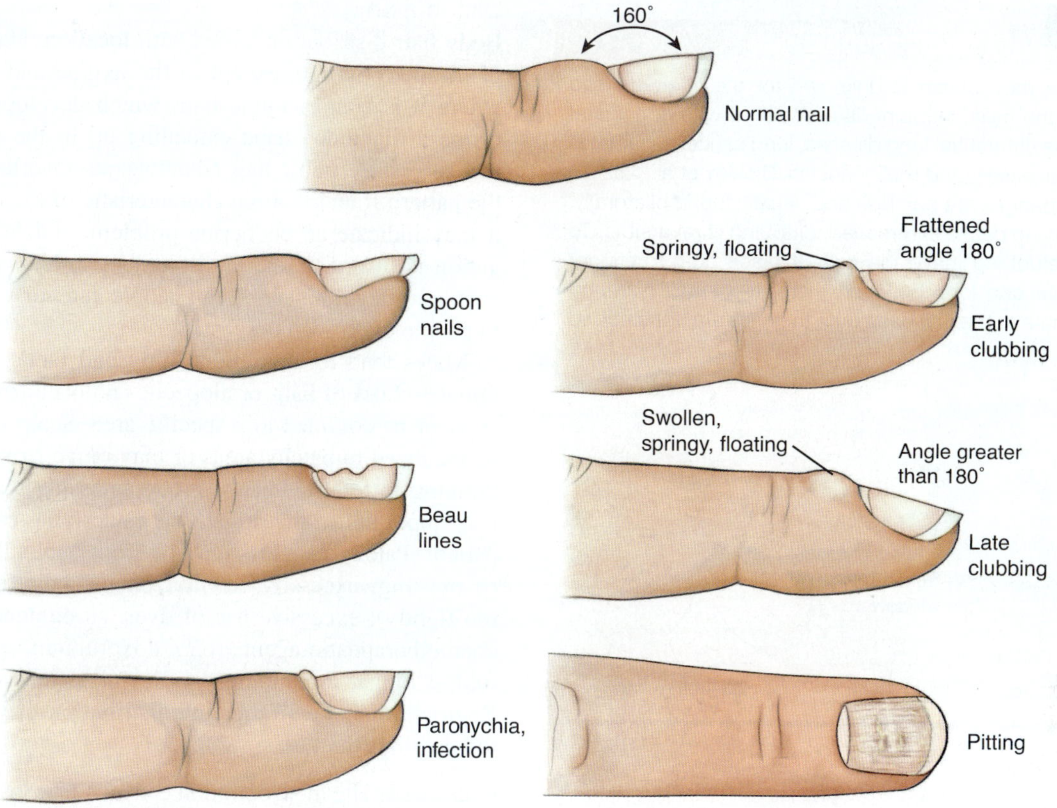

FIGURE 50-5 **Common nail disorders.**

- *Wound size:* Measure in centimeters (cm), as appropriate, to determine diameter and depth of the wound and surrounding erythema.
- *Surrounding skin:* Assess for color, suppleness and moisture, irritation, induration (abnormal firmness of tissue), and scaling.

Assessing Vascularity

After the color of the skin has been evaluated and lesions have been inspected, an assessment of vascular changes in the skin is performed. A description of vascular changes includes location, distribution, color, size, and the presence of pulsations. Common vascular changes include petechiae, ecchymoses, Telangiectasia (spider veins), angiomas, and venous stars. Petechiae are small (less than 2 mm in diameter) lesions that are red or purple in color. They are associated with broken capillaries or indicative of platelet abnormalities, specifically thrombocytopenia (low platelet counts).

Assessing Hydration

Skin moisture, temperature, and texture are assessed primarily by palpation. The turgor (i.e., elasticity) of the skin, which decreases in normal aging, may be a factor in assessing the hydration status of a patient. The forearm, sternum, or forehead is recommended for assessing turgor in the older population, rather than the hand, owing to the loss of elasticity with aging. The nurse pinches the skin of the sternum with the thumb and index finger, creating a tent of skin. Upon releasing it, normal turgid skin promptly resumes its shape, whereas a persistent fold or tent is associated with fluid volume deficit.

Assessing the Nails

A brief inspection of the nails includes observation of configuration, color, and consistency. Many alterations in the nail or nail bed reflect local or systemic abnormalities in progress or resulting from past events (Fig. 50-5). Transverse depressions known as *Beau lines* in the nails may reflect retarded growth of the nail matrix because of severe illness or, more commonly, local trauma. Ridging, hypertrophy, and other changes may also be visible with local trauma. Paronychia, an inflammation of the skin around the nail, is usually accompanied by tenderness and erythema. The angle between the normal nail and its base is 160 degrees. When palpated, the nail base is usually firm. Clubbing is manifested by a straightening of the normal angle (at least 180 degrees) and softening of the nail base (Box 50-4). The softened area feels sponge-like when palpated.

Assessing the Hair

Hair assessment involves inspection and palpation. Gloves are worn by the examiner, and the examination room should

BOX 50-4
Assessing for Clubbing

Although the mechanism is unknown for the characteristic changes to the nails, clubbing is associated with congenital heart disease, interstitial lung disease, lung cancer, inflammatory bowel diseases, and malignancies (Bickley et al., 2021).

The nail changes are painless and usually found bilaterally. If the underlying cause is removed, clubbing is reversible. To assess for clubbing, have the patient place both forefinger nails together and look between them. If a small diamond space is visible at the nail base then the nails are *not* clubbed (Schamroth sign).

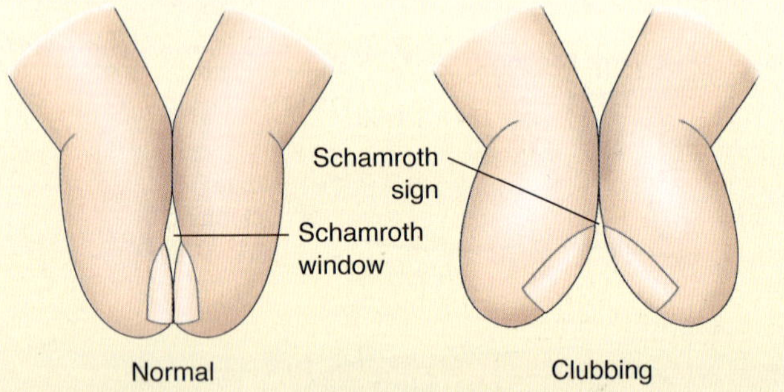

be well lighted. Separating the hair so that the condition of the skin underneath can be easily seen, the nurse assesses color, texture, and distribution. The wooden end of a cotton swab can be used to make small parts in the hair, so that the scalp can be inspected. Any abnormal lesions, evidence of itching, inflammation, scaling, or signs of infestation (i.e., lice or mites) are documented.

Color and Texture

Natural hair color ranges from white to black. Hair begins to turn gray with age, initially during the third decade of life, when the loss of melanin begins to become apparent. However, it is not unusual for the hair of younger people to turn gray as a result of hereditary traits. The person with albinism (i.e., partial or complete absence of pigmentation) has a genetic predisposition to white hair from birth. The natural state of the hair can be altered by using hair dyes, bleaches, and curling or relaxing products. The types of products used are identified in the assessment.

The texture of scalp hair ranges from fine to coarse, silky to brittle, oily to dry, and shiny to dull, and hair can be straight, curly, or kinky. Dry, brittle hair may result from overuse of hair dyes, hair dryers, and curling irons, or from endocrine disorders, such as thyroid dysfunction. Oily hair is usually caused by increased secretion from the sebaceous glands close to the scalp. If the patient reports a recent change in hair texture, the underlying reason is pursued; the alteration may arise simply from the overuse of commercial hair products or from changing to a new shampoo.

Distribution

Body hair distribution varies with location. Hair over most of the body is fine, except in the axillae and pubic areas, where it is coarse. Pubic hair, which develops at puberty, forms a diamond shape extending up to the umbilicus in males. Female pubic hair resembles an inverted triangle. If the pattern found is more characteristic of the opposite sex, it may indicate an endocrine problem, and further investigation is in order. Racial differences in hair are expected, such as straight hair in Asian people and curly, coarser hair in people of African descent.

Males tend to have more body and facial hair than do females. Loss of hair, or alopecia, can occur over the entire body or be confined to a specific area. Scalp hair loss may be localized to patchy areas or may range from generalized thinning to total baldness. When assessing scalp hair loss, it is important to investigate the underlying cause with the patient. Patchy hair loss may be from habitual hair pulling or twisting; excessive traction on the hair (e.g., braiding too tightly); excessive use of dyes, straighteners, and oils; chemotherapeutic agents (e.g., doxorubicin, cyclophosphamide); fungal infection; or moles or lesions on the scalp. Regrowth may be erratic, and distribution may never attain the previous thickness.

Hair Loss. The most common cause of hair loss is male pattern baldness, which affects more than one half of the male population and is believed to be related to heredity, aging, and androgen (male hormone) levels. Androgen is necessary for male pattern baldness to develop. The pattern of hair loss begins with receding of the hairline in the frontal-temporal area and progresses to gradual thinning and complete loss of hair over the top of the scalp and crown.

Other Changes. Male pattern hair distribution may be seen in some female patients at the time of menopause, when the hormone estrogen is no longer produced by the ovaries. In females with hirsutism, excessive hair may grow on the face, chest, shoulders, and pubic area. When menopause is ruled out as the underlying cause, hormonal abnormalities related to pituitary or adrenal dysfunction must be investigated.

Diagnostic Evaluation

Skin Biopsy

Performed to obtain tissue for microscopic examination, a skin biopsy may be obtained by scalpel excision or by a skin punch instrument that removes a small core of tissue. Biopsies are performed on skin nodules, plaques, blisters, ulcers, and other lesions to rule out malignancy and to establish an exact diagnosis.

Patch Testing

Performed to identify substances to which the patient has developed an allergy, patch testing involves applying the suspected allergens to normal skin under occlusive patches. The development of redness, fine elevations, or itching is considered a weak positive reaction; fine blisters, papules, and severe itching indicate a moderately positive reaction; and blisters, pain, and ulceration indicate a strong positive reaction.

Skin Scrapings

Tissue samples are scraped from suspected fungal lesions with a scalpel blade moistened with oil, so that the scraped skin adheres to the blade. The scraped material is transferred to a glass slide, covered with a coverslip, and examined microscopically. The spores and hyphae of dermatophyte infections, as well as infestations such as scabies, can be visualized.

Clinical Photographs

Photographs are taken to document the nature and extent of the skin condition and are used to determine progress or improvement resulting from treatment. They are sometimes used to track the status of moles to document if the characteristics of the mole are changing.

CHAPTER REVIEW

NCLEX-Style Review Questions

1. The clinic nurse assesses the skin of a patient. During the assessment, what does the nurse recognize as a normal function of the skin? Select all that apply.
   a. Thermal regulation
   b. Vitamin E production
   c. Synthesis of vitamin D
   d. Releasing of carbon dioxide
   e. Barrier to epidermal water loss

2. A 52-year-old patient has just returned to the room postoperatively. The nurse examines the patient's nail beds to assess for what condition? Select all that apply.
   a. Cyanosis
   b. Respiratory rate
   c. Edema
   d. Cellulitis
   e. Capillary refill

3. A patient is requesting to be evaluated today for a suspicious lesion that was noticed several weeks ago. When assessing the lesion, what characteristics are you looking for ? Select all that apply.
   a. Heat
   b. Claudication
   c. Size
   d. Erythema
   e. Pattern

4. Which of the following are associated with skin changes in older individuals? Select all that apply.
   a. Epidermis and dermis thin and flatten
   b. Hair growth gradually diminishes
   c. Subcutaneous fat increases in distal extremities
   d. Skin becomes fragile and transparent
   e. Increased remodeling and repairing skin

5. When considering clubbing of the digits, the nurse recognizes that it represents which of the following? Select all that apply.
   a. Clubbing is permanent change of the nailbed.
   b. Clubbing is only associated with hypoxemia.
   c. Clubbing may be associated with inflammatory bowel disorders.
   d. Clubbing is observed by a straightening of the normal angle of the nail and nail base as well as a softening of the nail base.
   e. The nails affected will be painful to touch.

REFERENCES AND SELECTED READINGS

References and selected readings associated with this chapter can be found on the website that accompanies the book. Visit **http://thepoint.lww.com/Honan3e** to access the references and other additional resources associated with this chapter.

CHAPTER 51

Nursing Management: Patients With Dermatologic Problems

Captain Patina S. Walton-Battle

Learning Objectives

After reading this chapter, you will be able to:

1. Describe the general management of the patient with an abnormal skin condition.
2. Describe general principles of wound care.
3. Identify stages of pressure ulcers.
4. Discuss the general management of a patient with pruritus.
5. Describe the health education needs of the patient with infections of the skin and parasitic skin diseases.
6. Discuss care of patients with noninfectious, inflammatory dermatoses, including psoriasis.
7. Describe nursing management of the patient with skin cancer.
8. Describe characteristics of the various types of Kaposi sarcoma.

Regardless of the environment where they work, nurses manage skin care. In addition, nurses predict patients who will be at risk for skin problems, assess skin changes, and intervene to prevent injury and maintain skin viability. As nurses, it is also important to utilize preventative practices to reduce transmission of infection or further injury and to maintain skin viability.

GENERAL MANAGEMENT OF SKIN DISORDERS

Nursing management of skin disorders includes protecting the skin, preventing infection, reversing inflammation, administering therapeutic baths, and administering medications.

PROVIDING SKIN CARE

Protecting the Skin

Some skin problems are aggravated by bathing. The essence of skin care in bathing a patient with skin problems is as follows:

- A mild, lipid-free soap or soap substitute is used.
- The area is rinsed completely and blotted dry with a soft cloth.
- Deodorant soaps are avoided.

Special care is necessary when changing dressings. Pledgets (small compress of material, usually cotton or gauze) saturated with oils, ointments, hydrogels, sterile saline or water, wound cleansers, or another prescribed solution help to loosen crusts, remove exudates, or free an adherent dry dressing.

Preventing Infection

Potentially infectious skin lesions should be regarded strictly as such, and proper precautions should be observed until the diagnosis is established. Most lesions with purulent drainage contain infectious material. The health care provider must adhere to standard contact precautions carried out according to Occupational Safety and Health Administration (OSHA) regulations.

Pearls for Practice

The most important interventions for preventing infection transmission are hand hygiene and use of standard precautions for all patients. Other precautions are based on how an organism is transmitted; these include contact, airborne, and droplet precautions (Link, 2019). The cornerstone of transmission-based precautions is appropriate use of personal protective equipment (PPE) to protect personnel and patients from infection. Donning and doffing of PPE is an important component of transmission-based precautions, and personnel who doff PPE incorrectly could become infected as a result

(CDC, 2017). Hand hygiene should be performed before gloves are donned, and gloves must be removed before hand hygiene is performed. Glove use does not replace the need for hand hygiene (CDC, 2017).

Reversing Inflammation

The type of skin lesion (e.g., oozing, infected, or dry) usually determines the type of local medication or treatment that is prescribed. As a rule, if the skin is acutely inflamed (i.e., hot), erythematous (red), and edematous (swollen) and draining, it is best to apply moist or specialty dressings and/or soothing lotions. For chronic conditions in which the skin surface is dry and scaly, water-soluble emulsions, creams, ointments, and pastes are used. The therapy is modified as the responses of the skin indicate. The patient and the nurse should note whether the medication or dressings seem to irritate the skin. The success or failure of therapy usually depends on adequate instruction and motivation of the patient and family, and the support of health care personnel promotes adherence to instructions.

Administering Therapeutic Baths (Balneotherapy)

Baths or soaks, known as **balneotherapy**, are useful when large areas of skin are affected. The baths remove crusts, scales, and old medications and relieve the inflammation and pruritus (itching) that accompany acute dermatoses. Additional information about therapeutic baths is given in Box 51-1.

BOX 51-1 **Therapeutic Baths**

Types of Therapeutic Baths

Bath Solution	Effects and Uses
Water	Same effect as wet dressings
Saline	Used for widely disseminated lesions
Colloidal (Aveeno, oatmeal)	Antipruritic, soothing
Sodium bicarbonate (baking soda)	Cooling
Starch	Soothing
Medicated tars	Psoriasis and chronic eczema
Bath oils	Antipruritic and emollient action; acute and subacute generalized eczematous eruptions

Nursing Interventions

- Fill the tub half full.
- Keep the water at a comfortable temperature.
- Do not allow the water to cool excessively.
- Use a bath mat because *medications added to the bath can cause the tub to be slippery.*
- Apply an emollient cream to damp skin after the bath if lubrication is desired.
- Because tars are volatile, the bath area should be well ventilated.
- Maintain a constant room temperature without drafts.
- Encourage the patient to wear light, loose clothing after the bath.

TABLE 51-1 **Common Topical Preparations and Medications**

Preparation	Product Name
Bath preparations	
With tar	Balnetar, Doak Oil, Lavatar
With colloidal oatmeal	Aveeno Oilated Bath Powder
With oatmeal and mineral oil	Aveeno Bath Oil, Nutra Soothe
With mineral oil	Nutraderm Bath Oil, Lubath, Alpha-Keri Bath Oil
Moisturizer creams	Acid Mantle Cream, Curel Cream, Dermasil, Eucerin, Lubriderm, Noxzema Skin Cream
Moisturizer ointments	Aquaphor Ointment, Eutra Swiss Skin Cream, Vaseline Ointment
Topical anesthetics	Anesthetic drugs such as lidocaine, tetracaine, benzocaine, and prilocaine in a cream, ointment, or gel. EMLA cream (lidocaine 2.5% and prilocaine 2.5%) is an example of one more commonly used.
Topical antibiotics	Bacitracin, polymyxin B), mupirocin 2% ointment or cream, erythromycin 2% clindamycin phosphate 1%, gentamicin sulfate 1% (cream or ointment), 1% silver sulfadiazine cream

Administering Pharmacologic Therapy

Topical Preparations

Table 51-1 lists some commonly used topical preparations.

Lotions

Lotions are used frequently to replenish lost skin oils or to relieve pruritus. They are usually applied directly to the skin, but a dressing soaked in the lotion can be placed on the affected area. The best time to apply a moisturizer is when the skin is already moistened such as immediately after a bath or shower (Sajwan et al., 2022). Lotions must be applied every 3 or 4 hours for sustained therapeutic effect because if left in place for a long period, they may crust and cake on the skin.

There are two types of lotions: suspensions and liniments. **Suspensions** are medicines that are mixed with a liquid, usually water, in which it cannot dissolve; therefore, the lotion remains intact in the form of small particles. The important thing to remember about suspensions is to shake the medication before giving each dose so that the medicine particles are evenly distributed throughout the liquid. An example is calamine lotion, which provides a rapid cooling and drying effect as it evaporates, leaving a thin, medicinal layer of powder on the affected skin. **Liniments** are lotions with oil added to prevent crusting. An example of a liniment is Ben-Gay for muscle aches.

Powders

Powders usually have a talc, zinc oxide, bentonite, or cornstarch base and are dusted on the skin with a shaker or applied with cotton sponges. Although their therapeutic action is brief, powders act as **hygroscopic** agents that absorb and retain moisture from the air and reduce friction between skin surfaces and clothing or bedding. Extra moisture in areas where skin rubs against skin can cause irritation and skin breakdown, particularly in areas of those body folds (intertriginous areas) where the environment tends to be warmer and moist. Commonly affected areas are between the toes or buttocks, in the armpits or groin, and under the breasts and abdominal skin folds. These warm moist areas also provide fertile breeding grounds for infections, especially with fungus and bacteria (Sajwan et al., 2022).

Creams and Emulsions

Creams may be suspensions of oil in water or emulsions of water in oil, with additional ingredients to prevent bacterial and fungal growth. Both may cause an allergic reaction, such as contact dermatitis (discussed on page 1234). Oil-in-water creams are easily applied and usually are the most cosmetically acceptable to the patient. Although they can be used on the face, they tend to have a drying effect. Water-in-oil emulsions are greasier and are preferred for drying and flaking dermatoses.

Gels

Gels are semisolid emulsions that become liquid when applied to the skin or scalp. The water-based gels appear to penetrate the skin more effectively, are greaseless and odorless, and cause less stinging on application. They are especially useful for acute dermatitis in which there is weeping exudate (e.g., poison ivy).

Pastes

Pastes are mixtures of powders and ointments and are used in inflammatory blistering conditions. They adhere to the skin and may be difficult to remove without using oil (e.g., olive oil or mineral oil). Pastes are applied with a wooden tongue depressor or gloved hand.

Ointments

Moisturizers make the skin smooth and soft and increase hydration. Ointments are better moisturizers or hydrators of the skin by improving and restoring skin integrity due to better adherence to the skin (Draelos, 2018). They are the preferred vehicle for delivering medication to patients with chronic or localized dry skin conditions, such as eczema or psoriasis (e.g., triamcinolone). Other ointments are used to aid in healing and treatment of pressure ulcers, varicose ulcers, and dehiscent wounds (e.g., Xenaderm). Ointments are applied with a wooden tongue depressor or gloved hand up to twice a day.

Sprays and Aerosols

Spray and aerosol preparations may be used on any widespread dermatologic condition e.g., 3M Cavilon Skin Protectant; Convatec Aloe Vesta Skin Protectant. They evaporate on contact and are used infrequently.

Corticosteroids

Corticosteroids are widely used in treating dermatologic conditions to provide anti-inflammatory, antipruritic, and vasoconstrictive effects. The patient is taught to apply the product sparingly and rub it into the prescribed area thoroughly. Absorption of topical corticosteroid is enhanced when the skin is hydrated or when the affected area is covered by an occlusive or moisture-retentive dressing. Inappropriate use of topical corticosteroids can result in local and systemic side effects, especially when the medication is absorbed through inflamed and excoriated skin or is used for long periods on sensitive areas. Local side effects may include skin atrophy and thinning, **striae** (bandlike streaks), and telangiectasia (small, dilated blood vessels on the surface of the skin). Thinning of the skin results from the ability of corticosteroids to inhibit the synthesis of skin collagen. The thinning process can be reversed by discontinuing the medication, but striae and telangiectasia are permanent. Systemic side effects may include hyperglycemia and symptoms of Cushing syndrome (refer to Chapter 30). Caution is required when applying corticosteroids around the eyes for two reasons: (1) long-term use may cause glaucoma or cataracts, and (2) the anti-inflammatory effect of corticosteroids may mask existing viral or fungal infections.

Concentrated (fluorinated) corticosteroids are never applied on the face or intertriginous areas (i.e., axilla and groin) because these areas have a thinner stratum corneum and absorb the medication much more quickly than do other areas of the body, such as the forearm or legs.

Pearls for Practice

It is important for the nurse to consider that penetration of a topical steroid depends on the skin site, which varies based upon the denseness of the stratum corneum, blood supply, and tissue integrity of the involved area. According to Brown et al. (2019), penetration of topical steroids applied to the eyelids or scrotum is 4 times greater than for the forehead and 36 times greater than the palms and soles. Thus, thinner and less intact skin has a higher absorption and thus poses a higher risk for side effects.

Intralesional Therapy

Intralesional therapy consists of injecting a sterile suspension of medication (usually a corticosteroid) into or just below a lesion. Although this treatment may have an anti-inflammatory effect, local atrophy may result if the medication is injected into subcutaneous fat. Skin lesions treated with intralesional therapy include psoriasis, keloids, and cystic acne.

Systemic Medications

Systemic medications are also prescribed for skin conditions. These include corticosteroids for short-term therapy for contact dermatitis or for long-term treatment of a chronic **dermatosis**. Other frequently used systemic medications include antibiotics, antifungals, antihistamines, sedatives, tranquilizers, analgesics, and **cytotoxic** (destructive of cells) agents.

CARING FOR WOUNDS

Wound Dressings

There are three types of wound dressings: primary, secondary, and active. Primary dressings have only a protective function and maintain a moist environment for natural healing. The balance of moisture is critical to wound healing. Evidence supports moist wound healing, and this continues to be the driving force in the development and the deciding factor on what type of dressing to use. Dressings include those that just cover the area (e.g., DuoDERM, Tegaderm) and may remain in place for several days. Secondary dressings are capable of absorbing wound exudate while (1) maintaining a moist environment in the area of the wound and (2) allowing the surrounding skin to remain dry. They include hydrocolloids, alginates, and hydrogels. Secondary dressings are able to modify the physiology of the wound environment by modulating and stimulating cellular activity and by releasing growth factor (Bryant & Nix, 2023; Weller & Team, 2019). Active dressings improve the healing process and decrease healing time. They include skin grafts and biologic skin substitutes. Both interactive and active dressings create a moist environment at the interface of the wound with the dressing.

Pearls for Practice

Knowledge of dressing products and experience with dressing selection are two major components in holistic wound management to ensure evidence-based wound care (Dowsett et al., 2017; Weller et al., 2020). Primary dressings are usually considered passive and provide protection to the wound, whereas interactive dressings create a moist wound environment and interact with the wound bed components to further enhance wound healing. Interactive dressings may reduce colonization count, reduce the level of exudate, improve wound bed moisture retention, improve wound collagen matrix, remove cellular products, and provide protection for the epithelializing bed (Bryant & Nix, 2023; Weller et al., 2020).

Because so many wound care products are available, it is often difficult to select the most appropriate product for a specific wound. Selection of products should be made carefully because of their expense. Both clinical efficacy and health-related outcomes (e.g., decreased pain, increased mobility) should be used to measure the success of a product for a wound. Even with the availability of a large variety of dressings, an appropriate selection can be made if certain principles are maintained. Table 51-2 is a guide to wound dressing functions and categories.

Occlusive Dressings

Occlusive dressings cover a topical medication that is applied to a skin lesion. The area is kept airtight by using plastic film (e.g., plastic wrap). Plastic film is thin and readily adapts to all sizes, body shapes, and skin surfaces. In general, plastic wrap should be used no more than 12 hours each day.

Transparent Films

Transparent films are thin, transparent, polyurethane, impermeable adhesive films that are used for partial thickness, minimally draining, or closed wounds. They permit visualization of the wound, promote autolysis, reduce friction, and are sometimes used as a secondary dressing. Examples are Op-Site and Tegaderm.

Specialty Absorptive Dressings

These are used for heavily exudating wounds. The dressings absorb copious amounts of drainage. Examples of these are Exudry and ABD pads.

Moisture-Retentive Dressings

Commercially produced moisture-retentive dressing can perform the same functions as wet dressings but are more efficient at removing exudate because of their higher moisture-vapor transmission rate; some have reservoirs that can hold excessive exudate. A number of moisture-retentive dressings are already impregnated with saline solution, petrolatum, zinc-saline solution, hydrogel, or antimicrobial agents, thereby eliminating the need to coat the skin to avoid maceration. Depending on the product used and the type of dermatologic problem encountered, most moisture-retentive dressings may remain in place from 12 to 24 hours; some can remain in place as long as a week.

Hydrogels

Hydrogels are polymers with a water content of 90% to 95%. They are available in impregnated sheets or as gel in a tube.

TABLE **51-2 Quick Guide to Wound Dressing Function and Categories**

Function	Action	Example
Absorption	Absorbs exudate	Alginates, composite dressings, foams, gauze, hydrocolloids, hydrogels
Cleansing	Removes purulent drainage, foreign debris, and devitalized tissue	Wound cleansers
Debridement	*Autolytic*: covers a wound and allows enzymes to self-digest sloughed skin	Absorption beads, pastes, powders; alginates; composite dressings; foams; hydrate gauze; hydrogels; hydrocolloids; transparent films; wound care systems
	Chemical or enzymatic: applied topically to break down devitalized tissue	Enzymatic debridement agents
	Mechanical: removes devitalized tissue with mechanical force	Wound cleansers, gauze (wet to dry), whirlpool
Diathermy	Produces electrical current to promote warmth and new tissue growth	Ultrasound and microwave (diathermy)
Hydration	Adds moisture to a wound	Gauze (saturated with saline solution), hydrogels, wound care systems
Maintain moist environment	Manages moisture levels in a wound and maintains a moist environment	Composites, contact layers, foams, gauze (impregnated or saturated), hydrogels, hydrocolloids, transparent films, wound care systems
Manage high-output wounds	Manages excessive quantities of exudate	Pouching systems
Pack or fill dead space	Prevents premature wound closure or fills shallow areas and provides absorption	Absorbent beads, powders, pastes; alginates, composites, foams, gauze (impregnated and nonimpregnated)
Protect and cover wound	Provides protection from the external environment	Composites, compression bandages/wraps, foams, gauze dressings, hydrogels, hydrocolloids, transparent film dressings
Protect periwound skin	Prevents moisture and mechanical trauma from damaging delicate tissue around the wound	Composites, foams, hydrocolloids, pouching systems, skin sealants, transparent film dressings
Provide therapeutic compression	Provides appropriate levels of support to the lower extremities in venous stasis disease	Compression bandages, wraps, support stockings

Their high moisture content makes them ideal for autolytic debridement of wounds. They are semitransparent, allowing for wound inspection without dressing removal. They are comfortable and soothing for the painful wound. They require a secondary dressing to keep them in place. Hydrogels are appropriate for superficial wounds with high serous output, such as abrasions, skin graft sites, and draining venous ulcers.

Hydrocolloids

Hydrocolloids are composed of a water-impermeable, polyurethane outer covering separated from the wound by a hydrocolloid material. They are adherent and nonpermeable to water vapor and oxygen. As water evaporates over the wound, it is absorbed into the dressing, which softens and discolors with the increased water content. The dressing can be removed without damage to the wound. As the dressing absorbs water, it produces a foul-smelling, yellowish covering over the wound. This is a normal chemical interaction between the dressing and wound exudate and should not be confused with purulent drainage from the wound. Most can be left in place for as long as 7 days.

Foam Dressings

Foam dressings are nonadherent and require a secondary dressing to keep them in place. Moisture is absorbed into the foam layer, decreasing maceration of surrounding tissue. A moist environment is maintained, and removal of the dressing does not damage the wound. Foams are a good choice for exudative wounds. They are especially helpful over bony prominences because they provide contoured cushioning.

Alginates

Calcium alginates (e.g., AlgiSite M, Kaltostat, Sorbsan, Algicell) are derived from brown seaweed and consist of very absorbent calcium alginate fibers that can absorb

20 times their weight (Bryant & Nix, 2023; Clark, 2018). They are useful in areas where the tissue is highly irritated or macerated. The alginate dressing forms a moist pocket over the wound while the surrounding skin stays dry. The dressing also reacts with wound fluid and forms a foul-smelling coating. Alginates work well when packed into a deep cavity, wound, or sinus tract with heavy drainage. They are nonadherent and require a secondary dressing.

Antimicrobial Dressings

Antimicrobial dressings are used for partial- and full-thickness wounds. They help to control or decrease the bioburden (the number of microorganisms living on the surface) and odor for minimal and heavy exudating wounds. They are a topical antifungal and antibiotic agent that come in ointments, gels, impregnated gauze, hydrofiber, and pads. Examples are Acticoat 7 and Aquacel Ag (hydrofiber).

Collagen Dressings

These dressings stimulate the wound and accelerate wound healing. Some forms can be left on for up to 7 days. They are used for minimal to moderate exudating wounds that are partial to full thickness. Examples are Promogran and ColActive.

Tissue-Engineered Skin

Apligraf and Dermagraft are dressings made up of a bioabsorbable matrix of collagen or suture material that contains living cytokines and fibroblasts. When applied to wounds, these agents stimulate platelet activity and potentially decrease wound-healing time (Bryant & Nix, 2023). Bioengineered skin works by maintaining wound moisture, providing a structure for regeneration of cells, and supplying beneficial cytokines.

Debridement

Debridement is the removal of nonviable tissue, biofilm (a thin film of microorganisms such as bacteria that adheres to a surface) and bioburden from pressure and vascular ulcers, burns, surgical or traumatic wounds, and other types of wounds to promote wound healing. The DIME approach to chronic wound management is used to bring about wound resolution. The four general steps to follow for better preparation are encompassed in the acronym DIME: D: Debridement of nonviable tissue within the wound. I: Management of inflammation and infection. M: Moisture control. E: Environmental and epithelialization assessment (Manna et al., 2018).

Autolytic Debridement

Autolytic **debridement** is a process that uses the body's own digestive enzymes to break down necrotic tissue. The wound is kept moist with occlusive dressings. Eschar and necrotic debris are softened, liquefied, and separated from the bed of the wound.

Enzymatic Debridement

Several commercially available products contain the same enzymes that the body produces naturally. These are called enzymatic debriding agents; an example is a collagenase. Application of these products speeds the rate at which necrotic tissue is removed. This method is slower and no more effective than surgical debridement.

Mechanical Debridement

Wet-to-dry dressings are still used, but not very much. It is considered a nonselective method of debridement, which removes necrotic tissue and absorbs small to large amounts of exudates. This method exposes healthy tissue in the wound and can damage it as well.

Wet dressings (e.g., wet open-weave cotton fabric for best results) are lightly packed into the wound bed and allowed to completely dry, trapping debris. This was traditionally used for acute, weeping, inflammatory lesions. Such dressings have become almost obsolete because of the many newer products available for wound care (Ramundo, 2016).

Negative Pressure Wound Therapy

In this therapy, an open-cell, reticulated foam, gauze, or specially designed dressing is placed into the wound, sealed with semi-occlusive drape, and exposed to subatmospheric pressure via an evacuation tube connected to a computerized pump. It is used for acute and chronic open wounds. It also can be used on partial- to full-thickness wounds and on partial-thickness burns.

Hyperbaric Oxygen Therapy

Hyperbaric oxygenation (HBO) is an adjunctive therapy that requires the patient to breathe 100% oxygen while under increased atmospheric pressure in a pressure chamber. It is recommended that hyperbaric therapy be utilized for limb-threatening diabetic wounds of the lower extremities and pressure ulcers. Also, it is used for hypoxic vascular wounds of the lower extremity. Those who received HBO as part of their wound care regimen healed faster than those who received standard treatment (Huang et al., 2019). HBO has been proposed as an adjuvant for clinical practice in severe patients, and also for recovery after SARS-CoV-2 infection. Results from clinical trials have already demonstrated the potential uses of this treatment to redirect O_2 diffusion avoided by hypoxemia and its ability to eliminate inflammatory cytokines (Ortega et al., 2021).

Pharmacologic Therapy

Pain management can be challenging. In caring for any patient with acute or chronic wounds, it is important to identify and measure the degree, site, and type of pain. This aids in utilizing the appropriate treatment for pain. Refer to Chapter 6 for additional information on pain management.

SKIN CONDITIONS

PRURITUS

While not a disorder but a manifestation, pruritus (itching) is one of the more common symptoms of patients with dermatologic disorders.

GENERAL PRURITUS

Pathophysiology

Itch receptors are unmyelinated, penicillate (brush-like) nerve endings that are found exclusively in the skin, mucous membranes, and cornea. Although pruritus is usually caused by a primary skin disease with resultant rash or lesions, it may occur without a rash or lesion. This is referred to as *essential pruritus*, which generally has a rapid onset, may be severe, and interferes with normal daily activities.

Pruritus may be the first indication of a systemic internal disease, such as diabetes mellitus, blood disorder, or cancer (occult malignancy of the breast or colon, Hodgkin disease, other lymphomas). It may also accompany kidney, liver, and thyroid diseases (Box 51-2). Some common oral medications, such as aspirin, antibiotics, hormones (e.g., estrogens, testosterone, or oral contraceptives), and opioids (e.g., morphine or cocaine) may cause pruritus directly or by increasing sensitivity to ultraviolet light. Certain soaps and chemicals, radiation therapy, prickly heat (miliaria), and contact with woolen garments are also associated with pruritus. Pruritus may also be caused by psychological factors, such as excessive stress in family or work situations.

Scratching the pruritic area causes the inflamed cells and nerve endings to release histamine, which produces more pruritus, generating a vicious itch–scratch cycle. If the patient responds to an itch by scratching, the integrity of the skin may be altered, and excoriation, erythema, raised areas (i.e., wheals), infection, or changes in pigmentation may result. Pruritus usually is more severe at night and is less frequently reported during waking hours, most likely because the person is distracted by daily activities. At night, when there are few distractions, even the slightest pruritus cannot be ignored easily. Severe itching can be debilitating.

Gerontologic Considerations

Pruritus occurs frequently in older people as a result of dry skin. Older people are also more likely to have a systemic illness that triggers pruritus, are at higher risk for occult malignancy, and are more likely to be taking multiple medications than younger people. All of these factors increase the incidence of pruritus in older people.

Medical and Nursing Management

A thorough history and physical examination usually provide clues to the underlying cause of the pruritus, such as hay fever, allergy, recent administration of a new medication, or a change of cosmetics or soaps. After the causative agent has been identified and removed (if possible), treatment of the condition should relieve the pruritus. Signs of infection and environmental clues, such as warm, dry air or irritating bed linens, should be identified. In general, washing with soap and hot water is avoided. Bath oils containing a surfactant that makes the oil mix with bath water (e.g., Alpha-Keri) may be sufficient for cleaning. A warm bath with a mild soap followed by application of a bland emollient to moist skin can control **xerosis** (dry skin). Applying a cold compress or cooling agents that contain menthol and camphor (which constrict blood vessels) may also help relieve pruritus. If baths have been prescribed, the nurse reminds the patient to use tepid (not hot) water and to shake off the excess water and blot between intertriginous areas (body folds) with a towel. Rubbing vigorously with the towel is avoided because this overstimulates the skin and causes more itching. It also removes water from the stratum corneum (horny layer or outermost layer of the epidermis). Immediately after bathing, the patient should lubricate the skin with an emollient to trap moisture. The nurse instructs the patient to avoid situations that cause vasodilation, such as exposure to an overly warm environment and ingestion of alcohol or hot foods and liquids. Activities that result in perspiration should be limited because perspiration may irritate and promote pruritus. If the patient is troubled at night with itching that interferes with sleep, the nurse can advise wearing cotton clothing next to the skin rather than synthetic materials. The room should be kept cool and humidified. Vigorous scratching should be avoided and nails kept trimmed to prevent skin damage and

BOX 51-2 Systemic Disorders Associated With Generalized Pruritus

- Chronic kidney disease
- Obstructive biliary disease (primary biliary cirrhosis, extrahepatic biliary obstruction, drug-induced cholestasis)
- Endocrine disease (thyrotoxicosis, hypothyroidism, diabetes mellitus)
- Psychiatric disorders (emotional stress, anxiety, neurosis, phobias)
- Malignancies (polycythemia vera; Hodgkin disease; lymphoma; leukemia; multiple myeloma; mycosis fungoides; and cancers of the lung, breast, central nervous system, and GI tract)
- Neurologic disorders (multiple sclerosis, brain abscess, brain tumor)
- Infestations (scabies, lice, other insects)
- Pruritus of pregnancy (pruritic urticarial papules of pregnancy [PUPP], cholestasis of pregnancy, pemphigoid of pregnancy)
- Folliculitis (bacterial, candidiasis, dermatophyte)
- Skin conditions (seborrheic dermatitis, folliculitis, iron deficiency anemia, atopic dermatitis)

infection. When the underlying cause of pruritus is unknown and further testing is required, the nurse explains each test and the expected outcome.

Topical corticosteroids may be beneficial as anti-inflammatory agents to decrease itching. Oral antihistamines are even more effective because they can overcome the effects of histamine released from damaged mast cells. An antihistamine, such as diphenhydramine or hydroxyzine, prescribed in a sedative dose at bedtime may be beneficial in producing a restful and comfortable sleep. Nonsedating antihistamine medications, such as fexofenadine, are more appropriate to relieve daytime pruritus. Tricyclic antidepressants may be prescribed for pruritus of neuropsychogenic origin. If pruritus continues, further investigation of a systemic problem is advised.

PERINEAL AND PERIANAL PRURITUS

Pathophysiology

Pruritus of the genital and anal regions may be caused by small particles of fecal material lodged in the perianal crevices or attached to anal hairs. Alternatively, it may result from perianal skin damage caused by scratching, moisture, and decreased skin resistance as a result of corticosteroid or antibiotic therapy. Other possible causes of perianal itching include local irritants such as scabies and lice, local lesions such as hemorrhoids, fungal or yeast infections, and pinworm infestation. Foods associated with anal pruritus include coffee, tea, cola, beer, chocolate, and tomatoes. Occasionally, no cause for genital and anal pruritus can be identified.

Medical and Nursing Management

The nurse instructs the patient to follow proper hygiene measures and to discontinue home and over-the-counter remedies. The perineal or anal area should be rinsed with lukewarm water and blotted dry with cotton balls. Premoistened tissues may be used after defecation. Cornstarch can be applied in the skinfold areas to absorb perspiration.

As part of health teaching, the nurse instructs the patient to avoid bathing in water that is too hot and to avoid using bubble baths, sodium bicarbonate, and detergent soaps, all of which aggravate dryness. To keep the perineal or perianal skin as dry as possible, patients should avoid wearing underwear made of synthetic fabrics. Local anesthetic agents should not be used because of possible allergic effects. The patient should also avoid vasodilating agents or stimulants (e.g., alcohol, caffeine) and mechanical irritants, such as rough or woolen clothing. A diet that includes adequate fiber may help maintain soft stools and prevent minor trauma to the anal mucosa.

ULCERATION

Superficial loss of surface tissue as a result of death of cells is called an ulceration. A simple **ulcer**, such as the kind found in a small, superficial, partial-thickness burn, tends to heal by granulation if kept clean and protected from injury. If exposed to the air, the serum that escapes will dry and form a scab, under which the epithelial cells grow and cover the surface completely. The four most common ulcers noted are arterial, venous, neuropathic/diabetic, and pressure ulcers (Table 51-3).

ARTERIAL ULCERS

Ulcers related to problems with arterial circulation are seen in older patients and patients with hypertension, diabetes, cigarette smoking, hypercholesterolemia, obesity, chronic kidney disease, family history of cardiovascular disease, persistent *Chlamydia pneumoniae* infection, periodontal disease, and a sedentary lifestyle. Arterial ulcers are caused by lower extremity arterial disease (LEAD), which is inadequate blood flow to the tissue, resulting in severe tissue ischemia, and which can create ulcers that are extremely painful (Bolognia et al., 2022). They are commonly found at the lateral malleolus, shin, toe tips, and web space of toes and heels. They can be caused by areas of exposed pressure, repetitive trauma, or rubbing footwear (Strauss et al., 2024). This condition is also referred to as peripheral arterial disease (PAD), peripheral vascular disease (PVD), or peripheral arterial occlusive disease (PAOD). In patients with LEAD and ulcers, treatment of the ulcers is concurrent with treatment of the arterial disease. Management includes the use of dressings and/or tissue perfusion improvement. Perfusion and tissue oxygenation can improve outcomes via surgical options (bypass graft, angioplasty), medications (antiplatelets, vasodilators, hemorheologics [decrease the viscosity of the blood], antilipemic [decrease lipid levels], analgesics), lifestyle changes, and adjunctive therapies (hyperbaric oxygen therapy) (Schneider et al., 2021). If these interventions are instituted early in the progression of an ulcer, the condition can often be effectively improved. Surgical amputation of an affected limb is a last resort. Refer to Chapter 17 for additional details on arterial and venous ulcers.

VENOUS ULCERS

Venous ulcers are more common than arterial ulcers. They occur due to impaired return of venous blood from the tissue to the heart, also known as chronic venous insufficiency (CVI) or lower extremity venous disease (LEVD). Risk factors are older age (>50), being female, obesity, multiple pregnancies, thrombophlebitis, leg trauma (deep vein thrombosis or fractures), and thrombophilic conditions (increased coagulability of the blood). Other risks factors include arthritis or calf muscle dysfunction, IV drug use involving the affected extremity, sedentary lifestyle, or prolonged standing. Typical location is superior to the medial malleolus but can be anywhere on the lower extremity (see Chapter 17). Healing can be affected by diabetes, smoking, nutrition, and medications. Management includes reduction of edema, prevention of complications, and appropriate topical therapy or specialty dressings (Schneider et al., 2021).

TABLE 51-3 **Characteristics of Ulcers**

Ulcer Type	Location	Description of Wound Bed	Exudate	Description of Wound Edges
Arterial 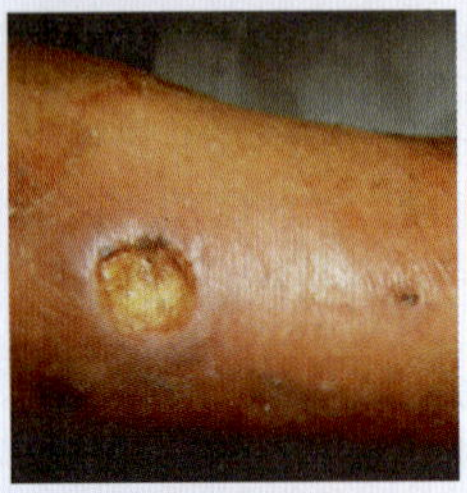	Tips of toes, pressure points, areas of trauma	Pale or necrotic	Minimal amount	Well defined
Venous 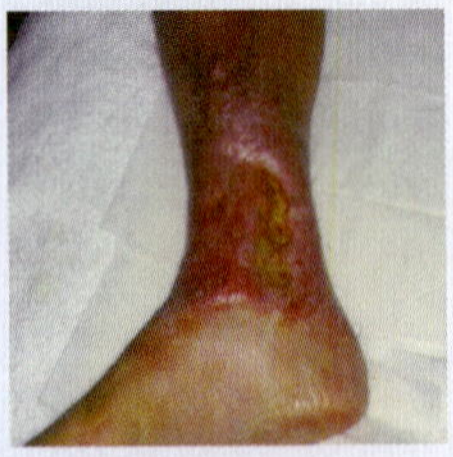	Commonly located in the lower leg just above the ankle (gaiter region)	Dark red, "ruddy"	Moderate to large amounts	Poorly defined; irregular
Neuropathic 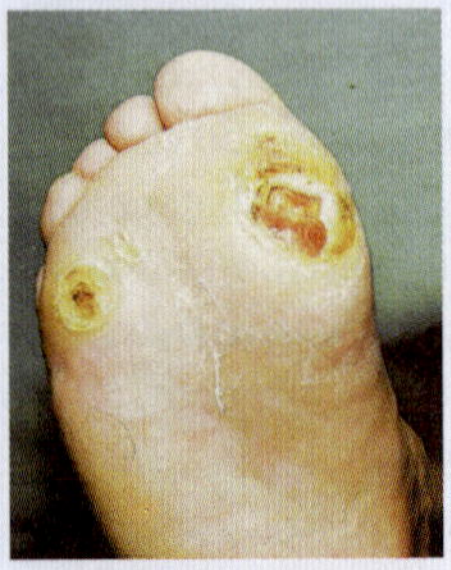	Plantar surface over metatarsal heads	Typically red (unless coexisting ischemia)	Moderate to large amounts	Well defined
Pressure 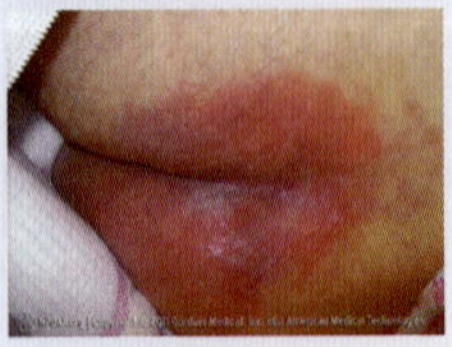	Any boney prominence	Erythremic or purplish in discoloration due to pressure	Minimal to large amounts	Poorly to well defined

Reprinted with permission from Goodheart, H. P. (2010). *Goodheart's same-site differential diagnosis: A rapid method of diagnosing and treating common skin disorders* (arterial ulcer). Lippincott, Williams, & Wilkins Nettina, S. M. (2001). *The Lippincott manual of nursing practice* (7th ed.). Lippincott, Williams & Wilkins (venous ulcer); Bickley, L. (2013). *A guide to physical examination and history taking* (11th ed.). J.B. Lippincott (neuropathic ulcer); and Doughty, D., & McNichol, L. (2015). *Wound, ostomy and continence nurses society core curriculum: Wound management*. Lippincott, Williams, and Wilkins (pressure ulcer).

NEUROPATHIC ULCERS

Diabetic foot ulcers are also known as neuropathic ulcers or lower extremity neuropathic disease (LEND). These ulcers occur due to reduced blood supply to the nerves, also known as microvascular damage, which can lead to neuropathy. Neuropathy is classified as a lack of sensorium, movement or autonomic function or feedback. Most neuropathic ulcerations occur on the lower extremity and affect prominent pedal surfaces, such as the heel and metatarsal heads, or areas of high friction that are prone to callus formation (Eastman & Dreyer, 2022). Risk factors include history of amputations or ulcers, long duration of diabetes and/or poor glucose control, limited joint mobility, long history of smoking, obesity, poor vision, poor footwear, vascular insufficiency, structural deformities and callus formation, absence of protective sensation, and autonomic neuropathy causing decreased sweating and dry feet (Driver et al., 2016; Oliver & Mutluoglu, 2022).

Early prevention can be achieved through comprehensive annual foot examinations (including monofilament testing for evidence of neuropathy), glycemic control, limiting other health complications, and offloading (pressure relief).

Nursing assessment includes determining the size and depth of the ulcer and inspecting the surrounding area for evidence of infection (pain, warmth, erythema, or induration [localized hardening of the soft tissue]) and vascular insufficiency (decreased pulses, loss of hair, muscle atrophy, gangrene) (Sumpio et al., 2020). Wound management may include revascularization to improve healing potential, debridement, callus removal, treatment of infection if needed, topical specialty wound care dressing, and/or adjunctive therapies (Driver et al., 2016; Oliver & Mutluoglu, 2022). For further information related to diabetic neuropathy, refer to Chapter 29.

PRESSURE ULCERS

Pathophysiology

Pressure ulcers involve the breakdown of the skin due to prolonged pressure, friction, and shear forces, and insufficient blood supply, usually at bony prominences. Pressure ulcers are localized areas of infarcted soft tissue that occur when pressure applied to the skin over time is greater than normal capillary closure pressure, which is about 32 mm Hg. Weight-bearing bony prominences are most susceptible to pressure ulcer development because they are covered only by skin and small amounts of subcutaneous tissue. Susceptible areas include the sacrum and coccygeal areas, ischial tuberosities (especially in people who sit for prolonged periods), greater trochanter, heel, knee, malleolus, medial condyle of the tibia, fibular head, scapula, and elbow (Fig. 51-1).

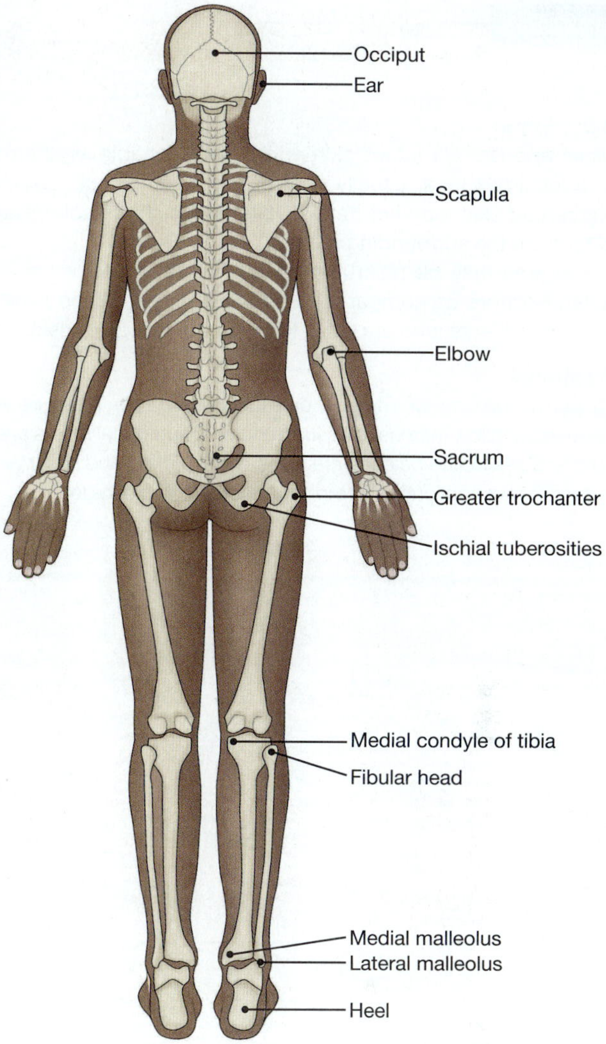

FIGURE 51-1 **Areas susceptible to pressure ulcers.**

Risk Factors

Box 51-3 summarizes risk factors for pressure ulcers.

Clinical Manifestations and Assessment

The initial sign of pressure is erythema (redness of the skin) caused by reactive hyperemia, which normally resolves in less than 1 hour. Unrelieved pressure results in tissue ischemia or anoxia. The cutaneous tissues become broken or destroyed, leading to progressive destruction and necrosis of underlying soft tissue, and the resulting pressure ulcer is painful and slow to heal. The nurse assesses the patient's mobility, sensory perception, cognitive abilities, tissue perfusion, nutritional status, friction and shear forces, sources of moisture on the skin, age, and skin condition. Scales such as the Braden or Norton scale may be used to facilitate systematic assessment and quantification of a patient's risk for pressure ulcers, although the nurse should recognize that the reliability of these scales is not well established for all patient populations. If a pressure area is observed, the nurse notes its size and location and uses a grading system to describe its severity (refer to Box 51-4 for current standards in assessing and staging pressure ulcers). Recent studies regarding tools for pressure ulcers reveal a lack of consensus regarding the key elements needed to conduct a comprehensive assessment, inconsistency in specific patient settings (critical care) and low quality of evidence. Many tools are currently undergoing revision; therefore, it is imperative that nurses use a consistent scale (Smet et al., 2021; Zhang et al., 2021).

BOX 51-3 **Risk Factors for Pressure Ulcers**

- Immobility, compromised mobility
- Prolonged pressure on tissue
- Altered skin moisture: excessively dry, excessively moist (perspiration, urine, feces, or drainage produces maceration [softening] of the skin)
- Equipment: Casts, traction, restraints, medical devices
- Impaired sensory perception or cognition
- Decreased tissue perfusion (seen with diabetes, obesity, and edema). Patients who are critically ill have a lower capillary closure pressure and, thus, higher risk.
- Decreased nutritional status (anemia, hypoalbuminemia, vitamin deficiency)
- Friction and shear forces

BOX 51-4

Stages of Pressure Ulcers

Stage I

Description

Ulcer appears as intact skin with nonblanchable erythema of a localized area, usually over a bony prominence. Darkly pigmented skin may not have visible blanching; its color may differ from the surrounding area.

The area may be painful, firm, soft, and warmer or cooler in temperature as compared to adjacent tissue. Stage I may indicate patients who are "at risk" (a heralding sign of risk).

Treatment

To permit healing of Stage I pressure ulcers, the pressure is removed to allow increased tissue perfusion; nutritional status and fluid and electrolyte balance are maintained; friction and shear are reduced; and application of moisture to the skin is avoided.

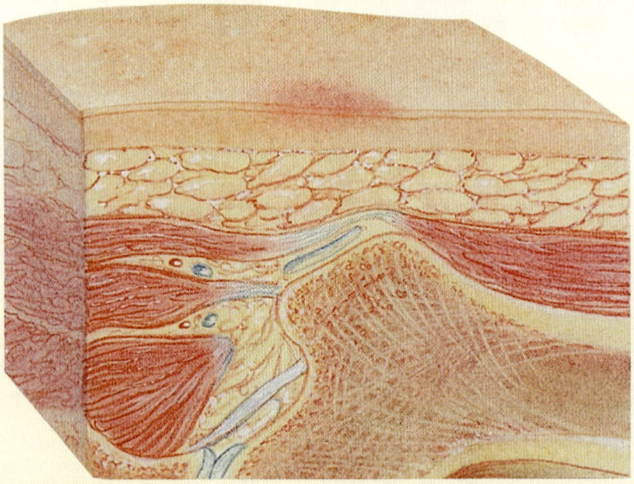

Stage II

Description

Ulcer appears as partial-thickness loss of dermis, presenting as a shallow open ulcer with a red or pink wound bed, without slough. It may also present as an intact or open/ruptured serum-filled blister.

It may be a shiny or dry shallow ulcer without slough or bruising (bruising indicates suspected deep tissue injury). This stage should not be used to describe skin tears, tape burns, perineal dermatitis, maceration, or excoriation.

Treatment

In addition to measures listed for Stage I pressure ulcers, a moist environment, in which migration of epidermal cells over the ulcer surface occurs more rapidly, should be provided to aid wound healing. The ulcer is gently cleansed with sterile saline solution. Use of a heat lamp to dry the open wound is avoided, as is the use of antiseptic solutions that damage healthy tissues and delay wound healing. Semipermeable occlusive dressings, hydrocolloid wafers, or wet saline dressings are helpful in providing a moist environment for healing and in minimizing the loss of fluids and proteins from the body.

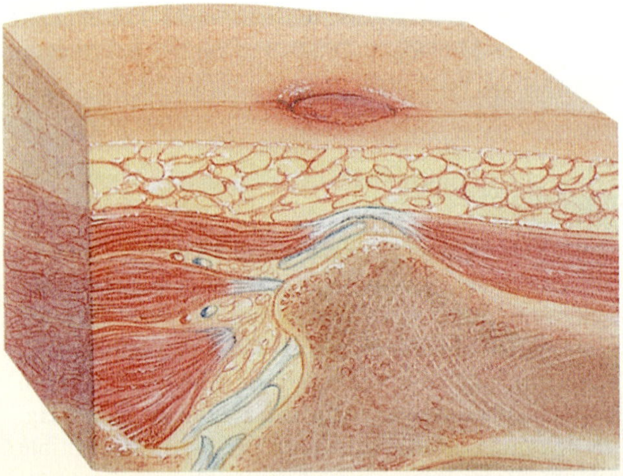

Stage III

Description

There is full-thickness tissue loss. Subcutaneous fat may be visible, but bone, tendon, or muscle is not exposed. Slough may be present but does not obscure the depth of tissue loss. The ulcer may include undermining and tunneling.

The depth of a Stage III pressure ulcer varies by anatomic location. The bridge of the nose, ear, occiput and malleolus do not have subcutaneous tissue, and Stage III ulcers here can be shallow. In contrast, areas of significant adiposity can develop Stage III pressure ulcers that are extremely deep. Bone/tendon is not visible or directly palpable.

Treatment

Stage III and IV pressure ulcers are characterized by extensive tissue damage. In addition to the measures listed for Stage II, these advanced, draining, necrotic pressure ulcers must be cleaned (debrided) to create an area that will heal. Necrotic, devitalized tissue favors bacterial growth, delays granulation, and inhibits healing. Wound cleaning and dressing are uncomfortable; therefore, the nurse must prepare the patient for the procedure by explaining what will occur and administering prescribed analgesia.

Debridement may be accomplished by wet-to-damp dressing changes, mechanical flushing of necrotic and infective exudate, application of prescribed enzyme preparations that dissolve necrotic tissue, or surgical dissection. If an eschar covers the ulcer, it is removed surgically to ensure a clean, vitalized wound. Exudate may be absorbed by dressings or special hydrophilic powders, beads, or gels. Cultures of infected pressure ulcers are obtained to guide the selection of antibiotic therapy.

After the pressure ulcer is clean, a topical treatment is prescribed to promote granulation. New granulation tissue must be protected from reinfection, drying, and damage, and care should be taken to prevent pressure and further trauma to the area. Dressings, solutions, and ointments applied to the ulcer should not disrupt the healing process. Multiple agents and protocols are used to treat pressure ulcers, but consistency is an important key to success. Objective evaluation of the pressure ulcer (e.g., measurement of the size and depth of the pressure ulcer, inspection for granulation tissue) for response to the treatment protocol must be made every 4–6 days. Taking photographs at weekly intervals is a reliable strategy for monitoring the healing process, which may take weeks to months.

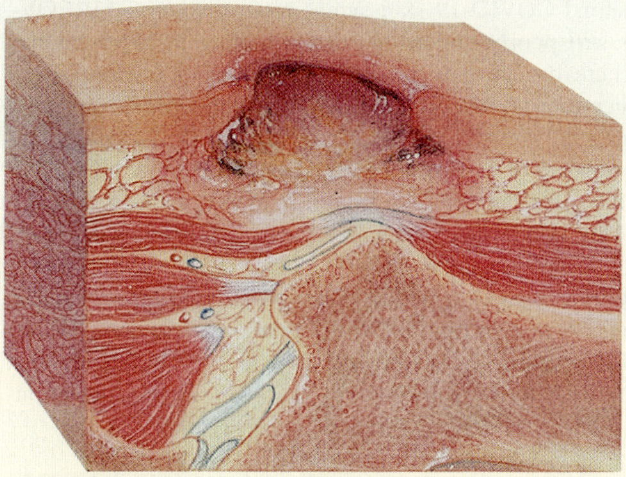

Stage IV

Description

There is full-thickness tissue loss with exposed bone, tendon, or muscle. Slough or eschar may be present on some parts of the wound bed. These ulcers often include undermining and tunneling.

The depth of a Stage IV pressure ulcer varies by anatomic location. The bridge of the nose, ear, occiput, and malleolus do not have subcutaneous tissue, and these ulcers can be shallow. Stage IV ulcers can extend into muscle and/or supporting structures (e.g., fascia, tendon, or joint capsule), making osteomyelitis possible. Exposed bone/tendon is visible or directly palpable.

Treatment

See Stage III treatment. In addition, surgical intervention may be necessary when the ulcer is extensive, when complications (e.g., fistula) exist, and when the ulcer does not respond to treatment. Surgical procedures include debridement, incision and drainage, bone resection, and skin grafting. Osteomyelitis is a common complication of wounds of Stage IV depth. See Chapter 40 for more information on osteomyelitis.

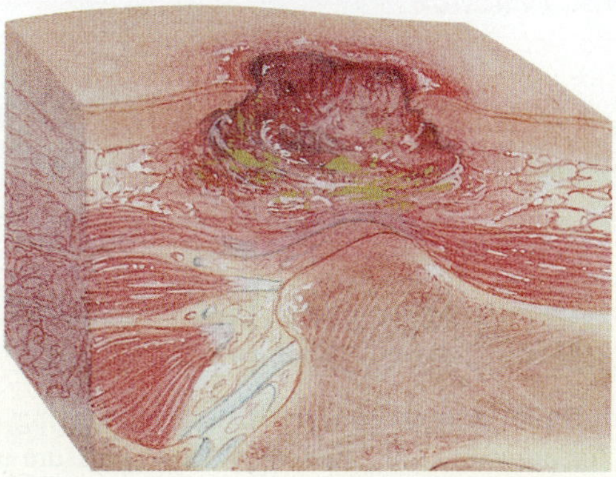

Unstageable

An unstageable lesion shows full-thickness tissue loss in which the base of the ulcer is covered by slough (yellow, tan, gray, green, or brown) and/or eschar (tan, brown or black) in the wound bed.

Until enough slough and/or eschar is removed to expose the base of the wound, the true depth and, therefore, stage cannot be determined. Stable (dry, adherent, intact without erythema or fluctuance) eschar on the heels serves as the body's natural (biologic) cover and should not be removed.

Suspected Deep Tissue Injury (DTI)

Suspected deep tissue injury (DTI) appears as a purple or maroon localized area of discolored intact skin or blood-filled blister due to damage of underlying soft tissue from pressure and/or shear. The area may be preceded by tissue that is painful, firm, mushy, boggy, warmer, or cooler as compared to adjacent tissue.

DTI may be difficult to detect in individuals with dark skin tones. Evolution may include a thin blister over a dark wound bed. The wound may further evolve and become covered by thin eschar. Evolution may be rapid, exposing additional layers of tissue even with optimal treatment.

Moisture-associated skin damage (MASD)

Inflammation or skin erosion can be caused by prolonged exposure to a source of moisture such as urine, stool, sweat, wound drainage, saliva, or mucus. It is proposed that for MASD to occur, another complicating factor is required in addition to moisture exposure.

The moisture barrier of the skin plays a critical role in maintaining homeostasis within the body, mainly by concurrently slowing the movement of water out of the body (transepidermal water loss, or TEWL) and regulating the absorption of water and solutes from outside the body.

Medical device–related pressure injuries (MDRPIs)

Medical device–related pressure injuries (MDRPIs) is a term utilized to describe a hospital-acquired pressure injury (HAPI) that occurs due to a particular medical device. Patients with a medical device are at risk for MDRPI due to impaired sensation, poor perfusion, altered tissue tolerance, poor nutrition, edema, and tendency to develop moisture under the devices. Respiratory devices such as oxygen tubing, endotracheal devices, tubes/drains such as urine catheters, and compression stockings/braces are the four most common types of devices that cause HAPIs in patients.

Pearls for Practice

As of 2008, Medicare regulations do not reimburse for treatment of pressure ulcers acquired in the hospital, even if the ulcer was present on admission but undocumented. Therefore, it is imperative that accurate recognition and staging of pressure ulcers occur in all patients.

Medical and Nursing Management

Treatment depends on stage (see Box 51-4). Nursing interventions for prevention and management of pressure ulcers include turning and repositioning the patient every 1 to 2 hours when in bed, and shifting of weight every 15 minutes while in a chair to allow the blood to flow into the ischemic areas to help tissues recover from the effects of pressure. The recumbent position is preferred to the semi-Fowler position because of increased support of body surface area (BSA) in this position, with careful attention paid to the repositioning of the patient's ankles, elbows, and shoulders. The nurse inspects the patient's skin at each position change and assesses for temperature elevation. If redness or heat is noted, or if the patient complains of discomfort, pressure on the area must be relieved.

A pillow or commercial heel protector may be used to support the heels off the bed when the patient is supine. Supporting the patient in a 30-degree side-lying position avoids pressure on the trochanter. At times, to help relieve the pressure on the skin, patients may need special beds and/or equipment, such as wheelchair cushions and static support devices (such as high-density foam, air, or liquid mattress overlays). Shear occurs when patients are pulled, are allowed to slump, or move by digging heels or elbows into the mattress. Raising the head of the bed by even a few centimeters increases the shearing force over the sacral area; therefore, the semireclining position is avoided in patients at risk. The patient is encouraged to remain active and is ambulated whenever possible. Exercise and repositioning improve tissue perfusion. Massage of erythematous areas is avoided because damage to the capillaries and deep tissue may occur.

Strategies to improve cognition and sensory perception may include stimulating the patient to increase awareness of self in the environment, encouraging the patient to participate in self-care, or supporting the patient's efforts toward active compensation for loss of sensation (e.g., a patient with paraplegia lifting up from the sitting position every 15 minutes).

Continuous moisture on the skin must be prevented by meticulous hygiene measures. Perspiration, urine, stool, and drainage must be removed from the skin promptly. The skin may be lubricated with a bland lotion to keep it soft and pliable. Drying agents and powders are avoided. Topical barrier ointments (e.g., petroleum jelly) may be helpful in protecting the skin of patients who are incontinent. Absorbent pads that wick moisture away from the body should be used to absorb drainage.

The patient's nutritional status must be adequate, and a positive nitrogen balance must be maintained because pressure ulcers develop more quickly and are more resistant to treatment in patients with nutritional disorders. A high-protein diet with protein supplements may be helpful. Iron preparations may be necessary to raise the hemoglobin concentration so that tissue oxygen levels can be maintained within acceptable limits. Ascorbic acid (vitamin C) is necessary for tissue healing. Other nutrients associated with healthy skin include vitamin A, B vitamins, zinc, and sulfur. See Box 51-5 for a systematic overview of research on preventing pressure ulcers.

COVID-19 Related Skin Manifestations

The COVID-19 pandemic has had a great impact on the integumentary system (skin, hair, nails). The pathology behind COVID-19 skin symptoms caused by SAR-COV-2 is still poorly understood and continues to be researched. There has been a tremendous amount of evidence-based literature to support the assessment, prevention, and treatment of pressure ulcers; it continues to be a challenge for providers to assess and identify the etiology of COVID-19 skin manifestations and formulate evidence-based treatment plans. There have been five cutaneous patterns identified among persons with COVID-19 that include chilblains-like lesions (e.g., COVID toes), purpuric lesions, urticarial rash, maculopapular/morbilliform lesions, and purpuric "vasculitic" pattern lesions (Freeman et al., 2020; Van Onselen, 2020). Box 51-6 summarizes COVID-19 skin manifestations.

Gerontologic Considerations

In older adults, the skin has diminished epidermal thickness, dermal collagen, and tissue elasticity. The skin is drier as a result of diminished activity of the sebaceous and sweat glands. Cardiovascular changes result in decreased tissue perfusion. Muscles atrophy, and bone structures become prominent. Diminished sensory perception and reduced ability to reposition oneself contribute to prolonged pressure on the skin. Therefore, older adults are more susceptible to pressure ulcers, which cause pain and suffering and reduce quality of life. Refer to Table 50-1 for age-related changes of the skin.

SEBORRHEIC DERMATITIS

Seborrhea is excessive production of sebum (secretion of sebaceous glands) in areas where sebaceous glands are normally found in large numbers, such as on the face, scalp, eyebrows, eyelids, sides of the nose and upper lip, malar regions (cheeks), ears, axillae, under the breasts, in the groin, and in the gluteal crease of the buttocks. Seborrheic dermatitis is a chronic inflammatory disease of the skin with a predilection for areas that are well supplied with sebaceous glands or lie between skin folds, where the bacteria count is high.

BOX 51-5

Nursing Research

Strategies to Prevent Hospital-Acquired Pressure Injuries in the Intensive Care Unit

Pomerleau, T. A. (2021). Strategies to prevent hospital acquired pressure injuries in the intensive care unit.

Purpose

Despite all the advances in health care, hospital-acquired pressure injuries (HAPIs) remain a worldwide public health problem related to patient safety (Gaspar et al., 2019). The hospital-acquired pressure injury rate in the medical surgical intensive care unit for the year 2019 at Hospital X was greater than the national benchmark. The global aim statement was to improve the quality of patient care by developing an evidence-based educational suite in collaboration with interdisciplinary team members for prevention of hospital-acquired pressure injuries.

Design

This Quality Improvement Project utilized the Plan Do Study Act Cycle to carry out the interventions and implementation. It took place in the intensive care unit of Hospital X. The educational session in a dedicated classroom followed a tandem integumentary assessment. The utilization of a standardized scale and the visual documentation of high-risk anatomy were logged on a daily basis.

The search strategy was designed to retrieve studies published in English across CINAHL, Medline, Cochrane Central Register of Controlled Trials, Embase, Scopus, and Mednar between 2000 and 2015. All adult ICU participants were aged 18 years or over. This review included randomized controlled trials, quasi-experimental studies, and comparative studies. The studies that were selected for retrieval were assessed by two independent reviewers for methodologic validity prior to inclusion in the review using standardized critical-appraisal instruments.

Findings

Among 48 nurses, 43 (90%) attended the evidence-based educational suite and performed a tandem integumentary assessment. Among 1,896 opportunities for a skin risk, 1,580 (83%) were completed. The visual documentation of high-risk anatomy by ICU staff went from 17% to 65% adherence.

Nursing Implications

A multidisciplinary team looked at the evidence-based care regarding hospital-acquired pressure injuries and assisted the care team to be able to work within the means of the technology and equipment that is available. Most of the nurses appeared to embrace the project. They were amenable to the idea of capturing the high-risk areas through wound photography. They were also amenable to utilizing the Braden Scale as a risk assessment tool.

Clinical Manifestations and Assessment

Two forms of seborrheic dermatitis can occur, an oily form and a dry form. Either form may start in childhood and continue throughout life. The oily form appears moist or "greasy." There may be patches of yellowish-red or gray-white, greasy skin, with white dry scaling macules and/or papules, with slight erythema, predominantly on the forehead; nasolabial folds; ears; retroauricular area (behind the auricle of the ear); beard area; scalp; sternum; and between adjacent skin surfaces in the regions of the axillae, groin, and breasts. Small pustules or papulopustules resembling acne may appear on the trunk. The dry form, consisting of flaky desquamation of the scalp with a profuse amount of fine, powdery scales, is commonly called dandruff. The mild forms of the disease are asymptomatic. When scaling occurs, it is often accompanied by pruritus, which may lead to scratching and secondary infections and excoriation.

Seborrheic dermatitis has a genetic predisposition. Hormones, nutritional status, infection, and emotional stress

BOX 51-6

COVID-19–Related Skin Manifestations

Pseudo-chilblains also referred to as pernio: Commonly presenting as "COVID toes," this is a local inflammatory skin disorder of acral surfaces (refers to the extremities and/or peripheral body parts such as ears) that presents as edema and discoloration of the affected area. The chilblains may present as erythematous-violaceous papules, macules, or nodules, accompanied by itching and pain. Unlike true chilblains, pseudo-chilblains are not associated with exposure to cold temperatures resulting in vasoconstriction (Young & Fernandez, 2020).

Morbilliform rash: This is an erythematous, maculopapular rash. It primarily involves the trunk but may extend to extremities. It is associated with viral exanthems (widespread rash). and is the most common skin manifestation observed in COVID-19 (Singh et al., 2021).

Urticaria: Commonly known as hives, urticaria presents as itchy raised, reddened, or skin-colored welts on the skin. It is triggered by an allergen resulting in release of high levels of histamine. These can vary in size and appearance and can disappear and reappear rapidly (Singh et al., 2021).

Petechiae/purpura lesions: This skin rash consists of red or purple spots caused by bleeding from small blood vessels. The lesions may also be seen on mucous membranes. It is associated with coagulation and vascular disorders (Singh et al., 2021; Young & Fernandez, 2020).

Vesicular rash: Small fluid-filled blisters are often seen with viral and less often with bacterial infections. Larger, tense lesions may be painful. This is a less common manifestation seen in COVID-19 (Singh et al., 2021).

Livedoid lesions including livedo racemosa and livedo reticularis lesions: These vascular lesions are often seen on the lower extremities and feet. Lesions may be erythematous or violaceous and present in a branched or irregular pattern. Lesions are often painful and may become necrotic (Sunderkötter, 2022).

influence its course. The remissions and exacerbations of this condition should be explained to the patient. If a person has not previously been diagnosed with this condition and suddenly appears with a severe outbreak, a complete history and physical examination should be considered.

Pearls for Practice

Children of color often do not experience the classic "cradle cap" appearance of seborrheic dermatitis and have erythema, flaking, and hypopigmentation of the affected areas and folds of skin. Skin of color may require a modified treatment approach that takes into account differences in hair texture and hair washing frequency (Elgash et al., 2019).

Medical and Nursing Management

Because there is no known cure for seborrhea, the objective of therapy is to control the disorder and allow the skin to repair itself. Seborrheic dermatitis of the body and face may respond to antifungals, keratolytics, antipruritics, and anti-inflammatories (topical corticosteroids and calcineurin inhibitors) (Tucker & Masood, 2022). However, if glucocorticoid creams or low potency topical steroids are used (since they decrease the inflammatory response), they should be used with caution near the eyelids because they can induce glaucoma and cataracts in predisposed patients. Patients with seborrheic dermatitis may develop a secondary candidal (yeast) infection in body creases or folds and may have to use a topical antifungal (e.g., topical 1% to 2% ketoconazole, 1% ciclopirox, 1% zinc pyrithione, and 1% hydrocortisone) (Tucker & Masood, 2020). To avoid this, patients should be advised to ensure maximum aeration of the skin and to clean carefully areas where there are creases or folds in the skin. Patients with persistent candidiasis should be evaluated for diabetes. Ultraviolet radiation therapy can be beneficial as a form of treatment as well.

The mainstay of dandruff treatment is proper, frequent shampooing (at least three times weekly) with medicated shampoos. Two or three different types of shampoo should be used in rotation to prevent the seborrhea from becoming resistant to a particular shampoo. The shampoo is left on at least 5 to 10 minutes. As the condition of the scalp improves, the treatment can be less frequent. Antiseborrheic shampoos include those containing selenium sulfide suspension, zinc pyrithione, salicylic acid, or sulfur compounds, and tar shampoo that contains sulfur or salicylic acid. Instructions for using medicated shampoos are reinforced for people with dandruff who require treatment. Frequent shampooing is contrary to some cultural practices; the nurse should be sensitive to these differences when teaching the patient about home care.

A person with seborrheic dermatitis is advised to avoid external irritants, excessive heat, and perspiration; rubbing and scratching prolong the disorder. To avoid secondary infection, the patient should air the skin and keep skin folds clean and dry.

The patient is cautioned that seborrheic dermatitis is a chronic problem that tends to reappear. The goal is to keep it under control. Patients need to be encouraged to adhere to the treatment program. Those who become discouraged and disheartened by the effect on body image should be treated with sensitivity and encouraged to express their feelings.

Research for seborrheic dermatitis and COVID-19 is ongoing. It is possible that the high temperature of the face induces abnormalities of microbiota and permeability of skin barrier and increases sweating with irritant action, and worsening of itching is caused by continuous mask use (Veraldi et al., 2020).

VIRAL SKIN INFECTIONS

HERPES ZOSTER

Herpes zoster, also called *shingles*, is an infection caused by the varicella-zoster virus, a member of a group of DNA viruses. The viruses causing chickenpox and herpes zoster are indistinguishable, hence the name varicella-zoster virus. The disease is characterized by a painful vesicular eruption along the area of distribution of the sensory nerves from one or more posterior ganglia.

Pathophysiology

After a case of chickenpox runs its course, the varicella-zoster viruses responsible for the outbreak lie dormant inside nerve cells near the brain and spinal cord. Later, when these latent viruses are reactivated because of declining cellular immunity, they travel by way of the peripheral nerves to the skin, where the viruses multiply and create a red rash of small, fluid-filled vesicles. About 10% of adults get shingles during their lifetimes, usually after 50 years of age. There is an increased frequency of herpes zoster infections among patients with weakened immune systems and cancers (especially leukemias and lymphomas), those on chemotherapy, and those who are HIV infected.

Clinical Manifestations and Assessment

The eruption is usually accompanied or preceded by pain, which may radiate over the entire region supplied by the affected nerves. The pain may be burning, lancinating (tearing or sharply cutting), stabbing, or aching. Some patients have no pain, but itching and tenderness may occur over the area. Sometimes, malaise and gastrointestinal (GI) disturbances precede the eruption. The patches of grouped vesicles appear on the red and swollen skin. The early vesicles, which contain serum, later may become purulent, rupture, and form crusts. The inflammation is usually unilateral, involving the thoracic, cervical, or cranial nerves in a band-like configuration. Usually the blisters are confined to a narrow region of the face or trunk (Fig. 51-2). The clinical course varies from 1 to 3 weeks. If an ophthalmic nerve is involved, the patient

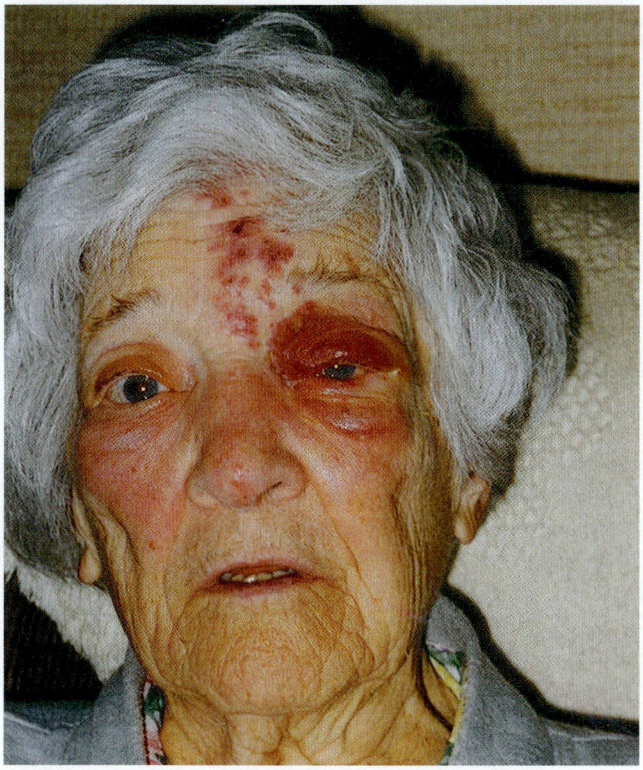

FIGURE 51-2 **Herpes zoster (shingles).**

may have eye pain. Inflammation and a rash on the trunk may cause pain with the slightest touch. The healing time varies from 7 to 26 days.

Herpes zoster in healthy adults is usually localized and benign. However, in patients who are immunosuppressed, the disease may be severe and disabling.

Medical and Nursing Management

There is evidence that infection is arrested if oral antiviral agents, such as acyclovir, valacyclovir, or famciclovir, are administered within 24 hours of the initial eruption. IV acyclovir, if started early, is effective in significantly reducing the pain and halting the progression of the disease. In older patients, the pain from herpes zoster may persist as postherpetic neuralgia (persistent pain of the affected nerve after healing) for months after the skin lesions disappear.

The goals of herpes zoster management are to relieve the pain and to reduce or avoid complications, which include infection, scarring, and postherpetic neuralgia and eye complications. Pain is controlled with analgesics because adequate pain control during the acute phase helps prevent persistent pain patterns. Systemic corticosteroids may be prescribed for patients older than 50 years of age to reduce the incidence and duration of postherpetic neuralgia. Healing usually occurs more quickly in those who have been treated with corticosteroids. Triamcinolone injected subcutaneously under painful areas is effective as an anti-inflammatory agent.

Ophthalmic herpes zoster occurs when an eye is involved. This is considered an ophthalmic emergency, and the patient should be referred to an ophthalmologist immediately to prevent the possible sequelae of keratitis, uveitis, ulceration, and blindness.

People who have been exposed to varicella by primary infection or by vaccination are not at risk for infection after exposure to patients with herpes zoster.

HERPES SIMPLEX

Herpes simplex is a common skin infection. There are two types of the causative virus, which are identified by viral typing. In general, herpes simplex type 1 occurs on the mouth and type 2 occurs in the genital area, but both viral types can be found in both locations. About 85% of adults worldwide are seropositive for herpes type 1. The prevalence of type 2 is lower; type 2 usually appears at the onset of sexual activity. Herpes simplex type 2 is discussed in detail in Chapter 34. Serologic testing shows that many more people are infected than have a history of clinical disease.

Herpes simplex infection is classified as a true primary infection, a nonprimary initial episode, or a recurrent episode. True primary infection is the initial exposure to the virus. A nonprimary initial episode is the initial episode of either type 1 or type 2 in a person previously infected with the other type. Recurrent episodes are subsequent episodes of the same viral type.

TINEA

Fungi—tiny members of a subdivision of the plant kingdom that feed on organic matter—are responsible for various common skin infections. In some cases, they affect only the skin and its appendages (hair and nails). In other cases, internal organs are involved, and the diseases may be life-threatening. However, superficial infections rarely cause even temporary disability and usually respond readily to treatment. Secondary infection with bacteria, *Candida*, or both organisms may occur.

The most common fungal skin infection is **tinea** (Fig. 51-3), which is also called *ringworm* because of its characteristic appearance of a ring or rounded tunnel under the skin. Tinea infections affect the head, body, groin, feet, and nails. Table 51-4 summarizes the tinea infections.

To obtain a specimen for diagnosis, the lesion is cleaned and a scalpel or glass slide is used to remove scales from the margin of the lesion. The scales are dropped onto a slide to which potassium hydroxide has been added. The diagnosis is made by microscopic examination of the infected scales for spores and hyphae or by isolating the organism in culture. Under Wood's light, a specimen of infected hair appears fluorescent; this may be helpful in diagnosing some cases of tinea capitis.

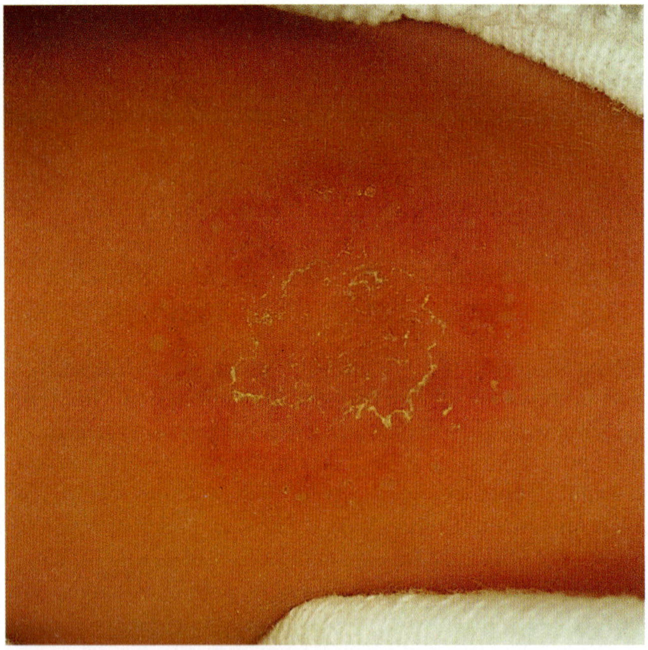

FIGURE 51-3 Tinea corporis. Tinea is one of several conditions (granuloma annulare, nummular eczema) that produces circular lesions. In tinea, the margin of the lesion contains microvesicles, which are best visualized by peering through the lens of a lighted otoscope, and is raised. The flat central area often shows fine scaling. (Reprinted with permission from Fleisher, G. R., Ludwig, S., & Baskin, M. N. [2004]. ***Atlas of pediatric emergency medicine*****. Lippincott Williams & Wilkins.)**

SCABIES

Scabies is an infestation of the skin by the itch mite *Sarcoptes scabiei.* The disease may be found in people living in substandard hygienic conditions, but it can occur in anyone. Infestations may or may not be associated with sexual activity. The mites frequently involve the fingers, and hand contact may produce infection. In children, overnight stays with friends or the exchange of clothes may be a source of infection.

Clinical Manifestations and Assessment

It takes approximately 4 weeks from the time of contact for the patient's symptoms to appear. The patient complains of severe itching caused by a delayed type of immunologic reaction to the mite or its fecal pellets. During examination, the nurse asks the patient where the pruritus is most severe. A magnifying glass and a penlight are held at an oblique angle to the skin while a search is made for the small, raised burrows created by the mites. The burrows may be multiple, straight or wavy, brown or black, thread-like lesions, most commonly observed between the fingers and on the wrists. Other sites are the extensor surfaces of the elbows; the knees; the edges of the feet; the points of the elbows; around the nipples; in the axillary folds; under pendulous breasts; and in or near the groin or gluteal fold, penis, or scrotum. Red, pruritic eruptions usually appear between adjacent skin areas. However, the burrow is not always visible. Any patient with a rash may have scabies.

One classic sign of scabies is the increased itching that occurs during the overnight hours, perhaps because the increased warmth of the skin has a stimulating effect on the parasite. Hypersensitivity to the organism and its products of excretion also may contribute to the pruritus. If the infection has spread, other members of the family and close friends also complain of pruritus about a month later.

Secondary lesions are quite common and include vesicles, papules, excoriations, and crusts. Bacterial superinfection

TABLE **51-4 Tinea (Ringworm) Infections**

Type and Location	Clinical Manifestations	Treatment
Tinea corporis (body)	• Begins with red macule, which spreads to a ring of papules or vesicles with central clearing. • Lesions are found in clusters. • Many spread to the hair, scalp, or nails. • Very pruritic. • An infected pet may be the source.	• Mild conditions: topical antifungal creams • Severe conditions: griseofulvin or terbinafine
Tinea cruris (groin area; "jock itch")	• Begins with small, red scaling patches, which spread to form circular elevated plaques. • Very pruritic. • Clusters of pustules may be seen around borders.	• Mild conditions: topical antifungal creams • Severe conditions: griseofulvin or terbinafine
Tinea pedis (foot; "athlete's foot")	• Soles of one or both feet have scaling and mild redness with maceration in the toe webs. • More acute infections may have clusters of clear vesicles on dusky base.	• Soak feet in vinegar and water solution • Resistant infections: griseofulvin or terbinafine • Terbinafine daily for 3 months
Tinea unguium (toenails; affects about 50% of adults)	• Nails thicken, crumble easily, and lack luster. • Whole nail may be destroyed.	• Itraconazole in pulses of 1 week a month for 3 months in cases of terbinafine failure

may result from constant excoriation of the burrows and papules.

The diagnosis is confirmed by recovering *S. scabiei* or the mites' byproducts from the skin. A sample of superficial epidermis is scraped from the top of the burrows or papules with a small scalpel blade. The scrapings are placed on a microscope slide and examined through a microscope at low power to demonstrate evidence of the mite; however, this method often misses the correct diagnosis because of the high chance of sampling error (Gilson & Crane, 2022).

Gerontologic Considerations

Older patients living in long-term care facilities are susceptible to outbreaks of scabies because of close living quarters, poor hygiene due to limited physical ability, and the potential for incidental spread of the organisms by staff members. Although pruritus may be severe in the older patient, the vivid inflammatory reaction seen in younger people seldom occurs. Scabies may not be recognized in the older person; the pruritus may be attributed erroneously to the dry skin of old age or to anxiety.

Health care personnel in extended-care facilities should wear gloves when providing hands-on care for a patient suspected of having scabies until the diagnosis is confirmed and treatment completed. It is advisable to treat all residents, staff, and families of patients at the same time to prevent reinfection. Because older patients may be more sensitive to side effects of the scabicides, they should be observed closely for reactions.

Medical and Nursing Management

The patient is instructed to take a warm, soapy bath or shower to remove the scaling debris from the crusts and then to dry thoroughly and allow the skin to cool. A prescription scabicide, such as lindane, crotamiton, or 5% permethrin, is applied thinly to the entire skin from the neck down, sparing only the face and scalp (which are not affected in scabies). The medication is left on for 12 to 24 hours, after which the patient is instructed to wash thoroughly. One application may be curative, but it is advisable to repeat the treatment in 1 week.

CONTACT DERMATITIS

Contact dermatitis is an inflammatory reaction of the skin to physical, chemical, or biologic agents.

Pathophysiology

The epidermis is damaged by repeated physical and chemical irritations. Contact dermatitis may be of the primary irritant type, in which a nonallergic reaction results from exposure to an irritating substance, or it may be an allergic reaction resulting from exposure of sensitized people to contact allergens. Common causes of irritant dermatitis are soaps, detergents, scouring compounds, and industrial chemicals. Predisposing factors include extremes of heat and cold, frequent contact with soap and water, and a pre-existing skin disease (Box 51-7).

BOX 51-7 **Patient Education**

Strategies for Avoiding Contact Dermatitis

The following precautions may help prevent repeated cases of contact dermatitis. Follow these instructions for at least 4 months after your skin appears to be completely healed:

- Study the pattern and location of your dermatitis and think about which things have touched your skin and which things may have caused the problem. Try to avoid contact with these materials.
- Avoid heat, soap, and rubbing, all of which are external irritants.
- Choose bath soaps, laundry detergents, and cosmetics that do not contain fragrance.
- Avoid using a fabric softener dryer sheet (Bounce, Cling Free). Fabric softeners that are added to the washer may be used.
- Avoid topical medications, lotions, or ointments, except those specifically prescribed for your condition.
- Wash your skin thoroughly immediately after exposure to possible irritants.
- When wearing gloves (e.g., for washing dishes or general cleaning), be sure they are cotton-lined. Do not wear them more than 15 or 20 minutes at a time.

Clinical Manifestations and Assessment

The eruptions begin when the causative agent contacts the skin. The first reactions include pruritus, burning, and erythema, followed closely by edema, papules, vesicles, and oozing or weeping. In the subacute phase, these vesicular changes are less marked, and they alternate with crusting, drying, fissuring, and peeling. If repeated reactions occur or if the patient continually scratches the skin, **lichenification** (thickening of the horny layer of the skin) and pigmentation occur. Secondary bacterial invasion may follow.

Medical and Nursing Management

The objectives of management are to rest the involved skin and protect it from further damage. The distribution pattern of the reaction is identified to differentiate allergic and irritant contact dermatitis. A detailed history is obtained. If possible, the offending irritant is removed. Local irritation should be avoided, and generally soap is not used until healing occurs.

Many preparations are advocated for relieving dermatitis. In general, a bland, unmedicated lotion is used for small patches of erythema. Cool, wet dressings also are applied over small areas of vesicular dermatitis. Finely cracked ice added to the water often enhances its antipruritic effect.

Wet dressings usually help clear the oozing eczematous lesions. Then a thin layer of cream or ointment containing a corticosteroid may be used. Medicated baths at room temperature are prescribed for larger areas of dermatitis. For severe, widespread conditions, a short course of systemic corticosteroids may be prescribed.

NONINFECTIOUS INFLAMMATORY DERMATOSES

PSORIASIS

Considered one of the most common skin diseases, psoriasis affects over 2% of the population, appearing more often in people of European ancestry. It is thought that this chronic, noninfectious, inflammatory disease stems from a hereditary defect that causes overproduction of keratin. Onset may occur at any age, but psoriasis is most common in people between 15 and 35 years of age. Individuals with psoriasis have an increased risk of developing other chronic diseases such as psoriatic arthritis, metabolic syndrome, depression, nonalcoholic fatty liver disease, Crohn disease, lymphoma, and cardiovascular disorders (Masson et al., 2020). Psoriasis has a tendency to improve and then recur periodically throughout life (Nair & Badri, 2022).

Pathophysiology

Although the primary cause of psoriasis is unknown, a combination of specific genetic makeup and environmental stimuli may trigger the onset of disease. Current evidence supports an immunologic basis for the disease mediated by T lymphocytes (Nair & Badri, 2022). Periods of emotional stress and anxiety aggravate the condition, and trauma, infections, and seasonal and hormonal changes also are trigger factors.

Epidermal cells are produced at a rate that is about six to nine times faster than normal. The cells in the basal layer of the skin divide too quickly, and the newly formed cells move so rapidly to the skin surface that they become evident as profuse scales or plaques of epidermal tissue. The psoriatic epidermal cell may travel from the basal cell layer of the epidermis to the stratum corneum and be cast off in 3 to 4 days, which is in sharp contrast to the normal 26 to 28 days. As a result of the increased number of basal cells and rapid cell passage, the normal events of cell maturation and growth cannot take place. This abnormal process does not allow the normal protective layers of the skin to form.

Clinical Manifestations and Assessment

Lesions appear as red, raised patches of skin covered with silvery scales. The scaly patches are formed by the buildup of living and dead skin resulting from the vast increase in the rate of skin cell growth and turnover (Fig. 51-4). If the scales are scraped away, the dark-red base of the lesion is exposed,

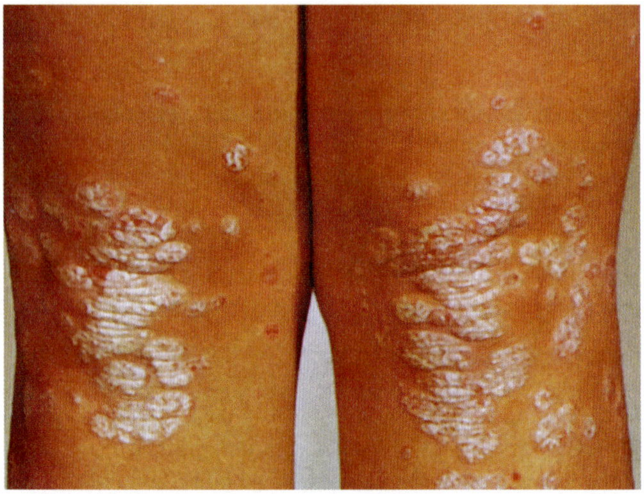

FIGURE 51-4 Psoriasis. (Reprinted with permission from Bickley, L. S. [2013]. *Bate's guide to physical examination and history taking*. Lippincott Williams & Wilkins.)

producing multiple bleeding points. These patches are not moist and may be pruritic. One variation of this condition is called *guttate* (in the shape of a drop) psoriasis because the lesions remain about 1 cm wide and are scattered like raindrops over the body. This variation is believed to be associated with a recent streptococcal throat infection. Psoriasis may range in severity from a cosmetic source of annoyance to a physically disabling and disfiguring disorder.

Particular sites of the body tend to be affected most by this condition; they include the scalp, the extensor surface of the elbows and knees, the lower part of the back, and the genitalia. Bilateral symmetry is a feature of psoriasis. In approximately one fourth to one half of patients, the nails are involved, with pitting, discoloration, crumbling beneath the free edges, and separation of the nail plate. When psoriasis occurs on the palms and soles, it can cause pustular lesions called *palmar pustular psoriasis.*

The presence of the classic plaque-type lesions generally confirms the diagnosis of psoriasis. Because the lesions tend to change histologically as they progress from early to chronic plaques, biopsy of the skin is of little diagnostic value. There are no specific blood tests for diagnosing the condition. When in doubt, the health care provider should assess for signs of nail and scalp involvement and for a positive family history.

Complications

Asymmetric rheumatoid factor–negative arthritis of multiple joints occurs in about 5% of people with psoriasis. The arthritic development can occur before or after the skin lesions appear. The relationship between arthritis and psoriasis is not understood, although an interplay among genetics, environmental factors, and the immune system is suspected; approximately 10% of patients develop severe deforming arthritis (Augustin & Radtke, 2016; Nair & Badri, 2022).

Erythrodermic psoriasis, an exfoliative psoriatic state, involves disease progression that affects the total body surface. The patient is acutely ill, with impaired temperature regulation and fluid and protein loss. Erythrodermic psoriasis often appears in people with chronic psoriasis after infections, after exposure to certain medications, or following withdrawal of systemic corticosteroids.

Medical and Nursing Management

The goals of management are to slow the rapid turnover of epidermis, to promote resolution of the psoriatic lesions, and to control the natural cycles of the disease. There is no known cure.

The therapeutic approach should be one that the patient understands; it should be cosmetically acceptable and minimally disruptive to the patient's lifestyle. Treatment involves the commitment of time and effort by the patient and possibly the family. First, any precipitating or aggravating factors are addressed. An assessment is made of lifestyle because psoriasis is significantly affected by stress. The patient is informed that treatment of severe psoriasis can be time-consuming, expensive, and aesthetically unappealing at times.

Removal of Scales

The most important principle of psoriasis treatment is gentle removal of scales. This can be accomplished with baths. Oils (e.g., olive oil, mineral oil, Aveeno Oilated Oatmeal Bath) or coal tar preparations can be added to the bath water and a soft brush used to scrub the psoriatic plaques gently. After bathing, the application of emollient creams containing alpha-hydroxy acids or salicylic acid continues to soften thick scales. The patient and family should be encouraged to establish a regular skin care routine that can be maintained even when the psoriasis is not in an acute stage.

Pharmacologic Therapy

With the recent addition of biologic medications, four types of therapy are now commonly used: topical, intralesional, oral, and injectable (Table 51-5).

Topical Agents

Topically applied agents are used to slow the overactive epidermis without affecting other tissues. These agents include lotions, ointments, pastes, creams, and shampoos. Topical corticosteroids may be applied for their anti-inflammatory effect. Choosing the correct strength of corticosteroid for the involved site and choosing the most effective vehicle base are important aspects of topical treatment. In general, high-potency topical corticosteroids should not be used on the face and intertriginous areas, and their use on other areas should be limited to a 4-week course of twice-daily applications. A 2-week break should be taken before repeating treatment with the high-potency corticosteroids. For long-term therapy, moderate-potency corticosteroids are used. On the face and intertriginous areas, only low-potency corticosteroids are appropriate for long-term use (see Table 51-6).

TABLE 51-5 Current Pharmacologic Treatment for Psoriasis

Topical Agents	Use	Selected Agents
Biologicals	Moderate to severe lesions	Cyclosporine, alefacept, etanercept, infliximab
Topical corticosteroids	Mild to moderate lesions Moderate to severe lesions Severe lesions Lesions on face and groin	Aristocort, Kenalog, Valisone Lidex, Psorcon, Cutivate Temovate, Diprolene, Ultravate Aclovate, DesOwen, Hytone 2.5%
Topical nonsteroidals	Mild to severe lesions	Retinoids, such as tazarotene Vitamin D_3 derivative calcipotriene
Coal tar products	Mild to moderate lesions	Coal tar and salicylic acid ointment; anthralin; Neutrogena T-Derm, Psori Gel
Medicated shampoos	Scalp lesions	Neutrogena T-Gel, T-Sal, Zetar, Head & Shoulders, Desenex, Selsun Blue, Bakers P&S (emulsifying agent with phenol, saline solution, and mineral oil)
Intralesional therapy	Thick plaques and nails	Kenalog, Cordran-impregnated tape, Fluoroplex
Systemic therapy	Extensive lesions and nails Psoriatic arthritis	Methotrexate; Hydroxyurea; retinoic acid (not to be used in patients who can become pregnant) Oral gold, etretinate, methotrexate
Photochemotherapy	Moderate to severe lesions	UVA or UVB light with or without topical medications PUVA (combines UVA light with oral psoralens, or topical Trisoralen)

TABLE 51-6 **Potency: Topical Corticosteroids**

Potency	Topical Corticosteroid
Over-the-counter	0.5–1.0% hydrocortisone
Lowest	Dexamethasone 0.1% Alclometasone 0.05% Hydrocortisone 2.5%
Low–Medium	Desonide 0.05% Fluocinolone acetonide 0.025% Hydrocortisone valerate 0.2% Betamethasone valerate 0.1% Fluticasone propionate 0.05%
Medium–High	Triamcinolone acetonide 0.1–0.5% Fluocinonide 0.05% Desoximetasone 0.05–0.25% Fluocinolone 0.2% Diflorasone diacetate 0.05%
Very high	Clobetasol propionate 0.05% Betamethasone dipropionate 0.05% Halobetasol propionate 0.05%

Occlusive dressings may be applied to increase the effectiveness of the corticosteroid. Large rolls of tubular plastic can be used to cover the arms and legs. Another option is a vinyl jogging suit. The medication is applied, and the suit is put on over it. The hands can be wrapped in gloves, the feet in plastic bags, and the head in a shower cap. Occlusive dressings should not remain in place longer than 8 hours. The skin should be inspected carefully for the appearance of atrophy, hypopigmentation, striae, and telangiectasias, all side effects of corticosteroids.

When psoriasis involves large areas of the body, topical corticosteroid treatment can be expensive and involve some systemic risk. The more potent corticosteroids, when applied to large areas of the body, have the potential to cause adrenal suppression through percutaneous absorption of the medication. In this event, other treatment modalities (e.g., nonsteroidal topical medications, ultraviolet light) may be used instead or in combination to decrease the need for corticosteroids.

Two topical nonsteroidal treatments introduced within the past few years are calcipotriene and tazarotene. Treatment with these agents tends to suppress **epidermopoiesis** (i.e., development of epidermal cells) and cause sloughing of the rapidly growing epidermal cells. Calcipotriene 0.05% is a derivative of vitamin D_2. It works by decreasing the mitotic turnover of the psoriatic plaques. Its most common side effect is local irritation. The intertriginous areas and face should be avoided when using this medication. The patient should be monitored for symptoms of hypercalcemia. Calcipotriene is available as a cream for use on the body and a solution for the scalp. It is not recommended for use by older patients because of their more fragile skin or by pregnant or lactating patients.

Tazarotene, a retinoid, causes sloughing of the scales covering psoriatic plaques. As with other retinoids, it causes increased sensitivity to sunlight by loss of the outermost layer of skin, so the patient should be cautioned to use an effective sunscreen and avoid other photosensitizers (e.g., tetracycline, antihistamines). Tazarotene is listed as a Category X drug in pregnancy; reports indicate evidence of fetal risk, and the risk of use in pregnant patients clearly outweighs any possible benefits. A negative result on a pregnancy test should be obtained before initiating this medication in patients who can become pregnant, and an effective contraceptive should be continued during treatment. Side effects include burning, erythema, or irritation at the site of application and worsening of psoriasis.

Intralesional Agents

Intralesional injections of the corticosteroid triamcinolone acetonide can be administered directly into highly visible or isolated patches of psoriasis that are resistant to other forms of therapy. Care must be taken to ensure that the medication is not injected into unaffected skin.

Systemic Agents

Although systemic corticosteroids may cause rapid improvement of psoriasis, their usual risks and the possibility of triggering a severe flare-up on withdrawal limit their use. Systemic cytotoxic preparations, such as methotrexate, have been used in treating extensive psoriasis that fails to respond to other forms of therapy.

Methotrexate appears to inhibit DNA synthesis in epidermal cells, thereby reducing the turnover time of the psoriatic epidermis. However, the medication can be toxic, especially to the liver, kidneys, and bone marrow. Laboratory studies must be monitored to ensure that the hepatic, hematopoietic, and renal systems are functioning adequately. The patient should avoid drinking alcohol while taking methotrexate because alcohol ingestion increases the possibility of liver damage. The medication is teratogenic (produces physical defects in the fetus) and thus should not be administered to pregnant patients.

Hydroxyurea also inhibits cell replication by affecting DNA synthesis. The patient is monitored for signs and symptoms of bone marrow depression.

Cyclosporine A, a cyclic peptide used to prevent rejection of transplanted organs, has shown some success in treating severe, therapy-resistant cases of psoriasis. However, its use is limited by side effects such as hypertension and nephrotoxicity.

Oral retinoids (i.e., synthetic derivatives of vitamin A and its metabolite, vitamin A acid) modulate the growth and differentiation of epithelial tissue. Etretinate is especially useful for severe pustular or erythrodermic psoriasis. Etretinate is a teratogen with a very long half-life; it cannot be used in patients who can become pregnant.

Photochemotherapy

One treatment for severely debilitating psoriasis is a psoralen (phototoxic) medication (e.g., methoxsalen) combined with ultraviolet-A (PUVA) light therapy. Ultraviolet light is the portion of the electromagnetic spectrum containing wavelengths ranging from 180 to 400 nm. In this treatment, the patient takes a photosensitizing medication (usually 8-methoxypsoralen) in a standard dose and is subsequently exposed to long-wave ultraviolet light as the medication plasma levels peak. Although the mechanism of action is not completely understood, it is thought that when psoralen-treated skin is exposed to ultraviolet-A light, the psoralen binds with DNA and decreases cellular proliferation. PUVA is not without its hazards; it has been associated with long-term risks of skin cancer, cataracts, and premature aging of the skin (Richard, 2022). The PUVA unit consists of a chamber that contains high-output black-light lamps and an external reflectance system. The exposure time is calibrated according to the specific unit in use and the anticipated tolerance of the patient's skin. The patient is usually treated two or three times each week until the psoriasis clears. An interim period of 48 hours between treatments is necessary; it takes this long for any burns resulting from PUVA therapy to become evident. In addition, NBUVB (Narrowband UVB light) is equally effective as PUVA without the side effects of psoralen (cataract formation, GI, and carcinogenic effects) and is safe in children, pregnant and lactating females, and even older patients (Nair & Badri, 2022).

After the psoriasis clears, the patient begins a maintenance program. Once little or no disease is active, less potent therapies are used to keep minor flare-ups under control.

Ultraviolet-B (UVB) light therapy is also used to treat generalized plaques. UVB light ranges from 270 to 350 nm, although research has shown that a narrow range, 310 to 312 nm, is the action spectrum. It is used alone or combined with topical coal tar. Side effects are similar to those of PUVA therapy. If access to a light treatment unit is not feasible, the patient can expose themself to sunlight. The risks of all light treatments are similar and include acute sunburn reaction; exacerbation of photosensitive disorders, such as lupus, rosacea, and polymorphic light eruption (a rash related to photosensitivity that can take on many forms); and other skin changes, such as increased wrinkles, thickening, and an increased risk for skin cancer.

EXFOLIATIVE DERMATITIS

Exfoliative dermatitis is a serious condition characterized by progressive inflammation in which generalized erythema and shedding of the skin occur. It may be associated with chills, fever, prostration, severe toxicity, and a pruritic scaling of the skin.

Pathophysiology

There is a profound loss of stratum corneum (i.e., outermost layer of the skin), which causes capillary leakage, hypoproteinemia, and negative nitrogen balance. Because of widespread dilation of cutaneous vessels, large amounts of body heat are lost, and exfoliative dermatitis has a marked effect on the entire body.

Exfoliative dermatitis has a variety of causes. It is considered to be a secondary or reactive process to an underlying skin or systemic disease. It may appear as a part of the lymphoma group of diseases and may precede the clinical manifestations of lymphoma.

Clinical Manifestations and Assessment

This condition starts acutely as a patchy or a generalized erythematous eruption accompanied by fever, malaise, and, occasionally, GI symptoms. The skin color changes from pink to dark red. Redness and other color changes are usually not noticed in patients with darker tones. It is recommended that the skin be compared with the adjacent or opposite area of the body to note skin color changes. The skin should also be assessed for firmness and bogginess when palpated as well as the presence of pain, edema, warmth, or cooler temperatures.

After a week, the characteristic exfoliation (i.e., scaling) begins, usually in the form of thin flakes that leave the underlying skin smooth and red, with new scales forming as the older ones come off. Hair loss may accompany this disorder. Relapses are common. The systemic effects include high-output heart failure, intestinal disturbances, breast enlargement, elevated levels of uric acid in the blood (i.e., hyperuricemia), and temperature disturbances.

Medical and Nursing Management

The objectives of management are to maintain fluid and electrolyte balance and to prevent infection. The treatment is individualized and supportive and should be initiated as soon as the condition is diagnosed.

The patient may be hospitalized and placed on bed rest. All medications that may be implicated are discontinued. A comfortable room temperature should be maintained because the patient does not have normal thermoregulatory control as a result of temperature fluctuations caused by vasodilation and evaporative water loss. Fluid and electrolyte balance must be maintained because there is considerable water and protein loss from the skin surface. Administration of plasma volume expanders may be indicated.

BLISTERING DISORDERS

PEMPHIGUS

Pemphigus is a group of serious diseases of the skin characterized by the appearance of bullae (blisters) of various sizes on apparently normal skin (Fig. 51-5) and mucous membranes.

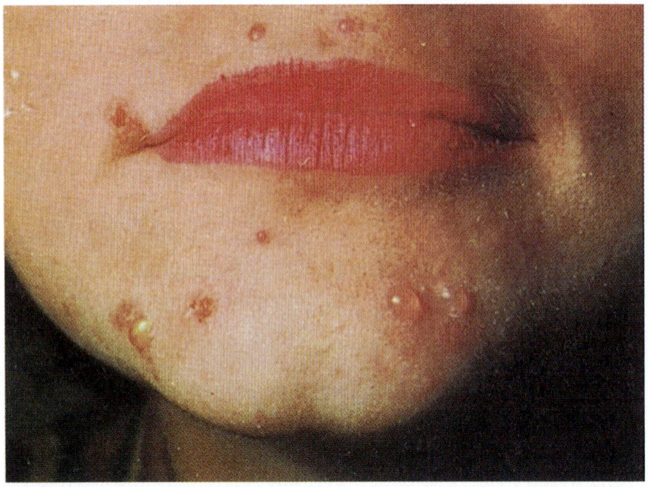

FIGURE 51-5 Vesicles on the chin (in pemphigus). (From Hall, J. C. [2006]. *Sauer's manual of skin diseases*. Lippincott Williams & Wilkins.)

Pathophysiology

Pemphigus is an autoimmune disease involving immunoglobulin G. It is thought that the pemphigus antibody is directed against a specific cell-surface antigen in epidermal cells. A blister forms from the antigen–antibody reaction. The level of serum antibody is predictive of disease severity.

Risk Factors

Genetic factors may also have a role in its development, with the highest incidence among those of Jewish or Mediterranean descent. This disorder usually occurs in middle and late adulthood. The condition may be associated with the use of penicillins and captopril and with the disorder myasthenia gravis.

Clinical Manifestations and Assessment

Most patients present with oral lesions appearing as irregularly shaped erosions that are painful, bleed easily, and heal slowly. The skin bullae enlarge; rupture; and leave large, painful, eroded areas that are accompanied by crusting and oozing. A characteristic offensive odor emanates from the bullae and the exuding serum. There is blistering or sloughing of uninvolved skin when minimal pressure is applied (Nikolsky sign). The eroded skin heals slowly, and large areas of the body eventually are involved. Bacterial superinfection is common.

Complications

The most common complications arise when the disease process is widespread. Before the advent of corticosteroid and immunosuppressive therapy, patients were very susceptible to secondary bacterial infection. Skin bacteria have relatively easy access to the bullae as they ooze, rupture, and leave denuded (loss of epidermis) areas exposed to the environment. Fluid and electrolyte imbalance results from fluid and protein loss as the bullae rupture. Hypoalbuminemia is common when the disease process includes extensive areas of the body's skin surface and mucous membranes.

Medical and Nursing Management

The goals of therapy are to bring the disease under control as rapidly as possible, to prevent loss of serum and the development of secondary infection, and to promote re-epithelization (i.e., renewal of epithelial tissue).

Corticosteroids are administered in high doses to control the disease and keep the skin free of blisters. The high dosage level is maintained until remission is apparent. In some cases, corticosteroid therapy must be maintained for life. High-dose corticosteroid therapy has serious toxic effects.

Immunosuppressive agents (e.g., azathioprine, cyclophosphamide, gold) may be prescribed to help control the disease and reduce the corticosteroid dose. **Plasmapheresis** temporarily decreases the serum antibody level and has been used with variable success, although it is generally reserved for life-threatening cases.

BULLOUS PEMPHIGOID

Bullous pemphigoid is an acquired disease of flaccid blisters appearing on normal or erythematous skin.

Clinical Manifestations and Assessment

Bullous pemphigoid appears more often on the flexor surfaces of the arms, legs, axilla, and groin. Oral lesions, if present, are usually transient and minimal. When the blisters break, the skin has shallow erosions that heal fairly quickly. Pruritus can be intense, even before the appearance of the blisters. Bullous pemphigoid is common in the older population, with a peak incidence at about 60 years of age. There is no gender or racial predilection, and the disease can be found in patients throughout the world.

Medical and Nursing Management

Medical treatment includes topical corticosteroids for localized eruptions and systemic corticosteroids for widespread involvement. Systemic corticosteroids (e.g., prednisone) may be continued for months, in alternative-day doses. The patient needs to understand the implications of long-term corticosteroid therapy.

Complications

Infection and Sepsis

The patient is susceptible to infection because the barrier function of the skin is compromised. Bullae are also susceptible to infection, and sepsis may follow. The skin is cleaned to remove debris and dead skin and to prevent infection.

Secondary infection may be accompanied by an unpleasant odor from skin or oral lesions. *Candida albicans* of the mouth (i.e., thrush) commonly affects patients receiving high-dose corticosteroid therapy. The oral cavity is inspected daily, and any changes are reported. Oral lesions are slow to heal.

Infection is the leading cause of death in patients with blistering diseases. Particular attention is given to assessment for signs and symptoms of local and systemic infection. Seemingly trivial complaints or minimal changes are investigated because corticosteroids can mask or alter typical signs and symptoms of infection. The patient's vital signs are monitored, and temperature fluctuations are documented. The patient is observed for chills, and all secretions and excretions are monitored for changes suggesting infection. Results of culture and sensitivity tests are monitored. Antimicrobial agents are administered as prescribed, and response to treatment is assessed. Health care personnel must perform effective hand hygiene and wear gloves.

In hospitalized patients, environmental contamination is reduced as much as possible. Protective isolation measures and standard precautions are warranted.

Fluid and Electrolyte Imbalance

Extensive denudation of the skin leads to fluid and electrolyte imbalance because of significant loss of fluids and sodium chloride from the skin, which is responsible for many of the systemic symptoms associated with the disease and is treated by IV administration of saline solution.

A large amount of protein and blood is also lost from the denuded skin areas. Blood component therapy may be prescribed to maintain the blood volume, hemoglobin level, and plasma protein concentration. Serum albumin, protein, hemoglobin, and hematocrit values are monitored.

The patient is encouraged to maintain adequate oral fluid intake. Cool, nonirritating fluids are encouraged to maintain hydration. Small, frequent meals or snacks of high-protein, high-calorie foods (e.g., oral nutritional supplements, eggnog, milkshakes) help maintain nutritional status. Parenteral nutrition is considered if the patient cannot eat an adequate diet.

TOXIC EPIDERMAL NECROLYSIS AND STEVENS–JOHNSON SYNDROME

Toxic epidermal necrolysis (TEN) and Stevens–Johnson syndrome (SJS) are potentially fatal skin disorders and the most severe forms of erythema multiforme.

These diseases are mucocutaneous reactions that constitute a spectrum of reactions, with TEN being the most severe. In SJS, the extensive blisters can progress to skin detachment usually affecting less than 10% of BSA, whereas in TEN, more than 30% of BSA is affected (Clinical Overview, 2021). The mortality rate ranges from approximately 10% for SJS to up to 50% for TEN (High, 2022). TEN and SJS are triggered by a reaction to medications in 75% to 85% of cases (Clinical Overview, 2021). Antibiotics, especially sulfonamides, antiseizure agents (phenytoin, carbamazepine, phenobarbital), nonsteroidal anti-inflammatory drugs (NSAIDs), are the medications implicated most frequently (Lee, 2022).

Risk Factors

These conditions occur in patients of all ages and sexes. The incidence is increased in older people because of their use of many medications. People who are immunosuppressed, including those with HIV infection and AIDS, have a high risk of SJS and TEN. Although the incidence of TEN and SJS in the general population is about 2 to 7 cases per 1 million people in the United States, the risk is much higher among HIV-positive individuals and patients with active cancer (High, 2022). Most patients with TEN have an abnormal metabolism of the medication; the mechanism leading to TEN seems to be a cell-mediated cytotoxic reaction.

Clinical Manifestations and Assessment

TEN and SJS may present as a viral syndrome with rash with symptoms such as conjunctival burning or itching, cutaneous tenderness, fever, cough, sore throat, headache, extreme malaise, and myalgias (i.e., aches and pains). These signs are followed by a rapid onset of erythema involving much of the skin surface and mucous membranes, including the oral mucosa, conjunctiva, and genitalia. In severe cases of mucosal involvement, there may be danger of damage to the larynx, bronchi, and esophagus from ulcerations. Large, flaccid bullae develop in some areas; in other areas, large sheets of epidermis are shed, exposing the underlying dermis. Fingernails, toenails, eyebrows, and eyelashes may be shed along with the surrounding epidermis. The skin is excruciatingly tender, and the loss of skin leaves a weeping surface similar to that of a total-body, partial-thickness burn; hence, the condition is also referred to as "scalded skin syndrome." There can be rapid clinical deterioration necessitating an ICU or burn unit admission.

A history of use of medications known to precipitate TEN or SJS may confirm medication reaction as the underlying cause. The timing of the start of suspected medication administration is an important factor in determining causality, since TEN or SJS usually begins within 8 weeks of initiation, most often within 4 weeks (with a mean of 15 days) (Clinical Overview, 2021). Punch biopsy analysis confirms diagnosis, showing necrotic epidermis and effects that involve all layers of skin (Clinical Overview, 2021).

Medical and Nursing Management

The goals of treatment include control of fluid and electrolyte balance, prevention of sepsis, and prevention of ophthalmic complications. Supportive care is the mainstay of treatment.

All nonessential medications are discontinued immediately. As noted earlier, the patient is treated in a regional burn center if possible because aggressive treatment similar to that for severe burns is required. Skin loss may approach 100% of the total BSA. Surgical debridement or hydrotherapy in a Hubbard tank (large steel tub) may be performed to remove involved skin. Meticulous wound care is performed, and nonadhesive dressings are applied to wounds and uninvolved skin (e.g., pressure points, friction sites) (Clinical Overview, 2021).

Tissue samples from the nasopharynx, eyes, ears, blood, urine, skin, and unruptured blisters are obtained for culture to identify pathogenic organisms. IV fluids are prescribed to maintain fluid and electrolyte balance, and potassium supplementation is often necessary, especially in the patient who has severe mucosal involvement and who cannot easily take oral nourishment. Because an indwelling IV catheter may be a site of infection, fluid replacement is carried out by nasogastric tube and then orally as soon as possible.

Initial treatment with systemic corticosteroids is controversial. Some experts argue for early high-dose corticosteroid treatment. However, in most cases, the risk of infection, the complication of fluid and electrolyte imbalance, the delay in the healing process, and the difficulty in initiating oral corticosteroids early in the course of the disease outweigh the perceived benefits. In patients with TEN thought to result from a medication reaction, corticosteroids may be administered; however, the patient should be monitored closely for adverse effects. Other treatment options include IV immunoglobulin; however, evidence of benefit is limited.

Protecting the skin with topical agents is crucial. Various topical antibacterial and anesthetic agents are used to prevent wound sepsis and to assist with pain management. Systemic antibiotic therapy is used with extreme caution. Temporary biologic dressings (e.g., pigskin, amniotic membrane) or plastic semi-permeable dressings (e.g., Vigilon) may be used to reduce pain, decrease evaporation, and prevent secondary infection until the epithelium regenerates. Meticulous oropharyngeal and eye care is essential when there is severe involvement of the mucous membranes and the eyes.

As the patient completes the acute inpatient stage of illness, the focus is directed toward rehabilitation and outpatient care or care in a rehabilitation center. Throughout this care, the patient and family members are involved in the care and are instructed in the procedures, such as wound care and dressing changes, that will need to be continued at home. The patient and family members are assisted in acquiring dressing supplies that will be needed at home.

The patient and family members are also provided with instructions about pain management; nutrition; measures to increase mobility; and prevention of complications, including prevention of infection. They are taught the signs and symptoms of complications and instructed when to notify the health care provider. When appropriate, instructions are provided in writing to the patient and family so they can refer to these instructions when necessary at later times.

Interdisciplinary follow-up care is imperative to ensure that the patient's progress continues. Some patients will require care in a rehabilitation center before returning home. Others will require outpatient physical and occupational therapy for an extended period. When the patient returns home, the home care nurse coordinates the care provided by the various members of the health care team (e.g., primary care provider, physical therapist, occupational therapist, and dietician). The nurse also monitors the patient's progress, provides ongoing assessment to identify complications, and monitors the patient's adherence to the plan of care. The patient's adaptation to the home care environment and the patient's and family's needs for support and assistance are also assessed. Referrals to community agencies are made as appropriate.

Complications

Sepsis

The major cause of death from TEN is infection, and the most common sites of infection are the skin and mucosal surfaces, lungs, and blood. The organisms involved most often are *Staphylococcus aureus, Pseudomonas, Klebsiella, Escherichia coli, Serratia*, and *Candida*. Monitoring vital signs closely and noticing changes in respiratory, renal, and GI function may quickly detect the beginning of an infection. Strict asepsis is always maintained during routine skin care measures. Hand hygiene and wearing sterile gloves when carrying out procedures are essential. When the condition involves a large portion of the body, the patient should be in a private room to prevent possible cross-infection from other patients. Visitors should wear protective garments and wash their hands before and after coming into contact with the patient. People with any infections or infectious disease should not visit the patient until they are no longer a danger to the patient. Refer to Chapter 53 for more details on sepsis.

Conjunctival Retraction, Scars, and Corneal Lesions

The nurse inspects the eyes daily for signs of pruritus, burning, and dryness, which may indicate progression to keratoconjunctivitis, the principal eye complication. Applying a cool, damp cloth over the eyes may relieve burning sensations. The eyes are kept clean and observed for signs of discharge or discomfort, and the progression of symptoms is documented and reported. Administering an eye lubricant, when prescribed, may alleviate dryness and prevent corneal abrasion. Using eye patches or reminding the patient to blink periodically may also counteract dryness. The patient is instructed to avoid rubbing the eyes or putting any medication into the eyes that has not been prescribed or approved by the provider.

BENIGN SKIN TUMORS

Table 51-7 provides descriptions of and treatments for common benign skin lesions.

TABLE **51-7 Benign Skin Lesions**

Lesion	Description	Treatment
Cysts	Cysts of the skin are epithelium-lined cavities that contain fluid or solid material.	
	Epidermal cysts (epidermoid cysts) occur frequently and are slow-growing, firm, elevated tumors frequently noted on the face, neck, upper chest, and back.	Removal of the cysts provides a cure.
	Pilar cysts (trichilemmal cysts), formerly called sebaceous cysts, frequently are found on the scalp. They originate from the middle portion of the hair follicle and from the cells of the outer hair root sheath.	Treatment is surgical removal.
Seborrheic and actinic keratoses	**Seborrheic keratoses** are benign, wartlike lesions of various sizes and colors, ranging from light tan to black, that are usually located on the face, shoulders, chest, and back.	Treatment is removal of the tumor tissue by excision, electrodesiccation, and curettage, or application of carbon dioxide or liquid nitrogen.
	Actinic keratoses are premalignant skin lesions that develop in chronically sun-exposed areas of the body. They appear as rough, scaly patches with underlying erythema. A small percentage of these lesions gradually transform into cutaneous squamous cell carcinoma.	They are usually removed by cryotherapy or shave excision.
Verrucae: Warts	**Warts** are common, benign skin tumors caused by infection with the human papillomavirus, which belongs to the DNA virus group. People of all ages may be affected, but the warts occur most frequently in patients between 12 and 16 years of age.	They may be treated with locally applied laser therapy, liquid nitrogen, salicylic acid plasters, or electrodesiccation.
	Genitalia and perianal warts are known as *condylomata acuminata*. They may be transmitted sexually. Condylomata that affect the uterine cervix predispose the patient to cervical cancer.	They are treated with liquid nitrogen, cryosurgery, electrosurgery, topically applied trichloroacetic acid, and curettage.
Angiomas	**Angiomas** are benign vascular tumors that involve the skin and the subcutaneous tissues. They are present at birth and may occur as flat, violet-red patches (port-wine angiomas) or as raised, bright-red, nodular lesions (strawberry angiomas). The latter tend to involute spontaneously within the first few years of life, but port-wine angiomas usually persist indefinitely.	Most patients use masking cosmetics (i.e., Covermark or Dermablend) to camouflage the lesions. The argon laser is being used on various angiomas with some success. Treatment of strawberry angiomas is more successful if undertaken as soon after birth as possible.
Pigmented nevi: Moles	**Moles** are common skin tumors of various sizes and shades, ranging from yellowish brown to black. They may be flat, macular lesions or elevated papules or nodules that occasionally contain hair. Most pigmented nevi are harmless lesions. However, in rare cases, malignant changes occur, and a melanoma develops at the site of the nevus.	Nevi that show a change in color or size, become symptomatic (e.g., itch), or develop irregular borders should be removed to determine if malignant changes have occurred. Moles that occur in unusual places (palms of the hands and soles of the feet) should be examined carefully for any irregularity and for notching of the border and variation in color. Nevi larger than 1 cm should be examined carefully. Excised nevi should be examined histologically.
Keloids	**Keloids** are benign overgrowths of fibrous tissue at the site of a scar or trauma. They appear to be more common among dark-skinned people. Keloids are asymptomatic but may cause disfigurement and cosmetic concern.	The treatment, which is not always satisfactory, consists of surgical excision, intralesional corticosteroid therapy, and radiation.

MALIGNANT SKIN TUMORS

Skin cancer is the most common cancer in the United States. If the incidence continues at the present rate, an estimated one of eight fair-skinned Americans will eventually develop skin cancer, especially basal cell carcinoma (BCC). Because the skin is easily inspected, skin cancer is readily seen and detected and is the type of cancer that is treated most successfully.

Exposure to the sun is the leading cause of skin cancer; incidence is related to the total amount of exposure to the sun. Sun damage is cumulative, and harmful effects may be severe by 20 years of age. The increase in skin cancer probably reflects changing lifestyles and the emphasis on sunbathing and related activities in light of changes in the environment, such as holes in Earth's ozone layer. Changes in the ozone layer from the effects of worldwide industrial air pollutants, such as chlorofluorocarbons, have prompted concern that the incidence of skin cancers, especially malignant melanoma, will increase. The ozone layer, a stratospheric blanket of bluish, explosive gas formed by the sun's ultraviolet radiation, varies in depth with the seasons and is thickest at the North and South Poles and thinnest at the equator. Scientists believe that it helps protect the earth from the effects of solar ultraviolet radiation. Proponents of this theory predict an increase in skin cancers as a consequence of changes in the ozone layer. Other skin cancer risk factors are summarized in Box 51-8. Protective measures should be used throughout life, and nurses should inform patients about risk factors associated with skin cancer.

BOX 51-8

Risk Factors for Skin Cancer

- Fair-skinned, fair-haired, blue-eyed people, particularly those of Celtic origin, with insufficient skin pigmentation to protect underlying tissues
- People who sustain sunburn and who do not tan
- Chronic sun exposure (certain occupations, such as farming, construction work)
- Exposure to chemical pollutants (industrial workers in arsenic, nitrates, coal, tar and pitch, oils and paraffins)
- Sun-damaged skin (older individuals)
- History of x-ray therapy for acne or benign lesions
- Scars from severe burns
- Chronic skin irritations
- Immunosuppression
- Genetic factors

BASAL CELL AND SQUAMOUS CELL CARCINOMA

The most common types of skin cancer are BCC and squamous cell (epidermoid) carcinoma (SCC). The third most common type, malignant melanoma, is discussed separately. Skin cancer is diagnosed by biopsy and histologic evaluation.

Clinical Manifestations and Assessment

BCC is the most common type of skin cancer. It generally appears on sun-exposed areas of the body and is more prevalent in regions where the population is subjected to intense and extensive exposure to the sun. The incidence is proportional to the age of the patient (average, 60 years of age) and the total amount of sun exposure, and it is inversely proportional to the amount of melanin in the skin.

BCC usually begins as a small, waxy nodule with rolled, translucent, pearly borders; telangiectatic vessels may be present. As it grows, it undergoes central ulceration and sometimes crusting (Fig. 51-6). The tumors appear most frequently on the face. BCC is characterized by invasion and erosion of contiguous (adjoining) tissues. It rarely metastasizes, but recurrence is common. However, a neglected

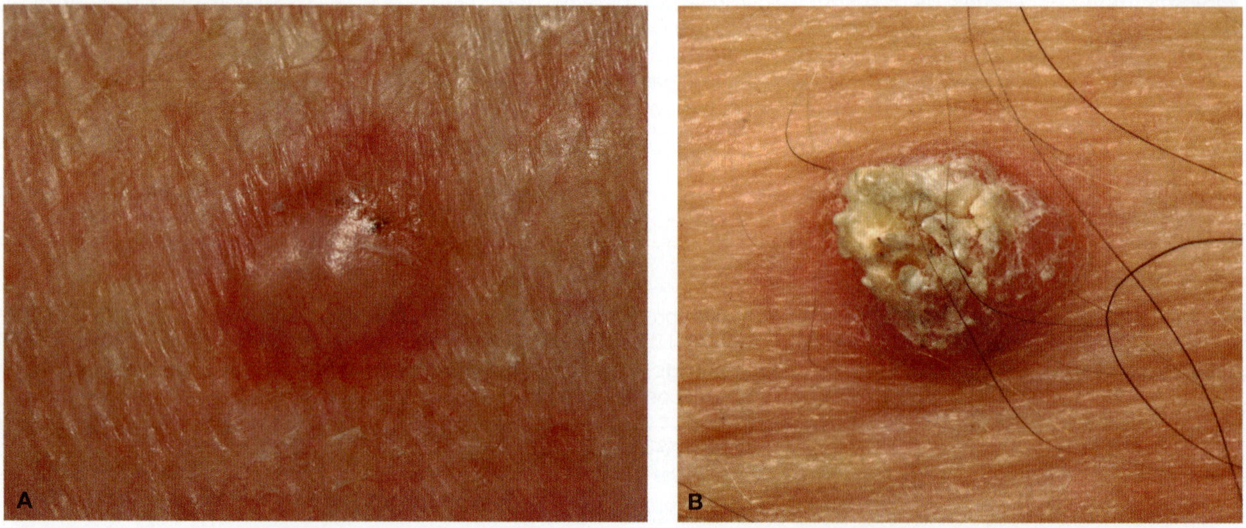

FIGURE 51-6 **Basal cell carcinoma (A) and squamous cell carcinoma (B). (Source: Shutterstock; Photo IDs: 1347741581 and 1347760484.)**

lesion can result in the loss of a nose, an ear, or a lip. Other variants of BCC may appear as shiny, flat, gray or yellowish plaques.

SCC is a malignant proliferation arising from the epidermis. Although it usually appears on sun-damaged skin, it may arise from normal skin or from pre-existing skin lesions. It is of greater concern than BCC because it is a truly invasive carcinoma, metastasizing by the blood or lymphatic system.

Metastases account for 75% of deaths from SCC. The lesions may be primary, arising on the skin and mucous membranes, or they may develop from a precancerous condition, such as actinic keratosis (lesions occurring in sun-exposed areas), leukoplakia (premalignant lesion of the mucous membrane), or scarred or ulcerated lesions. SCC appears as a rough, thickened, scaly tumor that may be asymptomatic or may involve bleeding (see Fig. 51-6). The border of an SCC lesion may be wider, more infiltrated, and more inflammatory than that of a BCC lesion. Secondary infection can occur. Exposed areas, especially of the upper extremities and of the face, lower lip, ears, nose, and forehead, are common sites.

The incidence of BCC and SCC is increased in all people who are immunocompromised, including those infected with HIV. Clinically, the tumors have the same appearance as in people who are not HIV infected; however, in patients with HIV, the tumors may grow more rapidly and recur more frequently. These tumors are managed the same as those for the general population. Frequent follow-up (every 4 to 6 months) is recommended to monitor for recurrence.

Medical Management

The goal of treatment is to eradicate the tumor. The treatment method depends on the tumor location; the cell type, location, and depth; the cosmetic desires of the patient; the history of previous treatment; whether the tumor is invasive; and whether metastatic nodes are present. The management of BCC and SCC includes surgical excision, Treatments include Mohs micrographic surgery, electrosurgery, cryosurgery, and radiation therapy.

Surgical Management

The primary goal is to remove the tumor entirely. The best way to maintain cosmetic appearance is to place the incision properly along natural skin tension lines and natural anatomic body lines. In this way, scars are less noticeable. The size of the incision depends on the tumor size and location but usually involves a length-to-width ratio of 3:1.

The adequacy of the surgical excision is verified by microscopic evaluation of sections of the specimen. When the tumor is large, reconstructive surgery with use of a skin flap or skin grafting may be required. The incision is closed in layers to enhance cosmetic effect. A pressure dressing applied over the wound provides support. Infection after a simple excision is uncommon if proper surgical asepsis is maintained.

Mohs Micrographic Surgery

Mohs micrographic surgery is the technique that is most accurate and that best conserves normal tissue. The procedure removes the tumor layer by layer. The first layer excised includes all evident tumor and a small margin of normal-appearing tissue. The specimen is frozen and analyzed by section to determine if the entire tumor has been removed. If not, additional layers of tissue are shaved and examined until all tissue margins are tumor-free. In this manner, only the tumor and a safe, normal-tissue margin are removed. Mohs surgery is the recommended tissue-sparing procedure, with extremely high cure rates for both BCC and SCC. It is the treatment of choice and the most effective for tumors around the eyes, nose, upper lip, and auricular and periauricular areas.

Electrosurgery

Electrosurgery is the destruction or removal of tissue by electrical energy. The current is converted to heat, which then passes to the tissue from a cold electrode. Electrosurgery may be preceded by curettage (excising the skin tumor by scraping its surface with a curette). Then electrodesiccation is implemented to achieve hemostasis and to destroy any viable malignant cells at the base of the wound or along its edges. Electrodesiccation is useful for lesions smaller than 1 to 2 cm (0.4 to 0.8 in) in diameter.

This method takes advantage of the fact that the tumor is softer than surrounding skin and, therefore, can be outlined by a curette, which "feels" the extent of the tumor. The tumor is removed and the base cauterized. The process is repeated twice. Usually, healing occurs within a month.

Cryosurgery

Cryosurgery destroys the tumor by deep-freezing the tissue. A thermocouple needle apparatus is inserted into the skin, and liquid nitrogen is directed to the center of the tumor until the tumor base is –40° to –60°C. Liquid nitrogen has the lowest boiling point of all cryogens, is inexpensive, and is easy to obtain. The tumor tissue is frozen, allowed to thaw, and then refrozen. The site thaws naturally and then becomes gelatinous and heals spontaneously. Swelling and edema follow the freezing. The appearance of the lesion varies. Normal healing, which may take 4 to 6 weeks, occurs faster in areas with a good blood supply.

Radiation Therapy

Frequently, radiation therapy is performed for cancer of the eyelid, the tip of the nose, and areas in or near vital structures (e.g., facial nerve). It is reserved for older patients because x-ray changes may be seen after 5 to 10 years, and malignant changes in scars may be induced by irradiation 15 to 30 years later.

The patient should be informed that the skin may become red and blistered. A bland skin ointment prescribed by the provider may be applied to relieve discomfort. Also the patient should be cautioned to avoid exposure to the sun. See Chapter 5 for more details on radiation therapy.

Nursing Management

Because many skin cancers are removed by excision, usually patients are treated in outpatient surgical units. The role of the nurse is to teach the patient about prevention of skin cancer and about self-care after treatment.

Teaching Self-Care

Usually the wound is covered with a dressing to protect the site from physical trauma, external irritants, and contaminants. The nurse instructs the patient about when to report for a dressing change or provides written and verbal information on how to change dressings, including the type of dressing to purchase, how to remove dressings and apply fresh ones, and the importance of hand hygiene before and after the procedure.

The patient watches for excessive bleeding and tight dressings that compromise circulation. If the lesion is in the perioral area, the patient is instructed to drink liquids through a straw and limit talking and facial movement. Dental work should be avoided until the area is completely healed.

After the sutures are removed, an emollient cream may be used to help reduce dryness. Applying a sunscreen over the wound is advised to prevent postoperative hyperpigmentation if the patient spends time outdoors.

Follow-up examinations should be at regular intervals, usually every 3 months for a year, and should include palpation of the adjacent lymph nodes. The nurse instructs the patient to seek treatment for any moles that are subject to repeated friction and irritation, and to watch for indications of potential malignancy in moles as described previously. The importance of life-long follow-up evaluations is emphasized.

Teaching Skin Cancer Prevention

Studies show that regular daily use of a sunscreen with a solar protection factor (SPF) of at least 15 can reduce the recurrence of skin cancer by as much as 40% (Box 51-9). The sunscreen should be applied to head, neck, arms, and hands every morning at least 30 minutes before leaving the house and reapplied every 4 hours if the skin perspires. Intermittent application of sunscreen only when exposure is anticipated has been shown to be less effective than daily use. Longer exposure is believed to contribute to the increasing incidence of melanoma. Although the evidence is insufficient, nurses should discuss the issues with patients who are at high risk of skin cancer. Nurses should also encourage skin self-examination (Box 51-10).

BOX 51-9 Health Promotion

Preventing Skin Cancer

- Teach patients that sunscreens are rated in strength from 4 (weakest) to 50 (strongest). The solar protection factor, or SPF, indicates how much longer a person can stay in the sun before the skin begins to redden. For example, if the person normally can stay in the sun for 10 minutes before reddening begins, an SPF of 4 will protect the person from reddening for about 40 minutes. A sunscreen with an SPF of 15 or greater is recommended under most conditions and indicates 93% protection; an SPF of 34 indicates 97% protection.
- Remind patients that up to 50% of ultraviolet rays can penetrate loosely woven clothing.
- Remind patients that ultraviolet light can penetrate cloud cover, and sunburn still can occur.
- Teach children to avoid all but modest sun exposure and to use a sunscreen regularly for life-long protection.
- Advise patients to:
  - Avoid tanning if their skin burns easily, never tans, or tans poorly.
  - Avoid unnecessary exposure to the sun, especially during the time of day when ultraviolet radiation (sunlight) is most intense (10 am to 3 pm).
  - Avoid sunburns.
  - Apply a sunscreen daily to block harmful sun rays.
  - Use a sunscreen with an SPF of 15 or higher that protects against both ultraviolet-A (UVA) and ultraviolet-B (UVB) light.
  - Reapply water-resistant sunscreens after swimming, if heavily sweating, and every 2–3 hours during prolonged periods of sun exposure.
  - Avoid applying oils before or during sun exposure (oils do not protect against sunlight or sun damage).
  - Use a lip balm that contains a sunscreen with an SPF of 15 or higher.
  - Wear protective clothing, such as a broad-brimmed hat and long sleeves.
  - Avoid using sun lamps for indoor tanning, and avoid commercial tanning booths.

MALIGNANT MELANOMA

A malignant melanoma is a cancerous neoplasm in which atypical melanocytes are present in the epidermis and the dermis (and sometimes the subcutaneous cells). It is the most lethal of all the skin cancers and is responsible for >7,000 deaths per year of all cancer deaths (Siegel et al., 2021). Malignant melanoma can occur in one of several forms: superficial spreading melanoma, lentigo-maligna melanoma, nodular melanoma, and acral-lentiginous melanoma. These types have specific clinical and histologic features as well as different biologic behaviors. Most melanomas arise from cutaneous epidermal melanocytes, but some appear in preexisting nevi (i.e., moles) in the skin or develop in the uveal tract of the eye. Melanomas occasionally appear simultaneously with cancer of other organs.

The worldwide incidence of melanoma doubles every 10 years, an increase that is probably related to increased recreational sun exposure, changes in the ozone layer, and

BOX 51-10

Patient Education

Periodic Self-Examination

Prevention of melanoma/skin cancer is the best weapon against these diseases, but if a melanoma should develop, it is almost always curable if caught in the early stages. Practice periodic self-examination to aid in early recognition of any new or developing lesion. The following is one way of self-examination that will ensure that no area of the body is neglected. To perform your self-examination, you will need a full-length mirror, a hand mirror, and a brightly lit room.

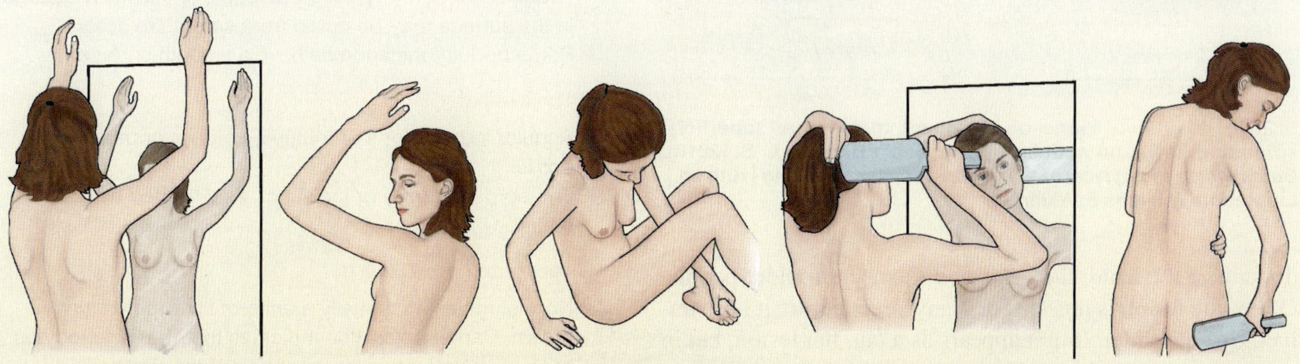

1. Examine the body front and back in the mirror, then the right and left sides, with the arms raised.
2. Bend the elbows, looking carefully at the forearms, back of the upper arms, and palms
3. Next, look at the back of the legs and feet, the spaces between the toes, and the soles of the feet.
4. Examine the back of the neck and the scalp with a hand-held mirror. Part the hair to lift.
5. Finally, check the back and buttocks with a hand mirror.

improved methods of early detection. Median age at diagnosis is 57 years of age; although melanoma affects all age groups, up to 75% of patients are younger than 70 years of age (Heistein et al., 2022). The incidence of melanoma is increasing faster than that of almost any other cancer, and the mortality rate is increasing faster than that of any other cancer except lung cancer. Survival rate is related to the stage at diagnosis, for example, the 5-year relative survival rate for patients with stage 0 is 97%, compared to <20% for those with metastatic disease (Heistein et al., 2022).

Risk Factors

The cause of malignant melanoma is unknown, but ultraviolet rays are strongly suspected based on indirect evidence, such as the increased incidence of melanoma in countries near the equator and in people younger than 30 years of age who have used a tanning bed more than 10 times per year. Race is a risk factor; in general, 1 in 100 White people acquires melanoma each year. As many as 10% of patients with melanoma are members of a family that is more melanoma-prone. They have multiple changing moles (dysplastic nevi), which are susceptible to malignant transformation. Patients with dysplastic nevus syndrome have been found to have unusual moles, larger and more numerous moles, lesions with irregular outlines, and pigmentation located all over the skin. Microscopic examination of dysplastic moles shows disordered, faulty growth. Box 51-11 lists risk factors for malignant melanoma.

Types

Superficial Spreading Melanoma

Superficial spreading melanoma occurs anywhere on the body and is the most common form of melanoma. It usually affects middle-aged people and occurs most frequently on the trunk and lower extremities. The lesion tends to be circular, with irregular outer portions. The margins of the lesion may be flat or elevated and palpable (Fig. 51-7). This type of melanoma may appear in a combination of colors, with hues of tan, brown, and black mixed with gray, blue-black, or white. Sometimes a dull pink rose color can be seen in a small area within the lesion.

Lentigo-Maligna Melanoma

Lentigo-maligna melanoma is a slowly evolving, pigmented lesion that occurs on exposed skin areas, especially the

BOX 51-11

Risk Factors for Malignant Melanoma

- Fair-skinned or freckled, blue-eyed, light-haired people of Celtic or Scandinavian origin
- People who burn and do not tan or who have a significant history of severe sunburn
- Environmental exposure to intense sunlight (older Americans retiring to the southwestern United States appear to have a higher incidence)
- History of melanoma (personal or family)
- Skin with giant congenital nevi

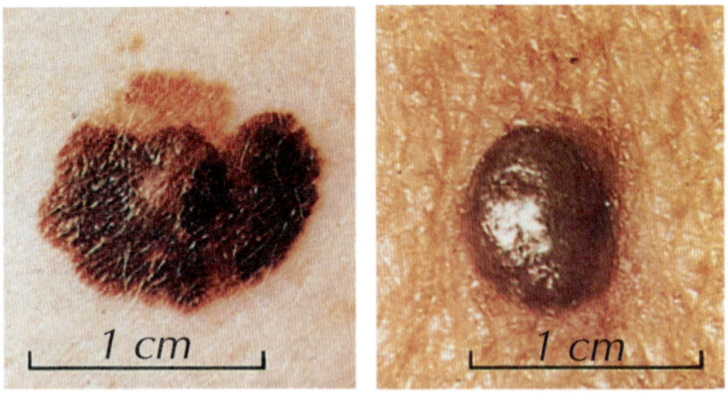

FIGURE 51-7 Two forms of malignant melanoma: superficial spreading (left) and nodular (right). (From Bickley, L. S. [2013]. *Bates' guide to physical examination and history taking* [10th ed.]. Lippincott Williams & Wilkins.)

dorsum of the hand, the head, and the neck in older people. Often, the lesion is present for many years before it is examined by a provider. It first appears as a tan, flat lesion, but in time it undergoes changes in size and color.

Nodular Melanoma

Nodular melanoma is a spherical, blueberry-like nodule with a relatively smooth surface and a relatively uniform, blue-black color (see Fig. 51-7). It may be dome-shaped with a smooth surface. It may have other shadings of red, gray, or purple. Sometimes, nodular melanomas appear as irregularly shaped plaques. The patient may describe this as a blood blister that fails to resolve. A nodular melanoma invades directly into the adjacent dermis (i.e., vertical growth) and therefore has a poorer prognosis.

Acral-Lentiginous Melanoma

Acral-lentiginous melanoma occurs in areas not excessively exposed to sunlight and where hair follicles are absent. It is found on the palms of the hands, on the soles, in the nail beds, and in the mucous membranes of people who are dark-skinned. These melanomas appear as irregular, pigmented macules that develop nodules. They may become invasive early.

Clinical Manifestations and Assessment

Biopsy results confirm the diagnosis of melanoma. An excisional biopsy specimen provides information on the type, level of invasion, and thickness of the lesion. An excisional biopsy specimen that includes a 1-cm margin of normal tissue and a portion of underlying subcutaneous fatty tissue is sufficient for staging a melanoma in situ or an early, noninvasive melanoma. Incisional biopsy should be performed when the suspicious lesion is too large to be removed safely without extensive scarring. Biopsy specimens obtained by shaving, curettage, or needle aspiration are not considered reliable histologic proof of disease.

A thorough history and physical examination should include a meticulous skin examination and palpation of regional lymph nodes that drain the lesional area. Box 51-12 discusses assessing moles. Because melanoma occurs in families, a positive family history of melanoma is investigated so that first-degree relatives, who may be at high risk for melanoma, can be evaluated for atypical lesions. After the diagnosis of melanoma has been confirmed, a chest x-ray, complete blood cell count, liver function tests, and radionuclide or computed tomography scans are usually performed to stage the extent of disease.

BOX 51-12 **Assessing the ABCDEs of Moles**

A for Asymmetry

- The lesion does not appear balanced on both sides. If an imaginary line were drawn down the middle, the two halves would not look alike.
- The lesion has an irregular surface with uneven elevations (irregular topography) either palpable or visible. A change in the surface may be noted from smooth to scaly.
- Some nodular melanomas have a smooth surface.

B for Irregular Border

- Angular indentations or multiple notches appear in the border.
- The border is fuzzy or indistinct, as if rubbed with an eraser.

C for Variegated Color

- Normal moles are usually a uniform light to medium brown. Darker coloration indicates that the melanocytes have penetrated to a deeper layer of the dermis.
- Colors that may indicate malignancy if found together within a single lesion are shades of red, white, and blue; shades of blue are ominous.
- White areas within a pigmented lesion are suspicious.
- Some malignant melanomas, however, are not variegated but are uniformly colored (bluish-black, bluish-gray, bluish-red).

D for Diameter

- A diameter exceeding 6 mm (about the size of a pencil eraser) is considered more suspicious, although this finding without other signs is not significant. Many benign skin growths are larger than 6 mm, whereas some early melanomas may be smaller.

E for Elevation, Enlargement, and/or Evolution

- The lesion is raised above the surface, enlarged, and/or has an uneven surface. *Evolution* refers to a lesion that has changed significantly (size, shape, symptoms [e.g., itching, tenderness, crusting, bleeding]) over time.

Medical and Nursing Management

Treatment depends on the level of invasion and the depth of the lesion. Surgical excision is the treatment of choice for small, superficial lesions. Deeper lesions require wide local excision, after which skin grafting may be necessary.

Sentinel node biopsy accurately identifies whether microscopic melanoma cells involve regional lymph nodes. The sentinel lymph node is the first node by which cancer is likely to spread from the primary tumor before spreading to other lymph nodes. This technique is used to sample the nodes nearest the tumor and to spare the patient the long-term sequelae of extensive removal of lymph nodes if the sample nodes are negative. If the sentinel node is positive, then lymph node dissection is performed.

Pearls for Practice: What Is a Sentinel Node?

The sentinel lymph nodes are the first lymph nodes that cancer cells are most likely to spread from a primary tumor. To locate the sentinel node(s), the provider will administer a radioactive substance, a blue dye, or both near the tumor and then observe for the presence of dye and/or use a device that detects the tracer activity. The node is then removed and sent to pathology to assess for cancer cells. If the sentinel node is positive, additional lymph nodes will be removed, and the pathologist will assess the subsequent nodes.

Additional therapies for metastatic disease include biologic response modifiers (e.g., interferon-alpha, interleukin-2), immunotherapy (i.e., lymphokine-activated killer cells, immune checkpoint inhibitors, high-dose IL-2, cancer vaccination, and adoptive T-cell transfer), monoclonal antibodies directed at melanoma antigens, chemotherapy, and radiation (Dinulos, 2021). Patients with metastatic disease should be referred to a cancer center with access to new adjuvant therapies and clinical trials (Dinulos, 2021). Refer to Chapter 5 for details on immunotherapy.

Further surgical intervention may be performed to debulk the tumor or to remove part of the organ involved (e.g., lung, liver, or colon). However, the rationale for more extensive surgery is for relief of symptoms, not for cure.

METASTATIC SKIN TUMORS

The skin is an important, although not a common, site of metastatic cancer. All types of cancer may metastasize to the skin, but carcinoma of the breast is the primary source of cutaneous metastases in females. Other sources include cancer of the large intestine, ovaries, and lungs. In males, the most common primary sites are the lungs, large intestine, oral cavity, kidneys, or stomach. Skin metastases from melanomas are found in both sexes. The clinical appearance of metastatic skin lesions is not distinctive, except perhaps in some cases of breast cancer in which diffuse, brawny hardening of the skin of the involved breast is seen. In most instances, metastatic lesions occur as multiple cutaneous or subcutaneous nodules of various sizes that may be skin-colored or different shades of red.

KAPOSI SARCOMA

Kaposi sarcoma (KS) is a malignancy of endothelial cells that line the small blood vessels. KS is manifested clinically by lesions of the skin, oral cavity, GI tract, and lungs. The skin lesions consist of reddish-purple to dark-blue macules, plaques, or nodules. KS is subdivided into three categories:

- **Classic KS** occurs predominantly in males of Mediterranean or Jewish ancestry between 40 and 70 years of age. Most patients have nodules or plaques on the lower extremities that rarely metastasize beyond this area. Classic KS is chronic, relatively benign, and rarely fatal.
- **Endemic (African) KS** affects people predominantly in the eastern half of Africa near the equator. Males are affected more often than females, and children can be affected as well. The disease may resemble classic KS, or it may infiltrate and progress to lymphadenopathic forms.
- **Immunosuppression-associated KS** occurs in transplant recipients and people with AIDS. This form of KS is characterized by local skin lesions and disseminated visceral and mucocutaneous diseases. The greater the degree of immunosuppression, the higher the incidence of KS. Immunosuppression-related KS that results from AIDS is an aggressive tumor that involves multiple body organs. Its presentation resembles that of KS associated with immunosuppressive therapy. Most patients are between 20 and 40 years of age. Refer to Chapter 36 for more information about KS and AIDS.

CHAPTER REVIEW

NCLEX-Style Review Questions

1. The health care provider has ordered collagenase for a patient with a left leg necrotic ulcer. What does the nurse understands about the use of collagenase? Select all that apply.

a. Removes necrotic tissue and absorbs small to large amounts of exudates

b. Uses the body's own digestive enzymes to break down necrotic tissue

c. Speeds the rate at which necrotic tissue is removed

d. Uses a high moisture-vapor transmission rate to remove exudate

e. Is slower than surgical debridement

2. Which of the following are risk factors for malignant melanoma? Select all that apply.
   a. Melanin-rich skin
   b. Family history of melanoma
   c. Sustained exposure to intense sunlight
   d. Fair-skinned people
   e. Significant history of severe sunburn

3. A patient who developed Stevens–Johnson syndrome 2 weeks after starting a sulfonamide medication has stabilized and is now being transferred from the intensive care unit to a medical unit with 2 beds per room. Select from the list below appropriate potential roommates for this patient.
   a. A patient with methicillin-resistant *Staphylococcus aureus* (MRSA)
   b. A patient with fever of unknown origin (FUO)
   c. A patient with heart failure (HF)
   d. A patient with asthma
   e. A patient with gastroenteritis

4. Topical corticosteroid therapy has been ordered for a patient with pruritus. What information should be incorporated into the plan of care for this patient? Select all that apply
   a. Apply liberally in the prescribed area.
   b. Absorption is enhanced when skin is dry.
   c. Local side effects may include skin atrophy and thinning.
   d. Absorption is decreased when covered with an occlusive dressing.
   e. Avoid applying near the eyes.

5. A 55-year-old patient with leukemia is being seen in the clinic for complaints of burning pain in the back. The patient has been diagnosed with shingles. The nurse would expect which medications might be ordered to reduce pain and halt the progression of the disease? Select all that apply.
   a. Cytotoxic agent
   b. Antiviral
   c. Antibiotic
   d. Antifungal
   e. Analgesic

REFERENCES AND SELECTED READINGS

References and selected readings associated with this chapter can be found on the website that accompanies the book. Visit **http://thepoint.lww.com/Honan3e** to access the references and other additional resources associated with this chapter.

CHAPTER 52

Nursing Management: Patients With Burn Injuries

Jacqueline Laird

Learning Objectives

After reading this chapter, you will be able to:

1. Discuss the classification system used for burn injuries.
2. Describe the local and systemic effects of a major burn injury.
3. Discuss the potential fluid and electrolyte alterations of the emergent/resuscitative and acute phases of burn management.
4. Describe nursing management of the patient with burn injuries.

In comparison to the larger health care picture, burn patients are few. However, according to the American Burn Association (ABA), yearly, there are more than 450,000 burn injuries occurring in the United States that are severe enough to require medical treatment (Herndon et al., 2018). Mortality rate of 3.3% is an overall average. For fire/flame injuries it rises to 5.8%; this is the most common cause of burn, and this rate increases dramatically with the presence of inhalation injury (Blyth & Murray, 2020). At the time of injury, at least 50% of burn fatalities occur because of massive hemorrhaging or a brain injury that is nonsurvivable (Sheridan, 2020). After severe injury people often face long-term physical and psychological sequelae. Impact to their functional abilities often results in long-term needs (Abouzeid et al., 2022).

Burns are categorized as thermal (including electrical burns), radiation, electrical, or chemical. The skin and the mucosa of the upper airways are the sites of tissue destruction. Disruption of the skin can lead to increased fluid loss; infection; hypothermia; compromised immunity; and changes in function, appearance, and body image. The nurse caring for the burn patient requires astute assessment skills and a high level of knowledge about physiologic changes after a major burn injury to detect subtle changes in the patient's condition.

OVERVIEW OF BURN INJURY

Incidence of Burn Injury

The two most common burn etiologies are flame burns at 43% and scald at 34%. The home remains the most common place of occurrence, accounting for 73% of burn injuries cared for in burn centers. Scald injuries are the most preventable burn injury in children under 5 years of age (ABA, 2018; Carey et al., 2021). A burn can affect any person at any time, in any place. Burns involve people of all ages and socioeconomic groups. Each year, approximately 486,000 people with burn injuries receive medical treatment, and just over 3,000 deaths occur annually from fire and smoke inhalation. Residential fires account for 2,745 of these deaths, with the remaining 310 from motor vehicle crash fires. Approximately 68% of all burn victims are males. For children under the age 14, burns are the third leading cause of death and burns are included in the top 10 causes of death for all age groups. Those at either extreme (the young and the aged) are particularly vulnerable because the skin is naturally thinner, resulting in the person sustaining a deeper burn at any temperature (Carey et al., 2021; Myers et al., 2022). Although prognosis can be influenced by several factors, the most important variables include severity of the burn, the presence of inhalation injury, associated injuries, the patient's age, and comorbid conditions.

People who are prone to burn injuries are older individuals; smokers; and people with disabilities, neurologic illness, substance use issues, and psychiatric illness.

Gerontologic Considerations

Representing an increasing population segment, older adults have an increased prevalence in the burned population; furthermore, mortality from burns increases with age (Herndon et al., 2018). Compared to their younger peers, older adults, aged 65 and above, experience more than twice as many deaths in housefires. Risk factors include reduced mobility, decreased sensory abilities, and potential cognitive decline which decreases reaction time, thereby increasing the risk for severe injury and death in a fire (Casteel et al., 2020). Thinning and loss of elasticity of the skin predispose them to deep injury from a thermal insult that might cause a less severe burn in a younger person. Furthermore, chronic illnesses decrease the older person's ability to withstand the multisystem stresses imposed by major burn injury. Mortality is nearly 90% in patients who are older than 60 years of age, have a burn that is greater than 40% of the total body surface area (TBSA), and have an inhalation injury (Sheridan, 2020). Successful prevention campaigns have been linked to smoke detectors, carbon monoxide detectors, fire extinguishers, escape plans, sprinkler systems, enforcement of fire codes, and fire-safe cigarettes. Scald injury prevention includes the use of an antiscald mixing valve for shower heads or tub faucets that stops or interrupts the flow of water when the temperature reaches a preset temperature (usually 110° to 114°F, but before it reaches 120°F) to reduce the frequency and severity of scald burns (Plummer, 2020). The nurse educates all patients about the importance of a working smoke alarm and, if possible, a working carbon monoxide detector.

Classification of Burns

Burn injuries are classified by the depth of the injury and the extent of the TBSA that is burned.

Depth

Burns are classified according to the depth of tissue destruction. Cell damage occurs at temperatures of at least 45°C (113°F). The depth depends on how much of the skin's dermis is affected. Burn depth determines whether spontaneous healing will occur and helps to determine the plan of care.

The following factors are considered in determining the depth of a burn:

- How the injury occurred
- Causative agent, such as flame, scald, chemical, or hot tar
- Temperature of the burning agent
- Duration of contact with the agent
- Thickness of the skin in the burned area

Burns are described as superficial, superficial partial-thickness, deep partial-thickness, or full-thickness injuries (Fig. 52-1; Table 52-1). Formerly referred to as a first-degree burn, a superficial burn damages only the **epidermis** (outer layer of the skin). The area is red and dry, with slight swelling but no blister, and painful, like a sunburn. These burns heal in about 7 days, usually with no scarring. In a superficial partial-thickness burn (one of two types of second-degree burns), the epidermis is destroyed and a small portion of the underlying **dermis** (deep, vascular inner portion of skin) is injured. The skin is blistered, the exposed dermis is red and moist, and hair follicles are intact. With appropriate wound care, these burns will heal in about 2 weeks without risk of scarring and therefore do not require surgical intervention; the chief symptom, which is pain, usually resolves within 72 hours (Brownson & Gibran, 2018; Myers et al., 2022).

A deep partial-thickness burn (the second of the two types of second-degree burns) extends into the reticular layer of the dermis (dense connective tissue that gives the skin strength and elasticity and houses sweat glands, lymph vessels, and hair follicles) and is hard to distinguish from a full-thickness burn. It is red or white, mottled, and can be moist or fairly dry. The patient is in severe pain. Deep partial burns usually take longer than 3 weeks to heal (3 to 8 weeks) and can heal with permanent scarring

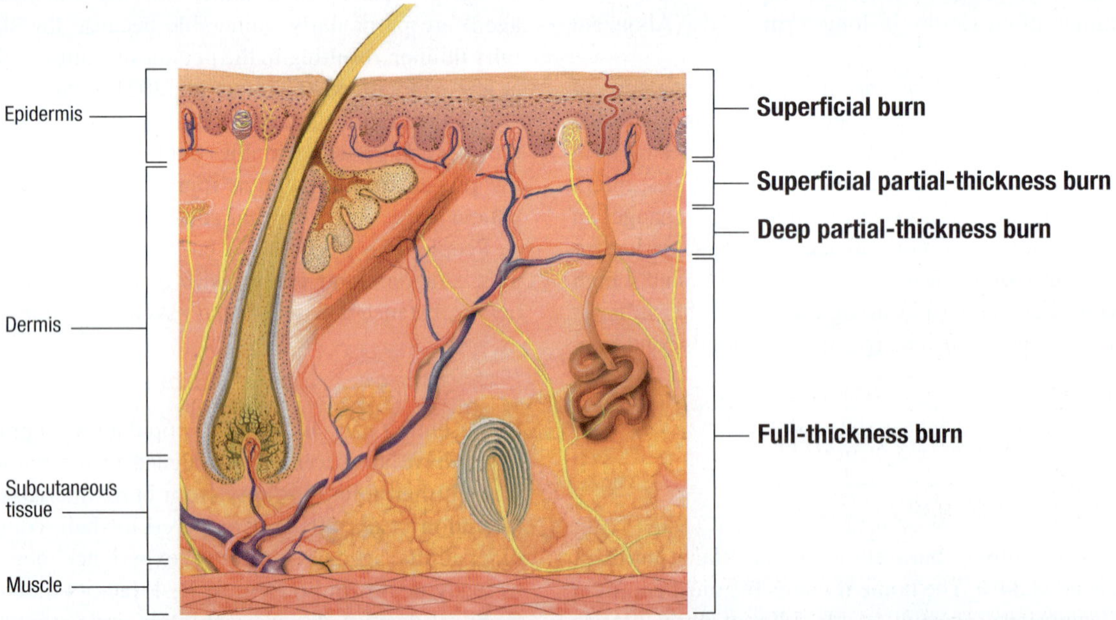

FIGURE 52-1 **Depth of burn injury.**

TABLE **52-1 Characteristics of Burns According to Depth**

Depth of Burn	Causes	Skin Involvement	Symptoms	Wound Appearance	Recuperative Course
Superficial	Thermal injury (heat/cold), electromagnetic energy, solar radiation, or topical caustic chemicals	Involves only the epidermis	Erythema and edema of skin	Redness, swelling, does not blister, pain	Three days or less
Superficial partial-thickness (similar to first-degree)	Sunburn Low-intensity flash	Epidermis; possibly a portion of dermis	Tingling Hyperesthesia (supersensitivity) Pain that is soothed by cooling	Reddened, blanches with pressure, dry Minimal or no edema Possible blisters	Complete recovery within 5–10 days; usually no scarring Peeling
Deep partial-thickness (similar to second-degree)	Scalds Flash flame Contact	Epidermis, upper dermis, portion of deeper dermis	Pain Hyperesthesia Sensitive to cold air	Blistered, mottled red base; broken epidermis; weeping surface Edema	Recovery in 3–8 weeks Some scarring and depigmentation contractures Infection may convert it to full thickness
Full-thickness (similar to third-degree)	Flame Prolonged exposure to hot liquids Electric current Chemical Contact	Epidermis, entire dermis, and sometimes subcutaneous tissue; may involve connective tissue, muscle, and bone	Pain free Shock Hematuria (blood in the urine) and possibly hemolysis (blood cell destruction) Possible entrance and exit wounds (electrical burn)	Dry; pale white, leathery, or charred Broken skin with fat exposed Edema	Eschar sloughs Grafting necessary Scarring and loss of contour and function; contractures Loss of digits or extremity possible

(some of these burns tend to have a better appearance when grafted). If there has not been healing by 3 weeks, as a rule the burn should be excised and grafted (Brownson & Gibran, 2018).

A full-thickness burn (formerly called a third- or fourth-degree burn) involves total destruction of the dermis and extends into the subcutaneous fat. It can also involve muscle and bone. It heals by contraction or epithelial migration. Wound color ranges widely from mottled white to red, brown, or black. It may be charred and appear leathery. It will look and feel dry, firm, and depressed when compared to nonburned tissue and will seldom blanch with pressure. In some instances, the burn tissue may look translucent with clotted vessels visible. These wounds are insensate to touch and pinprick. Hair follicles and sweat glands are destroyed. Most full-thickness burns should undergo early excision and grafting. Burns that are deeper, extending beyond subcutaneous tissue into fascia, muscle, tendon, and bone (formerly referred to as fourth-degree burns) will require excision and grafting (Brownson & Gibran, 2018; Myers et al., 2022).

Pearls for Practice

It is important for the nurse to acknowledge that even when skin is no longer in contact with the burn source, skin damage can continue. In the case of scald burns, 1 second of contact with hot tap water at 69°C (156°F) may result in a burn that destroys both the epidermis and the dermis, causing a full-thickness injury. A deep partial-thickness burn can convert to a full-thickness burn within 24 hours of injury; thus, immediate assessment and management, which includes the application of cool tap water for a minimum of 5 minutes, is important to decrease the risk of thermal injury (first-aid-fact-sheet.pdf [ameriburn.org]). It is imperative that the nurse remove all jewelry, rings, watches, or belts, which are typically made of metal, since they can retain heat, cause thermal injury, and act as a tourniquet with tissue swelling. Burning clothing must be removed immediately, and the wound should be covered with a sterile dressing or clean cloth that is loosely wrapped. If clothing has adhered to the wound, it should not

be removed. The use of ice water on large burns can result in hypothermia and can increase mortality. The best possible cooling temperature and duration of cooling is not known, but if excessive or prolonged, it may be harmful because of vasoconstriction and systemic hypothermia. The ABA's current guidelines recommend that cooling be limited to 30 minutes in the management of minor burns.

Extent of Body Surface Area Injured

Various methods are used to estimate the TBSA affected by burns; among them are the rule of nines and the Lund and Browder method.

Rule of Nines

The **rule of nines** (Fig. 52-2) is a simple and common way to estimate the extent of burns. The system assigns percentages in multiples of nine to major body surfaces, with the perineum forming the remaining 1%. This method must be modified in the pediatric population because of the proportionally larger heads and smaller limbs of children.

Lund and Browder Method

A more precise, age-specific method of estimating the extent of a burn is the Lund and Browder method, which recognizes the percentage of surface area of various anatomic parts, especially the head and legs, in relation to growth. Because of changes in body proportion with growth, the calculated TBSA changes with age as well (Myers et al., 2022). By dividing the body into very small areas and providing an estimate of the proportion of TBSA accounted for by each body part, one can obtain a reliable estimate of TBSA burned.

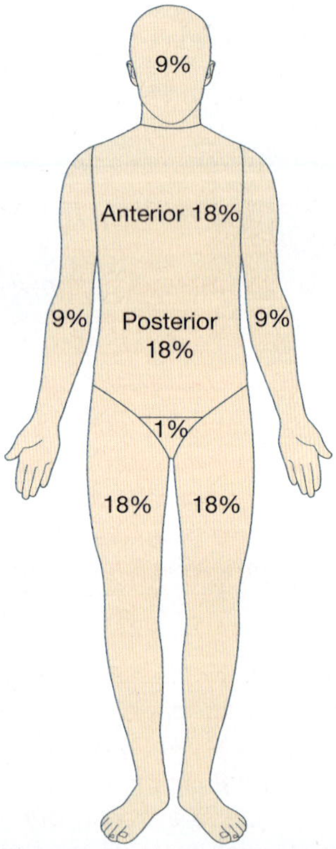

FIGURE 52-2 The rule of nines: Estimated percentage of total body surface area (TBSA) in the adult is arrived at by sectioning the body surface into areas with a numeric value related to nine. (Note: The anterior and posterior head total 9% of TBSA.)

Severity Grading System

The Severity Grading System (Box 52-1) adopted by the ABA includes minor, moderate, and major burns.

PATHOPHYSIOLOGY

Burns are a dynamic injury set that result in a cascade of local tissue and systemic inflammatory effects depending on the percentage of TBSA involved. Local effects of burns include the denaturation of protein (which results in the disruption and potential destruction of cells), liberation of vasoactive substances, and the formation of edema. As a result of the cellular injury, the osmotic and hydrostatic pressure gradients are disrupted, and intravascular fluid leaks into interstitial spaces. This damage is distributed throughout the injury as some cells die instantly, some are irreversibly

BOX 52-1 Classification of Extent of Burn Injury

Minor Burn Injury

- Second-degree burn of less than 15% total body surface area (TBSA) in adults or less than 10% TBSA in children
- Third-degree burn of less than 2% TBSA not involving special care areas (eyes, ears, face, hands, feet, perineum, joints)
- Excludes all patients with electrical injury, inhalation injury, or concurrent trauma and all at-risk patients (e.g., extremes of age, intercurrent disease)

Moderate, Uncomplicated Burn Injury

- Second-degree burns of 15–25% TBSA in adults or 10–20% in children
- Third-degree burns of less than 10% TBSA not involving special care areas
- Excludes all patients with electrical injury, inhalation injury, or concurrent trauma; all at-risk patients (e.g., extremes of age, intercurrent disease)

Major Burn Injury

- Second-degree burns of at least 25% TBSA in adults or at least 20% in children
- All third-degree burns 10% or more TBSA
- All burns involving eyes, ears, face, hands, feet, perineum, joints
- All patients with inhalation injury, electrical injury, or concurrent trauma; all at-risk patients

From Morton, P. G., & Fontaine, D. (2024). *Critical care nursing: A holistic approach* (12th ed.). Lippincott Williams & Wilkins.

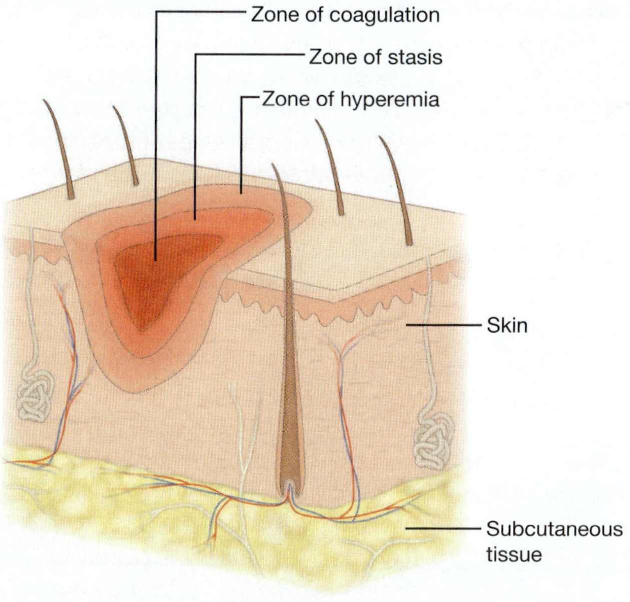

FIGURE 52-3 **Zones of burn injury. Each burned area has three zones of injury. The inner zone (known as the area of coagulation, in which cellular death occurs) sustains the most damage. The middle area, or zone of stasis, has a compromised blood supply, inflammation, and tissue injury. The outer zone—the zone of hyperemia—sustains the least damage.**

damaged, and some—if appropriate interventions occur—will survive. There are three distinct zones that appear in a bull's eye pattern. The zone of coagulation (in the center) is where the tissue is completely destroyed; the zone of stasis surrounds the nonviable tissue and is potentially viable; the zone of hyperemia has increased blood flow secondary to the natural inflammatory response (Fig. 52-3).

Burns that exceed 20% TBSA may produce a local and a systemic response and are considered major burn injuries. The incidence and significance of pathophysiologic changes are proportional to the extent of burn injury. In addition, burns of 60% TBSA cause depressed myocardial contractility; this, in combination with the loss of circulating plasma volume, hemoconcentration, and massive edema formation (Myers et al., 2022), results in both distributive and hypovolemic shock (see Chapter 53). Severe burns are marked by large losses of intravascular fluid, protein and electrolytes; these are greatest during the first 8 to 12 hours. Loss of fluid occurs as a result of the altered capillary permeability, significant hypoproteinemia, and shifts of sodium into the interstitial space. These severe fluid shifts decrease substantially by 24 hours post burn (Nitzschke, 2020). These patients are best served when transferred to a verified burn center, as they are at risk for the occurrence of burn shock.

Burn Shock: Cardiovascular Alterations

Burn shock develops from several abnormalities of the circulation. It can occur when more than 20% TBSA is involved; however, it can occur when a lower percentage is seen if the patient is medically fragile (Clinical Overview, 2023). The initial systemic event is hemodynamic instability, which results from loss of capillary integrity and a subsequent shift of fluid, sodium, and protein from the intravascular space into the interstitial spaces, producing blisters and edema. This leaky capillary syndrome increases cell permeability at the burn site, as well as throughout the body. In the major burn, this syndrome far exceeds the useful effect of the inflammatory response. Progressive edema develops in unburned tissue and organs, causing hypoperfusion and hypovolemic shock. As fluid loss continues from the burn wound(s) and the diffuse capillary leakage (from the intravascular space to the interstitial space), the blood volume decreases, the blood pressure (BP) falls, the cardiac output (CO) decreases, and urine output declines (Haglund & Phillips, 2023). This is the onset of burn shock. Burn shock is unique as it is a combination of hypovolemic and distributive shock indicated by intravascular volume depletion, increased pulmonary vascular resistance (PVR), elevated systemic vascular resistance, and depressed cardiac output (Myers et al., 2022). The systemic response is caused by the release of cytokines and other mediators into the systemic circulation. The outcome is a dramatic outpouring of fluids, electrolytes, and proteins into the interstitium; thus, burn shock is characterized by capillary leak, "third spacing" of fluid, severe hypovolemia, hemoconcentration, and decreased CO. If the burn patient is not resuscitated adequately, circulatory collapse ensues.

Pearls for Practice: Why Distributive Shock in Burns?

Distributive shock occurs when the blood volume is abnormally displaced within the body (e.g., when blood pools in peripheral blood vessels), causing a relative hypovolemia because not enough blood returns to the heart, which leads to inadequate tissue perfusion. It occurs primarily in conditions that cause vasodilation as in septic shock, neurogenic shock, or anaphylaxis. But in burn injury, there is systemic and pulmonary vasoconstriction (related to catecholaminergic release), so why distributive shock? It occurs due to the capillary leakage that causes the loss of fluid, electrolytes, and albumin from the blood into the interstitium. Thus, when the fluid is still retained in the body, just not where it is supposed to be, this is distributive shock. That is why you will see burn injury described as an actual fluid loss (hypovolemia) and fluid loss within the body (distributive).

Fluid and Electrolyte Alterations

Prompt fluid resuscitation maintains the BP in the low-normal range and improves CO. IV fluid resuscitation is based on the extent of burn injury and the patient's weight in kilograms (discussed shortly). In general, the greatest volume of fluid leak occurs in the first 24 to 36 hours after the burn. As the capillaries begin to regain their integrity, burn shock resolves and fluid returns to the vascular compartment. As fluid is reabsorbed from the interstitial tissue into the vascular compartment, blood volume increases. If kidney and cardiac function is adequate, urinary output increases. Lactated Ringer (LR) solution is the preferred IV fluid for burn resuscitation because of its physiologic similarity to the composition of extracellular fluid; for example, in LR sodium is 130 mEq/L and potassium (K^+) is 4 mEq/L, and normal intravascular levels are a sodium level of 135 to 145 mEq/L and K^+ of 3.5 to 5 mEq/L. LR also contains lactate (28 mEq/L), which can be converted by the liver to bicarbonate (the blood buffer) to aid in correcting the metabolic acidosis frequently seen in burn shock.

Patients with large burn wounds are at risk for abdominal compartment syndrome (ACS). This is one of the more life-threatening complications, with a mortality rate of 75% (Wurzer et al., 2018). With large burns, fluid shifts into the abdominal cavity, causing increased abdominal distention that interferes with pulmonary ventilation. The volume loss into the peritoneal space results in decreased CO, hypotension, and decreased urine output. When the intra-abdominal pressure exceeds 25 mm Hg or 34 cm H_2O (normally the intra-abdominal pressure ranges from 0 to 7 mm Hg, measured at end-expiration), the inferior vena cava is compressed, which restricts blood flow and perfusion to abdominal organs, further compromising renal, hepatic, and visceral organ function; the nurse observes for a tense abdomen, increased abdominal girth, oliguria (<400 mL/d), hypotension, and difficult ventilation and alerts the provider (Makic, 2021; Sheridan, 2020; Thurman, 2020). Decompression of the abdomen will be performed either in the ICU or in the operating room, and the patient will have an "open abdomen," that may be temporarily closed with a sterile perforated plastic sheet, clips, vacuum-assisted device, etc., and the skin and abdominal fascia are left open (Mondor, 2022). Later, the wound may be closed (depending on its size), or healed by secondary intention and eventual skin grafting (Mondor, 2022).

Pearls for Practice

The nurse recognizes that the clinical goal is to administer adequate but not excessive fluid while safeguarding that soft tissues are not rendered ischemic by increasing pressure beneath inelastic eschar or tense muscle compartments (Sheridan, 2020).

Pearls for Practice

Nurses measure intra-bladder pressure (IBP) using a bladder catheter (Foley), a pressure monitor or a manometer, room temperature saline solution, and a 60-mL syringe. A pressure monitor is set up and connected to the catheter drainage bag at the aspiration port via a Luer-lock or needle. Once the bladder is empty, 25 to 50 mL (depending on institutional policy) of saline solution is instilled through the bladder catheter using a 60-mL syringe, and it is clamped. The clamp must be on the drainage tubing below the aspiration port to allow measurement of bladder pressure. Patients must be in a supine position since head of bed elevation can have a significant impact on the reading (Mondor, 2022). The symphysis pubis (at the midaxillary line) is used as the zero reference point for the pressure bag at the midaxillary line. The pressure is recorded, the clamp released, and urine is allowed to flow into the drainage bag. The nurse remembers to subtract the amount of fluid instilled from the patient's urinary output to maintain an accurate intake and output (I&O) record (Fig. 52-4).

Patients with a major burn develop massive systemic edema. As fluid resuscitation proceeds, the edema worsens. As the taut, burned tissue becomes unyielding to the edema underneath its surface, it begins to act like a tourniquet, especially if the burn is circumferential. This complication is similar to a compartment syndrome. The provider may

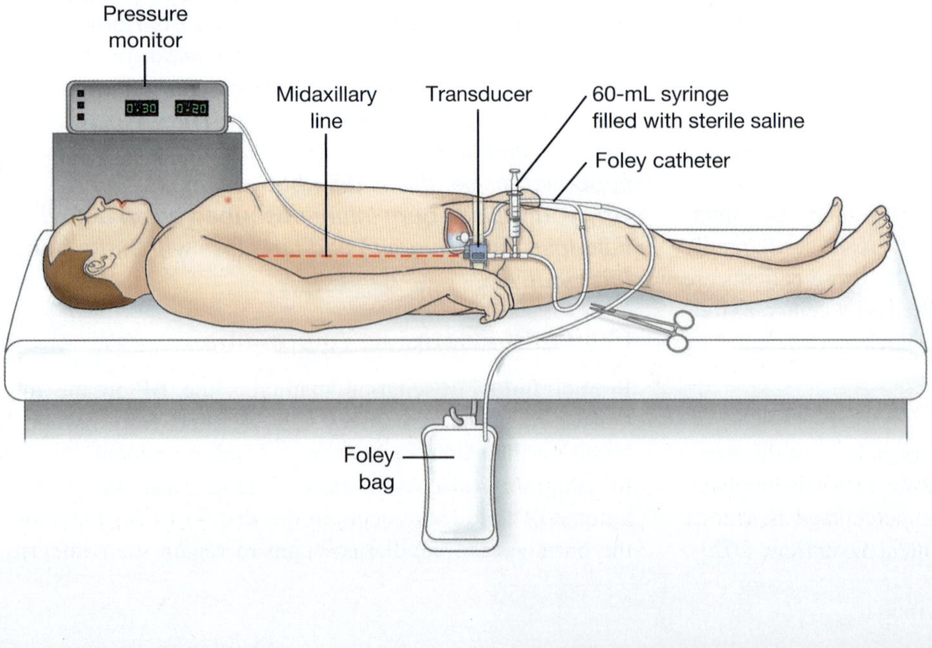

FIGURE 52-4 Measuring intra-bladder pressure. To assess for the development of abdominal compartment syndrome, the intra-bladder pressure may be monitored.

need to perform an **escharotomy**, a surgical incision into the **eschar** to relieve the constricting effect of the burned tissue. Refer to Chapter 41 for details on compartment syndrome.

Circulating blood volume decreases dramatically during burn shock due to severe capillary leak with variation of serum sodium levels in response to fluid resuscitation. Usually, hyponatremia (sodium depletion) is present during the resuscitation phase since sodium is lost directly through the burn wound, through the shifting of fluid and electrolytes into the interstitial space, and via the use of hypotonic salt solutions IV (recall LR sodium content is 130 mEq/L). Immediately after burn injury, hyperkalemia (excessive potassium) results from massive cell destruction, metabolic acidosis, and impaired kidney function caused by hemoglobinuria, myoglobinuria, or decreased renal perfusion (Myers et al., 2022). The loss of plasma, which begins almost immediately after the injury, reaches its peak within the first 48 hours, results in decreased circulating plasma volume, hemoconcentration, massive edema formation, decreased urine output, and depressed cardiovascular function (Meyers et al., 2022). Lactic acidosis is frequently seen in burn shock due to hypovolemia and hypoperfusion; thus, while the lactate in LR IV solution can be converted to base bicarbonate to correct the acidemia, the goal of treatment is aimed at reversing the hypoperfusion. Hypokalemia (potassium depletion) may occur later, with fluid shifts and inadequate potassium replacement. However, plasma lactate levels are significant markers of shock and resuscitation since they reflect tissue hypoperfusion and hypoxia and appear to be correlated to morbidity and outcome. A normal serum lactic acid level in venous blood is 0.5 to 2.2 mmol/L (0.5 to 2.2 mEq/L) (Fischbach et al., 2022). Lactic acidosis is defined by a serum lactate concentration >4 mmol/L (4 mEq/L) (Ferri, 2022); however, the nurse recognizes that values above 2.2 mmol/L are clearly consistent with hypoperfusion and shock (Angus, 2020). See discussion of fluid and electrolyte changes in the Emergent/Resuscitative Phase later in the chapter.

Pearls for Practice

The nurse is aware that severe lactic acidosis (pH less than 7.2) is associated with a high early mortality rate. There is a 28% mortality rate associated with a lactic acid level >4 mEq/L (Ferri, 2022).

Pearls for Practice

Ringer's lactate IV solution contains 28 mEq of lactate (28 mmol/L), which is metabolized into bicarbonate by the liver, aiding in correction of metabolic acidosis. However, the nurse is aware that liver function must be assessed to ensure adequate metabolism of this IV solution.

Pulmonary Alterations

Inhalation injury necessitates prolonged hospitalization and remains a major cause of morbidity and mortality and increases the amount of time the patient will spend on the ventilator (Wolf, 2022). An inhalation injury can occur when a person is trapped inside a burning structure or involved in an explosion that leads to the inhalation of superheated air, steam, and noxious gas. Inhalation injury is an independent risk factor for mortality (Woodson et al., 2018).

Clinical consequences can include increased mortality, impaired gas exchange, acute respiratory failure, acute respiratory distress syndrome (ARDS), upper airway edema, small airway occlusion, loss of ciliary clearance, increased dead space, intrapulmonary shunting, decreased lung compliance, decreased chest wall compliance, tracheobronchitis, and pneumonia (Woodson et al., 2018).

Pulmonary injuries fall into three major categories: (1) carbon monoxide poisoning, (2) upper airway obstruction, and (3) chemical pneumonitis (Myers et al., 2022). Carbon monoxide (CO) is probably the most common cause of inhalation injury because it is a byproduct of the combustion of organic materials and, therefore, is present in smoke. The pathophysiologic effects are caused by tissue hypoxia, a result of carbon monoxide combining with hemoglobin to form **carboxyhemoglobin (COHb or HbCO)**, which competes with oxygen for available hemoglobin-binding sites, which can quickly lead to anoxia and death. The affinity of hemoglobin for carbon monoxide is 200 to 250 times greater than that for oxygen. Refer to Table 52-2 for symptoms of CO poisoning (Anderson et al., 2019; Sheridan, 2020). It is reasonable for the nurse to assume that all burn patients are at risk for carbon monoxide poisoning when the patient was injured in an enclosed space such as a house fire.

Administering 100% oxygen is essential to accelerate the removal of carbon monoxide from the hemoglobin molecule and is the gold standard; this will reduce the half-life of CO from 250 minutes in room air to 40 to 60 minutes. Any cardiac or neurologic changes that are unexpected should raise suspicions and an arterial blood gas should be obtained to look for an elevated carboxyhemoglobin as the pulse oximetry can be falsely elevated. Monitor the oxygen saturation by pulse oximetry, but be aware that pulse oximetry readings

TABLE **52-2 Symptoms of Carbon Monoxide Toxicity**

Blood Carboxyhemoglobin Level (%)	Symptoms
Less than 15–20	Headache, dizziness, occasional confusion
20–40	Disorientation, visual impairment
40–60	Agitation, combativeness, hallucinations, coma, and shock
60	Death

Reprinted with permission from Barash, P., Cullen, B., & Stoelting, R. (2013). *Handbook of clinical anesthesia* (7th ed.). Lippincott Williams & Wilkins.

will be falsely elevated in patients with elevated carboxyhemoglobin levels. Fiberoptic bronchoscopy is often used as a diagnostic tool to view pulmonary insult.

Pearls for Practice

The pulse oximeter contains a light source (light-emitting diode [LED]) and a light detector, the sensor. The light source beams red and infrared light through the skin and blood, and the amount of light received by the detector is measured. The difference of the transmitted light during and between heart beats is calculated and converted to the percent of hemoglobin that is saturated with oxygen, the SpO_2. While the clinical usefulness of pulse oximeter cannot be disputed, there are at least three important limitations that the nurse needs to be aware of:

1. *Unfortunately, pulse oximeters cannot distinguish oxygenated Hb (HbO_2) from carbon monoxide-poisoned hemoglobin, aka carboxyhemoglobin (HbCO). Thus, falsely high SpO_2 saturations are seen in CO poisoning despite inadequate oxygenation of Hb. Moreover, the deficit in oxygen delivery to peripheral tissue is exacerbated by the ability of carbon monoxide to impair the release of oxygen that is bound to hemoglobin, often referred to as a decrease in the p50 (oxygen tension at which hemoglobin is 50% saturated).*
2. *While the SpO_2 accurately reflects the percentage of Hb saturation with O_2 under most conditions, it does not measure total O_2-carrying content of the blood. This can be particularly misleading in the anemic patient where the percent of Hb saturation may be normal but total oxygen delivery to tissues is markedly reduced as a consequence of the fall in red blood cell numbers.*
3. *The COVID pandemic revealed that pulse oximeters overestimate oxygen saturation measurements in patients with hypoxemia (when the oxygen saturation <90%), and that this error is larger across ethnic groups. For example, when an arterial blood gas demonstrated a true oxygen saturation of 85% to 89%; Black individuals had a mean pulse oximetry reading that was +3.9% higher, those of Asian ancestry 5.8% higher and White individuals +2.4% higher, when compared to arterial blood gas oxygenation (Crooks et al., 2022). Thus, the nurse recognizes that when concerned about a patient's respiratory status, arterial blood gases should be relied upon rather than pulse oximetry readings.*

Upper airway injury results from direct heat and edema or by chemical inflammation and necrosis (Myers et al., 2022). It is manifested by mechanical obstruction of the upper airway as small particles may reach the terminal bronchioles, causing bronchospasms and edema. The nurse observes for signs and symptoms of immediate or impending airway compromise (e.g., facial or oral burns, edema, hoarseness, stridor [which indicates a significant decrease in the diameter of the airway], dyspnea, wheezing). The head of the bed is elevated to >30 degrees to decrease airway edema; bronchodilators may assist in mobilizing secretions (Myers et al., 2022). Direct injury to the upper airway causes airway swelling that typically leads to maximal edema in the first 24 to 48 hours after injury and often requires a short course of endotracheal intubation for airway protection (before tracheal edema occurs) (Anderson et al., 2019).

Inhalation injury below the glottis results from inhaling noxious gases or steam. The injury results directly from chemical irritation of the pulmonary tissues at the alveolar level. These injuries cause loss of ciliary action, hypersecretion, severe mucosal edema, and possibly bronchospasm. The pulmonary surfactant is reduced, resulting in atelectasis (collapse of alveoli). Expectoration of carbon particles in the sputum is the cardinal sign of this injury.

Chemical pneumonitis is caused by the inhalation of various substances that results in the development of ARDS within days after a burn. The primary symptom is dyspnea, and there is increased work of breathing (tachypnea, nasal flaring, intercostal retractions, use of accessory muscles, crackles are auscultated as the fluid begins to leak into the alveolar interstitial space, and ABGs reveal hypoxemia). ARDS is common in these patients and can increase mortality to 66%. A 100% mortality was noted where the TBSA was greater than 60% in combination with inhalation injury and ARDS (Brownson & Gibran, 2018). Refer to Chapter 9 for management of ARDS. In summary, pulmonary abnormalities are not always immediately apparent. More than half of all patients with burn injuries with pulmonary involvement do not initially demonstrate pulmonary signs and symptoms. Any patient with possible inhalation injury must be observed for at least 24 hours for respiratory complications since upper airway edema may not be present until after the onset of fluid resuscitation (Myers et al., 2022). The nurse maintains a high degree of suspicion for possible pulmonary damage if the following indicators are present:

- History indicating that the burn occurred in an enclosed area
- Burns of the face or neck
- Singed nasal hair or eyebrows
- Hoarseness, voice change, dry cough, stridor
- Sooty (carbonaceous sputum) or bloody sputum
- Soot in or around the mouth
- Labored breathing or tachypnea (rapid breathing) and other signs of reduced oxygen levels (hypoxemia)
- Erythema and blistering of the oral or pharyngeal mucosa

Renal Alterations

Hypovolemia from insensible fluid losses, hypotension, nephrotoxic medications, and rhabdomyolysis (breakdown of skeletal muscles) are all significant factors of acute kidney injury (AKI). In burns, if skeletal muscle damage occurs, myoglobin and hemoglobin are released from the muscle cells and excreted by the kidney causing myoglobinuria; this is common in high-voltage injuries or deep thermal burns. A urinalysis is sent to the laboratory to determine the myoglobin level in those with burn injury. Myoglobinuria will have a pigmented appearance that may be described as brown, port-wine, cola, or coffee color. If there is inadequate blood flow through the kidneys, the hemoglobin and myoglobin occlude the renal tubules, resulting in AKI. Prevention of AKI is dependent on early and aggressive fluid resuscitation. Additional treatments in rhabdomyolysis include sodium bicarbonate to alkalize urine, which promotes myoglobin excretion, and diuretics such as mannitol to increase renal blood flow and glomerular filtration rate to facilitate myoglobin clearance; however, this is balanced against the risk of volume depletion (Myers et al., 2022). Blood urea nitrogen (BUN), serum creatinine levels, and strict measurement of intake and urinary output hourly are essential to evaluate kidney function. Urine output may be falsely elevated by use of diuretics, alcohol intoxication, hyperglycemia, or glucosuria (Cancio et al., 2018).

Immunologic Alterations

The immunologic defense of the body are greatly altered by a serious burn injury, as it diminishes resistance to infection. The loss of skin integrity is compounded by the release of abnormal inflammatory factors. There is a significant impairment of the production and release of granulocytes and macrophages from bone marrow; the resulting immunosuppression places the patient with burn injury at high risk for sepsis (see Chapter 53 for details on septicemia). In addition, while an indwelling urinary catheter is appropriate for the first 48 to 72 hours of a burn injury, it is removed as soon as possible due to infection risk (Myers et al., 2022).

Thermoregulatory Alterations

Loss of skin also results in an inability to regulate body temperature. Therefore, patients with burn injuries may exhibit low body temperatures in the early hours after injury. Then, as hypermetabolism resets core temperatures, the patient becomes hyperthermic for much of the post-burn period, even in the absence of infection.

Gastrointestinal Alterations

Two potential gastrointestinal (GI) complications may occur: paralytic ileus (absence of intestinal peristalsis) and Curling ulcer. Decreased peristalsis and bowel sounds are manifestations of paralytic ileus resulting from burn trauma where blood flow can decrease up to 60%, hypokalemia, or the sympathetic response to severe trauma (Myers et al., 2022). Gastric distention and nausea may lead to vomiting unless gastric decompression is initiated with the insertion of a nasogastric (NG) tube. Gastric bleeding secondary to massive physiologic stress may be signaled by occult blood in the stool, regurgitation of "coffee ground" material from the stomach, or bloody vomitus. These signs suggest gastric or duodenal erosion (Curling ulcer).

MANAGEMENT OF BURN INJURY

Burn care must be based on burn depth and local response, the extent of the injury, and the presence of a systemic response. Burn care is divided into three phases: emergent/resuscitative phase, acute/intermediate phase, and rehabilitation phase. Although priorities exist for each of the phases, they overlap, and assessment and management of specific problems and complications are not limited to these phases but take place throughout burn care. The three phases and the priorities for care are summarized in Table 52-3. Box 52-2 summarizes emergency care at the burn scene.

TABLE **52-3 Phases of Burn Care**

Phase	Duration	Priorities
Emergent/resuscitative	From onset of injury to completion of fluid resuscitation	• First aid • Prevention of shock • Prevention of respiratory distress • Detection and treatment of concomitant injuries • Wound assessment and initial care
Acute/intermediate	From beginning of diuresis to near completion of wound closure	• Wound care and closure • Prevention or treatment of complications, including infection • Nutritional support
Rehabilitation	From major wound closure to return to patient's optimal level of physical and psychosocial adjustment	• Prevention of scars and contractures • Physical, occupational, and vocational rehabilitation • Functional and cosmetic reconstruction • Psychosocial counseling

BOX 52-2

Emergency Procedures at the Burn Scene

- *Extinguish the flames:* When clothes catch fire, the flames can be extinguished if the person falls to the floor or ground and rolls ("stop, drop, and roll"); anything available to smother the flames, such as a blanket, rug, or coat, may be used. Standing still forces the person to breathe flames and smoke, and running fans the flames. If the burn source is electrical, the electrical source must be disconnected.
- *Cool the burn:* After the flames are extinguished, the burned area and adherent clothing are soaked with *cool* water, briefly, to cool the wound and halt the burning process. Once a burn has been sustained, the application of cool water is the best first-aid measure. Soaking the burn area intermittently in cool water or applying cool towels gives immediate and striking relief from pain and limits local tissue edema and damage. However, *never* apply ice directly to the burn, *never* wrap the person in ice, and *never* use cold soaks or dressings for longer than several minutes; such procedures may worsen the tissue damage and lead to hypothermia in people with large burns.
- *Remove restrictive objects:* If possible, remove clothing immediately. Adherent clothing may be left in place once cooled. Other clothing and all jewelry (especially rings), including all piercings, should be removed to allow for assessment and to prevent constriction secondary to rapidly developing edema.
- *Cover the wound:* The burn should be covered as quickly as possible to minimize bacterial contamination and decrease pain by preventing air from coming into contact with the injured surface. Sterile dressings are best, but any clean, dry cloth can be used as an emergency dressing. Ointments and salves should *not* be used. Other than the dressing, no medication or material should be applied to the burn wound.
- *Irrigate chemical burns:* Chemical burns resulting from contact with a corrosive material are irrigated immediately. Most chemical laboratories have a high-pressure shower for such emergencies. If such an injury occurs at home, brush off the chemical agent, remove clothes immediately, and rinse all areas of the body that have come in contact with the chemical. Rinsing can occur in the shower or any other source of continuous running water. If a chemical gets in or near the eyes, the eyes should be flushed with cool, clean water immediately. Outcomes for the patient with chemical burns are significantly improved by rapid, sustained flushing of the injury at the scene.

Emergent/Resuscitative Phase

Immediate Care

It is important to remember the CABD (circulation, airway, breathing, disability) steps (formerly called ABCs [Airway, Breathing, and Circulation]) of all trauma care during the early post-burn period. Refer to Chapter 55 for further details.

Circulation must be assessed quickly. The pulse (apical and radial) and BP are monitored frequently. Tachycardia (abnormally rapid heart rate, over 100 bpm) and slight hypotension are expected soon after the burn; however, with significant burns the patient may present in hypovolemic and distributive shock (discussed earlier). The nurse monitors the level of consciousness (LOC), which provides clues to cerebral perfusion. Recall that a mean arterial pressure (MAP) of >65 mm Hg is required for organ perfusion (normal range is 70 to 110 mm Hg). If the MAP drops below this point for an extended period, end-organ ischemia and infarction can occur. For example, a MAP >60 mm Hg is needed to perfuse the coronary arteries. If the MAP drops <60 mm Hg, blood will not be able to perfuse cerebral tissues as well and there will be a loss of consciousness, and neuronal death will quickly ensue (Lough et al., 2022). ECG monitoring is important, particularly with electrical burns, inhalation injury, or associated trauma; lead placement may be problematic, particularly with chest injuries, in which case nontraditional locations on nonburned skin should be selected (Myers et al., 2022). For major burns that are greater than 20% TBSA, a urinary catheter is inserted, and strict intake and hourly output is recorded. Monitoring of hourly urine output and daily weight provides clues about fluid volume status and fluid replacement. Any evidence of decreasing urine output or hemodynamic instability requires immediate notification of the provider. A large-bore (16- or 18-gauge) IV catheter should be inserted in a nonburned area for fluid replacement. An arterial line may be inserted to monitor BP continuously (see Chapter 54).

It is important to support the *airway* and protect the cervical spine. If edema of the airway develops, endotracheal intubation may be necessary.

The nurse assesses and promotes *breathing.* For mild pulmonary injury, 100% humidified oxygen is administered. Recall that the nurse assumes that all major burn should be suspected to have inhalation injury. The nurse monitors the respiratory rate, lung sounds, and oxygen saturation and notifies the provider if dyspnea, stridor, hoarseness, wheezing or changes in respiratory patterns (tachypnea) or saturation levels reflect declining ventilation and oxygenation. Early signs of hypoxemia include agitation and anxiety. Intubation and ventilation may be necessary.

Pearls for Practice

Breathing must be assessed and a patent airway established immediately during the initial minutes of emergency care. Immediate therapy is directed toward establishing an airway and administering humidified 100% oxygen. If qualified personnel and equipment are available and the victim has severe respiratory distress or airway edema, the rescuers can insert an endotracheal tube and initiate manual ventilation.

Pearls for Practice

In the event of a high-voltage electrical injury, spinal cord injury can result from the direct effect of electrical current or can occur secondary to trauma associated with blunt injury. Thus, the cervical spine should be immobilized. In addition, electrical injury interferes with cardiac conduction and can cause direct trauma to cardiac muscle fibers, resulting in a number of arrhythmias, including asystole, ventricular fibrillation, sinus tachycardia, and premature ventricular contractions (PVCs). Because the arrhythmias can present hours after the incident, cardiac monitoring for patients with all electrical injuries for at least 24 hours after cessation of arrhythmia is suggested.

In addition, related to *disability*, the neurologic status is assessed quickly in the patient with extensive burns. The nurse is aware that restlessness, confusion, difficulty attending to questions, or decreasing LOC may indicate cerebral hypoxia. Often, the patient is awake and alert initially, and vital information can be obtained at that time. A secondary head-to-toe survey of the patient is carried out to identify other potentially life-threatening injuries.

Assessment

After adequate circulatory and respiratory functions have been established, and the patient's condition is stable, attention is directed to the burn wound itself.

Information needs to include the time of the burn injury, the source of the burn, how the burn was treated at the scene, and any history of falling with the injury. A history of pre-existing diseases; allergies; medications; and the use of drugs, alcohol, and tobacco is obtained at this point to aid in planning the patient's care. Because poor tissue perfusion accompanies burn injuries, only IV analgesia (usually morphine) is administered, and it should be titrated according to patient need.

If the burn exceeds 20% TBSA, a nasogastric tube should be inserted and connected to low suction. All patients who are intubated should have a nasogastric tube inserted to decompress the abdomen and prevent vomiting.

Assessment of both the TBSA burned and the depth of the burn are completed. Careful attention is paid to keeping the patient warm during wound assessment. Baseline values for height, weight, arterial blood gases, carboxyhemoglobin, complete blood count, electrolyte values, BUN, creatinine, glucose, blood alcohol level, drug panel, blood screening, urinalysis, and baseline electrocardiogram (ECG) are obtained. In the case of an electrical burn injury, creatine kinase, urinalysis, and urine myoglobin are obtained to assess for rhabdomyolysis (Myers et al., 2022). Because burns are contaminated wounds, tetanus prophylaxis is administered if the patient's immunization status is not current (less than 5 years since last tetanus) or unknown (Myers et al., 2022).

Transfer to a Burn Center

The depth and extent of the burn are considered in determining whether the patient should be transferred to a burn center. However, if the patient's prognosis does not support transport to a burn center, nurses may contact burn center nurses via telephone and ask for support in patient management. Examples of criteria for referral to a burn unit can be found at https://ameriburn.org/resources/burn-center-referral-criteria/

Management of Fluid Loss and Shock

Next to managing respiratory difficulties, the most urgent need is preventing irreversible shock by replacing lost fluids and electrolytes (Table 52-4). The total volume and rate of IV fluid replacement are gauged by the patient's response and

TABLE 52-4 Fluid and Electrolyte Changes in the Emergent/Resuscitative Phase

Fluid accumulation phase (shock phase)
Plasma → interstitial fluid (edema at burn site)

Observation	Explanation
Generalized dehydration	Plasma leaks through damaged capillaries.
Reduction of blood volume	Secondary to plasma loss, fall of blood pressure, decreased MAP, narrow pulse pressure (PP), and diminished cardiac output.
Decreased urinary output	Secondary to: Fluid loss Decreased renal blood flow Sodium and water retention caused by increased adrenocortical activity Hemolysis of red blood cells, causing hemoglobinuria and myonecrosis or myoglobinuria
Potassium (K^+) excess	Massive cellular trauma causes release of K^+ into extracellular fluid (ordinarily, most K^+ is intracellular), metabolic acidosis, and impaired kidney function.
Sodium (Na^+) deficit	Large amount of Na^+ is lost in trapped edema fluid and exudate and by shift into cells as K^+ is released from cells (ordinarily, most Na^+ is extracellular) via the use of hypotonic salt solutions.
Metabolic acidosis (base–bicarbonate deficit)	Loss of bicarbonate ions accompanies sodium loss.
Hemoconcentration (elevated hematocrit)	Liquid blood component is lost into extravascular space.

guided by the resuscitation formula. Numerous fluid resuscitation formulas exist; the nurse needs to be familiar with current institutional protocols. The adequacy of fluid resuscitation is determined primarily by monitoring vital signs and urine output totals, an index of renal perfusion. The IV is titrated hourly to maintain a minimum urine output of 0.5 mL/kg/hr in adults and 1 mL/kg/hr in children as resuscitation goals (ABLS, 2018; Carey et al., 2021). If urine outputs are greater than 1 mL/kg/h, the IV fluids should be decreased by 20%, and the nurse continues to monitor hourly output. Urine output less than 0.5 mL/kg/h, should have the rate of IV fluid increased by 20%, with output monitored hourly (Briggs & Barth, 2022).

Use of advanced technology, such as monitoring with central venous pressures, pulmonary artery catheters, and esophageal echo-Doppler, to evaluate hemodynamic response in burn-shock resuscitation have utility but carry risks, such as infection and aspiration. Thus, traditional variables of hourly assessment of urinary output and vital signs are used to evaluate the adequacy of fluid replacement therapy.

Pearls for Practice: The Balance Between Hypervolemia and Hypovolemia

Patients that are at extremes of age, both the very young and the very old, have less tolerance for rapid changes in volume status; their ability to compensate for these "swings" in hypovolemia or hypervolemia is limited (Cancio et al., 2018). Although you will administer IV replacement fluid based on your burn protocol, you recognize that you will monitor the individual response of the patient by monitoring the urine output, heart rate, BP, and LOC. Underresuscitation results in decreased CO and increased risk of AKI, whereas overresuscitation results in pulmonary edema, heart failure, and compartment overload of the extremities and abdomen, which are all associated with higher mortality (Carey et al., 2021). You will be threading the needle of euvolemia (presence of a normal amount of blood) by meticulous recording of urinary output and administering and monitoring IV therapy.

The projected fluid requirements for the first 24 hours are calculated by the provider based on the extent of the burn injury. Formulas have been developed for estimating fluid loss based on the estimated percentage of burned TBSA and the weight of the patient. The length of time since the burn injury occurred is very important in calculating estimated fluid needs. Formulas must be adjusted so that initiation of fluid replacement reflects the time of injury. Resuscitation formulas are approximations only and are individualized to meet the requirements of each patient.

Pearls for Practice

Intravenous resuscitation formulas are to be used only as guides. The patient's response, evidenced by heart rate, blood pressure, and urine output, is the primary determinant of actual fluid therapy and must be assessed ***at least hourly.*** *You will adjust the IV rate to maintain adequate urine output, which is used to approximate perfusion of end organs (Carey et al., 2021).*

The ABA consensus formula, published in 2008, provides for the volume of an isotonic solution (e.g., LR) to be administered during the first 24 hours in a range of 2 to 4 mL/kg/% TBSA.

Adults and older children (over 14 years of age, weighing more than 40 kg) receive:

$$2 \text{ mL of LR} \times \text{kg} \times \text{the \% burn}$$

Patients with electrical injuries have LR administered:

$$4 \text{ mL} \times \text{kg} \times \text{the \% burn (ABLS, 2018).}$$

Another formula widely used is the Parkland formula, which is 4 mL/kg/% TBSA over 24 hours, using LR. It also administers half of the volume over the first 8 hours post-burn, and the remaining half is administered over the next 16 hours. The use of formulas and TBSA methods can improve the accuracy and ease of calculating fluid resuscitation requirements. Again, providers should take note that the resuscitation formula serves only as a guideline, and the patient's response to fluid therapy is the best parameter to use.

The following example illustrates use of the consensus formula in a 70-kg (154-lb) patient with a 50% TBSA burn:

1. Consensus formula: 2 to 4 mL/kg/% TBSA
2. $2 \times 70 \times 50 = 7{,}000$ mL/24 hr
3. Plan to administer: first 8 hours = 3,500 mL, or 437 mL/hr; next 16 hours = 3,500 mL, or 219 mL/hr

Factors that are associated with the increased fluid requirements include delayed resuscitation, scald burn injuries, inhalation injuries, high-voltage electrical injuries, hyperglycemia, alcohol intoxication, and chronic diuretic therapy.

Nursing Implications

Nursing assessment in the emergent phase of burn injury focuses on the major priorities for any trauma patient. Vital signs and respiratory status are monitored closely, and the monitoring of fluid intake and urinary output hourly is critical. Circulation, sensation, and mobility (CSM) of the burn area is assessed hourly. Refer to Chapter 39 for details on musculoskeletal assessment. Hourly, the nurse will assess warmth, capillary refill, pulses, sensation, and movement of the affected extremity using the unaffected extremity for comparison. A Doppler (ultrasound device) is useful to assess perfusion of the affected extremity. Elevation of burned extremities is crucial to decrease edema. Loss of pulse or sensation must be reported to the provider immediately. Burgundy-colored/pigmented urine suggests muscle damage, and the presence of oliguria may be associated with AKI or inadequate fluid resuscitation.

Pearls for Practice

If a blood pressure cuff is wrapped around a patient's arm, the cuff must be removed from the extremity between readings since it may act as a tourniquet as the extremity swells.

Pearls for Practice

Dressings impede circulation if they are wrapped too tightly. The peripheral pulses must be checked frequently, and burned extremities must be elevated on pillows.

Body temperature, body weight, current illnesses, and use of medications are assessed. A head-to-toe assessment is performed, focusing on signs and symptoms of concomitant illness, injury, or developing complications. Assessing the extent of the burn wound continues and is facilitated with anatomic diagrams (described previously).

Comorbid conditions coupled with the burn injury contribute to the high mortality rates of patients 60 years of age and older. Decreased function of the cardiovascular, renal, and pulmonary systems increases the need for close observation of older patients with even relatively minor burns during the emergent and acute phases. AKI is much more common in older patients than in those younger than 40 years of age. The margin of difference between hypovolemia and fluid overload is very small. Suppressed immunologic response, a high incidence of malnutrition, and an inability to withstand metabolic stressors further compromise the older person's ability to heal. As a result of these issues, close monitoring and prompt treatment of complications are mandatory. A plan of nursing care for a patient during the emergent/resuscitative phase of burn injury is available online at http://thepoint.lww.com/Honan3e.

Acute/Intermediate Phase

The acute or intermediate phase of burn care follows the emergent/resuscitative phase and begins 48 to 72 hours after the burn injury. During this phase, attention is directed toward continued assessment and maintenance of respiratory and circulatory status, fluid and electrolyte balance (Table 52-5), and GI function. Infection prevention, burn wound care, pain management, and nutritional support are priorities at this stage.

Maintenance of Circulatory and Respiratory Status

Changes may occur as the effects of resuscitative fluid and the chemical reactions of smoke ingredients with lung tissues become apparent. Pulmonary complications are not unusual.

The frequency of pneumonia and respiratory failure is much greater in patients with prolonged mechanical ventilation. Ideally, the best practice is to remove the endotracheal tube as soon as possible to decrease the risk of infection transmission. The standard of care is to perform protocolized daily sedation interruptions with spontaneous breathing trials. This has been shown to decrease ventilator days

TABLE **52-5 Fluid and Electrolyte Changes in the Acute Phase**

Fluid remobilization phase (state of diuresis)
Interstitial fluid → plasma

Observation	Explanation
Hemodilution (decreased hematocrit)	Blood cell concentration is diluted as fluid enters the intravascular compartment; loss of red blood cells destroyed at burn site occurs.
Increased urinary output	Fluid shift into intravascular compartment increases renal blood flow and causes increased urine formation.
Sodium (Na^+) deficit	With diuresis, sodium is lost with water; existing serum sodium is diluted by water influx.
Potassium (K^+) deficit (occurs occasionally in this phase)	Beginning on the fourth or fifth postburn day, K^+ shifts from extracellular fluid into cells.
Metabolic acidosis	Loss of sodium depletes fixed base; relative carbon dioxide content increases.

and mortality in randomized controlled trials (RCTs). An RCT has shown that for every seven patients that underwent this breathing trial protocol, one life was saved (Culnan et al., 2018). Refer to Chapter 54 for details on weaning from a ventilator.

The arterial blood gas values and other parameters determine the need for intubation and mechanical ventilation. Humidified oxygen is provided as necessary to maintain adequate oxygen saturation and provide moisture to injured tissues. The nurse assesses breath sounds; respiratory rate, rhythm, and depth; chest symmetry; and use of accessory muscles and notifies providers with concerns over pulmonary deterioration, such as increasing dyspnea or stridor and changes in respiratory patterns. As capillaries regain integrity, diuresis begins. If cardiac or renal function is inadequate, fluid overload occurs and symptoms of heart failure or pulmonary edema may result. Early detection allows for early intervention and carefully calculated fluid intake. Cautious administration of fluids and electrolytes continues during this phase of burn care. Blood components are administered as needed to treat blood loss and anemia.

Infection Prevention

When large numbers of bacteria accumulate in the burn wounds, those with high pathogenic capacity find their way into the adjacent tissue. This causes more necrosis and can further infiltrate circulation, leading to sepsis. Historically, burn wound sepsis has been the leading cause of death in burn patients. *Pseudomonas aeruginosa, Staphylococcus aureus,*

Klebsiella pneumoniae, Escherichia coli, Enterobacter spp., and *Candida* spp. are the most significant pathogens. Antibiotic-resistant Acinetobacter is now being seen as a cause of fatal sepsis (Hawkins, 2018).

The immunosuppression, absent epithelial barriers, and multiple invasive devices that accompany extensive burn injury place the patient at high risk of sepsis. Despite aseptic precautions and the use of topical antimicrobial agents, the burn wound is an excellent medium for bacterial growth and proliferation. While the wound is healing, it must be protected from infection. A primary source of bacterial infection is the patient's intestinal tract, the source of most microbes. A major secondary source of pathogenic microbes is the environment. Infection control is a major role of the burn team in providing wound care. Gown, mask, and gloves are worn while caring for the patient with open burn wounds. Clean technique is used when caring directly for burn wounds.

Antibiotics are seldom prescribed prophylactically because of the risk of promoting resistant strains of bacteria, and they do not seem to reduce the incidence of septic complications. Systemic antibiotics are administered when there is documentation of positive cultures in, for example, urine, sputum, or blood. Careful attention is paid to antibiotic use because inappropriate use of antibiotics significantly affects the microbial flora present and increases the risk of drug resistance.

One of the most significant ways to reduce mortality is to excise these burn wounds early; removal of the burn eschar and immediate wound closure provides the best chance for survival (Branski et al., 2018).

Wound Care

Wound care is the single most time-consuming element of burn care after the emergent phase. The nurse needs to make astute assessments of wound status, use creative approaches to wound dressing, and support the patient and family during the emotionally distressing and very painful experience of wound care.

Various measures are used to clean the burn wound. After the wounds are cleansed, the prescribed method of wound care is performed. Provider preferences, the availability of skilled nursing staff, and resources in terms of number of personnel, supplies, and time must be considered in choosing the best method. The goal is to protect the wound until either spontaneous healing or skin grafting can be achieved. Patient comfort and ability to participate in the prescribed treatment are also important considerations.

Topical Antibacterial Therapy

There is agreement that some form of antimicrobial therapy applied to the burn wound is the best method of local care. Topical antibacterial therapy does not sterilize the wound; it simply reduces the number of bacteria. For more than 50 years, it has been recognized that silver has bacteriostatic and bacteriocidal properties that make it an excellent treatment agent (Table 52-6).

Criteria for choice of topical agents include the following:

- They are effective against gram-negative organisms and even fungi.
- They are clinically effective.
- They penetrate the eschar but are not systemically toxic.
- They do not lose their effectiveness, allowing another infection to develop.
- They are cost-effective, available, and acceptable to the patient.
- They are easy to apply and remove, minimizing nursing care time.

Wound Debridement

As debris accumulates on the wound surface, it can delay the healing process. **Debridement** has two goals:

- To remove tissue contaminated by bacteria and foreign bodies
- To remove devitalized tissue or burn eschar in preparation for grafting and wound healing

Early surgical excision to remove devitalized tissue and with early burn wound closure are recognized as the most important factors contributing to survival of a patient with a major burn injury.

Wound Coverage

If wounds are full-thickness or extensive, spontaneous healing is not possible, and treatment of the wound is necessary until coverage with a graft of the patient's own skin (**autograft**) is possible. Autografts are the ideal covering for burn wounds because the grafts are the patient's own skin and therefore are not rejected by the patient's immune system.

The purposes of wound coverage are to decrease the risk of infection; prevent further loss of protein, fluid, and electrolytes through the wound; minimize heat loss through evaporation; and minimizing scarring. Once the wound is surgically excised, a wound covering is applied to keep the area moist and promote the granulation process.

Homograft is donor skin from a cadaver. It is a biologic dressing that has several uses. In extensive burns, it save lives by providing temporary wound coverage and protecting the granulation tissue until autografting is possible. Biologic dressings also provide temporary immediate coverage for clean, superficial burns and decrease the wound's evaporative water and protein loss. They decrease pain by protecting nerve endings and are an effective barrier against water loss and entry of bacteria. Biosynthetic and synthetic skin substitutes continue to be used as temporary wound coverings, and new ones are becoming available consistently.

In an attempt to develop the ideal burn wound covering product, dermal substitutes have been created. It is believed that skin substitutes enhance the healing process of an open wound when autologous skin is unavailable.

Care of the Graft Site. Occlusive dressings are commonly used initially after grafting to immobilize the graft. Synthetic

TABLE **52-6 Overview of Selected Topical Antibacterial Agents Used for Burn Wounds**

Agent	Indication	Application	Nursing Implications
Silver sulfadiazine 1% water-soluble cream	• Most bactericidal agent • Minimal penetration of eschar	Apply 1/16-in layer of cream with a sterile glove 1–3 times daily.	• Watch for leukopenia 2–3 days after initiation of therapy. (Leukopenia usually resolves within 2–3 days.) • Anticipate formation of pseudoeschar (proteinaceous gel), which is removed easily after 72 hours.
Mafenide acetate 5–10% hydrophilic-based cream	• Effective against gram-negative and gram-positive organisms • Diffuses rapidly through eschar • In 10% strength, the agent of choice for electrical burns because of its ability to penetrate thick eschar	Apply thin layer with sterile glove twice a day. Change the dressing every 12 hours as prescribed.	• Monitor arterial blood gas levels and discontinue as prescribed if acidosis occurs. Mafenide acetate is a strong carbonic anhydrase inhibitor that may reduce renal buffering and cause metabolic acidosis. • Premedicate the patient with an analgesic before applying mafenide acetate because this agent causes severe burning pain for up to 20 minutes after application.
Silver nitrate 0.5% aqueous solution	• Bacteriostatic and fungicidal • Does *not* penetrate eschar	Apply solution to gauze dressing and place over wound. Keep the dressing wet but covered with dry gauze and dry blankets to decrease vaporization. Remoisten every 2 hours, and re-dress wound daily as prescribed.	• Monitor serum sodium (Na^+) and potassium (K^+) levels and replace as prescribed. Silver nitrate solution is hypotonic and acts as a wick for sodium and potassium. • Protect bed linen and clothing from contact with silver nitrate, which stains everything it touches black.
Acticoat	• Effective against gram-negative and gram-positive organisms and some yeasts and molds • Delivers a uniform, antimicrobial concentration of silver to the burn wound	Moisten with sterile water only (*never* use normal saline as it will deactivate the silver in the dressing). Apply directly to wound. Cover with absorbent secondary dressing. Remoisten every 3–4 hours with sterile water.	• Do not use oil-based products or topical antimicrobials with Acticoat burn dressing. Keep Acticoat moist, not saturated. May produce a "pseudoeschar" from silver after application. • Can be left in place for 3–5 days. Also available in Acticoat 7, which can be left in place for up to 7 days without the need to change the dressing.

dressings may be used to protect grafts. The patient is positioned and turned carefully to avoid disturbing the graft or putting pressure on the graft site. If an extremity has been grafted, it is elevated to minimize edema.

Care of the Donor Site. A donor site requires careful management to support effective wound healing. Occlusive, adherent, alginate sheets or hydrocolloid dressings can be used depending on surgeon preference. With all types of covering, donor sites must remain clean, dry, and free from pressure. Because a donor site is usually a partial-thickness wound, it will heal spontaneously within 7 to 14 days with proper care. Donor sites are painful, and additional pain management must be a part of the patient's care.

Pain Management

A significant issue for burn-injured patients is pain, which has been described as one of the most intense and prolonged types of pain. It is complex given the physiology of injury, chronicity of pain, and the related psychological effect, making management challenging to providers (Joshi et al., 2022). Pain is related to tissue destruction of the dermis and to the inflammatory response and the release of cytokines and chemokines. The protective covering of the epidermis is damaged, and the associated inflammation leads to stimulation of the nerve endings. These injuries are painful to the affected areas and surrounding tissue. The pain starts immediately after injury and can last long into the recovery phase. Hyperalgesia (enhanced intensity of pain sensation) has been known to occur in burn patients; the pain threshold is lowered and pain can last minutes or hours; there may be **allodynia**, which is an exaggerated pain to no painful stimuli such as touch (He & Kim, 2021). Pain in patients with burn wounds can be divided into four types: (1) rest pain: constant background, dull pain; (2) breakthrough pain: intermittent, short duration, rapid onset, sometimes excruciating (3) procedural: short duration, greatest intensity (wound cleansing, therapy); and (4) psychogenic pain: anticipatory pain without stimulation (Joshi et al., 2022). The nurse should be aware that rest pain (background) is best handled by administering regularly scheduled long-acting opioids for continuous coverage; procedural pain requires premedication with analgesic medications before painful procedures. Range of motion of the affected limb(s) and routine activities contribute to background pain. Wound care, physical and occupational therapy, and the use of splints are examples of when procedural pain is expected (Myers et al., 2022). Breakthrough pain occurs when blood levels of analgesic agents decrease below the level required to control background pain. Psychogenic pain, which is pain that may be caused by an emotional issue (often fear, depression, stress, or anxiety), may be managed with early psychological evaluation and patient-specific treatment.

Pearls for Practice: Route for Pain Medication

Intramuscular or subcutaneous injections are not administered in burn-injured patients due to unpredictable absorption by these routes (Myers et al., 2022).

Pain changes in time as the wound is covered with new skin, healing takes place, and scars form. Management of this often severe pain is one of the most difficult challenges facing the burn team. Many factors contribute to the pain experience. These factors include the severity of the pain, the adequacy of the health care provider's assessment of the pain, appropriateness of pharmacologic treatment of pain, multiple procedures involved in burn care, and evaluation of the effectiveness of pain relief measures. Literature suggests that, despite advances in pain management, many burn patients are undertreated for pain. The outstanding features of burn pain are its intensity and long duration; thus, all medical providers should understand that opioid tolerance is not addiction, and pain should be managed when there is a clinical need. Furthermore, necessary wound care carries with it the anticipation of pain and anxiety. Refer to Chapter 6 for discussion of tolerance versus addiction.

In partial-thickness burns, the nerve endings are exposed, resulting in excruciating pain with exposure to air currents. Although nerve endings are destroyed in full-thickness burns, the margins of the burn wound are hypersensitive to pain, and there is pain in adjacent structures. Healing of full-thickness burns creates significant discomfort as regenerating nerve endings become entrapped in scar formation. Most severe burns are a combination of partial-thickness and full-thickness burns.

The patient's pain level must be assessed throughout the day because each type of pain is different, and various management strategies may be needed to address the different types of pain. The nurse uses a pain intensity scale to assess pain level (e.g., 1 to 10), and documents response to the treatment plan consistently. Opioid administration via the IV route, particularly in the emergent and acute phases of burn management, remains the mainstay for pharmacologic management. Titration of analgesic agents to obtain relief while minimizing side effects is crucial. The patient's requirements for analgesia are often high, but fear of addiction on the part of the patient and the health care provider hampers adequate opioid administration. Morphine sulfate remains the analgesic of choice. It is titrated to obtain pain relief based on the patient's self-report of pain.

Fentanyl is another useful opioid, particularly for procedural pain, because it has a rapid onset, high potency, and short duration, all of which make it effective for use with procedures.

Patient-controlled analgesia (PCA) maintains a steady level of opioid for pain relief and enables the patient to administer intermittent doses of medication.

Sustained-release opioids, such as MS Contin or oxycodone (OxyContin), have also been used successfully in the treatment of burn pain. These medications can effectively treat the resting pain that is associated with burn injury. Additional medications must be prescribed with these to cover breakthrough pain.

Also, nursing interventions, such as teaching the patient relaxation techniques, giving the patient some control over wound care and analgesia, and providing frequent reassurance, are helpful and should not be overlooked. Other pain-relieving approaches include distraction through video programs or video games, hypnosis, biofeedback, and behavioral modification. Providing the patient with some sense of control over pain management can reduce anxiety and the perception of pain, and the nurse reassures the patient that pain control issues will be addressed (Myers et al., 2022).

Anxiety and pain go hand in hand. The entire burn experience can produce severe anxiety, which can, in turn, exacerbate pain. Therefore, the ideal pain management regimen must incorporate the treatment of pain and anxiety and must be individualized for each patient.

It is important for the nurse to differentiate restlessness due to pain from restlessness due to hypoxia; a thorough respiratory assessment can help discriminate the etiology, noting oxygen saturation, lung sounds, chest expansion, and respiratory rate. The nurse also assesses the patient's sleep patterns since lack of sleep and rest interferes with healing, comfort, and restoration of energy. If necessary, sedatives are prescribed.

Nutritional Support

Burn injuries produce profound metabolic abnormalities fueled by the exaggerated stress response to the injury. The nurse recognizes the relationship between nutrition and healing; for example, a 10% loss of total body mass impacts immune dysfunction; 20% is linked with decreased wound healing; 30% leads to severe infections; a 40% loss is associated with death (Myers et al., 2022). It is essential to increase the anabolic process through adequate nutrition, decreasing heat loss from wounds, and maintaining a warm environment. Controlling secondary stress, such as pain and anxiety, also helps control the stress response.

The most important of these interventions is to provide adequate nutrition and calories. Healing of the burn wound consumes large quantities of energy. Several formulas exist for estimating the daily metabolic expenditure and caloric requirements. The enteral route of feeding is far superior to the parenteral route. Feedings are started as soon as possible. Vitamin and mineral supplements may be prescribed, and the nurse collaborates with the dietitian to plan a protein- and calorie-rich diet that is acceptable to the patient. Other treatment modalities include early excision and skin grafting of the burn wound, aggressive prevention or treatment of infections, and adequate exercise with physical therapy to lessen muscle wasting and increase strength.

Promoting Mobility

An early priority is to prevent complications of immobility. Deep breathing, turning, and proper positioning are essential nursing practices that prevent atelectasis and pneumonia, control edema, and prevent pressure ulcers and contractures. These interventions are modified to meet the patient's needs. Low–air-loss and rotation beds may be useful, and early sitting and ambulation are encouraged.

Psychological and Emotional Support

Family functioning is disrupted with burn injury. One of the nurse's responsibilities is to support the patient and family. Family members need to be instructed about ways that they can support the patient as adaptation to burn trauma occurs. The burn injury has tremendous psychological, economic, and practical impact on the patient and family. Referrals for social services or psychological counseling should be made as appropriate.

Rehabilitation Phase

Rehabilitation begins immediately after the burn has occurred and often extends for years after injury. In the aftermath of the acute stages of burn injury, the patient increasingly focuses on the alterations in self-image and lifestyle that may occur. Wound healing, psychosocial support, and restoration of maximal functional activity remain priorities so that the patient can have the best quality of life both personally and socially. The body goes through many changes as it heals. As the burn wound becomes a burn scar, the burn survivor may be faced with new complications. Often, reconstructive surgery to improve body appearance and function is needed.

Hypertrophic Scarring

The wound is in a dynamic state for 1.5 to 2 years after the burn occurs. If appropriate measures are instituted during this active period, the scar tissue can lose its redness and soften. Healed areas that are prone to hypertrophic scarring require the patient to wear a pressure garment. Pressure needs to be continuous. Gentle superficial massage aids in softening the connective tissue. Patients must be instructed about the need for lubrication and protection of the healing skin and the need to use pressure garments for at least 1 year after the injury. Treatment during rehabilitation is expected to include elastic pressure garments, splints, and exercise under the supervision of an experienced physical and occupational therapy team.

Continuing Care

Follow-up care by an interdisciplinary burn care team is necessary. Patients who receive care in a burn center usually return to the burn clinic for evaluation by the burn team, modification of home care instructions, and planning for reconstructive surgery. Many patients require outpatient physical or occupational therapy. It is often the nurse who is responsible for coordinating all aspects of care and ensuring that the patient's needs are met.

Patients who return home after a severe burn injury need referral for home care. Social services and community nursing services must be contacted to provide optimal care and supervision after hospital discharge. The home care nurse assesses the patient's physical and psychological status, as well as the adequacy of the home setting for safe and adequate care. The nurse monitors the plan of care and notes any problems that interfere with the patient's ability to carry out the care.

Patients who have survived burn injuries frequently suffer profound losses. These include not only a loss of body image due to disfigurement but also losses of personal property, homes, loved ones, and ability to work. The ABA has consistently advocated to help uninsured patients with disabling burn injuries receive care through Medicare and supported the Affordable Healthcare Act (ACA) offering all Americans the opportunity to secure health care insurance coverage.

The health care team must actively promote a healthy body image and self-concept so that patients can accept or challenge others' perceptions of those who are disfigured or disabled. Several burn patient support groups and other organizations throughout the United States offer services for burn survivors. They provide caring people (often people who have themselves recovered from burn injuries) who can visit the patient in the hospital or home or telephone the patient and family periodically to provide support and counseling about skin care, cosmetics, and problems related to psychosocial adjustment (www.phoenix-society.org). These organizations, and many regional burn centers, sponsor group meetings and social functions at which outpatients are welcome. Some also provide school-reentry programs and are active in burn prevention activities. If more information is needed regarding burn prevention, the ABA can help locate the nearest burn center and offer current burn prevention tips (www.ameriburn.org).

CHAPTER REVIEW

NCLEX-Style Review Questions

1. The nurse is caring for a 32-year-old patient with circumferential full-thickness burns to the trunk. Which cues are associated with abdominal compartment syndrome? Select all that apply.
   a. Increasing abdominal girth
   b. Hypertension
   c. Difficulty ventilating the patient
   d. Blisters on the burn area
   e. Tense abdomen

2. A patient with severe burn injuries to the abdomen and legs becomes anxious when it is time to change the dressings. What nursing intervention will be most helpful to this patient? Select all that apply.
   a. Allow the patient to participate in determining the time of dressing change.
   b. Premedicate the patient with pain and anxiety medications before dressing change.
   c. Tell the patient it is okay to cry during the dressing change.
   d. Explain the importance of dressing changes.
   e. Administer morphine sulfate SC 20 minutes before the dressing change.

3. A nurse would suspect an inhalation injury with which of the following findings? Select all that apply.
   a. History of burn occurring in an enclosed space
   b. Carbonaceous sputum
   c. Egophony
   d. Stridor
   e. Singeing of nasal hair

4. A patient who was burned at 10:00 am reports a pre-burn weight of 154 lb (70 kg). The estimated total body surface area (TBSA) burned is 60%. Using the Parkland/Baxter formula, the nurse verifies that the total amount of intravenous lactated Ringer solution to be infused by 6:00 pm on the day of the burn is which of the following?
   a. 5,200 mL
   b. 7,470 mL
   c. 8,400 mL
   d. 16,800 mL

5. A patient who suffered a burn injury this afternoon is now demonstrating hypovolemic and distributive shock. Select all patient assessment findings associated with shock.
   a. Mean arterial pressure (MAP) of 55 mm Hg
   b. Widening pulse pressure
   c. Elevated serum lactate
   d. Urine output of 1 mL/kg/hr
   e. Hypotension

REFERENCES AND SELECTED READINGS

References and selected readings associated with this chapter can be found on the website that accompanies the book. Visit **http://thepoint.lww.com/Honan3e** to access the references and other additional resources associated with this chapter.

UNIT FIFTEEN

Other Acute Problems

An 80-year-old patient developed acute kidney injury (AKI) and has been diagnosed with multiple organ dysfunction syndrome (MODS). The patient underwent a right hip replacement 2 days ago and currently has a temperature of 102.6°F.

- **What are treatment measures to reverse MODS?**
- **What patient populations are at increased risk for developing MODS?**
- **Discuss nursing care of patients with MODS.**

CHAPTER 53

Nursing Management: Shock and Multisystem Failure

Linda Honan • Philip R. Martinez, Jr.

Learning Objectives

After reading this chapter, you will be able to:

1. Describe shock and its underlying pathophysiology.
2. Compare clinical findings of the preshock, shock, and end-organ damage stages of shock.
3. Describe similarities and differences in hypovolemic, cardiogenic, distributive, and obstructive shock states.
4. Identify medical and nursing management priorities in treating patients in shock.
5. Identify vasoactive medications used in treating shock, and describe nursing implications associated with their use.

Shock is a life-threatening condition that results in cellular, metabolic, and hemodynamic alterations due to a variety of underlying causes. The progression of shock is neither linear nor predictable. Nurses caring for patients with shock and for those at risk for shock must understand the underlying mechanisms of shock and recognize its subtle as well as more obvious signs. Rapid assessment and response are essential to the patient's recovery.

OVERVIEW

Shock can best be defined as a condition in which tissue perfusion is inadequate to deliver oxygen and nutrients to support vital organs and cellular function. This definition differs from more traditional views of shock because it does **not** depend on absolute criteria for parameters, such as blood pressure (BP).

Pearls for Practice

By the time BP drops, damage has already been occurring at the cellular and tissue levels. Therefore, the patient at risk for shock must be assessed and monitored closely for more subtle clues of hemodynamic instability before the BP falls.

Adequate blood flow to the tissues and cells requires the following components: adequate cardiac pump, effective vasculature and circulatory system, and sufficient blood volume. If one or more components are impaired, perfusion to the tissues is threatened or compromised. Without treatment, inadequate delivery of oxygenated blood to the tissues results in poor delivery of oxygen and nutrients to the cells, cellular starvation, anaerobic metabolism and cell death, organ dysfunction progressing to organ failure, and eventual death.

Shock affects all body systems. It may develop rapidly or slowly, depending on the underlying cause. During shock, the body struggles to survive, utilizing a variety of homeostatic, compensatory mechanisms to restore blood flow. Any insult to the body can create a cascade of events resulting in poor tissue perfusion, which means that nurses should be vigilant about watching for signs of shock in all patients, regardless of their primary problem or diagnosis.

PATHOPHYSIOLOGY

Tissue perfusion is determined by cardiac output (CO) and systemic vascular resistance (SVR). CO is the amount of blood pumped by the heart in liters per minute (usual CO is about 4 to 8 L/min but varies greatly depending on the metabolic needs of the body). CO depends on stroke volume (the amount of blood ejected with each beat), determined by ventricular preload (volume), and heart rate, which is controlled in large part by the autonomic nervous system. Afterload is related closely to, and often equated with, the aortic pressure. It depends on the contractility of the right and/or left side of the heart and SVR (the resistance to the flow of blood out from the ventricles and a key determinant of aortic pressure). It is helpful to think of SVR as a vise grip on the

BOX 53-1

Classifications of Shock

- **Hypovolemic shock** is characterized by a decreased intravascular volume (decreased preload) secondary to loss of blood or fluids and electrolytes; it can be related to hemorrhagic or nonhemorrhagic causes.
- **Cardiogenic shock** occurs when the heart has an impaired pumping ability; it may be of coronary or noncoronary event origin.
- **Obstructive shock** occurs when there is impaired cardiac output due to a physical obstruction to blood flow either in the heart or major blood vessels, such as pericardial tamponade, tension pneumothorax, PE, or abdominal compartment syndrome.
- **Distributive shock** is a loss of vascular smooth muscle tone resulting in massive vasodilation, caused by nervous system injury (neurogenic shock), inflammatory release (septic or anaphylactic shock), or complications associated with medications such as epidural anesthesia.

aorta. If the vise is tightened, the SVR and aortic pressure rise, requiring more work for the ventricle to pump blood out. In contrast, if the vise grip is released from the aorta, there is little resistance to the outflow of blood and the work required of the heart muscle is diminished. Conventionally, the primary underlying pathophysiologic process is used to classify the shock state (Box 53-1 provides classifications). For example, if the heart (the pump) is the primary problem, cardiogenic shock occurs, whereas if the problem is primarily volume (decreased preload), hypovolemic shock occurs. In addition, the nurse considers that the CO is dependent on the volume received—it is a closed loop. The left ventricle can only eject the volume that is returned to the right heart from the venous system (King & Lowery, 2022). With constriction of the veins, more blood is returned to the heart, whereas with dilation of the veins, less blood is returned. It is good to remember that at any point, between 70% and 80% of blood is stored in veins and acts as a blood reservoir (Maiden & Peake, 2020). When considering possible causes of shock and potential interventions, nurses should remember that the interplay of these two factors (CO and SVR) is what determines the extent of the course of shock and the prognosis of the patient.

Pearls for Practice

The nurse is aware that cardiac output (CO) = stroke volume (SV) times heart rate (HR). Although often considered one concept, think about stroke volume as two separate concepts—stroke and volume. Stroke is dependent on the contractility of the heart, whereas volume relates to the amount of blood in the heart. The patient can have an adequate volume of blood in the heart but because of an inadequate pump (e.g., myocardial infarction, arrhythmia, septal defect), the CO falls. Likewise, the pump can be fine but if there is limited volume because of hemorrhage, third spacing, etc. the CO falls. Consider both aspects (stroke and volume) when evaluating risk for shock states in your patients.

In all types of shock, the cells lack an adequate blood supply and are inadequately oxygenated; therefore, they must produce energy through anaerobic metabolism. This results in an acidotic intracellular environment, along with a host of electrolyte derangements. In stress states such as shock, compensatory actions such as the release of catecholamines, cortisol, glucagon, and inflammatory cytokines and mediators occur, causing hyperglycemia and insulin resistance in an effort to mobilize glucose for cellular metabolism.

Pearls for Practice

A normal fasting blood glucose is <100 mg/dL (Fischbach et al., 2022). However, approximately 50% of critically ill patients present with stress hyperglycemia. In stress states the surging of catecholamines, cortisol, and glucagon increase the blood glucose level. Blood glucose levels >180 mg/dL may increase the risk of hospital complications, and glucose levels <110 mg/dL are associated with an increased risk of hypoglycemia (Pérez et al., 2020). While the optimal strategy for the management of hyperglycemia (also called stress hyperglycemia) in patients who are critically ill with and without diabetes is unknown, a target glucose range of 140 to 180 mg/dL may be appropriate for most critically ill patients and noncritically ill patients to avoid marked hyperglycemia while minimizing the risk of iatrogenic hypoglycemia (ADA, 2019; Pérez et al., 2020).

As the hypoxemia progresses and cellular metabolism becomes increasingly anaerobic, lactic acid levels begin to elevate as a response to the anaerobic metabolism. Excess levels of lactic acid limit the amount of adenosine triphosphate (ATP) produced, and normal cell function cannot be maintained. Recall ATP, which is in every cell, is responsible for storing and supplying needed energy to the cell. The impaired Na^+/K^+ and ATP membrane pump function results in intracellular accumulation of sodium and loss of K^+. Cellular edema results from the increased intracellular sodium and increased capillary permeability, further decreasing the CO. As the cell membrane becomes more permeable, allowing electrolytes and fluids to seep out of and into the cell, cell structures, primarily the mitochondria, are damaged and cell death results.

Pearls for Practice: Pathophysiology

Shock often affects the mitochondria within the cell, which normally function at the lowest oxygen

tensions in the body (mitochondrial pO_2 is about 5 mm Hg). However, they consume almost all the oxygen used by the body. More than 95% of aerobic chemical energy comes from mitochondrial work (aka oxidative phosphorylation), and the oxygen-dependent combustion of fuel substrates (primarily fats, amino acids, carbohydrates, ketones) into carbon dioxide (CO_2), water, and ATP. Because of this oxygen dependence, the mitochondria of patients in shock can be referred to as "canaries in the coal mine" since often they are affected first during inadequate tissue perfusion. Historically miners would carry canaries into the mine tunnels since the buildup of gases such as carbon monoxide would kill the canary before killing the miners; the canary's death was a warning to get out. Similarly, without sufficient oxygen, ATP is generated by potential mitochondrial fuels that are anaerobic. Thus, lactic acid accumulates in the blood and is a marker for anaerobic glycolysis. The higher the lactic acid level and the longer it takes to correct, the higher the mortality rate. Lactic acid is rapidly buffered, resulting in the formation of serum lactate; that is what you will use to evaluate the lactic acid level. Lactate levels greater than 4 mmol/L (normal value is 0.5 to 2.2 mmol/L) are associated with a fivefold increase in mortality) (Burger & Schaller, 2022; Kupchik, 2021).

STAGES OF SHOCK

Shock is believed to progress along a continuum. One way to understand the physiologic responses and subsequent clinical signs and symptoms is to divide the continuum into separate stages:

- Preshock stage (also called the *compensated stage*)
- Shock (also called the *uncompensated stage*)
- End-organ dysfunction (results in irreversible organ damage)

The earlier on this continuum that shock is recognized and interventions are initiated, the greater the patient's chance of survival. Table 53-1 compares clinical findings in the different stages of shock.

PRESHOCK OR COMPENSATED STAGE

Pathophysiology

In preshock, or the compensatory stage of shock, the BP often remains within normal limits. Compensatory responses, such as arterial and venous vasoconstriction, increased heart rate, and increased contractility of the heart, contribute to maintaining adequate CO and SVR. This results from stimulation of the sympathetic nervous system and subsequent release of catecholamines (epinephrine and norepinephrine). Activation of the renin–angiotensin–aldosterone system (RAAS) results in angiotensin II, which triggers vasoconstriction and the release of aldosterone and antidiuretic hormone (ADH), leading to sodium and water retention, and decreased urine output may become evident. Patients display the often-described "fight-or-flight" response. Thus, tachycardia or a modest change in systemic BP (increase or decrease) may be the only clinical sign of early shock. An elevated diastolic pressure with narrowed pulse pressure (difference between the systolic and diastolic pressure [normally 40 mm Hg])

TABLE **53-1 Clinical Findings in Stages of Shock**

	Stage		
Finding	*Compensated Stage* or Preshock	*Uncompensated Stage* or Shock	*Irreversible Stage* or End-Organ Dysfunction
Blood pressure	Near normal or normal	Systolic below 80–90 mm Hg; mean arterial pressure (MAP) less than 65 mm Hg	Requires mechanical or pharmacologic support
Heart rate	May be <100 or slightly >100 bpm	100–150 bpm	Erratic or asystole
Respiratory status	Fewer than 20 breaths/min	Rapid, shallow respirations; crackles	May require assisted ventilation
Skin	Cold, clammy	Mottled, petechiae	Jaundice
Urinary output	>30 mL/hr or mildly decreased	Severely decreased	Anuric, requires dialysis
Mentation	*Anxiety/impending feelings of doom*[a]	Lethargy	Unresponsive
Acid–base balance	Respiratory alkalosis	Metabolic acidosis	Profound acidosis

[a]Early indicator of decreased blood flow to the brain and should not be overlooked early in the clinical course of the patient.

may be seen due to the arteriole vasoconstriction (Carbino, 2020; Nicks & Gaillard, 2020). In order to provide energy to the cells, gluconeogenesis occurs, and the liver produces more glucose in response to the secretion of epinephrine, norepinephrine, glucagon, and cortisol resulting in hyperglycemia. Blood is shunted from the skin to vital organs (heart, brain), which can result in delayed capillary refill and cool temperature. The respiratory rate will increase to improve oxygenation and blow off CO_2 and a respiratory alkalosis may be seen. Adult patients can often compensate for <15% total volume loss through normal homeostatic mechanisms described above and have an HR <100, RR between 14–20, and a normal BP (Sharma & Sharma, 2022). Conversely, patients who have other medical problems or who take certain medications (such as beta blockers or calcium-channel blockers) may have a diminished ability to compensate.

Clinical Manifestations and Assessment

In the preshock stage, there are often no overt signs of organ dysfunction. The patient may show subtle clinical signs and symptoms indicating inadequate organ perfusion. Tachycardia, peripheral vasoconstriction, and anxiety are common. Anxiety and feelings of doom are common signs of shock during this early phase and should not be overlooked or attributed to something other than developing shock. Laboratory evaluation may demonstrate mild organ dysfunction (e.g., an increase in baseline creatinine, an increase in troponin, or a mild elevation of lactate); this sometimes precedes hypotension and serves as an early indicator of impaired tissue perfusion (Massaro, 2022).

Medical and Nursing Management

When appropriately identified at this nonprogressive stage, treatment is directed toward identifying the cause of shock, correcting the underlying disorder, and initiating aggressive measures aimed at not only correcting the cause of shock but also supporting the body's compensatory mechanisms. Because compensation cannot be maintained indefinitely, in addition to treating the underlying cause, measures such as aggressive fluid replacement and medication therapy must be initiated early to maintain an adequate BP and reestablish and maintain adequate tissue perfusion. *Early intervention along the continuum of shock is the key to improving the patient's prognosis.* Therefore, the nurse must assess the patient at risk for shock systematically to recognize the subtle clinical signs of the compensatory stage before the patient progresses to uncompensated shock. Box 53-2 highlights considerations for recognizing shock in older patients.

The role of the nurse at this stage is to monitor the patient's hemodynamic status, identify subtle signs of symptoms of organ dysfunction, and promptly report deviations to the provider to assist in identifying and treating the underlying disorder. In assessing tissue perfusion, the nurse specifically observes for changes in level of consciousness, vital signs, urinary output, skin, and laboratory values. Constant reassessment is warranted at this stage. Nurses should try to maintain a calm environment for both the patient's and family's sake and also ensure that assessments and interventions are rapid and ongoing. Providing brief explanations about the diagnostic and treatment procedures, supporting the patient during these procedures, and providing information about their outcomes reduces stress and anxiety and thus promotes the patient's physical and mental well-being. Speaking in a calm, reassuring voice and using gentle touch also help ease the patient's concerns.

BOX 53-2 **Highlighting Gerontology**

Recognizing Shock in Older Patients

The physiologic changes associated with aging, coupled with pathologic and chronic disease states, place older people at increased risk for developing a state of shock and possibly multiple organ dysfunction syndrome (MODS). The older patient can recover from shock if it is detected and treated early with aggressive and supportive therapies. Nurses play an essential role in assessing and interpreting subtle changes in older patients' responses to illness.

- During hypovolemic states, medications such as beta-blocking agents (metoprolol [Lopressor]) used to treat hypertension may mask tachycardia, a primary compensatory mechanism to increase CO.
- The aging immune system may not mount a truly febrile response, but an increasing trend in body temperature should be addressed.
- The heart does not function well in hypoxemic states, and the aging heart may respond to decreased myocardial oxygenation with arrhythmias that may be misinterpreted as a normal part of the aging process.
- Changes in mentation may be inappropriately misinterpreted as dementia. Older people with a sudden change in mentation should be aggressively treated for the presence of infection and organ hypoperfusion.

Pearls for Practice

For patients experiencing shock, if perfusion does not improve despite aggressive interventions, the nurse recognizes that the body will shunt blood from organs such as the skin, kidneys, and gastrointestinal (GI) tract to the brain and heart to ensure adequate blood supply to these vital organs. As a result, the skin is cool and clammy, bowel sounds are hypoactive, and urine output decreases.

UNCOMPENSATED STAGE OR SHOCK

In the uncompensated stage, the patient loses the ability to compensate for the insult, infection, or injury. It is during this stage that clinical signs become more obvious.

Pathophysiology

The heart and kidneys are among the first organs to show signs of dysfunction. Up until now on the continuum, the myocardium has kept pace by increasing CO, but this can only go on for a limited time. The body's inability to meet increased oxygen requirements produces ischemia, and biochemical mediators cause myocardial depression. This leads to failure of the cardiac pump, even if the underlying cause of the shock is not of cardiac origin.

The systemic impact of hypotension and thus hypoperfusion on the kidneys results in decreased urine output. The already narrowed pulse pressure will decrease further (Carbino, 2020). The patient becomes tachycardic, skin will become cool to the touch, and a decreased level of consciousness may also be seen. In addition, the inflammatory response to injury is activated, and proinflammatory and anti-inflammatory cytokines and mediators are released, which, in turn, activate the coagulation system in an effort to reestablish homeostasis. At the same time, worsening acidosis impairs all enzymatic functions, including coagulation. This can result in the development of disseminated intravascular coagulation (DIC), which is characterized by bleeding and thrombosis, resulting in the depletion of clotting factors, platelets, and RBCs (Carbino, 2020). Chapter 19 details DIC. A cascade of progressive organ failure resulting from poor tissue perfusion is illustrated in Figure 53-1. As the anaerobic metabolism continues, the serum lactate level will begin to rise. As a result of vasoconstriction and hypoperfusion to the gut, abdominal pain, ileus, gastrointestinal bleeding, and mesenteric ischemia can occur (Angus, 2020). Even if the underlying cause of the shock is reversed, the sequence of compensatory responses to the decrease in tissue perfusion perpetuates the shock state, and a vicious cycle ensues. It is believed that the body's appropriate or inappropriate response in this stage of shock may be the primary factor determining the patient's survival.

Clinical Manifestations and Assessment

Clinical manifestations that may be seen include symptomatic tachycardia, dyspnea, restlessness, diaphoresis, metabolic

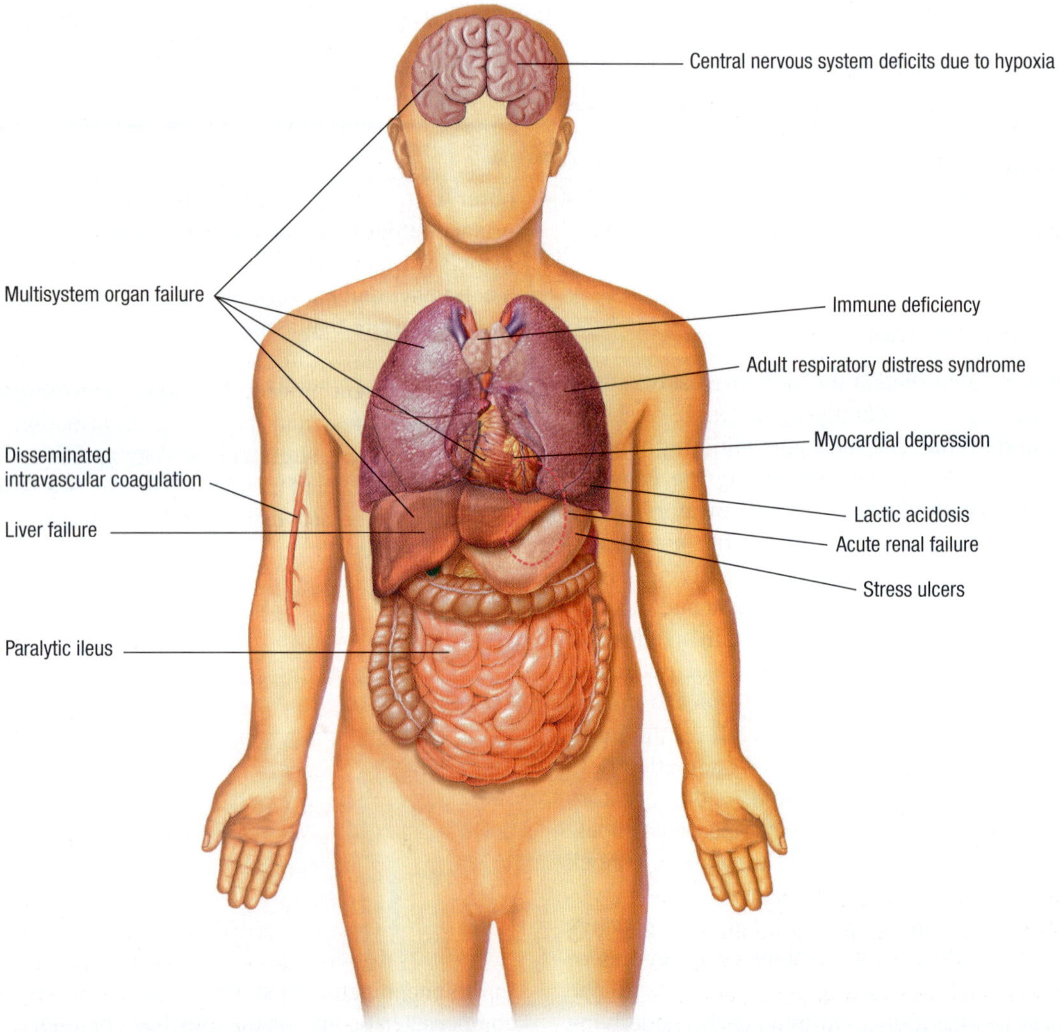

FIGURE 53-1 **Multiorgan system effects of shock.**

acidosis, prolonged capillary refill (more than 2 seconds), decreasing pulse pressure, and oliguria. The most frequent neurologic finding in patients with shock is alteration in the level of consciousness, ranging from confusion to unconsciousness (Carbino, 2020). Skin changes will depend on the type of shock and may include cool, clammy, mottled skin (related to vasoconstriction) or warm, pink skin (related to peripheral vasodilation of distributive shock); there can be a loss or decrease of peripheral pulses. In most cases, hypotension (a systolic blood pressure [SBP] <90 mm Hg or mean arterial pressure [MAP] <60 mm Hg), is seen with evidence of global tissue hypoperfusion (Graham, 2022). Recent studies suggest that patients with hypoperfusion can be considered to have shock (uncompensated stage), regardless of BP (Jentzer et al., 2021). When in doubt, the serum lactate level should be checked, and the nurse recognizes that values above 2 mmol/L are clearly consistent with hypoperfusion and shock (Angus, 2020).

Pearls for Practice

Pulse pressure is the difference between the systolic and diastolic pressure; for example, for a BP of 120/80 mm Hg, the pulse pressure is 40 mm Hg. In the seriously ill patient, hypotension is frequently associated with a narrow pulse pressure in an effort to maintain the MAP. For example, a BP of 90/70 mm Hg has a narrow pulse pressure of 20, but an MAP of 76, which provides perfusion to the organs (Lough, 2022). Recall the MAP = [(2 × diastolic pressure + systolic pressure)/3]). The diastolic pressure correlates with arteriolar vasoconstriction and may rise early in shock (as in the example above) and then falls when cardiovascular compensation fails (Angus, 2020). Pulse pressure rises when the stroke volume increases and narrows with decreased stroke volume and decreased rate of ventricular ejection (Suneja et al., 2020). The pulse pressure may decrease before the systolic pressure decreases, and in patients with shock pulse pressure less than 25 mm Hg. Nurses are key in identifying narrowing pulse pressures in patients early in the course of shock and should immediately report a pulse pressure of less than 25 mm Hg to the provider, even if other signs of shock have not yet manifested. Not all patients in shock have a narrow pulse pressure; for example in patients with sepsis, the vasodilatation that occurs can cause hypotension with a wide pulse pressure and inadequate organ perfusion (discussed later in this chapter).

Medical and Nursing Management

Early and aggressive interventions are essential to the survival of patients in shock; therefore, identifying patients who may be in shock and reporting subtle changes in assessment are imperative. Initially, two large-bore peripheral IVs (at least 16 gauge) are inserted to prepare for fluid administration and allow simultaneous administration of fluid, medications, and blood component therapy if required (Angus, 2020). However, central venous access may be necessary, as it is preferred for the administration of vasopressors, but this is balanced against the risk for infection and delay in care (Angus, 2020; Carbino, 2020). Patients in shock are often cared for in the intensive care unit (ICU) setting in order to:

- facilitate close monitoring (hemodynamic monitoring, arterial line insertion, electrocardiographic [ECG] monitoring, arterial blood gases [ABGs], oxygen saturation, serum electrolyte levels, lactate levels, physical examination and mental status changes);
- allow for rapid and frequent administration of various prescribed medications and fluids;
- provide access for strict measurement of intake and output (Foley catheter may be inserted, and urine output should be measured vigilantly; urine output of less than 30 mL/hr or < 0.5 mL/kg/hr is indicative of renal hypoperfusion and/or hypovolemia); and possibly
- provide interventions with supportive technologies, such as mechanical ventilation, dialysis, extracorporeal membrane oxygenation (ECMO), and intra-aortic balloon pump.

Nursing care of patients in shock requires expertise in assessing and understanding shock and the significance of changes in assessment data.

Specific management of shock depends on the type of shock and its underlying cause, but, in general, care is aimed at achieving the following goals using the acronym ASSESS:

A: Assess frequently the body's response to shock
S: Support the pumping action of the heart
S: Support the respiratory system
E: Encourage patient and family involvement in care, particularly in end-of-life discussions
S: Strengthen the competence of the vascular system
S: Significantly optimize intravascular volume

IRREVERSIBLE STAGE (END-ORGAN DYSFUNCTION)

Pathophysiology

If adequate tissue perfusion is not restored in a timely fashion, irreversible end-organ damage ensues. This represents the point along the shock continuum where end-organ damage is so severe that the patient does not respond to treatments and likely will not survive. As the damage increases, acidosis may become so severe that even aggressive therapies such as vasopressor support may not work. For example, kidney and liver failure, compounded by the release of necrotic tissue toxins, will create overwhelming metabolic acidosis. If the integrity of the gut barrier is compromised, bacteria and their toxins can be translocated into the bloodstream. With severe hypoperfusion of the liver, massive elevations in the enzyme aminotransferase and extensive hepatocellular damage occur. Anaerobic metabolism contributes to a worsening lactic acidosis. Respiratory system failure prevents adequate oxygenation and ventilation despite mechanical ventilatory support, and the cardiovascular system is ineffective in maintaining an adequate MAP for tissue perfusion. Multiple organ dysfunction progressing to complete organ failure has occurred, and death is imminent. Multiple organ dysfunction can occur as a progression along the shock continuum or as a syndrome unto itself and is described in more detail on page 1671.

Pearls for Practice

To optimize end-organ perfusion, the nurse monitors the MAP. Although a specific MAP goal has not been established for all shock states, an MAP of at least 65 mm Hg is a reasonable goal that represents adequate blood flow; however, depending on patient circumstances (e.g., chronic hypertension, head injury), variations will be seen (Maiden & Peake, 2020).

Medical and Nursing Management

Specific therapies in this stage are usually the same as for the other stages of shock. Although the patient may have progressed from shock to irreversible end-organ damage, the judgment that the shock is irreversible can be made only retrospectively on the basis of the patient's failure to respond to treatment. As in shock, the nurse focuses on carrying out prescribed treatments, monitoring the patient, preventing complications, protecting the patient from injury, and providing comfort.

Offering brief explanations to the patient about what is happening is essential even if there is no certainty that the patient hears or understands what is being said. Simple comfort measures, including reassuring touches, should continue to be provided despite the patient's nonresponsiveness to verbal stimuli. As it becomes obvious that the patient is unlikely to survive, the family must be informed about the prognosis and likely outcome. Clear, honest communication is imperative as families may not understand what is happening with the patient. Opportunities should be provided, throughout the patient's care, for the family to see, touch, and talk to the patient. Close family friends or spiritual advisors may be of comfort to the family members in dealing with the inevitable death of their loved one. Whenever possible, the patient's family should be approached regarding any living wills, advance directives, or other written or verbal wishes the patient may have shared in the event that they became unable to participate in end-of-life decisions. In some cases, ethics committees may assist families and health care teams in making difficult decisions.

GENERAL MANAGEMENT STRATEGIES IN SHOCK

As described previously, and in the discussion of types of shock to follow, management in all types and all phases of shock includes the following:

- Optimization of systemic oxygen delivery to improve tissue oxygenation
- Fluid replacement to restore intravascular volume
- **Vasoactive medications** to restore vasomotor tone and improve cardiac function
- Nutritional support to address the metabolic requirements that are often dramatically increased in shock
- Body positioning to optimize intravascular volume

Therapies described in this section require collaboration among all members of the health care team to ensure that the manifestations of shock are quickly identified and that adequate and timely treatment is instituted to achieve the best outcome possible (see Fig. 53-2).

Optimize Oxygen Delivery

The first step is to assess oxygenation and provide supplemental oxygen as needed. Oxygen is administered to increase the amount of oxygen carried by available hemoglobin in the blood. A patient who is confused may feel apprehensive with an oxygen mask or cannula in place, and frequent explanations about the need for the mask may reduce some of the patient's fear and anxiety. Frequent assessment of respiratory status is warranted since many patients with worsening shock may require intubation and ventilatory support. Continuous oxygen saturation monitoring is expected. It is important to consider that intubation and mechanical ventilation not only provide for delivery of oxygen and removal of carbon dioxide but also reduce the work of breathing, which, in the patient with hypoperfusion, further exacerbates lactic acidemia (Angus, 2020). Nurses understand that when patients are "working to breathe," this strenuous use of accessory respiratory muscles can increase oxygen consumption; thus, if the patient is struggling to breathe despite supplemental oxygen, intubation will decrease the work of breathing and facilitate gas exchange (Angus, 2020).

Pearls for Practice

While oxygen saturation as measured by pulse oximetry is important, the nurse recognizes that this data point does not provide information about acid–base balance or the patient's ventilation (hypoventilation or hyperventilation). Inaccuracies in pulse oximetry reading are discussed in Chapter 7; these can involve decreased perfusion (as in shock), patient movement, the presence of intravascular dyes, and dark skin tones (O_2 saturation overestimated by ~2%) (Kaczka et al., 2020; Torp et al., 2021).

Fluid Replacement

The fluids administered vary but may include **crystalloids** (electrolyte solutions that move freely between intravascular and interstitial spaces), **colloids** (large-molecule IV solutions such as albumin), and blood components (Table 53-2). In general, the patient is rehydrated with a fluid whose characteristics

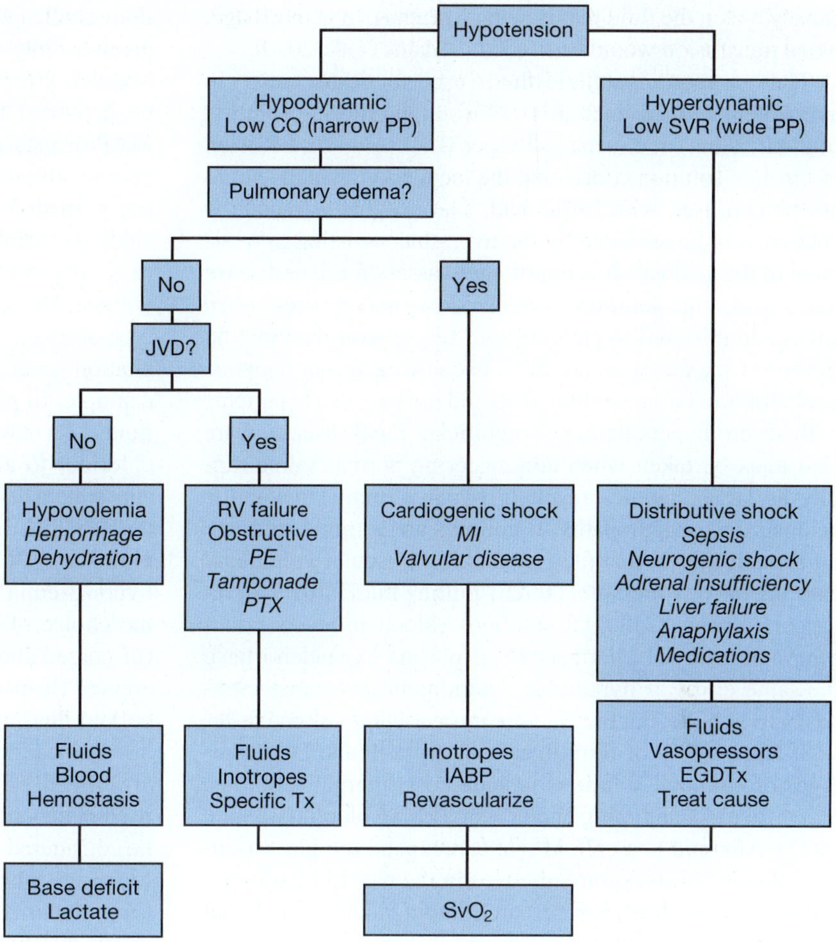

FIGURE 53-2 **Shock diagnosis, treatment, and monitoring. CO, cardiac output; PP, pulse pressure; SVR, systemic vascular resistance; JVD, jugular venous distention; PE, pulmonary embolism; PTX, pneumothorax; MI, myocardial infarction; Tx, treatment; IABP, intra-aortic balloon pump; EGDTx, early goal-directed therapy; SvO_2, mixed venous oxygen saturation (percent of oxygenated hemoglobin in blood returning to the right heart). (Reprinted with permission from Lawrence, P., Bell, R., Dayton, M., & Hebert, J. [2012]. *Essentials of general surgery* [5th ed.]. Lippincott Williams & Wilkins.)**

TABLE **53-2 Fluid Replacement in Shock**

Fluids	Advantages	Disadvantages
Crystalloids		
0.9% sodium chloride (normal saline solution)	Widely available, inexpensive	Requires large volume of infusion; can cause hyperchloremic metabolic acidosis, pulmonary edema
Lactated Ringer's (LR)	Lactate ion helps buffer metabolic acidosis	Requires large volume of infusion; it is mildly hypotonic, can cause pulmonary edema, cerebral edema; should not be used in patients with severe hyperkalemia or patients with severe liver dysfunction or traumatic brain injury; since it contains calcium it is contraindicated with citrated solutions (blood and blood products) due to risk of coagulation (Trinooson & Patel, 2023).
Hypertonic saline (3%, 5%, 7.5%)	Small volume needed to restore intravascular volume	Danger of hypernatremia; osmotic demyelination syndrome (ODS), formerly referred to as central pontine myelinolysis (see Chapter 3); and increased serum osmolality
Colloids		
Albumin (5%, 25%)	Rapidly expands plasma volume	Expensive; requires human donors; limited supply; can cause heart failure
Dextran (40, 70)	Synthetic plasma expander	Interferes with platelet aggregation; not recommended for patients with hemorrhagic shock

closely match the fluid that is being lost; thus, in hemorrhage, blood transfusion would be needed. (Adams et al., 2020).

The common crystalloid fluids used for resuscitation in hypovolemic shock include 0.9% sodium chloride solution (normal saline) and lactated Ringer (LR) solution. LR is an electrolyte solution containing the lactate ion, which should not be confused with lactic acid. The exogenous lactate is converted to bicarbonate by the liver, thus assisting in treatment of the acidosis. It is important to assess for liver disease when using this solution as the acidosis may worsen when LR is administered to patients with severe liver dysfunction (refer to Chapter 3). In addition, because each liter contains 4 mEq of potassium per liter, it should not be given to patients with severe hyperkalemia or significant renal disease. Care also must be taken when administering normal saline rapidly as large volumes result in hyperchloremic metabolic acidosis and coagulopathy. If colloids are administered, the nurse understands that they expand intravascular volume by exerting oncotic pressure, thereby pulling fluid into the intravascular space. Colloidal solutions (blood products, albumin, and artificial pharmaceutical plasma expanders) have the same effect as hypertonic solutions in increasing intravascular volume, but they restore intravascular volume faster with less volume of fluid than with crystalloids. Disadvantages of colloidal solutions include cost, allergic reactions, and difficulties in typing and crossmatching blood (Graham, 2022). Albumin is a colloid that can expand the intravascular volume. It was commonly used in the past to treat hypovolemic shock; however, research findings have not shown consistent benefit with its use as an initial resuscitation fluid compared with crystalloids (Mandel & Palevsky, 2022). Regardless of the solution administered, it is important to avoid "over resuscitation" and thus causing fluid volume excess, which may increase the risk of increased ventilator and ICU days, acute respiratory distress syndrome (ARDS) (see Chapter 9), abdominal compartment syndrome (ACS) (Chapter 52), AKI (Chapter 26), increased hospital length of stay, and mortality.

The best fluid to treat shock remains in debate. In emergencies, the "best" fluid is often the fluid that is readily available and is dependent on the type of shock and patient presentation. Of note, in those situations where there is concern over administering a fluid challenge IV (such as the critically ill older adult in cardiogenic shock), the passive leg raise (PLR) may be considered to assess response to fluid. When you raise the legs up, ~250 mL of venous blood from the lower body is diverted to the right heart—if the patient responds poorly to this volume increase (e.g., SOB, JVD), the legs can be placed down; thus, it is a "reversible" fluid challenge (Aswani & Ioannou, 2019). See Chapter 3 for more details on PLR.

Despite the risks described above, in almost all situations fluid resuscitation should be initiated early and aggressively in patients with shock to maximize intravascular volume. For example, in patients with septic shock, an intravenous fluid challenge of 30 mL/kg of crystalloid IV fluid may be given rapidly to improve intravascular volume (Schmidt & Mandel, 2022). Others recommend the IV fluid challenges be delivered by bolus of 500 mL (each time) titrated to MAP or measurement of preload and repeated based on the absence of pulmonary edema and evidence of improving tissue perfusion after each bolus (Schmidt & Mandel, 2022). Both crystalloids (e.g., saline and LR solution) and colloids (e.g., albumin) may be administered to restore intravascular volume. However, IV fluid choice remains dependent on the type of shock, patient chemistries, estimated volume of resuscitation needed, and on the specific patient presentation. For example, in patients with septic shock, balanced crystalloid fluid (LR) may be preferred over normal saline (0.9% sodium chloride) to avoid the development of hyperchloremia and subsequent hyperchloremic metabolic acidosis (see Chapter 3) which is associated when large volumes are infused. However, LR has potential side effects as well, including hyponatremia and/or hyperkalemia. The nurse is aware that the choice of solution is dependent on a variety of factors (discussed above) along with institutional and provider preference. Hespan (Hetastarch, Hydroxyethyl starch), a type of colloid fluid, has been shown to cause increased organ damage, acute kidney injury (AKI), and mortality in patients who are critically ill, including those with shock, and should not be used in the critically ill (Shepherd et al., 2021). Albumin may be considered over other colloidal fluids as there an immunologic anti-inflammatory effect not seen with artificial colloids (Townsend, 2021). Blood should be given for hypovolemic shock due to trauma and/or hemorrhage, although initially crystalloids may be given to patients to restore intravascular volume while waiting for blood products to transfuse.

The patient receiving fluid replacement in the context of shock must be monitored frequently for adequate urinary output, changes in mental status, skin perfusion, and changes in vital signs. Heart and lung sounds are auscultated frequently to detect signs of fluid volume excess (S3, S4, crackles, JVD, edema).

A central venous line may be inserted in order to measure central venous pressure (CVP). A normal CVP is 2 to 8 mm Hg and is used as an estimation of preload (volume returning to the right heart). However, it is dependent on the location of the catheter to the right atrium (RA), intrathoracic pressures, compliance of the veins, patient position, and competence of the tricuspid valve (between RA and right ventricle [RV]), and is affected by the ventilator and use of positive end-expiratory pressure (PEEP). Thus, the CVP may be used as a guide to right heart preload but not responsiveness to fluid administration (Kupchik, 2021).

Pearls for Practice

The nurse understands that the CVP represents the volume in the right atrium and therefore is reflective of the amount of preload to the right ventricle. But in patients with shock, because of the stiffening of the ventricles, the CVP cannot predict what is actually pumped out by the left ventricle; thus, the nurse considers parameters such as urinary output (increasing >1 mL/kg/hr), MAP (>65 mm Hg), and lactate concentrations (decreasing) as measures of improved hemodynamic response to treatment.

Hemodynamic catheters can be placed; these allow the monitoring of intravascular pressures and venous oxygen levels. Assessment of mixed venous oxygen saturation (SvO_2) or $ScvO_2$ (central venous oxygen saturation) is done with a CVP line or from a special pulmonary artery catheter that has fiber optics capable of calculating the oxygen saturation of hemoglobin. SvO_2 reflects the balance between oxygen delivery and oxygen consumption. Knowing the SvO_2 in conjunction with pulse oximetry is helpful in evaluating the adequacy of oxygenation; newer technology allows for continuous $SvO_2/ScvO_2$ measurements similar to the pulse oximetry. A normal $SvO_2/ScvO_2$ is 70% to 80% (i.e., when the blood is returning to the right side of the heart, it has lost only 20% to 30% of its oxygen). An $SvO_2/ScvO_2$ of 50% to 70% reveals that more oxygen is being extracted from the RBCs; when the $SvO_2/ScvO_2$ is at 30% to 50% the oxygen extraction is becoming exhausted and anaerobic metabolism and lactic acidosis begins, and at 25% to 30%, severe lactic acidosis exists. $SvO_2/ScvO_2$ below 25% is associated with cellular death (Shanmukhappa & Lokeshwaran, 2021). When the SvO_2 drops, it reflects the increased consumption of oxygen and the need for intervention.

When evaluating the intravascular volume and status of the patient in shock, there is no gold standard; rather, the nurse monitors multiple parameters including the BP (hypotension), PP (<25 mm Hg), MAP (<65 mm Hg), RR (tachypnea), urine output (<0.5 mL/kg/hr), ABGs (base deficit), physical examination findings (S3, S4, crackles, flat neck veins, JVD, edema, delayed capillary refill), sensorium (anxiety to unresponsiveness), ECG (arrhythmias, tachycardia, bradycardia), skin temperature (cool or warm in neurogenic shock), presence of mottling (lace-like purplish discoloration of skin), oxygen saturation (decreasing saturation), and lactate levels (>2 mmol/L) and alerts the provider to any evidence of clinical deterioration (Maiden & Peake, 2020). Hemodynamic monitoring with arterial and pulmonary artery lines may be implemented to allow close monitoring of the patient's perfusion and cardiac status, as well as response to therapy. For additional information about hemodynamic monitoring, see Chapter 54. When fluid administration alone fails to restore adequate perfusion, consideration moves to enhancing the circulation with medications (Maiden & Peake, 2020).

Pearls for Practice

Recall that in order to maintain a normal pH balance, 20 base bicarbonate (HCO_3^-) are needed for one carbonic acid (H_2CO_3). If the bicarbonate (base) level falls, there is an acidotic state, the pH falls, and there is a deficit of base. The normal base excess value is between +2 and −2. A negative value indicates too little base and too much acid; in the case of shock, metabolic acidosis is due to lactic acidosis.

Vasoactive Medication Therapy

Vasoactive medications can be used in patients with all forms of shock to improve the patient's hemodynamic stability when fluid therapy alone cannot maintain adequate MAP. Different medications work on different aspects of CO, and specific medications are selected depending on the underlying cause (see Chapter 54, Table 54-9). Although most of the medications have several effects, these medications are used to (1) increase the strength of myocardial contractility, (2) regulate the heart rate, (3) reduce myocardial resistance, and (4) initiate vasoconstriction.

Receptors in the sympathetic nervous system are known as alpha-adrenergic and beta-adrenergic receptors. Beta-adrenergic receptors are further classified as beta-1 and beta-2 adrenergic receptors. When alpha-adrenergic receptors are stimulated, blood vessels constrict in the cardiorespiratory and GI systems, skin, and kidneys. When beta-1 adrenergic receptors are stimulated, heart rate and myocardial contraction increase. When beta-2 adrenergic receptors are stimulated, vasodilation occurs in the heart and skeletal muscles, and the bronchioles relax. The medications used in treating shock consist of various combinations of vasoactive medications to maximize tissue perfusion by stimulating or blocking the alpha- and beta-adrenergic receptors.

When vasoactive medications are administered, the nurse must monitor vital signs frequently (at least every 15 minutes until stable, or more often if indicated) while actively titrating vasopressors to maintain the MAP. Vasoactive medications should be administered through a central venous line because infiltration and extravasation of some vasoactive medications can cause tissue necrosis and sloughing. Initiation of vasopressors should not be held while waiting for a central line to be placed. An IV pump must be used to ensure that the medications are delivered safely and accurately. Often, invasive monitoring of BP may occur using an arterial line; this is used to titrate medications accurately. Individual medication dosages are usually titrated by the nurse, who adjusts drip rates based on the prescribed dose and the patient's response. Dosages are changed to maintain the MAP at a physiologic level that ensures adequate tissue perfusion (usually above 65 mm Hg). Vasoactive medications should be tapered when possible, and the patient should be weaned from medication with frequent monitoring of BP (at least every 15 minutes).

Nutritional Support

Nutritional support is an important aspect of care for patients with shock. Increased metabolic rates during shock increase energy requirements and therefore caloric requirements. The release of catecholamines early in the shock continuum causes depletion of glycogen stores in about 8 to 10 hours. Nutritional energy requirements are then met by breaking down lean body mass. In this catabolic process, skeletal muscle mass is broken down even when the patient has large stores of fat or adipose tissue. Loss of skeletal muscle greatly prolongs the patient's recovery time. Parenteral or enteral nutritional support should be initiated within 24 to 48 hours, with some form of enteral nutrition being preferred when able to be tolerated (Graham, 2022). The integrity of the GI system depends on direct exposure to nutrients. When enteral nutrition is contraindicated, parenteral nutrition can be considered. In addition, if the patient is unable to meet more than 60% of energy and protein requirements by the enteral route alone, then supplemental PN should be considered after 7 to 10 days (Radovich, 2023). It is important to consider that nearly 30% of patients with enteral nutrition and 44% to 50% with parenteral nutrition (PN) experience hyperglycemia (Sangrador et al., 2020). The hyperglycemia is generally managed with insulin IV infusion, prepared at standard concentrations of 1 U/mL, and a target glucose range of 140 to 180 mg/dL is recommended in most protocols (refer to Chapter 29 for insulin infusion).

Body Positioning

In the early stage of shock, elevating the head of bed assists in breathing; however, because of blood redistribution with gravity the BP may fall. If the patient is significantly hypotensive, positioning the patient flat in bed with the legs elevated may be considered to increase venous pressure (see previous discussion on passive leg raise). This position also facilitates the insertion of central lines and intubation if required. However, patients in severe respiratory distress generally are unable to tolerate this position, and their hypoxemia may worsen. In addition, the risk for aspiration increases when the patient is flat. Once the patient is intubated, the head of the bed is elevated to a 30- to 45-degree angle to maximize inspiratory muscle length, maximize ventilation, and decrease aspiration risk (Güner & Kutlutürkan, 2021; Storzer, 2023; Wu et al., 2022). The nurse also considers positioning the patient to maximize oxygenation and ventilation by recognizing that perfusion is greatest in the dependent lung or dependent portions of the lung; thus, the goal is to match ventilation with perfusion. The "good lung down" is a position that will facilitate maximum oxygenation. However, maintaining any position for a prolonged period is associated with stagnation of secretions and pressure on the dependent lung, increasing the risk of atelectasis in the dependent lung. Therefore, the nurse turns the patient at regular intervals. Oxygenation in patients with ARDS (which is a complication of shock) is sometimes improved in the prone position, and research indicates this position reduces mortality in patients with moderate to severe ARDS (refer to Chapter 9 for details).

Pearls for Practice

Positioning the patient with their head down, known as the Trendelenburg position, had been thought to increase blood flow to vital organs by increasing preload. Evidence in fact reveals that it may worsen pulmonary gas exchange, increase the risk of aspiration, and increase intracranial and intraocular pressures (Thompson, 2023). An alternative is to keep the patient flat and elevate the patient's legs slightly to improve cerebral circulation and promote venous return to the heart, but this position is contraindicated in trauma of the hip, legs, or lumbar spine; deep venous thrombosis; and intracranial or abdominal hypertension (Critical Care Nurse, 2021).

TYPES OF SHOCK

HYPOVOLEMIC SHOCK

Hypovolemic shock, the most common type of shock, is characterized by a decreased intravascular volume (decreased preload) secondary to loss of blood or fluids and electrolytes. Hypovolemic shock occurs when there is a reduction in intravascular volume by 15% to 30%, which represents a loss of 750 to 1,500 mL of blood in a person who weighs 70 kg (154 lb) or higher (see Chapter 55, Table 55-1).

PATHOPHYSIOLOGY

Hypovolemic shock can be caused by hemorrhagic or nonhemorrhagic causes (Gaieski & Mikkelsen, 2022). It can also be the result of sudden fluid losses, such as in open fractures (femur, pelvis), abdominal aortic aneurysm (AAA) rupture, or postpartum hemorrhage, or by a gradual fluid loss, such as with dehydration (e.g., vomiting, diarrhea). The loss of fluid from the intravascular space leads to decreased preload and a decreased stroke volume. The body attempts to compensate for the decreased SV with an increased heart rate and vasoconstriction (sympathetic nervous system) as well as activation of RAAS. Ultimately, the CO falls and progressive tissue hypoxia ensues. Figure 53-3 depicts the sequence of events in hypovolemic shock. Box 53-3 discusses common causes of hypovolemic shock.

Pearls for Practice

Recall that bones are very vascular and when there are fractures there is blood loss. A closed femur fracture can result in blood loss of up to 3 L, whereas a pelvic fracture can result in the loss of 4 to 6 L (Walsh, 2020). The nurse needs to always be aware that mortality rate in pelvic fracture is high in those patients who present to the hospital in shock, and in open fractures the mortality rate may reach 45% (Tullington & Blecker, 2022).

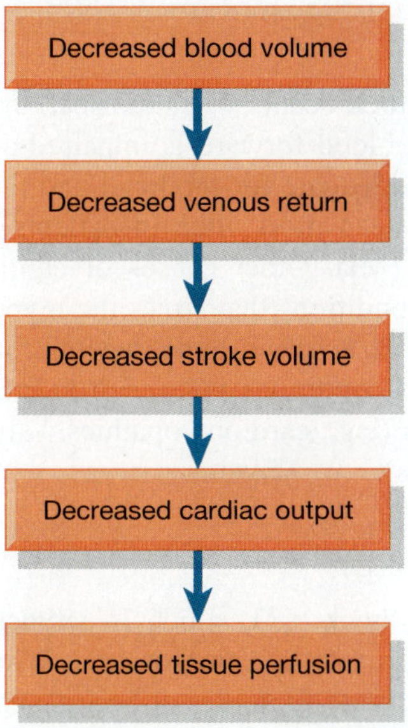

FIGURE 53-3 **Pathophysiologic sequence of events in hypovolemic shock.**

MEDICAL MANAGEMENT

Major goals in the treatment of hypovolemic shock are (1) to restore intravascular volume, (2) to reverse the sequence of events leading to inadequate tissue perfusion, and (3) to correct the underlying cause of the fluid loss as quickly as possible. Depending on the severity of shock and the patient's condition, it is likely that efforts will be made to address all three goals simultaneously.

If the patient is hemorrhaging, efforts are made to stop the bleeding. This may involve applying pressure to the bleeding site or a surgery or procedure to stop internal bleeding. If the cause of the hypovolemia is diarrhea or vomiting, medications to treat diarrhea and vomiting are administered while efforts are made to identify and treat the cause. In older patients, dehydration is a common cause of hypovolemia.

If the underlying cause of the hypovolemia is dehydration, medications are also administered to reverse the cause of the dehydration. For example, insulin is administered if dehydration is secondary to hyperglycemia (see Chapter 29), and desmopressin (DDAVP) is administered for patients with diabetes insipidus (see Chapter 30).

Beyond reversing the primary cause of the decreased intravascular volume, fluid replacement (also referred to as fluid resuscitation) is of primary concern. At least two large-gauge IV lines are inserted to establish access for fluid administration. Because the goal of the fluid replacement is to restore intravascular volume, it is necessary to administer fluids that will remain in the intravascular compartment in order to avoid fluid shifts from the intravascular compartment into the intracellular or interstitial compartment. Blood products may need to be administered, particularly if the cause of the hypovolemic shock is hemorrhage. Packed red blood cells are administered to replenish the patient's oxygen-carrying capacity, in conjunction with other fluids that will expand volume. Plasma and platelet transfusions can help with fluid resuscitation and also treat other underlying problems. The need for transfusions is based on the patient's individual perfusion needs, which are determined by vital signs, blood gas values, and clinical appearance rather than an arbitrary laboratory value. An area of active research is the development of synthetic forms of blood (i.e., compounds capable of carrying oxygen in the same way that blood does) as potential alternatives to blood component therapy. Risks inherent to administering blood include the possibility of a transfusion reaction. For nonhemorrhagic hypovolemic shock crystalloids are generally preferred for fluid resuscitation; for causes associated with decreased colloidal osmotic pressure (e.g., cirrhosis), albumin may be administered (Mandel & Palevsky, 2022).

BOX 53-3 Risk Factors for Hypovolemic Shock

Blood loss
- Traumatic hemorrhage
- Exsanguination
- Hemothorax
- Hemoperitoneum
- Fracture (femur and pelvis); open fractures increase blood loss

Nontraumatic hemorrhage
- GI bleed
- AAA rupture
- Ectopic pregnancy rupture

Volume loss
- Surgery
- Vomiting
- Diarrhea
- Burns
- Diuresis; polyuria (DKA, DI)
- NPO status
- Ascites
- Peritonitis
- Dehydration

DKA, diabetic ketoacidosis; DI, diabetes insipidus.
Adapted from Gasper, W. J., Iannuzzi, J. C., & Johnson, M. D. (2022). Shock. In M. A. Papadakis, S. J. McPhee, M. W. Rabow & K. R. McQuaid (Eds.), *Current Medical diagnosis & treatment* (Chapters 12–19). McGraw Hill. https://accessmedicine.mhmedical.com/content.aspx?bookid=3081&sectionid=258962688

NURSING MANAGEMENT

Primary prevention of shock is an essential focus of nursing care. Hypovolemic shock can be prevented in some instances by closely monitoring patients who are at risk for fluid deficits by monitoring I&O and daily weights and assisting with fluid replacement before intravascular volume is depleted. The nurse is alert to signs suggesting decreased intravascular volume including decreasing urine output (<0.5 mL/kg/hr), oliguria, hypotension, with decreased pulse pressure, flat neck veins, altered mental status (anxiety may be earliest symptom), delayed capillary refill, pallor, cool extremities, tachycardia, and tachypnea. Recall earlier discussion that hypotension may not be seen until there is 30% loss of the patient's total blood volume (Hannan, 2022). Hemodynamic findings include decreased CVP, pulmonary artery pressures (PAPs), pulmonary artery occlusion pressures (PAOPs), CO, and increased PVR and SVR. Nursing care focuses on assisting with treatment targeted at the cause of the shock and restoring intravascular volume.

General nursing measures include ensuring safe administration of prescribed fluids and medications (vasopressor agents may be used) and documenting response to their administration and effects. Administering blood transfusions safely is a vital nursing role. In emergency situations, it is important to acquire blood specimens quickly, to obtain a baseline complete blood count, and to type and cross-match the blood in anticipation of blood transfusions. A patient who receives a transfusion of blood products must be monitored closely for adverse effects (see Chapter 19). See Chapter 55 for nursing responsibilities with massive blood transfusion, which is defined as >4 units packed red blood cells (PRBCs) in 1 hour or 10 units of PRBCs in 24 hours.

Fluid replacement complications can occur, often when large volumes are administered rapidly. Therefore, the nurse monitors the patient closely for cardiovascular overload and edema. The risk of these complications is increased in the older population and in patients with pre-existing cardiac disease. Hemodynamic pressure, vital signs, ABGs, serum lactate levels, hemoglobin and hematocrit levels, and fluid I&O are among the parameters monitored. Temperature should also be monitored closely to ensure that rapid fluid resuscitation does not precipitate hypothermia. IV fluids may need to be warmed during the administration of large volumes. Physical assessment focuses on observing for "over resuscitation" by observing the jugular veins for distention; auscultation of the lungs for crackles; presence of S3, S4 gallop; displaced point of maximum impulse (PMI) in cardiac examination, and monitoring the CVP. CVP is typically low in hypovolemic shock; it increases with effective treatment and is significantly increased with fluid overload and heart failure. The nurse must monitor cardiac and respiratory status closely and report to the provider any changes in BP, pulse pressure, heart rate and rhythm, lung sounds, and urine output. Another important nursing role is monitoring for signs of complications and side effects of treatment and reporting these signs early in treatment. Complications include lactic acidosis; thus, the nurse monitors the serum lactate levels and alerts the provider when values are rising. Other complications include respiratory failure, kidney failure, decreased cerebral perfusion, and DIC (Efre & Boling, 2023).

CARDIOGENIC SHOCK

Cardiogenic shock occurs when the heart's ability to contract and pump blood forward is impaired and the supply of oxygen is inadequate for the heart and tissues. Cardiogenic shock is seen most often in patients with myocardial infarction (MI). Other causes of cardiogenic shock are related to conditions that stress the myocardium (e.g., severe hypoxemia, acidosis, hypoglycemia, and hypocalcemia), as well as conditions that result in ineffective myocardial function (e.g., cardiomyopathies, valvular damage, and arrhythmias).

Pathophysiology

In cardiogenic shock, CO, which is a function of stroke volume and heart rate, is compromised. When stroke volume and/or heart rate decreases or become erratic, BP falls (there is a decrease in the systolic BP from baseline of more than 30 mm Hg for more than 30 minutes or a decrease in the MAP <65 mm Hg), and systemic tissue perfusion is compromised (urine output decreases, skin becomes cool and mottled, mental status changes [sensorium becomes clouded], anxiety is obvious, capillary refill is delayed) (Graham, 2022). Blood supply for the heart muscle itself is inadequate, resulting in further decreases in CO (cardiac index is less than 2.2 L/min/m^2). In addition, diastolic dysfunction increases left atrial pressure, which leads to pulmonary congestion and hypoxemia that can further exacerbate myocardial ischemia and impair ventricular performance (pulmonary capillary wedge pressure is greater than 18 mm Hg [normal is 6 to 12 mm Hg]). This can occur rapidly or over a period of days. Patients in cardiogenic shock may experience angina and develop arrhythmias and hemodynamic instability. Figure 53-4 depicts the pathophysiology of cardiogenic shock.

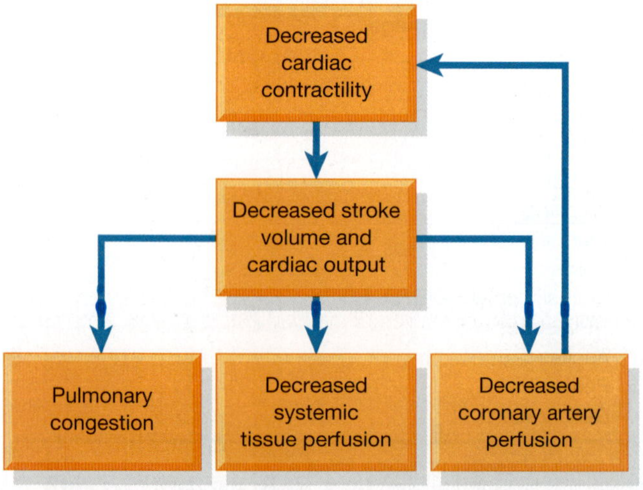

FIGURE 53-4 Pathophysiologic sequence of events in cardiogenic shock.

Pearls for Practice

In the case of heart failure resulting in cardiogenic shock, the nurse assesses for both left- and right-sided heart failure, which may include rales, shortness of breath, S_3 gallop, jugular vein distention (JVD), and dependent peripheral edema.

Medical Management

The goals of management in cardiogenic shock are (1) to limit further myocardial damage and preserve the healthy myocardium and (2) to improve the cardiac function by increasing cardiac contractility, decreasing ventricular afterload, or both. In general, these goals are achieved by increasing oxygen supply to the heart muscle while reducing oxygen demands.

As with all forms of shock, the underlying cause of cardiogenic shock must be corrected. It is necessary first to treat the oxygenation needs of the heart muscle to ensure its continued ability to pump blood to other organs. In the case of cardiogenic shock due to MI, the patient may require angioplasty, coronary artery bypass graft surgery, or thrombolytic therapy; bridge therapies such as intra-aortic balloon pump therapy or ventricular assist device (VAD); or some combination of these treatments. General interventions for cardiogenic shock include supplemental oxygen, controlling chest pain with pharmacologic therapies, providing selected fluid support, administering vasoactive medications (vasopressors, inotropic agents, and vasodilatory agents), controlling heart rate with medication or pacemaker, and using a mechanical assistive device if needed. Serial laboratory markers for ventricular dysfunction (e.g., BNP) and cardiac enzyme levels (i.e., troponin-I) are measured, serial 12-lead ECGs are obtained, and frequently an echocardiogram is ordered to assess the degree of myocardial damage or dysfunction.

Pharmacologic Therapy

Oxygen

In the early stages of shock, supplemental oxygen is administered at a rate sufficient to achieve an oxygen saturation exceeding 90%. Monitoring of ABG values and pulse oximetry values helps determine whether the patient requires a more invasive method of oxygen delivery such as high-flow nasal cannula, continuous or bilevel positive airway pressure ventilation, or intubation and mechanical ventilation.

Analgesia

If a patient experiences chest pain, an IV analgesic (commonly morphine sulfate) is administered for pain relief. In addition to relieving pain, morphine dilates the blood vessels. This reduces the workload of the heart by both decreasing the cardiac filling pressure (preload) and reducing the pressure against which the heart muscle has to eject blood (afterload). Nitrates may also be given to decrease preload and afterload, thereby reducing the myocardial demands on the heart and decreasing pain.

Antiplatelet Agents and Beta Blockers

Antiplatelet agents, such as aspirin, should be given in the case of a patient with acute MI. In addition, a beta blocker is used to decrease workload of the heart and preserve cardiac muscle. The use of these medications in the case of a patient with cardiogenic shock can be complicated since beta blockers will decrease BP. See Chapter 13 for acute treatment of chest pain and MI.

Pearls for Practice

During an acute MI, aspirin may be ordered to prevent worsening thrombosis in the coronary arteries. When administering aspirin in this acute situation, the nurse should ask the patient to chew the aspirin (162 to 325 mg) rather than swallow a whole enteric-coated aspirin. Chewing aspirin allows for a more rapid absorption rate than does swallowing it whole (Guo et al., 2022).

Vasoactive Medications

Vasoactive medication therapy consists of multiple pharmacologic strategies to restore and maintain adequate CO. In cardiogenic shock, the aims of vasoactive medication therapy are to improve cardiac contractility, optimize preload and afterload, reduce myocardial oxygen demand, and stabilize heart rate and rhythm. Medications commonly used to treat cardiogenic shock include dobutamine, dopamine, and nitroglycerin. See Table 54-9 for a review of common vasoactive medications.

Pearls for Practice

The nurse is vigilant in observing the patient's response to vasoactive agents because of the potential of worsening myocardial ischemia by increasing cardiac work. These agents should not be used for long periods of time or at high doses due to increased afterload and workload on the heart (Kaddoura et al., 2021).

Dopamine is a sympathomimetic agent. It acts as an inotrope (positive inotropes increase the strength of muscular contraction) and a vasopressor (at higher doses). It may be used with dobutamine and nitroglycerin to improve tissue perfusion. Sympathomimetic agents must be used with caution in patients with cardiogenic shock since they increase myocardial oxygen demand and can worsen failure. Also, in patients with severe metabolic acidosis, which occurs in the later stages of shock, the effectiveness of dopamine is diminished. Norepinephrine also may be considered as a first-line agent for hypotension in patients with cardiogenic shock; it is a vasoactive agent that acts primarily as a vasoconstrictor, has a mild inotropic effect, and increases coronary flow while having less of an effect on heart rate in patients with tachycardia (Kaddoura et al., 2021).

If tissue perfusion remains inadequate, inotropic therapy with dobutamine may be considered; this predominantly affects beta-1 adrenergic receptors (increases the strength of myocardial activity and improves CO). Dobutamine enhances the strength of cardiac contraction, improving stroke volume ejection and overall CO. Because it also has some beta-2 properties, vasodilation occurs (decreased afterload), and the bronchioles relax. The nurse is aware that dobutamine may exacerbate hypotension in some patients (related to vasodilatory effects) and can precipitate tachyarrhythmias (Kaddoura et al., 2021).

IV nitroglycerin in low doses acts as a venous vasodilator and therefore reduces preload. At higher doses, nitroglycerin causes arterial vasodilation and reduces afterload as well. These actions, in combination with dobutamine, increase CO while minimizing cardiac workload. In addition, vasodilation enhances blood flow to the myocardium, improving oxygen delivery to the weakened heart muscle. A combination of medications may be prescribed, depending on the patient's response to treatment. All vasoactive medications have adverse effects, making specific medications more useful than others at different stages of shock.

Pearls for Practice

Vasoactive medications should never be stopped abruptly because this could cause severe hemodynamic instability, perpetuating the shock state.

Diuretics

Diuretics such as furosemide may be administered to reduce the workload of the heart by reducing fluid accumulation. Diuretics must be used **cautiously** since they can lead to hypovolemia and worsening hypotension. In addition, aggressive diuresis can lead to metabolic alkalosis, often referred to as a *contraction alkalosis.* The use of diuretics can also lead to electrolyte abnormalities, the most common of which is hypokalemia.

Antiarrhythmic Medications

Multiple factors, such as hypoxemia, electrolyte imbalances, and acid–base imbalances, contribute to serious cardiac arrhythmias in all patients with shock. In addition, as a compensatory response to decreased CO and BP, the heart rate increases beyond normal limits. This impedes CO further by shortening diastole and thereby decreasing the time for ventricular filling. Consequently, antiarrhythmic medications are required to stabilize the heart rate. For a full discussion of cardiac arrhythmias, as well as commonly prescribed medications, see Chapter 16.

Fluid Status

Appropriate fluid administration is also necessary in the treatment of cardiogenic shock. Administration of fluids must be monitored closely to detect signs of fluid overload. Incremental IV fluid boluses are cautiously administered to determine optimal filling pressures for improving CO. Nurses should use caution when administering fluids rapidly because rapid fluid administration in patients with cardiac failure may result in acute pulmonary edema. Fluid overload and pulmonary edema are risks because of ineffective cardiac function and accumulation of fluid in the pulmonary tissues.

Mechanical Assistive Devices

If CO does not improve despite supplemental oxygen, vasoactive medications, and fluid boluses, mechanical assistive devices can sometimes be used temporarily to improve the heart's ability to pump. ECMO may be utilized to pump blood outside of the body to an oxygenator which can reoxygenate the blood and remove carbon dioxide replacing the workload of the heart and lungs. Intra-aortic balloon counter pulsation or left and right VADs and total temporary artificial hearts are means of providing temporary circulatory assistance and are reviewed in Chapters 15 and 54.

Nursing Management

Preventing Cardiogenic Shock

In many circumstances, identifying at-risk patients early, promoting adequate perfusion of the heart muscle, and decreasing cardiac workload can prevent cardiogenic shock. Risk factors include advanced age, anterior MI or previous MI, diabetes, hypertension, multivessel CAD, and peripheral vascular and cerebrovascular diseases (Provaznik et al., 2021). Patients who have decreased ejection fractions, larger infarctions, and echo results that demonstrate a lack of hyperkinesis in the myocardial remote from the infarction should be considered at risk for cardiogenic shock (Provaznik et al., 2021). Minimizing patient risk can be accomplished by conserving the patient's energy; promptly relieving angina; and administering supplemental oxygen, aspirin, and beta blockers. When cardiogenic shock is present, nursing management includes working with other members of the health care team to prevent shock from progressing and to restore adequate cardiac function and tissue perfusion.

Monitoring Hemodynamic Status

A major role of the nurse is monitoring the patient's hemodynamic and cardiac status. Arterial lines and ECG monitoring equipment must be well maintained and functioning properly. The nurse anticipates the medications, IV fluids, and equipment that might be used and is ready to assist in implementing these measures. Changes in hemodynamic, cardiac, pulmonary, and renal status and laboratory values are documented and reported promptly. In addition, adventitious breath sounds, changes in cardiac rhythm, and other abnormal physical assessment findings are reported immediately.

Administering Medications

The nurse documents and records medications and treatments that are administered, as well as the patient's response to treatment.

The nurse must be knowledgeable about the desired effects, as well as the side effects, of medications. For example, it is important to monitor the patient for decreased BP after administering morphine or nitroglycerin. Patients receiving thrombolytic therapy must be monitored for bleeding. Arterial and venous puncture sites must be observed for bleeding, and pressure must be applied at the sites if bleeding occurs. Frequent neurologic assessment is essential after the administration of thrombolytic therapy to assess for the potential complication of cerebral hemorrhage associated with the therapy. IV sites receiving infusions at risk of extravasation must be observed closely because tissue necrosis and sloughing may occur if vasopressor medications infiltrate the tissues. Urine output, blood urea nitrogen (BUN), and serum creatinine levels are closely monitored to detect decreased kidney function secondary to the effects of cardiogenic shock or its treatment.

Enhancing Safety and Comfort

Throughout care, the nurse must take an active role in safeguarding the patient, enhancing comfort, and reducing anxiety. This includes administering medication to relieve chest pain, preventing infection at the multiple arterial and venous line insertion sites, protecting the skin, and monitoring respiratory and kidney function. Proper positioning of the patient promotes effective breathing without decreasing BP and may also increase patient comfort while reducing anxiety.

Explanations about procedures that are being performed and the use of comforting touch often provide reassurance to the patient and family. The family is usually understandably anxious and benefits from opportunities to see and talk to the patient. Explanations of treatments and the patient's responses are often comforting to family members.

DISTRIBUTIVE SHOCK

Distributive shock, also sometimes called circulatory shock, occurs when the body's ability to adjust vascular tone is impaired and blood volume is therefore abnormally displaced in the vasculature (e.g., when blood volume pools in peripheral blood vessels). The displacement of blood volume causes a relative hypovolemia because not enough blood returns to the heart, which leads to subsequent inadequate tissue perfusion. The vascular tone is determined both by central regulatory mechanisms, as in BP regulation, and by local regulatory mechanisms, as in tissue demands for oxygen and nutrients. Therefore, distributive shock can be caused either by a loss of sympathetic tone or by release of biochemical mediators from cells.

The varied mechanisms leading to the initial vasodilation in distributive shock further subdivide this classification of shock into three types: (1) **septic shock**, (2) **neurogenic shock**, and (3) **anaphylactic shock**. Other causes of distributive shock are rare but include toxic shock syndrome, drug overdose, neurogenic insults, addisonian crisis, and myxedema coma (Smith et al., 2021). In all types of distributive shock, massive arterial and venous dilation allows blood to pool peripherally. The different types of shock cause variations in the pathophysiologic chain of events. Risk factors for distributive shock are summarized in Box 53-4.

BOX 53-4
Risk Factors for Distributive Shock

Septic shock:
- Immunosuppression
- Extremes of age (under 1 year of age and over 65 years of age)
- Malnourishment
- Chronic illness
- Invasive procedures

Neurogenic shock:
- Spinal cord injury
- Spinal anesthesia
- Depressant action of medications
- Glucose deficiency

Anaphylactic shock:
- Penicillin sensitivity
- Transfusion reaction
- Bee sting allergy
- Latex sensitivity
- Severe allergy to some foods or medications

SEPTIC SHOCK

Septic shock, the most common type of distributive shock, is caused by widespread, overwhelming infection in combination with a dysregulated host immune response. Because of the increased sophistication of antibiotic therapy and improved recognition of sepsis and initiation of intensive care management, the incidence of septic shock has declined. Approximately 1.7 million cases of severe sepsis or septic shock occur annually in the United States, with an estimated in-hospital mortality rate of 15.6% (Graham, 2022; Rhee et al., 2019). Finding and aggressively treating the source of infection, as well as providing aggressive cardiopulmonary support, are important determinants of the clinical outcome.

Risk Factors

Nosocomial infections (infections occurring in the hospital) in patients who are critically ill that may progress to septic shock commonly originate in the lungs (pneumonia) and urinary (pyelonephritis) and GI tract (peritonitis, intra-abdominal abscess, cholangitis), although they can originate anywhere in the body (refer to Table 53-3 for common sites related to sepsis). Organisms include gram-positive or negative bacteria; fungi; and, rarely, protozoa or rickettsiae. Commonly, gram-positive bacteria, especially methicillin-resistant *Staphylococcus aureus* (MRSA), vancomycin-resistant enterococci (VRE), penicillin-resistant *Streptococcus pneumoniae*, and resistant gram-negative bacilli are seen (Reddy, 2022). Additional risk factors are

TABLE 53-3 **Common Sites and Diseases Associated with Sepsis/Systemic Inflammatory Response Syndrome (SIRS)**

Organ System	Location	Disease
Respiratory	Upper respiratory tract	Sinusitis Mastoiditis
	Lower respiratory tract	Pneumonia Lung abscess Empyema Covid-19
Gastrointestinal	Mediastinum Hepatobiliary Intra-abdominal	Esophageal rupture/perforation Hepatic abscess Cholangitis Cholecystitis Intestinal infarction/perforation Pancreatitis Intra-abdominal/diverticular abscess Colitis Appendicitis
Cardiovascular	Mediastinum Native or prosthetic cardiac valve	Postoperative mediastinitis Endocarditis
Genitourinary	Kidney, ureter, and bladder	Perinephric abscess Pyelonephritis Cystitis
Neurologic	Brain and meninges	Meningitis Intracranial abscess
Dermatologic	Traumatic wound, surgical wound, or burn site	Soft tissue abscess Necrotizing fasciitis Infected decubitus ulcer Full- and partial-thickness burn
Prosthetic	IV catheters (central/peripheral venous catheter) Arterial catheter Ventriculoperitoneal shunt Dialysis catheter Articular prosthetic device Dialysis graft/shunt	Catheter infection Infected prosthesis
Other	Vascular system	Septic thrombophlebitis

Adapted with permission from Stenbit, A., & Serio, A. (2010). Sepsis. In R. Irwin & J. Rippe (Eds.), *Manual of intensive care management* (Chapter 123). Lippincott Williams & Wilkins.

age, immunocompromise due to malnutrition, alcohol use disorder, malignancy, diabetes mellitus, and AIDS, invasive procedures and indwelling medical devices, and the increased number of resistant microorganisms. Older patients continue to be at particular risk for sepsis because of decreased physiologic reserves and an aging immune system. The incidence of septic shock can be reduced by carrying out infection control practices, including the use of meticulous aseptic technique, properly cleaning and maintaining equipment, and using thorough hand hygiene techniques.

Pathophysiology

When microorganisms invade body tissues, patients exhibit an immune response. This immune response provokes the activation of biochemical cytokines and mediators associated with an inflammatory response and produces a complex cascade of physiologic events that leads to poor tissue perfusion. Widespread endothelial injury leads to increased capillary permeability, which triggers seepage of protein-rich fluid from the capillaries, and vasodilation, which occurs when injured endothelial cells release nitric acid (a potent vasodilator). These two effects interrupt the ability of the body to provide adequate perfusion, oxygen, and nutrients to the tissues and cells. In addition, proinflammatory and anti-inflammatory cytokines released during the inflammatory response activate the coagulation system, which begins to form clots in areas where a clot may or may not be needed, further compromising tissue perfusion. The imbalance of the inflammatory response and the clotting and fibrinolysis

gloves when possible, and patients at risk (patients with spina bifida, spinal cord injuries, and congenital abnormalities of the genitourinary tract) should be catheterized with nonlatex equipment when needed.

Pathophysiology

Anaphylactic shock is caused by a severe allergic reaction when patients who have already produced antibodies to a foreign substance (antigen) develop a systemic antigen–antibody reaction. This reaction provokes mast cells and basophils to release potent vasoactive substances, such as histamine or bradykinin, causing widespread vasodilation, capillary permeability, and potentially catastrophic vascular collapse. Mast cells in any organ system may be involved depending on the distribution of the instigating stimulus; in general, the principal targets include the cardiovascular, cutaneous, respiratory, and GI systems (where mast cells are most abundant) (Norris & Tuan, 2020). An equally important feature of anaphylactic shock is the onset of severe bronchospasm, which causes airway compromise (stridor, wheezing, shortness of breath) and urticaria. A delayed recurrence of the reaction, without re-exposure to the allergen, can sometimes occur. This has been termed a *biphasic reaction* and can occur 1 to 72 hours after the first reaction despite no further interaction with the trigger (Graham, 2022).

Clinical Manifestations and Assessment

The clinical manifestations are related to the potent vasoactive and smooth muscle contractile actions due to mast cell release of vasoactive substances. For example, the vasodilatation results in erythema, decreased venous return to the heart (up to 35% of the intravascular volume can be lost into the interstitial space within 10 minutes), and subsequent hypotension; activation of multiple inflammatory pathways causes fluid extravasation, seen as angioedema, tissue edema, and hypovolemia; whereas the smooth muscle contraction is associated with bronchospasm and abdominal and pelvic cramps (Graham, 2022). Thus, the nurse observes for generalized hives, pruritus or flushing, angioedema, swelling of the tongue and/or uvula, dyspnea, wheezing, stridor, hypoxemia, and reduced BP. GI symptoms, including nausea, vomiting, abdominal cramps, and diarrhea, may precede the more generalized clinical manifestations described previously after ingestion of an antigen (Kemp, 2020). Serum mast cell tryptase (MCT) is the only widely available assay used to confirm the diagnosis of anaphylaxis (Passia & Jandus, 2020).

Medical Management

Treatment of anaphylactic shock requires removing the causative antigen (e.g., discontinuing an antibiotic agent) and administering medications that restore vascular tone. In addition, the health care team will need to provide emergency airway support, position the patient in a supine position (see Pearls for Practice), administer oxygen, provide ventilation support (endotracheal intubation or tracheotomy may be necessary to establish an airway), perform external chest compressions if cardiac arrest occurs, and prepare for early administration of epinephrine. Epinephrine is usually given intramuscularly in the thigh in a dose of 0.01 mg/kg, with a usual dose of 0.2 to 0.5 mg for adults (maximum dose of 0.6 mg), which can be repeated every 5 to 30 minutes if the response is inadequate. Epinephrine is given for its vasoconstrictive action as well its effect of reducing bronchospasm (Dodd et al., 2021). When epinephrine is given early (before the onset of shock), systemic absorption of IM epinephrine is rapid, with a response seen in minutes. IV epinephrine carries more risks, and incorrect dosing has been associated with serious adverse events (Dodd et al., 2021). However, in patients with severe anaphylaxis, the nurse considers that decreased perfusion to the muscle may result in slow absorption of epinephrine into the circulation; therefore, IV epinephrine may be necessary. Diphenhydramine, given intramuscularly or intravenously, may be administered to reverse the urticaria and pruritus, but it is not likely to reduce the hypotension of tissue edema (Dodd et al., 2021). Nebulized medications, such as albuterol, may also be given to reverse histamine-induced bronchospasm. Glucocorticoids may be considered to prevent a rebound, biphasic reaction, although it is unlikely to be beneficial acutely because of the slow onset of action (Dodd et al., 2021). IV lines are inserted to provide access for administering fluids and medications. Aggressive IV fluid resuscitation is expected with hypotension. The patient's cardiac status is monitored, and the electrocardiogram is assessed because anaphylaxis and treatments can be associated with arrhythmias and cardiac ischemia. Pulse oximetry is also expected to monitor oxygenation status and response to treatment. Anaphylaxis and specific chemical mediators are discussed further in Chapter 37.

Pearls for Practice

It is important to note that Fowler (upright) or semi-Fowler (semirecumbent) position has been associated with fatal anaphylaxis. Changing the patient's position to one that is upright quickly reduces venous return to the heart and is proposed to exacerbate the pathophysiologic processes occurring in anaphylaxis; therefore, keeping a patient flat is suggested to improve venous return to the heart, a key aspect of the initial response to anaphylaxis, unless the patient is having difficulty breathing, at which point the patient may need to sit upright (slowly) to lessen respiratory distress (McLure et al., 2021).

Pearls for Practice

Nurses understand that epinephrine is typically supplied as 1 mg/mL (1:1,000 dilution). Most authorities recommend that 0.3 to 0.5 mg of the 1:1,000 solution (0.3 to 0.5 mL) be given intramuscularly in the anterolateral aspect of the thigh.

Nursing Management

The nurse plays an important role in preventing anaphylactic shock. The nurse must assess all patients for allergies or previous reactions to antigens (e.g., medications, blood products, foods, contrast agents, latex) and communicate the existence of these allergies or reactions to others. In addition, the nurse assesses the patient's understanding of previous reactions and the steps taken by the patient and family to prevent further exposure to antigens. When new allergies are identified, the nurse advises the patient to wear or carry identification that names the specific allergen or antigen.

When administering any new medication, the nurse observes all patients for allergic reactions. This is especially important with IV medications. Allergy to penicillin is one of the most common causes of anaphylactic shock. Patients who have a penicillin allergy may also develop an allergy to similar medications. For example, they may react to cefazolin sodium because it has a similar antimicrobial action of attaching to the penicillin-binding proteins found on the walls of infectious organisms. Previous adverse drug reactions increase the risk that the patient will develop an undesirable reaction to a new medication. If the patient reports an allergy to a medication, the nurse must be aware of the risks involved in the administration of similar medications.

In the hospital and outpatient diagnostic testing sites, the nurse must identify patients who are at risk for anaphylactic reactions to the contrast agents (radiocontrast media) that are used for diagnostic tests. These include patients with a known previous allergic reaction to contrast agents. This information must be conveyed to the staff at the diagnostic testing site, including radiology staff. The nurse anticipates that "pre-medication" regimens are likely to be administered in patients with known contrast allergies.

Pearls for Practice

Pre-medication with steroids and Benadryl may be recommended for patients who have had a previous reaction to a contrast agent when a similar contrast will be administered (Brockow, 2023).

The nurse must be knowledgeable about the clinical signs of anaphylaxis, must take immediate action if signs and symptoms occur, and must be prepared to begin cardiopulmonary resuscitation if cardiopulmonary arrest occurs. In addition to monitoring the patient's response to treatment, the nurse assists with intubation if needed, monitors the hemodynamic status, ensures IV access for administration of medications, administers prescribed medications and fluids, and documents treatments and their effects.

Pearls for Practice

If IV epinephrine is required, the nurse carefully titrates the medication to prevent a hypertensive surge. Symptoms of tachycardia, pallor, diaphoresis, and arrhythmias in a patient with normal or raised blood pressure are indicative of epinephrine toxicity. The provider should be notified and the infusion rate reduced (Dalal & Grujic, 2022). In addition, although there are no absolute contraindications to the administration of epinephrine, the nurse carefully observes the effect of epinephrine in patients with cerebrovascular or coronary artery disease, hypertension, diabetes, hyperthyroidism, cardiomyopathy, or narrow-angle glaucoma, in whom adverse events, such as MI, stroke, or pulmonary edema, can be precipitated (Dalal & Grujic, 2022).

Community health and home care nurses who administer medications, including antibiotic agents, in the patient's home or other settings, must be prepared to administer epinephrine intramuscularly in the event of an anaphylactic reaction. Prescriptions for prefilled epinephrine syringe (EpiPen or EpiPen Jr.) should be given, and the patient and significant others are instructed on how to administer the EpiPen and that the patient needs to carry it at all times (refer to Chapter 37). After recovery from anaphylaxis, the patient and family require an explanation of the event. Furthermore, the nurse provides instruction and counseling about avoiding future exposure to antigens and administering emergency medications to treat anaphylaxis.

OBSTRUCTIVE SHOCK

Obstructive shock is caused by a physical obstruction to blood flow, either in the heart or in major blood vessels. This causes a decrease in CO and thus a decrease in tissue perfusion. Common causes of obstructive shock include cardiac tamponade, tension pneumothorax, and pulmonary embolism (PE). Obstructive shock is common in the setting of trauma.

Pathophysiology

In the case of tension pneumothorax or hemothorax, air or blood has entered the pleural space and caused a restriction in lung expansion. If enough air or blood is trapped, then eventually pressure builds up and compresses the vessels and myocardium. This compression reduces preload (volume of blood) and increases afterload, in addition to restricting the expansion of the myocardium during filling. Clinical presentation may include JVD, crepitus (with pneumothorax), dyspnea, chest pain, tachycardia and tachypnea, tracheal shifting **away** from the tension pneumothorax, and decreased breath sounds on the affected side. Tension pneumothorax is common in trauma (rib fractures and bronchial tree injuries) but can also develop spontaneously or as a complication from a procedure such as central line placement, blockage of chest tubes with clots, or clamping or barotrauma (Dedeo, 2020). Patients who are mechanically ventilated are at higher risk of developing a clinically significant pneumothorax due to increased ventilatory pressures. In this situation, the barotrauma is commonly due to alveolar rupture, leading to an accumulation of air resulting in pneumothorax, pneumomediastinum, and subcutaneous emphysema (Diaz & Heller, 2022).

Cardiac tamponade results from excessive blood or fluid inside the pericardium, the sac that surrounds the heart. This can result from a traumatic or infectious cause with a resultant restricted filling of the atria and ventricles, leading to a reduction in CO (Carbino, 2020). Signs and symptoms of cardiac tamponade include narrowing pulse pressure (difference between the systolic and diastolic pressure, normally 40 mm Hg), chest pain, distant or muffled heart sounds, JVD, hypotension, and tachycardia.

A PE is a clot that gets lodged in the pulmonary vasculature and causes ischemia to the capillary beds. If large enough, the embolism interferes significantly with pulmonary blood flow, which causes blood to back up into the right side of the heart. As the clot increases the pressure in the pulmonary artery, the right heart must beat faster and harder to overcome the pressure. Overall, CO is decreased as the patient goes into right-sided heart failure. Clots that have traveled from the lower extremities or pelvic thrombus cause most PEs. Signs and symptoms of PE include pleuritic chest pain, shortness of breath, tachycardia, and hypoxia (refer to Chapter 9 for more details).

Medical Management

In the case of cardiac tamponade and tension pneumothorax, a procedure to relieve the obstruction should be performed immediately by a qualified provider. If the patient is experiencing obstructive shock, then the procedure is done emergently at the bedside. A chest radiograph is often used to diagnose a pneumothorax, although computed tomography (CT) scans and even ultrasound are more sensitive. A chest tube or needle decompression is the primary procedure to relieve tension pneumothorax. Cardiac tamponade is diagnosed similarly, with echocardiography being the most effective method. Pericardiocentesis is the treatment for cardiac tamponade and involves inserting a needle into the pericardium to draw off fluid or blood.

The treatment of PE is usually aimed toward preventing clot expansion, although if the patient is experiencing obstructive shock, then other treatments, such as thrombolytic drugs, catheter-directed ultrasound thrombolytic therapy, or surgical embolectomy, may be considered. Depending on the severity of the PE, mechanical ventilation and hemodynamic support may be needed to stabilize the patient. PE is usually diagnosed using a computed tomographic pulmonary angiography (CTPA) because it is sensitive and specific for the diagnosis of PE (Fu et al., 2020; Thompson et al., 2022). See Chapter 9 for additional details on PE.

Nursing Management

Because patients with tension pneumothorax and cardiac tamponade who are experiencing obstructive shock will need an emergent procedure, nurses should focus on facilitating that process. This includes collecting and setting up equipment, communicating effectively with staff, and helping gain consent from the patient and/or family. Careful monitoring of the patient prior to, during, and after the procedure is essential. If a chest tube is placed, then a chest drainage system will need to be set up and connected to suction as ordered. The chest tube setup needs to be monitored to ensure that it is functioning correctly and also to record output. A postprocedure chest radiograph will be ordered, and the results should be followed closely.

Nursing care of a patient with a PE that is causing obstructive shock involves monitoring and initiating ventilatory and hemodynamic support similar to what is done for patients with other types of shock. A primary function of the nurse in this situation is to facilitate diagnostic testing and imaging and then institute treatment in a timely manner. Patients with a PE large enough to cause obstructive shock have a very high mortality and often die within an hour of presentation.

Patients who experience obstructive shock are often quite suddenly acutely ill. This affects the entire health care team as decisions need to be made quickly, and the nurse should work hard to maintain a calm environment. Since obstructive shock usually has a sudden onset, families are quite often surprised when given news about massive PE or other causes of obstructive shock. Having other support personnel in place, such as a social worker or a chaplain, to provide support is advised.

MULTIPLE ORGAN DYSFUNCTION SYNDROME

MODS is altered organ function in patients who are acutely ill that requires medical intervention to support continued organ function. It is another phase in the progression of shock states. The actual incidence of MODS is difficult to determine because it develops with acute illnesses that compromise tissue perfusion. It is defined as severe organ dysfunction of two or more organ systems lasting at least 24 to 48 hours in the setting of sepsis, trauma, burns, or severe inflammatory conditions (Gourd & Nikitas, 2020). It is important to note that the definition includes the number of dysfunctional organs and duration. Mortality rates when two to four organ systems are involved are 10% to 40%, and persistent dysfunction (more than 72 hours) present in seven organ systems can result in a mortality risk as high as 100% (Gourd & Nikitas, 2020).

Pearls for Practice

*Providers may use the SOFA scale to rapidly identify adult patients with organ dysfunction and risk for poor outcomes. The acronym stands for **Sequential (Sepsis-related) Organ Failure Assessment** and includes parameters such as the PaO_2/FiO_2 ratio (respiratory system), the platelet count (coagulation), bilirubin level (hepatic system), MAP (cardiovascular system), Glasgow Coma Scale (CNS system), and creatinine and urine output (renal system). A higher SOFA score is associated with an increased probability of mortality (Gourd & Nikitas, 2020).*

PATHOPHYSIOLOGY

The inflammation, tissue injury, and other sequelae associated with MODS are thought to be caused by an unregulated host response. MODS may result from any form of shock because of inadequate tissue perfusion. As previously described, in patients with shock, all organ systems suffer damage from a lack of adequate perfusion, which can result in organ failure.

CLINICAL MANIFESTATIONS AND ASSESSMENT

Various causes of MODS have been identified, including dead or injured tissue, infection, and perfusion deficits. However, it is not possible as yet to predict which patients will develop MODS, partly because much of the organ damage occurs at the cellular level and therefore cannot be directly observed or measured. The most common types of organ dysfunction seen with MODS are acute kidney failure and ARDS. However, organ failure can affect the other body systems:

- Hepatic: jaundice, elevated liver function tests (LFTs), decreased albumin, elevated PT
- Hematologic: decreased platelets, elevated PT/APTT, increased D-dimer
- Central nervous system (CNS): altered level of consciousness (LOC), confusion, psychosis
- Respiratory: tachypnea, hypoxemia, PaO_2/FiO_2 greater than 300 (see Chapter 9)
- Cardiovascular: tachycardia, hypotension, altered CVP and PAP readings

Advanced age, malnutrition, and coexisting diseases appear to increase the risk of MODS in patients who are acutely ill.

Diagnosis	Systemic Blood Pressure	Heart Rate	Central Venous Pressure (CVP)	Pulmonary Artery Pressure	Cardiac Output (CO)	Systemic Vascular Resistance (SVR)
Cardiogenic: Myocardial Infarction (MI), Cardiac Tamponade, Pulmonary Emboli	↓	↑	↑	↑	↓	↑
Hypovolemic: Hemorrhage, Diarrhea, Burns, Dehydration	↓	↑	↓	↓	↓	↑
Septic: Severe Infection	↓	↑	↓	↓	↑↓	↓
Anaphylactic: Type 1 Hypersensitivity Reaction	↓	↑	↓	↓	↓	↓
Neurogenic: Brain Damage, Spinal Cord Injury	↓	↓	↓	↓	↓	↓

FIGURE 53-5 **Types of shock. Shock results from (*1*) an inability of the heart to pump adequately (cardiogenic shock); (*2*) decreased effective blood volume as a consequence of severely reduced blood or plasma volume (hypovolemic shock); or (*3*) widespread vasodilation (septic, anaphylactic, or neurogenic shock). Increased vascular permeability may complicate vasodilation by contributing to reduced effective blood volume. (Adapted from Lawrence, P., Bell, R., Dayton, M., & Hebert, J. [2012]. *Essentials of general surgery* [5th ed.]. Lippincott Williams & Wilkins.)**

MEDICAL MANAGEMENT

Prevention remains the top priority in managing MODS. Older patients are at increased risk for MODS because of the lack of physiologic reserve associated with aging and the natural degenerative process, especially immune compromise. Early detection and documentation of initial signs of infection are essential in managing MODS in older patients. Subtle changes in mentation and a gradual rise in temperature are early warning signs. Other patients at risk for MODS are those with chronic illness, malnutrition, immunosuppression, or surgical or traumatic wounds.

If preventive measures fail, treatment measures to reverse MODS are aimed at (1) controlling the initiating event, (2) promoting adequate organ perfusion, and (3) providing nutritional support.

NURSING MANAGEMENT

The general plan of nursing care for patients with MODS is the same as that for patients in septic shock. Primary nursing interventions are aimed at early and aggressive hemodynamic support until primary organ insults are halted. Providing information and support to family members is a critical role of the nurse. It is important that the health care team address end-of-life decisions to ensure that supportive therapies are congruent with the patient's wishes (see Chapter 2).

Refer to Figure 53-5 for a review of the various forms of shock.

CHAPTER REVIEW

NCLEX-Style Review Questions

1. Following spinal anesthesia, the post-anesthesia care unit (PACU) nurse's initial assessment reveals the patient's vital sign are as follows: BP 70/40, HR 46, RR 18, and Temp 98.4°F. The patient is awake and has loss of sensation and movement below the level of T4. The skin is warm. The surgery was uneventful with minimal blood loss. In Column 1 select all symptoms that are of concern, and in Column 2 select the problem the patient is experiencing.

Symptoms	Etiology
a. BP 70/40	1. Septic shock
b. HR 46	2. Neurogenic shock
c. RR 18	3. Hypovolemic shock
d. Temp 98.4°F	4. Cardiogenic shock
e. Warm, dry skin	

2. An older patient was admitted with a history of 5 days of diarrhea and is diagnosed with hypovolemic shock. Based upon this history, which of the following parameters would likely be expected? Select all that apply.

a. MAP of 59 mm Hg
b. MAP of 76 mm Hg
c. Narrow pulse pressure
d. Widening pulse pressure
e. Urine output of <0.5 mL/kg/hr
f. Urine output of 1 mL/kg/hr

3. You answer the call bell for a patient receiving an infusion of an IV antibiotic to treat a urinary tract infection. Upon your arrival to the room, the patient complains of their throat closing up and worsening shortness of breath. On your exam, you see redness and swelling all over their body and auscultate stridor over their trachea. Their vital signs are: heart rate 126 and regular, respiratory rate of 28, blood pressure of 82/60 mm Hg, and an O_2 sat of 87% on room air. Select all the appropriate interventions.

a. Place the patient in Trendelenburg position
b. Slow down the antibiotic infusion
c. Ensure the patient has IV access
d. Prepare for the administration of intramuscular epinephrine
e. Call a rapid response

4. Match the diagnosis with the type of shock that can occur:

1. Cardiac tamponade	Hypovolemic shock
2. Allergic reaction	Obstructive shock
3. Abdominal aortic aneurysm (AAA) rupture	Neurogenic shock
4. C4 spinal cord injury	Anaphylactic shock

5. A patient is brought into the emergency department after a motor vehicle collision. They are intubated and mechanically ventilated; the patient is unresponsive. On exam you appreciate no lung sounds to the left side, and the trachea is displaced to the right. Their vitals are: heart rate of 137 and regular, respiratory rate of 32, blood pressure of 72/50 mm Hg, and an O_2 sat of 86%. You suspect a tension pneumothorax. What interventions do you anticipate occurring? Select all that apply.

a. Possible emergent chest tube insertion
b. Chest x-ray to verify endotracheal tube placement and evaluation of a pneumothorax
c. Decreasing the oxygen to 40%
d. Administration of a beta blocker for the tachycardia
e. Calling the provider immediately to report the findings

REFERENCES AND SELECTED READINGS

References and selected readings associated with this chapter can be found on the website that accompanies the book. Visit **http://thepoint.lww.com/Honan3e** to access the references and other additional resources associated with this chapter.

CHAPTER 54

Nursing Management: Critical Care

Laura Kierol Andrews

Learning Objectives

After reading this chapter, you will be able to:

1. Describe the role of the critical care nurse in health care.
2. Describe nursing management of common problems in the critical care environment.
3. Understand common interventions and equipment used in the critical care environment.

The nurse's priority in caring for patients who are critically ill is to prevent harm and provide physical care, education, and emotional support to patients and families in an effort to return them to the highest possible state of health or to help them toward a peaceful death. Nurses are in the unique position of standing with the patient and family at the center of multisectoral activity. They are at the bedside to act as a care provider and liaison to other health care workers in an effort to coordinate said care. This chapter covers the role of the nurse in critical care and critical care responsibilities and modalities.

THE CRITICAL CARE ENVIRONMENT

The advent of critical care units evolved from Florence Nightingale's writings of the benefits of placing postoperative surgical patients in a separate area of the hospital (now known as post anesthesia care units). This led to the formation of critical care units where acutely and critically ill or injured patients would benefit from new biomedical technologies and care from specialized and trained nurses and providers (Urden, 2022). In 2000, the Institute of Medicine (IOM) challenged hospitals in their 100,000 Lives Campaign to prevent avoidable deaths and hospitals worldwide began developing Rapid Response Teams (RRTs) to address failure to recognize and rescue patients in early stages of deterioration (DeVita et al., 2006). These RRTs usually consist of a physician, an advanced practice registered nurse (APRN) or physician assistant (PA), a respiratory therapist, and a critical care nurse. These teams were established in hospitals to address the concerns of those patients outside of the intensive care unit (ICU) who were seen as requiring a higher level of care. The RRTs currently in place are able to provide the required higher level of care even when the patient is physically outside of the ICU and awaiting a bed inside the unit, thus making critical care a process and not a place.

NEUROLOGIC ISSUES

A neurologically healthy person is one who is awake, alert, and oriented, with the ability to respond appropriately to their environment without sensory or physical limitations. Whether or not a person is admitted with a specific neurologic or neurosurgical diagnosis, other medical problems or interventions may impact their neurologic status.

Altered Level of Consciousness

The causes of altered mental states are numerous and varied but can be remembered using the mnemonic in Table 54-1. Most ICU patients are at risk for mental status changes due to a myriad of potential factors: previously existing mental illness, increased age, severity of illness and comorbidities, sleep deprivation, and/or medications. Assessing changes in level of consciousness (LOC) alerts the nurse to neurologic impairment. A thorough review of possible causes and early intervention can impact a patient's long-term recovery. Refer to Chapter 42 for performing mental status assessment.

Delirium

Delirium is a common neuropsychiatric state that has a sudden onset and can last hours to days or weeks; it is characterized by hyper or hypoactivity and has the potential to be reversible. For example, the patient who quickly becomes confused and agitated while attempting to pull out IV lines and get out of bed may be experiencing hyperactive delirium. In addition, the patient who is somnolent or inattentive may

TABLE **54-1 Causes of Altered Mental Status**

	Cause	Example	Possible Nursing Interventions
A	Alcohol	Intoxication Withdrawal	Institute fall precautions Institute seizure precautions Institute ICU sedation protocol; Clinical Institute Withdrawal Assessment-Alcohol (CIWA-A) scale
E	Epilepsy Endocrine Electrolytes	New onset or low medication level Hypothyroidism Hyper or hyponatremia	Check medication level Check thyroid level IV fluids and serial sodium levels as ordered
I	Insulin	Hypoglycemia	Check glucose level Administer dextrose as ordered
O	Opiates and other drugs	Narcotic overdose	Administer reversal agent as ordered Airway protection with elevated head of bed
U	Uremia	Acute or chronic kidney failure	Follow trends of blood urea nitrogen and creatinine levels Ensure patency of dialysis access shunts and IV lines
T	Trauma Temperature	Hypothermia	Serial temperature measurements Blanket warmer Administer warm IV fluids as ordered
I	Infection	Sepsis	Obtain blood and body fluids for culture as ordered Administer antibiotics as ordered Ensure IV lines and Foley catheters have been changed according to hospital policy
P	Poison	Confusion, seizures, coma	Supportive care until poison is neutralized or removed
S	Shock Stroke Space-occupying lesion Subarachnoid hemorrhage	Hypovolemia Thrombolic or hemorrhagic Tumor Trauma or unmonitored anticoagulation use	IV fluids and cardiac pressors to support cerebral blood flow Call for stroke alert if found with acute symptoms Monitor for signs of increased intracranial pressure (ICP) Ensure functioning of ICP monitor or ventricular shunts

Emergency Medicine/Altered Mental Status. (2014). Retrieved May 13, 2015, from http://en.wikibooks.org/

be experiencing hypoactive delirium. These patients require extensive nursing time and often need someone to be present in the room with them at all times to prevent injury. The consequences of delirium cannot be underestimated. Though underdiagnosed, it has been found that delirium leads to a myriad of sequelae including: increased medicinal and restraint interventions, increased length of stay, delays in necessary treatments (surgeries, cancer therapies), persistent cognitive impairment with admission to chronic care facilities, and increased mortality (Keenan & Jain, 2022; Real et al., 2022).

Early identification of delirium in critical care patients can lead to prompt treatment in order to avoid complications. The Confusion Assessment Method for the intensive care unit (CAM-ICU) is a validated instrument that assigns scores based on onset, fluctuation of mental status, inattention, altered level of consciousness, and disorganized thinking and is easily accessed on a variety of websites (http://icudelirium.org/medical-professionals/delirium/monitoring-delirium-in-the-icu).

Pain and Anxiety

Pain and anxiety are interrelated and should be assessed together. For example, chest pain often produces great anxiety.

Pain

Critical care patients can experience pain as a result of their injury or disease as well as its treatment. It is well known that pain elicits a stress response, leading to a catabolic state with increased cardiac workload and an impaired immune response. Care must be taken to ensure that all ICU patients are assessed for any pain, whether or not they are able to communicate their pain level. Prevention and treatment of pain should include both pharmacologic and nonpharmacologic methods in collaboration with the patient (if able)

+4	Combative, violent, of immediate danger to himself and staff
+3	Very agitated, aggressive, pulls or removes tubes or catheters
+2	Agitated frequent nonpurposeful movement, dyssynchronous with the ventilator
+1	Restless, anxious but not aggressive
0	Alert and calm
−1	Drowsy, not fully alert, but has sustained eye-opening/eye contact to *voice* **(>10 s)**
−2	Light sedation-briefly awakens with eye contact to *voice* **(<10 s)**
−3	Moderate sedation—moves or opens eyes to *voice* **(but no eye contact)**
−4	Deep sedation. No response to voice. Movement or eye opening to *physical* stimulation
−5	Unarousable. No response to *voice or physical* stimulation

FIGURE 54-1 The Richmond Agitation and Sedation Scale (RASS). (Reprinted with permission from Bigatello, L. M., Alam, H., Allain, R. M., Bittner, E. A., Hess, D., Pino, R. M., & Schmidt, U. [Eds.] [2010]. *Critical care handbook of the Massachusetts General Hospital*. Lippincott Williams & Wilkins.)

and the medical team. Refer to Chapter 6 for details on pain assessment and management.

Anxiety

Anxiety has been defined as a universal experience with physical side effects and a subjective sense of danger or dread from real or perceived threats (Crocq, 2022). Each hospital also provides scales for objectifying signs and symptoms of anxiety, such as the Richmond Agitation and Sedation Scale (RASS), in order to standardize treatment and minimize its effects (see Fig. 54-1).

Table 54-2 summarizes assessment of anxiety. An ICU stay has inherent stressors of pain, lack of control over one's environment, decreased communication, and possible fears of imminent death, issues that are all causes for severe anxiety. It is estimated that up to 17% to 50%% of patients admitted to an ICU suffer from posttraumatic stress disorder (PTSD) as a result of their admission, and its prevention is of paramount importance when considering recovery and post discharge quality of life (Alonso-Fernandez-Gatta et al., 2021; Sayde et al., 2020).

Dependency and Withdrawal

Use of illegal and legal drugs is pervasive in the United States, with an estimated incidence of 20.7% (tobacco/nicotine), 50% (alcohol) and 21.4% (illicit drugs and marijuana) of the general population (SAMHSA, 2020) reporting use and abuse. It is important to realize that people of all ages may have a chemical dependence issue and that admission to the ICU will not "cure" this problem. It will more likely be that these patients require more pain and sedation medication to achieve desired effects, such as prevention of withdrawal and its sequelae.

Depression

Medical literature is filled with articles and studies demonstrating depression or depressed mood as a component of chronic and critical illness. It is also well known that many of the medications prescribed in the ICU, such as beta blockers, antibiotics, and steroids can cause depression. Patients admitted on antidepressive agents should continue them with the shortest interruption possible. Patients exhibiting signs of prolonged or exaggerated mood should be evaluated by a psychiatry provider for adequate diagnosis and treatment in order to facilitate the healing process.

Suicidal ideation, and actions taken with the intent to kill oneself, is another issue requiring assessment in the hospital setting. Suicide ranks as the 12th most common cause of death in the United States and a frequently reported sentinel event in health care institutions (Centers for Disease Control

TABLE **54-2 Anxiety Assessment**

Assessment	Possible Nursing Interventions
Does my patient have anxiety? If so, at what level?	Presume that all ICU patients are at risk for anxiety! Use appropriate scale to assess level of anxiety, such as the Richmond Agitation and Sedation Scale.
Why is the patient experiencing anxiety?	Provide any information for which the lack of information is the cause of anxiety.
What is the most appropriate medication?	Administer antianxiety medications if ordered.
What is the most appropriate method of delivery?	Assess the patient's ability to tolerate oral medication.
What nonpharmacologic methods of reducing anxiety are available?	Allow for visitation and distraction. Allow pet therapy if available and acceptable to patient.
Is our plan for anxiety relief working?	Reevaluate the patient regularly.
Does my patient have anxiety, and is unable to communicate this?	Observe nonverbal behavior including facial expressions, body language, gaze aversion; advocate for patients.

and Prevention [CDC], 2022c). The Joint Commission (2022) requires facilities to assess patients for suicidal ideation on admission and throughout their stay as it poses such a great risk. Admission to the ICU during a hospital stay does not diminish the need to assess patients for any suicidal thoughts or actions.

Sensory and Motor Function

Impairment of sensory and motor function (ability to feel and physically react to one's environment) can arise from various sources, including spinal cord injury, medications, peripheral vascular disease, and/or medical restraint devices. Alterations in sensation and motion can be viewed on a negative to positive continuum, ranging from insensate to numbness, normal, tingling, and then pain.

Communication

Communication allows patients and families to interact with health care system professionals in order to satisfy physical, emotional, and spiritual needs. The ICU environment and neurologic status deficits can make communication difficult. It is imperative that critical care nurses work to improve communication in order to satisfy the previously mentioned needs of their patients and families. Suggested methods may include:

- Asking yes or no questions to which the patient may nod their head
- Using an electronic tablet for texting
- Gaze-controlled computer devices
- Using a board with preprinted phrases to which the patient can point
- Using language and sign language interpreters (from within the hospital or interpreter services)
- Making a paper and writing utensil available

CARDIOVASCULAR ISSUES

Cardiovascular problems can be broadly categorized as those arising from the heart and vascular system and those affecting the heart and arterial and venous systems (Table 54-3). Patients may be admitted to critical care units for a number of concerns related to the cardiovascular system, including:

- a history of cardiovascular disease requiring careful observation, although not admitted specifically for cardiovascular disease, an active cardiac problem requiring advanced intervention, or
- another active medical problem affecting their cardiovascular status, such as hemorrhage, sepsis or postoperative cardiovascular surgeries

Monitoring the Patient

Depending upon the individual patient's condition, different levels of monitoring and intervention will be required.

TABLE **54-3** **Sources of Cardiac Disease**

Sources of Disease	Example
Cardiac	
Myocardial	Left ventricular hypertrophy, heart failure
Ischemic	Coronary artery disease, myocardial infarction
Conductive	Atrial fibrillation, heart blocks
Valvular	Mitral regurgitation, aortic stenosis
Other	
Infection	Pericarditis, sepsis, viral cardiomyopathy
Neurologic system	Spinal shock
Peripheral vascular system	Hypertension, deep vein thrombosis, pulmonary embolism
Respiratory system	Pulmonary hypertension
Renal system	Kidney failure leading to fluid overload
Trauma	Cardiac contusion, cardiac tamponade
Hemorrhage	Circulatory collapse

Table 54-4 provides a summary of the different levels of monitoring.

It is important to remember that monitors, invasive lines, and other devices are to assist in confirming or disproving physical examination results and clinical judgments, not replace them.

Intravenous Access in the Cardiac Patient

Peripheral Intravenous Access

At a minimum, peripheral intravenous (IV) access should be obtained on all patients in the critical care environment. Peripheral IVs give the health care team access the vascular system in case of emergency; a potential site for blood sampling; and the ability to provide fluids, medications, and nutrition (total parenteral nutrition [TPN], partial parenteral nutrition [PPN]). Contraindications to specific placements (right vs. left side) will include history of mastectomy, arterial-venous shunt placement, peripherally inserted central catheter (PICC) or midline placement, chronic kidney disease stage 3 or greater, thrombus, trauma, and other device placements, such as splints and casts. IV lines in the feet are reserved only for emergencies; they are to be removed as soon as possible and never inserted in the feet of patients with diabetes. Potential complications include bruising, infection, extravasation of fluids and medications, and air embolus.

TABLE 54-4 **Monitoring the Cardiac Patient**

Conditions and Circumstances	Related Monitoring and Interventions
• Patients who are expected to do well, but need additional monitoring in case unexpected complications, such as bleeding, or arrhythmias arise	Vital sign assessment Oxygen saturation Cardiac monitor Peripheral IV access in case of emergency
• Patients about to leave the critical care environment and who are awake, hemodynamically stable, and able to eat and drink	All of the above
• Patients admitted with singular issues, such as an elective surgery or uncomplicated medical diagnoses, who are expected to recover, but have a cardiac history (such patients may need IV fluids and medications for a limited time period).	All of the above + IV fluids, IV medications, or minimal blood products
• Patients who have a medical or surgical issue, in which recovery depends on the medical team's provision of more precise monitoring (such as heart failure)	All of the above + Central venous access and/or arterial line access
• Patients who are at risk for complications, or for whom basic monitoring and fluids have failed; patients requiring cardiac pressor support (these patients are often compromised due to sepsis).	All of the above + Vasoactive medications and/or further blood products
• Patients who have an unclear cardiac status, have not responded well to lesser interventions, or have undergone cardiac surgery	All of the above + Pulmonary artery catheterization
• Cardiac failure due to any cause	All of the above + Counterpulsation via intra-aortic balloon pump
• Complete cardiac failure	All of the above + Ventricular assist device

An arterial line is a peripheral IV in the arterial system used for frequent blood pressure monitoring when a patient requires vasoactive medications (such as norepinephrine), arterial blood gas, or frequent blood sampling. It is not for administration of fluids or medications. Potential complications include ischemia, thrombosis, infiltration, and exsanguination.

Central Intravenous Lines

Central IV lines (Fig. 54-2) are used for a number of reasons, including:

- Failure to obtain or maintain peripheral access
- Complication of peripheral access
- The patient requires numerous access sites, parenteral nutrition, or hypertonic fluid administration
- Treatment failure with IV fluids necessitates hemodynamic monitoring of central venous pressure (CVP) or pulmonary artery catheter (PAC) readings
- The patient requires vasoactive medications that place their limb at risk if an infiltrate occurs

The triple-lumen catheter is a central line that measures the CVP or the amount of fluid returning to the heart at the level of the right atrium (termed *preload*, see Table 54-5). See Chapter 11 for more information on CVP monitoring.

Pulmonary Artery Catheter

PACs are used when previous interventions have not yielded the expected outcome (increased urine output with increased IV fluid administration), for intra- and postoperative hemodynamic monitoring or when the patient has a complicating factor, such as kidney or heart failure or pulmonary hypertension, which makes clinical judgments difficult without additional information. After decades of its use in practice, there is still no consensus as to whether PACs improve patient outcomes. Without that evidence and because they increase the risk of complications, such as pneumothorax, cardiac arrhythmias, and pulmonary artery rupture, the use of PACs is decreasing. However, they still can be a helpful tool in assisting in the overall evaluation of a patient.

PACs allow the medical and nursing team to monitor, intervene upon, and evaluate:

- Blood volume status
- Blood flow
- Cardiac output/index
- Tissue oxygenation

Figure 54-3 illustrates components of the PAC system.

Blood Volume Status

Blood volume status is the amount of blood circulating in the enclosure of the arterial and venous systems. This fluid exerts or creates a pressure that can be monitored to determine preload: The greater the blood volume, the greater the pressure (assuming no confounding variables, such as severe hypertension). Using Starling's Law, the volume can be increased to give the heart a greater stretch or potential energy with which to pump blood to the body without causing overstretch and failure. It can be compared to a sling

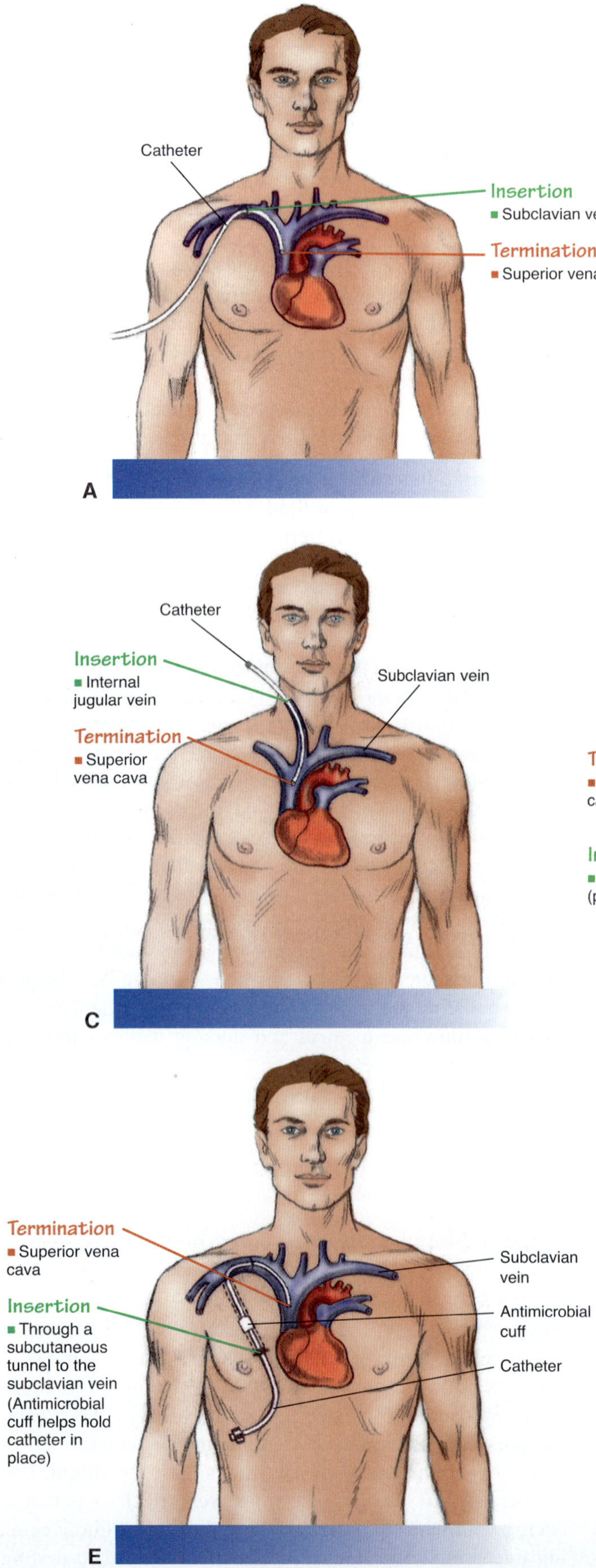

FIGURE 54-2 **Central vein catheter pathways showing various insertion and termination sites. Typically, a central vein catheter is inserted in the subclavian or internal jugular vein. (A) Subclavian insertion ending in Superior Vena Cava (SVC); (B) Subclavian insertion ending in the right atrium; (C) Jugular insertion ending in the SVC; (D) Peripherally inserted central catheter (PICC) ending in the SVE; € Hickman Catheter ending in the SVC. (From Lippincott Williams & Wilkins. [2010].** ***Hemodynamic monitoring made incredibly visual*** **[2nd ed.]. Lippincott Williams & Wilkins.)**

TABLE **54-5 Effects of Preload and Afterload on the Heart**

Factor	Possible Cause	Effects on Heart
Increased preload	Increased fluid volume Vasoconstriction	Increases stroke volume Increases ventricular work Increases myocardial oxygen requirements
Decreased preload	Hypovolemia Vasodilation	Decreases stroke volume Decreases ventricular work Decreases myocardial oxygen requirements
Increased afterload	Hypovolemia Vasoconstriction	Decreases stroke volume Increases ventricular work Increases myocardial oxygen requirements
Decreased afterload	Vasodilation	Increases stroke volume Decreases ventricular work Decreases myocardial oxygen requirements

From Lippincott Williams & Wilkins. (2010). Understanding the cardiac system. In *Hemodynamic monitoring made incredibly visual* (2nd ed., p. 15). Lippincott Williams & Wilkins.

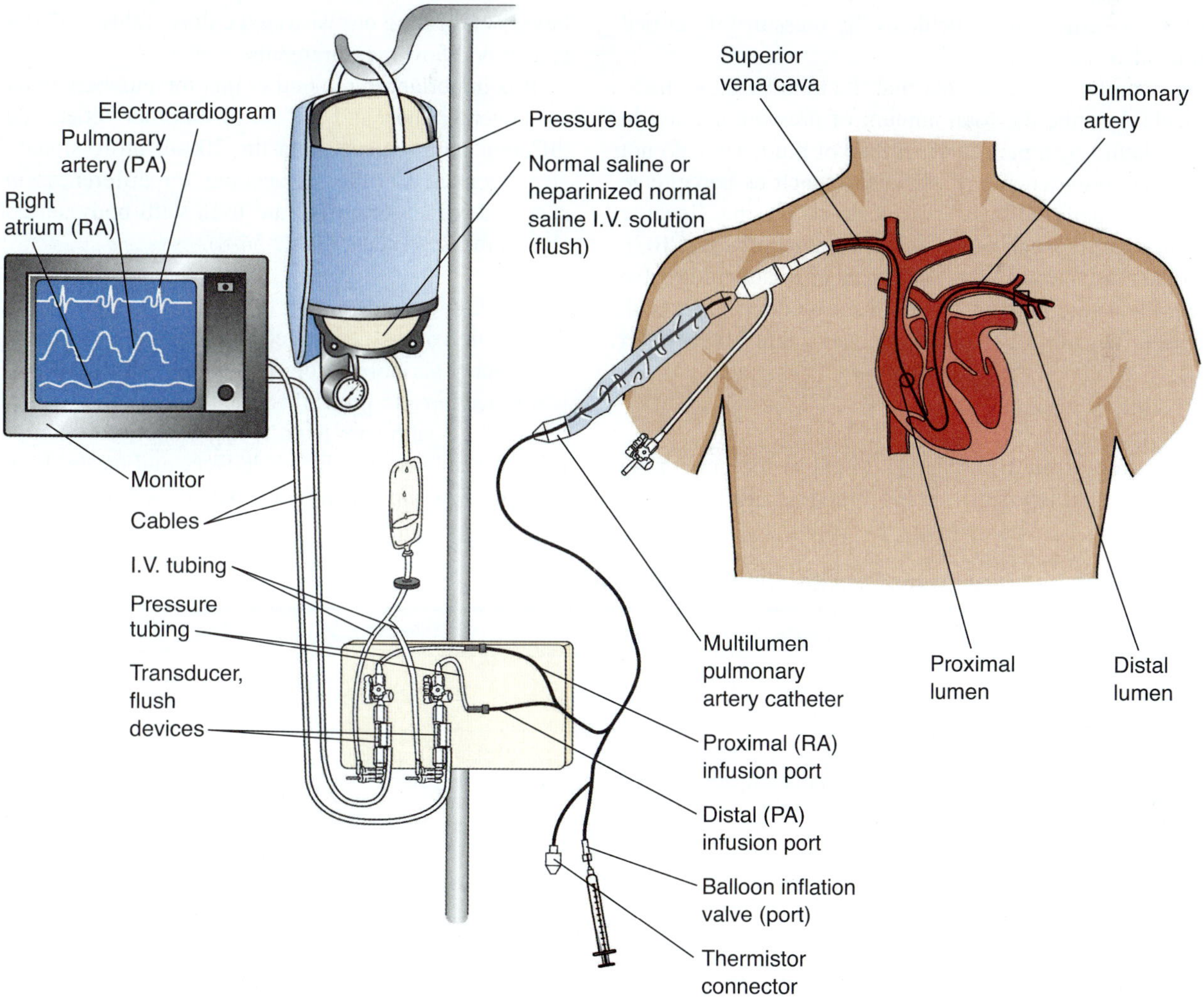

FIGURE 54-3 **Components of the pulmonary artery catheter (PAC) monitoring system. (From Lippincott Williams & Wilkins. [2010].** ***Hemodynamic monitoring made incredibly visual*** **[2nd ed.]. Lippincott Williams & Wilkins.)**

TABLE **54-6 Pulmonary Artery Catheter Pressure Measurements**

Measurement	Definition	Formula (If Applicable)	Normal Value (mm Hg)
Mean arterial pressure (MAP)	Average arterial pressure throughout the cardiac cycle	Systolic BP + 2(diastolic BP)/3	70–105
Right atrial pressure (RAP)	Pressure at the level of the right atrium		2–8
Pulmonary artery systolic pressure (PAS)	Pressure in pulmonary artery during systole		20–30
Pulmonary artery diastolic pressure (PAD)	Pressure in the pulmonary artery during diastole		8–15
Mean pulmonary artery pressure (MPAP)	Average pressure in the pulmonary artery throughout the cardiac cycle	PAS + 2(PAD)/3	10–15
Pulmonary artery wedge pressure	The indirect measurement of pressure in the left ventricle at the end of diastole		6–12

shot pulled back ever farther to throw a stone farther without stretching the sling to the point of breaking.

A PAC measures and calculates the pressures described in Table 54-6.

It is important to remember that the blood volume measurements describe the total amount of pressure exerted in the vasculature by a particular volume of fluid. They do not describe the components of the blood, such as percentage of red blood cells (RBCs; hematocrit) or plasma. Specific laboratory values, such as the complete blood count (CBC), determine these percentages. The goals of treatment involve restoring and maintaining an adequate blood volume with the right proportions of blood components that best support organ perfusion.

Blood Flow

The right side of the heart pumps blood to the pulmonary system, and the left side pumps blood to itself via the coronary arteries and the rest of the body via the aorta. The PAC measures how the heart is pumping and how the vasculature is receiving or resisting the flow. Table 54-7 describes PAC blood flow measurements.

It is important to remember that the numbers in the table are general values and that the 98-lb older patient will have different requirements than the 200-lb professional defensive lineman. In order to account for differences in body size, index measurements are used with body surface area (BSA) measurements (Table 54-8).

Tissue Oxygenation

The ability of tissues to receive and use oxygen depends upon many variables, from physiologic disorders and medical procedures to prescribed medications and their interactions. The health care team is responsible for manipulating these variables to maximize delivery and usage. In general, the following indicate how the patient is doing:

TABLE **54-7 Pulmonary Artery Catheter Blood Flow Measurements**

Measurement	Definition	Formula (If Applicable)	Normal Value
Heart rate (HR)	The number of beats per minute		60–100 bpm
Stroke volume (SV)	The amount of blood ejected from the left ventricle with each beat	End-diastolic volume–end systolic volume	Patient dependent
Cardiac output	The amount of blood pumped to the body each minute	HR × SV	4–8 L/min
Pulmonary vascular resistance (PVR)		PAM–PAWP/CO × 80	50–150 dynes/sec/cm^5
Systemic vascular resistance (SVR)		MAP–RAP/CO × 80	900–1,200 dynes/sec/cm^5

TABLE **54-8 Pulmonary Artery Catheter Indices**

Measurement	Definition	Formula	Normal Value
Stroke volume index	As above accounting for body surface area (BSA)		30–60 mL/beat/m^2
Cardiac index	As above accounting for BSA	CI/BSA	2.4–5 L/min/m^2
Pulmonary vascular resistance index (PVRI)	As above accounting for BSA	PAM–PAWP/CI × 80	200–350 dynes/sec/cm^5
Systemic vascular resistance index (SVRI)	As above accounting for BSA	MAP–RAP/CI × 80	1,800–2,800 dynes/sec/cm^5

- Arterial pH and partial pressure
- Venous pH and partial pressure
- End-organ function, such as urine production
- Lactic acid level
- Mixed venous oxygen saturation (MvO_2 or SvO_2) (obtained from a PAC)
- Central venous oxygen saturation ($ScvO_2$) (obtained from a triple lumen catheter)

Pearls for Practice

The lactic acid level represents the end product of anaerobic metabolism used by the body during times of insufficient oxygen supply. Lactic acidosis is considered to be present if the plasma lactate concentration is greater than 4 to 5 mEq/L (refer to your labs standard values). However, the nurse may see a rise in the lactic acid level as oxygen supplied via blood flow is initially restored. Consider a patient with a vascular blockage to their leg during which the extremity is not receiving enough oxygen and the limb is cold and pale without pulses. Lactic acid is building up in the leg, but this lactic acid is not measured because blood flow is blocked from flowing into the vascular system. Once vascular flow is restored, marked with a return of warmth and peripheral pulses, there will be an initial rise in lactic acid as the body releases it into the now flowing bloodstream. Thus, the nurse must consider the serum lactic level in conjunction with the patient's clinical situation.

Pearls for Practice

As bodies neither make nor store oxygen, humans have evolved and adapted with a safety mechanism to ensure oxygen delivery occurs in times of decreased supply and/or increased demand. The body only uses a portion of the oxygen delivered to the bloodstream during one circuit from the heart and lungs to the rest of the body and back. Consider a person experiencing cardiopulmonary arrest, when 4 to 6 minutes may pass without a heartbeat before brain damage occurs. This is because there is still oxygen in the blood from their last inspiration. The normal value for MvO_2 is 75%. Thus, the body used only 25% of delivered oxygen during the last lap through the body. A decrease in MvO_2 below 75% means the body is not receiving enough oxygen, extracting (septic shock) and/or has an increased demand for oxygen.

The various IV and intra-arterial lines discussed in the previous section are used to monitor cardiac function; they do not change it. To improve a patient's cardiac status, practitioners remove the root cause of the problem and provide support via the use of IV fluids, blood products, vasoactive medications, and medical devices.

Intravenous Fluids and Blood Products

IV fluids are given to obtain and help maintain a euvolemic and isotonic state within the body. The type and amount of fluid will be dependent upon each individual's medical situation. These crystalloid solutions in various concentrations and combinations contain electrolytes and sometimes sugars:

- Saline
- Lactated Ringer's
- 5% dextrose in water

IV solutions with larger molecules designed to expand IV volume with increased oncotic pressures include:

- Albumin (5% or 25%)
- Hespan or Hetastarch (rarely used due to increased risk of bleeding and hypersensitivity reactions)

Blood products can help with hydration and volume expansion, as well as provide additional or replacement oxygen-carrying capacity, clotting factors, and platelets:

- Packed red blood cells (PRBCs)
- Fresh-frozen plasma (FFP)
- Pooled platelets
- Cryoprecipitate

Cable et al. (2019) report that up to 50% of people admitted to the ICU receive at least one blood product transfusion. Current literature supports a restrictive transfusion strategy (hemoglobin <7 g/dL) in most ICU patients, except cardiovascular surgery (<7.5 g/dL) and possible higher in patients with acute coronary syndromes (<8 g/dL). Transfusion of blood products is costly, carries risks (infectious disease transmission, transfusion reactions [hemolytic, allergic]), transfusion-related acute lung injury (TRALI), and transfusion-associated circulatory overload (TACO). Refer to Chapter 19 for more details on blood transfusion complications.

Vasoactive Medications

Many medications are used to help support cardiovascular function. Vasoactive medications given in the ICU are designed to alter preload, afterload, contractility, and cardiac rhythm, as required by the patient's underlying disease and physiologic condition. These are potent drugs with a myriad of potential adverse effects necessitating close titration and monitoring in an ICU setting. Table 54-9 summarizes those IV medications most commonly used in the ICU.

Medical Devices

Patients in the ICU may require medical devices to assist with cardiac function.

Pacemakers

Pacemakers are medical devices generally used to treat cardiac disease caused by conduction problems. They can be placed temporarily or permanently in order to improve cardiac function with or without adjunct medications. Permanent pacemakers and implantable cardioverter defibrillators (ICDs) are discussed in Chapter 16.

Temporary pacemakers are used during cardiac surgery and medical emergencies. They can be placed in a variety of ways:

- *External pacemakers:* Involves placement of electrodes on the front and side or back of the chest to deliver repeated shocks
- *Transvenous pacemakers:* Involves placement of a wire into the right ventricle via a central IV catheter
- *Epicardial pacemaker:* Involves surgical placement of wires into the epicardium to prevent and treat postsurgical conduction defects
- *Transthoracic cardiac pacemakers:* Involves introduction of a wire into the right ventricle, which is attached to a surgically placed generator

TABLE **54-9 Vasoactive Medications**

Medication	Action or Effect	Indications	Dosing Range
Amiodarone	Decreased heart rate	Ventricular tachycardia Atrial fibrillation	Arrhythmia dependent
Diltiazem	Decreased heart rate and blood pressure	Atrial fibrillation Paroxysmal Supraventricular Tachycardia Hypertension	5–15 mg/hr
Dobutamine	Increased heart contractility Increased blood pressure	Congestive heart failure Low cardiac output	2.5–20 μg/kg/min
Dopamine	Increased heart rate and blood pressure	Bradycardia Hypotension	2–20 μg/kg/min
Epinephrine	Increased heart rate and blood pressure	Anaphylaxis Shock	1–40 μg/min
Esmolol	Decreased heart rate	Tachycardia Hypertension	500 μg/kg load 50–200 μg/kg/min
Nicardipine	Decreased blood pressure	Hypertension	5–15 mg/hr
Nitroglycerin	Decreased blood pressure Arterial vasodilatation	Myocardial ischemia Congestive heart failure Hypertension	10–200 μg/min
Nitroprusside	Decreased blood pressure	Congestive heart failure Hypertensive crisis	0.3–10 μg/kg/min
Norepinephrine	Increased blood pressure	Cardiac arrest Hypotension	1–30 μg/min
Phenylephrine	Increased blood pressure	Hypotension	40–400 μg/min
Vasopressin	Increased blood pressure	Diabetes insipidus Gastrointestinal bleed Septic shock	0.02–0.04 units/min

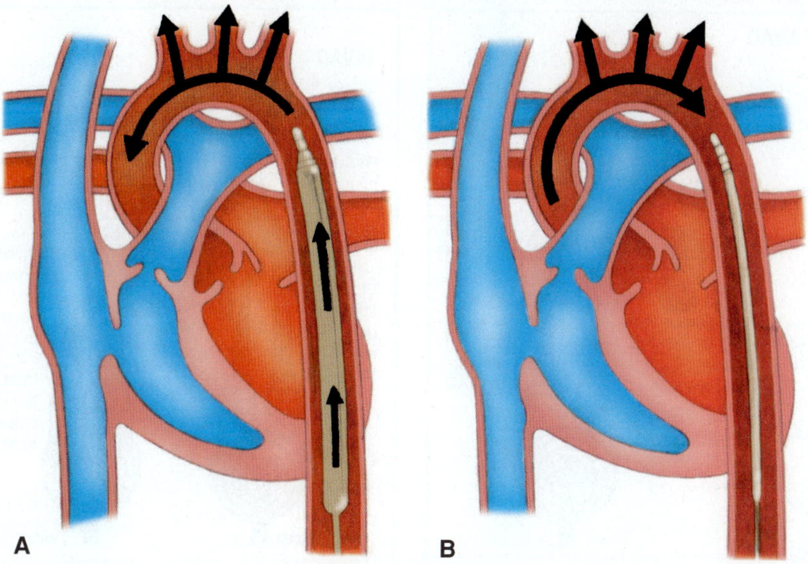

FIGURE 54-4 **Direction of blood flow when the pump inflates and deflates the balloon. A. Balloon inflation: The balloon inflates as the aortic valve closes and diastole begins. Diastole increases perfusion to the coronary arteries. B. Balloon deflation: The balloon deflates before ventricular ejection, when the aortic valve opens. This deflation permits ejection of blood from the left ventricle against a lowered resistance. As a result, aortic end-diastolic pressure and afterload decrease and cardiac output rises. (From Lippincott Williams & Wilkins. [2010].** ***Hemodynamic monitoring made incredibly visual*** **[2nd ed.]. Lippincott Williams & Wilkins.)**

Whether temporary or permanent, pacemakers necessitate that care for a patient with a pacemaker includes monitoring of the pacemaker's function and the patient's physical response to the pacing. This will include pain management and sedation for those with external pacers, infection control for newly inserted pacers, and physical assessment of cardiac, pulmonary, renal, and peripheral vascular function.

Intra-Aortic Balloon Pump

Patients with temporary or permanent heart muscle damage are unable to adequately perfuse their own heart and other organs. First attempts to improve cardiac muscle function include fluids and medications, but, at times, patients will require additional support in the form of an intra-aortic balloon pump (IABP). A balloon in placed in the descending aorta via a femoral artery. The balloon can be alternately inflated and deflated (Fig. 54-4). It is programmed to inflate during diastole, which pushes blood back toward the cardiac muscle itself, as well as toward the brain and into the coronary arteries. It deflates just before the ejection phase of systole and acts as a vacuum that pulls blood into the aorta with less effort from the left ventricle. An IABP essentially decreases the workload of the heart, allowing the heart muscle to rest and recover while improving organ perfusion. The machine itself can be programmed to assist with every heartbeat or every second, third, or fourth alternative beat, depending upon patient requirements. Care for patients on an IABP includes monitoring cardiac function with the use of a PAC and assessing peripheral circulation to the extremity below its insertion site.

Ventricular Assist Device

A ventricular assist device (VAD) is an implantable device in which cannulas are inserted into the atria or ventricles to support the right side of the heart, left side of the heart, or both sides by taking over the work of delivering blood to the pulmonary artery and/or aorta (see Fig. 54-5). There are three types of VADs. A right VAD (right ventricular assist device [RVAD]) provides pulmonary support by diverting blood from the right atrium or failing right ventricle to the VAD, which pumps the blood into the pulmonary circulation via the VAD connection to the left pulmonary artery.

With a left VAD (left ventricular assist device [LVAD]), blood flows from the left atrium or ventricle to the VAD, which then pumps blood back to the body via the VAD connection to the aorta. A RVAD and LVAD combination is referred to as *biventricular* (BiVAD) *support.*

VADs are reserved for patients who cannot be weaned from maximum volume/inotropic support or the IABP, are awaiting cardiac transplantation, or have class IV heart failure but are not candidates for transplantation. This intervention is the last-line treatment for cardiac failure and requires high-intensity nursing care to monitor cardiac function and the myriad of potential adverse effects, which range from infection, bleeding, and neurologic deficits to kidney and device failure. While usually deemed to be a temporary measure, VADs are gaining prominence due patients with refractory heart failure who cannot be transplanted who are creating a cohort of patients requiring long-term assistance without definitive cure. Thus, VAD support is the destination therapy. These patients are living in communities and should be known to emergency services in case of power outages (refer to Chapter 15 for further details).

Extracorporeal Membrane Oxygenation (ECMO)

ECMO is an invasive therapy that provides support for patients with respiratory and or cardiovascular failure. ECMO utilizes a centrifuge blood pump, membrane lung and

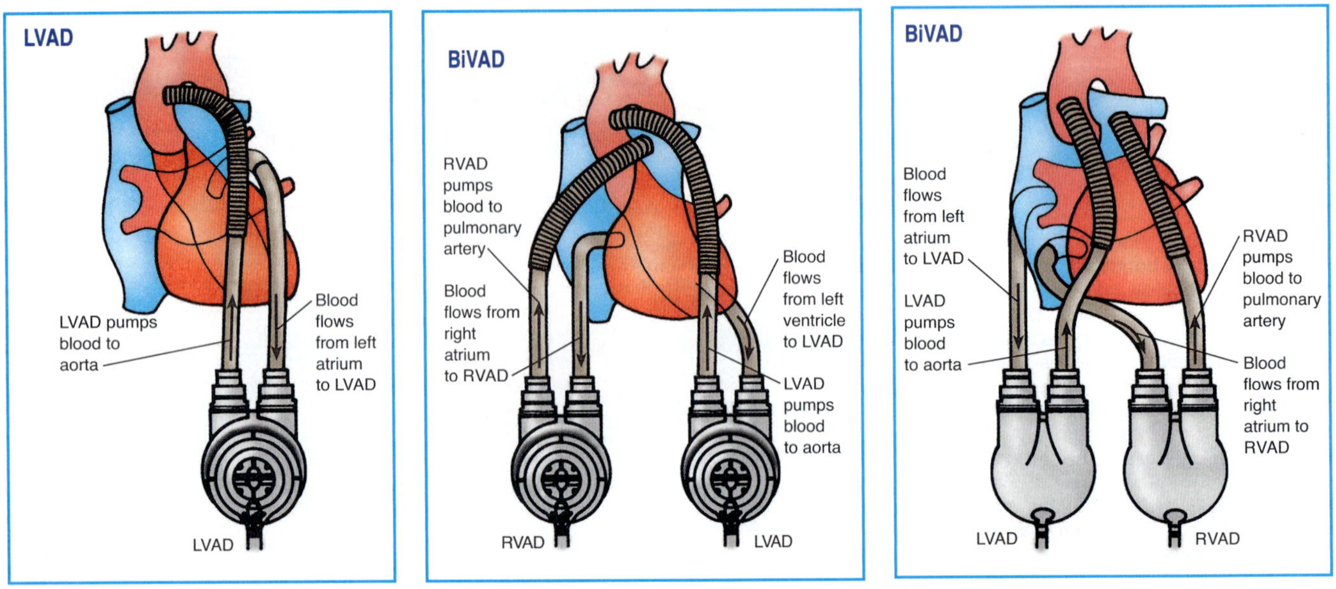

FIGURE 54-5 **Cannulation options. Ventricular assist devices (VADs) divert blood from failing ventricles to a pump that can effectively eject it. This diversion can occur by cannulation of either the atria or the ventricles. LVAD, left VAD; RVAD, right VAD; BiVAD, biventricular support. (From Lippincott Williams & Wilkins. [2010].** ***Hemodynamic monitoring made incredibly visual*** **[2nd ed.]. Lippincott Williams & Wilkins.)**

oxygen blender to support patients during severe hypoxic and/or hypercapnic (excessive carbon dioxide in the blood) respiratory failure, cardiogenic shock states, refractory ventricular fibrillation, cardiac arrest, bridge to heart and or lung transplants, or VAD placement. Configuration/placement of the ECMO cannulas is based on the patients need, with venovenous (VV ECMO) for respiratory failure and venoarterial (VA ECMO) for cardiac failure situation. ECMO programs are available at many large teaching hospitals, and in recent years are available to smaller hospitals with team being deployed, inserting cannulas and initiating ECMO therapy before transporting patients to the ECMO-center hospital. See Figure 54-6.

RESPIRATORY ISSUES

Respiratory Failure

Respiratory failure and the advent of mechanical ventilation led to the creation of critical care as a specialty service. As times change, so does technology. The use of noninvasive ventilator (NIV) support for respiratory complications is now a first line of treatment for an ever-increasing number of patient populations and care settings (Johnny, 2022). The number of patients needing ventilatory support is expected to grow over the next decades. Respiratory failure can generally be divided into two main categories (see Box 54-1).

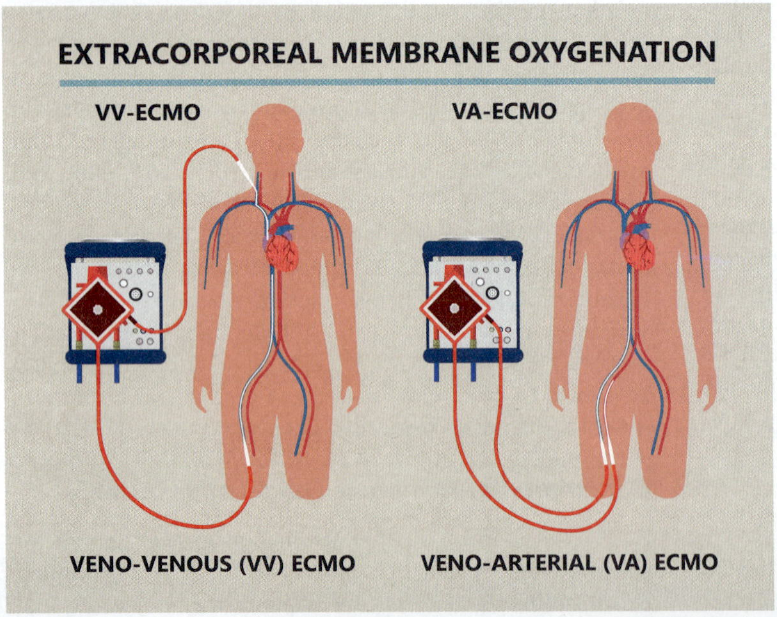

FIGURE 54-6 **Extracorporeal membrane oxygenation (ECMO) a life support system for respiratory failure. (From shutterstock.com. ID: 1810163059.)**

BOX 54-1 **Causes of Respiratory Failure**

Hypoxemic respiratory failure (too little oxygen reaches the tissues):
- Anemia
- Hemorrhage
- Intracardiac shunts
- Acute respiratory distress syndrome (ARDS)
- Pulmonary embolism

Ventilatory respiratory failure (too little oxygen is exchanged for carbon dioxide):
- Airway obstruction (chronic bronchitis, emphysema, cystic fibrosis)
- Weakness of breathing (acute intoxication, obesity with sleep apnea)
- Muscular weakness (spinal cord injury, muscular dystrophy)
- Lung disease (pneumonia, pulmonary edema)
- Chest wall abnormalities (scoliosis, severe kyphosis)

Oxygen Delivery

In the critical care environment, oxygen is treated as a drug, requiring a providers' order and nursing assessment of the patient's response to this prescription. The need for oxygen therapy and its specific method of delivery varies according to patient condition. Some patients will receive O_2 therapy as a preventative measure. Supplemental oxygen will assist some patients with extra oxygen delivery during acute episodes, such as in cases of myocardial infarction (MI). For the more critically ill, it will serve as an intervention to ensure oxygen delivery when they are unable to maintain their own ventilatory or respiratory function. Oxygen is the most commonly prescribed gas in the critical care environment and is commonly ordered in liters per minute (L/min), as a concentration of oxygen stated as a percentage (e.g., 30%), or as a fraction of inspired oxygen (FiO_2; e.g., 0.3). See Chapter 9 for detailed information on oxygen delivery systems, converting percentage of oxygen to L/min and nursing responsibilities.

Pearls for Practice

The nurse considers oxygen a drug, which has benefits and risks. The risks associated with oxygen increase as the FiO_2 increases. Healthy lungs may be able to tolerate FiO_2 levels of less than 60%; however, when lungs are damaged, FiO_2 that exceeds 50% may result in a toxic alveolar O_2 concentration (Stacy, 2022). In general, durations of FiO_2 >50% for >24 has resulted in oxygen toxicity, but it has occurred in as short as 6 hours (Christiani, 2020). Excessive O_2 concentrations have been associated with acute respiratory distress syndrome (ARDS), injury to the lung parenchyma, retinopathy (premature neonates), and resorptive atelectasis (see Chapter 9) (Hochber et al., 2021). Although the benefits of oxygen therapy typically outweigh the risks, the nurse is mindful that every intervention employed has to be evaluated for the risk/benefit balance.

Pearls for Practice: Cues to Oxygen Toxicity

Cues associated with oxygen toxicity include substernal chest pain that is exacerbated by deep breathing, a dry nonproductive cough, tachypnea, tracheal irritation progressing to pleuritic pain on inhalation, followed by dyspnea (Heiner, 2023). Additional complaints may include nasal stuffiness, sore throat, increased pressure sensation in the ears, headache, anorexia, and nausea (Stacy, 2022). The aim is to use the lowest FiO_2 that achieves adequate oxygenation (PaO_2 of 55 to 60 mm Hg and arterial oxygen saturation of 90%); however, treatment of hypoxemia is the priority over the possibility of oxygen toxicity (Christiani, 2020; Storzer, 2023).

Positive Airway Pressure

As explained by Meng et al. (2021) positive airway pressure machines, whether intermittent or continuous (CPAP), have been used for many years as a method of oxygen delivery in patients requiring assistance with keeping the upper airway open or improving intrathoracic pressure and lung volumes without invasive intubation of the trachea. When initiated for the first time, positive airway pressure is usually started in a highly monitored setting in order to assess for claustrophobia and nausea and vomiting (risk for gastric distention increases with positive pressures above 25 cm H_2O). This therapy requires patient cooperation and spontaneous ventilation, and the patient must also be able to tolerate some periods off the mask in order to eat and drink or perform mouth care and skin assessments. CPAP is most effective when there is a resilient seal around the airway to minimize air leak, but that poses a risk for skin irritation. The nurse assesses pressure areas and provides skin care as needed.

Noninvasive Ventilation

NIV appears similar to the methods of oxygen delivery discussed previously, but it is, in fact, not the same. NIV provides a greater pressure on the inspiratory phase than on expiration, unloading the work of the respiratory muscles and providing complete respiratory support (Meng et al., 2021).

Intubation and Mechanical Ventilation

Many patients in the ICU will require intubation and mechanical ventilation during their admission. It is hoped that this will be required for only a short time period to assist in supporting the patient's recovery from illness or injury. However, this advanced technology has moved from the acute care arena into chronic care facilities and even homes. Intubation and ventilation allow for:

- Airway protection in the event of neurologic deterioration or acute intoxication

- Airway protection during sedation for testing and procedures
- Airway clearance for those unable to manage their own secretions
- Management of respiratory function during surgery
- Rest for the patient with muscular fatigue
- Increased FiO_2 for the arterially hypoxic patient
- Increased flow, minute ventilation (tidal volume x's respiratory rate) and pressure to ensure adequate ventilation.

Caring for a patient on mechanical ventilation has become an integral part of nursing care in critical care and progressive care units. Positive patient outcomes depend on an understanding of the indications for and principles of mechanical ventilation, as well as the goals of therapy.

Pearls for Practice

It is important to remember that the right main bronchus is wider, shorter, and more vertical than the left. This physiologic difference may lead to inadvertent intubation of the right lung only. It is essential to listen to both sides of the chest for bilateral breath sounds, mark the correct endotracheal tube (ETT) placement at lip or nares, and monitor for high- and low-pressure alarms.

Types of Ventilators

Today's most commonly used ventilators are programmed to deliver oxygen through positive pressure. The ventilator pushes air into the lungs instead of creating a vacuum or negative pressure to pull air into the lungs when breathing spontaneously. Expiration occurs passively and endotracheal intubation or tracheotomy is necessary. Most ventilators are able to deliver breaths by varying modes. There are four common modes of positive pressure:

- *Time-cycled:* This terminates inspiration after a preset time. The volume of air the patient receives is regulated by the length of inspiration and the flow rate of the air.
- *Volume-cycled:* This is the used most commonly. The volume of air delivered with each inspiration is preset. Once this volume is delivered to the patient, the ventilator cycles off and exhalation occurs passively. The volume of air delivered by the ventilator is relatively constant, ensuring consistent, adequate breaths despite varying airway pressures.
- *Pressure-cycled:* This delivers a flow of air (inspiration) until it reaches a preset pressure and then cycles off to allow expiration to occur passively. The major limitation is that the volume of air or oxygen can vary as the patient's airway resistance or compliance changes. The tidal volume delivered may be inconsistent (the amount of air inhaled and exhaled with a normal breath).
- *Time- and pressure-cycled:* This delivers breaths at set inspiratory pressure and ends the breath at a preset time (in seconds). This mode is often used for severe hypoxic respiratory failure and allows for lung recruitment of diseased alveoli.

Ventilator Modes

Volume-Cycled Ventilators

Controlled Mandatory Ventilation. Controlled mandatory ventilation (CMV) delivers a set tidal volume at a set rate. It is used for the patient who is chemically paralyzed and sedated or whose neurologic status has deteriorated to the point that no drive to breathe exists. This mode is rarely used as a patient's intrinsic respiratory drive is ignored and can cause desynchrony between patient and ventilator.

Assist Control. Assist control (AC) also delivers a set tidal volume but allows patients to breath above the set number of breaths. When they take a breath, they receive the entire preset tidal volume, thus decreasing their work of breathing. If the rate is set high enough, it is essentially the same as CMV.

Synchronized Intermittent Mandatory Ventilation. Synchronized intermittent mandatory ventilation (SIMV) delivers a number of breaths at a preset tidal volume to ensure a minimum number of breaths with an adequate tidal volume. Patients may breathe spontaneously but will receive only the tidal volume they are able to inspire on their own.

High-Frequency Ventilation. High-frequency ventilation (HFV), or oscillating ventilators, deliver very small tidal volumes from 3 to 6 mL/kg or 50 to 80 mL in a range from 60 to over 540 times a minute. This works on the principle of oxygen diffusion gently pulsating throughout the lungs with less turbulent (more laminar) flow.

Pressure-Cycled Ventilators

Pressure Support Ventilation. Pressure support ventilation (PSV) is a mode of ventilation in which the patient breathes spontaneously but uses additional pressure during inspiration to increase airflow through the ventilator tubing and artificial airway. This decreases the work of breathing caused by a narrowed airway and the ventilator circuit. Patients using pressure support are often in the process of being weaned from the ventilator.

Continuous Positive Airway Pressure. Positive air flow is used via the ETT while the patient is on the ventilator (rather than using a mask, as discussed previously). It is also used as a method of decreasing the work of breathing while weaning the patient from the ventilator.

Airway Pressure Release Ventilation. Airway pressure release ventilation (APRV) is a newer mode of assistance that improves alveolar recruitment using pressure. It is essentially BiPAP on the ventilator using inverse ratio ventilation (IRV). It allows patients to breathe with the presence of end expiratory pressure in the alveoli, but this pressure is momentarily released to allow for gas release and ventilation.

Inverse Ratio Ventilation. IRV changes the normal inspiration to expiration ratios of 1 part inspiration to 3 parts expiration (1:3) to a ratio of 1:2 or more than 1:1 up to 2:1. Prolonging the inspiratory time allows alveolar recruitment (more alveoli used during respiration) at lower pressure levels, thus maintains or improves gas exchange at lower levels of PEEP. This is an uncomfortable way of breathing, and patients may need to be sedated and often on chemical neuromuscular blockade infusions.

Ventilator Settings

The primary provider will order individualized ventilator settings for the patient that will include the following:

Rate

The rate is the number of breaths the machine will give each minute.

Fraction of Inspired Air

Each breath will be given with a specified setting for inspired oxygen level, FiO_2. The goal for the FIO_2 is the lowest possible setting to provide adequate partial pressure of oxygen (PaO_2) in the bloodstream without the side effects of high oxygen percentages, such as oxygen toxicity, nitrogen washout and alveolar collapse.

Tidal Volume

The tidal volume (Tv) is the amount of air given in each breath. This is usually between 5 and 8 mL of air per kilogram of ideal body weight. This allows for air flow without overextending and damaging the alveoli. The Tv multiplied by the rate equals the minute volume (Mv). Patients with ARDS are generally managed with a low tidal volume (6 mL/kg of ideal body weight).

Positive End Expiratory Pressure

The theory behind positive end expiratory pressure (PEEP) is that it mimics the pressure left in the lungs by closure of the glottis, which is now interrupted by placement of an ETT. PEEP is used to keep alveoli open during exhalation, to allow more time for gas exchange, and to increase *functional residual capacity,* or the amount of air in the lungs at the end of expiration. Levels of PEEP above 10 cm H_2O put the patient at risk for alveolar rupture, pneumothorax, and decreased cardiac output via referred pressure counteracting forward blood flow from the heart. The ventilator-induced damage is termed *barotrauma.* In patients with severe ARDS, necessary PEEP levels can be as high as 25 cm H_2O.

Nursing Management

Nursing care of the patient who is mechanically ventilated requires expert technical skills.

Care is taken to simultaneously assess, intervene upon, and evaluate both the patient and the technology.

Assessing the Patient

The patient's physiologic response to illness or injury and particular indications for mechanical ventilation will determine the specific ventilator orders. The nurse should continually assess the patient's condition and resulting increase or decrease in ventilatory support required by said condition. For example, a patient with a recent decrease in neurologic function is no longer able to draw spontaneous breaths and will need an increase in the number of breaths provided by the ventilator.

Patients must be able to "allow" the ventilator to perform its function without interference caused by anxiety, biting the ETT, or problems with coughing or increased secretions. If the patient is able to let this happen and coordinate their own breaths with the machine, they are said to have *synchrony* with the ventilator. The nurse must assess the underlying cause of intolerance to mechanical ventilation and remove it in order to promote recovery of respiratory function. Common interventions include sedation, pain control, bronchodilators, and adequate suctioning.

Assessing the Equipment

The ventilator needs to be assessed to make sure that it is functioning properly and that the settings are appropriate. While not primarily responsible for the functioning of the ventilator, the nurse is responsible for the patient and, therefore, needs to evaluate how ventilator function affects the patient's overall status.

Ventilator alarms are designed to indicate that the ventilator is unable to deliver what it has been programmed to give the patient or that the patient is unable to tolerate the current settings.

Common problems with the ventilator include:

- Disconnection or kinking of tubing
- Disconnection of tubing from ETT or tracheostomy tube
- Water in the tubing
- Change in air temperature beyond set limits

Common problem with the settings includes:

- Limits set too high or too low, especially when exercising or weaning patients

Common problems with the patient include:

- Desynchronized breathing pattern between patient and ventilator
- Biting of the ETT
- Improper placement or inadvertent movement of ETT
- Coughing and/or sputum production interfering with air flow
- Lung or chest cavity fluid and pressure problems, as from heart failure, pulmonary edema, and pneumothorax

Pearls for Practice

Pressure limits is one of the ventilator settings with an alarm. Again, either patient condition or the equipment

may be the cause of an alarm. Pressure alarms on the ventilator may indicate a dangerous situation. Low-pressure alarms may indicate disconnection from the machine, ventilator circuit leak, endotracheal tube (ETT) cuff leakage, or migration of the ETT into the upper airway (the nurse assesses previous documented ETT placement marking at the lip or nares).

A high-pressure alarm usually indicates resistance to or obstruction of airflow from biting on the ETT, a kink in the tubing, buildup of secretions, patient coughing, or something as severe as bronchospasm or pneumothorax.

Preventing and Managing Adverse Effects of Mechanical Ventilation

As with many medical interventions, mechanical ventilation has the potential to cause complications or undesired secondary effects, and the nurse's priority is patient safety via a focus on preventing problems associated with any treatment modalities.

Ventilator-Associated Pneumonia. Currently, in the critical care world, ventilator-associated pneumonia (VAP) is receiving a lot of attention from patient advocacy groups, health care professionals, and regulatory bodies. It is caused by a patient being placed on a ventilator for a period of at least 48 hours whose oral and nasal secretions pooling above the ETT balloon fall into the lungs upon movement of the pliable balloon. Unfortunately, the mechanical ventilator is both a cause and an assistant in the treatment for pneumonia. The bacteriums found in patients with VAP are usually *Pseudomonas*, *Staphylococcus aureus*, *Escherichia coli*, *Klebsiella pneumoniae*, and *Acinetobacter* species, but any infection that is not present when a person is placed on a ventilator constitutes VAP.

This infection forces the hospital to develop, implement, and monitor a policy for its prevention. The most important intervention for infection control in the ICU remains handwashing and hand rubbing with alcohol-based solutions. Additional measures include avoiding intubation with the use of high-flow oxygen or NIV, minimizing sedation, daily tooth brushing (use of chlorhexidine mouth care is now controversial), head of bed elevated (30 to 45 degrees), early enteral nutrition and early tracheostomy (within 7 days of intubation) (Klompas et al., 2022).

Refer to Chapter 9 for more details on VAP.

Increased Intracranial Pressure. Upon receiving air, the positive pressure in the chest decreases venous return and may leave a higher volume of blood in the cranium. This can lead to altered LOC.

Altered Mental Status. Anxiety and discomfort from being placed on a ventilator, the frequent care in the form of suctioning, and persistent ventilator alarms can easily lead to sleep deprivation. Sleep deprivation, in turn, can affect changes in mental status and delay healing, as will be discussed further in this chapter.

Decreased Cardiac Output. The higher pressure in the pulmonary tree makes it difficult for blood to return to the heart from other areas of the body. If there is less blood returning, there is less blood to pump back to the body, causing hypotension and lower cardiac output.

Hypervolemia. The decreased pressure sensed by baroreceptors in the aorta may trick the body into believing hypovolemia exists; it reacts by stimulating production of antidiuretic hormone (ADH). Release of too much hormone may cause an overaccumulation of fluid in the vasculature, necessitating diuretics.

Venous Thromboembolism. Ventilated patients are prone to spending more time in bed due to instability or the practical difficulties of walking around when attached to the ventilator. Pooling of blood in the large veins of the legs (and upper extremities as well) while in bed can lead to clot formation and increase the possibility of pulmonary embolus (PE). With an incidence of 500,000 VTE among hospitalized patients (CDC, 2022a), deep venous thrombosis is an adverse effect with significant morbidity and potential mortality. Prophylaxis in the form of antiembolic stockings, sequential compression devices (SCDs), range-of-motion (ROM) activity, early mobility, and administration of anticoagulant medications (such as heparin) is advised for all patients who are intubated.

Barotrauma. As the name implies, barotrauma is damage to organs and vessels due to elevated pressures in the thoracic cavity. It is important to remember that this same trauma is possible in the abdominal cavity as well (further details on Abdominal Compartment Syndrome [ACS] are in Chapter 52; Fig. 52-4 details measuring intrabladder pressure).

Pneumothorax. Pneumothorax is a specific form of barotrauma resulting in the collapse of a lung (it is helpful to compare it to popping an overfilled balloon). Corrective action in the form of a chest tube is often required (Chapter 9 details this complication).

Gastrointestinal Bleeding. Critically ill patients are at risk for GI bleeding; severity of illness, use of circulatory support and renal replacement therapy are associated with higher likelihood of clinically important GI bleeding (Granholm et al., 2021). Stress ulceration usually occurs within 24 to 48 hours of onset of a critical illness and appears to be related to gastric erosions, rather than ulcers (Ferri, 2022). Although the reasons remain unclear, it is thought that gut ischemia and reperfusion injury leads to mucosal and/or deep tissue damage in the stomach and duodenum, which leads to ulcers and bleeding. The incidence of GI bleeding has decreased over the last few decades and is largely due to standard administration of proton pump inhibitors (PPIs, such as pantoprazole) or H_2-histamine antagonists (such as famotidine) in patients with previous or current GI bleeds. Although seen less frequently, the adverse effects of significant bleeding due to stress ulcers cannot be underestimated, and prophylaxis with the medications noted here remains the standard of care. However, recent research reveals that potential harm may be associated with stress ulcer prophylaxis, including increased risk of VAP (Klompas, 2019). In addition, further concerns include medication interactions, liver and bone marrow toxicity, and hypomagnesemia in ICU patients (Ferri, 2022). Guidelines for intervention are continuously evolving. It is up to the practitioner to keep up with the research findings and to apply the evidence to clinical practice.

Promoting Effective Airway Clearance

The presence of an ETT and continuous positive-pressure ventilation increases the production of secretions, regardless of the patient's underlying condition. Nursing interventions focus on maintaining a clear airway via turning and positioning, meticulous mouth care, and endotracheal/tracheal suctioning as needed.

Promoting Optimal Level of Mobility

The use of a mechanical ventilator limits the patient's mobility. The nurse helps the patient whose condition has become stable to get out of bed and move to a chair as soon as possible. Early mobility and muscle activity are beneficial because they stimulate respirations and improve patient psychological status. If the patient is unable to get out of bed, the nurse encourages performance of active ROM exercises every 6 to 8 hours. If the patient cannot perform these exercises, the nurse performs passive ROM exercises every 8 hours to prevent contractures and venous stasis. The nurse recalls that venous stasis which occurs in prolonged bed rest is a risk factor for deep vein thrombosis (DVT).

Promoting Optimal Communication

It is important to develop alternative methods of communication for the patient who is receiving mechanical ventilation. The nurse assesses the patient's communication abilities. Once the patient's limitations are known, the nurse offers several appropriate communication approaches: lip reading (use single key words), pad-and-pencil or erasable slate, communication board, electronic tablet, gesturing, sign language, or electric larynx. Use of a "talking" or fenestrated tracheostomy tube may be suggested to the provider; this allows the patient to talk while on the ventilator. The nurse makes sure that the patient's eyeglasses, hearing aid, sign interpreter, and language translator are available if needed to enhance the patient's ability to communicate.

Promoting Coping Ability

Encouraging the family to verbalize their feelings about the ventilator, the patient's condition, and the environment in general is beneficial. Explaining procedures helps reduce anxiety and familiarizes the patient with ventilator procedures. To restore a sense of control, the nurse encourages the patient to participate in decisions about care as appropriate. The patient may become withdrawn or depressed while receiving mechanical ventilation. It is important to provide diversions. Stress reduction techniques (e.g., a back rub, relaxation measures) help relieve tension and help the patient deal with anxieties and fears about the dependence on the ventilator.

Concept Mastery Alert

While tidal volume and vital capacity both describe the amount of air inhaled and exhaled, tidal volume is used for a normal breath, and vital capacity is used for the maximum amount of air that can be expelled after a maximum inhalation (measured as a forced vital capacity).

Weaning the Patient from the Ventilator

Mechanical ventilation is not a natural condition, and prolonged intubation carries a number of potentially serious side effects; therefore, every effort is made to make the need for this intervention as short as possible, with weaning from the ventilator initiated at the earliest possible time consistent with patient safety. The goal is to get the patient in the most optimal condition to succeed in weaning from the ventilator. While there are many indicators leading a practitioner to believe a patient is ready to wean, the following have proven the most predictive:

- Forced vital capacity (the maximum amount of air that can be expelled after a maximum inhalation) should be at least 10 mL/kg of ideal body weight.
- Negative inspiratory force (NIF, the ability to take a deep breath and to generate a cough strong enough to clear secretions; NIF should be at least –20 cm H_2O)
- Tidal volume (amount of air inhaled and exhaled in a normal breath; should be at least 5 mL/kg)
- Minute ventilation (total amount of air inhaled and exhaled in a minute; should be less than 10 L/min)
- Rapid shallow breathing index (RSBI, a ratio determined by the frequency of respirations [breaths per minute] divided by the tidal volume [measured in liters]); an RSBI less than 105 is considered criteria for weaning to extubation, while greater than 120 is considered as predictive of the continued necessity for ventilator support.

Other criteria to consider include:

- Cardiovascular stability
- Level of consciousness (Glasgow Coma Scale score >8)
- Adequate and stable arterial blood gas analysis (FiO_2 50% or less, PEEP 8 cm or less)
- Nutritional support with increasing or normal levels of phosphate, magnesium, and albumin
- Ability to swallow and manage saliva and secretions

ENDOCRINE ISSUES

The endocrine system participates along with the neurologic system to regulate bodily functions, such as growth and development, tissue function, metabolism, and even mood. Disorders of the endocrine system result from the secretion of too much or too little hormone, as well as from too much or too little sensitivity to a particular hormone.

This section covers hormones of particular importance in the critical care environment.

Problems Related to Antidiuretic Hormone

ADH is secreted from the posterior pituitary gland and helps to conserve water in the body. Head trauma and kidney disorders can decrease secretion, while trauma, various cancers, hemorrhage, and infection may lead to excessive secretion of ADH. Decreased secretion leads to diabetes insipidus (DI), while excessive secretion causes syndrome of inappropriate diuretic hormone (SIADH). Recall that DI or SIADH are commonly seen in TBI (see Chapters 30 and 44 for further discussion).

Patients at risk for altered ADH secretion should be monitored for neurologic changes as well as volume status via intake and output calculations, serum sodium levels, and serum and urine osmolality. Treatment for increased secretion involves water restriction, saline infusion, and use of demeclocycline, which blocks renal response to ADH. Treatment for decreased secretion is replacement of the hormone via one of the various forms of ADH, more commonly known as *arginine vasopressin*.

Problems Related to Thyroid Hormone

The thyroid gland uses iodine to make thyroxine (T_4) and triiodothyronine (T_3). These hormones are involved in body metabolism, alertness, mood, body temperature, and general energy and oxygen use. Disorders of secretion are viewed in relation to normal function; the trajectory ranges from:

Myxedema coma ↔ Hypothyroidism ↔ Normal function ↔ Hyperthyroidism ↔ Graves disease ↔ Thyroid storm

Critical illnesses, such as cancers and infections, can alter the secretion of these hormones. Metabolism is either adversely increased or decreased at a time when metabolic control is required. Too much hormone results in nervousness, anxiety, hyperthermia, tachycardia and eventual cardiac failure. Other patients with a history of thyroid disorders or surgery, or those not responding to a range of medical treatments, should have their thyroid hormone levels checked and supplemented, if necessary, to ensure assistance with increased metabolic demands.

Problems Related to Cortisol

Cortisol, secreted by the adrenal glands, is better known as the stress or fight-or-flight hormone. Levels are highest in the morning upon arising, in response to increased activity levels.

Problems related to too little or too much cortisol can be viewed on a continuum from:

Addison disease ↔ Normal function ↔ Cushing disease

At times, the level of this hormone is increased due to factors such as increased and prolonged stress; this leads to decreased cognition, hypertension, decreased thyroid and immune system function, hyperglycemia, and decreased bone density and muscle mass.

More commonly in the ICU, cortisol levels are low due to low perfusion states, infection, or adverse effects of medications. People with low levels of cortisol are unable to mount a physical response to bodily stressors and are likely to have fatigue, lower body temperature, hypoglycemia, and hypotension. Patients who meet clinical criteria for low cortisol levels are frequently given a cortisol stimulation test to determine if replacement is required to increase the body's metabolic response to illness.

Problems Related to Insulin

The beta cells of the pancreas secrete insulin to help move glucose into the cells to be used as an energy substrate. The majority of people with insulin disorders have type I or type II diabetes mellitus and are at particular risk for acute episodes of hyper- or hypoglycemia with the added stress of a critical illness. Patients with particularly brittle disease may be affected by sugar levels on this continuum:

Hypoglycemia ↔ Normal glucose level ↔ Diabetic ketoacidosis (DKA) or Hyperosmolar hyperglycemic nonketotic syndrome (HHNS), also called hyperglycemic hyperosmolar syndrome (HHS)

Patients with diabetes are frequently admitted to the ICU with complications of their illness, but it is also a disease frequently diagnosed for the first time while hospitalized. ICU patients are also at risk for "stress-induced" hyperglycemia due to release of stress hormones (cortisol, catecholamines), medications (epinephrine) and insulin resistance (refer to Chapter 29). All patients admitted to the ICU should have their blood glucose monitored three to four times a day to ensure they are able to maintain their glucose levels below each hospital's prescribed upper limit. For those who are unable to maintain a lower level of glucose, insulin therapy should be initiated according to hospital policy, with frequent monitoring of glucose levels to ensure lower levels without hypoglycemia. The most recent recommendations for insulin therapy target a glucose range of 140 to 180 mg/dL in most patients who are critically ill (Bohe et al., 2021).

GASTROINTESTINAL ISSUES

As with oxygen, food and drink becomes a medical prescription in the ICU. It is also regulated by practicalities such as kitchen schedules and nursing time to deliver food to or feed patients.

Nutritional Support

In the critical care unit, nutritional support is required to prevent catabolism of protein stores and provide the necessary elements for healing. The question in the ICU is not whether or not patients should be fed but, rather, when and how. Current trends in feeding include early initiation of enteral feedings whenever possible with increases to target energy needs within the first 48 hours of admission, with the preferred method being enteral (Compher et al., 2022).

Food

Because nature knows best, the optimal method of feeding patients is through oral intake of food and fluids. Specific diets will be altered depending on a patient's diagnoses. These may include altered content (low fat or low salt), altered consistency (soft or pureed), or with altered fluid (fluid restriction). The nurse ensures an environment and physical condition that makes the patient amenable to eating. Prevention of nausea and vomiting, pain relief, and proper positioning in a chair or upright in bed can all increase a person's appetite. At times, smaller more frequent meals consisting of something the patient likes to eat may help increase intake, maintain weight, and provide a diversion from the ICU environment.

Tube Feedings

A percentage of patients have a working GI tract but will not be able to take food orally due to their physiologic condition (dementia with dysphagia) or medical intervention (endotracheal intubation). These patients receive tube feedings. A particular liquid formula is recommended with collaboration of the dietician and medical practitioner. Again, the actual formula will depend upon the patient's diagnosis, current condition, and caloric or energy needs. Box 54-2 describes nursing responsibilities for patients receiving tube feedings. Tube feeding pumps deliver the nutrition via a variety of tubes that may include:

- *Nasogastric tube (NGT):* A tube inserted into the nares and ending in the stomach; used for gastric drainage or feeding (may be inserted orally [orogastric [OG] tube]) when nasal tubes are contraindicated or unable to be placed, for example, fracture of the cribriform plate, or has nasal or pharyngeal surgery (McGinnis, 2023).
- *Flexible feeding tube:* A synthetic tube of large or small bore (size) inserted into the nares to the stomach; softer, more flexible than the NGT, without the ability to convert to a drainage tube if needed.
- *Postpyloric tube:* A longer variety of the flexible feeding tube that reaches past the stomach into the duodenum, in order to use the small bowel when the stomach has the potential to not tolerate feeding or the risk of aspiration is high.
- *Percutaneous endoscopic gastrostomy (PEG) tube:* A tube inserted by the physician directly through the abdominal wall into the stomach; removes the discomfort, potential for accidental dislodgement, and potential for sinus infections caused by nasally inserted tubes.
- *Gastrojejunostomy (G-J) tube:* A tube that allows for simultaneous feeding of the small bowel and drainage of the stomach.

BOX 54-2

Caring for Patients Receiving Tube Feedings

With tube feeding patients, the nurse is responsible for:

- Noting that placement has been verified by the medical team via radiography, which is the gold standard for checking tube placement
- Assess patient's tolerance to medication and feeding administration (noting abdominal distention and complaints of abdominal pain, observing for passage of flatus and stool)
- Double-check placement by measurement of tube length, follow institutional procedures which may include assessing the pH measurement of aspirate (remains an area where further research is warranted) since measuring aspirate for pH is not a reliable method for distinguishing potential tube migration from the stomach to the esophagus (Bloom & Seckel, 2022); visual assessment of aspirate. In clinical practice, listening for air insufflation over the stomach may be seen, but this method is not accurate to determine placement (refer to Chapter 21)
- Assess skin circa the NG tube or G tube at routine time intervals for signs of pressure, erythema, rash, irritation, swelling, drainage and extra skin growth
- Preventing accidental dislodgement by patient or staff
- Maintaining patency of the tubes
- Monitoring for intolerance to feeding
- Monitoring for constipation and diarrhea

Pearls for Practice

Intolerance to feeding is a complicated issue with consequences for deteriorating nutritional status and aspiration pneumonia. Aspiration of GI contents into the lungs leads to increased morbidity and prolonged hospitalization. Risk factors for aspiration may include decreased mental status, placement of the head of the bed at less than 30 degrees, sedatives, vomiting, advanced age, mechanical ventilation, malpositioned feeding tube, major abdominal and thoracic surgery, neurologic disorders, diabetes mellitus, and high gastric residual volumes (Berta, 2022).

Parenteral Nutrition

Unfortunately, there are times when a patient is unable to tolerate enteral feeding and nutritional support must be given intravenously. Example of conditions where parenteral nutrition may include those patients with diminished absorption (e.g., short bowel syndrome, collagen vascular diseases such as scleroderma or Ehlers–Danlos syndrome, radiation enteritis), intestinal obstruction, peritonitis, or prolonged ileus (Berta, 2022). TPN or central parenteral nutrition (CPN) provides amino acids, dextrose, and fat. Because of its high osmolality, it must be given by a central catheter, such as a triple-lumen or Hickman catheter, or by a peripheral IV that terminates in a central vein, such as a PICC line. This type of support is used as a method to supplement or completely replace enteral feeding. However, it has numerous potential consequences, including pneumothorax during catheter insertion, catheter infection (due to high concentration of sugar in the solution), and liver failure. The goal is to use this support for as short a time as possible before returning to enteral feeds and eventually to having the patient provide their own oral intake. PPN may be administered via a peripheral IV because of the solution's lower osmolality. A number of metabolic complications are associated with parenteral nutrition, including hyperglycemia, electrolyte abnormalities, and irritation at the IV site. For more details on TPN/PPN refer to Chapter 21.

Immunonutrition

A deficit of nutrients can increase infection rates, length of hospital stay, and mortality. These nutrients are additional supplements to the various methods of feeding. Depending on patient diagnosis and condition, the nutrients in Table 54-10 should be considered.

Slow Motility

For a patient to tolerate feedings, the stomach must empty its contents into the small intestine, where nutrients are actually digested. This emptying is partially regulated by cholecystokinin (CCK) and polypeptide YY (PYY) levels that serve to slow gastric emptying. Unfortunately, it has been found that levels of these substances are elevated during critical illness, causing delayed emptying. Diabetes, gastroparesis (delayed gastric emptying), and slowed gut peristalsis due to

TABLE **54-10 Immunonutrition**

Element	Effects	Comment
Arginine (conditionally nonessential amino acid)	• Stimulation of growth hormone • Precursor in nitric oxide production • Improves immune function • Reduces healing time of injuries (particularly bone) • Increases muscle mass • Improved insulin sensitivity	Its use in septic patients remains controversial as the effects of sepsis on arginine metabolism or of arginine metabolism on sepsis are unclear.
Glutamine (conditionally nonessential amino acid)	• A substrate for DNA synthesis • Major role in protein synthesis • Primary source of fuel for enterocytes • Precursor for rapidly dividing immune cells, thus aiding in immune function • Regulation of acid–base balance in the kidney by producing ammonium • Alternative fuel source for the brain • Blocks cortisol-induced protein catabolism	It remains unclear whether outcomes are improved via enteral or IV administration.
Omega-3 fatty acids	• Reduced inflammation • Reduced lipid circulation in the bloodstream • Decreased platelet aggregation • Reduced cytokine production • Improved insulin sensitivity	
Copper	• Increased erythrocyte production • Increased absorption of iron • Maintenance of cytochrome p450 cycle • Vitamin C metabolism	
Selenium	• Maintenance of the cytochrome p450 system • DNA repair	
Zinc	• Increased growth hormone • Increased uptake of insulin • Increased cell division and promotion of wound healing • Treatment of diarrhea	

pain medications and calcium channel blockers are common causes of slow motility. This slow motility of gastric and intestinal contents can lead to nausea, vomiting, aspiration, and decreased nutritional status, which must be prevented or corrected as soon as possible. Current trends favor the use of promotility drugs, such as metoclopramide and/or erythromycin. It is not yet clear if these medications contribute to improved outcomes, and recommendations may change after future study. Adequate hydration and physical movement also assist in maintaining proper GI function.

If gastric motility cannot be improved, the general consensus dictates movement to small bowel feedings before adding or replacing enteral feeds with parenteral nutrition.

Diarrhea

Diarrhea is frequently seen in the ICU and has been found to be related to enteral therapy, hypoalbuminemia, antibiotic therapy, and sepsis. This makes the issue of diarrhea very difficult as enteral therapy is a treatment for low protein states and antibiotic therapy is required for treatment of overwhelming infections. Once diagnosed, the underlying cause, symptomatology, and potential adverse effects of diarrhea must be addressed and mitigated.

Causes

Enteral Therapy

The use of tube feedings is often required to prevent and treat malnutrition in the ICU. The clinical team needs to evaluate the composition of the prescribed feeding for possible changes required in the fiber or water content or osmolality. Current trends find that continuous feeding via a pump instead of intermittent feeding will decrease the amount of diarrhea. Patient care and testing often require changes of position, transfer, or NPO status, which interrupt feedings because it is considered unsafe to feed a patient while they are lying flat during turns and transfers. NPO status for individual medications (phenytoin, levothyroxine therapy) or tests also decreases nutritional intake. If possible, nursing needs to plan care in order to limit feeding interruptions. Fewer interruptions in feeding will maintain optimal caloric intake and reduce glucose fluctuations and the risk for diarrhea.

Hypoalbuminemia

Albumin is a protein responsible for maintaining oncotic pressure in the vascular system and, thus, distribution of fluids in the body. Low albumin levels cause water to leave the vasculature and accumulate in other parts of the body, such as the GI tract and tissues.

Antibiotics

The use of antibiotics changes normal gut flora depending upon the sensitivity of bacteria to the prescribed medications. The use of clindamycin, penicillins, cephalosporins, and fluoroquinolones are known to place patients at higher risk for overgrowth of *Clostridium difficile*, which forms a covering membrane inside the GI tract (pseudomembranes). The membrane acts to prevent absorption of fluid and nutrients and causes diarrhea. This particular infection requires yet another antibiotic treatment regimen with metronidazole and vancomycin.

Sepsis

Generalized infections not necessarily specific to the GI tract nonetheless have consequences for this system. Inflammation, cytokine release, and alterations in blood flow and the permeability of GI mucosa have also been found to cause diarrhea.

Symptoms and Adverse Effects

Diarrhea can be uncomfortable, painful, and embarrassing for the patient. It also requires extensive nursing time to keep patients clean and free of complications. The adverse effects of diarrhea are numerous and can impact outcomes. Hemodynamic instability due to fluid and electrolyte losses needs to be corrected with replacement of IV fluids, electrolytes, and minerals. This prevents cardiac arrhythmias and low perfusion states. Malnutrition due to poor absorption because of diarrhea, at a time when metabolic requirements are elevated, needs intervention with a possible change in feeding formula or supplementation with parenteral nutrition. Fecal contents and even skin cleansers change the normal pH of the skin and can lead to breakdown and the formation of pressure ulcers.

Prevention and Treatment of Diarrhea

The first goal is to prevent diarrhea. The second goal is to stop it as soon as possible if preventative efforts fail. Some of these efforts will be ordered by the provider, with patient response monitored by nursing. Interventions include:

- Change in feeding formula, with higher-fiber content or lower osmolality
- Prescription of probiotics, such as *Lactobacillus*, to alter gut flora
- Use of antidiarrheal medications, such as loperamide
- Frequent turning of patient to relieve pressure and enhance evaluation of skin
- Use of skin barrier lotions to prevent contact between skin and fecal contents

Constipation

Constipation, the infrequent or absence of bowel movements, is common in ICU patients and has been found to be related to use of opiates/opioids, enteral nutrition, bed rest, calcium channel blockers, GI dysmotility, and pseudo-obstruction. Constipation can lead to nausea, vomiting, intolerance of enteral feeds, distention, bloating and bowel perforation. Patients should be monitored for constipation, bowel movements (number and quality of) must be documented, and the use of bowel regimens considered in high-risk patients (Hay et al., 2019).

RENAL ISSUES

Many patients in a critical care unit are either at risk for or have pre-existing renal problems, particularly if they have a history of diabetes or hypertension. Damage to the renal system can be acute, chronic, or acute on chronic. Sources of kidney damage are classified as prerenal, intrarenal, and postrenal (refer to Chapter 26 for further details).

Promotion of Kidney Function

Despite the statistics given previously, many patients admitted to the ICU will have normal kidney function. However, admission to the ICU places patients at risk for kidney dysfunction; therefore, nurses need to monitor urine output and laboratory values such as serum creatinine, blood urea nitrogen, creatinine clearance, and glomerular filtration rates (GFRs) in order to ensure continued function or intervene as soon as possible in the event of declining function.

Spontaneous Voiding

The most comfortable method of urinating is to be able to go to the bathroom independently. The ability to do this necessitates functioning kidneys, the mental ability to recognize the need to void, and the physical strength and balance required for mobility. If patients are able to void spontaneously, the nurse should provide them every opportunity to do so. This eliminates the possibility of urinary catheter–related infections. It is important to note, however, that having to go to the bathroom is a very frequent reason for confused patients trying to get out of bed. The practice of toileting patients every few hours prevents the consequences of falls, incontinence, and skin breakdown.

External Urinary Catheters

Condom catheters are placed on penises and external suction catheters (PureWick) are placed between labial folds when patients are able to void spontaneously and strict hourly monitoring of urinary output is not required. In addition, if patients are confused, unable to realize the need to urinate, or lack the ability to use a bathroom or urinal, this provides an alternative to incontinence.

Urinary Catheters

Urinary catheters are inserted into the bladder by way of the urethra and are used to provide samples of urine for testing, a method of monitoring urine output when concerned with hemodynamic compromise, and as a means for controlling incontinence and skin breakdown. While convenient for staff, urinary catheters are associated the majority of all nosocomial infections in hospitalized patients (3.16/1,000 catheter days), known as catheter-associated urinary tract infections (CAUTIs) (Rosenthal et al., 2021). Standard practice should include aseptic insertion, daily preventative cleaning of the catheter with soap and water, wiping away from the urethra, episodic cleaning after bowel movements as noted previously, maintaining a closed system, ensuring the drainage bag is below the level of the bladder, and proper anchoring of the catheter on the leg to prevent undue strain on it.

According to the CDC, the most important risk factor for developing a CAUTI is prolonged use of the urinary catheter (CDC, 2015). Thus, the removal of the catheter at the earliest possible time is recommended.

Acute Kidney Injury

Acute kidney injury (AKI), an abrupt reduction in kidney function within a 7-day period or less, occurs in up to 50% of ICU patients and increases mortality, and the development of chronic kidney disease (CKD) and end-stage renal disease (ESRD) (Chawla et al., 2017). Patents' ability to filter and excrete metabolic waste is impaired; common causes of AKI in critically ill patients are sepsis (40%), hypovolemia (34%), drug or medication related (14%), and cardiogenic shock (13%) (Lough, 2022). Prevention of further deterioration of kidney function is critical. This will include hemodynamic support to maintain blood flow, as the kidneys require up to 20% of the cardiac output. In addition, the medical team and pharmacists have to evaluate drug dosages because the clearance of medications is impacted by renal excretion. Patients requiring IV contrast for radiographic studies are often prescribed "renal protection" in the form of IV normal saline, before their studies, along with using the lowest possible dose of contrast for the study since contrast-induced nephropathy (CIN) is a cause of AKI. The incidence of CIN–AKI ranges from 6% to 27%, and risk factors for CIN-AKI include pre-existing impaired renal function, diabetes, left ventricular dysfunction, and anemia (Efe et al., 2021). Medications that may increase risk of nephrotoxicity are withheld prior to contrast studies (e.g., nonsteroidal anti-inflammatory agents, metformin). Refer to Chapter 26 for additional details on CIN and AKI. Despite all efforts, some patients will progress from renal insufficiency to kidney failure, so the nurse must remain vigilant to deteriorating function.

Kidney Failure

Patients with AKI and worsening CKD have higher rates of morbidities and mortality; therefore, efforts to mimic normal renal mechanisms are accomplished via continuous renal replacement therapy (CRRT) or dialysis until kidney function resumes. Patients with ESRD, also termed end-stage kidney failure, have the option of complete renal replacement for extended periods of time.

Pearls for Practice

An insult to renal perfusion previously termed acute tubular necrosis (ATN), is now termed a form of AKI (Lough, 2022). It is commonly related to hypoperfusion and/or nephrotoxic agents, and is associated with patients who are critically ill. Nephrotoxins include hemoglobin (from hemolysis of RBCs) and myoglobin (from muscle breakdown or rhabdomyolysis) as occurs in crush injury, heatstroke, and seizure (Kallenbach, 2022). Therefore, the nurse monitors urinary output hourly in patients who are critically ill, assesses the serum peak and trough levels of nephrotoxic medications, and alerts the provider when urinary output is less than 30 mL/hr (or 0.5 mL/kg/hr) and/or abnormal peak and trough levels are seen. If recognized early, kidney function can be restored by improving renal blood flow, typically with IV fluids.

Renal Replacement

Renal replacement is accomplished via CRRT, hemodialysis, peritoneal dialysis, or kidney transplant through either cadaver or living donation. Dialysis can be provided for a short period of time, to allow the kidneys time to recover from an AKI; as a bridge to renal transplantation; or on a permanent basis. Other indications for starting renal replacement therapy include:

- Uremic encephalopathy: Confusion, asterixis, and seizures
- Pericarditis
- Bleeding
- Fluid overload unresponsive to diuretics
- Pleuritis
- Metabolic derangements: Metabolic acidosis, hyperkalemia, hyperphosphatemia, hyper- or hypocalcemia
- Overdose of medications/poisons that are dialyzable
- Contraindication to hemodialysis and peritoneal dialysis

Renal replacement therapies are discussed in detail in Chapter 26.

MUSCULOSKELETAL ISSUES

People admitted to critical care units are usually confined to bed for extended periods of time. Neurologic, cardiovascular, and respiratory instability are reasons why patients are restricted to bed rest in the ICU. Sometimes interventions (ICP monitors, balloon pumps) or the desire to prevent the increased oxygen demands of movement (heart failure, respiratory insufficiency/failure) necessitate bed rest. Other reasons for prolonged bed rest include conflicting priorities in the nursing staff ("Do I spend my time with my patient who is actively hemorrhaging, or with the one who needs to get out of bed?"), or lack of knowledge regarding the importance of physical activity. Being in the recumbent position is not a natural state, and prolonged bed rest has a plethora of adverse effects that are outlined in Table 54-11. Deconditioning is seen in patients after as few as 3 days of bed rest. This leads to a decline in overall ability to function and increases the need for admittance into rehabilitation centers after hospitalization. It is important for nurses to be aware of these potential complications and to create the opportunity for movement and limitation of bed rest activity whenever possible.

TABLE **54-11 Effects of Bed Rest**

System	Potential Effects
Neurologic	Anxiety Hallucinations
Cardiovascular	Hypovolemia Decreased carotid baroreceptor response Orthostatic hypotension Deep venous thrombosis
Respiratory	Atelectasis Pneumonia Pulmonary embolus
Gastrointestinal	Ileus Constipation
Genitourinary	Urinary stasis Renal calculi
Endocrine	Insulin resistance Hyperglycemia
Musculoskeletal	Muscular atrophy Bone demineralization Contractures
Skin	Decubitus ulcers Reduced skin integrity
Psychosocial	Depression
Other	Increased catabolism of immunoglobulin G Increased colonization with *Staphylococcus aureus*

Data from Timmerman, R. A. (2007). A mobility protocol for critically ill adults. *Dimensions of Critical Care Nursing*, *26*(5), 175–179; and Rubin, M. (1988). The physiology of bed rest. *The American Journal of Nursing*, *88*(1), 50–58.

ICU-Acquired Weakness

ICU-acquired weakness is an increasingly recognized disorder characterized by the inability of a patient to move against resistance. Gosselin et al. (2021) described this as "intensive care unit-acquired weakness (ICUAW)," a complication associated with increased short- and long-term morbidity and mortality. It encompasses both myopathy and neuropathy with multifactorial causes beyond the scope of this chapter. Patients at risk for this disorder include those with systemic inflammatory response syndrome (SIRS) and sepsis, hyperglycemia, as well as those receiving corticosteroids or neuromuscular blocking agents. Weakness can be difficult to diagnose in the ICU due to confounding issues, such as altered neurologic status, but is often first noticed when patients are unable to be removed from a ventilator. Preventative and rehabilitative measures generally include early identification and treatment of potential causes of multiple organ failure (in particular severe sepsis and septic shock), avoiding unnecessary deep sedation and hyperglycemia, promotion of early mobilization, and thoughtful decisions regarding the risks versus benefits of corticosteroids.

Contractures

Contractures are limitations in full active and passive ROM of a joint with resultant inability to perform activities of daily living. Dammeyer et al. (2013) noted shortening of muscle sarcomeres and the start of contractures begin with just 1 day of bed rest; immobilization also causes decreased muscle fiber diameter, reduces the capacity to synthesize proteins, and leads to an overall reduction in muscle volume (Stein & Chowdhury, 2019). Prevention is key by frequent active and passive ROM of the joint, early and frequent use of corrective splinting, and physical therapy. The use of transcutaneous electrical nerve stimulation (TENS) has been suggested to stretch the ankle joint to prevent the diminished range of ankle motion that occurs in patients admitted to the ICU; results revealed more improvement in ankle dorsiflexion and plantar flexion in prevention of ankle joint stiffness (Shamsi et al., 2019).

Foot drop (Fig. 54-7) is a specific type of contracture defined by the inability to lift the dorsum (anterior surface) of the foot and toes upward (dorsiflexion). It can be caused by neurologic or muscular diseases as well as by inactivity during bed rest. The inability to lift the feet impairs the person's ability to mobilize and improve overall functioning.

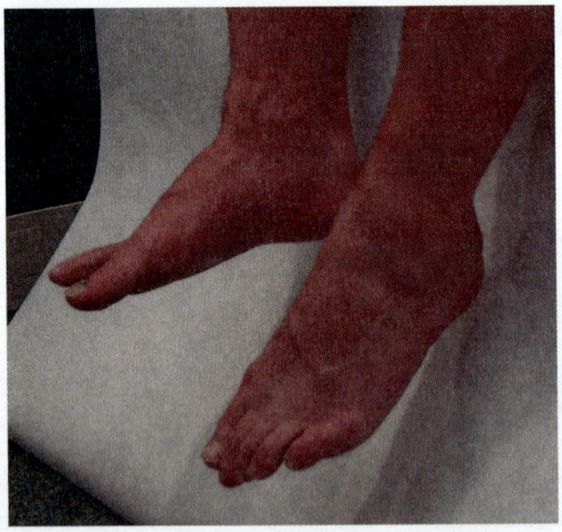

FIGURE 54-7 Foot drop is a consequence of weakened muscles for dorsiflexion, resulting in permanent plantarflexion. (From Lambert, H. W., & Wineski, L. E. [2010]. *Lippincott's illustrated Q&A review of anatomy and embryology* [2nd ed.]. Lippincott Williams & Wilkins.)

The use of multi-podus boots or foot drop boots to maintain dorsiflexion, are devises used to prevent foot drop. In addition, active and passive ROM and early ambulation are nursing interventions to prevent foot drop and improve post-ICU recovery.

Nitrogen Wasting

To maintain a healthy state, the body requires equilibrium between the amounts of protein supplied and muscle mass breakdown/turnover. Refer to Box 21-2, Establishing Positive Nitrogen Balance, for further details on attaining and maintaining a positive nitrogen balance. Critical illness often leads to increased requirements at a time when protein is either used for healing or lost at a higher rate due to immobility and/or disease processes.

Bone Demineralization

Weight-bearing contributes to calcium uptake by the bones, promoting continued strength and bone formation. When on bed rest, calcium is excreted from the bones at higher levels, while at the same time the patient may be at risk for decreased intake due to anorexia or intolerance to feedings.

Pearls for Practice

The variety of ill effects from bed rest demonstrated throughout the literature and in this book should alert every nurse to the need for their patients to move. If out of bed activity is restricted, active/passive ROM should be employed, at a minimum of every shift. It is important to note that while sitting in a chair is helpful, the need to walk is paramount in terms of improving cardiovascular, respiratory, GI, and musculoskeletal status. In short, if allowed, the nurse should encourage and help the patient to get out of bed.

INTEGUMENTARY ISSUES

Admission to the ICU places the patient's skin at risk. Because of decreased mental status or decreased ability to change position, hypoperfusion, fever, immobility, and restraint, a patient may not be able to move in response to discomfort. The state of a patient's skin should be documented on arrival to the unit, in order to follow changes. This documentation also has financial implications as Medicare is no longer reimbursing hospitals for hospital-acquired alterations in skin integrity, such as pressure ulcers.

Planned Medical Breaks in Skin Integrity

Intravenous Lines

The skin is normally one contiguous unit. The simple act of placing a peripheral IV in a patient disrupts skin continuity and serves as a planned medical break in the skin and a potential source of infection. All IV lines should be monitored for signs of infection (erythema [redness], warmth, and discharge at the IV site or an elevated temperature), and lines should be changed according to hospital policy.

Procedures

Minor procedures, such as pacemaker or PEG placement, are other examples of planned medical interventions that require breaks in the skin. Again, infection control is of paramount importance.

Surgery

Surgical procedures interrupt skin and tissue integrity. Postsurgical infections can arise from deep tissue and organs, but surgical incisions require specific care and attention to prevent infection and poor wound healing.

Unplanned Breaks in Skin Integrity

Skin Tears

A majority of patients in the ICU are older individuals and are affected by natural changes in the skin. More specifically, there is a flattening of the dermis and increased movement between the dermis and epidermis. When the two are separated, a skin tear occurs. ICU patients are prone to skin tears due to their age, medication history (chronic steroid use), immobility, shock states, use of vasopressors and altered mental status. ICU patients are also prone to skin tears due to nursing interventions, such as tape removal, as well as due to friction and shear forces when pulling patients up in bed. Protection of the limbs from skin tears requires vigilance and patience on the part of the nurse. This means asking for enough help to turn or move a large patient.

Pressure Injuries

A hospital-acquired pressure injury (HAPI) is a localized injury to the skin and/or underlying tissue, usually over a bony prominence, as a result of pressure alone or pressure in combination with shear and/or friction. These breaks in the skin can progress from the skin to subcutaneous tissue and bone. Because muscle and subcutaneous tissue are more susceptible to pressure-induced injury (also known as deep tissue injury), than skin, pressure ulcers are often worse than their initial appearance. Pressure ulcers are staged to guide clinical description of the depth of observable tissue destruction (see Chapter 51). Padula and Delarmente (2019) state that these wounds cost the U.S. health care system up to 26.8 billion dollars each year. See Chapter 51 for pressure ulcer staging and management.

Box 54-3 provides risk factors for pressure injuries development.

Unfortunately, many patients in critical care have one or more of these risk factors.

BOX 54-3 Risk Factors for Pressure Ulcer Development

- Malnutrition
- Hemodynamic instability
- Predisposing diseases, such as diabetes
- Advanced age
- Infection
- Motor/sensory deficits
- Decreased mental status
- Incontinence
- Mechanical ventilation
- Mobility/activity deficit

Medications, such as sedatives, vasoactive agents, neuromuscular blocking agents

- Contractures
- Spasms
- Prolonged ICU stay

Pearls for Practice

Nurses hold the vast majority of responsibility for patient skin assessment, frequent turning, and skin care for pressure ulcer prevention. Early identification of and aggressive treatment for such ulcers is required.

PSYCHOSOCIAL ISSUES

Entry into an ICU is stressful for patients and for their friends and families. Psychosocial issues can also play a part in the reason for ICU admission. Substance use disorder, violence, and reckless behaviors can all lead to serious accidents and illnesses. Nurses must always consider the possible psychosocial issues and disruptions that patients and families are confronting.

Fear

Every patient and family should be assessed to determine the presence of psychosocial issues. Fear or apprehension, awe, or anxiety due to perceived danger is a frequent entity in critical care. Patients and families can be afraid of death, permanent disability, fear of the unknown, and the critical care environment itself, where care of oneself or a loved one is entrusted to strangers. Lack of information regarding the plan of care and prognosis, as well as lack of understanding of the information provided, is also a common cause of fear. Patients who frequently use the call bell or call out for help and family members who are confrontational or demand constant nursing presence in the patient's room provide examples of not coping with the stress of ICU admission. Methods of decreasing fear for patients and families and decreasing the occurrence of PTSD and post-ICU syndrome are not complex, yet they require time and patience on the part of nursing staff (Sayde et al., 2020). Suggestions for allaying fear include:

- Introduction of staff and their roles in caring for the patient
- Explanation of what you are going to do to or with a patient and why
- Allowing family and friends to be present in the room
- Frequent updates to families
- Diary keeping
- Educating patients and families according to needs and desires
- Informing patients and families of progress or failure to progress

Grieving

Grieving is the process of coming to terms with loss: one's impending death, death of a loved one, loss of function and freedom, loss of self-image, and loss of future opportunities. The stages of grief are well defined throughout the literature, and all nurses should be aware of them. People will differ in their coping behaviors, and nurses should help people develop their best coping practices possible. This is a difficult and often time-consuming process. If nurses are unable to spend much time with grieving patients and families, it is imperative to find the patient alternative help: a colleague with more experience with grieving patients, a pastor, a social worker, hospital volunteers, family, or friends.

Violence

Violence in the home and workplace should never be tolerated, but it is a fact that critical care nurses must confront. Patients may have been a victim of past or recent injury. The sad fact is that many nurses can also report being a victim of violence at the hands of their patients or visitors at a 20% higher rate than other professions (Sarver et al., 2019). This included intimidation, verbal abuse, threats of physical violence, or actual violence. The nurse's goals are to identify patients at risk for being abused by others in their life, identify patients or families with a potential for violence against hospital staff, and establish a zero-tolerance workplace violence policy across the nation. The American Nurses Association (2019) notes that violence against health care worker is at "epidemic proportions," and encourages the reporting of workplace violence, the removal of barriers to reporting, and the creation of workplace culture that has "zero tolerance toward workplace violence."

Patient Safety

Many people live with violence in their home, either through neglect or outright physical abuse. The older population requiring significant time and resources from family members may be at increased risk for abuse as others become frustrated with their increasing disabilities. Assessing for a history of past injuries or evidence of current injury with appropriate referrals is warranted.

Patients with suicidal ideation also need to be protected in the acute care setting. This may include:

- A provider's order for one-to-one observation at all times
- A provider's order for chemical or mechanical restraint
- Removal of dangerous objects in the room
- Limit-setting and negotiation with the patient
- Family and/or friend intervention as appropriate

Staff Safety

Patients at risk for harming staff members require specific interventions:

- Notification of security and administration of the potential for violence
- Keeping the patient in view at all times
- Approaching the patient with a calm but firm demeanor only with support from colleagues (and security as required)

END-OF-LIFE ISSUES

The critical care nurse will encounter many patients of various ages who are facing the ends of their lives. Some of these deaths are unexpected, while others are anticipated. Each critical care nurse needs to be aware of their patient's medical prognosis and the patient's and family's response to a poor prognosis. Coping mechanisms will vary widely and range from sitting vigil by the patient to avoidance. An important component of care is providing patients with realistic information about their prognosis and end-of-life care while providing emotional support as they adjust to the idea of death. See Chapter 2 for more details on end-of-life care.

Unexpected Death

Society expects that young people will not die. Sadly, accidents, suicides, and illness do claim young lives. This requires nurses to be cognizant of these issues and support patients and families through anger, denial, and the other stages of grief. A number of studies have demonstrated that being with the patient at the end of life is important for many, and those who request it should have someone present whenever they wish—including during resuscitation efforts.

If there is to be any solace in the death of a young or relatively young person, it can be found in the arena of organ and tissue donation. Patients who meet the criteria for past health and current diagnosis of brain death are eligible to donate organs to those on the various transplant lists. This places nurses in a difficult position at times due to their simultaneous obligations to care for a particular patient and their family while informing organ donation services of a potential donor. When the diagnosis of brain death is made, it is usually up to the senior medical staff and organ procurement services to approach the family about the possibility of organ donation.

Expected Death

Patients with a severe chronic illness or those of an advanced age have most likely had a number of experiences with the health care system and may be somewhat more mentally and emotionally prepared for death. ICU nurses need to be aware of their patients' advanced directives and living wills in order to advocate for their wishes during hospital care. These patients may have placed limits on what treatments they will allow in the event they can no longer speak for themselves, and nurses need to support these wishes or changes in those wishes. At this stage of their patient's life, nurses can provide the means to make the patient as comfortable as possible while allowing family and friends to come to terms with the impending loss of a loved one.

OTHER ISSUES

Sleep

Sleep is an essential bodily function, with significant impact on recovery from illness. Critical care patients are known to become sleep deprived due to their illness, ICU admission, pain, medical procedures, and nursing care. No matter the cause, sleep deprivation has been associated with adverse effects in the ICU (Ortiz, 2020).

Nursing care interferes with patients' ability to move through the stages of sleep toward rapid eye movement (REM), the deepest form of sleep. It requires an average of 90 minutes to reach REM sleep. How often is a patient left comfortable and undisturbed for at least 90 minutes in an ICU? The answer is not often enough.

A number of interventions may assist in promoting sleep:

- Clustering care
- Adequate pain relief
- Ensuring synchrony with the ventilator
- Noise and light reduction (lights out/low, sleep eye masks, ear plugs)
- Day and night routines
- Sleep-promoting medications, such as melatonin
- Relaxation therapy, massage, and white noise
- Alarm limits (set limits appropriate to the individual patient, to minimize nuisance alarms)

Falls

It has been estimated that up to 40% of hospital adverse events are related to patient falls, with over one million occurrences annually, with up to 50% of those patients suffering bodily injury (de Freitas Luzia et al., 2020; Dolan et al., 2021). Despite the implementation of fall prevention programs, research reveals little impact on decreasing fall rates while a patient is hospitalized. Ideally, the only way to prevent falls is to have a mentally and physically strong enough person be with each patient at all times; something not financially feasible for most hospitals. Realistically, what can be done is to identify risk factors for falling and arrange the care environment as well as possible to reduce the possibility of falls occurring (Table 54-12).

Transport of the ICU Patient

Patients who are critically ill are often safest inside the ICU, where staff and equipment are available for monitoring as needed. New technology has led to the availability of an ever-increasing number of tests and interventions that are able to be done at the bedside. This includes portable x-rays, endoscopies, and ultrasounds and even minor surgical procedures, such as percutaneous tracheostomy and PEG tube placement. However, there are a number of times when a patient will require transportation from the ICU to the operating room or, more frequently, to the radiology department. The radiology department may be required for tests such as computed tomography (CT) scan or intervention such as cardiac stent placement. Intra-hospital movement of patients has long been known to be the cause of adverse effects: pain, increased intracranial pressure, hypotension, arrhythmia, hypoxia, VAP, decreased nutritional intake, hypo- and hyperglycemia, inadvertent disconnection from equipment, and falls.

Patients are placed at risk from transport due to decreased number of staff available to the patient, disruptions in continuity of care, decreased ability to monitor patients in places like the magnetic resonance imaging (MRI) suite, and possible adverse effects of the test itself. With these known risks to patient safety, a number of tools and guidelines have been developed to minimize adverse events associated with transport.

One communication tool, often called a "ticket to ride" using the Situation-Background-Assessment-Recommendation (SBAR; see Fig. 54-8), can be used to exchange information about a patient being transferred to the care of another health care professional. This tool ensures that all pertinent information required is up to date and available on one piece of paper as a reference for the person taking charge of the patient's care (Agency for Healthcare Research and Quality [AHRQ], 2021).

Transfer from the ICU

Eventually, all patients with some form of recovery will be discharged from the ICU. This usually occurs after morning provider rounds, when it is decided the patient is well enough to leave the unit for a lower level of care, such as a progressive care/step-down unit or other appropriate nursing unit. However, the need for ICU beds in the United States remains high, and many times, especially during the COVID-19 pandemic where ICU bed shortages required triaging and the least ill patient in the ICU to transfer out, to make room for someone more critically ill; and formulating surge plans with staff redeployment to newly instituted

TABLE **54-12 Minimizing Falls**

Risk Factors	Nursing Interventions to Decrease Risk for the Individual

History of falls	• Identify the patient as being at risk for falls.
	• Implement fall protocol.
	  • Use of hipsters or protective hip wear
	  • Use of helmets for the head, if at risk for head injury

Fear of falling	• Encourage patient to verbalize feelings. • Institute physical therapy consult to help patient demonstrate their ability to move safely.
Bowel and bladder incontinence	• Implement toileting routine. • Provide easy access to urinal/bedpan • Monitor bowel function to prevent diarrhea and constipation.
Cognitive impairment	• Evaluate patient for reversible causes of cognitive impairment/delirium and eliminate causes as possible. • Institute close observation by placing patient in view of nursing staff. • Start one-to-one observation. • Use monitoring devices, such as bed and chair exit alarms.
Mood	• Encourage verbalization of feelings. • Evaluate patient's ability to concentrate and learn new information. • Encourage engagement in daily activities. • Provide diversional activity. • Refer to geriatric psychiatry as appropriate.
Dizziness	• Monitor lying, sitting, and standing blood pressures, and continually evaluate for factors contributing to dizziness. • Dangle the patient for 5 minutes before rising with assistance • Set up environment to avoid movements that result in dizziness/vertigo. • If diabetic, monitor blood sugars and facilitate interventions to maintain appropriate blood sugars.
Functional impairment	• Encourage participation in personal care activities at highest level (i.e., if possible, encourage ambulation to bathroom rather than use of bedpan). • Use of rubber-soled heeled shoes or nonskid slippers • Use of corrective lenses for walking if appropriate • Refer to physical and occupational therapy as appropriate.
Medications	• Review medications with medical practitioner and determine need for each medication. • Ascertain that medications are being used at lowest dosages to obtain desired results.
Medical problems	• Assure patient that medical problems are not a reason to remain in bed and prevent participation in functional activities.
Environment	• Remove furniture if patient can't sit on it and have their feet reach the floor. • Remove clutter. • Make sure furniture and any assistive devices used are in good condition. • Make sure lighting is adequate. • Easy access to call light • *Avoid* the use of four side rails and other forms of restraint.

Data from Gray-Miceli, D. & Quigley, P. (2012). Preventing falls in acute care. In M. Boltz, E. Capezuti, T. Fulmer & D. Zwicker (Eds.), *Evidence-based geriatric nursing protocols for best practice* (4th ed.). Springer Publishing Company.

"ICU" beds (Wells et al., 2021). ICU discharges frequently happens late in the day or at night, when floor nursing staff levels are lower. It has been found that transfer from the ICU from 4:00 pm to 7:59 am pm is associated with readmission to the ICU and increased mortality (Vollam et al., 2022). More recently, an international panel of 27 intensive care experts reached consensus on a set of 28 intensive care discharge criteria for adult ICU patients, that reflect the patient's organ systems (respiratory [7], cardiovascular [9], central nervous [1], and urogenital system [2]), pain (1),

SBAR (Situation, Background, Assessment, Recommendation)*

NOTE: **Pronounced S-BAR** and first used by the military to improve the effectiveness of communication between care givers, the SBAR approach is recommended by patient safety experts. SBAR forms vary depending on purpose and setting. Some places use SBAR for giving hand-off situations (when one nurse transfers patient care to another). Some places use SBAR forms like the one below for calling physicians about a problem.

S **SITUATION:** Have the chart in hand before you make the phone call, and be sure you can readily communicate all the following: Briefly state the issue or problem: what it is, when it happened (or how it started) and how severe it is. Give the signs and symptoms that cause you concern.

B **BACKGROUND:** Give the date of admission and current medical diagnoses. Determine the pertinent medical history and give a brief synopsis of the treatment to date (eg, medications; oxygen use; nasogastric tube; IVs, code status).

A **ASSESSMENT:** Give most recent vital signs and any changes in the following:

- ❑ Mental status – neuro signs
- ❑ Respirations
- ❑ Pulse – skin color
- ❑ Comfort – Pain
- ❑ GI status (nausea-vomiting-diarrhea, distention)
- ❑ Urine Output
- ❑ Bleeding-Drainage
- ❑ Other: ________________

R **RECOMMENDATION:** State what you think should be done. For example:

- ❑ Come see the patient now
- ❑ Get a consultation
- ❑ Get additional studies (eg, CXR, ABG, EKG, CBC, other)
- ❑ Transfer the patient to ICU
- ❑ If the patient doesn't improve
- ❑ How frequent do you want vital signs.
- ❑ If there's no improvement, by when do you want us to call you?

*Data from: Haig, K, Sutton, S. and Whittington, J. (2006). SBAR: A Shared Mental Model for Improving Communication Between Clinicians. *Journal of Quality and Patient Safety, 32*(3), 167–175. Available: http://www.jcipatientsafety.org/fpfd/psp/SBAR.pdf

Source: R. Alfaro-LeFevre Handouts © 2007–2013 www.AlfaroTeachSmart.com

FIGURE 54-8 SBAR Tool promotes consistent communication. (From Alfaro-LeFevre, R. [2013]. *Applying nursing process*. Lippincott Williams & Wilkins.)

fluid loss and drainages (1), medication and nutrition (1), patient diagnosis, prognosis and preferences (2), and institution-specific criteria (4) (Hiller et al., 2022). Nursing workload at the discharging and the receiving unit, technical infrastructure, skill sets, patient/nurse ratios, protocols, and processes are included (Hiller et al., 2022). Further research will be needed to validate the criteria. While we know that the decision to transfer a patient is a medical and administrative one, nurses must either advocate for their patients to stay in the ICU or put their patients in the best position to do well outside of the ICU. Doing well outside of the ICU is the goal for all patients.

CHAPTER REVIEW

NCLEX-Style Review Questions

1. The nurse is caring for a 72-year-old patient admitted with pneumonia and is intubated on a ventilator. During assessment, the nurse finds the ventilator high airway pressure is alarming. What are the possible reasons for a high airway pressure to occur? Select all that apply.

a. Disconnection of ventilator from the endotracheal tube (ETT)
b. A buildup of pulmonary secretions
c. ETT cuff leakage
d. Check to see if the patient is agitated and biting the ET tube
e. Patient coughing

2. A patient, who underwent a total gastrectomy due to cancer, has just arrived from the operating room. The patient has a Salem sump tube (SST; double-lumen NG tube) in place. Care of this patient and the SST tube include which of the following actions? Select all that apply.

a. Placing the SST to low continuous wall suction
b. Frequent and vigorous flushing of the NG tube to ensure patency
c. Placing a sign at the head of the bed reminding staff not to alter the tube's position
d. Ensuring the NG tube is securely taped to the patient's nose and noting measurement in the plan of care
e. Head of bed should be flat to facilitate drainage

3. The nurse knows that the inability to wean from a ventilator is associated with which of the following laboratory or diagnostic studies? Select all that apply.

a. Albumin level of 4.0 g/dL
b. Tidal volume of 7 mL/kg
c. Normal sinus rhythm
d. Rapid Shallow Breathing Index of 130
e. Negative inspiratory force of –15 mm Hg

4. The nurse knows that complications associated with bed rest include which of the following? Select all that apply.

a. Hypertension
b. Constipation
c. Decubitus ulcer
d. Kidney stones
e. Venous stasis

5. You are admitting a 92-year-old patient to the ICU after a motor vehicle accident where the patient was unrestrained. The patient's GCS is 8, is currently intubated, vital signs are stable. The patient has a history of diabetes. Which of the following are risks for pressure-induced injury of the skin? Select all that apply.

a. Advancing age
b. Stable vital signs
c. GCS of 8
d. Mechanical ventilation
e. Recent admission to the ICU

REFERENCES AND SELECTED READINGS

References and selected readings associated with this chapter can be found on the website that accompanies the book. Visit **http://thepoint.lww.com/Honan3e** to access the references and other additional resources associated with this chapter.

CHAPTER 55

Nursing Management: Emergencies and Disasters

Deborah S. Adelman • Sharon Druce

Learning Objectives

After reading this chapter, you will be able to:

1. Describe primary and secondary survey content and assessment of the patient experiencing an emergency.
2. Discuss priority emergency measures instituted for any patient with an urgent condition.
3. Discuss the priorities and assessment of the patient experiencing traumatic injuries.
4. Describe the fundamental elements of a hospital disaster plan.
5. Discuss how triage in an emergency differs from triage in a disaster.
6. Identify the effects of prolonged stress on health care workers.
7. Identify resources and techniques for self-care for health care workers.
8. Evaluate the different levels of personal protection and decontamination procedures that may be necessary during an event involving mass casualties or weapons of mass destruction.
9. Identify the effects of chemical and nerve agents and the decontamination and treatment procedures that are necessary.

The emergency nurse has had specialized education, training, and experience, and has expertise in assessing and identifying patients' health care problems in crisis situations. The emergency nurse establishes priorities, monitors and continuously assesses patients of all ages who are acutely ill and injured, supports and attends to families, supervises allied health personnel, and teaches patients and families, all within a time-limited, high-pressured care environment. An additional component of emergency nursing is providing in-hospital care during disasters when local resources are overwhelmed.

EMERGENCY NURSING

The nursing process provides a logical framework for problem solving in the emergency department (ED). Patients in the ED have a wide variety of actual or potential problems, and their condition may change constantly. Therefore, nursing assessment must be continuous, and clinical decision making and interventions must adjust with the patient's condition. Emergency nursing requires an understanding of triage as well as assessment and management of common acute disorders and injuries.

FOUNDATIONS OF EMERGENCY NURSING

Triage

Triage is used to sort patients into groups based on the severity of their health problems and the immediacy with which these problems must be treated. All EDs share this characteristic of a hierarchy based on the potential for loss of life. A basic and widely used triage system that was in use for many years consisted of three categories: **emergent**, **urgent**, and **nonurgent** (The ESI Triage Research Team, LLC, 2020; Box 55-1). In this acuity system, patients who may have needed many resources yet had a lower acuity need might have been assigned a lower triage level, which did not reflect the care they needed. In addition, the three-category system did not address issues such as managing patient flow in EDs or issues of overcrowding and wait time, and it did not demonstrate consistent reliability and validity.

A more refined comprehensive triage system has been implemented to incorporate the changes in the use of the ED for both emergency and routine health care. The most effective triage systems are simple and require no complex

BOX 55-1

Traditional Triage Acuity System

Three categories:
- *Emergent:* Patients with the highest priority or life-threatening conditions
- *Urgent:* Patients with serious health problems that are not considered immediately life-threatening
- *Nonurgent:* Patients who do not have life-threatening illnesses or injuries

A fourth class was incorporated, termed "fast-track;" this includes patients who require simple first aid or basic primary care and may be treated in the emergency department or safely referred to a clinic or health provider's office.

BOX 55-2

Data Collected by the Triage Nurse

- Patient's presenting complaint of illness or injury
- Level of pain
- Level of consciousness
- Circumstances, precipitating events, location, and time of the injury or illness
- Treatment of injury or illness prior to arrival in the emergency department (ED)
- Method of arrival to ED
- Physician or health provider seen for nonemergent care
- Health status prior to injury or illness
- History of medical illness and previous surgeries
- Previous hospitalizations
- Allergies including medications, eggs, latex, nuts, etc.
- Current medications
- Use of recreational drugs
- Smoking history
- Evaluation of immunizations for currency (tetanus)
- Brief assessment of body systems, including behavioral health screening for depression or suicidal ideation
- Last menstrual period (for those who menstruate)
- Time of last meal or oral intake
- Focused assessment on system involved with presenting complaint
- Special circumstances or requests of patient, especially those related to limitations regarding treatments (e.g., resuscitation status or refusal of blood products)

scoring methodology. A four-level system is commonly used in the United States:

1. *Immediate (I—red)*: Patients have life-threatening injuries that are probably survivable with immediate treatment. Examples are tension pneumothorax, respiratory distress, major external hemorrhage, and airway injuries. With limited resources, ideally the only patients categorized as red will be those who would benefit from immediate short-duration treatment and then could be retriaged as yellow.
2. *Delayed (II—yellow)*: Patients require definitive treatment, but no immediate threat to life exists. Patients can wait for treatment without jeopardy. Examples include minor extremity fractures, laceration with hemorrhage controlled, and burns over less than 25% of body surface area.
3. *Minimal (III—green)*: Patients have minimal injuries, are ambulatory, and can self-treat or seek alternative medical attention independently. Examples include minor lacerations, contusions, and abrasions.
4. *Expectant (0—black)*: Patients have lethal injuries and usually will die despite treatment. Examples include devastating head injuries, major third-degree burns over most of the body, and destruction of vital organs. Retriage of this group may be done as resources become available (Ratcliff & Lincoln, 2017).

The increased number of triage levels assists the triage nurse with more precisely determining the needs of the patient and the urgency for treatment. There are alternative triage systems that are used in the United States; therefore, the nurse should follow institutional policies. For example, the Emergency Severity Index (ESI) has been endorsed by the American College of Emergency Physicians and the Emergency Nurses Association; it is a five-level triage algorithm that considers the patient's clinical presentation, vital signs, and the amount and type of resources (examples include laboratory, intravenous [IV] hydration, radiologic studies, simple or complex procedures, medications, consultation) needed to treat the patient (The ESI Triage Research Team, LLC, 2020). Nurses in the triage area collect baseline data like full vital signs including pain assessment, history of the current event and medical history, current medications, brief behavioral/mental status assessment, height, weight, allergies, and system review with a focus on the presenting complaint and clinical presentation. These data are recorded for reference by all health care team members treating the patient. Common assessment data are outlined in Box 55-2.

Primary and Secondary Surveys

A systematic approach to effectively establishing and treating health priorities is the primary survey/secondary survey approach. The primary survey focuses on stabilizing life-threatening conditions. The ED staff work collaboratively and follow the circulation, airway, breathing, and disability (CABD) method:

- Evaluate and restore cardiac output by controlling hemorrhage, preventing and treating shock, and maintaining or restoring effective circulation, including the prevention and management of hypothermia.
- Establish a patent airway.
- Provide adequate ventilation, employing resuscitation measures when necessary. Protection of the cervical spine in patients who have experienced trauma is mandatory when ventilating and resuscitation measures are needed.
- Determine neurologic disability by assessing neurologic function using the Glasgow Coma Scale (see Box 44-6 in Chapter 44). Evaluate for spinal cord injury if indicated.

After these priorities have been addressed, the ED team proceeds with the secondary survey. This includes:

- A complete health history and head-to-toe assessment
- Diagnostic and laboratory testing
- Insertion or application of monitoring devices, such as electrocardiogram (ECG) electrodes, arterial lines, or urinary catheters
- Splinting of suspected fractures
- Cleansing, closure, and dressing of wounds
- Performance of other necessary interventions based on the patient's condition

CARING FOR PATIENTS WITH LIFE-THREATENING CONDITIONS

Emergency nurses often confront airway obstruction and hemorrhage. These conditions are life-threatening and require immediate intervention to prevent death.

Airway Obstruction

Acute upper airway obstruction is a life-threatening medical emergency. The airway may be partially or completely occluded. Partial obstruction of the airway can lead to progressive hypoxia, hypercarbia (increased carbon dioxide levels in the blood), and respiratory and cardiac arrest. If the airway is completely obstructed, permanent brain injury or death will occur within 3 to 5 minutes secondary to hypoxia. Air movement is absent in the presence of complete airway obstruction. Oxygen saturation of the blood decreases rapidly because the obstructed airway prevents entry of air into the lungs. Oxygen deficit occurs in the brain, resulting in unconsciousness with death rapidly following.

Causes

Upper airway obstruction has a number of causes, including aspiration of foreign bodies, anaphylaxis, viral or bacterial infection, trauma, and inhalation or chemical burns. For older adult patients, especially those in extended-care facilities, sedatives and hypnotic medications, diseases affecting motor coordination (e.g., Parkinson disease), and mental dysfunction (e.g., dementia) are risk factors for asphyxiation by food. In adults, aspiration of a bolus of meat is the most common cause of airway obstruction. In children, small toys, buttons, coins, and other objects are commonly aspirated in addition to food. Peritonsillar abscesses, epiglottitis, and other acute infectious processes of the posterior pharynx can also result in airway obstruction.

Pearls for Practice

The nurse listens for severe stridor (loud, harsh, vibratory sound of variable pitch); if present and the patient has a persistent pulse, suspicion of aspiration of a foreign body or food should be considered. If this is suspected, a Heimlich maneuver (Box 55-3) may dislodge the obstructing body.

BOX 55-3 Managing a Foreign-Body Airway Obstruction

Heimlich Maneuver (Subdiaphragmatic Abdominal Thrusts)

For conscious patient (sitting or standing):

1. Stand behind the patient and wrap your arms around the patient's waist. If the victim is shorter than the rescuer, the rescuer may kneel behind the victim.
2. Make a fist with one hand.
3. Place the thumb side of the fist against the victim's abdomen, in the midline slightly above the navel and well below the breastbone.
4. Grasp your fist with the other hand and press your fist into the victim's abdomen with a quick upward thrust.
5. Repeat thrusts until the object is expelled from the airway or the victim becomes unresponsive.
6. Give each new thrust with a separate and distinct movement to relieve the obstruction.

Abdominal thrusts may be performed if the choking victim is responsive and lying down.

Chest Thrusts

For the patient who is conscious and sitting or standing and in advanced stages of pregnancy or has marked obesity:

1. Stand behind the patient with your arms under the patient's axillae to encircle the patient's chest.
2. Place the thumb side of your fist on the middle of the patient's sternum, taking care to avoid the xiphoid process and the margins of the rib cage.
3. Grasp your fist with the other hand and perform backward thrusts until the foreign body is expelled or the patient becomes unconscious. Each thrust should be administered with the intent of relieving the obstruction.

Unresponsive Choking, Adult Choking Victim Lying Down

If the choking victim becomes unresponsive, begin the sequence of cardiopulmonary resuscitation (CPR) by calling for support (or activating the emergency response system in a nonhospital setting). When opening the airway to deliver rescue breaths, open the victim's mouth wide, look for any foreign bodies, and remove any objects that can be seen. Be careful not to push any objects deeper into the airway. A blind finger sweep to search for foreign objects is not recommended. If the airway remains obstructed, reposition their head and attempt to deliver rescue breaths a second time. Begin compressions and continue with advanced life support measures.

Adapted from American Heart Association (AHA). (2021). *Part 5: Adult basic life support.* http://circ.ahajournals.org/content/122/18_suppl_3/S685.full

Clinical Manifestations and Assessment

Typically, a person with a foreign-body airway obstruction cannot speak, breathe, or cough. The patient may clutch the neck between the thumb and fingers (this is known as the *universal distress signal*). Other common signs and symptoms include choking, apprehensive appearance, inspiratory and expiratory stridor, labored breathing, use of accessory muscles (suprasternal and intercostal retraction), flaring nostrils, increasing anxiety, restlessness, and confusion. Cyanosis and loss of consciousness develop as hypoxia worsens.

Assessment of the patient who has a foreign object occluding the airway may simply involve asking the person whether they are choking and require help. If the person is unconscious, inspection of the oropharynx may reveal the offending object. X-rays, laryngoscopy, or bronchoscopy also may be required. If the patient can breathe and cough spontaneously, a partial obstruction should be suspected.

Medical and Nursing Management

For partial obstruction, the patient is encouraged to cough forcefully and to persist with spontaneous coughing and breathing efforts as long as adequate air exchange exists. Oxygen saturation should be monitored to evaluate oxygenation. Supplemental oxygen should be administered. There may be some wheezing between coughs. If the patient demonstrates a weak, ineffective cough, a high-pitched noise while inhaling, increased respiratory difficulty, or cyanosis, they should be managed as if there were complete airway obstruction.

After the obstruction is removed, rescue breathing is initiated if the patient has absent or inadequate respiratory effort. If the patient has no pulse, cardiac compressions are instituted. These measures provide oxygen to the brain, heart, and other vital organs until definitive medical treatment can restore and support normal heart and ventilatory activity.

Establishing an Airway

Establishing an airway may be as simple as repositioning the patient's head to prevent the tongue from obstructing the pharynx. Alternatively, other maneuvers, such as abdominal thrusts (also called subdiaphragmatic abdominal thrusts), the head-tilt–chin-lift maneuver, the jaw-thrust maneuver, or insertion of specialized equipment, may be needed to open the airway, remove a foreign body, or maintain the airway. Box 55-3 provides guidelines for performing the Heimlich maneuver and abdominal and chest thrusts. In all maneuvers, the cervical spine must be protected from injury. After these maneuvers are performed, the patient is assessed for breathing by watching for chest movement and listening and feeling for air movement.

The head-tilt–chin-lift maneuver is used only if there is no suspected injury to the cervical spine. It is performed as follows:

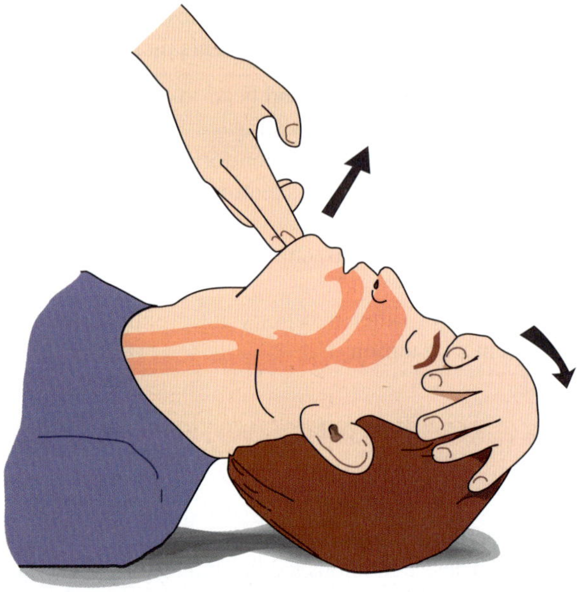

FIGURE 55-1 The head-tilt–chin-lift maneuver. (LifeART image © 2010. Lippincott Williams & Wilkins. All rights reserved.)

- The patient is placed supine on a firm, flat surface.
- If the patient is lying face down, the body is turned as a unit so that the head, shoulders, and torso move simultaneously with no twisting. This requires a minimum of two or preferably three staff members.
- Next, the airway is opened using either the head-tilt–chin-lift maneuver or the jaw-thrust maneuver:
  - In the head-tilt–chin-lift maneuver, one hand is placed on the patient's forehead, and firm backward pressure is applied with the palm to tilt the head back. This will move the tongue forward (away from the back of the throat). The fingers of the other hand are placed under the bony part of the lower jaw (mandible) near the chin and gently lifted up (Fig. 55-1). The chin and the teeth are lifted so that the teeth are almost brought together.
  - In the jaw-thrust maneuver, after one hand is placed on each side of the patient's jaw, the angles of the patient's lower jaw are grasped and lifted, displacing the mandible forward. This is a safe approach to opening the airway of a patient with suspected neck injury because it can be accomplished without extending the neck.

Oropharyngeal Airway

An oropharyngeal airway is a semicircular tube or tube-like plastic device that is inserted over the back of the tongue into the lower posterior pharynx in a patient who is breathing spontaneously but who is unconscious. This type of airway prevents the tongue from falling back against the posterior pharynx and obstructing the airway. It also allows health care providers to suction secretions. It should be reserved for unconscious patients without a gag reflex. A nasopharyngeal airway is tolerated better by patients who are not deeply unconscious, but it should be avoided in patients with craniofacial trauma (Carlson & Wang, 2020) (Box 55-4).

BOX 55-4

GUIDELINES FOR NURSING CARE

Inserting an Oropharyngeal Airway

Equipment

- Oropharyngeal airway
- Nonsterile gloves
- Protective eyewear if secretions are profuse or patient is coughing
- Equipment for suctioning

Implementation

ACTION	RATIONALE
1. Insert only in an unconscious patient who does not have a gag reflex with a risk of airway occlusion and no cervical spine injury, oral trauma, or recent oral surgery.	1. An oropharyngeal airway can prevent the tongue from occluding the airway against the posterior pharynx in an unconscious patient. Patients with known or suspected cervical spine injury may require emergent intubation for airway protection and ventilatory support. It is only used in an unconscious patient since vomiting and laryngospasm may be stimulated by the airway in a conscious or semiconscious patient. Oral trauma or recent oral surgery may be a contraindication to inserting an oropharyngeal airway.
2. Remove dentures, if present, before insertion.	2. Remove dentures to prevent them from causing an airway obstruction.
3. Measure the oral airway alongside the head. Correct size of the airway should extend from the corner of the mouth to the tip of the earlobe (Reardon et al., 2019).	3. Accurate measurement is needed to ensure the airway is appropriately sized to prevent the tongue from occluding the airway.
4. Extend the patient's head by placing one hand under the bony chin. With the other hand, tilt the head backward by applying pressure to the forehead while simultaneously lifting the chin forward. Open the patient's mouth.	4. When positioning the head for insertion, the head may be tilted back *only* if the patient has had the cervical spine cleared. In the patient with a potential cervical spine injury, use only the jaw-thrust maneuver to aid in positioning the head for airway insertion. Position facilitates insertion.
5. **A.** Insert the oropharyngeal airway with the tip facing up toward the roof of the mouth until it passes the uvula. **B.** Rotate the tip 180 degrees so that the tip is pointed down toward the pharynx.	5. This displaces the tongue anteriorly, and the patient then breathes through and around the airway.

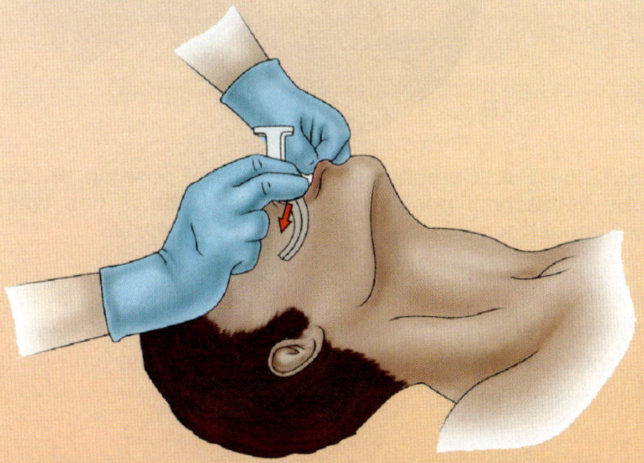

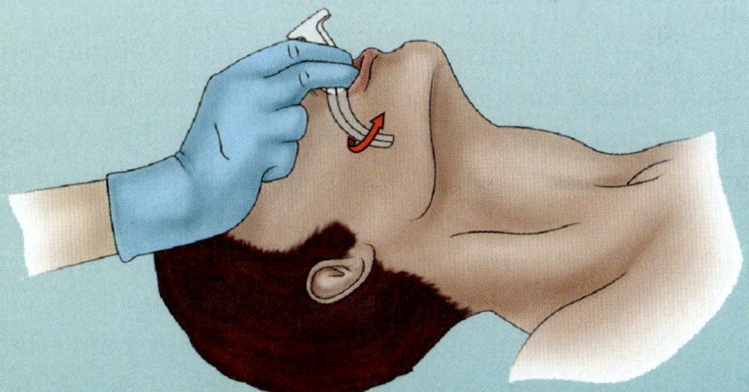

ACTION	RATIONALE
6. Ensure the distal end of the oropharyngeal airway is in the hypopharynx and the flange is approximately at the patient's lips. Make sure that the tongue has not been pushed into the airway.	6. An incorrectly placed airway can itself cause airway obstruction by pushing the tongue posteriorly into the hypopharynx.

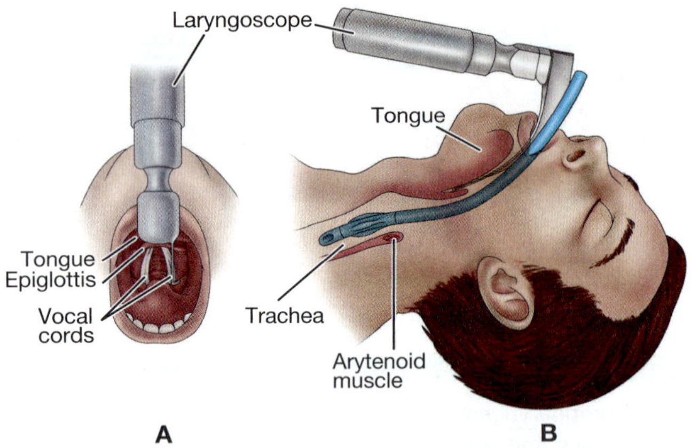

FIGURE 55-2 **Endotracheal intubation in a patient without a cervical spine injury. A. The primary glottis landmarks for tracheal intubation as visualized with proper placement of the laryngoscope. B. Positioning the endotracheal tube.**

Intubation

Endotracheal intubation is used to establish and maintain the airway in patients with respiratory insufficiency or hypoxia. Endotracheal intubation is indicated for the following reasons: (1) to establish an airway for a patient who cannot be adequately ventilated with an oropharyngeal airway; (2) to bypass an upper airway obstruction; (3) to prevent aspiration; (4) to permit connection of the patient to a resuscitation bag or mechanical ventilator; and (5) to facilitate the removal of tracheobronchial secretions. Because the procedure requires skill, endotracheal intubation is performed only by those who have had extensive training. However, the emergency nurse is commonly called on to assist with intubation (Fig. 55-2).

If the patient is not hospitalized and cannot be intubated in the field, emergency medical personnel may insert an esophagotracheal airway or a Combitube (The ESI Triage Research Team, LLC, 2020). The tube rapidly provides pharyngeal ventilation and is used in conjunction with a bag valve mask for ventilation. When the tube is inserted into the trachea, it functions like an endotracheal tube (Fig. 55-3).

The two balloons that surround the tube are inflated after the tube is inserted. One balloon is large and occludes the oropharynx. If a 41-French sized tube is used, 100 mL of air is used to inflate the oropharyngeal balloon, whereas for a 37-French, 85 mL is used. This permits ventilation by forcing air through the larynx. The smaller distal balloon, which is in the esophagus, is inflated with 15 mL of air and can occlude the trachea if it is inadvertently placed there (Laurin, 2020). Approximately 90% of the time, the distal tip of the tube will be in the esophagus. However, the nurse must assess breath sounds after balloon inflation to make sure that the oropharyngeal balloon (or cuff) does not obstruct the glottis. The patient can be ventilated through either one of the two ports (tracheal or esophageal) of the tube, depending on whether the tube is placed in the trachea or esophagus. If the distal balloon is in the esophagus, gastric contents can be aspirated and gastric decompression performed by passing the provided suction catheter through the distal balloon into the stomach (Laurin, 2020).

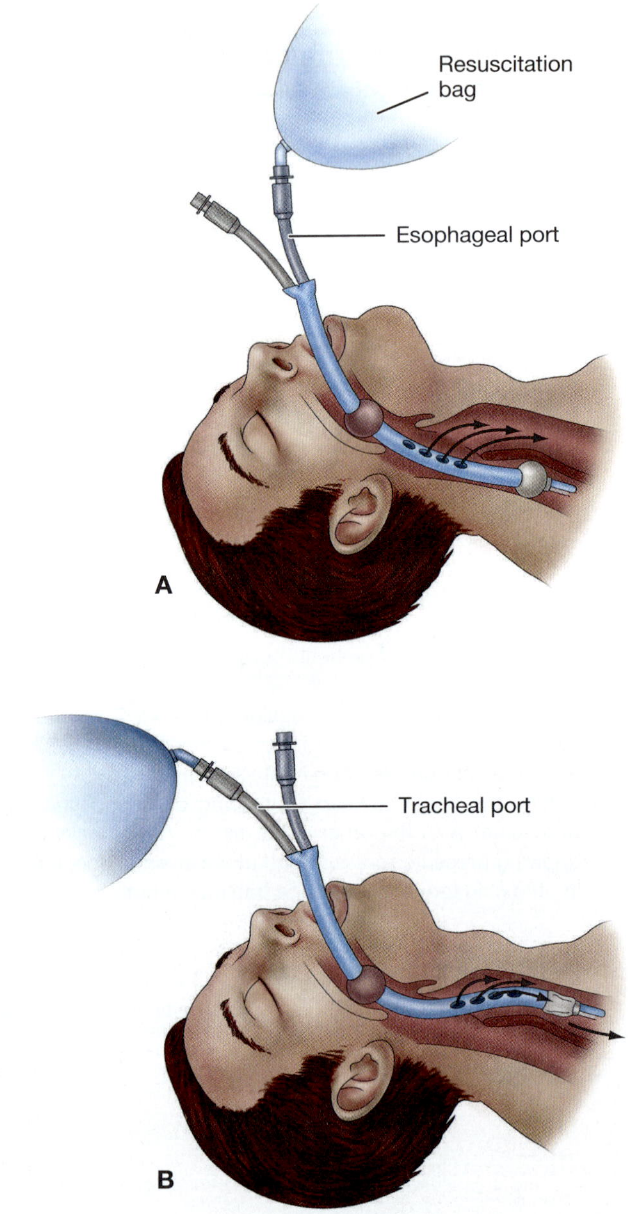

FIGURE 55-3 **A. Combitube in esophageal position. B. Combitube in tracheal position. Note: Combitube is one type of esophageal tracheal airway available on the market.**

Cricothyroidotomy

Cricothyroidotomy is the opening of the cricothyroid membrane to establish an airway. This procedure is used in emergency situations in which endotracheal intubation is either not possible or contraindicated, as in patients with airway obstruction from extensive maxillofacial trauma, cervical spine injuries, laryngospasm, laryngeal edema (after an allergic reaction or extubation), hemorrhage into neck tissue, or obstruction of the larynx.

Maintaining the Airway

After the airway is determined to be unobstructed, the nurse must ensure that adequate ventilation is maintained. Satisfactory management of ventilations may prevent hypoxia and hypercapnia (excessive carbon dioxide in the blood). The nurse must quickly assess for absent or diminished breath sounds as well as difficulty delivering artificial breaths for the patient. The nurse should monitor pulse oximetry, capnography (monitoring of the amount of exhaled carbon dioxide), and arterial blood gases (ABGs) if the patient requires airway or ventilatory assistance.

The nurse is aware that a tension pneumothorax can mimic hypovolemia, so ventilatory assessment precedes assessment for hemorrhage. A pneumothorax or sucking (open) chest wound is managed with a chest tube; immediate relief of the increasing positive intrapleural pressure (normally, the intrapleural pressure is negative) and maintenance of adequate ventilation should occur (refer to Chapter 9 for information on pneumothorax and chest tube insertion and management).

Pearls for Practice

Patients who have experienced trauma are kept on a stretcher to immobilize the spine. A backboard may be used for transporting the patient to the x-ray department, to the operating room, or to the intensive care unit. Cervical spine immobilization is maintained until cervical x-rays have been obtained and cervical spine injury has been ruled out. Ongoing neurologic examinations to assess for spinal cord impairment and change in level of consciousness (LOC) are essential.

Hemorrhage

Stopping bleeding is essential to the care and survival of patients in an emergency or disaster situation. Hemorrhage that results in the reduction of circulating blood volume is a primary cause of shock (see Chapter 53). Minor bleeding, which is usually venous, generally stops spontaneously unless the patient has a bleeding disorder or has been taking anticoagulants.

Clinical Manifestations and Assessment

The patient is assessed for signs and symptoms of shock, which may include cool, moist skin (resulting from poor peripheral perfusion); decreasing blood pressure; decreasing pulse pressure (difference between systolic and diastolic pressure); increasing heart rate; delayed capillary refill; and decreasing urine volume. These criteria are associated with an estimated blood loss of approximately 1,500 to 2,000 mL or 30% to 40% of blood volume; the nurse should assess for the earliest symptom of blood loss—increasing anxiety. Refer to Table 55-1 for estimated fluid and blood losses.

Pearls for Practice

If the patient is hemorrhaging, the nurse understands that the Trendelenburg position does not improve cardiopulmonary status, and it may predispose the patient to aspiration and worsening pulmonary gas exchange, as well as increasing intracranial pressures. The supine position with passive leg raising above the level of the heart may be effective. If passive leg raising results in an increase in blood pressure or cardiac output (CO), then fluid resuscitation is indicated (Nicks & Gaillard, 2020).

TABLE **55-1 Classes of Hemorrhagic Shock**

Class I Hemorrhage: Loss of up to 15% of Blood Volume (up to 750 mL in 70-kg Adult)	Class II Hemorrhage: Loss of 15–30% of Blood Volume (750–1,500 mL)	Class III Hemorrhage: Loss of 30–40% of Blood Volume (1,500–2,000 mL)	Class IV Hemorrhage: Loss of over 40% of Blood Volume (more than 2,000 mL)
Heart rate (HR) <100 bpm	HR >100 bpm	HR >120 bpm	HR >140 bpm
Systolic blood pressure (BP) normal	Systolic BP normal	Systolic BP decreased	Systolic BP markedly decreased
Respiratory rate (RR) 14–20 breaths per minute	RR 20–30 breaths per minute	RR 30–40 breaths per minute	RR greater than 35 breaths per minute
Increased or normal pulse pressure	Decreased pulse pressure	Decreased pulse pressure	Very narrow pulse pressure
Slight anxiety	Mildly anxious	Significant change in mental status: anxiety or confusion	Depressed mental status: confusion, lethargy, loss of consciousness
30 mL/hr	Small decrease in urine output (20–30 mL/hr)	Marked decrease in urine output (5–15 mL/hr)	Negligible urine output

Adapted from Chan, T. (2020). Hemorrhagic shock. In J. J. Schaider, R. M. Barkin, S. R. Hayden, R. E. Wolfe, A. Z. Barkin, & P. Shayne (Eds.), *Rosen & Barkin's 5-minute emergency medicine consult* (6th ed., pp. 508–509). Lippincott Williams & Wilkins.

Medical and Nursing Management

The goals of emergency management for patients with blood loss are to control bleeding, maintain adequate circulating blood volume for tissue oxygenation, and prevent shock. Patients who hemorrhage are at risk for cardiac arrest caused by hypovolemia with secondary anoxia (the absence or near absence of oxygen); therefore, continuous ECG monitoring is expected. Nursing interventions are carried out collaboratively with other members of the emergency health care team.

Fluid Replacement

Whenever a patient is experiencing hemorrhage, whether external or internal, a loss of circulating blood results in a fluid volume deficit and decreased CO. Therefore, fluid replacement is imperative to maintain circulation. Typically, two large-gauge IV catheters are inserted to provide a means for fluid and blood replacement, and blood samples are obtained for analysis, typing, and cross-matching. Replacement fluids are administered as prescribed, depending on clinical estimates of the type and volume of fluid lost. Replacement fluids may include isotonic electrolyte solutions (e.g., lactated Ringer's solution, normal saline), colloids, and blood component therapy.

Caution must be taken when infusing fluids. According to Advance Trauma Life Support revisions (Acker, 2019), fluids need to be warmed, and aggressive resuscitation of fluids prior to the identification and control of the source of bleeding should be avoided due to an increase in demonstrated mortality.

Hospitals should have written transfusion protocols and massive transfusion protocols. Massive transfusion protocols are defined as transfusion of more than 10 units of packed red blood cells (PRBCs) in 24 hours or more than 4 units in 1 hour. PRBCs are infused when there is massive blood loss. In emergencies, if typed and cross-matched blood is not available, then type O-negative blood should be reserved for females younger than 50 years of age; all others should receive type O-positive. In a situation with a patient requiring resuscitation with massive blood loss, there is no time to type and cross-match or type and screen blood. Type O-negative blood provides safe administration of blood immediately without sensitizing an Rh-negative patient to Rh-positive blood (sensitization can result in neonatal complications during a later pregnancy). Promoting homeostasis and restoring tissue oxygenation as fast as possible is necessary. However, PRBCs alone will not aid greatly in these processes and may worsen coagulopathies if plasma and platelets are not also infused. Administering PRBCs, fresh frozen plasma (FFP), and platelets in a 1:1:1 ratio has been shown to improve patient survival and decrease critical care and ventilator days (Motola et al., 2020). Tranexamic acid may be considered for patients with significant hemorrhage and may be considered in the prehospital area with additional follow-up when the patient is transferred to the hospital (Acker, 2019; Motola et al., 2020). Ongoing monitoring of the patient's hemoglobin, Hct, and coagulation factors will guide the administration of blood products.

Once the hemorrhage is controlled, transfusion should cease when the hemoglobin concentration is greater than 10 g/dL (100 g/L). Depending on the patient's comorbidities, lower end points may be considered and additional transfusion may be delayed if the patient is otherwise hemodynamically stable. "Consensus recommendations for transfusion are a hemoglobin concentration between 6 and 7 g/dL (60 to 70 g/L) for those without cardiopulmonary, cerebral, or peripheral vascular disease. [When the hemoglobin is] between 6 and 10 g/dL (60 to 100 g/L), use clinical judgment for transfusion" (Somand & Ward, 2020, para 1).

Controlling Blood Loss

If a patient is hemorrhaging externally (e.g., from a wound), a rapid physical assessment is performed as the patient's clothing is cut away in an attempt to identify the area of hemorrhage. Direct, firm pressure is applied over the bleeding area or the involved artery at a site that is proximal to (above) the wound (Fig. 55-4). Most bleeding can be stopped or at least controlled by application of direct pressure. Otherwise, unchecked arterial bleeding results in death. A firm pressure dressing is applied, and the injured part is elevated to stop venous and capillary bleeding if possible. If the injured area is an extremity, the extremity is immobilized to control blood loss.

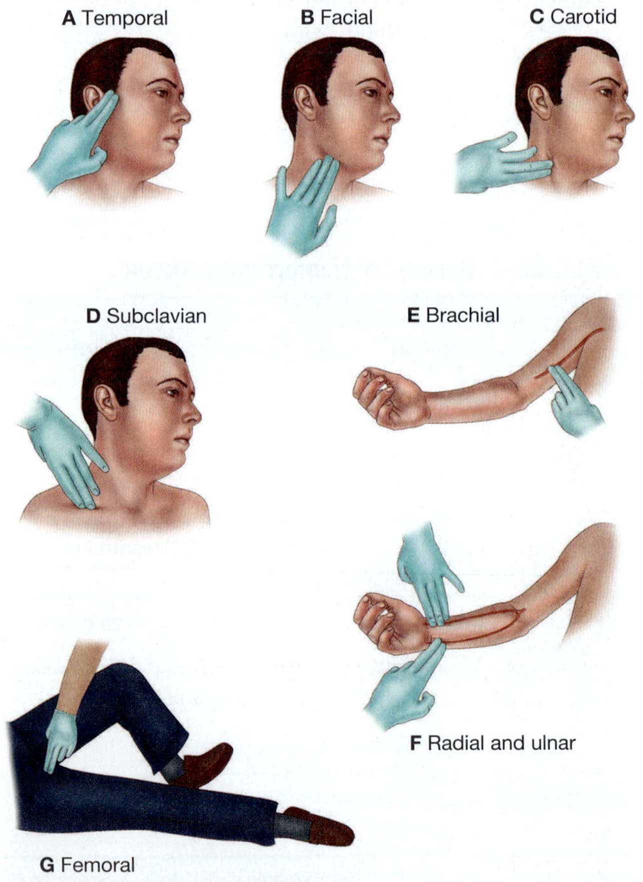

FIGURE 55-4 A–G. Pressure points for control of hemorrhage.

Pearls for Practice

In the event of amputated fingers or extremities, the nurse is aware that the body part should be wrapped with a moist, sterile, protective dressing, placed in a waterproof bag, and then placed in a container of ice water for preservation in the event that future reattachment is possible (Singer & Hollander, 2020a). It is important to note that the amputated limb should never be placed in ice or water directly as serious cellular damage may occur.

A tourniquet is applied to an extremity only as a *last resort* when the external hemorrhage cannot be controlled in any other way and immediate surgery is not feasible. Care must be taken when applying a tourniquet because of the risk for loss of the extremity. The tourniquet is applied just proximal to the wound and tied tightly enough to control arterial blood flow. Documentation of the application of the tourniquet is critical so that all providers are aware of the time and placement; suggestions include flow sheet documentation, use of a skin-marking pencil or adhesive tape on the forehead with a "T," and labeling the location of the tourniquet and application time. If there is no arterial bleeding, the tourniquet is removed and a pressure dressing is applied. *In general, tourniquets should not be used for more than 30 minutes* (Singer & Hollander, 2020b). If the patient has sustained a traumatic amputation with uncontrollable hemorrhage, the tourniquet remains in place until the patient is in the operating room.

If the patient shows no external signs of bleeding but exhibits tachycardia, falling blood pressure, thirst, apprehension, cool and moist skin, or delayed capillary refill, internal hemorrhage is suspected. Typically, PRBCs are administered at a rapid rate, and the patient is prepared for more definitive treatment (e.g., surgery, endoscopy, pharmacologic therapy). In addition, laboratory specimens, including complete blood count (CBC), electrolytes, coagulation studies, type and cross-match, and ABG specimens are obtained to evaluate pulmonary function and tissue perfusion and to establish baseline hemodynamic parameters, which are then used as an index for determining the amount of fluid replacement the patient can tolerate and the response to therapy. The patient is maintained in the supine position and monitored closely until hemodynamic or circulatory parameters improve or until transported for definitive therapy or continued treatment.

Failure to provide adequate fluid resuscitation and definitely control the source of hemorrhage may lead to hypovolemic (hemorrhagic) shock. This is the most common cause of postinjury death and should be suspected in any patient with hypotensive trauma until proven otherwise (Cowell & Moore, 2020). Hypovolemic shock should be anticipated in any emergency situation in which profound blood or fluid (vomiting or diarrhea) loss has occurred. The goals of treatment are to restore and maintain tissue perfusion and to correct physiologic abnormalities. Chapter 53 provides detailed information on the management of hypovolemic shock.

Ongoing nursing surveillance of the *total patient* is maintained. Blood pressure, heart and respiratory rates, skin temperature, color, pulse oximetry, neurologic status, central venous pressure (CVP), ABGs, ECG recordings, Hct, hemoglobin, coagulation profile, electrolytes, and urinary output are serially monitored to assess patient response to treatment. Commonly, a flow sheet is used to document these parameters, providing an analysis of trends rather than single values to reveal improvement or deterioration of the patient's condition.

In addition, the body's defense mechanisms are supported. The patient should be reassured and comforted. Sedation may be used judiciously to relieve apprehension. Analgesics are used cautiously to relieve pain. Body temperature is maintained within normal limits to prevent increasing metabolic demands that the body may be unable to meet. Administration of large volumes of IV crystalloids, blood products, or both can result in hypothermia. Hypothermia may be prevented by warming the fluids before they are administered.

CARING FOR PATIENTS WHO HAVE SUSTAINED TRAUMA

Trauma (an unintentional or intentional wound or injury inflicted on the body from a mechanism against which the body cannot protect itself) is the fourth leading cause of death in the United States (Centers for Disease Control and Prevention [CDC], 2021a). Alcohol and drug use are often implicated as factors in both blunt and penetrating trauma.

In assessing and managing any patient with an emergency condition, but especially the patient experiencing trauma, documentation, including descriptions of all wounds, mechanism of injury, and time of events, as well as collection of evidence, are essential. In trauma care, the nurse must be exceedingly careful with all potential evidence, handling and documenting it properly.

The basics of care management for patients with traumatic injury include an understanding that trauma in any patient (living or dead) has potential legal or forensic implications if criminal activity is suspected. Hence, proper management from both a medical and forensic perspective is essential. Box 55-5 describes collection of evidence.

Multiple trauma is caused by a single catastrophic event that causes life-threatening injuries to at least two distinct organs or organ systems. Mortality in patients with multiple trauma is related to the severity of the injuries and the number of systems and organs involved. Immediately after injury, the body is hypermetabolic, hypercoagulable, and severely stressed.

Care of the patient with multiple injuries requires a team approach, with one person responsible for coordinating the treatment. The nursing staff assumes responsibility for assessing and monitoring the patient, ensuring airway and

BOX 55-5
Collection of Forensic Evidence

When clothing is removed from the patient who has experienced trauma, the nurse must be careful not to cut through or disrupt any tears, holes, blood stains, or dirt present on the clothing if criminal activity is suspected. Each piece of clothing should be placed in an individual paper bag. If the clothing is wet, it should be hung to dry. Clothing should not be given to families. Valuables should be placed in the hospital safe or if given to a family member, clearly documented. If a police officer is present to collect clothing or any other items from the patient, each item is labeled. The transfer of custody to the officer, the officer's name, the date, and the time are documented.

If suicide or homicide is suspected in a patient who is deceased, the medical examiner examines the body onsite or has the body moved to the coroner's office for autopsy. All tubes and lines must remain in place. The patient's hands must be covered with paper bags to protect evidence on the hands or under the fingernails. In the patient who survives, tissue specimens may be swabbed from the hands and nails as potential evidence. Photographs of wounds or clothing are essential and should include a reference ruler in one photo and one photo without the ruler.

Documentation should also include any statements made by the patient in the patient's own words and surrounded by quotation marks. A chain of evidence is essential. If the patient's case is adjudicated in the future, clear documentation assists the judicial process and helps identify the activities that occurred in the emergency department.

IV access, administering prescribed medications, collecting laboratory specimens, and documenting activities and the patient's response.

Gross evidence of trauma may be slight or absent. Patients with multiple traumatic injuries should be assumed to have a spinal cord injury until it is proven otherwise. The injury regarded as the least significant in appearance may be the most lethal. For example, a pelvis fracture that goes unidentified until an x-ray is obtained may be the injury from which the patient is exsanguinating into the pelvic cavity. A tension pneumothorax may be insidiously increasing in size, eventually compressing both the heart and lungs, while the ED team is focused on repair of external lacerations. An obvious amputation of the arm may have already stopped bleeding from the body's normal response of vasoconstriction despite being an obvious and devastating injury; meanwhile, the patient may be dying from an internal, less visible, injury.

The goals of treatment are to determine the extent of injuries and to establish priorities of treatment. Any injury interfering with a vital physiologic function (i.e., airway, breathing, circulation) is an immediate threat to life and has the highest priority for immediate treatment. Essential life-saving procedures are performed simultaneously by the emergency team. As soon as the patient is resuscitated, clothes are usually cut off, and a rapid physical assessment is performed. Transfer from field management to the ED must be orderly and controlled, with attention given to the verbal report from emergency medical services (EMS). Treatment in a level I trauma center is appropriate for patients experiencing major trauma.

Wounds

Wounds involving injury to soft tissues can vary from minor tears to severe crushing injuries. The primary goal of treatment is to restore the physical integrity and function of the injured tissue while minimizing scarring and preventing infection. Proper documentation of the characteristics of the wound, using precise descriptions and correct terminology, is essential. Such information may be needed in the future for forensic evidence. Photographs are helpful because they provide an accurate, visible depiction of the wound. Photographs also become important for exigent wounds (wounds that will heal and later be unidentifiable). Patients whose injuries resulted from violence may need the photographs later to visually describe the extent of injury.

Determining *when* and *how* the wound occurred is important because a treatment delay increases infection risk. Using aseptic technique, the provider inspects the wound to determine the extent of damage to underlying structures. Visible contamination of the wound increases the risk of wound infection. In addition, the nurse is aware that bite wounds carry significant risk for infection owing to the high bacterial colonization in the mouth. Sensory, motor, and vascular function is evaluated for changes that might indicate complications.

Hair around the wound may be clipped if it is anticipated that the hairs will interfere with wound closure. Shaving should be avoided; it may result in an increased incidence of wound infection since many bacteria reside in hair follicles (Hollander & Singer, 2020b). Complete removal of eyebrow hairs is avoided as regrowth may not occur; clipping eyebrow hair to 1 to 2 mm above the wound is recommended if hair is interfering with wound care.

If indicated, the area is infiltrated with a local intradermal anesthetic through the wound margins or by regional block. Patients with soft tissue injuries usually have localized pain at the site of injury. The nurse then assists the physician, nurse practitioner, or physician's assistant in cleaning and debriding the wound.

Wound cleaning requires the selection of methods that minimize chemical and mechanical trauma to the wound tissue while removing surface debris and contaminants (Slotts & Schultz, 2020). Typically, the area around the wound is cleansed with normal saline solution or a polymer agent (e.g., Shur-Clens). Antibacterial agents, such as povidone–iodine (Betadine) or chlorhexidine, can be used to paint the intact skin surrounding the wound but should not be allowed to get into the wound since these solutions are associated with decreasing defense mechanisms and thus increase the risk of wound infection. With the emergence of antibiotic resistance, some researchers call for a reappraisal of the use of antiseptic solutions especially in the management of contaminated and infected wounds (Brown, 2018; Denke, 2020). At present, a standardized regimen for wound cleaning has yet to be established. Nurses should refer to their facility's protocol.

To decrease the incidence of wound infection, the nurse anticipates both the use of wound irrigation and debridement of dead wound tissue. The wound will be irrigated gently and copiously with sterile isotonic saline solution to remove surface dirt. The volume of irrigation fluid will vary based on the size of the wound and the potential for contamination. Although no standard recommended volume exists, a general guideline of 30 to 50 mL of irrigation per 1 cm of laceration is considered adequate for a clean wound without significant contamination (Thomsen et al., 2021). The nurse uses **personal protective equipment** (PPE) in the form of face shields. Devitalized tissue and foreign matter are removed by the provider because they impede healing and may encourage infection. Any small bleeding vessels are clamped or tied. Alternatively, hemostasis of small bleeding vessels is achieved by clamping, tying, or cauterization. After wound treatment, a nonadherent dressing is commonly applied to protect the wound. The dressing may serve as a splint and also as a reminder to the patient that the area is injured.

Pearls for Practice

The nurse is aware that irrigation may be high pressure or low pressure. High-pressure irrigation is used to clear debris and support reduction of infection. It is defined as approximately 7 psi (50 kPa) or greater and is achieved using any combination of a 30- to 65-mL syringe and a 19-gauge catheter or needle hub, or a commercially available splashguard, with forceful depression of the syringe piston. Conversely, low-pressure irrigation is defined as approximately 0.5 psi (3.5 kPa) or lower and is achieved with a slow, gentle wash. Low-pressure irrigation may be useful in simple, nonbite, uncontaminated wounds in highly vascular areas, such as the scalp and face (Singer & Hollander, 2020b).

The decision to suture a wound depends on the nature of the wound, the time since the injury was sustained, the degree of contamination, and the vascularity of tissues. If primary closure is indicated, the wound is sutured or stapled with the patient receiving either local anesthesia or moderate sedation. Sutures are placed near the wound edge, with the skin edges leveled carefully to promote optimal healing. Instead of sutures, sterile strips of reinforced microporous tape or a bonding agent (skin glue) may be used to close clean, superficial wounds.

Delayed primary closure may be indicated if tissue has been lost or there is a high potential for infection. A thin layer of gauze (to ensure drainage and prevent pooling of exudate), covered by an occlusive dressing, may be used. Other options include split-thickness cadaver allografts or porcine xenografts to simulate the function of epithelium. The wound is splinted in a functional position to prevent motion and decrease the possibility of contracture. Use of antibiotics to prevent infection depends on factors such as how the injury occurred, the age of the wound, the risk of contamination, and the presence of risk factors in the patient's medical history that decrease wound healing (diabetes, steroid use, chemotherapeutic agents, chronic kidney disease, peripheral vascular disease, advanced age, anemia, malnourishment). The site is immobilized and elevated to limit accumulation of fluid in the interstitial spaces of the wound.

Tetanus prophylaxis is administered as prescribed, based on the condition of the wound and the patient's immunization status. If the patient's last tetanus booster was given more than 5 years ago, or if the patient's immunization status is unknown, a tetanus booster must be given (CDC, 2020). The patient is educated about signs and symptoms of infection and is instructed to contact the health care provider or clinic if there is sudden or persistent pain, fever or chills, bleeding, rapid swelling, foul odor, drainage, or redness surrounding the wound.

Intra-Abdominal Injuries

Intra-abdominal injuries are categorized as penetrating or blunt trauma. Penetrating abdominal trauma (e.g., gunshot wounds, stab wounds) results in a high incidence of injury to hollow organs, particularly the small bowel; thus, they are serious and usually require surgery. The liver is the solid organ that is injured most frequently. In gunshot wounds, the most important factor is the velocity at which the missile (bullet) enters the body. The higher the velocity, the more extensive the tissue damage expected. All abdominal gunshot wounds that cross the peritoneum or are associated with peritoneal signs require surgical exploration. On the other hand, stab wounds may be managed nonoperatively. The nurse accurately documents the location and number of wounds. If abdominal viscera protrude, the area is immediately covered with sterile, moist saline dressings to keep the viscera from drying, and the patient is expected to go directly to the operating room for closure.

Pearls for Practice

The nurse is alert for the following signs of peritonitis: guarding or protecting of an exquisitely tender abdominal region and board-like abdominal rigidity. Pain with coughing is also a marker for peritoneal inflammation: The patient is asked to cough, and if the pain intensifies, it is considered positive for peritoneal involvement (Bickley, 2020).

Blunt trauma to the abdomen may result from motor vehicle crashes, falls, blows, or explosions. It is commonly associated with extra-abdominal injuries to the chest, head, or extremities. Blunt trauma injuries can be a challenge because they may be difficult to detect. The incidence of delayed and trauma-related complications is greater than that of penetrating injuries. This is especially true of blunt injuries involving the liver, kidneys, spleen, or blood vessels, which can lead to massive blood loss into the peritoneal cavity.

Clinical Manifestations and Assessment

As the history of the traumatic event is obtained, the abdomen is inspected for obvious signs of injury, including penetrating injuries, bruises, and abrasions. Abdominal assessment continues with auscultation of bowel sounds to provide baseline data from which changes can be noted. Absence of bowel sounds may be an early sign of intraperitoneal involvement. Further abdominal assessment may reveal progressive abdominal distention, involuntary guarding, tenderness, pain, muscular rigidity, or rebound tenderness, along with changes in bowel sounds, all of which are signs of peritoneal irritation (refer to Chapter 20 for further details of gastrointestinal [GI] assessment). Hypotension and signs and symptoms of shock may also be noted. In addition, the chest and other body systems are assessed for injuries that frequently accompany intra-abdominal injuries.

Studies that aid in assessment include:

- Urinalysis to detect hematuria (indicative of a urinary tract injury)
- Ultrasound of the abdomen to evaluate fluid collection (focused assessment with sonography in trauma, or *FAST*)
- Peritoneal lavage to evaluate abdominal fluid collection
- Radiology and/or computed tomography (CT) scan to evaluate abdominal organ injury, fluid, foreign particles
- Serial hemoglobin and Hct levels to evaluate trends reflecting the presence or absence of bleeding, coagulation studies (prothrombin time [PT], partial thromboplastin time [PTT], international normalized ratio [INR]), blood typing
- White blood cell (WBC) count to detect elevation (generally associated with trauma)
- Serum lipase analysis to detect increasing levels, which suggest pancreatic injury or perforation of the GI tract

Hemorrhage frequently accompanies abdominal injury, especially if the liver or spleen has been traumatized. Therefore, the patient is assessed continuously for signs and symptoms of external and internal bleeding. The front of the body, flanks, and back are inspected for bluish discoloration, asymmetry, abrasion, and contusion (see Chapter 20 for descriptions of Cullen and Grey–Turner signs). Abdominal CT scans permit detailed evaluation of abdominal contents and retroperitoneal examination. Abdominal ultrasound studies can rapidly assess hemodynamically unstable patients to detect intraperitoneal bleeding. This is referred to as the FAST examination.

The nurse suspects hemoperitoneum and splenic injuries if the patient complains of left shoulder pain. This symptom is termed *Kehr sign* and is referred pain due to diaphragmatic irritation associated with the splenic injury or intra-abdominal hemorrhaging. Pain in the right shoulder can result from laceration of the liver. Referred pain is a significant finding because it suggests intraperitoneal injury. The abdomen is assessed for tenderness, rebound tenderness, guarding, rigidity, spasm, increasing distention, and pain. To determine whether there is intraperitoneal injury and bleeding, the patient is usually prepared for diagnostic procedures, such as abdominal ultrasonography or abdominal CT scanning. FAST has rapidly replaced **diagnostic peritoneal lavage (DPL)**, owing to its sensitivity (90%), specificity (95%), and accuracy (99%) in determining the presence of intra-abdominal fluid (Jang, 2017; King & McDougall, 2019). In addition, because of their speed and detailed results, CT scans have largely replaced DPL in the stable patient. However, peritoneal lavage is useful in assessing hollow organ injury or when serial CT scans cannot be performed, as in patients with severe closed head injuries or high spinal cord injuries. It involves the instillation of 1 L of warmed lactated Ringer's solution or normal saline solution into the abdominal cavity. After a minimum of 400 mL has been returned, a fluid specimen is sent to the laboratory for analysis. Positive laboratory findings include a red blood cell (RBC) count greater than 100,000/mm^3; a WBC count greater than 500/mm^3; or the presence of bile, feces, or food.

In patients with stab wounds, the nurse anticipates that a surgeon will assess whether the peritoneal space has been punctured. Fluid resuscitation may be required, and if perforation is confirmed, exploration in the operating room is expected. The need for a tetanus booster will be evaluated, and antibiotics administration is anticipated.

Medical and Nursing Management

As indicated by the patient's condition, resuscitation procedures (restoration of circulation, airway, and breathing) are initiated. Circulating blood volume is maintained with IV fluid replacement, including blood component therapy, and the nurse monitors the patient's vital signs, oxygen saturation, urinary output, and mentation to detect stabilization or evidence of deterioration. A patent airway is maintained, and attempts to stabilize the respiratory, circulatory, and nervous systems are made. Bleeding is controlled by application of direct pressure to any external, bleeding wounds and by occlusion of any chest wounds.

Typically, when the patient presents with intra-abdominal injuries, oral fluids are withheld in anticipation of surgery and a nasogastric tube may be inserted to decompress the stomach and reduce the risk of aspiration. Tetanus prophylaxis and broad-spectrum antibiotics are administered as prescribed.

Throughout the stay in the ED, the patient's condition is continuously monitored for changes. If there is continuing evidence of shock, blood loss, free air under the diaphragm, evisceration, hematuria, severe head injury, or suspected or known abdominal injury, the patient is rapidly transported to surgery. In most cases, blunt injuries to the liver and spleen are managed nonsurgically.

Crush Injuries

Crush injuries occur when a person is caught between opposing forces (e.g., run over by a moving vehicle, compressed by machinery, crushed between two cars, crushed under a collapsed building).

Clinical Manifestations and Assessment

The patient who has sustained a crush injury is observed for:

- Hypovolemic shock resulting from extravasation of blood and plasma into injured tissues after compression has been released
- Paralysis of a body part
- Erythema and blistering of skin
- Damaged body part (usually an extremity) appearing swollen, tense, and hard
- Kidney dysfunction (prolonged hypotension causes kidney damage and acute kidney injury; myoglobinuria secondary to muscle damage can cause acute tubular necrosis and acute kidney failure). See Chapter 41, Box 41-9 for pathophysiology of rhabdomyolysis.

Medical and Nursing Management

In conjunction with maintaining the patient's circulation, airway, and breathing, the patient is observed for acute kidney injury. Injury to the back can cause severe kidney damage. Severe muscular damage may cause rhabdomyolysis, a significant release of myoglobin from ischemic skeletal muscle that can result in acute tubular necrosis. In addition, major soft tissue injuries are splinted early to control bleeding and pain. Fluid resuscitation, as discussed previously, is expected, and in addition to stabilization of vital signs, urine output, and hemodynamic parameters, the serum lactic acid level may be monitored as a parameter of successful resuscitation. Lactic acid levels are discussed in Chapter 54.

If an extremity is injured, it is elevated to relieve swelling and pressure. To restore neurovascular function, the provider may perform a **fasciotomy** (surgical incision to the level of the fascia). Refer to Chapter 41 for details on compartment syndrome. Medications for pain and anxiety are then administered as prescribed, and the patient is quickly transported to the operating suite for wound debridement and fracture repair. A hyperbaric chamber (if available) may be used for hyperoxygenation of the crushed tissue, if indicated.

Genitourinary Injury

A rectal or vaginal examination is performed by the primary provider to determine injury to the pelvis, bladder, or intestinal wall. To decompress the bladder and monitor urine output, an indwelling catheter is inserted after a visual examination of the genitourinary area and rectal examination has been completed (not before). A high-riding prostate gland (abnormal position) discovered during a rectal examination indicates a potential urethral injury. Coopernail sign, or ecchymosis (bruising) of the scrotum or labia, is associated with pelvic fracture or pelvic organ injury. Refer to Chapter 27 for details on genitourinary trauma.

Anaphylactic Reaction

An anaphylactic reaction is an acute systemic hypersensitivity reaction that occurs within seconds or minutes after exposure to certain foreign substances, such as medications and other agents like latex, insect stings, or foods. Repeated administration of parenteral or oral therapeutic agents (e.g., repeated exposures to penicillin) may also precipitate an anaphylactic reaction when initially only a mild allergic response occurred. See Chapter 37 for the pathophysiology and clinical manifestations of anaphylaxis.

With an anaphylactic reaction, establishing a patent airway and ventilation is essential. This is performed while another staff member administers epinephrine. Early endotracheal intubation is essential to preserve airway patency, and oropharyngeal suction may be necessary to remove excessive secretions. Resuscitative measures are used, especially for patients with stridor and progressive pulmonary edema. If glottal edema occurs, emergent cricothyroidotomy may be necessary to provide an airway.

Simultaneously with airway management, aqueous epinephrine is administered as prescribed to provide rapid relief of the hypersensitivity reaction. Epinephrine may be administered again if necessary and as prescribed. Judgment is used in choosing one of the following routes of administration:

- Subcutaneous injection for mild, generalized symptoms
- Intramuscular (IM) injection when the reaction is more severe and progressive and with the knowledge that vascular collapse will delay absorption of the medication
- IV route (aqueous epinephrine diluted in saline solution and administered *slowly*) used in rare instances in which there is complete loss of consciousness and severe cardiovascular collapse. This method may precipitate cardiac arrhythmias, so ECG monitoring with a readily available defibrillator is necessary. This method is controversial and is not usually recommended because it can lead to more distress than initially present. An IV infusion of saline solution is initiated to provide for emergency access to a vein and to treat hypotension.

Additional treatments may include:

- Antihistamines (e.g., diphenhydramine) to block further histamine binding at target cells
- Aminophylline titrated by IV drip for severe bronchospasm and wheezing refractory to other treatment
- Albuterol inhalers or humidified treatments to decrease bronchoconstriction; crystalloids, colloids, or vasopressors to treat prolonged hypotension
- Isoproterenol or dopamine for reduced cardiac output; oxygen to enhance tissue perfusion
- IV benzodiazepines (e.g., diazepam) for control of seizures, and corticosteroids (e.g., hydrocortisone) for prolonged reaction with persistent hypotension or bronchospasm

Depending on the severity of the acute symptoms, the patient may be admitted to the hospital for observation. The patient should be informed about ways to prevent anaphylactic reactions in the future.

Drug Alert

Epinephrine results in α- and β-adrenergic effects, resulting in vasoconstriction and bronchial smooth-muscle relaxation. Epinephrine works rapidly to reduce throat swelling, open the airways, and maintain blood pressure in patients. Age is not a barrier to IM epinephrine injections in patients with anaphylaxis (Rowe & Gaeta, 2020).

CARING FOR PATIENTS EXPERIENCING POISONING

A poison is any substance that when ingested, inhaled, absorbed, applied to the skin, or produced within the body in relatively small amounts, injures the body by its chemical action. Poisoning from inhalation and ingestion of toxic materials, both intentional and unintentional, constitutes a major health hazard and an emergency situation. Emergency treatment is initiated with the following goals:

- To remove or inactivate the poison before it is absorbed
- To provide supportive care in maintaining vital organ systems
- To administer a specific antidote to neutralize a specific poison
- To implement treatment that hastens the elimination of the absorbed poison

Ingested (Swallowed) Poisons

Swallowed poisons may be corrosive. **Corrosive poisons** include alkaline and acid agents that can cause tissue destruction after coming into contact with mucous membranes. Alkaline products include lye, drain cleaners, toilet bowl cleaners, bleach, nonphosphate detergents, oven cleaners, and button batteries (batteries used to power watches, calculators, or cameras). Acid products include toilet bowl cleaners, pool cleaners, metal cleaners, rust removers, and battery acid.

Medical and Nursing Management

Control of the airway, ventilation, and oxygenation are essential. In the absence of cerebral or kidney damage, the patient's prognosis depends largely on successful management of respiration and circulation. Measures are instituted to stabilize cardiovascular and other body functions. ECG, vital signs, and neurologic status are monitored closely for changes. Shock may result from the cardiodepressant action of the substance ingested, from venous pooling in the lower extremities, or from reduced circulating blood volume resulting from increased capillary permeability. An indwelling urinary catheter is inserted to monitor kidney function. Blood specimens are obtained to determine the concentration of the drug or poison.

Efforts are made to determine what substance was ingested; the amount of the substance; the time since ingestion; signs and symptoms, such as pain or burning sensations, any evidence of redness or burn in the mouth or throat, pain on swallowing or an inability to swallow, vomiting, or drooling; age and weight of the patient; and pertinent health history.

Measures are instituted to remove the toxin or decrease its absorption. Consultation with a Poison Control Center is strongly recommended for a definitive antidote and continued monitoring. The patient who has ingested a corrosive poison is given water or milk to drink for dilution. However, dilution is not attempted if the patient has acute airway edema or obstruction or if there is clinical evidence of esophageal, gastric, or intestinal burn or perforation. The following gastric emptying procedures may be used as prescribed:

- Syrup of ipecac to induce vomiting in the alert patient (*never* use with corrosive poisons)
- Gastric lavage for the obtunded patient. Gastric aspirate is saved and sent to the laboratory for toxicology screens.
- Activated charcoal administration if the poison is one that is absorbed by charcoal
- Cathartics, when appropriate

The specific chemical or physiologic antagonist (antidote) is administered as early as possible to reverse or diminish the effects of the toxin. If this measure is ineffective, procedures may be initiated to remove the ingested substance. These procedures include administration of multiple doses of charcoal, diuresis (for substances excreted by the kidneys), dialysis, or hemoperfusion once admitted to an appropriate inpatient setting. Hemoperfusion involves detoxification of the blood by processing it through an extracorporeal circuit and an adsorbent cartridge containing charcoal or resin, after which the cleansed blood is returned to the patient.

Throughout detoxification, the patient's vital signs, CVP, and fluid and electrolyte balance are monitored closely. Hypotension and cardiac arrhythmias are possible. Seizures are also possible because of central nervous system (CNS) excitement from the poison or from oxygen deprivation. If the patient complains of pain, analgesics are administered cautiously. Severe pain causes vasomotor collapse and reflex inhibition of normal physiologic functions.

Patients presenting with ingested poisoning need to be evaluated for accidental ingestion versus intentional ingestion due to suicide attempt or other psychiatric disturbance. After the patient's condition has stabilized, written material should be given to the patient indicating the signs and symptoms of potential problems related to the ingested poison and signs or symptoms requiring evaluation by the primary provider.

Carbon Monoxide Poisoning

Carbon monoxide poisoning may occur as a result of industrial or household incidents or attempted suicide. It is a colorless, odorless gas that is implicated in more deaths than any other toxin except alcohol.

When carbon monoxide poisoning occurs, the health department should be contacted so that the dwelling or building in question can be inspected. Carbon monoxide exerts its toxic effect by binding to circulating hemoglobin and thereby reducing the oxygen-carrying capacity of the blood.

Clinical Manifestations and Assessment

Because the CNS has a critical need for oxygen, CNS symptoms predominate with carbon monoxide toxicity. A person with carbon monoxide poisoning may appear intoxicated due to cerebral hypoxia. Other signs and symptoms include headache, muscular weakness, palpitation, dizziness, and confusion, which can progress rapidly to coma. Skin color, which can range from pink or cherry-red to cyanotic and pale, is not a reliable sign. Pulse oximetry is also not valid because the hemoglobin is well saturated. It is not saturated with oxygen, but the pulse oximeter only reads whether or not the hemoglobin is saturated; in this case, it is saturated with carbon monoxide rather than oxygen.

Medical and Nursing Management

Exposure to carbon monoxide requires immediate treatment. Goals of management are to reverse cerebral and myocardial hypoxia and to hasten elimination of carbon monoxide. Whenever a patient inhales a poison, the following general measures apply:

- Carry the patient to fresh air immediately; open all doors and windows.
- Loosen all tight clothing.
- Initiate cardiopulmonary resuscitation if required; administer 100% oxygen.
- Prevent chilling; wrap the patient in blankets.
- Keep the patient as quiet as possible.
- Do not give alcohol in any form or permit the patient to smoke.

In addition, for the patient with carbon monoxide poisoning, **carboxyhemoglobin** levels are analyzed on arrival at the ED and before treatment with oxygen if possible. Oxygen at 100% is administered at atmospheric or preferably hyperbaric pressures to reverse hypoxia and accelerate the elimination of carbon monoxide. Oxygen is administered until the carboxyhemoglobin level is less than 5%. The patient is monitored continuously. Psychoses, spastic paralysis, ataxia, visual disturbances, and deterioration of mental status and behavior may persist after resuscitation and may be symptoms of permanent brain damage.

DISASTER NURSING

Disasters are defined as any human-made or natural event that overwhelms the local community resources. Resources may be required from local, state, and federal agencies. International agency support may be required in cases in which extensive intervention is required. Acts of terrorism, warfare, air or rail accidents, epidemic and pandemic illness, weather-related events, toxic spills, or geologic events such as landslides and earthquakes are examples of some common disaster events that can result in casualties and tax the resources of health care facilities and communities (Adelman et al., 2019).

FEDERAL, STATE, AND LOCAL RESPONSES TO EMERGENCIES

When a **mass casualty incident (MCI)** occurs, the initial review and response occurs at the local level. Local emergency response agencies (including volunteer agencies) are typically the first responders. As the magnitude of the MCI is evaluated and scope of services needed is assessed, the progression to enlist aid from state and then federal resources may be made through official channels. Local and state offices of emergency management coordinate interagency efforts. These organizations maintain a corps of emergency management personnel, including responders, planners, and administrative and support staff. A request for federal resources is generally made when local resources have become or are expected to become depleted due to the magnitude of the event. Federal resources are available through several departments, though the intent is to support local and state efforts rather than assume responsibility for any disaster response. Table 55-2 lists federal resources.

The Incident Command System (ICS) is the local organization that coordinates personnel, facilities, equipment, and communication in any emergency situation. The ICS has a federal mandate and is an integral part of the National Incident Management System (NIMS). According to the Federal Emergency Management Agency (FEMA, 2021), the ICS can be used at all levels of disaster management to provide a standard management response that organizes and integrates

TABLE **55-2 Federal Disaster Resources**

Federal Disaster Resources	Type of Support Available
Department of Health and Human Services (DHHS)	
Centers for Disease Control and Prevention (CDC)	Collaborates to create the expertise, information, and tools needed to protect the health of the nation and the world
National Disaster Medical System (NDMS)	Has many medical support teams, such as Disaster Medical Assistance Teams (DMATs), Disaster Mortuary Response Teams (DMORTs), Veterinary Medical Assistance Teams (VMATs), and National Medical Response Teams for Weapons of Mass Destruction (NMRTs)
Department of Justice (DOJ)	
Federal Emergency Management Agency (FEMA)	Provides scene control and collection of forensic evidence
Department of Homeland Security	
Federal Bureau of Investigation (FBI)	Can activate teams such as the Urban Search and Rescue Teams (USRTs)

the coordination of response for personnel, facilities, and equipment. It establishes common responses for planning and managing resources at all response levels.

HOSPITAL EMERGENCY PREPAREDNESS PLANS

Health care facilities are required by the Joint Commission to create a plan for emergency preparedness that addresses both internal and external disasters. This plan should be developed with attention to the most likely internal and external disaster potentials. Disaster exercises are required to simulate mass casualty events with participation from multiple agencies.

Components

The Joint Commission has created accreditation standards that cover eight essential areas for disaster operation plans. These emergency management standards include expectations for plans for managing the consequences of emergencies, development and maintenance of an emergency operations plan (EOP), establishing emergency communication strategies, planning for managing resources and assets during emergencies, managing safety and security during emergencies, defining staff roles and responsibilities, establishing strategies for managing utilities during emergencies, and developing strategies for managing patient clinical and support activities during an emergency (The Joint Commission, 2021).

Initiating the Disaster Plan

Notification of a disaster situation to a health care facility varies with each situation. In general, the notification to the facility comes from outside sources unless the initial incident occurred at the facility. The disaster activation plan should clearly state how the EOP is to be initiated. If communication is functioning, field incident command will give notice of the approximate number of arriving patients, though the number of self-referring patients will not be known and may impact resource management.

Identifying Patients

Patient tracking is a critical component of casualty management. Disaster tags, which are numbered and include triage priority, name, address, age, location and description of injuries, and treatments or medications given, are used to communicate patient information. The tag should be securely placed on the patient and remain with the patient at all times. The tag number and the patient's name are recorded in a disaster log. The log is used by the command center to track patients, assign beds, and provide families with information.

Triage During Mass Casualty Incidents

In nondisaster situations, health care workers assign a high priority and allocate the most resources to those who are the most critically ill. However, in a disaster, when health care providers are faced with a large number of casualties, the fundamental principle guiding resource allocation is to do the greatest good for the greatest number of people. Decisions are based on the likelihood of survival and consumption of available resources. Therefore, patients with conditions associated with a high mortality rate would be assigned a low triage priority in a disaster situation, even if the person is conscious. Although this may sound uncaring, from an ethical standpoint the expenditure of limited resources on people with a low chance of survival, and denial of those resources to others with serious but treatable conditions, cannot be justified.

The triage officer rapidly assesses those injured at the disaster scene. Patients are immediately tagged and transported or given life-saving interventions. One person performs the initial triage while other EMS personnel perform life-saving measures (e.g., intubation) and transport patients. Although EMS personnel carry out initial field triage, secondary and continuous triage at all subsequent levels of care is essential.

Staff should control all entrances to the acute care facility so that incoming patients are directed to the triage area first. The triage area may be outside the entry or just at the door of the ED. This allows all patients, including those arriving by medical transport and those who walk in, to be triaged. Some patients already seen in the field may be reclassified in the triage area based on their current presentation.

Triage categories separate patients according to severity of injury. A special color-coded tagging system is used during an MCI so that the triage category is immediately obvious. There are several triage systems in use across the country, and every nurse should be aware of the system used by their facility and community. The North Atlantic Treaty Organization (NATO) triage system is one that is widely used and is presented here. It consists of four colors—red, yellow, green, and black (Table 55-3). Each color signifies a different level of priority, with red representing the most significant but potentially survivable injuries through green, representing minor injuries. Black designates "expected" death due to nonsurvivable injuries or patients for whom death appears to be imminent.

Communication With Media and Family

Communication is a key component of disaster management. Communication within the vast team of disaster responders is paramount; however, effective, informative communication with the media and worried family members is also crucial and must be addressed in the organization's disaster plan and communicated to staff.

Although the media have an obligation to report the news and can play a significant positive role in communication, the number of reporters and newscasters and their support teams can be overwhelming, possibly compromising operations and patient confidentiality. A clearly defined process for managing media requests that includes a designated spokesperson, a site for the dissemination of information (away from patient care areas), and a regular schedule for providing updates should be part of the disaster plan.

The disaster plan helps prevent the release of contradictory or inaccurate information. Initial statements should focus on current efforts and what is being done to better understand the scope and impact of the situation. Information about casualties should not be released. Security staff should not allow media personnel access to patient care areas.

Friends and family members converging on the scene must be cared for by the facility. They may be feeling intense anxiety, shock, or grief and should be provided with information and updates about their loved ones as soon as possible and regularly thereafter. They should not be in the

TABLE 55-3 NATO Triage Categories During a Mass Casualty Incident

Triage Category	Priority	Color	Typical Conditions
Immediate: Injuries are life-threatening but survivable with minimal intervention. Individuals in this group can progress rapidly to expectant category if treatment is delayed.	1	Red	Sucking chest wound, airway obstruction secondary to mechanical cause, shock, hemothorax, tension pneumothorax, asphyxia, unstable chest and abdominal wounds, incomplete amputations, open fractures of long bones, and second-/third-degree burns of 15–40% total body surface area
Delayed: Injuries are significant and require medical care but can wait hours without threat to life or limb. Individuals in this group receive treatment only after immediate casualties are treated.	2	Yellow	Stable abdominal wounds without evidence of significant hemorrhage; soft tissue injuries; maxillofacial wounds without airway compromise; vascular injuries with adequate collateral circulation; genitourinary tract disruption; fractures requiring open reduction, debridement, and external fixation; most eye and central nervous system injuries
Minimal: Injuries are minor and treatment can be delayed hours to days. Individuals in this group should be moved away from the main triage area.	3	Green	Upper extremity fractures, minor burns, sprains, small lacerations without significant bleeding, behavioral disorders or psychological disturbances
Expectant: Injuries are extensive, and chances of survival are unlikely even with definitive care. Persons in this group should be separated from other casualties but not abandoned. Comfort measures should be provided when possible.	4	Black	Unresponsive patients with penetrating head wounds, high spinal cord injuries, wounds involving multiple anatomic sites and organs, second-/third-degree burns in excess of 60% of body surface area, seizures or vomiting within 24 hours after radiation exposure, profound shock with multiple injuries, agonal respirations; no pulse, no blood pressure, pupils fixed and dilated

triage or treatment areas but in a designated area staffed by available social service workers, counselors, therapists, and/or clergy. Access to this area should be controlled to prevent families from being disturbed.

Emotional and behavioral effects vary among affected people. Factors that influence a person's response to a disaster include the degree and nature of the exposure to the disaster, loss of friends and loved ones, existing coping strategies, available resources and support, and the personal meaning attached to the event. Other factors, such as the loss of a home and valued possessions, extended exposure to danger, and exposure to toxic contamination, also influence response and increase the risk for adjustment problems. Those exposed to the dead and injured, those endangered by the event, older adults, children, emergency first responders, and health care personnel caring for victims are considered to be at higher risk of emotional sequelae.

Nurses can assist victims of disasters and their families through active listening and providing emotional support, giving information, and referring patients to therapists or social workers. Health care workers must refer people to mental health care services because few disaster victims seek these services, though early intervention can minimize psychological consequences. Nurses can also discourage victims from subjecting themselves to repeated exposure to the event through media replays and news articles and encourage them to return to normal activities and social roles when appropriate.

The Nurse's Role in Disaster Response Plans

The role of the nurse during a disaster varies. The nurse may be asked to perform duties outside their area of expertise and may take on responsibilities normally held by physicians or advanced practice nurses. Although the exact role of a nurse in disaster management depends on the specific needs of the facility at the time, it should be clear which nurse or physician is in charge of a given patient care area and which procedures each individual nurse may or may not perform. Assistance can be obtained through the incident command center, and nonmedical personnel can provide services where possible.

New settings and atypical roles for nurses arise during a disaster; for example, the nurse may facilitate shelter care in a temporary housing area or bereavement support and assistance with identification of deceased loved ones. People may require crisis intervention, or the nurse may participate in counseling other staff members and in critical incident stress management (CISM) (discussed later in this chapter). Special care may be warranted for at-risk populations during a disaster including people with disabilities, older adults, children, pregnant people, and members of other vulnerable populations.

Critical Incident Stress Management

CISM is an approach to preventing and treating the emotional trauma that can affect emergency responders as a consequence of their jobs and that can also occur to anyone involved in a disaster or MCI. CISM is handled by teams trained in the techniques.

Components of CISM plans include defusing, debriefing, demobilization, and follow-up care after the incident. *Defusing* is a process by which the person receives education about recognition of stress reactions and management strategies for handling stress. *Debriefing* is a more complicated intervention; it involves a 2- to 3-hour process during which participants are asked about their emotional reactions to the incident, what symptoms they may be experiencing (e.g., flashbacks, difficulty sleeping, intrusive thoughts), and other psychological ramifications. As an intervention, *demobilization* is usually reserved for large-scale events with large numbers of participants from different disciplines. If separate defusing interventions were attempted for each group, CISM resources might be overwhelmed. Similar to the defusing intervention, responders are presented with information regarding expected stress reactions that they might experience and how to manage them. The responders are also provided an opportunity to rest and eat before returning to their normal, preincident routines. In the event of large-scale disasters, it might be appropriate to participate in the demobilization process after each shift of work. In *follow-up*, members of the CISM team contact the participants of a debriefing and schedule a follow-up meeting if necessary. People with ongoing stress reactions are referred to mental health specialists.

PREPAREDNESS AND RESPONSE

As a health care provider, a nurse must be prepared for terrorism and other disasters; this includes awareness of the potential for covert use of weapons of mass destruction (WMD); self-protection; and early detection, containment, or **decontamination** of substances and agents that may affect others by secondary exposure. The strength of many toxins, today's mobile society, and long incubation periods for some organisms and diseases can result in an epidemic that can quickly and silently spread across the entire country. For example, there must be awareness that a formerly healthy person with a rapid onset of flu-like symptoms may have a dangerous illness, such as anthrax or severe acute respiratory syndrome (SARS), both of which are discussed in more detail later in this chapter.

Detection

Health care personnel should have a heightened awareness for trends that may suggest deliberate dispersal of toxic or infectious agents. Some general principles should be considered, such as:

- Awareness of an unusual increase in the number of people seeking care for fever, respiratory, or GI symptoms.

- Any clusters of patients presenting with the same unusual illness from a single location. Clusters can be from a specific geographic location, such as a city, or from a single sporting or entertainment event.
- Large number of rapidly fatal cases, especially when death occurs within 72 hours after hospital admission.
- Increase in disease incidence in a normally healthy population. These cases should be reported to the state health department and to the CDC, including information about recent travel and contact with others who have been ill or have recently died of an illness.

Suspicions or findings are reported to the appropriate unit in the facility and to proper authorities in the community. Resources for information can include the infection control department, material safety data sheets (MSDSs), the state health department, the CDC, the local poison control center, and many websites. Reporting furnishes data elements to those agencies responsible for epidemiology and response. Reporting also allows for sharing of information among facilities and jurisdictions and can help determine the source of infections or exposure and prevent further exposures and even deaths.

Personal Protection

Preparedness and response involve the protection of the health care provider by additional PPE prior to contact with a patient who is contaminated with hazardous material or infected with a contagion. The purpose of PPE is to shield health care workers from the chemical, physical, biologic, and radiologic hazards that may exist when caring for contaminated patients. The U.S. Environmental Protection Agency (EPA) has divided protective clothing and respiratory protection into four categories, level A through level D (Box 55-6; U.S. Environmental Protection Agency, 2020).

BOX 55-6 Environmental Protection Agency Categories of Protective Clothing and Respiratory Protection

- Level A protection is worn when the highest level of protection for the respiratory system, skin, eye, and mucous membrane is required. This includes a self-contained breathing apparatus (SCBA) and a fully encapsulating, vapor-tight, chemical-resistant suit with chemical-resistant gloves and boots.
- Level B protection requires the highest level of respiratory protection but a lesser level of skin and eye protection than with level A situations. This level of protection includes positive-pressure, full face-piece SCBA or positive-pressure supplied air respirator with escape SCBA, inner and outer chemical-resistant gloves, face shield, hooded chemical-resistant clothing, coveralls, and outer chemical-resistant boots.
- Level C protection requires the air-purified respirator, which uses filters or sorbent materials to remove harmful substances from the air. A chemical-resistant coverall with splash hood, chemical-resistant gloves, and boots are included in level C protection.
- Level D protection is the typical work uniform. Level D protective equipment may include gloves, safety glasses, or a face shield.

Decontamination

Decontamination, the process of removing accumulated contaminants, is critical to the health and safety of health care providers by preventing secondary contamination. The decontamination plan should establish procedures and educate employees about decontamination procedures, identify the equipment needed and methods to be used, and establish methods for disposal of contaminated materials.

Effective decontamination must include a minimum of two steps. The first step is removal of the patient's clothing and jewelry and then rinsing the patient with water. Depending on the type of exposure, this step alone can remove a large amount of the contaminant and decrease secondary contamination. Ideally, facilities should identify areas where patients can be decontaminated prior to entering the facility to prevent accidental contamination of the emergency services area, staff, and other hospital areas and personnel. The second step consists of a thorough soap-and-water wash and rinse. When patients arrive at the facility after being assessed and treated by a prehospital provider, it should not be assumed that they have been thoroughly decontaminated.

NATURAL DISASTERS

Natural disasters may result in mass casualties. Natural disasters can occur anywhere at any time and include events such as tornadoes, hurricanes, floods, avalanches, tidal waves (e.g., tsunamis), earthquakes, and volcanic eruptions. In many cases, preparation prior to the natural disaster is the best-laid plan. In the event of a natural disaster, loss of communications, potable water, and electricity are usually the greatest obstacles to a well-coordinated emergency response. Even wireless technology (e.g., mobile or cellular phones, computers, other communication devices) may not be functional.

The majority of the immediate casualties are trauma-related. These mass casualties tax the trauma system to its limits to provide triage, transport of patients (in poor weather and road conditions), and management within the trauma centers. Electrocution is also a common injury and can result in death.

Excessive exposure to the natural elements and the need for food and water (by both patients and emergency responders) are critical issues. Without cover (e.g., buildings may be unsafe or destroyed) or safe water (e.g., water may be either contaminated or unavailable), injuries from exposure to heat, cold, or contaminated food or water can occur.

Safety equipment that protects rescue workers from injury, exposure, and potentially dangerous animals must be readily available. Hypothermia can occur rapidly in workers who are exposed to water at temperatures of 75°F or less. As in all disasters, mental health workers and shelters are needed throughout the community. Veterinary assistance is also essential because pets may be lost, abandoned, or injured. After floods or water disasters, waterborne transmission of agents such as *Escherichia coli*, salmonella, shigella, typhoid, leptospirosis, malaria, and tularemia are common and cause widespread disease.

In some instances, early warning systems have assisted in decreasing the number of deaths from tornadoes and hurricanes. When buildings collapse, rapid response to identify and remove trapped victims is the only means of improving survivability. There is a direct relationship between time trapped and survival; survival is also related to the type of building construction and number of stories of the collapsed structure. Larger-scale issues that can cause significant later morbidity and mortality include the absence of water purification, waste removal, removal of human and animal remains, and vector control. Removal or disposal of biologic, chemical, and nuclear agents must also be considered.

BIOLOGIC AGENTS

Biologic weapons are weapons that spread disease among the general population or the military as part of **biologic warfare**. Biologic agents are delivered in either a liquid or dry state, applied to foods or water, or vaporized for inhalation or direct contact. Vaporization may be accomplished through spray or explosives loaded with the agent. Because of increases in global travel and interconnectedness, an agent could be released in one city and affect people in other cities thousands of miles away. The vector can be an insect, animal, or person, or there may be direct contact with the agent itself.

Anthrax and smallpox are the two agents most likely to be used or weaponized. Table 55-4 describes other easily weaponized biologic agents.

Anthrax

Inhaled anthrax is recognized as the most likely weaponized biologic agent available. *Bacillus anthracis* is a naturally occurring gram-positive, encapsulated rod that lives in the soil in the spore state throughout the world. The bacterium is liberated when exposed to air and is infective only in the spore form. Contact with infected animal products (raw meat) or inhalation of the spores results in infection.

Pathophysiology

Animal studies have suggested that small amounts of inhaled anthrax spores (as low as 50 to 98 spores) may be sufficient to cause death in 10% of the exposed human population (Center for Infectious Disease Research and Policy [CIDRAP], 2013; FDA, 2018). As an aerosol, anthrax is odorless and invisible and can travel a great distance before disseminating; hence, the site of release and the site of infection can be miles apart. Incubation of the inhaled spores can be as long as 7 days.

Clinical Manifestations

Initial symptoms may resemble a common cold. Anthrax does not present as pneumonia. After several days, the symptoms may progress to severe breathing problems and shock.

Medical and Nursing Management

Inhalation anthrax is frequently fatal, even with aggressive antibiotic and supportive therapy. Due to the presence of spores, antibiotic treatment is continued for 60 days. Anthrax cannot be spread from person to person, and standard level D universal precautions are sufficient (see Box 55-6).

Smallpox

Pathophysiology

Smallpox (variola) is classified as a DNA virus. It has an incubation period of 10 to 12 days. It is extremely contagious and is spread by direct contact, contact with clothing or linens, or inhaled droplets of saliva during contact with an infected person. During the incubation period, there are no symptoms. When the virus has multiplied sufficiently to cause the fever and characteristic rash, the affected person not only feels ill but is also at the most infectious period (CDC, 2017; De Laby, 2020). Aerosolization of the virus would result in widespread dissemination.

Clinical Manifestations and Assessment

Signs and symptoms of smallpox infection are similar to influenza and include high fever, malaise, headache, backache, and fatigue. After 2 to 3 days, a flat, red, lesioned rash appears, evolving at the same rate, beginning on the face, mouth, pharynx, and forearms. After several days, these lesions become filled with pus (Fig. 55-5) and form crusts in week 2. By week 3, these crusts have become scabs and begin to fall off (CDC, 2017; Conlon et al., 2019). There is a large amount of the virus in the saliva and pustules. Smallpox is contagious only after the appearance of the rash. There are two forms of smallpox, variola major and variola minor. Variola major is more common and results in a higher fever and more extensive rash. Variola major has a 30% case-fatality rate. Hemorrhagic smallpox, a subtype of variola major, includes all of the previously noted signs and symptoms plus a dusky erythema and petechiae to frank hemorrhage of the skin and mucous membranes, resulting in death by day 5 or 6.

TABLE **55-4 Examples of Biologic Agents That Can Be Used as Weapons**

Agent/ Organism	Contagion	Decontamination and Protective Equipment	Signs and Symptoms	Treatment (Mortality Rate)
Tularemia (*Francisella tularensis*): Gram-negative coccobacillus, one of the most infectious bacteria known	Direct contact with infected animals or aerosolized as a bioterror weapon; bites Not contagious through human-to-human contact	Standard barrier precautions Clothing and linens should be laundered under the usual hospital protocol.	*Initial:* Abrupt onset of fever, fatigue, chills, headache, lower backache, malaise, rigor, coryza (acute inflammation of the mucous membrane of the nasal cavities), dry cough, and sore throat without adenopathy. Nausea and vomiting or diarrhea possible. *As disease progresses:* Sweating, fever, progressive weakness, anorexia, and weight loss demonstrate continued illness. *Mortality secondary to:* Pneumonitis (if inhalation is the source) with copious watery or purulent sputum, hemoptysis, respiratory insufficiency, sepsis, and shock	Streptomycin or gentamicin/aminoglycoside for 10–14 days. Inhalation tularemia must be treated within 48 hours of onset. In mass casualty situations, doxycycline or ciprofloxacin is recommended. For persons exposed to tularemia, tetracycline or doxycycline is recommended for 14 days. (Mortality rate = 2%)
Botulism (*Clostridium botulinum*): Botulinum blocks acetylcholine-containing vesicles from fusing with the terminal membranes of the motor-neuron end-plate, resulting in a flaccid paralysis.	Direct contact Not contagious through human-to-human contact	Any skin exposure to the botulism toxin can be treated with soap and water or a 0.1% hypochlorite solution. Standard precautions are used when treating patients with botulism.	*Gastrointestinal botulism:* Abdominal cramps, nausea, vomiting, and diarrhea *Inhalation botulism:* Fever; symmetric descending flaccid paralysis with multiple cranial nerve palsies. Classic signs and symptoms include diplopia, dysphagia, dry mouth, lack of fever, and alert mental status. Other possible symptoms include ptosis of the eyelids, blurred vision, enlarged sluggish pupils, dysarthria, and dysphonia. *Mortality secondary to:* Airway obstruction and inadequate tidal volume	Supportive ventilatory therapy is necessary if respiratory infection occurs. Aminoglycosides and clindamycin are contraindicated because they exacerbate neuromuscular blockage. Equine antitoxin is used to minimize subsequent nerve damage. There is a 2% rate of anaphylaxis to the antitoxin; therefore, diphenhydramine (Benadryl) and epinephrine must be immediately available for use. Supportive care: Mechanical ventilation, nutrition, fluids, prevention of complications (Mortality rate = 5%)
Plague (*Yersinia pestis*): Nonsporulating gram-negative coccobacillus. The bacterium causes destruction and necrosis of the lymph nodes.	Contagious *Bubonic plague:* Transmitted through flea bites with no person-to-person transmission *Pneumonic plague:* Transmitted through respiratory droplet contact	Isolation barrier precautions with full face respirators. The patient should wear a mask. Rooms should receive a terminal cleaning. Clothing and linens with body fluids on them should be cleaned with the usual disinfectant. Routine precautions should be used in the case of death.	*Bubonic plague:* Sudden fever and chills, weakness, a swollen and tender lymph node (bubo) in the groin, axilla, or cervical area. The resultant bacteremia progresses to septicemia from the endotoxin and, finally, shock and death. *Primary septicemic plague:* Disseminated intravascular coagulation (DIC), necrosis of small vessels, purpura, and gangrene of the digits and nose (black death). *Pneumonic plague:* Severe bronchospasm, chest pain, dyspnea, cough, and hemoptysis. There is a 100% mortality associated with pneumonic plague if not treated within the first 24 hours.	Streptomycin or gentamicin for 10–14 days. Tetracycline or doxycycline is an acceptable alternative if an aminoglycoside cannot be given. People with close contact exposure (less than 2 m) require prophylaxis with doxycycline for 7 days. (Mortality rate = 50%)

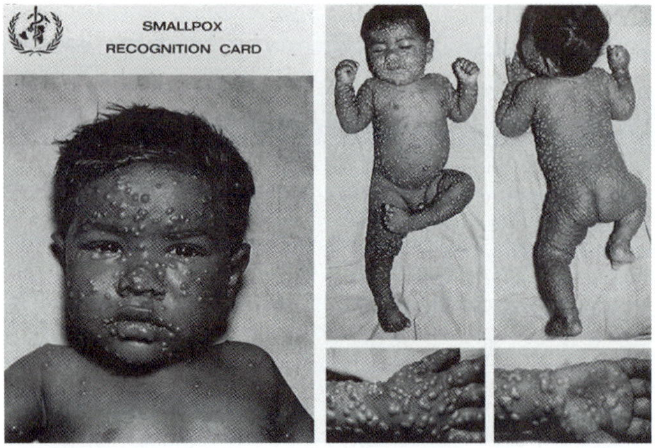

FIGURE 55-5 Patient with smallpox. (From Fenner, F., Henderson, D. A., Arita, I., Jezek, Z., & Ladnyi, I. D. [1988]. *Smallpox and its eradication*. World Health Organization, Geneva, with permission.)

Medical and Nursing Management

Patients with suspected or confirmed smallpox should be placed in a private negative airflow room with droplet and airborne precautions until all scabs have separated. Close contacts of the patient should isolate and check their temperature daily for 17 days after exposure. Any fever above 38°C (101°F) during the 17 days after exposure to a confirmed case would suggest the development of smallpox (National Library of Medicine, n.d.). Vaccination is preventative in staff or contacts exposed to smallpox and should be administered immediately; however, it must be administered prior to the signs of the smallpox rash. Treatment includes supportive care with antibiotics for any additional infection. Use of antiviral medications may be considered, though the current Food and Drug Administration (FDA)-approved antiviral drugs (tecovirimat and brincidofovir) for use in smallpox have only been tested in laboratory tests and have not been tested on people with smallpox infections (CDC, 2021b). Laundry and fabrics need to be placed in labeled bags per Occupational Safety and Health Administration (OSHA) guidelines. Laundry may be washed in hot water with detergents and bleach with hot air drying (National Library of Medicine, n.d.).

Public Health Emergencies: Epidemics and Pandemics

As noted by the American Association of Colleges of Nursing (2021), an important part of the nurse's role in disaster response is the focus on surveillance of community norms for wellness and illness to identify changes of concern, prevention of contributing factors or sequelae of the original event, and containment of the disaster or pandemic. Specific skills may be required to respond to any form of disaster or public health emergency. Disaster first responders and ED staff will especially focus on prevention and containment during the response. The goals of prevention and containment apply not only to the patients and communities involved but are also part of the expectations for responder health safety to prevent spread among themselves or to others in the communities.

Basic principles of public health epidemiology need to be understood to promote safe practices among responders and health care workers; recognize changes in customary disease patterns; and take appropriate measures to treat, mitigate, and contain outbreaks. Columbia University Mailman School of Public Health (2021) defined endemic diseases as a constant prevalence of a disease or infectious agent within a geographical community. This is not limited to acute infectious diseases; it may also include chronic diseases such as cardiovascular disease. When the level of the disease significantly exceeds baseline endemic levels, it may rise to an epidemic level. A rise in chronic or noninfectious disease is generally slower, and the ED does not experience massive, sudden changes in patients presenting with chronic diseases that overwhelms the resources necessary to provide care. Water, air, or soil contamination, unless the result of bioterrorism, are unlikely to cause significant impact to day-to-day operations of the ED. As the CDC (2013) notes, an endemic level of disease may not be desirable but it is the baseline level present in a community, state, or nation. This baseline level is used to measure the extent and progression of disease states.

The CDC (2013) defines epidemic as "an increase, often sudden, in the number of cases of a disease above what is normally expected in that population in that area." This definition is especially relevant to acute infectious diseases, but as with endemics, noninfectious diseases such as diabetes and obesity may also reach epidemic levels. Polio and smallpox are examples of acute disease epidemics that have occurred in the United States.

A pandemic is when a disease spans across continents and due to the extensive spread, affects a much larger number of people compared to an epidemic. The CDC (2013) notes four major factors that contribute to the development of a pandemic: a recent increase in the amount or virulence of an agent, the introduction of the agent into an area that has not been previously exposed to it, increased ability for the agent to be transmitted to others, and additional factors that increase exposure to susceptible hosts or a new method of transmission.

Disaster first responders may be required to respond to an endemic, epidemic, or pandemic disease that requires resources beyond what can be sourced from the geographic area. For example, in 2014, responders were called to Sierra Leone to mitigate spread and transmission of the Ebola virus endemic to prevent spread to other countries. In early 2020, health care workers, including state and federal resources, provided support to communities overwhelmed by the emerging COVID-19 pandemic. In most cases, the ED will be the primary source of care as patients seek health care for public health disease epidemics and pandemics.

A rapid surge in patients seeking emergency care coupled with a need for admission for continued care can rapidly overwhelm available hospital resources. ED operations can be heavily impacted by epidemic or pandemic conditions. The surge of patients, whether relatively short term or ongoing, can overwhelm resources in other nursing units as well due to a rapid influx of admissions coupled with a decrease in availability of staff to care for the admissions. Support services such as laboratory, housekeeping, and materials management may experience challenges in their ability to support the increased demands for supplies, rapid testing and cleaning, and preparation of surge containment areas. Increased utilization of ED and hospital resources due to epidemic or pandemic surges may also significantly affect access to necessary care for other diseases and illnesses.

When responding to epidemic and pandemic surges of acute infectious diseases, the role of the ED nurse focuses on assessment, mitigation, and treatment. The admitting history may provide clues to the nature of the illness based on symptoms, community prevalence, recent travel, and possible exposures to others who were in the same area or who had a known infection. Exposure to chemicals, infectious agents, or bioterrorism may be suspected based on an influx of patients with similar symptoms who attended the same event or were in the same area. Efforts should be made to recognize and segregate patients with acute infectious diseases from other ED patients to mitigate additional exposure and spread. All health care staff will need to wear PPE appropriate to the infectious disease suspected or confirmed. Definitive treatment will depend on the nature of the exposure or type of infectious disease identified.

As noted in Table 55-5, the influenza A variants responsible for the pandemics of 1918 and 2009, and SARS-CoV-2, the virus responsible for the COVID-19 pandemic demonstrate that pandemics are viral diseases that do not respond to treatment with antibiotics. Standard public health measures for cleaning (hands and surfaces), limiting exposure to groups of people, and wearing a mask to limit exposure to respiratory particles are measures used to mitigate the spread of the virus. Additional efforts to mitigate the spread of and exposure to the 2009 influenza A pandemic focused on influenza vaccine booster updates to the most at-risk populations. Because COVID-19 was a novel coronavirus, it presented challenges to rapidly produce and test new vaccines before release to the general public. In the United States, the vaccines initially released were first made available only to vulnerable populations under emergency use authorization due to the public health emergency. They were later made widely available and received final FDA approval. Vaccine hesitancy among U.S. residents became an ongoing challenge, contributing to viral mutation and further spread of the virus.

During surges in COVID-19 transmission, ED and hospital resources became significantly challenged compared to previous viral pandemics caused by influenza A and its variants. Staff shortages to handle the influx of patients,

TABLE 55-5 Comparison of Endemic, Epidemic, and Pandemic Acute Disease Processes

	Definition	Examples
Endemic	A constant prevalence of a disease or infectious agent within a geographical community	Malaria Hanta virus
Epidemic	An increase, often sudden, in the number of cases of a disease beyond what is normally expected in that population in that area	Smallpox Polio Ebola Zika
Pandemic	An epidemic that spans across continents and, due to the extensive spread, affects a much larger number of people compared to an epidemic	1918 Influenza (H1N1 virus) **1957-1958 Influenza (H2N2 virus)** **2003 SARS** 2009 Influenza A (H1N1pdm09 virus) 2019 Coronavirus COVID-19 (SARS-CoV-2 virus)

Adapted from Centers for Disease Control and Prevention (CDC). (2018). *Past pandemics*. https://www.cdc.gov/flu/pandemic-resources/basics/past-pandemics.html

insufficient or inadequate PPE, and a lack of initial understanding about the virus's transmission and produced effects in multiple body systems, especially the respiratory system, presented early challenges. Caring for patients prior to the release of vaccines under emergency use authorization for health care workers and vulnerable populations created additional stress for health care workers who worried about their own exposure and transmission to their contacts. ED holding or boarding of patients who needed to be admitted when no beds were available in critical care or other nursing units created additional strains on the usual care delivery processes and procedures. ED nurses and staff were confronted with rapidly changing care expectations, including infusions of monoclonal antibodies and rapid assessment and interventions for respiratory failure on a scale far beyond previous expectations. In order to avoid increased transmission, many areas limited or did not allow family members or support people to accompany patients in the ED. Communication among health care workers, patients, and family and support people was disrupted; updates via phone became challenging.

In any endemic, epidemic, or pandemic, communities can request assistance from the federal government, and this happened during the COVID-19 pandemic as different communities were affected at different times. Critical needs included additional medical and nursing staff to support exhausted and overwhelmed hospital staff as well as assistance with creating additional surge capacity through temporary structures including tents or transformation of conference rooms or parking structures into overflow assessment and treatment areas. However, additional resources were limited. Some states or geographic areas were forced to seek transfer of patients across state lines or to different areas. Alternatively, they were faced with initiating crisis standards of care due to limited availability of critical resources such as beds, ventilators, dialysis machines, and extra corporeal membrane oxygenation (ECMO) units as well as the highly specialized staff required to run some of the equipment.

Pearls for Practice: Lifting the Lens

You are entering the nursing profession as the nation and world navigate the first pandemic in a century. While most of your time in nursing school is dedicated to known disease, COVID-19 has reminded us that we must be alert to new emerging infectious diseases (EIDs). Many will likely have a zoonotic origin (natural transmission from animals to humans; Destoumieux-Garzón et al., 2021). It should also make you consider the importance of recognizing the interplay between planetary health (climate change, loss of biodiversity) and EID. A mindset that considers the human and ecologic factors associated with EID will be necessary, as will a recognition of the importance of a multidisciplinary approach in the face of global environmental change.

The Joint Commission surveys hospitals and other facilities as an accrediting agency in support of the Centers for Medicare & Medicaid Services (CMS). The Joint Commission defines standards expected for hospitals to care for patients during emergencies and disasters and focuses on planning and preparation (The Joint Commission, 2021). These standards support the CMS Emergency Preparedness Regulations Guidance. The purpose of the CMS emergency preparedness rules are to establish national emergency preparedness requirements to ensure adequate planning for both natural and human-made disasters and coordination with federal, state, tribal, regional, and local emergency preparedness systems (CMS, 2021).

According to the Joint Commission (2021), the three broad essentials that facilities need to meet to ensure access to health care during disasters or emergencies include safeguarding of human resources, maintaining business continuity, and protection of physical resources. Each hospital or facility will set specific policies and procedures around these key areas. Surveys of strengths and weaknesses of the facility's ability to manage these essentials are commonly performed at regular intervals, with policies and procedures revised as needed. The Joint Commission recognizes the need for facilities to be able to respond to local surge issues from a variety of sources including mass shootings, natural disasters, acts of terrorism, and disease outbreaks.

Safeguarding of human resources is a key requirement in the Joint Commission standards. Ensuring standards for employee safety including ventilation, ability to safely exit a building during an emergency if needed, and adequate worker health and safety protection through sufficient and appropriate use of PPE and monitoring of staff health are key elements of this standard. Hospitals may be hampered in securing sufficient PPE due to inadequate supply chains during significant epidemic and pandemic surges, but the facility is expected to meet their established policy guidelines for the amount and type of equipment to keep on hand.

In early 2021, OSHA was required to address existing standards that were deemed inadequate to protect workers from the biohazards of COVID-19. These emergency temporary orders addressed key areas to support health care worker safety and applied to health care facilities with more than 10 employees. These key areas included requirements to develop specific COVID-19 plans and policies to minimize the risk of transmission of COVID-19 to employees, to limit and monitor point of entry for patients along with procedures to screen employees and patients for COVID-19 symptoms; to implement patient management plans; to develop and implement policies and procedures for standard precautions based on CDC guidelines; and to set standards for the use of PPE when indoors, for use of respirators for aerosol-generating procedures, for disinfection, and for the number of personnel allowed in the room during procedures. Cleaning and disinfection of equipment was addressed to meet CDC standards, and access to handwashing stations and 60% alcohol-based hand sanitizers were included. In addition to the standards for protecting health care workers and patients, additional standards included access to vaccines as well as contact tracing and exposure notification and documentation protocols (OSHA, 2021),

Maintaining business continuity and protection of hospital resources according to the Joint Commission standards includes provisions to provide care under unexpected conditions. Assessments and policies created at the facility level include risk assessments for technology failures (including cybersecurity), loss of utilities, ventilation systems, hazardous materials such as those from chemical and radiologic accidents, and similar areas specific to hazards identified in the individual facility. Supply chain interruptions are part of the assessment, policies, and mitigation efforts. Facilities are expected to ensure supplies are available to support care needs of patients and staff during disaster situations.

Despite the efforts of facilities to ensure that business operations are maintained and supplies are adequate, a significant disaster may strain the system to the point of collapse. Difficult situations may need to be addressed for any other mitigation attempts or a move to a crisis standard of care. Crisis standards of care limit care received in an effort to provide the greatest good for the largest number of people. Care decisions may need to be implemented to provide care to patients who meet specific criteria or are most likely to benefit from treatment. These standards are created well in advance of need and implemented when the severity of the situation is so significant that failure to implement crisis standards has a high potential to increase comorbidity and death to a larger patient population. Triage decisions during a disaster may be considered disaster crisis standards of care when resuscitation efforts are not initiated in an MCI. In hospitals, care options for intubation, dialysis, or advanced technologies may be limited to those with a higher potential of survival. The emotional impact to first responders and facility staff cannot be ignored.

Severe Acute Respiratory Syndrome

Not all mass casualty biologic events are terrorist-based. The SARS outbreak in 2003 is a prime example of a non–terrorist-based mass casualty biologic event. The disease started as "atypical" pneumonia in China in February of that year, and it had spread to 29 countries throughout the world by July. Air travel and worldwide trade have increased the possibility that any contagious disease process may spread rapidly. The incubation period for SARS is 2 to 10 days.

Clinical Manifestations and Assessment

SARS should be considered in the cases of an outbreak of atypical pneumonia with travel to an area with a known SARS outbreak, a health care worker with direct patient contact, or a lab worker in a laboratory that contains live SARS-CoV. Early systemic signs are dry cough and shortness of breath with or without other respiratory symptoms. X-ray-confirmed pneumonia or acute respiratory distress syndrome (ARDS) is evident at 7 to 10 days along with fever and respiratory symptoms.

Medical and Nursing Management

Droplet precaution isolation and control of visits to the exposed patient are essential. Treatment is supportive. The overall case fatality rate is 10%, which increases to more than 50% in patients older than 60 years of age, putting frail older adults at higher risk.

Pearls for Practice

The goal of droplet precautions is to prevent the transmission of pathogens spread through close respiratory or mucous membrane contact with respiratory secretions. Because the pathogens do not remain infectious over long distances, special air handling and ventilation are not required to prevent transmission. A single-patient room is preferred for patients who require droplet precautions; however, if it is not available, consultation with infection control personnel is recommended regarding cohorting of patients. A mask is required for close contact (within 3 ft) with patients who are infectious; the mask is generally donned upon room entry. If the patient must be transported outside of the room, a mask should be applied (if tolerated), and the patient should be instructed in cough etiquette (covering the mouth and nose when coughing or sneezing, using and disposing of tissues). In addition, hand hygiene should be performed after hands have been in contact with respiratory secretions (Siegel et al., 2019; Wisconsin Department of Health Services, 2021).

CHEMICAL AGENTS

Agents that may be used in **chemical warfare** or terrorism are *overt* in that the effects are more apparent and occur more quickly than those caused by biologic weapons. Agents are available and well-known, result in major mortality and morbidity, and cause panic and social disruption. There are many agents, including those that affect nerves (sarin, soman), those that affect blood (cyanide), vesicants (lewisite, nitrogen and sulfur mustard, phosgene), heavy metals (arsenic, lead), volatile toxins (benzene, chloroform), pulmonary agents (chlorine), and corrosive acids (nitric acid, sulfuric acid) (Table 55-6).

Chemical agents vary in their absorption and effects. The *volatility* of chemical agents refers to the ability of the agent to become a vapor. Most chemicals are heavier than air, except for hydrogen cyanide, and heavier exposure occurs lower to the ground. *Persistence* of chemical agents means the chemical is less likely to vaporize and disperse. More volatile chemicals do not evaporate quickly and are more commonly used by military and terrorist agents than are industrial chemicals. *Toxicity* of the chemical agent is the ability to cause injury to the body. Toxicity is affected by concentration and length of exposure. *Latency* is the time from absorption to the appearance of symptoms. Sulfur mustards and pulmonary agents have the longest latency, whereas vesicants, nerve agents, and cyanide produce symptoms within seconds.

Nerve Agents

The most toxic agents in existence are the nerve agents, such as sarin, soman, tabun, venomous agent X (VX), and organophosphates (pesticides). They are inexpensive, effective in small quantities, and easily dispersed. In the liquid form, nerve agents evaporate into a colorless, odorless vapor. Organophosphates are similar in nature to the nerve agents used in warfare and are readily available. Nerve agents can be inhaled or absorbed percutaneously or subcutaneously. These agents bond with acetylcholinesterase, so that

TABLE 55-6 **Common Chemical Agents**

Agent	Action	Signs and Symptoms	Decontamination and Treatment
Nerve Agents			
Sarin Soman organophosphates	Inhibition of cholinesterase	Increased secretions, gastrointestinal motility, diarrhea, bronchospasm	Soap and water Supportive care Benzodiazepine Pralidoxime Atropine
Blood Agent			
Cyanide	Inhibition of aerobic metabolism	Inhalation—tachypnea, tachycardia, coma, seizures. Can progress to respiratory arrest, respiratory failure, cardiac arrest, death	Sodium nitrite Sodium thiocyanate Amyl nitrate Hydroxocobalamin
Vesicant Agents			
Lewisite Sulfur mustard Nitrogen mustard Phosgene	Blistering agents	Superficial to partial-thickness burn with vesicles that coalesce	Soap and water Blot; do not rub dry
Pulmonary Agents			
Phosgene Chlorine	Separation of alveoli from capillary bed	Pulmonary edema, bronchospasm	Airway management Ventilatory support Bronchoscopy

acetylcholine is not inactivated; the adverse result is continuous stimulation (hyperstimulation) of the nerve endings.

A very small drop of a nerve agent is enough to result in sweating and twitching at the site of exposure. A larger amount results in more systemic symptoms. Effects can begin anywhere from 30 minutes up to 18 hours after exposure. The more common organophosphates and carbamates (e.g., Sevin and malathion) that are used in agriculture result in less severe symptoms than do those used in warfare or in terrorist attacks. In an ordinary situation (e.g., non-warfare, non-terrorist attack situation), a patient could arrive at the ED having been exposed to organophosphates unintentionally, or intentionally in a suicide attempt.

Clinical Manifestations and Assessment

Signs and symptoms of nerve gas exposure are those of cholinergic crisis and include bilateral miosis (constriction of the pupil), visual disturbances, increased GI motility, nausea and vomiting, diarrhea, substernal spasm, indigestion, bradycardia and atrioventricular block, bronchoconstriction, laryngeal spasm, weakness, fasciculations (small, localized "twitching"), and incontinence. The patient must be examined in a dark area to truly identify miosis. Neurologic responses include insomnia, forgetfulness, impaired judgment, depression, and irritability. A lethal dose results in loss of consciousness, seizures, copious secretions, fasciculations, flaccid muscles, and apnea.

Medical and Nursing Management

Decontamination begins with removal of clothing and jewelry followed by washing with copious amounts of soap and water or saline solution for 8 to 20 minutes. It is estimated that up to 90% of chemical contamination is removed by disrobing alone (De Laby, 2020). The water is blotted, not wiped, off the skin. A 0.5% hypochlorite solution (bleach) can also be used (Agency for Toxic Substances and Disease Registry [ATSDR], 2017). The airway is maintained, and suctioning is frequently required. Plastic airway equipment will absorb sarin gas, which may result in continued exposure to the agent.

Atropine 2 to 4 mg is administered IV followed by 2 mg every 3 to 8 minutes for up to 24 hours of treatment. Alternatively, IV atropine 1 to 2 mg/hr may be administered until clear signs of anticholinergic activity have returned (decreased secretions, tachycardia, and decreased GI motility). Another medication that may serve as an antidote is pralidoxime, which allows cholinesterase to become active against acetylcholine. Pralidoxime 1 to 2 g in 100 to 150 mL of normal saline solution is administered over 15 to 30 minutes. Pralidoxime has no effect on secretions and may have side effects that include hypertension, tachycardia, weakness, dizziness, blurred vision, and diplopia.

Diazepam or other benzodiazepines should be administered to control seizures, decrease fasciculations, and alleviate apprehension and agitation. Military personnel believed to be at risk for chemical attack are provided with Mark I automatic injectors, which contain 2 mg of atropine and 600 mg of pralidoxime chloride. The automatic injectors can be self-administered. If additional doses are needed, or the person is unable to self-administer, then they could be administered by a medic or another in the field since all are trained on the use of the auto injector. Diazepam is provided in an auto injectable form and may be difficult to self-inject due to the severity of the symptoms. If the person is not able to administer their own injections, then the medic or another person can provide the injection.

Blood Agents

Blood agents, such as hydrogen cyanide and cyanogen chloride, have a direct effect on cellular metabolism, resulting in asphyxiation through alterations in hemoglobin. Cyanide is an agent that has profound systemic effects. It is commonly used in the mining of gold and silver and in the plastics and dye industries.

A cyanide release is often associated with the odor of bitter almonds. In house fires, cyanide is released during the combustion of plastics, rugs, silk, furniture, and other construction materials. There is a significant correlation between blood cyanide and carbon monoxide levels in patients who survive fires; in many cases, the cause of death is cyanide poisoning.

Clinical Manifestations and Assessment

Cyanide can be ingested, inhaled, or absorbed through the skin and mucous membranes. Cyanide is protein-bound and inhibits aerobic metabolism, leading to respiratory muscle failure, respiratory arrest, cardiac arrest, and death. Inhalation of cyanide results in flushing, tachypnea, tachycardia, nonspecific neurologic symptoms, stupor, coma, and seizure preceding respiratory arrest.

Medical and Nursing Management

Treatment of patients for cyanide poisoning includes rapid administration of amyl nitrate, sodium nitrite, and sodium thiosulfate, which is essential to the successful management of cyanide exposure. First, the patient is intubated and placed on a ventilator. Next, amyl nitrate pearls are crushed and placed in the ventilator reservoir to induce methemoglobinemia. Cyanide has a 20% to 25% higher affinity for methemoglobin than it does for hemoglobin; it binds with methemoglobin to form either cyanomethemoglobin or sulfmethemoglobin. The cyanomethemoglobin is then detoxified in the liver by the enzyme rhodanese. Next, IV sodium nitrite is administered to induce the rapid formation of methemoglobin. Sodium thiosulfate is then administered IV; it has a higher affinity for cyanide than methemoglobin does and stimulates the conversion of cyanide to sodium thiocyanate, which can be excreted by the kidneys. Although they may be life-saving, these emergency medications do have side effects; sodium nitrite can result in severe hypotension, and thiocyanate can cause vomiting, psychosis, arthralgia, and myalgia.

The production of methemoglobin is contraindicated in patients suffering from smoke inhalation because they already have decreased oxygen-carrying capacity secondary to the carboxyhemoglobin produced by smoke inhalation. In facilities where a hyperbaric chamber is available, it may be used to provide oxygenation while the previously discussed therapies are initiated. An alternative suggested treatment for cyanide poisoning is hydroxocobalamin (vitamin B_{12a}). Hydroxocobalamin binds cyanide to form cyanocobalamin (vitamin B_{12}). It must be administered IV in large doses. Administration of vitamin B_{12} can result in a transient pink discoloration of mucous membranes, skin, and urine. In high doses, tachycardia and hypertension can occur, but they usually resolve within 48 hours.

MORAL DISTRESS AND POSTTRAUMATIC STRESS AMONG EMERGENCY AND DISASTER RESPONDERS

Health care workers are commonly exposed to stress-producing events. ED staff and disaster responders are routinely required to perform at their best levels despite the sometimes chaotic work environment that includes sudden disruptions to work flow due to unplanned or unanticipated events. As has been discussed in the disaster response section, actions may include triage decisions to care for the victims who are most likely to survive. Basic life support for cardiac arrest is not provided in the field as it would most likely be in a hospital. Challenges to the routine care delivery models during prolonged events and the need to provide crisis standards of care, including limitations of care or decisions for the use of life-sustaining high-technology equipment, can cause moral distress.

Disasters can result in a disparity between the resources of the health care agency and the needs of those affected. This generates ethical dilemmas for nurses and other health care providers. Issues include conflicts related to:

- Rationing care and use of crisis standards of care: A substantial change in usual health care operations and the level of care it is possible to deliver
- Futile therapy: Beginning or continuing treatment that cannot cure, palliate, ameliorate, or restore a patient's quality of life
- Consent: Informing a patient about the risks, benefits, and alternatives of a given procedure or intervention; implicit to consent is that the patient is capable of understanding the information
- Duty: The professional and moral responsibilities of nurses (e.g., the duty of care toward a patient regardless of class, race, or religion)
- Confidentiality: Maintaining patient privacy

- Resuscitation: Attempts to restore proper blood circulation; ethical dilemmas may result from conflicts with futile therapy discussed previously

Disasters may be due to climate-related issues (e.g., typhoons, hurricanes, tornados) or human-caused events (e.g., terrorist attacks, transportation accidents). Some may be anticipated, such as impending critical weather events. Other disasters happen without advance warning (e.g., earthquakes, mass shootings, terrorist attacks). Critical events, whether over time as a cumulative effect (public health emergencies) or a single, large disaster event, have the potential to trigger posttraumatic stress symptoms (PTSSs). As noted by D'Ettorre et al. (2021), these symptoms include feelings of anxiety, guilt, helplessness, sleep disorders, depression, anger, and isolation in these feelings. Personal and work relationships may also be negatively impacted.

Triggers for experiencing these symptoms include self-identification with those affected; their age; and the circumstances, including the sight, sounds, and smells surrounding the emergency response. An inability to psychologically process a traumatic incident or the cumulative effect of frequent or continued exposure to stressful incidents may further impact health care workers and disaster responders, leading to posttraumatic stress disorder (PTSD). The International Classification of Diseases 10th Revision (ICD-10) criteria for PTSD indicate it may occur in response to physical injury or severe mental or emotional distress. PTSD can be an acute event (lasting 1 to 3 months) or a chronic anxiety disorder when the symptoms persist longer than 3 months. The symptoms of PTSD may also have a delayed onset, with symptoms developing more than 6 months after the incident. Unresolved symptoms of posttraumatic stress are major triggers for the progression to PTSD (ICDdata.com, 2021).

The nurse may be reluctant to share moral or emotional distress with coworkers in the belief that it would add to coworkers' distress or that the nurse may be perceived as weak and unable to work in emergency or disaster scenarios. When these feelings are unrelieved or denied, nontherapeutic behaviors, such as increased use of alcohol, illicit drugs, or prescription medications, may be attempted to relieve the symptoms experienced. Unrecognized moral distress or untreated effects of stress may increase the number of health care workers leaving the profession or seeking alternative work environments. In severe cases, especially without recognition of the cumulative effects and without the necessary support to manage emotional stress, suicidal ideations can follow.

The American Nurses Association (ANA) issued a foundational document for the practice of nursing (2015). Using the ANA *Code of Ethics for Nurses with Interpretive Statements* as a foundation for recognizing the need to care for oneself as well as others, Provision 5 of the code states: "the nurse owes the same duty to self as to others, including the responsibility to promote health and safety, preserve wholeness of character and integrity, maintain competence, and continue personal and professional growth" (ANA, 2015, p. 1). Owing the same duty to oneself as to others to promote health and safety may be a difficult goal for nurses. Caring for oneself is a moral imperative; attempting to ignore or failing to recognize symptoms of anxiety, stress, depression, or anger increases the potential for burnout, compassion fatigue, and care delivery below expected standards.

The ANA (2020a) recognized the competing priorities within Provision 2 that "the nurse's primary commitment is to the patient" and Provision 5 that "the nurse owes the same duty to self as to others." During periods of ongoing crisis, such as the COVD-19 pandemic, there can be ethical conflicts in caring for patients and caring for oneself. The ANA supports nurses who need to evaluate and weigh choices when deciding to work during crisis situations and when or if to volunteer for disaster response. As noted by the ANA (2020b, p. 5), "Nurses are never expected to sacrifice or trade their own safety for the benefit of others." Stepping back to care for oneself is not a sign of weakness. The nurse who cares for themself is physically and emotionally stronger to provide care for patients.

Emotional support of health care staff should be readily available. When there is an isolated traumatic event, CISM methods can be used to help affected team members process what occurred and the role each of them played (CISM International, 2021). Initially used for combat and military veterans, this formal process has been adapted for use with first responders, disaster responders, and health care staff. This is a formal debriefing process requiring trained facilitators that ideally occurs within a relatively short period of time (24 to 72 hours) following an incident. Facilitators assist the affected staff in processing feelings to mitigate the emotional impact of a critical incident to promote psychological recovery.

Longer-term crisis situations need ongoing options for physical and mental care for affected staff. Access to trained mental health professionals may be available through an employee assistance program or through personal health insurance benefits. Nurses and other health care professionals should strongly consider joining appropriate professional organizations. The Emergency Nurses Association (ENA) offers a wealth of mental health resources and can assist in providing free and reduced-cost mental health care (ENA, 2021). Although the listing is part of a larger collection of COVID-19 resources, the professional organization for ED nurses recognized the imperative to prioritize mental and emotional health for their members.

The ANA offers support and guidance for mental health care for nurses. In addition to providing mental health emergency resources for nurses in crisis, additional suggestions for self-care are offered. The critical step to healthy self-care includes being proactive to recognize when symptoms interfere with the ability to function to the best of one's ability at work and in life in general, including within family and social relationships. Meditation, exercise, yoga, mindfulness of the current moment, and recognizing the "normal" in life are among the many proactive methods that may reduce the effects of stress (ANA, n.d.).

Nurses may find it difficult to not provide medical care to people who are dying or to withhold information to avoid spreading fear and panic. Clinical scenarios that are unimaginable in normal circumstances confront the nurse in extreme instances. Other ethical dilemmas may arise out of health care providers' instinct for self-protection and protection of their families.

Nurses can plan for the ethical dilemmas they will face during disasters by establishing a framework for evaluating ethical questions before they arise and by identifying and exploring possible responses to difficult clinical situations. They can consider how the fundamental ethical principles of utilitarianism (actions are right if they are useful or for the benefit of a majority), beneficence (to act for the benefit of others), and justice (determining if actions are compatible with the law and the patient's rights and are fair and balanced when it comes to access to health care), will influence their decisions and care in disaster response. Education and practice of the disaster response plan can assist the nurse in achieving an understanding of the role changes and dilemmas that might impact job performance.

CHAPTER REVIEW

NCLEX-Style Review Questions

1. The nurse has been working in a busy ED for the past few years. In the past year, it has been increasingly common to work past the normal hours and receive calls during time off to work extra shifts. Recently, the nurse notices an increasing tendency to avoid activities with friends. Anticipating shifts is causing anxiety and a loss of sleep prior to work. What actions are appropriate to decrease the nurse's distress? Select all that apply.

a. Dismiss the feelings and continue to volunteer for extra work because the income is needed.
b. Discuss the feelings with a trusted coworker or supervisor.
c. Attend counseling sessions available through human resources, insurance, or professional organizations.
d. Look for job opportunities outside of health care because health care positions are too stressful.
e. Consider use of meditation, yoga, and exercise to promote self-care.

2. A patient contaminated by a chemical spill arrives in the ED. In which order will decontamination begin?

a. Rinse the patient with water, remove jewelry and clothing, and wash thoroughly with soap and water.
b. Remove jewelry and clothing, wash thoroughly with soap and water, and rinse the patient with water.
c. Remove jewelry and clothing, rinse the patient with water, and wash thoroughly with soap and water.
d. Rinse the patient with water, wash thoroughly with soap and water, and remove jewelry and clothing.

3. The hospital has received a large number of patients following a large-scale disaster. Emergency management plans and surge plans were initiated, but the hospital is now critically low on staffing, technology, and resources for providing the usual and customary standard of care. What resources and plans may be employed? Select all that apply.

a. Advertising for additional staff
b. Consideration for accessing the chain of command for emergency requests to state and federal agencies for additional support
c. Consideration of utilizing crisis care plans with state approval
d. Public service announcements to shelter in place and not come to the hospital
e. Utilizing volunteers from the community to be trained in providing emergency nursing care

4. A patient arrives at the ED via ambulance after falling off the roof. From the following table, select all parameters that are of concern, the condition the parameters represent, and all priority nursing actions.

Parameters of Concern	Potential Condition	Priority Nursing Actions
Capillary refill of 4 seconds	Septic shock	Insert two large-gauge IV catheters
Blood pressure (BP) 102/46 mm Hg	Anaphylaxis	Anticipate infusing IV solution of dextrose 5% in water (D5W).
Pulse pressure 28 mm Hg	Neurogenic shock	Anticipate obtaining laboratory specimens (CBC, electrolytes, coagulation studies, type and cross-match)
Heart rate (HR) 108 beats per minute (bpm)	Cardiac tamponade	Elevate the head of the bed (HOB)
Urinary output of 34 mL/hr	Hypovolemic shock	Monitor vital signs
Restlessness		Strict intake and output (I&O)

5. A patient arrives in the ED after a motorcycle collision. The patient is alert, restless, and complaining of chest and back pain, and their skin is cool and slightly clammy. Breath sounds are diminished over the left side. An upright chest x-ray reveals fractures of the left fifth through seventh ribs and a 25% left hemothorax. Pertinent data are BP 80/50 mm Hg; HR 125 bpm; CVP 2 mm Hg; respiratory rate 28 and slightly labored; oxygen saturation 93% on room air. Which measures are most likely to be included in this patient's initial care? Select all that apply.

a. Endotracheal intubation
b. Chest tube insertion
c. Oxygen administration
d. 0.9% NaCl or normal saline
e. Pericardiocentesis
f. D5W IV at a keep vein open rate

REFERENCES AND SELECTED READINGS

References and selected readings associated with this chapter can be found on the website that accompanies the book. Visit **http://thepoint.lww.com/Honan3e** to access the references and other additional resources associated with this chapter.

Appendix A
Major Fluid and Electrolyte Imbalances

Imbalance	Contributing Factors	Signs/Symptoms and Laboratory Findings
Fluid volume deficit (FVD) (hypovolemia)	Loss of water and electrolytes, as in vomiting, diarrhea, fistulas, fever, excess sweating, burns, acute blood loss, gastrointestinal suction, and third-space fluid shifts; and decreased intake, as in anorexia, nausea, and inability to gain access to fluid Diabetes insipidus and uncontrolled diabetes mellitus, causing conditions such as DKA or HHNS, may also contribute to a depletion of extracellular fluid volume.	Acute weight loss; decreased skin turgor; oliguria; concentrated urine; weak, rapid pulse; prolonged capillary filling time; low CVP; ↓ blood pressure; decreased mean arterial pressure (MAP); orthostatic hypotension; flattened neck veins; dizziness; weakness; thirst and confusion; ↑ pulse; muscle cramps; sunken eyes, decreased skin turgor (presence of skin tenting), dry buccal mucosa *Labs indicate:* ↑ hematocrit, ↑ serum and urine osmolality, and increased urine specific gravity, ↑ BUN out of proportion to serum creatinine
Fluid volume excess (FVE) (hypervolemia)	Compromised regulatory mechanisms, such as kidney failure, heart failure, and cirrhosis; overzealous administration of sodium-containing fluids; and fluid shifts (i.e., treatment of burns). Prolonged corticosteroid therapy, severe stress, hyperaldosteronism augment fluid volume excess.	Acute weight gain, peripheral edema and ascites, distended jugular veins, crackles, and elevated CVP, shortness of breath, ↑ blood pressure, increased MAP, bounding pulse, cough, ↑ respiratory rate, S3 heart sound, orthopnea *Labs indicate:* ↓ hematocrit, ↓ serum and urine osmolality, ↓ urine specific gravity, decreased BUN (due to plasma dilution)
Sodium deficit (hyponatremia) Serum sodium <135 mEq/L	May be related to an excess of fluid (dilutional hyponatremia); an excess loss of sodium with free water replacement; and rarely, inadequate sodium intake (Diepenbrock, 2020, p. 685). Loss of sodium, as in use of diuretics, loss of GI fluids, kidney disease, and adrenal insufficiency. Gain of water, as in excessive administration of D_5W and/or water supplements for patients receiving hypotonic tube feedings; disease states associated with SIADH, such as head trauma and oat-cell lung tumor; marked hyperglycemia, medications associated with water retention (oxytocin and certain tranquilizers); and psychogenic polydipsia. Patients with heart failure or liver disease may present with hyponatremia despite an excess of total body sodium.	Manifestations of hyponatremia depend on the cause, magnitude, and speed with which the deficit occurs. Symptoms include: Anorexia, nausea and vomiting, headache, lethargy, dizziness, confusion, muscle cramps and weakness, muscular twitching, seizures, papilledema, dry skin, ↑ pulse, ↓ BP, weight gain, edema *Labs indicate:* ↓ Serum sodium; urine sodium level varies depending on the etiology of the hyponatremia
Sodium excess (hypernatremia) Serum sodium >145 mEq/L	Occurs when water loss exceeds sodium or when H_2O intake is inadequate such as in patients unable to drink at will; hypertonic tube feedings without adequate water supplements; diabetes insipidus; heatstroke; hyperventilation; watery diarrhea; burns; and diaphoresis; excess corticosteroid, sodium bicarbonate, and sodium chloride administration; and salt water near-drowning victims.	Thirst, elevated body temperature, swollen dry tongue and sticky mucous membranes, hallucinations, lethargy, restlessness, agitation, irritability, focal or grand mal seizures, pulmonary edema, hyperreflexia, twitching, nausea, vomiting, anorexia, ↑ pulse, and ↑ BP *Labs indicate:* ↑ Serum sodium, increased serum osmolality; ↑ urine specific gravity and osmolality (provided the water loss is from a route other than the kidneys).

Imbalance	Contributing Factors	Signs/Symptoms and Laboratory Findings
Potassium deficit (hypokalemia) Serum potassium <3.5 mEq/L	Increased output of K^+ (diuretics, diarrhea, excess vomiting, gastric suction, recent ileostomy, colitis, intestinal drains, osmotic diuresis); decreased intake of K^+ (NPO, anorexia, vomiting, alcoholism, fasting diets); or redistribution of K^+ (metabolic alkalosis, insulin administration); adrenal disorders (aldosteronism, Cushing disease).	Fatigue, anorexia, nausea and vomiting, muscle weakness, decreased bowel motility, abdominal distention, ileus, ventricular arrhythmias, paresthesias, leg cramps, hypoactive reflexes, increased sensitivity to digitalis *ECG:* Flattened T waves, prominent U waves, ST depression, prolonged PR interval
Potassium excess (hyperkalemia) Serum potassium >5.0 mEq/L	Pseudohyperkalemia, oliguric kidney failure, use of potassium-conserving diuretics in patients with renal insufficiency, metabolic acidosis, Addison disease, stored bank blood transfusions, rapid IV administration of potassium, or massive cell damage (burns, crush injury)	Vague muscular weakness, lethargy, tachycardia → bradycardia, arrhythmias, ascending weakness (legs to trunk), flaccid paralysis, paresthesias, intestinal colic *ECG:* Tall tented T waves, prolonged PR interval and QRS duration, absent P waves, ST depression
Calcium deficit (hypocalcemia) Serum calcium <8.5 mg/dL	Hypoparathyroidism (may follow thyroid surgery or radical neck dissection), malabsorption, pancreatitis, alkalosis, vitamin D deficiency, massive subcutaneous infection, generalized peritonitis, massive transfusion of citrated blood, chronic diarrhea, decreased parathyroid hormone, kidney failure, ↑ PO_4, pancreatic and small bowel fistulas, hypomagnesemia, hypoalbuminemia	Numbness, tingling of fingers, toes, and circumoral region; positive Trousseau and Chvostek signs; tetany; seizures, carpopedal spasms, hyperactive deep tendon reflexes, irritability, laryngeal spasm, anxiety *ECG:* Prolonged QT interval and lengthened ST predisposing to torsades de pointes (form of ventricular tachycardia) *Labs indicate:* Serum calcium concentration is low; ionized serum calcium concentration is also low; ↓ Mg^{++} (inhibits PTH secretion)
Calcium excess (hypercalcemia) Serum calcium >10.5 mg/dL	Hyperparathyroidism, malignant neoplastic disease, prolonged immobilization, overuse of calcium supplements, vitamins A and D excess, oliguric phase of kidney failure, acidosis, thiazide diuretic use	Muscular weakness, confusion, constipation, anorexia, nausea and vomiting, polyuria and polydipsia, dehydration, hypoactive deep tendon reflexes, lethargy, deep bone pain, pathologic fractures, flank pain, and calcium stones. *ECG:* Shortened ST segment and QT interval, bradycardia, heart blocks
Magnesium deficit (hypomagnesemia) Serum magnesium <1.8 mg/dL	Inadequate dietary intake of magnesium, alcohol use disorder, hyperparathyroidism, hyperaldosteronism, diuretic phase of kidney failure, malabsorptive disorders, diabetic ketoacidosis, refeeding after starvation, parenteral nutrition, chronic laxative use, diarrhea, frequently exists with decreased serum K^+ and Ca^{++}, malignancy (hypomagnesemia associated with chemotherapy use), and certain pharmacologic agents (such as gentamicin, cisplatin, and cyclosporine)	Neuromuscular irritability, positive Trousseau and Chvostek signs, insomnia, mood changes, anorexia, vomiting, increased tendon reflexes, and potentiation of ventricular and supraventricular arrhythmias *ECG:* PVCs, flat or inverted T waves, depressed ST segment, prolonged PR and QTc intervals and widened QRS
Magnesium excess (hypermagnesemia) Serum magnesium >2.7 mg/dL	Renal insufficiency (particularly when magnesium-containing medications are administered IV or excessive ingestion of magnesium-containing antacids or laxatives), adrenal insufficiency	Nausea, vomiting, hypotension, drowsiness, hypoactive reflexes, depressed respirations leading to apnea, bradycardia and hypotension. *ECG:* Prolonged PR interval and QT interval.
Phosphorus deficit (hypophosphatemia) Serum phosphorus <2.5 mg/dL	Refeeding after starvation, alcohol withdrawal, diabetic ketoacidosis, respiratory alkalosis, ↓ magnesium, ↓ potassium, hyperparathyroidism, diarrhea, vitamin D deficiency associated with malabsorptive disorders, burns, acid–base disorders, parenteral nutrition, and diuretic and antacid use	Paresthesias, muscle weakness, bone pain and tenderness, chest pain, confusion, impaired myocardial contractility, cardiomyopathy, respiratory failure, seizures, tissue hypoxia, and increased susceptibility to infection

Imbalance	Contributing Factors	Signs/Symptoms and Laboratory Findings
Phosphorus excess (hyperphosphatemia) Serum phosphorus >4.5 mg/dL	Acute and chronic kidney failure, excessive intake of phosphorus, vitamin D excess, respiratory acidosis, hypoparathyroidism, volume depletion, leukemia/lymphoma treated with cytotoxic agents, increased tissue breakdown, rhabdomyolysis	Increased vulnerability to seizures, tetany, signs and symptoms of hypocalcemia; hyperactive reflexes; soft-tissue calcifications in lungs, heart, kidneys, and cornea
Chloride deficit (hypochloremia) Serum chloride <96 mEq/L	GI tube drainage and severe vomiting and diarrhea, laxatives, ileostomy, and fistulas; sodium and potassium deficiency; metabolic alkalosis; loop, osmotic, or thiazide diuretic use; overuse of bicarbonate; rapid removal of ascitic fluid with a high sodium content; intravenous fluids that lack chloride (dextrose and water); frequently associated with hyponatremia	Signs and symptoms of hypochloremia are associated with hyponatremia, hypokalemia, and metabolic alkalosis *Labs indicate:* ↓ Serum chloride, ↓ serum sodium, ↑ pH, ↑ serum bicarbonate, ↑ total carbon dioxide content, ↓ serum potassium
Chloride excess (hyperchloremia) Serum chloride >108 mEq/L	Excessive sodium chloride infusions with water loss; hypernatremia; kidney failure; corticosteroid use; dehydration; severe diarrhea (loss of bicarbonate); compensated respiratory alkalosis; administration of diuretics; overdose of salicylates; Kayexalate, acetazolamide, phenylbutazone, and ammonium chloride use; hyperparathyroidism; metabolic acidosis	Signs and symptoms of hyperchloremia are typically associated with metabolic acidosis (tachypnea, Kussmaul respirations, lethargy, diminished cognitive ability), and hypernatremia (fluid retention, dyspnea, tachycardia, hypertension) *Labs indicate:* ↑ Serum chloride, ↑ serum sodium, ↓ serum pH, ↓ serum bicarbonate, normal anion gap

↑ increased; ↓ decreased; BP, blood pressure; BUN, blood urea nitrogen; CVP, central venous pressure; DKA, diabetic ketoacidosis; GI, gastrointestinal; IV, intravenous; PVCs, premature ventricular contractions; SIADH, syndrome of inappropriate secretion of antidiuretic hormone.

HHNS, hyperglycemic hyperosmolar nonketotic syndrome.

Index

Page numbers followed by b indicate boxes; those followed by f indicate figures; those followed by t indicate tables.

B

C

E

F

H

M

O

P

T

U

W

X

Y

Z